AMERICAN COLLEGE OF SURGEONS

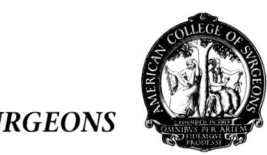

ACS SURGERY

Principles & Practice

2004

AMERICAN COLLEGE OF SURGEONS

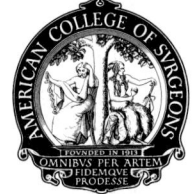

ACS SURGERY

Principles & Practice
2004

WILEY W. SOUBA, M.D., Sc.D., F.A.C.S.
John A. and Marian T. Waldhaun Professor of Surgery and Chair,
Department of Surgery, Penn State College of Medicine, and
Surgeon-in-Chief, Milton S. Hershey Medical Center
EDITORIAL CHAIRMAN

MITCHELL P. FINK, M.D., F.A.C.S.
Professor and Chairman, Department of Critical Care Medicine,
University of Pittsburgh School of Medicine
EDITOR

GREGORY J. JURKOVICH, M.D., F.A.C.S.
Professor of Surgery,
University of Washington School of Medicine
EDITOR

LARRY R. KAISER, M.D., F.A.C.S.
John Rhea Barton Professor and Chairman, Department of Surgery,
University of Pennsylvania School of Medicine
EDITOR

WILLIAM H. PEARCE, M.D., F.A.C.S.
Violet R. and Charles A. Baldwin Professor of Vascular Surgery,
Northwestern University Feinberg School of Medicine
EDITOR

JOHN H. PEMBERTON, M.D., F.A.C.S.
Professor of Surgery,
Mayo Graduate School of Medicine
EDITOR

NATHANIEL J. SOPER, M.D., F.A.C.S.
Professor of Surgery and Vice Chair of Clinical Affairs,
Northwestern University Feinberg School of Medicine
EDITOR

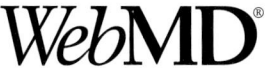

www.acssurgery.com

COUNCIL OF FOUNDING EDITORS

Library of Congress Cataloging-in-Publication Data

ACS surgery: principles and practice 2004/ Douglas W. Wilmore ... [et al.], editor.
    p. ; cm.
    Includes bibliographical references and index.
    ISBN 0-9703902-7-0 (2004)(alk. paper)
      1. Therapeutics, Surgical. 2. Surgery. I. Wilmore, Douglas W. (Douglas Wayne), date.
    II. American College of Surgeons.
    [DNLM: 1. Surgical Procedures, Operative—methods. 2. Perioperative Care—methods.
    WO 500 A187 2004
    RD49 .A275 2001
    617'.9—dc21

                                                                        2003024452

Vice President and Publisher	Nancy E. Chorpenning
Director, Electronic Publishing	Liz Pope
Managing Editor	Erin Michael Kelly
Development Editor	Richard P. Lindsey
Senior Copy Editor	John J. Anello
Copy Editor	David Terry
Editorial Coordinator	Stephen D'Agostino
Electronic Projects Manager	Janet Zinn
Art and Design Editor	Elizabeth Klarfeld
Associate Producers	Diane Joiner, Kelly Mercado, Jennifer Smith
Indexer	Julia Brooks Figures

Printed in the United States of America.
Published by WebMD Inc.

WebMD Professional Publishing
WebMD Inc.
224 West 30th Street, 4th Floor
New York, NY 10001

WO 500 A187 2004

ACS Surgery: Principles and Practice is sponsored by the American College of Surgeons and written by individuals who are recognized experts. The text represents the authors' approaches to clinical problems and to other important issues in surgical practice. It should be used as a general reference with other sources in the formation of an integrated care plan.

The authors, editors, and publisher have conscientiously and carefully tried to ensure that recommended measures and drug dosages in these pages are accurate and conform to the standards that prevailed at the time of publication. The reader is advised, however, to check the product information sheet accompanying each drug to be familiar with any changes in the dosage schedule or in the contraindications. This advice should be taken with particular seriousness if the agent to be administered is a new one or one that is infrequently used. *ACS Surgery: Principles and Practice* describes basic principles of diagnosis and therapy. Because of the uniqueness of each patient and the need to take into account a number of concurrent considerations, however, this information should be used by physicians only as a general guide to clinical decision making.

To better care for all surgical patients

CONTENTS

1. BASIC SURGICAL AND PERIOPERATIVE CONSIDERATIONS

2. BREAST, SKIN, SOFT TISSUE, AND NECK

4.   VASCULAR SYSTEM

Available Exclusively Online at www.acssurgery.com

ELEMENTS OF CONTEMPORARY PRACTICE

CARE IN SPECIAL SITUATIONS

NORMAL LABORATORY VALUES

See inside front cover to get started online.

CONTRIBUTORS

CAMERON M. AKBARI, M.D., F.A.C.S. Assistant Professor, Georgetown University School of Medicine, and Director, Vascular Diagnostic Laboratory, Washington Hospital Center

ELIAS J. ANAISSIE, M.D. Professor of Medicine, Department of Medicine, Myeloma and Transplantation Research Center, University of Arkansas College of Medicine; and Director, Department of Clinical Affairs, University Hospital of Arkansas, Little Rock

JOHN T. ANDERSON, M.D., F.A.C.S. Assistant Professor of Surgery, University of California, Davis, School of Medicine

FRANK R. ARKO, M.D. Postdoctoral Fellow/Endovascular Fellow, Division of Vascular Surgery, Department of Surgery, Stanford University School of Medicine

WALID S. ARNAOUT, M.D., F.A.C.S. Associate Director, Center for Liver Diseases and Transplantation, Cedars-Sinai Medical Center, Los Angeles

JYOTI ARYA, M.D. Assistant Professor, Department of Surgery, University of Colorado School of Medicine

STEVEN B. BACKMAN, M.D.C.M., Ph.D. Associate Professor, Department of Anesthesia, McGill University Faculty of Medicine

ALAN N. BARKUN, M.D. Associate Professor, Department of Medicine, McGill University Faculty of Medicine, and Director, Division of Gastroenterology, McGill University Health Centre

JEFFREY S. BARKUN, M.D., F.A.C.S. Associate Professor and Director, Division of Gastroenterology, Department of Surgery, McGill University Faculty of Medicine, and Department of Surgery, McGill University Health Centre

ROBERT H. BARTLETT, M.D., F.A.C.S. Professor, Division of General and Thoracic Surgery, University of Michigan Medical School

ROBERT W. BEART, JR., M.D., F.A.C.S. Chairman of Colon and Rectal Surgery and Costello Professor of Surgery, Division of Colorectal Surgery, Department of Surgery, Keck School of Medicine, University of Southern California

MICHAEL BELKIN, M.D., F.A.C.S. Associate Professor, Division of Vascular Surgery, Harvard Medical School

JOHN J. BERGAN, M.D., F.A.C.S. Professor, Department of Surgery, University of California, San Diego, School of Medicine, and Staff Surgeon, Scripps Memorial Hospital

RAMON BERGUER, M.D., F.A.C.S. Associate Professor of Surgery, University of California, Davis, School of Medicine

CLAUDIA BERMAN, M.D. Professor, Department of Radiology, University of South Florida College of Medicine, and Attending Radiologist, H. Lee Moffitt Cancer Center and Research Institute

PALMER Q. BESSEY, M.D., F.A.C.S. Professor, Department of Surgery, Weill Medical College of Cornell University, and Associate Director, William Randolph Hearst Burn Center, New York Presbyterian Hospital-Cornell Medical Center

A. GRISWOLD BEVIN, M.D. Professor Emeritus, Department of Plastic Surgery, University of North Carolina at Chapel Hill School of Medicine

ALBAIR B. BISHARA, M.D. Postdoctoral Fellow, Department of Surgery, University of Arkansas College of Medicine, Little Rock

ROBERT M. BLACK, M.D. Associate Professor, Department of Medicine, University of Massachusetts Medical School, and Director, Division of Renal Medicine, Worcester Medical Center

F. WILLIAM BLAISDELL, M.D., F.A.C.S. Professor and Chairman Emeritus, Department of Surgery, University of California, Davis, School of Medicine, and Chief of Surgical Services, Department of Surgery, Mather Veterans Affairs Hospital, Mather, California

LESLIE H. BLUMGART, M.D., F.A.C.S., F.R.C.S. Enid A. Haupt Chair in Surgery, and Chief, Hepatobiliary Services, Memorial Sloan-Kettering Cancer Center

RICHARD M. BONDY, M.D.C.M. Associate Professor, Department of Anesthesia, McGill University Faculty of Medicine

JULIAN BRITTON, M.S., F.R.C.S. Consultant Surgeon, Nuffield Department of Surgery, University of Oxford

DAVID C. BROOKS, M.D., F.A.C.S. Associate Professor, Department of Clinical Surgery, Harvard Medical School, and Senior Surgeon, Brigham and Women's Hospital

JON M. BURCH, M.D., F.A.C.S. Professor, Department of Surgery, University of Colorado Health Sciences Center, and Chief, Department of General and Vascular Surgery, Denver Health Medical Center

BRUCE A. CAIRNS, M.D., F.A.C.S. Assistant Professor, Department of Surgery, University of North Carolina School of Medicine

JOHN L. CAMERON, M.D., F.A.C.S. Alfred Blaylock Distinguished Service Professor of Surgery, Johns Hopkins University School of Medicine

E. RAMSAY CAMP, M.D. Adjunct Assistant Professor, Department of Surgery, University of Florida College of Medicine

KATHLEEN CASEY, M.D. Chief, Section of Infectious Disease, Jersey Shore Medical Center, and Clinical Professor of Medicine, University of Medicine and Dentistry of New Jersey Robert Wood Johnson Medical School

LAURENCE Y. CHEUNG, M.D., F.A.C.S. Professor and Chairman, Department of Surgery, University of Kansas School of Medicine, and Chief of Surgery, Department of Surgical Services, University of Kansas Hospital, Kansas City

TAE CHONG, M.D. Resident, Department of Surgery, University of Virginia Health System

NICOLAS V. CHRISTOU, M.D., Ph.D., F.A.C.S. Professor, Department of Surgery, McGill University Faculty of Medicine, and Head, Division of General Surgery, McGill University Health Centre

CLAUDIO S. CINÀ, M.D., Sp.Chir. (It.), M.Sc., F.R.S.C.(C) Assistant Clinical Professor, Department of Surgery, McMaster University Faculty of Health Sciences, Hamilton, Ontario

ORLO H. CLARK, M.D., F.A.C.S. Professor and Vice Chair, Department of Surgery, University of California, San Francisco, School of Medicine, and Chief, Department of Surgery, Mount Zion Medical Center of UC-San Francisco

CATHERINE M. CLASE, M.B., B.Chir., M.Sc. Assistant Professor, Department of Medicine, Dalhousie University Faculty of Medicine; Nephrologist, Department of Medicine, QE 2 Health Sciences Centre

ARNOLD G. CORAN, M.D., F.A.C.S. Professor, Division of Pediatric Surgery, Department of Surgery, University of Michigan Medical School, and Surgeon-in-Chief, Section of Pediatric Surgery, Department of Surgery, C. S. Mott Children's Hospital

CHARLES COX, M.D., F.A.C.S. Professor, Department of Surgery, University of South Florida College of Medicine, and Breast Cancer Program Leader, H. Lee Moffitt Cancer Center and Research Institute

JOHN MIHRAN DAVIS, M.D., F.A.C.S. Professor, Department of Surgery, University of Medicine and Dentistry of New Jersey Robert Wood Johnson Medical School, and Surgery Program Director, Jersey Shore Medical Center

ROMANO DELCORE, M.D., F.A.C.S. Professor, Department of Surgery, University of Kansas School of Medicine, and Medical Director, Department of Surgery, University of Kansas Medical Center

E. PATCHEN DELLINGER, M.D., F.A.C.S. Professor and Vice Chairman, Department of Surgery, University of Washington School of Medicine, and Chief and Associate Medical Director, Department of Surgery, University of Washington Medical Center

ERIC J. DEMARIA, M.D., F.A.C.S. Professor, Division of General/Trauma Surgery, Virginia Commonwealth University Medical College of Virginia, and Section Chief, General and Endoscopic Surgery, and Director, Medical College of Virginia's Hospital for Minimally Invasive Surgery

ACHILLES A. DEMETRIOU, M.D., Ph.D., F.A.C.S. Chairman, Department of Surgery, Cedars-Sinai Medical Center, Los Angeles

ROBERT H. DEMLING, M.D., F.A.C.S. Professor, Department of Surgery, Harvard Medical School, and Director, Burn Center, Brigham and Women's Hospital

ALAIN DESCHAMPS, M.D., Ph.D. Assistant Professor, Department of Anesthesia, McGill University Faculty of Medicine

JOSEPH J. DISA, M.D., F.A.C.S. Assistant Attending Surgeon, Department of Plastic and Reconstructive Surgery, Memorial Sloan-Kettering Cancer Center

BRIAN J. EASTRIDGE, M.D., F.A.C.S. Assistant Professor, Department of Surgery, University of Texas Southwestern Medical School

MARK K. ESKANDARI, M.D., F.A.C.S. Assistant Professor, Department of Surgery, Northwestern University Feinberg School of Medicine

DAVID C. EVANS, M.D., F.A.C.S. Assistant Professor, Department of Surgery, McGill University Faculty of Medicine, and Director, Trauma Unit, Montreal General Hospital

ALICIA FANNING, M.D. Laparoscopic/Endoscopic Fellow, Cleveland Clinic Foundation

SAMIR M. FAKHRY, M.D., F.A.C.S. Clinical Professor, Department of Surgery, Georgetown University School of Medicine, and Director, Trauma Services/Trauma Intensive Care Unit, Inova Fairfax Hospital, Falls Church, Virginia

LIANE S. FELDMAN, M.D., F.A.C.S. Assistant Professor, Department of Surgery, McGill University Faculty of Medicine, and Staff, Departments of Videoendoscopic Surgery and Surgery, McGill University Hospital Centre

DAVID V. FELICIANO, M.D., F.A.C.S. Professor, Department of Surgery, Emory University School of Medicine, and Chief of Surgery, Grady Memorial Hospital, Atlanta

WILLIAM R. FINKELMEIER, M.D., F.A.C.S. Director, VeinSolutions, Indianapolis

ANNA M. LEDGERWOOD, M.D., F.A.C.S.   Professor, Department of Surgery, Wayne State University School of Medicine, and General Surgeon, Detroit Receiving Hospital

RONALD T. LEWIS, M.B.B.S., M.Sc., F.A.C.S., F.R.C.S.(C)   Associate Professor, Department of Surgery, McGill University Faculty of Medicine, and Chief, Vascular Surgery, Department of Surgery, McGill University Health Centre

KEITH D. LILLEMOE, M.D., F.A.C.S.   Professor, Department of Surgery, Johns Hopkins University School of Medicine

FRANK W. LOGERFO, M.D., F.A.C.S.   William V. McDermott Professor of Surgery, Harvard Medical School

VIVIAN G. LOO, M.D., M.Sc.A.   Assistant Professor, Department of Medicine, McGill University Faculty of Medicine, and Director, Infection Control and Prevention Service, McGill University Health Centre

CHARLES E. LUCAS, M.D., F.A.C.S.   Professor, Department of Surgery, Wayne State University School of Medicine, and Surgeon, Detroit Receiving Hospital

THOMAS S. MALDONADO, M.D.   Clinical Instructor, Department of Surgery, New York University School of Medicine

JOSEPH MAMAZZA, M.D.   Assistant Professor, Department of Surgery, University of Toronto Faculty of Medicine; Medical Director of Minimal Access Therapeutics and Diseases of Digestive Systems and Director of Minimally Invasive Surgery, St. Michael's Hospital

JOHN C. MARSHALL, M.D., F.A.C.S., F.R.C.S.(C)   Professor, Department of Surgery, University of Toronto Faculty of Medicine, and Director of Research, Medical and Surgical Intensive Care Unit, and Staff Surgeon, Toronto General Hospital University Health Network

BYRON J. MASTERSON, M.D., F.A.C.S.   J. Wayne Reitz Professor of Gynecologic Surgery and Chairman Emeritus, University of Florida College of Medicine, Gainesville, and Professor, School of Public Health, University of South Florida (courtesy), Tampa

JON MATSUMURA, M.D., F.A.C.S.   Assistant Professor, Department of Surgery, Northwestern University Feinberg School of Medicine

KENNETH L. MATTOX, M.D., F.A.C.S.   Professor and Vice Chairman, Division of Thoracic Surgery, Department of Surgery, Baylor College of Medicine, and Chief of Staff and Chief of Surgery, Ben Taub General Hospital, Houston

JACK W. MCANINCH, M.D., F.A.C.S.   Professor, Department of Urology, University of California, San Francisco, School of Medicine, and Chief, Department of Urology, San Francisco General Hospital

JACQUELINE C. MCCLARAN, M.D.   Assistant Medical Director, John Radcliffe Trust, University of Oxford

DANIEL P. MCKELLAR, M.D., F.A.C.S.   Associate Clinical Professor, Department of Surgery, Wright State University School of Medicine

JONATHAN L. MEAKINS, M.D., D.Sc., F.A.C.S., F.R.C.S.(C)   Nuffield Professor and Head, Nuffield Department of Surgery, University of Oxford

TERRY J. MENGERT, M.D.   Associate Professor, Division of Emergency Medicine, Department of Medicine, University of Washington

JANE MESSINA, M.D.   Associate Professor, Department of Pathology, H. Lee Moffitt Cancer Center and Research Institute, University of South Florida College of Medicine

ANTHONY A. MEYER, M.D., Ph.D., F.A.C.S.   Professor, Vice Chairman, and Chief, Division of General Surgery, Department of Surgery, University of North Carolina at Chapel Hill School of Medicine, and Chief of General Surgery, North Carolina Jaycee Burn Center, University of North Carolina Hospitals and Clinics

RUSTY MILHOAN, M.D., F.A.C.S.   Trauma Surgeon, Department of Trauma Services, Christus St. Elizabeth Hospital, Beaumont, Texas

CHARLES M. MILLER, M.D., F.A.C.S.   Alfred and Florence Gross Professor of Surgery, Mount Sinai School of Medicine of the City University of New York, and Director, Recanati-Miller Transplantation Institute, Mount Sinai Medical Center, New York City

BERNARD MONTREUIL, M.D.   Assistant Professor, Division of Vascular Surgery, Department of Surgery, Royal Victoria Hospital, Montreal

ANNE MOORE, M.D.   Associate Professor, Department of Surgery, McGill University Faculty of Medicine

ERNEST E. MOORE, M.D., F.A.C.S.   Professor and Vice Chairman, Department of Surgery, University of Colorado Health Sciences Center, and Chief, Department of Surgery, Denver Health Medical Center

FREDERICK A. MOORE, M.D., F.A.C.S.   Professor and Vice Chairman, Department of Surgery, University of Texas Medical School at Houston, and Chief, Department of General Surgery, Trauma, and Critical Care, Memorial Hermann Hospital

WESLEY S. MOORE, M.D., F.A.C.S.   Professor, Division of Vascular Surgery, Department of Surgery, David Geffen School of Medicine, University of California, Los Angeles

LAURIE MORRISON, M.D.   Vascular Surgery and Technology, Bloomington, Indiana

J. PAUL MUIZELAAR, M.D., Ph.D.   Professor and Chairman, Department of Neurological Surgery, University of California, Davis, School of Medicine

LENA M. NAPOLITANO, M.D., F.A.C.S.   Associate Professor, Department of Surgery, University of Maryland Medical System, and Director of Surgical Critical Care, Surgical Care Center, VA Maryland Health Care System, Baltimore

CARL NOHR, M.D., Ph.D., F.A.C.S., F.R.C.S.(C)   Chief, Department of Surgery, Palliser Health Region, Alberta, Canada

RICHARD T. SCHLINKERT, M.D., F.A.C.S.   Professor, Department of Surgery, Mayo Graduate School of Medicine, and General Surgeon, Department of Surgery, Mayo Clinic Scottsdale

THOMAS SCHRICKER, M.D., Ph.D.   Assistant Professor, Department of Anesthesia, McGill University Faculty of Medicine

THEODORE R. SCHROCK, M.D., F.A.C.S.   Chairman, Associate Dean for Clinical Services, and J. Englebert Dunphy Professor, Department of Surgery, University of California, San Francisco, School of Medicine

PATRICIA C. SEIFERT, R.N.   Perioperative Cardiac Care Coordinator, Inova Fairfax Hospital, Falls Church, Virginia

ALAN E. SEYFER, M.D., F.A.C.S.   Distinguished Professor of Surgery and Distinguished Professor of Anatomy, Physiology, and Genetics, Uniformed Services University of the Health Sciences, Bethesda, Maryland

HIMANSU R. SHAH, M.D.   Clinical Instructor, Department of Surgery, University of Nevada School of Medicine

GEORGE F. SHELDON, M.D., F.A.C.S.   Zack D. Owens Distinguished Professor of Surgery, University of North Carolina at Chapel Hill School of Medicine

CYNTHIA K. SHORTELL, M.D., F.A.C.S.   Associate Professor, Department of Surgery, University of Rochester School of Medicine and Dentistry

BARBARA L. SMITH, M.D., Ph.D., F.A.C.S.   Assistant Professor, Department of Surgery, Harvard Medical School; Director, Comprehensive Breast Health Center, Massachusetts General Hospital; Co-Director, Women's Cancers Program, Dana Farber/Partner's Cancer Care; and Chief of Breast Surgical Services, Gillette Center at the Dana Farber Cancer Institute

ROBERT SMITH, M.D.   Surgical Research Fellow, University of Virginia School of Medicine

JOSEPH S. SOLOMKIN, M.D., F.A.C.S.   Professor, Department of Surgery, and Director, Surgical Infectious Diseases Division, University of Cincinnati College of Medicine

WILEY W. SOUBA, M.D., Sc.D., F.A.C.S.   John A. and Marian T. Waldhaun Professor of Surgery and Chair, Department of Surgery, Penn State College of Medicine, and Surgeon-in-Chief, Milton S. Hershey Medical Center

RENAE E. STAFFORD, M.D.   Assistant Professor of Trauma and Critical Care Surgery, Medical College of Wisconsin

THOMAS E. STARZL, M.D., Ph.D., F.A.C.S.   Professor, Department of Surgery, and Director, Thomas E. Starzl Transplantation Institute, University of Pittsburgh School of Medicine

RICHARD H. STERNS, M.D.   Professor of Medicine, University of Rochester School of Medicine and Dentistry, and Chief of Medicine, Rochester General Hospital and the Genesee Hospital

HARVEY J. SUGERMAN, M.D., F.A.C.S.   David M. Hume Professor and Head, Division of General and Trauma Surgery, Department of Surgery, Virginia Commonwealth University, Medical College of Virginia

WILLIAM D. SUGGS, M.D. , F.A.C.S.   Associate Professor, Department of Surgery, Albert Einstein College of Medicine of Yeshiva University

BRYCE R. TAYLOR, M.D., F.A.C.S., F.R.C.S.(C)   Professor and Associate Chair, Division of General Surgery, Department of Surgery, University of Toronto Faculty of Medicine, and McCutcheon Chair in Surgery, Surgeon-in-Chief, and Director of Surgical Services, University Health Network

ERWIN R. THAL, M.D., F.A.C.S.   Professor, Department of Surgery, University of Texas Southwestern Medical Center, Dallas

SETH THALLER, M.D., F.A.C.S.   Professor and Chief, Department of Plastic Surgery, University of Miami School of Medicine

GEORGE TZIMAS, M.D.   Chief of Surgical Services, Kypselis General Hospital, Athens, Greece

GILBERT R. UPCHURCH, JR., M.D., F.A.C.S.   Assistant Professor, Department of Surgery, University of Michigan Medical School

CAESAR URSIC, M.D.   Assistant Professor, Department of Surgery, UCSF–East Bay Surgery Program, University of California, San Francisco, School of Medicine

FRANK J. VEITH, M.D., F.A.C.S.   Professor, Department of Surgery, Albert Einstein College of Medicine of Yeshiva University

JOSEPH VIJUNGCO, M.D.   Vascular Surgery Fellow, Department of Surgery, Northwestern University Feinberg School of Medicine

JAMES M. WATTERS, M.D., F.A.C.S.   Professor, Department of Surgery, University of Ottawa Faculty of Medicine, and Attending Surgeon, Department of Surgery, Ottawa Hospital-Civic Campus

HUNTER WESSELLS, M.D., F.A.C.S.   Associate Professor, Department of Urology, University of Washington School of Medicine

MARVIN J. WEXLER, M.D., F.A.C.S.   Professor, Departments of Surgery and Oncology, McGill University Faculty of Medicine, and Senior Surgeon, Department of Surgery, Royal Victoria Hospital, Montreal

KAREN S. WILLIAMS, M.D.   Medical Director, St. Agnes Healthcare, Baltimore

DOUGLAS W. WILMORE, M.D., F.A.C.S.   Frank Sawyer Professor, Department of Surgery, Harvard Medical School, and Senior Staff Surgeon, Department of Surgery, Brigham and Women's Hospital

DAVID WISNER, M.D., F.A.C.S.   Professor and Chief, Division of Trauma Surgery, Department of Surgery, University of California, Davis, School of Medicine

JOHN YEE, M.D. Assistant Professor of Surgery, Division of
Thoracic Surgery, University of British Columbia Faculty of
Medicine, and Surgical Director of Transplant Surgery,
Vancouver Hopital and Health Sciences Centre

CHRISTOPHER K. ZARINS, M.D., F.A.C.S. Chidester Professor
of Surgery, Stanford University School of Medicine, and Chief,
Division of Vascular Surgery, Stanford University Medical
Center

MARIKE ZWIENENBERG-LEE, M.D. Research Fellow,
Department of Neurological Surgery, University of California,
Davis, School of Medicine

FOREWORD

As the call for health care reform has continued to go forth, surgeons remain in a leadership role in answering this challenge. We must provide not just better patient care, but more efficient patient care. Our collective best answer to this challenge lies in an aggressive approach to surgical education. The need for continual instruction and self-assessment, leading to a corresponding improvement in the care delivered, has long been one of the hallmark responsibilities of our profession. Patients, the government, professional organizations, and other health care providers all expect us to find innovative ways to bring the most benefit to the greatest number of patients. We certainly expect no less from ourselves.

ACS Surgery: Principles and Practice is a trailblazer in surgical education. Since its earliest days, it has approached the educational needs of surgeons by uniquely providing the most current instruction on state-of-the-art operative technique, as well as information on key professional issues outside the OR. What skills and techniques do I need to improve the care of this individual patient? What is the best global approach for me to take while away from the operating table that will improve the care of all of my patients?

Just as surgeons seek to continually self-improve, so does *ACS Surgery*. The 2004 edition features a new table of contents using an intuitive "body system" organization. And a new section online at www.acssurgery.com called "Elements of Contemporary Practice" brings together chapters that cut across the key professional and educational issues affecting surgical practice today, including patient safety, patient risk assessment, and professional liability. Three months of FREE access to this new online section, as well as to electronically updated chapters, is included with purchase of the book.

Thus, *ACS Surgery* again leads the way in surgical self-improvement. These efforts bring necessary support to the practicing surgeon as he or she answers the call for superlative patient care, and they are evidence of a commitment to providing quality surgical education that makes us at the American College of Surgeons very proud of our ongoing sponsorship of *ACS Surgery*.

Thomas R. Russell, MD, FACS
Executive Director, American College of Surgeons
acssurgery@webmd.net

PREFACE

Surgeons need a standard. In the face of the ongoing reforms taking place throughout organized medicine, surgeons need a standard against which they can measure their own knowledge of current surgical practice and with which they can meet the ever-rising goals for superior surgical care.

Since its beginnings as *Care of the Surgical Patient* in the 1980s, we have taken special pride in both the quality and the usability of the information presented in this surgical reference, now known as *ACS Surgery: Principles and Practice*—the only College-sponsored textbook of surgery. Because surgical standards are constantly evolving, we are continually updating our chapters. For what is now the third year in a row, at least 40% of the material in this book is either new or updated. We continue to improve upon how we present surgical knowledge as well. This year, we have introduced an intuitive "body system" organization for the chapters.

Our expert authors—often the very surgeons who are at the edge of surgical innovation—write their chapters with the needs of the practicing surgeon in mind. Thus, chapters that discuss operative procedures break down each operation into key steps, highlighting potential problem areas and providing strategies for preventing or managing them. Each chapter that covers a topic related to perioperative care begins with an algorithm that graphically depicts the surgeon's decision-making process. The chapter often also includes a discussion section, which explores basic science concepts and new theories as they apply to the field.

To further support the needs of the surgeon in practice, we have developed a third type of chapter, found in a new online section called *Elements of Contemporary Practice*. These chapters are found exclusively at www.acssurgery.com (the inside front cover of this book explains how to access them), and they bring together the latest thinking on the types of issues that health care reform is so focused on these days: • cost-effective care • malpractice • patient safety • risk stratification • infection control • outpatient surgery • fast track surgery.

ACS Surgery is available in three formats: print, CD-ROM, and online. Since many are still most comfortable with a traditional bound textbook, we keep the print version of *ACS Surgery* more current than any other surgery text. Our CD-ROM editions offer portability and ease of access, especially for those who travel frequently or who have limited access to the Internet. *ACS Surgery Online* is the most current surgical textbook available because we update it each month. Online readers can also benefit from our convenient CME service, which allows surgeons to earn up to 120 category 1 credits per year. And to inform readers of the newest chapters and updates on the Web site, we even provide a free e-mail alert service called *What's New in ACS Surgery*.

This is the first edition of *ACS Surgery* to be published under the able guidance of our new editorial board. Led by Editorial Chair Wiley W. Souba, M.D., F.A.C.S., they include Mitchell P. Fink, M.D., F.A.C.S., Gregory J. Jurkovich, M.D., F.A.C.S., William H. Pearce, M.D., F.A.C.S., Larry R. Kaiser, M.D., F.A.C.S., John H. Pemberton, M.D., F.A.C.S., and Nathaniel Soper, M.D., F.A.C.S. By involving new, young surgical leaders, we can continue to lead the field in improving contemporary surgical information. I know they have even greater enhancements in mind for the years to come.

I hope that you find *ACS Surgery* to be practical and informative in helping you provide superior surgical care.

Douglas W. Wilmore, M.D., F.A.C.S.
Founding Editor
douglaswilmoremd@webmd.net

1 BASIC SURGICAL AND PERIOPERATIVE CONSIDERATIONS

1 PREPARATION OF THE OPERATING ROOM

Rene Lafrenière, M.D., C.M., F.A.C.S., Ramon Berguer, M.D., F.A.C.S., Patricia C. Seifert, R.N., Michael Belkin, M.D., F.A.C.S., Stuart Roth, M.D., Ph.D., Karen S. Williams, M.D., Eric J. De Maria, M.D., F.A.C.S., and Lena M. Napolitano, M.D., F.A.C.S., for the American College of Surgeons Committee on Perioperative Care

Today's operating room is a complex environment wherein a variety of health care providers are engaged in the sacred ritual of surgery, controlling and modifying nature's complicated orchestra of disease entities. In what follows, we discuss certain key aspects of the OR environment—design, safety, efficiency, patient factors, and the multidisciplinary team—with the aim of improving surgeons' understanding and comprehension of this complex world. In particular, we focus on emerging technologies and the special OR requirements of the burgeoning fields of endovascular surgery and minimally invasive surgery.

General Principles of OR Design and Construction

PHYSICAL LAYOUT

The basic physical design and layout of the OR have not changed substantially over the past century. In the past few years, however, major changes have occurred in response to continuing technological developments in the areas of minimally invasive surgery, intraoperative imaging, invasive nonsurgical procedures (e.g., endoscopic, endovascular, and image-guided procedures), patient monitoring, and telemedicine.

The exact specifications for new construction and major remodeling of ORs in the United States depend, first and foremost, on state and local regulations, which often incorporate standards published by the Department of Health and Human Services.[1] The American Institute of Architects publishes a comprehensive set of guidelines for health care facility design that includes a detailed discussion of OR design.[2] The design of new ORs must also take into account recommendations generated by specialty associations and regulatory agencies.[3-6] Finally, there are numerous articles and books that can be consulted regarding various aspects of OR design.[7-11]

The architectural design process for modern ORs should include knowledgeable and committed representatives from hospital clinical services, support services, and administration. Important design considerations include the mix of inpatient and outpatient operations, patient flow into and out of the OR area, the transportation of supplies and waste materials to and from the OR, and flexibility to allow the incorporation of new technologies. This planning phase benefits greatly from the use of architectural drawings, flow diagrams, computer simulations, and physical mockups of the OR environment.

For an operation to be successful, multiple complex tasks must be carried out, both serially and in parallel, while care is exercised to ensure the safety of both the patient and OR personnel. To this end, it is vital that the OR be designed so as to permit patients, OR personnel, and equipment to move and be moved as necessary without being unduly hindered by overcrowding or by obstruction from cables, wires, tubes, or ceiling-mounted devices. Before and during the operation, critical devices must be positioned so that they can readily be brought into use for monitoring and life support. The supplies and instruments likely to be needed must be easily available. Effective communication must be in place among the members of the OR team, the OR front desk, and the rest of the hospital. Built-in computer, phone, imaging, and video systems can enhance efficiency and safety by facilitating access to clinical information and decision-making support. Finally, the design of the OR must facilitate cleaning and disinfection of the room as well as permit efficient turnover of needed equipment and supplies for the next procedure.

A modern OR must include adequate storage space for immediately needed supplies. Equally important, it must include adequate storage space for the multitude of equipment and devices required in current surgical practice. All too often, storage space is inadequate, with the result that equipment and supplies must be stored in hallways and in the ORs themselves, thereby creating obstructions and hazards for personnel and patients.

The basic design of today's OR consists of a quadrangular room with minimum dimensions of 20 × 20 ft. More often, the dimensions are closer to 30 × 30 ft to accommodate more specialized cardiac, neurosurgical, minimally invasive, or orthopedic procedures. Smaller rooms, however, are generally adequate for minor surgery and for procedures such as cystoscopy and eye surgery. Ceiling height should be at least 10 ft to allow mounting of operating lights, microscopes, and other equipment on the ceiling. An additional 1 to 2 ft of ceiling height may be needed if x-ray equipment is to be permanently mounted.

VOICE, VIDEO, AND DATA COMMUNICATION

The operating suite should be wired to provide two-way voice, video, and data communication between the OR and the rest of the health care facility. Teleconnection of the OR to other areas of the hospital (e.g., the pathology department, the radiology department, the emergency department, conference rooms, surgeons' offices, and wet/dry laboratories) can greatly enhance both patient care and teaching by improving the exchange of crucial information while keeping noncritical traffic out of the OR environment. Two-way audio and video teleconferencing can improve surgical management by facilitating proctoring of less experienced practitioners, real-time consultation with experienced specialists or the scientific literature, and immediate viewing of x-ray images, specimens, and histologic findings. Archiving of visual data also permits efficient sharing of information with other practitioners, to the point where even the most complex operative situation can be experienced on a nearly firsthand basis. It is largely true that our newfound technological ability to share the OR environment between institutions has greatly facilitated the rapid development of advanced laparoscopic surgical procedures on a global level. The superior educational value of a shared audio and visual environment for teaching and learning complex surgical procedures is now well established.

ACCOMMODATION OF NEW TECHNOLOGIES

In developing the OR of the future, it is essential to remain abreast of new technologies and incorporate them as appropriate; however, this should be done in such a way as to make the OR environment simpler rather than more complicated and less intimidating rather than more so. Any new technical development must undergo rigorous evaluation to ensure that the correct technology is introduced in the correct manner at the correct time.[12]

Properly utilized, technology can greatly facilitate surgical management. A potential example is the bar coding now seen in every facet of our daily lives. At a patient's first office visit, he or she can be given a bar code, which is entered into a computer. On the morning of surgery, the computer can give the patient a wake up call at 5:30 A.M. Upon arrival at the surgical center, the patient can be logged in by bar code. Each step in the process can be tracked: how many minutes it took for the patient to get to the OR, how long it took for the anesthesiologist and the resident to interview the patient in the preoperative holding area, and how long it took to position the patient. Essentially, this process is a variation on patient tracking and data acquisition that minimizes variability with respect to data entry. Tracking information can also be displayed on a video monitor, so that the patient's location and current status within the surgical care process are available on an ongoing basis.

MAXIMIZATION OF EFFICIENCY IN DESIGN AND PROCESS

With the proliferation of technology, the increased complexity of surgical procedures, and the ongoing advances in surgical capabilities, surgery today is a highly involved undertaking. As the number of potential processes and subprocesses in surgical care has increased, so too has the potential for inefficiency. Often, the organizational tendency to keep doing things the way they have always been done prevents necessary improvements from being made, even in the face of significant pressure from corporate interests to improve and simplify processes. Decreasing turnover time and increasing efficiency during procedures are essential and can be accomplished by simplifying rather than complicating the processes involved. An example of such an approach was documented in a 2002 article demonstrating that the redesign of a neurosurgical operating suite simplified processes and procedures related to neurosurgical operations, resulting in a 35% decrease in turnover time.[13] In addition, team efficiency was significantly increased, leading to further time savings. The time commitment required of the specialist and the team members to make the necessary changes was modest, but the presence of OR administrators, staff members, surgeons, and anesthesia personnel, all cooperating to make working conditions more productive and rewarding for everyone, was deemed crucial to the success of the experiment.

Environmental Issues in the OR

TEMPERATURE AND HUMIDITY

The ambient temperature of the OR often represents a compromise between the needs of the patient and those of the staff; the temperature desired by staff itself is a compromise between the needs of personnel who are dressed in surgical gowns and those who are not. In Europe and North America, OR temperatures range from 18° to 26° C (64.4° to 78.8° F). A higher temperature is necessary during operations on infants and burn patients because conservation of body heat is critical in these patients. Generally, surgeons who are actively working and fully gowned prefer a temperature of 18° C (64.4° F), but anesthesiologists prefer 21.5° C (70.7° F).[14]

Humidity in the OR is generally maintained at between 50% and 60%; humidity greater than 60% may cause condensation on cool surfaces, whereas humidity less than 50% may not suppress static electricity.

LIGHTING

Well-balanced illumination in the OR provides a surgeon with a clear view of the operative field, prevents eye strain, and provides appropriate light levels for nurses and anesthesiologists. Much of our factual knowledge of OR illumination has been gained through the efforts of Dr. William Beck and the Illuminating Engineering Society.[15,16] A general illumination brightness of up to 200 footcandles (ft-c) is desirable in new constructions. The lighting sources should not produce glare or undesirable reflection.

The amount of light required during an operation varies with the surgeon and the operative site. In one study, general surgeons operating on the common bile duct found 300 ft-c sufficient; because the reflectance of this tissue area is 15%, the required incident light level would be 2,000 ft-c.[17] Surgeons performing coronary bypass operations require a level of 3,500 ft-c.[17] Whether changes in the color of light can improve discrimination of different tissues is unknown.

Another facet of OR lighting is heat production. Heat may be produced by infrared light emitted either directly by the light source or via energy transformation of the illuminated object. However, most of the infrared light emitted by OR lights can be eliminated by filters or by heat-diverting dichroic reflectors.

Basic Safety Concerns in the OR

The OR presents a number of environmental hazards to both surgical personnel and patients. Chemical hazards exist from the use of trace anesthetic gases, flammable anesthetic agents, various detergents and antimicrobial solutions, medications, and latex products.[18] Other ever-present physical hazards include electrical shock and burns, exposure to radiation from x-ray equipment, and injuries caused by lasers.[19] In addition to causing injury directly, the use of lasers can expose OR personnel to papillomavirus in smoke plumes.[20] Hazards that are less often considered include noise pollution[21] and light hazards from high-intensity illumination.[22] The most effective way of minimizing the particular hazards in a given OR is to have an active in-hospital surveillance program run by a multidisciplinary team that includes surgeons.

MINIMIZATION OF HAZARDS TO PATIENT

Patient safety, the first order of business in the OR,[23] begins with proper handling of patients and their tissues, which is particularly important where patients are in direct contact with medical devices. It is imperative that physicians, nurses, and technicians protect patients from injuries caused by excessive pressure, heat, abrasion, electrical shock, chemicals, or trauma during their time in the OR. Equipment must be properly used and maintained because equipment malfunctions, especially in life-support or monitoring systems, can cause serious harm.

Anesthetic Considerations

Surgery, by its very nature, makes demands on the body's homeostatic mechanisms that, if unchecked, would be injurious. It is the role of the anesthesiologist to anticipate these demands, compensate for them, and protect the patient by supporting the body's own efforts to maintain homeostasis [see 1:3 Perioperative Considerations for Anesthesia]. Patient protection demands that concerned physicians understand the effects of their perioperative interventions, both positive and negative, and act to minimize the unintended consequences.

Even with straightforward surgical procedures, issues related to patient positioning can lead to unintended consequences. General, regional, and monitored anesthesia care render patients helpless to protect themselves from the stresses of an uncomfortable position. As the physician who renders the patient helpless, the anesthesiologist is responsible for protecting the patient from the results of the position. The surgeon, who chooses the position for the procedure that maximizes exposure and facilitates the operation, is responsible for the consequences of that choice. The OR team is responsible for procuring and maintaining whatever specialized equipment is needed to position the patient properly. The American Society of Anesthesiologists (ASA) Practice Advisory on the Prevention of Perioperative Peripheral Neuropathies recommends that when practical, the patient should be placed in the intended position before the procedure to see if it is comfortable.[24] If the position is uncomfortable when the patient is awake, it should be modified until it is comfortable.

The consequences of patient discomfort from positioning may include postoperative myalgias, neuropathies, and compartment syndromes. The greatest risk in the supine position, peripheral neuropathy, arises from the positioning of the upper extremity. The two most common peripheral neuropathies reported to the ASA Closed Claim Study as of 1999 were ulnar neuropathy and brachial plexopathy.[25] Approximately 28% of the closed claims for peripheral neuropathy were for ulnar neuropathy and 20% for brachial plexopathy.[25] With regard to upper-extremity positioning, the ASA Practice Advisory recommends that the arms be abducted no more than 90°.[24] The arms should also be positioned so as to decrease pressure on the postcondylar groove of the humerus. When the arms are tucked, the neutral position is recommended. Prolonged pressure on the radial nerve in the spiral groove of the humerus should be avoided. Finally, the elbows should not be extended beyond a comfortable range so as not to stretch the median nerve.

Approximately 80% of surgical procedures are performed with patients in the supine position.[26] Its ubiquity notwithstanding, the supine position has certain physiologic consequences for the patient, including gravitational effects on both the circulatory system and the pulmonary system.[27] The most immediate hemodynamic effect noted upon assumption of the supine position is increased cardiac output resulting from enhanced return of lower-extremity venous blood to the heart.[28] If this effect were unopposed, systemic blood pressure would rise. This rise does not occur, however, because baroreceptor afferent impulses lead to a reflexive change in the autonomic balance, which decreases stroke volume, heart rate, and contractility,[29] thereby serving to maintain blood pressure. Inhaled, I.V., and regional anesthetics all have the capacity to blunt or abolish these protective reflexes, thus causing hypotension in supine, anesthetized patients and necessitating the administration of additional fluids or, occasionally, pressors.

Immediate effects of the supine position on the respiratory system include cephalad and lateral shifting of the diaphragm and cephalad shifting of the abdominal contents, resulting in decreased functional residual capacity and total lung capacity.[27,28] In addition, perfusion of the lung changes as the supine position is assumed. When the patient is upright, the dependent portions of the lungs receive the bulk of the blood flow[23]; however, when the patient becomes supine, the blood flow becomes essentially uniform from apex to base.[29] During spontaneous ventilation in the supine position, the patient can compensate for the altered flow, but when he or she is anesthetized, paralyzed, and placed on positive pressure ventilation, the weight of the abdominal contents prevents the posterior diaphragm from moving as freely as the anterior diaphragm, thus contributing to a ventilation-perfusion mismatch.[30]

After the supine position, the lithotomy position is the next most common position for surgical procedures. Approximately 9% of operations are conducted with the patient in the lithotomy position.[26] Because the lithotomy position is basically a modification of the supine position, there is still a risk of upper-extremity neuropathy; however, the risk of lower-extremity neuropathy is significantly greater. The main hemodynamic consequence of the lithotomy position is increased cardiac output secondary to the gravity-induced increase in venous return to the heart caused by elevation of the lower extremities above the level of the heart.[28] Of greater concern is the effect on the lower extremity of the various devices used in positioning. Damage to the obturator, sciatic, lateral femoral cutaneous, and peroneal nerves after immobilization in the lithotomy position, though rare, has been reported.[31,32] Such complaints account for only 5% of all closed claims for nerve damage in the Closed Claims Data Base.[25]

Other patient positions can also lead to physiologic and neurologic complications, including the lateral decubitus, prone, sitting, Trendelenburg, and reverse Trendelenburg positions.

MINIMIZATION OF OCCUPATIONAL INJURIES TO HEALTH CARE TEAM

Work-related musculoskeletal injuries are a major cause of decreased productivity and increased litigation costs in the United States.[23] In the OR, occupational injuries can be caused by excessive lifting, improper posture, collision with devices, electrical or thermal injury, puncture by sharp instruments, or exposure to bodily tissues and fluids. Temporary musculoskeletal injuries resulting from poor posture (particularly static posture) or excessive straining are less commonly acknowledged by members of the surgical team but occur relatively frequently during some operations.

To reduce injuries from awkward posture and excessive straining, OR devices should be positioned in an ergonomically desirable manner, so that unnecessary bending, reaching, lifting, and twisting are minimized. Visual displays and monitors should be placed where the surgical team can view them comfortably. Devices that require adjustment during operations should be readily accessible. Placement of cables and tubes across the OR workspace should be avoided if possible. The patient and the operating table should be positioned so as to facilitate the surgeons' work while maintaining patient safety. Lifting injuries can be prevented by using proper transfer technique and obtaining adequate assistance when moving patients in the OR.

Equipment

Modern surgery uses an ever-increasing number of devices in the OR to support and protect the patient and to assist the work of the surgical team [see Table 1]. All OR equipment should be evaluated with respect to three basic concerns: maintenance of patient safety, maximization of surgical team efficiency, and prevention of occupational injuries.

ELECTROSURGICAL DEVICES

The electrosurgical device is a 500 W radio-frequency generator that is used to cut and coagulate tissue. Although it is both

Table 1 Devices Used in the OR

For support of patient	Anesthesia delivery devices Ventilator Physiologic monitoring devices Warming devices I.V. fluid warmers and infusers
For support of surgeon	Sources of mechanical, electrical, and internal power, including power tools and electrocautery, as well as laser and ultrasound instruments Mechanical retractors Lights mounted in various locations Suction devices and smoke evacuators Electromechanical and computerized assistive devices, such as robotic assistants Visualization equipment, including microscopes, endoscopic video cameras, and display devices such as video monitors, projection equipment, and head-mounted displays Data, sound, and video storage and transmission equipment Diagnostic imaging devices (e.g., for fluoroscopy, ultrasonography, MRI, and CT)
For support of OR team	Surgical instruments, usually packaged in case carts before each operation but occasionally stored in nearby fixed or mobile modules Tables for display of primary and secondary surgical instruments Containers for disposal of single-use equipment, gowns, drapes, etc. Workplace for charting and record keeping Communication equipment

common and necessary in the modern OR, it is also a constant hazard and therefore requires close attention.[33] When in use, the electrosurgical unit generates an electrical arc that has been associated with explosions. This risk has been lessened because explosive anesthetic agents are no longer used; however, explosion of hydrogen and methane gases in the large bowel is still a real—if rare—threat, especially when an operation is performed on an unprepared bowel.[34] Because the unit and its arc generate a broad band of radio frequencies, electrosurgical units interfere with monitoring devices, most notably the electrocardiographic monitor. Interference with cardiac pacemaker activity also has been reported.[35]

The most frequently reported hazard of the electrosurgical unit is a skin burn. Such burns are not often fatal, but they are painful, occasionally require skin grafts, and raise the possibility of litigation. The burn site can be at the dispersive electrode, ECG monitoring leads, esophageal or rectal temperature probes, or areas of body contact with grounded objects. The dispersive electrode should be firmly attached to a broad area of dry, hairless skin, preferably over a large muscle mass.[34]

LASERS

Lasers generate energy that is potentially detrimental. Lasers have caused injuries to both patients and staff, including skin burns, retinal injuries, injuries from endotracheal tube fires, pneumothorax, and damage to the colon and to arteries.[36] Some design changes in the OR are necessary to accommodate lasers. The OR should not have windows, and a sign should be posted indicating that a laser is in use. The walls and ceiling in the room should be nonreflective. Equipment used in the operative field should be nonreflective and nonflammable. The concentration of O_2 and N_2O in the inhaled gases should be reduced to decrease the possibility of fire. In addition, personnel should wear goggles of an appropriate type to protect the eyes from laser damage. A smoke evacuator should be attached to the laser to improve visualization, reduce objectionable odor, and decrease the potential for papillomavirus infection from the laser smoke plume.[37]

POWERED DEVICES

The most common powered device in the OR is the surgical table. Central to every operation, this device must be properly positioned and adjusted to ensure the safety of the patient and the efficient work of the surgical team. Manually adjustable tables are simple, but those with electrical controls are easier to manage. OR table attachments, such as the arm boards and leg stirrups used to position patients, must be properly maintained and secured to prevent injuries to patients or staff. During transfer to and from the OR table, care must be taken to ensure that the patient is not injured and that life-support, monitoring, and I.V. systems are not disconnected. Proper transfer technique, personnel assistance, and the use of devices such as rollers will help prevent musculoskeletal injuries to the OR staff during this maneuver.

Other powered surgical instruments common in the OR include those used to obtain skin grafts, open the sternum, and perform orthopedic procedures. Powered saws and drills can cause substantial aerosolization of body fluids, thereby creating a potential infectious hazard for OR personnel.[38,39]

VIEWING AND IMAGING DEVICES

OR microscopes are required for microsurgical procedures. Floor-mounted units are the most flexible, whereas built-in microscopes are best employed in rooms dedicated to this type of procedure.[40] Microscopes are bulky and heavy devices that can cause obstructions and collision hazards in the OR. All controls and displays must be properly positioned at or below the user's line of sight to allow comfortable and unobstructed viewing.

Today's less invasive operations require more accurate intraoperative assessment of the relevant surgical anatomy through the use of x-ray, computed tomography, magnetic resonance imaging, and ultrasonography. Intraoperative fluoroscopy and ultrasonography are most commonly used for this purpose. Intraoperative ultrasonography requires a high-quality portable ultrasound unit and specialized probes. Depending on the procedure and the training of the surgeon, the presence of a radiologist and an ultrasound technician may be required. The ultrasound unit must be positioned near the patient, and the surgical team must be able to view the image comfortably. In some cases, the image may be displayed on OR monitors by means of a video mixing device. Dedicated open radiologic units are usually installed either in the OR proper or immediately adjacent to the OR to permit intraoperative imaging of the selected body area. As image-guided procedures become more commonplace, OR designers will have to accommodate such devices within the OR workplace in a user-friendly manner.

ADDITIONAL DEVICES

The use of sequential compression stockings (SCDs), with or without additional medical anticoagulation, has become the standard of care for the prevention of venous thromboembolism in the majority of operations for which direct access to the lower extremities is not required [*see 4:6 Venous Thromboembolism*].[41] This is particularly true in operations lasting more than 4 hours for which the patient is in the lithotomy position. The pump often must be placed near the patient on the floor or on a nearby cart. The pressure tubing from the stockings to the pump must be routed out of the surgical team's way to prevent hazards and enlargements, particularly during operations for which perineal access is required.

Suction devices are ubiquitous in the OR, assisting the surgeon in the evacuation of blood and other fluids from the operative field. A typical suction apparatus consists of a set of canisters on a wheeled base that receive suction from a wall- or ceiling-mounted source. The surgeon's aspirating cannula is sterilely connected to these canisters. Suction tubing is a common tripping hazard in the OR, and the suction canisters fill rapidly enough to require repeated changing.

Portable OR lights or headlights are often used when the lighting provided by standard ceiling-mounted lights is insufficient or when hard-to-see body cavities prove difficult to illuminate. Headlights are usually preferred because the beam is aimed in the direction the surgeon is looking; however, these devices can be uncomfortable to wear for prolonged periods. The fiberoptic light cord from the headset tethers the surgeon to the light source, which can exacerbate crowding.

CASE CARTS AND STORAGE

In the case cart system, prepackaged sterile instruments and supplies for each scheduled operation are placed on a single open cart (or in an enclosed cart) and delivered from the central sterile supply area to the OR before the start of the procedure. Instrument sets should be sterilized according to facility policy. It is not recommended that instrument sets be flash sterilized immediately before use in order to avoid purchasing additional instrument sets.[42] Instruments that are used less frequently or are used as replacements for contaminated items can be kept in nearby fixed or mobile storage modules for ready access when required. Replacements for frequently used items that may become contaminated (e.g., dissecting scissors and hemostats) should be separately wrapped and sterile so that they are readily available if needed during an operation.

The Endovascular OR

The field of vascular surgery has rapidly expanded over the past decade to encompass a wide variety of both established and innovative endovascular procedures that are new to the OR environment. Such procedures include complex multilevel diagnostic arteriography, balloon angioplasty (with and without stenting), and endoluminal grafting of aortic aneurysms. Many of these procedures can be performed in the radiologic intervention suite as well as in the cardiac catheterization laboratory. However, the sterile environment, the option of performing combined open surgical and endovascular procedures, and the opportunity to provide one-stop diagnostic and therapeutic care make the OR the favored location for efficient and safe management. Although most OR personnel are familiar with fluoroscopic procedures as well as simple diagnostic arteriography, the development of a comprehensive and successful endovascular program in the OR requires significant personnel training, commitment of resources, and preparation. In what follows, we review certain basic considerations in the evolution of such a program, focusing primarily on space and equipment. Technical details of endovascular procedures are addressed in more detail elsewhere [see 4:7 Fundamentals of Endovascular Surgery].

RADIATION SAFETY

A detailed discussion of radiation physics and safety is beyond the scope of this chapter. There are, however, certain fundamental concerns that should be emphasized here to ensure the safety of patients and staff members.

Table 2 ICRP-Recommended Radiation Dose Limits[43]

	Dose Limit	
	Occupational	Public
Effective dose	20 mSv/yr averaged over defined periods of 5 yr	1 mSv/yr
Annual equivalent dose in Lens of the eye Skin Hands and feet	150 mSv 500 mSv 500 mSv	15 mSv 50 mSv —

ICRP—International Commission on Radiological Protection   mSv—millisievert

Units of Exposure

Radiation exposure is expressed in several ways. One of the most commonly used terms is the rad (radiation absorbed dose), defined as the amount of energy absorbed by tissue (100 erg/g = 1 rad). In the Système International, the gray (Gy) is used in place of the rad (1 Gy = 100 rad). The newest of the units in current use, the millisievert (mSv), was introduced as a measure of the effective absorbed dose to the entire body (accounting for different sensitivities of exposed tissues). The amount of radiation generated by the x-ray tube is determined by the energy generated by the beam, which in turn is determined both by the number of x-ray photons generated (measured in milliamperes [mA]) and by the power or penetration of the beam (measured in kilovolts [kV]). Most modern fluoroscopes automatically balance mA levels against kV levels on the basis of the contrast of the image so as to optimize image quality and minimize x-ray exposure.

Exposure of human beings to radiation is broadly categorized as either public (i.e., environmental exposure of the general public) or occupational. The International Commission on Radiological Protection (ICRP) has established recommended yearly limits of radiation exposure for these two categories [see Table 2].[43] A 2001 study determined that with appropriate protection, radiation exposure for busy endovascular surgeons fell between 5% and 8% of ICRP limits, whereas exposure for other OR personnel fell between 2% and 4%.[44] Average radiation exposure for patients undergoing endovascular aneurysm repair was 360 mSv/case (range, 120 to 860).[44]

Basic Safety Rules

A few simple rules and procedures can help ensure a safe environment for patients and OR staff. The simplest rule is to minimize the use of fluoroscopy. Inexperienced operators are notorious for excessive reliance on fluoroscopy. Such overutilization results both from needing more time to perform endovascular maneuvers than a more experienced surgeon would need and, more important, from performing excessive and unnecessary (and frequently unintentional) imaging between maneuvers. The use of pulsed fluoroscopy and effective collimation of the images will also minimize the dose of radiation administered. Minimal use of high-definition fluoroscopy and unnecessary cine runs (both of which boost radiation output) are desirable. Most important, surgeons and OR staff should maximize their working distance from radiation sources. Radiation scatter drops off rapidly with increasing distance from the fluoroscope.

Safety Equipment and Monitoring

All OR personnel should wear protective lead aprons (0.25 to

0.5 mm in thickness). Wraparound designs are preferred because members of the OR team will invariably turn their backs to the radiation source on occasion. The apron should include a thyroid shield. High-level users must wear protective lead-containing lenses. A mobile shield (e.g., of lead acrylic) is a useful adjunct that may be employed to reduce exposure during cine runs. All personnel should wear radiation safety badges. Although these badges afford no direct protection, they do allow direct monitoring of individual cumulative exposure on a monthly basis.

PHYSICAL LAYOUT

The design of the endovascular OR depends on the balance of institutional and programmatic needs. For large institutions with a significant endovascular volume, a dedicated endovascular OR may be desirable. Ideally, such a room would combine fixed ceiling-mounted imaging equipment with a dedicated "floating" fluoroscopy table. The main advantage of a dedicated endovascular OR is that it provides state-of-the-art imaging techniques and capabilities in the OR setting; the main disadvantage is that it is relatively inflexible and is not useful for other procedures. For many institutions, such a room may not be cost-effective. Fortunately, with careful design, a high-quality endovascular suite can be set up that is flexible enough to allow both complex endovascular procedures and conventional open vascular and nonvascular operations to be performed. Such a room should be at least 600 sq ft in area, with sufficient length and clearance for extension tables and angiographic wires and catheters.

EQUIPMENT

Imaging Equipment

There are two fundamental physical designs for OR imaging equipment. The first is the fixed ceiling-mounted system that is also employed in catheterization laboratories and dedicated radiologic interventional suites. The second is a system using portable C-arms with dedicated vascular software packages designed for optimal endovascular imaging. Each of these systems has advantages and disadvantages.

Notable benefits of the fixed ceiling-mounted system include higher power output and smaller focal spot size, resulting in the highest-quality images. Larger image intensifiers (up to 16 in.) make possible larger visual fields for diagnostic arteriograms; thus, fewer runs need be made, and injection of dye and exposure to radiation are reduced accordingly. The variable distance between the x-ray tube and the image intensifier allows the intensifier to be placed close to the patient if desired, thereby improving image quality and decreasing radiation scatter. Fixed systems are accompanied by floating angiography tables, which allow the surgeon to move the patient easily beneath the fixed image intensifier. It is generally accepted that such systems afford the surgeon the most control and permit the most effortless and efficient imaging of patients.

Unfortunately, fixed ceiling-mounted systems are quite expensive (typically $1 million to $1.5 million), and major structural renovations are often required for installation in a typical OR. Perhaps more important for most ORs, however, is that these systems are not particularly flexible. The floating angiography tables and the immobility of the image intensifiers render the rooms unsuitable for most conventional open surgical procedures. Consequently, fixed imaging systems are generally restricted to high-volume centers where utilization rates justify the construction of dedicated endovascular ORs.

As endovascular procedures in the OR have become increasingly common, the imaging capability and versatility of portable

Table 3 Standard Equipment for Endovascular ORs

Diagnostic arteriography	Entry needle (16-gauge beveled)
	Entry wire (J wire or floppy-tip wire)
	Arterial sheath (5 Fr)
	Catheters
	Multipurpose nonselective (pigtail, tennis racquet, straight, etc.)
	Selective (cobra head, shepherd's crook, etc.)
	Guide wires (floppy, steerable, angled, hydrophilic, etc.)
	Contrast agent (nonionic preferred)
	Power injector
Balloon stent angioplasty	Sheaths (various lengths and diameters)
	Guide catheters
	Balloons (various lengths and diameters)
	Stents
	Balloon expandable (various lengths and diameters)
	Self-expanding (various lengths and diameters)
	Inflation device
Endovascular aneurysm repair	Large-caliber sheaths (12–24 Fr)
	Super-stiff guide wires
	Endovascular stent grafts
	Main body and contralateral iliac limb
	Aortic and iliac extension grafts
	Endovascular arterial coils

digital C-arms have increased dramatically. State-of-the-art portable C-arms are considerably less expensive than fixed systems ($175,000 to $225,000) while retaining many of their advantages. The variable image intensifier size (from 6 to 12 in.) offers valuable flexibility, with excellent resolution at the smaller end and an adequate field of view at the larger end. With some portable C-arm systems, it is possible to vary the distance between the image intensifier and the x-ray tube, as with a fixed system (see above). Pulsed fluoroscopy, image collimation, and filtration are standard features for improving imaging and decreasing radiation exposure. Sophisticated software packages allow high-resolution digital subtraction angiography, variable magnification, road mapping (i.e., the superimposition of live fluoroscopy over a saved digital arteriogram), and a number of other useful features. Improvements in C-arm design allow the surgeon to use a foot pedal to select various imaging and recording modes as well as to play back selected images and sequences.

Unlike fixed systems, which require patients to be moved on a floating table to change the field of view, C-arm systems require the image intensifier to be moved from station to station over a fixed patient. Although more cumbersome than fixed systems, the newest C-arms have increased mobility and maneuverability. Patients must be placed on a special nonmetallic carbon fiber table. To provide a sufficient field of view and permit panning from head to toe, the tables must be supported at one end with complete clearance beneath. Although these tables do not flex, they are sufficient for most operations. Furthermore, they are mobile and may be replaced with conventional operating tables when the endovascular suite is being used for standard open surgical procedures.

Interventional Equipment

The performance of endovascular procedures in the OR requires familiarity with a wide range of devices that may be unfamiliar to OR personnel, such as guide wires, sheaths, specialized catheters, angioplasty balloons, stents, and stent grafts [*see Table 3*]. In a busy endovascular OR, much of this equipment must be

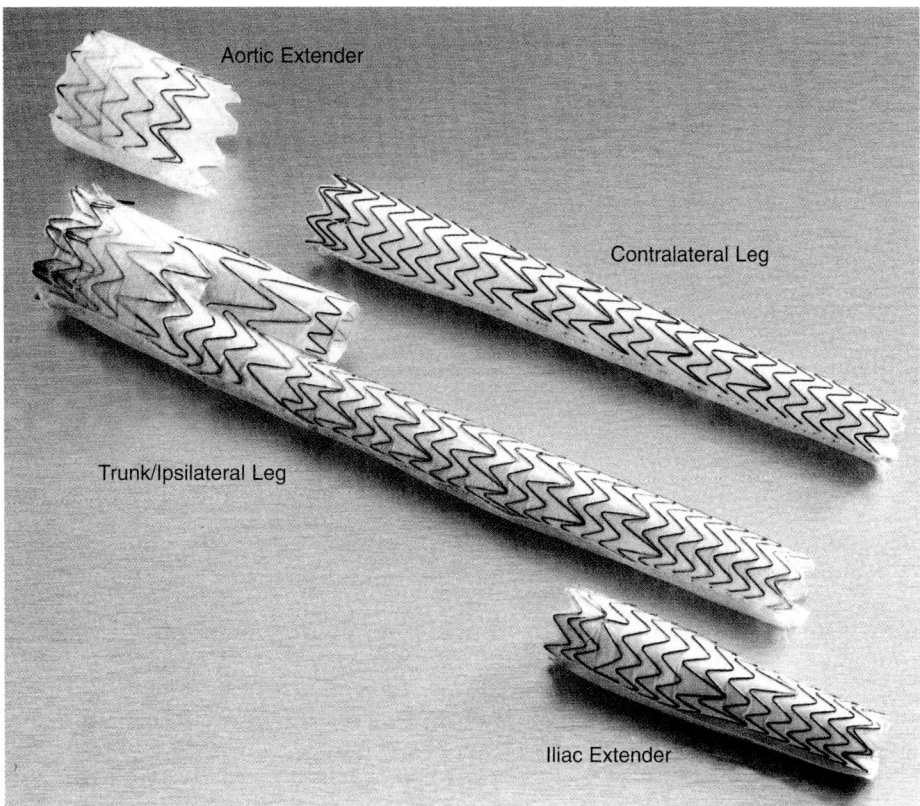

Figure 1   **Shown are the component parts of a modular aortic stent graft.**

stocked for everyday use, with the remainder ordered on a case-by-case basis. The expense of establishing the necessary inventory of equipment can be substantial and can place a considerable burden on smaller hospitals that are already spending sizable amounts on stocking similar devices for their catheterization laboratories and interventional suites. Fortunately, many companies are willing to supply equipment on a consignment basis, allowing hospitals to pay for devices as they are used.

Aortic Stent Grafts

Endovascular repair of an abdominal aortic aneurysm (EVAR) is the most common and important endovascular procedure performed in the OR [*see 4:9 Repair of Infrarenal Abdominal Aortic Aneurysms*]. As of spring 2003, three EVAR devices had been approved by the FDA for commercial use, with numerous others at various stages of the FDA approval process. All EVAR grafts are expensive (> $10,000). Although busy hospitals may maintain an inventory of devices, most grafts are ordered on a case-by-base basis. The favored devices are configured as bifurcated aortoiliac grafts. Most such grafts are modular in design, comprising two main pieces [*see Figure 1*], though one unibody device has been approved. Nonbifurcated grafts connecting the aorta to a single iliac artery are available for special circumstances. Grafts are constructed of either polyester or polytetrafluoroethelyne (PTFE) and have varying amounts of stent support. Proximal fixation is accomplished in different ways, ranging from friction fit to the use of hooks and barbs. Various extension components for both ends of the graft are available; in many cases, these components are necessary to complete the repair.

Endovascular therapy is a rapidly evolving field within the discipline of vascular surgery. Many operations traditionally performed as open surgical procedures are increasingly being sup-

planted by less invasive endovascular alternatives. Today's vascular surgery ORs must be prepared and equipped for a safe and efficient transition as this trend continues.

The Laparoscopic OR

PHYSICAL LAYOUT

With the advent of laparoscopy, it has become necessary to reevaluate traditional OR concepts with the aim of determining how best to design a surgical environment suitable for the demanding requirements of advanced minimally invasive surgical procedures.

As noted (see above), until the early 1990s, ORs were constructed in much the same way as they had been for nearly 100 years. The effect of the explosion in minimally invasive surgical procedures that occurred in that decade, along with the demonstration that patients benefited from significantly reduced recovery times, was to force OR personnel to move rapidly into a new age of technology, with little or no preparation. During the early days of laparoscopic surgery, surgeons noted significant increases in turnover time and procedural down time.[45] Adding to the problem was that the OR environment was becoming increasingly cluttered as a consequence of the addition of endoscopic video towers and other equipment. This equipment often proved to be complicated to use and expensive to repair. The increasing expenditure of money and time, coupled with an operating environment that increasingly promoted confusion rather than patient care, constituted a clear signal that the OR, as designed a century before, had been stretched beyond its capabilities and needed to be redesigned.

A key component of OR redesign for laparoscopic surgery is the placement of patient contact equipment on easily movable booms that are suspended from the ceiling. This arrangement makes rooms easier to clean and thus speeds turnover. All patient contact equipment and monitors are placed on these booms, and all other equipment is moved to the periphery of the surgical suite, usually in a nurse's command and control center. Thus, control of all equipment is at the fingertips of the circulating nurse, and the disruption and inconvenience of manipulating equipment on carts is avoided.

Rearranging monitors is much simpler with the easily movable booms than with carts, and there are no wires to trip OR personnel, because the wiring is done through the boom structure. Furthermore, because the wiring moves with the equipment, there is less risk that settings will be accidentally changed or wires unplugged—and thus less wear and tear on equipment and staff. The booms are easily moved to the periphery of the room, allowing the room to be used for multispecialty procedures, including non–minimally invasive procedures [see Figure 2].

LAPAROSCOPIC SURGICAL TEAM

The issue of time efficiency in the OR is at the heart of 21st-century surgical practice. Prolonged operating time, excessive setup time, and slow turnover can all affect productivity adversely. As managed care continues to evolve, less productive health care providers will be left behind. The right equipment and the right room design provide the basic foundation for a more productive OR. Without the right team, however, time efficiencies cannot be optimized. To achieve quick turnover time and efficient procedural flow in the laparoscopic OR, it is critical to inculcate a team orientation in all OR personnel.[46]

It is clear that a team of circulating nurses and scrub techs specially designated for minimally invasive surgical procedures can accomplish their tasks more quickly and efficiently than a random group of circulating nurses and scrub techs could. The time savings can be channeled into a larger volume of procedures and a more relaxed, patient care–driven OR environment.

Training seminars to improve the OR staff's familiarity with and performance of laparoscopic procedures should be given. Sessions in which surgeons present the technical issues involved in advanced laparoscopic procedures, including room setup, choice of equipment, and procedural steps, are beneficial. Video-tower setup and troubleshooting can be taught in small group sessions, with an emphasis on solving common technical problems by a process analogous to working through a differential diagnosis.

EQUIPMENT

In addition to having the correct room design, the laparoscopic OR must include equipment that provides the highest level of video quality and incorporates the latest developments in command and control systems.

Cameras and Scopes

No other device is as critical to the success of a laparoscopic procedure as the video camera. Without high-quality image capture and display, accurate identification and treatment of the disease process are impossible. The video cameras used for minimally invasive surgery contain solid-state light-sensitive receptors called charge-coupled devices (CCDs, or chips) that are able to detect differences in brightness at different points throughout an image. Generally, two types are available: one-chip cameras and three-chip cameras. Three-chip cameras provide the greatest resolution and light sensitivity; however, they are also the most expensive. One-chip cameras augment their single CCD with an overlay of millions of colored filters; electronics within the camera or the camera control unit then determine which filter the light hitting a specific point in the CCD is passing through. In this way, it is pos-

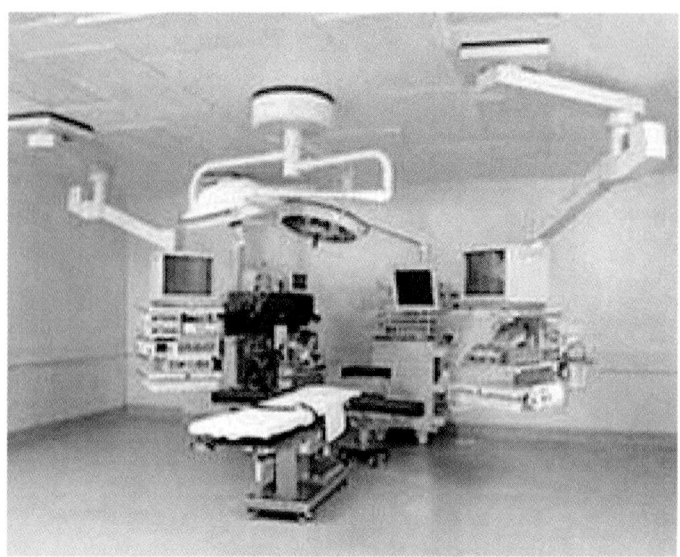

Figure 2 The new OR suites at the Medical College of Virginia incorporate the Endosuite design (Stryker Communications, San Jose, Calif.) for advanced laparoscopic procedures.

sible to produce cameras that are smaller and less expensive than three-chip cameras; however, resolution and sensitivity are both compromised.

The trend in laparoscopic surgery has been toward smaller scope diameters. In particular, there has been a large migration from 10 mm to 5 mm rigid scopes. As a result, it is essential to choose a camera that can perform under the reduced lighting conditions imposed by the use of 5 mm devices. The nature and intensity of the light source must be factored in as well. When a laparoscopic procedure is being performed through 5 mm ports, it is often preferable to use a xenon light source so as to maximize light throughput and optimize resolution.

Surgeon's Control of Equipment: Touch Panels, Voice Activation, and Robotics

There are some inherent shortcomings in the way OR equipment has traditionally been accessed, and those shortcomings have been exacerbated by the advent of minimally invasive procedures. Because most of the equipment needed for minimally invasive surgery resides outside the sterile field, the point person for critical controls became the circulating nurse. Often, the circulating nurse would be out of the room at the precise moment when an adjustment (e.g., in the level of the insufflator's CO_2) had to be made. Surgeons grew frustrated at the subsequent delays and at their inability to take their own steps to change things. Additionally, nurses grew weary of such responsibilities; these constant interactions with the video tower pulled them away from patient-related tasks and from necessary clerical and operational work. The answer was to improve surgeons' access to these critical devices via methods such as touchscreen control and, more recently, voice activation.

Development of voice activation began in the late 1960s. The goal was a simple, safe, and universally acceptable voice recognition system that flawlessly carried out the verbal requests of the user. However, attempts to construct a system capable of accurately recognizing a wide array of speech patterns faced formidable technological hurdles that only now are beginning to be overcome. Although voice recognition is not yet a mature technology, it is clearly here to stay, and it has begun to permeate many facets of everyday life.

In 1998, the first FDA-approved voice activation system, Hermes (Computer Motion, Santa Barbara, Calif.), was introduced into the OR. Designed to provide surgeons with direct access and control of surgical devices, Hermes is operated via either a handheld pendant or voice commands from the surgeon. The challenges of advanced laparoscopic surgery provide a fertile ground for demonstrating the benefits of voice activation [see Table 4]. Two-handed laparoscopic procedures make it very difficult for a surgeon to control ancillary equipment manually, even if touch-screens are sterile and within reach.

Voice activation gives surgeons immediate access to and direct control of surgical devices, and it provides the OR team with critical information. To operate a device, the surgeon must take approximately 20 minutes to train the recognition system to his or her voice patterns and must wear an audio headset to relay commands to the controller. The learning curve for voice control is minimal (two or three cases, on average). Many devices can now be controlled by voice activation software, including cameras, light sources, digital image capture and documentation devices, printers, insufflators, OR ambient and surgical lighting systems, operating tables, and electrocauteries.

In the future, more and more devices will be accessible to the surgeon through simple voice commands, and the time will soon arrive when telesurgical and telementoring capabilities will be an integral part of the system. The voice interface will allow surgeons to interact with the world at large in such a way that the performance of a surgical procedure is actively facilitated rather than interrupted. The OR will cease to be an environment of isolation.

Infection Control in the OR

Infection control is a major concern in health care in general, but it is a particularly important issue in the sterile environment of the OR, where patients undergo surgical procedures and are at significant risk for perioperative nosocomial infection. Even the best OR design will not compensate for improper surgical technique or failure to pay attention to infection prevention.

Surgical site infection (SSI) is a major cause of patient morbidity, mortality, and health care costs. In the United States, according to the Centers for Disease Control and Prevention (CDC), about 2.9% of nearly 30 million operations are complicated by SSIs each year. This percentage may in fact be an underestimate,

given the known inherent problems with surgeons' voluntary self-reporting of infections occurring in the ambulatory surgical setting.[47] Each infection is estimated to increase total hospital stay by an average of 7 days and add more than $3,000 in charges.

SSIs have been divided by the CDC into three broad categories: superficial incisional SSI, deep incisional SSI, and organ/space SSI [see Table 5 and 1:2 Prevention of Postoperative Infection].[48] Factors that contribute to the development of SSI include (1) those arising from the patient's health status, (2) those related to the physical environment where surgical care is provided, and (3) those resulting from clinical interventions that increase the patient's inherent risk. Careful patient selection and preparation, including judicious use of antibiotic prophylaxis, can decrease the overall risk of infection, especially after clean-contaminated and contaminated operations.

HAND HYGIENE

Hand antisepsis plays a significant role in preventing nosocomial infections. When outbreaks of infection occur in the perioperative period, careful assessment of the adequacy of hand hygiene among OR personnel is recommended. U.S. guidelines recommend that agents used for surgical hand scrubs should substantially reduce microorganisms on intact skin, contain a nonirritating antimicrobial preparation, possess broad-spectrum activity, and be fast-acting and persistent.[49] In October 2002, the CDC published the most recent version of its Guideline for Hand Hygiene in Health-Care Settings.[50] The Guideline's final recommendations regarding surgical hand antisepsis included the following:

- Surgical hand antisepsis using either an antimicrobial soap or an alcohol-based hand rub with persistent activity is recommended before donning sterile gloves when performing surgical procedures (evidence level IB).
- When performing surgical hand antisepsis using an antimicrobial soap, scrub hands and forearms for the length of time recommended by the manufacturer, usually 2 to 6 minutes. Long scrub times (e.g., 10 minutes) are not necessary (evidence level IB).
- When using an alcohol-based surgical hand-scrub product with persistent activity, follow the manufacturer's instructions. Before applying the alcohol solution, prewash hands and forearms with a nonantimicrobial soap, and dry hands and forearms completely. After application of the alcohol-based product, allow hands and forearms to dry thoroughly before donning sterile gloves.

GLOVES AND PROTECTIVE BARRIERS

Because of the invasive nature of surgery, there is a high risk of pathogen transfer during an operation, a risk from which both the patient and the surgical team must be protected. The risk can be reduced by using protective barriers, such as surgical gloves. Wearing two pairs of surgical gloves rather than a single pair is considered to provide an additional barrier and to further reduce the risk of contamination. A 2002 Cochrane review concluded that wearing two pairs of latex gloves significantly reduced the number of perforations of the innermost glove.[51] This evidence came from trials undertaken in low-risk surgical specialties—that is, specialties that did not include orthopedic joint surgery.

The Occupational Safety and Health Administration (OSHA) requires that personal protective equipment be available in the health care setting, and these requirements are spelled out in detail in the OSHA standard on Occupational Exposure to Bloodborne Pathogens, which went into effect in 1992. Among the require-

Table 4   Benefits of Voice Activation Technology in the Laparoscopic OR

Benefits to surgical team	Gives surgeons direct and immediate control of devices
	Frees nursing staff from dull, repetitive tasks
	Reduces miscommunication and frustration between surgeons and staff
	Increases OR efficiency
	Alerts staff when device is malfunctioning or setting off alarm
Benefits to hospital	Saves money, allowing shorter, more efficient operations
	Contributes to better OR utilization and, potentially, performance of more surgical procedures
	Lays foundation for expanded use of voice activation in ORs
	Allows seamless working environment
Benefit to patient	Reduces operating time, which—coupled with improved optics, ergonomics, and efficiency—leads to better surgical outcome

---

Table 5   Criteria for Defining a Surgical Site Infection (SSI)[71]

Superficial incisional SSI

Infection occurs within 30 days after the operation, *and* infection involves only skin or subcutaneous tissue of the incisions, *and* at least *one* of the following:

1. Purulent drainage, with or without laboratory confirmation, from the superficial incision
2. Organisms isolated from an aseptically obtained culture of fluid or tissue from the superficial incision
3. At least one of the following signs or symptoms of infection: pain or tenderness, localized swelling, redness, or heat; *and* superficial incision is deliberately opened by surgeon, *unless* incision is culture negative
4. Diagnosis of superficial incisional SSI by the surgeon or attending physician

Do *not* report the following conditions as SSI:

1. Stitch abscess (minimal inflammation and discharge confined to the points of suture penetration)
2. Infection of an episiotomy or newborn circumcision site
3. Infected burn wound
4. Incisional SSI that extends into the fascial and muscle layers (see deep incisional SSI)

Note: Specific criteria are used for identifying infected episiotomy and circumcision sites and burn wounds

Deep incisional SSI

Infection occurs within 30 days after the operation if no implant* is left in place or within 1 yr if implant is in place and the infection appears to be related to the operation, *and* infection involves deep soft tissues (e.g., fascial and muscle layers) on the incision, *and* at least *one* of the following:

1. Purulent drainage from the deep incision but not from the organ/space component of the surgical site
2. A deep incision spontaneously dehisces or is deliberately opened by a surgeon when the patient has at least one of the following signs or symptoms: fever (> 38° C [100.4° F]), localized pain, or tenderness, unless site is culture negative
3. An abscess or other evidence of infection involving the deep incision is found on direct examination, during reoperation, or by histopathologic or radiologic examination
4. Diagnosis of a deep incisional SSI by a surgeon or attending physician

Notes:

1. Report infection that involves both superficial and deep incision sites as deep incisional SSI
2. Report an organ/space SSI that drains through the incision as a deep incisional SSI

Organ/space SSI

Infection occurs within 30 days after the operation if no implant* is left in place or within 1 yr if implant is in place and the infection appears to be related to the operation, *and* infection involves any part of the anatomy (e.g., organs or spaces), other than the incision, which was opened or manipulated during an operation, *and* at least *one* of the following:

1. Purulent drainage from a drain that is placed through a stab wound† into the organ/space
2. Organisms isolated from an aseptically obtained culture of fluid or tissue in the organ/space
3. An abscess or other evidence of infection involving the organ/space that is found on direct examination, during reoperation, or by histopathologic or radiologic examination
4. Diagnosis of an organ/space SSI by a surgeon or attending physician

---

*National Nosocomial Infection Surveillance definition: a nonhuman-derived implantable foreign body (e.g., prosthetic heart valve, nonhuman vascular graft, mechanical heart, or hip prosthesis) that is permanantly placed in a patient during surgery.
†If the area around a stab wound becomes infected, it is not an SSI. It is considered a skin or soft tissue infection, depending on its depth.

---

ments is the implementation of the CDC's universal precautions,[52] designed to prevent transmission of human immunodeficiency virus, hepatitis B virus, and other bloodborne pathogens. These precautions involve the use of protective barriers (e.g., gloves, gowns, aprons, masks, and protective eyewear) to reduce the risk that the health care worker's skin or mucous membranes will be exposed to potentially infectious materials. Performance standards for protective barriers are the responsibility of the FDA's Center for Devices and Radiological Health. These standards define the performance properties that these products must exhibit, such as minimum strength, barrier protection, and fluid resistance. The current CDC recommendation is to use surgical gowns and drapes that resist liquid penetration and remain effective barriers when wet.

Compliance with universal precautions and barrier protection is notably difficult to achieve. A 2001 study, however, found that educational interventions aimed at OR personnel improved compliance significantly, particularly with regard to the use of protective eyewear and double-gloving. Furthermore, such interventions were associated with a reduced incidence of blood and body fluid exposure.[53]

INFECTION SURVEILLANCE PROGRAMS

Surveillance is an important part of infection control. The success of a surveillance program depends on the ability of the infection control team to form a partnership with the surgical staff. Creating a sense of ownership of the surveillance initiative among the members of the surgical staff enhances cooperation and ensures that the best use is made of the information generated. It is not possible to eliminate SSIs completely, but by sharing information and influencing subsequent behavior, it is certainly possible to reduce their incidence.

A 2002 study documented successful institution of a surveillance program after a period of high infection rates in an orthopedic surgical department.[54] This program contributed to a significant reduction in SSI rates after elective hip and knee replacement procedures and was successful in creating awareness of infection control practices among hospital staff members.

ANTIMICROBIAL PROPHYLAXIS

SSIs are established several hours after contamination.[55] Administration of antibiotics before contamination reduces the risk of infection but is subsequently of little value.[56] Selective use of short-duration, narrow-spectrum antibiotic agents should be considered for appropriate patients to cover the usual pathogens isolated from SSIs [*see Table 6*]. Optimal surgical antimicrobial prophylaxis is based on the following three principles: (1) appropriate choice of antimicrobial agent, (2) proper timing of antibiotic administration before incision, and (3) limited duration of antibiotic administration after operation.

Recommendations for antibiotic prophylaxis are addressed in more detail elsewhere [*see 1:2 Prevention of Postoperative Infection*]. When a preoperative antibiotic is indicated, a single dose of therapeutic strength, administered shortly before incision, usually suffices.[57] (The dose may have to be increased if the patient is morbidly obese.[58]) A second dose is indicated if the procedure is longer than two half-lives of the drug or if extensive blood loss occurs. Continuation of prophylaxis beyond 24 hours is not recommended.

With respect to redosing of the antimicrobial agent in lengthy procedures, consistency is important but can be difficult to obtain.

OR design can be helpful in this regard. In a 2003 study, significant improvement of intraoperative antibiotic prophylaxis in prolonged (> 4 hours) cardiac operations was achieved by employing an automated intraoperative alert system in the OR, with alarms both audible and visible on the OR computer console at 225 minutes after administration of preoperative antibiotics.[59] Intraoperative redosing of antibiotics was significantly more frequent in the reminder group (68%) than in the control group (40%; P < 0.0001). The use of an automatic reminder system in the OR improved compliance with guidelines on perioperative antibiotic prophylaxis.

NONPHARMACOLOGIC PREVENTIVE MEASURES

Several studies have confirmed that certain nonpharmacologic measures, including maintenance of perioperative normothermia and provision of supplemental perioperative oxygen, are efficacious in preventing SSIs.[60]

Perioperative Normothermia

A 1996 study showed that warming patients during colorectal surgery reduced infection rates.[61] A subsequent observational cohort study found that mild perioperative hypothermia was associated with a significantly increased incidence of SSI.[62] A randomized, controlled trial, published in 2001, was done to determine whether warming patients before short-duration clean procedures would have the same effect.[63] In this trial, 421 patients scheduled to undergo clean (breast, varicose vein, or hernia) procedures were randomly assigned either to a nonwarmed group or to one of two warmed groups (locally warmed and systemically warmed). Warming was applied for at least 30 minutes before surgery. Patients were followed, and masked outcome assessments were made at 2 and 6 weeks. SSIs occurred in 19 (14%) of 139

Table 6 Distribution of Pathogens Isolated from SSIs: National Nosocomial Infections Surveillance System, 1986–1996[48]

Pathogen	Percentage of Isolates*	
	1986–1989 (N=16,727)	1990–1996 (N=17,671)
Staphylococcus aureus	17	20
Coagulase-negative staphylococci	12	14
Enterococcus species	13	12
Escherichia coli	10	8
Pseudomonas aeruginosa	8	8
Enterobacter species	8	7
Proteus mirabilis	4	3
Klebsiella pneumoniae	3	3
Other Streptococcus species	3	3
Candida albicans	2	3
Group D streptococci (nonenterococci)	—	2
Other gram-positive aerobes	—	2
Bacteroides fragilis	—	2

*Pathogens representing less than 2% of isolates are excluded.

nonwarmed patients but in only 13 (5%) of 277 warmed patients (P = 0.001). Wound scores were also significantly lower in warmed patients (P = 0.007).

The safest and most effective way of protecting patients from hypothermia is to use forced-air warmers with specialized blankets placed over the upper or lower body. Alternatives include placing a warming water mattress under the patient and draping the patient with an aluminized blanket. Second-line therapy for maintaining normothermia is to warm all I.V. fluids. Any irrigation fluids used in a surgical procedure should be at or slightly above body temperature before use. Radiant heating devices placed above the operative field may be especially useful during operations on infants. Use of a warmer on the inhalation side of the anesthetic gas circuit can also help maintain the patient's body temperature during an operation.

Supplemental Perioperative Oxygen

Destruction by oxidation, or oxidative killing, is the body's most important defense against surgical pathogens. This defensive response depends on oxygen tension in contaminated tissue. An easy method of improving oxygen tension in adequately perfused tissue is to increase the fraction of inspired oxygen (F_IO_2). Supplemental perioperative oxygen (i.e., an F_IO_2 of 80% instead of 30%) significantly reduces postoperative nausea and vomiting and diminishes the decrease in phagocytosis and bacterial killing usually associated with anesthesia and surgery. Oxygen tension in wound tissue has been found to be a good predictor of SSI risk.[64]

Avoidance of Blood Transfusion

The association between blood transfusion and increased perioperative infection rates is well documented. In a 1997 study, geriatric hip fracture patients undergoing surgical repair who received blood transfusion had significantly higher rates of perioperative infection than those who did not (27% versus 15%), and this effect was present on multivariate analysis.[65] Another 1997 study, involving 697 patients undergoing surgery for colorectal cancer, yielded similar findings: 39% of transfused patients had bacterial infections, compared with 24% of nontransfused patients, and the relative risk of infection was 1.6 for transfusion of one to three units of blood and 3.6 for transfusion of more than three units.[66]

A large prospective cohort study published in 2003 evaluated the association between anemia, blood transfusion, and perioperative infection.[67] Logistic regression analysis confirmed that intraoperative transfusion of packed red blood cells was an independent risk factor for perioperative infection (odds ratio, 1.06; confidence interval, 1.01 to 1.11; P > 0.0001). Furthermore, transfusion of more than four units of packed red blood cells was associated with a 9.28-fold increased risk of infection (confidence interval, 5.74 to 15.00; P < 0.0001).

Housekeeping Procedures

FLOORS AND WALLS

Despite detailed recommendations for cleaning the OR [*see Table 7*],[68] the procedures that are optimal to provide a clean environment while still being cost-effective have not been critically analyzed.

Only a few studies have attempted to correlate surface contamination of the OR with SSI risk. In one study, for example, ORs were randomly assigned to either a control group or an experimental group.[69] The control rooms were cleaned with a germici-

Table 7 OR Cleaning Schedules

Areas requiring daily cleaning	Surgical lights and tracks Fixed ceiling-mounted equipment Furniture and mobile equipment, including wheels OR and hall floors Cabinet and push-plate handles Ventilation grills All horizontal surfaces Substerile areas Scrub and utility areas Scrub sinks
Areas requiring routinely scheduled cleaning	Ventilation ducts and filters Recessed tracks Cabinets and shelves Walls and ceilings Sterilizers, warming cabinets, refrigerators, and ice machines

dal agent and wet-vacuumed before the first case of the day and between cases; in the experimental rooms, cleaning consisted only of wiping up grossly visible contamination after clean and clean-contaminated cases. Both rooms had complete floor cleanup after contaminated or dirty and infected cases. The investigators found that bacterial colony counts obtained directly from the floors were lower in the control rooms but that counts obtained from other horizontal surfaces did not differ between the two OR groups. In addition, wound infection rates were the same in the control rooms and the experimental rooms and were comparable with rates reported in other series. Another study found that floor disinfectants decreased bacterial concentration on the floor for only 2 hours; colony counts then returned to pretreatment levels as personnel walked on the floor.[70] These investigators recommended discontinuing routine floor disinfection.

Even when an OR floor is contaminated, the rate of redispersal of bacteria into the air is low, and the clearance rate is high. It is unlikely, therefore, that bacteria from the floor contribute to SSI. Consequently, routine disinfection of the OR floor between clean or clean-contaminated cases appears unnecessary.

According to CDC guidelines for prevention of SSI, when visible soiling of surfaces or equipment occurs during an operation, an Environmental Protection Agency (EPA)–approved hospital disinfectant should be used to decontaminate the affected areas before the next operation.[71] This statement is in keeping with the OSHA requirement that all equipment and environmental surfaces be cleaned and decontaminated after contact with blood or other potentially infectious materials. Disinfection after a contaminated or dirty case and after the last case of the day is probably a reasonable practice, though it is not supported by directly pertinent data. Wet-vacuuming of the floor with an EPA-approved hospital disinfectant should be performed routinely after the last operation of the day or night.

DIRTY CASES

Operations are classified or stratified into four groups in relation to the epidemiology of SSIs [*see 1:2 Prevention of Postoperative Infection*].[72] Clean operations are those elective cases in which the GI tract or the respiratory tract is not entered and there are no major breaks in technique. The infection rate in this group should be less than 3%. Clean-contaminated operations are those elective cases in which the respiratory or the GI tract is entered or during which a break in aseptic technique has occurred. The infection rate in such cases should be less than 10%. Contaminated operations

are those cases in which a fresh traumatic wound is present or gross spillage of GI contents occurs. Dirty or infected operations include those in which bacterial inflammation occurs or in which pus is present. The infection rate may be as high as 40% in a contaminated or dirty operation.

Fear that bacteria from dirty or heavily contaminated cases could be transmitted to subsequent cases has resulted in the development of numerous and costly rituals of OR cleanup. However, there are no prospective studies and no large body of relevant data to support the usefulness of such rituals. In fact, one study found no significant difference in environmental bacterial counts after clean cases than after dirty ones.[73] Numerous authorities have recommended that there be only one standard of cleaning the OR after either clean or dirty cases.[68,73,74] This recommendation is reasonable because any patient may be a source of contamination caused by unrecognized bacterial or viral infection; more important, the other major source of OR contamination is the OR personnel.

Rituals applied to dirty cases include placing a germicide-soaked mat outside the OR door, allowing the OR to stand idle for an arbitrary period after cleanup of a dirty procedure, and using two circulating nurses, one inside the room and one outside. None of these practices has a sound theoretical or factual basis.

Traditionally, dirty cases have been scheduled after all the clean cases of the day. However, this restriction reduces the efficiency with which operations can be scheduled and may unnecessarily delay emergency cases. There are no data to support special cleaning procedures or closing of an OR after a contaminated or dirty operation has been performed.[75] Tacky mats placed outside the entrance to an OR suite have not been shown to reduce the number of organisms on shoes or stretcher wheels, nor do they reduce the risk of SSI.[76]

Data Management in the OR

In this era of capitated reimbursement and managed care, containment of health care costs is a prime concern; consequently, OR efficiency has become a higher priority for many institutions.[77] No OR environment can even function, let alone improve its efficiency, without data. Data control every facet of the activities within the OR environment. For evaluating procedural time, OR utilization and efficiency, OR scheduling, infection rates, injury prevention, and other key measures of organizational function, it is essential to have current, high-quality data.

To obtain good data, it is necessary first to determine what information is required. For example, assessment of OR utilization and efficiency depends on how utilization is measured. Before an OR can meaningfully be measured against a target figure, it is necessary to know exactly how the organization calculates utilization and how the parameters are defined. There is no accepted national standard. The future of the organization—not to mention the jobs of the people who work there—may depend on how well it understands and controls OR utilization.

It is generally agreed that 80% to 85% is the maximum utilization level that an OR can be expected to reach. At higher utilization levels, the OR loses flexibility, and the hospital should consider adding capacity. It is important that utilization of all OR resources by the various sectors of the institution be reasonable and balanced, because higher OR utilization can be achieved only when this is the case. To improve the use of OR time, it is important (1) to limit the number of ORs available to the number required to achieve good utilization, (2) to have nurses rather than attending surgeons control access to the surgical schedule, (3) to provide good scheduling systems that allow surgeons to follow themselves, and (4) to maintain systems that enable and enforce efficient turnover between cases.[78]

It has been estimated that 30% of all health care outlays are related to surgical expenditures.[79] Thus, it is likely that in a cost-conscious, competitive environment, the OR will be a major focus of change. Surgical costs are related to OR utilization, inventory levels, operative volume, supply usage, and equipment purchase, rental, and maintenance. Facility design also affects efficiency and thus the ability to reduce costs. All of these issues must be evaluated and monitored to ensure quality care at the lowest feasible cost.[80]

Once good data are available, the issue then becomes how practices and procedures should change as a result. Although new information, by itself, can often affect behavior, true behavior modification in the OR requires effective leadership from the chiefs of surgery, anesthesia, and nursing, all of whom should receive monthly performance reports.

DATA ACQUISITION

The necessary data must be not only available but also accessible in a rapid and convenient manner. Total automation of OR data management is critical for ascertaining patterns, managing productivity and resources, and providing solid informational bases for future decisions. Only through automation tools can relevant, timely, and accurate statistical data be generated to facilitate problem solving, trend spotting, forecasting, and revisioning.[81]

A long-standing question in OR utilization was how many historical data points were necessary or ideal to make appropriate decisions regarding OR staffing via statistical methods. In a 2002 study, statistical analysis of 30 workdays of data yielded staffing solutions that had, on average, 30% lower staffing costs and 27% higher staffing productivity than the existing staffing plans.[82] The productivity achieved in this way was 80%, and this figure was not significantly improved by increasing the number of workdays of data beyond 180. These findings suggest that in most OR environments, statistical methods of data acquisition and analysis can identify cost-lowering and productivity-enhancing staffing solutions by using 30 days of OR and anesthesia data.

OR SCHEDULING

For optimal OR utilization, it is important to have a system for releasing OR time efficiently and appropriately. Surgical services fill their OR time at different rates. In a 2002 study, the median period between the time when a patient was scheduled for surgery and the day of the operation ranged from 2 to 27 days, depending on the subspecialty.[83] Whereas ophthalmologic surgeons might schedule outpatient cases weeks beforehand, cardiac or thoracic surgeons might book cases the day before the operation. Consequently, it would not be logical to release allocated OR time for all services the same prespecified number of days before surgery.[84] A better approach would be to predict, as soon as a case is scheduled, which surgical service is likely to have the most underutilized OR time on the scheduled day of surgery. In practice, the OR information system would perform the forecasting and provide a recommendation to the OR scheduler. To produce reliable results, forecasting should be based on the previous 6 months of OR performance, with allowances made for vacations and meeting-related down time.

Perioperative costs can be reduced if cases are scheduled so that the workload evenly matches staffing schedules. Specifically, to minimize the cost per case, down time must be minimized. Appropriate choice of the day on which a patient will undergo surgery is the most important decision affecting OR labor costs.[84]

QUALITY IMPROVEMENT

The key to increased OR efficiency is increased productivity. Standardization and streamlining of internal procedures reduces bottlenecks, and computerization speeds the flow of information so that continuous improvement of the system becomes possible. Before a desired improvement can be implemented, the proposed change must be tested quickly so that its effect can be determined. This is accomplished by means of a collaborative effort, in which the group involved in the change learns how to plan, do, check and act—the so-called PDCA cycle, which is a classic quality initiative method. During the PDCA cycle, teams are encouraged to share ideas and talk about various solutions. A change is tested quickly, and if it works, implementation is expanded and tested further. The importance of the changes that can be implemented is often secondary to the progress made in building collaboration with fellow physicians and other health care professionals.[84]

References

1. Guidelines for construction and equipment of hospital and medical facilities. DHHS publication No. (HRS-M-HF) 84-1. US Department of Health and Human Services, Rockville, Maryland, 1984

2. The American Institute of Architects: Guidelines for Construction and Equipment of Hospital and Health Care Facilities. The American Institute of Architects Press, Washington, DC, 2001

3. Maloney ME: The dermatological surgical suite—design and materials. Practical Manuals in Dermatologic Surgery. Grekin M, Ed. Churchill Livingstone, New York, 1991

4. Jolesz FA, Shtern F: The operating room of the future. Report of the National Cancer Institute Workshop "Imaging-Guided Stereotactic Tumor Diagnosis and Treatment." Invest Radiol 27:326, 1992

5. Green FL, Taylor NC: Operating room configuration. Laparoscopic Surgery. Ballantyne G, Leahy PF, Modlin IR, Eds. WB Saunders Co, Philadelphia, 1994, p 34

6. Laufman H: Surgical hazard control: effect of architecture and engineering. Arch Surg 107:552, 1973

7. The Design and Utilization of Operating Theatres. Johnston D, Hunter A, Eds. London, Edward Arnold, 1984

8. Klebanoff G: Operating-room design: an introduction. Bull Am Coll Surg 64(11):6, 1979

9. Smith W: Planning the surgical suite. FW Dodge Corp, New York, 1960, p 459

10. Putsep E: Planning of surgical centres. Lloyd-Luke Ltd, London, 1973, p 249

11. A Bibliography of the Operating Room Environment. American College of Surgeons, Chicago, 1995

12. Mathius JM: OR of the future to be less complicated, more efficient. OR Manager 11:7, 1995

13. Mangum SS, Cutler K: Increased efficiency through OR redesign and process simplification. AORN J 76:1041, 2002

14. Chinyanga HM: Temperature regulation and anesthesia. Pharmacol Ther 26:147, 1984

15. Beck WC: Choosing surgical illumination. Am J Surg 140:327, 1980

16. Beck WC: Operating room illumination: the current state of the art. Bull Am Coll Surg 66(5):10, 1981

17. Kern KA: The National Patient Safety Foundation: what it offers surgeons. Bull Am Coll Surg 83(11):24, 1998

18. LoCicero J, Nichols RL: Environmental health hazards in the operating room. Bull Am Coll Surg 67(5):2, 1982

19. LoCicero J, Quebbeman EJ, Nichols RL: Health hazards in the operating room: an update. Bull Am Coll Surg 72(9):4, 1987

20. Garden JM, O'Banion MK, Shelnitz LS, et al: Papillomavirus in the vapor of carbon dioxide laser-treated verrucae. JAMA 259:1199, 1988

21. Ray CD, Levinson R: Noise pollution in the oper-

ating room: a hazard to surgeons, personnel, and patients. J Spinal Disord 5:485, 1992

22. Cowan C Jr: Light hazards in the operating room. J Natl Med Assoc 84:425, 1992

23. National Academy of Science/National Institute of Medicine/National Research Council: Work-related Musculoskeletal Disorders: A Review of the Evidence. National Academy Press, Washington, DC, 1998

24. Practice Advisory for the Prevention of Perioperative Peripheral Neuropathies. Anesthesiology 92:1168, 2000

25. Cheney FW, Domino KB, Caplan RA, et al: Nerve injury associated with anesthesia. Anesthesia 90:1062, 1999

26. Warner ME, LaMaster LM, Thoening AK, et al: Compartment syndrome in surgical patients. Anesthesiology 94:705, 2001

27. Martin JT: Patient positioning. Clinical Anesthesia. Barash PG, Cullen BT, Stoelting RK, Eds. JB Lippincott Co, Philadelphia, 1989

28. Cucciara RF, Faust RJ: Patient positioning. Anesthesia, 5th ed. Miller RD, Ed. Churchill Livingstone, Philadelphia, 2000

29. West JB: Respiratory Physiology, 2nd ed. Williams & Wilkins, Baltimore, 1979

30. Benumof JL: Respiratory physiology and respiratory function during anesthesia. Anesthesia, 5th ed. Miller RD, Ed. Churchill Livingstone, Philadelphia, 2000

31. Warner MA, Warner DO, Harper CM, et al: Lower extremity neuropathies associated with lithotomy positions. Anesthesiology 93:938, 2000

32. Pfeffer SD, Halliwell JR, Warner MA: Effects of lithotomy position and external compression on lower leg compartment pressure. Anesthesiology 95:632, 2001

33. AORN Recommended Practices Subcommittee: Recommended practices: electrosurgery. AORN J 41:633, 1985

34. Pearce J: Current electrosurgical practice: hazards. J Med Eng Technol 9:107, 1985

35. Bochenko WJ: A review of electrosurgical units in the operating room. J Clin Eng 2:313, 1977

36. Lobraico RB: Laser safety in health care facilities: an overview. Bull Am Coll Surg 76(8):16, 1991

37. Gloster HM Jr, Roenigk RK: Risk of acquiring human papillomavirus from the plume produced by the carbon dioxide laser in the treatment of warts. J Am Acad Dermatol 32:436, 1995

38. Wisniewski PM, Warhol MJ, Rando RF, et al: Studies on the transmission of viral disease via the CO_2 laser plume and ejecta. J Reprod Med 35:1117, 1990

39. Jewett DL, Heinsohn P, Bennett C, et al: Blood-containing aerosols generated by surgical techniques: a possible infectious hazard. Am Ind Hyg Assoc J 53:228, 1992

40. Patkin M: Ergonomics and the operating microscope. Adv Ophthalmol 37:53, 1978

41. Walenga JM, Fareed J: Current status on new anticoagulant and antithrombotic drugs and devices. Curr Opin Pulmon Med 3:291, 1997

42. Mangram AJ, Horan TC, Pearson ML, et al: The Hospital Infection Control Practices Advisory Committee. Guideline for prevention of surgical site infection, 1999. Am J Infect Control 27:98, 1999

43. Radiological Protection and Safety in Medicine: A report of the International Commission of Radiological Protection. Annals of the ICRP 26:1, 1996

44. Lipsitz EC, Veith FJ, Ohki T, et al: Does endovascular repair of aortoiliac aneurysms pose a radiation safety hazard to vascular surgeons? J Vasc Surg 32:702, 2000

45. Patterson P: Turnover time: is all the study worth the effort? OR Manager, 15(3):5, 1999

46. Fernsebner B: Building a staffing plan based on OR's needs. OR Manager 12(2):7, 1996

47. Barie PS: Surgical site infections: epidemiology and prevention. Surg Infect 3(suppl 1):S9, 2002

48. Mangram AJ, Horan TC, Pearson ML, et al: Guideline for the prevention of surgical site infection, 1999. Hospital Infection Practices Advisory Committee. Infect Control Hosp Epidemiol 20:250, 1999

49. AORN Recommended Practices Committee: Recommended practices for surgical hand scrubs. Fogg D, Parker N, Shevlin D, Eds. Standards, Recommended Practices, and Guidelines. AORN, Inc, Denver, 2001

50. Boyce JM, Pittet D, Healthcare Infection Control Practices Advisory Committee, HICPAC/SHEA/APIC/IDSA Hand Hygiene Task Force: Guideline for hand hygiene in health-care settings. Recommendations of the Healthcare Infection Control Practices Advisory Committee and the HICPA/SHEA/APIC/IDSA Hand Hygiene Task Force. MMWR Recomm Rep 51(RR-16):1, 2002

51. Tanner J, Parkinson H: Double-gloving to reduce surgical cross-infection (Cochrane Review). Cochrane Database Syst Rev 3:CD003087, 2002 www.cochrane.org

52. Universal precautions for prevention of transmission of human immunodeficiency virus, hepatitis B virus, and other bloodborne pathogens in health-care settings. MMWR Morbid Mortal Wkly Rept 37(24):377, 1988

53. Kim LE, Jeffe DB, Evanoff BA, et al: Improved compliance with universal precautions in the operating room following an educational intervention. Infect Control Hosp Epidemiol 22:522, 2001

54. Scheenberger PM, Smits MH, Zick RE, et al: Surveillance as a starting point to reduce surgical site infection rates in elective orthopedic surgery. Hosp Infect 51:179, 2002

55. Burke JF: The effective period of preventive antibiotic action in experimental incisions and dermal lesions. Surgery 50:161, 1961

56. Classen DC, Evans RS, Pestotnik SL, et al: The timing of prophylactic administration of antibiotics and the risk of surgical-wound infection. N Engl J Med 326:281, 1992

57. Antimicrobial prophylaxis in surgery. Med Lett Drugs Ther 43:92, 2001

58. Forse RA, Karam B, MacLean LD, et al: Antibiotic prophylaxis for surgery in morbidly obese patients. Surgery 106:750, 1989

59. Zanetti G, Flanagan HL Jr, Cohn LH, et al: Improvement of intraoperative antibiotic prophylaxis in prolonged cardiac surgery by automated alerts in the operating room. Infect Control Hosp Epidemiol 24:13, 2003

60. Sessler DI, Akca O: Nonpharmacological prevention of surgical wound infections. Clin Infect Dis 35:1397, 2002

61. Kurz A, Sessler DI, Lenhardt R: Perioperative normothermia to reduce the incidence of surgical wound infection and shorten hospitalization. Study of Wound Infection and Temperature Group. N Engl J Med 358:876, 1996

62. Flores-Maldonado A, Medine-Escobedo CE, Rios-Rodriguez HM, et al: Mild perioperative hypothermia and the risk of wound infection. Arch Med Res 32:227, 2001

63. Melling AC, Ali B, Scott EM, et al: Effects of preoperative warming on the incidence of wound infection after clean surgery: a randomized controlled trial. Lancet 358:876, 2001

64. Hopf HW, Hunt TK, West JM: Wound tissue oxygen tension predicts the risk of wound infection in surgical patients. Arch Surg 132:997, 1997

65. Koval KJ, Rosenberg AD, Zuckerman JD, et al: Does blood transfusion increase risk of infection after hip fracture? J Orthop Trauma 11:260, 1997

66. Houbiers JG, van de Velder CJ, van de Watering LM, et al: Transfusion of red cells is associated with increased incidence of bacterial infection after colorectal surgery: a prospective study. Transfusion 37:126, 1997

67. Dunne J, Malone D, Genuit T, et al: Perioperative anemia: an independent risk factor for infection and resource utilization in surgery. J Surg Res 102:237, 2002

68. Peers JG: Cleanup techniques in the operating room. Arch Surg 107:596, 1973

69. Weber DO, Gooch JJ, Wood WR, et al: Influence of operating room surface contamination on surgical wounds: a prospective study. Arch Surg 111:484, 1976

70. Daschner F: Patient-oriented hospital hygiene. Infection 39(suppl):243, 1980

71. Mangram AJ, Horan TC, Pearson ML, et al: Guideline for Prevention of Surgical Site Infection, 1999. The Hospital Infection Control Practices Advisory Committee. Am J Infect Control 27:98, 1999

72. Report of an Ad-Hoc Committee of the Committee of Trauma, Division of Medical Sciences, National Academy of Sciences-National Research Council. Postoperative Wound Infections: The influence of ultraviolet irradiation of the operating room and of various other factors. Ann Surg 160(suppl):1, 1964

73. Hambraeus A, Bengtsson S, Laurell G: Bacterial contamination in a modern operating suite: II. Effect of a zoning system on contamination of floors and other surfaces. J Hyg (Lond) 80:57, 1978

74. McWilliams RM: There should be only one way to clean up between all surgical procedures. J Hosp Infect Control 3:64, 1976

75. Nichols RL: The operating room. Hospital Infections, 3rd ed. Bennett JV, Brachman PS, Eds. Little, Brown & Co, Boston, 1992, p 461

76. Ayliffe GA: Role of the environment of the operating suite in surgical wound infection. Rev Infect Dis 13(suppl 10):S800, 1991

77. Overdyck FJ, Harvey SC, Fishman RL, et al: Successful strategies for improving operating room efficiency at academic institutions. Anesth Analg 86:896, 1998

78. Patterson P: Is an 80% to 85% utilization a realistic target for ORs? OR Manager 13(5):1, 1997

79. Munoz E, Tortella B, Jaker M: Surgical resources consumption in an academic health consortium. Surgery 115:411, 1994

80. Kanich DG, Byrd JR: How to increase efficiency in the operating room. Surg Clin North Am 76:161, 1996

81. Mueller J, Marinari B, Kunkel S: Flipping assumptions and revisioning perioperative services. J Nurs Admin 25:22, 1995

82. Epstein RH, Dexter F: Statistical power analysis to estimate how many months of data are required to identify operating room staffing solutions to reduce labor costs and increase productivity. Anesth Analg 94:640, 2002

83. Dexter F, Traub RD: How to schedule elective surgical cases into specific operating rooms to maximize the efficiency of use of operating room time. Anesth Analg 94:933, 2002

84. Surgery teams make strides on OR delays. OR Manager 14(1):1, 1998

Acknowledgment

Figure 1   Courtesy of W. L. Gore & Associates, Newark, Delaware.

2 PREVENTION OF POSTOPERATIVE INFECTION

Jonathan L. Meakins, M.D., D.Sc., F.A.C.S., and Byron J. Masterson, M.D., F.A.C.S.

Epidemiology of Surgical Site Infection

Historically, the control of wound infection depended on antiseptic and aseptic techniques directed at coping with the infecting organism. In the 19th century and the early part of the 20th century, wound infections had devastating consequences and a measurable mortality. Even in the 1960s, before the correct use of antibiotics and the advent of modern preoperative and postoperative care, as much as one quarter of a surgical ward might have been occupied by patients with wound complications. As a result, wound management, in itself, became an important component of ward care and of medical education. It is fortunate that many factors have intervened so that the so-called wound rounds have become a practice of the past. The epidemiology of wound infection has changed as surgeons have learned to control bacteria and the inoculum as well as to focus increasingly on the patient (the host) for measures that will continue to provide improved results.

The following three factors are the determinants of any infectious process:

1. The infecting organism (in surgical patients, usually bacteria).
2. The environment in which the infection takes place (the local response).
3. The host defense mechanisms, which deal systemically with the infectious process.[1]

Wounds are particularly appropriate for analysis of infection with respect to these three determinants. Because many components of the bacterial contribution to wound infection now are clearly understood and measures to control bacteria have been implemented, the host factors become more apparent. In addition, interactions between the three determinants play a critical role, and with limited exceptions (e.g., massive contamination), few infections will be the result of only one factor [*see Figure 1*].

Definition of Surgical Site Infection

Wound infections have traditionally been thought of as infections in a surgical wound occurring between the skin and the deep soft tissues—a view that fails to consider the operative site as a whole. As prevention of these wound infections has become more effective, it has become apparent that definitions of operation-related infection must take the entire operative field into account; obvious examples include sternal and mediastinal infections, vascular graft infections, and infections associated with implants (if occurring within 1 year of the procedure and

apparently related to it). Accordingly, the Centers for Disease Control and Prevention currently prefers to use the term surgical site infection (SSI). SSIs can be classified into three categories: superficial incisional SSIs (involving only skin and subcutaneous tissue), deep incisional SSIs (involving deep soft tissue), and organ/space SSIs (involving anatomic areas other than the incision itself that are opened or manipulated in the course of the procedure)[2,3] [*see Figure 2*].

Standardization in reporting will permit more effective surveillance and improve results as well as offer a painless way of achieving quality assurance. The natural tendency to deny that a surgical site has become infected contributes to the difficulty of defining SSI in a way that is both accurate and acceptable to surgeons. The surgical view of SSI recalls one judge's (probably apocryphal) remark about pornography: "It is hard to define, but I know it when I see it." SSIs are usually easy to identify. Nevertheless, there is a critical need for definitions of SSI that can be applied in different institutions. The criteria on which such definitions must be based are more detailed than the simple apocryphal remark just cited; they are outlined more fully elsewhere [*see 1:1 Preparation of the Operating Room*].

STRATIFICATION OF RISK FOR SSI

The National Academy of Sciences–National Research Council classification of wounds [*see Table 1*], published in 1964, was a

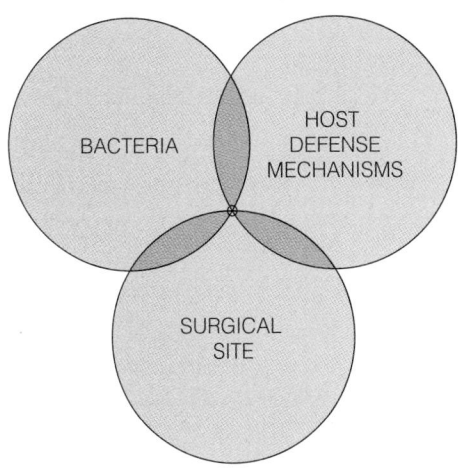

Figure 1 **In a homeostatic, normal state, the determinants of any infectious process—bacteria, the surgical site, and host defense mechanisms (represented by three circles)—intersect at a point indicating zero probability of sepsis.**

17

Epidemiology of Surgical Site Infection

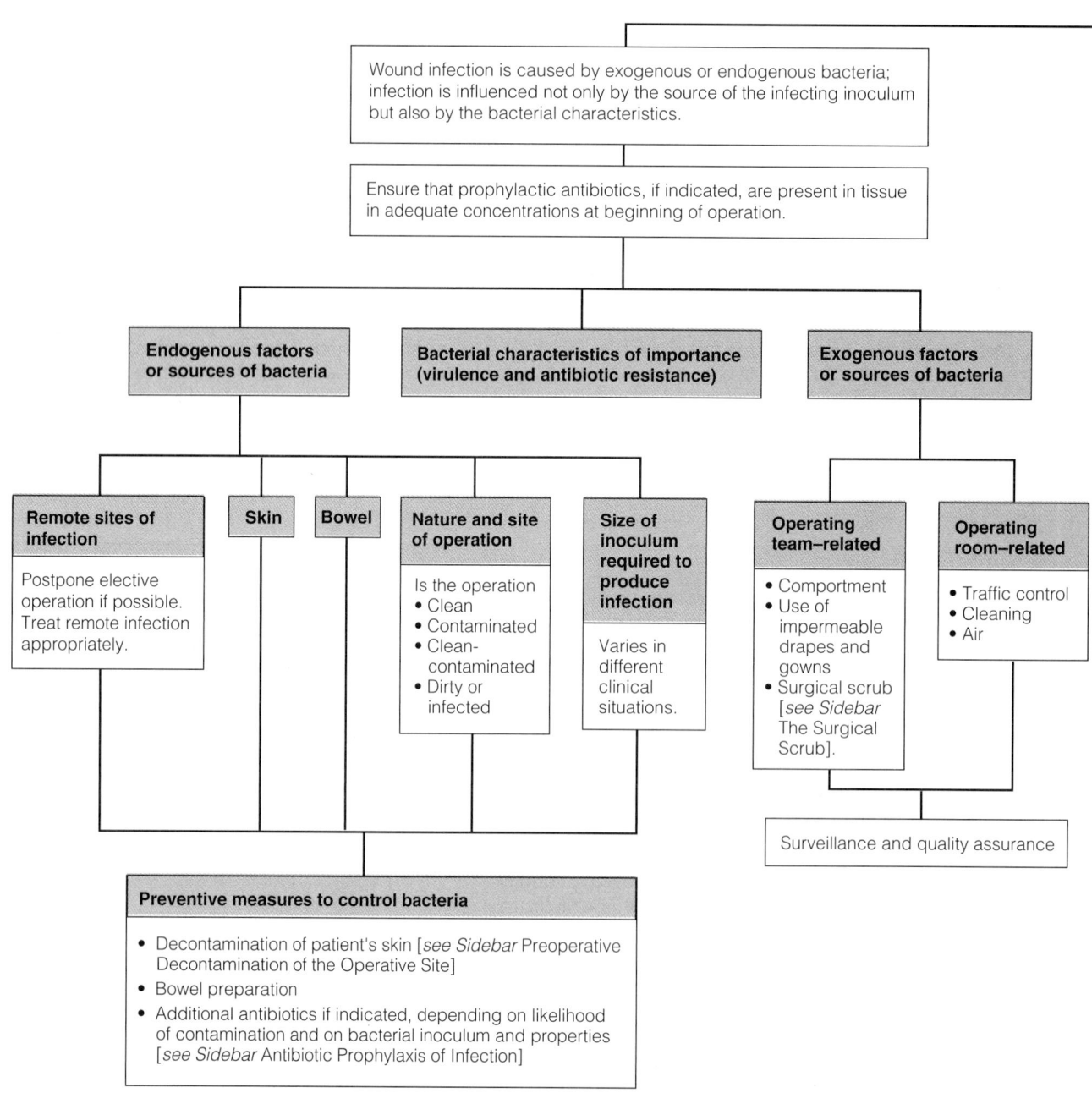

Wound infection is caused by exogenous or endogenous bacteria; infection is influenced not only by the source of the infecting inoculum but also by the bacterial characteristics.

Ensure that prophylactic antibiotics, if indicated, are present in tissue in adequate concentrations at beginning of operation.

Endogenous factors or sources of bacteria

Bacterial characteristics of importance (virulence and antibiotic resistance)

Exogenous factors or sources of bacteria

Remote sites of infection

Postpone elective operation if possible. Treat remote infection appropriately.

Skin

Bowel

Nature and site of operation

Is the operation
• Clean
• Contaminated
• Clean-contaminated
• Dirty or infected

Size of inoculum required to produce infection

Varies in different clinical situations.

Operating team–related

• Comportment
• Use of impermeable drapes and gowns
• Surgical scrub [*see Sidebar* The Surgical Scrub].

Operating room–related

• Traffic control
• Cleaning
• Air

Surveillance and quality assurance

Preventive measures to control bacteria

• Decontamination of patient's skin [*see Sidebar* Preoperative Decontamination of the Operative Site]
• Bowel preparation
• Additional antibiotics if indicated, depending on likelihood of contamination and on bacterial inoculum and properties [*see Sidebar* Antibiotic Prophylaxis of Infection]

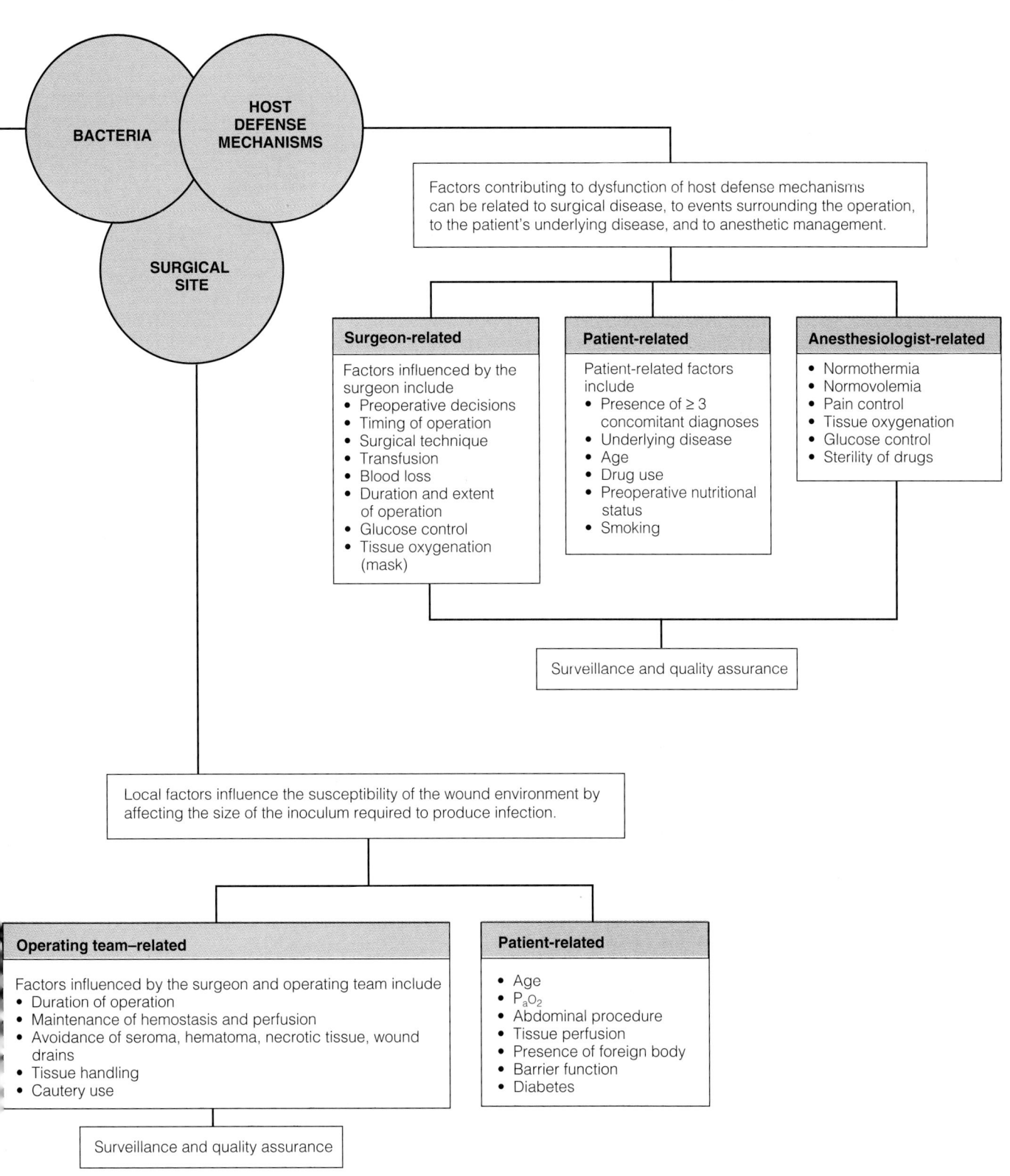

BACTERIA

HOST DEFENSE MECHANISMS

SURGICAL SITE

Factors contributing to dysfunction of host defense mechanisms can be related to surgical disease, to events surrounding the operation, to the patient's underlying disease, and to anesthetic management.

Surgeon-related

Factors influenced by the surgeon include
- Preoperative decisions
- Timing of operation
- Surgical technique
- Transfusion
- Blood loss
- Duration and extent of operation
- Glucose control
- Tissue oxygenation (mask)

Patient-related

Patient-related factors include
- Presence of ≥ 3 concomitant diagnoses
- Underlying disease
- Age
- Drug use
- Preoperative nutritional status
- Smoking

Anesthesiologist-related

- Normothermia
- Normovolemia
- Pain control
- Tissue oxygenation
- Glucose control
- Sterility of drugs

Surveillance and quality assurance

Local factors influence the susceptibility of the wound environment by affecting the size of the inoculum required to produce infection.

Operating team–related

Factors influenced by the surgeon and operating team include
- Duration of operation
- Maintenance of hemostasis and perfusion
- Avoidance of seroma, hematoma, necrotic tissue, wound drains
- Tissue handling
- Cautery use

Patient-related

- Age
- P_aO_2
- Abdominal procedure
- Tissue perfusion
- Presence of foreign body
- Barrier function
- Diabetes

Surveillance and quality assurance

19

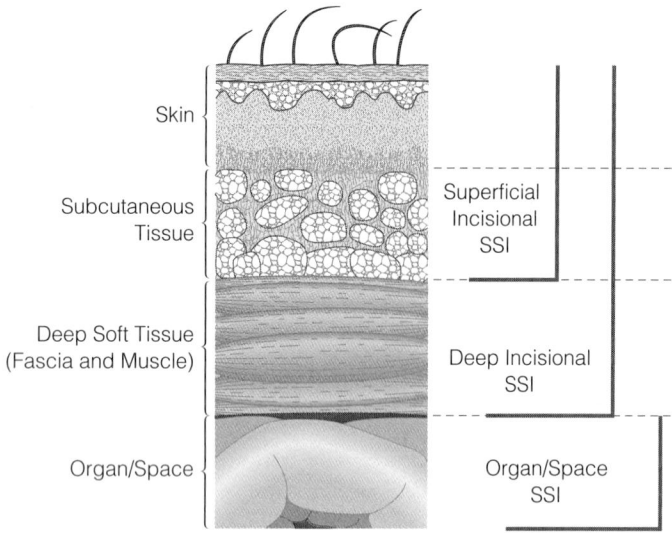

Figure 2 **Surgical site infections are classified into three cate-gories, depending on which anatomic areas are affected.**[3]

landmark in the field.[4] This report provided incontrovertible data to show that wounds could be classified as a function of probability of bacterial contamination (usually endogenous) in a consistent manner. Thus, wound infection rates could be validly compared from month to month, between services, and between hospitals. As surgery became more complex in the following decades, however, antibiotic use became more standardized and other risk variables began to assume greater prominence. In the early 1980s, the Study on the Efficacy of Nosocomial Infection Control (SENIC) study identified three risk factors in addition to wound class: location of operation (abdomen or chest), duration of operation, and patient clinical status (three or more diagnoses on discharge).[5] The National Nosocomial Infection Surveillance (NNIS) study reduced these four risk factors to three: wound classification, duration of operation, and American Society of Anesthesiologists (ASA) class III, IV or V.[6,7] Both risk assessments integrate the three determinants of infection: bacteria (wound class), local environment (duration), and systemic host defenses (one definition of patient health status), and they have been shown to be applicable outside the United States.[8] However, the SENIC and NNIS assessments do not integrate other known risk variables, such as smoking, tissue oxygen tension, glucose control, shock, and maintenance of normothermia, all of which are relevant for clinicians (though often hard to monitor and to fit into a manageable risk assessment).

Bacteria

Clearly, without an infecting agent, no infection will result. Accordingly, most of what is known about bacteria is put to use in major efforts directed at reducing their numbers by means of asepsis and antisepsis. The principal concept is based on the size of the bacterial inoculum.

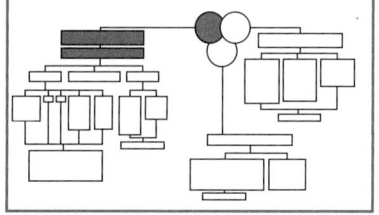

Wounds are traditionally classified according to whether the wound inoculum of bacteria is likely to be large enough to overwhelm local and systemic host defense mechanisms and produce an infection [*see Table 1*]. One study showed that the most impor-

tant factor in the development of a wound infection was the number of bacteria present in the wound at the end of an operative procedure.[9] Another study quantitated this relation and provided insight into how local environmental factors might be integrated into an understanding of the problem [*see Figure 3*].[10] In the years before prophylactic antibiotics as well as during the early phases of their use, there was a very clear relation between the classification of the operation (which is related to the probability of a significant inoculum) and the rate of wound infection.[4,11] This relation is now less dominant than it once was; therefore, other factors have come to play a significant role.[5,12]

CONTROL OF SOURCES OF BACTERIA

Endogenous bacteria are a more important cause of SSI than exogenous bacteria. In clean-contaminated, contaminated, and dirty-infected operations, the source

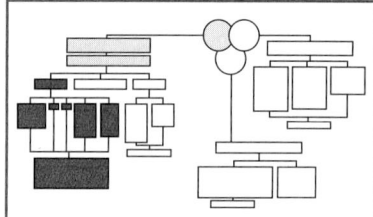

and the amount of bacteria are functions of the patient's disease and the specific organs being operated on.

Operations classified as infected are those in which infected tissue and pus are removed or drained, providing a guaranteed inoculum to the surgical site. The inoculum may be as high as 10^{10} bacteria/ml, some of which may already be producing an infection. In addition, some bacteria could be in the growth phase rather than the dormant or the lag phase and thus could be more pathogenic. The heavily contaminated wound is best managed by delayed primary closure. This type of management ensures that the wound is not closed over a bacterial inoculum that is almost certain to cause a wound infection, with attendant early and late consequences.

Patients should not have elective surgery in the presence of

Table 1 National Research Council Classification of Operative Wounds[4]

Clean (class I)	Nontraumatic
	No inflammation encountered
	No break in technique
	Respiratory, alimentary, or genitourinary tract not entered
Clean-contaminated (class II)	Gastrointestinal or respiratory tract entered without significant spillage
	Appendectomy
	Oropharynx entered
	Vagina entered
	Genitourinary tract entered in absence of infected urine
	Biliary tract entered in absence of infected bile
	Minor break in technique
Contaminated (class III)	Major break in technique
	Gross spillage from gastrointestinal tract
	Traumatic wound, fresh
	Entrance of genitourinary or biliary tracts in presence of infected urine or bile
Dirty and infected (class IV)	Acute bacterial inflammation encountered, without pus
	Transection of "clean" tissue for the purpose of surgical access to a collection of pus
	Traumatic wound with retained devitalized tissue, foreign bodies, fecal contamination, or delayed treatment, or all of these; or from dirty source

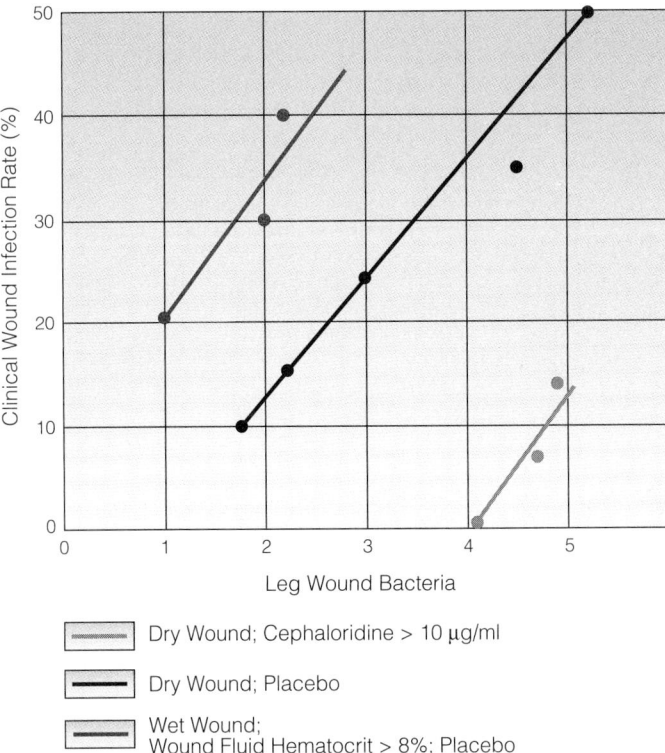

Dry Wound; Cephaloridine > 10 μg/ml

Dry Wound; Placebo

Wet Wound;
Wound Fluid Hematocrit > 8%; Placebo

Figure 3 **The wound infection rate is shown here as a function of bacterial inoculum in three different situations: a dry wound with an adequate concentration of antibiotic (cephaloridine > 10 μg/ml), a dry wound with no antibiotic (placebo), and a wet wound with no antibiotic (placebo, wound fluid hematocrit > 8%).[10]**

remote infection, which is associated with an increased incidence of wound infection.[4] In patients with urinary tract infections, wounds frequently become infected with the same organism. Remote infections should be treated appropriately, and the operation should proceed only under the best conditions possible. If operation cannot be appropriately delayed, the use of prophylactic and therapeutic antibiotics should be considered [*see Sidebar* Antibiotic Prophylaxis of Infection *and Tables 2 through 4*].

Preoperative techniques of reducing patient flora, especially endogenous bacteria, are of great concern. Bowel preparation, antimicrobial showers or baths, and preoperative skin decontamination have been proposed frequently. These techniques, particularly preoperative skin decontamination [*see Sidebar* Preoperative Decontamination of the Operative Site], may have specific roles in selected patients during epidemics or in units with high infection rates. As a routine for all patients, however, these techniques are unnecessary, time-consuming, and costly in institutions or units where infection rates are low.

The preoperative shave is a technique in need of reassessment. It is now clear that shaving the evening before an operation is associated with an increased wound infection rate. This increase is secondary to the trauma of the shave and the inevitable small areas of inflammation and infection. If hair removal is required,[13,14] clipping is preferable and should be done in the OR or the preparation room just before the operative procedure. Shaving, if ever performed, should not be done the night before operation.

Bowel preparation [*see Table 5*] has a clear role in colon and rectal surgery. The suggestion has been made that selective gut decontamination (SGD) may be useful in major elective procedures involving the upper GI tract and perhaps in other settings. At present, SGD for prevention of infection cannot be recommended in either the preoperative or the postoperative period.

When infection develops after clean operations, particularly those in which foreign bodies were implanted, endogenous infecting organisms are involved but the skin is the primary source of the infecting bacteria. The air in the operating room and other OR sources occasionally become significant in clean cases; the degree of endogenous contamination can be surpassed by that of exogenous contamination. Thus, both the operating team—surgeon, assistants, nurses, and anesthetists—and OR air have been reported as significant sources of bacteria [*see 1:1 Preparation of the Operating Room*]. In fact, personnel are the most important source of exogenous bacteria.[15-17] In the classic 1964 study by the National Academy of Sciences–National Research Council, ultraviolet light (UVL) was efficacious only in the limited situations of clean and ultraclean cases.[4] There were minimal numbers of endogenous bacteria, and UVL controlled one of the exogenous sources.

Clean air systems have very strong advocates, but they also have equally vociferous critics. It is possible to obtain excellent results in clean cases with implants without using these systems. However, clean air systems are here to stay. Nevertheless, the presence of a clean air system does not mean that basic principles of asepsis and antisepsis should be abandoned, because endogenous bacteria must still be controlled.

The use of impermeable drapes and gowns has received considerable attention. If bacteria can penetrate gown and drapes, they can gain access to the wound. The use of impermeable drapes may therefore be of clinical importance.[18,19] When wet, drapes of 140-thread-count cotton are permeable to bacteria. It is clear that some operations are wetter than others, but generally, much can be done to make drapes and gowns impermeable to bacteria. For example, drapes of 270-thread-count cotton that have been waterproofed are impermeable, but they can be washed only 75 times. Economics plays a role in the choice of drape fabric because entirely disposable drapes are expensive. Local institutional factors may be significant in the role of a specific type of drape in the prevention of SSI.

PROBABILITY OF CONTAMINATION

The probability of contamination is largely defined by the nature of the operation [*see Table 1*]. However, other factors contribute to the probability of contamination; the most obvious is the expected duration of the operative procedure, which, whenever examined, has been significant in the wound infection rate.[5,9,11] The longer the procedure lasts, the more bacteria accumulate in a wound; the sources of bacteria include the patient, the operating team (gowns, gloves with holes, wet drapes), the OR, and the equipment. In addition, the patient undergoing a longer operation is likely to be older, to have other diseases, and to have cancer of—or to be undergoing operation on—a structure with possible contamination. A longer duration, even of a clean operation, represents increased time at risk for contamination. These points, in addition to pharmacologic considerations, suggest that the surgeon should be alert to the need for a second dose of prophylactic antibiotics [*see Sidebar* Antibiotic Prophylaxis of Infection].

Abdominal operation is another risk factor not found in the NNIS risk assessment.[5,7] Significant disease and age play a role in outcome; however, because the major concentrations of endogenous bacteria are located in the abdomen, abdominal operations are more likely to involve bacterial contamination.

Antibiotic Prophylaxis of Infection

Selection

Spectrum. The antibiotic chosen should be active against the most likely pathogens. Single-agent therapy is almost always effective, except in colorectal operations, small-bowel procedures with stasis, emergency abdominal operations in the presence of a polymicrobial flora, and penetrating trauma; in such cases, a combination of antibiotics is usually used because anaerobic coverage is required.

Pharmacokinetics. The half-life of the antibiotic selected must be long enough to maintain adequate tissue levels throughout the operation.

Administration

Dosage, route, and timing. A single preoperative dose that is of the same strength as a full therapeutic dose is adequate in most instances. The single dose should be given I.V. immediately before skin incision. Administration by the anesthetist is most effective and efficient.

Duration. A second dose is warranted if the duration of the operation exceeds either 3 hours or twice the half-life of the antibiotic. No additional benefit has been demonstrated in continuing prophylaxis beyond the day of the operation, and mounting data suggest that the preoperative dose is sufficient. When massive hemorrhage has occurred (i.e., blood loss equal to or greater than blood volume), a second dose is warranted. Even in emergency or trauma cases, prolonged courses of antibiotics are not justified unless they are therapeutic.[66,67,71,112]

Indications

CLEAN CASES

Prophylactic antibiotics are not indicated in clean operations if the patient has no host risk factors or if the operation does not involve placement of prosthetic materials. Open heart operation and operations involving the aorta or the vessels in the groin require prophylaxis.

Patients in whom host factors suggest the need for prophylaxis include those who have more than three concomitant diagnoses, those whose operations are expected to last longer than 2 hours, and those whose operations are abdominal.[10] A patient who meets any two of these criteria is highly likely to benefit from prophylaxis. When host factors suggest that the probability of a surgical site infection is significant, administration of cefazolin at induction of anesthesia is appropriate prophylaxis. Vancomycin should be substituted in patients who are allergic to cephalosporins or who are susceptible to major immediate hypersensitivity reactions to penicillin.

When certain prostheses (e.g., heart valves, vascular grafts, and orthopedic hardware) are used, prophylaxis is justified when viewed in the light of the cost of a surgical site infection to the patient's health. Prophylaxis with either cefazolin or vancomycin is appropriate for cardiac, vascular, or orthopedic patients who receive prostheses.

Catheters for dialysis or nutrition, pacemakers, and shunts of various sorts are prone to infection mostly for technical reasons, and prophylaxis is not usually required. Meta-analysis indicates, however, that antimicrobial prophylaxis reduces the infection rate in CSF shunts by 50%.[113] Beneficial results may also be achievable for other permanently implanted shunts (e.g., peritoneovenous) and devices (e.g., long-term venous access catheters and pacemakers); however, the studies needed to confirm this possibility will never be done, because the infection rates are low and the sample sizes would have to be prohibitively large. The placement of such foreign bodies is a clean operation, and the use of antibiotics should be based on local experience.

CLEAN-CONTAMINATED CASES

Abdominal procedures. In biliary tract procedures (open or laparoscopic), prophylaxis is required only for patients at high risk: those whose common bile duct is likely to be explored (because of jaundice, bile duct obstruction, stones in the common bile duct, or a reoperative biliary procedure); those with acute cholecystitis; and those older than 70 years. A single dose of cefazolin is adequate. In hepatobiliary and pancreatic procedures, antibiotic prophylaxis is always warranted because these operations are clean-contaminated, because they are long, because they are abdominal, or for all of these reasons. Prophylaxis is also warranted for therapeutic endoscopic retrograde cholangiopancreatography.[11,12] In gastroduodenal procedures, patients whose gastric acidity is normal or high and in whom bleeding, cancer, gastric ulcer, and obstruction are absent are at low risk for infection and require no prophylaxis; all other patients are at high risk and require prophylaxis. Patients undergoing operation for morbid obesity should receive double the usual prophylactic dose[114]; cefazolin is an effective agent.

Operations on the head and neck (including the esophagus). Patients whose operations are of significance (i.e., involve entry into the oral cavity, the pharynx, or the esophagus) require prophylaxis.

Gynecologic procedures. Patients whose operation is either high-risk cesarean section, abortion, or vaginal or abdominal hysterectomy will benefit from cefazolin. Aqueous penicillin G or doxycycline may be preferable for first-trimester abortions in patients with a history of pelvic inflammatory disease. In patients with cephalosporin allergy, doxycycline is effective for those having hysterectomies and metronidazole for those having cesarean sections. Women delivering by cesarean section should be given the antibiotic immediately after cord clamping.

Urologic procedures. In principle, antibiotics are not required in patients with sterile urine. Patients with positive cultures should be treated. If an operative procedure is performed, a single dose of the appropriate antibiotic will suffice.

(continued)

For some years, postoperative contamination of the wound has been considered unlikely. However, one report of SSI in sternal incisions cleaned and redressed 4 hours postoperatively clearly shows that wounds can be contaminated and become infected in the postoperative period.[20] Accordingly, use of a dry dressing for 24 hours seems prudent.

BACTERIAL PROPERTIES

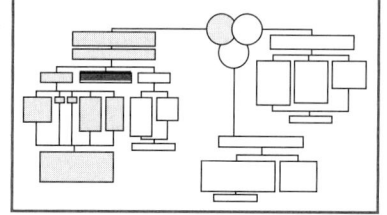

Not only is the size of the bacterial inoculum important; the bacterial properties of virulence and pathogenicity are also significant. The most obvious pathogenic bacteria in surgical patients are gram-positive cocci (e.g., *Staphylococcus aureus* and streptococci). With modern hygienic practice, it would be expected that *S. aureus* would be found mostly in clean cases,

with a wound infection incidence of 1% to 2%; however, it is in fact an increasingly common pathogen in SSIs. Surveillance can be very useful in identifying either wards or surgeons with increased rates. Operative procedures in infected areas have an increased infection rate because of the high inoculum with actively pathogenic bacteria.

The preoperative hospital stay has been found frequently to be an important contributing factor to wound infection rates.[11] The usual explanation is that during this stay, either more endogenous bacteria are present or commensal flora is replaced by hospital flora. With respect to bacterial changes, one must recognize that the patient's clinical picture is usually a complex one, often entailing exhaustive workup of more than one organ system, various complications, and a degree of illness that changes radically the host's ability to deal with an inoculum, however small. Therefore, multiple factors combine to transform the hospitalized preoperative patient into a susceptible host.

Bacteria with multiple antibiotic resistance (e.g., methicillin-

Antibiotic Prophylaxis of Infection (*continued*)

CONTAMINATED CASES

Abdominal procedures. In colorectal procedures, bowel preparation using antibiotics active against both aerobes and anaerobes, along with a parenteral cephalosporin, is recommended. In appendectomy, SSI prophylaxis requires an agent or combination of agents active against both aerobes and anaerobes; a single dose of cefoxitin, 2 g I.V., or, in patients who are allergic to β-lactam antibiotics, metronidazole, 500 mg I.V., is effective. A combination of an aminoglycoside and clindamycin is effective if the appendix is perforated; a therapeutic course of 3 to 5 days is appropriate but does not seem warranted unless the patient is particularly ill. A laparotomy without a precise diagnosis is usually an emergency procedure and demands preoperative prophylaxis. If the preoperative diagnosis is a ruptured viscus (e.g., the colon or the small bowel), both an agent active against aerobes and an agent active against anaerobes are required. Depending on operative findings, prophylaxis may be sufficient or may have to be supplemented with postoperative antibiotic therapy.

Trauma. The proper duration of antibiotic prophylaxis for trauma patients is a confusing issue—24 hours or less of prophylaxis is probably adequate, and more than 48 hours is certainly unwarranted. When laparotomy is performed for nonpenetrating injuries, prophylaxis should be administered. Coverage of both aerobes and anaerobes is mandatory. The duration of prophylaxis should be less than 24 hours. In cases of penetrating abdominal injury, prophylaxis with either cefoxitin or a combination of agents active against anaerobic and aerobic organisms is required. The duration of prophylaxis should be less than 24 hours, and in many cases, perioperative doses will be adequate. For open fractures, management should proceed as if a therapeutic course were required. For grade I or II injuries, a first-generation cephalosporin will suffice, whereas for grade III injuries, combination therapy is warranted; duration may vary. For operative repair of fractures, a single dose of cefazolin may be given preoperatively, with a second dose added if the procedure is long. Patients with major soft tissue injury with a danger of spreading infection will benefit from cefazolin, 1 g I.V. every 8 hours for 1 to 3 days.

DIRTY OR INFECTED CASES

Infected cases require therapeutic courses of antibiotics; prophylaxis is not appropriate in this context. In dirty cases, particularly those resulting from trauma, contamination and tissue destruction are usually so extensive that the wounds must be left open for delayed primary or secondary closure. Appropriate timing of wound closure is judged at the time of debridement. Antibiotics should be administered as part of resuscitation. Administration of antibiotics for 24 hours is probably adequate if infection is absent at the outset. However, a therapeutic course of antibiotics is warranted if infection is present from the outset or if more than 6 hours elapsed before treatment of the wounds was initiated.

Prophylaxis of Endocarditis

Studies of the incidence of endocarditis associated with dental procedures, endoscopy, or operations that may result in transient bacteremia are lacking. Nevertheless, the consensus is that patients with specific cardiac and vascular conditions are at risk for endocarditis or vascular prosthetic infection when undergoing certain procedures; these patients should receive prophylactic antibiotics.[115-119] A variety of organisms are dangerous, but viridans streptococci are most common after dental or oral procedures, and enterococci are most common if the portal of entry is the GU or GI tract. Oral amoxicillin now replaces penicillin V or ampicillin because of superior absorption and better serum levels. In penicillin-allergic patients, clindamycin is recommended; alternatives include cephalexin, cefadroxil, azithromycin, and clarithromycin. When there is a risk of exposure to bowel flora or enterococci, oral amoxicillin may be given; if an I.V. regimen is indicated, ampicillin may be given, with gentamicin added if the patient is at high risk for endocarditis. In patients allergic to penicillin, vancomycin is appropriate, with gentamicin added in high-risk patients. These parenteral regimens should be reserved for high-risk patients undergoing procedures with a significant probability of bacteremia.[119]

In patients receiving penicillin-based prophylaxis because of a history of rheumatic fever, erythromycin rather than amoxicillin should be used to protect against endocarditis.[115] There is no consensus concerning prophylaxis for orthopedic prostheses and acquired infection after transient bacteremia. In major procedures, where the risk of bacteremia is significant, the above recommendations are pertinent.

---

resistant *S. aureus* [MRSA], *S. epidermidis*, and vancomycin-resistant enterococci [VRE]) can be associated with significant SSI problems. In particular, staphylococci, with their natural virulence, present an important hazard if inappropriate prophylaxis is used. Many surgeons feel it is inappropriate or unnecessary to obtain good culture and sensitivity data on SSIs and instead simply drain infected wounds, believing that they will heal. However, there have been a number of reports of

Table 2 Parenteral Antibiotics Recommended
for Prophylaxis of Surgical Site Infection

	Antibiotic	Dose	Route of Administration
For coverage against aerobic gram-positive and gram-negative organisms	Cefazolin	1 g	I.V. or I.M. (I.V. preferred)
If patient is allergic to cephalosporins or if methicillin-resistant organisms are present	Vancomycin	1 g	I.V.
Combination regimens for coverage against gram-negative aerobes and anaerobes	Clindamycin *or*	600 mg	I.V.
	Metronidazole *plus*	500 mg	I.V.
	Tobramycin (or equivalent aminoglycoside)	1.5 mg/kg	I.V. or I.M. (I.V. preferred for first dose)
For single-agent coverage against gram-negative aerobes and anaerobes	Cefoxitin	1–2 g	I.V.
	Cefotetan	1–2 g	I.V.

Table 3 Conditions and Procedures
That Require Antibiotic Prophylaxis
against Endocarditis[115,116]

CONDITIONS

Cardiac
  Prosthetic cardiac valves (including biosynthetic valves)
  Most congenital cardiac malformations
  Surgically constructed systemic-pulmonary shunts
  Rheumatic and other acquired valvular dysfunction
  Idiopathic hypertrophic subaortic stenosis
  History of bacterial endocarditis
  Mitral valve prolapse causing mitral insufficiency
  Surgically repaired intracardiac lesions with residual hemodynamic
    abnormality or < 6 mo after operation

Vascular
  Synthetic vascular grafts

PROCEDURES

Dental or oropharyngeal
  Procedures that may induce bleeding
  Procedures that involve incision of the mucosa

Respiratory
  Rigid bronchoscopy

Incision and drainage or debridement of sites of infection

Urologic
  Cystoscopy with urethral dilatation
  Urinary tract procedures
  Catheterization in the presence of infected urine

Gynecologic
  Vaginal hysterectomy
  Vaginal delivery in the presence of infection

Gastrointestinal
  Procedures that involve incision or resection of mucosa
  Endoscopy that involves manipulation (e.g., biopsy, dilatation,
    or sclerotherapy) or ERCP

SSIs caused by unusual organisms[17,20,21]; these findings underscore the usefulness of culturing pus or fluid when an infection is being drained. SSIs caused by antibiotic-resistant organisms or unusual pathogens call for specific prophylaxis, perhaps other infection control efforts, and, if the problem persists, a search for a possible carrier or a common source.[15-17,20,21]

SURGEONS AND BACTERIA

The surgeon's perioperative rituals are designed to reduce or eliminate bacteria from the operative field. Many old habits are obsolete [*see Sidebar* The Surgical Scrub *and 1:1 Preparation of the Operating Room*].

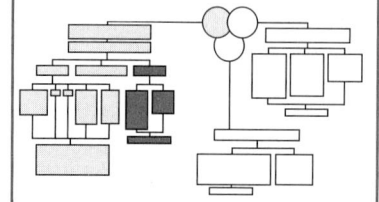

Nonetheless, it is clear that surgeons can influence SSI rates.[12] The refusal to use delayed primary closure or secondary closure is an example. Careful attention to the concepts of asepsis and antisepsis in the preparation and conduct of the operation is important. Although no single step in the ritual of preparing a patient for the operative procedure is indispensable, it is likely that certain critical standards of behavior must be maintained to achieve good results.

The measurement and publication of data about individuals or

hospitals with high SSI rates have been associated with a diminution of those rates [*see Table 6*].[11,12,22] It is uncertain by what process the diffusion of these data relates to the observed improvements. Although surveillance has unpleasant connotations, it provides objective data that individual surgeons are often too busy to acquire but that can contribute to improved patient care.

Environment: Local Factors

Local factors influence the development of an SSI because they affect the size of the bacterial inoculum that is required to produce an infection: in a susceptible wound, a smaller inoculum produces infection [*see Figure 2*].

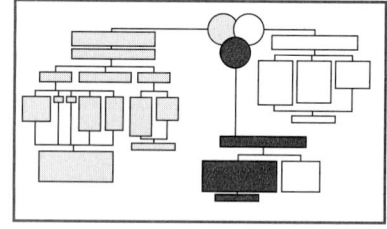

THE SURGEON'S INFLUENCE

Most of the local factors that make a surgical site favorable to bacteria are under the control of the surgeon. Although Halsted usually receives, deservedly so, the credit for having established the importance of technical excellence in the OR in preventing infection, individual surgeons in the distant past achieved remarkable results by careful attention to cleanliness and technique.[23] The Halstedian principles dealt with hemostasis, sharp dissection, fine sutures, anatomic dissection, and the gentle handling of tissues. Mass ligatures, large or braided nonabsorbable sutures, necrotic tissue, and the creation of hematomas or seromas must be avoided, and foreign materials must be judiciously used because these techniques and materials change the size of the inoculum required to initiate an infectious process. Logarithmically fewer bacteria are required to produce infection in the presence of a foreign body (e.g., suture, graft, metal, or pacemaker) or necrotic tissue (e.g., that caused by gross hemostasis or injudicious use of electrocautery).

The differences in inoculum required to produce wound infections can be seen in a model in which the two variables are wound hematocrit and the presence of antibiotic [*see Figure 3*]. Ten bacteria in the absence of an antibiotic and in the presence of wound fluid with a hematocrit of more than 8% yield a wound infection rate of 20%. In a technically good wound with no antibiotic, however, 1,000 bacteria produce a wound infection rate of 20%.[10] In the presence of an antibiotic, 10^5 to 10^6 bacteria are required.

Drains

The use of drains varies widely and is very subjective. All surgeons are certain that they understand when to use a drain. However, certain points are worth noting. It is now recognized that a simple Penrose drain can function not only as a drainage route but also as an access route for pathogens to the patient.[24] It is important that the operative site not be drained through the wound. The use of a closed suction drain further reduces the potential for contamination and infection.

Duration of Operation

In most studies,[5,9,11] contamination certainly increases with time (see above). Wound edges can dry out, become macerated, or in other ways be made more susceptible to infection (i.e., requiring fewer bacteria for development of infection). Speed and

Table 4 Antibiotics for Prevention of Endocarditis[75,115]

Manipulative Procedure	Prophylactic Regimen*	
	Usual	In Patients with Penicillin Allergy
Dental procedures likely to cause gingival bleeding; operations or instrumentation of the upper respiratory tract	*Oral* Amoxicillin, 2.0 g 1 hr before procedure *Parenteral* Ampicillin, 2.0 g I.M. or I.V. 30 min before procedure	*Oral* Clindamycin, 600 mg 1 hr before procedure *or* Cephalexin or cefadroxil,† 2.0 g 1 hr before procedure *or* Azithromycin or clarithromycin, 500 mg 1 hr before procedure *Parenteral* Clindamycin, 600 mg I.V. within 30 min before procedure *or* Cefazolin, 1.0 g I.M. or I.V. within 30 min before procedure
Gastrointestinal or genitourinary operation; abscess drainage	*Oral* Amoxicillin, 2.0 g 1 hr before procedure *Parenteral* Ampicillin, 2.0 g I.M. or I.V. within 30 min before procedure; if risk of endocarditis is considered high, add gentamicin, 1.5 mg/kg (to maximum of 120 mg) I.M. or I.V. 30 min before procedure‡	Vancomycin, 1.0 g I.V. infused slowly over 1 hr, beginning 1 hr before procedure; if risk of endocarditis is considered high, add gentamicin, 1.5 mg/kg (to maximum of 120 mg) I.M. or I.V. 30 min before procedure‡

*Pediatric dosages are as follows: oral amoxicillin, 50 mg/kg; oral or parenteral clindamycin, 20 mg/kg; oral cephalexin or cefadroxil, 50 mg/kg; oral azithromycin or clarithromycin, 15 mg/kg; parenteral ampicillin, 50 mg/kg; parenteral cefazolin, 25 mg/kg; parenteral gentamicin, 2 mg/kg; parenteral vancomycin, 20 mg/kg. *Total pediatric dose should not exceed total adult dose.*
†Patients with a history of immediate-type sensitivity to penicillin should not receive these agents.
‡High-risk patients should also receive ampicillin, 1.0 g I.M. or I.V., or amoxicillin, 1.0 g p.o., 6 hr after procedure.

poor technique are not suitable approaches; expeditious operation is appropriate.

Electrocautery

The use of electrocautery devices has been clearly associated with an increase in superficial SSI. However, when the unit is properly used to provide pinpoint coagulation (for which the bleeding vessels are best held by fine forceps) or to divide tissues under tension, there is minimal tissue destruction, no charring, and no change in the wound infection rate.[24]

PATIENT FACTORS

Local Blood Flow

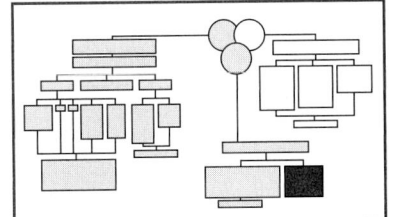

Local perfusion can greatly influence the development of infection, as is seen most easily in the tendency of the patient with peripheral vascular disease to acquire infection of an extremity. As a local problem, inadequate perfusion reduces the number of bacteria required for infection, in part because inadequate perfusion leads to decreased tissue levels of oxygen. Shock, by reducing local perfusion, also greatly enhances susceptibility to infection. Fewer organisms are required to produce infection during or immediately after shock [*see Figure 4*].

To counter these effects, the arterial oxygen tension (P_aO_2) must be translated into an adequate subcutaneous oxygen level (determined by measuring transcutaneous oxygen tension)[25]; this, together with adequate perfusion, will provide local protection by increasing the number of bacteria required to produce infection. It is now apparent that provision of supplemental oxygen in the perioperative period leads to a reduced SSI rate, probably as a consequence of increased tissue oxygen tension.[26] If the patient is not intubated, a mask, not nasal prongs, is required.[27]

Barrier Function

Inadequate perfusion may also affect the function of other organs, and the resulting dysfunction will, in turn, influence the patient's susceptibility to infection. For example, ischemia-reperfusion injury to the intestinal tract is a frequent consequence of hypovolemic shock and bloodstream infection. Inadequate perfusion of the GI tract may also occur during states of fluid and electrolyte imbalance or when cardiac output is marginal. Experimental studies have associated altered blood flow with breakdown of bowel barrier function—that is, inability of the intestinal tract to prevent bacteria, their toxins, or both from moving from the gut lumen into tissue at a rate too fast to permit clearance by the usual protective mechanisms. A variety of experimental approaches aimed at enhancing bowel barrier function have been studied; at present, however, the most clinically applicable method of bowel protection is initiation of enteral feeding (even if the quantity of nutrients provided does not satisfy all the nutrient requirements) and administration of the amino acid glutamine [*see 6:23 Nutritional Support*]. Glutamine is a specific fuel for enterocytes and colonocytes and has been found to aid recovery of damaged intestinal mucosa and enhance barrier function when administered either enterally or parenterally.

Advanced Age

Aging is associated with structural and functional changes that render the skin and subcutaneous tissues more susceptible to infection. These changes are immutable; however, they must be evaluated in advance and addressed by excellent surgical technique and, on occasion, prophylactic antibiotics [*see Sidebar Antibiotic Prophylaxis of Infection*].

Host Defense Mechanisms

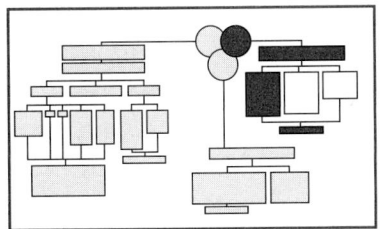

The systemic response is designed to control and eradicate infection. Many factors can inhibit systemic host defense mechanisms; some are related to

Preoperative Decontamination of the Operative Site

Preparation of Skin

The sole reason for preparing the patient's skin before an operation is to reduce the risk of wound infection. A preoperative antiseptic bath is not necessary for most surgical patients, but their personal hygiene must be assessed and preoperative cleanliness established. Multiple preoperative baths may prevent postoperative infection in selected patient groups, such as those who carry Staphylococcus aureus on their skin or who have infectious lesions. Chlorhexidine gluconate is the recommended agent for such baths.[120]

Hair should not be removed from the operative site unless it physically interferes with accurate anatomic approximation of the wound edges.[121] If hair must be removed, it should be clipped in the OR.[13] Shaving hair from the operative site, particularly on the evening before operation or immediately before wound incision in the OR, increases the risk of wound infection. Depilatories are not recommended, because they cause serious irritation and rashes in a significant number of patients, especially when used near the eyes and the genitalia.[122]

In emergency procedures, obvious dirt, grime, and dried blood should be mechanically cleansed from the operative site by using sufficient friction. In one study, cleansing of contaminated wounds by means of ultrasound debridement was compared with high-pressure irrigation and soaking. The experimental wounds were contaminated with a colloidal clay that potentiates infection 1,000-fold. The investigators irrigated wounds at pressures of 8 to 10 psi, a level obtained by using a 30 ml syringe with a 1.5 in. long 19-gauge needle and 300 ml of 0.85% sterile saline solution. High-pressure irrigation removed slightly more particulate matter (59%) than ultrasound debridement (48%), and both of these methods removed more matter than soaking (26%).[123] Both ultrasound debridement and high-pressure irrigation

were also effective in reducing the wound infection rate in experimental wounds contaminated with a subinfective dose of S. aureus.

For nonemergency procedures, the necessary reduction in microorganisms can be achieved by using povidone-iodine (10% available povidone-iodine and 1% available iodine) or chlorhexidine gluconate both for mechanical cleansing of the intertriginous folds and the umbilicus and for painting the operative site. The intertriginous folds and the umbilicus often require mechanical scrubbing to generate sufficient friction to remove entrapped microorganisms. In other areas of the skin, simply applying the agent (for example, by painting or spraying[124,125]) is an effective means of disinfection. Before the antiseptic is applied, the patient's history should be assessed for evidence of sensitivity to the antiseptic (particularly if the agent contains iodine) to minimize the risk of an allergic reaction. What some patients report as iodine allergies are actually iodine burns. Iodine in alcohol or in water is associated with an increased risk of skin irritation,[126] particularly at the edges of the operative field, where the iodine concentrates as the alcohol evaporates. Iodine should therefore be removed after sufficient contact time with the skin, especially at the edges. Iodophors do not irritate the skin and thus need not be removed.

Preparation of the Vagina

The purpose of preoperative preparation of the vagina is to reduce the number of bacteria and thereby decrease the risk of postoperative infection. The protocols for vaginal procedures almost always call for prophylactic antibiotics. Apparently, however, no additional benefit is gained from the preoperative use of a vaginal antiseptic.[127] Rather, the quantity of bacteria can be reduced by irrigating the vagina with saline solution.

---

the surgical disease, others to the patient's underlying disease or diseases and the events surrounding the operation.

SURGEON-RELATED FACTORS

There are a limited number of ways in which the surgeon

Table 5 **Parenteral Antibiotics Commonly Used for Broad-Spectrum Coverage of Colonic Microflora**

COMBINATION THERAPY OR PROPHYLAXIS

Aerobic Coverage
(to be combined with a drug having anaerobic activity)

Amikacin	Ciprofloxacin
Aztreonam	Gentamicin
Ceftriaxone	Tobramycin

Anaerobic Coverage
(to be combined with a drug having aerobic activity)

Chloramphenicol	Metronidazole
Clindamycin	

SINGLE-DRUG THERAPY OR PROPHYLAXIS

Aerobic-Anaerobic Coverage

Ampicillin-sulbactam	Imipenem-cilastatin*
Cefotetan	Piperacillin-tazobactam
Cefoxitin	Ticarcillin-clavulanate
Ceftizoxime	

*This agent should be used *only* for therapeutic purposes; it should not be used for prophylaxis.

can improve a patient's systemic responses to surgery. Nevertheless, when appropriate, attempts should be made to modify the host. The surgeon and the operation are both capable of reducing immunologic efficacy; hence, the operative procedure should be carried out in as judicious a manner as possible. Minimal blood loss, avoidance of shock, and maintenance of blood volume, tissue perfusion, and tissue oxygenation all will minimize trauma and will reduce the secondary, unintended immunologic effects of major procedures.

Diabetes has long been recognized as a risk factor for infection and for SSI in particular. Three studies from the past 5 years demonstrated the importance of glucose control for reducing SSI rates in both diabetic and nondiabetic patients who underwent operation,[28,29] as well as in critically ill ICU patients.[30] Glucose control is required throughout the entire perioperative period. The beneficial effect appears to lie in the enhancement of host defenses. The surgical team must also ensure maintenance of adequate tissue oxygen tension[25,26] and maintenance of normothermia.[31]

When abnormalities in host defenses are secondary to surgical disease, the timing of the operation is crucial to outcome. With acute and subacute inflammatory processes, early operation helps restore normal immune function. Deferral of definitive therapy frequently compounds problems.

PATIENT FACTORS

Surgeons have always known that the patient is a significant variable in the outcome of operation. Various clinical states are associated with altered resistance

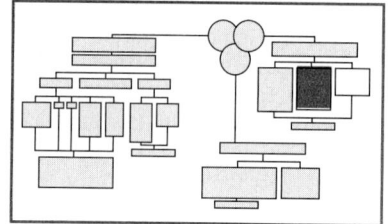

to infection. In all patients, but particularly those at high risk, SSI creates not only wound complications but also significant morbidity (e.g., reoperation, incisional hernia, secondary infection, impaired mobility, increased hospitalization, delayed rehabilitation, or permanent disability) and occasional mortality.[16] SENIC has proposed that the risk of wound infection be assessed not only in terms of probability of contamination but also in relation to host factors.[5,6,8] According to this study, patients most clearly at risk for wound infection are those with three or more concomitant diagnoses; others clearly at risk are those undergoing a clean-contaminated or contaminated abdominal procedure or any procedure expected to last longer than 2 hours. These past two risk groups are affected by a bacterial component, but all those patients who are undergoing major abdominal procedures or lengthy operations generally have a significant primary pathologic condition and are usually older, with an increased frequency of concomitant conditions. The NNIS system uses most of the same concepts but expresses them differently. In the NNIS study, host factors in the large study are evaluated in terms of the ASA score. Duration of operation is measured differently as well, with a lengthy operation being defined by the NNIS as one that is at or above the 75th percentile for operating time. Bacterial contami-

Table 6 Effect of Surveillance and Feedback on Wound Infection Rates in Two Hospitals[22]

		Period 1	Period 2*
Hospital A	Number of wounds	1,500	1,447
	Wound infection rate	8.4%	3.7%
Hospital B	Number of wounds	1,746	1,939
	Wound infection rate	5.7%	3.7%

*Periods 1 and 2 were separated by an interval during which feedback on wound infection rates was analyzed.

nation remains a risk factor, but operative site is eliminated.[7]

Shock has an influence on the incidence of wound infection [*see Figure 4*]. This influence is most obvious in cases of trauma, but there are significant implications for all patients in regard to maintenance of blood volume, hemostasis, and oxygen-carrying capacity. The effect of shock on the risk of infection appears to be not only immediate (i.e., its effect on local perfusion) but also late because systemic responses are blunted as local factors return to normal.

Advanced age, transfusion, and the use of steroids and other immunosuppressive drugs, including chemotherapeutic agents, are associated with an increased risk of SSI.[32,33] Often, these factors cannot be altered; however, the proper choice of operation, the appropriate use of prophylaxis, and meticulous surgical technique can reduce the risk of such infection by maintaining patient homeostasis, reducing the size of any infecting microbial inoculum, and creating a wound that is likely to heal primarily.

The basal nutritional state is known to affect immune response; this may be determined either by the patient (motivated by an interest in self-care, by socioeconomic conditions, or by underlying diseases) or by the surgeon. Of late, considerable attention has been focused on the beneficial effects of daily multivitamin supplements on infectious morbidity in individuals older than 65 years. In addition, there is some evidence that ingestion of certain antioxidants (e.g., β-carotene, vitamin C, and vitamin E) and trace metals (e.g., selenium and zinc) can enhance host responses to inflammation or infection. A large body of clinical data (particularly in patients with active rheumatoid arthritis) indicates that reducing the quantity of fat in the diet and substituting omega-3 fatty acids (found in high concentrations in fish oil) for omega-6 fatty acids reduces the clinical signs and symptoms of inflammation. Animal studies suggest that similar beneficial effects are observed in the presence of infection; human studies using this approach have yet to be performed. Dietary supplementation with arginine, glutamine, or both also appears to increase resistance to infectious challenge. Smoking, on the other hand, is associated with a striking increase in SSI incidence. As little as 1 week of abstinence from smoking will make a positive difference.[34]

Pharmacologic therapy can affect host response as well. Nonsteroidal anti-inflammatory drugs that attenuate the production of certain eicosanoids can greatly alter the adverse effects of infection by modifying fever and cardiovascular effects. Operative procedures involving inhalational anesthetics result in an immediate rise in plasma cortisol concentrations. The steroid response and the associated immunomodulation can be modified by using high epidural anesthesia as the method of choice; pituitary adrenal activation will be greatly attenuated. Some drugs that inhibit steroid elaboration (e.g., etomidate) have also been shown to be capable of modifying perioperative immune responses.

The Surgical Scrub

The purpose of cleansing the surgeon's hands is to reduce the numbers of resident flora and transient contaminants, thereby decreasing the risk of transmitting infection. Although the proper duration of the hand scrub is still subject to debate, evidence suggests that a 120-second scrub is sufficient, provided that a brush is used to remove the bacteria residing in the skin folds around the nails.[128] The nail folds, the nails, and the fingertips should receive the most attention because most bacteria are located around the nail folds and most glove punctures occur at the fingertips. Friction is required to remove resident microorganisms, which are attached by adhesion or adsorption, whereas transient bacteria are easily removed by simple hand washing.

Solutions containing either chlorhexidine gluconate or one of the iodophors are the most effective surgical scrub preparations and have the fewest problems with stability, contamination, and toxicity.[129] According to one review article, chlorhexidine gluconate (4%) in a sudsing base is the preferred agent because of its initial effectiveness, its residual activity, and its limited toxicity.[130] Another study showed that chlorhexidine gluconate achieves significant, immediate reduction of microorganisms and has persistent and residual efficacy.[131,132] In a comparative study of chlorhexidine gluconate, povidone-iodine, parachlorometaxylenol (PCMX or chloroxylenol), and alcohol, only chlorhexidine gluconate achieved significant antimicrobial efficacy in all parameters.

Alcohols applied to the skin are among the safest known antiseptics, and they produce the greatest and most rapid reduction in bacterial counts on clean skin.[126] A vigorous 1-minute scrub with enough alcohol to wet the hands completely has been shown to be the most effective method for hand antisepsis. A 1-minute immersion or scrub with alcohol is as effective as 4 to 7 minutes of skin preparation with other antiseptics, and washing with alcohol for 3 minutes is as effective as scrubbing for 20 minutes.[126] The main disadvantages of the alcohols are (1) their drying effects on the skin and (2) their volatility and flammability, which necessitate extreme caution when electrosurgery or laser procedures are performed. Although the alcohols are less commonly used in the United States, consistent, immediate, and effective reduction of skin flora makes them useful agents for preoperative skin cleansing.

All variables considered, chlorhexidine gluconate followed by an iodophor appears to be the best option.

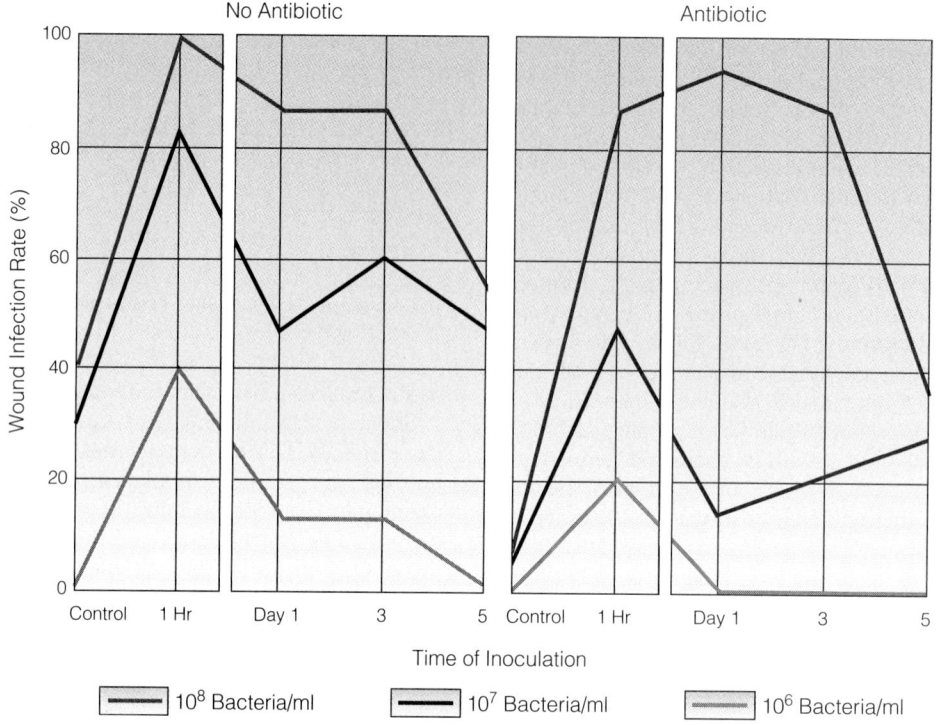

Figure 4 **Animals exposed to hemorrhagic shock followed by resuscitation show an early decreased resistance to wound infection. There is also a persistent influence of shock on the development of wound infection at different times of inoculation after shock. The importance of inoculum size (10^6/ml to 10^8/ml) and the effect of antibiotic on infection rates are evident at all times of inoculation.[107]**

ANESTHESIOLOGIST-RELATED FACTORS

A 2000 commentary in *The Lancet* by Donal Buggy considered the question of whether anesthetic management could influence surgical wound

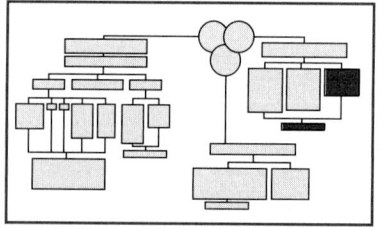

healing.[35] In addition to the surgeon- and patient-related factors already discussed (see above), Buggy cogently identified a number of anesthesiologist-related factors that could contribute to better wound healing and reduced wound infection. Some of these factors (e.g., pain control, epidural anesthesia, and autologous transfusion) are unproven at present but nonetheless make sense and should certainly be tested. Others (e.g., tissue perfusion, intravascular volume, and—significantly—maintenance of

Table 7 Determinants of Infection and Factors
That Influence Wound Infection Rates

Variable	Determinant of Infection		
	Bacteria	Wound Environment (Local Factors)	Host Defense Mechanisms (Systemic Factors)
Bacterial numbers in wound[9]	A		
Potential contamination[5,9,11]	A		
Preoperative shave[11]	A		
Presence of 3 or more diagnoses[5]			C
Age[9,11]		B	C
Duration of operation[5,9,11]	A	B	C
Abdominal operation[5]	A	B	C
ASA class III, IV, or V[7]			C
O₂ tension[25]		B	
Glucose control[28,29]			C
Normothermia[31]		B	C
Shock[107]		B	C
Smoking[34]		B	C

normal perioperative body temperature) have undergone formal evaluation. Very good studies have shown that dramatic reductions in SSI rates can be achieved through careful avoidance of hypothermia.[31,36] Patient-controlled analgesia pumps are known to be associated with increased SSI rates, through a mechanism that is currently unknown.[37] Infection control practices are required of all practitioners; contamination of anesthetic drugs by bacteria has resulted in numerous small outbreaks of SSI.[38,39]

As modern surgical practice has evolved and the variable of bacterial contamination has come to be generally well managed, the importance of all members of the surgical team in the prevention of SSI has become increasingly apparent. The crux of Buggy's commentary may be expressed as follows: details make a difference, and all of the participants in a patient's surgical journey can contribute to a continuing decrease in SSI. It is a systems issue.

INTEGRATION OF DETERMINANTS

As operative infection rates slowly fall, despite increasingly complex operations in patients at greater risk, surgeons are approaching the control of infection with a broader view than simply that of asepsis and antisepsis. This new, broader view must take into account many variables, of which some have no relation to bacteria but all play a role in SSI [see Table 7 and Figure 1].

To estimate risk, one must integrate the various determinants of infection in such a way that they can be applied to patient care. Much of this exercise is vague. In reality, the day-to-day practice of surgery includes a risk assessment that is essentially a form of logistic regression, though not recognized as such. Each surgeon's assessment of the probability of whether an SSI will occur takes into account the determining variables:

$$\text{Probability of SSI} =$$
$$x + a \text{ (bacteria)} + b \text{ (environment: local factors)}$$
$$+ c \text{ (host defense mechanisms: systemic factors)}$$

Discussion

Antibiotic Prophylaxis of Surgical Site Infection

It is difficult to understand why antibiotics have not always prevented SSI successfully. Certainly, surgeons were quick to appreciate the possibilities of antibiotics; nevertheless, the efficacy of antibiotic prophylaxis was not proved until the late 1960s.[10] Studies before then had major design flaws—principally, the administration of the antibiotic some time after the start of the operation, often in the recovery room. The failure of studies to demonstrate efficacy and the occasional finding that prophylactic antibiotics worsened rather than improved outcome led in the late 1950s to profound skepticism about prophylactic antibiotic use in any operation.

The principal reason for the apparent inefficacy was inadequate understanding of the biology of SSIs. Fruitful study of antibiotics and how they should be used began after physiologic groundwork established the importance of local blood flow, maintenance of local immune defenses, adjuvants, and local and systemic perfusion.[40]

The key antibiotic study, which was conducted in guinea pigs, unequivocally proved the following about antibiotics:

1. They are most effective when given before inoculation of bacteria.
2. They are ineffective if given 3 hours after inoculation.
3. They are of intermediate effectiveness when given in between these times [see Figure 5].[41]

Although efficacy with a complicated regimen was demonstrated in 1964,[42] the correct approach was not defined until 1969.[10] Established by these studies are the philosophical and practical bases of the principles of antibiotic prophylaxis of SSI in all surgical arenas[10,41]: that prophylactic antibiotics must be given preoperatively within 2 hours of the incision, in full dosage, parenterally, and for a very limited period. These principles remain essentially unchanged despite minor modifications from innumerable subsequent studies.[43-46] Prophylaxis for colorectal operations is discussed elsewhere [see Infection Prevention in Bowel Surgery, *below*].

PRINCIPLES OF PATIENT SELECTION

Patients must be selected for prophylaxis on the basis of either their risk for SSI or the cost to their health if an SSI develops (e.g., after implantation of a cardiac valve or another prosthesis). The most important criterion is the degree of bacterial contamination expected to occur during the operation. The traditional classification of such contamination was defined in 1964 by the historic National Academy of Sciences–National Research Council study.[4] The important features of the classification are its simplicity, ease of understanding, ease of coding, and reliability. Classification is dependent on only one variable—the bacterial inoculum—and the effects of this variable are now controllable by antimicrobial prophylaxis. Advances in operative technique, general care, antibiotic use, anesthesia, and surveillance have reduced SSI rates

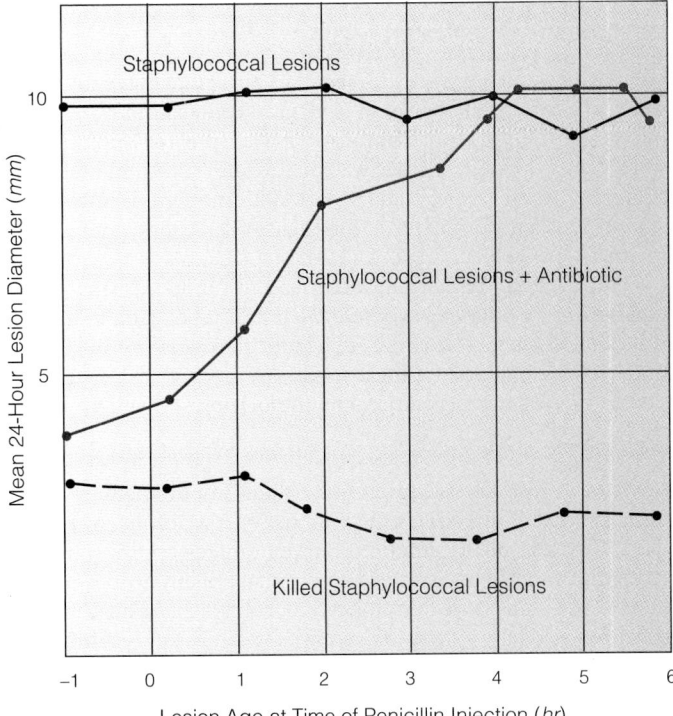

Figure 5 In a pioneer study of antibiotic prophylaxis,[41] the diameter of lesions induced by staphylococcal inoculation 24 hours earlier was observed to be critically affected by the timing of penicillin administration with respect to bacterial inoculation.

Table 8 Historical Rates of Wound Infection

Wound Classification	Infection Rate (%)				
	1960–1962[42] (15,613 patients)	1967–1977[11] (62,937 patients)	1975–1976[5] (59,353 patients)	1977–1981[12] (20,193 patients)	1982–1986[111] (20,703 patients)
Clean	5.1	1.5	2.9	1.8	1.3
Clean-contaminated	10.8	7.7	3.9	2.9	2.5
Contaminated	16.3	15.2	8.5	9.9	7.1
Dirty-infected	28.0	40.0	12.6	—	—
Overall	7.4	4.7	4.1	2.8	2.2

in all categories that were established by this classification [*see Table 8*].[5,11,12,42]

In 1960, after years of negative studies, it was said, "Nearly all surgeons now agree that the routine use of prophylaxis in clean operations is unnecessary and undesirable."[47] Since then, much has changed: there are now many clean operations for which no competent surgeon would omit the use of prophylactic antibiotics, particularly as procedures become increasingly complex and prosthetic materials are used in patients who are older, sicker, or immunocompromised.

A separate risk assessment that integrates host and bacterial variables (i.e., whether the operation is dirty or contaminated, is longer than 2 hours, or is an abdominal procedure and whether the patient has three or more concomitant diagnoses) segregates more effectively those patients who are prone to an increased incidence of SSI [*see* Integration of Determinants of Infection, *below*]. This approach enables the surgeon to identify those patients who are likely to require preventive measures, particularly in clean cases, in which antibiotics would normally not be used.[5]

It has been implied that antibiotic prophylaxis for two types of clean surgery—hernia repair and breast surgery—represents the standard of practice.[48] However, in the study from which these conclusions were drawn, SSI and urinary tract infection rates were higher than many would have predicted, sample sizes were not large, and potential hazards of widespread antibiotic use were not addressed; neither was the evolution to minimal excisions for breast surgery addressed. Without significantly more supportive data, prophylaxis for clean cases cannot be recommended unless specific risk factors are present.[5,49,50]

Data suggest that prophylactic use of antibiotics may contribute to secondary *Clostridium difficile* disease; caution should be exercised when widening the indications for prophylaxis is under consideration.[51] If local results are poor, surgical practice should be reassessed before antibiotics are prescribed.

ANTIBIOTIC SELECTION AND ADMINISTRATION

When antibiotics are given more than 2 hours before operation, the risk of infection is increased.[46,52] I.V. administration in the OR or the preanesthetic room guarantees appropriate levels at the time of incision. The organisms likely to be present dictate the choice of antibiotic for prophylaxis. The cephalosporins are ideally suited to prophylaxis: their features include a broad spectrum of activity, an excellent ratio of therapeutic to toxic dosages, a low rate of allergic responses, ease of administration, and attractive cost advantages. Mild allergic reactions to penicillin are not contraindications for the use of a cephalosporin.[53]

Physicians like new drugs and often tend to prescribe newer, more expensive antibiotics for simple tasks. First-generation cephalosporins (e.g., cefazolin) are ideal agents for prophylaxis. Third-generation cephalosporins are not: they cost more, are not more effective, and promote emergence of resistant strains.[54-56]

The most important first-generation cephalosporin for surgical patients continues to be cefazolin. Administered I.V. in the OR at the time of skin incision, it provides adequate tissue levels throughout most of the operation. A second dose administered in the OR after 3 hours will be beneficial if the procedure lasts longer than that.[57] Data on all operative site infections are imprecise, but SSIs can clearly be reduced by this regimen. No data suggest that further doses are required for prophylaxis.

Fortunately, cefazolin is effective against both gram-positive and gram-negative bacteria of importance, unless significant anaerobic organisms are encountered. The significance of anaerobic flora has been disputed,[58] but for elective colorectal operation,[59,60] abdominal trauma,[61,62] appendicitis,[63] or other circumstances in which penicillin-resistant anaerobic bacteria are likely to be encountered, coverage against both aerobic and anaerobic gram-negative organisms is strongly recommended and supported by the data.

Despite several decades of studies, prophylaxis is not always properly implemented. Unfortunately, didactic education is not always the best way to change behavior. Preprinted order forms[64] and a reminder sticker from the pharmacy[65] have proved to be effective methods of ensuring correct utilization.

The commonly heard decision "This case was tough, let's give an antibiotic for 3 to 5 days" has no data to support it and should be abandoned. Differentiation between prophylaxis and therapeusis is important. A therapeutic course for perforated diverticulitis or other types of peritoneal infection is appropriate. Data on casual contamination associated with trauma or with operative procedures suggest that 24 hours of prophylaxis or less is quite adequate.[66-70] Mounting evidence suggests that a single preoperative dose is good care and that additional doses are not required.[71]

Trauma Patients

The efficacy of antibiotic administration on arrival in the emergency department as an integral part of resuscitation has been clearly demonstrated.[61] The most common regimens have been (1) a combination of an aminoglycoside and clindamycin and (2) cefoxitin alone. These two regimens or variations thereof have been compared in a number of studies.[32,62,72-74] They appear to be equally effective, and either regimen can be recommended with confidence. For prophylaxis, there appears to be a trend toward using a single drug: cefoxitin[53] or cefotetan.[75] If therapy is required because of either a delay in surgery, terrible injury, or prolonged shock, the combination of an agent that is effective against anaerobes with an aminoglycoside seems to be favored. Because aminoglycosides are nephrotoxic, they must be used with care in the presence of shock.

In all the trauma studies just cited, antibiotic prophylaxis lasted for 48 hours or longer. Subsequent studies, however, indicated that prophylaxis lasting less than 24 hours is appropriate.[68-70,76] Single-dose prophylaxis is appropriate for patients with closed fractures.[77]

COMPLICATIONS

Complications of antibiotic prophylaxis are few. Although data linking prophylaxis to the development of resistant organisms are meager, resistant microbes have developed in every other situation in which antibiotics have been utilized, and it is reasonable to expect that prophylaxis in any ecosystem will have the same result,[78] particularly if selection of patients is poor, if prophylaxis lasts too long, or if too many late-generation agents are used.

A rare but important complication of antibiotic use is pseudomembranous enterocolitis, which is induced most commonly by clindamycin, the cephalosporins, and ampicillin [see 6:17 Nosocomial Infection].[51] The common denominator among different cases of pseudomembranous enterocolitis is hard to identify. Diarrhea and fever can develop after administration of single doses of prophylactic antibiotics. The condition is rare, but difficulties occur because of failure to make a rapid diagnosis.

CURRENT ISSUES

The most significant questions concerning prophylaxis of SSIs already have been answered. Important issues that remain are the proper duration of prophylaxis in complicated cases, trauma, and the presence of foreign bodies. No change in the criteria for antibiotic prophylaxis is required in laparoscopic procedures; the risk of infection is lower in such cases.[79,80] Cost factors are important and may justify the endless succession of studies that compare new drugs in competition for appropriate clinical niches.

Further advances in patient selection may take place but will require analysis of data from large numbers of patients and a distinction between approaches to infection of the wound, which is only a part of the operative field, and approaches to infections directly related to the operative site. These developments will define more clearly the prophylaxis requirements of patients whose operations are clean but whose risk of wound or operative site infection is increased.

A current issue of some concern is potential loss of infection surveillance capability. Infection control units have been shown to offer a number of benefits in the institutional setting, such as the following:

1. Identifying epidemics by common or uncommon organisms.[17,20,81]
2. Establishing correct use of prophylaxis (timing, dose, duration, and choice).[45,46]
3. Documenting costs, risk factors, and readmission rates.[82,83]
4. Monitoring postdischarge infections and secondary consequences.[84-86]
5. Ensuring patient safety.[87]
6. Managing MSRA and VRE.

These benefits notwithstanding, as the business of hospital care has become more expensive and financial control more rigid, the infection control unit is a hospital component that many administrators have come to consider a luxury and therefore expendable. Consequently, surveillance as a quality control and patient safety mechanism has been diminished.

It is apparent that SSIs have huge clinical and financial implications. Patients with infections tend to be sicker and to undergo more complex operations. Therefore, higher infection rates translate into higher morbidity and mortality as well as higher cost to the hospital, the patient, and society as a whole. With increasingly early discharge becoming the norm, delayed diagnosis of postdischarge SSI and the complications thereof is a growing problem.[84-86] Effective use of institutional databases may contribute greatly to identification of this problem.[85]

Clearly, the development of effective mechanisms for identifying and controlling SSIs is in the interests of all associated with the delivery of health care.[87] The identification of problems by means of surveillance and feedback can make a substantial contribution to reducing SSI rates [see Table 6].[11,87]

Skin Preparation

As the first line of defense against infection, the skin is remarkable in its complexity and efficiency. Surgeons must respect this organ and carefully manage preparation of both their own skin and their patients' skin. None of the topical antibacterial agents now in use are totally harmless; their destructive effect on the skin's natural defense mechanisms must be recognized and taken into account.

Although the importance of skin preparation cannot be denied, in healthy tissue, a wound contaminated with many microorganisms is amazingly resistant to infection. Admittedly, skin preparation has a relatively minor influence on wound infection as compared with surgical technique and host factors; nonetheless, it consumes OR time and the time of health care personnel, both of which are expensive. Therefore, choosing the most effective agent and method for skin preparation is an important economic decision as well as a surgical decision [see Table 9 and Sidebar The Surgical Scrub].

POSTOPERATIVE HAND WASHING

The purpose of washing the hands after surgery is to remove microorganisms that are resident, that flourished in the warm, wet environment created by wearing gloves, or that reached the hands by entering through puncture holes in the gloves. On the ward, even minimal contact with colonized patients has been demonstrated to transfer microorganisms.[88] As many as 1,000 organisms were transferred by simply touching the patient's hand, taking a pulse, or lifting the patient. The organisms survived for 20 to 150 minutes, making their transfer to the next patient clearly possible. Viruses have been shown to survive for 20 to 30 minutes on the hands.[89]

A return to the ancient practice of washing hands between each patient contact is warranted. Nosocomial spread of numerous organisms—including C. difficile; MRSA, VRE, and other antibiotic-resistant bacteria; and viruses—is a constant threat.

Hand washing on the ward is complicated by the fact that overwashing may actually increase bacterial counts. Dry, damaged skin harbors many more bacteria than healthy skin and is almost impossible to render even close to bacteria free. Although little is known about the physiologic changes in skin that result from frequent washings, the bacterial flora is certainly modified by alterations in the lipid or water content of the skin. The so-called dry hand syndrome was the impetus behind the development of the alcohol-based gels now available. These preparations make it easy for surgeons to clean their hands after every patient encounter with minimal damage to their skin.

Table 9   Characteristics of Three Topical Antimicrobial Agents Effective against
Both Gram-Positive and Gram-Negative Bacteria[126]

Agent	Mode of Action	Antifungal Activity	Comments
Chlorhexidine	Cell wall disruption	Fair	Poor activity against tuberculosis-causing organisms; can cause ototoxicity and eye irritation
Iodine/iodophors	Oxidation and substitution by free iodine	Good	Broad antibacterial spectrum; minimal skin residual activity; possible absorption toxicity and skin irritation
Alcohols	Denaturation of protein	Good	Rapid action but little residual activity; flammable

Infection Prevention in Bowel Surgery

The results of the numerous studies of antibiotic bowel preparation that have been done suggest that many different approaches may be equally effective in reducing infection after elective colonic resection. Certain features, however, appear to be common to most of the studies:

1. Oral antibiotic regimens with both aerobic and anaerobic activity (e.g., neomycin–erythromycin base and neomycin-metronidazole) were employed.
2. The oral agents were given in limited doses the day before operation.
3. Addition of systemic antibiotic agents without broad-spectrum coverage to the oral antibiotics generally did not improve the results.
4. Use of broad-spectrum parenteral antibiotic agents alone was associated with a lower infection rate than use of systemic agents with only limited coverage.
5. Addition of a broad-spectrum parenteral antibiotic to the oral antibiotics may further reduce the postoperative infection rate.
6. Parenteral or oral antibiotics should be administered only for short amounts of time during the perioperative period. A single parenteral dose given just before operation may be sufficient.[90-94]
7. A clean colon is associated with a lower infection rate.[94-96]

A 5-year cooperative Veterans Administration study of more than 1,000 patients undergoing elective colon operations compared two groups of patients receiving oral neomycin–erythromycin base: one group received only the oral preparation, whereas the other also received parenteral perioperative cephalothin.[95] The infection rates were not significantly different in the two groups and in fact were below 9% in both; however, there was a trend toward lower infection rates in patients receiving both oral and parenteral antibiotics.

The mechanical cleansing technique employed is very much a matter of preference. Traditional bowel preparation, if carried out for unnecessarily long periods (3 to 5 days), is associated with less patient compliance and a higher incidence of fatigue and other related symptoms than are other cleansing techniques. Whole gut irrigation with large amounts of fluid (10 to 15 L) has been recommended. Both of these approaches should be discouraged. Some authors recommend the use of mannitol in varying concentrations in lavage solutions.[97] Others emphasize that clinical dehydration may develop when 15% mannitol is used or that electrocautery may lead to colonic explosions when mannitol is used without oral antibiotics.[98] Lavage with polyethylene glycol–electrolyte solution appears to be the preferred cleansing method before elective colorectal surgery.[98,99] A study comparing the efficacy of 2-day routine mechanical cleansing with that of lavage performed once on the day before operation demonstrated no difference between the two approaches: 1-day lavage was both safe and economical, and the authors preferred it to 2-day mechanical cleansing.[100] Subsequent studies reported no differences in the adequacy of colon cleansing, whether bowel preparation was performed in the inpatient setting or the outpatient setting.[101,102] A 2003 study suggested that no bowel preparation is necessary in elective cases.[96] However, operating on a colon empty of liquid and stool makes sense and is supported by a considerable body of data.

Integration of Determinants of Infection

The significant advances in the control of wound infection during the past several decades are linked to a better understanding of the biology of wound infection, and this link has permitted the advance to the concept of SSI.[2] In all tissues at any time, there will be a critical inoculum of bacteria that would cause an infectious process [*see Figure 3*]. The standard definition of infection in urine and sputum has been 10^5 organisms/ml. In a clean dry wound, 10^5 bacteria produce a wound infection rate of 50% [*see Figure 3*].[10] Effective use of antibiotics reduces the infection rate to 10% with the same number of bacteria and thereby permits the wound to tolerate a much larger number of bacteria.

All of the clinical activities described are intended either to reduce the inoculum or to permit the host to manage the number of bacteria that would otherwise be pathologic. One study in guinea pigs showed how manipulation of local blood flow, shock, the local immune response, and foreign material can enhance the development of infection.[103] This study and two others defined an early decisive period of host antimicrobial activity that lasts for 3 to 6 hours after contamination.[41,103,104] Bacteria that remain after this period are the infecting inoculum. Processes that interfere with this early response (e.g., shock, altered perfusion, adjuvants, or foreign material) or support it (e.g., antibiotics or total care) have a major influence on outcome.

One investigation demonstrated that silk sutures decrease the number of bacteria required for infection.[105] Other investigators used a suture as the key adjuvant in studies of host manipulation,[106] whereas a separate study demonstrated persistent susceptibility to wound infection days after shock.[107] The common variable is the number of bacteria. This relation may be termed the inoculum effect, and it has great relevance in all aspects of infection control. Applying knowledge of this effect in practical terms involves the following three steps:

1. Keeping the bacterial contamination as low as possible via asepsis and antisepsis, preoperative preparation of patient and surgeon, and antibiotic prophylaxis.
2. Maintaining local factors in such a way that they can prevent the lodgment of bacteria and thereby provide a locally unreceptive environment.

Table 10   Comparison of Wound
Classification Systems[5]

Traditional Wound Classification System	Simplified Risk Index					
	Low Risk	Medium Risk	High Risk			All from Traditional Classification
	0	1	2	3	4	
Clean	1.1	3.9	8.4	15.8		2.9
Clean-contaminated	0.6	2.8	8.4	17.7		3.9
Contaminated		4.5	8.3	11.0	23.9	8.5
Dirty-infected		6.7	10.9	18.8	27.4	12.6
All from SENIC index	1.0	3.6	8.9	17.2	27.0	4.1

SENIC—Study of the Efficacy of Nosocomial Infection Control

3. Maintaining systemic responses at such a level that they can control the bacteria that become established.

These three steps are related to the determinants of infection and their applicability to daily practice. Year-by-year reductions in wound infection rates, when closely followed, indicate that it is possible for surgeons to continue improving results by attention to quality of clinical care and surgical technique, despite increasingly complex operations.[4,12,22-24] In particular, the measures involved in the first step (control of bacteria) have been progressively refined and are now well established.

The integration of determinants has significant effects [see Figures 3 and 4]. When wound closure was effected with a wound hematocrit of 8% or more, the inoculum required to produce a wound infection rate of 40% was 100 bacteria [see Figure 3]. Ten bacteria produced a wound infection rate of 20%. The shift in the number of organisms required to produce clinical infection is significant. It is obvious that this inoculum effect can be changed dramatically by good surgical technique and further altered by use of prophylactic antibiotics. If the inoculum is always slightly smaller than the number of organisms required to produce infection in any given setting, results are excellent. There is clearly a relation between the number of bacteria and the local environment. The local effect can also be seen secondary to systemic physiologic change, specifically shock. One study showed the low local perfusion in shock to be important in the development of an infection.[103,104]

One investigation has shown that shock can alter infection rates immediately after its occurrence [see Figure 4].[107] Furthermore, if the inoculum is large enough, antibiotics will not control bacteria. In addition, there is a late augmentation of infection lasting up to 3 days after restoration of blood volume. These early and late effects indicate that systemic determinants come into play after local effects are resolved. These observations call for further study, but obviously, it is the combined abnormalities that alter outcome.

Systemic host responses are important for the control of infection. The patient has been clearly implicated as one of the four critical variables in the development of wound infection.[5] In addition, the bacterial inoculum, the location of the procedure and its duration, and the coexistence of three or more diagnoses were found to give a more accurate prediction of the risk of wound infection. The spread of risk is defined better with the SENIC index (1% to 27%) than it is with the traditional classification (2.9% to 12.6%) [see

Table 10]. The importance of the number of bacteria is lessened if the other factors are considered in addition to inoculum. The inoculum effect has to be considered with respect to both the number of organisms and the local and systemic host factors that are in play. Certain variables were found to be significantly related to the risk of wound infection in three important prospective studies [see Table 10].[5,9,11] It is apparent that the problem of SSI cannot be examined only with respect to the management of bacteria. Host factors have become much more significant now that the bacterial inoculum can be maintained at low levels by means of asepsis, antisepsis, technique, and prophylactic antibiotics.[108]

Important host variables include the maintenance of normal homeostasis (physiology) and immune response. Maintenance of normal homeostasis in patients at risk is one of the great advances of surgical critical care.[108] The clearest improvements in this regard have come in maintenance of blood volume, oxygenation, and oxygen delivery.

One group demonstrated the importance of oxygen delivery, tissue perfusion, and P_aO_2 in the development of wound infection.[109] Oxygen can have as powerful a negative influence on the development of SSI as antibiotics can.[110] The influence is very similar to that seen in other investigations. Whereas a P_aO_2 equivalent to a true fractional concentration of oxygen in inspired gas (F_IO_2) of 45% is not feasible, maintenance, when appropriate, of an increased F_IO_2 in the postoperative period may prove an elementary and effective tool in managing the inoculum effect.

Modern surgical practice has reduced the rate of wound infection significantly. Consequently, it is more useful to think in terms of SSI, which is not limited to the incision but may occur anywhere in the operative field; this concept provides a global objective for control of infections associated with a surgical procedure. Surveillance is of great importance for quality assurance. Reports of recognized pathogens (e.g., *S. epidermidis* and group A streptococci) as well as unusual organisms (e.g., *Rhodococcus* [*Gordona*] *bronchialis*, *Mycoplasma hominis*, and *Legionella dumoffii*) in SSIs highlight the importance of infection control and epidemiology for quality assurance in surgical departments.[15-17,20,21] (Although these reports use the term wound infection, they are really addressing what we now call SSI.) The importance of surgeon-specific and service-specific SSI reports should be clear[11,12,111] [see Table 6], and their value in quality assurance evident.

References

1. Meakins JL: Host defence mechanisms: evaluation and roles of acquired defects and immunotherapy. Can J Surg 18:259, 1975

2. Consensus paper on the surveillance of surgical wound infections. The Society for Hospital Epidemiology of America; the Association for Practitioners in Infection Control; the Centers for Disease Control; the Surgical Infection Society. Infect Control Hosp Epidemiol 13:599, 1992

3. Horan TC, Gaynes RP, Martone WJ, et al: CDC definitions of nosocomial surgical site infections, 1992: a modification of CDC definitions of surgical wound infections. Infect Control Hosp Epidemiol 13:606, 1992

4. Report of an Ad Hoc Committee of the Committee on Trauma, Division of Medical Sciences, National Academy of Sciences–National Research Council: Postoperative wound infections: the influence of ultraviolet irradiation of the operating room and of various other factors. Ann Surg 160(suppl):1, 1964

5. Haley RW, Culver DH, Morgan WM, et al: Identifying patients at high risk of surgical wound infection: a simple multivariate index of patient susceptibility and wound contamination. Am J Epidemiol 121:206, 1985

6. Mangram AJ, Horan TC, Pearson ML, et al: The Hospital Infection Control Practices Advisory Committee: guideline for prevention of surgical site infection, 1999. Infect Control Hosp Epidemiol 20:247, 1999

7. Culver DH, Horan TC, Gaynes, RP, et al: Surgical wound infection rates by wound class, operative procedure and patient risk index. Am J Med 91(suppl 3B):153S, 1991

8. Fariñas-Álvarez C, Fariñas C, Prieto D, et al: Applicability of two surgical-site infection risk indices to risk of sepsis in surgical patients. Infect Control Hosp Epidemiol 21:633, 2000

9. Davidson AIG, Clark C, Smith G: Postoperative wound infection: a computer analysis. Br J Surg 58:333, 1971

10. Polk HC Jr, Lopez-Mayor JF: Postoperative wound infection: a prospective study of determinant factors and prevention. Surgery 66:97, 1969

11. Cruse PJE, Foord R: The epidemiology of wound infection: a 10-year prospective study of 62,939 wounds. Surg Clin North Am 60:27, 1980

12. Olson M, O'Connor M, Schwartz ML: Surgical wound infections: a 5-year prospective study of 20,193 wounds at the Minneapolis VA Medical Center. Ann Surg 199:253, 1984

13. Alexander JW, Fischer JE, Boyajian M, et al: The influence of hair-removal methods on wound infections. Arch Surg 118:347, 1983

14. Olson MM, MacCallum J, McQuarrie DG: Preoperative hair removal with clippers does not increase infection rate in clean surgical wounds. Surg Gynecol Obstet 162:181, 1986

15. Boyce JM, Potter-Bynoe G, Opal SM, et al: A common-source outbreak of Staphylococcus epidermidis infections among patients undergoing cardiac surgery. J Infect Dis 161:493, 1990

16. Mastro TD, Farley TA, Elliott JA, et al: An outbreak of surgical-wound infections due to group A Streptococcus carried on the scalp. N Engl J Med 323:968, 1990

17. Richet HM, Craven PC, Brown JM, et al: A cluster of Rhodococcus (Gordona) bronchialis sternal-wound infections after coronary-artery bypass surgery. N Engl J Med 324:104, 1991

18. Moylan JA, Kennedy BV: The importance of gown and drape barriers in the prevention of wound infection. Surg Gynecol Obstet 151:465, 1980

19. Garibaldi RA, Maglio S, Lerer T, et al: Comparison of nonwoven and woven gown and drape fabric to prevent intraoperative wound contamination and postoperative infection. Am J Surg 152:505, 1986

20. Lowry PW, Blankenship RJ, Gridley W, et al: A cluster of Legionella sternal-wound infections due to postoperative topical exposure to contaminated tap water. N Engl J Med 324:109, 1991

21. Wilson ME, Dietze C: Mycoplasma hominis surgical wound infection: a case report and discussion. Surgery 103:257, 1988

22. Cruse PJE: Surgical wound sepsis. Can Med Assoc J 102:251, 1970

23. Wangensteen OH, Wangensteen SD: The Rise of Surgery: Emergence from Empiric Craft to Scientific Discipline. University of Minnesota Press, Minneapolis, 1978

24. Cruse PJE: Wound infections: epidemiology and clinical characteristics. Surgical Infectious Disease, 2nd ed. Howard RJ, Simmons RL, Eds. Appleton and Lange, Norwalk, Connecticut, 1988

25. Hopf HW, Hunt TK, West JM, et al: Wound tissue oxygen tension predicts the risk of wound infection in surgical patients. Arch Surg 132:997, 1997

26. Greif R, Akca O, Horn EP, et al: Supplemental perioperative oxygen to reduce the incidence of surgical-wound infection. Outcomes Research Group. N Engl J Med 342:161, 2000

27. Gottrup F: Prevention of surgical-wound infections. N Engl J Med 342:202, 2000

28. Latham R, Lancaster AD, Covington JF, et al: The association of diabetes and glucose control with surgical-site infections among cardiothoracic surgery patients. Infect Control Hosp Epidemiol 22:607, 2001

29. Furnary AP, Zerr KJ, Grunkemeier GI, et al: Continuous intravenous insulin infusion reduces the incidence of deep sternal wound infection in diabetic patients after cardiac surgical procedures. Ann Thorac Surg 67:352, 1999

30. Van Den Berghe G, Wouters P, Weekers F, et al: Intensive insulin therapy in critically ill patients. N Engl J Med 345:1359, 2001

31. Kurz H, Sessler DI, Lenhardt R: Perioperative normothermia to reduce the incidence of surgical wound infection and shorten hospitalization. N Engl J Med 334:1209, 1996

32. Nichols RL, Smith JW, Klein DB, et al: Risk of infection after penetrating abdominal trauma. N Engl J Med 311:1065, 1984

33. Jensen LS, Andersen A, Fristup SC, et al: Comparison of one dose versus three doses of prophylactic antibiotics, and the influence of blood transfusion, on infectious complications in acute and elective colorectal surgery. Br J Surg 77:513, 1990

34. Møller AM, Villebro N, Pedersen T, et al: Effect of preoperative smoking intervention on postoperative complications: a randomised clinical trial. Lancet 359:114, 2002

35. Buggy D: Can anaesthetic management influence surgical wound healing? Lancet 356:355, 2000

36. Melling AC, Ali B, Scott EM, et al: Effects of preoperative warming on the incidence of wound infection after clean surgery: a randomised controlled trial. Lancet 358:876, 2001

37. Horn SD, Wright HL, Couperus JJ, et al: Association between patient-controlled analgesia pump use and postoperative surgical site infection in intestinal surgery patients. Surg Infect 3:109, 2002

38. Bennett SN, McNeil MM, Bland LA, et al: Postoperative infections traced to contamination of an intravenous anesthetic: propofol. N Engl J Med 333:147, 1995

39. Nichols RL, Smith JW: Bacterial contamination of an anesthetic agent. N Engl J Med 333:184, 1995

40. Miles AA, Miles EM, Burke J: The value and duration of defense reactions of the skin to the primary lodgment of bacteria. Br J Exp Pathol 38:79, 1957

41. Burke JF: The effective period of preventive antibiotic action in experimental incisions and dermal lesions. Surgery 50:161, 1961

42. Bernard HR, Cole WR: The prophylaxis of surgical infection: the effect of prophylactic antimicrobial drugs on incidence of infection following potentially contaminated wounds. Surgery 56:151, 1964

43. Chodak GW, Plaut ME: Use of systemic antibiotics for prophylaxis in surgery: a critical review. Arch Surg 112:326, 1977

44. Di Piro JT, Bivens BA, Record KE, et al: The prophylactic use of antimicrobials in surgery. Curr Probl Surg 20:72, 1983

45. Conte JE Jr, Polk HC Jr: Antibiotic Prophylaxis in Surgery: A Comprehensive Review. JB Lippincott Co, Philadelphia, 1984

46. Classen DC, Evans RS, Pestotnik SC, et al: The timing of prophylactic administration of antibiotics and the risk of surgical-wound infection. N Engl J Med 326: 282, 1992

47. Finland M: Antibacterial agents: uses and abuses in treatment and prophylaxis. RI Med J 43:499, 1960

48. Platt R, Zaleznik DF, Hopkins CC, et al: Perioperative antibiotic prophylaxis for herniorrhaphy and breast surgery. N Engl J Med 322:153, 1990

49. Taylor EW, Byrne DJ, Leaper DJ, et al: Antibiotic prophylaxis and open groin hernia repair. World J Surg 21:811, 1997

50. Platt R, Zucker JR, Zaleznik DF, et al: Prophylaxis against wound infection following hernia or breast surgery. J Infect Dis 166:556, 1992

51. Yee J, Dixon CM, McLean APH, et al: Clostridium difficile disease in a department of surgery: the significance of prophylactic antibiotics. Arch Surg 126:241, 1991

52. Burke JP. Maximising appropriate antibiotic prophylaxis for surgical patients: an update from LDS Hospital, Salt Lake City. Clin Infect Dis 33 (suppl):78, 2001

53. Kaiser AB: Antibiotic prophylaxis in surgery. N Engl J Med 315:1129, 1986

54. Meijer WS, Schmitz PI, Jeekel J: Meta-analysis of randomized, controlled clinical trials of antibiotic prophylaxis in biliary tract surgery. Br J Surg 77:283, 1990

55. Rotman N, Hay J-M, Lacaine F, et al: Prophylactic antibiotherapy in abdominal surgery: first- vs third-generation cephalosporins. Arch Surg 124:323, 1989

56. Choice of cephalosporins. Med Lett Drugs Ther 32:109, 1990

57. Shapiro M, Muñoz A, Tager IB, et al: Risk factors for infection at the operative site after abdominal or vaginal hysterectomy. N Engl J Med 307:1661, 1982

58. Polk HC Jr: Contributions of alimentary tract surgery to modern infection control. Am J Surg 153:2, 1987

59. Clarke JS, Condon RE, Bartlett JG, et al: Preoperative oral antibiotics reduce septic complications of colon operations: results of prospective, randomized, double-blind clinical study. Ann Surg 186:251, 1977

60. Washington JA III, Dearing WH, Judd ES, et al: Effect of preoperative antibiotic regimen on development of infection after intestinal surgery. Ann Surg 180:567, 1974

61. Fullen WD, Hunt J, Altemeier WA: Prophylactic antibiotics in penetrating wounds of the abdomen. J Trauma 12:282, 1972

62. Gentry LO, Feliciano DV, Lea AS, et al: Perioperative antibiotic therapy for penetrating injuries of the abdomen. Ann Surg 200:561, 1984

63. Heseltine PNR, Yellin AE, Appleman MD, et al: Perforated and gangrenous appendicitis: an analysis of antibiotic failures. J Infect Dis 148:322, 1983

64. Girotti MJ, Fodoruk S, Irvine-Meek J, et al: Antibiotic handbook and pre-printed perioperative order

forms for surgical prophylaxis: do they work? Can J Surg 33:385, 1990

65. Larsen RA, Evans RS, Burke JP, et al: Improved perioperative antibiotic use and reduced surgical wound infections through use of computer decision analysis. Infect Control Hosp Epidemiol 10:316, 1989

66. Stone HN, Haney BB, Kolb LD, et al: Prophylactic and preventive antibiotic therapy: timing duration and economics. Ann Surg 189:691, 1978

67. Rowlands BJ, Clark RG, Richards DG: Single-dose intraoperative antibiotic prophylaxis in emergency abdominal surgery. Arch Surg 117:195, 1982

68. Fabian TC, Croce MA, Payne LW, et al: Duration of antibiotic therapy for penetrating abdominal trauma: a prospective trial. Surgery 112:788, 1992

69. Sarmiento JM, Aristizabal G, Rubiano J, et al: Prophylactic antibiotics in abdominal trauma. J Trauma 37:803, 1994

70. Weigelt JA: Role of anaerobic bacteria in antibiotic prophylaxis for trauma. Infect Dis Clin Pract 5(suppl 3):S92, 1996

71. Di Piro JT, Cheung RPF, Bowden TA Jr, et al: Single dose systemic antibiotic prophylaxis of surgical wound infections. Am J Surg 152:552, 1986

72. Hofstetter SR, Pachter HL, Bailey AA, et al: A prospective comparison of two regimens of prophylactic antibiotics in abdominal trauma: cefoxitin versus triple drug. J Trauma 24:307, 1984

73. Heseltine PNR, Berne TV, Yellin AE, et al: The efficacy of cefoxitin vs clindamycin/gentamicin in surgically treated stab wounds of the bowel. J Trauma 26:241, 1986

74. Jones RC, Thal ER, Johnson NA, et al: Evaluation of antibiotic therapy following penetrating abdominal trauma. Ann Surg 201:576, 1985

75. Antimicrobial prophylaxis in surgery. Med Lett Drugs Ther 43:92, 2001

76. Dellinger EP: Antibiotic prophylaxis in trauma: penetrating abdominal injuries and open fractures. Rev Infect Dis 13:S847, 1991

77. Boxma H, Broekhuisen T, Patka P, et al: Randomized controlled trial of single-dose antibiotic prophylaxis in surgical treatment of closed fractures: the Dutch Trauma Trial. Lancet 347:1133, 1996

78. Archer GL, Armstrong BC: Alteration of staphylococcal flora in cardiac surgery patients receiving prophylaxis. J Infect Dis 147:642, 1983

79. Illig KA, Schmidt E, Cavanaugh J, et al: Are prophylactic antibiotics required for elective laparoscopic cholecystectomy? J Am Coll Surg 184:353, 1997

80. Richards C, Edwards J, Culver D, et al: Does using a laparoscopic approach to cholecystectomy decrease the risk of surgical site infection? Ann Surg 237:358, 2003

81. Kaiser AB: Surgical wound infection. N Eng J Med 324:123, 1991

82. Kirkland KB, Briggs JP, Trivette SL, et al: The impact of surgical-site infection in 1990's: attributable mortality, excess length of hospitalisation, and extra costs. Infect Control Hosp Epidemiol 20:725, 1999

83. Gaynes RP: Surveillance of surgical-site infections: the world coming together? Infect Control Hosp Epidemiol 21:309, 2000

84. Weiss CA, Statz CL, Dahms RA, et al: Six years of surgical wound infection surveillance at a tertiary care center. Arch Surg 134:1041, 1999

85. Sands K, Vineyard G, Livingston J, et al: Efficient identification of postdischarge surgical site infections: use of automated pharmacy dispensing information, administrative data, and medical record information. J Infect Dis 179:434, 1999

86. Platt R: Progress in surgical-site infection surveillance. Infect Control Hosp Epidemiol 23:361, 2002

87. Burke JP: Infection control—a problem for patient safety. N Engl J Med 348:651, 2003

88. Casewell M, Phillips I: Hands as route of transmission for Klebsiella species. Br Med J 2:1315, 1977

89. Schürmann W, Eggers HJ: Antiviral activity of an alcoholic hand disinfectant: comparison of the in vitro suspension test with in vivo experiments on hands, and on individual fingertips. Antiviral Res 3:25, 1983

90. Gorbach SL, Condon RE, Conte JE Jr, et al: General guidelines for the evaluation of new anti-infective drugs for prophylaxis of surgical infections. Clin Infect Dis 15(suppl 1):S313, 1992

91. Jagelman DG, Fabian TC, Nichols RL, et al: Single dose cefotetan versus multiple dose cefoxitin as prophylaxis in colorectal surgery. Am J Surg 155 (suppl 5A):71, 1988

92. Periti P, Mazzei T, Tonelli F, et al: Single dose cefotetan versus multiple dose cefoxitin—antimicrobial prophylaxis in colorectal surgery. Dis Colon Rectum 32:121, 1989

93. Norwegian Study Group for Colorectal Surgery: Should antimicrobial prophylaxis in colorectal surgery include agents effective against both anaerobic and aerobic microorganisms? A double-blind, multicenter study. Surgery 97:402, 1985

94. Song J, Glenny AM: Antimicrobial prophylaxis in colorectal surgery: a systematic review of randomized controlled trials. Br J Surg 85:1232, 1998

95. Condon RE, Bartlett JG, Greenlee H, et al: Efficacy of oral and systemic antibiotic prophylaxis in colorectal operations. Arch Surg 118:496, 1983

96. Zmora O, Mahajna A, Bar-Zakai B, et al: Colon and rectal surgery without mechanical bowel preparation: a randomised prospective trial. Ann Surg 237:363, 2003

97. Jagelman DG, Fazio VW, Lavery IC, et al: A prospective, randomized, double-blind study of 10% mannitol mechanical bowel preparation combined with oral neomycin and short-term, perioperative, intravenous Flagyl as prophylaxis in elective colorectal resections. Surgery 98:861, 1985

98. Beck DE, Harford FJ, DiPalma JA, et al: Bowel cleansing with polyethylene glycol electrolyte lavage solution. South Med J 78:1414, 1985

99. Fleites RA, Marshall JB, Eckhauser ML, et al: The efficacy of polyethylene glycol-electrolyte lavage solution versus traditional mechanical bowel preparation for elective colonic surgery: a randomized prospective, blinded clinical trial. Surgery 98:708, 1985

100. Wolff BG, Beart RW Jr, Dozois RR, et al: A new bowel preparation for elective colon and rectal surgery. Arch Surg 123:895, 1988

101. Frazee RC, Roberts J, Symmonds R, et al: Prospective, randomized trial of inpatient vs. outpatient bowel preparation for elective colorectal surgery. Dis Colon Rectum 35:223, 1992

102. Handelsman JC, Zeiler S, Coleman J, et al: Experience with ambulatory preoperative bowel preparation at the Johns Hopkins Hospital. Arch Surg 128:441, 1993

103. Miles AA, Miles EM, Burke J: The value and duration of defence reactions of the skin to the primary lodgement of bacteria. Br J Exp Pathol 38:79, 1957

104. Miles AA: The inflammatory response in relation to local infections. Surg Clin North Am 60:93, 1980

105. Alexander JW, Alexander WA: Penicillin prophylaxis of experimental staphylococcal wound infections. Surg Gynecol Obstet 120:243, 1965

106. Polk HC Jr: The enhancement of host defenses against infection: search for the holy grail. Surgery 99:1, 1986

107. Livingston DH, Malangoni MA: An experimental study of susceptibility to infection after hemorrhagic shock. Surg Gynecol Obstet 168:138, 1989

108. Meakins JL: Surgeons, surgery and immunomodulation. Arch Surg 126:494, 1991

109. Knighton D, Halliday B, Hunt TK: Oxygen as an antibiotic: a comparison of the effects of inspired oxygen concentration and antibiotic administration on in vivo bacterial clearance. Arch Surg 121:191, 1986

110. Rabkin J, Hunt TK: Infection and oxygen. Problem Wounds: The Role of Oxygen. Davis JC, Hunt TK, Eds. Elsevier, New York, 1987, p 1

111. Olson MM, Lee JT Jr: Continuous, 10-year wound infection surveillance: results, advantages, and unanswered questions. Arch Surg 125:794, 1990

112. Oreskovich MR, Dellinger EP, Lennard ES, et al: Duration of preventive antibiotic administration for penetrating abdominal trauma. Arch Surg 117:200, 1982

113. Langely JM, Le Blanc JC, Drake J, et al: Efficacy of antimicrobial prophylaxis in placement of cerebrospinal fluid shunts: meta-analysis. Clin Infect Dis 17:98, 1993

114. Forse RA, Karam B, MacLean LD, et al: Antibiotic prophylaxis for surgery in morbidly obese patients. Surgery 106:750, 1989

115. Dajani AS, Taubert KA, Wilson W, et al: Prevention of bacterial endocarditis: recommendations by the American Heart Association. JAMA 277:1794, 1997

116. Durack DT: Prevention of infective endocarditis. N Engl J Med 332:38, 1995

117. Prevention of bacterial endocarditis. Med Lett Drugs Ther 32:112, 1990

118. Kaye D: Prophylaxis for infective endocarditis: an update. Ann Intern Med 104:419, 1986

119. Petersen EA: Prevention of bacterial endocarditis. Arch Intern Med 150:2447, 1990

120. Hayek LJ, Emerson JM, Gardner AMN: A placebo-controlled trial of the effect of two preoperative baths or showers with chlorhexidine detergent on postoperative wound infection rates. J Hosp Infect 10:165, 1987

121. Garner JS: CDC guidelines for the prevention and control of nosocomial infections: guideline for prevention of surgical wound infections, 1985. Am J Infect Control 14:71, 1986

122. Hamilton HW, Hamilton KR, Lone FJ: Preoperative hair removal. Can J Surg 20:269, 1977

123. McDonald WS, Nichter LS: Debridement of bacterial and particulate-contaminated wounds. Ann Plast Surg 33:142, 1994

124. Brown TR, Ehrlich CE, Stehman FB, et al: A clinical evaluation of chlorhexidine gluconate spray as compared with iodophor scrub for preoperative skin preparation. Surg Gynecol Obstet 158:363, 1984

125. Ritter MA, French MLV, Eitzen HE, et al: The antimicrobial effectiveness of operative-site preparative agents: a microbiological and clinical study. J Bone Joint Surg [Am] 62A:826, 1980

126. Larson E: Guideline for use of topical antimicrobial agents. Am J Infect Control 16:253, 1988

127. Amstey MS, Jones AP: Preparation of the vagina for surgery: a comparison of povidone-iodine and saline solution. JAMA 245:839, 1981

128. Lowbury EJL, Lilly HA, Bull JP: Methods for disinfection of hands and operation sites. Br Med J 2:531, 1964

129. Aly R, Maibach HI: Comparative antibacterial efficacy of a 2-minute surgical scrub with chlorhexidine gluconate, povidone-iodine, and chloroxylenol sponge-brushes. Am J Infect Control 16:173, 1988

130. Kaul AF, Jewett JF: Agents and techniques for disinfection of the skin. Surg Gynecol Obstet 152:677, 1981

131. Paulson DS: Comparative evaluation of five surgical hand scrub preparations. AORN J 60:246, 1994

132. Proposed recommended practices for surgical hand scrubs. AORN Recommended Practices Committee. AORN J 60:270, 1994

Acknowledgment

Figures 3 and 4   Albert Miller.

3 PERIOPERATIVE CONSIDERATIONS FOR ANESTHESIA

Steven B. Backman, M.D.C.M., Ph.D., *Richard M. Bondy,* M.D.C.M., *Alain Deschamps,* M.D., Ph.D., *Anne Moore,* M.D., *and Thomas Schricker,* M.D., Ph.D.

Ongoing advancements in modern surgical care are being complemented by alterations in anesthetic management aimed at providing maximum patient benefit. Since the early 1990s, anesthesia practice has changed enormously—through the proliferation of airway devices, the routine employment of patient-controlled analgesia (PCA), the wider popularity of thoracic epidural anesthesia, the development of computer-controlled devices for infusing short-acting drugs, the growing use of quickly reversible inhalational drugs and muscle relaxants, the availability of online monitoring of CNS function, and the increased application of transesophageal echocardiography, to name but a few examples. Our aim in this chapter is to offer surgeons a current perspective on perioperative considerations for anesthesia so as to facilitate dialogue between the surgeon and the anesthesiologist and thereby help minimize patient risk. The primary focus is on the adult patient: the special issues involved in pediatric anesthesia are beyond the scope of our review. In addition, the ensuing discussion is necessarily selective; more comprehensive discussions may be found elsewhere.[1,2]

Perioperative Patient Management

Preoperative medical evaluation is an essential component of preoperative assessment for anesthesia. Of particular importance to the anesthesiologist is any history of personal or family problems with anesthesia. Information should be sought concerning difficulty with airway management or intubation, drug allergy, delayed awakening, significant postoperative nausea or vomiting (PONV), unexpected hospital or ICU admission, and postdural puncture headache (PDPH). Previous anesthetic records may be requested.

The airway must be carefully examined to identify patients at risk for difficult ventilation or intubation [see Special Scenarios, Difficult Airway, below], with particular attention paid to teeth, caps, crowns, dentures, and bridges. Patients must be informed about the risk of trauma associated with intubation and airway management. Anesthetic options [see Choice of Anesthesia, below] should be discussed, including the likelihood of postoperative ventilation and admission to the hospital or the intensive care unit. When relevant, the possibility of blood product administration should be raised, and the patient's acceptance or refusal of transfusion should be carefully documented. Postoperative pain management [see 1:5 Postoperative Pain] should be addressed, particularly when a major procedure is planned. The risks associated with general or regional anesthesia should be discussed in an informative and reassuring manner; a well-conducted preoperative anesthesia interview plays an important role in alleviating anxiety.

The medications the patient is taking can have a substantial impact on anesthetic management. Generally, patients should continue to take their regular medication up to the time of the operation. It is especially important not to abruptly discontinue medications that may result in withdrawal or rebound phenomena (e.g., beta blockers, alpha agonists, barbiturates, and opioids). With some medications (e.g., oral hypoglycemics, insulin, and corticosteroids), perioperative dosage adjustments may be necessary [see 6:11 Endocrine Problems]. Angiotensin-converting enzyme (ACE) inhibitors have been associated with intraoperative hypotension and may be withheld at the discretion of the anesthesiologist.[3] Drugs that should be discontinued preoperatively include monoamine oxidase inhibitors (MAOIs) and oral anticoagulants [see Table 1].

Many surgical patients are taking antiplatelet drugs. Careful consideration should be given to the withdrawal of these agents in the perioperative period [see Table 1] because of the possibility that discontinuance may lead to an acute coronary syndrome. If increased bleeding is a significant risk, longer-acting agents (e.g., aspirin, clopidogrel, and ticlopidine) can be replaced with nonsteroidal anti-inflammatory drugs (NSAIDs) that have shorter half-lives. Typically, these shorter-acting drugs are given for 10 days, stopped on the day of surgery, and then restarted 6 hours after operation. Platelet transfusion should be considered only in the presence of significant medical bleeding.[4]

The increasing use of herbal and alternative medicines has led to significant morbidity and mortality as a consequence of unexpected interactions with traditional drugs. Because many patients fail to mention such agents as part of their medication regimen during the preoperative assessment, it is advisable to question all patients directly about their use. Particular attention should be given to Chinese herbal teas, which include organic compounds and toxic contaminants that may produce renal fibrosis or failure, cholestasis, hepatitis, and thrombocytopenia. Specific recommendations for discontinuance for many of these agents have been developed [see Table 1].

Inpatient versus Outpatient Surgery

An ever-increasing number of operations are performed on an ambulatory basis. Operations considered appropriate for an ambulatory setting are associated with minimal physiologic trespass, low anesthetic complexity, and uncomplicated recovery.[5,6] The design of the ambulatory facility may impose limitations on the types of operations or patients that can be considered for ambulatory surgery. Such limitations may be secondary to availability of equipment, recovery room nursing expertise and access to consultants, and availability of ICU beds or hospital beds. Patients who are in class I or class II of the American Society of Anesthesiologists (ASA) physical status scale are ideally suited for ambulatory surgery; however, a subset of ASA class III patients may be at increased risk for prolonged recovery and hospital admission [see Table 2].

Table 1 Recommendations for Preoperative Discontinuance of Drugs and Medicines[51-64]

Type of Drug	Agent	Pharmacologic Effects	Adverse Effects	Discontinuance Recommendations
MAOIs	Isocarboxazid Phenelzine Pargyline Tranylcypromine Selegiline	Irreversible inhibition of mono-amine oxidase with the resultant increase in serotonin, norepinephrine, epinephrine, dopamine, and octamine neurotransmitters	Potentiation of sympathomimetic amines, possible hypertensive crisis May prolong and intensify effects of other CNS depressants Severe idiopathic hyperpyrexic reaction with meperidine and possibly other narcotics Potential catastrophic interaction with tricyclic antidepressants, characterized by high fever and excessive cerebral excitation and hypertension	*Elective surgery*: discontinue at least 2 wk in advance; consider potential for suicidal tendency—mental health specialist should be involved *Emergency surgery*: avoid meperidine; consider regional anesthesia
Oral anticoagulants	Warfarin	Inhibition of vitamin K–dependent clotting factors II, VII, IX, X	Bleeding	*Elective surgery*: discontinue 5–7 days in advance; replace with heparin if necessary
Antiplatelet agents	*Aspirin and NSAIDs* Aspirin Fenoprofen Ibuprofen Sodium meclofenamate Tolmetin Indomethacin Ketoprofen Diflunisal Naproxen Sulindac Piroxicam	Inhibition of thromboxane A_2 80% of platelets must be inhibited for therapeutic effect Susceptibility to aspirin varies between patients	May increase intraoperative and postoperative bleeding, but not transfusion requirement Perioperative hemorrhagic complications increase with increasing half-life of drug	Primary hemostasis normalizes in 48 hr in healthy persons; platelet activity fully recovered in 8–10 days Patients on long-term aspirin therapy for coronary or cerebrovascular pathology should *not* discontinue drug in perioperative period unless hemorrhagic complications of procedure outweigh risk of acute thrombotic event
	Thienopyridines Ticlopidine Clopidogrel	Inhibition of platelet aggregation Inhibition of platelet ADP–induced amplification	Synergistic antithrombotic effect with aspirin	Discontinue ticlopidine 2 wk in advance; discontinue clopidogrel 7–10 days in advance Patients with coronary artery stents must receive aspirin plus ticlopidine for 2–4 wk after angioplasty; stopping therapy considerably increases risk of coronary thrombosis; elective surgery should be delayed for 1–3 mo
	Antiglycoprotein agents Eptifibatide Tirofiban Abciximab	Competitive inhibition of GPIIb/IIIa receptors to prevent platelet aggregation Rapid onset of action Short half-lives Often combined with aspirin and/or heparin	Literature (mainly from cardiac surgery) shows increased hemorrhagic risk if surgery undertaken < 12 hr after discontinuance of abciximab Individual variability in recovery time of platelet function	Discontinue at least 12 hr in advance Transfuse platelets only if needed to correct clinically significant bleeding

(continued)

Premedication to produce anxiolysis, sedation, analgesia, amnesia, and reduction of PONV and aspiration may be considered for patients undergoing outpatient procedures, as it may for those undergoing inpatient procedures. Such premedication should not delay discharge. Fasting guidelines [*see Table 3*] and intraoperative monitoring standards for ambulatory surgery are identical to those for inpatient procedures [*see Patient Monitoring, below*].

A number of currently used anesthetics (e.g., propofol and desflurane), narcotics (e.g., alfentanil, fentanyl, sufentanil, and remifentanil), and muscle relaxants (e.g., atracurium, mivacurium, and rocuronium) demonstrate rapid recovery profiles. Nitrous oxide also has desirable pharmacokinetic properties, but it may be associated with increased PONV. Titration of anesthetics to indices of CNS activity (e.g., the bispectral index) may result in decreased drug dosages, faster recovery from anesthesia, and fewer complications.[7,8] Use of a laryngeal mask airway (LMA) rather than an endotracheal tube is ideal in the outpatient setting because lower doses of induction agent are required to blunt the hypertension and tachycardia associated with its insertion; in addition, it is associated with a decreased incidence of sore throat and does not require muscle paralysis for insertion. On the other hand, an LMA may not protect as well against aspiration.[5,9,10]

The benefits of regional anesthesia [*see Regional Anesthesia Techniques, below*] may include decreases in the incidence of aspiration, nausea, dizziness, and disorientation. Spinal and epidural anesthesia may be associated with PDPH and backache. Compared with spinal anesthesia, epidural anesthesia takes more time to perform, has a slower onset of action, and may not produce as profound a block; however, the duration of an epidural block can readily be extended intraoperatively or postoperatively if necessary. Care should be exercised in choosing a local anesthetic for neuraxial blockade: spinal lidocaine may be associated with a transient radicular irritation; bupivacaine may be associated with prolonged motor block; and narcotics may produce pruritus, urinary retention, nausea and vomiting, and respiratory depression. Various dosing regimens have been proposed to minimize these side effects.[11-14]

Monitored anesthesia care [*see Choice of Anesthesia, below*] achieves minimal CNS depression, so that the airway and sponta-

Table 1 (*continued*)

Type of Drug	Agent	Pharmacologic Effects	Adverse Effects	Discontinuance Recommendations
Herbal medicines	Garlic (*Allium sativum*)	Irreversible dose-dependent inhibition of platelet aggregation	Increased bleeding May potentiate other platelet inhibitors	Discontinue at least 7 days in advance
	Ginkgo (*Ginkgo biloba*)	Inhibition of platelet-activating factor Modulation of neurotransmitter receptor activity	Increased bleeding May potentiate other platelet inhibitors	Discontinue at least 36 hr in advance
	Ginger (*Zingiber officinale*)	Potent inhibitor of thromboxane synthase	Increased bleeding May potentiate effects of other anticoagulants	Discontinue at least 36 hr in advance
	Ginseng (*Panax ginseng*)	Inhibition of platelet aggregation, possibly irreversibly Antioxidant action Antihyperglycemic action "Steroid hormone"–like activity	Prolonged PT and PTT Hypoglycemia Reduced anticoagulation effect of warfarin Possible additive effect with other stimulants, with resultant hypertension and tachycardia	Discontinue at least 7 days in advance
	Ephedra/ma huang (*Ephedra sinica*)	Noncatecholamine sympatho-mimetic agent with α_1, β_1, and β_2 activity; both direct and indirect release of endogenous catecholamines	Dose-dependent increase in HR and BP, with potential for serious cardiac and CNS complications Possible adverse drug reactions: MAOIs (life-threatening hypertension, hyper-pyrexia, coma), oxytocin (hypertension), digoxin and volatile anesthetics (dysrhythmias), guanethedine (hypertension, tachycardia)	Discontinue at least 24 hr in advance
	Echinacea (*Echinacea purpurea*)	Immunostimulatory effect	Hepatotoxicity Allergic potential	Discontinue as far in advance as possible in any patient with hepatic dysfunction or surgery with possible hepatic blood flow compromise
	Licorice (*Glycyrrhiza glabra*)		Hypertension Hypokalemia Edema Contraindicated in chronic liver and renal insufficiency	
	Kava (*Piper methysticum*)	Dose-dependent potentiation of GABA-inhibitory neurotransmitter with sedative, anxiolytic, and antiepileptic effects	Potentiation of sedative anesthetics, including barbiturates and benzodi-azepines Possible potentiation of ethanol effects	
	Valerian (*Valeriana officinalis*)	Dose-dependent modulation of GABA neurotransmitter and receptor function	Possible potentiation of sedative anesthetics, including barbiturates and benzodiazepines	Discontinue at least 24 hr in advance
	St. John's wort (*Hypericum perforatum*)	Inhibits reuptake of serotonin, norepinephrine, and dopamine by neurons Increases metabolism of some P-450 isoforms	Possible interaction with MAOIs Evidence for reduced activity of cyclosporine, warfarin, calcium chan-nel blockers, lidocaine, midazolam, alfentanil, and NSAIDs	Discontinue on day of surgery; abrupt with-drawal in physically dependent patients may produce benzodiazepine-like with-drawal syndrome

ADP—adenosine diphosphate ETOH—ethyl alcohol GP—glycoprotein GABA—γ-aminobutyric acid MAOIs—monoamine oxidase inhibitors NSAIDs—nonsteroidal anti-inflammatory drugs
PT—prothrombin time PTT—partial thromboplastin time

neous ventilation are maintained and the patient is able to respond to verbal commands. Meticulous attention to monitoring is required to guard against airway obstruction, arterial desaturation, and pulmonary aspiration.

In the recovery room, the anesthetic plan is continued until discharge. Shorter-acting narcotics and NSAIDs are administered for pain relief, and any of several agents may be given for control of nausea and vomiting. Criteria for discharge from the recovery room have been established [*see Table 4*]. Recovery of normal muscle strength and sensation (including proprioception of the lower extremity, autonomic function, and ability to void) should be demonstrated after spinal or epidural anesthesia. Delays in discharge are usually the result of pain, PONV, hypotension, dizziness, unsteady gait, or lack of an escort.[15]

Elective versus Emergency Surgery

Surgical procedures performed on an emergency basis may range from relatively low priority (e.g., a previously cancelled case that was originally elective) to highly urgent (e.g., a case of impending airway obstruction). For trauma, specific evaluation and resuscitation sequences have been established to facilitate patient management [*see 5:1 Trauma Resuscitation*]. The urgency of the situation dictates how much time can be allotted to pre-operative patient assessment and optimization. When it is not possible to communicate with the patient, information obtained from family members and paramedics may be crucial. Information should be sought concerning allergies, current medications, significant past medical illnesses, nihil per os (NPO) status, personal or family problems with anesthesia, and recent ingestion

Table 2 Association between Preexisting Medical Conditions and Adverse Outcomes[65]

Medical Condition	Associated Adverse Outcome
Congestive heart failure	12% prolongation of postoperative stay
Hypertension	Twofold increase in risk of intraoperative cardiovascular events
Asthma	Fivefold increase in risk of postoperative respiratory events
Smoking	Fourfold increase in risk of postoperative respiratory events
Obesity	Fourfold increase in risk of intraoperative and postoperative respiratory events
Reflux	Eightfold increase in risk of intubation-related adverse events

of alcohol or drugs. Any factor that may complicate airway management should be noted (e.g., trauma to the face or the neck, a beard, a short and thick neck, obesity, or a full stomach). When appropriate, blood samples should be obtained as soon as possible for typing and crossmatching, as well as routine blood chemistries and a complete blood count. Arrangements for postoperative ICU monitoring, if appropriate, should be instituted early.

Clear communication must be established between the surgical team and anesthesia personnel so that an appropriate anesthetic management plan can be formulated and any specialized equipment required can be mobilized in the OR. The induction of anesthesia may coincide with resuscitation. Accordingly, the surgical team must be immediately available to help with difficult I.V. access, emergency tracheostomy, and cardiopulmonary resuscitation. Patients in shock may not tolerate standard anesthetics, which characteristically blunt sympathetic outflow. The anesthetic dose must be judiciously titrated, and definitive surgical treatment must not be unduly delayed by attempts to "get a line."

Choice of Anesthesia

Anesthesia may be classified into three broad categories: (1) general anesthesia, (2) regional anesthesia, and (3) monitored anesthesia care. General anesthesia can be defined as a state of

Table 3 Fasting Recommendations* to Reduce Risk of Pulmonary Aspiration[66]

Ingested Material	Minimum Fasting Period† (hr)
Clear liquids‡	2
Breast milk	4
Infant formula	6
Nonhuman milk§	6
Light meal¶	8

*These recommendations apply to healthy patients undergoing elective procedures; they are not intended for women in labor. Following the guidelines does not guarantee complete gastric emptying.

†These fasting periods apply to all ages.

‡Examples of clear liquids include water, fruit juices without pulp, carbonated beverages, clear tea, and black coffee.

§Because nonhuman milk is similar to solids in gastric emptying time, amount ingested must be considered in determining appropriate fasting period.

¶A light meal typically consists of toast and clear liquids. Meals that include fried or fatty foods or meat may prolong gastric emptying time. Both amount and type of foods ingested must be considered in determining appropriate fasting period.

insensibility characterized by loss of consciousness, amnesia, analgesia, and muscle relaxation. This state may be achieved either with a single anesthetic or, in a more balanced fashion, with a combination of several drugs that specifically induce hypnosis, analgesia, amnesia, and paralysis.

There is, at present, no consensus as to which general anesthetic regimen best preserves organ function. General anesthesia is employed when contraindications to regional anesthesia are present or when regional anesthesia or monitored anesthesia care fails to provide adequate intraoperative analgesia. In addition, there are a few situations that specifically mandate general anesthesia and controlled ventilation: the need for abdominal muscle paralysis, lung isolation, and hyperventilation; the presence of serious cardiorespiratory instability; and the lack of sufficient time to perform regional anesthesia. Alternatives to general surgery should be considered for patients who are susceptible to malignant hyperthermia, for those in whom intubation is likely to prove difficult or the risk of aspiration is high, and for those with pulmonary compromise that may worsen after intubation and positive pressure ventilation.

Regional anesthesia is achieved by interfering with afferent or efferent neural signaling at the level either of the spinal cord (neuraxial blockade) or of the peripheral nerves. Neuraxial anesthesia (i.e., epidural or spinal administration of local anesthetics) is commonly employed as the sole anesthetic technique for procedures involving the lower abdomen and the lower extremities; it also provides effective pain relief after intraperitoneal and intrathoracic procedures. Combining regional and general anesthesia has become increasingly popular.[16] Currently, some physicians are using neuraxial blockade as the sole anesthetic technique for procedures such as thoracotomy and coronary artery bypass grafting, which are traditionally thought to require general anesthesia and endotracheal intubation.[17]

Neuraxial blockade has several advantages over general anesthesia, including better dynamic pain control, shorter duration of paralytic ileus, reduced risk of pulmonary complications, and decreased transfusion requirements; it is also associated with a decreased incidence of renal failure and myocardial infarction [*see 1:5 Postoperative Pain*].[18-21] Contrary to conventional thinking, however, the type of anesthesia used (general or neuraxial) is not an independent risk factor for long-term cognitive dysfunction.[22] Neuraxial blockade is an essential component of multimodal rehabilitation programs aimed at optimization of perioperative care and acceleration of recovery.[23,24]

For short, superficial procedures, a wide variety of peripheral nerve blocks may be considered.[25] For procedures on the upper or lower extremity, an I.V. regional (Bier) block with diluted lidocaine is often useful. Anesthesia of the upper extremity and shoulder may be achieved with brachial plexus blocks. Anesthesia of the lower extremity may be achieved by blocking the femoral, obturator, and lateral femoral cutaneous nerves (for knee surgery) or the ankle and popliteal sciatic nerves (for foot surgery). Anesthesia of the thorax may be achieved with intercostal or intrapleural nerve blocks. Anesthesia of the abdomen may be achieved with celiac plexus and paravertebral blocks. Anesthesia of the head and neck may be achieved by blocking the trigeminal, supraorbital, supratrochlear, infraorbital, and mental nerves and the cervical plexus. Local infiltration of the operative site may provide intraoperative as well as postoperative analgesia.

Unlike the data on neuraxial blockade, the data on peripheral nerve blockade neither support nor discourage its use as a substitute for general anesthesia. Generally, however, we favor regional techniques when appropriate: such approaches maintain consciousness

Table 4 Postanesthetic Discharge
Scoring System (PADSS)[67]

Category	Score*	Explanation
Vital signs	2	Within 20% of preoperative value
	1	Within 20% to 40% of preoperative value
	0	Within 40% of preoperative value
Activity, mental status	2	Oriented and steady gait
	1	Oriented or steady gait
	0	Neither
Pain, nausea, vomiting	2	Minimal
	1	Moderate
	0	Severe
Surgical bleeding	2	Minimal
	1	Moderate
	0	Severe
Intake/output	2	Oral fluid intake and voiding
	1	Oral fluid intake or voiding
	0	Neither

*Total possible score is 10; patients scoring ≥ 9 are considered fit for discharge home.

and spontaneous breathing while causing only minimal depression of the CNS and the cardiorespiratory system, and they yield improved pain control in the immediate postoperative period.

Monitored anesthesia care involves the use of I.V. drugs to reduce anxiety, provide analgesia, and alleviate the discomfort of immobilization. This approach may be combined with local infiltration analgesia provided by the surgeon. Monitored anesthesia care requires monitoring of vital signs and the presence of an anesthesiologist who is prepared to convert to general anesthesia if necessary. Its benefits are substantially similar to those of regional anesthesia. These benefits are lost when attempts are made to overcome surgical pain with excessive doses of sedatives and analgesics.

Patient Monitoring

Patient monitoring is central to the practice of anesthesia. A trained, experienced physician is the only truly indispensable monitor; mechanical and electronic monitors, though useful, are, at most, aids to vigilance. Wherever anesthesia is administered, the proper equipment for pulse oximetry, blood pressure measurement, electrocardiography, and capnography should be available. At each anesthesia workstation, equipment for measuring temperature, a peripheral nerve stimulator, a stethoscope, and appropriate lighting must be immediately available. A spirometer must be available without undue delay.

Additional monitoring may be indicated, depending on the patient's health, the type of procedure to be performed, and the characteristics of the practice setting. Cardiopulmonary monitoring, including measurement of systemic arterial, central venous, pulmonary arterial, and wedge pressures, is covered in detail elsewhere [see 6:4 Cardiopulmonary Monitoring]. Additional information about the cardiovascular system may be obtained by means of transesophageal echocardiography.[26] Practice guidelines for this modality have been developed.[27] It may be particularly useful in patients who are undergoing valvular repair or who have persistent severe hypotension of unknown etiology.

The effects of anesthesia and surgery on the CNS may be monitored by recording processed EEG activity, as in the bispectral

index or the Patient State Index. These indices are used as measures of hypnosis to guide the administration of anesthetics.[28,29]

General Anesthesia Techniques

An ever-expanding armamentarium of drugs is available for premedication and for induction and maintenance of anesthesia. Selection of one agent over another is influenced by the patient's baseline condition, the procedure, and the predicted duration of hospitalization.

PREMEDICATION

Preoperative medications are given primarily to decrease anxiety, to reduce the incidence of nausea and vomiting, and to prevent aspiration. Other benefits include sedation, amnesia, analgesia, drying of oral secretions, and blunting of undesirable autonomic reflexes.

Sedatives and Analgesics

Benzodiazepines produce anxiolysis, sedation, hypnosis, amnesia, and muscle relaxation; they do not produce analgesia. They may be classified as short-acting (midazolam), intermediate-acting (lorazepam), or long-acting (diazepam). Adverse effects [see Table 5] may be marked in debilitated patients. Their central effects may be antagonized with flumazenil.

Muscarinic antagonists (e.g., scopolamine and atropine) were commonly administered at one time; this practice is not as popular today. They produce, to varying degrees, sedation, amnesia, lowered anesthetic requirements, diminished nausea and vomiting, reduced oral secretions, and decreased gastric hydrogen ion secretion. They blunt the cardiac parasympathetic reflex responses that may occur during certain procedures (e.g., ocular surgery, traction on the mesentery, and manipulation of the carotid body). Adverse effects include tachycardia, heat intolerance, inhibition of GI motility and micturition, and mydriasis.

Opioids are used when analgesia, in addition to sedation and anxiolysis, is required. With morphine and meperidine, the time of onset of action and the peak effect are unpredictable. Fentanyl has a rapid onset and a predictable time course, which make it more suitable for premedication immediately before operation. Adverse effects [see Table 6] can be reversed with full (naloxone) or partial (e.g., nalbuphine) antagonists.

The α_2-adrenergic agonists clonidine and dexmedetomidine are sympatholytic drugs that also exert sedative, anxiolytic, and analgesic effects. They reduce intraoperative anesthetic requirements, thus allowing faster recovery, and attenuate sympathetic activation

Table 5 Benzodiazepines: Doses
and Duration of Action[68]

Benzodiazepine	Dose (for Sedation)	Elimination Half-life	Comments
Midazolam	0.5–1.0 mg, repeated	1.7–2.6 hr	Respiratory depression, excessive sedation, hypotension, bradycardia, withdrawal Anticonvulsant activity
Lorazepam	0.25 mg, repeated	11–22 hr	See midazolam Venous thrombosis
Diazepam	2.0 mg, repeated	20–50 hr	See midazolam and lorazepam

Table 6 Opioids: Doses and Duration of Action[69]

Agent	Relative Analgesic Potency	Dose		Time to Peak Effect	Duration of Action	Comments
		Induction	Maintenance			
Morphine	1	1 mg/kg	For perioperative analgesia: 0.1 mg/kg I.V., I.M.	5–20 min	2–7 hr	Respiratory depression, nausea, vomiting, pruritus, constipation, urinary retention, biliary spasm, neuroexcitation ± seizure, tolerance Cough suppression, relief of dyspnea-induced anxiety (common to all opioids) Histamine release, orthostatic hypotension, prolonged emergence
Meperidine	0.1	NA	For perioperative analgesia: 0.5–1.5 mg/kg I.V., I.M., s.c.	2 hr (oral); 1 hr (s.c., I.M.)	2–4 hr	See morphine Orthostatic hypotension, myocardial depression, dry mouth, mild tachycardia, mydriasis, histamine release Attenuates shivering; to be avoided with MAOIs Local anesthetic–like effect
Remifentanil	250–300	1 µg/kg	0.25–0.4 µg/kg/min	3–5 min	5–10 min	See morphine Awareness, bradycardia, muscle rigidity Ideal for infusion; fast recovery, no postoperative analgesia
Alfentanil	7.5–25	50–300 µg/kg	1.25–8.0 µg/kg/min	1–2 min	10–15 min	See morphine Awareness, bradycardia, muscle rigidity
Fentanyl	75–125	5–30 µg/kg	0.25–0.5 µg/kg/min	5–15 min	30–60 min	See morphine and alfentanil
Sufentanil	525–625	2–20 µg/kg	0.05–0.1 µg/kg/min	3–5 min	20–45 min	See morphine and alfentanil Ideal for prolonged infusion

secondary to intubation and surgery, thus improving intraoperative hemodynamic stability. Major drawbacks are hypotension and bradycardia; rebound hypertensive crises may be precipitated by their discontinuance.[30,31]

Prevention of Aspiration

Aspiration of gastric contents is an extremely serious complication that is associated with significant morbidity and mortality. Fasting helps reduce the risk of this complication [see Table 3]. When the likelihood of aspiration is high, pharmacologic treatment may be helpful [see Table 7]. H_2 receptor antagonists (e.g., cimetidine, ranitidine, and famotidine) and proton pump inhibitors (e.g., omeprazole) reduce gastric acid secretion, thereby raising gastric pH without affecting gastric volume or emptying time. Nonparticulate antacids (e.g., sodium citrate) neutralize the acidity of gastric contents. Metoclopramide promotes gastric emptying (by stimulating propulsive GI motility) and decreases reflux

(by increasing the tone of the esophagogastric sphincter); it may also possess antiemetic properties.

In all patients at risk for aspiration who require general anesthesia, a rapid sequence induction is essential. This is achieved through adequate preoxygenation, administration of drugs to produce rapid loss of consciousness and paralysis, and exertion of pressure on the cricoid cartilage (the Sellick maneuver) as loss of consciousness occurs to occlude the esophagus and so limit reflux of gastric contents into the pharynx. An alternative is the so-called modified rapid sequence induction, which permits gentle mask ventilation during the application of cricoid pressure (thereby potentially reducing or abolishing insufflation of gas into the stomach). The advantages of the modified approach are that there is less risk of hypoxia and that there is more time to treat cardiovascular responses to induction agents before intubation. Regardless of which technique is used, consideration should be given to emptying the stomach via an orogastric or nasogastric tube before induction.

Table 7 Pharmacologic Prevention of Aspiration[70,71]

Agent	Dose	Timing of Administration before Operation	Comments
H_2 receptor antagonists		1–3 hr	
Cimetidine	300 mg, p.o.		Hypotension, bradycardia, heart block, increased airway resistance, CNS dysfunction, reduced hepatic metabolism of certain drugs
Ranitidine	50 mg I.V.		Bradycardia
Famotidine	20 mg I.V.		Rare CNS dysfunction
Sodium citrate	30 ml p.o.	20–30 min	Increased gastric fluid volume
Omeprazole	40 mg I.V.	40 min	Possible alteration of GI drug absorption, hepatic metabolism
Metoclopramide	10 mg I.V.	15–30 min	Extrapyramidal reactions, agitation, restlessness (large doses); to be avoided with MAOIs, pheochromocytoma, bowel obstruction

Table 8 Induction Agents: Doses and Duration of Action[68]

Agent	Induction Dose	Time to Peak Effect (sec)	Duration of Action (min)	Comments
Propofol	1.0–2.5 mg/kg	90–100	5–10	Hypotension, apnea, antiemetic (low dose), sexual fantasies and hallucinations, convulsions ± seizures (rare), pain on injection, thrombophlebitis
Thiopental	2.5–4.5 mg/kg	60	5–8	Hypotension, apnea, emergence delirium, prolonged somnolence, anaphylactoid reaction, injection pain, hyperalgesia Anticonvulsant effect Contraindicated with porphyria
Ketamine	0.5–2 mg/kg	30	10–15	Analgesia; increased BP, HR, CO; lacrimation and salivation; bronchial dilatation; elevated ICP Dreaming, illusions, excitement Preservation of respiration (apnea possible with high doses)
Etomidate	0.2–0.6 mg/kg	60	4–10	Minor effects on BP, HR, CO Adrenocortical suppression, injection pain and thrombophlebitis, myoclonus, nausea and vomiting

CO—cardiac output

INDUCTION

Induction of general anesthesia is produced by administering drugs to render the patient unconscious and secure the airway. It is one of the most crucial and potentially dangerous moments for the patient during general anesthesia. Various agents can be used for this purpose; the choice depends on the patient's baseline medical condition and fasting status, the state of the airway, the surgical procedure, and the expected length of the hospital stay. The agents most commonly employed for induction are propofol, sodium thiopental, ketamine, and etomidate [*see Table 8*]. The opioids alfentanil, fentanyl, sufentanil, and remifentanil are also used for this purpose; they are associated with a very stable hemodynamic profile during induction and operation [*see Table 6*].

Volatile agents [*see Table 9*] may be employed for induction of general anesthesia when maintenance of spontaneous ventilation is of paramount importance (e.g., with a difficult airway) or when bronchodilation is required (e.g., with severe hyperreactive airway disease). Inhalation induction is also popular for ambulatory surgery when paralysis is not required. Sevoflurane is well suited for this application because it is not irritating on inhalation, as most other volatile agents are, and it produces rapid loss of consciousness. Sevoflurane has mostly replaced halothane as the agent of choice for inhalation induction because it is less likely to cause dysrhythmias and is not hepatotoxic.

MAINTENANCE

Balanced general anesthesia is produced with a variety of drugs to maintain unconsciousness, prevent recall, and provide analgesia. Various combinations of volatile and I.V. agents may be employed to achieve these goals. The volatile agents isoflurane, desflurane, and sevoflurane are commonly used for maintenance [*see Table 9*]. Nitrous oxide is a strong analgesic and a weak anesthetic agent that possesses favorable pharmacokinetic properties. It cannot be used as the sole anesthetic agent unless it is administered in a hyperbaric chamber; it is usually administered with at least 30% oxygen to prevent hypoxia. Nitrous oxide is commonly used in combination with other volatile agents. All of the volatile agents can trigger malignant hyperthermia in susceptible patients.

The I.V. drugs currently used to maintain general anesthesia, whether partially or entirely, feature a short context-sensitive elimination half-life; thus, pharmacologically significant drug accumulation during prolonged infusion is avoided. Such agents (including propofol, midazolam, sufentanil, and remifentanil) are typically administered via computer-controlled infusion pumps that use population-based pharmacokinetic data to establish stable plasma (and CNS effector site) concentrations. Because of the extremely rapid hydrolysis of remifentanil, its administration may be labor intensive, necessitating frequent administration of boluses and constant vigilance. Its short half-life also limits its usefulness as an

Table 9 Volatile Drugs[72,73]

Agent	Oil/Gas Coefficient*	MAC† (atm)	Blood/Gas Coefficient‡	Rank Order (F_A/F_I)§
Halothane	224	0.0074	2.5	6
Enflurane	96.5	0.0168	1.8	5
Isoflurane	90.8	0.0115	1.4	4
Desflurane	18.7	0.060	0.45	2
Sevoflurane	47.2	0.0236	0.65	3
Nitrous oxide	1.4	1.04	0.47	1

*Lipid solubility correlates closely with anesthetic potency (Meyer-Overton rule).
†Correlates closely with lipid solubility.
‡Relative affinity of an anesthetic for blood compared to gas at equilibrium. The larger the coefficient, the greater the affinity of the drug for blood and hence the greater the quantity of drug contained in the blood.
§Rise in alveolar anesthetic concentration towards the inspired concentration is most rapid with the least soluble drugs and slowest with the most soluble.
F_A/F_I—alveolar concentration of gas/inspired concentration   MAC—minimum alveolar concentration to abolish purposeful movement in response to noxious stimulation in 50% of patients

Table 10 Neuromuscular Blocking Agents: Doses and Duration of Action[74]

Agent	Dose (mg/kg)	Duration of Action[1] (min)	Metabolism	Elimination	Comments
Succinylcholine chloride	0.7–2.5	5–10	Plasma cholinesterase	Renal < 2%, hepatic 0%	Fasciculations, elevation of serum potassium, increased ICP, bradycardia, MH trigger; prolonged effect in presence of atypical pseudocholinesterase
Pancuronium	0.04–0.1	60–120	Hepatic 10%–20%	Renal 85%, hepatic 15%	Muscarinic antagonist (vagolytic), prolonged paralysis (long-term use)
Rocuronium	0.6–1.2	35–75	None	Renal < 10%, hepatic > 70%	Minimal histamine release
Vecuronium	0.08–0.1	45–90	Hepatic 30%–40%	Renal 40%, hepatic 60%	Prolonged paralysis (long-term use)
Atracurium	0.3–0.5	30–45	Hoffman elimination, nonspecific ester hydrolysis	Renal 10%–40%, hepatic 0%	Histamine release; laudanosine metabolite (a CNS stimulant)
Cisatracurium	0.15–0.2	40–75	Hoffman elimination	Renal 16%, hepatic 0%	Negligible histamine release; laudanosine metabolite
Mivacurium	0.15–0.2	15–20	Plasma cholinesterase	Renal < 5%, hepatic 0%	Histamine release; prolonged effect in presence of atypical pseudocholinesterase

analgesic in the postoperative period. To circumvent this problem, various dosing regimens have been proposed in which the patient is switched from remifentanil to a longer-acting narcotic.

NEUROMUSCULAR BLOCKADE

The reversible paralysis produced by neuromuscular blockade improves conditions for endotracheal intubation and facilitates surgery. Neuromuscular blocking agents are classified as either depolarizing (succinylcholine) or nondepolarizing (pancuronium, rocuronium, vecuronium, atracurium, cisatracurium, and mivacurium) and may be further differentiated on the basis of chemical structure and duration of action [*see Table 10*]. The blocking effect of nondepolarizing muscle relaxants is enhanced by volatile drugs, hypothermia, acidosis, certain antibiotics, magnesium sulfate, and local anesthetics and is reduced by phenytoin and carbamazepine. Patients with weakness secondary to neuromuscular disorders (e.g., myasthenia gravis and Eaton-Lambert syndrome) may be particularly sensitive to nondepolarizing muscle relaxants.

EMERGENCE

General anesthesia is terminated by cessation of drug administration, reversal of paralysis, and extubation. During this period, close scrutiny of the patient is essential, and all OR personnel must coordinate their efforts to help ensure a smooth and safe emergence. In this phase, patients may demonstrate hemodynamic instability, retching and vomiting, respiratory compromise, and, occasionally, uncooperative or aggressive behavior.

Reversal of neuromuscular blockade is achieved by administering anticholinesterases such as neostigmine and edrophonium. These drugs should be given in conjunction with a muscarinic antagonist (atropine or glycopyrrolate) to block their unwanted parasympathomimetic side effects. Neostigmine is more potent than edrophonium in reversing profound neuromuscular blockade. It is imperative that paralysis be sufficiently reversed before extubation to ensure that spontaneous respiration is adequate and that the airway can be protected. Reversal can be clinically verified by confirming the patient's ability to lift the head for 5 seconds. Reversal can also be assessed by measuring muscle contraction in response to electrical nerve stimulation.

Causes of failure to emerge from anesthesia include residual neuromuscular blockade, a benzodiazepine or opioid overdose, the central anticholinergic syndrome, an intraoperative cerebrovascular accident, preexisting pathophysiologic conditions (e.g., CNS disorders, hepatic insufficiency, and drug or alcohol ingestion), electrolyte abnormalities, acidosis, hypercarbia, hypoxia, hypothermia, and hypothyroidism. As noted, the effects of narcotics and benzodiazepines can be reversed with naloxone and flumazenil, respectively. Physostigmine may be given to reverse the reduction in consciousness level produced by general anesthetics. Electrolyte, glucose, blood urea nitrogen, and creatinine levels should be measured; liver and thyroid function tests should be performed; and arterial blood gas values should be obtained. Patients should be normothermic. Unexplained failure to emerge from general anesthesia warrants immediate consultation with a neurologist.

Regional Anesthesia Techniques

Neuraxial (central) anesthesia techniques involve continuous or intermittent injection of drugs into the epidural or intrathecal space to produce sensory analgesia, motor blockade, and inhibition of sympathetic outflow. Peripheral nerve blockade involves inhibition of conduction in fibers of a single peripheral nerve or plexus (cervical, brachial, or lumbar) in the periphery. Intravenous regional anesthesia involves I.V. administration of a local anesthetic into a tourniquet-occluded extremity. Perioperative pain control may be facilitated by administering local anesthetics, either infiltrated into the wound or sprayed into the wound cavity.[32,33] Procedures performed solely under infiltration may be associated with patient dissatisfaction caused by intraoperative anxiety and pain.[34]

CONTRAINDICATIONS

Strong contraindications to regional (particularly neuraxial) anesthesia include patient refusal or inability to cooperate during the procedure, elevated intracranial pressure, anticoagulation, vascular malformation or infection at the needle insertion site, severe hemodynamic instability, and sepsis. Preexisting neurologic disease is a relative contraindication.

ANTICOAGULATION AND BLEEDING RISK

Although hemorrhagic complications can occur after any regional technique, bleeding associated with neuraxial blockade is the most serious because of its devastating consequences. Spinal hematoma may occur as a result of vascular trauma from placement of a needle or catheter into the subarachnoid or epidural

Table 11 Pharmacology of Anticoagulant Agents

Drug	Coagulation Tests		Time to Peak Effect	Time to Normal Hemostasis after Discontinuance
	INR	PTT		
Heparin				
I.V.	⇔	⇑	min	4–6 hr
s.c.	⇔	↑	1 hr	4–6 hr
LMWH	⇔	⇔	2–4 hr	12 hr
Warfarin	⇑	⇔	2–6 days	4–6 days
Aspirin	⇔	⇔	hr	5–8 days
Thrombolytic agents (t-PA, streptokinase)	⇔	⇑	min	1–2 days

⇑—clinically significant increase ↑—possibly clinically significant increase ⇔—clinically insignificant increase or no effect
LMWH—low-molecular-weight heparin t-PA—tissue plasminogen activator

space. Spinal hematoma may also occur spontaneously, even in the absence of antiplatelet or anticoagulant therapy. The actual incidence of spinal cord injury resulting from hemorrhagic complications is unknown; the reported incidence is estimated to be less than 1/150,000 for epidural anesthesia and 1/220,000 for spinal anesthesia.[35] With such low incidences, it is difficult to determine whether any increased risk can be attributed to anticoagulant use [see Table 11] without data from millions of patients, which are not currently available. Much of our clinical practice is based on small surveys and expert opinion.

Antiplatelet Agents

There is no universally accepted test that can guide antiplatelet therapy. Antiplatelet agents can be divided into four major classes: (1) aspirin and related cyclooxygenase inhibitors (nonsteroidal anti-inflammatory drugs, or NSAIDs); (2) ticlopidine and selective adenosine diphosphate antagonists; (3) direct thrombin inhibitors (e.g., hirudin); and (4) glycoprotein IIb/IIIa inhibitors. Only with aspirin is there sufficient experience to suggest that at clinical doses it does not increase the risk of spinal hematoma.[36] Caution should, however, be exercised when aspirin is used in conjunction with other anticoagulants.[37]

Oral Anticoagulants

Therapeutic anticoagulation with warfarin is a contraindication to regional anesthesia.[38] If regional anesthesia is planned, oral warfarin can be replaced with I.V. heparin (see below).

Heparin

There does not seem to be an increased risk of spinal bleeding in patients receiving subcutaneous low-dose (5,000 U) unfractionated heparin [see 4:6 Venous Thromboembolism] if the interval between administration of the drug and initiation of the procedure is greater than 4 hours.[39] Higher doses, however, are associated with increased risk. If neuraxial anesthesia or epidural catheter removal is planned, heparin infusion must be discontinued for at least 6 hours, and the partial thromboplastin time (PTT) should be measured. Recommendations for standard heparin cannot be extrapolated to low-molecular-weight heparin (LMWH), because the biologic actions of LMWH are different and the effects cannot be monitored by conventional coagulation measurements. After the release of LMWH for general use in the United States in 1993, more than 40 spinal hematomas were reported during a 5-year period. LMWH should be stopped at least 12 hours before regional blockade, and the first postoperative dose should be given no sooner than 4 hours afterward.[37]

COMPLICATIONS

Drug Toxicity

Systemic toxic reactions to local anesthetics primarily involve the CNS and the cardiovascular system [see Table 12]. The initial symptoms are light-headedness and dizziness, followed by visual and auditory disturbances. Convulsions and respiratory arrest may ensue and necessitate treatment and resuscitation.

Table 12 Local Anesthetics for Infiltration Anesthesia: Maximum Doses* and Duration of Action

Drug	Without Epinephrine		With Epinephrine (1:200,000)	
	Maximum Dose (mg)	Duration of Action (min)	Maximum Dose (mg)	Duration of Action (min)
Chloroprocaine	800	15–30	1000	3–90
Lidocaine	300	30–60	500	120–360
Mepivacaine	300	45–90	500	120–360
Prilocaine	500	30–90	600	120–360
Bupivacaine	175	120–240	225	180–420
Etidocaine	300	120–180	400	180–420

*Recommended maximum dose can be given to healthy, middle-aged, normal-sized adults without toxicity. Subsequent doses should not be given for at least 4 hr. Doses should be reduced during pregnancy.

Table 13 Pharmacologic Treatment of PONV[5]

Agent	Dose	Comments
Propofol	10 mg I.V., repeated dose	[See Table 8]
Ondansetron	4.0–8.0 mg I.V.	Highly effective, costly; headache, constipation, transiently increased LFTs
Dexamethasone	4.0–8.0 mg I.V.	Adrenocortical suppression, delayed wound healing, fluid retention, electrolyte disturbances, psychosis, osteoporosis
Droperidol	0.5–1.0 mg I.V.	Sedation, restlessness, dysphoria, ?dysrhythmia
Metoclopramide	10–20 mg I.V.	Avoid in bowel obstruction, extrapyramidal reactions
Scopolamine	0.1–0.6 mg s.c., I.M., I.V.	Muscarinic side effects, somnolence
Dimenhydrinate	25–50 mg I.V.	Drowsiness, dizziness

LFTs—liver function tests

The use of neuraxial analgesic adjuncts (e.g., opioids, clonidine, epinephrine, and neostigmine) decreases the dose of local anesthetic required, speeds recovery, and improves the quality of analgesia. The side effects of such adjuncts include respiratory depression (with morphine), tachycardia (with epinephrine), hypotension (with clonidine), and nausea and vomiting (with neostigmine and morphine).

Neurologic Complications

The incidence of neurologic complications ranges from 2/10,000 to 12/10,000 with epidural anesthesia and from 0.3/10,000 to 70/10,000 with spinal anesthesia.[40] The most common serious complication is neuropathy, followed by cranial nerve palsy, epidural abscess, epidural hematoma, anterior spinal artery syndrome, and cranial subdural hematoma. Vigilance and routine neurologic testing of sensory and motor function are of paramount importance for early detection and treatment of these potentially disastrous complications.

Transient neurologic symptoms The term transient neurologic symptoms (TNS) refers to backache with pain radiating into the buttocks or the lower extremities after spinal anesthesia. It occurs in 4% to 33% of patients, typically 12 to 36 hours after the resolution of spinal anesthesia, and lasts for 2 to 3 days.[41] TNS has been described after intrathecal use of all local anesthetics but is most commonly noted after administration of lidocaine, in the ambulatory surgical setting, and with the patient in the lithotomy position during operation. Discomfort from TNS is self-limited and can be effectively treated with NSAIDs.

Postdural Puncture Headache

Use of small-gauge pencil-point needles for spinal anesthesia is associated with a 1% incidence of PDPH. The incidence of PDPH after epidural analgesia varies substantially because the risk of inadvertent dural puncture with a Tuohy needle is directly dependent on the anesthesiologist's training. PDPH is characteristically aggravated by upright posture and may be associated with photophobia, neck stiffness, nausea, diplopia, and tinnitus. Meningitis should be considered in the differential diagnosis. Although PDPH is not life-threatening, it carries substantial morbidity in the form of restricted activity. Medical treatment with bed rest, I.V. fluids, NSAIDs, and caffeine is only moderately effective. An epidural blood patch is the treatment of choice: the success rate is approximately 70%.

Recovery

Admission to the postanesthetic care unit (PACU) is appropriate for patients whose vital signs are stable and whose pain is adequately controlled after emergence from anesthesia. Patients requiring hemodynamic or respiratory support may be admitted to the PACU if rapid improvement is expected and appropriate monitoring and personnel are available. Hemodynamic instability, the need for prolonged respiratory support, and poor baseline condition mandate admission to the ICU. Common complications encountered in the PACU include postoperative pulmonary insufficiency, cardiovascular instability, acute pain, and nausea and vomiting [*see Table 13*]. These complications are discussed in greater detail elsewhere [*see 6:5 Pulmonary Insufficiency, 6:2 Acute Dysrhythmia, and 1:5 Postoperative Pain*].

Special Scenarios

DIFFICULT AIRWAY

Airway management is a pivotal component of patient care because failure to maintain airway patency can lead to permanent disability, brain injury, or death. The difficult airway should be managed in accordance with contemporary airway guidelines, such as the protocols established by the ASA, to reduce the risk of adverse outcomes during attempts at ventilation and intubation. (The ASA protocols may be accessed on the organization's Web site: http://www.asahq.org/publicationsandservices/difficult%20airway.pdf.) The emphasis on preserving spontaneous ventilation and the focus on awake intubation options are central themes whose importance cannot be overemphasized.

It is crucial that all patients who are undergoing difficult or prolonged airway instrumentation be appropriately treated with topical anesthesia, sedation, and monitoring so as to ensure adequate ventilation and to attenuate, detect, and treat harmful neuroendocrine responses that can cause myocardial ischemia, bronchospasm, and intracranial hypertension. Extubation is stressful as well and may be associated with intense mucosal stimulation and exaggerated glottic closure reflexes resulting in laryngospasm and, possibly, pulmonary edema secondary to vigorous inspiratory efforts against an obstructed airway. Laryngeal incompetence and aspiration can also occur after extubation. Removal of an endotracheal tube from a known or suspected difficult airway should ideally be performed over a tube exchanger so as to facilitate emergency reintubation.

Alternatives to standard oral airways, masks, introducers, exchangers, laryngoscopes, and endotracheal tubes now exist that offer more options, greater safety, and better outcomes. It would be naive to believe that any single practitioner could master every new airway protocol and device. To keep up with technical and procedural advances, university hospital program directors should consider incorporating technical skill laboratories and simulator training sessions into their curricula.

MORBID OBESITY

Morbid obesity represents the extreme end of the overweight spectrum and is usually defined as a body-mass index higher than 40 kg/m² [see 3:3 Morbid Obesity].[42] It poses a formidable challenge to health care providers in the OR, the postoperative recovery ward, and the ICU. The major concerns in the surgical setting are the possibility of a difficult airway, the increased risk of known or occult cardiorespiratory compromise, and various serious technical problems related to positioning, monitoring, vascular access, and transport. Additional concerns are the potential for underlying hepatic and endocrine disease and the effects of altered drug pharmacokinetics and pharmacodynamics. For the morbidly obese patient, there is no such thing as minor surgery.

Initial management should be based on the assumptions that (1) a difficult airway is likely, (2) the patient will be predisposed to hiatal hernia, reflux, and aspiration, and (3) rapid arterial desaturation will occur with induction of anesthesia as a consequence of decreased functional residual capacity and high basal oxygen consumption. Often, the safest option is an awake fiberoptic intubation with appropriate topical anesthesia and light sedation.[43] In expert hands, this technique is extremely well tolerated and can usually be performed in less than 10 minutes. Morbidly obese patients often are hypoxemic at rest and have an abnormal alveolar-arterial oxygen gradient caused by ventilation-perfusion mismatching. The combination of general anesthesia and the supine position exacerbates alveolar collapse and airway closure. Mechanical ventilation, weaning, and extubation may be difficult and dangerous, especially in the presence of significant obstructive sleep apnea. Postoperative pulmonary complications (e.g., pneumonia, aspiration, atelectasis, and emboli) are common.

Morbid obesity imposes unusual loading conditions on both sides of the heart and the circulation, leading to the progressive development of insulin resistance, atherogenic dyslipidemias, systemic and pulmonary hypertension, ventricular hypertrophy, and a high risk of premature coronary artery disease and biventricular heart failure. Perioperative cardiac morbidity and mortality are therefore significant problems. Untoward events can happen suddenly, and resuscitation is extremely difficult. Cardiorespiratory compromise may be attenuated by effective postoperative pain control that permits early ambulation and effective ventilation. Surgical site infection and dehiscence may result in difficult reoperation and prolonged hospitalization.

MALIGNANT HYPERTHERMIA

Malignant hyperthermia (MH) is a rare but potentially fatal genetic condition characterized by life-threatening hypermetabolic reactions in susceptible individuals after the administration of volatile anesthetics or depolarizing muscle relaxants.[44] Abnormal function of the sarcoplasmic reticulum calcium release channel in skeletal muscle has been identified as a possible underlying cause.

In making the diagnosis of MH, it is important to consider other possible causes of postoperative temperature elevation. Such causes include inadequate anesthesia, equipment problems (e.g., misuse or malfunction of heating devices, ventilators, or breathing circuits), local or systemic inflammatory responses (either related or unrelated to infection), transfusion reaction, hypermetabolic endocrinopathy (e.g., thyroid storm or pheochromocytoma), neurologic catastrophe (e.g., intracranial hemorrhage), and reaction to or abuse of a drug.

Immediate recognition and treatment of a fulminant MH episode are essential for preventing morbidity and mortality. Therapy consists of discontinuing all triggers, instituting aggressive cooling measures, giving dantrolene in an initial dose of 2.5 mg/kg, and administering 100% oxygen to compensate for the tremendous increase in oxygen utilization and carbon dioxide production. An indwelling arterial line, central venous access, and bladder catheterization are indispensable for monitoring and resuscitation. Acidosis, hyperkalemia, and malignant dysrhythmias must be rapidly treated, with the caveat that calcium channel blockers are contraindicated in this setting. Maintenance of adequate urine output is of paramount importance and may be facilitated by the clinically significant amounts of mannitol contained in commercial dantrolene preparations. When the patient is stable and the surgical procedure is complete, monitoring and support are continued in the ICU, where repeat doses of dantrolene may be needed to prevent or treat recrudescence of the disease.

MASSIVE TRANSFUSION

Massive blood transfusion, defined as the replacement of a patient's entire circulating blood volume in less than 24 hours, is associated with significant morbidity and mortality. Management of massive transfusion requires an organized multidisciplinary team approach and a thorough understanding of associated hematologic and biochemical abnormalities and subsequent treatment options.

Patients suffering from shock as a result of massive blood loss often require transfusions of packed red blood cells, platelets, fresh frozen plasma, and cryoprecipitate to optimize oxygen-carrying capacity and address dilutional and consumptive loss of platelets and clotting factors [see 6:3 Shock and 1:4 Bleeding and Transfusion]. Transfusion of large amounts of blood products into a critically ill patient can lead to coagulopathies, hyperkalemia, acidosis, citrate intoxication, fluid overload, and hypothermia.[45] Therapy should be guided by vital signs, urine output, pulse oximetry, electrocardiography, capnography, invasive hemodynamic monitoring, serial arterial blood gases, biochemical profiles, and bedside coagulation screens. Fluids should be administered through large-bore cannulas connected to modern countercurrent warming devices. Shed blood should be salvaged and returned to the patient whenever possible. In refractory cases, transcatheter angiographic embolization techniques should be considered for control of bleeding.

Newer hemostatic agents, such as aprotinin and recombinant factor VIIa, should also be considered. Aprotinin is a serine protease inhibitor with unique antifibrinolytic and hemostatic properties. It is used during surgery to decrease blood loss and transfusion requirements as well as to attenuate potentially harmful inflammatory responses and minimize reperfusion injury. Recombinant factor VIIa was originally approved for hemophiliacs who developed antibodies against either factor VIII or factor IX; it may prove useful for managing uncontrolled hemorrhage deriving from trauma or surgery.

HYPOTHERMIA

Significant decreases in core temperature are common during anesthesia and surgery as a consequence of exposure to a cold OR environment and of disturbances in normal protective thermoregulatory responses. Patients lose heat through conduction, convection, radiation, and evaporation, especially from large wounds and during major intracavitary procedures. Moreover, effective vasoconstrictive reflexes and both shivering and nonshivering thermogenesis are severely blunted by anesthetics.[46] Neonates and the elderly are particularly vulnerable.

Hypothermia may confer some degree of organ preservation during ischemia and reperfusion. For example, in cardiac surgery, hypothermic cardiopulmonary bypass is a common strategy for protecting the myocardium and the CNS. Intentional hypothermia has also been shown to improve neurologic outcome and survival in comatose victims of cardiac arrest. Perioperative hypothermia can have significant deleterious effects as well, however, including myocardial ischemia, surgical site infection, increased blood loss and transfusion requirements, and prolonged anesthetic recovery and hospital stay.

The sensation of cold is highly uncomfortable for the patient, and shivering impedes monitoring, raises plasma catecholamine levels, and exacerbates imbalances between oxygen supply and demand by consuming valuable energy for involuntary muscular activity. It is therefore extremely important to measure the patient's temperature and maintain thermoneutrality. Increasing the ambient temperature of the OR and applying modern forced-air warming systems are the most effective techniques available. In addition, all I.V. and irrigation fluids should be heated. After the patient has been transferred from the OR, aggressive treatment of hypothermia with these techniques should be continued as necessary. Shivering may also be reduced by means of drugs such as meperidine, nefopam, tramadol, physostigmine, ketamine, methylphenidate, and doxapram.[47]

INTRAOPERATIVE AWARENESS

One of the goals of anesthesia is to produce a state of unconsciousness during which the patient neither perceives nor recalls noxious surgical stimuli. When this objective is not met, awareness occurs, and the patient will have explicit or implicit memory of intraoperative events. In some instances, intraoperative awareness develops because human error, machine malfunction, or technical problems result in an inappropriately light level of anesthesia. In others (e.g., when the patient is severely hemodynamically unstable or efforts are being made to avoid fetal depression during cesarean section), the light level of anesthesia may have been intentionally chosen. Regardless of the cause, intraoperative awareness is a terrifying experience for the patient and has been associated with serious long-term psychological sequelae.[48] Prevention of awareness depends on regular equipment maintenance, meticulous anesthetic technique, and close observation of the patient's movements and hemodynamic responses during operation. CNS monitoring may reduce the risk of intraoperative awareness.

ANAPHYLAXIS

Allergic reactions range in severity from mild pruritus and urticaria to anaphylactic shock and death. Inciting agents include antibiotics, contrast agents, blood products, volume expanders, protamine, aprotinin, narcotics, induction agents, muscle relaxants, latex,[49] and, rarely, local anesthetic solutions. Many drug additives and preservatives have also been implicated.

True anaphylaxis presents shortly after exposure to an allergen and is mediated by chemicals released from degranulated mast cells and basophils. Manifestations usually include dramatic hypotension, tachycardia, bronchospasm, arterial oxygen desaturation, and cutaneous changes. Laryngeal edema can occur within minutes, in which case the airway should be secured immediately. Anaphylaxis can mimic heart failure, asthma, pulmonary embolism, and tension pneumothorax. Treatment involves withdrawing the offending substance and administering oxygen, fluids, and epinephrine, followed by I.V. steroids, bronchodilators, and histamine antagonists. Prolonged intubation and ICU monitoring may be required until symptoms resolve. Appropriate skin and blood testing should be done to identify the causative agent.

PERIOPERATIVE DYSRHYTHMIAS

In 2000, current scientific developments in the treatment of stroke and coronary artery disease were merged with the evolving discipline of evidence-based medicine to produce the most comprehensive set of resuscitation standards ever created: a 12-part document from the American Heart Association entitled "Guidelines 2000 for Cardiopulmonary Resuscitation and Emergency Cardiovascular Care." This document addresses a wide array of key issues in both in-hospital and out-of-hospital resuscitation, including a recommendation for confirmation of tube position after endotracheal intubation and a warning about the danger associated with unintentional massive auto-PEEP.

As regards the impact the new guidelines have on management of dysrhythmias, the dominant role of amiodarone is undeniably the most visible and important development.[50] Amiodarone is a complex, powerful, and broad-spectrum agent that inhibits almost all of the drug receptors and ion channels conceivably responsible for the initiation and propagation of cardiac ectopy, irrespective of underlying ejection fraction, accessory pathway conduction, or anatomic substrate. It does, however, have potential drawbacks, such as its relatively long half-life, its toxicity to multiple organs, and its complicated administration scheme. Furthermore, amiodarone is a potent noncompetitive alpha and beta blocker, which has important implications for anesthetized, mechanically ventilated patients who may be debilitated and experiencing volume depletion, abnormal vasodilation, myocardial depression, and fluid, electrolyte, and acid-base abnormalities. That said, no other drug in its class has ever demonstrated a significant benefit in randomized trials addressing cardiac arrest in humans.

Amiodarone is effective in both children and adults, and it can be used for prophylaxis as well as treatment. The recommended cardiac arrest dose is a 300 mg I.V. bolus. In less acute situations, the initial 300 mg dose should be administered slowly over 15 to 20 minutes, and one or two additional boluses may be given similarly. A loading regimen is then initiated, first at 1 mg/min for 6 hours and then at 0.5 mg/min for 18 hours.

The inclusion of vasopressin (antidiuretic hormone) as an alternative to epinephrine in the revised ventricular tachycardia/ventricular fibrillation protocol represents another major change in drug therapy for advanced cardiac life support. Vasopressin is an integral component of the hypothalamic-pituitary-adrenal axis and the neuroendocrine stress response. The recommended dose for an adult in fibrillatory arrest is 40 units in a single bolus. For vasodilatory shock states associated with sepsis, hepatic failure, or vasomotor paralysis after cardiopulmonary bypass, infusion at a rate of 0.01 to 0.05 units/min may be particularly useful. Vasopressin is neither recommended nor forbidden in cases of pulseless electrical activity or asystolic arrest.

References

1. Clinical Anesthesia, 3rd ed. Barash PG, Cullen BF, Stoelting RK, Eds. Lippincott-Raven, Philadelphia, 2000

2. Anesthesia, 5th ed. Miller RD, Ed. Churchill Livingstone Inc, Philadelphia, 2000

3. Licker M, Neidhart P, Lustenberger S, et al: Long-term angiotensin-converting enzyme inhibitor attenuates adrenergic responsiveness without altering hemodynamic control in patients undergoing cardiac surgery. Anethesiology 84:789, 1996

4. Antiplatelet agents in the perioperative period: expert recommendations of the French Society of Anesthesiology and Intensive Care (SFAR) 2001—summary statement. Can J Anaesth 49:S26, 2002

5. Van Vlymen JM, White PF: Outpatient anesthesia. Anesthesia, 5th ed. Miller RD, Ed. Churchill Livingstone Inc, Philadelphia, 2000, p 2213

6. Dexter F, Macario A, Penning DH, et al: Development of an appropriate list of surgical procedures of a specified maximim anesthetic complexity to be performed at a new ambulatory surgery facility. Anesth Analg 95:78, 2002

7. Nelskyla KA, Yli-Hankala AM, Puro PH, et al: Sevoflurane titration using bispectral index decreases postoperative vomiting in phase II recovery after ambulatory surgery. Anesth Analg 93:1165, 2001

8. Song D, van Vlymen J, White PF: Is the bispectral index useful in predicting fast-track eligibility after ambulatory anesthesia with propofol and desflurane? Anesth Analg 87:1245, 1998

9. Brimacombe J, Brain AIJ, Berry A: The Laryngeal Mask Airway: Review and Practical Guide. WB Saunders Co, London, 1997

10. Joshi GP, Inagaki Y, White PF, et al: Use of the laryngeal mask airway as an alternative to the tracheal tube during ambulatory anesthesia. Anesth Analg 85:573, 1997

11. Tsen LC, Schultz R, Martin R, et al: Intrathecal low-dose bupivicaine versus lidocaine for in vitro fertilization procedures. Reg Anesth Pain Med 26:52, 2001

12. Frey K, Holman S, Mikat-Stevens M, et al: The recovery profile of hyperbaric spinal anesthesia with lidocaine, tetracaine, and bupivicaine. Reg Anesth Pain Med 23:159, 1998

13. Liguori GA, Zayas VM, Chisolm MF: Transient neurologic symptoms after spinal anesthesia with mepivacaine and lidocaine. Anesthesiology 88:619, 1998

14. Liu SS: Optimizing spinal anesthesia for ambulatory surgery. Reg Anesth 22:500, 1997

15. Chung F, Mezei G: Factors contributing to a prolonged stay after ambulatory surgery. Anesth Analg 89:1352, 1999

16. Kehlet H, Nolte K: Effect of postoperative analgesia on surgical outcome. Br J Anaesth 87:62, 2001

17. Kessler P, Neidhart G, Bremerich DH, et al: High thoracic epidural anesthesia for coronary artery bypass grafting using two different surgical approaches in conscious patients. Anesth Analg 95:791, 2002

18. Nolte K, Kehlet H: Postoperative ileus: a preventable event. Br J Surg 87:1480, 2000

19. Rodgers A, Walker N, Schug S, et al: Reduction of postoperative mortality and morbidity with epidural or spinal anaesthesia: results from overview of randomised trials. BMJ 321:1493, 2000

20. Beattie WS, Badner NH, Choi P: Epidural analgesia reduces postoperative myocardial infarction: a metaanalysis. Anesth Analg 93:853, 2001

21. Ballantyne JC, Carr DB, deFerranti S, et al: The comparative effects of postoperative analgesic therapies on pulmonary outcome: cumulative meta-analyses of randomized controlled trials. Anesth Analg 86:598, 1998

22. Moller JT, Cluitmans P, Houx P, et al: Long-term postoperative cognitive dysfunction in the elderly: ISPOCD1 study. Lancet 51:857, 1998

23. Kehlet H, Mogensen T: Hospital stay of 2 days after open sigmoidectomy with a multimodal rehabilitation programme. Br J Surg 86:227, 1999

24. Basse L, Jakobsen DH, Billesbolle P, et al: A clinical pathway to accelerate recovery after colonic resection. Ann Surg 232:51, 2000

25. Wedel DJ: Nerve blocks. Anesthesia, 5th ed. Miller RD, Ed. Churchill Livingstone Inc, Philadelphia, 2000, p 520

26. Cahalan MK: Transesophageal echocardiography. Anesthesia, 5th ed. Miller RD, Ed. Churchill Livingstone Inc, Philadelphia, 2000, p 1207

27. Practice Guidelines for Perioperative Transesophageal Echocardiography: a report by the American Society of Anesthesiologists and the Society of Cardiovascular Anesthesiologists Task Force on Transesophageal Echocardiography. Anesthesiology 84:986, 1996

28. Lehmann A, Boldt J, Thaler E, et al: Bispectral index in patients with target-controlled or manually controlled infusion of propofol. Anesth Analg 95:639, 2002

29. Drover DR, Lemmens HJ, Pierce ET, et al: Patient state index: titration of delivery and recovery from propofol, alfentanil and nitrous oxide anesthesia. Anesthesiology 97:82, 2002

30. Maze M, Tranquilli W: Alpha-2 adrenoceptor agonists: defining the role in clinical anesthesia. Anesthesiology 74:581, 1991

31. Peden CJ, Prys-Roberts C: Dexmedetomidine: a powerful new adjunct to anaesthesia? Br J Anaesth 68:123, 1992

32. Dahl JB, Moiniche S, Kehlet H: Wound infiltration with local anaesthetics for postoperative pain relief. Acta Anaesthesiol Scand 38:7, 1994

33. Labaille T, Mazoit JX, Paqueron X, et al: The clinical efficacy and pharmacokinetics of intraperitoneal ropivacaine for laparoscopic cholecystectomy. Anesth Analg 94:100, 2002

34. Callesen T, Bech K, Kehlet H: One-thousand consecutive inguinal hernia repairs under unmonitored local anesthesia. Anesth Analg 93:1373, 2001

35. Horlocker TT, Wedel DJ: Anticoagulation and neuraxial block: historical perspective, anesthetic implications, and risk management. Reg Anesth Pain Med 23:129, 1998

36. Horlocker TT, Wedel DJ, Schroeder DR, et al: Preoperative antiplatelet therapy does not increase the risk of spinal hematoma associated with regional anesthesia. Anesth Analg 80:303, 1995

37. Tryba M, Wedel DJ: Central neuraxial blockade and low molecular weight heparin (enoxaparine): lessons learned from different dosage regimes in two continents. Acta Anaesthesiol Scand 41:100, 1997

38. Tryba M: European practice guidelines: thromboembolism prophylaxis and regional anesthesia. Reg Anesth Pain Med 23:178, 1998

39. Horlocker TT, Wedel DJ: Neurological complications of spinal and epidural anesthesia. Reg Anesth Pain Med 25:83, 2000

40. Loo CC, Dahlgren G, Irestedt L: Neurological complications in obstetric regional anesthesia. Int J Obstet 9:99, 2000

41. Freedman JM, Li DK, Drasner K, et al: Transient neurologic symptoms after spinal anesthesia: an epidemiologic study of 1,863 patients. Anesthesiology 89:633, 1998

42. Yanovski SZ: Obesity. N Engl J Med 346:591, 2002

43. Simmons ST, Schleich AR: Airway regional anesthesia for awake fiberoptic intubation. Reg Anesth Pain Med 27:180, 2002

44. Hopkins PM: Malignant hyperthermia. Br J Anaesth 85:118, 2000

45. Desjardins G: Management of massive hemorrhage and transfusion. Semin Anesth 20:60, 2001

46. Sessler DI: Perioperative heat balance. Anesthesiology 92:578, 2000

47. de Witte J, Sessler DI: Perioperative shivering. Anesthesiology 96:467, 2002

48. Ghoneim MM: Awareness during anesthesia. Anesthesiology 92:597, 2000

49. Zucker-Pinchoff B: Latex allergy. Mt Sinai J Med 69:88, 2002

50. Guidelines 2000 for cardiopulmonary resuscitation and emergency cardiovascular care. The American Heart Association in Collaboration with the International Liaison Committee on Resuscitation. Circulation 102(8 suppl):I158, 2000

51. Baldessarini RJ: Drugs and the treatment of psychiatric disorders: depression and anxiety disorders. Goodman & Gilman's The Pharmacological Basis of Therapeutics, 10th ed. Hardman JG, Limbird LE, Gilman AG, Eds. McGraw-Hill, New York, 2001, p 447

52. Kearon C, Hirsh J: Management of anticoagulation before and after elective surgery. N Engl J Med 336:1506, 1997

53. Connelly CS, Panush RS: Should nonsteroidal anti-inflammatory drugs be stopped before elective surgery? Arch Intern Med 151:1963, 1991

54. Sonksen JR, Kong KL, Holder R: Magnitude and time course of impaired primary hemostasis after stopping chronic low and medium dose aspirin in healthy volunteers. Br J Anaesth 82:360, 1999

55. Gammic JS, Zenate M, Kormos RL, et al: Abciximab and excessive bleeding in patients undergoing emergency cardiac operations. Ann Thorac Surg 65:465, 1998

56. Hardy JF: Anticipated agents on perioperative bleeding. Anesthesiology Rounds 1(1):1, 2002

57. Majerus PW, Broze GJ Jr, Miletich JP, et al: Anticoagulant, thrombolytic, and antiplatelet drugs. Goodman & Gilman's The Pharmacological Basis of Therapeutics, 9th ed. Hardman JG, Limbird LE, Molinoff PB, et al, Eds. McGraw-Hill, New York, 1996, p 1341

58. Eisenberg DM, Davis RB, et al: Trends in alternative medicine use in the United States, 1990–1997: results of a follow-up national survey. JAMA 280:1569, 1998

59. Kaye AD, Clarke RC, Sabar R, et al: Herbal medicines: current trends in anesthesiology practice—a hospital survey. J Clin Anesth 12:468, 2000

60. Ang-Lee MK, Moss J, Yvan CS: Herbal medicines and perioperative care. JAMA 286:208, 2001

61. Vanderweghem JL, Depurreux M, Tielmans CH, et al: Rapidly progressive interstitial renal fibrosis in young women: association with summing regimen including Chinese herbs. Lancet 341:387, 1993

62. Jadont M, Plaen JF, Cosyns JP, et al: Adverse effects from traditional Chinese medicine. Lancet 347:892, 1995

63. Kao WF, Hung DZ, Lin KP: Podophylotoxin intoxication: toxic effect of Bajiaolian in herbal therapeutics. Hum Exp Toxicol 11:480, 1992

64. Edzard E: Harmless herbs? A review of the recent literature. Am J Med 104:170, 1998

65. Chung F, Mezei G: Adverse outcomes in ambulatory anesthesia. Can J Anesth 46:R18, 1999

66. ASA Task Force on Preoperative Fasting. Practice guidelines for preoperative fasting and the use of pharmacologic agents to reduce the risk of pulmonary aspiration: application to healthy patients undergoing elective procedures. Anesthesiology 90:896, 1999

67. Chung F: A post-anesthetic discharge scoring system for home readiness after ambulatory surgery. J Clin Anesth 7:500, 1995

68. Reves JG, Glass PSA, Lubarsky DA: Nonbarbiturate intravenous anesthetics. Anesthesia, 5th ed. Miller RD, Ed. Churchill Livingstone Inc, Philadelphia, 2000, p 228

69. Bailey PL, Egan TD, Stanley TH: Intravenous opioid anesthetics. Anesthesia, 5th ed. Miller RD, Ed. Churchill Livingstone Inc, Philadelphia, 2000, p 273

70. Stoelting RK: Histamine and histamine receptor antagonists. Pharmacology and Physiology in Anesthetic Practice, 3rd ed. Stoelting RK, Ed. Lippincott Williams & Wilkins, Philadelphia, p 385

71. Compendium of Pharmaceuticals and Specialties, Canadian Pharmacists Association. Webcom Limited, Toronto, 2002

72. Koblin DD: Mechanisms of action. Anesthesia, 5th ed. Miller RD, Ed. Churchill Livingstone Inc, Philadelphia, 2000, p 48

73. Eger EE II: Uptake and distribution. Anesthesia, 5th ed. Miller RD, Ed. Churchill Livingstone Inc, Philadelphia, 2000, p 74

74. Savarese JJ, Caldwell JE, Lien CA, et al: Pharmacology of muscle relaxants and their antagonists. Anesthesia, 5th ed. Miller RD, Ed. Churchill Livingstone Inc, Philadelphia, 2000, p 412

4 BLEEDING AND TRANSFUSION

John T. Owings, M.D., F.A.C.S., and Robert C. Gosselin, M.T.

Approach to the Patient with Ongoing Bleeding

A surgeon is often the first person to be called when a patient experiences ongoing bleeding. To treat such a patient appropriately, the surgeon must identify the cause or source of the bleeding. Causes fall into two main categories: (1) conditions leading to loss of vascular integrity, as in a postoperative patient with an unligated vessel that is bleeding or a trauma patient with a ruptured spleen, and (2) conditions leading to derangement of the hemostatic process. In this chapter, we focus on the latter category, which includes a broad spectrum of conditions ranging from aspirin-induced platelet dysfunction to von Willebrand disease (vWD) to disseminated intravascular coagulation (DIC) and even to hemophilia.

Coagulopathies are varied in their causes, treatments, and prognoses. Our aim is not to obviate the hematologic tests required for identification of rare congenital or acquired clotting abnormalities but to outline effective management approaches to the coagulopathies surgeons see most frequently. The vast majority of these coagulopathies can be diagnosed by means of a brief patient and family history, a review of medications, physical examination, and laboratory studies—in particular, activated partial thromboplastin time (aPTT), prothrombin time (PT, commonly expressed as an international normalized ratio [INR]), complete blood count (CBC), and D-dimer assay.

Exclusion of Technical Causes of Bleeding

It is critical for the surgeon to recognize that the most common causes of postoperative bleeding are technical: an unligated vessel or an unrecognized injury is much more likely to be the

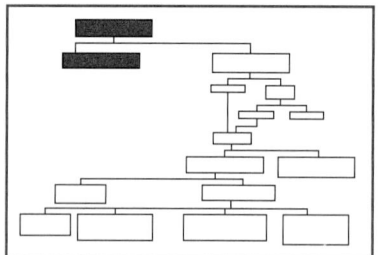

cause of a falling hematocrit than either a drug effect or an endogenous hemostatic defect. Furthermore, if an unligated vessel is treated as though it were an endogenous hemostatic defect (i.e., with transfusions), the outcome is likely to be disastrous. For these reasons, in all cases of ongoing bleeding, the first consideration must always be to exclude a surgically correctable cause.

Ongoing bleeding may be surprisingly difficult to diagnose. Healthy young patients can usually maintain a normal blood pressure until their blood loss exceeds 40% of their blood volume (roughly 2 L). If the bleeding is from a laceration to an extremity, it will be obvious; however, if the bleeding is occurring internally (e.g., from a ruptured spleen or an intraluminal GI source), there may be few physiologic signs [see 6:3 Shock]. For the purposes of the ensuing discussion, we assume that bleeding is known to have occurred or to be occurring.

Even when a technical cause of bleeding has seemingly been excluded, the possibility often must be reconsidered periodically throughout assessment. Patients who are either unresuscitated or underresuscitated undergo vasospasm, which may cause tamponade of the bleeding point.[1] As resuscitation proceeds, the catecholamine-induced vasospasm subsides and the bleeding may recur. For this reason, constant reassessment of the possibility of a technical cause of bleeding is appropriate. Only when the surgeon is confident that a missed injury or unligated vessel is not the cause of the bleeding should other potential causes be investigated.

Initial Assessment of Potential Coagulopathy

The first step in assessment of a patient with a potential coagulopathy is to draw a blood sample. The blood should be distributed into a tube containing ethylenediaminetetraacetic

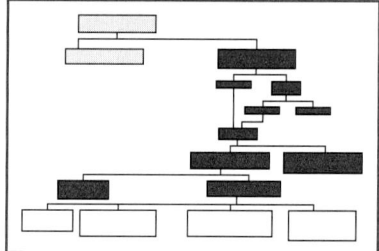

acid (EDTA) (for a CBC) and a citrated tube (for coagulation analysis).

At the same time, the patient's temperature should be noted. Because coagulation is a chemical reaction, it slows with increasing cold.[2] Thus, a patient with a temperature lower than 35° C (95° F) clots more slowly and less efficiently than one with a temperature of 37° C (98.6° F).[3] The resulting coagulatory abnormality is what is known as a hypothermic coagulopathy. Upon receipt of the drawn specimen, the laboratory warms the sample to 37° C to run the coagulation assays (aPTT and INR). In a patient with a purely hypothermic coagulopathy, this step results in normal coagulation parameters. Hypothermic patients should be actively rewarmed.[4] Typically, such patients cease to bleed after rewarming, and no further treatment is required. If the patient is normothermic and exhibits normal coagulation values but bleeding continues, attention should again be focused on the possibility of an unligated bleeding vessel or an uncontrolled occult bleeding source (e.g., the GI tract).

Ongoing bleeding in conjunction with abnormal coagulation parameters may have any of several underlying causes. In this setting, one of the most useful pieces of information to obtain is a personal and family history. A patient who has had dental extractions without major problems or who had a normal adolescence without any history of bleeding dyscrasias is very unlikely to have a congenital or hereditary bleeding disorder.[5] If there is a personal or family history of a specific bleeding disorder, appropriate steps should be taken to diagnose and treat the disorder [see Discussion, Bleeding Disorders, *below*].

Measurement of Coagulation Parameters

NORMAL INR, NORMAL aPTT

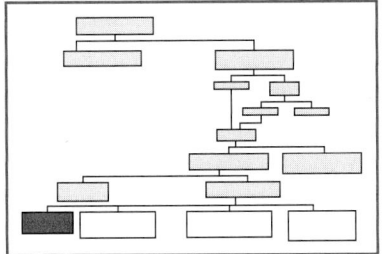

Patients with a normal INR and aPTT who exhibit ongoing bleeding may have impaired platelet activity. Inadequate platelet activity is frequently manifested as persistent oozing from wound edges or as low-volume bleeding. Such bleeding is rarely the cause of exsanguinating hemorrhage, though it may be life-threatening on occasion, depending on its location (e.g., the head or the pericardium). Inadequate platelet activity may be attributable either to an insufficient number of platelets or to platelet dysfunction. In the absence of a major surgical insult, a platelet count of 20,000/mm^3 or higher is usually adequate for normal coagulation.[6,7] There is some disagreement regarding the absolute level to which the platelet count must fall before platelet transfusion is justified in the absence of active bleeding. Patients undergoing procedures in which even capillary oozing is potentially life-threatening (e.g., craniotomy) should be maintained at a higher platelet count (i.e., > 20,000/mm^3). Patients without ongoing bleeding who are not specifically at increased risk for major complications from low-volume bleeding may be safely watched with platelet counts lower than 20,000/mm^3.

Oozing in a patient who has an adequate platelet count and normal coagulation parameters may be a signal of platelet dysfunction. The now-routine administration of aspirin to reduce the risk of myocardial infarction and stroke has led to a rise in the incidence of aspirin-induced platelet dysfunction. Aspirin causes irreversible platelet dysfunction through the cyclooxygenase pathway; the effect of aspirin can thus be expected to last for approximately 10 days. The platelet dysfunction caused by other nonsteroidal anti-inflammatory drugs (e.g., ibuprofen) is reversible and consequently does not last as long as that caused by aspirin. Newer platelet-blocking agents have been found to be effective in improving outcome after coronary angioplasty.[8] These drugs function predominantly by blocking the platelet surface receptor glycoprotein (GP) IIb-IIIa, which binds platelets to fibrinogen.

In patients with platelet dysfunction caused by an inhibitor of platelet function, such as an elevated blood urea nitrogen (BUN) level, 1-desamino-8-D-arginine vasopressin (DDAVP) is capable of partially reversing the dysfunction.[9] DDAVP has also been successful in partially reversing aspirin-induced platelet dysfunction.

Less common causes of bleeding in patients with a normal INR and a normal aPTT include factor XIII deficiency, hypofibrinogenemia or dysfibrinogenemia, and derangements in the fibrinolytic pathway [see Discussion, Mechanics of Hemostasis, below].

NORMAL INR, PROLONGED aPTT

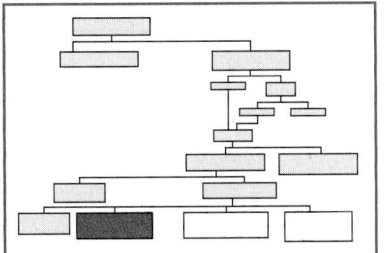

Patients with a normal INR and an abnormal aPTT are likely to have a drug-induced coagulation defect. The agent most commonly responsible is unfractionated heparin. Reversal of the heparin effect, if desired, can be accomplished by administering protamine sulfate. Protamine should be given with caution, however, because it has been reported to induce a hy-

percoagulable state.[10] It is likely that many of the thrombotic complications are related to simple reversal of a needed anticoagulant state. Protamine should also be used with caution in diabetic patients. These persons sometimes become sensitized to impurities in protamine through their exposure to similar impurities in insulin, and this sensitization may result in an anaphylactic reaction.

It should be remembered that the aPTT does not accurately measure the anticoagulant activity of low-molecular-weight heparins. Because such heparins exert the greater proportion of their anticoagulant effect by potentiating antithrombin to inactivate factor Xa rather than factor IIa, an assay that measures anti-Xa activity is needed to measure the anticoagulant effect. This effect, however, like that of unfractionated heparin, is reversible by protamine. A crucial point is that the administration of fresh frozen plasma (FFP) will not correct the anticoagulant effect of either unfractionated heparin or low-molecular-weight heparins. In fact, given that plasma contains antithrombin and that both unfractionated heparin and low-molecular-weight heparins act by potentiating antithrombin, administration of FFP could actually enhance the heparins' anticoagulant effect.

A variety of direct thrombin inhibitors (e.g., bivalirudin [Hirulog] and lepirudin) are currently available in Europe, Asia, and North America.[11] Many of them cause prolongation of the aPTT. One disadvantage shared by most of the direct thrombin inhibitors is that the effects are not reversible; if thrombin inhibition is no longer wanted, FFP must be given to correct the aPTT. Because the inhibitor that is circulating but not bound at the time of FFP administration will bind the prothrombin in the FFP, the amount of FFP required to correct the aPTT may be greater than would be needed with a simple factor deficiency.

von Willebrand disease is frequently, though not always, associated with a slight prolongation of the aPTT. Its clinical expression is variable. Confirmation of the diagnosis can be obtained by testing for circulating factor levels. Platelet function analysis will also show abnormal function. Correction is accomplished by administering directed therapy (von Willebrand factor [vWF]) [see Discussion, Bleeding Disorders, below], DDAVP, or cryoprecipitate.

Hemophilia may either cause spontaneous bleeding or lead to prolonged bleeding after a surgical or traumatic insult. As noted, hemophilia is rare in the absence of a personal or family history of the disorder. The most common forms of hemophilia involve deficiencies of factors VIII, IX, and XI (hemophilia A, hemophilia B, and hemophilia C, respectively). In contrast to depletion of natural anticoagulants such as antithrombin and protein C [see 4:6 Venous Thromboembolism], depletion of procoagulant factors rarely gives rise to significant manifestations until it is relatively severe. Typically, no laboratory abnormalities result from depletion of procoagulant factors until factor activity levels fall below 40% of normal, and clinical abnormalities are frequently absent even when factor activity levels fall to only 10% of normal. This tolerance for subcritical degrees of depletion is a reflection of the built-in redundancies in the procoagulant pathways.

If hemophilia is suspected, specific factor analysis is indicated. Appropriate therapy involves administering the deficient factor or factors [see Table 1]. Hemophiliac patients who have undergone extensive transfusion therapy may pose a particular challenge: massive transfusions frequently lead to the development of antibodies that make subsequent transfusion or even directed therapy impossible. Accordingly, several alternatives to transfusion or directed factor therapy (e.g., recombinant activated factor VII [rVIIa]) have been developed for use in this population.

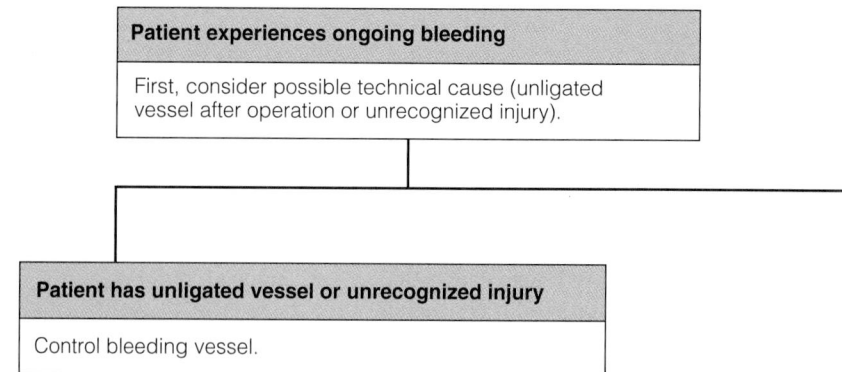

Approach to the Patient with Ongoing Bleeding

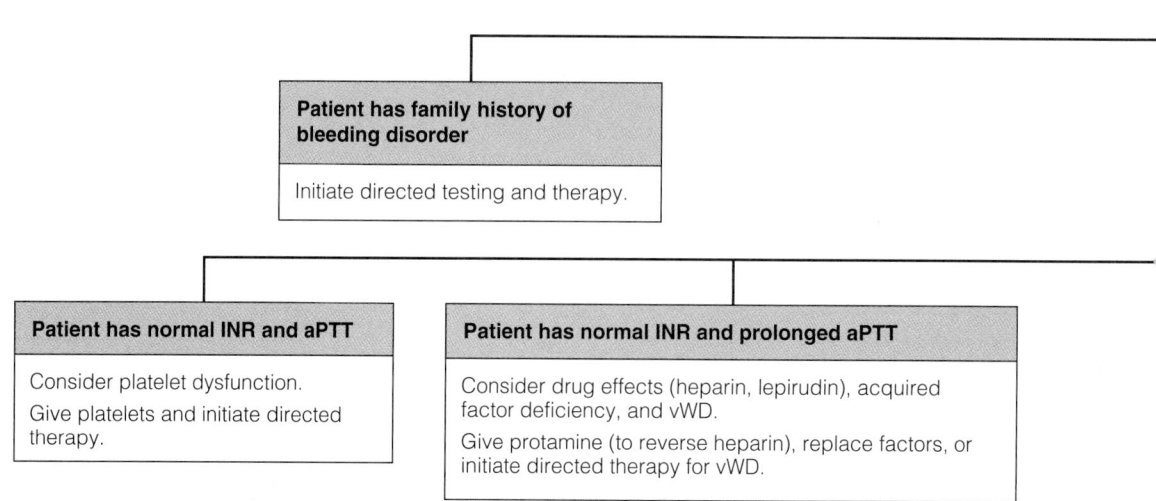

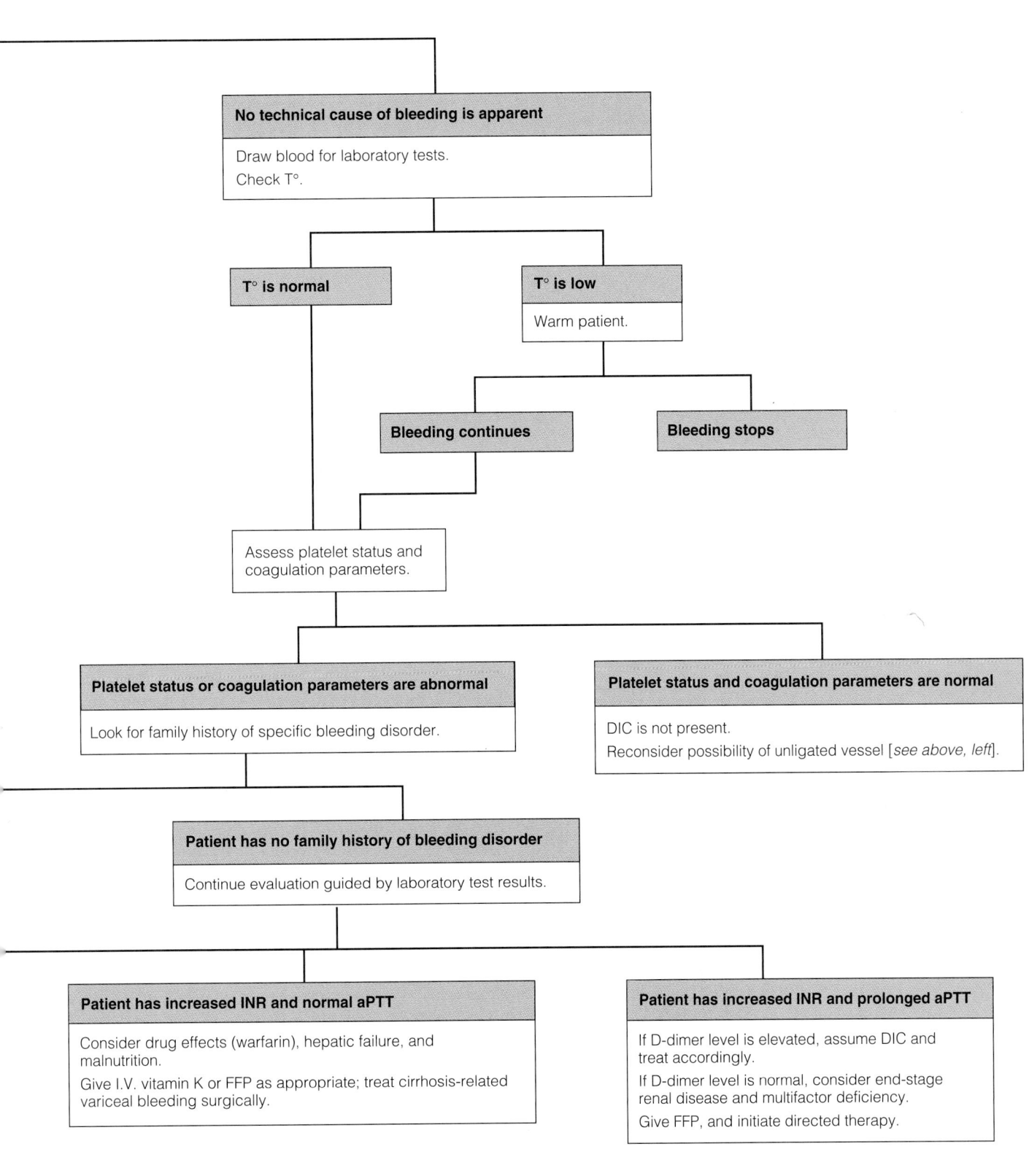

No technical cause of bleeding is apparent

Draw blood for laboratory tests.
Check T°.

T° is normal

T° is low

Warm patient.

Bleeding continues

Bleeding stops

Assess platelet status and coagulation parameters.

Platelet status or coagulation parameters are abnormal

Look for family history of specific bleeding disorder.

Platelet status and coagulation parameters are normal

DIC is not present.
Reconsider possibility of unligated vessel [*see above, left*].

Patient has no family history of bleeding disorder

Continue evaluation guided by laboratory test results.

Patient has increased INR and normal aPTT

Consider drug effects (warfarin), hepatic failure, and malnutrition.
Give I.V. vitamin K or FFP as appropriate; treat cirrhosis-related variceal bleeding surgically.

Patient has increased INR and prolonged aPTT

If D-dimer level is elevated, assume DIC and treat accordingly.
If D-dimer level is normal, consider end-stage renal disease and multifactor deficiency.
Give FFP, and initiate directed therapy.

Table 1   Preparations Used in Directed Therapy for Hemophilia

Product (Manufacturer)	Origin	Used to Compensate for Depletion of Factors		
		Factor VIII	Factor IX	vWF
Alphanate (Alpha Therapeutic)	Plasma	Yes	—	Yes
Monarc-M (American Red Cross)	Plasma	Yes	—	Yes
Hemofil M (Baxter Healthcare)	Plasma	Yes	—	Yes
Humate-P (Centeon)	Plasma	Yes	—	Yes
Koāte-HP (Bayer)	Plasma	Yes	—	Yes
Monoclate-P (Centeon)	Plasma	Yes	—	Yes
Recombinate (Baxter Healthcare)	Recombinant	Yes	—	—
Kogenate (Bayer)	Recombinant	Yes	—	—
Bioclate (Baxter Healthcare), Helixate (Centeon)	Recombinant	Yes	—	—
Hyate:C (Speywood)	Porcine plasma	Yes	—	—
Autoplex T (prothrombin complex concentrate) (NABI)	Plasma	—	Yes	—
Feiba VH Immuno (prothrombin complex concentrate) (Immuno-US)	Plasma	—	Yes	—
Mononine (Centeon)	Plasma	—	Yes	—
AlphaNine-SD (Alpha Therapeutic)	Plasma	—	Yes	—
Bebulin VH Immuno (Immuno-US)	Plasma	—	Yes	—
Proplex T (Baxter Healthcare)	Plasma	—	Yes	—
Konȳne 80 (Bayer)	Plasma	—	Yes	—
Profilnine SD (Alpha Therapeutic)	Plasma	—	Yes	—
BeneFix (Genetics Institute)	Recombinant	—	Yes	—
Novo Seven (Novo Nordisk)	Recombinant	Yes	Yes	—

INCREASED INR,
NORMAL aPTT

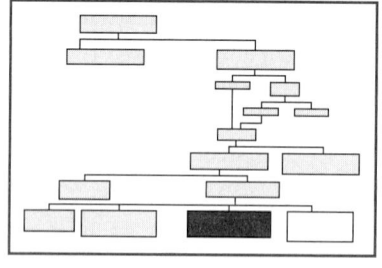

An increased INR in association with a normal aPTT is a more ominous finding in a patient with a coagulopathy. Any of a number of causes, all centering on factor deficiency, may be responsible.

Cirrhosis is arguably the most serious of the causes of an elevated INR. It is a major problem not so much because of the coagulopathy itself but because of the associated deficits in wound healing and immune function that result from the synthetic dysfunction and the loss of reticuloendothelial function. In all cases, factor replacement should be instituted with FFP. If the bleeding is a manifestation of the cirrhosis (as in variceal bleeding), emergency portal decompression should be accomplished before the coagulopathy worsens. Management of cirrhotic patients who have sustained injuries is particularly troublesome because such patients are at disproportionately high risk for subdural hematoma. The reason this risk is so high is that in addition to their pathologic autoanticoagulation, these patients often have some degree of cerebral atrophy as a result of one of the more frequent causes of cirrhosis—namely, alcoholism. As a result, the bridging intracranial veins are more vulnerable to tears and more likely to bleed. Modest elevations of the INR in patients who are not actively bleeding, have not recently undergone operation, and are not specifically at increased risk for life-threatening hemorrhage may be observed without correction.

An elevated INR with a normal aPTT may also be a consequence of warfarin administration. Such a coagulopathy is the result of a pure factor deficiency, and its degree is proportional to the prolongation of the INR. Because warfarin acts by disrupting vitamin K metabolism, the coagulopathy may be corrected by giving vitamin K [*see Table 2*].[12] If the patient is actively bleeding, vitamin K should still be given, but the primary corrective measure should be to administer FFP in an amount proportional to the patient's size and the relative increase in the INR. The INR should subsequently be rechecked to ensure that replacement therapy is adequate. Vitamin K replacement therapy has two main potential drawbacks: (1) if the patient is to be reanticoagulated with warfarin in the near future, dosing will be difficult because the patient will exhibit resistance to warfarin for a variable period; and (2) anaphylactic reactions have been reported when vitamin K is given I.V.

Table 2 Management of the Patient
with an Increased INR[12]

Indication	Recommended Treatment
INR above therapeutic range but < 5.0	If no bleeding is present or surgery is indicated, lower or hold next dose
INR > 5.0 but < 9.0	
Patient has no significant bleeding	In the absence of additional risk factors for bleeding, withhold next 1–2 doses; alternatively, withhold next dose and give vitamin K, 1.0–2.5 mg (oral route is acceptable)
Rapid reduction of INR is required	Give vitamin K, 2.0–4.0 mg p.o.; expected reduction of INR should occur within 24 hr
INR > 9.0	
Patient has no significant bleeding	Give vitamin K, 3.0–5.0 mg p.o.; expected reduction of INR should occur within 24 hr
Patient has serious bleeding or is overly anticoagulated (INR > 20.0)	Give vitamin K, 10 mg I.V., and FFP; further vitamin K supplementation may be required every 12 hr
Patient has life-threatening bleeding or is seriously overanticoagulated	Prothrombin complexes may be indicated, along with vitamin K, 10 mg I.V.

INCREASED INR,
PROLONGED aPTT

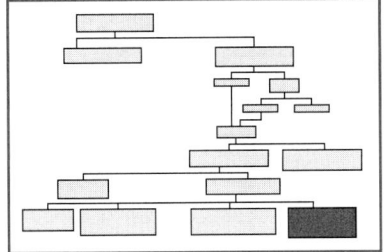

Increases in both the INR and the aPTT may be the most problematic finding of all. When both assays show increases, the patient is likely to have multiple factor deficiencies; possible causes include DIC, severe hemodilution, and renal failure with severe nephrotic syndrome. However, when dramatic elevations of the aPTT and the INR are observed in a seemingly asymptomatic patient, the problem may lie not in the patient's condition but in the laboratory analysis. If the tube in which the blood sample was placed for these tests was not adequately filled, the results of the coagulation assays may be inaccurate. In such cases, the blood sample should be redrawn and the tests repeated.

Hemodilution and nephrotic syndrome result in a coagulopathy that is attributable to decreased concentration of coagulation proteins. Dilutional coagulopathy may occur when a patient who is given a large volume of packed red blood cell (RBC) units is not also given coagulation factors.[13] Because of the tremendous redundancy of the hemostatic process, pure dilutional coagulopathy is rare. It is considered an unlikely diagnosis until after one full blood volume has been replaced (as when a patient requires 10 units of packed RBCs to maintain a stable hematocrit). Nephrotic syndrome is associated with loss of protein (coagulation proteins as well as other body proteins) from the kidneys.

Both hemodilution and nephrotic syndrome should be distinguished from DIC (which is a consumptive rather than a dilutional process[14]), though on occasion this distinction is a difficult one to make. A blood sample should be sent for D-dimer assay. If the D-dimer level is low (< 1,000 ng/ml), DIC is unlikely; if it is very high (> 2,000 ng/ml) and there is no other clear explanation (e.g., a complex unstable pelvic fracture), the diagnosis of DIC rather than dilution should be made. Treatment of dilutional coagulopathy should be directed at replacement of lost factors. FFP should be given first, followed by cryoprecipitate, calcium, and platelets. Transfusion

should be continued until the coagulation parameters are corrected and the bleeding stops.

DIC is a diffuse, disorganized activation of the clotting cascade within the vascular space. It may result either from intravascular presentation of an overwhelming clotting stimulus (e.g., massive crush injury or transfusion reaction) or from presentation of a moderate clotting stimulus in the context of shock. Different degrees of severity have been described. In the mildest form of DIC, acceleration of the clotting cascade is seen, and microthrombi are formed in the vascular space but are cleared effectively. Thus, mild DIC may be little more than an acceleration of the clotting cascade that escapes recognition. In the moderate form of DIC, the microthrombi are ineffectively lysed and cause occlusion of the microcirculation. This process is clinically manifested in the lungs as the acute respiratory distress syndrome (ARDS), in the kidneys as renal failure, and in the liver as hepatic failure.

Neither mild DIC nor moderate DIC is what surgeons traditionally think of as DIC. Severe DIC arises when congestion of the microvasculature with thrombi occurs, resulting in large-scale activation of the fibrinolytic system to restore circulation. This fibrinolytic activity results in breakdown of clot at previously hemostatic sites of microscopic injury (e.g., endothelial damage) and macroscopic injury (e.g., I.V. catheter sites, fractures, or surgical wounds). Bleeding and reexposure to tissue factor stimulate activation of factor VII with increased coagulation activity; thus, microthrombi are formed, and the vicious circle continues. The ultimate manifestation of severe DIC is bleeding from (1) fibrinolysis and (2) depletion (consumption) of coagulation factors.

Several scoring systems have been devised to assess the severity of DIC. These scoring systems are most useful for distinguishing DIC from other causes of coagulopathy (e.g., hypothermia, dilution, or drug effects) [see Table 3].[15]

DIC is a diagnosis of exclusion, largely because none of the various treatment strategies tried to date have been particularly successful. Heparin has been given in large doses in an attempt to break the cycle by stopping the clotting, thus allowing clotting factor levels to return to normal. Antifibrinolytic agents (e.g., ε-aminocaproic acid) have also been tried in an attempt to reduce fibrinolytic activity and thus slow the bleeding that stimulates subsequent clot formation. Antithrombotics (e.g., antithrombin and protein C) have been used as well; improvements have been noted in laboratory measures of DIC but not in survival.

Currently, the most appropriate way of treating a patient with severe DIC is to follow a multifaceted approach. First, the clotting stimulus, if still present, should be removed: dead or devitalized tissue should be amputated, abscesses drained, and suspect transfusions discontinued. Second, hypothermia, of any degree of severity, should be corrected. Third, both blood loss (as measured by the hematocrit) and clotting factor deficits (as measured by the INR) should be aggressively corrected (with blood and plasma, respec-

Table 3 Coagulopathy (DIC) Score

Score	INR (sec)	aPTT (sec)	Platelets (1,000/mm³)	Fibrinogen (mg/dl)	D-dimer (ng/ml)
0	< 1.2	< 34	> 150	> 200	< 1,000
1	> 1.2	> 34	< 150	< 200	< 2,000
2	> 1.4	> 39	< 100	< 150	< 4,000
3	> 1.6	> 54	< 60	< 100	> 4,000

DIC—disseminated intravascular coagulopathy   INR—international normalized ratio   aPTT—activated partial thromboplastin tively). This supportive approach is only modestly successful. For certain groups of patients in whom DIC develops (e.g., those who have sustained head injuries), mortality approaches 100%. This alarmingly high death rate is probably related more to the underlying pathology than to the hematologic derangement.

An increased INR with a prolonged aPTT may also be caused by various isolated factor deficiencies of the common pathway. Congenital deficiencies of factors X, V, and prothrombin are very rare. Acquired factor V deficiencies have been observed in patients with autoimmune disorders. Acquired hypoprothrombinemia has been documented in a small percentage of patients with lupus anticoagulants who exhibit abnormal bleeding. Factor X deficiencies have been noted in patients with amyloidosis.

Stabilized warfarin therapy will increase both the INR and the aPTT. Several current rodenticides (e.g., brodifacoum) exert the same effect on these parameters that warfarin does; however, because they have a considerably longer half-life than warfarin, the reversal of the anticoagulation effect with vitamin K or FFP may be correspondingly longer.[16] Animal venoms may also increase the INR and the aPTT.

Management of Anemia and Indications for Transfusion

Treatment of anemia has changed substantially since the early 1990s. Blood cell transfusions have been shown to have significant immunosuppressive potential, and transmission of fatal diseases through the blood supply has been extensively documented. Moreover, at least one large trial found that using a restrictive RBC transfusion protocol in place of a more traditional one improved survival.[17] These findings have led to a paradigm shift with respect to RBC transfusion: whereas the traditional view was that anemia by itself was a sufficient indication for transfusion, the current consensus is that a second indication must be present in addition to a decreased hemoglobin concentration.

The decision whether to transfuse should be based on the patient's current or predicted need for additional oxygen-carrying capacity [see Figure 1]. A major component of this decision is to determine as promptly as possible whether the patient is in a steady state with respect to hemoglobin supply (in which case transfusions are less likely to be needed) or not (in which case transfusions are usually indicated). Thus, there is no specific hemoglobin concentration or hematocrit (i.e., transfusion trigger) at which all patients should receive transfusions.

There are two large groups of patients who should be managed more aggressively than the general patient population with respect to RBC transfusion. Patients who are either actively bleeding or at high risk for active bleeding and patients who have significant coronary artery disease (CAD) should receive transfusions according to a more liberal protocol than that applied to other patients.

ACTIVE BLEEDING

Patients who are actively bleeding (e.g., those with GI hemorrhage) should receive transfusions up to a level sufficient to keep up with blood loss. Coagulation factors must also be replaced as necessary [see Measurement of Coagulation Parameters, Increased INR, Prolonged aPTT, above]. Patients at high risk for active bleeding (e.g., from massive liver injury) should receive transfusions up to a level at which, if bleeding occurs or recurs, enough reserve oxygen-carrying capacity is afforded to allow diagnosis and correction of the hemorrhage without significant compromise of oxygen delivery. In cases of major injury, we advocate a target hematocrit of 30%; however, this is not a fixed value but a rule-of-thumb figure

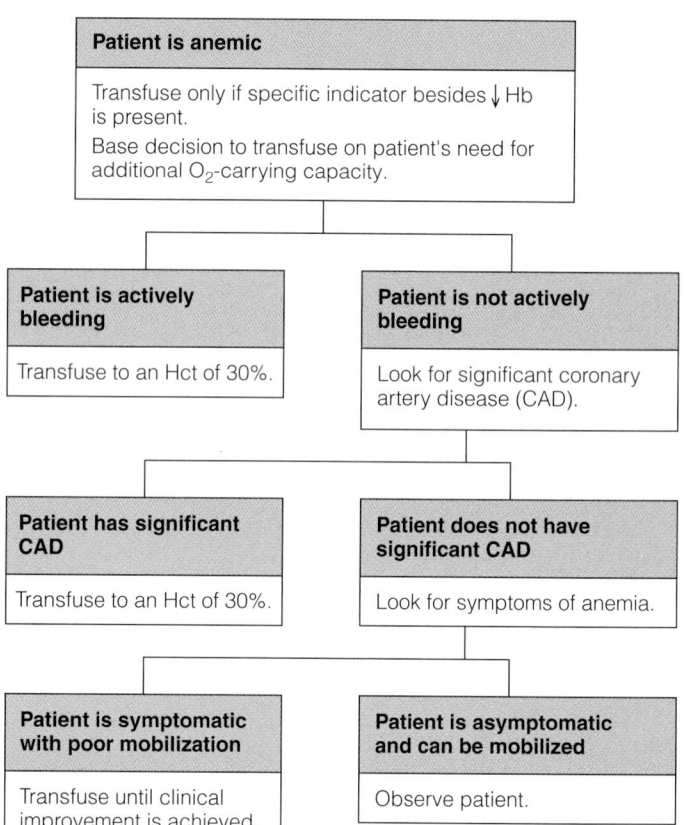

Figure 1 Algorithm depicts decision-making process for transfusion in anemic patients.

that may be increased or decreased as appropriate, depending on the individual patient's reserves and the individual surgical team's ability to diagnose and correct the underlying problem.

SIGNIFICANT CORONARY ARTERY DISEASE

Although no studies have conclusively shown that patients with significant CAD benefit from increased RBC mass, there is also no published evidence to support a restrictive transfusion policy.[17] The major trials that found most patients to benefit from a restrictive transfusion policy specifically excluded CAD patients out of concern that adverse cardiovascular events (e.g., myocardial infarction and cerebrovascular accidents) might increase in frequency at lower hematocrits. Studies evaluating the potential benefit of a more aggressive transfusion policy (i.e., to hematocrits > 30%) failed to show any benefit. Consequently, a target hematocrit of 30% is generally considered appropriate for patients with significant CAD.

SYMPTOMATIC ANEMIA

An additional indication for transfusion is oxygen-carrying capacity that is insufficient to support necessary activities (e.g., wound healing, mobilization, and physical therapy). Typical manifestations are light-headedness, tachycardia, and tachypnea either during the activity in question or at rest. Clearly, some degree of tachycardia is to be expected in any patient who has undergone a major operation or sustained a serious injury. The key point with respect to symptomatic anemia is that patients who have physiologically compensated for anemia must be distinguished from those whose health or recovery is compromised by anemia, and only the latter group should receive transfusions.

Table 4 Blood Substitutes[81]

Product (Manufacturer)	Source
PHP (Apex Bioscience)	Pyridoxylated human hemoglobin conjugated to polyoxyethylene
PEG-hemoglobin (Enzon)	Bovine hemoglobin conjugated to polyethylene glycol
PolyHeme (Northfield Laboratories)	Glutaraldehyde-polymerized pyridoxylated human hemoglobin
Hemopure (Biopure)	Glutaraldehyde-polymerized bovine hemoglobin
Hemolink (Hemosol)	Oxidized raffinose–crosslinked human hemoglobin from expired stored blood
Oxygent (Alliance Pharmaceutical)	Emulsified perflubron

OBSERVATION OF ANEMIA

It has become standard practice to observe patients with low hemoglobin concentrations that in the past would have triggered transfusion. The data currently available support this approach down to a hemoglobin concentration of 6 to 7 g/dl; below 6 g/dl, the data are not sufficient to support observation alone.

There does come a hemoglobin level below which life is not possible. Certain religions prohibit blood transfusion even when death is the probable or certain consequence. Such prohibitions have challenged the medical community to find techniques for supporting life at lower and lower hemoglobin concentrations. In addition, they have helped to define the limits beyond which a restrictive transfusion protocol may be fatal.

When RBC transfusion is not possible (whether for cultural reasons or because compatible blood is unavailable), there are a number of temporizing measures that can be used to support life. If oxygen-carrying capacity cannot be increased, one option is simply to decrease oxygen demand. Oxygen demand is directly proportional to metabolic activity; that is, as metabolic rate increases, so too does oxygen demand. Once unnecessary activity (e.g., assuming an upright posture or walking) has been eliminated, respiration becomes an activity that requires a significant amount of energy. Mechanical ventilation reduces the work of breathing and with it the oxygen requirements of the respiratory muscles. Even with full mechanical ventilation, however, most patients continue to initiate breaths on their own. This energy-requiring activity can be eliminated by administering a neuromuscular blocking agent, which dramatically reduces oxygen demand in essentially all skeletal muscle. The metabolic rate can be further reduced by inducing hypothermia. This measure should be used with caution, however, because hypothermia in the absence of neuromuscular blockade results in uncontrollable shivering, which actually increases the metabolic rate. In addition, trials addressing the use of hypothermia in head injury patients to reduce cerebral oxygen demand reported increased infection rates in the hypothermic groups.

A completely different approach to the issue of the unacceptability or unavailability of RBC transfusion involves the use of RBC substitutes to augment oxygen-carrying capacity. A variety of different substitutes are currently under investigation [*see Table 4*].[18] None have been approved for routine use by the United States Food and Drug Administration, but several have demonstrated promise in clinical trials. Without modification, the hemoglobin molecule is nephrotoxic. Accordingly, virtually all of the products now being studied depend on techniques for making an acellular hemoglobin molecule nontoxic for I.V. administration.

Acellular blood substitutes clearly possess a number of advantages, including greatly increased shelf life, reduced risk of viral transmission, availability that is not limited by donor supply, reduced or eliminated risk of incompatibility reactions, and—potentially, at least—reduced cultural and religious objections.[19] To what extent this approach is suited to the treatment of anemia in surgical patients should be clarified when the results of the trials now under way are published.[18]

Discussion

Mechanics of Hemostasis

Hemostasis is the term for the process by which cellular and plasma components interact in response to vessel injury in order to maintain vascular integrity and promote wound healing. The initial response to vascular injury (primary hemostasis) involves the recruitment and activation of platelets, which then adhere to the site of injury. Subsequently, plasma proteins, in concert with cellular components, begin to generate thrombin, which causes further activation of platelets and converts fibrinogen to fibrin monomers that polymerize into a fibrin clot. The final step is the release of plasminogen activators that induce clot lysis and tissue repair.

The cellular components of hemostasis include endothelium, white blood cells (WBCs), RBCs, and platelets. The plasma components include a number of procoagulant and regulatory proteins that, once activated, can accelerate or downregulate thrombin formation or clot lysis to facilitate wound healing. In normal individuals, these hemostatic components are in a regulatory balance; thus, any abnormality involving one or more of these components can result in a pathologic state, whether of uncontrolled clot formation (thrombosis) or of excessive bleeding (hemorrhage). These pathologies can result from either hereditary defects of protein synthesis or acquired deficiencies attributable to metabolic causes.

CELLULAR COMPONENTS

Endothelium

The endothelium has both procoagulant and anticoagulant properties. When vascular injury occurs, the endothelium serves as a nidus for recruitment of platelets, adhesion of platelets to the endothelial surface, platelet aggregation, migration of platelets across the endothelial surface, generation of fibrin, and expression of adhesion molecule receptors (E-selectin and P-selectin). Exposure of collagen fibrils and release of vWF from the Weibel-Palade bodies cause platelets to adhere to the cellular surface of the endothelium. The presence of interleukin-1β (IL-1β), tissue necrosis factor (TNF), interferon-8 (IFN-8), and thrombin promotes expression of tissue factor (TF) on the endothelium.[20,21] TF activates factors X and VII, and these activated factors generate additional thrombin, which increases both fibrin formation and platelet aggregation.

The endothelium also acts in numerous ways to downregulate coagulation.[22] Heparan sulfate and thrombomodulin are both downregulators of thrombin formation. In the presence of thrombin, the endothelium responds by (1) releasing thrombomodulin, which forms a complex with thrombin to activate protein C; (2) producing endothelium-derived relaxing factor (i.e., nitric oxide[23]) and prostacyclin, which have vasodilating and platelet aggregation–inhibiting effects, respectively; and (3) releasing tissue plasminogen activator (t-PA) or urokinase-type plasminogen activator (u-PA), either of which converts the zymogen plasminogen to an active form (i.e., plasmin) that degrades fibrin and fibrinogen.[20,24] Heparan sulfate, on the endothelium wall, forms a complex with plasma antithrombin to neutralize thrombin. The endothelium is also the source of tissue factor pathway inhibitor (TFPI), which downregulates TF-VIIa-Xa complexes.

Erythrocytes and Leukocytes

The nonplatelet cellular components of blood play indirect roles in hemostasis. RBCs contain thromboplastins that are potent stimulators of various procoagulant proteins. In addition, the concentration of RBCs within the bloodstream (expressed as the hematocrit) assists in primary hemostasis by physically forcing the platelets toward the endothelial surfaces. When the RBC count is low enough, the absence of this force results in inadequate endothelium-platelet interaction and a bleeding diathesis.

Leukocytes have several functions in the hemostatic process. The interaction between the adhesion molecules expressed on both leukocytes and endothelium results in cytokine production, initiation of inflammatory responses, and degradation of extracellular matrix to facilitate tissue healing. In the presence of thrombin, monocytes express TF, which is an integral procoagulant for thrombin generation. Neutrophils and activated monocytes bind to stimulated platelets and endothelial cells that express P-selectin. Adhesion and rolling of neutrophils, mediated by fibrinogen and selectins on the endothelium, appear to facilitate vessel integrity but may also lead to inflammatory responses.[25,26] Lymphocytes also adhere to endothelium via adhesion molecule receptors and appear to be responsible for cytokine production and inflammatory responses.

Platelets

The roles platelets play in hemostasis and subsequent fibrin formation rest on providing a phospholipid surface for localizing procoagulant activation. Activation of platelets by agonists such as adenosine triphosphate (ATP), adenosine diphosphate (ADP), epinephrine, thromboxane A_2, collagen, and thrombin causes platelets to undergo morphologic changes and degranulation. Degranulation of platelets results in the release of procoagulants that promote further platelet adhesion and aggregation (e.g., thrombospondin, vWF, fibrinogen, ADP, and ATP), vasodilation (e.g., serotonin), and surface expression of P-selectin, which induces cellular adhesion. Platelet degranulation also results in the release of β-thromboglobulin, platelet factor 4 (which has antiheparin properties), various growth factors, coagulation procoagulants, and calcium as well as the formation of platelet microparticles. Plasminogen activator inhibitor–I (PAI-I) released from degranulated platelets neutralizes the fibrinolytic pathway by forming a complex with t-PA.

Upon exposure to vascular injury, platelets adhere to the exposed endothelium via binding of vWF to the GPIb-IX-V complex.[27] Conformational changes in the GPIIb-IIIa complex on the activated platelet surface enhance fibrinogen binding, which results in platelet-to-platelet interaction (i.e., aggregation). The phospholipid surface of the platelet membranes anchors activated IXa-VIIIa and Xa-Va complexes, thereby localizing thrombin generation.[28]

PLASMA COMPONENTS

Procoagulants

Traditional diagrams of the coagulation cascade depict two distinct pathways for thrombin generation: the intrinsic pathway and the extrinsic pathway. The premise for the distinction between the

two is that the intrinsic pathway requires no extravascular source for initiation, whereas the extrinsic pathway requires an extravascular component (i.e., TF). This traditional depiction is useful in interpreting coagulation tests, but it is not an accurate reflection of the hemostatic process in vivo. Accordingly, our focus is not on this standard view but rather on the roles contact factors (within the intrinsic cascade) and TF play in coagulation. As noted, circulating plasma vWF is necessary for normal adhesion of platelets to the endothelium. Plasma vWF also serves as the carrier protein for factor VIII, preventing its neutralization by the protein C regulatory pathway.

Even in patients in whom laboratory tests strongly suggest a severe clotting abnormality (i.e., the aPTT is markedly prolonged), contact factors do not play a significant role in the generation of thrombin. However, contact factor activation does appear to play secondary roles that are essential to normal hemostasis and tissue repair. Factor XII, prekallikrein, and high-molecular-weight kininogen are bound to the endothelium to activate the bradykinin (BK) pathway. The BK pathway exerts profibrinolytic effects by stimulating endothelial release of plasminogen activators. It also stimulates endothelial production of nitric oxide and prostacyclin, which play vital regulatory roles in vasodilation and regulation of platelet activation.[29]

The key initiator of plasma procoagulant formation is the expression of TF on cell surfaces.[21,30] TF activates factor VII and binds with it to form the TF-VIIa complex, which activates factors X and IX. Factor Xa also enhances its own production by activating factor IX, which in turn activates factor X to form factor Xa. Factor Xa also produces minimal amounts of thrombin by cleaving the prothrombin molecule. The thrombin generated from this process cleaves the coagulation cofactors V and VIII to enhance production of the factor complexes IX-VIIIa (intrinsic tenase) and Xa-Va (prothrombinase), which catalyze conversion of prothrombin to thrombin [see Figure 2].[31]

Thrombin has numerous functions, including prothrombotic and regulatory functions. Its procoagulant properties include cleaving fibrinogen, activating the coagulation cofactors V and VIII, inducing platelet aggregation, inducing expression of TF on cell surfaces, and activating factor XIII. In cleaving fibrinogen, thrombin causes the release of fibrinopeptides A and B (fibrin monomer). The fibrin monomer undergoes conformational changes that expose the α and β chains of the molecule, which then polymerize with other fibrin monomers to form a fibrin mesh. Activated factor XIII cross-links the polymerized fibrin (between the α chains and the γ chains) to stabilize the fibrin clot and delay fibrinolysis.

Fibrin(ogen)olysis

Plasminogen is the primary fibrinolytic zymogen that circulates in plasma. In the presence of t-PA or u-PA (released from the endothelium), plasminogen is converted to the active form, plasmin. Plasmin cleaves fibrin (or fibrinogen) between the molecule's D and E domains, causing the formation of X, Y, D, and E fragments. The secondary function of the fibrinolytic pathway is the activation by u-PA of matrix metalloproteinases that degrade the extracellular matrix.[32]

Regulatory Factors

In persons with normal coagulation status, downregulation of hemostasis occurs simultaneously with the production of procoagulants (e.g., activated plasma factors, stimulated endothelium, and stimulated platelets). In addition to their procoagulant activity, both thrombin and contact factors stimulate downregulation of the coagulation process. Thrombin forms a complex with endothelium-bound thrombomodulin to activate protein C, which inhibits factors Va and VIIIa. The thrombin-thrombomodulin complex also regu-

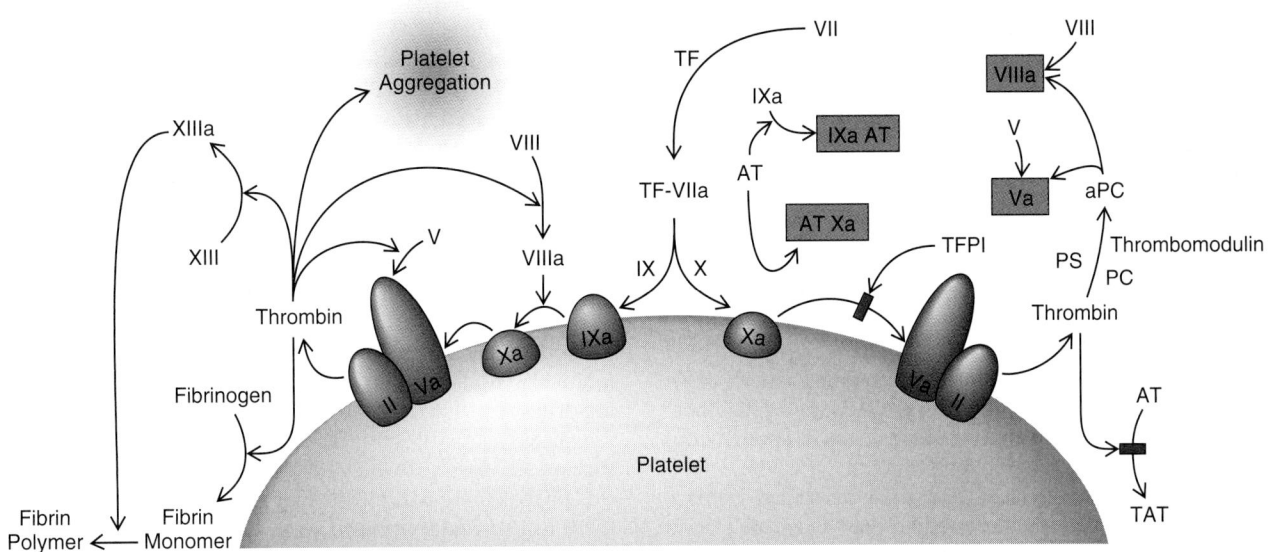

Figure 2   **Shown is a schematic representation of the procoagulant pathways.**

lates the fibrinolytic pathway by activating a circulating plasma protein known as thrombin-activatable fibrinolysis inhibitor (TAFI), which appears to suppress conversion of plasminogen to plasmin.[33] Contact factors are known to be required for normal surface-dependent fibrinolysis, and there is some evidence that contact factor deficiencies can lead to thromboembolism. Another plasma protein responsible for regulation of fibrinolysis is α_2-antiplasmin, which binds to circulating and bound plasmin to limit breakdown of fibrin.

Circulating downregulating proteins include antithrombin (a serine protease inhibitor of activated factors—especially factors IXa, Xa, and XIa—and thrombin[31]), proteins C and S (regulators of factors VIIIa and Va[34]), C1 inhibitor (a regulator of factor XIa), TFPI (a regulator of the TF-VIIa-Xa complex[35]), and α_2-macroglobulin (a thrombin inhibitor—the primary thrombin inhibitor in neonates[36]). Limitation of platelet activation occurs secondarily as a result of decreased levels of circulating agonists and endothelial release of prostacyclin [*see Figure 2*].

Bleeding Disorders

INHERITED COAGULOPATHIES

Numerous congenital abnormalities of the coagulation system have been identified. In particular, various abnormalities involving plasma proteins (e.g., hemophilia and vWD), platelet receptors (e.g., Glanzmann thrombasthenia and Bernard-Soulier syndrome), and endothelium (e.g., telangiectasia) have been described in detail. For the sake of brevity, we will refer to abnormal protein synthesis resulting in a dysfunctional coagulation protein as a defect and to abnormal protein synthesis resulting in decreased protein production as a deficiency.

Most of the coagulation defects associated with endothelium are closely related to thrombosis or atherosclerosis. Defects or deficiencies of thrombomodulin, TFPI, and t-PA, albeit rare, are associated with thrombosis.[37,38] Vascular defects (e.g., hemorrhagic telangiectasias) may carry an increased risk of bleeding as a consequence of dysfunctional fibrinolysis, concomitant platelet dysfunction, or coagulation factor deficiencies.[39]

Defects or deficiencies of RBCs and WBCs have other primary clinical manifestations that are not related to hemostasis. Alterations in the physical properties of blood (e.g., decreased blood flow from increased viscosity, polycythemia vera, leukocytosis, and sickle-cell anemia) have been reported to lead to thrombosis, but usually not to major bleeding.

Inherited platelet membrane receptor defects are relatively common. Of these, vWD is the one that most frequently causes bleeding.[40] The condition is characterized by vWF abnormalities, which may take three forms: vWF may be present in a reduced concentration (type I vWD), dysfunctional (type II vWD), or absent altogether (type III). Diagnosis of vWD is based on a combination of the patient history (e.g., previous mucosal bleeding) and laboratory parameters [*see Laboratory Assessment of Bleeding, below*]. It is necessary to identify the correct type or subtype of vWD: some treatments (e.g., DDAVP) are contraindicated in patients with type IIb vWD.[41]

Less common receptor defects include Glanzmann thrombasthenia (a defect in the GPIIb-IIIa complex), Bernard-Soulier syndrome (a defect in the GPIb-IX complex), and Scott syndrome (a defect in the platelet's activated surface that promotes thrombin formation); other agonist receptors on the platelet membrane may be affected as well.[42,43] Intracellular platelet defects are relatively rare but do occur; examples are gray platelet syndromes (e.g., alpha granule defects), Hermansky-Pudlak syndrome, dense granule defects, Wiskott-Aldrich syndrome, and various defects in intracellular production and signaling (involving defects of cyclooxygenase synthase and phospholipase C, respectively).[43]

Numerous pathologic states are also associated with deficiencies or defects of plasma procoagulants. Inherited sex-linked deficiencies of factor VIII (i.e., hemophilia A) and factor IX (i.e., hemophilia B and Christmas disease) are relatively common.[44-46] The clinical presentations of hemophilia A and hemophilia B are similar: hemarthroses are the most common clinical manifestations, ultimately leading to degenerative joint deformities. Spontaneous bleeding may also occur, resulting in intracranial hemorrhage, large hematomas in the muscles of extremities, hematuria, and GI bleeding. Factor XI deficiency is relatively common in Jewish persons but rarely results in spontaneous bleeding.[47,48] Such deficiency may result in bleeding after oral operations and trauma; however, there are a number of major procedures (e.g., cardiac bypass surgery) that do not result in postoperative bleeding in this population.[49]

Inherited deficiencies of the other coagulation factors are very rare. Factor XIII deficiencies result in delayed postoperative or posttraumatic bleeding. Congenital deficiencies of factor V, factor VII, factor X, prothrombin, and fibrinogen may become apparent in the neonatal period (presenting, for example, as umbilical stump bleeding); later in life, they result in clinical presentations such as epistaxis, intracranial bleeding, GI bleeding, deep and superficial bruising, and menorrhagia.

Defects or deficiencies in the fibrinolytic pathway are also rare and are most commonly associated with thromboembolic events. α_2-Antiplasmin deficiencies and primary fibrin(ogen)olysis are rare congenital coagulopathies with clinical presentations similar to those of factor deficiencies. In primary fibrin(ogen)olysis, failure of regulation of t-PA and u-PA leads to increases in circulating plasmin levels, which result in rapid degradation of clot and fibrinogen.[50,51]

ACQUIRED COAGULOPATHIES

A wide range of clinical conditions may cause deficiencies of the primary, secondary, or fibrinolytic pathways. Acquired coagulopathies are very common, and most do not result in spontaneous bleeding. (DIC is an exception [see below].)

As noted, coagulopathies related to the endothelium are primarily associated with thrombosis rather than bleeding. There are a number of disorders that may cause vascular injury, including sickle-cell anemia, hemolytic-uremic syndrome, and thrombotic thrombocytopenic purpura.

Acquired platelet abnormalities, both qualitative (i.e., dysfunction) and quantitative (i.e., decreases in absolute numbers), are common occurrences. Many acquired thrombocytopathies are attributable to either foods (e.g., fish oils, chocolate, red wine, garlic, and herbs) or drugs (e.g., aspirin, ibuprofen, other nonsteroidal anti-inflammatory drugs, ticlopidine, various antibiotics, certain antihistamines, and phenytoin).[52-56] Direct anti–platelet receptor drugs (e.g., abciximab and eptifibatide) block the GPIIb-IIIa complex, thereby preventing platelet aggregation.[57] Thrombocytopenia can be primary or secondary to a number of clinical conditions. Primary bone disorders (e.g., myelodysplastic or myelophthisic syndromes) and spontaneous bleeding may arise when platelet counts fall below 10,000/mm^3. Thrombocytopenia can be associated with immune causes (e.g., immune thrombocytopenic purpura or thrombotic thrombocytopenic purpura) or can occur secondary to administration of drugs (e.g., heparin). Acquired platelet dysfunction (e.g., acquired vWD) that is not related to dietary or pharmacologic causes has been observed in patients with immune disorders or cancer.

Acquired plasma factor deficiencies are common as well. Patients with severe renal disease typically exhibit platelet dysfunction (from excessive amounts of uremic metabolites), factor deficiencies associated with impaired synthesis or protein loss (as with increased urinary excretion), or thrombocytopenia (from diminished thrombopoietin production).[58,59] Patients with severe hepatic disease commonly have impairment of coagulation factor synthesis, increases in circulating levels of paraproteins, and splenic sequestration of platelets.

Hemodilution from massive RBC transfusions can occur if more than 10 packed RBC units are given within a short period without plasma supplementation. Immunologic reactions to ABO/Rh mismatches can induce immune-mediated hypercoagulation. Acquired multifactorial deficiencies associated with extracorporeal circuits (e.g., cardiopulmonary bypass, hemodialysis, and continuous venovenous dialysis) can arise as a consequence of hemodilution of circuit priming fluid or activation of procoagulants after exposure to thrombogenic surfaces.[60-62] Thrombocytopenia can result from platelet destruction and activation caused by circuit membrane exposure, or it can be secondary to the presence of heparin antibody.

Animal venoms can be either procoagulant or prothrombotic. The majority of the poisonous snakes in the United States (rattlesnakes in particular) have venom that works by activating prothrom-

bin, but cross-breeding has produced a number of new venoms with different hemostatic consequences. The clinical presentation of coagulopathies associated with snakebites generally mimics that of consumptive coagulopathies.[63]

Drug-induced factor deficiencies are common, particularly as a result of anticoagulant therapy. The most commonly used anticoagulants are heparin and warfarin. Heparin does not cause a factor deficiency; rather, it accelerates production of antithrombin, which inhibits factor IXa, factor Xa, and thrombin, thereby prolonging clot formation. Warfarin reduces procoagulant potential by inhibiting vitamin K synthesis, thereby reducing carboxylation of factor VII, factor IX, factor X, prothrombin, and proteins C and S. Newer drugs that may also cause factor deficiencies include direct thrombin inhibitors (e.g., lepirudin and bivalirudin[64]) and fibrinogen-degrading drugs (e.g., ancrod[65]).

Isolated acquired factor deficiencies are relatively rare. Clinically, they present in exactly the same way as inherited factor deficiencies, except that there is no history of earlier bleeding. In most cases, there is a secondary disease (e.g., lymphoma or an autoimmune disorder) that results in the development of antibody to a procoagulant (e.g., factor V, factor VIII, factor IX, vWF, prothrombin, or fibrinogen).[66-68]

Disseminated Intravascular Coagulation

DIC is a complex coagulation process that involves activation of the coagulation system with resultant activation of the fibrinolytic pathway and deposition of fibrin; the eventual consequence is the multiple organ dysfunction syndrome (MODS).[69] The activation occurs at all levels (platelets, endothelium, and procoagulants), but it is not known whether this process is initiated by a local stimulus or a systemic one. It is crucial to emphasize that DIC is an acquired disorder that occurs secondary to an underlying clinical event (e.g., a complicated birth, severe gram-negative infection, shock, major head injury, polytrauma, severe burns, or cancer. As noted [see Measurement of Coagulation Parameters, Increased INR, Prolonged aPTT, *above*], there is some controversy regarding the best approach to therapy, but there is no doubt that treating the underlying cause of DIC is paramount to patient recovery.

DIC is not always clinically evident: low-grade DIC may lack clinical symptoms altogether and manifest itself only through laboratory abnormalities, even when thrombin generation and fibrin deposition are occurring. In an attempt to facilitate recognition of DIC, the disorder has been divided into three phases, distinguished on the basis of clinical and laboratory evidence. In phase I DIC, there are no clinical symptoms, and the routine screening tests (i.e., INR, aPTT, fibrinogen level, and platelet count) are within normal limits.[70] Secondary testing (i.e., measurement of antithrombin, prothrombin fragment, thrombin-antithrombin complex, and soluble fibrin levels) may reveal subtle changes indicative of thrombin generation. In phase II DIC, there are usually clinical signs of bleeding around wounds, suture sites, I.V. sites, or venous puncture sites, and decreased function is noted in specific organs (e.g., lung, liver, and kidneys). The INR is increased, the aPTT is prolonged, and the fibrinogen level and platelet count are decreased or decreasing. Other markers of thrombin generation and fibrinolysis (e.g., D-dimer level) show sizable elevations. In phase III DIC, MODS is observed, the INR and the aPTT are markedly increased, and fibrinogen and D-dimer levels are markedly depressed. A peripheral blood smear would show large numbers of schistocytes, indicating RBC shearing resulting from fibrin deposition.

The activation of the coagulation system seen in DIC appears to be primarily caused by TF. The brain, the placenta, and solid tumors are all rich sources of TF. Gram-negative endotoxins also in-

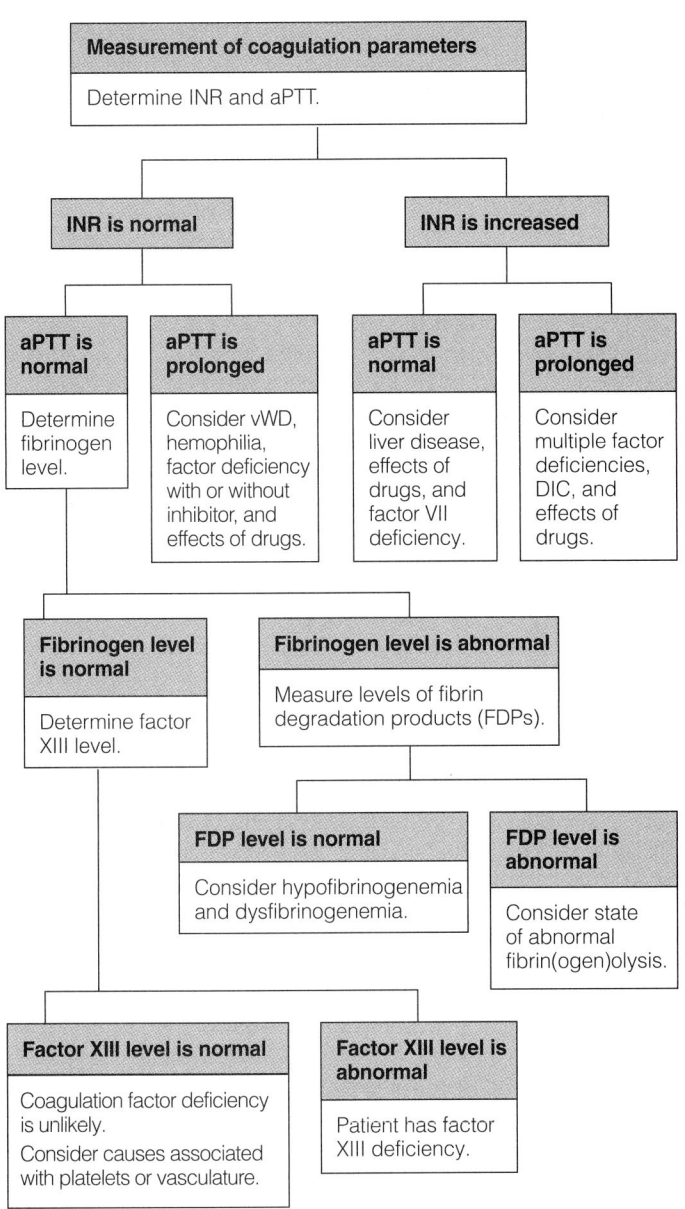

Figure 3 Algorithm depicts use of coagulation parameters in assessment of coagulopathies.

but it is imperative that blood samples for coagulation testing be drawn before therapy. The development of microprocessor technology has made it possible to perform diagnostic laboratory testing outside the confines of the clinical laboratory (so-called near-care testing). Whether near-care testing or clinical laboratory testing is employed, it is important to recognize that valuable as such testing is, it does not provide all of the needed diagnostic information.

In particular, the value of a careful patient history must not be underestimated. Previous bleeding events and a familial history of bleeding are both suggestive of a congenital coagulopathy. A thorough medication inventory is necessary to assess the possible impact of drugs on laboratory and clinical presentations. In the patient history query, it is advisable to ask explicitly about nonprescription drugs—using expressions such as "over-the-counter drugs," "cold medicines," and "Pepto-Bismol"—because unless specifically reminded, patients tend to equate the term medications with prescription drugs. If this is not done, many drugs that are capable of influencing hemostasis in vivo and in vitro (e.g., salicylates, cold and allergy medicines, and herbal supplements) may be missed. Mucosal and superficial bleeding is suggestive of platelet abnormalities, and deep bleeding is suggestive of factor deficiency.

It is important to be clear on the limitations of coagulation testing. At present, there are no laboratory or ex vivo methods capable of directly measuring the physiologic properties of the endothelium. Indirect assessments of endothelial damage can be obtained by

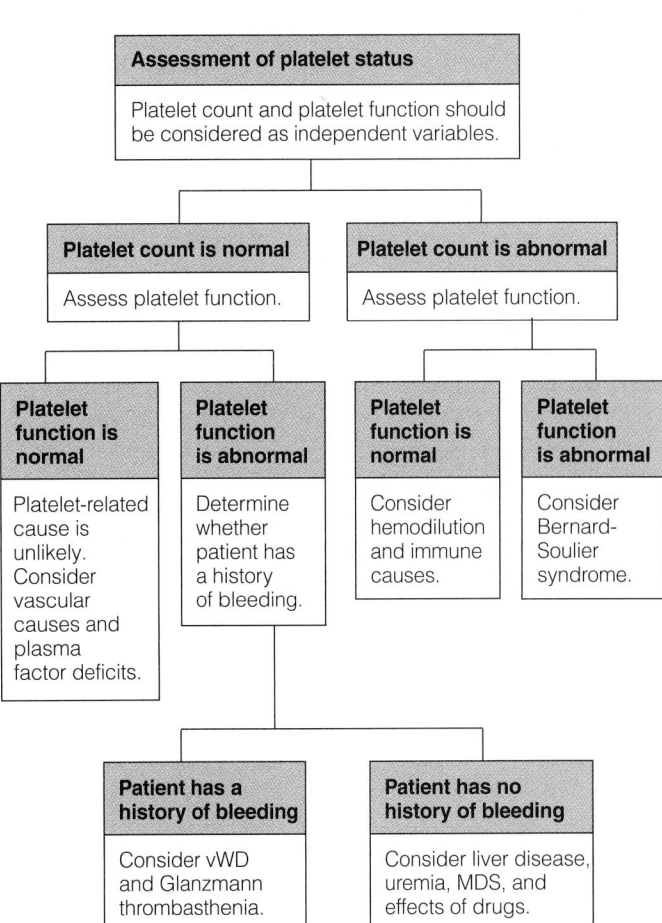

Figure 4 Algorithm depicts use of platelet count and platelet functional status in assessment of coagulopathies.

duce TF expression. The exposure of TF on cellular surfaces causes activation of factors VII and IX, which ultimately leads to thrombin generation. Circulating thrombin is rapidly cleared by antithrombin. Moreover, the coagulation pathway is downregulated by activated protein C and protein S. However, constant exposure of TF (as a result of underlying disorders) results in constant generation of thrombin, and these regulator proteins are rapidly consumed. TAFI and PAI also contribute to fibrin deposition by restricting fibrinolysis and subsequent fibrin degradation and clearance. Finally, it is likely that release of cytokines (e.g., IL-6, IL-10, and TNF) may play some role in causing the sequelae of DIC by modulating or activating the coagulation pathway.

Laboratory Assessment of Bleeding

Laboratory testing is an integral part of the diagnostic algorithm used in assessing the bleeding patient. It may not be prudent to wait for laboratory values before beginning treatment of acute bleeding,

Table 5 Tests of Platelet Function

Product (Manufacturer)	Method
PFA-100 (Dade Behring)	Measures time required to occlude aperture after exposure to platelet agonists at shear rates
hemoSTATUS (Medtronic)	Measures activated clotting time; platelet-activating factor is the platelet agonist
AggreStat (Centocor)	Measures changes in voltage (impedance) after addition of platelet agonist
Thromboelastograph (Haemascope)	Measures changes in the viscoelastic properties of clotting blood induced by a rotating piston
Sonoclot Analyzer (Sienco)	Measures changes in the viscoelastic properties of clotting blood induced by a vibrating probe
Clot Signature Analyzer (Xylum)	Measures changes in platelet function at shear rates
Ultegra Analyzer (Accumetrics)	Used primarily for measuring the effect of platelet glycoprotein blockers (e.g., abciximab and eptifibatide); thrombin receptor activator peptide is the agonist

measuring levels of several laboratory parameters (e.g., vWF, the soluble cytokines endothelian-1 and E-selectin, and thrombomodulin), but such measurements have no clinical utility in the assessment of a bleeding patient.

Another issue is that of bias resulting from technical factors. PT (i.e., INR) and aPTT testing involves adding activators, phospholipids, and calcium to plasma in a test tube (or the equivalent) and determining the time to clot formation. Time to clot formation is a relative value, in that it is compared with the time in a normal population. A perturbation within the coagulation cascade, an excess of calcium, or poor sampling techniques (e.g., inadequately filled coagulation tubes, excessive tourniquet time, and clotted or activated samples) can bias the results. Hemolysis from the drawing of blood can also bias results via the effects of thromboplastins released from RBC membranes to initiate the coagulation process. In addition, many coagulation factors are highly labile, and failure to process and run coagulation samples immediately can bias test results.

Finally, not all coagulation tests are functionally equivalent: different laboratory methods may yield differing results.[71] Coagulation reagents have been manufactured in such a way as to ensure that the coagulation screening tests are sensitive to factor VIII and IX deficiencies and the effects of anticoagulation with warfarin or heparin. Thus, a normal aPTT in a patient with an abnormal INR may not exclude the possibility of common pathway deficiencies (e.g., deficiencies of factors X, V, and II), and most current methods of determining the INR and the aPTT do not detect low fibrinogen levels. The approach we use assumes that the methods used to assess INR and aPTT can discriminate normal factor activity levels from abnormal levels (< 0.4 IU/ml).

The CBC (including platelet count and differential count), the INR, and the aPTT tests should be the primary laboratory tests for differentiating coagulopathies [*see Figure 3*].

Platelet count and platelet function should be considered as independent values [*see Figure 4*]. Patients with congenital thrombocytopathies often have normal platelet counts; therefore, assessment of platelet function is required as well. Historically, the bleeding time has been used to assess platelet function. This test is grossly inadequate, in that it may yield normal results in as many as 50% of patients with congenital thrombocytopathies.[72,73] Numerous rapid tests of platelet function are currently available that can be used to screen for platelet defects; these tests can and should be included in the diagnostic approach to the bleeding patient [*see Table 5*].[73-75]

Experimental Therapy for Bleeding

Novel approaches to controlling bleeding have been developed for use in two specific patient groups: (1) patients with uncontrolled exsanguinating hemorrhage and (2) elderly patients on warfarin therapy who have a therapeutic INR and who present with intracranial bleeding.

As noted [*see Measurement of Coagulation Parameters, Normal INR, Prolonged aPTT, above*], recombinant factor VIIa is currently used for control of bleeding in hemophilia A patients with antibodies to factors VIII as well as in hemophilia B patients with antibodies to factor IX, and it has received FDA approval for this indication. The remarkable success of rVIIa in this setting led many investigators to consider the possibility that giving this agent to actively bleeding patients would enhance the normal clotting mechanism and provide nonsurgical control or reduction of traumatic bleeding. Accordingly, rVIIa has been advocated for early use in injured patients with uncontrolled hemorrhage. Preliminary results from an Israeli study appeared promising in this regard.[76] The investigators found that patients had less need for transfusion and exhibited improved coagulation parameters after administration of rVIIa. Although the study was not controlled, the 43% mortality was judged to have been lower than would have been expected without the intervention. Several controlled trials have been done in animal models, with mixed results.[77-79] This experimental approach is currently being explored by the National Institutes of Health and the United States Department of Defense. Before rVIIa can be recommended as therapy for uncontrolled bleeding in trauma patients or patients with DIC, prospective controlled human trials must be done.

In elderly patients receiving therapeutic warfarin therapy, head injuries that would normally be inconsequential can result in life-threatening intracranial bleeding. Correction of the INR with either FFP or vitamin K may take so long that the patient becomes vegetative before the hemorrhage is controlled. Prothrombin complex concentrate appears to correct the INR more rapidly and effectively than FFP or vitamin K.[80] As with rVIIa, prospective controlled trials will have to be done before routine use of prothrombin complex for the correction of elevated INR in this patient population can be recommended.

References

1. Bickell WH, Wall MJ Jr, Pepe PE, et al: Immediate versus delayed fluid resuscitation for hypotensive patients with penetrating torso injuries. N Engl J Med 331: 1105, 1994

2. Gubler KD, Gentilello LM, Hassantash SA, et al: The impact of hypothermia on dilutional coagulopathy. J Trauma 36:847, 1994

3. Watts DD, Trask A, Soeken K, et al: Hypothermic coagulopathy in trauma: effect of varying levels of hypothermia on enzyme speed, platelet function, and fibrinolytic activity. J Trauma 44:846, 1998

4. Gentilello LM, Jurkovich GJ, Stark MS, et al: Is hypothermia in the victim of major trauma protective or harmful? A randomized, prospective study. Ann Surg 226:439, 1997

5. Rapaport SI: Blood coagulation and its alterations in hemorrhagic and thrombotic disorders. West J Med 158:153, 1993

6. Practice guidelines for blood component therapy: a report by the American Society of Anesthesiologists Task Force on Blood Component Therapy. Anesthesiology 84:732, 1996

7. Heckman KD, Weiner GJ, Davis CS, et al: Randomized study of prophylactic platelet transfusion threshold during induction therapy for adult acute leukemia: 10,000/μL versus 20,000/μL. J Clin Oncol 15:1143, 1997

8. Dyke CM, Bhatia D, Lorenz TJ, et al: Immediate coronary artery bypass surgery after platelet inhibition with eptifibatide: results from PURSUIT. Platelet Glycoprotein IIb/IIIa in Unstable Angina: Receptor Suppression Using Integrelin Therapy. Ann Thorac Surg 70:866, 2000

9. Despotis GJ, Levine V, Saleem R, et al: Use of point-of-care test in identification of patients who can benefit from desmopressin during cardiac surgery: a randomised controlled trial. Lancet 354:106, 1999

10. Levy JH, Schwieger IM, Zaidan JR, et al: Evaluation of patients at risk for protamine reactions. J Thorac Cardiovasc Surg 98:200, 1989

11. Fenton JW 2nd, Ofosu FA, Brezniak DV, et al: Thrombin and antithrombotics. Semin Thromb Hemost 24:87, 1998

12. Hirsh J, Dalen JE, Anderson DR, et al: Oral anticoagulants: mechanism of action, clinical effectiveness, and optimal therapeutic range. Chest 114(5 suppl):445S, 1998

13. Murray DJ, Pennell BJ, Weinstein SL, et al: Packed red cells in acute blood loss: dilutional coagulopathy as a cause of surgical bleeding. Anesth Analg 80:336, 1995

14. Holcroft JW, Blaisdell FW, Trunkey DD, et al: Intravascular coagulation and pulmonary edema in the septic baboon. J Surg Res 22:209, 1977

15. Owings JT, Bagley M, Gosselin R, et al: Effect of critical injury on plasma antithrombin activity: low antithrombin levels are associated with thromboembolic complications. J Trauma 41:396, 1996

16. Weitzel JN, Sadowski JA, Furie BC, et al: Surreptitious ingestion of a long-acting vitamin K antagonist/rodenticide, brodifacoum: clinical and metabolic studies of three cases. Blood 76:2555, 1990

17. Hébert PC, Wells G, Blajchman MA, et al: A multicenter, randomized, controlled clinical trial of transfusion requirements in critical care. Transfusion Requirements in Critical Care Investigators, Canadian Critical Care Trials Group. N Engl J Med 340:409, 1999

18. Maxwell RA, Gibson JB, Fabian TC, et al: Resuscitation of severe chest trauma with four different hemoglobin-based oxygen-carrying solutions. J Trauma 49: 200, 2000

19. Creteur J, Sibbald W, Vincent JL: Hemoglobin solutions—not just red blood cell substitutes. Crit Care Med 28:3025, 2000

20. Mantovani A, Sozzani S, Vecchi A, et al: Cytokine activation of endothelial cells: new molecules for an old paradigm. Thromb Haemost 78:406, 1997

21. Edington TS, Mackman N, Brand K, et al: The structural biology of expression and function of tissue factor. Thromb Haemost 66:67, 1991

22. Vane JR, Anggard EE, Botting RM: Regulatory function of the vascular endothelium. N Engl J Med 323: 27, 1990

23. Ignarro LJ, Buga GM, Wood KS, et al: Endothelium-derived relaxing factor produced and released from artery and vein is nitric oxide. Proc Natl Acad Sci 84:9265, 1987

24. ten Cate JW, van der Poll T, Levi M, et al: Cytokines: triggers of clinical thrombotic disease. Thromb Haemost 78:415, 1997

25. Cerletti C, Evangelista V, de Gaetano G: P-selectin-β2-integrin crosstalk: a molecular mechanism for polymorphonuclear leukocyte recruitment at the site of vascular damage. Thromb Haemost 82:787, 1999

26. Brunetti M, Martelli N, Manarini S, et al: Polymorphonuclear apoptosis is inhibited by platelet mediated-released mediators, role of TGFβ-1. Thromb Haemost 84:478, 2000

27. Stel HV, Sakariassen KS, de Groot PG, et al: Von-Willebrand factor in the vessel wall mediates platelet adherence. Blood 65:85, 1985

28. Michelson AD, Barnard MR: Thrombin-induced changes in platelet membrane glycoproteins Ib, IX, and IIb-IIIa complex. Blood 70:1673, 1987

29. Motta G, Rojkjaer R, Hasan AA, et al: High molecular weight kininogen regulates prekallikrein assembly and activation on endothelial cells: a novel mechanism for contact activation. Blood 91:516, 1998

30. Osterud B, Rappaport SI: Activation of factor IX by the reaction product of tissue factor and factor VII: additional pathway for initiating blood coagulation. Proc Natl Acad Sci USA 74:5260, 1997

31. Mann KG: Biochemistry and physiology of blood coagulation. Thromb Haemost 82:165, 1999

32. Collen D, Lijnen HR: Basic and clinical aspects of fibrinolysis and thrombolysis. Blood 78:3114, 1991

33. Chetaille P, Alessi MC, Kouassi D, et al: Plasma TAFI antigen variations in healthy subjects. Thromb Haemost 83:902, 2000

34. Esmon CT, Owen WG: Identification of an endothelial cell cofactor for thrombin-catalyzed activation of protein C. Proc Natl Acad Sci USA 78:2249, 1981

35. Broze GJ, Warren LA, Novotny WF, et al: The lipoprotein-associated coagulation inhibitor that inhibits factor Xa: insight into its possible mechanism of action. Blood 71:335, 1988

36. Schmidt B, Mitchell L, Ofosu FA, et al: Alpha-2-macroglobulin is an important progressive inhibitor of thrombin in neonatal and infant plasma. Thromb Haemost 62:1074, 1989

37. Juhan-Vague I, Valadier J, Alessi MC, et al: Deficient tPA release and elevated PA inhibitor levels on patients with spontaneous recurrent DVT. Thromb Haemost 57:67, 1987

38. Korninger C, Lechner K, Niessner H, et al: Impaired fibrinolytic capacity predisposes for recurrence of venous thrombosis. Thromb Haemost 52:127, 1984

39. Shovlin CL: Molecular defects in rare bleeding disorders: hereditary hemorrhagic telangiectasia. Thromb Haemost 78:145, 1997

40. Sadler JE, Mannucci PM, Berntop E, et al: Impact, diagnosis, and treatment of von Willebrand's disease. Thromb Haemost 84:160, 2000

41. Mannucci PM: Desmopressin: a nontransfusional form of treatment for congenital and acquired bleeding disorders. Blood 72:1449, 1988

42. Weiss HJ: Congenital disorders of platelet function. Semin Thromb Hemost 17:228, 1980

43. Nurden AT: Inherited abnormalities of platelets. Thromb Haemost 82:468, 1999

44. Ljung RC: Prenatal diagnosis of haemophilia. Haemophilia 5:84, 1999

45. Lillicrap D: Molecular diagnosis of inherited bleeding disorders and thrombophilia. Semin Hematol 36:340, 1999

46. Cawthern KM, van't Veer C, Lock JB, et al: Blood coagulation in hemophilia A and hemophilia C. Blood 91:4581, 1998

47. Rodriguez-Merchan EC: Common orthopaedic problems in haemophilia. Haemophilia 5[suppl 1]:53, 1999

48. Mannucci PM, Tuddenbam EG: The hemophilias: progress and problems. Semin Hematol 36[4 suppl 7]: 104, 1999

49. Bolton-Maggs PH: The management of factor XI deficiency. Haemophilia 4:683, 1998

50. Minowa H, Takahashi Y, Tanaka T, et al: Four cases of bleeding diathesis in children due to congenital plasminogen activator inhibitor-1 deficiency. Haemostasis 29:286, 1999

51. Lind B, Thorsen S: A novel missense mutation in the human plasmin inhibitor (alpha2-antiplasmin) gene associated with a bleeding tendency. Br J Haematol 107:317, 1999

52. Turpeinen AM, Mutanen M: Similar effects of diets high in oleic or linoleic acids on coagulation and fibrinolytic factors in healthy humans. Nutr Metab Cardiovasc Dis 9(2):65, 1999

53. Li D, Sinclair A, Mann N, et al: The association of diet and thrombotic risk factors in healthy male vegetarians and meat-eaters. Eur J Clin Nutr 53:612, 1999

54. Temme EH, Mensink RP, Hornstra G: Effects of diets enriched in lauric, palmitic or oleic acids on blood coagulation and fibrinolysis. Thromb Haemost 81:259, 1999

55. Rein D, Paglieroni T, Wun T, et al: Cocoa inhibits platelet activation and function. Am J Clin Nutr 72: 30, 2000

56. Rein D, Paglieroni T, Wun T, et al: Cocoa and wine polyphenols modulate platelet activation and function. J Nutr 130:2120S, 2000

57. Bhatt DL, Topol EJ: Current role of platelet glycoprotein IIb/IIIa inhibitors in acute coronary syndromes. JAMA 284:1549, 2000

58. Humphries JE: Transfusion therapy in acquired coagulopathies. Hematol Oncol Clin North Am 8:1181, 1994

59. Zachee P, Vermylen J, Boogaerts MA: Hematologic aspects of end-stage renal failure. Ann Hematol 69:33, 1994

60. Peek GJ, Firmin RK: The inflammatory and coagulative response to prolonged extracorporeal membrane oxygenation. ASAIO J 45:250, 1999

61. Hobisch-Hagen P, Wirleitner B, Mair J, et al: Consequences of acute normovolaemic haemodilution on haemostasis during major orthopaedic surgery. Br J Anaesth 82:503, 1999

62. Konrad C, Markl T, Schuepfer G, et al: The effects of in vitro hemodilution with gelatin, hydroxyethyl starch, and lactated Ringer's solution on markers of coagulation: an analysis using SONOCLOT. Anesth Analg 88:483, 1999

63. Boyer LV, Seifert SA, Clark RF, et al: Recurrent and persistent coagulopathy following pit viper envenomation. Arch Intern Med 159:706, 1999

64. Eriksson BI, Kalebo P, Ekman S, et al: Direct thrombin inhibition with rec-hirudin CGP 39393 as prophylaxis of thromboembolic complications after total hip replacement. Thromb Haemost 72:227, 1994

65. Sherman DG, Atkinson RP, Chippendale T, et al: Intravenous ancrod for treatment of acute ischemic stroke: the STAT study: a randomized controlled trial. Stroke Treatment with Ancrod Trial. JAMA 282:

2395, 2000

66. Oleksowicz L, Bhagwati N, DeLeon-Fernandez M: Deficient activity of von Willebrand's factor-cleaving protease in patients with disseminated malignancies. Cancer Res 59:2244, 1999

67. Francis JL, Biggerstaff J, Amirkhosravi A: Hemostasis and malignancy. Semin Thromb Hemost 24:93, 1998

68. Amirkhosravi M, Francis JL: Coagulation activation by MC28 fibrosarcoma cells facilitates lung tumor formation. Thromb Haemost 73:59, 1995

69. Williams EC, Moshen DF: Disseminated intravascular coagulation. Hematology: Basic Principles and Practice. Hoffman R, Benz EJ Sr, Shattil SJ, et al, Eds. Churchill-Livingstone, New York, 1995, p 1758

70. Muller-Berghaus G, ten Cate H, Levi M: Disseminated intravascular coagulation: clinical spectrum and established as well as new diagnostic approaches. Thromb Haemost 82:706, 1999

71. Lawrie AS, Kitchen S, Purdy G, et al: Assessment of Actin FS and Actin FSL sensitivity to specific clotting factor deficiencies. Clin Lab Haematol 20:179, 1998

72. Lind SE: The bleeding time does not predict surgical bleeding. Blood 77:2547, 1991

73. Mammen EF, Comp PC, Gosselin R, et al: PFA-100™ System: A new method for assessment of platelet dysfunction. Semin Thromb Hemost 24:195, 1998

74. Speiss BD: Coagulation function in the operating room. Anesth Clin North Am 8:481, 1990

75. LeForce WR, Bruno DS, Kanot WP, et al: Evaluation of the Sonoclot analyzer for the measurement of platelet function in whole blood. Am Clin Lab Sci 22:30, 1992

76. Martinowitz U, Kenet G, Segal E, et al: Recombinant activated factor VII for adjunctive hemorrhage control in trauma. J Trauma 51:431, 2001

77. Lynn M, Jerokhimov I, Jewelewicz D, et al: Early use of recombinant factor VIIa improves mean arterial pressure and may potentially decrease mortality in experimental hemorrhagic shock: a pilot study. J Trauma 52:703, 2002

78. Jeroukhimov I, Jewelewicz D, Zaias J, et al: Early injection of high-dose recombinant factor VIIa decreases blood loss and prolongs time from injury to death in experimental liver injury. J Trauma 53:1053, 2002

79. Schreiber MA, Holcomb JB, Hedner U, et al: The effect of recombinant factor VIIa on noncoagulopathic pigs with grade V liver injuries. J Am Coll Surg 196:691, 2003

80. Cartmill M, Dolan G, Byrne JL, et al: Prothrombin complex concentrate for oral anticoagulant reversal in neurosurgical emergencies. Br J Neurosurg 14:458, 2000

81. Winslow RM: Blood substitutes. Adv Drug Deliv Rev 40:131, 2000

Acknowledgments

Figures 1, 3, and 4   Marcia Kammerer.

Figure 2   Seward Hung.

5 POSTOPERATIVE PAIN

Henrik Kehlet, M.D., Ph.D., F.A.C.S. (Hon.)

Approach to the Patient with Postoperative Pain

Pain may usefully be classified into two varieties: acute and chronic. As a rule, postoperative pain is considered a form of acute pain, although it may become chronic if it is not effectively treated.

Postoperative pain consists of a constellation of unpleasant sensory, emotional, and mental experiences associated with autonomic, psychological, and behavioral responses precipitated by the surgical injury. Despite the considerable progress that has been made in medicine during the past few decades, the apparently simple problem of how to provide total or near total relief of postoperative pain remains largely unsolved. Pain management does not occupy an important place in academic surgery. However, government agencies have recently attempted to foster improved postoperative pain relief,[1,2] and guidelines have been published.[3,4] In 2001, the Joint Commission on Accreditation of Healthcare Organizations (JCAHO) introduced standards for pain management,[5] stating that patients have the right to appropriate assessment and management and that pain must be assessed.

Postoperative pain relief has two practical aims. The first is provision of subjective comfort, which is desirable for humanitarian reasons. The second is inhibition of trauma-induced nociceptive impulses to blunt autonomic and somatic reflex responses to pain and to enhance subsequent restoration of function by allowing the patient to breathe, cough, and move more easily. Because these effects reduce pulmonary, cardiovascular, thromboembolic, and other complications, they may lead secondarily to improved postoperative outcome.

Inadequate Treatment of Pain

A common misconception is that pain, no matter how severe, can always be effectively relieved by opioid analgesics. It has repeatedly been demonstrated, however, that in a high proportion of postoperative patients, pain is inadequately treated.[6] This discrepancy between what is possible and what is practiced can be attributed to a variety of causes [*see Table 1*], which to some extent can be ameliorated by increased teaching efforts. In general, however, the scientific approach to postoperative pain relief has not been a great help to surgical patients in the general ward, where intensive surveillance facilities may not be available.

Guidelines for Postoperative Pain Treatment

The recommendations provided below are aimed at surgeons working on the general surgical ward; superior regimens have been

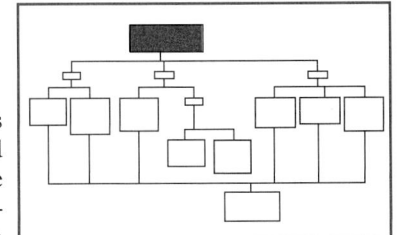

constructed by specialized groups interested in postoperative pain research, but these regimens are not currently applicable to the general surgical population, unless an acute pain service is available. Consideration is given to the efficiency of each analgesic technique, its safety versus its side effects, and the cost-efficiency problems arising from the need for intensive surveillance. For several analgesic techniques, evidence-based recommendations are now available.[7] For many others, however, there are not sufficient data in the literature to form a valid scientific database; accordingly, recommendations regarding their use are made on empirical grounds only.

THORACIC PROCEDURES

Pain after thoracotomy is severe, and pain therapy should therefore include a combination regimen, preferably of epidural local anesthetics and opioids plus systemic nonsteroidal anti-inflammatory drugs

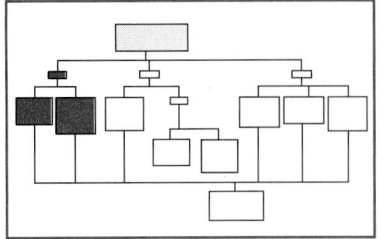

(NSAIDs) or cyclooxygenase-2 (COX-2) inhibitors.[8] If the epidural regimen is not available, NSAIDs and systemic opioids should be given to obtain the documented synergistic-additive effect. Cryoanalgesia is useful because it is moderately effective, easy to perform, free of significant side effects, and relatively inexpensive. Paravertebral blocks are also effective but necessitate continuous infusion. Acetaminophen is recommended as a basic analgesic for multimodal analgesia.

Pain after cardiac operation with sternotomy is less severe, and systemic opioids plus NSAIDs or COX-2 inhibitors are recommended. The combined regimen of epidural local anesthetics and opioids is recommended when more effective pain relief is necessary.

ABDOMINAL PROCEDURES

Pain after major and upper abdominal operations is severe, and a combined regimen of epidural local anesthetics and opioids plus systemic NSAIDs or COX-2 inhibitors is rec-

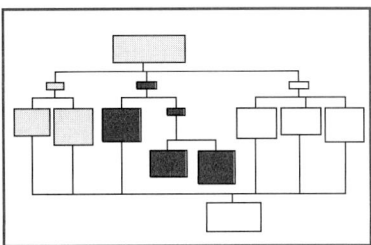

ommended because it has proved to be very effective and to have few and acceptable side effects.[9] Furthermore, the epidural regimen will reduce postoperative pulmonary complications and ileus, as compared with treatment with systemic opioids. Acetaminophen is recommended as a basic analgesic for multimodal analgesia.

After gynecologic operations, systemic opioids plus NSAIDs or COX-2 inhibitors are recommended except in patients in whom more effective pain relief is desirable. In such patients, the

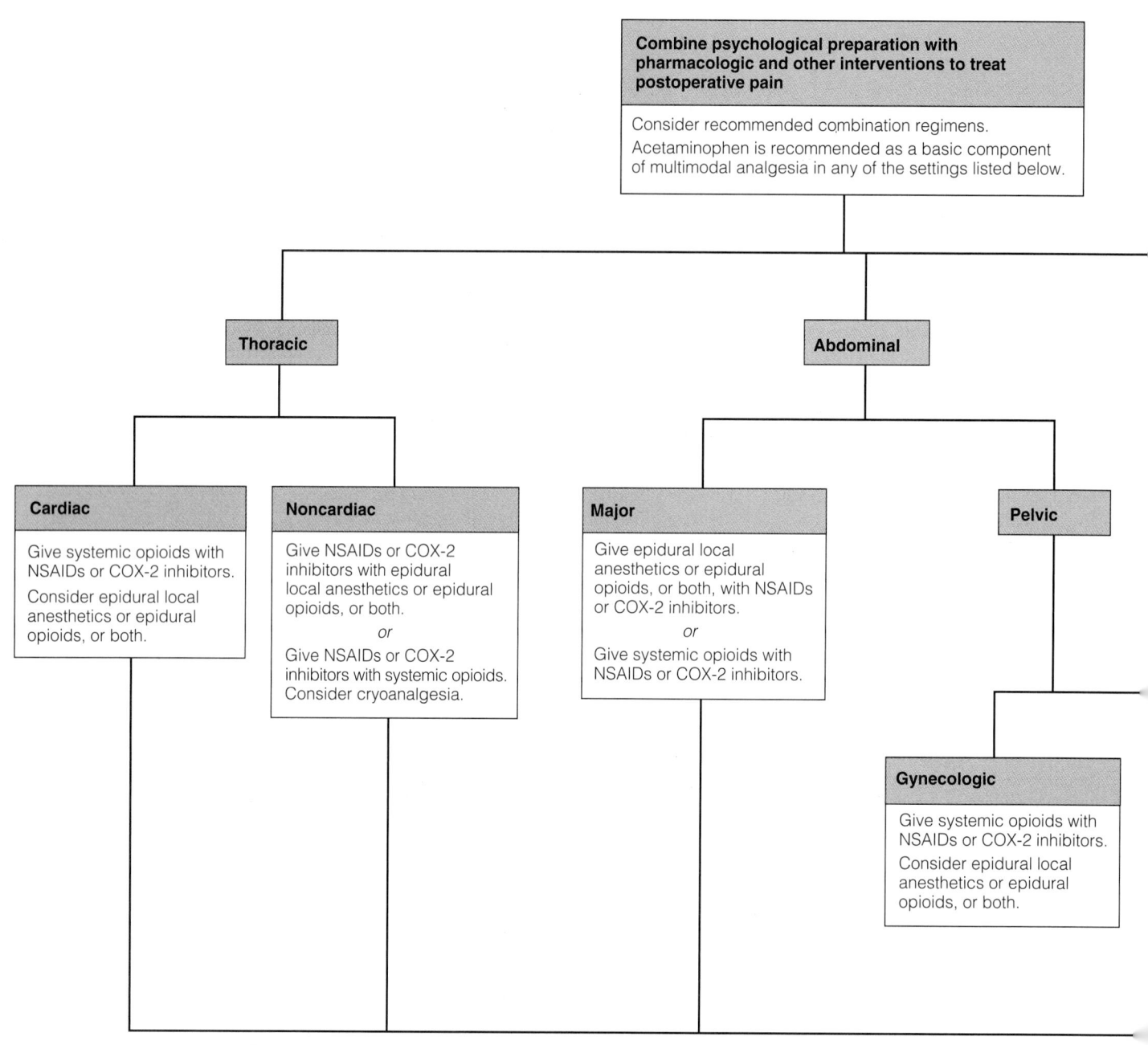

Combine psychological preparation with pharmacologic and other interventions to treat postoperative pain

Consider recommended combination regimens.
Acetaminophen is recommended as a basic component of multimodal analgesia in any of the settings listed below.

Thoracic

Abdominal

Cardiac

Give systemic opioids with NSAIDs or COX-2 inhibitors.

Consider epidural local anesthetics or epidural opioids, or both.

Noncardiac

Give NSAIDs or COX-2 inhibitors with epidural local anesthetics or epidural opioids, or both.

or

Give NSAIDs or COX-2 inhibitors with systemic opioids. Consider cryoanalgesia.

Major

Give epidural local anesthetics or epidural opioids, or both, with NSAIDs or COX-2 inhibitors.

or

Give systemic opioids with NSAIDs or COX-2 inhibitors.

Pelvic

Gynecologic

Give systemic opioids with NSAIDs or COX-2 inhibitors.

Consider epidural local anesthetics or epidural opioids, or both.

Approach to the Patient with Postoperative Pain

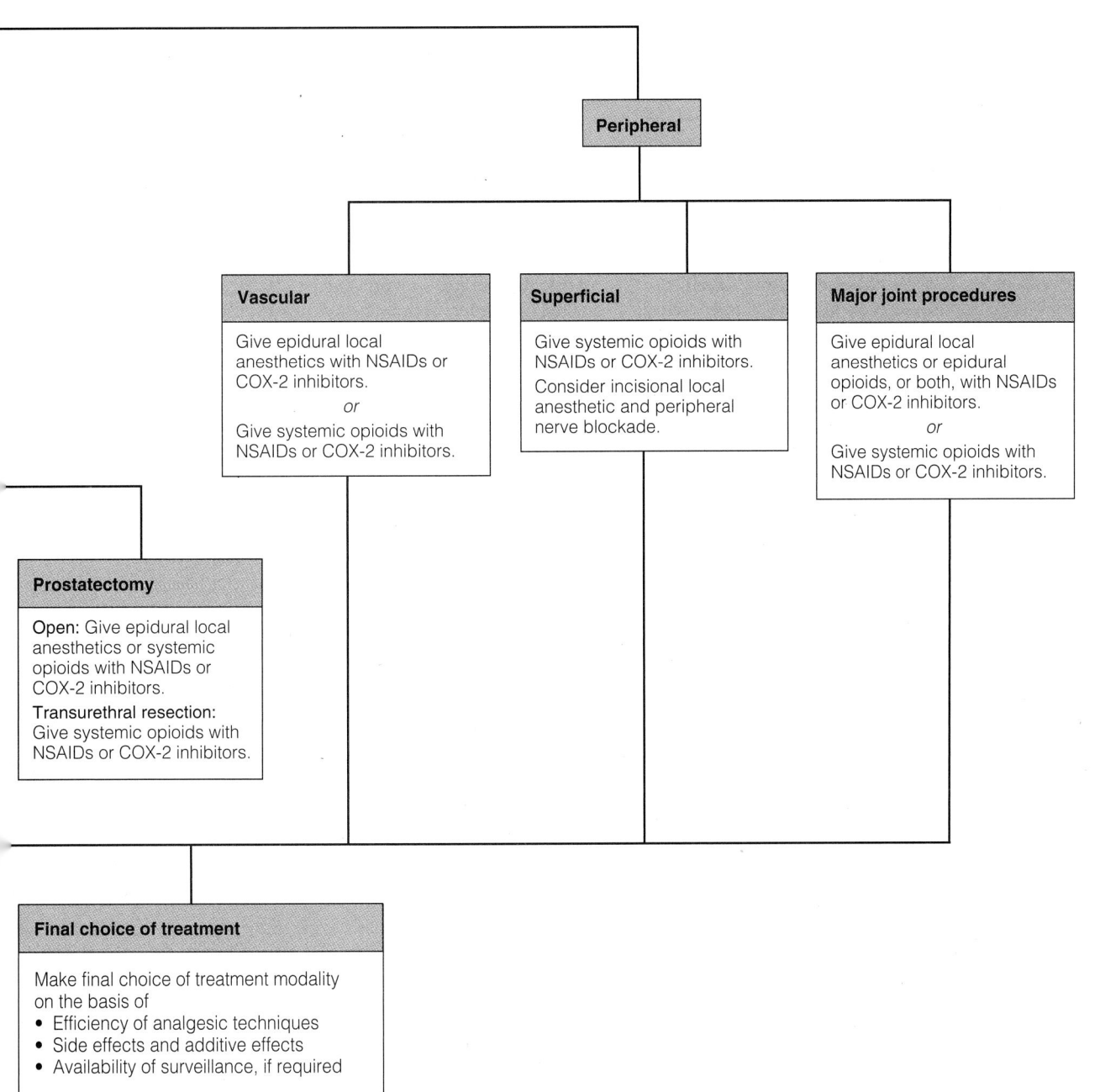

Peripheral

Vascular

Give epidural local anesthetics with NSAIDs or COX-2 inhibitors.

or

Give systemic opioids with NSAIDs or COX-2 inhibitors.

Superficial

Give systemic opioids with NSAIDs or COX-2 inhibitors.

Consider incisional local anesthetic and peripheral nerve blockade.

Major joint procedures

Give epidural local anesthetics or epidural opioids, or both, with NSAIDs or COX-2 inhibitors.

or

Give systemic opioids with NSAIDs or COX-2 inhibitors.

Prostatectomy

Open: Give epidural local anesthetics or systemic opioids with NSAIDs or COX-2 inhibitors.

Transurethral resection: Give systemic opioids with NSAIDs or COX-2 inhibitors.

Final choice of treatment

Make final choice of treatment modality on the basis of
- Efficiency of analgesic techniques
- Side effects and additive effects
- Availability of surveillance, if required

Table 1 Contributing Causes of Inadequate Pain Treatment

Insufficient knowledge of drug pharmacology among surgeons and nurses

Uniform (p.r.n.) prescriptions

Lack of concern for optimal pain relief

Failure to give prescribed analgesics

Fear of side effects

Fear of addiction

combined regimen of epidural local anesthetics and opioids is preferable, possibly in combination with systemic NSAIDs. Acetaminophen is recommended as a basic analgesic for multimodal analgesia.

Pain following prostatectomy is usually not severe and may be treated with systemic opioids combined with NSAIDs or COX-2 inhibitors and acetaminophen. However, blood loss and thromboembolic complications are reduced when epidural local anesthetics are administered. This method is therefore recommended intraoperatively and continued in selected high-risk patients for pain relief after open prostatectomy and transurethral resection. In low-risk patients, systemic opioids with NSAIDs or COX-2 inhibitors and acetaminophen alleviate postoperative pain.

PERIPHERAL PROCEDURES

After vascular procedures, postoperative pain control is probably best achieved with epidural local anesthetic–opioid mixtures, combined with systemic NSAIDs or COX-2 inhibi-

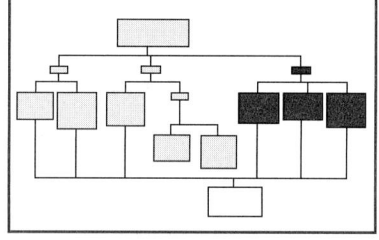

tors. Acetaminophen is recommended as a basic analgesic for multimodal analgesia. This regimen will be effective, and the increase in peripheral blood flow that is documented to occur with epidural local anesthetics may lower the risk of graft thrombosis.

Pain relief after major joint procedures (e.g., hip and knee operations) should also involve an epidural regimen because such

Table 2 Psychological Preparation of Surgical Patients

Procedural information Give a careful and relevant description of what will take place

Sensory information Describe the sensations that will be experienced either during or after the operation

Pain treatment information Outline the plan for administering sedative and analgesic medication, and encourage patients to communicate concerns and discomforts

Instructional information Teach patients postoperative exercises, such as leg exercises, and show them how to turn in bed or move so that pain is minimal

Reassurance Reassure those who are mentally, emotionally, or physically unable to cooperate that they are not expected to take an active role in coping with pain and will still receive sufficient analgesic treatment

regimens have been shown to reduce thromboembolic complications and intraoperative blood loss and to facilitate rehabilitation. The severe pain noted after knee replacement is probably best treated with epidural local anesthetics combined with opioids. If epidural regimens are not available, systemic opioids combined with NSAIDs or COX-2 inhibitors may provide moderately effective pain relief. Acetaminophen is provided as a basic analgesic for multimodal analgesia. After arthroscopic joint procedures, instillation of a local anesthetic and an opioid analgesic (e.g., morphine) provides effective early postoperative pain relief.

During superficial procedures, systemic opioids combined with NSAIDs or COX-2 inhibitors should suffice. Acetaminophen is provided as a basic analgesic for multimodal analgesia.

Treatment Modalities

PSYCHOLOGICAL INTERVENTIONS

Individuals differ considerably in how they respond to noxious stimuli; much of this variance

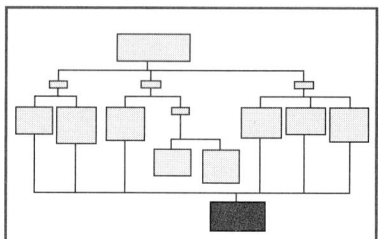

is accounted for by psychological factors. Cognitive, behavioral, or social interventions should be used in combination with pharmacologic therapies to prevent or control acute pain, with the goal of such interventions being to guide the patient toward partial or complete self-control of pain.[10,11] Sophisticated psychological techniques, such as biofeedback and hypnosis therapy, are not applicable to a busy surgical unit, but simple psychological techniques are a valuable part of good medical practice.

Psychological preparation in patients with postoperative pain has been demonstrated to shorten hospital stay and to reduce postoperative narcotic use [see Table 2].[12] Psychological techniques should be combined with pharmacologic or other interventions, but care must be taken to ensure that the pharmacologic treatment does not compromise the mental function necessary for the success of the planned psychological intervention.

SYSTEMIC OPIOIDS

The terminology associated with the pharmacology of the opioids is confusing, to say the least. Opiate is an appropriate term for any alkaloid derived from the juice of the plant (i.e., from opium). The proper term for the class of agents, whether exogenous, endogenous, natural, or synthetic, is opioid.

Mechanisms of Action

Opioids produce analgesia and other physiologic effects by binding to specific receptors in the peripheral and central nervous system [see Table 3]. These receptors normally bind a number of endogenous substances called opioid peptides. These receptor-binding interactions mediate a wide array of physiologic effects.[13] Five types of opioid receptors and their subtypes have been discovered: mu, delta, kappa, epsilon, and sigma receptors. Most commonly used opioids bind to mu receptors. The mu_1 receptor is responsible for the production of opioid-induced analgesia, whereas the mu_2 receptors appear to be related to the respiratory depression, cardiovascular effects, and inhibition of GI motility commonly seen with opioids. In a 2001 study, the investigators were able to reduce the GI side effects of morphine with a specific peripherally acting mu antagonist, without interfering with analgesia.[14]

The demonstration of the existence of peripheral opioid receptors has given rise to studies investigating the effect of adminis-

Table 3 Opioid Receptor Types and Physiologic Actions

Receptor Type	Prototypical Ligand		Physiologic Actions
	Endogenous	Exogenous	
Mu$_1$	β-Endorphin	Morphine	Supraspinal analgesia
Mu$_2$	β-Endorphin	Morphine	Respiratory depression
Delta	Enkephalin	—	Spinal analgesia
Kappa	Dynorphin	Ketocyclazocine	Spinal analgesia, sedation, ?visceral analgesia
Epsilon	β-Endorphin	—	?Hormone
Sigma	—	N-Allylnormetazocine	Psychotomimetic effect, dysphoria

tering small opioid doses at the surgical site. Unfortunately, incisional opioid administration has no significant beneficial effect[15]; however, intra-articular administration does yield a modest benefit.[16]

The relation between receptor binding and the intensity of the resultant physiologic effect is known as the intrinsic activity of an opioid. Most of the commonly used opioid analgesics are agonists. An agonist produces a maximal biologic response by binding to its receptor. Other opioids, such as naloxone, are termed antagonists because they compete with agonists for opioid receptor binding sites. Still other opioids are partial agonists because they produce a submaximal response after binding to the receptor. (An excellent example of a submaximal response produced by partial agonists is buprenorphine's action at the mu receptor.)

Drugs such as nalbuphine, butorphanol, and pentazocine are known as agonist-antagonists or mixed agonist-antagonists.[13] These opioids simultaneously act at different receptor sites: their action is agonistic at one receptor and antagonistic at another [see

Table 4]. The agonist-antagonists have certain pharmacologic properties that are distinct from those of the more common mu agonists: (1) they exhibit a ceiling effect and cause only submaximal analgesia as compared with mu agonists, and (2) administration of an agonist-antagonist and a complete agonist may cause a reduction in the effect of the complete agonist.[13]

Agents

Morphine Morphine is the opioid with which the most clinical experience has been gained. Sufficient pharmacokinetic and pharmacodynamic data are available. Use of this agent is recommended; it may be given orally, intravenously, or intramuscularly [see Table 5].

Meperidine Detailed and sufficient pharmacokinetic and pharmacodynamic data on meperidine are available. It is less suitable than morphine as an analgesic because its active metabolite, normeperidine, can accumulate, even in patients with nor-

Table 4 Intrinsic Activity of Opioids

Opioid	Receptor Type			
	Mu	Kappa	Delta	Sigma
Agonists				
Morphine	Agonist	—	—	—
Meperidine (Demerol)	Agonist	—	—	—
Hydromorphone (Dilaudid)	Agonist	—	—	—
Oxymorphone (Numorphan)	Agonist	—	—	—
Levorphanol (Levo-Dromoran)	Agonist	—	—	—
Fentanyl (Duragesic)	Agonist	—	—	—
Sufentanil (Sufenta)	Agonist	—	—	—
Alfentanil (Alfenta)	Agonist	—	—	—
Methadone (Dolophine)	Agonist	—	—	—
Agonist-Antagonists				
Buprenorphine (Buprenex)	Partial agonist	—	—	—
Butorphanol (Stadol)	Antagonist	Agonist	Agonist	—
Nalbuphine (Nubain)	Antagonist	Partial agonist	Agonist	—
Pentazocine (Talwin)	Antagonist	Agonist	Agonist	—
Dezocine (Dalgan)	Partial agonist	—	—	Agonist
Antagonists				
Naloxone (Narcan)	Antagonist	Antagonist	Antagonist	Antagonist

Table 5 Suggested Regimens for
Systemic Morphine Administration

	Intermittent Administration (Suggested Initial Dose)*			
	p.o.	I.M.	I.V.	Duration (hr)
Morphine	30–50 mg	10 mg	5–10 mg	3–4

	Continuous I.V. Infusion†
Morphine	≈ 3 mg/hr (loading dose: 5–10 mg)

*Number of doses to be given is calculated with the following formula:

$$\frac{24 \text{ hr}}{\text{actual duration of single effective dose (hr)}}$$

Single doses should be given at calculated fixed intervals approximately 30 min before expected recurrence of pain. Single dose should be readjusted daily. Elderly patients may be more susceptible to opioids.

†Dose should be adjusted according to effect and side effects.

mal renal clearance, and this accumulation can result in CNS excitation and seizures.[13] Other agents should be used before meperidine is considered. Like morphine, meperidine can be given orally, intravenously, or intramuscularly.

Side Effects

By depressing or stimulating the CNS, opioids cause a number of physiologic effects in addition to analgesia. The depressant effects of opioids include analgesia and altered respiration and mood; the excitatory effects include nausea, vomiting, and miosis.

All mu agonists produce a dose-dependent decrease in the responsiveness of brain-stem respiratory centers to increased carbon dioxide tension (PCO_2). This change is clinically manifested as an increase in resting PCO_2 and a shift in the CO_2 response curve. Agonist-antagonist opioids have a limited effect on the brain stem and appear to elicit a ceiling effect on increases in PCO_2.

Opioids also have effects on the GI tract. Nausea and vomiting are caused by stimulation of the chemoreceptor trigger zone of the medulla. Opioids enhance sphincteric tone and reduce peristaltic contraction. Delayed gastric emptying is caused by decreased motility, increased antral tone, and increased tone in the first part of the duodenum. Delay in passage of intestinal contents because of decreased peristalsis and increased sphincteric tone leads to greater absorption of water, increased viscosity, and desiccation of bowel contents, which cause constipation and contribute to postoperative ileus. Opioids also increase biliary tract pressure.

EPIDURAL AND SUBARACHNOID OPIOIDS

Opioids were first used in the epidural and subarachnoid space in 1979. Since that time, they have become the mainstay of postoperative management for severe pain. Epidural opioids may be administered in a single bolus or via continuous infusions. They are usually combined with local anesthetics in a continuous epidural infusion to enhance analgesia.[9]

Mechanisms of Action

Opioids injected into the epidural or subarachnoid space cause segmental (i.e., selective, spinally mediated) analgesia by binding to opioid receptors in the dorsal horn of the spinal cord.[17] The lipid solubility of an opioid, described by its partition coefficient, predicts its behavior when introduced into the epidural or subarachnoid space. Opioids with low lipid solubility (i.e., hydrophilic opioids) have a slow onset of action and a long dura-

tion of action. Opioids with high lipid solubility (i.e., lipophilic opioids) have a quick onset of action but a short duration of action. Thus, the lipid solubility of an opioid determines its access to the dorsal horn via (1) diffusion through the arachnoid granulations and (2) diffusion into spinal radicular artery blood flow.

Subarachnoid opioids should be used when the required duration of analgesia after surgery is relatively short. When protracted analgesia is required, epidural administration is preferred; repeated injections may be given through epidural catheters, or continuous infusions may be used. Smaller doses of subarachnoid opioids are generally required to produce analgesia. Ordinarily, no more than 0.1 to 0.25 mg of morphine should be used. These doses, which are about 10% to 20% of the size of comparably effective epidural doses, provide reliable pain relief with few side effects.[18] Fentanyl has also been extensively used in the subarachnoid space in a dose range of 6.25 to 50 µg. Pain relief after administration of subarachnoid fentanyl is as potent but not as prolonged as analgesia after administration of morphine.

Regimens for Acute Pain Relief

It is generally agreed that at least 2 mg of epidural morphine is needed to achieve a significant analgesic response, but the criteria used to assess this response have varied greatly in reported studies, and no firm conclusion can be derived from them.[17,19] Epidural opioids are less efficient in the earliest stages of the acute pain state than on subsequent days; moreover, they appear to be more successful at alleviating pain after procedures in the lower half of the body than at alleviating upper abdominal and thoracic pain. In general, 2 to 4 mg of morphine administered epidurally is sufficient after minor procedures, whereas about 4 mg is needed after vascular and gynecologic procedures and after major upper abdominal and thoracic procedures.[13,17,19] On postoperative day 1, however, such a regimen, even when repeated as many as three times, relieves pain completely in fewer than 50% of patients; on subsequent days, the success rate is substantially higher. The efficiency of this approach is lowest after major procedures.

There is evidence to suggest that continuous epidural administration of low-dosage morphine (0.1 to 0.3 mg/hr) or fentanyl (10 to 20 µg/hr) may lower the risk of late respiratory depression and may be more efficient than intermittent administration of higher dosages of morphine.[19] The continuous low-dosage approach is therefore recommended.

Side Effects

The chief side effects associated with epidural and subarachnoid opioids are respiratory depression, nausea and vomiting, pruritus, and urinary retention.[17-19] The poor lipid solubility of morphine is responsible for its protracted duration of action but also allows morphine to undergo cephalad migration in the cerebrospinal fluid. This migration can cause delayed respiratory depression, with a peak incidence 3 to 10 hours after an injection. The high lipid solubility of liphophilic opioids such as fentanyl allows them to be absorbed into lipids close to the site of administration. Consequently, the lipophilic opioids do not migrate rostrally in the CSF and cannot cause delayed respiratory depression. Of course, the high lipid solubility of liphophilic opioids allows them to be absorbed into blood vessels, which may cause early respiratory depression, as is commonly seen with systemic administration of opioids.

Naloxone reverses the depressive respiratory effects of spinal opioids. In an apneic patient, 0.4 mg I.V. will usually restore ventilation. If a patient has a depressed respiratory rate but is still breathing, small aliquots of naloxone (0.2 to 0.4 mg) can be given until the respiratory rate returns to normal.

Nausea and vomiting are caused by transport of opioids to the vomiting center and the chemoreceptor trigger zone in the medulla via CSF flow or the systemic circulation. Nausea can usually be treated with antiemetics or, if severe, with naloxone (in 0.2 mg increments, repeated if necessary).

Pruritus is probably the most common side effect of the spinal opioids. Histamine is released by certain opioids, but this mechanism probably plays a negligible role in the genesis of itching. Treatment of pruritus is similar to that of nausea.

The mechanism of spinal opioid–induced urinary retention involves inhibition of volume-induced bladder contractions and blockade of the vesical reflex. Naloxone administration is the treatment of choice, though bladder catheterization is sometimes required.

Table 6 Regimen for Pain Relief with Continuous Epidural Bupivacaine during Initial 24 Postoperative Hours

Type of Operation	Interspace for Catheter Insertion	Concentration (%)	Volume (ml/hr)
Thoracic procedures	T4–6	0.250–0.125	5–10
Upper laparotomy	T7–8	0.250–0.125	4–12
Gynecologic laparotomy	T10–12	0.250–0.125	4–10
Hip procedures	L2	0.125–0.0625	4–8
Vascular procedures	T10–12	0.250–0.125	4–10

Note: indications for postoperative epidural bupivacaine may be strengthened if this method is also indicated for intraoperative analgesia. Dosage requirements may vary and should be assessed 3 hr after the start of treatment, every 6 hr thereafter on the first day, and then every 12 hr (more often if pain occurs). The duration of treatment is 1–4 days, depending on the intensity of the pain. The concentration of bupivacaine employed should be the lowest possible and should be decreased with time postoperatively. Some patients, especially those who have undergone major upper abdominal operation, require 0.5% bupivacaine initially.

EPIDURAL LOCAL ANESTHETICS AND OTHER REGIONAL BLOCKS

Local anesthetics have become increasingly popular because of the growing familiarity with both epidural catheterization and regional nerve blockade. In addition, there is a great deal of experimental evidence that documents the benefits of blocking noxious impulses.[20] Local anesthetic neural blockade is unique among available analgesic techniques in that it may offer sufficient afferent neural blockade, resulting in relief of pain; avoidance of sedation, respiratory depression, and nausea; and, finally, efferent sympathetic blockade, resulting in increased blood flow to the region of neural blockade.[20] Despite the considerable scientific data documenting these beneficial effects, the place of epidural local anesthesia as a method of pain relief remains somewhat controversial in comparison with that of other analgesic techniques. Its side effects (e.g., hypotension, urinary retention, and motor blockade) and the need for trained staff for surveillance argue against its use; however, these side effects can be reduced by using combination regimens (see below).[19]

Mechanism of Action

Local anesthetic neural blockade is a nondepolarizing block that reduces the permeability of cell membranes to sodium ions.[21] Whether different local anesthetics have different effects on different nerve fibers is debatable.

Choice of Drug

For optimal management of postoperative pain, the anesthetic agent should provide excellent analgesia of rapid onset and long duration without inducing motor blockade. The various local anesthetic agents all meet one or more of these criteria; however, the ones that come closest to meeting all of the criteria are bupivacaine, ropivacaine, and levobupivacaine. This should not preclude the use of other agents, because their efficacy has also been demonstrated. Ropivacaine and levobupivacaine may have a better safety profile, but the improvement may be relevant only when high intraoperative doses are given.[21]

Continuous Epidural Analgesia

No regimen has been found that provides complete analgesia in all patients all of the time, and it is unlikely that one ever will be found. As a rule, the block should be limited to the area in which pain is felt. Care should be taken to avoid motor blockade and to spare autonomic function to the urinary bladder, as well as to formulate a regimen that requires only minimal attention from staff members and carries no significant toxicity. Given these requirements, continuous infusion [see Table 6] is more effective and reliable than intermittent injection.[19] Whether low hourly volume and high concentration approaches are preferable to high hourly volume and low concentration approaches remains to be determined.[19] The weaker solutions may produce less motor blockade while continuing to block smaller C and A-delta pain fibers and are recommended in lumbar epidural analgesia as a means of reducing the risk of orthostatic hypotension and lower-extremity motor blockade.[19]

Specific indications for continuous epidural analgesia that are supported by data from controlled morbidity studies include (1) pain relief and reduction of deep vein thrombosis, pulmonary embolism, and hypoxemia after total hip replacement and prostatectomy; (2) pain relief, facilitation of coughing, and reduction of chest infections after thoracic, abdominal, and orthopedic procedures; (3) pain relief, control of hypertension, and enhancement of graft flow after major vascular operations; and (4) pain relief and reduction of paralytic ileus after abdominal procedures.[22]

Side Effects

The main side effects of epidural local anesthesia are hypotension caused by sympathetic blockade, vagal overactivity, and decreased cardiac function (during a high thoracic block). Under no circumstances should epidural local anesthetics be used before a preexisting hypovolemic condition is treated. Hypotension may be treated with ephedrine, 10 to 15 mg I.V., and fluids, with the patient tilted in a head-down position. Atropine, 0.5 to 1.0 mg I.V., may be effective during vagal overactivity.

Urinary retention occurs in 20% to 100% of patients. Fortunately, urinary catheterization for only 24 to 48 hours in the course of a high-dose regimen probably has no important side effects, and many patients for whom epidural analgesia is indicated need an indwelling catheter for other reasons in any case. The incidence of urinary retention is probably below 10% when epidural local anesthetics are used in weak solutions.[23] Motor blockade may delay mobilization; however, its incidence can be reduced by using the weakest concentration of local anesthetic that is compatible with adequate sensory blockade. Cerebral and epidural analgesia should not be employed in patients already receiving anticoagulant therapy, but it may be started with catheter insertion before vascular or other procedures in which controlled heparin therapy is used. Epidural analgesia has been used in patients receiving thromboembolic prophylaxis with low-dose heparin and low-molecular-weight heparin without significant risk,[19] provided that current guidelines are followed.[24] The complications associated with the epidural catheter are minimal when proper nursing protocols are followed [see Table 7].[19] The decision to employ epidural local anesthetics in such patients should be made only after the risks are carefully compared with the documented advantages of such anesthetics.[19,22] It is important that the level of insertion into the epidural space correspond with the level of incision.

Other Nerve Blocks

The popularity of single-dose intercostal block and intrapleural regional analgesia has decreased in comparison with that of continuous epidural treatment. Intermittent or continuous administration of local anesthetics through a catheter inserted into the paravertebral space seems to be a promising approach to providing analgesia after thoracic and abdominal procedures,[8,25] but further data are needed. Intravenous and intraperitoneal administration of local anesthetics cannot be recommended for postoperative analgesia, because they are not efficacious.[26] Intraincisional administration of bupivacaine, which has negligible side effects and demands little or no surveillance, is recommended for patients undergoing relatively minor procedures.[27] Continuous peripheral nerve blocks are growing in popularity, and the analgesic treatment may be continued after discharge.[28,29] Before general recommendations can be formulated, however, further safety data are required. More detailed information on special blocks can be found in the anesthesiology literature. In general, despite its disadvantages, neural blockade with local anesthetics is recommended for relief of severe postoperative pain because of the advantageous physiologic effects it exerts and the reduction in postoperative morbidity it brings about.

CONVENTIONAL NSAIDS AND COX-2 INHIBITORS

NSAIDs are minor analgesics that, because of their anti-inflammatory effect, may be suitable for management of postop-

---

Table 7 Procedures for Maintenance of Epidural Anesthesia for Longer Than 24 Hours

1. Administer appropriate drug in appropriate dosage at selected infusion rate as determined by physician.
2. Nurse evaluates vital signs and intake and output as required for a postoperative patient.
3. Nurse checks infusion pump hourly to ensure that it is functioning properly, that infusion rate is proper, and that alarm is on.
4. Nurse also assesses
   - Bladder—for distention, if patient is not catheterized
   - Lower extremities—for status of motor function
   - CNS—for signs of toxicity or respiratory depression
   - Relief of pain (drug dosage may require modification)
   - Skin integrity on back (breakdown may occur if motor function is not present)
   - Tubing and dressing (disconnection of tubing or dislodgment of catheter may occur)
5. Every 48 hr, the catheter dressing should be removed, the catheter entrance site cleaned, and topical antibiotic applied (much as in care of a central venous catheter).

---

erative pain associated with a significant degree of inflammation (e.g., bone or soft tissue damage).[30] They may, however, have central analgesic effects as well and thus may have analgesic efficacy after all kinds of operations. Conventional NSAIDs inhibit both COX-1 and COX-2. A number of newer agents are now available that specifically inhibit COX-2. These agents have the potential to achieve analgesic efficacy comparable to that of conventional NSAIDs but with fewer side effects [see Table 8].[31,32]

Only a few of the NSAIDs may be given parenterally. The data now available on the use of NSAIDs for postoperative pain are insufficient to allow definitive recommendation of any agent or agents over the others, and selection may therefore depend on convenience of delivery, duration, and cost.[30] It is clear, however, that these agents may play a valuable role as adjuvants to other analgesics; accordingly, they have been recommended as basic analgesics for all operations in low-risk patients.[2] All of the NSAIDs have potentially serious side effects: GI and surgical site hemorrhage and renal failure. Fortunately, these effects are probably of minor importance during short-term postoperative treatment[33]; however, no information is available from high-risk surgical populations. COX-2 inhibitors have been shown to exert fewer GI side effects than conventional NSAIDs do, both during long-term treatment[31] and during acute treatment[34] (as assessed by endoscopy). These findings suggest that postoperative pain

Table 8 Recommended Dosages of NSAIDs or COX-2 Inhibitors for Relief of Postoperative Pain

NSAID	Dosage
Acetylsalicylic acid	500–1,000 mg q. 4–6 hr
Acetaminophen	500–1,000 mg q. 4–6 hr
Indomethacin	50–100 mg q. 6–8 hr
Ibuprofen	200–400 mg q. 4–6 hr
Ketorolac	30 mg q. 4–6 hr
Rofecoxib	12–25 mg q. 12 hr

treatment with COX-2 inhibitors may be appropriate in high-risk settings as well.

NSAIDs exert their anti-inflammatory effect by inhibiting prostaglandin synthesis at the surgical site and in the CNS, thereby decreasing the release of local inflammatory agents and pain mediators within the CNS.[35] Because prostaglandins are important for regulation of water and mineral homeostasis by the kidneys in the dehydrated patient,[32] perioperative treatment with NSAIDs may lead to postoperative renal failure.[30,33,36] So far, specific COX-2 inhibitors have not been demonstrated to be less nephrotoxic than conventional NSAIDs.[31,32] Although little systematic evaluation has been done, extensive clinical experience with NSAIDs suggests that the renal risk is not substantial.[33,36] Nonetheless, conventional NSAIDs and COX-2 inhibitors should be used with caution in patients who have preexisting renal dysfunction.

Although conventional NSAIDs prolong bleeding time and inhibit platelet aggregation, there generally does not seem to be a clinically significant risk of increased bleeding.[30,33] However, in procedures where strict hemostasis is critical (e.g., tonsillectomy, cosmetic surgery, and eye surgery), these drugs should be given with caution[37] or replaced with COX-2 inhibitors, which do not inhibit platelet aggregation.[38] The observation that prostaglandins are involved in bone and wound healing has given rise to concern about potential side effects in surgical patients. Although there is experimental evidence that both conventional NSAIDs and COX-2 inhibitors can impair bone healing,[39] the clinical data available at present are insufficient to document wound or bone healing failure with these drugs. This is a particularly important issue for future study in that many orthopedic surgeons remain reluctant to use NSAIDs.

Peripheral (i.e., surgical site) administration may have a slight additional analgesic effect compared with systemic administration,[40] but further data on safety are required.

Acetaminophen also possesses anti-inflammatory capability, both peripherally and centrally. Its analgesic effect is somewhat (about 20% to 30%) weaker than those of conventional NSAIDs and COX-2 inhibitors; however, it lacks the side effects typical of these agents.[41-43] Combining acetaminophen with NSAIDs may improve analgesia, especially in smaller and moderate-sized operations[41,42]; accordingly, this agent is recommended as a basic component of multimodal analgesia in all operations.

Despite the gaps in our current understanding of the working and differential effects of NSAIDs and COX-2 inhibitors, what is known is sufficiently encouraging to suggest that they should be recommended for baseline analgesic treatment after most operative procedures, with the exception that NSAIDs should not be given in the earliest part of the postoperative period immediately after heparinization during cardiovascular procedures or in high-risk patients. Indications for COX-2 inhibitors may be extended as a consequence of their superior safety profile with respect to the GI tract and platelet function. NSAIDs and COX-2 inhibitors are valuable components of multimodal pain treatment and may be of special value in patients undergoing short operations (e.g., laparoscopic procedures), in which opioid-sparing effects may reduce postoperative nausea and vomiting.

Glucocorticoids are powerful anti-inflammatory agents and have proven analgesic value in less extensive procedures,[44] especially dental, laparoscopic, and arthroscopic operations. Their profound antiemetic effects notwithstanding, concern over side effects has limited their use outside such settings.[44]

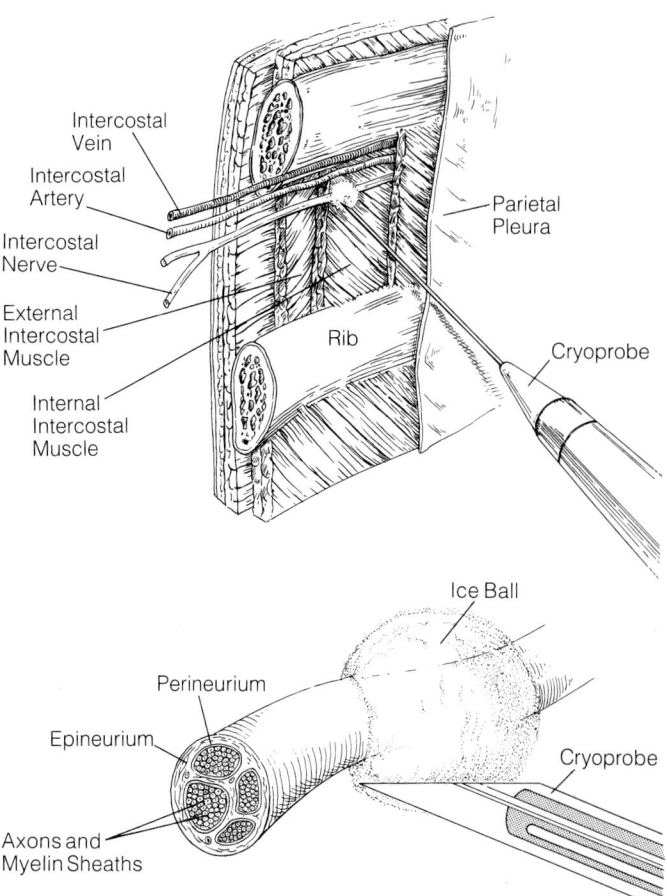

Figure 1 Illustrated is the procedure for performing cryoanalgesia in a thoracotomy. The intercostal nerve in the thoracotomy space is isolated, together with the two intercostal nerves above the space and the two below it, and the cryoprobe is applied to the nerves for 45 seconds. The probe is then defrosted and reapplied to the nerves for 45 seconds. The analgesia obtained lasts about 30 days.

OTHER ANALGESICS

Tramadol is a weak analgesic that has several relatively minor side effects (e.g., dizziness, nausea, and vomiting).[45,46] It can be combined with acetaminophen to yield analgesic activity comparable to that of NSAIDs.[46]

CRYOANALGESIA

Cryoanalgesia is the application of low temperatures (–20 to –29° C) to peripheral nerves with the goal of producing axonal degeneration and thus analgesia [*see Figure 1*]. Axonal regeneration takes place at a rate of 1 to 3 mm/day, which means that analgesia after intercostal blocks lasts about 30 days. Cryoanalgesia has no cardiac, respiratory, or cerebral side effects, and local side effects (e.g., neuroma formation) are extremely rare. In this context, it should be emphasized that postthoracotomy patients are at substantial risk (~30%) for chronic neuropathic pain without the use of cryoanalgesia[47]; however, this technique can be used only on sensory nerves or on nerves supplying muscles of no clinical importance.

At present, no information is available on the use of cryoanalgesia in operative procedures other than herniotomy and thoracotomy.[8] Cryoanalgesia is not efficacious after herniotomy.[48] The data on postthoracotomy cryoanalgesia, however, indicate improved pain alleviation and a concomitant reduction in the need for narcotics, which, in conjunction with the simplicity and low cost of the modality and the absence of side effects, present a strong argument for more extensive use of cryoanalgesia.

TRANSCUTANEOUS ELECTRICAL NERVE STIMULATION

Transcutaneous electrical nerve stimulation (TENS) is the application of a mild electrical current through the skin surface to a specific area, such as a surgical wound, to achieve pain relief; the exact mechanism whereby it achieves this effect is yet to be explained. Many TENS devices are available for clinical use, but the specific value and the proper use of the various stimulation frequencies, waveforms, and current intensities have not been determined. Unfortunately, the effect of TENS on acute pain is too small to warrant a recommendation for routine use.[49]

PATIENT-CONTROLLED ANALGESIA

Patient-controlled administration of opioids has experienced a dramatic increase in use. This increase may be attributed to (1) awareness of the inadequacy of traditional I.M. opioid regimens, (2) the development of effective and safe biotechnology, and (3) the widespread patient satisfaction with patient-controlled analgesia (PCA).[50,51] It must be emphasized, however, that the effect of PCA on movement-associated pain is limited in comparison with that of epidural local anesthesia.[9]

Mechanisms of Action

Traditional I.M. dosing of opioids does not result in consistent blood levels,[50,51] because opioids are absorbed at a variable rate from the vascular bed of muscle. Moreover, administration of traditional I.M. regimens results in opioid concentrations that exceed the concentrations required to produce analgesia only in about 30% of the time during any 4-hour dosing interval. PCA avoids these pitfalls by allowing repeated dosing on demand. PCA provides more constant and consistent plasma opioid levels and therefore better analgesia.[50,51]

Modes of Administration and Dosing Parameters

Several modes can be used to administer opioids under patient control. Intermittent delivery of a fixed dose is known as demand dosing. Background infusions have been used to supplement patient-administered doses, but this practice increases the risk of respiratory depression and should therefore be avoided.[50,51]

There are several basic prescription parameters for PCA: loading dose, demand dose, lockout interval, and 4-hour limits [see Table 9].[50,51] When PCA is used for postoperative care, it is usually initiated in the recovery room. The patient is made comfortable by administering as much opioid as is needed (i.e., a loading

Table 9 Prescription Guidelines for Intravenous Patient-Controlled Analgesia

Drug (Concentration)	Demand Dose	Lockout Interval (min)
Morphine (1 mg/ml)	0.5–3.0 mg	5–12
Meperdine (10 mg/ml)	5–30 mg	5–12
Fentanyl (10 µg/ml)	10–20 µg	5–10
Hydromorphone (0.2 mg/ml)	0.1–0.5 mg	5–10
Oxymorphone (0.25 mg/ml)	0.2–0.4 mg	8–10
Methadone (1 mg/ml)	0.5–2.5 mg	8–20
Nalbuphine (1 mg/ml)	1–5 mg	5–10

dose). When the patient is sufficiently recovered from the anesthetic, he or she may begin to use the infuser.

Side Effects

Minor side effects associated with PCA include nausea, vomiting, sweating, and pruritus. Clinically significant respiratory depression with PCA is rare. There is no evidence to suggest that PCA is associated with a higher incidence of side effects than are other routes of systemic opioid administration.[50,51] Side effects are the result of the pharmacologic properties of opioids, not the method of administration.[50,51]

COMBINATION REGIMENS

Because no single pain treatment modality is optimal, combination regimens (e.g., balanced analgesia or multimodal treatment) offer major advantages over single-modality regimens, whether by maintaining or improving analgesia, by reducing side effects, or by doing both.[52,53] Combinations of epidural local anesthetics and morphine,[9,19] of NSAIDs and opioids,[30,52,53] of NSAIDs and acetaminophen,[41,42] of acetaminophen and opioids,[43] and of acetaminophen and tramadol[46] have been reported to have additive effects. At present, information on other combinations (involving ketamine,[54] clonidine,[30] glucocorticoids,[44] and other agents) is too sparse to allow firm recommendations; however, multimodal analgesia is undoubtedly promising, and multidrug combinations should certainly be explored further.

Discussion

Physiologic Mechanisms of Acute Pain

The basic mechanisms of acute pain are (1) afferent transmission of nociceptive stimuli through the peripheral nervous system after tissue damage, (2) modulation of these injury signals by control systems in the dorsal horn, and (3) modulation of the ascending transmission of pain stimuli by a descending control system originating in the brain [see Figure 2].[55-57]

PERIPHERAL PAIN RECEPTORS AND NEURAL TRANSMISSION TO SPINAL CORD

Peripheral pain receptors (nociceptors) can be identified by function but cannot be distinguished anatomically. The responsiveness of peripheral pain receptors may be enhanced by endogenous analgesic substances (e.g., prostaglandins, serotonin, bradykinin, nerve growth factor, and histamine) as well

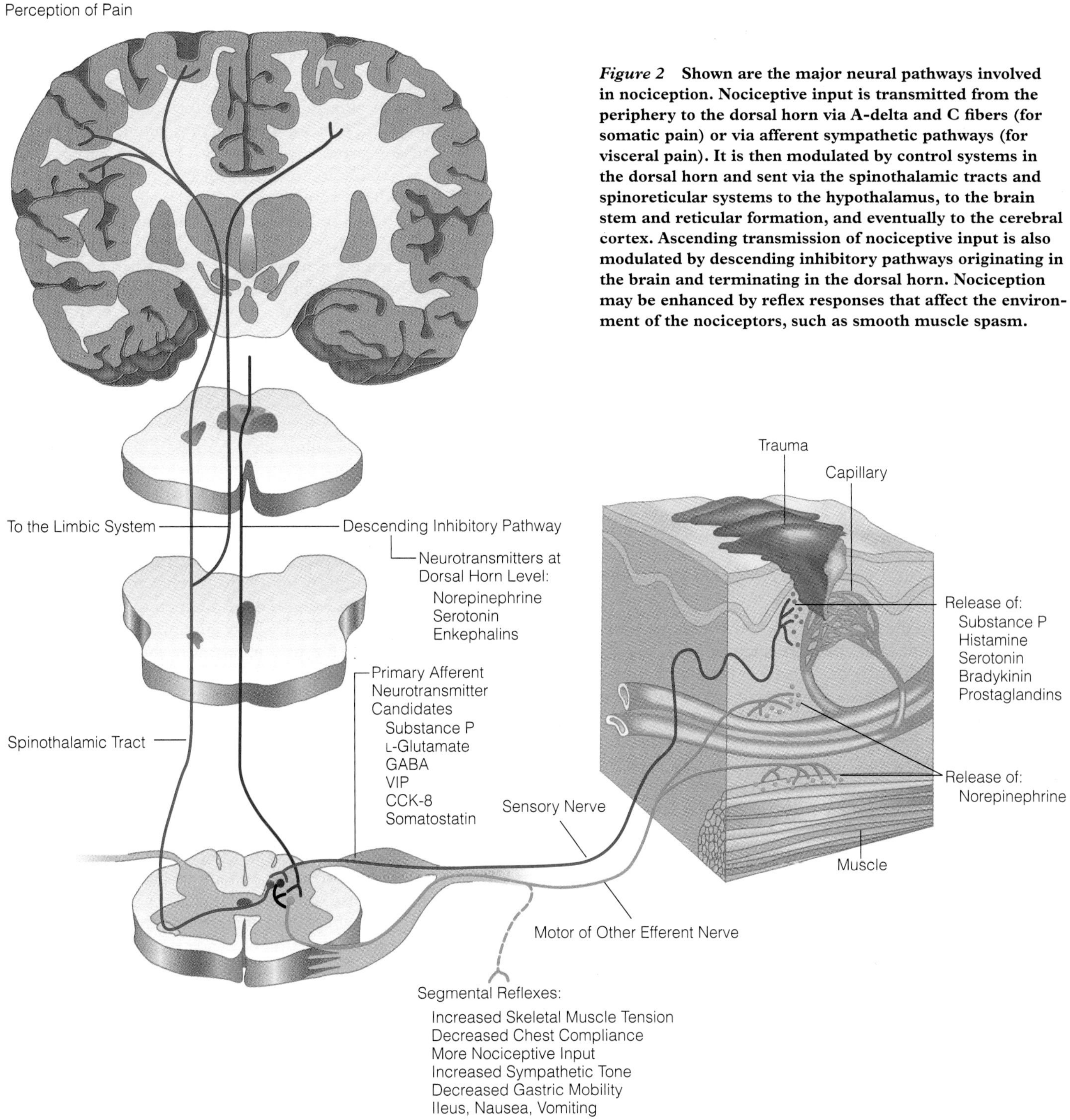

Perception of Pain

Figure 2 **Shown are the major neural pathways involved in nociception. Nociceptive input is transmitted from the periphery to the dorsal horn via A-delta and C fibers (for somatic pain) or via afferent sympathetic pathways (for visceral pain). It is then modulated by control systems in the dorsal horn and sent via the spinothalamic tracts and spinoreticular systems to the hypothalamus, to the brain stem and reticular formation, and eventually to the cerebral cortex. Ascending transmission of nociceptive input is also modulated by descending inhibitory pathways originating in the brain and terminating in the dorsal horn. Nociception may be enhanced by reflex responses that affect the environment of the nociceptors, such as smooth muscle spasm.**

To the Limbic System

Spinothalamic Tract

Descending Inhibitory Pathway

Neurotransmitters at Dorsal Horn Level:
Norepinephrine
Serotonin
Enkephalins

Primary Afferent Neurotransmitter Candidates
Substance P
L-Glutamate
GABA
VIP
CCK-8
Somatostatin

Trauma

Capillary

Release of:
Substance P
Histamine
Serotonin
Bradykinin
Prostaglandins

Release of:
Norepinephrine

Sensory Nerve

Muscle

Motor of Other Efferent Nerve

Segmental Reflexes:
Increased Skeletal Muscle Tension
Decreased Chest Compliance
More Nociceptive Input
Increased Sympathetic Tone
Decreased Gastric Mobility
Ileus, Nausea, Vomiting

as by increased efferent sympathetic activity.[55] Antidromic release of substance P may amplify the inflammatory response and thereby increase pain transmission. The peripheral mechanisms of visceral pain still are not well understood[56]—for example, no one has yet explained why cutting or burning may provoke pain in the skin but not provoke pain in visceral organs. Peripheral opioid receptors have been demonstrated to appear in inflammation on the peripheral nerve terminals, and clinical studies have demonstrated that there are analgesic effects from peripheral opioid administration during arthroscopic knee surgery.[16]

Somatic nociceptive input is transmitted to the CNS through A-delta and C fibers, which are small in diameter and either unmyelinated or thinly myelinated. Visceral pain is transmitted through afferent sympathetic pathways; the evidence that afferent parasympathetic pathways play a role in visceral nociception is inconclusive.[56]

DORSAL HORN CONTROL SYSTEMS AND MODULATION OF INCOMING SIGNALS

All incoming nociceptive traffic synapses in the gray matter of the dorsal horn (Rexed's laminae I to IV). Several substances may be involved in primary afferent transmission of nociceptive stimuli in the dorsal horn: substance P, enkephalins, somatostatin, neurotensin, γ-aminobutyric acid (GABA), glutamic acid, angiotensin II, vasoactive intestinal polypeptide (VIP), and cholecystokinin octapeptide (CCK-8).[57] From the dorsal horn, nociceptive information is transmitted through the spinothalamic tracts to the hypothalamus, through spinoreticular systems to the brain stem and reticular formation, and finally to the cerebral cortex.

DESCENDING PAIN CONTROL SYSTEM

A descending control system for sensory input originates in the brain stem and reticular formation and in certain higher brain areas. The main neurotransmitters in this system are norepinephrine, serotonin, and enkephalins. Epidural-intrathecal administration of alpha-adrenergic agonists (e.g., clonidine) may therefore provide pain relief.[57]

SPINAL REFLEXES

Nociception may be enhanced by spinal reflexes that affect the environment of the nociceptive nerve endings. Thus, tissue damage may provoke an afferent reflex that causes muscle spasm in the vicinity of the injury, thereby increasing nociception. Similarly, sympathetic reflexes may cause decreased microcirculation in injury tissue, thereby generating smooth muscle spasm, which amplifies the sensation.

POSTINJURY CHANGES IN PERIPHERAL AND CENTRAL NERVOUS SYSTEMS

After an injury, the afferent nociceptive pathways undergo physiologic, anatomic, and chemical changes.[57,58] These changes include increased sensitivity on the part of peripheral nociceptors as well as the growth of sprouts from damaged nerve fibers that become sensitive to mechanical and alpha-adrenergic stimuli and eventually begin to fire spontaneously. Moreover, excitability may be increased in the spinal cord, which leads to expansion of receptive fields in dorsal horn cells. Such changes may lower pain thresholds, may increase afferent barrage in the late postinjury state, and, if normal regression does not occur during convalescence, may contribute to a chronic pain state.[57]

Neural stimuli have generally been considered to be the main factor responsible for initiation of spinal neuroplasticity; however, it now appears that such neuroplasticity may also be mediated by cytokines released as a consequence of COX-2 induction.[35] Improved understanding of the mechanisms of pain may serve as a rational basis for future drug development.[59]

In experimental studies, acute pain behavior or hyperexcitability of dorsal horn neurons may be eliminated or reduced if the afferent barrage is prevented from reaching the CNS. Preinjury neural blockade with local anesthetics or opioids can suppress excitability of the CNS; this is called preemptive analgesia. Because similar antinociceptive procedures were less effective in experimental studies when applied after injury, timing of analgesia seems to be important in the treatment of postoperative pain; however, a critical analysis of controlled clinical studies that compared the efficacy of analgesic regimens administered preoperatively with the efficacy of the same regimens administered postoperatively concluded that preemptive analgesia does not provide a clinically significant increase in pain relief.[60] Nonetheless, it is important that pain treatment be initiated early to ensure that patients do not wake up with high-intensity pain. As long as the afferent input from the surgical wound continues, continuous treatment with multimodal or balanced analgesia may be the most effective method of treating postoperative pain.

Effects of Pain Relief

METABOLIC RESPONSE TO OPERATION

It still is not generally appreciated that acute pain in the postoperative period or after hospitalization for accidental injury not only serves no useful function but also may actually exert harmful physiologic and psychological effects. Therefore, except in the initial stage in acutely injured hypovolemic patients for whom increased sympathetic activity may provide cardiovascular support, the pain-induced reflex responses that may adversely affect respiratory function, increase cardiac demands, decrease intestinal motility, and initiate skeletal muscle spasm (thereby impairing mobilization) should be counteracted by all available means.

The traditional view of the physiologic role of the stress response to surgical injury is that it is a homeostatic defense mechanism that helps the body heal tissue and adapt to injury. However, the necessity for the stress response in modern anesthesiology and surgery has been questioned.[20] Thus, concern about the detrimental effects of operative procedures (e.g., myocardial infarction, pulmonary complications, and thromboembolism) that cannot be attributed solely to imperfections in surgical technique has led to the hypothesis that the unsupported continuous injury response may instead be a maladaptive response that erodes body mass and physiologic reserve.[20,61] Because neural stimuli play an important role in releasing the stress response to surgical injury, pain relief may modify this response, but this modulation is dependent on the mechanism of action of the pain treatment modality employed.[20]

Alleviation of pain through antagonism of peripheral pain mediators (i.e., through use of NSAIDs) has no important modifying effect on the response to operation.[20,22] The effects of blockade of afferent and efferent transmission of pain stimuli by means of regional anesthesia have been studied in detail.[20,62] Spinal or epidural analgesia with local anesthetics prevents the greater part of the classic endocrine metabolic response to operative procedures in the lower region of the body (e.g., gynecologic and urologic procedures and orthopedic procedures in the lower limbs) and improves protein economy; however, this effect is considerably weaker in major abdominal and thoracic procedures, probably because of insufficient afferent neural blockade. The modifying effect of epidural analgesia on the stress response is most pronounced if the neural blockade takes effect before the surgical insult. The optimal duration of neural blockade for attenuating the hypermetabolic response has not been established, but it should include at least the initial 24 to 48 hours.[20,62]

Alleviation of postoperative pain through administration of epidural-intrathecal opioids has a smaller modifying effect on the surgical stress response, in comparison with the degree of pain relief it provides[20,62]; furthermore, it does not provide efferent sympathetic blockade. Systemic administration of opioids, either according to a fixed administration regimen or according to a demand-based regimen, has no important modifying effect on the stress response.[20] The effects of pain relief by acetaminophen, tramadol, cryoanalgesia, or TENS on the stress response have not been established but probably are of no clinical significance. Further studies aimed at defining the effects of multimodal analgesia on the surgical stress response are required.

POSTOPERATIVE MORBIDITY

The effects of nociceptive blockade and pain relief on postoperative morbidity remain to be defined, except with respect to intraoperative spinal or epidural local anesthetics in lower-body procedures, about which the following four conclusions can be made.[20,63] First, intraoperative blood loss is reduced by about 30%. Second, thromboembolic and pulmonary complications are reduced by about 30% to 40%. Third, when epidural local anesthetics are continuously administered (with or without small doses of opioids) to patients undergoing abdominal or thoracic procedures, pulmonary infectious complications appear to be reduced by about 40%.[22] Fourth, the duration of postoperative ileus is reduced[22,62]; this effect may be of major significance in that reduction of ileus allows earlier oral nutrition,[62] which has been demonstrated to improve outcome.

The impact of continuous epidural analgesia on postoperative outcome after major operations remains the subject of some debate. Three large randomized trials from 2001 and 2002 found no positive effects except for improved pulmonary outcome.[64-66] One explanation for these negative findings may be the use of a predominantly opioid-based epidural analgesic regimen, which would hinder the normal physiologic responses supporting recovery to a greater extent than a local anesthetic regimen would.[20] Another explanation may be inadequate study design in some cases: most studies to date have focused on the effects of a single factor (i.e., epidural analgesia) on overall postoperative morbidity, which is probably too simplistic an approach, given that overall postoperative outcome is known to be determined by multiple factors.[67] Besides postoperative pain relief, reinforced psychological preparation of the patient, reduction of stress by performing neural blockade or opting for minimal invasive procedures, and enforcement of early oral postoperative feeding and mobilization may all play a significant role in determining outcome. Prevention of intraoperative hypothermia, avoidance of fluid overloading, and avoidance of hypoxemia may be important as well.[67]

Therefore, although adequate pain relief is obviously a prerequisite for good outcome, the best results are likely to be achieved by combining analgesia with all the aforementioned factors in a multimodal rehabilitation effort.[67] Observations from patients undergoing a variety of surgical procedures suggest that such a multimodal approach may lead to significant reductions in hospital stay, morbidity, and convalescence.[67] Admittedly, these preliminary observations require confirmation by randomized or multicenter trials. The role of the acute pain service[68] and the effect of establishing a postoperative rehabilitation unit should be assessed as well.

TOLERANCE, PHYSICAL DEPENDENCE, AND ADDICTION

Continued exposure of an opioid receptor to high concentrations of opioid will cause tolerance. Tolerance is the progressive decline in potency of an opioid with continuous use; higher and higher concentrations of the drug are required to cause the same analgesic effect. Physical dependence refers to the production of an abstinence syndrome when an opioid is withdrawn. It is defined by the World Health Organization as follows:

A state, psychic or sometimes also physical, resulting from interactions between a living organism and a drug, characterized by behavioural and other responses that always include a compulsion to take the drug on a continuous or periodic basis in order to experience its psychic effects, and sometimes to avoid discomfort from its absence.[69]

This definition is very close to the popular conception of addiction. It is important, however, to distinguish addiction (implying compulsive behavior and psychological dependence) from tolerance (a pharmacologic property) and from physical dependence (a characteristic physiologic effect of a group of drugs). Physical dependence does not imply addiction. Moreover, tolerance can occur without physical dependence; the converse does not appear to be true.

The possibility that the medical administration of opioids could result in a patient's becoming addicted has generated much debate about the use of opioids. In a prospective study of 12,000 hospitalized patients receiving at least one strong opioid for a protracted period, there were only four reasonably well documented cases of subsequent addiction, and in none of these was there a history of previous substance abuse.[70] Thus, the iatrogenic production of opioid addiction may be very rare.

CONCLUSION

The choice of therapeutic intervention for acute postoperative pain is determined largely by the nature of the patient's problem, the resources available, the efficacy of the various treatment techniques, the risks attendant on the procedures under consideration, and the cost to the patient. Whereas trauma has been the subject of intensive research, the mechanisms of the pain associated with trauma and surgical injury and the optimal methods of relieving such pain have received comparatively little attention from surgeons. It is to be hoped that our growing understanding of basic pain mechanisms and appropriate therapy, combined with the promising data supporting the idea that adequate inhibition of surgically induced nociceptive stimuli may reduce postoperative morbidity, will stimulate more surgeons to turn their attention to this area. Effective control of postoperative pain, combined with a high degree of surgical expertise and the judicious use of other perioperative therapeutic interventions within the context of multimodal postoperative rehabilitation, is certain to improve surgical outcome.

References

1. Report of a working party of the commission on the provision of surgical services. Pain after Surgery. The Royal College of Surgeons of England and the College of Anaesthetists, London, 1990

2. Agency for Health Care Policy and Research: Acute Pain Management and Trauma: Operative or Medical Procedures. Publication No 92-0032. US Department of Health and Human Services, Rockville, Maryland, 1992

3. American Pain Society Quality of Care Committee: Quality improved guidelines for the treatment of acute pain and cancer pain. JAMA 274:1874, 1995

4. Warfield CA, Kahn C: Acute pain management:

programs in U.S. hospitals and experiences and attitudes among U.S. adults. Anesthesiology 83:1090, 1995

5. Joint Commission on Accreditation of Healthcare Organizations: Pain management standards. www.jcaho.org/accredited+organizations/hospitals/standards/revisions/2001/pain+management1.htm

6. Huang N, Cunningham F, Laurito CE, et al: Can we do better with postoperative pain management? Am J Surg 182:440, 2001

7. McQuay H, Moore A: An Evidence-Based Resource for Pain Relief. Oxford University Press, Oxford, 1998

8. Kruger M, McRae K: Pain management in car-

dio-thoracic practice. Surg Clin North Am 79:387, 1999

9. Jørgensen H, Wetterslev J, Møiniche S, et al: Epidural local anesthetics versus opioid-based analgesic regimens on postoperative gastrointestinal paralysis, PONV and pain after abdominal surgery. Cochrane Library 4:1, 2000

10. Chapman CR: Psychological factors in postoperative pain. Acute Pain. Smith G, Covino BG. Eds. Butterworth Publishers, Stoneham, Massachusetts, 1985, p 22

11. Peck CL: Psychological factors in acute pain management. Acute Pain Management. Cousins MJ, Phillips GD, Eds. Churchill Livingstone, New York, 1986, p 251

12. Egbert LD, Battit GE, Welch SE, et al: Reduction of postoperative pain by encouragement and instruction of patients: a study of doctor-patient rapport. N Engl J Med 170:825, 1964

13. Austrup ML, Korean G: Analgesic agents for the postoperative period: opioids. Surg Clin North Am 79:253, 1999

14. Taguchi A, Sharma N, Saleem RM, et al: Selective postoperative inhibition of gastrointestinal opioid receptors. N Engl J Med 345:935, 2001

15. Picard PR, Tramèr MR, McQuay HJ, et al: Analgesic efficacy of peripheral opioids (all except intra-articular): a qualitative systematic review of randomized controlled trials. Pain 72:309, 1997

16. Gupta A, Bodin L, Holmström B, et al: A systematic review of the peripheral analgesic effects of intraarticular morphine. Anesth Analg 93:761, 2001

17. Rawal N: Epidural and spinal agents for postoperative analgesia. Surg Clin North Am 79:313, 1999

18. Dahl JB, Jeppesen IS, Jørgensen H, et al: Intraoperative and postoperative analgesic efficacy and adverse effects of intrathecal opioids in patients undergoing cesarean section with spinal anesthesia: a qualitative and quantitative systematic review of randomized controlled trials. Anesthesiology 91:1919, 1999

19. Wheatley RG, Schug SA, Watson D: Safety and efficacy of postoperative epidural analgesia. Br J Anaesth 87:47, 2001

20. Kehlet H: Modification of responses to surgery by neural blockade: clinical implications. Cousins MJ, Bridenbaugh, Eds. Neural Blockade in Clinical Anesthesia and Management of Pain, 3rd ed. Lippincott-Raven, Philadelphia, p 129, 1998

21. Whiteside JB, Wildsmith JAW: Developments in local anaesthetic drugs. Br J Anaesth 87:27, 2001

22. Kehlet H, Holte K: Effect of postoperative analgesia on surgical outcome. Br J Anaesth 87:62, 2001

23. Basse L, Werner M, Kehlet H: Is urinary drainage necessary during continuous epidural analgesia? Reg Anesth Pain Med 25:498, 2000

24. Horlocker TT, Wedel DJ: Spinal and epidural blockade and perioperative low molecular weight heparin: smooth sailing on the Titanic. Anesth Analg 86:1153, 1998

25. Peng PWH, Chan VWS: Local and regional block in postoperative pain control. Surg Clin North Am 79:345, 1999

26. Møiniche S, Jørgensen H, Wetterslev J, et al: Local anesthetic infiltration for postoperative pain relief after laparoscopy: a qualitative and quantitative systematic review of intraperitoneal, port-site infiltration and mesosalpinx block. Anesth Analg 90:899, 2000

27. Møiniche S, Mikkelsen S, Wetterslev J, et al: A qualitative systematic review of incisional local anaesthesia for postoperative pain relief after abdominal operations. Br J Anaesth 81:377, 1998

28. Rawal N, Allvin R, Axelsson K, et al: Patient-controlled regional analgesia (PCRA) at home. Anesthesiology 96:1290, 2002

29. Ilfeld B, Morey T, Enneking F: Continuous infraclaviculabrachial plexus block for postoperative pain control at home: a randomized, double-blinded placebo-controlled study. Anesthesiology 96:1297, 2002

30. Power I, Barratt S: Analgesic agents for the postoperative period: nonopioids. Surg Clin North Am 79:275, 1999

31. Fitzgeral GA, Patrono C: The coxibs, selective inhibitors of cyclooxygenase-2. N Engl J Med 345:433, 2001

32. McCrory CR, Lindahl SGE: Cyclooxygenase inhibition for postoperative analgesia. Anesth Analg 95:169, 2002

33. Ketorolac, diclofenac, and ketoprofen are equally safe for pain relief after major surgery. POINT Investigators. Br J Anaesth 88:227, 2002

34. Stoltz RR, Harris SI, Kuss ME, et al: Upper GI mucosal effects of parecoxib sodium in healthy elderly subjects. Am J Gastroenterol 97:65, 2002

35. Samad TA, Moore KA, Saphirstein A, et al: Intraleukin-1 β-mediated induction of COX-2 in the CNS contributes to inflammatory pain hypersensitivity. Nature 410:471, 2001

36. Lee A, Cooper MG, Craig JC, et al: The effects of non-steroidal anti-inflammatory drugs (NSAIDs) on postoperative renal function: a meta-analysis. Anesth Intensive Care 27: 574,1999

37. Møiniche S, Rømsing J, Dahl JB, et al: Nonsteroidal anti-inflammatory drugs and the risk of operative side bleeding after tonsillectomy: a quantitative, systematic review. Anesth Analg (in press)

38. Noveck RJ, Laurent A, Kuss M, et al: Parecoxib sodium does not impair platelet function in healthy elderly and non-elderly individuals: two randomized, controlled trials. Clin Drug Invest 21:465,2001

39. Einhorn TA: Do inhibitors of cyclooxygenase-2 impair bone healing? J Bone Mineral Res 17:977, 2002

40. Rømsing J, Møiniche S, Østergaard D, et al: Local infiltration with NSAIDs for postoperative analgesia: evidence for a peripheral analgesic action. Acta Anaesthesiol Scand 44:672, 2000

41. Rømsing J, Møiniche S, Dahl JB: Rectal and parenteral paracetamol, and paracetamol in combination with NSAID's for postoperative analgesia. Br J Anaesth 88:215, 2002

42. Hyllested M, Jones S, Pedersen JL, et al: Comparative effect of paracetamol, NSAID's or their combination in postoperative pain management: a qualitative review. Br J Anaesth 88:199, 2002

43. Moore A, Collins S, Carroll D, et al: Paracetamol with and without codeine in acute pain: a quantitative systematic review. Pain 70:193, 1997

44. Holte K, Kehlet H: Perioperative single-dose glucocorticoid administration: pathophysiological effects and clinical implications. J Am Coll Surg (in press)

45. Scott LJ, Perry CM: Tramadol: a review of its use in perioperative pain. Drugs 60:139, 2000

46. Edwards JE, McQuay HJ, Moore RA: Combination analgesic efficacy: individual patient data meta-analysis of single-dose oral tramadol plus acetaminophen in acute postoperative pain. J Pain Symptom Manage 23:121, 2002

47. Perkins FM, Kehlet H: Chronic pain as an outcome of surgery. Anesthesiology 93:1123, 2000

48. Callesen T, Bech K, Thorup J, et al: Cryoanalgesia: effect on postherniorrhaphy pain. Anesth Analg 87:896, 1998

49. Carroll D, Tramèr M, McQuay H, et al: Randomization is important in studies with pain outcomes: systematic review of transcutaneous electrical nerve stimulation in acute postoperative pain. Br J Anaesth 77:798, 1996

50. Etches RC: Patient-controlled analgesia. Surg Clin North Am 79:297, 1999

51. Macintyre PE: Safety and efficacy of patient-controlled analgesia. Br J Anaesth 87:36, 2001

52. Kehlet H, Werner M, Perkins F: Balanced analgesia: what is it and what are its advantages in postoperative pain? Drugs 58:793, 1999

53. Jin F, Chung F: Multimodal analgesia for postoperative pain control. J Clin Anesth 13:524, 2001

54. Schmid RL, Sandler AN, Katz J: Use and efficacy of low-dose ketamine in the management of acute postoperative pain: a review of current techniques and outcomes. Pain 82:111, 1999

55. Kidd BL, Urban LA: Mechanisms of inflammatory pain. Br J Anaesth 87:3, 2001

56. Cervero F, Laird JMA: Visceral pain. Lancet 353:2145, 1999

57. Carr DB, Goudas LC: Acute pain. Lancet 353:2051, 1999

58. Woolf CJ, Salter MW: Neural plasticity: increasing the gain in pain. Science 288:1765, 2000

59. Woolf CJ, Max MB: Mechanism-based pain diagnosis: issues for analgesic drug development. Anesthesiology 95:241, 2001

60. Møiniche S, Kehlet H, Dahl JB: A qualitative and quantitative systematic review of preemptive analgesia for postoperative pain relief. Anesthesiology 96:725, 2002

61. Wilmore DW: Metabolic response to severe surgical illness: overview. World J Surg 24:705, 2000

62. Holte K, Kehlet H: Epidural anaesthesia and analgesia: effects on surgical stress responses and implications for postoperative nutrition. Clin Nutr 21:199, 2002

63. Rodgers A, Walker N, Schug S, et al: Reduction of postoperative mortality and morbidity with epidural or spinal anaesthesia: results from overview or randomized trials. BMJ 321:1493, 2000

64. Effect of epidural anesthesia and analgesia on perioperative outcome: a randomized, controlled Veterans Affairs Cooperative study. Department of Veterans Affairs Cooperative Study #345 Study Group. Ann Surg 234:560, 2001

65. Norris EJ, Beattie C, Perler BA, et al: Double-masked randomized trial comparing alternate combinations of intraoperative anesthesia and postoperative analgesia in abdominal aortic surgery. Anesthesiology 95:1054, 2001

66. Epidural anaesthesia and analgesia and outcome of major surgery: a randomized trial. MASTER Anaesthesia Trial Study Group. Lancet 359:1276, 2002

67. Kehlet H, Wilmore DW: Multimodal strategies to improve surgical outcome. Am J Surg 183:630, 2002

68. Werner M, Søholm L, Rotbøll P, et al: Does an acute pain service improve postoperative outcome? Anesth Analg (in press)

69. World Health Organization: Expert committee on drug dependence, 16th report. Technical Report Series No. 407. World Health Organization, Geneva, 1969

70. Porter J, Jick H: Addiction is rare in patients treated with narcotics (letter). N Engl J Med 302:123, 1980

Acknowledgments

Figure 1 Carol Donner.

Figure 2 Dana Burns Pizer.

6 ROUTINE POSTOPERATIVE MANAGEMENT OF THE HOSPITALIZED PATIENT

Samir M. Fakhry, M.D., F.A.C.S., Edmund J. Rutherford, M.D., F.A.C.S., and George F. Sheldon, M.D., F.A.C.S.

Postoperative care is an integral part of complete surgical management. For a patient undergoing an elective operation, such care should be thought of within the context of perioperative care: that is, it should be considered as part of a continuum that ranges from evaluating and preparing the patient for a surgical procedure to minimizing the stress of the procedure to promoting a return to health after the procedure.

As a result of ongoing surgical and anesthetic advances and the growing application of minimally invasive surgical techniques, many procedures that once necessitated hospitalization are now commonly performed in day surgical units. Other procedures are proving to be amenable to a fast track surgical approach, in which postoperative care focuses on minimizing postoperative pain, enhancing mobility and exercise capacity, and encouraging enteral intake. Such programs typically reduce the length of stay after a major procedure to 1 to 4 days.

In what follows, we focus on postoperative management of more seriously ill patients undergoing major operations, for whom outpatient and fast track approaches generally are not well suited. Such patients may include those with comorbid conditions that prolong recovery, those who have sustained intraoperative complications, and those who are undergoing emergency operations. These patients are heavy users of hospital resources but benefit greatly from medical care available in the modern hospital setting (e.g., ventilatory support, continuous monitoring, and an extensive pharmacopoeia). A portion of this care is provided in the recovery room or the intensive care unit, and its efficient delivery depends on collaboration among physicians from several different disciplines. The surgeon brings balanced surgical judgment to this setting and interacts frequently with the patient and the family.

Postoperative Orders

The direction that postoperative management of a seriously ill patient will take is outlined in the surgeon's postoperative orders [see *Sidebar* Sample Postoperative Orders]. Through this document, the nursing staff is informed of (1) the diagnosis, (2) the operation performed, and (3) the patient's condition. Monitoring measures are listed, and the therapeutic measures to be employed (analgesia, antibiotics, wound care, I.V. fluid administration, and the handling of tubes, catheters, and drains) are detailed. Evidence-based analyses indicate that certain common therapies are indeed valuable (e.g., inhaled oxygen[1,2]), whereas others either are not of proven benefit (e.g., intermittent positive-pressure breathing [IPPB] and room humidification) or are indicated only in selected situations (e.g., for gastritis, which is appropriate only in patients who are undergoing mechanical ventilation or who have coagulopathies[3]).

Some uniformity in the postoperative orders is valuable because it allows a decrease in the floor stock of medications and increases the nursing staff's experience with specific medications and procedures. Physicians should become acquainted with the costs of the various treatments and medications at their institution. Choices made on the basis of both efficacy and expense will become increasingly common as hospital systems adapt to the changing health care environment.

Postoperative Monitoring

In the postoperative period, many patients return to the same room they occupied preoperatively. Some, however, require more advanced monitoring and care and will require admission to a monitored telemetry bed, an intermediate care unit, or a surgical critical care unit.

The selection of postoperative monitoring is guided by a thorough understanding of the patient's preoperative status and medical history, the diagnosis that led to the operation, the operation performed, and the circumstances of the operative procedure. The vital signs that are commonly monitored on a surgical ward include temperature, pulse rate, blood pressure, respiratory rate, urine output (hourly or at some other interval), weight (daily), and fluid intake and output. These can generally be obtained at intervals of 2 to 4 hours. If more frequent monitoring or nursing care (e.g., frequent suctioning) is required, admission to an intermediate care unit may be advisable. On a telemetry ward, continuous cardiac monitoring can be provided for patients who have significant cardiopulmonary disease or for those at risk for perioperative myocardial infarction or dysrhythmia. In a CCU, additional monitoring is provided, including both noninvasive and invasive monitoring with arterial lines, continuous monitoring of central venous pressure (CVP) and right-sided pulmonary arterial pressures via Swan-Ganz catheterization, continuous monitoring of arterial oxygen saturation via pulse oximetry, measurement of end-tidal carbon dioxide tension, and electrocardiographic monitoring [see *6:4 Cardiopulmonary Monitoring*]. Recommended criteria for ICU admission and discharge have been formulated.[4] When resources are limited, such guidelines may be useful in resolving triage difficulties, but each institution and each unit will have to develop its own approach to this sometimes thorny problem.

Controversy continues regarding what level of monitoring is most appropriate for each patient. In many hospitals, requests for ICU beds exceed the number of available critical care beds, and triage of patients is necessary. This sometimes means moving patients from the ICU before their primary physician feels they are ready for transfer, canceling or delaying operative procedures, and providing less than the requested level of postoperative monitoring for some patients. The increased use of intermediate or step-down units has provided some relief in these difficult situations, but appropriate allocation of resources continues to be a major issue in postoperative bed selection. It has been argued that in some clinical circumstances, our ability to monitor disease may have outpaced our ability to intervene therapeutically.[5] A

Sample Postoperative Orders

An otherwise healthy 50-year-old, 70 kg man was recently diagnosed with a cecal carcinoma. He has type 2 (adult-onset) diabetes, for which he takes an oral hypoglycemic. He has arrived in the postanesthesia care unit (PACU) in stable condition after an uneventful right hemicolectomy and primary reanastomosis of 2 hours' duration under general anesthesia. Intraoperative blood loss is estimated at 100 ml, fluid replacement was 2,500 ml of lactated Ringer solution, and urine output totaled 250 ml.

[Date and Time]
1. Admit to PACU; Service: surgery H; Attending: Sheldon; Resident: Fakhry
2. Diagnosis: colon cancer; status: post right hemicolectomy
3. Condition: stable
4. Vital signs per PACU routine, then every 4 hours on ward × 24 hours, then every shift
5. Activity: out of bed to chair three times a day, beginning this evening; walk hall three times a day
6. Diet: nothing by mouth, but may have sips of ice chips and hard candy
7. Allergies: no known drug allergies
8. [Daily weight]
9. Accurate intake and output
10. Foley catheter to gravity
11. Fluids: 5% dextrose in lactated Ringer solution at 125 ml/hr

12. Antithrombosis prophylaxis
13. Medications:
    patient-controlled analgesia (if indicated): morphine sulfate, 1 to 2 mg I.V. every 10 minutes on demand
    other medications as indicated (e.g., pain medication, acetaminophen, preoperative medications)
14. Insulin sliding scale (for diabetic patients): finger-stick glucose every 6 hours and cover as follows:
    < 60 ------------------ call physician
    60–180 ------------- no coverage
    180–240 ----------- 5 units subcutaneous regular insulin
    240–300 ----------- 10 units subcutaneous regular insulin
    > 300 -------------- 15 units subcutaneous regular insulin, and call physician
15. Morning laboratory tests: complete blood count and electrolyte panel (if indicated)
16. Call physician for
    systolic blood pressure > 180 mm Hg or < 90 mm Hg
    diastolic blood pressure > 100 mm Hg
    heart rate > 120 or < 60 a minute
    respirations > 32 or < 12 a minute
    temperature > 38.5° C (101.3° F)
    urine output < 200 ml every 4 hours

---

consensus conference sponsored by the National Institutes of Health in 1983 concluded that although the care provided in ICUs appears beneficial, the only area in which improved outcome could be documented was coronary care.[6] Acceptable indications for admission to CCUs and invasive monitoring with arterial lines and pulmonary arterial catheters have been proposed; they include myocardial infarction, shock, drug overdose, major cardiovascular surgery, acute respiratory distress syndrome (ARDS), and other forms of respiratory failure that call for mechanical ventilation [see 6:4 Cardiopulmonary Monitoring].[7]

The laboratory tests that are often obtained postoperatively may be thought of as another form of postoperative monitoring. Although such tests can be valuable, they are infrequently used to make important clinical judgments. Technological developments have made it possible for the nursing staff to monitor blood gas pressures, pH, and other biochemical indices at the bedside. For example, finger-stick blood glucose measurements are indicated in insulin-resistant patients and should be obtained every 6 hours (see below). Hematocrits should be obtained postoperatively only if serious bleeding is suspected. The white blood cell count routinely increases after the stress of operation and is therefore of little diagnostic value during the first few days after operation. Thrombocytopenia routinely accompanies major trauma, massive transfusion, and major operative procedures (e.g., cardiac bypass operation); platelet counts are necessary only if the patient shows evidence of bleeding.

In healthy individuals with normal renal function, serum electrolyte levels are usually well maintained despite major stress. In these patients, infrequent measurements of serum electrolytes are appropriate (every 2 or 3 days). By contrast, in patients with an underlying chronic disease, such as renal or hepatic disease or an illness that routinely results in electrolyte derangement, frequent measurements of electrolytes are indicated. The electrolyte

abnormalities that are the most serious and potentially the most immediately life threatening are hypokalemia and hyperkalemia. These abnormalities must be corrected rapidly; multiple potassium measurements to confirm this correction are required. Abnormal levels of sodium and chloride should be corrected over a period of days.

Serum calcium measurements reflect total serum calcium. Only the ionized fraction of serum calcium is active, however, and thus, total serum calcium levels are not reliable indicators of the need for calcium administration.[8] However, after parathyroid operation, measurements of calcium levels are valuable because the other factors that affect the level of ionized calcium are usually unchanged.

Coagulation studies are overused preoperatively and are unnecessary postoperatively, except to monitor anticoagulation therapy or to evaluate the bleeding patient. Arterial blood gas measurements are useful in ventilated or hypoxic patients but should be used judiciously.

Postoperative Pain Relief

Despite the considerable progress that has been made in understanding the pathophysiology of pain,[9] routine pain management is often unsatisfactory.[10] Many hospitals have established pain services that improve quality of care and optimize relief of pain,[11,12] which is a prerequisite for optimal recovery.[13]

Treatment of postoperative pain actually begins before the procedure, as the health care team educates the patient about the events that will occur before, during, and after the procedure. Classic studies demonstrated that such an educational approach reduced patients' requirements for analgesics and diminished their perception of pain.[14]

Preemptive anesthesia reduces the sensation of pain before the creation of the incision, thereby significantly decreasing pain per-

Table 1   Suggested Dosing of Opioid and Nonopioid Analgesics

Class	Drug	Oral Dosage	Parenteral Dosage	Comments
Opioid agonists	Morphine	10–30 mg q. 4 hr	0.05–0.1 mg/kg I.V. (maximum, 15 mg), followed by 4–6 mg/hr I.V. 5–20 mg I.M. q. 4 hr	—
	Heroin	—	—	Not available in United States
	Fentanyl	—	1–2 μg/kg I.V., followed by 1–2 μg/kg/hr I.V.	Transdermal patches available in 25, 50, 75, and 100 μg/hr release
	Sufentanil	—	0.2–0.6 μg/kg I.V., followed by 0.01–0.05 μg/kg/min I.V.	—
	Alfentanil	—	10–25 μg/kg I.V., followed by 0.5–3.0 μg/kg/min I.V.	Safe in renal insufficiency
	Remifentanil	—	0.0125–0.025 μg/kg/min I.V.	—
	Hydromorphone	2–4 mg q. 4–6 hr	0.5–2 mg I.V. q. 1–2 hr	—
	Oxymorphone	—	1–1.5 mg S.C. or I.M. q. 4–6 hr 0.5 mg I.V.	—
	Levorphanol	2–3 mg q. 4 hr	2–3 mg S.C. q. 4–6 hr	Optimal I.V. dose has not been established
	Methadone	5–20 mg q. 3–4 hr	2.5–10.0 mg S.C., I.M., or I.V. q. 3–4 hr	Excellent I.V.-to-oral bioavailability, 1:2 mg
	Meperidine	50–150 mg q. 3–4 hr	25–100 mg I.V. q. 3–4 hr	Generally not recommended, because of oral effectiveness and active metabolites; increased bioavailability in liver failure exacerbates action of the normeperidine metabolite
	Oxycodone	5–10 mg q. 4–6 hr	—	Certain preparations contain acetaminophen
	Hydrocodone	5–10 mg q. 4–6 hr	—	—
	Acetaminophen with codeine	15–60 mg q. 3–6 hr	15–60 mg S.C., I.M., or I.V. q. 4 hr	—
	Propoxyphene	32–65 mg q. 4 hr	—	—
Opioid agonist antagonists	Buprenorphine	—	0.3 mg I.M. or I.V. q. 6 hr	—
	Pentazocine	25 mg t.i.d.–q.i.d.	30 mg S.C., I.M., or I.V. q. 3–4 hr	—
	Nalbuphine	—	10 mg S.C., I.M., or I.V. q. 3–6 hr	Often used with epidural narcotics to decrease side-effect profile of itching and hypotension
	Butorphanol	—	1 mg I.V. q. 3–4 hr 2 mg I.M. q. 3–4 hr	—
	Dezocine	—	5–20 mg I.M. q. 3–6 hr 2.5–10.0 mg I.V. q. 2–4 hr	—
	Tramadol	50–100 mg q. 4–6 hr	—	—

COX—cyclooxygenase   OA—osteoarthritis   PDA—patent ductus arteriosus   RA—rheumatoid arthritis

(continued)

ception in the postoperative period. Techniques utilizing epidural anesthesia[15] or major field block[16] achieve a greater reduction in perceived pain than general anesthesia does, and they greatly reduce the need for postoperative analgesics while enhancing postdischarge activity. Epidural anesthesia and other regional techniques are being applied more frequently, now that a number of trials have found them to be superior to general anesthesia.[17] In the case of epidural anesthesia, the catheter can be used to provide sustained pain relief for several days after operation. This approach is particularly useful in patients who have undergone operations on the lower abdomen or the lower extremities: it can lead to earlier mobilization and return of bowel function after operation, thereby shortening hospital stay.[18]

Systemic medications used for postoperative pain relief include opioids, nonsteroidal anti-inflammatory drugs (NSAIDs), and other nonnarcotic agents [*see Table 1*]. Surgeons are currently moving away from systemic opioids: in addition to their well-recognized capacity for inducing respiratory depression, opioids prolong ileus and increase nausea and vomiting. Regional anesthesia coupled with NSAID administration appears to yield better results in terms of patient recovery.[18]

On occasion, however, systemically administered narcotics are still the best available choice. Studies addressing postoperative pain have shown that most cases of severe pain are not uniformly relieved by the current practice of narcotic prescription. According to one study, physicians prescribe inadequate doses of

Table 1   Suggested Dosing of Opioid and Nonopioid Analgesics (*continued*)

Class	Drug	Oral Dosage	Parenteral Dosage	Comments
Nonopioid analgesics	Acetaminophen	325–650 mg q. 4 hr	—	Maximum, 4 g/day
	Acetylated salicylate Aspirin	325–650 mg q. 4 hr	—	—
	Nonacetylated salicylates Diflunisal	Loading dose, 1,000 mg, then 500–1,000 mg/day	—	FDA indications: pain, OA, and RA
	Salsalate	1,500 mg b.i.d.	—	FDA indications: RA and OA
	Choline magnesium trisalicylate	1,000–2,000 mg b.i.d.	—	FDA indications: OA, RA, and acute painful shoulder
	Propionic acids Ibuprofen	400–800 mg t.i.d.–q.i.d.	—	FDA indications: RA, OA, pain, and dysmenorrhea
	Fenoprofen	200 mg q. 4–6 hr	—	FDA indications: RA, OA, and pain
	Ketoprofen	50–75 mg t.i.d. or q.i.d.	—	FDA indications: RA, OA, pain, and dysmenorrhea
	Naproxen	500 mg, followed by 250 mg q. 6 hr	—	FDA indications: pain, RA, OA, dysmenorrhea, juvenile arthritis, ankylosing spondylitis, tendinitis, bursitis, and gout
	Flurbiprofen	50–100 mg b.i.d. or t.i.d.	—	FDA indications: RA and OA
	Oxaprozin	1,200 mg q. day	—	FDA indications: OA and RA
	Acetic acids Indomethacin	25 mg b.i.d. or t.i.d.	I.V. used to close PDA	FDA indications: RA, OA, ankylosing spondylitis, acute painful shoulder, and gout
	Sulindac	200 mg b.i.d.	—	FDA indications: OA, RA, ankylosing spondylitis, acute painful shoulder, and gout
	Tolmetin	400 mg t.i.d.	—	FDA indications: RA and OA
	Diclofenac	50 mg t.i.d.	—	FDA indications: RA, OA, and ankylosing spondylitis
	Etodolac	200–400 mg q. 6–8 hr, to maximum of 1,200 mg/day	—	FDA indications: OA and pain
	Nabumetone	1,000 mg/day	—	FDA indications: OA and RA
	Ketorolac	10 mg q. 4 hr	30 mg I.V., followed by 15–30 mg I.V. q. 6 hr 60 mg deep I.M., followed by 30 mg I.V. q. 6 hr	Maximum, 120 mg/day
	Oxicam Piroxicam	20 mg/day	—	FDA indications: OA and RA
	Fenamates Meclofenamate	50 mg q. 4 hr	—	FDA indications: pain, dysmenorrhea, RA, and OA
	Mefenamic acid	500 mg, followed by 250 mg q. 6 hr	—	FDA indications: pain and dysmenorrhea
	COX-2 inhibitors Rofecoxib	12.5–25.0 mg/day	—	FDA indications: OA, pain, and dysmenorrhea
	Celecoxib	100–200 mg q. 12–24 hr	—	FDA indications: OA, RA, and familial adenomatous polyposis

narcotic analgesics for patients with moderate or severe pain, and nurses give only 40% to 50% of the amount prescribed.[19] In this study, the effective dose of narcotic required for pain relief was underestimated, the fear of respiratory depression was high, the duration of action was overestimated, and the danger of addic-tion was exaggerated. (Addiction usually does not develop unless narcotics are prescribed regularly for more than 2 weeks.)

NSAIDs, though safer than narcotics, have side effects of their own. In particular, they inhibit prostaglandin synthesis, thereby decreasing inflammation. This prostaglandin inhibition may

Table 2 Guidelines for I.V. Patient-Controlled Analgesia

Drug (Concentration)	Basal Dosage	Demand Dosage	Lockout Interval
Morphine (1–2 mg/ml)	0–0.5 mg/hr	0.5–3.0 mg	5–12 min
Meperidine (10 mg/ml)	0–5 mg/hr	5–30 mg	5–12 min
Fentanyl (10–20 µg/ml)	0–5 µg/hr	10–20 µg	5–10 min
Hydromorphone (0.2–0.5 mg/ml)	0–0.1 mg/hr	0.1–0.5 mg	5–10 min
Oxymorphone (0.25 mg/ml)	—	0.2–0.4 mg	8–10 min
Methadone (1 mg/ml)	0–0.5 mg/hr	0.5–2.5 mg	8–20 min
Nalbuphine (1 mg/ml)	—	1–5 mg	5–10 min

exacerbate renal insufficiency; for this reason, NSAIDs should be used with caution in patients with preexisting renal dysfunction. Other side effects include GI bleeding, inhibition of platelet aggregation, and prolonged bleeding time.

Patient-controlled analgesia (PCA) represents an important advance in pain management [see 1:5 Postoperative Pain].[20-22] This modality has gained widespread acceptance because it provides improved pain control and greater patient satisfaction, which are attributable both to more expedient administration of the drug and to more consistent plasma levels. PCA generally takes the form of intermittent drug doses administered on demand, with a minimal required interval between doses (the lockout interval). A constant background infusion (basal dosage) may be given to supplement the intermittent dose, but it should be used cautiously so as not to induce respiratory depression. The narcotics most commonly used for PCA are morphine, meperidine, and fentanyl. Methadone is rarely given in this setting because of its slow onset and long duration of action [see Table 2]. Nalbuphine, though possessing narcotic analgesic properties of its own, is generally used for its antagonist properties, which act against side effects such as pruritus. Other side effects seen with patient-controlled analgesia are nausea, vomiting, sweating, and the aforementioned respiratory depression.

Management of Fluid Imbalance, Electrolyte Abnormalities, and Acid-Base Disorders

Postoperative fluid therapy is guided by the patient's overall preoperative condition, the preoperative diagnosis, and the circumstances of the operative procedure. The presence of cardiac, pulmonary, renal, or hepatic disease will affect the type and rate of fluid required postoperatively. Similarly, peritonitis, the septic response, or other conditions that affect the patient's volume status and peripheral capillary permeability will influence the approach to fluid therapy. In an adequately hydrated patient who has undergone a minor procedure with minimal blood loss and for whom the postoperative recovery period is expected to be short, maintenance fluid administration alone is adequate. Maintenance requirements for a 70 kg patient are normally about 100 ml/hr of 5% dextrose in one-half normal saline, with approximately 20 mEq/L of potassium added. By contrast, in a patient with bowel obstruction, small bowel infarction, and bowel perforation, maintenance fluid administration alone is inadequate. In these patients, reequilibration and fluid loss from the intravascular space continue for many hours after operation; consequently, resuscitation must be continued postoperatively, and as much as 7 to 10 L of crystalloid may have to be given over 24 hours to maintain adequate perfusion.

In patients who require continued postoperative volume resuscitation, hypotonic fluids, even at an increased rate, are not appropriate. Isotonic fluid is required to maintain adequate intravascular volume. Administration of 5% dextrose in lactated Ringer solution at the rate of 150 ml/hr provides about six times as much intravascular volume resuscitation as the usual maintenance regimen. Adjustments in volume should be guided by careful monitoring of urine output, pulse rate, and BP. A common error in postoperative fluid therapy is to order hypotonic fluids at an increased rate of administration (i.e., 150 ml/hr of 5% dextrose in 0.5 N saline) after determining, on the basis of physical examination findings (i.e., tachycardia, decreased BP, and decreased urine output in the appropriate clinical situation), that a patient is relatively hypovolemic. Because fluid losses into the interstitium are isotonic, isotonic fluid replacement is indicated.

In addition, the use of isotonic fluids is important because of the presence of elevated levels of antidiuretic hormone (ADH) and other counterregulatory hormones. In a normal, unstressed person, free-water loading (e.g., the drinking of several glasses of water) results in a fall in ADH levels and excretion of very dilute urine by the kidney, thus allowing the serum sodium and osmolality to return to normal. Various stressful stimuli, including operative procedures, result in an inability to lower ADH levels and an inability to excrete free water.[23-25] The administration of hypotonic fluid, with its free-water content, can lead to hyponatremia in postoperative patients and others with elevated levels of counterregulatory stress hormones. The resultant hyponatremia may cause significant morbidity and mortality.[26,27] The use of isotonic fluid prevents this problem. In uncomplicated elective procedures of brief duration (e.g., hernia repair, cholecystectomy, and uncomplicated bowel surgery), the stress response is short-lived and the patient can be switched to maintenance fluids 24 hours after operation. Patients who undergo operation under local anesthesia do not experience a stress response and generally need little, if any, fluid.

Once recovery from a major insult has begun, the capillary leak closes and fluid is mobilized from the periphery into the vascular space. At this point, the fluid orders should be changed to maintenance rates or lower and from isotonic resuscitation fluid to hypotonic saline. An important sign that the capillary leak has reversed is the return of a brisk urine output. Such spontaneous diuresis is a significant marker of the patient's recovery. It is associated with a fall in levels of ADH, aldosterone, steroids, catecholamines, and other counterregulatory hormones and with a rise in atrial natriuretic factor.[28,29] The use of diuretics in an attempt to "diurese off" excess fluid masks this physiologic response; therefore, diuretics should be reserved for use in patients who have inadequate renal or cardiac function and should be administered only after the capillary leak has reversed, so as not to cause intravascular volume depletion.

Several I.V. fluids are commonly employed for maintenance and resuscitation [see Table 3]. Crystalloids are the fluids of choice for perioperative fluid replacement. The use of colloid solutions offers no clear advantages in perioperative care, and their very high cost makes it difficult to justify their use in the majority of surgical patients.[30-32] A meta-analysis of 30 randomized, controlled trials comparing albumin to either no albumin or crystalloid in critically ill patients with hypovolemia, burns, or hypoalbuminemia found strong evidence suggesting that use of albumin may increase mortality.[33]

In the first 24 hours after operation, potassium supplementation is unnecessary in most patients. Potassium levels in I.V. fluids should be adjusted according to serum potassium levels.

Unfortunately, the serum potassium level provides an extremely inaccurate estimate of total body potassium. A profound depletion may exist despite serum potassium levels in the low to normal range. The long-term use of diuretics such as furosemide and the thiazides is commonly associated with low body stores of potassium. Patients undergoing nutritional repletion will also tend to have low serum potassium levels. If the patient has questionable renal function, potassium should be withheld until a serum level is available. If renal function is normal and urine output is not compromised, we add 20 mEq/L of potassium to the I.V. fluids after the first 24 postoperative hours.

FLUID IMBALANCE

Patients who undergo uncomplicated elective procedures usually experience relatively inconsequential abnormalities of their intravascular volume. However, patients who undergo lengthy or complicated procedures or have abnormalities of intravascular volume preoperatively are more likely to manifest abnormalities of circulating volume and should be evaluated carefully in the postoperative period to assess their intravascular volume status and tissue perfusion.

Hypovolemia

Hypovolemia is a decrease in the effective intravascular volume, caused by losses incurred either externally (e.g., hemorrhage or loss of transcellular fluid) or internally (e.g., transcapillary leakage of fluid into traumatized tissue). Oxygen delivery and tissue perfusion are dependent on the ability to generate an adequate cardiac output in the presence of hemoglobin that is sufficiently saturated (arterial oxygen saturation [S_aO_2] more than 90%, arterial oxygen tension [P_aO_2] more than 60 mm Hg). An inadequate intravascular volume can lead to poor perfusion either because of a lowered preload that results in a depressed cardiac output or because of a low hemoglobin concentration (e.g., from bleeding). Younger patients usually tolerate a lowered hemoglobin

concentration by increasing cardiac output, provided that intravascular volume is adequate. Older patients with coronary artery disease are more likely to suffer deleterious effects if their intravascular volume, their hemoglobin concentration, or both are low, because such patients have a limited ability to augment cardiac output under these circumstances.

Standard monitoring of volume status includes vital signs, mental status, and urine output. Because of the effects of general anesthesia, unrecognized intravascular volume depletion may develop. If a Foley catheter has been inserted, a decrease in the urine output can be an early sign of such depletion. Hypovolemia with depletion of the intravascular compartment should not be confused with changes in total body water, which may or may not occur in hypovolemia. If body weight is used to assess total body water content, it is possible to assume that a patient is "fluid overloaded" because of an elevated body weight, though in fact the intravascular volume has been depleted and the patient is underperfused and hypovolemic. This is a common scenario in patients who have sustained significant losses of intravascular volume and blood with resulting shock, capillary leakage, and fluid accumulation in the interstitium and the intracellular compartment.[34]

It has been demonstrated that the volume status of an individual patient, especially if he or she has unstable vital signs or is critically ill in the ICU, cannot be easily estimated by means of clinical assessment alone.[35,36] The use of invasive monitoring is therefore important in determining the status of the intravascular compartment and the ability of the body to maintain tissue perfusion. The use of a pulmonary arterial catheter to determine cardiac filling pressures and cardiac output usually allows a more accurate assessment of the patient's intravascular volume status. In patients who are relatively stable hemodynamically but manifest signs of a contracted intravascular volume (e.g., low urine output, increased heart rate, low or borderline blood pressure, depressed mental status, poor capillary refill), an isotonic fluid challenge should be administered. At least 500 and preferably 1,000 ml of lactated Ringer solution or normal

Table 3 Commonly Used I.V. Fluids

Solution	Plasma Osmolality (mOsm/L)	pH	Na+ (mEq/L)	Cl− (mEq/L)	K+ (mEq/L)	Ca2+ (mEq/L)	Other Components	Cost* ($)	Comments
D5LR (1,000 ml)	525	5	130	109	4	3	Lactate 28 mEq/L, 50 g dextrose	6	Fluid of choice for initial resuscitation and postoperative replacement
D5NS (1,000 ml)	560	4	154	154	0	0	50 g dextrose	6	Alternative to D5LR, but large amounts may cause metabolic acidosis
D5½NS (1,000 ml)	406	4	77	77	0	0	50 g dextrose	6	Hypotonic maintenance fluid
D5¼NS (1,000 ml)	321	4	34	34	0	0	50 g dextrose	6	Hypotonic maintenance fluid
D5W (1,000 ml)	321	4.5	0	0	0	0	50 g dextrose	6	Free-water source, no role in resuscitation
25% Albumin (100 ml)	Equal to plasma	Equal to plasma	145	0	0	0	25 g albumin	67	Colloid, expensive
5% Plasma protein fraction (250 ml)	Equal to plasma	Equal to plasma	145	0	< 2	0	12.5 g protein	33	Colloid, expensive
6% Hetastarch in 0.9% NaCl (500 ml)	310	3.5–7.0	154	154	0	0	30 g hydroxyethyl starch	42	Use limited volume (500–1,000 ml); coagulation abnormalities with larger volumes

*Reflects sample cost to pharmacy at the University of North Carolina at Chapel Hill School of Medicine. Actual cost to the patient is likely to be significantly higher.
D5LR—5% dextrose in lactated Ringer solution D5NS—5% dextrose in normal saline solution D5½NS—5% dextrose in one-half normal saline solution D5¼NS—5% dextrose in one-quarter saline solution D5W—5% dextrose in water

saline solution should be given rapidly and the patient's response evaluated. If the vital signs normalize and the urine output rises, the patient is assumed to be responding to volume loading. Further observation will determine whether the patient requires more isotonic fluid administration. If the patient does not respond to the initial bolus of fluid or has significant renal or cardiopulmonary dysfunction, it is generally more prudent to employ invasive monitoring with a pulmonary arterial catheter to determine the status of the intravascular compartment. The use of diuretics in this setting should be limited to patients who have known severe cardiopulmonary dysfunction or advanced renal disease with a known dependency on diuretics. The administration of a diuretic to a patient with intravascular volume depletion can result in further depletion of the intravascular volume despite the production of urine.

Other techniques useful in the assessment of a patient's volume status include measurement of sodium in the urine sediment, cardiac echocardiography, and the determination of serum lactate levels. None of these techniques is entirely accurate or practical. The response to a fluid bolus remains a practical means of assessing the status of the intravascular compartment. Failure to respond to one or more fluid boluses should prompt further evaluation, including invasive monitoring if indicated.

Fluid Overload

Fluid overload in the postoperative surgical patient is reported to occur with varying frequency and has been associated with inferior outcomes.[37] The degree to which a patient may become "overloaded" with fluid is determined by the patient's preoperative status, age, and existing cardiopulmonary, renal, or hepatic disorders; the length of the operative procedure; the fluids administered; and the presence or absence of infection and inflammatory mediators. Although it is generally accepted that patients who require large amounts of fluid and who gain weight in the postoperative period are likely to have a less favorable outcome, it is difficult to separate the effect of large-volume resuscitation from the circumstances that prompt such therapy, most commonly shock, a septic response, or both.

Judicious use of fluids in the perioperative period and the application of the principles of invasive monitoring outlined above generally allow appropriate volume resuscitation without precipitating pulmonary edema or congestive heart failure. It should be recognized, however, that in patients who sustain shock or manifest a septic response (with or without bacterial infection), fluid will leak from the intravascular compartments and total body anasarca will develop. The resultant increase in body weight associated with an increased requirement for fluid infusion will give the impression that the patient is receiving excessive amounts of fluid. Although this may be the case, it is generally difficult to determine intravascular volume status in more seriously ill patients through simple observation alone.[35,36] The value of invasive monitoring in the ICU should again be emphasized. Patients suspected of being "fluid overloaded" should be carefully evaluated by an experienced clinician, and if they do not respond to preliminary measures to correct their volume status, they should undergo invasive monitoring.

ELECTROLYTE ABNORMALITIES

Disorders of Sodium Concentration

Hyponatremia Hyponatremia is caused by excess free water in the intravascular space [see 6:8 Disorders of Water and Sodium Balance]. The serum sodium concentration is not an accurate measure of total body sodium but rather reflects the concentration of sodium relative to the amount of free water in the intravascular compartment. The serum sodium concentration is not related to the volume state of the intravascular compartment. Patients may be normovolemic, hypovolemic, or hypervolemic in the presence of hyponatremia.

In the postoperative setting, hyponatremia usually results from an excess of free water. This occurs when hypotonic fluid is administered to patients whose ADH levels cannot fall because of the stress of operation or injury. In these patients, the free water administered as hypotonic fluid cannot be eliminated through the kidney, and hyponatremia results. In most cases, the stress subsides in 24 to 48 hours and the ADH levels fall, which allows the kidney to correct the free-water excess. Patients who continue to be ill or under stress and those who have poor renal function may experience difficulty in correcting the free-water excess. Significant morbidity and mortality can occur if the serum sodium concentration falls below 120 mEq/L.[26,27] Hyponatremia in the postoperative setting is best avoided by means of appropriate I.V. fluid management, including the use of isotonic fluid in the immediate postoperative period.

The treatment of hyponatremia depends on the serum sodium concentration and how long it took serum sodium to reach that level. Intravascular volume deficits, if present, should be corrected first. Patients who have chronically depressed serum sodium concentrations will tolerate slow correction with isotonic fluid (e.g., lactated Ringer solution or normal saline solution). Patients who experience an acute, rapid falloff of their serum sodium concentration or those who are symptomatic require correction with hypertonic (3%) saline over 24 to 48 hours.

Hypernatremia Hypernatremia reflects a relative deficiency of free water compared with sodium. Under normal circumstances, hypernatremia stimulates thirst, and the intake of free water returns the serum sodium concentration to normal. Hypernatremia may develop in patients who are unable to regulate fluid intake (e.g., obtunded patients) or do not have their fluids replaced appropriately. This is especially likely in patients with large free-water losses such as sweat and insensible losses. Patients with diabetes insipidus (e.g., as a result of head injury) develop hypernatremia because of large (> 10 L/day) losses of very dilute urine.

Treatment of hypernatremia consists of providing adequate volumes of free water to correct the deficit. Serum sodium concentration is a good indicator of the adequacy of replacement. In the case of diabetes insipidus, treatment with desmopressin acetate, either parenterally or by the nasal route, in concert with careful fluid management will generally alleviate the hypernatremia.

Disorders of Potassium Concentration

Hypokalemia Hypokalemia may have a number of causes in the postoperative patient. Chronic use of diuretics, poor nutrition with total body potassium depletion, and GI losses are all associated with varying degrees of hypokalemia. Among the most common causes is alkalosis, which brings about a shift of potassium into the intracellular compartment.

Since the serum potassium level does not accurately reflect the total body potassium pool, hypokalemia at levels of 3 mEq/L or less is associated with severe total body potassium depletion (usually in excess of 100 mEq). Such patients may require ECG monitoring and should receive I.V. potassium and have levels measured frequently to monitor their progress. Correction of the underlying cause of the problem is important. Potassium should be given only if there is reliable urine flow, however, as dangerously high potassium levels may result in anuric patients. Our practice is to deliver three doses of 10 mEq of potassium chloride in 50 to 100 ml of saline solution and then check serum levels.

Hyperkalemia Hyperkalemia is among the most dangerous of electrolyte abnormalities [see 6:9 Disorders of Acid-Base and Potassium Balance]. It is especially likely to occur in patients with renal dysfunction but can also result from crush injury, hemolysis, myonecrosis, and acidosis. Hyperkalemia can also occur in malignant hyperthermia and after the administration of succinylcholine to patients with spinal cord injury, burns, or neurologic disorders secondary to severe muscle contractions.

The most serious manifestations of hyperkalemia are cardiac in nature and include high-peaked T waves, absent P waves, widened QRS complexes, ventricular arrhythmias, and cardiac arrest (in diastole). Heart block can also occur. Cardiac effects begin at serum potassium levels of around 6.5 mEq/L; serious risk of death is associated with levels exceeding 8 mEq/L. Patients with serum levels above 6.5 mEq/L should be strongly considered for cardiac monitoring until their serum potassium level is under control.

Treatment consists of discontinuance of any exogenous potassium. If acidosis is present, sodium bicarbonate (50 mEq/L I.V.) should be administered. This dose can be repeated after 10 to 15 minutes. Since sodium bicarbonate is hypertonic saline, caution should be exercised in its use if hypernatremia or fluid overload is present. Calcium, 5 mmol I.V. over 5 minutes, will transiently depress the membrane threshold potential and antagonize the effect of potassium on the myocardium. Infusion of glucose and insulin will lower the serum potassium level by driving potassium into the cell. An ampule (50 ml) of 50% dextrose is administered intravenously along with 10 units of regular insulin. Administration of furosemide with or without a bolus of saline in patients with reasonable kidney function will also decrease potassium levels. The administration of cation-exchange resins (e.g., sodium polystyrene sulfonate) either orally or by enema will decrease potassium levels more slowly by binding to ions in the GI tract. If other measures fail, dialysis is highly effective in reducing potassium levels.

ACID-BASE DISORDERS

Respiratory Acidosis

Homeostatic mechanisms maintain arterial carbon dioxide tension (P_aCO_2) and serum pH within the normal range through the central regulation of minute ventilation (tidal volume × respiratory rate). Respiratory acidosis results when the ability to eliminate the produced CO_2 is exceeded [see 6:9 Disorders of Acid-Base and Potassium Balance]. A variety of causes of respiratory acidosis have been identified. They include central causes (e.g., excess sedation and neuromuscular disorders) as well as disorders of ventilation associated with respiratory failure and ventilatory malfunction. Patients with acute respiratory acidosis characteristically have an elevation in their P_aCO_2 associated with a decreased pH. Acute compensation is relatively limited; it is not until the respiratory acidosis has persisted for at least 12 to 24 hours that renal compensatory mechanisms are activated. Serum bicarbonate gradually rises over a period of several days and drives the pH back (but not completely) toward normal. It is thus possible to differentiate between patients with acute respiratory acidosis and those with chronic respiratory acidosis by the assessment of their serum bicarbonate level and pH. Patients should be assessed for potentially reversible factors. Those on mechanical ventilation should have an immediate increase in minute ventilation. If respiratory acidosis fails to resolve in a spontaneously breathing patient and respiratory distress develops, intubation and mechanical ventilation are necessary.

Respiratory Alkalosis

Respiratory alkalosis occurs when CO_2 elimination exceeds CO_2 production. This is usually caused by an increase in minute ventilation with a decrease in P_aCO_2 and an elevation of pH. Only small changes in the serum bicarbonate level occur in the acute form. If respiratory alkalosis persists, renal compensation will lead to a lowering of the serum bicarbonate level and a return of serum pH almost to normal. Patients with respiratory alkalosis generally have mild hypokalemia and hyperchloremia. The hypokalemia is related to the exchange of potassium for hydrogen ions between the intracellular and extracellular compartments in compensation for the alkalemia. In addition, potassium wasting occurs in the kidney. Hyperchloremia results from the renal retention of chloride to offset the gradually falling levels of serum bicarbonate.

The compensation that occurs in the first week of respiratory alkalosis is generally insufficient to return the pH to normal. More chronic forms of alkalosis will ultimately result in a normalization of the serum pH.

Metabolic Acidosis

Metabolic acidosis in the postoperative surgical patient is always worrisome. It occurs when there is either an increase in the production of H^+ or a significant loss of bicarbonate. Increased production of hydrogen ions is generally associated with underperfusion of tissues and the development of lactic acidosis. Although other conditions can result in metabolic acidosis, hypovolemia and poor tissue perfusion must be ruled out in the postoperative patient.

The initial compensatory response to metabolic acidosis in the spontaneously breathing patient is an increase in minute ventilation. Lactic acidosis exhibits a greater increase in minute ventilation than that seen in other forms of metabolic acidosis. If a patient is sedated or mechanically ventilated, this compensation may not occur, in which case the patient will continue to manifest a low serum pH. A pH of 7.2 or greater has not been associated with significant detrimental effects. Once the patient is known to have metabolic acidosis, assessment of the intravascular volume status should be undertaken immediately. If the metabolic acidosis does not resolve with preliminary maneuvers such as fluid bolus therapy, then invasive monitoring should be undertaken to establish the status of the intravascular circulation and the cardiopulmonary system. Persistent acidosis may signal myocardial ischemia, ischemic bowel, sepsis syndrome, or inadequate volume resuscitation in an injured or critically ill patient.

Determination of the anion gap [see 6:9 Disorders of Acid-Base and Potassium Balance], the base deficit, and the serum lactate level can be helpful in determining the cause of the metabolic acidosis. Besides poor tissue perfusion, causes may include renal failure, ketoacidosis, lactic acidosis, and poisoning (all associated with an increased anion gap) as well as renal tubular acidosis, diarrhea, ureteral diversion, and a variety of other conditions (all associated with a normal anion gap).

The base deficit has been shown to be a function of oxygen debt,[38] to correlate with mortality,[39,40] and to be a valuable guide to resuscitation.[40,41] In that the base deficit is a function of all unmeasured cations, it can also arise from types of acidosis other than lactic acidosis. The most common causes of a base deficit besides lactic acidosis are hyperchloremic acidosis and renal insufficiency.

The serum lactate level is a useful indicator of anaerobic metabolism. Clearance of lactate within 24 hours has been shown to correlate with survival.[42] Inadequate perfusion is a major cause of lactic acidosis, but other causes also exist that do not involve perfusion abnormalities. The administration of I.V. bicarbonate generally does not materially affect the outcome of patients who have metabolic acidosis related to inadequate tissue perfusion; the net effect of this measure is a temporary elevation of serum pH associated with an increase of CO_2 production. Bicarbonate combines with hydrogen ions to form carbonic acid and, subsequently, water and CO_2. It should be noted that this increased CO_2 production can result in a worsening of intracellular acidosis if minute ventilation is not increased to allow elimination of the excess CO_2. Furthermore, exogenous bicarbonate eliminates the utility of measuring the base deficit and may worsen oxygen delivery by causing an adverse shift in the oxygen dissociation curve.

Metabolic Alkalosis

Metabolic alkalosis is most often caused by a loss of hydrogen ions from the GI tract (e.g., through vomiting or nasogastric suction) or in the urine (e.g., as a result of diuretic therapy). The loss of hydrogen ions is associated with the liberation of bicarbonate, as shown in the following equation:

$$CO_2 + H_2O \rightarrow H_2CO_3 \rightarrow H^+ + HCO_3^-$$

Hypokalemia can result in metabolic alkalosis by causing a shift of hydrogen ions into the cell in exchange for potassium. Although perceived as extracellular metabolic alkalosis, this is in fact an intracellular metabolic acidosis because of the hydrogen ion shift. Prompt repletion of potassium in the hypokalemic patient can minimize the effect of these changes. Metabolic alkalosis can also result from contraction of the extracellular volume. This contraction alkalosis occurs when the lost fluid contains chloride but little or no bicarbonate, as occurs with diuretic therapy.

Of particular significance in the postoperative period is the development of hypokalemic, hypochloremic metabolic alkalosis associated with the loss of significant amounts of gastric secretions. This can occur either through nasogastric suction or with repeated vomiting. Patients develop intravascular volume contraction in addition to alkalosis and hypochloremia as they lose volume and HCl. This development is associated with an increase in sodium and water retention in the kidney, mediated by ADH and aldosterone. The volume deficit, hypochloremia, and hypokalemia all result in increased bicarbonate absorption by the kidney. Paradoxical aciduria will result as bicarbonate reabsorption, together with sodium and potassium retention, leads to an increased hydrogen ion concentration in the urine. Treatment of hypokalemic, hypochloremic metabolic alkalosis is directed at decreasing the fluid losses, if possible, and providing significant amounts of volume, potassium, and chloride.

Chloride repletion is important because chloride is the only reabsorbable anion in this setting. If adequate chloride is not given, electroneutrality in the distal nephron can be maintained only by the excretion of hydrogen ions. Since the patient is volume contracted, no excess sodium ions are available for excretion, and hypokalemia precludes the excretion of potassium ions. Bicarbonate is being reabsorbed avidly at this time. Thus, as sodium is reabsorbed in the hypovolemic state, hydrogen ions will of necessity be excreted in the urine. If chloride is provided in adequate amounts, it will be reabsorbed with sodium, thus obviating excretion of hydrogen ion (or potassium ions if they are available) to maintain electroneutrality.

Metabolic alkalosis can be divided into two varieties: saline responsive and saline resistant. Saline-responsive metabolic alkalosis is generally caused by GI losses or by diuresis, whereas saline-resistant metabolic alkalosis is usually a consequence of either severe hypokalemia or an edematous state such as cirrhosis. Patients with the saline-responsive variety generally respond well to volume expansion with sodium chloride.

Management of Tubes and Drains

Guidelines for the perioperative use of tubes and drains should be developed on the basis of scientific data. For the most part, current practices in this regard are not rigorously formulated and tested but are simply passed on to surgical trainees on little basis other than surgical tradition. With the development of evidence-based medicine, these approaches are being evaluated and challenged. As a result, this aspect of surgical care is evolving.

NASOGASTRIC TUBES

Traditionally, nasogastric tubes were routinely used in all patients undergoing GI surgery. In the past decade, however, the value of this routine practice for elective surgical patients has been questioned. A 1995 meta-analysis of 26 trials that included 3,964 patients concluded that nasogastric tubes are unnecessary in elective surgical patients and may even add to debility [*see Table 4*].[43] Nasogastric decompression is appropriate on a selective basis for any patient in whom severe nausea, vomiting, or gastric distention develops [*see Figure 1*]. Moreover, it is indicated in patients with intestinal obstruction or those with severe prolonged ileus, usually related to intra-abdominal sepsis.

FINE, PLIABLE FEEDING TUBES

The introduction of the Dobbhoff tube by Dobbie and Hoffmeister allowed routine intubation past the pylorus for feeding.[44] The Dobbhoff tube is a highly flexible No. 8 polyurethane tube with two distal side holes and a mercury-weighted tip. A steel wire is used to stent the tube during placement and is removed after the tube is positioned. The Dobbhoff tube and the Entriflex tube (a similar tube with a thin, elongated distal segment) are placed in a manner similar to that of a nasogastric tube [*see Figure 1*]. Once in the stomach, the tube can be advanced under fluoroscopic guidance into the duodenum. Alternatively, the tube can be allowed to pass spontaneously through the pylorus by placing the patient in the right lateral decubitus position and allowing enough slack externally. The use of metoclopramide can sometimes facilitate passage into the duodenum. A radiograph should always be obtained before the initiation of feedings through a nasoenteric small-bore catheter [*see Figure 2*]. These tubes can pass easily into the trachea even in intubated patients and can cause a pneumothorax or a pneumonic process if feedings are given without radiographic confirmation that the location of the tip is correct.[45,46]

LONG INTESTINAL TUBES

Long intestinal tubes (e.g., the Cantor tube and the Miller-Abbott tube) are occasionally used in patients with partial small-bowel obstruction early after operation, although mechanical bowel obstruction usually necessitates early operation. Use of long intestinal tubes should be reserved for selected patients who are not candidates for early reoperation. Because movement distally is dependent on peristalsis, these tubes are of little value in patients with paralytic ileus. The Cantor tube is made of silicone-coated polyvinyl chloride and has a small balloon tip. The tip is filled with mercury, passed through the nose, and allowed to advance into the small intestine either passively or under fluoroscopic guidance; there, it will aspirate fluid and gas. Removal of the tube is accomplished by pulling approximately 30 cm of tube out of the nose every 1 or 2 hours and either taping or clamping it to prevent slippage.

BILIARY DRAINAGE CATHETERS

Biliary tract drains include cholecystostomy tubes, percutaneous drains of the biliary tract placed under fluoroscopic control, T tubes, and endoscopically placed nasobiliary tubes. Cholecystostomy tubes may be placed with the help of local anesthesia in patients with advanced medical problems who cannot tolerate general anesthesia and formal cholecystectomy. Patients in whom dissection would be technically difficult and associated with a high risk of complications can also be treated by cholecystostomy tube placement. Ultrasonographically guided percutaneous cholecystostomy tube placement has gained acceptance for patients who are not considered good candidates for operation.

The use of T tubes is generally limited to operative exploration or repair of the common bile duct (CBD). In most cases, the CBD is explored for the presence of stones. The duct is then closed around the T-shaped end of the tube to stent the duct. The long end of the T tube is then brought out of an incision, sutured to the skin, and attached to a drainage bag. The exit site should be chosen to allow direct percutaneous access into the distal CBD should this become necessary for later stone extraction or duct manipulation. A T tube usually drains most of the bile produced (600 to 700 ml daily) initially. A decrease in the volume of bile drained indicates patency of the distal duct and free flow into the duodenum. At 7 to 10 days after the operation, a cholangiogram is obtained to assess the patency of the CBD and look for stones. I.V. antibiotics should be administered during cholangiography. A normal cholangiogram shows no stones; a patent, nondilated CBD without leakage; and free flow of contrast medium into the duodenum. The tube can be removed by gentle withdrawal; alternatively, the tube is clamped, and if the patient continues to do well, it is removed on an outpatient basis after 1 to 2 weeks. If the cholangiogram is abnormal, the T tube should be left to drain and the problem addressed either through the tract of the T tube or by means of endoscopic retrograde cholangiopancreatography.

Nasobiliary tubes are placed at the time of endoscopic evaluation of the biliary tree, usually to alleviate CBD obstruction. These tubes are left to drain by gravity and can otherwise be managed in much the same fashion as nasoenteric tubes.

DRAINS

Various tubes and associated devices have been used to drain purulent materials, blood, or serum from body cavities. These include Penrose drains (very soft rubber tubes with a gauze wick), closed suction drains (e.g., Jackson-Pratt or Hemovac drains), and sump drains (multiple-lumen tubes that draw air into one interior lumen and fluid from a companion tube). Controlled clinical trials in elective surgical patients indicate that routine use of drains does not improve outcome for patients undergoing cholecystectomy,[47] laminectomy,[48] colon surgery,[49]

Table 4 Meta-analysis of 26 Clinical Trials of Selective versus Routine Nasogastric Decompression[43]

	Selective Decompression	Routine Decompression	*P*
Total no. of patients	1,986	1,978	—
Patients with complications	833	1,084	< 0.03
Patients with pneumonia	53	119	< 0.0001
Patients with atelectasis	44	94	0.001
Patients with fever	108	212	0.02
Time to oral feeding (days)	3.53	4.59	0.04

or thyroid surgery.[50] Postoperative drainage does, however, reduce serum formation and other wound problems after mastectomy.[51] Postmastectomy wound drainage can be managed on an outpatient basis and thus need not hinder or delay discharge.

FOLEY CATHETERS

Foley catheters are routinely used after operation to drain the urinary bladder [*see Figure 3*]. Bladder catheterization alleviates the patient's discomfort and allows precise monitoring of urine output. When interpreted in the appropriate clinical situation, few measurements are more valuable than urine output. However, placement of a Foley catheter can lead to a number of complications, the most common of which is urinary tract infection.

Among general surgery patients, the overall infection rate is 10%, and 26% of these infections occur secondary to urinary tract infections[52]; for example, 49% of orthopedic infections and 75% of urologic and medical infections are related to urinary tract infections. The distal urethra is usually colonized with bacteria. Even one catheterization of the bladder will result in urinary tract infection in 1% of ambulatory patients.[52] Infection will develop within 3 to 4 days of catheterization in 95% of patients managed with indwelling catheters and open drainage systems.[52] A variety of organisms can cause urinary tract infection. *Escherichia coli* is by far the most common pathogen, although other Enterobacteriaceae are also common. Staphylococci, streptococci, and enterococci also frequently cause urinary tract infection. Dysuria can be a symptom of urinary tract infection; however, infection may often present only as fever or a septic response. Diagnosis is based on microscopic examination of the urine and urine culture [*see 6:17 Nosocomial Infection*]. Urinary tract infection can be prevented by (1) avoiding nonessential catheterization, (2) allowing only trained personnel to insert catheters, (3) using meticulous aseptic technique to avoid introduction of bacteria, (4) adequately securing the catheter after insertion so it does not move in and out of the urethra and the bladder, (5) maintaining proper drainage, and (6) removing the catheter at the earliest possible opportunity.

Few controlled studies have been published that address the optimal duration of bladder catheter drainage. One study suggests that such drainage should be limited to about 3 days after a major low-rectal operation and to about 1 day after other types of colon operations.[53] Epidural drug administration in the postoperative period should not be an indication for bladder drainage beyond 24 hours.[54]

Antinausea Prophylaxis

Postoperative nausea and vomiting are common problems and are best treated pharmacologically unless intestinal obstruction or severe ileus exists. For example, H_2-receptor antagonists and dexamethasone have been shown to be effective if given perioperatively. Droperidol may also be effective, and a 1999 randomized trial suggested that supplemental oxygen may also reduce nausea and vomiting.[2]

The use of local and regional anesthetic techniques reduces patient exposure to agents such as nitrous oxide, which predisposes to nausea. Administration of NSAIDs instead of a narcotic also reduces the incidence of this complication.

Ambulation and Nutrition

Traditional postoperative care generally included bed rest, which is now considered undesirable in that it increases muscle

a

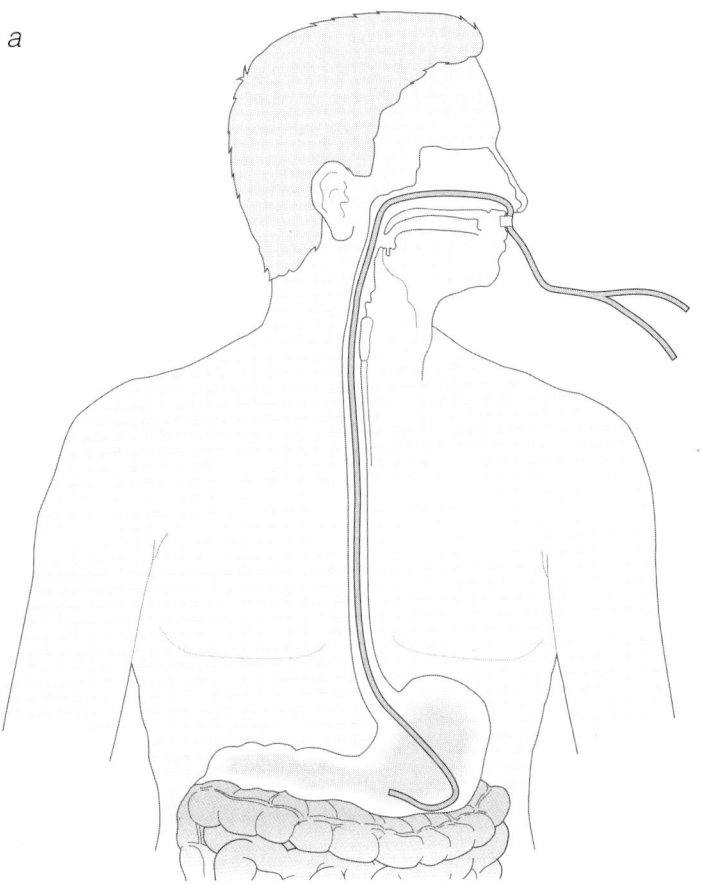

b

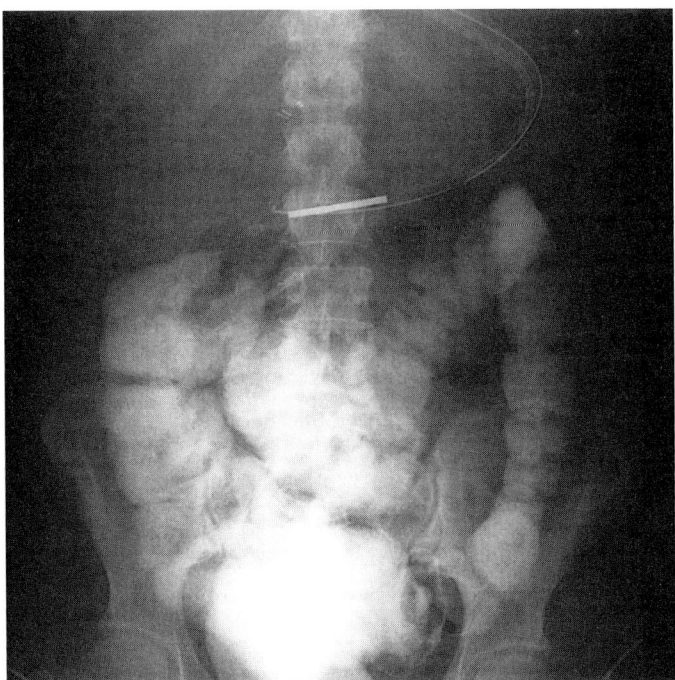

c

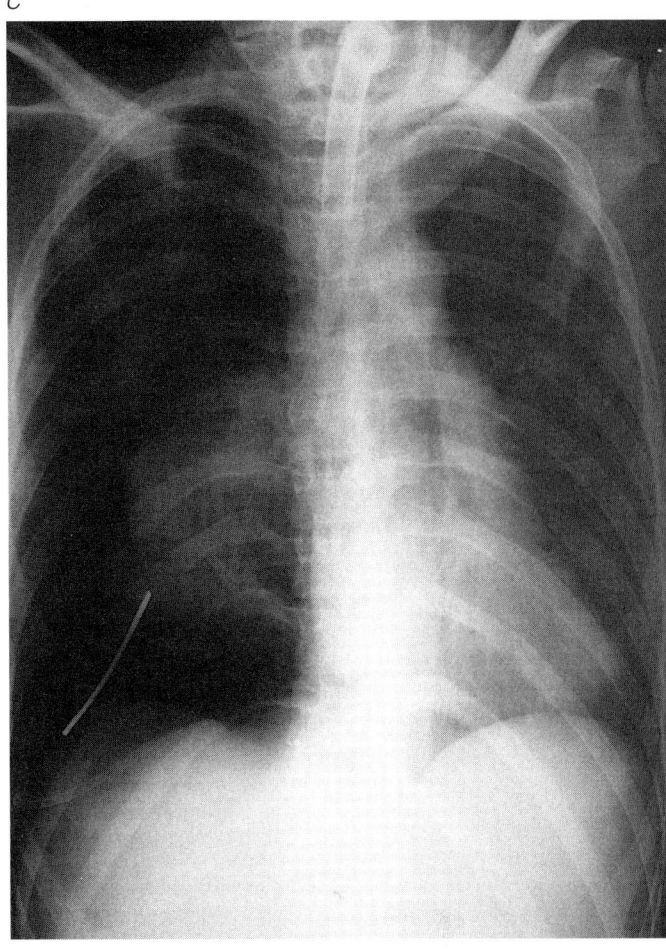

Figure 1   (*a*) The nasogastric tube (generally a No. 18 sump catheter) is passed through the nose to the posterior pharynx, at which point it must make a nearly 90° turn into the esophagus—a maneuver that should be executed gently and with extreme caution. Ideally, the patient should be in a sitting position with head forward and should be sipping liquids, which will help ease the progress of the tube into the stomach. The position of the tube is confirmed by rapid injection of 10 to 20 ml of air into the tube and auscultation over the gastric area of the abdomen. The exterior portion of the tube is gently secured with adhesive tape, preferably to the upper lip or to the nose, without tension or deviation of the alae or septum. If intubation does not drain fluid regularly, the tube may have to be irrigated or repositioned. If the position of the tube is in doubt, a radiograph should be taken (*b*) before feeding is initiated. Examples of inappropriate positioning include passage into the prevertebral fascia, which can cause mediastinitis, or into the lung, which can lead to pneumothorax (*c*) or pneumonia after feeding. At removal, the nasogastric tube is disconnected from the suction tubing and the adhesive tape removed. The patient is instructed to hold his or her breath, and the tube is then withdrawn gently but quickly. After removal, the tube is discarded.

Long intestinal tubes, most commonly a Cantor or Miller-Abbott tube, are passed through the nose and into the stomach in a manner similar to that of a nasogastric tube. Weighted by a balloon tip filled with 5 to 8 ml of mercury, the tube continues on through the stomach and into the small intestine either passively or with assistance under fluoroscopy. Once in the small intestine, it will aspirate fluid and gas as it proceeds. Removal of a long intestinal tube is accomplished gradually; approximately 30 cm of tubing is pulled out through the nose once every 1 or 2 hours and then taped or clamped to prevent slippage.

loss and weakness, impairs pulmonary function and tissue oxygenation, and predisposes to thromboembolic and pulmonary complications and orthostatic intolerance.[55,56] Every effort should be made to enforce postoperative mobilization, which is possible in most cases if effective pain relief is provided.

Oral intake is frequently limited in the postoperative period. When enteral feedings are provided, they are frequently given as

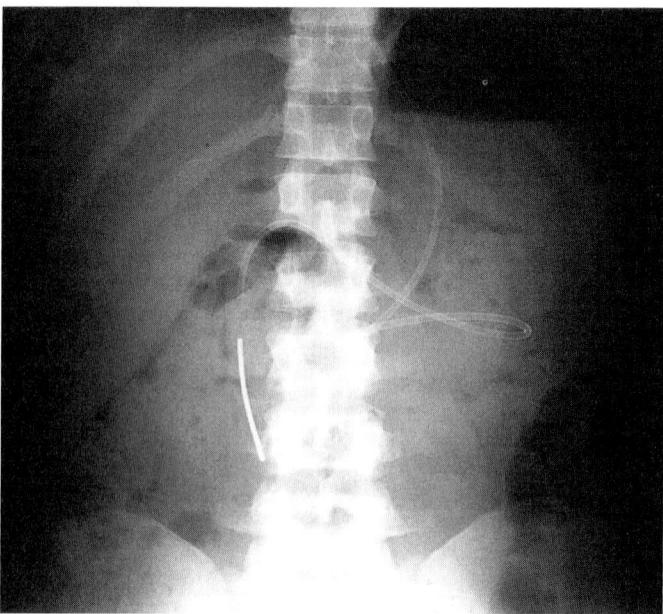

Figure 2 **Abdominal radiograph shows that the small-caliber feeding tube was passed into the stomach with its tip advanced into the duodenum, confirming that the tip of the feeding tube is safely positioned, so that feedings can be initiated.**

a dietary progression, starting with liquids and proceeding to soft food and finally to solid food. There is no scientific basis for this practice; in fact, several studies have shown that early oral feedings are safe in elective surgical patients even after colon procedures involving bowel anastomoses.[57] If nausea, vomiting, or ileus is present, pharmacologic treatment should be considered and feeding initiated. If a prolonged delay in initiating enteral nutrition is expected, parenteral nutrition should be considered [*see 6:23 Nutritional Support*]

Postoperative Complications

POSTOPERATIVE FEVER

A number of studies[58,59] have shown that postoperative fever is common. In one study, 72% of 153 postoperative patients had a temperature greater than 37° C (98.6° F), and 41% had a temperature greater than 38° C (100.4° F).[58] Postoperative fever usually is not associated with significant infection (only four of 256 febrile patients in one series had an infectious process[59]). Fever associated with infection usually occurs later than fever of noninfectious origin (2.7 versus 1.6 days after operation in one study[59]); fever associated with infection also lasts longer (5.4 versus 3.4 days). The absence of fever does not rule out infection; fever was experienced by only 50% of patients in whom an infection subsequently developed.[59]

Although fever is occasionally caused by serious underlying infection, the practice of routinely ordering a battery of expensive laboratory tests (e.g., chest x-ray, blood cultures, complete blood count, sputum culture, urinalysis, and urine culture) when fever is present should be avoided. The best way of differentiating between patients who have an infectious process and the vast majority who do not is via physical examination. The indiscriminate use of laboratory studies is costly and usually not diagnostic; by comparison, laboratory studies directed by physical examination are frequently valuable.

Factors that increase the risk of fever developing in the postoperative period include an operation more than 2 hours long, intraoperative transfusion, preexisting infection, and preoperative antibiotic prophylaxis (which implies contamination or potential operative contamination). Common causes of fever include atelectasis, pneumonia, urinary tract infection, septic and nonseptic phlebitis, drug allergies, wound infection, and other deep infections. Postoperative fever occurs more commonly in patients who have drains in place, even though infection may not subsequently develop.[60,61] Unusual causes of fever include delayed hemolytic reaction to transfusion (i.e., fever and anemia in a patient with a history of blood transfusion)[62] and other inflammatory disease processes such as systemic lupus erythematosus, rheumatoid arthritis, and gout. Other rare causes include hepatic toxicity resulting from anesthetic agents (e.g., halothane or enflurane[63]) or viral infections (e.g., cytomegalovirus or Epstein-Barr virus[64]). These complications generally occur late after the surgical procedure.

If the fever does reflect a serious underlying infection, the patient is at risk for multiple organ dysfunction syndrome (MODS). Various interventions aimed at preventing MODS by interrupting the cytokine cascade proved unsuccessful. In 2001, however, an international multicenter prospective, randomized, double-blind, placebo-controlled trial showed that activated protein C (drotrecogin alfa) caused a decrease in mortality (a mortality of 30.8% in the placebo group versus 24.7% in the treatment group.)[65]

HYPOTHERMIA

Mild hypothermia, a common postoperative complication, results from blockage of normal autoregulatory processes by the anesthetic agent, heat loss through the open abdomen or chest cavity, and the administration of cold fluids. Mild hypothermia is generally well tolerated and, except for the slight increase in peripheral vascular resistance and the decrease in total-body oxygen consumption that it causes, is of little concern. However, more marked hypothermia can cause a variety of serious complications, including marked elevation of peripheral vascular resistance, decreases in cardiac contractility and cardiac output, depressed neurologic status, and a coagulopathy with clotting system enzyme dysfunction. Profound hypothermia is frequently associated with major operations, particularly those performed after multiple trauma or those involving massive transfusion of cold stored blood and cold crystalloid.[66-70]

CARDIAC COMPLICATIONS

A variety of cardiovascular complications are commonly associated with general surgical procedures. These include dysrhythmias, myocardial infarction, ventricular failure, and hypertension.[71,72] As the average age of patients undergoing general surgical procedures has increased, so too has the incidence of significant heart disease in this population. Ideally, selective management to prevent significant cardiovascular complications is initiated preoperatively and is continued both intraoperatively and postoperatively. Specific measures should be taken to control congestive heart failure; such measures may include aggressive management with careful volume management as well as appropriate use of diuretics, digoxin, afterload reduction therapy, and oxygen therapy. There is a growing body of data supporting the use of prophylactic beta blockade in high-risk patients undergoing noncardiac surgery. Factors indicative of elevated risk include ischemic heart disease, congestive heart failure, major surgery (intraperitoneal, intrathoracic, and suprainguinal vascular procedures), diabetes mellitus, renal insufficiency, and poor function-

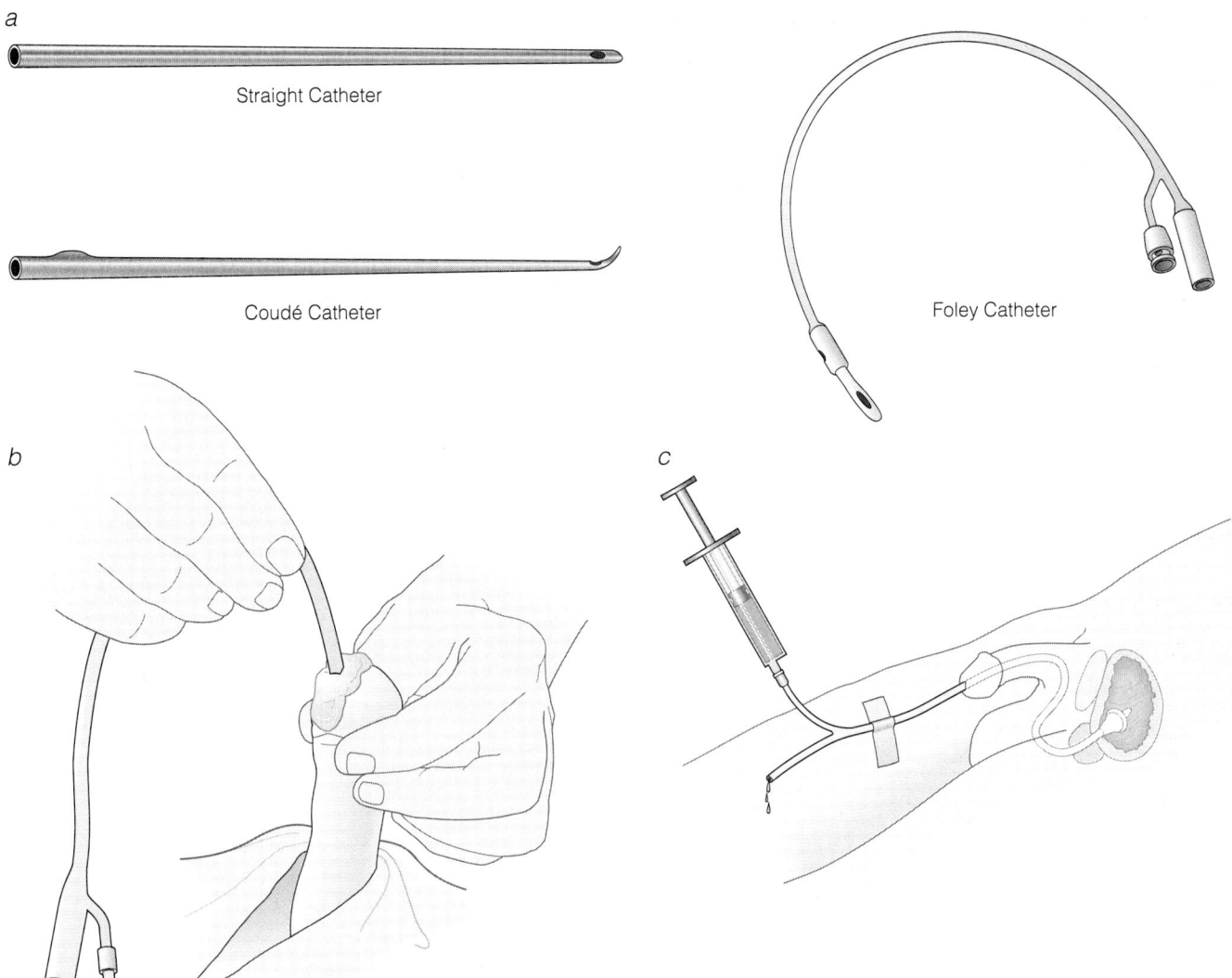

Figure 3 The Foley catheter is the primary type of catheter utilized for long-term bladder catheterization (*a*). If the bladder is to be catheterized a single time, however, a straight catheter without a balloon is used. When difficulty is encountered in passing a Foley catheter (often in men with an enlarged prostate gland), a curved-tip catheter, or coudé catheter, can often be passed by experienced personnel. The smallest-diameter catheter that will accomplish the task should be selected (16 French to 24 French for adult men, 16 French to 26 French for adult women). Before insertion, the balloon at the end of the Foley catheter should be tested, the patient's genital area cleansed, and the tip of the catheter well lubricated. In men, the penis should be held erect and the catheter inserted into the meatus and advanced gently until urine returns (*b*). In women, the labia should be gently spread, the urethral meatus located, and the catheter gently inserted until urine returns. In both men and women, once urine returns, the catheter is then advanced a little farther to ensure that the balloon does not lie in the urethra. The balloon is inflated by the injection of 5 to 10 ml of saline solution through the balloon port. After insertion is completed, the exterior portion of the catheter is taped to the patient's thigh (*c*). Once it is no longer necessary, the catheter should be removed. Removal consists of deflating the balloon and then withdrawing the catheter as gently as possible.

al status.[73] The surgeon should be alert for the presence of angina, cardiac valve disease, and arrhythmias, including heart block, ventricular arrhythmias, and supraventricular tachycardia.[74,75]

Hypertension in the postoperative period frequently occurs secondary to pain or hypoxia. Initial treatment, therefore, consists of administering adequate analgesia to control pain and ensuring adequate oxygenation. Once pain is alleviated and hypoxia corrected, drug treatment may be considered. A variety of agents are available for the treatment of hypertension [*see Table 5*].[76,77] The physician should generally become familiar with one or two medications and use them with confidence rather than try to master a large number of them.

RESPIRATORY COMPLICATIONS

Pulmonary complications are common after operative procedures. In one study, dependent atelectasis (3.4% of lung volume) developed in 100% of patients 5 to 10 minutes after administration of anesthesia[78]; 1 hour later, atelectasis was present in 90% of the patients, and 24 hours after operation, it was present in 50%. Up to 40% of obese patients show evidence of basal pulmonary atelectasis on initial postoperative x-ray.[79]

Postoperative respiratory complications include atelectasis, aspiration pneumonia, and other pneumonias. A variety of factors contribute to the development of these complications, and various approaches have been used to prevent and treat them. For example, abdominal incisions cause pain, which limits the patient's activity and shifts predominantly abdominal breathing to chest wall breathing. Fluoroscopy of the diaphragm after operation has demonstrated reduced diaphragmatic movement, with a shift from abdominal to rib cage breathing.[80] This shift begins to reverse after 24 hours. However, the placement of the incision can influence the risk of postoperative respiratory compromise. For example, lower abdominal and transverse incisions are associated with a lower rate of com-

Table 5 Drugs Used in Urgent and Emergency Treatment of Hypertension

Drug	Administration	Onset of Action	Mechanism of Action	Side Effects	Indications/Contraindications
Sodium nitroprusside	Prepare 50–100 mg/500 ml 5% dextrose in water; administer at rate of 25–50 µg/min and titrate (solution is light sensitive and should be covered with aluminum foil) Patient needs constant monitoring	Immediate	Vasodilatation	Nausea, restlessness, disorientation, severe hypotension, thiocyanate toxicity (check blood levels every 48 hr; discontinue if levels exceed 10 mg/dl), hypothyroidism or methemoglobinemia (rare), ↓ platelet adhesiveness, intracranial hypertension	Especially useful in patients with ischemic heart disease, aortic dissection (combined with a beta blocker), or intracranial hemorrhage
Trimethaphan	Prepare 500 mg/500 ml 5% dextrose in water; administer 1 mg/min initially and titrate Patient needs constant monitoring	Immediate	Ganglionic blockade	Severe hypotension, tachyphylaxis, orthostatic effect, sympathetic blockade (urinary retention, constipation, ileus, pupillary dilatation), respiratory arrest (> 5 mg/min)	Second-choice agent in patients with aortic dissection, intracranial hemorrhage, or ischemic heart disease when sodium nitroprusside cannot be used
Nifedipine	Administer 10–20 mg sublingually or orally as a broken or chewed capsule	5–30 min	Calcium channel blocker	Hypotension, tachycardia, flushing	Drug of choice for hypertensive emergencies when invasive monitoring is not required; contraindicated in patients with aortic dissection
Labetalol	Administer 20–80 mg I.V. at 10-min intervals (maximum cumulative dose 300 mg)	Immediate	Nonselective beta blocker and alpha$_1$ blocker	Pressor response after previous beta-blocker treatment, nausea, paresthesia, headache, hypotension, bradycardia, bronchospasm, urinary retention, ? congestive heart failure	Experience limited; contraindicated for patients with asthma, heart failure, heart block greater than first degree, or bradycardia
Diazoxide	Give 150–300 mg rapid I.V. push or 50–150 mg I.V. every 5 min; to minimize overshoot hypotension, use 7.5–30 mg/min constant I.V. infusion instead Each dose after the first 300 mg should be preceded by furosemide, 40 mg I.V.	Immediate	Vasodilatation	↑ CO, ↑ HR, ↑ blood glucose, ↑ uric acid, Na$^+$ retention; may precipitate angina and cardiac ischemia, nausea, postural hypotension, painful extravasation	Hypertensive encephalopathy, accelerated hypertension, eclampsia; not to be given to patients with ischemic heart disease, intracranial hemorrhage, or aortic dissection
Nicardipine	Administer 5 mg/hr by I.V. infusion and increase by 1–2 mg/hr every 15 min up to 15 mg/hr	1–5 min	Calcium channel blocker	Hypotension, headache, tachycardia, nausea, and vomiting	Similar to other calcium channel blockers; preferential vasodilatory effects; useful in patients who require careful detrition for the control of hypertension
Phentolamine mesylate	Administer 5–20 mg by I.V. bolus or 10–20 mg by I.M. injection	Immediate	Alpha blocker	Hypotension, tachycardia, vomiting, angina, nausea	Drug of choice in patients with pheochromocytoma and monoamine oxidase inhibitor–tyramine interaction; also useful for patients in whom severe hypertension develops after discontinuance of clonidine; short duration of action may require repeated boluses; can precipitate angina and myocardial ischemia in patients at risk
Hydralazine	Administer 5–10 mg I.V. or I.M.	15–30 min	Direct arteriolar vasodilatation	Tachycardia, flushing, angina	Associated with undesirable reflex tachycardia, which may be especially worrisome in patients with coronary artery disease; current usage restricted mostly to patients with renal insufficiency and toxemia
Clonidine	Initial dose 0.2 mg, then 0.1 mg every hr to a maximum of 0.7 mg	30–60 min	Central alpha-adrenergic agonist	Hypotension, sedation, dry mouth; blood pressure should be monitored for 4 hr after last dose	Especially useful in patients with severe hypertension (especially diastolic) without end-organ damage; useful in the emergency department and on the ward

CO—cardiac output   HR—heart rate

plications and a lower rate of respiratory compromise than longitudinal or midline incisions.[81] Other factors that increase the risk of postoperative pulmonary complications include age, underlying disease, malnutrition, and chronic obstructive pulmonary disease with subsequent colonization.[82,83]

A variety of preoperative, intraoperative, and postoperative respiratory treatments are available that may be valuable in preventing serious postoperative pulmonary complications. Preoperative treatment with incentive spirometry and chest physical therapy has been studied and appears to be of some value in improving patients' overall pulmonary status in preparation for operation.[84] Smoking should be discontinued, and underlying pulmonary infection such as bronchitis or pneumonia should always be treated and operation delayed if possible because the ciliary paralysis that occurs with the use of anesthetics has the potential for causing a severe pneumonia after operation.

Routine respiratory therapy is frequently used postoperatively to prevent pulmonary complications. Routine therapeutic measures include administration of bronchodilator aerosol or ultrasonic mist aerosol, IPPB, incentive spirometry, and oxygen therapy. However, some studies have questioned the value of many of these respiratory treatments.[85,86] One study demonstrated that a hospital-wide effort to reduce the use of specific respiratory therapy services did not adversely affect patient outcome.[87] For example, administration of beta agonists was successfully switched from air-driven aerosols to handheld nebulizers. The use of IPPB was almost completely eliminated, and treatment by incentive spirometry was reduced by 55%. The decrease in the use of incentive spirometry occurred in the late postoperative period, when, studies suggest, it is no longer of value. In patients at high risk, such as those undergoing upper abdominal operation, respiratory therapy is most beneficial when performed in the immediate postoperative period. Patients treated with incentive spirometry return more rapidly to preoperative pulmonary lung volumes than do untreated patients.[84] In this study, use of ultrasonic nebulization was also decreased markedly, whereas oxygen therapy was retained at about the same level.[87] Aerosol ultrasonic nebulization and mist aerosol are of little or no value.

Early mobilization after operation is believed to improve the patient's overall respiratory status. In several studies, early mobilization appeared to be as effective in improving overall respiratory status as chest physical therapy.[88,89] Early mobilization (i.e., turning every 2 hours) in coronary artery bypass patients was shown to decrease the incidence of atelectasis and pneumonia significantly. In high-risk patients, routine postoperative prophylactic chest physical therapy has been shown to decrease the frequency of pulmonary infection significantly.[90] However, in a study of children undergoing cardiac procedures, chest physical therapy had no effect on the development of pulmonary atelectasis.[91]

Atelectasis indicates pulmonary dysfunction and may also presage pneumonia. Postoperative pneumonia is an extremely serious complication and is a major cause of mortality on surgical services. Factors that increase the risk of postoperative pneumonia include advanced age, gram-negative bacterial infection, emergency operation, use of a ventilator, and postoperative peritonitis.

THROMBOEMBOLISM

Pulmonary Embolism

Pulmonary embolism is the most common fatal acute pulmonary disorder in hospitalized patients [see 4:6 *Venous Thromboembolism*]. In the United States, pulmonary embolism occurs in more than 250,00 patients each year[92]; mortality ranges from 8% to 23%.[93] Approximately one third of deaths occur in the first hour after embolism; however, as many as 90% of patients survive long enough to be evaluated and for therapeutic intervention to be considered. Aggressive early anticoagulation therapy is associated with 90% survival. Up to 95% of pulmonary emboli originate in the deep veins of the leg; a small percentage originate in pelvic veins and at other sites. There have been reports of pulmonary emboli originating in veins of the upper extremities, but such cases are exceedingly uncommon.

Dyspnea is the most common symptom of pulmonary embolism and is usually of sudden onset. Dyspnea can be transient. The most common physical finding is tachypnea. Rales are present in 50% of cases. Circulatory collapse characterized by shock or syncope occurs in 20% of patients with pulmonary embolism and correlates with larger emboli. Although most patients with pulmonary embolism are hypoxemic, a P_aO_2 greater than 80 mm Hg was found in 10% of patients in the urokinase-streptokinase pulmonary embolus trial. The chest x-ray, although it may be abnormal, is commonly nondiagnostic. The most common abnormalities evident on the electrocardiogram are T wave inversion, nonspecific ST segment elevation or depression, and sinus tachycardia. Ventilation-perfusion scans are frequently valuable in ruling out pulmonary embolism in a patient with a clear chest x-ray, but some data cast doubt on the utility of a ventilation-perfusion scan result of low or intermediate probability.[93,94] If the lung scan is equivocal, pulmonary angiography should be performed. Pulmonary arterial pressures are routinely elevated in patients with significant pulmonary embolism. The role of spiral CT in the detection of pulmonary embolism has not yet been fully defined; its specificity is good, but its sensitivity is poor as a consequence of its inability to detect subsegmental emboli.[95]

Treatment of pulmonary embolism is supportive and includes administration of oxygen, adequate maintenance of fluid resuscitation, and rapid I.V. anticoagulation. If heparin is used, it is given in an 80 U/kg bolus, then infused at a rate of 18 U/kg/hr.[96] The partial thromboplastin time (PTT) is then adjusted according to a nomogram.[97] Low-molecular-weight heparin can be used for prophylaxis and treatment of both deep vein thrombosis (DVT) and pulmonary embolism.[98] Patients who cannot receive heparin[99] or other forms of prophylaxis or who exhibit continued or recurrent signs and symptoms of pulmonary embolus should be strongly considered for vena caval filter placement.[100] Some patients may benefit from thrombolytic therapy administered early, but this option is generally not available for postoperative patients.[101]

Deep Vein Thrombosis

Some degree of DVT develops in approximately 30% of patients after abdominal or thoracic procedures and in up to 80% of patients after hip procedures [see 4:6 *Venous Thromboembolism*]. Some reviews suggest that routine prophylaxis is justified in all surgical patients who are at high risk for DVT (e.g., those older than 40 years, obese patients, patients with malignant disease, patients with prior DVT or pulmonary embolism, or patients undergoing long, complicated operative procedures). Low-dose unfractionated heparin (5,000 units subcutaneously every 12 hours) should be given until the patient is ambulatory. Increasing the frequency of administration does not decrease the incidence of emboli but does increase the risk of hemorrhagic complications. The addition of dihydroergotamine to heparin may improve efficacy, but the risk associated with its vasoconstrictor effects may outweigh its potential benefits. Dextran in an initial dose of 10 ml/kg appears to be equally effective in decreasing the risk of pulmonary embolism but is more expensive. Dextran 70 and dextran 40 appear to be equally efficacious. External pneumatic compression and gradient elastic stockings can also be employed to prevent DVT.

Findings from several reviews suggest that mortality from pulmonary embolism is decreasing and that effective prophylaxis with either subcutaneous heparin or pneumatic compression devices can decrease the risk of DVT and pulmonary embolism.[102-104] To achieve optimal results, prophylaxis must be started before the operative procedure begins.

CENTRAL VENOUS CATHETER COMPLICATIONS

Central venous catheters, arterial catheters, and triple-lumen catheters may be associated with such complications as perforation of the vascular system, thrombi, and infection. In one study, complications related to initial catheter placement occurred in 5.7% of patients, sepsis occurred in 6.5%, and mechanical complications occurred in 9%.[105,106] Complications of catheter placement are hemorrhage and pneumothorax. The most common late mechanical complications are major venous thrombosis and nursing mishaps. Central venous thrombophlebitis and sepsis usually necessitate immediate removal of the central venous catheter and antibiotic therapy. In some patients with Silastic catheters, treatment with I.V. antibiotics and anticoagulants and careful monitoring for potential exploration and drainage of perivascular infection or vein excision may be indicated.[105] Other studies have shown that administration of antibiotics through the indwelling catheter is effective. In one study of catheter-associated infections, 18 patients (86%) were cured without removal of the catheter. Absolute indications for catheter removal are lack of defervescence and continued positive blood cultures despite antibiotic therapy.[106] An effective method of assessing catheter contamination in patients with central lines in place is routine catheter exchange and culture [see 6:17 Nosocomial Infection]. Studies have shown a direct link between catheter infection and contamination of the site. To avoid mechanical complications, an x-ray should be obtained after insertion of any central line to document its position. The catheter should be evaluated every 2 to 7 days to ensure that it has not migrated or been displaced.

UPPER GASTROINTESTINAL BLEEDING

Before the advent of routine administration of antacids, life-threatening upper GI bleeding was a common problem in patients undergoing major stress, particularly in those with head injury, burns, or multiple trauma. A number of agents have been used for prophylaxis, including antacids, sucralfate, H_2 receptor antagonists, and proton pump inhibitors. The antacid regimen for bleeding prophylaxis is 30 to 60 ml by nasogastric tube every 1 to 2 hours to maintain gastric pH above 4. According to one study, sucralfate may also be effective for bleeding prophylaxis.[107] By comparison, H_2 receptor antagonists have not proved to be more effective than antacids in preventing major upper GI bleeding.[108,109] Agents that elevate gastric pH may increase the risk of nosocomial pneumonia by favoring gastric colonization.[110] Proton pump inhibitors significantly reduce rebleeding rates and offer an alternative to H_2 receptor antagonists.[111] With adequate prophylaxis, the incidence of massive upper GI bleeding is essentially zero.

POSTOPERATIVE TRANSFUSION AND ANEMIA

A decreased hematocrit and relative anemia occur very commonly after major operative procedures. In patients with these conditions, blood transfusion is often considered [see 1:4 Bleeding and Transfusion]. It is important, however, to avoid unnecessary transfusions because of the potential for transfusion-associated complications, which include hemolytic transfusion reactions, nonhemolytic transfusion reactions, and transmission of infection (e.g., hepatitis, AIDS, cytomegalovirus, and herpesvirus). In addition, blood transfusion itself may be a significant immunodepressant.[112-115] In the past, it was typically considered reasonable to order a blood transfusion when the hematocrit measured 30% or less. Today, however, there are few, if any, situations in which this practice should be followed. For example, in a young healthy patient who has no other disease and is expected to continue to improve, hematocrits in the low to middle 20s are acceptable. This restrictive approach to red blood cell transfusion is as effective as, and possibly superior to, a liberal transfusion approach in ICU patients.[116] In addition, patients with a variety of other chronic diseases that lead to persistently low hematocrits (e.g., chronic renal insufficiency) have been safely observed at relatively low hematocrit levels without transfusion.

Alternatives to transfusion include autologous donation, hemodilution, cell-saving techniques, oxygen-carrying solutions (both perfluorocarbon-based and hemoglobin-based), and recombinant erythropoietin. Autologous donation, hemodilution, and cell saver techniques require considerable advanced planning and are not cost-effective for widespread use. Perfluorocarbon-based and hemoglobin-based oxygen-carrying solutions are, at present, still investigational.[117] Recombinant erythropoietin has been used in anemic medical patients since 1989 and in surgical patients since 1997.[118] The indications and end points for its use have not yet been fully defined.

DIABETES MELLITUS

The diabetic patient presents a series of management problems in the postoperative period. Careful management of blood glucose levels is necessary to avoid hypoglycemia or hyperglycemia with associated complications such as diabetic ketoacidosis and dehydration secondary to glycosuria. Diabetes has a significant negative impact on wound healing. For patients whose disease is managed by diet alone, additional measures are usually unnecessary. In the postoperative period, careful monitoring, including finger-stick glucose measurements every 6 hours, is appropriate, with a sliding scale of regular insulin administered as needed. In patients who are receiving oral hypoglycemic agents, the medication should be discontinued on the day before operation, and insulin should be given as needed for hyperglycemia. Patients who require insulin should be given a dextrose infusion and one half of the total daily dose of insulin as regular insulin the morning of the operation. Glucose is administered throughout the operation, as guided by measured glucose levels. In patients who require major operations and massive fluid administration, blood glucose should be measured frequently during operation, and insulin should be given I.V. as needed. Postoperatively, glucose levels in some patients will be well controlled by administration of insulin on a sliding scale based on finger-stick glucose monitoring.

Shock, major trauma, or extremely prolonged operations can lead to hypoperfusion of the skin and subcutaneous tissue. In these patients, subcutaneous administration of insulin is inappropriate and dangerous. Instead, monitoring in the ICU, with frequent glucose measurements, and treatment with I.V. insulin should be undertaken. Dextrose should be included in postoperative administration of fluids.

OTHER ENDOCRINE COMPLICATIONS

Another postoperative endocrine complication is hypothyroidism, which usually occurs in the elderly. Hypothyroidism is frequently associated with (1) a low temperature and (2) a low blood pressure that does not respond to fluid management or pressors. The elderly are also at risk for hyponatremia, hypoventilation, and hypoglycemia. In these cases, thyroid levels should be measured and intravenous thyroxine (200 to 500 μg) given. This dose should provide adequate thyroid levels for several days.

Postoperative hypoadrenocorticism occurs in patients who have been receiving oral or parenteral steroids. The stress of operation necessitates replacement with hydrocortisone (300 to 400 mg/day) or its equivalent. The suggested regimen is 100 mg I.V. every 8 hours on postoperative day 1 or 2, which should be rapidly tapered if the level of stress and the length of preoperative therapy allow it. In patients who are treated with steroids, the wound healing process is slowed. This deleterious effect can be reversed by administration of vitamin A (25,000 units orally or by nasogastric tube).

Discharge from Hospital and Follow-up Care

Discharge from the hospital is an important milestone in the postoperative care of a patient. For many patients who return home after their hospitalization, discharge represents a marker of major improvement. For other patients who have more complex problems and require significant care after hospital discharge, it is the beginning of a long and often difficult journey through a rehabilitation system or a skilled nursing facility.

The vast majority of patients admitted for elective surgery and most patients admitted for emergency surgery are discharged from the hospital back to their preoperative domicile. Patients with complex injuries (especially head injury), advanced malignancy, or significant disabilities or elderly patients may require placement in a facility rather than being sent home. In some cases, support from agencies in their community, such as home health care groups, may obviate placement in a nursing facility. There is evidence to suggest that well-developed family networks contribute significantly to a decreased risk of institutionalization.[119] A continuum of care services exists but may vary from one community to another [see Table 6]. A qualified medical social worker or discharge planner is invaluable in providing access to the various available options in each particular locale.

Most patients are discharged once the physician determines that they have met certain criteria: they must be medically stable and afebrile, tolerant of oral intake, ambulatory, and reasonably comfortable, and they must have wounds or drains that require only minimal care. The physician should then write discharge orders in the hospital chart to notify the nursing staff and the hospital administration [see Sidebar Sample Discharge Orders]. The discharge summary, written or dictated by the physician, should

Sample Discharge Orders

[Date and Time]
1. Discharge patient home.
2. Return to clinic in 1 wk to see Dr. Smith. Patient may call 919-555-4343 for questions or problems.
3. Prescriptions for discharge medications on the chart.
4. Instructions regarding wound care or care of drains: as indicated.
5. Activity: ambulatory.
6. Patient may bathe or shower.
7. Diet: regular as tolerated.
8. Work status: to be determined at follow-up appointment.
9. Discharge summary dictated.
[Physician's signature and ID number]

include information from the patient's history; data from physical examinations, laboratory tests, and radiographs; details of the hospital course; and full discharge plans. A copy of the discharge summary may be sent to the referring or family physician, or a personal letter can be forwarded to inform the physician of the patient's progress and plans for follow-up.

Certain patients, however, require significantly more sophisticated discharge planning. These include patients with severe multiple injuries (especially head injury), elderly patients with limited ability to care for themselves, patients with significant disabilities and functional impairment, patients with advanced malignancy, and patients with one or more significant socioeconomic difficulties, including homelessness, a history of substance abuse, or AIDS. Such patients will require either significant levels of support at home or placement in a care facility [see Table 7]. Discharge planning for these patients should begin as soon as possible after admission. Once such a patient is identified, the physician should notify a medical social worker or other hospital employee with experience in discharge planning and placement. Such early notification will permit planning for discharge and placement to proceed more efficiently. This is especially relevant for patients with complex needs, such as those requiring placement into a rehabilitation facility or those who have no insurance and who can perhaps be enrolled in Medicaid to provide them with financial support for placement.

DISCHARGE PLANNING

With today's emphasis on decreasing the length of hospitalizations, discharge planning has become a crucial part of the management of patient care in the inpatient setting. Even for the most complicated patient, the issue of a patient's disposition can be addressed from the moment of admission. Comprehensive discharge planning can reduce readmissions, lengthen the interval between discharge and readmission, and decrease the cost of providing health care.[120]

Early in a patient's admission, discharge planning primarily takes the form of assessment. All health care workers involved in the patient's care may provide input based on their interactions with patient and family. How a patient and family cope initially in a crisis and throughout the course of recovery can indicate the strength or weakness of the existing support system. Once a patient progresses beyond the initial crisis, more concrete information pertaining to the patient's financial resources, living situation, physical and emotional supports, and family dynamics is essential. This information is most often obtained by a social worker or trained discharge planner. Once the complete picture of the numerous facets of a patient's life outside of the hospital

Table 6 Care Services

In-home services	Community services
Telephone reassurance	Congregate meals
Emergency response systems	Senior centers
Home-delivered meals	Day care
Respite care	Retirement communities
Housekeeping/shopping services	**Institutional services**
Congregate housing	Family care home
Home health care	Rest home
Hospice care	Nursing home
	Intermediate care facility
	Skilled nursing facility

comes into focus, it can be compared with the new limitations and needs that may have resulted from the illness or injury that necessitated the hospitalization. One should always remember that functioning well in the hospital setting and being independent at home, work, or school can be dramatically different.

A number of options are available for acute care placement for those patients who have special care needs after discharge [see Table 7]. They fall into two categories: in-home care and extended care facilities.

In-Home Care

In-home care consists of home health services, private duty nurses, and community resources such as Meals on Wheels and transportation services. For patients who can be discharged home but require assistance or support, home health services represent an excellent alternative to continued hospitalization. Home health agencies can provide skilled nursing care, assistance in the home (homemakers or aides), physical therapy services, speech therapy services, occupational therapy services, and medical social worker support [see Table 8]. These patients must be otherwise independent, as home health agencies do not provide long periods of custodial care. Patients who require greater assistance must therefore either hire private duty nurses or consider an extended care facility as an alternative after discharge.

Home health agencies charge per service per visit. Charges for skilled therapies, such as skilled nursing, occupational therapy, and physical therapy, may cost up to $100 a visit or an hour. These fees are comparable to those charged in acute care facilities. Charges for nonskilled assistance range from a few dollars an hour to as high as $15 an hour. Services offered through home health providers are time limited under Medicare and Medicaid rules.

The use of home health services has increased dramatically over the past decade. Medicare data indicate that $2.1 billion was spent in 1988, compared with $15 billion in 1999. Between 1980 and 1997, home health care costs increased from $842/recipient to $6,595/recipient.[121]

Extended Care Facilities

Extended care facilities, such as rest homes, nursing homes, and rehabilitation centers, are often very successful in maximizing a patient's potential for independence. They offer more intensive skilled therapies than are offered by home health agencies and provide supervision and assistance with activities of daily living that can be difficult for working family members to provide. Rehabilitation facilities are distinguished from skilled nursing facilities primarily by the amount of activity an individual patient can endure. The standard amount of activity for a rehabilitation center is 3 to 4 hours a day, though this need not be constant activity. Physical therapists, occupational therapists, and speech therapists can assist in making judgments about a patient's endurance, potential, and goals for independence.

Patients who require assistance with convalescence that cannot be provided in their home setting are most often referred to a rest home facility. This is a relatively cost-effective alternative and is generally an intermediate step before the patient returns to a home setting.

Patients who require a higher level of care than that provided in either a rest home or through home health care require admission to a nursing home. A nursing home is either an intermediate care facility or a skilled nursing facility. At an intermediate care facility, registered nurses or licensed practical nurses are on duty for at least 4 hours a day to tend to patients' special medical needs; additional care is provided full time by trained staff who are not registered or practical nurses. Patients who require round-the-clock care from either a registered nurse or a licensed practical nurse must be admitted to a skilled nursing facility. Such patients include those who are potentially unstable or who may have a special need such

Table 7 Options for Acute Care after Hospital Discharge

Facility	Approximate Daily Cost ($)	Insurance Coverage	Services Offered
Rest home	40–60*	Medicaid Private payment plans	Convalescent care
Intermediate care facility	85–135*	Medicaid Private payment plans Medicare will cover skilled services but not room and board	Skilled nursing, 4 hr a day Other skilled services (e.g., physical and occupational therapy) only on contractual basis
Skilled nursing facility	100–150*	Medicaid Medicare (for 100 days) Some insurance plans Private payment plans	Skilled nursing, 24 hr a day Other skilled services (e.g., physical and occupational therapy) only on contractual basis; some provide in-house physical therapy
Subacute care facility	400–600	Medicare (for 100 days) Medicaid Some insurance plans Private payment plans	Skilled nursing, 24 hr a day Other skilled services often provided in-house Specialize in complex wound care and ventilator-dependent patients
Rehabilitation facility	800–1,000	Medicare Medicaid Some insurance plans Private payment plans	All skilled services (physical, occupational, and speech therapy) provided in-house Intensive therapy provided 3–5 hr a day
Acute care facility	1,000+	All current payor sources	Therapies provided on less frequent basis and for shorter duration than at rehabilitation facilities

*Includes only room and board; additional fees required for therapies and medications.
Prices reflect average cost in 1998 based on semiprivate room rates.

Table 8 Services Offered by Home Health Professionals

Skilled nursing
Injections
Ostomy care
Dressing changes
Catheter care
Observation
Instruction in medication/disease process
In-home management training
Hospice care
Respiratory care
Tracheotomy
Post–cataract surgery care
Instruction in diabetes care and monitoring

Home health aide/homemaker
Bathing
Meal assistance
Personal grooming
Ambulation assistance

Physical therapy
Muscle strengthening
Gait or prosthesis training
Training in ambulation and transfer techniques (e.g., bed to wheelchair)
Pulmonary exercises
Ultrasound treatments

Speech therapy
Retraining speech and language function
Developing alternative communication skills
Swallowing therapy

Occupational therapy
Preparation for independence in activities of daily living
Motor coordination improvement
Increase in upper extremity function

Medical social services
Disability assistance
Coordination of community resources

team provides care in a structured, graded fashion. Most rehabilitation centers will send a member of their team to assess a patient while the patient is still in the hospital to determine whether he or she is a candidate for admission. In general, for admission to a rehabilitation facility, the following criteria must be met:

1. Patients must be medically stable.
2. Patients must require an intensive rehabilitation program as offered by the multidisciplinary team. An intensive rehabilitation program is one in which the patient has a demonstrated need for round-the-clock nursing care and is capable of receiving 3 to 4 hours of physical, occupational, or speech therapy.
3. Patients must be able to participate actively in the rehabilitation process and should be able to follow at least simple commands, except in cases of severe brain injury or stroke.
4. The patient must have the potential for attaining significant functional improvement, with the expectation that he or she will return to an acceptable level of functional recovery.

Current trends in posthospital care focus on providing patient care at home and on shortening the length of acute hospital stays. Some skilled nursing facilities are able to provide complex care without the high cost associated with a stay in an acute care hospital. Services provided include ventilator support, I.V. drug therapy, care of advanced decubitus ulcers, total parenteral nutrition, tracheostomy care, and dialysis. These advanced care facilities are often referred to as subacute facilities. If a patient has relatively complex needs, such as ongoing wound care or a need for mechanical ventilation, then admission to a subacute facility would be required. Medicare will cover up to 100 days at such a facility, as will some insurance companies. Because of the generally sophisticated level of care, these facilities tend to have long waiting lists, as do many nursing homes. It is therefore crucial to begin seeking placement for such patients as early as possible in their hospital course to ensure bed availability.

Other Options

Hospice programs provide care for patients who are no longer seeking a cure but rather require care near the end of life. The majority of patients admitted to hospices have terminal illnesses as a result of disseminated malignancy. Hospice care provides the opportunity for patients to gain greater control over decisions regarding their care and allows the family to become more closely involved with the day-to-day progress of the patient. Hospices offer such specialized services as pain management and grief counseling. They are designed to allow patients in the last phase of an incurable illness to live at home or in equally comfortable surroundings for as long as possible. The program strives to keep patients as active as possible and provides them outlets for expressing their feelings in a supportive environment. The hospice team includes members of the family, nurses, social workers, physicians, clergy, and volunteers. Help is available to the patient on a continuous basis. Many of the services provided through the hospice system are covered under Medicare as long as the patient's physician and the hospice medical director certify that the patient is terminally ill, with a life expectancy of less than 6 months, and the hospice providing care is certified by Medicare. Physician services unrelated to hospice care continue to be provided for under standard Medicare Part B coverage.

Some pharmaceutical companies and home health agencies combine skills and efforts to provide I.V. drug therapies at home for patients who are otherwise independent and have adequate family support and assistance. For patients who require more aggressive physical therapy than can be provided at home, outpa-

as I.V. fluid administration or oxygen therapy. In addition, such patients may require advanced comprehensive support services such as physical and occupational therapy. Although physical and occupational therapy and related services can be provided at an intermediate care facility, a skilled nursing facility provides a more comprehensive approach to such needs. Both intermediate care and skilled nursing facilities require physician involvement for admission evaluation and supervision of subsequent care. Payment arrangements may vary among different settings, and such information should be obtained with the assistance of a social worker or other discharge planner. In general, Medicare will cover nursing home costs for a period of up to 100 days.

Rehabilitation facilities are ideally suited for patients who have complex problems that require comprehensive care and graded rehabilitation. They offer nursing services as well as physical, occupational, and speech therapy. They can also provide complex care services in addition to general rehabilitation, and many specialize in areas such as head injury, spinal cord injury, respiratory rehabilitation, stroke, burns, or advanced neurologic disorders. The goal of such centers is to allow patients to attain their maximum level of independence and reintegration into society. An interdisciplinary tient physical therapy at a local hospital or clinic may be a good option to enable the patient to live at home. This option, however, requires extensive family support to provide transportation to therapy and care in the home.

Services for Indigent Patients

Patients without insurance and with no available financial resources can present a difficult problem for discharge planners. Most home health agencies are mandated to set aside funds for indigent clients, but the services provided tend to be the bare minimum. Nursing homes and rehabilitation facilities have no such mandate, however. They set aside a limited number of beds for Medicare and Medicaid patients, but these tend to be in high demand and may represent a resource drain for these facilities. Patients who are not eligible for Medicare can sometimes be enrolled in Medicaid programs. Patients who are not eligible for Medicaid assistance will have to spend their private funds until they qualify for Medicaid. In general, adults are eligible for Medicaid if they are disabled, have dependent children, or have inadequate financial resources.

References

1. Greif R, Akca O, Horn EP, et al: Supplemental perioperative oxygen to reduce the incidence of surgical wound infection. N Engl J Med 342:161, 2000

2. Greif P, Lucing S, Rapf B, et al: Supplemental oxygen reduces the incidence of nausea and vomiting. Anesthesiology 91:1246, 1999

3. Cook DJ, Fuller HD, Guyatt GH, et al: Risk factors for gastrointestinal bleeding in critically ill patients. N Engl J Med 330:377, 1994

4. Recommendations for intensive care unit admission and discharge criteria. Task Force on Guidelines, Society of Critical Care Medicine. Crit Care Med 16:807, 1988

5. Wiedemann HP, Matthay MA, Matthay RA: Cardiovascular-pulmonary monitoring in the intensive care unit (pt 1). Chest 85:537, 1984

6. Critical care medicine. NIH Consensus Conference. JAMA 250:798, 1983

7. Wiedemann HP, Matthay MA, Matthay RA: Cardiovascular-pulmonary monitoring in the intensive care unit (pt 2). Chest 85:656, 1984

8. Burchard KW, Gann DS, Colliton J, et al: Ionized calcium, parathormone, and mortality in critically ill surgical patients. Ann Surg 212:543, 1990

9. Carr DB, Goudas LC: Acute pain. Lancet 353:2051, 1999

10. McQuay HJ, Moore RA, Justins D: Treating acute pain in hospital. BMJ 314:1531, 1997

11. Warfield CA, Kahn CH: Acute pain management: programs in US hospitals and experiences and attitudes among US adults. Anesthesiology 83:1090, 1995

12. American Pain Society Quality of Care Committee: Quality improvement guidelines for the treatment of acute pain and cancer pain. JAMA 274:1874, 1995

13. Kehlet H: Acute pain control and accelerated postoperative surgical recovery. Surg Clin North Am 79:431, 1999

14. Egbert LD, Battit GE, Welch CE, et al: Reduction of postoperative pain by encouragement and instruction of patients: a study of doctor-patient rapport. N Engl J Med 270:825, 1964

15. Gottschalk A, Smith DS, Jobes DR, et al: Preemptive epidural analgesia and recovery from radical prostatectomy: a randomized controlled trial. JAMA 279:1076, 1998

16. Kato J, Ogawa S, Katz J, et al: Effects of presurgical local infiltration of bupivacaine in the surgical field on postsurgical wound pain in laparoscopic gynecologic examinations: a possible preemptive analgesic effect. Clin J Pain 16:12, 2000

17. Rogers A, Walker N, Schug S, et al: Reduction of post-operative mortality and morbidity with epidural or spinal anesthesia: results from an overview of randomized trials. BMJ 321:1, 2000

18. Kehlet H: Acute pain control and accelerated postoperative surgical recovery. Surg Clin Nutr Am 79:431, 1999

19. Marks RM, Sachar EJ: Undertreatment of medical inpatients with narcotic analgesics. Ann Intern Med 78:173, 1973

20. Bollish SJ, Collins CL, Kirking DM, et al: Efficacy of patient-controlled versus conventional analgesia for postoperative pain. Clin Pharm 4:48, 1985

21. Graves DA, Foster TS, Batenhorst RL, et al: Patient controlled analgesia. Ann Intern Med 99:360, 1983

22. Bennett RL, Batenhorst RL, Bivins BA, et al: Patient-controlled analgesia: a new concept of postoperative pain relief. Ann Surg 195:700, 1982

23. Moore FD: Common patterns of water and electrolyte change in injury, surgery and disease. N Engl J Med 258:277, 1958

24. Moran WH Jr, Miltenberger FW, Shuayb WA, et al: Relationship of antidiuretic hormone secretion to surgical stress. Surgery 56:99, 1964

25. Ukai M, Moran WH Jr, Zimmerman B: The role of visceral afferent pathways on vasopressin secretion and urinary excretory patterns during surgical stress. Ann Surg 168:16, 1968

26. Ayus JC, Krothapalli RK, Arieff AI: Treatment of symptomatic hyponatremia and its relation to brain damage. N Engl J Med 317:1190, 1987

27. Arieff AI: Hyponatremia, convulsions, respiratory arrest, and permanent brain damage after elective surgery in healthy women. N Engl J Med 314:1529, 1986

28. Needleman P, Greenwald JE: Atriopeptin: a cardiac hormone intimately involved in fluid, electrolyte, and blood-pressure homeostasis. N Engl J Med 314:828, 1986

29. Putensen C, Mutz N, Pomaroli A, et al: Atrial natriuretic factor release during hypovolemia and after volume replacement. Crit Care Med 20:984, 1992

30. Virgilio RW, Rice CL, Smith DE, et al: Crystalloid vs. colloid resuscitation: is one better? Surgery 85:129, 1979

31. Foley EF, Borlase BC, Dzik WH, et al: Albumin supplementation in the critically ill. Arch Surg 125:739, 1990

32. Golub R, Sorrento JJ Jr, Cantu R Jr, et al: Efficacy of albumin supplementation in the surgical intensive care unit: a prospective, randomized study. Crit Care Med 22:613, 1994

33. Cochrane Injuries Group Albumin Reviewers: Human albumin administration in critically ill patients: systematic review of randomized controlled trials. BMJ 317:235, 1998

34. Shires GT, Canizaro PC: Fluid resuscitation in the severely injured. Surg Clin North Am 53:1341, 1973

35. Eisenberg PR, Jaffe AS, Schuster DP: Clinical evaluation compared to pulmonary artery catheterization in the hemodynamic assessment of critically ill patients. Crit Care Med 12:549, 1984

36. Connors AF, McCaffree DR, Gray BA: Evaluation of right-heart catheterization in the critically ill patient without acute myocardial infarction. N Engl J Med 308:263, 1983

37. Lobo DN, Bostock KA, Neal KR, et al: Effect of salt and water balance on recovery of gastrointestinal function after elective colonic resection: a randomised controlled trial. Lancet 359:1812, 2002

38. Dunham CM, Siegel JH, Weireter L, et al: Oxygen debt and metabolic acidemia as quantitative predictors of mortality and the severity of the ischemic insult in hemorrhagic shock. Crit Care Med 19:231, 1991

39. Siegel JH, Rivkind AI, Dalal S, et al: Early physiologic predictors of injury severity and death in blunt multiple trauma. Arch Surg 125:498, 1990

40. Rutherford EJ, Morris Jr JA, Reed GW, et al: Base deficit stratifies mortality and determines therapy. J Trauma 33:417, 1992

41. Davis JW, Shachford SR, MacKersie RC, et al: Base deficit as a guide to volume resuscitation. J Trauma 28:1464, 1988

42. Abramson D, Scalea TM, Hitchcock R, et al: Lactate clearance and survival following injury. J Trauma 35:584, 1993

43. Cheatham ML, Chapman WC, Key SP, et al: A meta-analysis of selective versus routine nasogastric decompression after elective laparotomy. Ann Surg 221:469, 1995

44. Dobbie RP, Hoffmeister JA: Continuous pump-tube enteric hyperalimentation. Surg Gynecol Obstet 143:273, 1976

45. Roubenoff R, Ravich WJ: Pneumothorax due to nasogastric feeding tubes: report of four cases, review of the literature, and recommendations for prevention. Arch Intern Med 149:184, 1989

46. Harris MR, Huseby JS: Pulmonary complications from nasoenteral feeding tube insertion in an intensive care unit: incidence and prevention. Crit Care Med 17:917, 1989

47. Trowbridge PE: A randomized study of cholecystectomy with and without drainage. Surg Gynecol Obstet 155:171, 1982

48. Payne DH, Fishchgrund JS, Herkowitz HN, et al: Efficacy of closed wound suction drainage after single-level lumbar laminectomy. J Spinal Disord 9:401, 1996

49. Urbach DR, Kennedy ED, Cohen MM: Colon and rectal anastomosis do not require rectal drainage: a systematic review and meta-analysis. Ann Surg 229:174, 1999

50. Wihlborg O, Bergljung L, Martensson H: To drain or not to drain in thyroid surgery: a controlled clinical study. Arch Surg 123:40, 1988

51. Somers RG, Jablon LK, Kaplan MJ, et al: The use of closed suction drainage after lumpectomy and axillary node dissection for breast cancer: a prospective randomized trial. Ann Surg 215:146, 1992

52. Sobel JD, Kaye D: Urinary tract infections. Principles and Practice of Infectious Diseases, 2nd ed. Mandell GL, Douglas RG Jr, Bennett JE, Eds. John Wiley & Sons, New York, 1985

53. Benoist S, Panis Y, Denet C, et al: Optimal duration of urinary drainage after rectal resection: a randomized controlled trial. Surgery 125:135, 1999

54. Basse L, Werner M, Kehlet H: Is urinary drainage necessary during continuous epidural analgesia after colon resection? Reg Anesth Pain Med 25:498, 2000

55. Kovacevich GJ, Gaich SA, Lavin JP, et al: The prevalence of thromboembolic events among women with extended bed rest prescribed as part of the treatment for premature labor or preterm premature rupture of membranes. Am J Obstet Gynecol 182:1089, 2000

56. Convertino VA, Goldwater DJ, Sandler H: Effects of orthostatic stress on exercise performance after bedrest. Aviat Space Environ Med 53:652, 1982

57. Kehlet H, Mogensen T: Hospital stay of 2 days after open sigmoidectomy with a multimodal program. Br J Surg 86:227, 1999

58. Yeung RS, Buck JR, Filler RM: The significance of fever following operations in children. J Pediatr Surg 17:347, 1982

59. Galicier C, Richet H: A prospective study of postoperative fever in a general surgery department. Infect Control 6:487, 1985

60. Locker D, Norwood SH, Torma MJ, et al: A prospective randomized study of drained and undrained cholecystectomies. Am Surg 49:528, 1983

61. Trowbridge PE: A randomized study of cholecystectomy with and without drainage. Surg Gynecol Obstet 155:171, 1982

62. Soper DE: Delayed hemolytic transfusion reaction: a cause of late postoperative fever. Am J Obstet Gynecol 153:227, 1985

63. Lewis JH, Zimmerman HJ, Ishak KG, et al: Enflurane hepatotoxicity: a clinicopathologic study of 24 cases. Ann Intern Med 98:984, 1983

64. Siegman-Igra Y: Late postoperative fever-viral infection following multiple blood transfusion. Isr J Med Sci 19:267, 1983

65. Bernard GR, Vincent JL, Laterre PF, et al: Efficacy and safety of recombinant human activated protein C for severe sepsis. N Engl J Med 344:699, 2001

66. Slotman GJ, Jed EH, Burchard KW: Adverse effects of hypothermia in postoperative patients. Am J Surg 149:495, 1985

67. Valeri CR, Cassidy G, Khuri S, et al: Hypothermia-induced reversible platelet dysfunction. Ann Surg 205:175, 1987

68. Luna GK, Maier RV, Pavlin EG, et al: Incidence and effect of hypothermia in seriously injured patients. J Trauma 27:1014, 1987

69. Rutherford EJ, Fusco MA, Nunn CR, et al: Hypothermia in critically ill trauma patients. Injury 29:605, 1998

70. Ku J, Brasel KJ, Baker CC, et al: Triangle of death: hypothermia, acidosis, and coagulopathy. N Horizons 7:61, 1999

71. Lee TH, Marcantonio ER, Mangione CM, et al: Derivation and prospective validation of a simple index for prediction of cardiac risk of major noncardiac surgery. Circulation 100:1043, 1999

72. O'Kelly B, Browner WS, Massie B, et al: Ventricular arrhythmias in patients undergoing noncardiac surgery. JAMA 268:217, 1992

73. Fleisher LA, Eagle KA: Lowering cardiac risk in noncardiac surgery. N Engl J Med 345:1677, 2001

74. Pritchett ELC: Management of atrial fibrillation. N Engl J Med 326:1264, 1992

75. Salerno DM, Anderson B, Sharkey P, et al: Intravenous verapamil for treatment of multifocal atrial tachycardia with and without calcium pretreatment. Ann Intern Med 107:623, 1987

76. Calhoun DA, Oparil S: Treatment of hypertensive crisis. N Engl J Med 323:1177, 1990

77. Halpern NA, Goldberg M, Neely C, et al: Postoperative hypertension: a multicenter, prospective, randomized comparison between intravenous nicardipine and sodium nitroprusside. Crit Care Med 20:1637, 1992

78. Strandberg A, Tokics L, Brismar B, et al: Atelectasis during anaesthesia and in the postoperative period. Acta Anaesthesiol Scand 30:154, 1986

79. Ramsey-Stewart G: The perioperative management of morbidly obese patients (a surgeon's perspective). Anaesth Intensive Care 13:399, 1985

80. Ford GT, Whitelaw WA, Rosenal TW, et al: Diaphragm function after upper abdominal surgery in humans. Am Rev Respir Dis 127:431, 1983

81. Becquemin JP, Piquet J, Becquemin MH, et al: Pulmonary function after transverse or midline incision in patients with obstructive pulmonary disease. Intensive Care Med 11:247, 1985

82. Lawrence VA, Dhanda R, Hilsenbeck SG, et al: Risk of pulmonary complications after elective abdominal surgery. Chest 110:744, 1996

83. Mitchell CK, Smoger SH, Pfeifer MP, et al: Multivariate analysis of factors associated with postoperative pulmonary complications following general elective surgery. Arch Surg 133:194, 1998

84. Minschaert M, Vincent JL, Ros AM, et al: Influence of incentive spirometry on pulmonary volumes after laparotomy. Acta Anaesthesiol Belg 33:203, 1982

85. O'Donohue WJ Jr: National survey of the usage of lung expansion modalities for the prevention and treatment of postoperative atelectasis following abdominal and thoracic surgery. Chest 87:76, 1985

86. Pontoppidan H: Mechanical aids to lung expansion in non-intubated surgical patients. Am Rev Respir Dis 122:109, 1980

87. Zibrak JD, Rossetti P, Wood E: Effect of reductions in respiratory therapy on patient outcome. N Engl J Med 315:292, 1986

88. Morran CG, Finlay IG, Mathieson M, et al: Randomized controlled trial of physiotherapy for postoperative pulmonary complications. Br J Anaesth 55:1113, 1983

89. Castillo R, Haas A: Chest physical therapy: comparative efficacy of preoperative and postoperative in the elderly. Arch Phys Med Rehabil 66:376, 1985

90. Connors AF Jr, Hammon WE, Martin RJ, et al: Chest physical therapy: the immediate effect on oxygenation in acutely ill patients. Chest 78:559, 1980

91. Reines HD, Sade RM, Bradford BF, et al: Chest physiotherapy fails to prevent postoperative atelectasis in children after cardiac surgery. Ann Surg 195:451, 1982

92. Goldhaber SZ: Pulmonary embolism. N Engl J Med 339:93, 1998

93. Douketis JD, Kearon C, Bates S, et al: Risk of fatal pulmonary embolism in patients with treated venous thromboembolism. JAMA 279:458, 1998

94. Bone RC: Ventilation/perfusion scan in pulmonary embolism: "the emperor is incompletely attired" (editorial). JAMA 263:2794, 1990

95. Garg K: CT of pulmonary thromboembolic disease. Radiol Clin North Am 40:111, 2002

96. Hirsh J, Warkentin TE, Raschke R, et al: Heparin and low-molecular-weight heparin: mechanisms of action, pharmacokinetics, dosing considerations, monitoring, efficacy, and safety. Chest 114:489S, 1998

97. de Groot MR, Buller HR, ten Cate JW, et al: Use of a heparin nomogram for treatment of patients with venous thromboembolism in a community hospital. Thromb Haemost 80:70, 1998

98. Hirsh J, Warkentin TE, Shaughnessy SG, et al: Heparin and low-molecular-weight heparin: mechanisms of action, pharmacokinetics, dosing, monitoring, efficacy, and safety. Chest 119:64S, 2001

99. Laster J, Cikrit D, Walker N, et al: The heparin-induced thrombocytopenia syndrome: an update. Surgery 102:763, 1987

100. Greenfield LJ, Peyton R, Crute S, et al: Greenfield vena caval filter experience. Arch Surg 116:1451, 1981

101. Molina JE, Hunter DW, Yedlicka JW, et al: Thrombolytic therapy for postoperative pulmonary embolism. Am J Surg 163:375, 1992

102. Collins R, Scrimgeour A, Yusuf S, et al: Reduction in fatal pulmonary embolism and venous thrombosis by perioperative administration of subcutaneous heparin. N Engl J Med 318:1162, 1988

103. Clagett GP, Reisch JS: Prevention of venous thromboembolism in general surgical patients: a meta-analysis. Ann Surg 208:227, 1988

104. Geerts WH, Heit JA, Clagett GP, et al: Prevention of venous thromboembolism. Chest 119(1 suppl):132S, 2001

105. Wang EE, Prober CG, Ford-Jones L, et al: The management of central intravenous catheter infections. Pediatr Infect Dis 3:110, 1984

106. Verghese A, Widrich WC, Arbeit RD: Central venous septic thrombophlebitis—the role of medical therapy. Medicine (Baltimore) 64:394, 1985

107. Borrero E, Ciervo J, Chang JB: Antacid vs sucralfate in preventing acute gastrointestinal tract bleeding in abdominal aortic surgery: a randomized trial in 50 patients. Arch Surg 121:810, 1986

108. Shuman RB, Schuster DP, Zuckerman GR: Prophylactic therapy for stress ulcer bleeding: a reappraisal. Ann Intern Med 106:562, 1987

109. Cheung LY: Pathogenesis, prophylaxis, and treatment of stress gastritis. Am J Surg 156:437, 1988

110. Driks MR, Craven DE, Celli BR, et al: Nosocomial pneumonia in intubated patients given sucralfate as compared with antacids or histamine type 2 blockers. N Engl J Med 317:1376, 1987

111. Morgan D: Intravenous proton pump inhibitors in the critical care setting. Crit Care Med 30:S369, 2002

112. Opelz G, Terasaki PI: Dominant effect of transfusions on kidney graft survival. Transplantation 29:153, 1980

113. Blumberg N, Heal JM: Transfusion and host defenses against cancer recurrence and infection. Transfusion 29:236, 1989

114. Busch OR, Hop WC, Hoynck van Papendrecht MA, et al: Blood transfusions and prognosis in colorectal cancer. N Engl J Med 328:1372, 1993

115. Fong Y, Karpeh M, Mayer K, et al: Association of perioperative transfusions with poor outcome in resection of gastric adenocarcinoma. Am J Surg 167:256, 1994

116. Hebert PC, Wells G, Blajchman MA, et al: A multicenter, randomized, controlled clinical trial of transfusion requirements in critical care. N Engl J Med 340:409, 1999

117. Goodnough LT, Brecher ME, Kanter MH, et al: Transfusion medicine: blood conservation. N Engl J Med 340:525, 1999

118. Goodnough LT: Erythropoietin therapy versus red cell transfusion. Curr Opin Hematol 8:405, 2001

119. Freedman VA, Berkman LF, Rapp SR, et al: Family networks: predictors of nursing home entry. Am J Public Health 84:843, 1994

120. Naylor MD, Brooten D, Campbell R, et al: Comprehensive discharge planning and home follow-up of hospitalized elders: a randomized clinical trial. JAMA 281:613, 1999

121. Social Security Bulletin. Annual statistical supplement, 1997. Annu Stat Suppl Soc Secur Bull, Dec 1997, p 1

Acknowledgments

Figures 1a, 3   Tom Moore.
Figures 1b, 1c, 2   Courtesy of Samir M. Fakhry, M.D. The authors wish to thank Ms. Eva Powell, M.S.W., for her invaluable contributions to the section on hospital discharge planning.

7 ACUTE WOUND CARE

W. Thomas Lawrence, M.D., F.A.C.S., A. Griswold Bevin, M.D., and George F. Sheldon, M.D., F.A.C.S.

Approach to Acute Wound Management

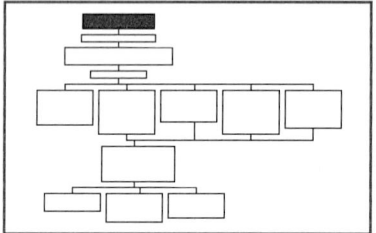

When a patient presents with an acute wound, the priorities are a careful, complete history and a thorough physical examination. Most cutaneous wounds are obvious and easily diagnosed but are not life threatening. However, the wounded patient may also have less apparent problems that are potentially lethal and demand immediate attention. The management of such potentially life-endangering problems takes precedence over wound management.

After more urgent problems have been ruled out or corrected, wound management can be addressed. Information about the time and mechanism of injury must be obtained. The patient should be asked about a coagulopathy and about conditions (e.g., diabetes, immune disorders, renal disease, hepatic dysfunction, and malignancies), practices (e.g., smoking), and medications (e.g., corticosteroids or chemotherapeutic agents) that could interfere with healing. The patient's nutritional status must be assessed, and the patient must be checked for signs of arterial or venous insufficiency in the wounded area.

The wound must then be carefully examined. Active hemorrhage must be noted. Wounded tissue must be assessed for viability, and foreign bodies must be sought. The possibility of damage to nerves, ducts, muscles, or bones in proximity to the injury must be assessed. X-rays and a careful motor and sensory examination may be required to rule out such coexistent injuries. It may be necessary to probe such ducts as the parotid or the lacrimal duct to assess them for injury. The patient's tetanus immunization status should be considered [*see* Tetanus Prophylaxis, *below*]. Antirabies treatment should be considered for patients who have been bitten by wild animals such as skunks, raccoons, foxes, and bats [*see 2:2 Soft Tissue Infection and 6:20 Viral Infection*].

Tetanus Prophylaxis

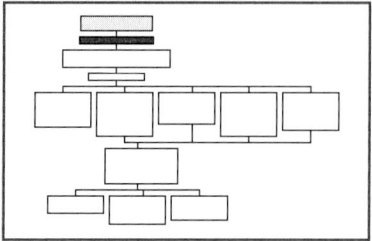

With any wound, it is important to consider the status of the patient's tetanus immunization.[1] The effectiveness of antibiotics for the prophylaxis of tetanus is uncertain.[2] Large, deep wounds with devitalized tissue are especially prone to tetanus infection and are defined as tetanus prone[3] [*see Tables 1 and 2*]. There is no one characteristic that defines a wound as tetanus prone: instead, wounds are considered tetanus prone if they have a significant number of the characteristics considered to define this state.

For non–tetanus-prone wounds, tetanus immune globulin (human) (TIG) is never indicated. If a patient with a non–tetanus-prone wound was never completely immunized or has not received a tetanus booster dose within the past 10 years, a booster dose of tetanus and diphtheria toxoids adsorbed (Td) is required. For a patient who has been previously immunized and has received a tetanus booster within the past 10 years, no further treatment is required.

For a patient with a tetanus-prone wound who has been completely immunized and has received a booster dose within the past 5 years, no treatment is indicated. If a previously immunized patient with a tetanus-prone wound has not been immunized within the past 5 years, a booster Td dose is administered. If a patient with a tetanus-prone wound either was not immunized or was incompletely immunized, TIG is given along with a dose of Td.

Antibiotic Prophylaxis

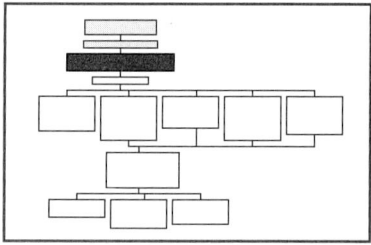

Prophylactic antibiotics are not indicated for most wounds. They are, however, indicated for contaminated wounds in immunocompromised or diabetic patients. They are also indicated for patients with extensive injuries to the central area of the face, to prevent spread of infection through the venous system to the meninges; for patients with valvular disease, to prevent endocarditis; and for patients with prostheses, to limit the chance of bacterial seeding of the prosthesis. Lymphedematous extremities

Table 1 Wound Classification[3]

Clinical Features	Tetanus-Prone Wounds	Non–Tetanus-Prone Wounds
Age of wound	> 6 hr	≤ 6 hr
Configuration	Stellate wound, avulsion, abrasion	Linear wound
Depth	> 1 cm	≤ 1 cm
Mechanism of injury	Missile, crush, burn, frostbite	Sharp surface (e.g., knife or glass)
Signs of infection	Present	Absent
Devitalized tissue	Present	Absent
Contaminants (e.g., dirt, feces, soil, or saliva)	Present	Absent

are particularly prone to cellulitis, and antibiotics are indicated when such extremities are wounded. Stool-contaminated wounds and human-bite wounds are considered infected from the moment of infliction and must be treated with antibiotics [see 2:2 Soft Tissue Infection].[4,5] As a rule, dog-bite wounds are less severely contaminated with bacteria; however, a 1994 meta-analysis suggested that prophylactic antibiotics are probably beneficial in this setting.[6] In addition, antibiotic prophylaxis is often indicated for wounds with extensive amounts of devitalized tissue (e.g., farm injuries).

When antibiotic prophylaxis is called for, the agent or agents to be used should be selected on the basis of the bacterial species believed to be present. Staphylococcus aureus, α-hemolytic streptococci, Eikenella corrodens, Haemophilus species, and anaerobes are often cultured from human-bite wounds.[4,5] To cover these species, a broad-spectrum antibiotic or combination of antibiotics should be administered; amoxicillin-clavulanate, a β-lactamase inhibitor, is a common choice.

Pasteurella multocida is the most common infecting organism in cat-bite wounds. P. multocida is also common in dog-bite wounds, though α-hemolytic streptococci and S. aureus are frequently isolated as well.[6,7] For cat-bite wounds, penicillin alone usually suffices, whereas for dog-bite wounds, a broad-spectrum agent (e.g., penicillin-clavulanate) is preferable. Mutilating injuries that are caused by farm equipment are often contaminated with a mixture of gram-positive organisms and gram-negative organisms, though not always excessively so.[8] When antibiotics are indicated for such injuries, broad-spectrum coverage is appropriate.

The anatomic location of a wound may also suggest whether oral flora, fecal flora, or some less aggressive bacterial contaminant is likely to be present. A Gram stain can provide an early clue to the type of bacteria present as well. The choice of prophylactic antibiotic to be given is ultimately based on the clinician's best judgment regarding which agent or combination of agents will cover the pathogens likely to be present in the wound on the basis of the information available.

Antibiotics are clearly indicated if cellulitis is present when an injured patient is first seen. The presence of infection suggests that there has been a significant delay between wounding and presentation for treatment. Routine soft tissue infections are usually caused by staphylococci or streptococci, and gram-positive coverage is generally indicated. The presence of crepitus or a foul smell suggests a possible anaerobic infection. Initial antibiotic choices are made empirically; more specific antibiotic treatment can be instituted when the results of bacterial culture and sensitivity studies become available.

Timing of Wound Closure

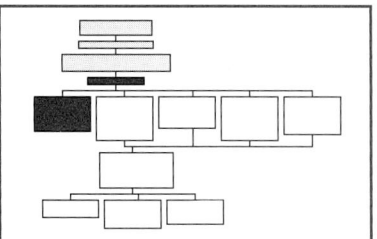

The goal of acute wound management should be a closed, healing wound. The first issue to address is the timing of closure. The choices are (1) primary closure, that is, to close the wound at the time of initial presentation; (2) secondary closure, that is, to allow the wound to heal on its own; and (3) tertiary closure, that is, to close the wound after a period of secondary healing. The proper choice depends on how the following questions are answered:

1. Must the wound be closed, or will secondary healing produce an acceptable result?
2. If closure is required,
   a. Can hemorrhage be easily controlled?
   b. Can all necrotic material and foreign bodies be clearly identified and excised?
   c. Is excessive bacterial contamination present?

Normal healing can proceed only if tissues are viable, the wound contains no foreign bodies, and tissues are free of excessive bacterial contamination.

SMALL OR SUPERFICIAL WOUNDS

Superficial wounds involving only the epidermis and a portion of the dermis will frequently heal secondarily within 1 to 2 weeks. In such wounds, the functional and aesthetic results of secondary healing are generally as good as or better than those obtained by primary or tertiary closure. For puncture wounds, secondary healing is preferred because it diminishes the likelihood of infection and produces an aesthetically acceptable scar. For wounds on concave surfaces such as the medial canthal region and the nasolabial region, secondary healing generally yields excellent aesthetic results.[9]

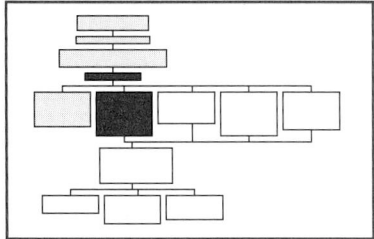

ACUTE WOUNDS WITHOUT BACTERIAL CONTAMINATION, FOREIGN BODIES, OR NECROTIC TISSUE

If wound closure is required, primary closure is preferred if it is feasible: it eliminates the need for extensive wound care; the wound reaches its final, healed state more quickly; and it minimizes patient discomfort. However, a wound with foreign bodies or necrotic tissue that cannot be removed by irrigation or debridement, or a wound with excessive bacterial contamination, should not be closed primarily (see below), nor should wounds in which hemostasis is incomplete. Hematomas,[10] necrotic tissue,[11] and foreign bodies[12] promote the growth of bacteria and provide a mechanical barrier between healing tissues.

Table 2   Immunization Schedule*

History of Tetanus Immunization (Doses)	Tetanus-Prone Wounds		Non–Tetanus-Prone Wounds	
	Td[†]	TIG	Td[†]	TIG
Unknown or < 3	Yes	Yes	Yes	No
3 or more	No[‡]	No	No[§]	No

Note: The only contraindication to tetanus and diphtheria toxoids for the wounded patient is a history of neurologic or severe hypersensitivity reaction to a previous dose. Local side effects alone do not preclude continued use. If a systemic reaction is suspected to represent allergic hypersensitivity, postpone immunization until appropriate skin testing is performed. If a contraindication to a tetanus toxoid–containing preparation exists, consider passive immunization against tetanus for a tetanus-prone wound.
*Modified from the recommendations of the Centers for Disease Control and Prevention.
†For children younger than 7 yr, diphtheria and tetanus toxoids and pertussis vaccine adsorbed (or diphtheria and tetanus toxoids adsorbed, if pertussis vaccine is contraindicated) is preferable to tetanus toxoid alone. For persons 7 yr of age and older, Td is preferable to tetanus toxoid alone.
‡Yes, if more than 5 yr since last dose.
§Yes, if more than 10 yr since last dose.
Td—tetanus and diphtheria toxoids adsorbed (for adult use)
TIG—tetanus immune globulin (human)

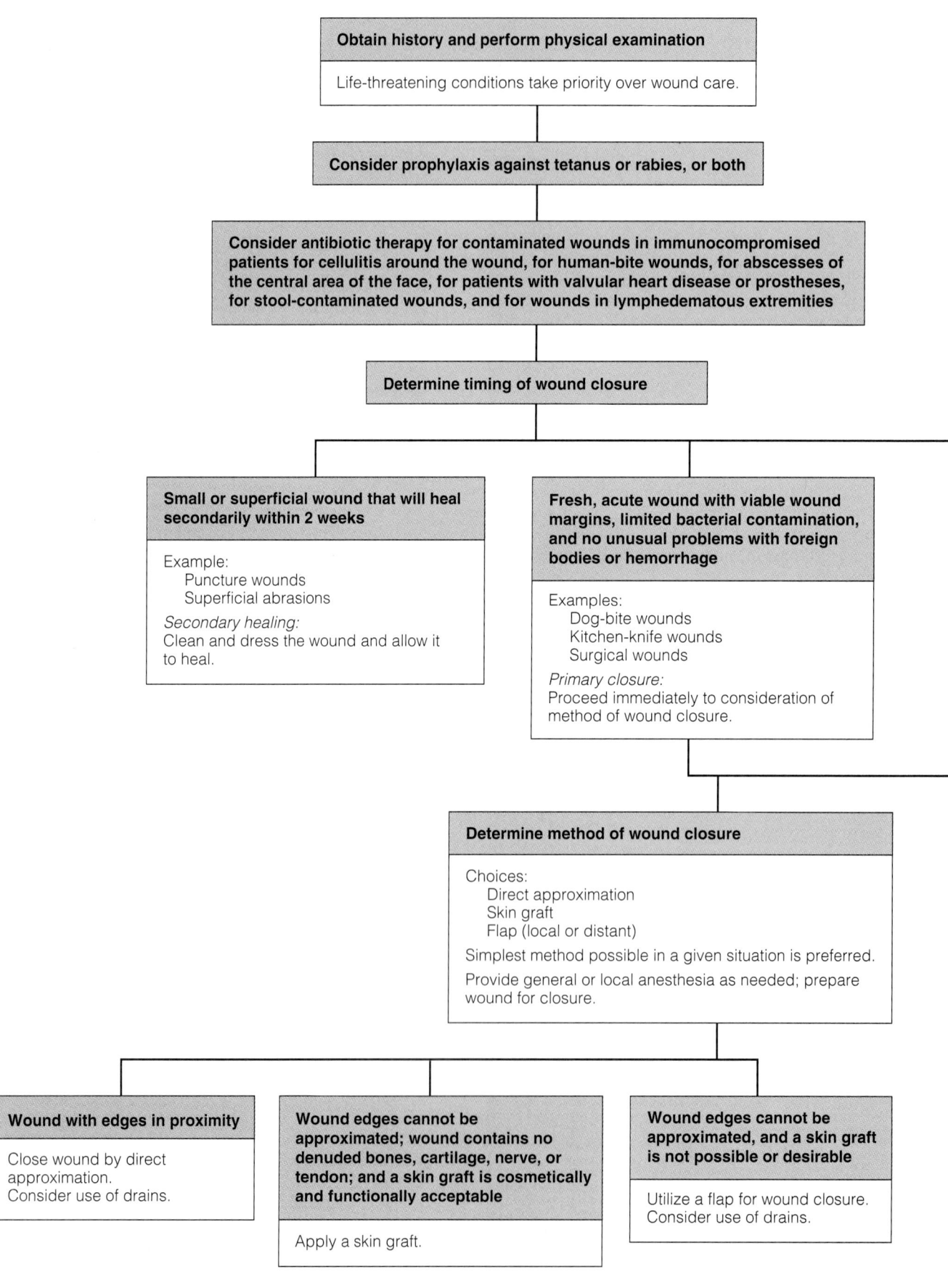

Obtain history and perform physical examination

Life-threatening conditions take priority over wound care.

Consider prophylaxis against tetanus or rabies, or both

Consider antibiotic therapy for contaminated wounds in immunocompromised patients for cellulitis around the wound, for human-bite wounds, for abscesses of the central area of the face, for patients with valvular heart disease or prostheses, for stool-contaminated wounds, and for wounds in lymphedematous extremities

Determine timing of wound closure

Small or superficial wound that will heal secondarily within 2 weeks

Example:
    Puncture wounds
    Superficial abrasions

Secondary healing:
Clean and dress the wound and allow it to heal.

Fresh, acute wound with viable wound margins, limited bacterial contamination, and no unusual problems with foreign bodies or hemorrhage

Examples:
    Dog-bite wounds
    Kitchen-knife wounds
    Surgical wounds

Primary closure:
Proceed immediately to consideration of method of wound closure.

Determine method of wound closure

Choices:
    Direct approximation
    Skin graft
    Flap (local or distant)

Simplest method possible in a given situation is preferred.

Provide general or local anesthesia as needed; prepare wound for closure.

Wound with edges in proximity

Close wound by direct approximation.
Consider use of drains.

Wound edges cannot be approximated; wound contains no denuded bones, cartilage, nerve, or tendon; and a skin graft is cosmetically and functionally acceptable

Apply a skin graft.

Wound edges cannot be approximated, and a skin graft is not possible or desirable

Utilize a flap for wound closure.
Consider use of drains.

Approach to Acute Wound Management

Acute wound with uncontrollable hemorrhage	Acute wound with questionably viable tissue or extreme contamination with foreign bodies	Acute or neglected wound with excessive bacterial contamination

Example:
   Wound in a hemophiliac
 	
Tertiary closure:
Pack or wrap wound tightly until bleeding is controlled; then proceed with closure.
	Examples:
	   Wounds with embedded road tar
	   Wounds with severely contused tissue
	
	Tertiary closure:
	Proceed with debridement of foreign bodies and necrotic tissue, and initiate dressing changes until wound is clean; then proceed with closure.
		Example:
		   Human-bite wounds
		
		Tertiary closure:
		Debride and irrigate wound and initiate dressing changes with antibacterial cream until bacterial count is $< 10^5$/g tissue; then proceed with closure.

ACUTE WOUNDS WITH
EXCESSIVE BLEEDING

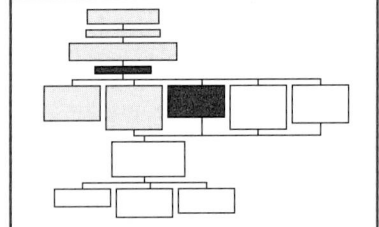

Hemorrhage can be readily controlled in most wounds with pressure, cauterization, or ligation. Occasionally, as with a patient with a bleeding diathesis, primary wound closure is precluded by inadequate hemostasis. In such cases, the wound should be packed or wrapped tightly and elevated if the anatomic site of the wound allows. The wound should then be reexamined within 24 hours to determine whether hemostasis is sufficient to allow safe closure. If bleeding within a wound occurs after closure, the course of action depends on the size of the resulting hematoma. Small hematomas, which will be resorbed, can be ignored. Larger hematomas, which provide a significant barrier to healing, require drainage.

ACUTE WOUNDS WITH
FOREIGN BODIES OR
NECROTIC TISSUE

Foreign Bodies

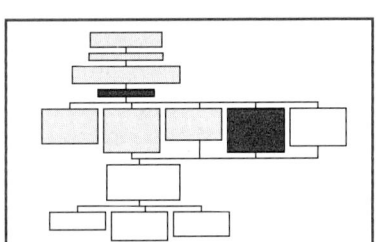

Most foreign bodies can be easily removed from wounds manually or debrided surgically. Patients injured in motorcycle accidents, however, frequently slide along asphalt pavements for long distances at high speeds, with the result that many small fragments of asphalt become embedded in and beneath the skin. Exploding gunpowder also causes many small pieces of foreign material to be embedded within the skin. These foreign bodies are often difficult to extract, but they should be removed as soon as possible after the injury. High-pressure irrigation with saline will remove many foreign bodies. Surgical debridement or vigorous scrubbing with a wire brush may be required for the removal of more firmly embedded foreign material. If too much time elapses between injury and treatment, the embedded material is gradually covered and encapsulated by advancing epithelium and thereby becomes sealed within the dermis. In such instances, surgical dermabrasion is necessary for the removal of the foreign material.[13,14]

Foreign materials such as paint, oil, and grease are sometimes inadvertently injected subcutaneously under pressure (600 to 12,000 psi) by the spray guns used for painting, automotive body work, or industrial purposes.[15,16] On initial examination, the injury may appear deceptively benign in that a punctate entry wound draining foreign material is often the only sign of injury other than edema. Nevertheless, these wounds must be treated aggressively if extensive tissue loss is to be avoided. With some injected materials, radiographs are useful for demonstrating the extent of distribution. The involved area, which is frequently the hand, should be incised, and as much of the foreign material as possible should be surgically debrided (preferably, if the hand is involved, by a surgeon who specializes in hand injuries). Because the foreign material is often widely distributed in the soft tissues, extensive incisions may be necessary. Antibiotics and tetanus prophylaxis are also recommended. The ultimate prognosis is at least partially determined by the type of material injected: paint is associated with a particularly poor prognosis, whereas water is associated with a good one.[17] Early aggressive therapy does not rule out the possibility of amputation, especially if the injected material is notably caustic.

High-velocity missiles such as bullets are rendered sterile by the explosion required for their propulsion; therefore, deeply embedded bullets can often be left safely where they have lodged. Center-fire rifle bullets and .44 magnum pistol bullets carry a large amount of kinetic energy and can produce extensive tissue damage. Wounds created by such high-velocity missiles may have to be debrided to permit excision of necrotic tissue. The mechanism of injury may suggest the possibility of a foreign body within the wound that is not immediately apparent. If a radiopaque material, such as metal or leaded glass, is being looked for, radiographs may detect its presence. For less opaque materials, xeroradiography, magnified radiographs, and computed tomographic scans are sometimes diagnostically useful.[18]

Identification and Debridement of Necrotic Tissue

The necrotic tissue in most wounds can be identified and surgically debrided at initial presentation. In some wounds, there may be a significant amount of tissue of questionable viability. If the amount of questionable material precludes acute debridement, dressing changes may be initiated. When all tissue has been identified as viable or necrotic, and when the necrotic tissue has been debrided surgically or by means of dressing changes, the wound can be closed.

Sometimes, a flap of tissue may be of questionable viability. Signs that suggest whether tissue is viable include color, bright-red arteriolar bleeding, and blanching on pressure followed by capillary refill. A flap can also be evaluated acutely by administering up to 15 mg/kg of fluorescein intravenously and observing the flap for fluorescence under an ultraviolet lamp after 10 to 15 minutes have elapsed.[19] Viable tissue fluoresces. Flap tissue that is thought to be devascularized, on the basis of physical examination or fluorescein examination, should be debrided. If the viability of a segment of tissue is in doubt, it may be sewn back in its anatomic location and allowed to define itself as viable or nonviable over time.

In burn wounds, it is impossible to assess the extent of final tissue damage at presentation because the injury can worsen during the first few days after the burn.[20] Closure of the burn wound is often delayed until the depth of the injury can be more precisely defined [see 5:14 *Burn Care after the First Postburn Week*].

Another type of wound in which the severity of the injury may not be readily apparent is the crush injury. With a crush injury, there may not be an external laceration, even though tissue damage may be extensive. The primary concern is whether muscle damage in the fascial compartments is severe enough to induce swelling sufficient to compromise the vascularity of the muscle. If pulses are diminished or paresthesias are developing, the pressure within the fascial compartment is clearly excessive, and fasciotomies are indicated. In less clear-cut cases, intracompartmental pressures may be assessed by percutaneous placement of catheters or wicks into the fascial compartments. The catheters or wicks are attached to pressure monitors or transducers. An intracompartmental pressure greater than 40 mm Hg indicates that capillary filling pressure has been exceeded and muscle perfusion is compromised. The fascial compartment must then be released to prevent ischemic muscle damage; the fasciotomies must be performed on an emergency basis. If the degree of damage is not severe enough to necessitate fasciotomy, the injured part should be elevated and dressed in a mildly compressive dressing to limit edema formation. If there is muscle damage, the possibility of crush syndrome with renal damage caused by rhabdomyolysis must be considered. If myoglobin is found in the urine, diuresis should be induced, and the urine should be alkalinized.

ACUTE OR NEGLECTED WOUNDS WITH BACTERIAL CONTAMINATION

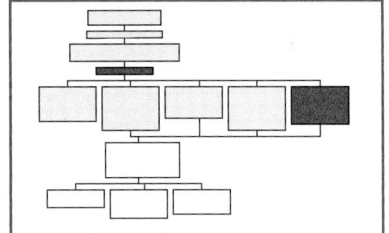

An infected wound is defined as one with bacterial concentrations greater than 10^5 organisms/g tissue.[21,22] β-Hemolytic streptococci are an exception to this rule and can produce clinical infections in lower concentrations.[23] It is often difficult to assess the degree of bacterial contamination of a wound solely through visual inspection. Ideally, quantitative cultures are ordered so that precise information about the type and numbers of bacteria present can be obtained. The rapid slide technique typically yields bacterial counts within 1 hour.[24] If this information cannot be obtained, the clinician must rely on more empirical information.

The age of the wound is one factor correlated with the degree of bacterial contamination. The initial 6 to 8 hours after wounding has been referred to as the golden period because closure can usually be accomplished safely during this period. In a clinical study in a civilian setting, most wounds less than 5 to 6 hours old were contaminated with fewer than 10^5 bacteria/g tissue and therefore could be safely closed primarily.[25] Experimental data suggest that bacteria trapped within the fibrinous exudate that forms over a wound's surface cause the infections seen in wounds closed after 6 to 8 hours.[26,27] The bacteria proliferate after wounding and generally take 6 to 8 hours to reach levels of 10^5/g tissue. The longer wounds remain open, the greater the likelihood that they will become infected.[25]

The location of the injury is also significant. Lacerations of the face, which has an abundant blood supply, are more likely to resist bacterial proliferation (and to do so for a longer time) than injuries to less adequately perfused areas, such as the lower extremities.[28] Immune status is also important. A wound is less likely to become infected in a young, healthy person than in an elderly, debilitated patient or a person receiving immunosuppressive medication.[29]

The mechanism of injury can suggest whether a wound may become infected and what species of bacteria are most likely to be present in the wound [see Antibiotic Prophylaxis, above]. Wounds with a high degree of bacterial contamination (e.g., human-bite wounds) generally should not be closed.

An infected wound can sometimes be excised to produce a fresh, less contaminated wound. A 1997 study of human facial bites reported successful wound closure when extensive debridement was performed before closure and patients were treated with antibiotics for 1 week.[30] An alternative approach to a contaminated wound is to close it over a drain and administer topical and systemic antibiotics; this approach has yielded low infection rates in some series.[31,32]

In situations in which the nature of the injury precludes complete wound excision or in which there is cellulitis of surrounding tissues, dressing changes should be initiated. The use of certain topical agents will lead to a decreased bacterial count. Silver sulfadiazine (Silvadene) is used frequently because its antibacterial spectrum is broad, it is comfortable for the patient, and it does not commonly lead to metabolic problems such as those seen with other agents, such as mafenide (Sulfamylon) or silver nitrate.[33,34] Silver sulfadiazine may also optimize the rate of epithelialization.[35] Parenteral antibiotics are not useful for killing bacteria in the wound itself, because they do not penetrate the wound directly.[36] In experiments on animals, parenteral antibiotics have proved useful for controlling bacteria within wounds when used in conjunction with proteolytic enzymes such as Travase.[26,37] This combination of treatments has not been widely used clinically.

Once bacterial control has been accomplished, the wound can be closed. In one series, tertiary closure was successful in more than 90% of cases when bacterial counts in tissue had diminished to less than 10^5/g.[38]

An alternative to either primary closure or dressing changes in these patients is delayed primary closure, a technique developed empirically during wartime.[39] Saline-soaked gauze is packed into the wound at the time of injury, and the wound is reexamined after several days. If the wound appears clean, the wound edges are then approximated. If the wound appears to be contaminated at follow-up, dressing changes are instituted. This approach limits the infection rate in potentially contaminated wounds.

When infection develops after closure of a wound, treatment involves removal of some or all of the sutures and initiation of dressing changes, often with use of topical antibacterials [see Dressings, below]. Any cellulitis surrounding the wound is treated with systemic antibiotics [see 2:2 Soft Tissue Infection].

Surgical Wounds

The American College of Surgeons has divided operative wounds into four major categories [see Table 3]. The likelihood of infection after any surgical procedure is correlated with the category of wound.[40] Wounds in classes I and II have low infection rates, whereas wounds in class IV have infection rates as high as 40%.

Wounds Resulting from Wild-Animal Bites: Special Considerations

Rabies prophylaxis must be considered for bite wounds from high-risk wild animals such as skunks, raccoons, foxes, coyotes, and bats.[41] Rabies is generally not a risk in bite wounds from rodents, rabbits, pets, and domestic animals unless the animal is acting unusually aggressive and is salivating excessively. If there is any possibility that the biting animal has rabies and the animal is available, it should be watched for symptoms of rabies for 10 days. If the biting animal can be killed and examined, rabies can be confirmed or excluded by means of an immunofluorescent antibody study of its brain. If rabies is confirmed or if the biting animal is not available for examination and rabies is suspected, the patient should be treated with both rabies immune globulin and human diploid cell vaccine. Specific schedules for administration appear elsewhere [see 2:2 Soft Tissue Infection].

With snakebite wounds, the possibility of envenomation must be considered. The poisonous snakes native to the United States are coral snakes and three species of pit vipers—namely, rattlesnakes, copperheads, and water moccasins.[42-44] The pit vipers can be identi-

Table 3 Classification and Infection Rates of Operative Wounds

Classification	Infection Rate (%)	Wound Characteristics
Clean (class I)	1.5–5.1	Atraumatic, uninfected; no entry of GU, GI, or respiratory tract
Clean-contaminated (class II)	7.7–10.8	Minor breaks in sterile technique; entry of GU, GI, or respiratory tract without significant spillage
Contaminated (class III)	15.2–16.3	Traumatic wounds; gross spillage from GI tract; entry into infected tissue, bone, urine, or bile
Dirty (class IV)	28.0–40.0	Drainage of abscess; debridement of soft tissue infection

fied by the pit between the eye and nostril on each side of the head, the vertical elliptic pupils, the triangular shape of the head, the single row of caudal plates, and the characteristic fang marks they inflict when they bite. Coral snakes have rounder heads and eyes and lack fangs; they are identified by their characteristic color pattern, consisting of red, yellow, and black vertical bands. Patients bitten by any of the pit vipers must be examined for massive swelling and pain, which, along with fang marks, suggest envenomation. The pain and swelling generally develop within 30 minutes of the bite, although they may take up to 4 hours to become manifest. Secondary local signs, such as erythema, petechiae, ecchymoses, and bullae, sometimes appear; if envenomation is extensive, systemic signs, such as disseminated intravascular coagulation (DIC), bleeding, shock, acute respiratory distress syndrome, and renal failure, may also be seen. Patients bitten by coral snakes, on the other hand, show no obvious local signs when envenomation has occurred. Consequently, the physician must look for systemic signs, such as paresthesias, increased salivation, fasciculations of the tongue, dysphagia, difficulty in speaking, visual disturbances, respiratory distress, convulsions, and shock. These symptoms may not develop until several hours after the bite.

No local care is necessary for coral snake bite wounds; however, a variety of techniques have been used for local care of pit viper bite wounds. Some groups have advocated surgical approaches, such as early incision with suction and wound excision, whereas others have suggested topical application of ice or use of tourniquets to limit the spread of venom. None of these treatments have been shown to provide a definite benefit. At present, topical application of ice is discouraged because it is more likely to lead to secondary injuries than to benefit the patient. Tight tourniquets cannot be left in place for long periods without risking damage to the extremity; however, loose tourniquets that slow lymphatic drainage may be of some value. Excision of the bite wound may be effective if it is performed within 1 to 2 hours of injury. To reduce the incidence of unintentional injuries, excision should be performed only by persons with medical training.

Antivenin is indicated if pain and swelling are substantial enough to suggest extensive envenomation. It should be administered only if it is clearly necessary because it is of equine origin and frequently produces serum sickness. Antivenin is almost never required for copperhead bites but is more commonly needed for rattlesnake bites.[45] When indicated, it should be administered as soon as possible because it is less effective when given after signs of envenomation have become severe.

Whenever there is any suggestion of envenomation, a battery of tests, including hematocrit, fibrinogen level, coagulation studies, platelet count, urinalysis, and serum chemistry values, should be performed. These tests should be repeated every 8 to 24 hours to evaluate any venom-induced changes. With severe envenomation, decreased fibrinogen levels, coagulopathies, and bleeding may be seen, as may myoglobinuria.

Envenomation is also a consideration with the bites of brown recluse spiders and black widow spiders.[44] The brown recluse spider has a violin-shaped mark on its dorsum; is found in dark, dry places; and is nocturnal. The symptoms of the bite may range from minor irritation to extreme tenderness associated with edema and erythema; the tenderness, erythema, and edema generally do not develop until 2 to 8 hours after the bite. In more severe cases, tissue necrosis can develop in as little as 12 hours, although more often the area of necrosis does not demarcate itself for weeks. Severe systemic reactions, including hemolysis and DIC, have been reported. The tissue necrosis resulting from the bite of the brown recluse can be minimized by the use of dapsone.[46] The black widow often has a red hourglass mark on its abdomen and lives in dark, dry, protected

areas.[44] The venom is a neurotoxin that produces severe local pain. Neurologic signs usually develop within 15 minutes and consist of muscle pain and cramps starting in the vicinity of the bite. The abdominal muscles frequently become involved. Other symptoms that may develop are vomiting, tremors, increased salivation, paresthesias, hyperreflexia, and, with severe envenomation, shock. In sensitive individuals, paralysis, hemolysis, renal failure, or coma may be seen. Treatment of black widow envenomation includes parenteral 10% calcium gluconate, parenteral methocarbamol, and one dose of parenteral antivenin.

Method of Wound Closure

When a wound is ready to be closed, the appropriate type of wound closure must be chosen. The types of wound closure are (1) direct approximation, (2) skin graft (autograft), (3) 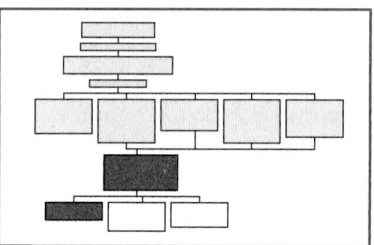 local flap, and (4) distant flap. In general, the simplest method possible in a given situation is preferred.

DIRECT WOUND APPROXIMATION

The most common surgical problem is the deep, relatively acute traumatic or surgical wound that is suitable for primary closure by direct approximation of the edges of the wound. In this setting, the goal is to provide the best possible chance for uncomplicated healing.

Adequate general or local anesthesia is an extremely important first step. If local anesthesia is indicated, as for small traumatic injuries, 0.5% or 1.0% lidocaine (Xylocaine) is generally injected directly into the wounded tissues. Although other local anesthetic agents can be used, lidocaine is the most popular choice because it acts quickly, it rarely provokes allergic reactions, and it provides local anesthesia for the 1 to 2 hours required for most wound closures. Epinephrine in a dilution of 1:100,000 or 1:200,000 is often used in combination with the lidocaine. Epinephrine prolongs the effectiveness of the anesthetic, increases the anesthetic dose that can be safely used, and aids hemostasis.[47] Lower concentrations of epinephrine can be effective, but it becomes unstable if stored for long periods at low concentrations. Traditionally, epinephrine has not been used in the fingers and toes out of concern that it might induce vasospasm, which could result in loss of one or more digits. In the first half of 2001, this guideline was questioned by a prospective study in which a series of digital blocks with epinephrine resulted in no reported morbidity.[48] In reviewing the literature, the authors of the study could not identify a single case in which local anesthesia alone resulted in digital loss. An experimental study from 1985 suggested that the use of epinephrine is associated with a higher incidence of infection[49]; however, this association has not been noted clinically.

The maximum safe doses of lidocaine traditionally cited are 4 mg/kg without epinephrine and 7 mg/kg with epinephrine. The upper limit of the maximum safe dose has been questioned. During liposuction procedures, up to 35 mg/kg of lidocaine has been administered in a 0.1% solution containing epinephrine in a 1:1,000,000 dilution without reaching toxic drug levels.[50,51] Given that some of the anesthetic is aspirated in the course of a liposuction procedure, caution should be exercised in extrapolating this finding to other types of procedures. The pain involved in injecting the local anesthetic can be minimized by using a small-caliber needle, warming the drug, injecting the drug slowly, using the subcutaneous rather than the intradermal route (even though the rate of onset is thereby slowed),[52] providing counterirritation, and buffering the agent with sodium bicarbonate to limit its acidity.[53]

Topical local anesthetics have been gaining in popularity. TAC (a solution of 0.5% tetracaine, 1:2,000 adrenaline [epinephrine], and 11.8% cocaine) has been demonstrated to be effective as injectable anesthetics when applied topically to an open wound, especially in the face or scalp.[54,55] Concerns have been expressed about the possible toxicity of the cocaine, and efforts have been made to identify alternative topical agents. Topical 5% lidocaine with 1:2,000 epinephrine,[56] topical 4% lidocaine with 0.1% epinephrine and 0.5% tetracaine,[57] 0.48% bupivicaine with 1:26,000 norepinephrine,[58] and 3.56% prilocaine with 0.10% phenylephrine[59] have all been demonstrated to be equivalent to TAC. EMLA (a eutectic mixture of lidocaine and prilocaine) has been used to induce local anesthesia in intact skin, often before venous cannulation,[60] and it has been evaluated in open wounds as well.[61] EMLA is a more effective local anesthetic than TAC for open wounds of the lower extremity. To induce sufficient anesthesia to be useful, however, EMLA must be in contact with the skin for 1 to 2 hours.

Hair may be clipped to facilitate exposure and wound closure, if necessary. Close shaving should be avoided, however, because it potentiates wound infections.[62] Clipping of eyebrows should also be avoided because they may not grow back.

The next step is to irrigate the wound with a high-pressure (≥ 8 psi) spray to decrease the number of bacteria in the wound.[63-65] A pressurized irrigation device is preferred, but if none is available, high-pressure irrigation may be performed by using (1) a 30 to 50 ml syringe and a 19-gauge needle or catheter or (2) a flexible bag of intravenous 0.9% saline attached to tubing and a 19-gauge catheter with a pressure device.[63] Low-pressure irrigation and scrubbing of the wound with a saline-soaked sponge have not been demonstrated to decrease the incidence of wound infections.[65,66] Irrigants that have been demonstrated to be nontoxic to tissues include 0.9% saline[67] and Pluronic F-68,[68,69] though lactated Ringer solution is also acceptable. Pluronic F-68 has surfactant properties that improve wound cleansing without damaging tissues. Antibiotics are sometimes added to irrigation solutions to increase their effectiveness at killing bacteria. Solutions of 1% neomycin sulfate and 2% kanamycin sulfate, which do not kill fibroblasts in culture,[70] have limited toxicity to tissues. There is some evidence[71] that antibiotic supplements are more effective than saline solution in decreasing bacterial counts in contaminated wounds.

There are a number of solutions that should never be placed on a wound. Povidone-iodine scrub and soaps containing hexachlorophene are especially damaging to normal tissues.[67,72,73] Chlorhexidine, which is found in various brands of soaps, has also been demonstrated to impede the healing process.[74,75] Alcohol is toxic to tissues and should not be placed in wounds.[76] A 0.5% solution of sodium hypochlorite (Dakin solution) has been demonstrated to be toxic to fibroblasts, to impair neutrophil function, and to slow epithelialization in open wounds.[70,77] A 0.25% solution of acetic acid has been demonstrated to kill fibroblasts in culture and to slow epithelialization in open wounds.[70] Hydrogen peroxide has been shown to kill fibroblasts in culture and to cause histologic damage to tissues.[67,70] Even standard hand soap can induce some tissue damage that is visible on histologic examination.[67,76] The dictum "Don't put in a wound what you wouldn't put in your eye" is a valid guideline.[78]

After adequate anesthesia has been achieved, hair has been clipped, and the wound has been irrigated, the tissue surrounding the wound is prepared with an antibacterial solution such as povidone-iodine,[79,80] and a sterile field is created by using sterile drapes. Skin preparation limits contamination of the wound by bacteria from adjacent skin. The wound is surgically debrided of any foreign bodies or necrotic material to limit the chances of postoperative infection.[81] If the wound edges are beveled and adequate local tissue is available, the wound edges should be excised by means of incisions perpendicular to the skin.

Although wound closure can usually proceed in a straightforward manner, special caution is necessary in certain situations. When a wound crosses tissues with different characteristics, such as at the vermilion border of the lip, at the eyebrow, or at the hairline of the scalp, great care must be taken to align the damaged structures accurately. Injured nerves or ducts should generally be repaired at the time of wound closure. In acute wounds, it is generally best to avoid more complex tissue rearrangements such as a Z-plasty or W-plasty. Actual reconstructive surgery in the face of trauma is rarely indicated [see 2:7 Surface Reconstruction Procedures]. Direct approximation of wounds does not always produce a uniform or aesthetically desirable result, particularly in extensive wounds, wounds lying outside normal skin folds or creases, wounds in children older than 2 years, wounds in the sternal and deltoid regions, U-shaped wounds, wounds with beveled edges, or wounds in regions of thick oily skin, such as the tip of the nose, where scars are often less acceptable. Wounds heal optimally when two perpendicular, well-vascularized wound edges are approximated in a tension-free manner.

An ideal method of wound closure would support the wound until it had nearly reached full strength (i.e., about 6 weeks), would not induce inflammation, would not induce ischemia, would not penetrate the epidermis and predispose to additional scars, and would not interfere with the healing process in any way. No existing method of wound closure accomplishes all of these goals: some sort of compromise is virtually always necessary.

Materials for Wound Closure

Materials available for wound closure are sutures, staples, tapes, and tissue adhesives. Of these, sutures are most commonly used. Absorbable sutures, such as those made of plain or chromic catgut, polyglactin 910 (Vicryl), polyglycolic acid (Dexon), polyglyconate (Maxon), or polydioxanone (PDS), are generally used for dermis, fat, muscle, or superficial fascia. Nonabsorbable sutures, such as those made of nylon, Ethibond, or polypropylene (Prolene), are most commonly used either for the skin (in which case they are removed) or for deeper structures that require prolonged wound support, such as the fascia of the abdominal wall or tendons.

The suture should be as small in diameter as possible while still being able to maintain approximation. The decision to remove skin sutures or staples involves balancing of optimal cosmesis with the need for wound support. Optimal cosmesis demands early removal of sutures, before inflammation can develop and before epithelialization can occur along the suture tracts. An epithelialized tract will develop around a suture or staple that remains in the skin for more than 7 to 10 days; after removal of the stitch, the tract will be replaced by an unwanted scar.[82] On the other hand, it takes a number of weeks for the wound to gain significant tensile strength, and early removal of wound support can lead to dehiscence of wounds subject to substantial tension. Wounds on the face and wounds along skin tension lines (e.g., incisions for thyroidectomy) are subject to limited tension, and sutures can be removed from these areas relatively early. Sutures are generally removed at day 4 or 5 from the face and generally by day 7 from other areas where skin tension is limited.

Sutures should remain longer in wounds subject to a greater amount of stress, such as wounds in the lower extremities and wounds closed under tension. Sutures also remain longer in wounds in persons with healing limitations, such as malnutrition. Less aesthetically pleasing consequences may have to be accepted in these cases.

One way of sustaining skin wound support while avoiding unwanted scars from skin sutures is to use buried dermal sutures. Synthetic materials, such as Vicryl, Dexon, PDS, or Maxon, are preferable to chromic or plain catgut because the former are absorbed by simple hydrolysis with little inflammatory response, whereas the latter provoke an active cellular inflammatory response that slows the healing process. Buried dermal sutures are often used in conjunction with either tapes (e.g., SteriStrips) or fine epidermal sutures to aid in precise epidermal alignment.

Closure with staples is more rapid than suture closure, although approximation may not be as precise.[83] Tape is easy to apply, is comfortable for the patient, and leaves no marks on the skin.[84-86] However, patients may inadvertently remove tapes, and approximation is less precise with tapes alone than with sutures. Furthermore, wound edema tends to cause inversion of taped wound edges. Supplemental dermal sutures can enhance the precision of the closure achieved with staples or tapes.

Cyanoacrylate tissue adhesives, used by surgeons for over 30 years, are strong, reasonably flexible, and biocompatible. When these compounds first became available, isobutyl cyanoacrylate and trifluoropropyl cyanoacrylate were placed between wound edges to hold them together. Adhesives used in this way created a mechanical barrier to healing and increased wound inflammation and infection rates. This use of cyanoacrylate tissue adhesives was abandoned relatively quickly.[87] Since then, cyanoacrylates have been applied topically to intact skin at the edge of wounds to hold injured surfaces together. Contact with open wounds is carefully avoided to limit toxicity. Hystoacryl Blue (n-butyl-2-cyanoacrylate) has been used extensively with good clinical results.[88] It creates limited wound strength during the first day after injury and should not be used in wounds subject to stress.[89]

Octylcyanoacrylate is stronger than Hystoacryl Blue. A prospective, randomized trial in Canada[90] compared octylcyanoacrylate to sutures for wound closure. There were few cases of dehiscence, and the aesthetic results of wounds assessed 3 months after closure were similar to those obtained with sutures. As would be expected, octylcyanoacrylate closures were faster for the surgeon and less painful to the patient. Octylcyanoacrylate was not used in deep wounds that penetrated fascia, and the authors also specifically recommended against its use on the hands and over joints where either washing or repetitive motion might lead to premature removal of the adhesive.[90]

Fibrin glue has been utilized to improve the adherence and take of skin grafts[91,92]; it has also been used with a limited number of sutures to close wounds subjected to limited tension (e.g., blepharoplasty incisions[93]) and to curtail seroma formation under flaps.[94] Although fibrin glue is helpful in these settings, it is not strong enough to be usable alone for the closure of wounds subject to even limited tension. Autologous fibrin can be produced from plasma, though the process is sufficiently laborious to discourage routine use. Homologous fibrin has been available in Europe for some time. As a result of its superb safety record, homologous fibrin has been approved by the Food and Drug Administration for general use in the United States.

The old surgical principle that dead space should be closed or obliterated seems to call for the closure of subcutaneous tissues. However, studies in both laboratory animals and humans have demonstrated that multiple layers of closure contribute to an increased incidence of infection.[95,96] Therefore, sutures should be avoided whenever possible in subcutaneous fat, which cannot hold them.

Deeper fascial layers that contribute to the structural integrity of areas such as the abdomen or the chest should be closed as a separate layer to prevent hernias or other structural deformities.

If there appears to be a potential risk of fluid collecting in an unclosed subcutaneous space, drains are a more suitable alternative than subcutaneous stitches. In addition to preventing the accumulation of blood or serum in the wound, suction drains also aid in the approximation of tissues. They are particularly useful in aiding tissue approximation under flaps. Most drains—especially those made of silicone rubber—are relatively inert. However, all drains tend to potentiate bacterial infections and should be removed from a wound as soon as possible.[97]

Drains can usually be safely removed when drainage reaches levels of 25 to 50 ml/day. If a seroma develops after drain removal, intermittent sterile aspirations followed by application of a compressive dressing are indicated. In the unusual case in which drainage is persistent and refractory to intermittent aspirations, a drain may be reintroduced. In unusual cases with prolonged drainage, drains have been left in place for weeks to avoid the development of a seroma.[98]

Occasionally, despite a surgeon's best efforts, a closed wound will dehisce. Dehiscence usually results from tension combined with local and systemic factors. Local factors include poor surgical technique and tissue damage by trauma, prior surgery, or radiation—or, in the case of the abdomen, increased intra-abdominal pressure. Systemic factors include malnutrition, obesity, and concurrent use of medications such as steroids or chemotherapeutic agents. If the dehiscence is noted within 6 to 8 hours and it involves only skin and superficial tissues, the wound can be reclosed or, alternatively, allowed to heal secondarily with dressing changes. Dehiscence of deeper structures such as the abdominal fascia can be a more serious problem. Fascial dehiscence in the abdomen is often heralded by serosanguineous discharge between sutures on days 5 to 8. Fascial separation of less than a few centimeters can be treated expectantly; if the dehiscence is larger, reoperation for fascial reclosure should be performed if the patient's condition permits.

SKIN GRAFTS

If a wound can be directly approximated without excessive tension or distortion of normal structures, that is almost always the method of choice. If a wound is so extensive that direct approximation is impossible, skin grafts should be considered [see 2:7

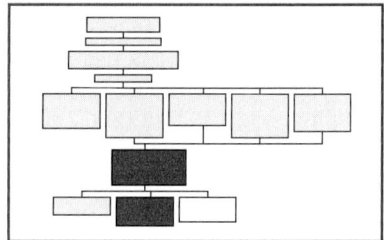

Surface Reconstruction Procedures]. However, skin grafts cannot be used to close injuries that involve bone denuded of periosteum, cartilage denuded of perichondrium, tendon denuded of paratenon, and nerve denuded of perineurium. Skin grafts will not heal over large areas (> 1.0 to 1.5 cm^2) of denuded bone, cartilage, nerve, or tendon, because these structures are relatively, if not totally, avascular, and blood vessels are not present to revascularize the graft. For such wounds, flaps must be considered (see below).

Skin grafts vary in thickness, from very thin split-thickness grafts that incorporate the epidermis and only a small portion of the dermis to full-thickness grafts that incorporate the entire dermis. (There are further variations within these two classifications.) The nature of the graft affects how readily the graft takes. Thin full-thickness skin grafts from areas such as the eyelid, the retroauricular area, or the medial surface of the upper arm take more reliably than thicker ones from other areas. Similarly, thin split-thickness grafts take more reliably than thicker ones. Grafts that incorporate most or all of the dermis maximally inhibit wound contraction. The ability to inhibit wound contraction is not dependent on the absolute thickness of the graft; rather, it is related to the amount of deeper dermis the graft contains.[99]

Skin grafting produces a second wound at the donor site. All donor sites for full-thickness grafts must be closed independently either by direct wound approximation or by application of an additional graft. Donor sites for split-thickness grafts generally heal secondarily. Donor sites for thicker grafts tend to heal more slowly; donor sites for very thick split-thickness grafts may require grafting for adequate closure.

Skin grafts can be meshed and expanded like a pantograph. This technique increases the area that can be covered and facilitates drainage of fluid through the resulting interstices. Meshed grafts conform well to irregular surfaces. However, the aesthetic result of a meshed graft is usually less satisfactory than that of an intact, unmeshed skin graft, especially if the meshed graft is expanded widely. Wound contraction is increased with an expanded meshed skin graft, which can be a problem around flexion and extension creases near joints.

A suitable donor site should provide a good color match for the wounded tissue and be as inconspicuous as possible.[100] Because humans are relatively symmetrical, the ideal graft tissue in terms of color and texture match is tissue from the contralateral structure. However, this type of graft is often impractical because the donor site is frequently too conspicuous. In general, skin anywhere above the clavicles resembles facial skin; the retroauricular and supraclavicular regions and the scalp are relatively inconspicuous donor sites for facial wounds. The buttocks and upper thighs are preferred donor sites for wounds of the trunk or the extremities.

Grafts will not take if bacterial contamination is excessive,[101] if a seroma or hematoma develops between the graft and the wound site, or if shearing occurs between the graft and the wound site. Infected wounds and wounds in which bleeding is inadequately controlled should not be grafted. Compressive, immobilizing dressing techniques and elevation can help prevent shearing and limit seroma formation. A graft must be protected to some extent until it reaches maturity, usually 6 months after placement.[102] Such measures are especially important for lower-extremity grafts, which may be more susceptible to trauma and dependent edema.

The color of grafted skin generally changes after transfer and is usually darker than it appeared in situ.[103] Hair is transferred only with full-thickness or very thick split-thickness skin grafts. In thicker split-thickness skin grafts, sebaceous activity is lost initially but resumes within 3 months. In the interim, the graft must be lubricated with skin creams. Sensibility in skin grafts is more like that of the recipient site than that of the area from which the graft was taken.[104] Perspiration returns with sensibility, and its pattern also is determined by that of the recipient site.[104] Full-thickness skin grafts have normal growth potential when they are placed during the early years of life, but the growth of split-thickness skin grafts is limited.[105] Skin grafts can be remarkably durable after complete healing and can be used effectively even on the soles of the feet.

FLAPS

Like skin grafts, flaps allow coverage of a wound that cannot be satisfactorily closed primarily; again, the cost is a secondary wound at the donor site. Flaps can be used to close any uninfect-

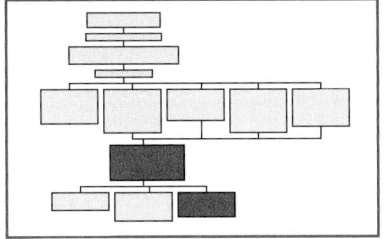

ed wound. They do not require as vascular a wound bed as grafts do, because they maintain their blood supply after transfer and do not depend on revascularization for survival. Flaps are indicated for wounds containing denuded bone, cartilage, tendon, or nerve that cannot be closed by direct approximation. Flaps may be used in some situations in which skin grafts are also a possible choice because they may provide tissue with desirable characteristics such as bulk or a more natural appearance. Flaps that include bone or muscle may also be indicated for functional purposes. Any flap creates at least some functional or aesthetic deficit, a consideration when deciding what type of flap should be used. When feasible, use of local flaps is generally preferred because they usually require a less complex operation and because local tissue is generally the most natural-looking substitute for the wounded tissue. Sometimes, however, specific tissue requirements mandate use of distant flaps.

A flap can be classified as either random or axial. A random flap is supplied with blood from the subdermal plexus but has no specific blood vessel supplying it. An axial flap must be supplied by a specific, predictable blood vessel. Generally, a flap that includes large amounts of tissue or specialized tissue such as muscle or bone is constructed as an axial flap. The most complex distant flap is an axial one that requires microvascular anastomoses of the primary blood vessels of the flap to appropriate recipient vessels in surrounding tissue [see 2:7 Surface Reconstruction Procedures].

The blood supply to the flap must not be impaired by poor design, kinking of the vascular pedicle, pressure from an ill-placed dressing, poor patient positioning, or hematoma formation. Drains are frequently placed under flaps both to encourage tissue approximation and to prevent collection of blood and serum under the flap. Flaps will retain their color, texture, hair-bearing characteristics, and sebaceous activity regardless of the recipient site. Sensibility and perspiration return to some extent between 6 weeks and 3 months after flap transfer. With certain axial flaps, sensibility and other neural functions are preserved from the outset. In children, flaps are also durable and have normal growth potential.

Dressings

Different types of dressings perform different functions. Therefore, for any wound, the purpose a dressing is to serve must be carefully considered before the dressing is applied.

Partial-thickness injuries, such as abrasions and skin graft donor sites, heal primarily by epithelialization and are best treated with dressings that maintain a warm, moist environment.[106,107] A variety of dressings can accomplish this goal, including biologic dressings (e.g., allograft,[108] amnion,[109] or xenograft[110]), synthetic biologic dressings (e.g., Biobrane[111]), hydrogel dressings, and dressings of semipermeable or nonpermeable membranes (e.g., Op-Site or Duoderm).[107] These dressings need not be changed as long as they remain adherent. Small, superficial wounds also heal readily when dressed with Xeroform or Scarlet Red; these dressings are often changed with greater regularity.[112] The traditional approach to partial-thickness injuries has been to apply gauze, often impregnated with a petrolatum-based antimicrobial such as bismuth tribromophenate (Xeroform), and to allow it to dry. Heat lamps have been used to accelerate the drying process. With this method, the gauze provides a matrix that facilitates scab formation.

A scab, which consists of dried fibrin, blood cells, and wound exudate, will protect a wound and limit desiccation and bacterial invasion. Epithelial cells advancing beneath a scab, however, must debride the scab-wound interface enzymatically to migrate across the wound surface beneath the scab.[113] Epithelialization is therefore slower under a scab than it would be under an occlusive dressing. Thus, wounds covered with a scab tend to cause the patient more discomfort than wounds covered with occlusive dressings as well.

For wounds containing necrotic tissue, foreign bodies, or other debris, wet-to-dry dressings are preferred. In this approach, saline-soaked, wide-meshed gauze dressings are applied, allowed to dry, and then changed every 4 to 6 hours. Granulation tissue (including necrotic tissue and other debris) and wound exudate become incorporated within the wide-meshed gauze; thus, a debriding effect is produced when the gauze is removed.[114,115] The disadvantage of this type of dressing is that some viable cells are damaged by the debridement process. Wet-to-wet dressing changes, in which the saline is not allowed to dry, minimize tissue damage but do not produce as much debridement. Enzymatic agents (e.g., Travase, Santyl, and Accuzyme) can debride wounds effectively and are a reasonable alternative to wet-to-dry or wet-to-wet dressings for wounds containing necrotic tissue.[116]

Virtually any type of dressing change will lower the bacterial count in infected wounds; however, application of antibacterial agents, which directly affect the infecting bacteria, generally decreases the bacterial count more quickly than other dressing-change regimens. Silver sulfadiazine is frequently used because in addition to its broad antibacterial spectrum and low incidence of side effects, it has the secondary benefits of maintaining the wound in a moist state and speeding epithelialization.[33]

For wounds with exposed tendons or nerves, it is particularly important to maintain a moist environment to prevent desiccation of the exposed vital structures. Although the biologic and membrane dressings mentioned accomplish this, they are difficult to use on deep or irregular wounds and wounds with a great deal of drainage. Consequently, wet-to-wet dressings or dressings including creams that contain agents such as silver sulfadiazine are often used.

For sutured wounds, the purpose of a dressing is to prevent bacterial contamination, protect the wound from trauma, manage any drainage, and facilitate epithelialization. One approach is to use a dressing with multiple layers, each of which serves a different purpose. The contact layer immediately adjacent to the wound must be sterile and nontoxic. An ideal contact layer does not stick to the wound or absorb fluid but instead facilitates drainage through itself to the overlying layers of the dressing. Materials with these characteristics include Xeroflo, a fine-meshed gauze impregnated with a hydrophilic substance, and N-terface, a synthetic fine-meshed gauze. The dressing layer directly over the contact layer should be absorptive and capable of conveying exudate or transudate away from the wound surface. Wide-meshed gauze facilitates capillary action and drainage.[117] Such absorptive layers must not be allowed to become soaked, because if they do, exudate collects on the wound surface, and maceration and bacterial contamination may occur. The outermost dressing layer is a binding layer, the purpose of which is to fix the dressing in place. Tape is most commonly used as a binding layer, though elastic wraps or other materials may sometimes be used instead.

With sutured wounds, dressings are required only until drainage from the wound ceases. With nondraining wounds, dressings may be removed after 48 hours, by which time epithelial cells will have sealed the superficial layers of the wound. An alternative method of treating minimally draining incisional wounds is to apply an antibacterial ointment. Such ointments are occlusive and maintain a sterile, moist environment for the 48 hours required for epithelialization.

Some physicians use occlusive dressings for incisional wounds. These dressings, as mentioned, create a warm, moist, sterile environment that is optimal for epithelialization. Some of these are transparent, allowing observation of the wound. The disadvantage of most of these dressings is their limited absorptive capacity, allowing drainage from the wound to collect under the dressing.

In certain small wounds in areas that are difficult to dress, such as the scalp, it may be reasonable to forgo a synthetic dressing and simply allow a scab to form on the wound surface.

Some novel approaches to wound management have been developed since the latter part of the 1990s. One such approach involves the use of skin substitutes, such as Alloderm, Integra, and Apligraf. Alloderm and Integra contain only dermal elements, whereas Apligraf and others contain cellular components, including epithelium. The cellular elements most likely do not remain in the wound for long, but they are thought to provide cytokines that may stimulate the healing process in the short term.

Discussion

Physiology of Wound Healing

Phylogenetically, humans have lost the ability of many lower animals, such as planaria and salamanders, to regenerate specialized structures in most of their tissues. Although the wound-healing process differs slightly from tissue to tissue, the process is similar throughout the body. The result in almost all tissues is scar, the so-called glue that repairs injuries. The goal of acute wound management is to facilitate the body's innate tendency to heal so that a strong but minimally apparent scar results. Generally, however, the normal wound-healing process cannot be accelerated.

The physiology of wound healing is usually described in phases [see Figure 1]. Although each of these phases will be discussed as a separate entity, the phases blend without distinct boundaries.

HEMOSTASIS

Most wounds extend into the dermis, injuring blood vessels and resulting in bleeding. This process stimulates vasoconstriction in the injured vessels, mediated by epinephrine from the peripheral circulation and norepinephrine from the sympathetic nervous system. Prostaglandins, such as prostaglandin $F_{2\alpha}$ ($PGF_{2\alpha}$), and thromboxane A_2 are also involved. As the vessels contract, platelets adhere to the collagen exposed by damage to the blood vessel endothelium and form a plug. Platelet aggregation during the hemostatic process results in the release of cytokines and other proteins from the alpha granules of the cytoplasm of platelet cells. These cytokines include platelet-derived growth factor (PDGF), transforming growth factor-β (TGF-β), transforming growth factor-α (TGF-α), basic fibroblast growth factor (bFGF, also called fibroblast growth factor 2 [FGF2]), platelet-derived epidermal growth factor (PD-EGF), and platelet-derived endothelial cell growth factor (PD-ECGF). Some of these cytokines have direct effects early in the healing process, and others are bound locally and play critical roles in later aspects of healing.

The extrinsic coagulation cascade is stimulated by a tissue factor released from the injured tissues and is essential for clot formation. The intrinsic cascade is triggered by exposure to factor XII and is

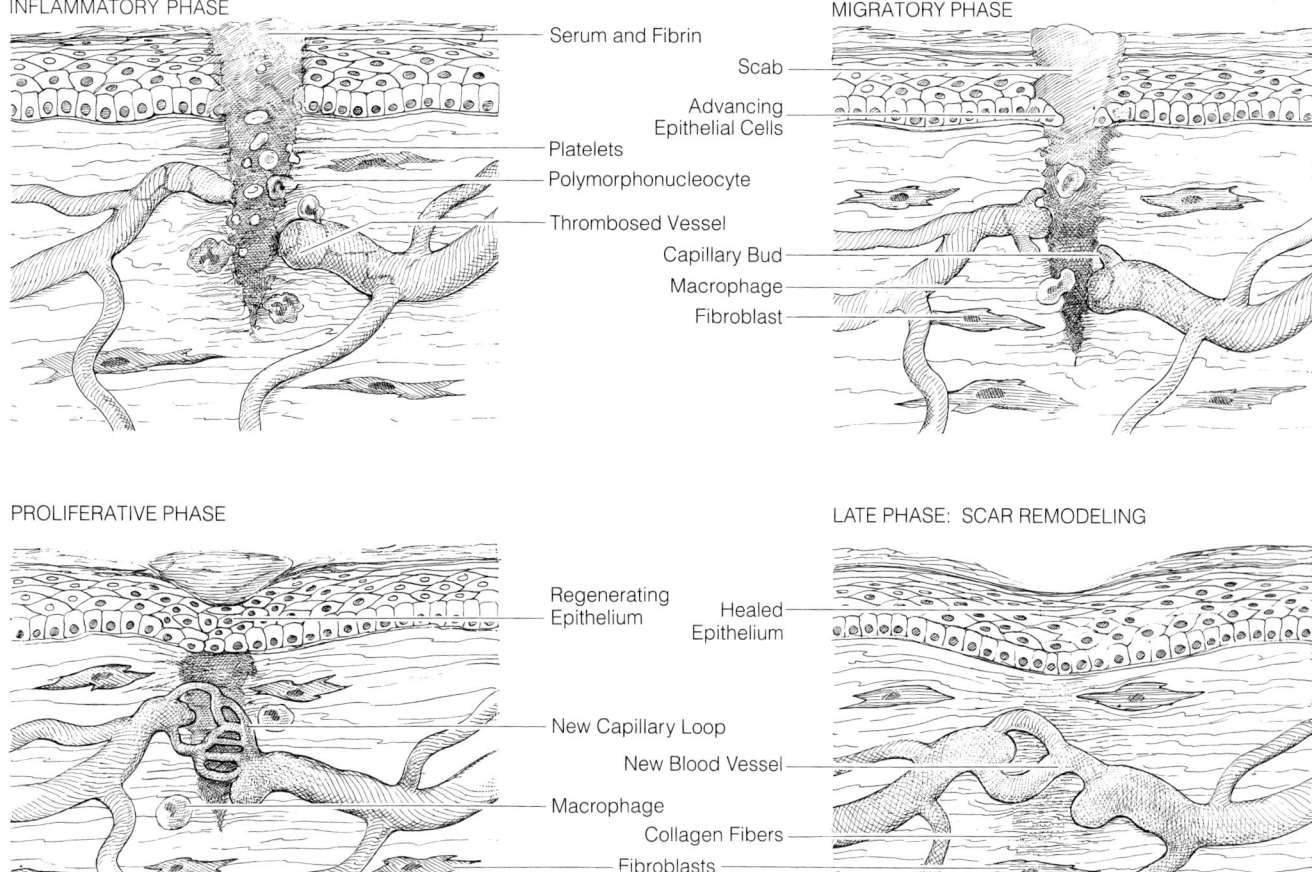

INFLAMMATORY PHASE
Serum and Fibrin
Platelets
Polymorphonucleocyte
Thrombosed Vessel

MIGRATORY PHASE
Scab
Advancing Epithelial Cells
Capillary Bud
Macrophage
Fibroblast

PROLIFERATIVE PHASE
Regenerating Epithelium
New Capillary Loop
Macrophage
Fibroblasts

LATE PHASE: SCAR REMODELING
Healed Epithelium
New Blood Vessel
Collagen Fibers

Figure 1 Depicted are the phases of wound healing. In the early phases (top, left), platelets adhere to collagen exposed by damage to blood vessels to form a plug. The intrinsic and extrinsic coagulation cascades generate fibrin, which combines with platelets to form a clot in the injured area. Initial local vasoconstriction is followed by vasodilatation mediated by histamine, PGE_2, PGI_2, serotonin, and kinins. Neutrophils are the predominant inflammatory cells (a polymorphonucleocyte is shown here). In the migratory phase (top, right), fibrin and fibronectin are the primary components of the provisional wound matrix. Additional inflammatory cells, as well as fibroblasts and other mesenchymal cells, migrate into the wound area. Gradually, macrophages replace neutrophils as the predominant inflammatory cells. Angiogenic factors induce the development of new blood vessels as capillaries. Epithelial cells advance across the wound area from the basal layer of the epidermis. The fibrin-platelet clot may dehydrate to form a scab. In the proliferative phase (bottom, left), the advancing epithelial cells have covered the wound area. New capillaries form. The wound's strength grows as a result of steadily increasing production of collagen and glycosaminoglycans by fibroblasts. Collagen replaces fibrin. Myofibroblasts induce wound contraction. In the late phase (bottom, right), scar remodeling occurs. The overall level of collagen in the wound plateaus; old collagen is broken down as new collagen is produced. The number of cross-links between collagen molecules increases, and the new collagen fibers are aligned so as to provide a gradual increase in wound tensile strength. New capillaries combine to form larger vessels. The epithelium is healed, although it never quite regains its normal architecture.

not essential. Both coagulation cascades generate fibrin, which acts with platelets to form a clot in the injured area [*see 1:4 Bleeding and Transfusion*]. In a large wound, the superficial portion of this clot may dehydrate over time to produce a scab.

In addition to contributing to hemostasis, fibrin is the primary component of the provisional matrix that forms in the wound during early healing. Fibrin becomes coated with vitronectin from the serum and fibronectin derived from both serum and aggregating platelets. Fibronectins are a class of glycoproteins that facilitate the attachment of migrating fibroblasts as well as other cell types to the fibrin lattice.[118] By influencing cellular attachment, fibronectin is a key modulator of the migration of various cell types in the wound.[119,120] In addition, the fibrin-fibronectin lattice binds various cytokines released at the time of injury and serves as a reservoir for these factors in the later stages of healing.[121]

INFLAMMATION

Tissue damage at the site of injury stimulates the inflammatory response. This response is most prominent during the first 24 hours after a wound is sustained. In clean wounds, signs of inflammation dissipate relatively quickly, and few if any inflammatory cells are seen after 5 to 7 days. In contaminated wounds, inflammation may persist for a prolonged period. The signs of inflammation, originally described by Hunter in 1794, include erythema, edema, heat, and pain.

The signs of inflammation are generated primarily by changes in the 20 to 30 μm diameter venules on the distal side of the capillary bed. In the first 5 to 10 minutes after wounding, the skin blanches as a result of the vasoconstriction that contributes to hemostasis. The initial vasoconstriction is followed by vasodilatation, which generates the characteristic erythema. The vasodilatation is mediated by (1) vasodilator prostaglandins such as PGE_2 and prostacyclin, released by injured cells; (2) histamine, released by mast cells and possibly by platelets to a lesser degree; (3) serotonin, also released by mast cells;

Table 4 Involvement of Cytokines in Wound-Healing Functions

Wound-Healing Function	Cytokines Involved
Neutrophil chemotaxis	PDGF IL-1
Macrophage chemotaxis	PDGF TGF-β IL-1
Fibroblast chemotaxis	EGF PDGF TGF-β
Fibroblast mitogenesis	EGF PDGF IGF TGF-β TGF-α IL-1 TNF-α
Angiogenesis, endothelial cell chemotaxis, mitogenesis	EGF Acidic and basic FGF (FGF1 and FGF2) TGF-β TGF-α TNF-α VEGF PD-ECGF
Epithelialization	EGF Basic FGF (FGF2) TGF-β TGF-α KGF IGF
Collagen synthesis	EGF Basic FGF (FGF2) PDGF TGF-β IL-1 TNF-α
Fibronectin synthesis	Basic FGF (FGF2) PDGF TGF-β EGF
Proteoglycan synthesis	Basic FGF (FGF2) PDGF TGF-β IL-1
Wound contraction	Basic FGF (FGF2) TGF-β
Scar remodeling, collagenase stimulation	EGF PDGF TGF-β IL-1 TNF-α

EGF—epidermal growth factor FGF—fibroblast growth factor IGF—insulinlike growth factor IL-1—interleukin-1 KGF—keratinocyte growth factor PD-ECGF—platelet-derived endothelial cell growth factor PDGF—platelet-derived growth factor TGF—transforming growth factor TNF—tumor necrosis factor VEGF—vascular endothelial growth factor

(4) kinins, the release of which is stimulated by the coagulation cascade; and possibly by other factors as well. As the blood vessels dilate, the endothelial cells lining the microvenules tend to contract and separate from one another, resulting in increased vascular permeability. Serum migrates into the extravascular space, giving rise to edema. Inflammatory cells initially adhere loosely to endothelial cells lining the capillaries and roll along the endothelial surface of the vessels. The inflammatory cells eventually adhere to the vessel wall, in a process mediated by the β2 class of integrins, and subsequently transmigrate into the extravascular space.[122] Chemoattractants stimulate the migration of inflammatory cells to the injured area. As monocytes migrate from the capillaries into the extravascular space, they transform into macrophages in a process mediated by serum factors and fibronectin.[123-125] After migration, the inflammatory cells must be activated before they can perform their biologic functions.

Neutrophils are the predominant inflammatory cell in the wound during the 2 to 3 days after wounding, but macrophages eventually become the predominant inflammatory cell in the wound. Because monocytes are present in the serum in much lower numbers than neutrophils, it is not unexpected that they are rarely seen in the wound area initially. After appearing in the wound, both neutrophils and macrophages engulf damaged tissue, digesting them in lysosomes. After neutrophils phagocytose damaged material, they cease to function and often release lysosomal contents, which can contribute to tissue damage and a prolonged inflammatory response. Inflammatory cells and liquefied tissue are the constituents of pus, which may or may not be sterile, depending on whether bacteria are present. Unlike neutrophils, macrophages survive after phagocytosing bacteria or damaged material. The shift in predominant inflammatory cell type within the wound from neutrophils to macrophages is at least in part due to macrophages' extended life span. Macrophage-specific chemoattractants may also selectively attract macrophages into the wound.

In addition to phagocytosis, macrophages are capable of secreting matrix metalloproteinases (MMPs) that break down damaged tis-

Table 5 Cell Sources of Cytokines

Cell Type	Cytokines
Platelet	EGF PDGF TGF-β TGF-α
Macrophage	FGF PDGF TGF-β TGF-α IL-1 TNF-α IGF-1
Lymphocyte	TGF-β IL-2
Endothelial cell	FGF PDGF
Epithelial cell	TGF-α PDGF TGF-β
Smooth muscle cell	PDGF

sue; they are also a primary source of cytokines that mediate other aspects of the healing process. Experimental studies have demonstrated that neutrophils are not essential to normal healing,[126] whereas macrophages are necessary.[127] These additional macrophage functions—especially their role as a cytokine source—most likely are what make them essential.

MIGRATORY PHASE

Many substances attract fibroblasts and other mesenchymal cells into the wound during the migratory phase, including many of the cytokines[118,128-130] [see Table 4]. It is not known which of them are most active biologically at different points after wounding. The fibroblasts migrate along the scaffold of fibrin and fibronectin, as mentioned. This migration involves the upregulation of integrin receptor sites on the cell membranes, which allows the cells to bind at different sites in the matrix and pull themselves through the scaffold. Migration through the provisional matrix is also facilitated by synthesis of MMPs, which help cleave a path for the cells. Additional cytokines stimulate the proliferation of mesenchymal cells important in the wound-healing process once these cells have been attracted into the wound area[131,132] [see Table 4].

Angiogenesis

Angiogenesis is also initiated in the migratory phase during the first 2 or 3 days after wounding. Before revascularization of the injured area, the wound microenvironment is hypoxic and is characterized by high lactic acid levels and a low pH. Angiogenic factors stimulate the process of neovascularization. Some of the more potent angiogenic factors are derived from platelets and macrophages[133,134] [see Tables 4 and 5]. New vessels develop from existing vessels as capillaries. The capillaries grow from the edges of the wound toward areas of inadequate perfusion within the provisional wound matrix, where lactate levels are increased and tissue oxygen tension is low. The generation of new vessels involves both migration and proliferation of cells. Both cellular activities are modulated by the angiogenic cytokines. A key aspect of endothelial cell migration is the upregulation of the α-β_3 integrin binding domain that facilitates the binding of the endothelial cells to the matrix. Migrating endothelial cells produce plasminogen activator, which catalyzes the breakdown of fibrin, as well as MMPs, which help create paths through the matrix for the developing blood vessels. When the budding capillaries meet other developing capillaries, they join and blood flow is initiated. As the wounded area becomes more vascularized, the capillaries consolidate to form larger blood vessels.

Epithelialization

Epithelialization of skin involves the migration of cells from the basal layer of the epidermis across the denuded wound area.[135] This migratory process begins approximately 24 hours after wounding. The migrating cells develop bands 40 to 80 Å wide that can be seen with electron microscopy and stained with antiactin antibodies. About 48 hours after wounding, the basal epidermal cells at the wound edge enlarge and begin to proliferate, producing more migratory cells. If the normal basement membrane is intact, the cells simply migrate over it; if it is not, they migrate over the provisional fibrin-fibronectin matrix.[136] As migration is initiated, desmosomes that link epithelial cells together and hemidesmosomes that link the cells to the basement membrane disappear.[137] Migrating cells express integrins on their cell membranes that facilitate migration. As they migrate, they secrete additional proteins that become part of the new basement membrane, including tenascin,[138] vitronectin, and collagen types I and V. In addition, they generate MMPs to facilitate migration, as noted.

When epithelial cells migrating from two areas meet, contact inhibition prevents further migration. The cells making up the epithelial monolayer then differentiate into basal cells and divide, eventually yielding a neoepidermis consisting of multiple cell layers. Epithelialization progresses both from wound edges and from epithelial appendages. Epithelial advancement is facilitated by adequate debridement and decreased bacterial counts, as well as by the flattening of rete pegs in the dermis adjacent to the wound area. The epithelium never returns to its previous state. The new epidermis at the edge of the wound remains somewhat hyperplastic and thickened, whereas the epidermis over the remainder of the wound is thinner and more fragile than normal. True rete pegs do not form in the healed area.

PROLIFERATIVE PHASE AND COLLAGEN SYNTHESIS

The proliferative phase of wound healing usually begins approximately 5 days after wounding. During this phase, the fibroblasts that have migrated into the wound begin to synthesize proteoglycans and collagen, and the wound gains strength. Until this point, fibrin has provided most of the wound's strength. Although a small amount of collagen is synthesized during the first 5 days of the healing process,[139] the rate of collagen synthesis increases greatly after the fifth day. Wound collagen content continually increases for 3 weeks, at which point it begins to plateau.[140]

Although there are at least 18 types of collagen, the ones of primary importance in skin are type I, which makes up 80% to 90% of the collagen in skin, and type III, which makes up the remaining 10% to 20%. A higher percentage of type III collagen is seen in embryologic skin and in early wound healing. A critical aspect of collagen synthesis is the hydroxylation of lysine and proline moieties within the collagen molecule. This process requires specific enzymes as well as oxygen, vitamin C, α-ketoglutarate, and ferrous iron, which function as cofactors. Hydroxyproline, which is found almost exclusively in collagen, serves as a marker of the quantity of collagen in tissue. Hydroxylysine is required for covalent cross-link formation between collagen molecules, which contributes greatly to wound strength. Deficiencies in oxygen or vitamin C or the suppression of enzymatic activity by corticosteroids may lead to underhydroxylated collagen incapable of generating strong crosslinks. Underhydroxylated collagen is easily broken down. After collagen molecules are synthesized by fibroblasts, they are released into the extracellular space. There, after enzymatic modification, they align

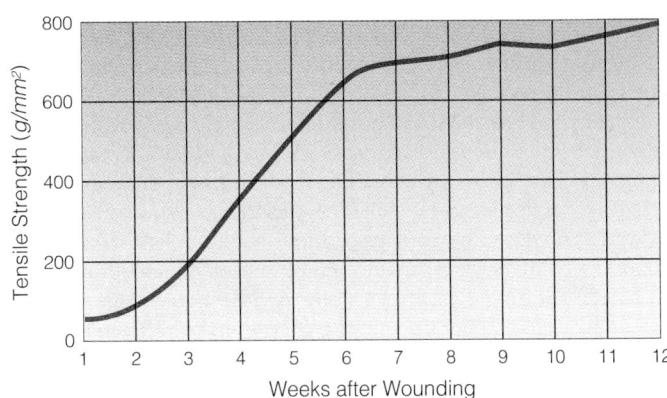

Figure 2 The tensile strength of skin wounds begins to increase gradually about 3 weeks after wounding. The collagen elaborated early in the healing process is replaced by stronger collagen that is aligned along the lines of stress in the tissue. Closer bonding and a greater number of cross-links between fibers augment the wound's tensile strength. The process of collagen replacement and scar remodeling continues for years.[248]

themselves into fibrils and fibers that give the wound strength. Initially, the collagen molecules are held together by electrostatic cross-links as fibrils form. These cross-links are subsequently replaced by more stable covalent bonds. The covalent bonds form between lysine and lysine, between lysine and hydroxylysine, and between hydroxylysine and hydroxylysine[141]; the strongest cross-links form between hydroxylysine and hydroxylysine.

Proteoglycans, also synthesized during the proliferative phase of healing, consist of a protein core linked to one or more glycosaminoglycans. Dermatan sulfate, heparin, heparan sulfate, keratan sulfate, and hyaluronic acid are the more common proteoglycans. The biologic effects of proteoglycans are less well understood than those of collagen. They generally anchor specific proteins in certain locations and affect the biologic activity of target proteins. Heparin is an important cofactor of bFGF during angiogenesis. Other proteoglycans most likely facilitate the alignment of collagen molecules into fibrils and fibers.

Wound Contraction

Collagen has no contractile properties, and its synthesis is not required for wound contraction. During the proliferative phase, myofibroblasts appear in the wound and probably contribute to its contraction.[142] Myofibroblasts are unique cells that resemble normal fibroblasts and may be derived from them. They have convoluted nuclei, vigorous rough endoplasmic reticula, and microfilament bundles 60 to 80 Å in diameter. These microfilaments can be stained with antiactin and antimyosin antibodies. Many authorities believe that the myofibroblasts pull the wound together from the edges of the wound; however, others believe, on the basis of observations in collagen lattices, that it is the fibroblasts within the center of the wound that generate the force of wound contraction. To date, this issue has not been resolved. TGF-β is a potent stimulant of wound contraction in experimental models.[143]

The wound edges are pulled together at a rate of 0.60 to 0.75 mm/day. The rate of contraction varies with tissue laxity. Contraction is greatest in anatomic sites where there is redundant tissue. Wound contraction generally continues most actively for 12 to 15 days or until wound edges meet.

LATE PHASE: SCAR REMODELING

Approximately 3 weeks after wounding, scar remodeling becomes the predominant feature of the healing process. Collagen synthesis is downregulated, and the wound becomes less cellular as apoptosis occurs. During this phase, there is continual turnover of collagen molecules as old collagen is broken down and new collagen is synthesized along lines of stress.[144,145] Collagen breakdown is mediated by several MMPs, found in scar tissue as well as in normal connective tissues.[146] At least 25 MMPs that affect different substrates have been identified. The more common of these include MMP-1 (collagenase-1), MMP-2 (gelatinase A), and MMP-3 (stromelysin-1). The activity of these collagenolytic enzymes is modulated by several tissue inhibitors of metalloproteinases (TIMPs). During this phase, there is little net change in total wound collagen,[144] but the number of cross-links between collagen strands increases.

The realigned, highly cross-linked collagen is much stronger than the collagen produced during the earlier phases of healing. The result is a steady, gradual growth in wound tensile strength that continues for 6 to 12 months after wounding [*see Figure 2*]. Scar tissue never reaches the tensile strength of unwounded tissue, however. The rate of gain in tensile strength begins to plateau at 6 weeks after injury. The common clinical recommendation that patients avoid heavy lifting or straining for 6 weeks after laparotomy, hernia repair, or many orthopedic procedures is based on the time required for increased tensile strength.

Role of Cytokines in Wound Healing

Wounding stimulates specific cellular activities in a consistent manner that is reproducible from wound to wound. Many, if not all, of these cellular activities appear to be mediated by cytokines. The predictability with which cellular activities start and stop after wounding suggests that the cytokines mediating them are released in a closely regulated fashion; however, the details of this process have not yet been elucidated.

Numerous cytokines are known to be capable of mediating the major biologic activities involved in wound healing [*see Table 4*]. Most of these activities can be mediated by more than one factor, and researchers have not yet been able to determine which factors are the most important stimulants of wound-healing functions in vivo. One possible explanation for the duplication in mediating functions is that factors with similar activities may act at different times in the course of the wound-healing process.

Cytokines are produced by platelets, macrophages, lymphocytes, endothelial cells, epithelial cells, and smooth muscle cells [*see Table 5*]. Some cytokines, such as PDGF, are produced by several cell types,[147-150] whereas others, such as interleukin-2 (IL-2), are produced by only one cell type.[151,152] The cell of origin is a key variable that determines the time at which a factor will be present after wounding. Platelets, for example, release PDGF,[147] TGF-β,[153] and epidermal growth factor (EGF),[154] and it would be expected that these cytokines would be found in a wound soon after injury. Factors produced by several different cell types may be released by individual cell types at different times. For example, PDGF[148,149] and TGF-β,[155] which are produced by both platelets and macrophages, might be released by platelets soon after wounding and by macrophages at a later stage in the healing process.

The names of cytokines are frequently misleading. In many cases, they derive from the first known cell of origin or from the first function discovered (or hypothesized) for the factor. As a result, a polyfunctional factor may have a name implying that it has only one function, a factor produced by multiple cell types may have a name suggesting that it is produced by a single cell type, or a factor's name may lay claim to a capability that the factor does not have. For example, TGF-β received its name because it was originally believed to be capable of transforming normal cells into malignant ones. Although it is now known that TGF-β does not have this capability, the name has not been altered.

Cytokines are also a promising tool in the biologic modification of the wound-healing process. Early experimental work was done with small quantities of factors extracted from biologic sources (e.g., platelets). Currently, recombinant technology can provide

Table 6 Factors Impairing Wound Healing

Local	Systemic
Infection	Malnutrition
Foreign bodies	Cancer
Ischemia/hypoxia	Diabetes mellitus
Venous insufficiency	Uremia
Toxins (e.g., spider venom)	Jaundice
Previous trauma	Old age
Radiation	Systemic corticosteroids
Cigarette smoking	Chemotherapeutic agents
	Alcoholism

large quantities of highly purified material that can be used clinically. It has been experimentally demonstrated that many of the cytokines are capable of accelerating wound healing in normal and healing-impaired models. TGF-β has markedly increased wound-breaking strength in incisional wounds in rats soon after wounding.[156] bFGF has increased the strength of incisional wounds when injected on day 3 after wounding.[157] EGF has accelerated the closure of partial-thickness wounds in pigs when applied topically,[158] and it has accelerated collagen accumulation in a wound chamber model.[159] PDGF has accelerated healing in incisional wounds in rats when administered in a slow-release vehicle at the time of wounding.[160] Cytokines have also been observed to reverse healing deficits produced by diabetes,[161] steroids,[162] doxorubicin,[163] and radiation[164] in experimental models.

The positive results of these experimental studies encouraged the use of cytokines in clinical trials in humans. In an early human study, EGF accelerated the healing of skin graft donor sites.[165] In another study, it was applied topically to chronic nonhealing wounds in an uncontrolled group of patients and was considered to contribute to improved healing in the majority.[166] Autogenous platelet extracts have been used on chronic nonhealing wounds as well, with good results.[167] In a better-controlled study, recombinant human PDGF-bb accelerated healing when applied topically to pressure sores in a randomized, double-blind, placebo-controlled fashion.[168] In another carefully controlled, randomized, prospective study, bFGF was also demonstrated to be efficacious as a topical wound-healing supplement for pressure sores.[169] PDGF-bb has been demonstrated to be efficacious and has been approved for use on diabetic ulcers.[170] It is being marketed as becaplermin (Regranex).

It is not known which factors will be most effective as healing adjuvants in either normal or impaired healing states. It would seem logical that addition of a combination of factors in a sequence mimicking that characteristic of normal healing would produce optimal effects when healing is unimpaired. When healing is impaired, it would seem logical to augment the quantity of whatever factors are lacking or present at reduced levels. However, much work remains to be done—first, to determine which factors are most critical in normal states and, second, to determine which factors are lacking in impaired states so that the best use can be made of the recombinant factors now available.

Physiology of Skin Graft Healing

Although the physiology of skin graft healing is similar to that of open wound healing, differences arise because the wound is covered by the graft and because the graft has its own intrinsic architectural nature. Initially, fibrin holds the graft on the recipient site. The strength of attachment increases rapidly for the first 8 hours after graft placement, after which the rate of increase tapers off slightly.[171] For the first 48 hours, the graft survives by serum imbibition[172]: plasmalike fluid is absorbed by the graft, which increases in weight by up to 30% during this period. The absorbed fluid supports only minimal metabolic activities and maintains cellular viability until revascularization occurs. After approximately 48 hours, new blood vessels begin to grow into the graft from the recipient site.[173] It is not known whether a new vascular network grows within the graft or whether vessels from the recipient site simply connect with existing vessels in the graft. Skin graft revascularization probably involves a combination of these two processes.[174] Blood flow in the graft reaches nearly normal levels approximately 7 days after grafting. The vascular system continues to mature, with smaller vessels merging into larger ones. By 21

days after grafting, the graft's vascular supply appears nearly normal on dye injection studies.[173]

Lymphatic channels begin to develop 4 to 5 days after grafting, and the lymphatic system gradually matures until it, too, is nearly normal after 21 days.[175] Epithelial cells and fibroblasts remain dormant for 3 days after placement of a skin graft and subsequently proliferate.[176] The epithelium remains hyperplastic for 6 weeks.[177] By 7 to 8 days after grafting, fibroblasts are more plentiful in the graft than in the surrounding skin, and new collagen is being synthesized.[176,177] Collagenolytic activity develops simultaneously and actually exceeds collagen synthesis for 2 weeks, leading to a net loss in graft collagen. However, during the third week after grafting, the net amount of collagen starts to increase as the rate of collagen synthesis begins to exceed the rate of collagenolysis. Active collagen synthesis continues for at least 20 weeks.[102]

Disturbances of Wound Healing

Healing does not always occur in a straightforward, undisturbed fashion. Both local and systemic factors can interfere with healing. Local factors include infection, foreign bodies, tissue hypoxia, venous insufficiency, local toxins, mechanical trauma, irradiation, and cigarette smoking. Systemic factors include malnutrition, cancer, diabetes mellitus, uremia, jaundice, old age, corticosteroids, chemotherapeutic agents, and alcoholism. Several of these local and systemic factors [see Table 6] will be discussed in more detail.

LOCAL FACTORS

Infection

The body maintains a symbiotic relationship with bacteria. Normal dry skin contains up to 1,000 bacteria/g,[4] and saliva contains 100 million bacteria/ml.[178] The bacterial population is kept in control by several mechanisms. Invasion is mechanically limited by an intact stratum corneum in the skin and intact oral mucosa.[5] Sebaceous secretions contain bactericidal and fungicidal fatty acids that modulate bacterial proliferation.[179] Edema dilutes these fatty acids, making edematous areas more infection prone. Lysozymes in skin hydrolyze bacterial cell membranes, further limiting bacterial proliferation.[180] The immune system augments local barriers to infection.

Infection occurs when the number or virulence of bacteria exceeds the ability of local tissue defenses to control them. Generally, as mentioned, infection exists when bacteria have proliferated to levels beyond 10^5 organisms/g tissue (β-hemolytic streptococci being the only exception). At this level, bacteria overwhelm host defenses and proliferate in an uncontrolled fashion. This number was defined by studies performed at the United States Army Institute of Surgical Research and elsewhere.[21,181-183] Local factors such as impaired circulation or radiation injury increase the risk of infection. Systemic diseases such as diabetes, AIDS, uremia, and cancer also increase the susceptibility to wound infection.

Hypoxia and Smoking

Delivery of oxygen to healing tissues is critical for prompt wound repair. Oxygen is necessary for cellular respiration as well as for hydroxylation of proline and lysine residues. Adequate tissue oxygenation requires an adequate circulating blood volume,[184] adequate cardiac function, and adequate local vasculature. Vascular disorders may be systemic, as in peripheral vascular disease, or localized, caused by scarring from trauma or prior surgery. Wound healing in ischemic extremities is directly correlated with transcutaneous oxygen tension.[185] Hyperbaric oxygen has been used in the treatment of many types of wounds in which tissue hypoxia may impair healing. Anemia, however, is not associated with impaired healing unless the anemia is severe enough to limit circulating blood volume.[186]

Smoking can impair tissue oxygenation. Smoking stimulates vasoconstriction acutely and contributes to the development of atherosclerosis and vascular disease over time.[187-189] Approximately 3% to 6% of cigarette smoke is carbon monoxide, which binds to hemoglobin, producing carboxyhemoglobin. Smokers have carboxyhemoglobin levels between 1% and 20%.[190] Carboxyhemoglobin limits the oxygen-carrying capacity of the blood, increases platelet adhesives,[191] and produces endothelial changes.[192,193]

Irradiation

Irradiation damages the DNA of cells in exposed areas. Some cells die, and others are rendered incapable of undergoing mitosis. When radiation is administered therapeutically, doses are fractionated and tangential fields are used to limit damage to normal cells while maximizing damage to tumor cells. Despite such techniques, normal cells are damaged by irradiation.

Radiation therapy initially produces inflammation and desquamation in a dose-dependent fashion.[194] After a course of irradiation, healing ensues if surrounding normal tissues have not been irreparably damaged. Additional cells must migrate into the treated area for adequate healing to occur. Fibroblasts migrating into irradiated tissue are often abnormal because of irradiation. These cells are characterized by multiple vacuoles, irregular rough endoplasmic reticulum, degenerating mitochondria, and cytoplasmic crystalline inclusion bodies. Increased levels of inflammatory mediators contribute to an abnormal healing response. Collagen is synthesized to an abnormal degree in irradiated tissue, causing characteristic fibrosis. The media of dermal blood vessels in irradiated areas thickens and some blood vessels become occluded, resulting in a decrease in the total number of blood vessels. Superficial telangiectasias may be seen. The epidermis becomes thinned, and changes in pigmentation often develop. Irradiated skin is dry because of damage to sebaceous and sweat glands, and it has little hair. The epidermal basement membrane is abnormal, and nuclear atypia is common in keratinocytes.

Abnormal healing is predictable after wounding of previously irradiated tissue. Decreased vascularity and increased fibrosis limit the ability of platelets and inflammatory cells to gain access to wounds in the area. The quantity of cytokines released is therefore limited in wounds in irradiated tissue. This relative cytokine deficiency causes impairment of virtually all cellular aspects of healing. Damaged fibroblasts and keratinocytes in the area may not respond normally to wound-healing stimulants. In addition, irradiated tissue is predisposed to infection, which can further slow the healing process.

Clinically, impaired healing is manifest by a higher rate of complications when an operation is performed on irradiated tissue.[195] Vitamin A has been used to reverse the healing impairment caused by radiation therapy.[196] Difficult wounds in irradiated tissue can often be managed surgically by bringing a new blood supply to the area with flaps from nonirradiated areas.

SYSTEMIC FACTORS

Malnutrition

Adequate amounts of protein, carbohydrates, fatty acids, vitamins, and other nutrients are required for wounds to heal. Malnutrition frequently contributes to suboptimal healing.[197] In experimental studies,[198] a loss of 15% to 20% of lean body mass has been associated with a decrease in wound-breaking strength and a decrease in colonic bursting pressure. Hypoproteinemia inhibits proper wound healing

by limiting the supply of critical amino acids required for synthesis of collagen and other proteins. Collagen synthesis essentially stops in the absence of protein intake,[199] resulting in impaired healing.[200,201] Arginine and glutamine appear to be particularly important amino acids. Cystine residues are found along the nonhelical peptide chain associated with procollagen; in the absence of these cystine residues, proper alignment of peptide chains into a triple helix is inhibited.[202]

Carbohydrates and fats provide energy for healing, and wound healing slows when carbohydrate or fat stores are limited. As an alternative energy source, protein is broken down instead of contributing primarily to tissue growth.[203] Fatty acids are also vital components of cell membranes.

Several vitamins are essential for normal healing. As mentioned, vitamin C is a necessary cofactor for hydroxylation of lysine and proline during collagen synthesis. The ability of fibroblasts to produce new, strongly cross-linked collagen is diminished if vitamin C is deficient. Clinically, existing scars dissolve because collagenolytic activity continues without adequate compensatory collagen synthesis, and new wounds fail to heal. Vitamin C deficiency is also associated with impaired resistance to infection.[203] Because vitamin A is essential for normal epithelialization, proteoglycan synthesis, and normal immune function,[204-206] healing is impaired when vitamin A is deficient. Thiamine deficiency has also been associated with impaired healing.[207] Vitamin D, required for normal calcium metabolism, is needed for bone healing. Exogenous vitamin E impairs wound healing in rats, most likely by influencing the inflammatory response in a corticosteroid-like manner.[208]

The minerals necessary for normal healing include the trace element zinc, a necessary cofactor for DNA polymerase and reverse transcriptase. Because zinc deficiency can result in an inhibition of cellular proliferation and deficient granulation tissue formation[209] and healing,[210] zinc replacement should be given if a deficiency is diagnosed. Pharmacologic overdosing with zinc does not accelerate wound healing and can have detrimental effects.[210]

Correction of generalized malnutrition requires refeeding. The amount of food ingested in the immediate preoperative period may have a greater influence than the overall degree of malnutrition, possibly by inducing positive nitrogen balance.[211] A prospective, randomized study of patients undergoing total parenteral nutrition prior to surgery demonstrated a significant reduction in postoperative morbidity and mortality.[212]

Cancer

Impaired wound healing associated with cancer has been demonstrated experimentally[213] and is often noted clinically. Cancer-bearing hosts may have impaired healing for a variety of reasons. Cancer-induced cachexia, manifest as weight loss, anorexia, and asthenia, significantly limits healing. Cachexia is a result of either decreased caloric intake, increased energy expenditure, or both.

Decreased oral intake may be due to anorexia or mechanical factors. Anorexia is mediated through as yet imperfectly defined circulating factors. Changes in taste perception, hypothalamic function, and tryptophan metabolism may contribute to anorexia. Tumors in the gastrointestinal tract can produce obstruction and generate fistulae that limit nutrient absorption. Other cancers generate peptides such as gastrin and vasoactive intestinal polypeptide (VIP) that alter transit times and interfere with absorption of nutrients.

Cancers alter host metabolism in dysfunctional ways as well. Glucose turnover may be increased, sometimes leading to glucose intolerance. The effect of increased glucose use is higher energy needs.[214] Protein catabolism may be accelerated. Protein breakdown in muscle is increased, as is hepatic utilization of amino acids. Such changes in protein metabolism produce a net loss of plasma protein. Unlike malnourished patients, cancer patients may not be able to alter their metabolism to rely on fat for most energy needs. In tumor-bearing animals, fat accumulates, while other, more vital tissues are broken down for energy. In addition, vitamin C may be taken up preferentially by some tumors, limiting availability of the vitamin for hydroxylation of proline and lysine moieties in collagen. All of these metabolic changes contribute to a negative energy balance and inefficient energy use.

Cancer patients may be relatively anergic, most likely because of abnormal inflammatory cell activity. Macrophages do not migrate or function normally in cancer patients. Inflammatory cell dysfunction may limit the availability of cytokines required for healing and may also predispose to infection.

Impaired healing must be anticipated in cancer patients because of the many alterations in metabolism and immune function. It has been suggested that vitamin A can improve healing in tumor-bearing mice,[215] but this effect has not been demonstrated in humans.

Old Age

The elderly heal less efficiently than younger persons. DuNuoy and Carrell,[216] who studied patients injured during World War I, demonstrated that wounds in 20-year-old patients contracted more rapidly than those in 30-year-old patients. In a blister epithelialization model,[217] younger patients also healed more rapidly than older patients. Another study[218] found that wound disruption occurred with less force in the elderly.

Diabetes

Diabetes mellitus is also associated with impaired healing. In a prospective study of 23,649 surgical wounds,[219] the risk of infection was five times greater in diabetic patients than in nondiabetic patients. This impairment has been demonstrated experimentally in several models.[220-222] A major contributor to this phenomenon is the impaired inflammatory response associated with hyperglycemia. Diabetes is associated with impaired granulocyte chemotaxis,[223] phagocytic function,[224-226] and humoral and cellular immunity. In addition, diabetes is associated with a microangiopathy that can limit blood supply to the healing wound, particularly in older diabetic patients.[227] Diabetic neuropathy impairs sensation, classically in a stocking or glove nerve distribution in extremities. Although this neuropathy does not limit healing directly, it can diminish an individual's ability to protect himself or herself from trauma. The diabetes-induced impairment in healing may be reduced by tight control of blood sugar levels with insulin.[228-230]

Uremia

Uremia has been associated with impaired healing, partially as a direct effect of urea and partially as the result of coexisting malnutrition. This healing impairment has been demonstrated experimentally in both incisional skin wounds and intestinal anastomoses in rats[231] and in an implantable Gore-Tex wound-healing model in humans.[232] This impairment may be ameliorated by regular dialysis.

Alcoholism

In mice chronically fed alcohol, cellular ingrowth and collagen accumulation were diminished in a sponge model.[233]

Steroids and Immunosuppression

Adrenocortical steroids inhibit all aspects of healing. In incisional wounds, steroids slow the development of breaking strength[234]; in open wounds healing secondarily, they impede wound contraction[235,236] and epithelialization.

This impaired healing results from derangements in cellular function induced by steroids. A primary feature of wounds in steroid-treated individuals is a deficiency in inflammatory cell function. As discussed, inflammatory cells, particularly macrophages, mediate essentially all aspects of healing through cytokines. By diminishing the supply of cytokines, steroids and other immunosuppressive agents profoundly impair all aspects of healing. Macrophage migration, fibroblast proliferation, collagen accumulation, and angiogenesis are among the processes diminished by steroid administration. Sandberg[237] demonstrated that the effects of steroids on healing are most pronounced when the drug is administered several days before or after wounding.

All aspects of steroid-induced healing impairment other than wound contraction can be reversed by supplemental vitamin A. The recommended dose is 25,000 IU/day. Topical vitamin A has also been found effective for open wounds.[238] Anabolic steroids and growth hormone–releasing factor have also reversed steroid-induced healing impairments.

Chemotherapeutic Agents

Chemotherapeutic agents impair healing primarily through inhibition of cellular proliferation. Many agents have been examined in experimental models, and virtually all agents impair healing.[239] Nitrogen mustard, cyclophosphamide, methotrexate, BCNU (carmustine), and doxorubicin are the most damaging to the healing process. Most chemotherapeutic regimens use a combination of agents, compounding their deleterious effects. Clinical trials with chemotherapeutic agents have not been associated with as high an incidence of complications as might be anticipated from experimental evidence. The timing of drug administration as well as the doses utilized may explain this apparent contradiction. Doxorubicin, for example, is a more potent inhibitor of wound healing when delivered preoperatively than postoperatively.[240]

Jaundice and Liver Failure

Liver dysfunction most likely impairs healing through the direct effect of hyperbilirubinemia and through metabolic impairments, such as hypoalbuminemia and hypoprothrombinemia, that develop when the synthetic functions of the liver are impaired. The effect of obstructive jaundice on wound healing has been examined experimentally by several investigators. Bayer and Ellis[241] demonstrated decreased wound-breaking strength in abdominal wounds in rats with obstructive jaundice. In jaundiced animals with gastric wounds, angiogenesis was subjectively diminished, but wound-breaking strength was normal. Arnaud and coworkers[242] demonstrated impaired healing with obstructive jaundice,[242] but Greaney and associates[243] could not duplicate their results in a similar model. Greaney did show diminished collagen accumulation, however, in the wounds of jaundiced animals. In humans, Ellis and Heddle[244] noted an increased incidence of wound dehiscence and hernias in patients undergoing surgery for relief of obstructive jaundice, although others have disagreed.

Clinicians must be aware of both local and systemic factors that can influence healing in an individual patient and take appropriate measures, whenever possible, to improve chances for optimal healing.

HYPERTROPHIC SCARS AND KELOIDS

The events involved in normal healing begin and end in a controlled fashion, producing flat, unobtrusive scars. Healing is a biologic process, and as with all biologic processes, it may occur to a greater or lesser degree. Disturbances that diminish healing have already been discussed. Excessive healing can result in a raised, thickened scar with both functional and cosmetic complications. If the scar is confined to the margins of the original wound, it is called a hypertrophic scar.[245] Keloids extend beyond the confines of the original injury, so that the original wound often can no longer be distinguished.

Certain patients and certain wounds are at higher risk for abnormal scarring. Dark-skinned persons and patients between the ages of 2 and 40 are at higher risk for the development of hypertrophic scars or keloids. Wounds in the presternal or deltoid area, wounds that cross skin tension lines, and wounds in thicker skin have a greater tendency to heal with a thickened scar. Some parts of the body, such as the genitalia, the eyelids, the palms of the hands, and the soles of the feet, almost never develop abnormal scars.

Certain patient and wound characteristics increase the relative likelihood of developing a hypertrophic scar as opposed to a keloid.[246] Keloids are more likely than hypertrophic scars to be familial. Hypertrophic scars are more likely to be seen in light-skinned people; both hypertrophic scars and keloids occur more frequently in dark-skinned people. Hypertrophic scars generally develop soon after injury, whereas keloids may develop up to a year after an injury. Hypertrophic scars may subside in time, whereas keloids rarely do. Hypertrophic scars are more likely to be associated with a contracture across a joint surface.

Keloids and hypertrophic scars result from a net increase in the quantity of collagen synthesized by fibroblasts in the wound area. The fibroblasts within keloids may be different in terms of their biologic responsiveness from those within normal dermis. Although many theories have been suggested, the etiology of keloids and hypertrophic scars is unknown. Treatment of hypertrophic scars and keloids has included surgical excision, steroid injection, pressure garments, topical Silastic gel, radiation therapy, and combinations of these approaches. The absence of a uniform treatment program accurately suggests that no specific treatment is predictably effective for these lesions.[247]

References

1. Committee on Trauma, American College of Surgeons: Early Care of the Injured Patient, 3rd ed. Walt AJ, Peltier LF, Pruitt BA Jr, et al, Eds. WB Saunders Co, Philadelphia, 1982, p 69

2. Grossman JAI, Adams JP, Kunec J: Prophylactic antibiotics in simple hand lacerations. JAMA 245:1055, 1981

3. Committee on Trauma, American College of Surgeons: A Guide to Prophylaxis against Tetanus in Wound Management, 1984 Revision. The American College of Surgeons, Chicago, 1984

4. Peeples C, Bowick JA Jr, Scott FA: Wounds of the hand contaminated by human or animal saliva. J Trauma 20:383, 1980

5. Edlich RF, Rodeheaver GT, Morgan RF, et al: Principles of emergency wound management. Ann Emerg Med 17:1284, 1988

6. Cummings P: Antibodies to prevent infection in patients with dog bite wounds: a meta-analysis of randomized trials. Ann Emerg Med 23:536, 1994

7. Brook I: Human and animal bite infections. J Fam Pract 28:713, 1989

8. Fitzgerald RH Jr, Cooney WP III, Washington JA II, et al: Bacterial colonization of mutilating hand injuries and its treatment. J Hand Surg [Am] 2:85, 1977

9. Zitelli JA: Wound healing by secondary intention: a cosmetic appraisal. J Am Acad Dermatol 9:407, 1983

10. Krizek TJ, Davis JH: The role of the red cell in subcutaneous infection. J Trauma 5:85, 1965

11. Howe CW: Experimental studies on determinants of wound infection. Surg Gynecol Obstet 123:507, 1966

12. Elek SD: Experimental staphylococcal infections in the skin of man. Ann NY Acad Sci 65:85, 1956

13. Iverson PC: Surgical removal of traumatic tattoos of the face. Plast Reconstr Surg 2:427, 1947

14. Agris J: Traumatic tattooing. J Trauma 16:798, 1976

15. Gelberman RH, Posch JL, Jurist JM: High-pressure injection injuries of the hand. J Bone Joint Surg [Am] 57:935, 1975

16. Mrvos RM, Dean BS, Krenzelok EP: High pressure injection injuries: a serious occupational hazard. J Toxicol Clin Toxicol 25:297, 1987

17. Weltmer JB Jr, Pack LL: High-pressure water-gun injection injuries to the extremities: a report of six cases. J Bone Joint Surg [Am] 70:1221, 1988

18. Lammers RL: Soft tissue foreign bodies. Ann Emerg Med 17:1336, 1988

19. Myers MB: Prediction of skin sloughs at the time of operation with the use of fluorescein dye. Surgery 51:158, 1962

20. Hinshaw JR: Progressive changes in the depth of burns. Arch Surg 87:993, 1963

21. Teplitz C, Davis D, Mason AD, et al: Pseudomonas burn wound sepsis: I. Pathogenesis of experimental burn wound sepsis. J Surg Res 4:200, 1964

22. Shuck JM, Moncreif JA: The management of burns: I. General considerations and the Sulfamylon method. Current Problems in Surgery. Year Book Medical Publishers, Inc, Chicago, 1969

23. Robson MC, Heggers JP: Surgical infection: II. The beta-hemolytic streptococcus. J Surg Res 9:289, 1969

24. Heggers JP, Robson MC, Ristroph JD: A rapid method of performing quantitative wound cultures. Milit Med 134:666, 1969

25. Robson MC, Duke WF, Krizek TJ: Rapid bacterial screening in the treatment of civilian wounds. J Surg Res 14:426, 1973

26. Rodeheaver GT, Rye DR, Rust R, et al: Mechanisms by which proteolytic enzymes prolong the golden period of antibiotic action. Am J Surg 136:379, 1978

27. Edlich RF, Smith OT, Edgerton MT: Resistance of the surgical wound to antimicrobial prophylaxis and its mechanism of development. Am J Surg 126:583, 1973

28. Kanthak FF, Dubrul EL: The immediate repair of war wound of the face. Plast Reconstr Surg 2:110, 1947

29. Ad Hoc Committee of the Committee on Trauma, Division of Medical Sciences, National Academy of Sciences–National Research Council: Postoperative wound infections: the influence of ultraviolet radiation of the operating room and of various other features. Ann Surg 160(suppl 1):1, 1964

30. Donkor P, Bankas DO: A study of primary closure of human bite injuries to the face. J Oral Maxillofac Surg 55:479, 1997

31. McIlrath DC, van Heerden JA, Edis AJ, et al: Closure of abdominal incisions with subcutaneous catheters. Surgery 60:411, 1976

32. Zelko JR, Moore EE: Primary closure of the contaminated wound: closed suction wound catheter. Am J Surg 142:704, 1981

33. Kucan JO, Robson MC, Heggers JP, et al: Comparison of silver sulfadiazine, povidone-iodine and physiologic saline in the treatment of chronic pressure ulcers. J Am Geriatr Soc 24:232, 1981

34. Moncrief JA: Topical therapy for control of bacteria in the burn wound. World J Surg 2:151, 1978

35. Geronemus RG, Mertz PM, Eaglstein WH: Wound healing: the effects of topical antimicrobial agents. Arch Dermatol 115:1311, 1979

36. Robson MC, Edstrom LE, Krizek TJ, et al: The efficacy of systemic antibiotics in the treatment of granulating wounds. J Surg Res 16:299, 1974

37. Rodeheaver G, Edgerton MT, Elliott MB, et al: Proteolytic enzymes as adjuncts to antibiotic prophylaxis of surgical wounds. Am J Surg 127:564, 1974

38. Robson MC, Heggers JP: Delayed wound closure based on bacterial counts. J Surg Oncol 2:379, 1970

39. Hepburn HH: Delayed primary suture of wounds. Br Med J 1:181, 1919

40. Cruise PJE, Foord R: The epidemiology of wound infection: a 10-year prospective study of 62,939 wounds. Surg Clin North Am 60:27, 1980

41. Klein M: Nondomestic mammalian bites. Am Fam Physician 32:137, 1985

42. Kurecki BA 3rd, Brownlee HJ Jr: Venomous snakebites in the United States. J Fam Pract 25:386, 1987

43. Sprenger TR, Bailey WJ: Snakebite treatment in the United States. Int J Dermatol 25:479, 1986

44. Pennell TC, Babu S-S, Meredith JW: The management of snake and spider bites in the southeastern United States. Am Surg 53:198, 1987

45. Lawrence WT, Giannopoulos A, Hansen A: Pit viper bites: rational management in locales in which copperheads and cottonmouths predominate. Ann Plast Surg 36:276, 1996

46. Rees RS, Altenbern P, Lynch JB, et al: Brown recluse spider bites: a comparison of early surgical excision versus dapsone and delayed surgical excision. Ann Surg 202:659, 1985

47. Siegel RJ, Vistnes LM, Iverson RE: Effective hemostasis with less epinephrine: an experimental and clinical study. Plast Reconstr Surg 51:129, 1973

48. Wilhelmi BJ, Blackwell SJ, Miller JH, et al: Do not use epinephrine in digital blocks: myth or truth? Plast Reconstr Surg 107:293, 2001

49. Tran D-T, Miller SH, Buck DS, et al: Potentiation of infection by epinephrine. Plast Reconstr Surg 76:933, 1985

50. Klein JA: Tumescent technique for local anesthesia improves safety in large-volume liposuction. Plast Reconstr Surg 92:1085, 1993

51. Samdal F, Amland PF, Bugge JF: Plasma lidocaine levels during suction-assisted lipectomy using large doses of dilute lidocaine with epinephrine. Plast Reconstr Surg 93:1217, 1994

52. Arndt KA, Burton C, Noe JM: Minimizing the pain of local anesthesia. Plast Reconstr Surg 72:676, 1983

53. Christoph RA, Buchanan L, Begalla K, et al: Pain reduction in local anesthesia administration through pH buffering. Ann Emerg Med 17:117, 1988

54. Anderson AB, Colecchi C, Baronoski R, et al: Local anesthesia in pediatric patients: topical TAC versus lidocaine. Ann Emerg Med 19:519, 1990

55. Hegenbarth MA, Allen MF, Hawk WH, et al: Comparison of topical tetracaine, adrenaline, and cocaine anesthesia with lidocaine infiltration for repair of lacerations in children. Ann Emerg Med 19:63, 1990

56. Blackburn PA, Butler KH, Hughes MJ, et al: Comparison of tetracaine-adrenaline-cocaine (TAC) with topical lidocaine-epinephrine (TLE): efficacy and cost. Am J Emerg Med 13:315, 1995

57. Schilling CG, Bank DE, Borchert BA, et al: Tetracaine, epinephrine (adrenalin) and cocaine (TAC) versus lidocaine, epinephrine and tetracaine (LET) for anesthesia of lacerations in children. Ann Emerg Med 25:203, 1995

58. Smith GA, Strausbaugh SD, Harbeck-Weber C, et al: Comparison of topical anesthetics without cocaine to tetracaine-adrenaline-cocaine and lidocaine infiltration during repair of lacerations: bupivicaine-norepinephrine is an effective topical anesthetic agent. Pediatrics 97:301, 1996

59. Smith GA, Strausbaugh SD, Harbeck-Weber C, et al: Prilocaine-phenylephrine and bupivicainephenyl-ephrine topical anesthetics compared with tetracaine-adrenaline-cocaine during repair of lacerations. Am J Emerg Med 16:121, 1998

60. Lander J, Hodgins M, Nazarali S, et al: Determinants of success and failure of EMLA. Pain 64:89, 1996

61. Zempsky WT, Karasic RB: EMLA versus TAC for topical anesthesia of extremity wounds in children. Ann Emerg Med 30:163, 1997

62. Alexander JW, Fischer JE, Boyajian M, et al: The influence of hair-removal methods on wound infections. Arch Surg 118:347, 1983

63. Madden H, Edlich RF, Schauerhamer R, et al: Application of principles of fluid dynamics to surgical wound irrigation. Current Topics in Surgical Research 3:85, 1971

64. Gross A, Cutright DE, Bhaskar SN: Effectiveness of pulsating water jet lavage in treatment of contaminated crushed wounds. Am J Surg 124:373, 1972

65. Hamer ML, Robson MC, Krizek TJ, et al: Quantitative bacterial analysis of comparative wound irrigations. Ann Surg 181:819, 1975

66. Schauerhamer RA, Edlich RF, Panek P, et al: Studies in the management of the contaminated wound: VII. Susceptibility of surgical wounds to postoperative surface contamination. Am J Surg 122:74, 1971

67. Branemark PI, Albrektsson B, Lindstrom J, et al: Local tissue effects of wound disinfectants. Acta Chir Scand 357(suppl):166, 1966

68. Rodeheaver GT, Smith SL, Thacker JG, et al: Mechanical cleansing of contaminated wounds with a surfactant. Am J Surg 129:241, 1975

69. Rodeheaver G, Turnbull V, Edgerton MT, et al: Pharmacokinetics of a new skin cleanser. Am J Surg 132:67, 1976

70. Lineaweaver W, Howard R, Soucy D, et al: Topical antimicrobial toxicity. Arch Surg 120:267, 1985

71. Dirschl DR, Wilson FC: Topical antibiotic irrigation in the prophylaxis of operative wound infections in orthopedic surgery. Ortho Clin North Am 22:419, 1991

72. Rodeheaver G, Bellamy W, Kody M, et al: Bactericidal activity and toxicity of iodine-containing solutions in wounds. Arch Surg 117:181, 1982

73. Custer J, Edlich RF, Prusak M, et al: Studies in the management of the contaminated wound: V. An assessment of the effectiveness of pHisoHex and beta-dine surgical scrub solutions. Am J Surg 121:572, 1971

74. Mobacken H, Wengstrom C: Interference with healing of rat skin incisions treated with chlorhexidine. Acta Derm Venereol (Stockh) 54:29, 1974

75. Saatman RA, Carlton WW, Hubben K, et al: A wound healing study of chlorhexidine digluconate in guinea pigs. Fundam Appl Toxicol 6:1, 1986

76. Branemark PI, Ekholm R: Tissue injury caused by wound disinfectants. J Bone Joint Surg [Am] 49:48, 1967

77. Kozol RA, Gillies C, Elgebaly SA: Effects of sodium hypochlorite (Dakin's solution) on cells of the wound module. Arch Surg 123:420, 1988

78. Rodeheaver G: Controversies in wound management. Wounds 1:19, 1989

79. Lowbury EJL, Lilly HA, Bull JP: Methods for disinfection of hands and operation sites. Br Med J 2:531, 1964

80. Saggers BA, Stewart GT: Polyvinyl-pyrrolidone-iodine: an assessment of antibacterial activity. J Hyg (Camb) 62:509, 1964

81. Haury B, Rodeheaver G, Vensko J, et al: Debridement: an essential component of traumatic wound care. Am J Surg 135:238, 1978

82. Ordman LJ, Gillman T: Studies in the healing of cutaneous wounds: II. The healing of epidermal, appendageal, and dermal injuries inflicted by suture needles and by suture material in the skin of pigs. Arch Surg 93:883, 1966

83. George TK, Simpson DC: Skin wound closure with staples in the accident and emergency department. J R Coll Surg Edinb 30:54, 1985

84. Golden T: Non-irritating, multipurpose surgical adhesive tape. Am J Surg 100:789, 1960

85. Golden T, Levy AH, O'Connor WT: Primary healing of skin wounds and incisions with a threadless suture. Am J Surg 104:603, 1962

86. Conolly WB, Hunt TK, Zederfeldt B, et al: Clinical comparison of surgical wounds closed by suture and adhesive tapes. Am J Surg 117:318, 1969

87. Edlich RF, Prusak M, Panek P, et al: Studies in the management of the contaminated wound: VIII. Assessment of tissue adhesives for repair of contaminated tissue. Am J Surg 122:394, 1971

88. Mizrahi S, Bicke A, Ben-Layisfh E: Use of tissue adhesives in the repair of lacerations in children. J Ped Surg 23:312, 1988

89. Yaron M, Halperin M, Huffler W, et al: Efficacy of tissue glue for laceration repair in an animal model. Acad Emerg Med 2:259, 1995

90. Quinn J, Wells G, Sutcliffe T, et al: A randomized trial comparing octylcyanoacrylate tissue adhesive and sutures in the management of lacerations. JAMA 277:1527, 1997

91. Saltz R, Sierra D, Feldman D, et al: Experimental and clinical applications of fibrin glue. Plast Reconstr Surg 88:1005, 1991

92. Jabs AD Jr, Wider TM, DeBellis J, et al: The effect of fibrin glue on skin grafts in infected sites. Plast Reconstr Surg 89:268, 1992

93. Mandel MA: Minimal suture blepharoplasty: closure of incisions with autologous fibrin glue. Aesthetic Plast Surg 16:269, 1992

94. Ersek RA, Schade K: Subcutaneous pseudobursa secondary to suction and surgery. Plast Reconstr Surg 85:442, 1991

95. Ferguson DJ: Clinical application of experimental relations between technique and wound infection. Surgery 63:377, 1968

96. DeHoll D, Rodeheaver G, Edgerton MT, et al: Potentiation of infection by suture closure of dead space. Am J Surg 127:716, 1974

97. Magee C, Rodeheaver GT, Golden GT, et al: Potentiation of wound infection by surgical drains. Am J Surg 131:547, 1976

98. Taldych L, Donegan WL: Postmastectomy seroma and wound drainage. Surg Gynecol Obstet 165:483, 1987

99. Rudolph R: The effect of skin graft preparation on wound contraction. Surg Gynecol Obstet 142:49, 1976

100. Edgerton MT, Hansen FC: Matching facial color with split thickness skin grafts from adjacent areas. Plast Reconstr Surg 25:455, 1960

101. Krizek TJ, Robson MC, Kho E: Bacterial growth and skin graft survival. Forum on Fundamental Surgical Problems 18:518, 1967

102. Klein L, Rudolph R: 3 H-Collagen turnover in skin grafts. Surg Gynecol Obstet 135:49, 1972

103. Mir y Mir L: The problem of pigmentation in the cutaneous graft. Br J Plast Surg 14:303, 1961

104. Ponten B: Grafted skin—observations on innervation and other qualities. Acta Chir Scand 257(suppl):1, 1960

105. Baran NK, Horton CE: Growth of skin grafts, flaps, and scars in young minipigs. Plast Reconstr Surg 50:487, 1972

106. Gimbel NS, Farris W: Skin grafting: the influence of surface temperature on the epithelialization rate of split thickness skin donor sites. Arch Surg 92:554, 1966

107. Alvarez OM, Mertz PM, Eaglstein WH: The effect of occlusive dressings on collagen synthesis and re-epithelialization in superficial wounds. J Surg Res 35:142, 1983

108. Shuck JM, Pruitt BA, Moncrief JA: Homograft skin for wound coverage: a study of versatility. Arch Surg 98:472, 1969

109. Robson MC, Krizek TJ, Koss N, et al: Amniotic membranes as a temporary wound dressing. Surg Gynecol Obstet 136:904, 1973

110. Bromberg BE, Song IC, Mohn MP: The use of pig skin as a temporary biologic dressing. Plast Reconstr Surg 36:80, 1965

111. Woodruff EA: Biobrane, a biosynthetic skin prosthesis. Burn Wound Coverings. Wise DL, Ed. CRC Press, New York, 1984

112. Salomon JC, Diegelman RF, Cohen IK: Effect of dressings on donor site epithelialization. Forum on Fundamental Surgical Problems 25:516, 1974

113. Winter GD, Scales JT: Effect of air drying and dressings on the surface of a wound. Nature 197:91, 1963

114. Noe JM, Kalish S: The problem of adherence in dressed wounds. Surg Gynecol Obstet 147:185, 1978

115. Noe JM, Kalish S: Wound Care. Chesebrough Pond's, Greenwich, Connecticut, 1976

116. Varma AO, Bugatch E, German FM: Debridement of dermal ulcers with collagenase. Surg Gynecol Obstet 136:281, 1973

117. Noe JM, Kalish S: The mechanism of capillarity in surgical dressings. Surg Gynecol Obstet 143:454, 1976

118. Grinnell F, Billingham RE, Burgess L: Distribution of fibronectin during wound healing in vivo. J Invest Dermatol 76:181, 1981

119. Clark RAF, Folkvord JM, Wertz RL: Fibronectin as well as other extracellular matrix proteins mediate human keratinocyte adherence. J Invest Dermatol 84:378, 1985

120. Grinnell F: Fibronectin and wound healing. J Cell Biochem 25:107, 1984

121. Wysocki AB, Grinnell F: Fibronectin profiles in normal and chronic wound fluid. Lab Invest 63:825, 1990

122. Ley K: Leukocyte adhesion to vascular endothelium. J Reconstr Microsurg 8:495, 1992

123. Newman SL, Henson JE, Henson PM: Phagocytosis of senescent neutrophils by human monocyte-derived macrophages and rabbit inflammatory macrophages. J Exp Med 156:430, 1982

124. Proveddini DM, Deftos LJ, Manolagas SC: 1,25-Dihydroxyvitamin D3 promotes in vitro morphologic and enzymatic changes in normal human

monocytes consistent with their differentiation into macrophages. Bone 7:23, 1986

125. Wright SD, Meyer BC: Fibronectin receptor of human macrophages recognizes sequence Arg-Gly-Asp-Ser. J Exp Med 162:762, 1985

126. Simpson DM, Ross R: Effects of heterologous anti-neutrophil serum in guinea pigs: hematologic and ultrastructural observations. Am J Pathol 65:79, 1971

127. Leibovich SJ, Ross R: The role of the macrophage in wound repair: a study with hydrocortisone and anti-macrophage serum. Am J Pathol 78:71, 1975

128. Seppa H, Grotendorst G, Seppa S, et al: Platelet-derived growth factor is chemotactic for fibroblasts. J Cell Biol 92:584, 1982

129. Gauss-Miller V, Kleinman H, Martin GR, et al: Role of attachment factors and attractants in fibroblast chemotaxis. J Lab Clin Med 96:1071, 1980

130. Grotendorst GR, Chang T, Seppa HEJ, et al: Platelet-derived growth factor is a chemoattractant for vascular smooth muscle cells. J Cell Physiol 113:261, 1982

131. Stiles CF, Capone GT, Scher CD, et al: Dual control of cell growth by somatomedins and platelet-derived growth factor. Proc Natl Acad Sci USA 76:1279, 1979

132. Leibovich SJ, Ross R: A macrophage-dependent factor that stimulates the proliferation of fibroblasts in vitro. Am J Pathol 84:501, 1976

133. Thakral KK, Goodson WH III, Hunt TK: Stimulation of wound blood vessel growth by wound macrophages. J Surg Res 26:430, 1979

134. Knighton DR, Hunt TK, Thakral KK, et al: Role of platelets and fibrin in the healing sequence: an in vivo study of angiogenesis and collagen synthesis. Ann Surg 196:379, 1982

135. Van Winkle W Jr: The epithelium in wound healing. Surg Gynecol Obstet 127:1089, 1968

136. Clark RAF, Lanigan JM, DellaPelle P, et al: Fibronectin and fibrin provide a provisional matrix for epidermal cell migration during wound reepithelialization. J Invest Dermatol 70:264, 1982

137. Gipson IK, Spurr-Michaud SJ, Tisdale AS: Hemidesmosomes and anchoring fibril collagen appear synchronously during development and wound healing. Dev Biol 126:253, 1988

138. Mackie EH, Halfter W, Liverani D: Induction of tenascin in healing wounds. J Cell Biol 107:2757, 1988

139. Cohen IK, Moore CD, Diegelman RF: Onset and localization of collagen synthesis during wound healing in open rat skin wounds. Proc Soc Exp Biol Med 160:458, 1979

140. Peacock EE Jr: Wound Repair, 3rd ed. WB Saunders Co, Philadelphia, 1984

141. Veis A, Averey J: Modes of intermolecular crosslinking in mature and insoluble collagen. J Biol Chem 240:3899, 1965

142. Rudolph R, Guber S, Suzuki M, et al: The life cycle of the myofibroblast. Surg Gynecol Obstet 145:389, 1977

143. Montesano R, Orci L: Transforming growth factor beta stimulates collagen-matrix contraction by fibroblasts: Implications for wound healing. Proc Natl Acad Sci USA 85:4894, 1988

144. Madden JW, Peacock EE Jr: Studies on the biology of collagen during wound healing: III. Dynamic metabolism of scar collagen and remodelling of dermal wounds. Ann Surg 174:511, 1971

145. Forrester JC, Zederfeldt BH, Hayes TL, et al: Wolff's law in relation to the healing skin wound. J Trauma 10:770, 1970

146. Riley WB Jr, Peacock EE Jr: Identification, distribution and significance of a collagenolytic enzyme in human tissue. Proc Soc Biol Med 214:207, 1967

147. Witte LD, Kaplan KL, Nossel HL, et al: Studies of the release from human platelets of the growth factor for cultured human arterial smooth muscle cells. Circ Res 42:402, 1978

148. Martinet Y, Bitterman PB, Mornex JF, et al: Activated human monocytes express the c-sis proto-oncogene and release a mediator showing PDGF-like activity. Nature 319:158, 1986

149. Shimokado K, Raines EW, Madtes DK, et al: A significant part of macrophage-derived growth factor consists of at least two forms of PDGF. Cell 43:277, 1985

150. Walker LN, Bowen-Pope DF, Ross R, et al: Production of platelet-derived growth factor-like molecules by cultured arterial smooth muscle cells accompanies proliferation after arterial injury. Proc Natl Acad Sci USA 83:7311, 1986

151. Barbul A, Knud-Hansen J, Wasserkrug HL, et al: Interleukin 2 enhances wound healing in rats. J Surg Res 40:315, 1986

152. DeCunzo LP, MacKenzie JW, Marafino BJ Jr, et al: The effect of interleukin-2 administration on wound healing in Adriamycin-treated rats. J Surg Res 49:419, 1990

153. Assoian RK, Komoriya A, Meyers CA, et al: Transforming growth factor-β in human platelets: identification of a major storage site, purification, and characterization. J Biol Chem 258:7155, 1983

154. Pesonen K, Viinikka L, Myllyla G, et al: Characterization of material with epidermal growth factor immunoreactivity in human serum and platelets. J Clin Endocrinol Metab 68:486, 1989

155. Assoian RK, Fleurdelys BE, Stevenson HC, et al: Expression and secretion of type β transforming growth factor by activated human macrophages. Proc Natl Acad Sci USA 84:6020, 1987

156. Mustoe TA, Pierce GF, Thomason A, et al: Accelerated healing of incisional wounds in rats induced by transforming growth factor-β. Science 237:1333, 1987

157. McGee GS, Davidson JM, Buckley A, et al: Recombinant basic fibroblast growth factor accelerates wound healing. J Surg Res 45:145, 1988

158. Brown GL, Curtsinger L III, Brightwell JR, et al: Enhancement of epidermal regeneration by biosynthetic epidermal growth factor. J Exp Med 163:1319, 1986

159. Laato M, Niinikoski J, Lebel L, et al: Stimulation of wound healing by epidermal growth factor: a dose-dependent effect. Ann Surg 203:379, 1986

160. Pierce GF, Mustoe TA, Senior RM, et al: In vivo incisional wound healing augmented by platelet-derived growth factor and recombinant c-sis gene homodimeric proteins. J Exp Med 167:974, 1988

161. Tsuboi R, Rifkin DB: Recombinant basic fibroblast growth factor stimulates wound healing in healing-impaired db/db mice. J Exp Med 172:245, 1990

162. Pierce GF, Mustoe TA, Lingelbach J, et al: Transforming growth factor-β reverses the glucocorticoid-induced wound-healing deficit in rats: possible regulation in macrophages by platelet-derived growth factor. Proc Natl Acad Sci USA 86:2229, 1989

163. Curtsinger LJ, Pietsch JD, Brown GL, et al: Reversal of Adriamycin-impaired wound healing by transforming growth factor-beta. Surg Gynecol Obstet 168:517, 1989

164. Mustoe TA, Purdy J, Gramates P, et al: Reversal of impaired wound healing in irradiated rats by platelet-derived growth factor-BB. Am J Surg 158:345, 1989

165. Brown GL, Nanney LB, Griffen J, et al: Enhancement of wound healing by topical treatment with epidermal growth factor. N Engl J Med 321:76, 1989

166. Brown GL, Curtsinger L, Jurkiewicz MJ, et al: Stimulation of healing of chronic wounds by epidermal growth factor. Plast Reconstr Surg 88:189, 1991

167. Knighton DR, Ciresi K, Fiegel VD, et al: Stimulation of repair in chronic, nonhealing, cutaneous ulcers using platelet-derived wound healing formula. Surg Gynecol Obstet 170:56, 1990

168. Robson MC, Phillips LG, Thomason A, et al: Recombinant human platelet-derived growth factor-BB for the treatment of chronic pressure ulcers. Ann Plast Surg 29:193, 1992

169. Robson MC, Phillips LG, Lawrence WT, et al: The safety and effect of topically applied recombinant basic fibroblast growth factor on the healing of chronic pressure sores. Ann Surg 216:401, 1992

170. Steed DL, Diabetic Ulcer Study Group: Clinical evaluation of recombinant human platelet derived growth factor for the treatment of lower extremity diabetic ulcers. J Vasc Surg 21:71, 1995

171. Polk HC: Adherence of thin skin grafts. Forum on Fundamental Surgical Problems 17:487, 1966

172. Converse JM, Uhlschmid GK, Ballantyne DL Jr: "Plasmatic circulation" in skin grafts: the phase of serum imbibition. Plast Reconstr Surg 43:495, 1969

173. Marckmann A: Autologous skin grafts in the rat: vital microscopic studies of the microcirculation. Angiology 17:475, 1966

174. Smahel J: The healing of skin grafts. Clin Plast Surg 4:409, 1977

175. Psillakis JM: Lymphatic vascularization of skin grafts. Plast Reconstr Surg 43:287, 1969

176. Converse JM, Ballantyne DL: Distribution of diphosphopyridine nucleotide diaphorase in rat skin autografts and homografts. Plast Reconstr Surg 30:415, 1962

177. Hinshaw JR, Miller ER: Histology of healing split-thickness, full-thickness autogenous skin grafts and donor sites. Arch Surg 91:658, 1965

178. Kligman AM: The bacteriology of normal skin. Skin Bacteria and Their Role in Infection. Wolcott BW, Rund DA, Eds. McGraw-Hill, New York, 1965, p 13

179. Ricketts CR, Squire JR, Topley E: Human skin lipids with particular reference to the self sterilising power of the skin. Clin Sci 10:89, 1951

180. Heggers JP: Natural host defense mechanisms. Clin Plast Surg 6:505, 1979

181. Lindberg RB, Moncrief JA, Switzer WE, et al: The successful control of burn wound sepsis. J Trauma 5:601, 1965

182. Kass EH: Asymptomatic infections of the urinary tract. Trans Assoc Am Physicians 69:56, 1956

183. Bendy RH, Nuccio PA, Wolfe E, et al.: Relationship of quantitative bacterial counts to healing of decubiti: effect of gentamycin. Antimicrob Agents Chemother 4:147, 1964

184. Hunt TK, Zederfeldt BH, Goldstick TK, et al: Tissue oxygen tensions during controlled hemorrhage. Surg Forum 18:3, 1967

185. Hauser CJ: Tissue salvage by mapping of skin transcutaneous oxygen tension index. Arch Surg 122:1128, 1987

186. Heughan C, Grislis G, Hunt TK: The effect of anemia on wound healing. Ann Surg 179:163, 1974

187. Roth GJ, McDonald JB, Sheard C: The effect of cigarettes and of intravenous injections of nicotine on the electrocardiogram, basal metabolic rate, cutaneous temperature, blood pressure, and pulse rate of normal persons. JAMA 125:761, 1944

188. Bruce JW, Miller JR, Hooker DR: The effect of smoking upon the blood pressures and upon the volume of the hand. Am J Physiol 24:104, 1909

189. Wright IS, Moffat D: The effects of tobacco on the peripheral vascular system. JAMA 103:315, 1934

190. Sackett DL, Gibson RW, Bross IDJ, et al: Relation between aortic atherosclerosis and the use of cigarettes and alcohol: an autopsy study. N Engl J Med 279:1413, 1968

191. Birnstingl MA, Brinson K, Chakrabarti R: The effect of short-term exposure to carbon monoxide on platelet stickiness. Br J Surg 58:837, 1971

192. Astrup P, Kjeldsen K: Carbon monoxide, smoking and atherosclerosis. Med Clin North Am 58:323, 1973

193. Kjeldsen K, Astrup P, Wanstrup J: Ultra-structural intimal changes in the rabbit aorta after a moderate

carbon monoxide exposure. Atherosclerosis 16:67, 1972

194. Fajardo LF, Berthong M: Radiation injury in surgical pathology. Part III. Salivary glands, pancreas and skin. Am J Surg Pathol 5:279, 1981

195. Rudolph R: Complications of surgery for radiotherapy skin damage. Plast Reconstr Surg 70:179, 1982

196. Levenson SM, Gruber CA, Rettura G, et al: Supplemental vitamin A prevents the acute radiation-induced defect in wound healing. Ann Surg 200:494, 1984

197. Howes EL, Briggs H, Shea R, et al: Effect of complete and partial starvation on the rate of fibroplasia in the healing wound. Arch Surg 27:846, 1933

198. Ward MW, Danzi M, Lewin MR, et al: The effects of subclinical malnutrition and refeeding on the healing of experimental colonic anastomoses. Br J Surg 69:308, 1982

199. Haydock DA, Hill GL: Impaired wound healing in surgical patients with varying degrees of malnutrition. JPEN J Parenter Enteral Nutr 10:550, 1986

200. Thompson WD, Ravdin IS, Frank IL: Effect of hypoproteinemia on wound disruption. Arch Surg 36:500, 1938

201. Devereux DF, Thistlewaite PA, Thibault LF, et al: Effect of tumor bearing and protein depletion on wound breaking strength in the rat. J Surg Res 27:233, 1979

202. Williamson MB, Fromm HJ: Effect of cystine and methionine on healing of experimental wounds. Proc Soc Exp Biol Med 80:623, 1957

203. Levenson SM, Seifter E: Dysnutrition, wound healing, and resistance to infection. Clin Plast Surg 4:375, 1977

204. Freiman M, Seifter E, Connerton C, et al: Vitamin A deficiency and surgical stress. Surg Forum 21:81, 1970

205. Shapiro SS, Mott DJ: Modulation of glycosaminoglycan synthesis by retinoids. Ann NY Acad Sci 359:306, 1981

206. Cohen BE, Till G, Cullen PR, et al: Reversal of postoperative immunosuppression in man by vitamin A. Surg Gynecol Obstet 149:658, 1979

207. Alvarez OM, Gilbreath RL: Effect of dietary thiamine on intermolecular collagen crosslinking during wound repair: a mechanical and biochemical assessment. J Trauma 22:20, 1982

208. Ehrlich HP, Tarver H, Hunt TK: Inhibitory effects of vitamin E on collagen synthesis and wound repair. Ann Surg 175:235, 1972

209. Fernandez-Madrid F, Prasad AS, Oberleas D: Effect of zinc deficiency on nucleic acids, collagen, and noncollagenous protein of the connective tissue. J Lab Clin Med 82:951, 1973

210. Haley JV: Zinc sulfate and wound healing. J Surg Res 27:168, 1979

211. Windsor JA, Knight GS, Hill GL: Wound healing response in surgical patients: recent food intake is more important than nutritional status. Br J Surg 75:135, 1988

212. Muller JM, Brenner U, Dienst C, et al: Preoperative parenteral nutrition in patients with gastrointestinal carcinomas. Lancet 1:68, 1982

213. Lawrence WT, Norton JA, Harvey AK, et al: Wound healing in sarcoma-bearing rats: tumor effects on cutaneous and deep wounds. J Surg Oncol 35:7, 1987

214. Chlebowski RT, Heber D: Metabolic abnormalities in cancer patients: carbohydrate metabolism. Surg Clin North Am 66:957, 1986

215. Weingweg J, Levenson SM, Rettura G, et al: Supplemental vitamin A prevents the tumor-induced defect in wound healing. Ann Surg 211:269, 1990

216. DuNuoy P, Carrell A: Cicatrization of wounds. J Exp Biol 34:339, 1921

217. Grove GL: Age-related differences in healing of superficial skin wounds in humans. Arch Dermatol Res 272:381, 1982

218. Sandblom P, Peterson P, Muren A: Determination of the tensile strength of the healing wound as a clinical test. Acta Chir Scand 105:252, 1953

219. Cruse PJE, Foord RA: A prospective study of 23,649 surgical wounds. Arch Surg 107:206, 1973

220. Goodson WH, Hunt TK: Studies of wound healing in experimental diabetes mellitus. J Surg Res 22:221, 1977

221. Prakash A, Pandit PN, Sharma LK: Studies in wound healing in experimental diabetes. Int Surg 59:25, 1974

222. Arquilla ER, Weringer EJ, Nakajo M: Wound healing: a model for the study of diabetic microangiopathy. Diabetes 25(suppl 2):811, 1976

223. Mowat AG, Baum J: Chemotaxis of polymorphonuclear leukocytes from patients with diabetes mellitus. N Engl J Med 284:621, 1971

224. Bybee JD, Rogers DE: The phagocytic activity of polymorphonuclear leukocytes obtained from patients with diabetes mellitus. J Lab Clin Med 64:1, 1964

225. Nolan CM, Beaty HN, Bagdade JD: Further characterization of the impaired bactericidal function of granulocytes in patients with poorly controlled diabetes. Diabetes 27:889, 1978

226. Bagdade JD, Root RK, Bugler RJ: Impaired leukocyte function in patients with poorly controlled diabetes. Diabetes 23:9, 1974

227. Duncan HJ, Faris IB: Skin vascular resistance and skin perfusion pressure as predictors of healing of ischemic lesions of the lower limb: influences of diabetes mellitus, hypertension, and age. Surgery 99:432, 1986

228. Gottrup F, Andreassen TT: Healing of incisional wounds in stomach and duodenum: the influence of experimental diabetes. J Surg Res 31:61, 1981

229. Weringer EJ, Kelso JM, Tamai IY, et al: Effects of insulin on wound healing in diabetic mice. Acta Endocrinol 99:101, 1982

230. Yue DK, McLennan S, Marsh M, et al: Effects of experimental diabetes, uremia, and malnutrition on wound healing. Diabetes 36:295, 1987

231. Colin JF, Elliot P, Ellis H: The effect of uremia upon wound healing: an experimental study. Br J Surg 66:793, 1979

232. Goodson WH III, Lindenfield SM, Omachi RS, et al: Chronic uremia causes poor healing. Surg Forum 33:54, 1982

233. Benveniste K, Thut P: The effect of chronic alcoholism on wound healing. Proc Soc Exp Biol Med 166:568, 1981

234. Howes EL, Plotz CM, Blunt JW, et al: Retardation of wound healing by cortisone. Surgery 28:177, 1950

235. Hunt TK, Ehrlich HP, Garcia JA, et al: The effect of vitamin A on reversing the inhibitory effect of cortisone on the healing of open wounds in animals. Ann Surg 170:633, 1969

236. Stephens FO, Dunphy JE, Hunt TK: Effect of delayed administration of corticosteroids on wound contraction. Ann Surg 173:214, 1971

237. Sandberg N: Time relationship between administration of cortisone and wound healing in rats. Acta Clin Scand 127:446, 1964

238. Hunt TK, Ehrlich HP, Garcia JA, et al: Effects of vitamin A on reversing the inhibitory effects of cortisone on healing of open wounds in animals and man. Ann Surg 170:633, 1969

239. Shamberger RC, Devereux DF, Brennan MF: The effect of chemotherapeutic agents on wound healing. Int Adv Surg Oncol 4:15, 1981

240. Lawrence WT, Talbot TL, Norton JA: Preoperative or postoperative doxorubicin hydrochloride (Adriamycin): which is better for wound healing? Surgery 100:9, 1986

241. Bayer I, Ellis HL: Jaundice and wound healing: an experimental study. Br J Surg 63:392, 1976

242. Arnaud J-P, Humbert W, Eloy M-R, et al: Effect of obstructive jaundice on wound healing. Am J Surg 141:593, 1981

243. Greaney MG, Van Noort R, Smythe A, et al: Does obstructive jaundice adversely affect wound healing? Br J Surg 66:478, 1979

244. Ellis H, Heddle R: Does the peritoneum need to be closed at laparotomy? Br J Surg 64:733, 1977

245. Peacock EE Jr, Madden JW, Trier WC: Biologic basis for the treatment of keloids and hypertrophic scars. South Med J 63:755, 1970

246. Brody GS, Peng STJ, Landel RF: The etiology of hypertrophic scar contracture: another view. Plast Reconstr Surg 67:673, 1981

247. Lawrence WT: In search of the optimal treatment of keloids: report of a series and a review of the literature. Ann Plast Surg 27:164, 1991

248. Levenson SM, Greever EF, Crowley LV, et al: The healing of rat skin wounds. Ann Surg 161:293, 1965

Acknowledgments

Figure 1   Carol Donner.
Figure 2   Janet Betries.

2 BREAST, SKIN, SOFT TISSUE, AND NECK

1 BREAST COMPLAINTS

Barbara L. Smith, M.D., Ph.D., F.A.C.S., and Wiley W. Souba, M.D., Sc.D., F.A.C.S.

Assessment and Management of Breast Complaints

One of every two women will consult her physician about a breast disorder at some point in her life. Although breast cancer is the most common malignancy of women in the United States, most breast disorders are nonmalignant: it is estimated that 80% to 90% of clinical presentations related to the breast are caused by benign disease. (The true incidence of benign diseases of the breast is difficult to estimate because of the blurred distinction between true breast disease and physiologic breast symptoms such as nodularity, lumpiness, and tenderness.) Because breast disorders are so common, it is important for the practicing general surgeon to be knowledgeable about the workup, diagnosis, and management of breast complaints.

Common Presenting Symptoms of Breast Disease

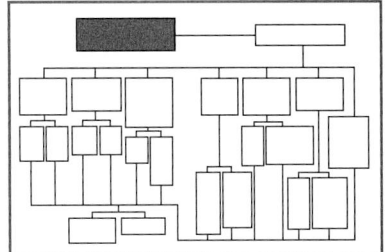

Most of the breast problems surgeons encounter in routine practice fall into six general categories, which are associated with varying degrees of risk for breast cancer [see Table 1]. Some presentations, such as a dominant mass in a postmenopausal woman, are clearly suggestive of malignancy, and their workup is relatively straightforward. Others, such as a tender thickening in a premenopausal woman, usually reflect benign disease. It is important to recognize, however, that any of these presenting symptoms can be associated with a malignancy, and thus all of them warrant a complete evaluation. In fact, it is the evaluation of the usually benign symptoms that places the greatest demands on the physician's clinical judgment. When such symptoms are the main presenting complaint of a breast cancer, their apparently benign nature may be misleadingly reassuring and delay the diagnosis of malignancy.

Risk Factors for Breast Cancer

The central task facing a physician examining a patient with a breast complaint is to determine whether the abnormality is benign or malignant. To this end, knowledge of the main risk factors for breast cancer is essential: prompt identification of the patients at highest risk for malignancy allows the physician to take an appropriately vigorous approach from the beginning of the diagnostic workup.

Various factors that place women at increased risk for breast carcinoma have been identified[1] [see Table 2]. These risk factors include increasing age; mutations in breast cancer risk genes (including *BRCA1* and *BRCA2, PTEN,* and *p53*) and other factors related to a family history of breast cancer[2]; hormonal and reproductive factors, including early menarche, late menopause, nulliparity, the absence of lactation, and the use of exogenous hormones[1,3-9]; environmental factors, including diet and the lifestyle characteristic of developed Western nations[10-12]; certain pathologic findings within breast tissue, including previous breast cancer and various premalignant lesions[13-15]; and certain nonbreast malignancies, including ovarian and endometrial carcinomas. There are also a number of molecular markers that can be correlated with prognosis.

Recognition of risk factors facilitates appropriate screening and clinical management of the individual patient. It is important to recognize, however, that in many women in whom breast cancer develops, known risk factors for breast carcinoma are entirely absent. The absence of these risk factors should not prevent full evaluation or biopsy of a suspicious breast lesion.

Workup of the Patient with a Breast Complaint

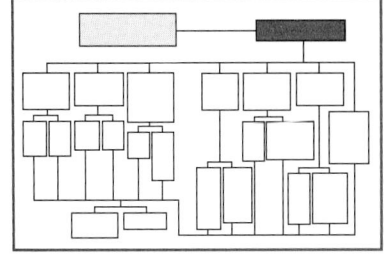

Evaluation of any breast problem should include a detailed history of the presenting complaint, previous breast problems, and any risk factors for breast carcinoma; a thorough physical examination of the breasts; appropriate imaging studies; and evaluation of the patient's general medical condition. Particular attention must be paid to any findings that increase the suspicion of malignancy.

HISTORY

The patient should be asked to describe when and how the problem was first identified. Changes in the size or tenderness of any palpable abnormalities since their initial discovery should be recorded, with particular attention paid to any changes that occurred during the menstrual cycle. Previous breast problems or breast operations should be documented, and pathology reports from any such operations should be obtained. All imaging studies or medical evaluations that have already been performed should be reviewed.

Next, those portions of the medical history that bear on the risk of breast cancer should be explored in detail. Age at menarche and either the date of the last menstrual period or, if applicable, age at menopause should be recorded. Parity, age at the first term pregnancy, and duration of lactation should be determined. Any use of exogenous hormones should be recorded, including use of oral contraceptives (with years of use before the first term pregnancy recorded separately), use of postmenopausal estrogen replacement therapy, and use of any other hormones as part of a fertility program or for other purposes.

In addition, any history of breast cancer in family members, up to and including third-degree relatives, should be detailed, and age at diagnosis should be recorded. Similarly, any family history of ovarian cancer or other cancers (particularly those that developed

Assessment and Management of Breast Complaints

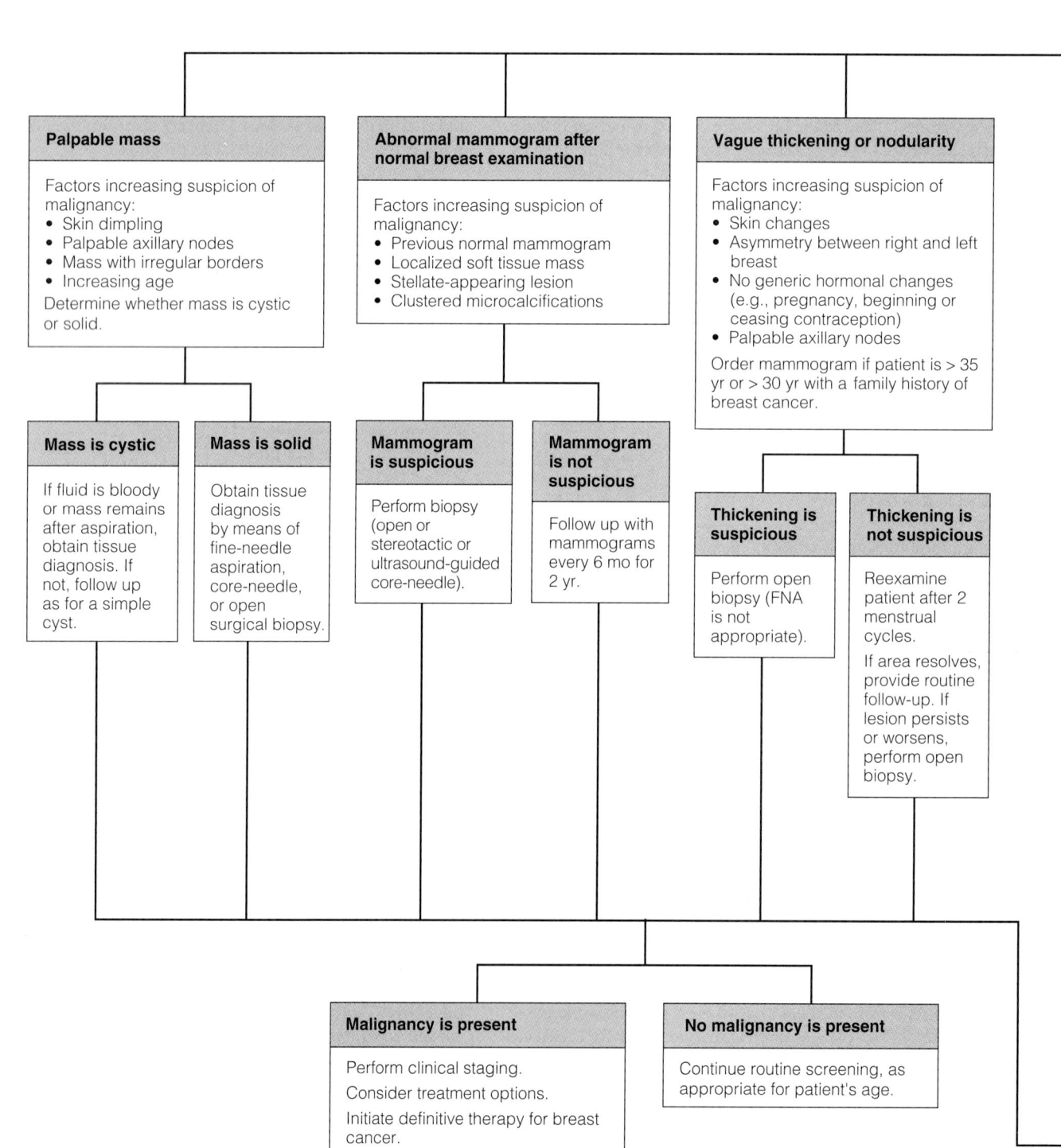

Patient presents with breast complaint

The most common presenting problems are
- Palpable mass
- Vague thickening or nodularity
- Breast infection or inflammation
- Normal physical examination with abnormal mammogram
- Nipple discharge
- Breast pain

Evaluate likelihood that lesion reflects cancer [*see Table 1*], and be aware of patient risk factors for cancer [*see Table 2*].

Palpable mass

Factors increasing suspicion of malignancy:
- Skin dimpling
- Palpable axillary nodes
- Mass with irregular borders
- Increasing age

Determine whether mass is cystic or solid.

Mass is cystic

If fluid is bloody or mass remains after aspiration, obtain tissue diagnosis. If not, follow up as for a simple cyst.

Mass is solid

Obtain tissue diagnosis by means of fine-needle aspiration, core-needle, or open surgical biopsy.

Abnormal mammogram after normal breast examination

Factors increasing suspicion of malignancy:
- Previous normal mammogram
- Localized soft tissue mass
- Stellate-appearing lesion
- Clustered microcalcifications

Mammogram is suspicious

Perform biopsy (open or stereotactic or ultrasound-guided core-needle).

Mammogram is not suspicious

Follow up with mammograms every 6 mo for 2 yr.

Vague thickening or nodularity

Factors increasing suspicion of malignancy:
- Skin changes
- Asymmetry between right and left breast
- No generic hormonal changes (e.g., pregnancy, beginning or ceasing contraception)
- Palpable axillary nodes

Order mammogram if patient is > 35 yr or > 30 yr with a family history of breast cancer.

Thickening is suspicious

Perform open biopsy (FNA is not appropriate).

Thickening is not suspicious

Reexamine patient after 2 menstrual cycles.

If area resolves, provide routine follow-up. If lesion persists or worsens, perform open biopsy.

Malignancy is present

Perform clinical staging.

Consider treatment options.

Initiate definitive therapy for breast cancer.

No malignancy is present

Continue routine screening, as appropriate for patient's age.

Work up patient:
- History, with particular attention to risk factors for breast cancer
- Physical examination
- Imaging studies (e.g., mammography)

Initiate evaluation of specific breast problem.

Nipple discharge

Factors increasing suspicion of malignancy:
- Bloody discharge
- Unilateral discharge
- Palpable mass (see facing page)
- Abnormal mammogram (see facing page)

Breast pain

Factors increasing suspicion of malignancy:
- Abnormal skin changes
- Noncyclic pain

Order mammogram if pain is noncyclic and patient is > 35 yr or > 30 yr with a family history of breast cancer.

Breast infection or inflammation

Factors increasing suspicion of malignancy:
- No elevation of white blood cell count
- No response to antibiotics
- Symptoms not associated with lactation

High-risk patients without symptons

Perform risk assessment (e.g., using Gail or Claus model).

Consider genetic testing for risk gene mutations.

Discuss risk with patient.

Select treatment option:
1. Close surveillance
2. Prophylactic mastectomy
3. Chemoprevention with tamoxifen or participation in chemoprevention trial

Mammogram is abnormal, or palpable mass is detected

Work up as indicated for palpable mass or abnormal mammogram.

Mammogram is normal, and physical examination yields normal results

Offer comfort, reassure, and perform follow-up examination in 2 mo.
If pain resolves or there is still no palpable abnormality, reassure further and follow up routinely. If there is a palpable abnormality, obtain tissue diagnosis.

Discharge is suspicious

Order mammogram. Perform biopsy of any lesions found.
If a single duct is the source of the pathologic discharge, excise duct. If source of discharge can only be localized to a quadrant, excise ducts in that quadrant.

Discharge is not suspicious (physiologic discharge or galactorrhea)

If discharge is physiologic, reassure patient; no further treatment is needed.
If galactorrhea is present, initiate appropriate workup (serum prolactin levels, thyroid function tests, and MRI if necessary).

Patient is lactating

Give oral antibiotics to cover gram-positive cocci, use warm soaks, and attempt to keep breast emptied.

If abscess forms, incise and drain.

Patient is not lactating

Incise and drain any abscesses, and give antibiotics to cover skin organisms (including anaerobes).

If there is no response to short course of antibiotics, rule out inflammatory carcinoma; perform biopsy, including skin.
If infection is chronic, excise subareolar duct complex.

127

Table 1 Common Presenting Symptoms of Breast Disease

Symptom	Likelihood of Malignancy	Risk of Missed Malignancy
Palpable mass	Highest	Lowest
Abnormal mammogram with normal breast examination	↑	
Vague thickening or nodularity		
Nipple discharge		
Breast pain		↓
Breast infection	Lowest	Highest

when the relative was young) should be recorded, along with age at diagnosis. Any personal history of cancer should be recorded, with particular attention paid to breast, ovarian, and endometrial cancers. Previous exposure to radiation, especially in the area of the chest wall, should be noted.

Finally, as with any surgical patient, an overview of the general medical history should be obtained that includes current medications, allergies, tobacco and alcohol use, previous surgical procedures, medical problems, and a brief social history.

PHYSICAL EXAMINATION

First, as the patient sits with her hands behind her head and her elbows back, the breasts should be inspected for asymmetry, dimpling of the skin, erythema, or edema. Each breast should then be carefully palpated from the clavicle to below the inframammary fold and from the sternum to the posterior axillary line, with pains taken to include the subareolar area. This is done with the patient both supine and sitting. If an abnormal area is identified, its size, contour, texture, tenderness, and position should be described; a diagram of the lesion is extremely useful for future reference.

Next, the nipples and areolae are inspected for skin breakdown and squeezed gently to check for discharge. The number and posi-

Table 2 Risk Factors for Breast Cancer

Increasing age
White race
Age at menarche ≤ 11 years
Age at menopause ≥ 55 years
Nulliparity
Age at first pregnancy ≥ 30 years
Absence of history of lactation
? Prolonged use of oral contraceptives before first pregnancy
Use of postmenopausal estrogen replacement, especially if prolonged
Use of other hormones, fertility regimens, or diethylstilbestrol
Mutations in breast cancer risk genes, including *BRCA1* and *BRCA2*, *PTEN*, and *p53*
Family history of breast cancer: multiple affected relatives, early onset, bilaterality
Family history of ovarian cancer: multiple affected relatives, early onset
Pathologic findings that indicate increased risk (e.g., atypical hyperplasia, lobular carcinoma in situ, proliferative fibrocystic disease)
Previous breast cancer
Previous breast problems
Previous breast operations
Previous exposure to radiation

tion of any ducts from which discharge is obtained should be recorded, and the color of the discharge (milky, green, yellow, clear, brown, or bloody) and its consistency (watery, sticky, or thick) should be noted. Discharge on one side calls for a careful search for discharge on the other side because unilateral, single-duct discharge is much more suspicious than bilateral, multiple-duct discharge. Any discharge obtained should be tested for occult blood. Cytologic study of nipple discharge generally is not indicated: it adds expense and rarely contributes significantly to the decision whether biopsy is needed.

Finally, the axillary and supraclavicular nodes are examined bilaterally. If enlarged nodes are discovered, their size, mobility, and number should be recorded. Any matting of nodes or fixation of nodes to the chest walls should also be recorded. Tenderness of enlarged nodes may suggest a reactive process and should therefore be recorded as well.

IMAGING STUDIES

Mammography

According to current recommendations, a baseline screening mammogram need not be performed until 40 (or possibly, as some suggest, until 50[16]) years of age; however, it is reasonable to perform a mammogram to rule out synchronous, nonpalpable lesions whenever a woman older than 35 years presents with a palpable breast mass or other specific symptoms. Approximately 4% to 5% of breast cancers occur in women younger than 40 years, and about 25% occur in women younger than 50 years.[17,18] On the other hand, mammography fails to detect 10% to 15% of all palpable malignant lesions, and its sensitivity is particularly decreased in women with lobular carcinoma or radiographically dense breast tissue. It must therefore be emphasized that a negative mammogram should not influence the decision to perform a biopsy of a clinically palpable lesion. The purpose of mammography is to look for synchronous lesions or nonpalpable calcifications surrounding the palpable abnormality, not to determine whether to perform a biopsy of the palpable lesion.

Ultrasonography

The main value of ultrasonography is in distinguishing cystic from solid lesions. If the lesion is palpable, this distinction is best made by direct needle aspiration, which is both diagnostic and therapeutic; if the lesion is not palpable, ultrasonography can determine whether the lesion is cystic and thus potentially eliminate the need for additional workup or treatment. Ultrasonography has not proved useful for screening: it fails to detect calcifications, misses a large number of malignancies, and identifies a great deal of normal breast texture as potential nodules. It is useful, however, for directing fine-needle or core-needle biopsy of the lesions that it does visualize: it permits real-time manipulation of the needle and direct confirmation of the position of the needle within the lesion. The use of advanced ultrasound technology for diagnostic purposes in the breast is currently being explored.

Magnetic Resonance Imaging

Magnetic resonance imaging after injection of gadolinium contrast enhances many malignant lesions in relation to normal breast parenchyma. Although some benign lesions (e.g., fibroadenomas) are also enhanced by gadolinium, the contrast agent appears to enhance malignant lesions more rapidly and often to a greater extent.

The sensitivity and specificity of MRI in distinguishing benign from malignant lesions are still being assessed. The main approved use of MRI in breast disease is for identification of leaks in silicone breast implants, because MRI can detect the ruptured silicone membrane within the silicone gel. MRI is also useful in identifying occult primary tumors in women who have palpable axillary nodes but no palpable or mammographically identified primary breast lesion. MRI appears to be effective for assessing the extent of vaguely defined tumors, identifying unsuspected multifocal disease, and helping identify patients who are not eligible for breast-conserving surgery. In addition, it appears that MRI can distinguish between a locally recurrent tumor and surgical scarring or radiation change after lumpectomy and radiation, although the technology may not provide reliable readings until 18 months or more after surgery or the completion of radiation therapy. The utility of MRI for screening of young high-risk women with mammographically dense breast tissue is being explored.

Nuclear medicine studies such as sestamibi scintimammography and positron emission tomography (PET) scanning remain primarily investigational tools. There is currently no role for thermography or xerography in the evaluation of breast problems.

Management of Specific Breast Problems

PALPABLE MASS

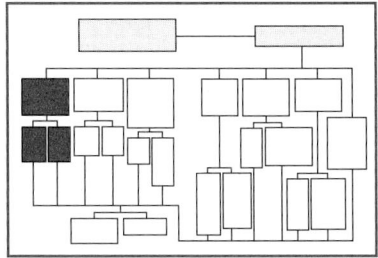

The workup and management of a discrete breast mass are governed by the age of the patient, the physical characteristics of the palpable lesion, and the patient's medical history.[19] The likelihood of malignancy is greater when the patient is 40 years of age or older, when the mass has irregular borders, or when skin dimpling or enlarged axillary nodes are present. A prebiopsy mammogram is indicated for women older than 35 years and for those younger than 35 years who have a strong family history of premenopausal breast cancer.

It is important to determine whether the mass is solid or cystic. Cysts are almost always benign; usually, aspiration is all that is required. Solid masses are more likely to be cancerous; a tissue diagnosis must be obtained to rule out malignancy. Clinical examination is not accurate in distinguishing cysts from a solid mass. In one study, only 58% of 66 palpable cysts were correctly identified on physical examination.[20]

Cystic Masses

If it is suspected that a palpable mass is a cyst, the suspicion should generally be confirmed by aspiration, even if ultrasound examination has already shown the mass to be a simple cyst. Aspiration verifies that the palpable mass corresponds to the lesion seen on ultrasonography; it also permits more thorough examination of the surrounding breast tissue. If the cyst fluid is bloody or a mass remains after aspiration, there is a significant chance of malignancy, and the aspirate should be sent for cytologic analysis.[21] At this point, excisional biopsy is generally indicated [see 2:5 Breast Procedures], even if the cytologic analysis reveals no malignancy. If the cyst fluid is not bloody and no mass remains after aspiration, there is little chance of malignancy, and the aspirate need not be sent for cytologic analysis.[22,23] In one study, there were no malignancies in 6,747 nonbloody cyst aspirates.[24]

If a cyst is aspirated without having been demonstrated to be a simple cyst by ultrasonography, the patient should be reexamined in 4 to 8 weeks. Fewer than 20% of simple cysts recur after a single aspiration, and fewer than 9% recur after two or three aspirations.[25] If a cyst recurs rapidly after aspiration, it should be reaspirated and its contents sent for cytologic analysis. If the results of

the analysis are suspicious or if the cyst recurs yet again, an excisional biopsy should be performed. If, however, a new cyst appears in a different area of breast tissue, this additional workup is not required, and the new cyst should be evaluated as a new problem. Additional cysts may be expected to occur in more than 50% of patients.[26]

Solid Masses

If a discrete mass in the breast is believed to be solid, either on the basis of ultrasonographic findings or because attempts at aspiration yield no fluid, a tissue diagnosis is necessary to rule out malignancy. Physical examination alone is insufficient: it correctly identifies masses as malignant in only 60% to 85% of cases.[27,28] Furthermore, experienced examiners often disagree on whether biopsy is needed for a particular lesion: in one study, four surgeons unanimously agreed on the necessity of biopsy for only 11 (73%) of 15 palpable masses that were later shown by biopsy to be malignant. Tissue diagnosis may be accomplished by fine-needle aspiration (FNA) biopsy, core-needle biopsy, or open surgical biopsy [see Sidebar Breast Biopsy and 2:5 Breast Procedures].

Phyllodes tumors The phyllodes tumor, a mesenchymal tumor limited to mammary tissue, is a rare condition. The tumor is typically smooth, round, firm, well defined, and mobile and causes no pain. It has no pathognomonic mammographic or ultrasonographic features and is difficult, if not impossible, to distinguish from a fibroadenoma on physical examination or radiologic evaluation unless it is quite large. Palpable axillary lymph nodes are encountered in 20% of patients with phyllodes tumors, but histologic evidence of malignancy is encountered in fewer than 5% of axillary lymph node dissections for clinically positive nodes. The remainder of the nodes are enlarged as a result of necrosis of the primary tumor.

Tumors are classified as low, intermediate, or high grade on the basis of five criteria: stromal cellularity, stromal atypia, the microscopic appearance of the tumor margin (infiltrating, effacing, or bulging), mitoses per 10 high-power fields, and the macroscopic size of the tumor. Structural[29] and cytogenetic[30] studies of constituent cells have demonstrated similarities between fibroadenomas and phyllodes tumors, and there is evidence[31] that certain fibroadenomas develop into phyllodes tumors. FNA is usually nondiagnostic, primarily because of the difficulty of obtaining adequate numbers of stromal cells for cytogenic analysis.[32] Although phyllodes tumors have minimal metastatic potential, they have a proclivity for local recurrence and should be excised with a 1 cm margin. Local recurrence has been correlated with excision margins but not with tumor grade or size.[33]

The diagnosis of phyllodes tumor should be considered in all patients with a history of a firm, rounded, well-circumscribed, solid (i.e., noncystic) lesion in the breast. Simple excisional biopsy should be performed if aspiration fails to return cyst fluid or if ultrasonography demonstrates a solid lesion. Because phyllodes tumors mimic fibroadenomas, they are often enucleated or excised with a close margin. If a 1 cm margin is not obtained after examination of the permanent section, the patient should undergo reexcision to obtain wider margins. Otherwise, a recurrence rate of 15% to 20% can be expected. If a simple excision cannot be accomplished without gross cosmetic deformity or if the tumor burden is too large, a simple mastectomy may be performed. Axillary lymph node dissection should be reserved for clinically palpable nodes. Radiation therapy may have a role in patients with chest wall invasion. Chemotherapy, which is reserved for patients with metastatic disease, is based on guidelines for the treatment of sarcomas, rather than breast adenocarcinomas.

Breast Biopsy

Techniques

FINE-NEEDLE ASPIRATION BIOPSY

Fine-needle aspiration (FNA) biopsy with a 22- to 25-gauge needle may be performed with minimal patient discomfort when a palpable mass is identified on physical examination; mammographically or ultrasonographically guided FNA biopsy may also be performed when a nonpalpable lesion is identified. The false negative rate with FNA biopsy ranges from 1% to 35% for palpable lesions[28,110] and may be as high as 68% for nonpalpable lesions.[111] The false positive rate generally ranges from 1% to 2%.[28,109] Nonspecific findings, such as normal or fibrocystic breast tissue, or any atypical findings on cytologic analysis should be evaluated further, usually by means of open surgical biopsy.

CORE-NEEDLE BIOPSY

A second nonsurgical form of breast biopsy is core-needle biopsy. This technique is more uncomfortable for the patient than FNA biopsy because a much larger needle is used and a small nick must be made in the skin. Core-needle biopsy obtains an 11- to 14-gauge cylinder of tissue from the mass being sampled, and the tissue is analyzed by conventional pathology rather than cytology.[112] Core-needle biopsy may be guided by palpation for palpable lesions or by stereotactic mammography or ultrasonography for nonpalpable lesions. As with FNA biopsy, the false positive rate is very low. False negative rates are lower than for FNA biopsy[111-113] but higher with needles smaller than 14 gauge,[112] with freehand rather than image-guided biopsy, and with less experienced operators.

The finding of atypical ductal hyperplasia (ADH) or any equivocal diagnosis with core-needle biopsy necessitates open surgical biopsy to rule out malignancy. A significant number of open biopsies find ductal carcinoma in situ (DCIS) after an initial core-needle biopsy indicates ADH. Core-needle biopsy findings that appear to contradict clinical or mammographic findings should be viewed with suspicion and followed with open surgical biopsy.

The use of core-needle biopsy instead of needle-localized open surgical biopsy for diagnosis of breast cancer can reduce the number of surgical procedures and the cost of diagnosis. In one series,[113] an average of 1.25 open surgical procedures were required for diagnosis of a nonpalpable breast malignancy by core-needle biopsy, compared with an average of nearly two surgical procedures per malignancy when open surgical biopsy was used for diagnosis.

OPEN BIOPSY

Open surgical biopsy remains the gold standard for diagnosis of breast lesions. It has a major advantage over FNA biopsy and core-needle biopsy in that it removes the lesion, thus allowing a more complete pathologic analysis, including analysis of the margins and the extent of intraductal disease in malignant lesions. However, open surgical biopsy costs more, takes more time, and causes more patient discomfort than either FNA or core-needle biopsy.

With palpable lesions, the surgeon should attempt to excise the lesion along with a narrow rim of normal-appearing breast tissue. Because most breast masses prove to be benign, it is important to avoid unnecessary distortion of the breast. With nonpalpable lesions, preoperative wire localization is performed to direct the surgeon to the appropriate area. The surgeon then removes tissue around the wire in such a way as to include the lesion along with a rim of normal-appearing breast tissue. A radiograph of the specimen should be obtained before the patient leaves the operating room to confirm that the lesion is contained within the specimen.

Most biopsies, including needle-localized biopsies of nonpalpable lesions, are now performed with the patient under local anesthesia or local anesthesia with sedation; general anesthesia is reserved for special circumstances, such as in cases in which multiple biopsies are necessary. The approach to surgical biopsy that once was standard—general anesthesia, frozen section diagnosis, and immediate definitive cancer surgery—has largely been abandoned. In addition to the logistical difficulties this approach poses for both patients and surgeons, it is clear that performing definitive surgery on the same day as biopsy does not improve survival or reduce the incidence of metastasis. Now that multiple treatment options are available for women with breast cancer, a staged approach that allows ample time for discussion of treatment options and decision making after a diagnosis of malignancy is preferred.

Analysis of Tissue

In addition to routine histologic analysis, a number of tests that provide prognostic or therapeutic information are now routinely performed on malignant breast tissue.

HORMONE RECEPTOR LEVELS

Determination of estrogen and progesterone receptor levels in breast carcinomas is essential because these levels predict response to hormone therapy. Furthermore, some studies suggest that patients with estrogen receptor–positive tumors have a better prognosis than patients with estrogen receptor–negative tumors. Receptor levels may be determined by using a competitive binding assay to measure cytosol receptor levels or by performing an immunohistochemical assay in which a monoclonal antibody binds to the receptor.

OTHER MOLECULAR MARKERS AND PROGNOSTIC FACTORS

A number of molecular markers have been identified that may eventually play a role in treating or determining the prognosis for patients with breast cancer. The true clinical value of these markers remains to be determined, but several of them have already been analyzed with the aim of assessing their relevance to the management of breast cancer.[114] At present, the marker with the greatest clinical relevance is HER-2-*neu*, a transmembrane protein thought to be involved in the control of cell growth. The overexpression of HER-2-*neu* appears to be an independent predictor of poor prognosis in breast cancer patients[115,116] and may be a predictor of a favorable response to chemotherapy in node-positive breast cancer patients.[117,118] Antibodies to HER-2-*neu* are available and are being evaluated in the treatment of breast cancers.

The density of neovascularization and the occurrence of cathepsin D, *myc*, *ras*, and *p53* have been measured in breast tumor specimens[114]; however, these studies are investigational, and their impact on clinical practice remains to be determined. Measurements of S-phase fraction and the proliferation marker Ki-67, used to estimate the growth rate of malignant tumors, may not be independent prognostic factors. The DNA content of tumor cells, measured by flow cytometry, does not appear to correlate well with prognosis.

ABNORMAL MAMMOGRAM WITH NORMAL FINDINGS ON PHYSICAL EXAMINATION

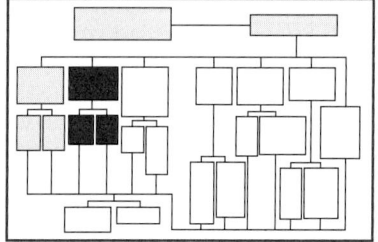

Routine mammographic screening has led to increased identification of nonpalpable lesions. The American College of Surgeons Commission on Cancer found that an abnormal screening mammogram was one of the presenting complaints for 56.1% of breast cancers in 1990, compared with 29.6% in 1983.[17] For two thirds of the cancers detected mammographically in 1990, an abnormal mammogram was the only abnormal finding.

Most mammographic abnormalities, however, are not associated with malignancy. In the United States, only 15% to 30% of mammographic lesions for which biopsy is recommended prove to be malignant.[34] Mammographic screening also identifies a number of abnormalities that are less suspicious for malignancy—so-called probably benign lesions. These lesions may be safely followed with mammograms at short intervals (e.g., every 6 months for 2 years), with biopsy reserved for lesions that become more suspicious during follow-up.[35-37] The decision whether to follow or to excise a particular mammographic lesion is based on (1) the mammographic appearance of the lesion, (2) assessment of the patient's risk factors for carcinoma, and (3) the patient's preferences.

In general, whenever the radiologist states that a lesion identified on mammography is suspicious, a tissue diagnosis should be obtained by means of either open needle-localized biopsy or mammographically guided stereotactic core-needle biopsy [*see 2:5 Breast Procedures*]. Findings especially suggestive of malignancy include the presence of a localized soft tissue mass within the breast that either is new or has changed in size or appearance, architectural distortion with irregular borders producing a stellate-appearing lesion, and clustered microcalcifications, with or without a new or changed mass or architectural distortion.

VAGUE THICKENING OR NODULARITY

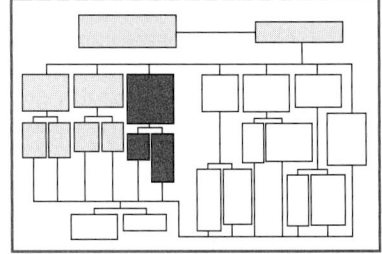

Normal breast texture is often heterogeneous, particularly in premenopausal women. Consequently, vague thickenings or areas of nodularity are frequently found in the breast, sometimes associated with tenderness and sometimes not. These areas must be distinguished from true masses.

In clinical practice, the first step in evaluating a nodular area is to compare it with the corresponding area of the opposite breast. Symmetrical areas of thickening—for example, in the upper outer quadrant of both breasts—are rarely pathologic, particularly those that are tender. These areas often represent fibrocystic changes and may resolve spontaneously. Asymmetrical areas of vague thickening in premenopausal women should be reexamined after one or two menstrual cycles. If the asymmetrical thickening resolves, it was probably caused by a benign process. If the asymmetrical thickening persists, however, the possibility of malignancy is increased, and biopsy should be performed to rule out malignancy. For any woman older than 35 years who has not had a mammogram in the past 6 months, a mammogram should be ordered at this point to rule out synchronous lesions. The value of a negative FNA biopsy in the presence of a vague thickening rather than a discrete mass is questionable. Open biopsy is generally required for adequate sampling.

NIPPLE DISCHARGE

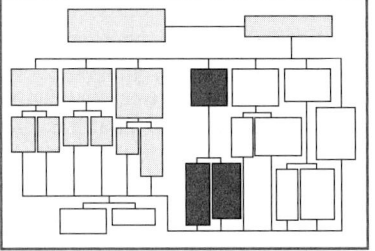

Nipple discharge may be classified as physiologic discharge, pathologic discharge, or galactorrhea. In most instances, it is physiologic—that is, bilateral, nonspontaneous, and arising from multiple ducts. The discharge is usually yellow to green and may be evoked by certain drugs, such as estrogen or tranquilizers, or by sexual stimulation. If physical examination and mammography do not identify a pathologic entity, the patient may be reassured that the discharge is benign, in which case no treatment or additional evaluation is necessary.

Pathologic discharge is spontaneous and is usually unilateral and localized to a single duct. It may be serous, bloody, or brownish. Although the most common causes of bloody nipple discharge are benign intraductal papillomas and duct ectasia, the presence of red blood cells and clusters of ductal cells may suggest malignancy.[38,39] The likelihood of malignancy is increased when the discharge arises in a postmenopausal woman. The workup should include mammography, careful physical examination, and biopsies of any lesions

found. Ductography is rarely useful: it almost never eliminates the need for a surgical procedure and rarely, if ever, changes the extent of the surgical procedure that is required. If a single duct can be identified as the source of the pathologic discharge, it should be excised flush with the nipple; if only the quadrant of the duct can be identified, excision of the major ducts in that quadrant is the procedure of choice [*see 2:5 Breast Procedures*].[40,41]

Galactorrhea is a bilateral discharge that is milky, contains fat, and arises from multiple ducts. As many as one third of women with galactorrhea have pituitary tumors; this is especially likely if they are also amenorrheic. Other causes of galactorrhea are hypothyroidism, chest wall trauma, and certain drugs. The evaluation of galactorrhea includes measurement of serum prolactin levels and thyroid function tests. If the prolactin level is elevated, a magnetic resonance imaging scan of the head, with particular attention to the sella turcica, should be obtained.

BREAST PAIN

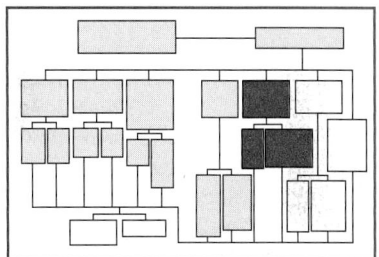

Breast pain, or mastalgia, is one of the most common breast symptoms for which patients consult physicians. At present, the causes of breast pain are poorly understood. Given that it is usually cyclic and typically resolves at menopause, there is reason to believe that it may be of hormonal origin. Several studies, however, have shown no differences in circulating estrogen levels between women with mastalgia and pain-free control subjects. It has been postulated that in women with breast pain, progesterone levels may be decreased or prolactin release may be increased in response to thyrotropin-releasing factor hormone.[42] Although histologic findings consistent with cysts, apocrine metaplasia, and ductal hyperplasia have been noted in the breasts of women with mastalgia, there is no convincing evidence that any of these pathologic changes actually cause breast pain.

In the examination of the patient with breast pain, it is worthwhile to attempt to differentiate between cyclic and noncyclic breast pain and to rule out causes of pain that do not arise from the breast itself. Cyclic breast pain generally is most severe shortly before the menses and is relieved with their onset. Noncyclic pain, on the other hand, bears no relation to the menstrual cycle. Both types of pain may be either intermittent or continuous and may be described by the patient as burning. Mammography and physical examination usually yield normal results in patients with breast pain. The likelihood of malignancy is increased when a patient with mastalgia is postmenopausal and not taking estrogens or when the pain is associated with skin changes or palpable abnormalities; however, these situations are uncommon.

For most women with breast pain, treatment consists of relieving symptoms and reassuring the patient that the workup has not identified an underlying breast carcinoma or another serious disorder. Nonsteroidal anti-inflammatory drugs and supportive bras are helpful. Elimination of caffeine, reduction of salt intake, and the use of diuretics, although generally harmless, have not been proved to be beneficial. Evening primrose oil, taken orally, has been reported to produce significant or complete pain relief in about 50% of women with cyclic mastalgia.[43]

For the rare patients who have severe pain that does not respond to conservative measures, administration of hormones or drugs may be appropriate. Danazol has been successful against breast pain and should be considered the first-line agent, although its androgenic effects may be troubling to many women.[44,45] Bromocriptine (a prolactin antagonist) and tamoxifen have also been used to treat mastalgia.[46,47] Pharmacotherapy for mastalgia is contraindicated in patients who are trying to become pregnant.

BREAST INFECTION OR INFLAMMATION

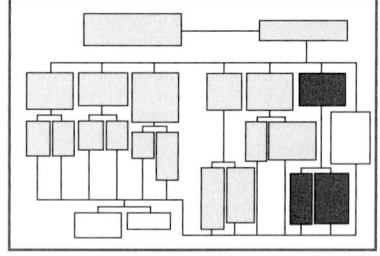

Infections of the breast fall into two general categories: (1) lactational infections and (2) chronic subareolar infections associated with duct ectasia. These benign infections must be distinguished from inflammatory carcinoma.

Both cellulitis and abscesses may occur in lactating women, often during weaning or at other times when engorgement occurs. In the early stages, infections are treated by giving oral antibiotics that cover gram-positive cocci, applying warm packs to the breast, and actively attempting to keep the breast emptied. Weaning is not necessary: the infant is not adversely affected by nursing from the infected breast.[48,49]

Once a breast abscess forms, however, surgical drainage is necessary, and the infant generally must be weaned. Because of the network of fibrous septa within the breast, breast abscesses in lactating women rarely form fluctuant masses.[48] The diagnosis is established by the clinical picture of fever, leukocytosis, and exquisite point tenderness in the breast. General anesthesia is almost always required for drainage of these abscesses, because of the tenderness of the affected area and the amount of manipulation necessary to break up the loculated abscess cavity adequately. The cavity should be packed open, as with any abscess.

Nonlactational infections of the breast often present as chronic relapsing infections of the subareolar ducts associated with periductal mastitis or duct ectasia. These infections usually involve multiple organisms, including skin anaerobes.[50,51] Retraction or inversion of the nipple, subareolar masses, recurrent periareolar abscesses, or a chronic fistula to the periareolar skin may result,[41,52] as may palpable masses and mammographic changes that mimic carcinoma. In the acute phase of infection, treatment entails incision, drainage, and administration of antibiotics that cover skin organisms, including anaerobes. In cases of repeated infection, the entire subareolar duct complex should be excised after the acute infection has completely resolved, with antibiotic coverage provided during the perioperative period. The necessity of drain placement is debated. Even after wide excision of the subareolar duct complex and intravenous antibiotic coverage, infections recur in some patients; these can be treated by excising the nipple and the areola.[40,53]

HIGH-RISK PATIENTS PRESENTING FOR SCREENING

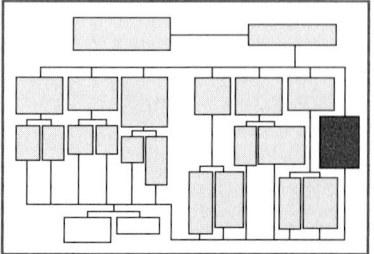

On the basis of established risk factors [see Risk Factors for Breast Cancer, above, and Table 2], certain asymptomatic women can be determined to be at increased risk for the development of breast cancer. The risk can be assessed by genetic testing for mutations in breast cancer risk genes or by the use of mathematical models to estimate risk. The Gail model,[54] which relies on data from the Breast Cancer Detection Demonstration Project, and the Claus model,[55] which relies on data from the Cancer and Steroid Hormone Project, are two of the tools that have

been used to make this determination. At present, there are three treatment options for women at high risk for breast cancer: (1) close surveillance, (2) prophylactic mastectomy, and (3) chemoprevention with tamoxifen or other agents in the setting of a clinical trial. Although most women at high risk choose the option of close surveillance, the growing body of data on chemoprevention and prophylactic mastectomy may increase selection of the other two options.

For women with a previous diagnosis of breast cancer, surveillance protocols are described elsewhere [see Management of the Patient with Breast Cancer, Follow-up after Treatment, below]. For women with lobular carcinoma in situ (LCIS) or a family history of breast carcinoma, surveillance should include twice-yearly physical examinations. Mammography should be performed annually after the diagnosis of LCIS or atypical hyperplasia. For women with a family history of breast cancer, mammography should be performed annually, beginning at least 5 years before the earliest age at which cancer was diagnosed in a relative and in any case no later than the age of 35 years.[56] For women who carry BRCA1 or BRCA2 mutations and other women from families with an autosomal dominant pattern of breast cancer transmission, annual mammographic screening should begin at least 10 years before the earliest age at which the cancer was diagnosed in a relative and no later than 25 years of age.[56]

Long-term results of prophylactic mastectomy in high-risk women[57] indicate that breast cancer risk was reduced by at least 90% in women at high or very high risk who underwent this procedure, compared with women who did not, with risk predicted by the Gail model.[54] Mathematical modeling suggests that prophylactic mastectomy could translate into improved survival for women at very high risk if it confers a 90% reduction in risk.[58]

Chemoprevention may be defined as the use of nutrients or pharmacologic agents to augment physiologic mechanisms that protect against the development of malignancy. Chemopreventive strategies are designed either to block the initiation of the carcinogenic process or to prevent (or reverse) the progression of the premalignant cell to an invasive cancer.[59] Chemoprevention began with the development of the antiestrogen tamoxifen. Whereas the efficacy of tamoxifen in estrogen receptor (ER)–positive breast cancer patients has been recognized for some time, its chemopreventive potential has only recently been established.

The first—and still the most extensive—study to be published on breast cancer chemoprevention was the National Surgical Adjuvant Breast and Bowel Project (NSABP) P-1 trial, in which women at increased risk for breast cancer were randomly assigned to receive either tamoxifen, 20 mg/day, or placebo.[60] Increased risk was determined on the basis of (1) age greater than 60 years, (2) a 5-year predicted incidence of breast cancer of at least 1.66% (determined according to Gail's criteria[54]), or (3) a personal history of lobular carcinoma in situ. After a median follow-up of 55 months, the overall risk of breast cancer was decreased by 49% in the tamoxifen group, and the risk of noninvasive breast cancer was decreased by 50%. The reduction in breast cancer risk was limited to ER-positive breast cancers. Several adverse side effects were noted in the tamoxifen group, the most worrisome of which were a threefold increase in the incidence of endometrial cancer, a higher incidence of deep vein thrombosis and pulmonary embolism, and a higher incidence of stroke. Although two subsequent trials, one from the United Kingdom[61] and one from Italy,[62] did not confirm these findings, the FDA found the results of the NSABP P-1 trial to be compelling enough to warrant approval of tamoxifen as a chemopreventive agent in high-risk women. As of June 2002, a fourth randomized trial of tamoxifen chemoprevention, the International Breast Cancer Intervention Study, was still in progress.

Concerns about the side effects of tamoxifen have generated growing interest in the use of selective estrogen receptor modulators (SERMs) as chemopreventive agents.[63] It appears possible that such so-called designer estrogens may have fewer side effects than tamoxifen while reducing the rate of new breast cancers and lowering the incidence of osteoporosis and cardiovascular disease. One of the SERMs, raloxifene, has been approved by the FDA for the treatment of postmenopausal osteoporosis and is known also to exert beneficial effects on lipid profiles. Unlike tamoxifen, raloxifene appears not to have stimulatory effects on the endometrium.[63] Moreover, the Multiple Outcomes of Raloxifene Evaluation (MORE) trial found that fewer breast cancers were noted in women treated with raloxifene than would have been expected without such treatment.[64]

On the basis of findings from osteoporosis trials, the NSABP incorporated raloxifene into an extensive multi-institutional chemoprevention trial that began enrolling patients in 1999. The Study of Tamoxifen and Raloxifene (STAR) trial is a randomized, double-blind trial whose purpose is to compare the effectiveness of raloxifene with that of tamoxifen in postmenopausal women at increased risk for breast cancer. Entry criteria are similar to those for the NSABP P-1 study. A total of 22,000 postmenopausal high-risk women will be randomly assigned to receive either tamoxifen, 20 mg/day orally, or raloxifene, 60 mg/day orally, for 5 years.

There are a number of newer agents that may possess some capacity for breast cancer chemoprevention. Aromatase inhibitors, which have been used as second-line therapies after tamoxifen in cases of advanced breast cancer, may exert chemopreventive effects by inhibiting parent estrogens and their catechol metabolites, thereby preventing cancer initation.[65] In addition, gonadotropin-releasing hormone agonists, monoterpenes, isoflavones, retinoids, rexinoids, vitamin D derivatives, and inhibitors of tyrosine kinase are all undergoing evaluation in clinical or preclinical studies with a view to assessing their potential chemopreventive activity.[66] Whether any of these compounds will play a clinically useful role in preventing breast cancer remains to be seen.

Management of the Patient with Breast Cancer

STAGING

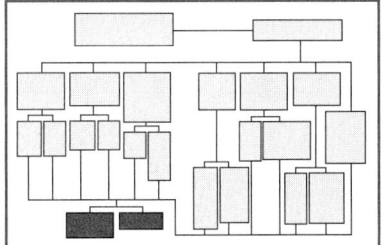

In patients with newly diagnosed breast cancer, it is important to determine the overall extent of disease before embarking on definitive therapy. This process, referred to as clinical staging, includes (1) physical examination to identify any areas of palpable disease in the breasts or the axillary and supraclavicular nodes, along with a detailed clinical history to identify symptoms that may suggest metastatic disease; (2) imaging studies, including mammography, chest x-ray, and, sometimes, bone scans or CT scans of the chest, the abdomen, or the head; and (3) laboratory studies, including a complete blood count (CBC) and liver function tests. Several clinical staging systems for breast cancer are currently in use [see Tables 3 and 4].

The extent of preoperative staging should be guided by the size and other characteristics of the primary tumor and by the patient's history and physical examination. For patients with early-stage cancer and a low probability of metastatic disease, extensive testing adds cost without offering much benefit and should therefore be discouraged. For patients with stage I or II disease, a CBC, liver function tests, and a chest x-ray should be performed before defini-

tive surgical therapy is initiated, and imaging studies should be reserved for patients who have abnormal test results or clinical symptoms that suggest metastatic disease (e.g., bone pain). For patients with higher-stage disease at presentation, the use of additional staging studies should be guided by the patient's clinical situation.

TREATMENT OPTIONS

Mastectomy versus Limited Surgery

Clinical trials in the 1970s and 1980s clearly demonstrated that in eligible women with stage I and II breast carcinoma, limited surgery—consisting of lumpectomy or quadrantectomy, axillary dissection, and radiation—yielded overall survival rates that were equivalent to those achieved with radical or modified radical mastectomy.[67-70] Certain categories of patients are now widely considered to be eligible for breast conservation and radiation therapy [see Table 5]: not only are long-term survival rates after breast conservation with limited surgery identical to those achieved with mastectomy in these groups, but local recurrence rates are low as well (5% to 10%). Approximately two thirds of all women with breast cancer are eligible for breast conservation. Nevertheless, many eligible women in the United States are still treated with mastectomy.[71-75] When a patient is eligible for limited surgery, the decision between mastectomy and breast conservation with radiation therapy is made on the basis of patient and physician preference, access or lack of access to radiation therapy, and the presence or absence of contraindications to breast conservation.

Contraindications to breast conservation There remain patients for whom mastectomy is still clearly the treatment of choice. These patients fall into four broad categories: (1) those in whom radiation therapy is contraindicated, (2) those in whom lumpectomy would have an unacceptable cosmetic result, (3) those for whom local recurrence is a concern, and (4) those high-risk patients in whom surgical prophylaxis is appropriate [see Management of Specific Breast Problems, High-Risk Patients Presenting for Screening, above].

Radiation therapy may be contraindicated for any of several reasons. Some patients choose not to undergo radiation therapy, either because it is inconvenient or because they are concerned about potential complications (including the induction of second malignancies). Some patients simply do not have access to radiation therapy, either because they live in a rural area or because they have physical conditions that make daily trips for therapy cumbersome. Other patients have medical or psychiatric disorders that would make it extremely difficult for them to comply with the daily treatment schedule. Still others have specific medical contraindications to radiation therapy, including pregnancy, collagen vascular disease, or previous irradiation of the chest wall (as in a woman with a local recurrence of a breast carcinoma that was treated with radiation therapy). Although there are some clinical data supporting the use of repeat local excision without further irradiation to treat local recurrence after radiation therapy, most authorities favor mastectomy.[76,77]

When resection of the primary tumor to clean margins would render the appearance of the remaining breast tissue cosmetically unacceptable, mastectomy with immediate reconstruction may be preferable. This is likely to be the case, for example, in patients with large primary tumors relative to their breast size: resection of the primary tumor would remove a substantial portion of the breast tissue. Another example is patients with multiple primary tumors, who would have not only an increased risk of local recurrence but also poor cosmetic results after multiple wide excisions. Patients with superficial central lesions, including Paget disease, are eligible for wide excision (including the nipple and areola) followed by radi-

Table 3 TNM Clinical Classification of Breast Cancer[119]

Tumor (T)

TX   Primary tumor cannot be assessed

T0   No evidence of primary tumor

Tis   Carcinoma in situ: intraductal carcinoma, lobular carcinoma in situ, or Paget disease of the nipple with no invasive tumor

T1   Tumor ≤ 2 cm in greatest dimension

      T1mic: Microinvasion ≤ 0.1 cm

         T1a: Tumor > 0.1 cm and ≤ 0.5 cm

         T1b: Tumor > 0.5 cm and ≤ 1.0 cm

         T1c: Tumor > 1 cm and ≤ 2 cm

T2   Tumor > 2 cm and ≤ 5 cm in greatest dimension

T3   Tumor > 5 cm in greatest dimension

T4   Tumor of any size; direct extension to chest wall or skin

T4a   Extension to chest wall

T4b   Edema (including *peau d'orange*) or ulceration of the skin of the breast or satellite skin nodules confined to the same breast

T4c   Both T4a and T4b

T4d   Inflammatory carcinoma

Nodes (N)

NX   Regional lymph nodes cannot be assessed (e.g., previously removed)

N0   No regional lymph node metastases

N1   Metastasis to movable ipsilateral axillary node(s)

N2   Metastasis to ipsilateral axillary node(s) fixed to one another or other structures

N3   Metastasis to ipsilateral internal mammary lymph node(s)

Metastasis (M)

MX   Presence of distant metastasis cannot be assessed

M0   No distant metastases

M1   Distant metastasis, including metastasis to ipsilateral supra-clavicular lymph node(s)

---

ation therapy, provided that clean margins are obtained. The survival and local recurrence rates in these patients are equivalent to those in other groups of patients undergoing lumpectomy and radiation.[78-80] In many cases, the cosmetic results of this procedure are preferable to those of immediate reconstruction, and there is always the option to reconstruct the nipple and areola later.

Patients who are at high risk for local recurrence often choose mastectomy as primary therapy. Features of primary tumors that are associated with higher local recurrence rates after limited surgery and radiation include gross residual disease after lumpectomy, multiple primary tumors within the breast, an extensive intraductal component, large tumor size, lymphatic vessel invasion, and lobular histologic findings.

In practice, obtaining clean margins is probably the most critical factor in decreasing the risk of local recurrence. The difficulty of obtaining microscopically clean margins in tumors with an extensive intraductal component and in lobular carcinomas may account for the higher local recurrence rates sometimes seen with these tumors. Histologic analysis of mastectomy specimens from patients with tumors with an extensive intraductal component has shown a high rate of multifocality within ipsilateral breast tissue; this residual disease is thought to be the nidus for local recurrence.[81]

The long-term benefits of choosing mastectomy to reduce local recurrences are not clear. Whereas the appearance of distant metastases typically heralds incurable and ultimately fatal disease, local recurrence after breast conservation appears to have little, if any, impact on overall survival. Prospective, randomized trials have had difficulty showing a statistically significant reduction in survival in women who have had a local recurrence after limited surgery and radiation. It has been suggested that additional follow-up may eventually confirm reduced survival in some patients with local recurrences.[82] Still, most of the evidence suggests that local recurrences are not the source of subsequent distant metastases. It is worthwhile to keep in mind, however, that even if mastectomy to prevent local recurrence does not actually improve survival, it may nevertheless provide significant benefit by reducing patient anxiety, the amount of follow-up testing required, and the need for subsequent treatment.

Options for axillary staging Axillary node status is one of the most powerful predictors of prognosis in breast cancer. Staging of the axilla, generally via a level I or II axillary dissection, has been a standard component of breast cancer surgery. Decisions about systemic and radiation therapy are often made on the basis of the number of axillary nodes involved by metastatic disease. The value of axillary dissection has been questioned, however, because of the increased use of systemic therapy even for many node-negative breast cancers as well as the morbidity associated with axillary dissection, including pain, reduced arm mobility, and the risk of lymphedema.

As an alternative to axillary dissection, sentinel lymph node (SLN) biopsy [*see 2:6 Lymphatic Mapping and Sentinel Lymph Node Biopsy*] has become increasingly popular as a way of assessing axillary node status with less morbidity.[83,84] The technique is technically demanding, however, and discussion continues as to the most appropriate way of implementing this approach in general practice.[85] SLN biopsy identifies an increased number of patients with micrometastases, with some identified by immunohistochemical staining alone. Treatment of patients with only micrometastases to axillary nodes remains a topic of debate, to be addressed in an ongoing clinical trial of SLN biopsy by the American College of Surgeons Oncology Group.

Breast reconstruction after mastectomy Breast reconstruction after mastectomy may provide both cosmetic and psychological benefits. In the past, reconstruction was generally delayed for

Table 4 Staging of Breast Cancer[119]

Stage	T	N	M
Stage 0	Tis	N0	M0
Stage I	T1	N0	M0
Stage IIA	T0	N1	M0
	T1	N1	M0
	T2	N0	M0
Stage IIB	T2	N1	M0
	T3	N0	M0
Stage IIIA	T0	N2	M0
	T1	N2	M0
	T2	N2	M0
	T3	N1, N2	M0
Stage IIIB	T4	Any N	M0
	Any T	N3	M0
Stage IV	Any T	Any N	M1

1 to 2 years after mastectomy; now, it is most often performed immediately after mastectomy.[17] This change has not been shown to have any serious adverse effects: it has not significantly increased recurrence or shortened survival, nor has it significantly delayed the detection of local recurrence or the administration of adjuvant chemotherapy.[86] Reconstruction options [*see 2:5 Breast Procedures*] include the placement of subpectoral saline implants (either immediately or after tissue expansion), latissimus dorsi myocutaneous flap reconstruction, and transverse rectus abdominis muscle myocutaneous flap reconstruction. Free flaps may also be employed under special circumstances.

Radiation Therapy

Current radiation therapy regimens consist of the delivery of approximately 5,000 cGy to the whole breast at a dosage of approximately 200 cGy/day, along with, in most cases, the delivery of an additional 1,000 to 1,500 cGy to the tumor bed, again at a dosage of 200 cGy/day. Axillary node fields are not irradiated unless there is evidence that the patient is at high risk for axillary relapse—namely, multiple (generally more than four) positive lymph nodes, extranodal extension of tumor, or bulky axillary disease (i.e., palpable nodes several centimeters in diameter). Because the combination of surgical therapy and radiation therapy increases the risk of lymphedema of the arm, it is appropriate only when there is sufficient risk of axillary relapse to justify the increased complication rate. As a rule, supraclavicular node fields are irradiated only in patients with multiple positive axillary nodes, who are at increased risk for supraclavicular disease. The internal mammary nodes are seldom irradiated prophylactically.

Postmastectomy radiation therapy involves the delivery of radiation to the chest wall after mastectomy; it is mainly reserved for patients with T3 or T4 primary tumors or multiple positive lymph nodes. Such therapy is recommended particularly when there are multiple positive axillary lymph nodes: significant axillary disease predicts higher rates of chest wall recurrence after mastectomy. Two series[87,88] have suggested that postmastectomy radiation therapy significantly improves survival in premenopausal women with any positive axillary nodes.

Irradiation of the breast or chest wall is generally well tolerated: most women experience only minor side effects, such as transient skin erythema, mild skin desquamation, and mild fatigue. Because a small amount of lung volume is included in the irradiated fields, there is usually a clinically insignificant but measurable reduction in pulmonary function. In addition, because the heart receives some radiation when the left breast or left chest wall is treated, there may be a slightly increased risk of future myocardial infarction. There is also a 1% to 2% chance that the radiation will induce a second malignancy (sarcoma, leukemia, or a second breast carcinoma). These radiation-induced malignancies appear after a long lag time, generally 7 to 15 years or longer.

Systemic Drug and Hormone Therapy

Despite the success of surgical treatment and radiation therapy in achieving local control of breast cancer, distant metastases still develop in many patients. Various drugs and hormones have therefore been used to treat both measurable and occult metastatic disease. It became clear in early trials that multiple-agent (or combination) chemotherapy was superior to single-agent chemotherapy.[89,90] It also became clear that chemotherapy and hormone therapy were limited in their ability to control large tumor masses, although on occasion, patients with large tumor masses showed dramatic partial responses or even complete responses to therapy.

Table 5 Determinants of Patient Eligibility for Lumpectomy and Radiation Therapy

Primary tumor ≤ 5 cm (may be larger in selected cases)

Tumor of lobular or ductal histology

Any location of primary within breast if lumpectomy to clean margins (including central lesions) will yield acceptable cosmetic results

Clinically suspicious but mobile axillary nodes

Tumor either positive or negative for estrogen and progesterone receptors

Any patient age

With the goal of eradicating breast cancer metastases while they are still microscopic, systemic therapy is now administered in a so-called adjuvant setting—that is, when there is no evidence of distant metastases but there is sufficient suspicion that metastasis may have occurred. Until the late 1980s, adjuvant chemotherapy was given primarily to women who had axillary node metastases but no other evidence of disease.[89,91,92] In node-positive premenopausal women, adjuvant chemotherapy appeared to be significantly more beneficial than adjuvant hormone therapy. In node-positive postmenopausal women, on the other hand, hormone therapy appeared to be as beneficial as chemotherapy and less toxic.[91]

This approach to adjuvant systemic therapy changed in 1988, when the National Cancer Institute issued a clinical alert stating that there was sufficient evidence of benefit to allow recommendation of adjuvant chemotherapy or hormone therapy for even node-negative breast cancer patients.[93] By that time, a number of studies had shown that adjuvant chemotherapy could improve survival in node-negative breast cancer patients.[92-95] A consensus conference of experts in the field suggested that such therapy be reserved for node-negative women with primary tumors larger than 1 cm in diameter.[96] In 1992, a meta-analysis that reviewed the treatment of 75,000 women in 133 randomized clinical trials of adjuvant therapy for breast cancer concluded that in node-negative premenopausal women, overall long-term survival was 20% to 30% higher in those who received chemotherapy than in those who did not.[97] This benefit also appeared to extend to postmenopausal women between 50 and 60 years of age. A 1998 overview of the use of adjuvant tamoxifen in randomized trials[98] demonstrated that in women with ER-positive tumors, those given tamoxifen for 5 years had a 47% reduction in tumor recurrence and a 26% reduction in mortality, compared with those women who were given placebo. In this analysis, the effects of tamoxifen on recurrence and survival were independent of age and menopausal status. Tamoxifen did not appear to improve survival, however, in women with ER-negative tumors. These results, together with data on the efficacy of tamoxifen for chemoprevention, have led to increased use of tamoxifen for premenopausal women and for women with small tumors.

TREATMENT OF NONINVASIVE CANCER

Ductal Carcinoma in Situ

Before mammographic screening was widely practiced, ductal carcinoma in situ (DCIS) was generally identified either as a palpable lesion (usually with comedo histology) or as an incidental finding on a biopsy performed for another lesion. With the increasing use of mammography, DCIS is accounting for a growing proportion of breast cancer cases. The diagnosis of DCIS is now made in 6.6% of all needle-localized breast biopsies and 1.4% of breast bi-

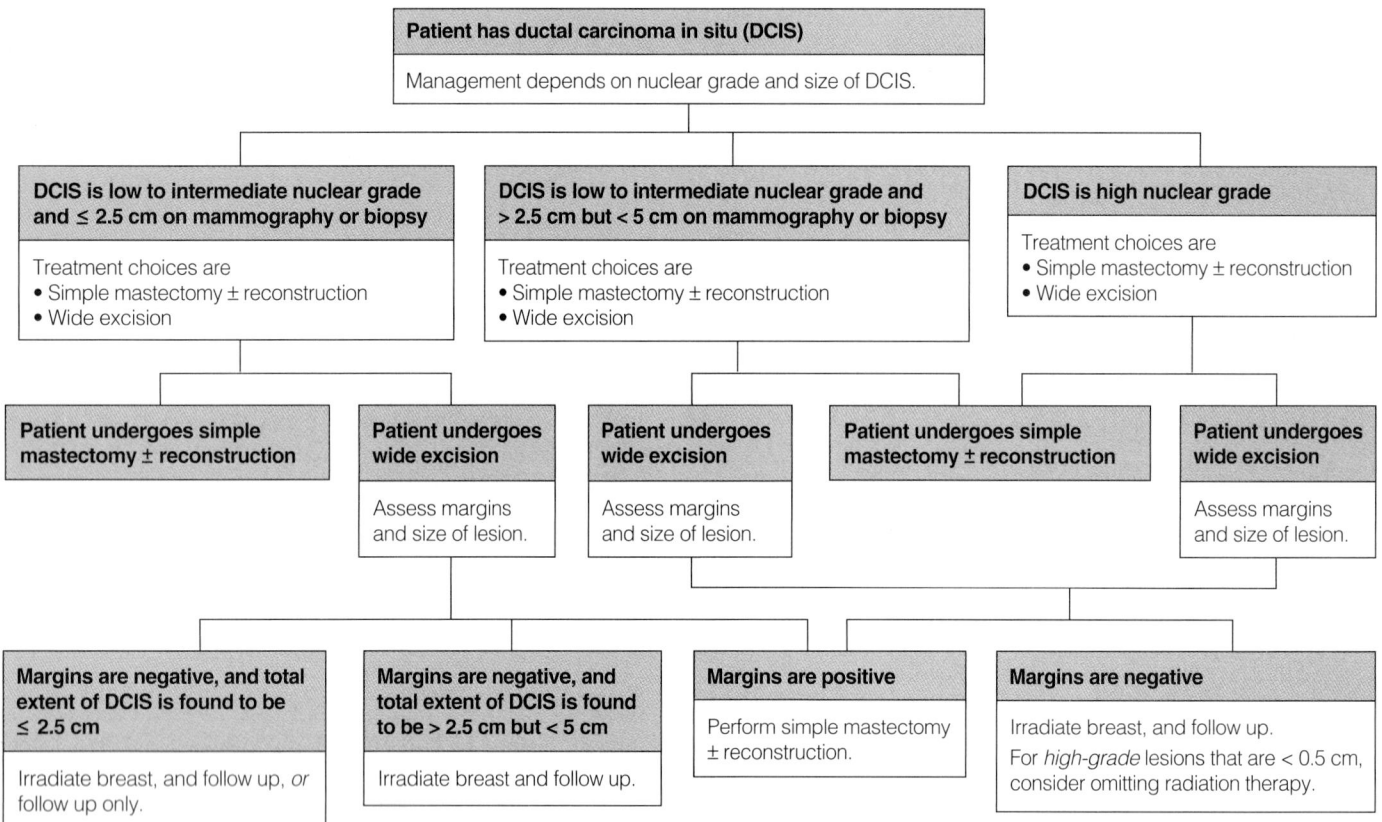

Figure 1 **Algorithm illustrates the approach to managing ductal carcinoma in situ.**

opsies for palpable lesions. About 30% of all mammographically detected malignancies are DCIS.[14]

It was recognized early on that DCIS had a very favorable prognosis compared with other forms of breast cancer: long-term survival approached 100% after treatment with mastectomy. Axillary lymph nodes were positive in only 1% to 2% of patients, most of whom had large or palpable lesions or comedo histology. The prognosis for DCIS continues to be very favorable in relation to that for invasive breast cancers. In theory, there is no potential for metastatic disease with a purely in situ lesion. In practice, however, axillary node metastases continue to be found in 1% to 2% of patients thought to have pure DCIS, presumably arising from a small area of invasion that was missed on pathologic evaluation.

DCIS is believed to be a true anatomic precursor of invasive breast cancer. There are at least two lines of evidence that support this conclusion. First, when DCIS is treated with biopsy alone (usually because it was missed on the initial biopsy and not found until subsequent review), invasive carcinoma develops in 25% to 50% of patients at the site of the initial biopsy; all these tumors appear within 10 years and are of ductal histology. Second, when DCIS recurs locally after breast conservation, invasive ductal carcinoma appears in about 50% of patients. The true relationship between DCIS and invasive ductal carcinoma awaits a better understanding of the molecular biology of breast cancer development.

The consequence of the view that DCIS is a precursor of invasive cancer is that treatment is required once the diagnosis is made. Treatment options for DCIS are similar to those for invasive breast cancer [*see Figure 1*]; however, it should be remembered that although the risk of local recurrence is greater after breast conservation for DCIS than after mastectomy, the likelihood of metastatic disease is very small. Wide excision to microscopically clean margins fol-

lowed by radiation therapy has become an accepted alternative to mastectomy. Smaller areas of DCIS, particularly of low to intermediate nuclear grade, are increasingly treated with wide excision without radiation.[99] If clean margins cannot be obtained or if the cosmetic result is expected to be poor after excision to clean margins, mastectomy should be performed. The NSABP B-17 study,[100] which examined the role of radiation in the treatment of DCIS, found that the addition of radiation therapy to wide excision reduced the recurrence rate at 43 months after operation by approximately half, from 16.4% with wide excision alone to 7.0% with wide excision and radiation. The report also suggested that the addition of radiation therapy may reduce the incidence of invasive recurrences.

Most patients in whom DCIS is identified mammographically can choose between mastectomy and wide excision with or without radiation, either of which yields excellent long-term survival. Given the lack of any significant difference in survival between the two options, the patient must weigh her feelings about the risk of a local, possibly invasive, recurrence after breast conservation against her feelings about the cosmetic and psychological effects of mastectomy. Mastectomy remains a reasonable treatment even for patients with very small DCIS lesions if the primary concern is to maximize local control of the cancer. Breast reconstruction after mastectomy for DCIS is an option that is open to most such patients.

Axillary dissection is not usually performed in conjunction with lumpectomy for DCIS, because the probability of positive nodes is low: it increases morbidity and expense while providing little prognostic information. On the other hand, low axillary dissection is often included in mastectomy for DCIS: a level I axillary dissection adds little morbidity to a mastectomy, and many surgeons believe that dissection must be carried into the low axilla to ensure that the entire axillary tail of the breast is removed.

In some patients with areas of mammographically detected DCIS lesions measuring less than 2.5 cm in diameter, it may be possible to omit radiation therapy, particularly if the lesions do not have comedo histology. Omission of radiation therapy is a complex decision that should be based on the individual patient's histology, the presence or absence of other risk factors, the presence or absence of contraindications to radiation therapy, and the degree to which the patient is willing to accept a higher local recurrence rate. This option is probably best pursued in the context of a clinical trial.

There are certain patients with DCIS for whom mastectomy remains the preferred treatment, such as those who have lesions larger than 5 cm in diameter. Some surgeons would also include those who have comedo lesions larger than 2.5 cm and those who present with palpable DCIS in this category. In these patients, the local recurrence rate after breast conservation, even in conjunction with radiation therapy, remains high. As many as half of these recurrences will contain invasive cancer with metastatic potential. These also are the DCIS patients who are at highest risk for positive axillary nodes. For this reason, an axillary node sampling is often performed in conjunction with the mastectomy.

Lobular Carcinoma in Situ

LCIS, also referred to as lobular neoplasia,[101] does not have the same clinical implications as DCIS, invasive ductal carcinoma, or invasive lobular carcinoma. It is now generally accepted that LCIS is a predictor of increased risk of subsequent invasive breast carcinoma rather than a marker of the site at which the subsequent carcinoma will arise.[13,14] Most of the carcinomas that develop after a biopsy showing LCIS are of ductal histology.[102-104] The increased risk of subsequent carcinoma is equally distributed between the biopsied breast and the contralateral breast and is thought to be between 20% and 25% in patients with LCIS and no other risk factors; it may be additive with other risk factors [see Risk Factors for Breast Cancer, above]. Because the two breasts are at equal risk for future carcinoma, unilateral mastectomy is inappropriate. Appropriate treatment options include (1) careful observation coupled with physical examination two or three times annually and mammograms annually, (2) prophylactic bilateral simple mastectomies with or without reconstruction, and (3) chemoprevention with tamoxifen or participation in chemoprevention trials with other agents. Most patients choose the first option, but there are some patients for whom prophylactic mastectomy is still preferable, either because of patient anxiety or because of concurrent risk factors.[105]

Management of tumors that contain LCIS mixed with invasive carcinoma of either lobular or ductal histology is dictated primarily by the features of the invasive carcinoma. Staging is not affected by the presence of LCIS.

TREATMENT OF INVASIVE CANCER

Although the optimal treatment regimen for breast cancer continues to be the subject of active investigation, there is at least a par-

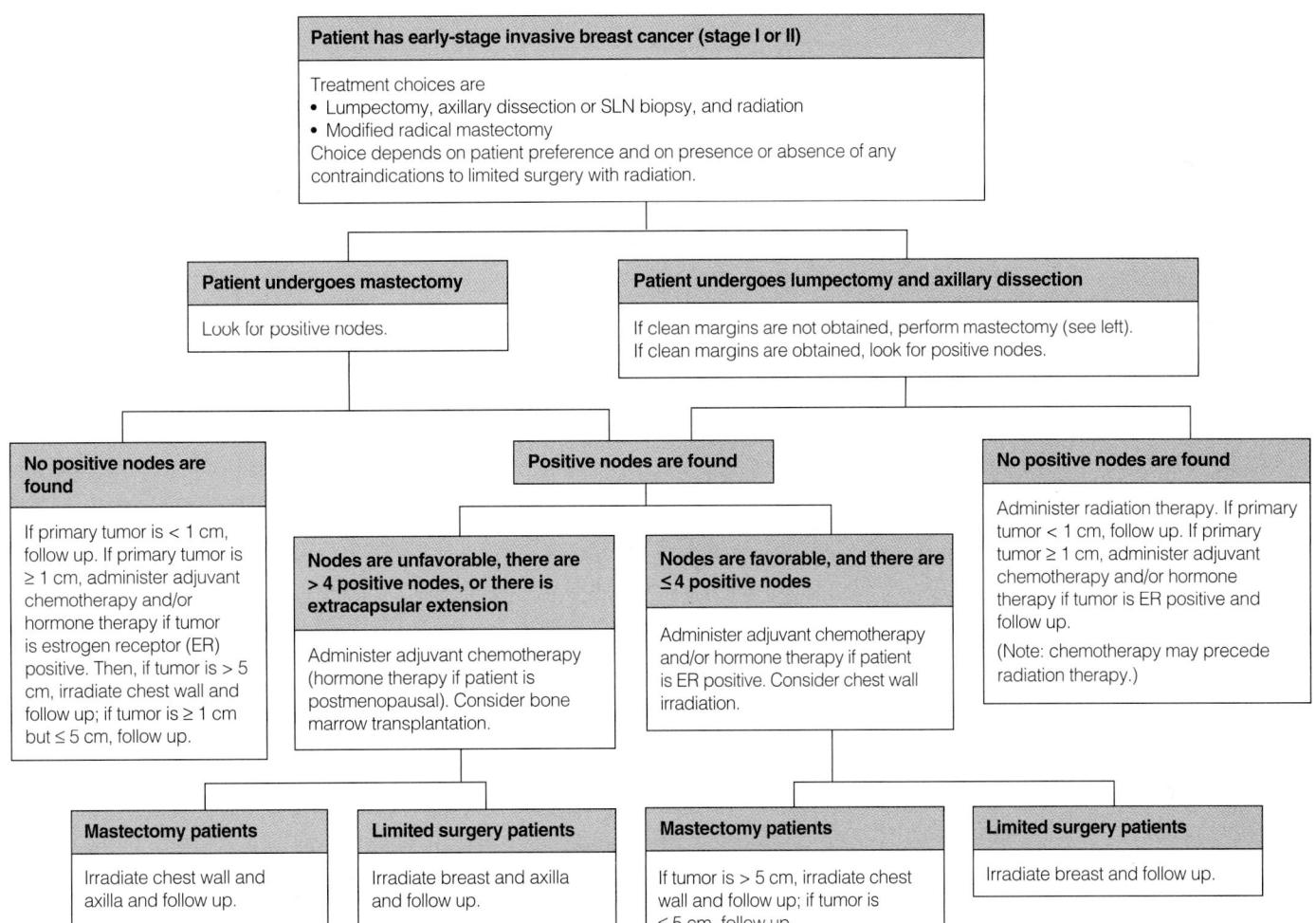

Figure 2 **Algorithm illustrates the approach to managing early-stage invasive breast cancer.**

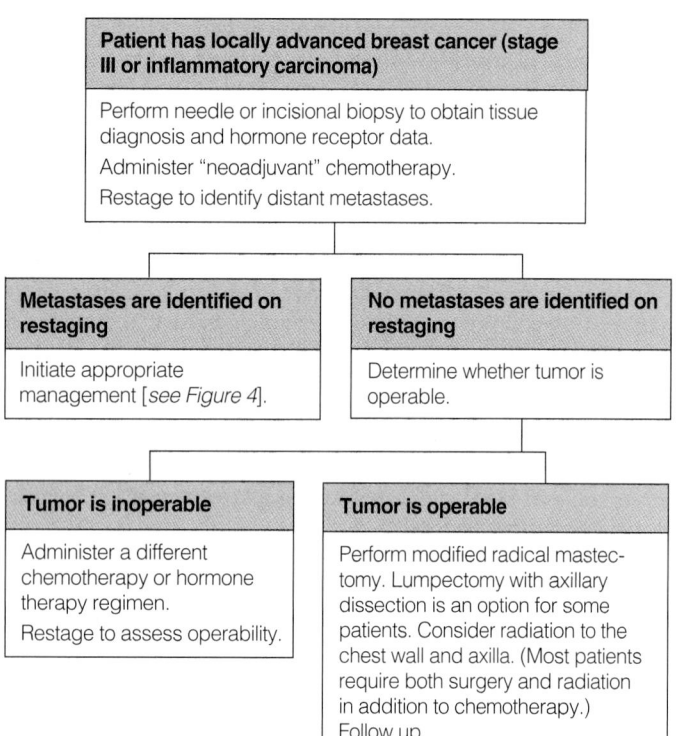

Patient has locally advanced breast cancer (stage III or inflammatory carcinoma)

Perform needle or incisional biopsy to obtain tissue diagnosis and hormone receptor data.
Administer "neoadjuvant" chemotherapy.
Restage to identify distant metastases.

Metastases are identified on restaging

Initiate appropriate management [*see Figure 4*].

No metastases are identified on restaging

Determine whether tumor is operable.

Tumor is inoperable

Administer a different chemotherapy or hormone therapy regimen.
Restage to assess operability.

Tumor is operable

Perform modified radical mastectomy. Lumpectomy with axillary dissection is an option for some patients. Consider radiation to the chest wall and axilla. (Most patients require both surgery and radiation in addition to chemotherapy.)
Follow up.

Figure 3 **Algorithm illustrates the approach to managing locally advanced breast cancer.**

tial consensus regarding current treatment options for the various stages of breast cancer.

Early-Stage Invasive Cancer

Local treatment In patients with stage I or II breast cancer, lumpectomy to microscopically clean margins combined with axillary dissection and radiation therapy [*see Figure 2*] appears to yield approximately the same long-term survival rates as mastectomy. Patients undergoing lumpectomy and radiation are, however, at risk for local recurrence in the treated breast as well as for the development of a new primary tumor in the remaining breast tissue. Local recurrences can generally be managed with mastectomy; overall survival is equivalent to that of women who underwent mastectomy at the time of initial diagnosis. There may, however, be a significant cost to the patient in terms of anxiety about recurrence, as well as the morbidity and potential mortality associated with undergoing a second surgical procedure.

On the other hand, patients who choose mastectomy as their initial surgical treatment face the psychological consequences of losing a breast. Although they are at lower risk for local recurrence than patients who choose lumpectomy, axillary node dissection, and radiation, their overall survival does not seem to be significantly improved. Each physician and each patient must weigh the inconvenience and potential complications of radiation therapy and the risk of local recurrence against the value of breast preservation, keeping in mind that the choice between procedures appears to have no significant effect on survival.

Adjuvant therapy It is generally agreed that adjuvant chemotherapy, adjuvant hormone therapy, or both should be considered for all women with tumors larger than 1 cm in diameter, even those with negative axillary lymph nodes.[96,97] For patients with tumors that have a very favorable prognosis (i.e., that are smaller than 1 cm or have a fa-

vorable histology), the potential benefits of adjuvant therapy are probably outweighed by its risks. Tamoxifen therapy is now being reconsidered for women with such low-risk tumors, given the data on the efficacy of this agent for both treatment and prevention of breast cancers.[98] In premenopausal women, adjuvant therapy should consist of combination chemotherapy, with hormone therapy reserved for clinical trials; in postmenopausal women, hormone therapy (generally consisting of tamoxifen, 10 mg twice daily) is the first-line treatment. Currently, however, the idea that menopause should be an absolute cutoff point for consideration of chemotherapy is being reassessed. For healthy postmenopausal women, particularly those between 50 and 60 years of age, the decision between hormone therapy and chemotherapy plus hormone therapy is made on an individual basis and takes into account the woman's overall health and the specifics of her tumor.

In cases of node-positive disease, combination chemotherapy is used for premenopausal women and for healthy postmenopausal women up to 60 years of age or even older. Hormone therapy is generally the treatment of choice in postmenopausal women who are older than 60 years and in poor health, particularly those with ER-positive tumors. There is currently renewed interest in other hormonal manipulations, such as oophorectomy and chemical castration, for premenopausal women who are at high risk for metastatic disease.[106]

Locally Advanced Cancer

Patients with locally advanced breast cancer include those with primary tumors larger than 5 cm (particularly those with palpable axillary lymph nodes), those with fixed or matted N2 axillary nodes, and those with inflammatory breast carcinoma. These patients are at high risk for systemic disease as well as for local failure after standard local therapy. Current practice is to administer multimodality therapy, with chemotherapy as the first treatment modality [*see Figure 3*]. This so-called neoadjuvant chemotherapy often has the effect of downstaging local disease, in some cases making inoperable tumors amenable to surgical resection. Patients are treated with FNA, core-needle, or open incisional biopsy to obtain a tissue diagnosis, hormone receptor data, and HER-2/*neu* status; they then undergo careful restaging after systemic therapy to identify any distant metastases. If the tumor responds to chemotherapy, the patient may then undergo radiation therapy, surgery, or both. Most patients require all three modalities for optimum local and systemic control.

The optimum treatment of patients with stage IIIa breast cancer remains controversial. Some practitioners favor neoadjuvant chemotherapy, whereas others favor surgery followed by chemotherapy and radiation therapy. The choice of surgical procedure for women with locally advanced breast cancer is also controversial. Whereas many surgeons favor mastectomy for all tumors larger than 5 cm, others offer wide excision with axillary dissection to patients in whom excision to clean margins will leave a cosmetically acceptable breast.

Stage IV Cancer

Patients who have distant metastases, whether at their initial presentation or after previous treatment for an earlier-stage breast cancer, are rarely cured. Before treatment begins, a tissue diagnosis consistent with breast cancer must be obtained from the primary lesion (at the initial presentation of the disease) or from a metastasis (if there is any doubt about the metastatic nature of the lesion or the source of the metastatic disease). Any tissue samples obtained should be sent for estrogen and progesterone receptor assays.

The usual first-line treatment for metastatic breast cancer is cytotoxic chemotherapy or hormone therapy [*see Figure 4*]. Radiation therapy may be used to relieve pain from bone metastases or to avert a pathologic fracture at a site of metastatic disease. There is also occasionally a role for so-called toilet mastectomy for patients who have metastatic disease and a locally advanced and ulcerated primary tumor if the condition of the primary tumor prevents the administration of needed chemotherapy.

Treatment for stage IV breast cancer should be on protocol whenever possible. For patients who are ineligible for therapy on protocol, palliative chemotherapy or hormone therapy may be the best treatment option.

FOLLOW-UP AFTER TREATMENT

Patients who have been treated for breast cancer remain at risk for both the recurrence of their original tumor and the development of a new primary breast cancer. The rate of recurrence of breast cancer is nearly linear over the first 10 years after treatment. After the first decade, recurrence becomes less likely, but it continues at a significant rate through the second decade and beyond. In patients who have undergone limited surgery and radiation therapy, radiation-induced breast and chest wall malignancies begin to appear 7 or more years after treatment and continue to appear for at least 20 years after treatment.

Follow-up of breast cancer patients thus includes screening of the breasts and nodal areas for locoregional recurrence or a new primary tumor by means of physical examination and mammography. There is no general agreement on the optimum intervals for follow-up. For patients treated with breast conservation, annual mammography is appropriate, beginning after any acute radiation reaction has resolved (generally 6 to 9 months after completion of radiation therapy). For patients treated with mastectomy, mammography should be continued on an annual basis for the contralateral breast. Physical examination and review of symptoms are generally performed at 3- to 6-month intervals for the first 5 years after completion of therapy, although these intervals have not yet been tested in a prospective fashion.

Although there has been little debate about the value of early detection of a local recurrence within the treated breast or of a new primary tumor in either breast, there has been a great deal of debate about the value of early detection of metastatic disease. Two prospective, randomized trials addressed this issue. In one, a group of breast cancer patients was intensively followed with blood tests every 3 months along with chest x-rays, bone scans, and liver ultrasonography annually.[107] There was no difference in survival or quality of life between this group and the control group, and metastatic disease was diagnosed, on average, less than 1 month earlier in the intensively followed group than in the control group. In the second study, a group of breast cancer patients received chest x-rays and bone scans every 6 months for 5 years.[108] Pulmonary and bone metastases were detected significantly earlier in this group than in the control group, but there was no improvement in survival. This study demonstrated that early detection of metastatic disease could be achieved with short-interval screening, but given current therapeutic options, early detection had no beneficial effect on survival. Both studies concluded that at present, there is no role for routine imaging studies in the follow-up of breast cancer patients and that imaging studies should be ordered only as prompted by clinical findings.

FUTURE DIRECTIONS IN TREATMENT

Efforts continue to be made to minimize the number and extent of invasive treatments for breast cancer without compromising survival or local control. Trials are now under way whose aim is to explore the need for radiation therapy for tumors in elderly women or tumors consisting of pure DCIS. The need for axillary dissection has been questioned, and the idea that features of the primary tumor rather than axillary node status should be

used to determine the prognosis and the need for adjuvant therapy is being discussed. Trials of SLN biopsy are under way.

Many current trials of chemotherapy for breast cancer focus on increasing the efficacy of treatment through dose intensification. Very high dose chemotherapy in conjunction with administration of growth factor or autologous bone marrow transplantation is being assessed in the hope that higher doses of chemotherapy will improve response rates and duration of response.

The early results from studies of bone marrow transplantation have been somewhat disappointing: median survival is prolonged by only 7 to 10 months beyond what is achievable with more standard chemotherapy.[109] There is, however, a small but significant group of long-term survivors who remain free of disease for more than 5 years after undergoing bone marrow transplantation to treat breast cancer with 10 or more positive lymph nodes at initial presentation.[108] Trials of improved bone marrow transplantation regimens continue in the hope that the toxicity and cost of the treatment can be reduced and the number of long-term survivors increased.

Immune therapy using antibodies to HER-2/*neu* protein, alone or in conjunction with chemotherapy, is being evaluated for tumors that overexpress the oncogene HER-2/*neu*. At present, there is no definitive evidence that the biologic therapies and immune therapies now available are of significant value in the treatment of breast cancer. These types of therapy continue to be actively explored.

Even more exciting than the prospect of improved therapy is the concept of chemoprevention—that is, the use of pharmacologic, hormonal, or other interventions to prevent the development or progression of a malignancy. Positive results of trials using tamoxifen for chemoprevention have raised hopes that many breast cancers can be prevented and have increased interest in identifying additional agents that can reduce breast cancer risk with minimal side effects. These results underscore the importance of understanding risk factors for breast cancer, including gene mutations, to better identify women who might benefit from chemoprevention.

MULTIDISCIPLINARY BREAST CANCER CARE

Care of even the earliest breast cancers now routinely entails consultation with and treatment by several specialists, including surgeons, radiation oncologists, medical oncologists, radiologists, and pathologists. The selection and timing of individual treatments are determined by this team of physicians in consultation with the patient. This process is greatly simplified when the physicians concerned are able

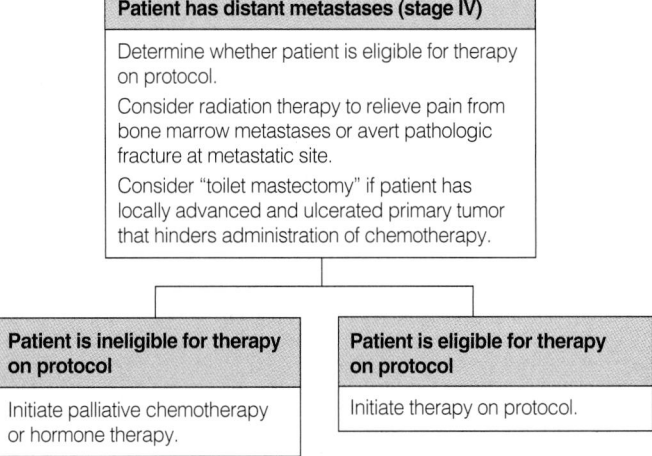

Figure 4 **Algorithm illustrates the approach to managing stage IV breast cancer.**

to coordinate their visits with the patient, thereby both saving time for the patient and facilitating decision making among the various specialists. A number of centers have established multidisciplinary breast centers that allow a patient to see all the specialists in a single visit while also allowing the physicians to consult with each other in reviewing the clinical data, imaging studies, and pathology and determining treatment options.

Patient education is also becoming more and more critical in the management of breast cancer. Patients are increasingly being asked to participate in decision making, and as hospital stays for breast cancer

treatments become shorter, they are also being asked to participate more actively in their own care. To participate effectively, patients must be educated about the advantages and disadvantages of the various aspects of cancer management. The shifting of a larger proportion of cancer care to the outpatient setting also necessitates the use of other support services, such as visiting nurses, social workers, and outpatient infusion services. How best to coordinate these complex services while maintaining a focus on the problems and needs of the individual patient remains one of the major challenges faced by physicians caring for patients with breast cancer.

References

1. Henderson IC: Risk factors for breast cancer development. Cancer 71(suppl):2127, 1993
2. Slattery ML, Kerber RA: A comprehensive evaluation of family history and breast cancer risk. JAMA 270:1563, 1993
3. Newcomb PA, Storer BE, Longnecker MP, et al: Lactation and a reduced risk of premenopausal breast cancer. N Engl J Med 330:81, 1994
4. Marchant DJ: Estrogen-replacement therapy after breast cancer: risk versus benefits. Cancer 71(suppl):2169, 1993
5. Squitieri R, Tartter PI, Ahmed S, et al: Carcinoma of the breast in postmenopausal hormone user and non-user control groups. J Am Coll Surg 178:167, 1994
6. Steinberg KK, Thacker SB, Smith SJ, et al: A meta-analysis of the effect of estrogen replacement therapy. JAMA 265:1985, 1991
7. Wingo PA, Lee NC, Ory H, et al: Age specific differences in the relationship between oral contraceptive use and breast cancer. Obstet Gynecol 78:161, 1991
8. Colditz GA, Stampfer MJ, Willett WC: Prospective study of estrogen replacement therapy and risk of breast cancer in post-menopausal women. JAMA 264:2648, 1990
9. Dupont WD, Page DL: Menopausal estrogen-replacement therapy and breast cancer. Arch Intern Med 151:67, 1991
10. Hunter DJ, Manson JE, Colditz GA, et al: A prospective study of the intake of vitamins C, E, and A and the risk of breast cancer. N Engl J Med 329:234, 1993
11. Willett WC, Hunter DJ, Stampfer MJ, et al: Dietary fat and fiber in relation to risk of breast cancer: an 8-year follow-up. JAMA 268:2037, 1992
12. Armstrong B, Doll R: Environmental factors and cancer incidence and mortality in different countries, with special reference to dietary practices. Int J Cancer 15:617, 1975
13. Page DL, Jensen RA: Evaluation and management of high risk and premalignant lesions of the breast. World J Surg 18:32, 1994
14. Frykberg ER, Bland KI: Management of in situ and minimally invasive breast carcinoma. World J Surg 18:45, 1994
15. Jacobs TJ, Byrne C, Colditz G, et al: Radial scars in benign breast-biopsy specimens and the risk of breast cancer. N Engl J Med 340:430, 1999
16. Fletcher SW, Black W, Harris R, et al: Report of the International Workshop on Screening for Breast Cancer. J Natl Cancer Inst 85:1644, 1989
17. Osteen RT, Cady B, Chmiel JS, et al: 1991 national survey of carcinoma of the breast by the Commission on Cancer. J Am Coll Surg 178:213, 1994
18. Surveillance, Epidemiology, and End Results: Incidence and Mortality Data, 1973-1977. DHEW Publ No. (NIH)81-2330. Public Health Service, Bethesda, Maryland, 1981

19. Donegan WL: Evaluation of a palpable breast mass. N Engl J Med 327:937, 1992
20. Rosner D, Blaird D: What ultrasonography can tell in breast masses that mammography and physical examination cannot. J Surg Oncol 28:308, 1985
21. Hamed H, Coady A, Chaudary MA, et al: Follow-up of patients with aspirated breast cysts is necessary. Arch Surg 124:253, 1989
22. Cowen PN, Benson GA: Cytological study of fluid from benign breast cysts. Br J Surg 66:209, 1979
23. Sartorius O, Smith H, Morris P, et al: Cytologic evaluation of breast fluid in the detection of breast disease. J Natl Cancer Inst 59:1073, 1977
24. Ciatto S, Cariaggi P, Bulgaresi P: The value of routine cytologic examination of breast cyst fluids. Acta Cytol 31:301, 1987
25. Leis HP Jr: Gross breast cysts: significance and management. Contemp Surg 39(2):13, 1991
26. Hughes LE, Bundred NJ: Breast macrocysts. World J Surg 13:711, 1989
27. Boyd NF, Sutherland HJ, Fish EB, et al: Prospective evaluation of physical examination of the breast. Am J Surg 142:331, 1981
28. Layfield LJ, Glasgow BJ, Cramer H: Fine-needle aspiration in the management of breast masses. Pathol Annu 24:23, 1989
29. Silverman JS, Tameness A: Mammary fibroadenoma and some phyllodes tumor stroma are composed of CD34+ fibroblasts and factor XIIIa+ dendrophages. Histopathology 29:411, 1996
30. Dietrich CU: Karyotypic changes in phyllodes tumors of the breast. Cancer Genet Cytogenet 78:200, 1994
31. Noguchi S, Yokouchi H, Aihara T, et al: Progression of fibroadenoma to phyllodes tumor demonstrated by clonal analysis. Cancer 76:1779, 1995
32. Shimizu K: Cytologic evaluation of phyllodes tumors as compared to fibroadenomas of breast. Acta Cytol 38:891, 1994
33. Mangi AA, Smith BL, Gadd MA, et al: Surgical management of phyllodes tumors. Arch Surg 134:487, 1999
34. Hall FM, Storella JM, Silverstone DZ, et al: Non-palpable breast lesions: recommendations for biopsy based on suspicion of carcinoma at mammography. Radiology 167:353, 1988
35. Sickles EA: Periodic mammographic follow-up of probably benign lesions: results in 3,184 consecutive cases. Radiology 179:463, 1991
36. Wolfe JN, Buck KA, Salane M, et al: Xeroradiography of the breast: overview of 21,057 consecutive cases. Radiology 165:305, 1987
37. Helvie MA, Pennes DR, Rebner M, et al: Mammographic follow-up of low-suspicion lesions: compliance rate and diagnostic yield. Radiology 178:155, 1991
38. Takeda T, Suzuki M, Sato Y, et al: Cytologic studies of nipple discharge. Acta Cytol 26:35, 1982

39. Chaudary M, Millis R, Davies G, et al: Nipple discharge: the diagnostic value of testing for occult blood. Ann Surg 196:651, 1982
40. Urban JA: Excision of the major duct system of the breast. Cancer 16:516, 1963
41. Passaro ME, Broughan TA, Sebek BA, et al: Lactiferous fistula. J Am Coll Surg 178:29, 1994
42. Watt-Boolsen S, Eskildsen P, Blaehr H: Release of prolactin, thyrotropin and growth hormone in women with cyclical mastalgia and fibrocystic disease of the breast. Cancer 56:500, 1985
43. Pashby NL, Mansel RE, Hughes LE, et al: A clinical trial of evening primrose oil in mastalgia. Br J Surg 68:801, 1981
44. Baker H, Snedecor P: Clinical trial of danazol for benign breast disease. Am Surg 45:727, 1979
45. Laursen N, Wilson K: The effect of danazol in the treatment of chronic cystic mastitis. Obstet Gynecol 48:93, 1976
46. Mansel R, Preece P, Hughes L: A double blind trial of the prolactin inhibitor bromocriptine in painful benign breast disease. Br J Surg 65:724, 1978
47. Fentiman I, Caleffi M, Brame K, et al: Double-blind controlled trial of tamoxifen therapy for mastalgia. Lancet 1:287, 1986
48. Benson EA: Management of breast abscesses. World J Surg 13:753, 1989
49. Niebyl JR, Spence MR, Parmley TH: Sporadic (nonepidemic) puerperal mastitis. J Reprod Med 20:97, 1978
50. Brook I: Microbiology of non-puerperal breast abscesses. J Infect Dis 157:377, 1988
51. Walker AP, Edmiston CE, Krepel CJ, et al: A prospective study of the microflora of nonpuerperal breast abscess. Arch Surg 123:908, 1988
52. Smith BL: Duct ectasia, periductal mastitis, and breast infections. Breast Diseases. Harris JR, Hellman S, Henderson IC, et al, Eds. JB Lippincott Co, Philadelphia, 1991, p 38
53. Hadfield J: Excision of the major duct system for benign disease of the breast. Br J Surg 47:472, 1960
54. Gail MG, Brinton LA, Byar DP, et al: Projecting individualized probabilities of developing breast cancer for white females who are being examined annually. J Natl Cancer Inst 81:1879, 1989
55. Claus EB, Risch N, Thompson WD: Autosomal dominant inheritance of early-onset breast cancer: implications for risk prediction. Cancer 73:643, 1994
56. Lynch HT, Marcus JN, Watson P, et al: Familial breast cancer, family cancer syndromes and predisposition to breast neoplasia. The Breast: Comprehensive Management of Benign and Malignant Diseases. Bland KI, Copeland EM, Eds. WB Saunders Co, Philadelphia, 1991, p 262
57. Hartmann LC, Schaid DJ, Woods JE, et al: Efficacy of bilateral prophylactic mastectomy in women with a family history of breast cancer. N Engl J Med 340: 77, 1999

58. Schrag D, Kuntz KM, Garber JE, et al: Decision analysis—effects of prophylactic mastectomy and oophorectomy on life expectancy among women with BRCA1 or BRCA2 mutations. N Engl J Med 336:1465, 1997

59. Zujewski J: Selective estrogen receptor modulators (SERMS) and retinoids in breast cancer chemoprevention. Environ Mol Mutagen 39:264, 2002

60. Fisher B, Costantino JP, Wickerham DL, et al: Tamoxifen for prevention of breast cancer: report of the National Surgical Adjuvant Breast and Bowel Project P-1 Study. J Natl Cancer Inst 90:1371, 1998

61. Powles T, Eeles R, Ashley S, et al: Interim analysis of the incidence of breast cancer in the Royal Marsden Hospital tamoxifen randomised chemoprevention trial. Lancet 352:98, 1998

62. Veronesi U, Maisonneuve P, Costs A, et al: Prevention of breast cancer with tamoxifen: preliminary findings from the Italian randomised trial among hysterectomised women. Lancet 352:93, 1998

63. Dalton R, Kallab A: Chemoprevention of breast cancer. South Med J 94:7, 2001

64. Cummings S, Eckert S, Kreuger K, et al: The effect of raloxifene on risk of breast cancer in postmenopausal women: results from the MORE randomized trial. Multiple Outcomes of Raloxifene Evaluation. JAMA 281:2189, 1999

65. Goss P, Strasser K: Chemoprevention with aromatase inhibitors—trial strategies. J Steroid Biochem Mol Biol 79:143, 2001

66. Fabian CJ: Breast cancer chemoprevention: beyond tamoxifen. Breast Cancer Res 3:99, 2001

67. Veronesi U, Banfi A, DelVecchio M, et al: Comparison of Halstead mastectomy with quadrantectomy, axillary dissection and radiotherapy in early breast cancer: long term results. Eur J Cancer Clin Oncol 22:1085, 1986

68. Sarrazin D, Le M, Rouesse J, et al: Conservative treatment versus mastectomy in breast cancer tumors with macroscopic diameter of 20 millimeters or less: the experience of the Institut Gustave Roussy. Cancer 53:1209, 1984

69. Fisher B, Bauer M, Margolese R, et al: Five-year results of a randomized clinical trial comparing total mastectomy and segmental mastectomy with or without radiation in the treatment of breast cancer. N Engl J Med 312:665, 1985

70. Fisher B, Redmond C, Poisson R, et al: Eight year results of a randomized clinical trial comparing total mastectomy and lumpectomy with or without irradiation in the treatment of breast cancer. N Engl J Med 320:822, 1989

71. Farrow DC, Hunt WC, Samot JM: Geographic variation in the treatment of localized breast cancer. N Engl J Med 326:1097, 1992

72. Nattinger AB, Gottlieb MS, Veum J, et al: Geographic variation in the use of breast-conserving treatment for breast cancer. N Engl J Med 326:1102, 1992

73. Osteen RT, Steele GD, Menck HR, et al: Regional differences in surgical management of breast cancer. Cancer 42:39, 1992

74. Lazovich D, White E, Thomas DB, et al: Underutilization of breast conserving surgery and radiation therapy among women with stage I or II breast cancer. JAMA 266:3433, 1991

75. Lee-Feldstein A, Anton-Culver H, Feldstein PJ: Treatment differences and other prognostic factors related to breast cancer survival: delivery systems and medical outcomes. JAMA 271:1163, 1994

76. Kurtz JM, Spitalier JM, Almaric R, et al: Results of wide excision for local recurrence after breast-conserving therapy. Cancer 61:1969, 1989

77. Haffty GB, Goldberg NB, Rose M, et al: Conservative surgery with radiation therapy in clinical stage I and II breast cancer: results of a 20 year experience. Arch Surg 124:1266, 1989

78. Harris JR, Hellman S, Kinne DW: Limited surgery and radiotherapy for early breast cancer. N Engl J Med 313:1365, 1985

79. Clarke DH, Le M, Sarrazin D, et al: Analysis of local regional relapses in patients with early breast cancers treated by excision and radiotherapy: experience of the Institut Gustave Roussy. Int J Radiat Oncol Biol Phys 11:137, 1985

80. Fisher B, Wolmark N: Limited surgical management for primary breast cancer: a commentary on the NSABP reports. World J Surg 9:682, 1985

81. Holland R, Connolly JL, Gelman R, et al: The presence of an extensive intraductal component following a limited excision correlates with prominent residual disease in the remainder of the breast. J Clin Oncol 8:113, 1990

82. Harris JR, Osteen RT: Patients with early breast cancer benefit from effective axillary treatment. Breast Cancer Res Treat 5:17, 1985

83. Krag D, Weaver D, Ashikaga T, et al: The sentinel node in breast cancer: a multicenter validation study. N Engl J Med 339:941, 1998

84. Giuliano AE, Jones RC, Brennan MM, et al: Sentinel lymphadenectomy in breast cancer. J Clin Oncol 15:2345, 1997

85. McMasters KM, Giuliano AE, Ross MI, et al: Sentinel-lymph node biopsy for breast cancer—not yet the standard of care. N Engl J Med 339:990, 1998

86. Eberlein TJ, Crespo LD, Smith BL, et al: Prospective evaluation of immediate reconstruction following mastectomy. Ann Surg 218:29, 1993

87. Overgaard M, Hansen PS, Overgaard J, et al: Postoperative radiotherapy in high-risk premenopausal women with breast cancer who receive adjuvant chemotherapy. N Engl J Med 337:949, 1997

88. Ragaz J, Jackson SM, Le N, et al: Adjuvant radiotherapy and chemotherapy in node-positive premenopausal women with breast cancer. N Engl J Med 337:956, 1997

89. Bonadonna G, Valagussa P, Tancini G, et al: Current status of Milan adjuvant chemotherapy trials for node-positive and node-negative breast cancer. J Natl Cancer Inst Monogr 1:45, 1986

90. Fisher B, Redmond C, Fisher E, et al: Systemic adjuvant therapy in treatment of primary operable breast cancer: NSABP experience. J Natl Cancer Inst Monogr 1:35, 1986

91. Consensus Conference: Adjuvant chemotherapy for breast cancer. JAMA 254:3461, 1985

92. Fisher B, Costantino J, Redmond C, et al: A randomized trial evaluating tamoxifen in the treatment of patients with node-negative breast cancer who have estrogen-receptor-positive tumors. N Engl J Med 320:479, 1989

93. Clinical Alert from the National Cancer Institute. Department of Human Services, National Cancer Institute, National Institutes of Health, May 16, 1988

94. Fisher B, Redmond C, Dimitrov NV, et al: A randomized clinical trial evaluating sequential methotrexate and fluorouracil in the treatment of patients with node-negative breast cancer who have estrogen-receptor-negative tumors. N Engl J Med 320:473, 1989

95. Mansour EG, Gray R, Shatila NH, et al: Efficacy of adjuvant chemotherapy in high-risk node-negative breast cancer. N Engl J Med 320:485, 1989

96. NIH Consensus Conference: Treatment of early-stage breast cancer. JAMA 265:391, 1991

97. Early Breast Cancer Trialists' Collaborative Group: Systemic treatment of early breast cancer by hormonal, cytotoxic, or immune therapy: 133 randomised trials involving 31,000 recurrences and 24,000 deaths among 75,000 women. Lancet 339:71, 1992

98. Tamoxifen for early breast cancer: an overview of the randomised trials. Early Breast Cancer Trialists' Collaborative Group. Lancet 351:1451, 1998

99. Silverstein MJ, Lagios MD, Groshen S, et al: The influence of margin width on local control of ductal carcinoma in situ of the breast. N Engl J Med 340:1455, 1999

100. Fisher B, Costantino J, Redmond C, et al: Lumpectomy compared with lumpectomy and radiation therapy for the treatment of intraductal breast cancer.

N Engl J Med 328:1581, 1993

101. Haagensen CD, Lane N, Lattes R, et al: Lobular neoplasia (so-called lobular carcinoma in situ) of the breast. Cancer 42:737, 1978

102. Rosen PP: Lobular carcinoma in situ and intraductal carcinoma of the breast. Monogr Pathol 25:59, 1984

103. Rosen PP, Kosloff C, Lieberman PH, et al: Lobular carcinoma in situ of the breast: detailed analysis of 99 patients with average follow-up of 24 years. Am J Surg Pathol 2:225, 1978

104. Fisher ER, Fisher B: Lobular carcinoma of the breast: an overview. Ann Surg 185:377, 1977

105. Kinne D: Clinical management of lobular carcinoma in situ. Breast Diseases. Harris JR, Hellman S, Henderson IC, et al, Eds. JB Lippincott Co, Philadelphia, 1991, p 239

106. Scottish Cancer Trials Breast Group: Adjuvant ovarian ablation versus CMF chemotherapy in premenopausal women with pathological stage II breast carcinoma: the Scottish trial. Lancet 341:1293, 1993

107. GIVIO Investigators: Impact of follow-up testing on survival and health-related quality of life in breast cancer patients. JAMA 271:1587, 1994

108. Del Turco MR, Palli D, Cariddi A, et al: National Research Council Project on Breast Cancer Follow-up. Intensive diagnostic follow-up after treatment of primary breast cancer: a randomized trial. JAMA 271:1593, 1994

109. Peters WP: High-dose chemotherapy and autologous bone marrow support for breast cancer. Important Advances in Oncology. DeVita VT Jr, Hellman S, Rosenberg SA, Eds. JB Lippincott Co, Philadelphia, 1991, p 135

110. Hammond S, Keyhani-Rofagha S, O'Toole RV: Statistical analysis of fine needle aspiration cytology of the breast: a review of 678 cases plus 4,265 cases from the literature. Acta Cytol 31:276, 1987

111. Dowlatshahi KD, Yaremko ML, Kluskens LF, et al: Nonpalpable breast lesions: findings of stereotaxic needle-core biopsy and fine-needle aspiration cytology. Radiology 181:745, 1991

112. Ballo MS, Sneige N: Can core needle biopsy replace fine needle aspiration cytology in the diagnosis of palpable breast carcinoma: a comparative study of 124 women. Cancer 78:773, 1996

113. Smith DN, Christian R, Meyer JE: Large-core needle biopsy of nonpalpable breast cancers: the impact on subsequent surgical excisions. Arch Surg 132:256, 1997

114. El-Ashry D, Lippman ME: Molecular biology of breast carcinoma. World J Surg 18:12, 1994

115. Slamon DJ, Godolphin W, Jones LA, et al: Studies of the HER-2/neu proto-oncogene in human breast and ovarian cancer. Science 244:707, 1989

116. Gusterson BA, Gelber RD, Goldhirsch A, et al: Prognostic importance of c-erbB-2 expression in breast cancer: International (Ludwig) Breast Cancer Study Group. J Clin Oncol 10:1049, 1992

117. Perren TJ: C-erbB-2 oncogene as a prognostic marker in breast cancer (editorial). Br J Cancer 63:328, 1991

118. Gullick WJ, Love SB, Wright C, et al: C-erbB-2 protein overexpression in breast cancer is a risk factor in patients with involved and uninvolved lymph nodes. Br J Cancer 63:434, 1991

119. American Joint Committee on Cancer: AJCC Cancer Staging Manual, 5th ed. Lippincott-Raven Publishers, Philadelphia, 1997, p 171

Acknowledgments

Figure 1   Marcia Kammerer.

Figures 2 through 4   Talar Agasyan.

2 SOFT TISSUE INFECTION

Ronald T. Lewis, M.B.B.S., M.Sc., F.A.C.S., F.R.C.S.(C)

Approach to the Patient with Soft Tissue Infection

The key to successful treatment of soft tissue infection is early recognition of infections that require prompt surgical drainage and debridement. It is convenient to classify lesions into those that are focal, such as cutaneous abscesses and pyoderma gangrenosum, and those that are diffuse and often require emergency treatment, such as cellulitis and necrotizing cellulitic infections. (There are also certain miscellaneous conditions, such as bite wound infections and purpura fulminans, that do not fit neatly into either category; these conditions are considered separately.) Many lesions appear deceptively innocent at first and are mistaken for nonspecific inflammation. To prompt recognition and effective treatment of any lesion, the answers to five questions should be sought:

1. Is infection present?
2. Is there an underlying systemic condition present that favors infection?
3. Should antibiotics be given?
4. Which antibiotics are most appropriate?
5. Is surgical treatment required?

Focal Inflammation

The history together with the clinical appearance of a focal lesion will indicate whether it is a minor, confined cutaneous abscess or a more serious, spreading focal lesion such as pyoderma gangrenosum. Cutaneous abscesses are very common and are readily recognized. Pyoderma gangrenosum, on the other hand, is a rare condition.

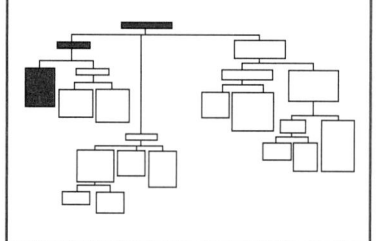

CONFINED CUTANEOUS ABSCESS

A cutaneous abscess is a walled-off collection of pus that presents as a painful fluctuant mass, usually with surrounding erythema and firm granulation tissue. It is treated by incision and drainage. Gram stain and culture of the pus are not done routinely, because antibiotics are not generally given. Antibiotics may be helpful, however, in immunocompromised patients and in patients with abscesses of the central area of the face. In such cases, the findings on Gram stain suggest appropriate antibiotic therapy. Gram-positive cocci in clusters indicate *Staphylococcus aureus*, which may be treated with an oral semisynthetic penicillin (e.g., cloxacillin, 0.5 to 1.0 g every 6 hours for 5 to 7 days). Mixed gram-positive and gram-negative bacilli represent an infection by aerobic and anaerobic organisms that can be treated with an oral cephalosporin (e.g., cephalexin, 0.5 g every 6 hours for 5 to 7 days). Occasionally, white blood cells but no organisms are seen. This finding confirms a sterile abscess, for which antibiotics are not needed.

SPREADING FOCAL LESION

Classic Pyoderma Gangrenosum

Classic pyoderma gangrenosum is characterized by a painful, raised pustular lesion that progresses to spreading ulceration with a

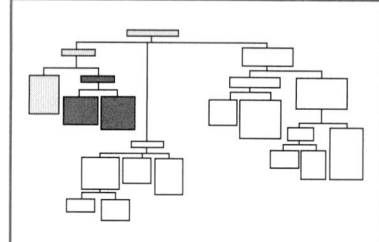

typical necrotic center, bluish undermined edges, and surrounding erythema [*see Figure 1*].[1] It occurs either singly or in groups, most often on the legs. The lesions may localize at sites of minor trauma (so-called pathergy). Fever, malaise, myalgias, and arthralgias are common. A biopsy is usually performed to rule out disorders that produce similar lesions: ischemic ulceration, vasculitis of periarteritis nodosa, and chronic bacterial, mycobacterial, or fungal disorders. Massive neutrophil infiltration and necrosis of the epidermis are typical. In contrast with vasculitis, only minor vessel wall infiltration is present with pyoderma gangrenosum. Underlying disease, often parainflammatory or hemoproliferative, is present in 60% to 80% of cases.[2] The most common concomitant conditions are inflammatory bowel disease (especially ulcerative colitis),[1] polyarthritis,[3] monoclonal gammopathy,[4] and malignant hematologic neoplasms (especially leukemia).[5] Four variants have been identified: peristomal (seen, for example, in Crohn disease); vulvar or penoscrotal, simulating the lesions of Behçet disease; oral (peristomatitis vegetans); and bullous. The skin lesion seen in leukemia is typically

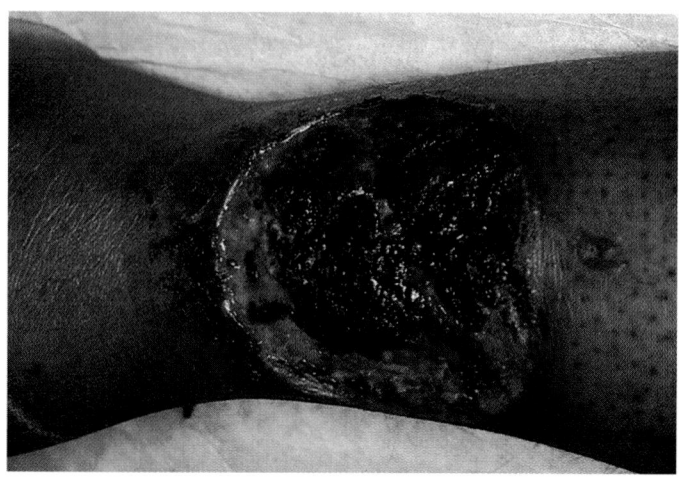

Figure 1 In this photograph of an advanced pyoderma gangrenosum lesion, the darker area surrounding the necrotic center corresponds to the violaceous zone of intense erythema.

142

the bullous variant: it remains superficial and exhibits more subdued colors than the classic lesion. About 30% of cases are idiopathic and remain so on follow-up of more than 2 years.[6]

Investigations should include Gram stain and culture of a biopsy specimen. Pyogenic organisms commonly grow from swabs of the central ulcer, but it is unlikely that these organisms are significant. Studies that should be performed to rule out underlying diseases include a complete blood count; blood chemistry studies; and immunologic tests, including assays for antinuclear antibody, rheumatoid factor, and serum protein as well as immunoglobulin electrophoresis. A chest x-ray, upper gastrointestinal series, and barium enema should also be done.

Treatment is controversial but should always include *specific therapy for the underlying disorder*. Thus, in patients with inflammatory bowel disease, colon resection may produce lasting remission of the skin lesions,[2] and in some patients with leukemia, pyoderma gangrenosum has improved or cleared completely after chemotherapy.[5]

Various antimicrobials have been used with success. They include sulfasalazine (4 g/day) and the antimycobacterial agent clofazimine (300 mg/day), as well as minocycline and rifampin. These agents, particularly sulfasalazine and clofazimine, may act not as antibiotics but by enhancing neutrophil phagocytosis and intracellular bacterial killing and by stimulating macrophage activity. Prednisone, 40 to 120 mg/day, and cyclosporin A, 5 mg/day, produce long-term remission in almost half of cases; however, 3 to 6 months of glucocorticoid treatment may be required before lesions heal, and fatal complications have been reported after such treatment.[3] Current theories suggest that the lesions of pyoderma gangrenosum may be caused by serum immune complexes or by defects in cellular or humoral immunity. Overexpression of interleukin-8 (IL-8) has been identified in subepidermal neutrophils. Cyclosporin A acts on T cells to limit production of interleukins, thereby reversing the ratio of T helper to T suppressor cells.[7] Resistant cases may respond to oral tacrolimus, 0.1 to 0.3 mg/kg/day, and topical tacrolimus, 0.1% in paraffin or beeswax.[8] This new immunosuppressive drug inhibits T-cell activation by blocking receptor-mediated signal transduction pathways. Intravenous immunoglobulin therapy may be helpful in cases of resistant disease.[9] Immunosuppressive therapy with azathioprine, cyclophosphamide, or dapsone is less effective[10] but is

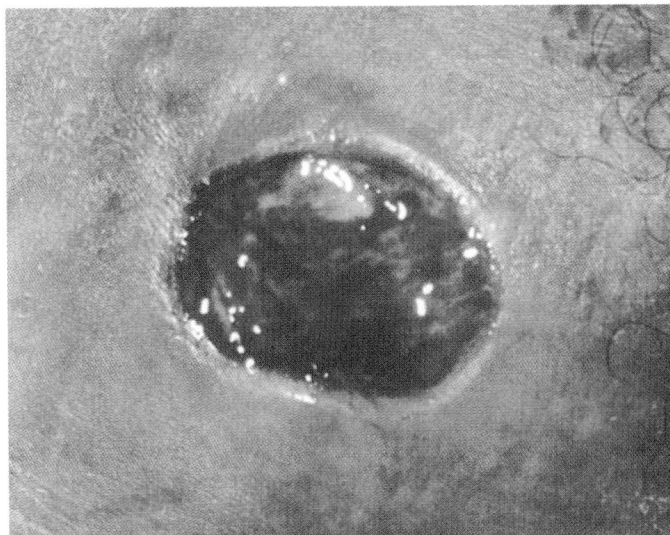

Figure 2 **This chronic ulcer of the lateral malleolus shows the violaceous discoloration, rolled edges, nongranulating base, and watery discharge characteristic of an atypical mycobacterial lesion.**

useful for maintenance purposes in patients with inflammatory bowel disease.

Topical measures include wet-to-dry dressings and intralesional injection or surface application of antibacterials and immune agents. Saline compresses provide some debridement. Aggressive debridement and skin grafting have been condemned,[2] but some workers[11] have reported dramatic improvement with surgical debridement. Heng has observed abundant formation of granulation tissue and arrest of extension of ulceration by a simplified topical application of hyperbaric oxygen (HBO).[12]

Superficial Atypical Mycobacterial Lesions

In cases of nonhealing extremity ulcers unresponsive to conventional surgical and antibiotic treatment, the possibility of an atypical mycobacterial infection should be considered. Although rare, indo-

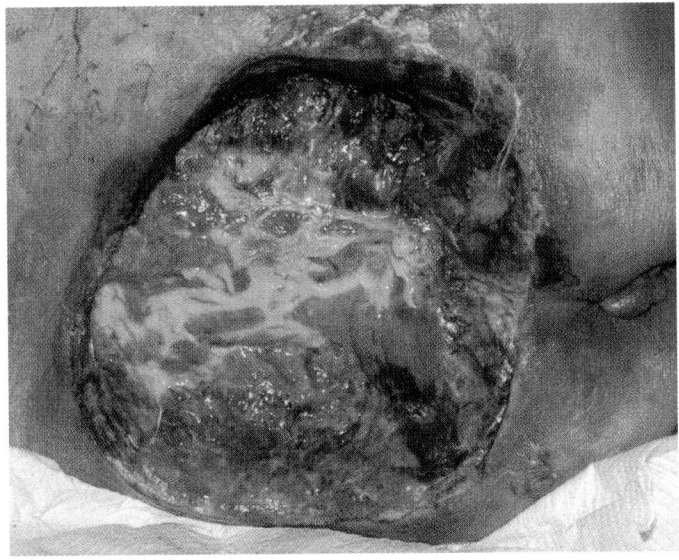

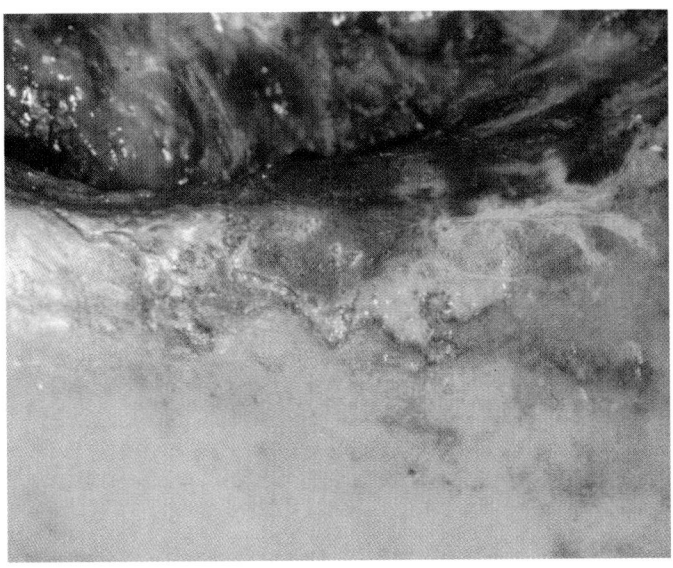

Figure 3 **Progressive bacterial gangrene has developed in the decubitus ulcer shown at left. The edge of the necrotic lesion shows the three characteristic zones of necrosis, discoloration, and erythema (right).**

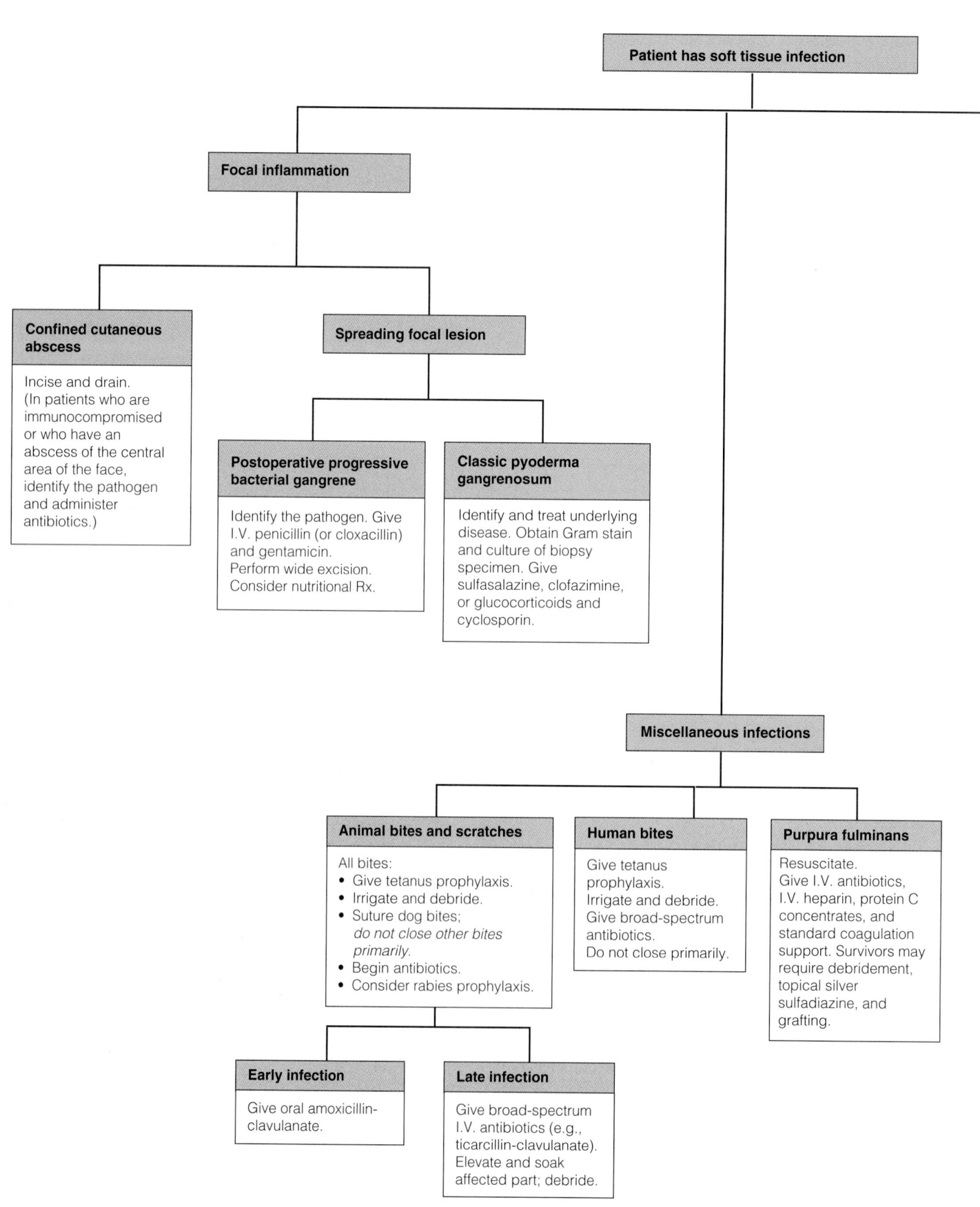

Patient has soft tissue infection

Focal inflammation

Confined cutaneous abscess

Incise and drain.
(In patients who are immunocompromised or who have an abscess of the central area of the face, identify the pathogen and administer antibiotics.)

Spreading focal lesion

Postoperative progressive bacterial gangrene

Identify the pathogen. Give I.V. penicillin (or cloxacillin) and gentamicin.
Perform wide excision.
Consider nutritional Rx.

Classic pyoderma gangrenosum

Identify and treat underlying disease. Obtain Gram stain and culture of biopsy specimen. Give sulfasalazine, clofazimine, or glucocorticoids and cyclosporin.

Miscellaneous infections

Animal bites and scratches

All bites:
• Give tetanus prophylaxis.
• Irrigate and debride.
• Suture dog bites;
  do not close other bites primarily.
• Begin antibiotics.
• Consider rabies prophylaxis.

Human bites

Give tetanus prophylaxis.
Irrigate and debride.
Give broad-spectrum antibiotics.
Do not close primarily.

Purpura fulminans

Resuscitate.
Give I.V. antibiotics, I.V. heparin, protein C concentrates, and standard coagulation support. Survivors may require debridement, topical silver sulfadiazine, and grafting.

Early infection

Give oral amoxicillin-clavulanate.

Late infection

Give broad-spectrum I.V. antibiotics (e.g., ticarcillin-clavulanate). Elevate and soak affected part; debride.

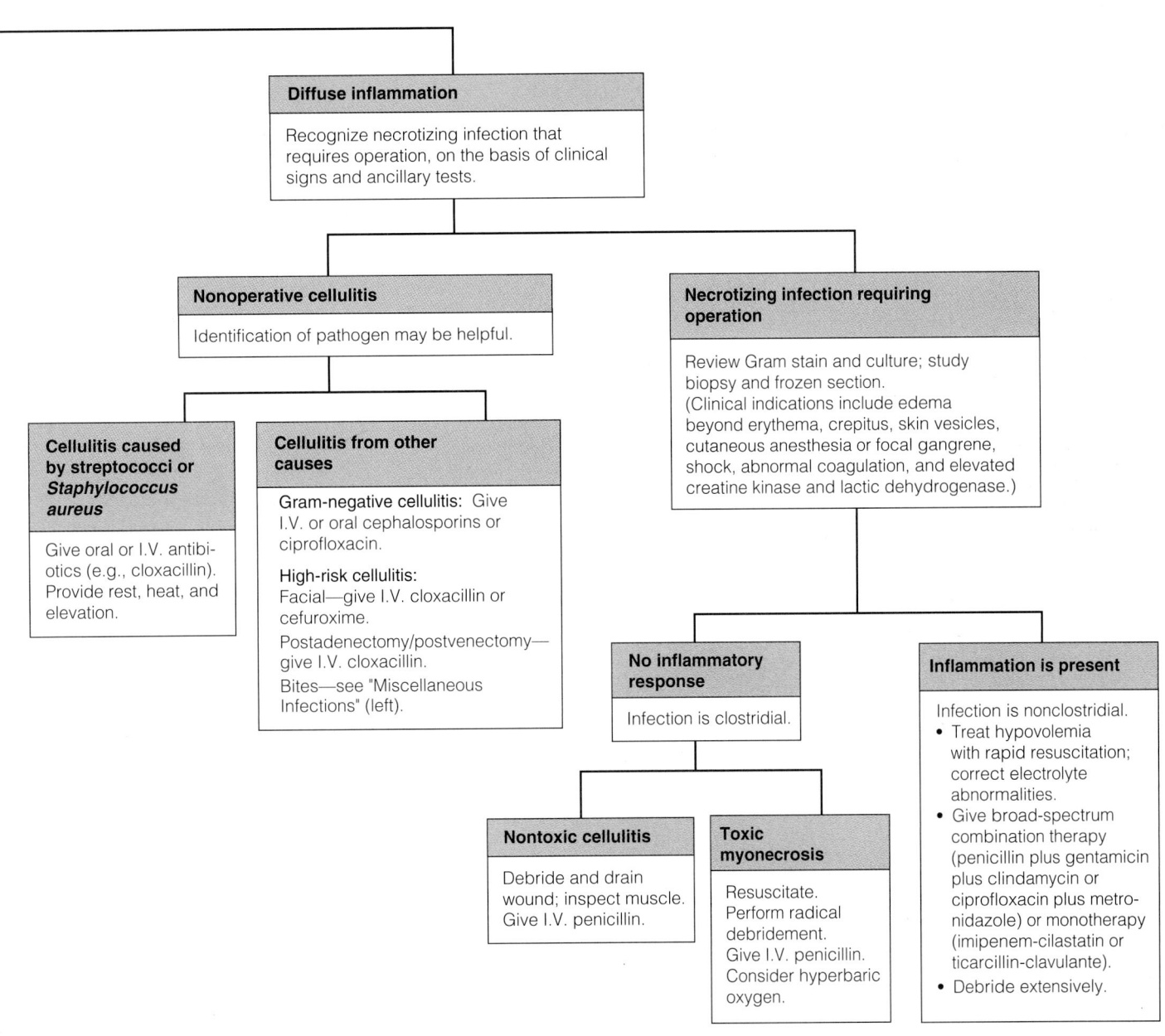

Diffuse inflammation

Recognize necrotizing infection that requires operation, on the basis of clinical signs and ancillary tests.

Nonoperative cellulitis

Identification of pathogen may be helpful.

Cellulitis caused by streptococci or *Staphylococcus aureus*

Give oral or I.V. antibiotics (e.g., cloxacillin). Provide rest, heat, and elevation.

Cellulitis from other causes

Gram-negative cellulitis: Give I.V. or oral cephalosporins or ciprofloxacin.

High-risk cellulitis: Facial—give I.V. cloxacillin or cefuroxime. Postadenectomy/postvenectomy—give I.V. cloxacillin. Bites—see "Miscellaneous Infections" (left).

Necrotizing infection requiring operation

Review Gram stain and culture; study biopsy and frozen section. (Clinical indications include edema beyond erythema, crepitus, skin vesicles, cutaneous anesthesia or focal gangrene, shock, abnormal coagulation, and elevated creatine kinase and lactic dehydrogenase.)

No inflammatory response

Infection is clostridial.

Nontoxic cellulitis

Debride and drain wound; inspect muscle. Give I.V. penicillin.

Toxic myonecrosis

Resuscitate. Perform radical debridement. Give I.V. penicillin. Consider hyperbaric oxygen.

Inflammation is present

Infection is nonclostridial.
• Treat hypovolemia with rapid resuscitation; correct electrolyte abnormalities.
• Give broad-spectrum combination therapy (penicillin plus gentamicin plus clindamycin or ciprofloxacin plus metronidazole) or monotherapy (imipenem-cilastatin or ticarcillin-clavulante).
• Debride extensively.

Approach to the Patient with Soft Tissue Infection

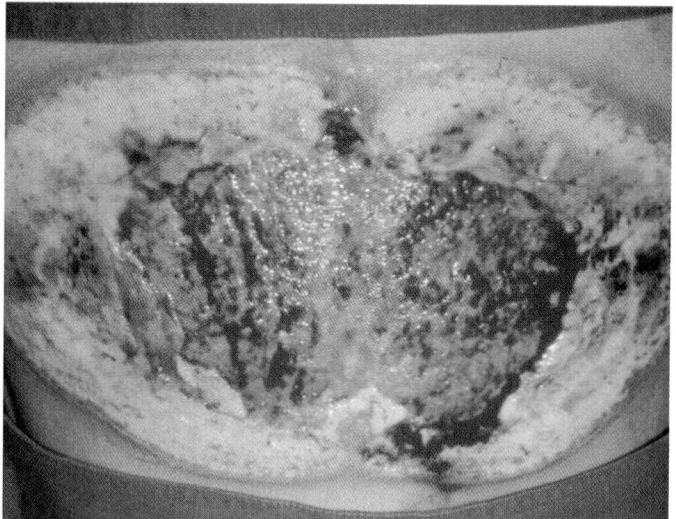

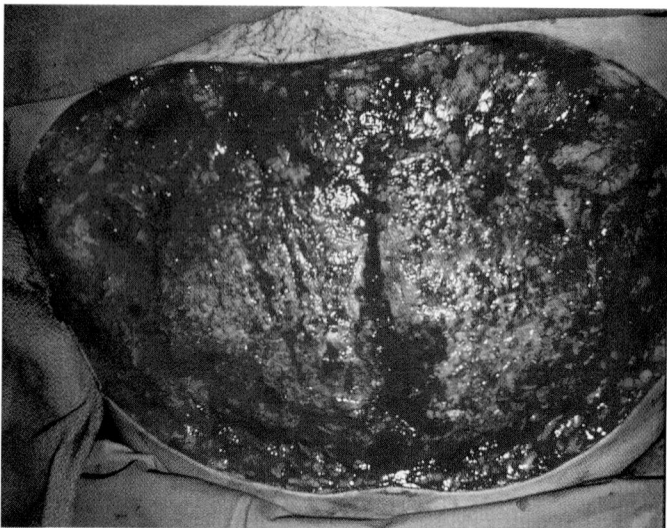

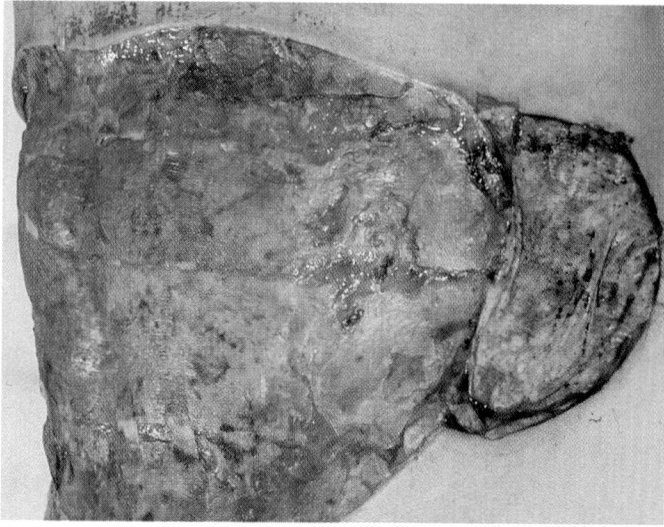

Figure 4 **Progressive bacterial gangrene developed in this patient's abdominal wall after cesarean section. In photograph at top, the lesion has been partially excised; extension of necrosis is evident. The lesion was widely excised (center). Extension of necrosis into the flank necessitated further excision and skin grafting (bottom); skin grafts done earlier on the central lesion are healing.**

lent mycobacterial lesions that closely resemble pyoderma gangrenosum have been observed. In one study, infected ulcers in four steroid-dependent patients yielded atypical mycobacteria upon culture of the excised tissue. Two ulcers contained *Mycobacterium smegmatis*, which rarely causes disease in humans; the third, *M. kansasii;* and the fourth, *M. chelonei.*[13] The lesions presented as chronic ulcerations with violaceous edges, rolled margins, a nongranulating base, and watery discharge [*see Figure 2*]. In three of the four patients, wide local excision and intravenous antibiotic therapy followed by oral antibiotic therapy were required for successful treatment. One patient was treated successfully with debridement and oral antibiotic therapy.

Because experience in treating these ulcers has been limited, the best antibiotic therapy is uncertain. *M. kansasii* is usually sensitive to rifampin, isoniazid, and ethambutol; and *M. chelonei* is sensitive to amikacin, cefoxitin, tetracycline, and erythromycin. All three species respond well to cefoxitin (1 g every 6 hours) or to quinolones (e.g., ciprofloxacin, 0.4 g every 12 hours); accordingly, these agents should be prescribed.

Postoperative Progressive Bacterial Gangrene

The postoperative progressive bacterial gangrene of Meleney[14] is considered to be a variant of classic pyoderma gangrenosum.[11] The lesion appears 2 weeks or more after accidental trauma or after operative management of purulent peritoneal or pleural infection; it is characterized by wound edema, redness, and tenderness that progress to the three characteristic zones of pyoderma gangrenosum: a necrotic center, bluish undermined edges, and surrounding erythema [*see Figure 3*]. Fever, muscle wasting, and toxicity are often present. A swab taken from the central necrotic area usually yields hemolytic *S. aureus* on culture; later in the course of the illness, it may show gram-negative bacilli. Needle aspirate from the outer zone may grow microaerophilic nonhemolytic streptococci.

Broad-spectrum parenteral antibiotics should be started promptly and are useful in reducing systemic toxicity. Penicillin, 1 to 2 million units I.V. every 6 hours, along with gentamicin, 1.5 mg/kg every 8 hours, may be given, but if *S. aureus* is found on Gram stain, cloxacillin, 1 to 2 g every 6 hours, is substituted for penicillin. Antibiotic therapy is followed by wide excision of the skin lesion [*see Figure 4*]. The wound is left open to granulate, and skin grafts are applied later. Researchers found that HBO reduced the extent of excision required,[15,16] but the value of HBO therapy is controversial in this and other necrotizing soft tissue infections [*see* Diffuse Inflammation, Inflammatory Response Is Absent (Clostridial Infection), *below*]. Because these patients have marked systemic manifestations and significant muscle wasting, supportive nutritional therapy may be of benefit [*see 6:23 Nutritional Support*].

Diffuse Inflammation

NECROTIZING INFECTION
REQUIRING OPERATION

In managing diffuse inflammatory lesions, it is crucial to recognize necrotizing infections promptly because they require surgical debridement. To spot a

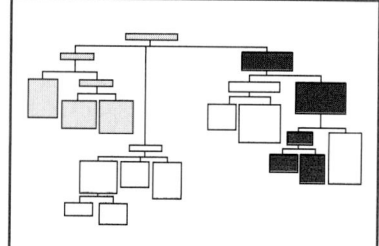

necrotizing infection, one must know the clinical setting in which it often occurs and must identify certain clinical clues. In some

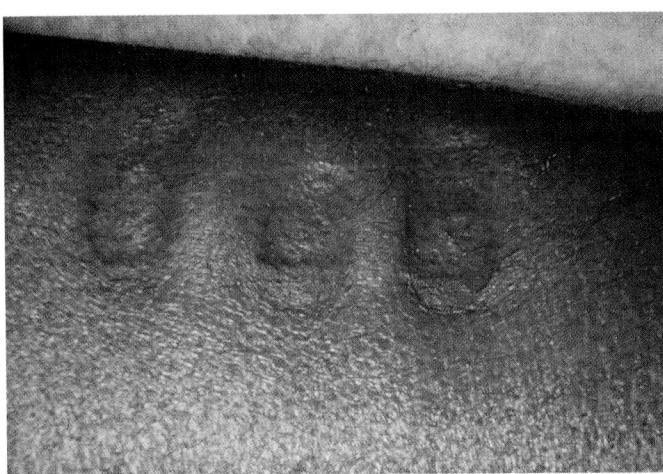

Figure 5 **Edema extending beyond the area of erythema is a marker of necrotizing soft tissue infection.**

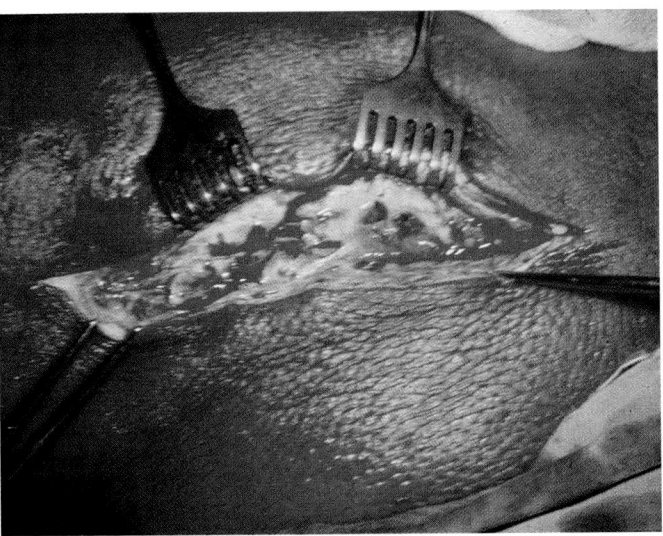

Figure 6 **In this patient with necrotizing fasciitis, edema is present without skin vesicles, and there is necrosis of the deep layer of the superficial fascia.**

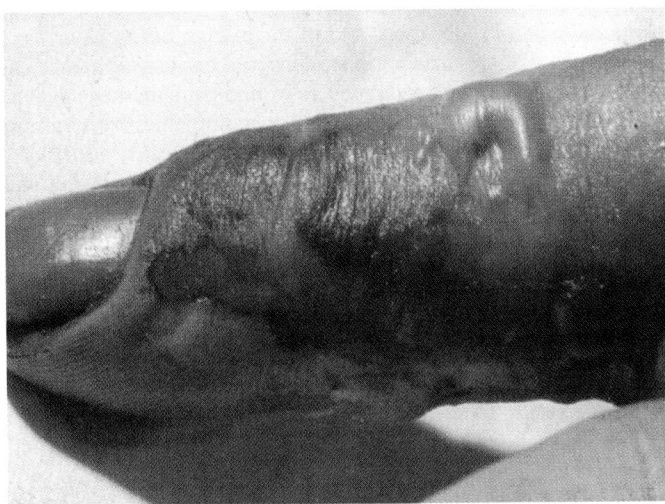

Figure 7 **Skin vesicles such as those on this patient's finger are seen early in streptococcal gangrene.**

cases, ancillary studies may help finalize the diagnosis. Necrotizing infections usually occur in patients with impaired host defense mechanisms, such as the elderly, those receiving immunosuppressive therapy, or those with an underlying systemic illness, such as cancer, chronic renal failure, chronic alcoholism, diabetes mellitus, or peripheral vascular disease. When cellulitis occurs in these patients, a necrotizing infection should be suspected. The initiating factor for necrotizing infections is often surprisingly minor, perhaps because of the poor host resistance. For example, necrotizing infections can occur in areas of blunt soft tissue contusion associated with a distant focus of infection.[17]

Important early clinical markers of necrotizing soft tissue infection include edema beyond the area of erythema, crepitus, and skin vesicles [*see Figures 5 through 7*]. The lymphangitis and lymphadenitis commonly seen in patients with nonoperative cellulitis are absent. In later stages of infection, cutaneous anesthesia, focal skin gangrene, shock, and impaired blood coagulation may occur.

Useful ancillary studies include soft tissue x-rays and blood chemistry studies. X-ray examination of the affected area may disclose soft tissue gas in patients in whom crepitus is not present on palpation [*see Figure 8*].[18] In addition, elevated blood levels of the muscle proteins creatine kinase and lactate dehydrogenase may suggest skeletal muscle breakdown.[19] Isoenzyme analysis may confirm the origin of these elevated enzymes.

Even in the initial absence of such clinical markers, a necrotizing infection should be suspected when cellulitis is refractory to appropriate antibiotic treatment. This is a signal to explore the wound.[20-23] On exploration, the diagnosis is almost always confirmed by the presence of gray necrotic fascia with little free pus and by easy dissection and undermining of the wound. Thrombosed blood vessels may also be seen. Incisional biopsies and frozen sections are favored for rapid diagnosis of necrotizing fasciitis.[24] The histologic criteria for diagnosis are the following:

1. Necrosis of the superficial fascia.
2. Infiltration of the dermis and of the fascia by polymorphic neutrophils.
3. Thrombosis of subcutaneous arteries and veins.
4. Angiitis and fibrinoid necrosis of arterial and venous walls.
5. Presence of microorganisms in the fascia and dermis on Gram stain.
6. Absence of muscle involvement.

In practice, the diagnosis of necrotizing infection is usually confirmed by the gross findings on surgical exploration. Histologic studies are not required for the initial diagnosis, although they are helpful in defining the cause of the infection [*see Inflammatory Response Is Absent (Clostridial Infection), below*].

Serial measurements of muscle compartment pressure have been used to confirm the need for operation.[19] Normal recumbent muscle compartment pressures are 0 to 8 mm Hg; pressures above 30 mm Hg are abnormal.[25]

Inflammatory Response Is Absent (Clostridial Infection)

On Gram stain or frozen section, histotoxic clostridial infection yields gram-positive rods without white blood cells [*see Figure 9*], whereas nonclostridial soft

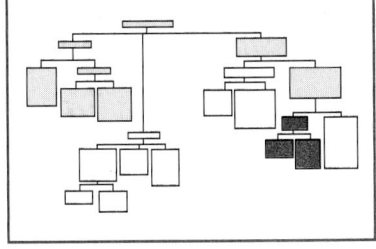

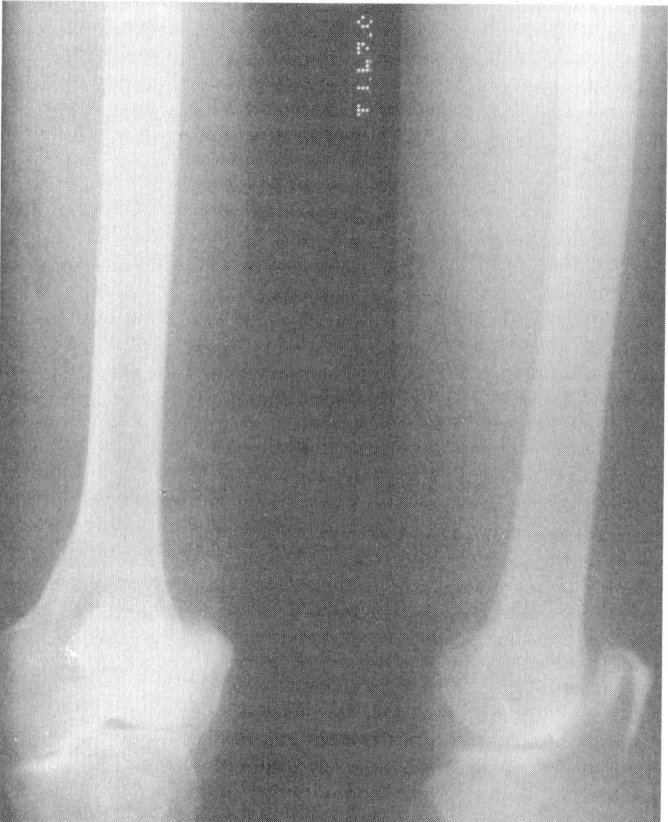

Figure 8 **In some patients with necrotizing soft tissue infection, air may be seen in the soft tissues on x-ray even in the absence of crepitus.**

tissue infection is associated with a significant number of white blood cells in the wound [*see Figure 10*].[26] Clostridial infection may present as a nontoxic cellulitis or toxic myonecrosis. Clostridial cellulitis develops 3 to 5 days after a wound is sustained. It is characterized by pain, a foul-smelling seropurulent discharge, skin vesicles that are small and flat, and limited systemic toxicity. Although pain may be severe, it does not compare to that experienced by patients with clostridial myonecrosis. Crepitus may be present. Effective treatment includes debridement and drainage of the wound and inspection of muscle to ensure that it is intact. Intravenous penicillin

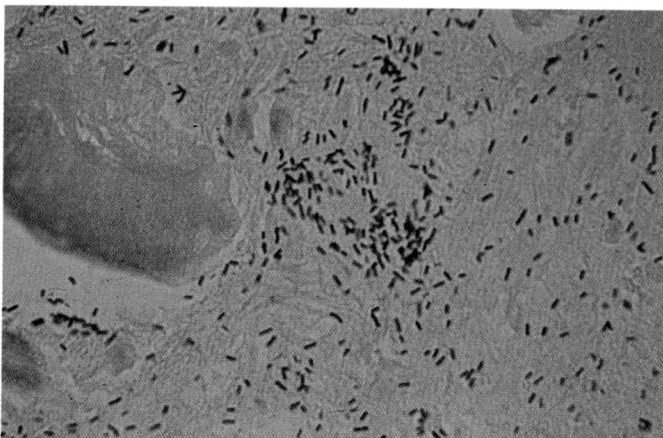

Figure 9 **In clostridial myonecrosis, there is no inflammatory response.**

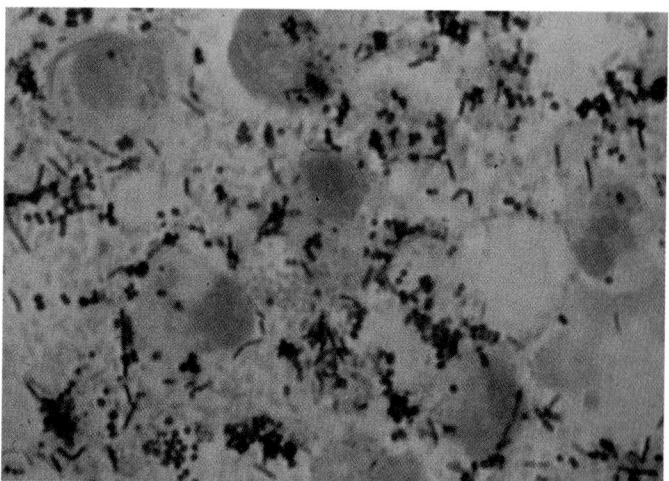

Figure 10 **In necrotizing fasciitis, an inflammatory response is present.**

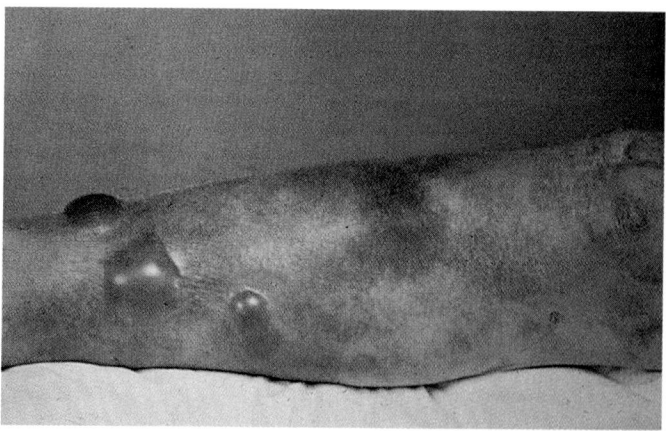

Figure 11 **Bronzing of the skin occurs early in gas gangrene. Skin vesicles, as seen on this patient with advanced gas gangrene, occur later.**

(6 to 12 million U/day for 7 to 10 days) decreases toxemia and limits the spread of infection.

Clostridial myonecrosis, also known as gas gangrene, occurs most commonly in the extremities of injured young men, in the abdominal wall of older men, and in the extremities of elderly patients with diabetes and peripheral arterial occlusive disease. The hallmarks of this infection are severe wound pain, marked swelling, and systemic toxicity. Hemolysis and coagulopathies are common. There may be a watery wound discharge with a musty odor, and a bronzing of the skin may occur. Skin vesicles, cutaneous gangrene, and crepitus, which may occur early in clostridial cellulitis, are late signs in myonecrosis [*see Figure 11*]. Resuscitation with I.V. fluids is required [*see 6:3 Shock*], and administration of I.V. penicillin (12 million U/day) is helpful, but radical surgical debridement is the mainstay of treatment.

The use of HBO in clostridial myonecrosis remains controversial; it inhibits production of exotoxins but does not neutralize those already present. However, edema is reduced, progression of necrosis may be halted,[27] and tissue may be spared.[28,29] It has been suggested that mortality may be decreased by HBO,[28,30] but no comparative controlled studies exist. HBO may be a useful adjunct, but it is not a substitute for surgical treatment and must not be allowed to delay surgical debridement.

Inflammatory Response Is Present (Nonclostridial Infection)

The nonclostridial diffuse necrotizing soft tissue infections seen most often are hemolytic streptococcal gangrene [*see Figure 7*], necrotizing fasciitis

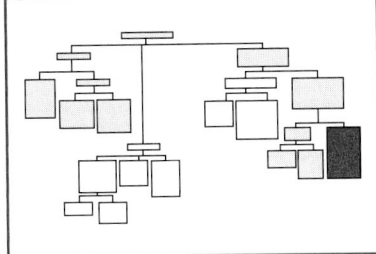

with or without streptococcal toxic-shock syndrome (TSS), gram-negative synergistic necrotizing cellulitis, and idiopathic scrotal gangrene. Much confusion has arisen from reports that merge these syndromes under the single name of necrotizing fasciitis; in fact, they are multiple entities requiring a common initial approach.[26] The specific final diagnosis can be made only in retrospect. Although this diagnosis is valuable for fine-tuning therapy, it is not required for effective empirical initial treatment. Factors that increase mortality include delay in making the diagnosis, immunocompromise, shock and organ failure, a polymicrobial flora, and disease of the trunk rather than of the extremities. The principles of treatment are rapid resuscitation of the hypovolemia and correction of the electrolyte abnormalities [*see 6:3 Shock and 6:8 Disorders of Water and Sodium Balance*], administration of broad-spectrum antibiotics, extensive surgical debridement of all necrotic tissue, and supportive care.

Broad-spectrum antibiotics are usually given initially to cover the variety of organisms that may cause similar syndromes. Combination therapy may be used, such as penicillin (6 to 12 million U/day) with gentamicin (1.5 mg/kg every 8 hours) and clindamycin (600 mg every 6 hours) or ciprofloxacin (400 mg every 12 hours) with metronidazole (500 mg every 8 hours). Alternatively, monotherapy that is effective against gram-negative bacilli, streptococci, and anaerobes may be given, such as imipenem-cilastatin (0.5 to 1.0 g I.V. every 6 hours) or ticarcillin-clavulanate (3.1 g I.V. every 6 hours). Later, when pathogens are identified in blood or tissue, antibiotic therapy should be tailored to the organisms identified.

The initial surgical debridement of the wound should be aggressive. The wound should be incised, and the necrotic tissue should be excised. Wherever possible, however, viable skin should be preserved, and skin incisions should be placed so as to minimize devascularization. The deep fascia should be incised to allow inspection of the muscle. Finally, the wound should be packed open. Further debridement of the wound is the rule and should be performed 24 to 48 hours after the initial debridement. The extent of further debridement depends on the findings during operation and on the evolving clinical syndrome.

Adjunctive fasciotomy has been recommended.[19] Temporary dressings with amniotic membrane[31] or porcine xenografts[32] may be helpful in minimizing colonization of debrided wounds and may promote the growth of granulation tissue, allowing early initiation of split-thickness skin grafts. In immunocompromised patients with perineal gangrene, a diverting colostomy[33] established early in treatment minimizes further contamination of the wound.

Supportive care includes nutritional therapy[21,34] [*see 6:23 Nutritional Support*] and the use of low-dose subcutaneous heparin in order to reduce the risk of venous thrombosis.[35] HBO is the approach favored by some researchers[19,36] but not by others.[21,37,38]

NONOPERATIVE CELLULITIS

In the absence of clinical clues or histologic findings indicating necrotizing infection, diffuse inflammation is probably simple nonoperative cellulitis. The classic lesion is a warm, erythema-

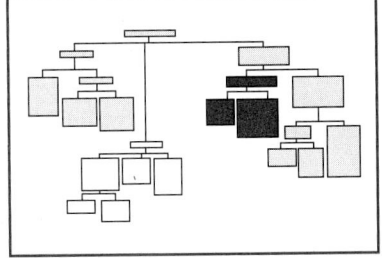

tous, edematous, painful spreading inflammation of the skin with nonelevated, poorly defined, advancing margins. Lymphangitis and lymphadenitis are often present in nonoperative cellulitis but not in necrotizing infection requiring operation [*see Figure 12*].

The identification of pathogens involved is not essential but may be helpful. If a primary lesion is found, swabs taken from it give the highest yields of positive cultures.[39] Needle aspiration of the advancing edge of cellulitis,[40] preferably without preliminary saline injection, yields positive cultures in only 20% to 40% of cases.[39,41,42] Blood cultures are positive in only 2% of cases, and false positive results are twice as common. Therefore, routine blood cultures are not cost-effective; however, blood cultures may be of value in cases where cellulitis of abrupt onset occurs in conjunction with high fever (> 38.4° C [101.1° F]), leukocytosis (> 13,500/mm³), or immunodeficiency.[43] Serologic tests are of limited value.[44]

Most cellulitis is caused by group A streptococci (occasionally by groups B, C, D, and G) or by *S. aureus*. Oral or intravenous antibiotics are the primary treatment. Because streptococcal and staphylococcal cellulitis often cannot be differentiated clinically, a semisynthetic penicillin is commonly used, such as cloxacillin (4 to 6 g/day). Nonspecific measures such as rest, elevation, and warm compresses are also helpful.

Although cellulitis in adults is rarely caused by organisms other than streptococci or *S. aureus,* gram-negative cellulitis and high-risk cellulitis are nonetheless important variants. Gram-negative bacilli, particularly *Proteus mirabilis* and *Klebsiella* species, may cause cellulitis in immunocompromised patients and in patients with underlying disease (e.g., cirrhosis and congestive heart failure). Fever is often absent, but the white blood cell count is typically higher than 13,500/mm³, and severe edema of the dermal papillae produces characteristic subepidermal vesicles or hemorrhagic bullae.[45] Similarly, cellulitis may develop in a laceration that has been exposed to soil or to water infested with *Aeromonas* species. These conditions all require broad-spectrum antibiotic therapy,[44] such as cefazolin or ce-

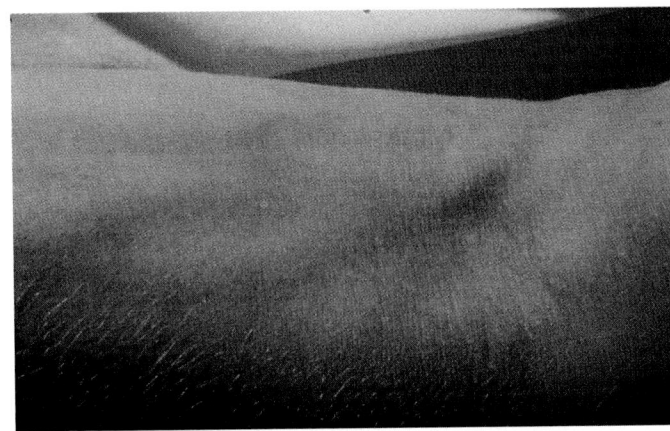

Figure 12 **Lymphangitis, as illustrated here, is commonly associated with nonoperative cellulitis but not with necrotizing infection requiring operation.**

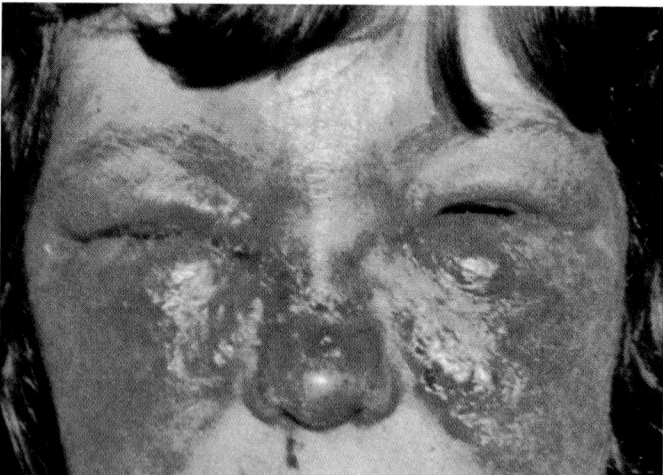

Figure 13 In this patient with late-stage erysipelas, bullae and induration of the cheeks are present along with well-demarcated erythema on the forehead.

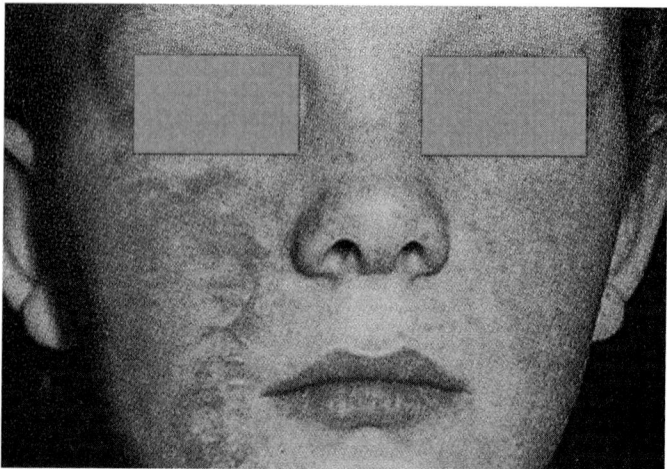

Figure 14 This child has *Haemophilus influenzae* type b cellulitis of the right cheek.

foxitin, 4 to 6 g/day in divided doses; oral ciprofloxacin, 500 mg twice daily; or oral cephalexin, 2 to 4 g/day.

High-risk cellulitis is often caused by unusual organisms. It occurs in critical locations, such as the face and the extremities (especially the hand), that are particularly vulnerable to serious complications. The term high-risk cellulitis includes several distinct conditions, namely, facial cellulitis, postadenectomy and postvenectomy cellulitis, and cellulitis after animal or human bites.

Facial cellulitis may be odontogenic, originating from the teeth and gums in older children, but most cases are nonodontogenic and occur in the upper face of infants and younger children. The best examples of facial cellulitis are erysipelas, *Haemophilus influenzae* type b (Hib) cellulitis, and orbital cellulitis. In erysipelas, a streptococcal upper respiratory infection invades the dermis and epidermis and produces a *peau d'orange* of the cheek [*see Figure 13*]. It responds to penicillin G, 1 million units I.V. four times daily. Hib cellulitis (now uncommon with the widespread use of *H. influenzae* vaccine) gives the cheek a bluish, bruised appearance [*see Figure 14*]. It is accompanied by severe respiratory infection, fever, leukocytosis, and Hib bacteremia.[46] A similar disorder occasionally occurs in adults.[47] Traditionally, ampicillin, 2 to 3 g/day I.V. in divided

doses, has been used for treatment, but currently, cefuroxime, 125 mg I.V. twice daily, is preferred. Orbital and periorbital cellulitis are characterized by pain, erythema, and swelling of the eyelids. Periorbital infections are common in children after minor trauma. Orbital cellulitis is a rare complication of acute sinusitis. The Chandler classification describes five stages of orbital cellulitis, determined on the basis of clinical findings and CT scanning: preseptal, postseptal, subperiosteal abscess, orbital abscess, and meningitis or brain abscess.[48] *S. aureus*, streptococci, and, occasionally, gram-negative aerobes are the usual causative organisms; accordingly, broad-spectrum antibiotics are the preferred agents. When an abscess is present, prompt orbital exploration and decompression are indicated if 36 hours of I.V. antibiotic therapy yields no improvement or if visual acuity or globe motion becomes impaired.[49]

Recurrent cellulitis may develop after adenectomy and in lymphedematous limbs after venectomy. Fever, toxic reactions, and chills are common. Non–group A streptococci (especially groups B, C, and G) are the usual causative organisms[50]; cloxacillin, 1 g I.V. every 4 to 6 hours, is the standard treatment. Similar syndromes related to lymphatic insufficiency have been reported in the breast after breast conservation therapy for carcinoma[51] and in the buttock after hip surgery.[52] In the former instance, *S. epidermidis*, *Streptococcus agalactiae*, and group B streptococci were incriminated. Initial treatment consists of oral cloxacillin or cephalexin, 500 mg to 1 g every 6 to 8 hours; if the infection does not respond to this regimen, specific therapy based on Gram staining or culture may be required. Patients with cellulitis of the buttock after hip surgery have been followed for several years, and no evidence of infection of the prosthetic implant has been found.

Animal and human bites may be complicated by severe infection, especially when they occur on the hands; they are discussed in more detail elsewhere (see below). Another high-risk infection of the hand is erysipeloid, in which cellulitis caused by a gram-positive rod, *Erysipelothrix rhusiopathae*, produces a purple-red infection of the finger or hand in fishers or butchers[53] [*see Figure 15*]. On rare occasions, erysipeloid is complicated by bacteremia or endocarditis. If the lesion is not recognized, diagnosis can be difficult, in that the organism lies deep in the skin and is hard to culture. A new PCR assay developed for diagnosis of swine erysipeloid has now been successfully applied in a human.[53] Erysipeloid responds to oral or parenteral penicillins (e.g., cloxacillin, 1 g every 6 hours).

Miscellaneous Infections

Of the miscellaneous soft tissue infections, only the common wound infections that occur after human and animal bites as well as the rare condition purpura fulminans are considered here. Established infection 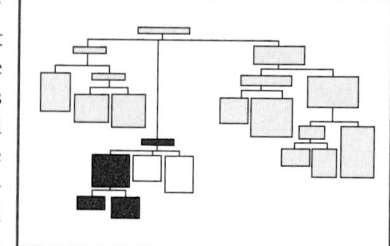 is more likely to occur when animal bites and scratches are seen late. When bites are seen early, infection is usually mild and responds well to treatment, which includes cleansing, tetanus prophylaxis [*see 1:7 Acute Wound Care*], rabies prophylaxis (see below), administration of antibiotics (see below), and surgical debridement.

INFECTION AFTER ANIMAL BITES

From 80% to 90% of reported animal bites are caused by dogs, 10% to 20% by cats, and 1% to 2% by nondomestic animals. About 50% of animal bites are trivial; 1% to 2% necessitate hospitaliza-

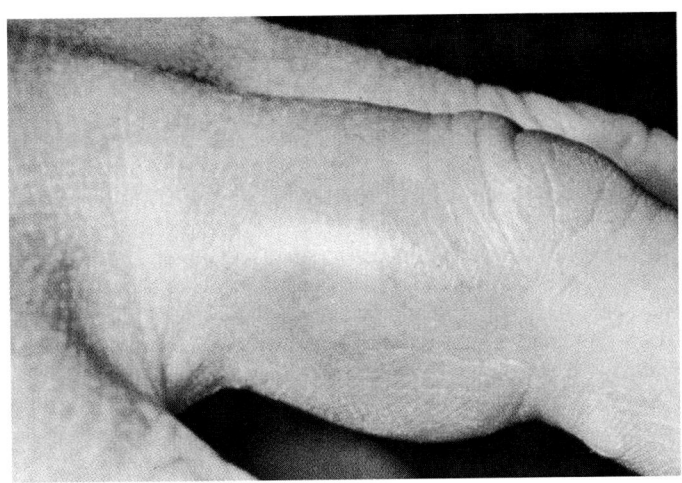

Figure 15 **Characteristic of erysipeloid is an indolent, purple, non-purulent swelling of the finger.**

tion.[54] Washing with soap and water is effective immediately after a bite; later, high-pressure jet irrigation with saline is best. Fresh puncture wounds should be cleansed but not irrigated, because irrigation may compound tissue injury. Older puncture wounds should be opened to allow irrigation. Local anesthetics should be infiltrated to facilitate cleansing and debridement. When seen early, dog bites may be debrided and closed; infection is unlikely provided that appropriate antibiotics are also given. Cat bites and monkey bites are better debrided and left open, except when they occur on the face. Infected wounds and wounds that are older than 24 hours should be left open. Tetanus prophylaxis is given by intramuscular injection [*see 1:7 Acute Wound Care*].

Another important consideration is rabies prophylaxis. Rabies is a viral infection transmitted in the saliva of infected animals. The virus enters the central nervous system of the host and results in encephalomyelitis that is nearly always fatal. Rabies prophylaxis is always indicated for bites by carnivorous wild animals (in particular, skunks, raccoons, foxes, and coyotes) and by bats but not for bites by a domestic animal unless the animal is thought to be rabid or unless it becomes rabid while confined. Prophylaxis is almost never indicated after bites by rodents such as mice, rats, or squirrels. In animal studies, wound cleansing and irrigation with virucidal agents such as povidone-iodine lowers the incidence of rabies markedly. Three rabies vaccines of comparable immunogenicity are available for commercial use: human diploid cell vaccine (HDCV); rabies vaccine adsorbed (RVA), and purified chick embryo vaccine (PCEC). Antibodies develop within 7 to 10 days of immunization; thus, passive protection with human rabies immune globulin (RIG) (half-life, 21 days) is also required.[54,55] Previously nonimmunized persons should receive five 1.0 ml doses of HDCV, RVA, or PCEC by intramuscular injection in the deltoid on days 0, 3, 7, 14, and 28. The recommended dose of human RIG is 20 IU/kg on day 0 or up to day 8; half of the dose should be infiltrated in the area of the wound, and the remainder should be given by intramuscular injection. The animal involved must be observed for rabies. A domestic animal should be confined for 10 days and killed only if it becomes rabid. A wild, stray, or unwanted animal—especially one that is behaving erratically—should be killed immediately, and its brain should be tested for evidence of rabies by means of immunofluorescence techniques.

About 85% of reported animal bites harbor pathogens, and about 15% to 20% of dog bites and 50% to 60% of cat bites become infected. The most common pathogens in animal bites are *Pasteurella multocida*, *S. aureus*, and viridans streptococci.[54] Infections that occur within 24 hours of a bite are usually caused by *P. multocida* and deserve special attention. This gram-negative coccobacillus occurs in the mouths of up to 54% of dogs and 70% of cats and is the most common source of infection in wounds from domestic animal bites and scratches.[56] Typically, it causes infection within 12 to 18 hours, with marked local pain and tenderness. A serosanguineous discharge, low-grade fever, and regional adenopathy are less common. Infections that develop later are most often caused by *S. aureus* and viridans streptococci.

The ideal antibiotic for outpatient treatment of domestic animal bites is amoxicillin-clavulanate, 500 mg amoxicillin with 125 mg potassium clavulanate, given for 5 to 7 days. For inpatient treatment of infected bites, ampicillin-sulbactam, 3 g I.V. every 6 hours, or ticarcillin-clavulanate, 3.1 g every 6 hours for 7 days, is best. For patients allergic to penicillin, either (1) trimethoprim-sulfamethoxazole plus clindamycin or (2) cefuroxime axetil or cefuroxime sodium plus metronidazole is recommended. Elevation of the affected part is also helpful. Obvious pus must be drained and necrotic tissue debrided; however, unnecessary surgical treatment can cause marked disability.

INFECTION AFTER HUMAN BITES

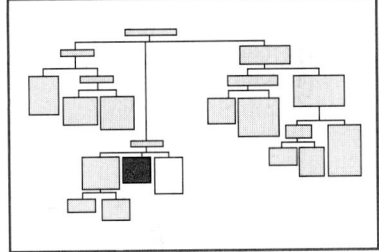

Human bites are rarely seen before infection is established,[54] and they therefore require more vigorous treatment than do animal bites. The minimum treatment of those presenting early includes tetanus prophylaxis [*see 1:7 Acute Wound Care*], high-pressure saline irrigation, broad-spectrum antibiotics, and local debridement without closure of the wounds. The severely infected wound must be treated in the hospital. Wide debridement is necessary, and broad-spectrum parenteral antibiotics are given. The largest percentage of human bite wound infections are attributable to anaerobic bacteria (50%), including *Bacteroides* species (40%); however, viridans streptococci (25%), *S. aureus* (25%), *Eikenella corrodens* (15%), and others are also common pathogens. Appropriate antibiotic therapy consists of cefoxitin, 2 g every 8 hours, ceftriaxone, 2 g every 24 hours, or ticarcillin-clavulanate, 3.1 g every 6 hours for 7 to 10 days. Bites to a clenched fist in which tendon sheaths and joint spaces are entered typically are seen late and often are severely infected at presentation. *E. corrodens* is often isolated from these wounds. Since *E. corrodens* is not sensitive to erythromycin, patients who are allergic to penicillin should receive a cephalosporin instead.

Transmission of HIV and hepatitis B is an additional concern. Transmission of HIV through a human bite is extremely unlikely because proteolytic enzymes in the saliva usually inactivate the virus; consequently, postexposure HIV prophylaxis is not recommended. Hepatitis B, on the other hand, may be transmitted through mucosal contact with blood or saliva from actively infected subjects. A hepatitis B surface antigen (HbsAg)–positive person who bites another person and breaks the skin may transmit the virus; likewise, a seronegative person who bites an HBsAg-positive subject and breaks the skin may acquire the virus. Accordingly, hepatitis B immunoglobulin should be given to all nonimmunized exposed persons.

PURPURA FULMINANS

Purpura fulminans is a rare, life-threatening condition associated with meningococcal or pneumococcal bacteremia. The clinical picture consists of bacteremia, shock, and disseminated intravascular coagulation

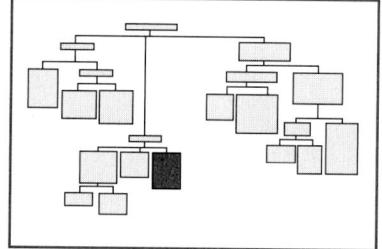

(DIC) causing symmetrical purpura in the skin and subcutaneous tissues of the distal extremities or the face.[57] Treatment includes immediate resuscitation for shock and sepsis and correction of the coagulation defects.[57] Complete volume replacement to establish a normal urine output, cardiotonic drugs, and specific antibiotic therapy are required. Heparin is advised for DIC. The heparin is given by continuous drip in sufficient dosage to maintain the activated partial thromboplastin time at twice the normal value; standard coagulation support is provided to keep the platelet count above 50,000/ mm^3 and the serum fibrinogen level above 2.0 g/L. DIC is known to be associated with a profound decrease in protein C levels; consequently, administration of protein C concentrates early in the course of DIC plays a central role in current therapy. Protein C concentrates are given first in a 10 IU/kg test dose, then in a 100 IU/kg bolus, and finally in a continuous infusion at a rate of 10 to 15 IU/kg/ hour to keep the protein C level between 80 and 120 IU/ml. Antithrombin III is administered when the plasma level falls to 35 IU/ml, below which point heparin is ineffective as an anticoagulant. A 25 IU/kg bolus is given every 6 hours while plasma levels are being monitored. Usually, this approach leads to reversal of DIC within 5 days. Protein C therapy is then withdrawn gradually over a period of 2 days while heparin infusion is maintained at 5 to 10 IU/kg/hour.

If the patient survives the first few days, organ failure is the main problem. Surgical treatment is seldom required early in the course of the disease. The initial mortality is 40%, but some patients who survive may need amputation; others require debridement, topical silver sulfadiazine dressing, and skin grafts.

Discussion

Recognizing the Disorder

In the management of soft tissue infection, success depends on early recognition and prompt treatment of the disorder. The primary treatment is often surgical operation, chosen empirically. When antibiotics are indicated, the initial selection of an antibiotic is also largely empirical. The first goal, then, is not to find the precise diagnosis but to decide whether the condition requires operation. This approach holds for focal lesions, for which diagnosis is easy and treatment of the usual cutaneous abscess is simple. It also holds for diffuse lesions, but the diagnosis of necrotizing infection is often difficult, and the management is challenging.

Value of Classification Systems

Although several classification systems for necrotizing soft tissue infections have been proposed, most are impractical, and some contribute to the confusion that surrounds these disorders. A practical classification system for diffuse necrotizing soft tissue infection is based on the clinical presentation, the anatomic site of primary tissue involvement, and the microbiology of the causative organisms [*see Table 1*]. These factors determine the course of the various clinical syndromes and are sufficiently predictable to influence the plan of treatment after the initial empirical approach.

Role of Operation

Operation is often the main treatment of soft tissue infection. Furthermore, in necrotizing infection, operation must be performed early to limit tissue damage. The extent of surgical debridement depends on operative findings and cannot be predicted before operation. Therefore, it is more important to recognize that operation is required than to identify exactly which procedure will be done. Incision and drainage suffice for cutaneous abscesses. Various modifications, such as primary closure,[58] excision, and marsupialization, have been shown to be effective and are well known to most surgeons, although they are practiced infrequently. These methods, compared with incision and drainage, result in shorter healing times but are associated with a higher rate of recurrence.[59,60] The role of operation in pyoderma gangrenosum is controversial,[2,10] but wide excision is generally required in the postoperative progressive bacterial gangrene of Meleney. In diffuse necrotizing infection, the wound is explored, by incision if necessary, to confirm the diagnosis. In necrotizing fasciitis, debridement of necrotic superficial fascia may create large, randomly based skin flaps that are poorly perfused. Some researchers have advocated preoperative planning of incisions by means of digital dermofluorometry.[61] Incision along a line joining the points of least fluorescence produces skin flaps with well-perfused bases. Thus, mutilation and disability are minimized.

In treating diffuse necrotizing soft tissue infections, reoperation is almost always required to inspect and debride the wound. The extent of debridement depends on the specific clinical syndrome,

Table 1 Classification and Characteristics of Diffuse Necrotizing Infections

Type	Characteristics
Clostridial	
Necrotizing cellulitis	Early local signs, moderate pain, and involvement of superficial tissue (skin and subcutaneous tissue)
Myonecrosis	Early systemic signs, severe pain, and involvement of deeper layers of tissue (primarily muscle)
Nonclostridial	
Monomicrobial necrotizing cellulitis Streptococcal gangrene *Vibrio* necrotizing infections	Rapid onset (1 to 3 days), single causative organism, and involvement of superficial tissue (skin and subcutaneous tissue)
Necrotizing fasciitis Classic bacteria Phycomycotic	Slower onset (4 to 7 days), bacterial synergy, some anaerobic activity, and involvement of deeper layers of tissue (Scarpa's fascia)
Synergistic necrotizing cellulitis caused by gram-negative bacteria	Slowest onset (5 to 10 days), bacterial synergy, greatest anaerobic activity, and involvement of deepest layers of tissue (deep fascia and possibly muscle)

which should be identifiable 24 to 48 hours after initial treatment on the basis of clinical, operative, and microbiological findings. Thus, in monomicrobial necrotizing cellulitis, only focal patchy areas of necrotic skin and subcutaneous tissue need to be excised. In necrotizing fasciitis, the superficial fascia requires further excision, whereas in synergistic necrotizing cellulitis and in clostridial myonecrosis, further debridement of muscle is required, and amputation of part or all of an extremity may be necessary.

Roles of Antibiotics and Pathogen Identification

Antibiotics play a limited role in treating focal soft tissue infection. They are not indicated in otherwise healthy patients with cutaneous abscesses.[62] In about 25% of patients,[63] however, systemic antibiotics are required because of the severity of associated systemic infection, because the patient is immunodeficient, or because a significant infection occurs in the central area of the face and carries a risk of cavernous sinus infection and thrombosis. The choice of antibiotics depends on the bacteria present. The anatomic site of the lesion, the duration of illness, the findings on Gram staining of specimens obtained by drainage or tissue aspiration, the odor of the pus, and the previous medical condition of the patient all provide clues to the likely pathogens.

Anaerobes are dominant in the perineum and rare on the hand. Swabs from cutaneous abscesses often initially yield *S. epidermidis* and streptococci; later, *S. aureus* may appear.[64] Pus that is foul smelling suggests anaerobic bacteria; *Clostridium* species, when present, cause a mousy odor. An abdominal wall abscess after bowel surgery may originate from an intestinal fistula. Gram stains obtained in these situations closely reflect the results of subsequent cultures.[63]

Only 4% of cutaneous abscesses are sterile. One third yield single isolates, usually *S. aureus* or occasionally *P. mirabilis;* the remainder yield a polymicrobial flora that includes many anaerobes.[63] *Bacteroides* species are the most common anaerobes. *B. melaninogenicus* and *B. ureolyticus* occur more frequently than *B. fragilis;* anaerobic gram-positive cocci occur less often, and *Clostridium* species are rare.

In patients with pyoderma gangrenosum, the significance of the pathogens obtained on primary lesion culture and needle aspirate culture is uncertain. A link between the pyogenic organisms found in the central lesion and the progressive destructive process of the skin has been proposed,[1] but this suggestion has not been substantiated, and the organisms are widely regarded as being merely opportunistic. The choice of antibiotics in classic pyoderma gangrenosum is not dictated by the pathogens identified. In his review of the postoperative variant of pyoderma gangrenosum, Meleney reported that when microaerophilic *Streptococcus* organisms and *S. aureus* were injected together into an experimental animal, cutaneous gangrene developed.[14] Injection of a pure culture of either organism failed to produce the skin lesion. These experiments confirmed the role of bacterial synergy in causing the clinical lesion. Gram-negative bacilli are sometimes found in the central area. Although the lesion must be excised for cure, broad-spectrum antibiotics are usually given empirically before surgery.

In diffuse necrotizing fasciitis, the initial antibiotic therapy is given empirically to manage the usual causative organisms. The best approaches are (1) combination therapy with I.V. penicillin, gentamicin, and clindamycin or with ciprofloxacin and metronidazole or (2) monotherapy with I.V. imipenem-cilastatin or ticarcillin-clavulanate [*see* Diffuse Inflammation, Inflammatory Response Is Present (Nonclostridial Infection), *above*]. Within 48 hours, the precise syndrome, whether clostridial or nonclostridial, may be defined by the results of Gram stain and culture of the tissue from the wound, by

the clinical findings and course, and by the anatomic and pathologic findings at operation. For monomicrobial necrotizing cellulitis or clostridial myonecrosis, treatment with penicillin (6 to 12 million U/day I.V.) is sufficient. In necrotizing fasciitis, use of antibiotics directed against *B. fragilis* may be eliminated if this organism is not found on culture. In necrotizing fasciitis with streptococcal TSS, penicillin (18 million U/day), clindamycin (2.7 g/day), and human immunoglobulin (400 mg/kg/day for 5 days) are recommended. Intravenous amphotericin B may be added if hyphae on Gram stain or histologic section suggest necrotizing fasciitis of phycomycotic origin. The initial broad-spectrum antibiotic therapy should be maintained if muscle necrosis and the presence of aerobic and anaerobic gram-negative bacilli, including *B. fragilis*, suggest synergistic necrotizing cellulitis caused by gram-negative bacteria.

In patients with nonoperative cellulitis, systemic antibiotics are the main mode of therapy. There is no indication for autogenous vaccine therapy or for operation, both of which were popular many years ago.[65] The choice of antibiotic is based on the knowledge that cellulitis is usually caused by group A streptococci or by *S. aureus*. A semisynthetic penicillin covers both organisms adequately. Significant improvement can be observed within 48 hours.

The causative bacteria in the usual case of cellulitis are not as predictable as in specifically identified conditions such as erysipelas, but there are three lines of evidence that suggest the role of streptococci and staphylococci. First, the role of streptococci in spontaneous cellulitis occurring in the lymphedematous extremity of the dog has been documented.[66] Second, a rising titer of antistreptolysins and antifibrinolysins has been demonstrated in patients recovering from acute attacks of recurrent tropical lymphangitis[67]; these titers fall again over time. Third, in the few cases in which pus is present, streptococci and staphylococci are often cultured from patients with cellulitis.[41,68] Thus, the usual case of cellulitis may be treated without identification of the pathogen. Moreover, attempts to find bacteria by means of needle aspiration culture, blood culture, or even tissue biopsy culture are often unrewarding.[39]

Although clinical evaluation for the presence of infection is fairly accurate in most instances, it lacks specificity for a variety of disorders within the spectrum of extremity infection. Accordingly, to identify necrosis of soft tissue or infections in bone—complications that may jeopardize the integrity of the limb—further evaluation is useful. For years, plain roentgenograms and scintigrams have been used to define musculoskeletal infection. Currently, however, magnetic resonance imaging with I.V. gadolinium contrast is becoming the preferred modality for evaluating and diagnosing complicated extremity infections because it accurately depicts the degree to which bone and soft tissue are involved and identifies areas of necrosis.[68] Thus, MRI yields superior anatomic delineation of the extent of infection; furthermore, visualization of the bone marrow and definition of bony changes such as cortical destruction allow sensitive detection of osteomyelitis. These findings may be the stimulus for prolonged antibiotic therapy or for surgical intervention.

Traditionally, severe and high-risk cellulitis have been treated in the hospital setting, both to ensure access to surgical debridement when necessary and to facilitate I.V. administration of antibiotics. Often, such treatment has necessitated prolonged hospital stays. With the technology and the antibiotics currently available, however, it is usually possible to discharge patients early and to offer them outpatient parenteral antibiotic therapy (OPAT) or conversion to oral antibiotic therapy. This change in practice derives from (1) the evolution of safe techniques of central venous access for outpatient use, (2) the development of effective antibiotics with long half-lives for daily or twice-daily administration, and (3) the development of antibiotics of such high bioavailability when taken orally that oral regimens match the effectiveness of parenteral regimens. In the United States, skin and soft tissue infection is now the most common indication for referral for outpatient antibiotic therapy.

The vascular access modalities currently in use include peripherally inserted central catheters (PICCs), tunneled central catheters, and implanted ports. Of these, implanted ports are the least likely to become infected, but PICCs are now the most widely used because they are safe and easy to insert and use and because they have proved dependable and durable for prolonged antibiotic administration both in and outside the hospital setting.[69] The delivery systems used with these catheters include (1) slow I.V. injection (so-called I.V. push), which is suitable for time-dependent antibiotics (e.g., cephalosporins) but not for antibiotics that must be given over longer periods of time for reasons of safety and that depend on peak levels or prolonged persistent effects for efficacy (e.g., aminoglycosides and antifungals); (2) minibag and tubing systems that are used with rate-controlling roller clamps to generate a premixed diluted drip; and (3) a variety of portable electronic pumps and specialized tubing that are simple to use but expensive.

A number of antibiotics with long half-lives (e.g., ceftriaxone) have been developed that may be given once daily and are ideal for OPAT. One study of children with preseptal orbital cellulitis concluded that the maximum time for resolution of inflammatory signs was 36 hours, after which time transition to oral antibiotic therapy was appropriate.[70] Other antibiotics (e.g., cefazolin) that are given twice daily, either alone or with probenecid, have also been shown to be effective for home parenteral treatment of moderate and severe cellulitis. In one prospective trial of 61 such episodes of cellulitis, 88% of patients were cured, all peak antibiotic concentrations were higher than 40 μg/ml, and all trough concentrations were above the minimum inhibitory concentration for the expected pathogens.[71]

Antibiotics that possess high bioavailability after oral administration (e.g., quinolones) have greatly facilitated oral therapy for moderate to severe cellulitis. Quinolones are effective against moderate wound infections[72]; combined with single-dose or short-term parenteral antibiotics, they may also be used to treat more severe infections. Oral semisynthetic penicillins and first- or second-generation cephalosporins have long been used alone to treat mild infections or to complete the treatment of moderate cellulitis. Current data suggest that compared with other antibiotics, cephalexin may have a relatively high failure rate (40%) in treating uncomplicated cellulitis and that concomitant acid-suppressive therapy may explain this failure in part.[73]

Pathogenesis of Necrotizing Infections

The pathogenesis of the necrotizing soft tissue infections has been well discussed in the literature,[37,74,75] particularly the pathogenesis of clostridial infections. However, what causes a necrotizing infection rather than nonoperative cellulitis to develop is poorly understood, and even less is known about why a particular type of necrotizing infection occurs. The following are the four known pathogenetic factors in necrotizing soft tissue infections:

1. An anaerobic wound environment.
2. The presence of toxic lytic enzymes.
3. Bacterial synergy.
4. Thrombosis of nutrient blood vessels to skin and subcutaneous tissue.

CLOSTRIDIAL NECROTIZING INFECTIONS

The role of clostridia in producing gas gangrene has been well studied. Six species of clostridia have been reported to cause gas

gangrene in humans: *C. perfringens, C. novyi, C. septicum, C. histolyticum, C. bifermentans,* and *C. fallax. C. perfringens* accounts for more than 80% of cases, *C. novyi* for 30% to 60%, and *C. septicum* for 5% to 20%. About 30% of trauma wounds are contaminated by *C. perfringens,*[74] but in only a few does gas gangrene develop. A fall in redox potential in contaminated puncture wounds or in limbs with ischemic muscle allows the spores to be converted to the vegetative, toxic form. The isolation of clostridia from the wound does not, however, establish the diagnosis of gas gangrene. Simple contamination and clostridial cellulitis must be differentiated from gas gangrene. The diagnosis is clinical.[75] Acceptable criteria for the diagnosis of gas gangrene are the presence of necrotic tissue with seropurulent exudate, gas bubbling from the wound or wound crepitus, and recovery of *C. perfringens* or gram-positive bacilli without spores from a symptomatic patient. In clostridial cellulitis, local signs of infection, including pus formation, predominate over systemic findings.

The hallmarks of gas gangrene—liquefaction of muscle fiber and systemic toxicity—are caused by the exotoxins of clostridia. *C. perfringens* produces at least 12 well-described exotoxins in infected wounds; *C. novyi,* eight; and *C. septicum,* four. The best known of these exotoxins is the α-toxin, lecithinase. It destroys cell membranes, alters capillary permeability, causes hemolysis, and is highly lethal. The θ-toxin causes hemolysis and necrosis and is cardiotoxic; the κ-toxin, a collagenase, lyses protein; the ν-toxin, a hyaluronidase, acts as a spreading factor; the μ-toxin affects cell DNA; and neuraminidase destroys immunologic receptors on erythrocytes. Prominent systemic signs of gas gangrene are apathy, tachycardia out of proportion to increased body temperature, and cardiovascular collapse. Renal failure resulting from the combined effects of cardiovascular collapse and hemolysis is the most common complication.

NONCLOSTRIDIAL NECROTIZING INFECTIONS

The four pathogenetic factors in necrotizing infections (i.e., an anaerobic wound environment, the presence of toxic lytic enzymes, bacterial synergy, and thrombosis of nutrient blood vessels supplying skin and subcutaneous tissue) are less well understood in nonclostridial than in clostridial infections. However, although the mechanisms of action of these factors are not well understood, their roles in infection are known. An anaerobic wound environment facilitates bacterial synergy, especially between aerobic and anaerobic bacteria, and may also explain why radiographs show subcutaneous gas in the wound in 90% of cases [see Gas in the Wound, below].[34] Local findings in the wound, such as skin necrosis, are caused by the action of lytic enzymes and by the thrombosis of nutrient blood vessels to the skin.

The range of clinical presentations of the nonclostridial necrotizing infections has changed since the original description of streptococcal gangrene by Meleney in 1924[76] and now includes necrotizing fasciitis and necrotizing fasciitis with TSS. These changes may be related to differences in pathogenesis.

Streptococcal Gangrene

Meleney emphasized the rapid development of streptococcal gangrene: the initial erythema appears within 24 hours and is associated with fever and toxicity; in 48 hours, blue-purple discoloration, blisters, and bullae appear; and by day 4 or 5, the purple patches become gangrenous[76] [see Table 2]. McCafferty attributed this rapid spread to proteolytic enzymes activated by streptokinase or staphylokinase. Skin necrosis appears early because of thrombosis of subcutaneous blood vessels [see Figure 7].[77]

Necrotizing Fasciitis

Necrotizing fasciitis was recognized in the 1950s.[78] It differs from

Table 2 Changes in Characteristics of Nonclostridial Necrotizing Soft Tissue Infections

Factor	Streptococcal Gangrene	Necrotizing Fasciitis	Necrotizing Fasciitis with Group A Streptococcal Toxic-Shock Syndrome
Historical description	Meleney (1924)[76]	Wilson (1952)[78]	Greenberg (1983)[87]
Patients	Healthy, minor trauma	Multiple medical problems	Healthy, minor trauma Elderly with diabetes
Bacteria	Hemolytic streptococci	Mixed organisms	Group A streptococci
Pathogenesis	Lytic toxins	Bacterial synergy plus lytic toxins	Toxins Virulence (because of superantigens, M proteins, or susceptibility)
Symptoms	Erythema within 24 hr Blisters Gangrene within 4–5 days	Pain Erythema Blisters in the second week	Pain Edema Fever Shock Organ failure
Mortality	20% (preantibiotic era)	20%	20%–60%

streptococcal gangrene in the preponderance of systemic over local findings and in the slower onset of symptoms [*see Table 2*]. No clear explanation is available for these differences. Although few toxic lytic enzymes have been identified during pathogenesis, clinical and experimental evidence of their role in necrotizing fasciitis is available. Meade and Mueller found in 1968 that a collagenase elaborated by *Pseudomonas* species causes the rapid progression of necrosis in the subcutaneous tissue and along the superficial fascia.[79] More recently, Talkington and coworkers found that necrotizing tissue lesions in streptococcal necrotizing fasciitis are associated with a protease elaborated by the bacteria.[80] Thrombosis of nutrient blood vessels occurs late and may also cause skin necrosis. Barker and coworkers reported that the incidence of thrombosis of nutrient blood vessels is higher in patients with acute skin necrosis than in those with subacute cases.[81]

There are two main bacteriologic types of necrotizing fasciitis.[82] Most cases are type I, in which synergy occurs between Enterobacteriaceae or non–group A β-hemolytic streptococci and anaerobic cocci or penicillin-sensitive *Bacteroides* organisms. Type II cases are far less frequent and include group A streptococci either alone or with staphylococci. The clinical features in patients with type I or type II bacteriologies are indistinguishable. The hemolytic streptococcus seen in necrotizing fasciitis may be a different strain from that which produces hemolytic streptococcal gangrene: Meleney noted that different strains of hemolytic streptococcus injected under the skin of rabbits caused different outcomes.[76]

Bacterial synergy is the rule in the pathogenesis of necrotizing fasciitis. Using an animal model, Seal and Kingston[83] studied the role of bacterial synergy and lytic toxin in promoting both local progression and systemic toxicity in necrotizing fasciitis. Intradermal injection of group A β-hemolytic streptococci produced spreading infection and toxicity in 12% of animals. However, when cultures of *S. aureus* were coinjected with β-hemolytic streptococci, spreading infection occurred in 50% of cases; and when the α-lysin of *S. aureus* was coinjected with β-hemolytic streptococci, spreading lesions occurred in 75%. The predominantly anaerobic wound environment in necrotizing fasciitis and gram-negative synergistic necrotizing cellulitis facilitates the bacterial synergy between aerobic and anaerobic bacteria that is important in the pathogenesis of these syndromes.

Necrotizing soft tissue infection caused by halophilic noncholera marine *Vibrio* bacteria has been described.[84] Such infection occurs in minor wounds that have been exposed to seawater or in puncture wounds or small lacerations sustained when the patient is cleaning seafood. The clinical presentation is similar to the presentations of other types of monomicrobial necrotizing cellulitis and is more like that of hemolytic streptococcal gangrene than that of necrotizing fasciitis, which has a slower course. The onset is abrupt and is marked by swelling, erythema, and toxemia. *V. vulnificus, V. parahaemolyticus,* and *V. alginolyticus* are the usual bacteria. The mechanism of pathogenicity is not well understood, but *V. vulnificus* can cause transmural acute necrotizing vasculitis, which leads to thrombosis of subcutaneous blood vessels.

A variant form of necrotizing fasciitis caused by phycomycoses has been described.[85,86] As in other forms of necrotizing fasciitis, the clinical presentation of this form is insidious. The main causative organisms are *Rhizopus arrhizus, Mucor* species, and *Absidia* species. Phycomycotic necrotizing fasciitis can be identified promptly only by histologic examination of the infected tissue. The recommended therapeutic measures are urgent radical excision and I.V. amphotericin B.

Necrotizing Fasciitis with Streptococcal Toxic-Shock Syndrome

Since the 1980s, a marked increase in cases of streptococcal TSS—highly invasive group A streptococcal soft tissue infections largely associated with shock and organ failure—has been noted.[87] Streptococcal TSS is still uncommon (approximately 10 to 20 cases per 100,000 persons), but the increase may be accurately described as epidemic. However, this does not mean that widespread dissemination of infection by these so-called flesh-eating bacteria is imminent. The characteristics of streptococcal gangrene, necrotizing fasciitis, and necrotizing fasciitis with streptococcal TSS differ [*see Table 2*].

The pathogenesis of group A streptococcal TSS is particularly interesting—especially the roles exotoxins play in producing shock and in enhancing virulence of the bacteria. Streptococcal pyrogenic exotoxins (SPEs), produced by specific strains of *S. pyogenes*, are responsible for the characteristic fever, shock, and tissue injury of streptococcal TSS. SPE-A is associated with most cases of streptococcal TSS in the United States, whereas SPE-B and SPE-C are more prevalent causes in Europe and Canada. Some workers have shown that SPE-A and SPE-B cause monocytes to produce monokines, especially tumor necrosis factor–α (TNF-α), a prominent mediator of fever, shock, and tissue injury; IL-1β; and IL-6. Other

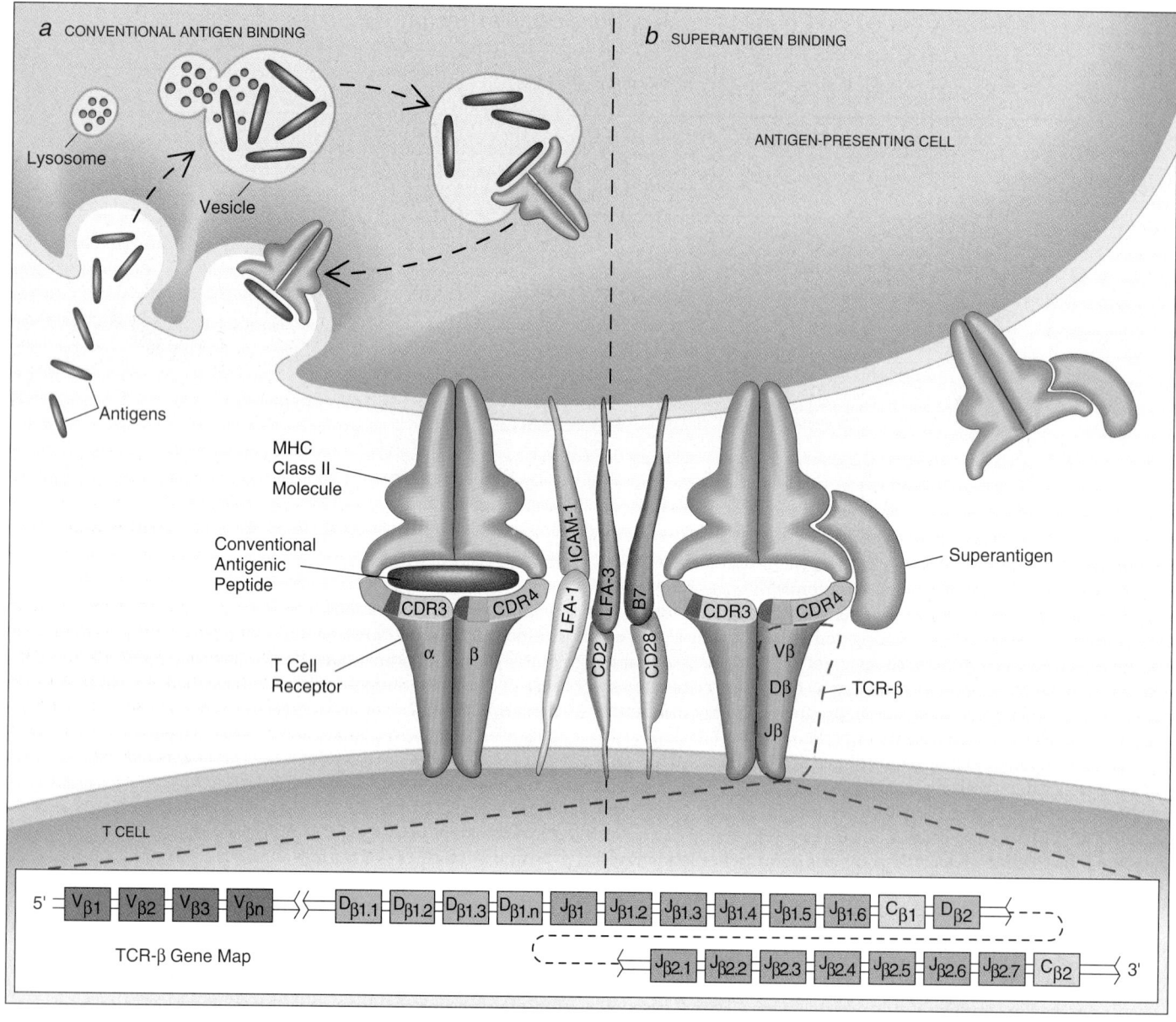

Figure 16 **Superantigens differ from conventional antigens in how they bind to and interact with T cells. A conventional antigen (*a*) is phagocytosed by an antigen-presenting cell (APC) and processed into an antigenic peptide in a lysosomal compartment. The processed peptide passes to a vesicle, where it binds to a major histocompatibility complex (MHC) class II molecule at the molecule's peptide-binding groove. The resultant MHC class II molecule–peptide complex travels to the surface of the APC to be sampled by T cells, whose specificity for the peptide is determined by the amino acid sequences of the five variable regions of the T cell receptor (TCR): the Vβ, Vα, Jβ, Jα, and Dβ segments. As a result, a conventional antigen is likely to be recognized by approximately 0.01% of T cells.**

Superantigens (*b*), by contrast, are not phagocytosed and are far less restricted to specific molecules. For example, binding occurs not in the peptide-binding groove of the MHC class II molecule but on the molecule's surface. Interaction between the MHC class II molecule–superantigen complex and the T cell is governed primarily by a single variable region of the TCR—the Vβ segment. The T cell is activated when the superantigen is recognized by the hypervariable complementarity-determining region CDR4 on the side of the Vβ chain rather than the CDR3 region employed by conventional antigens. Thus, superantigens are able to react with all T cells that have the same TCR-β chain, or between 5% and 20% of resting T cells.

exotoxins, such as streptolysin O, are also potent inducers of TNF-α and IL-1β. Peptidoglycan and lipotechoic acid also cause TNF-α release by monocytes. These mechanisms, added to the effects of the SPEs, result in shock.

Some investigators have tried to account for the increased virulence of group A streptococci in streptococcal TSS and for the dramatic morbidity of the syndrome by proposing that the SPEs also act as superantigens, which differ from conventional antigens in their interactions with T cells.

Conventional antigens interact with T cells in three phases: internalization and preprocessing (i.e., phagocytosis), binding, and T cell activation [*see Figure 16a*]. In phase 1—phagocytosis—antigens are internalized by monocytes and other antigen-presenting cells (APCs) and are processed into small peptide antigen determinants in the lysosomes. In phase 2, binding occurs: the peptides pass into special vesicles, where they form complexes with major histocompatibility complex (MHC) class II molecules at the molecules' peptide-binding groove. In phase 3, the MHC class II molecule–peptide complexes travel to the surface of the APC to be sampled by T cells that express the unique α and β T cell receptor (TCR) chains that are specific for those complexes. The α and β chains of each TCR contain constant (C), variable (V), joining (J), and diversity (D) regions. Specificity for an antigen is determined by the amino acid sequences of the five variable regions of the TCR: Vβ, Vα, Jβ, Jα, and Dβ. The region joining the α and β chains contains the hypervariable complementarity-determining region CDR3, which recognizes only specific MHC class II molecule–peptide complexes [see Figure 16a]. Thus, T cell activation by conventional antigens is restricted by the specificity of the TCR and the MHC class II molecule–peptide complexes. This limits the number of T cells that can be activated and, as a consequence, limits the magnitude of the resultant lymphokine response.

In contrast to conventional antigens, superantigens require no preprocessing and do not undergo phagocytosis [see Figure 16b]. They are less restricted to specific MHC class II molecules; binding occurs not in the peptide-binding groove but on the surface of the MHC class II molecules. The interaction of superantigens with T cells is governed primarily by the Vβ region of the TCR. In addition, T cell activation is triggered when the superantigen is recognized by the hypervariable region CDR4 on the side of the Vβ chain rather than the CDR3 region required by conventional antigens [see Figure 16b]. Superantigens are able to react with all T cells expressing those Vβ elements, or 5% to 20% of resting T cells, compared with conventional antigens, which evoke a response from only 0.01% of T cells. Therefore, if two of the 25 Vβ families recognize a particular superantigen, 8% of all T cells can be activated by that superantigen. Activation results in clonal proliferation of the entire T cell subset and in massive release of lymphokines—particularly IL-2, interferon gamma, and TNF-β. This massive response accounts for the greater virulence of group A streptococci in streptococcal TSS, for the extent and severity of the systemic manifestations, and for the increased mortality of the syndrome.

Although several studies support the concept that interaction of superantigens with MHC class II molecules and T cells triggers the biochemical events that initiate clonal expansion, the role of specific superantigens in streptococcal TSS remains unproven. The strongest evidence to date is the finding of selective depletion of Vβ-bearing T cells in the peripheral blood of patients with severe invasive group A streptococcal infection and TSS.[88] It is well known that exposure of T cells to superantigens can result either in proliferation or in deletion of target T cell subsets. When a superantigen, such as staphylococcal enterotoxin A (SEA), is injected into mice, an initial marked increase is seen in the number of circulating SEA-specific Vβ-bearing T cells for 4 days, after which a second phase ensues in which those T cells are deleted by the induction of anergy and programmed cell death, or apoptosis, and their numbers fall to very low levels for 1 to 4 months.[89] Other studies suggest that the amount of superantigen may determine whether T cell expansion or deletion occurs.[90] The activation of T cells by superantigens is facilitated by APC costimulatory molecules, such as B7 and intracellular adhesion molecule–1, and their respective ligands on the T cell, CD28 and leukocyte function–associated antigen–1. T cell–superantigen interaction may bring the costimulatory molecules and ligands closer together, allowing better transduction of the signals that direct T cell activation and proliferation. In the absence of costimulatory molecules, interaction of the TCR and superantigen may induce T cell anergy. On the other hand, when the interaction is primed by TNF-α or interferon gamma, preactivated T cells may undergo apoptosis and selective deletion when reexposed to a superantigen.

A further mechanism contributing to the syndrome of streptococcal TSS is an increased susceptibility to infection induced by M

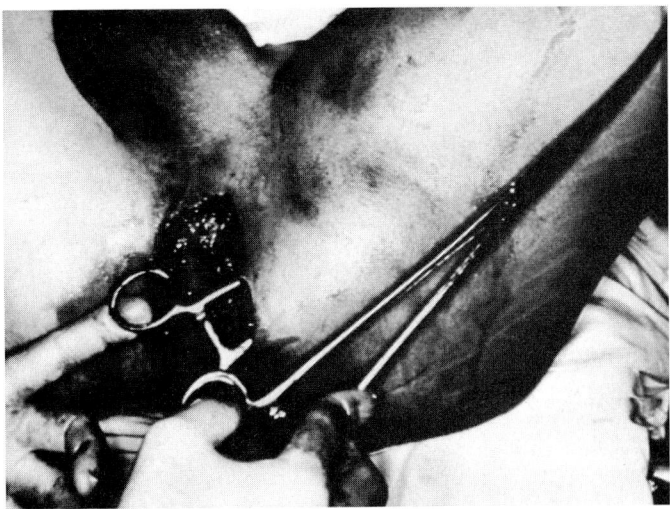

Figure 17   **The destruction of the deep layer of the superficial fascia accounts for the classic sign of unopposed dissection when a blunt instrument probes the plane of the superficial fascia, as illustrated here. The right-hand clamp points out the extent of dissection by the clamp in the left hand.**

proteins on streptococci. M proteins—particularly types 1 and 3—decrease phagocytosis of streptococci by polymorphonuclear leukocytes.[91] It is therefore of particular interest (1) that streptococcal strains that carry M protein types 1 and 3 have accounted for most cases of streptococcal TSS[92] and (2) that the specific antibody formed after infection by a group A streptococcus of a particular M protein type provides resistance to further infection by that strain. M proteins also enhance exotoxin production, thereby increasing tissue destruction. Clindamycin, which impairs M protein synthesis (and therefore suppresses exotoxin production), is particularly efficacious in the treatment of experimental *S. pyogenes* infections.

Knowledge of the pathogenesis and evolution of streptococcal TSS may suggest specific possible future modes of therapy. Such approaches may include the development of antimicrobials that kill the bacteria and suppress toxin formation at the initial stage (i.e., localized infection), antitoxins to neutralize circulating toxins at stage II, and agents that neutralize circulating cytokines at stage III to control the syndrome and prevent progression to the multiple organ dysfunction syndrome of stage IV. Takei and coworkers have shown that human immunoglobulin contains antibodies that inhibit activation of T cells by staphylococcal toxin superantigens in cases of staphylococcal TSS.[93]

Streptococcal Myositis

Neither muscle nor deep fascia is involved in hemolytic streptococcal gangrene or in necrotizing fasciitis. The term fasciitis refers to the constant involvement of the deep layer of superficial fascia.[78] The destruction of this layer accounts for the classic sign of unopposed dissection when a blunt instrument probes the plane of the superficial fascia [see Figure 17].[23] An interesting variant with muscle involvement is streptococcal myositis, which has been differentiated from gas gangrene.[94] Most patients present with bacteremia and severe pain, but crepitus or gas in the tissues is unusual.[95] In streptococcal myositis, a group A hemolytic streptococcus is associated with anaerobic streptococci, *S. aureus*, or gram-negative bacilli. The muscle is inflamed but shows no evidence of the necrosis typical of gas gangrene.

Myositis may also occur as one element of necrotizing fasciitis with streptococcal TSS.[95] This so-called gangrenous streptococcal

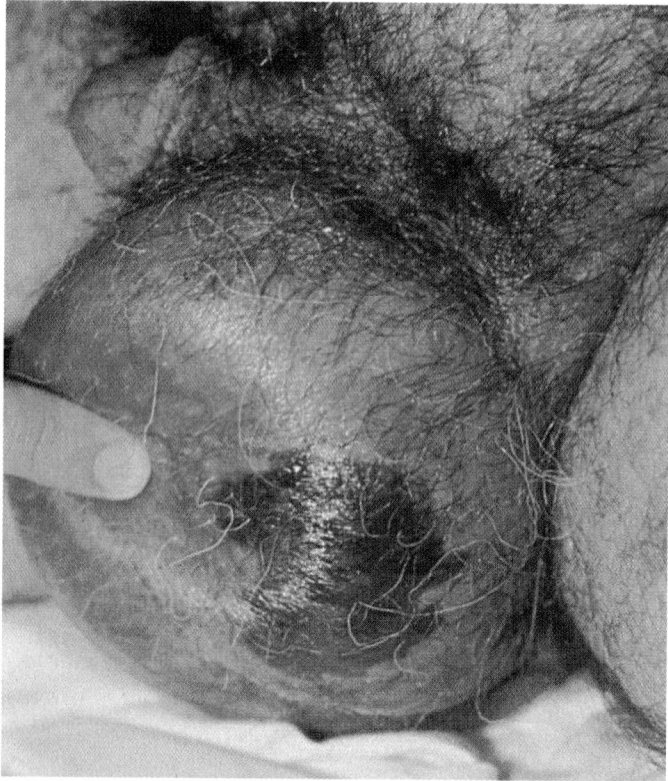

Figure 18 **Fournier's gangrene of the scrotum is shown in this photograph.**

myositis is similar to clostridial myonecrosis in abruptness of onset, severity of pain, and high mortality, but it differs in the absence of underlying disease or of recent trauma and in the lack of crepitus or gas in the tissues. It has been suggested that the bacteria reach the muscle by hematogenous dissemination; a prodromal viral myositis may predispose the involved muscle to localization of coincident streptococcal infection.

Gram-Negative Synergistic Necrotizing Cellulitis

True muscle necrosis also occurs in synergistic necrotizing cellulitis caused by gram-negative bacteria. In this condition, the slow onset of disease, the deep anatomic location, and the anaerobic environment favoring bacterial synergy produce more extensive tissue necrosis than is generally seen in monomicrobial necrotizing cellulitis or in necrotizing fasciitis.[96] Although the perineal form of synergistic necrotizing cellulitis caused by gram-negative bacteria has been called Fournier's gangrene,[97] it is quite different from the idiopathic scrotal gangrene described by Fournier [*see Figure 18*].[98,99] Indeed, the parallel between idiopathic scrotal gangrene and so-called Fournier's gangrene is similar to the parallel between hemolytic streptococcal gangrene and necrotizing fasciitis. Synergistic necrotizing cellulitis is caused by synergy between anaerobic and aerobic gram-negative bacteria—usually *B. fragilis* or peptostreptococci and Enterobacteriaciae. Thus, it is polymicrobial from the outset. In addition, unlike idiopathic scrotal gangrene, perineal synergistic necrotizing cellulitis caused by gram-negative bacteria may extend onto the abdominal wall, necessitating extensive and repeated debridement [*see Figures 19 and 20*].

Idiopathic Scrotal Gangrene

Idiopathic scrotal gangrene[98,99] is characterized by sudden onset of fever, rapid progressive gangrene of the scrotal skin within 24 to 30 hours, and quick separation of the slough from the testes. The main causative organisms are anaerobic streptococci,[100] but secondary overgrowth of gram-negative bacilli may occur later.[101] The tissue loss is more superficial than that which occurs in Fournier's gangrene. Prompt and repeated surgical debridement reduces mortality. The wound granulates rapidly, and skin grafting may be performed later.

Gas in the Wound

Gas in the wound is an ominous sign to most physicians, perhaps because of its association with gas gangrene.[102,103] The significance of gas in the wound, however, depends on its source.

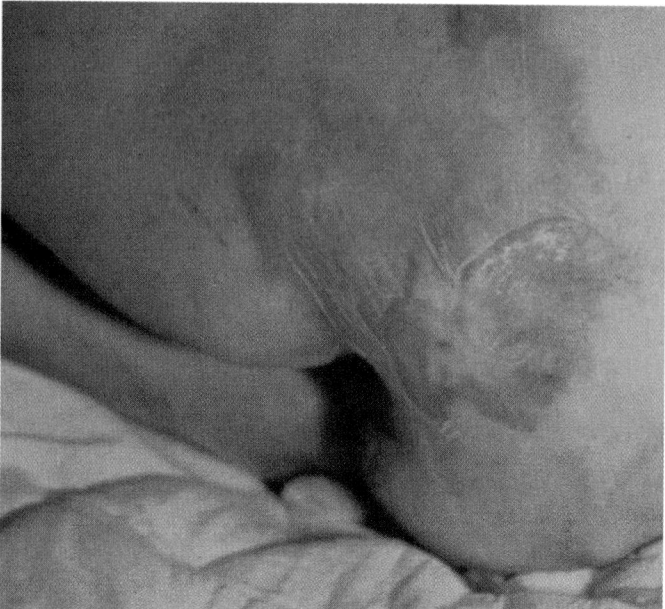

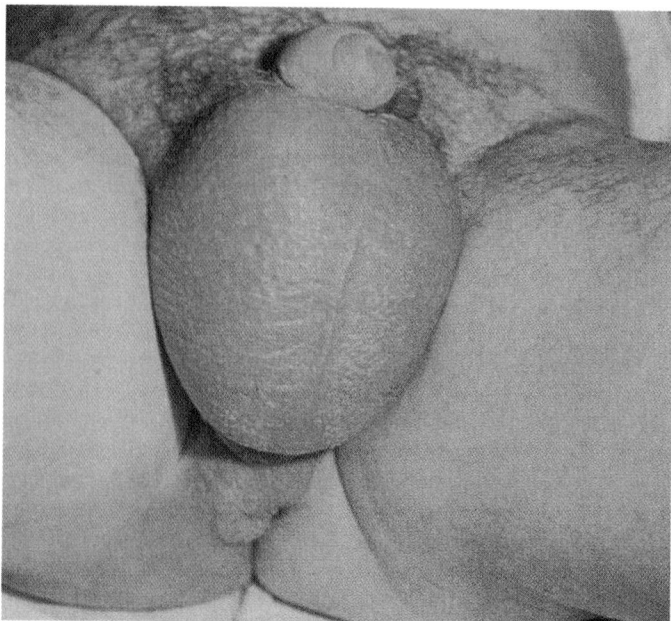

Figure 19 **Patients with synergistic necrotizing cellulitis caused by gram-negative bacteria may have necrotizing infection of the buttock (left). A perineal form is also seen (right).**

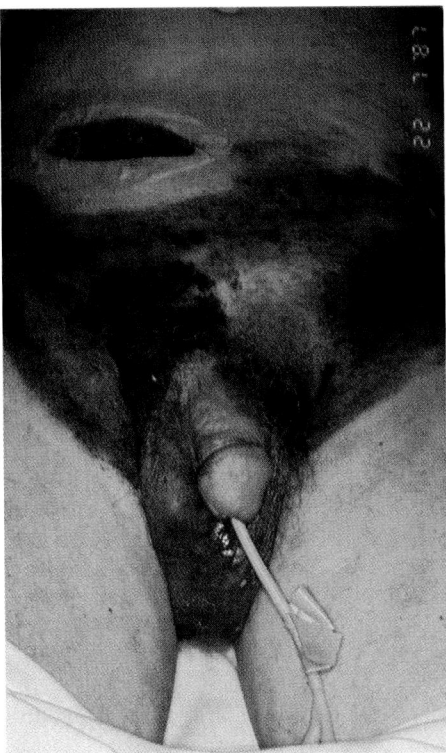
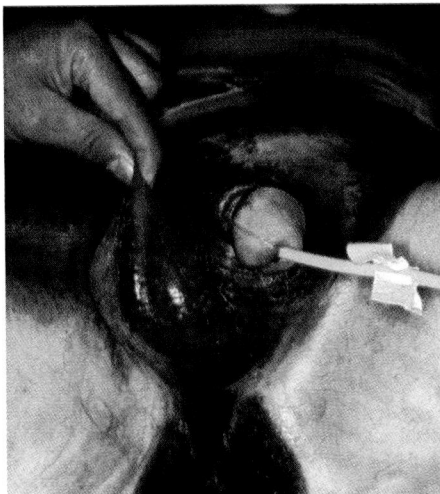
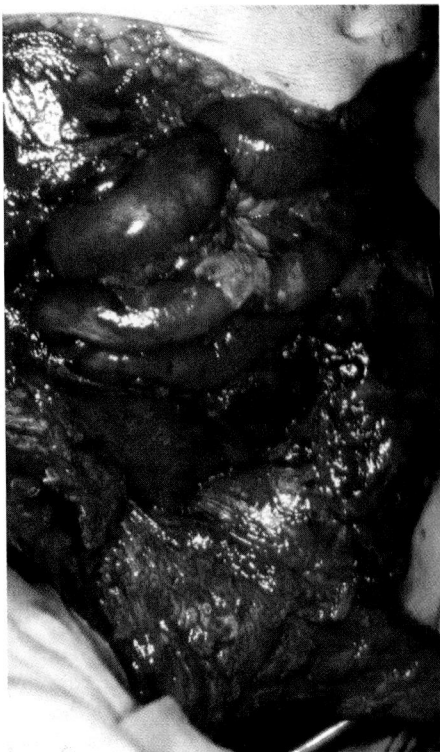

Figure 20 Synergistic necrotizing cellulitis caused by gram-negative bacteria on the anterior abdominal wall followed laparotomy for perforated carcinoma of the cecum in this patient. Ecchymosis and vesicles were present in the groin and anterior abdominal wall (left). Retroperitoneal dissection of infection and ecchymosis of the perianal region and scrotum are evident (center). Wide excision of the anterior abdominal wall revealed normal muscle in the flank but necrotic rectus abdominis and inguinal muscles in the lower abdomen (right).

Gas found in the wound may result from installation, leakage, or formation de novo. Installed gas is that left in the tissues in the course of tissue manipulation. It is characterized by the absence of other symptoms or signs and by gradual decrease in quantity over time.

Gas leakage into the tissues is characterized by a history of a predisposing event. It may occur after trauma—surgical or accidental—or after the violent retching and vomiting associated with spontaneous rupture of the esophagus. Air leakage from the esophagus, trachea, or lungs may follow blunt or penetrating trauma, and subcutaneous emphysema may follow tracheostomy or the insertion of a chest tube into the pleural space.

Gas formed in the tissues is truly spontaneous. It implies an anaerobic environment in which aerobic bacteria such as *E. coli, Klebsiella, Enterobacter,* or *Pseudomonas* or anaerobic bacteria such as peptostreptococci or *Bacteroides* species can produce gas. Usually, hydrogen and nitrogen are formed by processes of denitrification, fermentation, and deamination.[104] The volume of gas formed is quite variable. In some conditions, particularly synergistic necrotizing cellulitis caused by gram-negative bacteria, large volumes of gas may form, which dissect well beyond the area of infection. This occurrence, however, does not imply the need to excise or debride tissues beyond the area of infection. Simple incision will confirm that these tissues are not infected [*see Figure 21*].

Diagnosis and management of the patient with formed gas in the tissues is the same as that of the patient with a diffuse soft tissue infection. A search for telltale clinical features of necrotizing infection is combined with ancillary investigation—soft tissue x-ray, needle aspiration and Gram stain, blood culture, and serum muscle enzyme assay. The finding of gas within the muscle on x-ray is a telling sign of myonecrosis [*see Figure 22*].

Bite Wounds

Interesting differences between animal- and human-bite wounds should be noted because they affect management. Domestic animal bites and scratches occur far more often than human bites, but they are less serious. Only about half of all dog bites even receive medical attention. Human bites are more serious, in part because they usually present later, when infection is well established. In addition, the human oral cavity has a huge diversity of aerobic and anaerobic bac-

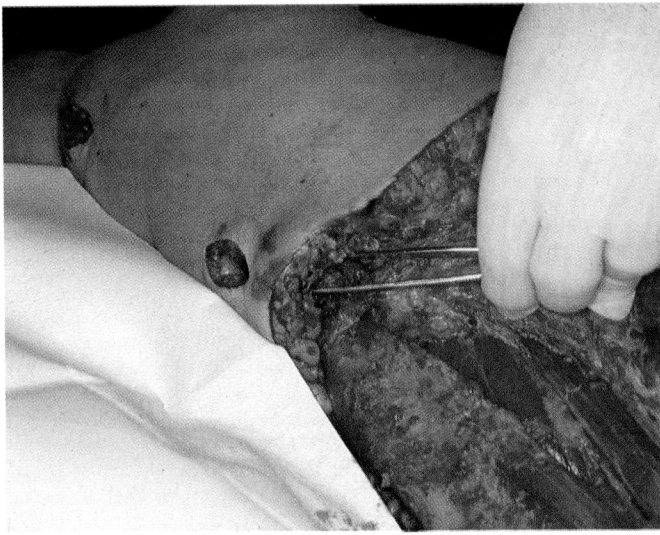

Figure 21 Exploratory incision must often be made to detect the presence of gas in the tissues beyond the area of necrosis.

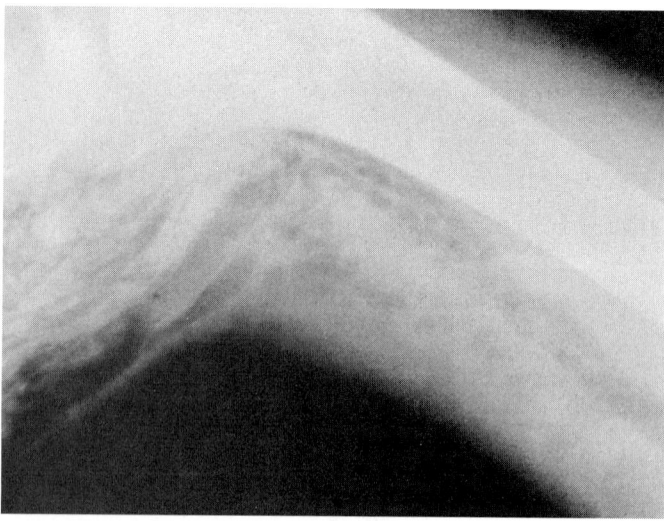

Figure 22 **Gas seen within the muscle on x-ray is a telling sign of myonecrosis.**

teria. All human-bite wounds should be considered infected; therefore, they call for a broader spectrum of antibiotic coverage and wider debridement than animal bites. Above all, the wounds must not be closed primarily. Of all animal wounds, dog bites have the lowest risk of infection. They may be debrided and closed primarily, provided antibiotics are given.[105]

Finally, the special risk of rabies after animal bites often raises questions about the need for prophylaxis. The risk of rabies depends on the species of animal involved, the circumstances of the bite, and the type of exposure. Bites by wild carnivorous animals involved in unprovoked attacks carry the highest risk. The HDCV is more immunogenic and better tolerated than the duck embryo vaccine used formerly. Pregnancy is not a contraindication to the use of HDCV. Patients with a history of hypersensitivity, however, should be given HDCV with caution: antihistamines may be used, epinephrine should be close at hand, and the patient should be observed carefully.

Pathogenesis of Purpura Fulminans

The pathogenesis of purpura fulminans is interesting but controversial. The earmarks of acute purpura fulminans, typically associated with meningococcemia, are purpuric skin and severe acute DIC. The skin changes differ from those characteristic of simple hemorrhage in that the lesions are raised, indurated, and circumferential and tend to coalesce, blister, and break. These changes are due to rapidly progressive microvascular thrombosis in the dermis, resulting in perivascular hemorrhage and necrosis with minimal inflammation. Acute purpura fulminans closely resembles the Shwartzman reaction, induced in experimental animals by two I.V. injections of endotoxin 12 to 24 hours apart.[106] Endotoxin damages endothelial cells and activates the Hageman factor (factor XII), thereby initiating intravascular thrombosis and causing ischemia, vessel wall damage, and bleeding.[107]

Endotoxin-induced microvascular thrombosis is also associated with severe DIC, which is particularly interesting because of the related profound and disproportionate fall in plasma concentration of protein C and the recently defined central role of protein C administration in therapy. Protein C is a vitamin K–dependent glycoprotein that acts as a natural anticoagulant. It combines with thrombomodulin and small amounts of thrombin on the endothelial surface to form activated protein C (APC), which with cofactor protein S blocks further generation of thrombin by inhibiting factors Va and VIIIa. Factor VIIIa normally activates factor X and acts in conjunction with factors Va and Xa in the prothrombinase complex that generates thrombin from prothrombin. By limiting thrombin generation, APC limits fibrin formation; moreover, by promoting fibrinolysis, it limits fibrin accumulation.

In meningococcemia, induced microvascular thrombosis initiates a vicious circle that triggers disproportionate consumption of protein C and produces severe DIC. The endotoxemia also promotes release of TNF-α and IL-1, resulting in elevated levels of plasminogen activator inhibitor–1, which blocks fibrinolysis. In addition, TNF-α increases vascular permeability and white blood cell trapping.[108] Through its anticoagulant and fibrinolytic actions, administered protein C decreases microvascular thrombosis. This effect is critical in preventing organ failure and digital gangrene.[108] Administered protein C is also anti-inflammatory because APC blocks release of TNF-α and IL-1. Steroid therapy has also been suggested for this condition but should not be used because the Shwartzman reaction can be primed with cortisone.[109]

Chronic purpura fulminans is seen only in children. It presents many days after a febrile illness, usually a viral upper respiratory tract infection. Antigen-antibody complexes are deposited in the skin and lead to patches of skin necrosis.

References

1. Brunsting LA, Goeckerm WH, O'Leary PA: Pyoderma (echthyma) gangrenosum: clinical and experimental observations in five cases occurring in adults. Archives of Dermatology and Syphilology 22:655, 1930

2. Newell LM, Malkinson FD: Commentary: pyoderma gangrenosum. Arch Dermatol 118:769, 1982

3. Holt PJA, Davies MG, Saunders KC, et al: Pyoderma gangrenosum. Medicine (Baltimore) 59:114, 1980

4. van der Sluis I: Two cases of pyoderma (ecthyma) gangraenosum associated with the presence of an abnormal serum protein (β₂ A-paraprotein). Dermatologica 132:409, 1966

5. Perry HO, Winkelmann RK: Bullous pyoderma gangrenosum and leukemia. Arch Dermatol 106:901, 1972

6. von den Driesch P: Pyoderma gangrenosum: a report of 44 cases with follow-up. Br J Dermatol 137:1000, 1997

7. Hughes JR, Smith E, Berry H, et al: Pyoderma gangrenosum in a patient with rheumatoid arthritis responding to treatment with cyclosporin A. Br J Rheumatol 33:680, 1994

8. Jolles S, Niclasse S, Benson E: Combination of oral and topical tacrolimus in therapy-resistant pyoderma gangrenosum. Br J Dermatol 140:564, 1999

9. Dirschka T, Kastner U, Behrens S, et al: Successful treatment of pyoderma gangrenosum with intravenous human immunoglobulin. J Am Acad Dermatol 39:789, 1998

10. Read AE: Pyoderma gangrenosum (editorial). Q J Med 55:99, 1985

11. Lewis SJ, Poh-Fitzpatrick MB, Walther RR: Atypical pyoderma gangrenosum with leukemia. JAMA 239:935, 1978

12. Heng MCY: Hyperbaric oxygen therapy for pyoderma gangrenosum. Aust NZ J Med 14:618, 1984

13. Plaus WJ, Hermann G: The surgical management of superficial infections caused by atypical mycobacteria. Surgery 110:99, 1991

14. Brewer GE, Meleney FL: Progressive gangrenous infection of the skin and subcutaneous tissues, following operation for acute perforative appendicitis. Ann Surg 84:438, 1926

15. Grainger RW, MacKenzie DA, McLachlin AD: Progressive bacterial synergistic gangrene: chronic undermining ulcer of Meleney. Can J Surg 10:439, 1967

16. Ledingham IMcA, Tehrani MA: Diagnosis, clinical course and treatment of acute dermal gangrene. Br J Surg 62:364, 1975

17. Svensson LG, Brookstone AJ, Wellsted M: Necrotizing fasciitis in contused areas. J Trauma 25:260, 1985

18. Fisher JR, Conway MJ, Takeshita RT, et al: Necrotizing fasciitis: importance of roentgenographic studies for soft-tissue gas. JAMA 241:803, 1979

19. Aitken DR, Mackett MCT, Smith LL: The changing pattern of hemolytic streptococcal gangrene. Arch Surg 117:561, 1982

20. Baxter CR: Surgical management of soft tissue infections. Surg Clin North Am 52:1483, 1972

21. Kaiser RE, Cerra FB: Progressive necrotizing surgical infections—a unified approach. J Trauma 21:349, 1981

22. Freischlag JA, Ajalat G, Busuttil RW: Treatment of necrotizing soft tissue infections: the need for a new approach. Am J Surg 149:751, 1985

23. Miller JD: The importance of early diagnosis and surgical treatment of necrotizing fasciitis. Surg Gynecol Obstet 157:197, 1983

24. Stamenkovic I, Lew PD: Early recognition of potentially fatal necrotizing fasciitis: the use of frozen-section biopsy. N Engl J Med 310:1689, 1984

25. Mubarak SJ, Hargens AR, Owen CA, et al: The wick catheter technique for measurement of intramuscular pressure: a new research and clinical tool. J Bone Joint Surg [Am] 58A:1016, 1976

26. Dellinger EP: Severe necrotizing soft-tissue infections: multiple disease entities requiring a common approach. JAMA 246:1717, 1981

27. Shupak A, Halpern P, Ziser A, et al: Hyperbaric oxygen therapy for gas gangrene casualties in the Lebanon War, 1982. Isr J Med Sci 20:323, 1984

28. Hitchcock CR, Demello FJ, Haglin JJ: Gangrene infection: new approaches to an old disease. Surg Clin North Am 55:1403, 1975

29. Hill GB, Osterhout S: Experimental effects of hyperbaric oxygen on selected clostridial species: II. In vivo studies in mice. J Infect Dis 125:26, 1972

30. Heimbach RD, Boerema I, Brummelkamp WH, et al: Current therapy of gas gangrene. Hyperbaric Oxygen Therapy. Davis JC, Hunt TK, Eds. Undersea Medical Society, Inc, Bethesda, Maryland, 1977, p 153

31. Zarutskie P, Silverberg F: Amniotic membranes as a temporary wound dressing in necrotizing fasciitis. Obstet Gynecol 64:284, 1984

32. Sutton GP, Smirz LR, Clark DH, et al: Group B streptococcal necrotizing fasciitis arising from an episiotomy. Obstet Gynecol 66:733, 1985

33. Hiatt JR, Kuchenbecker SL, Winston DJ: Perineal gangrene in the patient with granulocytopenia: the importance of early diverting colostomy. Surgery 100:912, 1986

34. Majeski JA, Alexander JW: Early diagnosis, nutritional support, and immediate extensive debridement improve survival in necrotizing fasciitis. Am J Surg 145:784, 1983

35. Hammar H, Wanger L: Erysipelas and necrotizing fasciitis. Br J Dermatol 96:409, 1977

36. Gozal D, Ziser A, Shupak A, et al: Necrotizing fasciitis. Arch Surg 121:233, 1986

37. Tehrani MA, Ledingham IMcA: Necrotizing fasciitis. Postgrad Med J 53:237, 1977

38. Barzilai A, Zaaroor M, Toledano C: Necrotizing fasciitis: early awareness and principles of treatment. Isr J Med Sci 21:127, 1985

39. Hook EW III, Hooton TM, Horton CA, et al: Microbiologic evaluation of cutaneous cellulitis in adults. Arch Intern Med 146:295, 1986

40. Uman SJ, Kunin CM: Needle aspiration in the diagnosis of soft tissue infections. Arch Intern Med 135:959, 1975

41. Ginsberg MB: Cellulitis: analysis of 101 cases and review of the literature. South Med J 74:530, 1981

42. Leppard BJ, Seal DV, Colman G, et al: The value of bacteriology and serology in the diagnosis of cellulitis and erysipelas. Br J Dermatol 112:559, 1985

43. Perl B, Gottehrer NP, Schlesinger Y, et al: Cost-effectiveness of blood cultures for adult patients with cellulitis. Clin Infect Dis 29:1483, 1999

44. Slutkin G, Marzouk J, Dall L, et al: Comparison of cefonicid and cefazolin for treatment of soft-tissue infections. Rev Infect Dis 6(suppl 4):S853, 1984

45. Yoon TY, Jung SK, Chang SH: Cellulitis due to Escherichia coli in three immunocompromised subjects. Br J Dermatol 139:885, 1998

46. Fleisher G, Heeger P, Topf P: Hemophilus influenzae cellulitis. Am J Emerg Med 3:274, 1983

47. Drapkin MS, Wilson ME, Shrager SM, et al: Bacteremic Hemophilus influenzae type B cellulitis in the adult. Am J Med 63:449, 1977

48. Chandler JR, Langenbrunner DJ, Stevens ER: The pathogenesis of orbital complications in acute sinusitis. Laryngoscope 80:1414, 1970

49. Goodwin WJ Jr, Weinshall M, Chandler JR: The role of high resolution computerized tomography and standardized ultrasound in the evaluation of orbital cellulitis. Laryngoscope 92:729, 1982

50. Baddour LM, Bisno AL: Non-group A beta-hemolytic streptococcal cellulitis: association with venous and lymphatic compromise. Am J Med 79:155, 1985

51. Mertz KB, Baddour LM, Bell JL: Breast cellulitis following breast conservation therapy: a novel complication of medical progress. Clin Infect Dis 26:481, 1998

52. Studer-Sachsenberg EM, Ruffieux PH, Saurat J-H: Cellulitis after hip surgery: long term follow-up of seven cases. Br J Dermatol 137:133, 1997

53. Brooke CJ, Riley TV: Erysipelothrix rhusiopathiae: bacteriology, epidemiology and clinical manifestations of an occupational pathogen. J Med Microbiol 48:789, 1999

54. Fleisher GR: The management of bite wounds. N Engl J Med 340:138, 1999

55. Advisory Committee on Immunization Practices: Human rabies prevention—United States 1999. Recommendations of the Advisory Committee on Immunization Practices. MMWR 48:1, 1999

56. Francis DP, Holmes MA, Brandon G: Pasteurella multocida: infections after domestic animal bites and scratches. JAMA 233:42, 1975

57. Smith OP, White B: Infectious purpura fulminans: diagnosis and treatment. Br J Haematol 104:202, 1999

58. Ellis M: Incision and primary suture of abscesses of the anal region. Proc R Soc Med 53:652, 1960

59. Macfie J, Harvey J: The treatment of acute superficial abscesses: a prospective clinical trial. Br J Surg 64:264, 1977

60. Sorensen C, Hjortrup A, Moesgaard F, et al: Linear incision and curettage vs deroofing and drainage in subcutaneous abscess: a randomized clinical trial. Acta Chir Scand 153:659, 1987

61. Bongard FS, Elings VB, Markison RE: New uses of fluorescence in the surgical management of necrotizing soft tissue infection. Am J Surg 150:281, 1985

62. Llera JL, Levy RC: Treatment of cutaneous abscess: a double-blind clinical study. Ann Emerg Med 14:15, 1985

63. Becker LE, Tschen E: Common bacterial infections of the skin. Primary Care 10:397, 1983

64. Meislin HW, Lerner SA, Graves MH, et al: Cutaneous abscesses: anaerobic and aerobic bacteriology and outpatient management. Ann Intern Med 87:145, 1977

65. Hughes B: The treatment of cellulitis with special reference to the hand and arm. Practitioner 89:142, 1912

66. Drinker CK, Field ME, Ward HK, et al: Increased susceptibility to local infection following blockage of lymph drainage. Am J Physiol 112:74, 1935

67. Morales-Otero P, Pomales-Lebrón A: The development of antistreptolysins and antifibrinolysins following acute attacks of recurrent tropical lymphangitis. Trans R Soc Trop Med Hyg 30:191, 1936

68. Towers JD: The use of intravenous contrast in MRI of extremity infection. Semin Ultrasound CT MR 18:269, 1997

69. Brown JM: An overview of vascular access for the alternate care setting. Infusion 1:11, 1995

70. Blumer J, O'Brien C, Lemon E, et al: Skin and soft tissue infections: pharmacologic approaches. Pediatr Infect Dis 4:336, 1985

71. Leder K, Turnidge JD, Grayson ML: Home-based treatment of cellulitis with twice-daily cefazolin. Med J Australia 169:519, 1998

72. Lipsky BA, Miller B, Schwartz R, et al: Sparfloxacin versus ciprofloxacin for the treatment of community-acquired complicated skin and skin-structure infections. Clin Therapeutics 21:675, 1999

73. Madaras-Kelly KJ, Arbogast R, Jue S: Increased therapeutic failure for cephalexin versus comparator antibiotics in the treatment of uncomplicated outpatient cellulitis. Pharmacotherapy 20:199, 2000

74. Altemeier WA, Fullen WD: Prevention and treatment of gas gangrene. JAMA 217:806, 1971

75. MacLennan JD: The histotoxic clostridial infections of man. Bact Review 26:177, 1962

76. Meleney FL: Hemolytic streptococcus gangrene. Arch Surg 9:317, 1924

77. McCafferty EL, Lyons C: Suppurative fasciitis as the essential feature of hemolytic streptococcus gangrene. Surgery 24:438, 1948

78. Wilson B: Necrotizing fasciitis. Am Surg 18:416, 1952

79. Meade JW, Mueller CB: Necrotizing infections of subcutaneous tissue and fascia. Ann Surg 168:274, 1968

80. Talkington DF, Schwartz B, Black CM, et al: Association of phenotypic and genotypic characteristics of invasive Streptococcus pyogenes isolates with clinical components of streptococcal toxic shock syndrome. Infect Immun 61:3369, 1993

81. Barker FG, Leppard BJ, Seal DV: Streptococcal necrotizing fasciitis: comparison between histological and clinical features. J Clin Pathol 40:335, 1987

82. Giuliano A, Lewis F, Hadley K, et al: Bacteriology of necrotizing fasciitis. Am J Surg 134:52, 1977

83. Seal DV, Kingston D: Streptococcal necrotizing fasciitis: development of an animal model to study its pathogenesis. Br J Exp Pathol 69:813, 1988

84. Howard RJ, Pesa ME, Brennaman BH, et al: Necrotizing soft tissue infections caused by marine vibrios. Surgery 98:126, 1985

85. Wilson CB, Siber GR, O'Brien TF, et al: Phycomycotic gangrenous cellulitis. Arch Surg 111:532, 1976

86. Patino JF, Castro D, Valencia A, et al: Necrotizing soft-tissue lesions after a volcanic cataclysm. World J Surg 15:240, 1991

87. Greenberg RN, Willoughby BG, Kennedy DJ, et al: Hypocalcemia and "toxic" syndrome associated with streptococcal fasciitis. South Med J 76:916, 1983

88. Watanabe-Ohnishi R, Low DE, McGeer A, et al: Selective depletion of Vβ-bearing T cells in patients with severe invasive group A streptococcal disease and streptococcal toxic shock syndrome: implications for a novel superantigen. J Infect Dis 171:74, 1995

89. Kawabe Y, Ochi A: Selective anergy of Vβ8+, CD4+ T cells in Staphylococcus enterotoxin B–primed mice. J Exp Med 172:1065, 1990

90. McCormack JE, Callahan JE, Kappler J, et al: Profound depletion of mature T cells in vivo by chronic exposure to exogenous superantigen. J Immunol 150:3785, 1993

91. Lancefield RC: Current knowledge of type-specific M antigens of group A streptococci. J Immunol 89:307, 1962

92. Schwartz B, Facklam RR, Brieman RF: Changing epidemiology of group A streptococcal infection in the USA. Lancet 336:1167, 1990

93. Takei S, Arora YK, Walker SM: Intravenous immunoglobulin contains specific antibodies inhibitory to activation of T cells by staphylococcal toxin superantigens. J Clin Invest 91:602, 1993

94. MacLennan JD: Streptococcal infection of muscle. Lancet 1:582, 1943

95. Yoder EL, Mendez J, Khatib R: Spontaneous gangrenous myositis induced by *Streptococcus pyogenes*: case report and review of the literature. Rev Infect Dis 9:382, 1987

96. Stone HH, Martin JD Jr: Synergistic necrotizing cellulitis. Ann Surg 129:702, 1972

97. Rouse TM, Malangoni MA, Schulte WJ: Necrotizing fasciitis: a preventable disaster. Surgery 92:765, 1982

98. Fournier JA: Gangrène foudroyante de la verge. La Semaine Médicale 3:345, 1883

99. Rudolf R, Soloway M, DePalma RG, et al: Fournier's syndrome: synergistic gangrene of the scrotum. Am J Surg 129:591, 1975

100. Coenen H, Przedborski J: Die gangrän des penis und scrotums. Beitrage zur Klinischen Chirurgie 75:136, 1911

101. Slater DN, Smith GT, Mundy K: Diabetes mellitus with ketoacidosis presenting as Fournier's gangrene. J R Soc Med 75:530, 1982

102. MacLennan JD: Anaerobic infections of war wounds in the Middle East. Lancet 2:63, 1943

103. Altemeier WA, Culbertson WR: Acute non-clostridial crepitant cellulitis. Surg Gynecol Obstet 87:207, 1948

104. Van Beek A, Zook E, Yaw P, et al: Nonclostridial gasforming infections: a collective review and report of seven cases. Arch Surg 108:552, 1974

105. Zook EG, Miller M, Van Beek AL, et al: Successful treatment protocol for canine fang injuries. J Trauma 20:243, 1980

106. Good RA, Thomas L: Studies on the generalized Shwartzman reaction: IV. Prevention of the local and generalized Shwartzman reactions with heparin. J Exp Med 97:871, 1953

107. Silbart S, Oppenheim W: Purpura fulminans: medical, surgical and rehabilitative considerations. Clin Orthop 193:206, 1985

108. Smith OP, White B, Vaughan D, et al: Use of protein C concentrate, heparin and haemofiltration in meningococcus induced purpura fulminans. Lancet 350:1590, 1997

109. Thomas L, Good RA: The effect of cortisone on the Shwartzman reaction: the production of lesions resembling the dermal and generalized Shwartzman reactions by a single injection of bacterial toxin in cortisone-treated rabbits. J Exp Med 95:409, 1952

Acknowledgments

Figure 1   Wolfin/Medichrome.

Figure 2   From "The Surgical Management of Superficial Infection Caused by Atypical Mycobacteria," by W. J. Plaus and G. Hermann, in *Surgery* 110:99, 1991.

Figures 5 through 8, 21, and 22   Courtesy of Jonathan L. Meakins, M.D., Royal Victoria Hospital, Montreal.

Figures 9 and 10   Courtesy of E. Patchen Dellinger, M.D., Harborview Medical Center, Seattle.

Figures 13 and 15   From *Infectious Diseases Illustrated,* by Harold Lambert and W. Edmund Farrar. Gower Medical Publishing Ltd., London, 1981.

Figure 14   From *Color Atlas of Paediatric Dermatology,* by Julian Verbow and Neil Morley. MTP Press, Lancaster, England, 1983.

Figure 16   Dimitry Schidlovsky.

Figure 17   Courtesy of Charles R. Baxter, M.D., University of Texas Health Science Center at Dallas.

Figures 18 and 19   From *A Visual Exploration of Anaerobic Infections,* by Charles A. Kallick. Merck-Frosst Canada, Inc., Kirkland, Quebec, 1978.

3 OPEN WOUND REQUIRING RECONSTRUCTION

Joseph J. Disa, M.D., F.A.C.S., and David A. Hidalgo, M.D., F.A.C.S.

Approach to Surgical Reconstruction

Acute Reconstruction

EVALUATION AND INITIAL TREATMENT OF OPEN WOUND

Problem wounds are characterized by one of the following: large size that precludes direct primary closure, gross infection or uncertain bacteriologic status, or threatened loss of critical structures exposed as a result of insufficient soft tissue coverage. Surgically created wounds, which generally pose less of a problem from a bacteriologic standpoint than traumatic wounds, are best managed by an immediate coverage procedure when direct closure is impossible.

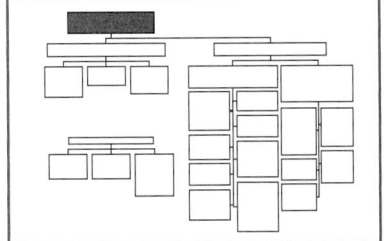

Traumatic wounds are more difficult to evaluate than surgical wounds for several reasons. First, in traumatic wounds, the potential for infection is high because of the environment in which the wound is created, the mechanism of injury, and the time that elapses before operative intervention. Second, the mechanism of injury (e.g., crush, avulsion, or gunshot) may extend the zone of injury beyond what is immediately apparent [*see Figure 1*]. Serious postoperative infection may develop in these cases if definitive wound coverage is provided in the absence of adequate debridement. Third, the long-term functional prospects for the injured part are a key determinant in selecting the method of acute treatment. However, accurate assessment of the chances for recovery of specific structures within the wound is often difficult immediately after injury.

Evaluation

The initial step in the management of problem wounds is to decide whether the wound is suitable for immediate soft tissue coverage. Wounds that are surgically created during the course of an elective procedure are almost always best treated with primary definitive coverage. Traumatic wounds that present within 1 or 2 hours of injury and have a minimal crush component are also best treated with a primary definitive coverage procedure after thorough operative debridement.

Injuries with a significant crush component and exposure of critical structures such as nerves, vessels, tendons, or bone are best treated more aggressively. In these cases, thorough debridement requires considerable surgical experience because the tendency is to debride inadequately. The degree of accuracy to which tissue viability can be assessed varies among different types of tissue. For example, skin can be evaluated by its color, the nature of its capillary refill, the quality of its dermal bleeding, or its bleeding response to pinprick. After I.V. fluorescein injection, skin viability can also be assessed qualitatively, with a Wood's light, or quantitatively, with a dermofluorometer. Muscle is the most difficult tissue to evaluate. Color, capillary bleeding, and contractile response to stimulation are not always reliable indicators of muscle viability. In

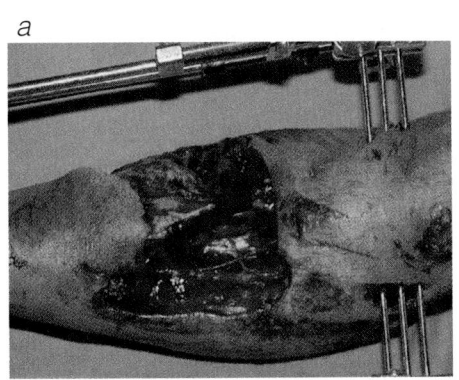 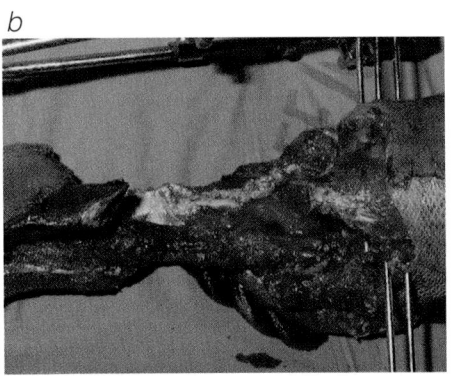 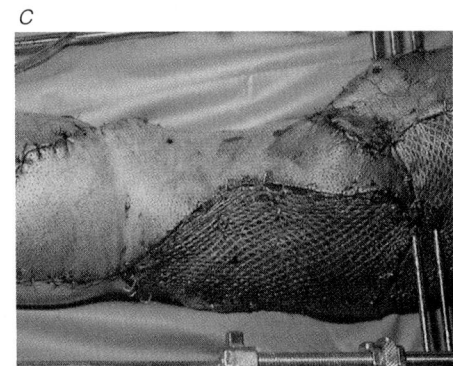

Figure 1 (*a*) A so-called bumper injury of the leg is shown after initial debridement and bony stabilization (2 days after injury). (*b*) After the second debridement, the true extent of devitalization of bone and soft tissue is apparent (4 days after injury). (*c*) A latissimus dorsi free flap has been used to reconstruct the soft tissue defect (5 days after injury).

Acute reconstruction is indicated

Evaluate and treat open wound.

Select coverage procedure to achieve healed wound and avoid infection.

Defer treatment of functional problems for secondary reconstruction.

Wound does not contain exposed bone, cartilage, nerve, or tendon but cannot be closed directly

Apply a skin graft.

Wound is a small defect but is in an area where graft contracture is not desirable (e.g., face, hand, or flexion crease)

Apply full-thickness skin graft; donor sites include the ear, upper eyelid, neck, and groin.

Wound has a large surface area or is a small wound in a noncritical area

Apply split-thickness skin graft.

Wound is known to be significantly contaminated

Apply meshed split-thickness skin graft or consider delayed skin graft replacement and open treatment of wound until bacteriologic status is clear.

Secondary reconstruction of chronic defect is indicated

Defect is a small localized scar or a focal scar contracture

Revise with Z-plasty or other local tissue rearrangement procedure.

There is a shortage of skin and subcutaneous tissue only, but skin graft coverage is not desirable

Use tissue expanders (except on hand or foot).

One or more of the following conditions is present:
• **Composite defect**
• **Functional defect of muscle or bone**
• **Contour deformity**
• **Unstable soft tissue coverage of vital structure**
• **Inadequate soft tissue coverage for bone or nerve grafting**

Repair with free or local flap.

Approach to Surgical Reconstruction

Bone, cartilage, nerve, or tendon is exposed and cannot be covered by direct wound closure

Perform flap coverage procedure.

Local donor site meets needs and is not involved in the primary process

Use local flap.
- *Small or clean wound:* use local skin flap if possible.
- *Large or contaminated wound:* use regional myocutaneous flap.

Local flap is not possible or would not provide appropriate tissue

Use free flap.
- If wound is clean and thin flap is desired, apply skin or fascial free flap.
- If wound is large or contaminated, apply muscle or myocutaneous free flap.

Muscle flaps require coverage with a meshed split-thickness skin graft.

Head or neck defect

- *Small facial defect with no facial features involved:* use Z-plasty, Limberg flap, or other advancement flap of cheek or forehead.
- *Large defect of neck or lower head:* use regional myocutaneous flap of trapezius, latissimus dorsi, or pectoralis major muscle.

Abdominal defect

Use regional flap (e.g., tensor fasciae latae, rectus femoris, or rectus abdominis muscle).

Gluteal or perineal defect

Use regional myocutaneous flap (e.g., gluteus maximus, gracilis, tensor fasciae latae, or biceps femoris).

Thigh, knee, or leg defect

- *Thigh defect:* use regional muscle flap (e.g., tensor fasciae latae, rectus femoris, vastus lateralis, or vastus medialis muscle).
- *Defect of knee or proximal leg:* use gastrocnemius muscle flap.
- *Proximal or midleg defect:* use soleus muscle flap.

Foot defect

- *Plantar:* close defect of weight-bearing heel or midsole with medially based skin rotation flap raised superficial to plantar fascia or with other myocutaneous or fasciocutaneous plantar flap. Cover limited defect of distal plantar surface with toe flap.
- *Posterior heel, Achilles tendon, malleoli:* use either extensor digitorum brevis muscle as pedicled flap or lateral calcaneal artery flap.

Chest or back defect

In most cases, use regional myocutaneous flap (e.g., pectoralis major, rectus abdominis, latissimus dorsi, or trapezius muscle).

Arm defect

Cover large wounds above the elbow with latissimus dorsi muscle transposed as a pedicled flap.

Hand defect

Free flaps are preferred, but pedicled distant skin flaps from the chest or abdomen are also acceptable. Defects of the digits can be covered with cross-finger flaps or, for tip injuries, with thenar flaps.

Head or neck defect

- *Large defect of scalp or upper face:* cover with latissimus dorsi, scapular, or rectus abdominis free flap.
- *Floor of the mouth:* replace with forearm free flap.
- *Mandible:* reconstruct with various composite free flaps of bone and skin.
- *Oropharynx or cervical esophagus:* use jejunum free flap or forearm flap.

Forearm defect

Cover large forearm wound with free flap of rectus abdominis, scapular, or latissimus dorsi muscle.

Hand defect

- *Exposed tendons on the dorsum:* cover with temporalis fascia free flap.
- *Defect of the web space:* correct with lateral arm free flap.

Knee or leg defect

- *Major wound of the popliteal fossa:* use free flap if the blood supply to the gastrocnemius muscle is compromised.
- *Defect of the lower third of the leg:* use latissimus dorsi, rectus abdominis, scapular, or gracilis free flap.

Foot defect

- *Plantar:* repair very large defect with muscle free flap covered with a skin graft.
- *Dorsum:* use fascial free flap and overlying skin graft, or use thin skin free flap.

severe injuries, they can be misleading. Inadequate debridement may lead to severe consequences resulting from infection. Therefore, serial debridement at 24- to 48-hour intervals is essential for accurately establishing the limits of muscle injury. Efforts should be made during debridement to preserve tissues such as major nerves and blood vessels unless they are severely contused. These structures are vital for function and are of small mass compared with other tissues (e.g., skin, fat, and muscle) at risk for necrosis and subsequent infection.

Wound debridement, therefore, should involve careful analysis of the injury from an anatomic point of view; debridement should not consist of indiscriminate excision of blocks of tissue. Between debridement procedures, the wound should be treated with sterile dressings but in an open manner (i.e., without closure by sutures and with wet-to-dry dressings changed three or four times a day). A definitive soft tissue coverage procedure should then be performed as soon after the initial injury as wound conditions permit. When thorough debridement and definitive coverage can be completed within less than a week, the wound will generally heal uneventfully. Inadequate debridement frequently results in the loss of any additional tissue invested to achieve acute soft tissue coverage. The wound becomes grossly infected, and important functional structures within the wound are reexposed.

Infected surgical wounds, neglected wounds, or other complex wounds in which initial wound management fails should be debrided and then treated by open methods. Proper care of these wounds is achieved by a multifaceted approach aimed at converting established gross infection to a much lower level of bacterial contamination, which is then compatible with successful secondary wound closure.

Initial Treatment

Debridement Devitalized tissue provides an ideal culture medium for bacteria and isolates them from host defense mechanisms. Surgical debridement must be performed as often as necessary to remove all necrotic tissue.

High-pressure irrigation A useful adjunct to debridement is high-pressure irrigation, which has been shown experimentally to decrease wound infection rates significantly.[1,2] The necessary pressure of 8 psi can be achieved by forceful irrigation through a 35 ml syringe fitted with a 19-gauge needle. Low-pressure irrigation with a bulb-type syringe, for example, has not proved to be beneficial.

Quantitative bacteriology The degree of bacterial wound contamination can be accurately quantified. The standard technique of quantitative bacteriology requires several days to complete. In addition to a count, it provides identification and antibiotic sensitivities of the organism. Quantitative bacteriology can also be performed by using the rapid slide technique, which provides valuable information about the wound within 20 minutes.[3,4] The level of bacterial contamination has been shown to be a significant predictor of outcome in wound closure by either skin-graft or flap-coverage techniques. According to the golden-period principle of wound closure, a minimum time interval is necessary for bacteria to proliferate to a certain threshold level. Contaminated wounds take a mean time of about 5 hours to reach a bacterial count of 10^5/g of tissue. Attempts to close wounds that have counts higher than 10^5/g of tissue will fail 75% to 100% of the time, whereas wounds with lower counts are successfully closed more than 90% of the time.[5] β-Hemolytic streptococci are an exception in that much lower concentrations of these organisms consistently result in failure of wound closure. When a β-hemolytic strepto-

coccus is the dominant isolate, the wound should generally be treated openly until cultures become negative.

Systemic antibiotics The role of systemic antibiotics in wound management is not clearly defined. Broad-spectrum antibiotics should be given in cases of severe trauma or established, uncontrolled infection. They may also be useful for minor wounds that cannot be closed within 3 hours of injury.

Topical antibiotics Certain antibiotics provide broad-spectrum activity when applied topically. Neomycin, 10 mg/ml, or a combination of bacitracin, 50 U/ml, and polymyxin B, 0.05 mg/ml, kills most common wound pathogens. These solutions can be used when wet dressings are indicated.

Topical antiseptics A variety of topical antiseptics have been used empirically in wound care. In the concentrations usually recommended, however, these solutions are detrimental to wound healing. Povidone-iodine (1%), hydrogen peroxide (3%), acetic acid (0.25%), and sodium hypochlorite (0.5%) all have been shown to be lethal to fibroblasts as well as to bacteria. More dilute concentrations of povidone-iodine (0.001%) and sodium hypochlorite (0.005%) are effective against bacteria while being safe for fibroblasts.[6] A number of these agents also inhibit normal white blood cell function in the wound.

Wet dressings Open wounds are treated with wet dressings, generally consisting of gauze soaked in saline or an acceptable topical antiseptic. Wet-to-wet dressings prevent desiccation of exposed vital structures or freshly placed skin grafts. Wet-to-dry dressings are useful for assisting in daily wound debridement. These dressings are allowed to dry on the wound; when they are removed, adherent fibrinous debris is removed with the dressing. Wet dressings of either type should be changed at least three times a day.

Small wounds can be expected to close by contraction and secondary epithelialization after appropriate open management with the techniques described. Large wounds will improve with aggressive open care but will then stabilize into a chronic state of wound colonization of varying degrees. A soft tissue coverage procedure is then necessary to complete closure in these cases.

SELECTION OF COVERAGE PROCEDURE

The goals of coverage procedures [see 2:7 Surface Reconstruction Procedures] in the management of acute as well as chronic wounds are to achieve a healed wound and to avoid infec-

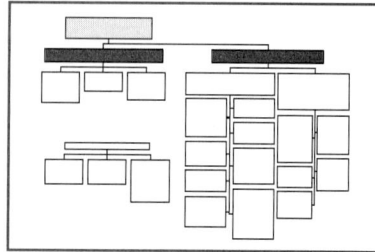

tion. The treatment of functional problems is generally deferred for secondary reconstruction.

The method of coverage depends on whether vital structures, such as vessels, tendons, nerves, and bone, are exposed in the wound. If no vital structures are exposed, skin-graft coverage is indicated. Skin grafts can also be used over tendon if the paratenon is intact, over nerve if the epineurium is intact, and over bone if the periosteum is intact. Skin grafts are the most expendable type of soft tissue available for the coverage of open wounds. They allow the wound to heal completely and set the stage for secondary reconstruction, during which more valuable tissue can be used to achieve other goals at minimal risk. When vital structures are exposed in the wound, a flap is preferred because it provides more substantial soft tissue coverage of the structure. The choice of flap depends on the location of the wound and on its overall size, depth, and topographic configuration (see below).

Skin Grafts

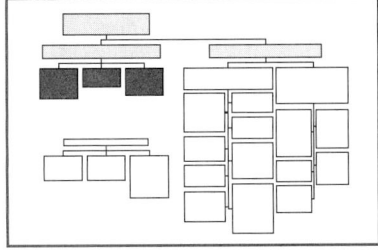

Skin grafts may be either partial thickness (i.e., split thickness) or full thickness [*see 2:7 Surface Reconstruction Procedures*]. Split-thickness grafts are preferred for wounds with a large surface area. Full-thickness grafts are suitable only for small defects because their donor sites must be closed primarily; the most common donor sites for full-thickness grafts are the ears, upper eyelids, neck, and groin. Full-thickness grafts contract less with time than split-thickness grafts and are therefore particularly suitable for wounds of the hands, extremity flexion creases, nose, eyelids, and other areas of the face.

Successful healing of skin grafts requires immobilization of the recipient site to prevent shearing in the plane between the graft and the wound bed. However, although complete immobilization is desirable, the required dressings may preclude observation of a wound that is known to be significantly contaminated. In such cases, a meshed split-thickness graft is indicated, and the wound should be treated in an open fashion. A meshed graft can be placed directly over the muscle of a flap and secured over its irregular contour with staples [*see Figure 2*]. Because the graft is meshed, serum can escape between the interstices and there is little risk of separation from the underlying tissue. A meshed graft is also less vulnerable to disruption by shear forces. An additional advantage of a meshed graft is that it permits the wound to be treated with wet dressings if there is still risk for infection. A mesh expansion ratio of 1.5:1.0 is generally preferred, except when the surface area of the wound is very large and the availability of donor sites is limited.

Flaps

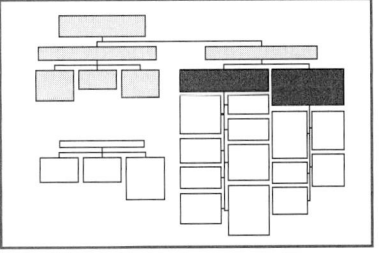

Flaps consist of tissues that have a self-contained vascular system [*see 2:7 Surface Reconstruction Procedures*]. They permit a more substantial transfer of tissue bulk than do skin grafts and may consist of either skin and subcutaneous tissue, fascia, muscle, bone, or a combination of several of these tissue types. Local flaps consist of tissue that is mostly detached from surrounding tissue but retains enough connection to preserve an adequate blood supply to the entire flap. Local flaps are either transposed, rotated, or advanced into adjacent defects for purposes of reconstruction. Free flaps are totally detached and have their blood supply reconnected at the recipient site by surgically performed microvascular anastomoses between recipient-site blood vessels and the major vessels that supply the flap.

Local flaps versus free flaps   The choice between a local flap and a free flap is determined by the amount and the type of tissue needed, as well as by the availability of flaps in the immediate area of the wound [*see Figure 3*]. Availability of local flaps, in turn, is determined by the nature of the regional blood supply. The vascular anatomy of a particular area determines the availability of arterialized skin flaps, fasciocutaneous flaps, myocutaneous flaps,

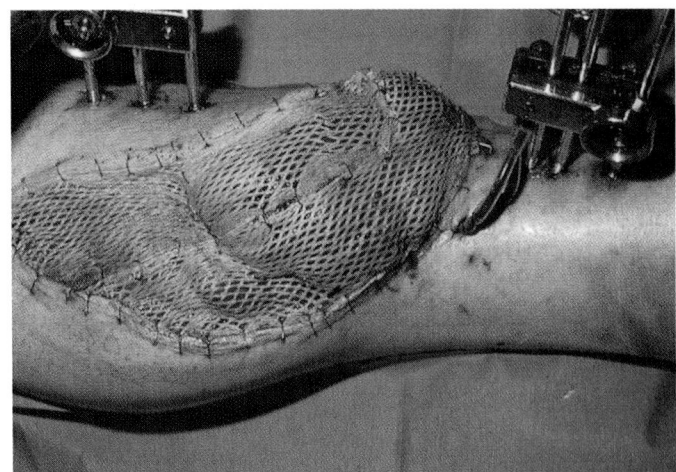

Figure 2   **A meshed (1.5-to-1.0 ratio) skin graft has been secured to the irregular contour of a muscle free flap with staples. No additional immobilization of the graft is needed. The interstices of the graft allow free drainage of serous exudate from the muscle.**

and other forms of composite flaps. Local flaps can be grouped regionally by the types of tissue that they provide [*see Table 1*].

A local flap is generally preferred over a free flap if the two provide similar tissue, primarily because of the additional effort required to move a free flap. A free-flap procedure commonly takes twice as long as a local-flap procedure. The preference for local flaps does not result from fear of performing microvascular anastomoses—experienced surgeons accomplish free tissue transfer with success rates higher than 95%.

Free flaps are indicated in areas where local flaps are unavailable, such as in the distal third of the leg, or when an extremely large flap is needed but is unavailable locally. When regional donor sites are affected by the primary process, free tissue transfer allows

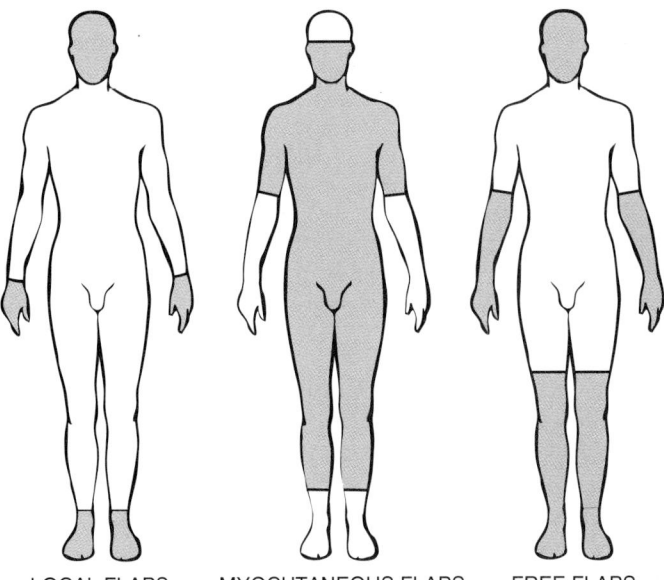

LOCAL FLAPS   MYOCUTANEOUS FLAPS   FREE FLAPS

Figure 3   **Regional alternatives in flap selection are illustrated. Defects in the central portion of the body are treated with myocutaneous flaps primarily; defects of the peripheral areas are treated with either local flaps or free flaps. In some areas, several options exist, and the choice is influenced by the size of the defect and the specific tissue requirements.**

Table 1 Selection of Local Flaps by Region and Tissue Type

Site	Skin Flaps	Muscle and Myocutaneous Flaps	Fascial and Fasciocutaneous Flaps
Head and neck	Scalp; forehead; nasolabial; cervico-facial; Mustardé; eyelid; lip	Trapezius; latissimus dorsi; pectoralis major	Superficial and deep temporal fascia
Chest and back	Lateral thoracic; deltopectoral	Trapezius; pectoralis major; latissimus dorsi; rectus abdominis (superiorly based)	Scapular
Arm	Medial arm (Tagliacozzi)	Latissimus dorsi; pectoralis major	Lateral arm; forearm
Hand	Cross-finger; thenar; neurovascular island; fingertip advancement	—	Forearm
Abdomen and perineum	Groin	Rectus abdominis (inferiorly based); tensor fasciae latae; rectus femoris; gracilis	Medial thigh
Gluteal area	Sacral; thoracolumbar	Gluteus maximus; gracilis; tensor fasciae latae; biceps femoris	Gluteal thigh
Thigh	—	Tensor fasciae latae; rectus femoris; vastus lateralis; vastus medialis; gracilis; biceps femoris; rectus abdominis	Anterior thigh; anteromedial thigh; posterior thigh
Knee and proximal leg	—	Gastrocnemius	Saphenous artery; posterior calf
Midleg	—	Soleus; tibialis anterior	Anterior leg; lateral leg; posterior leg
Distal leg	—	—	—
Foot	Dorsalis pedis; plantar rotation; lateral calcaneal artery; plantar V-Y	Flexor digitorum brevis; abductor hallucis; abductor digiti minimi; extensor digitorum brevis	—

healthy, well-vascularized tissue to be brought into the compromised area. Moreover, if free tissue is transferred, the size of the wound is not extended, because the donor site is not contiguous but instead is located at a distance from the wound.

If expertise in microvascular surgery is available, free flaps are frequently a first-line choice. Free flaps allow selection of the appropriate type of tissue in the most suitable size and configuration for the specific reconstructive problem. Compared with free flaps, local flaps are inefficient ways of moving tissue because only a small portion of a local flap actually reaches the defect itself. The choice of donor site is greater with free flaps because the limitations imposed by local availability are avoided.

Free flaps used in acute reconstruction can be grouped into three major types [see Table 2]. The soft tissue coverage requirements of most wounds can be met by so-called workhorse free flaps. These flaps typically have the advantages of large size, ease of dissection, and a vascular pedicle that is long and of large diameter. The disadvantages, such as awkward patient positioning for flap harvest, are minor. Most workhorse flaps consist of muscle with an optional skin component; they are the flaps of choice for contaminated wounds [see Figure 4]. A second group of free flaps is useful for acute reconstruction of unusually large wounds. These flaps consist of combined vascular territories supplied by a single vascular pedicle. A third category consists of smaller free

Table 2 Free Flap Selection for Soft Tissue Coverage*

Requirement	Specific Flap	Advantages	Disadvantages
Reliable workhorse flaps	Latissimus dorsi	Ideal pedicle[†]; ease of dissection	Awkward patient positioning
	Rectus abdominis	Ideal pedicle; supine position; ease of dissection	No major disadvantages
	Scapular	Ideal pedicle; skin flap only	Awkward patient positioning
Flaps of very large surface area	Combined latissimus dorsi and scapular	Independent component inset[‡]; primary donor-site closure possible; ideal pedicle	Awkward patient positioning
	Extended tensor fasciae latae and partial quadriceps	Supine position; large skin flap component	Donor-site healing[§]; pedicle configuration[‖]
Small flaps	Gracilis	Small muscle	Small vessels
	Lateral arm	Thin, sensate; convenient for hand trauma	Small vessels; donor-site scar
	Forearm	Thin skin flap; ideal pedicle	Minor hand morbidity; poor donor-site appearance
	Temporalis fascia	Thinnest flap; ideal coverage for exposed tendons[¶]; can transfer hair-bearing scalp	Variable donor-site scar alopecia

*Includes only the more commonly used free flaps for purposes of comparison.
[†]Characterized by large-diameter vessels and long pedicle length.
[‡]Each part can be arranged and sewn into the wound separately.
[§]Donor-site closure requires a skin graft, which may result in delayed healing.
[‖]Pedicle enters middle of undersurface of flap.
[¶]Permits tendon gliding underneath if used on dorsum of the hand or of the foot.

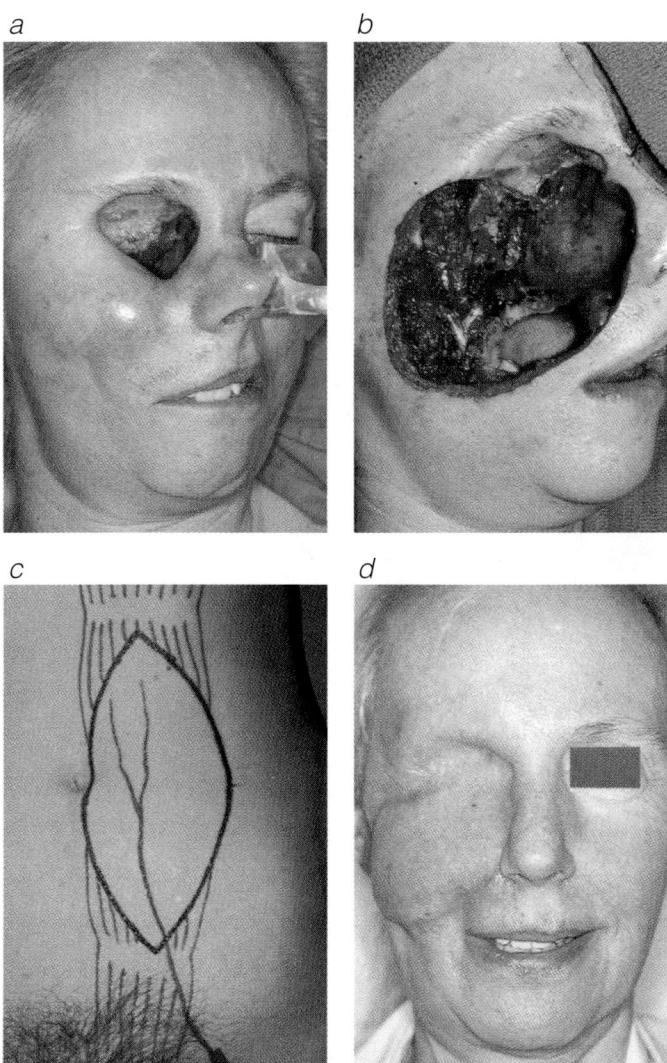

Figure 4 (*a*) **Shown is a facial tumor that has recurred after previous orbital exenteration. (*b*) The defect has been resected. Local flaps and regional myocutaneous flaps are not available for this defect. (*c*) A rectus abdominis myocutaneous free flap is designed. This flap can be designed in other sizes and configurations depending on specific needs. The vascular pedicle is long and of large diameter, and the flap is easily accessible in the supine patient. (*d*) After surgery, soft tissue coverage with a reasonable restoration of facial contour has been achieved.**

flaps that provide tissue that is superior in either amount or type to the local flaps that are otherwise available. An additional advantage of these flaps is that they tend not to be bulky. They are frequently used in areas such as the head, hands, distal third of the leg, and feet [*see Figure 5*].

Flap coverage procedures are illustrated in greater detail elsewhere [*see 2:7 Surface Reconstruction Procedures*].

Regional alternatives in flap selection

Head, neck. Facial defects of small to moderate size are best treated with local skin flaps. A variety of flaps are available for reconstruction of limited defects of the eyelids, cheeks, nose, and mouth.[7-9]

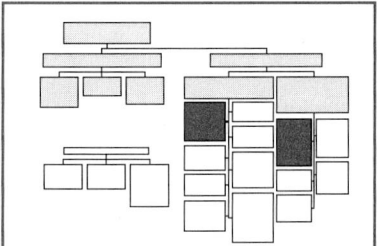

Small facial defects that do not directly involve the facial features can often be closed with several types of flaps that rearrange the existing tissue in the area—for example, Z-plasty or a Limberg flap. Tissues that are difficult to match, such as those of the eyelids or lips, can often be reconstructed with flaps that borrow tissue from their opposite, intact counterparts; the Abbe lip flap is such a flap.

For coverage of some large defects in the head and neck region, the trapezius, the latissimus dorsi, and the pectoralis major can be used. Each muscle can be raised with an optional skin island. These flaps are generally too bulky to be used on the face, and their reach is limited when used as pedicled flaps: none of them can cover major portions of the scalp or comfortably reach the upper face.

Latissimus dorsi, scapular, and rectus abdominis free flaps are useful for very large defects of the scalp or upper face. Smaller defects of the scalp are best treated with local scalp flaps.

Other free flaps of a specialized nature are superior for reconstruction of the floor of the mouth and mandible, even though local myocutaneous flaps will reach this area. For example, the forearm free flap based on the radial artery is quite thin and pliable and therefore provides an ideal replacement for the floor of the mouth. Composite free flaps that contain both bone and skin, such as those taken from the scapula, ilium, radius, and fibula, provide tissue of the appropriate type and proper configuration for defects of the lower face in which the mandible must be reconstructed along with the intraoral lining, the external skin, or both.

Chest, back. Most defects of the chest and back are amenable to treatment with local myocutaneous flaps because of the wide arc of rotation of muscles located in these areas.[10] Midline sternal wounds can be covered with either pectoralis

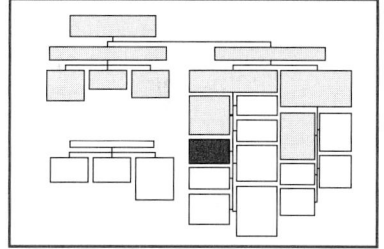

major or rectus abdominis flaps; lateral chest defects with latissimus dorsi or pectoralis major flaps; and midline back defects with latissimus dorsi or trapezius flaps. Both the pectoralis major and the latissimus dorsi can be divided from their primary vascular supply while retaining their intercostal supply and folded over as local flaps to cover midline defects anteriorly and posteriorly, respectively.

Arm, forearm. Large wounds above the elbow can be covered with a latissimus dorsi myocutaneous flap transposed as a pedicled flap, provided that the vascular pedicle of the muscle has not been affected by the injury. Forearm wounds

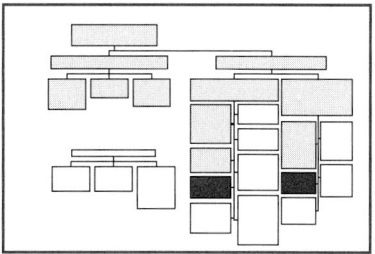

that require flap closure are best treated with free flaps. A rectus abdominis, scapular, or latissimus dorsi muscle flap can be used for large defects of the arm or forearm. Although soft tissue coverage with simultaneous functional forearm muscle replacement can be achieved with a single flap such as the gracilis muscle, this procedure is not generally recommended; rather, a skin flap such as a scapular free flap is preferred as a first stage of reconstruction to achieve wound healing.

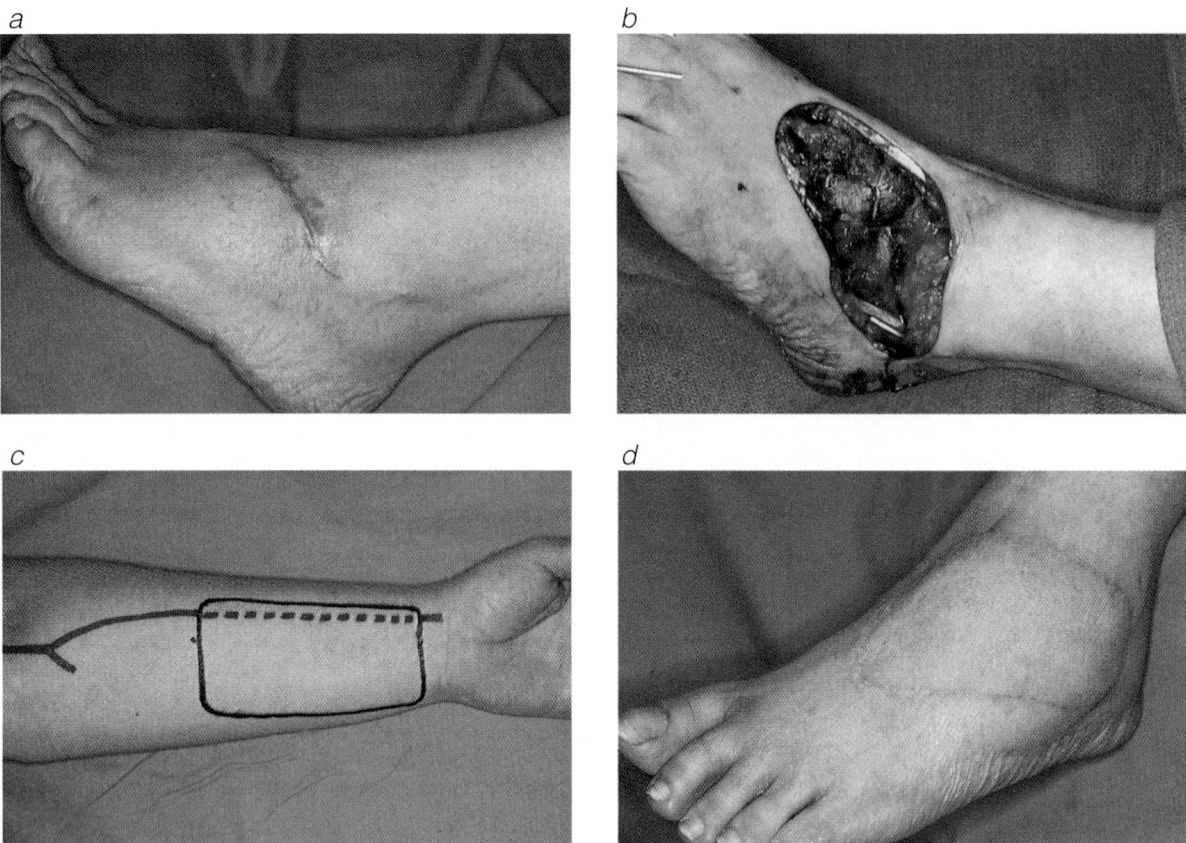

Figure 5 (*a*) **A soft tissue sarcoma has recurred in the scar of a previous excision. (*b*) Reexcision of the defect has exposed bone and tendons. No regional flaps are available for satisfactory coverage of this defect. (*c*) The forearm is a source of small, thin free flaps. (*d*) Flap transfer is complete. The radial artery and venae comitantes have been anastomosed to their dorsalis pedis counterparts.**

Hand. Both free flaps and pedicled skin flaps are useful for soft tissue coverage of hand wounds. The temporalis fascia free flap is particularly thin and is ideal for coverage of exposed tendons on the dorsum of the hand. The lateral arm

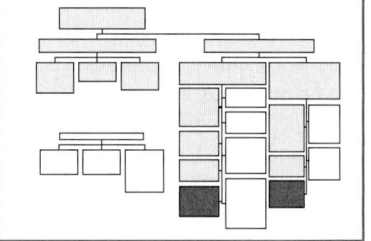

free flap is ideal for reconstruction of a large defect of the first web space; it has sensory potential because it contains a large sensory nerve. Both of these free flaps are small. Pedicled distant skin flaps from the chest or abdomen are available as an alternative form of coverage of sizable hand defects. However, pedicled skin flaps have major disadvantages: wound care is difficult, edema persists because elevation and movement of the hand are seldom possible while it is attached to the trunk, and a second procedure is needed to divide these flaps.

Digital injuries with exposed tendons can be closed with a variety of cross-finger flaps of skin and subcutaneous tissue raised from either the volar or extensor aspect of an adjacent digit. Because these flaps do not contain a great deal of subcutaneous tissue, they are preferred for coverage of digits proximally, where a thick subcutaneous pad is not essential. The thenar flap is useful for fingertip injuries in which the soft tissue pad of the fingertip is lost and bone is exposed. This flap provides an ideal pulp replacement as well as better sensory recovery than skin grafts. Fingertip injuries can also be closed with several types of V–Y advancement

flaps that can be raised from either the volar or lateral surfaces of the end of the finger.

Abdomen. Defects of the abdominal wall that require flap closure are best treated with local muscle flaps such as the tensor fasciae latae and the rectus femoris from the thigh. The rectus abdominis also can occasionally be transposed to cover an abdo-

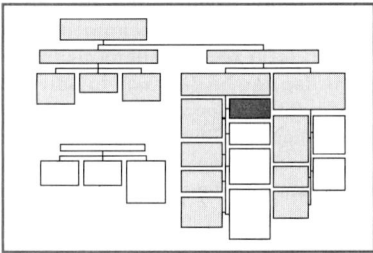

minal defect. Each of these flaps is harvested along with skin, although a large tensor fasciae latae flap will probably require skin-graft closure of the donor site. The tensor fasciae latae flap has the advantage of including the thickened deep fascia (iliotibial band) of the thigh, which can provide additional strength for abdominal wall closure.

Gluteal area, perineum. Local muscle flaps with or without skin are indicated for defects in this area. They are preferable to large, random-pattern advancement skin flaps from the posterior thigh and thoracolumbar rotation skin flaps. The glu-

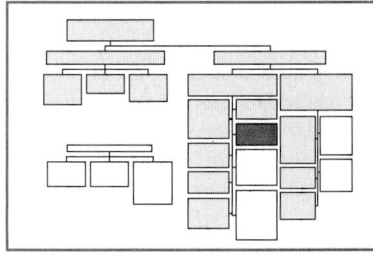

teus maximus, for example, can be used as a rotation, V–Y advancement, or turnover flap in the treatment of pressure sores. As a turnover flap, it can be proximally or distally based, or it can be split along its longitudinal axis so that only a portion of it is used. Also useful for covering defects in the gluteal area and the perineum is the myofasciocutaneous gluteal-thigh flap, a combination of a gluteus muscle flap and a fasciocutaneous flap from the posterior thigh that is supplied by an extension of the inferior gluteal artery. Because of its size and location, the gracilis is well suited for coverage of defects of the perineum. The gracilis and the biceps femoris are generally secondary choices for the treatment of pressure sores over the ischium. The tensor fasciae latae is frequently used for treating open wounds over the greater trochanter. The entire quadriceps can be used to close defects resulting from hemipelvectomy.

Thigh. Flaps are rarely required for soft tissue coverage in the thigh area, because critical vital structures are located deep within the thigh and are rarely exposed by injury or by surgical procedures. A number of regional muscle flaps are

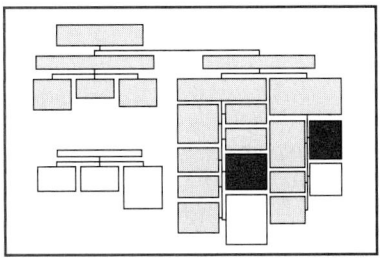

available, however, including the tensor fasciae latae, the rectus femoris, the vastus lateralis, and the vastus medialis. The gracilis and posterior thigh muscles are rarely used in this area. An anterior defect with exposure of the femoral vessels can be covered with either an ipsilateral or a contralateral rectus abdominis myocutaneous flap. A number of smaller local skin flaps that are supplied with blood from the deep fascia can be raised over portions of the thigh; except for the posterior thigh flap, however, the clinical usefulness of these flaps remains to be demonstrated.

Knee, proximal leg, midleg. The two heads of the gastrocnemius can be used either together or independently to cover defects of the knee and proximal leg. The soleus is useful for coverage of defects of the proximal leg and midleg. Local flaps should not be used for major leg wounds if the extent of the injury suggests involvement of the muscle donor site. Instead, a free flap should be used to bring healthy tissue into the area. Therefore, free flaps are a first choice, for example, for coverage of major wounds of the popliteal fossa, knee, and proximal leg that involve the sural artery blood supply to the gastrocnemius.

Skin flaps fed by the fascial blood supply can also be raised over the leg.[11] A number of fasciocutaneous flaps have been described in this area, but they tend to be smaller than muscle flaps and generally less reliable. These flaps are longitudinally oriented over the course of the anterior tibial artery or the peroneal artery. The maximum length at which such fasciocutaneous flaps are safe and their specific applications have not been well established.

Foot. The foot is as complex as the hand and the face in that it is composed of separate regions, each of which has a unique set of alternatives for reconstruction. These regions include the plantar surface; the dorsum; and the posterior

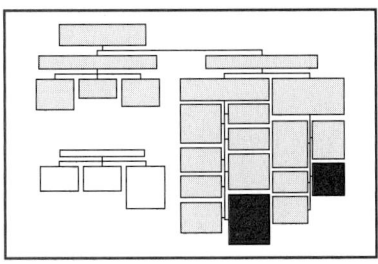

(non–weight-bearing) heel, Achilles tendon, and malleoli.

Superficial defects that lie completely within the non–weight-bearing portion of the midsole do not need flap coverage. Defects of the weight-bearing heel and midsole area that are less than 6 cm in diameter can be closed with a medially based skin rotation flap that is raised superficial to the plantar fascia.[12] This flap maintains plantar sensation. Limited defects of the distal plantar surface can be treated with local toe flaps that also maintain sensation. Very large plantar defects are best resurfaced with a muscle free flap (e.g., latissimus dorsi or rectus abdominis) covered with a skin graft. Although this type of flap lacks sensation, it appears to provide the most durable form of coverage because it resists shear forces well.[13]

Defects of the dorsum that require flap coverage are best covered either with a fascial free flap (e.g., temporalis fascia) and an overlying skin graft or with a skin free flap that is thin (e.g., from the forearm). The extensor digitorum brevis can be raised from the dorsum as a pedicled flap fed by the dorsalis pedis artery. This flap, which measures approximately 5 × 6 cm, has an arc of rotation that makes it useful for the coverage of defects of the malleolus or the Achilles tendon area. A narrow transposition skin flap fed by the lateral calcaneal artery is useful for coverage of defects approximately 3 cm in diameter that lie over the Achilles tendon or the non–weight-bearing posterior heel.

Secondary Reconstruction

Selection of the proper method for secondary reconstruction requires analysis of the type and extent of tissue deficiency that is present. Superficial defects may require replacement or supplementation of only skin and subcutaneous tissue, whereas more complex defects may require replacement of several types of tissue. Specialized tissue such as vascularized nerve (i.e., a nerve free flap) or intestine may be necessary to provide a functional reconstruction in some cases (see below).

SMALL LOCALIZED SCAR

When reconstruction is indicated for a small localized scar, soft tissue coverage is generally sufficient and poses no threat of breakdown leading to exposure of important structures. Instead, the recon-

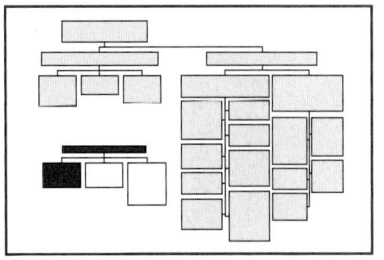

structive problem is generally functional in nature. An example is a tight scar band across a flexion crease, commonly seen after a burn injury. A local procedure that rearranges the existing tissue can relieve the tension by making more tissue available in one direction, though the amount of tissue in the area is not actually increased.

The Z-plasty is an example of such tissue rearrangement [*see 2:7 Surface Reconstruction Procedures*]. Multiple Z-plasties or other procedures, such as W-plasty, may be useful for some localized scars.

SHORTAGE OF SKIN AND SUBCUTANEOUS TISSUE

A shortage of skin and subcutaneous tissue may result from excision of a large scar or of a large congenital defect (e.g., a nevus). Mastectomy commonly leaves a shortage of skin that pre-

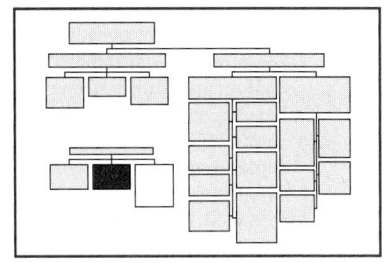

vents creation of a breast mound. In these cases, extra tissue can be created locally with the use of tissue expanders. These devices are inflatable plastic reservoirs of various shapes and volumes that are implanted under the skin. The skin over the expander is stretched during a period of several weeks as the expander is gradually filled by percutaneously injecting saline into an incorporated or remote fill port. The expander is then removed as a second procedure, and the expanded area of skin is advanced to cover the defect.

A number of important principles govern the use of tissue expanders. The expanders must be placed so as to allow expansion only in normal skin adjacent to the defect, not in the defect itself. A sufficiently large expander or multiple expanders must be used to ensure adequate expansion. Complications associated with the use of tissue expanders include infection, extrusion, deflation, flipped ports (remote type), and hematoma formation.[14]

Tissue expanders are used in secondary reconstruction only; they play no role in acute wound management. They are not indicated for contour defects (see below), because the tissue they provide is two-dimensional and lacking in bulk. Nor is expanded tissue adequate for coverage of chronically exposed structures (e.g., bone). Tissue expanders do not provide adequate replacement tissue to establish a suitable bed for nerve or bone grafting. Therefore, they are not a substitute for flaps in general.

The scalp is an ideal location for the use of tissue expanders because no equivalent substitute for this type of hair-bearing tissue exists. Expanders work effectively when implanted over the hard calvarium and are useful in cases of burn alopecia and large nevi involving the scalp. Expanders are also useful for breast reconstruction, for carefully selected large lesions of the face, and for certain scars of the limbs. They are generally not indicated for use in the hands or feet. Although some local flap donor sites, such as the forehead, can be expanded before flap transfer, there is a loss of tissue pliability that appears to limit the usefulness of this particular application.

a

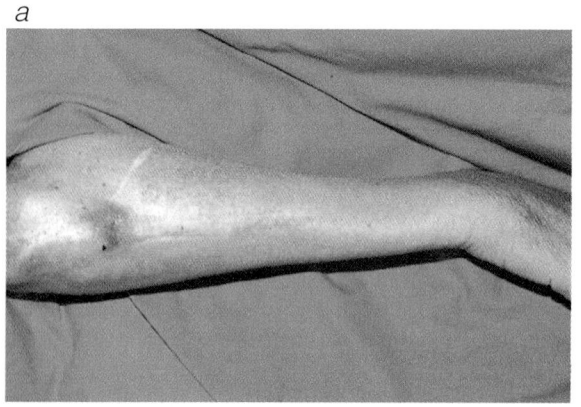

b

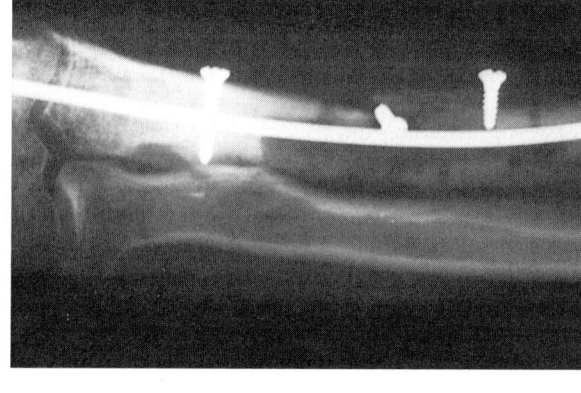

c

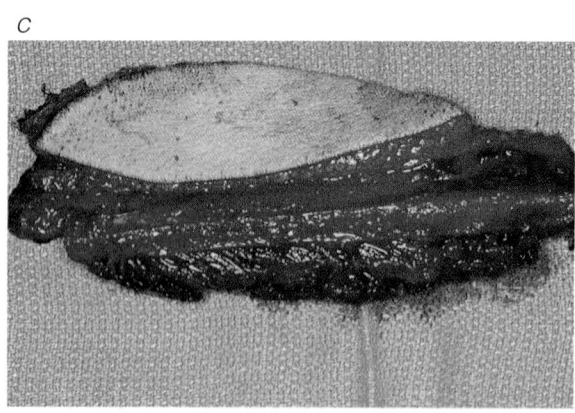

d

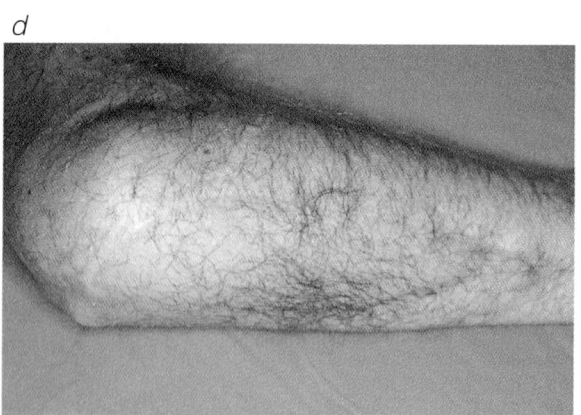

e

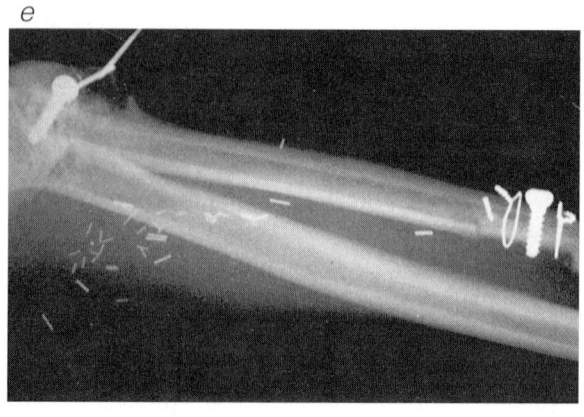

Figure 6 (*a*) **A chronic draining sinus of the ulna with poor overlying soft tissue coverage is shown. Simultaneous replacement of both bone and overlying soft tissue with a composite tissue flap is needed. (*b*) A radiograph shows nonunion of the ulna with orthopedic hardware. (*c*) A fibular free flap provides bone and skin in the appropriate amount and configuration for replacement of the affected tissues in a single stage. (*d*) The segment of ulna and overlying skin has been replaced. (*e*) A radiograph shows the vascularized fibula in place.**

COMPLEX DEFECTS

Certain reconstructive problems require substantial amounts of tissue of one or more types or of a very specialized type. Either local or free flaps are used to meet these tissue requirements.

Composite Defect

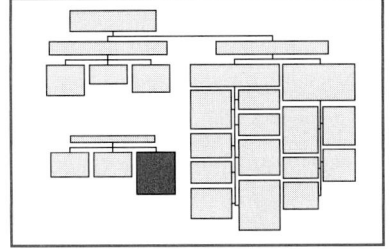

A composite defect may result from resection of an intraoral carcinoma with loss of the mandible and either the lining of the mouth or external skin. Another example is a crush injury of the leg with loss of soft tissue and a segment of weight-bearing bone. These defects require that a composite flap be brought to the area to meet more than one type of tissue deficiency. Local flaps generally do not provide the necessary types of tissue or permit the freedom of design possible with free flaps. The wide variety of free flap donor sites that exists allows tissue in the appropriate quantity and configuration to be selected for a particular defect [*see Figure 6*].

Functional Defect

Functional defects require repair with specialized flaps. Free flaps are frequently used because the specific tissue requirements usually cannot be satisfied by a local flap. A functional defect may result, for example, in the cervical esophagus from tumor resection or in the forearm from Volkmann's contracture. A segment of small intestine can repair the esophageal defect; transfer of a vascularized and innervated muscle (e.g., the gracilis) can replace forearm muscle.[15]

Contour Defect

Contour defects, such as those that result from mastectomy or from trauma to the lower extremity, can be reconstructed with either local or free flaps. A mastectomy defect, because of its location on the chest, is suitable for reconstruction with one of several myocutaneous flaps from either the back or the abdomen [*see 2:5 Breast Procedures*]. A free flap from the abdomen or the gluteal area is another alternative. The best reconstructive solution for a particular person is determined by variables such as body habitus and the size and configuration of the contralateral breast.

A contour defect of the lower extremity is best reconstructed with a large myocutaneous free flap that provides tissue of sufficient quantity and flexibility to allow sculpting into the appropriate shape.

Unstable Soft Tissue Coverage

Marginal soft tissue coverage (e.g., skin grafts) may break down after repeated minor trauma. Bones may become exposed and are then at risk for osteomyelitis. This situation can be avoided by elective replacement of the tissue at risk with a more substantial soft tissue covering. As in acute reconstruction, local flaps are the first choice for lesions of the trunk or the proximal extremities, whereas free flaps are often more appropriate for lesions of the distal extremities.

Soft tissue coverage is sometimes inadequate even in a healed wound. For example, certain procedures, such as nerve or bone grafting, require an ideal soft tissue bed to promote adequate graft revascularization. In some cases, it may be necessary first to replace the existing soft tissue coverage as a first-stage procedure before grafting a bone or nerve gap. A skin or muscle flap is most commonly used in these cases. This problem is most common in areas such as the distal extremities, where native soft tissue coverage is not overly abundant and is easily lost from trauma or tumor resection. Free flaps are usually chosen to provide a healthy, well-vascularized soft tissue bed before further functional reconstruction is undertaken.

Discussion

Wound Healing

The wound healing process consists of several identifiable phases [*see 1:7 Acute Wound Care*]. The first phase is an inflammatory response that includes both vascular and cellular components. The second stage is fibroplasia, during which collagen deposition by fibroblasts increases the tensile strength of the wound. The maturation phase of wound healing begins at about 3 weeks, when the rate of collagen degradation begins to balance the rate of collagen production. The previously random arrangement of collagen fibers becomes more organized, and the ratio of type I to type III collagen returns to normal. The wound gradually progresses from a raised, indurated, red scar to a mature form that is flat, soft, lighter in color, and of increased tensile strength. The maturation phase continues for more than a year.

Contraction of open, so-called granulating wounds is caused by myofibroblasts, modified fibroblasts that have smooth muscle characteristics. The number of myofibroblasts within the wound has been found to be proportional to the rate at which the wound contracts.[16,17] These cells are scattered throughout the wound and pull the edges of the wound toward the center. Skin grafts inhibit wound contraction, apparently by accelerating the life cycle of the myofibroblast.

Postoperative Management Issues

SKIN GRAFTS

Contraction and Reinnervation

Split-thickness skin grafts include the epidermis and only a portion of the dermis, whereas full-thickness skin grafts include the entire dermis. Skin grafts contract to a degree that is related to their thickness. After their harvest from donor sites, full-thickness grafts will contract to a surface area as small as 40% of their original surface area, whereas split-thickness grafts contract only about half as much. This reduction in area, referred to as primary contraction, is a passive phenomenon caused by elastic tissue within the graft. Secondary contraction occurs as a graft heals at the recipient site. Full-thickness grafts undergo minimal secondary contraction, whereas split-thickness grafts contract to a degree that is inversely proportional to their dermal content. In other words, thick split-thickness grafts contract less than thin split-thickness grafts.

Skin grafts gradually regain sensation by reinnervation from the wound bed. Thick grafts and healthy wound beds contribute to greater sensory recovery. However, the degree of sensation after healing is complete does not equal that of normal skin. Graft thickness also affects recovery of certain other functions of normal skin, such as secretion from sweat glands and sebaceous glands, and of hair growth. These processes will be active only in full-thickness and thick split-thickness grafts. Secretion from sweat glands depends on sympathetic reinnervation of the graft and follows the sweat pattern of the recipient site. Sebaceous glands, on the other hand, secrete independently of graft reinnervation by the recipient bed. Thin split-thickness skin grafts tend to be quite dry because they contain inadequate numbers of functioning sebaceous glands, which are more abundant in thicker grafts.

Revascularization

A phase of serum imbibition lasts for the first 2 days after placement of a skin graft. During this period, the graft is nourished by passive absorption of nutrients from serum in the recipient bed and not by direct vascular perfusion. The graft gains as much as 40% of extra weight because of fluid absorption. Vessels within the graft gradually dilate and fill with static columns of blood. A fibrin network in the wound bed causes graft adherence during this early phase.

The next phase in revascularization is a period of inosculation, during which anastomoses are formed between vessels in the graft and those in the wound bed. It is not clear, however, whether connections are established between existing vessels in the recipient bed and graft or whether new vessels grow into the graft from the recipient bed. Both processes may occur, and both may be important in graft revascularization. In any case, circulation is sluggish during postoperative days 3 and 4 but gradually increases during postoperative days 5 and 6 to become essentially normal by day 7.[18]

Lymphatic drainage from the graft is established at approximately the same rate as the circulation of blood. Lymphatic flow is present by postoperative day 5 or 6, and the graft starts losing the extra fluid weight it has gained. The graft begins to resume its normal weight by postoperative day 9.

Factors Affecting Graft Survival

Hematoma formation beneath a skin graft is the most common cause of graft failure. Blood accumulation interferes with graft adherence as well as with both imbibition and inosculation. Early evacuation of blood from beneath a skin graft can result in graft survival. Shear forces that result from inadequate immobilization cause graft failure by preventing or disrupting developing communications between vessels of the graft and the recipient bed. Infection of the recipient bed makes the bed unsuitable for grafting, and such infection is another major cause of graft failure. Proteolytic enzymes produced by microorganisms destroy the fibrin bond between the graft and recipient bed. Bacteria such as β-hemolytic streptococci and *Pseudomonas* are particularly virulent because they produce high levels of plasmin and other proteolytic enzymes. The type of organism present may actually be a more important factor in graft failure than the number of organisms.[19]

Healing of Donor Sites

Donor sites for split-thickness grafts heal by reepithelialization. Epithelial cells from remaining portions of skin appendages, such as hair follicles, sebaceous glands, and sweat glands, migrate across the exposed dermis to establish a new epidermis. Donor sites for thin grafts heal more rapidly and leave less of a scar than those for thick grafts, which take longer to heal and can be associated with significant scarring. The epidermis of a healed donor site is fully differentiated within 3 to 4 weeks. The dermis shows little evidence of regeneration, however. An occlusive dressing such as Op-Site promotes more rapid healing of the donor site than coverage with fine mesh gauze.[20]

FLAPS

Resistance to Infection

Skin flaps, myocutaneous flaps, and fasciocutaneous flaps have been shown experimentally to vary in their resistance to bacterial infection.[21] Random-pattern skin flaps are not as resistant as myocutaneous flaps. The cutaneous portions of myocutaneous and of fasciocutaneous flaps have similar levels of resistance, but the muscle component of myocutaneous flaps is more resistant than the fascial component of fasciocutaneous flaps in situations where the flap lies over a focus of infection within the wound. Muscle therefore appears to be the type of flap most resistant to infection. Such resistance is of clinical significance in cases of exposed bone with chronic osteomyelitis, for example. This condition can be successfully treated by debridement and immediate coverage with a muscle flap.

Free Flaps and Concept of No-Reflow

Free tissue transfer is unique in that the flap is completely ischemic for a given period. How long ischemia can be tolerated without resultant flap failure (despite technically satisfactory microvascular anastomoses) is an important clinical question. An increasing duration of ischemia has been associated experimentally with obstruction to blood flow in the microcirculation.[22,23] This obstruction results from cellular edema, increased interstitial fluid pressure, and sludging of blood and thrombus formation. This phenomenon is initially reversible but becomes irreversible as the duration of ischemia increases. After 12 hours of ischemia under experimental conditions, obstruction to blood flow has been demonstrated to be complete, preventing successful reperfusion of the flap. How long uninterrupted ischemia can safely continue is not precisely known clinically, and evidence suggests that the ischemic tolerance of specific types of tissue varies. For example, flaps that are primarily bone are more durable than muscle or bowel flaps. Evidence gained by clinical experience has shown that up to 4 hours of ischemia is safely tolerated by most free flaps.

Tissue Expansion

Histologic changes of expanded skin include thinning of the dermis but not of the epidermis,[24] suggesting a permanent net gain in epidermal tissue only. The mitotic rate in the epidermis has been shown to increase with expansion, but the mechanism for this increase is unclear.[25]

The circulation of expanded skin also changes. An increase in vascularity of expanded tissue is partially explained by the fact that tissue expansion is a form of delay procedure. However, experimental studies suggest that an increased potential for flap survivability is directly attributable to the expansion process and not merely to its delay component.[26-28] The fibrous capsule that forms around the prosthesis during expansion appears to contribute to the increased vascularity of these flaps, and the increased pressure around the expander may stimulate angiogenesis.

References

1. Edlich RF, Jones KC Jr, Buchanan L, et al: A disposable emergency wound treatment kit. J Emerg Med 10:463, 1992

2. Stevenson TR, Thacker JG, Rodeheaver GT, et al: Cleansing the traumatic wound by high pressure syringe irrigation. JACEP 5:17, 1976

3. Hollander JE, Singer AJ, Valentine SM, et al: Risk factors for infection in patients with traumatic lacerations. Acad Emerg Med 8:716, 2001

4. Edlich RF, Rodeheaver GT, Thacker JG: Technical factors in the prevention of wound infection. Surgical Infectious Diseases. Simmons R, Howard R, Eds. Appleton-Century-Croft, East Norwalk, Connecticut, 1981

5. Robson MC, Heggers JP: Delayed wound closures based on bacterial counts. J Surg Oncol 2:379, 1970

6. Teepe RG, Koebrugge EJ, Lowik CW, et al: Cytotoxic effects of topical antimicrobial and antiseptic agents on human keratinocytes in vitro. J Trauma 35:8, 1993

7. Jackson IT: Local Flaps in Head and Neck Reconstruction. CV Mosby, St Louis, 1985

8. Spinelli HM, Forman DL: Current treatment of post-traumatic deformities: residual orbital, adnexal, and soft-tissue abnormalities. Clin Plast Surg 24:519, 1997

9. Luce EA: Reconstruction of the lower lip. Clin Plast Surg 22:109, 1995

10. Mathes SJ, Nahai F: Reconstructive Surgery: Principles, Anatomy, Technique, Vol 1. Churchill Livingstone, New York, 1997, p 37

11. Taylor GI, Giantoutsos MP, Morris SF: The neurovascular territories of the skin and muscles: anatomic study and clinical implications. Plast Reconstr Surg 94:1, 1994

12. Hidalgo DA, Shaw WW: Reconstruction of foot injuries. Clin Plast Surg 13:663, 1986

13. May JW Jr, Halls MJ, Simon SR: Free microvascular muscle flaps with skin graft reconstruction of extensive defects of the foot: a clinical and gait analysis study. Plast Reconstr Surg 75:627, 1985

14. Bennett RG, Hirt M: A history of tissue expansion: concepts, controversies, and complications. J Dermatol Surg Oncol 19:1066, 1993

15. Hidalgo DA, Disa JJ, Cordeiro PG: A review of 716 consecutive free flaps for oncologic surgical defects: refinement in donor site selection and technique. Plast Reconstr Surg 102:722, 1998

16. McGrath MH, Hundahl SA: The spatial and temporal quantification of myofibroblasts. Plast Reconstr Surg 69:975, 1982

17. Rudolph R: Inhibition of myofibroblasts by skin grafts. Plast Reconstr Surg 63:473, 1979

18. Angel MF, Giesswein P, Hawner P: Skin grafting. Operative Plastic Surgery. Evans GRD, Ed. McGraw-Hill, New York, 2000, p 59

19. Teh BT: Why do skin grafts fail? Plast Reconstr Surg 63:323, 1979

20. Smith DJ Jr, Thomson PD, Bolton LL: Microbiology and healing of the occluded skin-graft donor site. Plast Reconstr Surg 91:1094, 1993

21. Gosain A, Chang N, Mathes S, et al: A study of the relationship between blood flow and bacterial inoculation in musculocutaneous and fasciocutaneous flaps. Plast Reconstr Surg 86:1152, 1990

22. Kerrigan CL, Stotland MA: Ischemia reperfusion injury: a review. Microsurgery 14:165, 1993

23. Kirschner RE, Fyfe BS, Hoffman LA, et al: Ischemia-reperfusion injury in myocutaneous flaps: role of leukocytes and leukotrienes. Plast Reconstr Surg 99: 1485, 1997

24. Johnson TM, Lowe L, Brown MD, et al: Histology and physiology of tissue expansion. J Dermatol Surg Oncol 19:1074, 1993

25. Olenius M, Johansson O: Variations in epidermal thickness in expanded human breast skin. Scand J Plast Reconstr Hand Surg 29:15, 1995

26. Babovic S, Angel MF, Im MJ, et al: Effects of tissue expansion on secondary ischemic tolerance in experimental free flaps. Ann Plast Surg 34:593, 1995

27. Matturri L, Azzolini A, Riberti C, et al: Long-term histopathologic evaluation of human expanded skin. Plast Reconstr Surg 90:636, 1992

28. Olenius M, Dalsgaard CJ, Wickman M: Mitotic activity in expanded human skin. Plast Reconstr Surg 91: 213, 1993

Acknowledgment

Figure 3 Carol Donner.

4 SKIN LESIONS

Alan E. Seyfer, M.D., F.A.C.S.

Assessment and Management of Skin Lesions

The clinical assessment and treatment of skin lesions can be challenging, since some skin lesions are capricious in their biologic behavior. History is of great importance. Recent changes in the appearance of a lesion usually indicate active growth, which increases the chance that the lesion is malignant. Likewise, a history of chronic sun exposure—particularly

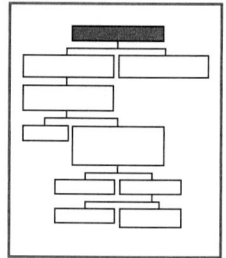

in a patient who has a fair complexion—multiplies the patient's risk of malignancy. Certain congenital lesions must also be viewed with suspicion, even though the incidence of malignancy in such lesions can be extremely variable. Any history that departs from the natural history of a simple nevus should raise suspicion of malignancy. In general, nevus tissue becomes apparent at 4 or 5 years of age. Nevi often darken with puberty and pregnancy and fade in the seventh to eighth decades of life. Malignancies usually differ from the characteristic clinical pattern of a simple nevus.

Nonsuspicious Lesions

In general, lesions are nonsuspicious if they remain stable and uniform in their physical characteristics (e.g., size, shape, color, profile, and texture). Nonsuspicious lesions may be safely monitored conservatively, especially if they are located in regions easily visible to the patient. Excisional biopsy is warranted if

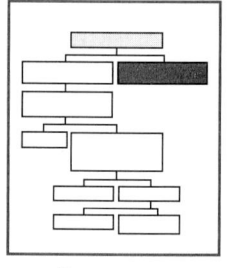

the lesions change in size, shape, color, profile, or texture. Cosmesis is always a subjective and relative indication for excision.

Suspicious Lesions

Changes and irregularities in the physical characteristics of a skin lesion (e.g., size, shape, color, profile, and texture) are important in helping determine whether the lesion is suspicious. For example, an irregular physical pattern, large size (1 to 2 cm or larger),

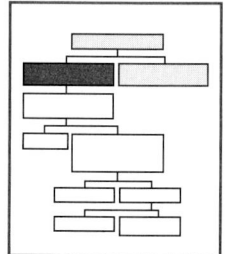

or unfavorable location (e.g., on skin that is unprotected from sun exposure) places the lesion in the suspicious category and is a relative indication for performing an excisional biopsy.

BIOPSY

If the lesion is suspicious, a biopsy is warranted. If the suspicious area is small, it should be completely excised with a 1 to 4 mm margin, depending on the clinical characteristics. The important principle is to include a margin of normal skin around the lesion. This helps the pathologist and may include occult areas of importance. Shave biopsies should never

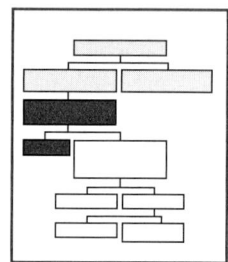

be performed, because the depth of the lesion is of great diagnostic importance, and lesion depth is destroyed by this technique. To provide a complete specimen for study, my preference is to include a full thickness of the dermis with subcutaneous fat. As noted above, a small margin of normal skin is helpful to the pathologist [see Surgical Technique, Excisional Biopsy, below].

If the lesion is found to be benign, further treatment is unwarranted. If the lesion proves to be malignant, further excision with an appropriate margin is usually necessary, and staging of the tumor becomes important (see below). Presentation of the biopsy to the tumor board is of great value both clinically and medicolegally. In cases of melanoma or other so-called liquid tumors that shed their cells readily in all tissue, ancillary treatment (e.g., with perfusion therapy, radiation therapy, or chemotherapy) may be reasonable before reexcision with wider margins.

CLINICAL STAGING OF MALIGNANCY

If a malignancy is suspected, regional node status is important, and the nodes that drain the region should be thoroughly examined. If nodes are palpable and the lesion proves to be a malignancy, a regional node dissection or sampling is necessary to stage the patient's tumor and plan for further treatment. Likewise, a node dissection may be ther-

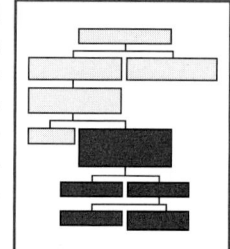

apeutic and may contribute to local control of the lesion. If the nodes are positive, it is reasonable to consider adjuvant therapy or ancillary treatment. If the nodes are negative microscopically, it is reasonable to follow the patient with serial examinations. Again, an interdisciplinary tumor board will assist in making the appropriate management decision once a malignancy is confirmed by biopsy.

A staging approach that is being increasingly widely used in certain patient groups is lymphatic mapping and sentinel lymph node (SLN) biopsy [see Discussion, Malignant Melanoma, Melanoma Staging, below].

Assessment and Management of Skin Lesions

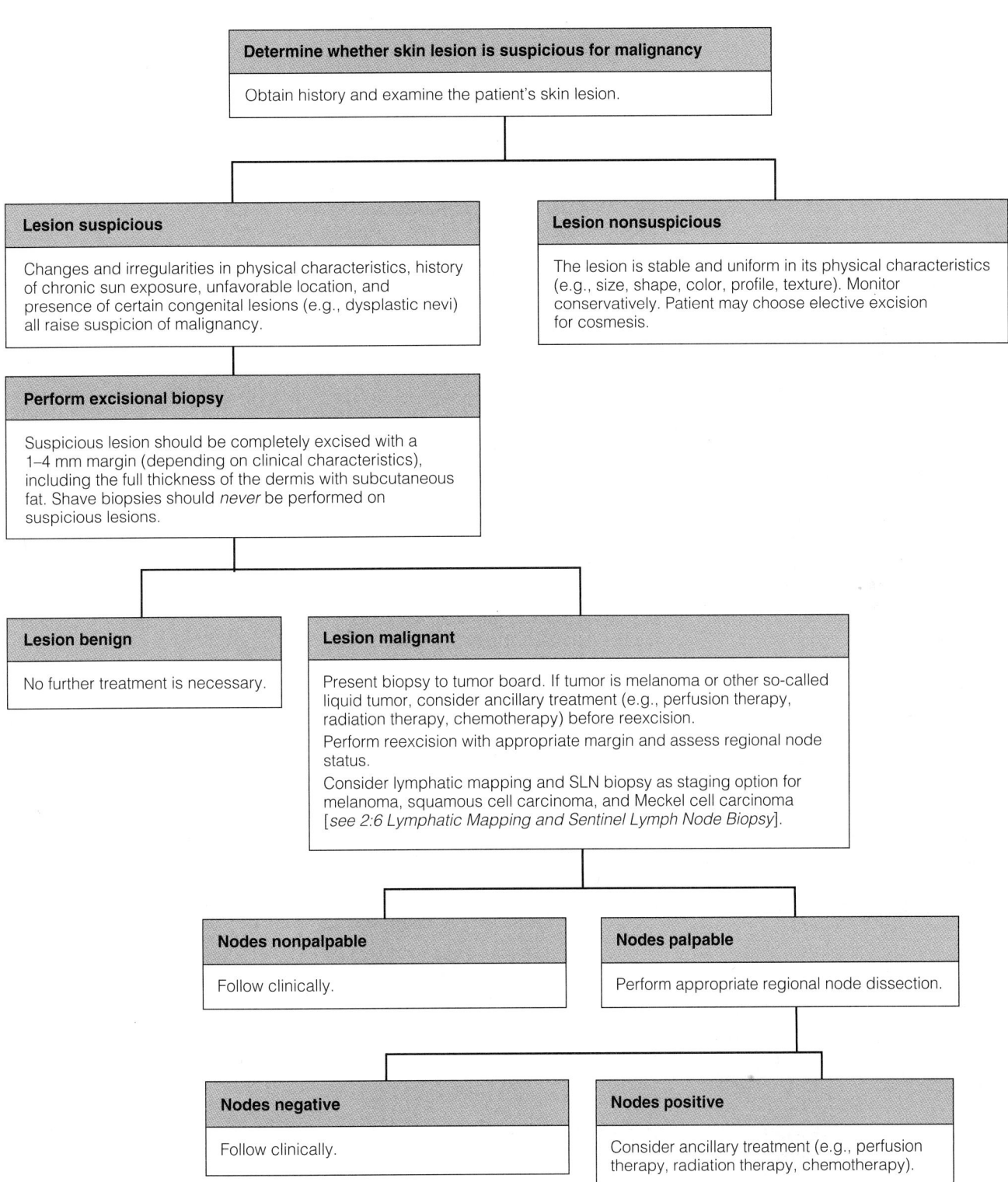

Determine whether skin lesion is suspicious for malignancy

Obtain history and examine the patient's skin lesion.

Lesion suspicious

Changes and irregularities in physical characteristics, history of chronic sun exposure, unfavorable location, and presence of certain congenital lesions (e.g., dysplastic nevi) all raise suspicion of malignancy.

Lesion nonsuspicious

The lesion is stable and uniform in its physical characteristics (e.g., size, shape, color, profile, texture). Monitor conservatively. Patient may choose elective excision for cosmesis.

Perform excisional biopsy

Suspicious lesion should be completely excised with a 1–4 mm margin (depending on clinical characteristics), including the full thickness of the dermis with subcutaneous fat. Shave biopsies should *never* be performed on suspicious lesions.

Lesion benign

No further treatment is necessary.

Lesion malignant

Present biopsy to tumor board. If tumor is melanoma or other so-called liquid tumor, consider ancillary treatment (e.g., perfusion therapy, radiation therapy, chemotherapy) before reexcision.

Perform reexcision with appropriate margin and assess regional node status.

Consider lymphatic mapping and SLN biopsy as staging option for melanoma, squamous cell carcinoma, and Meckel cell carcinoma [*see 2:6 Lymphatic Mapping and Sentinel Lymph Node Biopsy*].

Nodes nonpalpable

Follow clinically.

Nodes palpable

Perform appropriate regional node dissection.

Nodes negative

Follow clinically.

Nodes positive

Consider ancillary treatment (e.g., perfusion therapy, radiation therapy, chemotherapy).

Discussion

Nonmelanoma skin cancers are the most common cancers in the United States, accounting for about 35% of all cancers diagnosed every year.[1,2] Nonmelanoma skin cancers can be capricious, and it may be difficult to assess their biologic behavior from their appearance alone. Certainly, it is possible for a benign-looking papule to exhibit aggressive biologic behavior. Melanomas, at the more malignant end of the spectrum, can metastasize early and even present initially with cerebral metastasis.

Sun exposure with actinic changes in the skin is a predisposing factor for skin cancers of all types.[3-5] Fair-skinned persons lacking protective pigmentation are at much higher risk for the development of skin cancers.[6] Failure of the immunologic surveillance system, decreased cell-mediated immunity, and use of immunosuppressive agents have all been implicated as factors that may influence a patient's predisposition to malignant skin lesions.[7,8]

Basal Cell Carcinoma

Basal cell carcinomas originate in the pluripotential epithelial cells of the epidermis and skin adnexa.[1] These tumors tend to be characterized by slow growth and progressive morbidity by local extension. Their viability seems to depend on attachment to the dermis, and systemic metastases are therefore rare. However, certain types of basal cell carcinoma may be extremely aggressive, resulting in morbidity, mutilation, and death by local extension. This is particularly true of midface and sclerosing basal cell cancers.

Clinically, there are several types of basal cell carcinomas [see Figure 1]. The most common is the nodular type, which begins as a flesh-colored, raised, telangiectatic lesion that may be difficult to distinguish from a common nevus.[9] The nodular lesion is rounded in appearance during its early phase and characteristically assumes a raised rim with a craterlike central region, often with scaling of superficial skin cells at its center [see Figure 1a]. Perhaps the most dangerous type is the sclerosing, or morpheaform, basal cell carcinoma—a light, plaquelike lesion that can resemble a stellate scar [see Figure 1b]. Morpheaform basal cell carcinomas tend to be locally invasive, with multiple cancer projections, resembling tentacles, that penetrate toward the deep portions of the tissue. Therefore, it is possible—even likely—that tumor will be left behind after an excisional biopsy of the lesion.[10] Such tumors can also ulcerate and resemble pigmented melanomas [see Figure 1c].

The distribution of basal cell cancers is strongly weighted toward the midface, cheek, and ear regions.[11] Treatment is usually surgical, with removal of a rim of normal skin around the lesion. Morpheaform basal cell cancers should be treated with a wider margin of excision, and careful attention should be paid to the margins to confirm clearance of tumor cells. In most cases, closure can be accomplished by wide undermining of the skin and fat and direct closure. Otherwise, a skin graft is a useful alternative.

Radiation therapy for basal cell carcinomas claims an overall cure rate of over 90%.[12] This therapy can be offered to each patient, but the repeated treatments require multiple visits. Radiation therapy is a safe, noninvasive form of treatment that can be an attractive alternative for patients who are, for whatever reasons, considered bad candidates for surgical extirpation. Radiation is a particularly attractive alternative for the treatment of lesions in areas that are difficult to reconstruct, such as the medial canthal margin of the eyelids, certain external ear lesions, and the nostril rim.

Another therapeutic option is Mohs' micrographic surgical operation. Frederic Mohs, a general surgeon, developed the technique for lesions like basal cell carcinomas without metastatic potential that were of full thickness and involved the skin and the mucous membranes of the nose.[13] Perhaps the best indi-

a

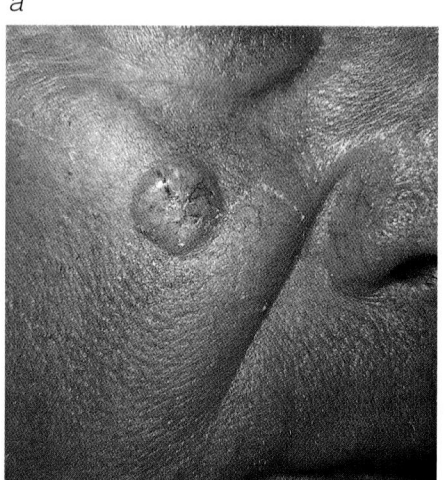

b

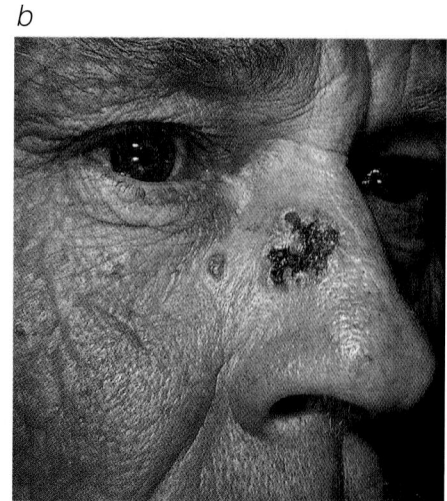

c

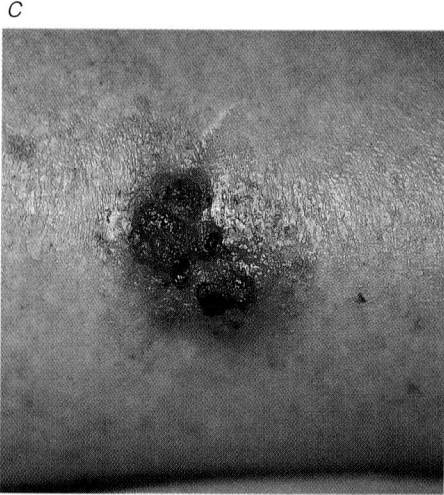

Figure 1   (*a*) A pearly luster and telangiectasias are evident in this typical basal cell carcinoma on the cheek of a 43-year-old man. (*b*) This sclerosing (morpheaform) basal cell carcinoma on the nose of a 55-year-old man was found to be deeply invasive and exhibited multidirectional growth. (*c*) This basal cell carcinoma on the lower leg of a 91-year-old woman showed ulceration and pigmentation similar to that of a melanoma.

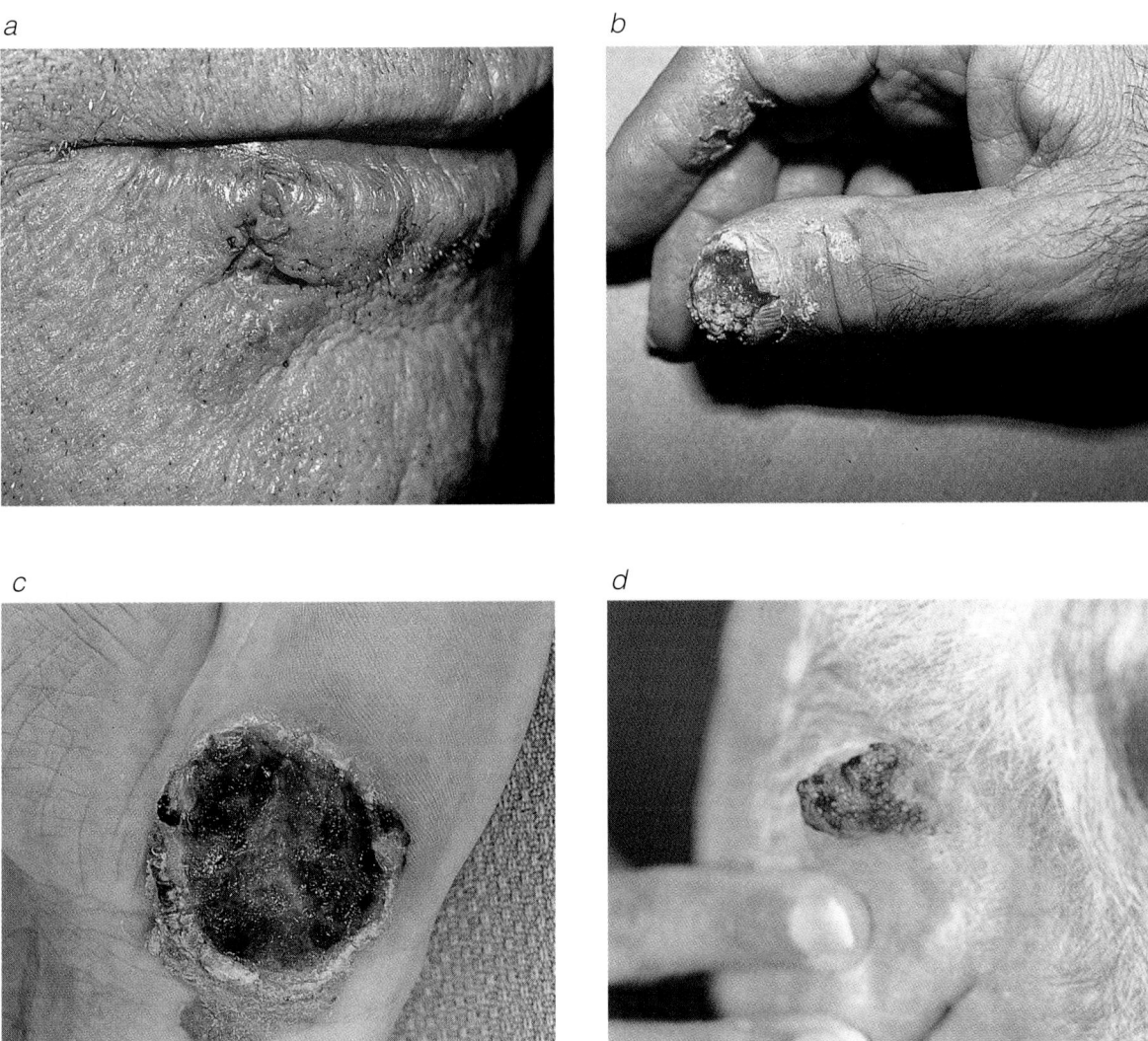

Figure 2 (*a*) **This squamous cell carcinoma on the lip of a 70-year-old man was related to sun exposure; the patient was a nonsmoker. (*b*) This squamous cell carcinoma involving the thumb and index finger of a 72-year-old man, a retired dentist, was related to exposure to occupational hazards; he had subjected these digits to repeated radiation exposures by holding dental x-rays against his patients' teeth. (*c*) The 61-year-old man who had this indolent, slow-growing squamous cell carcinoma on the hand also had a synchronous penile erythroplasia of Queyrat (localized)—a squamous cell carcinoma in situ; there was no evidence of metastasis from either lesion. (*d*) This squamous cell carcinoma on the helix of the external ear in a 73-year-old man can be seen extending to the scalp.**

cation for the Mohs procedure is recurrent basal cell carcinomas, especially those of the morpheaform type. The Mohs technique usually incorporates wide enough margins to ensure a reasonable cure rate. The Mohs technique may also be appropriate for microcystic adnexal carcinoma and dermatofibrosarcoma protuberans.[14] The drawbacks to the Mohs procedure are that it requires a considerable amount of time, exposure, and expense but has a cure rate similar to that of simple surgical excision.

Squamous Cell Carcinoma

Like basal cell cancers, squamous cell cancers are associated with actinic solar damage but may also arise out of old scars, radiation-damaged skin, or chronic, open wounds[15] [*see Figure 2*]. Chronic inflammation and irritation appear to be the common denominators. The biologic activity of squamous cell cancers is aggressive in comparison with that of basal cell cancers; fortunately, they are less common. Persons of fair complexion are at increased risk; all skin cancers are more likely to develop in sun-exposed regions[16] [*see Figure 2a*]. Certain occupational hazards have been associated with an increased risk for squamous cell cancer, including those experienced by dental personnel who habitually expose their hands to x-ray energy and technicians who paint radium watch dials [*see Figure 2b*].

Histologically, squamous cell lesions are characterized by masses of squamous epithelium that invade downward through the dermis in a palisade arrangement. The degree of epithelial differentiation determines the grade of the tumor. This grade is measured as a ratio of atypical cells to normal cells. In higher grades of tumor (i.e., those with a high degree of biologic aggressiveness), differentiation and keratinization are greatly diminished.[1] Anaplastic (i.e., undifferentiated) tumors may require further characterization. The presence of cytokeratin antibodies (indicative of squamous cells) or antibody to S100 protein (which may identify melanocytes, indicative of melanoma) may also help in assessing the more anaplastic tumors. Immunoperoxidase staining may help distinguish between the desmoplastic variety of melanoma and certain squamous cell cancers.[1,17] Differentiation of a squamous cell cancer, depth of invasion, and the presence of perineural invasion correlate with biologic aggressiveness.[1]

Clinically, the lesion may appear as a gradually enlarging, nonhealing, nontender sore [see Figure 2c], or it may present as an actinic patch—typically on the cheek or the external ear [see Figure 2d]. Tumors that arise in old scars or open wounds are characteristically aggressive. Squamous cell carcinomas that develop from Marjolin's ulcer (which arises in burn scars and open wounds such as osteomyelitis drainage sites) are characterized by extreme aggressiveness after surgical resection; this aggressive behavior may be attributable to the relatively immunologically privileged status of the tumors before extirpation. Surgical excision seems to activate certain lesions. Although the lesion may have remained indolent for many years, tumor recurrence and metastasis are common after treatment.[18,19]

Certain areas of the body are especially prone to early metastases and have a higher risk of regional nodal metastases. For example, squamous cell cancers of the scalp, nose, and extremities seem to metastasize early. Regional metastases are associated with a poorer prognosis.[1,20]

Bowen disease, a carcinoma in situ, presents as a red patch or plaque with small areas of crusting. The recommended treatment is wide-margin (0.5 to 1.0 cm) surgical excision.[16]

Malignant Melanoma

Although the clinical course of malignant melanoma is characteristically unpredictable, treatment strategies for primary lesions and nodal drainage systems can be developed with the assistance of some important prognostic markers: the thickness of the lesion (Breslow thickness) and the depth of tissue invasion (Clark level)[21] [see Melanoma Staging, below]. Melanomas tend to grow both vertically and radially; those that have a rapid onset in the vertical phase present as thicker lesions and have a worse prognosis.[22]

Over the past 40 years, the incidence of melanoma has increased; it is now the most rapidly increasing cancer among white males and the fourth most rapidly increasing cancer among white females.[23] Despite the poor prognosis associated with melanoma, survival after therapy has improved over the past 50 years. Some innovative and exciting immunotherapeutic strategies have been attempted, but the viable treatment options remain exclusively surgical.

As with other dermal neoplasms, a positive correlation is seen between sun exposure and the incidence of malignant melanoma. Some 98% of melanomas occur in whites, and within this population, the lighter-skinned persons are most at risk. Painful, blistering sunburns, early childhood exposure,[24] and sun-induced freckling are associated with a two to three times higher risk of cutaneous melanoma.[25]

DIFFERENTIAL CHARACTERISTICS OF BENIGN NEVI AND MALIGNANT MELANOMA

Unfortunately, the clinical presentation of malignant and benign pigmented lesions can be quite similar [see Figure 3]. However, certain differences do exist that can be helpful in making the distinction. For example, benign lesions tend to be less than 1 cm in diameter and have regular borders, a homogeneous color, and a smooth texture. Malignant lesions, on the other hand, are often larger, exhibit variable pigmentation and irregular borders, and are less orderly in their presentation.

Benign Nevi

Benign nevi, the most common pigmented lesions, are divided into three major histologic groups: (1) junctional, (2) compound, and (3) dermal. This classification, though arbitrary, refers to characteristic features of acquired melanocytic nevi.

Junctional nevi are the earliest stage of intraepidermal proliferation, the stage in which cells form nests along the dermal-

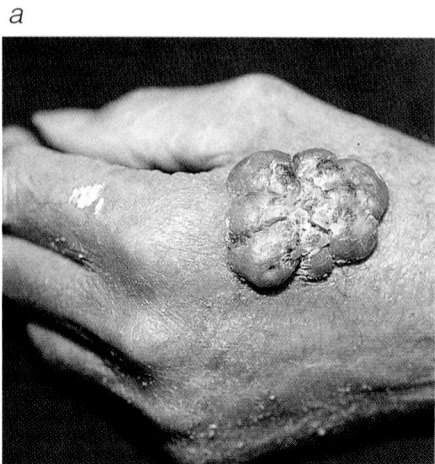
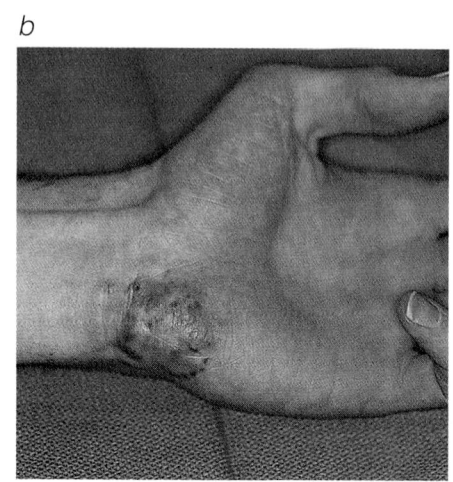
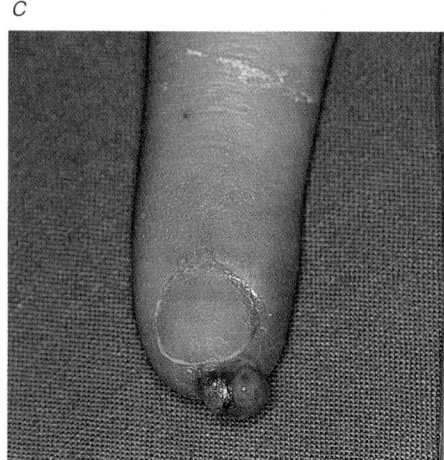

Figure 3 (*a*) **Benign keratoacanthoma, such as this one on the hand of a 67-year-old man, is a rapidly growing lesion that can be mistaken for a malignancy. (*b*) This dark lesion on the distal ulnar area of a 31-year-old man, a posttraumatic arteriovenous fistula, is similar in appearance to a pigmented dermal lesion. (*c*) This rapidly growing pyogenic granuloma on the index finger of a 24-year-old woman developed after a small skin wound; microscopically, the lesion represents granulation tissue.**

a

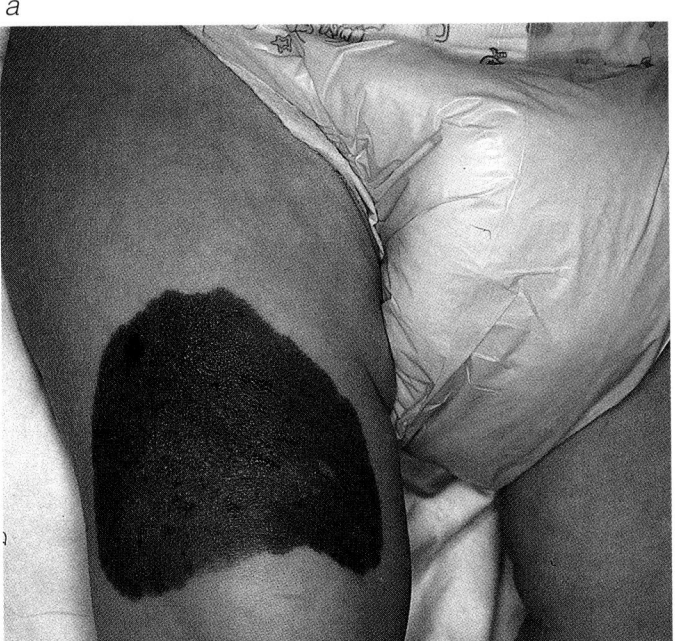

b

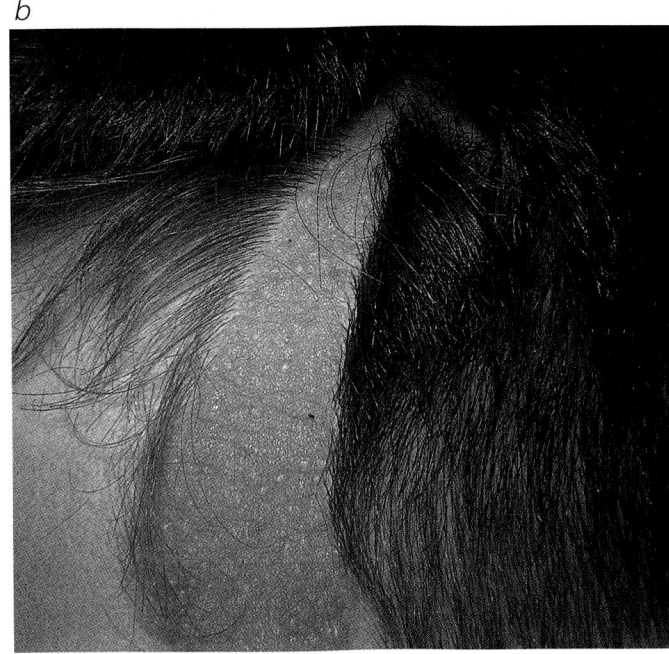

Figure 4 (*a*) **This nevus on the thigh of an infant is problematic because of its congenital nature. (*b*) This sebaceous nevus, or Jadassohn-Tièche nevus, involving the temporal scalp in a 19-year-old white man may undergo malignant change.**

epidermal junction. These lesions are relatively sessile and have a homogeneous, brownish pigmentation. Junctional nevi are characteristically smooth and have round or oval borders. They usually appear after 3 years of age and before adolescence, darken with the onset of puberty or pregnancy, and gradually fade in color and decrease in height in the later years of life. Compound nevi have junctional as well as dermal components. Dermal nevi are slightly raised, homogeneous in pigmentation, and well circumscribed, but they are confined to the dermis histologically.[26] Any lesion that tends to drift from this natural history should be regarded with suspicion, especially in the years after adolescence [*see Figure 4*].

Certain lesions, including dysplastic nevi, have a higher risk for malignant transformation.[27] The familial dysplastic nevus syndrome is characterized by an autosomal dominant pattern and a unique histologic appearance. Dysplastic nevi are typically larger than ordinary nevi, and significantly, their borders and color are irregular. Over time, dysplastic nevi progress to melanoma.

Malignant Melanoma

Malignant melanoma is characterized by radial and vertical growth phases.[21,22,26] During the radial growth phase, melanocytes within the epidermis and papillary dermis grow in all directions. The result is slow radial enlargement of the lesion. Vertical growth, which usually follows the radial growth phase, consists of growth perpendicular to the direction of growth that occurred in the radial phase. This pattern is characterized by deep invasion and subsequent development of metastases.

Three types of melanoma are clinically distinguishable [*see Figure 5*]. Superficial spreading melanoma is the most common type of melanoma, and it may arise in a preexisting nevus. The less common nodular melanoma usually exhibits more rapid and aggressive growth. Nodular melanoma is not usually associated with preexisting nevi, is more common in males, has a higher incidence in middle age, and typically presents over the trunk, head, and neck.[26] Lentigo malignant melanoma represents only 7% to 8% of all melanomas.[28,29] It presents in older patients and tends to be indolent. Lentigo malignant melanoma was originally described by Hutchinson in 1894, and although it has been termed Hutchinson's freckle—a name that implies benignity—the lesion does have clear malignant potential.

MELANOMA STAGING

The most common criteria for the staging of melanomas are the classification systems formulated by Clark and Breslow.

Clark categorized tumors according to their level of invasion into five separate regions [*see Figure 6*]. Clark level I, in which the tumor involves the epidermis, is essentially carcinoma in situ. Level II indicates extension of the tumor into the papillary dermis. Level III signifies a spreading of tumor cells along the papillary-reticular dermal interface. Level IV indicates invasion into the reticular dermis. Level V indicates extension into the subcutaneous tissue. According to Clark's criteria, survival decreases as the depth of invasion increases.[30]

Clark's dermal layers may be cumbersome, but the Breslow thickness provides comparable therapeutic and prognostic discrimination. Breslow classified the level of invasion by using an ocular micrometer to measure from the granular layer in the epidermis to the deepest point of invasion in the dermis. Under Breslow's criteria, thin melanomas invade 0.75 mm or less into the dermis (stage IA, T1). Intermediate-thickness melanomas invade 0.76 to 3.99 mm; these are further subdivided into thin intermediate melanomas of 0.76 to 1.49 mm (stage IB, T2), intermediate intermediate melanomas of 1.5 to 2.49 mm (stage IIA, T3a), and thick intermediate melanomas of 2.5 mm to 3.99 mm (stage IIA, T3b). Thick melanomas invade 4.0 mm and deeper (stage IIB, T4).[31]

It is important to note that any suspicious lesion should initially be removed by means of a full-thickness excisional biop-

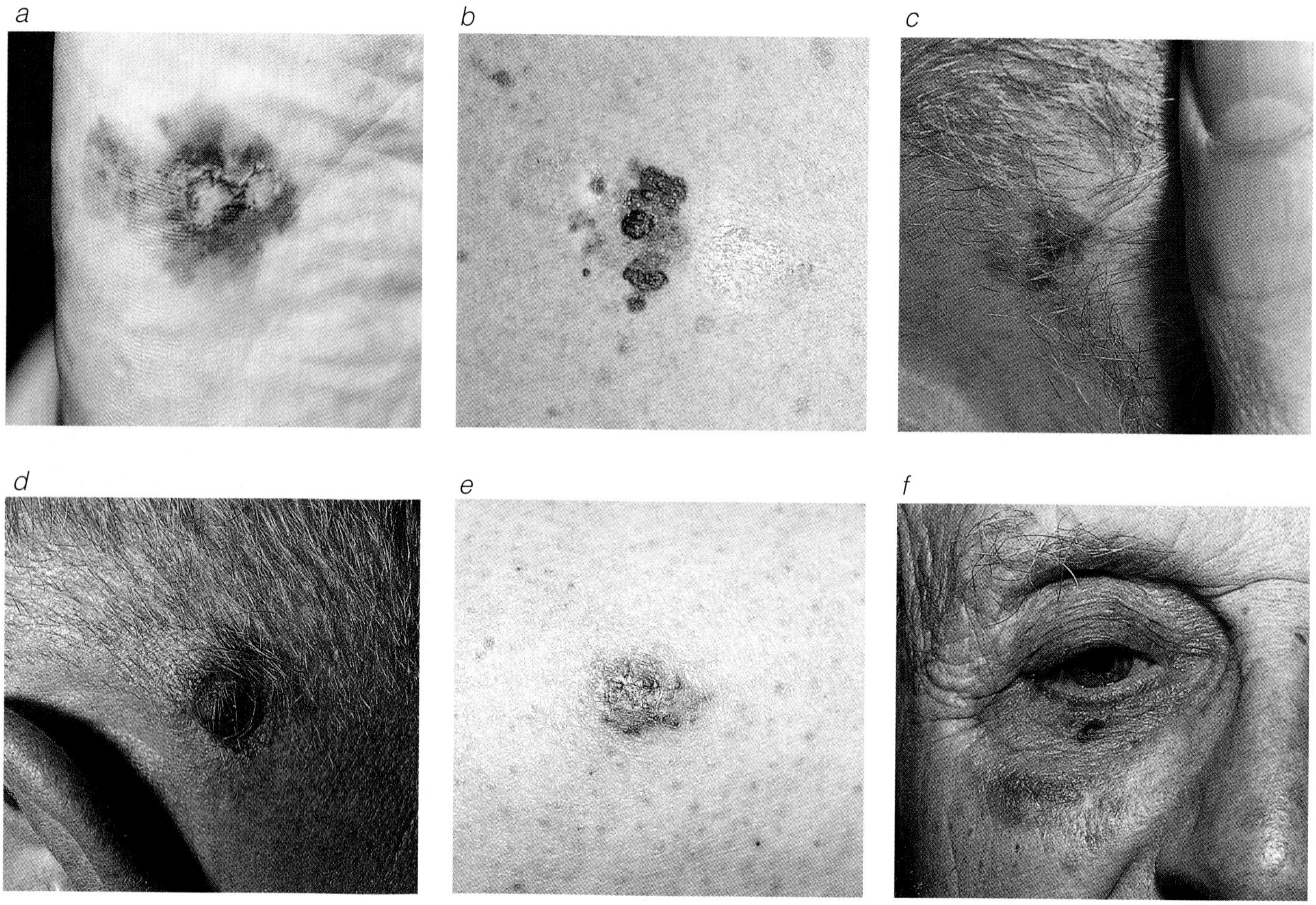

a

b

c

d

e

f

Figure 5 (*a*) This melanoma, on the sole of the foot of a 47-year-old black woman, shows irregularities in shape, contour, and pigmentation. (*b*) A so-called halo effect is visible along the left margin of this melanoma on the upper back of a 33-year-old white woman; irregularities in shape, contour, and pigmentation are also evident. (*c*) This melanoma of the postauricular scalp in a 56-year-old man exhibited ulceration and new growth (*d*) over the lower portion of the lesion 2 weeks later. (*e*) This melanoma on the thigh of a 31-year-old woman shows a slightly umbilicated center, irregular shape, and nonhomogeneous coloration. (*f*) This melanoma of the lower eyelid in another patient is visible as the darkly pigmented area just below the eyelashes.

Figure 6 Clark categorized skin tumors according to their level of invasion. Tumors of level I involve the epidermis and are essentially carcinoma in situ. In level II, the tumor has extended into the papillary dermis. Tumor cells at level III are spread along the papillary-reticular dermal interface. Invasion into the reticular dermis occurs at level IV. Level V tumors extend into the subcutaneous tissue. In general, survival decreases as the depth of invasion increases.

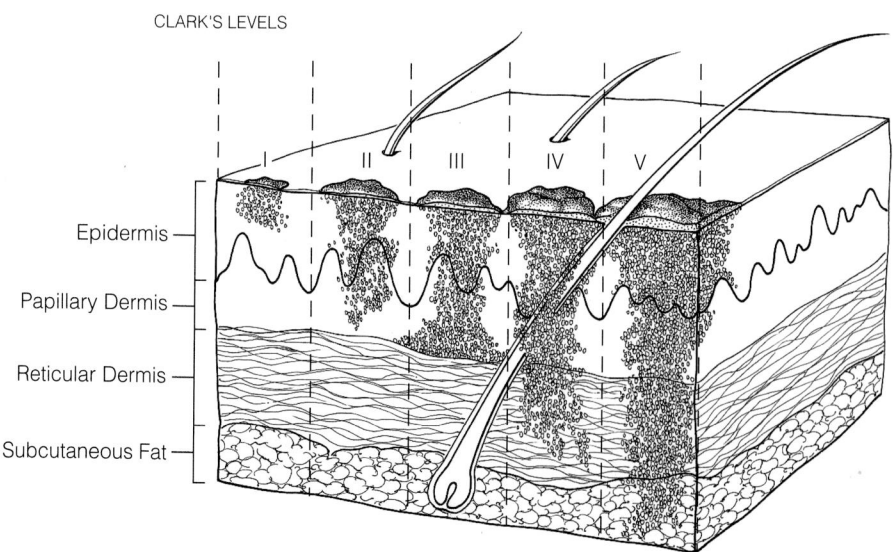

CLARK'S LEVELS

I II III IV V

Epidermis

Papillary Dermis

Reticular Dermis

Subcutaneous Fat

sy. This diagnostic excisional biopsy may be close, encompassing as little as a 1 mm margin of normal skin. Sharp dissection into and including a portion of subcutaneous fat will enable accurate histologic (depth and levels) staging. Shave biopsies must always be condemned because depth cannot be assessed.

Lymphatic Mapping and Sentinel Lymph Node Biopsy

Technological advances have made it possible for surgeons to identify the general characteristics of lymphatic flow and intercept early metastatic tissue by performing lymphatic mapping and SLN biopsy. The rationale, techniques, and indications for this valuable procedure are discussed more fully elsewhere [*see 2:6 Lymphatic Mapping and Sentinel Lymph Node Biopsy*], with particular reference to its use in patients with breast cancer or melanoma. In our unit, we now routinely employ lymphatic mapping and SLN biopsy for biopsy-proven melanomas, squamous cell carcinomas (especially large neurotropic ones), and Merkel cell carcinomas. Our usual practice is to use a combination of isosulfan blue dye and unfiltered technetium-labeled sulfur colloid.

TREATMENT

Effective treatment of melanoma remains exclusively surgical. Initial complete excision is the therapeutic goal. Thin melanomas can be safely excised with surgical margins of only 1 cm.[32,33] However, the appropriate margins for excision of intermediate-thickness lesions remain a matter of controversy.

The benefit of prophylactic regional node dissections in patients with intermediate-thickness lesions and nonpalpable nodes is also controversial. Prospective, randomized trials and a mathematical model indicate no survival benefit with elective lymph node dissection compared with subsequent so-called therapeutic regional lymphadenectomy only when nodes become palpable.[34,35] Intraoperative lymphatic mapping and selective lymphadenectomy may be warranted in a case-specific approach.[36]

Patients with intermediate-thickness tumors (between 0.76 and 3.99 mm) may benefit if an elective regional lymph node dissection (of nonpalpable nodes) is included in their initial surgical management. Benefit has also been shown with the use of elective regional lymph node dissection for the treatment of thick melanomas (4 mm and greater) and thin intermediate melanomas (between 0.76 mm and 1.49 mm) in men.[37] However, a clear understanding of the influence of other important factors, such as previous treatment, age, presence of comorbid disease, and location of the primary lesion, awaits the results of ongoing trials. In addition to providing local control, removal of lymph nodes may find its greatest utility in accurate pathologic staging.[38-40] Many aspects of this therapeutic approach remain controversial.[41]

Patients who have N1 or N2 regional node involvement traditionally have an unfavorable outcome but may benefit from isolated limb perfusion or limb infusion. Several investigators have reported increased survival rates in such patients with the use of isolated limb perfusion.[42] Perfusion with tumor necrosis factor–α appears to yield high local response rates, but the associated toxicity is high.[43] Intralesional immunotherapy, local radiation therapy, and systemic chemotherapy are options for the control of recurrent local lesions.[21] Unfortunately, regional disease develops within 3 years in all patients with thick melanomas (4 mm and greater) and stage IIIA disease, and distant metastases develop within 5 years in more than 60% of these patients.[30,31,37]

Although one might expect that patients with malignancies that have a high incidence of systemic involvement might benefit from adjuvant therapy, none has been proved to be uniformly effective. Allogeneic tumor vaccines (comprising a mixture of different tumor antigens) and other immunostimulation strategies are being studied in clinical trials.[21]

Trials of newer agents for the treatment of stage IV melanoma (involving distant metastases) have been disappointing. Studies of interleukin-2 (IL-2) immunotherapy for metastatic disease, both alone and with lymphokine-activated killer cells (LAK cells, or lymphocytes grown in IL-2), show potential rewards. IL-2 appears to have a 10% to 25% response rate in metastatic melanoma. Unfortunately, fewer than 50% of the responses are complete, and most are of limited duration. IL-2 is currently approved only for the treatment of renal cell cancer. IL-2 and other cytokines in combination with chemotherapeutic agents have generally shown little increase in benefit while carrying higher toxicity. IL-12, a macrophage-derived cytokine, enhances cellular immunity and may soon enter clinical trials.[21,44,45]

Certain melanoma surface antigens may be common to other tumors and may be recognized in an HLA class I molecule–restricted fashion. Melanoma patients who are HLA A1 positive (26% of all whites) and whose tumors contain *MAGE-1* (a tumor gene found in melanoma and other human tumors) could be immunized against their tumors with cytotoxic T cells sensitized to the melanoma cell surface antigen or against *MAGE-1* alone. Vaccinia recognizance (viral) vectors incorporating this *MAGE-1* gene are already being prepared for clinical trials.[21]

Surgical Technique

EXCISIONAL BIOPSY

The biopsy can often be performed in the clinic operating room with the patient under local anesthesia. Care should be taken to avoid injecting the lesion itself because the resulting bleeding may distort the histologic fixation of the specimen. A field block is usually sufficient.

Attention to proper surgical technique will prevent the spread of cancer cells and allow the pathologist sufficient tissue to make an accurate diagnosis. For the histologic diagnosis and staging of all skin lesions, the surgeon should submit at least a full-thickness portion of the lesion and preferably perform an excisional biopsy. With a larger tumor, it is important to incorporate a representative portion of the lesion with 1 mm of normal skin at the margin so that the pathologist can examine the skin adjacent to the neoplasm. Diagnostic biopsies should not be allowed to be damaged by electrocauterization. It is important to orient and mark the specimen properly so that the adequacy of the margins can be studied in relation to the overall anatomy.

Thus, the initial biopsy should include at least 1 mm of normal skin, and the surgeon should take care to perform a full-thickness excision into the fat. The tissue is gently retracted as the incision is continued around the lesion. Before the lesion is removed from the field, an orientation suture is placed. My preference is to make a small drawing on the pathology sheet, indicating where the suture is located in relation to the site on the body from which the lesion came. For example, a suture is placed at 12 o'clock, a small drawing is made of the patient's hand or face, and the specimen is sketched on the drawing itself. This allows the pathologist to identify and localize any margin that exhibits microscopic involvement with tumor cells. Similarly, excision of a segment of subcutaneous fat allows the pathologist to assess depth of invasion.

SUPERFICIAL AND RADICAL GROIN DISSECTIONS

The inguinal nodes drain the anterior and inferior abdominal wall, the perineum, the genitalia, the hips, the buttocks, and the thighs. A superficial groin dissection removes the inguinal nodes, whereas a radical dissection additionally incorporates the iliac and obturator nodes. Palpable nodes can be marked on the patient before operation. Photography can be very helpful for both orientation and documentation.

In cases of skin lesions overlying the anteromedial portion of the thigh, the primary excision can often incorporate an in-continuity groin dissection that is designed to eradicate the primary tumor along with the lymphatic drainage system.[46] As a general principle, the skin lesion, the subcutaneous fat, the lymphatic tissue, and the investing fascia are removed as a unit.

Technique

The patient is usually placed in a supine position on the operating table, with the hip slightly abducted and supported by a pillow and with the hip and knee slightly flexed. A Foley catheter is inserted, the patient is prepared and draped, and the drapes are stapled in position.

A wide ellipse (4 cm margin) incorporating the skin lesion is marked. The femoral artery is palpated and marked, and a diagonally oriented skin incision is planned. The incision will course from the region of the anterosuperior iliac spine, caudally over the central groin region, and through the femoral trigone, terminating at midthigh level on the anteromedial surface of the thigh. This incision interferes least with the musculocutaneous and cutaneous vascular territories of the skin, usually avoids ischemia to the skin, and promotes subsequent healing. The incision is made with a scalpel, and the electrocautery is employed sparingly. The initial incision should include the skin and subcutaneous fat and continue down through the deep investing fascia overlying the muscle. The dissection proceeds downward in a caudal direction, incorporating the fascia and exposing the inguinal ligament, the deep fascia, and the femoral vessels. Fat and nodal tissue are dissected off the external oblique aponeurosis, the spermatic cord, and the inguinal ligament [see Figure 7]. The superficial fascia over the vessels is removed, together with the fat and the contents of the femoral trigone, proceeding from lateral to medial. The femoral vessels and the femoral nerve are left undisturbed, and the dissection proceeds to the fossa ovalis femoris. The great saphenous vein is incorporated into the specimen, ligated by a suture at its junction with the femoral vein [see Figure 7]. The fascia is removed from the sartorius muscle, the adductor muscle

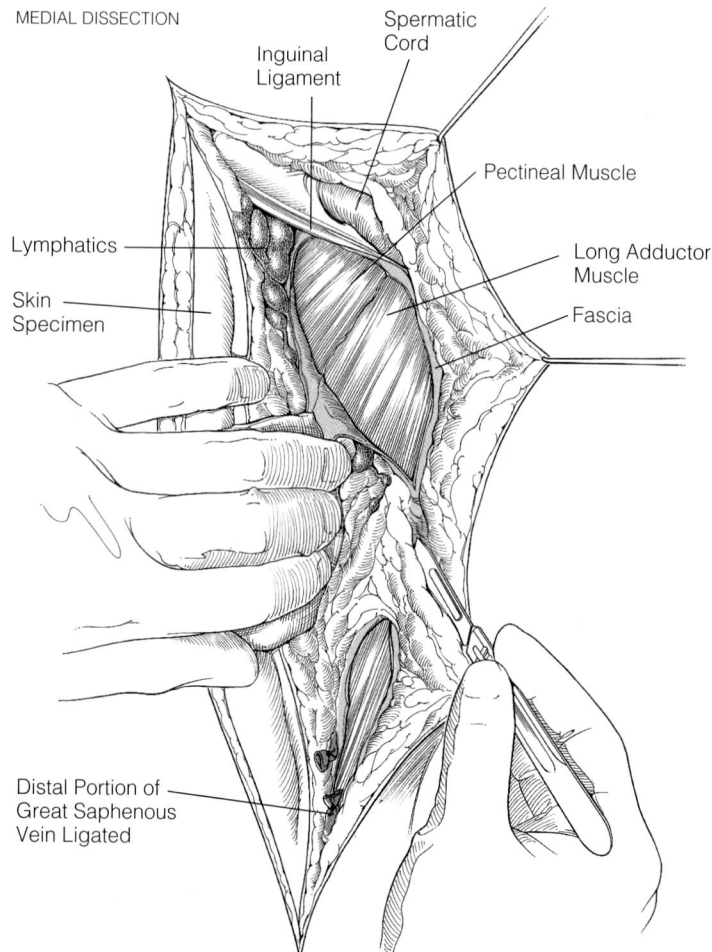

MEDIAL DISSECTION

Spermatic Cord
Inguinal Ligament
Pectineal Muscle
Lymphatics
Long Adductor Muscle
Skin Specimen
Fascia
Distal Portion of Great Saphenous Vein Ligated

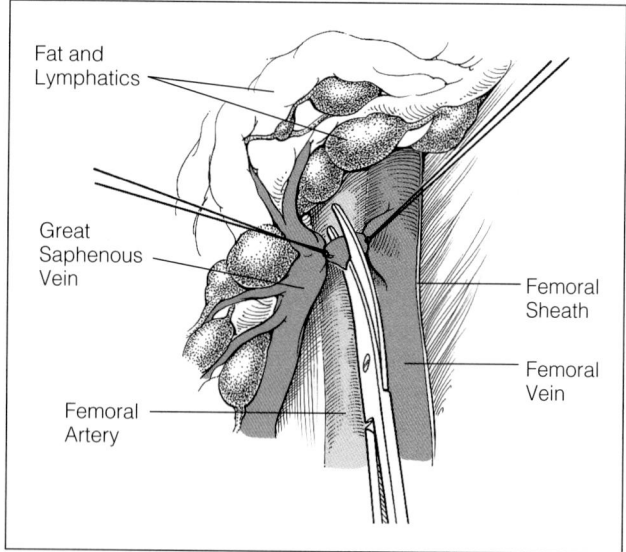

Fat and Lymphatics
Great Saphenous Vein
Femoral Sheath
Femoral Vein
Femoral Artery

Figure 7 In a superficial groin dissection, the incision is deepened to include the deep muscular fascia. The great saphenous vein is ligated and divided (inset).

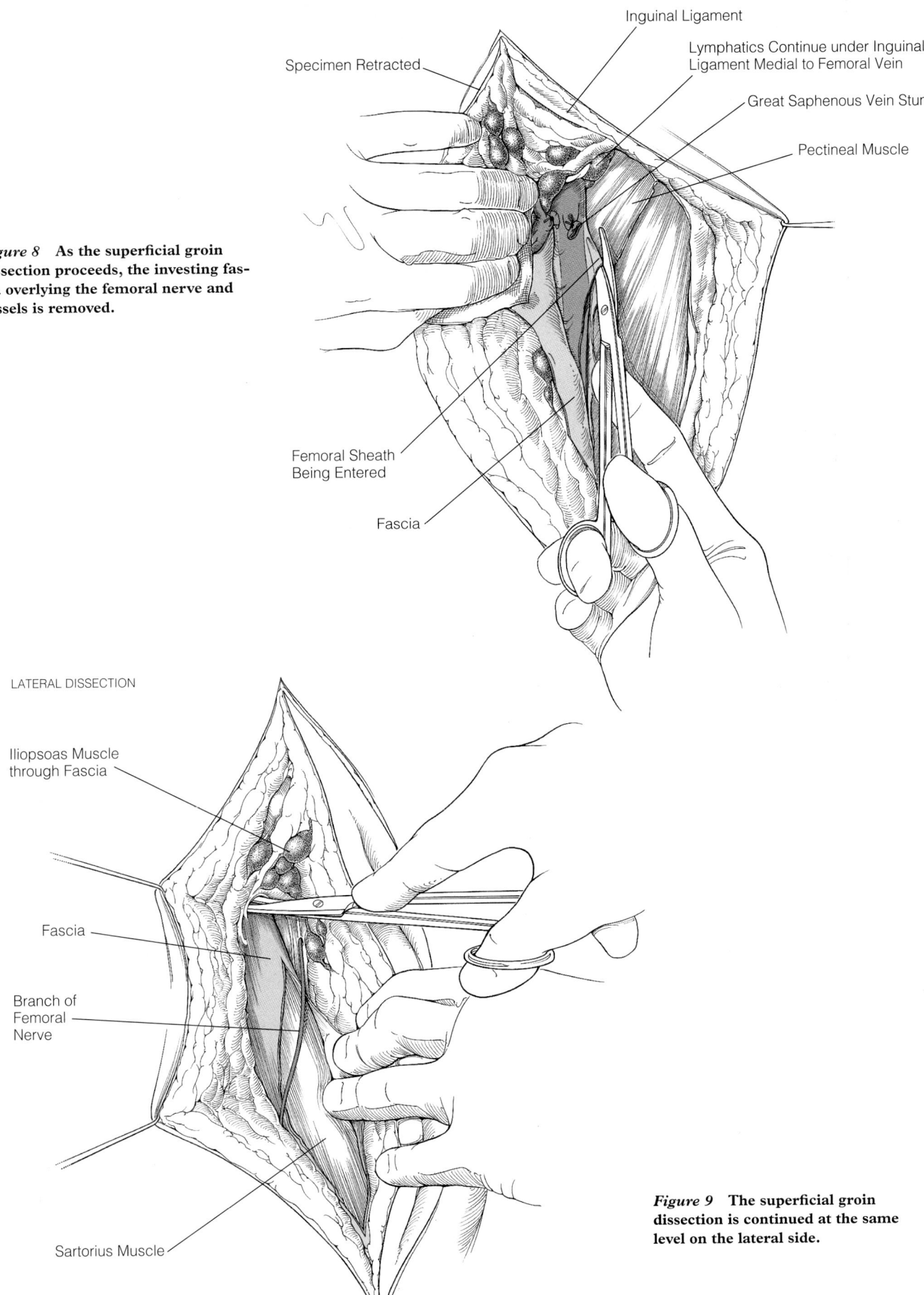

Inguinal Ligament

Lymphatics Continue under Inguinal
Ligament Medial to Femoral Vein

Great Saphenous Vein Stump

Pectineal Muscle

Specimen Retracted

Figure 8 **As the superficial groin
dissection proceeds, the investing fascia overlying the femoral nerve and
vessels is removed.**

Femoral Sheath
Being Entered

Fascia

LATERAL DISSECTION

Iliopsoas Muscle
through Fascia

Fascia

Branch of
Femoral
Nerve

Sartorius Muscle

Figure 9 **The superficial groin
dissection is continued at the same
level on the lateral side.**

group, and the rectus femoris, with all lymphatic tissue included in the surgical specimen [*see Figures 8 and 9*]. The dissection proceeds medially to the medial aspect of the femoral trigone. This completes the superficial portion of the groin dissection.

If the surgeon decides to perform a radical (ilioinguinal) node dissection, the incision is extended through the inguinal ligament, beginning medial to the anterosuperior iliac spine and continuing to a point approximately 2 cm lateral to the femoral artery. The inguinal canal is further exposed by releasing the internal oblique abdominal muscle, the transversus abdominis, and the fascia transversalis and dissecting into the retroperitoneal space. The deep circumflex iliac vessels are ligated, and blunt finger dissection separates the peritoneum from the preperitoneal fat and nodes.

Retractors are inserted to widen the retroperitoneal space, and the peritoneum and the abdominal viscera are retracted medially. The chain of lymph nodes, areolar tissue, and adventitial tissues along the external iliac vessels is dissected; the dissection proceeds proximally to the origins of the internal iliac vessels and incorporates the nodes overlying the obturator foramen by removing the internal obturator fascia. The deep epigastric vessels are usually ligated at their origins from the external iliac artery and vein. The lymph node–bearing specimen is then removed as a unit, oriented, and labeled appropriately with sutures. The inguinal canal is reconstructed to prevent a hernia, and the sartorius muscle is mobilized to the midportion of the wound to cover the femoral vessels. The skin and the subcutaneous tissues are then closed in layers over a soft suction drain.

References

1. Cottel WI: Skin tumors: basal cell and squamous cell carcinoma. Selected Readings in Plastic Surgery 7(6):1, 1992

2. Silverberg E, Lubera J: Cancer statistics. CA Cancer J Clin 39:3, 1989

3. Cancer of the Skin. Friedman RJ, Rigel DS, Kopf AW, et al, Eds. WB Saunders Co, Philadelphia, 1991

4. Koh HK, Kligler BE, Lew RA: Sunlight and cutaneous malignant melanoma: evidence for and against causation. Photochem Photobiol 51:765, 1990

5. Green HA, Drake L: Aging, sun damage, and sunscreens. Clin Plast Surg 20:1, 1993

6. Urbach F: Geographic distribution of skin cancer. J Surg Oncol 3:219, 1971

7. Dellon AL: Host-tumor relationship in basal cell and squamous cell cancer of the skin. Plast Reconstr Surg 62:37, 1978

8. Marshall V: Premalignant and malignant skin tumors in immunosuppressed patients. Transplantation 17: 272, 1974

9. Wade TR, Ackerman AB: The many faces of basal cell carcinoma. J Dermatol Surg Oncol 4:23, 1978

10. Salasche SJ, Amonette RA: Morpheaform basal cell epitheliomas: a study of subclinical extension in a series of 51 cases. J Dermatol Surg Oncol 7:387, 1981

11. Shanoff LB, Spira M, Hardy SB: Basal cell carcinoma: a statistical approach to rational management. Plast Reconstr Surg 39:619, 1967

12. Bart RS, Kopf AW, Peratos MA: X-ray therapy of skin cancer: evaluation of a "standardized" method for treating basal cell carcinoma. Fifth National Cancer Conference. JB Lippincott, Philadelphia, 1970, p 559

13. Mohs FE: Chemosurgery: microscopically controlled methods of cancer excision. Arch Surg 42:279, 1941

14. Robinson JK: Mohs micrographic surgery. Clin Plast Surg 20:149, 1993

15. Brownstein MH, Rabinowitz AD: The precursors of cutaneous squamous cell carcinoma. Int J Dermatol 18:1, 1979

16. Albricht SM: Treatment of malignant cutaneous tumors. Clin Plast Surg 20:167, 1993

17. Kohn H, Baumal R, From L: Role of immunohistochemistry in the diagnosis of undifferentiated tumors involving the skin. J Am Acad Dermatol 14:1063, 1986

18. Bostwick J, Pendergrast J, Vasconez L: Marjolin's ulcer: an immunologically privileged tumor? Plast Reconstr Surg 57:66, 1976

19. Traves N, Pack GT: The development of cancer in burn scars: analysis and report of 34 cases. Surg Gynecol Obstet 51:749, 1930

20. Ames FC, Hickey RC: Metastasis from squamous cell skin cancer of the extremities. South Med J 75: 920, 1982

21. Vetto J: Advances in the Therapy of Malignant Melanoma (monograph). Department of Surgery, Oregon Health Sciences University, Portland, Oregon, 1994

22. Morton DL, Dartyan DG, Wanek LA, et al: Multivariate analysis of the relationship between survival and the microstage of primary melanoma by Clark level and Breslow thickness. Cancer 71:3737, 1993

23. Koh HK: Cutaneous melanoma. N Engl J Med 325: 171, 1991

24. Armstrong BK: Epidemiology of malignant melanoma: intermittent or total accumulated exposure to the sun. J Dermatol Surg Oncol 14:835, 1988

25. Lew RA, Saber AJ, Cook N, et al: Sun exposure habits in patients with cutaneous melanoma: a case control study. J Dermatol Surg Oncol 9:981, 1983

26. Evans GR, Manson PN: Review and current perspectives of cutaneous malignant melanoma. J Am Coll Surg 178:523, 1994

27. Anderson RG: Skin tumors II: melanoma. Selected Readings in Plastic Surgery 7(7):1, 1992

28. Mihm MC, Clark WH, From L: The clinical diagnosis, classification, and histogenic concepts of the early stages of cutaneous melanoma. N Engl J Med 284: 1078, 1971

29. Friedman RJ, Rigel DS, Silverman MK, et al: Malignant melanoma in the 1990's: the continued importance of early detection and the role of physician examinations and self-examination of the skin. CA Cancer J Clin 41:201, 1991

30. Clark WH, From L, Bernardino EA, et al: The histogenesis and biologic behavior of primary human malignant melanomas of the skin. Cancer Res 29:705, 1969

31. Breslow A: Thickness, cross-sectional areas and depth of invasion in the prognosis of cutaneous melanoma. Ann Surg 172:902, 1970

32. Balch CM, Murad TM, Soong S, et al: Tumor thickness as a guide to surgical management of clinical stage I melanoma patients. Cancer 43:883, 1979

33. Veronisi U, Cascinelli N, Adamus J, et al: Thin stage I primary cutaneous malignant melanoma: comparison of excision with margins of 1 or 3 cm. N Engl J Med 318:1159, 1988

34. Sim FH, Taylor WF, Prichard DC, et al: Lymphadenectomy in the management of stage I malignant melanoma: a prospective randomized study. Mayo Clin Proc 61:697, 1986

35. Veronesi U, Adamus J, Bandiera DC, et al: Delayed regional lymph node dissection in stage I melanoma of the skin and lower extremities. Cancer 49:2420, 1982

36. Morton DL, Wen DR, Wong JH, et al: Technical details of intraoperative lymphatic mapping for early stage melanoma. Arch Surg 127:392, 1992

37. Balch CM, Soong SJ, Milton GW, et al: A comparison of prognostic factors and surgical results in 1,786 patients with localized (stage I) melanoma treated in Alabama, USA, and New South Wales, Australia. Ann Surg 196:677, 1982

38. Crowley NJ: The case against elective lymphadenectomy. Surg Oncol Clin North Am 1:223, 1992

39. Coates AS, Ingvar CI, Petersen-Schaefer K, et al: Elective lymph node dissection in patients with primary melanoma of the trunk and limbs treated at the Sydney melanoma unit from 1960 to 1991. J Am Coll Surg 180:402, 1995

40. Krag DN, Meijer SJ, Weaver DL, et al: Minimal-access surgery for staging of malignant melanoma. Arch Surg 130:654, 1995

41. Vetto J: Elective lymph node dissection for intermediate thickness melanoma: does it have a future? Clin Oncol Alert 11:6, 1996

42. Hartley JW, Fletcher WS: Improved survival of patients with stage II melanoma of the extremity using hyperthermic isolation perfusion with 1-phenylalanine mustard. J Surg Oncol 36:170, 1987

43. Lienard D, Lejeune FJ, Ewalenko P: In transit metastases of malignant melanoma treated by high dose rTNF-α in combination with interferon-gamma and melphalan isolation perfusion. World J Surg 16:234, 1992

44. Rosenberg SA, Lotze MT, Yang JC, et al: Prospective trial of high-dose interleukin-2 alone or in conjunction with lymphokine-activated killer cells for the treatment of patients with advanced cancer. J Natl Cancer Inst 85:622, 1993

45. Nastala CL, Edington HD, Storkus WJ, et al: Recombinant interleukin-12 (r-mil-12) mediates regression of both subcutaneous and metastatic murine tumors. Surg Forum 44:518, 1993

46. Karakousis CP: Technique of lymphadenectomy for melanoma. Surg Oncol Clin North Am 1:157, 1992

Recommended Reading

Cancer Facts and Figures—2003. American Cancer Society, New York, 2003

Hallock GG, Lutz DA: A prospective study of the accuracy of the surgeon's diagnosis and significance of positive margins in nonmelanoma skin cancers. Plast Reconstr Surg 107:942, 2001

Mathes SJ, Eriksson E, McGrath MH, et al: Management of cutaneous malignancies. Contemp Surg 49:307, 1996

Acknowledgments

Figures 7 through 9   Susan E. Brust, C.M.I.

The author is grateful to John Vetto, M.D., and Paul Manson, M.D., for their suggestions in the preparation of this chapter.

5 BREAST PROCEDURES

Barbara L. Smith, M.D., Ph.D., F.A.C.S., and Wiley W. Souba, M.D., Sc.D., F.A.C.S.

Since the 1970s, surgical procedures for cancer of the breast have become progressively less extensive while maintaining excellent control of local recurrence. Updates of multiple prospective, randomized trials continue to demonstrate that survival after lumpectomy, axillary dissection, and radiation therapy does not differ significantly from survival after mastectomy.[1-3] Local recurrence rates after lumpectomy and radiation therapy remain in the 10% range. At present, there are almost no remaining indications for the Halsted radical mastectomy.

The issue of the precise extent of surgical intervention necessary for evaluation and treatment of breast lesions continues to be reexamined. With the increased availability of screening mammography, a higher proportion of cancers are being detected at a nonpalpable stage (as in situ carcinomas or small invasive lesions), for which long-term survival rates range from 90% to 95% or higher. The efficacy of wide local excision without radiation in the treatment of in situ lesions is being investigated, and the need for axillary dissection in the treatment of small invasive cancers and cancers in elderly patients is being reconsidered. Improvements in imaging technology—including more refined mammographic techniques, improved breast ultrasonography, and the development of magnetic resonance imaging of the breast—are yielding enhanced diagnostic sensitivity and specificity. Stereotactic and ultrasound-guided core-needle biopsy of nonpalpable breast lesions has proved to be a less invasive and less costly alternative to open surgical biopsy that is appropriate for many patients. Fine-needle aspiration (FNA) biopsy is increasingly replacing open surgical biopsy in the diagnosis of palpable breast malignancies and is proving useful in the diagnosis of many palpable benign lesions as well.

In what follows, we describe our approach to selected common surgical procedures currently employed in the diagnosis and treatment of breast lesions, taking into account various technical and nontechnical issues raised by the growth of new technologies and the evolution of our understanding of the biology of breast diseases.

Breast Biopsy

OPTIONS FOR PALPABLE MASSES

Tissue diagnosis of a palpable breast mass may be obtained by means of FNA biopsy, core-needle biopsy, or open incisional or excisional biopsy. Needle biopsy techniques are less invasive and less costly than open biopsy but are significantly more likely to yield false negative results. The choice of a biopsy technique must be based on the clinical and radiographic features of the lesion.

Fine-Needle Aspiration Biopsy

FNA biopsy is best performed by an experienced operator. It is an appropriate first step in diagnosing most discrete palpable breast masses encountered in clinical practice. The procedure is less useful in evaluating areas of vague thickening or nodularity: such lesions often contain normal tissue mingled with malignant tissue, and the small samples obtained with FNA biopsy may not include any of the malignant cells. FNA biopsy also is not particularly useful for small masses: the mass must be large enough to permit the biopsy needle to be moved back and forth within the lesion without passing out into surrounding normal tissue and contaminating the specimen with excessive amounts of normal cells. FNA biopsy of lesions less than 1 cm in diameter is associated with an unacceptably high rate of sampling error. FNA biopsy is usually the diagnostic procedure of choice for T3 and T4 primary lesions and for chest wall and axillary recurrences for which systemic therapy or irradiation is indicated as the first treatment modality.

Discrete masses discovered on physical examination may be either cystic or solid. Unless previous ultrasonographic examination has shown the mass to be solid, the needle used should be large enough to permit aspiration of potentially viscous fluid if the lesion proves to be cystic (i.e., 20 or 21 gauge). If the mass is known to be solid, a smaller needle (22 to 25 gauge) is sufficient for obtaining diagnostic tissue and will cause the patient less discomfort. For sufficient suction to be generated, a syringe with a capacity no smaller than 10 ml should be used. A variety of syringe holders are available that facilitate application of suction with a single hand.

Technique The skin of the breast is prepared with alcohol or iodine, and the lesion to be biopsied is held steady between the thumb and the index finger of the nondominant hand. A local anesthetic is usually not necessary; if it is used, it should be injected so as to create only a small skin wheal, so that there will be minimal distortion of the approach to the lesion. To facilitate visualization of the collected sample, 1 to 2 ml of air is introduced into the biopsy syringe before the needle enters the skin. The tip of the needle is advanced into the lesion before any suction is applied to minimize collection of tissue outside the lesion. Once the tip is in place, strong suction is applied, and the needle is moved back and forth within the lesion repeatedly along a 5 to 10 mm long track to loosen and collect cells. (This oscillation of the needle along the same track is the most effective way of obtaining a cellular, diagnostic specimen.) The back-and-forth movement of the needle within the lesion is continued until tissue becomes visible in the hub of the needle. Suction is released while the needle is still within the lesion (again, to prevent collection of contaminating tissue from outside the lesion).

The needle is then withdrawn from the lesion, and its contents are expelled onto prepared glass slides, spread into a thin smear, and fixed according to the preferences of the cytology laboratory. Additional passes through the lesion may be made to ensure that a sufficiently cellular sample has been obtained, and the syringe may be rinsed so that a cell block can be prepared for further analysis. An adhesive bandage is applied to the biopsy site. If the lesion proves to be cystic, all fluid should be aspirated; this should cause the mass to disappear. The fluid need not be sent for analysis unless it is bloody or a palpable mass remains after as much fluid as possible has been aspirated.

The patient is reexamined 4 to 8 weeks after successful aspiration. If the same cyst has recurred, it should be aspirated again and the fluid sent for cytologic analysis.

Interpretation of results Analysis by an experienced cytologist is critical for accurate interpretation of FNA biopsy results. Many cytology laboratories are able to perform immunohistochemical analysis for hormone receptors on FNA specimens if an appropriate fixative has been used. In most cytology labs, the false positive rate for a diagnosis of malignancy in an FNA biopsy of a breast mass is only 1% to 2%. Thus, a diagnosis of malignancy that is based on cytologic analysis of an FNA specimen may generally be believed, and definitive surgery may be planned without further biopsy. It should be remembered, however, that FNA does not distinguish between invasive and in situ breast cancer; intraoperative frozen section should be performed if necessary to determine the need for axillary dissection.

The false negative rate for identifying breast malignancy, however, is high: FNA fails to diagnose as many as 40% of cancers. Any cellular atypia on FNA biopsy is an indication for open biopsy. A diagnosis of normal or fibrocystic breast tissue should also be viewed with suspicion; subsequent open biopsy is usually indicated if the physical examination or a mammogram of the biopsied lesion gives rise to even a minor degree of concern about malignancy. If the cytologic analysis is diagnostic of a specific benign lesion (e.g., a fibroadenoma or a lactating adenoma), it may generally be relied on if it is in keeping with the clinical features of the lesion, and no further workup is necessary. It has been suggested that no further workup is required when the so-called triple negative criteria (a physical examination suggestive of a benign lesion, a normal mammogram, and negative results from FNA biopsy) are present, particularly in younger women.

Core-Needle (Cutting-Needle) Biopsy

As its name suggests, a core-needle biopsy removes a narrow cylinder of tissue from the biopsied lesion. The tissue undergoes standard pathologic rather than cytologic analysis; consequently, this technique is preferable if a skilled cytologist is not available for interpretation of FNA biopsy specimens. Nonetheless, FNA biopsy has supplanted core-needle biopsy in the investigation of most palpable lesions. It should be noted that the false negative rate associated with core-needle biopsy for palpable lesions performed without ultrasonographic or stereotactic guidance is as high as or higher than that of FNA biopsy.[4] The technical difficulty of accurately placing and firing the core needle in small mobile lesions or in lesions surrounded by dense fibrocystic tissue makes FNA biopsy preferable in these set-

tings. Core-needle biopsy is, however, ideal for sampling large lesions or chest wall recurrences in which the larger samples permit more detailed pathologic analysis and easy determination of hormone receptor levels.

Technique If the mass is palpable, the surgeon can perform the core-needle biopsy in the office. A large needle (usually 14 gauge) is placed either by hand or with a biopsy gun device. Injection of a local anesthetic is usually required—again, in a quantity that will create only a small skin wheal. A nick is made in the skin with a No. 11 blade to permit easy entry of the biopsy needle into breast tissue and into the lesion. As with FNA biopsy (see above), the lesion is held steady in the nondominant hand while the biopsy needle is advanced into the lesion and a core sample obtained.

Interpretation of results Atypia on core-needle biopsy is an indication for open biopsy of the sampled lesion. In addition, any core-needle biopsy (especially one done without stereotactic or ultrasonographic guidance) that yields benign or fibrocystic tissue should be viewed with some suspicion because of the risk of technical or sampling error. Open biopsy should be considered if there is any discordance between a benign core-needle biopsy result and the clinical or mammographic features of the lesion.

Open Biopsy

The vast majority of open breast biopsies are now performed with either local anesthesia alone or the use of local anesthesia with intravenous sedation. General anesthesia is reserved for situations in which multiple lesions must be excised and the amount of local anesthetic required would exceed the maximum safe dose.

Technique Open biopsy incisions should generally be curvilinear and should be placed directly over the lesion to minimize tunneling through breast tissue [*see Figure 1*]. Because the possibility of malignancy must always be taken into account, all open biopsy incisions should also be oriented so that they will be included within any subsequent mastectomy incision. Accordingly, if an open biopsy is to be done at an extremely lateral or medial site, it may be best approached via a radial incision placed over the lesion rather than via a more vertical curvilinear incision.

The incision should be long enough to provide adequate exposure and to ensure that the mass can be excised as a single tissue fragment with a small margin of grossly normal tissue. Specimen margins should be inked by the pathologist. Meticulous hemostasis should be achieved before closure. Deep breast tissue should be approximated only if such approximation does not result in significant deformity of breast contour. A cosmetic subcuticular closure is preferred.

OPTIONS FOR NONPALPABLE MASSES

The increasingly widespread use of screening mammography has led to the identification of more and more nonpalpable breast masses for which tissue diagnosis is required. In most series,[5-7] 15% to 30% of such lesions prove to be malignant. Nonpalpable masses may be approached via core-needle biopsy or open biopsy with wire localization.

Image-Guided Core-Needle Biopsy

Needle biopsy techniques are increasingly being used to diagnose nonpalpable breast lesions. In general, FNA biopsy of nonpalpable lesions is inadvisable because of its high false negative rate. Little is lost by attempting an FNA biopsy of a palpable lesion in the office setting, but performing a stereotactic or ultrasound-guided FNA biopsy of a nonpalpable mass carries a significant cost in terms of time, patient discomfort, and expense. The diagnostic accuracy currently achievable with FNA biopsy in this setting does not justify this cost. Consequently, image-guided core-needle biopsy is the preferred approach for needle biopsy of nonpalpable lesions.

In choosing core-needle biopsy, both patient and physician must be comfortable with the fact that the lesion will only be sampled rather than excised, must recognize that the possibility of a sampling error that will cause the examiner to miss the lesion is higher with core-needle biopsy than with open biopsy, and must realize that equivocal findings will necessitate follow-up with open biopsy. The trade-off for these limitations is that core-needle biopsy generally costs less than open biopsy, takes less time, and leaves only a tiny scar. After a core-needle diagnosis of malignancy, the surgeon may proceed directly to wide local excision and will often be able to obtain clean margins with a single open procedure.[8]

Stereotactic versus ultrasound-guided biopsy Whenever feasible, core-needle biopsy is performed with ultrasonographic guidance, which permits real-time documentation of needle position within the lesion. Stereotactic mammography-guided core-needle biopsy is performed if the lesion is not visualized ultrasonographically. Stereotactic biopsy is appropriate for lesions that are favorably located within the breast (i.e., that can be stably positioned in the biopsy window of the machine). Lesions very close to the chest wall or the areola may not be accessible to stereotactic biopsy and are best approached via open biopsy with needle localization (see below).

Clustered microcalcifications may also be approached by stereotactic core-needle biopsy. If the cluster is not large enough for calcifications to remain to guide subsequent wide excision if a malignancy is found, a clip should be placed to mark the biopsy site.

Interpretation of results The introduction of large core-biopsy needles (11- and 14-gauge), coupled with the use of vacuum assistance to draw additional tissue into the needle, has markedly improved the false negative rate for core-needle biopsy. Currently, false negative rates for this procedure fall into the 1% to 2% range,[9,10] results that compare favorably with those reported for wire-localized open surgical biopsy. It is now routine to perform radiography of core-needle biopsy specimens to confirm that targeted calcifications have been removed. When the targeted lesion comprises dense tissue rather than calcifications, care must be taken to confirm that the lesion was adequately sampled and thus ensure that the findings can be interpreted reliably. Immediate postbiopsy radiography may be performed to demonstrate that a hole was made in the lesion. A finding of benign or fibrocystic tissue on such a biopsy should be viewed with some suspicion and interpreted in relation to the lesion sampled. One must decide whether the pathologic findings adequately account for the lesion visualized. If any concern remains, open biopsy is indicated.

Because false positive results are rare, a diagnosis of malignancy may be believed and acted upon without further biopsy. In planning treatment after core-needle biopsy that shows only carcinoma in situ, one should remember that the lesion was only sampled and that invasive tumor may still be found when

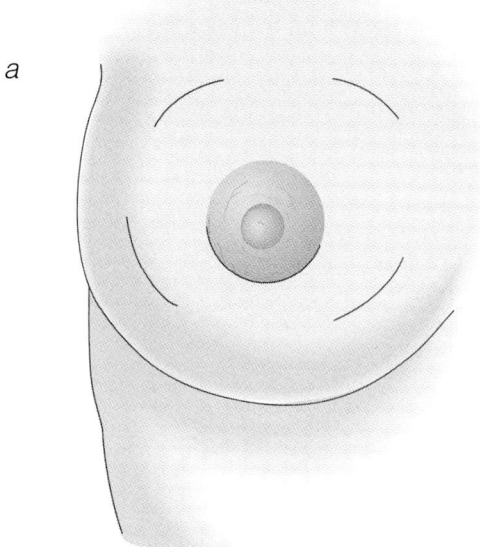

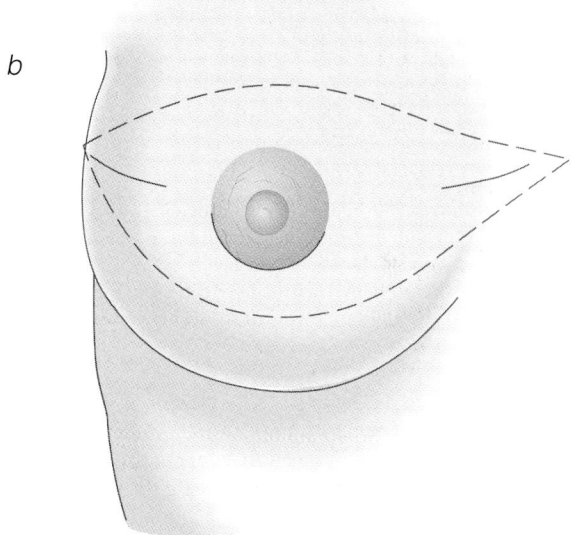

Figure 1 **Open breast biopsy. (*a*) In most cases, a curvilinear incision is preferred. If the mass is close to the areola, a periareolar incision may be used. (*b*) Extremely lateral or medial incisions may be radial. In any case, incisions should be placed directly over the lesion and should be oriented so that they will be included within a subsequent mastectomy incision if margins prove positive and mastectomy is indicated.**

the lesion is completely excised. The likelihood of finding invasive tumor on surgical excision after a core-needle biopsy indicative of ductal carcinoma may be as high as 20%.[10]

A finding of atypical ductal hyperplasia on core-needle biopsy is an indication for wire-localized open biopsy. Open biopsy after a core-needle biopsy indicative of atypical ductal hyperplasia may reveal ductal carcinoma in situ (DCIS) in as many as 50% of patients; this may be a less frequent finding when a larger (e.g., 11-gauge) needle was used for the core-needle biopsy.[10]

Follow-up Whether short-interval mammographic follow-up is necessary after core-needle biopsy depends on the patho-

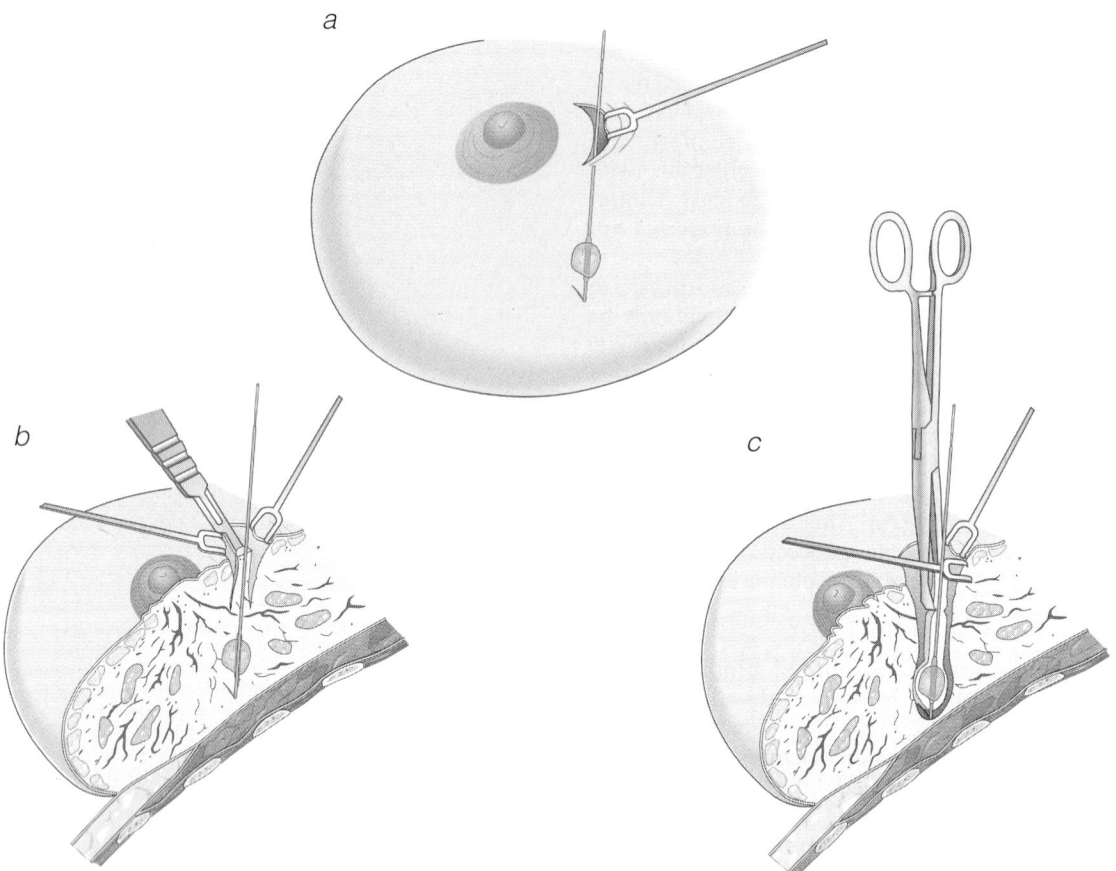

Figure 2 Needle-localized breast biopsy.[13] (*a*) **The mammographic abnormality is localized immediately before operation. The relation between the wire, the skin entry site, and the lesion is noted by the surgeon. (*b*) The skin incision is placed over the expected location of the mammographic abnormality. The dissection is accomplished with the wire as a guide. (*c*) The tissue around the wire is removed en bloc with the wire and sent for specimen mammography. Tunneling and piecemeal removal are to be avoided.**

logic findings and the mammographic appearance of the lesion. With a well-circumscribed lesion that pathologic evaluation shows to be a fibroadenoma or with calcifications that pathologic evaluation shows to be located in benign fibrocystic tissue, no special follow-up is required, and routine screening at normal intervals may be resumed. In general, if the pathologic findings are equivocal or discordant with the appearance of the lesion, immediate open excision is preferable to a 6-month repeat mammogram. To ensure appropriate follow-up, there should be close communication between the physician ordering the core-needle biopsy, the physician performing the biopsy, and the pathologist analyzing the specimen.

Open Biopsy with Needle (Wire) Localization

As is the case for open biopsy of palpable lesions, the vast majority of needle-localized breast biopsies are now performed with local anesthesia or local anesthesia with intravenous sedation. General anesthesia is reserved for excision of multiple lesions or other special circumstances.

Technique The lesion to be excised is localized by inserting a thin needle and a fine wire under mammographic or ultrasonographic guidance immediately before operation. To facilitate incision placement, images should be sent to the operating room with the wire entry site indicated on them. With superfi-

cial lesions, the wire entry site is usually close to the lesion and thus may be included in the incision. With some deeper lesions, the wire entry site is on the shortest path to the lesion and so may still be included in the incision. The incision is placed as directly as possible over the mass to minimize tunneling through breast tissue. Once the incision is made, a core of tissue is excised around and along the wire in such a way as to include the lesion [*see Figure 2*]. (This process is easier and involves less excision of tissue if the localizing wire has a thickened segment several centimeters in length that is placed adjacent to or within the lesion. One then follows the wire itself into breast tissue until the thick segment is reached and only then extends the excision away from the wire to include the lesion in a fairly small tissue fragment.)

With many lesions, the wire entry site is in a fairly peripheral location relative to the position of the lesion, which means that including the wire entry site in the incision would result in excessive tunneling within breast tissue. In such cases, the incision is placed over the expected position of the lesion [*see Figure 3*], the dissection is extended into breast tissue to identify the wire a few centimeters away from the lesion itself, and the free end of the wire is pulled up into the incision. A generous core of tissue is then excised around the wire. (Again, this process is easier if the thick segment of the localizing wire is placed adjacent to or within the lesion.)

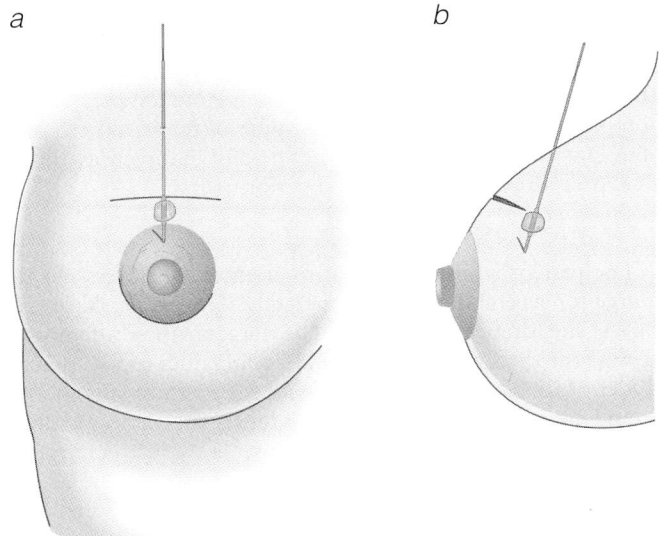

Figure 3 **Needle-localized breast biopsy.**[13] (*a*) **It is sometimes necessary to insert the localizing wire from a peripheral site to localize a deep or central lesion. The incision should be placed directly over the expected location of the lesion, not over the wire entry site. (*b*) Once the skin incision is made, the dissection is extended into breast tissue to identify the wire a short distance from the lesion. The free end of the wire is pulled into the wound, and the biopsy is performed as in Figure 2.**

Radiography should immediately be performed on all wire-localized biopsy specimens to confirm that the lesion has been excised. The patient should remain on the operating table with the sterile field preserved until such confirmation has been received. If the mass was missed and the surgeon has some idea of the likely location of the missed lesion, another tissue sample may be excised immediately. If, however, the surgeon suspects that the wire was dislodged before or during the procedure, the incision should be closed. After the patient has healed sufficiently to be able to tolerate repeat mammography, another mammogram is obtained, and repeat localization and biopsy are performed.

Directional Vacuum-Assisted Breast Biopsy (Mammotomy)

Directional vacuum-assisted biopsy (DVAB), or mammotomy, is a special procedure for obtaining specimens from single or multiple breast lesions (e.g., microcalcifications, circumscribed masses, and spiculated masses). DVAB is a diagnostic procedure and is not intended for therapeutic purposes. On the whole, it is safe, and the complication rate is acceptably low.

In comparison with core-needle biopsy, DVAB is more successful at removing microcalcifications, can obtain more specimens in the course of a single procedure, and is more sensitive in detecting ductal carcinoma in situ and atypical duct hyperplasia. DVAB also appears to diagnose nonpalpable breast lesions more effectively than stereotactically guided core-needle biopsy does. It may, in fact, be helpful to perform DVAB after core-needle biopsy when the diagnosis of atypical duct hyperplasia is being considered; this practice may lead to a decrease in the number of open biopsies performed.

Suitable candidates for DVAB include patients with nonpalpable but mammographically visible clusters of suspicious calcifications, those with well-defined masses that are likely to be benign, and those with suspicious masses. Target lesions must be clearly visible on digital images and identifiable on stereo-

tactic projections. DVAB is not recommended for patients with certain lesions located very posteriorly or very anteriorly in the breast, those with very small or very thin breasts, and those who, for one reason or another, cannot be properly positioned for the procedure or cannot cooperate with the surgeon. The procedure is done on an outpatient basis and usually can be completed in 1 hour or less. Patients are restricted from engaging in strenuous activity for 24 hours after DVAB.

The probe employed for the procedure consists of an outer trocar cannula, a sliding inner hollow coaxial cutter, a so-called knockout shaft, a distal sampling notch, and a proximal tissue retrieval chamber; in addition, it has a thumbwheel, which is used for manual advancement, cutting, and retrieval of biopsy specimens. It must be used under the guidance of an imaging modality (e.g., ultrasonography or roentgenography), and it may be either mounted or handheld. The device is connected to a suction machine, which acts first to draw the target tissue into the sampling notch and then to facilitate retrieval of tissue into the proximal collection chamber.

Stereotactic digital imaging is then performed to visualize the target and calculate its location in three dimensions, and a suitable trocar insertion site is identified. The skin is prepared, and a small amount of buffered 1% lidocaine with epinephrine (usually 10 ml or less) is administered. The skin at the insertion site is punctured with a No. 11 blade, the probe is manually advanced to the prefire site, and the position of the probe is confirmed by means of stereotactic imaging. The device is then fired, repeatedly cutting, rotating, and retrieving samples until the desired amount has been removed. If the lesions being removed are calcifications, the sufficiency of the sampling may be confirmed through x-rays of the specimens.

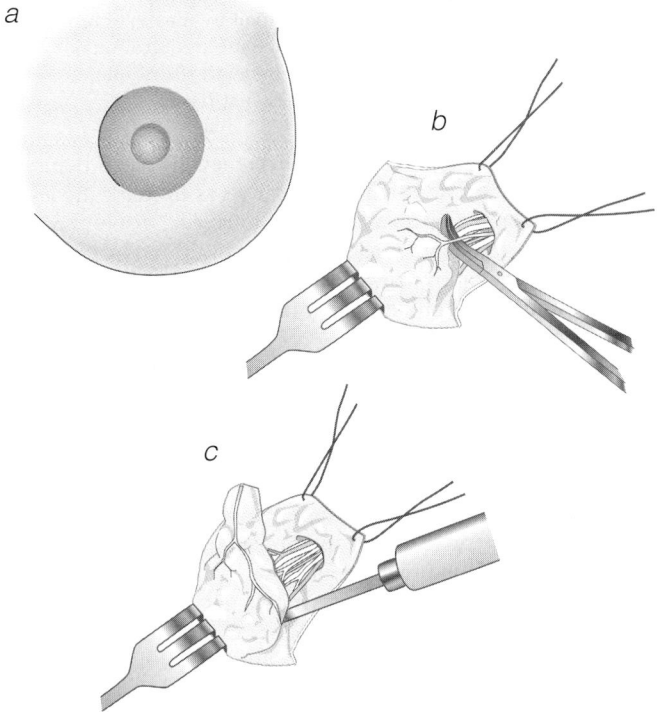

Figure 4 **Terminal duct excision (single duct).**[14] (*a*) **A periareolar incision is made. (*b*) The involved duct is identified by means of blunt dissection. (*c*) The duct is removed along with a core of breast tissue.**

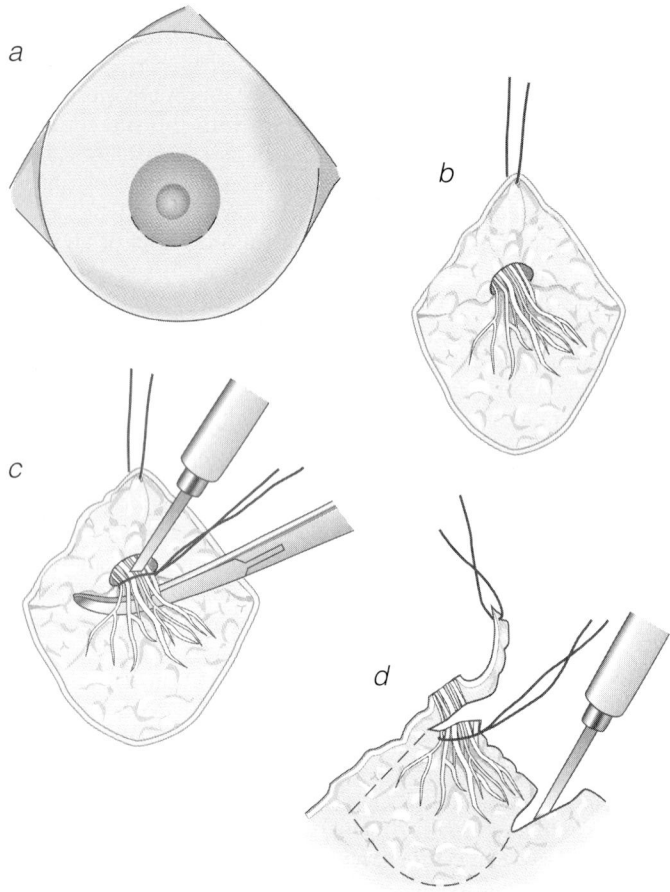

Figure 5 Terminal duct excision (entire ductal complex).[14] (*a*) A periareolar incision is made. (*b*) The nipple skin flap is raised. (*c*) The ductal complex is identified by means of blunt dissection and transected. (*d*) The entire subareolar ductal complex is excised from immediately beneath the nipple dermis to a depth of 4 to 5 cm within breast tissue.

Once the biopsy is complete, an inert metallic clip is deployed into the biopsy site through the trocar so as to mark the lesion for future reference in case it can no longer be visualized after biopsy; deployment and positioning are confirmed by stereotactic imaging. The biopsy device is then removed, the edges of the skin incision are approximated with Steri-Strips, and a compressive bandage is applied. Any bleeding occurring after removal of the biopsy device should be controlled by manual pressure before the final bandage is applied. Typically, 1 g of tissue (equivalent to approximately 10 to 12 samples with an 11-gauge probe) is sufficient for diagnosis of benign disease, atypical duct hyperplasia, or carcinoma.

Complications are uncommon. Brisk bleeding may occur during and immediately after the procedure. Bruising and discoloration may result but generally resolve within days. Less frequently still, hematomas may form, fat necrosis may occur, or the patient may note a palpable lump. Caution is advisable in women who are receiving anticoagulants. Surgical site infection has been reported as well, but it is rare.

Terminal Duct Excision

Terminal duct excision is the procedure of choice in the surgical treatment of nipple discharge. Local anesthesia with or without sedation (as for breast biopsy) is generally sufficient for this procedure. The goal is to excise the duct from which the discharge arises along with as little additional tissue as possible. To this end, the surgeon should carefully note the precise position of the discharging duct at the time of the initial examination. Ductograms generally are not helpful in directing the surgical procedure and need not be performed.

OPERATIVE TECHNIQUE

The patient is instructed not to attempt to express her discharge for several days before operation. The breast skin is prepared, and drapes are placed. The surgeon then attempts to express the discharge so that the offending duct can be precisely identified. If discharge is obtained, the mark for the incision should be made at the areolar border in the same quadrant, extending for about one third of the areola's circumference [*see Figure 4a*]. A local anesthetic is then administered, the edge of the nipple is grasped with a forceps, and a fine lacrimal duct probe (000 to 0000) is gently inserted into the discharging duct. An incision is then made as marked at the areolar border, the nipple skin flap is raised, and the duct containing the wire is excised with a margin of surrounding tissue from just below the nipple dermis into the deeper breast tissue [*see Figure 4b, c*].

If it is not possible to pass the lacrimal duct probe into the discharging duct, the skin incision is made and the nipple skin flap raised as described. The surgeon then bluntly dissects among the subareolar ducts to identify the dark, secretion-filled abnormal duct. If the duct is identified, it is excised along its length from the nipple dermis to a depth of 4 to 5 cm within breast tissue. An option at this point is to incise the duct and insert a lacrimal duct probe to facilitate identification of its course. If no single secretion-filled duct is identified, the entire subareolar duct complex must be excised from immediately beneath the nipple dermis to a depth of 4 to 5 cm within breast tissue [*see Figure 5*].

In all variants of this procedure, the electrocautery should not be used in the superficial portions of the dissection: it could cause devascularization of the nipple-areola complex and result in an electrocautery artifact that could interfere with pathologic analysis. If the patient has a history of periductal infection, the contents of the duct should be sent for culture and the area copiously irrigated with an antibiotic solution before wound closure. Good hemostasis should be obtained at the completion of the procedure. Breast tissue should be reapproximated beneath the nipple before skin closure to prevent retraction of the nipple or indentation of the areola.

Surgical Options for Breast Cancer

There are several surgical options for primary treatment of breast cancer; indications for selecting among them are reviewed elsewhere [*see 2:1 Breast Complaints*]. It should be emphasized that for most patients, wide local excision (lumpectomy) to microscopically clean margins coupled with axillary dissection and radiation therapy yields long-term survival equivalent to that associated with modified radical mastectomy. Currently, indications for mastectomy include patient preference, inability on the part of the surgeon to achieve clean margins without unacceptable deformation of the remaining breast tissue, the presence of multiple primary tumors, previous chest wall irradiation, pregnancy, and the presence of severe collagen vascular disease (e.g., scleroderma). Nonmedical indications for mastectomy include the lack of access to a radiation therapy facility and any other patient factors that would prevent completion of a full course of radiation therapy.

Lumpectomy

Lumpectomy—also referred to, more precisely, as wide local excision or partial mastectomy—involves excision of all cancerous tissue to microscopically clean margins. Reexcision or lumpectomy without axillary dissection may be performed with the patient under local anesthesia, but sedation or general anesthesia is usually advisable if a significant amount of tissue is to be excised or if there is tenderness from a previous biopsy. Lumpectomy with axillary dissection usually calls for general anesthesia, but it may be performed with thoracic epidural anesthesia supplemented by local anesthesia as needed.

OPERATIVE TECHNIQUE

Like open breast biopsy incisions [*see* Breast Biopsy, *above*], lumpectomy incisions should generally be curvilinear, should be placed directly over the lesion, and should also be oriented so as to be included within a subsequent mastectomy incision if margins prove positive [*see Figure 1*]. Extremely lateral or medial incisions may be better approached via a radial incision placed over the lesion. Because accurate assessment of margins is of central importance in a lumpectomy, it is critical that the incision be long enough to allow removal of the specimen in one piece rather than several.

Along with the mass itself, it is generally necessary to remove a 1 to 1.5 cm margin of normal-appearing tissue beyond the edge of the palpable tumor or, if excisional biopsy has already been performed, around the biopsy cavity. In the case of nonpalpable lesions diagnosed via needle biopsy, the position of the lesion must be determined by means of wire localization, and 2 to 3 cm of tissue should be excised around the wire to obtain an adequate margin. The specimen should be oriented by the surgeon and the margins inked by the pathologist; this orientation is useful if reexcision is required to achieve clean margins. Reexcision of any close margins may be performed during the same surgical procedure if the specimen margins are assessed immediately by the pathologist.

In the closure of the incision, hemostasis should be meticulous: a hematoma may delay administration of radiation therapy or chemotherapy. Deep breast tissue should be approximated only if such closure does not result in significant deformity of breast contour. A cosmetic subcuticular closure is preferred.

Lymphatic Mapping and Sentinel Lymph Node Biopsy

Lymphatic mapping and sentinel lymph node (SLN) biopsy [*see 2:6 Lymphatic Mapping and Sentinel Lymph Node Biopsy*] is a relatively new procedure that allows the surgeon to confirm or rule out axillary node involvement without performing a standard axillary dissection.[11,12] The technique is based on the theory that the lymphatic channels draining the primary breast tumor initially drain to a single SLN in the regional basin, which can be identified by means of intradermal injection of a vital blue dye, a radiocolloid, or both. A small incision is then made in the regional basin (which is usually the axilla in breast cancer patients), and the stained SLN is identified (either with a handheld gamma probe or by direct visualization), excised, and analyzed histologically.

Because SLN biopsy involves analysis of only one or two nodes, the pathologist can carry out a more detailed examina-

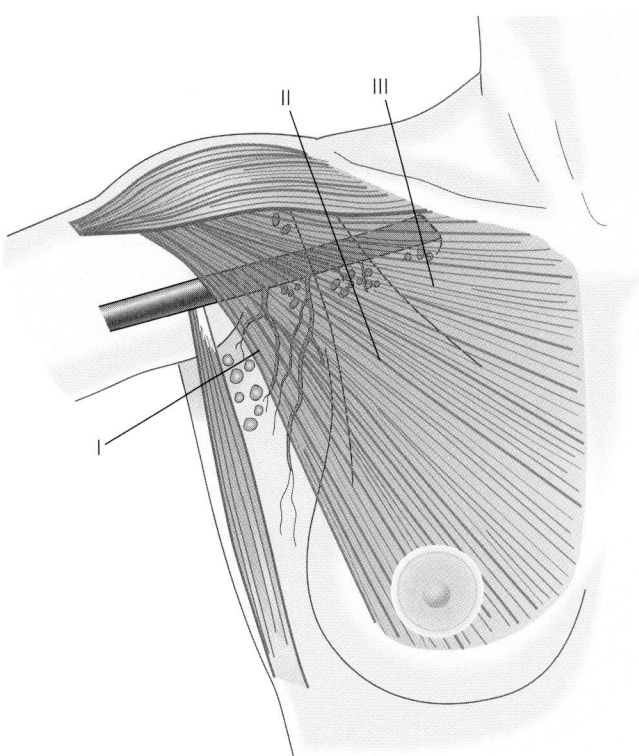

Figure 6 **Axillary dissection. Shown are axillary lymph node levels in relation to the axillary vein and the muscles of the axilla (I = low axilla, II = midaxilla, III = apex of axilla).**[15]

tion than would be possible with a standard axillary lymphadenectomy specimen, which contains multiple nodes. Newer techniques (e.g., immunohistochemical and molecular assays) can also be used to identify micrometastases that light microscopy would fail to detect, but the therapeutic and prognostic significance of tumor cells identified by such means remains unclear.

Although there is a significant learning curve for intraoperative lymphatic mapping, with sufficient experience, the SLN can be identified at least 80% to 90% of the time. Currently, standard axillary dissection is recommended for patients who have a positive SLN; however, prospective, randomized trials are now under way with a view to determining to what extent this step is necessary in node-positive patients. A number of studies have confirmed that the absence of metastases in the SLN reliably predicts the absence of metastases in the remaining axillary nodes.

Contraindications to SLN biopsy include the use of neoadjuvant chemotherapy, the presence of palpable axillary nodes suggestive of metastatic disease, the presence of large or locally advanced breast cancers, prior axillary surgery, and pregnancy or lactation.

Axillary Dissection

Axillary dissection for breast cancer includes resection of level I and level II lymph nodes and the fibrofatty tissue within which these nodes lie [*see Figure 6*]. The superior border of the dissection is formed by the axillary vein laterally and the upper extent of level II nodes medially; the lateral border of the dissection is formed by the latissimus dorsi muscle from the tail of

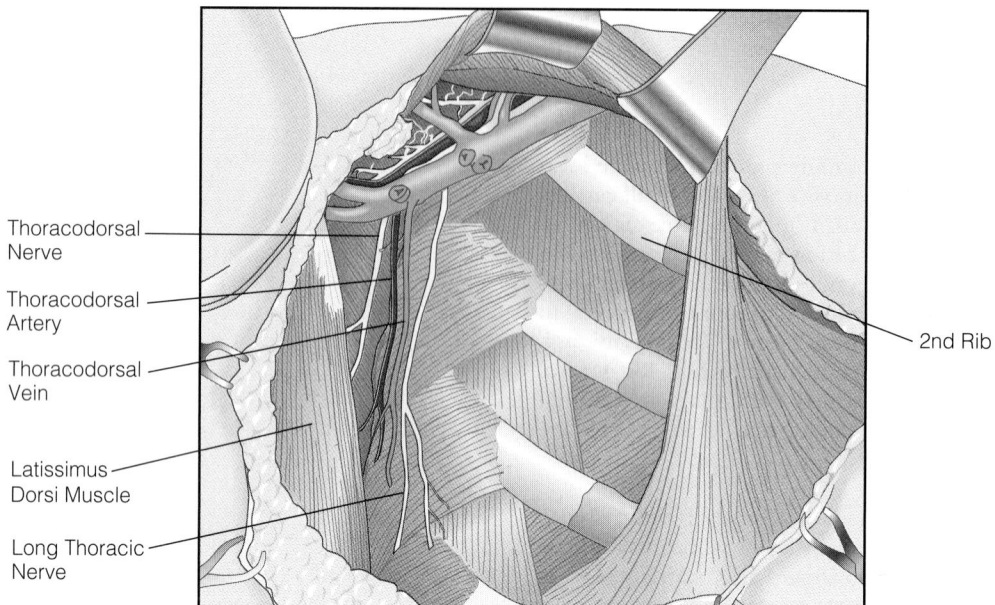

Figure 7 **Axillary dissection. Shown is a view of the structures of the axilla after completion of axillary dissection.**[16]

the breast to the crossing point of the axillary vein; the medial border is formed by the pectoral muscles and the anterior serratus muscle; and the inferior border is formed by the tail of the breast. Level II nodes are easily removed by retracting the greater and smaller pectoral muscles medially; it is not necessary to divide or remove the smaller pectoral muscle. In general, level III nodes are not removed unless palpable disease is present.

Axillary dissection, either alone or in conjunction with lumpectomy or mastectomy, usually calls for general anesthesia, but it may also be performed with thoracic epidural anesthesia supplemented by local anesthesia as needed. To facilitate identification and preservation of motor nerves that pass through the axilla, the anesthesiologist should refrain from using neuromuscular blocking agents. In the absence of neuromuscular blockade, any clamping of a motor nerve or too-close approach to a motor nerve with the electrocautery will be signaled by a visible muscle twitch.

STRUCTURES TO BE PRESERVED

There are a number of vascular structures and nerves passing through the axilla that must be preserved during axillary dissection [see Figure 7]. These structures include the axillary vein and artery; the brachial plexus; the long thoracic nerve, which innervates the anterior serratus muscle; the thoracodorsal nerve, artery, and vein, which supply the latissimus dorsi muscle; and the medial pectoral nerve, which innervates the lateral portion of the greater pectoral muscle.

The axillary artery and the brachial plexus should not be exposed during axillary dissection. If they are, the dissection has been carried too far superiorly, and proper orientation at a more inferior position should be established. In some patients, there may be sensory branches of the brachial plexus superficial (and, rarely, inferior) to the axillary vein laterally near the latissimus dorsi muscle; injury to these nerves results in numbness extending to the wrist. To prevent this complication, the axillary vein should initially be identified medially, under the greater pectoral

muscle. Medial to the thoracodorsal nerve and adherent to the chest wall is the long thoracic nerve of Bell. The medial pectoral nerve runs from superior to the axillary vein to the undersurface of the greater pectoral muscle, passing through the axillary fat pad and across the level II nodes; it has an accompanying vein whose blue color may be used to identify the nerve. If a submuscular implant reconstruction [see Breast Reconstruction after Mastectomy, below] is planned, preservation of the medial pectoral nerve is especially important to prevent atrophy of the muscle.

The intercostobrachial nerve provides sensation to the posterior portion of the upper arm. Sacrificing this nerve generally leads to numbness over the triceps region. In many women, the intercostobrachial nerve measures 2 mm in diameter and takes a fairly cephalad course near the axillary vein; when this is the case, preservation of the nerve will not interfere with node dissection. Sometimes, however, the nerve is tiny, has multiple branches, and is intermingled with nodal tissue that should be removed; when this is the case, one should not expend a great deal of time on attempting to preserve the nerve. If the intercostobrachial nerve is sacrificed, it should be transected with a knife or scissors rather than with the electrocautery, and the ends should be buried to reduce the likelihood of postoperative causalgia.

OPERATIVE TECHNIQUE

The incision for axillary dissection should be a transverse one made in the lower third of the hair-bearing skin of the axilla. For cosmetic reasons, it should not extend anteriorly onto the greater pectoral muscle; however, it may be extended posteriorly onto the latissimus dorsi muscle as necessary for exposure. Skin flaps are raised to the level of the axillary vein and to a point below the lowest extension of hair-bearing skin, either as an initial maneuver or after the initial identification of key structures.

The key to axillary dissection is obtaining and maintaining proper orientation with respect to the axillary vein, the thoracodorsal bundle, and the long thoracic nerve. After the incision has been made, the dissection is extended down into the true axillary fat pad through the overlying fascial layer. The fat of the axillary fat pad may be distinguished from subcutaneous fat on the basis of its smoother, lipomalike texture. There may be aberrant muscle slips from the latissimus dorsi muscle or the greater pectoral muscle; in addition, there may be an extremely dense fascial encasement around the axillary fat pad. It is important to divide these layers early in the dissection. The borders of the greater pectoral and latissimus dorsi muscles are then exposed, which clears the medial and lateral borders of the dissection.

The axillary vein and the thoracodorsal bundle are identified next. As discussed (see above), the initial identification of the axillary vein should be made medially, under the greater pectoral muscle, to prevent injury to low-lying branches of the brachial plexus. Sometimes, the axillary vein takes the form of several small branches rather than a single large vessel. If this is the case, all of the small branches should be preserved.

The thoracodorsal bundle may be identified either distally at its junction with the latissimus dorsi muscle or at its junction with the axillary vein. The junction with the latissimus dorsi muscle is within the axillary fat pad at a point two thirds of the way down the hair-bearing skin of the axilla, or approximately 4 cm below the inferior border of the axillary vein. Occasionally, the thoracodorsal bundle is bifurcated, with separate superior and inferior branches entering the latissimus dorsi muscle; this is particularly likely if the entry point appears very high. If the bundle is bifurcated, both branches should be preserved. The thoracodorsal bundle may be identified at its junction with the latissimus dorsi muscle by spreading within axillary fat parallel to the border of the muscle and looking for the blue of the thoracodorsal vein. The identification is also facilitated by lateral retraction of the latissimus dorsi muscle. The long thoracic nerve lies just medial to the thoracodorsal bundle on the chest wall at this point and at approximately the same anterior-posterior position. It may be identified by spreading tissue just medial to the thoracodorsal bundle and then running the index finger perpendicular to the course of the long thoracic nerve on the chest wall to identify the cordlike nerve as it moves under the finger. Once the nerve is identified, axillary tissue may be swept anteriorly away from the nerve by blunt dissection along the anterior serratus muscle; there are no significant vessels in this area.

The junction of the thoracodorsal bundle with the axillary vein is 1.5 to 2.0 cm medial to the point at which the axillary vein crosses the latissimus dorsi muscle. The thoracodorsal vein

enters the posterior surface of the axillary vein, and the nerve and the artery pass posterior to the axillary vein. There are generally one or two scapular veins that branch off the axillary vein medial to the junction with the thoracodorsal vein. These are divided during the dissection and should not be confused with the thoracodorsal bundle.

The axillary vein and the thoracodorsal bundle having been identified, the greater pectoral muscle is retracted medially at the level of the axillary vein, and the latissimus dorsi muscle is retracted laterally to place tension on the thoracodorsal bundle. Once this exposure is achieved, the axillary fat and the nodes are cleared away superficial and medial to the thoracodorsal bundle to the level of the axillary vein. Superiorly, dissection proceeds medially along the axillary vein to the point where the fat containing level II nodes crosses the axillary vein. To improve exposure, the fascia overlying the level II extension of the axillary fat pad should be incised to release tension and expose the lipomalike level II fat. As noted [see Structures to Be Preserved, above], the medial pectoral nerve passes onto the underside of the greater pectoral muscle in this area and should be preserved. One or more small venous branches may pass inferiorly from the medial pectoral bundle; particular attention should be paid to preserving the nerve when ligating these venous branches.

The next step in the dissection is to reflect the axillary fat pad inferiorly by dividing the medial attachments of the axillary fat pad along the anterior serratus muscle. Care must be taken to preserve the long thoracic nerve. Because there are no significant vessels or structures in the tissue anterior to the long thoracic nerve, this tissue may be divided sharply, with small perforating vessels either tied or cauterized. Finally, the axillary fat is freed from the tail of the breast with the electrocautery or a knife.

There is no need to orient the axillary specimen for the pathologist, because treatment is not affected by the anatomic level of node involvement. A closed suction drain is placed through a separate stab wound. (Some practitioners prefer not to place a drain and simply aspirate postoperative seromas as necessary.) A long-acting local anesthetic may be instilled into the axilla—a particularly helpful practice if the dissection was done as an outpatient procedure.

Mastectomy

The goal of a mastectomy is to remove all breast tissue, including the nipple and the areola, while leaving well-perfused, viable skin flaps for primary closure or reconstruction. This is

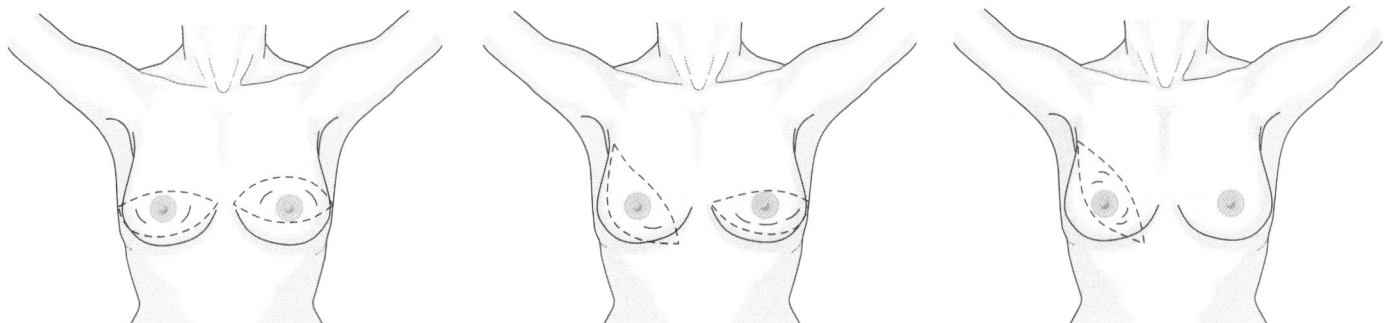

Figure 8 **Mastectomy. Shown are common incisions used for mastectomy.[13] Any previous biopsy incisions should have been done in such a way as to be included within the boundaries of the mastectomy incision.**

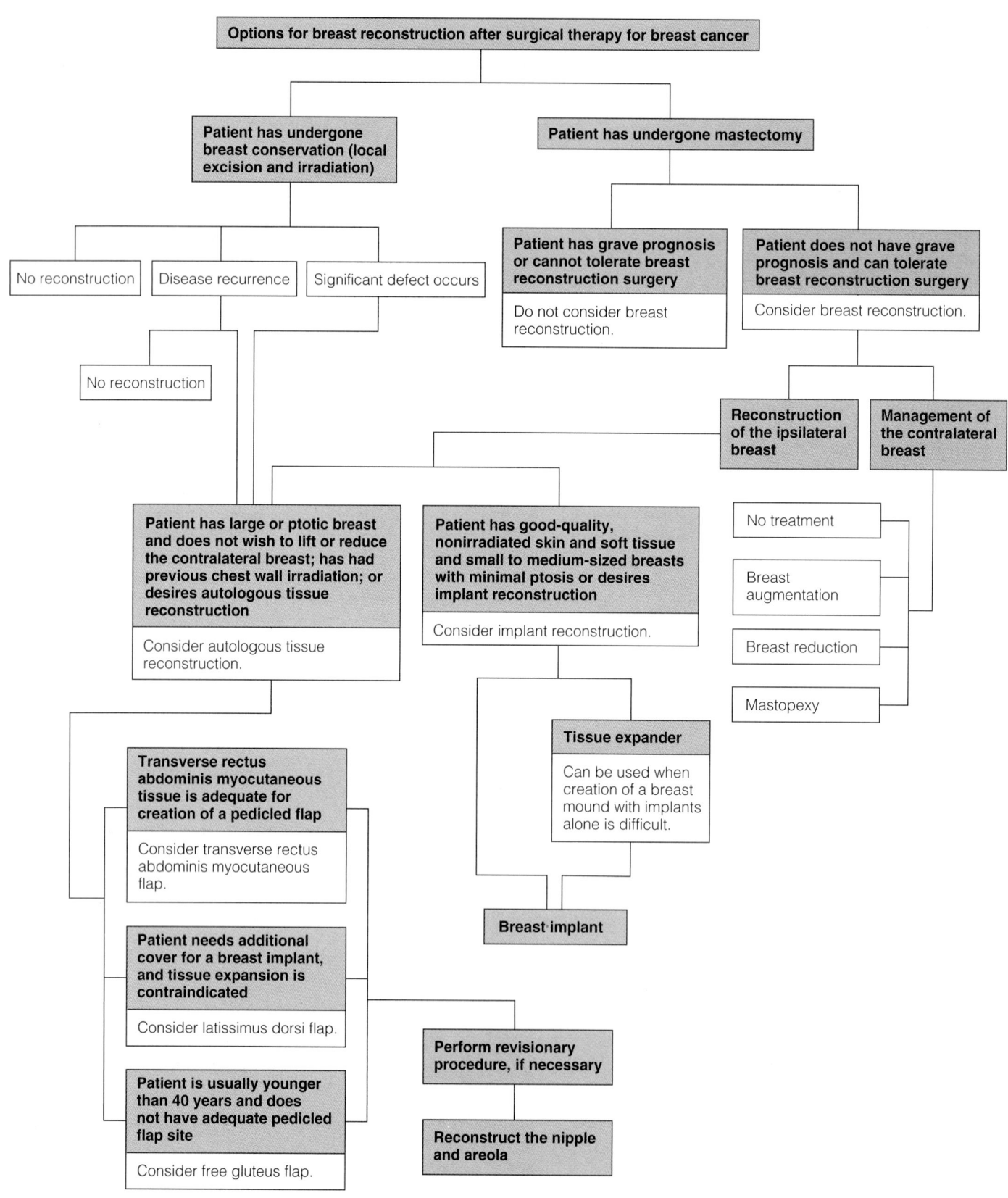

Figure 9 **Breast reconstruction after mastectomy. Shown is an algorithm outlining the major steps in breast reconstruction.**

the case whether the mastectomy is performed for treatment of breast cancer or for prophylaxis in high-risk patients. Proper skin incisions and good exposure throughout the procedure are the key components of a well-performed mastectomy. The borders of dissection extend superiorly to the clavicle, medially to the sternum, inferiorly to where breast tissue ends (on the costal margin, below the inframammary fold), and laterally to the border of the latissimus dorsi muscle. The fascia of the greater pectoral muscle forms the deep margin of the dissection and should be removed with the specimen.

Mastectomy usually calls for general anesthesia, but it may be performed with thoracic epidural anesthesia supplemented by local anesthesia as needed. When a simple mastectomy is to be performed in a frail patient for whom general anesthesia poses unacceptable risks (particularly if the patient is elderly and has a narrow-based, pendulous breast), local anesthesia with sedation is appropriate.

OPERATIVE TECHNIQUE

Skin-sparing mastectomy performed in conjunction with immediate reconstruction is discussed elsewhere [*see* Breast Reconstruction after Mastectomy, *below*]. In a modified radical or simple mastectomy without reconstruction, the goal is to leave a smooth chest wall that permits comfortable wearing of a bra and a prosthesis. It is important to remove a sufficient amount of skin to ensure that no dog-ears or lateral skin folds are left on the anterior chest wall. This undesirable result can be prevented by extending the incision far enough medially and laterally to remove all skin that contributes to the forward projection of the breast skin envelope.

The incision may be either transverse across the chest wall or angled upward toward the axilla as necessary to include the nipple-areola complex and any incisions from previous biopsies, and care should be taken to make the upper and lower skin flaps of similar length so that there is no redundant skin on either flap [*see Figure 8*]. The boundaries of the incision can be determined in the following five steps: (1) the lateral and medial end points of the incision are marked, (2) the breast is pulled firmly downward, (3) the upper incision is defined by drawing a straight line from one end point to the other across the upper surface of the breast, (4) the breast is pulled firmly upward, and (5) the lower incision is defined by drawing a straight line from one end point to the other across the lower surface of the breast. The outlined incision is then checked to ensure that it can be closed without either undue tension or redundant skin. (The closure should be fairly snug intraoperatively, when the patient's arm is positioned perpendicular to the torso for exposure, because a significant amount of slack is created when the arm is returned to a more normal position at the patient's side.) The medial and lateral end points of the incision may be adjusted upward or downward to include any previous biopsy incisions in the specimen.

Flaps

In most patients, there is a fairly well-defined avascular plane between subcutaneous fat and breast tissue. This plane is identified by pulling the edges of the incision upward with skin hooks and beginning a flap that is 8 to 10 mm thick and extends approximately 1 cm from the skin edge. After this initial release of the skin edge, the desired plane is developed by applying firm tension to pull breast tissue downward and away from the skin at a 45° angle. The fine fibrous attachments between breast tissue and subcutaneous fat (Cooper's ligaments) are then divided with the electrocautery or a blade, and crossing vessels are

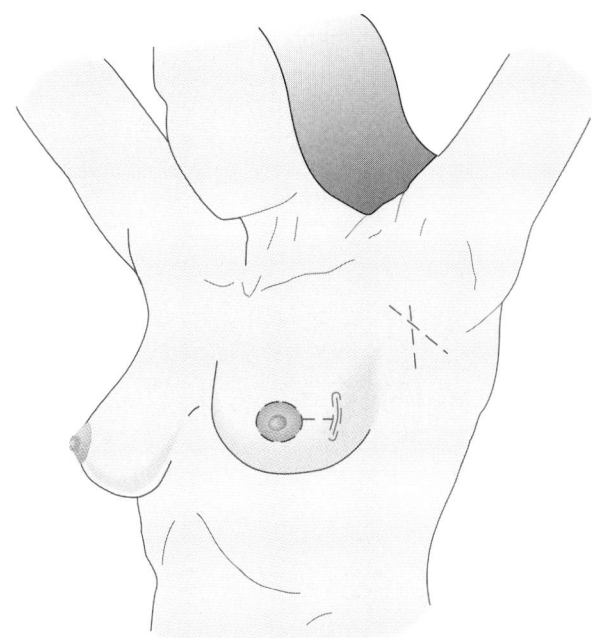

Figure 10 **Breast reconstruction after mastectomy. Shown is the recommended placement of incisions for skin-sparing mastectomy. T-shaped incisions extending from the areola to remove previous biopsy incisions may be used if necessary. A separate axillary incision may be necessary when axillary dissection is being done.**

coagulated or ligated as they appear. To protect both arterial supply to and venous drainage from the skin flap, one must refrain from excessive ligation or cauterization of vessels on the flap.

Completed mastectomy flaps are perfused through the network of fine subdermal vessels that remains after dissection. The viability of the flaps is determined by their length, the quality of the vessels they contain, the damage sustained by the vessels during the dissection, and the tension imposed by the final closure. For most women, flap viability is not an issue. It is, however, a serious consideration for diabetics and other patients with diffuse small vessel disease. In such patients, flaps should be carefully planned so that they are no longer than necessary and there is no excess tension, and extra care should be taken to preserve flap vessels. Patients should be warned that even with these additional efforts, there may be some necrosis along the edges of the incision. Such necrosis is best treated with gradual debridement of the dark eschar that forms as epithelialization proceeds from viable tissue.

Borders of Dissection

Flaps are raised superiorly to the clavicle, medially to the sternum, inferiorly to where breast tissue ends on the costal margin (generally below the inframammary fold), and laterally to the border of the latissimus dorsi muscle. The plane between breast tissue and subcutaneous fat is followed down to the greater pectoral muscle and through the pectoral fascia both superiorly and medially. Inferiorly, the fascia of the abdominal muscles is not divided. The greater pectoral muscle, the abdominal muscles, and the anterior serratus muscle form the deep border of the dissection. The pectoral fascia is removed with the breast specimen and may be separated from the muscle with either the electrocautery or a blade.

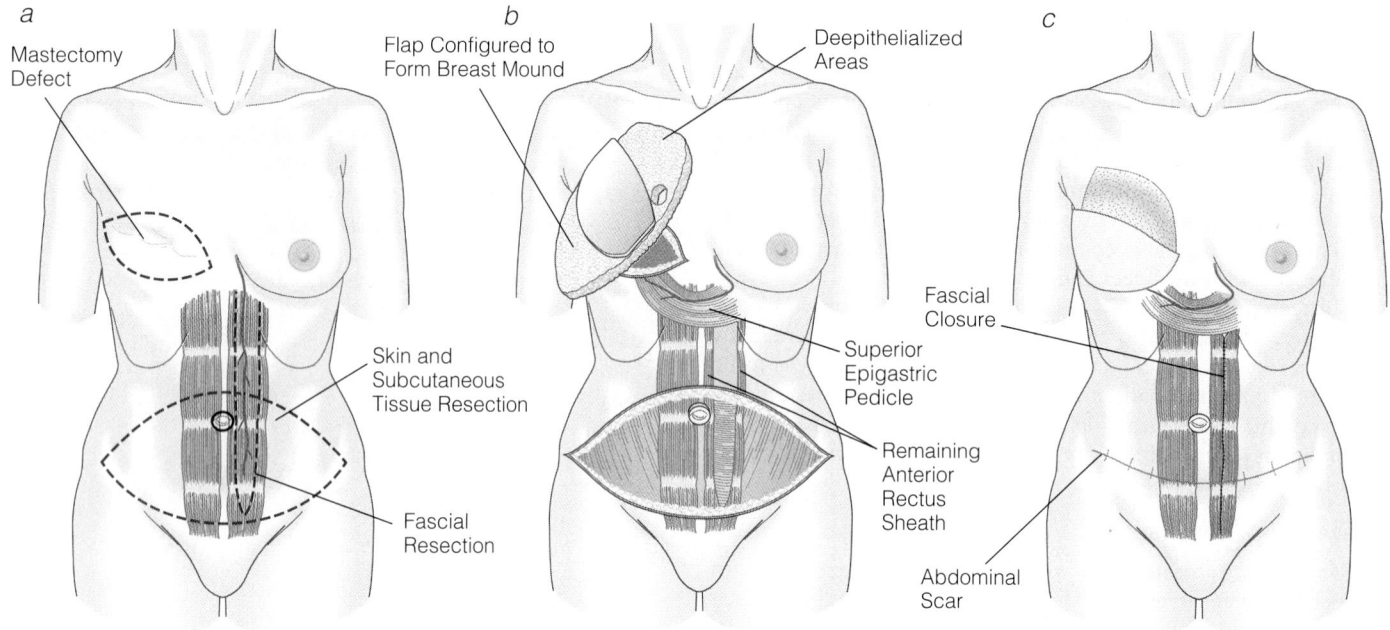

Figure 11 **Breast reconstruction after mastectomy. Shown is autologous tissue reconstruction with a transverse rectus abdominis myocutaneous (TRAM) flap. The infraumbilical flap is designed (*a*). The TRAM flap is tunneled subcutaneously into the chest wall cavity. Blood supply to the flap is maintained from the superior epigastric vessels of the rectus abdominis muscle. Subcutaneous fat and deepithelialized skin are positioned under the mastectomy flaps as needed to reconstruct the breast mound (*b*). The fascia of the anterior rectus sheath is approximated to achieve a tight closure of the abdominal wall defect and to prevent hernia formation. The umbilicus is sutured into its new position (*c*).**

To maintain the skin tension needed for the development of skin flaps, an assistant holds the flaps taut manually with skin hooks, dull-toothed rakes padded with damp sponges, or Deaver retractors. Care must be taken to obtain adequate tension and exposure so that as much breast tissue as possible can be removed without undue damage to the skin flaps.

Simple versus Modified Radical Mastectomy

Simple mastectomy is performed (1) to treat DCIS, (2) as a prophylactic measure, (3) as a follow-up to lumpectomy and axillary dissection if lumpectomy margins are positive for malignancy, (4) to treat local recurrence of breast cancer after lumpectomy, node dissection, and irradiation, and (5) in elderly patients in whom coexisting medical conditions or other factors constitute contraindications to axillary dissection. Simple mastectomy is also indicated for treatment of sarcomas of the breast: lymphatic spread to axillary nodes is not part of the natural history of this disease.

Modified radical mastectomy is performed to treat invasive breast cancer when (1) there are contraindications to breast preservation or (2) the patient or the physician prefers mastectomy. Simple mastectomy in conjunction with SLN biopsy is an increasingly common alternative to modified radical mastectomy for patients with clinically negative axillary nodes. If the nodes are positive for tumor on pathologic examination, the surgeon may then elect to perform a completion axillary dissection.

Simple mastectomy As described earlier (see above), a skin incision is made, and thin flaps are raised to allow removal of all breast tissue. Laterally, the dissection is extended to the border of the latissimus dorsi muscle, and breast tissue is removed anterior to the long thoracic nerve. The dissection proceeds around the lateral edge of the greater pectoral muscle but stops before entering the axillary fat pad. If one wishes to sample the low axillary nodes (as, for example, in a patient with extensive DCIS of comedo histology), one may remove the lower portion of the axillary fat pad between clamps. (In so doing, one must avoid the long thoracic nerve and the thoracodorsal nerve and keep the dissection low enough to ensure that the intercostobrachial sensory nerve is not damaged.) The breast is then taken off the underlying muscles, and the pectoral fascia is included with the specimen.

A single closed suction drain is placed through a separate stab wound laterally to extend under the lower flap and a short distance upward along the sternal border of the dissection. The skin is closed and a dressing applied according to the surgeon's preference. Early arm mobilization is encouraged.

Modified radical mastectomy The incision is placed and flaps are raised as for simple mastectomy. At the lateral edge of the dissection, the border of the latissimus dorsi muscle is exposed, as is the lateral border of the pectoral muscle. Some surgeons prefer to proceed with axillary dissection first, leaving the breast attached to the chest wall, whereas others prefer to remove the breast from the chest wall first and then use it to provide tension for the axillary dissection. In either case, mechanical or manual retraction of the latissimus dorsi muscle and the greater pectoral muscle generally provides excellent exposure for axillary dissection. The landmarks of the axillary dissection are identified as described earlier [*see* Axillary Dissection, *above*]. The thoracodorsal bundle can often be seen running along the latissimus dorsi muscle as the muscle is retracted laterally.

Once the axillary dissection has been completed and the breast has been removed from the chest wall, the incision is irrigated and two closed suction drains placed, one in the axilla and another under the lower flap to the midline. The skin is closed and a dressing applied according to the surgeon's preference. Early arm mobilization is encouraged.

Breast Reconstruction after Mastectomy

It is well recognized that immediate breast reconstruction after mastectomy is safe, does not significantly delay subsequent administration of chemotherapy or radiation therapy, and does not prevent detection of recurrent disease. Either implants or autologous tissue may be used in reconstruction. In most cases, the option of breast reconstruction is presented to the mastectomy patient by her breast surgeon during preoperative discussion of mastectomy or, in the case of delayed reconstruction, during follow-up after an earlier mastectomy. The patient, the plastic surgeon, and the oncologic or general surgeon will decide among the several reconstruction options available—implants with tissue expansion, the transverse rectus abdominis myocutaneous (TRAM) flap, the latissimus dorsi myocutaneous flap, and various free flaps—on the basis of patient preference and lifestyle, the availability of suitable autologous tissue, and the demands imposed by any additional cancer therapies required [*see Figure 9*]. Familiarity with the strengths and drawbacks of these reconstruction options facilitates this decision.

OPERATIVE TECHNIQUE

Placement of the incision for mastectomy with immediate reconstruction is determined in discussion with the plastic surgeon. The goal is to preserve as much viable skin as possible for the reconstruction without compromising complete resection of breast and axillary tissue. The nipple and the areola must be included in the resected skin, as must the biopsy incision through which the malignancy was diagnosed [*see Figure 10*]. (One option for removing biopsy incisions while leaving the maximal amount of unaffected skin is to place T-shaped incisions that extend outward from the areola.) FNA and core-needle biopsy incisions are generally not included in the excised skin segment; however, one may, if one wishes, excise a small amount of skin around a core-needle biopsy site. A linear incision should be made as far laterally as necessary to provide adequate exposure for axillary dissection and complete excision of breast tissue. A separate axillary incision may also be used when axillary dissection or SLN biopsy is being performed [*see Figure 10*]. The extent of dissection should never be compromised in any way for cosmetic reasons.

Reconstruction Options

Implants Perhaps the simplest method of reconstruction is to place a saline-filled implant beneath the greater pectoral muscle and the anterior serratus muscle to recreate a breast mound. Even after a skin-sparing mastectomy, the greater pectoral muscle is usually so tight that unless the patient is small-breasted, expansion of this muscle and the skin is necessary

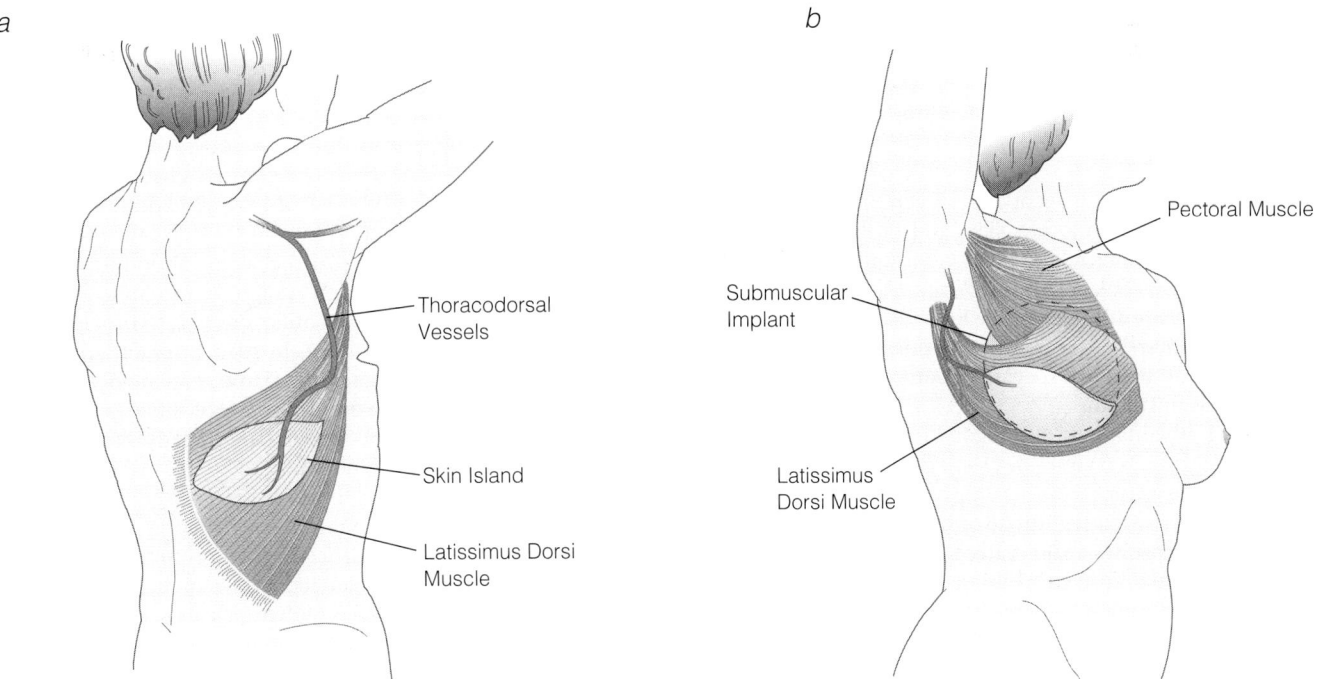

a

Thoracodorsal Vessels

Skin Island

Latissimus Dorsi Muscle

b

Pectoral Muscle

Submuscular Implant

Latissimus Dorsi Muscle

Figure 12 **Breast reconstruction after mastectomy. Shown is autologous tissue reconstruction with a latissimus dorsi myocutaneous flap in conjunction with a submuscular implant. (An implant is often required to provide the reconstructed breast with adequate volume and projection.) The myocutaneous flap is elevated; it is important to maintain the blood supply to the flap from the thoracodorsal vessels (*a*). The flap is tunneled subcutaneously to the mastectomy defect (*b*). The latissimus dorsi muscle is sutured to the greater pectoral muscle and the skin of the inframammary fold, so that the implant is completely covered by muscle.**

before an implant that matches the opposite breast can be inserted. Serial expansions are performed on an outpatient basis: saline is injected into the expander every 10 to 14 days until an appropriate size has been attained. A second operative procedure is then required to exchange the expander for a permanent implant. A nipple and an areola are constructed at a later date.

The major advantage of implant reconstruction is that there is no need to harvest autologous tissue, and thus the patient is spared the discomfort, scarring, and loss of muscle function that would occur at the donor site. Accordingly, implant reconstructions are commonly performed in patients who require bilateral mastectomies and reconstructions. The initial operative time is significantly shorter for implant reconstruction than for autologous tissue reconstruction, and there is no need for autologous blood donation or transfusion. Hospital stay and recuperation time are also significantly shorter. The main drawbacks are the prolonged time and the multiple office visits required to achieve a symmetrical reconstruction if tissue expansion is required and the necessity of a second surgical procedure to place the permanent implant. In addition, the final cosmetic result often is not as good as what can be achieved with autologous tissue reconstruction, and it may deteriorate over time as a consequence of capsule formation or implant migration. The implant-reconstructed breast is significantly firmer than the contralateral breast. The life expectancy of currently available saline implants has not been established, but it may be less than a decade, which means that many patients who have received or are receiving implants may need replacements at some point. Patients who have previously undergone irradiation of the breast or the chest wall may have tissue that cannot be adequately expanded and thus is unsuitable for implant reconstruction. If the final pathologic evaluation of the mastectomy specimen indicates that radiation therapy is needed for local control, one may consider irradiating the chest wall before expansion with an expander in place; however, this is not an ideal solution.

Autologous tissue   A second approach to reconstruction is to transfer vascularized muscle, skin, and fat from a donor site to the mastectomy defect. The most commonly used myocutaneous flaps are the TRAM flap [see Figure 11] and the latissimus dorsi flap [see Figure 12]. Use of the free TRAM flap is advocated by certain centers; other free-flap options, including the free gluteus flap, are used in special circumstances, when other donor sites are unsuitable.

The major advantage of autologous tissue reconstruction is that it generally yields a superior cosmetic result. Often, the size and shape of the opposite breast can be matched immediately, with no need for subsequent office or operative procedures. The reconstructed breast has a soft texture that is very similar to that of the contralateral breast. In addition, the cosmetic result is stable over time. The main drawbacks are the magnitude of the surgical procedure required for the reconstruction (involving both a prolonged operative time and longer inpatient hospital-

ization), the potential need for autologous blood donation or transfusion, and the pain, scarring, and loss of muscle function that arise at the donor site. Smokers and patients with significant vascular disease may not be ideal candidates for autologous tissue reconstruction. Partial necrosis of the transferred flap may create firm areas; on rare occasions, complete necrosis and consequent loss of the flap can occur.

A number of factors are considered in choosing between the TRAM flap and the latissimus dorsi flap. In a TRAM flap reconstruction, the contralateral rectus abdominis muscle is transferred along with overlying skin and fat to create a breast mound. This procedure yields a flatter abdominal contour but calls for a long transverse abdominal incision and necessitates repositioning of the umbilicus. A major advantage of the TRAM flap is that it can provide enough tissue to match all but the largest contralateral breasts. Some patients, however (e.g., those who have undergone an abdominal procedure that compromises the TRAM flap's vascular supply) are not ideal candidates for TRAM flap reconstruction. Postoperative discomfort is greater with TRAM flap reconstruction than with other flap reconstructions because of the extent of the abdominal portion of the procedure. In young, healthy, and motivated patients who require bilateral reconstructions, it is often possible to perform two TRAM flap procedures in the same operation.

In a latissimus dorsi myocutaneous flap reconstruction, the ipsilateral latissimus dorsi muscle is transferred along with overlying skin and fat to create a breast mound. Either a horizontal or a vertical donor site incision may be made on the back. The operative technique for the latissimus dorsi flap reconstruction is complex, requiring two intraoperative changes in patient position (from supine to lateral decubitus and from lateral decubitus back to supine for mastectomy, muscle harvest, and final inset of the flap). Patients who have undergone irradiation of the breast, chest wall, or axilla (including irradiation of the thoracodorsal vessels) may not be eligible for this procedure.

A major advantage of the latissimus dorsi flap is that its donor site is associated with less postoperative discomfort than the abdominal donor site of the TRAM flap. In addition, transfer of the latissimus dorsi muscle results in substantially less functional impairment than transfer of the rectus abdominis muscle. A drawback of the latissimus dorsi flap is that in many women, the latissimus dorsi muscle is not bulky enough to provide symmetry with the contralateral breast. In such cases, an implant must be added to the flap to match the size and shape of the opposite breast, which means that the drawback of the implant's limited life span is added to the drawbacks already associated with autologous tissue reconstruction.

Free-flap reconstruction options are utilized primarily when other autologous and implant reconstruction options are not available, do not provide sufficient tissue volume, or have failed. They are more complex procedures, requiring microvascular anastomoses and carrying a higher risk of total flap loss. The two most commonly employed free-flap options are the free TRAM flap and the free gluteus flap.

References

1. Fisher B, Redmond C, Poisson R, et al: Eight-year results of a randomized trial comparing total mastectomy and lumpectomy without irradiation in the treatment of breast cancer. N Engl J Med 320:822, 1989

2. Veronesi U, Luini A, Del Vecchio M, et al: Radiotherapy after breast-preserving surgery in women with localized cancer of the breast. N Engl J Med 328:1587, 1993

3. Sarrazin D, Le M, Rouesse J, et al: Conservative treatment versus mastectomy in breast cancer tumours with mascroscopic diameter of 20 millimetres or less. Cancer 53:1209, 1984

4. Shabot MM, Goldberg IM, Schick P, et al: Aspiration cytology is superior to "Tru-cut" needle biopsy in establishing the diagnosis of clinically suspicious breast masses. Ann Surg 196:122, 1982

5. Gisvold JJ, Martin JK: Prebiopsy localization of non-palpable breast lesions. AJR Am J Roentgenol 143:477, 1984

6. Meyer JE, Kopans DB, Stomper PC, et al: Occult breast abnormalities: percutaneous preoperative needle localization. Radiology 150:355, 1984

7. Rosenberg AL, Schwartz GF, Feig SA, et al: Clinically occult breast lesions: localization and significance. Radiology 162:167, 1987

8. Smith DN, Christian R, Meyer JE: Large-core needle biopsy of nonpalpable breast cancers: the impact on subsequent surgical excisions. Arch Surg 132:256, 1997

9. Parker SH, Lovin JD, Jobe WE, et al: Nonpalpable breast lesions: stereotactic automated large-core biopsies. Radiology 180:403, 1991

10. Meyer JE, Smith DN, Lester SC, et al: Large-core needle biopsy of nonpalpable breast lesions. JAMA 281:1638, 1999

11. Krag D, Weaver D, Ashikaga T, et al: The sentinel node in breast cancer: a multicenter validation study. N Engl J Med 339:941, 1998

12. Giuliano AE, Jones RC, Brennan M, et al: Sentinel lymphadenectomy in breast cancer. J Clin Oncol 15:2345, 1997

13. Souba WW, Bland KI: Indications and techniques for biopsy. The Breast: Comprehensive Management of Benign and Malignant Diseases. Bland KI, Copeland EM III, Eds. WB Saunders Co, Philadelphia, 1991, p 527

14. Morrow M: Management of common breast disorders. Breast Diseases, 2nd ed. Harris JR, Hellman S, Henderson IC, et al, Eds. JB Lippincott Co, Philadelphia, 1987

15. Kinne DW: Primary treatment of breast cancer. Breast Diseases, 2nd ed. Harris JR, Hellman S, Henderson IC, et al, Eds. JB Lippincott Co, Philadelphia, 1987

16. Kinne DW, DeCosse JJ: Modified radical mastectomy for carcinoma of the breast. Am Surg 48:543, 1982

Acknowledgments

The authors wish to thank David Van Hook, M.D., Chief of Mammography, Department of Radiology, Penn State Hershey Medical Center, Hershey, Pennsylvania, for his assistance in preparing the section on directional vacuum-assisted breast biopsy (mammotomy).

Figures 1 through 8, 10   Kerry G. Nicholson.

Figure 9   Marcia Kammerer.

Figures 11 and 12   Tom Moore.

6 LYMPHATIC MAPPING AND SENTINEL LYMPH NODE BIOPSY

Douglas Reintgen, M.D., F.A.C.S., Rosemary Giuliano, A.R.N.P., Claudia Berman, M.D., Frank Glass, M.D., Jane Messina, M.D., and Charles E. Cox, M.D., F.A.C.S.

There is an epidemic of melanoma in the United States: in 2000, 43,000 cases of invasive melanoma and 40,000 cases of melanoma in situ were diagnosed.[1] Moreover, melanoma affects young persons who are in the most productive years of their lives; accordingly, it constitutes a major public health problem. Since the early 1990s, the care of patients with melanoma has changed dramatically with the development of new lymphatic mapping techniques that reduce the cost and morbidity of nodal staging, the emergence of more sensitive assays for occult melanoma metastases, and the identification of interferon alfa-2b as an effective adjuvant therapy for melanoma patients who are at high risk for recurrence. Accurate staging of melanoma patients has become increasingly important in the light of a 1996 report[2] demonstrating improved survival in patients with T4 (tumor thickness > 4.0 mm) or stage III (nodal metastases) melanoma who were treated with adjuvant interferon alfa-2b.

Breast cancer is one of the most common of the malignancies that surgeons encounter in their practices: approximately 186,000 new cases are diagnosed each year in the United States, and the incidence is likely to increase in the next 10 years because the maturation of the baby-boomer population will result in a larger population at risk. It was one of the first tumors for which adjuvant therapy (i.e., treatment of patients who show no evidence of disease but who are at substantial risk for recurrence and death from the disease) was found to be effective. Most authorities believe that axillary nodal staging is an important part of primary breast cancer therapy in that it facilitates identification of patients who are candidates for more aggressive chemotherapy and enhances regional control of disease. Whether axillary node dissection contributes to survival remains controversial, however, and this issue is currently the subject of a national multicenter trial being performed by the American College of Surgeons. That most women with invasive breast cancers will receive either adjuvant chemotherapy or hormone therapy calls into question the necessity of axillary node dissection. Complete axillary node dissection is associated with significant morbidity, and physical problems resulting from the dissection are the complaints women voice most frequently after undergoing breast cancer surgery, once they have dealt with the psychological impact of having an incision on their breast or perhaps even losing the breast.

The development of intraoperative lymphatic mapping and selective lymphadenectomy has made it possible to map the lymphatic flow from a primary tumor and to identify its so-called sentinel lymph node (SLN) in the regional basin. Integration of this technique, in association with detailed pathologic examination of the SLN, into the surgical treatment of melanoma and breast cancer offers the potential for more conservative operations that not only result in lower morbidity but also permit more accurate staging. In what follows, we describe the technical aspects of this new approach, as well as certain related issues.

Lymphatic Mapping and SLN Biopsy for Melanoma

RATIONALE

Many factors are known to predict the risk for metastatic disease in melanoma patients. In evaluating treatments for melanoma, it is crucial to take into account prognostic factors that can accurately categorize patients into different risk groups for metastasis. If this is not done, it is difficult or impossible to determine whether differences between treatment regimens (or the absence thereof) are due to the treatments themselves or merely reflect imbalances of prognostic factors.

The presence or absence of lymph node metastases is the single most powerful predictor of recurrence and survival in melanoma patients: the 5-year survival rate is approximately 40% lower in patients who have lymph node metastases than in those who do not. A great deal of time, effort, and money has been expended on identifying prognostic factors based on primary tumor variables (e.g., Breslow's tumor thickness, ulceration, primary site, and sex); however, multiple regression analyses performed on many collected populations in the literature indicate that once melanoma metastasizes to the regional nodes, such prognostic factors contribute relatively little to the prognostic model compared with the patient's lymph node status. This finding suggests that many melanoma patients might benefit from an accurate nodal staging procedure.

Nodal Staging

Elective lymph node dissection Elective lymph node dissection (ELND) has been the mainstay of the surgeon's armamentarium for nodal staging of melanoma patients. ELND removes clinically negative nodes, as opposed to therapeutic dissection, which removes nodes with gross tumor involvement. Opinions are divided as to whether ELND actually extends survival or whether it is solely a staging procedure. Two prospective, randomized trials failed to demonstrate improved survival in melanoma patients treated with ELND in comparison with patients who underwent wide local excision (WLE) alone as primary surgical therapy.[3,4] Retrospective studies using large databases, however, suggested that there were subpopulations of melanoma patients who did benefit from ELND.[5,6]

The controversy may have been laid to rest by the results of the Intergroup Melanoma Trial, which was the first randomized study to prove enhanced survival after surgical treatment of clinically occult metastatic melanoma. Only patients with intermediate-thickness melanoma (tumor thickness, 1.0 to 4.0 mm) were eligible. In addition, the Intergroup Melanoma Trial was the first prospective study to require preoperative lymphoscintigraphy in all patients to identify and remove all basins at risk for metastasis. Without preoperative lymphoscintigraphy to provide a map for the surgeon, ELND may be misdirected in more than 50% of head and neck dissections and trunk dissections[7]; moreover, so-called in transit nodes (defined as nodes outside the classic anatomic basin between the primary site and the regional nodes), which are equally at risk for metastasis, may be missed in 5% of patients.[8]

In the Intergroup Melanoma Trial, overall survival was not significantly longer in patients who underwent WLE and ELND than in those who underwent WLE of the primary site coupled with observation of the regional basins. There were, however, two well-defined subsets of the ELND group that exhibited a significant increase in overall survival: patients with melanomas 1.1 to 2.0 mm thick and patients younger than 60 years.[9] Stratification by tumor thickness was part of the original design of the trial, but the age-related benefit only became apparent with retrospective subgroup analysis.

A subsequent report from the same group that included 10 years of follow-up indicated that the survival curves of the two groups continued to separate secondary to late recurrences and deaths in the group treated with WLE alone. In addition, the *P* value for survival differences across the entire study decreased from 0.25 to 0.09 over the longer follow-up period, suggesting that surgery in the regional nodal basin, in and of itself, may confer a survival benefit.[10]

Three national prospective, randomized trials—the Eastern Cooperative Oncology Group (ECOG) trials[2,11,12]—have investigated adjuvant interferon alfa-2b; the first of these, ECOG 1684,[2] was the impetus for FDA approval of interferon alfa-2b as the first effective adjuvant therapy for patients at high risk for recurrent melanoma. ECOG 1684 and ECOG 1694 reported significant overall survival benefits, but ECOG 1690 did not (though it did report a significant disease-free survival [DFS] benefit). Statistical analysis of the three ECOG trials shows that given three prospective, randomized trials with a predictive power of 0.8 and a statistical signif-

Choice of Radiocolloid and Vital Blue Dye for Lymphatic Mapping

Choice of Radiocolloid

Little work has been done to determine which radiocolloid is best suited to either preoperative or intraoperative mapping. The ideal radiocolloid for intraoperative SLN mapping would have small particles (< 100 nm) that are uniformly dispersed, would be highly stable, and would have a short half-life that would not complicate the handling of the excised specimen. Technetium (^{99m}Tc)-labeled compounds, being gamma emitters, satisfy most of these requirements. In a direct comparison between filtered (0.1 μm filter) ^{99m}Tc-labeled sulfur colloid (^{99m}Tc-SC) and ^{99m}Tc-labeled antimony trisulfide colloid (^{99m}Tc-ATC), which has a particle size of 3 to 30 nm, filtered ^{99m}Tc-SC was transported more quickly to the nodal basin and emitted less radiation to the liver, the spleen, and the whole body.[90] Unfiltered ^{99m}Tc-SC contains relatively large particles (100 to 1,000 nm), and some investigators have found it to migrate more slowly from the injection site; however, other investigators have found it to be slow to flow through the first SLN to higher secondary nodes, which is actually an advantage.

In comparisons between ^{99m}Tc-labeled human serum albumin (^{99m}Tc-HSA), ^{99m}Tc-labeled stannous phyate, and ^{99m}Tc-ATC with respect to lymphoscintigram quality, the last of these provided the best images for preoperative lymphoscintigraphy.[91] In an animal study comparing ^{99m}Tc-HSA and filtered ^{99m}Tc-SC, ^{99m}Tc-SC was actually concentrated in the SLN over a period of 1 to 2 hours, whereas ^{99m}Tc-HSA passed rapidly through the SLN.[34] As a result, ^{99m}Tc-SC yielded higher activity ratios at intraoperative mapping, improved the success rate of localization, made the technique easier, and thus was a superior reagent for this application.[33,34]

The Sydney Melanoma Unit (SMU) prefers to use ^{99m}Tc-ATC because it seems to have smaller, more uniform particles that rapidly migrate into the lymphatic channels but still are appropriately trapped and retained by the SLN.[92] At SMU, use of this compound allows injection of the radiocolloid and imaging to be performed the day before operation. These investigators find that hot spots in the regional basin are maintained even if 24 hours have elapsed from the time of the injection. The radioactivity in the basin over the hot spot (i.e., the SLN) is decreased because four half-lives of the technetium have been expended and because some of the radiocolloid has passed through, but the ex vivo activity ratio (i.e., SLN:neighboring non-SLN) is not substantially affected. In the United States, ^{99m}Tc-ATC has been removed from the market and is unavailable for clinical use.

Other investigators have obtained very good intraoperative mapping results with unfiltered ^{99m}Tc-SC; however, they have not obtained good planar images for lymphoscintigraphy and have been unable to identify cutaneous lymphatic flow to any basin in 10% of the patients.[21]

At MCC, we use filtered (0.2 μm filter) ^{99m}Tc-SC. This particle size gives good images on lymphoscintigraphy and is trapped and concentrated in the SLN over a significant period, so that the hot spot over the

SLN actually becomes hotter compared with surrounding tissue for 2 to 6 hours after injection, making the SLN easier to find. It also has an advantage over unfiltered ^{99m}Tc-SC in that it results in less shine-through of radioactivity from the primary site.

Choice of Vital Blue Dye

Several vital blue dyes have been investigated with an eye to their potential applicability to cutaneous lymphatic mapping. Among these are methylene blue (American Regent Lab, Shirley, New York); isosulfan blue, 1% in aqueous solution (Lymphazurin; United States Surgical Corporation, Norwalk, Connecticut); patent blue-V (Laboratoire Guerbert, France); Cyalume (American Cyanamid Company, Bound Brook, New Jersey); and fluorescein dye. All substances tested were known to be nontoxic in vivo and were injected intradermally as provided by the supplier. In a feline study,[13] patent blue-V and isosulfan blue were the most accurate in identifying the regional lymphatic drainage pattern. These dyes entered the lymphatics rapidly, with minimal diffusion into the surrounding tissue. Their bright-blue color was readily visible and allowed easy identification of the exposed lymphatics.

Isosulfan blue has worked extremely well for intraoperative SLN mapping. In some patients with thin skin, the afferent lymphatics can be seen through the skin after the injection of isosulfan blue. In addition, when the dye enters the SLN, it stains part of the node a pale blue, thus clearly distinguishing the SLN from the surrounding non-SLNs. The other dyes have largely been abandoned as unsatisfactory because they diffuse too rapidly into surrounding tissue and are not retained by the lymphatic channels in sufficient concentrations to stain the SLN. The fluorescent dyes fluorescein and Cyalume are readily visualized, but a dark room is necessary for optimal visualization; moreover, because of their diffusion into surrounding tissue, the background fluorescence is unacceptably high. Methylene blue is relatively poorly retained by the lymphatic vessels and thus stains the SLN too lightly.

Use of vital blue dyes has not given rise to any significant complications. Although allergic reactions, including anaphylactic reactions, have been reported on rare occasions in the literature, they have not occurred in large study populations.[17,18] Blue dye can be retained at the primary site for more than a year. The color gradually fades with time; however, patients can be left with a permanent tattoo if the injected dye is not removed with wide local excision (WLE) of the primary site or, in the case of breast cancer, with lumpectomy. Fortunately, in the head and neck area, where a permanent tattoo would be unacceptable, the richness of the cutaneous lymphatics allows rapid clearance of the blue dye from the skin and the subcutaneous tissues. A small amount of residual dye may be left behind after WLE, but this typically disappears rapidly and poses no real problem. All patients report the presence of dye in the urine and the stool during the first 24 hours. In some cases, the dye can interfere with transcutaneous oxygen monitoring during anesthesia.

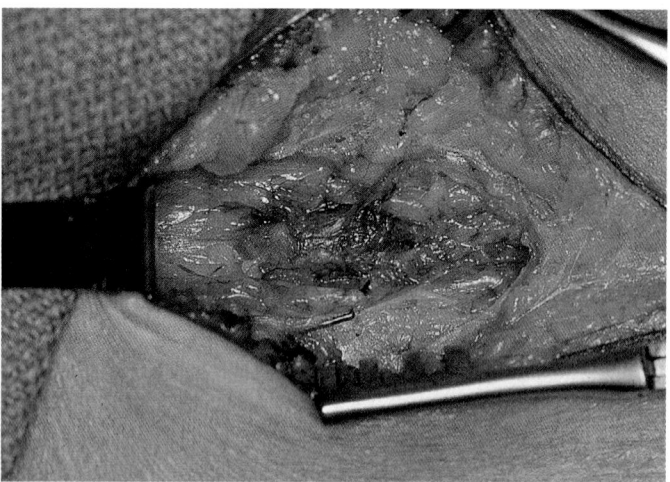

Figure 1 **Lymphatic mapping and SLN biopsy for melanoma. Primary sites for both melanoma and breast cancer may have four to six afferent lymphatics emerging from the tumor location, but as the lymphatics travel to the regional basin, they converge into one or two SLNs. Shown are four afferent lymphatics converging into one SLN.**

icance of 0.95, if two of them report a survival benefit and the third does not, the statistical probability that these results will be obtained with an effective therapy is 0.38. On the other hand, the statistical probability that these results will be obtained with an ineffective therapy is only 0.008. Thus, the evidence that high-dose interferon alfa-2b is an effective adjuvant therapy for patients with stage III melanoma is compelling.

Given the results from the Intergroup Melanoma Trial and the three ECOG trials,[9-12] one can make a strong argument that when the risk of nodal metastasis reaches a certain defined level, a nodal staging procedure should be done. At our institution (H. Lee Moffitt Cancer Center [MCC], Tampa, Florida), the level of primary melanoma thickness at which nodal staging is considered is 0.76 mm or greater. The nodal staging procedure we recommend and perform is lymphatic mapping and SLN biopsy.

Intraoperative lymphatic mapping and selective lymphadenectomy Intraoperative lymphatic mapping and selective lymphadenectomy was developed as a method of assessing regional lymph node status more accurately than ELND could while reducing both morbidity and expense. This technique relies on two concepts: first, that different regions of the skin have specific patterns of lymphatic drainage to the regional lymphatic basin; and second, that for a given skin region, there is a specific lymph node (i.e., an SLN) in the basin to which the cutaneous lymphatic vessels drain first. These concepts were borne out by initial animal studies using either vital blue dye[13] or radiocolloid[14] (which has been shown to map the same lymphatic pathways and label the same nodes as vital blue dye) [*see Sidebar* Choice of Radiocolloid and Vital Blue Dye for Lymphatic Mapping].

Intraoperative lymphatic mapping and selective lymphadenectomy was initially proposed by Morton and associates,[15,16] who used a vital blue dye method. These investigators showed that the SLN is the first node in the lymphatic basin into which the primary melanoma consistently drains (though not necessarily the closest to the primary). They also hypothesized that the status of the SLN, if it was negative for metastases, would reflect the status of higher nodes (i.e., nodes farther down the lymphatic drainage pathway, also termed second-tier nodes). Subsequent work on intraoperative

mapping and selective lymphadenectomy confirmed that the SLN is the first site of metastatic disease and demonstrated that if the SLN is histologically negative, then the remainder of the lymph nodes in the basin are histologically negative as well.[17,18] These findings suggest that melanoma patients can be accurately staged with procedures that are less extensive than complete dissection.

SLNs can be mapped from different primary site locations, and more than one node in the same basin can be an SLN, depending on the primary site. Fine dermal lymphatic vessels coalesce to form several major lymphatic trunks that eventually drain to the regional lymphatic basin. Because cutaneous lymphatic vessels converge rather than diverge [*see Figure 1*], one can perform intraoperative mapping from various skin sites and still harvest only one or two SLNs from the basin. The small number of specimens facilitates detailed pathologic examination: the pathologist can readily perform serial sections of the nodes and use immunohistochemical methods to look for micrometastatic disease. More intensive pathologic examination of one or two SLNs appears to identify patients with micrometastatic lymph node metastases more accurately than routine examination of all the regional lymph nodes.

Unusual or ambiguous drainage patterns. Lymphoscintigraphy has been used in live patients to map patterns of lymphatic drainage from various primary skin sites. Early assessments of lymphatic flow patterns, such as those of the 19th century anatomist Sappey,[19] were based on anatomic dissections of cadavers and do not accurately reflect lymphatic flow patterns in living humans. The watershed areas of the body are much larger than originally described by Sappey, and there is no clinically predictable lymphatic flow from a melanoma until it is located 10 cm off the midline or 10 cm off Sappey's line (a line running between the umbilicus and L2) [*see Figure 2*]. In addition, the entire head and neck region is a watershed area. Cutaneous lymphatic flow frequently cannot be predicted on the basis of anatomic site, and areas of ambiguous or multidirectional flow are

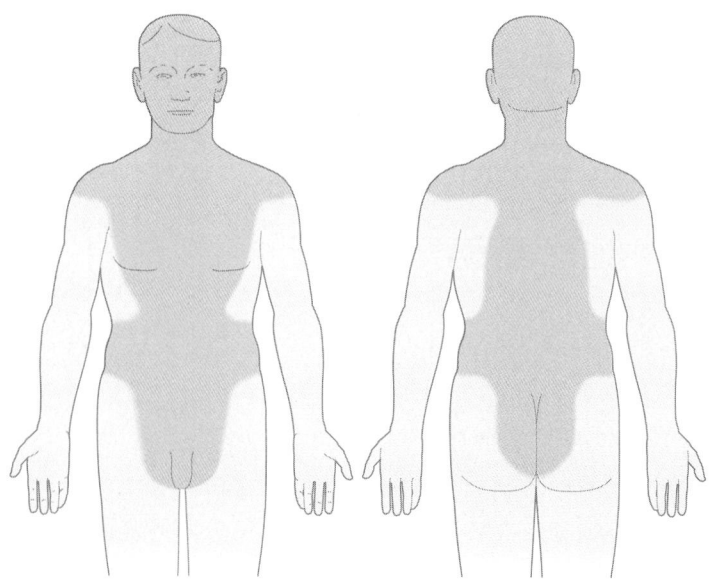

Figure 2 **Lymphatic mapping and SLN biopsy for melanoma. The watershed areas of the body where multidirectional cutaneous lymphatic flow is found are much more extensive than classical descriptions predicted. One does not find unidirectional cutaneous lymphatic flow until lesions are 10 cm off the midline or 10 cm off Sappey's line, which runs between the umbilicus and L2. The entire head and neck area is also unpredictable.**

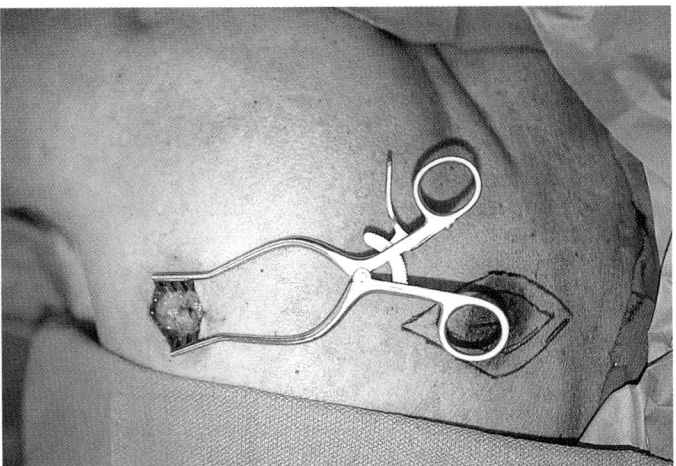

Figure 3 **Lymphatic mapping and SLN biopsy for melanoma. Shown is an intermediate-thickness melanoma of the left back in a 40-year-old man. Preoperative lymphoscintigraphy identified flow from the primary site into the left axilla and separate flow into an in transit node located at the tip of the left scapula. Vital blue dye was injected into the dermis around the primary site, and a small incision was made over the tattoo marking the location of the in transit node, which could then be visualized and harvested.**

significantly more extensive than classical descriptions predicted.[20]

A number of unusual drainage patterns and pathways have been noted in Australia[20]: 26% of melanomas on the back drained to an in transit node near the scapula in the intermuscular space [*see Figure 3*], 20% of melanomas near the umbilicus drained to an internal mammary node, some posterior scalp melanomas drained to lymph nodes at the base of the neck, and at least one forearm melanoma drained directly to a lymph node in the ipsilateral neck. Krag and coworkers[21,22] have also noted some unusual lymphatic drainage patterns: one melanoma on the right upper back drained directly to a node in the right midclavicular space, almost at the apex of the right lung; another melanoma on the lower back drained to an SLN along the neurovascular bundle under the 12th rib; and two lower extremity melanomas drained to SLNs in the popliteal fossa. A 2001 report from MCC documented 23 cases of primary cutaneous melanomas around the lower abdomen, the buttocks, and the lower extremities that drained directly to nodes in the deep pelvic area and to the iliac and hypogastric nodal groups.[23] In five of the 23 cases reported, metastatic melanoma was found in the deep pelvic nodes, and in three of these five, the deep pelvic nodes were the only site of disease (i.e., the SLN in the superficial groin area was negative). This finding confirmed that these skin sites had direct connections to the deep pelvic nodes and that the metastases did not reflect so-called pass-through.

PATIENT SELECTION

Selective lymphadenectomy and SLN biopsy are currently being evaluated in a randomized trial sponsored by the National Cancer Institute, the goal of which is to determine whether this surgical strategy by itself extends the survival of the melanoma patient [*see* Discussion, National Protocols, *below*]. Even if this trial demonstrates no inherent survival benefit, there are additional considerations that support use of the procedure in certain populations. Data from the interferon alfa-2b trial cited earlier[2] suggest that all patients whose melanoma is more than 1.0 mm thick should undergo a nodal staging procedure so that adjuvant therapy can be administered in a selective fashion. If T4N0 patients are removed from the analysis of this trial and only patients with lymph node metastases are considered, DFS increas-

es by 82% ($P = 0.0006$) with adjuvant therapy; overall survival increases by 24% as well ($P = 0.006$). Given such a substantial difference in both DFS and overall survival, one would naturally want to offer these patients interferon alfa-2b therapy. Accordingly, one would need to identify patients with nodal metastases who might benefit from such therapy. Lymphatic mapping and SLN biopsy is the least morbid and most cost-effective way of determining which melanoma patients have lymph node metastases.[24]

In female patients with melanomas less than 0.76 mm thick, the risk of nodal metastasis is less than 1%; thus, SLN biopsy is not indicated in this population. In male patients whose primary site is on the trunk, however, the incidence of occult nodal metastases may be as high as 9%, even if the primary lesion is less than 0.76 mm thick; lymphatic mapping may be considered in this population.

In patients whose tumor is 0.76 to 1.0 mm thick, the risk of nodal metastasis is less than 6%; the procedure can be offered as an option in this population. In our experience, these patients usually elect to undergo SLN biopsy despite the low risk of occult nodal metastasis: the morbidity of the procedure is low, and the finding of a positive SLN can radically affect subsequent treatment decisions. Several prognostic factors have been shown to identify patients with thin melanomas who are at higher risk (approximately 10%) for metastatic disease and death at 5 years: tumors at Clark level III or greater, ulcerated primaries, regressed lesions, male gender, and axial melanomas.[25] Patients with four or five of these five prognostic factors should be treated as if they have thicker lesions, and their SLNs should be harvested even if the primary lesions are less than 0.76 mm thick.

Patients whose melanoma is of intermediate thickness (1.0 to 4.0 mm) probably have the most to gain from lymphatic mapping and SLN biopsy. The procedure may be used for staging, so that patients can be offered adjuvant therapy in an appropriately selective fashion, and it may also increase survival, as the long-term follow-up data from the Intergroup Melanoma Trial suggest.[10]

In patients with thick (> 4.0 mm) melanomas, the rate of occult systemic metastasis is 70%, and that of occult nodal metastasis is 60% to 70%. Consequently, in the past, procedures involving the regional nodes (i.e., ELND) were not recommended, because there was no survival benefit. Now that effective adjuvant therapy is available, however, lymphatic mapping and SLN biopsy should be offered to these patients as a staging procedure. Survival is decreased in patients with thick melanomas and documented nodal microscopic disease compared with patients with thick melanomas and no sign of nodal spread[26]; accordingly, some medical oncologists observe T4 patients unless nodal metastasis is documented.

A crucial question to be answered is, what is the standard of surgical care for melanoma patients with tumors thicker than 1.0 mm? Given that the histology of the SLN has been shown to be indicative of the histology of the rest of the nodes in the basin, one can conclude that if the surgeon has adequate support from nuclear medicine and pathology services, there is no need to perform ELND. If such support is unavailable, if intraoperative mapping cannot be done (as, perhaps, when WLE of the primary melanoma has already been performed), or if the results of mapping are equivocal, then the ELND guidelines from the Intergroup Melanoma Surgical Trial[9] should be followed. If this approach is taken, ELND should be guided by preoperative lymphoscintigraphy for identification and dissection of all basins at risk for metastasis.

Finally, previous extensive primary site surgery constitutes a general technical contraindication to lymphatic mapping. Patients who have undergone rotational flap closure or Z-plasty reconstruction are considered ineligible for this procedure.

TECHNIQUE

The technique of intraoperative mapping varies considerably from center to center. We will describe the nuances of the technique as it is performed at MCC, detailing the steps that are important for successful mapping. It cannot be emphasized enough that successful intraoperative SLN mapping requires close collaboration between the surgeon, the nuclear radiologist, and the pathologist, with each member of the team playing a critical role.

An initial caveat regarding the timing of the procedure in relation to WLE is in order. Data from MCC indicate that when lymphatic mapping is done after WLE, the dissection tends to be more extensive than it need have been. More SLNs are removed and more regional basins dissected than when lymphatic mapping is done before WLE; moreover, the rate at which so-called skip metastases are detected appears to be increased. With lymphatic mapping and SLN biopsy becoming the standard of care in the United States for nodal staging to identify melanoma patients who are candidates for adjuvant therapy and a possible survival benefit, it is essential that patient care not be compromised by extensive primary site surgery before lymphatic mapping.

Step 1: Preoperative Lymphoscintigraphy

Patients come to the nuclear medicine suite early on the day of operation and undergo preoperative lymphoscintigraphy with the injection of 450 μCi in 1 ml of filtered technetium-99–labeled sulfur colloid (99mTc-SC) [*see Sidebar* Choice of Radiocolloid and Vital Blue Dye for Lymphatic Mapping]. Dynamic scans are performed 5 to 10 minutes after injection of the radiocolloid, and the location of the SLN in the basin is marked with an intradermal tattoo. All regional lymphatic basins at risk for metastatic spread, along with in transit nodes and SLNs, are identified and marked for harvesting.

Comment Preoperative lymphoscintigraphy serves as a road map for planning the surgical procedure and is used for four distinct reasons:

1. To identify all nodal basins at risk for metastatic disease.[7] This is especially important with melanomas of the trunk or the head and neck, whose lymphatic drainage patterns cannot be reliably predicted by clinical judgment or classic anatomic guidelines.[27]

2. To identify any in transit nodes that can be tattooed by the nuclear radiologist for later harvesting [*see Figure 4*]. An example is afforded by the case of a forearm lesion with an afferent lymphatic vessel flowing to an epitrochlear in transit node and a separate afferent vessel flowing from that node to the axillary basin [*see Figure 4a*]. The SLNs in both locations were harvested, and only the epitrochlear SLN was histologically positive. In this case, mapping with the blue dye alone would have yielded histologically negative axillary SLNs and understaged the patient. In addition, the tumor containing an epitrochlear in transit node would have been left in place and thus might later have seeded the axillary nodes or distant metastatic sites.

3. To identify the location of the SLN in relation to the rest of the nodes in the basin.[28-30] Because the location of the SLN may vary within a basin, it is important to mark the position of the SLN in reference to other nodes so that harvesting may be done with local anesthesia through a minimal incision. Preoperative lymphoscintigraphy can accomplish this task quite well, especially in the groin and the head and neck area, where the lymph nodes are more superficial. The axilla is the most difficult area to map: here, the best preoperative lymphoscintigraphy can do is to determine

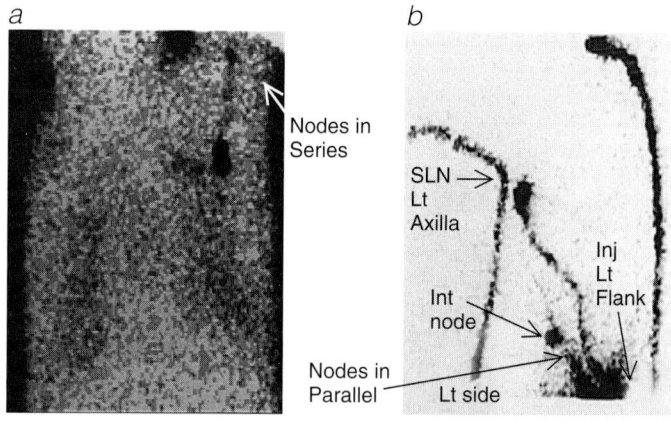

Lt Lat Chest W/M

Figure 4 **Lymphatic mapping and SLN biopsy for melanoma. In transit nodal areas are identified in 5% of melanoma patients; this is the reason why preoperative lymphoscintigraphy is performed for primary sites on either the upper or the lower extremity. In a patient with a melanoma on the left hand (*a*), the injection site and the left hand are raised above the head, and cutaneous lymphatic flow can be seen into an epitrochlear node. This in transit node then emits a lymphatic vessel flowing to the left axilla. By definition, the SLN is the first node in the chain that receives primary lymphatic flow. The epitrochlear node and any axillary nodes are nodes in series. Hence, the epitrochlear node is the SLN and thus is the only node that must be harvested. In a patient with a primary melanoma on the left flank (*b*), there are two separate afferent lymphatics, one leading to an SLN in the left axilla and the other leading to an in transit node on the left flank. These are nodes in parallel in that they both receive primary lymphatic flow from the skin site. Hence, the two nodes are equally at risk for metastatic disease, and both are considered SLNs and must be harvested.**

whether the node is located anteriorly, posteriorly, superiorly, or inferiorly in the basin. Use of hand-held gamma probes during SLN mapping has reduced the need to mark SLN locations during preoperative lymphoscintigraphy; however, intradermal tattooing to mark the location of the SLN can confirm the site and thereby make the surgical procedure more efficient.

4. To estimate the number of SLNs in the regional basin that will have to be harvested.

The timing of the injection of the mapping reagent has an impact on the success of the procedure. Whereas vital blue dyes typically travel to the regional basin within a matter of minutes, most radiocolloids are concentrated in the SLN over a period of hours. Activity ratios (see below) for 99mTc-SC are highest 2 to 6 hours after injection, which is helpful to the surgeon in three respects. First, the higher ratios make the SLN easier to locate. Second, the radiocolloid can be injected by the nuclear radiologist hours before the actual operation, and the surgeon does not need a special license for radioactivity handling. Third, cases are easier to schedule because there is a 2- to 6-hour window during which the intraoperative mapping can be easily accomplished.

Several groups have shown that lymphatic mapping for melanoma can still be effectively performed as long as 16 to 24 hours after injection of the radiocolloid.[31] Because of the short half-life of technetium (6 hours), the measured radioactivity around the injection site is substantially less when mapping is delayed to this extent. Nevertheless, it is usually possible to recognize the hot spot representing the concentration of radiocolloid in the SLN because once the radiocolloid enters the first node, it tends to be trapped there by the dendritic cells of the node, which means that very little of it passes through to second-tier nodes.

Step 2: Intraoperative Lymphatic Mapping and Identification of SLN

The patient is taken to the OR 2 to 24 hours later, and 1 ml of 1% isosulfan blue dye (Lymphazurin) [see Sidebar Choice of Radiocolloid and Vital Blue Dye for Lymphatic Mapping] per direction of drainage is injected around the primary site. The primary site and the regional basin are prepared and draped, and 10 minutes is allowed for the vital blue dye to travel to the SLN. Attention is then directed initially to the regional basin. The radioactive hot spot in the regional basin is identified with the hand-held gamma probe, and the in vivo activity ratio (see below) is noted. If shine-through from the radioactivity of the radiocolloid injected at the primary site is a problem, WLE of the primary may be performed first. An incision is made over the hot spot, and small flaps are created in all directions to allow identification of the blue-stained afferent lymphatic vessels. Surgical dissection is aided by visualization of the stained afferent lymphatic vessel leading down to the blue-stained node and by the use of the hand-held gamma probe to direct dissection down to the SLN. If, as is sometimes the case, one becomes confused as to what is proximal and what is distal on the afferent lymphatic vessel, the probe can be used to identify the direction of dissection.

Comment Radiocolloid and vital blue dye mapping techniques are complementary, and there is no reason why the two approaches should not be used simultaneously to improve the chances of locating the SLN successfully. Either may be crucial in a given instance, depending on the location of the primary in relation to the regional basin. If the primary site is close to, overlying, or in a direct line to the basin, so that the gamma probe is likely to encounter shine-through, use of vital blue dye may be the only technique that permits successful mapping. Only 1% to 5% of the injected radiocolloid dose is delivered to the regional basin; thus, even if the radioactivity from the primary site is reduced by performing WLE first, enough radioactivity may remain at that site (thanks to diffusion of the injectate) to increase the background level in the basin to the point where mapping with the radiocolloid alone is impossible. On the other hand, when one is mapping a fatty axilla or the head and neck region, it may be impossible to follow a wisp of blue-stained afferent lymphatic vessel to the SLN. Large flaps are especially to be avoided in the head and neck area because of the surrounding vital structures; in this setting, the ability of the gamma probe to locate the hot spot through the skin before the incision is made is a tremendous advantage.

A key issue with intraoperative radiocolloid mapping is how to define an SLN in terms of accumulated radioactivity. To do this, clinicians must use so-called activity (or localization) ratios. Measurement of the absolute level of radioactivity in a node is not sufficient, because in each harvest, there are a number of crucial variables: different radiocolloid doses are injected at the primary site, the injection is sometimes unevenly distributed around the primary site, the time interval between injection and harvest is not constant, the distance between the primary site and the regional basin is not always the same, and varying degrees of shine-through may be present. The effects of these variables can be eliminated by determining the in vivo activity ratio (i.e., the ratio of the radioactivity in the SLN to the background radioactivity). In vivo radioactivity is measured in counts/10 sec with the SLN fully exposed. Background activity is estimated by counting four areas in the basin equidistant from the injection site and away from the SLN. Perhaps more help-

ful is the ex vivo activity ratio (i.e., the ratio of the radioactivity in an excised SLN to that in an excised neighboring non-SLN), which has the virtue of eliminating all shine-through. At MCC, we define an SLN as a node with an activity ratio of 3:1 or higher in vivo or 10:1 or higher ex vivo. In our experience, 98% of SLNs exhibit these ratios.

Occasionally, pass-through of the blue dye or the radiocolloid occurs but rarely, if ever, to the point where it results in mistaken identification of a higher node as an SLN. That is, one typically does not see non-SLNs that are stained blue or that have activity ratios of 3:1 in vivo or 10:1 ex vivo. When the radiocolloid does pass through the SLN, it is distributed to multiple higher nodes, thereby helping to raise the background radiation level; however, it is not concentrated to any large extent in any one higher node.

Step 3: Removal of SLN

Once the SLN is identified, the entire node is removed by means of sharp dissection or the electrocautery. Afferent and efferent lymphatic vessels entering and exiting the SLN, some of which (i.e., the afferent vessels) are stained blue, are controlled with hemostatic clips because the electrocautery will not seal these vessels. This measure decreases the risk of postoperative wound seroma. If the opportunity presents itself without the risk of increased morbidity, a neighboring non-SLN may be removed to provide an internal control, and the ex vivo activity ratio may be calculated.

The radioactivity level in the excised SLN is checked with the hand-held gamma probe to confirm that the node has been correctly identified as the SLN. The residual radioactivity in the basin is then checked with the probe to verify that all SLNs have been removed. If radioactivity has not fallen to the background level, the probe should be used to direct additional dissection aimed at removing any additional SLNs present.

Comment The directed dissection achievable with the help of radio-guided mapping allows the surgeon to perform axillary and head and neck harvests without having to identify the motor nerves running through the basin. A series of 30 head and neck melanoma patients with SLN drainage to the parotid gland showed that the SLNs could be harvested with directed dissection without formal identification of fascial motor nerves.[32] The technique recommended by the authors—which may be adaptable to other basins where dissection passes close to a motor nerve—involved eliminating paralyzing agents with anesthesia, incising the parotid fascia, then, with blunt dissection under gamma-probe guidance, shelling out the SLN in the parotid gland. The success rate of SLN identification in the parotid gland was higher than 90%, and there were no instances of fascial nerve dysfunction. Likewise, in more than 2,000 axillary SLN mappings at MCC, there has been no evidence of prolonged postoperative thoracic or thoracodorsal dysfunction. Dissections in the posterior cervical triangle are performed similarly when in close proximity to the spinal accessory nerve.

A secondary benefit of radiocolloid mapping is its ability to provide immediate verification that all SLNs have been removed from the lymphatic basin: if all of the radiolabeled SLNs have in fact been excised, the radioactivity in the basin must return to its background level. When only vital blue dye is used for mapping, it often proves necessary to perform further dissection (and create more flaps) to locate additional blue-stained lymphatics and verify that all SLNs have been excised.

In addition, as noted [see Step 1: Preoperative Lymphoscintigraphy, above], the radiocolloid has a much longer retention time than the dye and tends to be concentrated in the SLN. When harvest occurs 2 to 24 hours after injection of the radiocolloid, activity ratios are double what they are when mapping is done immediately after injection.[33,34]

Step 4: Pathologic Examination of SLN

Once the SLN has been harvested, it is submitted for detailed pathologic examination. The examination may include serial sectioning, immunohistochemical staining with S-100 and HMB-45 monoclonal antibodies, and perhaps reverse transcriptase–polymerase chain reaction (RT-PCR) analysis.

COMPLICATIONS

Complications of lymphatic mapping are rare. All SLN harvests are performed without any postoperative drainage, and this contributes to the low morbidity of the procedure. A seroma develops in about 10% of patients, but it is easily handled with percutaneous aspiration. Surgical site infections are rare, and wound healing is better than with ELND because large flaps are not needed for the dissection.

In a 2001 report, investigators from the Sun Belt Melanoma Trial compared complication rates for lymphatic mapping in 1,202 patients who underwent SLN dissection alone with complication rates in 277 patients who required complete lymph node dissection (CLND) as part of the trial.[35] The incidences of seroma, lymphedema, and wound problems were 3%, 0.7%, and 1.7%, respectively, in the first group and 7.9%, 9.8%, and 11.9% in the second.

REPORTED RESULTS

In the initial report by Morton and associates,[15] in which mapping was done with vital blue dye alone, SLNs were successfully identified in 194 of 237 lymphatic basins, and 40 (21%) of the 194 specimens contained metastatic melanoma detected either by routine histologic examination with hematoxylin-eosin staining (12%) or by immunohistochemical staining exclusively (9%). Metastases were present in 47 (18%) of 259 SLNs, whereas non-SLNs were the exclusive site of metastasis in only two of 3,079 nodes from 194 dissections, for a false negative rate of 1% (with nodes rather than patients as the unit of analysis).

Given that lymphatic mapping can be evaluated only in patients with metastatic disease—because these are the only patients in whom a skip metastasis (i.e., a metastasis in which the SLN is histologically negative but nodes farther down the drainage pathway are histologically positive) could be documented—the investigators' findings in these patients are of considerable interest. Of 40 patients with histologically positive nodes, SLN mapping identified 38, for a 5% false negative rate. In 72% of basins, a particular primary site drained to a single SLN; in 20%, to two SLNs; and in 8%, to three or more SLNs. Surgeons successfully identified SLNs in 72% to 96% of attempts, depending on where the surgeons were on the learning curve. Overall, groin mappings were the most successful (89% of attempts); axillary mapping was generally successful as well (78% of attempts). The investigators concluded that a learning curve of 60 cases would be necessary, which meant that the procedure would have to be restricted to major medical centers that treat large numbers of melanoma patients. This caveat notwithstanding, the new technique clearly was capable of accurately identifying patients with occult lymph node metastases who might benefit from radical lymphadenectomy.[15,16]

Surgical trials at several other institutions confirmed two essential points.[8,17,18,21,22] First, nodal metastasis from cutaneous primary sites follows an orderly, nonrandom, progressive pattern. Second, SLNs in the lymphatic basins can be individually identified, and their status reflects the presence or absence of melanoma metastases in the remaining nodes in the basins. In an initial study of 42 patients with intermediate-thickness melanomas,[17] SLN harvesting

was followed by complete node dissection to confirm the low incidence of skip metastases in this population. None of the patients in this study had skip metastases: eight had a positive SLN, with the SLN as the only site of disease in seven of the eight, and 34 had a histologically negative SLN, with the rest of the nodes in the basin also histologically negative. Analysis of the results proved that the SLN was the first and favored site of metastatic disease. Preoperative lymphoscintigraphy was performed in this trial to define all basins at risk for metastatic disease, and intraoperative mapping was performed with isosulfan blue dye. The rate of technical failure was 10%.

A trial at the University of Vermont employed radiocolloid for intraoperative mapping after it was determined that in some cases, use of the vital blue dye was difficult if not impossible.[36] The investigators studied 100 patients with melanoma arising at a wide variety of primary sites. All of the patients underwent lymphoscintigraphy 1 to 24 hours before intraoperative mapping and SLN excision. A hand-held gamma probe was used to facilitate accurate identification and removal of the SLNs. Incisions were made directly over the hot spot to minimize dissection; further dissection, if needed, was guided by the probe. The SLNs were successfully located in 98% of the patients, a markedly better result than was obtained in previous reports.

Subsequently, this same melanoma consortium published updated findings.[21] Between February 1993 and October 1994, 121 patients with invasive melanomas and clinically negative nodes were enrolled in a study comparing two different approaches to intraoperative mapping. In one group (64% of patients), mapping involved only injection of a radiocolloid (unfiltered ^{99m}Tc-SC, ^{99m}Tc–human serum albumin [^{99m}Tc-HSA], or Microlite [Dupont, Billerica, Massachusetts]) around the primary site and use of a hand-held gamma probe; the SLN was successfully identified in 97.6% of the patients in this group. In the other group (36% of patients), both vital blue dye and radiocolloid were used. All of the blue-stained SLNs also yielded radioactive hot spots, and in four patients the blue dye was not identified in any of the lymph nodes, which meant that mapping would have been unsuccessful if blue-staining had been the only mapping technique applied. Preoperative lymphoscintigraphy was used in 93% of the patients, with a technical failure rate of 10%. The radiolabeled SLNs could not be successfully imaged in these 12 patients preoperatively, but with the help of the hand-held gamma probe, the SLNs could be identified intraoperatively. This result suggests that a hand-held gamma probe is more sensitive at identifying SLNs than a scintillation camera. The reason may be that the probe accumulates data for scanning the basin in seconds, compared with the 2 to 6 minutes needed for the camera to produce images. This difference probably also explains why multiple nodes are sometimes imaged on preoperative lymphoscintigraphy when 1 to 2 hours have elapsed between radiocolloid injection and imaging. Intraoperative mapping, on the other hand, readily identifies the SLN and does not find multiple nodes to be hot, even when it is done 2 to 24 hours after the lymphoscintigram—provided that ^{99m}Tc-SC is used as the mapping agent.[33] Micrometastatic disease was present in 15 (12.4%) of the 121 patients studied, and the SLN was the only metastatic site in 10 (8.3%). After a minimum follow-up of 220 days, one regional nodal recurrence was observed in an SLN-negative patient.

The addition of intraoperative radiolymphoscintigraphy to vital blue dye lymphatic mapping made SLN localization easier and more widely applicable.[21,33,37] The initial study from MCC on the use of this combined approach included 106 consecutive patients with cutaneous melanoma thicker than 0.75 mm at all primary site locations.[33] A total of 200 SLNs and 142 neighboring non-SLNs were harvested from 129 basins; 70% of the SLNs demonstrated blue staining, and 84% were identified as radioactive hot spots. When the two intraoperative mapping techniques were used in conjunction, the SLN could be identified in 96% of the nodal basins sampled. Routine histology identified SLN micrometastases in 15% of patients, and two patients had micrometastatic disease in nodes that were hot but not blue-stained. These data suggest that radiocolloid localization identifies more SLNs, some of which are clinically important in that they contain micrometastatic disease.[33]

In another study, a combination of vital blue dye and radiocolloid (^{99m}Tc-HSA) mapping was used in a series of 30 patients with melanoma from all primary sites.[37] The SLN stained blue and was the most radioactive site in 27 patients (90%). In five of 13 patients undergoing groin dissection, radiolymphoscintigraphy identified two SLNs in the drainage basin. In each case, the presence of the second inguinal SLN was suggested by the high residual radioactivity after removal of the first node, not by the blue dye; radioactivity decreased to background levels after excision of the second node. The investigators concluded that radiolymphoscintigraphy can be used not only to confirm blue-dye identification of an initial SLN but also to detect additional SLNs that are not easily identified with the dye technique alone.

In a subsequent MCC trial that used isosulfan blue dye and ^{99m}Tc-SC as mapping agents,[29] only patients with a positive SLN underwent complete node dissection. After 3 years of follow-up, two recurrences in regional basins were observed in patients whose previous SLN biopsy was negative. Serial sectioning and immunohistochemical staining of the SLN block found no abnormal cells; however, both patients' SLNs were RT-PCR–positive for messenger RNA (mRNA) for the tyrosinase gene,[38] which suggests the presence of micrometastatic disease that was missed by more conventional tests.

In another study, the Sydney Melanoma Unit reported an 87% success rate in identifying SLNs.[39] There was a pronounced learning curve, in that the success rate for the last 100 patients was 97%. Cutaneous lymphoscintigraphy was performed in 800 melanoma patients and was used to guide subsequent SLN harvesting; 23% of patients were found to have micrometastatic disease. Initially, the SLNs underwent frozen sectioning for occult metastases, but the 9% false negative rate led the investigators to switch to permanent sections, an approach that allowed the pathologist 2 to 5 days to perform a detailed examination. Patients found to have a positive SLN were returned to the OR for complete node dissection. When preoperative lymphoscintigraphy was followed by intraoperative mapping using vital blue-dye staining in conjunction with radiocolloid (^{99m}Tc-ATS) injection and a hand-held gamma probe, a 1.9% false negative rate was reported.

Finally, valuable findings are anticipated from the National Cancer Institute–sponsored prospective trial now under way [see Discussion, National Protocols, below]. Survival data from this trial are unlikely to be available before 2005.

Current data suggest that lymphatic mapping is applicable to all primary sites of the body, including the head and the neck (probably the most technically demanding sites).[31,40] The best results are achieved with a combination mapping approach that employs both vital blue dye and radiocolloid. The procedure is associated with slightly higher false negative rates in patients with head and neck melanoma than in those with extremity and trunk melanoma (10% versus 1% to 2%). Nevertheless, the false negative rates are still low enough to justify offering lymphatic mapping to patients with head and neck melanoma—especially given that the only alternative method of obtaining the nodal staging information is CLND, a more radical procedure that carries a higher morbidity.

Patterns of Failure after Negative SLN Biopsy

Several of the earlier studies found that SLN mapping had a false negative rate—defined as a negative SLN with positive higher nodes—of less than 4%, as determined by concomitant formal lymph node dissection[15-18]; however, they did not clearly establish the long-term risk of failure within the mapped nodal basin after a negative SLN alone. This issue was addressed by a joint study from MCC and the M. D. Anderson Cancer Center (Houston, Texas).[41] In this study, patients with cutaneous melanoma whose tumor was at least 1.0 mm thick or was categorized as Clark level IV or higher were eligible for mapping and SLN biopsy. All patients underwent preoperative lymphoscintigraphy, and only those with a histologically positive SLN underwent complete lymphadenectomy. A total of 618 patients underwent mapping with successful identification of at least one SLN; of these, 518 had histologically negative SLNs. After a minimum follow-up of 3 months and a median follow-up of 18 months, 32 (6%) of the 518 patients had recurrent disease; nine (1.7%) of the 518 had their first recurrence in a basin where the SLN was negative at the previous mapping. Patients with a histologically negative SLN had significantly better DFS (*P* < 0.001) and distant disease–free survival (*P* < 0.001) than those with a histologically positive SLN. When SLNs from the nine patients whose SLNs were determined to be free of metastatic disease on initial review were retrospectively reexamined by serial sectioning or immunohistochemistry, occult nodal metastases were present in seven (77%) of the nine. These data established the durable long-term accuracy of lymphatic mapping and SLN biopsy.

Optimal nodal staging requires not only accurate identification of the SLN but also careful examination of the SLN with special pathologic techniques. It is likely that many false negative SLN biopsies do not actually reflect true skip metastases but are the result of micrometastases missed on routine pathologic examination. In the study cited, it is clear, given the subsequent recurrences, that the missed micrometastases represented clinically relevant disease. The recurrences could have been prevented if the SLNs had undergone detailed histologic examination initially, the micrometastases had been found, and complete node dissection had been performed.

Other explanations of false positive SLN biopsies have been proposed. One is that after a negative SLN biopsy, some regional basins are seeded with metastatic cells from in transit metastases or local recurrences. In transit metastasis occurs in 2% to 3% of patients and could be a source of skip metastases.[8]

Clinical Implications

The information generated by all this experience is being used to change the standards for surgical management of melanoma so that only patients with evidence of nodal metastatic disease are subjected to the morbidity and expense of complete node dissection.[3-6] Initial studies showed the usefulness of lymphatic mapping with either vital blue dye or radiocolloid in obtaining such evidence; however, it is now clear that the success rate of SLN identification increases markedly when the two mapping approaches are combined as described [see Technique, above]. A combined mapping approach identifies SLNs both more accurately and more completely: it removes more SLNs and results in a lower incidence of positive nodes on subsequent CLND.

In 85% to 94% of melanoma patients, the SLN is the only site of metastasis. At MCC, we have seen no patients with melanomas less than 2.8 mm thick in whom nodes other than SLNs harbored metastases. It has been hypothesized that a melanoma must reach a certain thickness before it sheds enough cells to involve higher nodes beyond the SLN, and this hypothesis is supported by data from the M. D. Anderson Cancer Center showing no positive higher nodes after a positive SLN biopsy in patients with melanomas less than 2.5 mm thick. It appears that metastatic cells are concentrated in SLNs in much the same way that vital blue dyes and radiocolloids are. Thus, for many melanoma patients (in particular, those whose tumors have not reached the critical thickness just specified), to locate the SLN is essentially to define the limit of metastatic spread. Accordingly, lymphatic mapping, by identifying SLNs (and thus defining the extent of disease) with a high degree of accuracy, can be extremely useful in helping clinicians make more informed therapeutic decisions—for example, regarding eligibility for adjuvant therapy or the possibility of forgoing CLND.

On the basis of these data, a multicenter regional trial (the Florida Melanoma Trial II) has been initiated that will randomize patients with a microscopic positive SLN into either a group receiving adjuvant therapy alone or a group receiving CLND and adjuvant therapy. This trial will attempt to answer the question of what role CLND plays in the treatment of low-volume metastatic disease in a regional basin. It will also be the first trial to use molecular staging procedures (e.g., RT-PCR analysis) to define SLN-positive disease and to make treatment decisions on the basis of such staging procedures.

The findings of the studies cited demonstrate that intraoperative lymphatic mapping and SLN biopsy yields accurate pathologic staging, does not lower care standards, decreases morbidity (e.g., lymphedema is absent, and early return to work or normal activity is facilitated), makes possible rational yet less aggressive surgical and adjuvant medical approaches, and reduces costs.[24] A 2001 report examining a comprehensive database (including more than 25,000 melanoma patients) assembled from the major melanoma centers throughout the world by the AJCC melanoma staging committee lent support to these findings.[42] In this report, melanoma patients with intermediate-thickness (> 1.0 mm) melanomas who were determined to be node negative through clinical examination had a 5-year survival rate of 65%, and those who were determined to be node negative through ELND had a 5-year survival rate of 75%. In contrast, a similar population of melanoma patients who were determined to be node negative through lymphatic mapping and SLN biopsy had a 5-year survival rate of 90%. These statistically significant differences in survival suggest that lymphatic mapping misses less micrometastatic disease than either clinical examination of the nodal basin or ELND and hence identifies a purer population of truly node-negative patients. Accordingly, lymphatic mapping should be considered the preferred staging method for melanoma patients, particularly in clinical trial settings.

Additional improvements in survival rates can be expected for staged populations when the RT-PCR assay is added to the pathologic examination of the SLN. So-called ultrastaging may yield even further increases in survival for node-negative patients. The process involves serial examination and sampling of other immune compartments of the body besides the SLN, including peripheral blood and bone marrow, followed by analysis of the samples with very sensitive assays of occult metastases (based on RT-PCR technology). The potential value of ultrastaging is that it would allow monitoring of patient status as therapy is administered and might bring clinicians closer to being able to identify patients who have been surgically cured of their disease. That is to say, if both pathologic examination of the SLN and analysis of serial peripheral blood and bone marrow samples with sensitive RT-PCR assays determine that a melanoma patient is free of metastatic disease, that patient has been staged more accurately than would have been possible with ELND and superficial examination of all the nodes in the basin, and he or she is probably closer to being identified as a surgical cure.

The available staging data tend to support this hypothesis. In the literature, when melanoma patients were staged according to the traditional system—that is, by means of either clinical examination of the regional nodal basin or ELND—stage I patients had an 85% 5-year survival rate, stage II patients had a 70% survival rate, and stage III patients had a 47% survival rate. This older staging system yielded a reasonably good separation of the staging groups; however, a significant proportion of stage I and stage II patients (15% and 30%, respectively) experienced recurrences and died of their disease within 5 years of the initial diagnosis. It is instructive to compare these survival rates with those for melanoma patients who are staged by means of lymphatic mapping and RT-PCR assay, which typically approach 100%.

Lymphatic Mapping and SLN Biopsy for Breast Cancer

RATIONALE

For breast cancer, as for most solid tumors, the most powerful prognostic factor is the status of the regional nodes: the presence of regional metastases decreases 5-year survival by approximately 28% to 40%.[43,44] As for melanoma, many prognostic factors for breast cancer have been defined on the basis of primary tumor characteristics, yet regression analyses indicate that such factors add very little to the prognostic model once lymph node status is considered. Hence, the rationale for nodal staging is essentially the same as with melanoma.

Nodal Staging

Currently, surgical management of breast cancer is more conservative than it once was: breast conservation is now considered an acceptable alternative to modified radical mastectomy in as many as two thirds of patients. Management of the axilla in breast cancer patients remains controversial. It is generally accepted that axillary dissection is not indicated for patients with ductal carcinoma in situ (DCIS), because of the low likelihood of axillary node involvement.[45-47] The main point at issue is whether axillary dissection is indicated for patients with small invasive primary lesions. Some authors recommend that patients with T1a lesions be spared a dissection[48]; however, even when an invasive cancer is smaller than 1 cm, a significant percentage (14% to 37%) of patients have axillary nodal metastases.[49,50]

Breast tumors were once thought to have a random nodal metastatic pattern. Accordingly, investigators initially performed sampling procedures of anatomically defined first-station nodal basins in an effort to achieve accurate pathologic staging. These procedures were based on arbitrary assignment of node clusters in the axillary region to various levels (I, II, or III) rather than on intraoperative mapping of the SLN. Unfortunately, this approach led to a high (15%) prevalence of skip metastases (defined in this context as metastases to level II and III axillary nodes without involvement of level I nodes).[51] As a result, investigators abandoned sampling as a nodal staging technique for patients with breast cancer. Subsequent work demonstrated, however, that when lymphatic mapping is performed in patients with upper outer quadrant tumors, about 10% to 15% of them show direct drainage to level II axillary nodes, and skip metastases are not found. In previous studies, these patients would have been classified as having skip metastases; given the available data, it is likely that the earlier investigators simply were using insufficiently accurate staging techniques that were unable to map the SLNs or the levels of the axilla accurately.

More accurate staging involves more than just stage shifting[52]: it can improve survival in the breast cancer population by identifying patients who will gain a survival advantage associated with either the surgical procedure itself (complete axillary dissection)[53] or the accompanying adjuvant therapy.[44] In addition, it keeps a percentage of the population from being exposed to the complications of the more extensive surgical procedure or to the toxicities of the adjuvant therapy. In particular, the ability to limit full axillary lymph node dissection (ALND) to women with documented nodal metastases would be a major advance in the surgical treatment of breast cancer. Now that modern techniques have made breast conservation a viable option for so many women, the main physical complaints patients voice after operation have to do with the side effects of axillary dissection (i.e., lymphedema of the arm, reduced range of motion, and paresthesia). If node-negative patients could be protected from having to experience these side effects, that would be every bit as significant a therapeutic advance as the realization that breast cancer could be treated effectively with lumpectomy and radiation therapy.

PATIENT SELECTION

Any woman with invasive breast cancer is a potential candidate for lymphatic mapping and SLN biopsy. In patients with DCIS, the incidence of nodal metastasis on SLN biopsy with a more detailed examination of the node is 8.4%. In most cases, these apparent metastases are low-volume lesions that are discoverable only with cytokeratin staining of the SLN; there is disagreement as to whether they represent true viable metastases. In patients with invasive tumors more than 5 cm in diameter, the incidence of nodal metastasis on SLN biopsy with detailed examination is 75%. Clinicians must decide for themselves whether these patients should undergo nodal staging; however, at MCC, we routinely offer them the procedure because if nodal metastases are found, the subsequent treatment recommendations will be different.

Contraindications to the procedure are multifocal disease, inflammatory cancer, and extensive previous surgery or radiation therapy (e.g., breast reconstruction with implants above the pectoral muscle).

TECHNIQUE

Step 1: Preoperative Lymphoscintigraphy

Lymphoscintigraphy is performed in much the same way for breast cancer as for melanoma, except that the radiocolloid is injected into the breast parenchyma around the primary tumor. The radioactivity dose is the same as for melanoma (450 µCi), but larger volumes (6 ml) are administered because the breast lymphatics are not as rich as the cutaneous lymphatics. For this reason, the first images are not available until 30 to 40 minutes after injection [*see Figure 5*].

The injection must be diffuse enough around the tumor to allow the radiocolloid to be taken up by the breast lymphatics. If the tumor was detected mammographically, localization wires are placed under either mammographic or ultrasonographic guidance, and the radiocolloid is injected around the wire and the tumor. Injection must not be performed through the localization needle, because the needle will act as a wick, allowing the radiocolloid to flow back out and possibly contaminate the skin. The localization wire is left in place to guide subsequent injection of vital blue dye. If the tumor is palpable, injection is straightforward and is done tightly around the circumference of the tumor. If an excisional biopsy was performed, injection is done under ultrasonographic guidance so that the radiocolloid is placed in the breast parenchyma around the biopsy cavity. If the radiocolloid is placed in the tumor or the biopsy cavity, it will not migrate.

Alternative injection techniques have been described that include injecting the mapping agents either into the subareolar plexus (SAP) (because the breast lymphatics from all quadrants initially migrate to the SAP before traveling to the axilla) or into the skin above the tumor.[54,55] For axillary mapping, these alternative injection techniques seem to work as well as intraparenchymal injection. One potential disadvantage is that the breast lymphatics that drain into the internal mammary chain are located deep in the breast and pass through the pectoralis fascia, and these lymphatic vessels are not visualized with subareolar or intradermal injection. For most surgeons performing lymphatic mapping, successful axillary mapping is the most important aim, and the alternative injection techniques should make axillary mapping easier and its results more reproducible. In so doing, these newer techniques should effectively reduce the steepness of the learning curve.

Comment The timing of radiocolloid injection is not highly critical as long as enough time (2 to 24 hours) is allowed between injection and SLN harvesting for the mapping agent to migrate into the SLN. As the radiocolloid migrates, it is concentrated in the SLN. In most cases, this concentration results in an identifiable radioactive hot spot. When this happens, SLN harvesting becomes easier. Axillary hot spots have been identified up to 24 hours after radiocolloid injection. Harvesting can therefore be done as long as 24 hours after injection, provided that some level of radioactivity remains detectable in the axilla.[56,57]

One may question the need to image the patient after radiocolloid injection, given that the standard of care is to stage the patient according to the status of the axillary nodes alone. Lymphoscintigraphy can be used to identify women whose primary tumors drain bidirectionally to the axilla and to the internal mammary (IM) nodes (about 10% of patients, most of whom have inner-quadrant or central cancers). A 2001 report from MCC clinicians described a series of 30 breast cancer patients in whom lymphoscintigraphy showed bidirectional lymphatic drainage to both axillary and IM SLNs.[58] All axillary and IM SLNs were harvested. In five (16.7%) of the 30 patients, micrometastases were documented in the IM SLN; and in two of those five, the IM SLN was the only site of disease.[58] In two (6.6%) of the 30 patients, IM SLN sampling changed the staging. At MCC, patients whose IM SLN biopsy yields positive results subsequently undergo

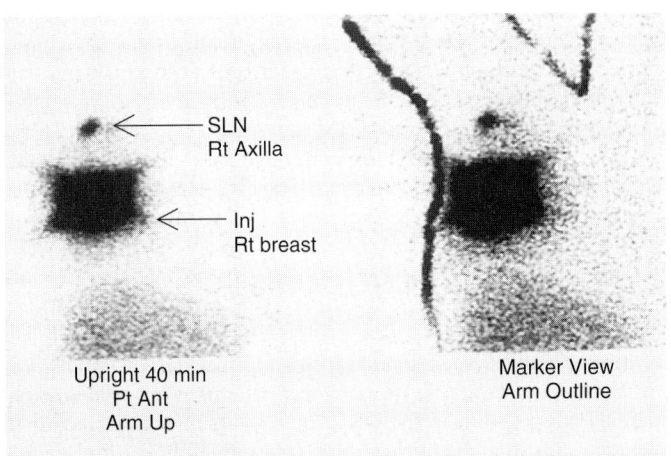

Figure 5 **Lymphatic mapping and SLN biopsy for breast cancer. Whereas flow of the radiocolloid to the SLN takes 5 to 10 minutes for melanoma mapping, it takes 30 to 40 minutes for breast cancer mapping. In addition, the primary site is usually closer to the regional basin in breast cancer than it is in melanoma, and shine-through from the primary site may be a problem. Invariably, the lumpectomy or mastectomy is performed first, followed by axillary SLN harvesting.**

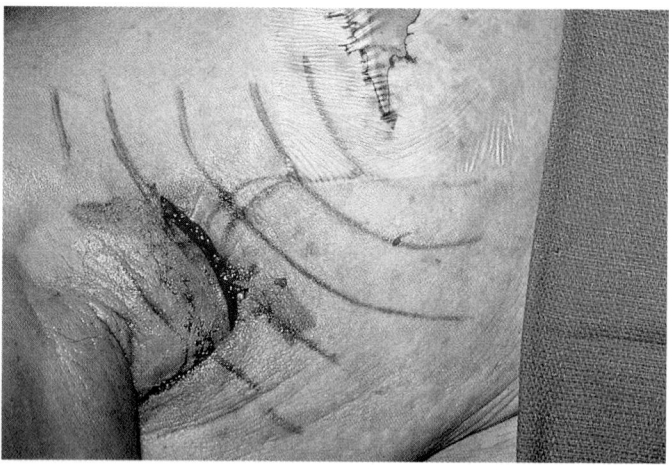

Figure 6 Lymphatic mapping and SLN biopsy for breast cancer. Isobars of radioactivity are drawn equidistant from the primary site (upper right), and hot spots are identified along each of the isobars. These hot spots represent the location of the afferent lymphatic leading to the SLN in the axilla.

irradiation of the remainder of the IM chain if they have chosen lumpectomy and radiation therapy to treat their primary breast cancer. Other groups take a broader approach, electing to irradiate the IM chain whenever bidirectional drainage is demonstrated on preoperative lymphoscintigraphy.

The importance of IM SLN harvesting is currently under investigation by a national trial being performed by the National Surgical Adjuvant Breast and Bowel Project (NSABP). Until the results of this trial are available, clinicians should concern themselves primarily with performing accurate mapping of axillary lymph nodes. Given proper training and enough cases to fill out the learning curve, surgeons have demonstrated that they can readily incorporate SLN biopsy into their breast cancer practices in the regional and community hospital setting.[59]

The variations in breast lymphatic drainage revealed by lymphatic mapping (e.g., to level II and III axillary lymph nodes, to subclavian and supraclavicular lymph nodes, and to IM SLNs) will inevitably lead to changes in breast cancer staging, much as has already occurred with melanoma staging. At present, breast cancer patients with micrometastatic disease in the axilla are classified as having stage II disease, those with disease in the IM nodes as having stage III disease, and those with micrometastases in the supraclavicular nodes as having stage IV disease. Lymphatic mapping data, however, suggest that in some patients, all of these scenarios may represent the same biologic phenomenon—that is, regional nodal spread of the breast cancer.

Step 2: Intraoperative Lymphatic Mapping and Identification of SLN

Intraoperative lymphatic mapping and SLN identification follow much the same course in breast cancer patients as in melanoma patients. Patients come to the OR 2 to 24 hours after the injection of the radiocolloid in the nuclear medicine suite. If the tumor is palpable, 5 ml of 1% isosulfan blue dye is injected around the circumference of the primary tumor 10 to 15 minutes before the surgical procedure. If the tumor is nonpalpable, the dye is injected around the localization wire left in place after preoperative lymphoscintigraphy. After injection of the vital blue dye, the breast is massaged for 5 minutes to facilitate migration of the mapping agents.

Given that the newer injection techniques described earlier appear to identify axillary SLNs as reliably as injection into the breast

parenchyma does, a reasonable alternative approach is to split the dose of vital blue dye between intraparenchymal injection around the tumor or the biopsy cavity and injection into the SAP. Injection into the SAP need only cover the 9 to 12 o'clock area in the right breast and the 12 to 3 o'clock area in the left breast because those are the areas where the main SAP lymphatic vessels leading to the axilla branch off.[60] SAP injection is more appealing than intradermal injection above the tumor in that the clinician does not have to know exactly where the tumor is located in the breast. In addition, SAP injection does not involve an injection around an excisional biopsy scar, which is occasionally a complicating factor with intradermal injection.

Before a skin incision is made, a hand-held gamma probe is used to identify the most radioactive area in the axilla. If there is sufficient distance between the primary site and the regional basin, isobar levels of radioactivity [see Figure 6] are drawn emanating from

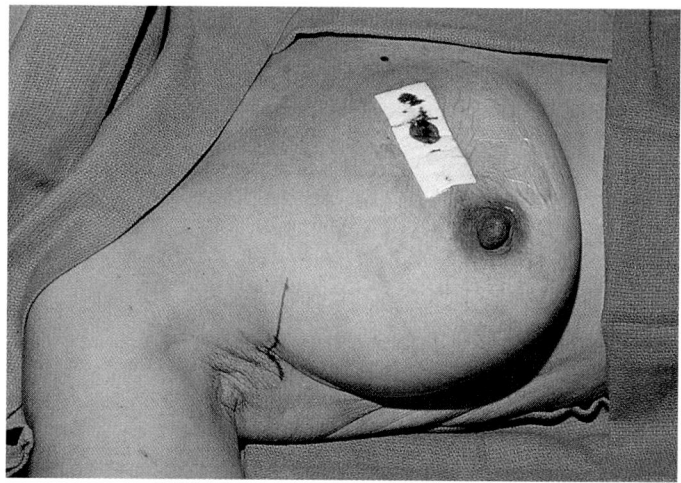

Figure 7 Lymphatic mapping and SLN biopsy for breast cancer. The hand-held gamma probe is used to trace the afferent lymphatic through the skin to a hot spot in the regional basin, under which the SLN is located.

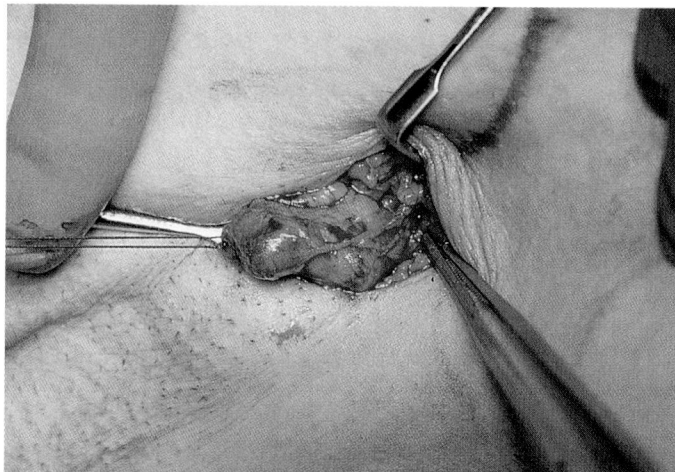

Figure 8 Lymphatic mapping and SLN biopsy for breast cancer. In the same patient as in Figure 7, a small incision is made in the axilla, and with the gamma probe directing the dissection, a blue-stained afferent lymphatic is seen leading into a blue-stained node. This node is hot as well as blue; it is the SLN and is the first site of metastatic disease.

the primary site, and hot spots of radioactivity are marked along each of the isobars. If possible, the afferent lymphatic is mapped and followed to a hot spot in the axilla that corresponds to the location of the SLN [see Figure 7]. A small (2 to 4 cm) axillary incision is made over the hot spot, dissection is directed through the axillary fat with the probe, and the SLN is identified [see Figure 8]. Ideally, the SLN should be both hot and blue. If the hot spot corresponds to a cluster of nodes, the blue staining will help distinguish the SLN from the non-SLNs. The in vivo activity ratio is determined to confirm that the node fulfills the criteria of an SLN. Care must be taken to ensure that the in vivo activity ratio is not being influenced by shine-through from the primary site or from other SLNs in the axilla. For this reason, the ex vivo activity ratio is more helpful in defining an SLN (though not particularly helpful when the surgeon is trying to decide whether to remove the axillary node or leave it in place). Careful dissection is performed to identify the blue-stained afferent lymphatics, which can then be followed to the pale blue–stained SLN or SLNs [see Figure 8].

Comment As with melanoma, mapping becomes simpler, more accurate, more complete, and more widely applicable when the vital blue dye method and the radiocolloid method are combined.[61,62] Either method may play a more important role in a given instance, depending on the circumstances. A unique feature of breast lymphatic mapping that makes it more technically demanding than melanoma mapping is that breast cancer primary sites are closer to their regional basins than most melanoma primaries are to theirs. As a result, there may be so much shine-through of radioactivity from the primary site that imaging of the axilla becomes impossible. This may also be the case intraoperatively, when one is trying to identify the axillary SLN, even if lumpectomy is performed first. In such circumstances, vital blue dye mapping takes on a more important role in finding the axillary SLN. On the other hand, radiocolloid mapping takes on a more important role when the blue dye is slow to travel to the regional basin or when the axillary SLN is full of tumor. In such instances, though one typically sees a dilated, blue-stained lymphatic vessel going into the SLN, the node itself may take up relatively little of the blue dye; however, a radioactive hot spot can usually be identified when the very sensitive handheld probe is placed directly at the level of the nodes in the basin.

When newer injection techniques (e.g., more diffuse injection of the radiocolloid around the primary tumor or biopsy cavity, intradermal injection, and subareolar injection) are used in conjunction with breast massage in the nuclear medicine suite, the axillary SLN is successfully imaged in as many as 85% to 90% of breast cancer patients. This is a significant improvement over the results cited in previous reports that examined only intraparenchymal injection, without breast massage. Surgeons may still be able to locate the SLN in the remaining 10% to 15% by using the handheld gamma probe (which is more sensitive than the camera) intraoperatively to find the axillary hot spot and direct dissection toward the SLN.

Activity (localization) ratios are used to eliminate uncontrolled variables that might affect identification of an SLN [see Lymphatic Mapping and SLN Biopsy for Melanoma, Technique, above]. The higher the activity ratio, the easier mapping will be and the more likely it is that SLN harvesting will be successful. A major reason for waiting 2 to 24 hours to allow the radiocolloid to migrate and become concentrated in the SLN before intraoperative mapping is that activity ratios are highest at this point. The alternative injection techniques described allow more of the radiocolloid to migrate to the SLN. As a result, SLN harvesting becomes easier, the axillary

SLN identification rate becomes closer to 100%, and the learning curve becomes less steep.[63]

A node is considered to be the SLN if it meets one of three criteria:

1. The node is blue.
2. The node has a blue-stained afferent lymphatic leading to it. Occasionally, a node is full of tumor and has a dilated blue-stained lymphatic vessel leading to it, but it does not take up the dye or the radiocolloid readily. This scenario is easily realized intraoperatively because the node is hard on direct palpation. Despite the lack of uptake of the mapping reagent, such nodes must be considered SLNs.
3. The node has an in vivo activity ratio of 3:1 or an ex vivo activity ratio of 10:1.

Step 3: Removal of SLN

Once the SLN is identified, it is removed. A neighboring non-SLN may also be removed so that the ex vivo activity ratio may be calculated. The blue-stained afferent lymphatics that have been visualized are clipped or tied off. The Bovie electrocautery does not seal lymphatic vessels, and the goal is to perform the dissection without the requirement for postoperative drainage. The central bed is then reexamined for radioactivity. If radioactivity is 150% of the background level or higher, dissection is continued in search of additional SLNs. The mean number of axillary SLNs removed in breast lymphatic mapping is 2.0/patient.

Step 4: Pathologic Examination of SLN

Once SLNs are dissected away from surrounding tissue, they are bivalved intraoperatively and examined for any gross evidence of metastatic disease. All of the excised nodal tissue is submitted for pathologic evaluation. Tissue contents are classified into three categories: SLNs, adjacent non-SLNs, and axillary contents. SLNs 5 mm or less in maximum diameter are bivalved, and those greater than 5 mm in diameter are serially sectioned at 2 to 3 mm intervals to maximize surface area for touch-print cytology and intraoperative immunohistochemistry (IHC). (To prevent loss of tissue in the cryostat, we do not perform frozen sections of the SLNs.) Imprints are made with a single gentle touch on each cut surface of the SLN. The slides are air-dried and stained with Diff-Quick stain, then sent for intraoperative interpretation. Approximately 5 to 8 minutes from the specimen's entry into the pathology laboratory, the intraoperative diagnosis (negative, indeterminate, or positive) is rendered. At MCC, we use an intraoperative IHC cytokeratin stain on the cytologic touch imprints as an adjunct to the Diff-Quick stain; this approach may enhance detection of micrometastases, especially with infiltrating lobular carcinoma or well-differentiated (low-grade) ductal carcinoma. If the diagnosis is positive, one can convert to CLND intraoperatively. Primary diagnoses are made and lumpectomy margins examined with the same touch-print cytology technique[64] [see Figure 9]. The utility of this intraoperative technique has been confirmed by the findings from a large series at the University of Arkansas.[65]

Each SLN is placed in a separate formalin container by the nuclear medicine department staff and quarantined in a dedicated refrigerator with the lumpectomy or mastectomy specimen for 48 hours (six half-lives of ^{99m}Tc) to allow decay of the radioisotope. After this period, the SLNs are catalogued, and one or two blocks of tissue per SLN are submitted for permanent histology. Each block is sectioned at one to three levels per slide, depending on the size of the tissue in each block. In addition, any SLNs that appear free of metastasis both grossly and on hematoxylin-eosin staining are stained with IHC using the avidin-biotin complex technique with diaminobenzidine chromogen.

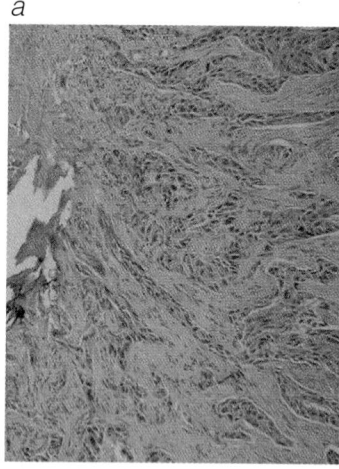 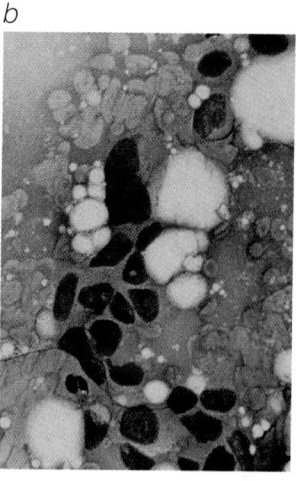

a *b*

Figure 9 **Lymphatic mapping and SLN biopsy for breast cancer. In touch-print cytology, slides are touched to tissue from a "hot" specimen, and cells on the section or the margin are exfoliated onto the slide for cytologic preparation. Shown are (*a*) permanent histology of an infiltrating ductal carcinoma extending down to an inked margin and (*b*) a touch preparation demonstrating bizarre malignant cells from the sampling of the margin. The advantages of this technique are that the entire margin can be sampled and that tissue is not lost in the cryostat.**

Comment One of the greatest advantages of lymphatic mapping is that the surgeon gives the pathologist only one or two SLNs, which allows more detailed examination with such procedures as serial sectioning, immunohistochemical staining, and perhaps RT-PCR analysis.[66,67] Incorporating a more detailed examination into routine practice enables clinicians to detect lesser degrees of disease and upstage a number of breast cancer patients. It was once believed that micrometastatic disease in a single lymph node was clinically unimportant in breast cancer patients because such patients were thought to have the same survival as node-negative patients. This belief has been challenged by studies demonstrating poorer survival in patients who are upstaged with serial sectioning,[68] immunohistochemical staining,[69-71] or RT-PCR analysis.[66,67] In fact, since 1996, immunohistochemical staining and new molecular biology assays for occult metastases have consistently been reported to upstage patients with melanoma,[38] breast cancer,[72] colon cancer,[73] neuroblastoma,[74] prostate cancer,[75] and stomach cancer,[76] and in most cases, this upstaging has proved clinically relevant.

In a series of 255 breast cancer patients who underwent SLN harvesting with detailed pathologic examination at MCC, intraoperative imprint cytology (IIC) with both Diff-Quick and cytokeratin staining was compared with the gold standard, permanent histology with both hematoxylin-eosin and IHC staining.[77] IIC identified only 50% of the patients with metastatic disease. Another way of stating this result, however, is to say that IIC enabled intraoperative conversion to CLND in 50% of patients with axillary metastatic disease, thereby sparing a substantial number of patients a second trip to the OR. Cytokeratin staining of permanent sections was responsible for the detection of disease in 36.2% of patients with metastases; this disease would have been missed by routine examination of one or two nodal sections and hematoxylin-eosin staining. Detailed examination of SLNs reveals nodal metastases in (i.e., upstages) 9.4% of histologically negative patients[77] [*see Figure 10*].

In another series from MCC, cytokeratin IHC staining was performed on 196 SLNs from 95 patients with comedo DCIS.[78] Eight of the 95 (8.4%) had positive SLNs. Routine histology identified the metastatic disease in only two (25%) of the eight patients, whereas cytokeratin IHC staining identified metastases in six (75%). CLND was performed in seven of the eight patients, and the SLN was the only site of disease in all of them. Previous studies have reported that when CLND is performed in DCIS patients, fewer than 1% turn out to have metastatic disease in the regional basin; accordingly, many clinics have eliminated CLND from primary surgical treatment of these patients. Review of these studies, however, shows that the pathologic examination of the nodes in the CLND specimen was superficial. Lymphatic mapping and SLN biopsy permits a more detailed examination of the one or two nodes most likely to contain disease and, consequently, yields a higher rate of identification of metastases: 2% (2/95) with hematoxylin-eosin staining and 6.2% (6/95) with IHC staining in this study.

A major reason to consider lymphatic mapping and SLN biopsy in patients with DCIS is that as many as 20% of cases of DCIS diagnosed by means of stereotactic breast biopsy are subsequently upstaged to invasive cancer when the formal lumpectomy is performed. In addition, lymphatic mapping and SLN biopsy is not as accurate after excisonal biopsy or lumpectomy, particularly for lesions in the upper outer quadrant, where the majority of breast cancers are found. At present, it is probably prudent for surgeons at regional and community hospitals to refrain from performing lymphatic mapping for DCIS patients (except under protocol) until the utility of the technique in this subgroup of patients is established by university centers and national trials.

Currently, the utility of cytokeratin staining of the SLN is being questioned in some quarters. Several breast pathologists (most notably David Page, M.D., of Vanderbilt University) have suggested that in some instances, isolated cytokeratin-positive cells in the SLN may in fact be benign ductal epithelial cells pushed into the afferent lymphatics and lodged in the SLN as a result of trauma to the breast (i.e., the manipulation and massage associated with lymphatic mapping). Nonetheless, at MCC, cytokeratin staining of the SLN is still considered potentially useful for directing the pathologist's search for metastatic disease. It is MCC's policy that before an SLN can be considered positive for metastatic disease, the cytokeratin-positive cells must be confirmed to be malignant through hematoxylin-eosin staining and cytologic evaluation. Only when malignancy has been verified in this way can the patient be classified as having stage II disease.

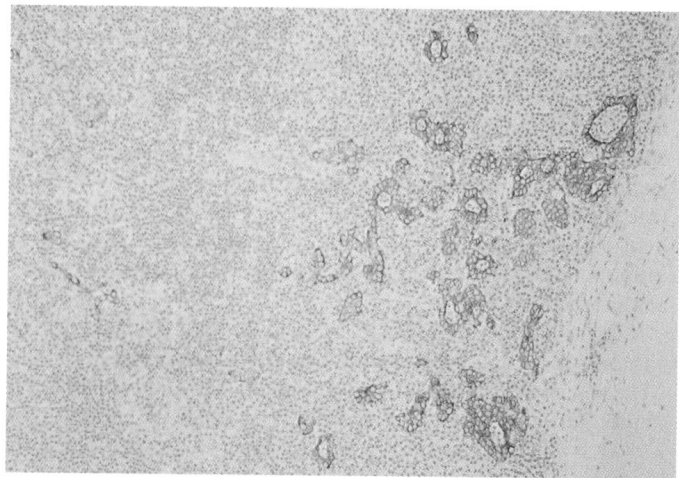

Figure 10 **Lymphatic mapping and SLN biopsy for breast cancer. Cytokeratin immunohistochemical staining finds metastatic cells in 9.4% of breast cancer patients whose SLNs are histologically negative on routine examination.**

COMPLICATIONS

The complications of the procedure are similar to those of melanoma mapping. Surgical site infections occur in fewer than 1% of cases; a seroma develops in about 10%. In our experience, no patients have complained of paresthesia or lymphedema after lymphatic mapping for breast cancer, in contrast to what is usually noted after CLND. Clearly, the complication rate is significantly lower after SLN biopsy alone than when CLND is required as well.[79] Discomfort, impaired mobility, paresthesias, lymphedema, and lancinating sensations are all less common in patients who undergo only SLN biopsy.

REPORTED RESULTS

MCC's initial experience with lymphatic mapping and SLN biopsy for breast cancer was gained between April 1994 and December 1995. All patients who presented to the Comprehensive Breast Cancer Program at MCC with suspected breast cancer were evaluated for enrollment into the study.[53] Enrollment criteria included invasive breast cancer documented by fine-needle aspiration (FNA) or core-needle biopsy [see 2:5 Breast Procedures] rather than excisional biopsy (which meant that the breast lymphatic vessels were unlikely to have been disrupted) and a clinically negative axilla on physical examination. Exclusion criteria included previous incisional or excisional biopsy of the breast cancer [see 2:5 Breast Procedures], a tumor that could not be adequately localized by palpation or stereotaxis, and pregnancy. A total of 62 women were enrolled in the study; their mean age was 60 years (range, 32 to 81 years). Axillary mapping was successful in 57. Of these 57 patients, 51 (89%) had a histologic diagnosis of invasive ductal carcinoma, four (7%) had invasive lobular carcinoma, one (2%) had invasive medullary carcinoma, and one (2%) had invasive tubular carcinoma. The mean tumor size was 2.2 cm (range, 0.4 to 8.0 cm).

All 62 patients were scheduled to undergo either lumpectomy and axillary node dissection (63%) or modified radical mastectomy (37%), depending on the clinical presentation and patient preference. Intraoperative lymphatic mapping with isosulfan blue dye and filtered ^{99m}Tc-SC was performed, followed by SLN biopsy and immediate complete axillary node dissection [see 2:5 Breast Procedures]. In this way, the skip metastasis rate (and hence the false negative rate) could be calculated. Shine-through from the primary site was handled by making a blind incision in the axilla (usually one fingerbreadth beneath the distal edge of the hair-bearing area of the axilla) and dissecting down to the level of the axillary nodes. The handheld gamma probe could then be positioned directly at the level of the nodes, as close as possible to the location of the SLNs and as far as possible from the primary site. This maneuver facilitated recognition of the SLN while reducing the effects of radioactivity from the primary site on the measurements. Accuracy was further enhanced by setting the energy threshold on the probe high enough to eliminate low-energy radioactivity from the primary site, which otherwise could have been redirected into the probe (the Compton effect).

The SLNs were identified and sent to the pathology laboratory as separate specimens. An average of 15.5 non-SLNs per patient and 2.2 SLNs per patient were obtained from the 57 women in whom lymphatic mapping was successful. Eighteen (32%) of the 57 had metastatic disease to the axilla; the number of nodes involved ranged from one to seven. In all 18, the SLNs were positive; thus, there were no skip metastases (i.e., no false negatives). In 12 of the 18, the SLN was the only metastatic site. The metastatic distribution was significantly in favor of SLN involvement ($P \leq 0.001$): 55% of the SLNs were positive for metastatic disease, compared with only 5% of the non-SLNs. The ex vivo activity ratio averaged 39.2. Addition of the radiocolloid technique to the vital blue dye tech-

nique improved the success rate of mapping from 73% to 92% and increased the average number of SLNs harvested per patient from 1.2 to 2.2. In none of the patients was metastatic disease documented in a hot SLN that was not also stained blue. In 12% of patients (mostly women with upper outer quadrant tumors), lymphatic drainage skipped level I nodes and proceeded directly to level II nodes; no direct drainage to level III nodes was observed in these patients.

In 1997, this experience was updated with a report of 466 women with breast cancer who underwent lymphatic mapping and SLN biopsy at MCC after any type of initial diagnostic procedure, including excisional biopsy.[80] Mapping was successful in 440 of the 466. An average of 1.92 SLNs per patient were harvested. One hundred five (23.8%) of the patients had metastases in the SLN; one patient, who had undergone an excisional biopsy, had a skip metastasis, for a false negative rate of less than 1%. Lymphatic mapping was performed in 87 patients with comedo DCIS, and four patients (4.6%) were found to have positive SLNs. As tumor size increased, the number of patients with a positive SLN also increased.

This series currently includes more than 2,000 patients. The success rate for identifying axillary SLNs remains high (about 98%), and the SLN is positive in 25.3% of patients. No additional skip metastases have been identified. For the last 1,850 patients, however, the false negative rate is being determined on the basis of nodal recurrence in long-term follow-up after a negative SLN; the reason is that these patients are not undergoing CLND when the SLN is negative. After a mean follow-up of 36 months, no axillary nodal recurrences have been observed in this patient group.[81]

If mapping fails in vivo, CLND is performed and an attempt is made to identify an axillary hot spot ex vivo. Occasionally, the SLN can be located when the axillary contents are removed and mapped on the back table to eliminate any shine-through. Although this approach exposes the patient to the morbidity of a CLND, it has an important advantage—namely, that if the SLN can be identified, it can be submitted separately to the pathology laboratory for detailed examination and more accurate staging.

At MCC, when excisional biopsy is done before lymphatic mapping, an average of 2.2 SLNs are removed per patient. In 26% of these cases, three or more SLNs are harvested, and this is the population in which the only skip metastasis has occurred. When lymphatic mapping is done with the tumor intact, an average of 1.8 SLNs are removed per patient. In only 16% of these cases are three or more SLNs excised. Excisional biopsy, whether for palpable tumors or for lesions detected mammographically with needle localization, may well become a thing of the past. In the future, when physical examination or mammography suggests the presence of breast cancer, the diagnosis is likely to be made with minimally invasive techniques, such as FNA or core-needle biopsy. Once the diagnosis is made, lymphatic mapping can be done to minimize unnecessary dissection.

Clinical Implications

It has been suggested that axillary dissection should no longer be performed in women with breast cancer[62,82,83]; however, given the importance of regional node status, it makes sense to continue to perform an axillary staging procedure. The problem is that axillary nodal dissection is associated with significant complications that can lengthen hospital stay, increase cost, and cause the patient considerable discomfort.[84-86] There are numerous reports in the literature suggesting that lymphatic mapping techniques can be used in breast cancer patients to reduce this morbidity.[53,87,88] Initial reports from the John Wayne Cancer Center in Santa Monica,

California,[87] (using blue dye only) and the University of Vermont[88] (using radiocolloid only) documented success rates of 65% and 71%, respectively, for SLN identification; combining the two mapping techniques, as is done at MCC, increases the success rate of SLN localization and makes the technique easier and more widely applicable. Those patients who are SLN negative (approximately 75% of all patients) can be spared having to undergo CLND.

Breast cancer centers across the world have now studied more than 10,000 women with breast cancer who have undergone lymphatic mapping and SLN harvesting. The mapping techniques vary slightly from center to center; however, most have attained similarly high success rates, which argues strongly for the viability of the procedure. Sensitivity and diagnostic accuracy rates for SLN identification have consistently been higher than 95%, and the false negative rate has ranged from 0% to 10%. This combined experience suggests that lymphatic mapping has the potential for changing the standards for surgical management of breast cancer in the same way that it has already changed the standards for surgical management of melanoma in the United States.

Discussion

Training and Credentialing

Credentialing criteria for new operative procedures have traditionally been under the jurisdiction of local hospital credentialing committees. When new technology becomes available, adequate training is essential, both to ensure that surgeons can perform the new procedure with confidence and to minimize any medicolegal problems. The American College of Surgeons has a committee (the Committee on Emerging Surgical Technology and Education) that monitors this activity. With some new techniques (e.g., laparoscopic cholecystectomy and image-guided breast biopsy), hospitals have required surgeons to attend formal training courses and to have their first cases proctored by surgeons experienced in the new technique before they are allowed to perform the procedure on their own.

National organizations continue to struggle with the problem of educating and credentialing surgeons to perform new procedures. This problem takes on increasing urgency as medicolegal issues proliferate, as other specialists begin to move into areas once generally considered to be the domain of surgeons (e.g., radiologists doing breast biopsies), and as new technical developments promise to revolutionize surgical care. In an effort to address this problem as it bears on lymphatic mapping, the American College of Surgeons, in association with MCC, has initiated a program designed to investigate how best to train teams (comprising surgeons, nuclear medicine physicians, radiologists, and pathologists) in the new technology. The formal training course is a 2-day session composed of didactic lectures, live surgery (including extensive surgeon-audience interaction during the procedure), and a hands-on animal laboratory. The program offers mentoring of initial cases as registrants go back to their institutions, maintains national registries on the World Wide Web so that different experiences with the technique can be compared, and, finally, facilitates the participation of other university and community physicians in national protocols [see National Protocols, below]. Further information may be obtained from the Center for Minimally Invasive Surgical Techniques (888-456-2840; www.slnmapping.org). Participation in programs such as this one provides a certain degree of protection against medicolegal risk as new technology and procedures are introduced.

The varied experience reported to date provides some idea of the learning curves associated with lymphatic mapping. For melanoma, the learning curve for mapping with vital blue dye alone is about 60 cases, which is more than many surgeons see in their entire career.[15,16] In contrast, gamma probe–guided resection of radiolabeled lymph nodes is readily mastered: even with minimal experience, the success rate of SLN localization approaches 98%. Combination mapping techniques further increase the success rate and abbreviate the learning curve.

For breast cancer, it has been suggested that the learning curve for lymphatic mapping is about 30 cases. In all of these first 30 patients, SLN harvesting should be followed by CLND; perhaps 10 of the 30 will have metastatic disease. The success rate for finding the axillary SLN should be 85% or higher, with no more than one skip metastasis identified in the first 10 patients with metastatic disease, before one can consider dropping CLND in SLN-negative patients. More than one surgeon can train on the same case, and the final decision as to when an institution is ready to drop full dissection after a negative SLN should be made in conjunction with the medical and radiation oncologists at the institution as well as with the credentialing committee. Clinicians at MCC examined the learning curves of five surgeons who performed more than 700 lymphatic mappings to find axillary SLNs in patients with breast cancer.[89] Learning curves were generated for each surgeon by plotting the failure rate against the number of cases. The failure rate was high (20% to 30%) in the first 20 patients but fell rapidly thereafter. The results of the study indicate that 23 cases and 53 cases are required to achieve success rates of 90% and 95%, respectively. The alternative (subareolar and intradermal) injection techniques mentioned earlier, by making SLNs easier to identify and harvest, should help make the learning curves somewhat less steep.

National Protocols

The first national multicenter study addressing lymphatic mapping for melanoma was the Multicenter Selective Lymphadenectomy Trial (Donald Morton, M.D., principal investigator), which began in 1998 and remains in progress under the sponsorship of the NCI (Grant No. PO1 CA29605-12). This trial focuses on the effect of lymphatic mapping and SLN biopsy on survival. Melanoma patients with intermediate or thick tumors (≥ 1.0 mm) are randomly selected to receive either WLE plus observation of the nodal basins or WLE plus SLN harvesting. The study differs from previous studies of ELND in that only some of the patients (i.e., those with a positive SLN) undergo CLND. If this study demonstrates a survival benefit, then there will be two good reasons to perform SLN: (1) to remove the node at highest risk for metastatic disease, so that CLND may be performed with a view to improving survival, and (2) to identify patients who are candidates for adjuvant therapy.

The second national trial that has been initiated to examine the role of this new procedure in treating melanoma is the industry-sponsored Sunbelt Melanoma Trial, in which 60 institutions across the country, equally divided between university centers and community hospitals, are participating. In this study, melanoma patients whose tumors are at least 1.0 mm thick are undergoing lymphatic mapping and SLN harvesting. SLNs are examined with routine histology, serial sectioning, and immunohistochemical staining. If an SLN is negative on the initial screen, an RT-PCR assay based on a panel of four melanoma-specific markers (at least two of which must be positive for a positive result) is performed. Patients whose SLNs are negative on histology and RT-PCR assay are observed; patients whose SLNs are histologically negative but positive on RT-PCR assay are randomly selected to undergo either observation, CLND, or CLND plus adjuvant interferon alfa-2b. It is conceivable that patients in the second category might have a very small volume of tumor that is confined to the SLN and thus might be cured with SLN harvesting alone, thereby avoiding the side effects attendant on CLND or adjuvant interferon therapy. Another arm of this trial is designed to focus on the role of adjuvant interferon alfa-2b in patients with microscopic nodal disease. In the cooperative group study that found interferon alfa-2b to be effective adjuvant therapy,[2] 85% of the patient population had gross nodal disease. It remains to be determined whether patients with minimal disease in the regional basin (i.e., those with only one positive microscopic SLN) benefit from this adjuvant therapy. This study has now enrolled more than 1,000 patients.

In July 2001, the Florida Melanoma Trial II was initiated (Douglas Reintgen, M.D., principal investigator). This trial involves the random selection of SLN-positive melanoma patients to undergo either observation of the remaining nodes in the basin plus adjuvant therapy or CLND plus adjuvant therapy. The data suggest that the SLN is the only site of disease in 80% to 94% of cases (depending on whether the initial SLN was harvested with a single-agent or a combination mapping technique); thus, the focus of this study would be on defining the role of CLND in patients with microscopic stage III disease documented by SLN biopsy. This trial is also the first national study to use molecular staging (through RT-PCR assay) to determine SLN status.

In fall 1998, the American College of Surgeons Oncology Group initiated a trial (Armando Giuliano, M.D., principal investigator) in which women with invasive breast cancer undergo lymphatic mapping and SLN biopsy. If the SLN is negative, patients are observed and a blinded cytokeratin analysis is performed; bone marrow staging is also investigated in this part of the study. If the SLN is positive, patients undergo either CLND or observation of the regional basin. It is assumed that all of these women will receive appropriate radiation therapy and postoperative adjuvant therapy. The aims of this trial are (1) to define the role of CLND in women with invasive breast cancer and (2) to begin to assess the clinical relevance of upstaging with IHC, not only in the SLN but also in the bone marrow of women with clinical stage I breast cancer.

In the North American Fareston Tamoxifen Adjuvant (NAFTA) trial (Michael Edwards, M.D., principal investigator), perimenopausal or postmenopausal women are staged with the lymphatic mapping technique; if the SLN is negative, no further surgery is performed. Those patients found to have estrogen receptor–positive or progesterone receptor–positive tumors are then eligible to be randomly selected to receive either tamoxifen or the newer antiestrogen toremifene (Fareston).

Finally, the NSABP (David Krag, M.D., principal investigator) will perform lymphatic mapping and SLN biopsy in women with invasive breast cancer who are undergoing breast conservation. Patients will be randomly selected to undergo either SLN biopsy, followed by CLND only if the SLN is positive, or CLND. Radiation therapy to the breast will be provided to all patients. The goal of the study is to determine whether lymphatic mapping coupled with selective use of CLND is as effective as the standard surgical approach to women with invasive breast cancer (i.e., axillary dissection including level I and II nodes).

Radiation Exposure Guidelines and Policies

The amount of radioactivity injected in the course of lymphatic mapping is minimal: about 450 μCi, on average. By comparison, the amount of radioactivity injected in the course of a typical bone scan is 20 mCi—44 times the lymphatic mapping dose. For the first 100 mappings done at MCC, surgeons and pathologists wore radiation detection badges and rings throughout the procedure, and nuclear medicine technicians swiped the relevant areas in the OR and the pathology laboratory after each case. No significant radiation exposure could be documented. Currently, MCC nuclear medicine technicians routinely come into the OR to calibrate and run the gamma probes, and once the specimen has been removed and processed by the surgeon, they handle the specimen and monitor the radioactivity in each one as it is transported from the OR into the pathology laboratory. A separate room is designated for intraoperative handling of specimens; this is particularly important with breast cancer specimens, for which diagnosis, lumpectomy margin, and SLN status may all be determined intraoperatively. In addition, fresh tissue specimens are removed and snap-frozen for RT-PCR assays and estrogen and progesterone receptor assays. As noted [see Lymphatic Mapping and SLN Biopsy for Breast Cancer, Technique, above], specimens are then placed in formalin for 48 hours, stored in a dedicated refrigerator, and later removed for routine processing.

Our experience in handling specimens at MCC notwithstanding, as investigators begin to create lymphatic mapping programs at their own institutions, state regulatory policies must be consulted and procedures put into place to meet each individual state's requirements. Clinicians may have to reinvent the wheel, in a sense, to convince their hospitals and their colleagues that lymphatic mapping and SLN biopsy can be performed safely and results in no significant radiation exposure or health risk.

Cost Considerations

A cost analysis was performed at MCC in an effort to ascertain the impact of lymphatic mapping on both cost and quality of care for patients with malignant melanoma.[24] A series of 98 consecutive patients registered at the Cutaneous Oncology Clinic from July 1993 to August 1994 were entered into the study and separated into four treatment groups, depending on their primary surgical therapy. Group 1 patients (29%) had thin melanomas (< 1.0 mm thick) and underwent 1.0 cm WLE under local anesthesia as outpatients in the clinic. Group 2 patients (13%) underwent WLE and nodal staging by ELND. Group 3 patients (47%) underwent WLE and nodal staging by lymphatic mapping and SLN biopsy under general anesthesia in the OR. As surgeons became comfortable with lymphatic mapping, it became evident that the procedure could be performed with straight local anesthesia, particularly for groin dissections. Group 4 patients (11%) underwent WLE and lymphatic mapping under local anesthesia. CLND was performed in SLN-positive group 3 and group 4 patients, and the costs of the additional surgery were entered into the analysis. The WLEs of the primary sites were closed primarily in all patients. Patients were discharged immediately after the procedure.

Significant cost savings were achieved in group 4 patients compared with group 3 patients ($t = 5.56$; $P = 0.001$); however, no significant cost savings were achieved in group 3 patients compared with group 2 patients ($t = 0.847$; $P = 0.40$). Morbidity was significantly lower in groups 3 and 4, with an earlier projected return to work or normal activity. The study findings suggest that, given an incidence of approximately 43,000 new cases of invasive melanoma in the United States each year, use of lymphatic mapping to stage the regional nodal basin could, by itself, save the health care system close to $120 million annually. This study illustrates that clinicians can maintain quality of care, reduce complications, and lower costs by incorporating this new technique into the care of melanoma patients. These benefits can be achieved without compromising the essential nodal staging data that are the criteria for entry into adjuvant therapy programs—a crucial point, in that adjuvant therapy is offered only to patients whom it has been proved to benefit.

For breast cancer, lymphatic mapping may yield more dramatic cost savings. It is conceivable that the combination of a number of emerging technologies and techniques (e.g., touch-print cytology for making the diagnosis and examining lumpectomy margins and lymphatic mapping and SLN harvesting for nodal staging) could lead to a scenario in which women with mammographic abnormalities can come to the clinic, have their breast lesion diagnosed, and receive at least surgical treatment (lumpectomy for clear margins and SLN biopsy) within a 3- to 4-hour period. With such "one-stop shopping," the patient need not be admitted to a hospital, enter a formal OR, be subjected to general anesthesia, or undergo axillary drainage after CLND.

References

1. Greenlee RT, Murray T, Bolden S, et al: Cancer statistics, 2000. CA Cancer J Clin 50:7, 2000
2. Kirkwood JM, Strawderman MH, Ernstoff MS, et al: Adjuvant therapy of high-risk resected cutaneous melanoma: the Eastern Cooperative Oncology Group Trial EST 1684. J Clin Oncol 14:7, 1996
3. Veronesi U, Adamus J, Bandiera DC, et al: Inefficacy of immediate node dissection in stage I melanoma of the limbs. N Engl J Med 297:627, l977
4. Sim FH, Taylor WF, Pritchard DJ, et al: Lymphadenectomy in the management of stage I malignant melanoma: a prospective randomized study. Mayo Clin Proc 61:697, l986
5. Balch CM, Soong SJ, Milton GW, et al: A comparison of prognostic factors and surgical results in l,786 patients with localized (stage I) melanoma treated in Alabama, USA, and New South Wales, Australia. Ann Surg 196:677, l982
6. Reintgen DS, Cox EB, McCarthy KS, et al: Efficacy of elective lymph node dissection in patients with intermediate thickness primary melanoma. Ann Surg 198:379, 1983
7. Norman J, Cruse CW, Wells K, et al: A redefinition of skin lymphatic drainage by lymphoscintigraphy for malignant melanoma. Am J Surg 162:432, 1991
8. Reintgen DS, Albertini J, Berman C, et al: Accurate nodal staging of malignant melanoma. Cancer Control: Journal of the Moffitt Cancer Center 2:405, 1995
9. Balch CM, Soong SJ, Bartolucci AA, et al: Efficacy of an elective regional lymph node dissection of 1 to 4 mm thick melanomas for patients 60 years of age and younger. Ann Surg 224:255, 1996
10. Balch CM, Soong SJ, Ross MI, et. al: Long-term results of a multi-institutional trial comparing prognostic factors and surgical results for intermediate thickness melanomas (1.0 to 4.0 mm). Intergroup Melanoma Surgical Trial. Ann Surg Oncol 7:87, 2000
11. Kirkwood J, Ibrahim JG, Sondak V, et al: High- and low-dose interferon alfa 2-b in high-risk melanoma: first analysis of intergroup trial E1690/S9111/C9190. J Clin Oncol 18:2444, 2000
12. Kirkwood J, Ibrahim JG, Sosmon JA, et al: High-dose interferon alfa-2b significantly prolongs relapse-free and overall survival compared with the GM2-KLH/QS-21 vaccine in patients with resected stage IIB-III melanoma: results of intergroup trial E1694/S9512/C509801. J Clin Oncol 19:2370, 2001
13. Wong JH, Cagle LA, Morton D: Lymphatic drainage of skin to a sentinel lymph node in a feline model. Ann Surg 214:637, 1991
14. Alex JC, Krag DN: Gamma-probe-guided localization of lymph nodes. Surg Oncol 2:137, 1993
15. Morton DL, Wen DR, Wong JH, et al: Technical details of intraoperative lymphatic mapping for early stage melanoma. Arch Surg 127:392, 1992
16. Morton DL, Wen DR, Cochran AJ: Management of early-stage melanoma by intraoperative lymphatic mapping and selective lymphadenectomy or "watch and wait." Surg Oncol Clin North Am 1:247, 1992
17. Reintgen DS, Cruse CW, Berman C, et al: An orderly progression of melanoma nodal metastases. Ann Surg 220:759, 1994
18. Ross M, Reintgen DS, Balch C: Selective lymphadenectomy: emerging role of lymphatic mapping and sentinel node biopsy in the management of early stage melanoma. Semin Surg Oncol 9:219, 1993
19. Sappey MPC: Injection, preparation et conservation des vaisseaux lymphatiques. Thèse pour le doctorat en médecine, No. 241. Paris, Rignoux Imprimeur de la Faculté de Médecine, 1843
20. Uren RF, Hoffman-Giles RB, Shaw HM, et al: Lymphoscintigraphy in high-risk melanoma of the trunk: predicting draining node groups, defining lymphatic channels and locating the sentinel node. J Nucl Med 34:1435, 1993
21. Krag DN, Meijer SJ, Weaver DL, et al: Minimal-access surgery for staging of melanoma. Arch Surg 130:654, 1995
22. Krag D, Meijer S, Weaver D, et al: Minimal access surgery for staging regional nodes in malignant melanoma (abstr). Presented at the 48th Cancer Symposium, Society of Surgical Oncology, Boston, 1995
23. Puleo C, Cruse CW, Lowe J, et al: Re-definition of pelvic cutaneous lymphatic drainage based on lymphatic mapping principles (abstr). Presented at the 54th Annual Cancer Symposium, Society of Surgical Oncology, Washington, DC, March 15–18, 2001
24. Reintgen DS, Einstein A: The role of research in cost containment. Cancer Control: Journal of the Moffitt Cancer Center 2:429, 1995
25. Slingluff C, Vollmer R, Reintgen D, et al: Lethal thin malignant melanoma. Ann Surg 208:150, 1988
26. Heaton KM, Sussman JJ, Gershenwald JE, et al: Surgical margins and prognostic factors in patients with thick (> 4 mm) primary melanoma. Ann Surg Oncol 5:322, 1998
27. Meyer CM, Lecklitner ML, Logie JR, et al: Technetium-99m sulfur-colloid cutaneous lymphoscintigraphy in the management of truncal melanoma. Radiology 131:205, 1979
28. Godellas CV, Berman C, Lyman G, et al: The identification and mapping of melanoma regional nodal metastases: minimally invasive surgery for the diagnosis of nodal metastases. Am Surg 61:97, 1995
29. Norman J, Wells K, Kearney R, et al: Identification of lymphatic basins in patients with cutaneous melanoma. Semin Surg Oncol 9:224, 1993
30. McCarthy WH, Thompson JF, Uren RF: Minimal access surgery for staging of malignant melanoma (invited commentary). Arch Surg 130:659, 1995
31. Byrd D, Nason K, Eary J, et al: Utility of sentinel lymph node dissection in patients with head and neck melanoma (abstr). Presented at the 54th Annual Cancer Symposium, Society of Surgical Oncology, Washington, DC, March 15–18, 2001
32. Wells K, Reintgen DS, Cruse CW, et al: Parotid gland sentinel lymphadenectomy in malignant melanoma (abstr). Presented at the International Congress on Melanoma, Sydney, Australia, 1997
33. Albertini J, Cruse CW, Rapaport D, et al: Intraoperative radiolymphoscintigraphy improves sentinel lymph node identification in melanoma patients. Ann Surg 223:217, 1996
34. Nathanson SD, Anaya P, Karvelis KC, et al: Sentinel lymph node uptake of two different technetium-labeled radiocolloids. Ann Surg Oncol 4:104, 1997
35. Wrightson WR, Reintgen DS, Edwards M, et al: Morbidity of sentinel lymph node biopsy (abstr). Presented at the 54th Annual Cancer Symposium, Society of Surgical Oncology, Washington, DC, March 15–18, 2001
36. Alex JC, Weaver DL, Fairbank JT, et al: Gamma-probe-guided lymph node localization in malignant melanoma. Surg Oncol 2:303, 1993
37. Essner R, Foshag L, Morton D: Intraoperative radiolymphoscintigraphy: a useful adjunct to intraoperative lymphatic mapping and selective lymphadenectomy in patients with clinical stage 1 melanoma (abstr). Presented at the 47th Cancer Symposium, Society of Surgical Oncology, Houston, Texas, 1994
38. Wang X, Heller R, VanVoorhis N, et al: Detection of submicroscopic metastases with polymerase chain reaction in patients with malignant melanoma. Ann Surg 220:768, 1994
39. Thompson JF, McCarthy WH, Robinson E, et al: Sentinel lymph node biopsy in 102 patients with clinical stage 1 melanoma undergoing elective lymph node dissection (abstr). Presented at the 47th Cancer Symposium, Society of Surgical Oncology, Houston, Texas, 1994
40. Medina-Franco H, Beenken S, Heslin M, et al: Sentinel lymph node biopsy for cutaneous melanoma of the head and neck (abstr). Presented at the 54th Annual Cancer Symposium, Society of Surgical Oncology, Washington, DC, March 15–18, 2001
41. Gershenwald J, Thompson W, Mansfield P, et al: Patterns of failure in melanoma patients after successful lymphatic mapping and negative sentinel node biopsy (abstr). Presented at the 49th Cancer Symposium, Society of Surgical Oncology, Atlanta, Georgia, 1996
42. Dessureault S, Soong S, Ross M, et al: Improved survival for node-negative patients with intermediate-to-thick melanomas (>1.0 mm) staged with sentinel lymph node (SLN) biopsy (abstr). Presented at the 54th Annual Cancer Symposium, Society of Surgical Oncology, Washington, DC, March 15–18, 2001
43. Haagensen CD: Treatment of curable carcinoma of the breast. Int J Radiat Oncol Biol Phys 2:975, 1977
44. Bonadonna G: Conceptual and practical advances in the management of breast cancer: Karnofsky Memorial Lecture. J Clin Oncol 7:1380, 1989

45. Balch CM, Singletary ES, Bland KI: Clinical decision-making in early breast cancer. Ann Surg 217:207, 1993

46. Frazier TG, Copeland EM, Gallaher HS, et al: Prognosis and treatment in minimal breast cancer. Am J Surg 133:697, 1977

47. Silverstein MJ, Rosser RJ, Gierson ED, et al: Axillary lymph node dissection for intraductal carcinoma: is it indicated? Cancer 59:1819, 1987

48. Silverstein MJ, Gierson ED, Waisman JR, et al: Axillary lymph node dissection for T1a breast carcinoma: is it indicated? Cancer 73:664, 1994

49. Baker LH: Breast Cancer Detection Demonstration Project: five-year summary report. CA 32:194, 1982

50. Dewar JA, Sarazin D, Benhamou E, et al: Management of the axilla in conservatively treated breast cancer: 592 patients treated at Institut Gustave-Roussy. Int J Radiat Oncol Biol Phys 13:475, 1987

51. Veronesi U, Rilke F, Luini A, et al: Distribution of axillary nodal metastases by level. Cancer 59:682, 1987

52. Feinstein AR, Sosin DM, Wells CK: The Will Rogers phenomenon: stage migration and new diagnostic techniques as a source of misleading statistics for survival in cancer. N Engl J Med 312:1604, 1985

53. Albertini J, Lyman G, Cantor A, et al: Lymphatic mapping and sentinel node biopsy in the breast cancer patient. JAMA 276:1818, 1996

54. Povoski SP, Dauway E, Ducatman BS: Sentinel lymph node mapping and biopsy for breast cancer at a rural-based university hospital: initial experience with intradermal and intraparenchymal injection routes (abstr). Presented at the 54th Annual Cancer Symposium, Society of Surgical Oncology, Washington, DC, March 15–18, 2001

55. Bauer TW, Bedrosian I, Spitz F, et al: Subareolar injection simplifies sentinel lymph node mapping for breast cancer (abstr). Presented at the 54th Annual Cancer Symposium, Society of Surgical Oncology, Washington, DC, March 15–18, 2001

56. McCarter M, Yeung H, Yeh S, et al: Radioisotope localization of the sentinel lymph node in breast cancer: identical results with same day vs day-before injection protocols (abstr). Presented at the 54th Annual Cancer Symposium, Society of Surgical Oncology, Washington, DC, March 15–18, 2001

57. Winchester DJ, Sener SF, Winchester DP, et al: Sentinel lymphadenectomy for breast cancer: experience with 180 consecutive patients: efficacy of filtered technetium 99m sulphur colloid with overnight migration time. J Am Coll Surg 188:597, 1999

58. Cox C, Dupont E, Peltz E, et al: Pre-operative detection of internal mammary lymph nodes using lymphoscintigraphy and intraoperative lymphatic mapping for breast cancer encourages excision (abstr). Presented at the 54th Annual Cancer Symposium, Society of Surgical Oncology, Washington, DC, March 15–18, 2001

59. Reintgen DS, Cox C, Shivers S, et al: Final results of the DoD multi-center breast lymphatic mapping trial (abstr). Presented at the 54th Annual Cancer Symposium, Society of Surgical Oncology, Washington, DC, March 15–18, 2001

60. Kern KA: Sentinel lymph node mapping in breast cancer using subareolar injection of blue dye. J Am Coll Surg 189:539, 1999

61. Nathanson SD, Nelson L, Karvelis KC: Rates of flow of technetium 99m-labeled human serum albumin from peripheral injection sites to sentinel nodes. Ann Surg Oncol 3:329, 1996

62. Cady B: The need to reexamine axillary lymph node dissection in invasive breast cancer. Cancer 73:505, 1994

63. Faddis D, Martin D, Recabaren J: The myth of the learning curve in breast sentinel node biopsy (abstr). Presented at the 54th Annual Cancer Symposium, Society of Surgical Oncology, Washington, DC, March 15–18, 2001

64. Cox C, Nicosia S, Ku NN, et al: Touch preparation cytology of breast lumpectomy margins. Arch Surg 126:490, 1991

65. Henry-Tillman R, Johnson A, Massoll N, et al: Intraoperative Touch Prep for Sentinel Lymph Node Biopsy (abstr). Presented at the 54th Annual Cancer Symposium, Society of Surgical Oncology, Washington, DC, March 15–18, 2001

66. Noguchi S, Aihara T, Motomura K, et al: Detection of breast cancer micrometastases in axillary lymph nodes by means of reverse transcriptase-polymerase chain reaction. Am J Pathol 148:649, 1996

67. Schoenfeld A, Lugmani Y, Smith D, et al: Detection of breast cancer micrometastases in axillary lymph nodes by using polymerase chain reaction. Cancer Res 54:2986, 1994

68. International Ludwig Breast Cancer Study: Prognostic importance of occult axillary lymph node micrometastases from breast cancers. Lancet 335:1565, 1990

69. Trojani M, de Mascarel I, Bonichon F, et al: Micrometastases to axillary lymph nodes from carcinoma of the breast: detection by immunohistochemistry and prognostic significance. Br J Cancer 55:303, 1987

70. Springall SJ, Rytina ERC, Millis RR: Incidence and significance of micrometastases in axillary lymph nodes detected by immunohistochemical techniques. J Pathol 160:174, 1990

71. Hainsworth PJ, Tjandra JJ, Stillwell RG, et al: Detection and significance of occult metastases in node negative breast cancer. Br J Surg 80:459, 1993

72. Fields K, Moscinski L, Trudeu W, et al: The use of polymerase chain reaction (PCR) for amplification of cytokeratin 19 (K19) to detect bone marrow micrometastases in breast cancer (abstr). Presented at the annual meeting of the American Society of Clinical Oncology, 1994

73. Greeson JK, Isenhart CE, Rice R, et al: Identification of occult micrometastases in pericolic lymph nodes of Duke's B colorectal cancer patients using monoclonal antibodies against cytokeratin and CC49: correlation with long-term survival. Cancer 73:563, 1994

74. Moss TJ, Reynolds CP, Sather HN, et al: Prognostic value of immunocytologic detection of bone marrow metastases in neuroblastoma. N Engl J Med 324:219, 1991

75. Moreno JG, Crose CM, Fisher R, et al: Detection of hematogenous micrometastases in patients with prostate cancer. Cancer Res 52:6110, 1992

76. Maehara Y, Oshiro T, Endo K, et al: Clinical significance of occult micrometastases in lymph nodes from patients with early gastric cancer who died of recurrence. Surgery 119:397, 1996

77. Ku NN: Pathologic examination of sentinel lymph nodes in breast cancer. Surg Oncol Clin North Am 8:469, 1999

78. Pendas S, Dauway E, Giuliano R, et al: Upstaging DCIS breast cancer patients using cytokeratin staining of the sentinel lymph nodes (abstr). Presented at the annual meeting of the American Society of Clinical Oncology, 1998

79. Temple LKF, Baron R, Fey J, et al: Postoperative symptoms in breast cancer patients are significantly fewer and less severe with SLN biopsy than with axillary lymph node dissection (ALND): baseline and 3-month results from a prospective study (abstr). Presented at the 54th Annual Cancer Symposium, Society of Surgical Oncology, Washington, DC, March 15–18, 2001

80. Cox C, Pendas S, Cox J, et al: Guidelines for sentinel node biopsy and lymphatic mapping of patients with breast cancer. Ann Surg 227:645, 1998

81. Dessureault S, Dupont E, Shons A, et al: Breast cancer patients with a negative sentinel lymph node (SLN) do not need a complete axillary lymph node dissection (CALND) for local control (abstr). Presented at the San Antonio Breast Cancer Conference, San Antonio, Texas, December 2000

82. Morrow M: Role of axillary dissection in breast cancer management. Ann Surg Oncol 3:233, 1996

83. Baxter N, McCready D, Chapman JA, et al: Clinical behavior of untreated axillary nodes after local treatment for primary cancer. Ann Surg Oncol 3:235, 1996

84. Lin PP, Allison DC, Wainstock J, et al: Impact of axillary node dissection on the therapy of breast cancer patients. J Clin Oncol 11:1536, 1993

85. Ivens D, Hoe AL, Podd TJ, et al: Assessment of morbidity from complete axillary dissection. Br J Cancer 66:136, 1992

86. Recht A, Houlihan MJ: Axillary lymph nodes and breast cancer: a review. Cancer 76:1491, 1995

87. Giuliano AE, Kirgan DM, Guenther MD, et al: Lymphatic mapping and sentinel lymphadenectomy for breast cancer. Ann Surg 220:391, 1994

88. Krag DN, Weaver DL, Alex JC, et al: Surgical resection and radio localization of the sentinel lymph node in breast cancer using a gamma probe. Ann Surg Oncol 6:553, 1999

89. Cox CE, Bass SS, Boulware D, et al: Implementation of a new surgical technology: outcome measures for lymphatic mapping of breast carcinoma. Ann Surg Oncol 6:553, 1999

90. Tanabe KK: Lymphatic mapping and epitrochlear node dissection for melanoma. Surgery 121:102, 1997

91. Hung JC, Wiseman GA, Wahner HW, et al: Filtered technetium-99m-sulfur colloid evaluated for lymphoscintigraphy. J Nucl Med 36:1895, 1995

92. Uren RF, Nowman RB, Thompson JF, et al: Lymphoscintigraphy in melanoma patients (abstr). Presented at the Sixth World Congress on Cancers of the Skin, Buenos Aires, Argentina, 1995

Acknowledgment

Figure 2 Tom Moore.

7 SURFACE RECONSTRUCTION PROCEDURES

Joseph J. Disa, M.D., F.A.C.S., Himansu R. Shah, M.D., and Gordon Kaplan, M.D.

General Technical Issues in Plastic Surgical Wound Repair

The key to achieving optimal results in wound closure is correct approximation of the wound edges.[1] Because remodeling scars contract downward, it is essential that the edges be maximally everted to prevent the development of a depression at the closure site.[2] Such eversion can easily be accomplished either with carefully placed simple sutures or with vertical or horizontal mattress sutures. It is also important that closure be performed in layers so as to eliminate dead space. Accurate realignment of wound edges is especially critical with facial injuries. In the case of a defect involving the vermilion border of the lip, it is very helpful to mark the exact position of the lip margin with a marking pen. For a full-thickness laceration of the lip, the mucous membrane should be repaired first with absorbable suture material. The muscle layer should then be repaired with absorbable suture material. Skin closure is performed last.

Fundamental to any plastic surgical wound repair is good suturing technique. Careful handling of tissues and placement of sutures facilitates optimal wound healing and minimizes scar formation. A curved cutting needle is typically used to repair skin. With the surgeon's forearm fully pronated, the point of the needle is passed through the skin and the dermis at right angles to the skin surface. As the forearm is supinated, the curve of the needle causes the point to penetrate the dermis on the opposite side of the wound. At every step, it is vital to cause as little tissue trauma as possible. Gentle pressure on the skin with a closed Adson forceps or a skin hook will achieve eversion of the wound margins and allow proper suture placement without crushing the skin edge. Excessive pressure on the forceps can lead to ischemia of the wound edge and diminish the quality of wound healing.

Plastic surgical repair of an open wound may involve any of the following types of sutures: (1) simple interrupted sutures, (2) vertical mattress sutures, (3) horizontal mattress sutures, (4) subcuticular continuous sutures, (5) half-buried horizontal mattress sutures, or (6) continuous over-and-over sutures [see Figure 1]. No single suturing technique is ideal for all contexts; clearly, individual surgeons have differing preferences depending on the clinical situation or on personal choice. In general, however, simple, subcuticular, and continuous sutures are preferred because they tend to produce less wound edge ischemia and ultimately result in better scars.

Simple interrupted sutures are useful for simple wounds without excess tension. Subcuticular continuous sutures are useful for approximating wound edges without tension after the dermis has been approximated with buried deep dermal sutures. Continuous over-and-over sutures are used for much the same purposes as simple sutures. They can be placed more quickly than interrupted sutures because knots are needed only at the beginning and the end; however, it is harder to distribute tension evenly over a nonlinear wound with a continuous over-and-over suture. When it is not possible to achieve a tension-free environment in which the dermis is properly apposed with buried sutures, mattress sutures may be preferred. These sutures generally provide better eversion of wound edges in areas where significant tension is present (e.g., on the lower extremities or over bony prominences); however, they tend to induce more wound edge ischemia and thus must be placed carefully. Half-buried mattress sutures are commonly employed for anchoring flaps and skin grafts, particularly at the corners.

The type of suture material used depends on personal preference to some extent; however, for the face, permanent suture material (e.g., 5-0 or 6-0 nylon) is generally preferred. Needle marks can be prevented by removing sutures earlier rather than later [see Table 1].

After a suture is placed, care should be taken to tie the knot properly. The knot should be brought to one side of the wound, and the tension should be adjusted so that the skin edges are apposed without compromising the blood supply. The optimal distance between sutures varies depending on the anatomic site undergoing repair; however, on the face, sutures should be approximately 3 to 4 mm apart and be placed 2 mm from the wound edge. Besides sutures, both staples and adhesive strips are currently used for wound closure.

Skin Grafts

Skin grafts are generally used to cover large open wounds that are not infected [see 2:3 Open Wound Requiring Reconstruction]. Healing requires a well-vascularized bed. Use of a skin graft is contraindicated in the presence of any of the following: (1) gross infection, (2) cortical bone denuded of periosteum, (3) a tendon denuded of paratenon, (4) cartilage denuded of perichondrium, and (5) heavily contaminated or irradiated areas (a relative rather than absolute contraindication).

CLASSIFICATION

Skin grafts are divided into two categories on the basis of thickness: (1) split-thickness (or partial-thickness) grafts and (2) full-thickness grafts. A full-thickness graft contains the entire epidermis and dermis, whereas a split-thickness graft contains the epidermis but only part of the dermis [see Figure 2]. Split-thickness grafts are further subdivided into thin and thick split-thickness grafts.

Full-thickness skin grafts can be harvested from the upper eyelid, the buttocks, the arms, the groin, and the postauricular and supraclavicular areas. Such grafts are more often associated with primary contraction than split-thickness grafts are but less often associated with secondary contraction. Full-thickness skin grafts are less likely to become hyperpigmented than split-thickness skin grafts are. Their size is limited by the dimensions of the sites from which they come.

Split-thickness skin grafts can be harvested from the thigh, the buttocks, the back, the abdomen, the chest, and the posterior neck. Split-thickness grafts are more readily available than full-thickness grafts and have better survival rates. Their main disad-

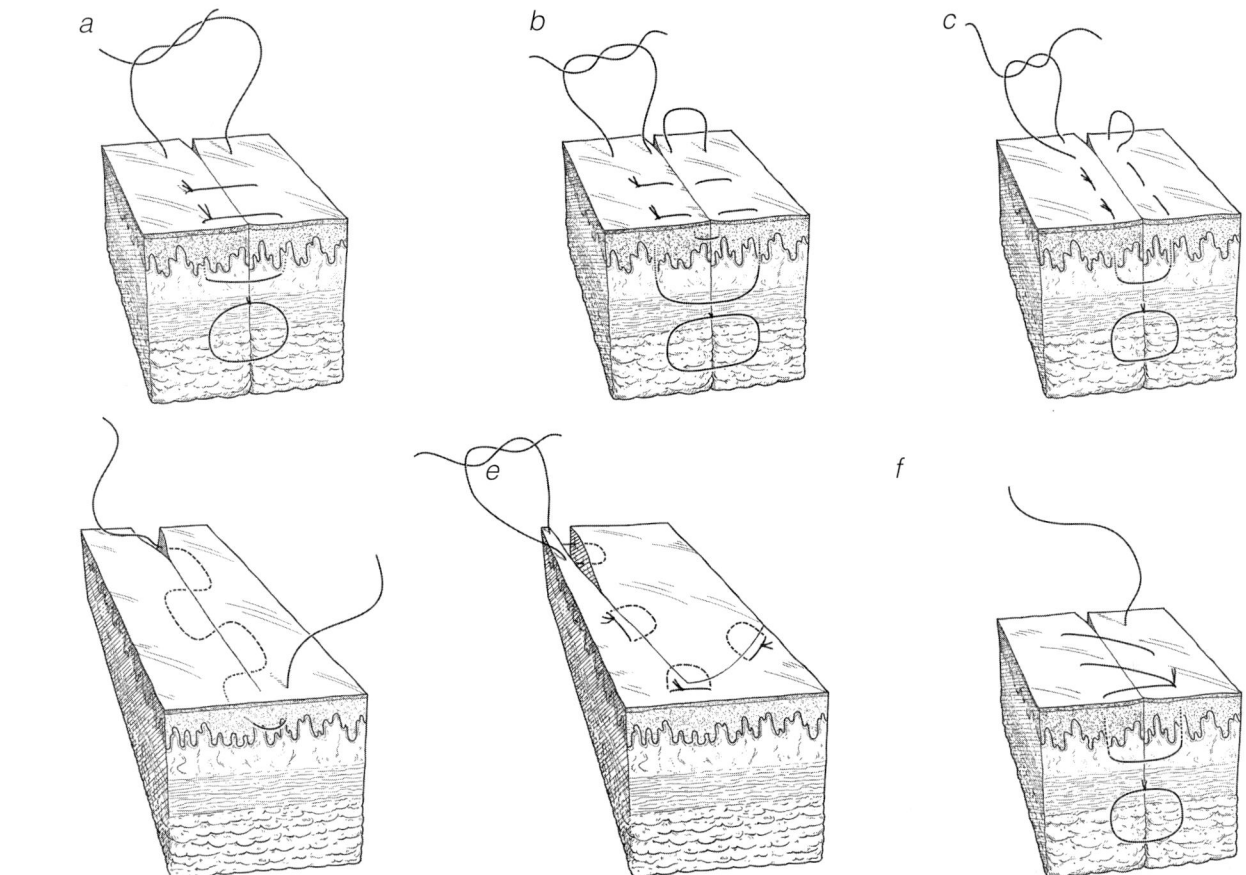

Figure 1 Shown are types of sutures used in plastic surgical wound repair. (*a*) Simple interrupted sutures. An equal bite of tissue is taken on each side of the wound; to ensure eversion of skin edges, a significant amount of deeper tissue is incorporated. (*b*) Vertical mattress sutures. Bites are taken either (1) first close to the wound and then distant from it or (2) vice versa. Bites on either side of the wound must be equally spaced from the skin edges. (*c*) Horizontal mattress sutures. As with vertical mattress sutures, all bites are equally spaced from the skin edges. (*d*) Subcuticular continuous suture. All bites, except for entrance and exit bites, are within the dermis at the same level; the suture should enter and exit the dermis at right angles. (*e*) Half-buried horizontal mattress sutures. These are similar to standard horizontal mattress sutures except that tissue opposite the side where the stitch enters the skin is grasped in the subcuticular level; thus, the needle passes into and out of the epidermis at only two locations. (*f*) Continuous over-and-over suture. This resembles a simple suture except that it is continuously passed through the wound until the desired terminus is reached.

vantages vis-à-vis full-thickness grafts are the increased secondary contraction and hyperpigmentation.

OPERATIVE TECHNIQUE

Full-Thickness Grafts

The recipient site is adequately debrided, and the defect is measured. An outline of the defect is made on the graft site. If the graft is circular, it may have to be converted to an ellipse for smooth closure [*see Figure 3a*]. An incision is made around the outline with a No. 10 or 15 blade. The edges of the graft are elevated with skin hooks. Meticulous dissection is performed in such a way that as little subcutaneous tissue as possible is included with the graft [*see Figure 3b*]. Once the graft is harvested, any subcutaneous tissue is sharply removed (a step known as defatting the graft). The graft is then wrapped in a saline-soaked sponge until ready for use.

The graft is properly positioned and secured with absorbable sutures [*see Figure 3c*]. A tie-over bolster dressing is applied—typically, Xeroform wrapped around cotton soaked with mineral oil

or saline [*see Figure 3d*]. The donor site closure is then closed, either in two layers (for thicker donor sites such as the groin) or in a single layer (for thinner donor sites such as the eyelid).

Table 1 Optimal Timing of Suture Removal after Wound Closure

Closure Site	Optimal Suture Removal Time (days after closure)
Eyelid	3–5
Face	5–7
Lip	5–7
Hands/feet	10–14
Trunk	7–10
Breast	7–10

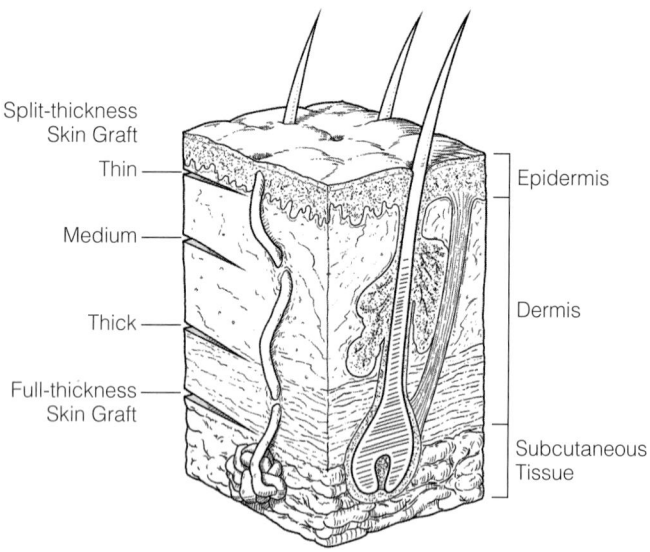

Figure 2 **Skin grafts. Shown are the layers of the skin in cross section. The levels at which split-thickness and full-thickness skin grafts are harvested are noted.**

Split-Thickness Grafts

A split-thickness graft may be harvested with a Humby knife, a Weck blade, or a power-driven dermatome. Currently, a power-driven dermatome is the most common choice.

Harvesting and placement of a split-thickness skin graft is a relatively simple technique; however, attention to detail is necessary to optimize graft take. The key to how well a skin graft takes is the quality of the recipient bed; the relevant contraindications should be kept in mind (see above).

The recipient wound is debrided until a uniform bleeding surface is encountered. Extra care should be taken to debride areas of nonviable tissue because the graft will not take in such areas. The defect is then measured [*see Figure 4a*], and the donor site is marked to indicate an appropriately sized graft. If the donor site is hairy, it is shaved before the graft is harvested. Any preparation solution remaining on the donor site is cleaned off, and mineral oil is applied to lubricate the skin.

Next, the dermatome is prepared by inserting the blade and securing it by tightening the screws [*see Figure 4b*]. The graft thickness is determined by the calibration gauge, which, for most split-thickness grafts, is typically set at 14 (a setting equivalent to 0.014 in. or approximately 0.356 mm). The skin surface is smoothed with gentle but steady traction to facilitate the harvest. Using an assistant for traction of the skin in all directions is very helpful [*see Figure 4c*]. The dermatome is turned on and placed to engage the skin either parallel to it or at a slight angle [*see Figure 4d*]. The dermatome is slowly advanced until an adequate amount of skin is harvested. The graft can then be applied to the recipient area either with or without meshing.

Meshing a skin graft can be advantageous, first, because it allows a smaller graft to cover a larger area, and second, because it provides interstices through which fluid can drain in exudative environments. Meshed grafts generally take longer to heal than nonmeshed grafts do because the interstices must

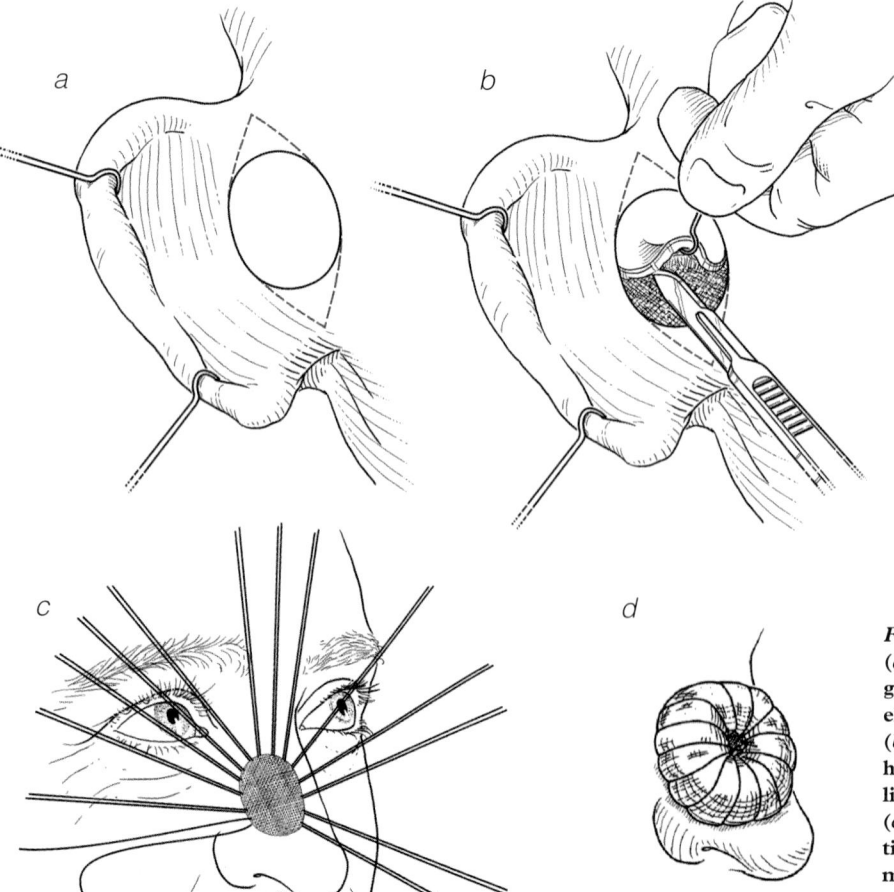

Figure 3 **Skin grafts: full thickness. (*a*) A retroauricular full-thickness skin graft is outlined; conversion to an elliptical shape may facilitate closure. (*b*) The graft is elevated with skin hooks, with care taken to include as little subcutaneous tissue as possible. (*c*) The graft is sutured in place. (*d*) A tie-over bolster dressing is applied to maintain pressure on the graft and ensure good contact between it and the recipient bed.**

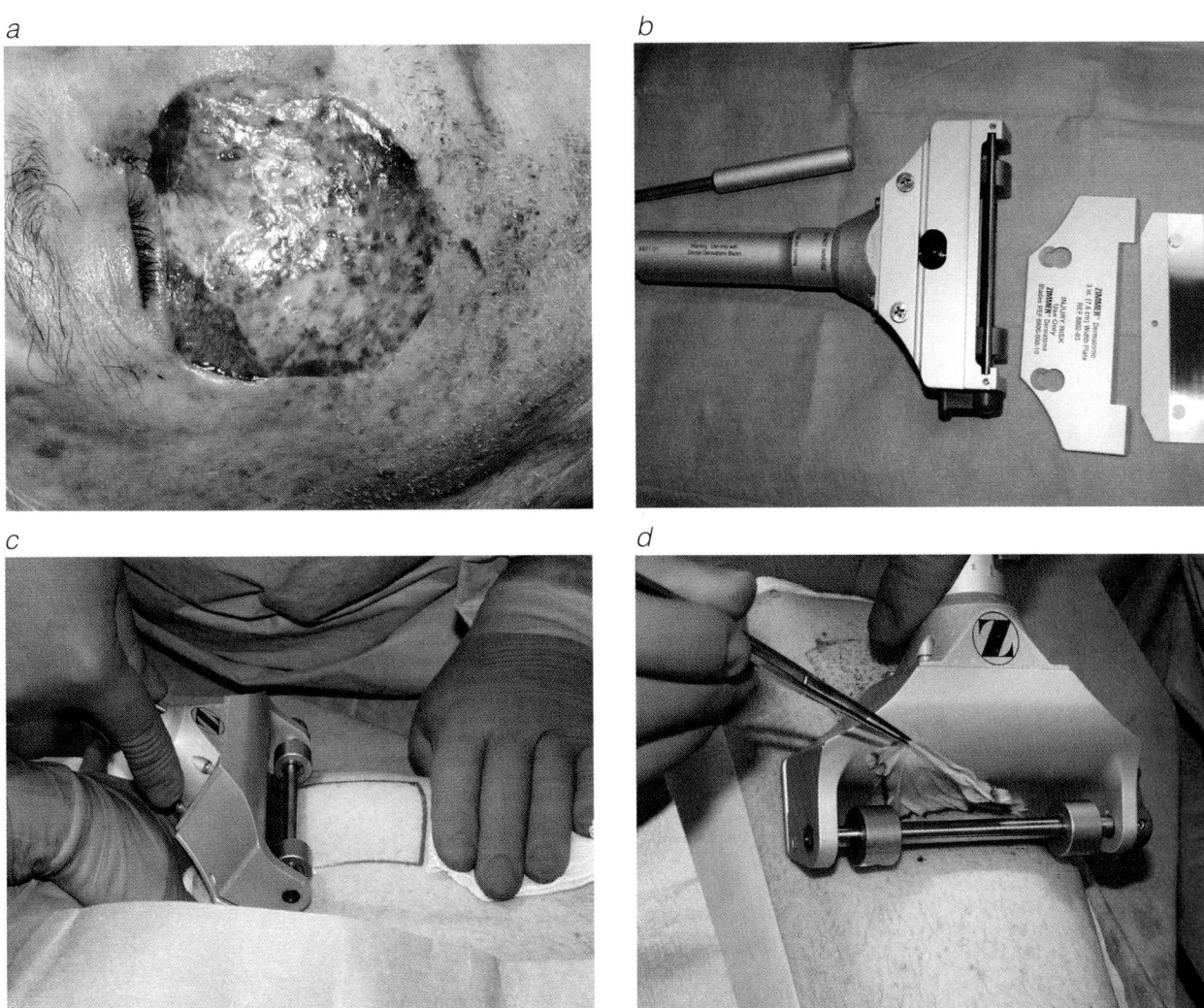

Figure 4 Skin grafts: split thickness. (*a*) Shown is a cheek defect after excision of a melanoma in situ. (*b*) A dermatome is used to harvest the graft. It is set to obtain a specific thickness of skin; 0.014 in. (0.356 mm) is a common setting. (*c*) The graft is harvested by applying steady pressure to the skin with the dermatome while advancing it forward. The assistant retracts the skin to optimize contact between blade and skin. (*d*) The skin is gently removed from the dermatome. If necessary, it can be meshed to increase its size.

contract and fill with scar tissue; in addition, meshed grafts often heal with a cobblestone appearance. There are two basic types of graft meshers, those that contain grooved meshing boards and those that do not. Expansion ratios range from 1.5:1 to 3:1. The desired ratio is selected by choosing either the appropriate meshing board or the appropriate cutting blade, depending on the type of mesher used. In most circumstances, an expansion ratio of 1.5:1, which increases surface area by 50%, is sufficient. On rare occasions, an expansion ratio of 3:1 is needed, depending on the availability of donor sites in relation to the requirements of the recipient area. The graft to be meshed is placed with the dermis side up on the grooved side of the meshing board. The meshing board is rolled through the mesher, and the meshed graft is ready for final placement over the recipient site.

The skin graft is secured to the recipient bed either with absorbable suture material or with staples [*see Figure 5a*]. A bolster dressing, made of Xeroform and of cotton soaked in saline or mineral oil, is applied over the graft. The bolster is fixed in place either by tying sutures over it (for broad, flat areas such as the trunk or the face) [*see Figure 5b*] or by wrapping gauze or an elastic bandage (or both) around it (for curved areas such as the extremities). For a graft on an extremity, splinting may be necessary for immobilization. The donor site is then dressed with an occlusive dressing such as Op-Site or a semiocclusive dressing such as Xeroform until reepithelialization occurs [*see Figure 5c*].

POSTOPERATIVE CARE

The postoperative fate of a skin graft is largely determined by the circumstances of the wound (especially the presence or absence of infection) and the technical execution of the grafting procedure.[3] Successful healing of skin grafts requires immobilization of the recipient site for 5 to 7 days. Immobilization can be accomplished with tie-over bolsters; on extremities, skin grafts can be further immobilized with plaster casts. Proper immobilization is critical for graft survival because it prevents shearing in the plane between the graft and the wound bed. After 5 to 7 days of immobilization, either a gauze dressing such as Xeroform or a lubricating antibiotic ointment should be applied for another 5 to 7 days.

a

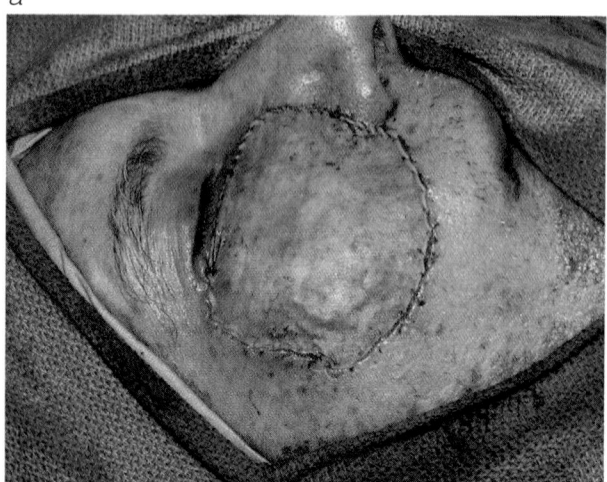

c

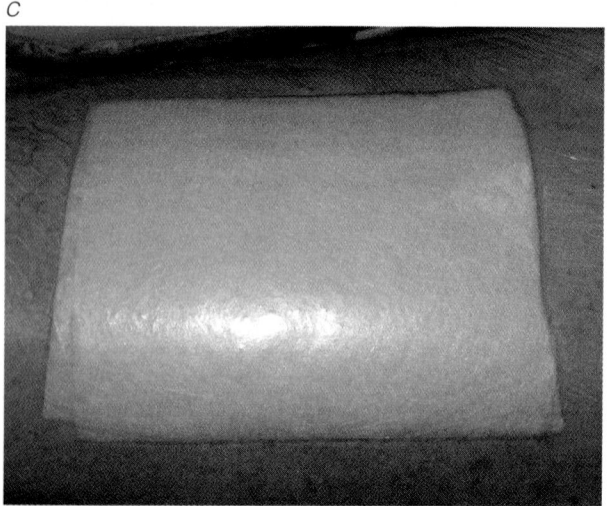

b

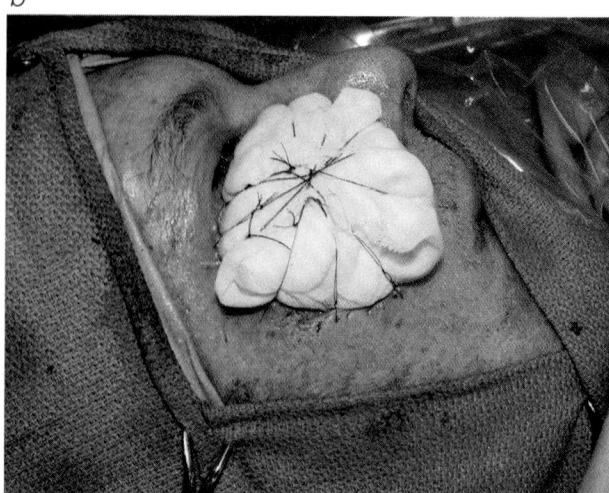

Figure 5 **Skin grafts: split thickness. (*a*) The skin graft is sutured in place. Care is taken to trim all excess skin and to ensure that the graft is in complete contact with the bed. (*b*) A tie-over bolster dressing is applied. (*c*) The donor site is dressed. In this case, calcium sodium alginate is applied to the bed, followed by a bio-occlusive dressing. The dressing is left intact until reepithelialization occurs (typically, 7 to 10 days).**

Grafts that are treated by closed methods (i.e., tie-over bolsters) are carefully observed for evidence of infection. Developing erythema or suppuration is an indication for immediate removal of the bolster dressing and inspection of the graft. A graft threatened by infection may be saved by switching to an open method of graft care with wet dressings changed three or four times a day.

Nonmeshed grafts may form a hematoma or seroma that will prevent the graft from taking. Fluid accumulation should be evacuated by puncturing the graft or by rolling cotton-tipped swabs over it until the fluid escapes from under its edges. Survival of the entire graft is possible if fluid is meticulously evacuated within the first few days after graft placement.

Meshed grafts are not subject to the problem of fluid accumulation, nor are they as vulnerable as nonmeshed grafts to the shear forces that can prevent graft survival. For meshed grafts, the postoperative goal is to prevent desiccation, because they are more exposed to the environment. Gauze dressings such as Xeroform should be placed over the graft and changed once a day. After 2 weeks, the dressings can be discontinued, but the graft should be kept well lubricated with either a skin cream or cocoa butter.

Meshed grafts that are placed over wounds at high risk for infection should be aggressively managed postoperatively with wet dressings changed three or four times a day. The dressing changes will not interfere with graft take and will maximize graft survival in the face of heavy bacterial contamination.

Extremities that are recipient sites for skin grafts should always be maintained above heart level for a minimum of 1 week postoperatively. Lower extremities with skin grafts, particularly below the knee, should remain elevated for a minimum of 10 days to 2 weeks. Patients should also be mobilized in a progressive manner, beginning with brief periods of limb dangling. Premature ambulation of patients with lower-extremity skin grafts can result in loss of the skin graft despite an early appearance of complete graft take.

Donor sites of split-thickness grafts heal by epithelialization. They are best managed by coverage with a gas-permeable polyurethane film dressing such as Op-Site. This dressing retains moisture underneath, which favors rapid reepithelialization. It is also impermeable to bacteria. The addition of calcium sodium alginate (Kaltostat) under the Op-Site facilitates the absorption of the fluid that tends to collect there, thus further simplifying donor site management.[4]

Local Flaps

CLASSIFICATION

Flaps are classified according to the types of tissue that they contain, their blood supply [*see Figure 6*], and the method by which they are moved from the donor to the recipient site.

Tissue Contents

Flaps commonly consist of skin and subcutaneous tissue alone. However, they may also consist of skin combined with muscle, fascia, or bone; in these cases, the flaps are called myocutaneous, fasciocutaneous, or osteocutaneous, respectively. If a flap composed of skin and subcutaneous tissue that contains a known major artery (an axial-pattern, or arterialized, skin flap [*see* Blood Supply, *below*]) is raised at the donor site and remains attached

RANDOM PATTERN   AXIAL PATTERN   MYOCUTANEOUS

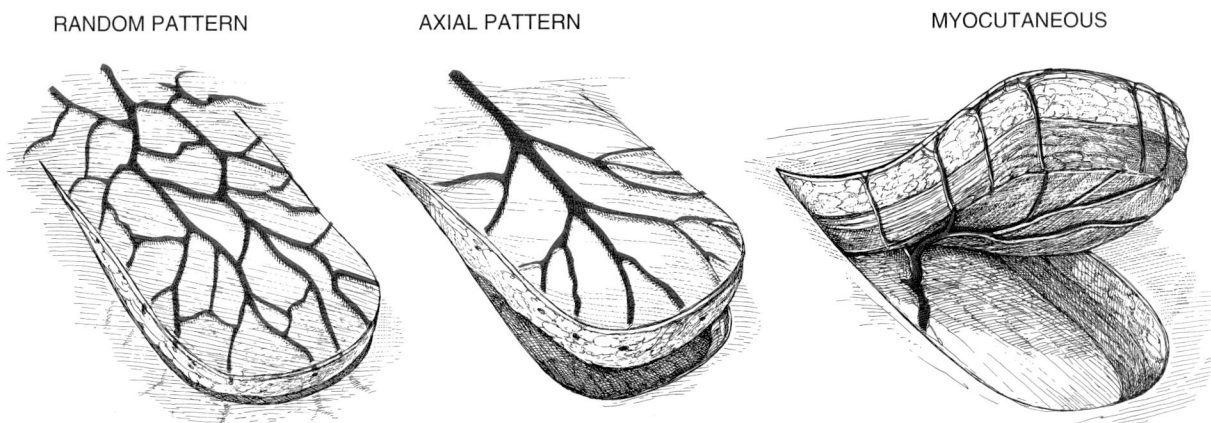

Figure 6   Local flaps. A random-pattern skin flap (left) is supplied by a subdermal plexus of small vessels that do not have an axial orientation. An axial-pattern skin flap (center) is designed parallel to the axis of a known major subcutaneous artery. It can have a greater length:width ratio because its blood supply is more reliable. A myocutaneous flap (right) derives the blood supply of its skin component from vertical perforators from the underlying muscle. The skin can be completely isolated over the muscle as an island.

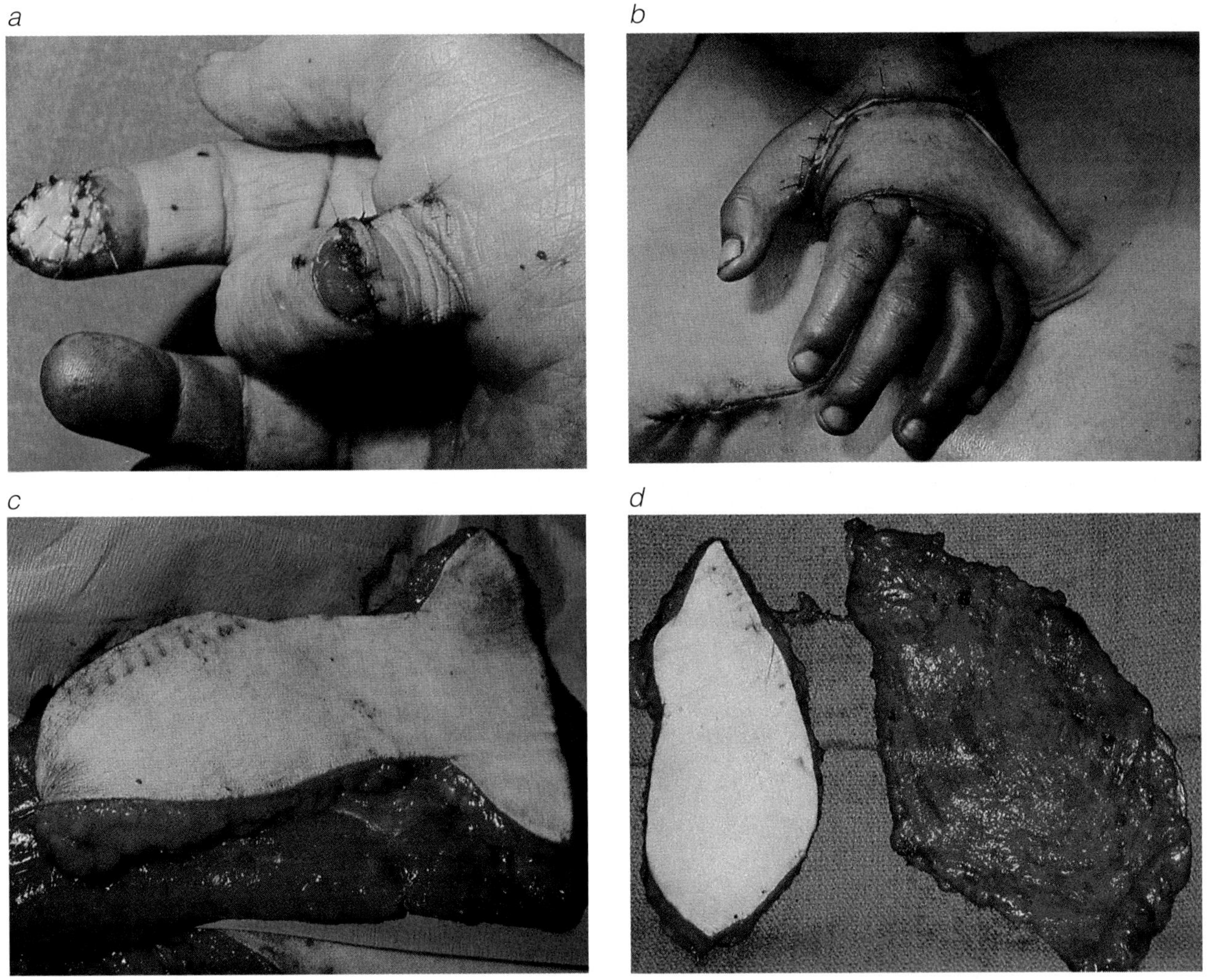

a   *b*

c   *d*

Figure 7   Local flaps. (*a*) The blood supply of random-pattern skin flaps is limited; only small flaps (e.g., thenar flaps, shown here), are consistently reliable. (*b*) Shown is an axial-pattern skin flap. (*c*) The skin and subcutaneous tissue of a myocutaneous flap can exist as a complete island because the blood supply is derived from vertical muscular perforators. (*d*) Shown are a large free flap of scapular area skin and the entire latissimus dorsi. The subscapular vessels that connect the two will supply both components of the flap after microvascular anastomoses.

only by the vascular pedicle, it is termed an island flap. The same flap is termed a free flap if the vascular pedicle is severed, the flap is transferred to a distant recipient site, and its circulation is restored by microvascular anastomoses.

Blood Supply

The earliest flaps in common use were skin flaps that had what is known as a random-pattern type of circulation [see Figure 7a], in which blood is supplied by the subdermal capillary plexus rather than by a major, named vessel.[5] The precarious nature of the blood supply of such flaps severely limited flap design and resulted in a preoccupation with suitable length:width ratios. Greater length:width ratios became possible after the empirical discovery that a more vigorous circulation develops in flaps raised in stages (the delay phenomenon).[6]

The next flaps to come into common use had an axial-pattern type of circulation, in which a sizable artery coursed directly to a specific cutaneous territory [see Figure 7b]. The groin was the first region where this arrangement was carefully described, and it remains a useful source of flaps for selected applications. Because longer flaps can be made in areas where the blood supply has an axial pattern, the length:width ratio and the delay phenomenon became less important issues.[7] Identification of an axial-pattern blood supply to a given graft allows so-called islanding of the graft from the donor site except for the vascular connection, which is preserved. Such island flaps have greater mobility than flaps with a less attenuated attachment to the donor site.

A third type of flap was based on the myocutaneous blood supply, a network of vessels that perforate muscles vertically and supply the overlying skin [see Figures 7c, d]. These vessels are not necessarily the exclusive supply to the skin in a specific region, but they are able to support the skin entirely when other sources of blood supply are eliminated. Investigation of the body musculature showed that there were at least five basic patterns of blood supply to muscle, distinguished by the existence of and balance between primary pedicles and secondary sources of supply [see Figure 8]. Some muscles can be rotated or transposed as myocutaneous flaps on the basis of either their dominant or secondary blood supply (e.g., pectoralis major and latissimus dorsi). Some muscles have two dominant supplies and can be transposed on either one (e.g., rectus abdominis). Other muscles do not reliably support skin territories supplied by minor pedicles (e.g., gracilis).

Other patterns of cutaneous blood supply are now well recognized. Fasciocutaneous flaps with high length:width ratios can be reliably raised on the trunk, arms, and legs. The blood supply of deep fascia appears to consist of both a deep and a superficial fascial plexus. These vessels connect both to perforating vessels from the underlying muscles and to the subcutaneous tissue vessels above them.[8] At least three types of fasciocutaneous flaps may be distinguished on the basis of the fascial blood supply to the skin [see Figure 9].[9]

In some areas, fascia supplies overlying subcutaneous tissue and skin more directly. Such a blood supply is most evident in the extremities, where direct branches from major vessels course through intermuscular septa to reach the deep fascia and supply the overlying skin and subcutaneous tissue. The forearm is a clinically important donor site because thin septocutaneous flaps fed by the radial artery can be raised as either pedicled or

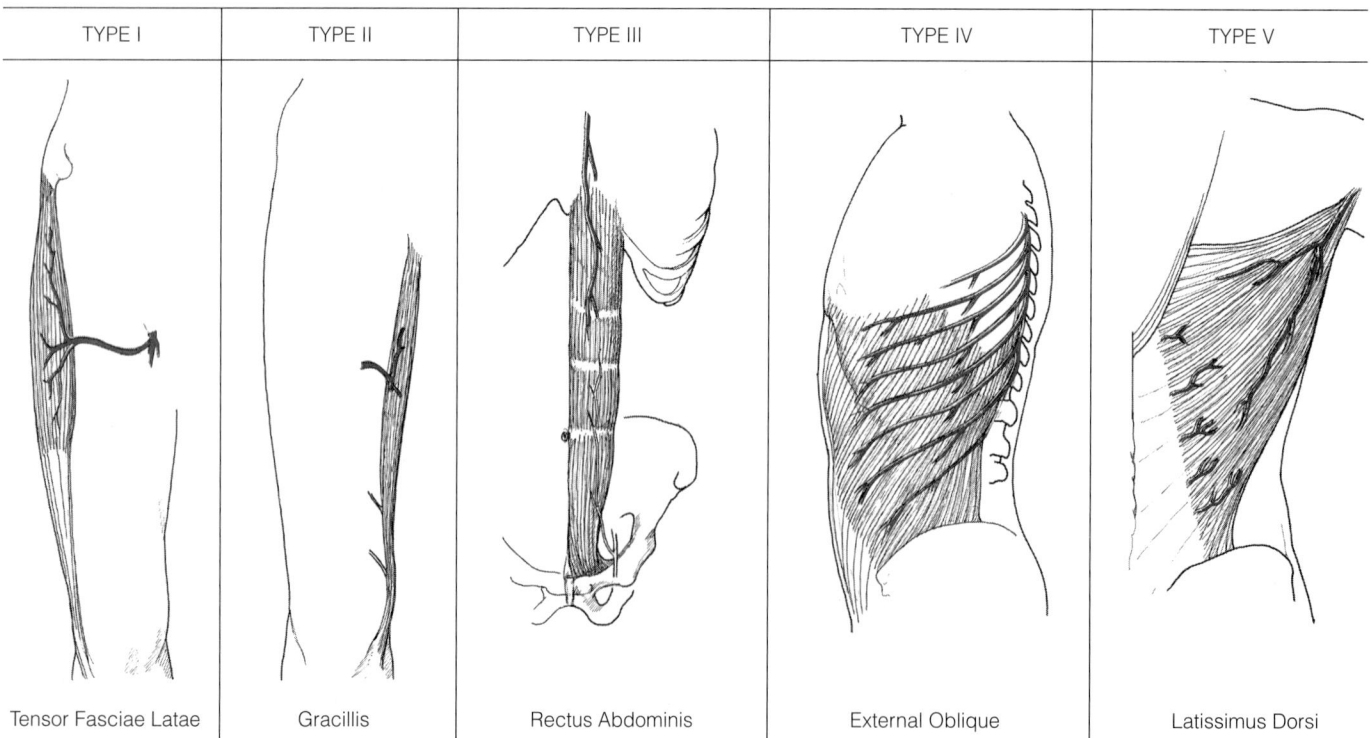

TYPE I	TYPE II	TYPE III	TYPE IV	TYPE V
Tensor Fasciae Latae	Gracillis	Rectus Abdominis	External Oblique	Latissimus Dorsi

Figure 8 **Local flaps. Schematized are the five basic patterns of blood supply to muscle. Individual muscles are classified on the basis of the dominance, number, and size of the vessels that supply them. Type I is supplied by a single dominant pedicle. Type II is supplied by one dominant vessel and several much smaller vessels. Type III is supplied by two dominant pedicles. Type IV is supplied by multiple vessels of similar size. Type V is supplied by one dominant pedicle and several smaller segmental vascular pedicles.**

TYPE A TYPE B TYPE C

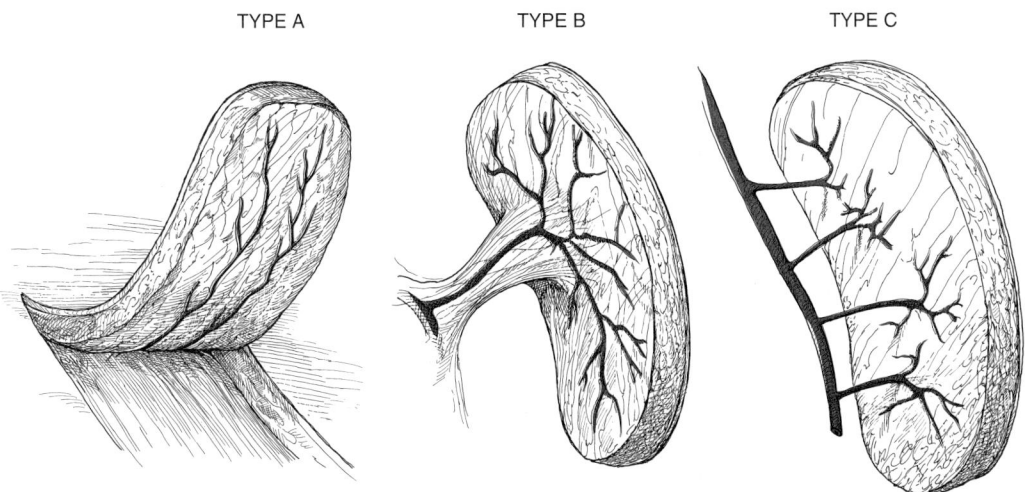

Figure 9 **Local flaps. At least three types of fasciocutaneous flaps exist, categorized by blood supply configuration. Type A is supplied by multiple small, longitudinal vessels coursing with the deep fascia. These flaps must retain a base of a certain width and cannot be raised as islands (e.g., longitudinally oriented flaps of skin and fascia on the lower leg). Type B is supplied by a single major vessel within the fascia (e.g., scapular flap). Type C is supplied by multiple perforating segments from a major vessel coursing through intermuscular septa (e.g., forearm flaps).**

free flaps. Other examples of fasciocutaneous flaps include the lateral arm septocutaneous flap, fed by the profunda brachii artery; the scapular flap, fed by the circumflex scapular artery [*see Figure 7d*]; and the fibular osteofasciocutaneous flap, fed by the peroneal artery.

Method of Movement to Recipient Site

Local flaps may be called either rotation, advancement, or transposition flaps, depending on how they are moved to reach their recipient sites.

A more complete characterization of flaps is achieved by combining all of the descriptive categories mentioned. For example, a muscle and skin flap that is rotated to cover an adjacent soft tissue defect is termed a myocutaneous rotation flap, and a skin and bone flap used to reconstruct a distant composite defect is termed an osteocutaneous free flap.

OPERATIVE TECHNIQUE

In all forms of plastic surgery, it is essential to cause as little tissue trauma as possible when raising a flap. Using skin hooks rather than forceps is helpful in this regard. The flap is marked and incised, and elevation is begun, first with a scalpel and then,

at the base of the flap, with a blunt scissors to keep from disrupting the blood supply. The electrocautery should be used judiciously in the elevation of skin flaps: although cauterization causes less bleeding, skin flaps often rely on the subdermal plexus for perfusion, and this plexus can be damaged by electrocautery dissection. Close attention to atraumatic technique throughout the procedure will result in less edema in the flap and, therefore, less circulatory compromise. Hemostasis is essential; in small flap procedures, bipolar coagulation controls bleeding with minimal damage to the flap's blood supply. Two-layer closure is recommended, with absorbable suture material in the deeper layer to decrease the tension and fine nylon for skin closure.

The recommendations just mentioned apply to local flap procedures in general. In what follows, we describe several different types of local flaps that are useful for the purposes of the general surgeon, and we summarize key technical points specific to each.

Transposition Flaps

A flap that is moved laterally into the primary defect is called a transposition flap. The essential concept in the design of such a flap is to ensure that the flap is long enough to cover the entire defect, so that the transfer can be done without tension [*see Figure 10*].

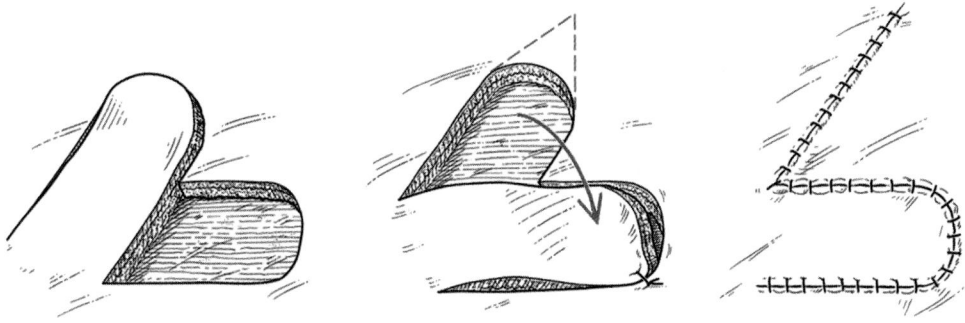

Figure 10 **Local flaps: transposition flap. After excision of the defect, a transposition flap of adequate length is designed and elevated in the subcutaneous plane. The flap is moved laterally into the defect and inset. It may be necessary to excise a dog-ear of excess skin at the tip of the flap harvest site.**

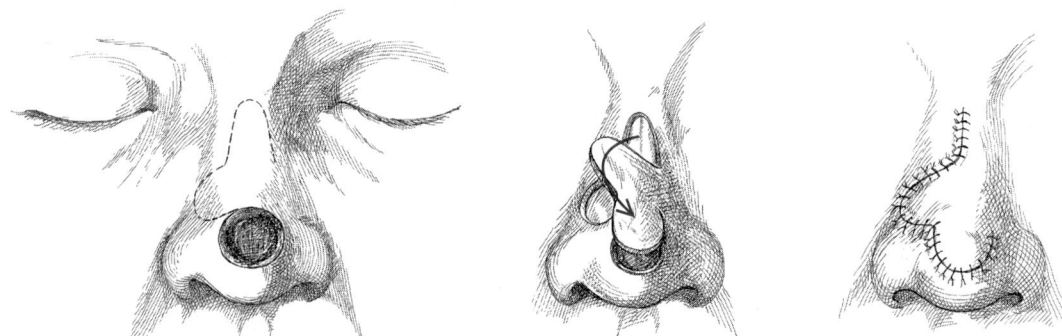

Figure 11 **Local flaps: bilobed flap. A flap with two lobes is created, with the first lobe the same size as the defect and the second lobe substantially (~50%) smaller than the first. The flap is elevated in the submuscular plane. Wide undermining at this level is necessary for tension-free transposition. The first lobe covers the initial defect, and the second covers the defect from the first. The second lobe is placed in an area of loose skin, and its area of origin is closed primarily.**

The skin is marked and incised with a scalpel, and dissection is carried through the subcutaneous fat. The flap is retracted with a skin hook, and dissection is performed with a blunt scissors until the flap is elevated sufficiently to allow it to be transposed into the defect without tension. The secondary defect is closed primarily; alternatively, depending on the location of the donor area and the degree of skin tension present there, a skin graft may be indicated. As with any local flap, wide undermining of the surrounding tissues may be necessary for closure of the defect and the donor site. Closure is then performed in two layers.

Bilobed flap A bilobed flap is a transposition flap consisting of two lobes of skin and subcutaneous tissue based on a common pedicle [*see Figure 11*]. It is often used to correct nasal defects involving the lateral aspect, the ala, or the tip. The keys to a successful bilobed flap are (1) accurate design and (2) wide undermining of the surrounding tissue in the submuscular plane to allow a smooth transposition. The primary lobe is usually at an angle of 45° or less to the defect; the secondary lobe is designed to achieve closure of the donor defect and is substantially smaller than the primary lobe. The angle between the two is 90° to 100°. Both flaps are raised simultaneously in the submuscular plane. Wide undermining of the area (also in the submuscular plane) minimizes tension. The primary lobe of the bilobed flap is transposed into the initial defect, the secondary lobe is transposed into the donor defect left by the primary lobe, and the defect left by the secondary lobe is closed primarily. Closure is accomplished with 5-0 or 6-0 nylon.

Rhomboid flap (Limberg flap) A rhomboid flap is a transposition flap that is designed in a specific geometric fashion [*see Figure 12*]. The initial defect is converted to a rhomboid, with care taken to plan the flap in an area with minimal skin tension. The rhomboid must be an equilateral parallelogram with angles of 60° and 120°; this design allows the surgeon to excise less tissue than would be needed for an elliptical flap. One face of the rhomboid constitutes the first side of the flap (YZ), which should be aligned along the line of maximum extensibility. The short diagonal of the rhomboid is then extended outward for a distance equal to its own length. This extension should be oriented along relaxed skin tension lines, perpendicular to the line of maximum extensibility; it constitutes the second side of the flap (XY). Next, a line parallel to YZ is drawn from X to outline the third side of the flap. Correct orientation of the rhomboid is vital for providing flap repair with minimal tension, particularly with respect to the line of maximum extensibility: it is along this base line that maximum tension results when the donor defect is closed. Once the flap has been correctly designed and elevated, it is transposed into the defect. Closure is done in two layers.

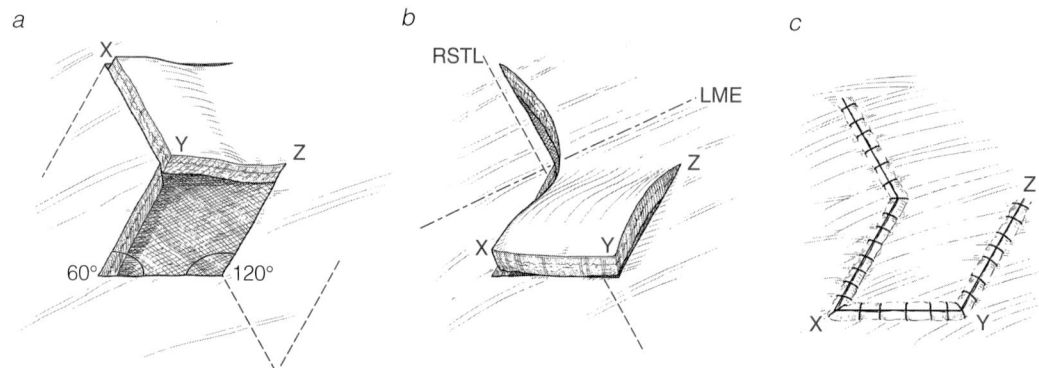

Figure 12 **Local flaps: rhomboid (Limberg) flap. (a) The defect is converted to a rhomboid, with all four sides of equal length and angles of 60° and 120°. An extension XY is made that is the same length as the short diagonal of the rhomboid, and a line of equal length is drawn from X paralleling YZ. (b) The flap is oriented so that XY follows the relaxed skin tension lines (RSTL) and YZ the line of maximum extensibility (LME). (c) The flap is inset.**

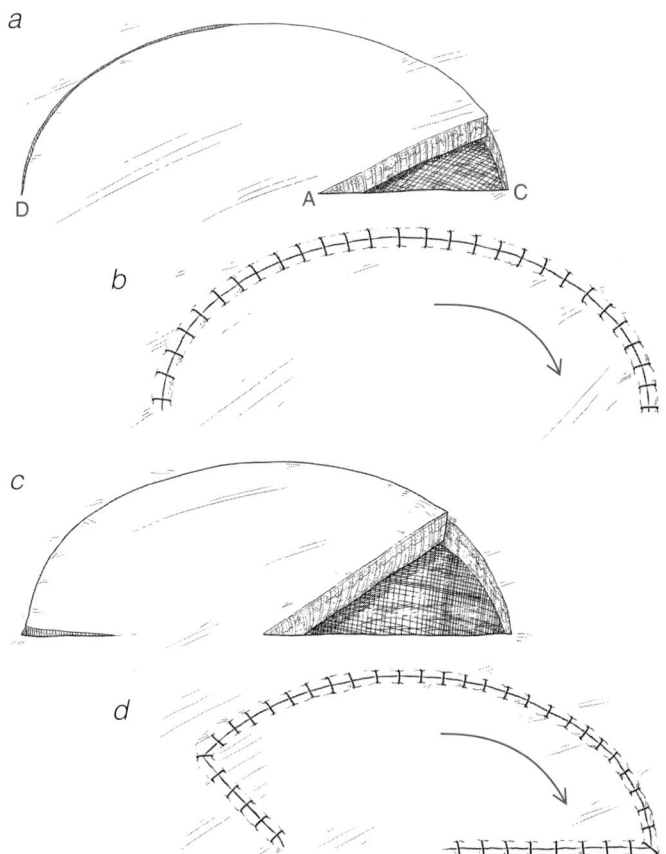

Figure 13 Local flaps: rotation flap. (*a*) The defect is converted into a wedge. One side (AC) is extended to a pivot point D, so that AD is at least 50% longer than AC. A semicircle from C to D is defined. (*b*) The flap is elevated, rotated, and inset. (*c, d*) If there is too much tension, a back cut may be necessary to release the flap and allow rotation. Care is taken not to make the back cut excessively long; to do so could devascularize the flap.

Rhomboid flaps work best on flat surfaces (e.g., the upper cheek and the temporal region). Extra attention to flap design is necessary when an attempt is made to close a defect over a convex surface with a rhomboid flap; improper flap design leads to excessive tension and potential flap necrosis.

Rotation Flaps

A flap that is rotated into the defect is called a rotation flap.[10,11] It takes the form of a semicircle of which the defect occupies a wedge-shaped segment [*see Figure 13*]. The original defect is converted to a triangular shape (ABC). One side of the triangular defect (AC) is extended to a point (D) that will serve as the pivot point for the flap. The distance between A and D should be at least 50% greater than that between A and C. A semicircular line extending from C to D is then defined.

The flap is incised with a scalpel, elevated, and rotated. As with all local skin flaps, wide undermining of the surrounding tissue may be necessary to allow tension-free rotation and wound closure. The flap is secured with a two-layer closure; the secondary defect may be closed primarily. Sometimes, a so-called back cut is required to gain adequate rotation. The most common technical error with rotation flaps is improper design: a flap that is too small will not cover the defect adequately.

Advancement Flaps

Advancement flaps are moved directly forward into a defect without either rotation or lateral movement. The single-pedicle advancement flap is a rectangular or square flap of skin and subcutaneous tissue that is stretched forward. The flap is oriented with respect to the local skin tension, with care taken to plan the advancement in an area where the skin is extensible. A rectangular defect is created, and the flap is elevated in an area of loose skin and advanced to cover the defect [*see Figure 14*]. When closure is performed, some excess skin (dog ears) at the base of the flap (Burow's triangles) may have to be excised.

V-Y advancement flap The V-Y advancement flap is a modification of a basic advancement flap [*see Figure 15*]. The use of a V-Y advancement flap eliminates the need to revise the dog-ears that sometimes result with rotation flaps. When possible, the flap should be oriented in accordance with the line of maximum extensibility. Its length should be 1.5 to 2 times that of the defect in the direction of the closure.

Incisions are made completely through skin. As with other flaps, skin hooks are used to retract the skin flap, and blunt scissors dissection is then performed. The point of the V on the flap is the area where tightness is most frequently encountered; this area may have to be released to facilitate advancement. Care must be taken not to undermine the advancing flap excessively: doing so may impair or interrupt the blood supply to the flap and result in necrosis. Once adequately advanced, the flap is sutured at the advancing edge and at the base of the Y.

Z-Plasty

When reconstruction is indicated for small, localized scars, soft tissue coverage is generally sufficient. With such coverage, there is no threat of breakdown leading to exposure of important structures; instead, the reconstructive problem is generally functional. An example is a tight scar band across a flexion crease, which is commonly seen after a burn injury. A local procedure that rearranges the existing tissue can relieve the tension by making more tissue available in one direction, even though the amount of tissue in the area is not actually increased.

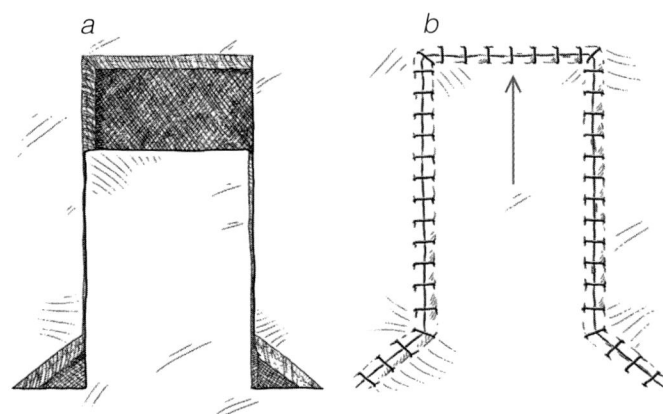

Figure 14 Local flaps: direct advancement flap. (*a*) A flap whose shape corresponds to that of the defect is elevated in the subcutaneous plane and advanced into the defect. (*b*) Excision of Burow's triangles (excess skin at the flap base) may be necessary to permit advancement.

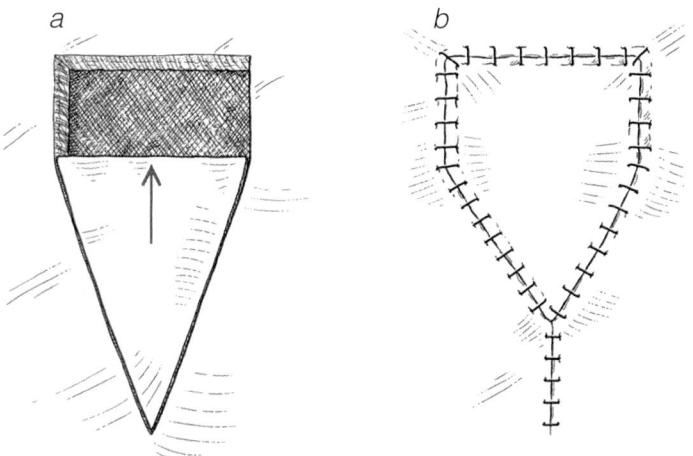

Figure 15 Local flaps: V-Y advancement flap. (*a*) A V-shaped flap is created whose length is 1.5 to 2 times that of the defect. With subcutaneous connections to the skin preserved (because these constitute the blood supply to the flap), the flap is advanced into the defect. (*b*) The V incision is converted to a Y as the base is closed primarily.

The Z-plasty [*see Figure 16*] is an example of such tissue rearrangement.[12] Two triangular flaps are designed so that they have in common a central limb aligned in the direction along which additional length is desired. For example, the limb may be placed along the line of a contracture. Two lines, approximately equal in length to the central limb, are drawn from either end of the limb, diverging from it at equal angles varying from 30° to 90°. The degree of lengthening obtained is determined by the size of this angle [*see Table 2*]. In theory, maximal length gain is achieved by using the largest angle possible, but in practice, the maximum usable angle is determined by the limits of skin elasticity. A 60° angle, which is commonly used, will result in a 75% gain in length along the central limb. Triangular flaps are elevated, and the fibrous tissue band responsible for the contracture is divided. The triangular flaps are transposed and inset, yielding increased length in the desired direction, with the original Z rotated 90° and reversed.

Although Z-plasty is conceptually simple, it is not necessarily easy: experience is necessary for the surgeon to realize the limi-

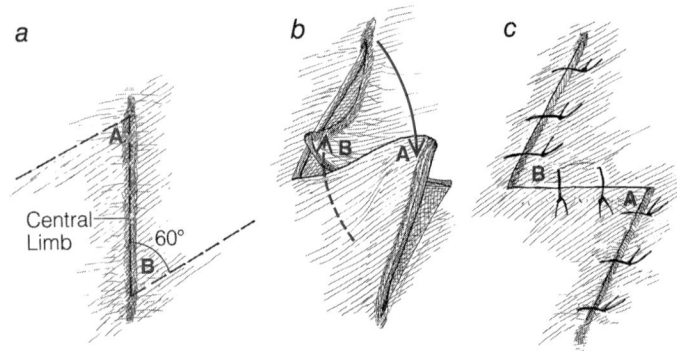

Figure 16 Local flaps: Z-plasty. (*a*) The central limb of the Z is placed along the line of contracture. Incisions diverging from the scar at a 60° angle will yield an increase of approximately 75% in the direction of the central limb. (*b*) The flaps are transposed. (*c*) The length has been increased in the desired direction, and the original Z design has been rotated 90° and reversed.

Table 2 Z-Plasty: Incision Angle and Degree of Lengthening Theoretically Possible

Incision Angle (degrees)	Theoretical Amount of Lengthening (%)
30	25
45	50
60	75
75	100
90	120

tations of technique and appreciate the subtleties of proper design. Important considerations in the use of Z-plasty include appropriate determination of the length of the central limb and correct orientation of the limbs so that the new central limb formed after transposition is parallel to skin tension lines. Multiple Z-plasties may be useful for some localized scars.

POSTOPERATIVE CARE

Local Flaps

The postoperative care of local flaps is not complex. Flap healing is supported by adequate nutrition and maintenance of a normal hemodynamic state, including normal blood volume. Tension must not be placed on the flap. Tension can develop in flaps on the trunk as a result of changes in patient position or in flaps on the limbs as a result of loss of immobilization. Generally, the tip of any local flap is not only its most valuable portion but also its most vulnerable area. At the tip, the blood supply is the most precarious, and the detrimental effects of tension are magnified. Unfortunately, no pharmacologic agents are of proven benefit in preventing necrosis of a flap with failing circulation. Any flap necrosis that might develop should be minimized by preventing infection of the necrotic tissue. Necrotic tissue must therefore be debrided after the extent of tissue loss becomes clear. Portions of the flap that are undergoing demarcation but do not appear actively infected can be protected by the application of a topical antibiotic such as silver sulfadiazine cream (Silvadene).

Extremities that are recipient sites for flaps, like those that are recipient sites for skin grafts, should be elevated after the operation until satisfactory wound healing has occurred.

Free Flaps

Survival of free flaps, unlike that of local flaps, tends to be an all-or-none phenomenon. Careful postoperative monitoring of flap circulation is essential because flap failure is likely to be the result of a problem at the vascular anastomoses. Flaps are usually monitored for 7 days. However, the most critical time for free-flap monitoring is the first 6 to 8 hours because the majority of vascular crises usually occur within this period. Early detection and aggressive investigation of such crises generally allow a flap to be salvaged. Maintenance of normal blood volume and treatment of hypothermia is particularly important in the early postoperative period to avoid vascular spasm. Spasm causes flaps to appear pale and to exhibit a significant temperature drop.

Free flaps exhibit venous engorgement when placed in a dependent position up to several weeks postoperatively. Such engorgement is generally not dangerous, though patients with free flaps below the knee should be gradually mobilized in the same fashion as patients with skin grafts in this location. These patients should also keep the lower extremity elevated for at least 10 to 14 days.

Free flaps in the head and neck area require that the patient's head motion be restricted somewhat for the first few days. It is important that electrocardiographic leads and tracheostomy tube ties not compress the external jugular vein if it was used as a recipient vessel for anastomosis. If central lines are used after operation, they should be placed on the contralateral side of the neck.

Free flaps should be monitored on an hourly basis during the early postoperative period. Most free flaps include an exposed skin island, which facilitates evaluation of the flap circulation. The flap is observed for color and for capillary refill. A pale flap generally indicates arterial insufficiency; however, the normal, lighter color of certain donor sites, such as the abdomen, can be misleading. Flaps with venous insufficiency are characteristically blue in color and exhibit rapid capillary refill. Bleeding from the edges of a flap is common in the presence of venous hypertension.

Surface temperature probes can be used to monitor free flaps that have a skin island. The advantages of this method are simplicity and reliability. One probe is placed on the flap and another on a nearby area to serve as a control. The flap surface temperature is generally less than the control temperature by 1.0° to 2.5° C. A progressive widening of the temperature difference is ominous and calls for critical assessment of the flap circulation. The absolute temperature of the flap probe is also significant: a flap temperature greater than 32° C indicates healthy circulation, whereas a temperature between 30° and 32° C indicates marginal circulation and a temperature less than 30° C often indicates a vascular problem. In a healthy flap, temperature fluctuations may be caused by a dislodged probe, an exogenous heat source (such as a lamp), cooling of one of the probes from an oxygen mist mask, or cleaning of the flap skin with alcohol (which results in a precipitous drop in skin temperature).

To confirm the presence of an anastomotic problem, flap circulation is assessed directly by a full-thickness puncture of the flap skin with a 20-, 22-, or 25-gauge needle. If flap circulation is healthy, a drop of bright-red blood should appear at the puncture site within a few seconds, and another drop should appear each time the previous drop is wiped away by an alcohol swab. The failure of blood to appear or the delayed appearance of a clear, serous ooze instead of blood is an indication of arterial insufficiency. Vigorous, dark bleeding confirms a venous problem. Flaps that are pale as a result of vascular spasm are difficult to assess because their bleeding response to needle puncture is poor despite intact anastomoses. Whenever uncertainty exists, however, surgical exploration should be undertaken because the entire flap may be in jeopardy.

Free flaps without skin islands are more difficult to monitor accurately. Muscle flaps can be followed in much the same way as skin free flaps by inserting needle temperature probes directly into the muscle belly. A healthy muscle free flap is red in color and typically has a serous ooze between the interstices of the overlying meshed skin graft. A flap with an arterial problem quickly becomes dry and dark in appearance. A muscle flap with a venous problem becomes dark and engorged with blood and exhibits bleeding from its surface and perimeter. A muscle free flap can be punctured with a needle to assess the quality of the bleeding if its circulatory status is unclear.

Fascial free flaps covered with skin grafts are more difficult to assess. They tend to transmit body core temperature readily because they are quite thin; therefore, needle temperature probes are generally unreliable. It is often possible in these cases either to observe the arterial pulsations in the flap directly or to monitor them with a conventional Doppler device.

Some free flaps are completely buried beneath the skin. Others, such as intraoral skin free flaps, are equally difficult to monitor postoperatively. Specialized transplants, such as jejunum, are particularly vulnerable to short periods of anoxia and are not likely to be salvageable by the time a problem is recognized. Alternative methods of monitoring buried free flaps are being developed, although they are not in wide clinical use. One example is the implantable Doppler monitor. This device is placed in direct contact with the artery distal to the anastomosis to obtain a continuous Doppler signal.[13]

References

1. Weinzweig N, Weinzweig J: Basic principles and techniques in plastic surgery. Mastery of Plastic and Reconstructive Surgery, Vol 1. Choen M, Ed. Little, Brown, and Co, Boston, 1994

2. Borges AF: Elective Incisions and Scar Revision. Little, Brown, and Co, Boston, 1973

3. Smahel J: The healing of skin grafts. Clin Plast Surg 4:409, 1977

4. Disa JJ, Alizadeh K, Smith JW, et al: Evaluation of a combined sodium alginate and bioocclusive membrane dressing in the management of split thickness skin graft donor sites. Ann Plast Surg 46:405, 2001

5. Daniel RK, Kerrigan CL: Skin flaps: an anatomical and hemodynamic approach. Clin Plast Surg 6:181, 1979

6. Cederna PS, Chang P, Pittet-Cuenod BM, et al: The effect of the delay phenomenon on the vascularity of rabbit abdominal cutaneous island flaps. Plast Reconstr Surg 99:183, 1997

7. Milton SH: Pedicled skin-flaps: the fallacy of the length:width ratio. Br J Surg 57:502, 1970

8. Lamberty BG, Cormack GC: Fasciocutaneous flaps. Clin Plast Surg 17:713, 1990

9. Cormack GC, Lamberty BG: Arterial Anatomy of Skin Flaps. Churchill Livingstone, Edinburgh, 1987

10. Jackson IT: Local rotational flaps. Operative Plastic Surgery. Evans GRD, Ed. McGraw-Hill, New York, 2000

11. Worthen EF: Scalp flaps and the rotation forehead flap. Grabb's Encyclopedia of Flaps, Vol 1. Strauch B, Vasconez LO, Hall-Findlay EJ, Eds. Lippincott-Raven Publishers, Philadelphia, 1998

12. McGregor IA, McGregor AD: The z-plasty. Fundamental Techniques of Plastic Surgery. Churchill Livingstone, Edinburgh, 1995

13. Kind GM, Buntic RF, Buncke GM, et al: The effect of an implantable Doppler probe on the salvage of microvascular tissue transplants. Plast Reconstr Surg 101:1268, 1998

Acknowledgments

Figures 1 through 3, 10, 12 through 15   Tom Moore.
Figures 6, 8, 9, 11, 16   Carol Donner.

8 THYROID AND PARATHYROID PROCEDURES

Gregg H. Jossart, M.D., F.A.C.S., and Orlo H. Clark, M.D., F.A.C.S.

Thyroidectomy

OPERATIVE PLANNING

If the patient has had any hoarseness or has undergone a neck operation before, indirect or direct (ideally, fiberoptic) laryngoscopy is essential to determine whether the vocal cords are functioning normally. All patients scheduled for thyroidectomy should be euthyroid at the time of operation; in all other respects, they should be prepared as they would be for any procedure calling for general anesthesia.

Optimum exposure of the thyroid is obtained by placing a sandbag between the scapula and a foam ring under the occiput; in this way, the neck is extended, and the thyroid can assume a more anterior position. The head must be well supported to prevent postoperative posterior neck pain. The patient is placed in a 20° reverse Trendelenburg position. The skin is prepared with 1% iodine or chlorhexidine.

OPERATIVE TECHNIQUE

General Troubleshooting

Thyroid and parathyroid operations should be performed in a blood-free field so that vital structures can be identified. Operating telescopes (magnification: ×2.5 or ×3.5) are also recommended because they make it easier to identify the normal parathyroid glands and the recurrent laryngeal nerve. If bleeding occurs, pressure should be applied. The vessel should be clamped only if (1) it can be precisely identified or (2) the recurrent laryngeal nerve has been identified and is not in close proximity to the vessel.

As a rule, dissection should always be done first on the side where the suspected tumor is; if there is a problem with the dissection on this side, a less than total thyroidectomy can be performed on the contralateral side to prevent complications. There is, however, one exception to this rule: if the tumor is very extensive, the surgeon will sometimes find it easier to do the dissection on the "easy" side first to facilitate orientation with respect to the trachea and the esophagus.

Step 1: Incision and Mobilization of Skin Layers

A Kocher transverse incision paralleling the normal skin lines of the neck is made 1 cm caudad to the cricoid cartilage [*see Figure 1*]. As a rule, the incision should be about 4 to 6 cm long and should extend from the anterior border of one sternocleidomastoid muscle to the anterior border of the other and through the platysma. Five straight Kelly clamps are placed on the dermis to facilitate dissection, which proceeds first cephalad in a subplatysmal plane anterior to the anterior jugular veins and posterior to the platysma to the level of the thyroid cartilage notch and then caudad to the suprasternal notch. Skin towels and a self-retaining retractor are then applied.

Troubleshooting Placing the incision 1 cm below the cricoid locates it precisely over the isthmus of the thyroid gland. The course of the incision should conform to the normal skin lines or creases. The length of the incision should be modified as necessary for good exposure. Patients with short, thick necks, low-lying thyroid glands, or large thyroid tumors require longer incisions than those with long, thin necks and small tumors. Patients whose necks do not extend also require longer incisions for adequate exposure. A sterile marking pen should be used to mark the midline of the neck, the level at which the incision should be made (i.e., 1 cm below the cricoid), and the lateral margins of the incision (which should be at equal distances from the midline so that the incision will be symmetrical). A scalpel should never be used to mark the neck: doing so will leave an unsightly scar in some patients. To mark the incision site itself, a 2-0 silk tie should be pressed against the neck [*see Figure 1*].

The upper flap is dissected first by placing five straight Kelly clamps on the dermis and retracting anteriorly and superiorly. Lateral traction with a vein retractor or an Army-Navy retractor

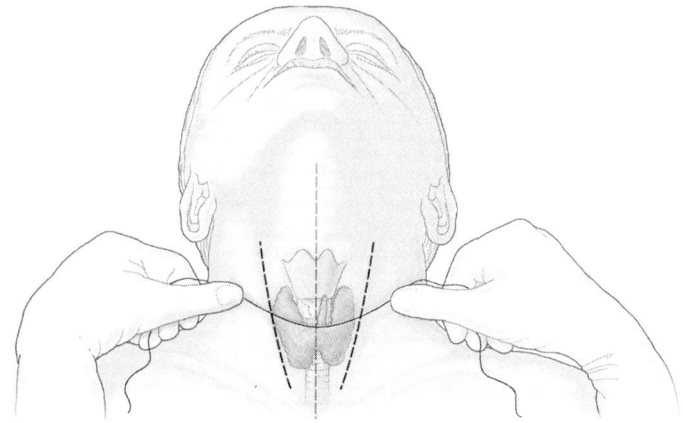

Figure 1 The initial incision in a thyroidectomy is made 1 cm below the cricoid cartilage and follows normal skin lines. A sterile marking pen is used to mark the midline of the neck, the level of the incision, and the lateral borders of the incision. A 2-0 silk tie is pressed against the neck to mark the incision site itself.[2]

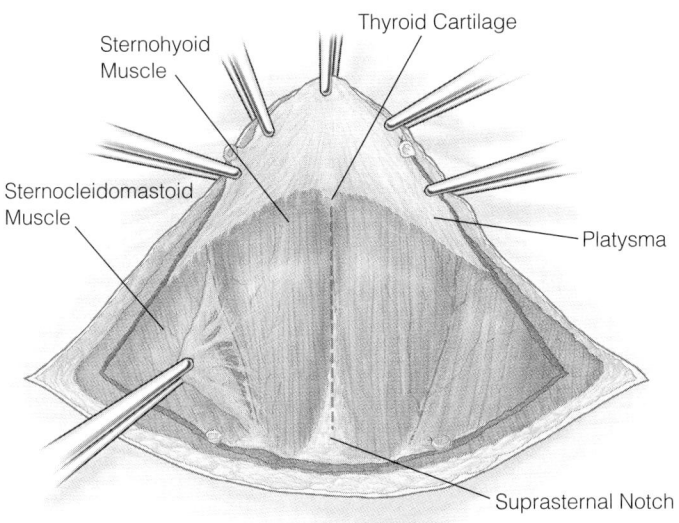

Figure 2 **To expose the thyroid, a midline incision is made through the superficial layer of deep cervical fascia between the strap muscles. The incision is begun at the suprasternal notch and extended to the thyroid cartilage.**[3]

helps identify the semilunar plane for dissection. This blood-free plane is deep to the platysma and superficial to the anterior jugular veins. Cephalad dissection can be done quickly with the electrocautery or a scalpel, and lateral dissection can be done bluntly. The same principles are applied to dissection of the lower flap. In thin patients, the surgeon must be careful not to dissect through the skin from within, especially at the level of the thyroid cartilage.

Step 2: Midline Dissection and Mobilization of Strap Muscles

The thyroid gland is exposed via a midline incision through the superficial layer of deep cervical fascia between the strap muscles. Because the strap muscles are farthest apart just above the suprasternal notch, the incision is begun at the notch and extended to the thyroid cartilage [*see Figure 2*].

On the side where the thyroid nodule or the suspected parathyroid adenoma is located, the more superficial sternohyoid muscle is separated from the underlying sternothyroid muscle by blunt dissection, which is extended laterally until the ansa cervicalis becomes visible on the lateral edge of the sternothyroid muscle and on the medial side of the internal jugular vein. The sternothyroid muscle is then dissected free from the thyroid and the prethyroidal fascia by blunt or sharp dissection until the middle thyroid vein or veins are encountered laterally.

A 2-0 silk suture is placed deeply through the thyroid lobe for retraction to facilitate exposure. This stitch should never be placed through the thyroid nodule: doing so could cause seeding of thyroid cancer cells. The thyroid is retracted anteriorly and medially and the carotid sheath laterally; this retraction places tension on the middle thyroid veins and helps expose the area posterolateral to the thyroid, where the parathyroid glands and the recurrent laryngeal nerves are situated. The middle thyroid veins are divided to give better exposure behind the upper lobe of the thyroid [*see Figure 3*].

Troubleshooting As a rule, it is not necessary to divide the strap muscles; however, if they are adherent to the underlying thyroid tumor, the portion of the muscle that is adhering to the

tumor should be sacrificed and allowed to remain attached to the thyroid. Separation of the sternohyoid muscle from the sternothyroid muscle provides better exposure of the operative field. The middle thyroid veins should be cleaned of adjacent tissues to prevent any injury to the recurrent laryngeal nerve when these veins are ligated and divided. It is always safest to mobilize tissues parallel to the recurrent laryngeal nerve.

Step 3: Division of Isthmus

When a thyroid lobectomy is to be performed, the isthmus of the thyroid gland is usually divided with Dandy or Colodny clamps at an early point in dissection to facilitate the subsequent mobilization of the thyroid gland. The thyroid tissue that is to remain is oversewn with a 2-0 silk ligature. To minimize the chance of invasion into the trachea or to avoid a visible mass in patients with compensatory thyroid hypertrophy, thyroid tissues should not be left anterior to the trachea.

Troubleshooting With larger glands, we divide the isthmus first. This step facilitates the lateral dissection by making the gland more mobile.

Step 4: Mobilization of Thyroid Gland and Identification of Upper Parathyroid Glands

Once the isthmus has been divided, dissection is continued superiorly, laterally, and posteriorly with a small sponge on a peanut clamp. The superior thyroid artery and veins are identified by retracting the thyroid inferiorly and medially. The tissues lateral to the upper lobe of the thyroid and medial to the carotid sheath can be mobilized caudally to the cricothyroid muscle; the recurrent laryngeal nerve enters the cricothyroid muscle at the level of the cricoid cartilage, first passing through Berry's ligament [*see Figure 4*]. The superior pole vessels are individually identified, skeletonized, double- or triple-clamped, ligated, and divided low on the thyroid gland [*see Figure 5*]. To prevent injury to the external laryngeal nerve, the vessels are divided and ligated on the thyroid surface, the thyroid is retracted laterally and caudally, and dissection is carried out on the medial edge of the thyroid gland and lateral to the cricothyroid muscle. The tis-

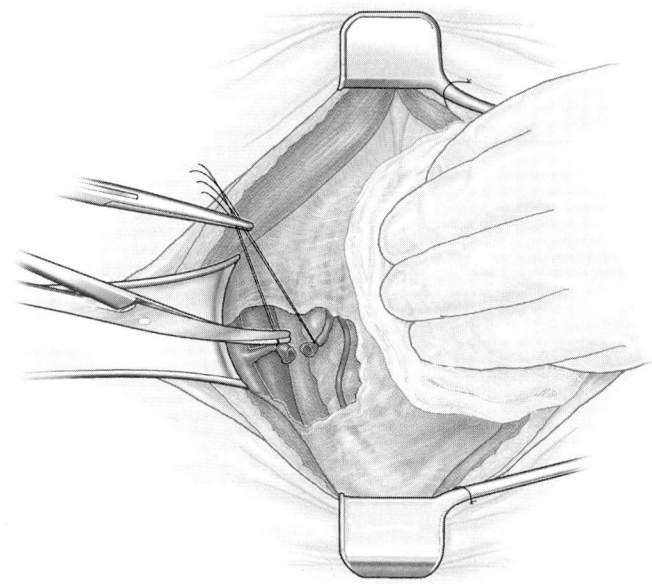

Figure 3 **The middle thyroid veins are divided to give better exposure behind the upper lobe of the thyroid.**[2]

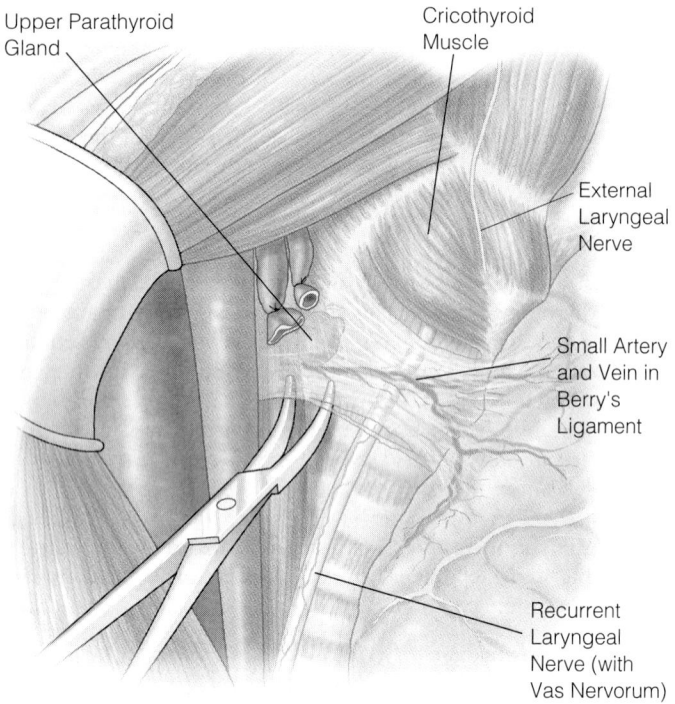

Figure 4 **The recurrent laryngeal nerve enters the cricothyroid muscle at the level of the cricoid cartilage, first passing through Berry's ligament.**[2]

sues posterior and lateral to the superior pole that have not already been mobilized can now be easily swept by blunt dissection away from the thyroid gland medially and anteriorly and away from the carotid sheath laterally. The upper parathyroid gland is often identified at this time at the level of the cricoid cartilage.

Troubleshooting It is essential to keep from injuring the external laryngeal nerve. This nerve is the motor branch of the superior laryngeal nerve and is responsible for tensing the vocal cords; it is also known as the high note nerve or the Amelita Galli-Curci nerve. In about 80% of patients, the external laryngeal nerve runs on the surface of the cricothyroid muscle; in about 10%, it runs with the superior pole vessels; and in the remaining 10%, it runs within the cricothyroid muscle. Given that this nerve is usually about the size of a single strand of a spider web, one should generally try to avoid it rather than to identify it. Injury to the external laryngeal nerve occurs in as many as 10% of patients undergoing thyroidectomy. The best ways of preventing such injury are (1) to provide gentle traction on the thyroid gland in a caudal and lateral direction and (2) to ligate the superior pole vessels directly on the capsule of the upper pole individually and low on the thyroid gland rather than to cross-clamp the entire superior pole pedicle.

The internal laryngeal nerve is the sensory branch of the superior laryngeal nerve; it provides sensory innervation to the posterior pharynx. Injury to this nerve can result in aspiration. Because the internal laryngeal nerve typically is cephalad to the area of dissection during thyroidectomy and runs cephalad to the lateral portion of the thyroid cartilage, it usually is at risk only when the surgeon dissects cephalad to the thyroid cartilage. Such dissection is necessary only when laryngeal mobilization is performed to relieve tension on the tracheal anastomosis after tracheal resection.

Step 5: Identification of Recurrent Laryngeal Nerves and Lower Parathyroid Glands

When the thyroid lobe is further mobilized, the lower parathyroid gland is usually seen; this gland is almost always located anterior to the recurrent laryngeal nerve and is usually located inferior to where the inferior thyroid artery crosses the recurrent laryngeal nerve [*see Figure 6*]. The carotid sheath is retracted laterally, and the thyroid gland is retracted anteriorly and medially. This retraction puts tension on the inferior thyroid artery and consequently on the recurrent laryngeal nerve, thereby facilitating the identification of the nerve. The recurrent laryngeal nerve is situated more medially on the left (running in the tracheoesophageal groove) and more obliquely on the right. Dissection should proceed cephalad along the lateral edge of the thyroid. Fatty and lymphatic tissues immediately adjacent to the thyroid gland are swept from it with a peanut clamp, and small vessels are ligated. No tissue should be transected until one is sure that it is not the recurrent laryngeal nerve.

Troubleshooting The upper parathyroid glands are usually situated on each side of the thyroid gland at the level where the recurrent laryngeal nerve enters the cricothyroid muscle [*see Figure 6*]. Because the recurrent laryngeal nerve enters the cricothyroid muscle at the level of the cricoid cartilage, the area cephalad to the cricoid cartilage is relatively safe.

The right and left recurrent laryngeal nerves must be preserved during every thyroid operation. Although both nerves enter at the posterior medial position of the larynx in the cricothyroid muscle, their courses vary considerably. The right recurrent laryngeal nerve takes a more oblique course than the left recurrent laryngeal nerve and may pass either anterior or posterior to the inferior thyroid artery. In about 0.5% of persons, the right recurrent laryngeal nerve is in fact nonrecurrent and may enter the thyroid from a superior or lateral direction.[1] On rare occasions, both a recurrent and a nonrecurrent laryn-

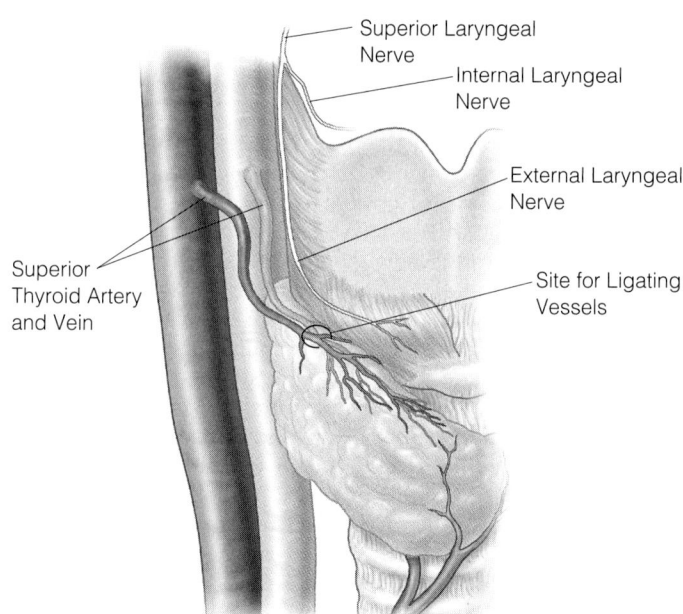

Figure 5 **The superior pole vessels should be individually identified and ligated low on the thyroid gland to minimize the chances of injury to the external laryngeal nerve.**[2]

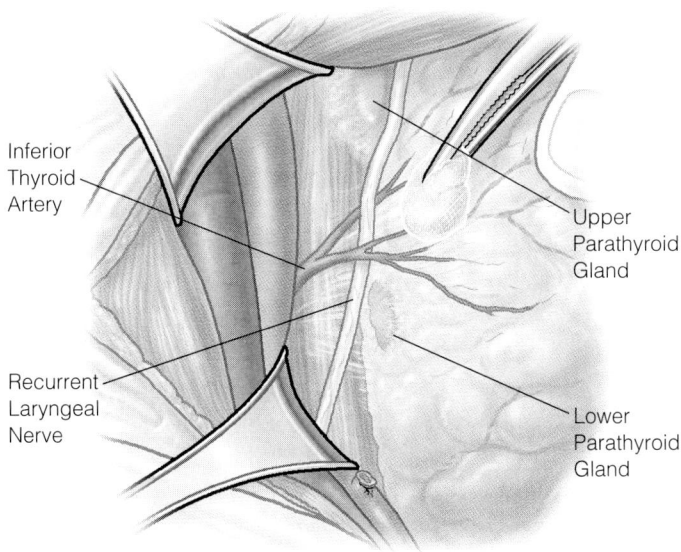

Figure 6 **The upper parathyroid glands are usually situated on either side of the thyroid at the level where the recurrent laryngeal nerve enters the cricothyroid muscle. The lower parathyroid glands are usually anterior to the recurrent laryngeal nerve and inferior to where the inferior thyroid artery crosses this nerve.**[2]

geal nerve may be present on the right. The left recurrent laryngeal nerve almost always runs in the tracheoesophageal groove because of its deeper origin within the thorax as it loops around the ductus arteriosus. Either recurrent laryngeal nerve may branch before entering the larynx; the left nerve is more likely to do this. Such branching is important to recognize because all of the motor fibers of the recurrent laryngeal nerve are usually in the most medial branch.

In identifying the recurrent laryngeal nerves, it is helpful to remember that they are supplied by a small vascular plexus and that a tiny vessel runs parallel to and directly on each nerve [*see Figures 4 and 6*]. In young persons, the artery usually is readily distinguished from the recurrent laryngeal nerve; however, in older persons with arteriosclerosis, the white-appearing artery may be mistaken for a nerve, and thus the nerve may be injured as a result of the misidentification. Lateral traction on the carotid sheath and medial and anterior traction on the thyroid gland place tension on the inferior thyroid artery; this maneuver often helps identify the recurrent laryngeal nerve where it courses lateral to the midportion of the thyroid gland. One should, however, be careful not to devascularize the inferior parathyroid glands by dividing the lateral vascular attachments: to remove the thyroid lobe, it is best to divide the vessels directly on the thyroid capsule to preserve the blood supply to the parathyroid glands. It is usually safest to identify the recurrent laryngeal nerve low in the neck and then to follow it to where it enters the cricothyroid muscle through Berry's ligament. The recurrent laryngeal nerves can usually be palpated through the surrounding tissue in the neck; they feel like a taut ligature of approximately 2-0 gauge.

Parathyroid glands should be swept from the thyroid gland on as broad a vascular pedicle as possible to prevent devascularization. When it is unclear whether a parathyroid gland can be saved on its own vascular pedicle, one should biopsy the gland to confirm that it is parathyroid and then autotransplant it in multiple 1 × 1 mm pieces into separate pockets in the ster-

nocleidomastoid muscle. At times, it is preferable to clip the blood vessels running from the thyroid to the parathyroid glands rather than to clamp and tie them. Clipping not only marks the parathyroid gland (which is useful if another operation subsequently becomes necessary) but also enables the gland to remain with minimal manipulation and with its remaining blood supply preserved.

In patients who have extensive thyroid tumors or who require reoperation, extensive scarring is often present. For some of these patients, it is preferable to identify the recurrent laryngeal nerve from a medial approach by dividing the isthmus with Colodny clamps and ligating and dividing the superior thyroid vessels. By carefully dissecting the thyroid away from the trachea, one can identify the recurrent laryngeal nerve at the point where its position is most consistent (i.e., at its entrance into the larynx immediately posterior to the cricothyroid muscle).

The most difficult part of dissection in a thyroidectomy is the part that involves Berry's ligament, which is situated at the posterior portion of the thyroid gland just caudal to the cricoid cartilage [*see Figure 4*]. A small branch of the inferior thyroid artery traverses the ligament, as do one or more veins from the thyroid gland. If bleeding occurs during this part of the dissection, it should be controlled by applying pressure with a gauze pad. Nothing should be clamped in this area until the recurrent laryngeal nerve is identified. In some patients (about 15%), the peduncle of Zuckerkandl, a small protuberance of thyroid tissue on the right, tends to obscure the recurrent laryngeal nerve at the level of Berry's ligament.

Step 6: Mobilization of Pyramidal Lobe

The pyramidal lobe is found in about 80% of patients. It extends in a cephalad direction, often through the notch in the thyroid cartilage to the hyoid bone. One or more lymph nodes are frequently found just cephalad to the isthmus of the thyroid gland over the cricothyroid membrane (so-called Delphian nodes) [*see Figure 7*]. The pyramidal lobe is mobilized by retracting it caudally and by dissecting immediately adjacent to it in a cephalad direction. Small vessels are coagulated or ligated.

Step 7: Thyroid Resection

Once the parathyroid glands have been carefully swept or dissected from the thyroid gland and the recurrent nerve has been identified, the thyroid lobe can be quickly resected. For total thyroidectomy, the same operation is done again on the other side.

Troubleshooting The thyroid lobe or gland should be carefully examined after removal. If a parathyroid gland is identified, a biopsy of it should be performed to confirm that it is parathyroid and then autotransplanted. In a thyroid procedure, every parathyroid gland should be treated as if it is the last one, and at least one parathyroid gland should be definitely identified. As a rule, biopsies should not be performed on normal parathyroid glands during a thyroid procedure.

Step 8: Closure

The sternothyroid muscles are approximated with 4-0 absorbable sutures, and a small opening is left in the midline at the suprasternal notch to make any bleeding that occurs more evident and to allow the blood to exit. The sternohyoid muscles are reapproximated in a similar fashion, as is the platysma. The skin is then closed with butterfly clips, which are hemostatic and inexpensive and permit precise alignment of the skin edges. (In children, the skin is closed with a subcuticular stitch and Steri-

Strips instead.) A sterile pressure dressing is applied.

Special Concerns

Invasion of the trachea or the esophagus On rare occasions, thyroid or parathyroid cancers may invade the trachea or the esophagus. As much as 5 cm of the trachea can be resected safely, without impairment of the patient's voice. If the invasion is not extensive and is confined to the anterior portion of the trachea, a small section of the trachea that contains the tumor should be excised, and a tracheostomy may be placed at the site of resection. If the invasion is more extensive or occurs in the lateral or posterior portion of the trachea, a segment of the trachea measuring several centimeters long is resected, and the remaining segments are reanastomosed. To prevent tension on the anastomosis, the trachea should be mobilized before resection, the recurrent laryngeal nerves should be preserved and mobilized from the trachea, and the mylohyoid fascia and muscles should be divided above the thyroid cartilage to drop the cartilage. Pains must be taken not to injure the internal laryngeal nerves during this dissection, given that these nerves course from lateral to medial just above the lateral aspects of the thyroid cartilage. After resection, the trachea is reapproximated with 3-0 Maxon sutures. One or two Penrose drains should be left near the resection site to allow air to exit. The drains are removed after several days, when there is no more evidence of air leakage.

If the esophagus is invaded by tumor, the muscular wall of the esophagus can be resected along with the tumor, with the inner esophageal layer left in place.

Neck dissection for nodal metastases Lymph nodes in the central neck (medial to the carotid sheath) are frequently involved in patients with papillary, medullary, and Hürthle cell cancer. These nodes should be removed without injury to the parathyroid glands or the recurrent laryngeal nerves. In most patients, it is relatively easy to remove all tissue between the carotid sheath and the trachea. In some patients with extensive lymphadenopathy, it is necessary to remove the parathyroids, perform biopsies on them to confirm that they are in fact parathyroid, and autotransplant them into the sternocleidomastoid muscle.

When lymph nodes are palpable in the lateral neck, a modified neck dissection is performed through a lateral extension of the Kocher collar incision to the anterior margin of the trapezius muscle (a MacFee incision). The jugular vein, the spinal accessory nerve, the phrenic nerve, the vagus nerve, the cervical sympathetic nerves, and the sternocleidomastoid muscle are preserved unless they are directly adherent to or invaded by tumor.

In patients with medullary thyroid cancer, a meticulous and thorough central neck dissection is necessary. When a primary medullary tumor is larger than 1 cm or the central neck nodes are obviously involved, these patients will also benefit from a lateral modified radical neck dissection (with the structures just mentioned preserved). During the dissection, all fibrofatty lymph node tissues should be removed from the level of the clavicle to the level of the hyoid bone. The deep dissection plane is developed anterior to the scalenus anticus muscle, the brachial plexus, and the scalenus medius muscle. The phrenic nerve runs obliquely on the scalenus anticus muscle. The cervical sensory nerves can usually be preserved unless there is extensive tumor involvement.

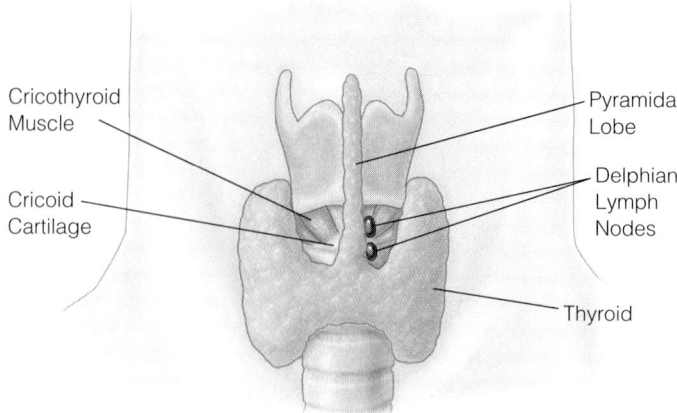

Figure 7 **Delphian lymph nodes may be found just cephalad to the isthmus over the cricothyroid membrane.**

Median sternotomy A median sternotomy is rarely necessary for removal of the thyroid gland because the blood supply to the thyroid gland, the thymus, and the lower parathyroid glands derives primarily from the inferior thyroid arteries in the neck. Metastatic lymph nodes frequently extend inferiorly in the tracheoesophageal groove into the superior mediastinum; these nodes can almost always be removed through a cervical incision without any need for a sternotomy. On rare occasions, metastatic nodes spread to the aortic pulmonary window and can be identified preoperatively on CT or MRI. If a median sternotomy proves necessary, the sternum should be divided to the level of the third intercostal space and then laterally on one side at the space between the third rib and the fourth. Median sternotomy provides excellent exposure of the upper anterior mediastinum and the lower neck.

COMPLICATIONS

The following are the most significant complications of thyroidectomy.

1. Injury to the recurrent laryngeal nerve. Bilateral injury to the recurrent laryngeal nerve may result in vocal cord paresis and stridor and may have to be treated with a tracheostomy.
2. Hypoparathyroidism. This complication may arise as the result of removal of, injury to, or devascularization of the parathyroid glands. As noted [*see* Operative Technique, *above*], we recommend leaving parathyroid glands on their own vascular pedicle; however, if one is concerned about possible devascularization of a parathyroid, biopsy should be performed on the gland to confirm its identity and then autotransplanted in 1 × 1 mm pieces into separate pockets in the sternocleidomastoid muscle.
3. Bleeding. Postoperative bleeding can be life threatening in that it can compromise the airway. Any postoperative respiratory distress can be thought of as attributable to a neck hematoma until proved otherwise. Most bleeding occurs within four hours of operation, and virtually all occurs within 24 hours.
4. Injury to the external laryngeal nerve [*see* Operative Technique, *above*].
5. Infection. This complication is quite rare after thyroidectomy. Any patient with acute pharyngitis should not undergo this procedure.

6. Seroma. Most seromas are small and resorb spontaneously; some must be aspirated.
7. Keloid. Keloid formation after thyroidectomy is most common in African-American patients and in patients with a history of keloids.
8. There are a number of miscellaneous complications that are somewhat less common.

OUTCOME EVALUATION

The duration of a thyroid operation is 1 to 3 hours, depending on the size and invasiveness of the tumor, its vascularity, and the location of the parathyroid glands. Postoperatively, the patient is kept in a low Fowler position with the head and shoulders elevated 10° to 20° for 6 to 12 hours to maintain negative pressure in the veins. The patient typically resumes eating within 3 to 4 hours, and an antiemetic is ordered as needed (many patients experience postoperative nausea and emesis).

The serum calcium level is measured approximately 5 to 8 hours after operation in patients who have undergone bilateral procedures; no tests are required in those who have undergone unilateral procedures. On the first morning after the thyroidectomy, the serum calcium and serum phosphate levels are measured. If the patient is still hospitalized on postoperative day 2, these tests are repeated on the second morning as well. Oral calcium supplements are given if the serum calcium is below 7.5 mg/dl or if the patient experiences perioral numbness or tingling. A low serum phosphate level (< 2.5 mg/dl) usually is a sign of so-called bone hunger and suggests that there is little reason to be concerned about permanent hypoparathyroidism, whereas a high level (> 4.5 mg/dl) should prompt concern about permanent hypoparathyroidism.

The surgical clips are removed on postoperative day 1, and Steri-Strips are applied to prevent tension on the healing wound. Patients usually are discharged on the first day, are given a prescription for thyroid hormone (L-thyroxine, 0.1 to 0.2 mg/day orally) if the procedure was more extensive than a thyroid lobectomy, and are told to take calcium tablets for any tingling or muscle cramps. Patients with papillary, follicular, or Hürthle cell cancer should receive enough L-thyroxine to keep their serum levels of thyroid-stimulating hormone (TSH) below 0.1 mIU/ml. The Steri-Strips are removed on day 10, the pathology is reviewed, and further management is discussed in the light of the pathologic findings. In patients with thyroid cancer, values for serum calcium, TSH, and thyroglobulin are obtained; in patients with coexisting hyperparathyroidism, values for serum calcium, phosphorus, and parathyroid hormone (PTH) are obtained.

Most patients can return to work or full activity in 1 to 2 weeks. Patients with benign lesions who have undergone hemithyroidectomy may or may not require thyroid hormone; those with multinodular goiter, thyroiditis, or occult papillary cancer typically do, whereas those with follicular adenoma typically do not. Patients who have undergone total or near-total thyroidectomy will require thyroid hormone. Patients with papillary or follicular cancer who have undergone total or near-total thyroidectomy appear to benefit from radioactive iodine scanning and therapy. (It is necessary to discontinue L-thyroxine for 6 to 8 weeks and L-triiodothyronine for 2 weeks before scanning.) Those considered to be at low risk (age < 45 years, tumor confined to the thyroid and not invasive, and tumor diameter < 4 cm) may receive radioactive iodine on an outpatient basis in a dose of approximately 30 mCi. Those who are considered to be at high risk should receive approximately 100 to 150 mCi. Long-term (20-year) mortality is about 4% in low-risk patients and about 40% in high-risk patients. Serum thyroglobulin levels should be determined before and after discontinuance of thyroid hormone; such levels are very sensitive indicators of persistent thyroid disease after total thyroidectomy.

Parathyroidectomy

OPERATIVE PLANNING

The preparation for parathyroidectomy is the same as that for thyroidectomy. Patients who have profound hypercalcemia (serum calcium ≥ 12.5 mg/dl) or mild to moderate renal failure should be vigorously hydrated and given furosemide before operation. On rare occasions, such patients require additional treatment—for example, administration of diphosphonates, mithramycin, or calcitonin. Any electrolyte abnormalities (e.g., hypokalemia) should be corrected.

We recommend bilateral exploration for most patients undergoing initial operations for primary or secondary hyperparathyroidism. For some patients with sporadic primary hyperparathyroidism in whom one abnormal gland has been identified by sestamibi scanning, a focused operation using intraoperative PTH assay is an acceptable alternative approach. Preoperative localization studies (e.g., ultrasonography, MRI, sestamibi scanning, and CT scanning) are generally unnecessary: they provide useful information in about 75% of patients, but they are not considered cost-effective, because an experienced surgeon can treat hyperparathyroidism successfully 95% to 98% of the time. Such studies are, however, essential when reoperation for persistent or recurrent hyperparathyroidism is indicated and when a focused approach with intraoperative PTH assay is to be used. We do not believe that using the gamma probe is any better than preoperative sestamibi scanning. All patients requiring reoperation should undergo direct or indirect laryngoscopy before operation for evaluation of vocal cord function.

OPERATIVE TECHNIQUE

Steps 1 through 4

Steps 1, 2, 3, and 4 of a parathyroidectomy are virtually identical to steps 1, 2, 4, and 5 of a thyroidectomy (see above), and essentially the same troubleshooting considerations apply.

Troubleshooting About 85% of people have four parathyroid glands, and in about 85% of these persons, the parathyroids are situated on the posterior lateral capsule of the thyroid. Normal parathyroid glands measure about 3 × 3 × 4 mm and are light brown in color. The upper parathyroid glands are more posterior (i.e., dorsal) and more constant in position (at the level of the cricoid cartilage) than the lower parathyroid glands, which typically are more anteriorly placed (on the posterior-lateral surface of the thyroid gland). Both the upper and the lower parathyroid glands are supplied by small branches of the inferior and superior thyroid arteries in most patients. About 15% of parathyroid glands are situated within the thymus gland, and about 1% are intrathyroidal. Other abnormal sites for the parathyroid glands are (1) the carotid sheath, (2) the anterior and posterior mediastinum, and (3) anterior to the carotid bulb or along the pharynx (undescended parathyroids).

The upper parathyroid glands are usually lateral to the recurrent laryngeal nerve at the level of Berry's ligament; their position makes them generally easier to preserve during thyroid-ectomy and easier to find during both parathyroid and thyroid surgery. When the upper parathyroids are not found at this site, they often can be found in the tracheoesophageal groove or in the posterior mediastinum along the esophagus. The lower parathyroid glands are almost always situated anterior to the recurrent laryngeal nerves and caudal to where the recurrent laryngeal nerve crosses the inferior thyroid artery; they may be surrounded by lymph nodes. When the lower parathyroids are not found at this site, they usually can be found in the anterior mediastinum (typically in the thymus or the thymic fat).

Step 5: Parathyroid Resection

Abnormal parathyroid glands are removed. In about 80% of patients with primary hyperparathyroidism, one parathyroid gland is abnormal; in about 15%, all glands are abnormal (diffuse hyperplasia); and in about 5%, two or three glands are abnormal and one or two normal. Parathyroid cancer occurs in about 1% of patients with primary hyperparathyroidism. About 50% of patients with parathyroid cancer have a palpable tumor, and most exhibit profound hypercalcemia (serum calcium ≥ 14.0 mg/dl).

Troubleshooting In some patients, parathyroid tumors and hyperplastic parathyroid glands are difficult to find. If this is the case, the first step is to explore the sites where parathyroids are usually located, near the posterolateral surface of the thyroid gland. (About 80% of parathyroid glands are situated within 1 cm of the point where the inferior thyroid artery crosses the recurrent laryngeal nerve.) When a lower gland is missing from the usual location, it is likely to be found in the thymus; this possibility can be confirmed by mobilizing the thymus from the anterior-superior mediastinum. In all, about 15% of parathyroid glands are found within the thymus. If an upper parathyroid gland cannot be located, one should look not only far behind the thyroid gland superiorly but also in a paraesophageal position down into the posterior mediastinum. A thyroid lobectomy or thyroidotomy should be done on the side where fewer than two parathyroid glands have been located and no abnormal parathyroid tissue has been identified. The carotid sheath and the area posterior to the carotid, as well as the retroesophageal area, should also be explored. In rare cases, there may be an undescended parathyroid tumor anterior to the carotid bulb.

Although we do not recommend routine biopsy of more than one normal-appearing parathyroid gland, we do recommend biopsy (not removal) and marking of all normal parathyroid glands that have been identified when no abnormal parathyroid tissue can be found. When four normal parathyroid glands are found in the neck, the fifth (abnormal) parathyroid gland is usually in the mediastinum. The surgeon's responsibility is to make sure during parathyroidectomy that the elusive parathyroid adenoma is not in or removable through the cervical incision used for the initial operation and to minimize complications. The risk of permanent hypoparathyroidism or injury to the recurrent nerve should be less than 2%.

Step 6: Closure

Closure is essentially the same for parathyroidectomy as for thyroidectomy.

COMPLICATIONS

The complications of parathyroidectomy are similar to those of thyroidectomy but occur less often. Patients with a very high serum alkaline phosphatase level and osteitis fibrosa cystica are prone to profound hypocalcemia after parathyroidectomy. In such patients, both serum calcium and serum phosphorus levels are low. In contrast, patients with hypoparathyroidism exhibit low serum calcium levels but high serum phosphorus levels.

OUTCOME EVALUATION

Outcome considerations are essentially the same as for thyroidectomy. The patient should have a normal voice and be normocalcemic. The overall complication rate should be less than 2%.

References

1. Henry JF, Audiffret J, Denizot A, et al: The nonrecurrent inferior laryngeal nerve: review of 33 cases, including two on the left side. Surgery 104:977, 1988

2. Clark OH: Endocrine Surgery of the Thyroid and Parathyroid Glands. CV Mosby, St Louis, 1985

3. Cady B, Rossi R: Surgery of thyroid gland. Surgery of the Thyroid and Parathyroid Glands. Cady B, Rossi R, Eds. WB Saunders Co, Philadelphia, 1991

Recommended Reading

Chen H, Sokol LJ, Udelsman R: Outpatient minimally invasive parathyroidectomy: a combination of sestamibi-spect localization, cervical block anesthesia, and intraoperative parathyroid hormone assay. Surgery 126:1016, 1999

Clark OH: Total thyroidectomy and lymph node dissection for cancer of the thyroid. Mastery of Surgery, 2nd ed. Nyhus LM, Baker RJ, Eds. Little, Brown and Co, Boston, 1992, p 204

Clark OH: Total thyroid lobectomy. Atlas of Surgical Oncology. Daly JM, Cady B, Low DW, Eds. CV Mosby Co, St. Louis, 1993, p 41

Gordon LL, Snyder WH, Wians JR, et al: The validity of quick intraoperative hormone assay: an evaluation of seventy-two patients based on gross morphology criteria. Surgery 126:1030, 1999

Irvin GL, Molinari AS, Figuero C, et al: Improved success rate in reoperative parathyroidectomy with intraoperative PTH assay. Ann Surg 229:874, 1999

Tezelman S, Shen W, Shaver JK, et al: Double parathyroid adenomas: clinical and biochemical characteristics before and after parathyroidectomy. Ann Surg 218:300, 1993

Acknowledgment

Figures 1 through 7 Tom Moore.

9 NECK MASS

Barry J. Roseman, M.D., and Orlo H. Clark, M.D., F.A.C.S.

Assessment of a Neck Mass

History

The evaluation of any neck mass begins with a careful history. The history should be taken with the differential diagnosis in mind [*see Table 1*] because directed questions can narrow down the diagnostic possibilities and focus subsequent investigations. For example, in younger patients, one would tend to look for congenital lesions, whereas in older adults, the first concern would always be neoplasia.

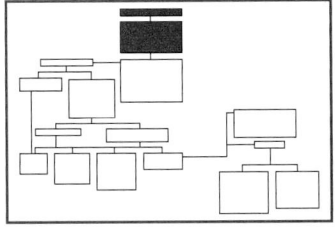

The duration and growth rate of the mass should be determined: malignant lesions are far more likely to exhibit rapid growth than benign ones, which may grow and shrink. Next, the location of the mass in the neck should be determined. This is particularly important for differentiating congenital masses from neoplastic or inflammatory ones because each type usually occurs consistently in particular locations. In addition, the location of a neoplasm is both diagnostically and prognostically significant. The possibility that the mass reflects an infectious or inflammatory process should also be assessed. One should check for evidence of infection or inflammation (e.g., fever, pain, or tenderness); a recent history of tuberculosis, sarcoidosis, or fungal infection; the presence of dental problems; and a history of trauma to the head and neck. Masses that appear inflamed or infected are far more likely to be benign.

Finally, factors suggestive of cancer should be sought: a previous malignancy elsewhere in the head and neck (e.g., a skin lesion or a head and neck tumor); night sweats (suggestive of lymphoma); excessive exposure to the sun (a risk factor for skin cancer); smoking or excessive alcohol consumption (risk factors for squamous cell carcinoma of the head and neck); nasal obstruction or bleeding, otalgia, odynophagia, dysphagia, or hoarseness (suggestive of a malignancy in the upper aerodigestive tract); or exposure to low-dose therapeutic radiation (a risk factor for thyroid cancer).

Physical Examination

Examination of the head and neck is challenging in that much of the area to be examined is not easily visualized. Patience and practice are necessary to master the special

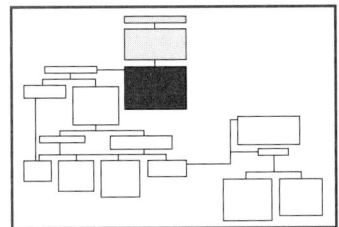

instruments and techniques of examination. A head and neck examination is usually performed with the patient sitting in front of the physician. Constant repositioning of the head is

Table 1 Etiology of Neck Mass

Inflammatory and infectious disorders	Acute lymphadenitis (bacterial or viral infection)
	Subcutaneous abscess (carbuncle)
	Infectious mononucleosis
	Cat-scratch fever
	AIDS
	Tuberculous lymphadenitis (scrofula)
	Fungal lymphadenitis (actinomycosis)
	Sarcoidosis
Congenital cystic lesions	Thyroglossal duct cyst
	Branchial cleft cyst
	Cystic hygroma (lymphangioma)
	Vascular malformation (hemangioma)
	Laryngocele
Benign neoplasms	Salivary gland tumor
	Thyroid nodules or goiter
	Soft tissue tumor (lipoma, sebaceous cyst)
	Chemodectoma (carotid body tumor)
	Neurogenic tumor (neurofibroma, neurilemoma)
	Laryngeal tumor (chondroma)
Malignant neoplasms	*Primary*
	Salivary gland tumor
	Thyroid cancer
	Upper aerodigestive tract cancer
	Soft tissue sarcoma
	Skin cancer (melanoma, squamous cell carcinoma, and basal cell carcinoma)
	Lymphoma
	Metastatic
	Upper aerodigestive tract cancer
	Skin cancer (melanoma, squamous cell carcinoma)
	Salivary gland tumor
	Thyroid cancer
	Adenocarcinoma (breast, GI tract, GU tract, lung)
	Unknown primary

239

Assessment of a Neck Mass

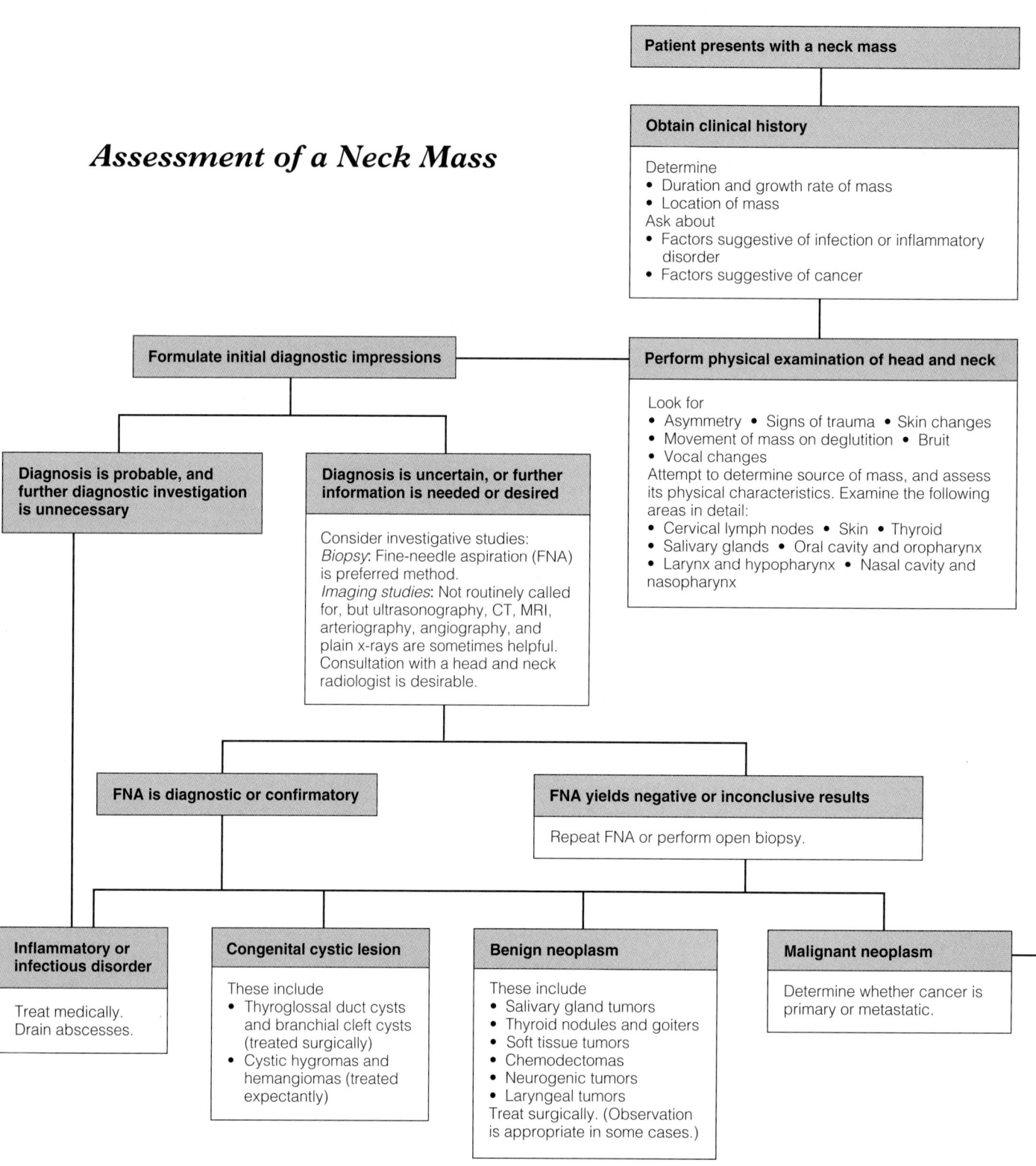

Patient presents with a neck mass

Obtain clinical history

Determine
- Duration and growth rate of mass
- Location of mass

Ask about
- Factors suggestive of infection or inflammatory disorder
- Factors suggestive of cancer

Perform physical examination of head and neck

Look for
- Asymmetry • Signs of trauma • Skin changes
- Movement of mass on deglutition • Bruit
- Vocal changes

Attempt to determine source of mass, and assess its physical characteristics. Examine the following areas in detail:
- Cervical lymph nodes • Skin • Thyroid
- Salivary glands • Oral cavity and oropharynx
- Larynx and hypopharynx • Nasal cavity and nasopharynx

Formulate initial diagnostic impressions

Diagnosis is probable, and further diagnostic investigation is unnecessary

Diagnosis is uncertain, or further information is needed or desired

Consider investigative studies:
Biopsy: Fine-needle aspiration (FNA) is preferred method.
Imaging studies: Not routinely called for, but ultrasonography, CT, MRI, arteriography, angiography, and plain x-rays are sometimes helpful. Consultation with a head and neck radiologist is desirable.

FNA is diagnostic or confirmatory

FNA yields negative or inconclusive results

Repeat FNA or perform open biopsy.

Inflammatory or infectious disorder

Treat medically.
Drain abscesses.

Congenital cystic lesion

These include
- Thyroglossal duct cysts and branchial cleft cysts (treated surgically)
- Cystic hygromas and hemangiomas (treated expectantly)

Benign neoplasm

These include
- Salivary gland tumors
- Thyroid nodules and goiters
- Soft tissue tumors
- Chemodectomas
- Neurogenic tumors
- Laryngeal tumors

Treat surgically. (Observation is appropriate in some cases.)

Malignant neoplasm

Determine whether cancer is primary or metastatic.

Primary neoplasm

These include
• Lymphoma • Thyroid cancer • Upper
aerodigestive tract cancer • Soft tissue sarcoma
• Skin cancer
Treat with surgery, radiation therapy, and/or
chemotherapy, as appropriate.

Metastatic tumor

Primary is known

Metastatic squamous cell carcinoma:
Perform selective neck dissection, and
consider adjuvant radiation therapy.
Metastatic adenocarcinoma: Perform
neck dissection (selective or other),
and consider adjuvant radiation
therapy.
Metastatic melanoma: Perform full-
thickness excision and SLN biopsy;
if there are positive SLNs or lymph
nodes are palpable, perform modified
neck dissection.

Primary is unknown

Evaluate nasopharynx, larynx,
esophagus, hypopharynx, and
tracheobronchial tree
endoscopically.
Biopsy nasopharynx, tonsils,
and hypopharynx.
Perform unilateral neck dissection
followed by irradiation of neck,
entire pharynx, and nasopharynx.

241

necessary to obtain adequate visualization of the various areas. Gloves must be worn during the examination, particularly if the mucous membranes are to be examined. Good illumination is essential. The time-honored but cumbersome head mirror has been largely supplanted by the headlight (usually a high-intensity halogen lamp). Fiberoptic endoscopy with a flexible laryngoscope and a nasopharyngoscope has become a common component of the physical examination for evaluating the larynx, the nasopharynx, and the paranasal sinuses, especially when these areas cannot be adequately visualized with more standard techniques.

The examination should begin with inspection for asymmetry, signs of trauma, and skin changes. One should ask the patient to swallow to see if the mass moves with deglutition. Palpation should be done both from the front and from behind. Auscultation is performed to detect audible bruits. One should also ask about the patient's voice, changes in which may suggest either a laryngeal tumor or recurrent nerve dysfunction from locally invasive thyroid cancer.

During the physical examination, one should be thinking about the following questions: What structure is the neck mass arising from? Is it a lymph node? Is the mass arising from a normally occurring structure, such as the thyroid gland, a nerve, a blood vessel, or a muscle? Or is it arising from an abnormal structure, such as a laryngocele, a branchial cleft cyst, or a cystic hygroma? Is the mass soft, fluctuant, easily mobile, well-encapsulated, and smooth? Or is it firm, poorly mobile, and fixed to surrounding structures? Does it pulsate? Is there a bruit? Does it appear to be superficial, or is it deeper in the neck? Is it attached to the skin? Is it tender?

The following areas of the head and neck are examined in some detail.

CERVICAL LYMPH NODES

Enlarged lymph nodes are by far the most common neck masses encountered. The cervical lymphatic system consists of interconnected groups or chains of nodes that parallel the major neurovascular structures in the head and neck. The skin and mucosal surfaces of the head and neck all have specific and predictable nodes associated with them. The classification of cervical lymph nodes has been standardized to comprise six levels [see Table 2 and Figure 1]. Accurate determination of lymph node level on physical examination and in surgical specimens not only helps establish a common language among clinicians but also permits comparison of data among different institutions.

The location, size, and consistency of lymph nodes furnish valuable clues to the nature of the primary disease. Other physical characteristics of the adenopathy should be noted as well, including the number of lymph nodes affected, their mobility, their degree of fixation, and their relation to surrounding anatomic structures. One can often establish a tentative diagnosis on the basis of these findings alone. For example, soft or tender nodes are more likely to derive from an inflammatory or infectious condition, whereas hard, fixed, painless nodes are more likely to represent metastatic cancer. Multiple regions of enlarged lymph nodes are usually a sign of systemic disease (e.g., lymphoma, tuberculosis, or infectious mononucleosis), whereas solitary nodes are more often due to malignancy. Firm, rubbery nodes are typical of lymphoma. Low cervical nodes are more likely to contain metastases from a primary source other than the head and neck, whereas upper cervical nodes are more likely to contain metastases from the head and neck.

The submental and submandibular nodes (level I) are palpated bimanually. Metastases to level I are commonly from the lips, the oral cavity, or the facial skin. The three levels of internal jugular chain nodes (levels II, III, and IV) are best examined by gently rolling the sternocleidomastoid muscle between the thumb and the index finger. Level II and level III lymph nodes are common sites for lymph node metastases from primary cancers of the oropharynx, the larynx, and the hypopharynx. Metastases in level IV lymph nodes can arise from cancers of the upper aerodigestive tract, from cancers of the thyroid gland, or from cancers arising below the clavicle (Virchow's node). The nodes in the posterior triangle (level V) are all palpated. Nodal metastases in this region can arise from nasopharyngeal and thyroid cancers as well as from squamous cell carcinoma or melanoma of the posterior scalp and the pinna of the ear. The tracheoesophageal groove nodes (level VI) are then palpated.

SKIN

Careful examination of the scalp, the ears, the face, and the neck will identify potentially malignant skin lesions, which may give rise to lymph node metastases.

THYROID GLAND

The thyroid gland is first observed as the patient swallows; it is then palpated and its size and consistency assessed with an eye to determining whether it is smooth, diffusely enlarged, or nodular and whether one nodule or several are present. If it is unclear whether the mass is truly thyroid, one can clarify the point by asking the patient to swallow and watching to see whether the mass moves. Signs of superior mediastinal syndrome (e.g., cervical venous engorgement and facial edema) suggest retrosternal extension of a thyroid goiter. The larynx and trachea are examined, with special attention to the cricothyroid membrane, over which Delphian nodes can be palpated. These nodes can be a harbinger of thyroid or laryngeal cancer.

MAJOR SALIVARY GLANDS

Examination of the paired parotid and submandibular glands involves not only palpation of the neck but also an intraoral examination to inspect the duct openings. The submandibular glands are best assessed by bimanual palpation, with one finger in the mouth and one in the neck. They are normally lower and more prominent in older patients. The parotid glands are often palpable in the neck, though the deep lobe cannot always be assessed. A mass in the region of the tail of the parotid must be

Table 2 Classification of Cervical Lymph Nodes

Level	Nodes
I	Submental nodes Submandibular nodes
II	Upper internal jugular chain nodes
III	Middle internal jugular chain nodes
IV	Lower internal jugular chain nodes
V	Spinal accessory nodes Transverse cervical nodes
VI	Tracheoesophageal groove nodes

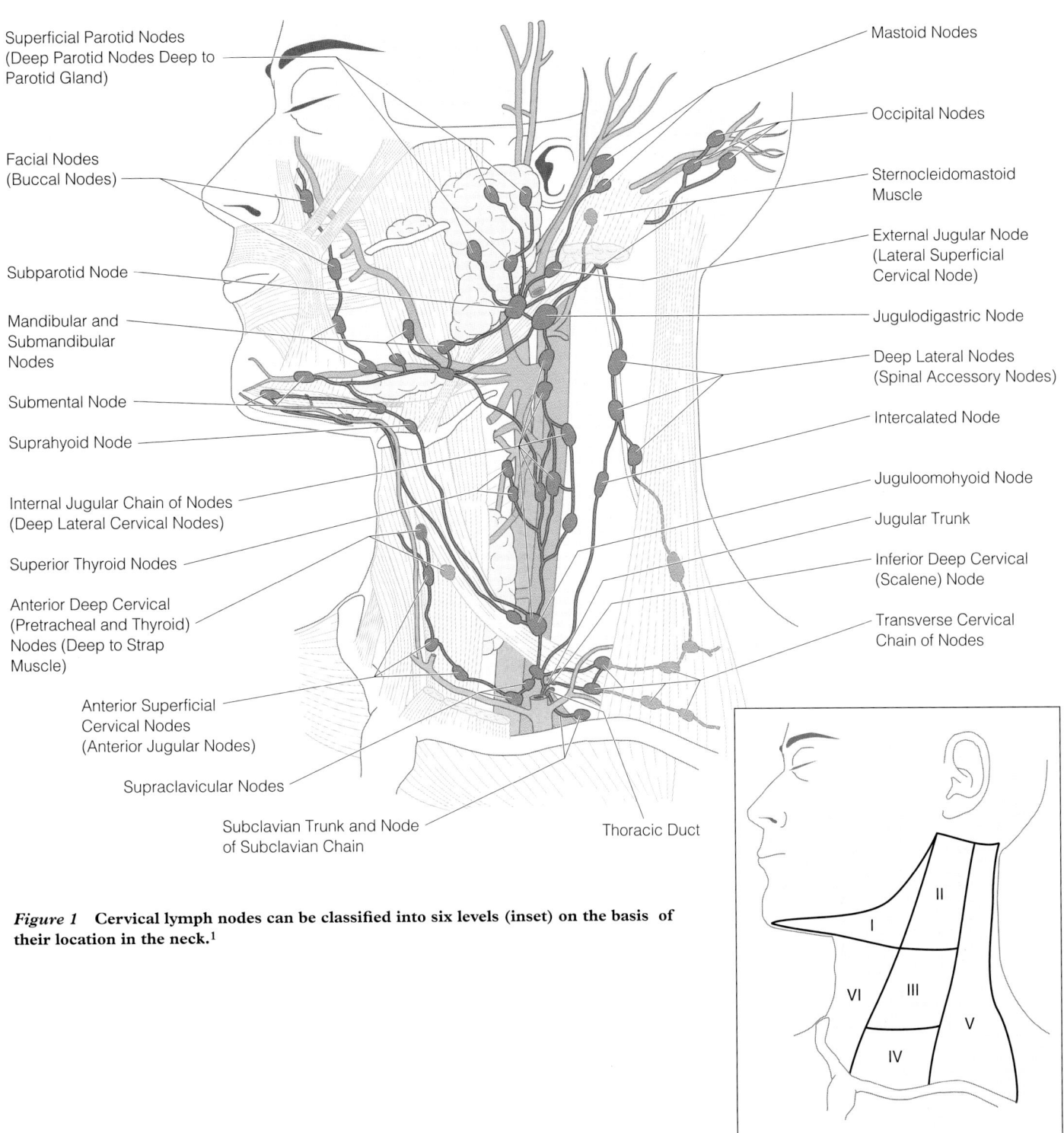

Superficial Parotid Nodes
(Deep Parotid Nodes Deep to
Parotid Gland)

Facial Nodes
(Buccal Nodes)

Subparotid Node

Mandibular and
Submandibular
Nodes

Submental Node

Suprahyoid Node

Internal Jugular Chain of Nodes
(Deep Lateral Cervical Nodes)

Superior Thyroid Nodes

Anterior Deep Cervical
(Pretracheal and Thyroid)
Nodes (Deep to Strap
Muscle)

Anterior Superficial
Cervical Nodes
(Anterior Jugular Nodes)

Supraclavicular Nodes

Subclavian Trunk and Node
of Subclavian Chain

Mastoid Nodes

Occipital Nodes

Sternocleidomastoid
Muscle

External Jugular Node
(Lateral Superficial
Cervical Node)

Jugulodigastric Node

Deep Lateral Nodes
(Spinal Accessory Nodes)

Intercalated Node

Juguloomohyoid Node

Jugular Trunk

Inferior Deep Cervical
(Scalene) Node

Transverse Cervical
Chain of Nodes

Thoracic Duct

Figure 1 **Cervical lymph nodes can be classified into six levels (inset) on the basis of their location in the neck.**[1]

distinguished from enlarged level II jugular nodes. The oropharynx is inspected for distortion of the lateral walls. The parotid (Stensen's) duct may be found opening into the buccal mucosa, opposite the second upper molar.

ORAL CAVITY AND OROPHARYNX

The lips should be inspected and palpated. Dentures should be removed before the mouth is examined. The buccal mucosa, the teeth, and the gingiva are then inspected. The patient should be asked to elevate the tongue so that the floor of the mouth can be examined and bimanual inspection performed. The tongue should be inspected both in its normal position in the mouth and during protrusion.

Most of the oropharyngeal contents are easily visualized if the tongue is depressed. Only the anterior two thirds of the tongue is clearly visible on examination, however. The base of the tongue is best visualized by using a mirror. In most persons, the tongue base can be palpated, at the cost of some discomfort to the patient. The ventral surface of the tongue must also be carefully inspected and palpated.

The hard palate is examined by gently tilting the patient's head backward, and the soft palate is inspected by gently depressing the tongue with a tongue blade. The movement of the palate is assessed by having the patient say "ahh."

The tonsils are then examined. They may vary substantially in size but are usually symmetrical. For example, in a young patient, hyperplastic tonsils may almost fill the oropharynx, but this is an uncommon finding in adults. Finally, the posterior pharyngeal wall is inspected.

LARYNX AND HYPOPHARYNX

The larynx and the hypopharynx are best examined by indirect or direct laryngoscopy. A mirror is warmed, and the patient's tongue is gently held forward to increase the space between the oropharyngeal structures. The mirror is carefully introduced into the oropharynx without touching the base of the tongue. The oropharynx, the larynx, and the hypopharynx can be visualized by changing the angle of the mirror.

The lingual and laryngeal surfaces of the epiglottis are examined. Often, the patient must be asked to phonate to bring the endolarynx into view. The aryepiglottic folds and the false and true vocal cords should be identified. The mobility of the true vocal cords is then assessed: their resting position is carefully noted, and their movement during inspiration is recorded. Normally, the vocal cords abduct during breathing and move to the median position during phonation. The larynx is elevated when the patient attempts to say "eeeee"; this allows one to observe vocal cord movement and to better visualize the piriform sinuses, the postcricoid hypopharynx, the laryngeal surface of the epiglottis, and the anterior commissure of the glottic larynx. Passage of a fiberoptic laryngoscope through the nose yields a clear view of the hypopharynx and the larynx. This procedure is well tolerated by almost all patients, particularly if a topical anesthetic is gently sprayed into the nose and swallowed, thereby anesthetizing both the nose and the pharynx.

NASAL CAVITY AND NASOPHARYNX

The nasopharynx is examined by depressing the tongue and inserting a small mirror behind the soft palate. The patient should be instructed to open the mouth widely and breathe through it to elevate the soft palate. With the patient relaxed, a warmed nasopharyngeal mirror should be carefully placed in the oropharynx behind the soft palate without touching the mucosa.

The nasal septum, the choanae, the turbinates, and the eustachian tube orifices are systematically assessed. The dorsum of the soft palate, the posterior nasopharyngeal wall, and the vault of the nasopharynx should also be assessed. The exterior of the nose should be carefully examined, and the septum should be inspected with a nasal speculum. Polyps or other neoplasms can be mistaken for turbinates.

Careful evaluation of the cranial nerves is essential, as is examination of the eyes (including assessment of ocular movement and visual activity), the external ear, and the tympanic membrane.

ADDITIONAL AREAS

The remainder of the physical examination is also important, particularly as regards the identification of a possible source of metastases to the neck. Other sets of lymph nodes—especially axillary and inguinal nodes—are examined for enlargement or tenderness. Women should undergo complete pelvic and rectal examinations. Men should undergo rectal, testicular, and prostate examinations; tumors from these organs occasionally metastasize to the neck. Appropriate blood tests should be ordered.

Initial Diagnostic Impressions

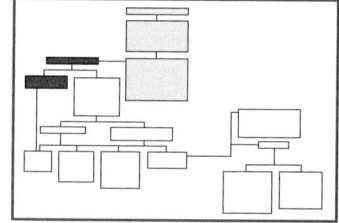

Having obtained a comprehensive history and performed a physical examination, one is likely to have a better idea of whether the neck mass is inflammatory, benign, or malignant. In some patients, the findings are clear enough to strongly suggest a specific disease entity. For example, a rapidly developing mass that is soft and tender to palpation is most likely a reactive lymph node from an acute bacterial or viral illness. A slow-growing facial mass associated with facial nerve deficits is probably a malignant parotid tumor. A thyroid nodule with an adjacent abnormal lymph node in a young patient probably represents thyroid cancer. In an elderly patient with a substantial history of smoking and alcohol use, a neck mass may well be a metastatic tumor (most likely from a squamous cell carcinoma in the aerodigestive tract).

One's initial diagnostic impressions and the degree of certainty one attaches to them determine the next steps in the workup and management of a neck mass; options include empirical therapy, ultrasonographic scanning, computed tomography, fine-needle aspiration (FNA), and observation alone. For example, in a patient with suspected bacterial lymphadenitis from an oral source, empirical antibiotic therapy with close follow-up is a reasonable approach. In a patient with a suspected parotid tumor, the best first test is a CT scan: the tumor probably must be removed, which means that one will have to ascertain the relation of the mass to adjacent structures. In a patient with suspected metastatic cancer, FNA is a sensible choice: it will confirm the presence of malignancy and may suggest a source of the primary cancer.

Investigative Studies

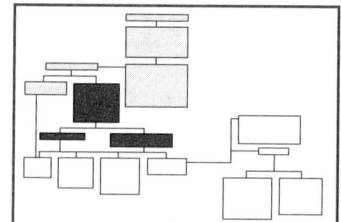

Neck masses of suspected infectious or inflammatory origin can be observed for short periods. Most neck masses in adults, however, are abnormal, and they are often manifestations of serious underlying conditions. In most cases, therefore, further diagnostic evaluation should be rigorously pursued.

BIOPSY

Whether or not the history and the physical examination strongly suggest a specific diagnosis, the information obtained by sampling tissue from the neck mass is often highly useful. In many cases, biopsy establishes the diagnosis; at the least, it may reduce the diagnostic possibilities. At present, the preferred method of obtaining material from a neck mass is FNA. FNA is the most important initial invasive diagnostic procedure in this setting. It is generally well tolerated and can usually be performed without local anesthesia. Although FNA is, on the whole, both safe and accurate, it is not completely free of potential problems (e.g., bleeding): it should therefore be done only if the results are likely to influence treatment.

FNA reliably distinguishes cystic from solid lesions and can often diagnose malignancy. It has in fact become the standard for making treatment decisions in patients with thyroid nodules and for confirming the clinical suspicion of a cystic lesion. FNA is also useful in patients with a known distant malignancy in whom confirmation of metastases is needed for staging and for planning therapy, as well as in patients with a primary tumor of the head and neck who are not candidates for operation but in whom a tissue diagnosis is necessary for appropriate nonsurgical therapy to be initiated. In addition, FNA is helpful in dealing with overly anxious patients in whom the clinical index of suspicion for a neoplasm is low and the head and neck examination is negative: negative biopsy results tend to reassure these patients and allow the surgeon time to follow the mass more confidently. (Of course, negative FNA results should not be considered the end point of any search and do not rule out cancer.)

Several studies have shown FNA to be approximately 90% accurate in establishing a definitive diagnosis. Lateral cystic neck masses that collapse on aspiration usually represent hygromas, branchial cleft cysts, or cystic degeneration of a metastatic papillary thyroid cancer. Fluid from these masses is sent for cytologic examination. If a palpable mass remains after cyst aspiration, a biopsy of the solid component should be done; the morphology of the cells will be better preserved.

If an extensive physical examination has been completed and the FNA is not diagnostic, one may have to perform an open biopsy to obtain a specimen for histologic sections and microbiologic studies. It is estimated that open biopsy eventually proves necessary in about 10% of patients with a malignant mass. In an open biopsy, it is important to orient skin incisions within the boundaries of a neck dissection; the incisions can then, if necessary, be extended for definitive therapy or reexcised if reoperation subsequently proves necessary. Crossing incisions should never be situated over vessels.

A suspected lymphoma constitutes a special situation. FNA alone is often incapable of determining the precise histologic subtype. Lymphoproliferative disease usually calls for open biopsy, frozen-section confirmation, and submission of fresh tissue to the pathologist. The intact node is placed in normal saline and sent directly to the pathologist for analysis of cellular content and nodal architecture and identification of lymphocyte markers. If infection is suspected, portions of the excised tissue are also sent for bacterial, fungal, mycobacterial, and viral cultures.

IMAGING STUDIES

Diagnostic imaging should be used selectively in the evaluation of a neck mass; imaging studies should be performed only if the results are likely to affect subsequent therapy. Such studies often supply useful information about the location and characteristics of the mass and its relation to adjacent structures. Diagnostic imaging is particularly useful when a biopsy has been performed and a malignant tumor identified. In such cases, these studies can help establish the extent of local disease and the presence or absence of metastases.

Ultrasonography reliably differentiates solid masses from cystic ones and is especially useful in assessing congenital and developmental cysts. It is a valuable noninvasive technique for vascular lesions and clearly delineates thyroid and parathyroid abnormalities. CT is also useful for differentiating cysts from solid lesions and for determining whether a mass is within or outside a gland or nodal chain. In addition, CT scanning can delineate small tongue-base or tonsillar tumors that have a min-

imal mucosal component. MRI provides much the same information as CT. T$_2$-weighted gadolinium-enhanced scans are particularly useful for delineating the invasion of soft tissue by tumor: endocrine tumors are often enhanced on such scans. Arteriography is useful mainly for evaluating vascular lesions and tumors fixed to the carotid artery. Angiography is helpful for evaluating the vascularity of a mass, its specific blood supply, or the status of the carotid artery, but it provides very little information about the physical characteristics of the mass. Plain radiographs of the neck are rarely helpful in differentiating neck masses, but a chest x-ray can often confirm a diagnosis (e.g., in patients with lymphoma, sarcoidosis, or metastatic lung cancer). A chest x-ray is required in any patient with a new diagnosis of cancer to determine if pulmonary metastases are present. It is also an important component of preoperative evaluation for any patient older than 40 years who requires an operation.

It is important to communicate with the radiologist: an experienced head and neck radiologist may be able to offer valuable guidance in choosing the best diagnostic test in a specific clinical scenario. Furthermore, providing the radiologist with a detailed clinical history facilitates interpretation of the images.

Management of Specific Disorders

INFLAMMATORY AND INFECTIOUS DISORDERS

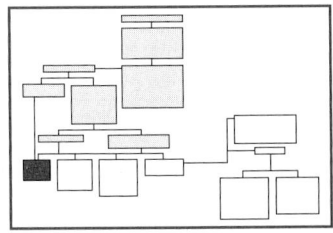

Acute infection of the neck (cervical adenitis) is most often the result of dental infection, tonsillitis, pharyngitis, viral upper respiratory tract infection, or skin infection. Lymph node enlargement is a frequent finding that may reflect any of a number of infectious disorders. The most common cause of this symptom is an acute infection of the mouth or pharynx. In this situation, the enlarged lymph nodes are usually just posterior and inferior to the angle of the mandible. Signs of acute infection (e.g., fever, malaise, and a sore mouth or throat) are usually present. A constitutional reaction, tenderness of the cervical mass, and the presence of an obvious infectious source confirm the diagnosis. Treatment should be directed toward the primary disease and should include a monospot test for infectious mononucleosis.

Neck masses may also derive from subcutaneous abscesses, infected sebaceous or inclusion cysts, or multiloculated carbuncles (most often occurring in the back of the neck in a patient with diabetes mellitus). The physical characteristics of abscesses make recognition of these problems relatively straightforward.

On occasion, primary head and neck bacterial infections can lead to infection of the fascial spaces of the neck. A high index of suspicion is required: such infections are sometimes difficult to diagnose. Aggressive treatment with antibiotics and drainage of closed spaces is indicated to prevent overwhelming fasciitis.

Various chronic infections (e.g., tuberculosis, fungal lymphadenitis, syphilis, cat-scratch fever, and AIDS) may also involve cervical lymph nodes. Certain chronic inflammatory disorders (e.g., sarcoidosis) may present with cervical lymphadenopathy as well. Because of the chronic lymph node involvement, these conditions are easily confused with neoplasms, especially lymphomas. Biopsy is occasionally necessary; however, skin tests and serologic studies are often more useful for establishing a diagnosis. Treatment of these conditions is primarily medical; surgery is reserved for complications.

CONGENITAL CYSTIC LESIONS

Thyroglossal Duct Cysts

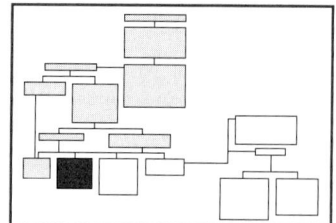

Thyroglossal duct cysts are remnants of the tract along which the thyroid gland descended into the neck from the foramen cecum [see Figure 2]. They account for about 70% of all congenital abnormalities of the neck. Thyroglossal duct cysts may be found in patients of any age but are most common in the first decade of life. They may take the form of a lone cyst, a cyst with a sinus tract, or a solid core of thyroid tissue. They may be so small as to be barely perceptible, as large as a grapefruit, or anything in between. Thyroglossal duct cysts are almost always found in the midline, at or below the level of the hyoid bone; however, they may be situated anywhere from the base of the tongue to the suprasternal notch. They occasionally present slightly lateral to the midline and are sometimes associated with an external fistula to the skin of the anterior neck. They are often ballotable and can usually be moved slightly from side to side but not up or down; however, they do move up and down when patients swallow or protrude the tongue.

Thyroglossal duct cysts must be differentiated from dermoid cysts, lymphadenomegaly in the anterior jugular chain, and cutaneous lesions (e.g., lipomas and sebaceous cysts). Operative treatment is almost always required, not only because of cosmetic considerations but also because of the high incidence of recurrent infection, including abscess formation. About 1% of thyroglossal duct cysts contain cancer; papillary cancer is the neoplasm most commonly encountered, followed by squamous cell carcinoma.

Branchial Cleft Cysts

Branchial cleft cysts are vestigial remnants of the fetal branchial apparatus from which all neck structures are derived. Early in embryonic development, there are five branchial arches and four grooves (or clefts) between them. The internal tract or opening of a branchial cleft cyst is situated at the embryologic derivative of the corresponding pharyngeal groove, such as the tonsil (second arch) or the piriform sinus (third and fourth arches). The second arch is the most common area of origin for such cysts. The position of the cyst tract is also determined by the embryologic relation of its arch to the derivatives of the arches on either side of it.

The majority of branchial cleft cysts (those that develop from the second, third, and fourth arches) tend to present as a bulge along the anterior border of the sternocleidomastoid muscle, with or without a sinus tract. Branchial cleft cysts may become symptomatic at any age, but most are diagnosed in the first two decades of life. They often present as a smooth, painless, slowly enlarging mass in the lateral neck. Frequently, there is a history of fluctuating size and intermittent tenderness. The diagnosis is more obvious when there is an external fistulous tract and there is a history of intermittent discharge. Infection of the cyst may be the reason for the first symptoms.

Treatment consists of complete surgical removal of the cyst and the sinus tract. Any infection or inflammation should be treated and allowed to resolve before the cyst and the tract are removed.

Cystic Hygromas (Lymphangiomas)

A cystic hygroma is a lymphangioma that arises from vestigial lymph channels in the neck. Almost always, this condition is first noted by the second year of life; on rare occasions, it is first diagnosed in adulthood. A cystic hygroma may present as a relatively simple thin-walled cyst in the floor of the mouth or may involve all the tissues from the floor of the mouth to the mediastinum. About 80% of the time, there is only a painless cyst in the posterior cervical triangle or in the supraclavicular area. A cystic hygroma can also occur, however, at the root of the neck, in the angle of the jaw (where it may involve the parotid gland), and in the midline (where it may involve the tongue, the floor of the mouth, or the larynx).

The typical clinical picture is of a diffuse, soft, doughy, irregular mass that is readily transilluminated. Cystic hygromas look and feel somewhat like lipomas but have less well defined margins. Aspiration of cystic hygromas yields straw-colored fluid. They may be confused with angiomas (which are compressible), pneumatoceles from the apex of the lung, or aneurysms. They can be distinguished from vascular lesions by means of arteriography. On occasion, a cystic hygroma grows suddenly as a result of an upper respiratory tract infection, infection of the hygroma itself, or hemorrhage into the tissues. If the mass becomes large enough, it can compress the trachea or hinder swallowing.

In the absence of pressure symptoms (i.e., obstruction of the airway or interference with swallowing) or gross deformity, cystic hygromas may be treated expectantly. They tend to regress spontaneously; if they do not, complete surgical excision is indicated. Excision can be difficult because of the numerous satellite extensions that often surround the main mass and because of the association of the tumor with vital structures such as the cranial nerves. Recurrences are common; staged resections for complete excision are often necessary.

Vascular Malformation (Hemangiomas)

Hemangiomas are usually considered congenital because they either are present at birth or appear within the first year of life. A number of characteristic findings—bluish-purple coloration, increased warmth, compressibility followed by refilling, bruit, and thrill—distinguish them from other head and neck masses. Angiography is diagnostic but is rarely indicated.

Given that most of these congenital lesions resolve spontaneously, the treatment approach of choice is observation alone unless there is rapid growth, thrombocytopenia, or involvement of vital structures.

BENIGN NEOPLASMS

Salivary Gland Tumors

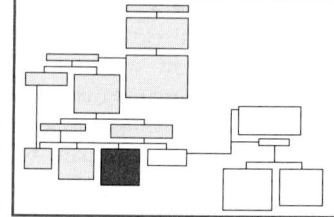

The possibility of a salivary gland neoplasm must be considered whenever an enlarging solid mass lies in front of and below the ear, at the angle of the mandible, or in the submandibular triangle. Benign salivary gland lesions are often asymptomatic; malignant ones are often associated with seventh cranial nerve symptoms or skin fixation. Diagnostic radiographic studies (CT or MRI) indicate whether the mass is salivary in origin but do not help classify it histologically. The diagnostic test of preference is open biopsy in the form of complete submandibular gland removal or superficial parotidectomy.

With any mass in or around the ear, one should be prepared to remove the superficial lobes of the parotid, the deep lobes, or both and to perform a careful facial nerve dissection. Any less complete approach reduces the chances of a cure: there is

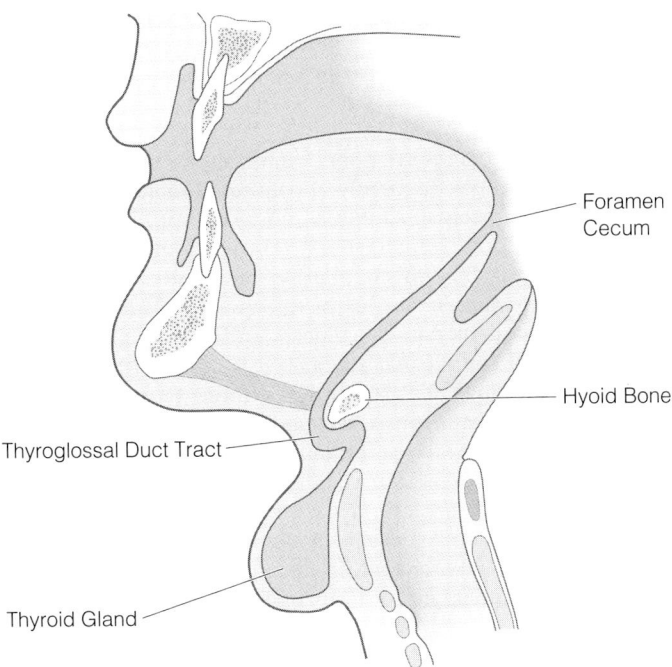

Figure 2 **Shown is the course of the thyroglossal duct tract from its origin in the area of the foramen cecum to the pyramidal lobe of the thyroid gland.[2] In the operative treatment of a thyroglossal duct cyst, the central portion of the hyoid bone must be removed to ensure complete removal of the tract and to prevent recurrence.**

Labels in figure:
Foramen Cecum
Hyoid Bone
Thyroglossal Duct Tract
Thyroid Gland

a high risk of implantation and seeding of malignant tumors. Benign mixed tumors make up two thirds of all salivary tumors; these must also be completely removed because recurrence is common after incomplete resection.

Benign Thyroid Nodules and Nodular Goiters

Thyroid disease is a relatively common cause of neck masses: in the United States, about 4% of women and 2% of men have a palpable thyroid nodule. Patients should be questioned about local symptoms (pain, dysphagia, pressure, hoarseness, or a change in the voice), about the duration of the nodule, and about systemic symptoms (from hyperthyroidism, hypothyroidism, or any other illness). Although most nodules are benign, malignancy is a significant concern. Nodules in children, young men, pregnant women, or persons with a history of radiation exposure or a family history of thyroid cancer are more likely to be malignant. Nodules that are truly solitary, feel firm or hard on examination, are growing rapidly, or are nonfunctional on scans are more likely to be malignant.

If physical examination suggests a discrete thyroid nodule, FNA should be done to ascertain whether malignancy is present within the nodule. If malignancy is confirmed or suspected, surgery is indicated. If the nodule is histologically benign or disappears with aspiration, thyroid suppression and observation are often sufficient. FNA often yields unrepresentative results in patients with a history of radiation exposure, in whom there is approximately a 40% chance that one of the nodules present contains cancer.

Surgery for thyroid nodules involves excisional biopsy consisting of at least total lobectomy; enucleation is almost never indicated. The surgical approach of choice for most patients with Graves disease or multinodular goiter is subtotal thy-

roidectomy or total lobectomy on one side and subtotal lobectomy on the other (Dunhill's operation). Treatment of thyroid cancer is discussed elsewhere [*see* Primary Malignant Neoplasms, Thyroid Cancer, *below*].

Soft Tissue Tumors (Lipomas, Sebaceous Cysts)

Superficial intracutaneous or subcutaneous masses may be sebaceous (or epidermal inclusion) cysts or lipomas. Final diagnosis and treatment usually involves simple surgical excision, often done as an office procedure with local anesthesia.

Chemodectomas (Carotid Body Tumors)

Carotid body tumors belong to a group of tumors known as chemodectomas (or, alternatively, as glomus tumors or nonchromaffin paragangliomas), which derive from the chemoreceptive tissue of the head and neck. In the head and neck, chemodectomas most often arise from the tympanic bodies in the middle ear, the glomus jugulare at the skull base, the vagal body near the skull base along the inferior ganglion of the vagus, and the carotid body at the carotid bifurcation. They are occasionally familial and sometimes occur bilaterally.

A carotid body tumor presents as a firm, round, slowly growing mass at the carotid bifurcation. Occasionally, a bruit is present. The tumor cannot be separated from the carotid artery by palpation and can usually be moved laterally and medially but not in a cephalocaudal plane. The differential diagnosis includes a carotid aneurysm, a branchial cleft cyst, a neurogenic tumor, and nodal metastases fixed to the carotid sheath. The diagnosis is made by means of CT scanning or arteriography, which demonstrate a characteristic highly vascular mass at the carotid bifurcation. Neurofibromas tend to displace, encircle, or compress a portion of the carotid artery system, events that are readily demonstrated by carotid angiography.

Biopsy should be avoided. Chemodectomas are sometimes malignant and should therefore be removed in most cases to prevent subsequent growth and pressure symptoms. Fortunately, even malignant chemodectomas are usually low grade; long-term results after removal are excellent on the whole. Some experience with vascular surgery is desirable: bleeding may occur, and clamping of the carotid artery may result in a stroke. Expectant treatment may be indicated in older or debilitated individuals. Radiotherapy may be appropriate for patients with unresectable tumors.

Neurogenic Tumors (Neurofibromas, Neurilemomas)

The large number of nerves in the head and neck renders the area susceptible to neurogenic tumors. The most common of such tumors, neurilemomas (schwannomas) and neurofibromas, arise from the neurilemma and usually present as painless, slowly growing masses in the lateral neck. Neurilemomas can be differentiated from neurofibromas only by means of histologic examination.

Given the potential these tumors possess for malignant degeneration and slow but progressive growth, surgical resection is indicated. This may include resection of the involved nerves, particularly with neurofibromas, which tend to be more invasive and less encapsulated than neurilemomas.

Laryngeal Tumors

In rare cases, a chondroma may arise from the thyroid cartilage or the cricoid cartilage. It is firmly fixed to the cartilage and may present as a mass in the neck or as the cause of a progressively compromised airway. Surgical excision is indicated.

PRIMARY MALIGNANT NEOPLASMS

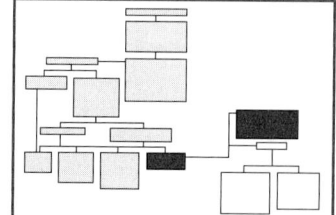

Lymphomas

Cervical adenopathy is one of the most common presenting symptoms in patients with Hodgkin and non-Hodgkin lymphoma. The nodes tend to be softer, smoother, more elastic, and more mobile than nodes containing metastatic carcinoma would be. Rapid growth is not unusual, particularly in non-Hodgkin lymphoma. Involvement of extranodal sites, particularly Waldeyer's tonsillar ring, is often seen in patients with non-Hodgkin lymphoma; enlargement of these sites may provide a clue to the diagnosis. The diagnosis is confirmed via excisional biopsy of an intact lymph node. As noted, the precise histologic subtype usually cannot be determined by FNA alone; open biopsy must be done, and fresh tissue must be submitted for surface marker and electron microscopic studies.

Lymphoma is treated by means of radiation therapy, chemotherapy, or both, depending on the disease's pathologic type and clinical stage.

Thyroid Cancer

The approach to suspected thyroid cancer differs in some respects from the approach to benign thyroid disease. The operation of choice for papillary thyroid cancer that is occult (< 1 cm in diameter) and confined to the thyroid gland and for minimally invasive follicular thyroid cancer (i.e., with only capsular invasion) is thyroid lobectomy; the prognosis is excellent. The procedure of choice for papillary, follicular, Hürthle cell, and medullary thyroid cancer is total or near-total thyroidectomy (when it can be done safely) [see 2:8 Thyroid and Parathyroid Procedures]. Patients who present with thyroid nodules and have a history of radiation exposure or a family history of thyroid cancer should also undergo total or near-total thyroidectomy because about 40% of them will have at least one focus of papillary thyroid cancer. Total thyroidectomy decreases recurrence and permits the use of iodine-131 (^{131}I) to scan for and treat residual disease; it also makes serum thyroglobulin and calcitonin assays more sensitive for diagnosing recurrent or persistent differentiated thyroid tumors of follicular or parafollicular cell origin.

Patients with medullary thyroid cancer should undergo meticulous elective (prophylactic) or therapeutic central neck dissection. They should be screened for ret proto-oncogene mutations on chromosome 10. Therapeutic modified neck dissection is indicated for all patients with thyroid cancer and palpable nodes laterally. Prophylactic modified neck dissection is indicated for patients with medullary thyroid cancer and either primary tumors larger than 1.5 cm or evidence of central neck node involvement.

Patients with anaplastic thyroid cancer are probably best treated with a combination of chemotherapy and radiation therapy, in conjunction with the removal of as much of the neoplasm as can safely be excised. Most patients with thyroid lymphoma should receive chemotherapy, radiation therapy, or both.

Upper Aerodigestive Tract Cancer

Deciding on the optimal therapeutic approach to tumors of the aerodigestive tract (i.e., surgery, radiation therapy, or some combination of the two) generally requires expertise beyond that of most general surgeons. Therefore, cancers involving the nose, the paranasal sinuses, the nasopharynx, the floor of the mouth, the tongue, the palate, the tonsils, the piriform sinus, the hypopharynx, or the larynx are best managed by an experienced head and neck oncologic surgeon in conjunction with a radiation therapist and a medical oncologist.

Soft Tissue Sarcomas

Malignant sarcomas are not common in the head and neck. The sarcomas most frequently encountered include the rhabdomyosarcoma seen in children, fibrosarcoma, liposarcoma, osteogenic sarcoma (which usually arises in young adults), and chondrosarcoma. The most common head and neck sarcoma, however, is malignant fibrous histiocytoma (MFH). MFH is seen most frequently in the elderly and extremely rarely in children, but it can arise at any age. It is often difficult to differentiate pathologically from other entities (e.g., fibrosarcoma). MFH can occur in the soft tissues of the neck or involve the bone of the maxilla or the mandible. The preferred treatment is wide surgical resection; adjuvant radiation therapy and chemotherapy are currently being studied in clinical trials.

Rhabdomyosarcoma, usually of the embryonic form, is the most common form of sarcoma in children. It generally occurs near the orbit, the nasopharynx, or the paranasal sinuses. The diagnosis is confirmed by biopsy. A thorough search for distal metastases is made before treatment—consisting of a combination of surgical resection, radiation therapy, and chemotherapy—is begun.

Skin Cancer

Basal cell carcinomas are the most common of the skin malignancies [see 2:4 Skin Lesions]. These lesions arise in areas that have been extensively exposed to sunlight (e.g., the nose, the forehead, the cheeks, and the ears). Treatment consists of local resection with adequate clear margins. Metastases are rare, and the prognosis is excellent. Inadequately excised and neglected basal cell carcinomas may ultimately spread to regional lymph nodes and can cause extensive local destruction of soft tissue and bone. For example, basal cell carcinoma of the medial canthus may invade the orbit, the ethmoid sinus, and even the brain. Periauricular basal cell carcinoma can spread across the cartilage of the ear canal or into the parotid gland.

Squamous cell carcinoma also arises in areas associated with extensive sunlight exposure; the lower lip and the pinna are the most common sites. Unlike basal cell carcinoma, however, squamous cell carcinoma tends to metastasize regionally and distally. This tumor must also be excised with an adequate margin.

Melanoma is classified on the basis of size, location, depth of invasion, and histologic subtype, although the prognosis is closely related to the thickness of the tumor [see Metastatic Tumors, Metastatic Melanomas, below]. In addition to the typical pigmented, irregularly shaped skin lesions [see 2:4 Skin Lesions], malignant melanoma may also arise on the mucous membranes of the nose or the throat, on the hard palate, or on the buccal mucosa. The treatment of choice is wide surgical resection. Radiation therapy, chemotherapy, and immunotherapy may also be considered.

METASTATIC TUMORS

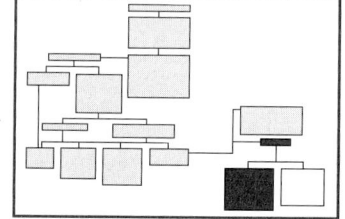

Any surgeon who is managing patients with head and neck cancers must have a thorough understanding of neck dissections and should have sufficient training and experience to perform these operations in the appropriate clinical circumstances.

Types of Neck Dissections

There are two classification systems for neck dissections. The first is based on the indications and goals of surgery. An *elective* (or *prophylactic*) neck dissection is done when the neck is clinically negative (that is, when no abnormal lymph nodes are palpable or visible on radiographic imaging). A *therapeutic* neck dissection is done to remove all palpable and occult disease in patients with suspicious lymph nodes discovered via physical examination or CT scanning.

The second system is based on the extent and type of dissection. *Comprehensive* neck dissections include the classic radical neck dissection as well as the modified radical (or functional) neck dissection [*see Figure 3*]. In a radical neck dissection, the sternocleidomastoid muscle, the internal and external jugular veins, the spinal accessory nerve, and the submaxillary gland are removed, along with all lymph node–bearing tissues. The modified radical or functional neck dissection is a modification of the radical neck dissection in which the lymphatic tissue from these areas is removed but the functional structures are preserved. *Selective* neck dissections involve the removal of specific levels of lymph nodes [*see Figure 1*]. The rationale for selective dissections is that several head and neck cancers consistently metastasize to specific localized lymph node regions. The following are examples of selective neck dissections: suprahyoid neck dissection (levels I and II); supraomohyoid neck dissection (levels I, II, and III); lateral neck dissection (levels II, III, and IV); and posterolateral neck dissection (levels II, III, IV, and V).

Metastatic Squamous Cell Carcinomas

The basic principle in the management of metastatic squamous cell carcinoma is to treat all regional lymph node groups at highest risk for metastases by means of surgery or radiation therapy, depending on the clinical circumstances. Selective lymph node dissection can be performed along with wide excision of the primary tumor at the time of initial operation. For example, carcinomas of the oral cavity are treated with supra-omohyoid neck dissection, and carcinomas of the oropharynx, the hypopharynx, and the larynx are treated with lateral neck dissection. If extranodal extension or the presence of multiple levels of positive nodes is confirmed by the pathologic findings, the patient should receive adjuvant bilateral neck radiation for 4 to 6 weeks after operation.

Metastatic Adenocarcinomas

Adenocarcinoma in a cervical node most frequently represents a metastasis from the thyroid gland, the salivary glands, or the GI tract. The primary tumor must therefore be sought through endoscopic and radiologic study of the bronchopulmonary tract, the GI tract, the genitourinary tract, the salivary glands, and the thyroid gland. Other possible primary malignancies to be considered include breast and pelvic tumors in women and prostate cancer in men.

If the primary site is controlled and the patient is potentially curable or if the primary site is not found and the neck disease is the only established site of malignancy, neck dissection is the appropriate treatment. Postoperative adjuvant radiation may also be considered. If the patient has thyroid cancer and palpable nodes, lateral neck dissection and ipsilateral central neck dissection are recommended.

Overall survival is low—about 20% at 2 years and 9% at 5 years—except for patients with papillary or follicular thyroid cancer, who have a good prognosis. Two factors associated with a better prognosis are unilateral neck involvement and limitation of disease to lymph nodes above the cricoid cartilage.

Metastatic Melanomas

If the patient has a thin melanoma (Breslow thickness < 1 mm; Clark level I, II, or III), full-thickness excision with 1 cm margins should be done. Intermediate-thickness melanomas (Breslow thickness 1 to 4 mm; Clark level IV) are also staged with lymphatic mapping and sentinel lymph node (SLN) biopsy [*see 2:6 Lymphatic Mapping and Sentinel Lymph Node Biopsy*]. All patients with intermediate-thickness melanomas and multiple positive SLNs and all melanoma patients with palpable lymph nodes should undergo modified neck dissection for adequate local disease control. Because these tumors may metastasize to nodes in the parotid region, superficial parotidectomy is often included in the neck dissection, particularly in the case of melanoma located on the upper face or the anterior scalp. Consultation with a medical oncologist is indicated for all patients with intermediate-thickness or thick (Breslow thickness > 4 mm; Clark level IV or V) melanomas; immunotherapy or chemotherapy may be considered. Radiation therapy is often considered in patients with extensive local or nodal disease.

Metastases from an Unknown Primary Malignancy

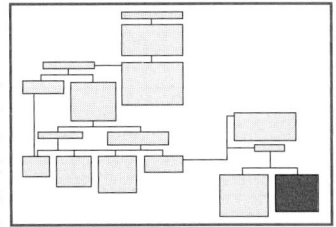

Management of patients with an unknown primary malignancy is challenging for the surgeon. It is helpful to know that when cervical lymph nodes are found to contain metastatic squamous cell carcinoma, the primary tumor is in the head and neck about 90% of the time. Typically, such patients are found to have squamous cell carcinoma on the basis of FNA of an abnormal cervical lymph node; this finding calls for an exhaustive review of systems as well as a detailed physical examination of the head and neck.

If no primary tumor is identified, the patient should undergo endoscopic evaluation of the nasopharynx, the hypopharynx, the esophagus, the larynx, and the tracheobronchial tree under gen-

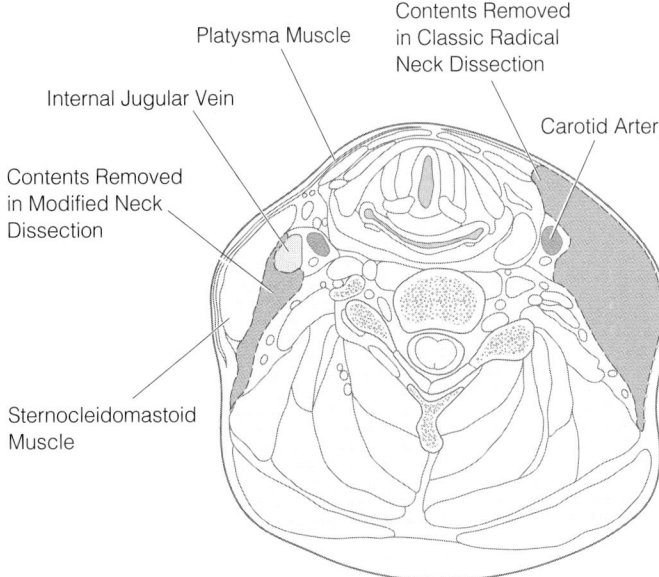

Figure 3 Cross section of the neck shows the structures removed in a classic radical neck dissection (right) and in a modified radical neck dissection (left).[3]

eral anesthesia. Biopsies of the nasopharynx, the tonsils, and the hypopharynx often identify the site of origin (although there is some debate on this point). If the biopsies do not reveal a primary source of cancer, the preferred treatment is unilateral neck dissection, followed by radiation therapy directed toward the neck, the entire pharynx, and the nasopharynx. In 15% to 20% of cases, the primary cancer is ultimately detected. Overall 5-year survival in such cases ranges from 25% to 50%.

If a malignant melanoma is found in a cervical lymph node but no primary tumor is evident, the patient should be asked about previous skin lesions, and a thorough repeat head and neck examination should be done, with particular attention to the scalp, the nose, the oral cavities, and the sinuses. An ophthalmologic exam-

ination is also required. If physical examination and radiographic studies find no evidence of metastases, modified neck dissection should be performed on the involved side.

Metastatic adenocarcinoma in a cervical lymph node with no known primary tumor is discussed elsewhere [see Metastatic Adenocarcinomas, above]. The most common primary sites in the head and neck are the salivary glands and the thyroid gland. The possibility of an isolated metastasis from the breast, the GI tract, or the genitourinary tract must also be rigorously investigated. If no primary site is identified, the patient should be considered for protocol-based chemotherapy and radiation therapy, directed according to what the primary site is most likely to be in that patient.

References

1. Fabian RL: Benign and malignant diseases of the head and neck. Current Practice of Surgery. Levine BA, Copeland EM III, Howard RJ, et al, Eds. Churchill Livingstone, New York, 1993, vol 2, sect VII, chap 1

2. Cohen JI: Benign neck masses. Boie's Fundamentals of Otolaryngology: A Textbook of Ear, Nose and Throat Disease, 6th ed. Adams GL, Boie LR Jr, Hilger PA, Eds. WB Saunders Co, Philadelphia, 1989

3. Coleman JJ III, Sultan MR: Tumors of the head and neck. Principles of Surgery, 6th ed. Schwartz SI, Shires GT, Spencer FC, Eds. McGraw-Hill Book Co, New York, 1994, p 595

Recommended Reading

Beenken SW, Maddox WA, Urist MM: Workup of a patient with a mass in the neck. Adv Surg 28:371, 1995

Byers RM: Neck dissection: concepts, controversies and technique. Semin Surg Oncol 7:9, 1991

Chandler JR, Mitchell B: Branchial cleft cysts, sinuses and fistulas. Otolaryngol Clin North Am 14:175, 1981

Clark O, Duh QY: Textbook of Endocrine Surgery. WB Saunders Co, Philadelphia, 1997

Clark OH, Noguchi S: Thyroid Cancer Diagnosis and Treatment. Quality Medical Publishing, St Louis, 2000

Davidson BJ, Spiro RH, Patel S, et al: Cervical metastases of occult origin: the impact of combined modality therapy. Am J Surg 168:195, 1994

Delbridge L, Guinea AL, Reeve TS: Total thyroidectomy for bilateral benign multinodular goiter: effect of changing practice. Arch Surg 134:1385, 1999

Hainsworth JD: Poorly differentiated carcinoma and poorly differentiated adenocarcinoma of unknown primary tumor site of the neck. Semin Oncol 20:279, 1993

Hoffman HT, Karnell LH, Funk GF, et al: The National Cancer Database report on cancer of the head and neck. Arch Otolaryngol Head Neck Surg 124:951, 1998

Jossart GH, Clark OH: Well-differentiated thyroid cancer. Curr Probl Surg 31:933, 1994

Lee NK, Byers RM, Abbruzzese JL, et al: Metastatic adenocarcinoma to the neck from an unknown primary source. Am J Surg 162:306, 1991

McGuirt WF: Diagnosis and management of masses in the neck, with special emphasis on metastatic disease. Oncology 4:85, 1990

Moley JF, De Beneditti MK: Patterns of nodal metastases in palpable medullary thyroid carcinoma: recommendations for extent of node dissection. Ann Surg 225:880, 1999

Montgomery WW: Surgery of the neck. Surgery of the Upper Respiratory System, 2nd ed. Lea & Febiger, Philadelphia, 1989, p 83

Nguyen TD, Malissard L, Theobald S, et al: Advanced carcinoma of the larynx: results of surgery and radiotherapy without induction chemotherapy (1980–1985): a multivariate analysis. Int J Radiat Oncol Biol Phys 36:1013, 1996

Shah JP, Medina JE, Shaha AR, et al: Cervical lymph node metastasis. Curr Probl Surg 30:1, 1993

Spiro RH: Management of malignant tumor of the salivary glands. Oncology 12:671, 1998

Van den Brekel MW, Castelijns JA: Surgery of lymph nodes in the neck. Semin Roentgenol 35:42, 2000

Wu HS, Young MT, Ituarte P, et al: Death from thyroid cancer of follicular cell origin. J Am Coll Surg 191:600, 2000

Acknowledgment

Figures 1 through 3   Tom Moore.

3 ALIMENTARY TRACT AND ABDOMEN

1 ACUTE ABDOMINAL PAIN

Romano Delcore, M.D., F.A.C.S., and Laurence Y. Cheung, M.D., F.A.C.S.

Assessment of Acute Abdominal Pain

The term acute abdominal pain generally refers to previously undiagnosed pain that arises suddenly and is of less than 7 days' (usually less than 48 hours') duration.[1] It may be caused by a great variety of intraperitoneal disorders, many of which call for surgical treatment, as well as many extraperitoneal disorders,[2] which typically do not call for surgical treatment [*see* Tentative Differential Diagnosis, *below*]. Abdominal pain that persists for 6 hours or longer is usually caused by disorders of surgical significance.[3] The primary goal in the management of patients with acute abdominal pain is to determine whether operative intervention is necessary and, if so, when the operation should be performed. Often, this determination is easy to make; on occasion, however, the evaluation of patients with acute abdominal pain can be one of the most difficult challenges in clinical surgery. It is essential to keep in mind that most (at least two thirds) of the patients who present with acute abdominal pain have disorders for which surgical intervention is not required.[2,4,5]

Making the correct decision regarding whether to operate on a patient with acute abdominal pain requires sound surgical judgment. The decision must be based on a detailed medical and surgical clinical history as well as a meticulous physical examination. These, in turn, must be based on experience, a thorough knowledge of the anatomy and physiology of the peritoneal cavity, and a clear understanding of the pathologic processes that occur within the abdomen. Much has been written about the diagnosis of acute abdominal pain since 1921, when Sir Zachary Cope first published his now classic paper.[3] Although the basic approach to assessment of acute abdominal pain remains much the same today, the introduction of new diagnostic technologies and better resuscitation methods, coupled with an aging population (in the United States and other developed countries) and new disease processes, necessitates periodic revision of the traditional approach as well as constant broadening of the differential diagnosis. For example, with the proliferation of less invasive surgery, the use of laparoscopy has expanded far beyond its initial application to cholecystectomy. Emergency laparoscopy has become more widely accepted in the treatment of acute surgical diseases (e.g., acute appendicitis and perforated peptic ulcer) as general surgeons gain competence in its use. Diagnostic laparoscopy has also proved valuable in the assessment of acute abdominal pain (see below).

Historically, diagnosis of the causes of acute abdominal pain has been based largely on pattern recognition, in which clinicians attempt to match new cases to preexisting stereotypes (so-called classic presentations) of various diseases. Certainly, knowledge of these classic presentations is basic to successful diagnosis, but it is crucial to remember that at least one third of patients with acute abdominal pain exhibit atypical features that render pattern recognition unreliable.[4,6,7]

Clinical History

A careful and methodical clinical history should be obtained that includes the mode of onset, duration, frequency, character, location, chronology, radiation, and intensity of the pain, as well as the presence or absence of any aggravating or alleviating factors and associated symptoms. Often, such a history is more valuable than any single laboratory or x-ray finding and determines the course of subsequent evaluation and management. Unfortunately, when the ability of clinicians to take an organized and accurate history has been studied, the results have been disappointing.[7] For this reason, the use of standardized history and physical forms, with or without the aid of diagnostic computer programs, has been recommended.

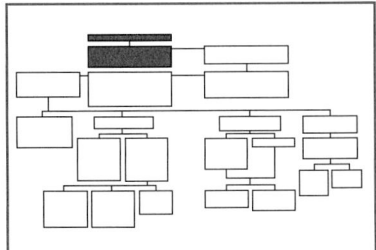

Computer-aided diagnosis has been extensively studied in England.[8-11] In these studies, physicians collected clinical data on structured data sheets and entered the information into a computer running a diagnostic program; the computer, which contained a large clinical database, then generated diagnostic probabilities. One such study demonstrated that integration of computer-aided diagnosis into the management of 16,737 patients with acute abdominal pain yielded a 20% improvement in diagnostic accuracy.[8] This improvement resulted in statistically significant reductions in inappropriate admissions, negative laparotomies, serious management errors (e.g., failure to operate on patients who require surgery), and length of hospital stay, as well as statistically significant increases in the number of patients who were immediately discharged home without adverse effects and the promptness with which those requiring surgery underwent operation. Although these impressive results are undoubtedly attributable to more than one cause, it is certain that the required use of a structured data sheet to record the patient's history for computer analysis played a crucial role. In fact, when the data sheets were used without the computer, diagnostic accuracy and overall decision making were still significantly improved.

There now appears to be more than sufficient evidence to support the routine use of structured data sheets in the initial stages of obtaining a history from a patient with acute abdominal pain.[9-11] An example of such a data sheet is the pain chart developed by the World Organization of Gastroenterology (OMGE) [*see Figure 1*]. The components of this data sheet represent the consensus of the more than 2,000 surgeons worldwide who contributed to its development and have used it to collect

Assessment of Acute Abdominal Pain

Patient presents with acute abdominal pain

Obtain clinical history

Assess mode of onset, duration, frequency, character, location, chronology, radiation, and intensity of pain.
Look for aggravating or alleviating factors and associated symptoms.
Use structured data sheets if possible.

Generate working diagnosis

Proceed with subsequent management on the basis of the working diagnosis.
Reevaluate patient repeatedly. If patient does not respond to treatment as expected, reassess working diagnosis and return to differential diagnosis.

Perform basic investigative studies

Laboratory: complete blood count, hematocrit, electrolytes, creatinine, blood urea nitrogen, glucose, liver function tests, amylase, lipase, urinalysis, pregnancy test, ECG (if patient is elderly or has atherosclerosis).

Radiologic: Plain abdominal films (upright and supine) and chest radiographs.
(Note: These studies are rarely diagnostic by themselves; their purpose is primarily confirmatory.)

Patient requires immediate laparotomy

Conditions necessitating immediate laparotomy include ruptured abdominal aortic or visceral aneurysm, ruptured ectopic pregnancy, spontaneous hepatic or splenic rupture, major blunt or penetrating abdominal trauma, and hemoperitoneum from various causes.
Severe hemodynamic instability is the essential indication.

Patient has suspected surgical abdomen

Determine whether urgent laparotomy is necessary.

Patient requires urgent laparotomy or laparoscopy

Conditions necessitating urgent laparotomy include perforated hollow viscus, appendicitis, Meckel diverticulitis, strangulated hernia, mesenteric ischemia, and ectopic pregnancy (unruptured).

Laparoscopy is recommended for acute appendicitis and perforated ulcers (provided that surgeon has sufficient experience and competence with the technique).

Patient should be hospitalized and observed

Observe patient carefully, and reevaluate condition periodically.
Consider additional investigative studies (e.g., CT, ultrasonography, diagnostic peritoneal lavage, radionuclide imaging, angiography, MRI, and GI endoscopy).

Diagnostic laparoscopy is recommended if pain persists after a period of observation.

Patient requires early laparotomy or laparoscopy

Early laparotomy or laparoscopy is reserved for patients whose conditions are unlikely to become life threatening if operation is delayed for 24–48 hr (e.g., those with uncomplicated intestinal obstruction, uncomplicated acute cholecystitis, uncomplicated acute diverticulitis, or nonstrangulated incarcerated hernia).

Patient is candidate for elective laparotomy or laparoscopy

Elective laparotomy or laparoscopy is reserved for patients who are highly likely to respond to conservative medical management or whose conditions are highly unlikely to become life threatening during prolonged evaluation (e.g., those with IBD, peptic ulcer disease, pancreatitis, or endometriosis).

Diagnosis is uncertain, or patient has suspected nonsurgical abdomen

Reevaluate patient as appropriate
(see facing page).

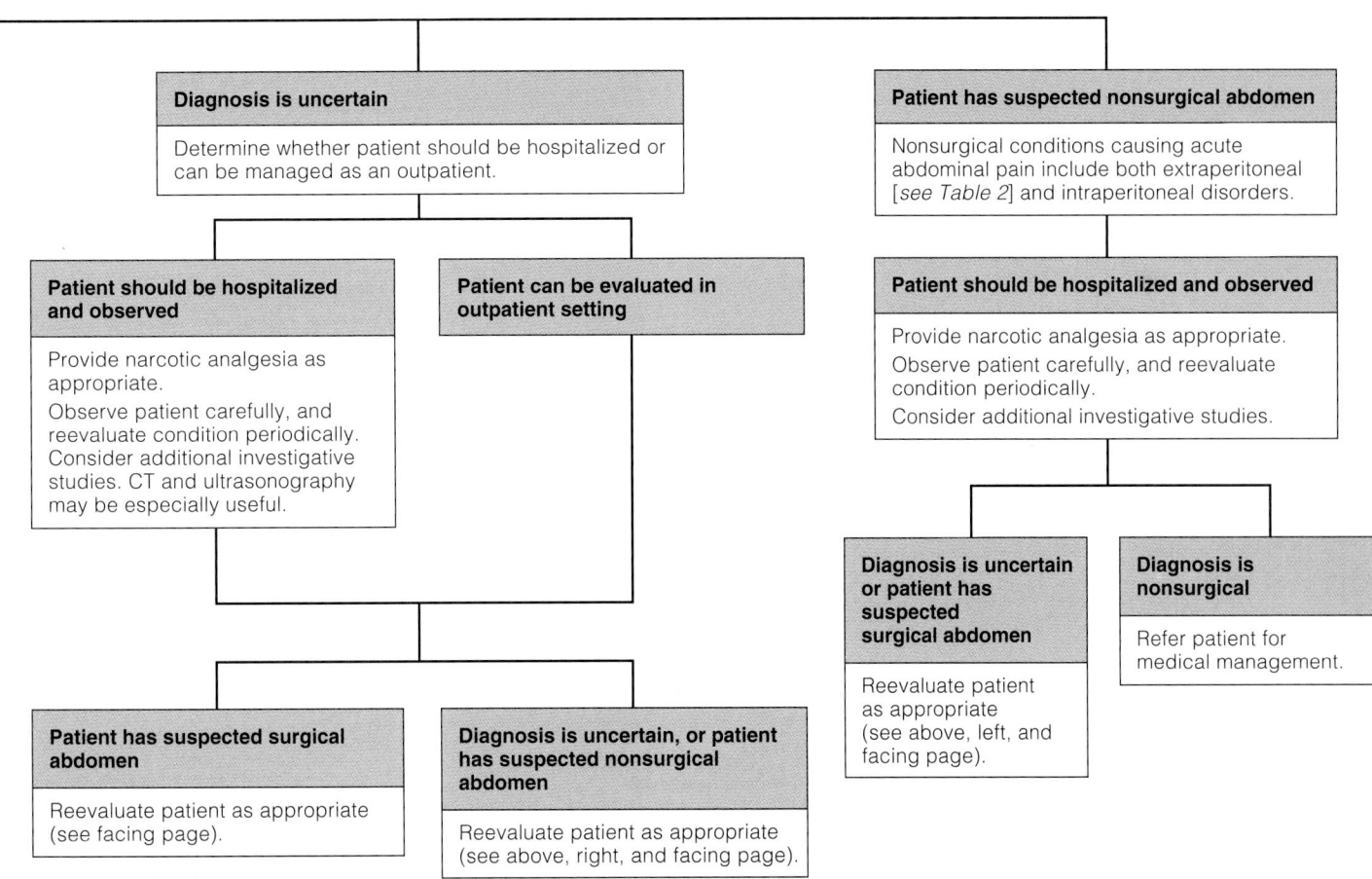

Generate tentative differential diagnosis

Remember that the majority of patients will turn out to have nonsurgical diagnoses.
Take into account effects of age and gender on diagnostic possibilities.

Perform physical examination

Evaluate general appearance and ability to answer questions; estimate degree of obvious pain; note position in bed; identify area of maximal pain; look for extra-abdominal causes of pain and signs of systemic illness.
Perform systematic abdominal examination: (1) inspection, (2) auscultation, (3) percussion, (4) palpation.
Perform rectal, genital, and pelvic examinations.

Diagnosis is uncertain

Determine whether patient should be hospitalized or can be managed as an outpatient.

Patient should be hospitalized and observed

Provide narcotic analgesia as appropriate.
Observe patient carefully, and reevaluate condition periodically.
Consider additional investigative studies. CT and ultrasonography may be especially useful.

Patient can be evaluated in outpatient setting

Patient has suspected surgical abdomen

Reevaluate patient as appropriate (see facing page).

Diagnosis is uncertain, or patient has suspected nonsurgical abdomen

Reevaluate patient as appropriate (see above, right, and facing page).

Patient has suspected nonsurgical abdomen

Nonsurgical conditions causing acute abdominal pain include both extraperitoneal [see Table 2] and intraperitoneal disorders.

Patient should be hospitalized and observed

Provide narcotic analgesia as appropriate.
Observe patient carefully, and reevaluate condition periodically.
Consider additional investigative studies.

Diagnosis is uncertain or patient has suspected surgical abdomen

Reevaluate patient as appropriate (see above, left, and facing page).

Diagnosis is nonsurgical

Refer patient for medical management.

ABDOMINAL PAIN CHART

NAME _____   REG. NUMBER _____

MALE _____ FEMALE _____ AGE _____   FORM FILLED BY _____

MODE OF ARRIVAL _____   DATE _____   TIME _____

PAIN

Site of Pain

At Onset

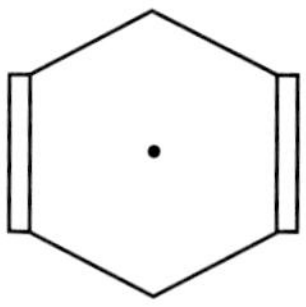

At Present

Radiation

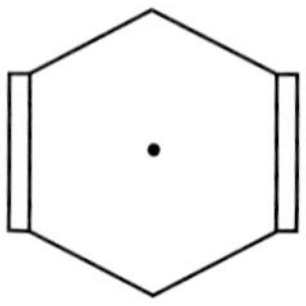

Aggravating Factors
  movement
  coughing
  respiration
  food
  other
  none

Relieving Factors
  lying still
  vomiting
  antacids
  food
  other
  none

Progression of Pain
  better
  same
  worse

Duration

Type
  intermittent
  steady
  colicky

Severity
  moderate
  severe

HISTORY

Nausea
  yes   no

Vomiting
  yes   no

Anorexia
  yes   no

Indigestion
  yes   no

Jaundice
  yes   no

Bowels
  normal
  constipation
  diarrhea
  blood
  mucus

Micturition
  normal
  frequency
  dysuria
  dark
  hematuria

Previous Similar Pain
  yes   no

Previous Abdominal Surgery
  yes   no

Drugs for Abdominal Pain
  yes   no

Female-LMP
  pregnant
  vaginal discharge
  dizzy/faint

EXAMINATION

Temp.   Pulse
BP

Mood
  normal
  upset
  anxious

Color
  normal
  pale
  flushed
  jaundiced
  cyanotic

Intestinal Movement
  normal
  poor/nil
  peristalsis

Scars
  yes   no

Distention
  yes   no

Location of Tenderness

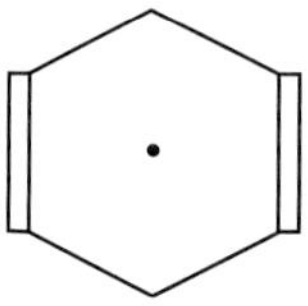

Rebound
  yes   no

Guarding
  yes   no

Rigidity
  yes   no

Mass
  yes   no

Murphy's Sign Present
  yes   no

Bowel Sounds
  normal
  absent
  increased

Rectal-Vaginal Tenderness
  left
  right
  general
  mass
  none

Initial Diagnosis & Plan

Results
  amylase
  blood count (WBC)
  urine
  x-ray

  other

Diagnosis & Plan after Investigation

(time   )

Discharge Diagnosis

History and examination of other systems on separate case notes.

Figure 1 **Shown is a data sheet modified from the abdominal pain chart developed by the OMGE.**[13]

information for the Research Committee of the OMGE and other groups studying acute abdominal pain.[12,13] Given that the data sheet is by no means exhaustive, individual surgeons may want to add to it; however, they would be well advised not to omit any of the symptoms and signs on the data sheet from their routine examination of patients with acute abdominal pain.[14]

When the surgeon obtains a complete clinical history with an open mind, the patient often provides important clues to the correct diagnosis. Patients should be allowed to relate the history in their own words, and examiners should refrain from suggesting specific symptoms, except as a last resort. Any questions that must be asked should be open-ended—for example, "What happens when you eat?" rather than "Does eating make the pain worse?" Leading questions should be avoided. When a leading question must be asked, it should be posed first as a negative question (i.e., one that calls for an answer in the negative), since a negative answer to a question is more likely to be honest and accurate. For example, if peritoneal inflammation is suspected, the question asked should be "Does coughing make the pain better?" rather than "Does coughing make the pain worse?"

The mode of onset of abdominal pain may help the examiner determine the severity of the underlying disease. Pain that has a sudden onset suggests an intra-abdominal catastrophe, such as a ruptured abdominal aortic aneurysm, a perforated viscus, or a ruptured ectopic pregnancy. Rapidly progressive pain that becomes intensely centered in a well-defined area within a period of a few minutes to an hour or two suggests a condition such as acute cholecystitis or pancreatitis. Pain that has a gradual onset over several hours, usually beginning as slight or vague discomfort and slowly progressing to steady and more localized pain, suggests a subacute process and is characteristic of peritoneal inflammation. Numerous disorders may be associated with this mode of onset, including acute appendicitis, diverticulitis, pelvic inflammatory disease (PID), and intestinal obstruction.

Pain can be either intermittent or continuous. Intermittent or cramping pain (colic) is pain that occurs for a short period (a few minutes), followed by longer periods (a few minutes to one-half hour) of complete remission during which there is no pain at all. Intermittent pain is characteristic of obstruction of a hollow viscus and results from vigorous peristalsis in the wall of the viscus proximal to the site of obstruction. This pain is perceived as deep in the abdomen and is poorly localized. The patient is restless, may writhe about incessantly in an effort to find a comfortable position, and often presses on the abdominal wall in an attempt to alleviate the pain. Whereas the intermittent pain associated with intestinal obstruction (typically described as gripping and mounting) is usually severe but bearable, the pain associated with obstruction of small conduits (e.g., the biliary tract, the ureters, and the uterine tubes) often becomes unbearable. Obstruction of the gallbladder or bile ducts gives rise to a type of pain often referred to as biliary colic; however, this term is a misnomer, in that biliary pain is usually constant because of the lack of a strong muscular coat in the biliary tree and the absence of regular peristalsis.

Continuous or constant pain is pain that is present for hours or days without any period of complete relief; it is more common than intermittent pain. Continuous pain is usually indicative of peritoneal inflammation or ischemia. It may be of steady intensity throughout, or it may be associated with intermittent pain. For example, the typical colicky pain associated with simple intestinal obstruction changes when strangulation occurs, becoming continuous pain that persists between episodes or waves of cramping pain.

Certain types of pain are generally held to be typical of certain pathologic states—for example, the general burning pain of a perforated gastric ulcer, the tearing pain of a dissecting aneurysm, and the gripping pain of intestinal obstruction. However, the character of the pain is not always a reliable clue to its cause.

For several reasons—atypical pain patterns, dual innervation by visceral and somatic afferents, normal variations in organ position, and widely diverse underlying pathologic states—the location of abdominal pain is only a rough guide to diagnosis. It is nevertheless true that in most disorders, the pain tends to occur in characteristic locations, such as the right upper quadrant (cholecystitis), the right lower quadrant (appendicitis), the epigastrium (pancreatitis), or the left lower quadrant (sigmoid diverticulitis) [see Figure 2]. It is important to determine the location of the pain at onset because this may differ from the location at the time of presentation (so-called shifting pain). In fact, the chronological sequence of events in the patient's history is often more important for diagnosis than the location of the pain alone. For example, the classic pain of appendicitis begins in the periumbilical region and settles in the right lower quadrant. A similar shift in location can occur when escaping gastroduodenal contents from a perforated ulcer pool in the right lower quadrant.

It is also important to take into account radiation or referral of the pain, which tends to occur in characteristic patterns [see Figure 3]. For example, biliary pain is referred to the right subscapular area, and the boring pain of pancreatitis typically radiates straight through to the back. The more severe the pain is, the more likely it is to be referred.

The intensity or severity of the pain is related to the magnitude of the underlying insult. It is important to distinguish between the intensity of the pain and the patient's reaction to it because there appear to be significant individual differences with respect to tolerance of and reaction to pain. Pain that is intense enough to awaken the patient from sleep usually indicates a significant underlying organic cause. Past episodes of pain and factors that aggravate or relieve the pain often provide useful diagnostic clues. For example, pain caused by peritonitis tends to be exacerbated by motion, deep breathing, coughing, or sneezing, and patients with peritonitis tend to lie quietly in bed and avoid any movement. The typical pain of acute pancreatitis is exacerbated by lying down and relieved by sitting up. Pain that is relieved by eating or taking antacids suggests duodenal ulcer disease, whereas diffuse abdominal pain that appears 30 minutes to 1 hour after meals suggests intestinal angina.

Associated gastrointestinal symptoms, such as nausea, vomiting, anorexia, diarrhea, and constipation, often accompany abdominal pain; however, these symptoms are nonspecific and therefore may not be of great value in the differential diagnosis. Vomiting in particular is common: when sufficiently stimulated by pain impulses traveling via secondary visceral afferent fibers, the medullary vomiting centers activate efferent fibers and cause reflex vomiting. Once again, the chronology of events is important, in that pain often precedes vomiting in patients with conditions necessitating operation, whereas the opposite is usually the case in patients with medical (i.e., nonsurgical) conditions.[4,6] This is particularly true for patients with acute appendicitis, in whom pain almost always precedes vomiting by several hours. Similarly, constipation may result from a reflex paralytic ileus when sufficiently stimulated visceral afferent fibers activate efferent sympathetic fibers (splanchnic nerves) to

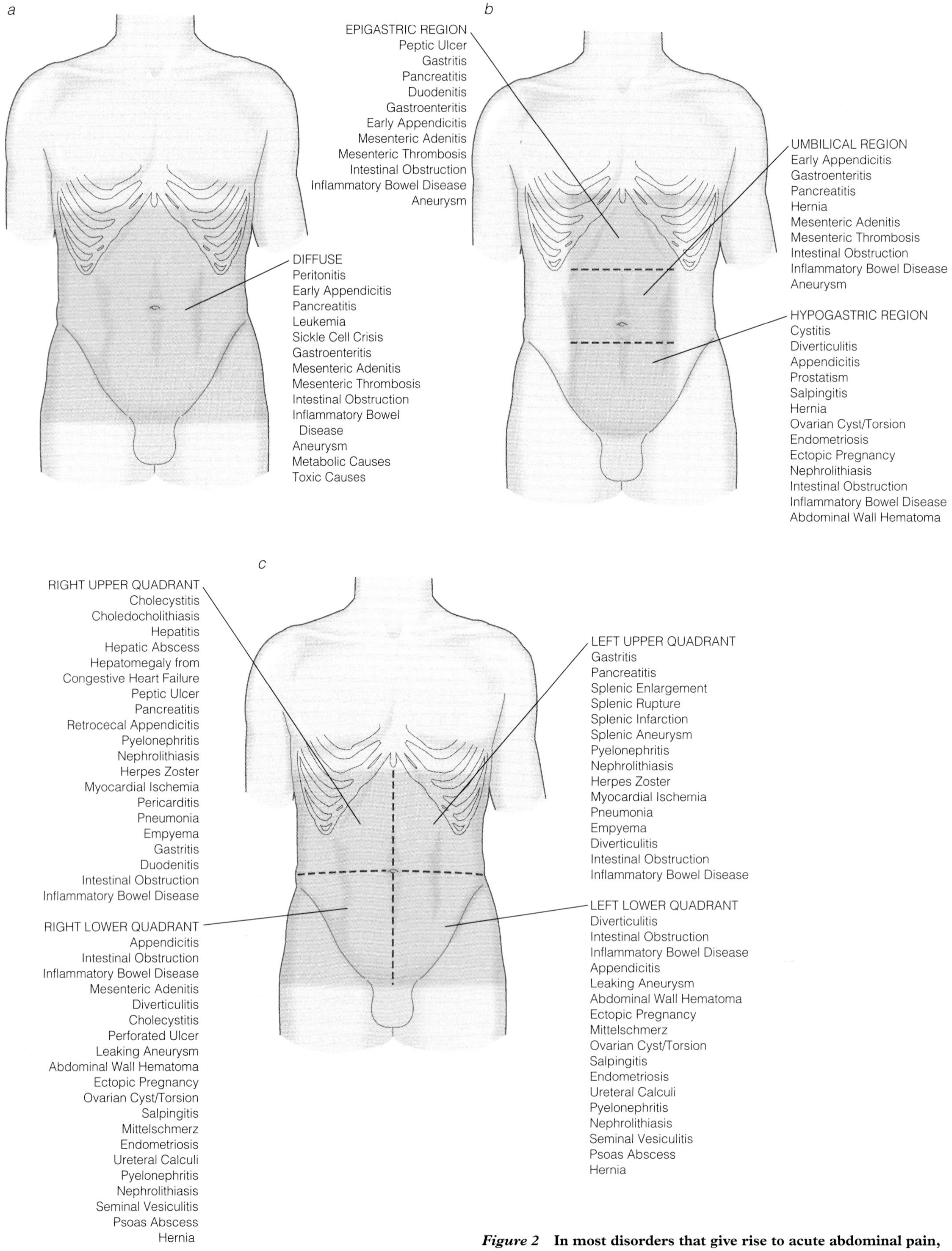

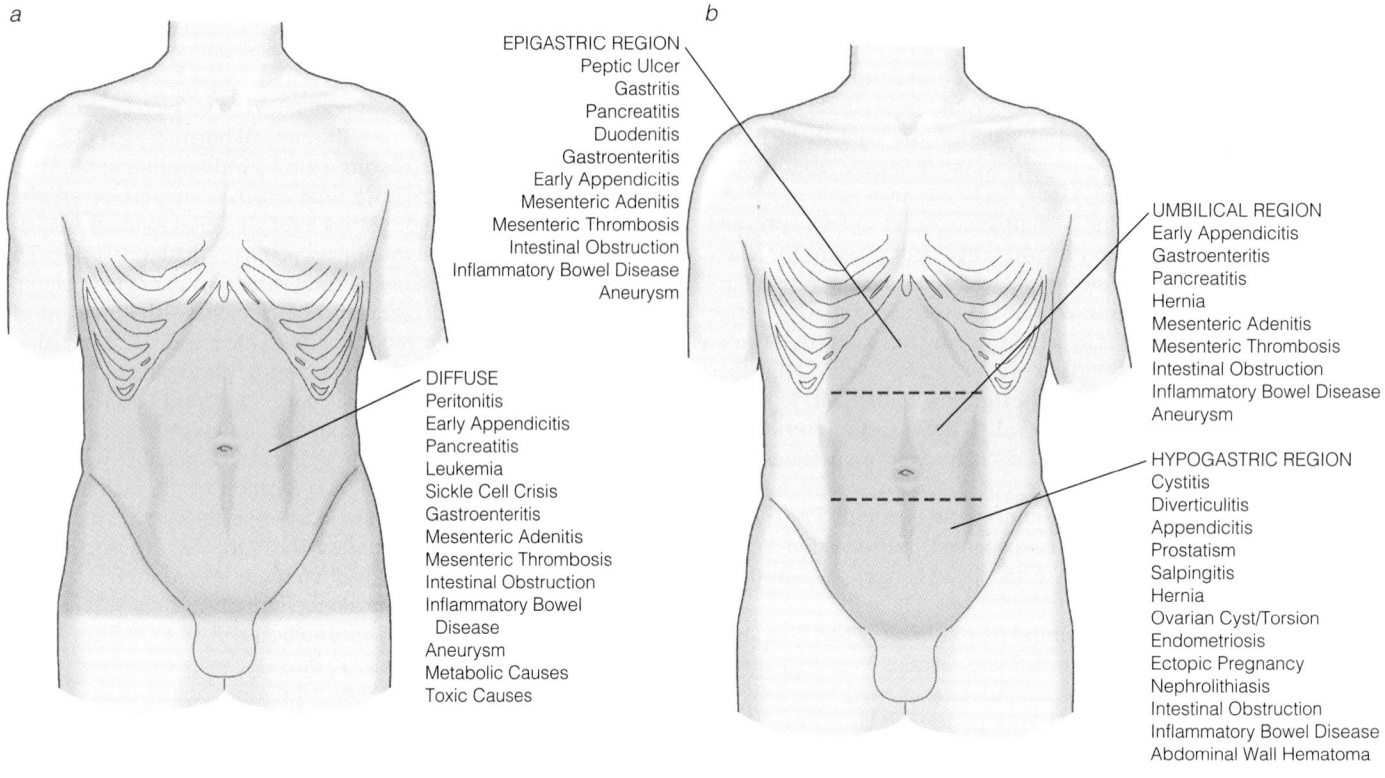

a

b

EPIGASTRIC REGION
Peptic Ulcer
Gastritis
Pancreatitis
Duodenitis
Gastroenteritis
Early Appendicitis
Mesenteric Adenitis
Mesenteric Thrombosis
Intestinal Obstruction
Inflammatory Bowel Disease
Aneurysm

DIFFUSE
Peritonitis
Early Appendicitis
Pancreatitis
Leukemia
Sickle Cell Crisis
Gastroenteritis
Mesenteric Adenitis
Mesenteric Thrombosis
Intestinal Obstruction
Inflammatory Bowel
 Disease
Aneurysm
Metabolic Causes
Toxic Causes

UMBILICAL REGION
Early Appendicitis
Gastroenteritis
Pancreatitis
Hernia
Mesenteric Adenitis
Mesenteric Thrombosis
Intestinal Obstruction
Inflammatory Bowel Disease
Aneurysm

HYPOGASTRIC REGION
Cystitis
Diverticulitis
Appendicitis
Prostatism
Salpingitis
Hernia
Ovarian Cyst/Torsion
Endometriosis
Ectopic Pregnancy
Nephrolithiasis
Intestinal Obstruction
Inflammatory Bowel Disease
Abdominal Wall Hematoma

c

RIGHT UPPER QUADRANT
Cholecystitis
Choledocholithiasis
Hepatitis
Hepatic Abscess
Hepatomegaly from
Congestive Heart Failure
Peptic Ulcer
Pancreatitis
Retrocecal Appendicitis
Pyelonephritis
Nephrolithiasis
Herpes Zoster
Myocardial Ischemia
Pericarditis
Pneumonia
Empyema
Gastritis
Duodenitis
Intestinal Obstruction
Inflammatory Bowel Disease

LEFT UPPER QUADRANT
Gastritis
Pancreatitis
Splenic Enlargement
Splenic Rupture
Splenic Infarction
Splenic Aneurysm
Pyelonephritis
Nephrolithiasis
Herpes Zoster
Myocardial Ischemia
Pneumonia
Empyema
Diverticulitis
Intestinal Obstruction
Inflammatory Bowel Disease

RIGHT LOWER QUADRANT
Appendicitis
Intestinal Obstruction
Inflammatory Bowel Disease
Mesenteric Adenitis
Diverticulitis
Cholecystitis
Perforated Ulcer
Leaking Aneurysm
Abdominal Wall Hematoma
Ectopic Pregnancy
Ovarian Cyst/Torsion
Salpingitis
Mittelschmerz
Endometriosis
Ureteral Calculi
Pyelonephritis
Nephrolithiasis
Seminal Vesiculitis
Psoas Abscess
Hernia

LEFT LOWER QUADRANT
Diverticulitis
Intestinal Obstruction
Inflammatory Bowel Disease
Appendicitis
Leaking Aneurysm
Abdominal Wall Hematoma
Ectopic Pregnancy
Mittelschmerz
Ovarian Cyst/Torsion
Salpingitis
Endometriosis
Ureteral Calculi
Pyelonephritis
Nephrolithiasis
Seminal Vesiculitis
Psoas Abscess
Hernia

Figure 2 **In most disorders that give rise to acute abdominal pain, the pain tends to occur in specific locations.**

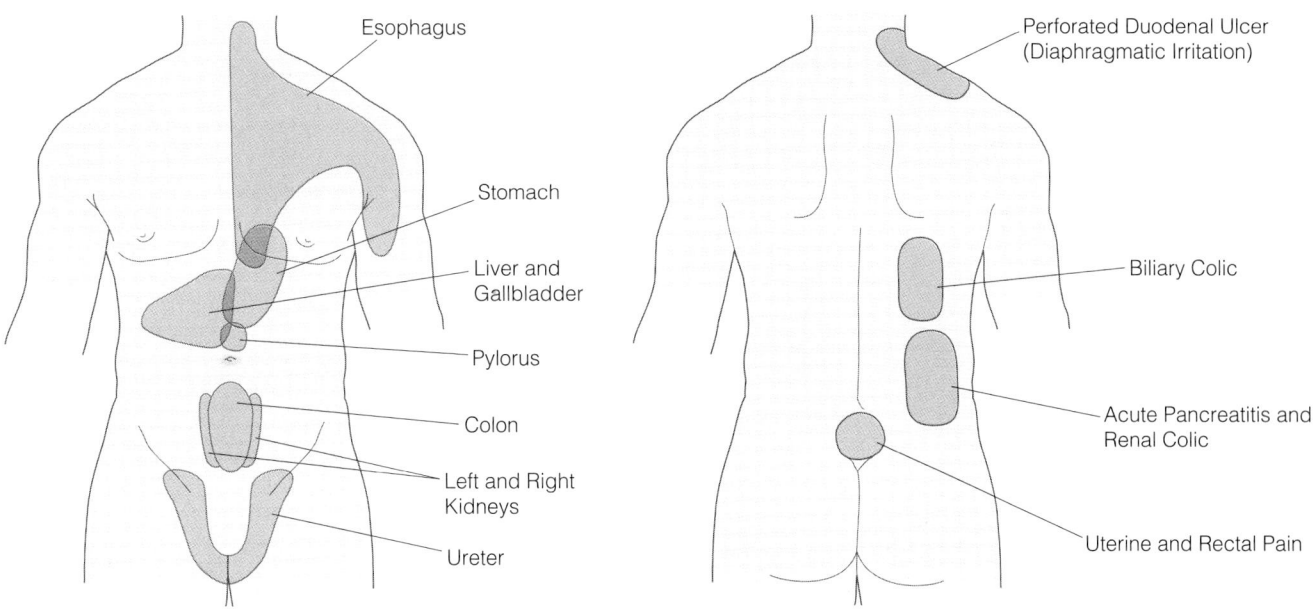

Figure 3 **Pain of abdominal origin tends to be referred in characteristic patterns.[43] The more severe the pain is, the more likely it is to be referred. Shown are anterior (left) and posterior (right) areas of referred pain.**

reduce intestinal peristalsis. Diarrhea is characteristic of gastroenteritis but may also accompany incomplete intestinal obstruction. More significant is a history of obstipation, because if it can be definitely established that a patient with acute abdominal pain has not passed gas or stool for 24 to 48 hours, it is certain that some degree of intestinal obstruction is present. Other associated symptoms that should be noted include jaundice, melena, hematochezia, hematemesis, and hematuria. These symptoms are much more specific than the ones just discussed and can be extremely valuable in the differential diagnosis. Most conditions that cause acute abdominal pain of surgical significance are associated with some degree of fever. Fever suggests an inflammatory process; however, it is usually low grade and often absent altogether, particularly in elderly and immunocompromised patients. The combination of a high fever with chills and rigors indicates bacteremia, and concomitant changes in mental status (e.g., agitation, disorientation, and lethargy) suggest impending septic shock.

A history of trauma (even if the patient considers the traumatic event trivial) should be actively sought in all cases of unexplained acute abdominal pain; such a history may not be readily volunteered (as is often the case with trauma resulting from domestic violence). With female patients, it is essential to obtain a detailed gynecologic history that includes the timing of symptoms within the menstrual cycle, the date of the last menses, previous and current use of contraception, any abnormal vaginal bleeding or discharge, an obstetric history, and any risk factors for ectopic pregnancy (e.g., PID, use of an intrauterine device, or previous ectopic or tubal surgery).

A complete history of previous medical conditions must be obtained because associated diseases of the cardiac, pulmonary, and renal systems may give rise to acute abdominal symptoms and may also significantly affect the morbidity and mortality associated with surgical intervention. Weight changes, past illnesses, recent travel, environmental exposure to toxins or infectious agents, and medications used should also be investigated. A history of previous abdominal operations should be obtained but should not be relied on too heavily in the absence of operative reports. A careful family history is important for detection of hereditary disorders that may

cause acute abdominal pain. A detailed social history should also be obtained that includes tobacco, alcohol, or illicit drug use as well as a sexual history.

Tentative Differential Diagnosis

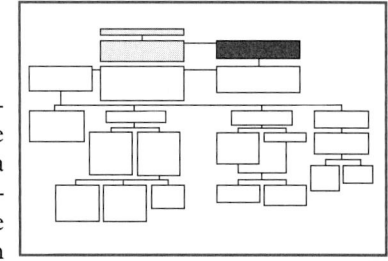

Once the patient's history has been obtained, the examiner should generate a tentative differential diagnosis and carry out the physical examination in search of specific signs or findings that either rule out or confirm the diagnostic possibilities. Given that the list of conditions that can cause acute abdominal pain is almost endless [*see Tables 1 and 2*], there is no substitute for some general knowledge of what the most common causes of acute abdominal pain are and how age, gender, and geography may affect the likelihood that any of these potential causes is present.

Ambulatory patients with acute abdominal pain as a chief complaint constitute 2% to 3% of all patients in an office practice and 5% to 10% of all patients seen in the emergency department.[4,13,15] At least two thirds of these patients have disorders that do not call for surgical intervention.[2,4,5] Although acute abdominal pain is the most common surgical emergency and most non–trauma-related surgical admissions (and 1% of all hospital admissions) are accounted for by patients complaining of abdominal pain, little information is available regarding the clinical spectrum of disease in these patients.[16] Nevertheless, detailed epidemiologic information can be an invaluable asset in the diagnosis and treatment of acute abdominal pain.

The most extensive information available comes from the ongoing survey begun in 1977 by the Research Committee of the OMGE. As of the last progress report on this survey, which was published in 1988,[12] more than 200 physicians at 26 centers in 17 countries had accumulated data on 10,320 patients with acute

Table 1 Intraperitoneal Causes of Acute Abdominal Pain[44]

Inflammatory
  Peritoneal
    Chemical and nonbacterial peritonitis
      Perforated peptic ulcer/biliary tree,
        pancreatitis, ruptured ovarian cyst,
        mittelschmerz
    Bacterial peritonitis
      Primary peritonitis
        Pneumococcal, streptococcal,
          tuberculous
        Spontaneous bacterial peritonitis
      Perforated hollow viscus
        Esophagus, stomach, duodenum, small
          intestine, bile duct, gallbladder, colon,
          urinary bladder
  Hollow visceral
    Appendicitis
    Cholecystitis
    Peptic ulcer
    Gastroenteritis
    Gastritis
    Duodenitis
    Inflammatory bowel disease
    Meckel diverticulitis
    Colitis (bacterial, amebic)
    Diverticulitis
  Solid visceral
    Pancreatitis
    Hepatitis

  Pancreatic abscess
  Hepatic abscess
  Splenic abscess
  Mesenteric
    Lymphadenitis (bacterial, viral)
    Epiploic appendagitis
  Pelvic
    Pelvic inflammatory disease (salpingitis)
    Tubo-ovarian abscess
    Endometritis

Mechanical (obstruction, acute distention)
  Hollow visceral
    Intestinal obstruction
      Adhesions, hernias, neoplasms, volvulus
      Intussusception, gallstone ileus, foreign
        bodies
      Bezoars, parasites
    Biliary obstruction
      Calculi, neoplasms, choledochal cyst,
        hemobilia
  Solid visceral
    Acute splenomegaly
    Acute hepatomegaly (congestive heart
      failure, Budd-Chiari syndrome)
  Mesenteric
    Omental torsion
  Pelvic
    Ovarian cyst

  Torsion or degeneration of fibroid
  Ectopic pregnancy

Hemoperitoneum
  Ruptured hepatic neoplasm
  Spontaneous splenic rupture
  Ruptured mesentery
  Ruptured uterus
  Ruptured graafian follicle
  Ruptured ectopic pregnancy
  Ruptured aortic or visceral aneurysm

Ischemic
  Mesenteric thrombosis
  Hepatic infarction (toxemia, purpura)
  Splenic infarction
  Omental ischemia
  Strangulated hernia

Neoplastic
  Primary or metastatic intraperitoneal
    neoplasms

Traumatic
  Blunt trauma
  Penetrating trauma
  Iatrogenic trauma
  Domestic violence

Miscellaneous
  Endometriosis

abdominal pain [*see Table 3*]. The most common diagnosis in these patients was nonspecific abdominal pain (NSAP)—that is, the retrospective diagnosis of exclusion in which no cause for the pain can be identified.[17,18] Nonspecific abdominal pain accounted for 34% of all patients seen; the four most common diagnoses accounted for more than 75%. The most common surgical diagnosis was acute appendicitis, followed by acute cholecystitis, small bowel obstruction, and gynecologic disorders. Relatively few patients had perforated peptic ulcer, a finding that confirms the recent downward trend in the incidence of this condition. Cancer was found to be a significant cause of acute abdominal pain. There was little variation in the geographic distribution of surgical causes of acute abdominal pain (i.e., conditions necessitating operation) among developed countries. In patients who required operation, the most common causes were acute appendicitis (42.6%), acute cholecystitis (14.7%), small bowel obstruction (6.2%), perforated peptic ulcer (3.7%), and acute pancreatitis (4.5%).[12]

The finding that NSAP is the most common diagnosis in patients with acute abdominal pain has been confirmed by several other clinical studies[4,5,16,19]; the finding that acute appendicitis, cholecystitis, and intestinal obstruction are the three most common diagnoses in patients with acute abdominal pain who require operation has also been amply confirmed[1,4,5,16,19] [*see Table 3*].

The data described so far provide a comprehensive picture of the most likely diagnoses for patients with acute abdominal pain in many centers around the world; however, this picture does not take into account the effect of age on the relative likelihood of the various potential diagnoses. It is well known that the disease spectrum of acute abdominal pain is different in different age groups, especially in the very old and the very young.[20] This variation is apparent

when the 10,320 patients from the OMGE study are segregated by age[21] [*see Table 4*]. In patients 50 years of age or older, cholecystitis was more common than either NSAP or acute appendicitis, and small bowel obstruction, diverticular disease, and pancreatitis were all approximately five times more common than in patients younger than 50 years. Hernias were also a much more common problem in older patients. In the entire group of patients, only one of every 10 instances of intestinal obstruction was attributable to a hernia, whereas in patients 50 years of age or older, one of every three instances was caused by an undiagnosed hernia. Cancer was 40 times more likely to be the cause of acute abdominal pain in patients 50 years of age or older; vascular diseases (including myocardial infarction, mesenteric ischemia, and ruptured abdominal aortic aneurysm) were 25 times more common in patients 50 years of age or older and 100 times more common in patients older than 70 years. What is more, outcome was clearly related to age: mortality was significantly higher in patients older than 70 years (5%) than in those younger than 50 years (less than 1%). Whereas the peak incidence of acute abdominal pain occurred in patients in their teens and 20s, the great majority of deaths occurred in patients older than 70 years.[22]

Further analysis of the data from the OMGE survey also makes it clear that the disease spectrum in children is different from that in adults: well over 90% of cases of acute abdominal pain in children are diagnosed as either acute appendicitis (32%) or nonspecific abdominal pain (62%).[22] Similar age-related differences in the spectrum of disease have been confirmed by other studies,[16] as have various gender-related differences.

Knowledge of the most common causes of acute abdominal pain and familiarity with the special circumstances that make particular causes more likely than others allow the surgeon to play the odds.[14] As has often been said, common things are common—or, to put it another way, most people get what most people get.

Physical Examination

In physical examination, as in history taking, there is no substitute for organization and patience; the amount of information that can be obtained is directly proportional to the gentleness and thoroughness of the examiner. The 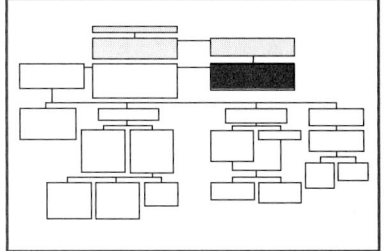 physical examination begins with a brief but thorough evaluation of the patient's general appearance and ability to answer questions. The degree of obvious pain should be estimated. The patient's position in bed should be noted: as an example, a patient who lies motionless with flexed hips and knees is more likely to have generalized peritonitis, whereas a restless patient who writhes about in bed is more likely to have colicky pain, which suggests different diagnoses. The area of maximal pain should be identified before the physical examination is begun.

The examiner can easily do this by simply asking the patient to cough and then to point with one finger to the area of maximal pain. This allows the examiner to avoid the area in the early stages of the examination and to confirm it at a later stage without causing the patient unnecessary discomfort in the meantime.

A complete physical examination should be performed and extra-abdominal causes of pain and signs of systemic illness should be sought before attention is directed to the patient's abdomen. Systemic signs of shock, such as diaphoresis, pallor, hypothermia, tachypnea, tachycardia with orthostasis, and frank hypotension, usually accompany a rapidly progressive or advanced intra-abdominal condition and, in the absence of extra-abdominal causes, are an indication for immediate laparotomy. The absence of any alteration in vital signs, however, does not necessarily exclude a serious intra-abdominal process.

The surgeon then begins the abdominal examination. This is done with the patient resting in a comfortable supine position. The examination should include inspection, auscultation, percussion, and palpation of all areas of the abdomen, the flanks, and the groin (including all hernia orifices) in addition to rectal and genital examinations (and, in female patients, a full gynecologic examination). A systematic approach is crucial: an examiner who methodically follows a set pattern of abdominal examination every time will be rewarded more frequently than one who improvises haphazardly with each patient.

Table 2   Extraperitoneal Causes of Acute Abdominal Pain

Genitourinary
Pyelonephritis
Perinephric abscess
Renal infarct
Nephrolithiasis
Ureteral obstruction (lithiasis, tumor)
Acute cystitis
Prostatitis
Seminal vesiculitis
Epididymitis
Orchitis
Testicular torsion
Dysmenorrhea
Threatened abortion

Pulmonary
Pneumonia
Empyema
Pulmonary embolus
Pulmonary infarction
Pneumothorax

Cardiac
Myocardial ischemia
Myocardial infarction
Acute rheumatic fever
Acute pericarditis

Metabolic
Acute intermittent porphyria
Familial Mediterranean fever
Hypolipoproteinemia
Hemochromatosis
Hereditary angioneurotic edema

Endocrine
Diabetic ketoacidosis
Hyperparathyroidism (hypercalcemia)
Acute adrenal insufficiency (Addisonian crisis)
Hyperthyroidism or hypothyroidism

Musculoskeletal
Rectus sheath hematoma
Arthritis/diskitis of thoracolumbar spine

Neurogenic
Herpes zoster
Tabes dorsalis
Nerve root compression
Spinal cord tumors
Osteomyelitis of the spine
Abdominal epilepsy
Abdominal migraine
Multiple sclerosis

Inflammatory
Schönlein-Henoch purpura
Systemic lupus erythematosus
Polyarteritis nodosa
Dermatomyositis
Scleroderma

Infectious
Bacterial
Parasitic (malaria)
Viral (measles, mumps, infectious mononucleosis)
Rickettsial (Rocky Mountain spotted fever)

Hematologic
Sickle cell crisis
Acute leukemia
Acute hemolytic states
Coagulopathies
Pernicious anemia
Other dyscrasias

Vascular
Vasculitis
Periarteritis

Toxins
Bacterial toxins (tetanus, staphylococcus)
Insect venom (black widow spider)
Animal venom
Heavy metals (lead, arsenic, mercury)
Poisonous mushrooms
Drugs
Withdrawal from narcotics

Retroperitoneal
Retroperitoneal hemorrhage (spontaneous adrenal hemorrhage)
Psoas abscess

Psychogenic
Hypochondriasis
Somatization disorders

Factitious
Munchausen syndrome
Malingering

Table 3 Frequency of Specific Diagnoses in Patients with Acute Abdominal Pain

Diagnosis	Frequency in Individual Studies (% of Patients)					
	OMGE[12] (N = 10,320)	Wilson[19] (N = 1,196)	Irvin[16] (N = 1,190)	Brewer[4] (N = 1,000)	de Dombal[1] (N = 552)	Hawthorn[5] (N = 496)
Nonspecific abdominal pain	34.0	45.6	34.9	41.3	50.5	36.0
Acute appendicitis	28.1	15.6	16.8	4.3	26.3	14.9
Acute cholecystitis	9.7	5.8	5.1	2.5	7.6	5.9
Small bowel obstruction	4.1	2.6	14.8	2.5	3.6	8.6
Acute gynecologic disease	4.0	4.0	1.1	8.5	—	—
Acute pancreatitis	2.9	1.3	2.4	—	2.9	2.1
Urologic disorders	2.9	4.7	5.9	11.4	—	12.8
Perforated peptic ulcer	2.5	2.3	2.5	2.0	3.1	—
Cancer	1.5	—	3.0	—	—	—
Diverticular disease	1.5	1.1	3.9	—	2.0	3.0
Dyspepsia	1.4	7.6	1.4	1.4	—	—
Gastroenteritis	—	—	0.3	6.9	—	5.1
Inflammatory bowel disease	—	—	0.8	—	—	2.1
Mesenteric adenitis	—	3.6	—	—	—	1.5
Gastritis	—	2.1	—	1.4	—	—
Constipation	—	2.4	—	2.3	—	—
Amebic hepatic abscess	1.2	—	1.9	—	—	—
Miscellaneous	6.3	1.3	5.2	15.5	4.0	8.0

The first step in the abdominal examination is careful inspection of the anterior and posterior abdominal walls, the flanks, the perineum, and the genitalia for previous surgical scars (possible adhesions), hernias (incarceration or strangulation), distention (intestinal obstruction), obvious masses (distended gallbladder, abscesses, or tumors), ecchymosis or abrasions (trauma), striae (pregnancy or ascites), everted umbilicus (increased intra-abdominal pressure), visible pulsations (aneurysm), visible peristalsis (obstruction), limitation of movement of the abdominal wall with ventilatory movements (peritonitis), or engorged veins (portal hypertension).

The next step in the abdominal examination is auscultation. Although it is important to note the presence (or absence) of bowel sounds and their quality, auscultation is probably the least rewarding aspect of the physical examination. Severe intra-abdominal conditions, even intra-abdominal catastrophes, may occur in patients with normal bowel sounds, and patients with silent abdomens may have no significant intra-abdominal pathology at all. In general, however, the absence of bowel sounds indicates a paralytic ileus; hyperactive or hypoactive bowel sounds often are variations of normal activity; and high-pitched bowel sounds with splashes, tinkles (echoing as in a large cavern), or rushes (prolonged, loud gurgles) indicate mechanical bowel obstruction.

The third step is percussion to search for any areas of dullness, fluid collections, sections of gas-filled bowel, or pockets of free air under the abdominal wall. Tympany may be present in patients with bowel obstruction or hollow viscus perforation. Percussion can be useful as a way of estimating organ size and of determining the presence of ascites (signaled by a fluid wave or shifting dullness). It is most useful, however, as a means of demonstrating peritoneal irritation (rebound tenderness). The customary technique is to dig the fingers deep into the patient's abdomen and then let go abruptly. This technique is a time-honored one, but it is painful and often misleads the examiner into assuming that an acute process is present when none exists. Gentle percussion over the four quadrants of the abdomen is much better tolerated by the patient; in addition, it is much more accurate in demonstrating rebound tenderness.

The last step, palpation, is the most informative aspect of the physical examination. Palpation of the abdomen must be done very gently to avoid causing additional pain early in the examination. It should begin as far as possible from the area of maximal pain and then should gradually advance toward this area, which should be the last to be palpated. The examiner should place the entire hand on the patient's abdomen with the fingers together and extended, applying pressure with the pulps (not the tips) of the fingers by flexing the wrists and the metacarpophalangeal joints. It is essential to determine whether true involuntary muscle guarding (muscle spasm) is present. This determination is made by means of gentle palpation over the abdominal wall while the patient takes a long, deep breath. If guarding is voluntary, the underlying muscle immediately relaxes under the gentle pressure of the palpating hand. If, however, the patient has true involuntary guarding, the muscle remains in spasm (i.e., taut and rigid) throughout the respiratory cycle (so-called boardlike abdomen). True involuntary guarding is indicative of localized or generalized peritonitis. It must be remembered that muscle rigidity is relative: for example, muscle guarding may be less pronounced or absent in debilitated and elderly patients who have poor abdominal musculature. In addition, the evaluation of muscle guarding is dependent on the patient's cooperation.

Palpation is also useful for determining the extent and severity of the patient's tenderness. Diffuse tenderness indicates generalized peritoneal inflammation. Mild diffuse tenderness without guarding usually indicates gastroenteritis or some other inflammatory intestinal process without peritoneal inflammation. Localized tenderness suggests an early stage of disease with limited peritoneal inflammation.

Careful palpation can elicit several specific signs [see Table 5]—such as the Rovsing sign (associated with acute appendicitis) and the Murphy sign (acute cholecystitis)—that are indicative of localized peritoneal inflammation. Similarly, specific maneuvers can elicit signs of localized peritoneal irritation, such as the psoas sign (associated with retrocecal appendicitis), the obturator sign (pelvic appendicitis), and the Kehr sign (diaphragmatic irritation). One very important maneuver is the Carnett test, in which the patient elevates his or her head off the bed, thus tensing the abdominal muscles. Tenderness to palpation persists when the pain is caused by abdominal wall conditions (e.g., rectal sheath hematoma) but decreases or disappears when the pain is caused by intraperitoneal conditions (the Carnett sign).

Rectal, genital, and (in women) pelvic examinations are an essential part of the evaluation in all patients with acute abdominal pain. The rectal examination should include evaluation of sphincter tone, tenderness (localized versus diffuse), and prostate size and tenderness, as well as a search for the presence of hemorrhoids, masses, fecal impaction, foreign bodies, and gross or occult blood. The genital examination should search for adenopathy, masses, discoloration, edema, and crepitus. The pelvic examination in women should check for vaginal discharge or bleeding, cervical discharge or bleeding, cervical mobility and tenderness, uterine tenderness, uterine size, and adnexal tenderness or masses. Although a carefully performed pelvic examination can be invaluable in differentiating nonsurgical conditions (e.g., PID) from conditions necessitating prompt operation (e.g., acute appendicitis), the possibility that a surgical condition is present should not be prematurely dismissed solely on the basis of a finding of tenderness on pelvic or rectal examination.

Basic Investigative Studies

Although laboratory and radiologic studies rarely, if ever, establish a definitive diagnosis by themselves, they are often useful for confirming the diagnosis suggested by the history and the physical examination.

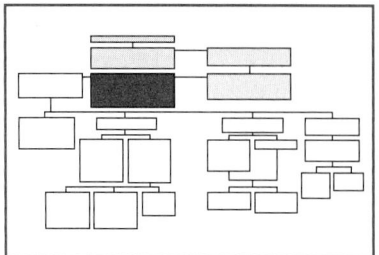

LABORATORY STUDIES

In all except extremely hemodynamically unstable patients, a complete blood count, blood chemistries, and a urinalysis are routinely obtained. The hematocrit is important in that it allows the surgeon to detect significant changes in plasma volume (e.g., dehydration caused by vomiting, diarrhea, or fluid loss into the peritoneum or the intestinal lumen), preexisting anemia, or bleeding. An elevated white blood cell count is indicative of an inflammatory process and is a particularly helpful finding if associated with a marked left shift; however, the presence or absence of leukocytosis should never be the single deciding factor as to whether the patient should undergo an operation. A low white blood cell count may be a feature of viral infections, gastroenteritis, or NSAP.

Serum electrolyte, blood urea nitrogen, and creatinine concentrations are useful in determining the nature and extent of fluid losses. Blood glucose and other blood chemistries may also be helpful. Liver function tests (serum bilirubin, alkaline phosphatase, and transaminase levels) are mandatory when abdominal pain is suspected to be hepatobiliary in origin. Similarly, amylase and lipase determinations are mandatory when pancreatitis is suspected, although it must be remembered that amylase levels may be low or normal in patients with pancreatitis and may be markedly elevated in patients with other conditions (e.g., intestinal obstruction, mesenteric thrombosis, and perforated ulcer).

Urinalysis may reveal red blood cells (suggestive of renal or ureteral calculi), white blood cells (urinary tract infection or inflammatory processes adjacent to the ureters, such as retrocecal appendicitis), increased specific gravity (dehydration), glucose, ketones (diabetes), or bilirubin (hepatitis). A pregnancy test should be considered in any woman of childbearing age with acute abdominal pain.

An electrocardiogram is mandatory in elderly patients and in patients with a history of atherosclerotic heart disease. Abdominal pain may be a manifestation of myocardial disease, and the physiologic stress of acute abdominal pain can increase myocardial oxygen demands and induce ischemia in patients with coronary artery disease.

RADIOLOGIC STUDIES

In most patients with acute abdominal pain, initial radiologic evaluation should include plain films of the abdomen in the

Table 4 **Frequency of Specific Diagnoses in Younger and Older Patients with Acute Abdominal Pain in the OMGE Study[12,21]**

Diagnosis	Frequency (% of Patients)	
	Age < 50 Yr (N = 6,317)	Age ≥ 50 Yr (N = 2,406)
Nonspecific abdominal pain	39.5	15.7
Appendicitis	32.0	15.2
Cholecystitis	6.3	20.9
Obstruction	2.5	12.3
Pancreatitis	1.6	7.3
Diverticular disease	< 0.1	5.5
Cancer	< 0.1	4.1
Hernia	< 0.1	3.1
Vascular disease	< 0.1	2.3

Table 5 Common Abdominal Signs and Findings Noted on Physical Examination[7]

Sign or Finding	Description	Associated Clinical Condition(s)
Aaron sign	Referred pain or feeling of distress in epigastrium or precordial region on continued firm pressure over the McBurney point	Acute appendicitis
Ballance sign	Presence of dull percussion note in both flanks, constant on left side but shifting with change of position on right side	Ruptured spleen
Bassler sign	Sharp pain elicited by pinching appendix between thumb of examiner and iliacus muscle	Chronic appendicitis
Beevor sign	Upward movement of umbilicus	Paralysis of lower portions of rectus abdominis muscles
Blumberg sign	Transient abdominal wall rebound tenderness	Peritoneal inflammation
Carnett sign	Disappearance of abdominal tenderness when anterior abdominal muscles are contracted	Abdominal pain of intra-abdominal origin
Chandelier sign	Intense lower abdominal and pelvic pain on manipulation of cervix	Pelvic inflammatory disease
Charcot sign	Intermittent right upper quadrant abdominal pain, jaundice, and fever	Choledocholithiasis
Chaussier sign	Severe epigastric pain in gravid female	Prodrome of eclampsia
Claybrook sign	Transmission of breath and heart sounds through abdominal wall	Ruptured abdominal viscus
Courvoisier sign	Palpable, nontender gallbladder in presence of clinical jaundice	Periampullary neoplasm
Cruveilhier sign	Varicose veins radiating from umbilicus (*caput medusae*)	Portal hypertension
Cullen sign	Periumbilical darkening of skin from blood	Hemoperitoneum (especially in ruptured ectopic pregnancy)
Cutaneous hyperesthesia	Increased abdominal wall sensation to light touch	Parietal peritoneal inflammation secondary to inflammatory intra-abdominal pathology
Dance sign	Slight retraction in area of right iliac fossa	Intussusception
Danforth sign	Shoulder pain on inspiration	Hemoperitoneum (especially in ruptured ectopic pregnancy)
Direct abdominal wall tenderness	—	Localized inflammation of abdominal wall, peritoneum, or an intra-abdominal viscus
Fothergill sign	Abdominal wall mass that does not cross midline and remains palpable when rectus muscle is tense	Rectus muscle hematoma

(continued)

supine and standing positions and chest radiographs.[23] If the patient is unable to stand, a left lateral decubitus radiograph should be obtained. Like the basic laboratory studies (see above), these plain radiographs may help confirm diagnoses suggested by the history and the physical examination, such as pneumonia (signaled by pulmonary infiltrates); intestinal obstruction (air-fluid levels and dilated loops of bowel); intestinal perforation (pneumoperitoneum); biliary, renal, or ureteral calculi (abnormal calcifications); appendicitis (fecalith); incarcerated hernia (bowel protruding beyond the confines of the peritoneal cavity); mesenteric infarction (air in the portal vein); chronic pancreatitis (pancreatic calcifications); acute pancreatitis (the so-called colon cutoff sign); visceral aneurysms (calcified rim); retroperitoneal hematoma or abscess (obliteration of the psoas shadow); and ischemic colitis (so-called thumbprinting on the colonic wall).

A prospective study published in 1999 evaluated the utility of routine plain abdominal radiographs in the management of adult patients with acute right lower quadrant abdominal pain.[24] The results seem to demonstrate that indiscriminate use of such radiographs in this patient subset is not helpful but that discriminating use in selected patients with clinically suspected small bowel obstruction or urinary symptoms may be worthwhile. Admittedly, plain abdominal radiographs cost relatively little; still, refraining from

routinely obtaining them in all patients with suspected acute appendicitis would help reduce the cost of medical care appreciably.

Working Diagnosis

Ideally, the tentative differential diagnosis list generated after the clinical history was obtained should be narrowed down to a working diagnosis by the physical examination and the information provided by the basic laboratory and radiologic studies. Once this working diagnosis has been established, subsequent management depends on the accepted treatment for the particular condition believed to be present. In general, the course of management follows four basic pathways (see below), depending on whether the patient (1) is in need of immediate laparotomy, (2) is believed to have an underlying surgical condition, (3) has an uncertain diagnosis, or (4) is believed to have an underlying nonsurgical condition.

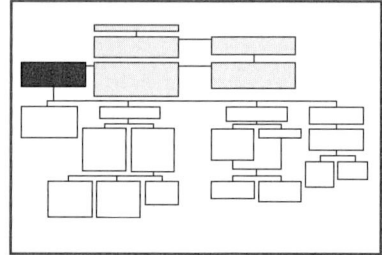

It must be emphasized that the patient must be constantly reevaluated (preferably by the same examiner) even after the working diagnosis has been established. If the patient does not

Table 5 *(continued)*

Sign or Finding	Description	Associated Clinical Condition(s)
Grey Turner sign	Local areas of discoloration around umbilicus and flanks	Acute hemorrhagic pancreatitis
Iliopsoas sign	Elevation and extension of leg against pressure of examiner's hand causes pain	Appendicitis (retrocecal) or an inflammatory mass in contact with psoas
Kehr sign	Left shoulder pain when patient is supine or in the Trendelenburg position (pain may occur spontaneously or after application of pressure to left subcostal region)	Hemoperitoneum (especially ruptured spleen)
Kustner sign	Palpable mass anterior to uterus	Dermoid cyst of ovary
Mannkopf sign	Acceleration of pulse when a painful point is pressed on by examiner	Absent in factitious abdominal pain
McClintock sign	Heart rate > 100 beats/min 1 hr post partum	Postpartum hemorrhage
Murphy sign	Palpation of right upper abdominal quadrant during deep inspiration results in right upper quadrant abdominal pain	Acute cholecystitis
Obturator sign	Flexion of right thigh at right angles to trunk and external rotation of same leg in supine position result in hypogastric pain	Appendicitis (pelvic appendix); pelvic abscess; an inflammatory mass in contact with muscle
Puddle sign	Alteration in intensity of transmitted sound in intra-abdominal cavity secondary to percussion when patient is positioned on all fours and stethoscope is gradually moved toward flank opposite percussion	Free peritoneal fluid
Ransohoff sign	Yellow pigmentation in umbilical region	Ruptured common bile duct
Rovsing sign	Pain referred to the McBurney point on application of pressure to descending colon	Acute appendicitis
Subcutaneous crepitance	Palpable crepitus in abdominal wall	Subcutaneous emphysema or gas gangrene
Summer sign	Increased abdominal muscle tone on exceedingly gentle palpation of right or left iliac fossa	Early appendicitis; nephrolithiasis; ureterolithiasis; ovarian torsion
Ten Horn sign	Pain caused by gentle traction on right spermatic cord	Acute appendicitis
Toma sign	Right-sided tympany and left-sided dullness in supine position as a result of peritoneal inflammation and subsequent mesenteric contraction of intestine to right side of abdominal cavity	Inflammatory ascites

respond to treatment as expected, the working diagnosis must be reassessed and the possibility that another condition exists must be immediately entertained and investigated by returning to the differential diagnosis list.

Indications for Immediate Laparotomy

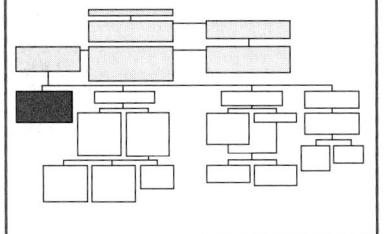

A systematic approach to patients with acute abdominal pain is essential because in some patients, action must be taken immediately and there is not enough time for an exhaustive evaluation. As outlined (see above), such an approach should include a brief initial assessment, a complete clinical history, a thorough physical examination, and basic laboratory and radiologic studies. These steps can usually be completed in less than 1 hour and should be insisted on in the evaluation of most patients.

There are, in fact, very few abdominal crises that mandate immediate operation, and even with these conditions, it is still necessary to spend a few minutes on assessing the seriousness of the problem and establishing a probable diagnosis. Among the most common of the abdominal catastrophes that necessitate immedi-

ate operation are ruptured abdominal aortic or visceral aneurysms, ruptured ectopic pregnancies, and spontaneous hepatic or splenic ruptures. The relative rarity of such conditions notwithstanding, it must always be remembered that patients with acute abdominal pain may have a progressive underlying intra-abdominal disorder causing the acute pain and that unnecessary delays in diagnosis and treatment can adversely affect outcome, often with catastrophic consequences.

When immediate operation is not called for, the physician must decide whether urgent or nonurgent but early operation is necessary, whether additional tests are required before a decision can be made, whether the patient should be admitted to the hospital for careful observation, or whether nonsurgical treatment is indicated [*see* Suspected Surgical Abdomen, Uncertain Diagnosis, *and* Suspected Nonsurgical Abdomen, *below*].

Suspected Surgical Abdomen

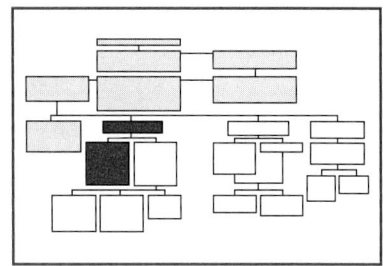

INDICATIONS FOR URGENT LAPAROTOMY OR LAPAROSCOPY

Once a definitive diagnosis has been made, it is easy to decide whether a patient should undergo operation. On occasion, however, a patient must be operated on before a precise diagnosis is reached. In contemporary clinical practice, the misuse or abuse of available technology frequently undermines the importance of sound surgical judgment at the bedside: in particular, too many patients with obvious surgical abdomens are subjected to time-consuming imaging studies before surgical consultation is obtained. *It cannot be emphasized too strongly that although diagnostic accuracy is intellectually satisfying and undoubtedly important, the primary goal in the management of patients with acute abdominal pain is not to arrive at an exact clinicopathologic diagnosis but rather to determine which patients require immediate or urgent surgical intervention.* Indications for immediate laparotomy (see above) are essentially limited to severe hemodynamic instability. Indications for urgent laparotomy are somewhat more numerous.

Urgent laparotomy implies operation within 1 to 2 hours of the patient's arrival; thus, there is usually sufficient time for adequate resuscitation, with proper rehydration and restoration of vital organ function, before the procedure. Indications for urgent laparotomy may be encountered during the physical examination, may be revealed by the basic laboratory and radiologic studies, or may not become apparent until other investigative studies are performed. Involuntary guarding or rigidity during the physical examination, particularly if spreading, is a strong indication for urgent laparotomy. Other indications include increasing severe localized tenderness, progressive tense distention, physical signs of sepsis (e.g., high fever, tachycardia, hypotension, and mental status changes), and physical signs of ischemia (e.g., fever and tachycardia). Basic laboratory and radiologic indications for urgent laparotomy include pneumoperitoneum, massive or progressive intestinal distention, signs of sepsis (e.g., marked or rising leukocytosis, increasing glucose intolerance, and acidosis), and signs of continued hemorrhage (e.g., a falling hematocrit). Additional findings that constitute indications for urgent laparotomy include free extravasation of radiologic contrast material, mesenteric occlusion on angiography, endoscopically uncontrollable bleeding, and positive results from peritoneal lavage (i.e., the presence of blood, pus, bile, urine, or gastrointestinal contents). Acute appendicitis, perforated hollow viscera, and strangulated hernias are examples of common conditions that necessitate urgent laparotomy.

Several studies from the 1990s suggest that laparoscopy is the procedure of choice when the primary clinical diagnosis is acute appendicitis or perforated peptic ulcer.[25-30] In a prospective, randomized trial,[26] Hansen and associates reported that laparoscopic appendectomy is as safe as open appendectomy. Although laparoscopic appendectomy requires a longer operating time (63 minutes versus 40 minutes), it has two advantages: the surgical site infection rate is lower, and patients return to normal activities earlier. Accordingly, we recommend laparoscopic appendectomy as a worthwhile alternative for patients with a clinical diagnosis of acute appendicitis. It has also been shown that diagnostic laparoscopy through the right lower abdominal incision is very helpful in establishing the correct diagnosis in patients who are operated on for suspected acute appendicitis but in whom the appendix is grossly normal.[27]

Laparoscopic treatment of perforated peptic ulcers—either with an omental patch or with sutures[28-30]—is becoming more popular as surgeons gain experience and competence with the technique. Compared with open approaches, laparoscopic repair results in reduced wound pain and respiratory complications as well as earlier return to normal activities.

HOSPITALIZATION AND ACTIVE OBSERVATION

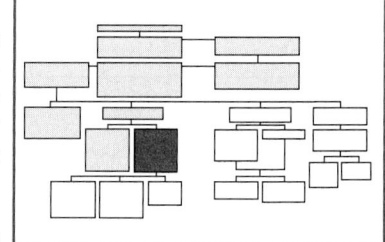

Numerous studies have shown that of all patients admitted for acute abdominal pain, only a minority require immediate or urgent operation.[2,4,5] It is therefore cost-effective as well as prudent to adopt a system of evaluation that allows for thought and investigation before definitive treatment in all patients with acute abdominal pain except those identified early on as needing immediate or urgent laparotomy. The traditional wisdom is that spending time on observation opens the door for complications (e.g., perforating appendicitis, intestinal perforation associated with bowel obstruction, or strangulation of an incarcerated hernia); however, careful clinical trials evaluating active in-hospital observation of patients with acute abdominal pain of uncertain origin have demonstrated that such observation is safe, is not accompanied by an increased incidence of complications, and results in fewer negative laparotomies.[31]

After the initial assessment has been completed, narcotic analgesia for pain relief should not be withheld.[32,33] In appropriately titrated doses, analgesics neither obscure important physical findings nor mask their subsequent development. In fact, some physical signs may be more easily identified after adequate pain relief.[34,35] Severe pain that persists in spite of adequate doses of narcotics suggests a serious condition that is likely to call for operative intervention.[33]

Active observation allows the surgeon to identify most of the patients whose acute abdominal pain is caused by NSAP or various specific nonsurgical conditions. It must be emphasized that active observation means something more than simply admitting the patient to the hospital: it implies an active process of thoughtful, discriminating, and meticulous reevaluation of the patient (preferably by the same examiner) at intervals ranging from minutes to a few hours, to be complemented by appropriately timed additional investigative studies.

Additional investigative studies beyond the basic ones already mentioned should be obtained only if the results are likely to alter or improve patient management significantly. Furthermore, the invasiveness, morbidity, and cost-effectiveness of each additional test must be carefully weighed. More liberal use of supplemental studies is justified in those patients in whom the history and physical findings tend to be less reliable (e.g., the very young, the elderly, the critically ill, or the immunocompromised).

Supplemental studies that may be considered include computed tomography, ultrasonography, diagnostic peritoneal lavage, radionuclide imaging, angiography, magnetic resonance imaging, gastrointestinal endoscopy [*see 3:8 Gastrointestinal Endoscopy*], and diagnostic laparoscopy. Diagnostic laparoscopy has been recommended when surgical disease is suspected but its probability is not high enough to warrant open laparotomy.[36] It is particularly valuable in young women of childbearing age, in whom gynecologic disorders frequently mimic acute appendicitis.[37] A report by Chung and coworkers showed that diagnostic laparoscopy had the same diagnostic yield as open laparotomy in 55 patients with acute abdomen[38]; 34 (62%) of these patients were safely managed with laparoscopy alone, with no increase in morbidity and with a shorter average hospital stay. Diagnostic laparoscopy has also been shown to be useful in the assessment of acute abdominal pain in ICU patients[39] and patients with AIDS.[40]

INDICATIONS FOR EARLY OR ELECTIVE LAPAROTOMY OR LAPAROSCOPY

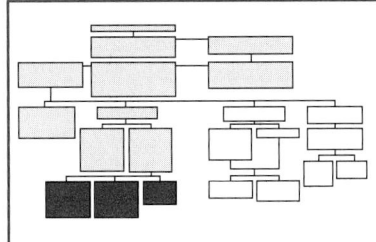

Early laparotomy or laparoscopy (within 24 to 48 hours of the initial evaluation) is reserved for patients whose conditions are not likely to become life threatening if operation is delayed to permit further resuscitation or additional investigative studies. It is often possible to perform early laparotomy or laparoscopy in patients with uncomplicated acute cholecystitis or diverticulitis and those with nonstrangulated incarcerated hernias, thereby preventing the increased patient risk that always accompanies unplanned emergency operations as well as avoiding the logistical impediments to unscheduled surgical procedures in the middle of the night or on weekends or holidays. Similarly, patients with simple uncomplicated intestinal obstructions often benefit from several hours of nasogastric tube decompression and fluid and electrolyte resuscitation.

Elective laparotomy or laparoscopy is reserved for patients whose condition is highly likely to respond to conservative medical management or highly unlikely to become life threatening during prolonged periods (several days or even weeks) of diagnostic evaluation.

Uncertain Diagnosis

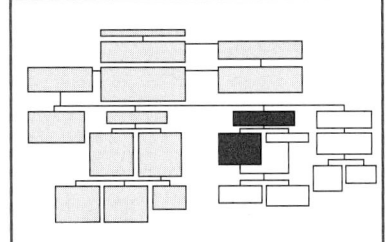

HOSPITALIZATION AND ACTIVE OBSERVATION

If the diagnosis is unclear, the surgeon's task is to determine whether hospitalization and active observation are necessary or whether outpatient evaluation is an option. All patients with acute abdominal pain and evidence of extracellular fluid deficits, electrolyte imbalances, or sepsis must be hospitalized. Furthermore, any patient with unexplained abdominal symptoms whose condition has not improved within 24 hours of the initial evaluation should be hospitalized.[41]

Supplemental studies are often required for further evaluation and complete workup of patients with uncertain diagnoses and for the exclusion of many medical conditions that do not call for operation. When the diagnosis is not obvious from the history and the physical examination, apparent on the plain radiographs, or suggested by the basic laboratory studies, ultrasonography and CT, both of which are now widely available, should be considered. CT is more useful in the early evaluation of patients with acute abdominal pain because it is not operator dependent, is not hampered by the presence of overlying gas (which transmits sound waves poorly and interferes with ultrasonography), and can be performed rapidly (a complete scan of the abdomen and pelvis takes less than 15 minutes). Although watchful observation with ongoing reexamination is a time-honored approach to the patient with acute abdominal pain of uncertain origin, excessive reliance on this practice or on esoteric physical diagnosis maneuvers (which most medical students have witnessed in awe at one time or another) suggests that the surgeon is unaware of how valuable, rapid, and accurate a CT scan can be in the early diagnosis of these patients.

Diagnostic peritoneal lavage, although most useful in the evaluation of blunt abdominal trauma, may be particularly helpful in obtunded or critically ill patients, whose condition is difficult to assess by means of history taking and physical examination.[42]

OUTPATIENT EVALUATION

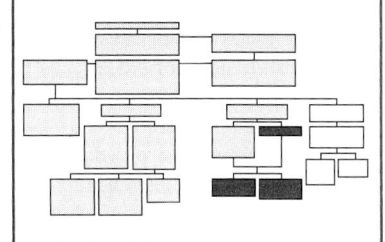

The epidemiology of acute abdominal pain is such that for every patient who requires hospitalization, there are at least two or three others who have self-limiting conditions for which neither operation nor hospitalization is necessary. Much or all of the evaluation of such patients, as well as any treatment that may be needed, can now be completed in the outpatient department. To treat acute abdominal pain cost-effectively and efficiently, the surgeon must be able not only to identify patients who need immediate or urgent laparotomy or laparoscopy but also to reliably identify those whose condition does not present a serious risk and who therefore can be managed without hospitalization. The reliability and intelligence of the patient, the proximity and availability of medical facilities, and the availability of responsible adults to observe and assist the patient at home are factors that should be carefully considered before the decision is made to evaluate or treat individuals with acute abdominal pain as outpatients.

Suspected Nonsurgical Abdomen

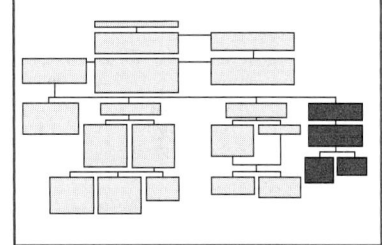

There are numerous disorders that cause acute abdominal pain but do not call for surgical intervention. These nonsurgical conditions are often extremely difficult to differentiate from surgical conditions that present with almost indistinguishable characteristics.[2] For example, the acute abdominal pain of lead poisoning or acute porphyria is difficult to differentiate from the intermittent pain of intestinal obstruction, in that marked hyperperistalsis is the hallmark of both. The pain of acute hypolipoproteinemia may be accompanied by pancreatitis, which, if not recognized, can lead to unnecessary laparotomy. Similarly, acute and prostrating abdominal pain accompanied by rigidity of the abdominal wall and a low hematocrit may lead to unnecessary urgent laparotomy in patients with sickle cell anemia crises. To further complicate the clinical picture, cholelithiasis is also often found in patients with sickle cell anemia.

In addition to numerous extraperitoneal disorders [see Table 2], nonsurgical causes of acute abdominal pain include a wide variety of intraperitoneal disorders, such as acute gastroenteritis (from enteric bacterial, viral, parasitic, or fungal infection), acute gastritis, acute duodenitis, hepatitis, mesenteric adenitis, salpingitis, Fitz-Hugh–Curtis syndrome, mittelschmerz, ovarian cyst, endometritis, endometriosis, threatened abortion, spontaneous bacterial peritonitis, and tuberculous peritonitis. Acute abdominal pain in immunosuppressed patients or patients with AIDS is now encountered with increasing frequency and can be caused by a number of unusual conditions (e.g., cytomegalovirus enterocolitis, opportunistic infections, lymphoma, and Kaposi sarcoma) as well as by the more usual ones.

As noted [*see* Tentative Differential Diagnosis, *above*], most patients with acute abdominal pain presenting to the office or the emergency department have an underlying nonsurgical condition and do not require operation.[2,4,5] Again, the single most common diagnosis in these patients is NSAP.[5,12,16-19] Although the natural history of NSAP has been well documented (harmless abdominal pain that is relieved in a few days without any treatment), there have been no prospective studies detailing the symptomatology and physical findings associated with this disorder. Furthermore, it remains unclear whether NSAP is in fact a single disease entity or is simply the presenting symptom complex for many different minor and self-limited conditions.[18] A complete clinical history and physical examination, coupled with careful in-hospital observation and a high index of suspicion, will in most cases prevent unnecessary laparotomy in patients with nonsurgical causes of acute abdominal pain. On rare occasions, diagnostic laparoscopy may be employed to prevent unnecessary laparotomy.

Conclusion

In the management of patients with acute abdominal pain, it occasionally happens that even with the aid of considerable clinical acumen and liberal use of diagnostic tests, the surgeon cannot readily determine whether a patient requires operation. In such cases, laparotomy or diagnostic laparoscopy may constitute the definitive, as well as the safest, approach to the evaluation of acute abdominal pain.

References

1. de Dombal FT: Diagnosis of Acute Abdominal Pain, 2nd ed. Churchill Livingstone, London, 1991

2. Purcell TB: Nonsurgical and extraperitoneal causes of abdominal pain. Emerg Med Clin North Am 7:721, 1989

3. Silen W: Cope's Early Diagnosis of the Acute Abdomen, 17th ed. Oxford University Press, New York, 1990

4. Brewer RJ, Golden GT, Hitch DC, et al: Abdominal pain: an analysis of 1,000 consecutive cases in a university hospital emergency room. Am J Surg 131: 219, 1976

5. Hawthorn IE: Abdominal pain as a cause of acute admission to hospital. J R Coll Surg Edinb 37:389, 1992

6. Staniland JR, Ditchburn J, de Dombal FT: Clinical presentation of acute abdomen: study of 600 patients. Br Med J 3:393, 1972

7. Hickey MS, Kiernan GJ, Weaver KE: Evaluation of abdominal pain. Emerg Med Clin North Am 7:437, 1989

8. Adams ID, Chan M, Clifford PC, et al: Computer aided diagnosis of acute abdominal pain: a multicentre study. Br Med J 293:800, 1986

9. Paterson-Brown S, Vipond MN: Modern aids to clinical decision-making in the acute abdomen. Br J Surg 77:13, 1990

10. Wellwood J, Johannessen S, Spiegelhalter DJ: How does computer-aided diagnosis improve the management of acute abdominal pain? Ann R Coll Surg Engl 74:40, 1992

11. de Dombal FT: Computers, diagnoses and patients with acute abdominal pain. Arch Emerg Med 9:267, 1992

12. de Dombal FT: The OMGE acute abdominal pain survey. Progress Report, 1986. Scand J Gastroenterol 144(suppl):35, 1988

13. American College of Emergency Physicians: Clinical policy for the initial approach to patients presenting with a chief complaint of nontraumatic acute abdominal pain. Ann Emerg Med 23:906, 1994

14. de Dombal FT: Surgical Decision Making in Practice: Acute Abdominal Pain. Butterworth-Heinemann Ltd, Oxford, 1993, p 65

15. Walters DT, Wendel HF: Abdominal pain. Prim Care 13:3, 1986

16. Irvin TT: Abdominal pain: a surgical audit of 1190 emergency admissions. Br J Surg 76:1121, 1989

17. Jess P, Bjerregaard B, Brynitz S, et al: Prognosis of acute nonspecific abdominal pain: a prospective study. Am J Surg 144:338, 1982

18. Gray DW, Collin J: Non-specific abdominal pain as a cause of acute admission to hospital. Br J Surg 74: 239, 1987

19. Wilson DH, Wilson PD, Walmsley RG, et al: Diagnosis of acute abdominal pain in the accident and emergency department. Br J Surg 64:249, 1977

20. Bender JS: Approach to the acute abdomen. Med Clin North Am 73:1413, 1989

21. Telfer S, Fenyo G, Holt PR, et al: Acute abdominal pain in patients over 50 years of age. Scand J Gastroenterol. Suppl 144:47, 1988

22. Dickson JAS, Jones A, Telfer S, et al: Acute abdominal pain in children. Progress Report, 1986. Scand J Gastroenterol. Suppl 144:43, 1988

23. Plewa MC: Emergency abdominal radiography. Emerg Med Clin North Am 9:827, 1991

24. Boleslawski E, Panis Y, Benoist S, et al: Plain abdominal radiography as a routine procedure for acute abdominal pain of the right lower quadrant: prospective evaluation. World J Surg 23:262, 1999

25. Fritts LL, Orlando R: Laparoscopic appendectomy: a safety and cost analysis. Arch Surg 128:521, 1993

26. Hansen JB, Smithers BM, Schache D, et al: Laparoscopic versus open appendectomy: prospective randomized trial. World J Surg 20:17, 1996

27. Schrenk P, Rieger R, Shamiyeh A, et al: Diagnostic laparoscopy through the right lower abdominal incision following open appendectomy. Surg Endosc 13: 133, 1999

28. Matsuda M, Nishiyama M, Hanai T, et al: Laparoscopic omental patch repair for the perforated peptic ulcer. Ann Surg 221:236, 1995

29. Tate JJ, Dawson JW, Lau WY, et al: Sutureless laparoscopic treatment of perforated duodenal ulcer. Br J Surg 80:235, 1993

30. Darzi A, Cheshire NJ, Somers SS, et al: Laparoscopic omental patch repair of perforated duodenal ulcer with an automated stapler. Br J Surg 80:1552, 1993

31. Thomson HJ, Jones PF: Active observation in acute abdominal pain. Am J Surg 152:522, 1986

32. Zoltie N, Cust MP: Analgesia in the acute abdomen. Ann R Coll Surg Engl 68:209, 1986

33. Boey JH: The acute abdomen. Current Surgical Diagnosis and Treatment, 10th ed. Way LW, Ed. Appleton & Lange, Norwalk, Connecticut, 1994, p 441

34. Cuschieri A: The acute abdomen and disorders of the peritoneal cavity. Essential Surgical Practice. Cuschieri A, Giles GT, Moosa AR, Eds. Wright PSG, Bristol, 1982, p 885

35. Attard AR, Corlett MJ, Kidner NJ, et al: Safety of early pain relief for acute abdominal pain. BMJ 305:554, 1992

36. Salky BA, Edye MB: The role of laparoscopy in the diagnosis and treatment of abdominal pain syndromes. Surg Endosc 12: 911, 1998

37. Borgstein PJ, Gordijn RV, Eijsbouts QA, et al: Acute appendicitis—a clear-cut case in men, a guessing game in young women: a prospective study on the role of laparoscopy. Surg Endosc 11:923, 1997

38. Chung RS, Diaz JJ, Chari V: Efficacy of routine laparoscopy for the acute abdomen. Surg Endosc 12:219, 1998

39. Orlando R, Crowell KL: Laparoscopy in the critically ill. Surg Endosc 11:1072, 1997

40. Box JC, Duncan T, Ramshaw B, et al: Laparoscopy in the evaluation and treatment of patients with AIDS and acute abdominal complaints. Surg Endosc 11: 1026, 1997

41. Hobsley M: An approach to the acute abdomen. Pathways in Surgical Management, 2nd ed. Edward Arnold Ltd, London, 1986

42. Larson FA, Haller CC, Delcore R, et al: Diagnostic peritoneal lavage in acute peritonitis. Am J Surg 164: 449, 1992

43. Cheung LY, Ballinger WF: Manifestations and diagnosis of gastrointestinal diseases. Hardy's Textbook of Surgery. Hardy JD, Ed. JB Lippincott Co, Philadelphia, 1983, p 445

44. McFadden DW, Zinner MJ: Manifestations of gastrointestinal disease. Principles of Surgery, 6th ed. Schwartz SI, Shires GT, Spencer FC, Eds. McGraw-Hill, New York, 1994, p 1015

Acknowledgment

Figures 2 and 3   Tom Moore.

2 ABDOMINAL MASS

Romano Delcore, M.D., F.A.C.S., and Laurence Y. Cheung, M.D., F.A.C.S.

Evaluation of Abdominal Masses

Abdominal masses are mentioned in some of the earliest known medical writings. The Papyrus Ebers (ca. 1500 B.C.) discusses the differential diagnosis of abdominal masses and describes methods of abdominal examination by palpation.[1] In his *Book of Prognostics* (ca. 400 B.C.), Hippocrates discussed the prognostic significance of abdominal masses:

> That state of the hypochondrium is best when it is free from pain, soft, and of equal size on the right side and the left. But if inflamed, or painful, or distended; or when the right and left sides are of disproportionate sizes; all these appearances are to be dreaded. . . . Such swellings as are soft, free from pain, and yield to the finger, occasion more protracted crises, and are less dangerous than the others .... Such, then, as are painful, hard, and large, indicate danger of speedy death.[2]

The term abdominal mass generally refers to a palpable mass that is anterior to the paraspinous muscles and is located anywhere between the costal margins, the iliac crests, and the pubic symphysis. An abdominal mass may be noticed initially by the patient or may be discovered by the surgeon as a new finding. In either case, the mass may have been present for days, months, or even years and may be caused by any of a great variety of intra-abdominal, pelvic, or retroperitoneal disorders, as well as by any of numerous different abdominal wall lesions.

Occasionally, after examining a patient with an abdominal mass, the surgeon is so certain about the diagnosis that no further investigation is necessary and appropriate management for the condition can be instituted immediately. Conditions that often can be readily diagnosed in this fashion include obesity, ascites, pregnancy, abdominal wall hernias, sebaceous cysts, and lipomas. It must be remembered, however, that even when an experienced clinician is convinced of the presence of a mass, it is still possible that no abnormality exists. In one study, 22% of patients thought to have a palpable mass on the basis of physical examination proved not to have any abnormalities on further investigation.[3]

Most often, the surgeon is confronted with a diagnostic challenge, in which assessing the origin and character of the abdominal mass proves difficult, time consuming, and expensive. This challenge involves not only establishing the correct diagnosis but also determining whether this can be accomplished without operative intervention. Making the correct decision regarding whether to operate on a patient with an abdominal mass requires sound surgical judgment. The decision must be based on a detailed medical and surgical history, as well as on a meticulous physical examination. These, in turn, must be guided by experience; a thorough knowledge of the anatomy and physiology of the abdominal wall, abdominal cavity, and retroperitoneum; and a clear understanding of the physiologic and pathologic processes within and around the abdomen. The arrival of new diseases, coupled with the continuous development of new diagnostic technologies, calls for constant broadening of the differential diagnosis and periodic revision of established approaches to the evaluation of abdominal masses.

Clinical History

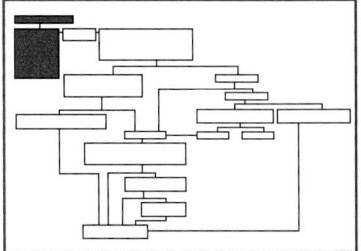

A careful and methodical clinical history should be obtained that includes the mode of onset, duration, character, location, and chronology of the abdominal mass, as well as the presence or absence of any associated symptoms. When the surgeon obtains an unhurried and complete clinical history, the patient often provides all the information needed for making the correct diagnosis. In addition, such a history is often more valuable than any single laboratory or radiologic finding and determines the course of subsequent evaluation and management. Patients should be allowed to relate the history in their own words, and examiners should refrain from suggesting specific chronologies or symptoms except as a last resort. Any questions that must be asked should be open-ended—for example, "When did you first notice a mass?" rather than "Did you just notice the mass?" Leading questions should be avoided. When a leading question must be asked, it should be posed first as a negative question (i.e., one that calls for an answer in the negative), since a negative answer to a question is more likely to be honest and accurate.

Various GI symptoms (e.g., nausea, vomiting, anorexia, diarrhea, constipation, and a decrease in stool caliber) often accompany an abdominal mass. These symptoms are nonspecific but may still be of some value in the differential diagnosis. Other associated symptoms that should be noted are jaundice, melena, hematochezia, hematemesis, hematuria, and menorrhagia. These symptoms are more specific and can be very valuable in the differential diagnosis. Urinary hesitancy or urgency in the presence of a lower abdominal mass may suggest bladder distention secondary to urethral obstruction or urinary retention caused by anticholinergic medications (e.g., phenothiazines). A female patient with a pelvic mass should be asked for a detailed gynecologic history that includes the timing of symptoms within the menstrual cycle, the date of the last menses, previous and current use of contraception, any abnormal vaginal bleeding or discharge, and a complete obstetric history. All patients with abdominal masses should also be asked about previous injuries, however minor: even a traumatic event the patient considers trivial can be diagnostically significant.

A complete history of previous medical conditions must be obtained because associated diseases may give rise to abdominal masses and may also significantly affect morbidity and mortality from subsequent surgical intervention. Weight changes suggesting carcinoma, past illnesses, previous abdominal operations, and recent travel (raising the possibility of amebic abscess or parasitic cyst) should also be investigated. A careful family history is important for detection of hereditary disorders that may cause abdominal masses.

Evaluation of Abdominal Masses

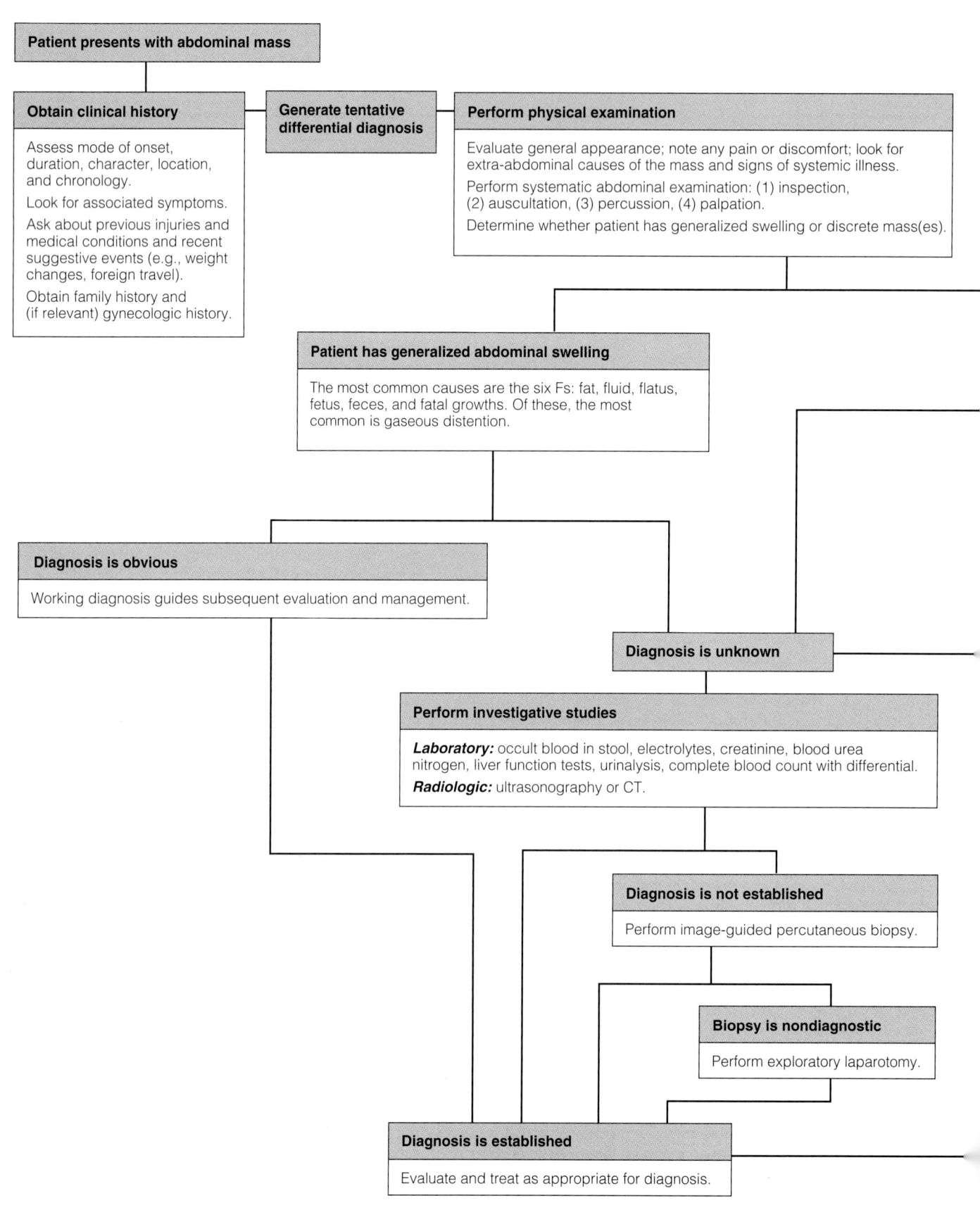

Patient presents with abdominal mass

Obtain clinical history

Assess mode of onset, duration, character, location, and chronology.

Look for associated symptoms.

Ask about previous injuries and medical conditions and recent suggestive events (e.g., weight changes, foreign travel).

Obtain family history and (if relevant) gynecologic history.

Generate tentative differential diagnosis

Perform physical examination

Evaluate general appearance; note any pain or discomfort; look for extra-abdominal causes of the mass and signs of systemic illness.

Perform systematic abdominal examination: (1) inspection, (2) auscultation, (3) percussion, (4) palpation.

Determine whether patient has generalized swelling or discrete mass(es).

Patient has generalized abdominal swelling

The most common causes are the six Fs: fat, fluid, flatus, fetus, feces, and fatal growths. Of these, the most common is gaseous distention.

Diagnosis is obvious

Working diagnosis guides subsequent evaluation and management.

Diagnosis is unknown

Perform investigative studies

Laboratory: occult blood in stool, electrolytes, creatinine, blood urea nitrogen, liver function tests, urinalysis, complete blood count with differential.
Radiologic: ultrasonography or CT.

Diagnosis is not established

Perform image-guided percutaneous biopsy.

Biopsy is nondiagnostic

Perform exploratory laparotomy.

Diagnosis is established

Evaluate and treat as appropriate for diagnosis.

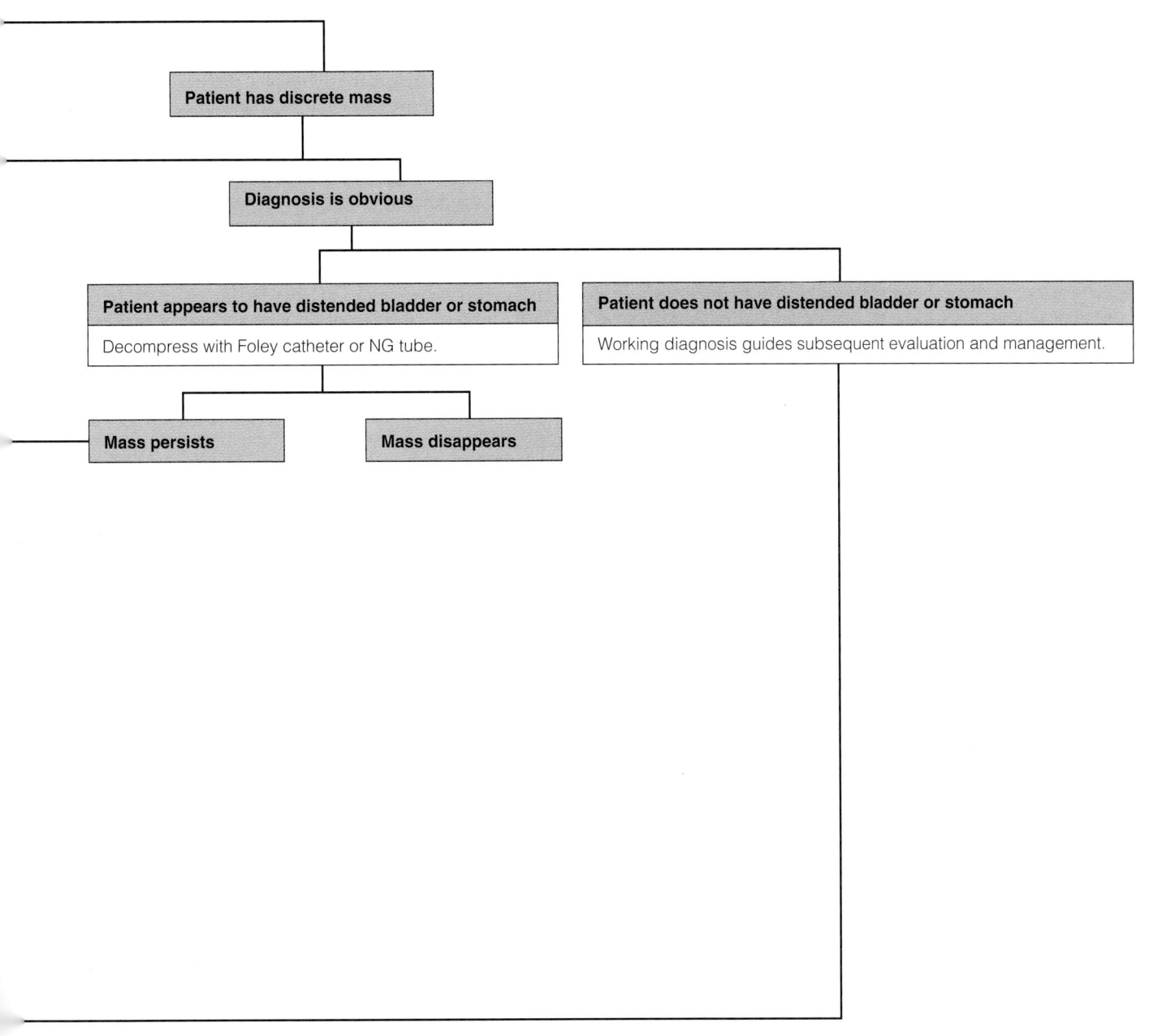

Patient has discrete mass

Diagnosis is obvious

Patient appears to have distended bladder or stomach
Decompress with Foley catheter or NG tube.

Patient does not have distended bladder or stomach
Working diagnosis guides subsequent evaluation and management.

Mass persists

Mass disappears

Tentative Differential Diagnosis

Once the history has been obtained, the examiner should generate a tentative differential diagnosis and carry out the physical examination in search of specific signs or findings that either

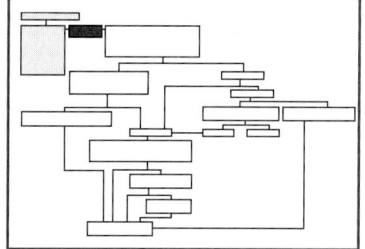

confirm or rule out the diagnostic possibilities. Failure to include a broad array of possibilities in the tentative differential diagnosis is a common and often costly mistake. For example, when urinary retention is not considered as part of the early differential diagnosis of a large lower abdominal mass, the patient may undergo needlessly extensive and expensive evaluations.

In the light of the large number of conditions that can give rise to an abdominal mass, the task of arriving at a specific diagnosis can appear overwhelming. To lessen the difficulty of this task, it would be invaluable to have some general knowledge of what the most common causes of abdominal masses are, as well as how age, gender, associated symptoms, and geography may affect the likelihood that any of these potential causes is present. Unfortunately, abdominal masses as such usually are not coded in the medical record; rather, specific diseases or definitive diagnoses are coded. Consequently, the true incidence of abdominal mass remains unknown, nor is there much information in the literature regarding the relative frequency with which specific diseases present with an abdominal mass.[4] Decades ago, two series were published that provided a differential diagnosis of abdominal masses based on statistical analysis and relative frequency.[1,5] These two series, however, have now been rendered hopelessly outdated by modern medical practice and the advent of newer diagnostic and therapeutic modalities. Nevertheless, knowledge of the most common disease processes associated with abdominal masses and familiarity with the characteristic signs and symptoms that accompany the most common causes of this presenting symptom can greatly facilitate and shorten the evaluation of patients presenting with abdominal masses.

Physical Examination

In physical examination, as in history taking, there is no substitute for organization and patience; the amount of information that can be obtained is directly proportional to the gentleness and thoroughness of the

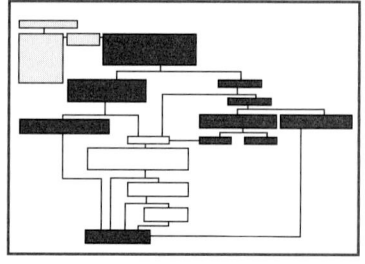

examiner. As in the evaluation of the acute abdomen [see 3:1 Acute Abdominal Pain], the physical examination begins with a brief but thorough evaluation of the patient's general appearance. Any obvious pain or associated discomfort should be noted. A complete physical examination should be performed, and possible extra-abdominal causes of the mass as well as signs of systemic illness should be sought before attention is directed to the mass. Systemic signs of shock, such as tachycardia, tachypnea, diaphoresis, pallor, orthostasis, and frank hypotension, usually accompany a rapidly progressive or advanced condition and are an indication for immediate resuscitation and laparotomy. Abdominal masses that may occur in association with systemic signs of shock and that must be recognized as soon as possible include abdominal aortic and other visceral aneurysms, hepatic

and splenic subcapsular hematomas, blood-filled pancreatic pseudocysts, and empyema of the gallbladder with associated ascending cholangitis. The abdominal examination should include inspection, auscultation, palpation, and percussion, generally in that order; these maneuvers are described in more detail elsewhere [see 3:1 Acute Abdominal Pain].

Inspection of the abdomen may reveal either generalized enlargement or distention of the entire abdomen or the presence of one or more discrete masses of varying sizes. Conditions that may give rise to generalized abdominal distention include obesity, tympanites or meteorism (swelling of the abdomen caused by gas within the intestine or peritoneal cavity), ascites, pregnancy, fecal impaction, and neoplasm. An easy way of remembering these conditions is to use the so-called six Fs mnemonic device: Fat, Fluid, Flatus, Fetus, Feces, and Fatal growths.[6-8]

The most common cause of transient generalized enlargement of the abdomen is intestinal gas or bloating. Gaseous distention may appear or disappear in minutes to hours and is usually accompanied by discomfort. Percussion of the abdomen elicits tympany. Because aerophagia and certain foods are common causes of gaseous distention, the differential diagnosis necessitates a detailed dietary history. Intestinal ileus and intestinal obstruction (in particular, distal obstruction) can present with generalized abdominal enlargement resulting from gaseous distention.

The most common cause of chronic abdominal enlargement is obesity. This condition is usually readily apparent on inspection and is confirmed on examination by the greatly increased skinfold thickness of the abdominal wall. When obesity results from adipose tissue in the mesentery, the omentum, and the extraperitoneal layer, the diagnosis may not be so readily apparent. In general, obesity makes evaluation of discrete abdominal masses by means of physical examination much more difficult, to the point where masses of remarkable size can be missed by even the most careful examiner. Massive enlargement of a single organ (e.g., the liver, the spleen, or the kidneys) or a large fluid-filled cyst can also cause generalized abdominal enlargement, as can accumulation of ascitic fluid in the peritoneal cavity. A common and often overlooked cause of an abdominal mass, particularly in elderly or institutionalized patients, is fecal impaction. Removal of the impaction causes the mass to disappear.

A distended urinary bladder may extend up to the level of the umbilicus; it is usually in the midline, and because of its extreme size, it is commonly mistaken for an abdominal mass. The swelling is fluctuant and resolves with catheterization. In cases of acute gastric dilatation, the distended stomach may also occasionally be large enough to all but fill the abdomen. Decompression with a nasogastric tube leads to complete resolution.

When the mass is discrete rather than generalized, the examiner should note whether it moves with respiration; such movement suggests that the mass is associated with a mobile organ in the abdominal cavity rather than located in the retroperitoneum or attached to the abdominal wall. Inspection should be followed by auscultation, before percussion and palpation stimulate the abdominal viscera to abnormal activity that may obscure vascular bruits.

The examination begins with light palpation of the entire abdomen, which may reveal regions of tenderness and increased resistance that should be examined later in detail. Light palpation can determine only the presence of a mass and its location; further information must be sought through deep palpation, which is done to confirm the findings from inspection and light palpation and to search for previously unsuspected masses. Frequently, a mass that is not visible on inspection is easily felt on palpation.

Normal structures felt during palpation must not be confused with abdominal masses. Prominent segments of the abdominal wall musculature, the abdominal aorta, and the sacral promontory may be mistaken for abdominal masses on a cursory examination. Masses must also be distinguished from muscle spasms.

During palpation of the mass, every effort should be made to determine as many of the following characteristics as possible: location, size, shape, consistency, surface (smooth or nodular), presence or absence of tenderness, temperature, the color of the overlying skin, degree of mobility, any fixation or attachments, pulsatility, fluctuation, response to ballottement, and appearance on transillumination. Clearly, it is not possible to determine all of these characteristics in every case. Knowing the location of the mass in the abdomen limits the number of possible organs to be considered and may give an insight into the nature and extent of the pathologic process.

Whether the mass is located within the abdominal cavity or in the wall of the abdomen is also an important diagnostic factor. A rectus sheath hematoma is an example of an abdominal wall lesion that is frequently mistaken for an intra-abdominal mass. Masses situated in the abdominal wall itself can be recognized on the basis of their superficial location; their adherence to skin, subcutaneous fascia, or muscles; or their failure to follow the movements of the viscera immediately underlying the abdominal wall. It may, however, be impossible to differentiate an intra-abdominal mass that has become attached to the abdominal wall (as either an inflammatory or a neoplastic process) from an abdominal wall lesion. A simple test that should be done with any patient who has an abdominal mass is to direct the patient to raise the head and shoulders or the legs from the examining table. This maneuver produces tightening of the abdominal muscles. If the mass is in the abdominal wall itself, it remains palpable, but if it is within or behind the abdominal cavity, it is obscured.

Some pathologic processes are suggested by the consistency of the mass and its resistance to pressure: for instance, carcinoma may be rock-hard, whereas an abscess may be soft and fluctuant. A smooth surface implies diffuse involvement, and a nodular surface suggests neoplastic metastases or granulomas. Tenderness may be caused by an acute inflammatory process or by distention of the capsule of a viscus. As noted, mobility with respiration tends to distinguish a peritoneal mass from an extraperitoneal one. Pulsatility should alert the examiner to the possibility that the mass is of vascular origin [see 4:3 Pulsatile Abdominal Mass]. Pulsation in the epigastrium of a thin patient is apparent almost routinely on palpation and usually results from the normal pulsation of the aorta lying over the vertebral bodies. In most cases, pulsation associated with an epigastric mass represents a pulsation transmitted through a pancreatic tumor or cyst or a gastric tumor. If, however, pulsation is associated with an expanding mass, it quite possibly represents an abdominal aortic aneurysm. Fluctuation may indicate a cyst, a pseudocyst, a hematoma, or an abscess.

Working Diagnosis

The tentative differential diagnosis list that is generated after the clinical history has been obtained can often be narrowed down to a working diagnosis on the basis of the physical examination. Once a working diagnosis has been established, subsequent management depends on the accepted methods of evaluation and treatment for the particular condition believed to be present. In a number of cases, however, the diagnosis remains unknown even after the physical examination. When this is the case, investigative studies are required. Often, basic investigative studies (e.g., laboratory testing, ultrasonography, or CT) are sufficient to establish the diagnosis. Occasionally, they are not, and further investigative studies are needed.

Investigative Studies

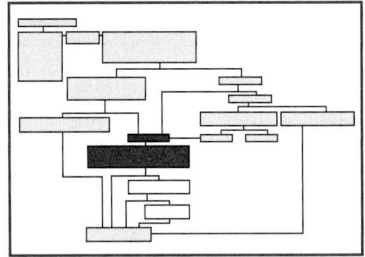

Integrating the information provided by one investigative test with that provided by preceding and subsequent tests yields a higher degree of diagnostic accuracy. Clearly, not every available mode of investigation should be used in each patient. The best evaluative approach in a given case depends somewhat on the preferences of the patient, the physician, and the institution as well as on consideration of relative costs. Most patients with abdominal masses can be evaluated as outpatients, but in making this decision, the examiner must be sure that the patient is both available and reliable. Investigative studies must be individualized so that the examiner can reach an accurate diagnosis in the shortest possible time using the fewest, least invasive, and (ideally) least expensive diagnostic tests possible.

LABORATORY STUDIES

If the cause of the mass can be determined without question on the basis of the history and the physical examination, laboratory evaluation may be unnecessary. If the cause of the abdominal mass remains unknown, the patient should undergo testing for occult blood in the stool, a chemistry profile (which should include at least electrolytes, blood urea nitrogen [BUN], creatinine, and liver function tests), a urinalysis, and a complete blood count with differential. An unexpected abnormal laboratory value may be the only finding that steers the surgeon toward the correct diagnosis. For example, an elevated alkaline phosphatase concentration may suggest metastasis to the liver, and an elevated serum amylase concentration may lead to the diagnosis of a pancreatic pseudocyst.

RADIOGRAPHIC STUDIES

Advances in cross-sectional imaging modalities, such as ultrasonography, CT, and magnetic resonance imaging, have made characterization of abdominal masses relatively simple and direct. The exquisite resolution of these imaging modalities permits accurate diagnosis, and when they are used to guide percutaneous biopsy, they make exploratory laparotomy solely for the purpose of diagnosis unnecessary in almost all instances.[9]

Each imaging modality has its unique strengths and weaknesses, and the American College of Radiology has issued guidelines for the appropriate use of different imaging modalities in the evaluation of abdominal masses.[10,11] The surgeon must correlate the clinical location of the mass with the history and the laboratory findings to determine which imaging modality is the most expeditious and cost-effective in a given instance. Of the currently available imaging procedures, ultrasonography [see 3:12 Ultrasonography: Surgical Applications] is the least expensive, the least invasive, and the most readily available. Proper interpretation of ultrasonograms is highly dependent on the skill and experience of the ultrasonographer; however, even examiners who lack great expertise with this modality generally are still able to obtain most of the information they need to evaluate an abdominal mass. The essential information available from the ultrasonogram includes where the mass is anatomically located, whether it is solid or cystic, and on what surrounding structures

a

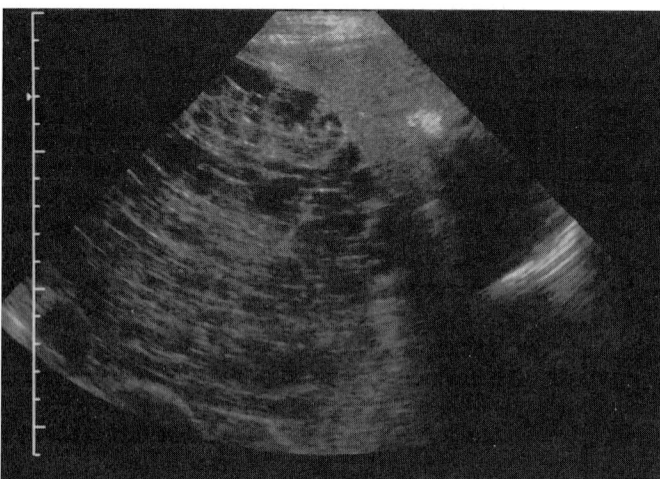

b

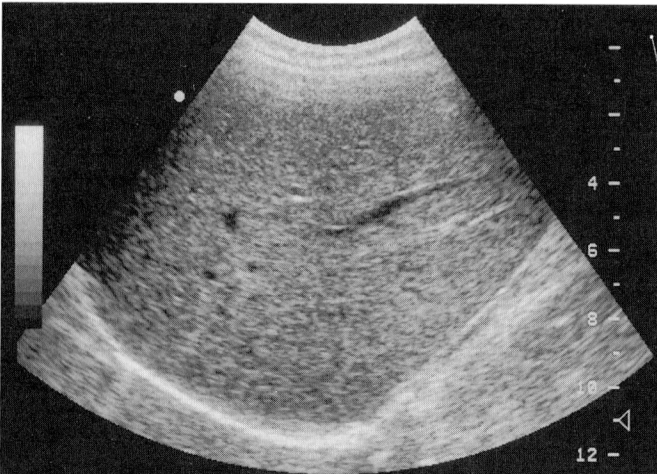

c

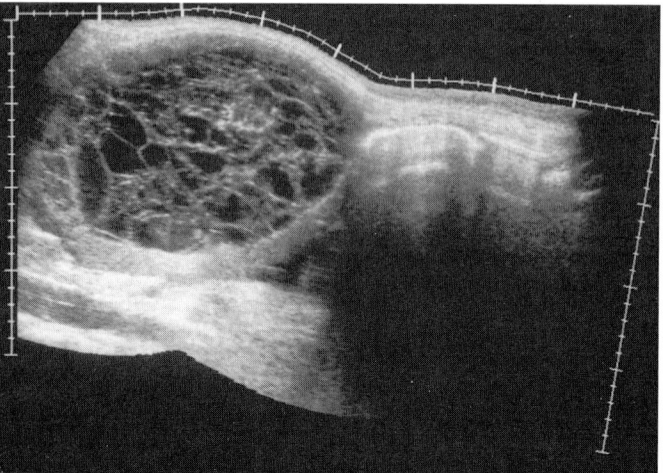

Figure 1 **A 51-year-old patient presented with a palpable abdominal mass. (*a*) A transverse ultrasonogram showed a complex, multiply septated peritoneal cyst. A normal transverse ultrasonogram of the same region (*b*) is provided for purposes of comparison. (*c*) A longitudinal ultrasonogram of the same patient shows the cyst from a different viewpoint.**

it impinges [*see Figure 1*]. Once this information is obtained, further imaging procedures are often unnecessary.

Plain Abdominal Radiographs

The plain abdominal radiograph (kidneys-ureters-bladder [KUB]) usually reveals only nonspecific and indirect evidence of a mass, such as alteration in the size or density of an organ or displacement of normal structures or fat planes. Occasionally, however, this low-cost technique can make specific diagnoses, such as a calcified aortic aneurysm, acute gastric distention, fecal impaction, or an enlarged porcelain gallbladder.

Conventional Barium Studies

At one time, barium studies were the best noninvasive method for evaluating abdominal masses. The advent of cross-sectional imaging has relegated barium studies to an adjunctive role in the evaluation of upper abdominal and midabdominal masses because unless a mass arises directly from the alimentary tract, barium studies yield only indirect signs of its presence. Barium studies still play an important role in the evaluation of adult patients with lower abdominal masses whose history suggests GI pathology (e.g., anemia and weight loss, suggesting a colonic neoplasm, or fever and leukocytosis, suggesting a diverticular inflammatory mass).

Excretory Urography

Excretory urography is not recommended as an initial examination in the evaluation of abdominal masses, because unless the mass originates directly from the kidney or bladder, this technique yields only indirect signs, such as displacement or obstruction of the kidney, the ureter, or the bladder.

Angiography

Cross-sectional imaging modalities have relegated arteriography and venography to secondary roles in the evaluation of abdominal masses. The major role of these techniques is to provide a vascular road map for the surgeon before operation.

Radionucleotide Scanning

Cross-sectional imaging has essentially eliminated the use of radionucleotide studies in the evaluation of abdominal masses.

Magnetic Resonance Imaging

MRI can display abdominal masses directly and is excellent at discriminating varying degrees of density in soft tissue. Because MRI is not as widely available as ultrasonography or CT and because its cost-effectiveness in relation to these modalities has not been demonstrated, MRI is not used as a primary imaging modality for abdominal masses.

Ultrasonography

Ultrasonography has several advantages in the evaluation of abdominal masses: widespread availability, speed, absence of ionizing radiation, portability, low cost, and the ability to document a mass's size, consistency, and (usually) origin in real time.[12,13] In addition, the necessary equipment can be transported to the patient's bedside, and the test requires no patient preparation and only minimal patient cooperation.

Ultrasonography can readily differentiate solid from cystic masses, but its ability to visualize the abdominal cavity is limited by the acoustic barriers presented by intestinal gas and bone, which prevent the evaluation of underlying structures. Another limitation is that spatial resolution decreases as depth of penetra-

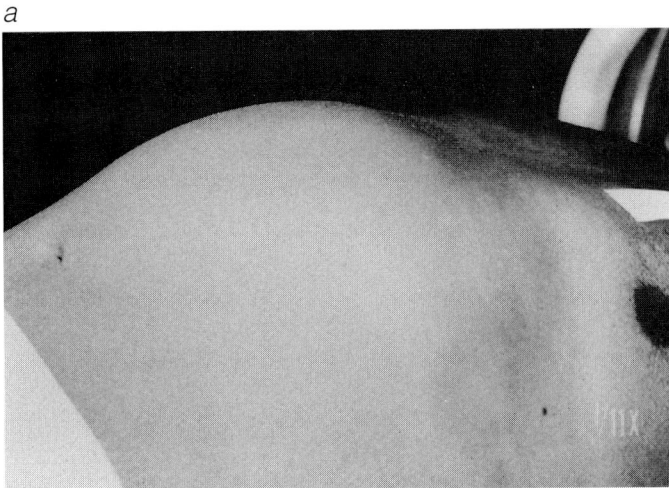
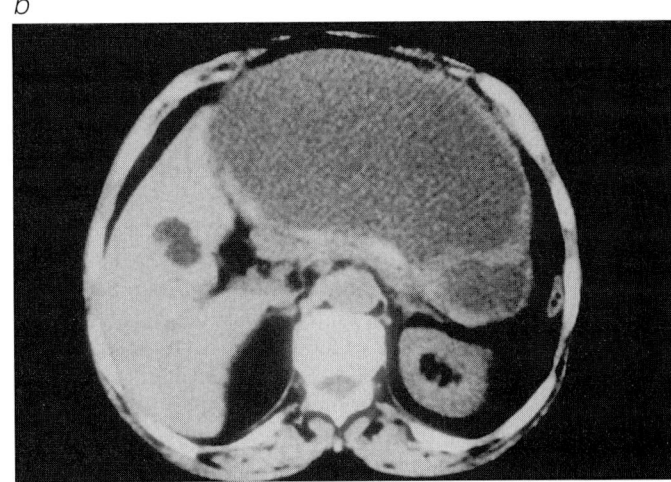

Figure 2 A 58-year-old male patient presented with a palpable, visible (*a*) abdominal mass. (*b*) A CT scan showed a mass arising from the omentum. An omental leiomyosarcoma was surgically resected.

tion increases [*see 3:12 Ultrasonography: Surgical Applications*]. For these reasons, ultrasonography is most effective in regions where an acoustic window exists, such as the right upper quadrant, the pelvis, and the left upper quadrant.

The principal disadvantage of ultrasonography is its dependence on the technical proficiency of the operator. Because ultrasonography is so operator dependent, it is quite possible that in the hands of an inexperienced ultrasonographer, it can contribute to misdiagnosis. The experience level of the ultrasonographer must always be taken into account when ultrasonography is used in the evaluation of an abdominal mass.

Computed Tomography

Currently, CT is the most efficient imaging modality available for the evaluation of abdominal masses[3,9,14]: it has excellent spatial resolution and exquisite density discrimination, and it provides cross-sectional images that are unaffected by bowel gas, bone, excessive abdominal fat, or unusually large body size [*see Figures 2 and 3*]. CT yields excellent visualization of vascular structures and can assess the vascularity of an abdominal mass after intravenous administration of contrast material. It routinely visualizes retroperitoneal and abdominal wall structures and perfectly displays the peritoneal compartments, clearly defining tissue planes and illustrating relations

between masses and adjacent organs and structures.[15-17] If, however, the bowel is not opacified, the accuracy of CT in evaluating abdominal masses is significantly reduced because unopacified intestinal loops can simulate a mass or an abscess.

When the examiner suspects that an abdominal mass is neoplastic, CT is the initial imaging procedure of choice because in addition to imaging the mass itself directly, CT provides invaluable information for staging purposes (e.g., evidence of contiguous spread or the presence of distant metastases).

BIOPSY

Image-Guided Percutaneous Biopsy

The value of image-guided percutaneous biopsy in the evaluation of abdominal masses is now firmly established.[18,19] Recent improvements in imaging techniques (in particular, developments

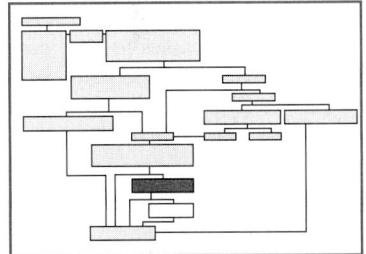

in high-resolution cross-sectional imaging), advances in cytologic methods (in terms of both performance technique and inter-

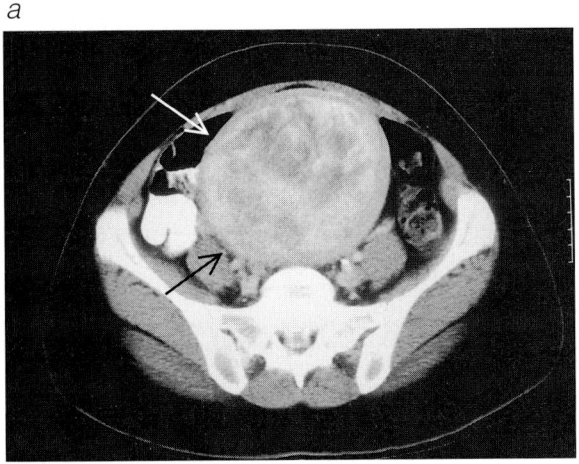
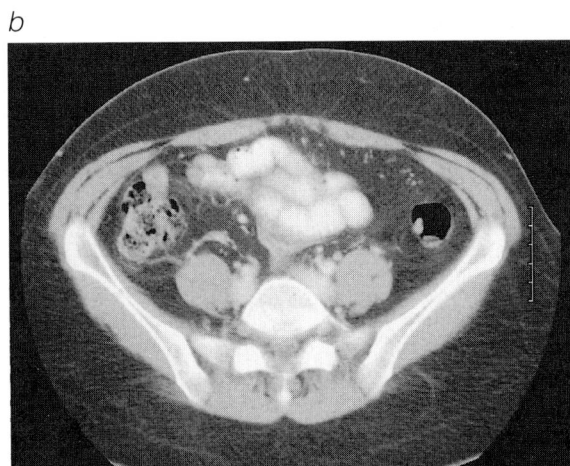

Figure 3 A 49-year-old female patient presented with an abdominal mass. (*a*) A CT scan revealed a uterine fibroid presenting as a pelvic mass. A normal CT of the same region (*b*) is provided for purposes of comparison.

pretation of findings) that permit accurate evaluation of minute quantities of aspirated material, and the availability of fine flexible needles for obtaining tissue specimens have all contributed to the rapid growth in the use of this diagnostic method.[20]

Both ultrasonography and CT can be used to guide percutaneous needle insertion.[21-25] The choice between the two depends on several factors, including how large the mass is, where it is, whether it is better visualized with one imaging modality than with the other, and which modality is more readily available. With many masses, either ultrasound guidance or CT guidance will yield good results; in these cases, the choice depends largely on the personal preference and experience of the radiologist performing the biopsy. MRI can also be used to guide needle biopsy, but it has not yet been thoroughly evaluated against ultrasonography and CT in this role.

Traditionally, ultrasound guidance has been used for biopsy of large, superficial, and cystic masses. Currently, however, because of improvements in instrumentation and biopsy techniques, ultrasonography can also accurately guide biopsy of small, deep, and solid masses. The greatest advantage ultrasonography possesses as a guidance modality is that it enables real-time visualization of the needle tip as it passes through tissue planes into the mass. This real-time visualization allows the examiner to place the needle with considerable precision and to avoid important intervening structures. Another advantage ultrasonography has is that it facilitates angled approaches to the mass, in that it is capable of providing guidance in multiple transverse, longitudinal, or oblique planes. In addition, color flow Doppler imaging can identify blood vessels in and around a mass and can prevent complications by helping the examiner to avoid any vascular structures lying in the path of the needle. Theoretically, any mass that is well visualized on an ultrasonogram is amenable to ultrasound-guided biopsy; in practice, however, this technique probably is still best suited to masses located superficially or at moderate depth in thin or average-sized patients.

CT is well established as an accurate guidance method for percutaneous biopsy of most regions of the body. In the abdomen, CT provides excellent spatial resolution of all structures between the skin and the lesion, regardless of how large the patient is or how deep the mass is. Its only limitation is that it does not provide continuous visualization of the needle during insertion and biopsy. In most cases, however, the direction and depth of the needle can be established reliably with CT guidance [see Figure 4]; substantial repositioning of the needle is rarely necessary.

Numerous different needles of varying caliber, length, and tip design have been used for percutaneous image-guided biopsy. They can be grouped into two general categories: small caliber (20 to 25 gauge) and large caliber (14 to 19 gauge). Small-caliber needles are employed primarily to obtain specimens for cytologic analysis but may also be employed to obtain small pieces of tissue for histologic examination. Their flexible shafts permit movement of the needle during respiration and minimize the risk of tissue or organ laceration and damage from tearing. The main advantage of these smaller needles is that biopsies of masses situated behind loops of bowel can be done with minimal risk of infection. Large-caliber needles are employed to obtain greater amounts of material for histologic as well as cytologic analysis.

The following three events are relative contraindications to percutaneous biopsy:

1. Uncorrectable coagulopathy. Although postbiopsy embolization of the needle tract is capable of controlling hemorrhage in

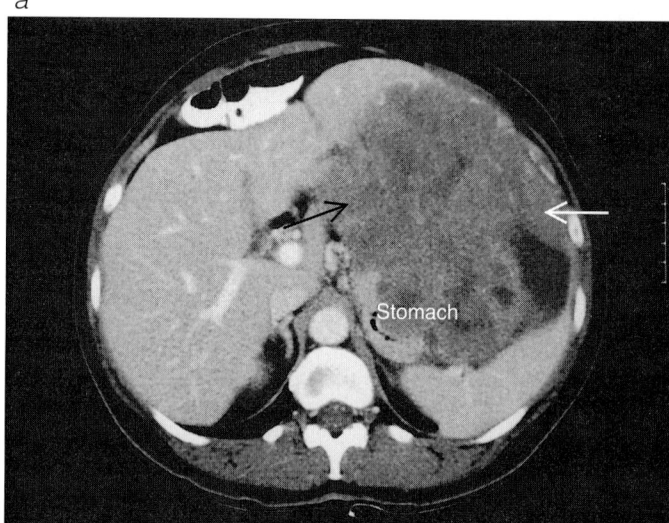

a

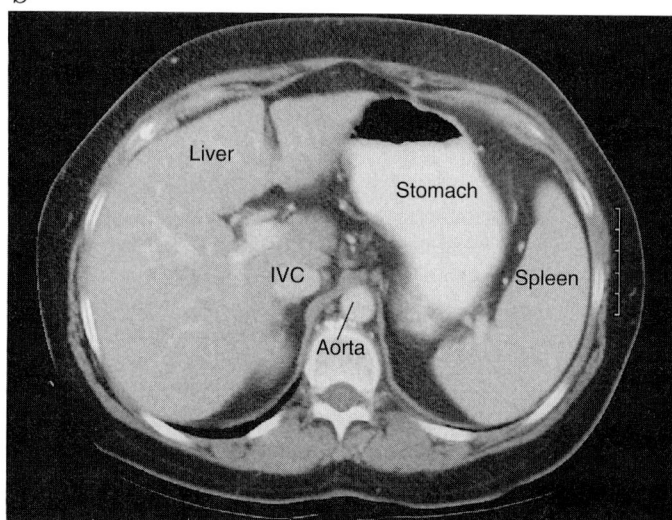

b

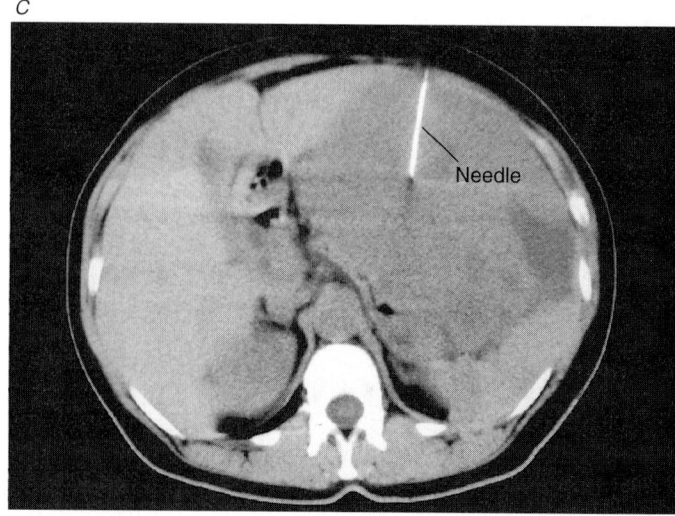

c

Figure 4 A 51-year-old woman presented with a palpable abdominal mass. (*a*) A CT scan located a suspicious lesion. A normal CT scan of the same region (*b*) is provided for purposes of comparison. (IVC—inferior vena cava) (*c*) A CT-guided needle biopsy was performed, and the results indicated that the lesion was a gastric leiomyosarcoma.

patients with uncorrectable coagulopathy, special expertise and equipment are required.

2. Absence of a safe biopsy route. When the location of the mass necessitates that the biopsy path extend through a large blood vessel, the stomach, or an intestinal loop, the potential for hemorrhage or infection increases; however, neither potential complication is a contraindication if a small-caliber needle is used. Biopsies done through collections of ascitic fluid have also proved safe.

3. Lack of cooperation on the part of the patient. An uncooperative patient's uncontrolled motion during needle placement can substantially increase the risk of tissue laceration and hemorrhage; in such cases, sedation or anesthesia may be necessary.

The safety of image-guided percutaneous biopsy is well attested.[20,26] Several large multi-institutional reviews have reported mortalities ranging from 0.008% to 0.031% and major complication rates ranging from 0.05% to 0.18%.[27-29] A review of 11,700 patients who underwent percutaneous abdominal biopsy with 20- to 23-gauge needles between 1969 and 1982 found a total complication rate of only 0.05% and a mortality of only 0.008%.[27] Another study, involving 63,180 patients, demonstrated a complication rate of 0.16%.[30] A single-institution review of 8,000 ultrasound-guided needle biopsies done with both large- and small-caliber needles reported similar results: a mortality of 0.038% and a major complication rate of 0.187%.[31] A prospective study of 3,393 biopsies (1,825 ultrasound-guided and 1,568 CT-guided) showed a mortality of 0.06% and a complication rate of 0.34% (0.3% for ultrasound-guided biopsies and 0.5% for CT-guided biopsies).[26]

Of the major complications, hemorrhage is the most commonly reported. Other major complications reported are pneumothorax, pancreatitis, bile leakage, peritonitis, and needle-track seeding. Although needle-track seeding is an important theoretical consideration when a mass seems likely to be of malignant neoplastic origin, it remains an exceedingly rare complication: fewer than 100 cases have been reported in the literature, for an estimated frequency of only 0.005%.[30,32,33] Because seeding is so rare, it should affect the decision to perform percutaneous biopsy only when the surgeon is convinced the lesion is amenable to curative surgical resection. Most cases of needle-track seeding have occurred after biopsy of a pancreatic carcinoma; however, it has also been reported after biopsy of hepatic and retroperitoneal lesions. There is some evidence to suggest that with masses in solid organs, using large-caliber needles or cutting needles does not lead to a significantly higher complication rate than fine-needle aspiration biopsy does, provided that there is a direct path to the mass.[26,34,35]

The reported accuracy of ultrasound-guided biopsy ranges from 66% to 97%, depending on the location, size, and histologic origin of the mass.[26] In one series of ultrasound-guided biopsies of 126 consecutive small (< 3 cm) solid masses in various anatomic locations and of various histologic types, the overall accuracy of biopsy was 91%.[36] Results improved as the size of the mass increased, rising from 79% in masses 1 cm or less in diameter to 98% in masses 2 to 3 cm in diameter. The accuracy of biopsy for hepatic masses of any size was 96%.[36] Another report found ultrasound-guided biopsy to be 91% accurate for small (< 2.5 cm) abdominal masses.[37] Two organ-specific reviews demonstrated 94% accuracy for ultrasound-guided liver biopsy[38] and 95% accuracy for ultrasound-guided biopsy of pancreatic masses.[39]

The reported accuracy of CT-guided biopsy ranges from 80% to 100%, depending on the location, size, and histologic origin of the mass.[23,24,35] In a study of 200 consecutive CT-guided needle biopsies, the overall accuracy for all sites was 95%. Accuracy of diagnosis was very high for hepatic (99%) and renal (100%) biopsies and for characterization of fluid collections (100%) but somewhat lower for retroperitoneal (87.5%) and pancreatic (82%) biopsies.[21] In a prospective study of 1,000 consecutive CT-guided biopsies, the procedure was 91.8% sensitive and 98.9% specific.[35]

Endoscopic Ultrasound-Guided Biopsy

Endoscopic ultrasonography (EUS) is a relatively new cross-sectional imaging modality that allows accurate visualization of the gastrointestinal wall and surrounding structures with greater spatial resolution and better anatomic detail than transcutaneous ultrasonography or CT. In fact, EUS provides unique imaging information currently unavailable with any other technology.[40] Because depth of ultrasound penetration is inversely related to frequency (whereas image resolution is directly related to frequency), endoscopic placement of an ultrasound transducer immediately adjacent to an area of interest allows the use of higher ultrasound frequencies than is possible with transcutaneous ultrasonography. Thus, EUS can detect much smaller masses than is possible with conventional transcutaneous ultrasonography. For evaluation of some organs, such as the pancreas, EUS is the most sensitive diagnostic tool currently available, demonstrating greater sensitivity for small masses than CT.[40,41] EUS also avoids the problem of intervening bowel gas that often limits the use of transcutaneous ultrasonography as an adjunct to percutaneous biopsy. EUS-guided biopsy is therefore well suited for the evaluation of abdominal masses that are too small for visualization by other cross-sectional imaging modalities or inaccessible for percutaneous biopsy.[40]

EUS-guided biopsy became widely available as a diagnostic tool only recently because the original radial scanning systems utilized for EUS, although efficient for diagnostic imaging, did not allow safe and direct guidance of needles for biopsy. With radial scanning echoendoscopes, a rotating transducer produces a 360° view perpendicular to the axis of the endoscope and the needle exiting the biopsy channel appears only as a dot on the ultrasound image. In the early 1990s, the linear scanning system was introduced, with a plane of ultrasound imaging parallel to the shaft of the endoscope that allows direct, real-time visualization of the biopsy needle throughout its entire course. The linear array instrument also has color flow Doppler capability that allows the endoscopist to avoid any vascular structures lying in the path of the biopsy needle. EUS-guided biopsy with the linear scanning system offers clear and consistent visualization of the biopsy needle along its entire path in real time, excellent delineation of intervening tissues, and no interference by intestinal gas.

Compared with other cross-sectional imaging modalities, EUS has proved superior for detection of pancreatic masses and nodal metastases, as well as for local tumor staging of other gastrointestinal neoplasms.[40-43] With EUS-guided biopsy, the risk of seeding the needle track with malignant cells is minimized and becomes irrelevant in many patients with potentially curable lesions because the needle tract is later removed as part of the surgical specimen (e.g., resection of a mass in the head of the pancreas by pancreatoduodenectomy). EUS-guided biopsy can now be considered a first-line modality for obtaining tissue diagnoses, particularly in the evaluation of extraintestinal and pancreatic masses.

In a large single-institution study, 327 abdominal masses were sampled by EUS-guided biopsy, with an overall accuracy for the diagnosis of malignancy of 86%, a sensitivity of 84%, and a specificity of 96%. Only one patient (0.3%) suffered a complication.[43] Multiple other studies have confirmed the high sensitivity and specificity of EUS-guided biopsy, especially for the diagnosis of extraluminal abdominal masses, and confirmed the safety of the procedure; reported complication rates are between 0.3% and 2%.[40-44] This complication rate, while slightly higher than that of diagnostic upper gastrointestinal endoscopy, appears to be lower than the complication rate encountered with other advanced endoscopic procedures, such as therapeutic endoscopic retrograde cholangiopancreatography.

Currently, the most frequent application for EUS-guided biopsy is in the diagnosis and staging of pancreatic masses. EUS-guided biopsy should also be considered for the diagnosis of abdominal masses that are not readily accessible to percutaneous biopsy, because it may obviate more invasive procedures, such as laparoscopy or laparotomy. In a 10-year study of the impact of EUS on patient management, 86% of patients avoided further imaging and 25% avoided unnecessary laparotomy. Overall, EUS was found to significantly change clinical management in up to one third of the 537 patients studied.[44]

As is the case with transcutaneous ultrasonography, the principal disadvantage of EUS-guided biopsy is its dependence on the proficiency of the ultrasonographer. Moreover, EUS-guided biopsy is one of the most technically demanding of all GI endoscopic procedures, requiring an operator who is not only an experienced ultrasonographer but also an expert endoscopist.

Laparoscopic Biopsy

Even though laparoscopy provides excellent visualization of the inside of the abdominal cavity and now plays an important role in the staging of some abdominal neoplasms, its role in the evaluation of abdominal masses is limited.[45] Laparoscopic biopsy specimens are best obtained under direct vision with a biopsy needle introduced at an independent site rather than with a biopsy forceps: forceps biopsy usually produces superficial, small, squeezed, and distorted specimens. Although percutaneous biopsies of this type can be especially useful when bleeding from the biopsy site is a concern, image-guided percutaneous biopsy usually offers a more expedient, less invasive, cheaper, and often safer means of obtaining the diagnosis. More important, in the presence of adhesions, laparoscopic biopsy is much less effective and typically fails to make a diagnosis altogether unless the mass is clearly visible on the anterior surface of the viscera.

Exploratory Laparotomy

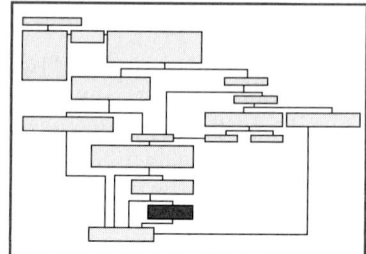

Despite recent advances in diagnostic imaging and laparoscopic procedures, it still occasionally proves necessary to perform an exploratory laparotomy for the sole purpose of establishing a diagnosis in the patient with an abdominal mass. It is essential to keep in mind, however, that many patients with abdominal masses have disorders for which operative intervention is not required. In addition, although exploratory laparotomy can yield crucial information and may be, in a sense, the "ultimate diagnostic test" (as some have referred to it), it is not infallible. Errors in the intra-abdominal surgical diagnosis of abdominal masses can and do occur. For example, in six instances observed during an 18-month period at a single institution, exploratory laparotomy failed to reveal abdominal masses that had already been demonstrated by preoperative evaluation and were subsequently confirmed during the postoperative period.[46]

References

1. Butler DB, Bargen JA: Abdominal masses. Gastroenterology 19:1, 1951
2. Hippocrates: The Book of Prognostics, part 7. The Internet Classics Archives, http://classics.mit.edu/Hippocrates/prognost.7.7.html
3. Dixon AK, Kingham JGC, Fry IK, et al: Computed tomography in patients with an abdominal mass: effective and efficient? A controlled trial. Lancet 1:1199, 1981
4. Cassidy D: Abdominal mass. The Clinical Practice of Emergency Medicine, 2nd ed. Harwood-Nuss AL, Linden CH, Luten RC, et al, Eds. Lippincott-Raven, Philadelphia, 1996, p 133
5. Cabot RC: Differential Diagnosis, Presented Through an Analysis of 317 Cases, 2nd ed. WB Saunders Co, Philadelphia, 1915, vol 2, p 709
6. Schaffner F: Abdominal enlargement and masses. Gastroenterology. Haubrich WS, Schaffner F, Berk JE, Eds. WB Saunders Co, Philadelphia, 1998, p 138
7. Morales TG, Fennerty MB: Abdominal distention. Clinical Medicine, 2nd ed. Greene HL, Fincher RME, Johnson WP, et al, Eds. Mosby, St. Louis, 1996, p 290
8. DeGowin EL, DeGowin RL: Bedside Diagnostic Examination. Macmillan Publishing Co, New York, 1976, p 471
9. Gore RM: Palpable abdominal masses. Diagnostic Imaging: An Algorithmic Approach. Eisenberg RL, Ed. JB Lippincott Co, Philadelphia, 1988, p 214
10. DiSantis DJ, Ralls PW, Balfe DM, et al: Imaging evaluation of the palpable abdominal mass. American College of Radiology. ACR Appropriateness Criteria. Radiology 215(suppl):201, 2000
11. Grollman J, Bettmann MA, Boxt LM, et al: Pulsatile abdominal mass. American College of Radiology. ACR Appropriateness Criteria. Radiology 215(suppl):55, 2000
12. Aspelin P, Hildell J, Karlsson S, et al: Ultrasonic evaluation of palpable abdominal masses. Acta Chir Scand 156:501, 1980
13. Barker CS, Lindsell DRM: Ultrasound of the palpable abdominal mass. Clin Radiol 41:98, 1990
14. Williams MP, Scott IHK, Dixon AK: Computed tomography in 101 patients with a palpable abdominal mass. Clin Radiol 35:293, 1984
15. Engel IA, Auh YH, Rubenstein WA, et al: Large posterior abdominal masses: computed tomographic localization. Radiology 149:203, 1983
16. Pistolesi GF, Procacci C, Caudana R, et al: C.T. criteria of the differential diagnosis in primary retroperitoneal masses. Eur J Radiol 4:127, 1984
17. Pandolfo I, Blandino A, Gaeta M, et al: CT findings in palpable lesions of the anterior abdominal wall. J Comput Assist Tomogr 10:629, 1986
18. Gazelle GS, Haaga JR: Guided percutaneous biopsy of intraabdominal lesions. AJR Am J Radiol 153:929, 1989
19. Welch TJ, Reading CC: Imaging-guided biopsy. Mayo Clin Proc 64:1295, 1989
20. Grainger RG, Allison D: Interventional radiology. Diagnostic Radiology: A Textbook of Medical Imaging. Grainger RG, Allison D, Eds. Churchill Livingstone, New York, 1997, p 2485
21. Staab EV, Jaques PF, Partain CL: Percutaneous biopsy in the management of solid intra-abdominal masses of unknown etiology. Radiol Clin North Am 17:435, 1979
22. Ennis MG, MacErlean DP: Percutaneous aspiration biopsy of abdomen and retroperitoneum. Clin Radiol 31:611, 1980
23. Sundaram M, Wolverson MK, Heiberg E, et al: Utility of CT-guided abdominal aspiration procedures. AJR Am J Radiol 139:1111, 1982
24. Smith C, Butler JA: Efficacy of directed percutaneous fine-needle aspiration cytology in the diagnosis of intra-abdominal masses. Arch Surg 123:820, 1988
25. Jaeger HJ, MacFie J, Mitchell CJ, et al: Diagnosis of abdominal masses with percutaneous biopsy guided by ultrasound. Br Med J 301:1188, 1990
26. Rumack CM, Wilson SR, Charboneau JW: Ultrasound-guided biopsy and drainage of the abdomen and pelvis. Diagnostic Ultrasound. Rumack CM, Wilson SR, Charboneau JW, Eds. Mosby-Year Book, New York, 1998, p 600
27. Livraghi R, Damascelli B, Lombardi C, et al: Risk in fine needle abdominal biopsy. J Clin Ultrasound 11:77, 1983

28. Fornari F, Civardi G, Cavanna L, et al: Complications of ultrasonically guided fine needle abdominal biopsy: results of a multi-centre Italian study and a review of the literature (The Cooperative Italian Study Group). Scand J Gastroenterol 24:949, 1989

29. Smith EH: Complications of percutaneous abdominal fine needle biopsy. Review Radiology 178:253, 1991

30. Smith EH: The hazards of fine needle aspiration biopsy. Ultrasound Med Biol 10:629, 1984

31. Nolsoe C, Nielsen L, Torp-Pedersen S, et al: Major complications and deaths due to interventional ultrasonography: a review of 8000 cases. J Clin Ultrasound 18:179, 1990

32. Engzell U, Esposti PL, Rubio C, et al: Investigation on tumour spread in connection with aspiration biopsy. Acta Radiol Ther Phys Biol 10:385, 1971

33. Smith FP, Macdonald JS, Schein PS, et al: Cutaneous seeding of pancreatic cancer by skinny-needle aspiration biopsy. Arch Intern Med 140:855, 1980

34. Martino CR, Haaga JR, Bryan PJ, et al: CT-guided liver biopsies: eight years' experience. Radiology 152:755, 1984

35. Welch TJ, Sheedy PF, Johnson CD, et al: CT-guided biopsy: prospective analysis of 1,000 procedures. Radiology 171:493, 1989

36. Reading CC, Charboneau JW, James EM, et al: Sonographically guided percutaneous biopsy of small (3 cm or less) masses. AJR Am J Radiol 151:189, 1988

37. Downey DB, Wilson SR: Ultrasonographically guided biopsy of small intra-abdominal masses. Can Assoc Radiol J 44:350, 1993

38. Buscarini L, Fornari F, Bolondi L, et al: Ultrasound-guided fine-needle biopsy of focal liver lesions: technique, diagnostic accuracy and complications: a retrospective study on 2091 biopsies. J Hepatol 11:344, 1990

39. Brandt KR, Charboneau JW, Stephens DH, et al: CT- and US-guided biopsy of the pancreas. Radiology 187:99, 1993

40. Pfau PR, Chak A: Endoscopic ultrasonography. Endoscopy 34:21, 2002

41. Harewood GC, Wiersema MJ: Endosonography-guided fine needle aspiration biopsy in the evaluation of pancreatic masses. Am J Gastroenterol 97:1386, 2002

42. Catalano MF, Sial S, Chak A, et al: EUS-guided fine needle aspiration of idiopathic abdominal masses. Gastrointest Endosc 55:854, 2002

43. Williams DB, Sahai AV, Aabakken L, et al: Endoscopic ultrasound guided fine needle aspiration biopsy: a large single centre experience. Gut 44:720, 1999

44. Kaffes AJ, Mishra A, Simpson SB, et al: Upper gastrointestinal endoscopic ultrasound and its impact on patient management: 1990–2000. Intern Med J 32:372, 2002

45. Sackier JM, Berci G, Paz-Partlow M: Elective diagnostic laparoscopy. Am J Surg 161:326, 1991

46. Harbin WP, Wittenberg J, Ferrucci JT, et al: Fallibility of exploratory laparotomy in detection of hepatic and retroperitoneal masses. AJR Am J Roentgenol 135:115, 1980

3 MORBID OBESITY

Harvey J. Sugerman, M.D., F.A.C.S.

Approach to the Morbidly Obese Patient

Many surgeons are afraid to operate on the morbidly obese patient (i.e., a patient whose weight is 100 lb greater than ideal body weight or who has a body mass index [BMI] greater than 35 kg/mg2) because they presuppose a marked increase in perioperative morbidity and mortality. Although the morbidly obese patient is certainly at greater risk, this risk can be markedly reduced by paying careful attention to detail in preoperative and post-

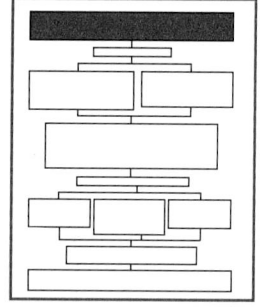

operative care. The increased risks encountered in these patients include wound infection, dehiscence, thrombophlebitis, pulmonary embolism, anesthetic calamities, acute postoperative asphyxia in patients with obstructive sleep apnea syndrome (SAS), acute respiratory failure, right ventricular or biventricular cardiac failure, and missed acute catastrophes of the abdomen, such as an anastomotic leak. In a series of about 3,000 gastric procedures for morbid obesity itself, we have observed the following incidence of complications: wound infection that delayed hospital discharge, 5%, as well as minor infections or seromas in an additional 10%; clinically apparent phlebitis, 0.4%; clinically diagnosed fatal pulmonary embolism, 0.2%; and pneumonia, 0.5%. We have observed a 1% operative mortality. Although many of these patients had severe preoperative morbidity (respiratory insufficiency, pseudotumor cerebri, or insulin-dependent diabetes), the risks of complications approach the risks associated with major abdominal operation in nonobese patients. In what follows, the focus is on issues that the surgeon should carefully consider when operating on an extremely overweight patient.

Cardiac Dysfunction

Morbidly obese patients are at significant risk of coronary artery disease as a result of an increased incidence of systemic hypertension, hypercholesterolemia, and diabetes. Because of this increased risk for cardiac dysfunction, preoperative electrocardiography probably should be performed on all obese patients 30 years of age or older.

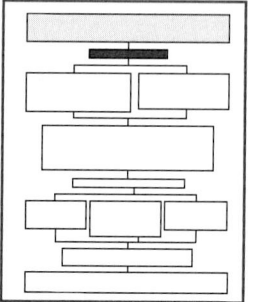

Most morbidly obese patients have minimal evidence of cardiac dysfunction as detected by Swan-Ganz catheterization. Markedly elevated pulmonary arterial pressure (PAP) and pulmonary arterial

wedge pressure (PAWP) values will frequently be noted in patients with the respiratory insufficiency of obesity, especially those with obesity hypoventilation syndrome (OHS) [*see* Respiratory Insufficiency, Obesity Hypoventilation Syndrome, *below*].[1] Intubation and ventilation in these patients will often be followed by a vigorous diuresis, and it is not unusual for a patient to lose 50 lb or more of retained fluid. In a few obese patients, acute respiratory insufficiency will be caused by a greatly expanded central blood volume and heart failure. Abnormal blood gas values in these individuals will be corrected by vigorous diuresis alone. As with most other abnormalities related to morbid obesity, weight loss will also correct cardiac dysfunction.

Respiratory Insufficiency

Morbidly obese patients may suffer from obstructive SAS or OHS. The simultaneous presence of SAS and OHS is known as the pickwickian syndrome [*see* Discussion, Respiratory Insufficiency of Obesity, *below*].[2-4]

SLEEP APNEA SYNDROME

SAS is a potentially fatal complication of morbid obesity. A diagnosis of SAS should be suspected when there is a history of loud snoring, frequent nocturnal awakening with shortness of breath, and daytime somnolence. It is estimated that 2% of middle-aged women and 4% of middle-aged men in the United States workforce have SAS, and the incidence is markedly higher in the severely obese.[5]

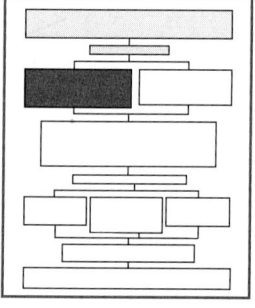

Patients will often admit to falling asleep while driving and waking up with their car on the road's median strip or bumping its guardrail. It is extremely important that trauma surgeons be aware of the relation between obesity and somnolence should a morbidly obese patient be seen in the emergency room after an automobile accident in which he or she fell asleep at the wheel. Elective patients with suspected sleep apnea syndrome should undergo preoperative polysomnography at a sleep center to confirm the diagnosis. Medications are usually ineffective. Stimulants, such as methylphenidate hydrochloride (Ritalin), should not be used. If a patient has a respiratory disturbance index (RDI) greater than 25—indicating more than 25 apneic or hypopneic episodes per hour of sleep—or has cardiac arrhythmias in association with apnea, treatment by nocturnal nasal continuous positive airway pres-

Approach to the Morbidly Obese Patient

Patient is morbidly obese (current weight at least 100 lb > ideal body weight, body mass index $\geq$ 35 kg/m², or both)

Increased risks include
- Missed abdominal catastrophe
- Respiratory failure
- Cardiac failure

- Anesthetic calamities
- Pulmonary embolism
- Internal hernia
- Acute gastric distention

- Wound infection
- Postoperative asphyxia
- Dehiscence
- Thrombophlebitis

Evaluate cardiopulmonary status preoperatively

Patient reports loud snoring, frequent nocturnal awakening, and daytime somnolence, or trauma victim has fallen asleep at the wheel

Suspect sleep apnea syndrome (SAS).

Confirm SAS by polysomnography in elective patients. Provide nocturnal nasal CPAP if apneic episodes are $\geq$ 25/hr of sleep or are associated with arrhythmias. If patient does not respond to — or does not tolerate — CPAP, perform tracheostomy with extra-long tube.

Patient has heart failure or extreme shortness of breath

Suspect obesity hypoventilation syndrome (OHS).
OHS is confirmed by $P_aO_2 \leq 55$ mm Hg or $P_aO_2 \geq 47$ mm Hg
- If PAWP $\geq$ 18 mm Hg, try I.V. furosemide.
- If PAP $\geq$ 40 mm Hg, consider insertion of Greenfield vena caval filter.
- If Hb $\geq$ 16 g/dl, phlebotomize to Hb of 15 g/dl.

Give prophylaxis against thromboembolism, induce anesthesia, and intubate

Administer regular or low-molecular-weight heparin 30 min preoperatively and at appropriate intervals thereafter until the patient is ambulatory.

Use intermittent sequential venous compression boots during anesthesia induction and throughout operation.

Two anesthesia personnel are required for induction and intubation of patients with SAS or OHS (one to hold the mask and one to squeeze the ventilation bag).

Insert oral airway after administration of succinylcholine and sodium pentobarbital. Ventilate with 100% O_2 for several minutes before intubation. If intubation is unsuccessful, reinsert oral airway and ventilate with a mask. Patient should be in reverse Trendelenburg position.

In the recovery room, keep patient in reverse Trendelenburg position

Patient does not have respiratory insufficiency of obesity

Extubate in recovery room when patient is fully alert and ventilatory effort is adequate; return patient to room.

Patient has SAS

In the absence of OHS, wean and extubate the day after operation. If patient was on nasal CPAP before operation, reinstitute on second night after operation. Monitor for prolonged apnea or arrhythmia; if either occurs, awaken patient.

Patient has OHS

Continue mechanical ventilation after operation until pain of breathing resolves. Wean to preoperative arterial blood gas levels; several days may be required.

Encourage early postoperative ambulation

Use intermittent sequential venous compression boots until patient is fully ambulatory.

Maintain high index of suspicion for recognition of abdominal catastrophes

Guarding, tenderness, and rigidity may be absent. Signs of infection (fever, tachypnea, tachycardia) may be absent. Acute respiratory failure may be secondary to peritonitis. Radiographic contrast studies and laparotomy may be indicated even when clinical signs are few.

sure (nasal CPAP) should be provided. If the patient has severe SAS with an RDI greater than 40 and does not respond with elimination of the apneic episodes or cannot tolerate nasal CPAP, a tracheostomy should be considered. An extra-long tracheostomy tube is usually necessary because of the depth of the trachea in the morbidly obese patient.

OBESITY HYPOVENTILATION SYNDROME

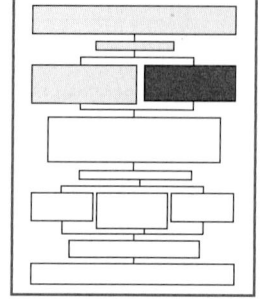

OHS should be suspected in patients who present with heart failure or extreme shortness of breath. Patients who have a BMI of 50 kg/m² or greater or who have a history of pulmonary problems (e.g., smoking, chronic obstructive pulmonary disease, sarcoidosis, pulmonary fibrosis, or asthma) should undergo a baseline arterial blood gas (ABG) determination before operation. Diagnosis of OHS is confirmed when the patient's arterial oxygen tension (P_aO_2) is 55 mm Hg or less or the arterial carbon dioxide tension (P_aCO_2) is 47 mm Hg or greater. These patients often have marked elevations in mean PAP, mean PAWP, or both, as well as severe polycythemia. In patients with obesity hypoventilation syndrome, a Swan-Ganz catheter should be inserted as part of the preoperative evaluation. If PAWP is 18 mm Hg or greater, diuresis with intravenous furosemide is indicated. In many of these patients, however, an elevated PAWP reflects an increased intrathoracic pressure and is necessary to maintain adequate cardiac output; such patients do not have congestive heart failure, despite a markedly elevated filling pressure [see Discussion, below]. Little can be done for the pulmonary hypertension that is seen in many of these patients; raising the P_aO_2 above 60 mm Hg usually will not lower PAP acutely.

Polycythemia can significantly increase the incidence of phlebothrombosis. If the hemoglobin (Hb) concentration is 16 g/dl or greater, phlebotomy to a concentration of 15 g/dl should be performed to reduce the postoperative risk of venous thrombosis. If PAP is 40 mm Hg or greater, consideration should be given to prophylactic insertion of a Greenfield vena caval filter because of the high risk of a fatal pulmonary embolism in these patients.[6] Placement of this filter can be a challenge because the appropriate landmarks cannot be identified in the operating room with fluoroscopy. It is necessary before operation to tape a quarter to the patient's back over the second lumbar vertebra with the aid of fixed radiographs and then during operation to aim for the quarter with the insertion catheter, using fluoroscopy. Because these patients are usually too heavy for angiography tables, the Greenfield filter usually cannot be inserted percutaneously in the radiology department.

Embolism

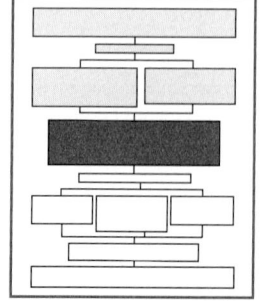

The risk of deep vein thrombosis [see 4:6 Venous Thromboembolism] increases with a prolonged operation or a postoperative period of immobilization, and it increases even further in the morbidly obese patient. Standard or low-molecular-weight heparin should be administered subcutaneously 30 minutes before operation and at appropriate intervals thereafter (depending on the type of heparin used) for at least 2 days or until the patient is ambulatory. Because respiratory function in the morbidly obese patient is greatly enhanced with the reverse Trendelenburg position, intermittent sequential venous compression boots should be used to counteract the increased venous stasis and the propensity for clotting. It is important that the intermittent venous compression boots be used before induction of anesthesia and throughout the operative procedure. Compression boots are usually part of a standard preoperative protocol in gastric procedures for weight control; their use should not be unintentionally neglected in preparation for other elective or emergency procedures on morbidly obese patients. Patients with severe venous stasis disease (e.g., pretibial stasis ulcers or bronze edema) are at significantly increased risk for fatal pulmonary embolism (PE).[7] Prophylactic insertion of a Greenfield vena cava filter should be considered in both patients with severe venous stasis disease and patients with OHS and a high PAP. Bariatric surgery–induced weight loss will correct the venous stasis disease in most cases.[7]

Anesthesia in Patients with Respiratory Insufficiency

Morbidly obese patients can be intimidating to the anesthesiologist because they are at significant risk for complications from anesthesia, especially during induction. The risk is particularly great for obese patients with respiratory insufficiency. An obese patient often has a short, fat neck and a heavy chest wall, which make intubation and ventilation a challenge. If endotracheal intubation proves difficult, however, these patients can usually be well ventilated with a mask. Awake intubation can be performed, with or without fiberoptic aids, but is quite unpleasant and rarely necessary.

It is extremely important that at least two anesthesia personnel be present during induction and intubation for patients with respiratory insufficiency of obesity. An oral airway is inserted after muscle paralysis with succinylcholine and sodium pentobarbital induction. One person elevates the jaw, hyperextends the neck, and ensures a tight fit of the mask, using both hands. To ensure adequate oxygen delivery, a second person compresses the ventilation reservoir bag, using two hands because of the resistance to air flow from the poorly compliant, heavy chest wall. After ventilation with 100% oxygen for several minutes, intubation is attempted. If difficulties are encountered within 30 seconds, the steps above should be repeated until the patient has been successfully intubated. A volume ventilator is required during operation. Placing the patient in the reverse Trendelenburg position expands total lung volume and facilitates ventilation[8]; however, the reverse Trendelenburg position increases lower extremity venous pressure and therefore mandates the use of intermittent sequential venous compression boots [see Embolism, above]. It is helpful to monitor blood gases through a radial arterial line or digital pulse oximeter.

Postoperative Management

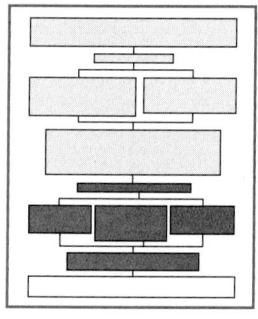

After operation, the obese patient should be kept in the reverse Trendelenburg position and should not be extubated until he or she is fully alert and showing evidence of adequate ventilatory effort [see 6:6 Use of the Mechanical Ventilator]. In the absence of respiratory insufficiency, most obese patients can be extubated in the OR or the recovery room and returned to a standard hospital room.

Patients with SAS, however, should be managed with overnight mechanical ventilation in the ICU. In the absence of concomitant OHS, they can usually be weaned and extubated the day after operation. Patients who were receiving ventilatory support with nasal CPAP before operation should have this treatment reinstituted the second night after operation; monitoring for prolonged apnea should be continued in the ICU or in a stepdown unit with digital oximetry. If apnea occurs, simply waking the patient should correct the problem. Patients who required tracheostomy can also usually be weaned from the ventilator the morning after operation.

Patients with OHS require prolonged mechanical volume ventilation until the pain of breathing resolves. One cannot expect such patients to manifest normal ABG levels, and they should be weaned to their preoperative values. This is why baseline ABG values are obtained preoperatively. The weaning process may require several days. It is important that these patients remain in the reverse Trendelenburg position to maximize diaphragmatic excursion. Positive end-expiratory pressure (PEEP) ventilation may be detrimental in patients with OHS because it can overdistend alveoli, thereby leading to capillary compression, decreased cardiac output, and increased dead space, all of which can exacerbate retention of carbon dioxide.

Swan-Ganz catheters, inserted preoperatively in patients with severe OHS, are useful in monitoring postoperative intravascular volume and oxygen delivery status. Excessive diuresis or restriction of fluids should be avoided [see Discussion, below].

It is extremely important to encourage early postoperative ambulation for the morbidly obese patient. These patients have surprisingly little pain, and it is not unusual to see them walking in the afternoon or early evening after a major abdominal procedure. If the patients have been advised preoperatively of the merits of early postoperative ambulation and know it is for their own welfare, they are usually willing to cooperate.

Complications of Gastric Surgery for Obesity

Current gastric procedures for obesity include open and laparoscopic gastric bypass (GBP), gastroplasty, and laparoscopic adjustable gastric banding. The procedures themselves are described in more detail elsewhere [see 3:14 Gastric Procedures for Morbid Obesity]; the following are some of the main complications associated with any abdominal operation in a severely obese patient.

ABDOMINAL CATASTROPHE

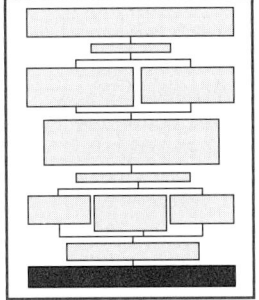

It may be very difficult to recognize an abdominal catastrophe in patients who are very young, very old, or morbidly obese or who are receiving high doses of steroids. The obese patient, for example, may present in the emergency room with a perforated duodenal ulcer or a ruptured diverticulum, complaining of abdominal pain, and yet on abdominal examination have no evidence of peritoneal irritation (no guarding, tenderness, or rigidity). This situation has been well documented in patients in whom an anastomotic or gastric leak has developed after operation for morbid obesity.[9] Symptoms include shoulder pain, pelvic or scrotal pain, back pain, tenesmus, urinary frequency, and, of great importance, marked anxiety. Signs of infection (e.g., fever, tachypnea, and tachycardia) may be absent, though tachycardia is often the first sign of a significant problem. Patients with peritonitis often have clinical symptoms and signs suggesting a massive pulmonary embolus: severe tachypnea, tachycardia, and sudden hypotension. Such acute pulmonary failure is probably secondary to sepsis-induced acute respiratory dis-

tress syndrome (ARDS). Thus, peritonitis must be suspected in any morbidly obese patient with acute respiratory failure. Patients who have undergone a laparoscopic bariatric procedure may be reexplored without much difficulty if there is concern about a possible leak.

Because a high index of suspicion of peritonitis is required to detect the condition in morbidly obese patients, radiographic contrast studies with water-soluble agents such as diatrizoate meglumine (Gastrografin) may be indicated even when there are few clinical signs. If a perforated viscus is suspected, an exploratory laparotomy may be necessary despite normal findings on radiographic contrast study.

INTERNAL HERNIA

GBP places patients at risk for internal hernia with a closed-loop obstruction, leading to bowel strangulation. There are three potential locations for these internal hernias: the Roux-en-Y anastomosis; the opening in the transverse mesocolon through which the retrocolic Roux limb is brought; and the Petersen hernia, which is located behind the retrocolic Roux limb. The primary symptom of an internal hernia is periumbilical pain, usually in the form of cramping consistent with visceral colic. These internal hernias may be very difficult to diagnose. Upper gastrointestinal radiographic series and abdominal CT scans are often normal, providing a false sense of security. The resulting assumption that no problem exists may be devastating for the patient should bowel infarction occur as a consequence of closed-loop obstruction. One should always carefully inspect the plain abdominal radiograph for the abnormal placement or spreading of the Roux-en-Y anastomotic staples. The safest course of action in patients with recurrent attacks of cramping periumbilical pain is abdominal surgical exploration. The frequency of this complication seems to have increased with the advent of laparoscopic GBP, presumably because of the difficulty of closing the potential hernia spaces completely. Some attribute the problem to the decreased tendency toward adhesion formation after laparoscopic surgery.

ACUTE GASTRIC DISTENTION

After GBP, massive gaseous distention occasionally develops in the distal bypassed stomach; this can lead to a gastric perforation or disruption of the gastrojejunostomy. The primary symptoms of this complication are hiccups and a bloated feeling. Massive gastric dilatation can lead to severe left shoulder pain and shock. The problem is usually secondary to edema at the Roux-en-Y anastomosis but can also be secondary to a mechanical problem. The diagnosis is made by means of an urgent upright abdominal radiograph, which reveals the markedly dilated and air-filled bypassed stomach. Occasionally, the stomach is filled with fluid, and the diagnosis may be more difficult. In those few cases in which the dilatation is primarily caused by air, the problem can be relieved by percutaneous transabdominal skinny-needle decompression with subsequent passage of gas and gastric and biliopancreatic juices through the Roux-en-Y anastomosis. Should the dilatation recur or the patient be in serious difficulty, an emergency laparotomy with insertion of a gastrostomy tube should be performed and the jejunojejunostomy evaluated. If a patient has extensive adhesions from previous abdominal surgery, a gastrostomy tube should be inserted at the time of GBP to prevent gastric dilatation.

Diabetes Mellitus

Type 2 (non–insulin-dependent) diabetes mellitus, a nonketotic form of diabetes that is usually noted after age 40, is markedly exacerbated by obesity. Patients with this type of diabetes often require large amounts of insulin for blood glucose control because of a significant reduction in insulin receptors. It is not unusual, however, to note a complete absence of the requirement for insulin in the immediate postoperative period in morbidly obese patients. Therefore, insulin should be withheld on the morning of operation. There is often a marked reduction in the requirement for insulin throughout the postoperative period and even at discharge in morbidly obese patients who have undergone GBP, probably because of increased release of gastric inhibitory peptide (GIP) from the proximal small bowel. Therefore, regular subcutaneous insulin should be administered to GBP patients according to a sliding scale after operation until insulin requirements can be determined. Before discharge, the patient should be taking an appropriate dose of neutral protamine Hagedorn (NPH) or Lente insulin but must perform frequent finger-stick blood glucose determinations afterward, given that the need for insulin will decrease progressively with weight loss.

In one study of 23 patients with diabetes mellitus who underwent gastric bariatric operation, the average requirement for insulin decreased from 74 units/day before operation to 8 units/day after operation.[10] Fourteen of the 23 patients were able to discontinue insulin completely, 11 by the time of discharge from the hospital 1 week after operation. These benefits were maintained during long-term follow-up to 39 months and were a result of a major decrease in insulin resistance that was associated with decreased food intake as well as weight loss.

Wound Care

Morbidly obese patients have been reported to have an increased risk of wound infection and dehiscence. However, the incidence of these complications in this group of patients can be very low. In a randomized, prospective trial comparing a running, continuous absorbable No. 2 polyglycolic acid suture with a No. 28 stainless-steel wire in morbidly obese patients who weighed an average of 320 lb, there was no significant difference in complications, including the incidence of incisional hernia, between the types of closure.[11] However, the running absorbable suture closure required significantly less time. Similar results comparing continuous with interrupted sutures have been noted by others.[12] Subcutaneous sutures should not be used, because the subcutaneous fat becomes reapproximated during skin closure, and subcutaneous sutures have been found to increase the risk of wound infection.[13] Obese patients undergoing clean-contaminated intestinal procedures should be given a parenteral antibiotic immediately before the operation and for only 24 hours after the operation[14]; it is important to note that morbidly obese patients should receive a double dose of prophylactic antibiotics because of the increased volume of distribution. If a gastric or gallbladder operation is planned, only aerobic bacterial coverage is necessary; a colon operation will necessitate anaerobic coverage as well.

It has been our experience that the incidence of incisional hernia is much higher in morbidly obese patients than in thin patients with ulcerative colitis who are taking large doses of corticosteroids and who undergo the same fascial wound closure with running No. 2 polyglycolic acid sutures.[15] This increased risk in morbidly

obese patients is probably secondary to the increased intra-abdominal pressures (IAP) present in patients with central, or android, obesity.[16]

Obese diabetic patients are at risk for rapidly spreading panniculitis secondary to mixed aerobic and anaerobic organisms.[17] Subcutaneous gas and extensive necrosis, which usually does not involve the underlying muscle, are often present. It is uncommon to culture clostridia from these wounds. Even after extensive and repeated debridement, mortality remains high [see 2:2 Soft Tissue Infection].

Other Obesity-Related Diseases

GALLSTONES

Approximately one third of morbidly obese patients either have had a cholecystectomy or may have had gallstones noted at the time of another intra-abdominal operative procedure, such as gastric operation for morbid obesity. Preoperative evaluation of the gallbladder may be technically quite difficult in morbidly obese patients because gallstones may be missed with either ultrasonography or oral cholecystography. Intraoperative sonography is probably much more accurate. Should stones be present in a patient undergoing gastric operation for obesity, the gallbladder should be removed. In the past, obese patients with intermittent attacks of biliary colic were told to lose weight before an elective cholecystectomy for fear of significant morbidity and mortality from an elective operation. This attitude is no longer valid, because among the large numbers of obese patients who now undergo major elective abdominal procedures, morbidity is similar to that seen in thin patients if appropriate precautions are taken. Furthermore, obese patients have great difficulty losing large amounts of weight by diet alone and should be allowed to undergo definitive corrective operative procedures before weight reduction.

Rapid weight loss may lead to the development of gallstones in 25% to 40% of patients who undergo GBP. The risk of cholelithiasis in this setting can be reduced to 2% by administering ursodeoxycholic acid, 300 mg orally twice daily.[18]

PSEUDOTUMOR CEREBRI

Pseudotumor cerebri is an unusual complication of morbid obesity that is associated with benign intracranial hypertension, papilledema, blurred vision, headache, and elevated cerebrospinal fluid pressures.[19] It has been our experience that patients with pseudotumor cerebri are not at any additional perioperative risk and that cerebrospinal fluid does not have to be removed before anesthesia and major abdominal operation. Weight reduction will cure pseudotumor cerebri.[20,21]

DEGENERATIVE OSTEOARTHRITIS

Degenerative osteoarthritis of the knees, hips, and back is a common complication of morbid obesity. Weight reduction alone may greatly reduce the pain and immobility that afflict these patients, although the damage may be so extensive that a total joint replacement may be desirable. However, joint replacement in patients who weigh more than 250 lb is associated with an unacceptable incidence of loosening.[22] Weight reduction by means of a gastric bariatric operation may be the most sensible initial approach, to be followed by joint replacement after weight loss if pain and dysfunction persist.

Discussion

Morbidity Associated with Central Fat Deposition

Much has been written about the increased health risks inherent in central, or android, fat deposition as compared with peripheral, or gynoid, fat deposition. It is thought that in the former, the increased metabolic activity of mesenteric fat is associated with increased metabolism of amino acids to sugar, which leads to hyperglycemia and hyperinsulinism. Hyperinsulinism gives rise to increased sodium absorption and hypertension. Furthermore, central obesity has been linked to hypercholesterolemia. Hence, these patients have a significantly higher incidence of diabetes, hypertension, hypercholesterolemia, and gallstones[23]—which explains the higher mortality of the apple distribution of body fat as compared with the pear distribution. In the past, fat distribution was measured on the basis of the waist-to-hip ratio; however, computed tomography scans have shown that abdominal circumference is a more accurate measurement of central fat distribution.[24] We have found that morbidly obese women have significantly increased IAP and that this is associated with stress and urge overflow urinary incontinence.[25] With weight loss comes a significant decrease in bladder pressure and correction of incontinence. We have found IAP, as reflected in bladder pressure, to be closely correlated with sagittal abdominal diameter and waist circumference but not with waist-to-hip ratio (many morbidly obese patients have both central and peripheral obesity). We have also found that the increased IAP associated with central obesity may cause additional comorbid factors, including venous stasis ulcers, OHS, gastroesophageal reflux, and inguinal and incisional hernias.

Respiratory Insufficiency of Obesity

Obese patients are at risk for respiratory difficulties, which may be present before operation or may be exacerbated by an operation. The term pickwickian syndrome (which derives from *The Posthumous Papers of the Pickwick Club*, by Charles Dickens) was resurrected from the late 1800s to describe a morbidly obese man 52 years of age who fell asleep in a poker game while holding a hand containing a full house.[2] He was taken to the hospital by friends who presumed he was ill. The pickwickian syndrome is now known to comprise two pulmonary syndromes associated with morbid obesity: obstructive SAS and OHS.[3]

Patients with SAS suffer from repeated attacks of upper airway obstruction during sleep. The cause is probably related to a large, fat tongue as well as to excessive fat deposition in the uvula, pharynx, and hypopharynx. The normal genioglossus reflex is depressed, but this depression may be secondary to the excessive weight of the tongue. These patients are notorious snorers. As a result of inadequate stage IV and rapid eye movement (REM) sleep, they are markedly somnolent during the day.

Patients with SAS are at great risk for acute upper airway obstruction and respiratory arrest after operation and general anesthesia. A high index of suspicion is necessary before operation. Patients with severe SAS often have ventricular arrhythmias and sinus arrest during their apneic episodes, thereby placing them at even greater risk. A history of heavy snoring, early morning headaches, frequent awakening at night with shortness of breath, severe daytime somnolence (including falling asleep at the wheel), and frequent headaches should prompt further study. The syndrome is confirmed by sleep polysomnography, which is available at sleep centers in most major cities.

In most instances, severe SAS can be treated with nocturnal nasal CPAP. With this technique, air flowing through a nasal mask against a constant airway resistance enters the nasal pharynx and pushes the tongue forward to prevent recurrent obstruction.[26] The pressure can be adjusted for each patient. Unfortunately, many patients cannot tolerate the device, because it is cumbersome and noisy and tends to dry out the upper airway, although dryness can be prevented with an inexpensive room humidifier. If nasal CPAP cannot be tolerated by the patient, or if it is ineffective and the problem is severe (i.e., causing cardiac arrhythmias or severe hypoxia), tracheostomy is indicated. This procedure can be very difficult and dangerous and therefore should not be relegated to the youngest house officer in a surgical residency program. Because of the extremely deep neck in obese patients, a standard tracheostomy tube is usually inadequate, and a special tube with a deep bend should be used.

OHS is a condition associated with morbid obesity in which an individual suffers from hypoxemia and hypercapnia when breathing room air while awake but resting.[27] Spirometry reveals decreases in forced vital capacity, residual lung volume, expiratory reserve volume, functional residual capacity, and maximum minute volume ventilation, usually without obstruction to airflow [*see Figure 1*]. The most profound decrease is that in expiratory reserve volume; it is probably secondary to increased intra-abdominal pressure and a high-riding diaphragm. Thus, these patients have a restrictive rather than an obstructive pulmonary disease. The decreased expiratory reserve volume implies that many alveolar units are collapsed at end-expiration, which leads to perfusion of unventilated alveoli, or shunting. Patients with OHS often are heavy smokers or have additional pulmonary problems, such as asthma, sarcoidosis, idiopathic pulmonary fibrosis, or recurrent pulmonary emboli. One study of patients who underwent operation for morbid obesity showed no statistically significant difference in weight between those who had OHS and those who did not.[3]

As a result of chronic and severe hypoxemia, patients with OHS are often markedly polycythemic. The polycythemia further increases their already significant risk for venous thrombosis and pulmonary embolism. Because we have had several patients who later had a subclavian venous thrombosis and one patient who probably had a transient sagittal sinus thrombosis, patients with OHS should probably undergo phlebotomy to a hemoglobin concentration of 15 g/dl before elective operation.

Chronic hypoxemia also leads to pulmonary arterial vasoconstriction and severe pulmonary hypertension[1,28] and eventually to

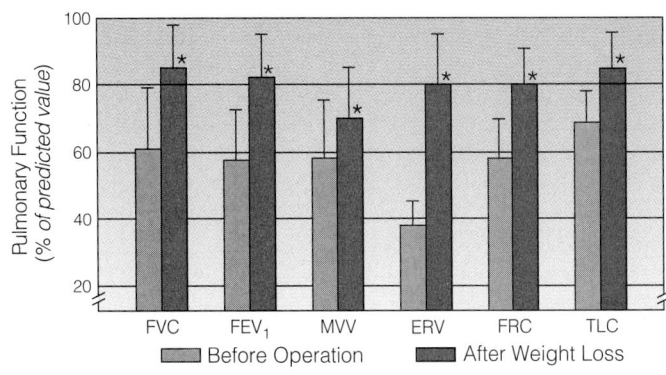

*P < 0.01 Compared with Preoperative Values

Figure 1 **Impaired pulmonary function in the morbidly obese improved significantly after weight loss induced by gastric operation.**[3]

right-sided heart failure or cor pulmonale with neck vein distention, tricuspid valvular insufficiency, right upper quadrant tenderness secondary to acute hepatic engorgement, and massive peripheral edema. Such patients may also have significantly elevated PAWP, which suggests left ventricular dysfunction.[1] Morbidly obese patients with a history of pulmonary disease or a BMI higher than 50 kg/m[2] should have preoperative determinations of blood gas values. If ABG measurement reveals severe hypoxemia (i.e., $P_aO_2 \leq 55$ mm Hg), severe hypercapnia ($P_aCO_2 \geq 47$ mm Hg), or both, the patient should undergo Swan-Ganz catheterization. If PAWP is 18 mm Hg or greater, intravenous furosemide should be administered for diuresis before elective operation. However, some patients may require a high ventricular filling pressure. A low cardiac output and hypotension may follow diuresis, necessitating volume reexpansion. If mean PAP is 40 mm Hg or greater, consideration should be given to the prophylactic insertion of a Greenfield inferior vena caval filter [see Thrombophlebitis, Venous Stasis Ulcers, and Pulmonary Embolism in the Morbidly Obese Patient, below].

It is highly probable that some of the elevated PAP and PAWP measurements are caused by the increased IAP in the morbidly obese [see Figure 2].[16,29] This leads to an elevated diaphragm, which in turn increases intrapleural pressure and thereby PAP and PAWP; if the pleural pressure is measured with an esophageal transducer, the transmyocardial pressure can be estimated. For this reason, these patients may require a markedly elevated PAWP to maintain an adequate cardiac output, and excessive diuresis may lead to hypotension. The same reasoning may be applied to a patient with a distended abdomen resulting from peritonitis and pancreatitis in whom what seem to be unusually high cardiac filling pressures are necessary. Therefore, one must rely on relative changes in cardiac output in response to either volume challenge or diuresis to determine the optimal PAWP in morbidly obese patients.

Patients with OHS respond rapidly to supplemental oxygen. However, oxygen administration is occasionally associated with significant CO_2 retention, which necessitates intubation and mechanical ventilation. Because their pulmonary disease is restrictive rather than obstructive, these patients are usually easy to ventilate without high peak airway pressures. Arterial blood gases need not return to normal before extubation; it is only necessary that they return to their preoperative values. These values are achieved, on average, 4 days after major upper abdominal operation, when the patients no longer have abdominal pain.[3]

It is important to emphasize that morbidly obese patients, especially those with respiratory insufficiency, should be placed in the reverse Trendelenburg's position to maximize diaphragmatic excursion and to increase residual lung volume.[8] These patients will often complain of air hunger and respiratory distress when they lie supine. So-called breaking of the bed at the waist may exacerbate the problem by pushing the abdominal contents into the chest, thereby raising the diaphragm and further reducing lung volumes. Placing these patients in the leg-down position may predispose them to venous stasis, phlebitis, and pulmonary embolism, which should be offset with intermittent venous compression boots [see Thrombophlebitis, Venous Stasis Ulcers, and Pulmonary Embolism in the Morbidly Obese Patient, below].[30]

Both SAS and OHS can be completely corrected with weight reduction after gastric operation for morbid obesity: the nocturnal apneas resolve, the P_aO_2 rises, and the P_aCO_2 falls to normal as lung volumes improve.[3]

Cardiac Dysfunction in the Morbidly Obese Patient

Cardiac dysfunction in the morbidly obese patient is usually as-

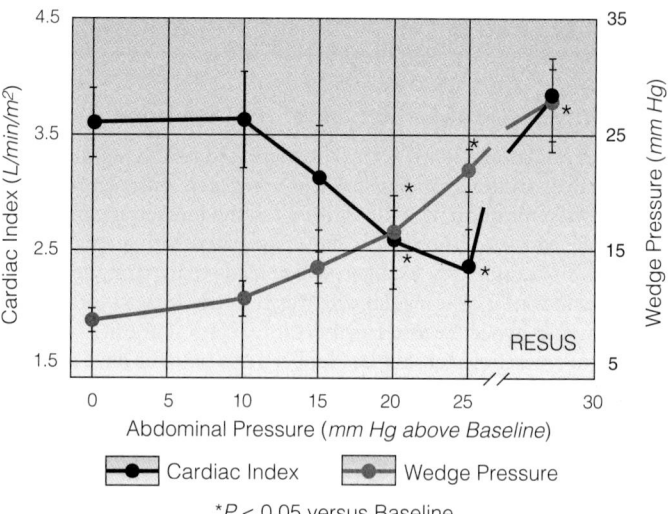

Figure 2 In a porcine model,[29] raising IAP caused cardiac index to fall and PAWP to rise. At an IAP of 25 mm Hg, saline was given to restore intravascular volume; cardiac index returned to baseline levels, but PAWP remained elevated. (IAP—intra-abdominal pressure; PAWP—pulmonary arterial wedge pressure)

sociated with respiratory insufficiency of obesity, especially OHS.[2] Elevated PAP in these patients may be secondary to hypoxemia-induced pulmonary arterial vasoconstriction, to elevated left atrial pressures secondary to left ventricular dysfunction, or to a combination of these; they may also be secondary to the increased pleural pressures arising from an elevated diaphragm secondary to increased IAP.[1,29,30] It is unusual for morbidly obese patients without respiratory insufficiency to experience significant cardiac dysfunction in the absence of severe coronary artery disease. Morbidly obese patients often have systemic hypertension, which can aggravate left ventricular dysfunction; however, mild left ventricular dysfunction can be documented in many morbidly obese patients in the absence of systemic hypertension.[31,32] Circulating blood volume, plasma volume, and cardiac output increase in proportion to body weight.[32] Massively obese patients may occasionally present with acute heart failure: it is reasonable to assume that the enormous metabolic requirements of such patients can present a greater

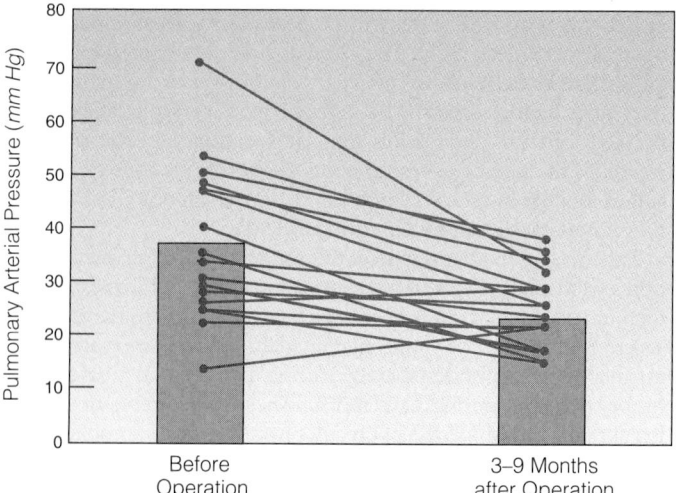

Figure 3 Mean pulmonary arterial pressure was significantly improved in 18 patients 3 to 9 months after gastric surgery–induced weight loss of 42% ± 19% of excess weight.[1]

demand for blood flow than the heart can provide. Vigorous diuresis will often correct such acute heart failure. Significant weight loss will correct pulmonary hypertension [*see Figure 3*] as well as left ventricular dysfunction associated with respiratory insufficiency.[1,33]

Thrombophlebitis, Venous Stasis Ulcers, and Pulmonary Embolism in the Morbidly Obese Patient

Morbidly obese individuals have difficulty walking; tend to be sedentary; have a large amount of abdominal weight resting on their inferior vena cava; and have increased intrapleural pressure, which impedes venous return.[28,29] All of these conditions increase the tendency toward phlebothrombosis. Patients are most at risk when immobilized in the supine position for long periods in the OR. These patients have also been shown to have low levels of antithrombin, which may increase their tendency toward venous thrombosis.[34] It has also been suggested that starvation, particularly in the postoperative period, may be associated with high levels of free fatty acids,[35] which may predispose to perioperative thrombotic complications.[35]

Intermittent venous compression boots have been shown in randomized trials to reduce the incidence of deep vein thrombosis.[30] Administration of low-dose subcutaneous heparin must be started immediately before operation. However, because morbidly obese patients show a significant improvement in pulmonary function when placed in the reverse Trendelenburg position,[8] and because this position further increases venous pressure in the legs and the tendency toward stasis, it is preferable to use this position and intermittent venous compression boots. All patients, but especially the morbidly obese, should make every attempt to walk during the evening after operation.

Because pulmonary embolism is quite unusual when the appropriate precautions have been taken, acute air hunger, tachypnea, and hypoxemia should suggest the equal likelihood that sepsis-induced ARDS is present secondary to an intra-abdominal anastomotic leak.

Patients with severe OHS often have noticeably elevated PAP, which can lead to right-sided heart failure and can increase the risk of venous stasis and thrombosis. Investigators have noted that patients with primary idiopathic pulmonary hypertension are at significant risk for fatal PE.[5] For this reason, it has been our policy to place a prophylactic Greenfield vena caval filter in patients with respiratory insufficiency of obesity and a mean PAP of 40 mm Hg or greater. With this approach (in which a vena caval filter was used in 15 patients), we have had one fatal pulmonary embolus in 156 patients with respiratory insufficiency of obesity who have undergone gastric bariatric procedures. The fatality was a patient whose mean PAP was initially 40 mm Hg but fell to 35 mm Hg with diuresis and who was not considered to require a filter.

Venous stasis ulcers can be quite difficult to treat in a thin individual; they are almost impossible to cure in a patient with morbid obesity [*see Figure 4*]. The most important goal in management of these ulcers is weight loss, which almost invariably leads to healing of the ulcer, probably as a result of decreased IAP.[7] Patients with venous stasis ulcers also are at high risk for fatal PE and should be considered for prophylactic placement of a vena caval filter.

Pseudotumor Cerebri in the Morbidly Obese Patient

Pseudotumor cerebri (also known as idiopathic intracranial hypertension) associated with obesity is almost certainly secondary to increased IAP. The rise in IAP causes a rise in intrathoracic pressure, which in turn raises central venous pressure and PAWP [*see Figure 2*], thus decreasing venous drainage from the brain.[29] This se-

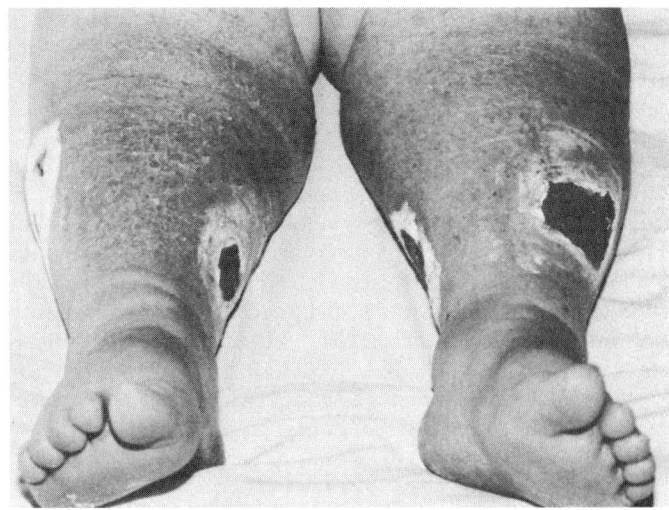

Figure 4 This chronic venous stasis ulcer was present for several years in a morbidly obese patient. Healing promptly followed weight loss induced by a gastric operation.

quence of events has been reproduced in a porcine model.[36] The elevated intracranial pressure (ICP) can be prevented by means of median sternotomy and pleuropericardiotomy [*see Figure 5*].[37] In humans studied 3 years after weight-reduction surgery, surgically induced weight loss was associated with a significant decrease in ICP (from 353 ± 35 mm H_2O to 168 ± 12 mm H_2O; $P < 0.001$) and with relief of headache and pulsatile tinnitus.[20,21]

Conclusion

Although the morbidly obese patient is potentially at risk for significant perioperative morbidity and mortality, attention to detail in preoperative preparation as well as in postoperative management

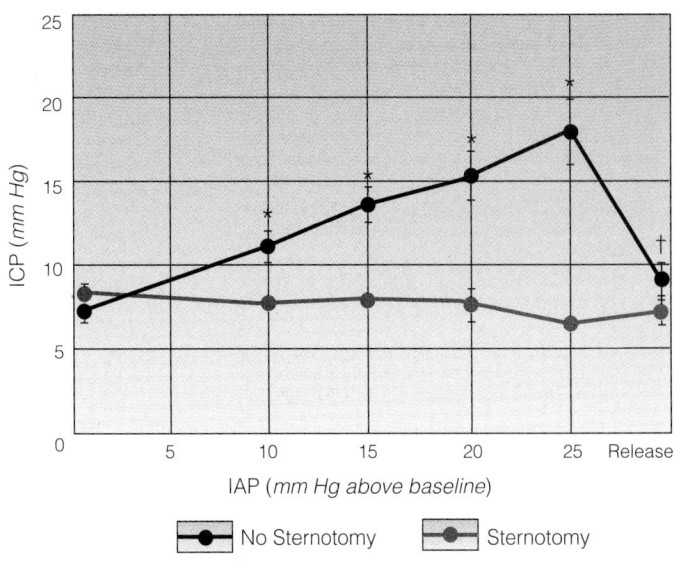

Figure 5 In a porcine model,[37] IAP was increased to 25 mm Hg in 12 animals, of which three underwent median sternotomy and pleuropericardiotomy (red line) and nine did not (black line). Sternotomy and pleuropericardiotomy prevented the expected increase in ICP. (ICP—intracranial pressure)

should reduce this risk almost to that of the general population. A high index of suspicion for peritonitis must be maintained after an intra-abdominal procedure or when the patient complains of abdominal pain in the emergency room. Awareness of the problems associated with respiratory insufficiency in obese patients should enable the surgeon to avoid pitfalls when managing the patient with obstructive SAS or OHS. These patients may require preoperative pulmonary arterial catheterization for optimal fluid management before and after operation. The risks of venous thrombosis and PE are high, but the use of intermittent compression boots and early ambulation can minimize the dangers. The obese patient with non–insulin-dependent diabetes has been surprisingly easy to manage after major operation.

Weight reduction by diet is associated with a 95% incidence of recidivism. The average morbidly obese patient can be expected to lose two thirds of the excess weight within 1 year after a standard GBP or, if superobese, after a long-limb gastric bypass. Furthermore, recent reports note that this weight loss is long-lasting and averages 60% of excess weight at 5 years and more than 50% of excess weight up to 10 years after operation. This weight loss is associated with the correction of insulin-dependent diabetes, obstructive SAS, OHS, pseudotumor cerebri, hypertension, chronic venous stasis ulcers, stress incontinence, gastroesophageal reflux, and female sex hormone abnormalities, which may be related to dysmenorrhea, infertility, hirsutism, and an increased risk of endometrial carcinoma. Weight loss can markedly improve the patient's self-image and employability. Because techniques for operation for morbid obesity continue to change as understanding of pathophysiology improves, it is important for surgeons to keep abreast of the latest developments.

References

1. Sugerman HJ, Baron PL, Fairman RP, et al: Hemodynamic dysfunction in obesity hypoventilation syndrome and the effects of treatment with surgically induced weight loss. Ann Surg 207:604, 1988

2. Burwell CS, Robin ED, Whaley RD, et al: Extreme obesity associated with alveolar hypoventilation—a pickwickian syndrome. Am J Med 21:811, 1956

3. Sugerman HJ, Fairman RP, Baron PL, et al: Gastric surgery for respiratory insufficiency of obesity. Chest 89:81, 1986

4. Sugerman HJ, Fairman RP, Sood RK, et al: Long-term effects of gastric surgery for treating respiratory insufficiency of obesity. Am J Clin Nutr 55(2 suppl): 597S, 1992

5. Young T, Palta M, Dempsey J, et al: The occurrence of sleep-disordered breathing among middle-aged adults. N Engl J Med 328:1230, 1993

6. Greenfield LJ, Scher LA, Elkins RC: KMA-Greenfield® filter placement for chronic pulmonary hypertension. Ann Surg 189:560, 1979

7. Sugerman HJ, Sugerman EL, Wolfe L, et al: Risks/benefits of gastric bypass in morbidly obese patients with severe venous stasis disease. Ann Surg 234:41, 2001

8. Vaughan RW, Bauer S, Wise L: Effect of position (semirecumbent versus supine) on postoperative oxygenation in markedly obese subjects. Anesth Analg 55:37, 1976

9. Mason EE, Printen KJ, Barron P, et al: Risk reduction in gastric operations for obesity. Ann Surg 190:158, 1979

10. Herbst CA, Hughes TA, Gwynne JT, et al: Gastric bariatric operation in insulin-treated adults. Surgery 95:209, 1984

11. McNeill PM, Sugerman HJ: Continuous absorbable vs interrupted nonabsorbable fascial closure: a prospective, randomized comparison. Arch Surg 121:821, 1986

12. Richards PC, Balch CM, Aldrete JS: Abdominal wound closure: a randomized prospective study of 571 patients comparing continuous vs. interrupted suture techniques. Ann Surg 197:238, 1983

13. De Holl D, Rodeheaver G, Edgerton MT, et al: Potentiation of infection by suture closure of dead space. Am J Surg 127:716, 1974

14. Stone HH, Hooper CA, Kolb LD, et al: Antibiotic prophylaxis in gastric, biliary, and colonic surgery. Ann Surg 184:443, 1976

15. Sugerman HJ, Kellum JM, Reines HD, et al: Incisional hernia: greater risk with morbidly obese than steroid dependent patients; low recurrence rate with prefascial polypropylene mesh repair. Am J Surg 171:80, 1996

16. Sugerman H, Windsor A, Bessos M, et al: Intra-abdominal pressure, sagittal abdominal diameter, and obesity co-morbidity. J Intern Med 241:71, 1997

17. Rouse TM, Malangoni MA, Schulte WJ: Necrotizing fasciitis: a preventable disaster. Surgery 92:765, 1982

18. Sugerman HJ, Brewer WH, Shiffman ML, et al: A multicenter, placebo-controlled, randomized, double-blind, prospective trial of prophylactic ursodiol for the prevention of gallstone formation following gastric-bypass-induced rapid weight loss. Am J Surg 169:91, 1995

19. Corbett JJ, Mehta MP: Cerebrospinal fluid pressure in normal obese subjects and patients with pseudotumor cerebri. Neurology 33:1386, 1983

20. Sugerman HJ, Felton WL, Salvant JB, et al: Effects of surgically induced weight loss on pseudotumor cerebri in morbid obesity. Neurology 45:1655, 1995

21. Sugerman HJ, Felton WL III, Sismanis A, et al: Gastric surgery for pseudotumor cerebri associated with severe obesity. Ann Surg 229:634, 1999

22. Goldin RH, McAdam L, Louie JS, et al: Clinical and radiologic survey of the incidence of osteoarthritis among obese patients. Ann Rheum Dis 35:349, 1976

23. Kissebah AH, Vydelingum N, Murray R, et al: Relation of body fat distribution to metabolic complications of obesity. J Clin Endocrinol Metab 54:254, 1982

24. Kvist H, Chowdhury B, Grangard U, et al: Total and visceral adipose-tissue volumes derived from measurements with computed tomography in adult men and women: predictive equations. Am J Clin Nutr 48:1351, 1988

25. Bump RC, Sugerman HJ, Fantl JA, et al: Obesity and lower urinary tract function in women: effect of surgically induced weight loss. Am J Obstet Gynecol 167:392, 1992

26. Sullivan CE, Issa FG, Berthon-Jones M, et al: Reversal of obstructive sleep apnoea by continuous positive airway pressure applied through the nares. Lancet 1:862, 1981

27. Rochester DR, Enson Y: Current concepts in the pathogenesis of the obesity hypoventilation syndrome: mechanical and circulatory factors. Am J Med 57:402, 1974

28. Alexander JK, Amad KH, Cole VW: Observations on some clinical features of extreme obesity, with particular reference to cardiorespiratory effects. Am J Med 32:512, 1962

29. Ridings PC, Bloomfield GL, Blocher CR, et al: Cardiopulmonary effects of raised intra-abdominal pressure before and after volume expansion. J Trauma 39:1168, 1995

30. Coe NP, Collins RE, Klein LA, et al: Prevention of deep vein thrombosis in urological patients: a controlled, randomized trial of low-dose heparin and external pneumatic compression boots. Surgery 83:230, 1978

31. Kaltman AJ, Goldring RM: Role of circulatory congestion in the cardiorespiratory failure of obesity. Am J Med 60:645, 1976

32. De Divitiis O, Fazio S, Petitto M, et al: Obesity and cardiac function. Circulation 64:477, 1981

33. Alpert MA, Terry BE, Kelly DL: Effect of weight loss on cardiac chamber size, wall thickness and left ventricular function in morbid obesity. Am J Cardiol 55:783, 1985

34. Batist G, Bothe A, Bern M, et al: Low antithrombin III in morbid obesity: return to normal with weight reduction. JPEN 7:447, 1983

35. Printen HJ, Miller EV, Mason EE, et al: Venous thromboembolism in the morbidly obese. Surg Gynecol Obstet 147:63, 1978

36. Bloomfield GL, Ridings PC, Blocher CR, et al: Effects of increased intra-abdominal pressure upon intracranial and cerebral perfusion before and after volume expansion. J Trauma 40:936, 1996

37. Bloomfield GL, Ridings PC, Blocher CR, et al: A proposed relationship between increased intra-abdominal, intrathoracic, and intracranial pressure. Crit Care Med 25:496, 1997

Acknowledgments

Figures 1 and 3   Albert Miller.
Figures 2 and 5   Marcia Kammerer.

4 JAUNDICE

Jeffrey S. Barkun, M.D., F.A.C.S., and Alan N. Barkun, M.D.

Approach to the Jaundiced Patient

The term jaundice refers to the yellowish discoloration of skin, sclerae, and mucous membranes that results from excessive deposition of bilirubin in tissues. It usually is unmistakable but on occasion may manifest itself subtly. It is generally held that jaundice develops when serum bilirubin levels rise above 34.2 μmol/L (2 mg/dl)[1]; however, the appearance of jaundice also depends on whether it is conjugated or unconjugated bilirubin that is elevated and on how long the episode of jaundice lasts.

In what follows, we outline a problem-based approach to the jaundiced patient that involves assessing the incremental information provided by successive clinical and laboratory investigations as well as the information obtained by means of modern imaging modalities. We also propose a classification of jaundice that stresses the therapeutic options most pertinent to surgeons. We have not attempted a detailed review of bilirubin metabolism and the various pediatric disorders that cause jaundice; such issues are beyond the scope of this chapter. Finally, we emphasize that modern decision making in the approach to the jaundiced patient includes not only careful evaluation of anatomic issues but also close attention to patient morbidity and quality-of-life concerns, as well as a focus on working up the patient in a cost-effective fashion. For optimal treatment, in our view, an integrated approach that involves the surgeon, the gastroenterologist, and the radiologist is essential.

Clinical Assessment

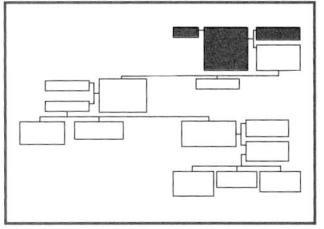

When a patient presents with a skin discoloration suggestive of jaundice, the first step is to confirm that icterus is indeed present. To this end, the mucous membranes of the mouth, the palms, the soles, and the sclerae should be examined in natural light. Because such areas are protected from the sun, photodegradation of bile is minimized; thus, the yellowish discoloration of elastic tissues may be more easily detected. Occasionally, deposition of a yellowish pigment on skin may mimic jaundice but may in fact be related to the consumption of large quantities of food containing lycopene or carotene or drugs such as rifampin or quinacrine. In these cases, the skin is usually the only site of coloration, and careful inspection of sclerae and mucous membranes generally reveals no icteric pigmentation. In certain cultures, long-term application of tea bags to the eyes may lead to a brownish discoloration of the sclerae that can mimic jaundice.[2]

DIRECT VERSUS INDIRECT HYPERBILIRUBINEMIA

Once the presence of jaundice has been confirmed, further clinical assessment determines whether the hyperbilirubinemia is predominantly direct or indirect. This distinction is based on the division of bilirubin into conjugated and unconjugated fractions, which are also known, respectively, as direct and indirect fractions on the basis of their behavior in the van den Bergh (diazo) reaction.[3] If the patient has normal-colored urine and stools, unconjugated bilirubin [*see Sidebar* Unconjugated (Indirect) Bilirubin] is predominant [*see Table 1*]. If the patient has dark urine, pale stools, or any other signs or symptoms of a cholestatic syndrome (see below), the serum bilirubin fractionation usually indicates that conjugated bilirubin is

---

Unconjugated (Indirect) Bilirubin

The breakdown of heme leads to the production of unconjugated bilirubin, which is water insoluble, is tightly bound to albumin, and does not pass into the urine. Excessive production of unconjugated bilirubin typically follows an episode of hemolysis. In the absence of concomitant liver disease or biliary obstruction, the liver can usually handle the extra bilirubin, and only a modest rise in serum levels is observed. There is a substantial increase in bile pigment excretion, leading to large quantities of stercobilinogen in the stool. A patient with hemolysis may therefore be slightly jaundiced with normal-colored urine and stools. Blood tests reveal that 60% to 85% of bilirubin is indirect.[105]

Possible causes of indirect hyperbilirubinemia include a variety of disorders that result in significant hemolysis or ineffective erythropoiesis. The diagnosis of indirect hyperbilirubinemia attributable to hemolysis is confirmed by an elevated serum lactate dehydrogenase (LDH) level, a decreased serum haptoglobin level, and evidence of hemolysis on microscopic examination of the blood smear.

Disorders associated with defects in hepatic bilirubin uptake or conjugation can also produce unconjugated hyperbilirubinemia. The most common of these, Gilbert syndrome, is a benign condition affecting up to 7% of the general population.[106,107] It is not a single disease but a heterogeneous group of disorders, all of which are characterized by a homozygosity for a defect in the promoter controlling the transcription of the UDP glucuronyl transferase I gene.[108] The consequent impairment of bilirubin glucuronidation presents as a mild unconjugated hyperbilirubinemia. The elevated bilirubin level is usually detected on routine blood testing, and affected patients may report that their skin turns yellow when they are fatigued or at stressful times (e.g., after missing meals, after vomiting, or in the presence of an infection). Other causes of an unconjugated hyperbilirubinemia are beyond the scope of this chapter.

Approach to the Jaundiced Patient

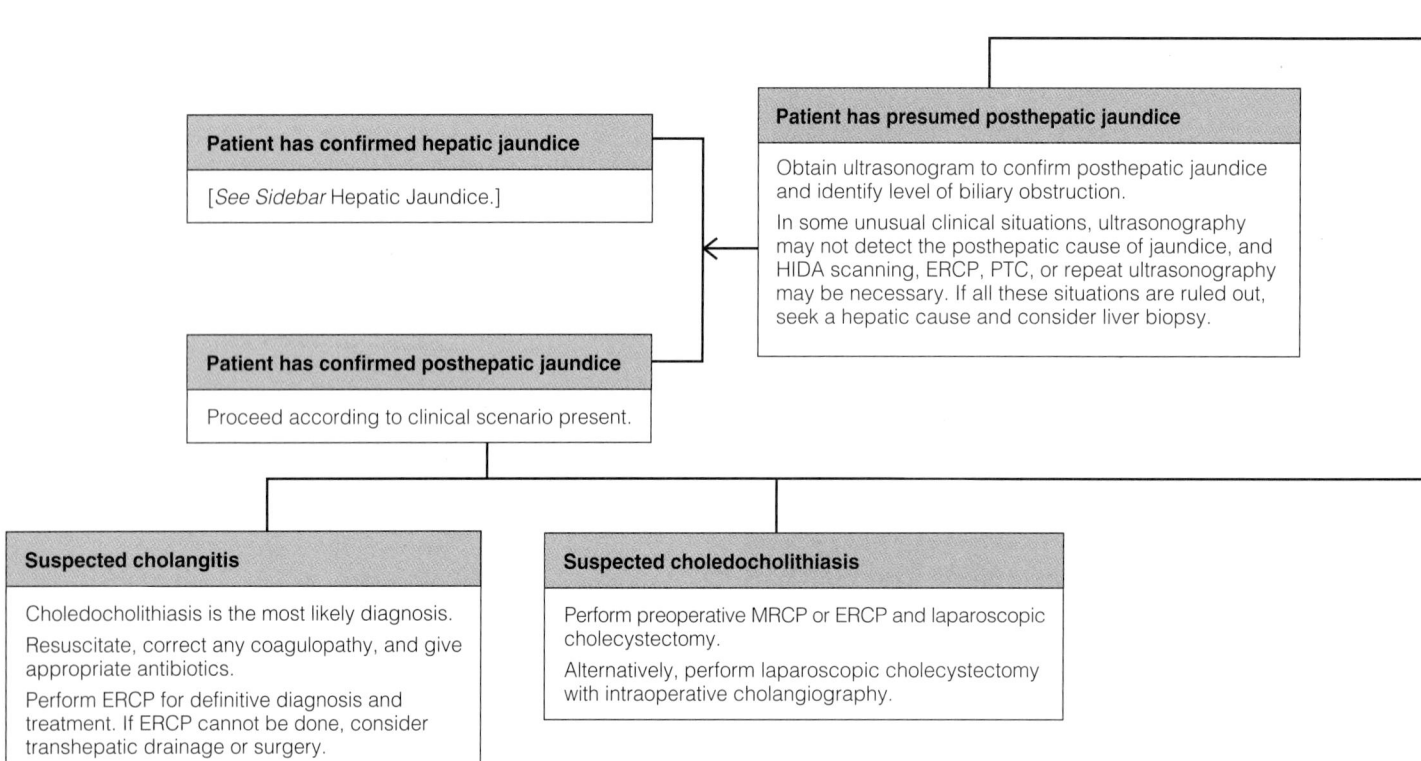

Patient has confirmed hepatic jaundice

[*See Sidebar* Hepatic Jaundice.]

Patient has presumed posthepatic jaundice

Obtain ultrasonogram to confirm posthepatic jaundice and identify level of biliary obstruction.

In some unusual clinical situations, ultrasonography may not detect the posthepatic cause of jaundice, and HIDA scanning, ERCP, PTC, or repeat ultrasonography may be necessary. If all these situations are ruled out, seek a hepatic cause and consider liver biopsy.

Patient has confirmed posthepatic jaundice

Proceed according to clinical scenario present.

Suspected cholangitis

Choledocholithiasis is the most likely diagnosis.

Resuscitate, correct any coagulopathy, and give appropriate antibiotics.

Perform ERCP for definitive diagnosis and treatment. If ERCP cannot be done, consider transhepatic drainage or surgery.

Suspected choledocholithiasis

Perform preoperative MRCP or ERCP and laparoscopic cholecystectomy.

Alternatively, perform laparoscopic cholecystectomy with intraoperative cholangiography.

Patient presents with skin discoloration suggestive of jaundice

Perform clinical assessment

Perform physical exam and obtain history.

Confirm icterus by examining oral mucous membranes, palms, soles, and sclerae in natural light.

Distinguish indirect (unconjugated) from direct (conjugated) hyperbilirubinemia:

- Normal-colored urine and stools suggest indirect hyperbilirubinemia
- Dark urine, pale stools, and signs or symptoms of a cholestatic syndrome suggest direct hyperbilirubinemia

Measure total serum bilirubin and percentage of conjugated bilirubin.

Patient has indirect hyperbilirubinemia

[*See Sidebar* Unconjugated (Indirect) Bilirubin.]

Patient has direct hyperbilirubinemia

Distinguish hepatic ("medical") jaundice from posthepatic ("surgical") jaundice.

- Acute hepatitis, alcohol abuse, and physical evidence of cirrhosis or portal hypertension suggest hepatic jaundice
- Abdominal pain, rigors, itching, and a palpable liver > 2 cm below costal margin suggest posthepatic jaundice

Patient has presumed hepatic jaundice

[*See Sidebar* Hepatic Jaundice.]

Suspected lesion other than choledocholithiasis

The most common single cause is pancreatic cancer; many of the other possible causes also involve malignancy.

Perform spiral CT or MRI with MRCP to diagnose lesion and assess resectability.

Consider EUS for distal-third obstruction.

Perform Doppler ultrasonography to stage lesion further; CT angiography or MRA may be considered if ultrasonogram is abnormal.

Perform MRCP to assess intrahepatic biliary system in patients with middle-third or upper-third obstruction.

Lesion appears unresectable, and surgical palliation is not indicated

Treat with ERCP or PTC and drainage. For advanced malignant disease, supportive care alone may be indicated.

Lesion appears resectable, or surgical palliation is indicated

Treat with surgical bypass or resection as appropriate for level of obstruction.

Perform laparoscopy to confirm resectability before laparotomy.

Upper-third obstruction

Palliation: bypass with left (segment III) hepaticojejunostomy.

Resection for cure: resection of tumor, possibly with hepatectomy or segmentectomy, and reconstruction with hepaticojejunostomy or cholangiojejunostomy.

Middle-third obstruction

Palliation: bypass with hepaticojejunostomy.

Resection for cure: resection of tumor and reconstruction with hepaticojejunostomy.

Lower-third obstruction

Palliation: bypass with Roux-en-Y choledochojejunostomy.

Resection for cure: resection of tumor with pancreaticoduodenectomy or local ampullary excision.

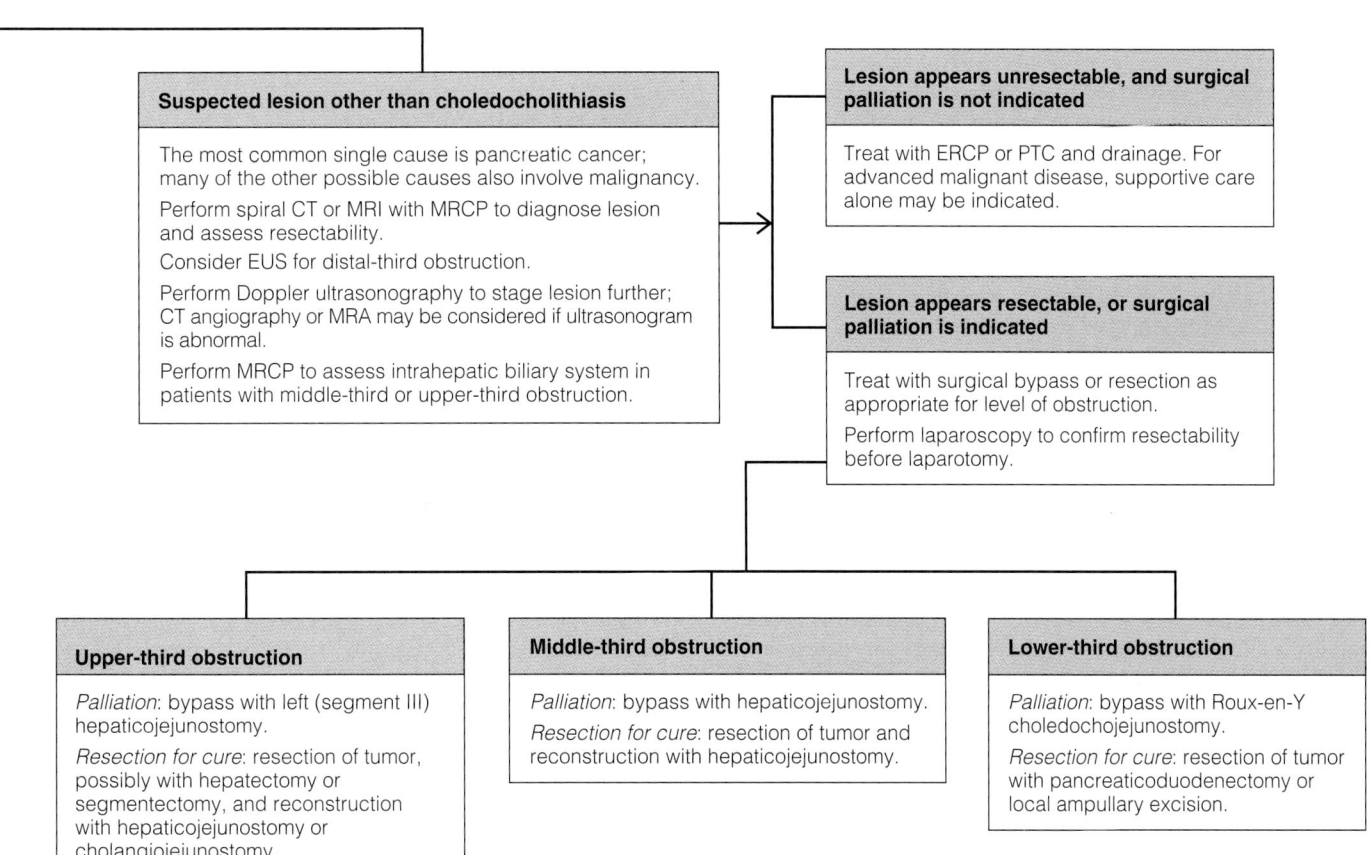

Table 1   Causes of Unconjugated Hyperbilirubinemia

Increased RBC breakdown
  Acute hemolysis
  Chronic hemolytic disorders
  Large hematoma resorption, multiple blood transfusions
  Gilbert syndrome

Decreased hepatic bilirubin conjugation
  Gilbert syndrome
  Crigler-Najjar syndrome types I and II
  Familial unconjugated hyperbilirubinemia

predominant. Rarely, the clinical picture may be secondary to a massive increase in both direct and indirect bilirubin production after the latter has overcome the ability of the hepatocytes to secrete conjugated bilirubin.

It is nearly always possible to distinguish between direct and indirect hyperbilirubinemia on clinical grounds alone.[4] Our emphasis here is on direct hyperbilirubinemia, which is the type that is more relevant to general surgeons.

Cholestatic Syndrome

The term cholestasis refers to decreased delivery of bilirubin into the intestine (and subsequent accumulation in the hepatocytes and in blood), irrespective of the underlying cause. When cholestasis is mild, it may not be associated with clinical jaundice. As it worsens, a conjugated hyperbilirubinemia develops that presents as jaundice. The conjugated hyperbilirubinemia may derive either from a defect in hepatocellular function (hepatic jaundice, also referred to as nonobstructive or medical jaundice) or from a blockage somewhere in the biliary tree (posthepatic jaundice, also referred to as obstructive or surgical jaundice). In this chapter, we refer to hepatic and posthepatic causes of jaundice, reserving the term cholestasis for the specific clinical syndrome that is attributable to a chronic lack of delivery of bile into the intestine. This syndrome is characterized by signs and symptoms that are related either to the conjugated hyperbilirubinemia or to chronic malabsorption of fat-soluble vitamins (i.e., vitamins A, D, E, and K): jaundice, dark urine, pale stools, pruritus, bruising, steatorrhea, night blindness, osteomalacia, and neuromuscular weakness.[5]

HEPATIC VERSUS POSTHEPATIC JAUNDICE

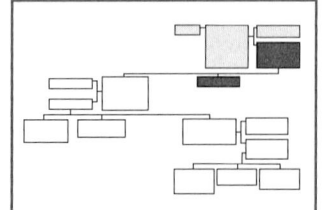

Once the presence of direct hyperbilirubinemia is confirmed, the next step is to determine whether the jaundice is hepatic or posthepatic. A number of authors have studied the reliability of clinical assessment for making this determination.[6-17] The sensitivities of history, physical examination, and blood tests alone range from 70% to 95%,[6-11] whereas the specificities are approximately 75%.[10,11] The overall accuracy of clinical assessment of hepatic and posthepatic causes of jaundice ranges from 87% to 97%.[8,12] Clinically, hepatic jaundice is most often signaled by acute hepatitis, a history of alco-

hol abuse, or physical findings reflecting cirrhosis or portal hypertension[13]; posthepatic jaundice is most often signaled by abdominal pain, rigors, itching, or a palpable liver more than 2 cm below the costal margin.[14]

By using discriminant analysis in a pediatric patient population, two investigators[15] were able to isolate three biochemical tests that differentiated between biliary atresia and intrahepatic cholestasis with an accuracy of 95%: total serum bilirubin concentration, alkaline phosphatase level, and γ-glutamyltranspeptidase level. Serum transaminase levels added no independent information of significance to the model. Another multivariate analysis model[16] demonstrated that patients with posthepatic jaundice were younger, had a longer history of jaundice, were more likely to present with fever, and had greater elevations of serum protein concentrations and shorter coagulation times than patients with hepatic jaundice. This model, however, despite its 96% sensitivity (greater than that of any single radiologic diagnostic modality), could not accurately predict the level of a biliary obstruction. Other investigators[8,12,13] have reported similar findings, and most agree that strategies that omit ultrasonography are clearly inferior.[17]

In summary, a clinical approach supported by simple biochemical evaluation displays good predictive ability to distinguish hepatic from posthepatic jaundice; however, a clinical approach alone does not accurately identify the level of biliary obstruction in a patient with posthepatic jaundice.

The remainder of this chapter focuses primarily on management of posthepatic jaundice; hepatic jaundice is less often seen and dealt with by general surgeons [*see Table 2 and Sidebar Hepatic Jaundice*].

Imaging

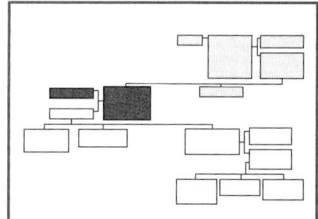

Once the history has been obtained and bedside and laboratory assessments have been completed, the next step is imaging, the goals of which are (1) to confirm the presence of an extrahepatic obstruction (i.e., to verify that the jaundice is indeed posthepatic rather than hepatic), (2) to determine the level of the obstruction, (3) to identify the specific cause of the obstruction, and (4) to provide complementary information relating to the underlying diagnosis (e.g., staging information in cases of malignancy).

Of the many imaging methods available today, the gold standard for defining the level of a biliary obstruction before operation in a jaundiced patient remains direct cholangiography, which can be performed either via endoscopic retrograde cholangiopancreatography (ERCP) [*see 3:8 Gastrointestinal Endoscopy*] or via percutaneous transhepatic cholangiography (PTC). Unlike other imaging modalities, direct cholangiography poses significant risks to the patient: there is a 4% to 7% incidence of pancreatitis or cholangitis after ERCP[18,19] and a 4% incidence of bile leakage, cholangitis, or bleeding after PTC.[20] There are also several risks that are particular to the manipulation of an obstructed biliary system (see below). For these reasons and because both modalities have therapeutic capability, it is important to gather as much imaging information as possible on the likely cause of the jaundice before performing ERCP or PTC. We have found the following approach to be an efficacious, cost-effective,[21] and safe way of obtaining such

---

Table 2 Causes of Hepatic Jaundice[113]

Hepatitis
  Viral
  Autoimmune
  Alcoholic
Drugs and hormones
Diseases of intrahepatic bile ducts
Liver infiltration and storage disorders
Systemic infections
Total parenteral nutrition
Postoperative intrahepatic cholestasis
Cholestasis of pregnancy
Benign recurrent intrahepatic cholestasis
Infantile cholestatic syndromes
Inherited metabolic defects
No identifiable cause (idiopathic hepatic jaundice)

---

information in a patient with presumed posthepatic jaundice.

The presence of ductal dilatation of the intrahepatic or extrahepatic biliary system confirms that a posthepatic cause is responsible for the jaundice. Ultrasonography detects ductal dilatation with an accuracy of 95%, although results are to some extent operator-dependent.[22] If ultrasonography does not reveal bile duct dilatation, it is unlikely that an obstructing lesion is present. In some cases, although ductal dilatation is absent,

other ultrasonographic findings may still point to a specific hepatic cause of jaundice (e.g., multiple liver metastases, cirrhosis, or infiltration of the liver by tumor).

There are a few specific instances in which ultrasonography may fail to detect a posthepatic cause of jaundice. For instance, very early in the course of an obstructive process, not enough time may have elapsed for biliary dilatation to occur. In this setting, a hepato-iminodiacetic acid (HIDA) scan may help identify bile duct blockage.[23] The yield from this test is highest when the serum bilirubin level is lower than 100 μmol/L, and it diminishes as the serum bilirubin level rises.[1] Occasionally, the intrahepatic biliary tree is unable to dilate; possible causes of such inability include extensive hepatic fibrosis, cirrhosis, sclerosing cholangitis, and recent liver transplantation. If one of these diagnoses is suspected, either ERCP or PTC will eventually be required to confirm the diagnosis of biliary obstruction. Occasionally, the biliary tree dilatation may be intermittent; possible causes of this condition include choledocholithiasis and some biliary tumors. In a patient with gallstones, transient liver test abnormalities by themselves may suggest an intermediate to high likelihood of common bile duct (CBD) stones, even if there is no biliary ductal dilatation.[24,25] If one of these diagnoses is suspected, ultrasonography may be repeated after a short period of observation (when clinically applicable); biliary ductal dilatation then generally becomes apparent. If all of these unusual clinical situations have been ruled out, a hepatic cause for the jaundice should be sought [see Table 2] and a liver biopsy considered.[26,27]

Besides being able to identify the presence of extrahepatic ductal obstruction with a high degree of reliability, ultrasonography can accurately determine the level of the obstruction in 90% of cases.[28] For example, a dilated gallbladder suggests

Hepatic Jaundice

Hepatic jaundice may be either acute or chronic and may be caused by a variety of conditions [see Table 2].

Acute hepatic jaundice may arise de novo or in the setting of ongoing liver disease. Historical clues may suggest a particular cause, such as medications or viral hepatitis. Physical examination usually reveals little; however, an enlarged liver is sometimes palpated. In the presence of preexisting chronic liver disease, bedside stigmata (e.g., ascites, spider nevi, caput medusae, palmar erythema, gynecomastia, or Dupuytren contracture) may be present. Although specific therapies exist for certain clinical problems (e.g., acetylcysteine for acetaminophen ingestion and penicillin plus silibinin for *Amanita phalloides* poisoning), treatment in most cases remains supportive. Patients in whom encephalopathy develops within 2 to 8 weeks of the onset of jaundice are usually classified as having fulminant hepatic failure [see 6:10 Hepatic Failure]: Evidence of encephalopathy, renal failure, or a severe coagulopathy is predictive of poor outcome in this setting.[109] The most common causes of fulminant hepatic failure are viral hepatitis and drug toxicity. The mortality from fulminant hepatic failure remains high even though liver transplantation has favorably affected the prognosis.[110]

In cases of chronic hepatic jaundice, the patient may have chronic hepatitis or cholestasis, with or without cirrhosis. The cause usually is determined on the basis of the history in conjunction with the results of serology, biochemistry, and, occasionally, histology. Causes include viral infection, drug-induced chronic hepatitis, autoimmune liver disease, genetic disorders (e.g., Wilson disease and α₁-antitrypsin deficiency), chronic cholestatic disorders, alcoholic liver disease, and steatohepatitis.[111] Physical examination reveals the stigmata of chronic liver disease and occasionally suggests a specific cause (e.g., Kayser-Fleischer rings on slit-lamp examination in Wilson disease).

Treatment, once again, is usually supportive, depending on the clinical presentation; whether more specific therapy is needed and what form it takes depend on the cause of liver disease. Although physiologic tests have been developed to quantify hepatic reserve, the most widely used and best-validated prognostic index remains the Child-Pugh classification (see below), which correlates with individual survival and has been shown to predict operative risk.[112] Liver transplantation is the treatment of choice in most cases of end-stage liver disease.

The Child-Pugh Classification[112]
Numerical Score (*points*)

Variable	1	2	3
Encephalopathy	Nil (0)	Slight to moderate (1, 2)	Moderate to severe (3–5)
Ascites	Nil	Slight	Moderate to severe
Bilirubin, mg/dl (μmol/L*)	< 2 (< 34)	2–3 (34–51)	> 3 (> 51)
Albumin, g/dl (g/L*)	> 3.5 (> 35)	2.8–3.5 (28–35)	< 2.8 (< 28)
Prothrombin index	> 70%	40%–70%	< 40%

Modified Child's risk grade (depending on total score): 5 or 6 points, grade A; 7 to 9 points, grade B; 10 to 15 points, grade C.
*Système International d'Unités, or SI units.

that the obstruction is probably located in the middle third or the distal third of the CBD.

Some centers prefer CT to ultrasonography as the initial imaging modality,[29] but we, like a number of other authors,[30] find ultrasonography to be the most expedient, most readily available, least invasive, and most economical imaging method for differentiating between hepatic and posthepatic causes of jaundice as well as for suggesting the level of obstruction.[31] Traditional imaging techniques, such as oral or intravenous cholangiography, have a negligible role to play in this setting because of their very poor accuracy and safety, especially in jaundiced patients.

Magnetic resonance cholangiopancreatography (MRCP) [see Figure 1] and endoscopic ultrasonography (EUS) have been used to visualize the biliary and pancreatic trees in a variety of populations of patients with obstructive jaundice,[32-36] and experience with these newer imaging modalities is accumulating rapidly. Compared with direct cholangiography, both MRCP and EUS appear to be excellent at diagnosing biliary obstruction and establishing its location and nature.[37,38] MRCP exhibits more modest detection rates when diagnosing small CBD stones.[39] Helical, or spiral, CT scanning is also useful in diagnosing biliary obstruction and determining its cause, though concomitant oral or I.V. cholangiography is required to detect choledocholithiasis.[40,41]

In addition to their ability to detect choledocholithiasis, spiral CT, EUS, and MRCP in combination with abdominal magnetic resonance imaging (e.g., of the pancreas) are very useful in diagnosing and staging biliopancreatic tumors.[42-44] Cytology specimens are readily obtained via fine-needle aspiration (FNA) during CT or EUS.[43]

It is our current practice to employ these modalities as second-line tests after the initial abdominal ultrasonographic examination. We favor EUS for periampullary pathologic conditions and MRI with MRCP for more proximal diseases of the biliary tree.

In making the choice among the various available second-line tests, cost-effectiveness becomes an important consideration. Several of these imaging modalities, individually or in combination with others, have been evaluated for their cost-effectiveness in the workup of patients with obstructive jaundice. Unfortunately, the reports published to date have been flawed, suffering either from limited assumptions (when the methodology involved decision modeling) or from the lack of an effectiveness-type design (when the methodology involved allocation of patients).

Workup and Management of Posthepatic Jaundice

Once ultrasonography has confirmed that ductal obstruction is present, there are three possible clinical scenarios: suspected cholangitis, suspected choledocholithiasis without cholangitis, and a suspected lesion other than choledocholithiasis. The direction of the subsequent workup depends on which of the three appears most likely.

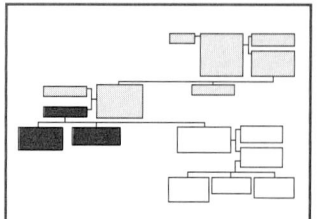

SUSPECTED CHOLANGITIS

If a jaundiced patient exhibits a clinical picture compatible with acute suppurative cholangitis (Charcot's triad or Raynaud's pentad), the most likely diagnosis is choledocholithiasis. After

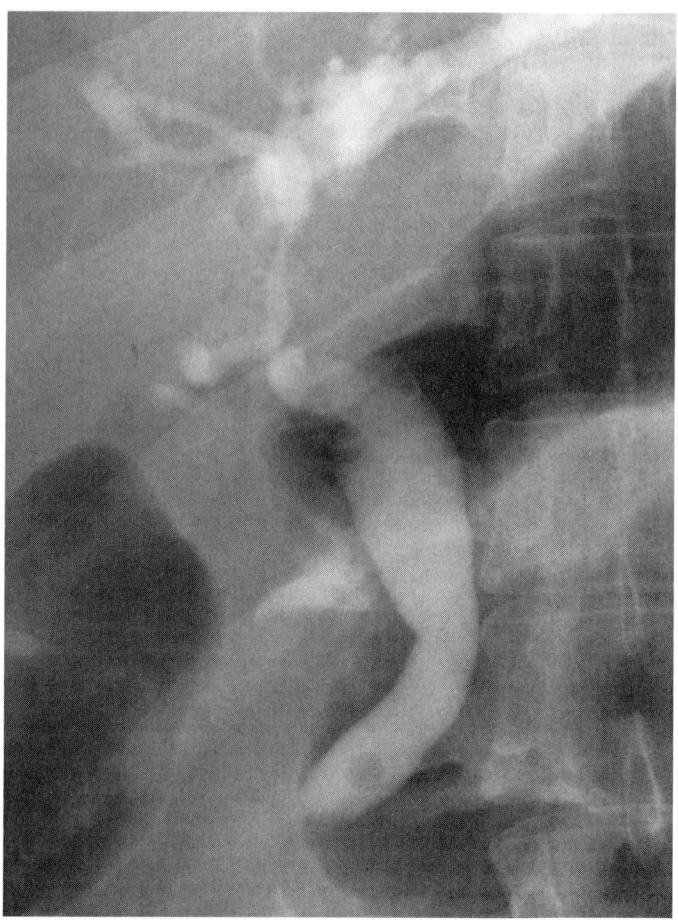

a

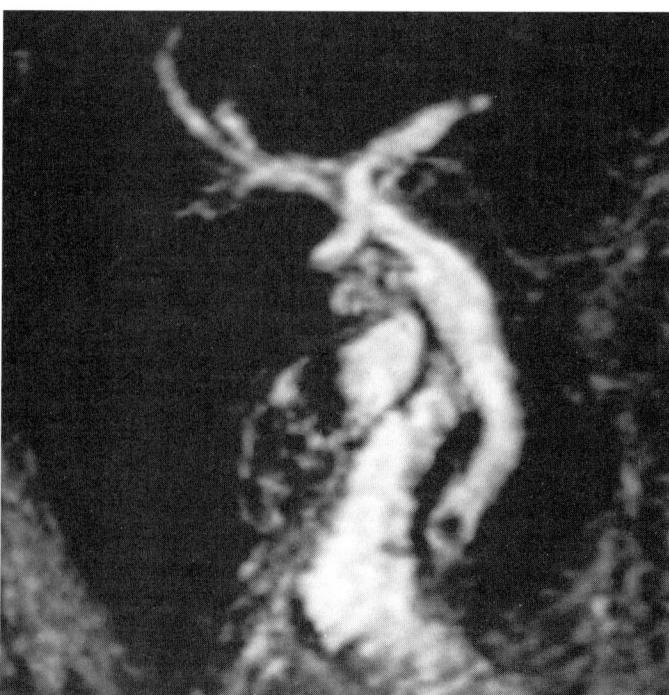

b

Figure 1 ERCP (*a*) and corresponding MRCP (*b*) demonstrate the presence of a stone in the distal CBD.

appropriate resuscitation, correction of any coagulopathies present, and administration of antibiotics, ERCP is indicated for diagnosis and treatment.[45] If ERCP is unavailable or is not feasible (e.g., because of previous Roux-en-Y reconstruction), transhepatic drainage or surgery may be necessary. It is important to emphasize here that the mainstay of treatment of severe cholangitis is not just the administration of appropriate antibiotics but rather the establishment of adequate biliary drainage.

SUSPECTED CHOLEDOCHOLITHIASIS WITHOUT CHOLANGITIS

Choledocholithiasis is the most common cause of biliary obstruction[13,14] and should be strongly suspected if the jaundice is episodic or painful or if ultrasonography has demonstrated the presence of gallstones or bile duct stones. Patients with suspected choledocholithiasis should be referred for laparoscopic cholecystectomy with either preoperative ERCP or intraoperative cholangiography [see 3:15 Laparoscopic Cholecystectomy]. We favor preoperative ERCP in this setting of jaundice because its diagnostic yield is high,[46] it allows confirmation of the diagnosis preoperatively (thus obviating intraoperative surprises), and it is capable of clearing the CBD of stones in 95% of cases. Decision analyses appear to confirm the utility of this strategy when laparoscopic CBD exploration is not an option.[47-50] Many authors, however, favor a fully laparoscopic approach, in which choledocholithiasis is detected in the OR by means of intraoperative cholangiography[51,52] or ultrasonography[53-55] and laparoscopic biliary clearance is performed when choledocholithiasis is confirmed. Given that both the ERCP approach and the fully laparoscopic approach have advantages and limitations, one may reasonably maintain that the optimal approach in a particular setting should be dictated by local expertise.

SUSPECTED LESION OTHER THAN CHOLEDOCHOLITHIASIS

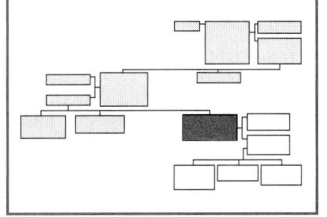

If no gallstones are identified, if the clinical presentation is less acute (e.g., constant abdominal or back pain), or if there are associated constitutional symptoms (e.g., weight loss, fatigue, and long-standing anorexia), the presence of a lesion other than choledocholithiasis should be suspected. In such cases, another imaging modality besides the ultrasonography already performed must be considered before the decision is made to proceed to cholangiography or operation.

Possible causes of posthepatic obstruction (other than choledocholithiasis) may be classified into three categories depending on the location of the obstructing lesion (as suggested by the pattern of gallbladder and biliary tree dilatation on the ultrasonogram): the upper third of the biliary tree, the middle third, or the lower (distal) third [see Table 3]. Once it has been determined that choledocholithias is unlikely, the most common cause of such obstruction is pancreatic cancer.[13,14] In adults, many of the other possible causes also involve malignant processes. Consequently, the next step in the workup of the patient is typically the assessment of resectability and operability [see 3:16 Biliary Tract Procedures].

Diagnosis and Assessment of Resectability

Because surgery is the only chance for definitive treatment of a biliary or pancreatic malignancy, it is important not to deny a patient this chance. Assessment of the resectability of a

Table 3 Causes of Posthepatic Jaundice

Upper-third obstruction
 Polycystic liver disease
 Caroli disease
 Hepatocellular carcinoma
 Oriental cholangiohepatitis
 Hepatic arterial thrombosis (e.g., after liver transplantation or chemotherapy)
 Hemobilia (e.g., after biliary manipulation)
 Iatrogenic bile duct injury (e.g., after laparoscopic cholecystectomy)
 Cholangiocarcinoma (Klatskin tumor)
 Sclerosing cholangitis
 Papillomas of the bile duct

Middle-third obstruction
 Cholangiocarcinoma
 Sclerosing cholangitis
 Papillomas of the bile duct
 Gallbladder cancer
 Choledochal cyst
 Intrabiliary parasites
 Mirizzi syndrome
 Extrinsic nodal compression (e.g., from breast cancer or lymphoma)
 Iatrogenic bile duct injury (e.g., after open cholecystectomy)
 Cystic fibrosis
 Benign idiopathic bile duct stricture

Lower-third obstruction
 Cholangiocarcinoma
 Sclerosing cholangitis
 Papillomas of the bile duct
 Pancreatic tumors
 Ampullary tumors
 Chronic pancreatitis
 Sphincter of Oddi dysfunction
 Papillary stenosis
 Duodenal diverticula
 Penetrating duodenal ulcer
 Retroduodenal adenopathy (e.g., lymphoma, carcinoid)

tumor usually hinges on whether the superior mesenteric vein, the portal vein, the superior mesenteric artery, and the porta hepatis are free of tumor and on whether there is evidence of significant local adenopathy or extrapancreatic extension of tumor. Unfortunately, the majority of lesions will be clearly unresectable, either because of tumor extension or because of the presence of hepatic or peritoneal metastases.

Many imaging modalities are currently being used to determine resectability, and several of these have been established as effective alternatives to direct cholangiography because they involve little if any morbidity. Their accuracy varies according to the underlying pathology and the expertise of the user. They have been studied mostly with respect to the staging and diagnosis of pancreatic, periampullary, and biliary hilar cancers.

For determining resectability and staging lesions before operation, we rely mainly on spiral CT, which allows good definition of the nature and extent of the lesion. At present, this modality is thought to be superior for the diagnosis and staging of lesions such as pancreatic cancer.[42,56-58] Spiral CT exhibits a high negative predictive value and has a false positive rate of less than

10%; its sensitivity is optimal for pancreatic lesions larger than 1.5 cm in diameter. The presence of ascites, liver metastases, lymph nodes larger than 2 cm in diameter, and invasion into adjacent organs are all signs of advanced disease.[59] On the basis of these criteria, spiral CT can predict that a lesion will not be resectable with an accuracy approaching 95%; however, as many as 33% of tumors that appear to be resectable on CT are found to be unresectable at operation.[57,58] Occasionally, spiral CT does not yield sufficient information, and as a result, supplementary imaging studies are required.

MRI has also been shown to be helpful in determining the nature of the malignant obstruction, and MRI-based staging, along with MRCP, can further dictate the subsequent choice of therapy.[59-62] MRI may be particularly useful for following up patients in whom clip artifacts interfere with a CT image.[59] It also appears to be successful in detecting cholangiocarcinoma spreading along the proximal biliary tree.[63]

Only in a few very rare instances is traditional angiography used to assess resectability or stage a hepatobiliary or pancreatic neoplasm. Increasingly, it is being replaced by CT angiography or duplex Doppler ultrasonography, which can confirm the presence of flow in the hepatic arterial or portal venous systems and occasionally can demonstrate invasion of these vessels by tumor.[64] Magnetic resonance angiography (MRA) has also been used with excellent results. As yet, none of these noninvasive modalities has been shown to be clearly superior to any of the others.[65]

EUS appears to be a highly promising modality, particularly with respect to assessment of the resectability of pancreatic tumors.[43,66,67] In a large study comprising 232 patients, EUS was found to be superior to CT and to standard ultrasonography in detecting venous and gastric invasion by cancers measuring 3 cm or less in diameter.[68] In another large series, it was reported to be more accurate than CT in the comparative staging of pancreatic and ampullary cancers.[69] EUS is also useful for identifying small (< 2 cm) pancreatic tumors, which may be suspected in a patient with an obstruction of the distal third of the bile duct and whose CT scan is normal.[67] An additional benefit is that one can perform guided FNA at the time of EUS. Furthermore, EUS is currently the dominant technique for staging ampullary tumors.[70]

At this point in the evaluation, patients can be referred for direct cholangiography (usually ERCP) to better delineate the proximal biliary anatomy (for upper-third lesions) or to clarify a still-unclear diagnosis. There is, however, a growing body of evidence suggesting that in patients with either pancreatic[71,72] or hepatic[73] malignancies, routine preoperative direct cholangiography with decompression may be associated with a higher incidence of postoperative complications when tumor resection is ultimately carried out.

If a biliary stricture is detected at cholangiography, brush cytology or biopsy is mandatory. Biliary cytology, however, has been disappointing, particularly at ERCP: diagnostic accuracy ranges from 40% to 85%,[74,75] mostly because the negative predictive value is poor. Accuracy improves with multiple sampling and when a biliary rather than a pancreatic malignancy is detected. In addition, biopsy tends to be more accurate than brush cytology.[74]

If a pancreatic tumor is suspected, percutaneous FNA cytology may be helpful; the yield is best for larger tumors. Direct FNA of the lesion at EUS is also an increasingly attractive option. In the case of potentially resectable lesions, however, this measure adds very little to the decision-making process.

The limited data currently available suggest that assays of tumor markers in serum and pancreatic fluid are useful, particularly for cystic lesions of the pancreas.[76]

Nonoperative Management: Drainage and Cholangiography

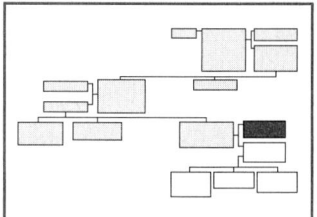

In the majority of patients with malignant obstructions, treatment is palliative rather than curative. It is therefore especially important to recognize and minimize the iatrogenic risks related to the manipulation of an obstructed biliary system; this is why staging and cholangiography are currently being performed with less invasive methods.

Cholangiography and decompression of obstructed biliary system   As a rule, we favor ERCP, although PTC may be preferable for obstructions near the hepatic duct bifurcation. Whichever imaging modality is used, the following four principles apply.

1. In the absence of preexisting or concomitant hepatocellular dysfunction, drainage of one half of the liver is generally sufficient for resolution of jaundice.
2. Because of its external diameter, a transhepatic drain, once inserted, does not necessarily permit equal drainage of all segments of the liver, particularly if there are a number of intrahepatic ductal stenoses. Accordingly, some patients with conditions such as sclerosing cholangitis or a growing tumor may experience persistent sepsis from an infected excluded liver segment even when the prosthesis is patent [*see Figure 2*]. An excluded segment may even be responsible for severe persistent pruritus.
3. Any attempt at opacifying an obstructed biliary tree introduces a significant risk of subsequent cholangitis, even when appropriate antibiotic prophylaxis is provided. Accordingly, when one elects to perform direct cholangiography, there should be a plan for biliary drainage either at the time of ERCP or PTC or soon thereafter.
4. Even though jaundice is believed to be associated with multiple adverse systemic effects (e.g., renal failure, sepsis, and impaired wound healing),[77,78] routine preoperative drainage of an obstructed biliary system does not benefit patients who will soon undergo operative correction.[79,80] In fact, as noted (see above), routine preoperative drainage of subsequently resected hepatic or pancreatic malignancies may be deleterious.

When direct cholangiography is ordered, it should be thought of as more than just a diagnostic test: it is the ideal setting for cytology, biopsy, or even drainage of the obstructed bile duct via a sphincterotomy, a nasobiliary tube, or a catheter or stent. Accordingly, it is essential that the surgeon, the gastroenterologist, and the radiologist discuss the possible need for drainage well before it is required. Early, open communication among all the members of the treating team is a hallmark of the modern management of biliary obstruction.

Palliation in patients with advanced malignant disease
When a patient has advanced malignant disease, drainage of the biliary system for palliation is not routinely indicated,

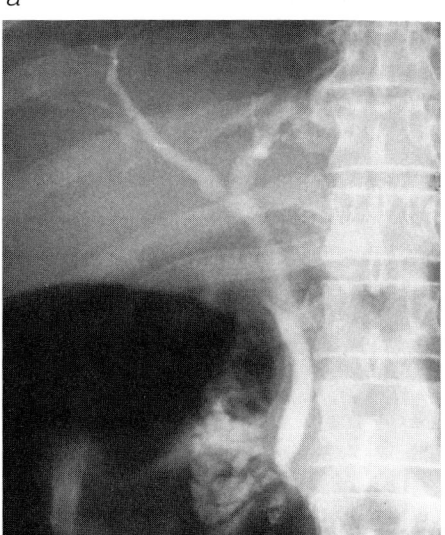
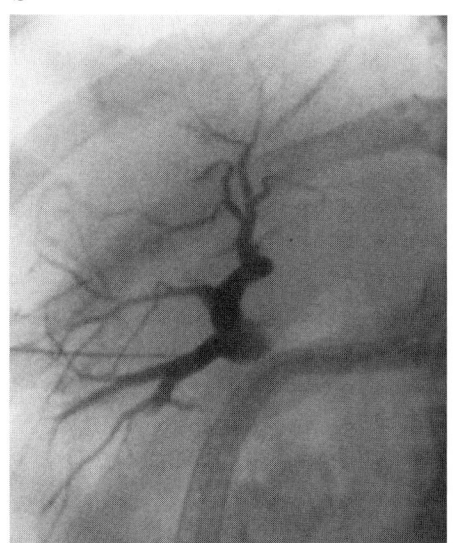
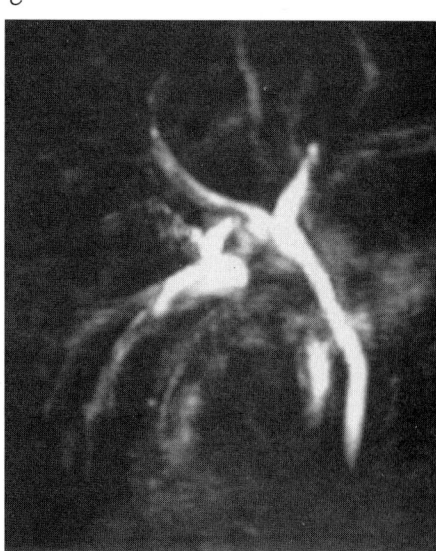

a *b* *c*

Figure 2 **ERCP (*a*) demonstrates missing liver segments. Transhepatic cholangiography (*b*) of segment VI reveals excluded liver ductal system. MRCP (*c*) shows the excluded liver segments as well as the biliary system, which still communicates with the common hepatic duct.**

because the risk of complications related to the procedure may outweigh the potential benefit. Indeed, the best treatment for a patient with asymptomatic obstructive jaundice and liver metastases may be supportive care alone.[81] Biliary decompression is indicated if cholangitis or severe pruritus that interferes with quality of life is present.

We, like others,[21] consider a stent placed with ERCP to be the palliative modality of choice for advanced disease, although upper-third lesions may be managed most easily through the initial placement of an internal/external catheter at the time of PTC. Metal expandable stents remain patent longer than large conventional plastic stents,[82,83] but the high price of the metal stents has kept them from being widely used, and their overall cost-effectiveness has yet to be clearly demonstrated. Whether plastic biliary stents should be replaced prophylactically or only after obstruction has occurred remains controversial; however, results from a randomized trial favor the former approach.[84]

Randomized controlled trials suggest that surgical biliary bypass should be reserved for patients who are expected to survive for prolonged periods because bypass is associated with more prolonged palliation at the cost of greater initial morbidity.[85]

The role of prophylactic gastric drainage at the time of operative biliary drainage remains controversial.[86] However, jaundiced patients with unresectable lesions who also present with duodenal or jejunal obstruction should be referred for gastrojejunostomy at the time of biliary bypass surgery. There is evidence to suggest that when a pancreatic malignancy is present, intraoperative celiac ganglion injection should be performed for either prophylactic or therapeutic pain control.[87]

Operative Management at Specific Sites: Bypass and Resection

Surgical treatment of tumors causing biliary obstruction is determined primarily by the level of the biliary obstruction. There is a growing body of evidence

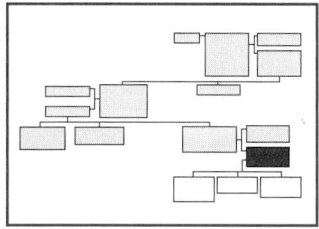

indicating that modern surgical approaches are resulting in lower postoperative morbidity and, possibly, improved 5-year survival[88]; however, the prognosis is still uniformly poor, except for patients with ampullary tumors. In fact, the surgical procedure rarely proves curative, even after meticulous preoperative patient selection.

The first step toward potential resection of a jaundice-causing cancer should be laparoscopy to determine resectability and to prevent the hospital stay and prolonged convalescence associated with an unnecessary laparotomy. Laparoscopy is used mostly to detect peritoneal carcinomatosis, liver metastases, malignant ascites, and gross hilar adenopathy.[89,90] In a trial involving 115 patients with potentially resectable peripancreatic tumors, full laparoscopic staging could be performed in 94%, and the overall resectability rate was 76%.[89] In several studies, a combined approach including both laparoscopy and laparoscopic ultrasonography was associated with shorter hospital stays and lower costs.[90-92] The main limitation of such an approach appears to be that it does not accurately detect the spread of tumors to lymph nodes or the vascular system.[92]

Once laparoscopy confirms that there is no obvious advanced disease, the patient should undergo a full laparotomy, usually in the same setting but occasionally in a different operative session.

In what follows, only the general principles of resection or bypass at each level of obstruction are discussed; operative technical details are addressed elsewhere [*see 3:16 Biliary Tract Procedures*]. Our preferred method of biliary anastomosis, for either reconstruction or bypass, involves the fashioning of a Roux-en-Y loop, followed by a mucosa-to-mucosa anastomosis. In all cases, a cholecystectomy is performed to facilitate access to the biliary tree.

Upper-third obstruction

Palliation. In the absence of liver compromise, drainage of one half of the liver usually leads to clearance of jaundice.[93] Because the left hepatic duct has a long extrahepatic segment that makes it more accessible,

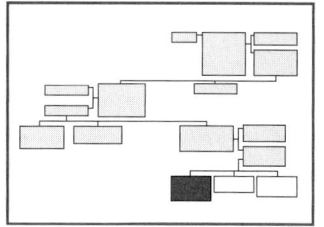

the preferred bypass technique for an obstructing upper-third lesion is a left (or segment 3) hepaticojejunostomy. This operation has superseded the Longmire procedure because it does not involve formal resection of liver parenchyma. Laparoscopic bypass techniques that make use of segment 3 have been developed, but their performance has yet to be formally assessed.[94,95]

Resection for cure. The hilar plate is taken down to lengthen the hepatic duct segment available for subsequent anastomosis. Often, a formal hepatectomy or segmentectomy is required to ensure an adequate margin of resection. If the resection must be carried out proximal to the hepatic duct bifurcation, several cholangiojejunostomies will have to be done to anastomose individual hepatic biliary branches. Frozen section examination of the proximal and distal resection margins is important because of the propensity of tumors such as cholangiocarcinoma to spread in a submucosal or perineural plane.

The results of aggressive hilar tumor resections that included as much liver tissue as was necessary to obtain a negative margin appear to justify this approach.[96] In cases of left hepatic involvement, resection of the caudate lobe (segment 1) is indicated as well.[97]

Middle-third obstruction

Palliation. Surgical bypass of middle-third lesions is technically simpler because a hepaticojejunostomy can often be performed distal to the hepatic duct bifurcation, which means that exposure of the hilar plate or the intrahepatic ducts is unnecessary.

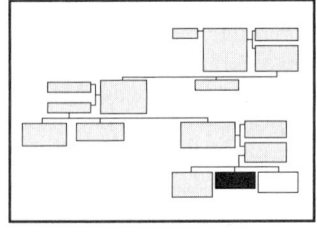

Resection for cure. Discrete tumors in this part of the bile duct, though uncommon, are usually quite amenable to resection along with the lymphatic chains in the porta hepatis. Resection of an early gallbladder cancer may, on occasion, necessitate the concomitant resection of segment 5, although the value of resecting this segment prophylactically has not been conclusively demonstrated. Sometimes, jaundice from a suspected middle-third lesion is in fact caused by a case of Mirizzi syndrome [*see Figure 3*]. In such cases, a gallstone is responsible for extrinsic obstruction of the CBD, either by causing inflammation of the gallbladder wall or via direct impingement. Proper treatment of this syndrome may involve hepaticojejunostomy in addition to cholecystectomy if a cholecystocholedochal fistula is present.[98]

Lower-third obstruction

Palliation. The preferred bypass technique for lower-third lesions is a Roux-en-Y choledochojejunostomy. Cholecystojejunostomy carries a higher risk of complications and subsequent development of jaundice[99]; this remains true even when it is performed laparoscopically.[94] Occasionally, it may be done as a temporizing measure before a more definitive procedure in the context of an upcoming transfer to a specialized center.

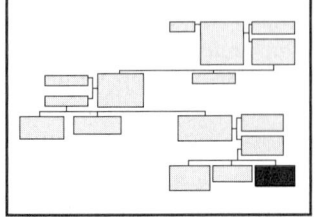

Resection for cure. Occasionally, an impacted CBD stone at the duodenal ampulla mimics a tumor and is not clearly identified

preoperatively. In this situation, intraoperative choledochoscopy before resection helps confirm the diagnosis and may even permit removal of the stone. Because of the growing use of EUS and MRCP, such a situation is increasingly uncommon. Resection of a lower-third lesion usually involves a pancreaticoduodenectomy [*see 3:18 Pancreatic Procedures*], although local ampullary resection may be an acceptable alternative for a small adenoma of the ampulla; local duodenal resection with removal of the head of the pancreas has also been described. For optimal results, pancreaticoduodenectomy is best performed in specialized centers.[100]

It has been suggested that postoperative adjuvant therapy may improve the prognosis after resection of a pancreatic adenocarcinoma,[88] but this debate falls outside the scope of our discussion.

Postoperative Jaundice

A clinical scenario of particular pertinence to surgeons that we have not yet addressed is the development of jaundice in the postoperative setting.

Jaundice develops in approximately 1% of all surgical patients after operation.[101] When jaundice occurs after a hepatobiliary procedure, it may be attributable to specific biliary causes, such

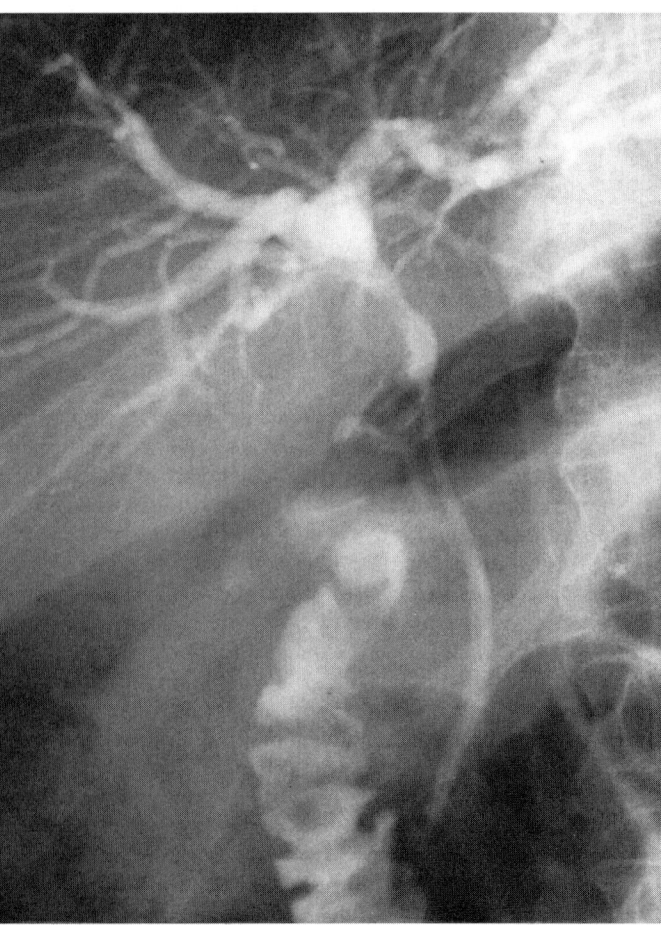

Figure 3 **ERCP demonstrates extrinsic compression of the common hepatic duct by a stone in Hartmann's pouch. A biliary stent has been inserted for drainage.**

as retained CBD stones, postoperative biliary leakage (through reabsorption of bile leaking into the peritoneum) [*see Figure 4*], injury to the CBD, and the subsequent development of biliary strictures. In most instances, however, the jaundice derives from a combination of disease processes, and only rarely is invasive testing or active treatment required.[102]

A diagnostic approach similar to the one outlined earlier (see above) is applicable to postoperative jaundice; however, another useful approach is to consider the possible causes in the light of the time interval between the operation and the subsequent development of jaundice.

- Jaundice may develop within 48 hours of the operation; this is most often the result of the breakdown of red blood cells, occurring in the context of multiple blood transfusions (particularly with stored blood), the resorption of a large hematoma, or a transfusion reaction. Hemolysis may also develop in a patient with a known underlying hemolytic anemia and may be precipitated by the administration of specific drugs (e.g., sulfa drugs in a patient who has glucose-6-phosphate dehydrogenase deficiency).[103] Cardiopulmonary bypass or the insertion of a prosthetic valve may be associated with the development of early postoperative jaundice as well. Gilbert syndrome [*see Sidebar* Hepatic Jaundice] may first manifest itself early in the postoperative period. Occasionally, a mild conjugated hyperbilirubinemia may be related to Dubin-Johnson syndrome, which is an inherited disorder of bilirubin metabolism. This condition is usually self-limited and is characterized by the presence of a melaninlike pigment in the liver.

- Intraoperative hypotension or hypoxemia or the early development of heart failure can lead to conjugated hyperbilirubinemia within 5 to 10 days after operation. The hyperbilirubinemia may be associated with other end-organ damage (e.g., acute tubular necrosis). In fact, any impairment of renal function causes a decrease in bilirubin excretion and can be responsible for a mild hyperbilirubinemia.

- Jaundice may develop 7 to 10 days after operation in association with a medication-induced hepatitis attributable to an anesthetic agent. This syndrome has an estimated incidence of one in 10,000 after an initial exposure.[103] More commonly, the jaundice is related to the administration of antibiotics or other medications used in the perioperative setting.[103]

- After the first week, jaundice associated with intrahepatic cholestasis is often a manifestation of a septic response and usually presents in the setting of overt infection, particularly in patients with multiple organ dysfunction syndrome. Gram-negative sepsis from an intra-abdominal source is typical; if it persists, the outcome is likely to be poor. Jaundice may occur in as many as 30% of patients receiving total parenteral nutrition (TPN). It may be attributable to steatosis, particularly with formulas containing large amounts of carbohydrates. In addition, decreased export of bilirubin from the hepatocytes may lead to cholestasis, the severity of which appears to be related to the duration of TPN administration. Acalculous cholecystitis or even ductal obstruction may develop as a result of sludge in the gall-

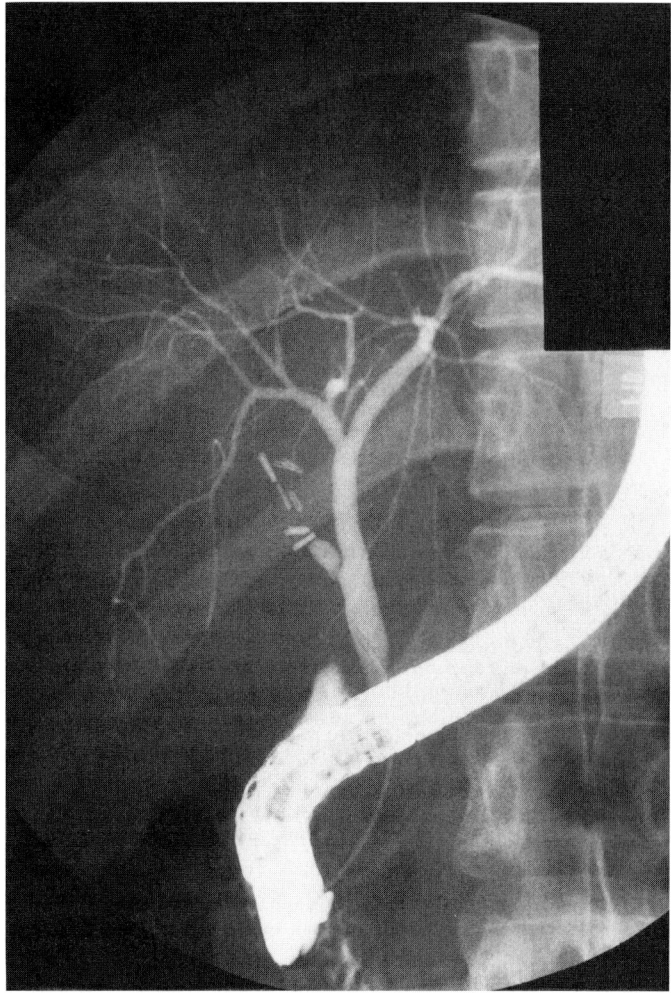

Figure 4 **Jaundice has occurred after laparoscopic cholecystectomy as a result of bile leakage from a distal biliary tributary. A stent has been inserted to decrease bile duct luminal pressure and foster spontaneous resolution.**

bladder and the CBD. An elevated postoperative bilirubin level at any time may also result from unsuspected hepatic or posthepatic causes (e.g., occult cirrhosis, choledocholithiasis, or cholecystitis). A rare cause of postoperative jaundice is the development of thyrotoxicosis. Another entity to consider (as a diagnosis of exclusion) is so-called benign postoperative cholestasis, a primarily cholestatic, self-limited process with no clearly demonstrable cause that typically arises within 2 to 10 days after operation. Benign postoperative cholestasis may be attributable to a combination of mechanisms, including an increased pigment load, impaired liver function resulting from hypoxemia and hypotension, and decreased renal bilirubin excretion caused by varying degrees of tubular necrosis.[104] The predominantly conjugated hyperbilirubinemia may reach 40 mg/dl and remain elevated for as long as 3 weeks.[103] This is a diagnosis of exclusion.

- In the late postoperative period, the development of non-A, non-B, non-C viral hepatitis after transfusion of blood products will usually occur within 5 to 12 weeks of operation.

References

1. Schiff L: Jaundice: a clinical approach. Diseases of the Liver, 7th ed. Schiff L, Schiff ER, Eds. JB Lippincott Co, Philadelphia, 1993, p 334

2. Jabbari M: Personal communication

3. Scharschmidt BF, Gollan JL: Current concepts of bilirubin metabolism and hereditary hyperbilirubinemia. Progress in Liver Diseases. Popper H, Schaffner F, Eds. Grune & Stratton, New York, 1979, p 187

4. Frank BB: Clinical evaluation of jaundice: a guideline of the Patient Care Committee of the American Gastroenterological Association. JAMA 262:3031, 1989

5. Schiff's Diseases of the Liver, 8th ed. Schiff ER, Sorrell MF, Maddrey WC, Eds. Lippincott-Raven, Philadelphia, 1999, p 119

6. Lindberg G, Björkman A, Helmers C: A description of diagnostic strategies in jaundice. Scand J Gastroenterol 18:257, 1983

7. Lumeng L, Snodgrass PJ, Swonder JW: Final report of a blinded prospective study comparing current non-invasive approaches in the differential diagnosis of medical and surgical jaundice. Gastroenterology 78:1312, 1980

8. Martin W, Apostolakos PC, Roazen H: Clinical versus actuarial prediction in the differential diagnosis of jaundice. Am J Med Sci 240:571, 1960

9. Matzen P, Malchow-Möller A, Hilden J, et al: Differential diagnosis of jaundice: a pocket diagnostic chart. Liver 4:360, 1984

10. O'Connor K, Snodgrass PJ, Swonder JE, et al: A blinded prospective study comparing four current non-invasive approaches in the differential diagnosis of medical versus surgical jaundice. Gastroenterology 84:1498, 1983

11. Schenker S, Balint J, Schiff L: Differential diagnosis of jaundice: report of a prospective study of 61 proved cases. Am J Dig Dis 7:449, 1962

12. Theodossi A, Spiegelhalter D, Portmann B, et al: The value of clinical, biochemical, ultrasound and liver biopsy data in assessing patients with liver disease. Liver 3:315, 1983

13. Pasanen PA, Pikkarainen P, Alhava E, et al: The value of clinical assessment in the diagnosis of icterus and cholestasis. Ital J Gastroenterol Hepatol 24:313, 1992

14. Theodossi A: The value of symptoms and signs in the assessment of jaundiced patients. Clin Gastroenterol 14:545, 1985

15. Fung KP, Lau SP: Differentiation between extrahepatic and intrahepatic cholestasis by discriminant analysis. J Paediatr Child Health 26:132, 1990

16. Pasanen PA, Pikkarainen P, Alhava E, et al: Evaluation of a computer-based diagnostic score system in the diagnosis of jaundice and cholestasis. Scand J Gastroenterol 28:732, 1993

17. Malchow-Möller A, Gronvall S, Hilden J, et al: Ultrasound examination in jaundiced patients: is computer-assisted preclassification helpful? J Hepatol 12:321, 1991

18. Loperfido S, Angelini G, Benedetti G, et al: Major early complications from diagnostic and therapeutic ERCP: a prospective multicenter study. Gastrointest Endosc 48:1, 1998

19. Freeman ML, DiSario JA, Nelson DB, et al: Risk factors for post-ERCP pancreatitis: a prospective, multicenter study. Gastrointest Endosc 54:425, 2001

20. Lillemoe KD: Surgical treatment of biliary tract infections. Am Surg 66:138, 2000

21. Rossi LR, Traverso W, Pimentel F: Malignant obstructive jaundice: evaluation and management. Surg Clin North Am 76:63, 1996

22. Taylor KJW, Rosenfield A: Grey-scale ultrasonography in the differential diagnosis of jaundice. Arch Surg 112:820, 1977

23. Kaplun L, Weissman HS, Rosenblatt RR, et al: The early diagnosis of common bile duct obstruction using cholescintigraphy. JAMA 254:2431, 1985

24. Abboud PA, Malet PF, Berlin JA, et al: Predictors of common bile duct stones prior to cholecystectomy: a meta-analysis. Gastrointest Endosc 44:450, 1996

25. Roston AD, Jacobson IM: Evaluation of the pattern of liver tests and yield of cholangiography in symptomatic choledocholithiasis: a prospective study. Gastrointest Endosc 45:394, 1997

26. Richter JM, Silverstein MD, Schapiro R: Suspected obstructive jaundice: a decision analysis of diagnostic strategies. Ann Intern Med 99:46, 1983

27. Bravo AA, Sheth SG, Chopra S: Liver biopsy. N Engl J Med 344:495, 2001

28. Blackbourne LH, Earnhardt RC, Sistrom CL, et al: The sensitivity and role of ultrasound in the evaluation of biliary obstruction. Am Surg 60:683, 1994

29. Sherlock S: Ultrasound (US), computerized axial tomography (CT) and magnetic resonance imaging (MRI). Diseases of the Liver and Biliary System 5:70, 1989

30. Cosgrove DO: Ultrasound in surgery of the liver and biliary tract. Surgery of the Liver and Biliary Tract, 2nd ed, Vol 1. Blumgart LH, Ed. New York, Churchill Livingstone, 1994, p 189

31. Lindsell DRM: Ultrasound imaging of pancreas and biliary tract. Lancet 335:390, 1990

32. Gillams A, Gardener J, Richards R, et al: Three-dimensional computed tomography cholangiography: a new technique for biliary tract imaging. Br J Radiol 67:445, 1994

33. Low RN, Sigeti JS, Francis IR, et al: Evaluation of malignant biliary obstruction: efficacy of fast multiplanar spoiled gradient-recalled MR imaging vs spin-echo MR imaging, CT, and cholangiography. AJR Am J Roentgenol 162:315, 1994

34. Amouyal P, Amouyal G, Levy P, et al: Diagnosis of choledocholithiasis by endoscopic ultrasonography. Gastroenterology 106:1062, 1994

35. Guibaud L, Bret PM, Reinhold C, et al: Bile duct obstruction and choledocholithiasis: diagnosis with MR cholangiography. Radiology 197:109, 1995

36. Ishizaki Y, Wakayama T, Okada Y, et al: MR cholangiography for evaluation of obstructed jaundice. Am J Gastroenterol 88:2072, 1993

37. Bardou M, Romagnuolo J, Barkun AN, et al: Magnetic resonance cholangiopancreatography, a new gold standard for pancreatico-biliary disease? a systematic review of literature. Can J Gastroenterol (in press)

38. Mallery S, Van Dam J: Current status of diagnostic and therapeutic endoscopic ultrasonography. Radiol Clin North Am 39:449, 2001

39. Sugiyama M, Atomi Y, Hachiya J: Magnetic resonance cholangiography using half-Fourier acquisition for diagnosing choledocholithiasis. Am J Gastroenterol 93:1886, 1998

40. Soto JA, Alvarez O, Munera F, et al: Diagnosing bile duct stones: comparison of unenhanced helical CT, oral contrast-enhanced CT cholangiography, and MR cholangiography. AJR Am J Roentgenol 175:1127, 2000

41. Soto JA, Velez SM, Guzman J: Choledocholithiasis: diagnosis with oral-contrast-enhanced CT cholangiography. AJR Am J Roentgenol 172:943, 1999

42. Freeny PC: Computed tomography in the diagnosis and staging of cholangiocarcinoma and pancreatic carcinoma. Ann Oncol 10(suppl 4):12, 1999

43. Hawes RH, Xiong Q, Waxman I, et al: A multispecialty approach to the diagnosis and management of pancreatic cancer. Am J Gastroenterol 95:17, 2000

44. Megibow AJ, Lavelle MT, Rofsky NM: MR imaging of the pancreas. Surg Clin North Am 81:307, 2001

45. Lai EC, Mok FP, Tan ES, et al: Endoscopic biliary drainage for severe acute cholangitis. N Engl J Med 326:1582, 1992

46. Barkun JS, Fried GM, Barkun AN, et al: Cholecystectomy without operative cholangiography: implications for bile duct injury and common bile duct stones. Ann Surg 218:371, 1993

47. Sahai AV, Mauldin PD, Marsi V, et al: Bile duct stones and laparoscopic cholecystectomy: a decision analysis to assess the roles of intraoperative cholangiography, EUS, and ERCP. Gastrointest Endosc 49(3 pt 1):334, 1999

48. Abraham N, Barkun AN, Barkun JS, et al: What is the optimal management of patients with suspected choledocholithiasis in the era of laparoscopic cholecystectomy? a decision analysis. Gastroenterology 116:G0012, 1999

49. Erickson RA, Carlson B: The role of endoscopic retrograde cholangiopancreatography in patients with laparoscopic cholecystectomies. Gastroenterology 109:252, 1995

50. Urbach DR, Khajanchee YS, Jobe BA, et al: Cost-effective management of common bile duct stones: a decision analysis of the use of endoscopic retrograde cholangiopancreatography (ERCP), intraoperative cholangiography, and laparoscopic bile duct exploration. Surg Endosc 15:4, 2001

51. Memon MA, Hassaballa H, Memon MI: Laparoscopic common bile duct exploration: the past, the present, and the future. Am J Surg 179:309, 2000

52. Crawford DL, Phillips EH: Laparoscopic common bile duct exploration. World J Surg 23:343, 1999

53. Falcone RA Jr, Fegelman EJ, Nussbaum MS, et al: A prospective comparison of laparoscopic ultrasound vs intraoperative cholangiogram during laparoscopic cholecystectomy. Surg Endosc 13:784, 1999

54. Thompson DM, Arregui ME, Tetik C, et al: A comparison of laparoscopic ultrasound with digital fluorocholangiography for detecting choledocholithiasis during laparoscopic cholecystectomy. Surg Endosc 12:929, 1998

55. Wu JS, Dunnegan DL, Soper NJ: The utility of intracorporeal ultrasonography for screening of the bile duct during laparoscopic cholecystectomy. J Gastrointest Surg 2:50, 1998

56. Freeny PC, Traverso LW, Ryan JA: Diagnosis and staging of pancreatic adenocarcinoma with dynamic computed tomography. Am J Surg 165:600, 1993

57. Freeny PC, Marks WM, Ryan JA, et al: Pancreatic ductal adenocarcinoma: diagnosis and staging with dynamic CT. Radiology 166:125, 1988

58. Moosa AR, Gamagami RA: Diagnosis and staging of pancreatic neoplasms. Surg Clin North Am 75:871, 1995

59. Megibow AJ, Zhou XH, Rotterdam H, et al: Pancreatic carcinoma: CT vs MR imaging in the evaluation of resectability. Radiology 195:327, 1995

60. Hann LE, Winston CB, Brown KT, et al: Diagnostic imaging approaches and relationship to hepatobiliary cancer staging and therapy. Semin Surg Oncol 19:94, 2000

61. Zidi SH, Prat F, Le Guen O, et al: Performance characteristics of magnetic resonance cholangiography in the staging of malignant hilar strictures. Gut 46:103, 2000

62. Kim MJ, Mitchell DG, Ito K, et al: Biliary dilatation: differentiation of benign from malignant causes--value of adding conventional MR imaging to MR cholangiopancreatography. Radiology 214:173, 2000

63. Georgopoulos SK, Schwartz LH, Jarnagin WR, et al: Comparison of magnetic resonance and endoscopic retrograde cholangiopancreatography in malignant pancreaticobiliary obstruction. Arch Surg 134:1002, 1999

64. Smits NJ, Reeders JW: Current applicability of duplex Doppler ultrasonography in pancreatic head and biliary malignancies. Baillieres Clin Gastroenterol 9:153, 1995

65. Arslan A, Buanes T, Geitung JT: Pancreatic carcinoma: MR, MR angiography and dynamic helical CT in the evaluation of vascular invasion. Eur J Radiol 38:151, 2001

66. Giovannini M, Seitz JF: Endoscopic ultrasonography with a linear-type echoendoscope in the evaluation of 94 patients with pancreatobiliary disease. Endoscopy 26:579, 1994

67. Snady H, Cooperman A, Siegel J: Endoscopic ultrasonography compared with computed tomography and E.R.C.P. in patients with obstructive jaundice or small peri-pancreatic mass. Gastrointest Endoscopy 38:27, 1992

68. Nakaizumi A, Uehara H, Iishi H, et al: Endoscopic ultrasonography in diagnosis and staging of pancreatic cancer. Dig Dis Sci 40:696, 1995

69. Bakkevold KE, Arnesjo B, Kambestad B: Carcinoma of the pancreas and papilla of Vater—assessment of resectability and factors influencing resectability in stage I carcinomas: a prospective multicentre trial in 472 patients. Eur J Surg Oncol 18:494, 1992

70. Cannon ME, Carpenter SL, Elta GH, et al: EUS compared with CT, magnetic resonance imaging, and angiography and the influence of biliary stenting on staging accuracy of ampullary neoplasms. Gastrointest Endosc 50:27, 1999

71. Povoski SP, Karpeh MS Jr, Conlon KC, et al: Preoperative biliary drainage: impact on intraoperative bile cultures and infectious morbidity and mortality after pancreaticoduodenectomy. J Gastrointest Surg 3:496, 1999

72. Sohn TA, Yeo CJ, Cameron JL, et al: Do preoperative biliary stents increase postpancreaticoduodenectomy complications? J Gastrointest Surg 4:258, 2000

73. Jarnagin WR, Bodniewicz J, Dougherty E, et al: A prospective analysis of staging laparoscopy in patients with primary and secondary hepatobiliary malignancies. J Gastrointest Surg 4:34, 2000

74. Davidson BR: Progress in determining the nature of biliary strictures. Gut 34:725, 1993

75. Hawes RH: Endoscopy and non-calculus biliary obstruction. Annuals of Gastrointestinal Endoscopy, 8th ed. Cotton PB, Tytgat GNJ, Williams CB, Eds. Current Science, England, 1995, p 101

76. Fernandez Del Castillo C, Warshaw AL: Cystic tumors of the pancreas. Surg Clin North Am 75:1001, 1995

77. Rege RV: Adverse effects of biliary obstruction: implications for treatment of patients with obstructive jaundice. AJR Am J Roentgenol 164:287, 1995

78. Grande L, Garcia-Valdecasas JC, Fuster J, et al: Obstructive jaundice and wound healing. Br J Surg 77:440, 1990

79. Pitt HA, Gomes AS, Lois JF: Does preoperative percutaneous biliary drainage reduce operative risk or increase hospital cost? Ann Surg 201:545, 1985

80. McPherson GA, Benjamin IS, Hodgson HJ, et al: Preoperative percutaneous transhepatic biliary drainage: results of a controlled trial. Br J Surg 71:371, 1984

81. Abraham N, Barkun J, Barkun AN, et al: Clinical risk factors of plastic biliary stent obstruction: a prospective trial. Am J Gastroenterol 95:2471, 2000

82. Knyrim K, Wagner HJ, Pausch J, et al: A prospective, randomized controlled trial of metal stents for malignant obstruction of the common bile duct. Endoscopy 25:207, 1993

83. Davids P, Groen A, Rauws E, et al: Randomized trial of self-expanding metal stents versus polyethylene stents for distal malignant biliary obstruction. Lancet 340:1488, 1992

84. Prat F, Chapat O, Ducot B, et al: A randomized trial of endoscopic drainage methods for inoperable malignant strictures of the common bile duct. Gastrointest Endosc 47:1, 1998

85. Smith AC, Dowsett JF, Russell RC, et al: Randomized trial of endoscopic stenting vs surgical bypass in malignant low bile duct obstruction. Lancet 344:1655, 1994

86. Lillemoe KD, Sauter P, Pitt HA, et al: Current status of surgical palliation of periampullary carcinoma. Surg Gynecol Obstet 176:1, 1993

87. Lillemoe KD, Cameron JL, Kaufman HS, et al: Chemical splanchnicectomy in patients with unresectable pancreatic cancer: a prospective randomized trial. Ann Surg 217:447, 1993

88. Lillemoe KD, Cameron JL, Yeo CJ, et al: Pancreaticoduodenectomy: does it have a role in the palliation of pancreatic cancer? Ann Surg 223:718, 1996

89. Conlon KC, Dougherty E, Klimstra DS, et al: The value of minimal access surgery in the staging of patients with potentially resectable pancreatic malignancy. Ann Surg 223:134, 1996

90. John TG, Greig JD, Carter DC, et al: Carcinoma of the pancreatic head and periampullary region: tumor staging with laparoscopy and laparoscopic ultrasonography. Ann Surg 221:156, 1995

91. Hunerbein M, Rau B, Schlag PM: Laparoscopic ultrasound for staging of upper gastrointestinal tumours. Eur J Surg Oncol 21:50, 1995

92. Jarnagin WR, Bodniewicz J, Dougherty E, et al: A prospective analysis of staging laparoscopy in patients with primary and secondary hepatobiliary malignancies. J Gastrointest Surg 4:34, 2000

93. Baer HU, Rhyner M, Stain SC, et al: The effect of communication between the right and left liver on the outcome of surgical drainage from jaundice due to malignant obstruction at the hilus of the liver. HPB Surg 8:27, 1994

94. Gagner M: Personal communication

95. Scott-Conner CE: Laparoscopic biliary bypass for inoperable pancreatic cancer. Semin Laparosc Surg 5:185, 1998

96. Chamberlain RS, Blumgart LH: Hilar cholangiocarcinoma: a review and commentary. Ann Surg Oncol 7:55, 2000

97. Ogura Y, Kawarada Y: Surgical strategies for carcinoma of the hepatic duct confluence. Br J Surg 85:20, 1998

98. Baer HU, Matthews JB, Schweizer WP, et al: Management of the Mirizzi syndrome and the surgical implications of cholecystocholedochal fistula. Br J Surg 77:743, 1990

99. Sarfeh MG, Rypins EB, Jakowatz JG, et al: A prospective, randomized clinical investigation of cholecystoenterostomy and choledochoenterostomy. Am J Surg 155:411, 1988

100. Lieberman MD, Kilburn H, Lindsey M, et al: Relation of perioperative deaths to hospital volume among patients undergoing pancreatic resection for malignancy. Ann Surg 222:638, 1995

101. Lamont JT, Isselbacher KJ: Current concepts of postoperative hepatic dysfunction. Conn Med 39:461, 1975

102. Matlof DS, Kaplan MM: Postoperative jaundice. Orthop Clin North Am 9:799, 1978

103. Moody FG, Potts JR III: Postoperative jaundice. Diseases of the Liver, 7th ed. Schiff L, Schiff ER, Eds. JB Lippincott Co, Philadelphia, 1993, p 370

104. Isselbacher KJ: Bilirubin metabolism and hyperbilirubinemia. Harrison's Principles of Internal Medicine, 12th ed. Wilson JD, Braunwald E, Isselbacher KJ, et al, Eds. McGraw-Hill, New York, 1991, p 1320

105. Watson CJ: Prognosis and treatment of hepatic insufficiency. Ann Intern Med 31:405, 1959

106. Sherlock S: Jaundice. Diseases of the Liver and Biliary System, 8th ed. Sherlock S, Ed. Blackwell Scientific Publications, Oxford, 1989, p 230

107. Gollan JL, Keefe EB, Scharschmidt BF: Cholestasis and hyperbilirubinemia. Current Hepatology, Vol I. Gitnick G, Ed. Houghton Mifflin, Boston, 1980, p 277

108. Bosma PJ, Chowdhury JR, Bakker C, et al: The genetic basis of the reduced expression of bilirubin UCP-glucuronosyltransferase 1 in Gilbert's syndrome. N Engl J Med 333:1171, 1995

109. O'Grady JG, Portmann B, Williams R: Fulminant hepatic failure. Diseases of the Liver, 7th ed. Schiff L, Schiff ER, Eds. JB Lippincott Co, Philadelphia, 1993, p 1077

110. Bismuth H, Samuel D, Castaing D, et al: Orthotopic liver transplantation in fulminant and subfulminant hepatitis. Ann Surg 222:109, 1995

111. Boyer JL, Reuben A: Chronic hepatitis. Diseases of the Liver, 7th ed. Schiff L, Schiff ER, Eds. JB Lippincott Co, Philadelphia, 1993, p 586

112. Pugh RN, Murray-Lyon IM, Dawson JL, et al: Transection of the esophagus for bleeding esophageal varices. Br J Surg 60:646, 1973

113. Fallon MB, Anderson JM, Boyer JL: Intrahepatic cholestasis. Diseases of the Liver, 7th ed. Schiff L, Schiff ER, Eds. JB Lippincott Co, Philadelphia, 1993, p 343

Acknowledgment

Figure 2c From *MRI of the Abdomen and Pelvis: A Text-Atlas*, by R. C. Semelka, S. M. Asher, and C. Reinhold. John Wiley and Sons, New York, 1997. Used with permission.

5 INTESTINAL OBSTRUCTION

W. Scott Helton, M.D., F.A.C.S.

Assessment of Intestinal Obstruction

Intestinal obstruction is a common medical problem and accounts for a large percentage of surgical admissions for acute abdominal pain [*see 3:1 Acute Abdominal Pain*].[1] It develops when air and secretions are prevented from passing aborally as a result of either intrinsic or extrinsic compression (i.e., mechanical obstruction) or gastrointestinal paralysis (i.e., non-mechanical obstruction in the form of ileus or pseudo-obstruction). Small intestinal ileus is the most common form of intestinal obstruction; it occurs after most abdominal operations and is a common response to acute extra-abdominal medical conditions and intra-abdominal inflammatory conditions [*see Table 1*]. Mechanical small bowel obstruction is somewhat less common; such obstruction is secondary to intra-abdominal adhesions, hernias, or cancer in about 90% of cases [*see Table 2*]. Mechanical colonic obstruction accounts for only 10% to 15% of all cases of mechanical obstruction and most often develops in response to obstructing carcinoma, diverticulitis, or volvulus [*see Table 3*]. Acute colonic pseudo-obstruction occurs most frequently in the postoperative period or in response to another acute medical illness.

In what follows, several different methods of classifying mechanical obstruction are used: acute versus chronic, partial versus complete, simple versus closed-loop, and gangrenous versus nongangrenous. The importance of these classifications is that the natural history of the condition, its response to treatment, and the associated morbidity and mortality all vary according to which type of obstruction is present.

When chyme and gas can traverse the point of obstruction, obstruction is partial; when this is not the case, obstruction is complete. When the bowel is occluded at a single point along the intestinal tract, leading to intestinal dilatation, hypersecretion, and bacterial overgrowth proximal to the obstruction and decompression distal to the obstruction, simple obstruction is present. When a segment of bowel is occluded at two points along its course by a single constrictive lesion that occludes both the proximal and the distal end of the intestinal loop as well as traps the bowel's mesentery, closed-loop obstruction is present. When the blood supply to a closed-loop segment of bowel becomes compromised, leading to ischemia and eventually to bowel wall necrosis and perforation, strangulation is present. The most common causes of simple obstruction are intra-abdominal adhesions, tumors, and strictures; the most common causes of closed-loop obstruction are hernias, adhesions, and volvulus.

One of the most difficult tasks in general surgery is deciding when to operate on a patient with intestinal obstruction. The purpose of the following discussion is to outline a safe, efficient, and cost-effective stepwise approach to making this often difficult decision and to optimizing the management of patients with this problem. Absolutes are few and far between: treatment must always be highly individualized. Consequently, the following recommendations are intended only as guidelines, not as surgical dicta.

History and Clinical Setting

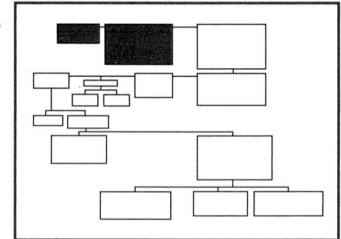

When a patient complains of acute obstipation, abdominal pain and distention, nausea, and vomiting, the probability that either mechanical bowel obstruction or ileus is present is very high.[2] Mechanical obstruction can often be distinguished from ileus or pseudo-obstruction on the basis of the location, character, and severity of abdominal pain. Pain from mechanical obstruction is usually located in the middle of the abdomen, whereas pain from ileus and pseudo-obstruction is diffuse. Pain from ileus is usually mild, and pain from obstruction is typically more severe. In general, pain increases in severity and depth over time as obstruction progresses; however, in mechanical obstruction, pain severity may decrease over time as a result of bowel fatigue and atony. The periodicity of pain can help localize the level of obstruction: pain from proximal intestinal obstruction has a short periodicity (3 to 4 minutes), and distal small bowel or colonic pain has longer intervals (15 to 20 minutes) between episodes of nausea, cramping, and vomiting.

Abdominal distention, nausea, and vomiting usually develop after pain has already been felt for some time. The patient should be asked what degree of abdominal distention is present and whether there has been a sudden or rapid change. Distention developing over many weeks suggests a chronic process or progressive partial obstruction. Massive abdominal distention coupled with minimal crampy pain, nausea, and vomiting suggests long-standing intermittent mechanical obstruction or some form of chronic intestinal pseudo-obstruction. The combination of a gradual change in bowel habits, progressive abdominal distention, early satiety, mild crampy pain after meals, and weight loss also suggests chronic partial mechanical bowel obstruction. If the patient has undergone evaluation for similar symptoms before, any previous abdominal radiographs or contrast studies should be reviewed. The patient should be asked when flatus was last passed: failure to pass flatus may signal a transition from partial to complete bowel obstruction. Patients with an intestinal

Table 1 Causes of Ileus

Intra-abdominal causes
  Intraperitoneal problems
    Peritonitis or abscess
    Inflammatory condition
      Mechanical: operation, foreign body
      Chemical: gastric juice, bile, blood
      Autoimmune: serositis, vasculitis
    Intestinal ischemia: arterial or venous, sickle-cell disease
  Retroperitoneal problems
    Pancreatitis
    Retroperitoneal hematoma
    Spine fracture
    Aortic operation
    Renal colic
    Pyelonephritis
    Metastasis

Extra-abdominal causes
  Thoracic problems
    Myocardial infarction
    Pneumonia
    Congestive heart failure
    Rib fractures
  Metabolic abnormalities
    Electrolyte imbalance (e.g., hypokalemia)
    Sepsis
    Lead poisoning
    Porphyria
    Hypothyroidism
    Hypoparathyroidism
    Uremia
  Medicines
    Opiates
    Anticholinergics
    Alpha agonists
    Antihistamines
    Catecholamines
  Spinal cord injury or operations
  Head, thoracic, or retroperitoneal trauma
  Chemotherapy, radiation therapy

read the operative report, which can provide a great deal of helpful information (e.g., description of adhesions, assessment of their severity, and evaluation of intra-abdominal pathology and anatomy). If abdominal cancer was present, one should find out what operation was performed and attempt to determine the likelihood of intra-abdominal recurrence.

The clinical setting often provides clues to the cause and type of bowel obstruction. In hospitalized patients, there is likely to be an associated medical condition or metabolic derangement that led to obstruction. A thorough review of the patient's medical history and hospital course should be undertaken to identify precipitating events that could have led to intestinal obstipation. One should ask the patient about any previous abdominal irradiation and should note and take into account all medications the patient is taking, especially anticoagulants and agents with anticholinergic side effects. Patients who are receiving chemotherapy or have undergone abdominal radiation therapy are prone to ileus. Severe infection, fluid and electrolyte imbalances, narcotic and anticholinergic medications, and intra-abdominal inflammation of any origin may be implicated. Acute massive abdominal distention in a hospitalized patient usually results from acute gastric distention, small bowel ileus, or acute colonic pseudo-obstruction. Excessive anticoagulation can lead to retroperitoneal, intra-abdominal, or intramural hematoma that can cause mechanical obstruction or ileus. Finally, there are specific problems that tend to arise in the postoperative period; these are discussed more fully elsewhere [*see* Urgent Operation, Early Postoperative Technical Complications, *and* No Operation, Early Postoperative Obstruction, *below*].

Table 2 Causes of Small Bowel Obstruction in Adults

Extrinsic causes
  Adhesions*
  Hernias (external, internal, incisional)*
  Metastatic cancer*
  Volvulus
  Intra-abdominal abscess
  Intra-abdominal hematoma
  Pancreatic pseudocyst
  Intra-abdominal drains
  Tight fascial opening at stoma

Intraluminal causes
  Tumors*
  Gallstones
  Foreign body
  Worms
  Bezoars

Intramural abnormalities
  Tumors
  Strictures
  Hematoma
  Intussusception
  Regional enteritis
  Radiation enteritis

*Approximately 85% of all small bowel obstructions are secondary to adhesions, hernias, or tumors.

stoma (ileostomy or colostomy) who present with signs and symptoms of obstruction often report abdominal distention and pain after a sudden change in stomal output of stool, liquid, or air.

The patient should also be asked about (1) previous episodes of bowel obstruction, (2) previous abdominal or pelvic operations, (3) a history of abdominal cancer, and (4) a history of intra-abdominal inflammation (e.g., inflammatory bowel disease, cholecystitis, pancreatitis, pelvic inflammatory disease, or abdominal trauma). Any of these factors increases the chance that the obstruction is secondary to an adhesion or recurrent cancer. Obstructive symptoms that come and go suddenly over several days in a patient older than 65 years should increase the index of suspicion for gallstone ileus.[3] If the patient has experienced episodes of obstruction before, one should ask about the etiology and the response to treatment. If the patient has ever undergone an abdominal operation, one should try to obtain and

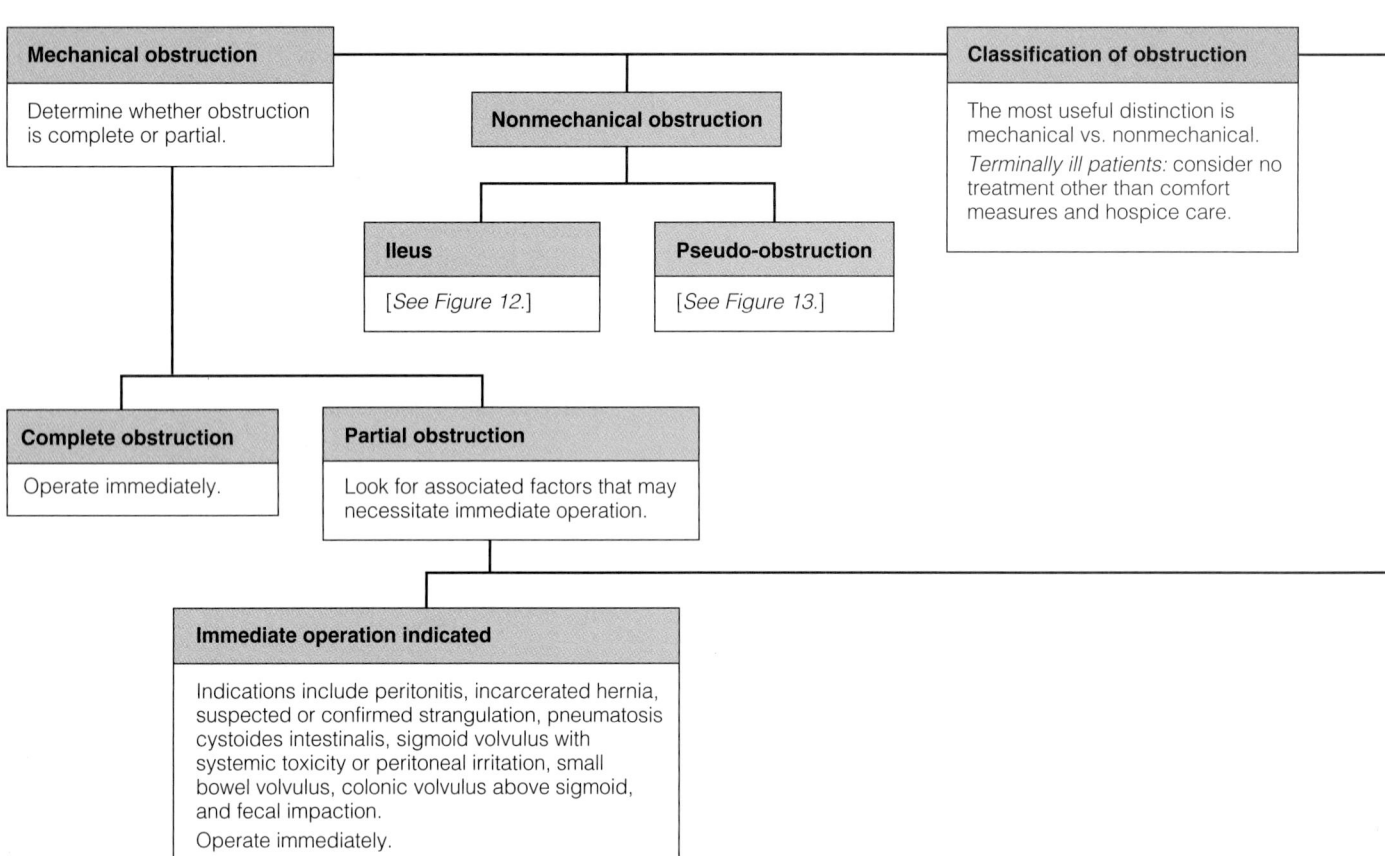

Signs and symptoms of intestinal obstruction

Signs and symptoms include abdominal pain or distention, nausea, vomiting, and obstipation.

Clinical history

Assess character, severity, location, and periodicity of pain.

Assess degree of abdominal distention, and ask about any sudden or rapid changes.

Ask about changes in bowel habits, weight loss, and last passage of flatus.

Ask about (1) previous obstruction, (2) previous abdominal or pelvic procedures, (3) abdominal cancer, (4) intra-abdominal inflammation.

Consider clinical setting: ask about medical conditions or metabolic derangements, exposure to radiation, all medications. Immediate postoperative state is special situation.

Mechanical obstruction

Determine whether obstruction is complete or partial.

Nonmechanical obstruction

Classification of obstruction

The most useful distinction is mechanical vs. nonmechanical.

Terminally ill patients: consider no treatment other than comfort measures and hospice care.

Ileus

[*See Figure 12.*]

Pseudo-obstruction

[*See Figure 13.*]

Complete obstruction

Operate immediately.

Partial obstruction

Look for associated factors that may necessitate immediate operation.

Immediate operation indicated

Indications include peritonitis, incarcerated hernia, suspected or confirmed strangulation, pneumatosis cystoides intestinalis, sigmoid volvulus with systemic toxicity or peritoneal irritation, small bowel volvulus, colonic volvulus above sigmoid, and fecal impaction.

Operate immediately.

Assessment of Intestinal Obstruction

Urgent operation

Indications include
- Lack of response to 24–48 hr of nonoperative therapy (increasing abdominal pain, distention, or tenderness; NG aspirate changing from nonfeculent to feculent; ↑ proximal small bowel distention with ↓ distal gas).
- Early technical complications of operation (abscess, phlegmon, hematoma, hernia, intussusception, anastomotic obstruction).

Physical exam and resuscitate as necessary

Develop gestalt of patient's illness, and assess patient's vital signs, hydration, and cardiopulmonary system.

Place NG tube, Foley catheter, and I.V. line immediately. Assess volume and character of NG aspirate, and measure urine output.

Replace lost fluid with isotonic saline or lactated Ringer solution. Look for signs of abscess, pneumonia, or myocardial infarction, and be alert for dyspnea, labored breathing, or jaundice.

Perform systematic abdominal examination: observation → auscultation → palpation and percussion. Look for abdominal masses, tenderness, incisions, and hernias; assess bowel sounds; examine rectum for masses, fecal impaction, and occult blood.

Investigative studies

Obtain chest x-rays and abdominal films.

If uncertainty about presence or nature of colonic obstruction remains, perform sigmoidoscopy and barium enema examination.

Measure serum electrolytes and creatinine, determine hematocrit, and order coagulation profile. If ileus is suspected, measure serum magnesium and calcium and order urinalysis.

Perform CT (with oral or I.V. contrast agents), abdominal ultrasonography, or both.

Immediate operation not indicated

Manage initially with nonoperative measures.

Reassess patient every 4 hours.

For partial obstruction, consider administering oral diatrizoate meglumine.

Look for changes in pain, abdominal findings, and volume and character of NG aspirate.

Repeat abdominal x-rays, and look for changes in gas distribution, pneumatosis cystoides intestinalis, and free intraperitoneal air.

Classify patient's condition as improved, unchanged, or worse.

Decide whether operative treatment is necessary and, if so, whether it should be done on urgent or elective basis.

Arrival of contrast agent in right colon within 24 hr is highly predictive of successful resolution of adhesive obstruction without operation.

No operation

Conditions that typically resolve with nonoperative therapy include adhesive obstruction (unless it does not improve in 12 hr), early postoperative obstruction (unless it does not improve in 2 wk), and various inflammatory conditions (IBD, radiation enteritis, diverticulitis, acute Crohn disease).

Elective operation

Indications include nontoxic, nontender sigmoid volvulus with sigmoidoscopically managed obstruction; recurrent adhesive or stricture-related small bowel obstruction; partial colonic obstruction unresponsive to 24 hr of nonoperative therapy; development and resolution of small bowel obstruction in patient who has never undergone abdominal operation.

305

Table 3 Causes of Colonic Obstruction

Common causes
- Cancer (primary, anastomotic, metastatic)
- Volvulus
- Diverticulitis
- Pseudo-obstruction
- Hernia
- Anastomotic stricture

Unusual causes
- Intussusception
- Fecal impaction
- Strictures (from one of the following)
  - Inflammatory bowel disease
  - Endometriosis
  - Radiation therapy
  - Ischemia
- Foreign body
- Extrinsic compression by a mass
  - Pancreatic pseudocyst
  - Hematoma
  - Metastasis
  - Primary tumors

Physical Examination and Resuscitation

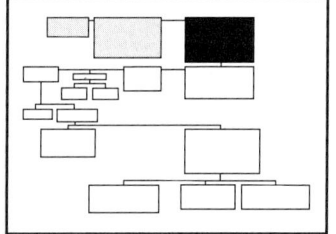

The initial steps in the physical examination are (1) developing a gestalt of the patient's illness and (2) assessing the patient's vital signs, hydration status, and cardiopulmonary system. A nasogastric tube, a Foley catheter, and an I.V. line are placed immediately while the physical examination is in progress. The volume and character of the gastric aspirate and urine are noted. A clear, gastric effluent is suggestive of gastric outlet obstruction. A bilious, nonfeculent aspirate is a typical sign of medial to proximal small bowel obstruction or colonic obstruction with a competent ileocecal valve. A feculent aspirate is a typical sign of distal small bowel obstruction. Volume replacement, if necessary, is initiated with isotonic saline solution or lactated Ringer solution. Urine output must be adequate (at least 0.5 ml/kg/hr) before the patient can be taken to the OR; supplemental potassium chloride (40 mEq/L) is administered once this is achieved.

Fever may be present, suggesting that the obstruction may be a manifestation of an intra-abdominal abscess. Signs of pneumonia or myocardial infarction should be sought: these conditions, like intestinal obstruction, can have upper abdominal pain, distention, nausea, and vomiting as presenting symptoms. Dyspnea and labored breathing may occur secondary to severe abdominal distention or pain, in which case immediate relief should be provided by placing the patient in the lateral decubitus position and offering narcotics as soon as the initial physical examination is performed. Jaundice raises the possibility of gallstone ileus or metastatic cancer.

Examination of the abdomen proceeds in an orderly manner from observation to auscultation to palpation and percussion. The patient is placed in the supine position with the legs flexed at the hip to decrease tension on the rectus muscles. The degree of abdominal distention observed varies, depending on the level of obstruction: proximal obstructions may cause little or no distention. Abdominal scars should be noted. Abdominal asymmetry or a protruding mass suggests an underlying malignancy, an abscess, or closed-loop obstruction. The abdominal wall should be observed for evidence of peristaltic waves, which are indicative of acute small bowel obstruction.

Auscultation should be performed for at least 3 to 4 minutes to determine the presence and quality of bowel sounds. High-pitched bowel tones, tingles, and rushes are suggestive of an obstructive process, especially when temporally associated with waves of crampy pain, nausea, or vomiting. The absence of bowel tones is typical of intestinal paralysis but may also indicate intestinal fatigue from long-standing obstruction, closed-loop obstruction, or pseudo-obstruction.

Approximately 70% of patients with bowel obstruction have symmetric tenderness, whereas fewer than 50% have rebound tenderness, guarding, or rigidity.[2] The traditional teaching is that localized tenderness and guarding indicate underlying strangulated bowel; however, prospective studies have demonstrated that these physical findings are neither specific nor sensitive for detecting underlying strangulation[4] or even obstruction.[2] Nevertheless, most surgeons still believe that guarding, rebound tenderness, and localized tenderness reflect underlying strangulation and therefore are indications for operation. Patients with ileus tend to have generalized abdominal tenderness that cannot be distinguished from the tenderness of mechanical obstruction. Gentle percussion is performed over all quadrants of the abdomen to search for areas of dullness (suggestive of an underlying mass), tympany (suggestive of underlying distended bowel), and peritoneal irritation.

A thorough search is made for inguinal, femoral, umbilical, and incisional hernias. The rectum is examined for masses, fecal impaction, and occult blood. If the patient has an ileostomy or a colostomy, the stoma is examined digitally to make sure that there is no obstruction at the level of the fascia.

Investigative Studies

IMAGING STUDIES

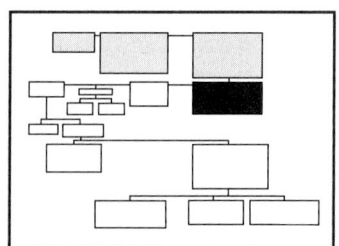

One should obtain a chest x-ray in all patients with bowel obstruction to exclude a pneumonic process and to look for subdiaphragmatic air. In most cases, supine, upright, or lateral decubitus films of the abdomen can distinguish the type of obstruction present (mechanical or nonmechanical, partial or complete) and establish the location of the obstruction (stomach, small bowel, or colon). A useful technique for evaluating abdominal radiographs is to look systematically for intestinal gas along the normal route of the GI tract, beginning at the stomach, continuing through the small bowel, and, finally, following the course of the colon to the rectum. The following questions should be kept in mind as this is done.

- Are there abnormally dilated loops of bowel, signs of small bowel dilatation, or air-fluid levels?

- Are air-fluid levels and bowel loops in the same place on supine and upright films?

- Is there gas throughout the entire length of the colon (suggestive of ileus or partial mechanical obstruction)?

- Is there a paucity of distal colonic gas or an abrupt cutoff of colonic gas with proximal colonic distention and air-fluid levels (suggestive of complete or near-complete colonic obstruction)?

- Is there evidence of strangulation (e.g., thickened small bowel loops, mucosal thumb printing, pneumatosis cystoides intestinalis, or free peritoneal air)?

- Is there massive distention of the colon, especially of the cecum or sigmoid (suggestive of either volvulus or pseudo-obstruction)?

- Are there any biliary or renal calculi, and is there any air in the biliary tree (suggestive of gallstone ileus[5] or a renal stone that could be causing ileus)?

It is important to be able to distinguish between small and large bowel gas. Gas in a distended small bowel outlines the valvulae conniventes, which traverse the entire diameter of the bowel lumen [see Figure 1]. Gas in a distended colon, on the other hand, outlines the colonic haustral markings, which cross only part of the bowel lumen and typically interdigitate [see Figures 2 and 3]. Distended small bowel loops usually occupy the central abdomen [see Figure 1], whereas distended large bowel loops are typically seen around the periphery [see Figure 2]. In patients with ileus, distention usually extends uniformly throughout the stomach, the small bowel, and the colon [see Figure 3], and air-fluid levels may be found in the colon and the small intestine.

Patients with gastric outlet obstruction or gastric atony typically have a giant gastric bubble if no nasogastric tube has been placed, with little or no air in the small bowel or the colon. Patients with mechanical small bowel obstruction usually have multiple air-fluid levels, with distended bowel loops of varying sizes arranged in an inverted U configuration [see Figure 4]. A dilated loop of small bowel appearing in the same location on supine and upright films suggests obstruction of a fixed segment of bowel by an adhesion [see Figures 1 and 4]. Small bowel obstruction is often accompanied by a paucity of gas in the colon. The complete absence of colonic gas is strongly suggestive of complete small bowel obstruction; however, the presence of colonic gas does not exclude complete small bowel obstruction, in that there may have been unevacuated gas distal to a point of complete obstruction before the radiograph was taken. On the other hand, if repeat radiographs demonstrate decreased or absent colonic or rectal gas in a patient with small bowel obstruction who previously had more colonic or rectal gas, it is probable that partial obstruction has become complete, and immediate operation is almost always indicated. High-grade obstruction of the colon with an incompetent ileocecal valve may manifest itself as distended small bowel loops with air-fluid levels, thereby mimicking small bowel obstruction. Hence, it is sometimes necessary to perform a barium enema to exclude colonic obstruction.

Massive gaseous distention of the colon is usually secondary to distal colonic or rectal obstruction, volvulus, or pseudo-obstruction [see Figures 2, 5a, 5b, 6a, 6b, and 7]. There are well-defined radiographic criteria that are highly sensitive and specific for sigmoid volvulus.[5] If there is any uncertainty regarding the presence, type, or level of colonic obstruction, immediate sigmoidoscopy followed by barium enema is diagnostic.

LABORATORY STUDIES

Serum electrolyte concentrations, the hematocrit, the serum creatinine concentration, and the coagulation profile (prothrombin time [or international normalized ratio—INR] and platelet count) are helpful in determining the severity of volume

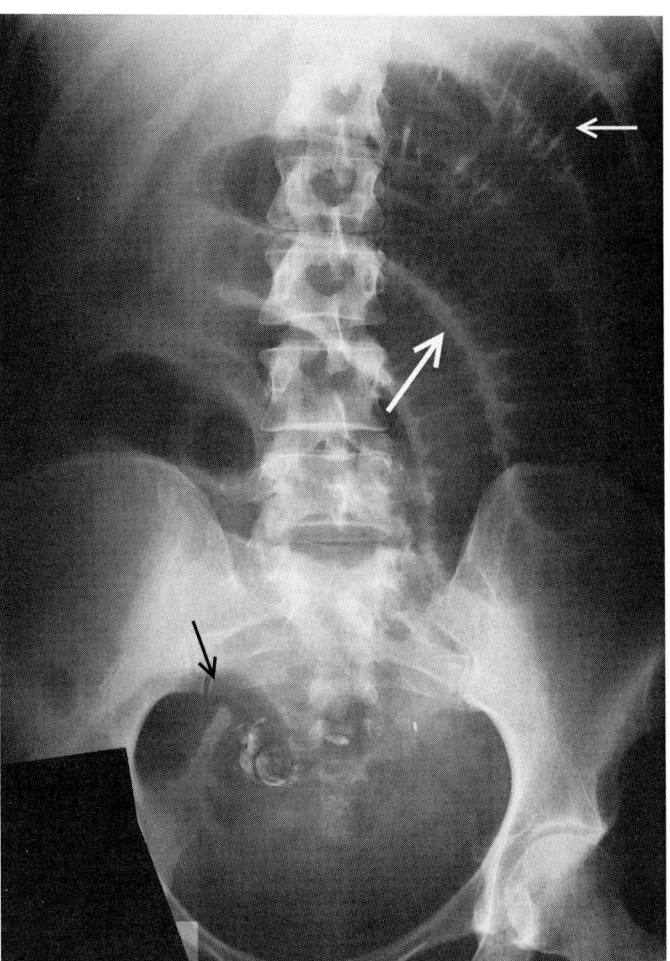

Figure 1 Supine radiograph from a patient with complete small bowel obstruction shows distended small bowel loops in the central abdomen with prominent valvulae conniventes (small white arrow). Bowel wall between the loops is thickened and edematous (large white arrow). No air is seen in the colon or the rectum. Note the presence of an isolated small bowel loop in the right lower quadrant (black arrow), which is seen fixed in the same location on upright films, as shown in Figure 4.

depletion and guiding resuscitative efforts. If ileus is suspected, serum magnesium and calcium levels should be measured, and urinalysis should be done to check for hematuria.

Determination of Need for Operation and Classification of Obstruction

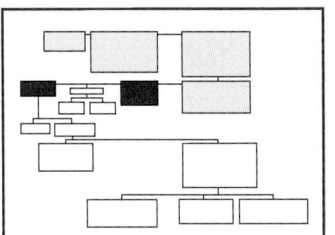

The combination of a thorough history, a carefully performed physical examination, and correctly interpreted abdominal radiographs usually allows one to identify the type of bowel obstruction present and to decide whether a patient requires immediate, urgent, or delayed operation [see Table 4] or can safely be treated initially with nonoperative measures. To this end, it is particularly important and useful to stratify patients into those with mechanical obstruction and those with nonmechanical obstruction. In patients with mechanical bowel obstruction,

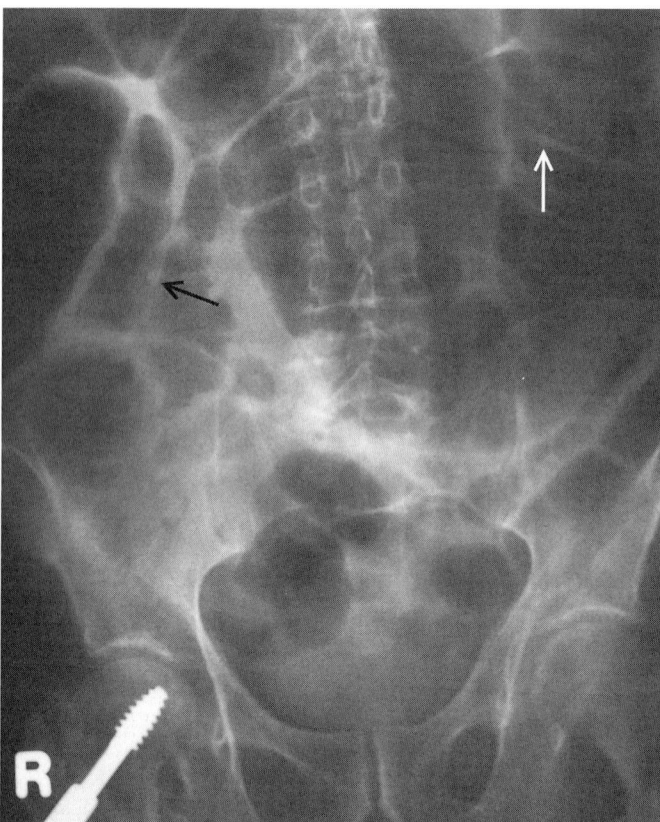

Figure 2 Radiograph from a patient with acute colonic pseudo-obstruction shows a dilated colon with haustral markings (white arrow) and edematous small bowel loops (black arrow). Air extends down to the distal sigmoid. This picture is also consistent with rectal obstruction, which could have been excluded by rigid sigmoidoscopy.

an effort should be made to determine whether the obstruction is complete or partial. Except for a few clinical situations, patients with complete bowel obstruction require immediate operation; conversely, patients with partial bowel obstruction rarely do. Finally, an effort should be made to establish the level and cause of obstruction because these factors often help guide therapy and affect the probability of success in response to specific therapeutic intervention. Patients with nonmechanical obstruction, which derives from ileus or pseudo-obstruction [*see* Ileus and Pseudo-obstruction, *below*], do not require immediate operation.

ADJUNCTIVE TESTS FOR EQUIVOCAL SITUATIONS

Sigmoidoscopy

When one is uncertain whether the obstruction is mechanical or not on the basis of the information in hand, additional diagnostic measures are immediately indicated. When large amounts of colonic air extend down to the rectum, flexible or rigid sigmoidoscopy will readily exclude a rectal or distal sigmoid obstruction. If sigmoidoscopy yields normal findings and partial colonic obstruction is the most likely diagnosis, a barium enema with

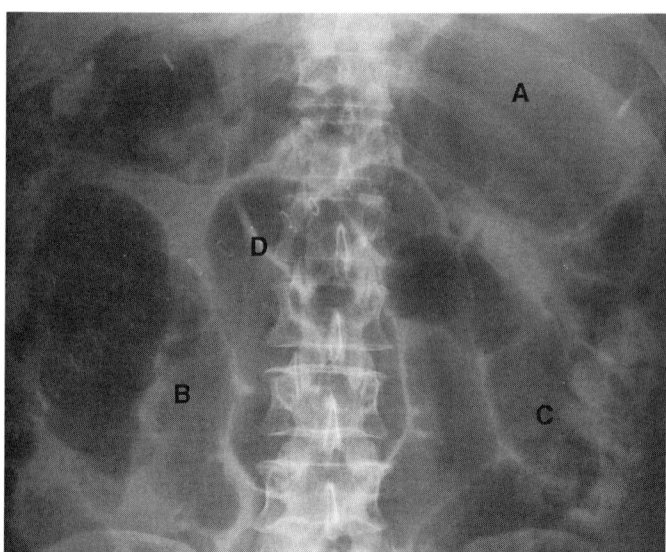

Figure 3 Radiograph from a patient with postoperative ileus shows massive gastric distention (A), distended small bowel loops (B), air throughout the colon, mild dilatation of the sigmoid colon (C) with air mixed with stool, and a haustral fold in the apex of the sigmoid colon (D).

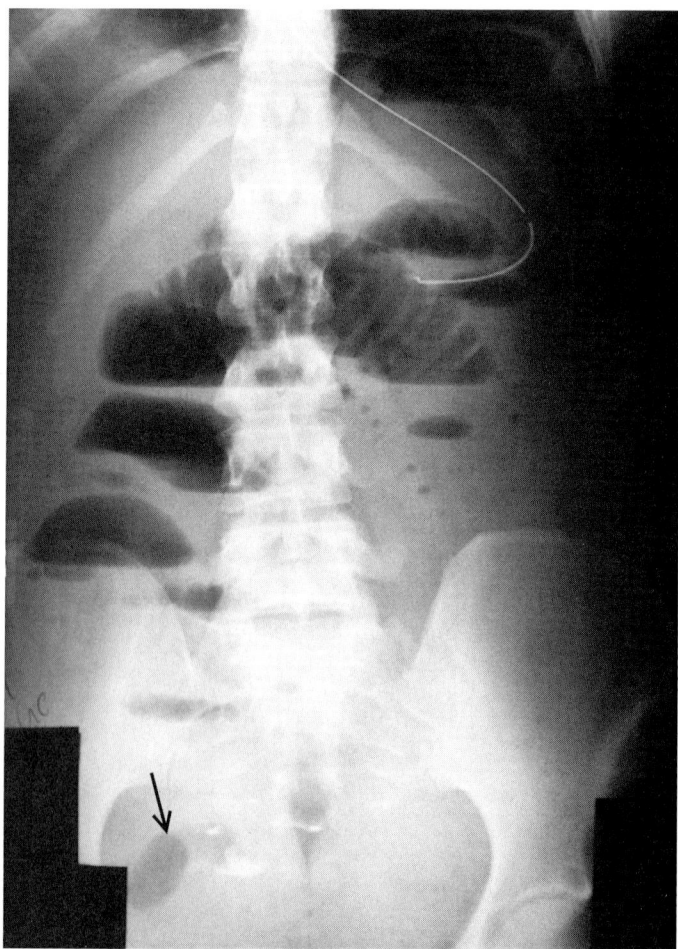

Figure 4 Upright radiograph from the same patient as the supine radiograph in Figure 1 shows multiple air-fluid levels of varying size arranged in inverted U's. In the right lower pelvis, a loop of small bowel is seen in exactly the same location as on the supine abdominal film (black arrow), a finding suggestive of adhesive obstruction.

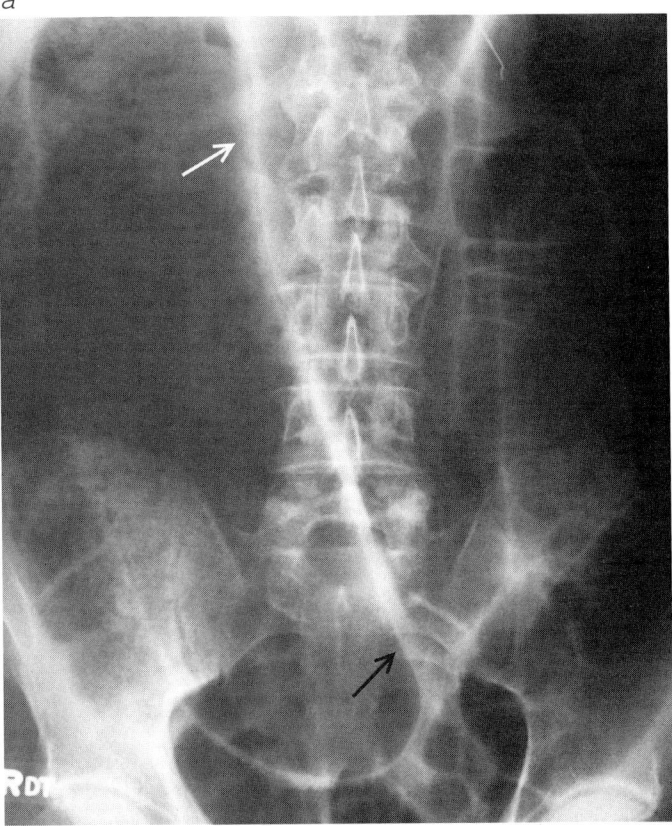

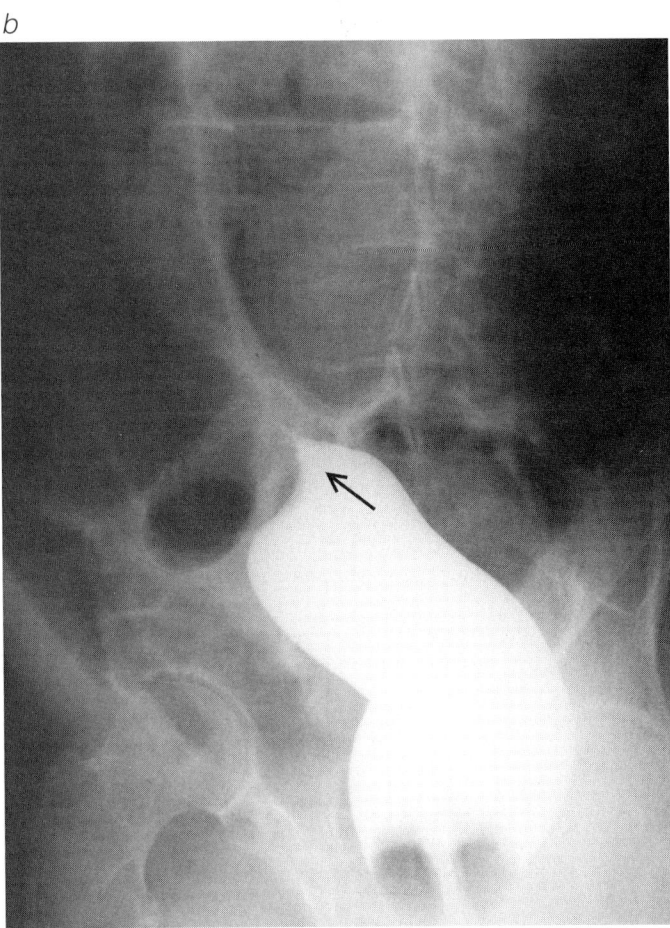

water-soluble contrast material should immediately be performed.[6] Abdominal ultrasonography, though not as definitive as a contrast examination, is also able to diagnose suspected colonic obstruction in 85% of patients.[7]

Ultrasonography and CT Scanning

Abdominal radiographs can be entirely normal in patients with complete, closed-loop, or strangulation obstruction.[8] Therefore, if the patient's clinical profile and the results of physical examination are consistent with intestinal obstruction despite normal abdominal radiographs, abdominal ultrasonography or CT scanning should be performed immediately.[8-15] Both of these imaging modalities are highly sensitive and specific for intestinal obstruction when performed properly and interpreted by experienced clinicians. Two prospective clinical trials found ultrasonography to be as sensitive as and more specific than abdominal radiography in diagnosing intestinal obstruction.[16,17] Both ultrasonography and CT are capable of detecting the cause of the obstruction as well as the presence of closed-loop or strangulation obstruction.[7,9,14,15,18-21] Sonographic criteria have been established for small bowel and colonic obstruction[7,18,19]: (1) simultaneous observation of distended and collapsed bowel segments, (2) free peritoneal fluid, (3) inspissated intestinal contents, (4) paradoxical pendulating peristalsis, (5) highly reflective fluid within the bowel lumen, (6) bowel wall edema between serosa and mucosa, and (7) a fixed mass of aperistaltic, fluid-filled, dilated intestinal loops. One group of authors has recommended that when abdominal radiographs are inconclusive or normal in patients with suspected colonic obstruction, ultrasonography, rather than CT or barium enema, should be the next diagnostic step.[7] Ultrasonography is well suited to critically ill patients: because it can be performed at the bedside, the risk associated with transport to the radiology suite is avoided. Given that ultrasonography is relatively inexpensive, is easy and quick to perform, and often can provide a great deal of information about the location, nature, and severity of the obstruction, it should be employed early on in the evaluation of all patients with intestinal obstruction.[16]

Several authors have recommended that patients with suspected small bowel obstruction and equivocal plain abdominal films undergo CT scanning before a small bowel contrast series is ordered.[10-13] CT scanning has several advantages over a small bowel contrast examination in this setting: (1) it can ascertain the level of obstruction, (2) it can assess the severity of the obstruction and determine its cause, and (3) it can detect closed-loop obstruction and early strangulation [*see Figures 8, 9, 10, and 11*]. CT can also detect inflammatory or neoplastic processes both outside and inside the peritoneal cavity and can visualize small amounts of intraperitoneal air or pneumatosis cystoides intestinalis not seen on conventional films [*see Figure 10*]. Prospective studies have demonstrated that the accuracy of CT in diagnosing bowel obstruction is higher than 95% and its sensitivity and specificity are each higher than 94%.[20,21] When CT scanning is nondiagnostic in a patient with suspected bowel obstruction, a small bowel follow-through examination with dilute barium is often useful.[13]

Figure 5 (*a*) **Radiograph from a patient with massive sigmoid volvulus shows a distended ahaustral sigmoid loop (white arrow), inferior convergence of the walls of the sigmoid loop to the left of the midline, and approximation of the medial walls of the sigmoid loop as a summation line (black arrow). (*b*) Barium enema of the colon shows a tapered obstruction at the rectosigmoid junction with a typical bird's-beak deformity (black arrow).**

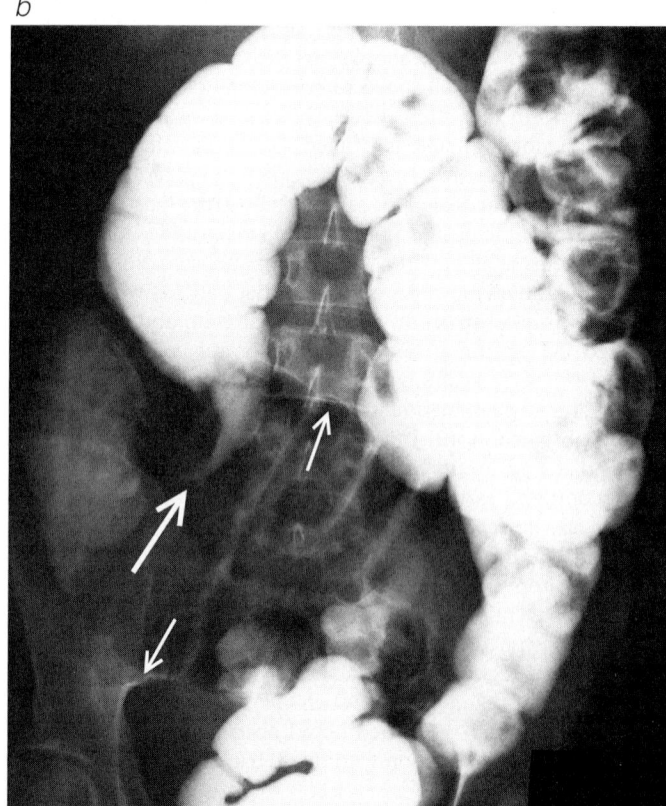

a

b

Figure 6 (*a*) Radiograph from a patient with cecal volvulus shows a dilated cecum with no air distally in the colorectum. Convergence of the medial walls of the loop (black arrow) points to the right, a typical finding in cecal volvulus. (*b*) Barium examination demonstrates a bird's-beak deformity tapering at the point of volvulus (large white arrow). Note walls of dilated cecum (small white arrows).

Contrast Studies

Enteroclysis (direct injection of BaSO₄ into the small bowel) is generally considered the most sensitive method of distinguishing between ileus and partial mechanical small bowel obstruction: it has a diagnostic sensitivity of 87% for adhesive obstruction.[22,23] Many surgeons are concerned that injection of barium might cause partial obstruction to progress to complete obstruction; however, there is no evidence that this ever occurs, and one therefore should not refrain from using barium to diagnose partial small bowel obstruction.[24-27] If complete obstruction is identified, the patient should undergo immediate operation. If partial obstruction is identified in either the small or the large bowel, the patient is treated accordingly. If (1) mechanical obstruction is not identified and (2) a point of obstruction, as evidenced by the finding of both dilated and decompressed intestinal loops, cannot be identified through abdominal ultrasonography, CT scanning, or both, then the diagnosis is almost certainly ileus, in which case one's attention is directed toward identifying and correcting the underlying precipitating cause [*see Table 1 and* Mechanical Obstruction, No Operation, Adhesive Partial Small Bowel Obstruction, *below*].

Mechanical Obstruction

TERMINAL ILLNESS

Patients with a terminal illness (e.g., AIDS or advanced carcinomatosis) to whom surgical treatment offers little hope of improved quality or duration of life may choose not to undergo operative intervention for acute bowel obstruction. These patients should be offered comfort measures, including continuous morphine infusion, rehydration, and administration of antisecretory agents.[28-30] In some of these patients, endoscopic deployment of plastic stents may relieve high-grade partial obstruction, thus rendering laparotomy unnecessary.[31,32] Patients who do not wish to die of malignant bowel obstruction in a hospital should be offered hospice care or home visiting nurse services with continuous octreotide infusion, I.V. rehydration and gastrostomy decompression.[33,34] Two prospective, randomized clinical trials demonstrated that octreotide significantly attenuated the severity of nausea and vomiting and the degree of subjective discomfort in patients with inoperable obstruction and permitted the discontinuation of nasogastric tube decompression.[29,30] When long-term gastric decompression is required for palliation in a terminally ill patient, percutaneous endoscopic gastrostomy or jejunostomy should be considered [*see 3:8 Gastrointestinal Endoscopy*].[35] It is essential to always pay attention to quality-of-life issues and to the patient's potential interest in pursuing nonoperative forms of palliation. For many terminally ill or incurable patients with bowel obstruction, the most humane and sensible treatment comprises nothing more than instituting palliative measures such as those described.

IMMEDIATE OPERATION

All patients with complete bowel obstruction, whether of the small intestine or the large, should undergo immediate operation unless extraordinary circumstances (e.g., diffuse carcinomatosis, terminal illness, or sigmoid volvulus that responds

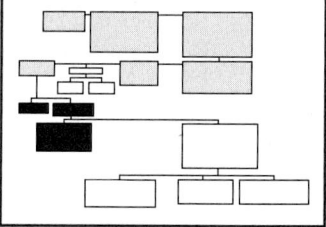

to sigmoidoscopic decompression) are present. If one attempts to manage complete intestinal obstruction nonoperatively, one risks delaying definitive treatment of patients with intestinal ischemia and subjecting them to significantly increased morbidity and mortality should perforation or severe infection develop.[4,36]

Immediate operation is also indicated when bowel obstruction is associated with peritonitis; incarcerated strangulated hernias; suspected or confirmed strangulation; pneumatosis cystoides intestinalis; sigmoid volvulus accompanied by systemic toxicity or peritoneal irritation; colonic volvulus above the sigmoid colon; or fecal impaction. These conditions will not resolve without operation and are associated with increased morbidity, mortality, and cost if diagnosis and treatment are delayed. The only time one would not operate immediately on any patient with one of these diagnoses is when the patient requires cardiopulmonary stabilization, additional resuscitation, or both. Whenever there is any doubt as to the presence of any of these conditions, additional diagnostic tests (e.g., ultrasonography, CT, or contrast studies) are indicated to confirm or exclude them.

Strangulation and Closed-Loop Obstruction

Morbidity and mortality from intestinal obstruction vary significantly and depend primarily on the presence of strangulation and subsequent infection. Strangulation obstruction occurs in approximately 10% of all patients with small intestinal obstruction. It carries a mortality of 10% to 37%, whereas simple obstruction carries a mortality of less than 5%.[4,24,37,38] Early recognition and immediate operative treatment of strangulation obstruction are the only current means of decreasing this mortality. Strangulation obstruction occurs most frequently in patients with incarcerated hernias, closed-loop obstruction, volvulus, or complete bowel obstruction; hence, identification of any of these specific causes of obstruction is an important and clear indication for immediate operation. Radiographic evidence of pneumatosis cystoides intestinalis or free intraperitoneal air in a patient with a clinical picture of bowel obstruction is indicative of strangulation, perforation, or both and constitutes an indication for operation. High-quality abdominal CT with I.V. contrast can detect advanced strangulation as well as identify early, reversible strangulation [see Figure 11].[12,14,15]

Abdominal ultrasonography can also identify edematous, hemorrhagic loops of intestine. Accordingly, whenever one is concerned about possible strangulation or closed-loop obstruction but is not yet committed to taking the patient immediately to the OR, an ultrasonogram or a CT scan should be obtained. In fact, given that ultrasonography and CT are the only well-established means of diagnosing strangulation obstruction short of exploratory laparotomy or laparoscopy, an argument can be made that one or the other should be performed in all patients who have been admitted to the hospital with bowel obstruction and are initially being treated nonoperatively.

Many surgeons base the decision whether to operate on patients with bowel obstruction on the presence or absence of the so-called classic signs of strangulation obstruction—continuous abdominal pain, fever, tachycardia, peritoneal signs, and leukocytosis—and on their clinical experience. Unfortunately, these classically taught signs, even in conjunction with abdominal x-rays and clinical judgment, are incapable of reliably detecting closed-loop or gangrenous bowel obstruction.[4,24,36,39] In fact, one prospective clinical trial concluded that the five classic signs of strangulation obstruction and experienced clinical judgment were not sensitive for, specific for, or predictive of strangulation[4]: in more than 50% of the patients who had intestinal strangulation, the condition was not recognized preoperatively. Such findings suggest that early nonoperative recognition of intestinal strangulation is not feasible without ultrasonography or CT.

Incarcerated or Strangulated Hernias

A hernia that is incarcerated, tender, erythematous, warm, or edematous is an indication for immediate operation. Primary or incisional hernias may not be palpable in obese patients, in which case ultrasonography or CT scanning should be performed.

Nonsigmoid Volvulus and Sigmoid Volvulus with Systemic Toxicity or Peritoneal Signs

All intestinal volvuli are closed-loop obstructions and thus carry a high risk of intestinal strangulation, infarction, and perforation. Patients typically present with acute, colicky abdominal pain, massive distention, nausea, and vomiting. Sigmoid volvulus is the most common form of colonic volvulus, followed by cecal volvulus. Abdominal radiographs are fairly diagnostic for colonic volvulus [see Figures 5a, 5b, 6a, and 6b]. In contrast, small bowel volvulus may not be visualized on plain radiographs, because the closed loop fills completely with fluid and no air-fluid level can be seen. Small bowel volvulus is readily detected by ultrasonography or CT scanning; one or both of these procedures should be performed in patients presenting with signs and symptoms of bowel obstruction and normal abdominal radiographs. Small bowel volvulus is an indication for immediate operation.

If one observes signs of systemic toxicity, a bloody rectal discharge, fever, leukocytosis, or peritoneal irritation in a patient with sigmoid volvulus, the patient should undergo immediate operation; if all of these signs are absent, the patient should undergo sigmoidoscopy. When there are no signs of peritonitis or generalized toxicity, sigmoidoscopic decompression is safe and effective in more than 95% of patients with sigmoid volvulus.[40] If mucosal gangrene or a bloody effluent is noted at the time of sigmoidoscopy, immediate operative intervention is nec-

---

Table 4 Guidelines for Operative and Nonoperative Therapy

Situations necessitating emergent operation
  Incarcerated, strangulated hernias
  Peritonitis
  Pneumatosis cystoides intestinalis
  Pneumoperitoneum
  Suspected or proven intestinal strangulation
  Closed-loop obstruction
  Nonsigmoid colonic volvulus
  Sigmoid volvulus associated with toxicity or peritoneal signs
  Complete bowel obstruction

Situations necessitating urgent operation
  Progressive bowel obstruction at any time after nonoperative measures are started
  Failure to improve with conservative therapy within 24–48 hr
  Early postoperative technical complications

Situations in which delayed operation is usually safe
  Immediate postoperative obstruction
  Sigmoid volvulus successfully decompressed by sigmoidoscopy
  Acute exacerbation of Crohn disease, diverticulitis, or radiation enteritis
  Chronic, recurrent partial obstruction
  Gastric outlet obstruction
  Postoperative adhesions
  Resolved partial colonic obstruction

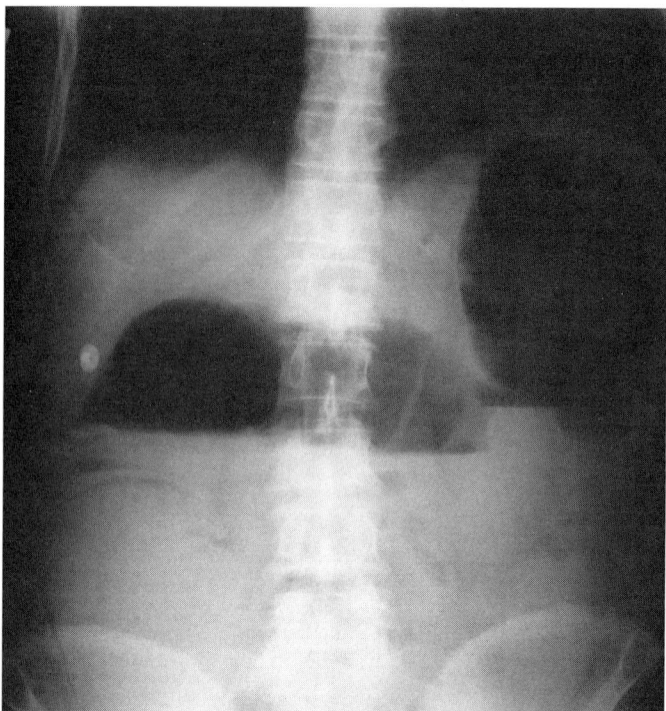

Figure 7 Shown is a radiograph from a patient with complete colonic obstruction from an obstructing carcinoma in the descending left colon with proximal air-fluid levels. The absence of air distally in the rectum or the sigmoid is suggestive of complete obstruction. The ileocecal valve is competent, and thus, there is no small bowel air.

elective bowel preparation and a single-stage sigmoid resection before being discharged from the hospital. If, however, clinical toxicity, a bloody rectal discharge, fever, or peritoneal irritation arises at any time after sigmoidoscopic decompression while the patient is being prepared for elective operation, immediate operation is indicated.

Patients with volvulus proximal to the sigmoid colon should undergo immediate operation regardless of whether peritoneal irritation is present. The incidence of strangulation infarction is high in such patients, and nonoperative therapy often fails. If the diagnosis of nonsigmoid colonic volvulus is in doubt, a barium enema is indicated to exclude colonic pseudo-obstruction.

Fecal Impaction

Complete colonic obstruction secondary to fecal impaction in the rectum can sometimes be successfully relieved through disimpaction at the bedside; however, this can be difficult and extremely uncomfortable for the patient. The most expeditious and successful method of relieving the obstruction is to disimpact the patient while he or she is under general or spinal anesthesia.

URGENT OPERATION

Lack of Response to Nonoperative Therapy within 24 to 48 Hours

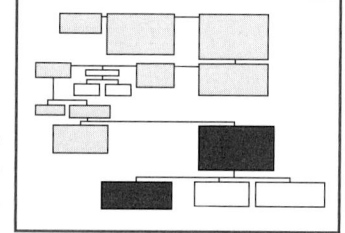

It is usually safe to manage partial bowel obstruction initially by nonoperative means: a nihil per os (NPO) regimen, nasogastric decompression, analgesics, and octreotide. Such therapy is successful in most cases, especially if the cause of

essary even in the absence of any clinical signs or symptoms of strangulation. After sigmoidoscopy, the patient can undergo

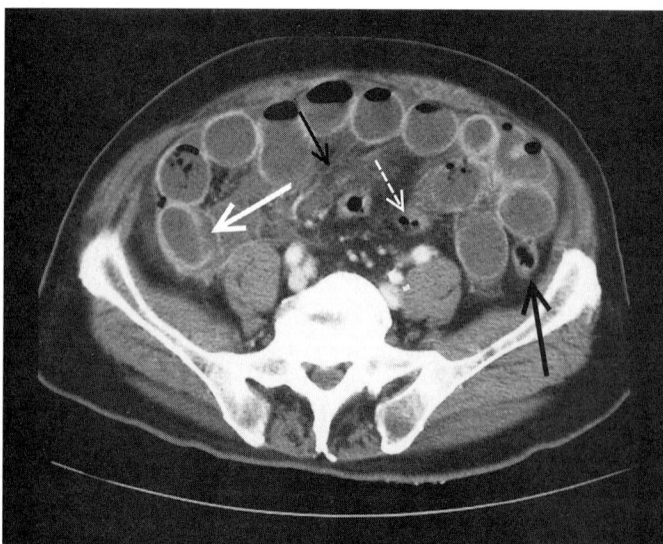

Figure 8 CT scan from a patient with partial small bowel obstruction shows distended, fluid-filled loops of small bowel with air-fluid levels, hyperemia, and bowel wall thickening (large white arrow). Note the discrepancy in caliber between dilated small bowel and decompressed small bowel (dashed white arrow) and the stranding (small black arrow) in the small bowel mesentery. Air in a decompressed descending colon (large black arrow) is indicative of partial obstruction.

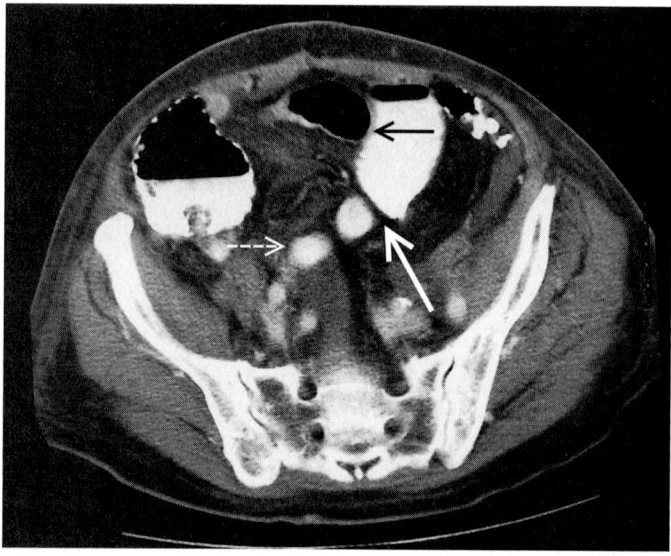

Figure 9 CT scan from a patient with adhesive partial small bowel obstruction shows massively dilated small intestine (black arrow) proximal to a thick adhesive band (large white arrow) and decompressed small bowel distal to the adhesion (dashed white arrow). The patient was operated on because of the low probability that this obstruction would resolve with conservative management.

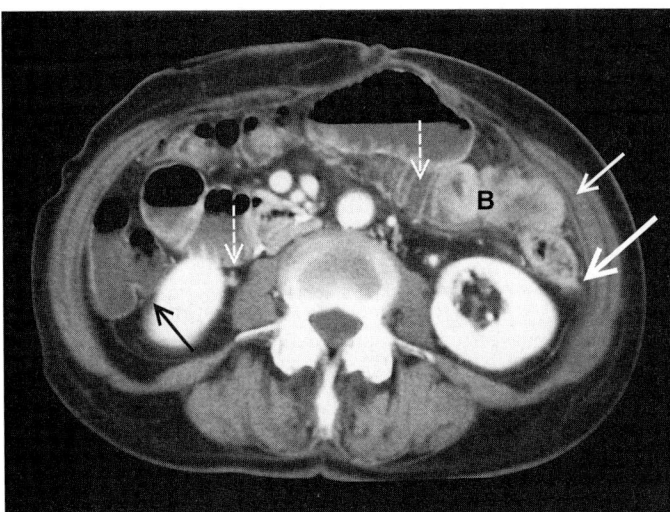

Figure 10 CT scan from a patient with partial small bowel obstruction from cancer shows distended small bowel (dashed white arrows) proximal to a mass (small white arrow). There is air in the cecum (black arrow), the transverse colon, and the descending colon (large white arrow). The small bowel is maximally dilated, with hyperemic, edematous bowel wall (B) just proximal to an obstructing recurrent colon carcinoma. Even though plain radiographs showed partial small bowel obstruction, this CT scan led to early operation because continued nonoperative management would not resolve the problem.

obstruction is from postoperative adhesions, but there is always the risk that complete bowel obstruction or strangulation already exists but is undetected. Furthermore, there is the risk that while the patient is being observed, partial obstruction will progress to complete obstruction or strangulation and perforation will develop. It is therefore crucial to be alert to changes in the patient's condition.

Repeated examination of the abdomen by the same clinician is the most sensitive way of detecting progressive obstruction. Examinations should be performed no less frequently than every 3 hours. If abdominal pain, tenderness, or distention increases or the gastric aspirate changes from nonfeculent to feculent, abdominal exploration is usually indicated. Abdominal radiographs should be repeated every 6 hours after nasogastric decompression and reviewed by the surgeon who is following the patient. If proximal small bowel distention increases or distal intestinal gas decreases, nonoperative therapy is less likely to be successful; in these circumstances, early operative intervention should be seriously considered. Conversely, if the patient's condition appears stable or improved and x-rays indicate that the obstruction either has resolved somewhat or at least is no worse, it is generally safe to continue nonoperative care for another 12 to 24 hours. If the clinical picture is stable after 24 hours of observation, one must decide whether to operate or to continue nonoperative therapy. One's clinical judgment and experience, coupled with a thorough and accurate assessment of the patient's underlying diagnosis and clinical condition, have traditionally been the most reliable guides for making this decision. Currently, however, it appears that the decision whether to operate can be made more cost-effectively and reliably on the basis of CT scans and contrast studies [*see* No Operation, Adhesive Partial Small Bowel Obstruction, *below*].

Early Postoperative Technical Complications

When normal bowel function initially returns after an abdominal operation but then is replaced by a clinical picture suggestive of early postoperative mechanical obstruction, the explanation may be a technical complication of the operation (e.g., phlegmon, abscess, intussusception, a narrow anastomosis, an internal hernia, or obstruction at the level of a stoma). An early, aggressive diagnostic workup should be performed to identify or exclude these problems because they are unlikely to respond to nasogastric decompression or other forms of conservative management. It is critical to know exactly what was done within the abdomen in the course of the operation. To this end, one should try to speak directly with the operating surgeon rather than attempt to deduce the needed information from the operative report.

If the patient had peritonitis or a colonic anastomosis at the initial operation, one should order a CT scan to look for an intra-abdominal abscess. An abscess or a phlegmon at the site of an anastomosis is usually secondary to anastomotic leakage and is an indication for reoperation. CT scanning can also identify intra-abdominal hematomas, which should be evacuated through early reoperation. In patients recovering from a proctectomy, herniation of the small bowel through a defect in the pelvic floor is a common cause of intestinal obstruction. Oral contrast studies can help identify patients with an internal hernia, intussusception, or anastomotic obstruction and should be performed after the CT scan. A retrograde barium examination should be performed in patients thought to have a problem related to a stoma or an intestinal anastomosis. When none of the above factors appears to be the cause of the postoperative obstruction, it is reasonable for the surgeon to assume that the obstruction is secondary to postoperative adhesions, which are best treated conservatively (see below).

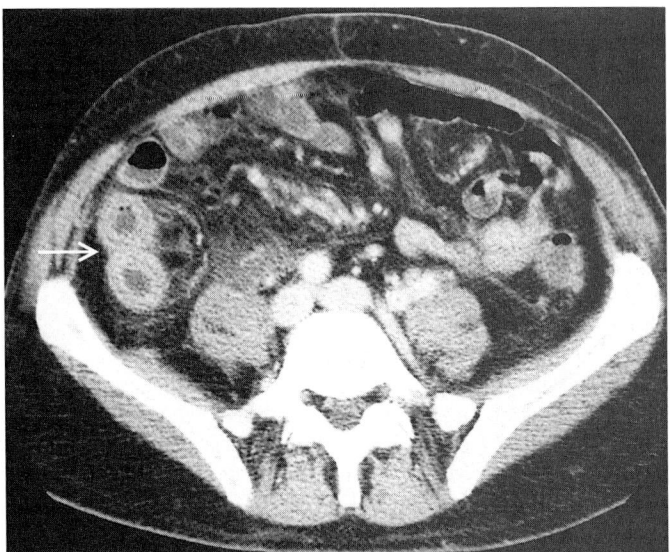

Figure 11 Early closed-loop small bowel obstruction CT scan from a patient with early closed-loop obstruction of the small intestine shows markedly edematous, hyperemic small bowel, a finding indicative of early strangulation (white arrow). The patient had minimal symptoms, and there was air in the transverse colon and the descending colon (a finding indicative of partial small bowel obstruction); however, the finding of gangrenous, nonperforated small bowel on this CT scan led to early operation.

NO OPERATION

In selected patients, nonoperative management of partial small bowel obstruction is highly successful and carries an acceptably low mortality. Such patients include those whose partial obstruction is secondary to intra-abdominal adhesions,

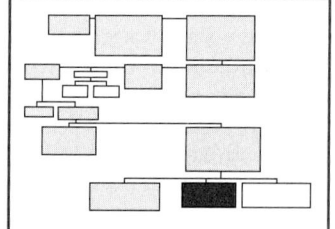

occurs in the immediate postoperative period, or derives from an inflammatory condition (e.g., inflammatory bowel disease, radiation enteritis, or diverticulitis).

Adhesive Partial Small Bowel Obstruction

Adhesive partial small bowel obstruction is treated initially with nasogastric decompression, I.V. rehydration, and analgesia. Parenteral nutrition should be begun if one believes that oral or enteral nutrition will not be adequate within 5 days. Nonoperative therapy leads to resolution of adhesive partial obstruction in as many as 90% of patients.[41] Some studies suggest that the nature of the previous abdominal operation or the type of adhesions present may influence the probability that the obstruction will not respond to medical therapy.[42] Operations associated with a lower likelihood of response to medical therapy include those performed through a midline incision; those involving the aorta, the colon, the rectum, the appendix, or the pelvic adnexa; and those done to relieve previous carcinomatous obstruction. Matted adhesions, which are more common in patients who have undergone midline incisions or colorectal procedures, are less amenable to conservative management than a simple obstructive band is.[42] In the context of this kind of operative history, strong consideration should be given to surgical intervention if the obstruction does not resolve within 24 hours—unless comorbid medical conditions tip the risk-benefit balance in the direction of nonoperative therapy.

There is an ongoing debate regarding how long patients with partial adhesive obstruction should be treated conservatively. After 48 hours of nonoperative management, the risk of complications increases substantially, and the probability that the obstruction will resolve diminishes.[38] Generally, if the obstruction is going to resolve with nonoperative therapy, there will be a fairly prompt response within the first 8 to 12 hours. Therefore, if a patient's condition has deteriorated or has not significantly improved by 12 hours after the operation, exploratory laparotomy is advisable. During this observation period, the patient must be constantly reevaluated, ideally by the same examiner. Analgesics can be safely administered, and repeat abdominal examinations should be performed at 3-hour intervals when the influence of narcotics has waned. Repeat abdominal x-rays should be obtained no later than 6 hours after nasogastric decompression, and the pattern of gas distribution should be compared with that seen on the admission films. A decrease in intestinal gas distal to a point of obstruction coupled with an increase in proximal dilatation suggests that the obstruction is worsening; conversely, a decrease in intestinal distention coupled with the appearance of more gas distally in the colon suggests that the obstruction is being reduced. The degree of abdominal distention, the passage of flatus, and the nature of the nasogastric aspirate should be evaluated periodically. If abdominal distention does not decrease or the gastric aspirate changes from bilious to feculent, the patient should be operated on.

Experimental and clinical studies suggest that patients undergoing nonoperative treatment for bowel obstruction may benefit

from the administration of somatostatin analogues as a result of the potent effects these substances exert on intestinal sodium, chloride, and water absorption.[43] In one study, animals with either complete or closed-loop partial small bowel obstruction were given either long-acting somatostatin or saline; the treatment group had significantly less intestinal distention, less infarction, and longer survival than the control group.[43,44] In a prospective, randomized clinical trial evaluating the use of somatostatin in patients who had complete small bowel obstruction without clinical or radiologic evidence of strangulation, the treatment group was less likely to need operation, had less proximal intestinal distention, and exhibited decreased mucosal necrosis proximal to the point of obstruction.[45] In other trials, long-acting somatostatin analogues and other nonsecretagogues significantly decreased the amount of gastric contents aspirated and alleviated the symptoms of intestinal obstruction in terminally ill patients with nonoperable malignant disease.[28,29,33-35]

It should be possible to determine with a high degree of accuracy and safety which patients will require operation for adhesive small bowel obstruction within 24 hours of admission to the hospital. As a rule, patients with closed loop or complete bowel obstruction, who require immediate or urgent operation, can be readily identified by means of abdominal CT scanning.[11-13] For the remaining patients, who have some degree of partial obstruction, it is possible to make highly accurate predictions regarding whether conservative management will succeed or fail by recording the arrival of contrast material (either a water-soluble agent or a mixed barium preparation) in the right colon within a defined period of time.[13,26,46,47] One prospective study evaluated the arrival of diatrizoate meglumine–diatrizoate sodium in the colon within 24 hours as a predictor of successful nonoperative treatment and found this measure to have a sensitivity of 98%, a specificity of 100%, an accuracy of 99%, a positive predictive value of 100%, and a negative predictive value of 96%.[48] Other studies have used shorter arrival times (as early as 4 or 8 hours), with comparable results.[13,47,49]

Several prospective, randomized clinical trials have addressed the issue of whether administration of contrast material can itself be therapeutic with respect to resolving adhesive small bowel obstruction. Two such studies examined small bowel follow-through with barium, either alone or mixed with diatrizoate meglumine.[26,27] Both found that the intervals between admission and operation were shorter for patients randomized to the contrast arm than for those in the control group but that contrast examination did not lead to more expeditious resolution of obstruction. Both studies also demonstrated that barium could be administered to patients with small bowel obstruction safely and without complications.

Two prospective, randomized trials investigated the effects of administering water-soluble hyperosmolar contrast agents to patients with small bowel obstruction.[46,50] In one study, administration of diatrizoate meglumine (1,900 mOsm/L) promoted resolution of adhesive partial obstruction and shortened hospital stay but had no effect on whether laparotomy was required.[46] The mean interval between operation and the first stool was 23.3 hours in the control group and 6.2 hours in the trial group ($P < 0.00001$). Ten (21%) of the 48 obstructive episodes in the control group necessitated operation, compared with six (10%) of the 59 in the trial group ($P = 0.12$). The mean hospital stay for patients who responded to conservative treatment was 4.4 days in the control group and 2.2 days in the trial group ($P < 0.00001$). No contrast-related complications were observed. This study demonstrated that oral administration of diatrizoate meglumine was safe in patients with partial adhesive obstruction, facilitated early identification of patients who required operation, and shortened hospital stay. In the second study, administration of a different water-soluble hyperosmolar contrast agent, ioxitalamate meglumine (1,500 mOsm/L), had no therapeutic effect on patients with partial small bowel obstruction.[50] Again, no contrast-related complications were observed. The disparate results of these two clinical trials notwithstanding, the significant treatment effect reported in the first trial and the absence of any deleterious consequences in either one constitute sufficient evidence to support the administration of 100 ml of diatrizoate meglumine to patients with adhesive partial small bowel obstruction.

By accelerating the resolution of partial small bowel obstruction and ileus, administration of water-soluble contrast agents can shorten the expected hospital stay and thereby also reduce the cost of care. Thus, it is reasonable that the first step in managing suspected partial small bowel obstruction from adhesions or postoperative ileus is to administer water-soluble contrast material intragastrically. If bowel function does not return within 24 hours, then the obstruction is less likely to resolve with nonoperative therapy, and early operation, especially when performed laparoscopically, may be the best option for shortening hospital stay. If ileus persists after intragastric administration of the contrast material and mechanical obstruction is excluded, then continued observation is warranted, with close attention paid to factors that may be causing the ileus. Prospective trials will be necessary to assess this potentially cost-effective strategy.

Laparoscopic adhesiolysis Laparoscopic or laparoscopic-assisted lysis of adhesions relieves bowel obstruction in more than 50% of patients and is associated with lower morbidity, earlier return of bowel function, quicker resumption of normal diet, and a shorter hospital stay than open operative lysis of adhesions.[51-54] A 2000 study found that despite a reduction in median length of stay (from 8 days to 3), patients treated laparoscopically were at increased risk for early unplanned reoperation.[54] Nevertheless, the preponderance of the published experience with laparoscopic adhesiolysis in patients with small bowel obstruction suggests that a minimal-access approach should be employed before laparotomy. If such an approach fails to identify and relieve an obvious point of obstruction or if adhesiolysis is inadequate or unsafe, conversion to an open approach is indicated.

Early Postoperative Obstruction

Early postoperative mechanical small bowel obstruction is often difficult to diagnose because it gives rise to many of the same signs and symptoms as postoperative ileus: obstipation, distention, nausea, vomiting, abdominal pain, and altered bowel sounds. In most cases, there are roentgenographic signs indicative of small bowel obstruction rather than ileus; however, in some cases, abdominal x-rays fail to diagnose the obstruction.[55] Traditionally, when plain radiographs are equivocal, an upper GI barium study with follow-through views is the next test performed to distinguish ileus from partial or complete small bowel obstruction[56]; however, such studies may yield the wrong diagnosis in as many as 30% of cases.[22,55,57] A number of authorities believe that abdominal ultrasonography is excellent at distinguishing postoperative ileus from mechanical obstruction and recommend that it be done before any contrast study.[19]

Early postoperative obstruction is caused by adhesions in about 90% of patients.[55,58] When there are no signs of toxicity and no acute abdominal signs, such obstruction can usually be managed safely with nasogastric decompression.[55,57,58] As many as 75% of patients respond to nasogastric suction within 2 weeks. About 70% of the patients who respond to nonoperative treatment do so within 1 week, and an additional 25% respond during the following 7 days. If postoperative obstruction does not resolve in the first 2 weeks, it is unlikely to do so with continued nonoperative therapy, and reoperation is probably indicated[55,58]; about 25% of patients whose postoperative obstruction was initially treated nonoperatively eventually require reoperation. An exception to this guideline arises in patients known to have severe dense adhesions (sometimes referred to as obliterative peritonitis) in response to multiple sequential laparotomies. These patients may have a combination of mechanical obstruction and diffuse small bowel and colonic ileus. The risk of closed-loop obstruction, volvulus, or strangulation in this group of patients is low. Repeat laparotomies and attempts to lyse adhesions may lead to complications, the development of enterocutaneous fistulae, or exacerbation of the adhesions. Often, the best approach to managing these patients is observation for prolonged periods (i.e., months). Total parenteral nutrition (TPN) is indicated in these patients. The addition of octreotide to the TPN solution may be helpful.

Because the risk of intestinal strangulation in patients with postoperative adhesive obstruction is extremely low (< 1%),[55,59] one can generally treat these patients nonoperatively for longer periods. In fact, the conservative approach is often the wise one: reoperation may do more harm than good (e.g., by causing enterotomies and inducing denser adhesions). The traditional indications for operation in patients with early postoperative obstruction include (1) deteriorating clinical status, (2) worsening obstructive symptoms, and (3) failure to respond to nonoperative management within 2 weeks. With the rising cost of hospitalization, it might in fact be more cost-effective to reoperate on patients who have persistent obstruction after 7 days. This speculation would have to be tested by a well-organized cost-benefit study conducted in a prospective fashion.

Long intestinal tubes have no beneficial role in the management of postoperative bowel obstruction; in fact, some authorities have reported that the use of such tubes increases morbidity.[24,38,39] One prospective randomized clinical trial compared the utility of long intestinal tubes with that of nasogastric tubes for the resolution of small bowel obstruction.[60] There were no differences between the two groups with respect to the percentage of patients who were able to avoid operation, the incidence of complications, the time between admission and operation, or the duration of postoperative ileus.

Inflammatory Conditions

Partial bowel obstruction secondary to inflammatory bowel disease, radiation enteritis, or diverticulitis usually resolves with nonoperative therapy. Bowel obstruction accompanying an acute exacerbation of Crohn disease usually resolves with nasogastric suction, I.V. antibiotics, and anti-inflammatory agents. If, however, CT scanning detects intra-abdominal abscess, there is evidence of a chronic stricture, or the patient exhibits persistent obstructive symptoms, operation may be necessary. Similarly, bowel obstruction arising from acute enteritis caused by radiation exposure or chemotherapy usually resolves with supportive care. Chronic radiation-induced strictures are problematic; astute clinical judgment must be exercised to determine when operative treatment is the best option.

Patients with acute diverticulitis typically present with a history of altered bowel movements, fever, leukocytosis, localized pain, tenderness, and guarding in the left lower quadrant of the abdomen. Approximately 20% of patients with colonic diverticulitis also present with signs and symptoms of partial colonic obstruction. A CT scan should be obtained early in all patients with diverticulitis to ascertain whether there is a pericolic abscess that could be drained percutaneously.[61] Partial colonic obstruction in these patients usually resolves with antibiotic therapy, an NPO regimen, and nasogastric decompression. If obstructive symptoms persist for more than 7 days or if obstructive symptoms from a documented stricture recur, operation is indicated.

ELECTIVE OPERATION

Nontoxic, Nontender Sigmoid Volvulus

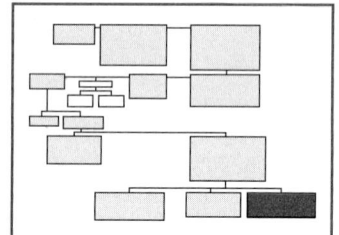

Patients with nontoxic, nontender sigmoid volvulus whose bowel obstruction is initially treated successfully with sigmoidoscopic decompression are at risk for recurrent colonic obstruction. Accordingly, these patients should undergo elective sigmoid resection after complete bowel preparation.

Recurrent Adhesive or Stricture-Related Partial Small Bowel Obstruction

Many patients whose adhesive bowel obstruction resolves experience no further obstructive episodes. If a patient does present with recurrent obstruction from presumed adhesions, either a contrast examination of the bowel or CT scanning is indicated to determine whether there is a surgically correctable point of stenosis. A strong argument can be made that non–high-risk patients should undergo elective operation after presenting with their second episode of mechanical obstruction. Similarly, patients with recurrent obstruction from strictures of any sort should undergo elective operation, given that these lesions are unlikely to resolve.

Partial Colonic Obstruction

The most common causes of partial colonic obstruction are colon cancer, strictures, and diverticulitis. Cancer and strictures usually must be managed surgically because they generally go on to cause obstruction later. Strictures from ischemia or endometriosis usually call for elective colonic resection. Inflammatory strictures from diverticulitis may resolve; however, if obstructive symptoms persist or if barium enema examination continues to yield evidence of colonic narrowing, elective resection is warranted.

When abdominal x-rays suggest distal colonic obstruction, digital examination and rigid sigmoidoscopy are performed to exclude fecal impaction, tumors, strictures, and sigmoid volvulus. If obstruction is proximal to the sigmoidoscope, barium contrast examination is indicated. If barium examination does not demonstrate mechanical obstruction, a presumptive diagnosis of colonic pseudo-obstruction is made.

The morbidity and mortality associated with elective colorectal procedures are significantly lower than those associated with emergency colonic surgery. Furthermore, immediate operation for left-side colonic obstruction almost always necessitates the creation of a diverting colostomy. If a colostomy takedown subsequently proves necessary, the overall cost of caring for the patient will be significantly higher than it would have been had a single-stage procedure been performed. For these reasons, one

should initially treat patients with partial colonic obstruction with nasogastric suction, enemas, and I.V. rehydration in the hope that the obstruction will resolve and that the patient thus can undergo mechanical and antibiotic bowel preparation and a single-stage procedure comprising resection and primary anastomosis. Patients who do not respond to nonoperative measures within 24 hours should undergo operation within 12 hours with the aim of preventing perforation.

In patients with partially obstructing rectal or distal sigmoid tumors or strictures that can be traversed with a radiologic guide wire, balloon dilatation can be performed and a self-expanding stent deployed.[32,62-65] Clinical improvement and resolution of obstruction occur in more than 90% of patients within 96 hours.[32,64] With restoration of the bowel lumen, patients can be prepared for elective surgery, can be spared the creation of a diverting colostomy, and can avoid the extra expense and morbidity associated with the performance of two operations.[64,65] This approach is also highly successful as primary therapy for bowel obstruction in patients who are not surgical candidates.[32] In patients with large, fixed rectal masses, one should obtain CT scans of the pelvis to assess the extent of the tumor. Transrectal laser fulguration and endoluminal stenting are palliative options for restoring bowel lumen patency that may be considered for patients with nonresectable recurrent rectal cancer or radiation strictures in whom operative risk is prohibitively high.

Bowel Obstruction without Previous Abdominal Operation

When partial small bowel obstruction develops and resolves in a patient who has not previously undergone an abdominal operation, one should perform a diagnostic workup to identify the cause of the obstruction; there may be an underlying condition that is likely to cause recurrent obstruction (e.g., an internal hernia, a tumor, malrotation, or metastatic cancer). The first diagnostic test to be ordered should be a CT scan, followed by an upper GI barium study with follow-through views and a barium enema.[66] If a pathologic lesion is identified, elective operation is indicated. An argument can be made that no additional diagnostic tests should be performed in these patients and that diagnostic laparoscopy should be performed instead to enable laparoscopic surgery in case a cause of obstruction is identified that can be treated with a minimally invasive procedure. If no cause of obstruction is found at laparoscopy, open laparotomy is performed.

Nonmechanical Obstruction

ILEUS

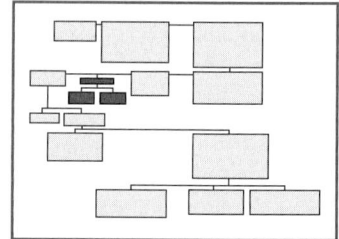

Ileus, or intestinal paralysis, is most common after abdominal operations but can also occur in response to any acute medical condition or metabolic derangement [see Table 1].

The pathophysiologic mechanisms that cause ileus are incompletely understood but appear to involve disruption of normal neurohumoral responses.[67] Ileus may be classified into two broad categories: postoperative ileus and ileus without antecedent abdominal operation. Postoperative ileus is manifested by atony of the stomach, the small intestine, and the colon and usually resolves spontaneously within a few days as normal bowel motility returns. Typically, the small bowel regains its motility within 24 hours of operation, followed 3 to 4 days later by the stomach and the colon. Initial therapy of ileus is directed at identifying and correcting the presumed cause [see Figure 12]. If the patient experiences abdominal distention, abdominal pain, nausea, or vomiting, then nasogastric decompression, placement of a Foley catheter, and I.V. rehydration are indicated. In postoperative patients, it is best not to use strong narcotics for analgesia and instead to rely on epidural anesthesia and nonsteroidal anti-inflammatory drugs. When ileus develops in patients who have not recently undergone an operation, a thorough history, a careful physical examination, and well-chosen laboratory tests are necessary to identify the possible causes.

When ileus persists for what is, in one's best clinical judgment, an inordinate length of time for the operation performed (typically, longer than 3 to 4 days), the possibility of partial mechanical obstruction, possibly associated with an intra-abdominal abscess or another source of infection, must be considered. If an abscess is suspected, an abdominal CT scan should be obtained. Abdominal ultrasonography has been reported to distinguish postoperative ileus from mechanical obstruction reliably.[19] A small bowel contrast examination with barium identifies partial mechanical small bowel obstruction in about 75% of patients.[22,24] CT scanning distinguishes ileus from obstruction in about 80% of patients.

Intragastric administration of a water-soluble contrast agent has recently shown great potential in the treatment of ileus.[68,69] In one study, administration of 120 ml of diatrizoate meglumine or diatrizoate sodium via nasogastric tube to 40 adults with postoperative small bowel ileus led to restored intestinal motility within 6 hours in all 40, allowing them to resume oral alimentation within 24 hours.[68] Given these results, a prospective, randomized trial that addresses cost-management end points is warranted.

PSEUDO-OBSTRUCTION

Pseudo-obstruction [see Figure 13] can exist in the small bowel or the colon and can be either acute or chronic. Acute colonic pseudo-obstruction, also known as Ogilvie syndrome, is the most common form. Colonic pseudo-obstruction occurs most commonly in hospitalized patients in the postoperative period or in response to a nonsurgical acute illness (e.g., pneumonia, myocardial infarction, hypoxia, shock, intestinal ischemia, or electrolyte imbalance). The pathophysiologic mechanisms underlying idiopathic pseudo-obstruction appear to be related to an imbalance in the parasympathetic and sympathetic influences on colonic motility. The presenting symptoms of acute colonic pseudo-obstruction are massive dilatation of the colon (with the cecum more dilated than the distal colon), crampy pain, nausea, and

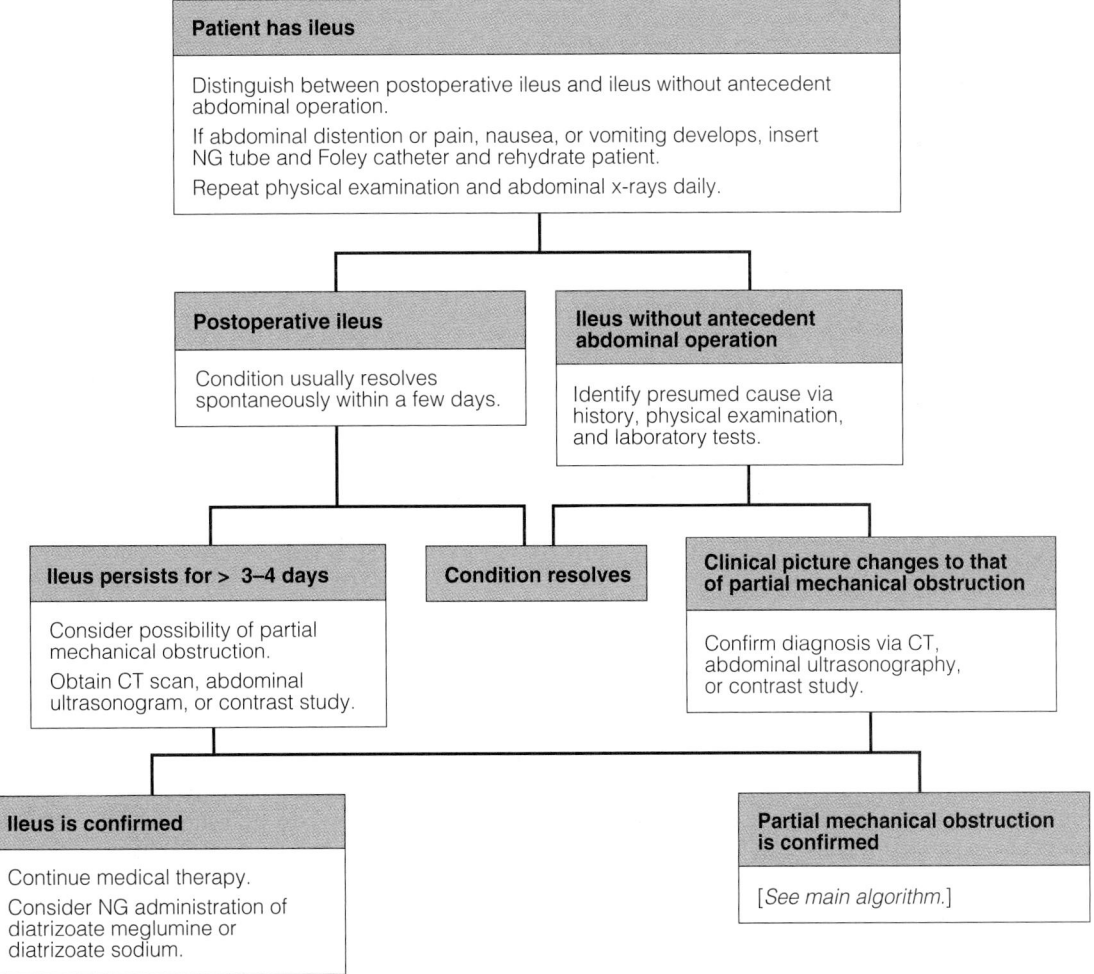

Figure 12 Shown is an algorithm outlining an approach to management of ileus.

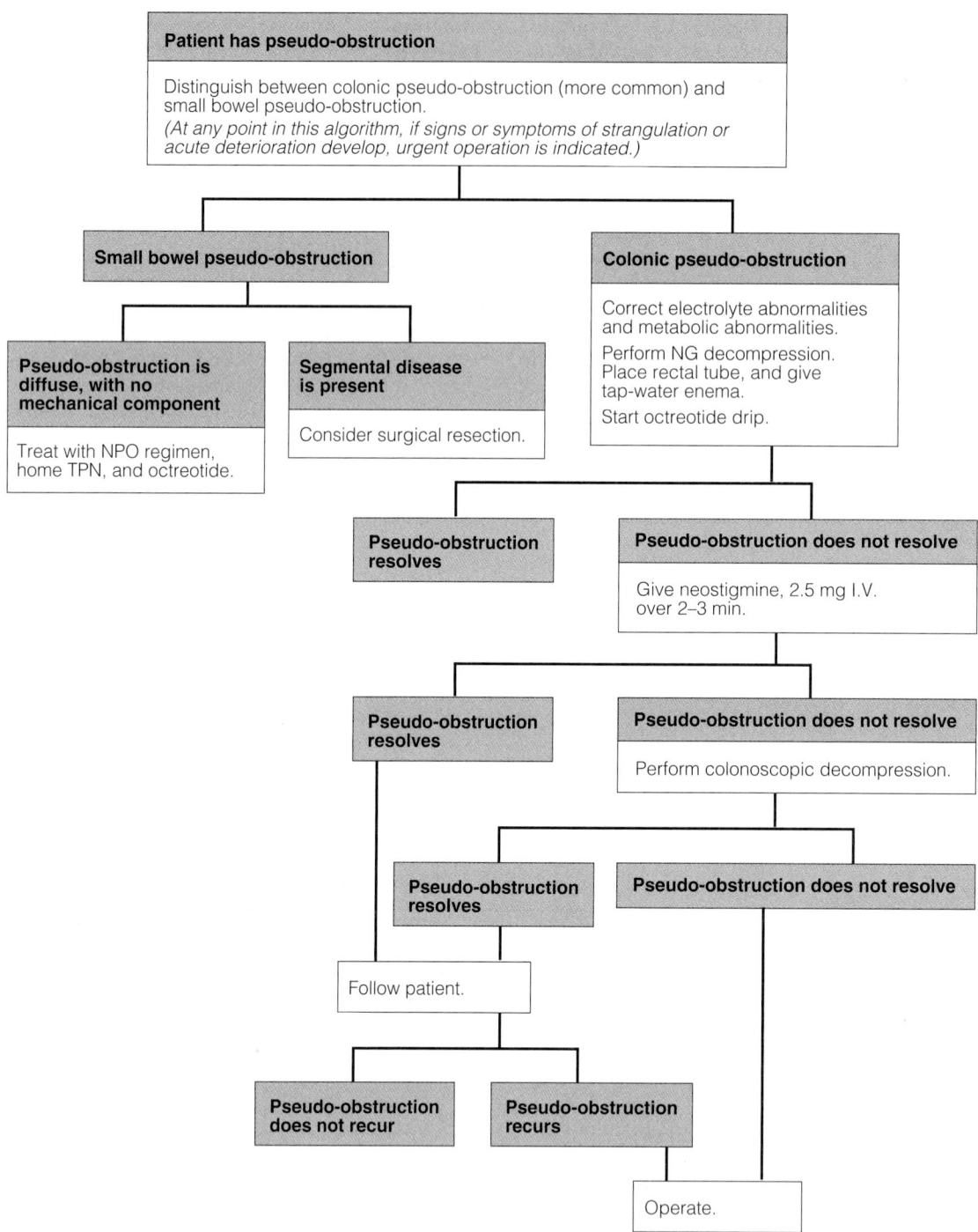

Figure 13 Shown is an algorithm outlining an approach to management of pseudo-obstruction.

vomiting.[70] If peritoneal irritation or systemic toxicity is present, immediate laparotomy is indicated; if not, treatment involves nasogastric decompression, placement of a rectal tube, tap-water enemas, correction of any underlying metabolic disturbances, and avoidance of narcotic and anticholinergic medications. With conservative management, acute colonic pseudo-obstruction resolves within 4 days in more than 80% of cases.[71] Colonoscopy was previously the method of choice for decompression in this setting.[72] More recently, however, it has been shown that I.V. administration of neostigmine, 2.5 mg over 2 to 3 minutes, leads to prompt resolution of acute colonic pseudo-obstruction within

minutes in nearly all cases.[73,74] Now that this previously difficult and potentially lethal problem can readily be treated pharmacologically, one should reserve colonoscopic decompression and surgical intervention for cases in which pharmacologic measures fail.

Chronic intestinal pseudo-obstruction is a rare acquired disorder that is caused by various diseases involving gastrointestinal smooth muscle, the enteric nervous system, or the extrinsic autonomic nerve supply to the gut.[75] These disorders are treated with an NPO regimen, home TPN, and octreotide. Patients with chronic intestinal pseudo-obstruction should be followed closely for long periods and should undergo repeat contrast studies: there are times when a condition will develop that can cause mechanical obstruction and that may be surgically correctable.[76,77]

Cost Considerations

Cost considerations are exerting an ever-growing influence on surgical care in general and on the decision whether to operate in particular. A large percentage of the high total cost of caring for patients with ileus or mechanical intestinal obstruction is accounted for by the cost of hospitalization or need for laparotomy.

Strategies for reducing the overall cost of managing patients with bowel obstruction may take several forms: the development of diagnostic and therapeutic methods that lead to more rapid diagnosis and resolution of ileus and partial small bowel obstruction; the development of techniques for rapid identification of patients with complete or closed-loop obstruction and early reversible strangulation, which would permit earlier operative intervention and thereby reduce the incidence of complications; the development of therapeutic approaches that prevent postoperative ileus; and the development of methods for preventing intra-abdominal adhesions, which would significantly reduce the overall incidence of bowel obstruction.

From a management viewpoint, if a specific diagnostic test, medication, or approach (e.g., laparoscopy) costs less than a day of hospitalization does, it immediately becomes cost-effective if it reduces complications and shortens length of stay by 1 day. Intragastric administration of a water-soluble contrast agent to relieve small bowel ileus or partial adhesive obstruction is an example of an innovative, cost-effective therapeutic strategy. Diagnostic laparoscopy, abdominal ultrasonography, and CT scanning have all been successfully used to make earlier definitive management decisions and to prevent gangrenous obstruction. Laparoscopic adhesiolysis also leads to earlier hospital discharge. On the basis of the collective experience reported in a substantial number of studies (see above), a logical proposal for cost-effective management of patients with bowel obstruction would be to perform ultrasonography or abdominal CT scanning immediately after initial resuscitation, then to perform laparoscopic surgery on those patients in whom the contrast agent does not arrive in the right colon within 24 hours. However, prospective, randomized clinical trials are needed to evaluate the cost-effectiveness of this and other newer management strategies.

References

1. Irvin T: Abdominal pain: a surgical audit of 1190 emergency admissions. Br J Surg 76:1121, 1989
2. Eskelinen M, Ikonen J, Lipponen P: Contributions of history-taking, physical examination, and computer assistance to diagnosis of acute small-bowel obstruction: a prospective study of 1333 patients with acute abdominal pain. Scand J Gastroenterol 29:715, 1994
3. Reisner R, Cohen J: Gallstone ileus: a review of 1001 reported cases. Am Surg 60:441, 1994
4. Sarr M, Bulkley G, Zuidema G: Preoperative recognition of intestinal strangulation obstruction: prospective evaluation of diagnostic capability. Am J Surg 145:176, 1983
5. Burrell H, Baker D, Wardrop P, et al: Significant plain film findings in sigmoid volvulus. Clin Radiol 49:317, 1994
6. Fatarr S, Schulman A: Small bowel obstruction masking synchronous large bowel obstruction: a need for emergency barium enema. AJR Am J Roentgenol 140:1159, 1983
7. Lim J, Ko Y, Lee D, et al: Determining the site and causes of colonic obstruction with sonography. AJR Am J Roentgenol 163:113, 1994
8. Gough I: Strangulating adhesive small bowel obstruction with normal radiographs. Br J Surg 65:431, 1978
9. Ko Y, Lim J, Le D, et al: Small bowel obstruction: sonographic evaluation. Radiology 188:649, 1993
10. Balthazar E: For suspected small-bowel obstruction and an equivocal plain film, should we perform CT or a small-bowel series? AJR Am J Roentgenol 163:1260, 1994
11. Daneshmand S, Hedley C, Stain S: The utility and reliability of computed tomography scan in the diagnosis of small bowel obstruction. Am Surg 65:922, 1999
12. Donckier V, Closset J, Van Gansbeke D, et al: Contribution of computed tomography to decision making in the management of adhesive small bowel obstruction. Br J Surg 85:1071, 1998
13. Peck J, Milleson T, Phelan J: The role of computed tomography with contrast and small bowel follow-through in management of small bowel obstruction. Am J Surg 177:375, 1999
14. Zalcman M, Sy M, Donckier V, et al: Helical CT signs in the diagnosis of intestinal ischemia in small-bowel obstruction. AJR Am J Roentgenol 175:1601, 2000
15. Ha H: CT in the early detection of strangulation in intestinal obstruction. Semin Ultrasound CT MRI 16:141, 1995
16. Ogata M, Mateer J, Condon R: Prospective evaluation of abdominal sonography for the diagnosis of bowel obstruction. Ann Surg 223:237, 1996
17. Grunshaw N, Renwick IG, Scarisbrick G, et al: Prospective evaluation of ultrasound in distal ileal and colonic obstruction. Clin Radiol 55:356, 2000
18. Meiser G, Meissner K: Intermittent incomplete intestinal obstruction: a frequently mistaken identity. Ultrasonographic diagnosis and management. Surg Endosc 3:46, 1989
19. Meiser G, Meissner K: Ileus and intestinal obstruction—ultrasonographic findings as a guideline to therapy. Hepatogastroenterology 34:194, 1987
20. Megibow A: Bowel obstruction: evaluation with CT. Radiol Clin North Am 32:861, 1994
21. Balthazar E: CT of small-bowel obstruction. AJR Am J Roentgenol 162:255, 1994
22. Dunn JT, Halls JM, Berne TV: Roentgenographic contrast studies in acute small-bowel obstruction. Arch Surg 119:1305, 1984
23. Caroline DF, Herlinger H, Laufer I, et al: Small bowel enema in the diagnosis of adhesive obstructions. AJR Am J Roentgenol 142:1133, 1984
24. Brolin R: Partial small bowel obstruction. Surgery 95:145, 1984
25. Maglinte D, Peterson D, Vahey T, et al: Enteroclysis in partial small bowel obstruction. Am J Surg 147:325, 1984
26. Anderson C, Humphry W: Contrast radiography in small bowel obstruction: a prospective randomized trial. Mil Med 162:749, 1997
27. Fevang BT, Jensen D, Fevang J, et al: Upper gastrointestinal contrast study in the management of small bowel obstruction—a prospective randomised study. Eur J Surg 166:39, 2000
28. Muir J, von Gunten C: Antisecretory agents in gastrointestinal obstruction. Clin Geriatr Med 16:327, 2000
29. Mercadante S, Ripamonti C, Casuccio A, et al: Comparison of octreotide and hyoscine butylbromide in controlling gastrointestinal symptoms due to malignant inoperable bowel obstruction. Support Care Cancer 8:188, 2000
30. Ripamonti C, Mercadante S, Groff L, et al: Role of octreotide, scopolamine butylbromide, and hydration in symptom control of patients with inoperable bowel obstruction and nasogastric tubes: a prospective randomized trial. J Pain Symptom Manage 19:23, 2000
31. Matsushita M, Hajiro K, Takukawa H, et al: Plastic prosthesis in the palliation of small bowel stenosis secondary to recurrent gastric cancer: initial cost savings. Gastrointest Endosc 52:571, 2000
32. de Gregorio MA, Mainar A, Tejero E, et al: Acute colorectal obstruction: stent placement for palliative treatment—results of a multicenter study. Radiology 209:117, 1998
33. Khoo D, Hall E, Motson R, et al: Palliation of malignant intestinal obstruction using octreotide. Eur J Cancer 30A:28, 1994
34. Stiefel F, Morant R: Vapreotide, a new somatostatin analogue in the palliative management of obstructive ileus in advanced cancer. Support Care Cancer 1:57, 1993
35. Scheidbach H, Horbach T, Groitl H, et al: Percutaneous endoscopic gastrostomy/jejunostomy (PEG/PEJ) for decompression in the upper gastrointestinal tract. Initial experience with palliative treatment of gastrointestinal obstruction in terminally ill patients with advanced carcinomas. Surg Endosc 13:1103, 1999
36. Silen W, Hein MF, Goldman L: Strangulation obstruction of the small intestine. Arch Surg 85:137, 1962

37. Laws H, Aldrete J: Small bowel obstruction: a review of 465 cases. South Med J 69:733, 1976

38. Sosa J, Gardner B: Management of patients diagnosed as acute intestinal obstruction secondary to adhesions. Am Surg 59:125, 1993

39. Snyder EN, McCranie D: Closed loop obstruction of the small bowel. Am J Surg 111:398, 1966

40. Mangiante E, Croce M, Fabian T, et al: Sigmoid volvulus: a four-decade experience. Am Surg 55:41, 1989

41. Bizer L, Liebling R, Delany H, et al: Small bowel obstruction: the role of non-operative treatment in simple intestinal obstruction and predictive criteria for strangulation obstruction. Surgery 89:407, 1981

42. Miller G, Boman J, Shrier I, et al: Natural history of patients with adhesive small bowel obstruction. Br J Surg 87:1240, 2000

43. Mulvihill S, Pappas T, Fonkalsrud Z, et al: The effect of somatostatin on experimental intestinal obstruction. Ann Surg 207:169, 1988

44. Gittes G, Nelson M, Debas H, et al: Improvement in survival of mice with proximal small bowel obstruction treated with octreotide. Am J Surg 163:231, 1992

45. Bastounis E, Hadjinikolaou L, Ioannou N, et al: Somatostatin as adjuvant therapy in the management of obstructive ileus. Hepatogastroenterology 36:538, 1989

46. Assalia A, Schein M, Kopelman D, et al: Therapeutic effect of oral Gastrografin in adhesive, partial small-bowel obstruction: a prospective randomized trial. Surgery 115:433, 1994

47. Blackmon S, Lucius C, Wilson JP, et al: The use of water-soluble contrast in evaluating clinically equivocal small bowel obstruction. Am Surg 66:238, 2000

48. Chen SC, Chang KJ, Lee PH, et al: Oral urografin in postoperative small bowel obstruction. World J Surg 23:1051, 1999

49. Chen SC, Lin FY, Lee PH, et al: Water-soluble contrast study predicts the need for early surgery in adhesive small bowel obstruction. Br J Surg 85:1692, 1998

50. Feigin E, Seror D, Szold A, et al: Water-soluble contrast material has no therapeutic effect on postoperative small-bowel obstruction: results of a prospective, randomized clinical trial. Am J Surg 171:227, 1996

51. Leon EL, Metzger A, Tsiotos GG, et al: Laparoscopic management of small bowel obstruction: indications and outcome. J Gastrointest Surg 2:132, 1998

52. Strickland P, Lourie DJ, Suddleson EA, et al: Is laparoscopy safe and effective for treatment of acute small-bowel obstruction? Surg Endosc 13:695, 1999

53. Suter M, Zermatten P, Halkic N, et al: Laparoscopic management of mechanical small bowel obstruction; are there predictors of success or failure? Surg Endosc 14:478, 2000

54. Bailey IS, Rhodes M, O'Rourke N, et al: Laparoscopic management of acute small bowel obstruction. Br J Surg 85:84, 1998

55. Pickleman J, Lee R: The management of patients with suspected early postoperative small bowel obstruction. Ann Surg 212:216, 1989

56. Brolin R: The role of gastrointestinal tube decompression in the treatment of mechanical intestinal obstruction. Am Surg 49:131, 1983

57. Quatromoni J, Rosoff L, Halls J, et al: Early postoperative small bowel obstruction. Ann Surg 191:72, 1980

58. Stewart R, Page C, Brender J, et al: The incidence and risk of early postoperative small bowel obstruction. Am J Surg 154:643, 1987

59. Spears H, Petrelli N, Herrera L, et al: Treatment of small bowel obstruction after colorectal carcinoma. Am J Surg 155:383, 1988

60. Fleshner PR, Siegman MG, Slater GI, et al: A prospective, randomized trial of short versus long tubes in adhesive small-bowel obstruction. Am J Surg 170:366, 1995

61. Hulnick D, Megibow A, Balthazar E, et al: Computed tomography in the evaluation of diverticulitis. Radiology 152:491, 1984

62. Tejero E, Mainar A, Fernández L, et al: New procedure for the treatment of colorectal neoplastic obstructions. Dis Colon Rectum 37:1158, 1994

63. Itabashi M, Hamano K, Kameoka S, et al: Self-expanding stainless steel stent application in rectosigmoid stricture. Dis Colon Rectum 36:508, 1993

64. Binkert C, Ledermann H, Jost R, et al: Acute colonic obstruction: clinical aspects and cost-effectiveness of preoperative and palliative treatment with self-expanding metallic stents—a preliminary report. Radiology 206:199, 1998

65. Mainar A, DeGregorio Ariza MA, Tejero E, et al: Acute colorectal obstruction: treatment with self-expandable metallic stents before scheduled surgery—results of a multicenter study. Radiology 210:65, 1999

66. Stelmach W, Cass A: Small bowel obstructions: the case for investigation for occult large bowel carcinoma. Aust NZ J Surg 59:181, 1989

67. Fromm D: Ileus and obstruction. Surgery: Scientific Principles and Practice. Greenfield LJ, Mulholland MW, Oldham KT, et al, Eds. JB Lippincott Co, Philadelphia, 1993, p 731

68. Watkins D, Robertson C: Water-soluble radiocontrast material in the treatment of the postoperative ileus. Am J Obstet Gynecol 152:450, 1985

69. Zer M, Kanzenelson D, Feigenberg Z, et al: The value of Gastrografin in the differential diagnosis of paralytic ileus and mechanical obstruction. Dis Colon Rectum 20:573, 1977

70. Vanek V, Al-Salti M: Acute pseudo-obstruction of the colon (Ogilvie's syndrome): an analysis of 400 cases. Dis Colon Rectum 29:203, 1986

71. Sloyer A, Panella V, Demas B: Ogilvie's syndrome: successful management with colonoscopy. Dig Dis Sci 33:1391, 1988

72. Nakhgevany KB: Colonoscopic decompression of the colon in patients with Ogilvie's syndrome. Am J Surg 148:317, 1984

73. Hutchinson R, Griffiths C: Acute colonic pseudo-obstruction: a pharmacological approach. Ann R Coll Surg Engl 74:364, 1992

74. Ponec RJ, Saunders MD, Kimmey MB: Neostigmine for the treatment of acute colonic pseudo-obstruction. N Engl J Med 341:137, 1999

75. Faulk D, Anuras S, Christensen J: Chronic intestinal pseudo-obstruction. Gastroenterology 74:922, 1978

76. Schuffler M, Deitch E: Chronic idiopathic intestinal pseudo-obstruction: a surgical approach. Ann Surg 192:752, 1980

77. Knoll RF Jr, Schuffler MD, Helton WS: Small bowel resection for relief of chronic intestinal pseudo-obstruction. Am J Gastroenterol 90:1142, 1995

Acknowledgment

Figures 12 and 13 Marcia Kammerer.

6 UPPER GASTROINTESTINAL BLEEDING

Richard T. Schlinkert, M.D., F.A.C.S., and Keith A. Kelly, M.D., F.A.C.S.

Assessment and Management of Upper Gastrointestinal Bleeding

The most common causes of upper gastrointestinal bleeding are chronic duodenal ulcers, chronic gastric ulcers, esophageal varices, gastric varices, Mallory-Weiss tears, acute hemorrhagic gastritis, and gastric neoplasms [*see* Management of Specific Sources of Upper GI Bleeding, *below*]. Less common causes include various other gastrointestinal conditions as well as certain hepatobiliary and pancreatic disorders.

Presentation and Initial Management

INITIAL ASSESSMENT AND MANAGEMENT

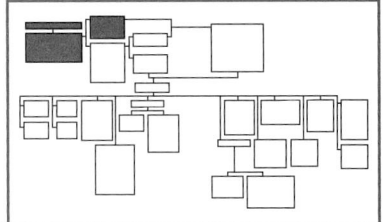

Upper gastrointestinal hemorrhage may present as severe bleeding with hematemesis, hematochezia, and hypotension; as gradual bleeding with melena; or as occult bleeding detected by positive tests for blood in the stool. The initial steps in the evaluation of patients with upper GI bleeding are based on the perceived rate of bleeding and the degree of hemodynamic stability. Hemodynamically stable patients who show no evidence of active bleeding or comorbidities and in whom endoscopic findings are favorable may be treated on an outpatient basis, whereas patients who show evidence of serious bleeding should be managed aggressively and hospitalized.

The airway, breathing, and circulation should be rapidly assessed, and the examiner should note whether the patient has a history of or currently exhibits hematemesis, melena, or hematochezia. Blood should be drawn for a complete blood count, blood chemistries (including tests of liver function and renal function), and measurement of the prothrombin time (PT) and the partial thromboplastin time (PTT). Blood should be sent to the blood bank for typing and crossmatching.

If the patient is stable and shows no evidence of recent or active hemorrhage, the surgeon may proceed with the workup.

If, however, the patient is stable but shows evidence of recent or active bleeding, a large-bore intravenous line should be placed before workup is begun; the presence of the line ensures immediate I.V. access should the patient subsequently become unstable.

If the patient is unstable, resuscitation should be begun immediately.

RESUSCITATION

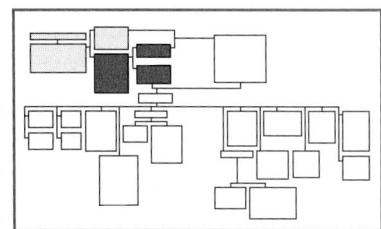

Resuscitation of an unstable patient is begun by establishing a secure airway and ensuring adequate ventilation. Oxygen should be given as necessary, either by mask or by endotracheal tube and ventilator. A large-bore I.V. line should then be placed, through which lactated Ringer solution should be infused at a rate high enough to maintain tissue perfusion. A urinary catheter should be inserted and urine output monitored. Blood should be given as necessary, and any coagulopathies should be corrected if possible. It is all too easy to forget these basic steps in a desire to evaluate and manage massive GI hemorrhage.

If the patient remains unstable and continues to bleed despite supportive measures, he or she should be taken to the operating room for intraoperative diagnosis. The abdomen should be opened through an upper midline incision, and an anterior gastrotomy should be performed. If inspection does not reveal the source of the bleeding or if bleeding is observed beyond the pylorus, a duodenotomy is made, with care taken to preserve the pylorus if possible. Bleeding from the proximal stomach may be difficult to verify, but it should be actively sought if no other bleeding site is identified.

Workup

HISTORY

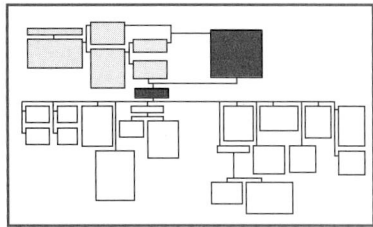

Only after the initial measures to protect the airway and stabilize the patient have been completed should an attempt be made to establish the cause of the bleeding. The history should focus on known causes of upper GI bleeding (e.g., ulcers, recent trauma or stress, liver disease, varices, alcoholism, and vomiting) and on the possible use of medications that interfere with coagulation (e.g., aspirin, nonsteroidal anti-inflammatory drugs [NSAIDs], and dipyridamole) or alter hemodynamics (e.g., beta blockers and antihypertensive agents). The cardiac history is particularly important for assessing the patient's ability to withstand varying degrees of anemia.

321

Assessment and Management of Upper Gastrointestinal Bleeding

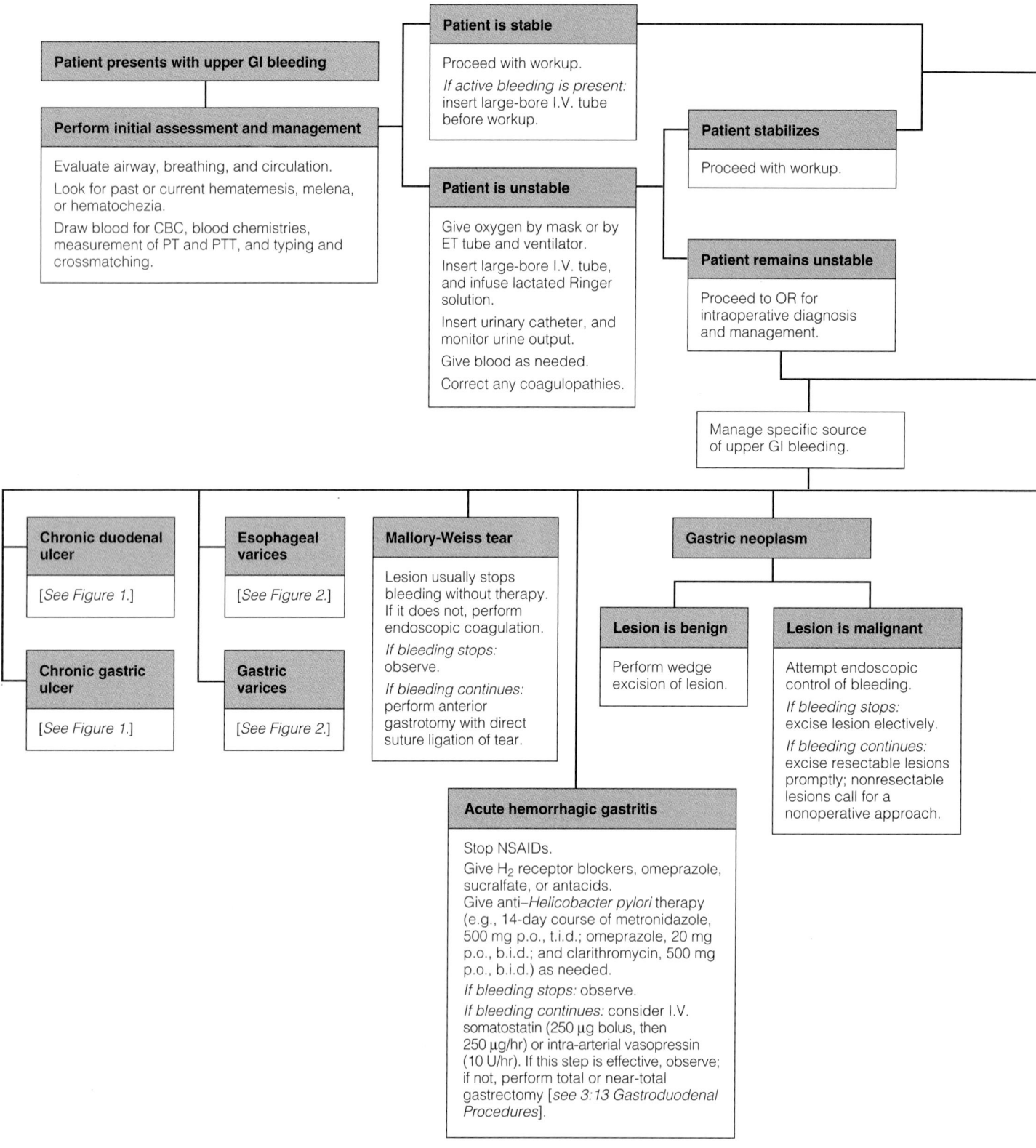

Patient presents with upper GI bleeding

Perform initial assessment and management

Evaluate airway, breathing, and circulation.

Look for past or current hematemesis, melena, or hematochezia.

Draw blood for CBC, blood chemistries, measurement of PT and PTT, and typing and crossmatching.

Patient is stable

Proceed with workup.

If active bleeding is present: insert large-bore I.V. tube before workup.

Patient is unstable

Give oxygen by mask or by ET tube and ventilator.

Insert large-bore I.V. tube, and infuse lactated Ringer solution.

Insert urinary catheter, and monitor urine output.

Give blood as needed.

Correct any coagulopathies.

Patient stabilizes

Proceed with workup.

Patient remains unstable

Proceed to OR for intraoperative diagnosis and management.

Manage specific source of upper GI bleeding.

Chronic duodenal ulcer

[*See Figure 1.*]

Chronic gastric ulcer

[*See Figure 1.*]

Esophageal varices

[*See Figure 2.*]

Gastric varices

[*See Figure 2.*]

Mallory-Weiss tear

Lesion usually stops bleeding without therapy. If it does not, perform endoscopic coagulation.

If bleeding stops: observe.

If bleeding continues: perform anterior gastrotomy with direct suture ligation of tear.

Gastric neoplasm

Lesion is benign

Perform wedge excision of lesion.

Lesion is malignant

Attempt endoscopic control of bleeding.

If bleeding stops: excise lesion electively.

If bleeding continues: excise resectable lesions promptly; nonresectable lesions call for a nonoperative approach.

Acute hemorrhagic gastritis

Stop NSAIDs.

Give H_2 receptor blockers, omeprazole, sucralfate, or antacids.

Give anti–*Helicobacter pylori* therapy (e.g., 14-day course of metronidazole, 500 mg p.o., t.i.d.; omeprazole, 20 mg p.o., b.i.d.; and clarithromycin, 500 mg p.o., b.i.d.) as needed.

If bleeding stops: observe.

If bleeding continues: consider I.V. somatostatin (250 µg bolus, then 250 µg/hr) or intra-arterial vasopressin (10 U/hr). If this step is effective, observe; if not, perform total or near-total gastrectomy [*see 3:13 Gastroduodenal Procedures*].

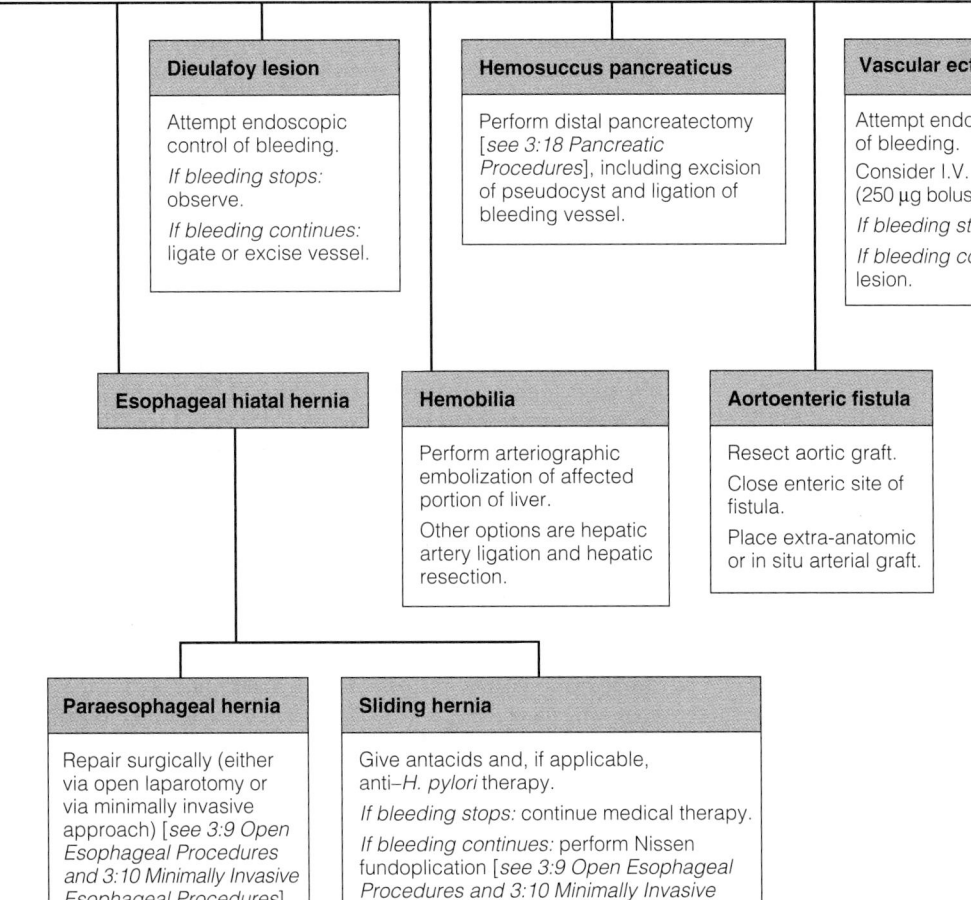

Work up patient

Obtain history, focusing on known causes of upper GI bleeding and suspect medications.

Perform physical examination.

Perform NG aspiration.

Perform esophagogastroduodenoscopy [*see 3:8 Gastrointestinal Endoscopy*].

Use other tests as appropriate:
- tagged red cell scans
- arteriography
- roentgenography with BaSO₄
- intraoperative endoscopic exploration

Dieulafoy lesion

Attempt endoscopic control of bleeding.

If bleeding stops: observe.

If bleeding continues: ligate or excise vessel.

Hemosuccus pancreaticus

Perform distal pancreatectomy [*see 3:18 Pancreatic Procedures*], including excision of pseudocyst and ligation of bleeding vessel.

Vascular ectases

Attempt endoscopic control of bleeding.

Consider I.V. somatostatin (250 μg bolus, then 250 μg/hr).

If bleeding stops: observe.

If bleeding continues: resect lesion.

Jejunal ulcer

Manage underlying causes if known (e.g., medications, infections, or gastrinomas).

If bleeding stops: observe.

If bleeding continues: excise bleeding segment of jejunum.

Esophageal hiatal hernia

Hemobilia

Perform arteriographic embolization of affected portion of liver.

Other options are hepatic artery ligation and hepatic resection.

Aortoenteric fistula

Resect aortic graft.

Close enteric site of fistula.

Place extra-anatomic or in situ arterial graft.

Duodenal or jejunal diverticula

Excise lesion, with or without the aid of intraoperative endoscopy.

Paraesophageal hernia

Repair surgically (either via open laparotomy or via minimally invasive approach) [*see 3:9 Open Esophageal Procedures and 3:10 Minimally Invasive Esophageal Procedures*].

Sliding hernia

Give antacids and, if applicable, anti–*H. pylori* therapy.

If bleeding stops: continue medical therapy.

If bleeding continues: perform Nissen fundoplication [*see 3:9 Open Esophageal Procedures and 3:10 Minimally Invasive Esophageal Procedures*].

PHYSICAL EXAMINATION

The physical examination is seldom of much help in determining the exact site of bleeding, but it may reveal jaundice, ascites, or other signs of hepatic disease; a tumor mass; or a bruit from an abdominal vascular lesion.

NASOGASTRIC ASPIRATION

The next step is nasogastric aspiration. A bloody aspirate is an indication for esophagogastroduodenoscopy (EGD), as is a clear, nonbilious aspirate if a bleeding site distal to the pylorus has not been excluded. If the aspirate is clear and bile-stained, the source of the bleeding is unlikely to be the stomach, the duodenum, the liver, the biliary tree, or the pancreas. Nonetheless, if subsequent evaluation of the lower GI tract for the source of the bleeding is unrewarding, an upper GI site that had stopped bleeding when the nasogastric tube was passed or that was distal to the ligament of Treitz should still be considered.

UPPER GI ENDOSCOPY (ESOPHAGOGASTRODUODENOSCOPY)

EGD [*see 3:8 Gastrointestinal Endoscopy*] almost always reveals the source of upper GI bleeding; its utility and accuracy have been well documented in the literature. This procedure requires considerable skill: identification of bleeding sites in a blood-filled stomach is far from easy. Hematemesis is an indication for emergent EGD, usually within 1 hour of presentation. If the rate of bleeding is high, saline lavage may be performed to clear the stomach of blood and clots. If the rate of bleeding is moderate or low, as is often the case in patients with melena, urgent EGD is indicated.

EGD is not only an excellent diagnostic tool but also a valuable therapeutic modality. Indeed, most upper GI hemorrhages may be controlled endoscopically, though the degree of success to be expected in individual cases varies according to the expertise of the endoscopist and the specific cause of the bleeding. Therapeutic endoscopic maneuvers include injection, thermal coagulation, and mechanical occlusion of bleeding sites. The choice of therapy depends on the cause, the site, and the rate of bleeding.

OTHER TESTS

If endoscopic examination reveals no lesions in the stomach or the duodenum and bleeding has ceased, enteroclysis (direct introduction of $BaSO_4$ into the small bowel) and roentgenography of the duodenum and the jejunum should be done next. This is probably a more sensitive radiologic test than a standard small bowel roentgenogram. Nonetheless, the absence of a lesion on this test does not rule out the small bowel as the source of the hemorrhage; not uncommonly, the x-ray is negative when a bleeding small bowel lesion is present.

Tagged red cell scans may confirm the presence of an active bleeding site; however, scans are fairly nonspecific with respect to determining the anatomic location of the bleeding. Arteriography may demonstrate that a lesion is present, but it cannot reliably identify a bleeding site unless the bleeding is brisk (> 1 ml/min). Occasionally, arteriography reveals the cause of the bleeding even if the bleeding has stopped.

When a patient has recurrent bleeding that is believed to originate in the small bowel, intraoperative endoscopic exploration may prove useful. Before the small bowel is manipulated, a pediatric colonoscope is introduced either orally or through a distal jejunal enterotomy; the latter method allows easier viewing of the entire small bowel. The mucosal detail is

examined as the surgeon guides the scope through the small bowel. The bowel must be handled gently to avoid a mucosal injury, which could mimic a significant lesion.

These tests, in conjunction with EGD, should allow the surgeon to establish the cause of upper GI bleeding at least 90% of the time.

Management of Specific Sources of Upper GI Bleeding

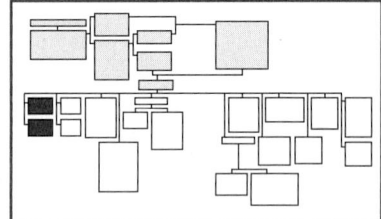

CHRONIC DUODENAL ULCER

The development of effective medical regimens for controlling uncomplicated duodenal ulcers has led to a drastic reduction in the number of elective surgical procedures performed for this purpose. Nevertheless, the incidence of bleeding from duodenal ulcers that is severe enough to necessitate emergency endoscopic or operative intervention has not decreased.

Once EGD has demonstrated that a duodenal ulcer is the source of the bleeding, the first question that must be addressed is whether active bleeding is present. If it is, an attempt should be made to control the hemorrhage endoscopically [*see Figure 1*]. Because ongoing blood loss eventually leads to coagulopathies, the surgeon must exercise good judgment in deciding how long to pursue endoscopic treatment before concluding that such treatment has failed and that surgical treatment is necessary. In general, substantial bleeding (four to six units or more) that is not easily controlled endoscopically is an indication for immediate surgical intervention. Likewise, ongoing hemorrhage in a hemodynamically unstable patient (especially an elderly one) calls for immediate surgical therapy.

If bleeding is controlled endoscopically, then an H_2 receptor blocker should be given intravenously. In addition, antibiotic therapy directed against *Helicobacter pylori* (e.g., a 14-day course of metronidazole, 500 mg p.o., t.i.d.; omeprazole, 20 mg p.o., b.i.d.; and clarithromycin, 500 mg p.o., b.i.d.) should be considered if the organism is present; such therapy has been shown to decrease rebleeding rates after antacid medication has been stopped. Food need not be withheld unless the likelihood of rebleeding is high, in which case operation or repeat endoscopy would be necessary. Resumption of oral feeding does not appear to affect rebleeding rates. Early oral intake also allows earlier initiation of therapy with a proton pump inhibitor.

If bleeding continues despite medical and endoscopic therapy, it should be managed surgically. In addition, certain patients whose bleeding was controlled endoscopically—such as those with a visible gastroduodenal artery and a clot in the base of the ulcer, those who experience rebleeding despite medical and endoscopic therapy, and those with giant ulcers—should be strongly considered for surgical therapy.

At operation, an upper midline incision is made. The duodenum is mobilized and an anterior longitudinal duodenotomy performed over the site of the ulcer. The bleeding vessel, which is usually on the posterior wall of the first portion of the duodenum, is ligated with nonabsorbable sutures at sites proximal and distal to the bleeding point. A third stitch is placed posterior to the bleeding vessel. Pains must be taken to avoid injury to the common bile duct during the placement of these sutures. The duodenotomy is then closed.

Patient has bleeding from chronic duodenal or gastric ulcer

Attempt to control hemorrhage endoscopically.

If bleeding stops: manage patient medically.

If bleeding continues: perform suture ligation of bleeding vessel.

Duodenal ulcer

Administer aggressive acid-suppressive therapy (proton pump inhibitor or H₂ receptor antagonist) and, if indicated, anti–*H. pylori* therapy (e.g., a 14-day course of metronidazole, 500 mg p.o., t.i.d.; omeprazole, 20 mg p.o., b.i.d.; and clarithromycin, 500 mg p.o., b.i.d) postoperatively.

Gastric ulcer

Perform wedge excision.

Administer aggressive acid-suppressive therapy (proton pump inhibitor or H₂ receptor antagonist) and, if indicated, anti–*H. pylori* therapy (e.g., a 14-day course of metronidazole, 500 mg p.o., t.i.d.; omeprazole, 20 mg p.o., b.i.d.; and clarithromycin, 500 mg p.o., b.i.d) postoperatively.

Figure 1 **Shown is an algorithm for management of bleeding from chronic duodenal or gastric ulcers.**

The role of vagotomy in the management of bleeding duodenal ulcers has been called into question. Previously, proximal gastric vagotomy was recommended for stable patients. It was considered preferable to truncal vagotomy because it is less likely to result in gastric atony, alkaline reflux gastritis, dumping, and diarrhea. In unstable patients, truncal vagotomy was typically performed in conjunction with pyloroplasty [*see 3:13 Gastroduodenal Procedures*]. Frozen section to confirm the presence of nerve tissue is helpful for ensuring that the vagotomy is complete.

The recommendation for truncal vagotomy was based on data from studies done before proton pump inhibitor and anti–*H. pylori* therapy came into use. Subsequent studies that evaluated rebleeding rates with current medical regimens, however, demonstrated much lower rebleeding rates. Furthermore, it seems probable that long-term proton pump inhibitor therapy (e.g., omeprazole, 20 mg p.o., q.d.)—the medical equivalent of vagotomy—in conjunction with eradication of *H. pylori* and avoidance of NSAIDs, should decrease rebleeding rates significantly. Therefore, one may consider an alternative treatment approach in patients who had not been receiving ulcer therapy before the bleeding began—namely, ligation of the bleeding vessel, postoperative administration of H₂ receptor blockers, and anti–*H. pylori* therapy. This approach avoids the complications associated with truncal vagotomy.

CHRONIC GASTRIC ULCER

Initially, bleeding from a chronic gastric ulcer is managed in much the same way as that from a chronic duodenal ulcer (i.e., endoscopically) [*see Figure 1*]. To prevent aggravation of the bleeding, early biopsy generally is not recommended; repeat endoscopy and biopsy are done at a later date. Emergent surgical indications for gastric ulcers are the same as those for duodenal ulcers. In addition, if a gastric ulcer does not resolve after 6 weeks of medical therapy, surgical excision is often indicated.

In stable patients, surgical management of a nonhealing chronic gastric ulcer generally consists of a hemigastrectomy that includes the ulcer site; if the ulcer is located more proximally, wedge excision of the ulcer, antrectomy, and gastroduodenostomy or gastrojejunostomy are done [*see 3:13 Gastroduodenal Procedures*]. Excision of the ulcer should be immediately followed by frozen section to rule out cancer. There is no need for a vagotomy in these instances. In unstable patients, hemigastrectomy should probably be avoided because of the increased morbidity and mortality that can follow it. Wedge excision can be combined with either truncal vagotomy and pyloroplasty or aggressive acid suppressive therapy (proton pump inhibitors or H₂ receptor antagonists), followed by anti–*H. pylori* treatment.

ESOPHAGEAL VARICES

The value of endoscopy in the diagnosis and management of variceal bleeding cannot be overemphasized. Even in patients with known varices, the site of bleed-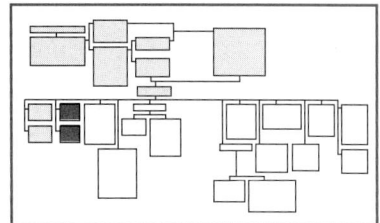ing is frequently nonvariceal; endoscopy is therefore essential. If bleeding varices are identified, rubber banding or intravariceal sclerotherapy with 1.5% sodium tetradecyl sulfate is performed [*see Figure 2*]. If these measures do not control the hemorrhage, balloon tamponade is indicated. Patients who are to undergo this procedure should have an endotracheal tube in place. The tube we prefer to use for balloon tamponade is the four-port Minnesota tube, although the Sengstaken-Blakemore tube is also acceptable. The Minnesota tube has a gastric balloon, an esophageal balloon, and aspiration ports for the esophagus and the stomach. The gastric balloon is inflated first and placed on traction. If the bleeding is not controlled, the esophageal balloon is then

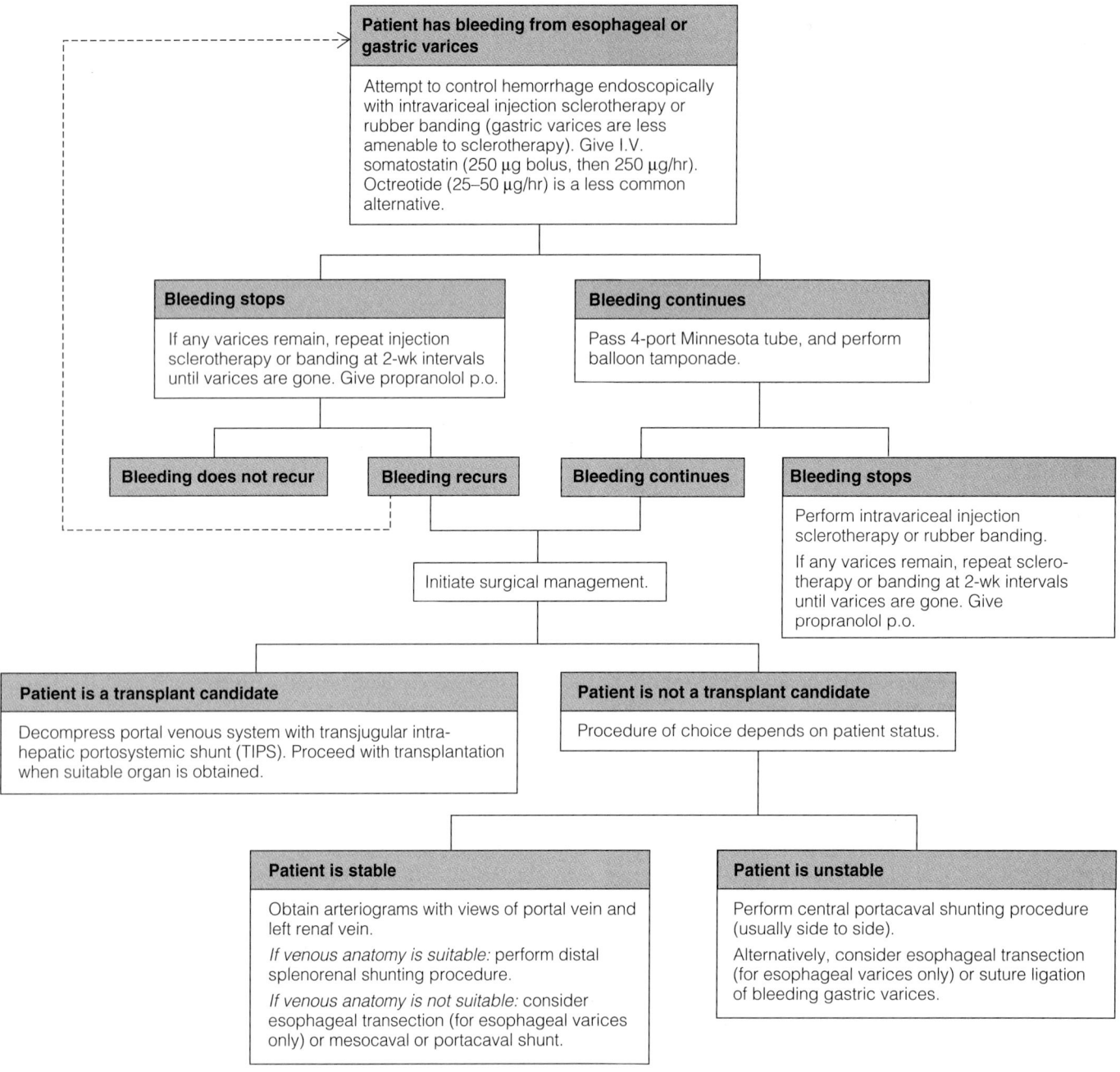

Patient has bleeding from esophageal or gastric varices

Attempt to control hemorrhage endoscopically with intravariceal injection sclerotherapy or rubber banding (gastric varices are less amenable to sclerotherapy). Give I.V. somatostatin (250 µg bolus, then 250 µg/hr). Octreotide (25–50 µg/hr) is a less common alternative.

Bleeding stops

If any varices remain, repeat injection sclerotherapy or banding at 2-wk intervals until varices are gone. Give propranolol p.o.

Bleeding continues

Pass 4-port Minnesota tube, and perform balloon tamponade.

Bleeding does not recur

Bleeding recurs

Bleeding continues

Bleeding stops

Perform intravariceal injection sclerotherapy or rubber banding.

If any varices remain, repeat sclerotherapy or banding at 2-wk intervals until varices are gone. Give propranolol p.o.

Initiate surgical management.

Patient is a transplant candidate

Decompress portal venous system with transjugular intra-hepatic portosystemic shunt (TIPS). Proceed with transplantation when suitable organ is obtained.

Patient is not a transplant candidate

Procedure of choice depends on patient status.

Patient is stable

Obtain arteriograms with views of portal vein and left renal vein.

If venous anatomy is suitable: perform distal splenorenal shunting procedure.

If venous anatomy is not suitable: consider esophageal transection (for esophageal varices only) or mesocaval or portacaval shunt.

Patient is unstable

Perform central portacaval shunting procedure (usually side to side).

Alternatively, consider esophageal transection (for esophageal varices only) or suture ligation of bleeding gastric varices.

Figure 2   Shown is an algorithm for management of bleeding from esophageal or gastric varices.

inflated. The pressure in the balloons should be released in 24 to 48 hours to prevent necrosis of the esophageal or the gastric wall. Successful balloon tamponade is followed by endoscopic variceal injection or variceal banding.

I.V. somatostatin (250 µg bolus, followed by infusion of 250 µg/hr) should be administered in conjunction with the above-mentioned steps. Vasopressin (10 U/hr) may also be given; however, it causes diffuse vasoconstriction, and nitroglycerin is required to alleviate cardiac side effects. Somatostatin has proved superior to placebo in controlling variceal hemorrhage when used in conjunction with endoscopic sclerotherapy. It is as effective as vasopressin while giving rise to fewer side effects. Octreotide shares many of the properties of somatostatin but perhaps not all. Both agents decrease secretion of gastric acid and pepsin; to date, however, the decreased gastric blood flow observed with somato-

statin administration has not been reported with octreotide administration. Nevertheless, some clinicians elect to use octreotide (25 to 50 µg/hr) in place of I.V. somatostatin.

Multiple prospective, randomized trials have shown that propranolol (40 mg b.i.d., p.o.) decreases the incidence of first-time variceal bleeding as well as the incidence of recurrent variceal bleeding. Propranolol should not be used during active bleeding but should be started once bleeding stops.

After the acute variceal bleeding has been controlled, any remaining varices should be subjected to injection sclerotherapy or banding at 2-week intervals until they too are obliterated.

The main indications for surgical intervention in patients with bleeding esophageal varices are uncontrolled hemorrhage and persistent rebleeding despite endoscopic and medical therapy. When surgical intervention is planned, it is essential to determine whether the patient is a transplant candidate. If so, operation should be avoided and bleeding managed by decompressing the portal venous system with a transjugular intrahepatic portosystemic shunt (TIPS). TIPS yields excellent short-term results with respect to stopping bleeding and providing time to locate a liver suitable for transplantation; however, it has not been shown to have the capacity to control hemorrhage by itself over the long term. Thus, its use in patients who are not transplant candidates is questionable.

If the patient is not a transplant candidate and is not actively bleeding, a distal splenorenal shunt is preferable. Arteriograms with views of the portal vein and the left renal vein are obtained. Alternatively, computed tomographic angiography with three-dimensional reconstruction may be performed. If the venous anatomy is suitable—that is, if the diameter of the splenic vein is greater than 0.75 cm (preferably greater than 1.0 cm) and the vein is within one vertebral body of the renal vein on venography—a distal splenorenal shunting procedure should be feasible. If the venous anatomy is not suitable, then esophageal transection, a mesocaval venous graft, or a portacaval shunt is required.

In the emergency setting, we prefer a central portacaval shunt, usually in a side-to-side fashion. Esophageal transection is also a reasonable choice. This procedure is associated with a lower incidence of encephalopathy than a portacaval shunting procedure; however, it is associated with higher rates of rebleeding (particularly late rebleeding), and it can be difficult to perform when active bleeding is present. Suture ligation of the bleeding varices with devascularization (the Segura procedure) should also be considered.

In general, prognosis is related to the underlying liver disease. For example, patients with varices that are secondary to chronic extrahepatic portal venous or splenic venous occlusion generally have a much better prognosis than those whose portal hypertension is secondary to hepatic parenchymal causes. The severity of the cirrhosis also determines short-term and long-term survival and may influence the decision whether to perform a shunting procedure.

Varices in children are generally secondary to portal vein thrombosis. A conservative, nonoperative approach is preferred. If operation is required, either a portacaval shunt, a distal splenorenal shunt, or a devascularization procedure is performed. In children or adults with varices that are secondary to splenic vein thrombosis (sinistral portal hypertension), a splenectomy is usually curative.

GASTRIC VARICES

Gastric varices are managed in much the same way as esophageal varices [see Figure 2], though they are less amenable to sclerotherapy. The surgical options are the same, except that esophageal transection is not a good choice. If bleeding from gastric varices is not controlled by sclerotherapy, suture ligation is indicated.

MALLORY-WEISS TEARS

Mallory-Weiss tears are linear tears at the esophagogastric junction that are usually caused by vomiting. Any patient who presents with vomiting that initially was not

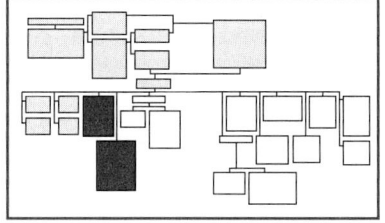

bloody but later turns so should be suspected of having a Mallory-Weiss tear. As a rule, these lesions stop bleeding without therapy. If bleeding is substantial or persistent, however, endoscopic coagulation may be necessary. In rare instances, the tear will have to be oversewn at operation. This is accomplished via an anterior gastrotomy and direct suture ligation of the tear.

ACUTE HEMORRHAGIC GASTRITIS

Bleeding from gastritis is virtually always managed medically with H_2 receptor blockers, omeprazole, sucralfate, or antacids (either alone or in combination), along with antibiotics if *H. pylori* is present. Somatostatin may be beneficial. Sometimes, administration of vasopressin via the left gastric artery is needed to control bleeding. In rare cases, total or near-total gastrectomy [see 3:13 Gastroduodenal Procedures] is required; however, the mortality associated with this operation in this setting is high. Stress ulcer prophylaxis in severely ill or traumatized patients is essential to prevent this problem. The gastric pH should be kept as close to neutral as possible. If the gastritis is relatively mild, a biopsy specimen should be obtained and tested for *H. pylori*. Treatment consists of acid reduction and anti–*H. pylori* therapy.

NEOPLASMS

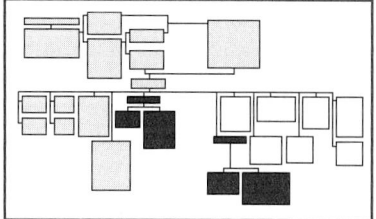

Benign tumors of the upper GI tract (e.g., leiomyomas, hamartomas, and hemangiomas) bleed at times. Wedge excision of the offending lesion is the procedure of choice.

Bleeding from malignant neoplasms, whether early stage or late stage, generally can be controlled initially by endoscopic means; however, rebleeding rates are high. If the lesion is resectable, it should be excised promptly once the patient is stable and any coagulopathies have been corrected. If disease is advanced, however, surgical options are limited, and a nonoperative approach, though necessarily imperfect, is preferable.

ESOPHAGEAL HIATAL HERNIA

Not infrequently, the source of chronic enteric blood loss is an esophageal hiatal hernia. Major bleeding is rare in this condition but may occur as a result of linear erosions at the level of the diaphragm (Cameron lesions), gastritis within the hernia, or torsion of a paraesophageal hernia. Endoscopy is generally diagnostic, though the sources of chronic blood loss are not always obvious. Recognition that the bleeding derives from a Cameron lesion should incline the surgeon toward operative intervention: this lesion is usually mechanically induced and therefore tends to be less responsive to antacid therapy.

Chronic bleeding from a sliding esophageal hiatal hernia should be treated initially with a proton pump inhibitor; anti–*H. pylori* therapy should be added if biopsy shows this organism to be present. Operation (i.e., laparoscopic Nissen fundoplication [see 3:10 Minimally Invasive Esophageal Procedures]) should be considered for fit patients who have complications associated with their hiatal hernia. A para-esophageal hernia should be repaired surgically. This repair may be performed via either a laparoscopic or an open approach; neither has yet been shown to be clearly superior.

DIEULAFOY LESION

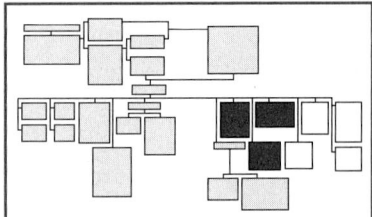

Dieulafoy lesion (also referred to as exulceratio simplex) is the rupturing of a 1 to 3 mm bleeding vessel through the gastric mucosa (usually in the proximal stomach) without surrounding ulceration. This lesion tends to be found high on the lesser curvature, but it can also occur in other locations. Histologic studies have not revealed any intrinsic abnormalities either of the mucosa or of the vessel.

Initial treatment consists of either coagulation of the bleeding vessel with a heater probe or mechanical control with clips or rubber bands; local injection of epinephrine may help control acute hemorrhage while this is being done. In skilled hands, endoscopic therapy has a 95% success rate, and long-term control is excellent. If endoscopic therapy fails, surgical options, including ligation or excision of the vessel involved, come into play. Arteriographic embolization may be employed in patients who are too ill to tolerate surgical intervention.

HEMOBILIA

Hemobilia should be suspected in all patients who present with the classic triad of epigastric and right upper quadrant pain, GI bleeding, and jaundice; however, only about 40% of patients with hemobilia present with the entire triad. Endoscopy demonstrating blood coming from the ampulla of Vater points to a source in the biliary tree or the pancreas (hemosuccus pancreaticus).

Arteriography may provide the definitive diagnosis: a bleeding tumor, a ruptured artery from trauma, or another cause. Arteriographic embolization of the affected portion of the liver is the preferred treatment option; hepatic artery ligation (selective if possible) or hepatic resection may be required.

HEMOSUCCUS PANCREATICUS

Bleeding into the pancreatic duct, generally from erosion of a pancreatic pseudocyst into the splenic artery, is signaled by upper abdominal pain followed by hematochezia. If endoscopy is performed when hematochezia is present, the bleeding site may not be seen; however, if endoscopy is performed when pain is first noted, blood may be seen coming from the ampulla of Vater. The combination of significant GI bleeding, abdominal pain, a history of alcohol abuse or pancreatitis, and hyperamylasemia should suggest the diagnosis. Distal pancreatectomy [see 3:18 Pancreatic Procedures], including excision of the pseudocyst and ligation of the splenic artery, is the preferred treatment and generally leads to cure.

AORTOENTERIC FISTULA

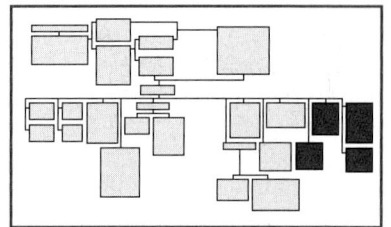

Aortoenteric fistulas may occur spontaneously as a result of rupture of an aortic aneurysm or perforation of a duodenal lesion; more often, they arise after aortic surgery. A common initial manifestation of an aortoenteric fistula is a small herald bleed that is followed a few days later by a massive hemorrhage. Patients often present with the triad of GI hemorrhage, a pulsatile mass, and infection; however, not all of these symptoms are invariably present. A high index of suspicion facilitates diagnosis. Endoscopy may show an aortic graft eroding into the enteric lumen, but this is an uncommon finding. CT scanning is the procedure of choice for diagnosis. The finding of air around the aorta or the aortic graft is diagnostic and is an indication for emergency exploration. The preferred surgical treatment is resection of the graft with extra-abdominal bypass. Some authorities, however, advocate resection of the graft with in situ graft replacement.

VASCULAR ECTASES

Vascular ectases (also referred to as vascular dysplasia, angiodysplasia, angiomata, telangiectasia, and arteriovenous malformations) may bleed briskly. As a rule, gastric lesions are readily identified and the bleeding controlled by endoscopic means. Lesions that continue to bleed, either acutely or chronically, despite endoscopic measures should be excised. Some patients have multiple and extensive lesions that necessitate resection of large portions of the stomach or the small intestine. Pharmacotherapy and hormonal therapy have been tried; the results have been mixed.

DUODENAL AND JEJUNAL DIVERTICULA

Duodenal and jejunal diverticula are rare causes of upper GI bleeding. Accurate identification of a bleeding site within a given diverticulum is difficult, but an attempt should be made to accomplish this by means of peroral enteroscopy. Excision is the preferred treatment. Great care must be taken in the treatment of duodenal diverticula in the region of the ampulla of Vater to ensure that the pancreatic duct and the bile ducts are not injured during excision.

JEJUNAL ULCER

Ulcerations of the jejunum are also rare. They may be secondary to medication, infection, a gastrinoma, or idiopathic causes. Offending medications should be stopped, infections should be treated, and gastrinomas should be excised. If these measures do not control the hemorrhage, the bleeding segment of the jejunum should be excised.

Recommended Reading

PROSPECTIVE, RANDOMIZED, CONTROLLED TRIALS

Avgerinos A, Nevens F, Raptis S, et al: Early administration of somatostatin and efficacy of sclerotherapy in acute oesophageal variceal bleeds: the European Acute Bleeding Oesophageal Variceal Episodes (ABOVE) randomised trial. Lancet 350:1495, 1997

Cello JP, Grendell JH, Crass RA, et al: Endoscopic sclerotherapy versus portacaval shunt in patients with severe cirrhosis and variceal hemorrhage. N Engl J Med 311:1589, 1984

Clark AW, Westaby D, Silk DBA, et al: Prospective controlled trial of injection sclerotherapy in patients with cirrhosis and recent variceal hemorrhage. Lancet 2:552, 1980

Conn HO, Grace ND, Bosch J, et al: Propranolol in the prevention of the first hemorrhage from esophagogastric varices: a multicenter, randomized clinical trial. Hepatology 13:902, 1991

Garcia-Pagan JC, Feu F, Bosch J, et al: Propranolol compared with propranolol plus isosorbide-5-mononitrate for portal hypertension in cirrhosis: a randomized controlled study. Ann Intern Med 114:869, 1991

Graham DY, Hepps KS, Ramirez FC, et al: Treatment of

Helicobacter pylori reduces the rate of rebleeding in peptic ulcer disease. Scand J Gastroenterol 28:939, 1993

Gregory PB: Prophylactic sclerotherapy for esophageal varices in men with alcoholic liver disease: a randomized, single-blind, multicenter trial. N Engl J Med 324:1779, 1991

Groszmann RJ, Bosch J, Grace ND, et al: Hemodynamic events in a prospective randomized trial of propranolol versus placebo in the prevention of a first variceal hemorrhage. Gastroenterology 99:1401, 1990

Hartigan PM, Gebhard RL, Gregory PB: Sclerotherapy for actively bleeding esophageal varices in male alcoholics with cirrhosis. Gastrointest Endosc 46:1, 1997

Krejs GJ, Little KH, Westergaard H, et al: Laser photocoagulation for the treatment of acute peptic-ulcer bleeding: a randomized controlled clinical trial. N Engl J Med 316:1618, 1987

Laine L: Multipolar electrocoagulation versus injection therapy in the treatment of bleeding peptic ulcers: a prospective, randomized trial. Gastroenterology 99:1303, 1990

Laine L, Cohen H, Brodhead J, et al: Prospective evaluation of immediate versus delayed refeeding and prognostic value of endoscopy in patients with upper gastrointestinal hemorrhage. Gastroenterology 102:314, 1992

Metz CA, Livingston DH, Smith JS, et al: Impact of multiple risk factors and ranitidine prophylaxis on the development of stress-related upper gastrointestinal bleeding: a prospective, multicenter, double-blind, randomized trial. Crit Care Med 21:1844, 1993

Pascal JP, Cales P: Propranolol in the prevention of first upper gastrointestinal tract hemorrhage in patients with cirrhosis of the liver and esophageal varices. N Engl J Med 317:856, 1987

Saeed ZA, Winchester CB, Michaletz PA, et al: A scoring system to predict rebleeding after endoscopic therapy of nonvariceal upper gastrointestinal hemorrhage, with a comparison of heat probe and ethanol injection. Am J Gastroenterol 88:1842, 1993

Vinel JP, Lamouliatte H, Cales P, et al: Propranolol reduces the rebleeding rate during endoscopic sclerotherapy before variceal obliteration. Gastroenterology 102:1760, 1992

Warren WD, Henderson JM, Millikan WJ, et al: Distal splenorenal shunt versus endoscopic sclerotherapy for long-term management of variceal bleeding: preliminary report of a prospective, randomized trial. Ann Surg 203:454, 1986

META-ANALYSES

Cook DJ, Guyatt GH, Salena BJ, et al: Endoscopic therapy for acute nonvariceal upper gastrointestinal hemorrhage: a meta-analysis. Gastroenterology 102:139, 1992

Poynard T, Cales P, Pasta L, et al: Beta-adrenergic-antagonist drugs in the prevention of gastrointestinal bleeding in patients with cirrhosis and esophageal varices. N Engl J Med 324:1532, 1991

Tryba M: Prophylaxis of stress ulcer bleeding: a meta-analysis. J Clin Gastroenterol 13(suppl 2):S44, 1991

PROSPECTIVE STUDIES

Barkun AN, Cockeram AW, Plourde V, et al: Review article: acid suppression in non-variceal acute upper gastrointestinal bleeding. Aliment Pharmacol Ther 13:1565, 1999

Branicki FJ, Coleman SY, Pritchett CJ, et al: Emergency surgical treatment for nonvariceal bleeding of the upper part of the gastrointestinal tract. Surg Gynecol Obstet 172:113, 1991

Cebollero-Santamaria F, Smith J, Gioe S, et al: Selective outpatient management of upper gastrointestinal bleeding in the elderly. Am J Gastroenteral 94:1242, 1999

Gostout CJ, Wang KK, Ahlquist DA, et al: Acute gastrointestinal bleeding: experience of a specialized management team. J Clin Gastroenterol 14:260, 1992

Hunt PS, Fracs MS, Korman MG, et al: An 8-year prospective experience with balloon tamponade in emergency control of bleeding esophageal varices. Dig Dis Sci 27:413, 1982

Loftus EV, Alexander GL, Ahlquist DA, et al: Endoscopic treatment of major bleeding from advanced gastroduodenal malignant lesions. Mayo Clin Proc 69:736, 1994

Rockey DC, Cello JP: Evaluation of the gastrointestinal tract in patients with iron-deficiency anemia. N Engl J Med 329:1691, 1993

Terblanche J, Northoever JMA, Bornman P, et al: A prospective evaluation of injection sclerotherapy in the treatment of acute bleeding from esophageal varices. Surgery 85:239, 1979

Wilcox CM, Alexander LN, Straub RF, et al: A prospective endoscopic evaluation of the causes of upper GI hemorrhage in alcoholics: a focus on alcoholic gastropathy. Am J Gastroenteral 91:1343, 1996

Zuckerman G, Benitez J: A prospective study of bidirectional endoscopy (colonoscopy and upper endoscopy) in the evaluation of patients with occult gastrointestinal bleeding. Am J Gastroenterol 87:62, 1992

RETROSPECTIVE STUDIES

Corley DA, Stefan AM, Wolf M, et al: Early indicators of prognosis in upper gastrointestinal hemorrhage. Am J Gastroenterol 93:336, 1998

Cotton PB, Rosenberg MT, Waldram RPL, et al: Early endoscopy of oesophagus, stomach, and duodenal bulb in patients with haematemesis and melaena. Br Med J 2:505, 1973

Dempsey DT, Burke DR, Reilly RS, et al: Angiography in poor-risk patients with massive nonvariceal upper gastrointestinal bleeding. Am J Surg 159:282, 1990

Fox JG, Hunt PS: Management of acute bleeding gastric malignancy. Aust NZ J Surg 63:462, 1993

Gaisford WD: Endoscopic electrohemostasis of active upper gastrointestinal bleeding. Am J Surg 137:47, 1979

Henriksson AE, Svensson J-O: Upper gastrointestinal bleeding (with special reference to blood transfusion). Eur J Surg 157:193, 1991

Himal HS, Perrault C, Mzabi R: Upper gastrointestinal hemorrhage: aggressive management decreases mortality. Surgery 84:448, 1978

Jacobson AR, Cerqueira MD: Prognostic significance of late imaging results in technetium-99m-labeled red blood cell gastrointestinal bleeding studies with early negative images. J Nucl Med 33:202, 1992

Jim G, Rikkers LF: Cause and management of upper gastrointestinal bleeding after distal splenorenal shunt. Surgery 112:719, 1992

Kaye GL, McCormick A, Siringo S, et al: Bleeding from staple line erosion after esophageal transection: effect of omeprazole. Hepatology 15:1031, 1992

Kollef MH, O'Brien JD, Zuckerman GR, et al: Bleed: a classification tool to predict outcomes in patients with acute upper and lower gastrointestinal hemorrhage. Crit Care Med 25:1125, 1997

Liebler JM, Benner K, Putnam T, et al: Respiratory complications in critically ill medical patients with acute upper gastrointestinal bleeding. Crit Care Med 19:1152, 1991

Lipper B, Simon D, Cerrone F: Pulmonary aspiration during emergency endoscopy in patients with upper gastrointestinal hemorrhage. Crit Care Med 19:330, 1991

Miller AR, Farnell MB, Kelly KA, et al: The impact of therapeutic endoscopy on the treatment of bleeding duodenal ulcers, 1980–90. World J Surg 19:89, 1995

Norton ID, Petersen BT, Sorbi D, et al: Management and long-term prognosis of Dieulafoy lesion. Gastrointest Endosc 50:762, 1999

Sakorafas GH, Sarr MG, Farley DR: Hemosuccus pancreaticus complicating chronic pancreatitis: an obscure cause of upper gastrointestinal bleeding. Langenbeck Arch Surg 385:124, 2000

Sugawa C, Benishek D, Walt AJ: Mallory-Weiss syndrome: a study of 224 patients. Am J Surg 145:30, 1983

Sugawa C, Steffes CP, Nakamura R, et al: Upper gastrointestinal bleeding in an urban hospital: etiology, recurrence, and prognosis. Ann Surg 212:521, 1990

Wilairatana S, Sriussadaporn S, Tanphaiphat C: A review of 1338 patients with acute upper gastrointestinal bleeding at Chulalongkorn University Hospital, Bangkok. Gastroenterologia Japonica 26:58, 1991

Reviews

De Franchis R: Emerging strategies in the management of upper gastrointestinal bleeding. Digestion 60(suppl 3):17, 1999

Groszmann RJ, Grace ND: Complications of portal hypertension: esophagogastric varices and ascites. Gastroenterol Clin North Am 21:103, 1992

Jenkins SA: Drug therapy for non-variceal upper gastrointestinal bleeding. Digestion 60(suppl 3):39, 1999

Kankaria AG, Fleischer DE: The critical care management of nonvariceal upper gastrointestinal bleeding. Crit Care Clin 11:347, 1995

Katz PO, Salas L: Less frequent causes of upper gastrointestinal bleeding. Gastroenterol Clin North Am 22:875, 1993

Montgomery RS, Wilson SE: Surgical management of gastrointestinal fistulas. Surg Clin North Am 76:1148, 1996

Savides TJ, Jensen DM: Therapeutic endoscopy for nonvariceal upper gastrointestinal bleeding. Gastroenterol Clin North Am 29:465, 2000

Weiner FR, Simon DM: Gastric vascular ectases. Gastrointest Endosc Clin North Am 6:681, 1996

Zoller WG, Gross M: Beta-blockers for prophylaxis of bleeding from esophageal varices in cirrhotic portal hypertension: review of the literature. Eur J Med Res 1:407, 1995/96

7 LOWER GASTROINTESTINAL BLEEDING

Michael Rosen, M.D., and Jeffrey L. Ponsky, M.D., F.A.C.S.

Approach to Lower GI Bleeding

Lower gastrointestinal bleeding is defined as abnormal hemorrhage into the lumen of the bowel from a source distal to the ligament of Treitz. In the majority of cases, lower GI bleeding derives from the colon; however, the small bowel is identified as the source of bleeding in as many as one third of cases,[1,2] and the upper GI tract is identified as the source in as many as 11% of patients presenting with bright red blood per rectum.[3]

Lower GI bleeding is more common in men than in women. The incidence rises steeply with advancing age, exhibiting a greater than 200-fold increase from the third decade of life to the ninth. This increase is largely attributable to the various colonic disorders commonly associated with aging (e.g., diverticulosis and angiodysplasia).[4-6] The exact incidence of lower GI bleeding is not known, because there is no standardized technique for localizing it. Several investigators, however, estimate the incidence to be in the range of 20 to 27 cases per 100,000 adults.[4,7] A 1997 survey of GI bleeding from the American College of Gastroenterology found that lower GI hemorrhage accounted for 24% of all GI bleeding events.[8] Another study published the same year found that 0.7% of 17,941 discharges from a Veterans Affairs Hospital were for patients who had had lower GI bleeding.[9]

The basic components of management are (1) initial hemodynamic stabilization, (2) localization of the bleeding site, and (3) site-specific therapeutic intervention. There are many conditions that can cause lower GI hemorrhage [*see* Discussion, Etiology of Lower GI Bleeding, *below*]; accordingly, successful localization depends on timely and appropriate use of a variety of diagnostic tests. Despite the abundance of diagnostic modalities available, attempts to localize the source of the hemorrhage fail in as many as 8% to 12% of patients.[10,11] Once the bleeding site is localized, the appropriate therapeutic intervention must be carried out as expeditiously as possible.

Lower GI bleeding can be acute and life-threatening, chronic, or even occult. In what follows, we focus on severe, life-threatening hematochezia, reviewing the wide array of possible causes of lower GI bleeding and outlining the diagnostic and therapeutic modalities available for treating this difficult clinical problem.

Initial Evaluation and Resuscitation

Initial evaluation of a patient with lower GI bleeding should include a focused history and physical examination, to be carried out simultaneously with resuscitation. Of particular importance in

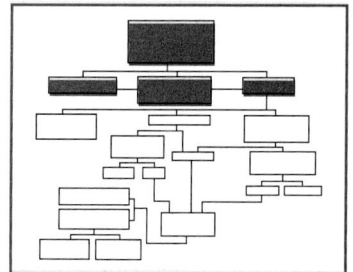

taking the history is to ascertain the nature and duration of the bleeding, including stool color and frequency. The patient should also be asked about any associated symptoms of potential significance (e.g., abdominal pain, changes in bowel habits, fever, urgency, tenesmus, or weight loss) as well as about relevant past medical events (e.g., previous GI bleeding episodes, injuries, surgical procedures, peptic ulcer disease, inflammatory bowel disease, and exposure to abdominal or pelvic radiation). Any complicating comorbid conditions (e.g., heart or liver disease and clotting disorders) should be investigated. A comprehensive review of medications—in particular, nonsteroidal anti-inflammatory drugs (NSAIDs) and anticoagulants—is mandatory.[12]

The physical examination should include determination of postural vital signs so that intravascular volume status can be accurately estimated. A drop in the orthostatic blood pressure greater than 10 mm Hg or an increase in the pulse rate greater than 10 beats/min indicates that more than 800 ml of blood (> 15% of the total circulating blood volume) has been lost. Marked tachycardia and tachypnea in association with hypotension and depressed mental status indicates that more than 1,500 ml of blood (> 30% of the total circulating blood volume) has been lost.[13] A complete abdominal examination, including digital rectal examination and anoscopy, should be performed.

Laboratory evaluation should include a complete blood count, measurement of serum electrolyte concentrations, a coagulation profile (prothrombin time and partial thromboplastin time) [*see 1:4 Bleeding and Transfusion*], and typing and crossmatching.

A nasogastric tube should be placed for gastric lavage. If lavage yields positive results (i.e., the aspirate contains gross blood or so-called coffee grounds), esophagogastroduodenoscopy (EGD) is indicated [*see 3:8 Gastrointestinal Endoscopy*]. An aspirate that contains copious amounts of bile is strongly suggestive of a lower GI source of bleeding, and the workup proceeds accordingly [*see* Diagnostic Testing, *below*]. The choice is less clear-cut with a clear aspirate. In the absence of bile, such an aspirate cannot rule out a duodenal source for the bleeding. Accordingly, there is some degree of latitude for clinical judgment: depending on the overall clinical picture, the surgeon may choose either to perform EGD to rule out a duodenal bleeding source or to proceed with colonoscopy on the assumption that the source of the bleeding is in the lower GI tract.

Resuscitative efforts should begin immediately, with the aim of maintaining the patient in a euvolemic state. Two large-bore peripheral intravenous catheters should be inserted and isotonic I.V. fluid administered. A Foley catheter should be placed to facilitate monitoring of intravascular volume status. Whether and in what form to administer blood products is determined on an individual basis, with appropriate weight given to the presence or absence of comorbid conditions, the rate of blood loss, and the degree of hemodynamic stability. Severe hemodynamic instability may necessitate monitoring in the intensive care unit.

Diagnostic Testing

A number of diagnostic techniques are available for determining the source of lower GI hemorrhage, the most useful of which are colonoscopy [see *3:8 Gastrointestinal Endoscopy*], radionuclide scanning, and angiography (in the form of selective mesenteric arteriography). The goal of these tests is accurate localization of the site of bleeding so that definitive therapy can be properly directed. Which diagnostic test is chosen for a specific patient depends on several factors, including the hemodynamic stability of the patient, the bleeding rate, the comorbid conditions present, and the local expertise available at the physician's hospital.

COLONOSCOPY

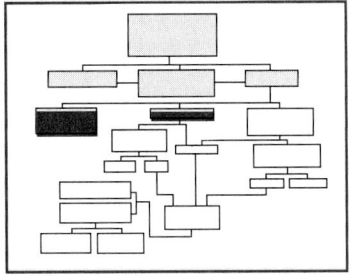

Several large series that evaluated the diagnostic utility of colonoscopy in patients with lower GI bleeding found this modality to be moderately to highly accurate, with overall diagnostic yields ranging from 53% to 97% [see Table 1].[3,14-19] Those studies that reported morbidity found colonoscopy to be safe as well, with an average complication rate of 0.5%. Colonoscopy has both a higher diagnostic yield and a lower complication rate than arteriography in this setting and thus would appear to be a more attractive initial test in most circumstances.[3,20] An argument has been made—one with which we agree—that colonoscopy should be considered the procedure of choice for structural evaluation of lower GI bleeding and that arteriography should be reserved for patients with massive, ongoing bleeding in whom endoscopy is not feasible or colonoscopy fails to reveal the source of the hemorrhage.[12]

The merits of colonic purging have been extensively debated in the literature.[3,15,21] Although no firm conclusion has been reached, we feel that adequate colonic purging can improve both the diagnostic yield and the safety of colonoscopy. Given the absence of any definitive data suggesting that colonic purging either reactivates or increases bleeding,[12] it is our practice to administer an oral purge after the patient has been adequately resuscitated.

If the entire colon has been adequately visualized and no source for the bleeding has been identified, the ileum should be intubated; fresh blood in this region suggests a possible small bowel source. If no active bleeding is observed in the ileum, upper GI endoscopy should be performed to rule out an upper GI bleeding site.

RADIOLABELED RED BLOOD CELL SCANNING

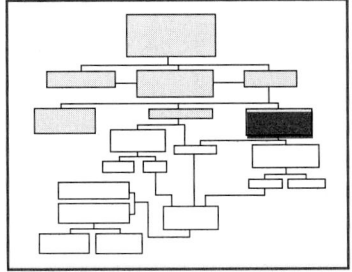

Radionuclide scanning is highly sensitive for lower GI hemorrhage: it is capable of detecting bleeding at rates as slow as 0.1 to 0.4 ml/min.[22] Two imaging tracers, both labeled with technetium-99m (99mTc), are currently avail-

Table 1 Diagnostic Accuracy of Colonoscopy in Localizing Source of Lower GI Hemorrhage

Study	No. of Patients	Diagnostic Yield (%)
Richter[14]	78	70 (90%)
Jensen[3]	80	68 (85%)
Rossini[15]	409	311 (76%)
Geller[16]	524	280 (53%)
Goenka[17]	166	141 (85%)
Ohyama[18]	345	307 (89%)
Chaudhry[19]	85	82 (97%)
Total	1,687	1,259 (75%)

able for radionuclide scanning in this setting: 99mTc-labeled sulfur colloid (99mTc-SC) and 99mTc-labeled red blood cells. 99mTc-SC requires no preparation time and can be injected immediately into the patient; however, its rapid absorption into the liver and the spleen can often hinder accurate localization of overlying bleeding sites.[9] At our institution, we prefer to use 99mTc-labeled RBCs. This agent requires some preparation time, but it has a much longer half-life than 99mTc-SC does, it is not taken up by the liver and spleen, and it can be detected on images as long as 24 to 48 hours after injection [see Figure 1].[23,24]

One study directly compared these two techniques and found 99mTc-labeled RBC scanning to have an accuracy of 93%, compared with an accuracy of only 12% for 99mTc-SC scanning.[25] The high sensitivity of 99mTc-labeled RBC scanning—80% to 98%—is well attested, but there is considerable disagreement in the literature with regard to its specificity in identifying the anatomic site of bleeding.[26-31] For example, on one hand, a 1996 study found radiolabeled RBC scanning to be 97% accurate for localiz-

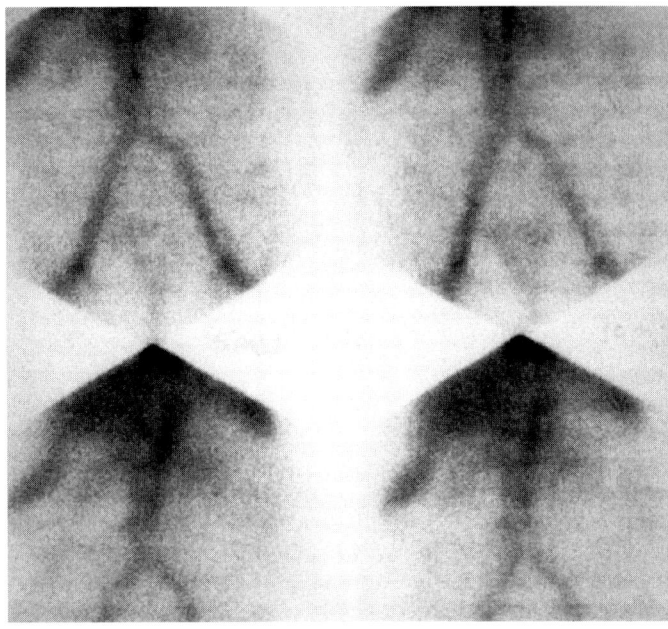

Figure 1 **99mTechnetium-labeled RBC scan demonstrates collection of tracer at hepatic flexure.**

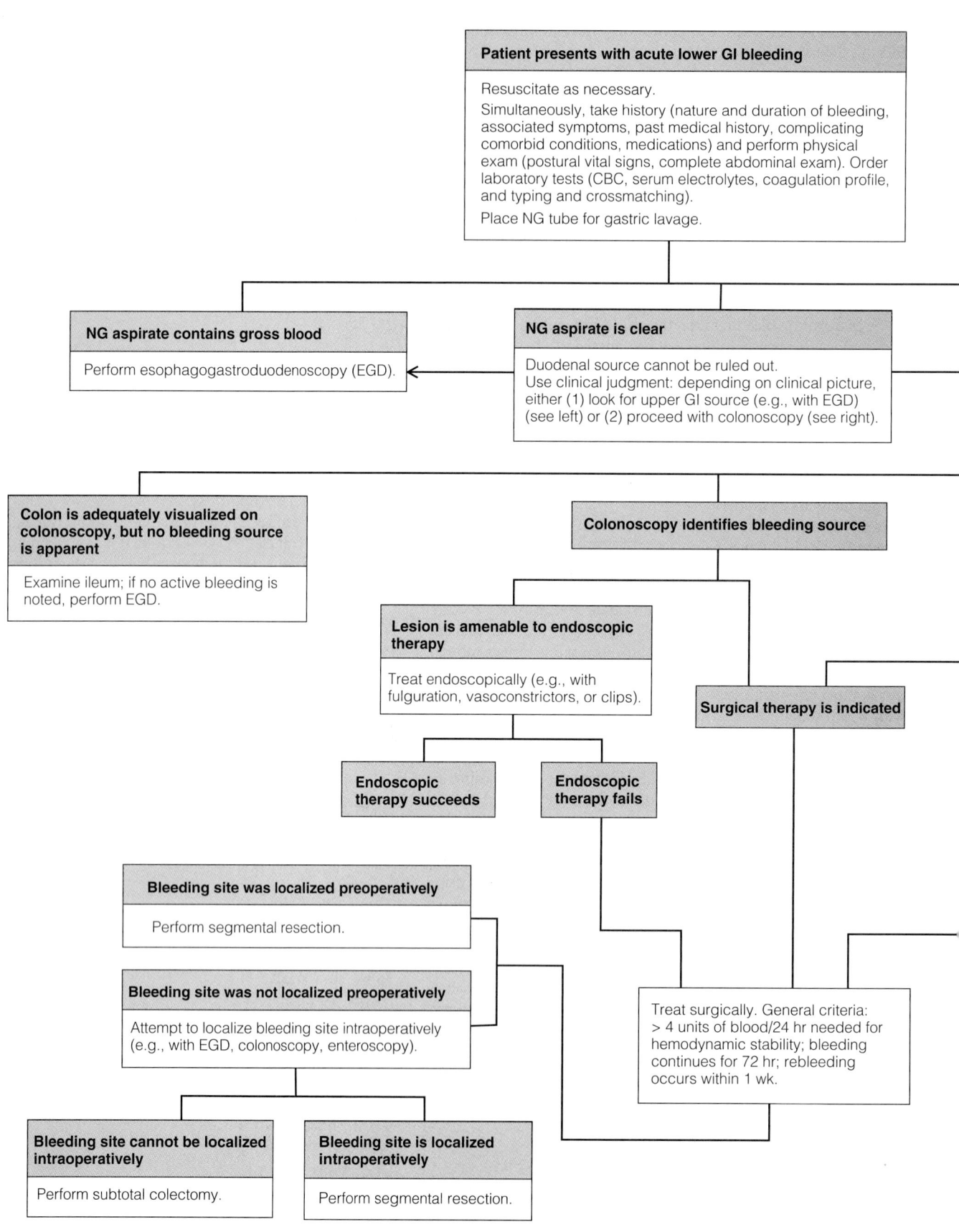

Patient presents with acute lower GI bleeding

Resuscitate as necessary.

Simultaneously, take history (nature and duration of bleeding, associated symptoms, past medical history, complicating comorbid conditions, medications) and perform physical exam (postural vital signs, complete abdominal exam). Order laboratory tests (CBC, serum electrolytes, coagulation profile, and typing and crossmatching).

Place NG tube for gastric lavage.

NG aspirate contains gross blood

Perform esophagogastroduodenoscopy (EGD).

NG aspirate is clear

Duodenal source cannot be ruled out.
Use clinical judgment: depending on clinical picture, either (1) look for upper GI source (e.g., with EGD) (see left) or (2) proceed with colonoscopy (see right).

Colon is adequately visualized on colonoscopy, but no bleeding source is apparent

Examine ileum; if no active bleeding is noted, perform EGD.

Colonoscopy identifies bleeding source

Lesion is amenable to endoscopic therapy

Treat endoscopically (e.g., with fulguration, vasoconstrictors, or clips).

Surgical therapy is indicated

Endoscopic therapy succeeds

Endoscopic therapy fails

Bleeding site was localized preoperatively

Perform segmental resection.

Bleeding site was not localized preoperatively

Attempt to localize bleeding site intraoperatively (e.g., with EGD, colonoscopy, enteroscopy).

Treat surgically. General criteria: > 4 units of blood/24 hr needed for hemodynamic stability; bleeding continues for 72 hr; rebleeding occurs within 1 wk.

Bleeding site cannot be localized intraoperatively

Perform subtotal colectomy.

Bleeding site is localized intraoperatively

Perform segmental resection.

Approach to Lower GI Bleeding

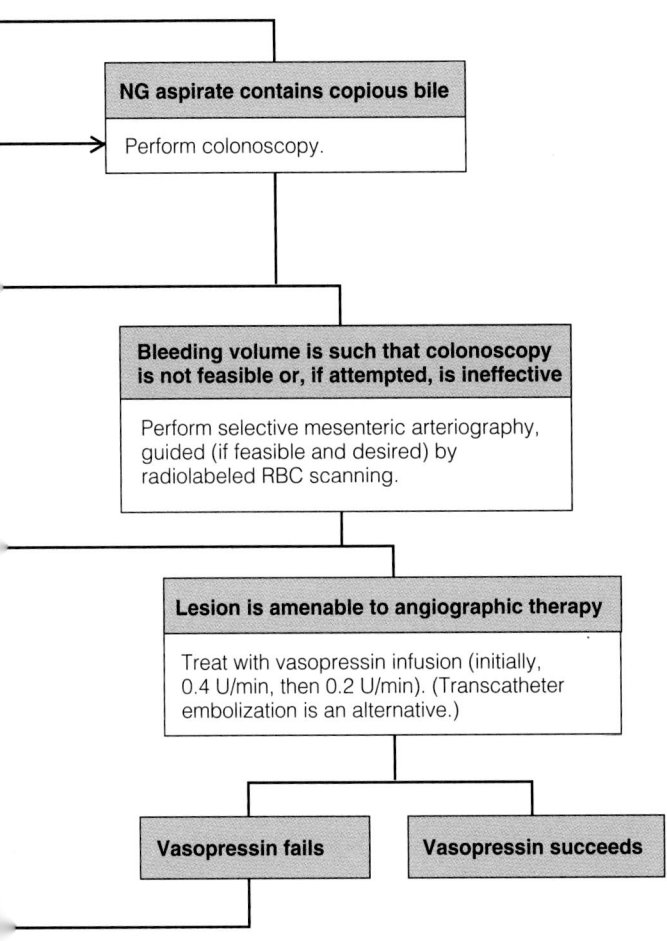

NG aspirate contains copious bile

Perform colonoscopy.

Bleeding volume is such that colonoscopy is not feasible or, if attempted, is ineffective

Perform selective mesenteric arteriography, guided (if feasible and desired) by radiolabeled RBC scanning.

Lesion is amenable to angiographic therapy

Treat with vasopressin infusion (initially, 0.4 U/min, then 0.2 U/min). (Transcatheter embolization is an alternative.)

Vasopressin fails

Vasopressin succeeds

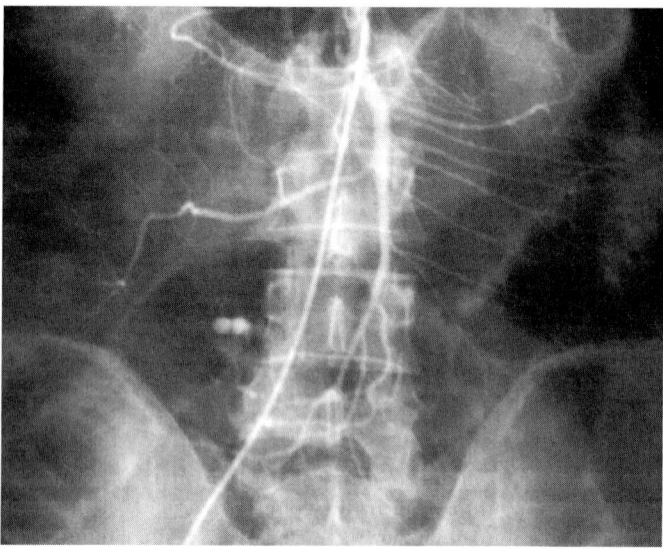

Figure 2 Angiographic study documents extravasation of contrast into small bowel.

ing bleeding in 37 patients undergoing surgical resection[27]; on the other hand, a 1990 study reported a 42% rate of incorrect resection when surgical therapy was based solely on this modality.[28]

To date, no prospective randomized trials have compared radionuclide scanning with colonoscopy as the initial diagnostic procedure for patients with lower GI hemorrhage. In our view, however, given that radionuclide scanning, unlike colonoscopy and angiography, has no therapeutic intervention capabilities, its best use is in patients with non–life-threatening lower GI bleeding as a prelude and a guide to mesenteric angiography after active hemorrhage has been confirmed.

ANGIOGRAPHY

Selective Mesenteric Arteriography

Selective mesenteric arteriography is somewhat less sensitive than radionuclide scanning for lower GI hemorrhage: bleeding

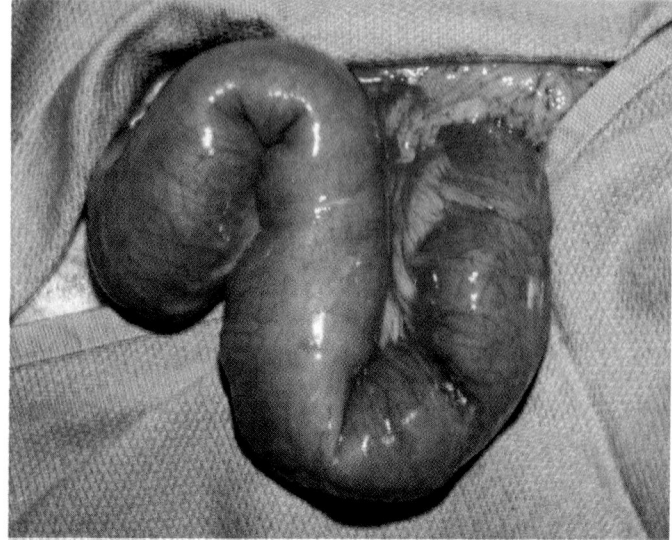

Figure 3 Intraoperative examination of bowel is aided by injection of methlyene blue dye, which facilitates localization of bleeding site and thereby helps direct surgical resection.

Table 2 Diagnostic Accuracy of Mesenteric Angiography in Localizing Source of Lower GI Hemorrhage

Study	No. of Patients	No. of Positive Angiograms (%)
Pennoyer[35]	131	37 (28%)
Ng[29]	49	22 (45%)
Rantis[36]	30	8 (27%)
Leitman[37]	68	27 (40%)
Casarella[38]	69	46 (67%)
Colacchio[39]	98	40 (41%)
Total	445	180 (40%)

must be occurring at a rate of at least 1.0 to 1.5 ml/min to be detectable with this test.[32] The procedure involves percutaneous placement of a transfemoral arterial catheter for evaluation of the superior mesenteric, inferior mesenteric, and celiac arteries. A positive test result is defined as extravasation of contrast into the lumen of the bowel [*see Figure 2*]. Once the bleeding vessel has been localized angiographically, the area must be marked so that it can be successfully identified intraoperatively; this is commonly accomplished by infusing methylene blue into the bleeding artery [*see Figure 3*].[33,34]

In several large series [*see Table 2*], the overall diagnostic yield of arteriography ranged from 27% to 67%.[29,35-39] The complication rate for arteriography performed for lower GI bleeding ranges from 2% to 4%.[2,39] Reported complications include contrast allergy, renal failure, bleeding from arterial puncture, and embolism from dislodged thrombus.[12]

Unlike radionuclide scanning, arteriography provides several therapeutic options, including vasopressin infusion and embolization of bleeding vessels. Nonetheless, given that arteriography has a lower diagnostic yield and a higher complication rate than colonoscopy does, it is reasonable to attempt colonoscopy first in patients with lower GI hemorrhage and to reserve angiography for patients in whom the volume of bleeding is such that colonoscopy would be neither safe nor accurate.

Provocative Angiography for Continued Obscure Bleeding

In a minority of patients, obscure bleeding persists despite negative findings from endoscopy, mesenteric arteriography, and radiolabeled RBC scanning. This obscure bleeding presents a considerable diagnostic challenge, which some investigators have proposed addressing by means of so-called provocative angiography.[40,41] Provocative angiography involves the use of short-acting anticoagulant agents (unfractionated heparin, vasodilators, thrombolytics, or combinations thereof) in association with angiography. Once the bleeding point has been localized, methylene blue is injected and the patient is immediately brought to the OR for surgical treatment. To date, unfortunately, little has been published on this technique, but it does appear to be a promising approach to this difficult problem.

Therapeutic Intervention

Although in the majority of cases, lower GI bleeding stops spontaneously, in a significant number of cases, hemorrhage continues and necessitates therapeutic intervention. Treatment options include endoscopic therapy, angiographic therapy, and surgical resection.

ENDOSCOPIC THERAPY

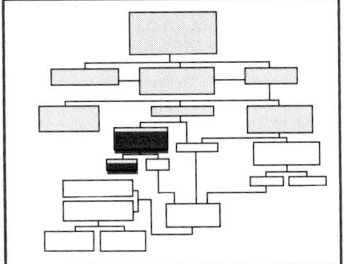

When colonoscopy identifies a bleeding source, endoscopic treatment may be an option [see 3:8 Gastrointestinal Endoscopy]. Endoscopic modalities used to treat lower GI bleeding include use of thermal contact probes,[42,43] laser photocoagulation,[44] electrocauterization,[45] injection of vasoconstrictors, application of metallic clips,[46] and injection sclerotherapy.[47] The choice of a specific modality often depends on the nature of the offending lesion and on the expertise and resources available locally. A 1995 survey of members of the American College of Gastroenterology found that endoscopic therapy was used in 27% of patients presenting with lower GI bleeding.[8]

Diverticular hemorrhage can be difficult to treat endoscopically because of the high bleeding rate and the location of the bleeding point within the diverticulum. In 2000, one group of investigators reported their experience with endoscopic therapy for severe hematochezia and diverticulosis in a prospective series of 121 patients.[48] In this series, none of the patients treated endoscopically with epinephrine injections, bipolar coagulation, or both required surgery and none experienced recurrent bleeding episodes. A 2001 study from another group, however, reported high rates of recurrent bleeding episodes in both the early and the late posttreatment periods.[49] In the absence of prospective, randomized trials, it is difficult to draw definitive conclusions about the utility of endoscopic therapy in treating diverticular hemorrhage.

Angiodysplasias resulting in GI hemorrhage typically are amenable to endoscopic treatment. That these lesions are frequently found in the right colon makes perforation a concern; this complication is reported in approximately 2% of patients.[50] Good success rates have been reported with both injection and thermal methods.[51] In one series, endoscopic fulguration was successful in 87% of patients, and no rebleeding episodes occurred over a 1- to 7-year follow-up period.[51] Bleeding from multiple telangiectatic lesions in the distal colon resulting from radiation injury can be treated with thermal contact probes, lasers, or noncontact devices such as the argon plasma coagulator.[52]

Postpolypectomy hemorrhage can often be successfully treated by endoscopic means. Methods used include simple resnaring of the stalk while pressure is maintained[53]; electrocauterization, with or without epinephrine injection; endoscopic band ligation; and placement of metallic clips. For patients whose bleeding is attributable to benign anorectal causes, endoscopic therapy may include epinephrine injection, sclerosant injection, or band ligation of internal hemorrhoids.[54]

ANGIOGRAPHIC THERAPY

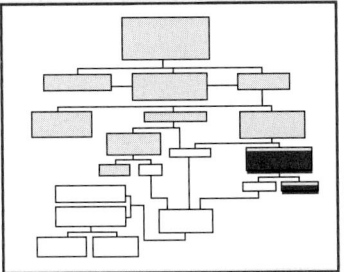

Diagnostic use of angiography in patients with lower GI bleeding can often be followed by angiographic therapy. The two main angiographic treatment options are intra-arterial injection of vasopressin and transcatheter embolization.

Vasopressin acts to control bleeding by causing arteriolar vasoconstriction and bowel wall contraction.[9] Once the bleeding site has been localized angiographically, the catheter is positioned in the main trunk of the vessel. Infusion of vasopressin is initiated at a rate of 0.2 U/min and can be increased to a rate of 0.4 U/min. Within 20 to 30 minutes, another angiogram is performed to determine whether the bleeding has ceased. If the bleeding is under control, the catheter is left in place and vasopressin is continuously infused for 6 to 12 hours. If the bleeding continues to be controlled, infusion is continued for an additional 6 to 12 hours at 50% of the previous rate. Finally, vasopressin infusion is replaced by continuous saline infusion, and if bleeding does not recur, the catheter is removed.[55,56]

The vasoconstrictive action of vasopressin can have deleterious systemic side effects, including myocardial ischemia, peripheral ischemia, hypertension, dysrhythmias, mesenteric thrombosis, intestinal infarction, and death.[9,37] Occasionally, simultaneous I.V. administration of nitroglycerine is necessary to counteract these systemic effects. The reported success rate of vasopressin in controlling lower GI bleeding ranges from 60% to 100%, and the incidence of major complications ranges from 10% to 20%.[57-60] Rebleeding rates as high as 50% have been reported.[59,60]

An alternative for patients with coronary vascular disease, severe peripheral vascular disease, or other comorbidities that prevent safe administration of vasopressin is transcatheter embolization. In this technique, a catheter is superselectively placed into the identified bleeding vessel and an embolizing agent (e.g., a gelatin sponge, a microcoil, polyvinyl alcohol particles, or a balloon) is injected. Several small series found this technique to be 90% to 100% successful at stopping bleeding.[61-64] Equally impressive was the finding that the rebleeding rates in these series were 0%. The complication rates of this procedure are generally reasonable as well; however, intestinal infarction has been reported.[37,65]

SURGICAL THERAPY

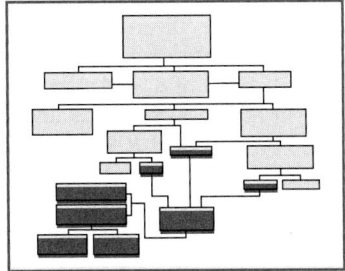

Although there are no absolute criteria for surgery, there are several factors—including hemodynamic status, associated comorbidities, transfusion requirements, and persistent bleeding—that are instrumental in making an appropriate and timely decision whether to operate. In general, patients who require more than 4 units of blood in a 24-hour period to remain hemodynamically stable, whose bleeding has not stopped after 72 hours, or who experience rebleeding within 1 week of an initial episode should undergo surgery.[9]

If the patient's hemodynamic status permits, surgical treatment should be undertaken after accurate localization of the bleeding site. When possible, directed segmental resection is the procedure of choice: it is associated with rebleeding rates ranging from 0% to 14% and mortalities ranging from 0% to 13%.[10,37,66] Blind segmental colectomy should never be performed: it is associated with rebleeding rates as high as 75% and mortalities as high as 50%.[67] If hemodynamic compromise and ongoing hemorrhage make it necessary to perform surgical exploration before the bleeding site can be localized, every effort should be made to identify the source of bleeding intraoperatively before embarking on resection. Intraoperative options for bleeding site localization include colonoscopy (to allow for this option, patients should always be placed in the lithotomy position), EGD, and transoral passage of a pediatric colonoscope for enteroscopy with simultaneous intraperitoneal assistance for small bowel manipulation.[9] If the bleeding site still cannot be accurately localized, subtotal colectomy is the procedure of choice. This procedure is associated with mortalities ranging from 5% to 33%,[68,69] which underscores the importance of accurate preoperative localization of bleeding before surgical intervention.

Discussion

Etiology of Lower GI Bleeding

As noted, lower GI bleeding has a wide array of possible causes [*see Table 3*].[9,70] Of these, diverticular disease is the most common, accounting for 30% to 40% of all cases.[21,71] Arteriovenous malformations (AVMs), though extensively described in the literature, are considerably less common causes, accounting for 1% to 4% of cases.[72-74] Other significant causative conditions are inflammatory bowel disease (IBD), benign and malignant neoplasms, ischemia, infectious colitis, anorectal disease, coagulopathy, use of NSAIDs, radiation proctitis, AIDS, and small bowel disorders.

DIVERTICULAR DISEASE

The reported prevalence of colonic diverticulosis in Western societies is 37% to 45%.[75] The vast majority of colonic diverticula are actually false diverticula (pseudodiverticula) that contain only serosa and mucosa. They occur at weak points in the colonic wall where the vasa recta penetrate the muscularis to supply the mucosa[9]; as the diverticulum expands, these vessels are displaced. A 1976 anatomical study of colonic specimens from patients with diverticular bleeding used angiography to demonstrate that in all cases, the vasa recta overlying the diverticulum ruptured into the lumen of the diverticulum, not into the peritoneum [*see Figure 4*].[76]

It has been estimated that approximately 17% of patients with colonic diverticulosis experience bleeding, which may range from minor to severe and life-threatening.[77] As many as 80% to 85% of diverticular hemorrhages stop spontaneously.[78] In one series, surgery was unlikely to be necessary if fewer than 4 units of packed RBCs were transfused in a 24-hour period, whereas 60% of patients receiving more than 4 units of packed RBCs in a 24-hour period required surgical intervention.[79] The risk of a second bleeding episode is approximately 25%.[3] Semielective surgical therapy is usually offered after a second diverticular bleeding episode because once a second such episode has occurred, the risk that a third will follow exceeds 50%.[80] In a series of 83 conservatively managed cases of diverticular disease, the predicted yearly recurrence rates were 9% at 1 year, 10% at 2 years, 19% at 3 years, and 25% at 4 years.[4]

COLITIS

The broad term colitis includes IBD, infectious colitis, radiation colitis, and idiopathic ulcers. IBD, in turn, includes Crohn disease and ulcerative colitis. Patients with IBD usually present with bloody diarrhea that is not life-threatening; however, 6% to 10% of patients with ulcerative colitis have lower GI bleeding severe enough to necessitate emergency surgical resection,[81,82] and 0.6% to 1.3% of patients with Crohn disease have acute life-threatening lower GI bleeding.[81,83] In one review, 50% of patients with intestinal hemorrhage from IBD experienced spontaneous cessation of bleeding.[81] Approximately 35% of patients whose bleeding stops without intervention will have another bleeding episode. Because of this high recurrence rate, semielective surgery is recommended after the first episode of severe GI bleeding secondary to IBD.

Colitis caused by various infectious agents (e.g., *Salmonella typhi*,[84,85] *Escherichia coli* O157:H7,[86] *Clostridium difficile*,[87] and cytomegalovirus[88]) can result in severe lower GI bleeding, but this is a relatively rare occurrence.

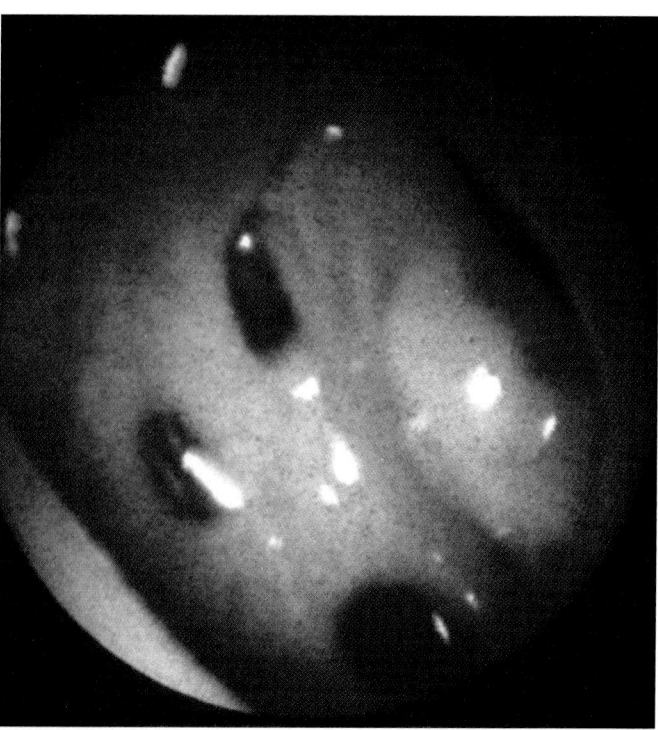

Figure 4 **Shown is the appearance of a bleeding diverticulum on colonoscopy.**

Table 3 Common Causes of Lower GI Hemorrhage

Cause of Bleeding	Frequency
Diverticulosis	17%–40%
Arteriovenous malformation	2%–30%
Colitis	9%–21%
Neoplasia (including postpolypectomy bleeding)	7%–33%
Benign anorectal disease	4%–10%
Upper GI source	0%–11%
Small bowel source	2%–9%

Increasing use of radiation therapy to treat pelvic malignancies has led to a corresponding increase in the incidence of chronic radiation proctitis.[89] Radiation therapy damages bowel mucosa, resulting in the formation of vascular telangiectases that are prone to bleeding.[90] From 1% to 5% of cases of acute lower GI bleeding from radiation-induced proctocolitis are severe enough to necessitate hospitalization.[4,15] In a survey of patients with prostate cancer who underwent pelvic irradiation, 5% of the subjects reported hematochezia daily.[91] Initial therapy for clinically significant hematochezia related to radiation proctitis should include some form of endoscopic treatment (e.g., argon beam coagulation). Surgery should be reserved for unstoppable hemorrhage or other major complications, such as fistulas and strictures.[89]

NEOPLASIA

Significant GI bleeding from colorectal neoplasia accounts for 7% to 33% of cases of severe lower GI hemorrhage.[3,15,21,37,92] Such bleeding is believed to result from erosions on the luminal surface.[93] One report identified ulcerated cancers as the cause in 21% of cases of hematochezia.[15] Adenomatous polyps are implicated in 5% to 11% of cases of acute lower GI bleeding.[7,8,15,94,95] Lower GI hemorrhage, either immediate or delayed, is the most common reported complication after endoscopic polypectomy, occurring in 0.2% to 6% of cases.[3,4,96,97] Immediate postpolypectomy bleeding is believed to result from incomplete coagulation of the stalk before transection.[53] Delayed bleeding has been reported as long as 15 days after polypectomy and is thought to be secondary to sloughing of the coagulum; it is less common than immediate bleeding, occurring in only 0.3% of cases.[15,53]

COAGULOPATHY

Lower GI bleeding can be a presenting symptom both for patients with iatrogenic coagulopathy from heparin or warfarin therapy and for patients with a hematologic coagulopathy from thrombocytopenia. It is unclear, however, whether severe coagulopathy leads to spontaneous hemorrhage or whether it predisposes to bleeding from an existing lesion.[98,99] In an early series of leukemic patients with thrombocytopenia and severe GI hemorrhage, 50% of bleeding patients had platelet counts lower than 20,000/mm³ without any identifiable mucosal lesions; furthermore, when the platelet count rose above 20,000/mm³, the incidence of bleeding decreased to 0.8%.[98] The investigator concluded that severe thrombocytopenia led to spontaneous GI hemorrhage. Other investigators subsequently challenged this conclusion, arguing that spontaneous bleeding from coagulopathy is in fact rare.[100,101] In one report, the distribution of pathologic lesions in patients with GI bleeding who were taking heparin or warfarin was essentially equivalent to that in the general population.[100] Regardless of what the precise relation between coagulopathy and GI hemorrhage may be, a thorough investigation for an anatomic lesion is imperative in the workup of patients with lower GI bleeding even in the face of coagulopathy or thrombocytopenia.

BENIGN ANORECTAL DISEASE

Hemorrhoids, ulcer/fissure disease, and fistula in ano must not be overlooked as causes of GI hemorrhage: in one review comprising almost 18,000 cases of lower GI bleeding, 11% were attributable to anorectal pathology.[72] It is crucial to remember that identification of a benign anorectal lesion does not eliminate the possibility of a more proximal cause of hemorrhage. In general, patients with hemorrhoids identified on physical exam-

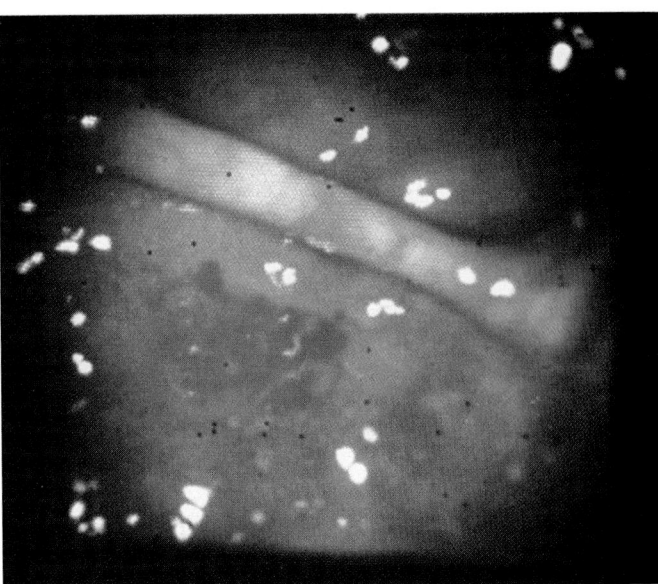

Figure 5 **Shown is the appearance of an arteriovenous malformation on colonoscopy.**

ination should still undergo thorough endoscopic evaluation of the colon to rule out other pathologic conditions.

Portal hypertension, congestive heart failure, and splenic vein thrombosis can cause colonic or anorectal varices, which can result in massive lower GI hemorrhage.[102] The reported incidence of anorectal varices in patients with portal hypertension ranges from 78% to 89%.[103-105] If local measures fail to control hemorrhage, some form of portosystemic shunting is indicated.

COLONIC ARTERIOVENOUS MALFORMATIONS

The term arteriovenous malformation includes vascular ectasias, angiomas, and angiodysplasias. AVMs are ectatic blood vessels seen in the mucosa and submucosa of the GI tract. They are degenerative lesions of the GI tract, occurring more frequently with advancing age.[9] In autopsy series, the reported incidence of colonic AVMs is 1% to 2%.[106] In patients older than 50 years, the incidence of colonic AVMs is estimated to range from 2% to 30%.[107-110] In healthy asymptomatic adults, the prevalence is estimated to be approximately 0.8%.[111]

Colonic AVMs are believed to derive from chronic colonic wall muscle contraction, which leads to chronic partial obstruction of the submucosal veins, causing the vessels to become dilated and tortuous. This process eventually renders the precapillary sphincters incompetent, resulting in direct arterial-venous communication.[112,113] Colonic AVMs are most commonly found in the cecum.[10] They have been associated with several systemic diseases, including atherosclerotic cardiovascular disease, aortic stenosis, chronic renal disease, collagen vascular disease, von Willebrand disease, chronic obstructive pulmonary disease, and cirrhosis of the liver; to date, however, no definite causal relationship to any of these conditions has been established.[6,23,45,114]

The diagnosis of a colonic AVM is made at the time of angiography or colonoscopy. During angiography, visualization of ectatic, slow-emptying veins, vascular tufts, or early-filling veins establishes the diagnosis.[115] During endoscopy, angiodysplasias appear as red, flat lesions about 2 to 10 mm in diameter, sometimes accompanied by a feeding vessel [*see Figure 5*].[6,42,45,111]

COLONIC ISCHEMIA

Acute lower GI bleeding can also be a presenting symptom of colonic ischemia. In several large series, colonic ischemia accounted for 3% to 9% of cases of acute lower GI hemorrhage.[4,8,15,94,117] Other vascular diseases reported as potential causes are polyarteritis nodosa, Wegener granulomatosis, and rheumatoid vasculitis.[118,119] The resultant vasculitis can cause ulceration, necrosis, and ultimately hemorrhage.[120]

SMALL INTESTINAL SOURCES

Small intestinal sources account for 0.7% to 9% of cases of acute lower GI bleeding.[3,4,121-123] About 70% to 80% of cases of small bowel hemorrhage are attributable to AVMs[124]; other, less common causes are jejunoileal diverticula, Meckel's diverticulum,[125] neoplasia, regional enteritis, and aortoenteric fistulas [see Figure 6].[92,126,127] Accurate localization of a bleeding site in the small intestine can be highly challenging: the length and the free intraperitoneal position of the small bowel make endoscopic examination difficult, and the nature of the overlying loops makes angiographic localization imprecise. For these reasons, the small intestine is usually left for last in the attempt to localize the source of lower GI bleeding and is examined only after sources in the colon, the upper GI tract, and the anorectum have been ruled out.[9]

AIDS

The etiology of lower GI bleeding in patients with AIDS differs from that in the general population.[93] In AIDS patients, lower GI bleeding is caused predominantly by conditions related to the underlying HIV infection. Cytomegalovirus colitis is the most common cause of such bleeding in this population, occurring in 39% of cases.[128] AIDS patients with hemorrhoids or anal fissures often experience significant bleeding as a result of HIV-induced thrombocytopenia.[128] A 1998 study reported that in 23% of AIDS patients hospitalized for lower GI bleeding, benign anorectal disease was the cause.[129] Other significant causes of lower GI hemorrhage in this population are colonic histoplasmosis, Kaposi sarcoma of the colon, and bacterial colitis.[129,130]

NSAIDS

The association between NSAID use and upper GI hemorrhage is well known.[131] Current data suggest that NSAIDs have a toxic effect on colonic mucosa as well.[132] An epidemiologic study estimated the incidence of NSAID-associated large-bowel bleeding to be 7/100,000.[133] A retrospective review found that patients who had experienced lower GI bleeding were twice as likely to have taken NSAIDs as those who had not.[134] NSAIDs have also been linked to diverticular hemorrhage: in one study, 92% of patients with diverticular bleeding were taking NSAIDs.[71] Although the exact mechanism of NSAID-induced colonic injury is unknown, however, heightened clinical awareness of this potential cause of lower GI bleeding is warranted.[93]

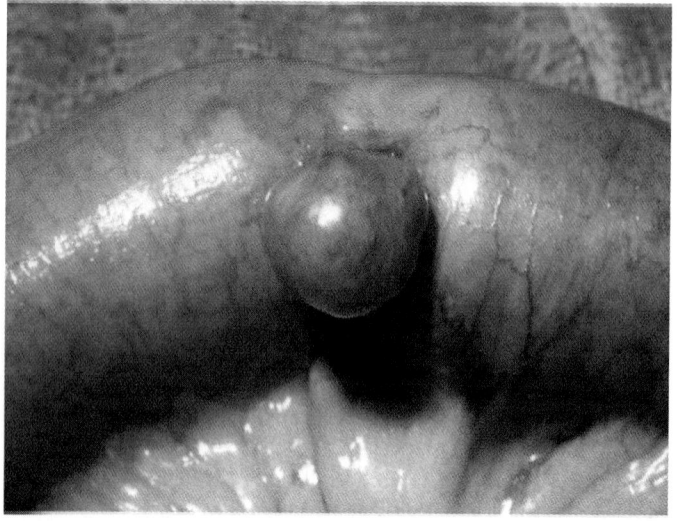
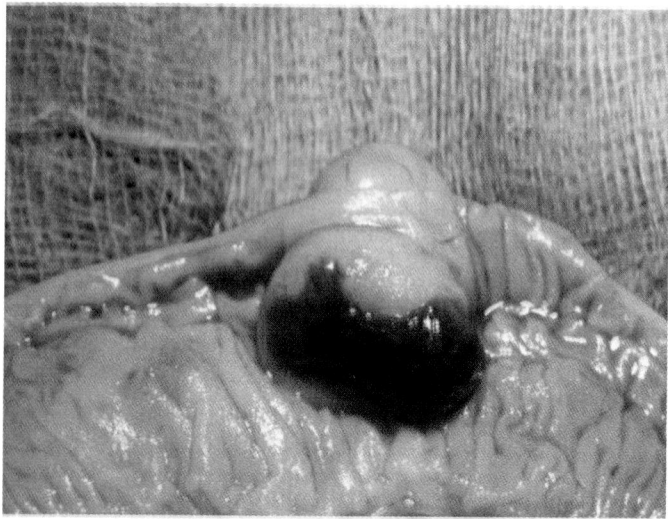

Figure 6 **Shown are intraoperative specimens of small-bowel tumors causing lower GI hemorrhage.**

Typically, the bleeding caused by colonic AVMs is chronic, slow, and intermittent.[9] Although these lesions can cause severe lower GI hemorrhage, they are a relatively uncommon cause: in most large series, they account for only about 2% of cases of acute bleeding.[74,108] The bleeding stops spontaneously in 85% to 90% of cases,[10] but it recurs in 25% to 85%.[116] Accordingly, definitive surgical or colonoscopic treatment should be rendered once the lesion has been identified.

References

1. Briley CA, Jackson DC, Johnsrude IS, et al: Acute gastrointestinal hemorrhage of small-bowel origin. Radiology 136:317, 1980

2. Koval G, Benner KG, Rosch J, et al: Aggressive angiographic diagnosis in acute lower gastrointestinal hemorrhage. Dig Dis Sci 32:248, 1987

3. Jensen DM, Machicado GA: Diagnosis and treatment of severe hematochezia: the role of urgent colonoscopy after purge. Gastroenterology 95:1569, 1988

4. Longstreth GF: Epidemiology and outcome of patients hospitalized with acute lower gastrointestinal hemorrhage: a population-based study. Am J Gastroenterol 92:419, 1997

5. McGuire H: Bleeding colonic diverticula: a reappraisal of natural history and management. Ann Surg 220:653, 1994

6. Foutch PG: Angiodysplasia of the gastrointestinal tract. Am J Gastroenterol 88:807, 1993

7. Bramely P, Masson J, McKnight G, et al: The role of an open-access bleeding unit in the manage-

ment of colonic hemorrhage. A 2 year prospective study. Scand J Gastroenterol 31:764, 1996

8. Peura DA, Lanza FL, Gostout CJ, et al: The American College of Gastroenterology Bleeding Registry: preliminary findings. Am J Gastroenterol 92:924, 1997

9. Vernava AM, Moore BA, Longo WE, et al: Lower gastrointestinal bleeding. Dis Colon Rectum 40:846, 1997

10. Boley SJ, DiBiase A, Brandt LJ, et al: Lower intestinal bleeding in the elderly. Am J Surg 137:57, 1979

11. Caos A, Benner K, Manier J, et al: Colonoscopy after Golytely preparation in acute rectal bleeding. J Clin Gastroenterol 8:46, 1986

12. Zuccaro G Jr: Management of the adult patient with acute lower gastrointestinal bleeding. American College of Gastroenterology. Practice Parameters Committee. Am J Gastroenterol 93:1202, 1998

13. Committee on Trauma ACS: Advanced Trauma Life Support, 5th ed. American College of Surgeons, Chicago, 1993, p 84

14. Richter JM, Christensen MR, Kaplan LM, et al: Effectiveness of current technology in the diagnosis and management of lower gastrointestinal hemorrhage. Gastrointest Endosc 41:93, 1995

15. Rossini FP, Ferrari A, Spandre M, et al: Emergency colonoscopy. World J Surg 13:190, 1989

16. Geller AJ, Mayoral W, Balm R, et al: Colonoscopy in acute lower gastrointestinal bleeding (abstract). Gastrointest Endosc 45:AB107, 1997

17. Goenka MK, Kochhar R, Mehta SK: Spectrum of lower gastrointestinal hemorrhage: an endoscopic study of 166 patients. Indian J Gastroenterol 12:129, 1993

18. Ohyama T, Sakurai Y, Ito M, et al: Analysis of urgent colonoscopy for lower gastrointestinal tract bleeding. Digestion 61:189, 2000

19. Chaudhry V, Hyser MJ, Gracias VH, et al: Colonoscopy: the initial test for acute lower gastrointestinal bleeding. Am Surg 64:723, 1998

20. Cohn SM, Moller BA, Zieg PM, et al: Angiography for preoperative evaluation in patients with lower gastrointestinal bleeding: are the benefits worth the risks? Arch Surg 133:50, 1998

21. Caos A, Benner KG, Manier J, et al: Colonoscopy after Golytely preparation in acute rectal bleeding. J Clin Gastroenterol 8:46, 1986

22. Alavi A, Dann RW, Baum S, et al: Scintigraphic detection of acute gastrointestinal bleeding. Radiology 124:753, 1977

23. Gupta N, Longo W, Vernava A: Angiodysplasia of the lower gastrointestinal tract: an entity readily diagnosed by colonoscopy and primarily managed nonoperatively. Dis Colon Rectum 38:979, 1995

24. McKusick KA, Froelich J, Callahan RJ, et al: ^{99m}Tc red blood cells for detection of gastrointestinal bleeding: experience with 80 patients. AJR Am J Roentgenol 137:1113, 1981

25. Bunker SR, Lull RJ, Hattner RS, et al: The ideal radiotracer in gastrointestinal bleeding detection. AJR Am J Roentgenol 138:982, 1982

26. Kester RR, Welch JP, Sziklas JP: The ^{99m}Tc-labeled RBC scan: a diagnostic method for lower gastrointestinal bleeding. Dis Colon Rectum 27:47, 1984

27. Suzman MS, Talmor M, Jennis R, et al: Accurate localization and surgical management of active lower gastrointestinal hemorrhage with technetium-labeled erythrocyte scintigraphy. Ann Surg 224:29, 1996

28. Hunter JM, Pezim ME: Limited value of technetium 99m-labeled red cell scintigraphy in localization of lower gastrointestinal bleeding. Am J Surg 159:504, 1990

29. Ng D, Opelka F, Beck D, et al: Predictive value of technetium Tc 99m labeled red blood cell scintigraphy for positive angiogram in massive lower gastrointestinal hemorrhage. Dis Colon Rectum 40:471, 1997

30. Wadwa KS, Kalloo AN: Bleeding scans in patients with lower gastrointestinal bleeding of undetermined cause: are they useful? [abstract]. Gastrointest Endosc 45:AB120, 1997

31. Prakash C, Sreenarasimhaih J, Royal H, et al: A varied diagnostic approach to acute lower gastrointestinal bleeding [abstract]. Am J Gastroenterol 92:1685, 1997

32. Baum S, Athanasoulis CA, Waltman AC: Angiographic diagnosis and control of large-bowel bleeding. Dis Colon Rectum 17:447, 1974

33. Athanasoulis CA, Moncure AC, Greenfield AJ, et al: Intraoperative localization of small bowel bleeding sites with combined use of angiographic methods and methylene blue injection. Surgery 87:77, 1980

34. Schrodt JF, Bradford WR: Presurgical angiographic localization of small bowel bleeding site with methylene blue injection. J Ky Med Assoc 94:192, 1996

35. Pennoyer WP, Vignati PV, Cohen JL: Management of angiogram positive lower gastrointestinal hemorrhage: long term follow-up of non-operative treatments. Int J Colorectal Dis 11:279, 1996

36. Rantis PC, Harford FJ, Wagner RH, et al: Technetium-labelled red blood cell scintigraphy: is it useful in acute lower gastrointestinal bleeding? Int J Colorectal Dis 10:210, 1995

37. Leitman IM, Paull DE, Shires GT 3rd: Evaluation and management of massive lower gastrointestinal hemorrhage. Ann Surg 209:175, 1989

38. Casarella WJ, Galloway SJ, Taxin RN: Lower gastrointestinal tract hemorrhage: new concepts based on arteriography. AJR Am J Roentgenol 121:357, 1974

39. Colacchio TA, Forde KA, Patsos TJ, et al: Impact of modern diagnostic methods on the management of active rectal bleeding: ten year experience. Am J Surg 143:607, 1982

40. Bloomfeld RS, Smith TP, Schneider AM, et al: Provocative angiography in patients with gastrointestinal hemorrhage of obscure origin. Am J Gastroenterol 95:2807, 2000

41. Shetzline MA, Suhocki P, Dash R, et al: Provocative angiography in obscure gastrointestinal bleeding. South Med J 93:1205, 2000

42. Krevsky B: Detection and treatment of angiodysplasia. Gastrointest Endosc 7:509, 1997

43. Foutch PG: Colonic angiodysplasia. Gastroenterologist 5:148, 1997

44. Rutgeerts P, Van Gompel F, Geboes K, et al: Long term results of treatment of vascular malformations of the gastrointestinal tract by neodymium Yag laser photocoagulation. Gut 26:586, 1985

45. Rogers BH: Endoscopic diagnosis and therapy of mucosal vascular abnormalities of the gastrointestinal tract occurring in elderly patients and associated with cardiac, vascular, and pulmonary disease. Gastrointest Endosc 26:134, 1980

46. Binmoeller KF, Thonke F, Soehendra N: Endoscopic hemoclip treatment for gastrointestinal bleeding. Endoscopy 25:167, 1993

47. Jaspersen D, Korner T, Schorr W, et al: Diagnosis and treatment control of bleeding intestinal angiodysplasias with an endoscopic Doppler device. Bildgebung 62:14, 1995

48. Jensen DM, Machicado GA, Jutabha R, et al: Urgent colonoscopy for the diagnosis and treatment of severe diverticular hemorrhage. N Engl J Med 342:78, 2000

49. Bloomfeld RS, Rockey DC, Shetzline MA: Endoscopic therapy of acute diverticular hemorrhage. Am J Gastroenterol 96:2367, 2001

50. Naveau S, Aubert A, Poynard T, et al: Long-term results of treatment of vascular malformations of the gastrointestinal tract by neodymium YAG laser photocoagulation. Dig Dis Sci 35:821, 1990

51. Santos JC, Aprilli F, Guimaraes AS, et al: Angiodysplasia of the colon: endoscopic diagnosis and treatment. Br J Surg 75:256, 1988

52. Eisen GM, Dominitz JA, Faigel DO, et al: An annotated algorithmic approach to upper gastrointestinal bleeding. Gastrointest Endosc 53:853, 2001

53. Habr-Gama A, Waye J: Complications and hazards of gastrointestinal endoscopy. World J Surg 13:193, 1989

54. Trowers E, Ganga U, Hodges D: Endoscopic hemorrhoidal ligation: preliminary clinical experience. Gastrointest Endosc 48:49, 1998

55. Athanasoulis CA, Baum S, Rosch J, et al: Mesenteric arterial infusions of vasopressin for hemorrhage from colonic diverticulosis. Am J Surg 129:212, 1975

56. Rahn NH 3rd, Tishler JM, Han SY, et al: Diagnostic and interventional angiography in acute gastrointestinal hemorrhage. Radiology 143:361, 1982

57. Levinson SL, Powell DW, Callahan WT, et al: A current approach to rectal bleeding. J Clin Gastroenterol 3(suppl 1):9, 1981

58. Lichtiger S, Karnbluth A, Salomon P, et al: Lower gastrointestinal bleeding. Gastrointestinal Emergencies. Taylor MB, Gollan JL, Peppercorn MA, et al, Eds. Baltimore, Williams & Wilkins, 1992, p 358

59. Clark RA, Colley DP, Eggers FM: Acute arterial gastrointestinal hemorrhage: efficacy of transcatheter control. AJR Am J Roentgenol 136:1185, 1981

60. Browder W, Cerise EJ, Litwin MS: Impact of emergency angiography in massive lower gastrointestinal bleeding. Ann Surg 204:530, 1986

61. Matolo NM, Link DP: Selective embolization for control of gastrointestinal hemorrhage. Am J Surg 138:840, 1979

62. Encarnacion CE, Kadir S, Beam CA, et al: Gastrointestinal bleeding: treatment with gastrointestinal arterial embolization. Radiology 183:505, 1992

63. Bookstein JJ, Chlosta EM, Foley D, et al: Transcatheter hemostasis of gastrointestinal bleeding using modified autogenous clot. Radiology 113:277, 1974

64. Peck DJ, McLoughlin RF, Hughson MN, et al: Percutaneous embolotherapy of lower gastrointestinal hemorrhage. J Vasc Interv Radiol 9:747, 1998

65. Gomes AS, Lois JF, McCoy RD: Angiographic treatment of gastrointestinal hemorrhage: comparison of vasopressin infusion and embolization. AJR Am J Roentgenol 146:1031, 1986

66. Wright HK, Pelliccia O, Higgins EF, et al: Controlled, semielective, segmental resection for massive colonic hemorrhage. Am J Surg 139:535, 1980

67. Eaton AC: Emergency surgery for acute colonic haemorrhage—a retrospective study. Br J Surg 68:109, 1981

68. McGuire HH, Haynes BW: Massive hemorrhage for diverticulosis of the colon: guidelines for therapy based on bleeding patterns observed in fifty cases. Ann Surg 175:847, 1972

69. Setya V, Singer JA, Minken SL: Subtotal colectomy as a last resort for unrelenting, unlocalized, lower gastrointestinal hemorrhage: experience with 12 cases. Am Surg 58:295, 1992

70. Jensen DM, Machicado GA: Colonoscopy for diagnosis and treatment of severe lower gastrointestinal bleeding: routine outcomes and cost

analysis. Gastrointest Endosc Clin N Am 7:477, 1997

71. Foutch PG: Diverticular bleeding: are non-steroidal anti-inflammatory drugs risk factors for hemorrhage and can colonoscopy predict outcome for patients? Am J Gastroenterol 90:1779, 1995

72. Vernava A, Longo W, Virgo K, et al: A nationwide study of the incidence and etiology of lower gastrointestinal bleeding. Surg Res Commun 18:113, 1996

73. Heer M, Ammann R, Buhler H: Die klinische Bedeutung der Angiodysplasien im Kolon. Schweiz Med Wochenschr 114:1416, 1984

74. Sebastian JJ, Lucia F, Botella MT, et al: Angiodisplasia gastrointestinal difusa asociada a cirrosis hepática criptogenética y coagulopatia que simulaba una enfermedad de von Willebrand. Rev Esp Enferm Dig 88:631, 1996

75. Hughes L: Postmortem survey of diverticular disease of the colon. Gut 10:336, 1969

76. Meyers MA, Alonso DR, Gray GF, et al: Pathogenesis of bleeding colonic diverticulosis. Gastroenterology 71:577, 1976

77. Rushford A: The significance of bleeding as a symptom in diverticulitis. J R Soc Med 49:577, 1956

78. Bokhari M, Vernava AM, Ure T, et al: Diverticular hemorrhage in the elderly—is it well tolerated? Dis Colon Rectum 39:191, 1996

79. McGuire HH: Bleeding colonic diverticula: a reappraisal of natural history and management. Ann Surg 220:653, 1994

80. Luk GD, Bynum TE, Hendrix TR: Gastric aspiration in localization of gastrointestinal hemorrhage. JAMA 241:576, 1979

81. Robert JR, Sachar DB, Greenstein AJ: Severe gastrointestinal hemorrhage in Crohn's disease. Ann Surg 213:207, 1991

82. Binder S, Miller H, Deterling R: Emergency and urgent operations for ulcerative colitis. Arch Surg 110:281, 1975

83. Cirocco WC, Reilly JC, Rusin LC: Life-threatening hemorrhage and exsanguination from Crohn's disease: report of four cases. Dis Colon Rectum 38:85, 1995

84. Reyes E, Hernandez J, Gonzalez A: Typhoid colitis with massive lower gastrointestinal bleeding: an unexpected behavior of Salmonella typhi. Dis Colon Rectum 29:511, 1986

85. Maguire TM, Wensel RH, Malcolm N, et al: Massive gastrointestinal hemorrhage cecal ulcers and salmonella colitis. J Clin Gastroenterol 7:249, 1985

86. Cohen M, Fianella R: Hemorrhagic colitis associated with Escherichia coli O157:H7. Adv Intern Med 37:173, 1992

87. Gould O, Khawaja FI, Rosenthal W: Antibiotic associated hemorrhagic colitis. Am J Gastroenterol 77:491, 1982

88. Escudero-Faber A, Cummings OW, Kirklin J, et al: Cytomegalovirus colitis presenting as hematochezia and requiring resection. Arch Surg 127:102, 1992

89. Tagkalidis PP, Tjandra JJ: Chronic radiation proctitis. Aust NZ J Surg 71:230, 2001

90. Den Harog Jager F, Van Haastert M, Batterman J, et al: The endoscopic spectrum of late radiation damage of the rectosigmoid colon. Endoscopy 17:214, 1985

91. Crook J, Esche J, Futter N: Effect of pelvic radiotherapy for prostate cancer on bowel, bladder, and sexual function: the patient's perspective. Urology 47:387, 1996

92. Ellis DJ, Reinus JF: Lower intestinal hemorrhage. Crit Care Clin 11:369, 1995

93. Zuckerman GR, Prakash C: Acute lower intestinal bleeding. Part II: etiology, therapy, and outcomes. Gastrointest Endosc 49:228, 1999

94. Wagner HE, Stain SC, Gilg M, et al: Systematic assessment of massive bleeding of the lower part of the gastrointestinal tract. Surg Gynecol Obstet 175:445, 1992

95. Makela JT, Kiviniemi H, Laitinen S, et al: Diagnosis and treatment of acute lower gastrointestinal bleeding. Scand J Gastroenterol 28:1062, 1993

96. Greenen J, Schmitt M, Wu W: Major complications of colonoscopy: bleeding and perforation. Am J Dig Dis 20:231, 1975

97. Macrae JF, Tan K, Williams C: Towards safer colonoscopy: a report on the complications of 5000 diagnostic or therapeutic colonoscopies. Gut 24:376, 1983

98. Gaydos J, Freireich J, Mantel N: The quantitative relationship between platelet count and hemorrhage in patients with acute leukemia. N Engl J Med 266:905, 1962

99. Wilkson J, Nour-Edlin F, Israels M, et al: Hemophilic syndromes: a survey of 267 patients. Lancet 2:947, 1961

100. Coon W, Willis JP: Hemorrhagic complications of anticoagulant therapy. Arch Intern Med 133:386, 1974

101. Mittal R, Spero JA, Lewis JH, et al: Patterns of gastrointestinal hemorrhage in hemophilia. Gastroenterology 88:515, 1985

102. Cappel M, Price J: Characterization of the syndrome of small and large intestinal variceal bleeding. Dig Dis Sci 32:422, 1987

103. Strong J: Colonic, anorectal and peristomal varices. Semin Colon Rectal Surg 5:50, 1994

104. Chawla Y, Dilawari J: Anorectal varices—their frequency in cirrhotic and non-cirrhotic portal hypertension. Gut 32:309, 1991

105. Goenka MK, Kochhar R, Nagi B, et al: Rectosigmoid varices and other mucosal changes in patients with portal hypertension. Am J Gastroenterol 86:1185, 1991

106. Baer JW, Ryan S: Analysis of cecal vasculature in the search for vascular malformations. Am J Roentgenol 126:394, 1976

107. Danesh BJ, Spiliadis C, Williams CB, et al: Angiodysplasia—an uncommon cause of colonic bleeding: colonoscopic evaluation of 1,050 patients with rectal bleeding and anaemia. Int J Colorectal Dis 2:218, 1987

108. Heer M, Sulser H, Hany A: Angiodysplasia of the colon: an expression of occlusive vascular disease. Hepatogastroenterology 34:127, 1987

109. Richter JM, Hedberg SE, Athanasoulis CA, et al: Angiodysplasia: clinical presentation and colonoscopic diagnosis. Dig Dis Sci 29:481, 1984

110. Zuckerman G, Benitez J: A prospective study of bidirectional endoscopy (colonoscopy and upper endoscopy) in the evaluation of patients with occult gastrointestinal bleeding. Am J Gastroenterol 87:62, 1992

111. Foutch PG, Rex DK, Lieberman D: Prevalance and natural history of colonic angiodysplasias among healthy asymptomatic adults. Am J Gastroenterol 90:564, 1995

112. Boley SJ, Sammartano R, Adams A, et al: On the nature and etiology of vascular ectasias of the colon: degenerative lesions of aging. Gastroenterology 72:650, 1977

113. Mitsudo SM, Boley SJ, Brandt LJ, et al: Vascular ectasias of the right colon in the elderly: a distinct pathologic entity. Hum Pathol 10:585, 1979

114. Imperiale TF, Ransohoff DF: Aortic stenosis, idiopathic gastrointestinal bleeding, and angiodysplasia: is there an association? A methodologic critique of the literature. Gastroenterology 95:1670, 1988

115. Boley SJ, Sprayragen S, Sammartano R, et al: The pathophysiologic basis for the angiographic signs of vascular ectasias of the colon. Radiology 125:615, 1977

116. Helmrich GA, Stallworth JR, Brown JJ: Angiodysplasia: characterization, diagnosis, and advances in treatment. South Med J 83:1450, 1990

117. Bramley PN, Masson JW, McKnight G, et al: The role of an open-access bleeding unit in the management of colonic haemorrhage: a 2-year prospective study. Scand J Gastroenterol 31:764, 1996

118. Moses FM: Gastrointestinal bleeding and the athlete. Am J Gastroenterol 88:1157, 1993

119. Burt R, Berenson M, Samuelson C, et al: Rheumatoid vasculitis of the colon presenting as pancolitis. Dig Dis Sci 28:183, 1983

120. Sokol R, Farrell M, McAdams A: An unusual presentation of Wegener's granulomatosis mimicking inflammatory bowel disease. Gastroenterology 87:426, 1984

121. Klinvimol T, Ho YH, Parry BR, et al: Small bowel causes of per rectum haemorrhage. Ann Acad Med Singapore 23:866, 1994

122. Gilmore PR: Angiodysplasia of the upper gastrointestinal tract. J Clin Gastroenterol 10:386, 1988

123. Netterville R, Hardy J, Martin R: Small bowel hemorrhage. Ann Surg 167:949, 1968

124. Lewis B, Waye J: Bleeding from the small intestine. Gastrointestinal Bleeding. Sugawa C, Schuman BM, Lucas CE, Eds. Igaku-Shoin, New York, 1992, p 178

125. Lu CL, Chen CY, Chiu ST, et al: Adult intussuscepted Meckel's diverticulum presenting mainly lower gastrointestinal bleeding. J Gastroenterol Hepatol 16:478, 2001

126. Longo WE, Vernava AM 3rd: Clinical implications of jejunoileal diverticular disease. Dis Colon Rectum 35:381, 1992

127. Buchman TG, Bulkley GB: Current management of patients with lower gastrointestinal bleeding. Surg Clin North Am 67:651, 1987

128. Chalasani N, Wilcox CM: Gastrointestinal hemorrhage in patients with AIDS. AIDS Patient Care STDS 13:343, 1999

129. Chalasani N, Wilcox CM: Etiology and outcome of lower gastrointestinal bleeding in patients with AIDS. Am J Gastroenterol 93:175, 1998

130. Becherer PR, Sokol-Anderson M, Joist JH, et al: Gastrointestinal histoplasmosis presenting as hematochezia in human immunodeficiency virus–infected hemophilic patients. Am J Hematol 47:229, 1994

131. Allison M, Howatson A, Torrance C, et al: Gastrointestinal damage associated with the use of nonsteroidal antiinflammatory drugs. N Engl J Med 327:749, 1992

132. Davies NM: Toxicity of nonsteroidal anti-inflammatory drugs in the large intestine. Dis Colon Rectum 38:1311, 1995

133. Langman MJ, Morgan LR, Worral J: Use of anti-inflammatory drugs by patients admitted with small or large bowel perforations and hemorrhage. BMJ 290:347, 1985

134. Holt S, Rigoglioso V, Sidhu M, et al: Nonsteroidal antiinflammatory drugs and lower gastrointestinal bleeding. Dig Dis Sci 38:1619, 1993

8 GASTROINTESTINAL ENDOSCOPY

Alicia Fanning, M.D., and Jeffrey L. Ponsky, M.D., F.A.C.S.

Since the beginning of the 1970s, flexible endoscopy of the gastrointestinal tract has been the dominant modality for the diagnosis of gastrointestinal disease. Over the same period, developments in technology and methodology have made possible the use of endoscopy to treat a host of conditions that once were considered to be manageable only by means of open surgical procedures. The integration of flexible endoscopic techniques into the armamentarium of the GI surgeon permits a more multidimensional approach to the treatment of digestive disease. The modern GI surgeon should be conversant in and adept at many of these procedures.

Diagnostic Esophagogastroduodenoscopy

Diagnostic esophagogastroduodenoscopy (EGD) is indicated when a patient has abnormal findings on traditional GI x-ray series, dysphagia, odynophagia, epigastric pain that does not respond to medical therapy, persistent heartburn, or upper GI bleeding; it is also indicated for surveillance of patients at high risk for malignancy and for sampling of GI tissue or fluid. One prepares for the examination by ensuring the patient's hemodynamic stability, having the patient fast for 6 to 8 hours beforehand, and performing conscious sedation, which generally involves applying a topical anesthetic to the posterior pharynx and administering a narcotic and a benzodiazepine intravenously. Monitoring of arterial blood pressure and oxygen saturation throughout the procedure is now standard practice.

TECHNIQUE

With the patient in the left lateral decubitus position, a topical anesthetic is applied to the posterior pharynx and an intravenous sedative administered. The forward-viewing panendoscope—a small-caliber instrument that is long enough to permit examination of the foregut from the mouth to the third portion of the duodenum—is employed.

The endoscope may be introduced either blindly, via finger-guided palpation of the pharynx, or under direct vision. The latter approach is preferable. In this approach, the instrument is advanced slowly until the epiglottis and vocal cords are visualized [see Figure 1]; it is then angled posteriorly to the esophageal introitus and gently advanced as the patient is asked to swallow. Insufflation of air is begun to distend the esophagus, which appears as a long, round tube. Frequent peristaltic waves are seen; these are normal. Mucosal surfaces must be closely inspected for signs of ulceration, stricture, tumor, or Barrett's (columnar) epithelium, which manifests itself as orange patches in otherwise pale salmon-pink esophageal (squamous) mucosa. When abnormalities are noted, biopsy, brushing for cytologic evaluation, or both should be performed. Staining of the esophagus with methylene blue may be useful in the search for Barrett's mucosa: the blue dye is avidly absorbed by the intestinal absorptive cells of the columnar epithelium. Darkly stained areas may be biopsied for confirmation.

As the endoscope is advanced, insufflation is continued, and the curve of the lumen is followed to the left as the esophagus traverses the diaphragm to enter the stomach. There is a pinched area where the diaphragm compresses the esophagus; the pinching is exaggerated when the patient is asked to sniff. If gastric folds are seen above this pinched area, a hiatal hernia is present. When the stomach is entered, the tip of the endoscope is elevated so as to center it within the gastric lumen. It should be noted that with the patient lying in the left lateral decubitus position, the stomach is also on its side, with the greater curvature at 6 o'clock, the lesser curvature at 12 o'clock, the posterior wall at 3 o'clock, and the anterior wall at 9 o'clock. Air should be insufflated to distend the stomach fully and permit careful inspection of the mucosal surfaces.

As the instrument is advanced toward the gastric antrum, its tip should be slightly elevated because the stomach has a J shape and the prepyloric region curves upward. The pylorus is normally round and may be seen to open and close with gastric peristalsis. With the tip of the endoscope positioned at the proximal gastric antrum, just under the incisura angularis, a retroflex view of the cardia and the fundus is obtained by elevating the tip of the scope and rotating the shaft to the left. This maneuver provides visual and therapeutic access to the proximal stomach.

After the stomach has been viewed, the instrument is advanced under direct vision through the pylorus and into the duodenal bulb. Insufflation of air should continue as the scope is

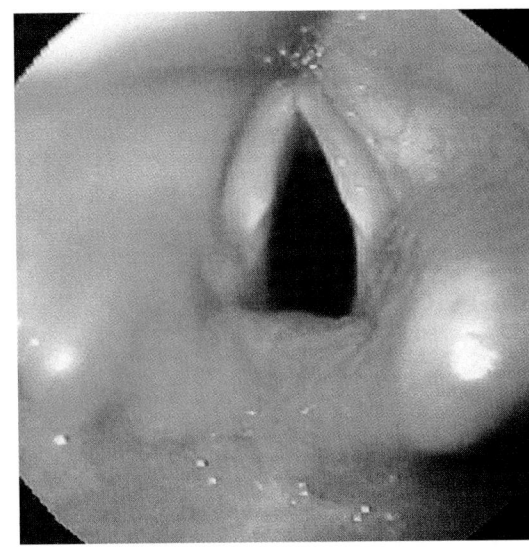

Figure 1 **Diagnostic esophagogastroduodenoscopy. As the endoscope is introduced under direct vision, the vocal cords are clearly noted. The esophageal opening is posterior to the cords.**

pressed against the pylorus to facilitate passage of the instrument. The scope tends to pop into the duodenal bulb rather than slide smoothly; it should be pulled back slightly to allow one to observe the mucosal surfaces of the bulb before moving ahead. Unlike the rest of the small bowel, the duodenal bulb has no semicircular folds. The tip of the scope must be rotated slightly to permit examination of the walls of the bulb. It is advisable to pull the instrument back into the stomach while observing the walls of the bulb and the pyloric channel for lesions; several such withdrawals may be required for full assessment of this area.

Once the duodenal bulb has been examined, the endoscope is advanced just past the bulb to the point where the first duodenal folds are observed. Here, the duodenum turns sharply to the rear and downward as it becomes retroperitoneal. Advancement of the scope into the second portion of the duodenum is one of the few endoscopic maneuvers that cannot be accomplished under direct vision. Because of the sharp angle of the turn, one will experience a moment of so-called red out as the tip of the endoscope touches the mucosa during the turn. To ensure that the turn is accomplished safely, the instrument is advanced as far through the bulb as is possible under direct vision. The control handle of the scope is then rotated approximately 90° to the right as the tip of the scope is turned to the right and angled first upward, then downward. As the second portion of the duodenum appears, the scope is rotated back to its neutral position. When done correctly, the turn is actually quite easy. It should never be forced: if the instrument does not proceed easily into the descending duodenum, the scope should be pulled back and the attempt repeated. Pushing against resistance may result in perforation.

Entering the descending duodenum causes the scope to form a large loop in the stomach. Therefore, once the second portion of the duodenum is successfully entered, the shaft of the instrument is pulled back. Paradoxically, as this movement straightens the gastric loop, it also advances the tip of the instrument deeper into the duodenum. Further advancement of the instrument under direct vision often permits entry into the third or even the fourth portion of the duodenum. Once the distal limit of intubation is reached, the scope is withdrawn and the luminal surfaces are carefully examined. Rotating the scope with small right-left movements of the controls and side-to-side movements of the control handle itself will help demonstrate the more subtle details of duodenal anatomy. Often, the upper GI tract is inspected more completely while the instrument is being withdrawn than while it is being advanced.

Mucosal abnormalities should be biopsied; liberal use of brush cytology in combination with biopsy enhances the yield.

COMPLICATIONS

EGD is an extremely safe procedure. Perhaps the most common problems associated with the technique arise from the preparatory sedation and analgesia. Respiratory depression and aspiration may occur during the procedure. Careful attention must be paid to the patient's state of consciousness and airway during the endoscopic procedure, appropriate drugs must be available to reverse sedative effects, and a suction apparatus must be ready for use at all times. Blind advancement of the endoscope by force may lead to perforation of the esophagus; this problem may be avoided by taking care never to advance the instrument against resistance.

Therapeutic Esophagogastroduodenoscopy

CONTROL OF VARICEAL HEMORRHAGE

In patients with massive upper GI hemorrhage, the first priori-

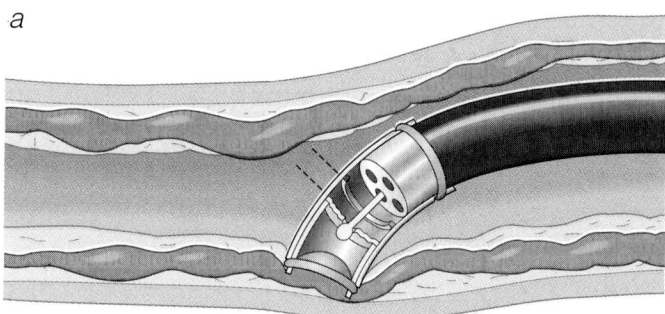

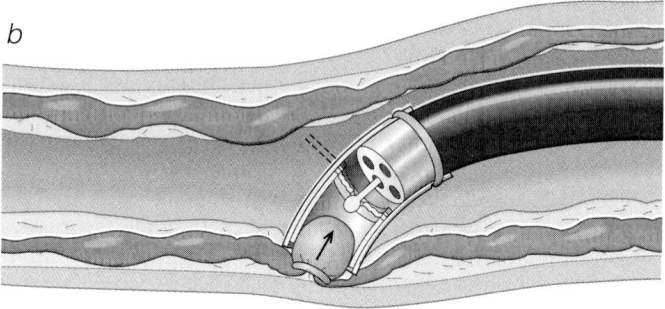

Figure 2 **Therapeutic esophagogastroduodenoscopy: control of variceal hemorrhage. (*a*) A plastic tip on the endoscope is used to create a chamber. (*b*) An esophageal varix is suctioned into the chamber, and a rubber band is released around it.**

ties are to establish a secure airway and to ensure hemodynamic stability. These priorities must be addressed before endoscopy is attempted. If the bleeding is thought to be coming from esophageal varices, it is frequently useful to perform endotracheal intubation for control of the airway before the endoscopic intervention.

Technique

A rapid but complete diagnostic upper GI endoscopic procedure is performed to determine whether varices are present and to identify the exact site of hemorrhage. Endoscopic therapy for variceal disease is then delivered by means of either sclerotherapy or rubber band ligation.

Sclerotherapy is commenced in the distal esophagus at the site of active or suspected bleeding: 2 to 3 ml of a sclerosant solution (e.g., sodium tetradecyl sulfate) is injected directly into the lumen of the varix. Additional varices can be treated in the same fashion. After the bleeding has stopped, further therapy is usually delivered at weekly intervals until total variceal obliteration is achieved.

Rubber band ligation of varices has become extremely popular in recent years and has been shown to possess some clear advantages over sclerotherapy [*see Figure 2*]. Originally, multiple passages of the endoscope were required to allow for reloading of the bands; however, newer ligating devices permit ligation of as many as 10 varices with a single passage of the endoscope. As with sclerotherapy, the site of active or suspected bleeding is attacked first; it is most often near the esophagogastric junction. The offending varix is centered in the field of view, and suction is applied to pull it into the ligator cup, which sits on the end of the endoscope. When the varix is deep within the cup, the trigger string on the ligator is pulled, and a rubber band is released around the varix. Suction is then released, and the ligated varix is visualized. Additional ligations may be performed at the initial session; follow-up sessions are usually held at weekly intervals until total variceal obliteration is achieved.

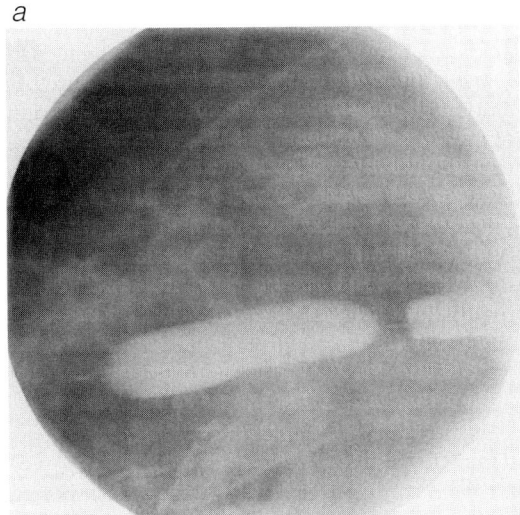
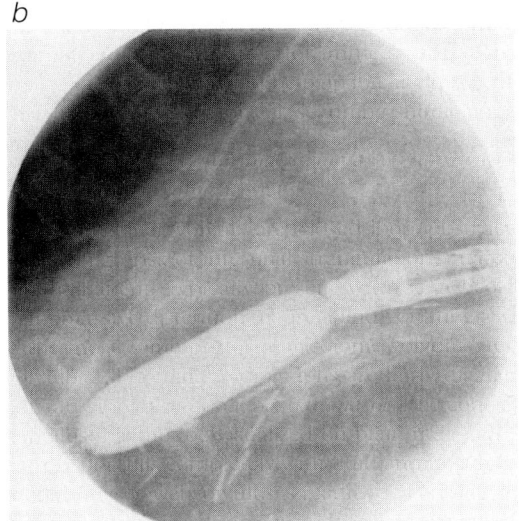

a   *b*

Figure 3   Therapeutic esophagogastroduodenoscopy: dilation of esophageal strictures. (*a*) A hydrostatic dilating balloon filled with a contrast agent is inflated within the stricture under fluoroscopic guidance. Initially, a "waist" appears at the stricture site. (*b*) Inflation of the balloon is continued until the waist is ablated, which indicates complete dilation of the stricture.

Complications

Because aspiration of blood and gastric contents may occur during endoscopic control of variceal hemorrhage, endotracheal intubation must be considered when bleeding is massive. In many cases, general anesthesia will permit adequate airway control and a quiet operating field. Violent patient motion when the injection needle is in a varix may result in perforation of the esophagus. This is a rare complication, however; tearing of the varix, with resultant hemorrhage, is more frequent. Injection of excessive amounts of sclerosant may lead to significant ulceration and necrosis of esophageal tissue. Fever, severe infection, pleural effusion, and subsequent esophageal stricture occasionally occur after sclerotherapy. Ulceration and necrosis of tissue, with subsequent stricture, occur after rubber band ligation as well, but severe infection is less common in this setting.

CONTROL OF NONVARICEAL HEMORRHAGE

Bleeding from peptic ulcer disease, gastritis, or vascular malformations is a common indication for EGD. Once the patient has been adequately resuscitated, endoscopy should be performed, and the entire esophagus, stomach, and duodenum should be examined thoroughly. Before the procedure is begun, the stomach should be vigorously irrigated through a large-bore tube so that as much clotted blood as possible can be evacuated. If a pool of blood is noted in the stomach, the position of the patient should be changed so as to move the pool and permit complete examination of the stomach.

The therapeutic modalities available for control of nonvariceal bleeding include (1) the injection of hypertonic saline, epinephrine (in a 1:10,000 solution), or 98% alcohol, (2) bipolar electrocoagulation, (3) the use of heater probes, (4) argon beam coagulation, (5) the application of acrylic glue, (6) the application of hemostatic clips, and (7) the use of the neodynium:yttrium-aluminum-garnet (Nd:YAG) laser.

Technique

The most popular therapeutic modalities are injection therapy, bipolar coagulation, and the use of the heater probe. Injection

therapy is performed around the bleeding lesion to create edema and vasospasm in the area. The bipolar coagulator or the heater probe is applied directly to the bleeding lesion in an attempt to coapt the bleeding vessel as heat is delivered. Frequently, injection therapy is employed in conjunction with coagulation; this combination is very effective.

If there is a clot covering the ulcer base, it must be removed with suction or a snare before coagulation is attempted. If a rapidly bleeding lesion is present, the best approach often is injection therapy in adjacent areas to slow or stop the bleeding, followed by coagulation by direct coaptation. Vascular lesions are often multiple or diffuse, as in so-called watermelon stomach. Such lesions are most effectively treated by means of modalities that can be applied in a spraying fashion, such as the Nd:YAG laser or the argon beam coagulator.

Complications

Nonvariceal hemorrhage is successfully controlled by endoscopic means in more than 90% of cases. At times, however, attempts at endoscopic control may exacerbate the bleeding. Several therapeutic modalities should always be available: one may succeed when another fails. Excessive injection therapy or persistent attempts at coagulation may lead to tissue necrosis and subsequent perforation. Although the argon beam coagulator can injure tissue only to a depth of several millimeters, excessive application may result in massive distention of the bowel if care is not taken to aspirate the constantly infused argon gas frequently. The Nd:YAG laser has the potential to cause full-thickness injury to the gastric wall.

DILATION OF ESOPHAGEAL STRICTURES

When patients complain of dysphagia or odynophagia, prompt endoscopic investigation is warranted. Strictures may be secondary to reflux disease, secondary to caustic burns, or of neoplastic origin.

Technique

Endoscopy is performed in the usual fashion. It is imperative that the endoscope be advanced only under direct vision. When a stricture is encountered, its location, morphology, and length should be determined. Biopsy and cytology specimens should be gathered from the circumference of the stricture. When a stricture is present at the esophagogastric junction and the scope can easily be passed by the stricture, it is helpful to view the area from below with the tip of the scope retroflexed.

Stricture dilation can be accomplished in several different ways and with several different kinds of dilators. One commonly employed method is to use the endoscope to guide the passage of a soft-tipped guide wire through the stricture; the scope is then removed, leaving the wire in place. Subsequently, dilators are passed over the guide wire, usually under fluoroscopic control. Another method for endoscopic dilation of strictures is the use of through-the-scope (TTS) hydrostatic dilating balloons. A balloon of the appropriate inflated diameter (usually no larger than 18 mm or 54 French) is selected, passed through the biopsy channel of the endoscope, and advanced under direct vision until its middle portion passes through the stricture. At the stricture site, the balloon is compressed, giving the appearance of a waist. The balloon is then inflated until the waist is fully expanded [see Figure 3]. Full expansion is verified by fluoroscopic surveillance and the use of contrast to inflate the balloon. This second method is extremely useful for initial dilation of tight strictures in preparation for the use of other, nonendoscopic dilators or the placement of an esophageal stent.

Complications

Dilation of esophageal strictures may result in bleeding (usually minor) or perforation of the esophagus. When a patient experiences severe pain after dilation, a chest x-ray is imperative. The finding of mediastinal or subcutaneous air should prompt the immediate performance of a contrast study with a water-soluble agent to determine whether a perforation is present. Some small perforations can be managed with intravenous antibiotics and observation, but most must be managed surgically. The incidence of perforation can be minimized by avoiding excessive or forceful dilation.

STENTING OF ESOPHAGEAL TUMORS

Under optimal circumstances, esophageal tumors should be treated by means of extirpative surgery. When surgical cure or palliation seems to have little to offer, placement of an esophageal prosthesis by endoscopic means is a reasonable approach.

Technique

Modern esophageal prostheses are placed under fluoroscopic guidance, frequently after endoscopic balloon dilation of the tumor. During the endoscopic examination, it is useful to inject a small amount of water-soluble contrast material into the muscular wall of the esophagus just above and below the tumor; this enables one to measure the length of the tumor and select the correct stent. Once the tumor has been dilated and marked endoscopically, the scope is removed, and the expandable stent is passed into the esophagus and positioned between the endoscopic injection markings seen on fluoroscopy. The stent is then deployed and allowed to expand [see Figure 4]. The endoscope may then be reintroduced to ensure that the prosthesis is patent and is correctly placed.

Complications

Incorrect positioning of the prosthesis is a frequent problem. Attention to the details of endoscopic marking is very important. Also crucial is correct selection of a stent: stents shorten from both ends as they are deployed, and this must be taken into account in selecting the correct stent length. On occasion, the stent may migrate as a result of tumor-related necrosis or incorrect placement. If it migrates into the stomach, it can usually be captured in a snare and retrieved.

RETRIEVAL OF FOREIGN BODIES

Many ingested foreign bodies pass through the GI tract uneventfully, but a good number must be removed by endoscopic means—in particular, foreign bodies in the esophagus, sharp objects that are likely to perforate the bowel, and objects that do not progress from the stomach.

If the ingested object is of an unfamiliar type, it is an extremely good idea to practice with a similar object outside the patient before attempting endoscopic retrieval. This preparatory step allows one to select the most appropriate accessory and technique for removing the object.

Technique

Objects with sharp edges should be removed with the sharp end trailing to prevent perforation. In some cases, this means that the object must be pushed into the stomach and turned

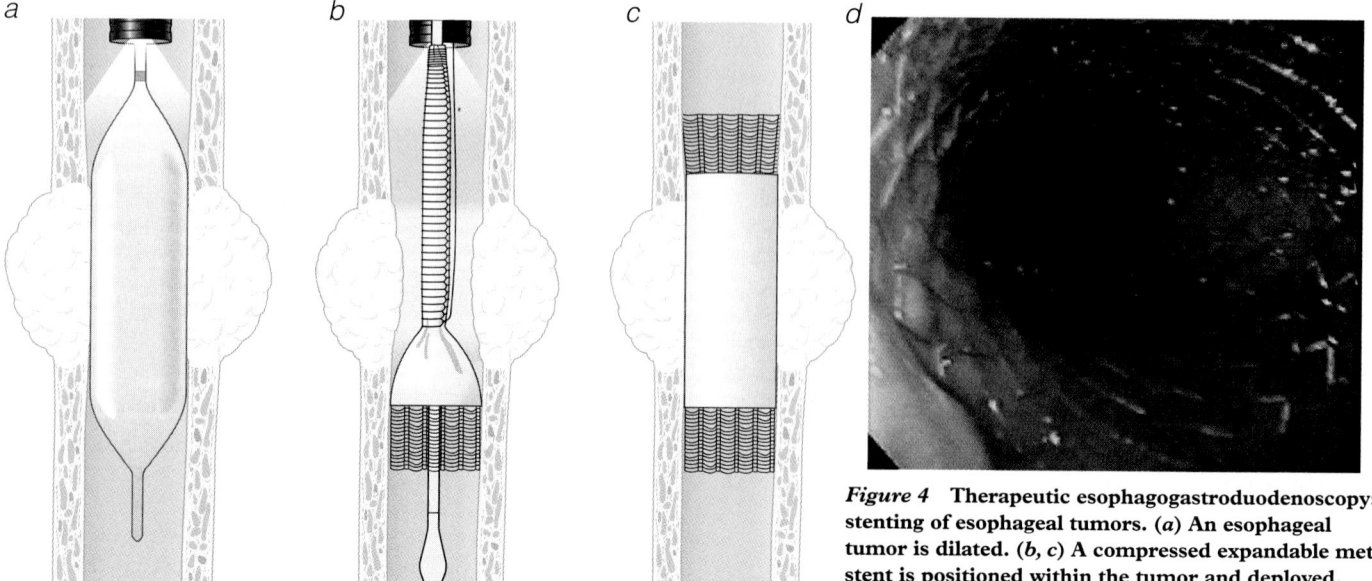

a *b* *c* *d*

Figure 4 Therapeutic esophagogastroduodenoscopy: stenting of esophageal tumors. (*a*) An esophageal tumor is dilated. (*b, c*) A compressed expandable metal stent is positioned within the tumor and deployed. (*d*) The expanded stent yields a large enough lumen to permit the patient to continue oral alimentation.

around before being removed. If multiple foreign bodies are present or if it is highly likely that the foreign body will injure the esophagus if removed in the standard manner, an overtube should be placed over the scope before insertion. The overtube enables one to pass the instrument several times and retrieve any sharp objects without injuring the esophagus; it also helps ensure that the object is not aspirated into the airway. If the patient is a child, general anesthesia may be advisable.

Perhaps the best method of removing foreign bodies is to surround them with a simple polypectomy snare and secure them in the endoscope's grasp. Meat boluses that form in the esophagus or proximal to a gastric band may be extremely difficult to dislodge; the use of a variceal ligator cap to produce a suction chamber can be helpful in such situations.

Complications

Endoscopic removal of foreign bodies is extremely safe and effective. Care must be taken to ensure that the esophagus is not injured during removal of the object. If the object is deeply embedded or refractory to removal, a surgical approach is preferred.

PERCUTANEOUS ENDOSCOPIC GASTROSTOMY

Since 1980, endoscopically guided placement of a tube gastrostomy has been widely employed to provide access to the GI tract for feeding or decompression. Indications for percutaneous endoscopic gastrostomy (PEG) include various disease processes that interfere with swallowing, such as severe neurologic impairment, oropharyngeal tumors, and facial trauma. PEG has also been employed to establish a route for recycling bile in patients with malignant biliary obstruction, to provide supplemental feeding in selected patients with inflammatory bowel disease, and to accomplish gastric decompression in patients with conditions such as carcinomatosis, radiation enteritis, and diabetic gastropathy.

Technique

The patient fasts for 8 hours beforehand, and a single prophylactic dose of an antibiotic is administered just before the procedure is begun. The patient is placed in the supine position, a topical anesthetic is applied to the posterior pharynx, and intravenous sedation is begun. A forward-viewing endoscope is passed into the esophagus and advanced into the stomach. The abdomen is prepared in a sterile fashion and draped. The stomach and the duodenum are then inspected.

The room lights are dimmed, and the light of the endoscope is used to transilluminate the abdominal wall so as to indicate a point where the gastric wall and the abdominal wall are in close proximity. Finger pressure is applied to various areas of the abdomen until a spot is identified at which such pressure produces clear indentation of the gastric wall. An endoscopic snare is deployed through the biopsy channel of the endoscope to cover this spot, and a local anesthetic is infiltrated into the overlying skin [see Figure 5]. A 1 cm skin incision is made at the chosen spot, and a needle is passed through the incision and into the gastric lumen. The endoscopic snare is tightened around the needle, and a wire is passed through the needle and into the gastric lumen. The snare is moved so as to surround the wire, which is then pulled out of the patient's mouth. The gastrostomy tube is fastened to the wire and pulled in a retrograde manner down the esophagus and into the stomach. The gastroscope is subsequently reinserted to ensure that the head of the catheter is correctly positioned against the gastric mucosa [see Figure 6].

An outer crossbar is put in place to prevent inward migration of the tube and to hold the stomach in approximation to the

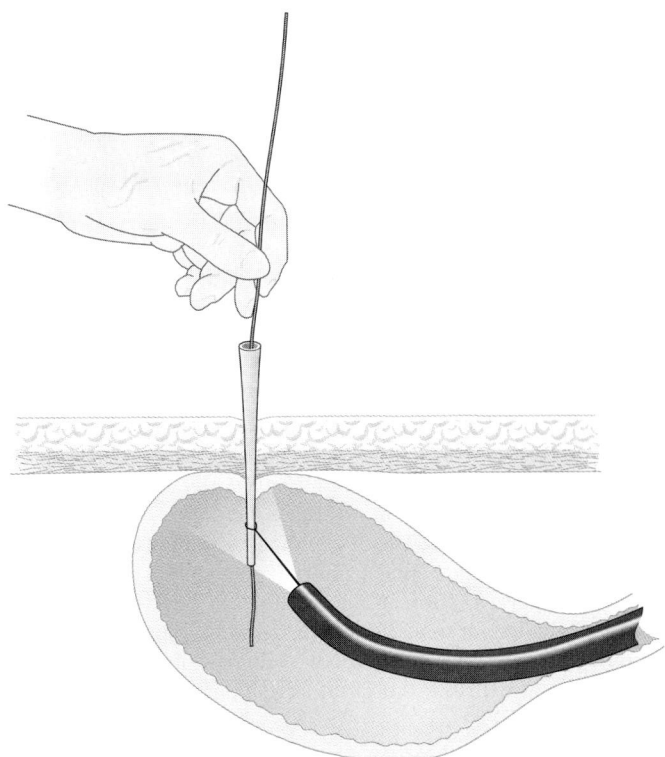

Figure 5 Therapeutic esophagogastroduodenoscopy: percutaneous endoscopic gastrostomy. The first steps in the procedure involve selecting a proper site in the stomach and using a snare to surround a needle that has been passed through the abdominal and gastric walls.

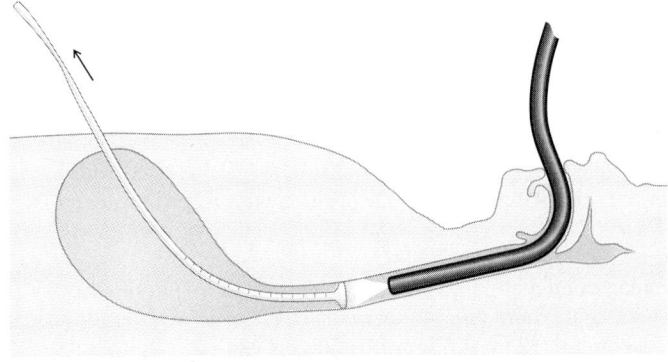

Figure 6 Therapeutic esophagogastroduodenoscopy: percutaneous endoscopic gastrostomy. After the suture is retrieved from the stomach, it is affixed to the gastrostomy tube and used to pull the tube back into the stomach and out the abdominal wall. The gastroscope is reinserted to follow the process and ensure that the final position of the tube is correct.

abdominal wall. The crossbar should remain several millimeters from the skin to prevent excessive tension, which would cause ischemic necrosis of the underlying tissue.

Complications

Local wound infections are the most common complications of PEG. They can be minimized by administering preoperative antibiotics and ensuring that excessive tension is not applied to the crossbar at the end of the procedure. When such infections do occur, they can usually be treated via simple drainage and local wound care; sacrifice of the gastrostomy is rarely necessary. Several other complications, such as early extrusion of the tube, progressive enlargement of the tract, and separation of the gastric and abdominal walls with leakage of feedings into the abdominal cavity, are also most often attributable to excessive crossbar tension and subsequent ischemia. Gastrocolic fistula can occur after PEG. This problem may not be obvious for months afterward, but severe diarrhea after feedings is grounds for suspicion. Once the PEG tract is mature, gastrocolic fistulas usually close quickly after simple removal of the gastrostomy tube.

Diagnostic Endoscopic Retrograde Cholangiopancreatography

Endoscopic retrograde cholangiopancreatography (ERCP) is an advanced procedure that is technically more challenging than standard upper GI endoscopy; however, it can be mastered by most endoscopists who are willing to dedicate sufficient time to learning the method. ERCP yields a radiologic image of the pancreatic and biliary trees, and in many cases, it provides access for therapy. Indications for ERCP include suspected benign or malignant maladies of the common bile duct (CBD), the ampulla of Vater, or the pancreas. Cholelithiasis per se is not an indication for ERCP unless choledocholithiasis is suspected.

TECHNIQUE

As with standard upper GI endoscopy, the patient fasts for 6 to 8 hours beforehand. Intravenous sedation is administered, and prophylactic antibiotics are given when biliary obstruction is suspected. The patient is initially placed in the left lateral decubitus position but is later rotated to the prone position after the scope is in place in the second portion of the duodenum. A side-viewing endoscope is employed because it allows the best visualization of the ampulla of Vater. The instrument is passed into the esophagus and maneuvered through the stomach, across the pylorus, and into the duodenum. Manipulation of a side-viewing instrument is a bit awkward for the novice but is easily learned.

Once the endoscope is in the second portion of the duodenum, it is pulled back so that the gastric loop is straightened and the tip of the scope occupies a better position with regard to the papilla. This so-called short scope position is generally best for work in the CBD [see Figure 7]. The papilla of Vater (also known as the major duodenal papilla) appears as a small longitudinal nubbin crossing the horizontal semicircular folds of the duodenum, generally in the 12 to 1 o'clock position. At its tip, a small, soft, reticulated area may be noted; this is the papillary orifice. Often, a small mucosal protuberance is seen just proximal and to the right of the papilla of Vater; this is the minor duodenal papilla.

A small plastic cannula is passed through the channel of the endoscope and introduced into the ampullary orifice, and contrast material is injected under fluoroscopic control to provide visualization of the CBD and the pancreatic duct. The two may share a single orifice within the ampulla or may have separate orifices. The CBD exits the papilla in a cephalad direction, tangential to the duodenal wall. The bulge of the ampulla within the duodenum represents the intramural segment of the duct. The orifice of the CBD is typically found at the 11 o'clock position in the ampulla. The pancreatic duct leaves the papilla in a perpendicular fashion. Its orifice is usually in the 1 o'clock area of the papilla [see Figure 8].

COMPLICATIONS

When contrast material is being injected into the pancreatic ductal system, care must be taken to avoid overfilling, which can

lead to acinarization, or rupture of the small ductules, with extravasation of contrast material into the pancreatic parenchyma; pancreatitis is a frequent consequence of acinarization. Cholangitis may result when contrast is injected proximal to an obstruction of the biliary tree. When obstruction is demonstrated, drainage of the system by means of stone extraction, stenting, or nasobiliary intubation is important to prevent cholangitis.

Therapeutic Endoscopic Retrograde Cholangiopancreatography

Therapeutic interventions that may be accomplished at the time of ERCP include sphincterotomy for ductal access or ampullary stenosis, removal of CBD stones, dilation of benign and malignant biliary strictures, and insertion of stents to maintain ductal patency. Pancreatic duct interventions include removal of stones, bridging of ductal disruptions, and drainage of pseudocysts.

TECHNIQUE

All therapeutic applications of ERCP must begin with selective cannulation of the duct being treated. Frequently, a guide wire is then introduced deep into the duct to provide a means of obtaining access to the duct on an ongoing basis and to ensure correct

a

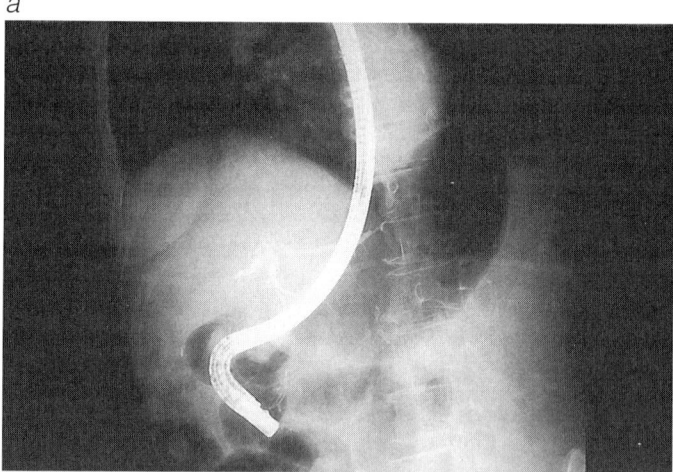

b

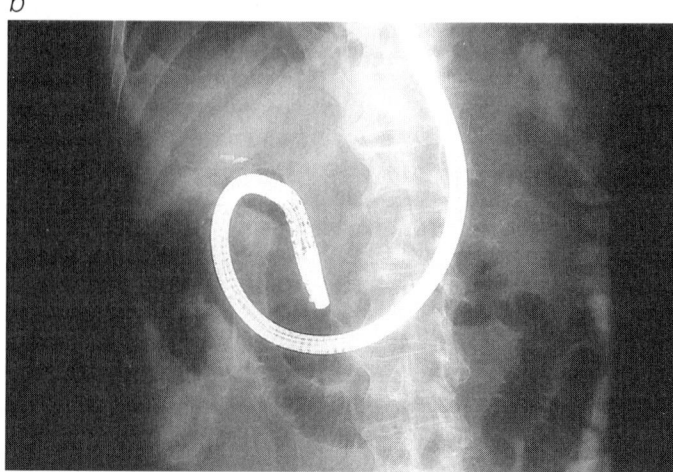

Figure 7 **Diagnostic endoscopic retrograde cholangiopancreatography. (*a*) The so-called short scope position, along the lesser curve of the stomach, is usually the most effective in biliary interventions. (*b*) The so-called long scope position may be necessary at times.**

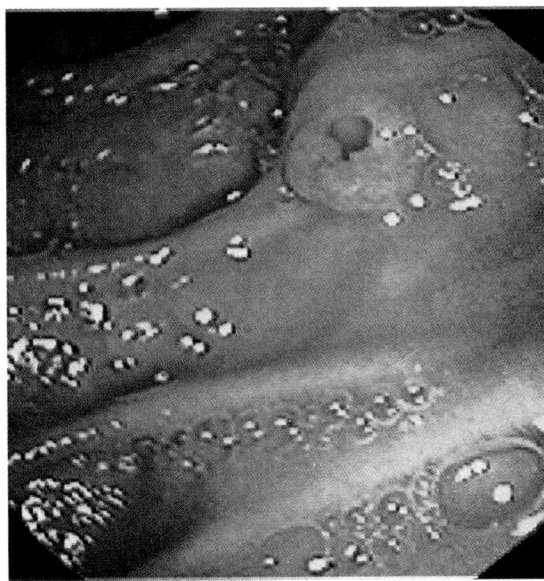

Figure 8 Diagnostic endoscopic retrograde cholangiopancreatography. The so-called long scope position, along the greater curve of the stomach, may be useful in some pancreatic interventions; shown is the pancreatic duct orifice.

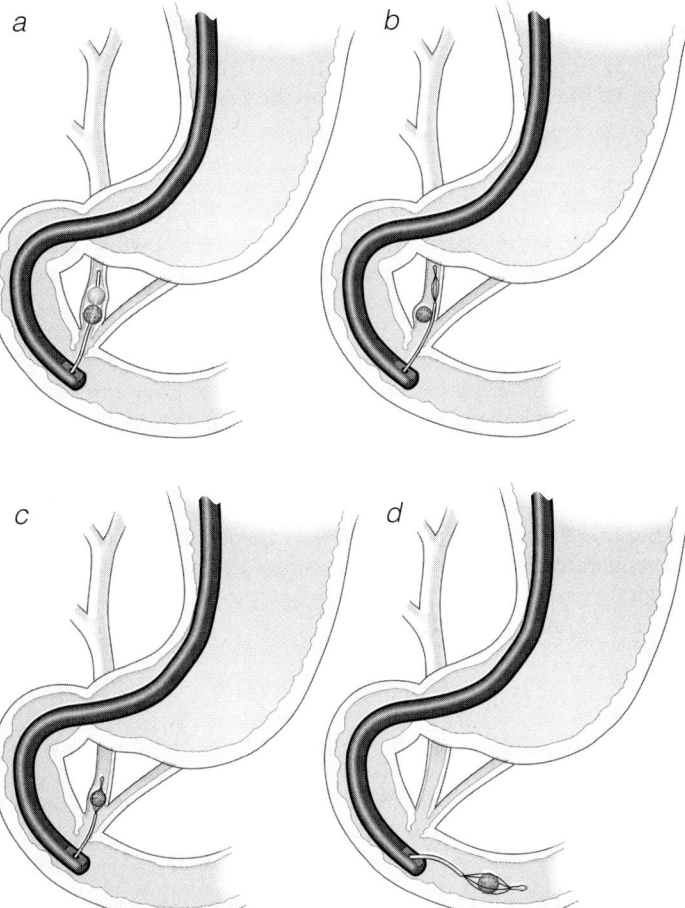

Figure 9 Therapeutic endoscopic retrograde cholangiopancreatography. After endoscopic sphincterotomy, CBD stones may be retrieved with balloons (*a*) or baskets (*b, c, d*).

positioning for intraductal manipulations. After electrosurgical division of the papilla, biliary stones are retrieved with balloon or baskets [*see Figure 9*]. Often, large stones can be captured within the duct in mechanical lithotripsy baskets and crushed before removal.

Strictures should be brushed for cytologic evaluation once they have been traversed by a wire. They may then be dilated with hydrostatic balloons under fluoroscopic guidance and stented [*see Figure 10*]. Plastic stents are used for most benign and many malignant strictures; however, self-expanding metal stents are now being used more frequently for malignant strictures because they remain patent longer [*see Figure 11*].

COMPLICATIONS

Perforation can occur during endoscopic sphincterotomy as a result of extension or tearing of the papilla beyond the junction of the CBD with the duodenal wall. Retroperitoneal or free intraperitoneal air may be seen. In many cases, intravenous antibiotics, hydration, and avoidance of oral intake are sufficient to manage such complications. If the patient's condition deteriorates, surgical exploration is indicated.

Bleeding may also occur with sphincterotomy. It is usually controllable with injection of epinephrine solution (1:10,000), electrocoagulation, or balloon tamponade. Arteriographic embolization of the gastroduodenal artery may be helpful in some cases. As with diagnostic ERCP, pancreatitis may occur; it usually responds to conservative measures.

Diagnostic Colonoscopy

Colonoscopy has become one of the most frequently performed endoscopic examinations. It has revolutionized the diagnosis and treatment of colonic disease and offers the promise of reducing the occurrence of colon cancer. Indications for colonoscopy include iron deficiency anemia, frank or occult rectal bleeding, a history of colonic cancer in the patient or in first-degree family members, a history or suspicion of colonic polyps, inflammatory bowel disease, and a persistent change in bowel habits. Preparation involves purging the bowel mechanically by placing the patient on a clear liquid diet for several days, then giving cathartics and enemas; alternatively, one may use osmotic lavage, in which 1 gal of lavage fluid is administered orally over a period of 4 hours. It is often helpful to administer 10 mg of metoclopramide to enhance gastric motility as preparation begins.

TECHNIQUE

Sedation is accomplished as for upper GI endoscopy, and the patient fasts for 6 to 8 hours before the procedure. With the patient in the left lateral decubitus position, a rectal examination is performed. This step helps relax the anal sphincter in preparation for insertion of the scope and ensures that low-lying rectal lesions are not overlooked.

The colonoscope is introduced into the rectal vault, and insufflation of air is commenced. The instrument is advanced only when the lumen is clearly apparent. At times, only a portion of the lumen may be visible, but this is usually enough to guide advancement of the scope. Frequently, when the lumen itself is not visible, light reflected onto the colonic folds can guide one to the lumen, with the concavity of the fold indicating the direction of the lumen. In contrast with upper GI endoscopy, in which torsion on the shaft of the endoscope is rarely necessary, such torsion is the rule in colonoscopy. The shaft of the instrument is rotated with the right hand to facilitate

a

b

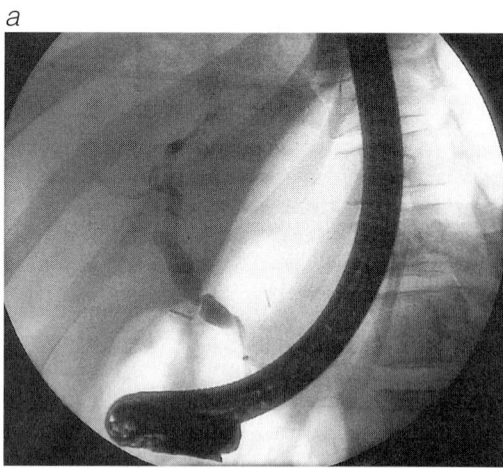
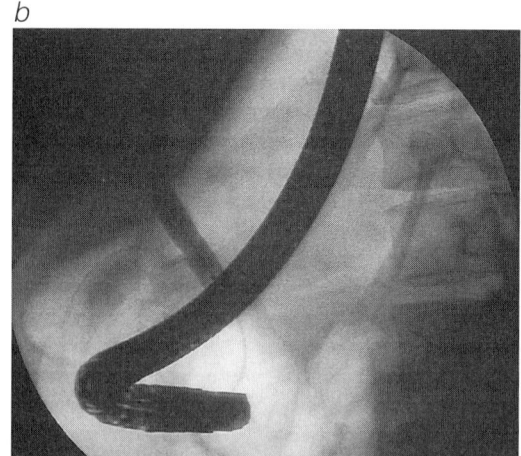

Figure 10   **Therapeutic endoscopic retrograde cholangiopancreatography. CBD strictures (*a*), whether benign or malignant, may be dilated effectively with hydrostatic balloons under fluoroscopic guidance (*b*).**

straightening and intubation of the colon. By applying torsion to the shaft frequently and pulling back the scope as necessary, one can pleat the colon on the instrument as it is advanced. Pulling back is one of the most useful techniques for advancing the colonoscope through the colon.

The colon exhibits a number of characteristic anatomic features that are readily observed during colonoscopy. The sigmoid colon, because of its frequent turns, yields elliptical views of the lumen. The descending colon appears as a long, round tunnel with little haustration. The transverse colon has well-defined triangular folds, and the hepatic flexure may exhibit a blue hue resulting from the proximity of the liver. The cecum is recognized on the basis of the appearance of the ileocecal valve on the lateral wall, the convergence of the colonic taenia to form the cecal strap (the so-called Mercedes sign), and the presence of the appendiceal orifice.

Insertion of the colonoscope as far as the hepatic flexure is rarely difficult. Occasionally, the sigmoid colon presents a chal-

lenge, in which case placement of the patient on the back or the abdomen to change the orientation may be helpful. Once again, pulling back and straightening the scope is a highly useful maneuver. Once the scope is in the hepatic flexure looking down the right colon, pulling back, counterclockwise torsion, and the application of suction may all assist in advancing the instrument into the cecum. Changing the patient's position or applying pressure to various points in the abdomen may also be helpful. Once the cecum is reached, the instrument is slowly withdrawn while the colonic parietes are carefully examined. Biopsy and cytologic brushing may be done as appropriate, and colonic contents may be aspirated into a suction trap for examination.

COMPLICATIONS

Perforation is the most common complication of diagnostic colonoscopy. It may result from direct tip pressure, bowing of the shaft of the scope while a large loop is being formed, blowout of a diverticulum secondary to air insufflation, or tearing of an adhesion of the colon to an adjacent structure. The risk of perforation can be minimized by observing the lumen directly as the scope is advanced, avoiding excessive insufflation, and minimizing loop formation. Close attention to patient discomfort is important. If the patient feels poorly after the procedure, an upright chest x-ray, an upright abdominal x-ray, or a lateral decubitus abdominal x-ray should be obtained to determine whether there is any free air, which would indicate a perforation. Such situations have been successfully managed by nonoperative means in some cases, but in most cases, prompt operative intervention with primary repair of the perforation is the best approach.

Therapeutic Colonoscopy

By far the most common use of therapeutic colonoscopy is for the excision of polyps. Other applications include control of bleeding, dilation of strictures, and placement of enteral stents.

TECHNIQUE

The development of colonoscopic polypectomy—electrosurgical excision of the polyp with a wire snare—has rendered operative colotomy unnecessary in the management of colonic polyps. Pedunculated polyps are approached by placing the snare over the polyp's head and tightening the loop around the

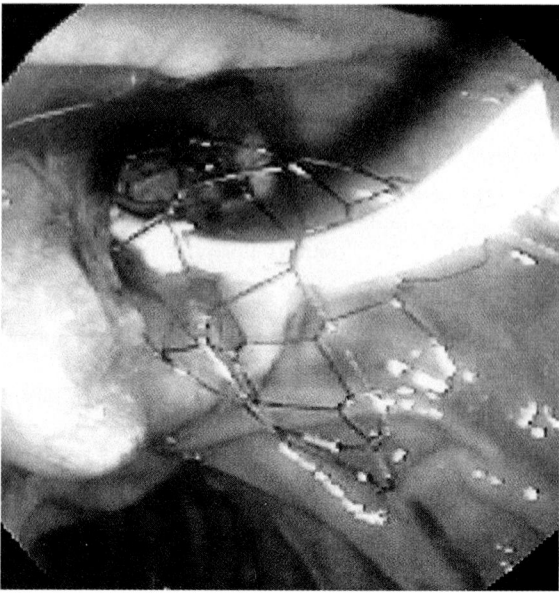

Figure 11   **Therapeutic endoscopic retrograde cholangiopancreatography. Self-expanding metal stents may provide effective long-term palliation of malignant biliary obstruction.**

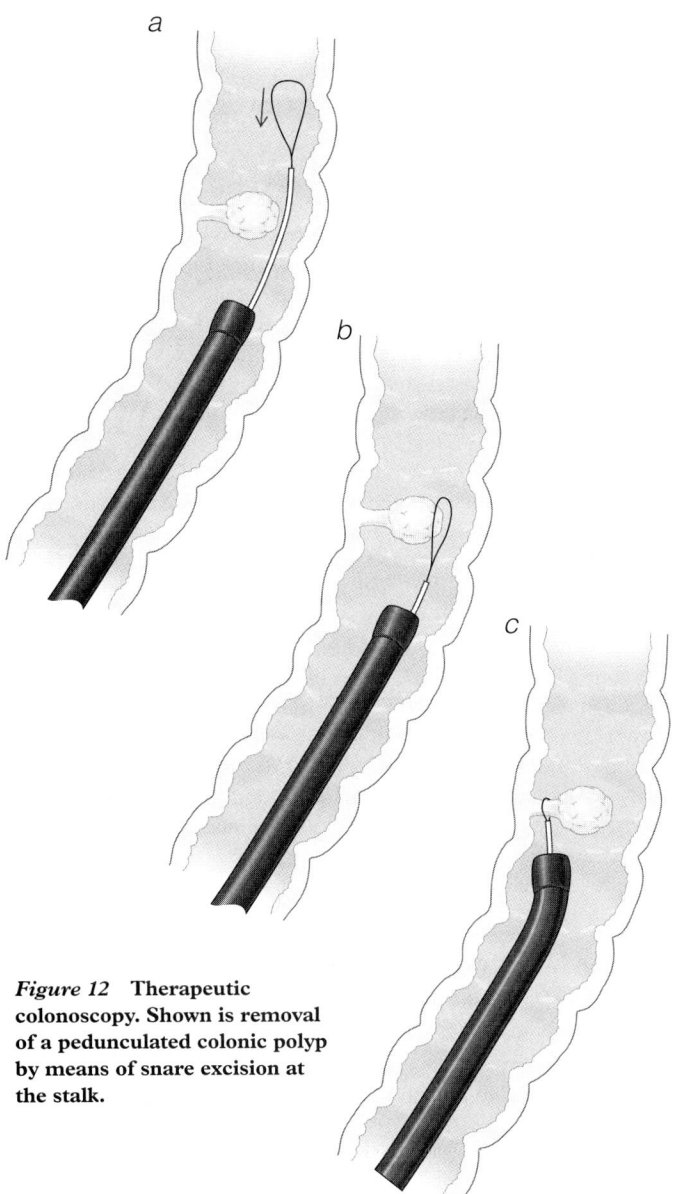

Figure 12 **Therapeutic colonoscopy. Shown is removal of a pedunculated colonic polyp by means of snare excision at the stalk.**

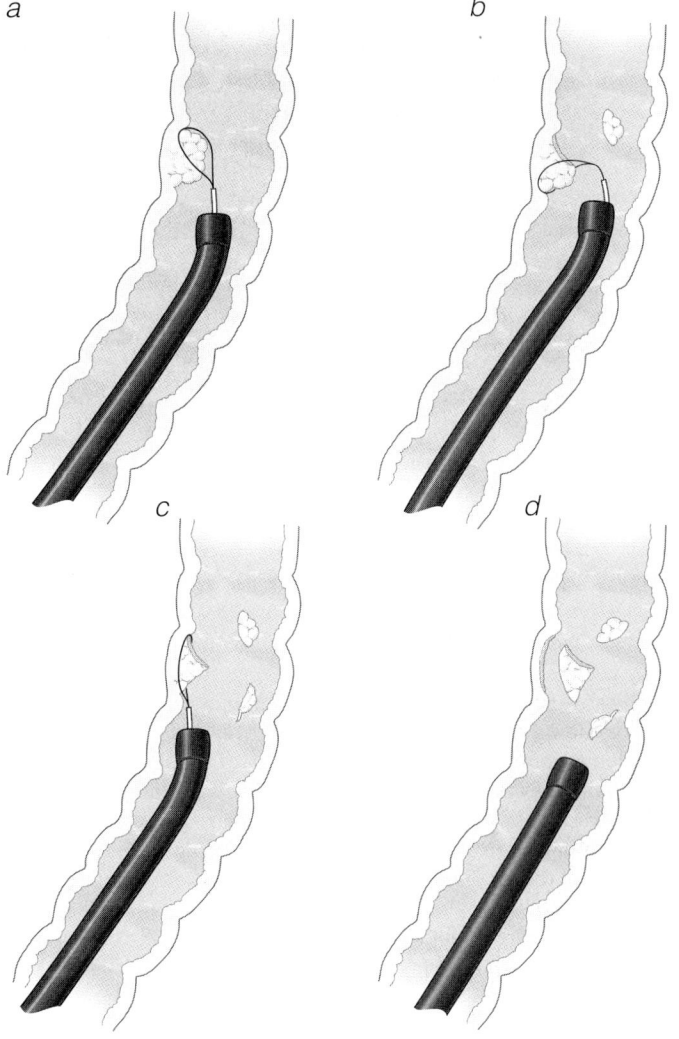

Figure 13   **Therapeutic colonoscopy. Illustrated is piecemeal excision of a sessile colonic polyp.**

stalk near the junction of the head and the stalk [*see Figure 12*]. Because the stalk is an extension of normal mucosa, it is unnecessary—and often unwise—to excise the stalk close to the colonic wall; excision near the head of the polyp is usually sufficient. Short bursts of coagulating current are applied to transect the stalk. During excision, the polyps must be moved around to prevent conduction burns to the opposing colonic wall. Once transection is complete, if the polyp is small, it may be suctioned into a trap; if it is large, it may be suctioned onto the tip of the scope and retrieved or captured in a snare or basket. Sessile polyps are more challenging and risky to excise. Accordingly, it is often preferable to excise such polyps in a piecemeal fashion [*see Figure 13*]. The snare is applied several times to successive portions of the polyp until it is excised down to the colonic wall. The excised fragments are then retrieved. Difficult or large sessile polyps may be elevated before excision by injecting epinephrine solution or saline submucosally into the polyp or the surrounding tissue. This maneuver makes transmural injury less likely (see below).

Although the use of colonoscopy to define the site of colonic bleeding is commonplace, its use to treat such bleeding is not.

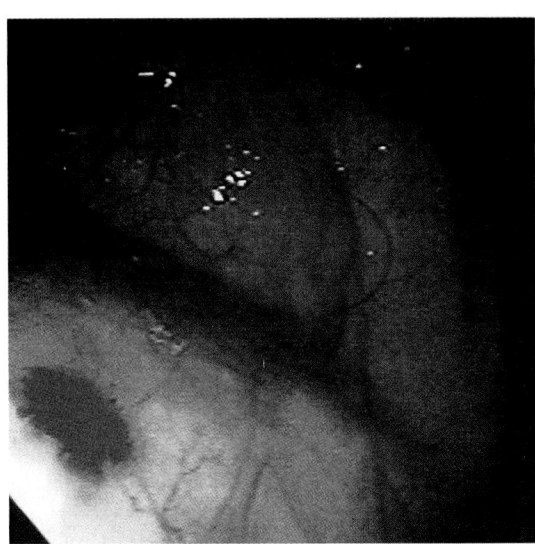

Figure 14   **Therapeutic colonoscopy. Shown is an angiodysplasia of the right colon, a frequent cause of lower GI hemorrhage.**

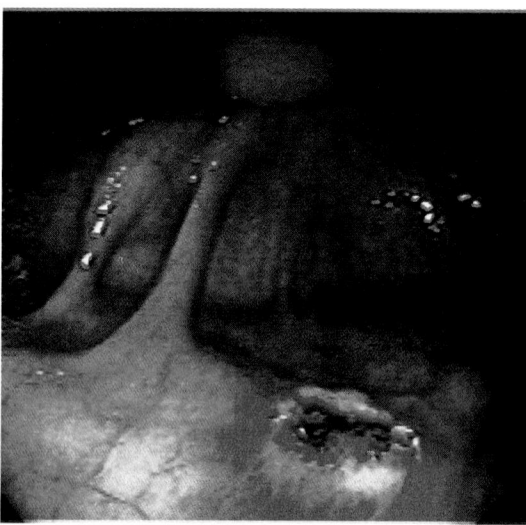

Figure 15 **Therapeutic colonoscopy. Shown is a right colonic angiodysplasia after treatment with bipolar electrocoagulation.**

Diverticular bleeding often stops when colonoscopy is done, and only in rare instances is the actual bleeding diverticulum seen. In such cases, injection of epinephrine solution around the mouth of the offending diverticulum is often effective. Angiodysplasias are frequently found in the right colon, though they are rarely identified while they are bleeding [*see Figure 14*]. They may be treated with a variety of modalities, including bipolar electrocoagulation, injection of a sclerosant solution, and laser therapy [*see Figure 15*]. Currently, the argon plasma coagulator is often employed for obliteration of these lesions. This device has the advantage of being able to obliterate angiodysplasias with minimal wall penetration, thereby increasing the safety of this intervention in the thin-walled right colon.

Strictures may occur in the colon, as in the rest of the GI tract. Colonic strictures usually develop at an anastomosis, though they may also be the result of ischemia. Hydrostatic balloon dilation is very effective in treating such strictures. The balloon is introduced through the lumen of the endoscope, and dilation is carried out under direct vision, often in conjunction with fluoroscopic observation to confirm that dilation is complete. In patients with fully or almost fully obstructing tumors of the colon, self-expanding metal stents may be placed to provide decompression and at least temporary relief of obstruction. This step may avert emergency surgery or, if the tumor is inoperable, provide palliation.

COMPLICATIONS

Perforation may occur as a result of transmural thermal injury during polypectomy. Some perforations are immediately apparent, but others may not be noticed for several days. When perforation is documented, surgical exploration is indicated. Occasionally, a patient may present with fever and abdominal tenderness several days after polypectomy but show no free air on abdominal films. Such a patient may have a thermal injury to the bowel wall or so-called postpolypectomy syndrome and can usually be treated with intravenous fluids, antibiotics, and observation. Bleeding from the stalk of a pedunculated polyp may occur after excision; it may present immediately or may be delayed until the coagulum on the stalk separates 3 to 5 days after polypectomy. Such bleeding is a rare occurrence. When it does occur, it can be treated by injecting epinephrine solution (1:10,000) into the stalk.

Chromoendoscopy

The development of extirpative endoscopy has allowed physicians to treat several conditions that previously required open or laparoscopic surgical procedures. However, it is not always possible to see the difference between diseased and healthy tissue on endoscopy, and this limitation has precluded one-stage procedures. Identification of tissue types required biopsy, and lesion margins were impossible to determine at the time of the procedure.

Chromoendoscopy can help to identify diseased tissue and define lesion borders. This process is essentially an in vivo staining technique in which a variety of specialized stains are applied to tissues to improve their characterization. This differs from carbon-dye injection (tattooing), a technique that is used for later surgical identification, in that the stains used for chromoendoscopy are specific to the anatomic area being examined. Several chromoendoscopic dyes are commercially available in the United States [*see Table 1*]. Selection of a particular agent is based on the type of tissue being studied, the disease state, and physician familiarity.

One of the first agents used for chromoendoscopy was methylene blue. It was initially used in Japan in the 1970s to detect intestinal metaplasia in the stomach. Subsequent studies in the United States, Japan, and Europe independently demonstrated that methylene blue will selectively stain metaplasia in Barrett's esophagus (see above). On routine screening endoscopy in patients with Barrett's esophagus, methylene blue chromoendoscopy offers improved detection of dysplasia and early malignancy compared with four-quadrant random biopsy studies. Other reported applications include esophageal carcinoma, gastric metaplasia, oropharyngeal cancer, mucosal lesions, and heterotopic gastric mucosa.

Endoscopic Mucosal Resection

Endoscopic polypectomy marked the beginning of extirpative procedures. Subsequently, endoscopic resection techniques have continued to advance, as a result of improvements in imaging and instrumentation, along with the development of chromoendoscopy and specific techniques designed as adjuncts to tissue removal. One such technique is endoscopic mucosal resection (EMR).

EMR has its basis in the anatomy of the GI tract. Histologically, the GI tract has three layers: a superficial mucosal, a middle submucosal, and an outer muscular layer. EMR is designed to help the endoscopist remove superficial mucosal tissue while leaving the deeper submucosal and muscular layers intact. These layers can be relatively easily separated from each other by injecting a liquid that spreads within the plane of injection. This step elevates the layers superficial to the injection, thus facilitating the resection of those layers. Advantages over other resection techniques include the preservation of histologic architecture (in contrast to electrocautery or laser ablation), which allows improved pathologic assessment; the ease with which EMR can be combined with endoscopic ultrasonography; and its safety and minimal invasiveness.

EMR was first described in 1955, when submucosal saline injections through a rigid sigmoidoscope were used in the resection of rectal and sigmoid polyps. In 1973, a submucosal saline injection was employed to assist with the removal of sessile polyps throughout the colon. Additional development was accomplished in Japan in 1983, when mucosal resection was used in the treatment of early gastric carcinoma in a technique termed strip-off biopsy. The technique has been refined and is now routinely used for lesions in the esophagus, stomach, duodenum, colon, and rectum. It is widely incorporated into aggressive screening programs designed to detect early GI cancers.

EMR can be used to treat dysplastic and other premalignant lesions, as well as superficial cancers of the GI tract. One must be careful to comply with all standard principles of cancer resection, including knowledge of the depth of the lesion, its radial extent, and staging. Consequently, several criteria must be fulfilled before EMR can be viewed as a curative intervention. Classification of lesions on the basis of their endoscopic appearance can be combined with information obtained through the use of chromoendoscopy and EUS to determine the potential for EMR.

Lesion location within the GI tract is important with respect to long-term outcomes. For example, EMR can be used to treat circumferential colonic lesions but is inappropriate for esophageal lesions that extend beyond one third of the circumference, because of the risk of a late stricture.

Although specific methods differ among practitioners, several generalizations about the technical aspects can be made. First, a liquid must be injected deep to the mucosal layer, allowing separation of the wall components. Although the ideal solution for injection has not been determined, the liquid chosen must be biodegradable, biocompatible, noninflammatory, and have viscoelastic properties allowing the development of an adequate bleb. Saline, hypertonic saline, epinephrine, hyaluronic acid, and glycerol solutions are all in current use. The elevated tissue is then held in place with a grasper or suction mechanism, and snares, needle knives, or lasers are used to cut the tissue at its base. Optimal results are obtained on nonulcerated lesions that are less than 2 cm after elevation; other lesions have a high probability of submucosal lymphatic and vascular invasion.

Although complications can occur, with proper patient selection and procedural refinement they are relatively rare. Perforation has been noted, particularly when submucosal bleb formation is suboptimal. Inadequate blebs may result from insufficient liquid being injected, improper needle depth, or severe scarring of the local tissues. Bleeding has been reported to occur in 1.6% of EMR cases. This complication is relatively easily handled with a combination of electrocautery and epinephrine injection. Infection in the absence of perforation is uncommon.

Overall, EMR provides a minimally invasive means to treat early cancers in favorable locations. Patients must understand that additional resection may be required if histopathologic assessment does not show curative margins. Future development of endoscopic instruments and injection liquids will likely broaden the applicability of the procedure.

Endoscopic Ultrasonography

The 1980s saw the introduction of EUS. Extracavitary ultrasonographic methods have been hampered by the presence of air within the GI tract, which precludes high-resolution imaging. Consequently, they had been relegated to gross estimates of disease and detection of displacement of other tissues or fluid accumulation proximal to stenoses, such as ductal dilation in patients with common bile duct stones.

Three advances have proven invaluable in allowing EUS to carve out a niche in the field of GI diagnosis. First is the improvement in endoscopes that allows transducer and receiver channels to traverse a tortuous path. Second is the development of multiple frequency options in conjunction with circumferential visualization. Higher frequencies provide higher resolutions, allowing useful differentiation of the various layers of the intestinal tract. Third is the evolution of treatment protocols keyed to the accu-

Table 1 Special Stains Used in Endoscopy

Stain	Site of Use	Comment
Lugol solution (2% iodine)	Esophagus	Normal mucosa stains green-brown (as a result of intracellular glycogen); dysplastic cells do not stain
Indigo carmine (0.4% solution)	Stomach, colon	Enhances contour of mucosa, giving tissue a three-dimensional appearance
Toluidine blue	Oropharynx, esophagus	Absorbed by the nucleic acid component of malignant epithelial cells
Congo red	Acid-secreting areas of gastric mucosa	Turns a blue-black color when pH < 3
Methylene blue (0.5% solution)	Intestinal metaplasia, Barrett's esophagus	Absorbed only by dysplastic tissue; however, absorption decreases as severe dysplasia develops

rate staging of tumors—information that is sometimes unobtainable from other imaging techniques.

This technology has now been firmly established as an accurate way to identify carcinoma. More recent developments are allowing EUS to expand from the field of diagnosis into the realm of intervention. Examples of EUS-guided procedures include fine-needle aspiration, lymph node sampling, and drainage of pancreatic pseudocysts.

EUS devices come in both linear and radial transducers. Radial transducers have the advantage of providing circumferential visualization that parallels the standard modes of perceiving the GI tract. Linear images allow EUS-directed biopsies and have the potential to provide color and pulsed Doppler imaging. Probes can be mounted on the top of an oblique viewing fiberoptic scope, or come in an over-the-wire format for use in the pancreaticobiliary tree. A series of frequencies is available, with the higher frequencies providing greater resolution but less tissue depth penetration. Lower-frequency probes allow deeper tissue assessment and a broader view, but at the price of reduced resolution. Nevertheless, any form of EUS will provide better resolution than transcutaneous ultrasonography, allowing markedly improved two-point discrimination and hence more accurate tissue diagnosis.

The benefits of accurate staging of GI tumors paved the way for EUS development. Tissue sampling techniques are further benefited by this technology. The sensitivity of EUS makes it one of the best modalities for the evaluation and detection of pancreatic tumors. Its sensitivity, which is in excess of 95%, contrasts favorably with those of other modalities, including ultrasonography (75%), computed tomography (80%), and angiography (89%). The accuracy of T staging by EUS in esophageal cancer (80% to 90%) is greater than that of staging determined by CT scanning (50% to 60%). This finding has led to the development of several staging schemes that are based solely on EUS findings. EUS has established a role in the identification of early pancreatitis; the detection of common bile duct stones and mediastinal masses; and the assessment of anastomotic strictures, thickened gastric folds, and the integrity of the anal sphincter. It has also proved a useful adjunct in the determination of whether a tumor is amenable to EMR techniques or is better served by adjuvant therapies or surgical interventions.

The sensitivity of EUS is rooted in its ability to delineate the various layers of the alimentary canal. Experienced endoscopists can easily evaluate the submucosa and differentiate intramural from extrinsic masses. Characteristic patterns are readily learned and rapidly recognized, obviating tissue diagnoses in straightforward cases. Criteria have also been established to aid in the differentiation of benign and malignant lesions. With the continued use of this technique, additional algorithms will be established in conjunction with more innovative interventional adjuncts. However, two limitations have caused many practitioners to remain skeptical: cost and training issues. Other imaging modalities, such as CT and magnetic resonance imaging, have also made tremendous strides in the recent past. Although these various modalities are often considered competitors—a view arising from the perceived need for a single imaging modality—the issue of which is superior to the others pales in comparison to the benefits that can be gained from combining imaging techniques in appropriate circumstances.

Endoscopic Suturing

The ability to suture through an endoscope would open up an entire arena of new possibilities, including antireflux procedures, morbid obesity surgery, and advances in the control of acute hemorrhage, as well as improved ability to manage complications of other endoscopic techniques. Despite the development and commercial availability of numerous devices, however, design problems have relegated most applications to investigational status. For such devices to enter clinical practice, they must encompass fundamental surgical techniques: the ability to cut, suture, tie knots, and staple. These are critical for maintaining hemostasis and constructing durable anastomoses. Although these techniques are plausible with modern devices, continued innovation and experience in conjunction with a new paradigm of disease management will direct the future of endoscopic interventions.

Recommended Reading

Abi-Hanna D, Williams SJ: Advances in gastrointestinal endoscopy. Med J Aust 170:131, 1999

Acosta MM, Boyce HW Jr: Chromoendoscopy—where is it useful? J Clin Gastroenterol 27:13, 1998

Brugge WR: Endoscopic ultrasonography: the current status. Gastroenterology 115:1577, 1998

Canto M: Methylene blue chromoendoscopy for Barrett's esophagus: coming soon to your GI unit? Gastrointest Endosc 54:403, 2001

Cotton PB, Williams CB: Practical Gastrointestinal Endoscopy, 3rd ed. Blackwell Scientific, Oxford, 1990

Hawes RH: Endoscopic ultrasound. Gastrointest Endosc Clin N Am 10:161, 2000

Hawes RH: Perspectives in endoscopic mucosal resection. Gastrointest Endosc Clin N Am 11:549, 2001

Inoue H: Endoscopic mucosal resection for the entire gastrointestinal mucosal lesions. Gastrointest Endosc Clin N Am 11:459, 2001

Matsuda K: Introduction to endoscopic mucosal resection. Gastrointest Endosc Clin N Am 11:439, 2001

Ponchon T: Endoscopic mucosal resection. J Clin Gastroenterol 32:6, 2001

Ponsky JL: Atlas of Surgical Endoscopy. Mosby–Year Book, St. Louis, 1992

Ponsky JL, King JF: Endoscopic marking of colonic lesions. Gastrointest Endosc 22:42, 1975

Rosch T, Lightdale CJ, Botel JF, et al: Localization of pancreatic endocrine tumors by endoscopic ultrasound. N Engl J Med 326:1721, 1992

Rosen M, Ponsky JL: Endoscopic therapy for gastroesophageal reflux disease. Semin Laparosc Surg 8:207, 2001

Schrock T: Colon and rectum: diagnostic techniques. Shackelford's Surgery of the Alimentary Tract. Vol 4: Colon and Anorectum, 3rd ed. Condon R, Ed. Philadelphia, WB Saunders Co, 1991, p 22

Schuman BM, Sugawa C: Diagnostic endoscopy of upper gastrointestinal bleeding. Gastrointestinal Bleeding. Sugawa C, Schuman BM, Lucas CE, Eds. Igaku Shoin, New York, 1992, p 222

Soetikno R, Inoue H, Chang KJ: Endoscopic muscosal resection: current concepts. Gastrointest Endosc Clin N Am 10:595, 2000

Swain CP: Endoscopic sewing and stapling machines. Endoscopy 29:205, 1997

Venu RP, Geenen JE: Overview of endoscopic sphincterotomy for common bile duct stone. Endoscopic Approach to Biliary Stones. Kozarek RA, Ed. Gastrointest Endosc Clin N Am 1:3, 1991

Acknowledgment

Figures 2, 4a, 4b, 4c, 5, 6, 9 12, 13   Tom Moore.

9 OPEN ESOPHAGEAL PROCEDURES

John Yee, M.D., and Richard J. Finley, M.D., F.A.C.S.

The remarkable advances in diagnosis, imaging, and surgical treatment of esophageal diseases over the past decade have resulted in markedly better patient outcomes. Ciné barium swallow remains the most cost-effective method of defining abnormal esophageal anatomy; however, high-quality endoscopic ultrasonography and computed tomography are now widely used to obtain information regarding mass lesions not only in the esophageal wall but also in the surrounding tissues. High-resolution endoscopy combined with photodynamic imaging or vital staining allows accurate diagnosis of dysplastic or malignant esophageal lesions in their earliest stages. Positron emission tomography (PET) and high-resolution CT scanning greatly facilitate identification of metastatic esophageal cancer. Refinements in the use of esophageal manometry, 24-hour esophageal pH tests, and esophageal and gastric nuclear transit studies, combined with improvements in endoscopic and ciné barium swallow techniques, permit more accurate diagnosis and more effective treatment of gastroesophageal reflux disease (GERD) and of functional abnormalities of the esophagus.

In particular, operative techniques for treating esophageal disease have advanced considerably in recent years, as a result of our improved understanding of esophageal anatomy and physiology and the successful introduction of minimally invasive approaches to the esophagus [*see 3:10 Minimally Invasive Esophageal Procedures*]. For a number of diseases (e.g., achalasia), minimally invasive procedures have proved to be as effective as their open counterparts while causing less postoperative morbidity. Nevertheless, the growing stature of minimally invasive approaches does not diminish the importance of the equivalent open approaches. In what follows, we describe common open operations performed to excise Zenker's diverticulum, to manage complex GERD, and to resect esophageal and proximal gastric tumors.

General Preoperative Considerations

Patients with obstructing esophageal diseases are often elderly, debilitated, and malnourished. Although months of insufficient nutrition cannot be corrected in the space of a few hours, anemia, dehydration, and electrolyte abnormalities can be mitigated by means of intravenous support and appropriate laboratory monitoring. If esophageal obstruction prevents oral intake, endoscopic dilatation of the stricture accompanied by either nasogastric intubation or percutaneous endoscopic gastrostomy (PEG) [*see 3:8 Gastrointestinal Endoscopy*] is indicated. Enteral nutrition, comprising at least 2,000 kcal/day of a high-protein liquid diet, should be administered for at least 10 days before the operation. Cardiovascular, renal, hepatic, and respiratory function should be documented and optimized. If the patient is aspirating, the esophagus should be evacuated and the patient should be given nothing by mouth until after the operation. Aspiration pneumonia should always be corrected preoperatively.

Cricopharyngeal Myotomy and Excision of Zenker's Diverticulum

PREOPERATIVE EVALUATION

Patients who are candidates for cricopharyngeal myotomy usually present with difficulty initiating swallowing, dysphagia or odynophagia, and symptoms of pulmonary aspiration. These symptoms of cricopharyngeal dysfunction may or may not be associated with a Zenker's diverticulum. Ciné barium swallow studies may reveal poor pharyngeal contractility, pulmonary or nasal aspiration, abnormalities of the upper esophageal sphincter, pharyngeal pouches, or structural abnormalities. Zenker's diverticulum is a pulsion diverticulum that arises within the inferior pharyngeal constrictor, between the oblique fibers of the posterior pharyngeal constrictors and the cricopharyngeus muscle. This mucosal outpouching results from a transient incomplete opening of the upper esophageal sphincter: the diverticulum enlarges, drapes over the cricopharyngeus, and dissects behind the esophagus into the prevertebral space. The pouch usually deviates to one side or the other; accordingly, the side on which the deviation occurs must be determined by means of a barium swallow so that the appropriate operative approach can be selected. Esophageal motility studies may show either incomplete upper esophageal relaxation on swallowing or discoordination of the upper esophageal relaxation phase with pharyngeal contractions. Upper GI endoscopy is performed preoperatively to exclude the presence of a pharyngeal or esophageal carcinoma and to assess upper GI anatomy. If there is evidence of GERD, proton pump inhibitors are given.

In symptomatic patients (e.g., those with dysphagia, nocturnal cough, or recurrent pneumonia from aspiration), surgical therapy is indicated regardless of whether a pouch is present or how large it may be. Such treatment involves correcting the underlying cricopharyngeal muscle dysfunction with a cricopharyngeal myotomy. If there is a diverticulum larger than 2 cm, it should be excised in addition to the cricopharyngeal myotomy. Alternatively, the diverticulum can be managed via endoscopic obliteration of the common wall between the pharyngeal pouch and the esophagus with either a stapler or a laser. Cricopharyngeal discoordination may be temporarily relieved by injecting botulinum toxin into the cricopharyngeus muscle.

OPERATIVE PLANNING

The patient is placed on a clear fluid diet for 2 days before the operation. With the patient under general anesthesia, the trachea is intubated with a single-lumen endotracheal tube. A soft roll is placed behind the shoulders to extend the neck. The patient is placed in a 20° reverse Trendelenburg position, and the legs are wrapped with pneumatic calf compressors to prevent deep vein thrombosis (DVT). With the endotracheal tube placed to the left side of the mouth, a preliminary flexible esophagogastroscopy is performed to empty the diverticulum of food and to examine the esophagus and the stomach. The scope is then brought back up

353

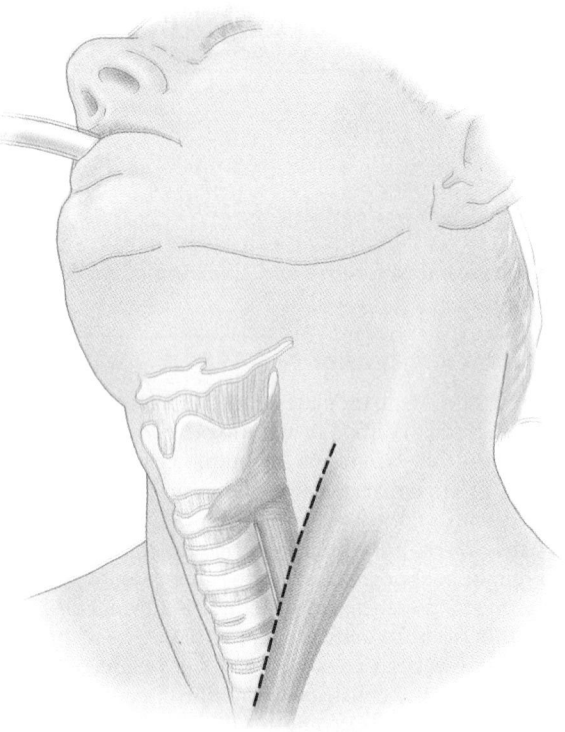

Figure 1 **Cricopharyngeal myotomy and excision of Zenker's diverticulum. A soft roll is placed behind the shoulders to extend the neck. The head is turned to the side opposite the incision. The cricoid cartilage is palpated and marked. The skin is incised obliquely along the sternocleidomastoid muscle, as shown, or transversely in a skin crease at the level of the cricoid.**

into the oropharynx and moved into the pouch. The location of the diverticulum (left or right side) is confirmed by turning the room lights off and noting the light coming from the gastroscope.

OPERATIVE TECHNIQUE

Step 1: Incision and Dissection of Pharyngeal Pouch

The patient lies with the head turned away from the side on which the incision is made. The cricoid cartilage is palpated and marked. A 5 cm skin incision is made, either obliquely along the sternocleidomastoid muscle [*see Figure 1*] or transversely in a skin crease at the level of the cricoid. The platysma is divided in the same line. Self-retaining retractors are inserted. The anterior border of the sternocleidomastoid muscle is incised throughout its length. The omohyoid muscle and the sternohyoid and sternothyroid muscles are retracted [*see Figure 2*]. The sternocleidomastoid muscle is retracted laterally to expose the carotid sheath and the internal jugular vein. The middle thyroid vein is ligated and divided, and the thyroid gland and the trachea are retracted medially by the assistant's finger to minimize the risk of injury to the underlying recurrent laryngeal nerve. The deep cervical fascia is divided. The inferior thyroid artery is divided as laterally as possible. The carotid sheath is retracted laterally, and dissection is carried down to the prevertebral fascia [*see Figure 2*]. The endoscope placed in the diverticulum is palpated, and the pouch is dissected away from the cervical esophagus up as far as the pharyngoesophageal junction. The flexible endoscope is then removed from the pouch and

advanced into the thoracic esophagus so that it can be used as a stent for the cricopharyngeal myotomy. Dissection of the pharyngeal pouch is then completed.

Step 2: Myotomy

The esophageal myotomy is started approximately 3 cm below the cricopharyngeus muscle on the posterolateral esophageal wall [*see Figure 3a*]. The esophageal muscle is divided down to the mucosa, which is recognizable from its bluish coloration with the submucosal plexus overlying it. The esophageal muscle is dissected away from the mucosa with a right-angle dissector and divided with a low-intensity diathermy unit. The myotomy is then continued proximally through the cricopharyngeus muscle and up into the muscular wall of the hypopharynx for 2 cm if there is no diverticulum present. The hypopharynx is distinguished by a pronounced submucosal venous plexus. The muscle is then swept off the mucosa for 120°.

Step 3: Freeing or Excision of Diverticulum

If there is a diverticulum less than 2 cm in diameter, the cricopharyngeus is transected and the muscularis around the diverticulum is freed. The myotomy is extended onto the hypopharynx for 2 cm. The diverticulum may be suspended to the back wall of the pharynx. It should not be sutured to the prevertebral fascia, because the passage of sutures through the diverticulum can contaminate the fascia, leading to an increased risk of fascial infection.

If the diverticulum is more than 2 cm in diameter, it is excised with a linear stapler, which is placed at the base of the sac and pressed firmly against the esophagoscope [*see Figure 3b*]. Particular care must be taken at this point so as not to injure the recurrent laryngeal nerve. The stapler is fired, and the divertic-

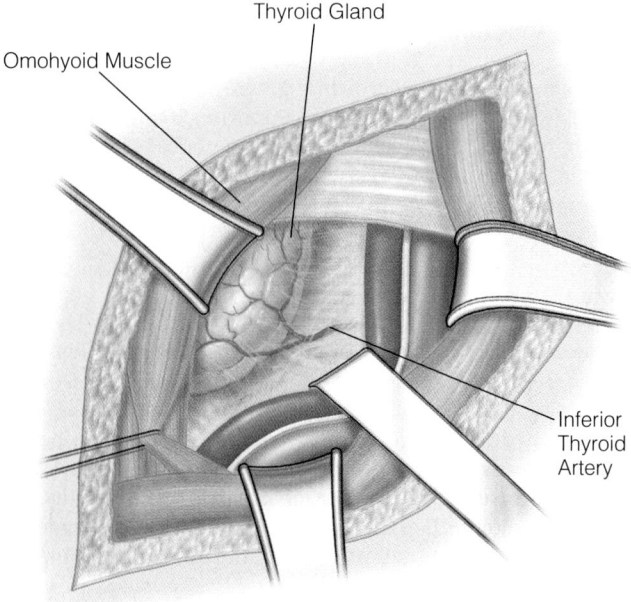

Thyroid Gland

Omohyoid Muscle

Inferior Thyroid Artery

Figure 2 **Cricopharyngeal myotomy and excision of Zenker's diverticulum. The sternocleidomastoid is incised along the anterior border so as to expose the omohyoid muscle and the sternohyoid and sternothyroid muscles, which are retracted. The thyroid gland and the trachea are retracted medially by the assistant's finger, and the inferior thyroid artery is ligated and divided laterally to avoid injury to the recurrent laryngeal nerve.**

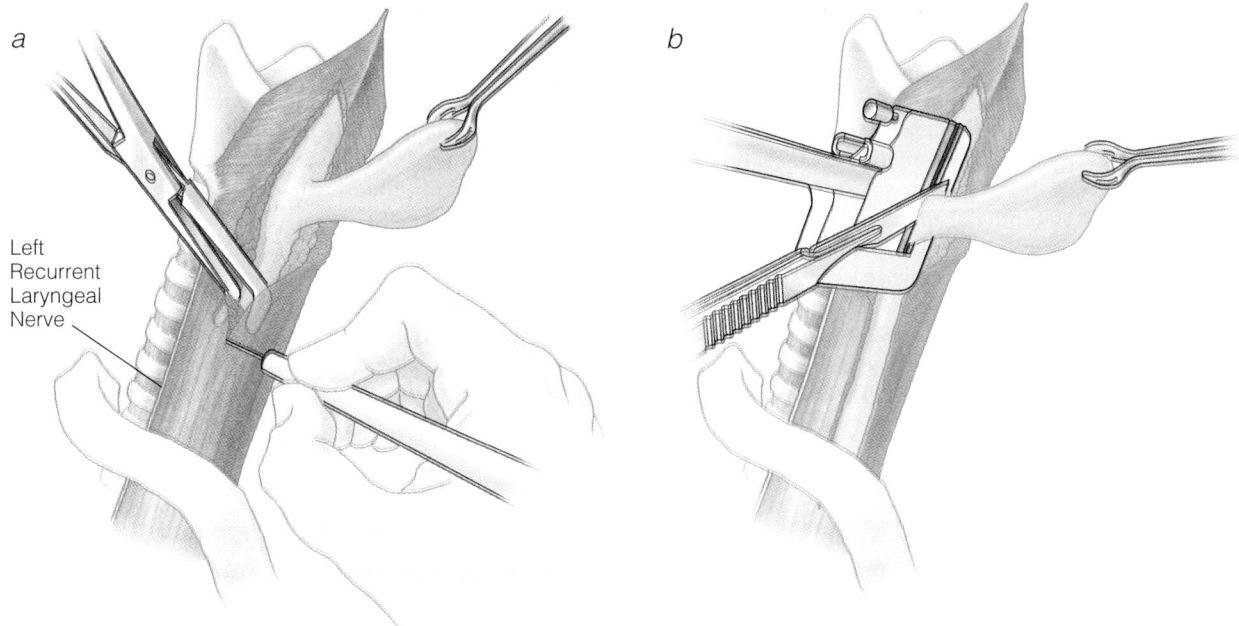

Figure 3 Cricopharyngeal myotomy and excision of Zenker's diverticulum. (*a*) The diverticulum is dissected away from the esophagus, and an esophageal myotomy is started approximately 3 cm below the cricopharyngeus muscle. The myotomy is continued proximally through the cricopharyngeus, and the muscle around the diverticulum is freed. (*b*) A linear stapler is placed at the base of the sac and pressed firmly against the esophagoscope. The stapler is fired, and the diverticulum is excised.

ulum is excised. The staple line is cleaned with an antiseptic solution, and the incision is filled with saline. The esophagus is insufflated with air to determine whether mucosal leakage has occurred, and the esophagoscope is removed; any mucosal leaks found are closed with fine absorbable sutures. In the absence of a stapler, the best way of excising the sac is to make a series of short incisions through the neck of the sac with scissors, suturing the edges after each cut with absorbable monofilament sutures (the so-called cut-and-sew technique). The esophagoscope ensures that the esophageal lumen is not narrowed.

Step 4: Drainage and Closure

Once hemostasis has been achieved, a short vacuum drain is placed through the skin into the retroesophageal space. The platysma is repaired with absorbable sutures, and the skin is closed with a subcuticular absorbable suture. Nasogastric intubation is unnecessary. Prokinetic agents and proton pump inhibitors are administered to prevent gastroesophageal reflux. A water-soluble contrast study is done on the day of the operation. If the results are normal, the patient is started on a liquid diet, and the drain is removed on postoperative day 1, when the patient is discharged.

COMPLICATIONS

The main complications associated with cricopharyngeal myotomy are recurrent laryngeal nerve trauma (0.5%), hematoma formation, infection (2%), aspiration, and recurrence (4%). Hematomas and infections must be drained promptly. Fistulas usually close once the prevertebral space is drained and the associated infection controlled. Aspiration is the most serious complication after cricopharyngeal myotomy. Gastroesophageal reflux may contribute to oropharyngeal dysphagia. Division of the upper esophageal sphincter in a patient with an incompetent esophagogastric junction may lead to massive tracheobronchial

aspiration. Therefore, documented gastroesophageal reflux, gastroesophageal regurgitation, and severe distal esophagitis may be relative contraindications to cricopharyngeal myotomy until the lower esophageal sphincter defect has been remedied with an antireflux operation.

OUTCOME EVALUATION

Of patients with a Zenker's diverticulum, at least 90% experience excellent results from surgical treatment. Of patients without a Zenker's diverticulum, one third experience excellent results, another third show moderate improvement, and the remaining third show no improvement.[1] Patients with poor pharyngeal contractility in conjunction with normal upper esophageal sphincter function show little improvement with cricopharyngeal myotomy. Patients with oropharyngeal dysphagia secondary to neurologic involvement who have intact voluntary deglutination, adequate pulsion of the tongue, and normal phonation may show improvement with cricopharyngeal myotomy. Appropriate selection of patients for cricopharyngeal myotomy leads to better surgical outcomes.

Transthoracic Hiatal Hernia Repair

Unlike most operations on the esophagus, which are extirpative procedures, hiatal hernia repair with fundoplication is a reconstructive procedure. Currently, this repair is often accomplished via minimally invasive approaches; however, such approaches may be hampered by significant perceptual and motor limitations, such as loss of stereosis, reduced tactile feedback, and decreased range of motion for the instruments. In certain patients, laparoscopic reconstruction of a competent gastroesophageal high-pressure zone may be very difficult and may demand a degree of tactile sensitivity that is not yet achievable via videoendoscopy.

The long-term success of antireflux surgery, whether done transthoracically or laparoscopically, depends on three factors: (1) a tension-free repair that maintains a 4 cm long segment of esophagus in the intra-abdominal position, (2) durable approximation of the diaphragmatic crura, and (3) correct matching of the fundoplication technique chosen to the peristaltic function of the esophagus. The transthoracic approach should be considered whenever the standard abdominal approaches carry an increased risk of failure or complication—for instance, in patients who have a foreshortened esophagus, peptic strictures of the esophagus, an associated esophageal motility disorder, or a massive hiatal hernia with the stomach elevated into the chest; those who are morbidly obese; and those who have undergone multiple previous abdominal operations or in whom earlier antireflux procedures have failed.

PREOPERATIVE EVALUATION

Symptomatic Evaluation

All patients being considered for fundoplication to treat GERD must undergo a comprehensive evaluation to determine whether there is indeed an anatomic substrate for their symptoms and what the most appropriate form of repair is. Specifically, a history of heartburn and effortless regurgitation should be sought. Dysphagia and odynophagia are not typical and may reflect the presence of a stricture or a neoplasm. Atypical pain from cholelithiasis, peptic ulcer, or coronary artery disease may also confound the diagnosis.

Imaging

Radiographic investigation should begin with a ciné barium swallow, which may yield valuable information regarding the length of the esophagus, its peristaltic function, and the integrity of the mucosal surface. The gastric views can be used for qualitative assessment of emptying. Next, esophagogastroscopy should be performed to examine the mucosa for the presence of esophagitis, Barrett's mucosa, stricture, or malignancy. The locations of any lesions observed, along with the position of the squamocolumnar junction, should be carefully documented in terms of distance from the incisors. All strictures must undergo brush biopsy to rule out an occult malignancy. The presence of severe esophagitis raises the possibility of acquired shortening of the esophagus secondary to transmural inflammation and contraction scarring. Every effort should be made to measure the length of the esophagus accurately.

Dilatation

If a stricture is found during esophagoscopy, a decision must be made about whether to attempt esophageal dilatation. This procedure carries substantial risk and should only be done after careful consideration. If the stricture is diagnosed at the time of the initial endoscopic examination, it is advisable to perform only the brush biopsy at this point, deferring dilatation to a subsequent visit. Delaying dilatation gives the surgeon time to reassess the anatomy depicted on the barium swallow, to decide whether wire-guided or blind dilatation is indicated, to obtain informed consent, to assemble the requisite equipment, and to plan sedation for what is often an uncomfortable procedure.

The standard adult esophagoscope is approximately 32 French in caliber. In advancing the scope into the stricture, only very gentle pressure should be necessary. The weight of the dilator alone should be sufficient to effect its passage, with little or no forward force applied. As a rule, a mild stricture that is not associated with steep angulation of the esophagus will readily accept passage of the endoscope and will be amenable to subsequent blind dilation with Hurst-Maloney bougies. After successful passage, the scope is removed, and sequential insertion of progressively larger dilators (starting at 32 French) into the stricture is attempted. Although the patient will be able to swallow comfortably only after satisfactory passage of a dilator at least 48 French in caliber, it is essential never to try to force passage. To this end, the surgeon must take careful note of the subtle signs of increasing resistance transmitted through the dilator. Sequential dilation should be stopped whenever significant resistance is encountered or blood streaks appear on the dilator. Sudden pain during dilatation is an ominous sign that calls for immediate investigation with a water-soluble contrast swallow study. Perforation must be definitively ruled out before the patient can be discharged.

Highly stenotic strictures that do not allow the passage of a standard adult endoscope may be associated with a distorted and a steeply angulated esophagus. In such cases, the use of a pediatric endoscope may permit directed placement of a guide wire through the stricture; fluoroscopy is a useful adjunct for this purpose. A series of progressively larger Savary-Gillard dilators may then be passed over the guide wire to enlarge the lumen and allow subsequent endoscopic biopsy. The caveats that apply to blind dilation also apply to wire-guided dilation.

Patients whose esophagus can be dilated to 48 French and who are candidates for antireflux surgery may undergo subsequent intraoperative dilation to 54 to 60 French. Patients who cannot be dilated to 48 French and fail to achieve comfortable swallowing should be classified as having a nondilatable stricture and should be considered for transhiatal esophagectomy [*see* Resection of Esophagus and Proximal Stomach, *below*].

Functional Evaluation

Esophageal manometry permits quantitative assessment of peristalsis, a capability that is critically important for determining which type of fundoplication is most suitable for reconstructing a nonoccluding high-pressure zone at the esophagogastric junction. Stationary pH tests measure the capacity of the esophagus to clear acid, its sensitivity to instilled acid, the relationship of reflux episodes to body position, and the correlation between changes in esophageal pH and the subjective symptoms of heartburn. Ambulatory 24-hour pH testing allows further quantification of reflux episodes with respect to duration, frequency, and association with patient symptoms.

OPERATIVE PLANNING

Either a partial fundoplication (as in the 240° Belsey Mark IV procedure) or a complete fundoplication (as in the 360° Nissen procedure) may be performed. The extent of the wrap aside, the two procedures are essentially identical. Acquired shortening of the esophagus may necessitate lengthening of the esophagus by means of a Collis gastroplasty, in which the portion of the gastric cardia along the lesser curvature and directly contiguous to the distal esophagus is fashioned into a tube [*see* Operative Technique, Step 6a, *below*].

A thoracic epidural catheter is placed for regional analgesia. General anesthesia is administered, and flexible esophagoscopy is performed by the operating team. Insufflation should be done with the minimum amount of air practical, particularly in the case of large paraesophageal hernias. The extent of the pathologic condition is documented and the absence of malignancy verified. The stomach is decompressed and the endoscope removed. Tracheal intubation is then performed with either a standard single-lumen endotracheal tube or a double-lumen tube. The former requires that the ventilated left lung be retracted cephalad with moist packs during the procedure; the latter allows lung isolation and is preferred by some surgeons. A Foley catheter is placed; central venous access and arterial lines are generally not required. Subcutaneous heparin is administered for prophylaxis against deep vein thrombosis (DVT), and pneumatic calf compression devices are applied. Antibiotic prophylaxis is provided [*see 1:2 Prevention of Postoperative Infection*].

The patient is positioned for a left thoracotomy. The table is flexed to distract the ribs. An axillary roll is placed to protect the right brachial plexus. The right leg is bent at hip and knee while the left leg is kept straight. Pillows are placed between the legs, and all pressure points are padded. The arms are positioned so that the humeri are at right angles to the chest and the elbows bent 90°.

OPERATIVE TECHNIQUE

Step 1: Incision and Entry into Chest

A standard left posterolateral thoracotomy is performed. The latissimus dorsi muscle is divided. The serratus fascia is incised, but the muscle itself can generally be preserved. The paraspinal muscles are elevated away from the posterior aspect of the ribs, and a 1 cm segment of the seventh rib is resected to facilitate exposure. The chest is entered through the sixth interspace, and the lung and the pleural space are thoroughly inspected. The leaves of the retractor are spread slowly over a period of several minutes so as not to cause iatrogenic rib fractures.

Step 2: Exposure and Mobilization of Esophagus and Vagi

The inferior pulmonary ligament is divided with the electrocautery to the level of the inferior pulmonary vein [*see Figure 4*]. The mediastinal pleura overlying the esophagus is incised to expose the esophagus from the level of the carina to the diaphragm. Particular care is taken to avoid injury to the vagi. Vessels supplying the esophagus and arising from the adjacent aorta are ligated and divided. The esophagus is encircled just below the inferior pulmonary vein with a Penrose drain [*see Figure 4*]. The two vagi are mobilized and carried with the esophagus. (The right vagus is located along the right anterior border of the descending aorta and can easily be missed.)

The esophagus is then elevated, and mobilization is circumferentially completed in the direction of the diaphragm. The right pleura is closely approximated to the esophagus for 2 to 5 cm above the diaphragm; in the presence of a substantial hiatal hernia and its sac, it may be difficult to identify. The right pleura should be dissected away from the esophagus without entry into the right chest. If a tear occurs, it should be closed with absorbable suture material to prevent accumulation of blood and fluid on the right side during the operation. Dissection is continued to expose the right and left crura.

Step 3: Division of Phrenoesophageal Membrane and Gastrohepatic Ligament

The esophagus is retracted anteriorly to expose the posteriorly located phrenoesophageal membrane, which is then divided to yield entry into the peritoneum and exposure of the lesser sac. The remainder of the phrenoesophageal membrane is elevated with a right-angle clamp as it courses anteriorly, yielding a view of the spleen below. The esophagus is then mobilized from the left crus. The esophageal branch of the left phrenic artery, visible near the left vagus, is divided near the crus. Dissection proceeds

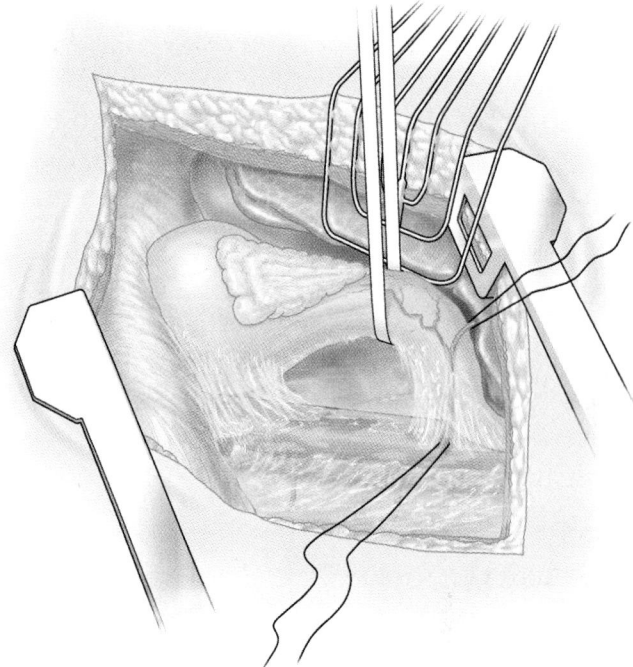

Figure 4 **Transthoracic hiatal hernia repair. The lung is retracted, and the inferior pulmonary ligament is divided to the level of the inferior pulmonary vein. The mediastinal pleura overlying the esophagus is incised to expose the esophagus from the level of the carina to the diaphragm. The esophagus and both vagi are encircled just below the inferior pulmonary vein with a Penrose drain. Vessels supplying the esophagus and arising from the adjacent aorta are ligated and divided.**

anteriorly until the distal end of the right crus is encountered at the apex of the hiatus; the right crus is then exposed posteriorly.

The uppermost portion of the gastrohepatic ligament is divided with the electrocautery. Belsey's artery, a communicating branch between the left gastric artery and the inferior phrenic artery, lies in this area and generally must be directly ligated. It is vital to divide the gastrohepatic ligament down to the level of the left gastric artery. The caudate lobe of the liver must be clearly visible. This opening is essential for subsequent passage of the fundoplication wrap behind the esophagus.

Step 4: Completion of Hiatal Dissection, Excision of Hernia Sac, and Ligation of Short Gastric Vessels

Dissection of the hiatus is completed along the right crus to the apex of the hiatus, thus joining the line of incision. Any hernia sac found is then excised. The highest short gastric arteries are ligated between ties to permit mobilization of the fundus. Excessive traction must be avoided to prevent splenic injury. Three or four vessels are usually divided. The esophagogastric junction is then elevated into the chest.

Step 5: Closure of Crura

Because the right crus is often quite attenuated, it is crucial to incorporate an adequate amount of tissue into the repair. An Allis clamp is placed at the apex of the hiatus and into the central tendon so that the crura can be placed under tension. The esophagus is retracted anteriorly, and a No. 1 silk suture is passed through the most posterior aspect of the right crus, with care taken to avoid the adjacent inferior vena cava [*see Figure 5*]. A notched spoon retractor is placed through the hiatus and into

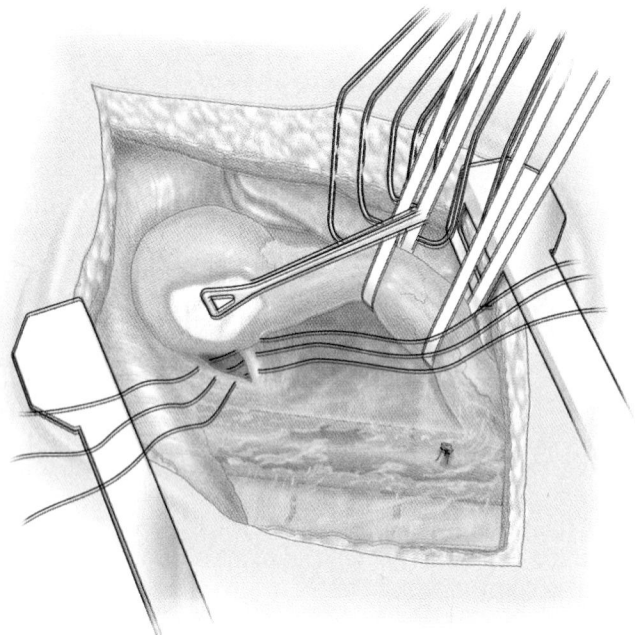

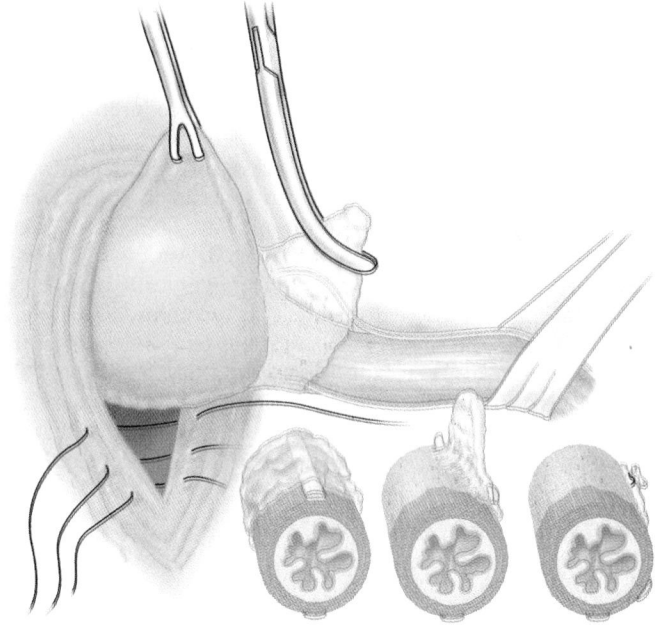

Figure 5   **Transthoracic hiatal hernia repair. The esophagogastric junction is mobilized by dividing the phrenoesophageal ligament and some short gastric vessels. No. 1 silk sutures are passed through the exterior aspect of the right crus (with care taken to avoid the adjacent inferior vena cava) and through the left crus (with care taken to avoid the spleen).**

Figure 6   **Transthoracic hiatal hernia repair. The anterior fat pad is removed from the esophagus with sharp dissection, with care taken to avoid injury to the vagi.**

the abdomen behind the left crus. The spleen is thus protected while the suture is brought through the left crus. Three or four crural repair stitches are then placed at 1 cm intervals, from posterior to anterior. The sutures are held together with hemostats but left untied for the time being. Placement of traction on the last suture should close the defect while still allowing easy passage of one finger along the esophagus. The final decision on whether to tie this last suture or cut it out is made later, after construction of the fundoplication.

Step 6: Assessment of Esophageal Length and Removal of Anterior Fat Pad

After placement of the crural stitches, an assessment of the esophageal length is made. Ideally, the stomach can easily be reduced into the abdomen without placing tension on the thoracic esophagus. When esophageal foreshortening is found, a Collis gastroplasty is performed [*see* Step 6a, *below*].

If an esophageal stricture is present, the assistant performs dilatation by passing a tapered bougie per os while the surgeon supports the esophagus. The anterior fat pad is removed via sharp dissection so as not to injure the vagi located on either side [*see Figure 6*].

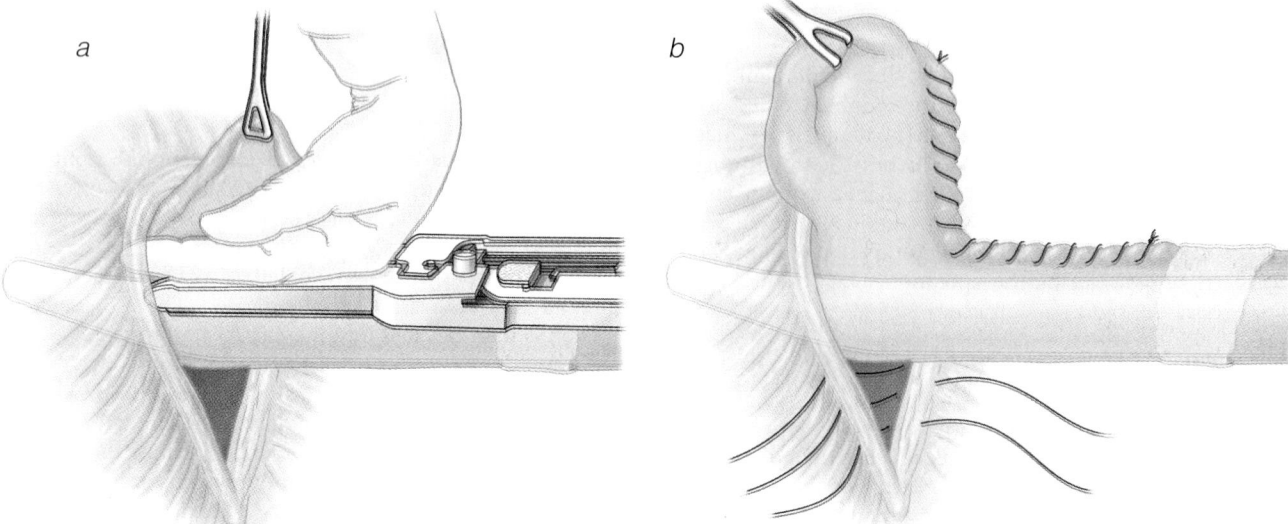

Figure 7   **Transthoracic hiatal hernia repair. (*a*) If esophageal foreshortening is present, a Collis gastroplasty is performed. A 54 French Maloney bougie is inserted through the esophagogastric junction. A 4 to 5 cm neoesophagus is formed with a 60 mm GIA stapler loaded with 3.5 mm staples. (*b*) Both the fundal staple line and the lesser curvature staple line are oversewn with nonabsorbable monofilament suture.**

Step 6a: Collis Gastroplasty

In a Collis gastroplasty for a short esophagus, a stapler is used to form a 4 to 5 cm neoesophagus out of the proximal stomach, thereby effectively lengthening the esophagus and transposing the esophagogastric junction more distally. A large-caliber Maloney bougie (54 French for women, 56 French for men) is placed in the esophagus to prevent narrowing of the lumen. The bougie is advanced well into the stomach, so that its widest portion rests at the esophagogastric junction. The bougie is held against the lesser curvature, and the fundus is retracted away at a right angle to the esophagus. A 60 mm gastrointestinal anastomosis (GIA) stapler loaded with 3.5 mm staples is applied immediately alongside the bougie on the greater curvature side [see Figure 7a] and fired, simultaneously cutting and stapling the cardia. The staple line is oversewn with nonabsorbable monofilament suture material on both sides [see Figure 7b]. Two metal clips are placed to mark the distal extent of the gastroplasty tube, denoting the new esophagogastric junction.

Step 7: Fundoplication and Reduction of Wrap into Abdomen

The fundus is passed posteriorly behind the esophagus and brought up against the anterior stomach, with care taken to avoid torsion of the fundal wrap. The fundus is then wrapped either over the lower 2 cm of the esophagus, if no gastroplasty was done, or over 2 cm of the length of the gastroplasty tube while the bougie is in place. The seromuscular layer of the fundus is approximated to that of the esophagus or the gastroplasty tube and that of the adjacent anterior stomach with interrupted 2-0 silk sutures [see Figure 8]. When tied, the wrap should still be loose enough to accommodate a finger alongside the esophagus. The fundoplication sutures are again oversewn with a continuous seromuscular nonabsorbable monofilament suture. Two clips are placed at the superior aspect of the wrap. These, along with the previously placed clips, will help confirm both the length and the location of the wrap on chest x-ray.

Once the fundoplication is complete, the wrap is reduced into the abdomen. Two mattress sutures of 2-0 silk are placed to secure the top of the fundoplication to the underside of the diaphragm. The crural sutures are then sequentially tied, from the most posterior one to the most anterior. When the final suture is tied, one finger should still be able to pass through the hiatus alongside the esophagus. The dilator is then removed and the mattress sutures tied.

Step 8: Drainage and Closure

A nasogastric tube is passed into the stomach and secured. Hemostasis is verified, and a single thoracostomy tube is placed. The wound is closed in layers. A chest x-ray is performed to verify the position of the tubes and the location of the clips marking the wrap. The patient is then extubated in the OR and transported to the recovery area.

POSTOPERATIVE CARE

Patients typically remain in the hospital for 5 days. The nasogastric tube is left on low suction and removed on postoperative day 3. Patients then begin liquid oral intake, advancing to a full fluid diet as tolerated. Early ambulation is encouraged to prevent respiratory complications. Judicious use of analgesics and antiemetics minimizes nausea and vomiting. The thoracostomy tube is removed as drainage subsides. A barium swallow is performed on postoperative day 5 to verify the position of the wrap, to ensure that no significant obstruction has developed, and to provide a qualitative impression of gastric emptying.

Once patients can tolerate a soft solid diet, they are generally discharged home with instructions about the gradual resumption of a normal diet at home. Large meals and carbonated beverages must be avoided in the early postoperative period.

COMPLICATIONS

The root causes of the complications arising after transthoracic hiatal hernia repair are often technical; thus, the best prevention, in most cases, is meticulous surgical technique. Mobilization of the stomach with ligation of short gastric vessels may result in injury to the spleen. Injury to the vagi predisposes to gastric dysfunction, early satiety, and so-called gas-bloat syndrome. Poor crural approximation increases the chances that the repair will fail. Dehiscence allows upward migration of the wrap into the chest or the development of a paraesophageal hernia. The gastroplasty may leak at the staple line. Overzealous dissection along the lesser curvature can devascularize the cardia and cause ischemic stenosis of the gastroplasty tube. Torsion of the fundus results in perforation and sepsis. Excessive distraction of the ribs can lead to pain, atelectasis, or pneumonia. Inadequate mobilization of the fundus may place excessive tension on the wrap and promote later disruption and recurrent reflux. A so-called slipped Nissen—in which the wrap is inadequately fixed to the esophagus or the gastroplasty tube, and the stomach telescopes through the intact fundoplication and assumes an hourglass configuration—results in heartburn, regurgitation, and dysphagia to varying degrees. A wrap that is too tight or too long results in persistent dysphagia.

Recurrent heartburn and regurgitation call for evaluation with contrast studies and esophagoscopy. If there is an anatomic condition that is responsible for disruption of the fundoplication or failure of the crural repair, reoperation is usually necessary; in such cases, maximal medical treatment for symptoms of reflux has invariably failed already. Dysphagia that is not related to recurrent reflux or ulceration usually responds to dilatation and does not necessitate reoperation.

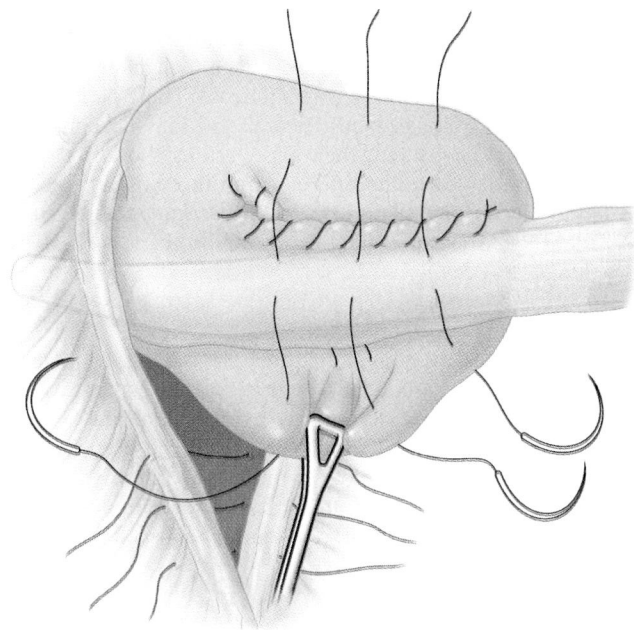

Figure 8 **Transthoracic hiatal hernia repair. The fundus is passed behind the esophagus and sewn to the neoesophagus and the anterior stomach over a 2 cm length with interrupted 2.0 silk sutures.**

Transthoracic hiatal hernia repair yields good to excellent results in more than 85% of patients undergoing a primary repair. Approximately 75% of patients who have previously undergone hiatal hernia repair experience symptomatic improvement.[2]

Resection of Esophagus and Proximal Stomach

In the remainder of the chapter, we describe the standard open techniques for resection of the esophagus and the esophagogastric junction. Transhiatal esophagectomy is commonly performed to treat end-stage benign esophageal disease and carcinomas of the cardia and the lower esophagus. Esophageal resection through a combined laparotomy–right thoracotomy approach is ideal for cancers of the middle and upper esophagus. The gastric conduit may be anastomosed to the cervical esophagus either high in the right chest (as in an Ivor-Lewis esophagectomy) or in the neck (as in a transhiatal esophagectomy). The left thoracoabdominal approach is indicated for resection of the distal esophagus and the proximal stomach when removal of the stomach necessitates the use of an intestinal substitute to restore swallowing.

PREOPERATIVE EVALUATION

Thorough preoperative preparation is essential for good postoperative outcome. Smoking cessation and a graded regimen of home exercise will help minimize postoperative complications and encourage early mobilization. Schematic diagrams have proved useful for educating patients and shaping their expectations about quality of life and ability to swallow after esophagectomy. Illustrations, by emphasizing the anatomic relations, greatly facilitate discussion of potential complications (e.g., hoarseness from recurrent laryngeal nerve injury, pneumothorax, anastomotic leakage, mediastinal bleeding, and splenic injury).

Potential postoperative problems (e.g., reflux, regurgitation, early satiety, dumping, and dysphagia) must be discussed before operation. Such discussion is particularly relevant for patients undergoing esophagectomy for early-stage malignant tumors or for high-grade dysplasia in Barrett's mucosa. These patients generally have no esophageal obstruction and may be completely asymptomatic; accordingly, their expectations about postoperative function may be quite different from those of patients with profound dysphagia secondary to near-complete esophageal occlusion. Realistic expectations improve the chances of satisfactory outcome.

Evaluation of Operative Risk

Preoperative assessment should include a thorough review of the patient's cardiopulmonary reserve and an estimate of the level of operative risk. Spirometry, arterial blood gas analysis, and exercise stress testing should be considered. Patients must be able to tolerate a thoracotomy and a laparotomy. Thoracic epidural analgesia should be administered for pain control, and a double-lumen endotracheal tube should be placed for separate lung ventilation.

Imaging

Contrast esophagography, esophagoscopy with biopsy, and contrast-enhanced CT of the chest and the upper abdomen are required before esophagectomy. The esophagogram identifies the location of the tumor and may indicate whether it extends into the proximal stomach. Esophagoscopy allows direct assessment of the mucosa, precise localization of the tumor, and collection of tissue for histologic study. Retroflexion views of the stomach, after distention with air, are particularly important if proximal gastric invasion is suspected, in which case esophagogastrectomy with reconstruction of alimentary continuity by means of intestinal interposition may be required. Thoracic and abdominal CT scans yield information on the extent of any celiac or mediastinal adenopathy, the degree of esophageal thickening, and the possibility of invasion of the adjacent aorta or tracheobronchial tree. The lung parenchyma is assessed for metastatic nodules, as are the liver and the adrenal glands. Suspicious areas may be further assessed by means of either PET scanning or needle biopsy. Invasion of mediastinal structures and distant metastases are contraindications to transhiatal esophagectomy.

Endoscopic ultrasonography, though quite sensitive for detection of paraesophageal adenopathy, is currently incapable of differentiating reactive lymph nodes from nodes invaded by malignancy.

Chemoradiation Therapy

Patients with esophageal cancer who are candidates for resection may benefit from neoadjuvant chemotherapy and concurrent radiation therapy. In particular, patients with good performance status and bulky disease should be considered for such therapy. There are, as yet, no randomized trials that conclusively demonstrate a survival benefit with this approach, but several series have documented a 20% to 30% rate of complete response with no viable tumor found at the time of resection. After chemoradiation, patients are restaged with a barium swallow and CT. If no contraindications to surgical treatment are noted, resection is scheduled 2 weeks later. Previous chemoradiation does not make transhiatal esophagectomy significantly more difficult or complicated. In centers with experience in this approach, the rates of bleeding and anastomotic leakage remain low.

OPERATIVE PLANNING

Transhiatal Esophagectomy

In transhiatal esophagectomy, the stomach is mobilized through a short upper midline laparotomy, the esophagus is mobilized from adjacent mediastinal structures via dissection through the hiatus without the use of a thoracotomy, and the stomach is transposed through the posterior mediastinum and anastomosed to the cervical esophagus at the level of the clavicles. The main advantages of this approach are (1) a proximal surgical margin that is well away from the tumor site, (2) an extrathoracic esophagogastric anastomosis that is easily accessible in the event of complications, and (3) reduced overall operative trauma. Single-center studies throughout the world have shown transhiatal esophagectomy to be safe and well tolerated, even in patients who may have significantly reduced cardiopulmonary reserve. Long-term survival is equivalent to that reported after transthoracic esophagectomy.

Although transhiatal esophagectomy has been used for resection of tumors at any location in the esophagus, it is best suited for resection of tumors in the lower esophagus and at the esophagogastric junction. It should also be considered the operation of choice for certain advanced nonmalignant conditions of the esophagus. Nondilatable strictures of the esophagus may occur as an end-stage complication of gastroesophageal reflux.

Intractable reflux after failed hiatal hernia repair may not be amenable to further attempts at reconstruction of the esophagogastric junction and thus may call for esophagectomy. Because of the high cervical anastomosis, a transhiatal esophagectomy is less likely to predispose to postoperative reflux and recurrent stricture formation than a transthoracic esophagectomy would be. Achalasia may result in megaesophagus and dysphagia that cannot be managed without removal of the esophagus. Transhiatal esophagectomy permits complete removal of the thoracic esophagus and, in the majority of patients, restoration of comfortable swallowing without the need for a thoracotomy.

Generally, patients are admitted to the hospital on the day of the operation. Thoracic epidural analgesia is administered, both intraoperatively and postoperatively, and appropriate antibiotic prophylaxis is provided [see 1:2 Prevention of Postoperative Infection]. Heparin, 5,000 U subcutaneously, is given before induction, and pneumatic calf compression devices are applied. A radial artery catheter is placed to permit continuous monitoring of blood pressure. Central venous access is rarely required. General anesthesia is administered via an uncut single-lumen endotracheal tube. Flexible esophagoscopy is performed by the surgical team. A nasogastric tube is placed before final positioning and draping.

The patient is placed in the supine position with a small rolled sheet between the shoulders. The arms are secured to the sides, and the head is rotated to the right with the neck extended. The neck, the chest, and the abdomen are prepared as a single sterile field. The drapes are placed so as to expose the patient from the left ear to the pubis. The operative field is extended laterally to the anterior axillary lines to permit placement of thoracostomy tubes as needed. A self-retaining table-mounted retractor is used to facilitate upward and lateral traction along the costal margin.

Ivor-Lewis Esophagectomy

At many institutions, Ivor-Lewis esophagectomy is preferred because of the excellent direct exposure it affords for dissection of the intrathoracic esophagus. This procedure should be considered when there is concern regarding the extent of esophageal fixation within the mediastinum. An extensive local lymphadenectomy is easily performed through a right thoracotomy. Whether any regional lymph node dissection is necessary is highly controversial; no significant survival advantage has yet been demonstrated. Long-term survival after Ivor-Lewis resection is equivalent to that after transhiatal esophagectomy.[3]

The main disadvantages of the Ivor-Lewis procedure are (1) the physiologic impact of the two major access incisions employed (a right thoracotomy and a midline laparotomy) and (2) the location of the anastomosis (in the chest, at the level of the azygos vein). Incision-related pain may hinder deep breathing and the clearing of bronchial secretions, resulting in atelectasis and pneumonia. Complications of the intrathoracic anastomosis may be hard to manage. If the anastomosis leaks, drainage will be difficult, empyema may result, and reoperation may prove necessary.

Left Thoracoabdominal Esophagogastrectomy

The left thoracoabdominal approach is indicated for resection of the distal esophagus and the proximal stomach when removal of the stomach necessitates the use of an intestinal substitute to restore swallowing. If the proximal stomach must be resected for adequate resection margins to be obtained, then the distal stomach may be anastomosed to the esophagus in the chest. This operation is frequently associated with significant esophagitis

from bile reflux. Consequently, many surgeons prefer to resect the entire stomach and the distal esophagus and then to restore swallowing with a Roux-en-Y jejunal interposition anastomosed to the residual thoracic esophagus.

OPERATIVE TECHNIQUE

Transhiatal Esophagectomy

Transhiatal esophagectomy is best understood as consisting of three components: abdominal, mediastinal, and cervical. The abdominal portion involves mobilization of the stomach, pyloromyotomy, and a temporary feeding jejunostomy.

Step 1: incision and entry into peritoneum A midline laparotomy is performed from the tip of the xiphoid to the umbilicus. The peritoneum is opened to the left of the midline so that the falciform and the preperitoneal fat may be retracted en bloc to the right. Body wall retractors are placed at 45° angles from the midline to elevate and distract both costal margins. The abdomen is then inspected for metastases.

Step 2: division of gastrohepatic ligament and mobilization of distal esophagus The left lobe of the liver is mobilized by dividing the triangular ligament, then folded to the right and held in this position with a moist laparotomy pad and a deep-bladed self-retaining retractor. Next, the gastrohepatic ligament is divided. Occasionally, there is an aberrant left hepatic artery arising from the left gastric artery [see Figure 9]. The peritoneum over the right crus is incised, and the hiatus is palpated; the extent and mobility of any tumor may then be assessed. The esophagus is encircled with a Penrose drain, and gentle traction is applied to draw the esophagogastric junction upward and to the right.

Step 3: mobilization of duodenum and pyloromyotomy The duodenum is mobilized with a Kocher maneuver. Careful attention to the superior extent of this dissection is critical. Adhesions to either the porta hepatis or the gallbladder must be divided to ensure that the pylorus is sufficiently freed for later migration to the diaphragmatic hiatus.

Gastric drainage is provided by a pyloromyotomy. Two figure-eight traction sutures of 2-0 cardiovascular silk are placed deeply through both the superior and the inferior border of the pylorus; traction is then placed on these sutures to provide both exposure and some degree of hemostasis. The pyloromyotomy is begun 2 to 3 cm on the gastric side of the pylorus. The serosa and the muscle are divided with a needle-tipped electrocautery to expose the submucosa; generally, these layers of the stomach are robust, making the proper plane easy to find. Dissection is extended toward the duodenum with the aid of a fine-tipped right-angle clamp. The duodenal submucosa, recognizable by its fatty deposits and yellow coloration, is exposed for approximately 0.5 cm. The duodenal submucosa is usually much more superficial than expected, and accidental entry into the duodenum often occurs just past the left edge of the circular muscle of the pylorus. Releasing the tension on the traction sutures helps the surgeon visualize the proper depth of dissection. Should entry into the lumen occur, a simple repair using interrupted fine monofilament sutures to close the mucosa is performed. Small metal clips are applied to the knots of the traction sutures before removal of the ends; these clips serve to indicate the level of the pyloromyotomy on subsequent radiographic studies.

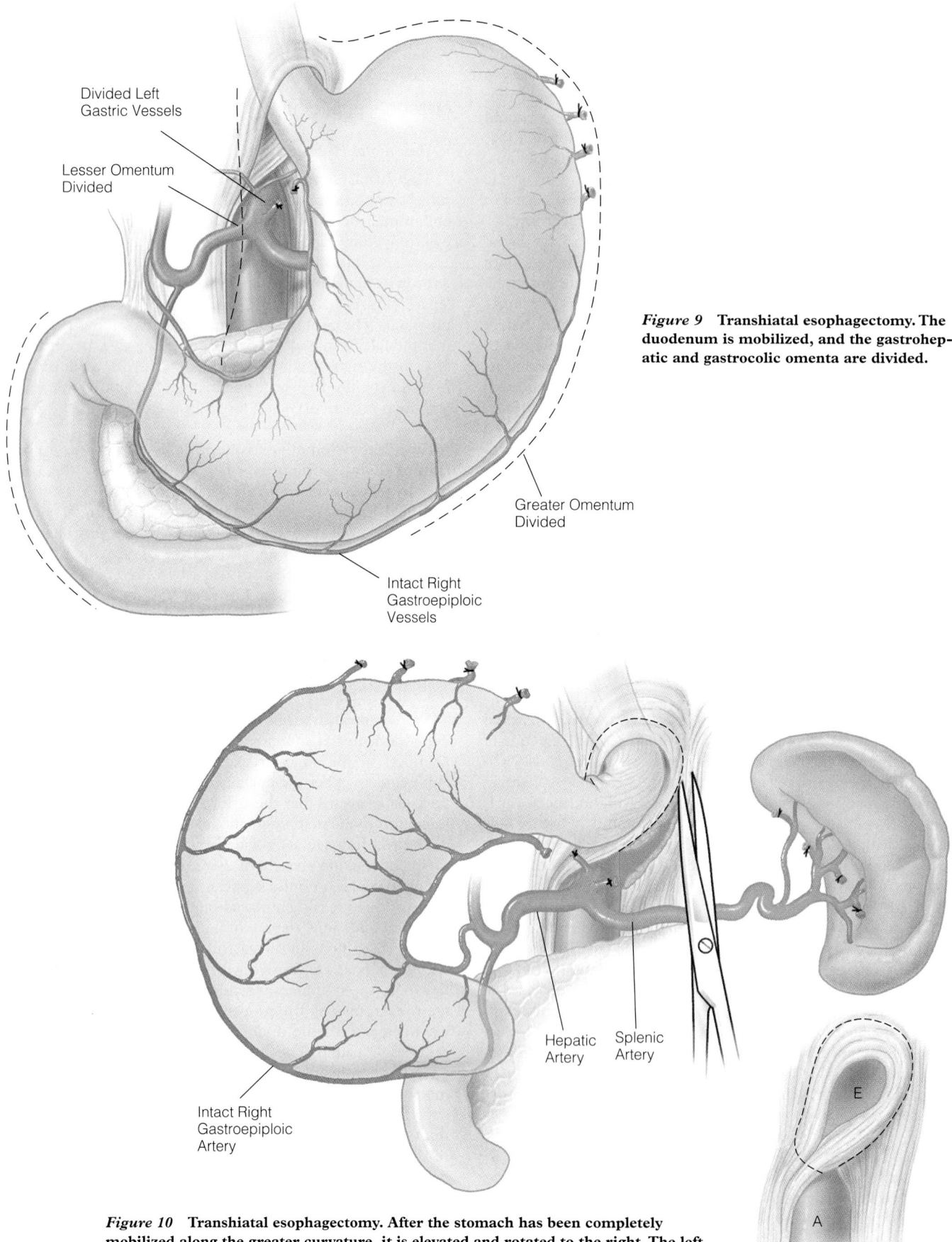

Divided Left
Gastric Vessels

Lesser Omentum
Divided

Figure 9 **Transhiatal esophagectomy. The
duodenum is mobilized, and the gastrohepatic and gastrocolic omenta are divided.**

Greater Omentum
Divided

Intact Right
Gastroepiploic
Vessels

Hepatic
Artery

Splenic
Artery

Intact Right
Gastroepiploic
Artery

E

A

Figure 10 **Transhiatal esophagectomy. After the stomach has been completely
mobilized along the greater curvature, it is elevated and rotated to the right. The left
gastric vessels are suture-ligated and divided. A 1 cm margin of the diaphragmatic
crura is taken in continuity with the esophagogastric junction, providing ample
clearance of the tumor and improved exposure of the lower mediastinum.**

Step 4: mobilization of stomach The greater curvature of the stomach is inspected and the right gastroepiploic artery palpated. The lesser sac is generally entered near the midpoint of the greater curvature. The transition zone between the right gastroepiploic arcade and the short gastric arteries is usually devoid of blood vessels.

Dissection then proceeds along the greater curvature toward the pylorus. The omentum is mobilized from the right gastroepiploic artery. Vessels are ligated between 2-0 silk ties, and great care is exercised to avoid placing excessive traction on the arterial arcade. A 1 cm margin is always maintained between the line of dissection and the right gastroepiploic artery. Venous injuries, in particular, can occur with injudicious handling of tissue. The ultrasonic scalpel is particularly efficient and effective for mobilization of the stomach; again, this instrument must be applied well away from the gastroepiploic arcade. Dissection is continued rightward to the level of the pylorus. It should be noted that the location of the gastroepiploic artery in this area may vary; often, it is at some unexpected distance from the stomach wall. Posterior adhesions between the stomach and the pancreas are lysed so that the lesser sac can be completely opened.

The assistant's left hand is then placed into the lesser sac to retract the stomach gently to the right and place the short gastric vessels on tension. Dissection along the greater curvature proceeds cephalad. The vessels are divided well away from the wall of the stomach to prevent injury to the fundus. Clamps should never be placed on the stomach. A high short gastric artery is typically encountered just adjacent to the left crus. Precise technique is required to prevent injury to the spleen. The previously placed Penrose drain [see Step 2, above] is exposed as the peritoneum is opened over the left crus.

Once the stomach has been completely mobilized along the greater curvature, it is elevated and rotated to the right [see Figure 10]; the left gastric artery and associated nodal tissues can then be visualized via the lesser sac. The superior edge of the pancreas is visible, and the remaining posterior attachments of the stomach are divided along the hiatus and the left crus.

If the operation is being done for malignant disease, a final determination of resectability can be made at this point. Tumor fixation to the aorta or the retroperitoneum can be assessed. Celiac and paraortic lymph nodes can be palpated and, if necessary, sent for biopsy. The left gastric artery and vein are then ligated proximally. All nodal tissue is dissected free in anticipation of subsequent removal en bloc with the specimen.

Step 5: feeding jejunostomy A standard Weitzel jejunostomy completes the abdominal portion of the transhiatal esophagectomy.

Step 6: exposure and encirclement of cervical esophagus The cervical esophagus is exposed through a 6 cm incision along the anterior edge of the left sternocleidomastoid muscle [see Figure 1] that is centered over the level of the cricoid cartilage. The platysma is divided to expose the omohyoid, which is divided at its tendon. The strap muscles are divided low in the neck. The esophagus and its indwelling nasogastric tube can be palpated.

The carotid sheath is retracted laterally, and blunt dissection is employed to reach the prevertebral fascia. The inferior thyroid artery is ligated laterally; the recurrent laryngeal nerve is visible just deep and medial to this vessel. No retractor other than the surgeon's finger should be applied medially: traction injury to

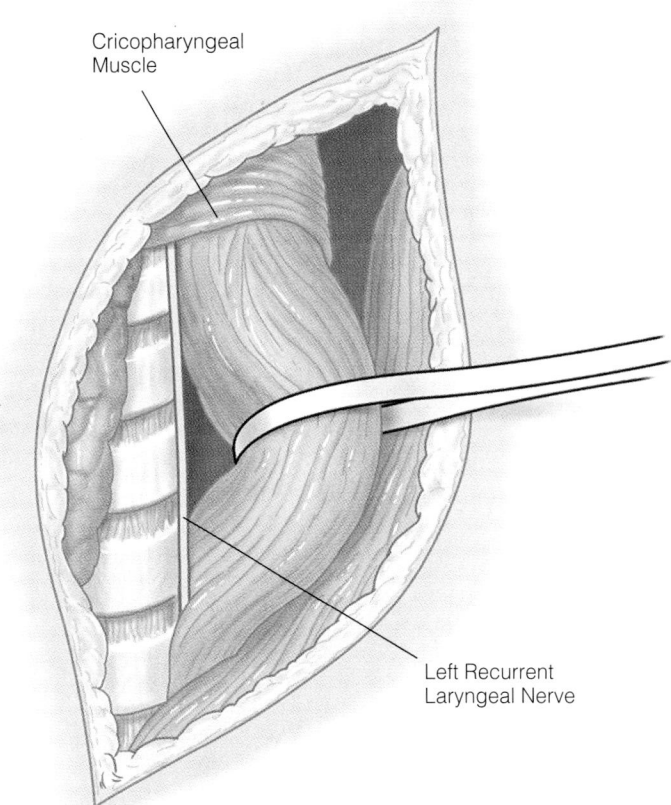

Cricopharyngeal Muscle

Left Recurrent Laryngeal Nerve

Figure 11 **Transhiatal esophagectomy. Once the cervical esophagus is exposed through an incision along the left sternocleidomastoid muscle, strap muscles are divided and retracted, and the cervical esophagus is dissected away from the left and right recurrent laryngeal nerves.**

the recurrent laryngeal nerve will result in both vocal cord palsy and uncoordinated swallowing with aspiration. The tracheoesophageal groove is incised close to the esophageal wall while gentle finger traction is applied cephalad to elevate the thyroid cartilage toward the right. This measure usually suffices to define the location of the nerve.

The esophagus is then encircled by passing a right-angle clamp posteriorly from left to right while the surgeon's finger remains in the tracheoesophageal groove. The tip of the clamp is brought into the pulp of the fingertip. The medially located recurrent laryngeal nerve and the membranous trachea are thereby protected from injury. The clamp is brought around, and a narrow Penrose drain is passed around the esophagus [see Figure 11]. Blunt finger dissection is employed to develop the anterior and posterior planes around the esophagus at the level of the thoracic inlet.

Step 7: mediastinal dissection Three specific maneuvers are now carried out. First, the plane posterior to the esophagus is developed [see Figure 12]. The surgeon's right hand is advanced palm upward into the hiatus, with the fingers closely applied to the esophagus. The volar aspects of the fingers run along the prevertebral fascia, elevating the esophagus off the spine. A moist sponge stick is placed through the cervical incision, also posterior to the esophagus. The sponge is advanced toward the right hand, which is positioned within the mediastinum. As the sponge is advanced into the right palm, the posterior plane is completed. A 28 French mediastinal sump is then passed from the cervical incision into the abdomen along the

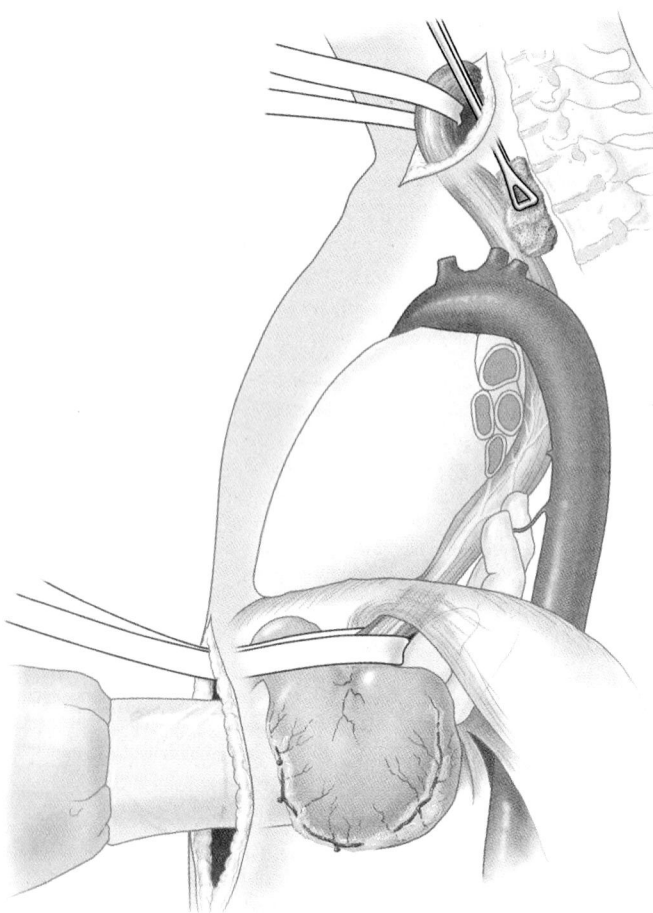

Figure 12 **Transhiatal esophagectomy. The plane posterior to the esophagus is developed by placing the surgeon's right hand into the hiatus along the prevertebral fascia. A moist sponge-stick is placed through the cervical incision posterior to the esophagus, and the posterior plane is completed.**

posterior esophageal wall and attached to suction. Any blood loss from the mediastinum is collected and monitored.

Second, the anterior plane is developed [*see Figure 13*]. This is often much more difficult than developing the posterior plane because the left mainstem bronchus may be quite close to the esophagus. Again, the surgeon's right hand is placed through the hiatus, but it is now palm down and anterior to the esophagus. The fingertips enter the space between the esophagus and the left mainstem bronchus. The hand is gently advanced, and the airway is displaced anteriorly. A blunt curved suction handle is employed from above as a substitute finger. It is advanced along the anterior aspect of the esophagus through the cervical incision. The right hand guides the tip of the suction handle beneath the bronchus. Lateral displacement of the handle allows further mobilization of the bronchus away from the esophagus. Completion of the anterior and posterior planes usually results in a highly mobile esophagus.

Third, the lateral attachments of the esophagus are divided. Upward traction is applied with the previously placed encircling Penrose drain, allowing further dissection at the level of the thoracic inlet. Lateral attachments are pushed caudally into the mediastinum, and traction applied to the esophagus from below allows these attachments to be visualized through the hiatus, then isolated with long right-angle clamps and divided with the electrocautery. Caution must be exercised so as not to injure the

azygos vein. Dissection on the right side must therefore be kept close to the esophagus. Once the last lateral attachment is divided, the esophagus is completely free and can be advanced into the cervical wound.

Step 8: proximal transection of esophagus and delivery into abdomen The nasogastric tube is retracted to the level of the cricopharyngeus muscle, and the esophagus is divided with a cutting stapler 5 to 6 cm distal to the muscle. The esophagus is then removed via the abdomen [*see Figure 14*]. Narrow curved Harrington retractors are placed into the hiatus and used to elevate the pericardium. Caudal traction is placed on the esophagus, allowing excellent visualization of the hiatus and the distal esophagus. Paraesophageal lymph nodes are removed either en bloc or as separate specimens. Dissection is continued cephalad with the electrocautery and a long-handled right-angle clamp. The two vagi are divided, the remaining periesophageal adhesions are lysed, and the esophagus is delivered into the abdomen.

Close monitoring of arterial blood pressure is maintained throughout. Transient hypotension may occur as a result of mediastinal compression and temporary impairment of cardiac venous return. Vasopressors are never required for management: simple repositioning of the retractors or removal of the dissecting hand usually results in prompt restoration of normal BP.

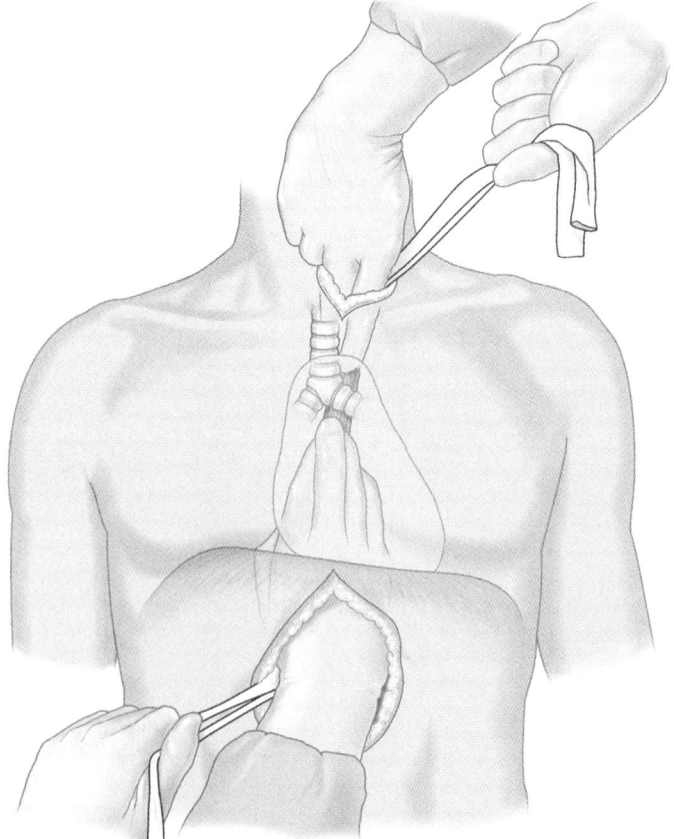

Figure 13 **Transhiatal esophagectomy. The anterior plane is developed by placing the surgeon's right hand through the hiatus anterior to the esophagus. The fingertips enter the space between the esophagus and the left mainstem bronchus, to be met by a blunt suction handle passed downward through the cervical incision. The lateral attachments of the esophagus are divided from above downward as far as the aortic arch.**

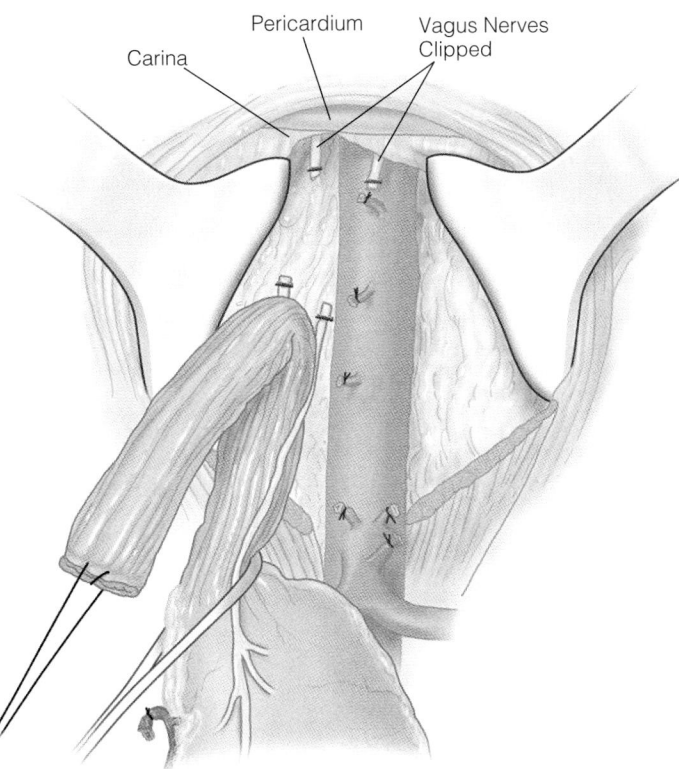

Figure 14 Transhiatal esophagectomy. The esophagus is divided in the neck and delivered into the abdomen. Retractors are placed in the hiatus, and any vessels entering into the esophagus are clipped and divided. The vagi are also clipped and divided.

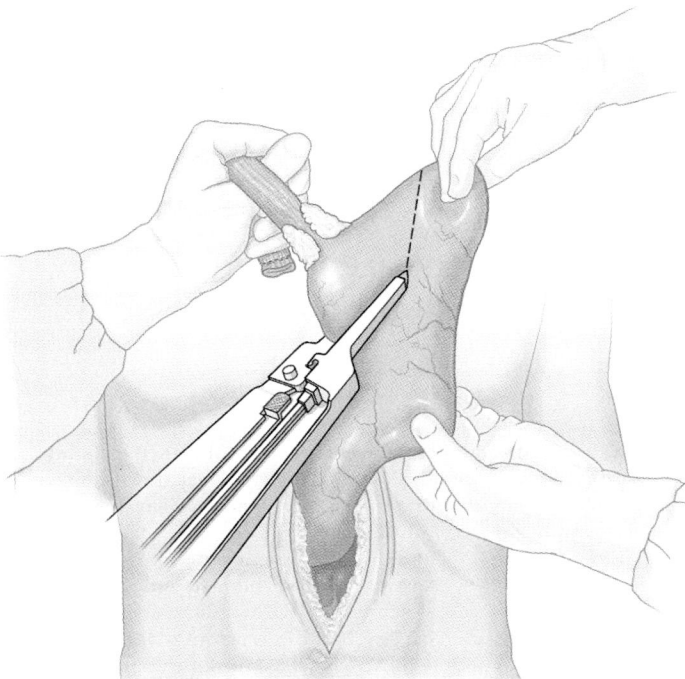

Figure 15 Transhiatal esophagectomy. A gastric tube is formed by stapling along the lesser curvature of the stomach from the junction of the right and left gastric vessels to the top of the fundus. This staple line is oversewn with a continuous 3-0 suture, with care taken not to foreshorten the gastric tube.

Placement of the patient in a slight Trendelenburg position is often helpful. Retractors are placed in the hiatus, and the mediastinum is inspected for hemostasis. The sump is removed. Both pleurae are inspected. The lungs are inflated so that it can be determined which pleural space requires thoracostomy drainage. The mediastinum is packed with dry laparotomy pads from below. A narrow pack is placed into the thoracic inlet from above. Chest tubes are then placed as required along the inframammary crease in the anterior axillary line.

Step 9: excision of specimen and formation of gastric tube The gastric fundus is grasped, and gentle tension is applied along the length of the stomach. The esophagus is held at right angles to the body of the stomach, and the fat in the gastrohepatic ligament is elevated off the lesser curvature; all lymph nodes are thus mobilized. A point approximately midway along the lesser curvature is selected. The blood vessels traversing this area from the right gastric artery are ligated to expose the lesser curvature. The distal resection margin is then determined; it should be 4 to 6 cm from the esophagogastric junction, extending from the selected point on the lesser curvature to a point medial to the fundus. A 60 mm GIA stapler loaded with 3.5 mm staples is then used to transect the proximal stomach, proceeding from the lesser curvature toward the fundus [*see Figure 15*]. Resection of the cardia along with the adjacent portion of the lesser curvature effectively converts a J-shaped stomach into a straight tube.

For maximizing the length of the gastric tube, there are several technical points that are critical. Tension must be maintained on the stomach as the stapler is serially applied cephalad. The stapler should be simply placed on the stomach and fired: no attempt should be made to telescope tissue into the jaws, because to do so would effectively reconstitute the curve of the stomach and diminish its upward reach. Multiple staple loads will be required.

The specimen is removed, and frozen section examination is done on the distal margin. The completed staple line is then oversewn with a continuous Lembert suture of 4-0 polypropylene. Once again, tension is maintained along the stomach to prevent any foreshortening of the lesser curvature. The use of two separate sutures, each reinforcing half of the staple line, is helpful in this regard.

Step 10: advancement of stomach into chest or neck The mediastinal packs are removed, and hemostasis is verified in the chest. The stomach is inspected as well. The ends of any short gastric vessels that were divided with the ultrasonic scalpel are now tied so that subsequent manipulation does not precipitate bleeding. The stomach is oriented so that the greater curvature is to the patient's left. There must be no torsion. The stomach can usually be advanced through the posterior mediastinum without any traction sutures or clamps. The surgeon's hand is placed palm down on the anterior surface of the stomach, with the fingertips about 5 cm proximal to the tip of the fundus. The hand is then gently advanced through the chest, pushing the stomach ahead of itself. The tip of the fundus is gently grasped with a Babcock clamp as it appears in the neck. To prevent trauma at this most distant aspect of the gastric tube, the clamp should not be ratcheted closed.

No attempt should be made to pull the stomach up into the neck: the position of the fundus is simply maintained as the surgeon's hand is removed from the mediastinum. Further length in the neck can usually be gained by gently readvancing the hand along the anterior aspect of the stomach. This measure uniformly distributes tension along the tube and ensures proper torsion-free orientation in the chest. The stomach is pushed up into the neck rather than drawn up by the clamp.

A useful alternate approach for positioning the gastric tube involves passing a large-bore Foley catheter through the mediastinum from the neck incision. The balloon is inflated, and a 50 cm section of a narrow plastic laparoscopic camera bag is tied onto the catheter just above the balloon. The gastric tube is positioned within the bag, and suction is applied through the catheter, creating an atraumatic seal between the stomach and the surrounding plastic bag. As the bag is drawn upward through the neck with gentle traction on the Foley catheter, the stomach advances through the mediastinum. A small dry pack is placed in the neck behind the fundus to prevent retraction into the chest. The stomach is not secured to the prevertebral fascia in any way. The viability of the fundus is checked periodically as the feeding jejunostomy is brought out through the abdomen and the laparotomy incision is closed.

Step 11: esophagogastrostomy The construction of the esophagogastric anastomosis is the most important part of the entire operation: any anastomotic complication will greatly compromise the patient's ability to swallow comfortably. Accordingly, meticulous technique is essential.

A seromuscular traction suture of 4-0 Vicryl is placed through the anterior stomach at the level of the clavicle and drawn upward, thus elevating the fundus into the neck wound and greatly facilitating the anastomosis. The pack behind the fundus is then removed.

The site of the anterior gastrotomy is then carefully selected: it should be midway between the oversewn lesser curvature staple line and the greater curvature of the fundus (marked by the ligated ends of the short gastric vessels). The staple line on the cervical esophagus is removed, and the anterior aspect of the esophagus is grasped with a fine-toothed forceps at the level of the planned gastrotomy. A straight DeBakey forceps is then applied across the full width of the esophagus to act as a guide for division. The esophagus is cut with a scalpel at a 45° angle so that the anterior wall is slightly longer than the posterior wall; the anterior wall then forms the hood of the anastomosis. The fine-toothed forceps is used to maintain orientation of the esophagus throughout. Two full-thickness stay sutures of 4-0 Vicryl are placed, one at the midpoint of the anterior cut edge of the esophagus and one at the corresponding location posteriorly. The posterior stitch is placed from inside the lumen, and the needle is left on the suture for later use.

A 2 cm gastrotomy is then performed with a needle-tipped electrocautery using cutting current. The incision is obliquely oriented, with the cephalad extent proceeding medially. The needle from the stay suture previously placed on the posterior wall of the esophagus is then passed the full thickness of the cephalad aspect of the gastrotomy [see Figure 16a]. Traction on this untied suture brings the esophagus toward the stomach. An endoscopic stapler loaded with 3.5 mm staples is used to form the back wall of the anastomosis. The thicker portion of the device (the cartridge) is advanced cephalad into the stomach, with the narrower portion (the anvil) in the esophageal lumen [see Figure 16b]. The tip of the stapler should be aimed toward the patient's right ear. Tension is applied to the stay suture holding the esophagus and stomach together so as to bring tissue into the jaws of the device. The portion of the fundus extending beyond the stapler is then rotated medially to ensure that the

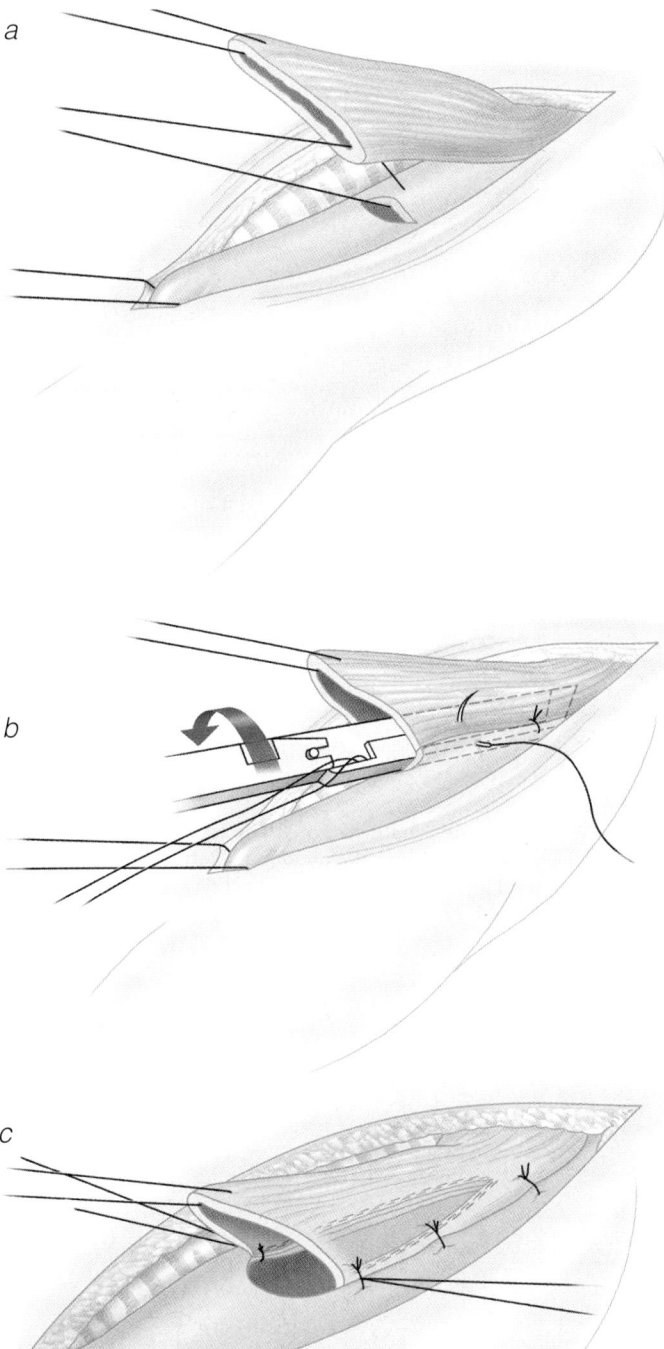

Figure 16 **Transhiatal esophagectomy. (*a*) After the proximal end of the stomach tube is delivered into the neck, the esophagus is cut at a 45% angle so that the anterior wall is longer than the posterior wall. A gastrotomy is placed between the oversewn lesser curvature staple line and the greater curvature of the fundus. A full-thickness suture is placed through all layers of the esophagus and all layers of the gastrotomy. (*b*) An endoscopic GIA stapler is used to form the back wall of the anastomosis. The thicker (cartridge) portion of the device is placed into the stomach, while the narrow (anvil) portion is placed into the esophageal lumen. The tip of the stapler should be aimed toward the patient's right ear. The staple line must be well away from the lesser curvature staple line. Two suspension sutures are placed on either side of the closed stapler, one toward the tip and the other near the heel of the jaws. (*c*) The stapler is fired to complete the posterior portion of the anastomosis.**

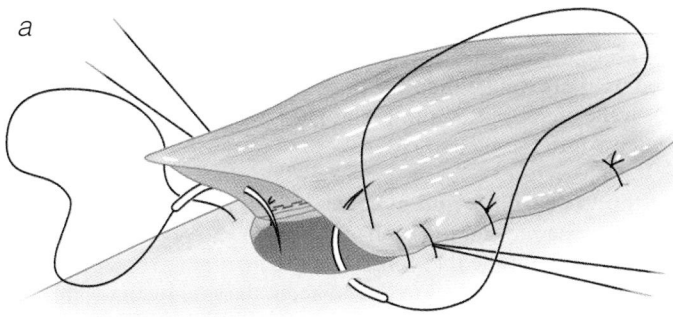

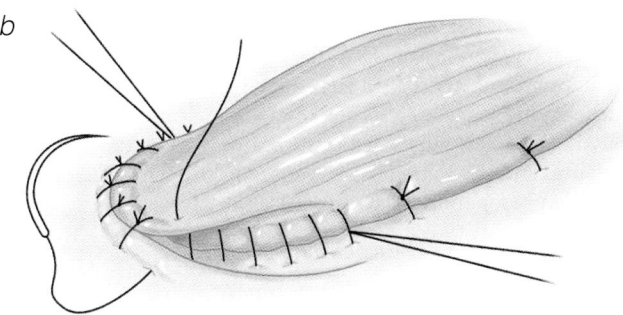

Figure 17 **Transhiatal esophagectomy. The anterior portion of the anastomosis is completed with (*a*) an inner layer consisting of a continuous 4.0 PDS suture and (*b*) an outer layer consisting of interrupted sutures.**

new staple line is well away from the one previously placed along the lesser curvature. This is a crucial point: crossing of the two staple lines may create an ischemic area that can give rise to a large leak in the postoperative period.

The stapler is then closed, holding the esophagus and stomach together, but not yet fired. Two suspension sutures are placed on either side of the closed stapler, one toward the tip and the other near the heel of the jaws. These sutures alleviate any potential tension on the staple line by approximating the muscular layer of the esophagus to the seromuscular layer of the stomach. The suspension sutures are tied, and the stapler is fired, thereby completing the posterior portion of the anastomosis [*see Figure 16c*].

The anterior portion of the anastomosis is closed in two layers. The inner layer consists of a continuous 4-0 polydioxane (PDS) suture placed as full-thickness inverting stitches, and the second layer consists of interrupted seromuscular Lembert sutures [*see Figure 17*]. The lateral and medial corners of the anastomosis, where the staple line meets the hand-sewn portion, merit extra attention. These corners are quite fragile, and excessive traction may result in dehiscence progressing cephalad along the staple line in a zipperlike fashion. The inner layer should therefore be started at each corner. Once several stitches have been placed from the two corners, the nasogastric tube can be passed through the anastomosis. The inner layer is then completed as the two sutures are tied at the midpoint.

Step 12: drainage, closure, and completion x-ray A small Penrose drain is placed in the thoracic inlet below the anastomosis and brought out through the inferior end of the neck incision. The drain is secured, and the incision is irrigated. The strap muscles are not reapproximated but are merely

attached loosely to the underside of the sternocleidomastoid muscle with two interrupted 4-0 Vicryl sutures. The platysma is reconstituted with interrupted 4-0 Vicryl sutures. The nasogastric tube is secured. A chest x-ray is obtained in the OR to verify the position of the drains and the absence of any abnormal collections in the chest. Patients are extubated in the OR and transported to the anesthetic recovery area. Once they are awake and alert, which is usually 3 to 4 hours after the operation, they are taken to the general ward.

In certain patients, a stapled anastomosis may be impractical. In patients with a bull-neck habitus, for example, a partial sternal split may be required for adequate exposure of the cervical esophagus, and a hand-sewn true end-to-end anastomosis may be necessary. In addition, patients who have previously undergone antireflux surgery may have a relatively short gastric tube that will necessitate an end-to-end reconstruction.

Ivor-Lewis Esophagectomy

Steps 1 through 5 Esophagoscopy is performed to confirm the location of the tumor. Steps 1, 2, 3, 4, and 5 of an Ivor-Lewis esophagectomy are virtually identical to the first five steps (i.e., the abdominal portion) of a transhiatal esophagectomy. Once complete mobilization of the stomach is verified, the pylorus is manually advanced to the level of the diaphragm to ensure that it is not being tethered by the duodenum or the greater omentum. The stomach is then placed back into the anatomic position, and the laparotomy is closed.

Step 6: exposure and mobilization of esophagus The patient is shifted to the left lateral decubitus position and redraped. Single-lung ventilation is instituted, and the chest is entered through a right fifth or sixth interspace thoracotomy. The inferior pulmonary ligament is divided, and the lung is retracted cephalad. The esophagus is mobilized from the level of the diaphragm to a point above the azygos vein [*see Figure 18*], which is typically divided with a vascular stapler. The pleura overlying the esophagus is divided to the level of the thoracic inlet, superior to the azygos vein. The esophagus is encircled with a Penrose drain in the retrotracheal region. The pleura is then divided to the level of the diaphragm, with care taken to stay close to the right bronchus and the pericardium and avoid injury to the thoracic duct. The soft tissue between the esophagus and the aorta posteriorly and between the esophagus and the trachea or the pericardium anteriorly is dissected free and maintained en bloc with the esophagus. Periesophageal and subcarinal nodes are thereby mobilized.

Step 7: excision and removal of specimen The hiatus is incised and the abdomen entered. The stomach is drawn up into the chest, with care taken not to place excessive traction on the gastroepiploic pedicle. The esophagus is divided with a stapler proximally at least 5 cm away from any grossly evident tumor. A margin is sent for frozen section examination. The distal resection margin is completed in a similar manner, and the esophageal specimen is removed from the operative field [*see Figure 19*]. The gastric staple line is oversewn, and the stomach is positioned in the posterior mediastinum.

Step 8: esophagogastrostomy The site of the esophagogastric anastomosis should be about 2 cm above the divided azygos vein. Several interrupted sutures are used to secure the transposed stomach to the adjacent pleura. The staple line on the esophagus is removed, and a gastrotomy is performed in

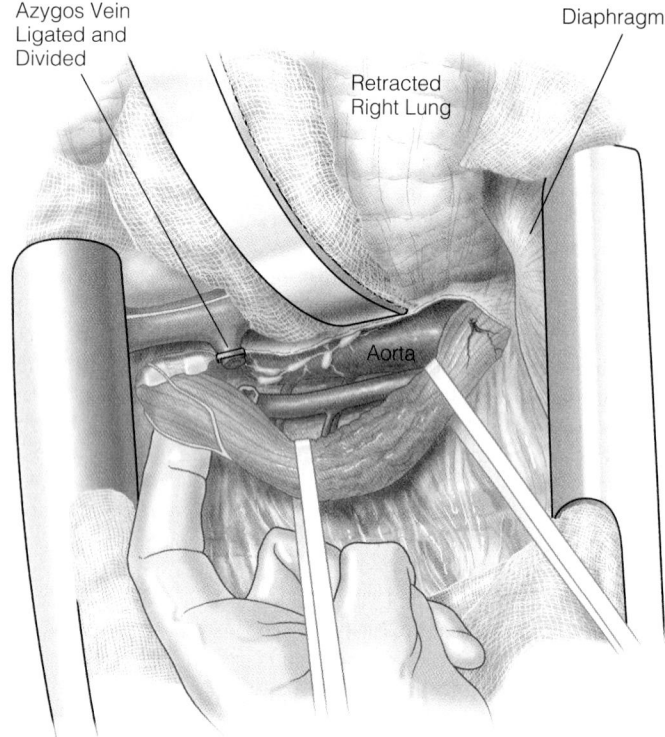

Azygos Vein
Ligated and
Divided

Retracted
Right Lung

Diaphragm

Aorta

Figure 18 **Ivor-Lewis esophagectomy. The lung is retracted, and the azygos vein is stapled and divided. The esophagus and the vagi are mobilized from the level of the diaphragm to the thoracic inlet.**

preparation for a side-to-side functional end-to-end anastomosis [*see Figure 20*]. With the aid of full-thickness traction sutures, the esophagus is positioned along the surface of the stomach and well away from the oversewn staple line defining the gastric resection margin. The posterior aspect of the anastomosis is completed with an endoscopic GIA stapler as described earlier [*see* Transhiatal Esophagectomy, Step 11, *above, and Figures 16 and 17*]. A nasogastric tube is passed, and the anterior wall is completed in two layers. The first layer consists of a full-thickness continuous 3-0 PDS suture; the second consists of interrupted absorbable sutures approximating the seromuscular layer of the stomach to the muscular layer of the esophagus.

Two alternative methods of anastomosis are sometimes used: (1) a totally hand-sewn end-to-side anastomosis and (2) a totally stapled end-to-end anastomosis. The latter technique involves opening the previously placed gastric staple line and advancing the handle of an end-to-end anastomosis (EEA) stapler through the stomach. The proximal esophagus is dilated sufficiently to accommodate at least a 25 mm head. The anvil is placed into the distal esophagus and secured with a purse-string suture. The tip of the stapler is brought out through the apical wall of the stomach and attached to the anvil. The stapler is then fired to create the end-to-end anastomosis, and the gastrotomy is closed. The advantages of this technique are its relative simplicity and the theoretical security of a completely stapled anastomosis; the main potential disadvantage is the risk of postoperative dysphagia resulting from an overly narrow anastomotic ring.

After completion of the anastomosis, the stomach is inspected for any potential redundancy or torsion in the chest. To prevent torsion, the stomach is anchored to the pericardium with non-absorbable sutures. The diaphragmatic hiatus is then inspected:

it should allow easy passage of two fingers into the abdomen alongside the transposed stomach. Interrupted sutures may be used to approximate the edge of the crura to the adjacent stomach wall, thereby preventing any later herniation of abdominal contents into the pleural space.

Step 9: drainage and closure Two chest tubes are placed through separate stab incisions. The tip of the posterior drain is positioned alongside the stomach at the level of the anastomosis. Fine gut sutures secured to the adjacent parietal pleura will help maintain the position of the tube. The thoracotomy is then closed in the standard fashion.

Patients should begin walking on postoperative day 1. The nasogastric tube is generally removed on postoperative day 3. Oral intake is not begun at this point; feeding is accomplished via the temporary jejunostomy. A barium contrast study is performed approximately 5 to 7 days after the operation. If there is no anastomotic leakage, oral intake is initiated and advanced as tolerated. The chest tubes are removed only after the reinstitution of oral intake. Patients are generally discharged from the hospital by postoperative day 8 to 10.

Left Thoracoabdominal Esophagogastrectomy

Step 1: incision and entry into peritoneum The patient is placed in the right lateral position, with the hips rotated backward about 30°. An exploratory laparotomy is performed through an oblique incision extending from the tip of the sixth costal cartilage to a point about halfway between the sternum and the umbilicus. The peritoneal cavity is carefully examined to rule out peritoneal and hepatic metastases. The region of the cardia is palpated and the mobility of the tumor assessed. If there is minor involvement of the crura or the tail of the pancreas, resection may still be possible; however, if the tumor is firmly fixed or there are peritoneal or hepatic metastases, resection should be

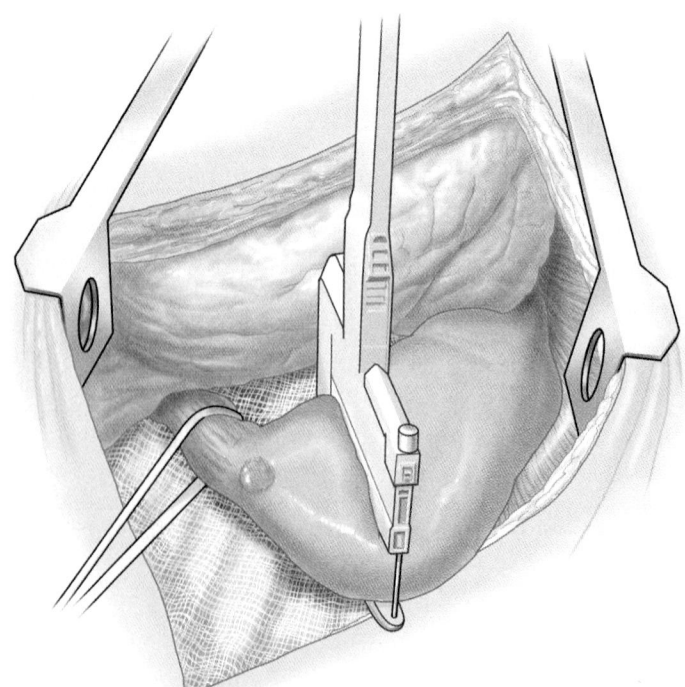

Figure 19 **Ivor-Lewis esophagectomy. The esophagus and the proximal stomach are divided and stapled at least 5 cm away from the gross tumor.**

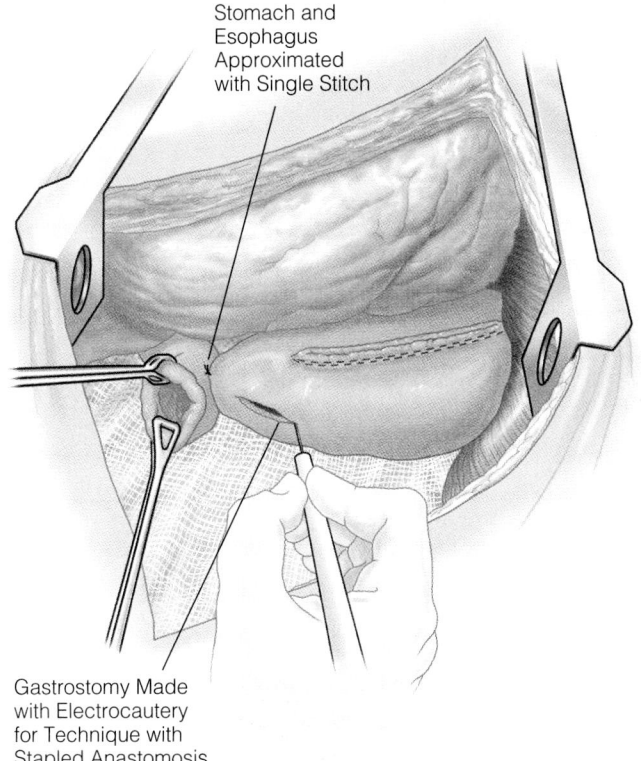

Stomach and
Esophagus
Approximated
with Single Stitch

Gastrostomy Made
with Electrocautery
for Technique with
Stapled Anastomosis

Figure 20 **Ivor-Lewis esophagectomy. The transposed stomach is sutured to the adjacent pericardium, and a gastrotomy is carried out halfway between the lesser curvature staple line and the greater curvature. The anastomosis is completed as in a transhiatal esophagectomy [*see Figures 16 and 17*].**

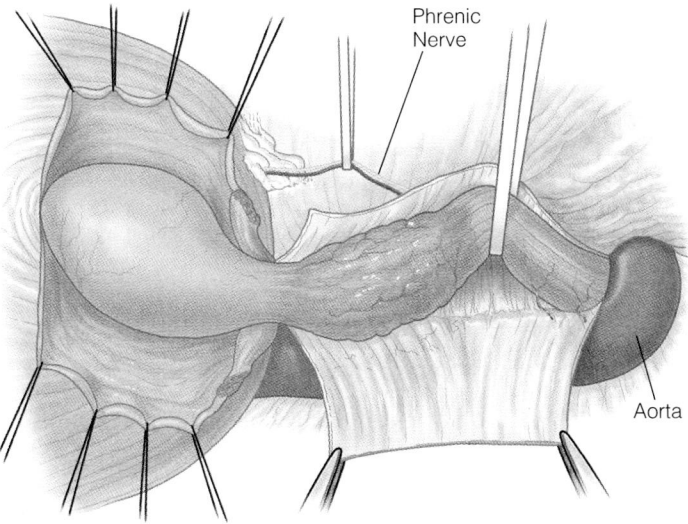

Phrenic
Nerve

Aorta

Diaphragm Sutures

Figure 21 **Left thoracoabdominal esophagogastrectomy. The diaphragm is incised radially. The branches of the pericardial phrenic artery are suture-ligated, and the sutures are left long to be used as diaphragmatic retractors. The pulmonary ligament is divided, and the esophagus is mobilized above the tumor and retracted with a Penrose drain. The esophageal vessels are ligated and divided. The tumor and the esophagus are mobilized off the aorta down to the hiatus; 1 cm of the diaphragmatic crura is taken in continuity with the tumor to provide local clearance. The stomach is then mobilized in much the same way as in a transhiatal esophagectomy [*see Figure 9*].**

abandoned. A feeding jejunostomy, an esophageal stent, or both may be inserted to improve swallowing and allow nutrition.

Step 2: assessment of gastric involvement and incision of diaphragm The extent to which the tumor involves the stomach determines whether a total gastrectomy or a proximal gastrectomy is indicated along with the distal esophagectomy. If no metastases are found, the incision is extended and the chest is opened with a left posterolateral incision through the sixth interspace. If the thoracic component of the tumor appears to be resectable, the costal margin is divided. It is advisable to remove a 1 to 2 cm segment of the costal margin to facilitate repair of the diaphragm at the end of the operation and reduce postoperative costal margin pain. The diaphragm is incised radially [*see Figure 21*]. Branches of the pericardiophrenic artery are suture-ligated, and the sutures are left long so that they can be used as diaphragmatic retractors. Alternatively, a circumferential incision may be made about 2 cm from the costal margin to reduce the risk of postoperative diaphragmatic paralysis.

Step 3: division of pulmonary ligament and mobilization of esophagus and stomach The pulmonary ligament is divided, and the mediastinal pleura is incised over the esophagus as far as the aortic arch. The esophagus is mobilized above the tumor and is retracted by a Penrose drain [*see Figure 21*]. The esophageal vessels are carefully dissected, ligated, and divided. The tumor is then mobilized; the plane of the dissection is kept close to the aorta on the left, and if necessary, the right parietal pleura is taken in continuity with the lesion. About 1 cm of the crura is taken in continuity with the tumor to provide good local clearance. The stomach is then mobilized in much the same way as in a transhiatal esophagectomy [*see Figure 9*].

Step 4: assessment of pancreatic involvement and hepatic viability The lesser sac is opened through the greater omentum so that it can be determined whether the primary tumor involves the distal pancreas. If so, it is reasonable to resect the distal pancreas, the spleen, or both in continuity with the stomach; if not, the short gastric vessels are ligated and divided, with the spleen preserved. The lesser omentum is detached from the right side of the esophagus and the hilum of the liver, then divided down to the area of the pylorus, with the right gastric artery and vein preserved. There is often a hepatic branch from the left gastric artery running through the gastrohepatic omentum. If this hepatic branch is of significant size, a soft vascular clamp should be placed on the artery for 20 minutes so that the viability of the liver can be assessed. If the liver is viable, the artery is suture-ligated and divided.

Step 5: division of greater omentum and short gastric vessels The greater omentum is divided, with care taken to preserve the right gastroepiploic artery and vein. These two vessels are suture-ligated and divided well away from the stomach. Ligation and division of the short gastric vessels allow complete mobilization of the greater curvature of the stomach. Dissection is extended downward as far as the pylorus. The stomach is turned upward, and the left gastric vessels are exposed through the lesser sac [*see Figure 10*]. The lymph nodes along the celiac axis and the left gastric artery are swept up into the specimen, and the gastric vessels are either suture-ligated or stapled.

Step 6: choice of partial or total gastrectomy At this time, the surgeon determines whether the whole stomach must be resected to remove the gastric part of the cancer or whether a partial (i.e., proximal) gastrectomy will suffice.

Proximal esophagogastrectomy with esophagogastrostomy. If the surgeon decides that resection of the proximal stomach will remove all of the tumor while leaving at least 5 cm of tumor-free stomach, a proximal esophagogastrectomy is performed [*see Figure 22*]. A gastric tube is fashioned with a linear stapler [*see Transhiatal Esophagectomy, Step 9, above, and Figure 15*]. The staple line is oversewn with inverting 3-0 sutures. Because the vagus nerves are divided and gastric stasis may result, a pyloromyotomy is performed, much as in a transhiatal esophagectomy.

The proximal gastric resection margin is covered with a sponge and turned upward over the costal margin. The stomach tube is then brought up through the hiatus and into the thorax behind the proximal esophageal resection margin. The margin should be at least 10 cm from the proximal end of the esophagogastric cancer. If the esophageal resection margin is not adequate, the stomach tube is mobilized and brought to the left neck, then anastomosed to the cervical esophagus through a left neck incision; alternatively, the left colon is interposed between the gastric stump and the cervical esophagus. If the resection margin is adequate, the tip of the stomach tube is sewn to the posterior wall of the esophagus [*see Figure 23*].

The anastomosis is then performed with the stapling technique previously described for transhiatal esophagectomy [*see Figures 16 and 17*]. A nasogastric tube is passed down into the gastric remnant. The tube is sewn to the pericardium and the endothoracic fascia to prevent anastomotic dehiscence.

Total gastrectomy with Roux-en-Y esophagojejunostomy. If the surgeon decides that a total gastrectomy is necessary, the right gastroepiploic and right gastric vessels are suture-ligated and divided distal to the pylorus. The duodenum is divided just distal to the pylorus with a linear stapler. The staple line is inverted with interrupted 3-0 nonabsorbable sutures and covered with omentum to prevent duodenal stump blowout.

The esophagus is then mobilized up to the level of the inferior pulmonary vein. Two retaining sutures are placed in the esophageal wall. A monofilament nylon purse-string suture is placed around the circumferance of the proximal esophagus in preparation for stapling. A No. 24 Foley catheter with a 20 ml balloon is advanced into the esophagus and gently inflated to distend the esophageal lumen. The resected specimen is sent to the pathologist for examination of the margins.

A jejunal interposition is then fashioned by using the Roux-en-Y technique. One or two jejunal arteriovenous arcades are divided to mobilize enough jejunum to allow anastomosis to the thoracic esophagus [*see Figure 24*]. After removal of the Foley catheter, a 25 or 28 mm EEA stapler is passed through the jejunum into the esophagus, fired, and removed. The jejunum is anchored to the pericardium and the proximal esophagus. The duodenal loop is anastomosed to the jejunum at least 45 to 50 cm distal to the esophageal jejunal anastomosis to minimize bile reflux [*see Figure 24*]. The blind end of the jejunal loop is then stapled closed.

After careful irrigation of the chest, the first step in the closure is to repair the diaphragm around the hiatus. The gastric or jejunal interposition is sewn to the crura with interrupted nonabsorbable sutures. The remainder of the diaphragm is closed with interrupted nonabsorbable 0 mattress sutures. A chest tube is placed into the pleural space close to but not touching the anastomosis. The final sutures in the peripheral part of the

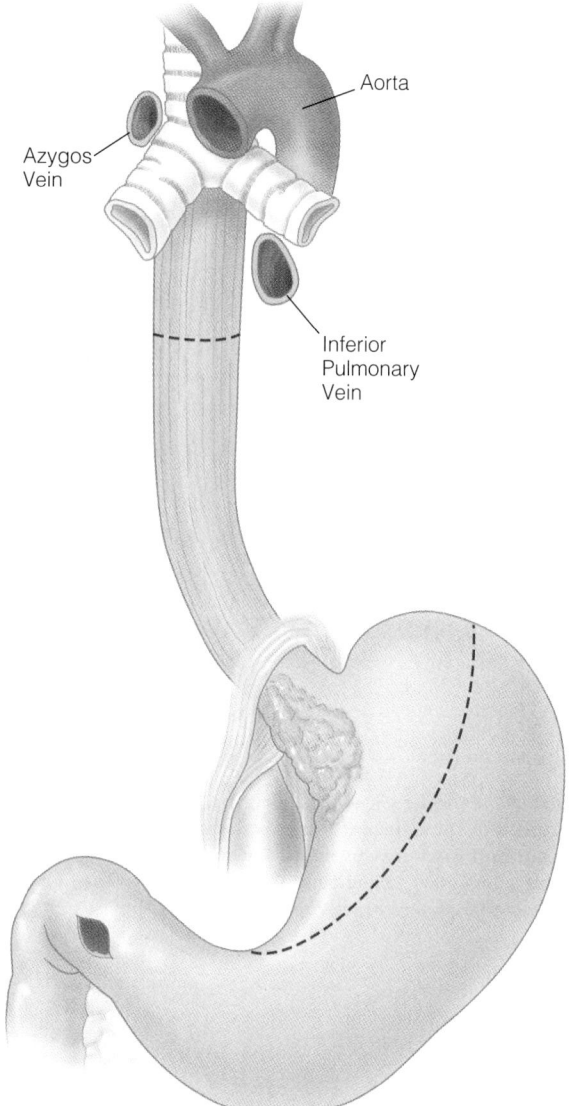

Figure 22 **Left thoracoabdominal esophagogastrectomy: proximal esophagogastrectomy with esophagogastrostomy. If the tumor can be completely resected by removing the proximal stomach, a proximal esophagogastrectomy is carried out.**

diaphragm are placed but are not tied until the ribs are brought together with pericostal sutures. The left lung is reexpanded. The costal cartilages are not approximated but are left to float free. If the ends of the costal margin are abutting, another 2 cm of costal cartilage should be removed to reduce postoperative pain. Thoracic and abdominal skin layers are closed with a continuous absorbable suture. The skin and the subcutaneous tissue are closed in the usual fashion.

POSTOPERATIVE CARE

As a rule, patients are not routinely admitted to the ICU after esophagectomy; however, individual practices depend on the distribution of skilled nursing and physiotherapy personnel. Early ambulation is the mainstay of postoperative care. As a rule, patients are able to walk slowly, with assistance, on postoperative day 1. Patient-controlled epidural analgesia is particularly useful in facilitating good pulmonary toilet and minimizing the risk of atelectasis or pneumonia.

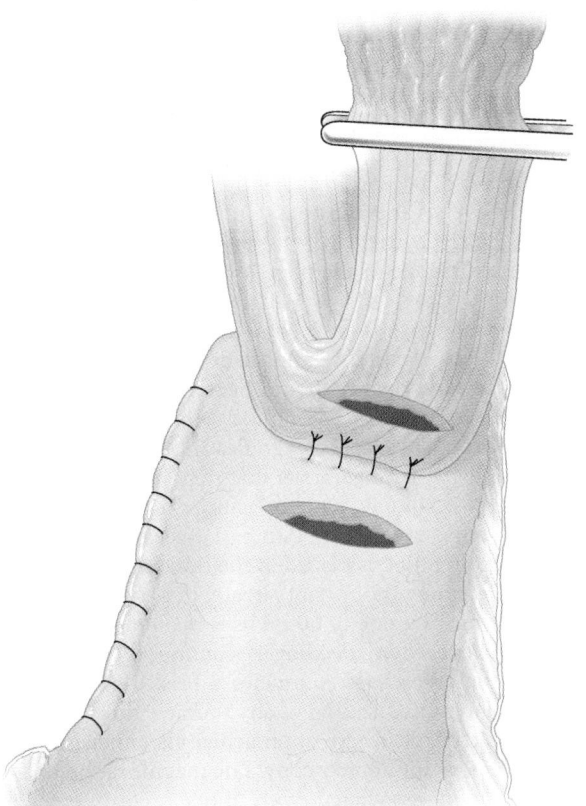

Figure 23 **Left thoracoabdominal esophagogastrectomy: proximal esophagogastrectomy with esophagogastrostomy. The esophagus is sewn to the tip of the stomach tube, halfway between the lesser curvature suture line and the greater curvature. An anastomosis is then fashioned with the stapling technique used in transhiatal esophagectomy [*see Figures 16 and 17*].**

The nasogastric tube is removed on postoperative day 3; jejunostomy tube feedings are gradually started at the same time. Once bowel function normalizes, patients are allowed small sips of liquids. Chest tubes are removed as pleural drainage subsides. By postoperative day 6, most patients have progressed to a soft solid diet. Dietary education is provided, focusing primarily on eating smaller and more frequent meals, avoiding bulky foods (e.g., meat and bread) in the early postoperative period, and taking measures to minimize postprandial dumping. Patients are also taught how to care for their temporary feeding jejunostomy. Consumption of caffeine and carbonated beverages is usually limited during the first few weeks after discharge.

A barium swallow is performed on postoperative day 7 to verify the integrity of the anastomosis and the patency of the pyloromyotomy. Patients are usually discharged on postoperative day 7 or 8. The feeding jejunostomy is left in place until the first postoperative evaluation, which usually takes place 2 to 3 weeks after the operation. The feeding tube is removed during that visit if oral intake and weight are stable.

COMPLICATIONS OF ESOPHAGECTOMY

Pulmonary Impairment

Atelectasis and pneumonia should be considered preventable complications of esophagectomy. Patients with recognized pre-

operative impairment of pulmonary reserve should be considered for transhiatal esophagectomy. Existing pulmonary function can be optimized through incentive spirometry, use of bronchodilators, and physical rehabilitation. Chronic nocturnal aspiration from esophageal obstruction should be watched for in the preoperative patient. Effective pain control is essential to prevent postoperative atelectasis. Routine use of patient-controlled thoracic epidural analgesia should be considered. Deep breathing, early ambulation, and chest physiotherapy encourage the clearing of bronchial secretions. Certain patients will require nasotracheal aspiration or bronchoscopy for pulmonary toilet.

Tracheobronchial Injury

Laceration of the membranous trachea or the left mainstem bronchus may occur during esophagectomy. When such injuries occur during transthoracic resection, management is relatively simple, thanks to the already excellent operative exposure. Direct suture repair and tissue reinforcement with adjacent pleura or a

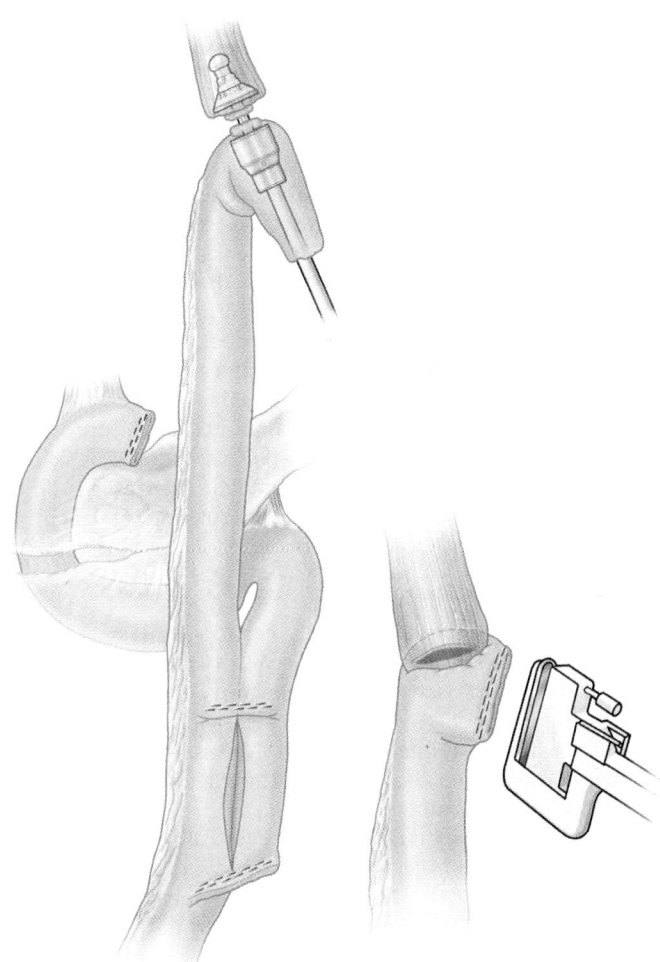

Figure 24 **Left thoracoabdominal esophagogastrectomy: total gastrectomy with Roux-en-Y esophagojejunostomy. A jejunal interposition is fashioned with the Roux-en-Y technique. One or two jejunal arteriovenous arcades are divided to mobilize enough jejunum for anastomosis to the thoracic esophagus. A 25 or 28 mm EEA stapler is passed through the jejunum into the esophagus. The jejunum is anchored to the pericardium and the proximal esophagus. The duodenal loop is anastomosed to the jejunum at least 45 to 50 cm distal to the esophageal-jejunal anastomosis. The blind end of the jejunal loop is then stapled closed.**

pedicle of intercostal muscle provide safe closure in almost all cases. When tracheobronchial injuries occur during transhiatal esophagectomy, they are less obvious but no less urgent. This rare complication arises during mediastinal dissection. Typically, the anesthetic team notes a loss of ventilatory volume, and the surgeon may detect the smell of inhalational agents in the operative field. Bronchoscopy should be promptly performed to identify the site of the injury. The uncut endotracheal tube is then advanced past the site of the laceration to restore proper ventilation. High tracheal injuries can usually be repaired by extending the cervical incision and adding a partial sternotomy. Injury to the carina or the left mainstem bronchus must be repaired via a right thoracotomy.

Bleeding

Hemorrhage should be rare during esophagectomy. The blood supply to the esophagus consists of small branches coming from the aorta, which are easily controlled and generally constrict if left untied. Splenic injuries sometimes occur during mobilization of the stomach. The resultant hemorrhage can be immediate or delayed; blood loss may be significant, and splenectomy is usually required. Precise dissection around the left gastric artery is vital: the bleeding vessels may retract, and attempts at control may result in injury to the celiac artery or its hepatic branches.

Bleeding that arises during the mediastinal stage of the transhiatal esophagectomy generally subsides with packing if it derives from periesophageal arterial branches. Brisk loss of dark blood usually signifies injury to the azygos vein. The first step in addressing such injuries is to pack the mediastinum quickly so as to allow the anesthetic team to stabilize the patient and infuse fluid. Chest tubes are immediately placed to allow detection of any free hemorrhage into the pleural space. Precise localization of the bleeding site may then follow. Injury to the azygos vein may be addressed via an upper sternal split; however, when the exposure is poor, the surgeon should not hesitate to proceed to a full sternotomy. Bleeding from the subcarinal area is usually bright red and may involve bronchial arteries or small periesophageal vessels arising from the aorta, both of which can usually be controlled through the hiatus.

Laryngeal Nerve Injury

Injury to the recurrent laryngeal nerve is a major potential complication of transhiatal esophagectomy. Traction neuropraxia may be temporary and require no specific treatment. Permanent injury will lead to hoarseness and impaired protection of the airway during deglutition. Meticulous protection of the nerve during the cervical stage should minimize the incidence of this complication.

Of particular concern is the risk of bilateral nerve injury after a transthoracic esophagectomy with a cervical esophagogastric anastomosis (i.e., a so-called three-hole esophagectomy). Any dissection of the upper esophagus performed through the right chest should be done as close to the esophagus as possible to avoid placing traction on the right recurrent laryngeal nerve; the subsequent left cervical dissection may put the left recurrent laryngeal nerve at risk for damage. Bilateral paralysis of the vocal cords is very poorly tolerated and has a devastating impact on quality of life.

Chylothorax

Thoracic duct injuries typically present by postoperative day 3 or 4. Dyspnea and pleural effusion may be noted if thoracostomy tubes are not in place. Thoracocentesis yields an opaque,

milky fluid. In patients who already have a chest drain in place, there is typically a high volume of serous drainage in the first 2 postoperative days. As enteral nutrition is established and dietary fat reintroduced, the fluid assumes a characteristic milky appearance. In most cases, the gross appearance is diagnostic, and there is rarely a need to confirm the diagnosis by measuring the triglyceride level. A thoracostomy drain is placed to monitor the volume of the chyle leak. Chest x-rays should be obtained to verify complete drainage of the pleural space and full expansion of the lung.

Patients with chylothorax should be converted to fat-free enteral nutrition. Persistent drainage exceeding 500 ml/8 hr is an indication for early operation and ligation of the thoracic duct; high-volume chyle leaks are unlikely to close spontaneously. Prolonged loss of chyle causes significant electrolyte, nutritional, and immunologic derangements that may prove fatal if allowed to progress. Accordingly, patients with persistent chyle leakage should undergo operation within 1 week of diagnosis. A Dobbhoff feeding tube is placed in the duodenum before operation if a jejunostomy tube is not already in place. Jejunal feeding with 35% cream at a rate of 60 ml/hr is maintained for at least 4 hours before operation. Feeding is continued even during the procedure: the enteral fat stimulates a brisk flow of chyle and greatly facilitates visualization of any thoracic duct injury.

Right-side chyle leaks are approached via either a thoracotomy or video-assisted thoracoscopy. The magnification and excellent illumination associated with thoracoscopy are partially counterbalanced by the constraints imposed by port placement and limited tissue retraction. The inferior pulmonary ligament is divided, and the posterior mediastinum is inspected for extravasation of milky fluid. Any visible sources of chyle leakage can be controlled with clips or suture ligatures. In some cases, mass ligation of the thoracic duct at the level of the diaphragm, incorporating all the soft tissue between the aorta and the azygos vein, may be required.

Left-side leaks can be difficult to manage. The subcarinal area is typically involved; this is the level at which the thoracic duct crosses over from the right. Exploration should begin on the left side. If the leak cannot be visualized, a right-side approach may be necessary to control the thoracic duct as it first enters the chest.

Anastomotic Leakage

The consequences of anastomotic complications after esophagectomy vary considerably in severity, depending on their location and their cause. The cervical anastomotic leaks that may develop after transhiatal esophagectomy are generally simple to treat. Leaks in the early postoperative period are usually related to technical factors, such as excessive tension across the anastomosis. Any possibility of ischemia in the transposed stomach must be addressed promptly, given that a nonviable stomach may not give rise to obvious signs. Tachycardia, confusion, leukocytosis, cervical wound drainage, and neck tenderness may or may not be present.

The morbidity of an open cervical wound is not great—certainly less than that of an untreated leak. Accordingly, any clinical suspicion of a leak should prompt a diagnostic contrast swallow study using dilute barium. Large leaks are manifested as persistent collections of contrast material outside the esophagus. Although such leaks rarely extend into the pleural space, any fluid in the chest must be drained so that its nature can be determined. The neck wound is opened by removing the sutures and performing gentle digital exploration of the prevertebral space behind the esophagus as the finger is advanced into the mediastinum; this is usually done at the bedside and requires little, if any, patient sedation.

Saline-moistened gauze packing is changed three or four times a day. Prolonged or copious cervical drainage may call for supplemental deep wound aspiration with a Yankauer suction handle. Administering water per os during aspiration facilitates removal of any necrotic debris. A fetid, malodorous breath associated with sanguineous discharge from the nasogastric tube and purulent fluid in the opened neck incision are ominous signs that should prompt early esophagoscopy. Diffuse mucosal ischemia may indicate the presence of a nonviable stomach; reoperation with completion gastrectomy and proximal esophagostomy is required to treat this catastrophic complication.

Generally, leaks that occur more than 7 days after operation are small and are related to some degree of late ischemic disruption along the anastomosis. They can usually be managed by opening the cervical wound at the bedside and packing the site with gauze. Oral diet is advanced as tolerated. It may be noted that the volume of the leak is markedly greater or less depending on the position of the head during swallowing. Accordingly, before discharge, patients are taught how to temporarily adjust their swallowing as well as how to manage their dressing changes. Applying gentle pressure to the neck wound and turning the head to the left may help the patient ingest liquids with minimal soiling of the open neck incision. Dysphagia, even with an opened neck incision, should be treated by passing tapered esophageal dilators per os between 2 and 4 weeks after surgery. When a bougie at least 48 French in caliber can be passed through the anastomosis, the patient can usually swallow comfortably. The size of the leak often decreases after dilatation as food is allowed to proceed preferentially into the stomach.

When a routine predischarge barium swallow after transhiatal esophagectomy raises the possibility of an anastomotic leak in an asymptomatic patient, the question arises of whether the wound should be opened at all. For small, contained leaks associated with preferential flow of contrast material into the stomach, observation alone may suffice in selected cases. Patients must be closely watched for fever or other signs of major infection. Given that cervical wound exploration carries quite a low morbidity, the surgeon should not hesitate to drain the neck should the patient's condition change.

The incidence of anastomotic leakage is low after Ivor-Lewis resection, but the consequences are significant. Leaks presenting early in the postoperative period are usually related to technical problems and are difficult to manage; those presenting later are generally related to some degree of ischemic tissue loss. Patients who have received radiation therapy or are nutritionally depleted may be especially vulnerable to problems with anastomotic healing. A contrast swallow with dilute barium is the best method of evaluating the anastomosis. Leaks may be manifested either as a free flow of contrast into the pleural space or as a contained fluid collection.

Small leaks that drain immediately into properly placed thoracostomy tubes can usually be managed by giving antibiotics and withholding oral intake. Local control of infection generally results in spontaneous healing. Anastomotic disruptions that are large or are associated with a major pleural collection typically necessitate open drainage with decortication; percutaneous drainage may be considered as a preliminary approach in selected patients. Persistent soiling of the mediastinum and the pleural space is fatal if untreated.

Early esophagoscopy is strongly advised to evaluate the viability of the gastric remnant. Ischemic necrosis of the stomach necessitates reexploration, decortication, takedown of the anastomosis, gastric debridement, return of any viable stomach into the abdomen, closure of the hiatus, and proximal diversion with a cervical esophagostomy. Repair or revision of the anastomosis in an infected field is certain to fail and should never be considered. In certain cases, diversion via a cervical esophagostomy and a completion gastrectomy may be required.

Late Complications

At every postoperative visit, symptoms of reflux, regurgitation, dumping, poor gastric emptying, and dysphagia must be specifically sought: these are the major quality-of-life issues for postesophagectomy patients.[4] Reflux and regurgitation may complicate any form of alimentary reconstruction after esophagectomy, though cervical anastomoses are less likely to be associated with symptomatic reflux than intrathoracic anastomoses are. Reflux symptoms generally respond to dietary modifications, such as smaller and more frequent meals. Regurgitation is usually related to the supine position and thus tends to be worse at night; elevating the bed and avoiding late meals may suffice for symptom control. Dumping is exacerbated by foods with high fat or sugar content. Dysphagia may be related to narrowing at the anastomosis or, rarely, to poor emptying of the transposed stomach. Anastomotic strictures are most commonly encountered as a sequel to postoperative leakage, resulting either from anatomic distortion of the transposed stomach or from simple atony. Specific tests for gastric atony include nuclear medicine gastric emptying studies using radiolabeled food.

Any form of anastomotic leak will increase the incidence of late stricture. Dysphagia may be treated by means of progressive dilatation with Maloney bougies. This procedure is performed in the outpatient clinic and does not require sedation or any other special patient preparation. Complications are rare if due care is exercised during the procedure. As noted elsewhere [*see* Transthoracic Hiatal Hernia Repair, Preoperative Evaluation, Dilatation, *above*], it is essential that the caliber of the dilators be increased gradually and that little or no force be applied in advancing them. The appearance of blood on a withdrawn dilator signals a breach of the mucosa; further dilatation should be done cautiously lest a transmural injury result. Comfortable swallowing is usually achieved after the successful passage of a 48 French bougie. For late strictures that are particularly difficult to dilate, endoscopic examination and histologic evaluation may be required to rule out a recurrent tumor. CT of the chest should also be performed whenever there is unexplained weight loss late after esophagectomy.

The Savary system of wire-guided dilators has been particularly helpful in the management of tight or eccentric strictures. Patients are generally treated in the endoscopy suite. Temporary sedation with I.V. fentanyl and midazolam is required. Fluoroscopy is used to confirm proper placement of a flexible-tip wire across the stricture. Serial wire-guided dilation can then be performed with confidence and increased patient safety.

OUTCOME EVALUATION

Transhiatal Esophagectomy

A 1999 study from the University of Michigan presented data on 1,085 patients who underwent transhiatal esophagectomy without thoracotomy, of whom 74% had carcinoma and 26% had nonmalignant disease.[5] Transhiatal esophagectomy was completed in 98.6% of the patients; the remaining 1.4% were converted to a transthoracic esophagectomy as a result of either thoracic esophageal fixation or bleeding. Previous chemotherapy or radiation therapy did not preclude performance of a transhiatal esophagectomy. Nine patients experienced inordinate intraoperative blood loss; three died as a result. The overall hospital mortality was 4%. The overall 5-year survival rate for patients undergoing transhiatal esophagectomy is approximately 20% for adenocarcinoma of the cardia and the esophagus and 30% for squamous cell carcinoma of the esophagus.

The stapled anastomosis described earlier [see Operative Technique, Transhiatal Esophagectomy, Step 8, above] reflects numerous refinements introduced at the University of Michigan. The endoscopic GIA stapler has a low-profile head that is ideally suited to the tight confines of the neck, enabling the surgeon to fashion a widely patent side-to-side functional end-to-end anastomosis with three rows of staples along the back wall. The rate of anastomotic stricture is markedly lower with this anastomosis than with a totally hand-sewn anastomosis. As regards postoperative function, stomach interposition through the posterior mediastinum after transhiatal esophagectomy is associated with low rates of aspiration and regurgitation. Esophageal reflux and esophagitis—commonly seen with intrathoracic esophagogastric anastomoses—are usually not clinically significant problems with this approach. Patients are advised to elevate the head of their bed and to continue taking proton pump inhibitors for about 3 months after the operation. Approximately one third will require esophageal dilatation for dysphagia after the operation. Some 7% to 10% experience postvagotomy dumping symptoms, which in most cases can be controlled by simply avoiding high-carbohydrate foods and dairy products.

Ivor-Lewis Esophagectomy

Ivor-Lewis esophagectomy is associated with anastomotic leakage rates and operative mortalities of less than 3%.[3,6] Approximately 5% of patients will require anastomotic dilatation. Again, patients are advised to elevate the head of the bed and to continue taking proton pump inhibitors. In some patients, the gastric interposition rotates into the right posterolateral thoracic gutter, resulting in postprandial gastric tension and rendering them more susceptible to aspiration. The 3-year survival rate is approximately 18% to 25%.

Left Thoracoabdominal Esophagectomy

Left thoracoabdominal esophagogastrectomy is also associated with anastomotic leakage rates and operative mortalities of less than 3%.[7] Approximately 5% of patients will require esophageal dilatation. Reconstructions involving anastomosis of the distal stomach to the esophagus are associated with a high incidence of delayed gastric emptying and bile gastritis and esophagitis. Of all the operations we have described, this one results in the lowest postoperative quality of life. Accordingly, most surgeons prefer to carry out a total gastrectomy. Swallowing is restored with a Roux-en-Y jejunal interposition.

References

1. Lahey FH, Warren K: Esophageal diverticula. Surg Gynecol Obstet 98:1, 1954

2. Stirling MC, Orringer MB: Continued assessment of the combined Collis-Nissen operation. Ann Thorac Surg 47:224, 1989

3. Mathiesen DJ, Grillo HC, Wilkens EW Jr: Transthoracic esophagectomy: a safe approach to carcinoma of the esophagus. Ann Thorac Surg 45:137, 1988

4. Finley RJ, Lamy A, Clifton J, et al: Gastrointestinal function following esophagectomy for malignancy. Am J Surg 169:471, 1995

5. Orringer MB, Marshall B, Iannettoni MD: Transhiatal esophagectomy: clinical experience and refinements. Ann Surg 230:392, 1999

6. King RM, Pairolero PC, Trastek VF, et al: Ivor Lewis esophagogastrectomy for carcinoma of the esophagus: early and long-term results. Ann Thorac Surg 44:119, 1987

7. Akiyama H, Miyazono H, Tsurumaru M, et al: Thoracoabdominal approach for carcinoma of the cardia of the stomach. Am J Surg 137:345, 1979

Acknowledgment

Figures 1 through 24   Tom Moore.

10 MINIMALLY INVASIVE ESOPHAGEAL PROCEDURES

Marco G. Patti, M.D., F.A.C.S., and Piero M. Fisichella, M.D.

During the 1970s and the 1980s, operations for benign esophageal disorders were often withheld or delayed in favor of less effective forms of treatment in an effort to prevent the postoperative discomfort, the long hospital stay, and the recovery time associated with open surgical procedures. For instance, pneumatic dilatation became the first line of treatment for achalasia, even though studies had shown that surgical management was clearly superior.[1]

Since the beginning of the 1990s, thanks to the advent of minimally invasive techniques, there has been a revolution in the field of general surgery and, in particular, in the management of benign esophageal disorders. In the first part of the 1990s, it became clear that treatment of these conditions with minimally invasive procedures yielded results comparable to those of treatment with traditional operations while causing minimal postoperative discomfort, reducing the duration of hospitalization, shortening recovery time, and permitting earlier return to work.[2,3] Consequently, minimally invasive surgery was increasingly considered as first-line treatment for achalasia, and laparoscopic fundoplication was considered more readily and at an earlier stage in the management of gastroesophageal reflux disease (GERD).

In the latter part of the 1990s and the first few years of the 21st century, minimally invasive esophageal procedures continued to evolve, thanks to better instrumentation and improved surgical expertise. In addition, as experience with these procedures accumulates and the follow-up period lengthens, it becomes possible to analyze techniques and their results more rigorously. For instance, whereas a few years ago a left thoracoscopic Heller myotomy was considered the procedure of choice for achalasia, the current procedure of choice is a laparoscopic Heller myotomy with partial fundoplication, which is now known to be better at relieving dysphagia and controlling postoperative reflux.[4-7] Similarly, whereas total fundoplication and partial fundoplication were initially considered equally effective in treating GERD,[8] long-term follow-up indicates that total fundoplication is clearly superior in controlling reflux and should be used whenever feasible.[9]

In what follows, we do not address the standard open esophageal operations, which are described elsewhere [*see 3:9 Open Esophageal Procedures*]. Instead, we focus on minimally invasive techniques for the treatment of abnormal gastroesophageal reflux and motility disorders of the esophagus.

Laparoscopic Nissen Fundoplication

PREOPERATIVE EVALUATION

All patients who are candidates for a laparoscopic fundoplication should undergo a preoperative evaluation that includes the following: (1) symptomatic evaluation, (2) an upper GI series, (3) endoscopy, (4) esophageal manometry, and (5) ambulatory pH monitoring.

Symptomatic Evaluation

The presence of both typical symptoms (heartburn, regurgitation, and dysphagia) and atypical symptoms of GERD (cough, wheezing, chest pain, and hoarseness) should be investigated, and symptoms should be graded with respect to their intensity both before and after operation. Nonetheless, a diagnosis of GERD should never be based solely on symptomatic evaluation. Many authorities assert that the diagnosis of GERD can be made reliably from the clinical history,[10] so that a complaint of heartburn should lead to the presumption that acid reflux is present; however, testing of this diagnostic strategy demonstrates that symptoms are far less sensitive and specific than is usually believed.[11] For instance, our group found that of 822 consecutive patients referred for esophageal function tests with a clinical diagnosis of GERD (based on symptoms and endoscopic findings), only 70% had abnormal reflux on pH monitoring.[12] Heartburn and regurgitation were no more frequent in patients who had genuine reflux than in those who did not; thus, symptomatic evaluation, by itself, could not distinguish between the two groups.

The response to proton pump inhibitors is a better predictor of abnormal reflux. For example, in our study, 75% of patients with GERD reported a good or excellent response to these agents, compared with only 26% of patients without GERD.[12] Similarly, a 1999 multivariate analysis of factors predicting outcome after laparoscopic fundoplication concluded that a clinical response to acid suppression therapy was one of three factors predictive of a successful outcome, the other two being an abnormal 24-hour pH score and the presence of a typical primary symptom (e.g., heartburn).[13]

Upper Gastrointestinal Series

An upper GI series is useful for diagnosing and characterizing an existing hiatal hernia. The size of the hiatal hernia helps predict how difficult it will be to reduce the esophagogastric junction below the diaphragm. In addition, large hiatal hernias are associated with more severe disturbances of esophageal peristalsis and esophageal acid clearance.[14] Esophagograms are also useful for determining the location, shape, and size of a stricture and detecting a short esophagus.

Endoscopy

Endoscopy is typically the first test performed to confirm a symptom-based diagnosis of GERD. This approach has two pitfalls, however. First, even though the goal of endoscopy is to assess the mucosal damage caused by reflux, mucosal changes are absent in about 50% of GERD patients.[12] Second, major interobserver variations have been reported with esophageal

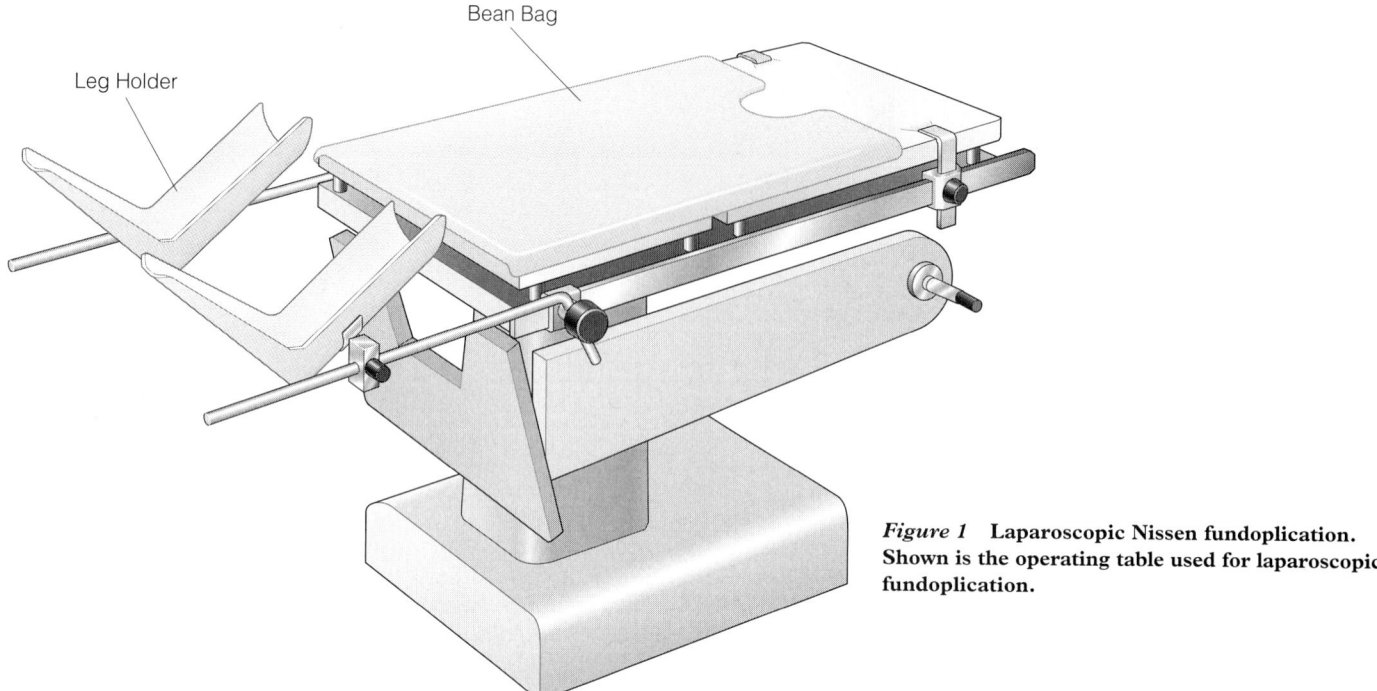

Figure 1   **Laparoscopic Nissen fundoplication. Shown is the operating table used for laparoscopic fundoplication.**

endoscopy, particularly for low-grade esophagitis.[15] For instance, our group found that of 247 patients with negative results on pH monitoring, 60 (24%) had been diagnosed as having grade I or II esophagitis.[12] Accordingly, we believe that endoscopy is most valuable for excluding gastric and duodenal pathology and for detecting the presence of Barrett's esophagus.

Esophageal Manometry

Esophageal manometry provides useful information about the motor function of the esophagus by determining the length and resting pressure of the lower esophageal sphincter (LES) and assessing the quality (i.e., the amplitude and propagation) of esophageal peristalsis. In addition, it allows proper placement of the pH probe for ambulatory pH monitoring (5 cm above the upper border of the LES).

Ambulatory pH Monitoring

Ambulatory pH monitoring is the most reliable test for the diagnosis of GERD, with a sensitivity and specificity of about 92%.[16] It is of key importance in the workup for the following four reasons:

1. It determines whether abnormal reflux is present. In our study, pH monitoring yielded normal results in 30% of patients with a clinical diagnosis of GERD,[12] thereby obviating the continuation of inappropriate and expensive drugs (e.g., proton pump inhibitors) or the performance of a fundoplication. In addition, pH monitoring prompted further investigation that in a number of cases pointed to other diseases, such as cholelithiasis and irritable bowel syndrome.

2. It establishes a temporal correlation between symptoms and episodes of reflux. Such a correlation is particularly important when atypical symptoms (e.g., cough and wheezing) are present because 50% of these patients experience no heartburn and 50% do not have esophagitis on endoscopy.[17]

3. It allows staging of patients according to disease severity. Specifically, pH monitoring identifies a subgroup of patients characterized by worse esophageal motor function (manifest-

ed by a defective LES or by abnormal esophageal peristalsis), more acid reflux in the distal and proximal esophagus, and slower acid clearance. These patients more frequently experience stricture formation and Barrett metaplasia and thus might benefit from early antireflux surgery.[18]

4. It provides baseline data that may prove very useful postoperatively if symptoms do not respond to the procedure.

OPERATIVE PLANNING

The patient is placed under general anesthesia and intubated with a single-lumen endotracheal tube. Abdominal wall relaxation is ensured by the administration of a nondepolarizing muscle relaxant, the action of which is rapidly reversed at the end of the operation. Adequate muscle relaxation is essential because increased abdominal wall compliance allows increased pneumoperitoneum, which yields better exposure. An orogastric tube is inserted at the beginning of the operation to keep the stomach decompressed; it is removed at the end of the procedure.

The patient is placed in a steep reverse Trendelenburg position, with the legs extended on stirrups. The surgeon stands between the patient's legs. To keep the patient from sliding as a result of the steep position used during the operation, a bean bag is inflated under the patient [*see Figure 1*], and the knees are flexed only 20° to 30°. A Foley catheter is inserted at the beginning of the procedure and usually is removed in the postoperative period. Because increased abdominal pressure from pneumoperitoneum and the steep reverse Trendelenburg position decrease venous return, pneumatic compression stockings are always used as prophylaxis against deep vein thrombosis.

The equipment required for a laparoscopic Nissen fundoplication includes five 10 mm trocars, a 30° laparoscope, a hook cautery, and various other instruments [*see Table 1*]. In addition, we use a three-chip camera system that is separate from the laparoscope.

OPERATIVE TECHNIQUE

In all patients except those with very poor esophageal motility—for whom partial fundoplication [*see* Laparoscopic Partial

(Guarner) Fundoplication, *below*] is preferable—we advocate performing a 360° wrap of the gastric fundus around the lower esophagus as described by Nissen, but we always take down the short gastric vessels to achieve what is called a floppy fundoplication. This type of wrap is very effective in controlling gastroesophageal reflux.[1] The operation can be divided into nine key steps as follows.

Step 1: Insertion of Trocars

Five 10 mm trocars are used for the operation [*see Figure 2*]. Port A is placed about 14 cm below the xiphoid process; it can also be placed slightly (2 to 3 cm) to the left of the midline to be in line with the hiatus. This port is used for insertion of the scope. Port B is placed at the same level as port A, but in the left midclavicular line. It is used for insertion of the Babcock clamp; insertion of a grasper to hold the Penrose drain once it is in place surrounding the esophagus; or insertion of the clip applier, the ultrasonic coagulating shears (LaparoSonic Coagulating Shears [LCS], Ethicon Endo-Surgery, Inc.), or both to take down the short gastric vessels. Port C is placed at the same level as the previous two ports but in the right midclavicular line. It is used for insertion of the fan retractor, the purpose of which is to lift the lateral segment of the left lobe of the liver and expose the esophagogastric junction. We do not divide the left triangular ligament. The fan retractor can be held in place by a self-retaining system fixed to the operating table. Ports D and E are placed as high as possible under the costal margin and about 5 to 6 cm to the right and the left of the midline, so that they are about 15 cm from the esophageal hiatus; in addition, they should be placed in such a way that their axes form an angle of 60° to 120°. These ports are used for insertion of the graspers, the electrocautery, and the suturing instruments.

Troubleshooting   A common mistake is to place the ports too low in the abdomen, thereby making the operation more difficult. If port C is too low, the fan retractor will not retract the lateral segment of the left lobe of the liver well, and the esophagogastric junction will not be exposed. If port B is too low, the Babcock clamp will not reach the esophagogastric junction, and when the LCS or the clip applier is placed through the same

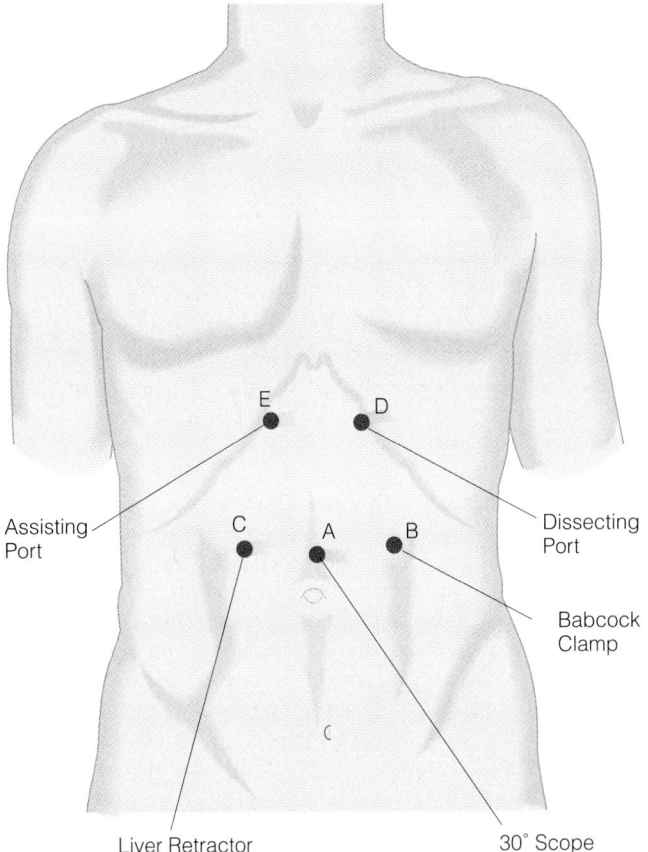

Figure 2   **Laparoscopic Nissen fundoplication. Illustrated is the recommended placement of the trocars.**

port, it will not reach the upper short gastric vessels. If ports D and E are too low, the dissection at the beginning of the case and the suturing at the end are problematic.

Other mistakes of positioning must be avoided as well. It is important not to place port C too medially, because the fan retractor may clash with the left-hand instrument; the gallbladder fossa is a good landmark for positioning this port. Port A must be placed with extreme caution in the supraumbilical area: its insertion site is just above the aorta, before its bifurcation. Accordingly, we recommend initially inflating the abdomen to a pressure of 18 mm Hg just for placement of port A; increasing the distance between the abdominal wall and the aorta reduces the risk of aortic injury. We also recommend directing the port toward the coccyx. A Hasson cannula can be used in this location, particularly if the patient has already had one or more midline incisions. Maintaining the proper angle (60° to 120°) between the axes of the two suturing instruments inserted through ports D and E is also important: if the angle is smaller, the instruments will cover part of the operating field, whereas if it is larger, depth perception may be impaired. Finally, if a trocar is not in the ideal position, it is better to insert another one than to operate through an inconveniently placed port.

If the surgeon spears the epigastric vessels with a trocar, bleeding will occur, in which case there are two options. The first option is to pull the port out, insert a 24 French Foley catheter with a 30 ml balloon through the site, inflate the balloon, and apply traction with a clamp. The advantage of this maneuver is that the vessel need not be sutured; the disadvan-

---

Table 1   Instrumentation for Laparoscopic Nissen Fundoplication

Five 10 mm trocars

30° scope

Graspers

Babcock clamp

L-shaped hook cautery with suction-irrigation capacity

Scissors

Laparoscopic clip applier

Ultrasonic coagulating shears

Fan retractor

Needle holder

Penrose drain

2-0 silk sutures

56 French esophageal bougie

tage is that the surgeon must then choose another insertion site. At the end of the case, the balloon is deflated. If some bleeding is still present, it must be controlled with sutures placed from outside under direct vision. The second option is to use a long needle with a suture, with which one can rapidly place two U-shaped stitches, one above the clamp and one below. The suture is tied outside over a sponge and left in place for 2 or 3 days.

Step 2: Division of Gastrohepatic Ligament; Identification of Right Crus of Diaphragm and Posterior Vagus Nerve

Once the ports are in place, the gastrohepatic ligament is divided. Dissection begins above the caudate lobe of the liver, where this ligament usually is very thin, and continues toward the diaphragm until the right crus is identified. The crus is then separated from the right side of the esophagus by blunt dissection, and the posterior vagus nerve is identified. The right crus is dissected inferiorly toward the junction with the left crus.

Troubleshooting   An accessory left hepatic artery originating from the left gastric artery is frequently encountered in the gastrohepatic ligament. If this vessel creates problems of exposure, we divide it; to date, its division has not caused problems. When dissecting the right crus from the esophagus, we try to use the electrocautery with particular caution. Because the monopolar current tends to spread laterally, the posterior vagus nerve can sustain damage simply from being in proximity to the device, even when there is no direct contact. The risk of neuropraxia can be reduced by using the cut mode rather than the coagulation mode when the electrocautery is close to the nerve. The cut mode has problems of its own, however, and is not recommended in most laparoscopic procedures. A better alternative is to use bipolar scissors.

Step 3: Division of Peritoneum and Phrenoesophageal Membrane above Esophagus; Identification of Left Crus of Diaphragm and Anterior Vagus Nerve

The peritoneum and the phrenicoesophageal membrane above the esophagus are divided with the electrocautery, and the anterior vagus nerve is identified. The left crus of the diaphragm is dissected downward toward the junction with the right crus.

Troubleshooting   During this part of the dissection, pains should be taken not to damage the anterior vagus nerve or the esophageal wall. To this end, the nerve should be left attached to the esophageal wall, and the peritoneum and the phrenicoesophageal membrane should be lifted from the wall by blunt dissection before they are divided.

Step 4: Creation of Window between Gastric Fundus, Esophagus, and Diaphragmatic Crura; Placement of Penrose Drain around Esophagus

The esophagus is retracted upward by means of a Babcock clamp applied at the level of the esophagogastric junction. Via blunt and sharp dissection, a window is created under the esophagus between the gastric fundus, the esophagus, and the diaphragmatic crura. The window is enlarged with the cautery. Sometimes, one or two short gastric vessels can be divided via this exposure. A Penrose drain is then passed around the esophagus. This drain is used for traction instead of the Babcock clamp from this point on to decrease the chances of damage to the gastric wall.

Troubleshooting   There are two main problems to watch for during this part of the procedure: (1) creation of a left pneumothorax and (2) perforation of the gastric fundus.

A left pneumothorax is usually caused by dissection done above the left crus in the mediastinum rather than between the crus and the gastric fundus. This problem can be avoided by properly dissecting and identifying the left crus; the use of curved instruments is also helpful.

Perforation of the gastric fundus is usually caused by pushing a blunt instrument under the esophagus and below the left crus without having done enough dissection. Care must be exercised in taking down small vessels from the gastric fundus when the area behind the esophagus is approached from the right: the anatomy is not as clear from this viewpoint, and perforation can easily occur. Sometimes, perforation is caused by the use of a monopolar electrocautery for dissection. An electrocautery burn can go unrecognized during dissection and manifest itself in the form of a leak during the first 48 hours after operation.

Step 5: Division of Short Gastric Vessels

The clip applier or the LCS is introduced through port B. A grasper is introduced by the surgeon through port D, and an assistant applies traction on the greater curvature of the stomach through port E. Dissection begins at the level of the middle portion of the gastric body and continues upward until the most proximal short gastric vessel is divided and the Penrose drain is reached.

Troubleshooting   Again, there are two main problems to watch for during this part of the procedure: (1) bleeding, either from the gastric vessels or from the spleen, and (2) damage to the gastric wall.

Bleeding from the gastric vessels is usually caused by excessive traction or by division of a vessel when the clips are not completely occluding the vessel on both sides. Vessels up to 5 mm in diameter can be taken down with the LCS; this process requires about half of the amount of time needed when only clips are used. The lower blade has a sharp, oscillating inferior edge that must always be kept in view to prevent damage to other structures (e.g., the pancreas, the splenic artery and vein, and the spleen).

Damage to the gastric wall can be caused by a burn from the electrocautery used to dissect between vessels or by traction applied via the graspers or the Babcock clamp.

Step 6: Closure of Crura

The diaphragmatic crura are closed with interrupted 2-0 silk sutures on a curved needle; the sutures are tied intracorporeally. Exposure during this phase is provided by retracting the esophagus upward and toward the patient's left with the Penrose drain. The lens of the 30° laparoscope is angled slightly to the left by moving the light cable of the scope to the patient's right. The first stitch should be placed just above the junction of the two crura. Additional stitches are placed 1 cm apart, and a space of about 1 cm is left between the uppermost stitch and the esophagus.

Troubleshooting   Pains must be taken not to spear the posterior wall of the esophagus with either the tip or the back of the needle. We do not place the bougie inside the esophagus during this part of the procedure; to do so would limit the space available for suturing.

Step 7: Insertion of Bougie into Esophagus and through Esophagogastric Junction

The esophageal stethoscope and the orogastric tube are removed, and a 56 French bougie is inserted by the anesthesiologist. The bougie is passed through the esophagogastric junction under the view provided by the laparoscope. The crura must be snug around the esophagus but not too tight: a closed grasper should be able to slide easily between the esophagus and the crura.

Troubleshooting The most worrisome complication during this step is perforation of the esophagus. This can be prevented by lubricating the bougie and instructing the anesthesiologist to advance the bougie slowly and to stop if any resistance is encountered. In addition, it is essential to remove any instruments from the esophagogastric junction and to open the Penrose drain; these measures prevent the creation of an angle between the stomach and the esophagus, which can increase the likelihood of perforation. The position of the bougie can be confirmed by pressing with a grasper over the esophagus, which will feel full when the bougie is in place.

Step 8: Wrapping of Gastric Fundus around Lower Esophagus

The gastric fundus is gently pulled under the esophagus with the graspers. The left and right sides of the fundus are wrapped above the fat pad (which lies above the esophagogastric junction) and held together in place with a Babcock clamp introduced through port B. (The Penrose drain should be removed at this point because it is in the way.) Usually, three 2-0 silk sutures are used to secure the two ends of the wrap to each other. The first stitch does not include the esophagus and is used for traction; the second and the third include a bite of the esophageal muscle. Two coronal stitches are then placed between the top of the wrap and the esophagus, one on the right and one on the left. Finally, two additional sutures are placed between the right side of the wrap and the closed crura. It is important to pass the bougie into the stomach after the first stitch is placed to gauge the size of the wrap. If the wrap seems at all tight, the stitch is removed and repositioned more laterally.

To avoid the risk of injuring the inferior vena cava at the beginning of the dissection, some surgeons use a different method—the so-called left crus approach.[19] In this approach, the operation begins with identification of the left crus of the diaphragm and division of the peritoneum and the phrenicoesophageal membrane overlying it. The next step is division of the short gastric vessels, starting midway along the greater curvature of the stomach and continuing upward to join the area of the previous dissection. When the fundus has been thoroughly mobilized, the peritoneum is divided from the left to the right crus, and the right crus is dissected downward to expose the junction of the right and left crura. With this technique, the vena cava is never at risk. In addition, the branches of the anterior vagus nerve and the left gastric artery are less exposed to danger. We feel that this technique is very useful, particularly for management of very large paraesophageal hernias and for second antireflux operations [see Reoperation for GERD, *below*].

Troubleshooting To determine whether the wrap is going to be floppy, the surgeon must deliver the fundus of the stomach under the esophagus, making sure that the origins of the short gastric vessels that have been transected are seen.

Essentially, the posterior wall of the fundus is being used for the wrap. If the wrap remains to the right of the esophagus without retracting back to the left, then it is floppy, and suturing can proceed. If not, the surgeon must make sure that the upper short gastric vessels have been transected. If tension is still present after these maneuvers, it is probably best to perform a partial wrap [see Laparoscopic Partial (Guarner) Fundoplication, *below*].

Damage to the gastric wall may occur during the delivery of the fundus. Atraumatic graspers must be used, and the gastric fundus must be pulled gently and passed from one grasper to the other. Sometimes, it is helpful to push the gastric fundus under the esophagus from the left. The wrap should measure no more than 2 to 2.5 cm in length and, as noted, should be done with no more than three sutures. The first stitch is usually the lowest one; it must be placed just above the fat pad where the esophagogastric junction is thought to be.

If the anesthesiologist observes that peak airway pressure has increased (because of a pneumothorax) or that neck emphysema is present (because of pneumomediastinum), the pneumoperitoneum should be reduced from 15 mm Hg to 7 to 8 mm Hg until the end of the procedure. Pneumomediastinum tends to resolve without intervention within a few hours of the end of the procedure. Small pneumothoraces (usually on the left side) tend to reabsorb spontaneously, and thus, the insertion of a chest tube is unnecessary. Larger pneumothoraces (> 20%) call for the insertion of a small chest tube (18 to 20 French).

Step 9: Final Inspection and Removal of Instruments and Ports from Abdomen

After hemostasis is obtained, the instruments and the ports are removed from the abdomen under direct vision.

Troubleshooting If any areas of oozing were observed during the procedure, they should be irrigated and dried with sponges rolled into a cigarettelike shape before the ports are removed. In addition, if some grounds for concern remain, the oozing areas should be examined after the pneumoperitoneum is decreased to an intra-abdominal pressure of 7 to 8 mm Hg to abolish the tamponading effect exerted by the high intra-abdominal pressure.

All the ports should be removed from the abdomen under direct vision so that any bleeding from the abdominal wall can be readily detected. Such bleeding is easily controlled, either from inside or from outside.

COMPLICATIONS

A feared complication of laparoscopic Nissen fundoplication is esophageal or gastric perforation. As noted, this complication is caused by traction applied with the Babcock clamp or a grasper to the esophagus or the stomach (particularly when the stomach is pulled under the esophagus) or by inadvertent electrocautery burns during any part of the dissection. A leak will manifest itself during the first 48 hours. Peritoneal signs will be noted if the spillage is limited to the abdomen; shortness of breath and a pleural effusion will be noted if spillage also occurs in the chest. The site of the leak should always be confirmed by a contrast study with barium or a water-soluble contrast agent. Perforation is best handled by means of laparotomy and direct repair. If a perforation is detected intraoperatively, it may be closed laparoscopically.

About 50% of patients experience mild dysphagia postoperatively. This problem usually resolves after 4 to 6 weeks, during which period patients receive pain medications in an elixir form and are advised to avoid eating meat and bread. If, however, dysphagia persists beyond this period, one or more of the following causes is responsible.

1. A wrap that is too tight or too long. The wrap should be performed without tension over a 56 French bougie. The total length of the wrap should not exceed 2.5 cm.
2. Lateral torsion with corkscrew effect. If the wrap rotates toward the right (either because of tension from intact short gastric vessels or because the fundus is small), a corkscrew effect is created.
3. A wrap made with the body of the stomach rather than the fundus. The relaxation of the LES and the gastric fundus is controlled by vasoactive intestinal polypeptide and nitric oxide[20,21]; after fundoplication, the two structures relax simultaneously with swallowing. If part of the body of the stomach rather than the fundus is used for the wrap, it will not relax as the LES does on arrival of the food bolus.
4. Choice of the wrong procedure. In patients who have severely abnormal esophageal peristalsis (as in end-stage connective tissue disorders), a partial wrap should be performed. A 360° wrap will control reflux, but it may cause postoperative dysphagia and gas bloat syndrome.

If the wrap slips into the chest, the patient becomes unable to eat and prone to vomiting. A chest radiograph shows a gastric bubble above the diaphragm, and the diagnosis is confirmed by means of a barium swallow. This problem can be prevented by using coronal sutures and by ensuring that the crura are closed securely.

Paraesophageal hernia may occur if the crura have not been closed or if the closure is too loose. In our view, closure of the crura not only is essential for preventing paraesophageal hernia but also is important from a physiologic point of view, in that it acts synergistically with the LES against stress reflux. Sometimes, it is possible to reduce the stomach and close the crura laparoscopically. More often, however, because the crural opening is very tight and the gastric wall is edematous, laparoscopic repair is impossible and laparotomy is preferable.

OUTCOME EVALUATION

Outcome evaluation of laparoscopic Nissen fundoplication is discussed elsewhere in conjunction with outcome evaluation of partial fundoplication [see Laparoscopic Partial (Guarner) Fundoplication, Outcome Evaluation, below].

Laparoscopic Partial (Guarner) Fundoplication

PREOPERATIVE EVALUATION AND OPERATIVE PLANNING

Preoperative evaluation and operative planning are essentially the same for partial (Guarner) fundoplication as for Nissen fundoplication. This operation should be performed only in patients with the most severe abnormalities of esophageal peristalsis: it has been shown to be less effective than a 360° wrap for long-term control of reflux.[9] In addition, laparoscopic partial fundoplication may be performed after laparoscopic Heller myotomy for achalasia.[22]

OPERATIVE TECHNIQUE

The first seven steps in a Guarner fundoplication are identical to the first seven in a Nissen fundoplication. The wrap, however, differs in that it extends around only 240° to 280° of the esophageal circumference. Once the gastric fundus is delivered under the esophagus, the two sides are not approximated over the esophagus. Instead, 80° to 120° of the anterior esophagus is left uncovered, and each of the two sides of the wrap (right and left) is separately affixed to the esophagus with three 2-0 silk sutures, with each stitch including the muscle layer of the esophageal wall. The remaining stitches (i.e., the coronal stitches and those between the right side of the wrap and the closed crura) are identical to those placed in a Nissen fundoplication.

OUTCOME EVALUATION

Initially, our average OR time for a laparoscopic fundoplication was about 3 hours. As we gained more experience and began using the LCS to take down the short gastric vessels, the average operating time decreased: it is now some 60 minutes shorter. We start patients on a soft mechanical diet on the morning of postoperative day 1 and usually discharge them after 23 to 48 hours. The recovery time for the operation is about 7 to 10 days. Long-term follow-up indicates that whereas total fundoplication controls reflux symptoms in about 90% of patients, partial fundoplication has a success rate of about 60% to 70%.

Laparoscopic Heller Myotomy with Partial Fundoplication

It has been demonstrated that minimally invasive surgical procedures for primary esophageal motility disorders (achalasia, diffuse esophageal spasm, and nutcracker esophagus) yield results that are comparable to those of open procedures but are associated with less postoperative pain and with a shorter recovery time.[23] Today, laparoscopic Heller myotomy with partial fundoplication is considered the procedure of choice for esophageal achalasia, replacing the left thoracoscopic approach that was initially favored.[4-7] Long-term studies demonstrated that even though left thoracoscopic myotomy led to resolution of dysphagia in about 85% to 90% of patients, it had the following four drawbacks:

1. Gastroesophageal reflux developed postoperatively in about 60% of patients because no fundoplication was performed in conjunction with the myotomy.[4] With the laparoscopic approach, in contrast, a partial fundoplication can easily be performed, and this prevents reflux in the majority of patients[4,5] as well as corrects many instances of preexisting reflux arising from pneumatic dilatation.[4]
2. The extension of the myotomy onto the gastric wall (clearly the most critical and challenging part of the operation) proved difficult because of poor exposure, with the consequent risk of a short myotomy and persistent dysphagia. With the laparoscopic approach, in contrast, excellent exposure of the esophagogastric junction is easily achieved, and the myotomy can be extended onto the gastric wall for about 2 cm.[4]
3. Double-lumen endotracheal intubation and single-lung ventilation were required, with the patient in the right lateral decubitus position. In contrast, the setting for a laparoscopic myotomy, being the same as that for a laparoscopic fundoplication, is much easier for the patient, the anesthesiologist, and the OR personnel. In addition, most surgeons have by now acquired substantial experience with laparoscopic antireflux procedures and thus are more familiar and comfortable with laparoscopic exposure of the distal esophagus and the esophagogastric junction.

4. After a thoracoscopic myotomy, patients remained in the hospital for about 3 days because of the chest tube left in place at the time of the operation and the discomfort arising from the thoracic incisions. After a laparoscopic Heller myotomy, the hospital stay is only 1 or 2 days; there is no need for a chest tube, and patients are more comfortable.

Because of these drawbacks, left thoracoscopic myotomy is now largely reserved for patients with achalasia who have undergone multiple abdominal operations (which may rule out a laparoscopic approach) and for patients with diffuse esophageal spasm or nutcracker esophagus involving the lower half of the esophagus.

PREOPERATIVE EVALUATION

All candidates for a laparoscopic Heller myotomy should undergo a thorough and careful evaluation to establish the diagnosis and characterize the disease.[24]

An upper GI series is a useful diagnostic test. A characteristic so-called bird beak is usually seen in patients with achalasia. A dilated, sigmoid esophagus may be present in patients with long-standing achalasia. A corkscrew esophagus is often seen in patients with diffuse esophageal spasm.

Endoscopy is performed to rule out a tumor of the esophagogastric junction and gastroduodenal pathology.

Esophageal manometry is the key test for establishing the diagnosis of esophageal achalasia. The classic manometric findings are (1) absence of esophageal peristalsis and (2) a hypertensive LES that fails to relax appropriately in response to swallowing.

Ambulatory pH monitoring should always be done in patients who have undergone pneumatic dilatation to rule out abnormal gastroesophageal reflux. In addition, pH monitoring should be performed postoperatively to detect abnormal reflux, which, if present, should be treated with acid-reducing medications.[24]

In patients older than 60 years who have experienced the recent onset of dysphagia and excessive weight loss, secondary achalasia or pseudoachalasia from cancer of the esophagogastric junction should be ruled out. Endoscopic ultrasonography or computed tomography can help establish the diagnosis.[25]

OPERATIVE PLANNING

Patient preparation (i.e., anesthesia, positioning, and instrumentation) is identical to that for laparoscopic fundoplication.

OPERATIVE TECHNIQUE

Many of the steps in a laparoscopic Heller myotomy are the same as the corresponding steps in a laparoscopic fundoplication. In the ensuing description, we focus on those steps that differ significantly.

To prevent the development of gastroesophageal reflux, a Dor or Guarner fundoplication [see Laparoscopic Partial (Guarner) Fundoplication, above] is often performed in conjunction with a Heller myotomy. The Dor fundoplication is an anterior 180° wrap. Its advantages are that (1) it does not require posterior dissection and the creation of a window between the esophagus, the stomach, and the left pillar of the crus; (2) it covers the exposed esophageal mucosa after completion of the myotomy; and (3) it is effective even in patients with GERD.[26] Its main disadvantage is that achieving the proper geometry can be difficult, and a wrong configuration

can lead to dysphagia even after a properly performed myotomy.[27] The advantages of the Guarner fundoplication are that (1) it is easier to perform; (2) it keeps the edges of the myotomy well separated; and (3) it might be more effective than a Dor procedure in preventing reflux. Its main disadvantages are that (1) it requires more dissection for the creation of a posterior window and (2) it leaves the esophageal mucosa exposed.

Steps 1 through 6

Steps 1, 2, 3, 4, 5, and 6 of a laparoscopic Heller myotomy are essentially identical to the first six steps of a laparoscopic fundoplication. Steps 4 and 6, however, are necessary only if a posterior partial fundoplication is to be performed. Care must be taken not to narrow the esophageal hiatus too much and push the esophagus anteriorly.

Step 7: Intraoperative Endoscopy

The esophageal stethoscope and the orogastric tube are removed, and an endoscope is inserted. The endoscopic view allows easy identification of the squamocolumnar junction, so that the myotomy can be extended downward onto the gastric wall for about 2 cm distal to this point. In addition, if possible mucosal perforation is a concern, the esophagus can be covered with water from outside while air is insufflated from inside; bubbling will be observed over the site of any perforation present.

At the beginning of a surgeon's experience with laparoscopic Heller myotomy, intraoperative endoscopy is a very important and helpful step; however, once the surgeon has gained adequate experience with this procedure and has become familiar with the landmarks between esophageal and gastric musculature from a laparoscopic perspective, it can be omitted.

Troubleshooting The most worrisome complication during this step is perforation of the esophagus. This complication can be prevented by having an experienced endoscopist who is familiar with achalasia perform the procedure intraoperatively.

Step 8: Initiation of Myotomy and Entry into Submucosal Plane at Single Point

The fat pad is removed with the LCS to provide clear exposure of the esophagogastric junction. A Babcock clamp is then applied over the junction, and the esophagus is pulled downward and to the left; this maneuver exposes the right side of the esophagus. The myotomy is performed at the 11 o'clock position. It is helpful to mark the surface of the esophagus along the line through which the myotomy will be carried out [see Figure 3]. The myotomy is started about 3 cm above the esophagogastric junction. Before it is extended upward and downward, the proper submucosal plane should be reached at a single point; in this way, the likelihood of subsequent mucosal perforation can be reduced.

Troubleshooting The myotomy should not be started close to the esophagogastric junction, because at this level the layers often are poorly defined, particularly if multiple dilatations or injections of botulinum toxin have been performed. It is easier to start about 3 cm above the esophagogastric junction, where the esophageal wall is usually normal. As a rule, we do not open the entire longitudinal layer first and then the circular layer; we find it easier and safer to try to reach the submucosal plane at one point and then move upward and down-

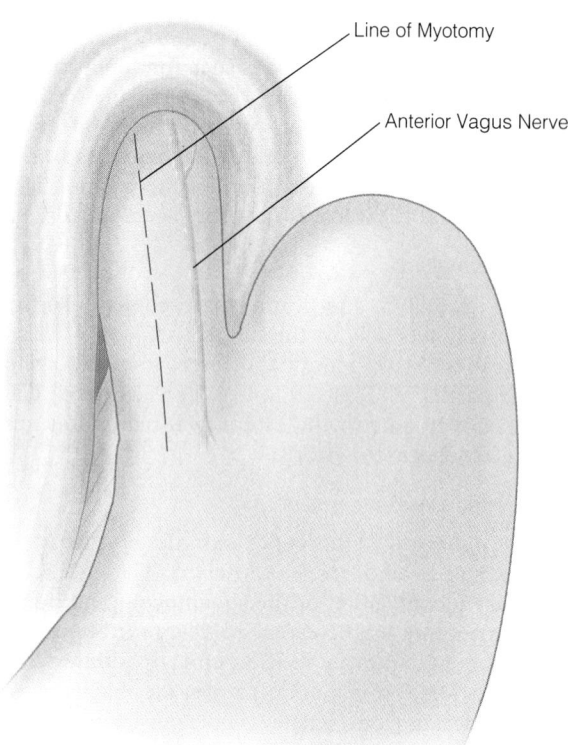

Figure 3 **Laparoscopic Heller myotomy with partial fundoplication. The proposed myotomy line is marked on the surface of the esophagus.**

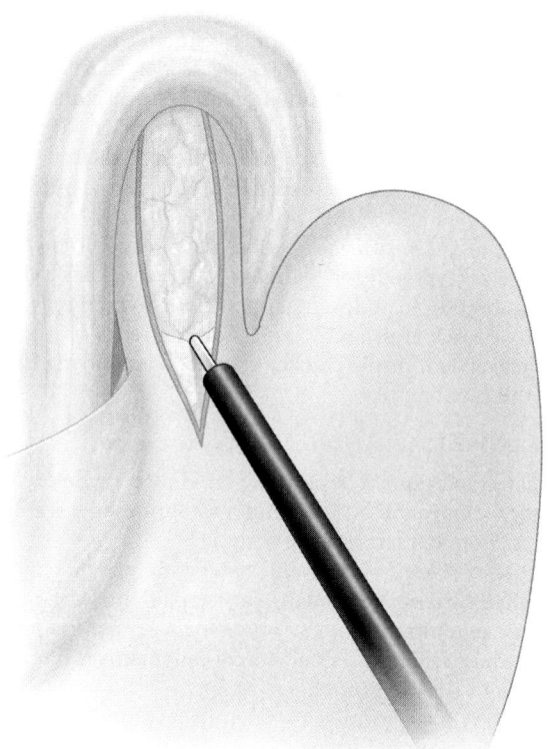

Figure 4 **Laparoscopic Heller myotomy with partial fundoplication. The myotomy is extended proximally and distally.**

ward from there. In the course of the myotomy, there is always some bleeding from the cut muscle fibers, particularly if the esophagus is dilated and the wall is very thick. After the source of the bleeding is identified by irrigation, the electrocautery must be used with caution. The most troublesome bleeding comes from the submucosal veins (which are usually large) encountered at the esophagogastric junction. In most instances, gentle compression is preferable to electrocautery. A sponge introduced through one of the ports facilitates the application of direct pressure.

Step 9: Proximal and Distal Extension of Myotomy

Once the mucosa has been exposed, the myotomy can safely be extended proximally and distally [*see Figure 4*]. Distally, we extend the myotomy for about 2 cm onto the gastric wall. Proximally, we extend it for about 6 cm above the esophagogastric junction. Thus, the total length of the myotomy is typically about 8 cm [*see Figure 5*].

Troubleshooting   It is vital to identify the course of the anterior vagus nerve before the myotomy is started. If this nerve crosses the line of the myotomy, it must be lifted away from the esophageal wall, and the muscle layers must then be cut under it. In addition, care must be taken not to injure the anterior vagus nerve while removing the fat pad. Treatment with botulinum toxin occasionally results in fibrosis with scarring and loss of the normal anatomic planes; this occurs more frequently at the level of the esophagogastric junction.

If a perforation seems possible or likely, it should be sought as described earlier [*see Step 7, above*]. Any perforation found should be repaired with 5-0 absorbable suture material, with interrupted sutures employed for a small perforation and a

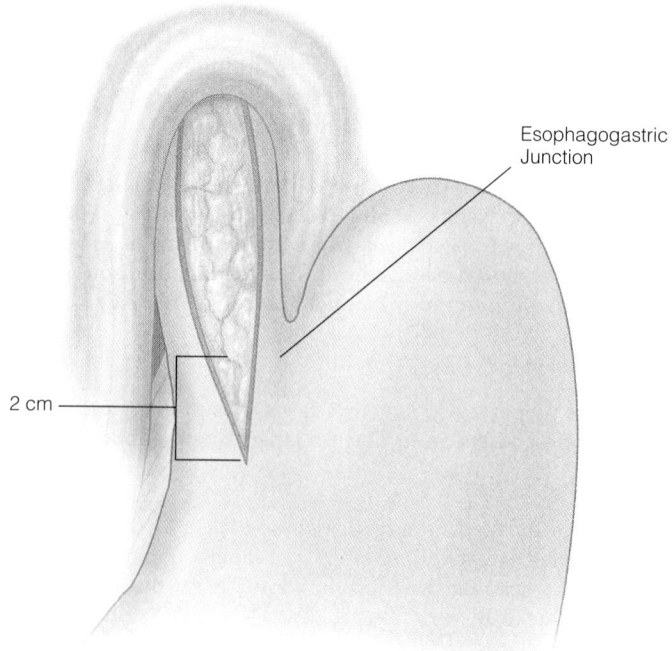

Figure 5 **Laparoscopic Heller myotomy with partial fundoplication. The myotomy is approximately 8 cm long, extending distally for about 2 cm onto the gastric wall and proximally for about 6 cm above the esophagogastric junction.**

continuous suture for a larger one. When a perforation has occurred, an anterior fundoplication is usually chosen in preference to a posterior one because the stomach will offer further protection against a leak.

Step 10 (Dor Procedure): Anterior Partial Fundoplication

Two rows of sutures are placed. The first row (on the left side) comprises three stitches: the uppermost stitch incorporates the gastric fundus, the esophageal wall, and the left pillar of the crus [*see Figure 6*], and the other two incorporate only the gastric fundus and the left side of the esophageal wall [*see Figure 7*]. The gastric fundus is then folded over the myotomy, and the second row (also comprising three stitches) is placed

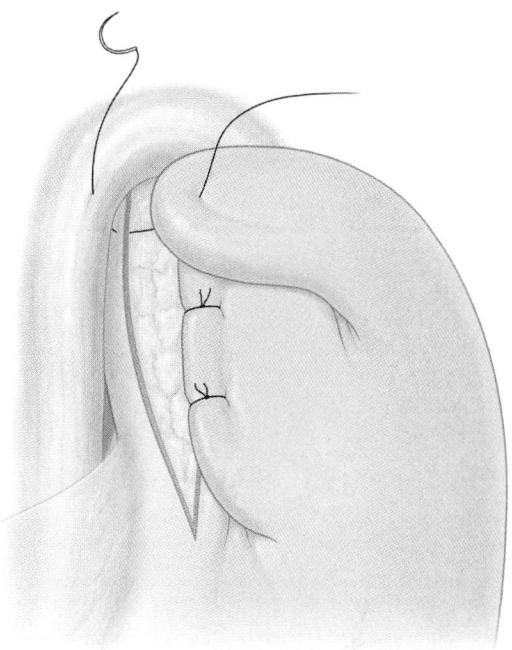

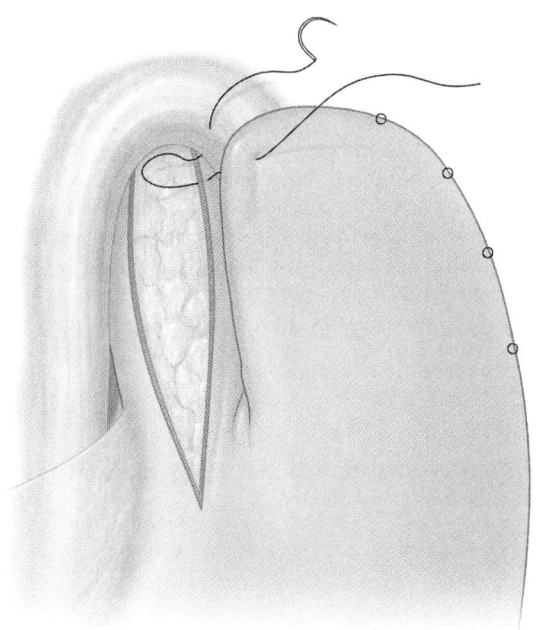

Figure 6 Laparoscopic Heller myotomy with anterior partial fundoplication (Dor procedure). The uppermost stitch in the first row incorporates the fundus, the esophageal wall, and the left pillar of the crus.

Figure 8 Laparoscopic Heller myotomy with anterior partial fundoplication (Dor procedure). The uppermost stitch in the second row incorporates the fundus, the esophageal wall, and the right crus.

on the right side between the fundus and the right side of the esophageal wall, with only the uppermost stitch incorporating the right crus [*see Figures 8 and 9*]. Finally, two additional stitches are placed between the anterior rim of the hiatus and the superior aspect of the fundoplication [*see Figure 10*].

Troubleshooting Efforts must be made to ensure that the fundoplication does not become a cause of postoperative dysphagia. To this end, we always take down the short gastric vessels, even though some authorities suggest that this step can be omitted.[5,26] In addition, the gastric fundus rather than the body of the stomach should be used for the wrap, and only the uppermost stitch of the right row of sutures should incorporate the right pillar of the crus.[27]

Step 10 (Guarner Procedure): Posterior Partial Fundoplication

Alternatively, a posterior 220° fundoplication may be performed. The gastric fundus is delivered under the esophagus, and each side of the wrap (right and left) is attached to the esophageal wall, lateral to the myotomy, with three sutures [*see Figure 11*].

Step 11: Final Inspection and Removal of Instruments and Ports from Abdomen

Step 11 of a laparoscopic Heller myotomy is identical to step 9 of a laparoscopic Nissen fundoplication.

POSTOPERATIVE COMPLICATIONS

Delayed esophageal leakage, which is most often the result of an electrocautery burn to the esophageal mucosa, may occur during the first 24 to 36 hours after operation. The characteristic signals are chest pain, fever, and a pleural effusion on the chest x-ray. The diagnosis is confirmed by an esophagogram. Treatment options depend on the time of diagnosis and on the

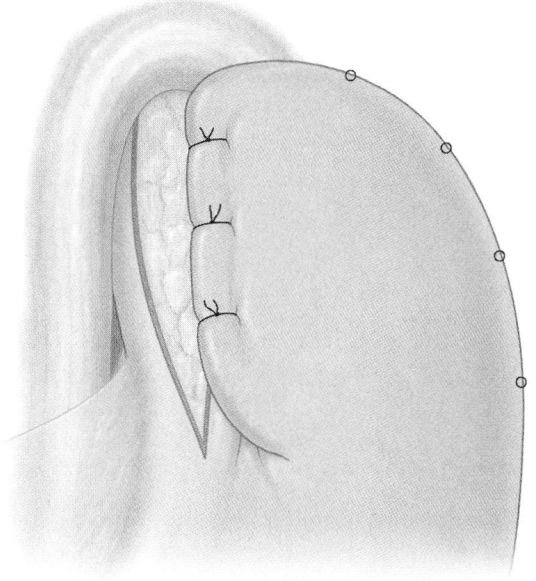

Figure 7 Laparoscopic Heller myotomy with anterior partial fundoplication (Dor procedure). The second and third stitches in the first row incorporate only the fundus and the left side of the esophageal wall.

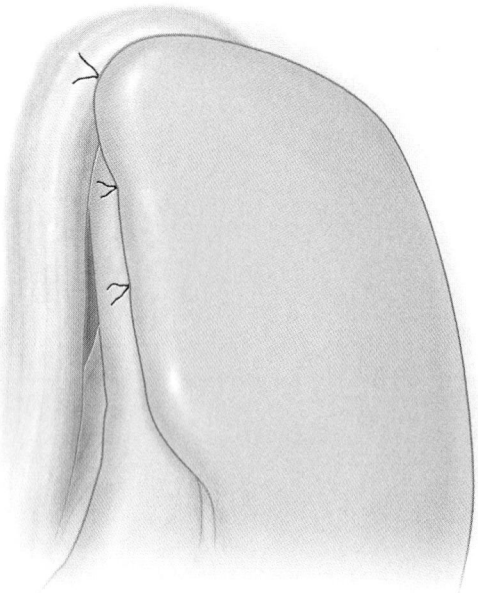

Figure 9 **Laparoscopic Heller myotomy with anterior partial fundoplication (Dor procedure). The second and third stitches in the second row incorporate only the fundus and the right side of the esophageal wall.**

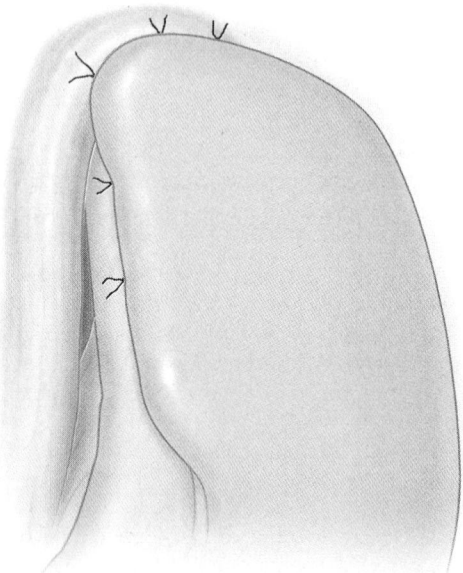

Figure 10 **Laparoscopic Heller myotomy with anterior partial fundoplication (Dor procedure). Two final stitches are placed between the superior portion of the wrap and the anterior rim of the hiatus.**

size and location of the leak. Early, small leaks can be repaired directly. If the site of the leak is high in the chest, a thoracotomy provides the best approach for the repair; if the site is at the level of the esophagogastric junction, a laparotomy provides the best approach, and the stomach can be used to reinforce the repair. If the damage to the esophagus is too extensive to permit repair, a transhiatal esophagectomy [see *3:9 Open Esophageal Procedures*] is indicated.

Dysphagia may either persist after the operation or recur after a symptom-free interval. In either case, a complete

workup is necessary, and treatment is individualized on the basis of the specific cause of dysphagia. Reoperation may be indicated [*see* Reoperation for Esophageal Achalasia, *below*].

Abnormal gastroesophageal reflux occurs in 7% to 20% of patients after operation.[4,5] Because most patients are asymptomatic, it is essential to try to evaluate all patients postoperatively with manometry and prolonged pH monitoring. Reflux should be treated with acid-reducing medications.

OUTCOME EVALUATION

We do not routinely obtain an esophagogram before initiating feeding. We start patients on a soft mechanical diet on the morning of postoperative day 1, and this diet is continued for the rest of the first week. Patients are discharged after 24 to 48 hours and are able to resume regular activities in 7 to 14 days.

The results obtained to date with laparoscopic Heller myotomy and partial fundoplication are excellent and are generally comparable to those obtained with the corresponding open surgical procedures: dysphagia is reduced or eliminated in more than 90% of patients.[4-7]

Left Thoracoscopic Myotomy

PREOPERATIVE EVALUATION

Preoperative evaluation is essentially the same as that for laparoscopic Heller myotomy.

OPERATIVE PLANNING

The patient is placed under general anesthesia and intubated with a double-lumen endotracheal tube so that the left lung can be deflated during the procedure.

The patient is placed in the right lateral decubitus position over an inflated bean bag, as for a left thoracotomy.

The instrumentation for this procedure is similar to that for a laparoscopic Nissen or Guarner fundoplication. Instead of

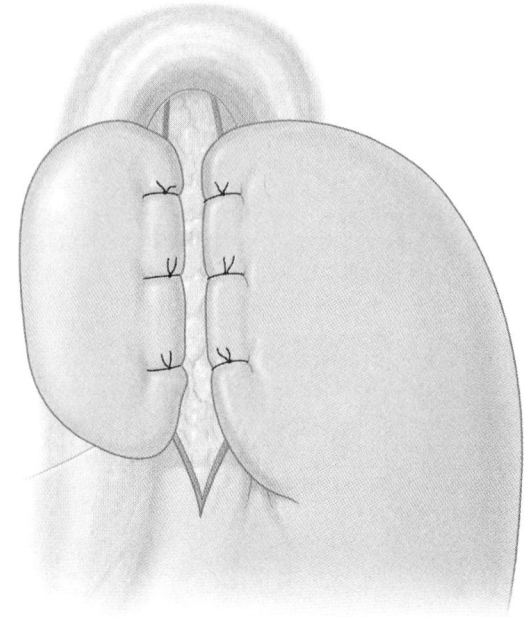

Figure 11 **Laparoscopic Heller myotomy with posterior partial fundoplication (Guarner procedure). Each side of the posterior 220° wrap is attached to the esophageal wall with three sutures.**

conventional trocars, we use four or five thoracoports with blunt obturators because insufflation of the thoracic cavity is not required. The myotomy can be performed with a monopolar hook cautery, bipolar scissors, or an ultrasonic scalpel (e.g., the Harmonic Scalpel, Ethicon Endo-Surgery, Inc.). A 30° scope and a 45° scope are essential instruments for the performance of thoracoscopic procedures. In addition, an endoscope is used for intraoperative endoscopy.

OPERATIVE TECHNIQUE

Step 1: Insertion of Thoracoports

Five ports are usually placed [*see Figure 12*]. Port A is inserted in the sixth intercostal space about 3.5 to 5 cm behind the posterior axillary line. This port is used for the 30° scope. Port B is placed in the third intercostal space about 1.25 to 2.5 cm anterior to the posterior axillary line. This port is used for the lung retractor. Port C is placed in the sixth intercostal space in the anterior axillary line. It is used for insertion of a grasper. Port D is placed in the seventh intercostal space in the midaxillary line. It is used for insertion of the instrument used for the myotomy. Port E is placed in the eighth intercostal space between the anterior axillary line and the midaxillary line. This port is optional: it is needed in about 30% of cases to allow the surgeon to obtain further exposure of the esophagogastric junction through retraction of the diaphragm.

Troubleshooting   A common mistake is to insert port A too anteriorly. This port must be placed well beyond the posterior axillary line to provide the best angle for the 30° scope. Often, the other ports are placed one or two intercostal spaces too high. This mistake hampers the performance of the most delicate portion of the operation, the myotomy of the distal portion of the esophagus and the stomach.

Sometimes, bleeding occurs from the chest wall as a result of the insertion of the ports. The dripping blood will obscure the operating field, and consequently, it is essential to stop the bleeding before the intrathoracic portion of the procedure is begun. Bleeding can be stopped either by using the cautery from the inside or by applying a stitch from the outside if an intercostal vessel has been damaged.

Step 2: Retraction of Left Lung and Division of Inferior Pulmonary Ligament

Once the ports are in place, the deflated left lung is retracted cephalad with a fan retractor introduced through port B. This maneuver places tension on the inferior pulmonary ligament, which is then divided. After the ligament is divided, the fan retractor can be held in place by a self-retaining system fixed to the operating table.

Troubleshooting   Before the inferior pulmonary ligament is divided, the inferior pulmonary vein must be identified to prevent a life-threatening injury to this vessel. If oxygen saturation decreases, particularly in patients with lung disease, the retractor should be removed and the lung inflated intermittently.

Step 3: Division of Mediastinal Pleura and Dissection of Periesophageal Tissues

The mediastinal pleura is divided, and the tissues overlying the esophageal wall are dissected until the wall of the esophagus is visible. This maneuver varies in difficulty depending on

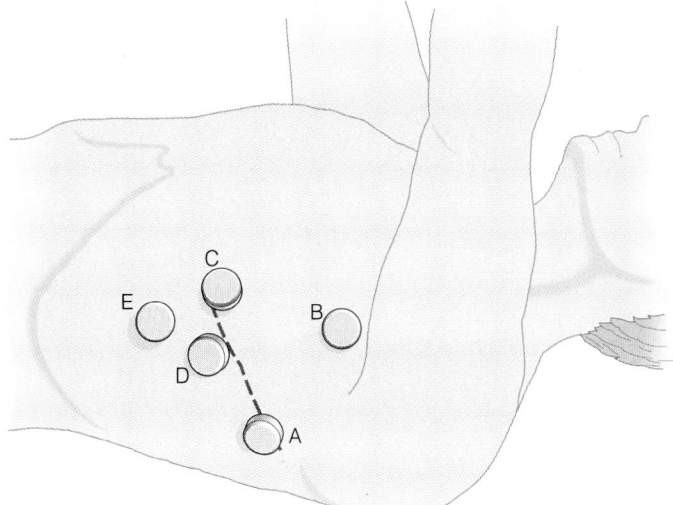

Figure 12   **Left thoracoscopic myotomy. Illustrated is the recommended placement of the thoracoports.**

the width of the space between the aorta and the pericardium (which sometimes is very small) and on the size and shape of the esophagus. Large (sigmoid) esophagi tend to curve to the right, which makes identification of the wall difficult. If the esophagus is not immediately apparent, it can be easily identified in the groove between the heart and the aorta by means of transillumination provided by an endoscope [*see Figure 13*].

Troubleshooting   The endoscope placed inside the esophagus at the beginning of the procedure plays an important role. In the early stages of the procedure, it allows identification of the esophagus via transillumination. When the light intensity of the 30° scope is turned down, the esophagus appears as a bright structure. In addition, tilting the tip of the endoscope brings the esophagus into view as it is lifted from the groove between the aorta and the heart.

Step 4: Initiation of Myotomy and Entry into Submucosal Plane at Single Point

As in a laparoscopic Heller myotomy, it is helpful to mark the surface of the esophagus along the line through which the myotomy will be carried out. The myotomy is started halfway between the diaphragm and the inferior pulmonary vein. Again, the proper submucosal plane should be reached at a single point before the myotomy is extended upward and downward.

Troubleshooting   Troubleshooting for this step is essentially the same as that for step 8 of a laparoscopic Heller myotomy, with the exception that here the myotomy is started 4 to 5 cm (rather than 3 cm) above the esophagogastric junction.

Step 5: Proximal and Distal Extension of Myotomy

Once the mucosa has been exposed, the myotomy can safely be extended proximally and distally [*see Figure 14*]. We usually extend the myotomy for about 5 mm onto the gastric wall, without adding an antireflux procedure.[3,4] Typically, the total length of the myotomy is about 6 cm for patients with achalasia.

Troubleshooting   Proximally, we extend the myotomy all the way to the inferior pulmonary vein only in cases of vigorous

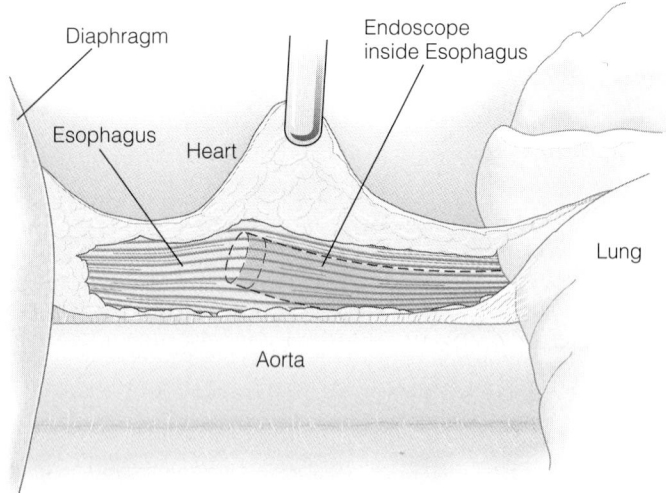

Figure 13   **Left thoracoscopic myotomy. The esophagus may be identified by means of transillumination from the endoscope.**

achalasia (high-amplitude simultaneous contractions associated with chest pain in addition to dysphagia) or diffuse esophageal spasm; otherwise, we limit the myotomy to the distal 5 to 6 cm of the esophagus. If a longer myotomy is needed, the lung is displaced anteriorly and the myotomy extended to the aortic arch.

Distally, we continue the myotomy for 5 mm past the esophagogastric junction. We use the endoluminal view provided by the endoscope to assess the location of the esophagogastric junction. Often, the stomach is distended by the air insufflated by the endoscope and pushes the diaphragm upward, thereby limiting the view of the esophagogastric junction. If sucking air out of the stomach does not resolve this problem, an additional port (i.e., port E) may be placed in the eighth intercostal space, and a fan retractor may be introduced through this port to push the diaphragm down.

Because the myotomy of the gastric wall is the most challenging part of the operation, good exposure is essential. It is at

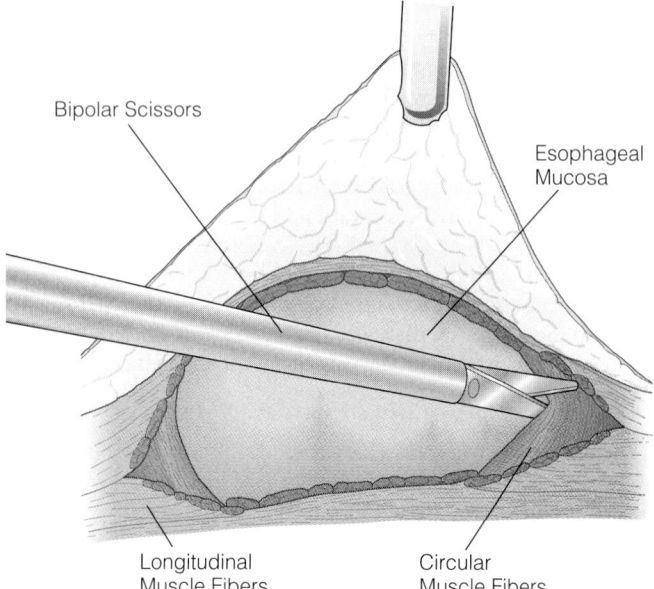

Figure 14   **Left thoracoscopic myotomy. Shown are the distal and proximal extensions of the myotomy.**

this level that an esophageal perforation is most likely to occur. The risk is particularly high in patients who have undergone pneumatic dilatation or injection of botulinum toxin, both of which may lead to the replacement of muscle layers by scar tissue and the consequent loss of the regular planes. Perforations recognized in the OR can be repaired by thoracoscopic intracorporeal suturing or, if this fails, by thoracotomy and open repair. The gastric fundus can be used to buttress the repair. If it is unclear whether a perforation has occurred, the esophagus should be covered with water and air insufflated through the endoscope as described earlier [*see* Laparoscopic Heller Myotomy with Partial Fundoplication, Operative Technique, Step 7, *above*].

Step 6: Insertion of Chest Tube and Removal of Thoracoports

A 24 French angled chest tube is inserted under direct vision through port D or port E. The ports are removed under direct vision, and the thoracic wall is inspected for bleeding.

POSTOPERATIVE COMPLICATIONS

As with laparoscopic Heller myotomy, delayed esophageal leakage is a common postoperative complication, and treatment options are similar.

If the myotomy is not extended far enough onto the gastric wall, residual dysphagia occurs. To prevent this problem, the distal extent of the myotomy should be assessed by the endoscopist, who will confirm that the myotomy includes 5 mm of the gastric wall. Patients with residual dysphagia must be evaluated by means of esophageal manometry, which will document the extent of and the pressure in the residual high-pressure zone. The myotomy can be easily extended by a laparoscopic approach, and a Dor fundoplication can be added.

If, on the other hand, the myotomy is extended too far onto the gastric wall, abnormal gastroesophageal reflux occurs. Some patients present with heartburn; others are asymptomatic. It is essential to evaluate patients postoperatively with manometry and prolonged pH monitoring. Mild reflux can be treated with acid-reducing medications, particularly in elderly patients. In younger patients, abnormal reflux should be corrected by means of a laparoscopic partial fundoplication (e.g., Dor fundoplication).

OUTCOME EVALUATION

We start patients on a liquid diet the morning of postoperative day 1; on postoperative day 2, we start them on a soft mechanical diet, which is continued for the rest of the first week. We do not routinely obtain an esophagogram before starting feedings. The chest tube is removed after 24 hours if the lung is fully expanded and there is no air leak. Patients are discharged after 48 to 72 hours and are able to resume regular activities in 7 to 10 days.

The results obtained with thoracoscopic esophageal myotomy are generally comparable to those obtained with open surgical procedures. Of the first 30 patients with achalasia whom we treated in this fashion, 26 (87%) experienced good or excellent results [*see Table 2*].[4]

Right Thoracoscopic Myotomy

A long myotomy from the diaphragm to the thoracic inlet, performed via a right thoracoscopic approach, is the preferred procedure for patients who have nutcracker esophagus or dif-

Table 2 Results of Thoracoscopic Myotomy in 30 Patients with Achalasia

Results	Patients (% of Total)
Excellent (no dysphagia)	21 (70)
Good (dysphagia < once/wk)	5 (17)
Fair (dysphagia > once/wk)	3 (10)
Poor (persistent dysphagia)	1 (3)

fuse esophageal spasm involving the entire length of the esophagus but who have normal LES function. On the whole, this procedure is technically simpler than a left thoracoscopic myotomy: because there is no need to go through the esophagogastric junction, perforation, postoperative dysphagia, and abnormal gastroesophageal reflux are largely prevented.

PREOPERATIVE EVALUATION

Preoperative evaluation of patients being considered for right thoracoscopic myotomy is essentially the same as that of patients being considered for left thoracoscopic myotomy.

OPERATIVE PLANNING

Operative planning is similar to that for a left thoracoscopic myotomy. The double-lumen tube is used to deflate the right lung rather than the left.

The patient is placed in the left lateral decubitus position over an inflated bean bag, as for a right thoracotomy.

The instrumentation is identical except for the endovascular 30 mm stapler used to transect the azygos vein. It is essential to have a thoracotomy tray ready in case an emergency thoracotomy is necessary to control bleeding.

OPERATIVE TECHNIQUE

Step 1: Insertion of Thoracoports

Only port B is inserted where it would be for a left thoracoscopic myotomy. All the other ports are inserted one intercostal space higher because the myotomy need not be extended all the way to the stomach but must be extended to the thoracic inlet. Usually, only four ports are used; however, an additional port can be placed in the fourth intercostal space in the anterior axillary line to facilitate the proximal extension of the myotomy.

Step 2: Dissection of Periesophageal Tissues and Division of Azygos Vein

The periesophageal tissues above and below the azygos vein are dissected away from the esophagus. A tunnel is created between the azygos vein and the esophagus with a dissector, a right-angle clamp, or both. The azygos vein is then transected with an endovascular 30 mm stapler. (Alternatively, the azygos vein can be spared and simply lifted off the esophagus with umbilical tape.)

Troubleshooting Dissection of the azygos vein is the most critical part of this procedure. We have found that it is easier to transect the azygos vein than to keep the vein lifted away from the esophagus and perform the myotomy under it.

Steps 3, 4, and 5

Steps 3, 4, and 5 of a right thoracoscopic myotomy are virtually identical to steps 4, 5, and 6 of a left thoracoscopic myotomy, with a few minor exceptions. Once the submucosal plane is reached, the myotomy is extended distally to the diaphragm and proximally to the thoracic inlet. The endoscope plays a less critical role in this procedure than in a left thoracoscopic myotomy because the esophagus is easily identified and because the myotomy is not extended through the esophagogastric junction. Instead, we place a 52 to 56 French bougie inside the esophagus. This facilitates the division of the circular fibers and separates the edges of the myotomy nicely.

COMPLICATIONS

A delayed esophageal leak is the most common postoperative complication. It should be handled as described earlier [*see* Laparoscopic Heller Myotomy with Partial Fundoplication, Postoperative Complications, *above*].

OUTCOME EVALUATION

The postoperative course of patients who have undergone this procedure is usually identical to that of patients operated on for achalasia. Complete relief of chest pain is obtained in about 75% to 80% of patients.[23]

Reoperation for GERD

Over the past 10 years, we have seen an increasing number of patients being referred to the UCSF Swallowing Center for evaluation and treatment of foregut symptoms after laparoscopic antireflux surgery. In what follows, we describe our approach to this highly challenging group of patients.

PREOPERATIVE EVALUATION

Some degree of dysphagia, bloating, and abdominal discomfort is common during the first 6 to 8 weeks after a fundoplication. If these symptoms persist or heartburn and regurgitation occur, a thorough evaluation (with barium swallow, endoscopy, esophageal manometry, and pH monitoring) is carried out with the aim of answering the following three questions:

1. Are the symptoms attributable to persistent gastroesophageal reflux?
2. Are the symptoms attributable to the fundoplication itself?
3. Can the cause of the failure of the first operation be identified and corrected by a second operation?

Many patients report heartburn after a fundoplication. It is often assumed that this symptom must be the result of a failed operation and that acid-reducing medications should be restarted. In the majority of patients, however, this assumption is mistaken: postoperative pH monitoring yields abnormal results in only about 20% of patients.[28] The value of manometry lies in its ability to document the changes caused by the operation at the level of the LES and the esophageal body. The pH monitoring assesses the reflux status and determines whether there is a correlation between symptoms experienced by the patient and actual episodes of reflux. If abnormal reflux is in fact present, the therapeutic choice is between medical therapy and a second operation.

Other patients complain of dysphagia arising de novo after the operation. This symptom is usually attributable to the operation itself, and it can occur in the absence of abnormal reflux. In addition to manometry and pH monitoring, a barium swallow is essential to define the anatomy of the esophagogastric junction. As shown by investigators from the University of Washington,[29] the anatomic configurations observed can generally be divided into three main types: (1) type I hernia, in which the esophagogastric junction is above the diaphragm (further subdivided into type IA, in which both the esophagogastric junction and the wrap are above the diaphragm, and type IB, in which only the esophagogastric junction is above the diaphragm); (2) type II hernia, a paraesophageal configuration; and (3) type III hernia, in which the esophagogastric junction is below the diaphragm and there is no evidence of hernia but in which the body of the stomach rather than the gastric fundus is used to perform the wrap. In 10% of patients, however, the investigators could not identify the cause of the failure preoperatively.[29]

Some patients present with a mix of postprandial bloating, nausea, and diarrhea. These symptoms may be the result of damage to the vagus nerves. Radionuclide evaluation of gastric emptying of solids and liquids often helps quantify the problem.

OPERATIVE PLANNING

Patient preparation (i.e., anesthesia, positioning, and instrumentation) for operations for reflux is identical to that for the initial laparoscopic fundoplication.

OPERATIVE TECHNIQUE

We routinely attempt a second antireflux operation laparoscopically; however, if the dissection does not proceed smoothly, a laparotomy is performed. To provide a stepwise technical description that would be suitable for all reoperations for reflux is impossible because the optimal procedure depends on the original approach (open versus laparoscopic), the severity of the adhesions, and the specific technique used for the first operation (total or partial fundoplication). The key goals of reoperation for reflux are as follows:

1. To dissect the wrap and the esophagus away from the crura. This is the most difficult part of the operation. The major complications seen during this part of the procedure are damage to the vagus nerves and perforation of the esophagus and the gastric fundus.
2. To take down the previous repair. The earlier repair must be completely undone and the gastric fundus returned to its natural position. If the short gastric vessels were not taken down during the first procedure, they must be taken down during the second.
3. To dissect the esophagus in the posterior mediastinum so as to have enough esophageal length below the diaphragm and avoid placing tension on the repair.
4. To reconstruct the cardia. We follow the same steps described for a first time repair. If, after extensive esophageal mobilization, the esophagogastric junction remains above the diaphragm (short esophagus), esophageal lengthening can be accomplished by adding a thoracoscopic Collis gastroplasty to the fundoplication. In our entire laparoscopic experience to date, however, we have not yet found this step to be necessary.

POSTOPERATIVE COMPLICATIONS

The risk of gastric or esophageal perforation or of damage to the vagus nerves is much higher during a second antireflux operation. Accordingly, the surgeon must stand ready to convert to a laparotomy if the dissection proves too cumbersome or the structures are not properly identified. Most perforations are recognized and repaired intraoperatively. A leak will manifest itself during the first 48 hours. Peritoneal signs will be noted if the spillage is limited to the abdomen; shortness of breath and a pleural effusion will be noted if spillage also occurs in the chest. The site of the leak should always be confirmed by means of a contrast study with barium or a water-soluble contrast agent. Perforation is best handled through laparotomy and direct repair.

OUTCOME EVALUATION

Whereas the success rate is around 90% for a first antireflux operation, it falls to 75% to 80% for a second such operation. In our opinion, a second operation should be attempted by an expert team only if medical management fails to control heartburn or pneumatic dilatation has not relieved dysphagia.

Reoperation for Esophageal Achalasia

Laparoscopic Heller myotomy improves swallowing in more than 90% of patients. What causes the relatively few failures reported is still incompletely understood. Typically, a failed Heller myotomy is signaled either by persistent dysphagia or by recurrent dysphagia that develops after a variable symptom-free interval following the original operation.

A complete workup (routinely including barium swallow, endoscopy, manometry, and pH monitoring) is required before treatment is planned. In addition, it is our practice to review the video of the first operation to search for technical errors that might have been responsible for the poor outcome. Such errors typically fall into one of the following three categories.

1. A too-short myotomy. The myotomy can be too short either distally or proximally. If the myotomy is too short distally, a barium swallow shows persistent distal esophageal narrowing and manometry shows a residual high-pressure zone. If the myotomy is too short proximally, it will be apparent from the barium swallow.
2. A constricting Dor fundoplication. Often, manometry and pH monitoring yield normal results, but a barium swallow shows slow passage of contrast media from the esophagus into the stomach. In our own experience,[27] problems with Dor fundoplications occurred in four (4%) of 102 patients. Analysis of the video records of the first operations showed that in three of the four patients, all the stitches in the right suture row had incorporated the esophagus, the right pillar of the crus, and the stomach, thereby constricting the myotomy. In one patient, the short gastric vessels had not been taken down, and the body of the stomach rather than the gastric fundus had been used for the fundoplication.
3. Transmural scarring caused by previous treatment. In patients treated with intrasphincteric injection of botulinum toxin, transmural fibrosis can sometimes be found at the level of the esophagogastric junction. This unwelcome finding makes the myotomy more difficult and the results less reliable.

There are two treatment options for persistent or recurrent dysphagia after Heller myotomy: (1) pneumatic dilatation and (2) a second operation tailored to the results of preoperative evaluation. In a 2002 study,[30] pneumatic dilatation was successfully used to treat seven of 10 patients who experienced dysphagia postoperatively; of the remaining three patients, two required a second operation and one refused any treatment.

Our own experience has been different: we found pneumatic dilatation to be effective in only one (short distal myotomy) of the eight patients in whom it was tried.[27] The only one of our patients who was helped by dilatation was the one with a short distal myotomy; none of the four patients with dysphagia resulting from a poorly constructed Dor fundoplication derived any benefit. In two patients who had a short proximal myotomy, we successfully extended the myotomy to the inferior pulmonary vein through a left thoracoscopic approach. Of the four patients with a constricting Dor fundoplication, two underwent a second operation during which the Dor was taken down, and one of these two had a second myotomy. Both patients are free of dysphagia; however, they experience abnormal reflux and are currently being treated with acid-reducing medications.

Reoperation for achalasia is a technically challenging procedure. It is of paramount importance to avoid perforating the exposed esophageal mucosa during the dissection. A small hole can be repaired, but a larger laceration might necessitate an esophagectomy. This option should always be discussed with the patient before the operation.

Overall, about 10% of patients have some degree of dysphagia after a Heller myotomy. Pneumatic dilatation, a second operation, or both should always be tried before a radical procedure such as esophagectomy is decided on.

References

1. Csendes A, Braghetto I, Henriquez A, et al: Late results of a prospective randomized study comparing forceful dilatation and oesophagomyotomy in patients with achalasia. Gut 30:299, 1989
2. Hinder RA, Filipi CJ, Wetscher G, et al: Laparoscopic Nissen fundoplication is an effective treatment for gastroesophageal reflux disease. Ann Surg 220:472, 1994
3. Pellegrini CA, Wetter LA, Patti MG, et al: Thoracoscopic esophagomyotomy: initial experience with a new approach for the treatment of achalasia. Ann Surg 216:291, 1992
4. Patti MG, Pellegrini CA, Horgan S, et al: Minimally invasive surgery for achalasia. An 8 year experience with 168 patients. Ann Surg 587:230, 1999
5. Zaninotto G, Costantini M, Molena D, et al: Treatment of esophageal achalasia with laparoscopic Heller myotomy and Dor partial anterior fundoplication: prospective evaluation of 100 consecutive patients. J Gastrointest Surg 282:4, 2000
6. Ackroyd R, Watson DI, Devitt PG, et al: Laparoscopic cardiomyotomy and anterior partial fundoplication for achalasia. Surg Endosc 683:15, 2001
7. Finley RJ, Clifton JC, Stewart KC, et al: Laparoscopic Heller myotomy improves esophageal emptying and the symptoms of achalasia. Arch Surg 892:136, 2001
8. Patti MG, Arcerito M, Feo CV, et al: An analysis of operations for gastroesophageal reflux disease: identifying the important technical elements. Arch Surg 600:133, 2001
9. Horvath KD, Jobe BA, Herron DM, et al: Laparoscopic Toupet fundoplication is an inadequate procedure for patients with severe reflux disease. J Gastrointest Surg 583:3, 1999
10. Sonnenberg A, Delco F, El-Serag HB: Empirical therapy versus diagnostic tests in gastroesophageal reflux disease: a medical decision analysis. Dig Dis Sci 1001:43, 1998
11. Johnsson F, Joelsson B, Gudmundsson K, et al: Symptoms and endoscopic findings in the diagnosis of gastroesophageal reflux disease. Scan J Gastroenterol 714:22, 1987
12. Patti MG, Diener U, Tamburini A, et al: Role of esophageal function tests in the diagnosis of gastroesophageal reflux disease. Dig Dis Sci 597:46, 2001
13. Campos GM, Peters JH, DeMeester TR, et al: Multivariate analysis of factors predicting outcome after laparoscopic Nissen fundoplication. J Gastrointest Surg 292:3, 1999
14. Patti MG, Goldberg HI, Arcerito M, et al: Hiatal hernia size affects the lower esophageal sphincter function, esophageal acid exposure, and the degree of mucosal injury. Am J Surg 182:171, 1996
15. Bytzer P, Havelund T, Moller Hansen J: Interobserver variation in the endoscopic diagnosis of reflux esophagitis. Scan J Gastroenterol 119:28, 1993
16. Fuchs KH, DeMeester TR, Albertucci M: Specificity and sensitivity of objective diagnosis of gastroesophageal reflux disease. Surgery 575:102, 1987
17. Patti MG, Arcerito M, Tamburini A, et al: Effect of laparoscopic fundoplication on GERD-induced respiratory symptoms. J Gastrointest Surg 143:4, 2000
18. Diener U, Patti MG, Molena D, et al: Esophageal dysmotility and gastroesophageal reflux disease. J Gastrointest Surg 260:5, 2001
19. Horgan S, Pellegrini CA: Surgical treatment of gastroesophageal reflux disease. Surg Clin North Am 1063:77, 1997
20. Guelrud M, Rossiter A, Souney PF, et al: The effect of vasoactive intestinal polypeptide on the lower esophageal sphincter in achalasia. Gastroenterology 103:377, 1992
21. Tottrup A, Svane D, Forman A: Nitric oxide mediating NANC inhibition in opossum lower esophageal sphincter. Am J Physiol 260:385, 1991
22. Champion JK, Delisle N, Hunt T: Laparoscopic esophagomyotomy with posterior partial fundoplication for primary esophageal motility disorders. Surg Endosc 746:14, 2000
23. Patti MG, Pellegrini CA, Arcerito M, et al: Comparison of medical and minimally invasive surgical therapy for primary esophageal motility disorders. Arch Surg 130:609, 1995
24. Patti MG, Diener U, Molena D: Esophageal achalasia: preoperative assessment and postoperative follow-up. J Gastrointest Surg 11:5, 2001
25. Moonka R, Patti MG, Feo CV, et al: Clinical presentation and evaluation of malignant pseudoachalasia. J Gastrointest Surg 456:3, 1999
26. Watson DI, Liu JF, Devitt PG, et al: Outcome of laparoscopic anterior 180-degree partial fundoplication for gastroesophageal reflux disease. J Gastrointest Surg 486:4, 2000
27. Patti MG, Molena D, Fisichella PM, et al: Laparoscopic Heller myotomy and Dor fundoplication for achalasia: analysis of successes and failures. Arch Surg 870:136, 2001
28. Lord RVN, Kaminski A, Oberg S, et al: Absence of gastroesophageal reflux disease in a majority of patients taking acid suppression medications after Nissen fundoplication. J Gastrointest Surg 6:3, 2002.
29. Horgan S, Pohl D, Bogetti D, et al: Failed antireflux surgery: what have we learned from reoperations? Arch Surg 809:13, 1999
30. Zaninotto G, Costantini M, Portale G, et al: Etiology, diagnosis and treatment of failures after laparoscopic Heller myotomy for achalasia. Ann Surg 186:235, 2002.

Acknowledgment

Figures 1 through 14 Tom Moore.

11 VIDEO-ASSISTED THORACIC SURGERY

Raja M. Flores, M.D., and Valerie W. Rusch, M.D., F.A.C.S.

The technique of thoracoscopy was first described in 1910 by Jacobeus, a Swedish physician who used a cystoscope to examine the pleural space.[1] Although thoracoscopy was initially performed for diagnostic purposes, it later evolved into a therapeutic procedure. During the 1930s and 1940s, it was used to lyse intrapleural adhesions after collapse therapy for tuberculosis. During the 1950s, when effective antituberculous chemotherapy became available, thoracoscopy fell into disuse in the United States[2]; however, it remained popular in Europe, where it was employed in diagnosing and treating problems such as pleural effusion, empyema, traumatic hemothorax, persistent air leak after pulmonary resection, and spontaneous pneumothorax.[3-5] During the 1970s and 1980s, a few North American surgeons revived the practice of thoracoscopy, both to manage pleural disease and to perform small peripheral lung biopsies in patients with diffuse pneumonitis.

In the first stages of its revival, thoracoscopy was often performed with open endoscopes that were originally designed for other procedures (e.g., mediastinoscopes).[6,7] As optics and lighting systems improved, smaller-caliber endoscopes were created specifically for thoracoscopic applications[8]; however, these instruments were limited in that only one person could visualize the operative field at a given time. In 1991, the application of video technology to thoracoscopy revolutionized the procedure because it allowed several persons to see the operative field simultaneously and to operate together as they would during an open procedure. In addition, the development of endoscopic instruments, particularly endoscopic staplers, enabled surgeons to perform major operations using minimally invasive techniques. The impact of this new technology was so profound that within a 2-year period, traditional thoracoscopic techniques were abandoned in favor of video-assisted thoracic surgery (VATS).[9,10] In what follows, therefore, we focus on current VATS procedures rather than traditional thoracoscopic techniques. There are numerous accepted diagnostic and therapeutic indications for VATS [see Table 1]. Accordingly, there are numerous operations that can be performed by VATS; we describe the most important of these, with the exception of esophageal myotomy and fundoplication, which are covered elsewhere [see 3:10 *Minimally Invasive Esophageal Procedures*].

A major force driving surgeons to perform VATS procedures has been patient demand. Unfortunately, the application of VATS has not always been accompanied by careful evaluation of outcomes. Feasibility has sometimes been confused with success. Although VATS appears to have beneficial effects in terms of cosmesis and postoperative pain in the short term, it has not yet been proved to have beneficial effects on pulmonary function and return to normal activity in the long term.[11,12]

Questions remain about the oncologic soundness of some VATS procedures. It appears that levels of cytokines and other acute-phase reactants are lower with minimally invasive procedures than with the corresponding open procedures[13,14]; however, it remains to be determined whether this decrease will ultimately result in decreased tumor growth or reduced recurrence rates. Rigorous evaluation in the setting of well-designed clinical trials is needed to determine how VATS may be most appropriately and safely employed, especially in cancer patients.

Table 1 Indications and Contraindications for VATS Procedures

Diagnostic indications
  Undiagnosed pleural effusion
  Indeterminate pulmonary nodule
  Undiagnosed interstitial lung disease
  Pulmonary infection in the immunosuppressed patient
  To define cell type in known thoracic malignancy
  To define extent of a primary thoracic tumor
  Nodal staging of a primary thoracic tumor
  Diagnosis of intrathoracic pathology to stage a primary extrathoracic tumor
  Evaluation of intrapleural infection

Therapeutic indications
  Lung
    Spontaneous pneumothorax
    Bullous disease
    Lung volume reduction
    Persistent parenchymal air leak
    Benign pulmonary nodule
    Resection of pulmonary metastases (in highly selected cases)
    Resection of primary lung tumor (in highly selected cases)
  Mediastinum
    Drainage of pericardial effusion
    Excision of bronchogenic or pericardial cyst
    Resection of selected primary mediastinal tumors
    Esophageal myotomy
    Facilitation of transhiatal esophagectomy
    ? Resection of primary esophageal tumors
    ? Thymic resection
    Ligation of thoracic duct
  Pleura
    Drainage of a multiloculated effusion
    Drainage of an early empyema
    Pleurodesis

Contraindications
  Extensive intrapleural adhesions
  Inability to sustain single-lung ventilation
  Extensive involvement of hilar structures
  Preoperative induction chemotherapy or chemoradiotherapy
  Severe coagulopathy

Operative Planning

PATIENT PREPARATION AND INTRAOPERATIVE CARE

Patient preparation and positioning are much the same for most VATS procedures. As a rule, the lateral decubitus position offers the best exposure, and it permits easy conversion to a thoracotomy if necessary. There are occasional exceptions to this rule, however, and in such cases the choice of position is dictated by the procedure planned. For instance, if a cervical mediastinoscopy or a Chamberlain procedure is being performed for lung cancer staging and the pleura must be examined to rule out the presence of metastases, the patient can be left in the supine position and the videothoracoscope introduced through the parasternal incision or a separate inferior incision.[15]

Port placement, the use of so-called access incisions (utility thoracotomies), and instrumentation vary from one procedure to the next. In approximately 20% of patients undergoing VATS, intraoperative conversion to a standard thoracotomy will be necessary for any of several reasons, including extensive pleural adhesions and pulmonary lesions that cannot be located thoracoscopically or require a more extensive resection than can be accomplished endosurgically. With experience, one can learn to predict the likelihood of such conversion in a given case. It is important to discuss this possibility with the patient before operation and to obtain informed consent to conversion. Any patient who is likely to require conversion to a thoracotomy or who may be undergoing lobectomy or pneumonectomy should receive the cardiopulmonary evaluation that is usual for such procedures before VATS is performed.

VATS procedures are performed with the patient under general anesthesia. Very limited operations (e.g., pleural biopsies) can be done with a single-lumen endotracheal tube in place, but most procedures should be performed with single-lung ventilation using a double-lumen endotracheal tube or a bronchial blocker. The degree of intraoperative monitoring needed depends on the extent of the planned procedure and on the patient's general medical condition. Standard monitoring techniques, including pulse oximetry, are always used, but arterial lines are placed selectively. A central venous catheter or a Swan-Ganz catheter is inserted only when the patient's baseline cardiac status demands precise hemodynamic monitoring. A Foley catheter is inserted at the beginning of all VATS procedures to monitor urine output because it is not always possible to predict how long the operation will take or whether conversion to thoracotomy will prove necessary.

INSTRUMENTATION

Instrumentation for VATS comprises (1) video equipment, (2) endoscopes and thoracoports, (3) staplers, (4) thoracic instruments (e.g., lung clamps and retractors) modified for endoscopic use, and (5) various devices for tissue cauterization, including lasers. Because immediate conversion to thoracotomy is occasionally necessary, a basic set of thoracotomy instruments should be an integral part of a VATS instrument tray.[16]

Video Equipment

Several companies manufacture excellent video equipment for thoracoscopy. Minor variations in lighting and optics aside, the basic components of all of these systems are similar: a large-screen (21 in.) video monitor, a xenon light source, a video recorder, and a printer for still photography, mounted together on a cart. A second video monitor, also mounted on a cart, is connected by cable to the main monitor and is placed across from it at the head of the operating table. By using two monitors placed in this manner, both the surgeon and the first assistant can look directly at a video display without having to turn away from the surgical field. Alternatively, a single monitor can be placed at the head of the operating table. The only additional item of equipment necessary for laparoscopy is an insufflator. To maximize cost-efficiency, therefore, hospitals acquiring video monitors and endoscopes should coordinate the choice of this expensive equipment among the specialties using it, including thoracic surgery, general surgery, gynecology, and urology. Hospitals performing many endoscopic procedures may find it advisable to dedicate one or more rooms to video endoscopic surgery and to mount video equipment on the ceilings or walls.

Endoscopes and Thoracoports

Most procedures are performed with a forward-viewing (0°) rigid scope; 30°-angled scopes are useful for visualizing the sulci and the superior and posterior mediastinum. In addition to the standard 10 mm thoracoscopes, there are now 5 mm thoracoscopes, whose resolution is nearly as good. The scope is attached to the light source by a light cable and is coupled to the video-monitor system by a camera cable [see Figure 1]. Although camera cables can be sterilized, it is best to cover the camera head and cable with a clear plastic bag so that the camera cable can remain in the OR at all times. Newer videoscopes are now available in which the camera chip is located at the tip of the scope rather than in the connecting camera cable; these will eventually replace the older endoscopes because they provide a sharper image. Flexible thoracoscopes are also available; these look like a short, heavy version of a flexible bronchoscope but have a more rigid distal end. Some surgeons feel that flexible thoracoscopes enhance their ability to visualize the entire pleural space, but these devices are very expensive and thus continue to be premium purchases for most hospitals.

0° Rigid Scope

Detachable Camera
Cable

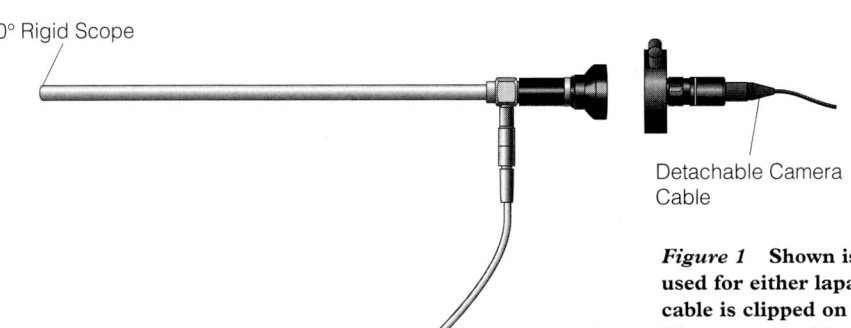

Figure 1 **Shown is a forward-viewing (0°) rigid scope that can be used for either laparoscopy or thoracoscopy. A detachable camera cable is clipped on to the eyepiece of the scope for video endoscopy. The camera cable can be sterilized or enclosed within a plastic sheath if it is used frequently.**

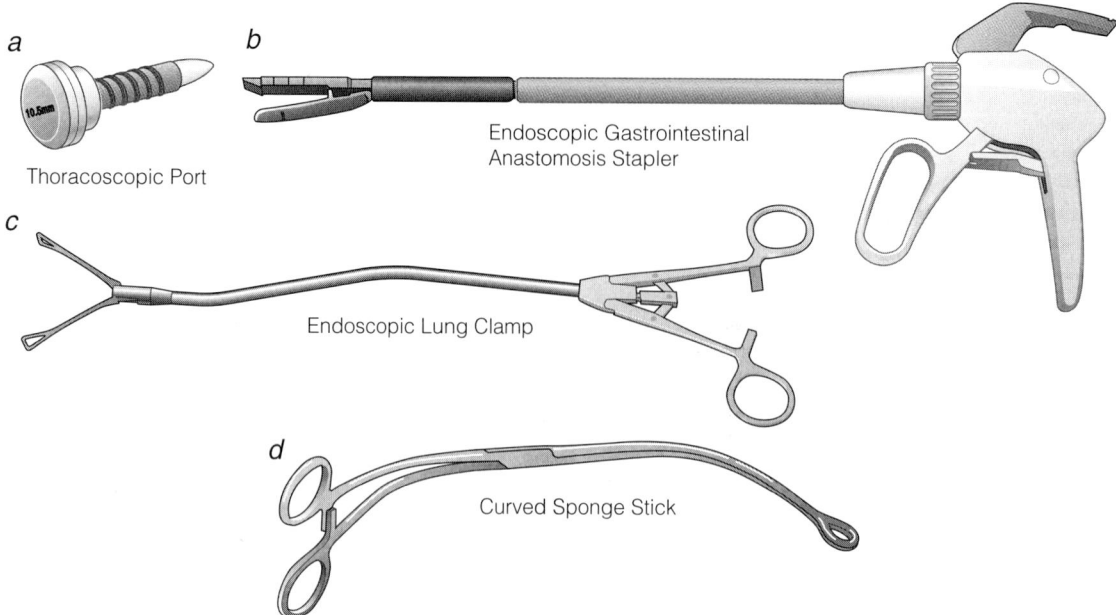

Figure 2 **Shown are instruments commonly used during VATS. Modified trocar cannulas, called thoraco-ports (*a*), facilitate access to the pleural space. They are shorter than the cannulas used in laparoscopy and have a corkscrew configuration on the outside that maintains their position on the chest wall. The trocar is a blunt-tipped plastic obturator that facilitates passage of the cannula through the chest wall. A thin plastic diaphragm stabilizes the position of the instruments or can be removed to facilitate access to the pleural space. Endoscopic GIA staplers that make incisions between two triple rows of staples (*b*) can be inserted through these ports. Like staplers designed for open procedures, endoscopic GIA staplers are disposable multifire instruments that hold three replacements of the staple cartridge. Another instrument that can be inserted through these ports is the nondisposable endoscopic lung clamp (*c*), which is available in various shapes with serrations at the end or along the full length of the clamp. Finally, the port allows insertion of curved sponge sticks (*d*), which have been modified for endoscopic use as lung clamps or lymph node holders.**

Originally, thoracoscopy made use of trocar cannulas designed for laparoscopy to access the pleural space. These devices are too long and have sharp ends that can injure the lung. Because patients undergoing thoracoscopy are under general anesthesia and have a double-lumen endotracheal tube in place, the cannulas need not maintain an airtight seal, as they do in laparoscopy. Accordingly, modified trocar cannulas called thoracoports, which are shorter than laparoscopy cannulas and have a corkscrew configuration on the outside that stabilizes them within the chest wall, are now routinely used. The trocar is simply a blunt-tip obturator that facilitates passage of the cannula through the chest wall [*see Figure 2a*]. Thoracoports are available in several sizes (5, 10.5, 12.0, and 15 mm in diameter) to accommodate various instruments.

Staplers

Endoscopic staplers that cut between two simultaneously applied triple rows of staples (gastrointestinal anastomosis [GIA] staplers) are available in lengths of 30 and 60 mm and in staple depths of 2.5, 3.5, and 4.8 mm [*see Figure 2b*]. Like their counterparts designed for open procedures, they are disposable multicartridge instruments. The endoscopic GIA stapler with 2.5 mm staples is designed for division of pulmonary vessels. Some surgeons are reluctant to use it on hilar vessels because if the stapler fails mechanically (e.g., cuts without applying both staple lines properly), life-threatening hemorrhage can ensue. Endoscopic staplers that do not cut (transverse anastomosis [TA] staplers) are also available. Endoscopic GIA staplers have revolutionized surgeons' ability to perform minimally invasive pulmonary resections. These devices are highly reliable, and because they apply triple rows of staples instead of double rows, they provide excellent hemostasis and closure of air leaks. There are also stapler cartridges that buttress the staple line with Gore-Tex (W. L. Gore, Boulder, Colorado) to reduce postoperative air leakage in patients with emphysematous lung tissue.

Standard stapling instruments are also used during some VATS procedures. They are unnecessary for most pulmonary wedge resections but may be helpful for more complex procedures, such as lobectomies. Standard GIA and roticulator TA staplers are the most practical devices for VATS because they can be inserted and positioned through an access incision.

Instruments

Various types of Pennington and Duval clamps are available [*see Figure 2c*]. Sponge sticks modified by the introduction of various curves and a line of DeBakey-type teeth on the end can also be used as lung clamps or lymph node holders [*see Figure 2d*].

Several retractors have been developed for endoscopic surgery. One such device is a modified Finochietto retractor with long, narrow blades, which is particularly helpful for retracting the chest wall soft tissues in an access incision. Others are the disposable vein retractor [*see Figure 3a*], the tip of which can be withdrawn into the straight instrument shaft, and the fan retractor, which can be opened and closed like a fan by turning a knob on the end of the retractor [*see Figure 3b*]. Of these, the fan retractor is the most useful general retractor for thoracoscopic procedures. Vein retractors are best suited for gentle retraction of hilar or mediastinal structures (e.g., vessels, bronchi, esophagus, or lymph nodes).

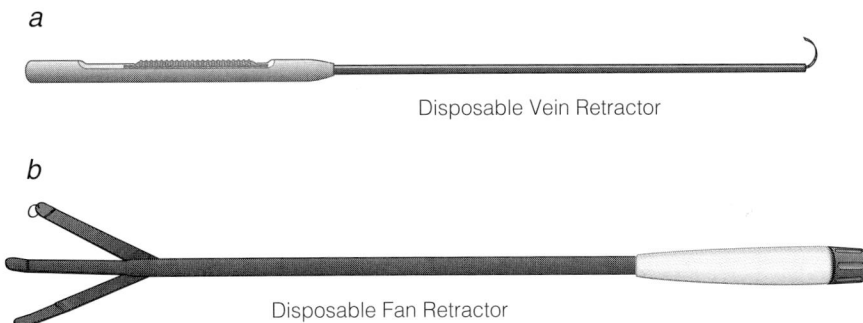

a

Disposable Vein Retractor

b

Disposable Fan Retractor

Figure 3 Shown are retractors used for VATS. Vein retractors are best suited for the gentle retraction of hilar or mediastinal structures, such as the vessels, bronchi, esophagus, and lymph nodes. The tip of the disposable vein retractor (*a*) can be extended from or withdrawn into the shaft to allow insertion of the retractor through a 12 mm port. The most useful retractor for general purposes is the fan retractor (*b*). A knob on the end of the handle opens and closes the fan, so that the retractor can be inserted through a port and opened for retraction in the pleural space.

Although biopsy forceps have been specifically created for laparoscopy and thoracoscopy, those used for mediastinoscopy are, in fact, well suited for thoracoscopy. Because laparoscopy instruments were developed before thoracoscopy instruments, many types of grasping forceps are available; however, most are too traumatizing for thoracic surgery. DeBakey forceps, modified for endoscopic use, are the gentlest type available. Various curved and right-angle dissecting clamps, needle holders, and scissors [*see Figure 4*] have been developed. In addition, standard thoracotomy instruments can be inserted through a minithoracotomy incision and used just as they would be in an open procedure.

Devices for Tissue Cauterization

Most scissors have an electrocautery attachment that permits simultaneous cutting and cauterizing. The neodymium:yttrium-aluminum-garnet (Nd:YAG) laser is sometimes applied to VATS resection of pulmonary lesions. This is done by inserting the YAG laser-fiber through angled or straight handpieces [*see Figure 5*]. Laser-assisted pulmonary resection is helpful in removing

lesions on the flat surface of the lung, where a stapler cannot be easily applied.[17]

The argon beam electrocoagulator (ABC) (Birtcher Corporation, Englewood, Colorado) is a noncontact form of electrocautery that provides superb hemostasis on raw surfaces, such as denuded pulmonary parenchyma or the chest wall after pleurectomy, and helps seal air leaks from the surface of the lung.[18] The standard disposable ABC handpiece used for open procedures is narrow enough to pass through a thoracoport and thus may be used for VATS. Both the YAG laser and the ABC can be used to cauterize the pleural surface for pleurodesis and to ablate bullous disease, though neither has proved as effective as endoscopic stapling for lung volume reduction surgery (LVRS).

Instrumentation for videothoracoscopy continues to evolve, especially as minimally invasive cardiac surgical procedures become commonplace. Nevertheless, to put together the best set of instruments, it still is necessary to combine disposable and nondisposable instruments from different manufacturers and to borrow instruments originally designed for other procedures, such as mediastinoscopy and thoracotomy. Rather than create separate instrument trays for different VATS procedures, it is best to maintain a single standard tray that includes the basic instruments required for most operations and to add instruments as needed. Again, this tray should also include the instruments needed for conversion to thoracotomy.

Basic Operative Technique

VATS procedures include both true videothoracoscopies and video-assisted procedures that are really a cross between videothoracoscopies and standard thoracotomies. Because VATS procedures are still evolving, there is no firm consensus among surgeons with respect to the number, size, and location of incisions.

The basic videothoracoscopy techniques have been well described.[19] The primary strategy is to place the instruments and the thoracoscope so that all are oriented in the same direction, facing the target disease within a 180° arc [*see Figure 6*]; this posi-

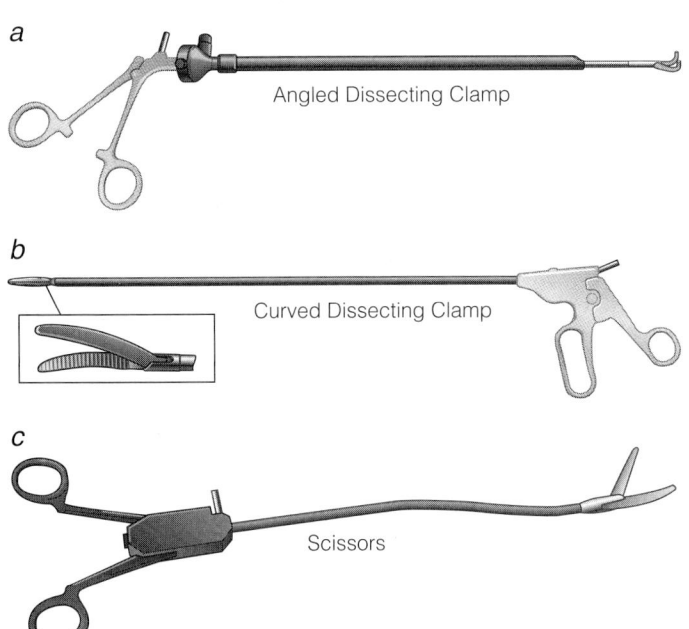

a

Angled Dissecting Clamp

b

Curved Dissecting Clamp

c

Scissors

Figure 4 Various right-angle (*a*) and curved (*b*) dissecting clamps are available. On the angled model shown (*a*), the knob close to the handle rotates the shaft of the clamp 360°. Finally, many types of endoscopic scissors (*c*) are available. Some scissors incorporate an attachment for electrocautery so that the surgeon can cut and cauterize simultaneously.

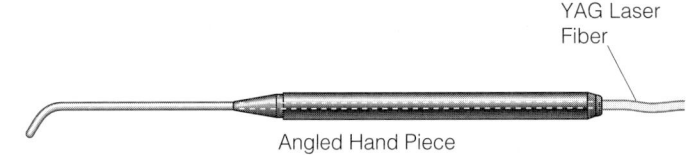

YAG Laser Fiber

Angled Hand Piece

Figure 5 Shown is an angled handpiece through which an yttrium-aluminum-garnet (YAG) laser can be placed during VATS. The handpiece is narrow enough to be used during thoracoscopy as well as during open procedures.

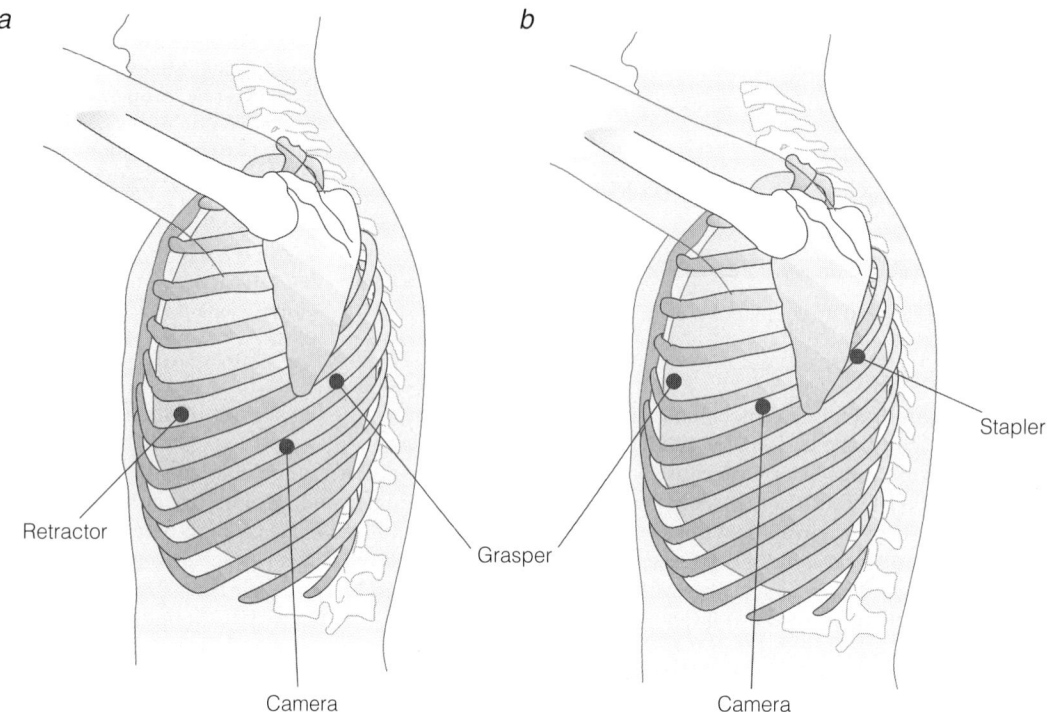

Figure 6 **Basic operative technique. Shown is the typical positioning of instruments and the video camera for patients undergoing VATS for a lesion in the superior segment of the left lower lobe of the lung. Instruments are introduced through two port incisions made anteriorly at approximately the fifth intercostal space in the anterior axillary line and posteriorly parallel to and 2 to 3 cm away from the border of the scapula (*a*). For patients undergoing thoracoscopy for apical bullous disease in the left upper lobe of the lung, the camera port can be placed at the fifth or sixth intercostal space, and one instrument port can be inserted in the axilla and the other port inserted higher on the posterior chest wall at approximately the third intercostal space (*b*).**

tioning prevents mirror imaging. The incisions should also be placed widely distant from each other so that the instruments do not crowd one another.

For most procedures [*see Figure 6a*], the videothoracoscope is inserted through a thoracoport placed in the midaxillary line at the seventh or eighth intercostal space. Instruments are introduced through two thoracoports, one placed at approximately the fifth intercostal space in the anterior axillary line, and the other placed at the fifth space, parallel to and about 2 to 3 cm away from the posterior border of the scapula. If the procedure is converted to a thoracotomy, the two upper incisions can be incorporated into the thoracotomy incision, and the lower incision can be used as a chest tube site. When a patient is being operated upon for an apical lesion (e.g., bullae causing a spontaneous pneumothorax) [*see Figure 6b*], the camera port can be placed at the fifth or sixth intercostal space, and the instrument ports are also moved higher: one in the axilla and the other higher on the posterior chest wall at approximately the third intercostal space. Depending on the location of the lesion being removed, a fourth port incision may be helpful to permit the introduction of additional instruments.

When the lung has to be palpated so that a small or deep-seated lesion can be located or when complex video-assisted procedures are being performed, a small (about 5 cm) intercostal incision is added to the three port incisions. This utility thoracotomy, or access incision, is usually placed in the midaxillary line or in the auscultatory triangle. An infant Finochietto retractor or a

Weitlaner retractor is used to retract the soft tissues without actually spreading the ribs [*see Figure 7*].

These basic concepts regarding incision placement are modified as necessary to accommodate the procedure being performed and the location of the lesion being removed (see below).

VATS Procedures for Pleural Disease

OPERATIVE TECHNIQUE

A double-lumen endotracheal tube is inserted, and the patient is placed in the lateral decubitus position. Two 1.5 cm incisions are made, one for the videothoracoscope and one for the instruments. The videothoracoscope is inserted through a 10.5 mm thoracoport at the seventh or eighth intercostal space in the midaxillary line; the instruments are inserted through a port placed a couple of interspaces higher in the anterior axillary line. If a talc poudrage is performed, both incisions are reused for placement of chest tubes, with a right-angle tube inserted on the diaphragm through the lower incision and a straight tube up to the apex of the pleural space through the upper incision. The addition of a diaphragmatic chest tube helps prevent loculated basilar fluid collections after a talc pleurodesis. If a thoracotomy is subsequently performed, the upper port site is incorporated into the anterior aspect of the incision, and the lower site can be reused as a chest tube site. Proper placement of port incisions is especially important in patients with suspected malignant

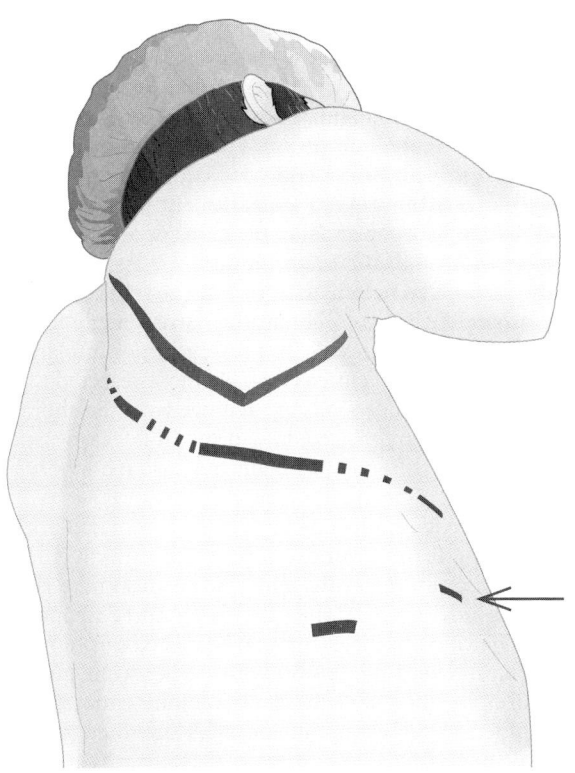

Figure 7 **Basic operative technique. Shown are the incisions used for common VATS procedures. The thoracoscope is inserted through the bottom incision. Anterior and posterior incisions are used for the introduction of instruments. Only one additional low anterior incision (arrow) is needed for thoracoscopic pleural procedures. A so-called utility thoracotomy (dotted line) can be added at the fifth intercostal space, if necessary. The tip of the scapula is outlined. These incisions can be incorporated into a standard thoracotomy incision if the VATS procedure is converted to an open procedure.**

mesothelioma because of the propensity of this tumor to implant in incisions and needle tracks.[8,20,21]

Once the videothoracoscope has been inserted, pleural biopsies are obtained under direct vision by introducing a biopsy forceps through a port placed in the upper incision. The mediastinoscopy biopsy forceps is well suited to this task. Pleural fluid is evacuated with a Yankauer or pool-tip suction device. Fibrinous debris can be removed by irrigating the pleural space with a pulsating water jet lavage device (e.g., Water-Pik, Orthotec, Stryker, Kalamazoo, Michigan) designed for debridement of orthopedic wounds. This technique is particularly useful for the debridement and drainage of loculated fibrinopurulent empyemas.[22] At the end of the procedure, intercostal blocks are performed by using a mediastinoscopy aspiration needle, and talc can be insufflated for pleurodesis, if indicated. All of these instruments are introduced sequentially through the upper incision.[23]

An alternative approach is to make a single incision in the midaxillary line at the sixth or seventh intercostal space and to use an operating thoracoscope that incorporates a biopsy forceps. This approach has the advantage of requiring only one incision; however, it does not allow as much latitude in draining or debriding the pleural space. Moreover, the biopsy forceps in an operating thoracoscope is of a smaller caliber than a mediastinoscopy biopsy forceps and thus cannot obtain as large a biopsy specimen.

TROUBLESHOOTING

In patients with loculated effusion, thoracoport placement sometimes must be modified. The preoperative chest computed tomographic scan and chest x-ray should help ensure that the ports are placed in areas when the lung is not adherent to the chest wall.

In some cases, the pleural space is obliterated by adhesions or tumor. This event occurs most frequently in patients who have had severe inflammatory disease (e.g., pneumonia, empyema, or tuberculosis) or extensive pleural malignancy (e.g., locally advanced malignant mesothelioma). In these circumstances, the anterior thoracoport incision can be extended to a length of 5 to 6 cm, the underlying rib section can be resected, and the parietal pleura can be biopsied directly; a full thoracotomy is not required. If thoracotomy is subsequently warranted for therapeutic reasons (e.g, for pleurectomy, decortication, or extrapleural pneumonectomy for mesothelioma), this small incision can be incorporated into the thoracotomy incision.

VATS Pulmonary Wedge Resection

VATS pulmonary wedge resection has become a standard approach to diagnosing small indeterminate pulmonary nodules, especially those not technically amenable to transthoracic needle biopsy.[24,25] It is also an accepted method of diagnosing pulmonary infiltrates of uncertain origin, particularly in immunocompromised patients in whom transbronchial biopsy is either unsafe or inappropriate.[26,27]

The role of VATS wedge resection is less well defined in the management of primary lung cancers. It is an appropriate compromise operation for primary lung cancers in patients whose cardiac or pulmonary function status rules out lobectomy. However, it remains a highly controversial approach to the treatment of pulmonary metastases.[28] In an often-quoted 1993 study,[29] patients with CT-documented pulmonary metastases underwent first thoracoscopic resection and then thoracotomy in the same setting. Many additional lesions, both benign and malignant, were found at thoracotomy that were missed by VATS. The study was terminated early because of the failure of thoracoscopy to identify these lesions. One criticism of the study is that the preoperative CT scans were not comparable to the spiral, or helical, CT scans currently available and therefore probably missed many pulmonary nodules that modern scanning methods would have caught.

A 2000 multicenter study of patients undergoing VATS metastasectomy for colon cancer suggested that minimal residual disease not identified by helical CT and not resected by VATS may not affect survival significantly[30]; however, this conclusion is completely at odds with all of the previously published surgical literature on pulmonary metastasectomy. Improved survival in patients with pulmonary metastases appears to be directly linked to the ability to remove all gross tumor, and VATS does not allow the careful bimanual palpation that is critical to detecting pulmonary metastases that are too small or too deep to be visible endoscopically.[29,31,32] Accordingly, most centers reserve VATS for the diagnosis rather than the treatment of pulmonary metastases. Until a well-designed prospective, randomized trial is conducted with survival as an end point, the standard of care remains thoracotomy and metastasectomy.

Anecdotal reports of port-site recurrence have also raised concerns about VATS as a treatment method in patients with malignancies; however, a 2001 study of 410 patients from a prospective VATS database at the Memorial Sloan-Kettering Cancer

Center (MSKCC) found only one case of port-site recurrence.[33] The authors concluded that the incidence of such recurrences can be kept low if surgical oncologic principles are respected. At MSKCC, these principles include (1) reserving VATS for lesions that can be widely excised, (2) conversion to an open thoracotomy for definitive or extensive operations, and (3) meticulous technique for extraction of specimens from the pleural space, with small specimens removed directly through a thoracoport and larger specimens through specimen bags.

OPERATIVE TECHNIQUE

Once general anesthesia has been induced and a double-lumen endotracheal tube inserted, the patient is placed in the full lateral decubitus position. It is important to stop ventilation to the lung being operated on as soon as the patient is rotated into the lateral decubitus position, so that the lung will be thoroughly collapsed by the time the videothoracoscope is inserted into the pleural space. Small subpleural pulmonary nodules are most easily identified in a fully atelectatic lung because they protrude

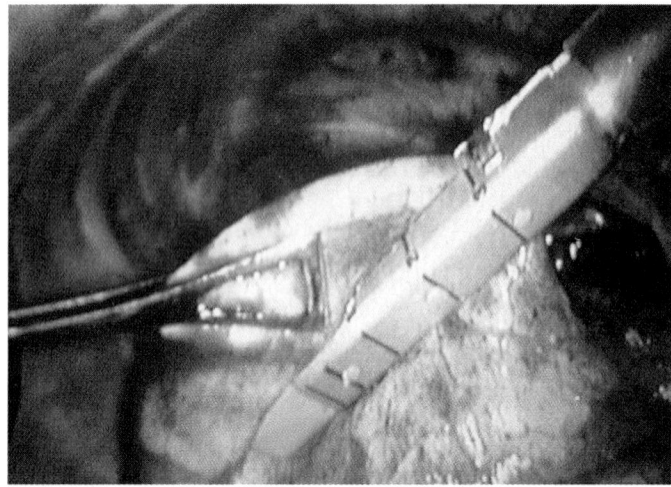

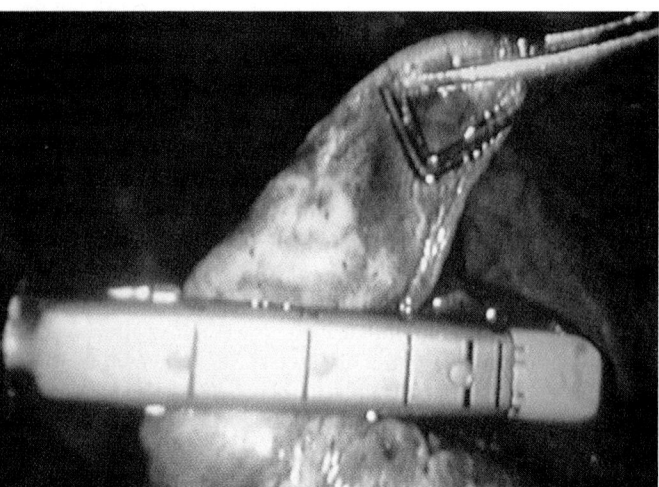

Figure 8 **VATS pulmonary wedge resection. A double-lumen endotracheal tube is used to render the lung partially atelectatic. The pulmonary nodule is lifted upward with a lung clamp, and the endoscopic GIA stapler is applied to the lung underneath (top). During the wedge resection, the lung clamp and the endoscopic GIA stapler are alternately inserted through opposite ports to obtain the correct angle for performance of the wedge resection (bottom).**

from the surrounding collapsed pulmonary parenchyma, which is softer.[19,20] Most pulmonary wedge resections are performed as true videothoracoscopic procedures using just three port incisions placed in the triangulated manner already described [*see* Basic Operative Technique, *above*]. The pulmonary nodules to be removed are grasped with an endoscopic lung clamp (Pennington or Duval) inserted through one instrument port, and wedge resection is done with repeated applications of an endoscopic stapler inserted through the opposite port.[24,34] As the resection is performed, it is often helpful to introduce the stapler through each of two instrument ports to obtain the correct angle for application to the lung [*see Figure 8*]. To prevent tumor implantation in the chest wall, small specimens (usually those resected with three or fewer stapler applications) are removed via the thoracoport. Larger specimens are placed in a disposable plastic specimen retrieval bag, which is then brought out through a very slightly enlarged anterior thoracoport incision.

When the wedge resections have been completed, intercostal blocks are performed under direct vision via the mediastinoscopy aspiration needle, and a single chest tube is inserted through the inferior port after the videothoracoscope is withdrawn.[35] The videothoracoscope can be placed through the anterior incision to check the position of the chest tube and confirm reinflation of the lung after the double-lumen endotracheal tube is unclamped. The remaining incisions are then closed with sutures.

TROUBLESHOOTING

Four techniques can be used to locate pulmonary nodules that are either too deep or too small to be easily visible on simple inspection of the lung. All of these should be used in conjunction with a high-quality preoperative chest CT scan to identify the lung segment in which the nodule is located. First, an endoscopic lung clamp can be gently run across the surface of the lung as an extension of digital palpation.[20,36] With some patience and experience, one can achieve considerable success with this technique. Second, ultrasonographic examination of the collapsed lung can also locate deep pulmonary nodules; at present, however, experience with this approach remains very limited.[37] Third, CT-guided needle localization can be used preoperatively if a nodule is likely to be difficult to locate. Localization is accomplished by injecting methylene blue or by inserting a barbed mammography localization needle, which is then cut off at the skin exit site and later retrieved thoracoscopically.[38] Needle localization techniques are effective, but they are also costly and time-consuming and hence not used by most surgeons. Finally, if careful endoscopic examination of the lung does not reveal the location of a nodule, an access incision is added to the videothoracoscopy.[24,39] Each lobe of the lung is sequentially rotated up to this non–rib-spreading utility thoracotomy for direct digital palpation. This technique almost always allows identification of a nodule when other techniques fail. As the endoscopist gains experience with these techniques, conversion to thoracotomy just for the purpose of locating a pulmonary nodule is rarely necessary.[40]

Pulmonary nodules located on the broad surface of the lung may not be amenable to a wedge resection with an endoscopic stapler. Such nodules can be removed by means of electrocauterization, just as in an open thoracotomy. An extension is placed on the handle of the electrocautery, which is then introduced into the pleural space through either a port or an access incision. Another approach is to resect the pulmonary nodule with a laser in either a contact or a noncontact mode. The potassium-titanyl-phosphate

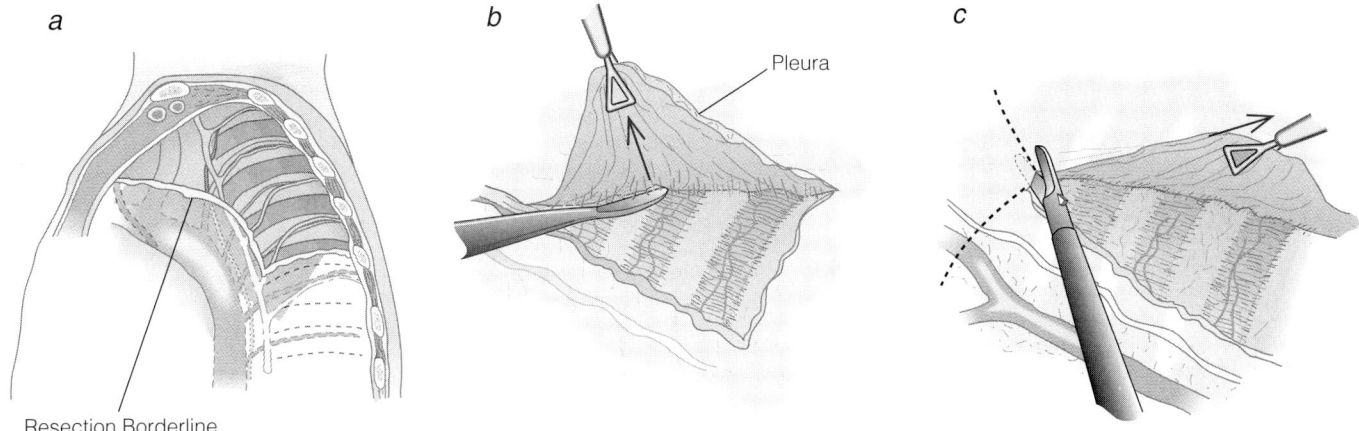

Figure 9 **VATS procedures for spontaneous pneumothorax and bullous disease. Limited apical pleurectomy is a useful alternative to chemical pleurodesis in young patients with spontaneous pneumothorax because these patients may need to undergo thoracotomy later in life. Shown is an outline of the pleural resection (*a*) performed in this procedure. The pleura is grasped at the inferior border with forceps and lifted in the avascular layer in a cranial or ventral direction (*b*). A T-shaped incision is made in the pleura at the level of the subclavian artery or the truncus brachiocephalicus. The dissection of the pleural flap thus created is extended in either the ventral or the parasternal direction and in either the apical or the mediastinal direction (*c*).**

(KTP)/YAG laser is particularly suited to this task because it is capable of both cutting and coagulation. To minimize bleeding and air leakage, raw pulmonary surfaces can be cauterized with either the Nd:YAG laser or the ABC.[17] Numerous types of absorbable sealant patches or materials are also available to control air leaks from areas of raw pulmonary parenchyma.

Occasionally, after a wedge resection, it is necessary to suture together the pleural edges over an area of raw pulmonary parenchyma. The suturing can be done directly through a non–rib-spreading minithoracotomy incision or through port sites. In the latter case, the ports are removed, and a 3-0 Prolene suture is passed through the anterior port site with a standard needle holder. A second needle holder is introduced via the posterior port site and used in place of a forceps to pick up and reposition the needle as it is passed through the lung. The surgeon and the first assistant work together to oversew the lung, in contrast with the normal practice for an open procedure, in which the surgeon uses a needle holder and a forceps to place the sutures.

VATS Procedures for Spontaneous Pneumothorax and Bullous Disease

OPERATIVE TECHNIQUE

VATS is now frequently performed for the management of recurrent spontaneous pneumothorax and for bullous disease.[41,42] The approach is similar to that followed in a wedge resection. Three or four port sites are used. The videothoracoscope is inserted at the fifth intercostal space in the midaxillary line. Two other port sites are added at the fourth intercostal space in the anterior and posterior axillary lines.

In patients with spontaneous pneumothorax, the responsible bulla (which is usually apical in location) is identified, and wedge resection is done with an endoscopic stapler.[43,44] Bullae can be excised by applying the stapler across the base of the area of bullous disease. They can also be ablated with the ABC or the Nd:YAG laser, then suture-plicated if necessary; however, this approach may not be as successful over the long term.[45,46]

Some surgeons, noting the lower rate of recurrence, the short-

er hospital stay, and the relative cost-effectiveness, advocate performing VATS for the first episode of spontaneous pneumothorax.[47,48] To justify this approach in patients with primary spontaneous pneumothorax, however, well-designed clinical trials rather than retrospective reviews will be required.

TROUBLESHOOTING

The placement of port incisions should be determined by the location of the bullae. Because bullous disease is generally apical, port sites are correspondingly higher than for the average wedge resection (i.e., at the fourth and sixth intercostal spaces rather than at the fifth or sixth and eighth spaces). The precise placement should, however, be determined by pinpointing the disease site or sites on the preoperative chest x-ray and CT scans.

The main problem after resection for bullous disease is prolonged leakage of air from the staple line. This problem can be minimized by applying commercially available sleeves made of bovine pericardium or Gore-Tex over the arms of the stapler to reinforce the staple line and by performing some form of pleurodesis. Mechanical pleurodesis is done with a small gauze sponge passed through a port site. Some surgeons scarify the pleura by cauterizing it with the ABC or the Nd:YAG laser, but this is not as successful as a mechanical pleurodesis. Chemical pleurodesis by talc poudrage is an appropriate option for older patients with emphysema and bullous disease but is unwise in young patients with spontaneous pneumothorax, who might require a thoracotomy later in life.[49] Another option in younger patients is a limited apical pleurectomy [see Figure 9]. Special angulated instruments and blunt dissectors have been designed for this procedure; however, a parietal pleurectomy is also easily performed with combinations of standard blunt and sharp instruments.[50]

VATS Lung Volume Reduction Surgery

OPERATIVE TECHNIQUE

VATS may also be applied to the performance of LVRS. Many candidates for LVRS are receiving steroids and thus are at risk for sternal wound infection; the thoracoscopic approach reduces this risk substantially. If unilateral LVRS is planned, the patient is placed in the lateral decubitus position, and port placement is similar to that for a patient undergoing a wedge resection of the upper lobe. Most patients undergoing LVRS, however, benefit from bilateral LVRS. For this procedure, the patient is placed in the standard supine bilateral lung transplant position, with shoulder rolls placed vertically in an I fashion behind the back and with the arms positioned above the head. The camera port is placed in the anterior axillary line at the sixth interspace. A lung compression clamp is placed on the area that will be resected. A Gore-Tex–reinforced stapler is then inserted into the chest and fired sequentially until the desired area is excised [see Figure 10a].

Another approach used to help buttress the tenuous staple line in emphysematous lung tissue is lung plication [see Figure 10b].[51] In this method, the defunctionalized, bullous lung tissue is stapled to itself to form a plicated autologous buttress [see Figure 11]. Because the diseased bullous lung is not cut, the risk of postoperative air leakage is minimized.

TROUBLESHOOTING

A major cause of morbidity and mortality with this procedure is the occurrence of air leaks, which sometimes are large enough to compromise ventilation significantly. Thus, once LVRS has been done on one side, the lung is reexpanded and any air leaks carefully assessed. If the leak is small, the other side is operated on in the same setting; if the leak is large, the contralateral procedure is put off to a later date. The use of fibrin glue or another commercially available pneumostatic sealant along the staple line should be considered to minimize postoperative air leakage.

VATS Lobectomy and Pneumonectomy

Although VATS lobectomy is much less frequently performed than VATS pulmonary wedge resection, standard techniques have been developed for it.[52] VATS pneumonectomy, on the other hand, is less well accepted. Both operations are done as video-assisted procedures using a utility thoracotomy, which facilitates the insertion of standard thoracotomy instruments, the extraction of the resected specimen from the pleural space, and the performance of the technically complex aspects of the procedure, including dissection of the hilar vessels and of the mediastinal lymph nodes.

A 1998 retrospective study addressing the adequacy of VATS lobectomy as an oncologic procedure reported on 298 patients who underwent VATS lobectomy with mediastinal lymph node dissection for primary non–small cell lung cancer.[53] On the basis of a 70% 4-year survival rate for stage I tumors, the investigators concluded that outcome after VATS lobectomy is comparable to that after open thoracotomy. At 5 years, however, survival rates after VATS are inferior, stage for stage, to the rates generally reported after thoracotomy. Such differences could reflect either inaccurate staging or true oncologic differences between VATS and thoracotomy; additional prospective studies are needed to clarify these issues.

Although VATS lobectomy has not been proved to be an oncologically sound procedure in the long term, there is good evidence that it is safe in acute settings.[54] Therefore, it should certainly be performed to treat benign diseases (e.g., bronchiectasis).[55] As with all minimally invasive procedures, conversion to open thoracotomy is indicated if technical issues require it. Some authors advocate VATS lobectomy for low-grade malignancies (e.g., carcinoids) as well.[56] It must be recognized, however, that although carcinoids have a lower malignant potential than non–small cell lung cancer, they are still malignancies and must be treated appropriately for optimal long-term outcome.

Two approaches to lobectomy have been developed. One involves sequential anatomic ligation of the hilar structures, much as in a standard lobectomy,[57,58] and the other involves mass ligation of the pulmonary vessels and the bronchus. Both approaches require at least two port incisions in addition to the utility thoracotomy. The sequential anatomic ligation approach has been well described.[57]

OPERATIVE TECHNIQUE

Lobectomy

Right-side resections The specific operative approach taken in performing a VATS lobectomy may vary depending on the patient's body habitus and the intraoperative pathology. In our view, however, it is generally the safest strategy to leave the bronchial resection until last, regardless of which lobe is to be resected. When the bronchus is transected first, it may be difficult to gauge the amount of traction placed on the hilum, and accidental traction injury to the pulmonary artery may result in significant hemorrhage.

a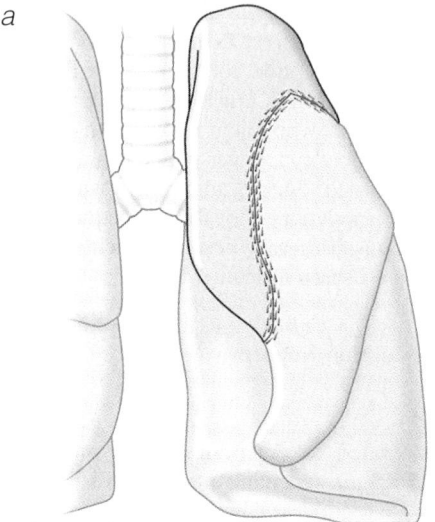

b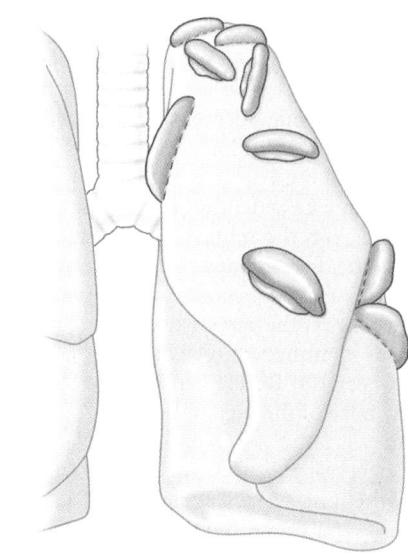

Figure 10 **VATS lung volume reduction surgery. Thoracoscopic lung volume reduction can be accomplished through either (*a*) resection or (*b*) plication without cutting.**

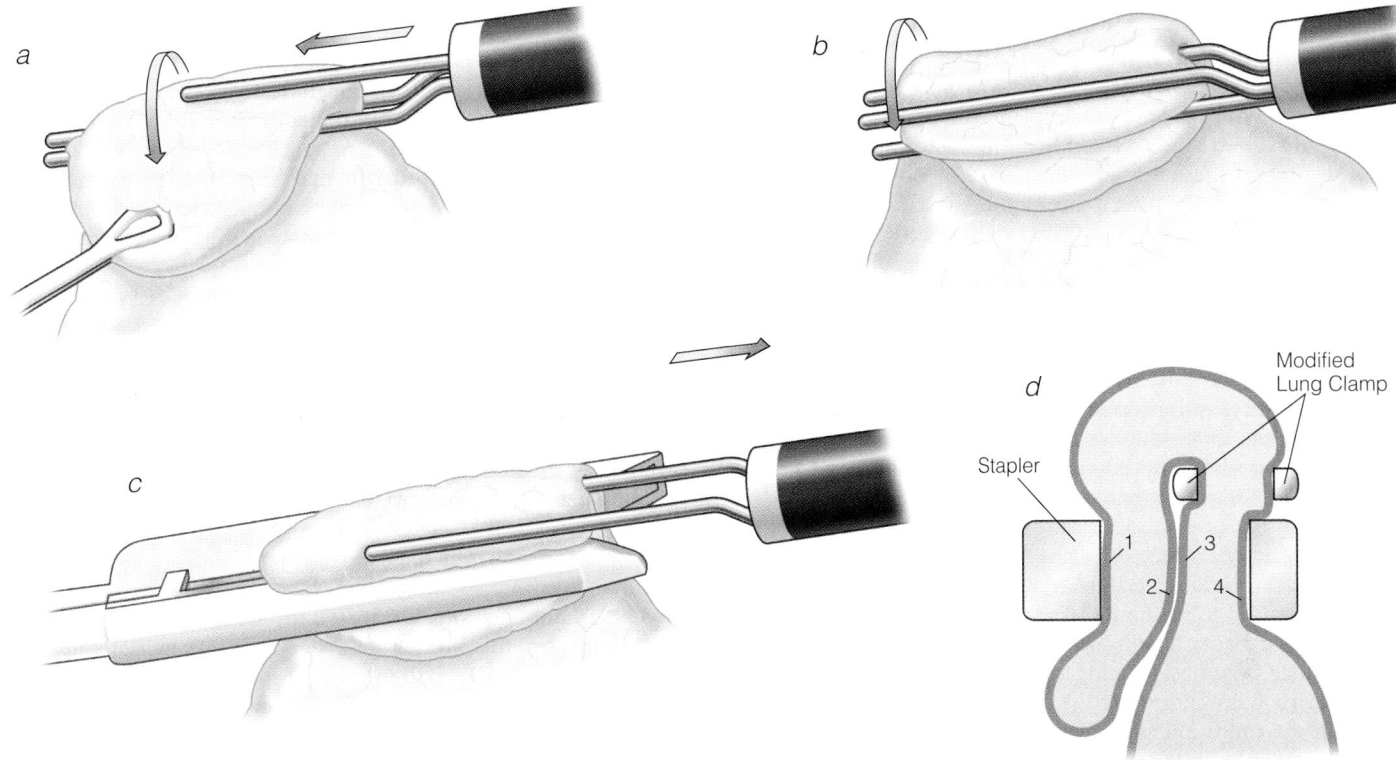

Figure 11 **VATS lung volume reduction surgery. Shown are the key steps in the plication method of LVRS. (*a*) The apex of the lung area selected for plication is drawn to one side over a lung plication clamp, and the retractable guidebar of the clamp is extended into position. (*b*) The clamp is rotated 180° to fold the lung over itself. (*c*) The guidebar is retracted, a stapler is positioned with its jaws around the folded lung (but not yet closed), and the plication clamp is removed. (*d*) Shown is a cross-section of the folded lung after the stapler has been positioned but before the clamp has been removed. The stapler is then fired to complete the plication.**

The first step is to place a camera port at the sixth or seventh interspace between the anterior axillary line and the midaxillary line. Once the camera is inserted and the lung and the pleura have been thoroughly examined for metastatic disease, the access incision is placed under thoracoscopic guidance directly over the interspace that gives the best exposure to the pulmonary hilum; usually the best location is at the fifth interspace in the anterior axillary line. A second thoracoport is placed at the same interspace as the camera port, usually several inches posteriorly but in some cases (depending on patient anatomy) anteriorly. The inferior pulmonary ligament is then divided. A finger is placed through the utility thoracotomy, and an empty sponge stick is placed through the lower thoracoport, thereby allowing digital palpation of the entire lung.

If no other lesions have been identified, the posterior mediastinal pleura is opened to expose the subcarinal (level 7) lymph nodes and the bifurcation of the mainstem bronchus. This maneuver facilitates subsequent division of the major fissure.

The right pulmonary artery is then identified within the fissure by meticulous dissection through the utility thoracotomy. Even when the fissure is incomplete, careful use of the electrocautery can keep bleeding to a minimum. The technique used for dissection of the pulmonary artery in VATS is exactly the same as that in a thoracotomy. The key structures to identify within the fissure are the right pulmonary artery trunk, the right middle lobe artery, the apical posterior segmental artery to the right upper lobe (the recurrent artery), and the artery to the superior segment of the lower lobe. Once these structures have been identified, the various lobes are resected as follows.

Right upper lobe. The superior pulmonary vein is dissected via the access incision in the same manner as in an open lobectomy. The vein is then encircled with a silk tie, and a No. 10 red rubber catheter is placed behind it, with its open end at the inferior portion of the vein. An endovascular stapler is placed via one of the lower thoracoports; to provide the optimal angle for directing the stapler behind the vein, the camera may have to be switched to the posterior port. Once the stapler is inside the chest, it is positioned via the utility thoracotomy so that its open jaw is in the opening of the red rubber catheter. The catheter is then pulled to lead the stapler safely behind the pulmonary vein. Once the stapler is behind the vein, the catheter is removed via the access incision with a DeBakey forceps and the stapler is fired, thereby transecting the superior pulmonary vein.

Once the pulmonary vein has been divided, the pulmonary artery behind the divided vein is dissected, with the middle lobe retracted laterally and posteriorly until the right middle lobe artery is visualized. A tape is then placed around the fissure, just above the right middle lobe artery, and pulled through one of the lower thoracoports. The middle lobe is pulled up to the lateral chest wall with a lung clamp. With the middle lobe vein used as a guide, the minor fissure is completed with an endoscopic GIA stapler. The middle lobe is then moved anteriorly and the lower lobe retracted inferiorly so that a Harken clamp can be placed between the superior segmental artery to the right lower lobe and the recurrent branch to the right upper lobe; the clamp should be aimed toward the area at the bifurcation of the right upper lobe and the bronchus intermedius posteriorly. It may be useful to retract the entire lung anteriorly and dissect this area posteriorly with a peanut sponge to allow better visualization of the bronchial bifurcation. A tape is then passed around the fissure, and an endoscopic GIA stapler is used to complete the fissure.

Once the entire fissure is complete, the recurrent branch is further dissected and stapled with an endovascular stapler passed through the lower anterior port. If it is difficult to place the stapler behind the artery, a red rubber catheter may be used to guide the stapler behind it. The right upper lobe is retracted laterally, and the endovascular stapler is placed via the inferior anterior port and used to divide the truncus anterior. At this point, the only structure remaining to be addressed is the right upper lobe bronchus. This structure is freed of all peribronchial nodal tissue by means of sharp and blunt dissection via the access incision and transected with an endoscopic stapler inserted through the lower anterior port. The specimen is placed in a specimen bag and removed via the access incision, and level 4 and level 7 nodes are either sampled or dissected.

Right lower lobe. Once the right middle lobe artery has been identified, the right lower lobe is retracted posteriorly and laterally to expose the superior aspect of the inferior pulmonary vein. Blunt dissection with a peanut sponge is used to clear the perivascular tissue by pushing up on the lung just superior to the inferior pulmonary vein. A Harken clamp is then placed through the utility thoracotomy, starting at the inferior border of the right middle lobe artery and extending to the area just above the lower lobe vein. The fissure is encircled with a tape and divided with an endoscopic GIA stapler. The lower lobe is retracted via the utility thoracotomy, and an endovascular stapler placed via the lower anterior port is used to transect the vein; the artery is then divided through the same port. Sometimes, the basilar segmental pulmonary artery and the superior segmental artery must be taken separately. The posterior aspect of the major fissure is then completed, and the lower lobe bronchus is transected last.

Right middle lobe. The fissures are completed essentially as already described (see above), with several modifications. The anterior aspect of the major fissure is completed first, as in a lower lobectomy. Next, the middle lobe vein is transected with an endovascular stapler inserted through the inferior thoracoport. The right middle artery is transected from below as well. A peanut sponge is then used to free the superior portion of the right middle lobe bronchus. With the superior pulmonary vein as a guide, the minor fissure is completed, separating the upper and middle lobes. Finally, the bronchus is divided.

Left-side resections The left side is approached somewhat differently. The initial placement of the camera port should be in the midaxillary line because the apex of the heart prevents good visualization if the camera is inserted in the anterior axillary line. The pulmonary artery is usually easier to identify on the left side than on the right. The lung is retracted anteriorly, and the posterior mediastinal pleura is opened to expose the left main pulmonary artery, the subcarinal space, and the inferior pulmonary vein. The left pulmonary artery, the superior segmental artery to the left lower lobe, and the lingular artery should be clearly identified. The lung is retracted posteriorly, and the bronchial bifurcation between the superior and inferior pulmonary veins is clearly identified by means of sharp and blunt dissection. Once this identification has been made, the fissure between the lingula and the lower lobe is divided with an endoscopic GIA stapler.

Left upper lobe. The fissure having been completed, the superior pulmonary vein is transected. The lingular branches are then transected, usually via the inferior midaxillary port, and the apicoposterior branches of the pulmonary artery are transected via the posterior port, with the camera placed through the utility thoracotomy. The anterior segmental branch of the pulmonary artery may be transected either via the utility thoracotomy or via an extra posterior port placed in the line of the thoracotomy. The bronchus is divided last.

Left lower lobe. The fissure having been completed, the inferior pulmonary vein is transected via either the utility thoracotomy or the most posterior port incision. The lower lobe pulmonary artery is transected via the utility thoracotomy, with the end of the stapler visualized via a lower thoracoport. The bronchus is divided last. Again, a No. 10 red rubber catheter can facilitate passage of endovascular staplers around the vessels.

Mass ligation The mass ligation approach, or so-called SIS (simultaneous individual stapling) lobectomy, has its advocates as well.[59] Four incisions are made: an incision for the camera port at the seventh intercostal space, a 2 cm incision in the midaxillary line at the sixth intercostal space for the insertion of staplers, and two 3 cm incisions at the fourth intercostal space in the anterior and posterior axillary lines for the insertion of additional instruments. In the initial report of this technique, the bronchus and the pulmonary vessels were ligated separately, but the vessels were stapled en masse.[60] Subsequently, the technique was refined so that the bronchus and the vessels were stapled simultaneously by applying the stapler twice, the first time loosely to obtain closure of the bronchus and the second time more tightly to obtain hemostatic closure of the vessels. Although the early results were satisfactory,[61] concern about the long-term risks of bronchovascular or arteriovenous fistula formation resulting from mass ligation of the hilar structures has prevented universal acceptance of this approach.

Pneumonectomy

A similar approach has been used for VATS pneumonectomy. The thoracoscope is inserted at the seventh intercostal space in the midaxillary line, and a utility thoracotomy is performed at the fourth intercostal space in the same line. Two port sites are then created at the sixth intercostal space in the anterior and posterior axillary lines. The hilar vessels are sequentially isolated, ligated, and divided with endoscopic or standard staplers. The inferior pulmonary vein is done first, followed by the superior pulmonary vein and the pulmonary artery. The bronchus is stapled and divided last.[62,63]

TROUBLESHOOTING

The endoscopic GIA stapler should never be used to divide the hilar vessels: if it fails to fire staples properly, the vessels retract into the pericardium, causing exsanguinating hemorrhage. The hilar vessels can be ligated proximally with a TA stapler, then ligated and divided distally with an endoscopic GIA stapler; alternatively, they can be divided with the scissors after two TA staple rows have been applied. Another option is to doubly ligate or suture-ligate the vessels via the utility thoracotomy, just as is traditionally done during an open procedure.

Most of the reported VATS lobectomies have been performed in patients with stage I lung cancer. If the tumor is invading the chest wall or the mediastinum or if the resection is being performed after induction chemotherapy or chemoradiotherapy,

VATS is inappropriate because it does not provide adequate exposure for complex resections, particularly when significant perihilar fibrosis is present. Since a randomized trial comparing VATS lobectomy to lobectomy performed through a standard muscle-sparing thoracotomy incision failed to show any significant difference between the two with respect to hospital stay or perioperative morbidity, enthusiasm for VATS lobectomy has diminished.[64-66] It is never wise to compromise the quality of a cancer resection for the perceived benefits of a shorter hospital stay or less pain.

Proper specimen extraction is critical. Tumor implantation in the chest wall is now a recognized complication of VATS procedures. Steps should be taken to prevent intrapleural fragmentation of the tumor, and all specimens should be carefully placed in a plastic bag before being withdrawn through the utility thoracotomy incision or a port site.[67,68]

VATS Mediastinal Lymph Node Dissection

OPERATIVE TECHNIQUE

VATS mediastinal lymph node dissection (MLND) can be performed as an alternative to a Chamberlain procedure for biopsy of the aortopulmonary window nodes or anterior mediastinal masses and is thought by some surgeons to provide better exposure and a superior cosmetic result.[69] The thoracoscope is inserted at the fifth or sixth intercostal space in the posterior axillary line. Instruments for retracting the lung inferiorly are introduced via a port at the seventh intercostal space in the midaxillary line. Instruments for dissecting nodes are introduced through ports placed at the fourth intercostal space in the anterior axillary line and in the auscultatory triangle. The lymph nodes are dissected free with graspers, scissors, the electrocautery, and endoscopic hemostatic clips. Curved sponge sticks are ideal lymph node graspers. A similar approach can be used for biopsy of other mediastinal nodes, including the paratracheal and periesophageal nodes. This method has become an accepted approach to the surgical staging of esophageal cancer.[70,71] It is harder to do a complete en bloc subcarinal lymph node dissection, though nodal sampling of this region by VATS is certainly feasible, especially when an access incision is used.

TROUBLESHOOTING

Care should be taken not to injure the phrenic nerve as it courses along the superior vena cava on the right and across the anterior aspect of the aortopulmonary window on the left. The vagus nerve should be visualized, and the origin of the recurrent laryngeal nerve should be avoided during dissection. The recurrent laryngeal nerve is easily injured on the left side, where it passes around the ligamentum arteriosum before traveling under the aortic arch; however, it can also be injured on the right side if MLND is carried too high superiorly along the origin of the innominate artery.

It is unwise to perform a VATS MLND after induction chemotherapy or chemoradiotherapy because the lymph nodes are often densely adherent to surrounding structures. This is especially true on the right side, where the superior mediastinal lymph nodes are usually densely adherent to the superior vena cava, the azygos vein, and the right main pulmonary artery. A thoracotomy, with extensive exposure and sharp dissection, is usually required for a safe and complete MLND.

All lymphatic branches should be ligated during node biopsy or dissection to prevent leakage of chyle. Often, there are large lymphatic branches in the distal right paratracheal area. The thoracic duct can be injured if periesophageal or posterior mediastinal lymph nodes are being removed.

VATS Esophagectomy

OPERATIVE TECHNIQUE

To date, surgeons' experience with thoracoscopic esophageal resection has been limited. VATS esophagectomy can take either a transhiatal or a transthoracic approach.

Transhiatal Approach

The technique for VATS transhiatal esophagectomy[72] is a modification of the open technique advocated by Orringer[73] [see 3:9 Open Esophageal Procedures] and allows the esophagectomy to be performed completely under direct vision with the help of a specially designed operating mediastinoscope. This instrument has a partially concave olive tip that distracts the mediastinal tissues away from the mediastinoscope and cradles the esophagus in a stable position during the dissection. The mediastinoscope incorporates an optical system, an irrigation canal, and an operating channel for insertion of scissors, suction devices, and monopolar and bipolar cautery forceps.

The mediastinoscope is introduced through the neck incision used to expose the cervical esophagus after the stomach and the distal esophagus have been mobilized via a laparotomy. The thoracic esophagus is circumferentially freed from the surrounding mediastinal structures, beginning at the thoracic inlet and moving inferiorly to the hiatus, primarily by means of blunt dissection with the suction device. Vessels are cauterized or clipped. Dissection is performed first along the posterior wall of the esophagus, then along both lateral walls, and finally on the anterior surface of the esophagus. At the level of the primary tumor, periesophageal soft tissues are resected en bloc to ensure complete removal of the cancer.

When the esophagus has been fully mobilized down to the diaphragmatic hiatus, a plastic tube is passed into the hiatus, where it is grasped by the mediastinoscope. Both the mediastinoscope and the plastic tube are then withdrawn to the cervical incision. The cervical esophagus is transected at the sternal notch with the GIA stapler, and the plastic tube is sutured to the distal end of the divided esophagus. The tube is then gently pulled back down to the diaphragmatic hiatus, and in the process, the thoracic esophagus is folded onto itself. The mediastinoscope is reintroduced and used to follow the esophagus as it is removed from the mediastinum. Any undivided vessels or lymphatics are easily visualized and are either ligated or cauterized. After the esophagus is extracted, the stomach is passed up to the neck via the posterior mediastinum, and the esophagogastric anastomosis is performed in the standard manner for a transhiatal esophagectomy [see Figure 12].

Transthoracic Approach

The transthoracic thoracoscopic technique for esophagectomy has been described by several authors.[74-76] One group has refined a clinical VATS technique that is based on results from animal studies.[77] A double-lumen endotracheal tube is inserted, the patient is placed in the left lateral decubitus position, and six thoracoports are placed [see Figure 13]. The soft tissue is dissected with endoscopic instruments, including a 10 mm scissors, 5 mm grasping forceps, and a cherry dissector. The mediastinal pleura is opened widely, and the anterior edge is retracted with two stay

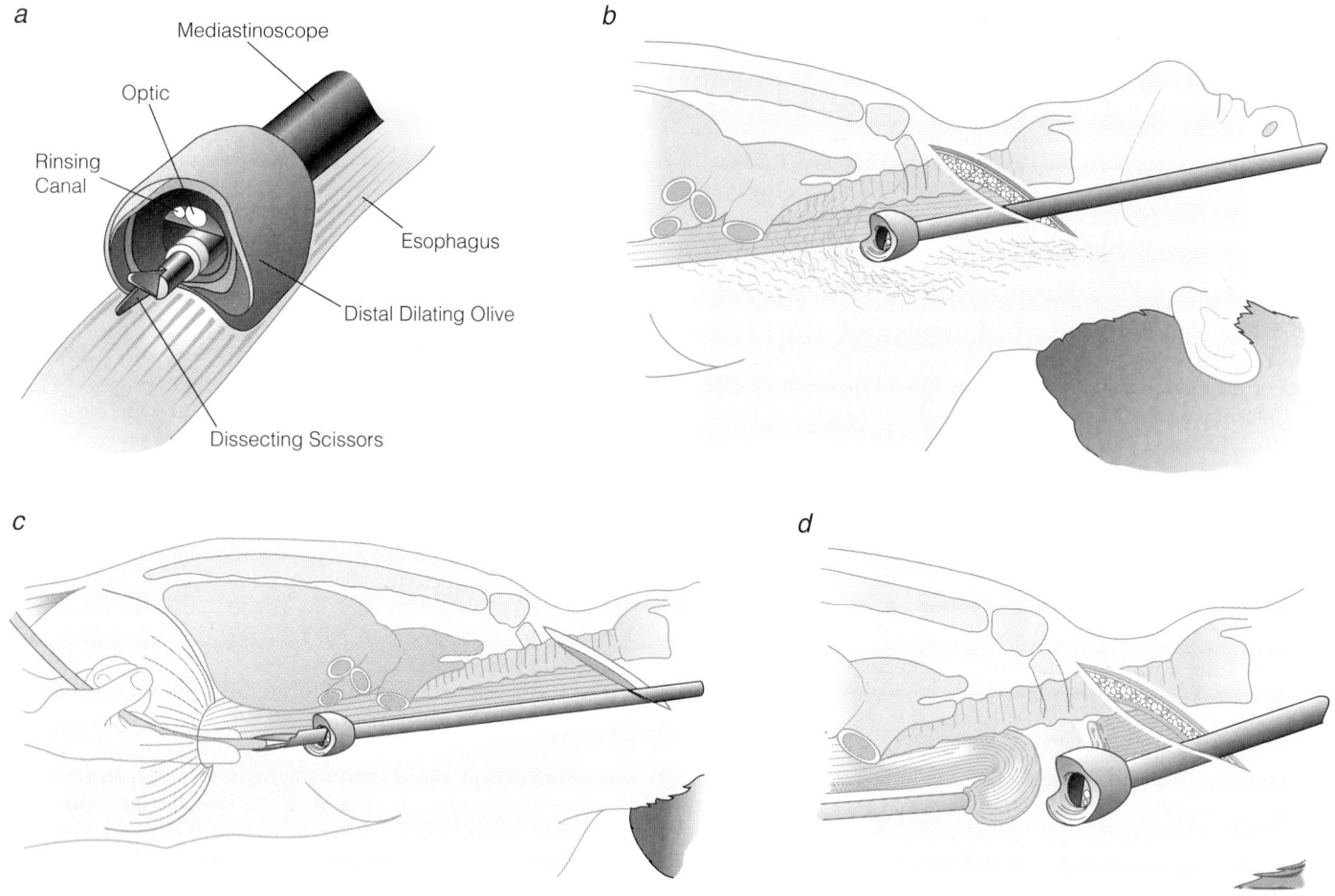

Figure 12 **VATS esophagectomy. In the transhiatal approach, a specially designed operating mediastinoscope with an olive-shaped tip (*a*) is used. This tip mechanically distracts the mediastinal tissues away from the mediastinoscope and keeps the esophagus in a stable position during dissection. The scope is shown cradling the esophagus with the dissecting scissors inserted. During periesophageal dissection, the distal dilating olive of the mediastinoscope is placed behind the esophagus (*b*). The olive creates and maintains space by careful probing of the periesophageal areolar tissue. When the esophagus has been fully mobilized down to the diaphragmatic hiatus, a plastic tube is passed into the hiatus, where it is grasped by the mediastinoscope. Both the mediastinoscope and the plastic tube are pulled up from the hiatus (*c*). After esophageal resection with an endoscopic GIA stapler, the esophagus is folded over by using endoscopic control (*d*). Structures still attached to the esophagus are placed in traction, coagulated, and divided.**

sutures. The azygos vein is divided with an endoscopic stapler. The inferior half of the thoracic esophagus is mobilized away from the aorta and pericardium. The subcarinal lymph nodes are removed en bloc. The upper third of the thoracic esophagus is mobilized away from the trachea, and the right paratracheal lymph nodes are removed, with care taken not to injure the recurrent laryngeal nerve. Once the esophagus has been fully mobilized, the pleural traction sutures are removed, two chest tubes inserted through port sites, and the other port incisions closed. The patient is then moved to the supine position. The stomach is mobilized through a laparotomy and brought up to the neck, where a cervical anastomosis is performed.

TROUBLESHOOTING

The technical problems associated with VATS esophagectomy are similar to those associated with open thoracic esophagectomy, including thoracic duct injury, recurrent nerve palsy, bleeding from the intercostal vessels, and anastomotic leakage [*see 3:9 Open Esophageal Procedures*]. These problems are best prevented by obtaining good visualization of the superior and posterior mediastinum, which can be achieved by using a 30° angled thoracoscope. The most common reason for conversion to thoracotomy is the presence of a locally advanced tumor that necessitates extensive dissection for safe mobilization away from adjacent mediastinal structures.

To date, comparison of the results of VATS esophagectomy with those of open esophagectomy has not shown VATS to yield a significant decrease in major complications, especially postoperative respiratory insufficiency and cardiac arrhythmias. These findings may be attributable in part to the number of port sites required to accomplish a complicated resection and to the necessity of combining VATS with an upper midline laparotomy for mobilization of the stomach.[78,79] As a result, most centers still prefer the standard open transhiatal or transthoracic approaches to esophagectomy.

VATS also plays a useful role in the management of postoperative chylothorax.[80] The thoracic duct can be ligated thoracoscopically, though it is sometimes difficult to identify and ligate

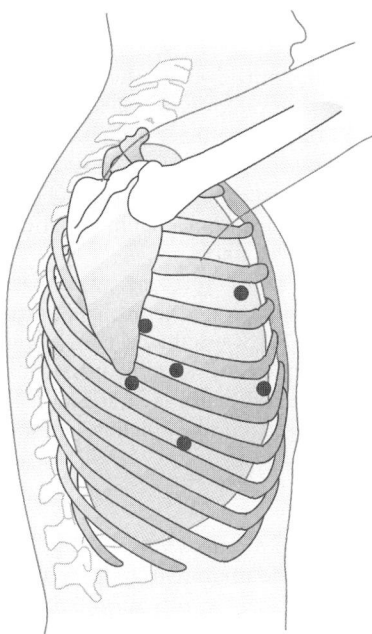

Figure 13 **VATS esophagectomy. Shown are trocar sites for the transthoracic approach.**[77]

the primary site of a postoperative lymphatic leak without reopening the thoracotomy.

VATS Pericardial Window

OPERATIVE TECHNIQUE

Some surgeons create a pericardial window by means of VATS as an alternative to taking the subxiphoid approach or the left anterior thoracotomy approach.[81,82] A double-lumen endotracheal tube is inserted with the patient under general anesthesia, and the patient is rotated into the right lateral decubitus position. Three access sites are used, with the thoracoscope inserted at the seventh intercostal space in the posterior axillary line and instruments introduced through two ports, one at the tip of the scapula and the other at the sixth intercostal space in the axillary line [*see Figure 14a*]. The pericardium is retracted with a grasper forceps, and scissors are used to resect 8 to 10 cm² areas of pericardium both anterior and posterior to the phrenic nerve. If indicated, talc pleurodesis can be performed to control an associated pleural effusion. One or two chest tubes are then inserted through the port-site incisions.

TROUBLESHOOTING

When a pericardial effusion causes cardiac tamponade, a subxiphoid approach is preferable to VATS for creating a pericardial window because it is safer to perform in a hemodynamically unstable patient. A VATS pericardial window is also inadvisable in patients with constrictive physiology or with intrapericardial adhesions discovered at the time of operation. Conversion to an open procedure with formal pericardiectomy is advisable under these circumstances.

VATS Procedures for Mediastinal Masses

A 1998 multicenter trial aimed at defining the role of VATS in the management of mediastinal tumors suggested that VATS can

be used safely to diagnose and resect most middle and posterior mediastinal masses, especially in view of the typically benign nature of these tumors.[83]

VATS thymectomy has been employed to treat myasthenia gravis and thymoma.[84] To date, only anecdotal experience is available, and no studies examining long-term outcome have been published. Although a VATS approach to myasthenia gravis may appear attractive at first, it is not the least invasive approach to the thymus. Transcervical thymectomy is a minimally invasive approach to the thymus that does not require a chest incision, does not violate the pleural space, and allows most patients to be discharged home the next day.[85] There is still a degree of controversy as to whether complete thymic resection, including all ectopic thymic tissue, is necessary to obtain clinical remission in patients with myasthenia gravis.[86] For patients with a thymic mass, we prefer a transsternal approach. For patients with myasthenia gravis who do not have a thymoma, however, we believe that there is a need for prospective studies comparing VATS with other surgical approaches to thymectomy.

OPERATIVE TECHNIQUE

VATS has been used to resect masses in all of the mediastinal compartments. VATS resection is an ideal approach to posterior neurogenic tumors that do not extend into the neural canal.[87,88] With the patient in the lateral decubitus position, the operating table is rotated anteriorly so that the lung falls away from the paravertebral region. The port sites are placed anteriorly; the thoracoscope is inserted at the fifth intercostal space in the midaxillary line, a lung retractor is inserted at the sixth intercostal space in the anterior axillary line, and dissecting instruments are inserted at the second and fourth intercostal spaces in the anterior axillary line [*see Figure 14b*]. The mass is manipulated with a grasper to expose the posteriorly located pedicle, which is then dissected, ligated, and divided with the scissors, clip appliers, and the electrocautery.[89,90]

For removal of anterior mediastinal masses, the port sites are placed in more posterior locations. The thoracoscope is introduced at the fifth intercostal space in the midaxillary or posterior axillary line, and instruments are inserted through two ports, one at the second intercostal space at the midaxillary line and the other at the fifth or sixth intercostal space in the anterior axillary line [*see Figure 14c*]. The mass is retracted with a grasper and dissected free with a combination of sharp and blunt dissection, clip appliers, and the electrocautery.[91,92]

A similar technique is used to resect middle mediastinal masses, most of which are pericardial or bronchogenic cysts.[93,94] The access sites should be chosen according to the location of the mass on the preoperative CT scan. Generally, however, the triangulated site placement used for pulmonary wedge resections provides more suitable exposure than the site placement used for anterior or posterior mediastinal masses.

TROUBLESHOOTING

The placement of the thoracoports and the positioning of the operative team for the resection of posterior mediastinal tumors or for thoracic diskectomy differ significantly from the usual practice in most other VATS procedures. In place of the standard arrangement of trocars in an inverted triangle, the viewing port is placed in the posterior axillary line and the operating ports in the anterior axillary line. The thoracic surgeon and the neurosurgeon both stand on the anterior side of the patient, each viewing a monitor on the opposite side. In addition, a 30° scope is essential for visualizing the intervertebral disk space.[88,90]

Removal of dumbbell neurogenic tumors can be accomplished thoracoscopically if immediately preceded by posterior surgical removal of the spinal component of the tumor via laminectomy and intervertebral foraminotomy. Preoperative MRI scanning is crucial for defining the extent of tumor within the spinal canal.[89] Resection of posterior mediastinal tumors is sometimes associated with significant bleeding from intercostal or spinal arteries; should such bleeding occur, there should be no hesitation in converting to a thoracotomy.

Ideally, anterior mediastinal cysts should be resected in toto to avoid recurrence; however, if the cysts are firmly adherent to vital mediastinal structures, partial excision with cauterization of the endothelial lining may be safer.

VATS Management of Thoracic Trauma

The major contraindication to thoracoscopy in thoracic trauma is hemodynamic instability. For major life-threatening injuries involving the great vessels and the mediastinum, thoracotomy is required to obtain expeditious control of injured structures. However, hemodynamically stable patients with certain thoracic problems—such as diaphragmatic injury, slow continued intrathoracic bleeding, persistent air leakage, and empyema—can be diagnosed and often treated by means of VATS.[95,96]

In the assessment of a trauma patient with a potential diaphragmatic injury, it is important not to ignore the high incidence of associated intra-abdominal injury. If intra-abdominal injury has been ruled out and there is concern about the presence of a diaphragmatic tear, thoracoscopic assessment of the diaphragm is justified. Such assessment allows a more thorough evaluation of the entire diaphragm than the laparoscopic approach, which is limited by the liver on the right side. In the largest series published to date, 60 of 171 patients who underwent thoracoscopy for penetrating chest injuries had diaphragmatic injuries that necessitated repair.[97] For hemodynamically stable patients with suspected diaphragmatic injuries, the VATS approach appears reasonable.

When a patient has an ongoing intrathoracic problem such as persistent bleeding or a large air leak 24 to 48 hours after a traumatic injury, VATS should be considered before a thoracotomy is done because most problems encountered at this time (e.g., chest wall bleeding and laceration of the lung parenchyma) can be managed endoscopically, without the need for a thoracotomy.

TROUBLESHOOTING

The main pitfall in thoracoscopic evaluation of the diaphragm is failure to assess the abdomen appropriately and consequent failure to recognize an occult intra-abdominal injury. When laparoscopy is performed in a patient with a diaphragmatic injury, CO_2 insufflation can cause a tension pneumothorax to develop on the side of the diaphragmatic injury; accordingly, whenever diaphragmatic injury is a possibility, the chest should be included in the operative field to allow chest tube insertion if required. Because thoracoscopy does not require CO_2 insufflation, it is safer in such situations.

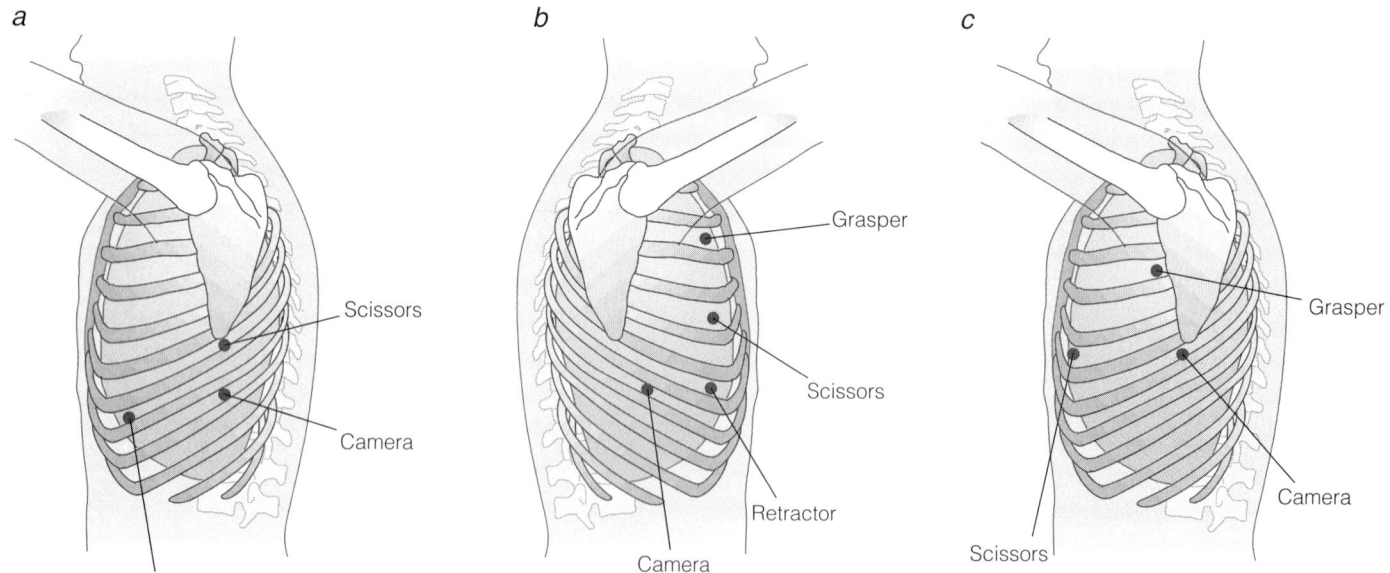

Figure 14 (*a*) **VATS pericardial window. Three access sites are used. The thoracoscope is inserted in the posterior axillary line at the seventh intercostal space, the endoscopic scissors are inserted through one port at the tip of the scapula, and the grasper forceps is inserted through another port in the anterior axillary line at the sixth intercostal space.** (*b, c*) **VATS procedures for mediastinal masses. For posterior masses, the port sites are placed anteriorly** (*b*), **and the thoracoscope is inserted at the fifth intercostal space in the midaxillary line. A lung retractor is inserted at the sixth intercostal space in the anterior axillary line, and dissecting instruments are inserted at the second and fourth intercostal spaces in the anterior axillary line. For anterior mediastinal masses and thymectomy, the port sites are placed in more posterior locations** (*c*). **The thoracoscope is introduced at the fifth intercostal space in the midaxillary or the posterior axillary line, and instruments are inserted through one port at the second intercostal space in the midaxillary line and another at the fifth or sixth intercostal space in the anterior axillary line.**

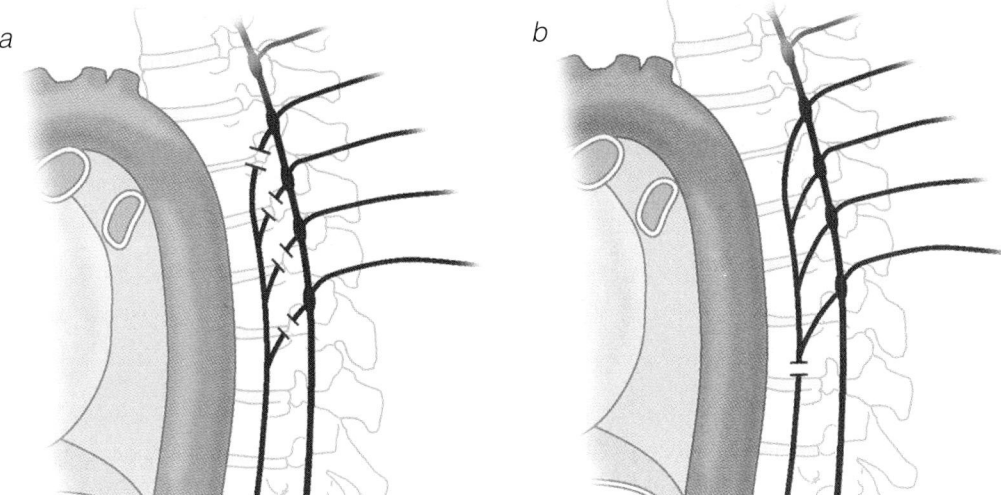

Figure 15 **VATS splanchnicectomy. Splanchnicectomy may be accomplished by either (*a*) dividing the roots of the splanchnic nerves or (*b*) dividing the splanchnic nerve itself.**

VATS Sympathectomy and Splanchnicectomy

Thoracic sympathectomy is known to be the most effective treatment for upper limb hyperhidrosis, and VATS is now an accepted approach to this operation.

The main indication for splanchnicectomy is intractable abdominal pain from unresectable malignancies (e.g., pancreatic or gastric carcinoma) and chronic pancreatitis. The effects of celiac ganglion blocks are transient, and surgical manipulation of this area is usually very difficult because of the primary disease process, previous operations, or both. In the past, thoracotomy was generally considered too invasive an approach to splanchnic denervation in these patients. Currently, however, because of the less invasive nature of thoracoscopy and the quicker recovery time associated with it, thoracoscopic splanchnicectomy is an attractive therapeutic option.[98]

OPERATIVE TECHNIQUE

Sympathectomy

VATS sympathectomy is performed with the patient under general anesthesia and a double-lumen tube in place. Three port sites are used: one for the thoracoscope at the third intercostal space in the midaxillary line, one at the third intercostal space in the anterior axillary line, and one at the tip of the scapula. The pleura is incised and divided from T2 to T5, and the sympathetic chain is dissected free with scissors. For complete control of upper limb hyperhidrosis, VATS must be done bilaterally.[99,100]

Splanchnicectomy

The technical aspects of VATS splanchnicectomy are quite simple: a sound knowledge of the splanchnic anatomy and a basic set of thoracoscopic instruments are all that is needed. Single-lung ventilation is required. Three thoracoports are placed. A silk stitch is placed in the central tendon of the diaphragm and pulled through the most anterior and inferior port to allow better visualization of the splanchnic nerves. The camera is also placed though this port. An endoscopic grasper and an endoscopic scissors with an electrocautery attachment are used to remove the nerve segment from T5 to T9. The greater

and lesser splanchnic nerves are resected [*see Figure 15*]. The least splanchnic nerve is rarely visualized.

TROUBLESHOOTING

Care should be taken to identify the first and second ribs. Division of the sympathetic trunk at the level of the first rib causes Horner syndrome and does not reduce palmar hyperhidrosis.

Division of the rami communicantes rather than the main sympathetic trunk reduces the incidence of undesirable side effects, especially compensatory hyperhidrosis of the trunk, but its overall success rate in controlling upper limb hyperhidrosis is lower.[99] Abolition of only the T2 and T3 ganglia may control palmar hyperhidrosis without being as likely to result in unacceptable compensatory truncal sweating. Target areas for axillary sweating also include T4 and T5. In addition, an accessory sympathetic nerve fiber that runs lateral to the sympathetic chain (known as the nerve of Kuntz) should be sought and, if identified, divided. Compensatory hyperhidrosis of the inner thighs is a not uncommon complication.

Neuralgia is frequent after VATS sympathectomy. Some authors advocate a 2-day postoperative course of dexamethasone to reduce the incidence of this problem.[100]

Miscellaneous VATS Procedures

Several other procedures have been performed by VATS, including ligation of the thoracic duct[101] and resection of the adrenal gland.[102] For adrenal resection, three incisions are placed at the 9th or 10th intercostal space, extending from the anterior axillary line to the posterior axillary line. A fan retractor is inserted through a radial incision in the diaphragm and used to retract the perirenal fat. The adrenal gland is dissected free and removed, and the associated vessels are clipped or cauterized.[102]

Clinical Considerations

Minimally invasive surgery is currently in high demand, largely as a result of patient preferences. This growing popularity, however, must not be allowed to override clinical concerns. In particular, extreme care must be taken in the treatment of malignant disease because the consequences of cancer surgery are far greater than the consequences of surgery for benign disease. Whether a VATS procedure has good or acceptable long-term results is at least as important as whether it is technically feasible. It is our responsibility as thoracic surgeons to perform these procedures selectively rather than indiscriminately, either in settings where the effectiveness of VATS is clearly proved or, where the role of VATS has not been fully established, within the context of well-designed clinical trials.

Cost Considerations

It is hard to estimate the cost-effectiveness of VATS procedures because the instrumentation, the types of procedures performed, and the surgical expertise with these operations are all still evolving. Initially, VATS procedures proved expensive, for several reasons (e.g., the cost of purchasing video and endoscopic equipment, the cost of disposable instrumentation, and the need for long operating times as surgeons and nursing staff gained experience performing these procedures). Soon after VATS was introduced, a study from the Mayo Clinic compared the cost of performing VATS pulmonary wedge resections with that of the same operation done by thoracotomy.[103] The VATS approach was associated with substantially shorter hospital stays but also with increased OR costs; hence, the use of VATS did not result in any significant overall savings. Since that study, however, as some VATS procedures (e.g., pulmonary wedge resection) have become standard operations and more reusable instrumentation has become available, the cost of VATS has undoubtedly decreased. Whether other, more complex VATS procedures (e.g., thoracoscopic esophagectomy) are cost-effective remains to be determined.

Training and Certification in VATS

Thoracoscopy is most frequently performed by thoracic surgeons.[2] In some centers, however, particularly in Europe, pulmonologists became highly experienced in the application of traditional thoracoscopic techniques for the diagnosis of pleural disease. The experience of Boutin epitomizes the involvement of physicians who do not have specific surgical training.[4,8] The development of small-caliber endoscopes that could be used with local anesthesia outside the OR made it easy for nonsurgeons to perform thoracoscopy.

After the 1950s, thoracoscopy was largely forgotten by surgeons and pulmonologists in the United States until the advent of VATS. The dramatic initial popularity of this technique generated considerable debate about whether nonsurgeons should perform VATS in the same way as they perform other invasive endoscopic procedures.[104-106] During this same period, laparoscopic cholecystectomy became widely practiced, often by persons who lacked adequate training, and reports of serious complications emerged.

Within this context, the Society of Thoracic Surgeons (STS) and the American Association for Thoracic Surgery (AATS) formed a joint committee to establish standards and guidelines for training and certification in VATS [see Sidebar Statement of AATS/STS Joint Committee on Thoracoscopy and Video Assisted Thoracic Surgery].[107] As a result of the educational efforts of this committee, many surgeons were trained within a short time, and VATS was quickly incorporated into thoracic surgical practice and residency training.

The important considerations with respect to the training and practice of VATS have been well articulated.[106,107] VATS is not a minor procedure: it is minimally invasive, complex intrathoracic surgery that should be performed only by persons who are familiar with intrathoracic anatomy and pathology and are fully competent to manage complications and make intraoperative decisions in such a way as to ensure safe outcomes for thoracic surgical patients. The complications encountered during thoracoscopic operations are potentially immediately life-threatening, whereas those encountered during other endoscopic procedures usually are not. For that reason, VATS procedures should not be performed by anyone—surgeon or nonsurgeon—who lacks the training and experience to perform immediate thoracotomy and repair of intrathoracic injuries.

VATS is now an integral part of the practice of thoracic surgery.[108] The direct involvement of the major thoracic societies in the dispersion of this technology has discouraged the casual and unsafe application of VATS and has promoted an ongoing critical appraisal of VATS procedures.

Statement of AATS/STS Joint Committee on Thoracoscopy and Video Assisted Thoracic Surgery[107]

The Councils of the American Association for Thoracic Surgery and the Society of Thoracic Surgeons have formed a Joint Committee on Thoracoscopy and Video Assisted Thoracic Surgery. The purpose of this Committee is to facilitate the education of thoracic surgeons in this new technology and to provide guidelines for appropriate training in and performance of thoracoscopy and video assisted, minimally invasive thoracic surgery.

The following guidelines are recommended by the Joint Committee:

1. In order to ensure optimal quality patient care, thoracoscopy and video assisted thoracic surgery (TVATS) should be performed only by thoracic surgeons who are qualified, through documented training and experience, to perform open thoracic surgical procedures and manage their potential complications. The surgeon must have the judgment, training, and capability to proceed immediately to a standard open thoracic procedure if necessary.

   The preoperative and postoperative care of patients treated by TVATS should be the responsibility of the operating surgeon.

2. It is recommended that TVATS techniques be learned through appropriate instruction:

   a. As part of a formal approved thoracic surgical residency or fellowship program which includes structured and documented experience in these procedures.

   b. For the practicing thoracic surgeon, completion of a course that follows the guidelines approved by the Joint Committee, with hands-on laboratory experience, plus observation of these techniques performed by thoracic surgeons experienced in such procedures.

3. The granting of privileges to perform TVATS remains the responsibility of the credentialing body of individual hospitals.

For the AATS/STS Joint Committee on Thoracoscopy and Video Assisted Thoracic Surgery: Martin F. McKneally, M.D., and Ralph J. Lewis, M.D., co-chairmen; Richard P. Anderson, M.D., Richard G. Fosburg, M.D., William A. Gay, Jr., M.D., Robert H. Jones, M.D., and Mark B. Orringer, M.D.

References

1. Jacobeus HC: The practical importance of thoracoscopy in surgery of the chest. Surg Gynecol Obstet 34:289, 1922

2. Bloomberg AE: Thoracoscopy in perspective. Surg Gynecol Obstet 147:433, 1978

3. Weissberg D, Kaufman M: Diagnostic and therapeutic pleuroscopy: experience with 127 patients. Chest 78:732, 1980

4. Boutin C, Viallat JR, Cargnino P, et al: Thoracoscopy in malignant pleural effusions. Am Rev Respir Dis 124:588, 1981

5. Wihlm JM, Roeslin N, Morand G, et al: Résultats comparés de la ponction, de la biopsie à l'aiguille, de la pleuroscopie et de la thoracotomie dans le diagnostic des pleurésies chroniques. Poumon Coeur 37:57, 1981

6. Rodgers BM, Ryckman FC, Moazam F, et al: Thoracoscopy for intrathoracic tumors. Ann Thorac Surg 31:414, 1981

7. Rusch VW, Mountain C: Thoracoscopy under regional anesthesia for the diagnosis and management of pleural disease. Am J Surg 154:274, 1987

8. Boutin C, Viallat JR, Aelony Y: Practical Thoracoscopy. Berlin, Springer-Verlag, 1991

9. Hazelrigg SR, Nunchuck SK, LoCicero JI: Video Assisted Thoracic Surgery Study Group data. Ann Thorac Surg 56:1039, 1993

10. Krasna MJ, Deshmukh S, McLaughlin JS: Complications of thoracoscopy. Ann Thorac Surg 61:1066, 1996

11. Nakata M, Saeki H, Yokoyama N, et al: Pulmonary function after lobectomy: video-assisted thoracic surgery versus thoracotomy. Ann Thorac Surg 70:938, 2000

12. Kaseda S, Aoki T, Hangai N, et al: Better pulmonary function and prognosis with video-assisted thoracic surgery than with thoracotomy. Ann Thorac Surg 70:1644, 2000

13. Craig SR, Leaver HA, Yap PL, et al: Acute phase responses following minimal access and conventional thoracic surgery. Eur J Cardiothorac Surg 20:455, 2001

14. Yim AP, Wan S, Lee TW, et al: VATS lobectomy reduces cytokine responses compared with conventional surgery. Ann Thorac Surg 70:243, 2000

15. Deslauriers J, Beaulieu M, Dufour C, et al: Mediastinopleuroscopy: a new approach to the diagnosis of intrathoracic diseases. Ann Thorac Surg 22:265, 1976

16. Rusch VW: Instrumentation for video-assisted thoracic surgery. Chest Surg Clin North Am 3:215, 1993

17. Landreneau RJ, Herlan DB, Johnson JA, et al: Thoracoscopic neodymium:yttrium-aluminum garnet laser-assisted pulmonary resection. Ann Thorac Surg 52:1176, 1991

18. Rusch VW, Schmidt R, Shoji Y, et al: Use of the argon beam electrocoagulator for performing pulmonary wedge resections. Ann Thorac Surg 49:287, 1990

19. Landreneau RJ, Mack MJ, Hazelrigg SR, et al: Video-assisted thoracic surgery: basic technical concepts and intercostal approach strategies. Ann Thorac Surg 54:800, 1992

20. Rusch VW, Bains MS, Burt ME, et al: Contribution of videothoracoscopy to the management of the cancer patient. Ann Surg Oncol 1:94, 1994

21. Ohri SK, Oswal SK, Townsend ER, et al: Early and late outcome after diagnostic thoracoscopy and talc pleurodesis. Ann Thorac Surg 53:1038, 1992

22. Angelillo Mackinlay TA, Lyons GA, Chimondeguy DJ, et al: VATS debridement versus thoracotomy in the treatment of loculated postpneumonia empyema. Ann Thorac Surg 61:1626, 1996

23. Hartman DL, Gaither JM, Kesler KA, et al: Comparison of insufflated talc under thoracoscopic guidance with standard tetracycline and bleomycin pleurodesis for control of malignant pleural effusions. J Thorac Cardiovasc Surg 105:743, 1993

24. Landreneau RJ, Hazelrigg SR, Ferson PF, et al: Thoracoscopic resection of 85 pulmonary lesions. Ann Thorac Surg 54:415, 1992

25. Jimenez MF, The Spanish Video-Assisted Thoracic Surgery Group: Prospective study on video-assisted thoracoscopic surgery in the resection of pulmonary nodules: 209 cases from the Spanish Video-Assisted Thoracic Surgery Group. Eur J Cardiothorac Surg 19:562, 2001

26. Ferson PF, Landreneau RJ, Dowling RD, et al: Comparison of open versus thoracoscopic lung biopsy for diffuse infiltrative pulmonary disease. J Thorac Cardiovasc Surg 106:194, 1993

27. Miller JD, Urschel JD, Cox G, et al: A randomized, controlled trial comparing thoracoscopy and limited thoracotomy for lung biopsy in interstitial lung disease. Ann Thorac Surg 70:1647, 2000

28. Dowling RD, Keenan RJ, Ferson PF, et al: Video-assisted thoracoscopic resection of pulmonary metastases. Ann Thorac Surg 56:772, 1993

29. Landreneau RJ, De Giacomo T, Mack MJ, et al: Therapeutic video-assisted thoracoscopic surgical resection of colorectal pulmonary metastases. Eur J Cardiothorac Surg 18:671, 2000

30. McCormack PM, Ginsberg KB, Bains MS, et al: Accuracy of lung imaging in metastases with implications for the role of thoracoscopy. Ann Thorac Surg 56:863, 1993

31. Dowling RD, Ferson PF, Landreneau RJ: Thoracoscopic resection of pulmonary metastases. Chest 102:1450, 1992

32. McCormack PM, Bains MS, Begg CB, et al: Role of video-assisted thoracic surgery in the treatment of pulmonary metastases: Results of a prospective trial. Ann Thorac Surg 62:213, 1996

33. Parekh K, Rusch V, Bains M, et al: VATS port site recurrence: a technique dependent problem. Ann Surg Oncol 8:175, 2001

34. Miller DL, Allen MS, Trastek VF, et al: Videothoracoscopic wedge excision of the lung. Ann Thorac Surg 54:410, 1992

35. Bolotin G, Lazarovici H, Uretzky G, et al: The efficacy of intraoperative internal intercostal nerve block during video-assisted thoracic surgery on postoperative pain. Ann Thorac Surg 70:1872, 2000

36. Normori H, Horio H: Endofinger for tactile localization of pulmonary nodules during thoracoscopic resection. Thorac Cardiovasc Surg 44:50, 1996

37. Shennib H, Bret P: Intraoperative transthoracic ultrasonographic localization of occult lung lesions. Ann Thorac Surg 55:767, 1993

38. Plunkett MB, Peterson MS, Landreneau RJ, et al: Peripheral pulmonary nodules: preoperative percutaneous needle localization with CT guidance. Radiology 185:274, 1992

39. Lewis RJ, Caccavale RJ, Sisler GE, et al: One hundred consecutive patients undergoing video-assisted thoracic operations. Ann Thorac Surg 54:421, 1992

40. Demmy TL, Nielson D, Curtis JJ: Improved method for deep thoracoscopic lung nodule excision. Missouri Med 93:86, 1996

41. Mouroux J, Elkaïm D, Padovani B, et al: Video-assisted thoracoscopic treatment of spontaneous pneumothorax: technique and results of one hundred cases. J Thorac Cardiovasc Surg 112:385, 1996

42. Schrmael FMNH, Sutedja TG, Braber JCE, et al: Cost-effectiveness of video-assisted thoracoscopic surgery versus conservative treatment for first time or recurrent spontaneous pneumothorax. Eur Respir J 9:1821, 1996

43. Hazelrigg SR, Landreneau RJ, Mack M, et al: Thoracoscopic stapled resection for spontaneous pneumothorax. J Thorac Cardiovasc Surg 105:389, 1993

44. Cole FH, Jr, Cole FH, Khandekar A, et al: Video-assisted thoracic surgery: primary therapy for spontaneous pneumothorax? Ann Thorac Surg 60:931, 1995

45. Wakabayashi A: Expanded applications of diagnostic and therapeutic thoracoscopy. J Thorac Cardiovasc Surg 102:721, 1991

46. Wakabayashi A: Thoracoscopic laser pneumoplasty in the treatment of diffuse bullous emphysema. Ann Thorac Surg 60:936, 1995

47. Torresini G, Vaccarili M, Divisi D, et al: Is video-assisted thoracic surgery justified at first spontaneous pneumothorax? Eur J Cardiothorac Surg 20:42, 2001

48. Yim AP: Video-assisted thoracoscopic management of primary spontaneous pneumothorax. Ann Acad Med Singapore 25:668, 1996

49. Colt HG, Russack V, Chiu Y, et al: A comparison of thoracoscopic talc insufflation, slurry, and mechanical abrasion pleurodesis. Chest 111:442, 1997

50. Inderbitzi RGC, Furrer M, Striffeler H, et al: Thoracoscopic pleurectomy for treatment of complicated spontaneous pneumothorax. J Thorac Cardiovasc Surg 105:84, 1993

51. Swanson SJ, Mentzer SJ, DeCamp MM, et al: No-cut thoracoscopic lung plication: a new technique for lung volume reduction surgery. J Am Coll Surg 185:25, 1997

52. Yim APC, Ko K-M, Ma C-C, et al: Thoracoscopic lobectomy for benign diseases. Chest 109:554, 1996

53. McKenna RJ Jr, Wolf RK, Brenner M, et al: Is lobectomy by video-assisted thoracic surgery an adequate cancer operation? Ann Thorac Surg 66:1903, 1998

54. Demmy TL, Curtis JJ: Minimally invasive lobectomy directed toward frail and high-risk patients: a case-control study. Ann Thorac Surg 68:194, 1999

55. Weber A, Stammberger U, Inci I, et al: Thoracoscopic lobectomy for benign disease—a single centre study on 64 cases. Eur J Cardiothorac Surg 20:443, 2001

56. Solaini L, Prusciano F, Bagioni P, et al: Video-assisted thoracic surgery major pulmonary resections: present experience. Eur J Cardiothorac Surg 20:437, 2001

57. Kirby TJ, Mack MJ, Landreneau RJ, et al: Initial experience with video-assisted thoracoscopic lobectomy. Ann Thorac Surg 56:1248, 1993

58. Kohno T, Murakami T, Wakabayashi A: Anatomic lobectomy of the lung by means of thoracoscopy: an experimental study. J Thorac Cardiovasc Surg 105:729, 1993

59. Lewis RJ: Simultaneously stapled lobectomy: a safe technique for video-assisted thoracic surgery. J Thorac Cardiovasc Surg 109:619, 1995

60. Lewis RJ, Sisler GE, Caccavale RJ: Imaged thoracic lobectomy: should it be done? Ann Thorac Surg 54:80, 1992

61. Lewis RJ: Personal communication, 1993

62. Roviaro GC, Rebuffat C, Varoli F, et al: Video-endoscopic thoracic surgery. Int Surg 78:4, 1993

63. Roviaro GC, Varoli F, Rebuffat C, et al: Video-thoracoscopic staging and treatment of lung cancer. Ann Thorac Surg 59:971, 1995

64. Landreneau RJ, Hazelrigg SR, Mack MJ, et al: Postoperative pain-related morbidity: video-assisted thoracic surgery versus thoracotomy. Ann Thorac Surg 56:1285, 1993

65. Kirby TJ, Mack MJ, Landreneau RJ, et al: Lobectomy—video-assisted thoracic surgery versus muscle-sparing thoracotomy: a randomized trial. J Thorac Cardiovasc Surg 109:997, 1995

66. Landreneau RJ, Mack MJ, Hazelrigg SR, et al: Prevalence of chronic pain after pulmonary resection by thoracotomy or video-assisted thoracic surgery. J Thorac Cardiovasc Surg 107:1079, 1994

67. Downey RJ, McCormack P, LoCicero JI, et al: Dissemination of malignant tumors after video-assisted thoracic surgery: a report of twenty-one cases. J Thorac Cardiovasc Surg 111:954, 1996

68. Johnstone PAS, Rohde DC, Swartz SE, et al: Port site recurrences after laparoscopic and thoracoscopic procedures in malignancy. J Clin Oncol 14:1950, 1996

69. Landreneau RJ, Hazelrigg SR, Mack MJ, et al: Thoracoscopic mediastinal lymph node sampling: useful for mediastinal lymph node stations inaccessible by cervical mediastinoscopy. J Thorac Cardiovasc Surg 106:554, 1993

70. Krasna MJ: Minimally invasive staging for esophageal cancer. Chest 112:191S, 1997

71. Krasna MJ, Flowers JL, Attar S, et al: Combined thoracoscopic/laparoscopic staging of esophageal cancer. J Thorac Cardiovasc Surg 111:800, 1996

72. Buess G, Becker HD, Lenz G: Perivisceral endoscopic oesophagectomy. Operative Manual of Endoscopic Surgery. Cuschieri A, Ed. Springer-Verlag, Berlin, 1992, p 149

73. Orringer MB: Transhiatal esophagectomy without thoracotomy for carcinoma of the thoracic esophagus. Ann Surg 200:282, 1984

74. Law S, Fok M, Chu KM, et al: Thoracoscopic esophagectomy for esophageal cancer. Surgery 122:8, 1997

75. Collard J-M, Lengele B, Otte J-B, et al: En bloc and standard esophagectomies by thoracoscopy. Ann Thorac Surg 56:675, 1993

76. Gossot D, Fourquier P, Celerier M: Thoracoscopic oesophagectomy. Ann Chir Gyn Fenniae 83:162, 1994

77. Akaishi T, Kaneda I, Higuchi N, et al: Thoracoscopic en bloc total esophagectomy with radical mediastinal lymphadenectomy. J Thorac Cardiovasc Surg 112:1533, 1996

78. Collard J-M: En bloc and standard esophagectomies by thoracoscopy: update. Ann Thorac Surg 61:769, 1996

79. Peracchia A, Rosati R, Fumagalli U, et al: Thoracoscopic esophagectomy: are there benefits? Sem Surg Onc 13:259, 1997

80. Fahimi H, Casselman FP, Mariani MA, et al: Current management of postoperative chylothorax. Ann Thorac Surg 71:448, 2001

81. Mack MJ, Landreneau RJ, Hazelrigg SR, et al: Video thoracoscopic management of benign and malignant pericardial effusions. Chest 103:390S, 1993

82. Flores RM, Jaklitsch MT, DeCamp MM Jr, et al: Video-assisted thoracic surgery pericardial resection for effusive disease. Chest Surg Clin North Am 8:835, 1998

83. Demmy TL, Krasna MJ, Detterbeck FC, et al: Multicenter VATS experience with mediastinal tumors. Ann Thorac Surg 66:187, 1998

84. Mack MJ, Landreneau RJ, Yim AP, et al: Results of video-assisted thymectomy in patients with myasthenia gravis. J Thorac Cardiovasc Surg 112:1352, 1996

85. Cooper JD, Al-Jilaihawi AN, Pearson FG, et al: An improved technique to facilitate transcervical thymectomy for myasthenia gravis. Ann Thorac Surg 45:242, 1988

86. Jaretzki A, III, Wolff M: "Maximal" thymectomy for myasthenia gravis: surgical anatomy and operative technique. J Thorac Cardiovasc Surg 96:711, 1988

87. Riquet M, Mouroux J, Pons F, et al: Videothoracoscopic excision of thoracic neurogenic tumors. Ann Thorac Surg 60:943, 1995

88. Bousamra M, II, Haasler GB, Patterson GA, et al: A comparative study of thoracoscopic vs open removal of benign neurogenic mediastinal tumors. Chest 109:1461, 1996

89. Vallières E, Findlay JM, Fraser RE: Combined microneurosurgical and thoracoscopic removal of neurogenic dumbbell tumors. Ann Thorac Surg 59:469, 1995

90. Mack MJ, Regan JJ, McAfee PC, et al: Video-assisted thoracic surgery for the anterior approach to the thoracic spine. Ann Thorac Surg 59:1100, 1995

91. Yim APC, Kay RLC, Ho JKS: Video-assisted thoracoscopic thymectomy for myasthenia gravis. Chest 108:1440, 1995

92. Knight R, Ratzer ER, Fenoglio ME, et al: Thoracoscopic excision of mediastinal parathyroid adenomas: a report of two cases and review of the literature. J Am Coll Surg 185:481, 1997

93. Hazelrigg SR, Landreneau RJ, Mack MJ, et al: Thoracoscopic resection of mediastinal cysts. Ann Thorac Surg 56:659, 1993

94. Lewis RJ, Caccavale RJ, Sisler GE: Imaged thoracoscopic surgery: a new thoracic technique for resection of mediastinal cysts. Ann Thorac Surg 53:318, 1992

95. Lang-Lazdunski L, Mouroux J, Pons F, et al: Role of videothoracoscopy in chest trauma. Ann Thorac Surg 63:327, 1997

96. Spann JC, Nwariaku FE, Wait M: Evaluation of video-assisted thoracoscopic surgery in the diagnosis of diaphragmatic injuries. Am J Surg 170:628, 1995

97. Freeman RK, Al-Dossari G, Hutcheson KA, et al: Indications for using video-assisted thoracoscopic surgery to diagnose diaphragmatic injuries after penetrating chest trauma. Ann Thorac Surg 72:342, 2001

98. Le Pimpec-Barthes F, Chapuis O, Riquet M, et al: Thoracoscopic splanchinicectomy for control of intractable pain in pancreatic cancer. Ann Thorac Surg 65:810, 1998

99. Gossot D, Toledo L, Fritsch S, et al: Thoracoscopic sympathectomy for upper limb hyperhidrosis: looking for the right operation. Ann Thorac Surg 64:975, 1997

100. Wong C-W: Transthoracic video endoscopic electrocautery of sympathetic ganglia for hyperhidrosis palmaris: special reference to localization of the first and second ribs. Surg Neurol 47:224, 1997

101. Shirai T, Amano J, Takabe K: Thoracoscopic diagnosis and treatment of chylothorax after pneumonectomy. Ann Thorac Surg 52:306, 1991

102. Mack MJ, Aronoff RJ, Acuff TE, et al: Thoracoscopic transdiaphragmatic approach for adrenal biopsy. Ann Thorac Surg 55:772, 1993

103. Allen MS, Deschamps C, Lee RE, et al: Video-assisted thoracoscopic stapled wedge excision for indeterminate pulmonary nodules. J Thorac Cardiovasc Surg 106:1048, 1993

104. Mathur P, Martin WJ Jr: Clinical utility of thoracoscopy. Chest 102:2, 1992

105. Forum: Who should perform thoracoscopy? Chest 102:1553, 1992

106. Thoracoscopy forum, continuing dialogue. Chest 102:1915, 1992

107. McKneally MF, Lewis RJ, Anderson RP, et al: Statement of the AATS/STS Joint Committee on Thoracoscopy and Video Assisted Thoracic Surgery. J Thorac Cardiovasc Surg 104:1, 1992

108. Mack MJ, Scruggs GR, Kelly KM, et al: Video-assisted thoracic surgery: has technology found its place? Ann Thorac Surg 64:211, 1997

Acknowledgment

Figures 1 through 7 and 9 through 15   Tom Moore.

12 ULTRASONOGRAPHY: SURGICAL APPLICATIONS

Grace S. Rozycki, M.D., F.A.C.S.

Although the scientific principles underlying ultrasonography first began to be elucidated in the 19th century, it was not until the second half of the 20th century that this technology could be effectively applied to medicine. In particular, surgeons in the United States have now embraced ultrasonography as a key diagnostic tool in many areas of clinical practice. Because ultrasonography is noninvasive, portable, rapid, and easily repeatable, it is especially well suited to surgical practice. In addition, computer-enhanced high-resolution imaging and multifrequency specialized transducers have made ultrasonography increasingly user friendly, enhancing its applicability to a variety of surgical settings.

Physics and Instrumentation

Before the application of ultrasound devices to patient evaluation is addressed, it is worthwhile to briefly review certain basic physical principles and terminology associated with ultrasonography [see Tables 1, 2, and 3].[1-5] Nowhere in diagnostic imaging is the understanding of wave physics more important than in ultrasound diagnostic imaging, because ultrasonography is highly operator dependent. To perform an ultrasound examination correctly, a surgeon must be able to interpret echo patterns, determine artifacts, and adjust the machine appropriately so as to obtain the best images.

In diagnostic ultrasonography, the transducer or probe interconverts electrical and acoustic energy [see Figure 1].[6] To accomplish this interconversion, the transducer contains the following essential components:

1. An active element. Electrical energy is applied to the piezoelectric crystals within the transducer, and an ultrasound

pulse is thereby generated via the piezoelectric effect. The pulse distorts the crystals, and an electrical signal is produced. This signal causes an ultrasound image to form on the screen via the reverse piezoelectric effect.
2. Damping or backing material. An epoxy resin absorbs the vibrations and reduces the number of cycles in a pulse, thereby improving the resolution of the ultrasound image.
3. A matching layer. This substance reduces the reflection that occurs at the transducer-tissue interface. The great difference in density (i.e., the impedance mismatch) between the soft tissue and the transducer results in reflection of the ultrasound waves. The matching material decreases this reflection and facilitates the transit of the ultrasound waves through the body and into the target organ.

Transducers are classified according to (1) the arrangement of the active elements (array) contained within the transducer and (2) the frequency of the ultrasound wave produced. Transducer arrays contain closely packed piezoelectric elements, each with its own electrical connection to the ultrasound instrument.[7] These elements can be excited individually or in groups to produce the ultrasound beam. There are four main transducer arrays: (1) the rectangular linear array, which yields a rectangular image, (2) the curved array, which yields a trapezoidal image, (3) the phased array, a small transducer in which the sound pulses are generated by activating all of the elements in the array, and (4) the annular array, in which the elements are arranged in a circular fashion. The advantage of transducer arrays is that the ultrasound beam can be electronically steered without any moving mechanical parts (except for the annular array) and focused.[7,8] In the clinical set-

Table 1 Ultrasound Physics Terminology Relevant to Ultrasonographic Imaging[4-6]

Term	Definition	Significance
Ultrasound	High-frequency (> 20 kHz) mechanical radiant energy transmitted through a medium	
Frequency	Number of cycles/sec (10^6 cycles/sec = 1 MHz) Diagnostic ultrasound: 1–20 MHz	Increasing frequency improves resolution
Wavelength	Distance traveled by wave per cycle: as frequency becomes higher, wavelength becomes smaller	Wavelength is related to spatial resolution of object: shorter wavelengths yield better resolution but poorer penetration
Amplitude Attenuation Absorption Scattering Reflection	Strength or height of wave Decrease in amplitude and intensity of wave as it travels through a medium; attenuation is affected by absorption, scattering, and reflection Conversion of sound energy into heat Redirection of wave as it strikes a rough or small boundary Return of wave toward transducer	Amplitude and intensity are reduced (attenuated) as waves travel through tissue; time-gain compensation circuit compensates for this attenuation
Propagation speed	Speed with which wave travels through soft tissue (1,540 m/sec)	Propagation speed (determined by density and stiffness of medium) is greater in solids than in liquids and greater in liquids than in gases

Table 2 Essential Principles of Ultrasound

Principle	Explanation
Piezoelectric effect	Piezoelectric crystals expand and contract to interconvert electrical and mechanical energy
Pulse-echo principle	When ultrasound wave contacts tissue, some of signal is reflected while some is transmitted into tissue; these waves are then reflected to crystals within transducer, generating electrical impulse comparable to strength of returning wave
Acoustic impedance	Acoustic impedance = density of tissue × speed of sound in tissue Strength of returning echo depends on difference in density between two structures imaged: structures of different acoustic impedance (e.g., bile and gallstone) are relatively easy to distinguish from one another, whereas those of similar acoustic impedance (e.g., spleen and kidney) are more difficult to distinguish

ting, this arrangement allows the operator to adjust the focal zone so that he or she can accurately image a large organ (e.g., the liver) while still being able to obtain fine details of a lesion.

The frequency of the transducer is determined by the thickness of the piezoelectric elements within the transducer: the thinner the piezoelectric elements, the higher the frequency.[7,8] Although diagnostic ultrasonography makes use of transducer frequencies ranging from 1 MHz to 20 MHz, the most commonly used frequencies for medical diagnostic imaging are those between 2.5 and 10 MHz [see Table 4]. Ultrasound beams of different frequencies have different characteristics: higher frequencies penetrate tissue poorly but yield excellent resolution, whereas lower frequencies penetrate well but at the cost of compromised resolution. Accordingly, transducers are generally chosen on the basis of the depth of the structure to be imaged.[9] For example, a 7.5 MHz transducer is a suitable choice for imaging a superficial organ such as the thyroid, but a 3.5 MHz transducer would be preferable for imaging a deep structure such as the abdominal aorta.

Ultrasound machines vary in complexity, but each has the following essential components:

1. A monitor (for displaying the ultrasound image).
2. A keyboard (for labeling the image and making adjustments to produce a quality image).
3. A transducer (for interconverting electrical and acoustic energy).

Table 3 Terminology Used in Assessment of Ultrasonograms[3,108]

Term	Definition
Echogenicity	Degree to which tissue echoes ultrasonic waves (generally reflected in ultrasound image as degree of brightness)
Anechoic	Showing no internal echoes, appearing dark or black
Isoechoic	Having appearance similar to that of surrounding tissue
Hypoechoic	Less echoic or darker than surrounding tissue
Hyperechoic	More echoic or whiter than surrounding tissue
Resolution	Ability to distinguish between two different structures; spatial resolution improves as frequency increases
Lateral	Resolution transverse to ultrasound wave; relates to width of structure
Axial	Resolution parallel to ultrasound wave; relates to depth of structure

4. An image recorder (for producing copies of the ultrasound images).

Finally, there are three scanning modes, A, B, and M; these modes evolved over several years.[10] A mode (amplitude modulation), the most basic form of diagnostic ultrasonography, yields a one-dimensional image that displays the amplitude or strength of the wave along the vertical axis and the time along the horizontal axis. Therefore, the greater the signal returning to the transducer, the higher the "spike." B mode (brightness modulation), the mode most commonly used today, relates the brightness of the image to the amplitude of the ultrasound wave. Thus, denser structures appear brighter (i.e., whiter, more echogenic) on the image because they reflect the ultrasound waves better. M mode relates the amplitude of the ultrasound wave to the imaging of moving structures, such as cardiac muscle. Before real-time imaging became available, M-mode scanning formed the basis for echocardiography.[10,11]

Clinical Applications of Ultrasonography in Surgical Practice

As an extension of the physical examination, ultrasonography is a valuable adjunct to surgical practice in the office, the emergency department, the OR, and the SICU. Once surgeons have learned the essential principles of ultrasonography, they can readily build on this experience and extend the use of this technology to various specific aspects of surgery. In what follows, I list and briefly describe several clinical areas in which surgeon-performed ultrasonography has proved to be an effective diagnostic and interventional tool.

BREAST

Ultrasound-directed biopsy of breast lesions is now a common office procedure for general surgeons. The increase in the number of screening mammograms performed since the late 1970s has led to the detection of more nonpalpable breast lesions. The traditional choice for further evaluation of such masses has been open surgical excision, but the yield of malignancies with this approach has been only about 20%.[12-14] Advances in ultrasound technology, including automated biopsy needles, high-resolution transducers,[15] and computer-aided diagnosis programs,[16] have prompted a surge of interest in fine-needle and core biopsy tissue sampling as an alternative to open biopsy. Such procedures are appealing because they are minimally invasive, are about as accurate as open biopsy,[17] and can be performed by the surgeon in the office setting.[18] Essentially, surgeons use ultrasound to evaluate the breast for the presence of a solid or cystic lesion and to identify those characteristics of a lesion that suggest whether it is benign or malignant.

Current indications for breast ultrasonography include (1) evaluation of mammographically detected microcalcifications or nonpalpable, new, or growing masses, (2) evaluation of duct size in the presence of nipple discharge, (3) assessment of a dense breast or a vaguely palpable mass, (4) differentiation between a solid palpable mass and a cystic one, and (5) guidance of percutaneous drainage of an abscess.[19-24] Additional uses include postoperative follow-up for hematomas, seromas, and prostheses.

Ultrasound-guided interventions now in clinical use include cyst aspiration, biopsy of solid lesions, preoperative needle localization, axillary lymph node fine-needle aspiration (FNA), and peritumoral injection for sentinel lymph node biopsy [see 2:6 Lymphatic Mapping and Sentinel Lymph Node Biopsy].[25] Reports suggest that high-resolution ultrasonography can accurately detect intraductal spread of

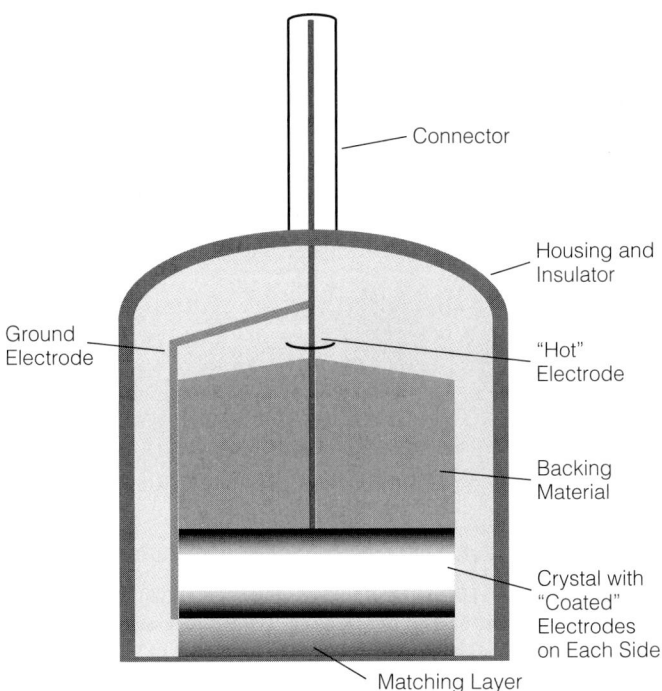

Figure 1 Shown are the basic components of an ultrasound transducer.

Connector

Housing and Insulator

Ground Electrode

"Hot" Electrode

Backing Material

Crystal with "Coated" Electrodes on Each Side

Matching Layer

tumors and delineate their multiple foci. Ongoing developments in imaging technology and contrast agents have given perfusion studies an enhanced contrast resolution that increases the sensitivity of ultrasonography for small nodal metastases. Accordingly, the use of breast ultrasonography in the office setting has become considerably more sophisticated and sensitive, allowing more patients to be screened for microdisease.[18]

GASTROINTESTINAL TRACT

Endoscopic and endorectal ultrasonography have added a new dimension to the preoperative assessment and treatment of many GI lesions. Endoscopic ultrasonography (EUS) involves the visualization of the GI tract via a high-frequency (12 to 20 MHz) ultrasound transducer placed through an endoscope. With the transducer near the target organ, images of the gut wall and the surrounding parenchymal organs can be obtained that are detailed enough to define the depth of tumor penetration with precision and to detect the presence of involved lymph nodes as small as 2 mm. When done preoperatively, EUS is 80% to 90%

accurate at predicting the stage of the tumor; if an endoscopically directed biopsy attachment is used, the diagnostic potential is even higher.[26]

Indications for EUS include (1) preoperative staging of GI malignancies, (2) preoperative localization of pancreatic endocrine tumors, particularly insulinomas, (3) evaluation of submucosal lesions of the GI tract, and (4) guidance of imaging during interventional procedures (e.g., tissue sampling and drainage of a pancreatic pseudocyst).[27-30] Currently, EUS is being used in conjunction with FNA biopsy to evaluate submucosal lesions of the GI tract as well as lesions of the pancreas. This combination is especially useful for pancreatic lesions: EUS-guided FNA accurately detects neoplastic pancreatic cysts and therefore may be helpful in determining whether medical or surgical treatment is indicated.[31,32]

Endorectal ultrasonography is used in the evaluation of patients with benign and malignant rectal conditions.[33-41] It is commonly performed with an axial 7.0 or 10.0 MHz rotating transducer that produces a 360° horizontal cross-sectional view of the rectal wall. This special transducer is 24 cm long and is covered with a water-filled latex balloon. After the transducer is advanced above the rectal lesion, the balloon that surrounds the transducer is filled with degassed water to create an acoustic window for ultrasound imaging. The transducer is gradually withdrawn while the examiner views the layers of the rectal wall [see Figure 2] by means of real-time imaging.[42,43] These layers are important landmarks in ultrasonographic staging, just as they are in postoperative pathologic staging. For example, if the middle white line (i.e., the submucosa) is intact, a benign lesion may be removed via a submucosal resection. A classification of preoperative tumor staging called uTNM has been proposed that is analogous to the TNM classification for tumor staging.[44] This classification is based on ultrasonographic determination of the infiltrative tumor depth (the prefix *u* stands for ultrasonography).

The sensitivity of ultrasonography in determining the depth of tumor invasion is about 85% to 90%; however, it can sometimes overestimate the extent of invasion in the presence of tissue inflammation and edema.[35] Further research is needed to assess the accuracy of ultrasonography in detecting recurrent cancer after surgery.[45] Errors in staging are likely to occur with tumors that invade the lamina muscularis mucosae or are associated with inflammation of the lamina propria mucosae.[46] In addition, lesions characterized by ultramicroscopic invasion of the submucosa may be misstaged because the technology currently available cannot

Table 4 Clinical Applications of Selected Transducer Frequencies

Frequency	Applications
2.5–3.5 MHz	Renal Aortic General abdominal
5.0 MHz	Transvaginal Pediatric abdominal Testicular
7.5 MHz	Vascular Foreign body in soft tissue Thyroid

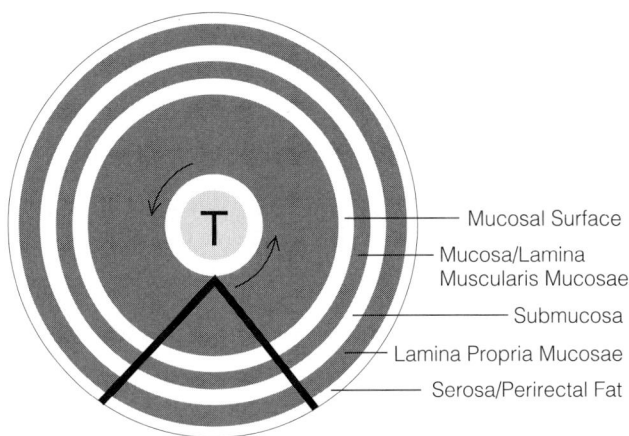

T

Mucosal Surface

Mucosa/Lamina Muscularis Mucosae

Submucosa

Lamina Propria Mucosae

Serosa/Perirectal Fat

Figure 2 Depicted is the five-layer model of rectal wall anatomy as delineated by endorectal ultrasonography.[109]

provide the fine resolution necessary to assess such invasion.[35,47] Flexible 360° rotating transducers are now available for the evaluation of rectal lesions. Investigators from Madigan Army Medical Center found that whereas rigid endoscopic transducers were slightly more sensitive than flexible transducers in detecting lesions, the flexible devices were highly accurate (77%) in staging rectal cancers; learning curves were comparable for the two types of transducers.[48]

Endoanal ultrasonography is an important part of the evaluation of anal incontinence because it is capable of detecting defects in the internal and external sphincters.[49-53] It is done in much the same way as endorectal ultrasonography, except that the 10 MHz transducer is covered with a sonolucent hard plastic cone instead of a water-filled balloon. Although endoanal ultrasonography does not measure sphincter function, ultrasound-detected sphincter disruption correlates well with pressure measurements[54,55] and operative findings.[53,56] Additional indications for endoanal ultrasonography include evaluation of patients with an exophytic distal rectal tumor (e.g., a villous adenoma) and assessment of patients who have a perianal abscess, fistula in ano, a presacral cyst, or a rectal ulcer.

ACUTE CONDITIONS

Traumatic

The FAST (*F*ocused *A*ssessment for the *S*onographic examination of the *T*rauma patient) is a rapid diagnostic test developed for the evaluation of patients with potential truncal injuries. Historically, its development is rooted in several fundamental studies that demonstrated the high sensitivity of ultrasonography in detecting small degrees of ascites,[57] splenic injury,[58] and hemoperitoneum in the hepatorenal space and the pelvis.[59] The FAST determines the presence or absence of blood in the pericardial sac and three dependent abdominal regions, including Morison's pouch, the splenorenal recess, and the pelvis.

Ultrasonography may also be used in traumatic settings to detect hemothorax, sternal fracture, and pneumothorax.[60-62]

Nontraumatic

In the acute nontraumatic setting, surgeons are currently using ultrasonography for the following purposes:

1. Assessment for multiple loculations and drainage of a soft tissue abscess.[63,64]
2. Early diagnosis of wound dehiscence through visualization of the fascial defect [see Figure 3].
3. Detection of a foreign body in soft tissue.[65-67]
4. Evaluation of a patient with abdominal pain (e.g., from gallstones).[63,64,68,69]
5. Confirmation of the reduction of an incarcerated hernia through identification of the fascial defect and observation of the reduction occurring with real-time imaging [see Figure 4].[70]
6. Identification of an abdominal aortic aneurysm in a patient who presents with back pain and hypotension. Intramural calcification and intraluminal thrombus are common findings [see Figure 5]. If the aortic aneurysm ruptures into the peritoneal cavity, the FAST can detect the presence of hemoperitoneum.

LAPAROSCOPY AND INTRAOPERATIVE USE

Examination with intraoperative or laparoscopic ultrasonography is an integral part of many hepatic, biliary, and pancreatic surgical procedures. With this tool, surgeons can detect previously

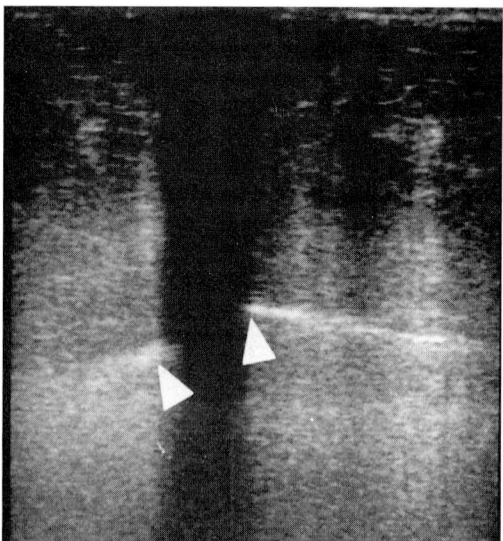

Figure 3 **Ultrasound image shows midline abdominal wound dehiscence. Transducer orientation is sagittal with respect to long axis of wound. Interruption in horizontal white line (arrows) represents separation of fascia.**

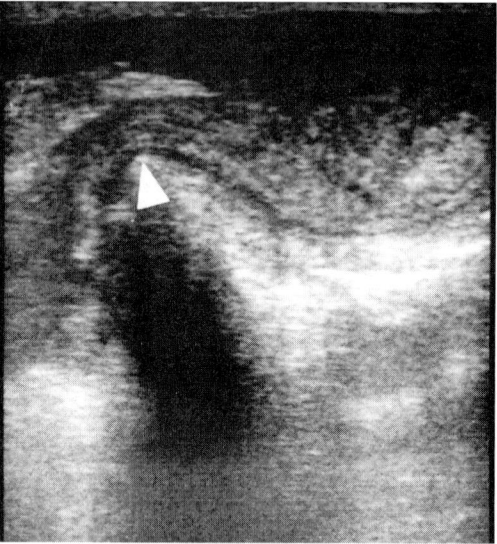

Figure 4 **Sagittal ultrasound image shows ventral hernia with fascial defect (arrow).**

undiagnosed lesions or bile duct stones,[71] avoid unnecessary dissection of vessels or ducts, clarify tumor margins, and perform biopsy and cryoablation procedures.[72] Compared with preoperative imaging modalities, intraoperative ultrasonography is much more sensitive in detecting malignant or benign lesions.[73] The precision with which intraoperative ultrasonography can delineate small lesions (5 mm) and define their relationship to other structures facilitates resection, reduces operative time, and frequently alters the surgeon's operative strategy.[73-76]

Intraoperative ultrasonography makes use of both contact scanning and so-called standoff scanning for imaging.[77] In contact scanning, the transducer is directly applied to the organ so that the deepest part of the organ is accurately depicted. This technique is most often used for imaging large organs (e.g., the liver). In standoff scanning, the transducer is placed about 1 to 2 cm away from

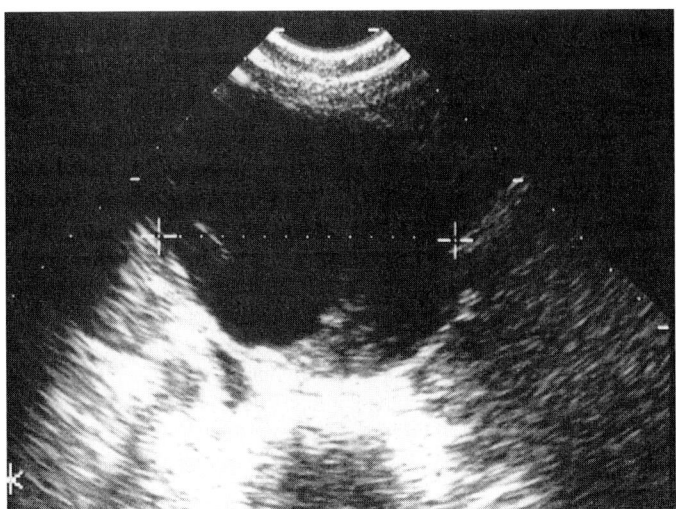

Figure 5 **Transverse ultrasound image shows abdominal aortic aneurysm with intraluminal thrombus.**

the structure in a pool of sterile saline solution that permits the transmission of ultrasound waves. This technique is often used to image blood vessels, bile ducts, or the spinal cord; it allows good visualization of the structure without compression by the transducer. The size, shape, and type of ultrasound transducer used for intraoperative scanning depend on the anatomic structure to be examined. For example, a pencillike 7.5 MHz transducer is used for scanning the common bile duct, whereas a side-viewing T-shaped 5 MHz transducer is preferable for imaging a cirrhotic liver. Intraoperative ultrasound examinations are conducted systematically to ensure that no subtle pathology is missed and that the examination is reproducible. For example, the liver is imaged sequentially according to a system based on Couinaud's anatomic segments [*see 3:17 Hepatic Resection*].[78]

Similar principles apply to laparoscopic ultrasonography, except that the transducers are made to adapt to the laparoscopic equipment.[79,80] Indications for this modality include detection of common bile duct stones, staging of pancreatic cancer to prevent unnecessary celiotomy, and resection or cryoablation of hepatic metastases.[80]

VASCULAR SYSTEM

Color flow duplex imaging and endoluminal ultrasonography have significantly expanded the diagnostic and therapeutic aspects of vascular imaging. Vascular diagnostic imaging is commonly used for diagnosing arterial disease or deep vein thrombosis (DVT); however, it is also helpful for diagnosing other disorders, such as Raynaud disease and thoracic outlet syndrome. In the office setting, surgeons use ultrasonography to screen for abdominal aortic aneurysm or to follow patients with a diagnosed aneurysm, because it is capable of detecting change in aortic diameter as small as a few millimeters.[81] In patients who have undergone repair of an abdominal aortic aneurysm, color flow duplex imaging is highly specific for the diagnosis of anastomotic false aneurysms. In one study, this modality was compared with B-mode ultrasonography, CT, digital subtraction arteriography, and magnetic resonance imaging and emerged as the diagnostic test of choice when the accuracy, cost, safety, and availability of each method were assessed.[82]

Color flow duplex scanning is also used to examine the patency and size of the portal vein and the hepatic artery in patients who have undergone liver transplantation, to assess the resectability of pancreatic tumors, to diagnose superior mesenteric artery occlu-

sion, and to diagnose a pseudoaneurysm or an arteriovenous fistula after percutaneous arterial catheterization.[83,84] In the acute setting, several investigators have found color flow duplex imaging to be a reliable, time-saving, noninvasive alternative to arteriography for the detection of arterial injury.[85-89]

Duplex imaging of the lower extremity is used to assess the patency of the deep venous system and is capable of detecting DVT reliably.[90] The addition of color flow imaging facilitates the examination by making the artery and its associated vein easier to identify. By performing serial duplex venous ultrasound imaging to detect DVT, one group of investigators was able to identify a subgroup of injured patients who were at highest risk for pulmonary embolism; they suggested that these patients be given DVT prophylaxis and undergo close surveillance with duplex imaging.[90]

Intraoperative duplex imaging can be used to detect technical errors in vascular anastomoses as well as abnormalities in flow.[91] Arteriography assesses the patency of an anastomosis and measures distal arterial runoff, but it is invasive. Intraoperative duplex imaging, on the other hand, permits rapid visualization of the anatomic and hemodynamic aspects of a vascular reconstruction, and it is noninvasive, easily repeatable, and less time-consuming than arteriography.

SURGICAL INTENSIVE CARE UNIT

Indications for surgeon-performed ultrasonography in the SICU include localization of a central vein or an artery for hemodynamic monitoring[92] and detection of a pleural effusion [*see Figure 6*]. Not only are fewer lateral decubitus x-rays ordered when ultrasonography is done in the SICU, but the safety of thoracentesis is also enhanced when it is performed under ultrasound guidance.[93,94]

General Considerations for Diagnostic Ultrasound Examinations

INSTRUMENTATION

Before an ultrasound examination is performed, the following three steps should be observed:

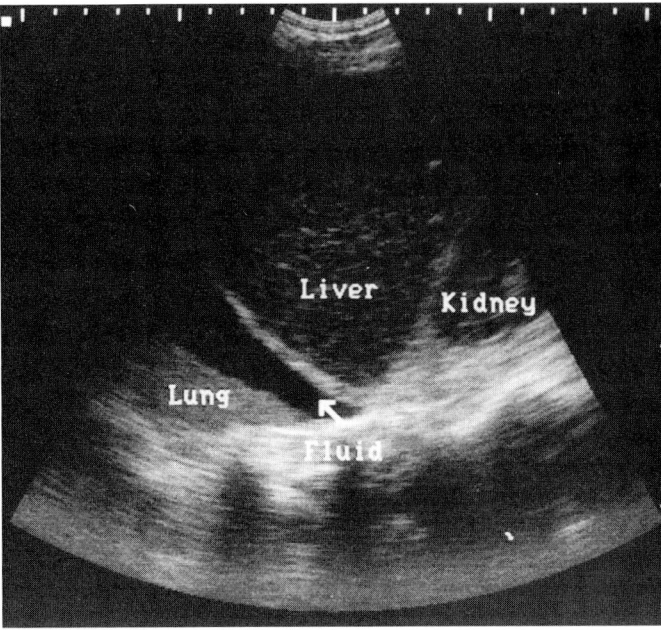

Figure 6 **Sagittal ultrasound image demonstrates pleural effusion.**

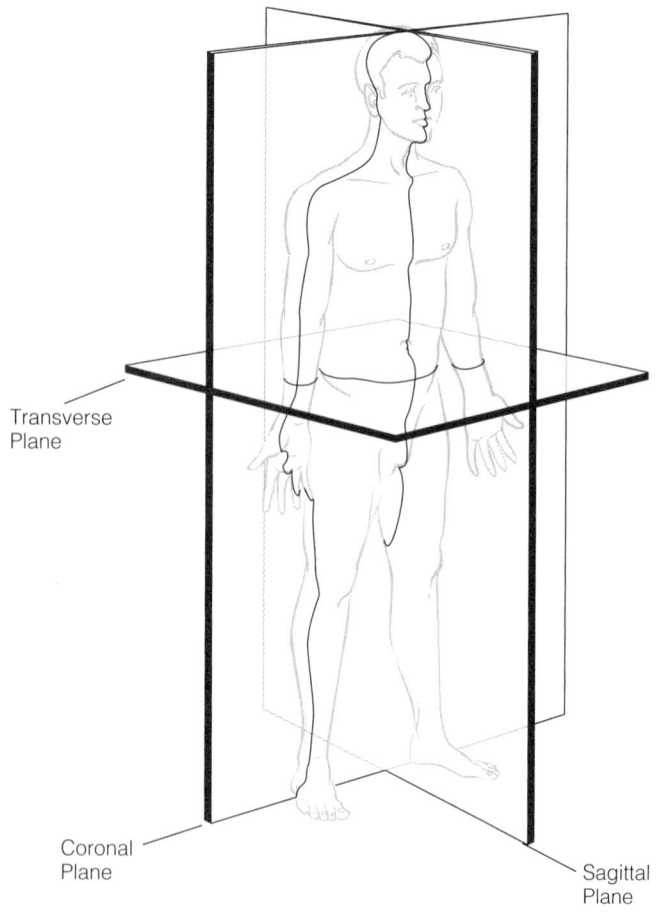

Figure 7 **Depicted are scanning planes used in ultrasonography.**

1. The correct ultrasound machine and transducer should be chosen for the specific type of examination to be done. For example, if a vascular study is to be performed, the machine should have Doppler capability and, ideally, color flow capability as well.
2. The transducer should be chosen according to the structure or organ to be imaged. It must provide both sufficient depth of penetration to image the entire organ and sufficient resolution to allow the examiner to distinguish the details of lesions.
3. Although many machines have preset controls for power and gain, a standard image should be obtained to confirm that the settings are correct for the specific examination being done. For example, the FAST begins with an image of the heart so that blood can be identified and the gain controls adjusted (if necessary) to permit accurate detection of hemoperitoneum.

PATIENT POSITIONING

The patient should be positioned so that all of the images required for a particular examination can be readily obtained. The surgeon should take time to review the scanning planes [*see Figure 7*] and understand the orientation of the patient on the monitor screen in relation to the transducer. It is also important to follow conventional scanning protocols so that when the images are reviewed, a lesion can be accurately located and the scan can be reproduced even by another ultrasonographer. An example of such a protocol is the radial-scanning technique recommended for

examination of the breast [*see* Technique for Selected Surgical Applications of Ultrasonography, Breast Examination, *below*].

DOCUMENTATION

The machine's annotation keys are used to record the patient's name and identification number, the area of interest, and the scanning plane. Most machines have function keys that automate the recording of these data. Furthermore, the internal clock automatically labels each image with the date and time (accurate to 0.01 second).

Any hard copies of the ultrasound images that may be required should be printed, saved, and reviewed. Ideally, the ultrasound images should be videotaped, because the dynamic real-time image provides more information than still images, thereby increasing the confidence level associated with each observation.

CONTINUOUS PERFORMANCE IMPROVEMENT

As part of the performance improvement process, ultrasound images should be routinely reviewed, with special attention paid to false positive or false negative examinations. The goal of this process is to help identify any correctable factors associated with such examinations and thereby minimize or prevent their recurrence. Some studies have noted the presence of a pronounced learning curve, as a result of which the sensitivity and specificity initially achieved by new surgeon-ultrasonographers have been relatively low[68,95-97]; however, there is evidence that surgeons' performance may be improved with the help of an ultrasound training course that focuses on those pitfalls of imaging that were found to be problems in the clinical setting. For example, in one study, surgeons learned both to perform

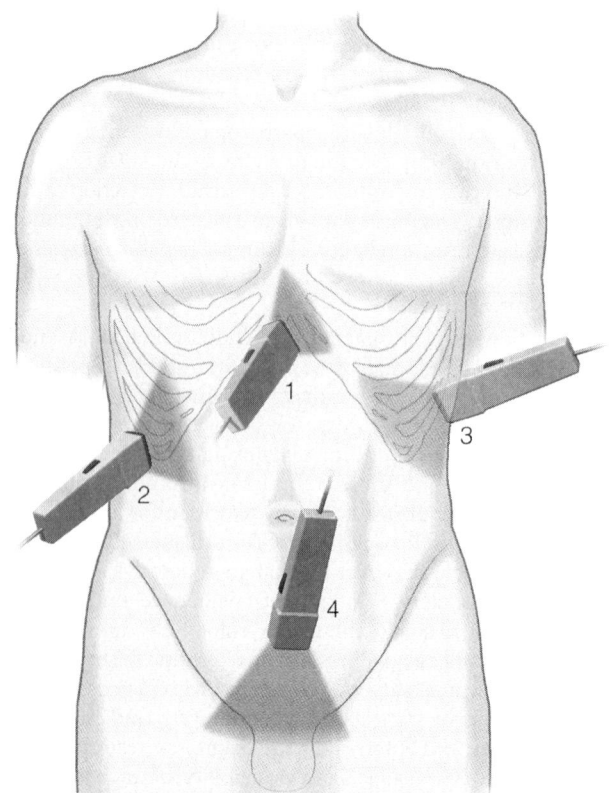

Figure 8 **FAST. Shown are four transducer positions used in FAST: (1) pericardial area, (2) right upper quadrant, (3) left upper quadrant, and (4) pelvis.**[95]

examinations correctly and to interpret positive results accurately in patients with minimal as well as pronounced ascites; as a result, they were better able to distinguish relatively subtle differences within the spectrum of positive FAST results.[97] Other suggestions for improving performance are (1) to perform the ultrasound examination initially on normal tissue (as in evaluation of a breast mass) and (2) to perform the examinations on patients with known disease (e.g., a palpable breast mass, ascites, gallstones, or benign pericardial effusion). The rationale for the latter suggestion is that it should help the surgeon learn more rapidly how to recognize lesions with varying degrees of pathology.

TECHNICAL TIPS

The following general technical tips should prove useful in a wide range of ultrasonographic applications:

1. The ultrasound machine should be inspected according to the guidelines of the institution's department of biomedical engineering to ensure that it is functioning properly.

2. The patient's orientation on the monitor or screen relative to the position of the transducer should be checked by applying gel to the transducer's footprint (i.e., the part of the transducer that is in contact with the patient's skin) and then rubbing the footprint with a finger near the indicator line of the transducer. Motion on the left side of the screen indicates that the transducer is properly oriented.

3. Liberal amounts of gel should be applied to the area being examined. The gel acts as an acoustic coupler, helping to transmit the ultrasound waves and reduce their reflection. If not enough gel has been applied, the waves will not be transmitted properly, and a dark area will appear on the ultrasound image.

4. The transducer should be manipulated with small movements (not wide sweeps), and gentle pressure should be applied initially. This second point is especially important in imaging the breast or the thyroid: the tissues are superficial, and too much pressure can easily compress them and distort the ultrasound image.

5. The gain and time-gain compensation settings should be rechecked for each new examination. For example, after completing a breast examination, the sonographer should not begin an examination of the carotid vessels without confirming that these settings are correct.

6. Normal tissue should be examined ultrasonographically before the sonographer turns to the area of interest. For example, if the goal is to assess an abscess or DVT in one extremity, the first step should be to inspect the other extremity to see what the corresponding normal tissue looks like. This helps to sensitize the examiner to subtle pathologic changes in the abnormal tissue.

7. The patient should be asked to take a deep breath so that the motion of the diaphragm and the organs can be observed. If the motion of these structures is impaired, inflammation or an abscess may be present.

8. If the left upper quadrant is difficult to examine (as is sometimes the case in the FAST), a nasogastric tube should be inserted to decompress the stomach and minimize the presence of air so that it does not interfere with the transmission of the ultrasound waves.

9. Although B-mode ultrasound is usually sufficient to identify blood vessels, it sometimes is unable to distinguish the artery from the vein because of pulsations transmitted from the artery. In such cases, use of the Doppler mode, compression of the vessel (veins compress very easily), or having the patient perform the Valsalva maneuver can help differentiate arterial from venous anatomy. In addition, the vena cava is more readily identified as the patient completes inspiration.

10. A full bladder is needed for pelvic ultrasound examinations: it acts as an acoustic window, facilitating visualization of the pelvic structures. It should not, however, be so full that it is overdistended. If the bladder is not full enough, the urinary catheter can be clamped to allow it to fill; if it is too full, the catheter can be unclamped to allow it to drain. In this way, hematomas in the pelvis can be more easily detected.

a

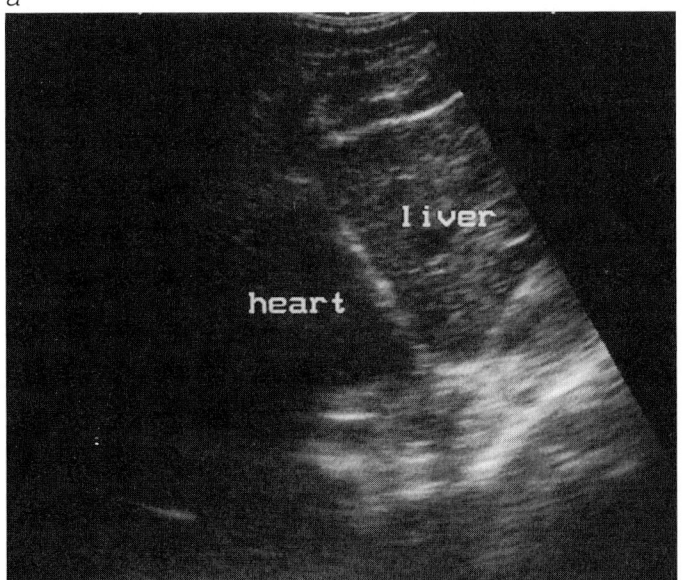

b

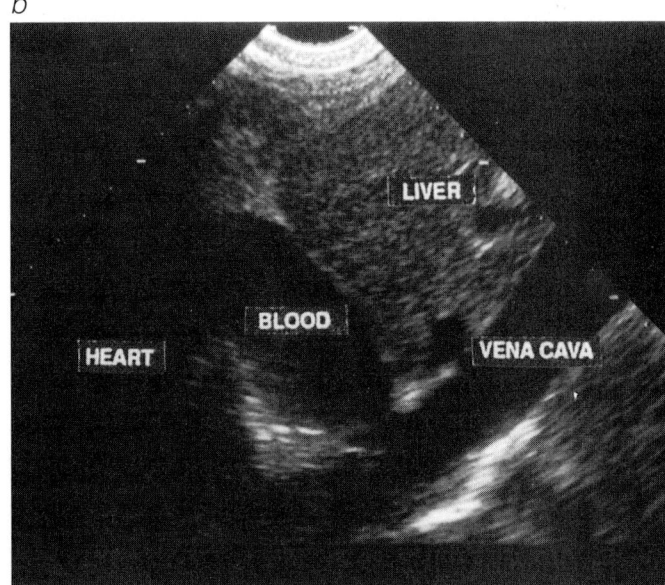

Figure 9 **FAST. (*a*) Sagittal ultrasound image of heart shows pericardium as single echogenic (white) line; normal findings. (*b*) Sagittal ultrasound image of heart shows separation of pericardial layers by blood.**

a

b

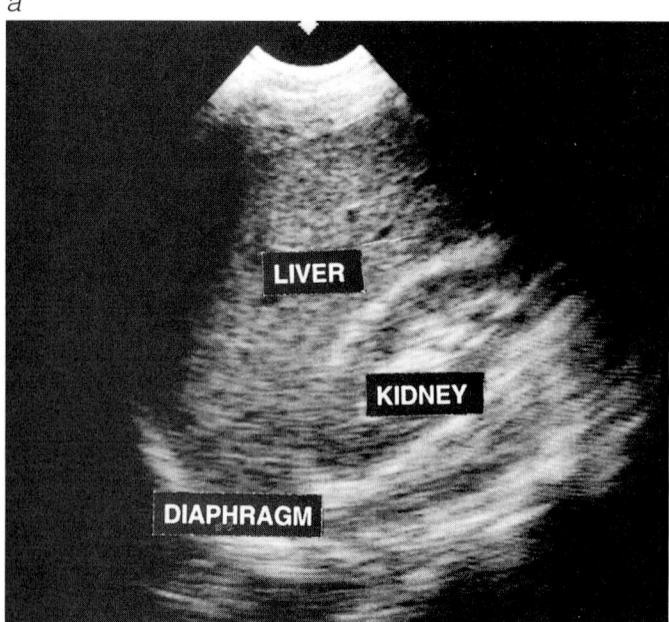
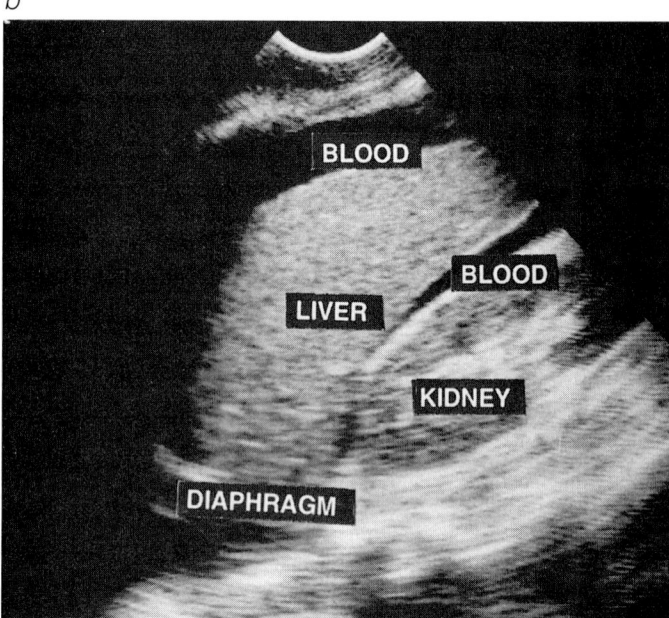

Figure 10   FAST. (*a*) Sagittal ultrasound image of liver, kidney, and diaphragm yields normal findings. (*b*) Sagittal ultrasound image of right upper quadrant shows blood between liver and kidney and between liver and diaphragm.

Technique for Selected Surgical Applications of Ultrasonography

FOCUSED ASSESSMENT FOR THE SONOGRAPHIC EXAMINATION OF THE TRAUMA PATIENT

The FAST is performed during the Advanced Trauma Life Support secondary survey while the patient is in the supine position [*see 5:1 Trauma Resuscitation*]. With the thoracoabdominal area exposed, warmed hypoallergenic, water-soluble ultrasound transmission gel is applied to the abdomen in four specific areas. A focused, limited ex-

amination for the detection of blood in these four regions is conducted in sequence as follows: (1) the pericardial area, (2) the right upper abdominal quadrant, (3) the left upper abdominal quadrant, and (4) the pouch of Douglas [*see Figure 8*].

The transducer is oriented for sagittal sections and placed in the subxiphoid region. The heart is then identified, with the density of blood used as a standard. The subxiphoid approach through the longitudinal axis is taken to enable the examiner to identify the heart and to look for blood in the pericardial region [*see Figure 9*].

a

b

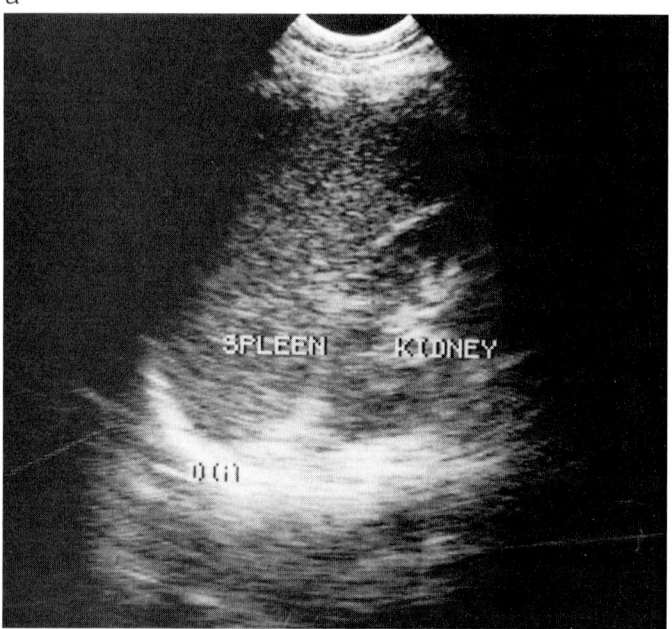
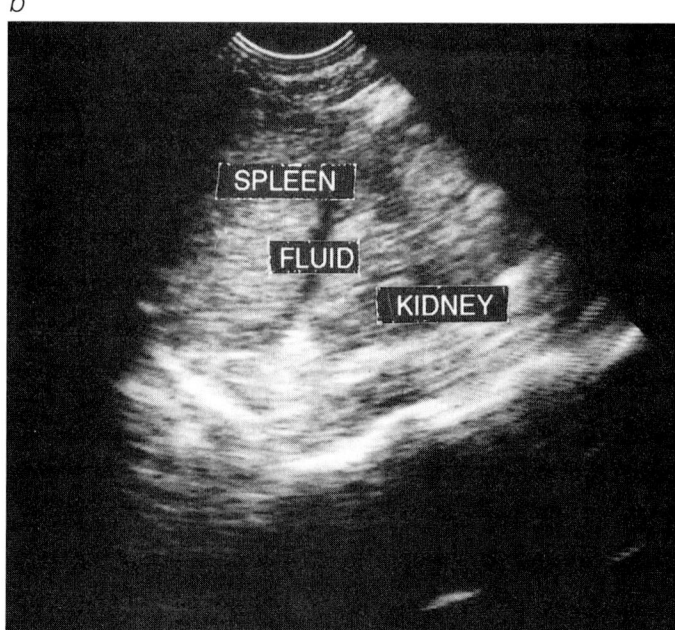

Figure 11   FAST. (*a*) Sagittal ultrasound image of spleen and kidney yields normal findings. (*b*) Sagittal ultrasound image of left upper quadrant shows blood between spleen and kidney.

a

b

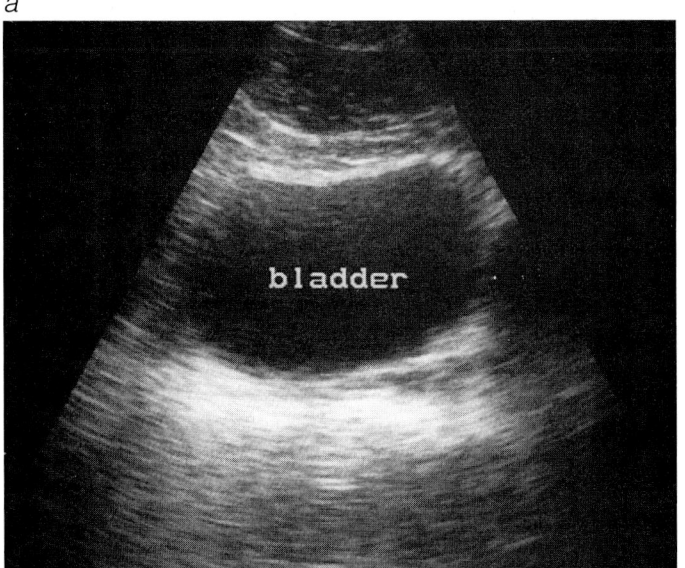
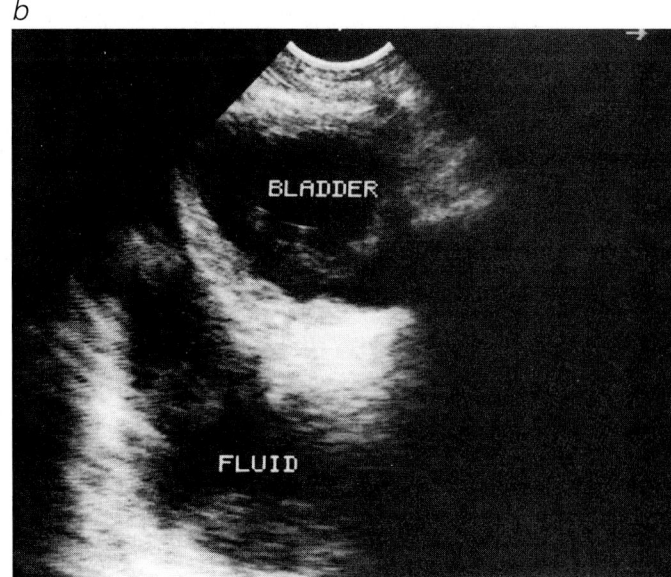

Figure 12 FAST. (*a*) Coronal ultrasound image of pelvis shows full bladder; normal findings. (*b*) Coronal ultrasound image of pelvis shows full bladder surrounded by blood.

The transducer is then placed in the right midaxillary line region between the 11th and 12th ribs to enable the examiner to identify the liver, the kidney, and the diaphragm and to look for blood in Morison's pouch [*see Figure 10*].

Next, the transducer is positioned on the left posterior axillary line between the 10th and 11th ribs to enable the examiner to visualize the spleen and the kidney and to look for blood in the space between these organs and posterior to the spleen [*see Figure 11*].

The transducer is then oriented for transverse sections and placed in the midline approximately 4 cm superior to the symphysis pubis to determine whether there is blood around the full bladder [*see Figure 12*].

An analysis of 1,540 injured patients undergoing FAST examinations performed by surgeon-ultrasonographers reached the following conclusions[97]:

1. Ultrasonography should be the initial diagnostic adjunct for the evaluation of patients with precordial wounds and blunt truncal injuries because it is rapid and accurate and augments the surgeon's diagnostic capabilities.
2. Surgeon-performed FAST is most accurate when used for the evaluation of patients with precordial or transthoracic wounds and a possible hemopericardium and for the evaluation of hypotensive patients with blunt torso trauma.
3. Because of the high sensitivity and specificity of ultrasonography when it is used for the evaluation of patients

with precordial or transthoracic wounds and hypotensive patients with blunt torso trauma, immediate operative intervention is justified in these patients when the ultrasound examination is positive [*see Figures 13 and 14*].

Although the FAST accurately detects the presence or absence of hemoperitoneum in patients with blunt trauma, it does not readily identify intraparenchymal or retroperitoneal injuries. Therefore, a computed tomographic scan of the abdomen may be needed to complement the FAST and reduce the incidence of missed injuries.[95,97-100] There is some evidence that false negative results are more common in patients with pelvic ring fractures, which suggests that CT of the abdomen is routinely indicated in such patients.[101]

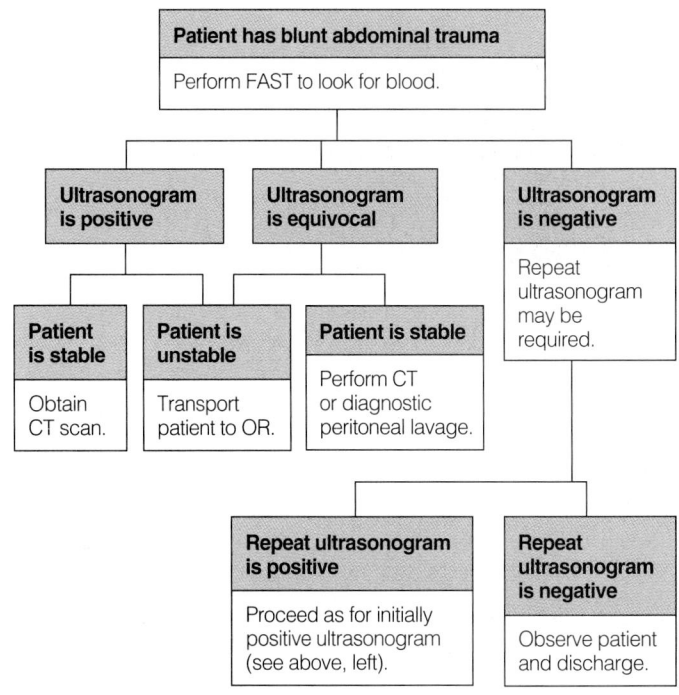
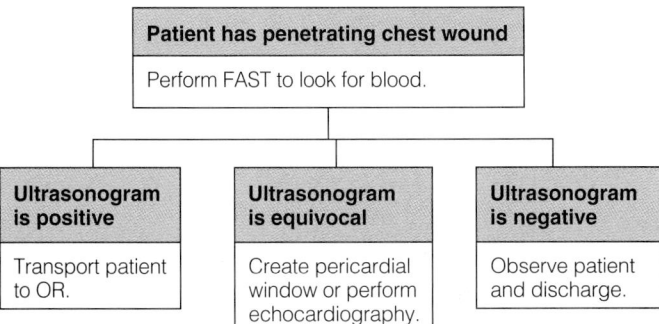

Figure 13 FAST. Shown is an algorithm for use of ultrasonography in evaluation of patients with penetrating precordial wounds.[110]

Figure 14 FAST. Shown is an algorithm for use of ultrasonography in evaluation of patients with blunt abdominal trauma.[110]

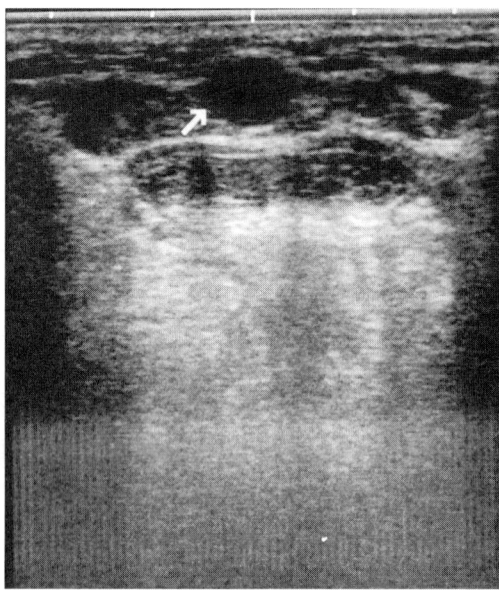

Figure 15 **Breast examination. Ultrasound image shows simple cyst (arrow) of breast characterized by sharp, smooth margins and homogeneous, anechoic interior.**

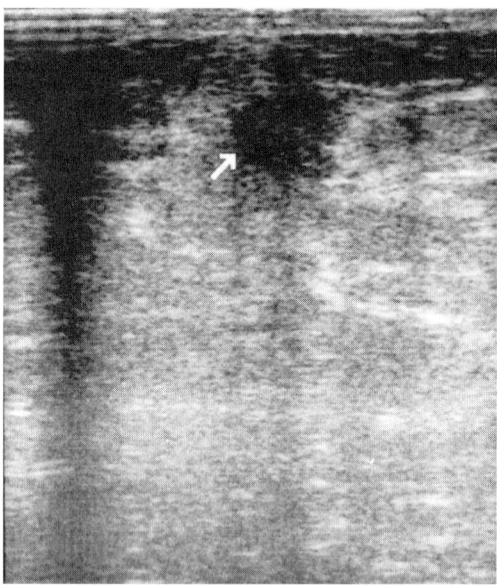

Figure 16 **Breast examination. Ultrasound image shows malignant breast lesion (arrow) with indistinct, jagged margins, few internal echoes, and slight posterior shadowing.**

The increase in surgeon-performed ultrasound examinations has led to decreased performance of diagnostic peritoneal lavage and CT scanning in the trauma setting. It has become apparent that the FAST can replace central venous pressure monitoring in the diagnosis of hemopericardium and can replace diagnostic peritoneal lavage in the detection of hemoperitoneum in many injured patients. Although CT scanning remains a valuable diagnostic test, the indications for its use in the evaluation of injured patients are now narrower than they once were.

BREAST EXAMINATION

The surgeon must be thoroughly familiar with the ultrasonographic anatomy of normal breast tissue to be able to recognize a mass, discern its ultrasonographic characteristics, and determine whether it is likely to be benign [*see Figure 15*] or malignant [*see Figure 16*].[102,103] Analytic criteria for the interpretation of focal lesions detected on breast ultrasound examinations have been well described and depicted elsewhere [*see Figure 17*].[102]

As noted, breast examination should be done according to a specific scanning protocol. The recommended approach is the radial-scanning technique reported by Teboul.[104] A 7.5 MHz linear-array transducer is used, and the patient is placed in the supine position with the ipsilateral arm behind the head. The transducer is placed at the 6 o'clock position; the breast tissue is scanned, and the transducer is then advanced toward the periphery beyond the breast tissue. Next, the 5 o'clock region is evaluated in the same manner. Each sector (or "hour") of the breast

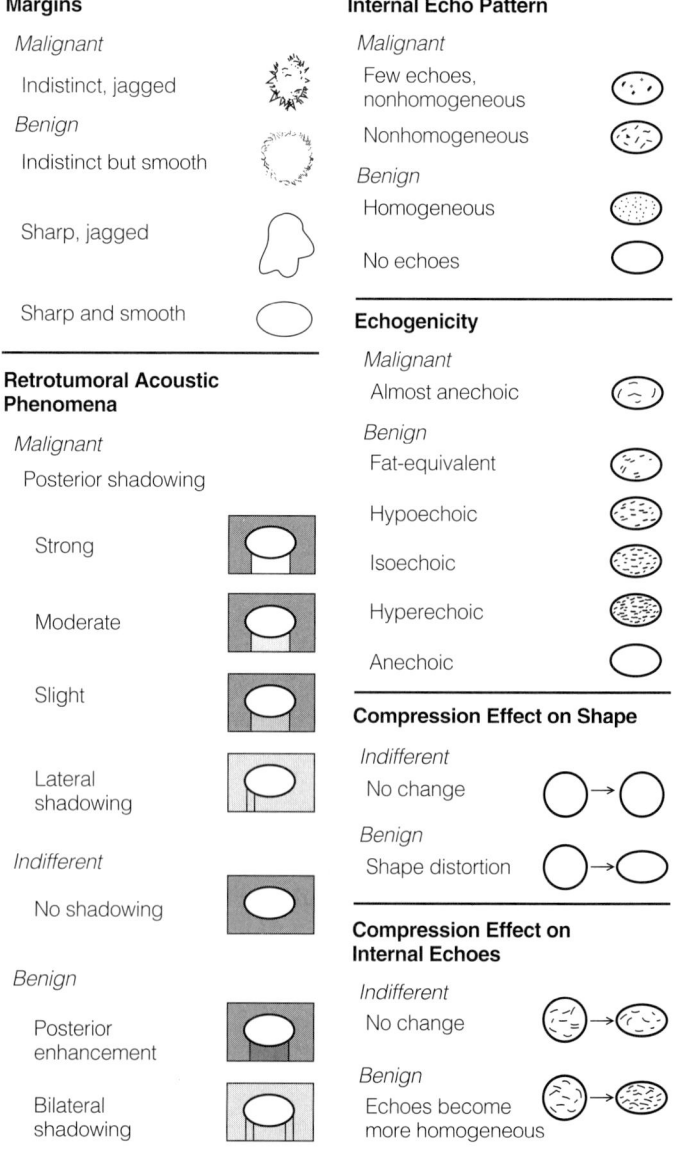

Figure 17 **Breast examination. Shown is a schematic representation of analytic criteria for the interpretation of breast sonograms.[102]**

is then scanned in a sequential counterclockwise fashion until the process is completed. Some experts recommend that the nipple be used as a visual pivot point during scanning, remaining in the upper left corner of the monitor throughout the ultrasound examination.[105]

To image the nipple-areola complex, the transducer is placed next to the nipple and angled toward the retroareolar area. Several transverse scans are performed to assess the uniformity of the ligamentous structures and to detect any small tumor that may be present between these structures. Finally, the axilla is scanned with transverse and longitudinal sweeps of the transducer to inspect for lymph nodes.[105]

An important principle in the performance of breast ultrasonography is that the examination must be performed in a consistent and methodical manner so that findings can be accurately described and reproduced. If this principle is followed, a trained examiner can probably identify 80% to 90% of mammographically detected nonpalpable breast masses.[106] One important drawback to remember, however, is that ultrasonography generally will not reveal lesions less than 5 mm in diameter or lesions with an isoechoic appearance.[107]

References

1. Maggio M, Sanders RC: Basic physics. Clinical Sonography: A Practical Guide. Sanders RC, Ed. Little, Brown and Co, Boston, 1991, p 4

2. Hedrick WR, Hykes L, Starchman DE: Ultrasound Physics and Instrumentation. Mosby, St. Louis, 1995, chap 1, p 23

3. Miner NS: Basic principles. Clinical Sonography: A Practical Guide. Sanders RC, Ed. Little, Brown and Co, Boston, 1991, p 33

4. Kremkau F: Diagnostic Ultrasound: Principles, Instrumentation and Exercises. WB Saunders Co, Philadelphia, 1984, chap 2, p 6

5. Hedrick WR, Hykes L, Starchman DE: Ultrasound Physics and Instrumentation. Mosby, St. Louis, 1995, chap 1, p 8

6. Dubinsky T, Horii S, Odwin CS: Ultrasonic physics and instrumentation. Appleton & Lange's Review for the Ultrasonography Examination. Odwin CS, Dubinsky T, Fleischer AC, Eds. Appleton & Lange, Norwalk, Connecticut, 1993, p 8

7. Zagzebski JA: Physics of diagnostic ultrasound. Essentials of Ultrasound Physics. Zagzebski JA, Ed. Mosby, St. Louis, 1996, p 20

8. Hedrick WR, Hykes L, Starchman DE: Ultrasound Physics and Instrumentation. Mosby, St. Louis, 1995, chap 4, p 96

9. Hedrick WR, Hykes L, Starchman DE: Ultrasound Physics and Instrumentation. Mosby, St. Louis, 1995, chap 2, p 55

10. Sanders RC, Miner NS: Introduction. Clinical Sonography: A Practical Guide. Sanders RC, Ed. Little, Brown and Co, Boston, 1991, p 10

11. Kremkau F: Doppler ultrasound: principles and instruments. Ultrasound: Principles, Instrumentation and Exercises. WB Saunders Co, Philadelphia, 1995, chap 7, p 123

12. Sailors DM, Crabtree JD, Land RL, et al: Needle localization for nonpalpable breast lesions. Am Surg 60:186, 1984

13. Wilhelm NC, DeParedes ES, Pope T: The changing mammogram: a primary indication for needle localization biopsy. Arch Surg 121:1311, 1986

14. Miller RS, Adelman RW, Espinosa MH: The early detection of non-palpable breast carcinoma with needle localization: experience with 500 patients in a community hospital. Am Surg 58:193, 1992

15. Schlecht L, Hadijuana J, Hosten N, et al: Ultrasonography of the female breast: comparison 7.5 MHz versus 13 MHz. Akt Radiol 6:69, 1996

16. Chang R, Kuo W, Chen D, et al: Computer-aided diagnosis for surgical office-based breast ultrasound. Arch Surg 135:696, 2000

17. Saarela AO, Kiviniemi HO, Rissanen TJ, et al: Nonpalpable breast lesions: pathologic correlation of ultrasonographically guided fine-needle aspiration biopsy. J Ultrasound Med 15:549, 1996

18. Rizzatto G: Towards a more sophisticated use of breast ultrasound. Eur Radiol 11:2423, 2000

19. Jackson VP: The role of ultrasound in breast imaging. Radiology 177:305, 1990

20. Muttarak M: Abscess in the non-lactating breast: radiodiagnostic aspects. Australas Radiol 40:223, 1996

21. Dempsey PJ: Breast sonography: historical perspective, clinical application, and image interpretation. Ultrasound Q 6:69, 1988

22. Guyer PB, Dewbury KC: Ultrasound of the breast in the symptomatic and x-ray dense breast. Clin Radiol 36:69, 1985

23. Jackson VP, Hendrick RE, Feit SA, et al: Imaging of the radiographically dense breast. Radiology 188:297, 1993

24. Gufler H, Buitrago-Tellez C, Madjar H, et al: Ultrasound demonstration of mammographically detected microcalcifications. Acta Radiol 41:217, 2000

25. Harness JK, Gittleman MA: Breast ultrasound. Ultrasound in Surgical Practice: Basic Principles and Clinical Applications. Harness JK, Wisher D, Eds. Wiley-Liss & Sons, Inc, New York, 2002, p 159

26. Vilmann P, Jacobsen GK, Henriksen FW, et al: Endoscopic ultrasonography with guided fine needle aspiration biopsy in pancreatic disease. Gastrointest Endosc 38:172, 1992

27. Rosch T, Lightdale CJ, Botet JF: Localization of pancreatic endocrine tumors by endoscopic ultrasonography. N Engl J Med 326:1721, 1992

28. Scheiman JM: Endosonography: is it sound for the masses? J Clin Gastroenterol 19:2, 1994

29. Wiersema MJ, Kochman ML, Cramer HM, et al: Real-time endoscopic ultrasound-guided fine-needle aspiration of a mediastinal lymph node. Gastrointest Endosc 39: 429, 1993

30. Chen C, Yang C, Yeh Y: Preoperative staging of gastric cancer by endoscopic ultrasound: the prognostic usefulness of ascites detected by endoscopic ultrasound. J Clin Gastroenterol 35:321, 2002

31. Fu K, Eloubeidi M, Jhala N, et al: Diagnosis of gastrointestinal stromal tumor by endoscopic ultrasound-guided fine needle aspiration biopsy-apotential pitfall. Ann Diagn Radiol 6:294, 2002

32. Hernandez L, Mishra G, Forsmarck C, et al: Role of endoscopic ultrasound (EUS) and EUS-guided fine needle aspiration in the diagnosis and treatment of cystic lesions of the pancreas. Pancreas 25:222, 2002

33. de Lange EE: Staging rectal carcinoma with endorectal imaging: how much detail do we really need? Radiology 190:633, 1994

34. Waizer A, Powsner E, Russo I: Prospective comparative study of magnetic resonance imaging versus transrectal ultrasound for preoperative staging and follow-up of rectal cancer: preliminary report. Dis Colon Rectum 34:1068, 1991

35. Herzog U, von Flue M, Tondelli P, et al: How accurate is endorectal ultrasound in the preoperative staging of rectal cancer? Dis Colon Rectum 36:127, 1993

36. Glaser F, Friedl P, Schlag P, et al: Influence of endorectal ultrasound on surgical treatment of rectal cancer. Eur J Oncol 16:304, 1990

37. Solomon MJ, McLeod RS, Cohen EK: Reliability and validity studies of endoluminal ultrasonography for anorectal disorders. Dis Colon Rectum 37:546, 1994

38. Kusunoki M, Yanagi H, Gondoh N, et al: Use of transrectal ultrasonography to select type of surgery for villous tumors in the lower two thirds of the rectum. Arch Surg 131:714, 1996

39. Beynon J: An evaluation of the role of rectal endosonography in rectal cancer. Ann R Coll Surg Engl 71:131, 1989

40. Milsom JW, Lavery I, Stolfi V, et al: The expanding utility of endoluminal ultrasonography in the management of rectal cancer. Surgery 112:832, 1992

41. Anderson B, Hann L, Enker W, et al: Transrectal ultrasonography and operative selection for early carcinoma of the rectum. J Am Coll Surg 179:513, 1994

42. Saclarides TJ: Endorectal ultrasonography for malignant disease. Ultrasound for the Surgeon. Staren ED, Arregui ME, Eds. Lippincott-Raven, Philadelphia, 1997, p 75

43. Beynon J, Foy DM, Temple LN, et al: The endosonic appearances of normal colon and rectum. Dis Colon Rectum 29:810, 1986

44. Hildebrandt U, Feifel G: Preoperative staging of rectal cancer by intrarectal ultrasound. Dis Colon Rectum 28:42, 1985

45. Romano G, Escercizio L, Santangelo M, et al: Impact of computed tomography vs. intrarectal ultrasound on the diagnosis, resectability, and prognosis of locally recurrent rectal cancer. Dis Colon Rectum 36:261, 1993

46. Hulsmans F, Tio TL, Fockens P, et al: Assessment of tumor infiltration depth in rectal cancer with transrectal sonography: caution is necessary. Radiology 190: 715, 1994

47. Sentovitch SM, Blatchford GJ, Falk PM, et al: Transrectal ultrasound of rectal tumors. Am J Surg 166:638, 1993

48. Steele S, Martin M, Platt RJ: Flexible endorectal ultrasound for predicting pathologic stage of rectal cancers. Am J Surg 184:126, 2002

49. Burnett S, Bartram C: Endosonographic variations in the normal internal anal sphincter. Int J Colorect Dis 6:2, 1991

50. Gantke B, Schafer A, Enck P, et al: Sonographic, manometric and myographic evaluation of the anal sphincter's morphology and function. Dis Colon Rectum 36:1037, 1993

51. Law PJ, Kamm MA, Bartram CI: Anal endosonography in the investigation of faecal incontinence. Br J Surg 78:312, 1991

52. Burnett S, Speakman CT, Kamm MA, et al:

Confirmation of endosonographic detection of external anal sphincter defects by simultaneous electromyographic mapping. Br J Surg 78:448, 1991

53. Deen KI, Kumar D, Williams JG: Anal sphincter defects: correlation between endoanal ultrasound and surgery. Ann Surg 218:201, 1993

54. Felt-Bersma RJ, Cuesta MA, Koorevaar M: Anal endosonography: relationship with anal manometry and neurophysiologic tests. Dis Colon Rectum 37:468, 1992

55. Falk PM, Blatchford GJ, Cali RL: Transanal ultrasound and manometry in the evaluation of fecal incontinence. Dis Colon Rectum 37:468, 1994

56. Sultan AH, Kamm MA, Talbot IC: Anal endosonography for identifying external sphincter defects confirmed histologically. Br J Surg 81:463, 1994

57. Goldberg BB, Goodman GA, Clearfield HR: Evaluation of ascites by ultrasound. Radiology 96:15, 1970

58. Asher WM, Parvin S, Virgillo RW, et al: Echographic evaluation of splenic injury after blunt trauma. Radiology 118:411, 1976

59. Chambers JA, Pilbrow WJ: Ultrasound in abdominal trauma: an alternative to peritoneal lavage. Arch Emerg Med 5:26, 1988

60. Sisley AC, Rozycki GS, Ballard RB, et al: Rapid detection of traumatic effusion using surgeon-performed ultrasound. J Trauma 44:291, 1998

61. Fenkl R, von Garrel T, Knaepler H: Emergency diagnosis of sternum fracture with ultrasound. Unfallchirurg 95:375, 1992

62. Dulchavsky SA, Schwarz KL, Kirkpatrick A, et al: Prospective evaluation of thoracic ultrasound in the detection of pneumothorax. J Trauma 50:201, 2001

63. Parys BT, Barr H, Chantarasak ND, et al: Use of ultrasound scan as a bedside diagnostic aid. Br J Surg 74:611, 1987

64. Peiper HJ, Schmid A, Steffens H, et al: Ultrasound diagnosis in acute abdomen and blunt abdominal trauma. Chirurg 58:189, 1987

65. Blyme PJH, Lind T, Schantz K: Ultrasonographic detection of foreign bodies in soft tissue. Arch Ortho Trauma Surg 110:24, 1990

66. Schlager D, Sanders A, Wiggins D: Ultrasound for the detection of foreign bodies. Ann Emerg Med 20:189, 1991

67. Manthey DE, Storrow AB, Milbourn JM, et al: Ultrasound versus radiography in the detection of soft-tissue foreign bodies. Ann Emerg Med 28:7, 1996

68. Williams RJ, Windsor AC, Rosin RD, et al: Ultrasound scanning of the acute abdomen by surgeons in training. Ann R Coll Surg Engl 76:228, 1994

69. Imhof M, Raunest J, Rauen U, et al: Acute acalculous cholecystitis in severely traumatized patients: a prospective sonographic study. Surg Endosc 6:68, 1992

70. Yokoyama T, Munakata Y, Ogiwara M, et al: Preoperative diagnosis of strangulated obturator hernia using ultrasonography. Am J Surg 174:76, 1997

71. Barteau JA, Castro D, Arregui ME, et al: A comparison of intraoperative ultrasound versus cholangiography in the evaluation of the common bile duct during laparoscopic cholecystectomy. Surg Endosc 9:490, 1995

72. Ravikumar TS, Kane R, Cady B: Hepatic cryosurgery with intraoperative ultrasound monitoring for metastatic colon carcinoma. Arch Surg 102:403, 1987

73. Rafaelsen SR, Kronborg O, Larsen C, et al: Intraoperative ultrasonography in detection of hepatic metastases from colorectal cancer. Dis Colon Rectum 38:355, 1995

74. Machi J, Isomoto H, Kurohiji T, et al: Detection of unrecognized liver metastases from colorectal cancers by routine use of operative ultrasonography. Dis Colon Rectum 29: 405, 1986

75. Castaing D, Emond J, Kunstlinger F, et al: Utility of operative ultrasound in the surgical management of liver tumors. Ann Surg 204:600, 1986

76. Kern KA, Shawker TH, Doppman JL, et al: The use of high-resolution ultrasound to locate parathyroid tumors during reoperations for primary hyperparathyroidism. World J Surg 11:579, 1987

77. Machi J, Sigel B: Operative ultrasonography in general surgery. Am J Surg 172:15, 1996

78. Couinaud C: Le Foie, Etudes Anatomiques et Chirurgicales. Masson et Cie, Paris, 1957

79. Schirmer B: Laparoscopic ultrasonography: enhancing minimally invasive surgery. Ann Surg 220:709, 1994

80. John TG: Superior staging of liver tumors with laparoscopy and laparoscopic ultrasound. Ann Surg 220:711, 1994

81. Cook TA, Galland RB: A prospective study to define the optimum rescreening interval for small abdominal aneurysm. Cardiovasc Surg 4:441, 1996

82. Bastounis E, Georgopoulos S, Maltezos C, et al: The validity of current vascular imaging methods in the evaluation of aortic anastomotic aneurysms developing after abdominal aortic aneurysm repair. Ann Vasc Surg 10:537, 1996

83. Turetschek K, Nasel C, Wunderbaldinger P, et al: Power Doppler versus imaging in renal allograft evaluation. J Ultrasound Med 15:517, 1996

84. Wren SM, Ralls PW, Stain SC, et al: Assessment of resectability of pancreatic head and periampullary tumors by color flow Doppler sonography. Arch Surg 131:812, 1996

85. Klyachkin ML, Rohmiller M, Charash WE, et al: Penetrating injuries of the neck: selective management evolving. Am Surg 63:189, 1997

86. Ginzburg E, Montalvo B, LeBlang S, et al: The use of duplex ultrasonography in penetrating neck trauma. Arch Surg 131:691, 1996

87. Demetriades D, Theodorou D, Cornwell E, et al: Evaluation of penetrating injuries of the neck: prospective study of 223 patients. World J Surg 21:41, 1997

88. Knudson MM, Lewis FR, Atkinson K, et al: The role of duplex ultrasound arterial imaging in patients with penetrating extremity trauma. Arch Surg 128:1033, 1993

89. Bergstein JM, Blair JF, Edwards J, et al: Pitfalls in the use of color-flow duplex ultrasound for screening of suspected arterial injuries in penetrating extremities. J Trauma 33:395, 1992

90. Knudson MM, Collins JA, Goodman SB, et al: Thromboembolism following multiple trauma. J Trauma 32:2, 1992

91. Bandyk DF, Mills JL, Gahtan V, et al: Intraoperative duplex scanning of arterial reconstructions: fate of repaired and unrepaired defects. J Vasc Surg 20:426, 1994

92. Gualtieri E, Deppe SA, Sipperly ME, et al: Subclavian venous catheterization: greater success rate for less experienced operators using ultrasound guidance. Crit Care Med 23:692, 1995

93. Sisley AC, Rozycki GS, Ballard RB, et al: Rapid detection of traumatic effusion using surgeon-performed ultrasound. J Trauma 44:291, 1998

94. Kohan JM, Poe RH, Israel RH: Value of chest ultrasonography versus decubitus roentgenography for thoracentesis. Am Rev Respir Dis 133:1124, 1986

95. Rozycki GS, Ochsner MG, Jaffin JH, et al: Prospective evaluation of surgeons' use of ultrasound in the evaluation of trauma patients. J Trauma 34:516, 1993

96. Tso P, Rodriguez A, Cooper C, et al: Sonography in blunt abdominal trauma: a preliminary progress report. J Trauma 33:39, 1992

97. Rozycki GS, Ballard RB, Feliciano DV, et al: Surgeon-performed ultrasound for the assessment of truncal injuries: lessons learned from 1,540 patients. Ann Surg 228:557, 1998

98. Rozycki GS, Ochsner MG, Schmidt JA, et al: A prospective study of surgeon-performed ultrasound as the primary adjuvant modality for injured patient assessment. J Trauma 39:492, 1995

99. Boulanger BR, Brenneman FD, McLellan BA, et al: A prospective study of emergent abdominal sonography after blunt trauma. J Trauma 39:325, 1995

100. Chiu WC, Cushing BM, Rodriguez A, et al: Abdominal injuries without hemoperitoneum: a potential limitation of focused abdominal sonography for trauma (FAST). J Trauma 42:617, 1997

101. Ballard RB, Rozycki GS, Newman PG, et al: The efficacy of an algorithm to reduce the incidence of false negative FAST examination in patients at high-risk for occult injury. J Am Coll Surg (in press)

102. Leucht W: Analytic criteria for the interpretation of focal sonographic lesions. Teaching Atlas of Breast Ultrasound. Leucht D, Madjar H, Eds. Thieme, New York, 1996, p 23

103. Staren ED: Physics and principles of breast ultrasound. Am Surg 62:103, 1996

104. Teboul M: A new concept in breast investigation: echo-histological acino-ductal 13-analysis or analytic echography. Biomed Pharmacother 42:289, 1988

105. Khattar S, Staren ED: Diagnostic breast ultrasound. Ultrasound for the Surgeon. Staren ED, Arregui ME, Eds. Philadelphia, Lippincott-Raven, 1997, p 85

106. Staren ED: Surgical office-based ultrasound of the breast. Am Surg 61:619, 1995

107. Staren ED, Fine R: Breast ultrasound for surgeons. Am Surg 62:108, 1996

108. Sanders RC, Topper IW: Equipment care and quality control. Clinical Sonography: A Practical Guide. Sanders RC, Ed. Little, Brown and Co, Boston, 1991, p 475

109. Wong WK: Endorectal ultrasonography for benign disease. Ultrasound for the Surgeon. Staren ED, Arregui ME, Eds. Lippincott-Raven, Philadelphia, 1997, p 66

110. Rozycki GS, Shackford SR: Ultrasound: what every trauma surgeon should know. J Trauma 40:1, 1996

Acknowledgments

Figures 1 and 7   Dimitry Schidlovsky.
Figures 2, 13, 14, and 17   Marcia Kammerer.
Figure 8   Tom Moore.

13 GASTRODUODENAL PROCEDURES

E. Ramsay Camp, M.D., and Steven N. Hochwald, M.D., F.A.C.S.

Gastroduodenal Procedures for Benign Disorders

PREOPERATIVE EVALUATION

The improvements in medical treatment of peptic ulcer disease and the discovery of *Helicobacter pylori* have dramatically altered the role of surgery in the management of peptic ulcer disease. Currently, surgery for intractable or chronic ulcer disease is rarely necessary; as a consequence, such complex procedures as vagotomy with antrectomy and highly selective vagotomy are virtually nonexistent today. Surgery is now reserved for the treatment of complications of the acute ulcer (e.g., bleeding, perforation, and obstruction). In general, treatment of peptic ulcer disease should be aimed at correcting complications and managing *H. pylori*. Nonsteroidal anti-inflammatory drugs (NSAIDs), which can be associated with ulcers, should be discontinued as well.

Hemorrhage is the leading cause of death associated with peptic ulcer disease. In many patients, GI endoscopy can effectively identify the source of the bleeding and treat the lesion. Operative therapy is indicated in the presence of hemorrhage associated with hemodynamic instability, blood loss necessitating transfusion of more than 6 units, or rebleeding during hospitalization. For patients in whom surgical management is contraindicated, angiographic embolization may be an effective alternative.

Perforation of a duodenal ulcer is usually signaled by an acute abdomen, and the decision to operate is typically straightforward. By far the most common operative treatment is an omental (Graham) patch; more definitive management is rarely necessary.

In its acute phase, gastric outlet obstruction often resolves with conservative therapy. In its chronic phase, typically associated with significant stenosis, surgery is indicated. The most common surgical treatment is vagotomy with antrectomy or a drainage procedure.

For emergency surgical treatment of a gastric ulcer, distal gastrectomy incorporating the ulcer in conjunction with vagotomy is ideal. In high-risk unstable patients, either oversewing the ulcer or wedge resection is acceptable. For elective surgical treatment of a gastric ulcer, the choice of operation largely depends on the location of the ulcer. The most common indications for resection are failure of an ulcer to heal after 12 weeks of optimal medical therapy and recurrence after previous healing with medical therapy. In addition to a definitive ulcer operation, a histologic evaluation must be performed to rule out an underlying malignancy. With prepyloric ulcers, vagotomy should be included in the procedure.

Laparoscopy has now been used successfully in many procedures related to benign gastroduodenal disorders. Preoperative evaluation should be the same for laparoscopic procedures as for their open equivalents; however, because of their longer operating times, laparoscopic gastroduodenal procedures should not be done in patients in extreme shock.

OPERATIVE PLANNING

Operative planning for open gastric procedures for benign dis-

ease is generally straightforward. The patient is always under general anesthesia and supine. Once the patient is intubated, a nasogastric tube and a Foley catheter are placed. Most surgeons elect to perform gastric operations through an upper midline incision; however, in obese patients or those with a thick body habitus, a bilateral subcostal incision may provide better exposure. A ringed retractor may then be placed to allow further exposure. Given the easy accessibility of the stomach to endoscopy, the surgeon should consider liberal use of this modality during the procedure as an aid to operative management.

OMENTAL PATCH OF DUODENAL PERFORATION (GRAHAM PATCH)

Operative Technique

The emergency operative repair of a perforated duodenal ulcer described by Graham some 60 years ago is still done today, essentially unchanged. The anterior duodenal wall ulcer is visualized and carefully debrided. Three or four interrupted sutures (silk or absorbable) are placed along the length of the ulcer in an effort to close the perforation [*see Figure 1*]. An omental pedicle with an adequate blood supply is then placed over the perforation and secured in place by tying the sutures over it. Thus, a well-vascularized region is brought in contact with the duodenal serosa.

Troubleshooting

If exposure proves difficult, the suture ends should be placed on hemostats one by one and kept in order. The most superior suture should be tied first to ensure that sufficient omentum is available to patch the perforation. To keep from devascularizing the omental pedicle, the sutures should not be tied too tightly. If the perforation is large (> 1 cm), the surgeon should consider incorporating the perforation into a pyloroplasty.

Complications

Incomplete closure of the perforation can result in persistent leakage and continued peritonitis. It may be useful—though it is necessary in only a minority of cases before abdominal closure—to assess the adequacy of the repair intraoperatively by instilling saline with methylene blue through the nasogastric tube near the perforation, then compressing the duodenum beyond the perforation and looking for any fluid leakage from the repaired hole. If operative closure proves very difficult and there are serious concerns about possible continued leakage, a Jackson-Pratt drain may be placed close to the repair before abdominal closure. The drain can provide early notification of an ongoing leak, but it will be of minimal help in managing the problem. In most cases, continued leakage should be treated with reoperation and antrectomy.

Outcome

Until relatively recently, the consensus was that two thirds of

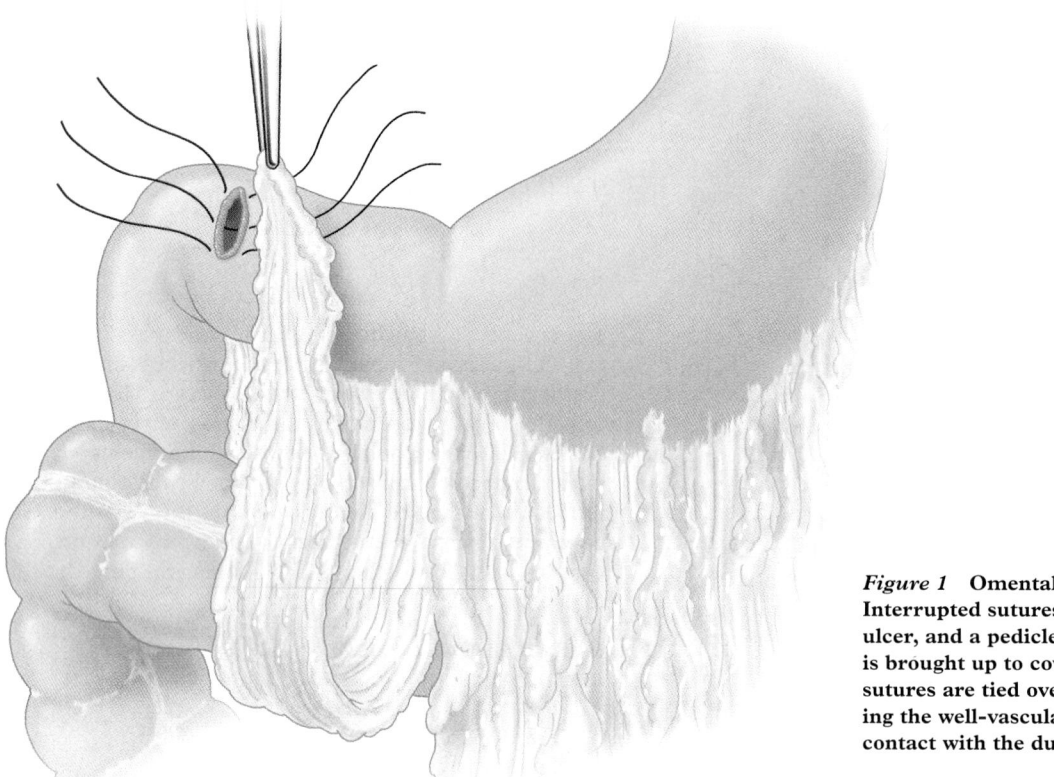

Figure 1 **Omental (Graham) patch. Interrupted sutures are placed along the ulcer, and a pedicle of greater omentum is brought up to cover the defect. The sutures are tied over the pedicle, bringing the well-vascularized omentum in contact with the duodenal wall.**

patients would have symptomatic recurrence of ulcer disease and one third would need additional surgical treatment of ulcer disease after a Graham patch. Today, with the ability to eradicate *H. pylori* and the wide availability of acid suppressants, ulcers should recur in only a minority of patients. A randomized study in which patients with perforated duodenal ulcers received either anti–*H. pylori* therapy or omeprazole alone after patch repair found that the ulcer recurrence rate at 1 year was 4.8% in those receiving anti–*H. pylori* therapy, compared with 38.1% in those receiving omeprazole alone.[1]

VAGOTOMY AND PYLOROPLASTY

Operative Technique

Step 1: division of pyloric ring   Once adequate exposure is obtained, the pyloric ring is opened in such a way as to incorporate any perforated ulcer present. Two sutures are placed on the anterior portion of the pylorus, one superiorly and the other inferiorly. With traction placed on these sutures, a longitudinal opening in the anterior pylorus is created between the sutures with the electrocautery [*see Figure 2a*]. This opening is extended proximal-

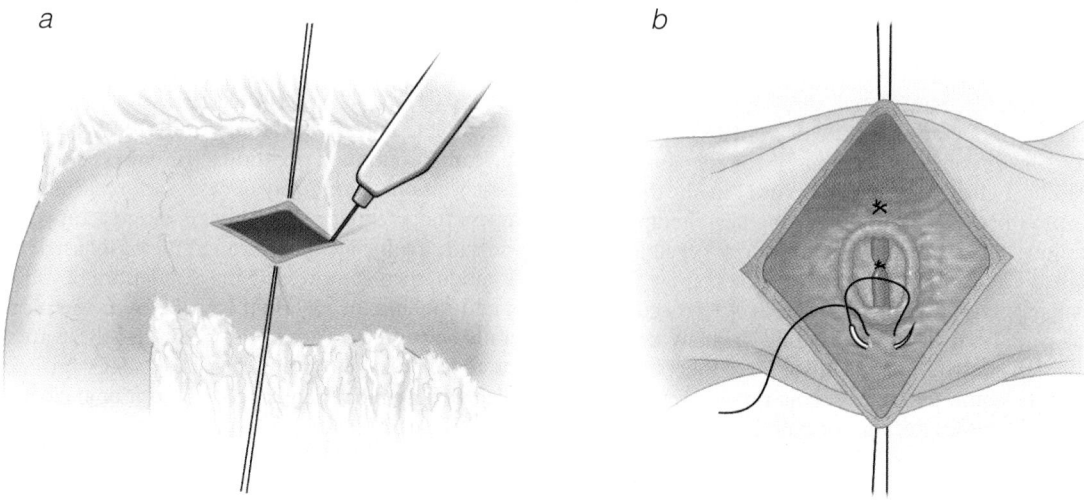

Figure 2   **Pyloroplasty. (*a*) With gentle retraction on the stay sutures, the pylorus is opened longitudinally. (*b*) Once the bleeding vessel is exposed, deep sutures are placed above and below the bleeding site to ligate the gastroduodenal artery, and the longitudinal opening is closed transversely with interrupted sutures. Alternatively, a TA stapler can be used to close the pyloric opening.**

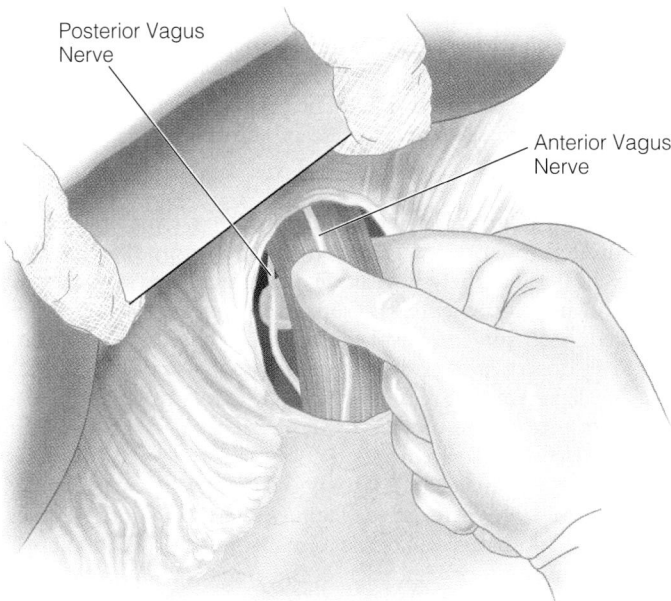

Posterior Vagus
Nerve

Anterior Vagus
Nerve

Figure 3 **Vagotomy. The peritoneum is incised sharply, and the esophagus is encircled. With gentle traction placed on the stomach, the posterior and anterior vagus nerves should be felt as bowstrings. The anterior vagus nerve is located on the anterior esophageal wall; the posterior vagus is located to the right and posteriorly.**

ly onto the anterior gastric wall for approximately 2 to 3 cm and distally on the duodenal side of the pylorus for approximately 1 cm, for a total length of 3 to 4 cm.

Step 2: ligation of bleeding vessel A small, malleable retractor is placed inside the duodenal lumen to allow exposure of the bleeding ulcer and the gastroduodenal artery. If no ongoing bleeding is apparent, any clot present on the ulcer should be removed to permit identification of the bleeding site. Once the arterial bleeding site is located, deep figure-eight sutures are placed above, below, and on either side of the lesion. To prevent further hemorrhage, care must be taken not to injure the common bile duct (CBD) in the course of suture placement.

Step 3: pyloroplasty Once the hemorrhage is under control, the longitudinal opening is closed transversely in a single layer with full-thickness bites of an absorbable or nonabsorbable suture material (Heineke-Mikulicz pyloroplasty) [*see Figure 2b*]. Alternatively, the opening may be closed with a transverse anastomosis (TA) stapler. The edges of the duodenal wall are brought together with Allis clamps, with care taken to incorporate all layers of the wall. The TA stapler is then fired below the Allis clamps to complete the pyloroplasty.

Step 4: vagotomy With adequate exposure of the esophagogastric junction, vagotomy may be attempted. If necessary, the left triangular ligament may be divided to facilitate retraction of the liver. Caudal traction is placed on the stomach, and the peritoneum overlying the esophagus is incised with the electrocautery. The stomach is retracted in the direction of the spleen to prevent damage to the short gastric vessels. When this is done, the nerves can generally be appreciated both anteriorly and posteriorly proximal to the esophagogastric junction; they are typically described

as feeling like bowstrings [*see Figure 3*]. The anterior vagal trunk is identified and dissected into the lower mediastinum, with all branches divided as they pass inferiorly. Finally, approximately 5 cm of the main anterior trunk is resected between surgical clips.

The posterior vagus nerve has a more variable location. In most cases, it is located directly behind the esophagus, but on occasion, it may course more medially, next to the aorta or in the areolar tissue just medial to the right crus of the diaphragm. As with the anterior vagus nerve, caudal retraction of the stomach facilitates identification, and approximately 5 cm of the nerve is resected between clips.

Troubleshooting

If the location of the pylorus is difficult to determine, a small incision should be made in the nearby surrounding area. Once entry into the stomach or the duodenum is achieved, the pyloric ring can usually be located by palpation from the inside. Upward traction on stitches placed on the superior and inferior portions of the anterior pylorus facilitates identification and division of the pyloric ring without injuring the posterior wall. Alternatively, the pylorus can be grasped between the thumb and the index finger, and the anterior ring can then be palpated and divided. If simple full-thickness sutures are used to close the pyloroplasty, they should be placed close together (3 to 4 mm apart).

Particular care must be taken in closing the opening with the TA stapler because the thickness of the pyloric musculature may hinder staple closure. If staples are used, sutures should be placed to reinforce the staple line. The presence of significant inflammation is a contraindication to staple closure: the presence of edematous tissue and excessive tension increases the risk that the closure will fail. Routine coverage of the pyloroplasty closure with omentum or retroperitoneal fat should be considered.

Complications

Leakage from the pyloroplasty is rare but not unknown. It may occur as a consequence of technical mishaps or of poor healing of edematous or inflamed tissue. If potential leakage is a significant concern at the time of operation and if the more distal duodenum appears less involved, antrectomy with careful duodenal stump closure should be considered.

Outcome

Rebleeding and ulcer recurrence rates should be low if sutures are correctly placed and anti–*H. pylori* treatment is administered.

ANTRECTOMY

Operative Technique

Step 1: mobilization of stomach Exposure is obtained as described earlier [*see Operative Planning, above*]. Generally, dissection is begun in the avascular portion of the greater omentum to gain exposure to the posterior wall of the stomach. The stomach is separated from the pancreas through blunt and electrocautery dissection. The greater omentum is dissected away from the stomach from the pylorus to the midportion of the stomach. In a similar manner, the lesser omentum is opened completely; this can be done relatively quickly if no replaced left gastric artery is present.

The points of division on the stomach are then selected. Because the antrum extends more proximally on the lesser curvature, dissection on this aspect must be continued several centimeters proximal to the incisura. In the course of this dissection, the

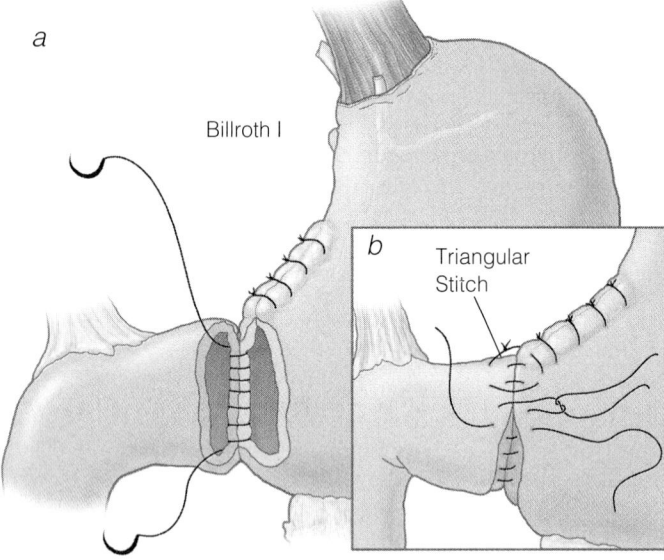

Figure 4 **Billroth I gastroduodenostomy. (a) A two-layer anastomosis is fashioned with continuous or interrupted absorbable sutures. A Lembert seromuscular suture is used to bring together the posterior gastric and duodenal walls. The second layer approximates the full thickness of the gastric and duodenal walls with a suture that commences in the midline with two separate needles. The suture is continued anteriorly, the opposing anterior walls are inverted with an over-and-over suture (or, alternatively, a Connell inverting suture), and the suture ends are tied in the midline. (b) An outer layer of continuous or interrupted absorbable Lembert sutures is placed, and the angle of sorrow—the potential weak spot—is closed with a triangular stitch.**

descending branch of the left gastric artery is secured and divided. On the greater curvature, the antrum extends to a point approximately halfway between the pylorus and the fundus.

Step 2: division of stomach   Once the dissection is completed, the stomach is divided with a gastrointestinal anastomosis (GIA)–90 stapler. The remaining portion of the antrum may be retracted anteriorly to facilitate dissection of the duodenum. Just distal to the pylorus and on the inferior portion of the duodenum are the right gastroepiploic artery and vein, which are divided between clamps. The plane underneath the duodenum is then entered. Along the superior portion of the duodenum is the right gastric artery, which is divided between clamps. When the duodenum has been mobilized, a TA-55 stapler is placed on the specimen side, fired, and released. The stapler is then applied to the duodenal stump side, fired again, and left in place; the duodenum is divided close to this staple line. Resection of the pylorus in the specimen must be confirmed to ensure that there is no retained antrum.

Step 3a: reconstruction (Billroth I)   For establishing GI continuity, either a Billroth I reconstruction (gastroduodenostomy) or a Billroth II reconstruction (gastrojejunostomy) may be performed. Billroth I reconstruction has the advantage of maintaining duodenal antegrade nutrient flow, thereby helping to support physiologic digestion and reducing the incidence of reflux gastritis. Accordingly, in situations where the disease process does not involve the duodenum, many surgeons would favor a gastroduodenostomy. For extended resections, however, a gastrojejunostomy would be preferable to minimize tension on the anastomosis and avoid excessive dissection.

A Kocher maneuver is performed. With the colon retracted inferiorly and to the left, the lateral surface of the duodenum is exposed, and the avascular attachments to the retroperitoneum can easily be seen and divided. The gastroduodenostomy is fashioned as a hand-sewn end-to-side or end-to-end anastomosis in two layers [*see Figure 4*].

Step 3b: reconstruction (Billroth II)   A gastrojejunostomy is indicated when technical reasons make a gastroduodenostomy difficult. Because there now are few indications for surgical treatment of ulcer disease, the Billroth I reconstruction is rarely performed. Most surgeons favor the Billroth II anastomosis, which is typically done as a stapled or hand-sewn side-to-side anastomosis.

The ligament of Treitz is identified, and a proximal loop of jejunum that can be mobilized without tension is brought up to the stomach. Generally, this is best done posterior to the transverse colon, but an antecolic anastomosis is sometimes performed. Enterotomies are made on the antimesenteric wall of the jejunum and on the posterior wall of the remaining stomach approximately 2 cm from the divided edge of the stomach. The arms of the GIA stapler are inserted through the enterotomies and fired to create the side-to-side anastomosis [*see Figure 5a*]. The opening may be extended 3 to 4 cm with an endoscopic GIA stapler placed at the distal end of the new stapled anastomosis.

For a hand-sewn gastrojejunostomy, the antimesenteric side of the jejunum at the planned site of the enterotomy is scored with the electrocautery. The posterior wall of the jejunum is approximated to the posterior wall of the stomach just below the staple line on the greater curvature with a continuous 3-0 polydioxanone Lembert suture taking seromuscular bites. A portion of the staple line on the greater curvature is then removed with the electrocautery. The enterotomy is completed on the jejunum [*see Figure 5b*]. Two more continuous 3-0 polydioxanone sutures are placed to form the posterior wall of the anastomosis by bringing together the full thickness of the jejunum and the stomach. These two sutures are continued onto the anterior side of the anastomosis in a Connell stitch and tied in the midline anteriorly. A fourth continuous 3-0 polydioxanone Lembert suture is placed to reinforce the anterior portion of the anastomosis. A so-called angle of sorrow stitch can be placed at the convergence of the staple line on the lesser curvature and the sutured gastrojejunostomy.

Once the gastrojejunostomy is complete, a Braun enteroenterostomy may be added to decrease bile reflux and help decompress the duodenal stump [*see Figure 5c*]. Approximately 25 cm downstream from the completed gastrojejunostomy, the afferent and efferent limbs of the gastrojejunostomy are sutured or stapled together.

Troubleshooting

Difficult duodenal stump   Various techniques are used to address the difficult closure of the duodenal stump. Of these, the one most frequently employed is a lateral T tube duodenostomy, which helps to decompress the stump by placing a drainage catheter through viable noninflamed tissue. After extensive mobilization of the duodenum, the T tube is placed in the third portion of the duodenum, beyond the ampulla. The duodenum is tacked to the abdominal wall at the site of the T tube in several places (much as in a Stamm gastrostomy). An alternative (albeit less desirable) approach is to place a duodenostomy tube into the end of the duodenal stump and suture it to the duodenal wall with purse-string sutures.

It is imperative to cover the duodenal stump with an omental patch. Also, it is helpful to pass the nasogastric tube through the gastrojejunostomy into the afferent limb; this stabilizes the limb and decompresses the stump. Finally, if a lateral duodenostomy tube is not possible, a jejunostomy tube can be placed in the proximal jejunum. This tube can be directed into the duodenum in a retrograde manner and used to decompress the stump.

Staples versus sutures for duodenal closure Although some authors advocate division of the duodenum with the GIA stapler, we prefer to use the TA stapler for this purpose. Because of its unique shape, the TA stapler is easier to use when the patient is obese or has a deep body cavity and when exposure is limited. Attempts to use the GIA stapler in these settings often result in excessive pulling on the duodenum to position the stapler properly, as well as poor apposition of the duodenal walls.

In general, if the duodenum is soft where the staples are applied, no additional sutures are necessary to reinforce the duodenal stump closure. If, however, the stump is inflamed, stapled closure should be avoided. Every effort should be made to mobilize the stump sufficiently to allow full-thickness suture closure. In addition, the stump end should be inverted with seromuscular bites to help reinforce the closure.

Whichever closure method is employed, the stump should be carefully evaluated for evidence of ischemia at the suture line. If ischemia is present, the duodenal stump sutures should be removed or the duodenum mobilized back to healthy tissue, the ischemic areas should be debrided, and the stump should be reclosed. If there is only a small ischemic segment at the suture or staple line, it can simply be inverted with seromuscular bites of the duodenal wall.

Gastric Procedures for Cancer

Surgery remains the primary means by which a patient with gastric cancer can be cured. Unfortunately, most patients present with advanced lesions, and survival with surgical treatment alone is suboptimal. Accordingly, the use of adjuvant and neoadjuvant chemotherapy and radiation treatment in an effort to improve outcome is on the rise.[2] In what follows, we address selection of the appropriate procedures for various types of gastric cancer and describe key steps in the performance of the procedures.

PREOPERATIVE EVALUATION

Before the operation, endoscopy—with or without endoscopic ultrasonography—should be done for diagnosis and assessment of the primary lesion. It is critical to determine how far proximally the tumor extends. A CT scan should be obtained for further assessment of the extent of the local disease and to search for metastases. The presence of metastatic disease should direct the surgeon either to perform a conservative palliative procedure or to treat the patient nonoperatively. Laparoscopy has also been used to stage gastric cancer patients before resection [*see* Laparoscopic Staging for Gastric Cancer, *below*]. For patients with dysplastic lesions, preoperative counseling should include a discussion of the possibility that the resected lesion could harbor an invasive malignancy and that further resection with lymphadenectomy may be necessary.

Finally, the surgeon must decide whether the patient is medically fit to undergo operation. Malnutrition is often an issue in gastric cancer patients. In select cases, preoperative total parenteral nutrition (TPN) may be helpful [*see* 6:23 Nutritional Support].

RESECTION OF HIGH-GRADE DYSPLASIA OR CARCINOMA IN SITU

Operative Planning

High-grade dysplasia of the stomach should be considered a premalignant lesion because if left untreated, it frequently leads to invasive malignancy.[3] At the time of the initial evaluation, the area of concern in the stomach should be extensively sampled by an experienced endoscopist, and the biopsy specimens should be

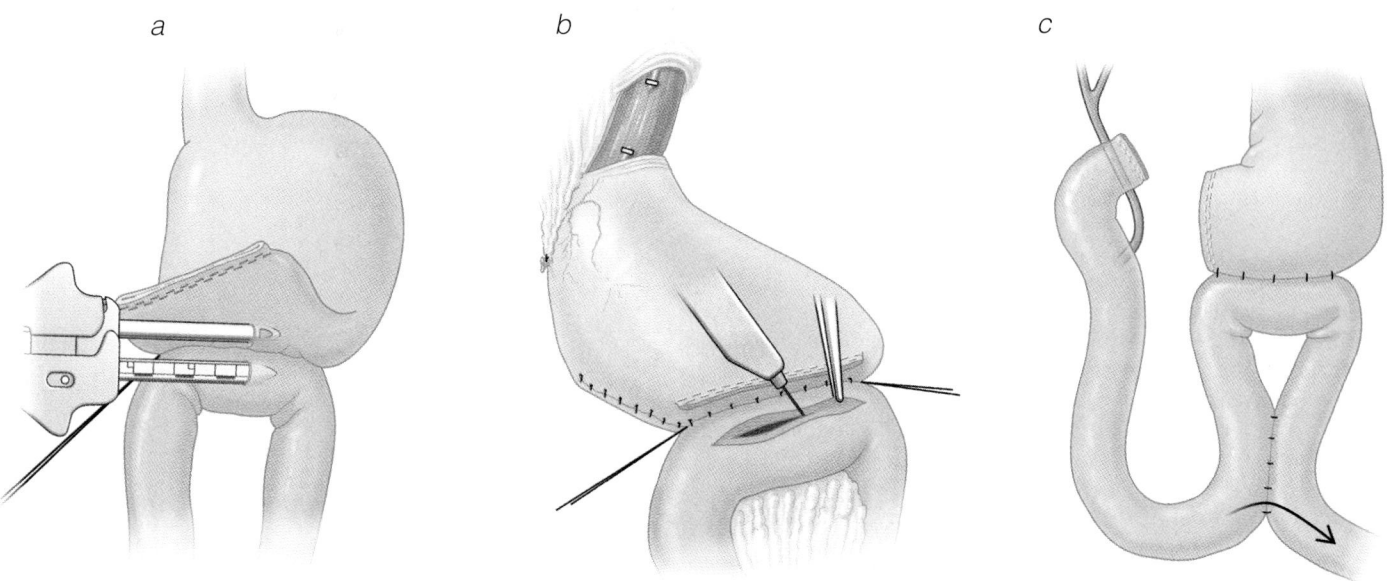

a *b* *c*

Figure 5 **Billroth II gastrojejunostomy. (*a*) A GIA stapler is inserted and fired through enterotomies made on the posterior wall of the stomach and in the jejunum. A TA stapler is then used to close the enterotomies. (*b*) During the hand-sewn procedure, once the posterior wall of Lembert sutures is completed, the jejunum is opened with the electrocautery to the desired length for the gastrojejunostomy. A portion of the gastric staple line approximately as long as the jejunostomy is removed. The continuous inner layer of the anastomosis is then completed. (*c*) A Braun enteroenterostomy may be added to help decompress the duodenal stump.**

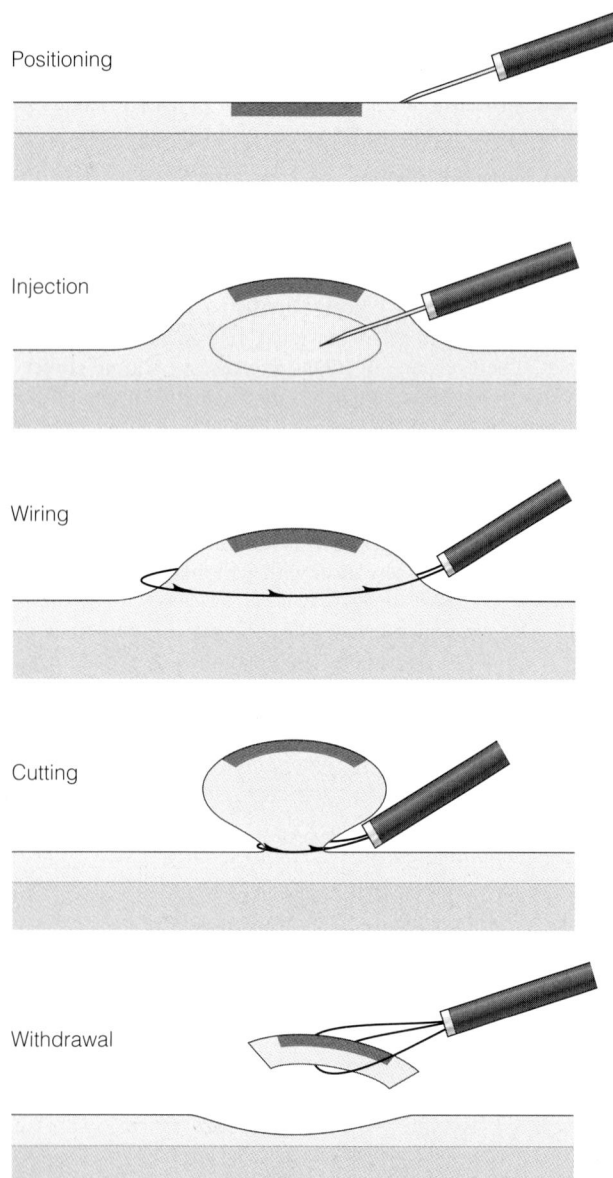

Positioning

Injection

Wiring

Cutting

Withdrawal

Figure 6 Endoscopic mucosal resection. Injecting saline into the submucosa lifts the lesion away from the gastric wall, thereby facilitating endoscopic resection.

interpreted by one or more pathologists who are experts in GI pathology. Histologic interpretation of the specimens is of crucial importance in helping determine the surgeon's treatment recommendations. The critical distinction is between high-grade dysplasia and lesser-grade dysplasia.

The recommended treatment for high-grade dysplasia is resection. Generally, patients with lesser-grade dysplasia may be followed with serial endoscopy and biopsy to rule out histologic progression; however, gastrectomy should be considered if there is a strong family history of gastric cancer. Small areas of high-grade dysplasia or carcinoma in situ can be removed by means of endoscopic mucosal resection (EMR)[4] or wedge resection of the stomach without lymphadenectomy. Larger areas of high-grade dysplasia in the distal stomach should be treated with an antrectomy, and extensive areas of high-grade dysplasia in the proximal stomach should be treated with a total gastrectomy. If a patient with high-grade dysplasia has a strong family history of

gastric cancer, a total gastrectomy should be considered regardless of lesion location.

Operative Technique

EMR Endoscopic mucosal resection [*see 3:8 Gastrointestinal Endoscopy*] is performed in the endoscopy suite by someone skilled in this procedure [*see Figure 6*]. EMR is more difficult to perform for tumors in the gastric body than in the antrum or the incisura region.[5] If EMR is not possible, then wedge resection is indicated. This procedure can frequently be performed laparoscopically with the assistance of intraoperative endoscopy.

Laparoscopic wedge resection with intraoperative endoscopy This procedure is best suited for anteriorly situated small tumors or lesions along the greater curvature. For lesions on the posterior stomach or along the lesser curvature, extensive mobilization of the stomach may be required before laparoscopic removal.

An umbilical port is inserted for insufflation and for passage of a 30° scope. Four upper abdominal ports are placed, two on each side of the midline [*see Figure 7*]. It is important that the lesion be easy to identify in the OR. The preferred method of accomplishing this is intraoperative endoscopy with direct visualization and marking of the lesion. Alternatively, India ink can be injected into the submucosa at the lesion before the operation; the ink should be injected in sufficient amount to be visible on the serosal surface of the stomach.

Once the lesion is located, the so-called lesion-lifting technique is employed. Sutures are placed in the normal tissue around the tumor, and traction is applied superiorly, causing the portion of

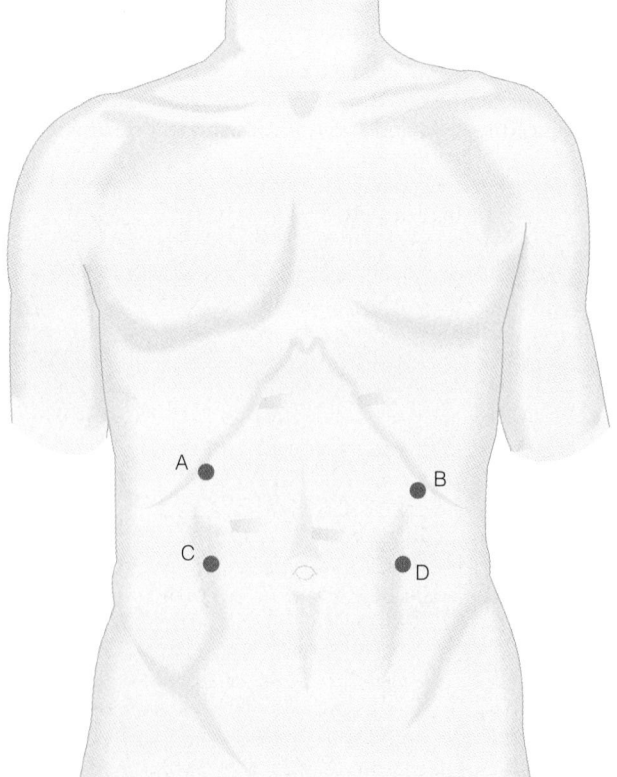

Figure 7 Laparoscopic wedge resection. In addition to the umbilical port, four ports are placed to the right and left of the midline in the upper abdomen. Port placement is similar for laparoscopic staging, except that often, only ports A and B are needed. If necessary for adequate exposure, the other two ports may be added.

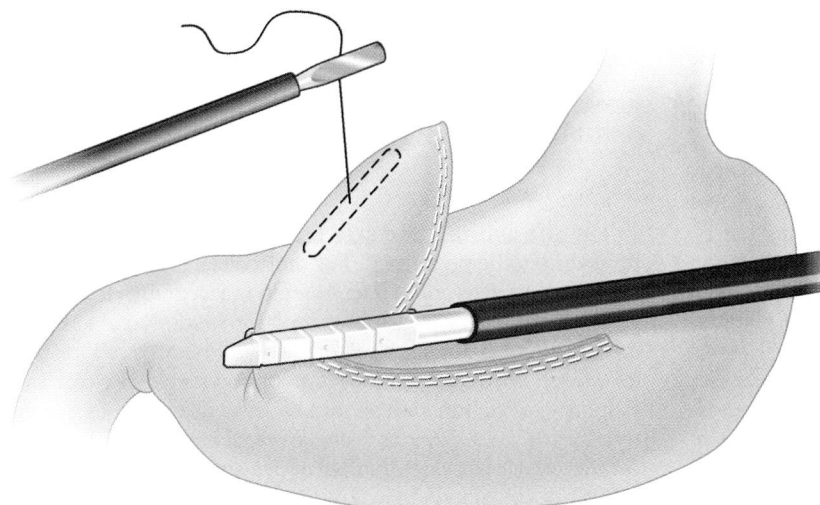

Figure 8 **Laparoscopic wedge resection. Sutures are placed in the normal tissue around the tumor, then retracted upward so that the portion of the gastric wall with the lesion is tented up. A wedge resection is then performed with an endoscopic stapler.**

the gastric wall containing the tumor to be tented upward; a wedge resection is then performed with a multifire endoscopic stapler [*see Figure 8*]. Before completion of the procedure, endoscopy is employed to confirm that the lesion has been removed, hemostasis is adequate, and the gastric outlet has not been significantly narrowed. For posterior tumors, the same basic approach applies, though exposure is gained through the avascular portion of the lesser sac. In this variant of the procedure, the greater curvature is retracted anteriorly, and the tumor is tented posteriorly.

As an alternative to laparoscopy, if necessary, wedge resection can be performed during a laparotomy by applying Allis clamps to the stomach wall and using the TA stapler.

Troubleshooting

Preoperative injection of India ink to identify the lesion may be problematic, either because the dye is insufficiently visible on the serosal surface of the stomach or because the staining of the serosal surface is excessively diffuse. Therefore, an experienced endoscopist should be available at the time of operation in case it proves necessary to perform an intraoperative examination.

Frequently, the gastroepiploic vessels or portions of the omentum will have to be divided to provide adequate exposure. The gastroepiploic vessels should be doubly clipped and divided; the omentum can be divided with the ultrasonic scalpel or another laparoscopic coagulating device. It is also helpful to place at least two sutures at the site of the lesion, positioned so that they can be used to elevate the entire lesion away from the rest of the stomach.

In general, resected lesions should be sent to the pathologist immediately for assessment of the margins. In some cases, the margins are clearly delineated, and this step may not be necessary. Certainly, with laparoscopic removal, the ability to obtain generous margins may be limited. Liberal use of pathologic frozen section evaluation to ensure negative margins is advisable.

Complications

In general, the stomach is durable and very well vascularized. Therefore, provided that patients are properly selected for laparoscopic wedge resection, postoperative leakage from the stomach should be comparatively rare, occurring no more often than after open resection. If leakage does occur, prompt reoperation and revision of the gastric closure are indicated. Delayed gastric emptying may occur after wedge resection secondary to division of vagal nerve fibers to the stomach. This problem may be alleviated by drugs that stimulate GI motility (e.g., erythromycin). Laparo-

scopic wedge resection may be associated with a lower incidence of pneumonia than open resection.

Outcome

Survival should be excellent after resection of high-grade dysplasia or carcinoma in situ. If there is a stomach remnant after the procedure, follow-up serial endoscopy is appropriate. The follow-up schedule should be individualized for each patient, but generally, examinations should not be necessary more often than every 6 months. The interval between examinations may be lengthened if the results of initial follow-up examinations are encouraging.

Laparoscopic wedge resection may be associated with a slightly shorter hospital stay than laparotomy; however, this difference depends in part on factors other than the procedure itself, including policies regarding resumption of oral diet in those undergoing laparotomy. With laparoscopic resection, significantly better scores on quality of life indices would be expected, as would significantly quicker return to preoperative status.

At present, in Western countries, laparoscopic resections are mostly limited to benign lesions. Early malignant lesions are treated laparoscopically in Japan but in few other countries; more advanced lesions are laparoscopically resected in only a few centers around the world. For the foreseeable future, given the technical complexity of laparoscopic gastric resections and the low prevalence of gastric tumors in Western countries, it is unlikely that these procedures will receive full endorsement from randomized, controlled trials.[6]

RESECTION OF EARLY GASTRIC CANCER

Operative Planning

In the United States, early gastric cancer accounts for a minority (< 15%) of gastric cancers; however, with the increased use of endoscopy, this number may be on the rise. The term early gastric cancer encompasses a heterogeneous group of lesions that are confined to the mucosa or submucosa (T1, NX, M0). With T1 lesions limited to the mucosa, the risk of lymph node metastases is less than 5%. With lesions that invade the submucosa, the risk may be as high as 20%. Because the incidence of lymph node metastases is low in early gastric cancer, some authorities advocate selective lymphadenectomy[7]; however, during preoperative evaluation, it can be difficult to distinguish between lesions with a very low risk of lymph node metastases and those with a higher risk.

Early gastric cancer is relatively common in Japan. As a consequence, early detection methods are well developed there, and the disease has been very well characterized. In Japanese centers, preoperative evaluation is based on the size and macroscopic appearance of the lesion.[8] Protruded-type carcinomas (type I and type IIA) with diameters smaller than 25 mm and excavated-type lesions with diameters smaller than 20 mm are almost always free of lymph node metastases; in fact, many of these lesions can be treated with EMR.[9] Histologic differentiation is also used in Japan to select patients for EMR: undifferentiated carcinomas often show diffuse, ill-defined superficial growth and thus are not suitable for EMR.

At present, Western countries have relatively little experience with the macroscopic classification system used in Japan for categorizing patients with early gastric cancer. This system requires an experienced endoscopist who has significant experience with gastric cancer, and findings are subjective. More objective findings may be achievable with endoluminal ultrasonography. If ultrasonography indicates that a tumor is limited to the mucosa, is small in diameter, shows no evidence of venous invasion, and is not poorly differentiated, the patient should be initially considered for limited resection without lymphadenectomy.[7]

Operative Technique

In Western countries, carefully selected patients with early gastric cancer can undergo limited resection. However, because of the usual stage at presentation and the biology of the disease, only a minority are suitable candidates for wedge resection (laparoscopic or open) without lymphadenectomy according to strict Japanese surgical guidelines. For most early gastric cancer patients in the United States, gastrectomy with removal of perigastric lymph nodes (D1 lymphadenectomy) is indicated. For patients with distal gastric lesions, the recommended treatment is distal gastrectomy with removal of the infrapyloric and suprapyloric nodes along with some of the nodes along the greater and lesser curvatures. For patients with lesions in the middle portion of the stomach, the appropriate procedure is subtotal gastrectomy with removal of the infrapyloric and suprapyloric nodes along with all of the lesser and greater curvature nodes. For patients with lesions in the proximal stomach, the operation of choice is total gastrectomy with removal of all of the nodes previously mentioned, as well as the right and left pericardial nodes near the esophagogastric junction. These techniques are discussed in greater detail in the context of more advanced gastric cancer [see Resection of Advanced Gastric Cancer: Total Gastrectomy with D2 Lymphadenectomy *and* Resection of Advanced Gastric Cancer: Subtotal or Distal Gastrectomy, *below*].

Troubleshooting

An experienced endoscopist and pathologist are critical for successful selective resection. If a wedge resection is to be performed, careful intraoperative evaluation of the margins is necessary.

Complications

Generally, the complications of resection of early gastric cancer are similar to those of wedge resection [see Resection of High-Grade Dysplasia and Carcinoma in Situ, *above*]. They are also somewhat similar to the complications of more extensive resections for advanced gastric cancer (see below), but they tend to arise less frequently.

Outcome

In appropriate patients, limited resection for early gastric cancer should result in low rates of recurrence. In a study of 711 patients with early gastric cancer in Japan, the recurrence rate was 4%.[10]

RESECTION OF ADVANCED GASTRIC CANCER: TOTAL GASTRECTOMY WITH D2 LYMPHADENECTOMY

Operative Planning

The site and the extent of the cancer determine the surgical procedure to be performed. For more distal lesions, a limited gastric resection with only a 5 cm margin is acceptable, in that no survival benefit has been demonstrated for routine total gastrectomy in this setting.[11] Total gastrectomy should be reserved for patients in whom adequate margins are unobtainable. Lesions at the esophagogastric junction should be treated with an esophagogastrectomy [see 3:9 Open Esophageal Procedures].

The extent to which lymph nodes should be dissected is the subject of ongoing debate. To date, 16 different lymph node stations have been associated with gastric cancer. Lymph node dissections are classified as either D1 or D2. A D1 dissection includes resection of the immediate lesser and greater curvature nodes along with the gastrectomy. This is the minimal dissection that should be considered in patients who are not judged to have early

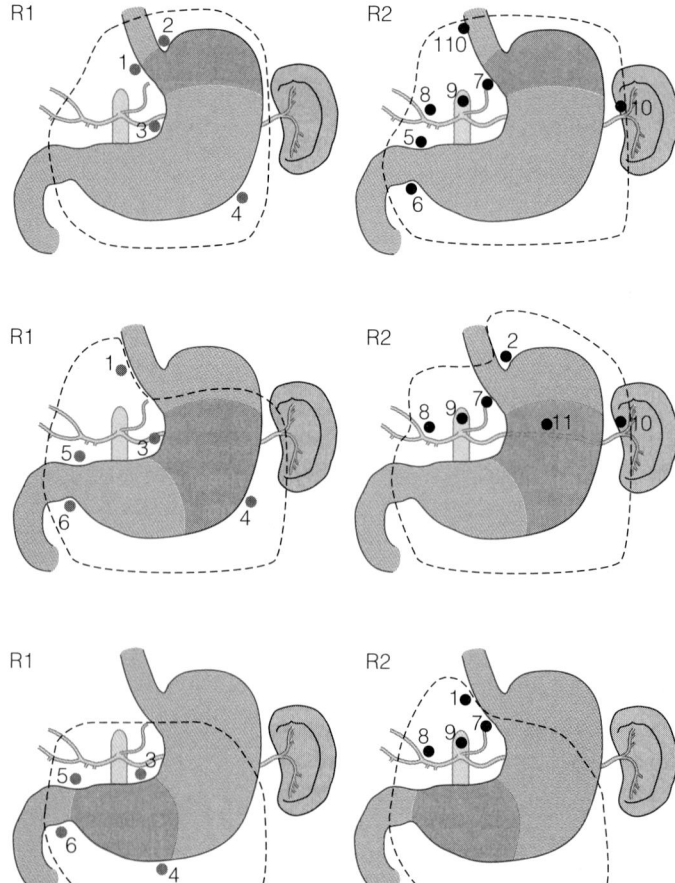

Figure 9 **Illustrated are recommended gastric resections and lymphadenectomies for lesions within the shaded areas.**[14] **Dotted line demonstrates extent of lymph node dissection; extent of gastric resection is based on lesion location. Dots represent node groups. (1—right cardiac; 2—left cardiac; 3—lesser curvature; 4—greater curvature [and short gastric]; 5—suprapyloric; 6—infrapyloric; 7—left gastric; 8—hepatic; 9—celiac; 10—splenic hilar; 11—splenic; 110—paracardial)**

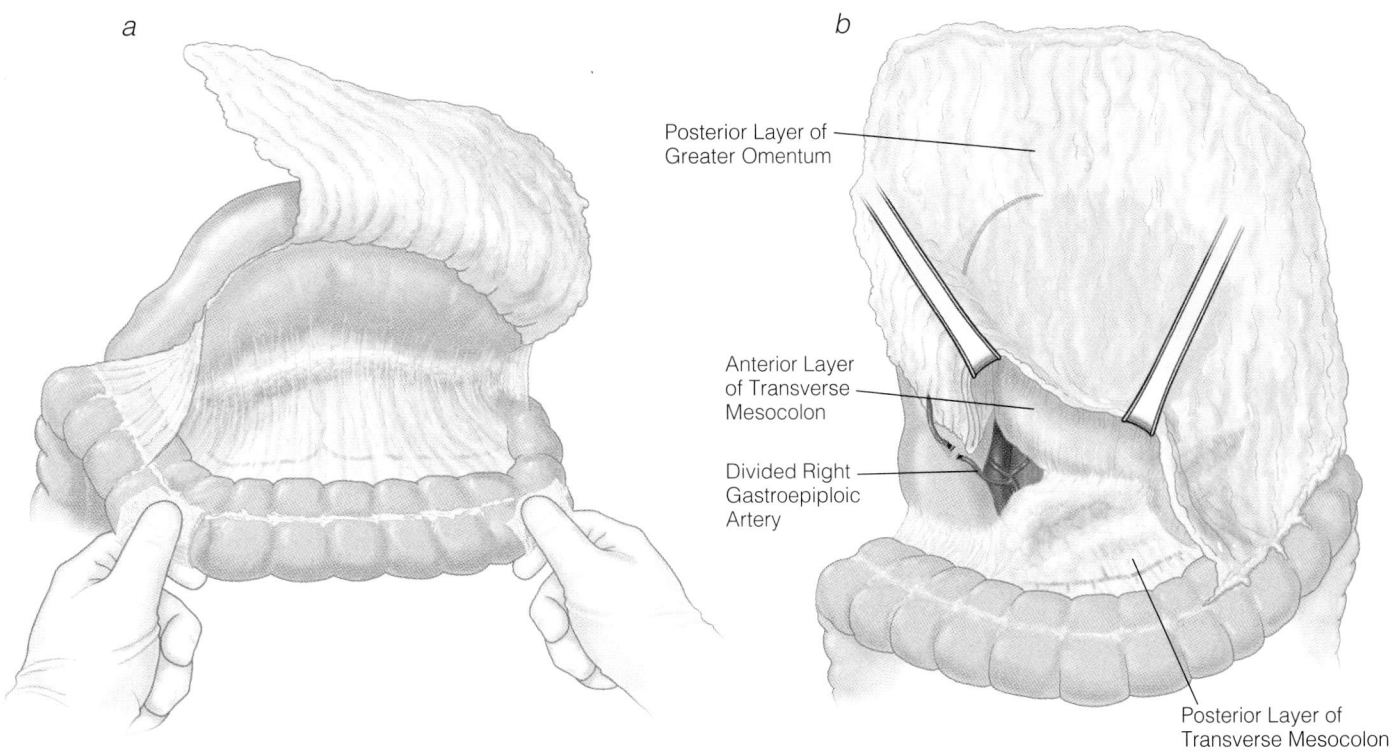

a

b

Posterior Layer of
Greater Omentum

Anterior Layer
of Transverse
Mesocolon

Divided Right
Gastroepiploic
Artery

Posterior Layer of
Transverse Mesocolon

Figure 10 **Total gastrectomy with D2 lymphadenectomy. (*a*) The greater omentum is carefully separated from the transverse colon; gentle retraction of the colon and greater omentum helps to expose the correct plane of dissection. Particular care should be taken in the region of the middle colic vessels. (*b*) With continued dissection, the gastroepiploic vessels are exposed and ligated. The anterior capsule of the pancreas is resected with the specimen.**

gastric cancer. A D2 dissection incorporates the omental bursa, the anterior leaf of the transverse colon, and all nodes related to the location of the tumor. This extended lymphadenectomy is beneficial for staging T2 and T3 lesions and may improve survival in a small subset of patients with limited lymph node metastasis. With T3 tumors, the risk of metastatic disease involving the level 2 nodes is greater than 40%. Japanese investigators have found that extensive lymph node dissection confers a significant survival advantage, though these results have been difficult to duplicate elsewhere.[12,13] Long-term follow-up data from a multi-institutional randomized Dutch study comparing D1 and D2 lymph node dissection suggest that patients undergoing a D2 lymphadenectomy may survive longer.[14]

The extent of the lymph node dissection also depends on the location of the tumor [*see Figure 9*]. For proximal lesions, a total gastrectomy with a D2 lymphadenectomy encompassing the splenic, celiac, hepatic, pericardial, and left gastric nodes should be performed. For middle gastric lesions, a total or subtotal gastrectomy, depending on the location of the lesion and the obtainability of 5 cm margins, can be performed in conjunction with a D2 lymphadenectomy encompassing the splenic, celiac, hepatic, left gastric, and right pericardial nodes. For distal lesions, a distal gastrectomy should be performed with dissection of the celiac, hepatic, right pericardial, and left gastric nodes.[15,16]

Routine splenectomy appears to confer no survival benefit. In fact, including a routine splenectomy with the resection significantly increases morbidity. Accordingly, splenectomy should be incorporated in the dissection only when there is direct spread of tumor to the spleen.[17]

Preoperative bowel preparation is indicated because of the extensive dissection of the omentum from the transverse mesocolon.

Operative Technique

If there is no active tumor bleeding or evidence of gastric outlet obstruction, then laparoscopy may be performed in an effort to detect metastatic disease that would preclude operative resection.[18] If metastatic disease is found, palliative resection must be done with caution. Such resection can lead to significant postoperative morbidity,[19] thereby delaying or preventing chemotherapy, which is of proven benefit in this setting.

Step 1: incision and exposure A total gastrectomy is commonly done through a midline incision, though a bilateral subcostal incision may provide better exposure in obese or deep patients. Once the peritoneal cavity has been opened, a thorough exploration is undertaken to assess the extent of the cancer and look for metastatic lesions. In women, the ovaries should be examined for the presence of a Krukenberg tumor.

Step 2: separation of omental bursa The omental bursa is separated from the transverse mesocolon with the electrocautery [*see Figure 10*]. This step can be simplified by retracting the omentum anteriorly and placing gentle inferior traction on the colon. This area should be avascular for the most part. In the course of the dissection, the right gastroepiploic vein and artery are ligated near their origin on the inferior aspect of the antrum.

Troubleshooting. Separation of the omental bursa from the transverse mesocolon requires meticulous dissection and patience. A hole in the omentum signifies entry into the wrong field of dissection. Particular care must be taken in the region of the middle colic vessels, which run just posterior to the plane of dissection. The correct plane may be easier to identify on the left

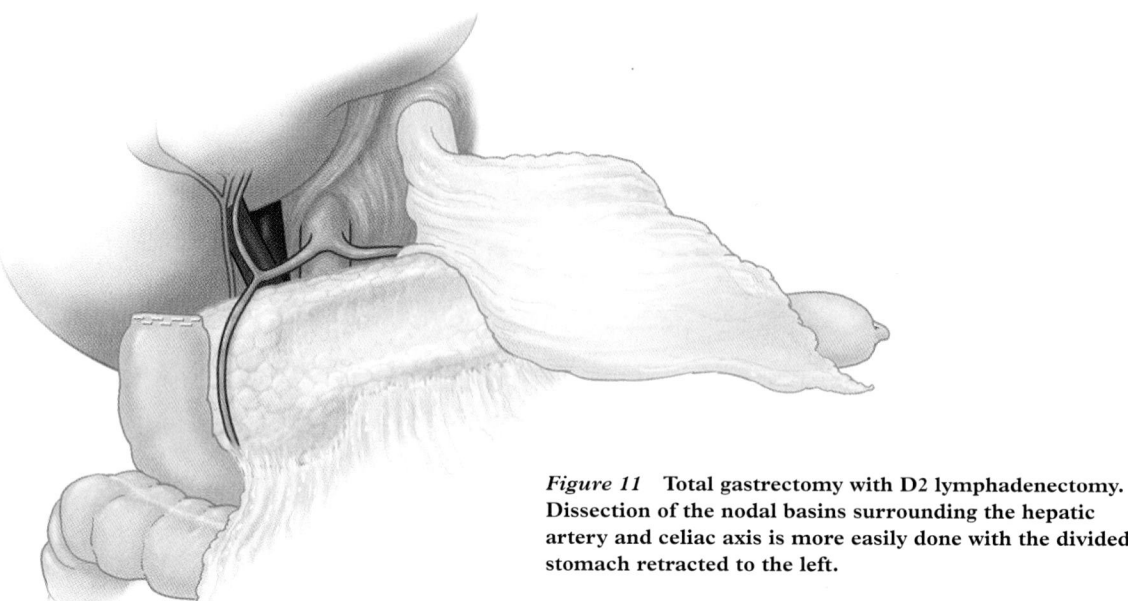

Figure 11 Total gastrectomy with D2 lymphadenectomy. Dissection of the nodal basins surrounding the hepatic artery and celiac axis is more easily done with the divided stomach retracted to the left.

and right aspects of the omental attachments to the colon than in the middle.

Step 3: mobilization and division of duodenum The duodenum is then freed just beyond the pylorus by dividing the right gastric artery. The suprapyloric lymph nodes are swept toward the specimen. The duodenum is then divided with the stapler. Dissection continues to the inferior border of the pancreas, and the pancreatic capsule is freed and elevated superiorly.

Troubleshooting. Often, the duodenum can be safely divided with a GIA stapler; however, if the patient has a deep body cavity or if exposure is difficult, it is best to divide the duodenum flush with a TA stapler. Duodenal staple lines are never cauterized to stop hemorrhage, but they may be reinforced with sutures to obtain hemostasis. If there is any doubt about the integrity of the stapled duodenal closure, the staple line should be inverted.

Step 4: dissection around porta hepatis and celiac axis With the stomach retracted anteriorly and to the patient's left, the major structures in the porta hepatis (i.e., the hepatic artery and ducts) are carefully identified, and the surrounding lymph nodes are removed [*see Figure 11*]. Dissection then proceeds along the hepatic artery in a distal-to-proximal manner toward the celiac axis. All soft tissue surrounding the common hepatic, left gastric, and splenic arteries should be included. The left gastric vein is encountered during this dissection and is divided. The splenic artery is cleared of nodal tissue from its origin throughout most of its path to the splenic hilum.

Troubleshooting. Clearance of nodal tissue along the celiac vessels should begin with identification of the right gastroepiploic artery as it arises from the gastroduodenal artery. The gastroduodenal artery should be traced to the hepatic artery, which can then be traced proximally to the celiac axis.

Step 5: dissection along greater curvature The left gastric artery is encircled near its origin and divided. Dissection then continues along greater curvature; anterior retraction of the stomach helps to expose this region. The left gastroepiploic artery and

the short gastric vessels are carefully ligated. If possible, the left gastroepiploic artery should be ligated near its origin from the splenic artery in the hilum of the spleen. The spleen can usually be spared unless direct extension of the tumor is apparent in this area.

Step 6: division of lesser omentum The lesser omentum is divided close to the liver from the esophageal hiatus to the hepatoduodenal ligament. Gentle inferior retraction of the stomach improves exposure of the lesser omentum. If an accessory or replaced left hepatic artery is encountered, it should be carefully ligated. The right and left diaphragmatic crura are identified and skeletonized.

Step 7: mobilization and division of esophagus The esophagus is completely mobilized, and the vagus nerves are sharply divided. The esophagus is then divided, the specimen removed, and reconstruction performed. Reconstruction options include stapled or hand-sewn end-to-side esophagojejunostomy, side-to-side esophagojejunostomy, and jejunal pouch reconstruction [*see Step 8a through 8d, below*].

Alternatively, the specimen can be left attached and used as a handle, the anastomosis performed next, and the specimen removed last; however, this alternative should be considered only when the proximal margin is not an issue. If there is any doubt about the proximal margin, the specimen should be removed first and the proximal margin evaluated. In this setting, an end-to-side esophagojejunostomy may be the best reconstruction option.

Before completion of the operation, a feeding jejunostomy is placed.

Troubleshooting. Any concerns about margins should be addressed intraoperatively with frozen section analysis. Some gastric cancers (e.g., poorly differentiated lesions) are associated with submucosal spread. Thus, tumor may be present in the stomach wall well above the termination of the palpable mass.

Step 8a: reconstruction (stapled Roux-en-Y end-to-side esophagojejunostomy) With the stomach retracted inferiorly, the esophagus is mobilized, and a Satinsky clamp is placed on it well above the level of division to keep it from retracting after transection [*see Figure 12a*]. A purse-string is created on the esophageal wall, either with a hand-placed 2-0 polypropylene suture or with an automatic purse-string device. The esophagus is then sharply divided. The specimen, including the stomach, lymph nodes, and omentum, is removed.

A Roux jejunal limb is fashioned and brought up behind the colon to the esophagus. To minimize biliary reflux, this limb should be 40 to 50 cm long. The esophagojejunostomy is created on the antimesenteric portion of the jejunum rather than at the divided end because of the superior blood supply to the former [see Figure 12b, c]. The anvil of the stapler is placed in the end of the esophagus, and the purse-string suture is tied around it. The stapler is placed through the end of the Roux limb and brought out on the antimesenteric border approximately 10 cm distally. It is then connected to the anvil and fired to create the anastomosis. Finally, the open end of the jejunal limb is closed with a TA stapler. A nasogastric tube is carefully positioned just above the anastomosis; it is removed early in the postoperative period.

Troubleshooting. The distal esophagus should be mobilized for at least 6 to 8 cm into the mediastinum before the anastomosis is attempted. The Satinsky clamp should be placed several centimeters above the end of the esophagus so as not to interfere with the placement of the anvil in the esophagus. Before the EEA stapler is introduced into the end of the jejunum, the last several centimeters of the limb should be devascularized by dividing its mesentery. Care should be taken not to incorporate the mesentery when the EEA stapler is closed: if the mesentery is brought into the staple line, the diameter of the anastomosis will be significantly decreased and hemorrhage may ensue. If there is any concern about possible hemorrhage, the anastomosis should be reinforced with additional interrupted sutures. To ensure that the anastomosis is tension free, the jejunal limb should be sutured to the phrenoesophageal ligament. In closing the open end of the jejunum, the TA stapler should be applied at a point where the bowel is vascularized, a few centimeters away from the anastomosis.

Step 8b: reconstruction (hand-sewn end-to-side esophagojejunostomy)   As in a stapled end-to-side esophagojejunostomy, the esophagus is mobilized, a Satinsky clamp placed, and the esophagus divided. A location on the antimesenteric portion of the jejunal limb, 5 cm from the end, is used for the anastomosis. Stay sutures of 3-0 absorbable material are placed (with the needle left on) at the 3 o'clock and 9 o'clock positions on the esophagus. The jejunum is opened. The posterior wall of the jejunum is sutured to the posterior wall of the esophagus with interrupted 3-0 absorbable sutures. Usually, this is done by starting in the midline and working toward each corner, with the knots placed on the inside. Once the corners are reached, the stay sutures are used to begin the anterior row. When all of the anterior row sutures have been placed, the knots are tied on the outside.

Troubleshooting. Suture placement will be more accurate if the knots are not tied until all of the posterior row sutures have been placed. The same is true for the anterior row sutures.

Step 8c: reconstruction (side-to-side esophagojejunostomy)   If no significant concern exists about the status of the proximal margin, a side-to-side anastomosis is a reasonable alternative [see Figure 13]. The advantage of this approach is that the new anastomosis is well away from the divided end of the esophagus, at a spot where the blood supply is uninterrupted. In addition, the anastomosis can readily be lengthened to allow improved oral intake, and unlike an end-to-side anastomosis, its size is not limited by the size of the EEA stapler used.

The lower end of the esophagus is extensively mobilized. With the stomach retracted to draw the esophagus into the abdomen, openings are made in the esophagus and the jejunum. A GIA-55 or GIA-80 stapler is inserted with one arm in the esophagotomy and the other in the jejunotomy, then fired to create the anastomosis. If a longer anastomosis is desired, additional length can be

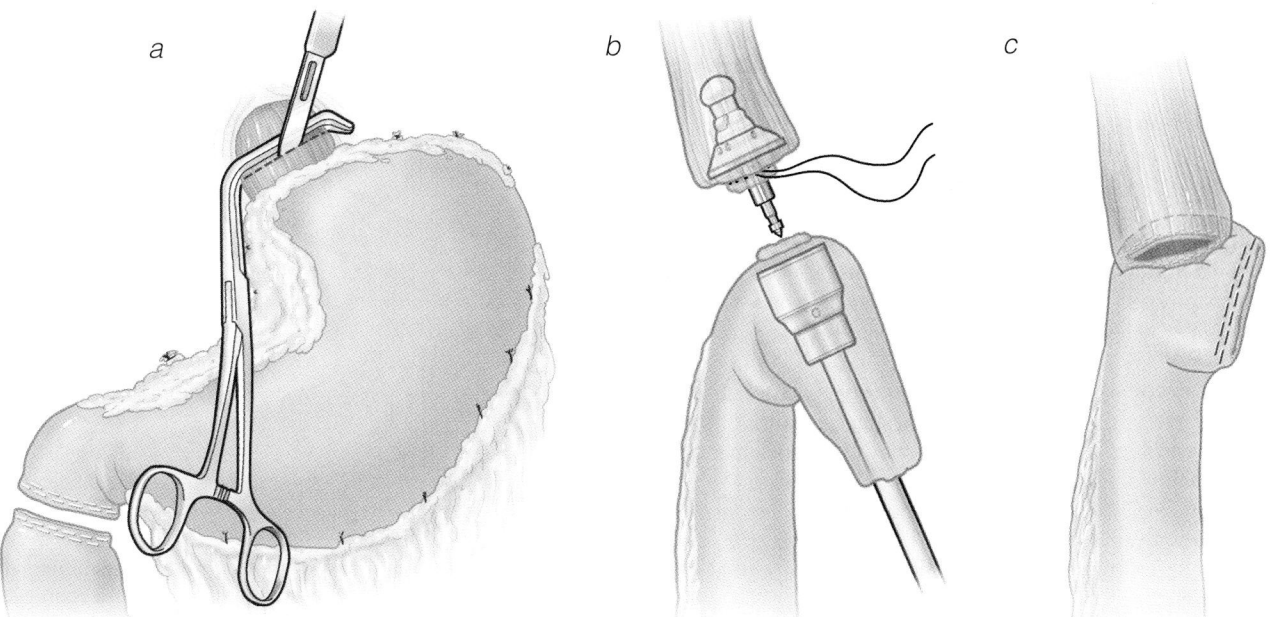

Figure 12   **Total gastrectomy with D2 lymphadenectomy: end-to-side esophagojejunostomy. (*a*) A Satinsky clamp is placed on the esophagus before division of the stomach. (*b*) A purse-string suture is placed at the divided end of the esophagus. The EEA stapler is inserted through the distal end of the Roux limb, and the tip is brought out 10 cm distally on the antimesenteric border. The anvil of the stapler is secured in the esophagus with the purse-string suture. (*c*) The EEA stapler is connected and fired, completing the anastomosis.**

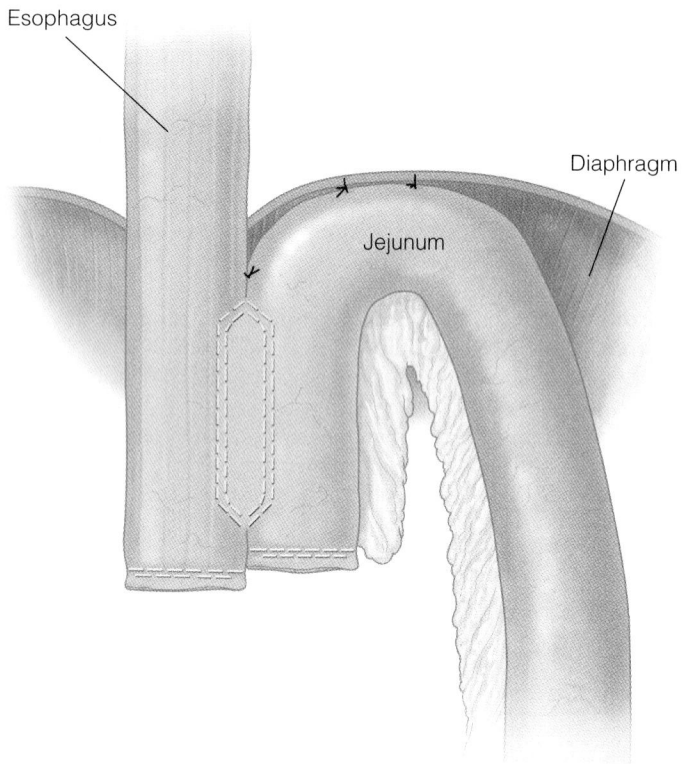

Esophagus

Diaphragm

Jejunum

end of the Roux limb for a length of 15 cm. The antimesenteric borders are apposed with three interrupted sutures. An enterotomy is made at the apex of the proposed pouch, and a GIA-55 stapler is inserted with one arm of the device in each side of the doubled-over limb. The stapler is fired, then advanced and fired again to create an appropriately sized pouch. A purse-string suture of 2-0 polypropylene is placed in the jejunal wall at the site of the enterotomy. The EEA stapler is then introduced through the proximal end of the jejunal limb, advanced through the pouch, and brought out through the site of the previous enterotomy. The purse-string suture is tied around the stapler, and the stapler is then attached to the anvil in the esophagus and fired to create the anastomosis. The end of the jejunum is closed by applying a TA stapler at a point where the bowel is viable.

In the second method, two enterotomies are created, one at the proximal end of the divided jejunum and the other at a corresponding location on the doubled loop [*see Figure 14*]. A GIA stapler is inserted with one arm in each enterotomy and fired. To complete the pouch, a second GIA stapler or a laparoscopic GIA stapler is fired in the same orientation as the first stapler. Once this pouch is created, an EEA stapler is easily inserted through its open end to complete the anastomosis. The anvil of the stapler is placed within the divided esophagus, and a purse-string suture is secured around it, either manually or with an automatic purse-string device. Next, the EEA stapler is placed in the open end created by the GIA stapler, and the tip is brought out at the apex of the

Figure 13 **Total gastrectomy with D2 lymphadenectomy: side-to-side esophagojejunostomy. A GIA stapler is used to fashion an anastomosis between the antimesenteric border of the Roux jejunal limb and the side of the divided esophagus. The enterotomy is closed with a TA stapler. The distal esophagus is then closed with the TA stapler, and the specimen is removed.**

obtained by using an endoscopic GIA stapler to extend the opening. The enterotomies are closed with a TA stapler. The TA stapler is applied a second time to occlude the end of the esophagus, and the specimen is freed by cutting along the TA staple line.

Troubleshooting. The jejunum should be placed along the esophagus in a side-to-side (functional end-to-end) fashion. A seromuscular suture between esophagus and jejunum should be placed just proximal to the anastomosis to remove tension from the apex of the anastomosis. The jejunum should also be sutured to the phrenoesophageal ligament to relieve tension on the anastomosis.

Step 8d: reconstruction (jejunal pouch) Although only limited data are available, there is some suggestion that pouch reconstruction after total gastrectomy may be associated with improved quality of life in the early postoperative period.[20,21] For most patients with advanced gastric cancer, pouch reconstruction offers no advantage; however, for some patients with early stage disease or extensive carcinoma in situ, it is an option worth considering.

Once the specimen has been removed, the esophagus is prepared for placement of the anvil from the EEA stapler as described earlier (see above). A jejunal pouch is then fashioned for anastomosis to the esophagus. This can be done in several different ways; we will describe two of the most commonly used methods.

In the first method, the pouch is created by doubling over the

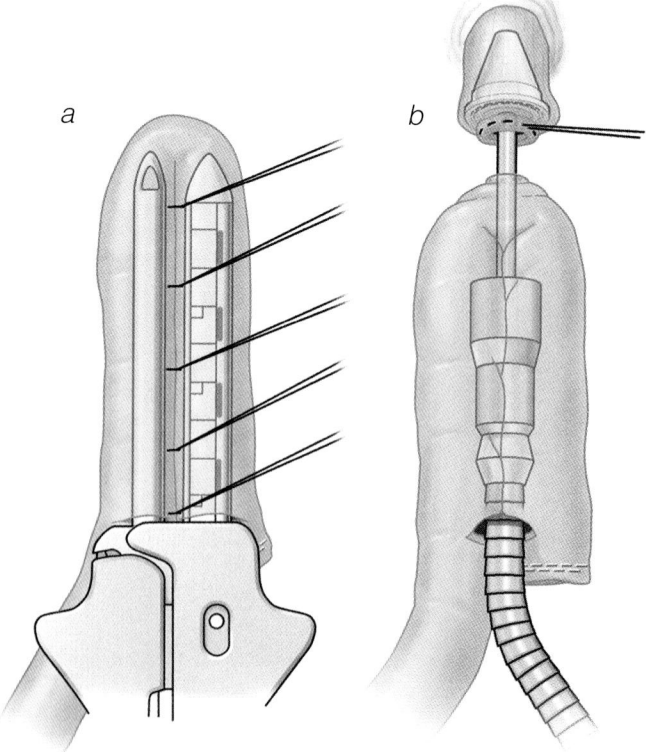

a

b

Figure 14 **Total gastrectomy with D2 lymphadenectomy: jejunal pouch reconstruction. (*a*) The stomach having been removed, the free end of the jejunum is brought up behind the colon into the upper abdomen. This free end is doubled over to create a loop about 15 cm long, and the two sides of the loop are apposed with sutures. A GIA stapler is inserted with one arm in each side of the loop and fired to create the pouch. (*b*) An EEA stapler is inserted within the pouch and connected to the anvil previously secured in the esophagus, then fired to create the anastomosis.**

pouch. The EEA stapler is fired to complete the anastomosis. The open end of the pouch can be closed with a TA stapler.

Troubleshooting. Pouch reconstruction is technically demanding and can be difficult in deep or obese patients. Careful planning is necessary to ensure that an appropriately sized pouch is created, that the EEA stapler can pass easily through the end of the jejunum, and that the jejunum can be closed without undue difficulty. The end of the jejunum through which the EEA is inserted should be carefully closed with a TA stapler at a viable location upon completion of the anastomosis.

Complications

Lymphadenectomy-related Certainly, the operating time is longer and the potential for complications greater with a D2 lymphadenectomy than with a D1 lymphadenectomy. Major complications may include operative blood loss and postoperative hemorrhage related to more extensive dissection, colonic injury resulting from skeletonization of the transverse mesocolon, postoperative pancreatitis caused by manipulation of the pancreas, intra-abdominal infection related to all of the above, and erosion into celiac vessels that have been stripped clean of protective fibroglandular tissue. There are, however, several reports indicating that in experienced hands, D2 lymphadenectomy (without distal pancreatectomy or splenectomy) is not associated with significantly more complications than D1 lymphadenectomy is. In our experience, operating time and intraoperative blood loss are slightly greater with D2 lymphadenectomy, but otherwise, complications are not significantly increased. For most surgeons who are not experienced with this technique, additional training is recommended to enhance outcome.

Anastomosis-related Despite the relatively poor blood supply to the end of the esophagus, the risk of leakage after an end-to-side esophagojejunal anastomosis is low. Moreover, given that a long-defunctionalized jejunal limb is used for the anastomosis, leakage, though undesirable, is not often life-threatening. Patients with an anastomotic leak may show evidence of sepsis as a consequence of bacterial colonization of the esophagus via drainage of secretions. A nasogastric tube should be positioned above the anastomosis, broad-spectrum antibiotics initiated, and fluid collections drained. Aggressive nutritional support via either a feeding jejunostomy or TPN is indicated. Other complications (e.g., anastomotic strictures) are uncommon with either stapled or hand-sewn end-to-side anastomoses; however, the size of the anastomosis is limited by the diameter of the end of the esophagus.

Our experience with side-to-side esophagojejunostomy suggests that anastomotic leakage rates are minimal and that early oral intake is well tolerated. To date, however, no randomized comparisons between end-to-side and side-to-side reconstruction have been performed.

Outcome

Randomized, prospective trials have not found survival to be better after a D2 lymphadenectomy than after a D1 lymphadenectomy in patients with advanced gastric cancer. As noted, however, long-term follow-up from one of these trials does suggest a survival advantage with D2 lymphadenectomy.[14] Certainly, many surgeons who have treated numerous gastric cancer patients have seen long-term survivors who had node-positive disease removed in a D2 lymphadenectomy.

Fat and protein malabsorption caused by failure of adequate food intake is often seen after total gastrectomy. This condition abates with time. Initially, patients must eat a number of small meals in the course of the day, but after a few months, they can usually resume eating three regular meals a day. With a Roux-en-Y esophagojejunostomy, transit of food through the small intestine is slower than normal. The proximal jejunal limb does not act as a reservoir, but because it may empty rapidly during eating, patients are able to eat a normal-sized meal. The only nutrient that must be replaced on a continuing basis after total gastrectomy is vitamin B_{12}, which is given to prevent megaloblastic anemia.

RESECTION OF ADVANCED GASTRIC CANCER: SUBTOTAL OR DISTAL GASTRECTOMY

Gastric cancers of the antrum or the distal third of the stomach are potentially resectable by means of a distal or subtotal gastrectomy. The dissection begins in much the same fashion as in a total gastrectomy, though the short gastric arteries are not ligated. The greater omentum, the lesser omentum, the left gastric artery, and the lymph nodes in the region of the hepatic and celiac artery are all removed; the right pericardial lymph nodes are also included with the specimen. The stomach is divided 5 cm proximal to the tumor. A common point of division is just inferior to the short gastric vessels and proximal to the incisura. The aims are to obtain adequate margins and remove the antrum completely. GI continuity should be restored by means of a Billroth II anastomosis [see Antrectomy, *above*].

LAPAROSCOPIC STAGING FOR GASTRIC CANCER

Discovery of metastatic peritoneal or liver disease through laparoscopy may spare a patient a laparotomy. In addition, laparoscopic staging allows uniform classification when patients are being enrolled into trials investigating the benefits of neoadjuvant therapy. Staging laparoscopy is not necessary for early gastric cancer. It should be reserved for malignant lesions at high risk for peritoneal seeding (i.e., T2 to T4 tumors). In this setting, laparoscopic staging has been shown to detect occult metastatic disease in 20% to 30% of patients who were considered to have local-regional disease on the basis of preoperative imaging.[18] Laparoscopic ultrasonography can also be incorporated to establish the T stage of the tumor and to help determine whether it is resectable.

Operative Technique

After insufflation through an umbilical port, a 30° degree telescope is inserted. The peritoneum, the liver, the diaphragm, the omentum, and all serosal surfaces are carefully inspected. A second port is placed in the right upper quadrant for exploration, palpation, and possible biopsy of any suspicious lesions. A third port is placed on the left side to facilitate evaluation of the ligament of Treitz and the porta hepatis for possible disease [see Figure 7]. If laparoscopic ultrasonography is not being performed, the right and left ports can be 5 mm. In the absence of obvious peritoneal disease, peritoneal washings are obtained from the left hemidiaphragm, the right hemidiaphragm, and the pelvis. Immediate cytologic analysis is frequently unavailable; therefore, specimens should be sent for routine cytologic analysis. In a few patients with T2 to T4 gastric cancers, cytology yields positive results, and such findings aid in predicting clinical outcome. Positive cytologic results are associated with survival rates similar to those seen with metastatic gastric cancer. After peritoneal washings are performed, suspicious lesions are sampled and the specimens sent for frozen section evaluation.

Troubleshooting

If possible, port sites should be placed in such a way that a laparotomy incision would encompass them. A laparoscopic biopsy instrument is very helpful in obtaining tissue samples from peritoneal and liver surfaces. If such an instrument is not available, a biopsy instrument from a bronchoscopy set may be used instead.

Complications

Complication rates should be low to nonexistent with laparoscopic staging. Port site metastases are not a significant issue: large series have shown that the rate of such metastases is equivalent to that observed with open procedures.[22] In the absence of any contraindications, patients can be discharged home on the day of the laparoscopic procedure.

Duodenal Procedures for Cancer

LOCAL RESECTION OF DUODENAL TUMORS

Preoperative Evaluation

Tumor type, size, and location are the key determinants of appropriate surgical treatment. Lesions that are often amenable to local duodenal wall resection without mesenteric resection include small neuroendocrine tumors and gastrointestinal stromal tumors (GISTs). It is important to locate the tumor with respect to the ampulla and the pancreatic head; whereas lesions on the lateral side of the duodenum are relatively easy to remove, lesions on the medial wall, which is covered by the head of the pancreas, are much less accessible. Preoperative endoscopy with tumor localization and biopsy is critical before resection is attempted.

Operative Planning

Operative planning for open duodenal procedures is generally straightforward. The operation is always performed with the patient under general anesthesia and supine. Once the patient is intubated, a nasogastric tube and a Foley catheter are placed. Most surgeons elect to perform duodenal surgery through an upper midline incision, though in obese or deep patients, a right subcostal incision may yield better exposure.

Operative Technique

The duodenum and the head of the pancreas are extensively mobilized by dividing the retroperitoneal attachments. Any small tumor that is palpable on the lateral aspect of any portion of the duodenum can be resected. A longitudinal duodenotomy is made 0.5 cm away from the tumor. The tumor is grasped and everted. A full-thickness portion of the duodenal wall is resected with the tumor. Stay sutures may be placed on the duodenum as the wall is being resected to preserve orientation for closure.

Frequently, the duodenum can be closed transversely so as not to narrow the lumen. Stay sutures are placed at the ends of the duodenotomy, which is then held transversely. The walls are approximated with Allis clamps, and a TA stapler is applied to close the duodenal wall below the clamps. Alternatively, the duodenal wall may be closed longitudinally with a single layer of interrupted 3-0 absorbable sutures. If the duodenal opening is large, transverse closure may be impossible because there would be too much tension on the suture line. In this situation, the duodenal wall is closed longitudinally with the TA stapler. Omentum is placed over the duodenal closure.

Troubleshooting

Small duodenal lesions may not be palpable, in which case intraoperative endoscopy may be required for localization. This possibility should be prepared for in advance of the operation. Lesions on the medial side of the duodenum can still be resected locally if the head of the pancreas can be mobilized away from the duodenal wall. Fine blood vessels running between the head of the pancreas and the medial duodenal wall should be carefully divided to allow exposure of the duodenum. During this dissection, the location of the ampulla can be determined more accurately by inserting a Fogarty catheter into the cystic duct, down the CBD, and through the ampulla into the duodenum. This step requires that the gallbladder be removed and the cystic duct isolated.

RESECTION OF DISTAL DUODENAL TUMORS

Preoperative Evaluation

On rare occasion, resection of the fourth portion of the duodenum and part of the third without pancreaticoduodenectomy is called for. This approach is indicated for lesions that are distal to the ampulla and are not invading the pancreatic head, the superior mesenteric vein (SMV), or the superior mesenteric artery (SMA). Such lesions may include carcinoids and GISTs that are located on the medial duodenal wall or even duodenal adenocarcinomas when mesenteric resection is necessary. Careful localization with upper GI endoscopy is essential, with particular attention paid to how the lesion is situated with respect to the ampulla. Preoperative CT scanning and endoscopic ultrasonography (EUS) should be performed. In our experience, EUS, when done by an experienced endoscopist, can be very helpful in assessing the extent of tumor invasion. Ultimately, however, the surgical procedure is determined by the intraoperative findings.

Operative Planning

Operative planning for resection of distal duodenal tumors is similar to that for a possible pancreaticoduodenectomy.

Operative Technique

The duodenum and the head of the pancreas are extensively mobilized by dividing the retroperitoneal attachments, and the ligament of Treitz is identified. The distal duodenum and the proximal jejunum are mobilized upward into the field by dissecting the ligament of Treitz away from their antimesenteric borders. Care must be taken not to injure the inferior mesenteric vein at this location.

A window is made in the mesentery, and the proximal jejunum is divided with a stapler. The mesentery of the proximal jejunum and the distal duodenum is serially divided between clamps and tied. After extensive mobilization and division of the mesentery to the left of the SMV and the SMA, the duodenum is passed under these vessels and brought out on the patient's right. If necessary for mobilization of the duodenum from the head of the pancreas, The mesentery may be further divided. The duodenum is then transected with a GIA stapler, and the specimen is removed.

A window is made in an avascular portion of the transverse mesocolon. The proximal jejunum is brought up to the duodenal wall, and a side-to-side duodenojejunostomy is fashioned in two layers with four continuous 3-0 polydioxanone sutures. Finally, the anastomosis is covered with omentum.

Troubleshooting

The location of the ampulla must be known at all times during the mobilization of the duodenum and its separation from the pancreat-

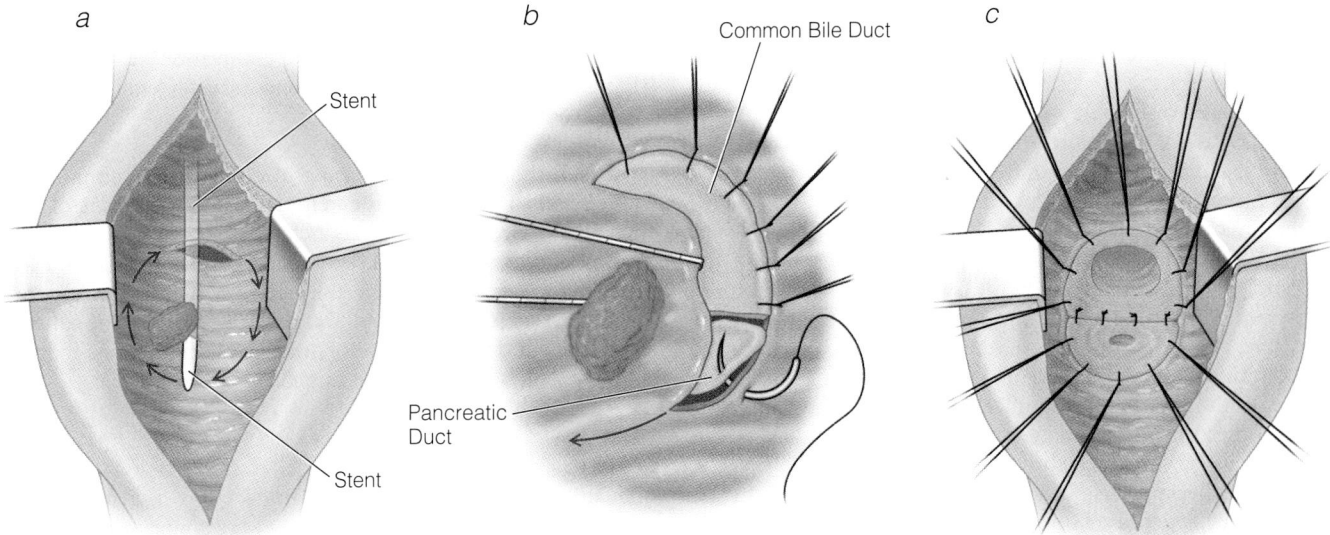

Figure 15 **Ampullectomy.** (*a*) **A transverse incision is made at the 11 to 12 o'clock position over the stent in the distal CBD.** (*b*) **As the tumor and the ampulla are pulled anteriorly and downward with a stay suture, the posterior duodenal wall and underlying distal CBD are cut in small increments and sutured together. This process continues circumferentially in a clockwise direction. At the 3 o'clock position, the pancreatic duct must be divided and sutured to the bile duct anteriorly and the duodenal wall laterally and inferiorly.** (*c*) **Once the specimen has been removed, the CBD and the pancreatic duct are reimplanted into the posterior duodenal wall.**

ic head. To this end, it is helpful to pass a Fogarty balloon catheter down the cystic duct, through the ampulla, and into the duodenum. If the jejunum cannot easily reach the duodenum through an opening in the transverse mesocolon, then it may be brought to it via a more direct route: the small bowel is elevated, and the jejunum is passed under the SMV and the SMA and placed in a manner similar to the placement of the resected duodenum.

AMPULLECTOMY

Preoperative Evaluation

Ampullectomy is indicated for benign tumors (e.g., lipomas, neurogenic tumors, lymphangiomas, leiomyofibromas, and adenomatous polyps) and for some small neuroendocrine tumors of the ampulla of Vater. The malignant potential of adenomatous polyps of the ampulla has been well documented and may be determined on the basis of the size and histologic features of the polyp. The risk of malignancy seems higher in villous than in tubular adenomas. With large (> 2 cm) lesions that show evidence of severe dysplasia, there is a significant risk that they harbor foci of adenocarcinoma; accordingly, caution is advised in attempting local resection in this setting. If there is evidence of overt adenocarcinoma, ampullectomy is not recommended, because the recurrence rates are too high. Biopsy specimens should be reviewed by an experienced pathologist before treatment is planned. In as many as 25% of cases, however, endoscopic biopsy may fail to establish the diagnosis; therefore, patterns of presentation, including evidence of weight loss or obstructive jaundice, the presence of a mass on CT, and suggestive findings from endoscopic retrograde cholangiopancreatography, should be taken into account in formulating treatment recommendations.

Preoperative investigations should be carried to establish the diagnosis and stage the tumor. Transabdominal ultrasonography and CT are usually the first examinations to be performed in the presence of altered liver function tests or obstructive jaundice. Dilatation of the CBD down to the ampullary region may be

observed, as may dilatation of the pancreatic duct on occasion. Visualization of the papilla and collection of biopsy specimens are done via endoscopy. Frequently, an endoscopic sphincterotomy must be performed to gain direct access to the tumor. Some endoscopists have found that EUS reliably and accurately detects malignancy in ampullary tumors; others have not. Given that EUS is user dependent, an experienced operator is essential.

The ampulla and the intraduodenal portion of the CBD should be easily identifiable at the time of surgery. Preoperative placement of a biliary stent may facilitate rapid identification of these structures; alternatively, intraoperative cannulation of the distal CBD from above via the cystic duct or from below with a probe through the ampulla may be performed. During operation, an undilated pancreatic duct may be difficult to locate. Administration of secretin can stimulate pancreatic duct flow and allow rapid identification of the duct; accordingly, secretin should be made available at the time of surgery.

Operative Planning

Operative planning for ampullectomy is similar to that for possible pancreaticoduodenectomy. Patients should be prepared for pancreaticoduodenectomy if ampullectomy proves inadequate.

Operative Technique

The operation involves complete resection of the ampulla of Vater, the distal CBD, and the pancreatic duct along with surrounding pancreatic tissue [*see Figure 15*].[23] The duodenum is mobilized by means of the Kocher maneuver, and a longitudinal duodenotomy is performed opposite the ampulla of Vater. The stent or catheter in the bile duct is palpated at the 11 o'clock position. A stay suture is placed on the ampullary lesion. At a point above the lesion, the posterior duodenal wall and the underlying lower CBD are opened transversely over the stent with the electrocautery.

A 4-0 absorbable suture is used to bring together the cut posterior duodenal wall and the new end of the CBD. The duodenal wall and the CBD are then further divided in small segments, progressing clockwise in a circular manner from 11 o'clock to 3 o'clock. The cut duodenal wall and CBD are serially approximated with interrupted sutures that are not tied. At the 3 o'clock position, the pancreatic duct is encountered, and this structure is carefully divided and sutured to the duodenal wall. As noted (see above), if the pancreatic duct is difficult to identify, secretin can be given to stimulate pancreatic fluid release. Once the pancreatic duct is divided, the inferior portion of the CBD and the superior portion of the pancreatic duct are sutured together to create a new common opening for these two structures. The clockwise division of the duodenal wall continues around to the starting point at the 11 o'clock position. During this part of the procedure, the inferior portion of the pancreatic duct is sutured to the duodenal wall after the ampulla is separated from its posterior attachments.

Once the specimen has been removed, additional sutures are placed to complete the reimplantation of the ducts into the duodenal wall. The sutures are then tied. The gallbladder is removed because of the risk of cholecystitis after ampullectomy as a result of chronic duodenobiliary reflux. If the CBD or the pancreatic duct is not dilated, a stent may be left in one or both ducts and remain in the duodenum after the completion of the procedure. Finally, the duodenum is closed longitudinally with a TA stapler.

Troubleshooting

Given the risk of troublesome bleeding during ampullectomy, meticulous dissection with careful hemostasis is crucial. Use of a needle-tip electrocautery may help minimize this risk. Upon removal of the lesion, frozen section analysis is indicated to rule out malignancy and to evaluate the margins. If the margins are not clear, further resection should be performed before the sutures are tied and cut. In the absence of ductal dilatation, loupe magnification facilitates precise reconstruction.

Outcome

In properly selected patients (i.e., those with premalignant and benign lesions of the ampulla), ampullectomy is generally safe. It is well suited for selected patients with significant comorbidities and for elderly patients. The hospital stay is significantly shorter and the return to baseline activity significantly quicker with ampullectomy than with pancreaticoduodenectomy.

References

1. Ng EK, Lam YH, Sung JJ, et al: Eradication of *Helicobacter pylori* prevents recurrence of ulcer after simple closure of duodenal ulcer perforation: randomized controlled trial. Ann Surg 231:153, 2000

2. MacDonald JS, Smalley SR, Benedetti J, et al: Chemoradiotherapy after surgery compared with surgery alone for adenocarcioma of the stomach or gastroesophageal junction. N Engl J Med 345:725, 2001

3. Lansdown M, Quirke P, Dixon MF, et al: High grade dysplasia of the gastric mucosa: a marker for gastric carcinoma. Gut 31:977, 1990

4. Inoue H, Fukami N, Yoshida T, et al: Endoscopic mucosal resection for esophageal and gastric cancers. J Gastroenterol Hepatol 17:382, 2002

5. Ohyama T, Kobayashi Y, Mori K, et al: Factors affecting complete resection of gastric tumors by the endoscopic resection procedure. J Gastroenterol Hepatol 17:844, 2002

6. Rosin D, Brasesco O, Rosenthal RJ: Laparoscopy for gastric tumors. Surg Oncol Clin North Am 10:511, 2001

7. Hochwald SN, Brennan MF, Klimstra DS, et al: Is lymphadenectomy necessary for early gastric cancer. Ann Surg Oncol 6:664, 1999

8. Nishi M, Ishihara S, Nakajima T, et al: Chronological changes of characteristics of early gastric cancer and therapy: experience in the Cancer Institute Hospital of Tokyo, 1950–1994. J Cancer Res Clin Oncol 121:535, 1995

9. Sano T, Kobori O, Muto T: Lymph node metastasis from early gastric cancer: endoscopic resection of tumour. Br J Surg 79:241, 1992

10. Suzuki S, Kosugi S, Kuwabara S, et al: Tumor recurrence in patients with early gastric cancer: a clinicopathologic evaluation. J Exp Clin Cancer Res 17:187, 1998

11. Bozzetti F, Marubini E, Bonfanti G, et al: Subtotal versus total gastrectomy for gastric cancer: five-year survival rates in a multicenter randomized Italian trial. Ann Surg 230:170, 1999

12. Bonenkamp JJ, Hermans J, Sasako M, et al: Extended lymph-node dissection for gastric cancer. N Engl J Med 340:908, 1999

13. Cuschieri A, Weeden S, Fielding J, et al: Patient survival after D1 and D2 resections for gastric cancer: long-term results of the MRC randomized surgical trial. Br J Cancer 79:1522, 1999

14. Hartgrink HH, van de Velde CJH, Dutch Gastric Cancer Group: Update of the Dutch D1 vs D2 gastric cancer trial (abstr). International Gastric Cancer Congress Abstract Book, 2001, p 665

15. Smith JW, Shiu MH, Kelsey L, et al: Morbidity of radical lymphadenectomy in the curative resection of gastric carcinoma. Arch Surg 126:1469, 1991

16. Smith JW, Brennan MF: Surgical treatment of gastric cancer: proximal, mid, and distal stomach. Surg Clin North Am 72:381, 1992

17. Cuschieri A, Fayers P, Fielding J, et al: Postoperative morbidity and mortality after D1 and D2 resections for gastric cancer: preliminary results of the MRC randomized controlled surgical trial. Lancet 347:995, 1996

18. Burke EC, Karpeh MS, Brennan MF: Laparoscopy in the management of gastric adenocarcinoma. Ann Surg 225:262, 1997

19. Hartgrink HH, Putter H, Klein Kranenbarg E, et al: Value of palliative resection in gastric cancer. Br J Surg 89:1438, 2002

20. Jivonen MK, Koskinen MO, Ikonen TJ, et al: Emptying of the jejunal pouch and roux-en-Y limb after total gastrectomy—a randomized, prospective study. Eur J Surg 165:742, 1999

21. Svedlund J, Sullivan M, Liedman B, et al: Long term consequences of gastrectomy for patients' quality of life: the impact of reconstructive techniques. Am J Gastroenterol 94:438, 1999

22. Shoup M, Brennan MF, Karpeh MS, et al: Port site metastasis after diagnostic laparoscopy for upper gastrointestinal tract malignancies: an uncommon entity. Ann Surg Oncol 9:632, 2002

23. Gertsch P, Blumgart LH: Transduodenal resection of the papilla of Vater. Surgery of the Liver and Biliary Tract, 3rd ed. Blumgart LH, Fong Y, Eds. WB Saunders Co, Edinburgh, 2000, p 1091

Acknowledgment

Figures 1 through 15   Tom Moore.

14 GASTRIC PROCEDURES FOR MORBID OBESITY

Eric J. DeMaria, M.D., F.A.C.S., and Harvey J. Sugerman, M.D., F.A.C.S.

It is clear that severe obesity is associated with a significant increase in morbidity[1] and a decreased life expectancy.[2] Morbid obesity has been shown to have a significant genetic basis.[3,4] To date, attempts to manage morbid obesity with medical weight reduction programs have met with an unacceptably high incidence of recidivism.[5] The approach that has had the greatest and longest-lasting success in achieving weight loss is bariatric surgery.

Choice between Gastric Bypass and Gastric Restriction

The gastric operations performed for morbid obesity include gastric bypass (GBP) procedures and gastric restrictive procedures (i.e., gastroplasty). Randomized, prospective trials have conclusively shown that GBP is as effective for weight control as jejunoileal (JI) bypass and results in significantly fewer complications.[6,7] JI bypass is associated with a substantial incidence of both early complications (e.g., acute cirrhosis, electrolyte imbalance, and fulminant diarrhea)[8] and late complications (e.g., cirrhosis, interstitial nephritis, arthritis, enteritis, nephrocalcinosis, and recurrent oxalate renal stones).[9] If evidence of cirrhosis, renal failure secondary to interstitial nephritis, or other complications mandates reversal of a JI bypass, the patient, if not extremely ill, should be converted to a GBP; otherwise, all the lost weight is sure to be regained, and the obesity-related comorbidity will return. Admittedly, however, many patients have done well after JI bypass and do not need to have the operation reversed.

Several randomized, prospective trials have found that horizontal gastroplasty yields poorer results than GBP.[10-12] Failure of horizontal gastroplasty has generally been attributed to technical causes, such as enlargement of the proximal pouch or the stoma or disruption of the staple line. Vertical banded gastroplasty (VBG) was developed by Mason in the hope that it would solve these technical problems and yield weight loss comparable to that seen after GBP without incurring the significant risk of iron, calcium, and vitamin B_{12} deficiencies associated with GBP. Although VBG appears to be an excellent procedure from a technical point of view,[13] one randomized, prospective trial found it to be significantly less effective than standard GBP.[14] In this trial, patients addicted to sweets lost much more weight after GBP than after VBG because they experienced symptoms of dumping syndrome when ingesting sweets. The failure rate was high after VBG because these patients experienced no difficulties when eating candy or drinking nondietetic sodas.

Two subsequent randomized, prospective trials confirmed the superiority of GBP.[15,16] Furthermore, weight loss after GBP appears to continue for as long as 10 years after operation: in the average patient, weight loss amounts to about two thirds of excess weight at 1 to 3 years after operation, three fifths at 5 years, and more than half in years 5 through 10.[17,18] It has been suggested that standard, or proximal, GBP will fail in 10% to 15% of patients because these patients will frequently nibble on high-fat snacks (e.g., corn chips, potato chips, and buttered popcorn). Such patients may have to be converted to a combined restrictive and malabsorptive procedure, such as partial biliopancreatic bypass (BPB).[19]

The original BPB involves hemigastrectomy and anastomosis of the distal 250 cm of intestine to the stomach; the bypassed small intestine is reanastomosed to the ileum 50 cm from the ileocecal valve. However, BPB has been associated with a high incidence of deficiencies of fat-soluble vitamins, hypocalcemia-induced osteoporosis, and protein-calorie malnutrition.[20] These nutritional deficiencies may be more common in the United States, where fat intake is high, than in many other countries. In Italy, for example, starch intake (as in pasta) probably outstrips fat intake; still, a number of Italian patients have had to be readmitted for parenteral nutrition and extension of the common absorptive intestinal tract because of refractory malnutrition. In some patients, it might be possible to convert a failed proximal GBP into a modified BPB with a 150 cm absorptive ileal limb; however, these patients also must be monitored carefully for deficiencies of fat-soluble vitamins, osteoporosis, and malnutrition.

Superobese patients, defined as those whose weight is 225% of ideal body weight or greater or whose body mass index (BMI) is 50 kg/m² or higher, will lose, on average, only about half of their excess weight, rather than two thirds, after standard GBP. In these patients, a 150 cm proximal Roux-en-Y procedure (so-called long-limb GBP [see Proximal Gastric Bypass, Operative Technique, *below*]) has been found to increase weight loss to two thirds of excess weight without causing an increase in nutritional complications.[21]

Preparation for Operation

Many surgeons, fearing increased perioperative morbidity and mortality, hesitate to operate on morbidly obese patients. It is true that such patients are at greater risk for complications and adverse results. Nevertheless, severely obese patients can undergo major abdominal surgery for weight loss with a remarkably low complication rate and a low mortality. These results, however, can only be achieved if a comprehensive program for preoperative and postoperative surgical care is rigorously planned and followed. The key elements of preparation for operation in the morbidly obese patient are discussed in greater detail elsewhere [see 3:3 *Morbid Obesity*].

Vertical Banded Gastroplasty

OPERATIVE TECHNIQUE

The first step in VBG is to make a circular stapled opening in the stomach 5 cm from the esophagogastric junction. A 90 mm

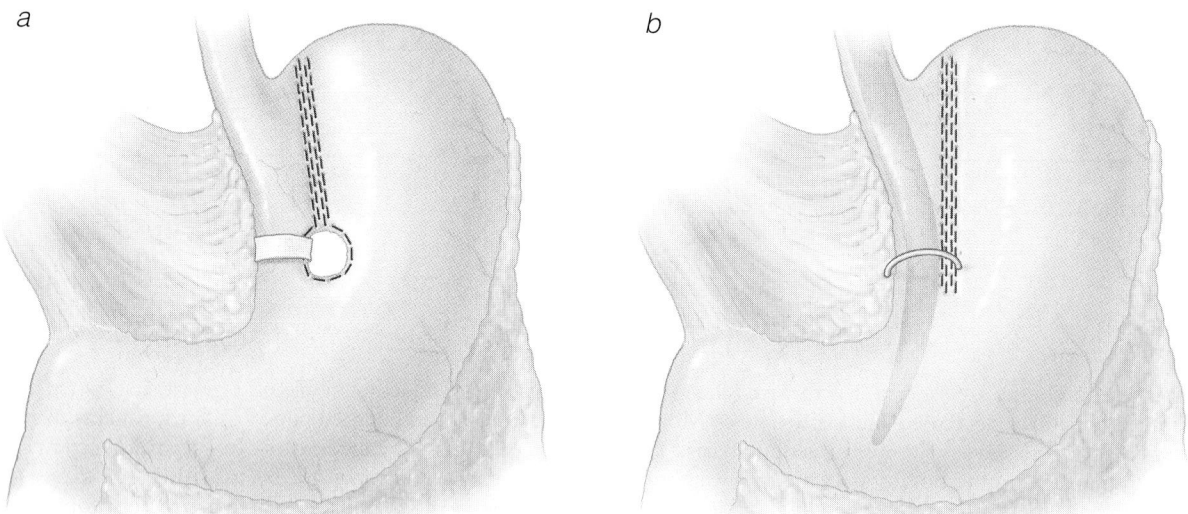

a *b*

Figure 1 **Vertical banded gastroplasty. Depicted are (*a*) standard VBG and (*b*) Silastic ring gastroplasty, a variant of VBG in which the stoma is reinforced with a Silastic tube.**

bariatric stapler with four parallel rows of staples is then applied once between this opening and the angle of His. (At this point, according to Mason, the originator of the procedure, the volume of the pouch should be measured by means of an Ewald tube placed by the anesthetist; ideally, pouch volume should be 15 ml.) Next, a strip of polypropylene mesh is wrapped around the gastrogastric outlet on the lesser curvature and sutured to itself—but not to the stomach—in such a way as to create an outlet with a circumference of 5 cm for the small upper gastric pouch [*see Figure 1a*]. Some surgeons have used a stomal outlet 4.5 cm in circumference, but this smaller outlet has not led to better weight loss; in fact, many patients with the 4.5 cm outlet exhibit maladaptive eating behavior, drinking high-calorie liquids because meat tends to get caught in the small stoma.

Silastic ring gastroplasty [*see Figure 1b*] is a variant of VBG that uses a vertical staple line and a stoma reinforced with Silastic tubing.

COMPLICATIONS

Complications of VBG include erosion of the polypropylene mesh used to restrict the gastroplasty stoma into the gastric lumen, enlargement of the pouch, stomal stenosis, reflux esophagitis, and mild vitamin deficiencies.[22] To date, mesh erosion has been infrequently observed after VBG. Pouch enlargement is fairly common with horizontal gastroplasty but is much less likely to occur with VBG, in which the vertical staple line is placed in the thicker, more muscular part of the stomach. In addition, stomal diameter remains fixed with the mesh band. If mesh erosion, pouch enlargement, stomal stenosis, disabling GI reflux, or recurrent vomiting occurs, it is probably best to convert the patient to GBP. In particular, patients with a Silastic ring VBG may exhibit intractable vomiting of solid foods with no evidence of mechanical obstruction. In our experience, conversion of these patients to GBP yields good results and eliminates the vomiting problem. Finally, vitamin deficiencies may be prevented by having VBG patients take a multivitamin daily for life.

Laparoscopic Adjustable Gastric Banding

Gastric banding is another form of gastroplasty, in which a

polypropylene or Silastic band is placed around the stomach just below the esophagogastric junction. In several series, gastric banding has had markedly variable results with respect to achievement of weight loss. Furthermore, it has been associated with slipping or kinking of the banded stoma, obstruction at the band, and intractable vomiting.

In the past few years, laparoscopic approaches to gastric banding have been developed and brought into use at a number of centers around the world. Laparoscopic adjustable gastric banding is potentially a significant advance over open gastric banding procedures, primarily because of the adjustability of the band. Open gastric banding procedures have used a variety of materials to constrict the gastric lumen and carry a recognized risk of postoperative nausea and vomiting that do not respond to any treatment short of reoperation. The adjustable gastric band (BioEnterics, Carpinteria, California) used in the laparoscopic procedure [*see Figure 2*] is a silicone device with an inflatable reservoir that can be inflated or deflated postoperatively through a subcutaneous port placed deep in the abdominal wall for percutaneous access. Saline is injected into or withdrawn from the reservoir through the port to adjust gastric luminal diameter, as measured by barium contrast evaluations. Thus, if intractable vomiting develops, saline can

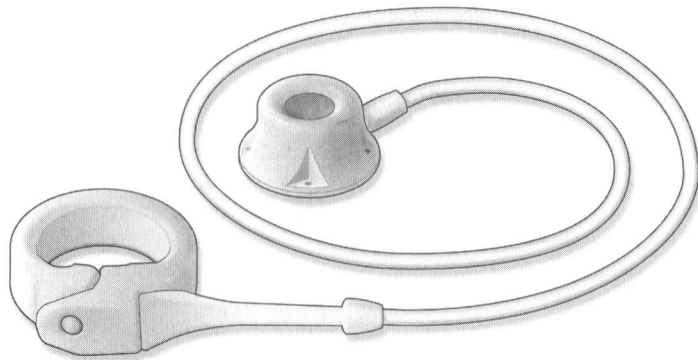

Figure 2 **Laparoscopic adjustable gastric banding. Shown is the adjustable gastric banding device used in the procedure.**

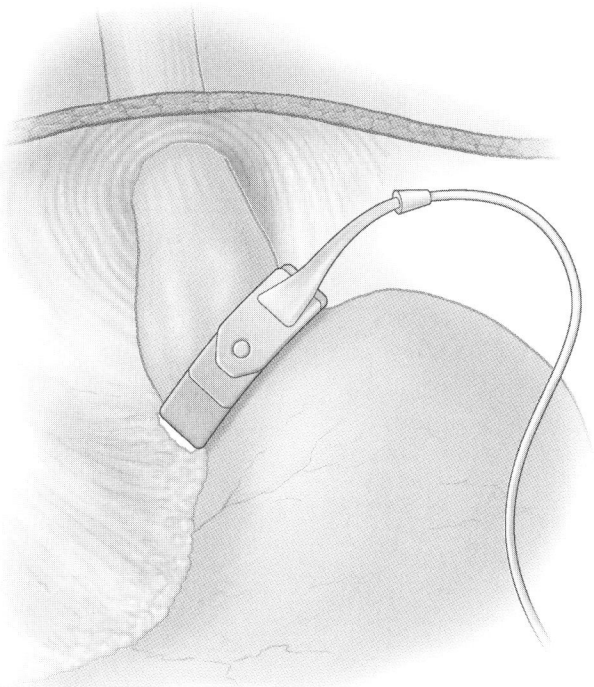

Figure 3 **Laparoscopic adjustable gastric banding. Once in the correct position on the proximal stomach, the adjustable band is locked into place.**

easily be removed from the band to alleviate the problem; similarly, if the patient fails to lose weight after operation, additional saline may be injected into the band to narrow the gastric lumen further.

In June 2001, use of the laparoscopically placed adjustable gastric band was approved by the Food and Drug Administration (FDA). Key data on safety and effectiveness were provided by a prospective, single-arm trial involving 299 patients at eight cen-

ters in the United States. In this study, patients who completed 36 months of follow-up achieved a mean excess weight loss of 36% and a mean overall weight loss of 18%. More than half (62%) of these patients lost more than 25% of their excess weight. Most patients (89%) experienced at least one adverse event, however, and 25% of patients required removal of the banding system.

OPERATIVE TECHNIQUE

Laparoscopic adjustable gastric banding is performed by using a six-port technique. Initial abdominal access is obtained via a supraumbilical trocar, and the remaining five ports are placed sequentially along the right and left costal margins. The liver is retracted via the right lateral port, and the proximal stomach is visualized via a laparoscope inserted through the subxiphoid port. A 20 ml balloon catheter is placed perorally into the proximal stomach to define an appropriately small pouch size. Dissection is then begun at the equator of the balloon with a hook electrocautery placed immediately alongside the gastric wall. The retrogastric tunnel should be above the posterior peritoneal reflection so that the free space of the lesser sac posterior to the stomach is not entered. Additional dissection is carried out laterally at the angle of His to open the peritoneum and start clearing a plane behind the proximal stomach. Once the plane is completely cleared from the lesser curve to the angle of His, a specially designed implement is inserted behind the stomach and used to grasp the tubing of the banding device and pull it around the stomach. The banding device is then locked into place at a spot overlying a pressure-sensitive location on the specially designed balloon catheter; this step allows one to confirm that the band is properly closed in the correct position and that the lumen is sufficiently tightened [*see Figure 3*]. The band tubing is then brought through the left midcla-vicular trocar port, which is placed via the left midclavicular line subcostal trocar incision and fixed to the abdominal wall fascia with sutures. The tubing is connected to the reservoir, which is filled with saline.

a

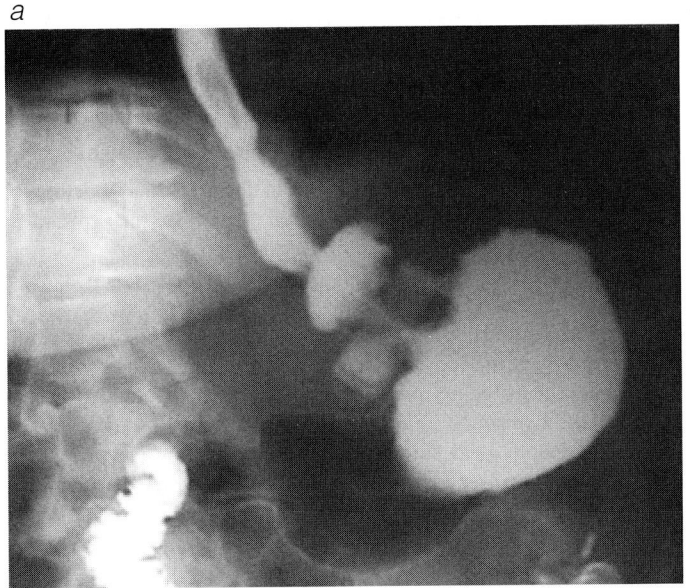

b

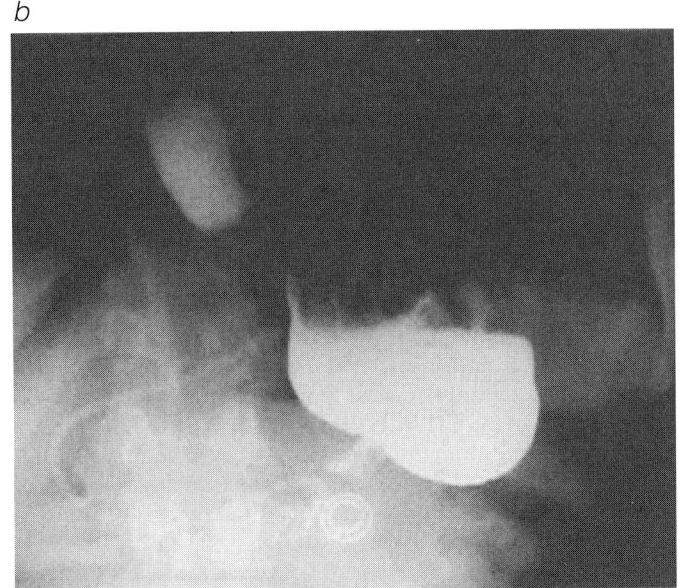

Figure 4 **Laparoscopic adjustable gastric banding. Contrast studies illustrate (*a*) a normally positioned laparoscopic adjustable gastric band and (*b*) a slipped band.**

TROUBLESHOOTING

It is essential to place the band properly during the initial procedure. Early results suggest that the proximal pouch must be very small to optimize weight loss. In addition, proper placement minimizes—though it does not eliminate—the risk of band slippage and the complications thereof.

It remains controversial whether posterior fixation of the band is necessary to prevent band slippage. Anterior fixation is routinely performed, with interrupted sutures of nonabsorbable material placed between the distal and the proximal stomach to allow tissue to be apposed over the band and held in place. Several techniques have been suggested for posterior fixation of the band, but they are more difficult than anterior fixation techniques. If, as recommended (see above), the band is tunneled above the peritoneal reflection posteriorly, posterior fixation may not be necessary.

Although laparoscopic adjustable gastric banding appears easier than many of the procedures done to treat obesity, there is a definite learning curve. A number of surgical misadventures have been reported, including gastric perforation, splenic injury, and malposition of the band.

COMPLICATIONS

Band slippage (usually posterior rather than anterior) may occur even after proper placement, resulting in intolerance of oral intake and vomiting. Such complaints are an indication for an upper GI series, which usually reveals dilatation of the proximal pouch and rotation of the band [see Figure 4]. Initial treatment consists of evacuating all saline from the band. Frequently, however, the proximal pouch does not return to its normal size, and symptoms recur or fail to resolve. Laparoscopic or open revision of the banding procedure is then required; if the patient also has not lost a sufficient amount of weight, conversion to GBP may be recommended. It is noteworthy that band erosion into the stomach, a not infrequent complication of the use of mesh in VBG or in the Angelchik prosthesis for gastroesophageal reflux treatment, has not been frequently reported to date. Longer follow-up will be necessary to evaluate the true extent of this risk.

As after any form of gastroplasty, the patient may fail to lose weight or may regain lost weight. Inappropriate eating behaviors (e.g., intake of high-calorie sweets) are the most likely cause. If obesity-related comorbid conditions persist, conversion to proximal GBP is appropriate.

OUTCOME EVALUATION

How successful laparoscopic adjustable gastric banding is at achieving weight loss over the long term remains unclear. The adjustability and reversibility of the operation, as well as the decreased disability that results, make it attractive to both patients and physicians. The procedure appears to avoid some of the major postoperative complications associated with open gastric bypass procedures (e.g., incisional hernia, marginal ulcer, and stomal stenosis. Band slippage remains a major postoperative concern, however, though the incidence of slippage does appear to decrease as one's experience with the procedure increases. More significant, there appears to be a high frequency of failed weight loss—as high as 15% to 20% of all patients undergoing the procedure and possibly even higher. European and Australian data confirm that there is a significant failure rate but also suggest that the remaining patients achieve a degree of weight loss approaching that seen with proximal GBP. Whether these reports will withstand the scrutiny of long-term follow-up remains to be seen.

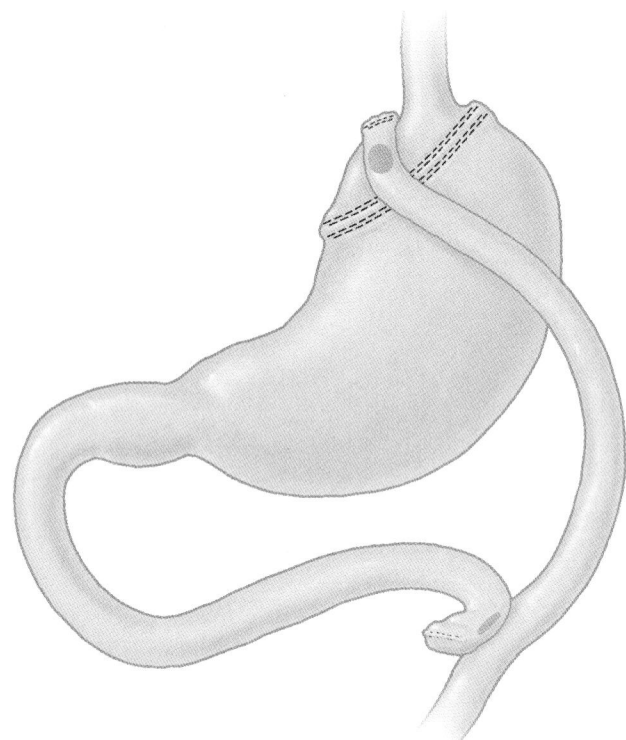

Figure 5 **Proximal gastric bypass. Depicted is the completed procedure.**

Now that the laparoscopic adjustable gastric band has received the approval of the FDA, this procedure may come to play an important role in the management of some morbidly obese patients in the United States.

Proximal Gastric Bypass

Proximal GBP results in greater weight loss than the gastric restrictive procedures (see above) and carries a lower incidence of weight regain; consequently we consider it the superior procedure. Our focus since the beginning of the 1990s has been on developing techniques for minimizing complications after proximal GBP. In our view, any surgeon currently performing this procedure ought to be able to achieve a gastrojejunal anastomotic leakage rate lower than 5%; many groups, in fact, report rates lower than 3%. In addition, we believe that other postoperative complications (e.g., acute dilatation of the excluded portion of the stomach) are usually preventable if strict attention is paid to mastering the technical aspects of the operation.

Compared with the version of GBP we perform at our institution, the original GBP created a much larger proximal gastric pouch and a much wider anastomotic opening, and it was often associated with inadequate weight loss. In our version of GBP, three superimposed 55 or 90 mm staple lines are placed across the proximal stomach in such a way as to create a gastric pouch no larger than 30 ml with a 45 cm Roux limb and a stoma no larger than 1 cm [see Figure 5].

OPERATIVE TECHNIQUE

Step 1: Initial Incision and Abdominal Exploration

Once the patient is anesthetized, the abdomen receives a thorough, careful cleansing with Betadine and is draped in a sterile fashion. An upper midline incision is made and extended through the fascia alongside the xiphoid process to facilitate cephalad exposure. We routinely carry the incision down to the supraumbilical area. The deep layer of subcutaneous fat can often be separated bluntly with aggressive lateral traction applied by the surgeon and the assistant, and the midline usually can then be identified for fascial incision. We use the electrocautery to enter the abdominal cavity and often encounter a thick layer of subfascial preperitoneal fat before entry into the peritoneal cavity. Abdominal exploration is undertaken in every patient, including examination of the liver for possible signs of liver disease. Other incidental findings may become apparent as well.

Troubleshooting   On a number of occasions, we have discovered unexpected significant liver disease at the time of operation. If the patient has cirrhosis without portal hypertension, one should perhaps proceed with bypass if the patient's comorbid conditions make it mandatory; liver transplantation carries increased risk in morbidly obese patients. The gallbladder should be palpated for gallstones, which, if found, we consider an indication for cholecystectomy at the time of the bypass procedure. If there are no visual or palpable gallbladder abnormalities, we use intraoperative ultrasonography to examine the gallbladder and perform cholecystectomy if small stones, sludge, or polyps are identified.

It is not unusual to discover previously unrecognized conditions during GBP, primarily because symptoms may not be obvious in morbidly obese patients and because their large size tends to make radiologic imaging difficult or even impossible. For example, intraoperative discovery of pelvic cysts and tumors is not uncommon in obese female patients. Such lesions may be excised during GBP; on occasion, if they appear benign and their location prevents safe excision, they may be managed with careful follow-up.

Step 2: Mobilization of the Esophagus

The bypass procedure itself is begun by mobilizing the distal esophagus and encircling it with a soft rubber drain 0.5 in. in diameter. The gastrohepatic omentum is bluntly entered at a point overlying the caudate lobe, with care taken to look for and avoid injury to an aberrant left hepatic artery. The phrenoesophageal ligament overlying the anterior and lateral distal esophagus is sharply incised to facilitate subsequent blunt mobilization of the distal esophagus. To prevent esophageal injury, the nasogastric tube is carefully palpated within the lumen of the esophagus during mobilization, and blunt dissection proceeds widely around this important landmark. Laterally, dissection must be at the level of the esophagus or higher.

Troubleshooting   If dissection is too low laterally, it may result in blunt injury to the short gastric vessels, bleeding, and the need for urgent splenectomy, which is no easy task in a morbidly obese patient. In addition, it may lead to creation of an inappropriately large pouch by keeping the surgeon from recognizing that some of the stomach is above the level at which the encircling rubber drain is placed.

Step 3: Division of the Mesentery and Dissection around the Stomach

Once the esophagus is mobilized, the assistant's left hand is placed through the gastrohepatic omental opening behind the stomach wall on the lesser curvature. The space between the first and second branches of the left gastric artery is then identified as a landmark for location of the gastric staple line, both to ensure that the pouch created is no larger than 30 ml and to prevent

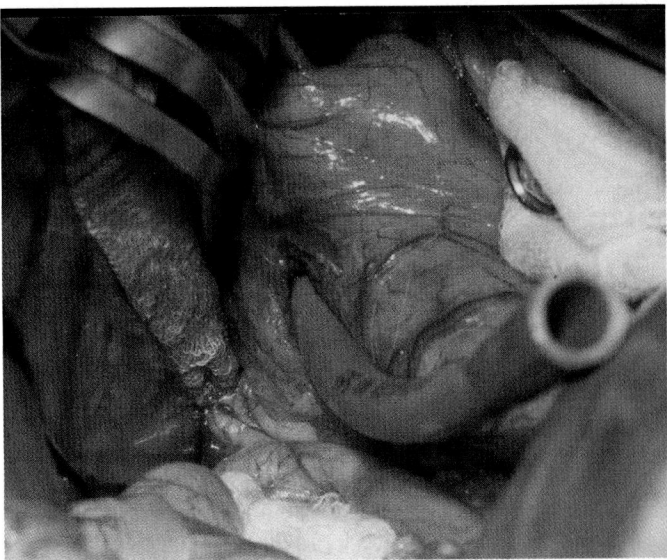

Figure 6   **Proximal gastric bypass. After dissection of the avascular tissue on the posterior gastric wall, a red rubber catheter is passed through the resulting space to encircle the stomach.**

injury to the left gastric artery, which usually runs cephalad to this location. With the surgeon's posterior finger pressing anteriorly to place tension on the tissue, a fine-tip right-angle clamp and the electrocautery pencil are used to divide the mesentery carefully at this level immediately alongside the stomach wall so as to create a mesenteric opening that will admit a large right-angle clamp. The avascular tissue on the posterior wall of the stomach is then bluntly dissected between the opening in the gastrohepatic omentum and the lateral angle of His, which is identified by the encircling rubber drain. The blunt tip of a large 28 French red rubber tube is placed behind the stomach in a medial-to-lateral direction along this dissected path to encircle the stomach [see Figure 6]. The open end of the red rubber tube is subsequently brought through the previously created mesenteric opening with a large right-angle clamp. The stomach is now ready for stapling, and the red rubber tube serves as a guide for introduction of the stapler. At this point, all intraluminal tubes and devices (e.g., the nasogastric tube and the esophageal stethoscope) are removed from the esophagus by the anesthetist.

Troubleshooting   When a tube is inadvertently stapled within the stomach, excising it from the staple line can become a technical nightmare. To remove the stapled tube, it is usually necessary to transect the stomach, thereby creating the potential for significant injury to the gastric tissue and possibly compromising the eventual anastomosis.

Step 4: Creation and Mobilization of the Roux Limb and Jejunojejunostomy

The ligament of Treitz is identified, and the jejunum is measured to a point 45 cm beyond the ligament, where the jejunum is divided with a stapler. An 8 to 12 cm segment of jejunum is resected at this point to create a larger mesenteric defect, which we believe facilitates mobilization of the limb to the proximal stomach. Mesenteric dissection is carried posteriorly in fat with the sequential application of clamps until further dissection appears either unnecessary for mobilization or unwise (i.e., likely to cause mesenteric vascular injury).

A side-to-side jejunojejunostomy is then created with a 60 mm linear stapler either 45 cm beyond the initial point of jejunal division, for standard proximal GBP, or 150 cm downstream, for the long-limb modification of the procedure used in superobese patients [see Choice between Gastric Bypass and Gastric Restriction, above]. It is important not to narrow the efferent lumen at the jejunojejunostomy site, particularly with the long-limb modification, in which the lumen at the distal end of the Roux limb may be quite small. The enterotomies made to allow placement of the stapler can usually be closed with a 55 mm stapler loaded with 3.5 mm staples; however, if stapling would cause undue narrowing of the lumen, the closures should be handsewn instead.

Troubleshooting We generally proceed to mobilization of the Roux limb before committing to stapling the stomach so that we can determine whether the limb can be extended to reach the proximal stomach without tension being placed on it. In those rare cases in which the mesentery is too foreshortened to permit the limb to reach the proximal stomach, we advocate changing the procedure to VBG rather than creating a gastrojejunal anastomosis under tension and incurring the increased risk of leakage.

Step 5: Gastric Stapling and Gastrojejunostomy

The Roux limb is brought through the mesentery of the transverse colon with blunt dissection and then brought up to the proximal stomach. The 55 or 90 mm stapler, loaded with 4.8 mm staples, is guided behind the stomach by inserting its open-mouthed end into the lumen of the previously positioned red rubber tube. Once it is determined that the staple line will reach completely across the stomach and that the stomach is not folded on itself, the stomach is stapled three times in such a way that the three staple lines are superimposed [see Figure 7].

A 1 cm anastomosis is created between the proximal stomach pouch and the Roux limb, with an outer layer composed of interrupted 3-0 silk sutures and an inner layer composed of a continuous absorbable 2-0 polyglycolic acid (Dexon) suture. When the posterior aspect of the anastomosis is complete, a 30 French dilator is placed with the patient under anesthesia and is guided through the anastomosis by the surgeon to ensure that the stoma has the appropriate diameter [see Figure 8]. The anterior aspect of the anastomosis is then completed.

Troubleshooting A significant concern for many bariatric surgeons has been a high incidence of staple line disruption causing failed weight loss or weight regain; in one series, the incidence of such disruption was 35%. To minimize this risk, some surgeons advocate transecting the stomach. This is done by inserting two parallel TA-90 staplers and cutting between them with a scalpel after the staplers are fired. Other surgeons, however, prefer to oversew the staple line. By using the technique of three superimposed staple lines, we have decreased the incidence of staple line disruption to less than 2%; consequently, we believe that gastric transection is unnecessary on a routine basis (though occasionally useful in selected cases) and may increase the risk of the procedure. Another advantage of gastric transection besides reduction of staple line disruption is that it allows the Roux limb to be brought up to the gastric pouch via a retrocolic and retrogastric tract, which is significantly shorter and places less tension on the limb. This approach is particularly helpful in severely obese patients with a fatty and foreshortened mesentery, in whom it is difficult to free the Roux limb sufficiently to reach the proximal stomach without tension. The possibility that gastric transection may prove helpful in a specific patient is another reason why it is advisable to delay stapling the stomach until the Roux limb is mobilized.

Step 6: Assessment of the Anastomosis

When the entire anastomosis is complete, the dilator is removed and the tip of an 18 French nasogastric tube is advanced by the anesthetist and carefully guided through the anastomosis by the surgeon. The Roux limb is occluded with the assistant's left hand or with an atraumatic intestinal clamp, and the anesthetist injects a series of 10 ml aliquots of methylene blue dye through the nasogastric tube to determine whether the anastomosis is leaking. A total of 30 to 60 ml of methylene blue must usually be injected; lesser amounts will not stress the suture line enough to constitute an adequate test.

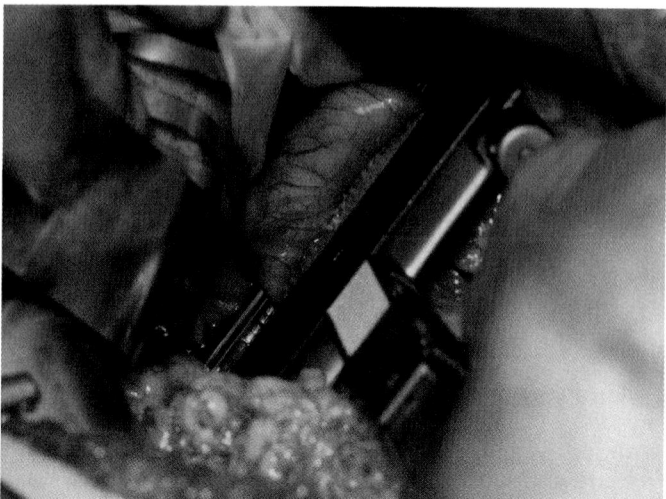

Figure 7 Proximal gastric bypass. The stomach is stapled to create the small proximal pouch. The stapler is fired three times to create three superimposed staple lines, thereby decreasing the risk of staple line disruption.

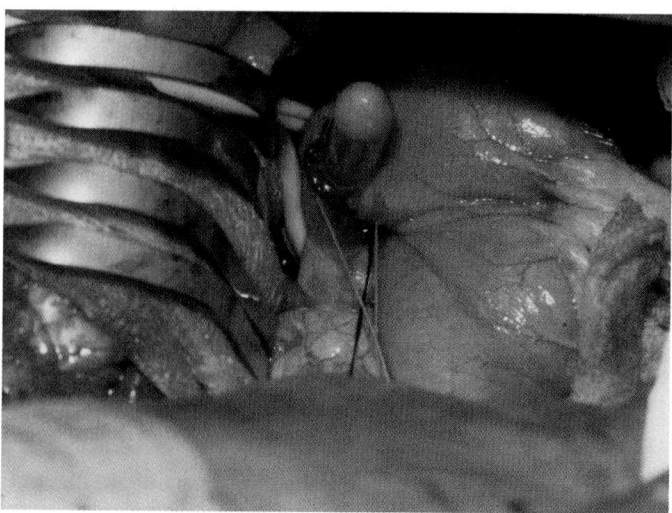

Figure 8 Proximal gastric bypass. When the posterior aspect of the gastrojejunal anastomosis has been completed, a 30 French dilator is placed through the stoma to confirm that the opening is correctly sized.

Troubleshooting When an intraoperative leak is identified, we oversew the area of leakage with silk sutures until injection of additional methylene blue dye via the nasogastric tube yields no further leakage. The most difficult area to repair is the posterior suture line, which is quite close to the gastric staple line. Posterior leaks are usually repaired by reinforcing the posterior suture line with additional sutures between the excluded stomach and the jejunal limb; often, we oversew the entire posterior suture line. In addition, a viable pedicle of omentum may be mobilized and placed around the anastomosis for additional reinforcement. Closed suction drains may also be placed in this area, both to detect possible postoperative leakage and to control a postoperative fistula.

Finally, a gastrostomy tube is placed in the excluded portion of the stomach. This measure provides postoperative decompression, which should prevent the development of undue tension on the Roux limb as a result of gastric distention, and establishes a route for enteral feeding if a fistula develops. Fortunately, such fistulas are rare. When they do occur, they often heal if (1) they are well drained, (2) there is no distal obstruction or local abscess, and (3) the patient is receiving nutritional support with no oral intake. A gastrostomy tube should also be placed in the distal gastric pouch when extensive adhesions from a previous procedure or a difficult gastric reoperation prevents postoperative dilatation of the pouch.

Step 7: Closure

When the absence of leakage is confirmed or when any leaks identified have been controlled, the tip of the nasogastric tube can be positioned further down in the Roux limb and left to continuous suction overnight. All mesenteric defects—at the jejunojejunostomy, at the mesocolon, and behind the Roux limb—are then closed to prevent a Petersen hernia. The abdominal fascia is reapproximated with a continuous No. 2 nonabsorbable suture, subcutaneous tissues are irrigated with a crystalloid solution containing 1% neomycin, and the skin is closed with skin staples. No subcutaneous sutures or drains are used in routine cases.

COMPLICATIONS

Proximal GBP is associated with a significant incidence of stomal stenosis and with marginal ulcer.[23] The former responds to endoscopic stomal dilatation, and the latter usually responds to H_2 receptor blocker or proton pump inhibitor therapy.

Iron, vitamin B_{12}, and folic acid deficiencies may occur but can usually be corrected with oral supplements[22]; accordingly, GBP patients, like VBG patients, should be advised to take a multivitamin daily for life. Compared with VBG, GBP results in significantly lower serum hemoglobin and iron concentrations. This is primarily a problem in menstruating women. All menstruating women who have undergone GBP should be treated prophylactically with supplemental oral ferrous sulfate, 325 mg/day. As many as six iron tablets a day may be required if menstrual bleeding is heavy. On occasion, intramuscular iron injections or, rarely, hysterectomy may be necessary. The risk of vitamin B_{12} deficiency is higher after GBP than after VBG, but this condition can be prevented with supplemental oral vitamin B_{12}, 500 mg/day. A few patients may require (or prefer) monthly B_{12} injections, which they can learn to administer themselves.

Concerns have been expressed that GBP can lead to other divalent cation deficiencies. We have not encountered zinc deficiencies 5 to 9 years after GBP. We have, however, observed calcium deficiencies leading to osteoporosis, which may take many years to become manifest and may not be biochemically evident because of normal serum calcium levels. We therefore recommend that all our GBP patients take oral calcium supplements. Magnesium deficiencies should be treated with $MgSO_4$ supplementation.

Nutritional deficiencies do not appear to be a greater problem with long-limb GBP than with standard proximal GBP. We do monitor patients for possible malabsorption of the fat-soluble vitamins A, D, and E after long-limb GBP.

BPB may be associated with all of the complications seen after GBP. In addition, patients who undergo BPB may experience diarrhea, severe protein malnutrition (manifested as hypoalbuminemia), and deficiencies of vitamins A (manifested as severe night blindness), D (manifested as severe osteoporosis), and E.[20] Hypoalbuminemia may respond to oral pancreatic enzymes but often must be treated with total parenteral nutrition. In some patients, it may prove necessary to lengthen the absorptive intestinal tract from 50 cm to 200 cm.

OUTCOME EVALUATION

In our series of 672 open proximal GBP procedures,[17] we reported a 1.2% incidence of anastomotic leak with peritonitis, a 4.4% incidence of severe wound infection (defined as infection serious enough to delay hospital discharge), an 11.4% incidence of minor wound infections and seromas (which were easily treated at home), a less than 1% incidence of gastric staple line disruption with the use of three superimposed applications of a 90 mm linear stapler, a 15% incidence of stomal stenosis, a 13% incidence of marginal ulcer, a 16.9% incidence of incisional hernia, and a 10% incidence of cholecystitis necessitating cholecystectomy. Gallstones developed in 32% of the GBP patients who had a normal intraoperative gallbladder ultrasonogram within 6 months of surgery, and sludge was observed in another 10%. In a multicenter randomized prospective trial,[24] we and others were able to reduce the incidence of gallstones within 6 months of GBP from 32% to 2% by giving patients ursodeoxycholic acid, 300 mg twice daily. Gallstone formation is very rare beyond 6 months. The operative mortality in our series was less than 1%. Patients with respiratory insufficiency of obesity had a 2.2% operative mortality, whereas those without pulmonary dysfunction had a 0.4% mortality.

Neither the data from our randomized, prospective trial nor the data from selective studies support the contention that VBG is safer than GBP. Although GBP includes one more anastomosis than VBG, complications such as leaks and peritonitis occur with both operations. A common criticism of GBP is that it is difficult to evaluate the distal gastric pouch and duodenum after the operation. Such evaluation, however, can be done in 75% of patients by means of retrograde passage of an endoscope into the duodenum and the stomach and in others by means of percutaneous distal distention gastrography (DeMaria EJ, Sugerman HJ, unpublished data, 2000). To our knowledge, bleeding from either the distal gastric pouch or a duodenal ulcer has occurred in only one of our more than 1,200 GBP patients. In one patient, a perforation of the proximal gastric pouch developed after administration of high-dose nonsteroidal anti-inflammatory medication. Gastric mucosal metaplasia of the bypassed portion of the stomach was noted in 5% of patients after retrograde endoscopy, a finding that has raised concerns regarding the risk of carcinoma arising at that location. However, tens of thousands of these procedures have been performed since 1967, and only one case of cancer in the bypassed stomach has been reported to date. We have also had one such case but have not published it.

Laparoscopic Gastric Bypass

Laparoscopic gastric bypass is a relatively new alternative to standard open GBP. One would anticipate that laparoscopic GBP would yield much the same weight loss results as open

GBP but with less pain, reduced disability, and a shorter hospitalization period. In addition, one would anticipate a decrease in major wound infections as well as fewer incisional hernias. On the face of it, it seems likely that the laparoscopic procedure, though more expensive, would be cost-effective, but proving it is so will probably require an analysis of long-term follow-up that documents decreased subsequent hospitalizations for wound infections, hernia repairs, and complications of intra-abdominal adhesions (e.g., bowel obstruction), given that early results cannot demonstrate a dramatic reduction in the length of hospitalization after the procedure. If the additional benefit of reduced disability-related absence from work is realized, this would help reduce overall costs as well.

TOTAL INTRACORPOREAL LAPAROSCOPIC GASTRIC BYPASS

Laparoscopic GBP poses significant technical challenges, even for surgeons with advanced laparoscopic skills. Most of the variations seen at different institutions are related to creation of the gastrojejunal anastomosis, with most groups favoring the use of a circular rather than a linear stapler. The anvil of the circular stapler may be placed within the proximal gastric pouch either by means of flexible upper GI endoscopy, through an approach similar to the snare-and-wire technique used for placement of a percutaneous endoscopic gastrostomy (PEG) tube, or by means of a gastrotomy of the pouch for intra-abdominal anvil placement followed by staple closure of the gastrotomy. Peroral placement of the stapler's anvil can be problematic: even the small 21 French anvil is hard to pass through the proximal esophagus in some patients. Nevertheless, we will describe this approach in some detail because it seems to be favored by most surgeons at present and it is easier to perform.

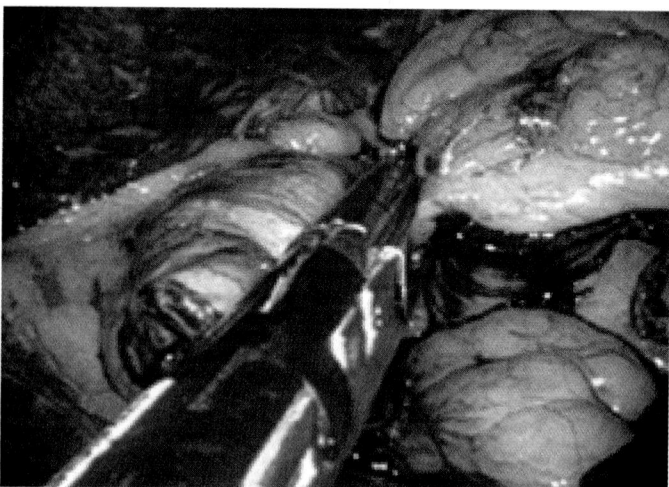

Figure 10 **Laparoscopic gastric bypass: total intracorporeal approach. Much as in open GBP, a linear endoscopic GIA stapler is fired three times to transect the stomach and create the gastric pouch.**

Operative Technique

Step 1: initial access and trocar placement Initial access to the abdomen is obtained through a left subcostal incision with either a Veress needle or a commercially available device that allows direct vision through the scope while a 12 mm trocar is inserted. Gas is then insufflated into the abdomen to a pressure of 15 mm Hg; on occasion, a pressure of 18 mm Hg may be necessary. Additional trocars are placed in specific locations [*see Figure 9*]. To retract the liver, we employ a metal Nathanson liver retraction device anchored to the bed, which is inserted after a 5 mm sharp trocar is used to enter the abdominal cavity and peritoneum and removed. If the left lateral segment of the liver is very large (as in patients with steatosis), additional liver retraction may be necessary.

The falciform ligament is then dissected from the anterior abdominal wall with an ultrasonic scalpel. This dissection allows the trocar incision to be placed quite high in the epigastrium, which facilitates proximal gastric exposure. A 12 mm port placed in the right paramedian position near the costal margin serves as the surgeon's primary operative port; two lateral subcostal 5 mm ports allow both surgeon and assistant to employ two-handed techniques for the entire procedure.

Step 2: dissection around the stomach and creation of the gastric pouch Dissection is performed along the lesser curvature of the stomach between the neurovascular bundle and the gastric wall; the ultrasonic scalpel is the best instrument for this purpose. Dissection posterior to the stomach is performed in the avascular free plane of the lesser sac. Additional dissection along the lesser curvature is not recommended, because it may increase the devascularization of the pouch. Further dissection is done with the ultrasonic scalpel at the angle of His to create a connection with the posterior gastric space. A linear endoscopic gastrointestinal anastomosis (GIA) stapler loaded with 3.5 mm staples in 60 mm cartridges is then used to transect the stomach and create the proximal gastric pouch; three firings are usually necessary [*see Figure 10*].

Step 3 (circular stapling): placement of the stapler in the gastric pouch As noted (see above), surgeons use several different techniques to complete the gastrojejunal anastomosis.

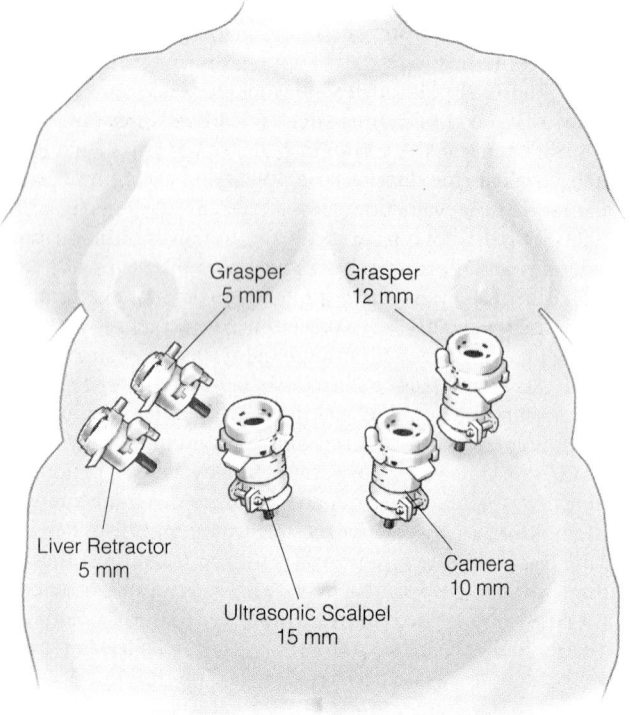

Figure 9 **Laparoscopic gastric bypass: total intracorporeal approach. Shown are the trocar incision sites for laparoscopic GBP.**

Initially, we employed the technique reported in Wittgrove's original description of the procedure,[25] which involved passing the anvil of a circular stapler down the patient's esophagus in a manner resembling placement of a PEG tube. With this approach, the next step in the procedure is to have an assistant perform flexible upper GI endoscopy of the gastric pouch. The pouch wall is transilluminated by the endoscope light, and a site is chosen for the gastrojejunostomy. The endoscopist then places an endoscopic snare, which can be seen pressing against the tissue of the pouch wall. A small opening is made in the pouch with the electrocautery scissors so that the snare can be pushed through the gastric wall at this location. The snare is then used to grasp a wire placed through a needle across the abdominal wall in the left abdomen, and snare and wire are withdrawn through the mouth along with the scope.

The anvil of the stapler is attached to the end of the wire that was drawn through the mouth, and the surgeon pulls on the other end of the wire to deliver the anvil through the mouth, down the esophagus, and into the gastric pouch, where it can be visualized. The electrocautery attached to the scissors is used to enlarge the opening in the gastric wall slightly, and the stem of the stapler is then brought through the gastrotomy. To prevent anastomotic leakage after stapling, the gastrotomy should be no larger than the diameter of the stem; if it is too large, it can be closed around the stem by placing one or two simple sutures.

Troubleshooting. Difficulty in passing the anvil perorally may arise at the level where the trachea separates from the esophagus in the deep pharynx. This difficulty can usually be overcome either by having the endoscopist perform a jaw-thrust maneuver or by placing a large laryngoscope blade deep in the pharynx to make the anvil visible in the proximal esophagus and then nudging the anvil forward with either the tip of the blade or a McGill forceps. Deflating the endotracheal tube balloon may also help. Occasionally, we use the large esophageal dilator to place pressure on the tip of the anvil. Given the potential for esophageal injury if the anvil will not advance, it is important not to apply excessive force. We have seen a case in which the anvil became lodged in the proximal esophagus beyond the laryngoscopic view and the long suture holding it broke; retrograde passage of an esophageal dilator was required to dislodge the anvil. Other surgeons who use wire to draw the anvil down the esophagus have identified nontransmural esophageal injuries on postoperative contrast studies or have seen subcutaneous emphysema in the neck after operation.

Step 3 (linear stapling)   Currently, we prefer a technique in which a linear stapler, rather than a circular one, is used to create the gastrojejunal anastomosis. In this approach, therefore, we proceed directly from creation of the gastric pouch to creation of the Roux limb for subsequent anastomosis to the pouch.

Step 4: creation and mobilization of the Roux limb and jejunojejunostomy   In most reports of laparoscopic GBP, regardless of how the gastrojejunostomy is done, the approach to creating the Roux limb is essentially the same. The patient is placed in a supine position, and graspers are used to bring the omentum upward into the upper abdomen so that the transverse colon and the underlying mesocolon are exposed. Graspers are then placed on the transverse mesocolon and used to elevate it anteriorly so that the ligament of Treitz is exposed. The position of the ligament of Treitz is confirmed by careful manipulation and verification that the bowel is attached to the retroperitoneum at

this location; this may be a more difficult task in patients who have previously undergone abdominal procedures.

With the help of a measuring instrument inserted into the abdomen, the small bowel is measured to a point 30 to 40 cm from the ligament of Treitz, where it is transected with the endoscopic GIA stapler, loaded with 2.5 mm staples. A 0.5 in. Penrose rubber drain is sutured to the cut end of the Roux limb so that it is not confused with the other cut end of the bowel. The Roux limb is then measured to a length of 45 to 60 cm. (As in open GBP, the Roux limb may have to be significantly longer—up to 150 cm—if the long-limb modification is being performed.) The afferent side of the previously transected small bowel is then attached with a simple absorbable suture to the proposed jejunojejunostomy site on the Roux limb. Intracorporeal suturing is facilitated by using an automatic suturing device. Positioning is important: the afferent limb should be kept to the patient's left, with the Roux limb more medial.

A small enterotomy is then made in preparation for passage of the linear stapler, loaded with 2.5 mm staples in a 60 mm cartridge, into the bowel. Two sutures are placed, one anterior to the enterotomy and the other posterior, to help manipulate the bowel onto the stapler. The stapler is then fired, creating a 60 mm side-to-side anastomosis. A third suture is placed at the midpoint of the enterotomy, and all three sutures are grasped to facilitate closure of the enterotomy with another application of the linear stapler. Once completed, the anastomosis is inspected both for integrity and for possible narrowing. At this point, anterior traction is applied to the three sutures to facilitate placement of interrupted or continuous sutures to close the mesenteric defect.

Next, a retrocolic, retrogastric tunnel (which we consider clearly superior to an antecolic approach) is created so that the Roux limb can be advanced to the proximal stomach for anastomosis. The ligament of Treitz is once again identified by lifting the transverse mesocolon anteriorly, and a spot 1 to 2 cm anterior and to the left of the ligament is chosen as the starting point for dissection with the ultrasonic scalpel. The middle colic artery should be visualized medial to this point of entry into the mesocolon. The goal of the dissection is to identify the posterior wall of the stomach, which may be difficult in patients who are extremely obese, have a fatty, foreshortened mesocolon, or have previously undergone abdominal surgery. Once the stomach is visible, it is grasped and elevated through the mesocolic window, and the end of the Penrose drain is grasped and brought through the mesocolic defect into the lesser sac. When the Penrose is in place in the lesser sac, the omentum is pulled down from the epigastrium to allow visualization of the drain, now posterior to the divided distal stomach. The Penrose drain is grasped, and the patient is placed back into a steep reverse Trendelenburg position. Traction is applied to the Penrose drain to deliver the cut end of the Roux limb up into the lesser sac for anastomosis.

Troubleshooting. Some surgeons place the Roux limb in the antecolic position and divide the fatty omentum with the ultrasonic scalpel to decrease the tension on the limb. This technique appears to be inferior to the retrocolic approach, in that it does not decrease the tension on the limb and the anastomosis sufficiently and it necessitates more aggressive transection of the small bowel mesentery to achieve adequate mobilization. For these very reasons, many bariatric surgeons do not favor the antecolic approach during open GBP; thus, to use this approach during laparoscopic GBP violates a basic principle of modern surgery, according to which the application of minimally invasive techniques to an operation must not compromise the quality of the procedure. There are also some surgeons who prefer to create a loop gastrojejunostomy, thus avoiding the technical challenges of creating a Roux limb laparoscopically. This approach was abandoned years ago in open GBP because of postoperative bile reflux and an increased severity of complications resulting from high output of digestive juices when a leak occurs at the gastrojejunal anastomosis; it should be abandoned in laparoscopic GBP as well. We firmly believe that the practice of using such suboptimal methods for the purpose of performing this complex operation more expeditiously is poorly conceived and is to be condemned.

Step 5 (circular stapling): gastrojejunostomy In the circular stapling technique, the stapled end of the Roux limb is open to permit introduction of the stapler. The 12 mm trocar site in the left upper quadrant is dilated so that the circular stapler can be inserted through the abdominal wall without the need for a trocar; lubrication is helpful for this step. The stapler then cannulates the Roux limb. This step is facilitated by holding the open mouth of the limb in three locations, with one of the three holds involving traction on the Penrose drain previously sutured to the bowel. The stapler is advanced 3 to 4 cm down the limb, and the spike on the stapler is brought through the antimesenteric portion of the bowel by unscrewing the stapler under direct vision. Once the stapler has been opened completely, it is laparoscopically joined to the anvil and the gastric pouch, then closed and fired.

Once fired, the stapler is removed from the abdominal wall, and a balloon trocar device is used to close the dilated abdominal wall opening. A single firing of the endoscopic GIA stapler, loaded with 2.5 mm staples, is often all that is required to reclose the cut end of the small bowel. Interrupted or continuous absorbable sutures are then placed around the stapled anastomosis for added security.

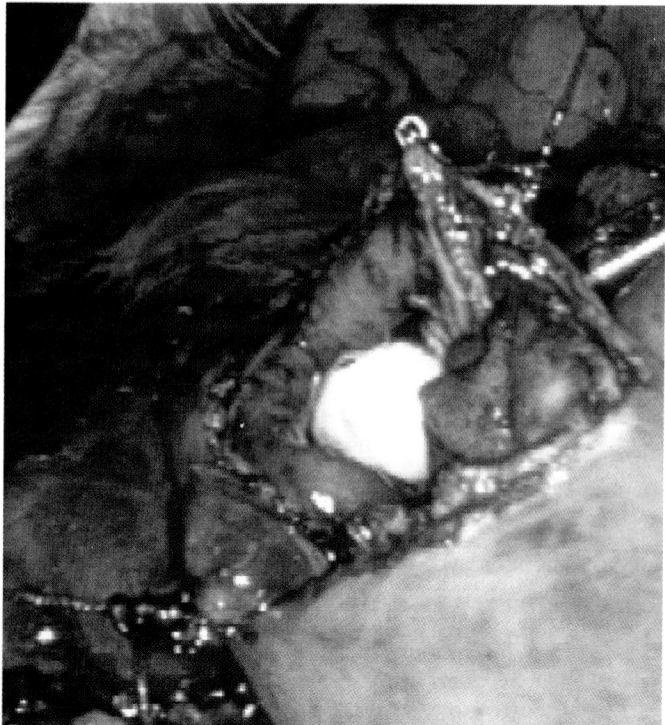

Figure 11 **Laparoscopic gastric bypass: total intracorporeal approach. A 30 French dilator is placed into the proximal gastric pouch before closure of the gastrojejunal anastomosis with the endoscopic GIA stapler.**

Step 5 (linear stapling): gastrojejunostomy For the linear stapling technique that we currently prefer, it is not necessary to dilate a trocar site, which appears to increase postoperative pain. Two holding sutures are placed to secure the antimesenteric Roux limb to the posterior gastric pouch toward the lesser curvature. Between the two sutures, an enterotomy and a gastrotomy are performed that are large enough to admit the jaws of the endoscopic GIA stapler, which is loaded with 3.5 mm staples in a 30 mm cartridge for a side-to-side anastomosis [*see Figure 11*]. Applying traction to the sutures facilitates placement of the stapler into the lumen of the bowel and the stomach by means of the same techniques employed in creation of the jejunojejunostomy. A 30 French dilator is then passed into the pouch by the anesthetist and guided through the anastomosis by the surgeon under direct vision to maintain the appropriate stomal diameter (10 to 12 mm) during closure of the open end. Placement of a third suture between the first two holding sutures allows anterior traction and facilitates amputation of the tissue to close the openings. The stapler, loaded with 3.5 mm staples in a 60 mm cartridge, should be placed so as to amputate a significant amount of tissue during this closure; the esophageal dilator preserves the stomal diameter.

We have found that using the linear GIA stapler simplifies the procedure, decreases operative time, and eliminates the concerns about injury to the body of the esophagus that arise with passage of the circular stapler.

Step 6: assessment of the anastomosis In every case, regardless of which stapling technique is employed, flexible upper GI endoscopy is performed to assess the anastomosis. The Roux limb is occluded with an intestinal clamp to prevent excessive bowel and distal gastric dilatation. The patient is placed in the supine position, and the area around the anastomosis is irrigated with saline; the presence of air bubbles, easily detectable in the irrigant, indicates that the anastomosis is leaking. In most cases, we are able to distend the pouch and the Roux limb tightly, and we reinforce even tiny air leaks with additional sutures. The anastomosis and the staple lines are visualized, and the endoscope is navigated through the anastomosis into the Roux limb whenever possible. After adequate visualization and testing, the gas is suctioned from the intestine, the Roux limb is unclamped, and the endoscope is removed.

Step 7: closure Finally, a 10 mm closed suction drainage tube is placed adjacent to the anastomosis to permit monitoring for postoperative leaks. This drain is removed after the patient begins oral intake if an upper GI series reveals no postoperative leakage [*see Figure 12*]. The liver retractor is removed under direct vision to ensure that no bleeding occurs. Trocar sites 10 mm in diameter or larger are closed by using a needle suture passer to place 0 absorbable sutures under direct endoscopic visualization. Skin wounds are closed with skin staples or absorbable subcutaneous sutures.

HAND-ASSISTED LAPAROSCOPIC GASTRIC BYPASS

Because total intracorporeal laparoscopic GBP is such a challenging technical adventure, we initially developed a technique for a hand-assisted version of the procedure based on work done by others.[26] We viewed this technique as a bridge to the total intracorporeal approach, in that it enabled us to learn the technical aspects of a difficult, highly advanced laparoscopic procedure while enjoying the security provided by the presence of an intraabdominal hand for palpation and manipulation during the procedure. This added security is the major advantage of the hand-

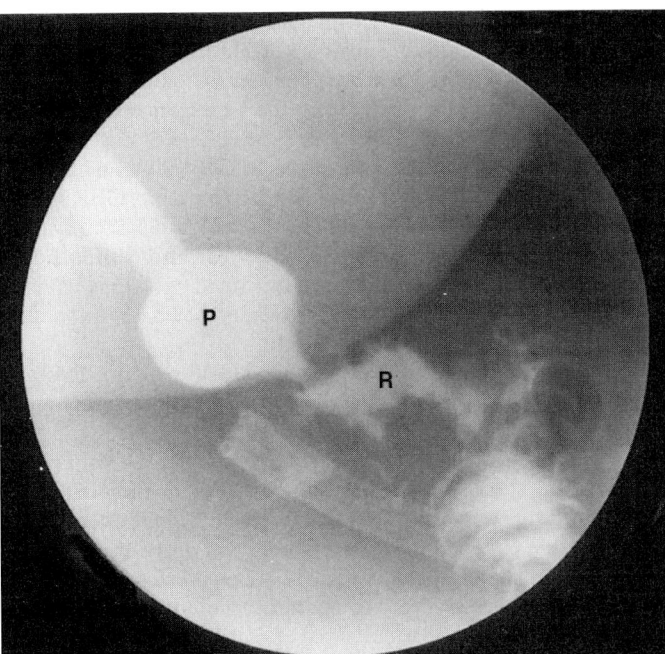

Figure 12 **Laparoscopic gastric bypass: total intracorporeal approach. Flexible upper GI endoscopy is performed to assess the completed anastomosis.**

assisted approach. The major disadvantage is the potential for complications at the incision used for manual access. The complications seen at this site are reminiscent of those seen after open GBP, including major wound infection, dehiscence, and hernia formation. In our series of hand-assisted laparoscopic GBP procedures, we have seen one major wound infection in the hand incision and one instance of postoperative fascial dehiscence.

Operative Technique

Step 1: initial access and placement of the hand-assisted device A left subcostal incision is made, a Veress needle is inserted, and gas is insufflated into the abdomen to a pressure of 15 mm Hg. A periumbilical location for a midline incision is then identified. This incision will allow insertion of the hand at a later point in the procedure; thus, its length in centimeters should roughly correspond to the surgeon's glove size. To provide the assisting hand with access to the abdomen, we use a device called the Pneumo Sleeve (Dexterity Surgical, Inc., Roswell, Georgia). This device includes a ring system at one end. Once pneumoperitoneum is obtained, the ring is glued to the skin of the abdominal wall in such a way that the proposed line of incision is in the middle of the ring.

Step 2: creation and mobilization of the Roux limb, jejunojejunostomy, and creation of the gastric pouch With the ring of the Pneumo Sleeve secured to the skin, the small midline incision is opened and extended directly through the midline fascia. The pneumoperitoneum is released as this incision is opened, and the ligament of Treitz is identified by palpation. Retractors are placed into the incision, and the Roux limb is constructed with an open surgical technique. The small bowel is mobilized into the wound to the extent possible and is transected 20 to 30 cm from the ligament of Treitz. A side-to-side stapled jejunojejunostomy is then constructed with an open technique. In our experience, using an endoscopic GIA stapler rather than a

traditional surgical stapler for this step is both technically superior and more cost-efficient.

Once the anastomosis is created and the enterotomy is closed, the mesenteric defect is sutured in the usual fashion with an open technique. A Penrose drain is sutured to the cut end of the Roux limb. The surgeon, standing on the patient's left side, attaches the Pneumo Sleeve to the nondominant hand and places this into the abdominal cavity. Pneumoperitoneum is reestablished. The ligament of Treitz can then be manually identified, and a blunt mesocolic dissection into the retrogastric space can be performed. This manipulation can be visualized through a laparoscope with the placement of additional trocars, including two in the right subcostal area (as in total intracorporeal laparoscopic GBP); we usually place the laparoscope through a left subcostal trocar site. The Penrose drain is then grasped with the surgeon's fingers and advanced through the mesocolic tunnel into the retrogastric space. The hand is then brought anterior to the stomach, and the patient is placed in a steep reverse Trendelenburg position.

The Nathanson liver retractor is inserted through a subxiphoid puncture as described earlier [*see* Total Intracorporeal Laparoscopic Gastric Bypass, *above*] and positioned to allow visualization of the esophagogastric junction and proximal stomach. The gastrohepatic ligament is bluntly opened, and the surgeon's hand is extended behind the stomach into the lesser sac to retrieve the Penrose drain. The hand is then used to facilitate the mesenteric dissection on the lesser curvature of the stomach 2 to 3 cm from the esophagogastric junction. An endoscopic GIA stapler loaded with 3.5 mm staples in 60 mm cartridges is fired three times to create the gastric pouch (as in total intracorporeal laparoscopic GBP).

Step 3: gastrojejunostomy Again, the gastrojejunal anastomosis can be created with either a circular stapler or a linear stapler [*see* Total Intracorporeal Laparoscopic Gastric Bypass, *above*]. The Roux limb is manipulated into view with the surgeon's hand. In the circular stapling technique, the stapler is placed into the Roux limb with the help of the intra-abdominal hand so that it can be opened, penetrating the antimesenteric portion of the bowel, and joined to the anvil in the gastric pouch. The hand also facilitates removal of the circular stapler, which is occasionally difficult.

Step 4: assessment of the anastomosis The open end of the Roux limb is then stapled closed, and flexible upper GI endoscopy is performed as in total intracorporeal laparoscopic GBP, with the hand (rather than an intestinal clamp) occluding the limb to allow insufflation and testing of the anastomosis. Additional absorbable sutures can be placed around the anastomosis for added security; we use an automatic suturing device such as the Endostitch (United States Surgical, Norwalk, Connecticut) for this purpose. If the sutures are left long, the surgeon can actually tie knots intra-abdominally, using the sleeved hand in a one-handed technique.

Step 5: closure Except for the hand incision, closure is accomplished in the same way as for total laparoscopic GBP. Although the hand incision is small, it may be difficult to close in severely obese patients who have a thick layer of subcutaneous fat. We use a continuous fascial closure with a heavy No. 1 or 2 nonabsorbable suture.

POSTOPERATIVE CARE

The basic principles of care after bariatric surgery [*see* Postoperative Management, *below*] generally apply to laparoscopic cases as well, but with some differences. Unlike patients who have undergone open GBP, those who have undergone laparoscopic GBP do not have a nasogastric tube left in place. In addition, a contrast study of both the pouch and the anastomosis is ordered on postoperative day 1. A water-soluble contrast agent is initially used for this study, followed by barium if no leak or abnormality is identified. The patient may then begin to drink small amounts of liquids and may advance to a pureed diet with no sugar or concentrated sweets as soon as he or she can tolerate it. Discharge usually takes place 2 or 3 days after operation.

COMPLICATIONS

The complications observed to date after laparoscopic GBP include the usual problems that occur in some patients after open GBP, including marginal ulcer and stenosis at the gastrojejunal anastomosis necessitating dilatation. We have seen one gastrogastric fistula leading to a treatment-resistant marginal ulcer. The major advantage of laparoscopic GBP over open GBP is likely to be reduced wound complications (e.g., major wound infection and incisional hernia). We have seen several relatively minor trocar site infections but none carrying the long wound care disability characteristic of a major wound infection after open GBP. In our experience to date, weight loss with laparoscopic GBP is identical to that with open GBP.

Postoperative Management

For optimal results after bariatric surgery, postoperative management must be as well planned as preoperative preparation. The basic principles of postoperative care, including intubation, ambulation, feeding, and monitoring for complications (e.g., anastomotic leakage, abdominal catastrophe, acute gastric distention, and internal hernia), are discussed more fully elsewhere [see *3:3 Morbid Obesity*].

FAILED WEIGHT LOSS AND WEIGHT REGAIN

A postoperative problem that deserves special mention is the risk of failed weight loss or weight regain. This is one of the greatest problems associated with bariatric surgery and may arise after any gastric procedure for morbid obesity. Approximately 20% of VBG patients have difficulty with solid foods and come to exhibit a maladaptive eating behavior involving frequent ingestion of high-calorie liquid carbohydrates; in about 10% of VBG patients, the procedure fails for this reason. We have converted 53 VBG patients to GBP.[27] After VBG, the average loss of excess weight was $31 \pm 5\%$; 2 years after conversion to GBP, it was $67 \pm 2\%$, a value virtually identical to that in our primary GBP group. Thirteen patients became sweets eaters and had lost only $15 \pm 5\%$ of their excess weight more than 1 year after VBG, though there were no radiographically demonstrated problems with the procedure; 1 year after conversion to GBP, they had lost an average of $78 \pm 11\%$ of their excess weight.

Inadequate weight loss is also seen in GBP patients. In some, stomal dilatation eventually develops after the procedure; however, no correlation between stomal size and weight loss has been demonstrated for GBP patients, and reoperation to make the pouch or the stoma smaller has not yielded any benefit when the initial procedure has failed. In our experience, failure of GBP is generally due either to the loss or absence of dumping syndrome symptoms in a small percentage of patients, leading to resumption of high-calorie sweets ingestion, or, more often, to frequent ingestion of high-fat junk foods (e.g., potato or corn chips, microwave popcorn, or peanut butter crackers) that crumble easily and empty quickly from the pouch, thereby keeping the patient from feeling full. Repeated dietary counseling over a period of years is required to educate patients to eat low-calorie, high-fiber foods (e.g., raw carrots, broccoli, cauliflower, apples, and oranges) that will stay in the small gastric pouch longer and provide a sensation of early satiety.

Our philosophy is to make clear to patients, well in advance of the operation, that bariatric surgery is designed to help them help themselves. Obesity is easily beaten by surgical treatment, but to maintain the victory, patients must continue to make good food choices and exercise appropriately for the rest of their lives. In our experience, patients who begin to eat more than 1,100 kcal/day will begin to gain weight; even if weight gain is only 0.5 lb/month, this amounts to 6 lb/year, or 60 lb in 10 years. We strongly believe, therefore, that bariatric surgical patients need lifelong nutritional counseling to optimize the results of surgical management of morbid obesity.

References

1. Van Itallie TB: Obesity: adverse effects on health and longevity. Am J Clin Nutr 32:2723, 1979

2. Drenick EJ, Bale GS, Seltzer F, et al: Excessive mortality and causes of death in morbidly obese men. JAMA 243:443, 1980

3. Stunkard AJ, Foch TT, Hrubec Z: A twin study of human obesity. JAMA 256:51, 1986

4. Stunkard AJ, Sorensen TIA, Hanis C, et al: An adoption study of human obesity. N Engl J Med 314:193, 1986

5. Johnson D, Drenick EJ: Therapeutic fasting in morbid obesity: long-term follow-up. Arch Intern Med 137:1381, 1977

6. Griffen WO, Young VL, Stevenson CC: A prospective comparison of gastric and jejunoileal bypass procedures for morbid obesity. Ann Surg 186:500, 1977

7. Buckwalter JA: A prospective comparison of the jejunoileal and gastric bypass operations for morbid obesity. World J Surg 1:757, 1977

8. Halverson JD, Wise L, Wazna MF, et al: Jejunoileal bypass for morbid obesity: a critical appraisal. Am J Med 64:461, 1978

9. Hocking MP, Duerson MC, O'Leary PJ, et al: Jejunoileal bypass for morbid obesity: late follow-up in 100 cases. N Engl J Med 308:995, 1983

10. Pories WJ, Flicinger EG, Meelheim D, et al: The effectiveness of gastric bypass over gastric partition in morbid obesity: consequences of distal gastric and duodenal exclusion. Ann Surg 196:389, 1982

11. Lechner GW, Elliott DW: Comparison of weight loss after gastric exclusion and partitioning. Arch Surg 118:685, 1983

12. Linner JH: Comparative effectiveness of gastric bypass and gastroplasty: a clinical study. Arch Surg 117:695, 1982

13. Mason EE: Vertical banded gastroplasty for obesity. Arch Surg 117:701, 1982

14. Sugerman HJ, Starkey JV, Birkenhauer R: A randomized prospective trial of gastric bypass versus vertical banded gastroplasty for morbid obesity and their effects on sweets versus non-sweets eaters. Ann Surg 205:613, 1987

15. Hall JC, Watts JM, O'Brien PE, et al: Gastric surgery for morbid obesity: the Adelaide Study. Ann Surg 211:419, 1990

16. MacLean LD, Rhode BM, Sampalis J, et al: Results of the surgical treatment of obesity. Am J Surg 165:155, 1993

17. Sugerman HJ, Kellum JM, Engle KM, et al: Gastric bypass for treating severe obesity. Am J Clin Nutr 55(suppl 2):560S, 1992

18. Pories WJ, MacDonald KG Jr, Morgan EJ, et al: Surgical treatment of obesity and its effect on diabetes: 10-year follow-up. Am J Clin Nutr 55(suppl 2):582S, 1992

19. Scopinaro N, Bachi V: Evoluzione del bypass biliopancreatico parziale per l'obesita. Minerva Chir 39:1299, 1984

20. Liszka TG, Sugerman HJ, Kellum JM, et al: Risk/benefit considerations of distal gastric bypass. Int J

Obes 12(suppl A):604, 1988

21. Brolin RE, Kenler HA, Gorman JH, et al: Long-limb gastric bypass in the superobese: a prospective randomized study. Ann Surg 215:387, 1992

22. MacLean LD, Rhode BM, Shizgal HM: Nutrition following gastric operations for morbid obesity. Ann Surg 198:347, 1983

23. Sanyal AJ, Sugerman HJ, Kellum JM, et al: Stomal complications of gastric bypass: incidence and outcome of therapy. Am J Gastroenterol 87:1165, 1992

24. Sugerman HJ, Brewer WH, Shiffman ML, et al. A multi-center, placebo-controlled, randomized, double-blind, prospective trial of prophylactic ursodiol for the prevention of gallstone formation following gastric bypass-induced rapid weight loss. Am J Surg 169:91, 1995

25. Wittgrove AC, Clark GW, Schubert KR: Laparoscopic gastric bypass: Roux-en-Y technique and results in 75 patients with 3-30 month follow-up. Obes Surg 6:500, 1996

26. Naihoth T, Gagner M: Laparoscopically assisted gastric bypass surgery using Dexterity Pneumo Sleeve. Surg Endosc 11:830, 1997

27. Sugerman HJ, Kellum JM, DeMaria EJ, et al: Conversion of failed or complicated vertical banded gastroplasty to gastric bypass in morbid obesity. Am J Surg 171:263, 1996

Acknowledgment

Figures 1, 2, 3, 5, and 9   Tom Moore.

15 LAPAROSCOPIC CHOLECYSTECTOMY

Gerald M. Fried, M.D., F.A.C.S., Liane S. Feldman, M.D., F.A.C.S., and Dennis R. Klassen, M.D.

Cholecystectomy is the treatment of choice for symptomatic gallstones because it removes the organ that contributes to both the formation of gallstones and the complications ensuing from them. The morbidity associated with cholecystectomy is attributable to injury to the abdominal wall in the process of gaining access to the gallbladder (i.e., the incision in the abdominal wall and its closure) or to inadvertent injury to surrounding structures during dissection of the gallbladder. Efforts to diminish the morbidity of open cholecystectomy have led to the development of laparoscopic cholecystectomy, made possible by modern optics and video technology.

Erich Mühe performed the first laparoscopic cholecystectomy in Germany in 1985; by 1992, 90% of cholecystectomies in the United States were being performed laparoscopically. Compared with open cholecystectomy, the laparoscopic approach has dramatically reduced hospital stay, postoperative pain, and convalescent time. However, rapid adoption of laparoscopic cholecystectomy as the so-called gold standard for treatment of symptomatic gallstone disease was associated with complications, including an increased incidence of major bile duct injuries.

Since the early 1990s, considerable advances have been made in instrumentation and equipment, and a great deal of experience with laparoscopic cholecystectomy has been amassed worldwide. Of particular significance is the miniaturization of optics and instruments, the aim of which is to reduce the morbidity of the procedure by making possible ever smaller incisions. With proper patient selection and preparation, laparoscopic cholecystectomy is being safely performed on an outpatient basis in many centers.

The primary goal of laparoscopic cholecystectomy is removal of the gallbladder with minimal risk of injury to the bile ducts and surrounding structures. Our approach is designed to maximize the safety of both routine and complicated laparoscopic cholecystectomies. In what follows, we describe our approach and discuss current indications and techniques for imaging and exploring the common bile duct (CBD).

Preoperative Evaluation

To plan the surgical procedure, assess the likelihood of conversion to open cholecystectomy, and determine which patients are at high risk for CBD stones, the surgeon must obtain certain data preoperatively. Useful information can be obtained from the patient's history, from imaging studies, and from laboratory tests.

PREOPERATIVE DATA

History and Physical Examination

A good medical history provides information about associated medical problems that may affect the patient's tolerance of pneumoperitoneum. Patients with cardiorespiratory disease may have difficulty with the effects of CO_2 pneumoperitoneum on cardiac output, lung inflation pressure, acid-base balance, and the ability of the lungs to eliminate CO_2. Most bleeding disorders can also be identified through the history. A disease-specific history is important in identifying patients in whom previous episodes of acute cholecystitis may make laparoscopic cholecystectomy more difficult, as well as those at increased risk for choledocholithiasis (e.g., those who have had jaundice, pancreatitis, or cholangitis).

Physical examination identifies patients whose body habitus is likely to make laparoscopic cholecystectomy difficult and is helpful for determining optimal trocar placement. Abdominal examination also reveals any scars, stomas, or hernias that are likely to necessitate the use of special techniques for trocar insertion.

Imaging Studies

Ultrasonography is highly operator dependent, but in capable hands, it can provide useful information. It is the best test for diagnosing cholelithiasis, and it can usually determine the size and number of stones. Large stones indicate that a larger incision in the skin and the fascia will be necessary to retrieve the gallbladder. Multiple small stones suggest that the patient is more likely to require operative cholangiography (if a policy of selective cholangiography is practiced) [see Operative Technique, Step 5, *below*]. A shrunken gallbladder, a thickened gallbladder wall, and pericholecystic fluid on ultrasonographic examination are significant predictors of conversion to open cholecystectomy. The presence of a dilated CBD or CBD stones preoperatively is predictive of choledocholithiasis. Other intra-abdominal pathologic conditions, either related to or separate from the hepatic-biliary-pancreatic system, may influence operative planning.

Preoperative imaging studies of the CBD may allow the surgeon to identify patients with CBD stones before operation. Such imaging may involve endoscopic retrograde cholangiopancreatography (ERCP) [see 3:8 Gastrointestinal Endoscopy], magnetic resonance cholangiopancreatography (MRCP) [see Figure 1], or endoscopic ultrasonography (EUS). These imaging modalities also provide an anatomic map of the extrahepatic biliary tree, identifying unusual anatomy preoperatively and helping the surgeon plan a safe operation. Endoscopic sphincterotomy (ES) is performed during ERCP if stones are identified in the CBD. MRCP has an advantage over ERCP and EUS in that it is noninvasive and does not make use of injected iodinated contrast solutions. Most surgeons would probably recommend that preoperative cholangiography be performed selectively in patients with clinical or biochemical features associated with a high risk of choledocholithiasis. The specific modality used in such a case varies with the technology and expertise available locally.

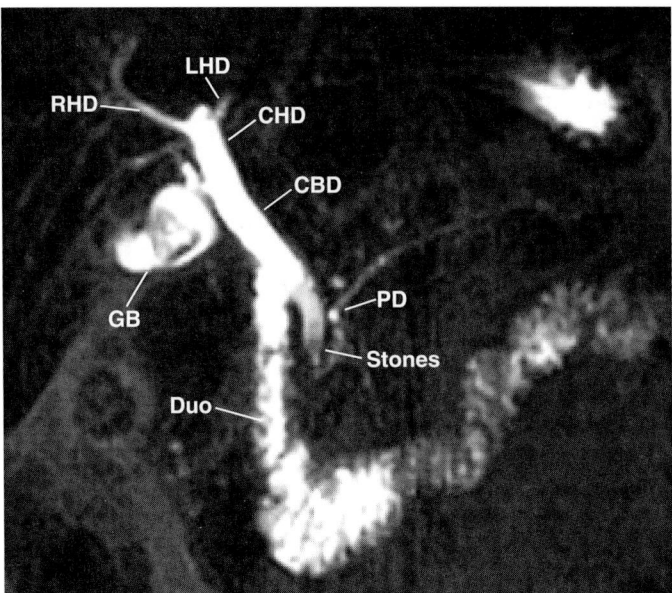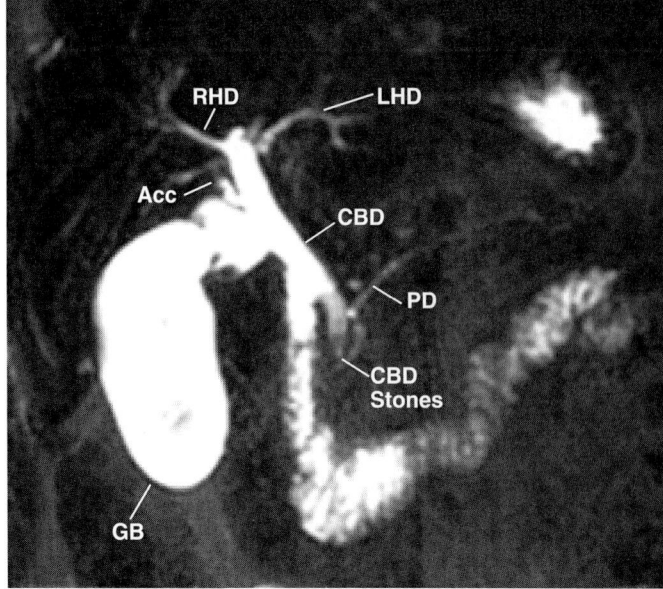

Figure 1 **Laparoscopic cholecystectomy. Preoperative MRCP alerts the surgeon to abnormal anatomy and the presence of stones in the distal CBD. (GB—gallbladder, containing stones; RHD—right hepatic duct; LHD—left hepatic duct; CHD—common hepatic duct; Acc—accessory duct entering common hepatic duct near neck of gall-bladder; PD—pancreatic duct; Duo—duodenum)**

Laboratory Tests

Preoperative blood tests are important for evaluation of liver function and for detection of unsuspected abnormalities of renal function, electrolyte balance, or coagulation. Abnormal liver function test results may reflect choledocholithiasis or primary hepatic dysfunction.

SELECTION OF PATIENTS

Patients Eligible for Outpatient Cholecystectomy

Patients in good general health who have a reasonable amount of support from family or friends and who do not live too far away from adequate medical facilities are eligible for outpatient cholecystectomy, especially if they are at low risk for conversion to laparotomy [*see* Special Problems, Conversion to Laparotomy, *below*]. These patients can generally be discharged home from the recovery room 6 to 12 hours after surgery, provided that the operation went smoothly, their vital signs are stable, they are able to void, they can manage at least a liquid diet without vomiting, and their pain can be controlled with oral analgesics.

Technically Challenging Patients

Before performing laparoscopic cholecystectomy, the surgeon can predict which patients are likely to be technically challenging. These include patients who have a particularly unsuitable body habitus, those who are at high risk for multiple and dense peritoneal adhesions, and those who are likely to have distorted anatomy in the region of the gallbladder.

Morbidly obese patients present specific difficulties [*see* Operative Technique, Step 1, Special Considerations in Obese Patients, *below*]. Small, muscular patients have a noncompliant abdominal wall, resulting in a small working space in the abdomen and necessitating high inflation pressures to obtain reasonable exposure.

Patients with a history of multiple abdominal operations, especially in the upper abdomen, and those who have a history of peritonitis are likely to pose difficulties because of peritoneal adhesions. These adhesions make access to the abdomen more risky and exposure of the gallbladder more difficult.

Patients who have undergone gastroduodenal surgery, those who have any history of acute cholecystitis, those who have a long history of recurrent gallbladder attacks, and those who have recently had severe pancreatitis are particularly difficult candidates for laparoscopic cholecystectomy. These patients may have dense adhesions in the region of the gallbladder, the anatomy may be distorted, the cystic duct may be foreshortened, and the CBD may be very closely and densely adherent to the gallbladder. Such patients are a challenge to the most experienced laparoscopic surgeon. When such problems are encountered, conversion to open cholecystectomy should be considered early in the operation.

Predictors of Choledocholithiasis

CBD stones may be discovered preoperatively, intraoperatively, or postoperatively. The surgeon's goal is to clear the ducts but to use the smallest number of procedures with the lowest risk of morbidity. Thus, before elective laparoscopic cholecystectomy, it is desirable to classify patients into one of three groups: high risk (those who have clinical jaundice or cholangitis, visible choledocholithiasis, or a dilated CBD on ultrasonography), moderate risk (those who have hyperbilirubinemia, elevated alkaline phosphatase levels, pancreatitis, or multiple small gallstones), and low risk.

In our institution, where MRCP and EUS are available and reliable and where ERCP achieves stone clearance rates higher than 90%, we recommend the following approach: (1) preoperative ERCP and sphincterotomy (if required) for high-risk patients and (2) MRCP, EUS, or intraoperative fluoroscopic cholangiography for moderate-risk patients. Patients at low risk for CBD stones do not routinely undergo cholangiography [*see Figure 2*]. Laparoscopic CBD exploration and postoperative ERCP appear to be equally effective in clearing stones from the CBD.

Ultimately, surgeons and institutions must establish a reasonable approach to choledocholithiasis that takes into account the expertise and equipment locally available.

Contraindications

There are few absolute contraindications to laparoscopic cholecystectomy. Certainly, no patient who poses an unacceptable risk for open cholecystectomy should be considered for laparoscopic cholecystectomy, because it is always possible that conversion will become necessary. Of the relative contraindications, surgical inexperience is the most important.

Neither ascites nor hernia is a contraindication to laparoscopic cholecystectomy. Ascites can be drained and the gallbladder visualized. Large hernias may present a problem, however, because with insufflation, the gas preferentially fills the hernia. Patients with large inguinal hernias may require an external support to minimize this problem and the discomfort related to pneumoscrotum. Patients with umbilical hernias can have their hernias repaired while they are undergoing laparoscopic cholecystectomy. For such patients, the initial trocar should be placed by open insertion according to the Hasson technique [*see* Operative Technique, Step 1, *below*], with care taken to avoid injury to the contents of the hernia. The sutures required to close the hernia defect can be placed before insertion of the initial trocar. A similar technique can be applied to patients with incisional hernias, although for large incisional hernias, laparoscopic cholecystectomy may have no advantages over open cholecystectomy if a large incision and dissection of adhesions are required. Patients with stomas may also undergo laparoscopic cholecystectomy, provided that the appropriate steps are taken to prevent injury to the bowel during placement of trocars and division of adhesions.

Patients with cirrhosis or portal hypertension are at high risk for morbidity and mortality with open cholecystectomy. If absolutely necessary, laparoscopic cholecystectomy may be attempted by an experienced surgeon. The risk of bleeding can be minimized by rigorous preoperative preparation, meticulous

dissection with the help of magnification available through the laparoscope, and use of the electrocautery.

Patients with bleeding diatheses, such as hemophilia, von Willebrand disease, and thrombocytopenia, may undergo laparoscopic cholecystectomy. They require appropriate preoperative and postoperative care and monitoring, and a hematologist should be consulted.

Questions have been raised about whether laparoscopic cholecystectomy should be performed in pregnant patients; it has been argued that the increased intra-abdominal pressure may pose a risk to the fetus. Because of the enlarged uterus, open insertion of the initial trocar is mandatory, and the positioning of other trocars may have to be modified according to the position of the uterus. Inflation pressures should be kept as low as possible, and prophylaxis of deep vein thrombosis (DVT) is recommended. Despite these potential problems, safe performance of laparoscopic cholecystectomy and other laparoscopic procedures in pregnant patients is increasingly being described in the literature. If cholecystectomy is necessary before delivery, the second trimester is the best time for it.

Patients in whom preoperative imaging gives rise to a strong suspicion of gallbladder cancer should probably undergo open surgical management.

Operative Planning

ANTIBIOTIC PROPHYLAXIS

Some surgeons recommend routine preoperative administration of antibiotics to all patients undergoing laparoscopic cholecystectomy, on the grounds that inadvertent entry into the gallbladder is not uncommon and can lead to spillage of bile or stones into the peritoneal cavity. Other surgeons, however, recommend using the same guidelines for antibiotic prophylaxis in patients undergoing laparoscopic cholecystectomy as in those undergoing open cholecystectomy. Resolution of this controversy awaits proper prospective trials. We recommend selective use

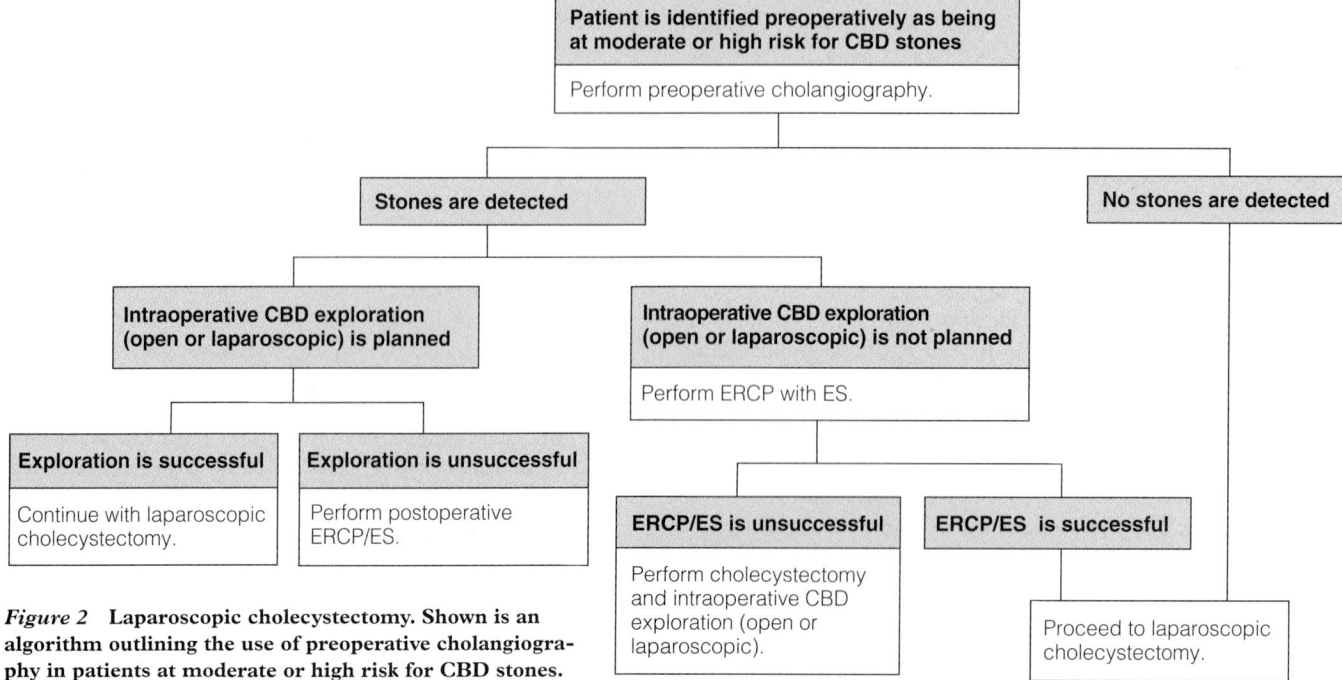

Figure 2 **Laparoscopic cholecystectomy. Shown is an algorithm outlining the use of preoperative cholangiography in patients at moderate or high risk for CBD stones.**

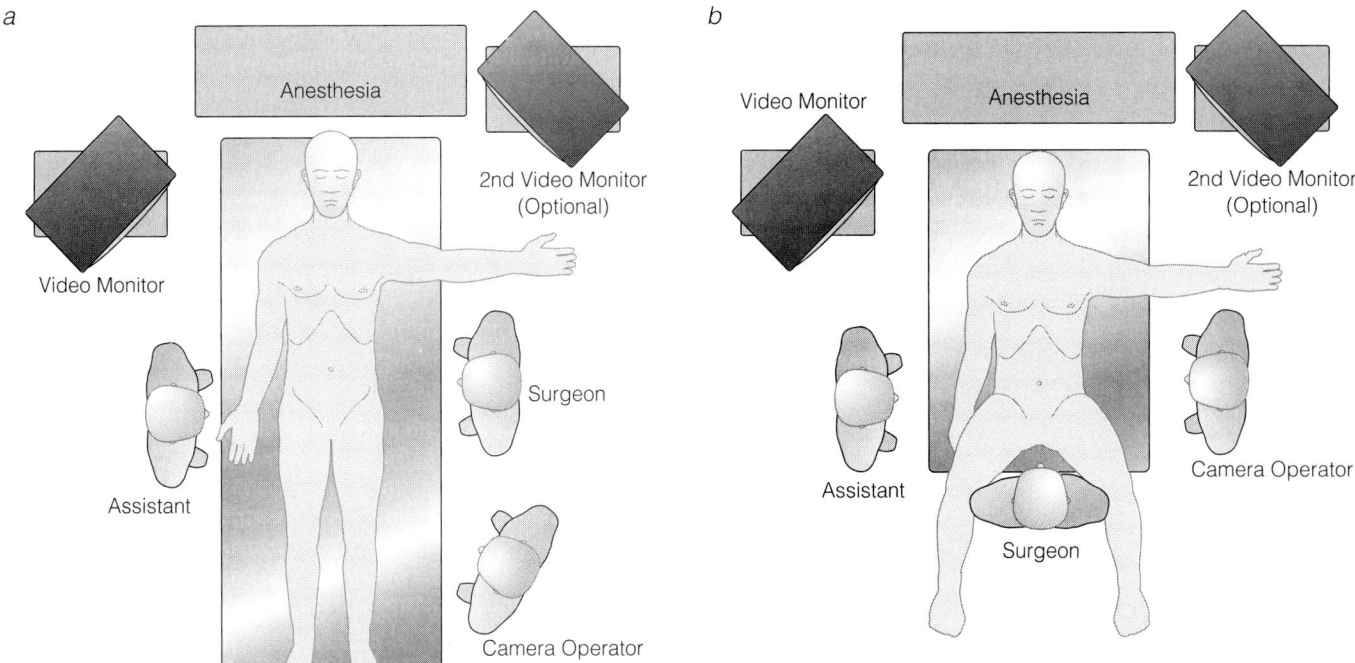

a

b

Figure 3 Laparoscopic cholecystectomy. A patient undergoing laparoscopic cholecystectomy should be positioned so as to allow easy access to the gallbladder and a clear view of the monitors. Shown are the positions of the surgeon, the camera operator, and the assistant in the OR according to (*a*) North American positioning and (*b*) European positioning.

of antibiotic prophylaxis for patients at highest risk for bacteria in the bile (including those with acute cholecystitis or CBD stones, those who have previously undergone instrumentation of the biliary tree, and those older than 70 years) and for patients with prosthetic heart valves and joint prostheses.

PROPHYLAXIS OF DVT

The reverse Trendelenburg position used during laparoscopic cholecystectomy, coupled with the positive intra-abdominal pressure generated by CO_2 pneumoperitoneum and the vasodilatation induced by general anesthesia, leads to venous pooling in the lower extremities. This consequence may be minimized by using antiembolic stockings or by wrapping the legs with elastic bandages. Subcutaneous heparin and pneumatic compression devices may be employed for patients at increased risk for DVT [*see 4:6 Venous Thromboembolism*]. As yet, however, there is no convincing evidence that the incidence of DVT is higher with laparoscopy than with open surgery.

PATIENT POSITIONING

The patient should be positioned so as to optimize exposure of the gallbladder and to give the surgeon, the camera operator, and the assistant easy access to the patient and a clear view of the video monitor or monitors. There should be a direct line from the surgeon to the laparoscope to the gallbladder. This can be accomplished with the patient in the supine position and the surgeon on the patient's left (North American positioning) [*see Figure 3a*] or with the patient in low stirrups and the surgeon on the patient's left or between the patient's legs (European positioning) [*see Figure 3b*].

With North American positioning, in which the patient is supine, the camera operator usually stands on the patient's left to the left of the surgeon, while the assistant stands on the patient's right. The video monitor is positioned on the patient's right above

the level of the costal margin. If a second monitor is available, it should be positioned on the patient's left to the right of the surgeon, where the assistant can have an unobstructed and comfortable view. Exposure can be improved by tilting the patient in the reverse Trendelenburg position and rotating the table with the patient's right side up. Gravity pulls the duodenum, the colon, and the omentum away from the gallbladder, thereby increasing the working space available in the upper abdomen.

The OR table should allow easy access for a fluoroscopic C arm, to facilitate intraoperative cholangiography. The table cover should be radiolucent.

EQUIPMENT

The equipment required for laparoscopic cholecystectomy [*see Table 1*] includes an optical system, an electronic insufflator, trocars (cannulas), surgical instruments, and hemostatic devices.

Optical System

The optical system consists of a laparoscope, a high-intensity light source, a miniature video camera and camera box, and a high-resolution video monitor. A videotape recording system is desirable but not essential. A video printing system and a digital-image capturing system are also valuable for documenting operative findings.

The laparoscope can provide either a straight, end-on (0°) view or an angled (30° or 45°) view. Scopes that provide an end-on view are easier to learn to use, but angled scopes are more versatile. Scopes with a 30° angle cause less disorientation than those with a 45° angle and are ideal for laparoscopic cholecystectomy. Excellent 30° scopes are currently available in diameters of 10 mm, 5 mm, and 3.5 mm.

Illumination in the abdomen is provided by a separate high-intensity light source (usually xenon or metal halide) that generates 150 to 300 watts. Most light sources have an automatic brightness-control system that reduces light output the closer the scope is to the operative field, thereby diminishing reflective glare. Some cameras also have a control that can be used for regulating light output.

The high-resolution miniature video camera systems now in use typically use charge-coupled devices (CCDs) in a one-chip or three-chip configuration. In one-chip systems, a single chip is responsible for all colors, whereas in three-chip systems, a prism splits the light into red, green, and blue, with each color acquired by a separate chip. In most cases, three-chip systems provide better images, albeit at a higher cost. Systems are available in both analog and digital formats.

High-resolution video monitors are available in various sizes; generally, larger monitors are preferred. Fully digital flat-panel displays are now available that yield improved resolution, take up less space, are less subject to signal interference, and require less power.

The resolution and quality of the final image depend on (1) the brightness of the light source; (2) the integrity of the fiberoptic cord used to convey the light; (3) clean and secure connections between the light source and the scope; (4) the quality of the laparoscope (glass-rod lens systems are preferred), the camera, and the monitor; and (5) correct wiring of the components. The distal end of the scope must be kept clean and free of condensation: bile, blood, or fat will reduce brightness and distort the image. Lens fogging can be prevented by immersion in heated water or by antifogging solutions.

The camera will last longer if it is not sterilized. During the operation, it can be placed in a sterile, disposable plastic bag.

Insufflator

For laparoscopic procedures, a working space must be created within the abdomen by insufflating gas under positive pressure. CO_2 is preferred because it is highly soluble in water and

Table 1 Equipment for Laparoscopic Cholecystectomy

Instrument/Device	Number	Size	Comments

Laparoscopic cart
  High-intensity halogen light source (150–300 watts)
  High-flow electronic insufflator (minimum flow rate of 6 L/min)
  Laparoscopic camera box
  Videocassette recorder (optional)
  Digital still image capture system (optional)			

Laparoscope	1	3.5–10 mm	Available in 0° and angled views; we prefer to use a 30° 5 mm diameter laparoscope
Atraumatic grasping forceps	2–4	2–10 mm	Selection of graspers should allow surgeon choice appropriate to thickness and consistency of gallbladder wall; insulation is unnecessary
Large-tooth grasping forceps	1	10 mm	Used to extract gallbladder at end of procedure
Curved dissector	1	2–5 mm	Should have a rotatable shaft; insulation is required
Scissors	2–3	2–5 mm	One curved and one straight scissors with rotating shaft and insulation; additional microscissors may be helpful for incising cystic duct
Clip appliers	1–2	5–10 mm	Either disposable multiple clip applier or 2 manually loaded reusable single clip appliers for small and medium-to-large clips
Dissecting electrocautery hook or spatula	1	5 mm	Available in various shapes according to surgeon's preference; instrument should have channel for suction and irrigation controlled by trumpet valve(s); insulation required
High-frequency electrical cord	1		Cord should be designed with appropriate connectors for electrosurgical unit and instruments being used
Suction-irrigation probe	1	5–10 mm	Probe should have trumpet valve controls for suction and irrigation; may be used with pump for hydrodissection
10–to–5 mm reducers	2		Allow use of 5 mm instruments in 10 mm trocar without loss of pneumoperitoneum; these are often unnecessary with newer disposable trocars and may be built into some reusable trocars
5–to–3 mm reducer	1		Allows use of 2–3 mm instruments and ligating loops in 5 mm trocars
Ligating loops			
Endoscopic needle holders	1–2	5 mm	
Cholangiogram clamp with catheter	1	5 mm	Allows passage of catheter and clamping of catheter in cystic duct
Veress needle	1		Used if initial trocar is inserted by percutaneous technique
Allis or Babcock forceps	1–2	5 mm	Allow atraumatic grasping of bowel or gallbladder
Long spinal needle	1	14-gauge	Useful for aspirating gallbladder percutaneously in cases of acute cholecystitis or hydrops
Retrieval bag	1		Useful for preventing spillage of bile or stones in removal of inflamed or friable gallbladder; facilitates retrieval of spilled stones

because it does not support combustion when the electrocautery is used. The CO_2 should be insufflated with an electronic pump capable of a flow rate of at least 6 L/min; most current systems have a maximum flow rate of 20 L/min or higher. The insufflator is connected to one of the trocars by means of a flexible tube and a stopcock.

When intra-abdominal pressure drops below a preset value (usually 12 to 15 mm Hg), gas flow begins at the preset rate. The insufflator should provide digital readouts of the actual gas flow rate, the actual intra-abdominal pressure, and the total amount of CO_2 used during the procedure. It should also have a control for adjusting maximum flow rate and a control for setting the pressure above which gas flow is automatically shut off. An audible alarm should sound when the measured pressure exceeds a certain preset value.

Whenever multiple trocars are used, there is a certain unavoidable loss of gas around and through the trocars. The insufflator rapidly replaces this gas. Because the rate of gas flow is influenced by the diameter of the port through which the gas is infused, insufflators capable of flow rates higher than 6 L/min are rarely used to their full potential. Insufflators that can provide heated gas minimize heat loss and fogging and may offer hemodynamic benefits.

Trocars

The trocars through which access to the abdominal cavity is gained are available in a variety of sizes; selection depends on the external diameter of the instruments to be placed through them.

For cholecystectomy, at least one trocar site must be large enough to allow passage of the gallbladder and any stones removed. Most surgeons prefer to use a 10/12 mm trocar at the umbilicus for this purpose. The other trocars can range from 2 to 12 mm, depending on the size of the laparoscope, the grasping forceps, and the clip appliers being used. The conventional approach is to use 10/12 mm trocars at the umbilicus and the operating port site and 5 mm trocars for the other instruments; however, if a 5 mm laparoscope and a 5 mm clip applier are used, the operating port size can be reduced to 5 mm.

Currently, 2 mm instrumentation is growing in popularity. It must be remembered, however, that as a rule, the smaller the working port, the less versatile the instruments. In our experience, the combination of a 10 mm umbilical trocar, a 5 mm operating port, and 2 mm ports for grasping forceps is a good one: optical quality is maintained, little flexibility is lost with respect to selecting operating instruments, trocar size is minimized, and the cosmetic result is excellent.

Surgical Instruments

The choice of surgical instruments from the large array now available is clearly a personal one. Many instruments are available in both disposable and reusable forms. Reusable instruments tend to be sturdier and better designed, but their design may rapidly become obsolete, and like reusable trocars, they must be checked periodically. Disposables are more current in design, are consistently sharp, and are excellent to have as backups in case nondisposables break down. Instruments are also available in both insulated versions (to allow use of the electrocautery) or noninsulated versions (to reduce maintenance costs).

A minimal set of instruments for laparoscopic cholecystectomy would include graspers, dissectors, clip appliers, scissors, a dissecting electrocautery hook or spatula (or both), probes, reducers, ligating loops, a Veress needle, needle holders, and a cholangiography catheter system [see Table 1]; other instruments may be considered as options.

For clip appliers, curved scissors, and curved dissectors, a rotatable shaft can afford the surgeon more comfortable and convenient working angles. The shaft should be easily locked once it is at the appropriate angle so that it does not rotate during use.

Suction and irrigation probes are available with either trumpet valves or stopcock attachments. Reusable instruments must be checked periodically to ensure that the valves do not stick or leak. Irrigation can be provided under pressure by means of a commercial pump system, a system that uses high-pressure gas, or a pressure bag like those used for infusion of blood products. If a pressure bag is used, it should be pressurized to approximately 300 mm Hg, and either normal saline or lactated Ringer solution can be used as an irrigant.

A retrieval bag system is also useful. When the gallbladder has been perforated, it and any spilled stones should be placed into a bag before removal. This measure minimizes further bile spillage and stone loss and greatly simplifies removal. Although special self-opening retrieval bags are available, many surgeons take a less expensive approach and simply use sterilized food storage bags.

Hemostatic Devices

Hemostasis can be achieved with monopolar or bipolar electrocauterization. Electrocautery units are widely available, safe, inexpensive, and familiar to all surgeons, and they provide excellent hemostasis. A monopolar electrocautery can be connected to most available instruments; however, it is likely that bipolar electrocauterization will eventually prove safer. With a monopolar electrocautery, depth of burn is less predictable, current can be conducted through noninsulated instruments and trocars, and any area of the instrument that is stripped of insulation may conduct current and result in a burn. Caution is essential when the electrocautery is used near hemostatic clips because delayed sloughing may occur.

Electrocauterization should be avoided near the CBD because delayed bile duct injuries and leaks may occur as a result of sloughing from a burned area and devascularization of the duct. Care must be exercised when a cautery is employed near the bowel and when intra-abdominal adhesions are being taken down. The electrocautery can be used with a forceps, scissors, hooks (L or J shaped), a spatula, and other instruments. Some cautery probes incorporate nonsticking surfaces to prevent buildup of eschar. The use of hand-activated cautery probes and the presence of a channel that allows suction and irrigation through the cautery probes are especially convenient.

More advanced energy sources and instruments are also available. Bipolar devices designed to weld tissues have proved capable of achieving superb hemostasis. Ultrasonic dissecting shears can also be used to dissect and coagulate tissues effectively and precisely. For laparoscopic cholecystectomy, however, such advanced—and costly—devices are rarely needed.

Operative Technique

STEP 1: PLACEMENT OF TROCARS AND ACCESSORY PORTS

Placement of Initial Trocar

The first step in laparoscopic cholecystectomy is the creation of pneumoperitoneum and the insertion of an initial trocar through which the laparoscope can be passed. This step is critical because complications resulting from improper placement may cause serious morbidity and death. The surgeon may use either a percuta-

a 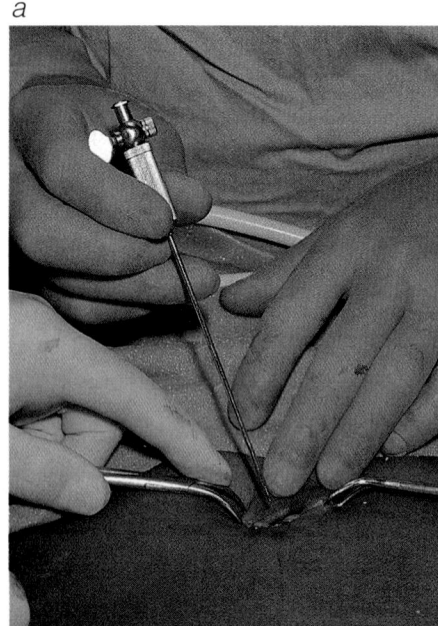   *b* 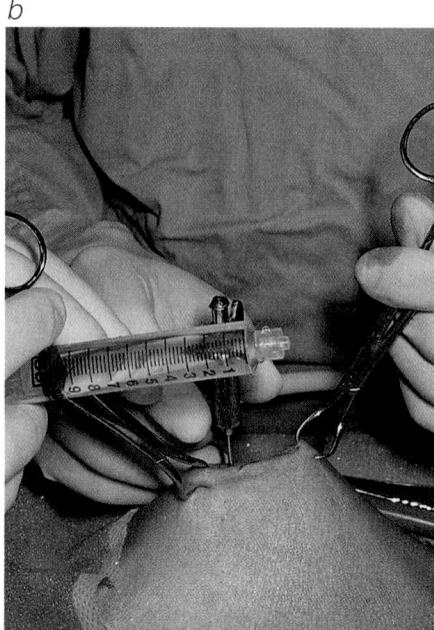   *c*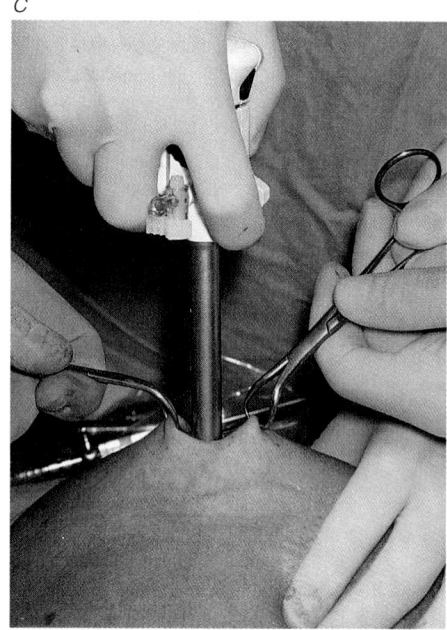

Figure 4 **Laparoscopic cholecystectomy. Illustrated is percutaneous placement of the initial trocar. (*a*) A Veress needle is used for percutaneous entry into the peritoneal cavity. It is angled toward the sacral hollow (where the distance from the anterior to the posterior abdominal wall is greatest) and toward an area below the bifurcation of the aorta. This space can be enlarged by tilting the patient in the Trendelenburg position, allowing the free intestinal loops to fall cephalad. (*b*) With the stopcock on the Veress needle in the closed position, a drop of saline is placed into the hub of the needle. The stopcock is then opened and the abdominal wall elevated. Lifting the abdominal wall creates negative pressure in the peritoneal cavity. Thus, if the tip of the needle is properly positioned within the cavity, the drop of saline should be drawn into the abdomen. (*c*) The abdominal wall is elevated, and a sharp 10/12 mm trocar is inserted into the peritoneal cavity along the same path as the Veress needle. Disposable trocars with a retracting plastic sheath provide further protection against perforation of viscera or vessels.**

neous technique or an open technique. We prefer the open technique, which eliminates the risks inherent in the blind puncture.

Percutaneous technique   For percutaneous trocar insertion, a small curvilinear incision is made in the area of the umbilicus and extended downward through the subcutaneous fat. A Veress needle is then inserted through the fascia and the peritoneum into the abdominal cavity [*see Figure 4a*]. This is best accomplished by elevating the abdominal wall and slightly angling the needle toward the pelvis, with the patient in the Trendelenburg position. The tip of the needle should be directed toward the hollow of the sacrum. Entry of the needle into the peritoneal cavity can usually be confirmed by a popping sensation as the resistance of the peritoneum is overcome. A 10 ml syringe is then attached to the needle and aspiration attempted. If the aspirate contains any blood or bowel contents, the needle is clearly in an inappropriate position.

If the aspirate is clear, the next step is to confirm proper positioning by means of the saline drop test [*see Figure 4b*]. The surgeon then attaches the insufflator to the needle and begins inflating the abdomen at a rate of approximately 1 L/min. The intra-abdominal pressure should be very low when insufflation is started, usually about 2 to 5 mm Hg; high pressure suggests improper needle placement. As the abdomen is distended with CO_2, the surgeon percusses the abdomen to ensure even distribution of the gas. When a pressure of approximately 15 mm Hg is reached (which requires about 5 L of gas in an average-sized patient), the Veress needle is withdrawn, and a sharp 10/12 mm trocar is percutaneously inserted through the same incision into the abdominal cavity, following the same route as the needle.

Because this procedure is done blindly, it may be advisable to enhance its safety by using disposable trocars with a spring-loaded protective plastic mechanism [*see Figure 4c*]. Once the initial trocar is inserted, proper positioning is confirmed by placing the laparoscope. Insufflation of CO_2 through the trocar then resumes, maintaining pneumoperitoneum.

Open insertion technique   The advantage of the open technique is that the trocar is inserted into the peritoneal cavity under direct vision; no Veress needle is required. Although it is certainly possible to injure the bowel inadvertently when placing the trocar, the injury almost always can be identified immediately and usually can be repaired easily through the same incision. Injury to the blood vessels or the bladder should virtually never occur with the open technique.

The umbilical skin is elevated with a sharp towel clip, and a 1 cm incision is made just inferior to the umbilicus [*see Figure 5a*]. Dissection is carried down through the subcutaneous tissue. The skin flap is raised, and a raphe can be seen connecting its undersurface to the midline fascia of the abdominal wall. The raphe is followed down to the fascia, which is then elevated between vertically placed forceps and incised [*see Figure 5b*]. The peritoneum is grasped next and pulled up into the wound, where it is incised. Entry into the abdominal cavity is easily confirmed by inserting a finger or a blunt instrument into the peritoneum [*see Figure 5c*]. Stay sutures are then placed on either side of the fascial incision, and a blunt olive-tipped 10/12 mm trocar, designed to occlude the fascial defect around it, is placed into the abdomen under direct vision. These sutures are then used to fasten the trocar to the wound and to prevent any leakage of gas. Because proper

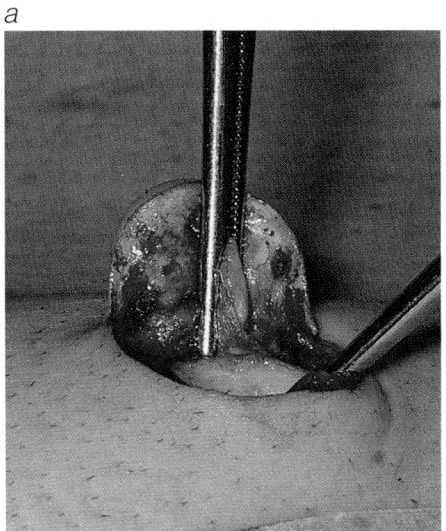 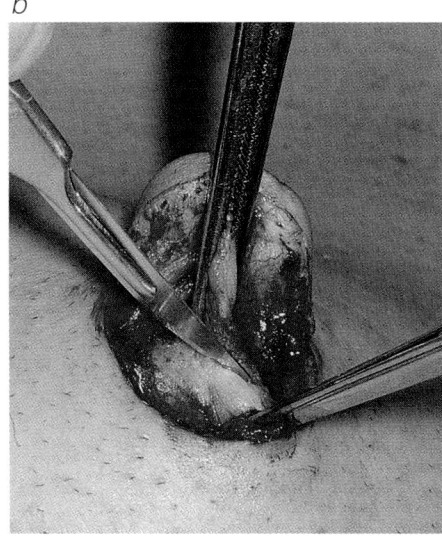 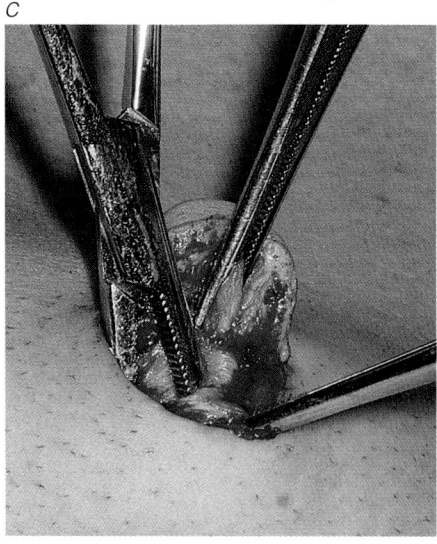

Figure 5 **Laparoscopic cholecystectomy. With the open insertion technique, the initial trocar is placed under direct vision. (*a*) The umbilical skin is elevated with a sharp towel clip. A curvilinear incision is made in the inferior umbilical fold. The skin flap is elevated, and the raphe leading from the dermis to the fascia is thereby exposed. (*b*) The fascia is grasped in the midline between forceps and elevated. The fascia and the underlying peritoneum are incised under direct vision. (*c*) A blunt instrument is placed into the peritoneum to ensure that the undersurface of the peritoneum is free of adhesions. The opening can be enlarged sufficiently to allow placement of a blunt 10/11 mm trocar.**

positioning of the trocar is obvious and needs no further confirmation, pneumoperitoneum can be created rapidly. The additional time expended on the dissection needed for insertion of the trocar is more than outweighed by the increased speed with which pneumoperitoneum is created and facilitates removal of the gallbladder at the end of the procedure. The stay sutures can also be used at the end of the procedure to close the fascial defect.

Scars

Patients who have previously undergone abdominal surgery are at risk for adhesions, both to the undersurface of the abdominal wall and intra-abdominally. Adhesions to the undersurface of the abdominal wall make access to the abdominal cavity potentially hazardous, particularly when the percutaneous method is used for placement of the initial trocar. Scars from previous operations may affect insertion of the initial trocar, depending on its orientation and location. If a patient has a scar in the lower abdomen (e.g., from a Pfannenstiel incision or an incision in the right lower quadrant for an appendectomy), the position of the initial trocar need not be changed. If the scar is in the upper abdomen, the initial trocar may be inserted below the umbilicus in the midline. If there is a long midline scar that is impossible to avoid, careful dissection of the peritoneum through a somewhat longer vertical incision than usual affords safe access to the peritoneum in most cases.

An alternative is to insert the initial trocar high in the epigastrium or in the right anterior axillary line, where bowel adhesions are less common. The laparoscope is inserted through this trocar and used to examine the undersurface of the old scar for a clear site near the umbilicus where a 10 mm trocar can be placed. Previous laparoscopy, which rarely creates significant intra-abdominal adhesions, rarely necessitates modification of trocar insertion.

The surgeon should also consider the reason for the previous surgery. For example, a patient who underwent an appendectomy for perforating appendicitis may have had diffuse peritonitis and may have adhesions well away from the old scar.

Placement of Accessory Ports

In most cases, four ports are necessary. The first port is for the laparoscope; the remaining ports are for grasping forceps, dissectors, and clip appliers. The precise position of the accessory ports depends on the surgeon's preference, the patient's body habitus, and the presence or absence of previous scars or intra-abdominal adhesions. A rigid approach to port placement is inappropriate: trocar placement determines operative exposure, and improper placement will haunt the surgeon throughout the procedure. In some cases, a fifth trocar is required to elevate a floppy liver or to depress or retract the omentum or a bulky hepatic flexure of the colon. In trocar placement, as in patient positioning, European practice tends to differ from North American practice [*see Figure 6*].

Most surgeons elect to place one of the grasping forceps on the fundus of the gallbladder through an accessory port placed approximately in the anterior axillary line below the level of the gallbladder. Because the level of the gallbladder varies from patient to patient, the placement of this accessory port should not be decided on until the gallbladder is visualized. If the gallbladder is low lying and the trocar is placed too high, it is difficult for the surgeon to achieve the appropriate angle of retraction. As a general rule, positioning the trocar in the anterior axillary line approximately halfway between the costal margin and the anterosuperior iliac spine provides the appropriate exposure. A 2 to 5 mm port usually suffices at this site because its only likely function is to allow retraction of the gallbladder. In some cases of acute cholecystitis, however, a larger port may be preferable, so that a larger grasper can be inserted and used to hold the gallbladder without tearing it.

A second accessory port (also 2 to 5 mm) allows the surgeon to grasp the gallbladder in the area of Hartmann's pouch for retraction. This port is usually positioned just beneath the right costal margin. Some surgeons prefer it to be approximately at the midclavicular line; others prefer it to be higher and more medial, just to the right of the falciform ligament.

The main operating port should be 5 or 10 mm in diameter, so that clip appliers can be readily placed through it and the laparoscope can be moved to this port at the end of the procedure. The positioning of this port is determined by the surgeon's preference and, in particular, by the patient's body habitus. The optimum placement is at about the same horizontal level as the gallbladder or slightly higher, so that during the operation, the laparoscope and the operating instrument form an angle of about 90°. Some surgeons prefer to place the operative port in the midline, to the right of the falciform ligament; others prefer to place it to the left of the falciform, passing the trocar underneath the ligament and elevating it with the trocar.

Surgeons should be encouraged to use both hands when performing laparoscopic cholecystectomy. One hand should control the grasping forceps holding Hartmann's pouch, so that the gallbladder can be moved to provide the best possible exposure. The other hand should control the dissecting instruments placed through the operating port.

Special Considerations in Obese Patients

Obese patients pose specific problems that affect port placement. The problems may be related to the thick abdominal wall, the large amount of intra-abdominal fat, or both. A thick abdominal wall makes it more difficult to rotate the trocar around the normal fulcrum point in the abdominal wall. Consequently, it is essential to place the trocar at the angle most likely to be used during the procedure. When a trocar is tunneled through the abdominal wall, more of the cannula is within the abdominal wall than if the trocar had been placed perpendicularly; accordingly, the trocar is less mobile. If the trocars are not easily rotated, the instruments placed through them will be difficult to manipulate smoothly. Thus, in the patient with a very thick pannus, a standard-length trocar may be too short. Displacement of

trocars can lead to insufflation into the abdominal wall and consequently to subcutaneous emphysema, which further thickens the abdominal wall and hinders exposure.

To prevent such problems, special extra-length trocars designed for morbidly obese patients have been developed. It may also be necessary to place the trocars closer to the area of the gallbladder to ensure that the operating instruments can reach the gallbladder. For example, the initial port may have to be placed above the umbilicus.

In obese patients, the bulky falciform ligament and the large omentum may adversely affect exposure. A 30° laparoscope may help the surgeon see over the omentum and the high-lying hepatic flexure of the colon. In some cases, it is useful to place a fifth port so that the surgeon can retract the hepatic flexure downward. Fat may envelop the cystic duct and artery and the portal structures, obscuring normal anatomic landmarks. When the electrocautery is used, the heat melts the fat and causes it to sizzle and spray onto the lens of the laparoscope, resulting in a blurry image. To prevent this, the camera operator should pull the scope slightly away from the operative field during electrocauterization, then advance the scope during dissection. This should also be done when an ultrasonic dissector is being used.

Given that obese patients are more difficult candidates for open cholecystectomy and have a higher complication rate with laparotomy, the advantages of laparoscopic cholecystectomy in these individuals justify the effort needed to overcome the technical problems.

STEP 2: EXPOSURE OF GALLBLADDER AND CALOT'S TRIANGLE

Dissection of Adhesions

Adhesions must be dissected to provide an unimpeded view of the gallbladder through the laparoscope. Not all intra-abdominal

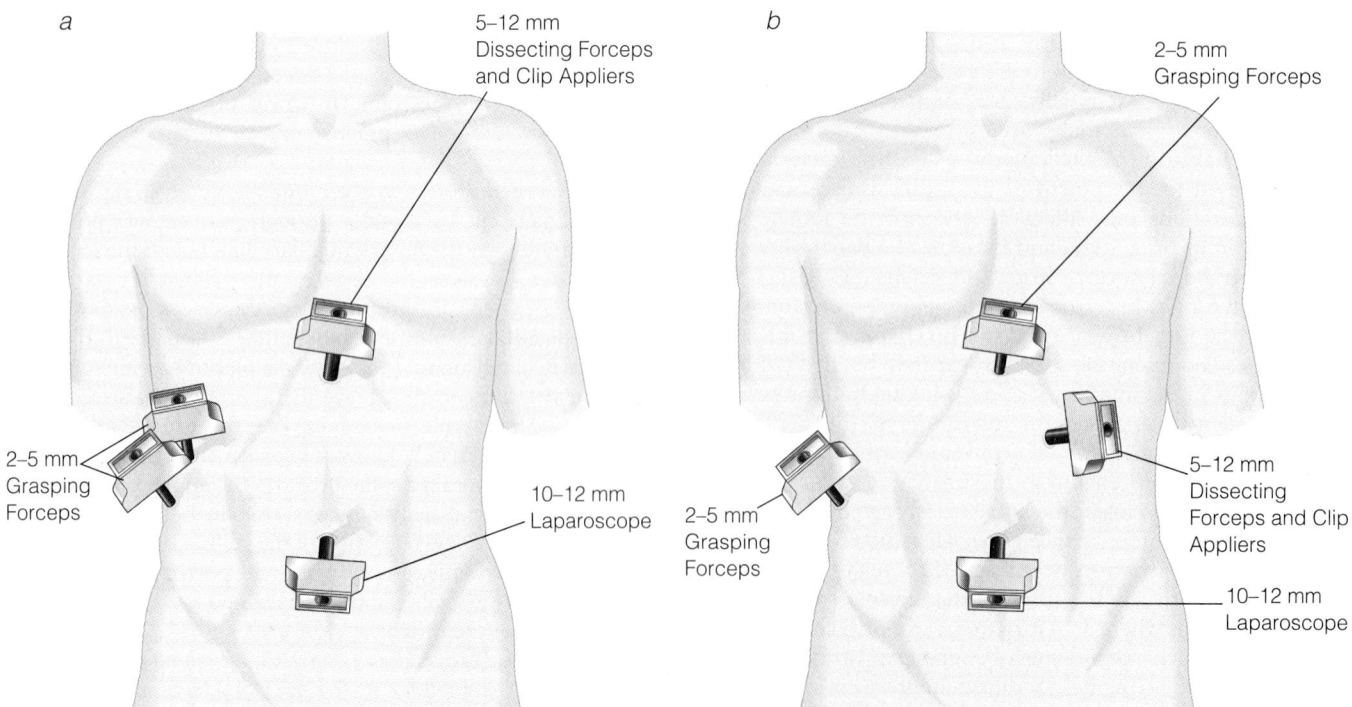

Figure 6 **Laparoscopic cholecystectomy. Illustrated are the differences between typical North American practice (*a*) and typical European practice (*b*) with respect to the placement of the trocars and the instruments inserted through each port.**

adhesions must be taken down, just enough to allow entry of accessory trocars under direct vision and thus permit access to the gallbladder. This process is facilitated by pneumoperitoneum, which provides traction on adhesions to the abdominal wall, and by the magnification provided by the optical system, which allows identification of the avascular plane of attachment.

The most difficult problem is positioning the dissecting instruments so that they can reach the undersurface of the anterior abdominal wall. A rigid trocar inserted through the anterior abdominal wall cannot be rotated enough to allow scissors passed through this port to cut adhesions to the anterior abdominal wall. In such cases, one or two trocars should be placed laterally, near the anterior axillary or midaxillary line. Instruments passed through these ports can easily be angled parallel to the anterior abdominal wall, and the adhesions can then be dissected without difficulty.

Bowel adhesions should be taken down with endoscopic scissors at their insertion to the abdominal wall, where they are least vascular. Electrocauterization, generally unnecessary, should be avoided because of the risk of thermal injury to the bowel. Interloop adhesions, which rarely interfere with exposure of the gallbladder, need not be dissected. Frequently, adhesions to the gallbladder occur as a reaction to inflammatory attacks [*see Figure 7*]. They are usually relatively avascular. Dissection of these adhesions should begin at the fundus of the gallbladder and should then proceed down toward the neck of the gallbladder. The best way to take them down is to grasp the gallbladder with one grasping forceps at the site where the adhesions attach, gradually placing traction on the adhesions with the other hand. Usually, the adhesions peel down in an avascular plane. Dissection should continue until all adhesions to the inferolateral aspect of the gallbladder have been taken down. It is not necessary to divide adhesions between the superior surface of the liver and the undersurface of the diaphragm unless they impede superior retraction of the liver.

Exposing Calot's Triangle

Obtaining adequate exposure of Calot's triangle is a key step. First, the patient is placed in a reverse Trendelenburg position,

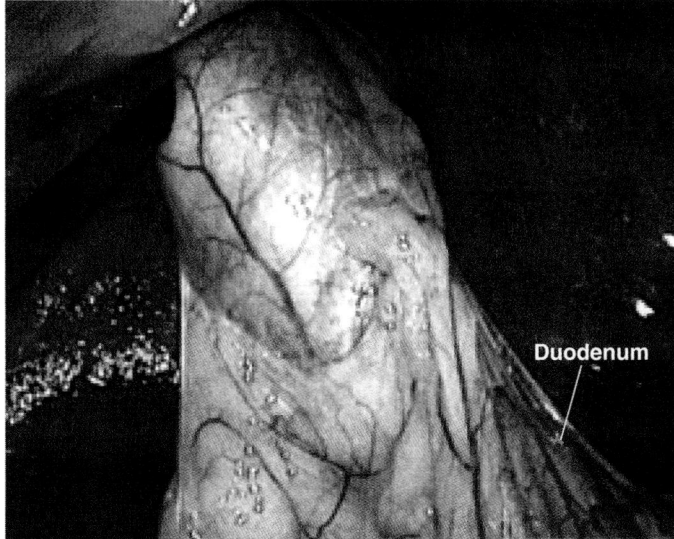

Figure 7 **Laparoscopic cholecystectomy. Adhesions of duodenum and omentum to gallbladder wall obscure view of structures of Calot's triangle.**

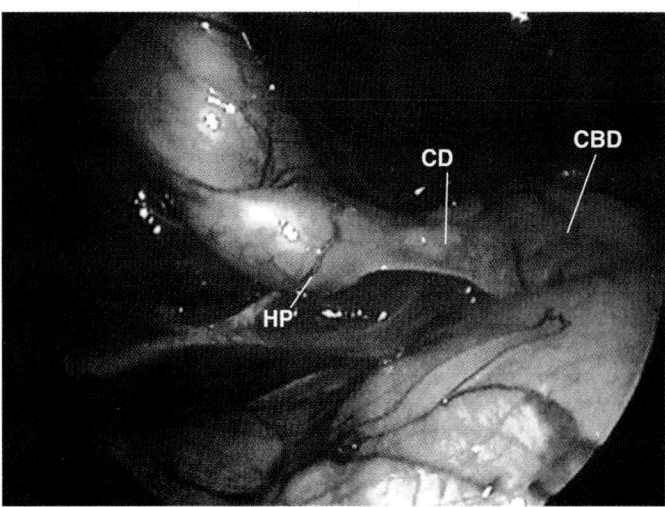

Figure 8 **Laparoscopic cholecystectomy. Initial view of gallbladder and related structures is facilitated by appropriate tilting of the operating table. Hartmann's pouch (HP), the cystic duct (CD), and the common bile duct (CBD) can be readily identified before any dissection.**

with the table rotated toward the left side. Next, the fundus of the gallbladder and the right lobe of the liver are elevated toward the patient's right shoulder. One grasping forceps, inserted through the most lateral right-side port and held by an assistant, is placed on the fundus of the gallbladder [*see Figure 8*], and the gallbladder is retracted superiorly and laterally above the right hepatic lobe. This maneuver straightens out folds in the body of the gallbladder and permits initial visualization of the area of Calot's triangle. If Calot's triangle is still obscured, the patient can be placed in a steeper reverse Trendelenburg position, the stomach can be emptied of air via an orogastric tube inserted by the anesthetist, or, if necessary, a fifth trocar can be inserted on the patient's right side to push down the duodenum.

In some patients, such as those with acute cholecystitis and hydrops of the gallbladder, the gallbladder is tense and distended, making it difficult to grasp and easy to tear. In these patients, retraction of the fundus is difficult, and exposure of Calot's triangle is unsatisfactory. This problem is best managed by aspirating the contents of the gallbladder either percutaneously with a 14- or 16-gauge needle inserted into the fundus of the gallbladder under laparoscopic vision or by using the 5 mm trocar in the right upper abdomen to puncture the fundus and then aspirate with the suction irrigator. After the needle is withdrawn, a large atraumatic grasping forceps can be used to hold the gallbladder and occlude the hole; a 10 mm forceps may be preferred if the wall is markedly thickened. An alternative is to place a stitch or a ligating loop around the fundus of the collapsed gallbladder; the tail of the suture can then be grasped with a forceps to achieve a secure grip and also prevent further leakage of gallbladder contents from the needle hole.

Once the fundus of the gallbladder is retracted superiorly by the assistant, the surgeon places a grasping forceps in the area of Hartmann's pouch. Using both hands, the surgeon controls the grasper on Hartmann's pouch as well as the operating instrument. The surgeon maneuvers Hartmann's pouch to provide various angles for safe dissection of Calot's triangle. Initially, lateral and inferior traction are placed on Hartmann's pouch, opening up the angle between the cystic duct and the common ducts [*see Figure 9*], avoiding their alignment [*see Figure 10*].

A large stone impacted in the gallbladder neck may impede the surgeon's ability to place the forceps on Hartmann's pouch. This problem can usually be managed by dislodging the stone early in the operation, as follows: the gallbladder is grasped as low as possible with one grasping forceps; a widely opening dissecting instrument, such as a right-angle dissector, a Babcock forceps, or a curved dissector, is used to dislodge the stone and milk it up toward the fundus; with the same forceps or another large grasper, the stone is held up and away from the neck of the gallbladder, and appropriate retraction is provided.

If the stone cannot be disimpacted, an instrument can be used to elevate the infundibulum of the gallbladder superiorly, allowing exposure of Calot's triangle. Alternatively, one can attempt to crush the stone, but small pieces of the stone may fall into the cystic duct. A third option is to place a stitch in Hartmann's pouch and grasp the end of the stitch to provide exposure.

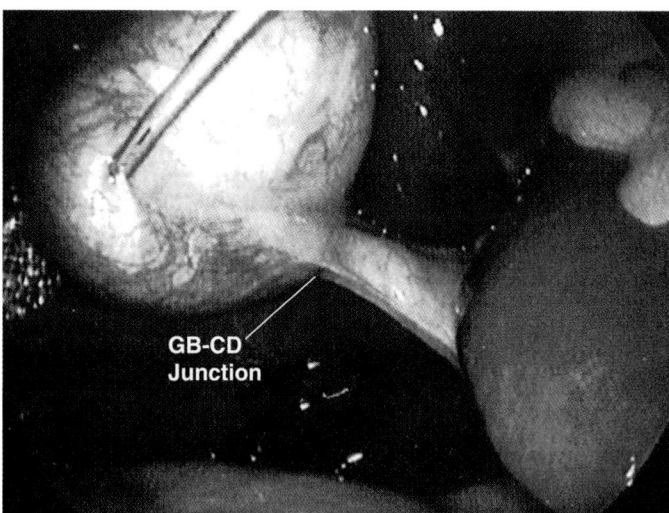

Figure 11 **Laparoscopic cholecystectomy. The gallbladder–cystic duct (GB-CD) junction can be identified as lateral traction is applied to the area of Hartmann's pouch.**

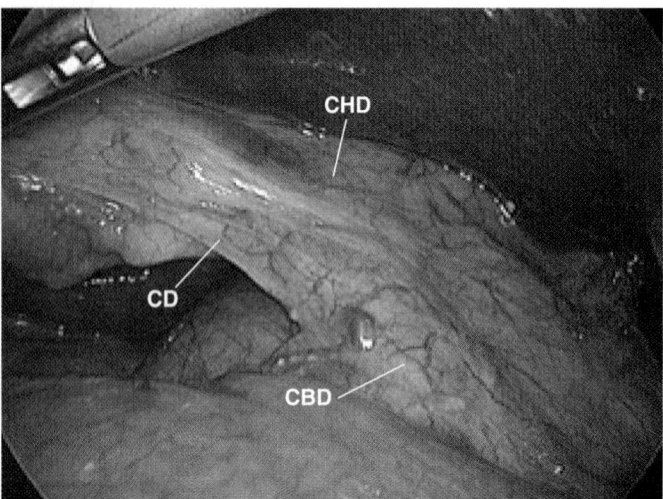

Figure 9 **Laparoscopic cholecystectomy. The area of Hartmann's pouch is retracted laterally. The cystic duct (CD) is seen at an angle to the common hepatic duct (CHD) and the common bile duct (CBD).**

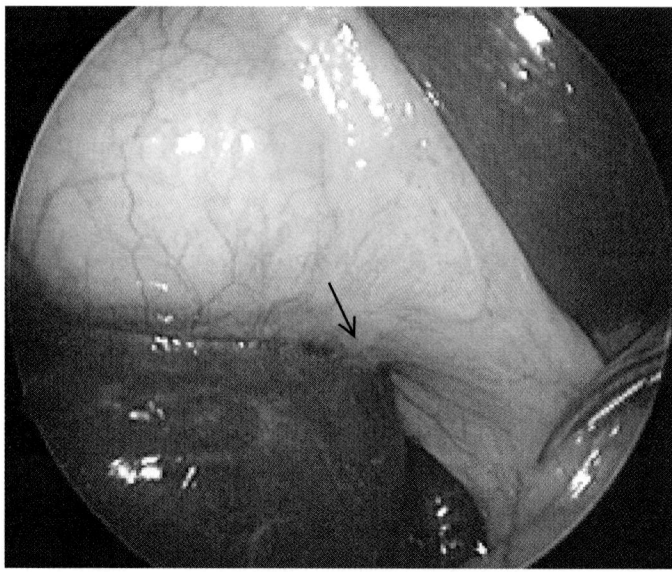

Figure 12 **Laparoscopic cholecystectomy. A view from below with a 30° laparoscope demonstrates the point for beginning dissection (arrow), where the gallbladder funnels down to its junction with the cystic duct. Just below this point can be seen a cleft in the liver known as Rouvier's sulcus. This cleft, present in 70% to 80% of livers, reliably indicates the plane of the CBD.**

STEP 3: STRIPPING OF PERITONEUM

The key to avoiding injury to the major ducts during laparoscopic cholecystectomy is accurate identification of the junction between the gallbladder and the cystic duct [*see Figure 11*]. Unless the gallbladder–cystic duct junction is immediately obvious upon examination of Calot's triangle anteriorly, our approach is to begin dissection of Calot's triangle posteriorly [*see Figure 12*]. From this approach, the insertion of the gallbladder neck into the cystic duct is usually more clearly identified, especially with the aid of a 30° laparoscope. Exposure is obtained by retracting Hartmann's pouch superomedially and is facilitated by looking from below with a 30° scope.

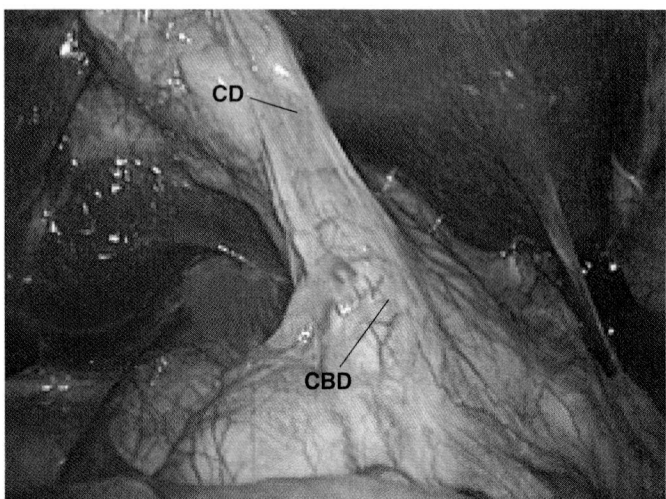

Figure 10 **Laparoscopic cholecystectomy. In this case, the gallbladder is retracted cephalad. The cystic duct (CD) can be seen running in the same direction as the common bile duct (CBD). The CBD may be misinterpreted as being the cystic duct and consequently is at risk for injury.**

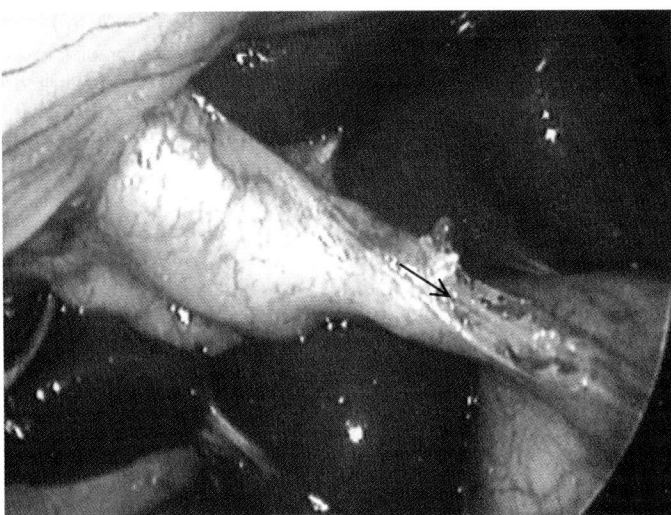

Figure 13 **Laparoscopic cholecystectomy. The peritoneum is dissected from the gallbladder–cystic duct junction (arrow), as seen from below through a 30° angled laparoscope.**

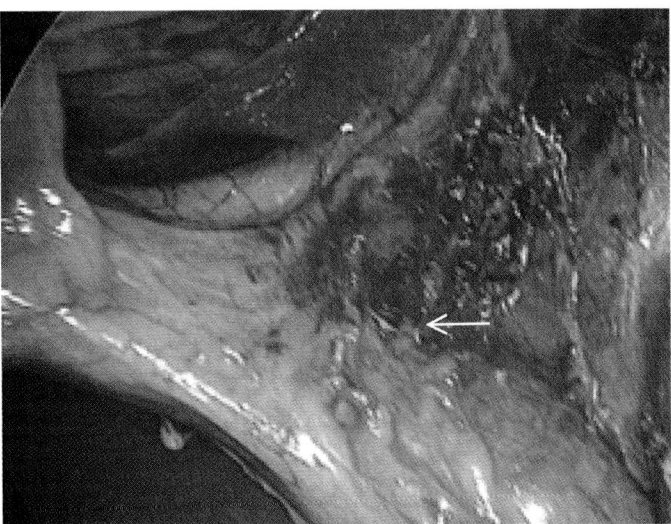

Figure 14 **Laparoscopic cholecystectomy. Arterial bleeding can be seen (arrow) from a branch of the cystic artery injured during dissection from the posterior approach.**

Dissection should always start high on the gallbladder and hug the gallbladder closely until the anatomy is identified clearly. Using a curved dissector, the surgeon gently teases away peritoneum attaching the neck of gallbladder to the liver posterolaterally to visualize the funneling of the neck of the gallbladder into the cystic duct [*see Figure 13*]. Only the posterior layer of peritoneum is dissected; care must be taken not to dissect deeply in this area because of the risk of injury to the cystic artery [*see Figure 14*].

In some problem cases, edema, fibrosis, and adhesions make identification of the gallbladder–cystic duct junction very difficult. An anatomic landmark on the liver known as Rouvier's sulcus may be helpful in such circumstances [*see Figure 12*]. This sulcus, or the remnant of it, is present in 70% to 80% of livers and usually contains the right portal triad or its branches. Its location is consistently to the right of the hepatic hilum and anterior to the caudate process (Couinaud segment 1). This landmark reliably indicates the plane of the CBD. Therefore, dissection dorsal to it should be done with caution.

Once the funneling of the gallbladder into the cystic duct has been identified, the area of Hartmann's pouch should be again pulled laterally and inferiorly so that the anterior peritoneum can be dissected, while the 30° scope is angled to view the area. The two-handed technique facilitates the surgeon's movement between the posterior and anterior aspects of Calot's triangle, providing complete visualization. Dissection should always take place at the gallbladder–cystic duct junction, staying close to the gallbladder to avoid inadvertent injury to the CBD. A curved dissecting forceps is used to strip the fibroareolar tissue just superior to the cystic duct. The superior border of the cystic duct can then be identified and the cystic duct gently and gradually dissected [*see Figure 15*]. The cystic duct lymph node is a useful landmark at this location and may facilitate identification of the gallbladder–cystic duct junction.

When traction is placed as described, the cystic artery tends to run parallel and somewhat cephalad to the cystic duct. This artery can often be identified by noting its close relation to the cystic duct lymph node. Complete dissection of the area between the cystic duct and the artery develops a window through which the liver should be visible. The cystic duct is then encircled with a curved dissecting instrument or an L-shaped hook. Downward traction should be applied to the cystic duct to open this window and ensure that there is no ductal structure running through this space in Calot's triangle to join the cystic duct (i.e., the right hepatic duct).

Dissection of Calot's triangle should be completed before the cystic duct is clipped or divided. This is best accomplished by dissecting the neck of the gallbladder from the liver bed. Unequivocal identification of the gallbladder–cystic duct junction is imperative. The cystic duct should be dissected for a length sufficient to permit secure placement of two clips; it is not necessary, and indeed may be hazardous, to attempt to dissect the cystic duct–CBD junction.

The cystic artery is exposed next [*see Figure 16*]. A small vein can usually be identified in the space between the cystic duct and the cystic artery; it can usually be pulled up anteriorly and cauterized. Because dissection is done near the gallbladder, it is not unusual to encounter more than one branch of the cystic artery. Each of these branches should be dissected free of the fibroareolar tissue. Care should also be taken to ensure that the right hepatic artery is not inadvertently injured as a result of being mistaken for the cystic artery.

STEP 4: CONTROL AND DIVISION OF CYSTIC DUCT AND CYSTIC ARTERY

At this point, the cystic duct is clipped on the gallbladder side, and a cholangiogram is obtained if desired [*see Step 5, below*]. If a cholangiogram is not desired, three or four clips should be placed on the cystic duct and the cystic duct divided between them. Two or three hemostatic clips are placed on the cystic artery, and the vessel is divided. It is prudent to incise the artery partially before transecting it completely to ensure that the clips are secure and that there is no pulsatile bleeding. Once the artery is completely divided, the proximal end will retract medially, making it more difficult to expose and control the artery safely if bleeding occurs. Electrocauterization should be avoided near the cystic duct and all metallic clips. Electrical current will be conducted through metallic clips and may result in delayed sloughing of the duct or a clip. Delayed injuries to the CBD may be caused by a direct burn to the duct or by sparking from noninsulated instruments or clips during dissection. As an alternative, locking polymer clips that fit through 5 mm ports, clip across a greater width of tissue, and do not conduct electricity may be used.

Control of Short or Wide Cystic Duct

Edema and acute inflammation may lead to thickening and foreshortening of the cystic duct, with subsequent difficulties in dissection and ligation. If the duct is edematous, clips may cut through it; if the duct is too wide, the clip may not occlude it completely. A modified clipping technique can be employed, with placement of an initial clip to occlude as much of the duct as possible. The occluded portion of the duct is then incised, and

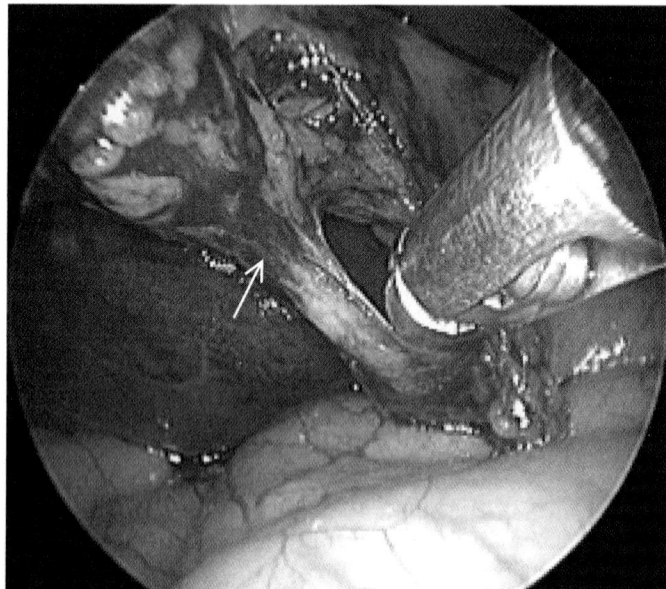

Figure 15 **Laparoscopic cholecystectomy. The superior border of the cystic duct has been dissected. Funneling of the gallbladder into the cystic duct is clearly seen (arrow).**

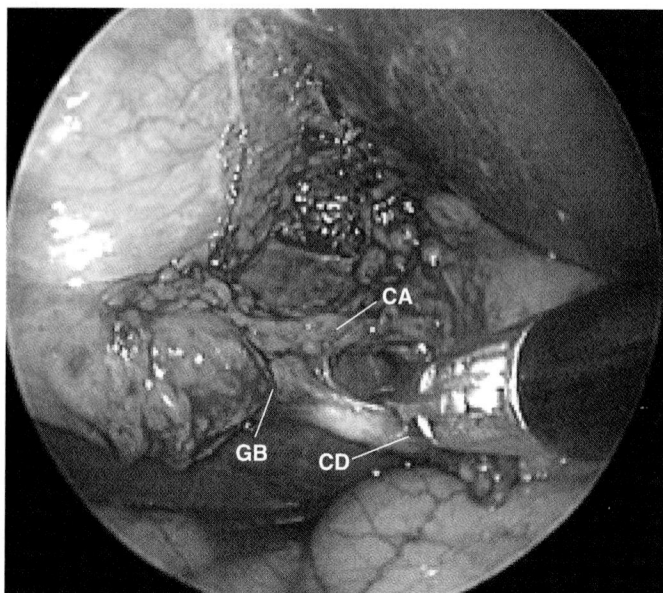

Figure 16 **Laparoscopic cholecystectomy. Dissection of Calot's triangle further exposes the cystic duct (CD) and the cystic artery (CA) near their entry into the gallbladder (GB) in preparation for clipping and division.**

a second clip is placed flush with the first so as to occlude the rest of the duct. Alternatively, wider polymer clips may be used.

Because this technique is not always possible, the surgeon should be familiar with techniques for ligating the duct with either intracorporeal or extracorporeal ties. It is extremely helpful to know how to tie extracorporeal ties so that the cystic duct can be ligated in continuity before it is divided. In some cases, the duct can be divided, held with a forceps, and controlled with a ligating loop. If there is concern about secure closure of the cystic duct, a closed suction drain may be placed. If inflammation, as in cholecystitis, has caused the duct to be shorter than usual, dissection must be kept close to the gallbladder to avoid inadvertent injury to the CBD. A short cystic duct is often associated with acute cholecystitis. Patient blunt dissection with the suction-irrigation device may be the safest technique.

Cystic Duct Stones

Stones in the cystic duct may be visualized or felt during laparoscopic cholecystectomy. Every effort should be made to milk them into the gallbladder before applying clips. Placing a clip across a stone may push a fragment of the stone into the CBD and will increase the risk that the clip will become displaced, leading to a bile leak. If the stone cannot be milked into the gallbladder, a small incision can be made in the cystic duct (as is done for cholangiography), and the stone can usually be expressed and retrieved. Given that cystic duct stones are predictive of CBD stones, cholangiography or intraoperative ultrasonography is indicated.

STEP 5: INTRAOPERATIVE CHOLANGIOGRAPHY

Whether intraoperative cholangiography should be performed routinely is still controversial. Advocates believe that this technique enhances understanding of the biliary anatomy, thus reducing the risk of bile duct injury; at present, however, there are no objective data to confirm this impression. Cholangiography is not a substitute for meticulous dissection, and injuries to the CBD can occur before cystic duct dissection reaches the point at which cholangiography can be performed. Catheter-induced injuries and perforations of the biliary tree have been reported, and cholangiograms have been misinterpreted. On the other hand, one of the main advantages of cholangiography is that injuries can be recognized during the operation and promptly repaired. Another advantage of routine cholangiography is that it helps develop the skills required for more complex biliary tract procedures, such as transcystic CBD exploration.

The two methods of laparoscopic cholangiography differ in their technique for introducing the cholangiogram catheter into the cystic duct. In both approaches, a clip is placed at the gallbladder–cystic duct junction and a small incision made in the anterior wall of the cystic duct. In the first technique, a specially designed 5 mm cholangiogram clamp (the Olsen clamp) with a 5 French catheter is inserted via a subcostal trocar. For easy guidance of the catheter into the incision in the cystic duct, the catheter should be parallel, rather than perpendicular, to the cystic duct. This angle is facilitated by placing the subcostal port directly below the costal margin, near the anterior axillary line. A fifth trocar may occasionally be needed if exposure is lost when one of the grasping forceps is removed to allow passage of the cholangiogram clamp. The clamp and the catheter are then brought to the cystic duct under direct vision, and the catheter is steered into the duct [*see Figure 17*]. The clamp is then closed, holding the catheter in position and sealing the duct to avoid extravasation of dye.

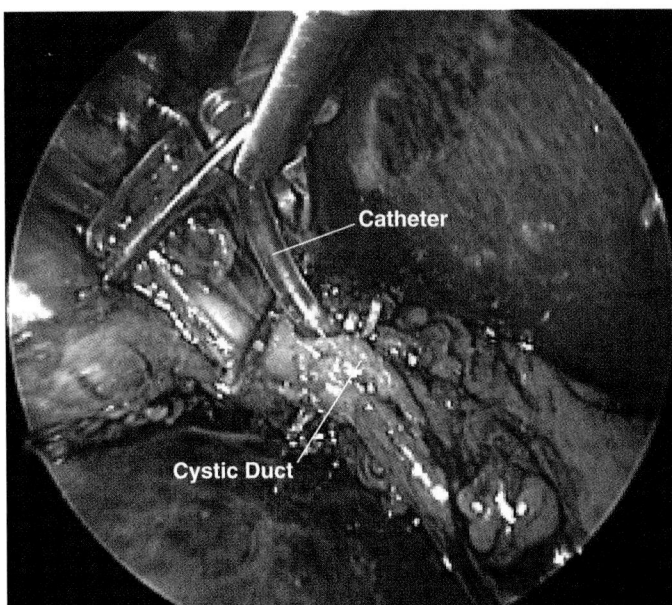

Figure 17 **Laparoscopic cholecystectomy. The cystic duct has been clipped, a small incision has been made for placement of the cholangiogram catheter, and the catheter has been advanced through the specialized cholangiogram clamp into the cystic duct.**

In the second method, the cholangiogram catheter is introduced percutaneously through a 12- to 14-gauge catheter, inserted subcostally as described (see above). The surgeon then grasps the cholangiogram catheter and directs it into the cystic duct. A hemostatic clip is applied to secure the catheter in place. If passage of the catheter into the cystic duct is prevented by Heister's valve, a guide wire can be passed initially.

If the cystic duct is tiny and it is anticipated that cannulation will be difficult or impossible, the gallbladder can be punctured, bile aspirated, and contrast material injected through the gallbladder until the biliary tree is filled.

The cannulas and operating instruments should be positioned so as not to obstruct the view of the biliary tree. If the cannulas cannot be positioned outside the x-ray window, radiolucent cannulas should be used, or the cannulas should be removed and replaced after the cholangiogram. A cholangiogram that does not visualize the biliary tree from the liver to the duodenum is inadequate.

Fluoroscopic cholangiography [*see Figure 18*] may be performed either with hard-copy film or with digital imaging and storage. After the C arm is positioned, with the operating staff protected behind a lead screen, full-strength contrast is slowly injected under fluoroscopic control. The goal is to visualize the biliary tree in its entirety, including the right and left hepatic ductal systems as well as the distal duct. Once the cholangiogram is obtained, the catheter is removed, and the cystic duct is double-clipped and transected.

Laparoscopic Ultrasonography

An emerging alternative for evaluation of the biliary tree is intraoperative laparoscopic ultrasonography, which appears to be as accurate as intraoperative fluorocholangiography in identifying biliary stones. This modality has several advantages over conventional cholangiography: it does not expose patients and staff to radiation; contrast agents are unnecessary; there is no need to cannulate the cystic duct; significantly less time is required; the capital cost of most ultrasound units is less than that of fluoroscopic equipment; and disposable cholangiogram catheters are not needed.

Most of the laparoscopic ultrasound devices in use at present are 7.5 MHz linear-array rigid probes 10 mm in diameter. Flexible probes capable of multiple frequencies are also currently available, and it is likely that future probes will be increasingly versatile. The probe is inserted through a 10/12 mm port (usually a periumbilical or epigastric port) and placed directly on the porta hepatis, perpendicular to the structures of the hepatoduodenal ligament. The probe is then moved to the cystic duct–CBD junction. The transverse image obtained should show the three tubular structures of the hepatoduodenal ligament in the so-called Mickey Mouse head configuration: the CBD, the portal vein, and the hepatic artery [*see Figure 19*]. As the probe is moved distally, it is rotated clockwise to allow identification of the distal CBD and the pancreatic duct where they unite at the papilla. Instillation of saline into the right upper quadrant can enhance acoustic coupling and improve visualization.

Because of its many advantages, intraoperative laparoscopic ultrasonography may eventually replace fluorocholangiography in this setting, particularly for surgeons who practice routine intraoperative evaluation of the CBD. Although the learning curve for effective performance of laparoscopic ultrasound examination is not long, surgeons should receive expert mentoring and formal instruction in ultrasonography before attempting it. During the first few attempts, it may be instructive to perform intraoperative laparoscopic ultrasonography in conjunction with fluorocholangiography.

It should be emphasized that intraoperative laparoscopic ultrasonography is not a replacement for intraoperative cholangiography if the purpose of the examination is to define an anomalous anatomy or to evaluate a suspected injury or leak.

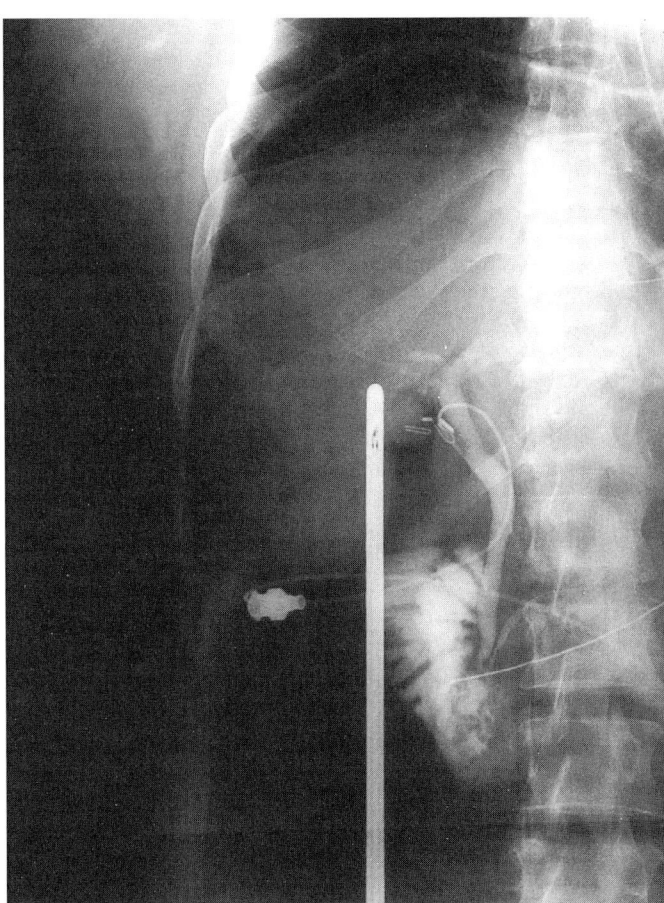

Figure 18 **Laparoscopic cholecystectomy. Shown is a normal intraoperative cholangiogram.**

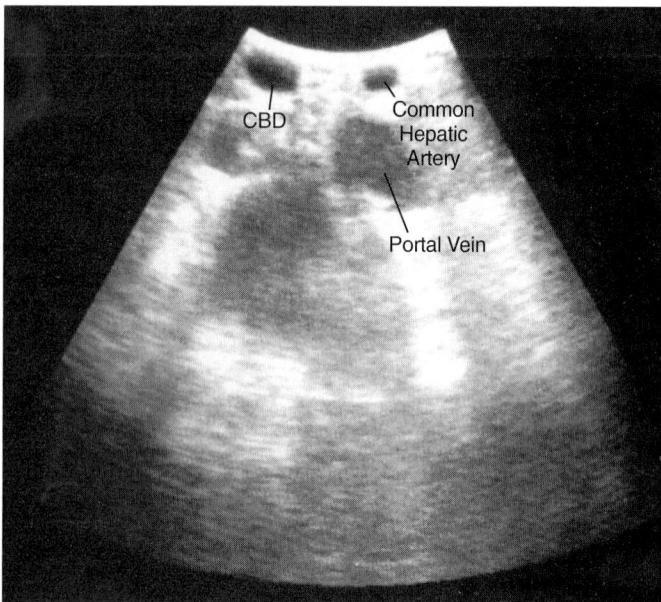

Figure 19 **Laparoscopic cholecystectomy. A transverse intraoperative ultrasound scan of the hepatoduodenal ligament reveals a typical "Mickey Mouse head" appearance. Visible are the CBD, the common hepatic artery, and the portal vein.**

STEP 6: DISSECTION OF GALLBLADDER FROM LIVER BED

The gallbladder is grasped near the cystic duct insertion and pulled down toward the right anterosuperior iliac spine, placing the areolar tissue between the gallbladder and liver anteriorly under tension. The areolar tissue is cauterized with an L-shaped hook dissector or spatula, and dissection is carried upward as far as possible for as long as there is sufficient exposure. When exposure begins to diminish, the cystic duct end of the gallbladder should be pulled up toward or over the left lobe of the liver to expose the posteroinferior attachments of the gallbladder. A two-handed approach by the surgeon facilitates this dissection. It is sometimes helpful to apply downward and lateral traction on the forceps grasping the fundus. Bleeding during this stage generally indicates that the surgeon has entered the wrong plane and dissection has entered the liver. Bleeding can usually be readily controlled with the electrocautery. In some difficult cases (e.g., an intrahepatic gallbladder), it may be prudent to leave some of the posterior wall of the gallbladder in situ and cauterize it rather than persist with an excessively bloody dissection.

Dissection continues until the gallbladder is attached only by a small piece of peritoneum at the fundus. Before the last attachment to the gallbladder is completely divided, the vital clips are reinspected to ensure that they have not slipped off, and the operative field is checked for hemostasis and the presence of any bile leakage. The final attachment to the gallbladder is then divided. The gallbladder is placed over the right lobe of the liver and laterally so that it can be found again to be retrieved. The grasping forceps on the gallbladder should not be removed.

Perforation of Gallbladder

The gallbladder may be accidentally breached at some point in the operation, with the result that bile and stones are spilled into the peritoneal cavity. Efforts should be made to suction the spilled bile, which accumulates in the suprahepatic space, the right subhepatic space, and the lower abdomen because of the patient's position. Each of these areas should be irrigated and the effluent aspirated until it is clear.

Stones should be located and removed whenever possible. An effective way of removing small stones is to irrigate the subhepatic space copiously. Cholesterol stones usually float on the irrigation fluid and can then be suctioned through a 10 mm suction probe or through a 32 French chest tube passed through the 10 mm operating port. Unfortunately, small stones may be lost in the omentum or between bowel loops. In such cases, it is probably appropriate to leave the stones within the peritoneum rather than perform a laparotomy to attempt to retrieve them. However, there have been reports of serious morbidity, including intra-abdominal abscess, fistula, empyema, and bowel obstruction, resulting from lost stones.

If the gallbladder is perforated and it seems likely that multiple stones will be spilled, the surgeon should introduce a sterile bag into the peritoneal cavity, placing it close to the perforation. Spilled stones can then be transferred immediately into the bag. After the gallbladder is removed from the liver bed, it too is placed in the bag, affording some protection to the wound when it is removed from the abdominal cavity.

STEP 7: EXTRACTION OF GALLBLADDER

The laparoscope is moved to the epigastric port, and a large-tooth grasping forceps is inserted through the umbilical port to grasp the gallbladder at the area of the cystic duct. Under direct vision, the gallbladder is then retrieved and pulled out as far as possible through the umbilical port. If the gallbladder is small enough, it can be drawn right into the trocar sleeve, and it and the trocar can then be removed together. It is sometimes necessary to stretch the fascial opening with a Kelly clamp or to aspirate bile from the gallbladder. It is far preferable to enlarge the incision than to have stones or bile spill into the abdominal cavity from a ripped gallbladder. Enlargement of this incision is easier if initial access was obtained via the Hasson technique. All of the other ports are then removed from the abdominal wall under direct vision to ensure that there is no bleeding. All residual CO_2 should be removed to prevent postoperative shoulder pain. The fascial opening at the umbilicus should be sutured closed to prevent subsequent herniation, and all skin incisions should be closed.

Need for Drainage

The decision to place a drain after laparoscopic cholecystectomy should be governed by the same principles applied to patients undergoing open cholecystectomy. There are two main indications for drainage: (1) the cystic duct was not closed securely, and (2) the CBD was explored by either a direct or a transcystic approach.

Drain placement is easily accomplished. A closed suction drain is inserted intra-abdominally through the 10 mm operative port. A grasping forceps placed through the right lateral port is used to pull one end of the drain out through the abdominal wall. The other end is then positioned according to the surgeon's preference, usually in the subhepatic space.

Complications

INTRAOPERATIVE

Veress Needle Injury

A syringe must always be attached to the Veress needle, and fluid must be aspirated before insufflation is initiated: failure to do so may lead to insufflation into a vessel and consequently to massive gas embolism. If the aspirate from the syringe attached to the Veress needle contains copious amounts of blood, a major vascular injury may have occurred, and immediate laparotomy is indicated. Because the problem at this point is a needle injury, it can usually be repaired easily and without serious sequelae.

Puncture of the bowel by a Veress needle is usually signaled by aspiration of bowel contents through the needle. If this occurs, the needle should be withdrawn and the approximate course and direction of the puncture remembered. The initial trocar should then be inserted by means of the open technique, under direct vision, to ensure that the undersurface of the abdominal wall is free of adherent bowel. Once pneumoperitoneum is created, careful examination of the abdomen through the laparoscope is undertaken. In most cases, either further leakage of bowel contents, staining of the serosal surface with bowel contents, or an ecchymosis on the serosal surface of the bowel helps the surgeon locate the site of the bowel injury. If ecchymosis is present without spillage of bowel contents, the bowel loop should be marked with a suture and reinspected at the end of the procedure. If ongoing leakage of bowel contents is noted, the injured loop of bowel can be either repaired by means of laparoscopic suturing or grasped with an atraumatic forceps and gently withdrawn through an enlarged umbilical incision for suture repair. The bowel is returned to the peritoneal cavity and the laparoscopic cholecystectomy completed.

Improper placement of the Veress needle into the omentum, the retroperitoneum, or the preperitoneal space may be signaled by high inflation pressures, uneven distribution of the gas on percussion, or marked subcutaneous emphysema. If such misplacement goes unrecognized, creation of a safe intraperitoneal space is impossible, and subsequent blind insertion of the trocar may result in injury to an intraperitoneal structure.

Trocar Injury

Trocar injury to blood vessels or bowel is much more dangerous than Veress needle injury to the same structures. Major vascular injuries virtually never occur when trocars are placed under direct vision; however, they remain a potentially lethal—though rare—complication of percutaneous trocar insertion. If active bleeding follows removal of the trocar from the cannula, prompt laparotomy is mandatory; if bleeding passes unnoticed and insufflation begins, massive air embolism will result. At the time of laparotomy, both the anterior and the posterior wall of the vessel must be examined after proximal and distal control of the vessel have been obtained.

Bowel injuries can result from either percutaneous or open insertion of the initial trocar. With open insertion, the bowel injury should be immediately obvious and can be repaired after the injured bowel is pulled through an enlarged umbilical incision; laparoscopic cholecystectomy can then proceed. Bowel injuries caused by percutaneous insertion may occur even in the absence of abdominal wall adhesions and can be managed in the same way as those caused by open insertion. The one caveat is that it is possible to spear the bowel in a through-and-through fashion so that when the laparoscope is inserted through the trocar, the view is normal and the injury is not recognized. This type of injury can be diagnosed only if the laparoscope is repositioned to the operating port at some time during the procedure and the undersurface of the umbilical site is carefully examined. This step is mandatory during the course of the operation, preferably early.

Bleeding

Abdominal wall Bleeding from the abdominal wall can usually be prevented by careful trocar placement. The abdominal wall should be transilluminated before percutaneous trocar insertion and the larger vessels avoided. If a vessel is speared, the cannula usually tamponades the bleeding reasonably effectively during the procedure.

Once the procedure is completed, each trocar is removed under direct vision. If bleeding follows the removal of a trocar, the puncture hole can be occluded with digital pressure to maintain pneumoperitoneum and the bleeding controlled by cauterization or suture repair. Alternatively, the surgeon may place a Foley catheter through the trocar site with a stylet, inflate the balloon, and place traction on the catheter for 4 to 6 hours; however, tissue ischemia can make this technique quite painful.

Omental or mesenteric adhesions Generally, omental adhesions can be bluntly teased from their attachments to the gallbladder, with the plane of dissection kept close to the gallbladder, where the adhesions are less vascular. Adhesions to the liver should be taken down with the electrocautery to prevent capsular tears. Persistent bleeding from omental adhesions is unusual but can be managed by means of electrocauterization (with care taken to avoid damage to the duodenum or colon) or the application of hemostatic clips or a pretied ligating loop.

Cystic artery branch Arterial bleeding encountered during dissection in Calot's triangle is usually due to loss of control of the cystic artery or one of its branches. Biliary surgeons must be aware of the many anatomic variations in the vasculature of the gallbladder and the liver. Because the main cystic artery frequently branches, it is common to find more than one artery if dissection is maintained close to the gallbladder. If what seems to be the main cystic artery is small, a posterior cystic artery may be present and may have to be clipped during the dissection.

Prevention of arterial bleeding begins by dissecting the artery carefully and completely before clipping and by inspecting of the clips to ensure that they are placed completely across the artery without incorporating additional tissue (e.g., a posterior cystic artery or right hepatic artery). When arterial bleeding is encountered, it is essential to maintain adequate exposure and to avoid blind application of hemostatic clips or cauterization. The laparoscope should be withdrawn slightly so that the lens is not spattered with blood. The surgeon should then pass an atraumatic grasping forceps through a port other than the operating port and attempt to grasp the bleeding vessel. An additional trocar may have to be inserted for simultaneous suction-irrigation. Once proximal control is obtained, the operative field should be suctioned and irrigated to improve exposure. Hemostatic clips are then applied under direct vision; in addition, a sponge may be introduced to apply pressure to the bleeding vessel. Conversion to open cholecystectomy is indicated whenever bleeding cannot be promptly controlled laparoscopically.

Liver bed Bleeding from the liver bed may be encountered when the wrong plane is developed during dissection of the gallbladder. Patients who have portal hypertension, cirrhosis, or coagulation disorders are at particularly high risk. Control of bleeding requires good exposure, accomplished via lateral and superior retraction of the gallbladder; hence, all bleeding should be controlled before the gallbladder is detached from the liver bed. Most liver bed bleeding can be controlled with the electrocautery, and

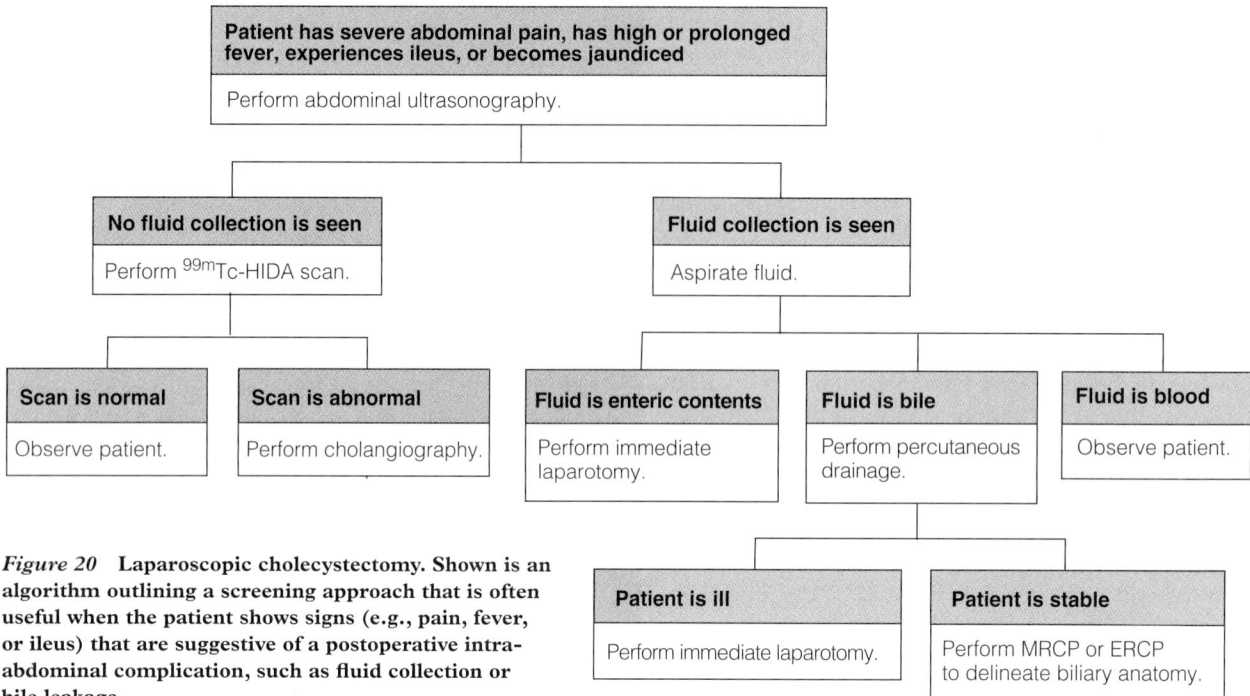

Figure 20 Laparoscopic cholecystectomy. Shown is an algorithm outlining a screening approach that is often useful when the patient shows signs (e.g., pain, fever, or ileus) that are suggestive of a postoperative intra-abdominal complication, such as fluid collection or bile leakage.

it should be controlled as it is encountered to allow exposure of the specific bleeding site. Either a hook-shaped or a spatula-shaped coagulation electrode is effective. If oozing continues, oxidized cellulose can be placed as a pack through the operative port and pressure applied on the raw surface of the liver. If needed, fibrin glue can be applied to the bleeding raw surface.

POSTOPERATIVE

If a patient (1) complains of a great deal of abdominal pain necessitating systemic narcotics, (2) has a high or prolonged fever, (3) experiences ileus, or (4) becomes jaundiced, an intra-abdominal complication may have occurred. Blood should be drawn so that the white blood cell count, the hemoglobin concentration, liver function, and the serum amylase level can be assessed. Abdominal ultrasonography may help diagnose dilated intrahepatic ducts and subhepatic fluid collections [see Figure 20].

Fluid Collection or Bile Leakage

When a significant fluid collection is seen, it should be aspirated percutaneously under ultrasonographic guidance. If the fluid is blood and the patient is hemodynamically stable and requires no transfusion, observation of the patient and culture of the fluid are usually sufficient. If the fluid is enteric contents, immediate laparotomy is indicated. If the fluid is bile and the patient is ill, immediate laparotomy should be considered; if the patient is stable and the appropriate facilities are available, MRCP or ERCP may be performed to identify the site of bile leakage, determine whether obstruction is also present, and assess the integrity of the extrahepatic biliary tree. If the bile ducts are in continuity and the bile is coming from the cystic duct stump or a small lateral tear in the bile duct, ES, with or without stenting, usually controls the leak. Percutaneous placement of a drain under ultrasonographic guidance allows control of the bile leakage and measurement of the quantity of fluid present.

Fever

Postoperative fever is a common complication of laparoscopic cholecystectomy. As noted, it may be indicative of a postopera-

tive complication such as a bile collection or bile leakage. Other common reasons for postoperative fever (e.g., atelectasis) should also be considered.

Abnormal Liver Function

When postoperative blood tests indicate significantly abnormal liver function, possible causes include injury to the biliary tree and retained CBD stones [see Figure 21]. Cholangiography is required, even if it was performed intraoperatively. If MRCP or ERCP yields normal results, observation is sufficient; the abnormalities may be attributable to a passed stone or drug-related cholestasis. If stones are present, ES can usually solve the problem. If ERCP demonstrates extravasation of bile, it is important to establish whether the CBD is in continuity. If the duct is interrupted, early reoperation, ideally at a specialized center, is the best option. If the duct is in continuity, endoscopic and radiologic techniques may successfully resolve the problem without substantial morbidity. Percutaneous drainage is instituted to control the fistula, and sphincterotomy or stenting is useful to overcome any resistance at the sphincter of Oddi. Any retained stones causing distal obstruction should also be removed.

Major ductal injuries usually call for operative repair. When such an injury is identified at operation, the surgeon must decide whether to attempt repair immediately or not; this decision should be based on the surgeon's experience with reconstructive biliary surgery and on the local expertise available. At a minimum, adequate drainage must be established. Most major ductal injuries are not in fact identified intraoperatively. When such an injury is identified postoperatively, adequate drainage must be established and the anatomy of the injury clarified as well as possible before repair. MRCP or transhepatic cholangiography may be required to delineate the anatomy of the proximal biliary tree when ERCP does not opacify the biliary tract above the injury. If surgical repair is indicated, it should be performed by a surgeon experienced in complex biliary tract procedures. Often, referral to a specialized center is the most appropriate decision, especially in the case of more proximal biliary injuries.

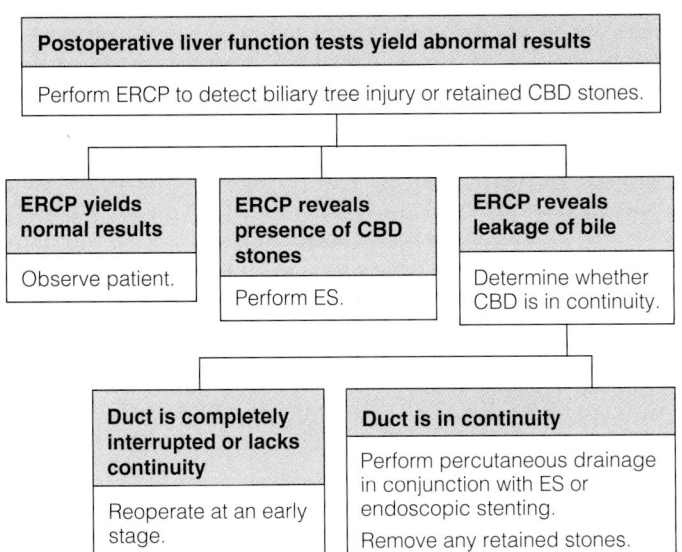

Postoperative liver function tests yield abnormal results

Perform ERCP to detect biliary tree injury or retained CBD stones.

ERCP yields normal results

Observe patient.

ERCP reveals presence of CBD stones

Perform ES.

ERCP reveals leakage of bile

Determine whether CBD is in continuity.

Duct is completely interrupted or lacks continuity

Reoperate at an early stage.

Duct is in continuity

Perform percutaneous drainage in conjunction with ES or endoscopic stenting. Remove any retained stones.

Figure 21 **Laparoscopic cholecystectomy. Shown is an algorithm outlining an approach to abnormal liver function test results after laparoscopic cholecystectomy.**

Special Problems

CONVERSION TO LAPAROTOMY

Conversion from laparoscopy to laparotomy may be required in any laparoscopic cholecystectomy, in accordance with the judgment of the surgeon. The most common reason for such conversion is the inability to identify important anatomic structures in the region of the gallbladder. Distorted anatomy may be the result of previous operations, inflammation, or anatomic variations. Conversion may also be required because of an intraoperative complication [*see* Complications, Postoperative, *above*]. Ideally, the surgeon would wish to convert before any complication occurs. It must be emphasized that conversion to open surgery should not be considered a failure or a complication. Rather, it should be considered a prudent maneuver for achieving the desired objective—namely, safe removal of the gallbladder. Accordingly, every patient consent obtained for a laparoscopic cholecystectomy must explicitly allow for the possibility of conversion to an open procedure.

Attempts have been made to predict the probability of conversion on the basis of preoperative information. It is clearly useful to stratify patients according to likelihood of conversion. This information is helpful in selecting patients for laparoscopic cholecystectomy in an outpatient versus hospital setting, in determining the resources required in the OR, and in assisting patients in planning their work and family needs around the time of surgery.

Factors found to be predictive of an increased probability of conversion include acute cholecystitis, either at the time of surgery or at any point in the past; age greater than 65 years; male sex; and thickening of the gallbladder wall to more than 3 mm as measured by ultrasonography. Other factors more variably associated with an increased likelihood of conversion are obesity, previous upper abdominal operations (especially gastroduodenal), multiple gallbladder attacks over a long period, and severe pancreatitis. Factors not associated with an increased likelihood of conversion are jaundice, previous ES, previous lower abdominal procedures, stomas, mild pancreatitis, and diabetes.

On the basis of our data, a 45-year-old woman with no history of acute cholecystitis and no gallbladder wall thickening has a probability of conversion lower than 1%; such a patient is a good candidate for laparoscopic cholecystectomy in an outpatient setting. Conversely, a 70-year-old man with acute cholecystitis and ultrasonographic evidence of gallbladder wall thickening has a probability of conversion of about 30%; such a patient would be better managed in a traditional hospital environment.

ACUTE CHOLECYSTITIS

Laparoscopic cholecystectomy has been shown to be safe and effective for treating acute cholecystitis. There are, however, several technical problems in this setting that must be addressed if the procedure is to be performed with minimal risk. It should also be recognized that the probability of conversion to laparotomy is greatly increased in these circumstances. There appears to be no advantage to delaying surgery in patients with acute cholecystitis, even if rapid improvement is noted with nonoperative management. Many patients return within a short time with recurrent attacks, and delaying surgery does not reduce the probability of conversion.

Technical difficulties associated with cholecystectomy for acute cholecystitis include dense adhesions, the increased vascularity of tissues, difficulty in grasping the gallbladder, an impacted stone in the gallbladder neck or the cystic duct, shortening and thickening of the cystic duct, and close approximation of the CBD to the gallbladder wall.

The surgeon should not hesitate to insert additional ports (e.g., for a suction-irrigation apparatus) if necessary. Because the tense, distended gallbladder is difficult to grasp reliably, it should be aspirated through the fundus early in the procedure, as previously described. If the graspers fail to grasp the wall or cause it to tear, exposure of Calot's triangle can be achieved by propping up or levering the neck of the gallbladder and the right liver with a blunt instrument. A sponge can be used for this purpose, thereby reducing the potential trauma of the retraction. This maneuver is also useful when an impacted stone in the neck of the gallbladder prevents the surgeon from grasping the gallbladder in the area of Hartmann's pouch. Dense adhesions that may be present between the gallbladder and the omentum, duodenum, or colon should be dissected bluntly (e.g., with a suction tip). Because the tissues are friable and vascular, oozing may be encountered. Electrocauterization should be only sparingly employed until the vital structures in Calot's triangle are identified. Instead, the surgeon should move to another area of dissection, allowing most of the oozing to coagulate on its own. Liberal use of suction and irrigation will keep the operative field free of blood.

In the identification of anatomic structures, it is important to keep dissection close to the gallbladder wall, working down from the gallbladder toward Calot's triangle. Dissection of the lower part of the gallbladder from the liver bed early in the operation may aid in identification of the gallbladder neck–cystic duct junction (analogous to an open, retrograde dissection). The surgeon should be aware that edema and acute inflammation may cause foreshortening of the cystic duct. If the anatomy cannot be identified, preliminary cholangiography through the emptied gallbladder may indicate the position of the cystic duct and the CBD.

Often, the obstructing stone responsible for the acute attack is in the neck of the gallbladder; thus, the cystic duct will be normal and easily secured with clips. If the stone is in the cystic duct, it must be removed before the duct is clipped or ligated. A thickened, edematous cystic duct is better controlled by ligation with an extracorporeal tie or a ligating loop than by clipping. If closure of the cystic duct is tenuous, closed suction drainage is advisable. Obviously, conversion to open cholecystectomy is indicated if the anatomy remains obscure. Conversion should also be considered if no progress is made after a predesignated period (e.g., 15 minutes) because at this point, the surgeon is unlikely to make any headway.

CBD STONES

Identification of Patients at Risk

About 10% of all patients undergoing cholecystectomy for gallstones will also have choledocholithiasis. To select from the various diagnostic and therapeutic options for managing choledocholithiasis, it is helpful to know preoperatively whether the patient is at high, moderate, or low risk for stones. Patients with obvious clinical jaundice or cholangitis, a dilated CBD, or stones visualized in the CBD on preoperative ultrasonography are likely to have choledocholithiasis (risk > 50%). Patients who have a history of jaundice or pancreatitis, elevated preoperative levels of alkaline phosphatase or bilirubin, or ultrasonographic evidence of multiple small gallstones are somewhat less likely to have choledocholithiasis (risk, 10% to 50%). Patients with large gallstones, no history of jaundice or pancreatitis, and normal liver function are unlikely to have choledocholithiasis (risk < 5%).

Diagnostic and Therapeutic Options

One argument for routine intraoperative cholangiography is that it is a good way of identifying unsuspected CBD stones. However, more selective approaches to diagnosing choledocholithiasis make use of preoperative cholangiography via MRCP, EUS, or, more invasively, ERCP [*see 3:8 Gastrointestinal Endoscopy*]. Preoperative identification of choledocholithiasis allows the surgeon to attempt preoperative clearance of the CBD by means of ES or intraoperative clearance during laparoscopy, depending on his or her expertise. Preoperative cholangiography is suggested when the patient's history and the results of laboratory and diagnostic tests suggest that there is a moderate or high risk of CBD stones. It is our practice to have patients at high risk for CBD stones undergo ERCP and ES if warranted. For patients at moderate risk, MRCP or EUS is done first, followed by therapeutic ERCP if CBD stones are identified. Intraoperative cholangiography can also be used to identify choledocholithiasis. ERCP with ES may result in pancreatitis, perforation, or bleeding and carries a mortality of approximately 0.2%.

When stones are detected during the operation, the options include laparoscopic transcystic duct exploration, laparoscopic choledochotomy and CBD exploration, open CBD exploration, and postoperative ERCP/ES. If a single small (2 mm) stone is visualized, it can probably be flushed into the duodenum by flushing the CBD via the cholangiogram catheter and administering glucagons 1 to 2 mg I.V., to relax the sphincter of Oddi. Even if a stone of this size does not pass intraoperatively, it will usually pass on its own postoperatively.

Laparoscopic Transcystic CBD Exploration

Access to biliary tree The cholangiogram is reviewed; the size of the cystic duct, the site where the cystic duct inserts into the CBD, and the size and location of the CBD stones all contribute to the success or failure of transcystic CBD exploration. For example, transcystic exploration is extremely challenging in a patient who has a long, spiraling cystic duct with a medial insertion. The size of the stones to be removed dictates the approach to the CBD: stones smaller than 4 mm can usually be

retrieved in fluoroscopically directed baskets and generally do not necessitate cystic duct dilatation; larger stones (4 to 8 mm) are retrieved under direct vision with the choledochoscope.

A hydrophilic guide wire is inserted through the cholangiogram catheter into the CBD under fluoroscopic guidance. The cholangiogram catheter is then removed. If the largest stone is larger than the cystic duct, dilatation of the duct is necessary, not only for passage of the stone but also to allow passage of the choledochoscope, which may be 3 to 5 mm in diameter.

Dilatation is accomplished with either a balloon dilator or sequential plastic dilators. Because plastic dilators may cause the cystic duct to split, balloon dilatation is recommended. A balloon 3 to 5 cm in length is passed over the guide wire and positioned with its distal end just inside the CBD and its proximal end just outside the incision in the cystic duct. The balloon is then inflated to the pressure recommended by the manufacturer and observed closely for evidence of shearing of the cystic duct. The cystic duct should not be dilated to a diameter greater than 8 mm. Larger stones in the CBD may be either fragmented with electrohydraulic or mechanical lithotripsy, if available, or removed via choledochotomy.

Once dilatation is complete, the guide wire may be removed or left in place to guide passage of a choledochoscope or baskets. When the choledochoscope is used, a second incision in the cystic duct, close to the CBD, avoids Heister's valve and allows removal of the guide wire. If baskets are used, a 6 French plastic introducer sheath may be inserted through the trocar used for cholangiography into the cystic duct. This sheath is especially useful if multiple stones must be removed.

Fluoroscopic wire basket transcystic CBD exploration Stones smaller than 2 to 4 mm that do not pass with irrigation through the cholangiocatheter after injection of glucagon can usually be retrieved by using a 4 French or 5 French helical stone basket passed into the CBD over a guide wire under fluoroscopic guidance. The baskets can be passed alongside the cholangiocatheter or inserted via a plastic sheath replacing the cholangiocatheter. The basket is opened in the ampulla of Vater, pulled back into the CBD, and rotated clockwise until the stone is entrapped. The stone and basket are then removed together. A Fogarty catheter should not be used, because the stones are likely to be pulled up into the hepatic ducts, where they are much more difficult to remove.

Endoscopic transcystic CBD exploration When stones are 4 to 8 mm in diameter, the helical stone basket wires are generally too close together to permit retrieval. Hence, choledochoscopic basketing is utilized. A 7 to 10 French choledochoscope with a working channel is either passed over the guide wire or inserted directly into the cystic duct. Because the usual grasping forceps may damage the choledochoscope, forceps with rubber-covered jaws should be used. A separate camera should be inserted onto the choledochoscope, and the image it produces can be displayed on the monitor by means of an audiovisual mixer (i.e., a picture within a picture) or displayed on a separate monitor.

Once the choledochoscope enters the cystic duct, warm saline irrigation is begun under low pressure to distend the CBD and provide a working space. The choledochoscope usually enters the CBD rather than the common hepatic duct. When a stone is seen, a 2.4 French straight four-wire basket is inserted through the operating port. The stones closest to the cystic duct are removed first, by advancing the closed basket beyond each stone, opening the basket, and pulling the basket back, thereby trapping the stone. The basket is then closed and pulled up against the choledochoscope so that they can be withdrawn as a unit. Multiple passes may be required until the duct is clear. A completion cholangiogram is done to ensure that the duct is clear and to rule out proximal stones. The dilated, traumatized cystic duct is ligated with a ligating loop rather than a hemostatic clip. If drainage is required, a red rubber catheter can be inserted into the CBD via the cystic duct.

Because of the angle created by the cephalad and superior retraction of the gallbladder, it may be difficult to pass the choledochoscope into the proximal ducts. If a common hepatic duct stone is seen on the cholangiogram, the patient is placed in a steep reverse Trendelenburg position. In this position, any nonimpacted stones may fall into the distal duct for retrieval. It may be possible to pass the choledochoscope into the proximal ducts by applying caudal traction to the cystic duct so as to align it with the common hepatic duct. An additional access port in the right upper quadrant may be needed. If the cystic duct is long or spiraling or inserts medially, this measure may not be feasible, in which case access must be obtained by means of choledochotomy.

Laparoscopic CBD Exploration

Large stones (> 1 cm), as well as most stones in the common hepatic ducts, are not retrievable with the techniques described above. Ductal clearance can be achieved via choledochotomy if the duct is dilated and the surgeon is sufficiently experienced.

The anterior wall of the CBD is bluntly dissected for a distance of 1 to 2 cm. When small vessels are encountered, it is preferable to apply pressure and wait for hemostasis rather than use the electrocautery in this area. Two stay sutures are placed in the CBD. An additional 5 mm trocar is placed in the right lower quadrant for insertion of an additional needle driver. A small longitudinal choledochotomy (a few millimeters longer than the circumference of the largest stone) is made with curved microscissors on the anterior aspect of the duct while the stay sutures are elevated. A choledochoscope is then inserted and warm saline irrigation initiated. In most cases, baskets should suffice for stone retrieval; however, lithotriptor probes and lasers are available for use through the working channel of the choledochoscope. The choice of approach depends on availability and individual surgical experience.

Subsequently, a 12 or 14 French latex T tube is fashioned with short limbs, placed entirely intraperitoneally to prevent CO_2 from escaping, and positioned in the CBD. The choledochotomy is then closed with fine interrupted absorbable sutures. The first suture is placed right next to the T tube, securing it distally, and the second is placed at the most proximal end of the choledochotomy; lifting these two sutures facilitates placement of additional sutures. Intracorporeal knots are preferred to avoid sawing of the delicate tissues. The end of the T tube is then pulled out through a trocar, and cholangiography is performed after completion of the procedure.

Bibliography

GENERAL REFERENCES

Asbun HJ, Rossi RL: Techniques of laparoscopic cholecystectomy: the difficult operation. Surg Clin North Am 74:755, 1994

Barkun JS, Barkun AN, Sampalis JS, et al: Randomised controlled trial of laparoscopic versus mini cholecystectomy. The McGill Gallstone Treatment Group. Lancet 340:1116, 1992

Bass EB, Pitt HA, Lillemoe KD: Cost-effectiveness of laparoscopic cholecystectomy versus open cholecystectomy. Am J Surg 165:466, 1993

Crist DW, Gadacz TR: Laparoscopic anatomy of the biliary tree. Surg Clin North Am 73:785, 1993

Deziel D: Complications of cholecystectomy: incidence, clinical manifestations and diagnosis. Surg Clin North Am 74:809, 1994

Kane RL, Lurie N, Borbas C, et al: The outcomes of elective laparoscopic and open cholecystectomies. J Am Coll Surg 180:136, 1995

Lam D, Miranda R, Hom SJ: Laparoscopic cholecystectomy as an outpatient procedure. J Am Coll Surg 185:152, 1997

Management of the complicated gallbladder. Semin Laparosc Surg Vol 5 No 2. Cuschieri A, MacFadyen BV Jr, Eds, 1998

Mühe E: Die erste: cholecystecktomie durch das laparoskop. Langenbecks Arch Klin Chir 369:804, 1986

National Institutes of Health Consensus Development Conference Statement on Gallstones and Laparoscopic Cholecystectomy. Am J Surg 165:390, 1993

Society of American Gastrointestinal Endoscopic Surgeons: Guidelines for the clinical application of laparoscopic biliary tract surgery. Surg Endosc 8:1457, 1994

Traverso LW, Hargrave K: A prospective cost analysis of laparoscopic cholecystectomy. Am J Surg 169:503, 1995

Wherry DC, Rob CG, Marohn MR, et al: An external audit of laparoscopic cholecystectomy performed in

medical treatment facilities of the Department of Defense. Ann Surg 220:626, 1994

PATIENT SELECTION

Amos JD, Schorr SJ, Norman PF, et al: Laparoscopic surgery during pregnancy. Am J Surg 171:435, 1996

Angrisani L, Lorenzo M, De Palma G, et al: Laparoscopic cholecystectomy in obese patients compared with nonobese patients. Surg Laparosc Endosc 5:197, 1995

Curet MJ: Special problems in laparoscopic surgery: previous abdominal surgery, obesity, and pregnancy. Surg Clin North Am 80:1093, 2000

Curet MJ, Allen D, Josloff RK, et al: Laparoscopy during pregnancy. Arch Surg 131:546, 1996

Fried GM, Clas D, Meakins JL: Minimally invasive surgery in the elderly patient. Surg Clin North Am 74:375, 1994

Lacy AM, Balaguer C, Andrade E, et al: Laparoscopic cholecystectomy in cirrhotic patients: indication or contraindication? Surg Endosc 9:407, 1995

SAGES Committee on Standards of Practice. SAGES Guidelines for Laparoscopic Surgery During Pregnancy. SAGES Publication #0023. Society of American Gastrointestinal Endoscopic Surgeons (SAGES), Santa Monica, California, 2000

Steinbrook RA, Brooks DC, Datta S: Laparoscopic cholecystectomy during pregnancy: review of anesthetic management, surgical considerations. Surg Endosc 10:511, 1996

Tanner AG, Hartley JE, Darzi A, et al: Laparoscopic surgery in patients with human immunodeficiency virus. Br J Surg 81:1647, 1994

ESTABLISHMENT OF PNEUMOPERITONEUM

Bhoyrul S, Vierra MA, Nezhat CR, et al: Trocar injuries in laparoscopic surgery. J Am Coll Surg 192:677, 2001

Sigman HH, Fried GM, Garzon J, et al: Risks of blind

versus open approach to celiotomy for laparoscopic surgery. Surg Laparosc Endosc 3:296, 1993

CHOLANGIOGRAPHY AND THE MANAGEMENT OF COMMON BILE DUCT STONES

Abboud PC, Malet PF, Berlin JA, et al: Predictors of common bile duct stones prior to cholecystectomy: a meta-analysis. Gastrointest Endosc 44:450, 1996

Barkun AN, Barkun JS, Fried GM, et al: Useful predictors of bile duct stones in patients undergoing laparoscopic cholecystectomy. McGill Gallstone Treatment Group. Ann Surg 220:32, 1994

Barkun JS, Fried GM, Barkun AN, et al: Cholecystectomy without operative cholangiography: implications for common bile duct injury and retained common bile duct stones. Ann Surg 218:371, 1993

Clair DG, Brooks DC: Laparoscopic cholangiography: the case for a selective approach. Surg Clin North Am 74:961, 1994

Cotton PB: Endoscopic retrograde cholangiopancreatography and laparoscopic cholecystectomy. Am J Surg 165:474, 1993

Crawford DL, Phillips EH: Laparoscopic common duct exploration. World J Surg 23:343, 1999

Cuschieri A, Lezoche E, Morino M, et al: E.A.E.S. multicenter prospective randomised trial comparing two-stage vs single-stage management of patients with gallstone disease and ductal calculi. Surg Endosc 13:952, 1999

Freeman ML, Nelson DB, Sherman S, et al: Complications of endoscopic biliary sphincterotomy. N Engl J Med 335:909, 1996

Guibaud L, Bret PM, Reinhold C, et al: Bile duct obstruction and choledocholithiasis: diagnosis with MR cholangiography. Radiology 197:109, 1995

Halpin VJ, Dunnegan D, Soper NJ: Laparoscopic intracorporeal ultrasound vs fluoroscopic intraoperative cholangiography. Surg Endosc 16:336, 2002

Hunter JG, Trus T: Laparoscopic cholecystectomy,

intraoperative cholangiography, and common bile duct exploration. Mastery of Surgery, 3rd ed, Nyhus LM, Baker RJ, Fischer JE, Eds. Little, Brown & Co, New York, 1997

Hunter JG: Laparoscopic transcystic common bile duct exploration. Am J Surg 163:53, 1992

Hunter JG, Soper NJ: Laparoscopic management of bile duct stones. Surg Clin North Am 72:1077, 1992

Jones DB, Soper NJ: Common duct stones. Current Surgical Therapy, 5th ed, Cameron JL, Ed. Mosby-Year Book, St. Louis, 1995

Korman J, Cosgrove J, Furman M, et al: The role of endoscopic retrograde cholangiopancreatography and cholangiography in the laparoscopic era. Ann Surg 223:212, 1996

Liberman MA, Phillips EH, Carroll BJ, et al: Cost-effective management of complicated choledocholithiasis: laparoscopic transcystic duct exploration or endoscopic sphincterotomy. J Am Coll Surg 182:488, 1996

Mahmud S, Hamza Y, Nassar AHM: The significance of cystic duct stones encountered during laparoscopic cholecystectomy. Surg Endosc 15:460,2001

Menack MJ, Arregui ME: Laparoscopic sonography of the biliary tree and pancreas. Surg Clin North Am 80:1151, 2000

Musella M, Barbalace G, Capparelli G, et al: Magnetic resonance imaging in evaluation of the common bile duct. Br J Surg 85:16, 1998

National Institute of Health State-Of-The-Science Conference statement. Endoscopic retrograde cholangiopancreatography (ERCP) for diagnosis and therapy. Draft statement, January 14–16, 2002

Ohtani T, Kawai C, Shirai Y, et al: Intraoperative ultrasonography versus cholangiography during laparoscopic cholecystectomy: a prospective comparative study. J Am Coll Surg 185:274, 1997

Park AE, Mastrangelo MJ: Endoscopic retrograde cholangiopancreatography in the management of choledocholitiasis. Surg Endosc 14:219, 2000

Paul A, Millat B, Holthhausen U, et al: Diagnosis and treatment of common bile duct stones (CBDS): results of a consensus development conference. Surg Endosc 12:856, 1998

Petelin JB: Laparoscopic approach to common duct pathology. Am J Surg 165:487, 1993

Phillips EH: Choledochotomy in laparoscopy. Operative Laparoscopy and Thoracoscopy. MacFadyen BV, Ponsky JL, Eds. Lippincott-Raven Publishers, Philadelphia, 1996

Phillips EH: Laparoscopic transcystic duct common bile duct exploration-outcome and costs. Surg Endosc 9:1240, 1995

Phillips EH: Controversies in the management of common duct calculi. Surg Clin North Am 74:931, 1994

Phillips EH, Carroll BJ, Pearlstein AR, et al: Laparoscopic choledochoscopy and extraction of common bile duct stones. World J Surg 17:22, 1993

Rhodes M, Sussman L, Cohen L, et al: Randomized trial of laparoscopic exploration of common bile duct versus postoperative endoscopic retrograde cholangiography for common bile duct stones. Lancet 351:159, 1998

Soper NJ, Brunt LM: The case for routine operative cholangiography during laparoscopic cholecystectomy. Surg Clin North Am 74:953, 1994

Voyles CR, Sanders DL, Hogan R: Common bile duct evaluation in the era of laparoscopic cholecystectomy: 1050 cases later. Ann Surg 219:744,1994

Wu JS, Dunnegan DL, Soper NJ: The utility of intracorporeal ultrasonography for screening of the bile duct during laparoscopic cholecystectomy. J Gastrointest Surg 2:50, 1998

Zucker KA, Josloff RK: Transcystic common bile duct exploration. Operative Laparoscopy and Thoracoscopy. MacFadyen BV, Ponsky JL, Eds. Lippincott-Raven Publishers, Philadelphia, 1996

CONVERSION TO OPEN CHOLECYSTECTOMY

Fried GM, Barkun JS, Sigman HH, et al: Factors determining conversion to laparotomy in patients undergoing laparoscopic cholecystectomy. Am J Surg 167:35, 1994

Sanabria JR, Gallinger S, Croxford R, et al: Risk factors in elective laparoscopic cholecystectomy for conversion to open cholecystectomy. J Am Coll Surg 179:696, 1994

Schrenk P, Woisetschlager R, Wayand WU: Laparoscopic cholecystectomy: cause of conversions in 1300 patients and analysis of risk factors. Surg Endosc 9:25, 1995

COMPLICATIONS OF LAPAROSCOPIC CHOLECYSTECTOMY

Bernard HR, Hartman TW: Complications after laparoscopic cholecystectomy. Am J Surg 165:533, 1993

Branum G, Schmitt C, Baillie J, et al: Management of major biliary complications after laparoscopic cholecystectomy. Ann Surg 217:532, 1993

Deziel DJ: Complications of cholecystectomy: incidence, clinical manifestations, and diagnosis. Surg Clin North Am 74:809, 1994

Deziel DJ, Millikan KW, Economou SG, et al: Complications of laparoscopic cholecystectomy: a national survey of 4,292 hospitals and an analysis of 77,604 cases. Am J Surg 165:9, 1993

Fletcher DR, Hobbs MST, Tan P, et al: Complications of cholecystectomy: risks of the laparoscopic approach and protective effects of operative cholangiography. Ann Surg 229:449, 1999

Halevy A, Gold-Deutch R, Negri M, et al: Are elevated liver enzymes and bilirubin levels significant after laparoscopic cholecystectomy in the absence of bile duct injury? Ann Surg 219:362, 1994

Hunter JG: Avoidance of bile duct injury during laparoscopic cholecystectomy. Am J Surg 162:71, 1991

Jatzko GR, Lisborg PH, Pertl AM, et al: Multivariate comparison of complications after laparoscopic cholecystectomy and open cholecystectomy. Ann Surg 221:381, 1995

Lillemoe KD, Martin SA, Cameron JL, et al: Major bile duct injuries during laparoscopic cholecystectomy: follow-up after combined surgical and radiologic management. Ann Surg 225:459, 1997

MacFadyen BV, Vecchio R, Ricardo AE, et al: Bile duct injury after laparoscopic cholecystectomy: the United States experience. Surg Endosc 12:315, 1998

Martin RF, Rossi RL: Bile duct injuries: spectrum, mechanisms of injury, and their prevention. Surg Clin North Am 74:781, 1994

McGahan JP, Stein M: Complications of laparoscopic cholecystectomy: imaging and intervention. AJR Am J Roentgenol 165:1089, 1995

Millitz K, Moote DJ, Sparrow RK, et al: Pneumoperitoneum after laparoscopic cholecystectomy: frequency and duration as seen on upright chest radiographs. AJR Am J Roentgenol 163:837, 1994

Olsen D: Bile duct injuries during laparoscopic cholecystectomy. Surg Endosc 11:133, 1997

Ponsky JL: Endoscopic approaches to common bile duct injuries. Surg Clin North Am 76:505, 1996

Ress AM, Sarr MG, Nagorney DM, et al: Spectrum and management of major complications of laparoscopic cholecystectomy. Am J Surg 165:655, 1993

Soper NJ, Flye MW, Brunt LM, et al: Diagnosis and management of biliary complications of laparoscopic cholecystectomy. Am J Surg 165:663, 1993

Strasberg SM, Hertl M, Soper NJ: An analysis of the problem of biliary injury during laparoscopic cholecystectomy. J Am Coll Surg 180:101, 1995

Woods MS, Traverso LW, Kozarek RA, et al: Characteristics of biliary tract complications during laparoscopic cholecystectomy: a multi-institutional study. Am J Surg 167:27, 1994

ACUTE CHOLECYSTITIS

Koo KP, Thirlby RC: Laparoscopic cholecystectomy in acute cholecystitis: what is the optimal timing for operation? Arch Surg 131:540, 1996

Lo CM, Liu CL, Lai EC, et al: Early versus delayed laparoscopic cholecystectomy for treatment of acute cholecystitis. Ann Surg 223:37, 1996

Rattner DW, Ferguson C, Warshaw AL: Factors associated with successful laparoscopic cholecystectomy for acute cholecystitis. Ann Surg 217:233, 1993

Zucker KA, Flowers JL, Bailey RW, et al: Laparoscopic management of acute cholecystitis. Am J Surg 165:508, 1993

Acknowledgments

Figures 2, 3, 6 Tom Moore.
Figure 19 Courtesy of Nathaniel J. Soper, M.D., Northwestern University Feinberg School of Medicine, Chicago.

16 BILIARY TRACT PROCEDURES

Bryce R. Taylor, M.D., F.A.C.S., F.R.C.S.(C), and Bernard Langer, M.D., F.A.C.S., F.R.C.S.(C)

Over the past few decades, remarkable advances in imaging technology have been made that allow more accurate diagnosis of biliary tract diseases and better planning of surgical procedures and other interventions aimed at managing these conditions. Operative techniques have also improved as a result of a better understanding of biliary and hepatic anatomy and physiology. In what follows, we describe common operations performed to treat diseases of the biliary tract, emphasizing details of operative planning and intraoperative technique and suggesting specific strategies for preventing common problems. It should be remembered that complex biliary tract procedures are best done in specialized units where surgeons, anesthetists, intensivists, and nursing staff all are accustomed to handling the special problems and requirements of patients undergoing such procedures.

Preoperative Evaluation

IMAGING STUDIES

It is essential to define the pathologic anatomy accurately before embarking on any operation on the biliary tract. Extensive familiarity with the numerous variations of ductal and vascular anatomy in this region is crucial. High-quality ultrasonography and computed tomography are noninvasive and usually provide excellent information regarding mass lesions, the presence or absence of ductal dilatation, the extent and level of duct obstruction, and the extent of vessel involvement. Cholangiography—percutaneous transhepatic cholangiography (PTC), endoscopic retrograde cholangiopancreatography (ERCP), or magnetic resonance cholangiopancreatography (MRCP) [see 3:4 Jaundice]—can supply more detailed information about ductal anatomy and is used when CT and ultrasonography yield insufficient information. Angiography is rarely required to determine resectability. Magnetic resonance imaging and MRCP, which are noninvasive, are preferred where available. As newer MRCP technology becomes available, further improvements in definition of biliary anatomy appear to be obtainable. In the near future, it may prove possible to avoid the complications associated with ERCP (a more invasive alternative), at least for diagnostic indications.

MANAGEMENT OF BILIARY OBSTRUCTION

Although jaundice by itself does not increase operative risk, biliary obstruction has secondary effects that may increase operative mortality and the incidence of complications. There is little evidence to support the practice of routine preoperative biliary drainage in all jaundiced patients, but there are some elective situations in which preoperative drainage is required.

Infection

Patients with clinical cholangitis, whether spontaneous or induced by duct intubation (via PTC or ERCP), should be treated with biliary drainage and appropriate antibiotics until they are infection free; the recommended duration of treatment is at least 3 weeks. In addition, perioperative antibiotic prophylaxis with cefazolin or another agent with a comparable spectrum of activity should be employed routinely before any intervention or operation involving the biliary tract. For certain patients with biliary tract infection (e.g., associated with choledocholithiasis), urgent surgical decompression may be necessary, especially if antibiotics and endoscopic or transhepatic drainage are not immediately effective.

Renal Dysfunction

The combination of a high bilirubin level and hypovolemia is a significant risk factor for acute renal failure, which can occur in the presence of a number of additional factors, such as acute infection, hypotension, and the infusion of contrast material. Patients with biliary obstruction should therefore be well hydrated before receiving I.V. contrast agents or undergoing operative procedures. In patients with acute renal dysfunction secondary to biliary obstruction, decompression of the bile duct until renal function returns to normal is advisable before any major elective procedure for malignant disease.

Impaired Immunologic Function or Malnutrition

Patients with long-standing biliary obstruction have impaired immune function and may become malnourished. Decompression of the bile duct until immune function and nutritional status are restored to normal is indicated before any major elective procedure is undertaken; this may take as long as 4 to 6 weeks.

Coagulation Dysfunction

Prolonged bile duct obstruction may lead to significant deficits in clotting factors. These deficits should be corrected with fresh frozen plasma and vitamin K before an operative procedure is begun. Even if there is no measurable coagulation dysfunction, vitamin K should be given to all patients with obstructive jaundice at least 24 hours before operation to replenish their depleted vitamin K stores.

Projected Major Liver Resection

If resection of an obstructing bile duct tumor is likely to necessitate major liver resection (e.g., a right trisegmentectomy), it may be advisable to decompress the liver segments that are to be retained for approximately 4 to 6 weeks.

Operative Planning

PATIENT POSITIONING

The patient is placed in the supine position on an operating table that can be rotated and elevated. An x-ray cassette and machine should be available during major resections. Slight elevation of the right portion of the chest with an I.V. bag facilitates exposure of the liver and the biliary structures. A choledochoscope and equipment for intraoperative ultrasonography should also be available. Access to a pathology department that can perform cytologic or frozen section examination of tissue is essential in operations intended as treatment of malignant disease.

GENERAL TECHNICAL CONSIDERATIONS

Exposure of Subhepatic Field

A right subcostal incision provides excellent exposure for most open procedures on the gallbladder and biliary tract. For more extensive resections or reconstructions, the right subcostal incision can be extended laterally below the costal margin and across the midline to the left as a chevron incision. In patients with very narrow costal margins, a vertical midline incision may be more suitable for limited operations on the gallbladder and biliary tract, and a combination of a unilateral or bilateral subcostal incision and a midline vertical extension to the xiphoid may be required for more extensive operations. In any case, the incision must be long enough to allow sufficient visualization for safe performance of the procedure.

Adequate exposure and lighting are essential. The best retractors are those that can be fixed to the table while remaining flexible in terms of placement and angles of retraction. Modern high-intensity lights with focusing capabilities and headlamps are especially useful when the surgeon wears magnifying glasses.

Good access to the hepatoduodenal ligament and the structures in the porta hepatis is critical. In patients who have never undergone an abdominal procedure, identification of these structures is straightforward. In patients who have undergone previous operations or have a local inflammatory process, however, there may be considerable obliteration of planes. If this is the case, the following techniques may be useful in defining the anatomy.

1. *Using the falciform ligament as a landmark.* In reoperative surgery, the key to opening up the upper abdomen is the falciform ligament. This structure should be found immediately after the opening of the abdominal wall and retracted superiorly. The omentum, the colon, and the stomach are then dissected inferiorly, and a plane that leads to the hepatoduodenal ligament and the porta hepatis is thereby opened.
2. *Taking the right posterolateral approach.* When the colon and the duodenum are adherent to the undersurface of the right lobe of the liver, separation may be difficult. In most patients, an open space remains that can be approached by sliding the left hand posteriorly to the right of these adhesions and into the (usually open) subhepatic space in front of the kidney and behind the adhesions. Anterior retraction allows identification of the adherent structures by palpation and permits dissection of the adhesions in a lateral-to-medial direction. The undersurface of the liver is thus cleared, and the hepatoduodenal ligament can be approached.
3. *Taking the lesser sac approach.* Ordinarily, the foramen of Winslow is open, and the left index finger can be passed through it from the right subhepatic space. When the foramen of Winslow is obliterated, however, one should approach it from the left, dividing the lesser omentum and passing an index finger from the lesser sac behind the hepatoduodenal ligament to reopen the foramen of Winslow by blunt dissection.
4. *Using the round ligament to find the true porta hepatis.* Patients who have already undergone one or more operations on the

bile duct often have adhesions between the hepatoduodenal ligament and segment 4 of the liver. If one dissects this area via the anterior approach, one may think that the actual porta hepatis has been reached but notice that the hepatoduodenal ligament looks unusually short. In most cases, one can find the true porta more easily by tracing the round ligament to the point where it joins the left portal pedicle (including the ascending branch of the left portal vein) and then following that to the right along the true porta. The adhesions between the hepatoduodenal ligament and segment 4 can then be more easily divided from the left than from the front.

5. *Using aids to dissection.* Usually, structures in the hepatoduodenal ligament can be identified by inspection and palpation, especially if there is a biliary stent in place. In cases in which such identification is not easily accomplished, an intraoperative Doppler flow detector may be useful in identifying the hepatic artery and the portal vein, intraoperative ultrasonography may be helpful in identifying the bile duct as well as vessels, and needle aspiration may also be used before the duct is incised if there is any doubt about its location. Either blunt or sharp dissection is effective in this area. Our preference is to use a long right-angle clamp (Mixter) to obtain exposure in a layer-by-layer fashion; we then electrocoagulate or ligate and divide the exposed tissue.

Guidelines for Biliary Anastomosis

As a rule, biliary anastomoses, whether of duct to bowel or of duct to duct, heal very well provided that the principles of preservation of adequate blood supply, avoidance of tension, and accurate placement of sutures are followed. In preparing the bile duct for anastomosis, it is essential to define adequate margins while avoiding excessive dissection that might compromise the blood supply to the duct. In repairs that follow acute injuries, it is important to resect crushed or devascularized tissue; however, in late repairs, it is not necessary to resect all scar tissue as long as an adequate opening can be made in the proximal obstructed duct through normal healthy tissue and as long as mucosa, rather than granulation tissue, is present at the duct margin. The length of the corresponding opening in the jejunal loop should be significantly smaller than the bile duct opening because the bowel opening tends to enlarge during the procedure.

Mucosa-to-mucosa apposition is essential for good healing and the prevention of late stricture. Sutures should be of a monofilament synthetic material (preferably absorbable) and should be as fine as is practical (e.g., 5-0 for a normal duct and 4-0 for a thickened duct). Because the bile duct wall has only one layer, biliary anastomoses should all be single layer. Sutures should pass through all layers of the bowel, taking sizable bites of the seromuscular layer and much smaller bites of the mucosa, and should take moderate-sized (1 to 3 mm, depending on duct diameter) bites in the bile duct. Interrupted sutures are used when access is difficult or the duct is small; continuous sutures, when access is easy and the duct is larger. Sutures should be securely placed but should not be so tight as to injure the tissues. It is sometimes wise to vary the spacing of the stitches: placing many stitches close together may cause ischemia of the suture line in a postage-stamp pattern. Magnification with loupes is particularly useful in anastomosing small ducts. Stents are not routinely required for biliary anastomoses, and drainage of the operative field is seldom necessary.

There are several principles of suture placement that can be applied to most biliary anastomoses, whether end to side or side to side. When the bile duct opening has a vertical configuration (as in side-to-side choledochoduodenostomy or choledochojejunostomy), stay sutures are placed inferiorly and superiorly in the duct and at corresponding points in the intestine. Traction is placed on these sutures to line up the adjacent walls. The right side of the anastomosis is done first; the bowel is then rotated 180°, and the other side is completed [see Figure 1]. This maneuver may be facilitated by retracting the first interrupted posterior stitch leftward to serve as a pivotal stitch. It is advisable to sew about two thirds of the right wall and two thirds of the left wall, leaving the anterior third of the circumference (the easiest part) to be closed last. This technique can also be used for end-to-side choledochojejunostomy and allows all the knots to be tied outside the lumen. When the bile duct opening lies transversely, as in bifurcation reconstruction, lateral stay sutures are placed first, and the posterior wall stitches are placed from inside the lumen. If interrupted sutures are used, they are all placed individually before any of them are tied, with the untied tails carefully arranged in order. When the posterior wall sutures have been tied, the anterior wall can then be sutured with either continuous or interrupted sutures [see Figure 2].

When the intended anastomosis is intrahepatic and access is particularly difficult because of some combination of an unfavorable position, a previous scar, or, perhaps, a stiff liver that is difficult to retract, another technique may be useful. All of the anterior wall stitches are placed into the duct, grouped together on a single retracting forceps with the needles left attached, and retracted superiorly to promote better exposure of the posterior duct wall [see Figure 2c]. The posterior stitches are placed into the duct and the bowel as described, tied in order, and cut; the anterior wall stitches are then completed by being placed into the bowel and tied.

When the duct is small, there are three techniques that may be useful for increasing the size of the lumen.

1. An anterior longitudinal incision can be made in a small common bile duct (CBD), and the sharp corners can be trimmed to enlarge the opening [see Figure 3a].
2. If the cystic duct is present alongside a divided CBD, an incision can be made in the shared wall to create a single larger lumen [see Figure 3b].
3. If the bifurcation has been resected, two small ducts can be brought together and sutures placed into their adjoining walls to form a single larger lumen [see Figure 3c].

Construction of Roux Loop

When the jejunum is used for long-term biliary drainage, a Roux loop is used to prevent reflux of small bowel content into the biliary system. In the creation of the loop, it is important to select a segment of jejunum with a well-defined vascular arcade that will be long enough to support a tension-free anastomosis. If access to the biliary system will be required in the future (e.g., in an operation for recurrent intrahepatic stones), the loop

a

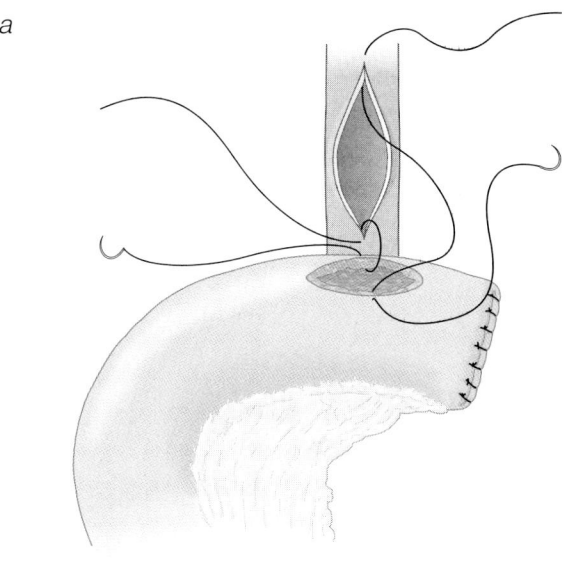

b

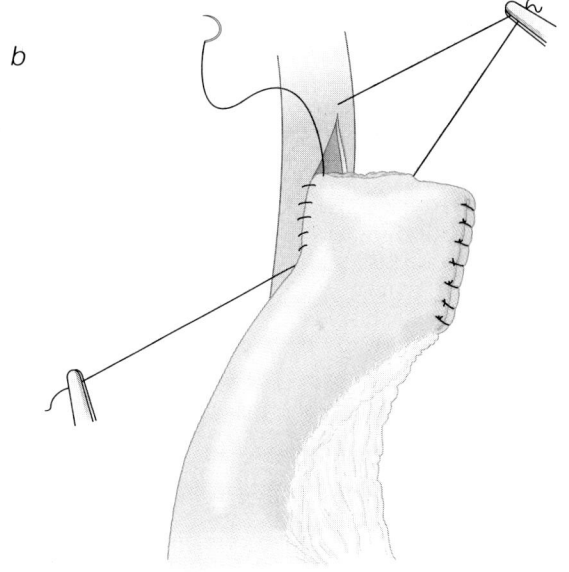

c

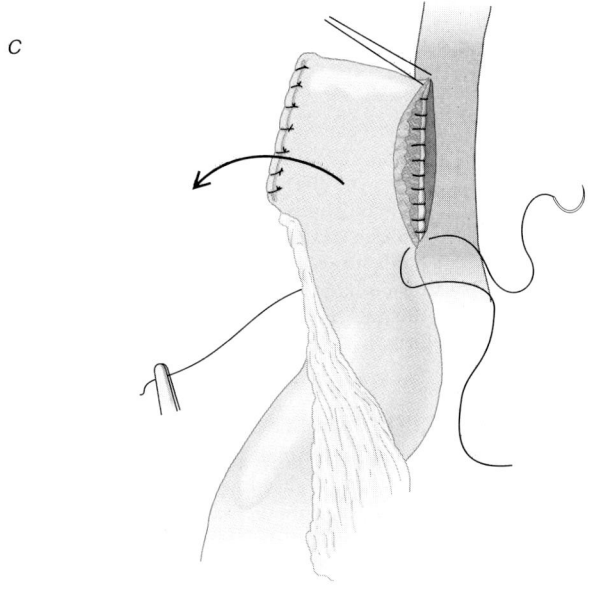

Figure 1 Technical issues in biliary anastomosis. Shown is a side-to-side choledochojejunostomy using a vertical incision in the bile duct. The same technique can be used for choledochoduodenostomy or end-to-side choledochojejunostomy. (*a*) Inferior and superior corner continuous sutures are placed. (*b*) The right side of the anastomosis is sewn. (*c*) The bowel is rotated 180° so that the left side is exposed. The left side of the anastomosis is then sewn.

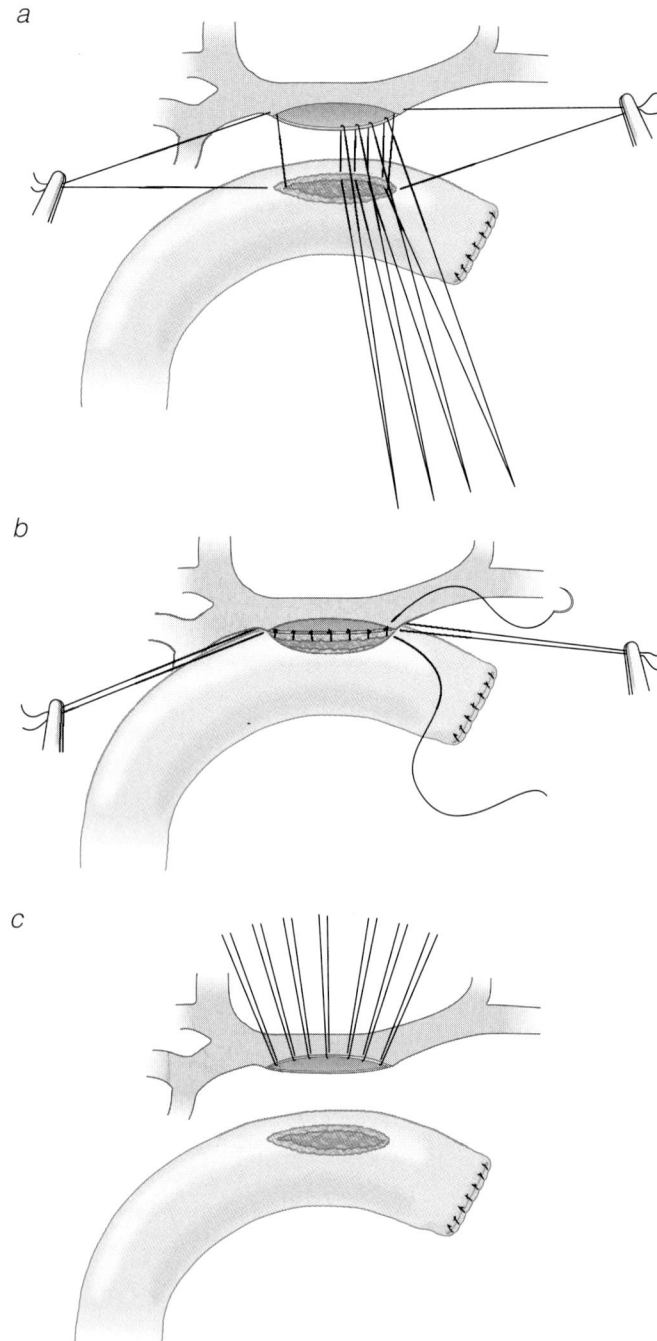

a

b

c

Figure 2 **Technical issues in biliary anastomosis. Shown is an end-to-side choledochojejunostomy using a transverse opening in the bile duct. This technique can be used at any level. (*a*) Corner sutures and posterior wall sutures are all placed before being tied. (*b*) The posterior wall is completed, and the anterior wall is sewn. (*c*) In difficult cases, the anterior wall sutures may be placed first, then retracted superiorly.**

should be long enough to allow one to place a tube jejunostomy, fixing the loop to the abdominal wall with nonabsorbable sutures. The site of attachment should be marked with metallic clips to facilitate future percutaneous puncture and cannulation and removal of recurrent or persistent stones. The tube can be removed after postoperative imaging studies confirm that the biliary tree is free of stones.

Open Cholecystectomy

Most of the cholecystectomies done for gallstone disease are performed laparoscopically [see *3:15 Laparoscopic Cholecystectomy*]. The decision between the laparoscopic approach and the open approach is based largely on operator experience and the technology available. The open method is more likely to be used in pregnant patients and patients with acute cholecystitis or multiple adhesions; sometimes, it is used as part of a major open procedure (e.g., resection of the stomach or the colon or major hepatic lobectomy). It is also used when the presence of a gallbladder tumor is suspected, when a cholecystostomy has already been done, or when there is a recognized cholecystenteric fistula. Surgeons should not be reluctant to choose the open approach whenever they feel, for any reason, that it is safer in a given situation than the laparoscopic approach; conversion of a laparoscopic procedure to the open method for any reason should not be regarded as a complication.

OPERATIVE TECHNIQUE

Step 1: Identification of Anatomic Structures

The important anatomic structures must be identified and the common anatomic variations kept in mind. The cystic duct and the cystic artery are identified by retracting the duodenum to the left and retracting Hartmann's pouch downward and to the right [see *Figure 4*]. The cystic node is the landmark for the position of the cystic artery. The window in Calot's triangle can then be opened between the cystic artery and the liver bed, and the fatty and areolar tissue can be cleared away from the cystic duct and the cystic artery via sharp and blunt dissection. Verification of the identity of the cystic duct is more safely accomplished by dissecting proximally to the duct's junction with the gallbladder neck than by dissecting distally to its junction with the CBD.

Step 2: Cholangiography

Cystic duct cholangiography is ordered routinely by some surgeons and selectively by others. It is mandatory if there is any question about local anatomy or if CBD exploration is contemplated (e.g., for possible choledocholithiasis). Visualization of the CBD on cholangiography is facilitated by elevating the patient's left side on an I.V. fluid bag to prevent superimposition of the bile duct image on the lumbar spine.

Step 3: Excision of Gallbladder

The gallbladder can be removed in either a prograde or a retrograde fashion. The dissection must stay close to the gallbladder wall to minimize the risk of injury to the right hepatic artery (which may be coursing close to Hartmann's pouch) and prevent entry into the subcapsular plane of the liver (which results in bleeding, especially in cirrhotic patients). The cystic artery and the cystic duct must be cleared around their entire circumference before being divided. Once divided, they can be either ligated or occluded with a carefully applied clip. Postoperative drainage is not routinely used.

TROUBLESHOOTING

In the face of chronic inflammation, the planes may be obscured, rendering dissection difficult. The cystic duct may be shortened and the relationship to the CBD poorly defined. In this situation, manual palpation of the cystic duct may allow identification of the relevant structures, especially after one has rolled the tissues between finger and thumb to squeeze out the liquefied fat and edema fluid [see *Figure 5*]. This technique is

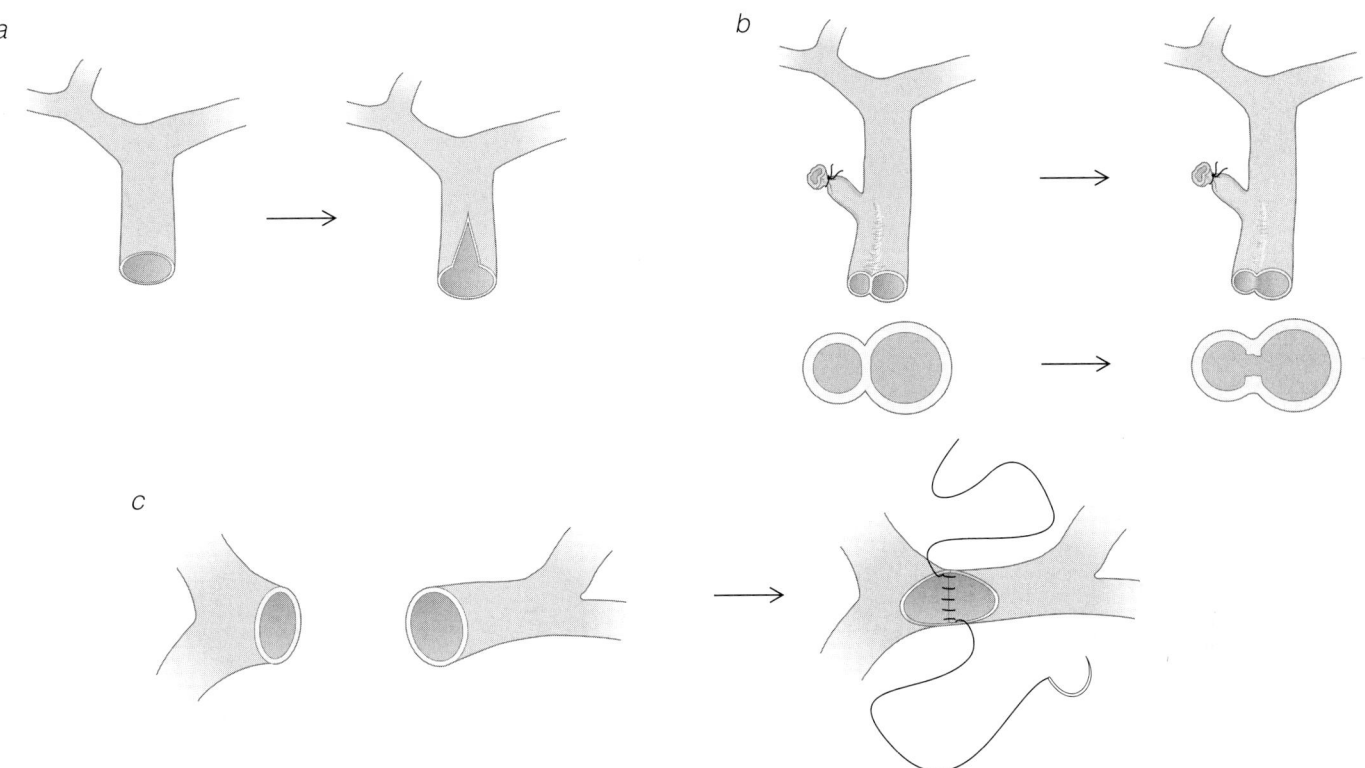

Figure 3 **Technical issues in biliary anastomosis. Shown are three methods of enlarging a small duct. (*a*) An anterior longitudinal incision can be made in the duct wall. (*b*) A wall shared by the CBD and the cystic duct can be divided. (*c*) Adjoining walls of two small ducts can be sutured together to make a single opening for anastomosis.**

especially useful in the presence of acute cholecystitis. When chronic fibrosis is present and the structures cannot be readily identified either visually or with palpation, it may be better to open the gallbladder, remove the stones, and then identify the cystic duct by using a sound in the gallbladder. In the face of extensive scarring or inflammation of the gallbladder neck, removal of the gallstones accompanied by cholecystostomy may be safer than continued dissection without landmarks.

On occasion, it may not be possible to cannulate the cystic duct. In this situation, the cystic duct can be dissected distally, with care taken to ensure that there are no cystic duct stones, and the incision in the duct can be enlarged and dilated gently with sounds. If cannulation is not possible and cholangiography is mandatory, needle cholangiography directly into the CBD should be considered.

Chronic scarring or severe inflammation may make identification of the correct plane between the gallbladder and the liver

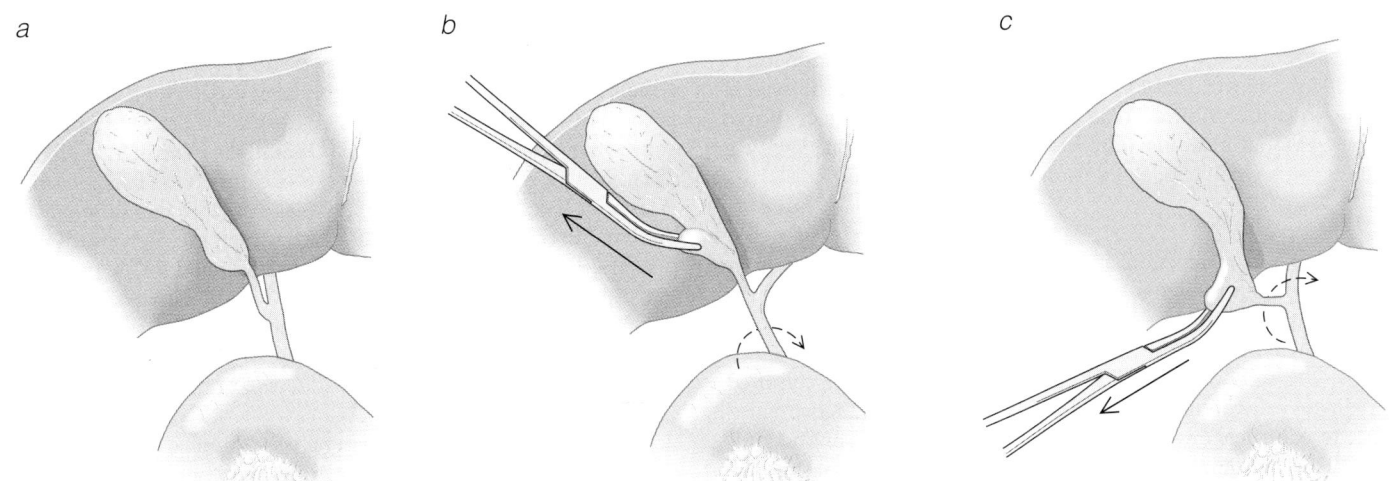

Figure 4 **Open cholecystectomy. (*a*) Shown are the resting positions of the cystic duct and the CBD (with Calot's triangle closed). (*b*) Improper upward retraction of Hartmann's pouch lines up the CBD and the cystic duct so that one can easily encircle the CBD or clamp the cystic duct and the CBD. (*c*) Correct downward and rightward retraction opens Calot's triangle; dissection proceeds lateral to the CBD.**

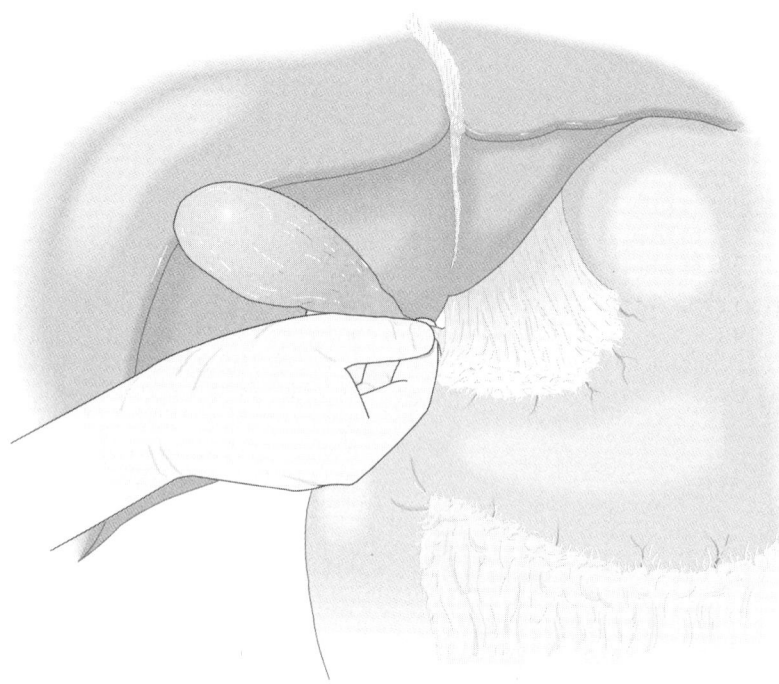

Figure 5 **Open cholecystectomy. Shown is the right finger-thumb technique for identifying the cystic duct and the cystic artery.**

impossible. In this situation, the gallbladder may be opened and the stones removed. Then, with the surgeon's finger in the gallbladder lumen, the gallbladder wall is dissected away from the liver, with the finger used for control. Alternatively, the free portion of the gallbladder wall may be resected, with the part adjacent to the liver left in situ, or the gallbladder may be left in place and a cholecystostomy performed if the cystic duct and the cystic artery are still patent.

As noted, dissection in the subcapsular liver plane may lead to bleeding from the gallbladder bed, especially in cirrhotic patients. This problem can be largely prevented by proper operative technique (see above). If bleeding does occur, however, it usually can be managed without great difficulty. If the bleeding is venous and comes from the liver parenchyma, local pressure should be applied, along with Surgicel or Avitene packing. Surface cauterization is appropriate for smaller vessels, and sutures may be required in cirrhotic patients. If the bleeding is arterial, one should not use the electrocautery or clamps indiscriminately until the source of the bleeding has been accurately identified. A Pringle maneuver should be performed, initially with the fingers and then with a noncrushing clamp, to identify the exact source of the arterial bleeding. The bleeding is then controlled with a hemostat, a small clip, or fine sutures, as appropriate.

COMPLICATIONS

Postoperative infection and bleeding are uncommon complications unless problems were encountered in the course of the operation. Injury to the biliary tract is also an uncommon complication; it can almost always be prevented if the anatomic landmarks are carefully identified before any structures are clamped or divided. Ligation of the CBD will result in obstructive jaundice within a few days. In the case of a transected but not occluded CBD, abdominal symptoms may be mild and nonspecific, and the development of jaundice may be delayed as bile accumulates in the peritoneal cavity. The most useful initial test in a patient with suspected CBD injury is a radiolabeled biliary scan. If a CBD injury is diagnosed, ERCP (with or without PTC) should be performed to define the nature and extent of the injury

before any corrective intervention is initiated. As MRCP continues to evolve, it may prove useful in this setting as well.

Common Bile Duct Exploration (Open)

Most CBD explorations are performed in patients known or believed to have common duct stones; a minority are done in patients with undiagnosed distal bile duct obstruction. Whenever possible, the nature of the pathologic process should be confirmed via cholangiography before exploration is begun.

OPERATIVE TECHNIQUE

Step 1: Identification of Anatomic Structures and Evaluation of CBD

All of the important anatomic structures, including the CBD, the hepatic artery, and the duodenum, must be clearly seen. In a patient undergoing CBD exploration for the first time, the duct usually is easily identified by its slightly greenish-blue color, which is visible through the peritoneum, especially if the patient is thin. In a reoperative situation, exposure of the CBD may be somewhat more involved [*see* Operative Planning, General Technical Considerations, Exposure of Subhepatic Field, *above*]. A limited Kocher maneuver allows the surgeon, standing on the patient's left and using the left hand, to palpate the distal CBD between the fingers behind the pancreatic head and the thumb in front of it. Preoperative evaluation of the duct is desirable; if it is not possible, preexploration cholangiography is advisable, especially in the case of stone disease.

Step 2: Entry into CBD

The CBD is opened by making a vertical incision on its anterior surface to avoid the main arterial blood supply, which runs vertically at the 3 o'clock and 9 o'clock positions. The incision may be facilitated by placing two stay sutures in the duct wall. The opening is then enlarged with scissors to accommodate the largest palpable stone and any exploring instruments required. If the duct is small, care must be taken to avoid the back wall.

Step 3: Extraction of Stones

Many stones can be removed with gentle manual manipulation of the duct. This is done first, and the duct is then irrigated proximally and distally through a 12 or 14 French catheter to wash out mobile stones before any instruments are inserted. Stone forceps, baskets, and balloon catheters are used to retrieve stones identified via palpation, cholangiography, or choledochoscopy. Care must always be taken with these maneuvers: smaller sounds can perforate thin intrahepatic ducts or the lower end of the CBD, and vigorous proximal irrigation can lead to impaction of small stones. The patency of the ampulla is confirmed by gentle passage of a 3 French sound or a filiform catheter through the ampulla and into the duodenum. Dilation of the ampulla with sounds is potentially dangerous and is never indicated.

Step 4: Choledochoscopy

Choledochoscopy facilitates stone extraction with a Fogarty balloon catheter or a Dormia basket and is the most reliable method of verifying complete removal. A flexible fiberoptic choledochoscope yields a good view of the intrahepatic ducts and the distal CBD; in most patients, a rigid right-angle choledochoscope or nephroscope also provides adequate visualization.

Step 5: Closure and Postoperative Care

The incision in the CBD is usually closed over a T tube so that immediate cholangiography can be done to confirm that the duct is clear. If there is concern that some stones might have been left behind, a 14 French T tube should be left in place to allow extraction of stones through the tube tract at a later date. The T tube should take a slightly curved route from the CBD to the abdominal wall—that is, curved enough to prevent dislodgment from the duct by abdominal wall movement but not so curved as to make subsequent percutaneous stone removal difficult [see Figure 6].

The T tube is left to free drainage until GI function has resumed. The follow-up cholangiogram is obtained on postoperative day 4 or 5, and if there is free passage of contrast material into the duodenum with gravity flow only, the tube can be clamped. The T tube may be removed after 14 days (4 weeks if the patient is receiving steroids or immunosuppressive agents), provided that the follow-up cholangiogram is normal. If retained stones are discovered on follow-up cholangiography, the T tube should be left in place for a total of 4 weeks, and the stones should then be removed through the T tube tract or, if this approach fails, via ERCP.

Drainage of the subhepatic space is not routinely required; however, a drain may be left in place if the CBD closure is insecure or if there is concern about persistent distal CBD obstruction.

TROUBLESHOOTING

Impacted stones, either at the ampulla or in the intrahepatic ducts, may resist the usual removal techniques (i.e., manipulation, baskets, and balloon catheters). Distal stones should be removed via transduodenal sphincterotomy at the time of the open operation; proximal stones may be left behind for later retrieval via the T tube tract under direct fluoroscopic control, sometimes with additional help via the transhepatic route.

Instrument injuries can result from excessively vigorous or persistent efforts to retrieve or dislodge impacted stones. For example, a Fogarty balloon catheter can rupture an intrahepatic duct if overinflated, and it can strip duct mucosa if traction is applied when it is overinflated. A Dormia basket can perforate a duct wall if forced past an impacted stone. A CBD sound can make a false passage into the duodenum, the pancreas, or the retroperitoneum if it is forced past an impacted stone or through a tight ampulla of Vater. The primary solution to these problems is simple prevention. All instrument manipulations in the CBD must be done gently. The maxim "If it doesn't go easily, you're in the wrong place" is appropriate here.

The T tube may migrate out of the CBD if there is not enough slack in the tube between the anchoring stitches in the CBD and the abdominal wall as a result of patient movement or abdominal distention. Accordingly, it is important, as noted [see Operative Technique, above], to ensure that the course the tube follows is slightly curved (but not too much so) [see Figure 6].

Choledochoduodenostomy

Choledochoduodenostomy is a relatively straightforward side-to-side biliary-enteric bypass procedure that is effective in certain restricted circumstances and has the advantage of being simpler and safer than transduodenal sphincteroplasty. It is most commonly used in patients with multiple bile duct stones when there is concern about leaving residual stones at the time of CBD exploration as well as in patients with recurrent bile duct stones when endoscopic papillotomy either cannot be done or has been unsuccessful. It is also used in patients with benign distal biliary obstruction (e.g., from chronic pancreatitis) and occasionally in patients with malignant distal CBD obstruction

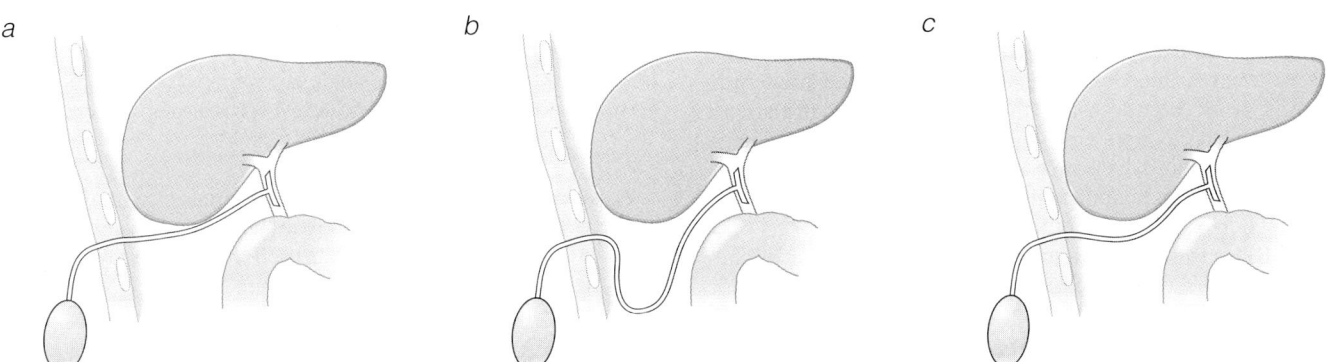

a   *b*   *c*

Figure 6 **CBD exploration (open). Proper placement of a T tube is shown. The route the tube takes should be neither straight (*a*) nor very curved (*b*) but only slightly curved (*c*).**

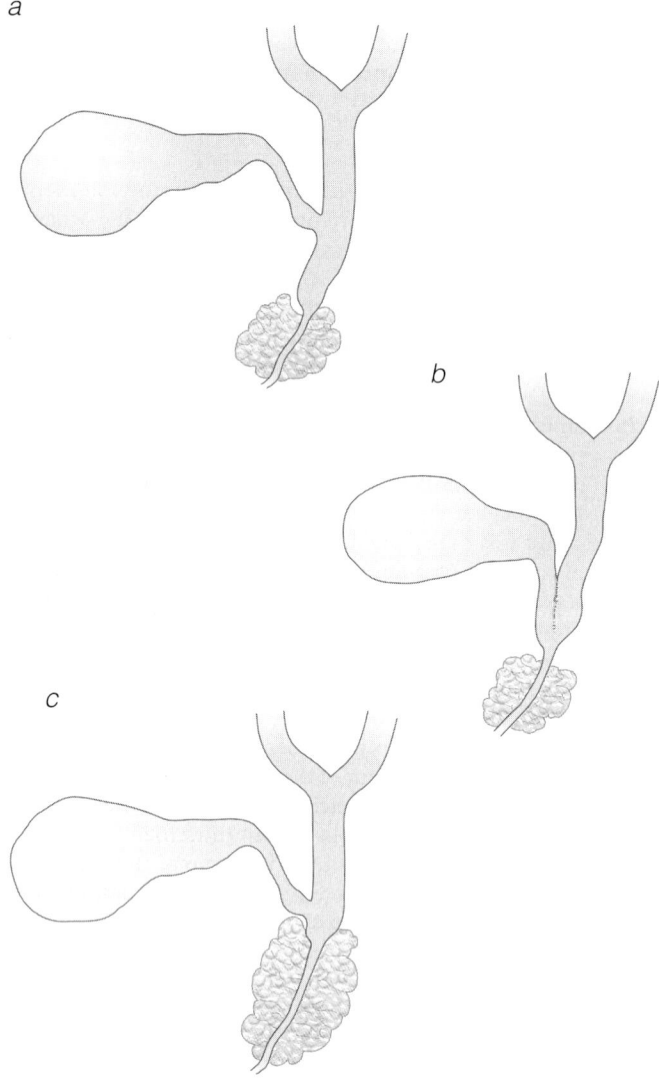

a

b

c

Figure 7 **Cholecystojejunostomy. Cholangiography is essential for determining whether the anatomy is suitable (*a*) or unsuitable (*b*, *c*) for the procedure.**

whose life expectancy is short. Choledochoduodenostomy works best if the CBD is at least 1 cm in diameter; it should not be used in patients with actual or potential duodenal obstruction.

OPERATIVE TECHNIQUE

The duodenum is mobilized to allow approximation to the CBD without tension. Ordinarily, the first part of the duodenum can easily be rolled up against the CBD; however, in patients who have chronic pancreatitis or have previously undergone an abdominal procedure, extensive kocherization may be required. If satisfactory approximation is not achieved with this maneuver, a choledochojejunostomy should be performed.

The CBD is exposed as described earlier [*see* Operative Planning, General Technical Considerations, Exposure of Subhepatic Field, *above*]. Longitudinal incisions are made in both the duodenum and the duct [*see Figure 1*], and the anastomosis is carried out as described previously [*see* Operative Planning, General Technical Considerations, Guidelines for Biliary Anastomosis, *above*].

COMPLICATIONS

Late closure or stricture of the anastomosis may occur if the CBD is small or malignant disease is present. Alternative methods of biliary decompression should be considered in these situations.

Cholangitis related to the presence of food in the CBD distal to the anastomosis (so-called sump syndrome) is an uncommon occurrence. The larger the anastomosis, the smaller the likelihood that this complication will occur.

Cholecystojejunostomy

Cholecystojejunostomy may be performed to treat malignant biliary obstruction in selected patients who are found to be unresectable at operation and whose life expectancy is expected to be short. Occasionally, it is indicated for patients in whom endoscopic or percutaneous stenting has been unsuccessful. This operation is not the preferred procedure for long-term decompression.

Laparoscopic cholecystojejunostomies and choledochojejunostomies have been performed; however, these procedures are still evolving and should be attempted only by surgeons with a high level of laparoscopic expertise.

OPERATIVE TECHNIQUE

Step 1: Verification of Feasibility of Procedure

The cystic duct must be patent. Its junction with the CBD must be at least 1 cm above the tumor obstruction [*see Figure 7*]. The suitability of the anatomy for cholecystojejunostomy may have been verified by cholangiography preoperatively; if not, intraoperative cholangiography via the gallbladder or the CBD is mandatory. If one still cannot be certain that the operation is feasible, the CBD should be opened and a choledochoenterostomy performed. The finding of a bile-filled gallbladder is not sufficient evidence that the patient is a suitable candidate for a cholecystojejunostomy. The gallbladder should be normal: there should be no evidence of cholecystitis or stones. Normal status is verified by inspection, palpation, and, if necessary, needle cholecystography. Finally, for the anastomosis to be feasible, one should be able to approximate the jejunum to the gallbladder easily.

Step 2: Preparation for Anastomosis

A site near the fundus is selected for the anastomosis, and an appropriate segment of proximal jejunum is anchored to the gallbladder with two fine stay sutures in anticipation of a transverse incision in the gallbladder and a longitudinal incision in the antimesenteric border of the bowel.

Step 3: Anastomosis

A 2 cm opening is made in the gallbladder and the adjacent segment of the jejunum, and a single-layer anastomosis is constructed with a continuous monofilament absorbable suture or a stapler.

Step 4: Optional Additional Procedures

A Roux loop, rather than a simple jejunal loop, may be used in the construction of the choledochojejunostomy, and a gastrojejunostomy [*see 3:13 Gastroduodenal Procedures*] may be added in patients with pancreatic head cancer in whom duodenal obstruction is either present or anticipated in the near future.

COMPLICATIONS

Bile leakage may occur if there is excessive tension on the anastomosis. In addition, jaundice may persist if there is unrecognized cystic duct obstruction resulting from inflammation or an unnoticed stone in the cystic duct or the gallbladder. Recurrent jaundice is usually the result of extension from an obstructing tumor that has involved the cystic duct–CBD junction.

Choledochojejunostomy

Choledochojejunostomy, one of the most commonly performed biliary tract procedures, is done to provide biliary drainage after CBD resection, repair of ductal injury, or relief of benign or malignant stricture. To reduce the likelihood of reflux of intestinal contents into the biliary tract, a Roux-en-Y jejunal loop is usually used for the anastomosis [see Operative Planning, General Technical Considerations, Construction of Roux Loop, above]. If long-term access to the biliary tract is required (e.g., in patients with recurrent intrahepatic strictures or stones), the Roux limb may be anchored to the abdominal wall rather than left free in the abdominal cavity.

When the operation is performed after CBD resection, an end-to-side choledochojejunostomy using the proximal transected duct is made. When the operation is performed for bile duct obstruction resulting from tumor or stricture and no resection has been performed, a side-to-side anastomosis is constructed. If a stent has already been placed endoscopically or percutaneously, the bile duct is often thickened.

OPERATIVE TECHNIQUE

Step 1: Preparation for Anastomosis

Preparation for an end-to-side anastomosis includes resection of any crushed or devitalized tissue. The CBD should be trimmed back to healthy, viable, bleeding duct wall. If the lumen of the duct is small, a short incision on the anterior wall will effectively increase its circumference to facilitate the anastomosis [see Figure 3a]. If the CBD has been transected at the level of the cystic duct, the lumina of the CBD and the cystic duct may be combined by incising and oversewing their common wall [see Figure 3b].

If a side-to-side anastomosis is being performed for stricture or tumor, the proximal duct is almost always dilated and has thicker walls, and thus a vertical incision is made on the anterior surface. When the procedure is being done for malignant disease, the incision should be made as high as possible above the malignancy to delay the eventual obstruction of the anastomosis by tumor growth.

Step 2: Anastomosis

When the duct is large, a secure, tension-free anastomosis can be constructed by means of the techniques previously illustrated [see Figures 1 and 2]. When the duct is small, extra effort must be made to place sutures carefully to prevent narrowing of the lumen.

TROUBLESHOOTING

It is essential to preserve the blood supply to the CBD. Adequate debridement of injured ducts is mandatory even if this means extending the resection of the duct to the bifurcation. Incisions should not be made in the medial or lateral portions of the CBD, where the major longitudinal blood supply is found. Finally, extensive mobilization of the duct from the surrounding tissues should be avoided so as to preserve the ductal blood supply.

Meticulous surgical technique is critical for ensuring good healing and preventing stricture. The finest suture material that will do the job should be employed, and magnifying devices should be used to facilitate the accurate placement of sutures. In very small ducts, the temporary placement of a small T tube at the anastomosis will allow most of the circumference to be completed without the risk of either picking up the opposite wall or placing sutures incorrectly. The T tube is then removed and the anastomosis completed. Routine use of postoperative stents is unnecessary but may be helpful in those rare cases in which mucosal apposition cannot be accomplished. In these situations, sutures may have to be placed in surrounding liver or scar tissue in much the same way as in a Kasai procedure. In difficult cases of proximal stricture, the surgeon may incise the liver plate and seek out viable duct above the bifurcation.

COMPLICATIONS

The main complications of choledochojejunostomy are bile leakage, late stricture, and recurrent jaundice as a result of tumor extension [see Cholecystojejunostomy and Choledochoduodenostomy, above].

Transduodenal Sphincteroplasty

Transduodenal sphincteroplasty is often indicated when an impacted stone at the ampulla of Vater cannot be removed via choledochotomy. It is also sometimes useful for clarifying the nature of an obstructive process at the ampulla, definitively treating ampullary stenosis, and gaining access to the main pancreatic duct if ERCP has been unsuccessful. Pancreatic sphincteroplasty may be added in selected cases.

OPERATIVE TECHNIQUE

Step 1: Exposure of Ampulla

Mobilization of the duodenum and the pancreatic head is necessary for obtaining exposure of the lateral portion of the second part of the duodenum. The ampulla is located by palpation, which may be facilitated by passage of a sound down the CBD, out the ampulla, and into the duodenum. A longitudinal incision is made on the lateral surface of the duodenum; it should be at least 3 cm long to ensure good exposure. The duodenal edges are retracted gently. Crushing forceps should not be used; they may cause hematomas.

Step 2: Cannulation

If the bile duct has been opened, cannulation of the CBD is done from above. A metal sound may be used; alternatively, a filiform catheter with a flexible follower may be inserted, and the ampulla can then be gently cannulated and elevated into the field [see Figure 8]. This step facilitates accurate placement of an incision in the ampulla. If the duct has not been opened, cannulation is accomplished from below with a sound. Use of a grooved director may simplify the sphincterotomy.

Step 3: Sphincteroplasty

To prevent injury to the pancreatic duct, the incision in the ampulla is placed at the 11 o'clock position with either scissors or a scalpel rather than the electrocautery. A so-called cut-and-sew approach, using interrupted 5-0 monofilament absorbable sutures placed 2 mm apart, is followed. The incision is started at the papillary orifice and extended above the ampullary sphinc-

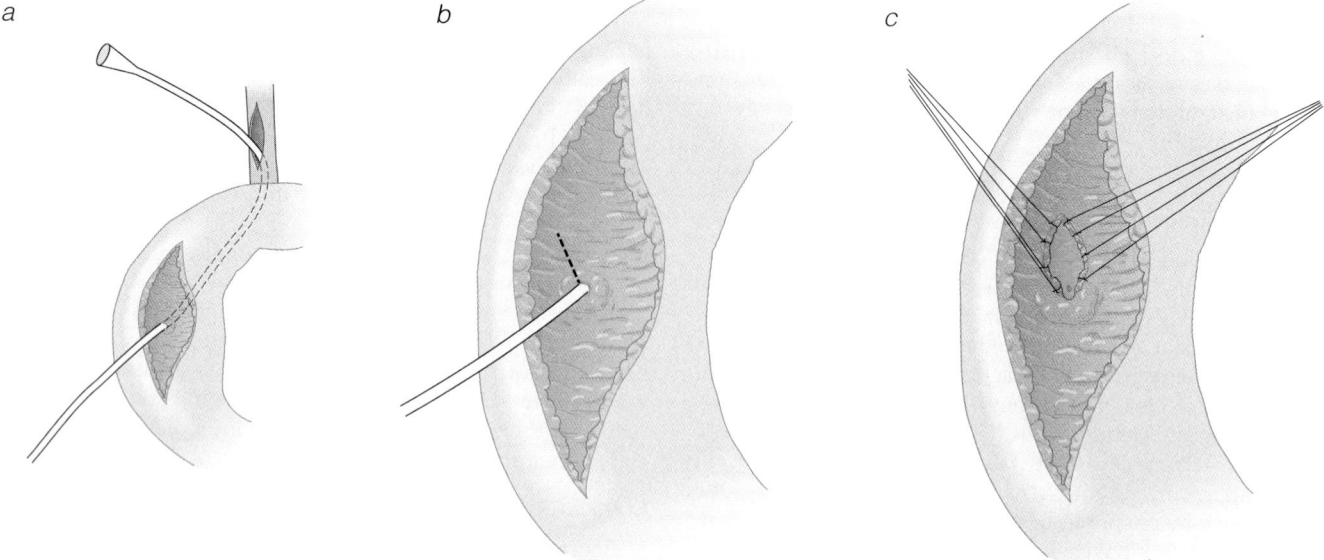

Figure 8 **Transduodenal sphincteroplasty. (*a*) A longitudinal incision is made in the duodenum, and a fili-form catheter and a follower are used to find and elevate the ampulla. (*b*) An incision is made at the 11 o'clock position with scissors or a scalpel. (*c*) Interrupted sutures are placed through the bile duct wall and the duodenal wall. Lateral traction is applied.**

ter. The sutures should include both the bile duct and the duo-denal wall. Once the sutures have been placed, lateral traction is applied to provide exposure of the bile duct lumen and to make each subsequent step in the cut-and-sew procedure easier. The pancreatic duct opening (usually found at the 4 o'clock position) must be identified and protected from being incorporated in the sutures.

Step 4: Exploration of CBD

Exploration of the bile duct should be completed from below with sounds and choledochoscopy to ensure that all stones are removed. If the presence of a tumor is suspected, biopsies of any suspicious areas should be performed.

Step 5: Closure and Postoperative Care

The duodenum is then closed in the direction in which the incision was made. This can be done in either one or two layers, provided that care is taken to prevent inversion and preserve the luminal diameter. Routine drainage is not necessary unless there is concern about the duodenotomy closure or the choledochoto-my closure. If a T tube has been left in place, a cholangiogram should be obtained before it is removed.

TROUBLESHOOTING

There may be an impacted stone at the distal end of the CBD that prevents cannulation from either above or below. Such a stone can usually be felt through the duodenal wall, in which case a vertical incision can be made in the medial duodenal wall directly onto the stone. Once the stone has been extracted, the incision can be extended down through the ampulla with a sound used as a guide.

Occasionally (e.g., in some patients with chronic pancreatitis), a long stricture of the CBD may extend above the ampulla. In such cases, the sphincteroplasty may have to be extended proxi-mally to the point where it communicates with the retroperi-toneal space. This will not be a problem as long as the duode-num-to-CBD repair is carefully executed. If the obstruction cannot be managed with an extended sphincteroplasty, a differ-

ent decompressive procedure, such as choledochojejunostomy or choledochoduodenostomy, must be chosen.

Postoperative pancreatitis may develop if there was excessive manipulation of the ampulla, if the electrocautery was used at the ampulla, or if the pancreatic duct orifice is occluded by one of the sphincteroplasty sutures.

Choledochal Cyst Resection

Choledochal cysts are generally categorized according to the Todani classification [*see Figure 9*]. More than 80% are type I cysts that involve the CBD in its accessible portion. The follow-ing discussion addresses the resection of type I cysts and those type IV cysts that include the proximal right or left hepatic ducts.

Most choledochal cysts are related to an abnormal junction of the pancreatic duct and the distal CBD. Preoperative cholan-giography to clarify the anatomy is important for preventing injury to the pancreatic duct, especially when an intrapancreat-ic resection may be required. Occasionally, intraoperative cholangiography is required to clarify abnormal anatomy. Patients may be symptomatic as a result of stones within the cyst, infection, or malignancy, any of which is an indication for operation. Because of the high incidence of such conditions and the extremely high mortality associated with carcinoma in this setting, prophylactic cyst resection seems justified even in asymptomatic patients.

The objectives of treatment are (1) to remove the cyst com-pletely, along with the gallbladder and any stones that remain in the bile ducts proximal to the cyst, and (2) to achieve free biliary drainage. Resection of a choledochal cyst may be made more dif-ficult by several factors, such as previous operations, recurrent bouts of infection and inflammation in the cyst, and portal hypertension, which may develop as a result of long-standing cholangitis or portal vein thrombosis.

OPERATIVE TECHNIQUE

Resection of a choledochal cyst may be difficult and bloody, especially if inflammation is present. In addition, dissection of a

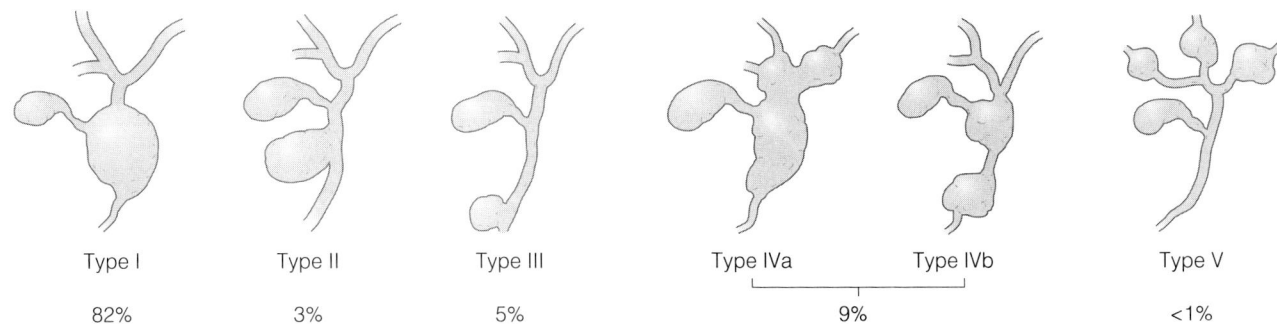

Figure 9   **Choledochal cyst resection. Illustrated is the Todani classification of choledochal cysts.**

choledochal cyst in its intrapancreatic portion may be hazardous because of the vascularity of this region and the difficulty of identifying anatomic structures.

Step 1: Clarification of Anatomy

The proximal and distal extent of the cyst and the presence or absence of stones or tumor may be determined preoperatively, as noted, but in many cases, intraoperative verification of the findings is necessary. Intraoperative cholangiography can be carried out by inserting a catheter through the gallbladder, by directly needling the cyst, or both. If cholangiography does not yield an accurate definition of the anatomy of the cyst, the cyst may then be opened and digital exploration and choledochoscopy used to clarify the anatomy.

Step 2: Initial Dissection

If the gallbladder is still in place, it is dissected free of the liver and left attached to the cyst via the cystic duct, then retracted to the right. If the patient has already undergone a cystoenteric anastomosis, this should be taken down at the beginning of the procedure, and the opening in the bowel should be carefully closed.

Step 3: Mobilization of Cyst

As noted, the vascularity of the region and the presence of inflammation may render dissection difficult. Rather than cleaning off the hepatic artery and the portal vein and dissecting them off the cyst, the surgeon should find a plane immediately adjacent to the wall of the cyst and remain close to it [*see Figure 10*]. This approach differs significantly from the corresponding approach in resection of a bile duct malignancy [*see* Resection of Middle-Third and Proximal Bile Duct Tumors, Operative Technique, *below*]. If necessary, the cyst may be opened and the dissection continued with a finger inside the cyst to yield a more accurate definition of its boundaries. The cyst should be cleared circumferentially in the middle third of the CBD so that a tape can be passed around it and traction applied to separate the cyst from the hepatic artery, the portal vein, and any remaining soft tissue in the hepatoduodenal ligament.

Step 4: Distal Dissection

Dissection then proceeds distally along the wall of the cyst until the junction of the cyst with the normal portion of the CBD is reached. If the intrapancreatic portion of the CBD is involved, the cyst must be separated from pancreatic tissue. There are a number of small vessels that must be individually identified and ligated to minimize the risk of early or delayed bleeding. If the cyst is close to the pancreatic duct junction, considerable care must be exercised not to injure the pancreatic duct.

Step 5: Proximal Dissection

If the proximal common hepatic duct is normal (as in a type I cyst), it is transected above the cyst. If the cystic dilatation includes the bifurcation (as in a type IVa cyst), a small button of proximal cyst is usually left attached to the intrahepatic ducts [*see Figure 11*].

Step 6: Reconstruction

Reconstruction is accomplished via an end-to-side anastomosis to a Roux jejunal loop to minimize the likelihood of reflux of enteric contents into the biliary tract.

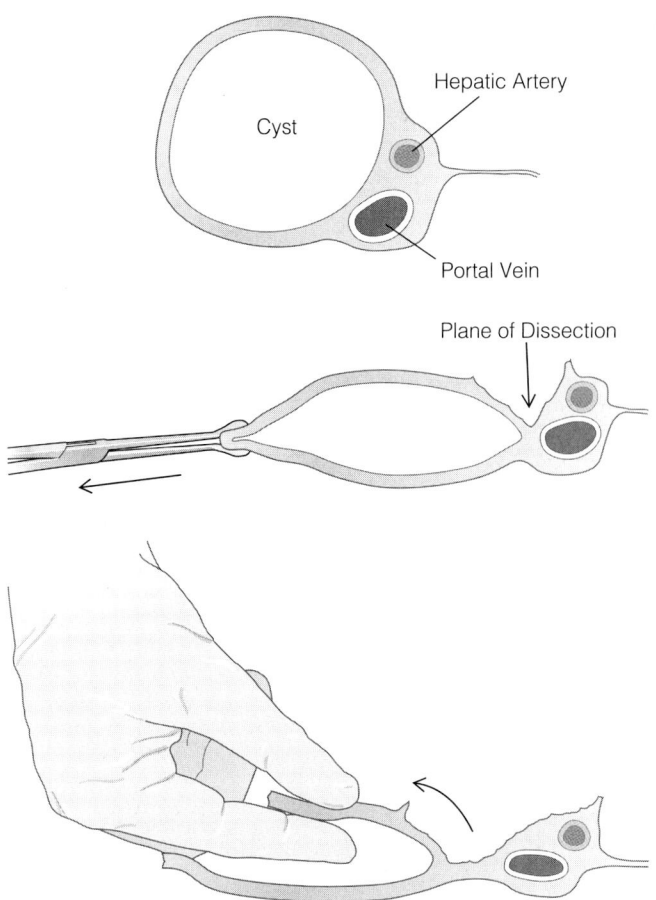

Figure 10   **Choledochal cyst resection. Illustrated is the proper plane of dissection in removal of a choledochal cyst. If necessary, dissection can be done with a finger inside the cyst.**

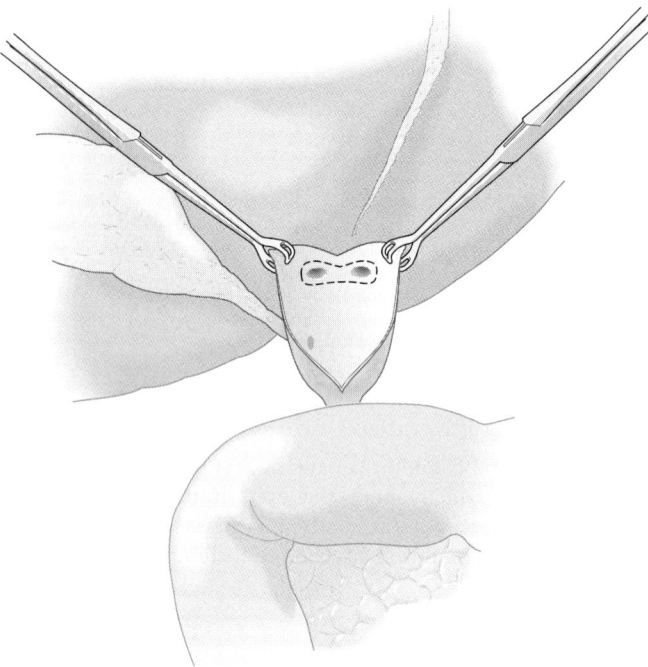

Figure 11 **Choledochal cyst resection. If a cyst extends proximally past the bifurcation (e.g., a type IVa cyst), it may be necessary to open the cyst widely to identify the hepatic duct orifices. A small button of cyst wall is left attached to the hepatic ducts.**

Step 7: Closure

The abdomen is closed in the standard fashion. Stenting is not required, but the area should be drained with closed suction drains if an intrapancreatic resection has been done.

TROUBLESHOOTING

If dissection of the cyst is carried distally into the pancreas, care must be taken to keep from injuring the pancreatic duct. The cyst should be transected as distally as possible, and the end should be carefully oversewn with absorbable sutures. Somatostatin, 100 µg subcutaneously during the operation and every 8 hours for 5 days afterward, should be given to reduce the likelihood of pancreatitis and pancreatic fistula. Occasionally, intraoperative cholangiography is useful to confirm the relationship of the cyst and the CBD to the pancreatic duct.

If the cystic process extends to include the bifurcation (type IVa), the hepatic ducts should be identified from within the cyst and their orifices preserved by leaving a small button of cyst wall in situ; this is preferable to performing an intrahepatic dissection to remove the entire cyst. The presence of this button simplifies and facilitates the anastomosis to the Roux loop.

COMPLICATIONS

Bleeding and pancreatitis are the main early complications of cystectomy. These can be largely prevented by meticulous dissection and ligation of all fine bleeding vessels as well as tissue adjacent to an intrapancreatic cyst. Late stricture of the anastomosis is an uncommon complication but may occur, especially if a small button of proximal cyst is left in place for the anastomosis; this particular complication is considered an acceptable hazard in a difficult situation.

OUTCOME EVALUATION

The immediate expected outcome is the relief of pain, jaundice, and cholangitis and the return of liver function to normal. The long-term expected outcome is the absence of any recurrence of symptoms of stone disease, cholangitis, or malignancy. Because of the rarity of this condition, no good data on the recurrence rate of problems are available.

Resection of Middle-Third and Proximal Bile Duct Tumors

The most common bile duct tumor is adenocarcinoma. Because this tumor responds poorly to irradiation and chemotherapy, surgical resection offers the best opportunity for cure. The appropriate operative approach depends on the location and extent of the tumor [*see Figure 12*]. Tumors in the distal third of the CBD (the pancreatic portion) are treated by means of a Whipple procedure that includes bile duct and periductal tissues right up to the bifurcation [*see 3:18 Pancreatic Procedures*]. Those in the middle third or the proximal third are treated by means of bile duct resection, with or without liver resection (see below).

There are certain basic principles underlying bile duct resection for tumor that must be followed. First, the proximal extent of the tumor must be identified so that the correct procedure can be planned. Preoperative PTC is usually not required for staging if high-quality ultrasonography and MRCP are available. Some authorities advocate bilateral percutaneous drainage to facilitate intraoperative dissection. We do not routinely use preoperative drainage tubes, because of the risk of cholangitis.

Second, given that bile duct tumors spread by local extension to lymphatics, along perineural spaces, and along the bile radicles themselves directly into the liver, wide local excision beyond the visible edges of the tumor is required in the performance of curative resections. In proximal tumors, such excision necessitates resection of the adjacent segments of the liver. The principles of en bloc resection beyond tumor margins must be closely adhered to: dissection into or even close to the tumor must be avoided.

Third, intraoperative biopsy of the tumor should not be done, because of the difficulty of making a firm pathologic diagnosis on the basis of frozen section examination and because of the risk of tumor dissemination.

Finally, given that liver resection is required in most cases, one must be careful to preserve enough healthy liver tissue to allow regeneration of the remnant. If there has been long-standing obstruction, biliary drainage on the side to be preserved is important for recovery of function in that portion of the liver. Some authors advocate preoperative portal vein embolization on the contralateral side to stimulate hepatic regeneration in the segments to be preserved, especially if the future remnant is marginal in size.

In recent years, we have generally become more aggressive in treating proximal tumors, for two main reasons: (1) the accompanying liver resection can now be done with greater safety, and (2) this more radical approach has been shown to yield improved long-term results. For middle-third or type I proximal tumors, we favor resection of the bifurcation in conjunction with intrahepatic cholangiojejunostomy. For types II, IIIa, and IV, we recommend additional liver resection: a right trisegmentectomy (segments 5, 6, 7, 8, 4A, 4B, and 1) for types II, IIIb, and IV and a formal left hepatic lobectomy (segments 1, 2, 3, 4A, and 4B) for type IIIb.

OPERATIVE TECHNIQUE

Step 1: Assessment of Resectability

Before any dissection of the tumor or the CBD is done, a careful search for peritoneal metastases is undertaken. Spread within the liver is evaluated via palpation and intraoperative ultrasonography. Lymph nodes are assessed in the immediate and secondary drainage areas. Biopsies of any suspicious areas outside the planned resection margins are carried out. If tumor is found, stenting or a bypass procedure is indicated.

During dissection, determination of resectability is often difficult, especially with respect to assessment of tumor extension into the liver and the degree of vessel involvement. Therefore, any firm commitment to resection (e.g., dividing the blood supply) should be deferred until resectability is confirmed.

The gallbladder is mobilized from the liver bed by entering the usual plane superficial to the liver capsule without dissecting or dividing the cystic artery and the cystic duct. Exposure is improved by mobilizing the gallbladder and, if necessary, emptying the gallbladder of bile. The gallbladder can also be used as a retractor on the bile duct.

Dissection is then begun from below. The common hepatic artery and the portal vein are identified just above the neck of the pancreas and circumferentially cleared of all tissue. Dissection then proceeds proximally, with the hepatic artery retracted to the left and the portal vein to the right. Adjacent areolar tissue, nerve trunks, and lymph nodes are left in place around the CBD and the tumor [see Figure 13]. As noted, this approach differs from that used in resection of choledochal cysts [see Choledochal Cyst Resection, Operative Technique, above].

Step 2: Division of CBD

Once resectability is confirmed, the CBD is divided at the level of the pancreas. A clamp is placed on the upper end of the divided duct, which is then used as a retractor to facilitate the most proximal dissection of the CBD and the tumor away from the hepatic artery and the portal vein [see Figure 14].

Step 3: Proximal Dissection

With middle-third tumors or Bismuth type I proximal tumors, it is usually possible to palpate the proximal tumor margin and identify uninvolved right and left hepatic ducts. If this is not the case, the possibility of a type II or III tumor should be considered, and complete excision of the bifurcation, with or without part of the liver, should be planned.

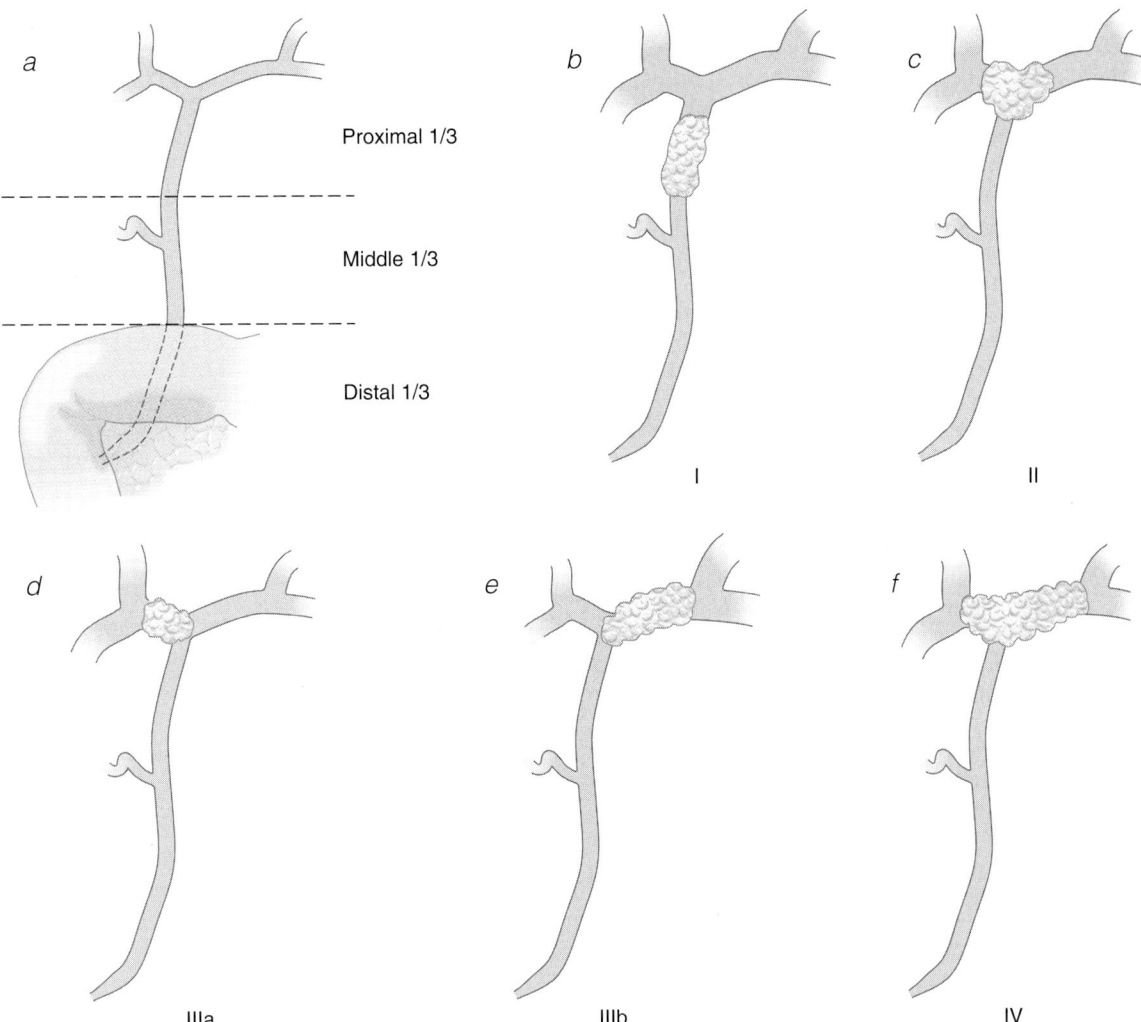

Figure 12 Resection of middle-third and proximal bile duct tumors. The appropriate operation depends on the location and extent of the tumor. (*a*) Broadly, tumors may be localized to the proximal third, the middle third, or the distal third of the biliary tract. (*b* through *f*) Proximal tumors may be further categorized according to the Bismuth classification.

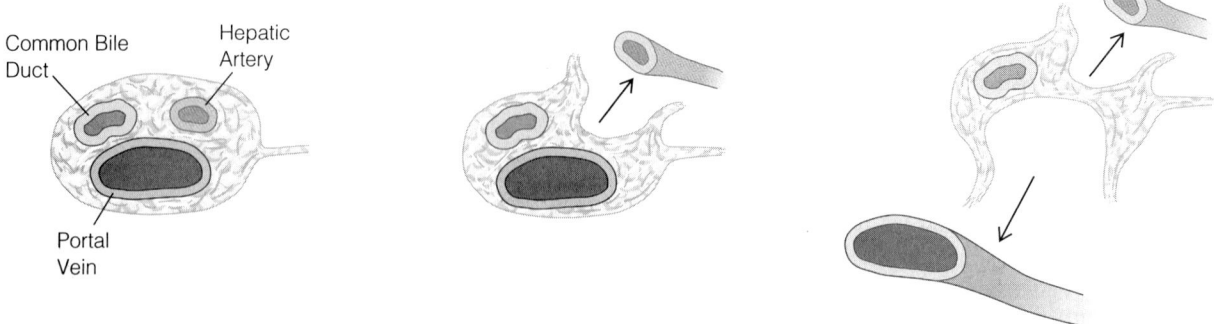

Figure 13 Resection of middle-third and proximal bile duct tumors. Shown is the proper plane of dissection in the removal of a bile duct cancer. Except for the hepatic artery and the portal vein, all tissue stays with the CBD to be resected.

The hepatic artery is dissected by retracting the vessel anteriorly and to the left, dividing and ligating the cystic artery where it originates from the right hepatic artery, and clearing all tissue off the right and left branches at least 1 cm proximal to the proximal margin of the tumor. Involvement of the right or left hepatic artery by tumor is almost always a sign of extensive spread on the corresponding side and an indication for resection of that half of the liver.

The portal vein is dissected by retracting the bile duct and the tumor anteriorly and the hepatic artery to the left. All tissue is then cleanly dissected away from the portal vein to expose the bifurcation and the region proximal to it [*see Figure 14*]. At this point, the duct may be found to be tethered down to the caudate lobe by several small branches. If these branches are clearly proximal to the tumor, they are divided and carefully ligated, and the caudate lobe is preserved. If there is tumor in this area, the caudate lobe is resected along with the bifurcation tumor.

The level at which the proximal bile ducts are transected depends on the proximal extent of the tumor. For all **middle**-third or proximal tumors that are at least 1 cm beyond the bifurcation, proximal resection should usually be above the level of the bifurcation. For type I or type II proximal tumors, proximal resection should always include all of the bifurcation along with the proximal right and left bile ducts out as far as the first major branch [*see Figure 15*]. With type III or IV proximal tumors, the proximal extent of the tumor cannot be determined in both right and left ducts unless the main pedicles are dissected out of the liver. Because these tumors tend to infiltrate locally, such dissection is not advisable. A decision on whether liver resection is indicated should be made at an early stage so that the chances of a cure are not compromised. Intraoperative ultrasonography may help verify the extent of tumor at this point in the operation. Any major liver resection for type III or IV bile duct cancer should include the caudate lobe [*see Figure 16*].

Once the decision to resect part of the liver has been made, the operation consists of dissecting the hepatic artery and the portal vein branch to the part of the liver to be saved away from the tumor area. The hepatic artery and the portal vein branch to the side to be resected are then divided; this allows the tumor to be retracted further and provides better exposure of the duct to the side to be preserved [*see Figures 17 and 18*]. In selected cases, resection of an involved portal vein bifurcation may be carried out at this point [*see Figure 19*]; an end-to-end anastomosis is then fashioned.

The point at which the hepatic parenchyma will be divided is marked, and the parenchymal transection is performed. Division of the hepatic duct (or ducts) to the part of the liver being preserved is done as far from the tumor as possible.

Step 4: Reconstruction

After resection of the bifurcation or intrahepatic bile ducts, an intrahepatic cholangiojejunostomy is performed [*see* Intrahepatic Cholangiojejunostomy, *below*]. The duct tissue is usually healthy enough and the duct lumen large enough to allow mucosa-to-

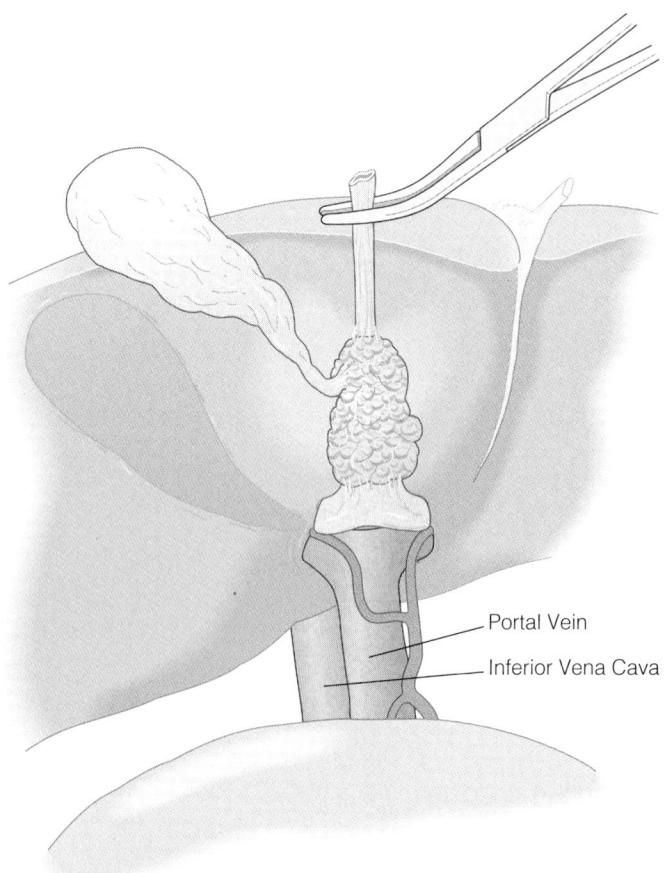

Figure 14 Resection of middle-third and proximal bile duct tumors. When resectability is confirmed, the CBD is transected at the duodenum. The proximal portion of the divided duct is retracted anteriorly, and the CBD is cleaned off the portal vein up to a point above the bifurcation.

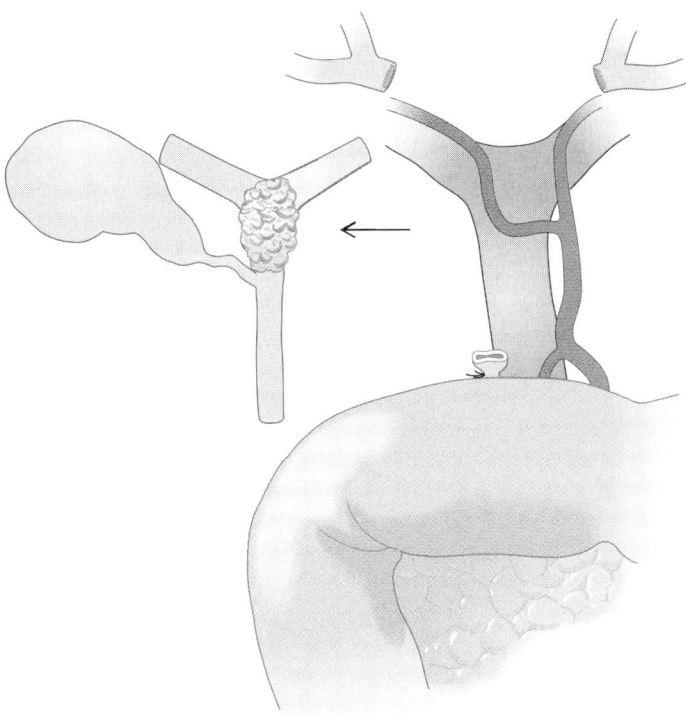

Figure 15 **Resection of middle-third and proximal bile duct tumors. Illustrated is the level of resection for middle-third and type I proximal tumors. The CBD is resected from the pancreas to a point above the bifurcation. Reconstruction is accomplished via Roux-en-Y hepaticojejunostomy (involving either one or two separate anastomoses).**

mucosa repair without stenting. Some authors place transhepatic tubes through these anastomoses to facilitate postoperative treatment with internal radiation sources; however, there is no evidence that this practice reduces local recurrence or prolongs survival.

Step 5: Closure and Postoperative Care

The abdomen is closed in the standard fashion, and closed suction drains are placed. Liver function is monitored, particularly when a major liver resection has been done. Mild abnormalities in coagulation test results are common, and soluble coagulation factors are given only if there is evidence of bleeding.

COMPLICATIONS

Bile leakage, bleeding, and infection are the most important complications of bile duct resection for tumor. Parahepatic collections are treated with percutaneous drainage, and significant early bleeding is usually best managed by reexploration.

Intrahepatic Cholangiojejunostomy

Intrahepatic cholangiojejunostomy is commonly performed after resection of the bifurcation for a more proximal tumor; it is also performed to manage injury or stricture at the level of the bifurcation and to bypass an unresectable bifurcation tumor.

Because the ducts are smaller, have thinner walls, and are more adherent to the areolar tissue of the pedicles than either the portal vein branches or the hepatic artery branches, dissec-

tion of the ducts must be more meticulous. Magnification is an important aid, particularly in dealing with undilated ducts. Good exposure is essential; if necessary, the liver may be split to allow adequate visualization, access, and lighting. Anatomic mucosal suturing can be achieved in most situations. In rare instances, excessive inflammation, scarring, or tumor makes such suturing impossible, in which case periductal sutures are used and a stent is placed. As described [*see* General Considerations, Technical Issues in Biliary Anastomosis, *above*], separate ducts that are close together can be first sutured together at their adjacent walls to create a single larger proximal duct lumen so that a safer anastomosis can be created [*see Figure 3c*].

OPERATIVE TECHNIQUE

Step 1: Definition of Tissues for Anastomosis

In the case of injury, crushed, cauterized, or devitalized tissue must be debrided back to normal healthy tissue before reconstruction is begun. In the case of bile duct resection for tumor, there should be no attempt to clear a length of duct from surrounding areolar or liver tissue; the suturing should take place in situ, with the stitches passed through the duct wall and the areolar tissue of the portal pedicles. In the case of bypass for unresectable cancer, the duct being used should be opened as far from the tumor as possible. The left main hepatic duct can be approached between the bifurcation and the umbilical fis-

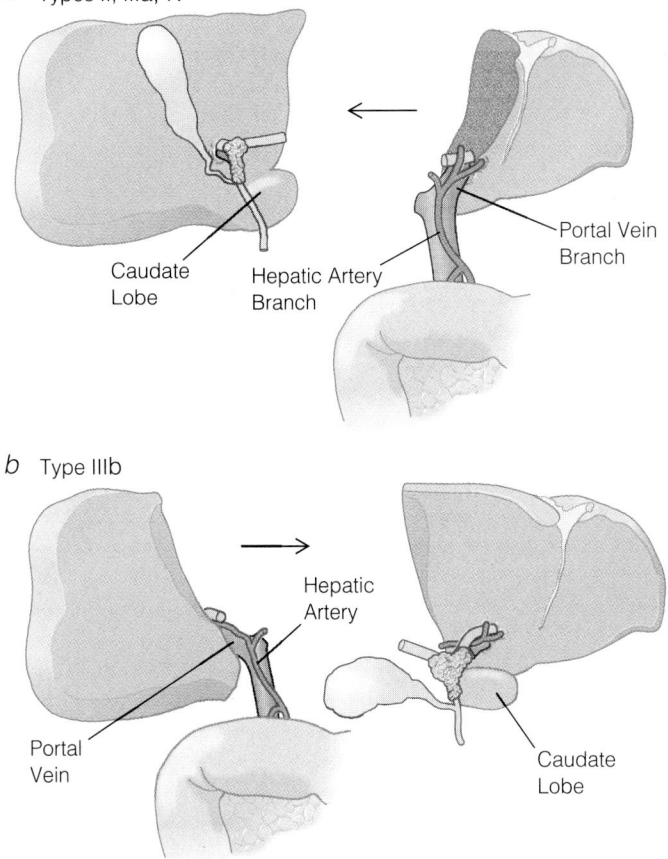

Figure 16 **Resection of middle-third and proximal bile duct tumors. Illustrated are (*a*) a right trisegmentectomy for types II, IIIa, and IV tumors and (*b*) a left hepatic lobectomy (including the caudate lobe) for type IIIb tumors.**

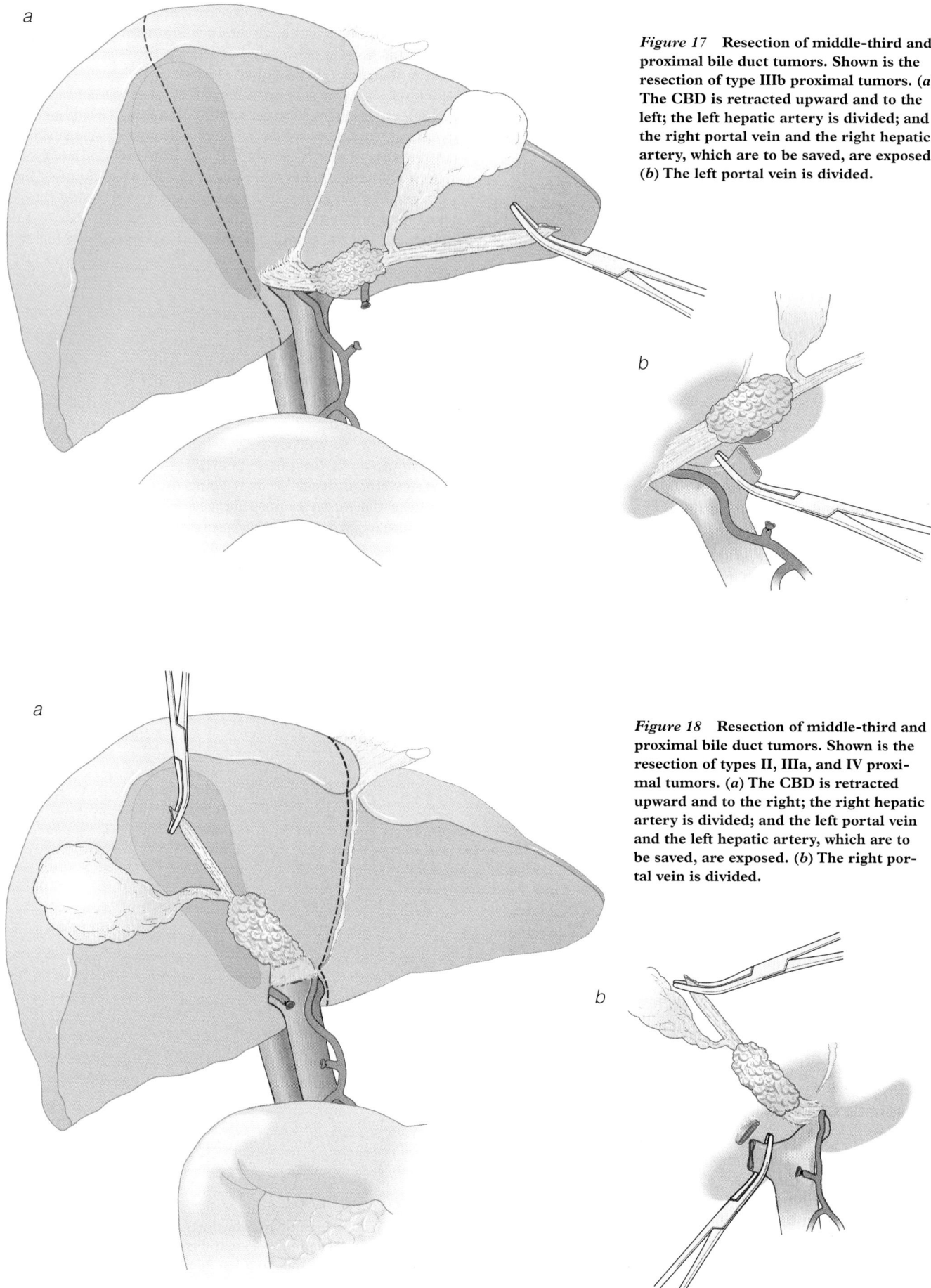

Figure 17 Resection of middle-third and proximal bile duct tumors. Shown is the resection of type IIIb proximal tumors. (*a*) The CBD is retracted upward and to the left; the left hepatic artery is divided; and the right portal vein and the right hepatic artery, which are to be saved, are exposed. (*b*) The left portal vein is divided.

Figure 18 Resection of middle-third and proximal bile duct tumors. Shown is the resection of types II, IIIa, and IV proximal tumors. (*a*) The CBD is retracted upward and to the right; the right hepatic artery is divided; and the left portal vein and the left hepatic artery, which are to be saved, are exposed. (*b*) The right portal vein is divided.

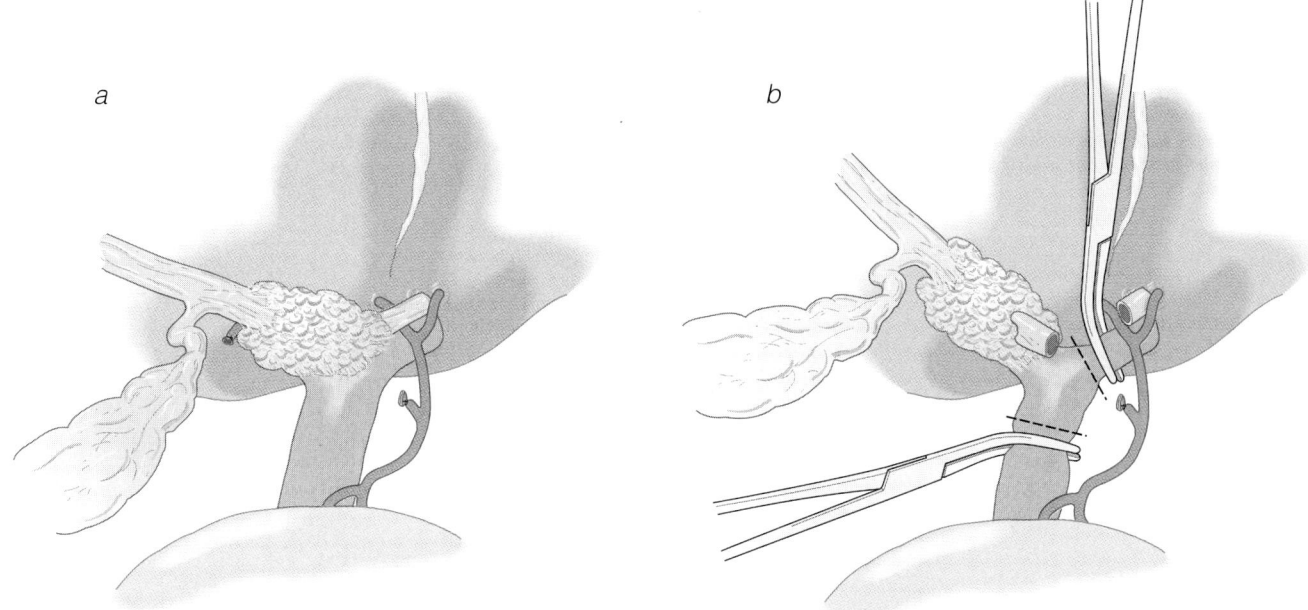

Figure 19 **Resection of middle-third and proximal bile duct tumors. (*a*) Occasionally, a type III or IV proximal tumor will involve the portal vein bifurcation. (*b*) Shown is the resection of an involved portal vein bifurcation. Reconstruction is accomplished in an end-to-end fashion.**

sure. If the tumor involves the left main hepatic duct, the branch to segment 3 of the liver can be used instead; it can be approached in the umbilical fissure, above the round ligament. Occasionally, incision into the liver or excision of a wedge of liver tissue is necessary to provide adequate exposure [*see Figure 20*]. If an intrahepatic anastomosis is required for a bifurcation stricture, resection of the stricture is not necessary; however, it is important to identify a normal duct above the level of the bifurcation. If there is no communication from right to left, a horizontal incision can be made in the left duct and carried across into the right duct just above or through the bifurcation

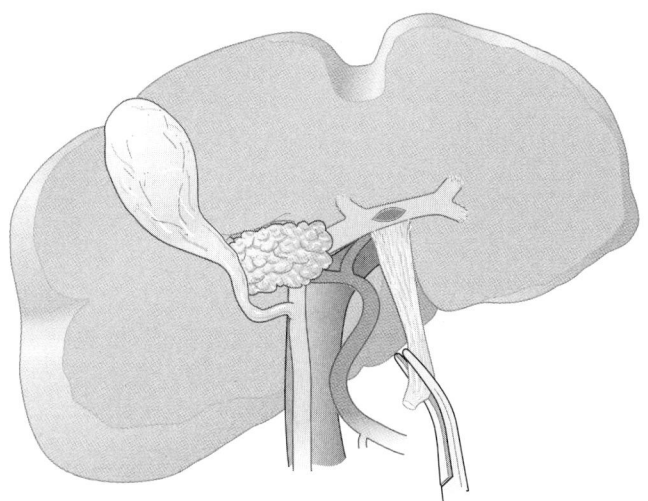

Figure 20 **Intrahepatic cholangiojejunostomy. If a tumor involves the left main hepatic duct, the branch of the duct that supplies segment 3 of the liver may be used instead for anastomosis to the jejunum. This branch may be approached in the umbilical fissure, above the round ligament. Incision into the liver or wedge excision may be necessary to ensure adequate exposure.**

stricture, so that a single anastomosis can be made that incorporates both ducts. Duct openings can be enlarged by making a small longitudinal incision in the most accessible portion of the duct. This is easier to accomplish in the left hepatic duct (because of its extrahepatic transverse position) than in the right hepatic duct (which tends to run laterally and posteriorly directly in the liver substance).

Step 2: Anastomosis

A Roux loop of sufficient length to make a tension-free anastomosis is constructed. A biliary-enteric anastomosis is then performed. When adequate access is difficult to obtain, interrupted sutures are first placed in the anterior wall of the bile duct to allow retraction of that wall and facilitate accurate placement of interrupted sutures in the back wall.

Postoperative Care

In a patient with impaired liver function or following major liver resection, the results of liver function tests, particularly coagulation studies, should be carefully monitored postoperatively. Transient worsening of these results is not unusual, especially if the procedure was long. Moderately elevated results from coagulation studies (e.g., international normalized ratio [INR] < 2.0) are not an indication for treatment with fresh frozen plasma or concentrated coagulation factors unless clinical bleeding is evident.

Postoperative infections may occur as a result of biliary tract contamination, especially if a bile duct stent was placed preoperatively. Antibiotic prophylaxis with broad-spectrum agents for periods longer than usual for perioperative treatment may be appropriate in such cases. If postoperative fever occurs, especially if it is accompanied by unusual pain and tenderness, imaging studies should be promptly obtained and fluid collections sought. In most cases, bile or pus can be drained satisfactorily through percutaneously placed tubes.

Recommended Reading

Bismuth H, Nakache R, Diamond T: Management strategies in resection for hilar cholangiocarcinoma. Ann Surg 215:31, 1992

Bornman PC, Terblanche J: Subtotal cholecystectomy: for the difficult gallbladder in portal hypertension and cholecystitis. Surgery 98:1, 1985

Braasch JW, Rossi RL: Reconstruction of the biliary tract. Surg Clin North Am 65:273, 1985

Fry DE: Surgical techniques in the management of distal biliary tract obstruction. American Surgeon 49:138, 1983

Gallinger S, Gluckman D, Langer B: Proximal bile duct cancer. Advances in Surgery, vol 23. Cameron JL, Ed. Year Book Medical Publishers, St. Louis, 1990, p 89

Lillemoe KD, Pitt HA, Cameron JL: Current management of benign bile duct strictures. Advances in Surgery, vol 25. Cameron JL, Ed. Year Book Medical Publishers, St. Louis, 1992, p 119

Russell E, Hutson DG, Guerra JJ Jr: Dilatation of biliary strictures through a stomatized jejunal limb. Acta Radiologica: Diagnosis 26:283, 1985

Smadja C, Blumgart LH: The biliary tract and the anatomy of biliary exposure. Surgery of the Liver and Biliary Tract. Blumgart LH, Ed. Churchill Livingstone, New York, 1988, p 11

Stain SC, Guthrie CR, Yellin AE, et al: Choledochal cyst in the adult. Ann Surg 222:128, 1995

Strom PR, Stone HH: A technique for transduodenal sphincteroplasty. Surgery 92:546, 1982

Acknowledgment

Figures 1 through 20   Tom Moore.

17 HEPATIC RESECTION

Yuman Fong, M.D., F.A.C.S., and Leslie H. Blumgart, M.D., F.A.C.S., F.R.C.S.

Liver resections were first described centuries ago, but until the latter half of the 20th century, the majority of such resections were performed for management of either injuries or infections. Today, these procedures are performed not only for treatment of acute emergencies (e.g., traumatic injuries or abscesses) but also as potentially curative therapy for a variety of benign and malignant hepatic lesions.

The first planned anatomic resection of a lobe of a liver is credited to Lortat-Jacob, who in 1952 performed a right lobectomy as treatment for metastatic colon cancer.[1] Major hepatectomies, however, did not become commonplace until the 1980s. Since then, the safety of these operations has improved dramatically, and as safety has improved, the indications for hepatic resection have become better refined as well. Currently, resection of as much as 85% of the functional liver parenchyma is being performed at numerous centers with an operative mortality of less than 2%. The duration of hospitalization is typically less than 2 weeks, and almost all individuals regain normal hepatic function.

In what follows, we focus on the technical aspects of hepatic resection, emphasizing efficiency and safety and taking into account recent developments, current controversies, and special operative considerations (e.g., the cirrhotic patient and repeat liver resection). Detailed discussions of the indications for hepatic resection are available elsewhere.[2-4]

Hepatic Anatomy

Familiarity with the surgical anatomy of the liver is essential for safe performance of a partial hepatectomy. The liver can be divided into two lobes (right and left) comprising eight segments [*see Figure 1*]. Each of these segments is a discrete anatomic unit that possesses its own nutrient blood supply and its own venous and biliary drainage. The right lobe consists of segments 5 through 8 and is nourished by the right hepatic artery and the right portal vein; the left lobe consists of segments 1 through 4 and is nourished by the left hepatic artery and the left portal vein. The anatomic division between the right lobe and the left is not at the falciform ligament (the most readily apparent visual landmark on the anterior liver) but follows a line projected through a plane (the principal plane, or Cantlie's line) that runs posterosuperiorly from the medial margin of the gallbladder to the left side of the vena cava.

The venous drainage of the liver consists of multiple small veins draining directly from the back of the right lobe and the caudate lobe to the vena cava, along with three major hepatic veins. These major hepatic veins occupy three planes, known as portal scissurae. The three scissurae divide the liver into four sectors, each of which is supplied by a portal pedicle; further branching of the pedicles subdivides the sectors into the eight segments [*see Figure 1*].[5-7] (Some surgeons refer to these sectors

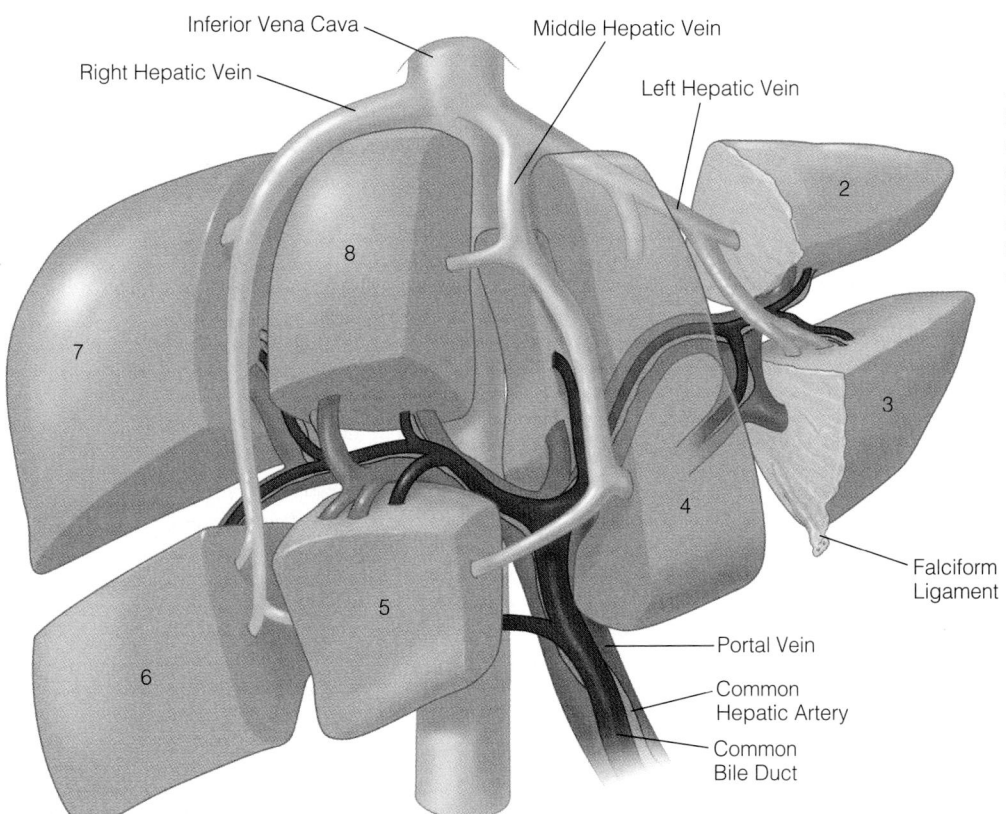

Figure 1 **The liver is separated into eight anatomic segments, each with an independent nutrient blood supply and venous and biliary drainage. Appreciation of this segmental anatomy is the basis of anatomic resection of the liver.**

a   *b*

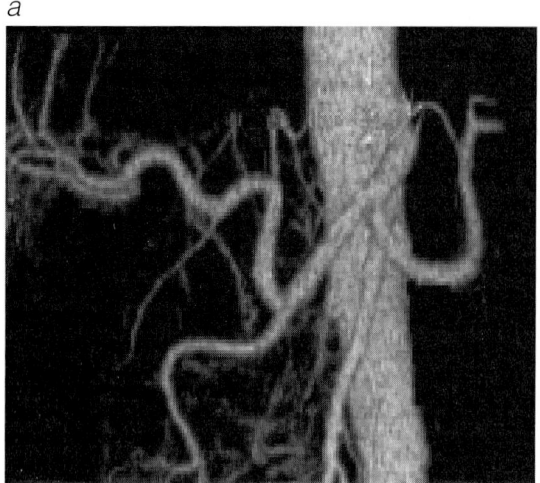
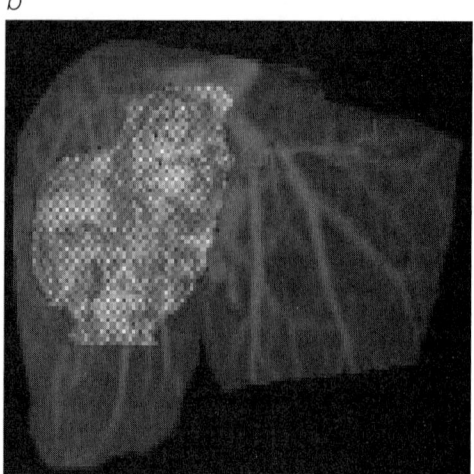

Figure 2 (*a*) **The arterial anatomy of the celiac axis is reconstructed from thin-slice CT images. (*b*) The hepatic venous anatomy is similarly reconstructed, with the tumor superimposed on the vascular reconstruction.**

as segments—hence the term trisegmentectomy.) The right hepatic vein passes between the right anterior sector (segments 5 and 8) and the right posterior sector (segments 6 and 7) in the right scissura. This vein empties directly into the vena cava near the atriocaval junction. The middle hepatic vein passes between the right anterior sector and the left medial sector (segment 4) in the central, or principal, scissura, which represents the division between the right lobe and the left. The left hepatic vein runs in the left scissura between segments 2 and 3. In most persons, the left and middle hepatic veins join to form a common trunk before entering the vena cava. Occasionally, a large inferior right hepatic vein is present that may provide adequate drainage of the right lobe after resection of the left even when all three major hepatic veins are ligated.[8]

The portal vein and the hepatic artery divide into left and right branches below the hilus of the liver. Unlike the hepatic veins, which run between segments, the portal venous and hepatic arterial branches, along with the hepatic ducts, typically run centrally within segments [*see Figure 1*]. On the right side, the hepatic artery and the portal vein enter the liver substance almost immediately after branching. The short course of the right-side extrahepatic vessels and the variable anatomy of the biliary tree make these vessels vulnerable to damage during dissection.[9] In contrast, the left branch of the portal vein and the left hepatic duct take a long extrahepatic course after branching beneath segment 4. When these vessels reach the base of the umbilical fissure, they are joined by the left hepatic artery to form a triad, which then enters the left liver substance at this point. It must be emphasized that proximal to the base of the umbilical fissure, the left-side structures are not a triad. A consequence of the long extrahepatic course of the left-side structures is that for tumors that involve the hilus (e.g., Klatskin tumors), when a choice exists between an extended right hepatectomy or an extended left hepatectomy, most surgeons choose the former because the greater ease of dissection on the left side facilitates preservation of the left-side structures. Knowledge of the relative anatomic courses of the portal veins, the hepatic arteries, and the hepatic ducts is the basis of the classical extrahepatic dissection for control of hepatic inflow [*see* Operative Technique, Right Lobectomy, Step 6 (Extrahepatic Dissection and Ligation), *below*].

The fibrous capsule surrounding the liver substance was described by Glisson in 1654.[10] It was Couinaud,[6] however, who demonstrated that this fibrous capsule extends to envelop the portal triads as they pass into the liver substance. Thus, within the liver, the portal vein, the hepatic artery, and the hepatic duct running to each segment of the liver lie within a substantial sheath. This dense sheath allows rapid control of inflow vessels to specific anatomic units within the liver and permits en masse ligation of these vascular structures in a maneuver known as pedicle ligation [*see* Operative Technique, Right Lobectomy, Step 6—Alternative (Intrahepatic Pedicle Ligation), *below*].[11]

Preoperative Evaluation

Cross-sectional imaging modalities such as computed tomography, magnetic resonance imaging, and ultrasonography play an important role in enhancing the safety and efficacy of hepatic resection. These modalities, along with biologic scanning techniques such as positron emission tomography (PET), are also invaluable for staging malignancies so as to improve patient selection and thereby optimize long-term surgical outcome.

At a minimum, all candidates for hepatic resection should undergo either CT or MRI. These imaging tests not only identify the number and size of any mass lesions within the liver but also delineate the relations of the lesions to the major vasculature—data that are crucial for deciding whether to operate and which operative approach to follow.

Use of contrast enhancement during CT scanning is vital for accurate definition of the vascular anatomy. In fact, data from thin-slice (1 to 2 mm) images captured by current spiral, or helical, CT scanners can be reconstructed to provide angiographic pictures whose level of detail rivals that of direct angiograms [*see Figure 2*]. Triple-phase scans (including a noncontrast phase, an arterial phase, and a venous phase) are recommended: these yield the best definition and characterization of intrahepatic lesions. For example, some vascular tumors become isodense with liver parenchyma after contrast injection. By first obtaining noncontrast scans and then obtaining contrast scans at two different times after contrast injection, the examiner stands a better chance of visualizing such tumors.

For small tumors, a CT variant known as CT portography is recommended. In this technique, contrast material is injected through the superior mesenteric artery, and images are obtained during the portal venous phase. The normal liver receives the majority of its nutrient blood from the portal vein and is therefore contrast-enhanced in this phase. Tumors, on the other hand, usually derive their nutrient blood from the hepatic artery and therefore appear as exaggerated perfusion defects. CT portography is the most sensitive test available for identifying small hepatic tumors.[12]

MRI may also be valuable for characterizing lesions and defining them vis-à-vis the vasculature. It is particularly helpful in diagnosing benign lesions such as hemangiomas, fibronodular hyperplasia, and adenomas. Whenever any of these benign lesions is suspected, MRI is usually indicated. With regard to surgical planning, MRI angiographic images are useful for identifying the major hepatic veins and clarifying their relations to any tumor masses.[13]

Imaging recommendations may be summed up as follows. A triple-phase CT should be obtained for most patients under consideration for hepatic resection. If diagnostic doubt remains after CT, particularly if the differential diagnosis includes an asymptomatic benign tumor, MRI should be performed. If questions remain after CT as to the extent of hepatic venous or major biliary involvement, MRI or duplex ultrasonography should be considered.[14] If small tumors are encountered, CT portography should be performed. Duplex ultrasonography, by demonstrating the vascular hilar structures, the hepatic veins, and the inferior vena cava, renders angiography unnecessary in many cases.[13,15] Currently, direct hepatic angiography is rarely required, and inferior vena cavography is almost never needed.

Operative Planning

PREPARATION

In general, preparation for hepatic resection is much the same as that for other major abdominal procedures. All patients who are older than 65 years or have a history of cardiopulmonary disease undergo a full cardiopulmonary assessment. It was once commonly believed that patients 70 years of age or older were poor candidates for major liver resection,[16,17] but this notion has been dispelled by more recent data.[18-20] Advanced chronologic age is not a complete contraindication to hepatectomy.

Anemia and coagulopathy, if present, are corrected. All patients are now encouraged to donate two units of autologous blood before a major hepatectomy. Appropriate single-dose antibiotic prophylaxis is administered [see 1:2 Prevention of Postoperative Infection].

ANESTHESIA

Decisions regarding anesthesia should take into account the possibility of baseline hepatic parenchymal dysfunction as well as the postoperative hepatic functional deficits resulting from resection of a major portion of the hepatic parenchyma.

The most important consideration, however, is the possibility of major intraoperative hemorrhage. Suitable monitoring and sufficient vascular access to permit rapid transfusion should be in place. At some centers, fluid resuscitation and blood transfusion are begun early in the course of resection to increase intravascular volume as a buffer against sudden blood loss. At the Memorial Sloan-Kettering Cancer Center (MSKCC), however, we favor the opposite approach, whereby a low central venous pressure is maintained during resection. The rationale for our preference is that generally, most of the blood lost during hepatic resection comes from the major hepatic veins or the vena cava.[21,22] If central venous pressure is kept below 5 mm Hg, there is less bleeding from the hepatic venous radicles during dissection.

Reduction of intrahepatic venous pressure can be facilitated by performing the dissection with the patient in a 15° Trendelenburg position, which increases venous return to the heart and enhances cardiac output. Central venous pressure is maintained at the desired level through a combination of anesthesia and early intraoperative fluid restriction. The minimal acceptable intraoperative urine output is 25 ml/hr.

The need for intraoperative blood transfusion can be minimized by accepting hematocrits lower than the common target figure of 30%: 24% in patients without antecedent cardiac disease and 29% in patients with cardiac disease. If blood loss is estimated to reach or exceed 20% of total volume or the patient becomes hemodynamically unstable, transfusion is indicated.[21]

PATIENT POSITIONING

The patient should be supine: to date, we have not found a lateral position to be necessary even for the largest of tumors. Electrocardiographic leads should be kept clear of the right chest wall and the presternal area in case a thoracoabdominal incision is necessitated by the position of a tumor or by intraoperative hemorrhage. Preparation and draping should therefore also allow for exposure of the lower chest and the entire upper abdomen down past the umbilicus. A crossbar or a similar device that holds self-retaining retractors should be used to elevate the costal margin. Some surgeons prefer ring-based self-retaining retractors. In our experience, although these retractors are adequate for most resections, the rings tend to restrict lateral access, thereby potentially hindering posterior dissection, particularly of the vena cava.

ANATOMIC VERSUS NONANATOMIC RESECTION

The key decision in planning a hepatectomy is whether the resection should be anatomic or nonanatomic. For treatment of malignant disease, anatomic resection is usually favored because the long-term outcome is better. Anatomic resections permit excision of parenchymal areas distal to the index tumors, where there is a high incidence of vascular micrometastases. In addition, they are significantly less likely to have positive margins than nonanatomic resections are. In a large series of hepatectomies for metastatic colorectal cancer, wedge or nonanatomic resections were associated with a 19% rate of positive margins.[23] In a recent examination of our increasing preference for anatomic resections over wedge resections, wedge resections were associated with a 16% rate of positive margins, compared with a 2% rate for anatomic resections.[24]

There are two oncologic settings where nonanatomic resections are favored. In patients with hepatocellular carcinoma, viral hepatitis and cirrhosis are often complicating factors. Cirrhotic patients tolerate resection of more than two segments of functional parenchyma poorly. Accordingly, for these patients, the smallest resection that will achieve complete tumor excision is favored, even if it is a wedge resection. For management of metastatic neuroendocrine tumors, in which resections are merely debulking procedures designed to alleviate symptoms, nonanatomic resections are accepted because cure is highly unlikely.

Hepatic resections for benign hepatic tumors are usually performed for one of three reasons: (1) to relieve symptoms (e.g., pain or early satiety), (2) because the diagnosis is uncertain, or (3) to prevent malignant transformation. A goal of such resections should be to spare as much normal parenchyma as possible. Consequently, lesions such as hemangiomas, adenomas, complex cysts, and fibronodular hyperplasia are often excised by means of enucleation or another nonanatomic resection with limited margins.

Operative Technique

Theoretically, any hepatic segment can be resected in isolation. For practical purposes, however, there are five types of major anatomic resections [*see Figure 3*]. We follow the most commonly used terminology, that of Goldsmith and Woodburne.[25] Some authors prefer other systems of nomenclature, based on the anatomic descriptions of Couinaud[6] or Bismuth.[7]

The essential principles of all anatomic hepatectomies are the same: (1) control of inflow vessels, (2) control of outflow vessels, and (3) parenchymal transection. To illustrate these principles, we begin by outlining the steps in a right lobectomy [*see Figure 3a*] in some detail, describing both extrahepatic vascular dissection and ligation and the alternative approach to inflow control, intrahepatic pedicle ligation. Left lobectomy [*see Figure 3b*] and other common anatomic resections share a number of steps with right lobectomy; accordingly, we discuss them in somewhat less detail. Further detail on these procedures is available in other sources.[26,27]

RIGHT LOBECTOMY

Step 1: Laparoscopic Inspection

Experience from MSKCC[28,29] and other centers[30,31] indicates that laparoscopy allows detection of unresectable disease and prevents the morbidity associated with a nontherapeutic laparotomy. We generally perform laparoscopy immediately before laparotomy during the same period of anesthesia. The laparoscopic port sites are placed in the upper abdomen along the line of the intended incision [*see* Step 2, *below*]. The first two ports are usually 10 mm ports placed in the right subcostal area along the midclavicular line and along the anterior axillary line. These

ports allow inspection of the abdomen and of the entire liver, including the dome and segment 7. The port along the right anterior axillary line is particularly suitable for laparoscopic ultrasound devices. If additional ports are necessary, a left subcostal midclavicular port is usually the best choice.

Step 2: Incision

For the majority of hepatic resections, most surgeons use a bilateral subcostal incision extended vertically to the xiphisternum [*see Figure 4*]. Our own preference, however, is to use an upper midline incision extending to a point approximately 2 cm above the umbilicus, with a rightward extension from that point to a point in the midaxillary line halfway between the lowest rib and the iliac crest [*see Figure 4*]. We find that this incision provides superb access for either right- or left-side resection, without the wound complications often encountered with trifurcated incisions (e.g., ascitic leakage and incisional hernia). On rare occasions (e.g., in the resection of large, rigid posterior tumors of the right lobe), a right thoracoabdominal incision may be required. In a recent series of nearly 2,000 resections at MSKCC, however, a thoracoabdominal incision proved necessary in only 3% of patients; the most common indication was repeat liver resection after previous right hepatic lobectomy [*see* Repeat Hepatic Resection, *below*].

Step 3: Abdominal Exploration and Intraoperative Ultrasonography

The liver is palpated bimanually. Intraoperative ultrasonography is systematically performed to identify all possible lesions and their relations to the major vascular structures. This modality is capable of identifying small lesions that preoperative imaging studies and palpation of the liver may miss.[32] The lesser omentum is incised to allow palpation of the caudate lobe and inspection of the celiac region for nodal metastases. A finger is passed from the lesser sac inferior to the caudate lobe through the foramen of Winslow to permit identification of the portal vein and palpation of the portocaval lymph nodes. The hilar lymph nodes are palpated, and any suspicious nodes are removed for frozen section examination. If the operation is being done for cancer, the entire abdomen is inspected for evidence of extrahepatic tumor.

Step 4: Mobilization of Liver

Once the decision is made to proceed with hepatic resection, the liver is fully mobilized by detaching all ligamentous attachments on the side to be resected. (Some surgeons defer completion of mobilization to a later stage in the procedure.) In particular, the suprahepatic inferior vena cava and the hepatic veins above the liver are dissected to facilitate the subsequent approach to the hepatic veins [*see* Step 7, *below*]. Once the liver is mobilized, further palpation is done to detect any small lesions that may have been obscured initially. This additional palpation is particularly important on the right side because before mobilization, the posterior parts of the liver cannot be effectively palpated, and intraoperative ultrasonography may fail to detect small lesions in this area.[32]

If, in the course of mobilization, tumor is found to be attached to the diaphragm, the affected area of the diaphragm may be excised and subsequently repaired.

Step 5: Identification of Arterial Anomalies

Any hepatic arterial anomalies present should be identified before resection is begun. With good preoperative imaging, the arterial anatomy is usually defined with sufficient exactitude before

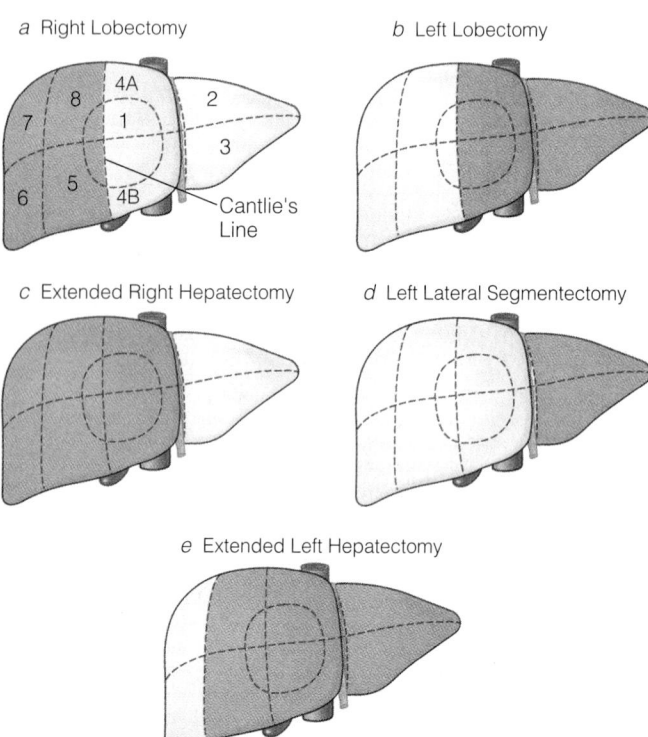

Figure 3 **Shown are schematic illustrations of standard hepatic resections, with the shaded areas representing the resected portions: (*a*) right lobectomy, (*b*) left lobectomy, (*c*) extended right hepatectomy (or right trisegmentectomy), (*d*) left lateral segmentectomy, and (*e*) extended left hepatectomy (or left trisegmentectomy).**

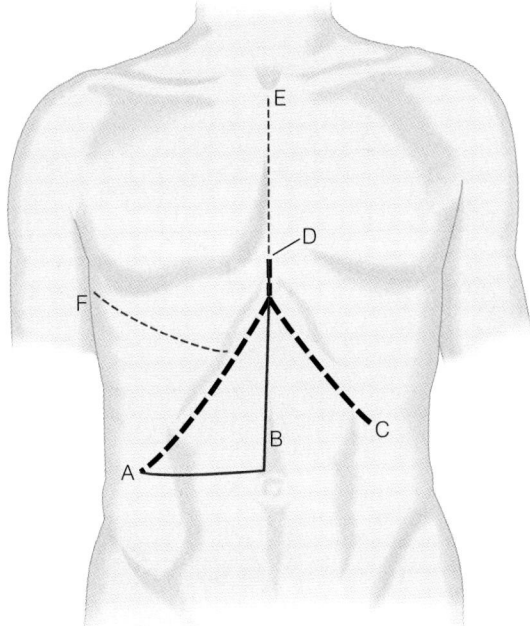

Figure 4 **Right lobectomy. A right subcostal incision (A) with a midline extension to the xiphoid (D) is the most common choice; an extension to the left subcostal area (C) is sometimes added to provide further operative exposure. We prefer a long midline incision from the xiphoid (D) to a point approximately 3 cm above the umbilicus (B) along with a rightward extension (A) because this incision provides superb exposure of both the right side and the left without the wound complications of a trifurcated incision. The chest can be entered through either a median sternotomy (E) or an anterolateral right thoracoabdominal incision (F).**

laparotomy. It is also possible to gain a clear picture of the arterial anatomy intraoperatively by means of simple maneuvers that do not involve major dissection.

The lesser omentum should be examined to determine whether there is a vessel coursing through its middle to the base of the umbilical fissure, and the hepatoduodenal ligament should be palpated with an index finger within the foramen of Winslow to see whether there is an artery in the gastropancreatic fold on its medial aspect. The usual bifurcation of the hepatic arteries occurs low and medially in the hepatoduodenal ligament, and the left hepatic artery normally travels on the medial aspect of the ligament to reach the base of the umbilical fissure. Thus, if an artery is palpable in the medial upper portion of the hepatoduodenal ligament, it is the main left hepatic artery. Any vessel seen in the lesser omentum must therefore be an accessory left artery. If, however, no pulse is found in the medial upper portion of the hepatoduodenal ligament, the vessel in the lesser omentum must be a replaced left hepatic artery. The right hepatic artery usually travels transversely behind the common bile duct (CBD) to reach the base of the cystic plate. A vertically traveling artery on the lateral hepatoduodenal ligament must therefore be either a replaced or an accessory right hepatic artery, probably arising from the superior mesenteric artery.

Step 6 (Extrahepatic Dissection and Ligation): Control of Inflow Vessels

The classic approach to extrahepatic control of the inflow vessels in a right lobectomy involves extrahepatic dissection and ligation [see Figure 5]. The cystic duct and the cystic artery are li-

gated and divided. The gallbladder may be either removed or left attached to the right liver, according to the surgeon's preference. The usual practice is first to ligate the right hepatic duct, then the right hepatic artery, and finally the right portal vein, working from anterior to posterior. Our preference, however, is to work from posterior to anterior, as follows.

The sheath of the porta hepatis is opened laterally. Dissection is then performed in the plane between the CBD and the portal vein. To facilitate this dissection, the CBD is elevated by applying forward traction to the ligated cystic duct. The portal vein is then followed cephalad until its bifurcation into the left and right portal veins is visible. In a small percentage of patients, the left portal vein arises from the right anterior branch of the portal vein. If the main right portal vein is ligated in a patient who exhibits this anatomic variant, the portion of the liver remaining after resection will lack any portal flow. There is usually a small portal branch that passes from the main right portal vein to the caudate process. Ligation of this branch untethers another 1 to 2 cm of the right portal vein, thereby allowing safer dissection and ligation. The right portal vein is usually clamped with vascular clamps, divided, and oversewn with nonabsorbable sutures. Once this is done, the right hepatic artery is visible behind the CBD and can easily be secured and ligated with nonabsorbable sutures. Because of the multitude of biliary anatomic variations, we usually leave the right hepatic duct intact until parenchymal dissection [see Step 8, *below*] is begun, when this structure can be secured higher within the hepatic parenchyma and divided with greater safety.

Staple ligation Vascular staplers may be used for stapling the right or the left portal vein during extrahepatic vascular dissection[33,34]; however, suture ligation of the extrahepatic portal veins is such a straightforward technical exercise that staplers add little except cost.

Step 6—Alternative (Intrahepatic Pedicle Ligation): Control of Inflow Vessels

The observations of Glisson and Couinard (see above) that the nutrient vessels to the liver are contained within a thick connective tissue capsule [see Figure 6] were the basis for the initial proposal by Launois and Jamieson[11] that intrahepatic vascular pedicle ligation could serve as an alternative to extrahepatic dissection and ligation for controlling vascular inflow to the liver. This alternative technique has the advantages of being rapid and of being unlikely to cause injury to the vasculature or the biliary drainage of the contralateral liver. Given adequate intrahepatic definition and control of the portal triads supplying the area of the liver to be resected, one can readily isolate the various major pedicles by using simple combinations of hepatotomies at specific sites on the inferior surface of the liver [see Figure 7].

The right liver is completely mobilized from the retroperitoneum. The most inferior small hepatic veins are ligated, and the inferior right liver is mobilized off the vena cava. Incisions are then made in the liver capsule at hepatotomy sites A and B [see Figure 7]. The first incision is made though the caudate process. The full thickness of the caudate process is divided with a combination of diathermy, crushing, and ligation. The second incision is made almost vertically in the medial part of the gallbladder bed. Both incisions must be fairly substantial and reasonably deep. Care must be taken to avoid the terminal branches of the middle hepatic vein, which are the most common source of significant bleeding. By means of either finger dissection or the passage of a large curved clamp, a tape is then placed around the right main sheath [see Figure 8]. This tape can be pulled medial-

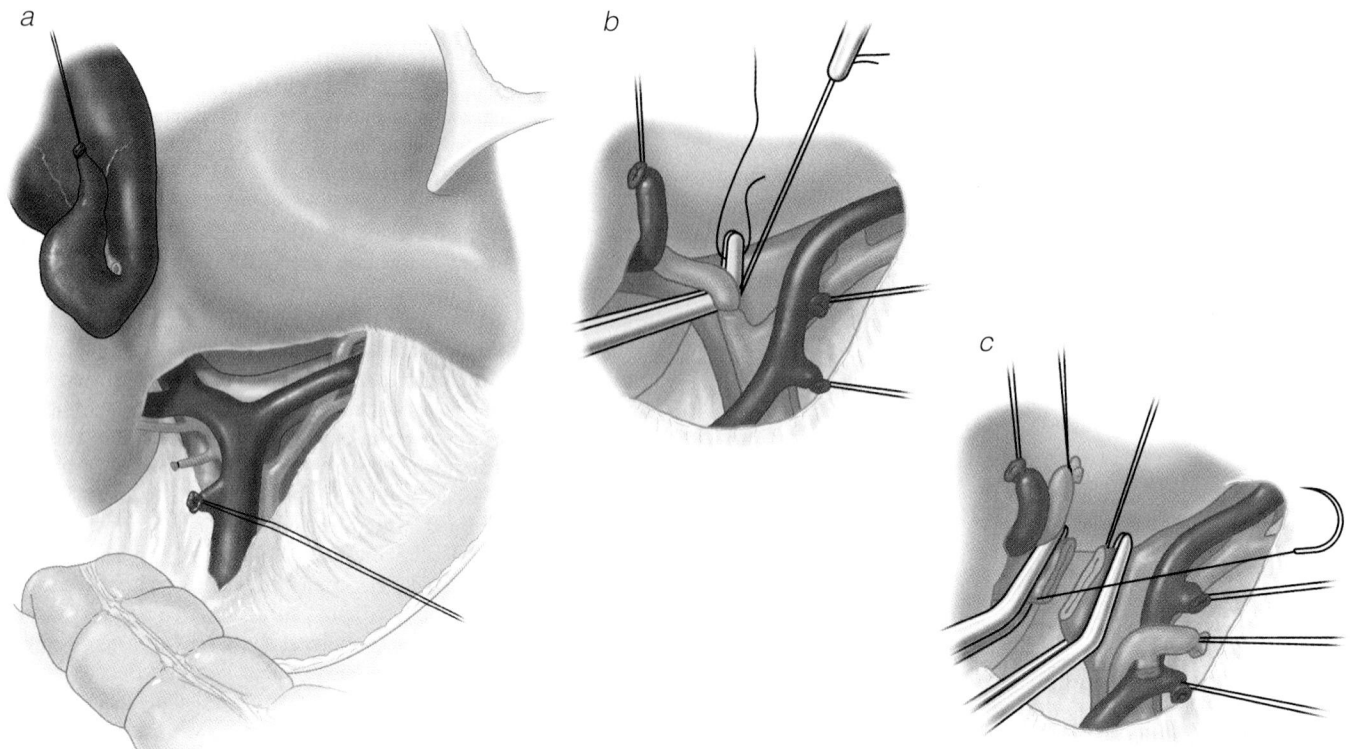

Figure 5 **Right lobectomy. For control of the inflow vessels of the right liver, the liver is retracted cephalad to allow exposure of the porta hepatis. (*a*) The gallbladder is resected to allow access to the bile duct and hepatic vessels. (*b*) The right hepatic duct is ligated to allow access to the hepatic artery and the portal vein. (*c*) After the right hepatic artery is divided, the right portal vein is controlled and divided. Alternatively, the vessels may be approached from a posterolateral direction and the portal vein and hepatic artery may be divided first, with the hepatic duct left intact until the parenchymal transection.**

ly to provide better exposure of the intrahepatic right pedicle and to retract the left biliary tree and portal vein away from the area to be clamped and divided. Clamps are then applied, the right pedicle is divided, and the stumps are suture-ligated.

In practice, for right lobectomies, we prefer to isolate the right anterior and posterior pedicles separately [*see Figure 8*] and ligate them individually. This measure ensures that the left-side structures cannot be injured. Any minor bleeding from a hepatotomy

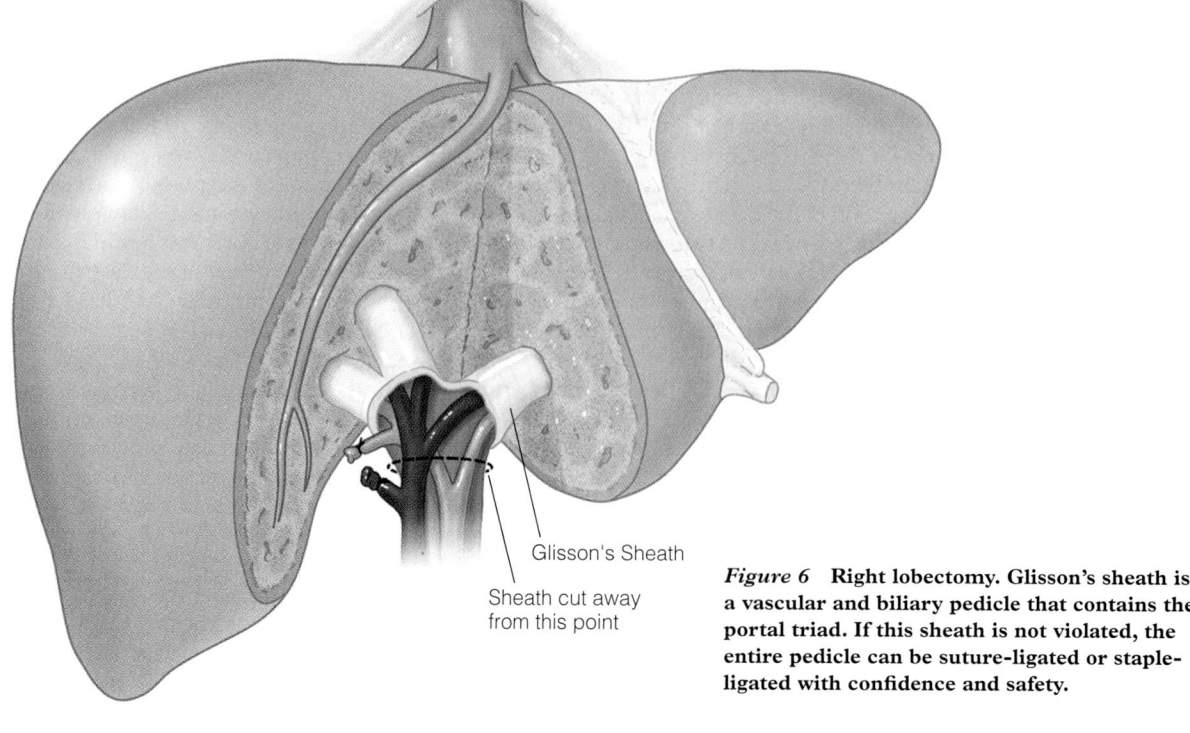

Glisson's Sheath

Sheath cut away
from this point

Figure 6 **Right lobectomy. Glisson's sheath is a vascular and biliary pedicle that contains the portal triad. If this sheath is not violated, the entire pedicle can be suture-ligated or staple-ligated with confidence and safety.**

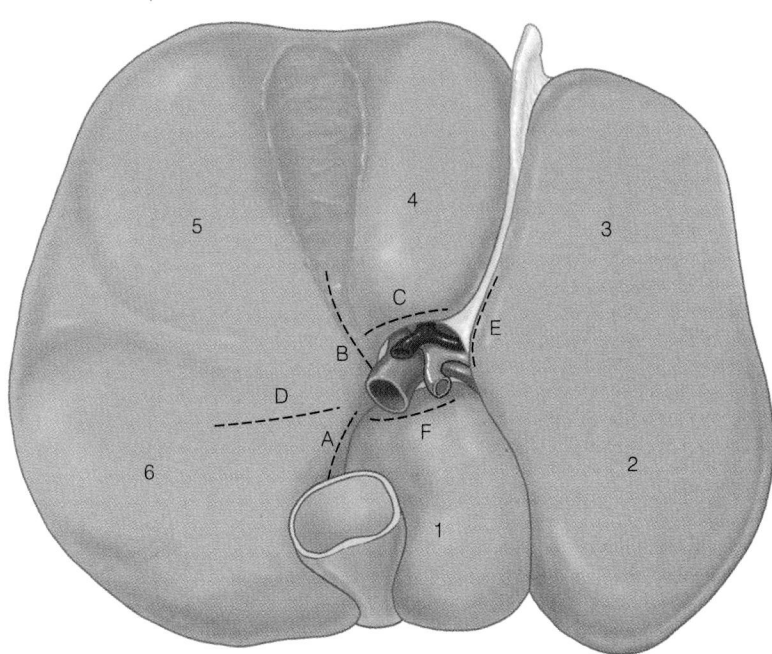

Figure 7 **Right lobectomy. Depicted are sites where hepatotomies can be made to permit isolation of various vascular pedicles. Incisions at sites A and B allow isolation of the right main portal pedicle. Incisions at sites A and D allow isolation of the right posterior portal pedicle. Incisions at sites B and D allow isolation of the right anterior pedicle. Incisions at sites C and E allow isolation of the left main portal pedicle; if the caudate is to be removed, incisions are made at sites C and F.**

usually ceases spontaneously or else stops when Surgicel is placed into the wound.

Staple ligation   The use of staplers is now well established for liver resections,[33-38] and we find that staple ligation greatly increases the speed with which intrahepatic portal pedicle ligations can be performed. To control the intrahepatic portal pedicles for a right lobectomy, incisions are made at hepatotomy sites A and B [*see Figure 7*]. Ultrasonography directed from the inferior aspect of the liver helps determine the depth at which the right pedicle lies, which is usually 1 to 2 cm from the inferior surface. The right main pedicle is then secured either digitally or with a curved blunt clamp (e.g., a renal pedicle clamp), and an umbilical tape is placed around it [*see Figure 9a*]. The hilar plate in the back of segment 4 is lowered via an incision at hepatotomy site C [*see Figure 7*] to ensure that the left-side vascular and biliary structures are mobilized well away from the area of staple ligation. A transverse anastomosis (TA) vascular stapler is applied to the right main pedicle while firm countertraction is being applied to the umbilical tape to pull the hilus to the left [*see Figure 9a*]. The stapler is fired, and the pedicle is divided [*see Figure 9b*].

Troubleshooting   There are several important guiding principles that should be followed in deciding on and performing intrahepatic pedicle ligation. The most important principle is that in patients undergoing operation for cancer, an intrahepatic pedicle approach should not be used when a tumor is within 2 cm of the hepatic hilus. In such cases, extrahepatic dissection should be performed to avoid violation of the tumor margin.

From a technical standpoint, removal of the gallbladder greatly facilitates isolation and control of right-side vascular pedicles in a right lobectomy. Application of the Pringle maneuver decreases bleeding during hepatotomy and isolation of the pedicle. Finally, the lowest hepatic veins behind the liver should be dissected before any attempt is made to isolate the right-side portal pedicles: incising the caudate process without dividing the small hepatic veins draining this portion of the liver to the vena cava can lead to significant hemorrhage.

Step 7: Control of Outflow Vessels

Control of the outflow vasculature begins with division of the hepatic veins passing from the posterior aspect of the right liver directly to the vena cava. After the right lobe is completely mobilized off the retroperitoneum by dividing the right triangular ligament, it is carefully dissected off the vena cava. Dissection proceeds upward from the inferior border of the liver until the right hepatic vein is exposed. Complete mobilization of the right liver

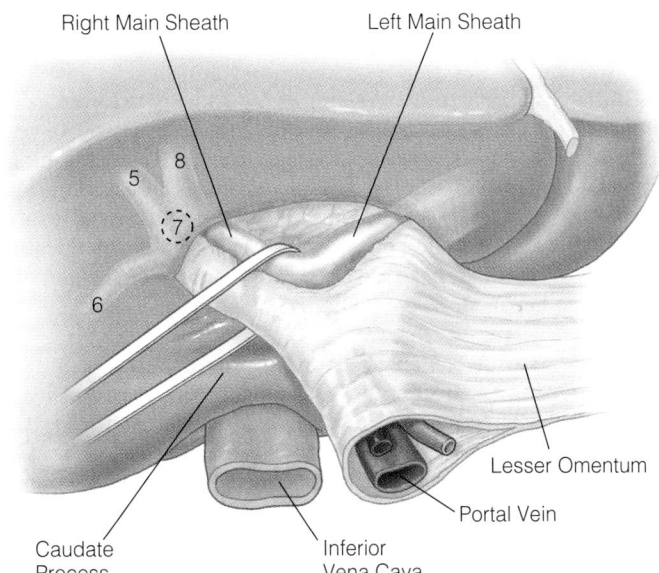

Figure 8 **Right lobectomy. Depicted is isolation of the main right portal pedicle. The pedicle is controlled with a vascular tape and retracted from within the liver substance. This tape can be used for countertraction when a vascular clamp or stapler is applied. The main right portal pedicle has anterior and posterior branches. The right anterior pedicle consists of pedicles to segments 5 and 8. The right posterior pedicle usually consists of only the segment 6 pedicle but may also give rise to the segment 7 pedicle.**

a

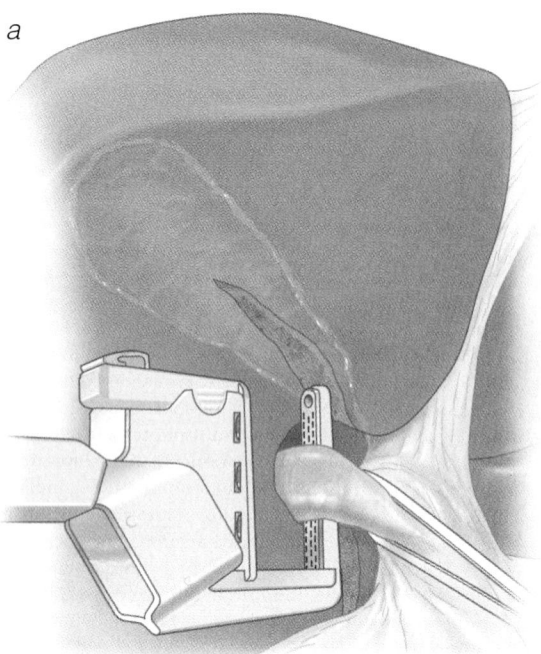

b

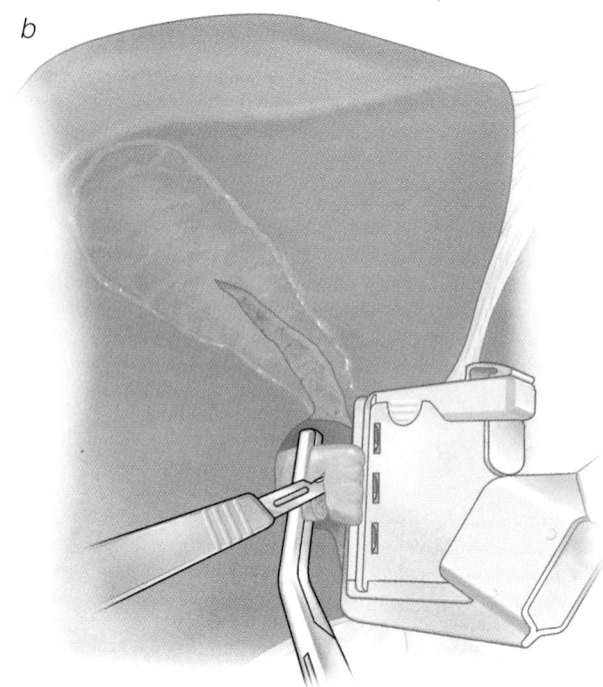

Figure 9 **Right lobectomy. Shown is staple ligation of the right portal pedicle. (*a*) After the liver is incised across the caudate process and along the gallbladder bed, the right main pedicle is isolated and held with an umbilical tape. Countertraction is placed on the umbilical tape while a TA vascular stapler is placed across the pedicle, allowing the left hepatic duct and the left vascular structures to be retracted away from the line of stapling. (*b*) After the stapler is fired, the pedicle is clamped and divided.**

is particularly critical for tumors close to the vena cava. The right hepatic vein is then isolated, cross-clamped, divided, and over-sewn [*see Figure 10*]. Unless the tumor or lesion involves the middle hepatic vein close to its junction with the vena cava, the middle hepatic vein usually is not controlled extrahepatically for right-side resections and is easily secured during parenchymal transection.

If there is a large tumor residing at the dome of the liver, gaining control of the hepatic veins and the vena cava may prove very difficult. If so, one should not hesitate to extend the incision to the chest by means of a right thoracoabdominal extension. The morbidity of a thoracoabdominal incision is preferable to the potentially catastrophic hemorrhage that is sometimes encountered when the right hepatic vein is torn during mobilization of a rigid right hepatic lobe containing a large tumor.

Staple ligation   Staple ligation has proved useful for outflow control during hepatectomy. When the tumor is in proximity to the hepatic vein–vena cava junction, extrahepatic control of the hepatic veins is essential for excision of the tumor with clear margins, and it limits blood loss during parenchymal transection.[39] Ligating the hepatic veins, particularly with a large and rigid tumor in the vicinity, can be a technically demanding and dangerous exercise. Tearing the hepatic vein or the vena cava during this maneuver is the most common cause of major intraoperative hemorrhage.[27] The endoscopic gastrointestinal anastomosis (GIA) stapler is well suited for ligation of the major hepatic veins in that it has a low profile and is capable of simultaneously sealing both the hepatic vein stump on the vena cava side and the one on the specimen side.

For staple ligation of the right hepatic vein, the right liver is mobilized off the vena cava. Any large accessory right hepatic

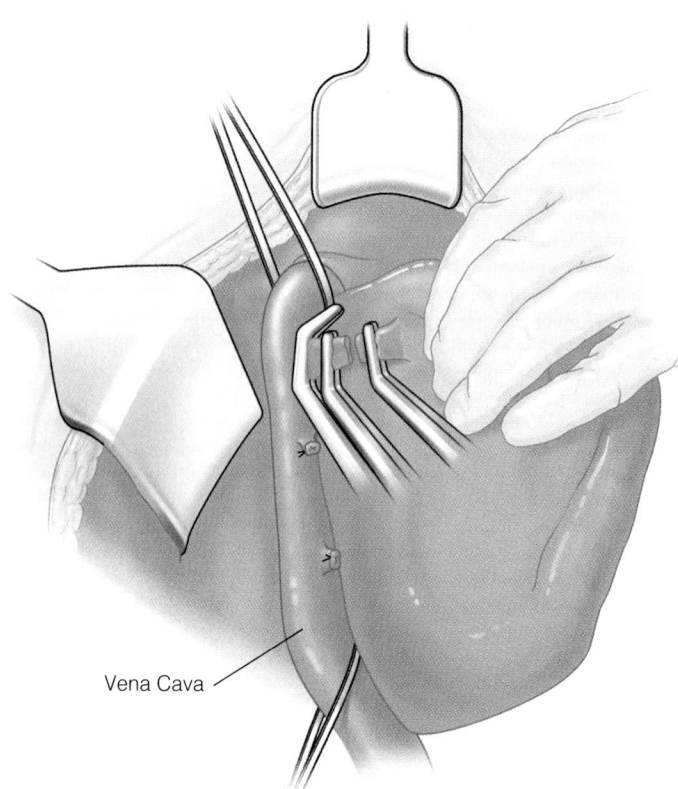

Vena Cava

Figure 10   **Right lobectomy. Once the small perforating vessels to the vena cava have been ligated, further dissection cephalad leads to the right hepatic vein. This vessel is controlled with vascular clamps and divided.**

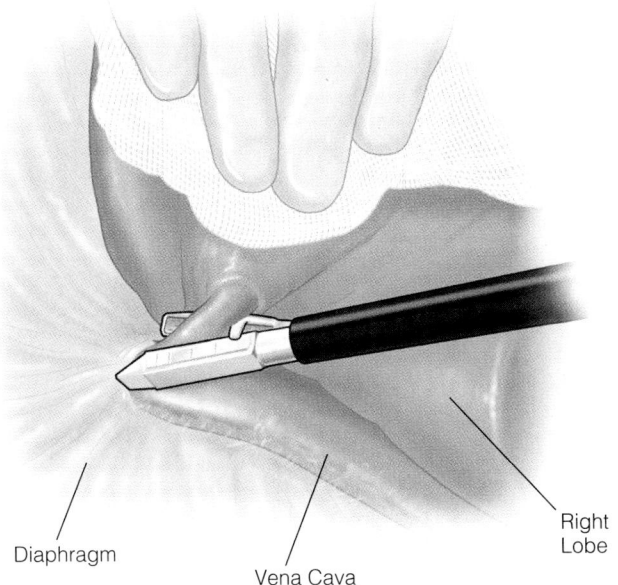

Diaphragm

Vena Cava

Right Lobe

Figure 11 **Right lobectomy. As an alternative to clamping and division, the right hepatic vein may be staple-ligated. Once the small perforating tributaries from the right liver to the vena cava have been divided, the right hepatic vein is isolated and ligated with an endoscopic GIA vascular stapler. The safest method for introducing this stapler is to retract the liver cephalad and to the left while advancing the stapler cephalad in the direction of the vena cava.**

vein encountered can be staple-ligated, as can the tongue of liver tissue that often passes from the right lobe behind the vena cava to the caudate lobe. The right hepatic vein is then identified and isolated. It is the practice of some authors to introduce the stapler from the top of the liver downward,[34] but we find that in most patients, the liver is sufficiently high in the surgical wound to render this angle of introduction technically impracticable. Accordingly, we introduce the stapler parallel to the vena cava and direct it from below upward [see Figure 11]. To ensure that the stapler does not misfire, care should be taken to confirm that no vascular clips are near the site where the stapler is applied.

Step 8: Parenchymal Transection

Inflow to the left liver is temporarily interrupted by clamping the hepatoduodenal ligament (the Pringle maneuver) [see 5:6 *Injuries to the Liver, Biliary Tract, Spleen, and Diaphragm*]. The safety of temporary occlusion of the vessels supplying the hepatic remnant is well documented. Even in patients with cirrhosis, the warm ischemia produced by continuous application of the Pringle maneuver is well tolerated for as long as 1 hour.[40] Our practice is to apply the Pringle maneuver intermittently for periods of 10 minutes, with 2 to 5 minutes of perfusion between applications to allow decompression of the gut.

Parenchymal division is then begun along the line demarcated by the devascularization of the right liver. The line of transection along the principal plane is marked with the electrocautery and then cut with scissors. Stay sutures of 0 chromic catgut are placed on either side of the plane of transection and used for traction, separation, and elevation as dissection proceeds.

Many special instruments have been proposed for use in parenchymal transection, including electrocauteries, ultrasonic dissectors, and water-jet dissectors. We find that for the majority of hepatic resections, blunt clamp dissection is the most rapid method and is quite safe. In essence, a large Kelly clamp is used to crush the liver parenchyma [see Figure 12]. The relatively soft liver substance dissects away, leaving behind the vascular and biliary structures, which are then ligated. With this technique, the principal plane of the liver can usually be transected in less than 30 minutes.

In cirrhotic patients, the clamp-crushing technique may not work as well because of the firmness of the liver substance: the vessels often tear before the parenchyma does. Accordingly, in

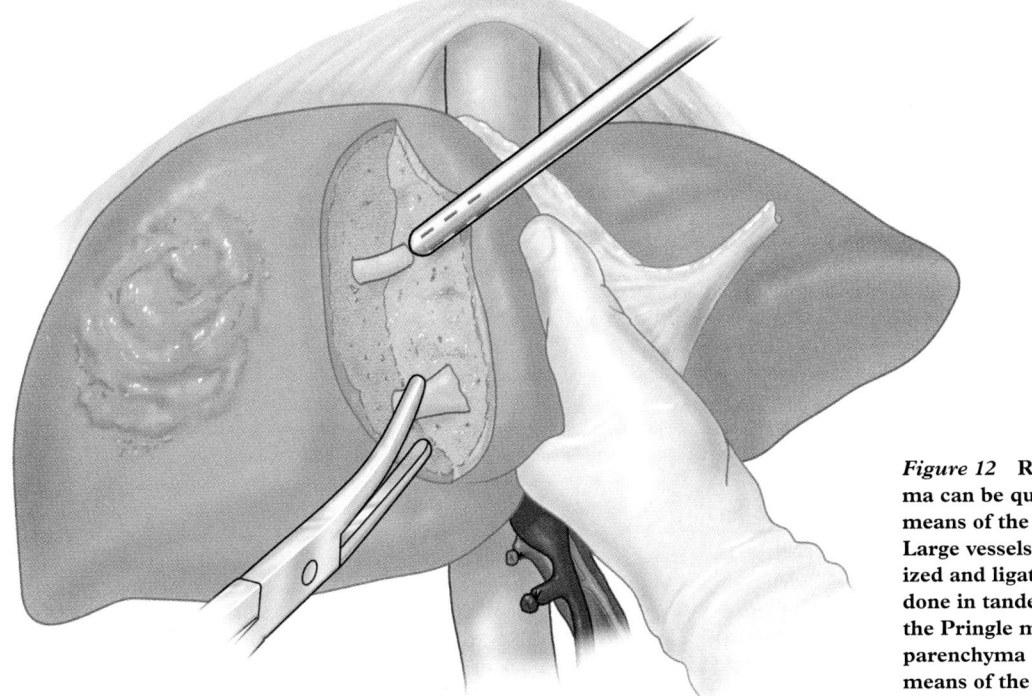

Figure 12 **Right lobectomy. The parenchyma can be quickly and safely transected by means of the clamp-crushing technique. Large vessels and biliary radicles are visualized and ligated or clipped. This is usually done in tandem with inflow occlusion (i.e., the Pringle maneuver). Alternatively, the parenchyma can be bluntly dissected away by means of the finger-fracture technique.**

cirrhotic patients, ultrasonic dissectors that coagulate while transecting the parenchyma may be a better choice. Water-jet dissectors may be useful in defining the major intrahepatic vascular pedicles or the junction of the hepatic vein and the vena cava, particularly if tumor is in close proximity.

After the specimen is removed, the raw surface of the hepatic remnant is carefully examined for hemostasis and bile leaks. Any oozing from the raw surface may be controlled with the argon beam coagulator. Biliary leaks should be controlled with clipping or suture ligation. The retroperitoneal surfaces should also be examined carefully for hemostasis, and the argon beam coagulator should be used where necessary.

Step 9: Closure and Drainage

The abdominal wall is closed in one or two layers with continuous absorbable monofilament sutures. The skin is closed with staples or with subcuticular sutures. Drains are unnecessary in most routine cases[41]; sometimes, in fact, they may exert harmful effects by leading to ascending infection or fluid management problems if ascites develops. There are four clinical situations in which we will routinely place a drain: (1) clear biliary leakage, (2) an infected operative field, (3) a thoracoabdominal incision, and (4) biliary reconstruction. In the case of the thoracoabdominal incision, a drain is placed to ensure that biliary leakage does not develop into a fistula into the chest.

LEFT LOBECTOMY

Steps 1 through 5

Left lobectomy involves removal of segments 2, 3, 4, and sometimes 1. The first five steps of the procedure are much the same as those of a right lobectomy.

Step 6 (Extrahepatic Dissection and Ligation): Control of Inflow Vessels

Extrahepatic control of vascular inflow vessels can be achieved in essentially the same fashion in a right-side resection. Our preference is to start the dissection at the base of the umbilical fissure. The left hepatic artery is divided first. The left branch of the portal vein is then easily identified at the base of the umbilical fissure. The point at which the left portal vein is to be divided depends on the extent of the planned parenchymal resection [see Figure 13]: if the caudate lobe is to be preserved, the left portal vein is ligated just distal to its caudate branch (line B); if the caudate lobe is to be removed, the left portal vein is ligated proximal to the origins of the portal venous branches to this lobe (line A).

Step 6—Alternative (Intrahepatic Pedicle Ligation): Control of Inflow Vessels

If the hepatectomy is being done to treat benign disease or to remove a malignancy that is remote from the base of the umbilical fissure, we highly recommend performing stapler-assisted pedicle ligation in preference to extrahepatic dissection and ligation.

The left portal pedicle is identified at the base of the umbilical fissure. The hilar plate is lowered through an incision at hepatotomy site C [see Figure 7], and a second incision is made in the back of segment 2 at hepatotomy site E [see Figure 7], thereby allowing isolation of the left portal pedicle with minimal risk of injury to the hilus. If the caudate lobe is to be removed as well, incisions should be made at hepatotomy sites C and F [see Figure 7] to allow isolation of the main left portal pedicle proximal to the vessels nourishing the caudate. The portal pedicle is isolated and secured with an umbilical tape. There is some risk that in the

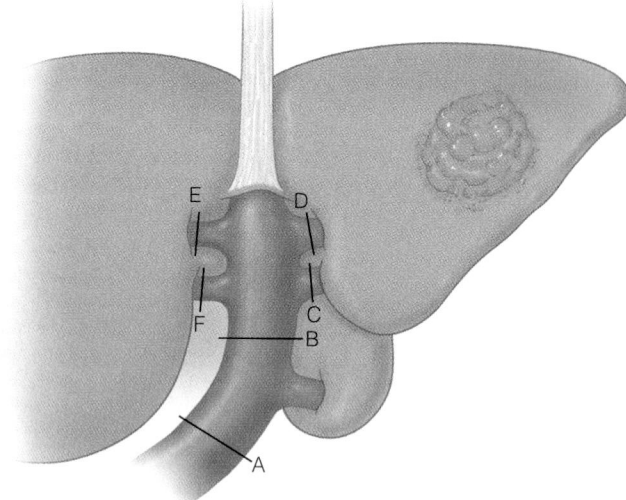

Figure 13 Left lobectomy. Ligation of vascular pedicles at specific sites in the left liver interrupts inflow to specific areas. Ligation at A interrupts inflow to the entire left liver, including the caudate lobe. Ligation at B interrupts blood flow to the left liver while sparing the caudate lobe. Ligation at C devascularizes segment 2, and ligation at D devascularizes segment 3. Ligation at E and F devascularizes segment 4.

course of securing the left portal pedicle, the middle hepatic vein, which lies immediately lateral to the left portal pedicle, may be injured. To minimize this risk, firm downward traction is applied to the umbilical tape, and a TA-30 vascular stapler is placed across the left portal pedicle [see Figure 14]. The pedicle is then stapled and divided.

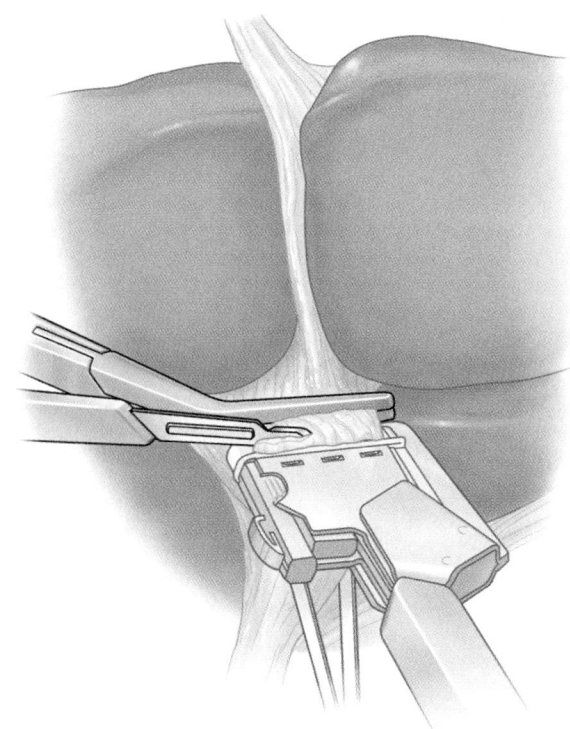

Figure 14 Left lobectomy. After hepatotomies in segment 4 and in the back of segment 2, the left portal pedicle is isolated, stapled, and divided.

Step 7: Control of Outflow Vessels

The left liver is retracted to the patient's right, and the entire lesser omentum is divided. The ligamentum venosum is identified between the caudate lobe and the back of segment 2 and is then divided near its attachment to the left hepatic vein; this measure facilitates identification and dissection of the left and middle hepatic veins anterior to the inferior vena cava. The left and middle hepatic veins are isolated in preparation for division.

Control of the left hepatic vein is quickly and safely accomplished by means of stapled ligation. In approximately 60% of patients, the left and middle hepatic veins join to form a single trunk before entering the vena cava. In a left lobectomy, the middle hepatic vein is often left intact; accordingly, if this is the surgeon's intent, it is vital to protect the middle hepatic vein while ligating the left. After the left hepatic vein is identified, an endoscopic GIA-30 vascular stapler is directed from above downward [*see Figure 15*] to ligate this vessel. The liver is retracted to the right to permit visualization of the junction of the left and middle hepatic veins. If ligation of the middle hepatic vein is desired as well, as is the case when there is tumor in proximity to the vessel, this can be accomplished with a stapler directed along the same path used for left hepatic vein ligation.

Steps 8 and 9

Parenchymal transection and closure are accomplished in much the same manner in a left lobectomy as in a right lobectomy (see above).

OTHER ANATOMIC RESECTIONS

In the ensuing discussion of the other major anatomic resections, we focus primarily on the major points in which they differ from right and left lobectomy. More detailed discussions of these operations are available in specialty texts on liver resection.[26,27]

Extended Right Hepatectomy (Right Trisegmentectomy)

An extended right hepatectomy involves removal of the right lobe along with segment 4—that is, all liver tissue to the right of the falciform ligament [*see Figure 3c*]. The initial steps of this operation are the same as those of a right lobectomy, up through division of the right inflow vessels and the right hepatic vein.

The next step is devascularization of segment 4. The umbilical fissure is dissected to permit identification of the vascular pedicles to segments 2, 3, and 4, which lie within this fissure [*see Figure 13*]. In most cases, the lower part of the umbilical fissure is concealed by a bridge of liver tissue fusing segments 2 and 3 to segment 4. After this tissue bridge is divided with diathermy, the ligamentum teres is retracted caudally to reveal the vascular pedicles from the umbilical fissure to segment 4 (lines E and F [*see Figure 13*]). We generally suture-ligate these pedicles before dividing them.

The liver tissue is then transected immediately to the right of the falciform ligament, from the anterior surface back toward the divided right hepatic vein. The middle hepatic vein is generally left intact until it is encountered in the upper part of the dissection, at which point it is controlled and either suture- or staple-ligated.

Left Lateral Segmentectomy

A left lateral segmentectomy involves removal of only segments 2 and 3—that is, all liver tissue to the left of the falciform ligament [*see Figure 3d*]. These segments are mobilized by dividing the left falciform and triangular ligaments. As this is done, care

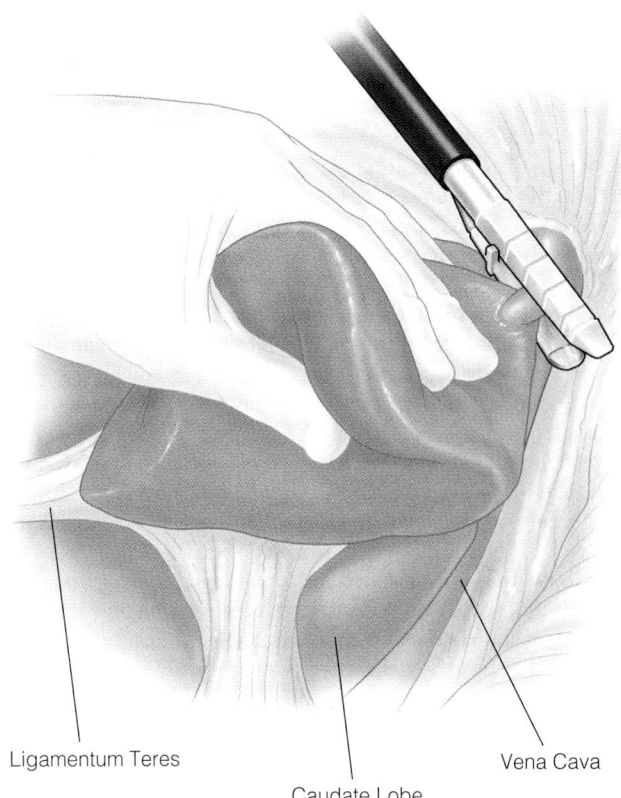

Ligamentum Teres

Caudate Lobe

Vena Cava

Figure 15 **Left lobectomy. Staple ligation of the left hepatic vein. After the left lobe is completely mobilized through division of the left triangular ligament and the lesser omentum, the left hepatic vein is isolated and ligated with an endoscopic GIA vascular stapler. The best angle for introducing the stapler is from the xiphoid posteriorly and caudad.**

must be taken not to injure the left hepatic and phrenic veins, which lie on the medial portion of the left triangular ligament.

The falciform ligament is retracted caudally, and the bridge of liver tissue between segment 4 and segments 2 and 3 is divided with diathermy. Dissection is then performed within the umbilical fissure to the left of the main triad. The vascular pedicles to segments 2 and 3 usually are then readily dissected and controlled (lines C and D [*see Figure 13*]). Control of these pedicles within the umbilical fissure is particularly important for tumor clearance if tumor is in proximity to the umbilical fissure: if the condition is benign or if tumor is remote from the umbilical fissure, the liver may be split anteroposteriorly just to the left of the ligamentum teres and the falciform ligament, and the vascular pedicles may be identified and ligated as they are encountered in the course of parenchymal transection.

Once the inflow vessels have been ligated, the left hepatic vein is identified and then divided either before parenchymal transection or as the vessel is encountered near the completion of parenchymal transection. If there is tumor near the dome, it is particularly important for tumor clearance that the left hepatic vein be controlled and ligated early and outside the liver.

Extended Left Hepatectomy (Left Trisegmentectomy)

An extended left hepatectomy involves resection of segments 2, 3, 4, 5, 8, and sometimes 1 [*see Figure 3e*]. In essence, it is a left lobectomy combined with a right anterior sectorectomy; it may or may not include excision of the caudate lobe. This complex resection is usually undertaken to excise large tumors that occupy the left lobe and cross the principal scissura into the right anterior sector.

In this procedure, it is essential to preserve the right hepatic vein, which constitutes the sole venous drainage of the hepatic remnant. Usually, however, parenchymal transection must be performed along the course of this vein; thus, the major potential danger in the operation is injury to the vessel, which could lead to hemorrhage or hepatic failure from venous congestion of the hepatic remnant. In addition, because the blood supply to segment 7 often arises from the right anterior portal pedicle or from the junction of the right anterior and posterior pedicles [see Figure 8], there is a risk that the operation may result in devascularization of a large portion of the hepatic remnant. Finally, because of the great variability of the biliary anatomy and the extensive intrahepatic dissection required in this procedure, there is a significant risk of biliary complications.[42] For all of these reasons, extended left hepatectomies are rarely performed outside major centers.[43]

In the planning of an extended left hepatectomy, particularly close attention must be paid to preoperative imaging investigations so that the right-side intrahepatic vessels and biliary structures can be accurately delineated. Thin-slice CT or MRI images in the form of arterial, portal venous, and hepatic venous reconstructions [see Figure 2] are quite helpful in this regard. For large tumors encroaching on the hepatic hilum or on the junction of the right anterior and posterior pedicles, direct angiography may still be necessary.

The liver is fully mobilized by dividing not only the left triangular ligament but also the ligaments on the right. This step is essential for identifying the correct plane of parenchymal dissection and for ensuring safe dissection along the right hepatic vein.

The initial dissection is the same as for a left lobectomy. The liver is turned to the right side and the portal triad approached. The inflow vessels to the left liver are ligated, and the left hepatic vein and the subdiaphragmatic inferior vena cava are dissected free. The left and middle hepatic veins are controlled and ligated in the extrahepatic portions of their courses.[43] The left liver is thereby freed, and dissection on the right liver is greatly facilitated.

Next, the plane of transection within the right liver is defined. This plane is horizontal and lies lateral to the gallbladder fossa and just anterior to the main right hepatic venous trunk in the right scissura, halfway between the right anterior pedicle and the right posterior pedicle. The plane can be approximated by drawing a line from just anterior to the right hepatic vein at its insertion into the vena cava to a point immediately behind the fissure of Gans. This line can be accurately defined by clamping the portal pedicle to the anterior right sector of the liver.[43] If the tumor is remote from the junction of the right anterior and posterior portal pedicles, the anterior pedicle is controlled as outlined earlier [see Right Lobectomy, Step 6—Alternative (Intrahepatic Pedicle Ligation), above]. A vascular clamp is placed on the pedicle and the line of demarcation on the liver surface inspected before the pedicle is divided. If segment 7 appears to be ischemic as well, further dissection must be done to identify and protect the origins of the vessels supplying segment 7.

Parenchymal dissection is then carried out from below upward, with bleeding controlled by means of low central venous pressure anesthesia and intermittent application of the Pringle maneuver. If the caudate lobe is to be removed as part of the total resection, the veins draining the caudate must be controlled before parenchymal transection.

Segment-Oriented Resection

Each segment of the liver can be resected independently. In addition, resections involving only the right posterior sector (segments 6 and 7) or the right anterior sector (segments 5 and 8) are not uncommon. Extensive and excellent descriptions of so-called segment-oriented hepatic resection are available elsewhere.[44,45]

Postoperative Care

I.V. fluids administered postoperatively should include phosphorus for support of liver regeneration. For large-volume hepatic resections, electrolyte levels, blood count, and prothrombin time (PT) are checked after the operation and then daily for 3 to 4 days. Packed red blood cells are administered if the hemoglobin level falls to 8 mg/dl or lower, and fresh frozen plasma is given if the PT is longer than 17 seconds. Postoperative pain control is best achieved with patient-controlled analgesia (PCA). Because of the decreased clearance of liver-metabolized drugs after a major hepatectomy, selection and dosing of pain medications should be adjusted accordingly. An oral diet can be resumed as early as postoperative day 3 unless a biliary-enteric anastomosis was performed.

Peripheral edema is common after major hepatic resections and may be treated with spironolactone. If an unexplained fever occurs or the bilirubin level rises when other hepatic function parameters are normal, an intra-abdominal bile collection may be present, and a CT scan should be obtained. Percutaneous drain placement usually brings about resolution of such collections after a few days; reoperation is rarely necessary.

Special Considerations

TOTAL VASCULAR ISOLATION FOR CONTROL OF BLEEDING

For control of bleeding during liver parenchymal transection, a technique known as total vascular isolation can be used as an alternative to the Pringle maneuver. In this technique, the liver is isolated by controlling the inferior vena cava (both above and below the liver), the portal vein, and the hepatic artery. This approach is based on techniques developed for liver transplantation and on the observation that the liver is capable of tolerating total normothermic ischemia for as long as 1 hour.[46] Its primary advantage is that while the liver is isolated, little or no bleeding occurs. It does, however, have disadvantages as well. In some patients, temporary occlusion of the inferior vena cava causes hemodynamic instability as a consequence of reduced cardiac output coupled with increased systemic vascular resistance.[47] Cardiac failure with marked hypotension, cardiac arrhythmia, and even cardiac arrest may ensue. In addition, when hepatic perfusion is restored, the sudden return of stagnant potassium-rich blood to the systemic circulation can aggravate the situation. For these reasons and because bleeding is generally well controlled with low central venous pressure anesthesia, we believe that total vascular isolation is useful only in rare cases. The clinical data published to date support this view. A prospective study from 1996 found that total vascular isolation had no major advantages over the approach described earlier [see Operative Technique, Right Lobectomy, Step 8, above] and was actually associated with greater blood loss.[39]

The one setting where we believe that total vascular isolation may have a significant role to play is in the surgical management of hepatic tumors, particularly very large tumors that compromise the vena cava or the hepatic veins. To extend the duration of vascular isolation in this setting, a venovenous bypass that vents the splanchnic blood into the systemic circulation may be used.[48] To further minimize parenchymal injury during vascular isolation, the liver may be perfused with cold organ preservation solutions. For extensive vascular invasion that necessitates major vena caval or hepatic venous reconstruction, some authors have suggested that the liver can be removed during venovenous bypass and resection and reconstruction performed extracorporeally.[49]

Although there are clinical situations that call for venovenous bypass and ex vivo resection, in practice, these techniques are very rarely necessary: short-length vena caval resection and reconstruction can be performed quite safely without resort to them. In fact, involvement of the retrohepatic vena cava at a level below the major hepatic veins can generally be treated with simple excision of the affected segment without replacement,[50] particularly if complete obstruction at this level has already led to established collateral circulation.

THE CIRRHOTIC PATIENT

Cirrhotic patients, by definition, have reduced hepatic functional capacity and reserve. Accordingly, these patients are at higher risk from hepatectomy and require careful assessment of liver function, appropriate selection for surgery and choice of operation, and greater attention to perioperative care.

Operative Planning

Selection of patients Hepatic failure is the major cause of hospital death and long-term morbidity after hepatic resection in cirrhotic patients.[51-55] Consequently, determination of a cirrhotic patient's candidacy for hepatectomy is based on preoperative assessment of baseline liver function.

A variety of tests have been proposed for assessment of hepatic reserve, including measurement of clearance of various dyes and metabolic substrates (e.g., indocyanine green[56,57] and aminopyrine[51]). Measurement of the urea-nitrogen synthesis rate has also been suggested as a way of predicting outcome after resection.[54] Another functional test involves administering lidocaine and measuring levels of monethylglycinexylidide (a metabolite of lidocaine that is generated mostly through the cytochrome P-450 enzyme system in the liver) as a gauge of liver function.[58] Measurement of the hepatic portal venous pressure gradient via invasive radiologic techniques has been found to predict postoperative hepatic failure.[59] Assessment of portal venous hemodynamics by means of noninvasive Doppler ultrasonography has also been found to predict outcome after hepatectomy.[60]

Currently, none of these functional tests are routinely done at most major liver resection centers. In practice, the Child-Pugh score [*see 3:4 Jaundice*] is the most commonly employed clinical tool for selection of surgical candidates. A Child-Pugh score higher than 8 is generally accepted as a contraindication to major hepatic resection.[53,55,61-64]

Choice of procedure The appropriate extent of resection for cirrhotic patients may be quite different from that for noncirrhotic patients. In cirrhotic patients, the majority of hepatectomies are performed to eradicate hepatocellular carcinoma. A prime consideration in such resections is the margin needed to ensure tumor clearance. Most clinicians aim for a tumor-free margin of 1 cm. A 1989 study, however, found that in cirrhotic patients with hepatocellular carcinoma, as long as the tumor margin was microscopically clear of cancer, the exact size of the margin was not correlated with the incidence of recurrence.[65] In fact, the acceptance

of limited margins, coupled with the acceptance of nonanatomic resections aimed at preserving as much functional parenchyma as possible, is the single change in technical practice that is most responsible for the great improvements in the safety of hepatic resection observed worldwide in cirrhotic patients.

The guiding principle for hepatectomy in cirrhotic patients is that limited resections should be favored, with as much functional parenchyma spared as possible. In general, even for patients with well-compensated Child's grade A cirrhosis, we try to limit resections to less than two segments of functional liver. Patients with large tumors are more likely to tolerate a major resection because little functional parenchyma must be removed along with the tumor. Major hepatic resections involving removal of at least one lobe are now reported to carry an operative mortality of less than 10% in cirrhotic patients.[66,67] Such procedures are usually performed in cirrhotic patients who have large tumors replacing most of one lobe, acceptable liver function, and no atrophy of the uninvolved lobe. Small tumors are often more difficult to manage. For patients with small, deeply placed tumors whose resection would necessitate removal of a large amount of functional parenchyma, an ablative alternative or even transplantation might be more suitable.

In an attempt to preserve as much functional liver as possible, many surgeons resort to more technically challenging operations. Most will perform multiple limited resections in order to avoid performing a full lobectomy.[68,69] Some go so far as to reconstruct the right hepatic vein for the purpose of preserving venous outflow in segments 5 and 6 after resection of segments 7 and 8.

Operative Technique

Hepatic resection in cirrhotic patients is associated with certain specific technical difficulties that substantially increase the complexity of the operation. The liver parenchyma is hard, which makes retraction of the liver difficult. In addition, anatomic landmarks are distorted and difficult to find as a consequence of fibrosis and atrophy-hypertrophy. Finally, portal hypertension and tissue friability contribute to increased blood loss during mobilization and parenchymal transection.

Exposure and mobilization Trifurcated incisions and thoracoabdominal incisions should be avoided in cirrhotic patients because of the potential for ascitic leakage externally or into the chest. The increased firmness of the cirrhotic liver and the consequent difficulty of retraction can lead to significant blood loss from retroperitoneal or phrenic collateral vessels during mobilization. To prevent such bleeding, it may be preferable to use an anterior approach in which the liver parenchyma is split within the principal interlobar plane down to the anterior surface of the vena cava before the right liver is mobilized off the retroperitoneum.[70] The right lobe is then mobilized in a medial-to-lateral direction, and the right hepatic vein is secured during mobilization of the right lobe off the vena cava.

Inflow control At one time, it was widely doubted whether the Pringle maneuver was safe in cirrhotic patients. Subsequently, however, many studies verified that this maneuver can be performed for extended periods in cirrhotic patients without increasing either morbidity or mortality.[71-76] Nevertheless, it is advisable to employ the Pringle maneuver sparingly in this population so as to minimize ischemic stress. Our practice is to clamp the portal triad with a vessel loop tourniquet for 10-minute periods with 5-minute breaks in between. We have not found additional protective maneuvers (e.g., topical cooling[77,78]) to be necessary.

a   *b*

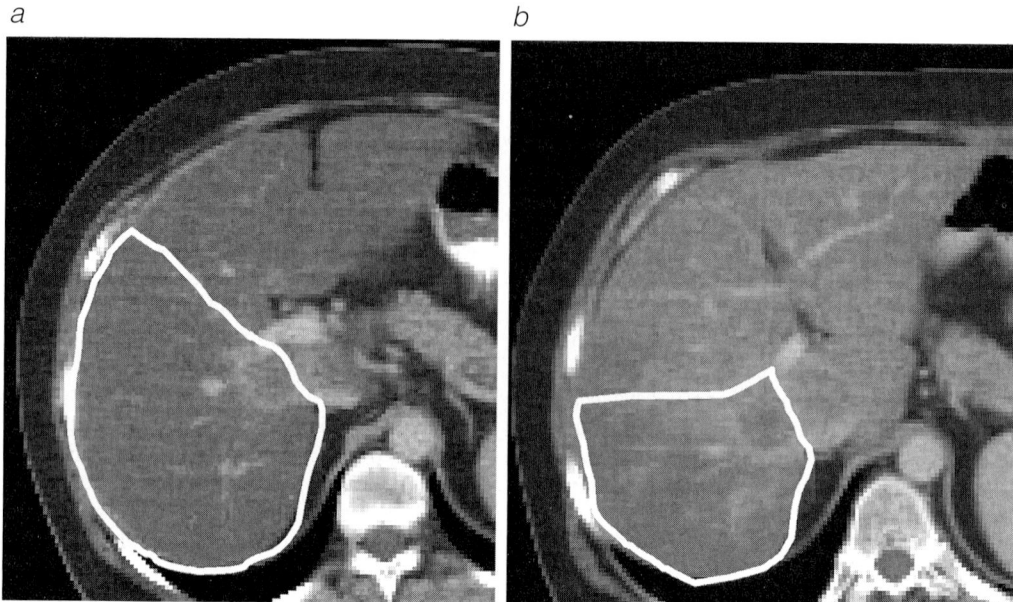

Figure 16   Liver atrophy and hypertrophy occur after right portal vein embolization. Shown are images of the liver (*a*) at baseline and (*b*) 6 weeks after PVE. The right liver is outlined in white.

Parenchymal transection   In patients with normal liver parenchyma, most experienced hepatic surgeons use blunt dissection, with either the clamp-crushing technique or the finger-fracture technique, to transect the liver tissue.[79] In patients with cirrhosis, however, the firmness of the parenchyma makes the clamp-crushing technique less than ideal: because the parenchyma is often harder than the underlying vasculature and biliary radicles, blunt dissection is likely to tear these vessels. Accordingly, ultrasonic dissectors that coagulate and seal vessels during dissection are more suitable for parenchymal transection in this population.

Closure and drainage   Because of the likelihood of postoperative ascites, the abdominal wall is closed with a heavy continuous absorbable monofilament suture to create a watertight closure. To prevent major fluid and protein losses and ascending infections, abdominal drains generally are not used.[41] Reports specifically examining the role of drainage in cirrhotic patients documented a much lower incidence of postoperative complications and a shorter hospital stay for patients in whom no drains were placed.[80,81]

Postoperative Care

The focus of postoperative care in cirrhotic patients is on management of cirrhosis and portal hypertension. In most such patients who undergo hepatic resection, transient hepatic insufficiency develops postoperatively, with hyperbilirubinemia, ascites formation, hypoalbuminemia, edema, and worsening of the baseline coagulopathy.

In the first 24 hours after the procedure, crystalloid must be administered at a level sufficient to maintain adequate portal perfusion.[82] If patients are stable after the first 24 hours, they are subjected to water and sodium restriction and receive liberal amounts of salt-poor albumin for volume expansion if needed. Spironolactone is started in all patients as soon as oral diet is resumed; furosemide is added as needed. On rare occasions, a peritoneovenous shunt may have to be employed to control postoperative ascites,[83] but this measure is usually unnecessary if patients were properly selected. The PT is checked twice daily

during the immediate postoperative period: a PT longer than 17 seconds is corrected by administering fresh frozen plasma.

Preoperative Portal Vein Embolization

Most liver surgeons would be reluctant to resect more than the equivalent of two segments of functional liver in a patient with documented cirrhosis.[84] Consequently, many cirrhotic patients with technically resectable tumors are relegated to noncurative ablative therapy out of concern over possible postoperative hepatic failure. The situation may be changing, however, with the growing use of preoperative portal vein embolization (PVE), a technique that may extend surgeons' ability to resect tumor in cirrhotic patients.

In PVE, access to the portal vein on the side of the liver to be resected is gained via a percutaneous transhepatic approach. The vein is embolized approximately 1 month before the planned resection so as to produce ipsilateral atrophy along with compensatory hypertrophy of the contralateral future hepatic remnant.[85] The degree of compensatory hypertrophy can be dramatic [*see Figure 16*] and may modulate postoperative hepatic dysfunction. PVE is also employed in patients with normal parenchyma in whom extensive resection may result in a very small hepatic remnant. In patients undergoing extended right hepatectomy, particularly those with congenitally small left lateral sectors, the entire area of the extended hepatectomy, including the main right portal vein and the segmental branches supplying segment 4, can be embolized.[86]

There is substantial evidence that preoperative PVE can be successfully used in patients with cirrhotic livers or impaired liver function and that such use is generally well tolerated.[87-90] This technique can also serve as a test of the regenerative capacity of the hepatic remnant. If no compensatory hypertrophy is seen 4 weeks after PVE, the decision to perform a major hepatectomy should be reconsidered.

Repeat Hepatic Resection

Since 1984, when one of the first reports of repeat hepatic resection was published,[91] a number of reports from around the world have demonstrated that repeat resection can be done safely and with good long-term results even for recurrent malignancies. The morbidity rates and mortalities reported after repeat hepatectomy for metastatic colorectal cancer[92-104] and hepatocellular carcinoma[105-112] are comparable to those reported after initial hepatectomy. Extended survival has been demonstrated, and in some cases, the survival rate is equivalent to or even better than that observed after initial resection.[93,100,107,113] In the following section, we concentrate on the key technical aspects of repeat hepatic resection. Discussions of indications, patient selection, and outcome are available in other sources.[93,100,107,113]

Repeat hepatic resection poses certain technical difficulties that are not commonly encountered during initial resection.[92,114,115] First, adhesions at the previous line of parenchymal transection can make reexposure of the liver difficult. Mobilizing the liver off the vena cava and reexposing the porta hepatis and the hepatic veins can be extremely hazardous if dissection was previously done in these areas. Second, liver regeneration and systemic chemotherapy can induce accumulation of fat within the liver, thereby rendering it more friable[93]; the increased friability further increases the difficulties of reexposure and predisposes to tearing of Glisson's capsule.[114] Third, regeneration alters the normal anatomic configuration of the portal structures [*see Figure 17*].[116] For example, after a right hepatectomy, the porta hepatis is rotated posteriorly and to the right. The normal relationship among the portal structures is altered, with the bile duct displaced posteriorly and the portal vein displaced anteriorly.

Preoperative imaging is even more important for repeat resections than for primary resections. This is because scarring limits access to the liver for intraoperative assessment via palpation or ultrasonography. Before embarking on a repeat resection, it is essential to know the exact number and locations of the lesions to be treated within the regenerated parenchyma. Preoperative imaging also facilitates operative planning by accurately delineating the vasculature within the regenerated liver.

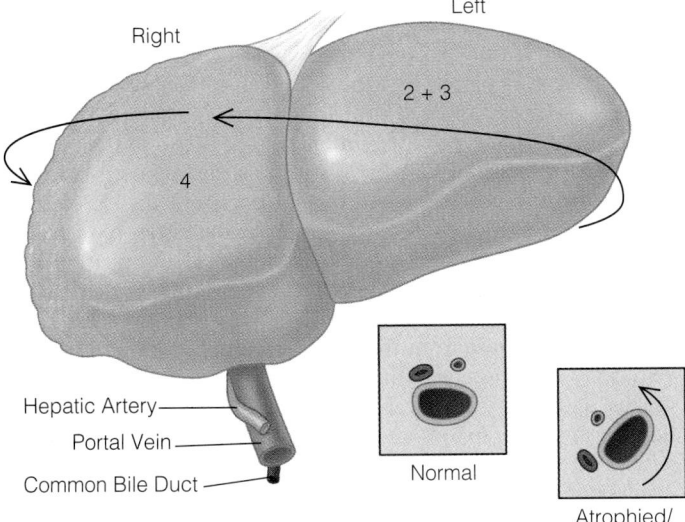

Right

Left

2 + 3

4

Hepatic Artery

Portal Vein

Common Bile Duct

Normal

Atrophied/ Hypertrophied

Figure 17 **Repeat hepatic resection. Depicted are the changes in the relations of the portal structures that occur as a result of right liver atrophy or resection and left-side hypertrophy. The structures in the porta hepatis rotate to the right, with the CBD coming to rest laterally rather than anteriorly.**

In a repeat resection after a previous major right hepatectomy, it is important to be prepared to convert the incision into a thoracoabdominal incision if necessary. Access through the right chest may be required for mobilization of the liver because of adherence of the previous resection margin to the diaphragm, or it may be required for access to the rotated CBD and portal vasculature at the porta hepatis.

In the dissection of the right upper quadrant after a previous right hepatectomy, three landmarks are particularly helpful in defining the anatomic structures within the regenerated left liver. The first landmark is remnants of the ligamentum teres, which defines the demarcation between the left lateral segment and segment 4; these should be found early on. The ligamentum teres may be followed to the base of the umbilical fissure to define the location of the left hepatic artery. Whether this artery arises from the common hepatic artery or from the left gastric artery, it passes into the liver parenchyma at the base of the umbilical fissure. The second landmark is the caudate lobe. The lesser omentum should be opened early on to reveal this lobe. An index finger should then be passed in front of the caudate toward the obliterated foramen of Winslow to define the porta hepatis and the location of the portal vein. The third landmark is the vena cava. Performing the Kocher maneuver to mobilize the duodenum off the vena cava allows this vessel to be dissected, thus further defining the portocaval plane. Definition of this plane leads to the correct plane for dissection and mobilization of the liver off the vena cava; it also allows isolation of the hepatoduodenal ligament for application of the Pringle maneuver and for extrahepatic dissection of the inflow vessels.

In a repeat resection after a previous left hepatectomy, the main concern with regard to mobilization of the liver is the anterior position of the portal vasculature after right-side hypertrophy. It is therefore prudent to mobilize the right liver, perform a Kocher maneuver, and follow the vena cava caudally to identify the portal vein from the right. The stomach and the colon usually are adherent to the edge of the previous resection and must be carefully dissected free to allow access to the liver. If the middle hepatic vein was preserved in the earlier left hepatectomy, it will lie immediately deep to the plane of the stomach or the colon and thus may be a source of hemorrhage during dissection.

Control of the inflow or outflow vasculature may be compromised by the scarring resulting from the previous operation. If extensive extrahepatic dissection was performed for control of inflow vasculature in the earlier procedure, control of these vessels in the repeat resection is more safely accomplished via intrahepatic pedicle ligation [*see* Operative Technique, Right Lobectomy, Step 6—Alternative (Intrahepatic Pedicle Ligation), *above*].

A major concern with repeat hepatectomy is that it is sometimes necessary to perform more limited resections than would otherwise be indicated. Normally, for removal of liver tumors, we avoid wedge excisions because these nonanatomic resections are more often associated with greater blood loss and positive margins than anatomic resections are.[99,117] In a repeat hepatectomy, however, anatomic considerations arising in the regenerated liver may make a wedge resection the best choice.

With appropriate patient selection and careful operative planning, very favorable perioperative and long-term results can be achieved after repeat hepatic resection. It is noteworthy that studies addressing repeat resection have not documented any substantial increases in blood loss, duration of operation, or rate of complications in comparison with the initial resection.[93-97,118]

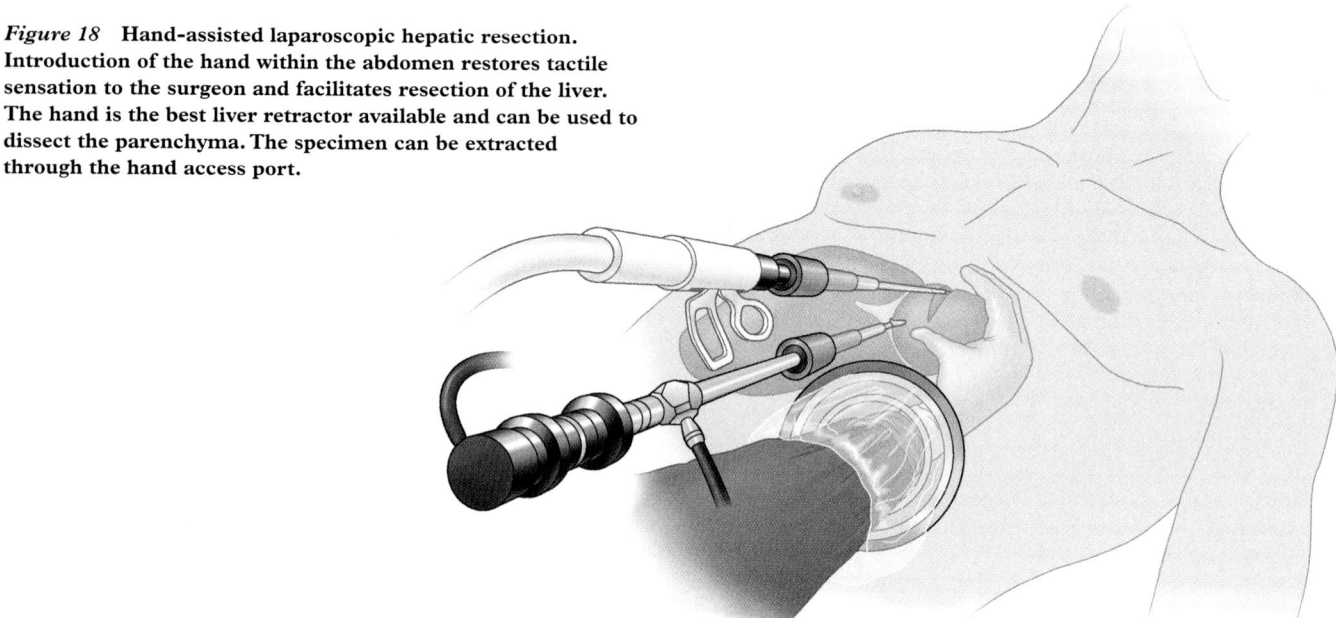

Figure 18 **Hand-assisted laparoscopic hepatic resection. Introduction of the hand within the abdomen restores tactile sensation to the surgeon and facilitates resection of the liver. The hand is the best liver retractor available and can be used to dissect the parenchyma. The specimen can be extracted through the hand access port.**

Hand-Assisted Laparoscopic Hepatic Resection

In addition to revolutionizing treatment of gallstone disease,[119] laparoscopic techniques are increasingly used for fenestration of benign cysts of the liver[120,121] and for staging of hepatobiliary malignancies to prevent unnecessary laparotomies.[29,122,123] Until recently, however, laparoscopic resection of liver tumors was described only in case reports or small series.[120,124-128] Perhaps the main reason for the strong resistance to laparoscopic hepatic resection has been fear of catastrophic bleeding. If inadvertent damage to a major hepatic vein or the vena cava occurs during an open operation, the bleeding can be controlled with direct manual compression until the vessel is repaired; however, if such damage occurs during a laparoscopic operation, control of the bleeding is considerably more difficult. In addition, damage to a hepatic vein or the vena cava during a laparoscopic procedure can theoretically result in CO_2 embolism. Another concern is that the loss of tactile sensation characteristic of laparoscopic surgery may lead to inadequate tumor clearance. Finally, whereas there are many liver retractors designed to hold the liver in one position, there is no good retractor for repeatedly moving the liver from side to side, as would be necessary during a laparoscopic hepatectomy. The human hand is still the best tool for this purpose.

Laparoscopic hepatic resection has been greatly facilitated by several recent technologic advances, including laparoscopic staplers[129] and ultrasonic dissectors,[130] which can be used for ligation of the hepatic vasculature and transection of liver parenchyma. The most important advance, however, is the hand access port, a small port through which one hand can be introduced into the abdomen for a hand-assisted laparoscopic resection [*see Figure 18*].[131-133] With this approach, the surgeon not only regains a measure of tactile sensation but also is able to employ the best liver retractor available. Moreover, direct manual compression of any bleeding vessels is once again possible, and the incision made for the hand access port is also used for extraction of the resected specimen.

Patient selection is essential for safe laparoscopic resection of liver tumors. Resection of any two segments along the lower edge of the liver is easily accomplished laparoscopically. At MSKCC, we have laparoscopically resected lesions from all segments.[38]

The procedure starts with the placement of a 10 mm port, usually in the right or left upper quadrant on the side opposite that on which the hand access port will be placed. After staging is performed to ensure that the lesion is resectable, a 5 to 6 cm incision is made for placement of the hand access port. The port site should be chosen so as to allow manual retraction of the part of the liver to be resected, with the falciform and triangular ligaments used to provide countertraction. Once the access port is in place, the abdomen is fully palpated under laparoscopic vision. A laparotomy sponge is placed into the abdomen to facilitate retraction and absorb blood, and a long bulldog clamp is inserted for use in the Pringle maneuver. A long umbilical tape is tied to the bulldog clamp beforehand so that the instrument can be easily located throughout the procedure. Additional ports are then placed as necessary for introduction of the stapler or the ultrasonic scalpel.

The area to be resected is outlined with the electrocautery. The liver is manually retracted, intermittent application of the Pringle maneuver is initiated, and the parenchyma is transected. Liver parenchyma remote from the major portal pedicles and hepatic veins may be transected either with the ultrasonic dissector or by means of finger fracture. Near the major portal pedicles and hepatic veins, an endoscopic GIA vascular stapler may be used. After removal of the specimen, the laparoscopic argon beam coagulator (Conmed Corporation, Utica, New York) and hemostatic agents may be used.

The laparoscopic approach is suitable for minor as well as major hepatic resections. At present, however, it is unclear whether this approach constitutes a significant advance in liver surgery. To clarify this issue, further study of laparoscopic hepatic resection with respect to perioperative outcome, quality of life, and long-term survival is required.

References

1. Lortat-Jacob JL, Robert HG: Hepatectomie droite reglee. Presse Med 60:549, 1952

2. Fong Y: Hepatic colorectal metastasis: current surgical therapy, selection criteria for hepatectomy, and role for adjuvant therapy. Adv Surg 34:351, 2000

3. Jarnagin WR, Fong Y, Blumgart LH: The current management of hilar cholangiocarcinoma. Adv Surg 33:345, 1999

4. Fong Y, Sun RL, Jarnagin W, et al: An analysis of 412 cases of hepatocellular carcinoma at a Western center. Ann Surg 229:790, 1999

5. Couinaud C: Bases anatomiques des hepatectomies gauche et droite reglées. J Chir 70:933, 1954

6. Couinaud C: Le Foie: Etudes Anatomiques et Chirurgicales. Masson, Paris, 1957

7. Bismuth H: Surgical anatomy and anatomic surgery of the liver. World J Surg 6:3, 1982

8. Baer HU, Dennison AR, Maddern GJ, et al: Subtotal hepatectomy: a new procedure based on the inferior right hepatic vein. Br J Surg 78:1221, 1991

9. Smadja C, Blumgart LH: The biliary tract and the anatomy of biliary exposure. Surgery of the Liver and Biliary Tract, 2nd ed. Blumgart LH, Ed. Churchill Livingstone, London, 1994

10. Glisson F: Anatomia Hepatis. O Pullein, London, 1654

11. Launois B, Jamieson GG: The importance of Glisson's capsule and its sheaths in the intrahepatic approach to resection of the liver. Surg Gynecol Obstet 174:7, 1992

12. Soyer P, Levesque M, Elias D, et al: Preoperative assessment of resectability of hepatic metastases from colonic carcinoma: CT portography vs sonography and dynamic CT. AJR Am J Roentgenol 159:741, 1992

13. Hann LE, Schwartz LH, Panicek DM, et al: Tumor involvement in hepatic veins: comparison of MR imaging and US for preoperative assessment. Radiology 206:651, 1998

14. Hann LE, Fong Y, Shriver CD, et al: Malignant hepatic hilar tumors: can ultrasonography be used as an alternative to angiography with CT arterial portography for determination of resectability? J Ultrasound Med 15:37, 1996

15. Gibson RN, Yeung E, Thompson JN, et al: Bile duct obstruction: radiologic evaluation of level, cause and tumor resectability. Radiology 160:43, 1986

16. Fortner JG, Lincer RM: Hepatic resection in the elderly. Ann Surg 211:141, 1990

17. Karl RC, Smith SK, Fabri PJ: Validity of major cancer operations in elderly patients. Ann Surg Oncol 2:107, 1995

18. Fong Y, Blumgart LH, Fortner JG, et al: Pancreatic or liver resection for malignancy is safe and effective for the elderly. Ann Surg 222:426, 1995

19. Hanazaki K, Kajikawa S, Shimozawa N, et al: Hepatic resection for hepatocellular carcinoma in the elderly. J Am Coll Surg 192:38, 2001

20. Fong Y, Brennan MF, Cohen AM, et al: Liver resection in the elderly. Br J Surg 84:1386, 1997

21. Cunningham JD, Fong Y, Shriver C, et al: One hundred consecutive hepatic resections: blood loss, transfusion and operative technique. Arch Surg 129:1050, 1994

22. Melendez J, Ferri E, Zwillman M, et al: Extended hepatic resection: a 6-year retrospective study of risk factors for perioperative mortality. J Am Coll Surg 192:47, 2001

23. Scheele J, Stangl R, Altendorf-Hofmann A, et al: Indicators of prognosis after hepatic resection for colorectal secondaries. Surgery 110:13, 1991

24. Weber SM, Jarnagin WR, DeMatteo RP, et al: Survival after resection of multiple hepatic colorectal metastases. Ann Surg Oncol 7:643, 2000

25. Goldsmith NA, Woodburne RT: The surgical anatomy pertaining to liver resection. Surg Gynecol Obstet 105:310, 1957

26. Blumgart LH, Jarnagin W, Fong Y: Liver resection for benign disease and for liver and biliary tumors. Surgery of the Liver and Biliary Tract, 3rd ed. Blumgart LH, Fong Y, Eds. WB Saunders, London, 2000, p 1639

27. Blumgart LH, Fong Y: Surgical management of colorectal metastases to the liver. Curr Probl Surg 5:333, 1995

28. Jarnagin WR, Conlon K, Bodniewicz J, et al: A clinical scoring system predicts the yield of diagnostic laparoscopy in patients with potentially resectable hepatic colorectal metastases. Cancer 91:1121, 2001

29. Jarnagin WR, Bodniewicz J, Dougherty E, et al: A prospective analysis of staging laparoscopy in patients with primary and secondary hepatobiliary malignancies. J Gastrointest Surg 4:34, 2000

30. Lo CM, Lai EC, Liu CL, et al: Laparoscopy and laparoscopic ultrasonography avoid exploratory laparotomy in patients with hepatocellular carcinoma. Ann Surg 227:527, 1998

31. Callery MP, Strasberg SM, Doherty GM, et al: Staging laparoscopy with laparoscopic ultrasonography: optimizing resectability in hepatobiliary and pancreatic malingnancy. J Am Coll Surg 185:33, 1997

32. Castaing D, Kunstlinger F, Habib N: Intraoperative ultrasound study of the liver: methodology and anatomical results. Am J Surg 149:676, 1985

33. McEntee GP, Nagorney DM: Use of hepatic staplers in major hepatic resections. Br J Surg 78:40, 1991

34. Cohen AM: Use of laparoscopic vascular stapler at laparotomy for colorectal cancer. Dis Colon Rectum 35:910, 1992

35. Jurim O, Colonna II JO, Colquhoun SD, et al: A stapling technique for hepatic resection. J Am Coll Surg 178:510, 1994

36. Yanaga K, Nishizaki T, Yamamoto K, et al: Simplified inflow control using stapling devices for major hepatic resection. Arch Surg 131:104, 1996

37. Lefor AT, Flowers JL: Laparoscopic wedge biopsy of the liver. J Am Coll Surg 178:307, 1994

38. Fong Y, Jarnagin W, Conlon KC, et al: Hand-assisted laparoscopic liver resection: lessons from an initial experience. Arch Surg 135:854, 2000

39. Belghiti J, Noun R, Zante E, et al: Portal triad clamping or hepatic vascular exclusion for major liver resection. Ann Surg 224:155, 1996

40. Bothe AJ, Steele G Jr: Is there a role for perioperative nutritional support in liver resection? HPB Surgery 10:177, 1997

41. Fong Y, Brennan MF, Brown K, et al: Drainage is unnecessary after elective liver resection. Am J Surg 171:158, 1996

42. Starzl TE, Iwatsuki S, Shaw BW, et al: Left hepatic trisegmentectomy. Surg Gynecol Obstet 155:21, 1982

43. Blumgart LH, Baer HU, Czerniak A, et al: Extended left hepatectomy: technical aspects of an evolving procedure. Br J Surg 80:903, 1993

44. Scheele J: Segment oriented resection of the liver: rationale and technique in hepato-biliary and pancreatic malignancies. Lygidakis NJ, Tytgat GNJ, Eds. Thieme, Stuttgart, 1989

45. Scheele J, Stangl R: Segment oriented anatomical liver resections. Surgery of the Liver and Biliary Tract. Blumgart LH, Ed. Churchill Livingstone, London, 1994

46. Huguet C, Nordlinger B, Gallopin JJ, et al: Normothermic hepatic vascular occlusion for extensive hepatectomy. Surg Gynecol Obstet 147:689, 1978

47. Pappas G, Palmer WM, Martineau GL, et al: Hemodynamic alterations caused during orthotopic liver transplantation in humans. Surgery 70:872, 1971

48. Shaw BW, Martin DJ, Marquez JM, et al: Venous bypass in clinical liver transplantation. Ann Surg 200:524, 1984

49. Pichlmayr R, Grosse H, Hauss J, et al: Technique and preliminary results of extracorporeal liver surgery (bench procedure) and of surgery on the in situ perfused liver. Br J Surg 77:21, 1990

50. Cunci O, Coste T, Vacher B, et al: Resection de la veine cave inferieure retro-hepatique au cours d'une hepatectomie pour tumeur. Ann Chir 37:197, 1983

51. Lau H, Man K, Fan ST, et al: Evaluation of preoperative hepatic function in patients with hepatocellular carcinoma undergoing hepatectomy. Br J Surg 84:1255, 1997

52. Takenaka K, Kanematsu T, Fukuzawa K, et al: Can hepatic failure after surgery for hepatocellular carcinoma in cirrhotic patients be prevented? World J Surg 14:123, 1990

53. Nagasue N, Yukaya H, Kohno H, et al: Morbidity and mortality after major hepatic resection in cirrhotic patients with hepatocellular carcinoma. HPB Surg 1:45, 1988

54. Paquet KJ, Koussouris P, Mercado MA, et al: Limited hepatic resection for selected cirrhotic patients with hepatocellular or cholangiocellular carcinoma: a prospective study. Br J Surg 78:459, 1991

55. Fan ST, Lai EC, Lo CM, et al: Hospital mortality of major hepatectomy for hepatocellular carcinoma associated with cirrhosis. Arch Surg 130:198, 1995

56. Hasegawa H, Yamazaki S, Makuuchi M, et al: [Hepatectomy for hepatocarcinoma on a cirrhotic liver: decision plans and principles of perioperative resuscitation. Experience with 204 cases.] J Chir (Paris) 124:425, 1987

57. Makuuchi M, Kosuge T, Takayama T, et al: Surgery for small liver cancers. Semin Surg Oncol 9:298, 1993

58. Ercolani G, Grazi GL, Calliva R, et al: The lidocaine (MEGX) test as an index of hepatic function: its clinical usefulness in liver surgery. Surgery 127:464, 2000

59. Bruix J, Castells A, Bosch J, et al: Surgical resection of hepatocellular carcinoma in cirrhotic patients: prognostic value of preoperative portal pressure. Gastroenterology 111:1018, 1996

60. Yin XY, Lu MD, Huang JF, et al: Significance of portal hemodynamic investigation in prediction of hepatic functional reserve in patients with hepatocellular carcinoma undergoing operative treatment. Hepatogastroenterology 48:1701, 2001

61. Franco D, Capussotti L, Smadja C, et al: Resection of hepatocellular carcinomas: results in 72 European patients with cirrhosis. Gastroenterology 98:733, 1990

62. Wu CC, Ho WL, Yeh DC, et al: Hepatic resection of hepatocellular carcinoma in cirrhotic livers: is it unjustified in impaired liver function? Surgery 120:34, 1996

63. Noun R, Jagot P, Farges O, et al: High preoperative serum alanine transferase levels: effect on

the risk of liver resection in Child grade A cirrhotic patients. World J Surg 21:390, 1997

64. Capussotti L, Borgonovo G, Bouzari H, et al: Results of major hepatectomy for large primary liver cancer in patients with cirrhosis. Br J Surg 81:427, 1994

65. Yoshida Y, Kanematsu T, Matsumata T, et al: Surgical margin and recurrence after resection of hepatocellular carcinoma in patients with cirrhosis: further evaluation of limited hepatic resection. Ann Surg 209:297, 1989

66. Vauthey JN, Klimstra D, Franceschi D, et al: Factors affecting long-term outcome after hepatic resection for hepatocellular carcinoma. Am J Surg 169:28, 1995

67. Poon RT, Fan ST, Lo CM, et al: Intrahepatic recurrence after curative resection of hepatocellular carcinoma: long-term results of treatment and prognostic factors. Ann Surg 229:216, 1999

68. Makuuchi M, Hasegawa H, Yamazaki S, et al: Four new hepatectomy procedures for resection of the right hepatic vein and preservation of the inferior right hepatic vein. Surg Gynecol Obstet 164:68, 1987

69. Makuuchi M, Mori T, Gunven P, et al: Safety of hemihepatic vascular occlusion during resection of the liver. Surg Gynecol Obstet 164:155, 1987

70. Lai EC, Fan ST, Lo CM, et al: Anterior approach for difficult major right hepatectomy. World J Surg 20:314, 1996

71. Nagasue N, Uchida M, Kubota H, et al: Cirrhotic livers can tolerate 30 minutes ischaemia at normal environmental temperature. Eur J Surg 161:181, 1995

72. Wu CC, Hwang CR, Liu TJ, et al: Effects and limitations of prolonged intermittent ischaemia for hepatic resection of the cirrhotic liver. Br J Surg 83:121, 1996

73. Kim YI, Kobayashi M, Aramaki M, et al: "Early-stage" cirrhotic liver can withstand 75 minutes of inflow occlusion during resection. Hepatogastroenterology 41:355, 1994

74. Kim YI, Nakashima K, Tada I, et al: Prolonged normothermic ischaemia of human cirrhotic liver during hepatectomy: a preliminary report. Br J Surg 80:1566, 1993

75. Smadja C, Kahwaji F, Berthoux L, et al: [Value of total pedicle clamping in hepatic excision for hepatocellular carcinoma in cirrhotic patients.] Ann Chir 41:639, 1987

76. Elias D, Desruennes E, Lasser P: Prolonged intermittent clamping of the portal triad during hepatectomy. Br J Surg 78:42, 1991

77. Yamanaka N, Furukawa K, Tanaka T, et al: Topical cooling-assisted hepatic segmentectomy for cirrhotic liver with hepatocellular carcinoma. J Am Coll Surg 184:290, 1997

78. Kim YI, Kobayashi M, Nakashima K, et al: In situ and surface liver cooling with prolonged inflow occlusion during hepatectomy in patients with chronic liver disease. Arch Surg 129:620, 1994

79. Lin TY: A simplified technique for hepatic resection: the crush method. Ann Surg 180:285, 1974

80. Smadja C, Berthoux L, Meakins JL, et al: Patterns of improvement in resection of hepatocellular carcinoma in cirrhotic patients: results of a non drainage policy. HPB Surg 1:141, 1989

81. Franco D, Smadja C, Meakins JL, et al: Improved early results of elective hepatic resection for liver tumors: one hundred consecutive hepatectomies in cirrhotic and noncirrhotic patients. Arch Surg 124:1033, 1989

82. Tsuge H, Mimura H, Orita K, et al: Evaluation of preoperative and postoperative sodium and water loading in patients undergoing hepatectomy for liver cirrhosis complicated by hepatocellular carcinoma. Hepatogastroenterology 38(suppl 1):56, 1991

83. Maeda T, Shimada M, Shirabe K, et al: Strategies for intractable ascites after hepatic resection: analysis of two cases. Br J Clin Pract 49:149, 1995

84. Shirabe K, Shimada M, Gion T, et al: Postoperative liver failure after major hepatic resection for hepatocellular carcinoma in the modern era with special reference to remnant liver volume. J Am Coll Surg 188:304, 1999

85. Makuuchi M, Thai BL, Takayasu K, et al: Preoperative portal embolization to increase safety of major hepatectomy for hilar bile duct carcinoma: a preliminary report. Surgery 107:521, 1990

86. Nagino M, Nimura Y, Kamiya J, et al: Right or left trisegmental portal vein embolization before hepatic trisegmentectomy for hilar bile duct carcinoma. Surgery 117:677, 1995

87. Shimamura T, Nakajima Y, Une Y, et al: Efficacy and safety of preoperative percutaneous transhepatic portal embolization with absolute ethanol: a clinical study. Surgery 121:135, 1997

88. Lee KC, Kinoshita H, Hirohashi K, et al: Extension of surgical indications for hepatocellular carcinoma by portal vein embolization. World J Surg 17:109, 1993

89. Wakabayashi H, Okada S, Maeba T, et al: Effect of preoperative portal vein embolization on major hepatectomy for advanced-stage hepatocellular carcinomas in injured livers: a preliminary report. Surg Today 27:403, 1997

90. Azoulay D, Castaing D, Krissat J, et al: Percutaneous portal vein embolization increases the feasibility and safety of major liver resection for hepatocellular carcinoma in injured liver. Ann Surg 232:665, 2000

91. Tomas de la Vega JE, Donahue EJ, Doolas A, et al: A ten year experience with hepatic resection. Surg Gynecol Obstet 159:223, 1984

92. Bismuth H, Adam R, Navarro F: Re-resection for colorectal liver metastasis. Surg Oncol Clin North Am 5:353, 1996

93. Adam R, Bismuth H, Castaing D, et al: Repeat hepatectomy for colorectal liver metastases. Ann Surg 225:51, 1997

94. Fong Y, Blumgart LH, Cohen A, et al: Repeat hepatic resections for metastatic colorectal cancer. Ann Surg 220:657, 1994

95. Petrowsky H, Gonen M, Jarnagin W, et al: Second liver resections are safe and effective treatment for recurrent hepatic metastases from colorectal cancer: a bi-institutional analysis. Ann Surg 235:863, 2002

96. Pinson CW, Wright JK, Chapman WC, et al: Repeat hepatic surgery for colorectal cancer metastases to the liver. Ann Surg 223:765, 1996

97. Tuttle TM, Curley SA, Roh MS: Repeat hepatic resection as effective treatment for recurrent colorectal liver metastases. Ann Surg Oncol 4:125, 1997

98. Nordlinger B, Vaillant JC, Guiguet M, et al: Survival benefit of repeat liver resections for recurrent colorectal metastases: 143 cases. J Clin Oncol 12:1491, 1994

99. Fernandez-Trigo V, Sharmsa F, Sugarbaker PH, et al: Repeat liver resections from colorectal metastasis. Surgery 117:296, 1995

100. Yamamoto J, Kosuge T, Shimada K, et al: Repeat liver resection for recurrent colorectal liver metastases. Am J Surg 178:275, 1999

101. Muratore A, Polastri R, Bouzari H, et al: Repeat hepatectomy for colorectal liver metastases: a worthwhile operation? J Surg Oncol 76:127, 2001

102. Suzuki S, Sakaguchi T, Yokoi Y, et al: Impact of repeat hepatectomy on recurrent colorectal liver metastases. Surgery 129:421, 2001

103. Riesener K-P, Kasperk R, Winkeltau G, et al: Repeat resection of recurrent hepatic metastases: improvement in prognosis? Eur J Surg 162:709, 1996

104. Kin T, Nakajima Y, Kanehiro H, et al: Repeat hepatectomy for recurrent colorectal metastases. World J Surg 22:1087, 1998

105. Farges O, Regimbeau JM, Belghiti J: Aggressive management of recurrence following surgical resection of hepatocellular carcinoma. Hepatogastroenterology 45(suppl 3):1275, 1998

106. Nagasue N, Kohno H, Hayashi T, et al: Repeat hepatectomy for recurrent hepatocellular carcinoma. Br J Surg 83:127, 1996

107. Neeleman N, Andersson R: Repeated liver resection for recurrent liver cancer. Br J Surg 83:893, 1996

108. Lee PH, Lin WJ, Tsang YM, et al: Clinical management of recurrent hepatocellular carcinoma. Ann Surg 222:670, 1995

109. Hu RH, Lee PH, Yu SC, et al: Surgical resection for recurrent hepatocellular carcinoma: prognosis and analysis of risk factors. Surgery 120:23, 1996

110. Shimada M, Takenaka K, Gion T, et al: Prognosis of recurrent hepatocellular carcinoma: a 10-year surgical experience in Japan. Gastroenterology 111:720, 1996

111. Shuto T, Kinoshita H, Hirohashi K, et al: Indications for, and effectiveness of, a second hepatic resection for recurrent hepatocellular carcinoma. Hepatogastroenterology 43:932, 1996

112. Shimada M, Takenaka K, Taguchi K, et al: Prognostic factors after repeat hepatectomy for recurrent hepatocellular carcinoma. Ann Surg 227:80, 1998

113. Sugimachi K, Maehara S, Tanaka S, et al: Repeat hepatectomy is the most useful treatment for recurrent hepatocellular carcinoma. J Hepatobiliary Pancreat Surg 8:410, 2001

114. Elias D, Lasser P, Hoang JM, et al: Repeat hepatectomy for cancer. Br J Surg 80:1557, 1993

115. Hemming AW, Langer B: Repeat resection of recurrent hepatic colorectal metastases. Br J Surg 81:1553, 1994

116. Blumgart LH, Baer HU: Hilar and intrahepatic biliary-enteric anastomosis. Surgery of the Liver and Biliary Tract. Blumgart LH, Ed. Churchill Livingstone, London, 1994, p 1051

117. Polk W, Fong Y, Karpeh M, et al: A technique for the use of cryosurgery to assist hepatectomy. J Am Coll Surg 180:171, 1995

118. Chu QD, Vezeridis MP, Avradopoulos KA, et al: Repeat hepatic resection for recurrent colorectal cancer. World J Surg 21:292, 1997

119. The Southern Surgeons Club: A prospective analysis of 1518 laparoscopic cholecystectomies. N Engl J Med 324:1073, 1991

120. Katkhouda N, Hurwitz M, Gugenheim J, et al: Laparoscopic management of benign solid and cycstic lesions of the liver. Ann Surg 229:460, 1999

121. Jeng KS, Yang FS, Kao CR, et al: Management of symptomatic polycystic liver disease: laparoscopy adjuvant with alcohol sclerotherapy. J Gastroenterol Hepatol 10:359, 1995

122. Cuesta MA, Meijer S, Borgstein PJ, et al: Laparoscopic ultrasonography for hepatobiliary and pancreatic malignancy. Br J Surg 80:1571, 1993

123. Ravikumar TS: Laparoscopic staging and intraoperative ultrasonography for liver tumor management. Surg Oncol Clin North Am 5:271, 1996

124. Asahara T, Dohi K, Nakahara H, et al: Laparoscopy-assisted hepatectomy for a large tumor of the liver. Hiroshima J Med Sci 47:163, 1998

125. Huscher CGS, Lirici MM, Chiodini S: Laparoscopic liver resections. Semin Laparosc Surg 5:204, 1998

126. Kaneko H, Takagi S, Shiba T: Laparoscopic partial hepatectomy and left lateral segmentectomy: technique and results of a clinical series. Surgery 120:468, 1996

127. Rau HG, Meyer G, Cohnert TU, et al: Laparoscopic liver resection with the water-jet dissector. Surg Endosc 9:1009, 1995

128. Yamanaka N, Tanaka T, Tanaka W, et al: Laparoscopic partial hepatectomy. Hepatogastroenterology 45:29, 1998

129. Fong Y, Blumgart LH: Useful stapling techniques in liver surgery. J Am Coll Surg 185:93, 1997

130. Jackman SV, Cadeddu JA, Chen RN, et al: Utility of the harmonic scalpel for laparoscopic partial nephrectomy. J Endourol 12:441, 1998

131. Wolf JSJ, Moon TD, Nakada SY: Hand assisted laparoscopic nephrectomy: comparison to standard laparoscopic nephrectomy. J Urol 160:22, 1998

132. Klingler PJ, Hinder RA, Menke DM, et al: Hand-assisted laparoscopic distal pancreatectomy for pancreatic cystadenoma. Surg Laparosc Endosc 8:180, 1998

133. Nakada SY, Moon TD, Gist M, et al: Use of the pneumo sleeve as an adjunct in laparoscopic nephrectomy. Urology 49:612, 1997

Acknowledgment

Figures 1, 3 through 15, 17, 18   Tom Moore.

18 PANCREATIC PROCEDURES

Keith D. Lillemoe, M.D., F.A.C.S., and John L. Cameron, M.D., F.A.C.S.

Pylorus-Preserving Pancreaticoduodenectomy (Whipple Procedure)

Surgical resection of a periampullary carcinoma can be accomplished by means of either a pylorus-preserving pancreaticoduodenectomy or the classic resection (including an antrectomy). The decision is usually made on the basis of individual surgeon preference (unless there is obvious tumor encroachment on the first portion of the duodenum). Neither approach appears to have a proven advantage in terms of either relative ease of performance or short- or long-term outcome (including survival). In the ensuing technical description, we focus primarily on the pylorus-preserving modification but also refer to certain important components of the classic Whipple resection.

The peritoneal cavity is entered through either an upper midline or a bilateral subcostal incision, and the abdomen is thoroughly explored. The head of the pancreas and the duodenum are extensively mobilized out of the retroperitoneum via the Kocher maneuver. (This extensive kocherization allows one to palpate the superior mesenteric artery to confirm that the tumor has not extended from the uncinate process to involve the vessel. It is distinctly unusual for the tumor to extend directly posteriorly into the aorta or the inferior vena cava.) If there is no evidence of local or regional spread to serosal surfaces or the liver, the gallbladder is mobilized out of the liver bed. The common hepatic duct is identified, circumferentially dissected, and then divided [*see Figure 1*]. A complete rim of the duct is sent for frozen section examination.

Once the common hepatic duct has been divided, the anterior surface of the portal vein is easily and quickly identified. The lymph node tissue lateral to the hepatic duct and the portal vein should be dissected off the structures to be included in the surgical specimen. A replaced right hepatic artery is a commonly found anatomic variant in this location; if present, it must be recognized and preserved. If one finds the appropriate plane directly on the anterior surface of the portal vein, one can use a combination of sharp and blunt dissection to develop a plane between the vein and the first portion of the duodenum and the neck of the pancreas; usually, there are no veins joining the anterior surface of the portal vein, and the maneuver can be carried out with no resistance. If this maneuver is difficult, the gastroduodenal artery should be identified where it comes off the common hepatic artery. This artery should first be clamped with a nonoccluding vascular clamp to ensure that the pulse in the hepatic artery is preserved. (Loss of a hepatic artery pulse may suggest misidentification of the vessel or an aberrant blood flow pattern attributable to a congenital variant or to acquired celiac stenosis.) If the hepatic artery pulse is preserved, the gastroduodenal artery is divided between 2-0 silk ties, with a Prolene suture placed on the proximal stump. This step, by providing improved access, often facilitates dissection of the portal vein from the undersurface of the pancreas.

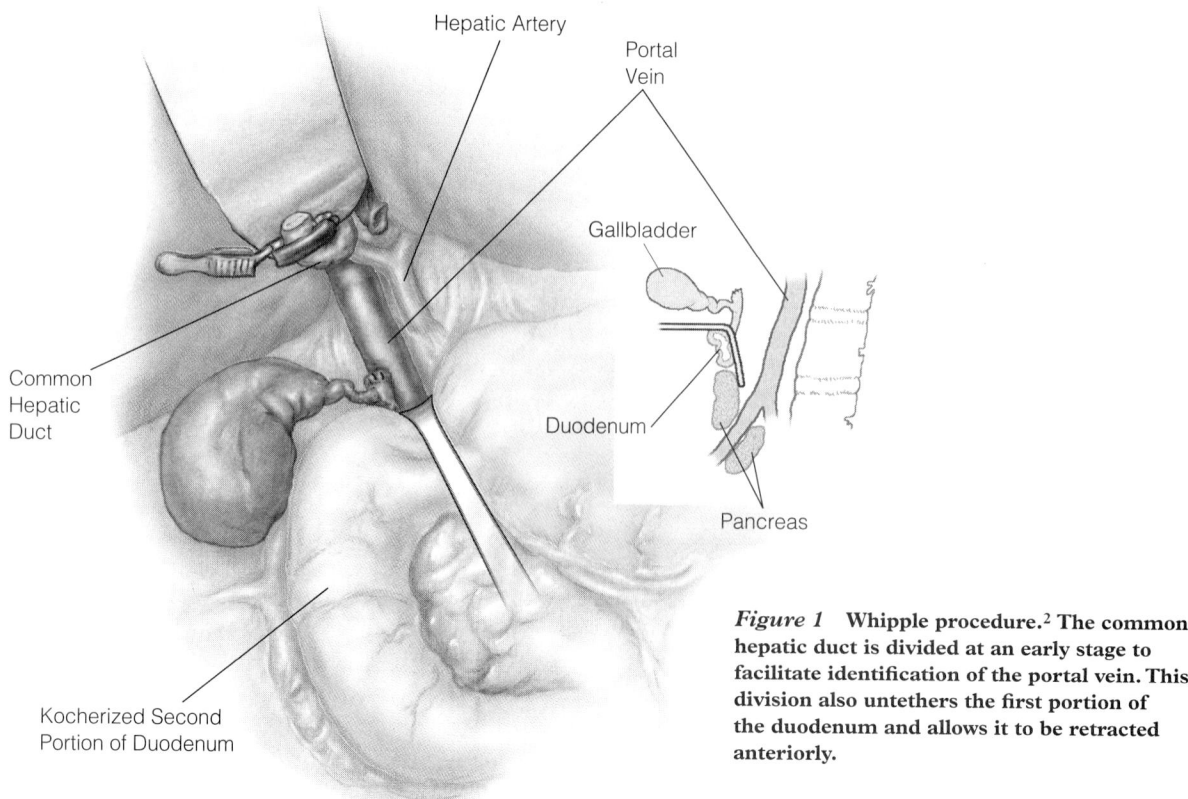

Figure 1 Whipple procedure.[2] The common hepatic duct is divided at an early stage to facilitate identification of the portal vein. This division also untethers the first portion of the duodenum and allows it to be retracted anteriorly.

508

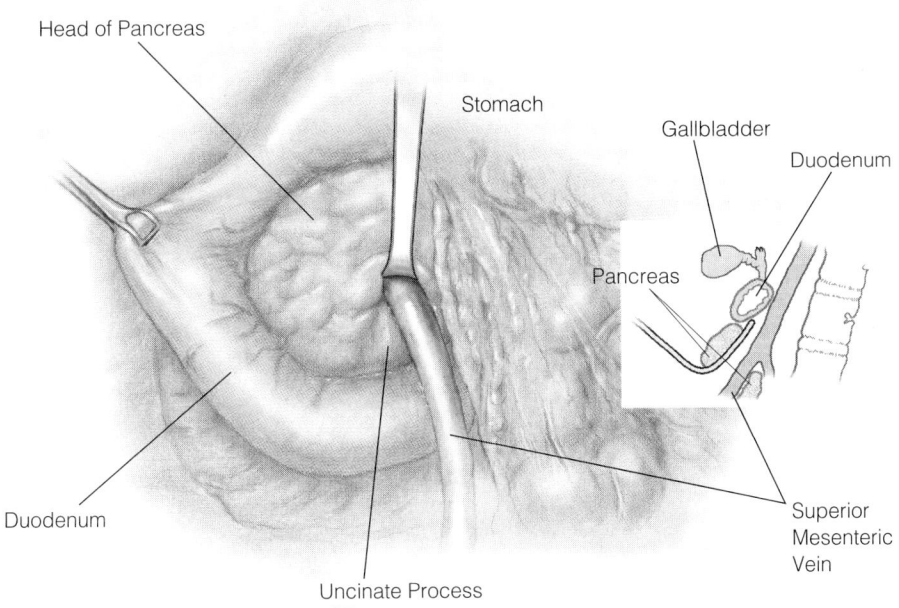

Head of Pancreas

Stomach

Gallbladder

Duodenum

Pancreas

Duodenum

Uncinate Process
of Pancreas

Superior
Mesenteric
Vein

Figure 2 **Whipple procedure.[2]
Kocherization of the duodenum is continued along the third portion until the
superior mesenteric vein is reached. This
vein can then be easily cleaned up to its
connection with the portal vein.**

The third portion of the duodenum is then further kocherized until the superior mesenteric vein is identified [*see Figure
2*]. The superior mesenteric vein is cleaned along its anterior
surface under the neck of the pancreas up to its connection
with the portal vein. (Identification of the superior mesenteric
vein is far easier by this anterior approach than by the traditional route through the lesser sac and is associated with virtually no blood loss.) Once this anterior plane is fully developed,
the right lateral surface of the vein should be assessed for tumor
involvement. This step, in conjunction with preoperative spiral
CT assessment of arterial and venous involvement, helps confirm that the tumor can be resected with negative margins.

The first portion of the duodenum is mobilized from the
neck of the pancreas and divided with a gastrointestinal anastomosis (GIA) stapler approximately 2 cm distal to the pylorus.
If the surgeon chooses to carry out a classic pancreaticoduodenectomy, an antrectomy is performed. The right gastroepiploic arcade and the right gastric vessels are divided to permit
mobilization of the antrum. The stomach is then divided with a
GIA stapler, usually at the level of the incisura. A Babcock
clamp is then placed on the proximal first portion of the duodenum, which is reflected medially. The posterior surface of the
proximal first portion of the duodenum is dissected until the
lesser sac is entered. At this point, the soft tissue attachments
from the inferior border of the duodenum to the inferior border of the pancreas are divided; the right gastroepiploic vessels,
which can be sizable, are clamped, divided, and ligated with 2-
0 silk. In a similar fashion, the soft tissue areolar attachments
found superiorly are divided with the electrocautery or else
clamped, divided, and ligated with 2-0 silk. (Care must be
taken to identify and preserve the right gastric artery, which
comes off the common hepatic artery and actually joins the
foregut along the proximal part of the first portion of the duodenum.) If the gastroduodenal artery was not divided earlier, it
is now identified and divided as described earlier (see above).

The neck of the pancreas is divided with the electrocautery.
A rush of pancreatic juice is the signal that the enlarged pancreatic duct has been divided. A 1 mm thick complete cross
section of the pancreas is taken at this time and sent for frozen

section examination. (Margins should be sent for frozen section
as they become available so that one is not delayed in proceeding with the reconstruction while the pathologist takes the margin off the pancreaticoduodenectomy specimen at the end of
the formal resection.)

The portal vein and the superior mesenteric vein are mobilized from the uncinate process of the pancreas. It is often necessary to place vessel loops around one or both of these veins so
that one can retract them far enough medially to remove them
completely from the uncinate process. (There are amazingly few
veins that must be ligated and divided in this region.) Dissection
should proceed until the superior mesenteric artery, clearly palpable with the index finger of the left hand, is visualized. The
uncinate process is divided between Reinhoff clamps and ligated with 2-0 silk ties. The uncinate process should be divided
flush with the superior mesenteric artery [*see Figure 3*]. The
superior mesenteric artery is completely exposed during this
dissection, which proceeds from cephalad to caudad. Generally,
there are two large veins joining the superior mesenteric vein
inferiorly (the superior and inferior pancreaticoduodenal veins)
that one must dissect free, doubly ligate, and divide.

After the uncinate process has been completely divided, the
specimen is attached only by the third portion of the duodenum.
At this point, the upper abdomen is copiously irrigated with an
antibiotic solution and packed. The transverse colon, along
with the greater omentum, is reflected cephalad. The proximal
jejunum and the ligament of Treitz, along with the fourth portion of the duodenum, are dissected free, and the dissection is
continued until it meets the right-side upper abdominal dissection. At a convenient point where there is a wide vascular arcade,
the proximal jejunum is divided with a GIA stapler approximately 10 to 12 cm from the ligament of Treitz. The proximal
jejunum is then grasped with a Babcock clamp and retracted
cephalad. The mesentery to the proximal jejunum is divided
between Reinhoff clamps and ligated with 2-0 silk. When the
mesentery is completely divided, the specimen is free and can be
removed from the operative field.

The proximal jejunum is then brought up through a rent in
the transverse mesocolon. In our technique of choice, end-to-

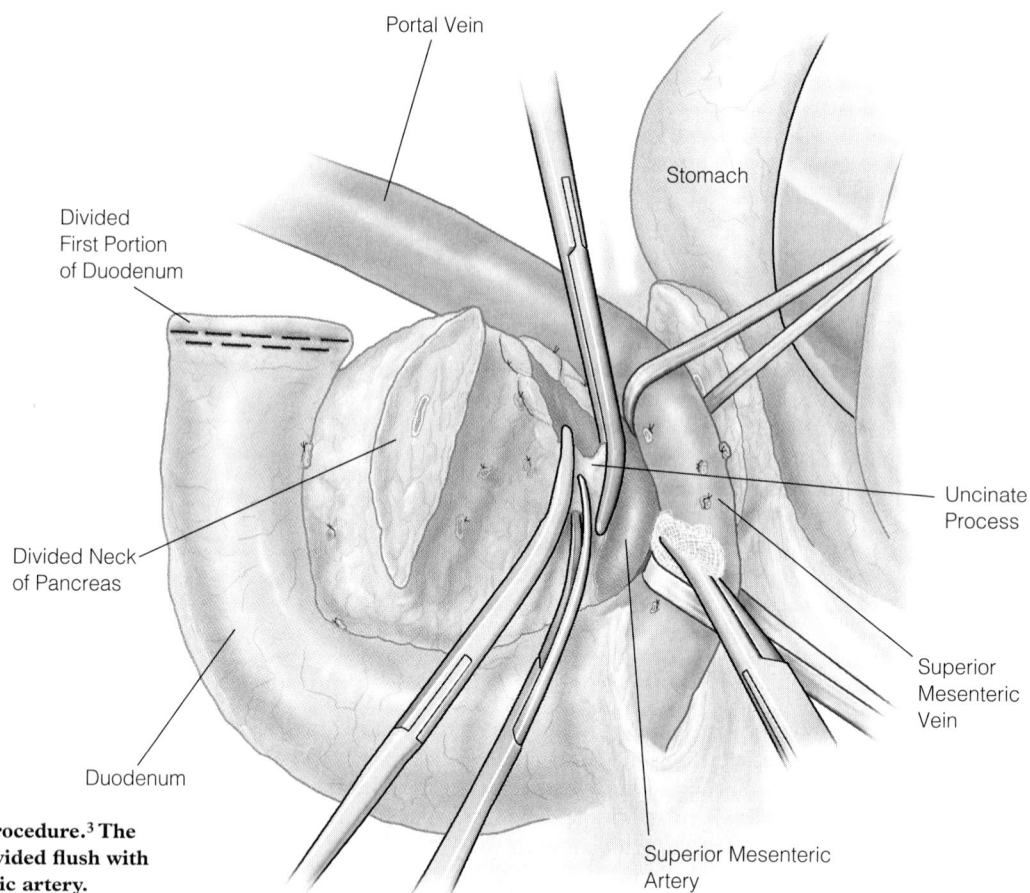

Portal Vein

Stomach

Divided
First Portion
of Duodenum

Uncinate
Process

Divided Neck
of Pancreas

Superior
Mesenteric
Vein

Duodenum

Superior Mesenteric
Artery

Figure 3 **Whipple procedure.**[3] **The uncinate process is divided flush with the superior mesenteric artery.**

end or end-to-side pancreaticojejunostomy is performed. In our technique of choice, the end of the pancreas is invaginated into the jejunum for approximately 2 cm. This anastomosis is performed with an outer interrupted layer of 3-0 silk and an inner continuous layer of 3-0 absorbable synthetic suture material [*see Figure 4a*]. The inner layer incorporates the dilated pancreatic duct with several throws, both posteriorly and anteriorly. This

invagination technique may be performed in either an end-to-end or an end-to-side manner. As an alternative, an end-to-side mucosa-to-mucosa anastomosis may be performed [*see Figure 4b*]. An outer layer of interrupted 3-0 silk sutures is placed between the capsule of the gland and the seromuscular layer of the bowel. An inner layer of interrupted 4-0 absorbable synthetic sutures is then placed between the pancreatic duct and a

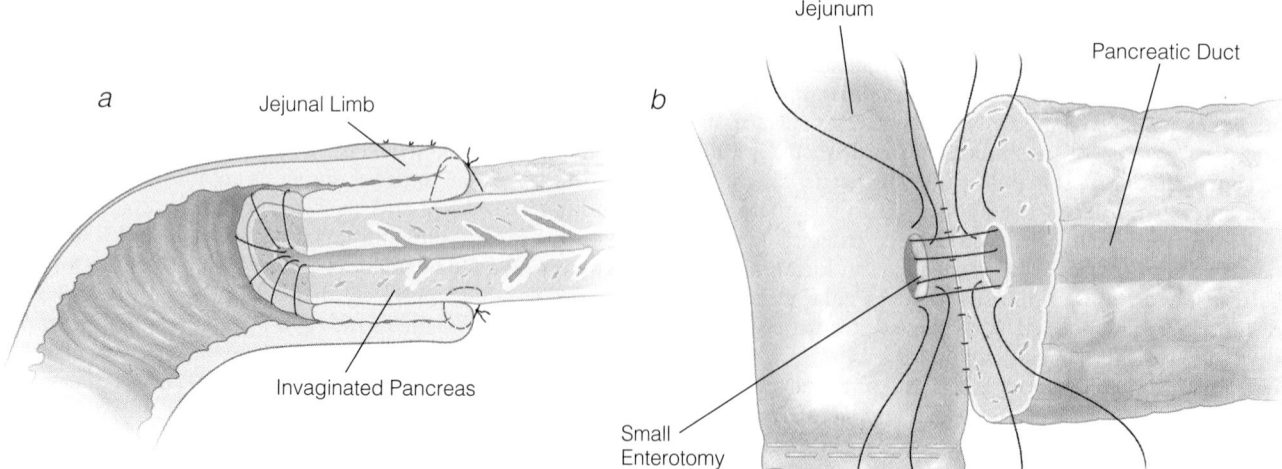

Jejunum

Pancreatic Duct

a

Jejunal Limb

b

Invaginated Pancreas

Small
Enterotomy

Figure 4 **Whipple procedure.**[3] **(*a*) In the authors' preferred approach to pancreaticojejunostomy, the end of the pancreas is invaginated into the end of the jejunum for approximately 2 cm. The anastomosis is done with an outer interrupted layer of 3-0 silk and an inner continuous layer of 3-0 absorbable synthetic suture material. (*b*) In an alternative approach, an end-to-end mucosa-to-mucosa pancreaticojejunostomy is again done in two layers with an outer layer of interrupted 3-0 silk sutures and an inner layer of interrupted 4-0 absorbable synthetic sutures.**

small enterotomy in the jejunum, either with or without a pancreatic duct stent.

Approximately 4 to 6 cm distal to the pancreaticojejunostomy, an end-to-side hepaticojejunostomy (common hepatic duct to jejunum) is performed with a single interrupted layer of 4-0 absorbable synthetic suture material [see Figure 5]. The anastomosis is generally performed without either a transanastomotic stent or a T tube. If a percutaneous transhepatic biliary catheter was placed preoperatively for decompression of the obstructed biliary tree, it may be placed across the anastomosis and left to gravity drainage during the early postoperative period.

Approximately 20 cm distal to the biliary-enteric anastomosis, an end-to-side duodenojejunostomy is performed with an inner continuous layer of 3-0 absorbable synthetic suture material and an outer interrupted layer of 3-0 silk [see Figure 6]. If an antrectomy has been performed, the medial half of the gastric staple line is reinforced with interrupted 3-0 silk seromuscular Lembert sutures. The gastrojejunal anastomosis is completed to the lateral (greater curvature) aspect of the staple line as a two-layer Hofmeister-style anastomosis.

The abdomen is copiously irrigated with an antibiotic solution. The jejunal loop is tacked to the rent in the transverse mesocolon with interrupted 3-0 silk sutures. The defect in the retroperitoneum previously occupied by the third portion of the duodenum is closed with a continuous 3-0 silk suture. Closed suction Silastic drains (two, as a rule) are placed adjacent to both the pancreatic and the biliary anastomosis. The abdomen is closed with multiple interrupted No. 1 monofilament sutures placed through and through all muscle and fascial layers. The subcutaneous tissues are irrigated with an antibiotic solution and closed with a continuous 3-0 absorbable synthetic suture. The subcuticular layer is closed with a continuous 4-0 absorbable synthetic suture. Steri-Strips are applied.

Distal Pancreatectomy for Chronic Pancreatitis

The peritoneal cavity is entered through an upper midline incision, and the abdomen is thoroughly explored. The omentum is taken off the transverse colon, and the lesser sac is exposed widely. (One can enter the lesser sac by dividing the middle portion of the omentum instead of removing it from the colon; however, so much of the omentum must be divided during a distal pancreatectomy that one runs the risk of devascularizing some of the distal omentum.)

The tail, body, neck, and head of the pancreas are exposed and examined. (In some patients who have chronic pancreatitis, the posterior wall of the stomach is adherent to the body and tail of the pancreas because of repeated bouts of inflammation. If this is the case, the posterior wall of the stomach is mobilized via both sharp and blunt dissection. If the distal pancreatectomy were being done to remove a tumor, one would also have to be certain that vital structures such as the celiac axis and the superior mesenteric vessels were not involved; such involvement might render the lesion unresectable.) The duodenum is kocherized, and the head and the uncinate process of the pancreas are palpated and visualized.

The splenic artery is identified as it comes off the celiac axis, and a vessel loop is placed around it. This step gives one control of the splenic artery and allows one to ligate it early in the procedure if bleeding should occur. Occasionally, patients with chronic pancreatitis have a thrombosed splenic vein and left-

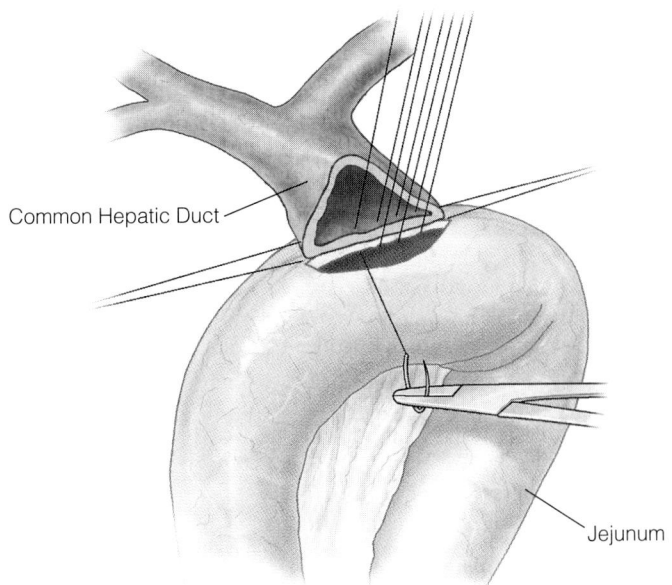

Figure 5 **Whipple procedure.[3] The common hepatic duct is anastomosed to the jejunum in an end-to-side fashion with a single layer of 4-0 interrupted absorbable synthetic sutures.**

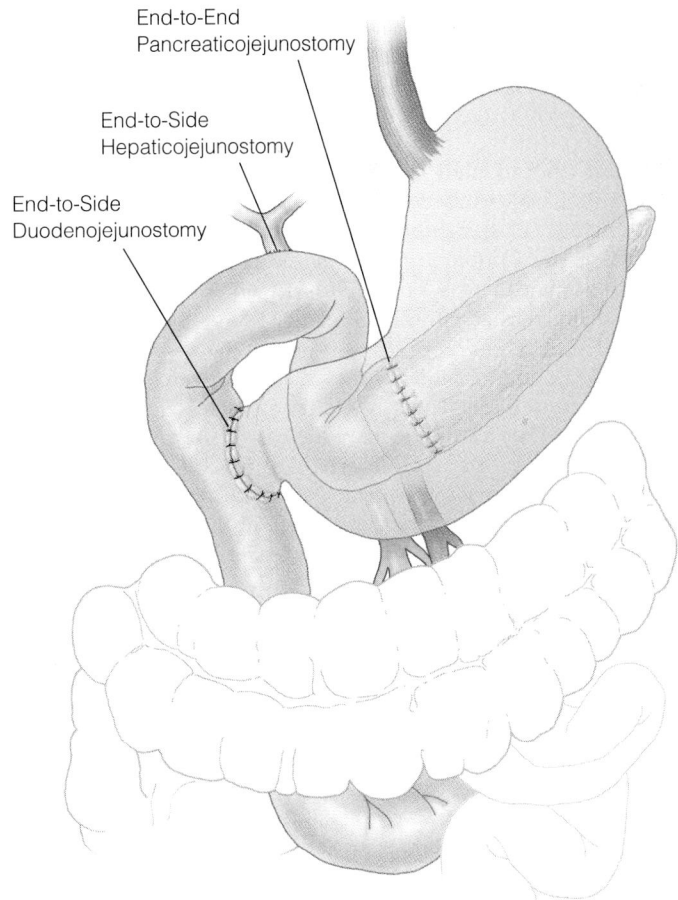

Figure 6 **Whipple procedure.[3] After the end-to-end pancreaticojejunostomy and the end-to-side hepaticojejunostomy, the duodenum is anastomosed to the jejunum in an end-to-side fashion with an inner continuous layer of 3-0 absorbable suture material and an outer interrupted layer of 3-0 silk.**

side portal hypertension. If this is the case, there are usually multiple collateral vessels leading from the spleen to the stomach via the vasa brevia and involving the omentum. In such circumstances, it is usually preferable to ligate and divide the splenic artery early in the procedure.

The spleen is mobilized out of the retroperitoneum. This task is made easier if a splenic pack has been placed beneath the left flank of the patient to elevate the left retroperitoneum before preparation and draping. The spleen is retracted toward the midline with the left hand; it should be compressed medially toward the spine rather than retracted anteriorly. As one opens up the retroperitoneum with the electrocautery, the assistant, standing to the left of the patient, grasps the retroperitoneal serosa. Once the serosa has been divided, the retroperitoneum usually consists of loose areolar tissue that is easily mobilized. One must be careful not to dissect too deeply and injure the kidney or its vessels.

The tail of the pancreas is mobilized out of the retroperitoneum via both sharp and blunt dissection. The omental attachments anterior to the hilum of the spleen are divided between Kelly clamps and ligated with 2-0 silk. (The line of division is easily determined if the omentum has previously been completely taken off the transverse colon. As the division extends up toward and then along the greater curvature of the stomach, the vasa brevia are encountered and are doubly clamped, divided, and ligated.) The splenic flexure of the colon is carefully dissected away from the inferior pole of the spleen, and the peritoneal attachments that make up the splenocolic ligament are divided.

The tail and body of the pancreas are further mobilized out of the retroperitoneum by retracting the spleen and the tail of the pancreas medially. (In the course of this mobilization, one must be careful not to injure the left adrenal gland, which often occupies a fairly superficial position in the retroperitoneum, anterior and medial to the superior pole of the left kidney.) The splenic vein is easily identified in the middle portion of the posterior aspect of the pancreas. The inferior mesenteric vein, which joins the splenic vein at the middle of the body of the pancreas, is identified in the retroperitoneum just lateral to the ligament of Treitz. (Although the inferior mesenteric vein can be divided and ligated with impunity, one should try to preserve it.)

Further mobilization of the pancreas to the midline exposes the point where the splenic artery comes off the celiac axis. (Whereas the splenic vein invariably resides in a groove in the middle portion of the posterior surface of the gland, the splenic artery usually runs along the superior aspect of the gland and is easily identified by palpation where it arises from the celiac axis.) The splenic artery is clamped and divided with 2-0 silk ties and a 3-0 Prolene suture ligature on the proximal stump of the vessel.

The junction of the inferior mesenteric vein and the splenic vein is identified, and the splenic vein is mobilized just distal to this junction. (Because the splenic vein resides in a groove or trough on the posterior aspect of the pancreas, one must be careful when mobilizing the splenic vein out of the pancreatic parenchyma. There are several small venous branches that can be injured if the mobilization is not done fastidiously.) The splenic vein is triply clamped and divided just distal to its junction with the inferior mesenteric vein. The splenic vein is then mobilized from the posterior surface of the pancreas from this point onward to its junction with the superior mesenteric vein and the portal vein [see Figure 7]. If there is a pancreatic tumor arising from the proximal body of the gland, the splenic vein may be ligated flush with the superior mesenteric vein. At this location, it is best to

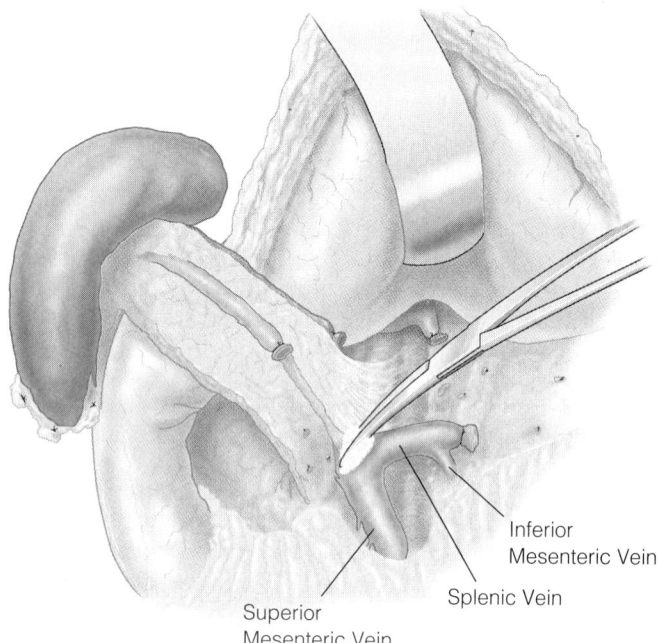

Superior
Mesenteric Vein

Inferior
Mesenteric Vein

Splenic Vein

Figure 7 **Distal pancreatectomy.**[3] **The splenic vein is divided just distal to its junction with the inferior mesenteric vein and then dissected away from the posterior surface of the pancreas from this point up to where it joins the superior mesenteric vein to form the portal vein.**

oversew the vein with a continuous 3-0 Prolene suture so as not to compromise the superior mesenteric vein–portal vein complex.

The portal vein and the superior mesenteric vein are carefully dissected away from the undersurface of the neck of the pancreas. (At the neck, the pancreas is often very thinned out and narrow before expanding into the substantially thicker head and uncinate process.) A row of overlapping horizontal mattress sutures of 3-0 absorbable synthetic material is placed in the neck of the pancreas just proximal to the point where it is to be divided. (Using large needles that have been straightened makes this task simple even if the head-neck junction through which the needles are passed is thickened.) The neck of the pancreas is then divided with the electrocautery. A row of figure-eight sutures of 3-0 absorbable synthetic suture material is placed over the end of the pancreas [see Figure 8]. If the pancreatic duct can be identified, it should be separately oversewn with a figure-eight or mattress suture (again, of 3-0 absorbable synthetic suture material).

The abdomen is copiously irrigated with an antibiotic solution. The pancreatic remnant is drained with a closed suction Silastic drain brought out through a stab wound in the left upper quadrant. There is no need to drain the splenic bed. The abdominal wall is closed with a single layer of interrupted No. 1 nonabsorbable synthetic monofilament sutures placed through and through all muscle and fascial layers. The subcutaneous tissues are irrigated with an antibiotic solution and closed with a continuous 3-0 absorbable synthetic suture. The subcuticular layer is closed with a continuous 4-0 absorbable synthetic suture. Steri-Strips are applied.

Longitudinal Pancreaticojejunostomy (Puestow Procedure)

The abdomen is entered through an upper midline incision. The lesser sac is entered by removing the greater omentum

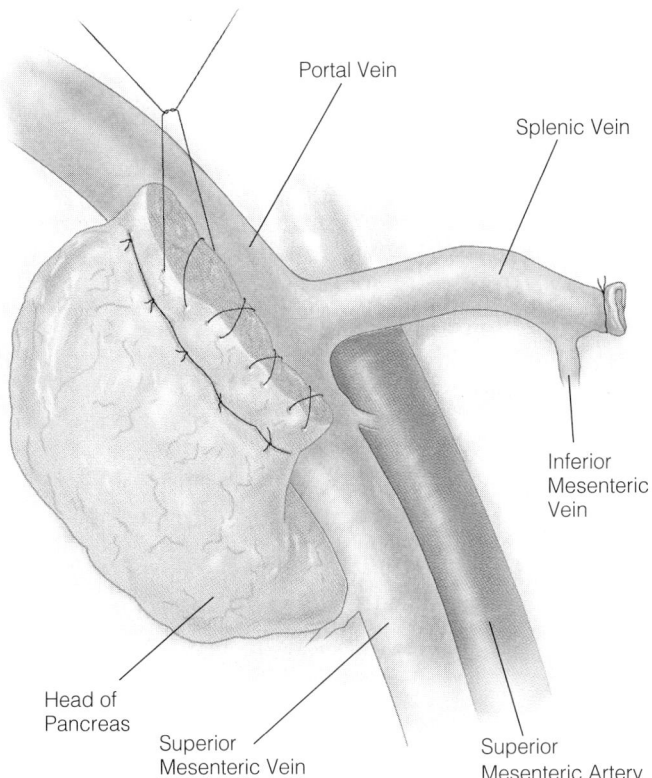

Figure 8 **Distal pancreatectomy.[3] A row of overlapping horizontal mattress sutures is placed in the neck of the pancreas just proximal to where it is to be divided, the neck is divided with the electrocautery, and a row of figure-eight sutures of 3-0 absorbable synthetic suture material is placed over the end of the pancreas.**

from the transverse colon along virtually its entire length, thereby exposing the entire tail, body, neck, and head of the pancreas. The pancreas often appears markedly fibrotic and scarred. The posterior wall of the stomach may be adherent to a portion of the body of the pancreas as a result of multiple episodes of inflammation; if it is adherent, it is easily dissected free. The duodenum is kocherized, and the head and the uncinate process of the pancreas are palpated from both an anterior and a posterior direction. In many cases, the pancreatic duct is markedly dilated and can actually be palpated through the anterior surface in the middle portion of the body of the pancreas. The rest of the abdomen is explored to check for the presence of other pathologic conditions. To confirm the position of the dilated pancreatic duct, a 20-gauge needle on a 10 ml syringe is used to aspirate the duct. Once pancreatic juice is obtained, the syringe is removed from the needle hub, with the needle left in place.

The pancreatic duct is entered by dividing the pancreatic parenchyma with the electrocautery on either side of the needle. A large right-angle clamp is then inserted, and the duct is filleted open with the electrocautery both proximally and distally [*see Figure 9*]. Small pancreatic ductal concretions are carefully removed. (Experience has demonstrated that at least 6 cm of the duct must be opened to yield a good chance of long-term success. Ideally, if the duct is dilated all the way out to the tail, it can be filleted open virtually to the tip of the pancreas. In the proximal direction, the duct can easily be opened as far as the neck of the pancreas. Beyond this point, however, the duct passes posteriorly and inferiorly into the head of the pancreas;

because the head can be very thick, opening up the duct any further can be difficult.)

A Bakes dilator is carefully passed proximally through the open pancreatic duct, down through the pancreatic duct in the unopened head, through the ampulla of Vater, and into the duodenum. (If a Bakes dilator cannot be passed into the duodenum, some surgeons elect to open the duodenum and perform a sphincteroplasty, so that by working both from within the duodenum and from within the open pancreatic duct, they can ensure the patency of the entire pancreatic duct.)

A Roux-en-Y jejunal loop approximately 60 cm long is constructed. The most proximal loop of jejunum in which there is a good vascular arcade is selected. A 2 cm segment of this loop is cleaned and divided with a GIA stapler. The small bowel mesentery is divided between clamps down through the arcade vessel and is ligated with 3-0 silk. The end of the distal jejunum is oversewn with a layer of 3-0 silk Lembert sutures. A 60 cm length is then measured. Alimentary tract continuity is reestablished by means of an end-to-side jejunojejunostomy, in which the most proximal portion of the divided jejunum is anastomosed to the side of the Roux-en-Y jejunal loop 60 cm distally with an inner continuous layer of 3-0 absorbable synthetic suture material and an outer interrupted layer of 3-0 silk. The defect in the small bowel mesentery is closed with a continuous 4-0 silk suture.

The Roux-en-Y jejunal loop is brought up into the lesser sac in a retrocolic position through a small rent in the transverse mesocolon. A side-to-side pancreaticojejunostomy is performed in two layers. Before the Roux loop is opened, an outer interrupted layer of 3-0 silk is placed between the jejunal loop and the pancreatotomy, passing through the capsule of the pancreas and out through the opened pancreatic parenchyma along the inferior border of the pancreas. When this layer is complete, an enterotomy approximately 2 mm from the jejunal suture line is

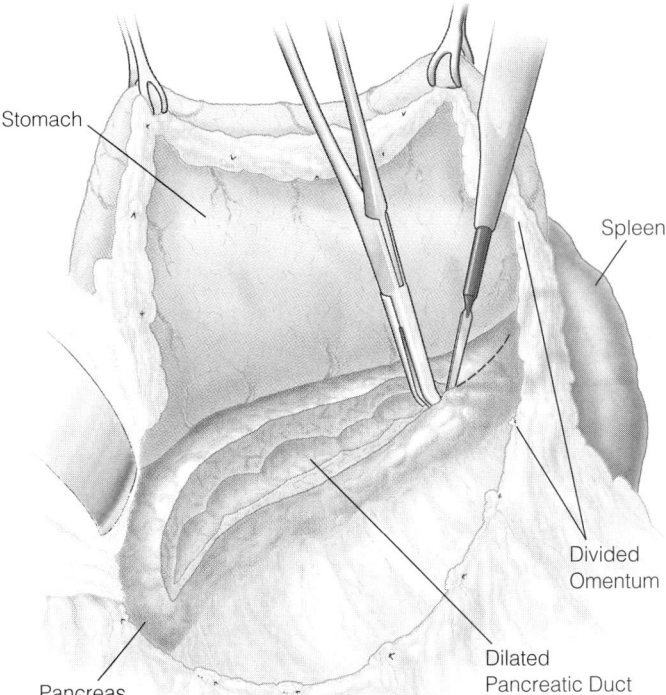

Figure 9 **Puestow procedure.[3] The dilated pancreatic duct is filleted open with the electrocautery both proximally and distally. At least 6 cm of the duct should be opened.**

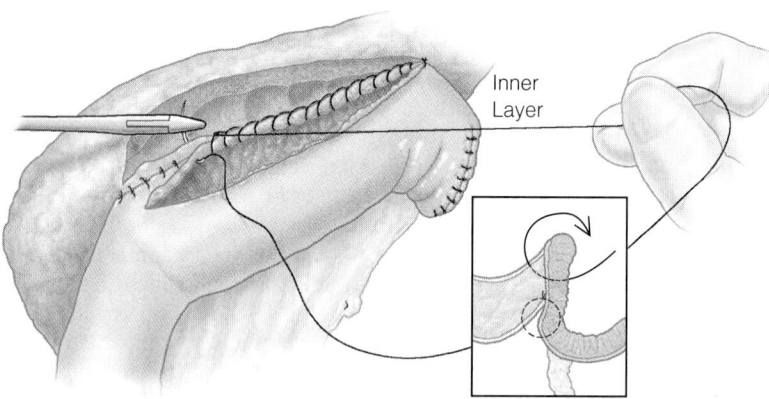

Inner
Layer

Figure 10 Puestow procedure.[3] When the diameter of the dilated pancreatic duct is 1 cm or wider, a side-to-side pancreaticojejunostomy should be done in two layers. Once an outer layer of interrupted 3-0 silk sutures is placed between the jejunal loop and the pancreatotomy, an enterotomy is made along the entire length of the jejunal suture line, and an inner layer consisting of a continuous 3-0 absorbable synthetic suture is placed.

made along the entire length of this line. Starting at the distal pancreatic tail, an inner continuous layer of 3-0 absorbable synthetic suture material is placed in an over-and-over locking fashion through the entire wall of the jejunum and the entire divided surface of the pancreas and into the duct [*see Figure 10*]. The inner layer of the superior suture line is placed in an over-and-over fashion without locking, again with a continuous 3-0 absorbable synthetic suture. The outer layer of the superior suture line consists of interrupted 3-0 silk sutures placed in a Lembert fashion. (When the pancreatic duct is dilated to a diameter of 1 cm or greater, a two-layer anastomosis is possible and is in fact preferred. However, when the diameter of the duct is between 5 mm and 1 cm, a two-layer anastomosis is generally difficult, and a one-layer anastomosis is preferred. A single layer of interrupted 3-0 silk sutures is placed so that the knots are tied on the outside. This is easily accomplished with the superior suture line. With the inferior suture line, which is placed first, the suture passes from outside inward on the pancreas and then from inside outward on the jejunum. In a single-layer side-to-side pancreaticojejunostomy, the jejunotomy must be performed before any sutures are placed.) The Roux-en-Y jejunal loop is then tacked to the rent in the transverse mesocolon with interrupted 3-0 silk sutures.

The longitudinal pancreaticojejunostomy anastomosis is drained with closed suction Silastic drains that are placed on either side of the anastomosis and brought out through separate stab wounds in the left upper quadrant. The abdomen is copiously irrigated with an antibiotic solution. The midline incision is closed with a single interrupted layer of No. 1 nonabsorbable synthetic monofilament sutures passed through and through all muscle and fascial layers. The subcutaneous tissues are irrigated with an antibiotic solution and closed with a continuous 3-0 absorbable synthetic suture. The subcuticular layer is closed with a continuous 4-0 absorbable synthetic suture. Steri-Strips are applied.

Drainage of Pancreatic Pseudocyst into a Roux-en-Y Jejunal Loop

The peritoneal cavity is entered through a midline incision, and the abdomen is explored. Typically, a substantial mass that is cystic and easily ballotable is palpable posterior to the stomach. The duodenum and the head of the pancreas are kocherized so that the head may be palpated both anteriorly and posteriorly. The physical characteristics of chronic pancreatitis are usually present. The body and the tail of the pancreas are palpated as well; the pancreas is usually fibrotic, firm, and somewhat enlarged. The rest of the abdomen is explored to check for the presence of other pathologic conditions. (At this point, the size

and configuration of the cyst are compared with the size and configuration on the preoperative CT scan. If the CT scan shows a unilocular solitary cyst and if, at the time of laparotomy, there appears to be a mass that coincides exactly with what is seen on the CT scan, there is no need to enter the lesser sac. The lesion can be drained into a Roux-en-Y jejunal loop through the transverse mesocolon, and the lesser sac need not be explored. Most pseudocysts are formed by anterior disruptions of the main pancreatic duct. When pancreatic secretions leak out into the lesser sac, the body walls off the leak through its inflammatory response. The transverse mesocolon becomes adherent to the posterior wall of the stomach, which in turn becomes adherent to other adjacent structures in and around the retroperitoneum, and the leak is sealed off. Thus, the transverse mesocolon is usually the inferior and most dependent portion of the pseudocyst, and this site is the ideal location for drainage [*see Figure 11*].)

The transverse colon is retracted cephalad, and the cyst is easily visualized and palpated through the transverse mesocolon. The location of the cyst is confirmed by aspirating pancreatic juice through the transverse mesocolon with a 10 ml syringe and a 20-gauge needle. (One must be careful to identify and avoid the middle colic vessels.) A 60 cm long Roux-en-Y jejunal loop is constructed. The proximal jejunum is divided with a GIA stapler at the first convenient arcade. The small bowel mesentery is divided down through the arcade. The distal end of the jejunum is inverted with an interrupted layer of 3-0 silk Lembert sutures.

Alimentary tract continuity is reestablished by means of an end-to-side jejunojejunostomy, in which the proximal jejunum is anastomosed to the side of the Roux-en-Y jejunal loop 60 cm from the inverted end. This anastomosis is performed with an inner continuous layer of 3-0 absorbable synthetic suture material and an outer interrupted layer of 3-0 silk. The rent in the small bowel mesentery is closed with a continuous 3-0 silk suture.

A side-to-side cystojejunostomy is performed with an outer interrupted layer of 3-0 silk and an inner continuous layer of 3-0 absorbable synthetic suture material. The posterior outer layer of the anastomosis consists of a series of 3-0 silk sutures passed through and through the jejunal loop and through and through the transverse mesocolon (which is the inferior wall of the pseudocyst) [*see Figure 12*]. The suture line should be approximately 2.5 to 5 cm long. After the posterior layer has been secured, a cystotomy is performed with the electrocautery. An ellipse of cyst wall is removed and sent for frozen section examination. (No matter how convinced one is that one is dealing with a pseudocyst, a specimen from the cyst wall should always be sent for frozen section examination. Some cystic

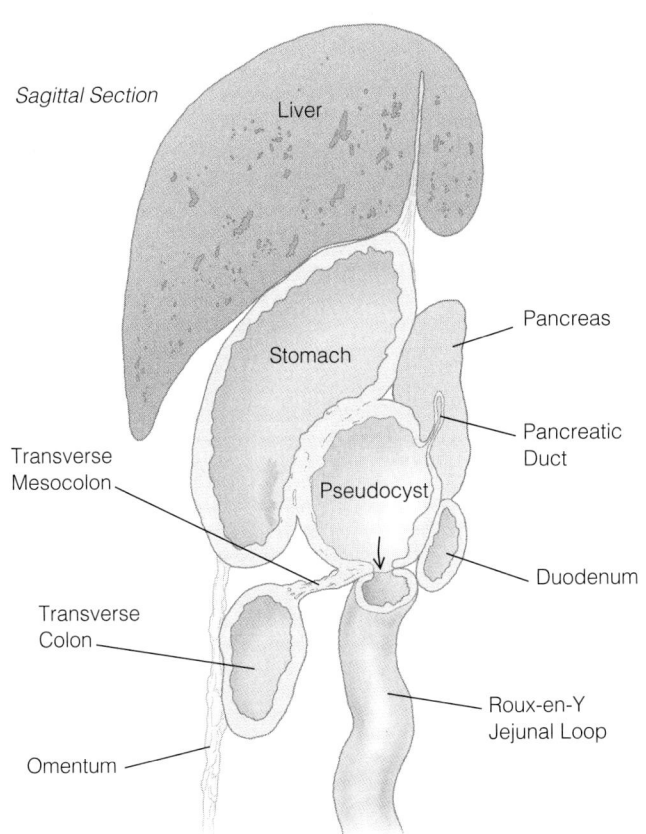

Figure 11 Drainage of pancreatic pseudocyst into Roux-en-Y jejunal loop.[3] The transverse mesocolon is usually the most inferior and dependent part of a pancreatic pseudocyst; thus, drainage through the transverse mesocolon into a Roux loop is usually the ideal approach.

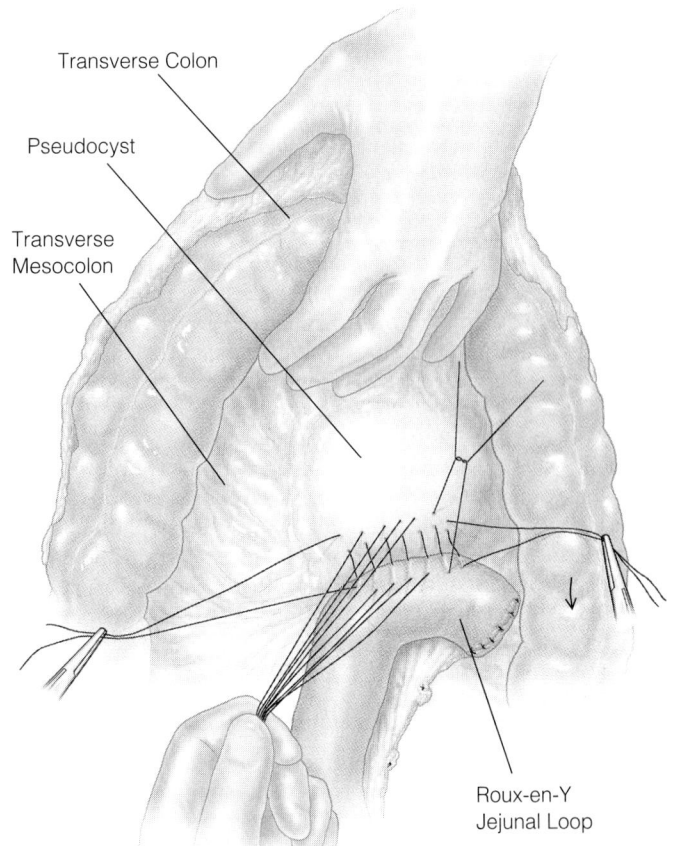

Figure 12 Drainage of pancreatic pseudocyst into Roux-en-Y jejunal loop.[3] The outer posterior layer of the side-to-side cystojejunostomy comprises a series of 3-0 silk sutures placed through and through the jejunal loop and the transverse mesocolon.

lesions of the pancreas are cystic neoplasms, which must be resected rather than drained. If no epithelial lining is found on frozen section examination, one can assume that the lesion is not a cystic neoplasm but a pancreatic pseudocyst and may proceed accordingly.) A parallel enterotomy is made in the jejunum. An inner continuous layer of 3-0 absorbable synthetic suture material is placed inferiorly in a locking fashion and then brought around superiorly in a Connell stitch. An outer interrupted layer of 3-0 silk is placed superiorly. With the cyst decompressed, one should easily be able to palpate a sizable lumen in the anastomosis between the cyst and the jejunal loop.

A closed suction Silastic drain is left near the anastomosis and brought out through a stab wound in the left upper quadrant. The abdomen is copiously irrigated with an antibiotic solution. The wound is closed with multiple interrupted No. 1 nonabsorbable synthetic monofilament sutures placed through and through all muscle and fascial layers. The subcutaneous tissues are irrigated with an antibiotic solution and closed with a continuous 3-0 absorbable synthetic suture. The subcuticular layer is closed with a continuous 4-0 absorbable synthetic suture. Steri-Strips are applied.

Drainage of Pancreatic Pseudocyst into the Stomach

The peritoneal cavity is entered through an upper midline incision, and the abdomen is explored. Typically, a pseudocyst that is not amenable to drainage through the transverse mesocolon presents as a mass that is cystic and is palpable through the anterior wall of the stomach and the lesser omentum in the upper

abdomen; the mass generally is not palpable through the root of the transverse mesocolon with the transverse mesocolon reflected cephalad and thus is not easily drained into a Roux-en-Y jejunal loop. The duodenum and the head of the pancreas are kocherized and the head of the pancreas is palpated. Signs of chronic pancreatitis are invariably present. The body and tail of the pancreas are palpated through the transverse mesocolon and show changes characteristic of chronic inflammation. The rest of the abdomen is explored to check for the presence of other pathologic conditions. (A cyst that is situated high in the abdomen and presents more through the lesser omentum is not accessible to dependent drainage with a Roux-en-Y loop through the transverse mesocolon. Because bringing a Roux-en-Y loop anterior to the stomach to drain the cyst through the lesser omentum is unsatisfactory, such cysts are best drained into the stomach.)

Stay sutures of 3-0 silk are placed in the body of the stomach. A transverse gastrotomy is made with the electrocautery. The cyst wall is easily palpable through the posterior wall of the stomach. The location of the cyst is confirmed by aspirating pancreatic juice through the back wall of the stomach with a 10 ml syringe and a 20-gauge needle [see Figure 13]. (The mass palpated at the time of operation is compared with the cyst as it appears on the preoperative CT scan. If the CT scan shows a solitary unilocular cyst that corresponds to the palpable mass identified at the time of laparotomy, one can be certain that the cyst is solitary and can be drained effectively into the stomach.)

A transverse incision is made with the electrocautery through the posterior wall of the stomach, through the cyst wall, and into the pseudocyst. It is often desirable to leave the 20-gauge needle in place and to perform the posterior wall gastrotomy on either side of the needle. An ellipse of cyst wall is sent for frozen section examination. (Again, no matter how obvious it seems that one is dealing with an inflammatory cyst, a portion of the cyst wall should always be sent for frozen section examination to rule out a neoplasm.) A continuous locking suture of 3-0 absorbable synthetic material is placed through and through the posterior wall of the stomach and the anterior wall of the cyst [see Figure 14]. (This step may or may not actually be important for achieving long-term patency of the opening between the cyst and the posterior wall of the stomach, but it does ensure good hemostasis.) The anterior gastrotomy is closed with an inner continuous layer of 3-0 absorbable synthetic suture material in a Connell stitch and an outer interrupted layer of 3-0 silk.

The abdomen is copiously irrigated with an antibiotic solution. The wound is closed with a single layer of interrupted No. 1 nonabsorbable synthetic monofilament sutures. The subcutaneous tissues are irrigated with an antibiotic solution and closed with a continuous 3-0 absorbable synthetic suture. The subcuticular layer is closed with a continuous 4-0 absorbable synthetic suture. Steri-Strips are applied.

Palliative Bypass for Unresectable Pancreatic Cancer

The peritoneal cavity is entered through an upper midline incision. The head of the pancreas (containing a mass) and the duodenum are mobilized out of the retroperitoneum via the Kocher maneuver. The rest of the abdomen is examined for evidence of liver metastases or serosal spread. (Such evidence may

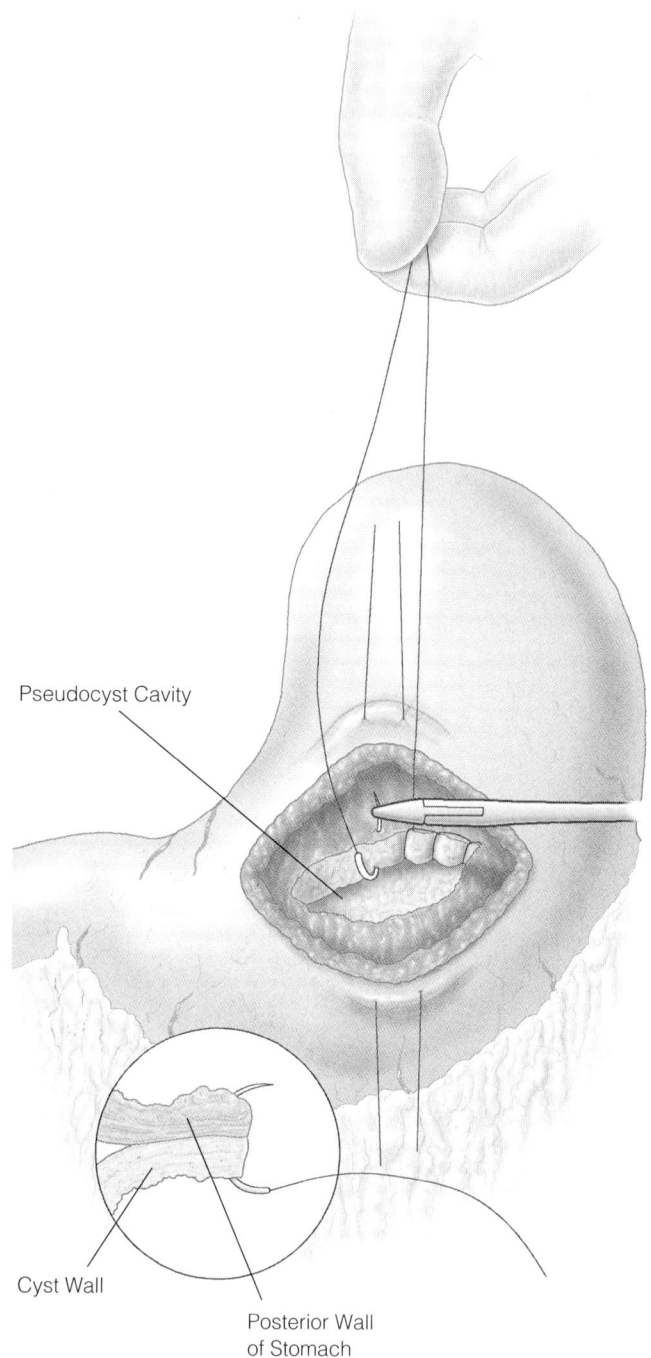

Figure 14 **Drainage of pancreatic pseudocyst into stomach.[3] Once an incision has been made through the posterior wall of the stomach, through the cyst wall, and into the pseudocyst, a continuous locking 3-0 absorbable synthetic suture is placed through and through the posterior wall of the stomach and the cyst wall.**

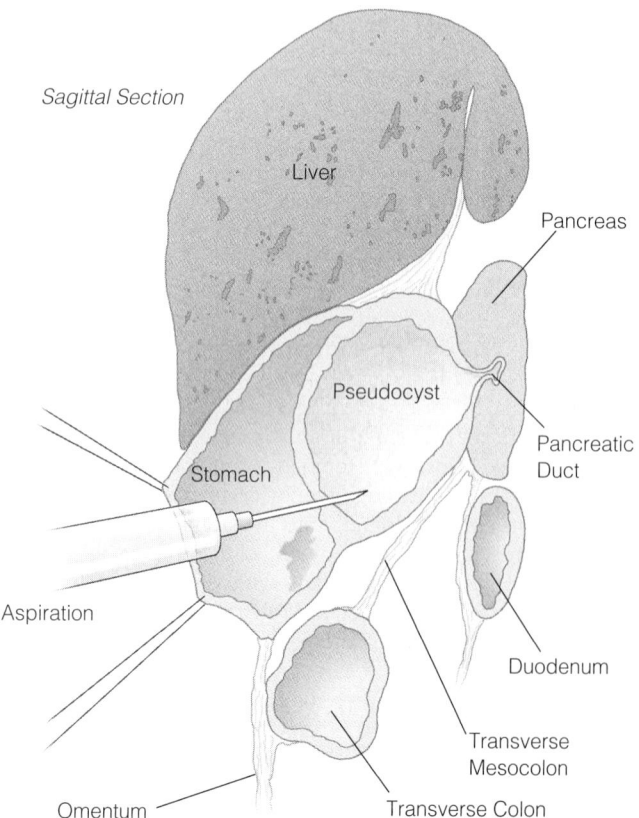

Figure 13 **Drainage of pancreatic pseudocyst into stomach.[3] The location of the pseudocyst is confirmed by aspirating pancreatic juice through the back wall of the stomach.**

be absent; thus, at this stage, the lesion may appear to be resectable.) The gallbladder is mobilized out of the liver bed. The common hepatic duct is circumferentially mobilized and divided. (Dividing the common hepatic duct early often facilitates identification and dissection of the portal vein. Even if the lesion proves to be unresectable, the gallbladder would not be used for the biliary bypass, given that we consider a hepaticojejunostomy preferable to a cholecystojejunostomy.)

Once the common hepatic duct is divided, the portal vein is easily identified. The anterior surface of the vein is cleaned

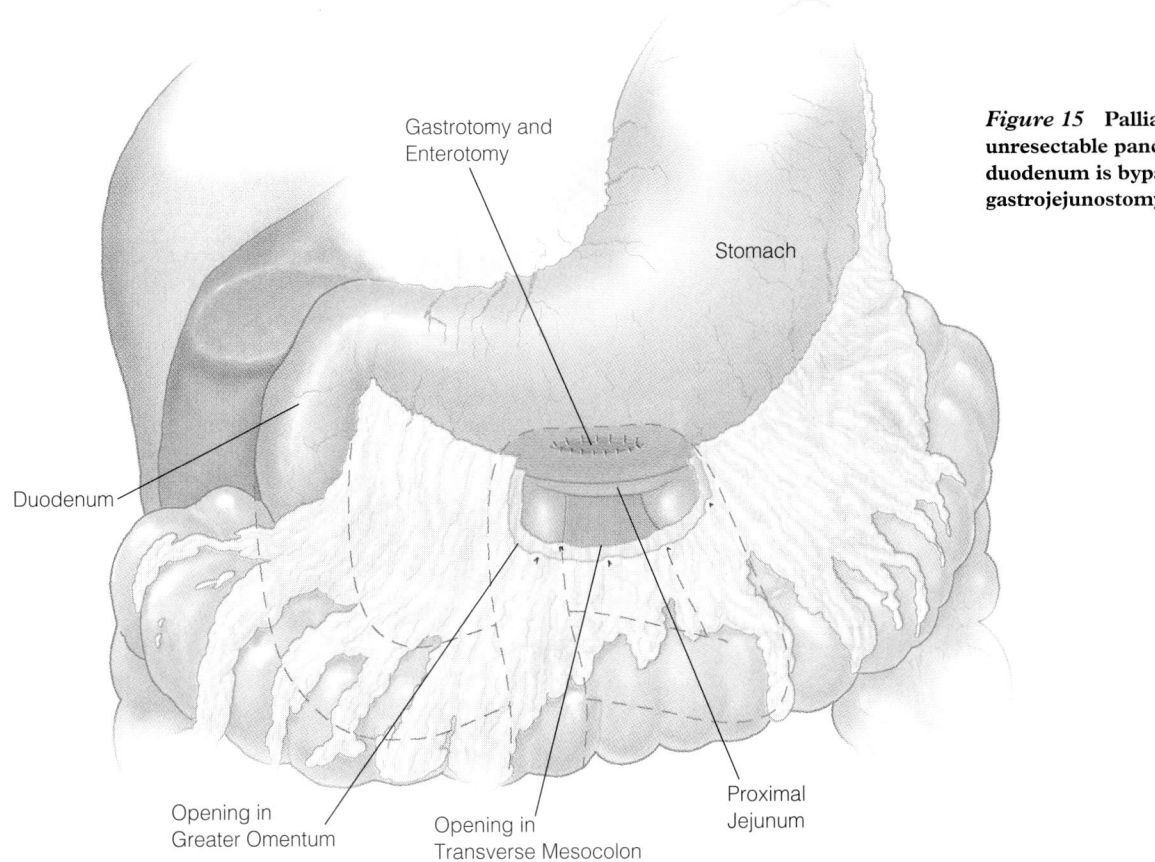

Gastrotomy and
Enterotomy

Stomach

Duodenum

Opening in
Greater Omentum

Opening in
Transverse Mesocolon

Proximal
Jejunum

Figure 15 **Palliative double bypass for unresectable pancreatic cancer.[3] The duodenum is bypassed with a retrocolic gastrojejunostomy.**

under the first portion of the duodenum. An attempt is made to separate the head and neck of the pancreas from the portal vein. In many cases, it is not until this point that the lesion is ascertained to be unresectable. (As an example, the tumor may be found to be directly invading the portal vein, but the invasion was not apparent from the preoperative staging tests.) Once it is clear that the tumor is unresectable, a palliative double bypass procedure is begun, in which the duodenum is bypassed with a retrocolic gastrojejunostomy [*see Figure 15*] and the distally obstructed biliary tree with a hepaticojejunostomy.

Approximately 4 cm of the most dependent portion of the greater curvature of the stomach is cleaned by doubly clamping, dividing, and ligating attachments of the greater omentum. Once this is accomplished, a small rent is made in the transverse mesocolon, and a proximal loop of jejunum is brought up through this rent and anastomosed to the greater curvature of the stomach in a side-to-side fashion. The anastomosis is performed with an outer interrupted layer of 3-0 silk and an inner continuous layer of 3-0 absorbable synthetic suture material. (In the past, palliative duodenal bypasses for pancreatic cancer were performed by carrying out an anterior antecolic gastrojejunostomy. Unfortunately, delayed gastric emptying is frequent after an anterior gastrojejunostomy. A posterior retrocolic gastroenterostomy virtually eliminates this complication. Historically, surgeons have been reluctant to perform retrocolic

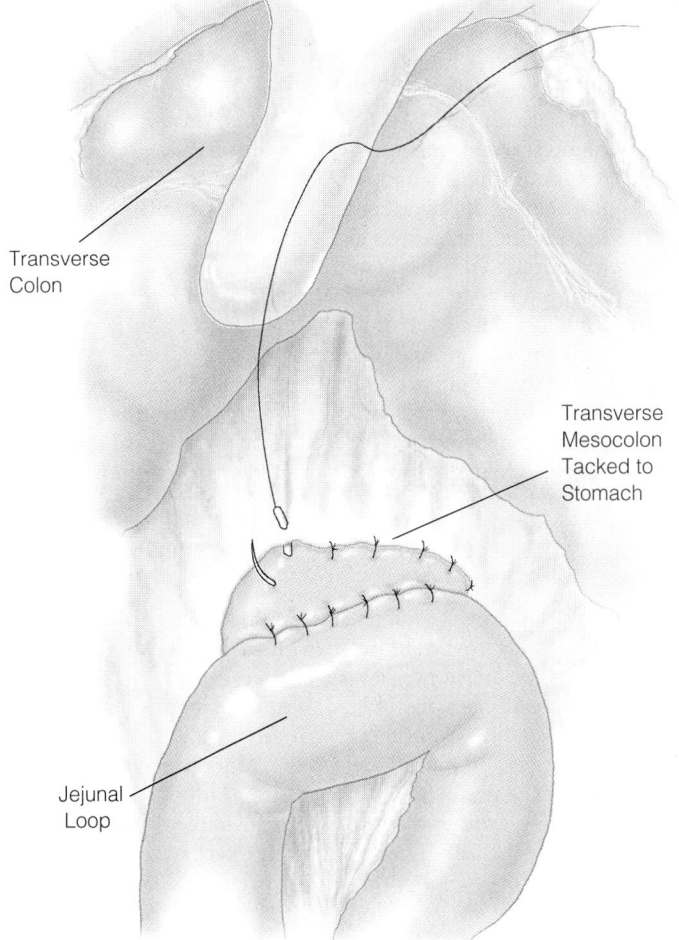

Transverse
Colon

Transverse
Mesocolon
Tacked to
Stomach

Jejunal
Loop

Figure 16 **Palliative double bypass for unresectable pancreatic cancer.[3] Once the retrocolic gastrojejunostomy is complete, the anastomosis is tacked to the rent in the transverse mesocolon on the gastric side with interrupted 3-0 silk sutures.**

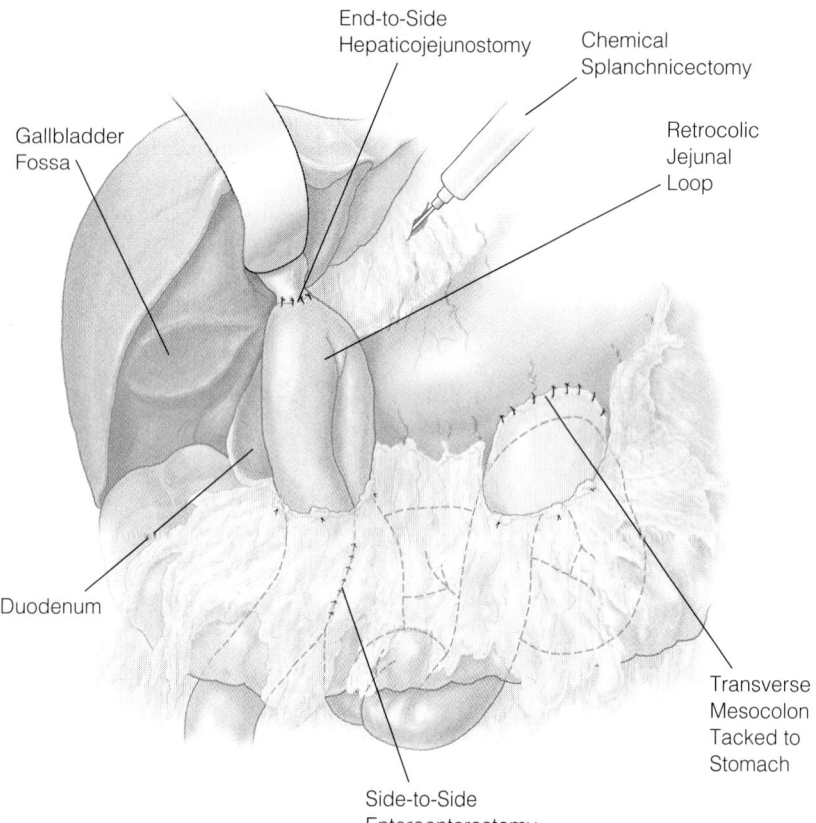

Gallbladder Fossa

End-to-Side Hepaticojejunostomy

Chemical Splanchnicectomy

Retrocolic Jejunal Loop

Duodenum

Transverse Mesocolon Tacked to Stomach

Side-to-Side Enteroenterostomy

Figure 17   **Palliative double bypass for unresectable pancreatic cancer.[3] An end-to-side hepaticojejunostomy is performed, followed by a side-to-side jejunojejunostomy between the afferent loop leading to the biliary anastomosis and the efferent loop leading from it. An opening is made in the lesser omentum, and a chemical splanchnicectomy is performed by injecting alcohol into the celiac plexus.**

gastroenterostomies for pancreatic cancer, fearing that tumor growth would occlude the anastomosis; however, at our institution, we have performed well over 200 such posterior retrocolic gastroenterostomies in this setting and have yet to demonstrate any tumor ingrowth into the anastomosis.) Once the posterior gastroenterostomy is complete, the anastomosis is tacked to the rent in the transverse mesocolon on the gastric side with multiple interrupted 3-0 silk sutures [*see Figure 16*]. (The purpose of this step is to prevent the afferent and efferent jejunal limbs from herniating up through the rent in the transverse mesocolon and becoming obstructed.)

The gallbladder is removed, and the distal biliary segment is oversewn with interrupted 3-0 silk sutures. (The distal biliary segment is routinely oversewn because there is a possibility that if a common channel is present, pancreatic secretions might reflux up the distal biliary tree and out into the peritoneal cavity.)

Approximately 30 cm distal to the gastrojejunostomy, a loop of jejunum is brought up into the right upper quadrant through a second rent in the transverse mesocolon. An end-to-side hepaticojejunostomy is performed with one layer of interrupted 4-0 absorbable synthetic sutures [*see Figure 17*].

A side-to-side anastomosis is performed between the afferent jejunal loop leading to the biliary anastomosis and the efferent jejunal loop leading from it [*see Figure 17*]. This short side-to-side anastomosis is placed below the rent in the transverse mesocolon. It is performed with an inner continuous layer of 3-0 absorbable synthetic suture material and an outer interrupted layer of 3-0 silk. The two limbs are tacked to the rent in the transverse mesocolon to prevent herniation. Alternatively, a Roux limb may be used to provide a conduit for biliary drainage.

The lesser omentum is divided, and a chemical splanchnicectomy is performed by injecting 20 ml of 50% alcohol into the celiac plexus on either side of the aorta at the level of the celiac axis [*see Figure 17*]. The level of the celiac axis is easily determined by palpating the thrill that is invariably present in the common hepatic artery as it comes off the celiac axis. (A prospective, randomized, double-blind study performed at our institution[1] demonstrated that chemical splanchnicectomies performed in this fashion in patients with unresectable pancreatic cancer were, in most cases, markedly effective in decreasing or eliminating pain for the remaining months of life. In addition, this procedure decreased or eliminated patients' narcotic requirements. Moreover, patients who underwent chemical splanchnicectomy actually survived significantly longer than those who did not. The improved survival was attributed to better nutritional intake in the pain-free patients.)

A closed suction Silastic drain is left posterior to the area of the hepaticojejunostomy and brought out through a stab wound in the right upper quadrant. If tissue confirmation of the presence of adenocarcinoma of the head of the pancreas was not obtained preoperatively, it should be obtained during operation. As a rule, this is most easily accomplished by performing a needle biopsy with a Tru-Cut needle transduodenally. The abdomen is irrigated with an antibiotic solution and then closed with multiple interrupted No. 1 nonabsorbable synthetic sutures placed through and through all muscle and fascial layers. The subcutaneous tissues are irrigated with an antibiotic-containing saline solution and closed with a continuous 3-0 absorbable synthetic suture. The subcuticular layer is closed with a continuous 4-0 absorbable synthetic suture. Steri-Strips are applied.

References

1. Lillemoe KD, Cameron JL, Kaufman HS, et al: Chemical splanchnicectomy in patients with unresectable pancreatic cancer: a prospective randomized trial. Ann Surg 217:447, 1993
2. Cameron JL: Rapid exposure of the portal and superior mesenteric veins. Surg Gynecol Obstet 176:395, 1995
3. Cameron JL: Atlas of Surgery. Mosby-Year Book, Inc., St. Louis, 1994

Selected Readings

Cameron JL, Pitt HA, Yeo CJ, et al: One hundred and forty-five consecutive pancreaticoduodenectomies without mortality. Ann Surg 217:430, 1993

Fernandez-del Castillo C, Rattner DW, Warshaw AL: Standards for pancreatic resection in the 1990s. Arch Surg 130:295, 1995

Lillemoe KD, Cameron JL, Hardacre JM, et al: Is prophylactic gastrojejunostomy indicated for unresectable periampullary cancer? a prospective randomized trial. Ann Surg 230:322, 1999

Lillemoe KD, Yeo CJ, Cameron JL: Pancreatic cancer: state-of-the-art care. CA Cancer J Clin 50:241, 2000

Sohn TA, Lillemoe KD, Cameron JL, et al: Surgical palliation of unresectable periampullary adenocarcinoma in the 1990s. J Am Coll Surg 188:658, 1999

Trede M, Schwall G, Saeger HD: Survival after pancreatoduodenectomy: 118 consecutive resections without an operative mortality. Ann Surg 211:447, 1990

Yeo CJ, Cameron JL, Lillemoe KD, et al: Does prophylactic octreotide decrease the rates of pancreatic fistula and other complications after pancreaticoduodenectomy? results of a prospective randomized placebo-controlled trial. Ann Surg 232:419, 2000

Yeo CJ, Cameron JL, Lillemoe KD, et al: Pancreaticoduodenectomy for cancer of the head of the pancreas: 201 patients. Ann Surg 221:721, 1995

Yeo CJ, Cameron JL, Sohn TA, et al: Six hundred fifty consecutive pancreaticoduodenectomies in the 1990s: pathology, complications, and outcomes. Ann Surg 226:248, 1997

Acknowledgments

Figures 1, 2, and 4   Tom Moore.
Figures 3 and 5 through 17   Tom Moore. Adapted from original illustrations by Corinne Sandone.

19 LAPAROSCOPIC SPLENECTOMY

Eric C. Poulin, M.D., M.Sc., F.R.C.S.(C), Christopher M. Schlachta, M.D., F.A.C.S., and Joseph Mamazza, M.D.

Medicine is not an exact science, and nowhere is this observation more appropriate than in the operating room when a spleen is being removed.[1]

The first reported splenectomy in the western world was performed by Zacarello in 1549, though the veracity of his operative description has been questioned. Between this initial report and the 1800s, very few cases were recorded. The first reported splenectomy in North America was performed by O'Brien in 1816. The patient was in the act of committing a rape when his victim plunged a large knife into his left side. As in this case, most early splenectomies were done in patients who had undergone penetrating trauma; often, the spleen was protruding from the wound and the surgeon proceeded with en masse ligation. The first elective splenectomy was performed by Quittenbaum in 1826 for sequelae of portal hypertension, and soon afterward, Wells performed one of the first splenectomies using general anesthesia; both patients died. In 1866, Bryant was the first to attempt splenectomy in a patient with leukemia. Over the following 15 years, 14 splenectomies were attempted as therapy for leukemia; none of the patients survived. In a 1908 review of 49 similar cases, Johnston reported a mortality of 87.7%.[2] These dismal results led to the abandonment of splenectomy for leukemia. In 1916, Kaznelson, of Prague, was the first to report good results from splenectomy in patients with thrombocytopenic purpura.

As the 20th century progressed, splenectomy became more common in direct proportion to the increase in the use of the automobile. The eventual recognition of the syndrome known as overwhelming postsplenectomy sepsis (OPSS) made splenic conservation an important consideration. Partial splenectomy had initially been described by the French surgeon Péan in the 19th century. This procedure received little further study until almost 100 years later, when the Brazilian surgeon Campos Cristo reevaluated Péan's technique in his report of eight trauma patients treated with partial splenectomy.[3] Simpson's report on 16 children admitted for splenic trauma to the Hospital for Sick Children in Toronto between 1948 and 1955 was instrumental in establishing the validity of nonoperative treatment of splenic trauma[4] [*see 5:6 Injuries to the Liver, Biliary Tract, Spleen, and Diaphragm*].

In late 1991 and early 1992, four groups working independently—Delaître in Paris, Carroll in Los Angeles, Cushieri in the United Kingdom, and our group in Canada—published the first reports of laparoscopic splenectomy in patients with hematologic disorders.[5-7] Since then, the development of operative techniques for partial laparoscopic splenectomy has tested the limits of minimally invasive surgery and encouraged clinical research regarding methods of simplifying the execution of the operation.[8,9] With the benefit of years of experience with laparoscopic splenectomy, it is possible to articulate a rational approach to this procedure that takes into account the technical lessons learned so far.

Preoperative Evaluation

Currently, we consider all patients evaluated for elective splenectomy to be potential candidates for laparoscopic splenectomy. Contraindications to a laparoscopic approach include severe portal hypertension, uncorrectable coagulopathy, severe ascites, and most traumatic injuries to the spleen. Extreme splenomegaly remains a relative contraindication as well. Because most patients scheduled for laparoscopic splenectomy have hematologic disorders, they undergo the same hematologic preparation that patients scheduled for open surgery do—namely, steroids and γ-globulins (when required). Ultrasonography is performed to determine the size of the spleen. Spleen size is expressed in terms of the maximum interpole length (i.e., the length of the line joining the two organ poles) and is generally classified into three categories: (1) normal spleen size (< 11 cm), (2) moderate splenomegaly (11 to 20 cm), and (3) severe splenomegaly (> 20 cm).[10] Because extremely large spleens present special technical problems that test the current limits of laparoscopic surgery, we make use of a fourth category for spleens longer than 30 cm, which we call megaspleens [*see Table 1*]. The ultrasonographer is also asked to try to identify any accessory spleens that may be present. The results of the ultrasound examination often determine whether the surgeon employs the anterior or the lateral approach to the procedure. Computed tomography is done when there is doubt about the exactness of the ultrasonographic measurement; such measurement is sometimes inaccurate at the upper pole and with spleens longer than 16 cm.

Patients receive thorough counseling about the consequences of the asplenic state. Polyvalent pneumococcal vaccine is administered at least 2 weeks before operation in all cases; preoperative *Haemophilus influenzae* vaccination is also advisable. Heparin prophylaxis for thrombophlebitis is administered according to standard guidelines, provided that there is no hematologic contraindication [*see 4:6 Venous Thromboembolism*]. Nonsteroidal anti-inflammatory drugs (NSAIDs) are often given in suppository form before operation to minimize postoperative pain; however, on empirical grounds, NSAIDs are not used when heparin prophylaxis is employed. Platelets are rarely, if ever, required when laparoscopic splenectomy is performed for idiopathic (immune) thrombocytopenic purpura (ITP).

Operative Planning

Laparoscopic splenectomy presents special problems, such as the necessity of dealing with a fragile and richly vascularized organ that is situated close to the stomach, the colon, and the pancreas and the difficulty of devising an extraction strategy that is compatible with

Table 1 Classification of Spleens According to Spleen Length*

Spleen Class	Spleen Length
Normal-size spleen	7–11 cm
Moderate splenomegaly	12–20 cm
Massive splenomegaly	21–30 cm
Megaspleen	> 30 cm

*Spleen length is defined as interpole length, measured along a straight line connecting the two poles.

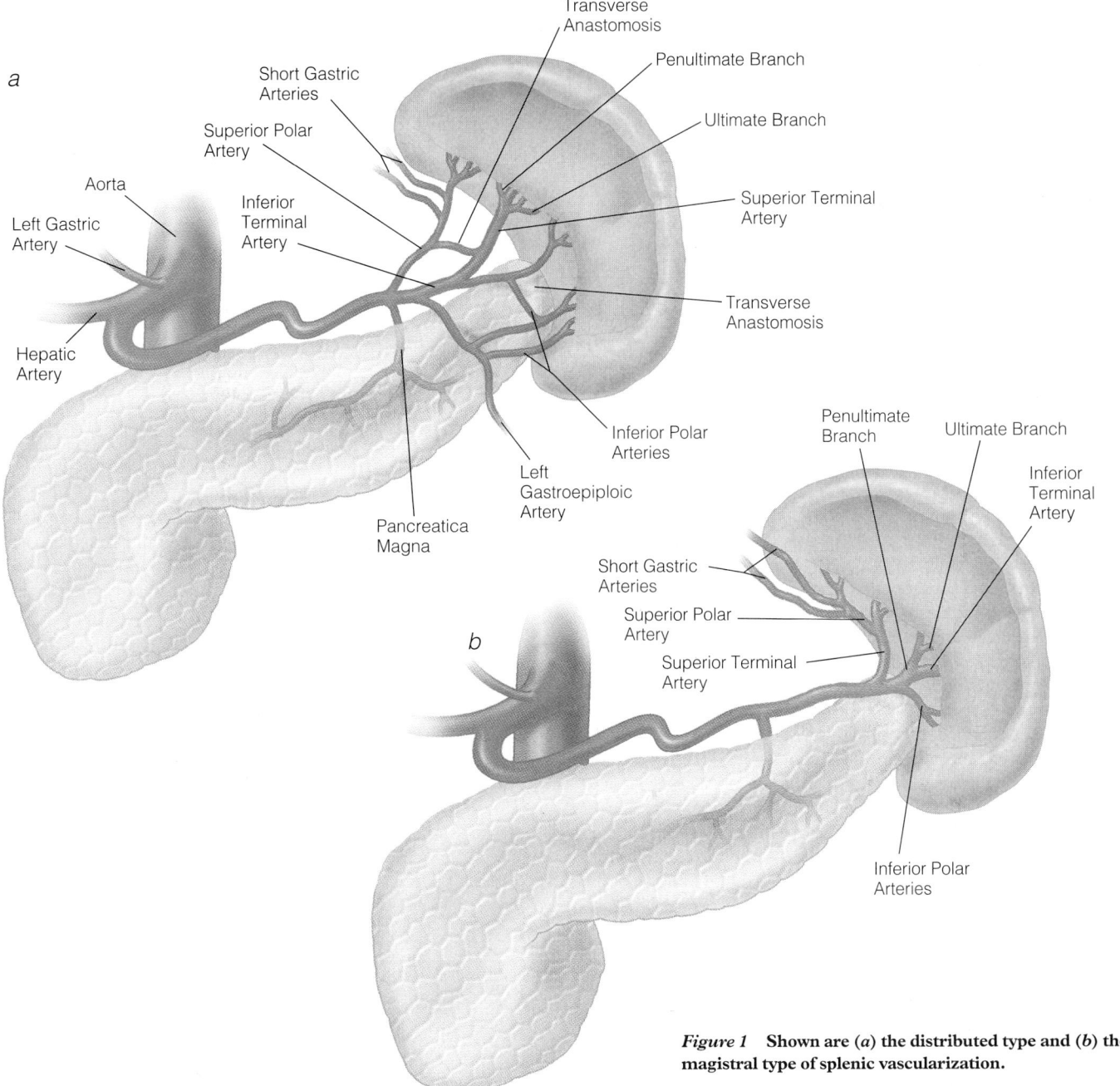

Figure 1 **Shown are (*a*) the distributed type and (*b*) the magistral type of splenic vascularization.**

proper histologic confirmation of the pathologic process while maintaining the advantages of minimal access surgery. For successful performance of laparoscopic splenectomy, a detailed knowledge of both splenic anatomy and potential complications is essential. It is the anatomic features—which may vary considerably from patient to patient (see below)—that largely determine the operative strategy.[11]

ANATOMIC CONSIDERATIONS

Most anatomy texts suggest that the splenic artery is constant in its course and branches; however, as the classic essay by Michels made clear, each spleen has its own peculiar pattern of terminal artery branches.[12]

Splenic Artery

The celiac axis is the largest but shortest branch of the abdominal aorta: it is only 15 to 20 mm long. The celiac axis arises above the body of the pancreas and, in 82% of specimens, divides into three primary branches: the left gastric artery, which is the first branch, and the hepatic and splenic arteries, which derive from a common stem. In rare instances, the splenic artery originates directly from the aorta; even less often, a second splenic artery arises from the celiac axis. There are numerous other possible variations, in which the splenic artery may originate from the aorta, the superior mesenteric artery, the middle colic artery, the left gastric artery, the left hepatic artery, or the accessory right hepatic artery. As a rule, however, the splenic artery arises from the celiac axis to the right of the midline, which means that the aorta must be crossed to reach the spleen and that selective angiography is likely to be difficult at times. The splenic artery can take a very tortuous course, particularly in patients who are elderly patients or who have a longer artery.

In his study of 100 cadaver spleens,[12] Michels divided splenic arterial geography into two types, distributed and magistral [*see Figure 1*]. In the distributed type, found in 70% of dissections, the splenic trunk is short, and six to 12 long branches enter the spleen over approximately 75% of its medial surface. The branches originate between 3 and 13 cm from the hilum [see Figure 1a]. In the magistral type, found in the remaining 30% of dissections, there is a long main splenic artery that divides near the hilum into three or four large, short terminal branches that enter the spleen over only 25% to 35% of its medial surface. These short splenic branches originate, on average, 3.5 cm from the spleen, and they reach the center of the organ as a compact bundle [see Figure 1b]. Early identification of the type of splenic blood supply present can help the surgeon estimate how difficult a particular splenectomy is likely to be. Operation on a spleen with a distributed vascular anatomy usually involves dissection of more blood vessels; however, the vessels, being spread over a wider area of the splenic hilum, are relatively easy to deal with. Operation on a spleen with a magistral-type blood supply typically involves dissection of fewer vessels; however, because the hilum is narrower and more compact, dissection and separation of the vessels are more difficult.

Branches of Splenic Artery

The splenic branches vary so markedly in length, size, and origin that no two spleens have the same anatomy. Outside the spleen, the arteries also frequently form transverse anastomoses with each other that, like most collaterals, arise at a 90° angle to the vessels involved [see Figure 1].[13] As a consequence, attempts to occlude a branch of the splenic artery by means of clips or embolization, if carried out proximal to such an anastomosis, may fail to devascularize the corresponding splenic segment. Before the splenic trunk divides, it usually gives off a few slender branches to the tail of the pancreas. The most important of these is called the pancreatica magna (a vessel familiar to vascular radiologists); occlusion of this branch with embolic materiel has been reported to result in pancreatitis. Next, the splenic artery divides into two to six first and second terminal branches, and these branches undergo two further levels of division into two to 12 penultimate and ultimate branches. Segmental and subsegmental division can occur either outside or inside the spleen. The number of arteries entering the spleen ranges from six to 36. The size of the spleen does not determine the number of arteries entering it; how-

ever, the presence of notches and tubercles usually correlates well with a higher number of entering arteries.

A reasonable general scheme of splenic artery branches might include as many as seven principal branches at various division levels and in various anatomic arrangements: (1) the superior terminal artery, (2) the inferior terminal artery, (3) the medial terminal artery, (4) the short gastric arteries, (5) the left gastroepiploic artery, (6) the inferior polar artery, and (7) the superior polar artery [see Figure 2]. Veins are usually located behind the corresponding arteries, except at the ultimate level of division, where they may be either anterior or posterior.

First terminal division branches   A classic study from 1917 found that 72% of specimens had three terminal branches (superior polar, superior terminal, and inferior terminal) and 28% had two[14]; the medial terminal artery was observed in only 20% of cases. When the superior terminal artery is excessively large, the inferior terminal is rudimentary, with an added blood supply often coming from the left gastroepiploic and polar vessels.

Second terminal division branches   *Superior polar artery.* The superior polar artery is present in 65% of patients. It usually arises from the main splenic trunk (75% of cases) or the superior terminal artery (20% of cases), but on occasion, it may originate from the inferior terminal artery or separately from the celiac axis (thus providing the spleen with a double splenic artery). In most instances, the superior polar artery gives rise to one or two short gastric branches; rarely, it gives rise to the left inferior phrenic and pancreatic rami. The presence and size of this artery appear to be correlated with tubercle formation, in that it is more prominent in spleens with large tubercles. The superior polar artery is frequently very long and slender and thus easily torn during splenectomy; accordingly, it was suggested in 1928 that ligation of splenic branches be started from the inferior pole of the spleen.[15]

Inferior polar artery. The inferior polar artery is present in 82% of cases. As many as five collateral branches may arise from the

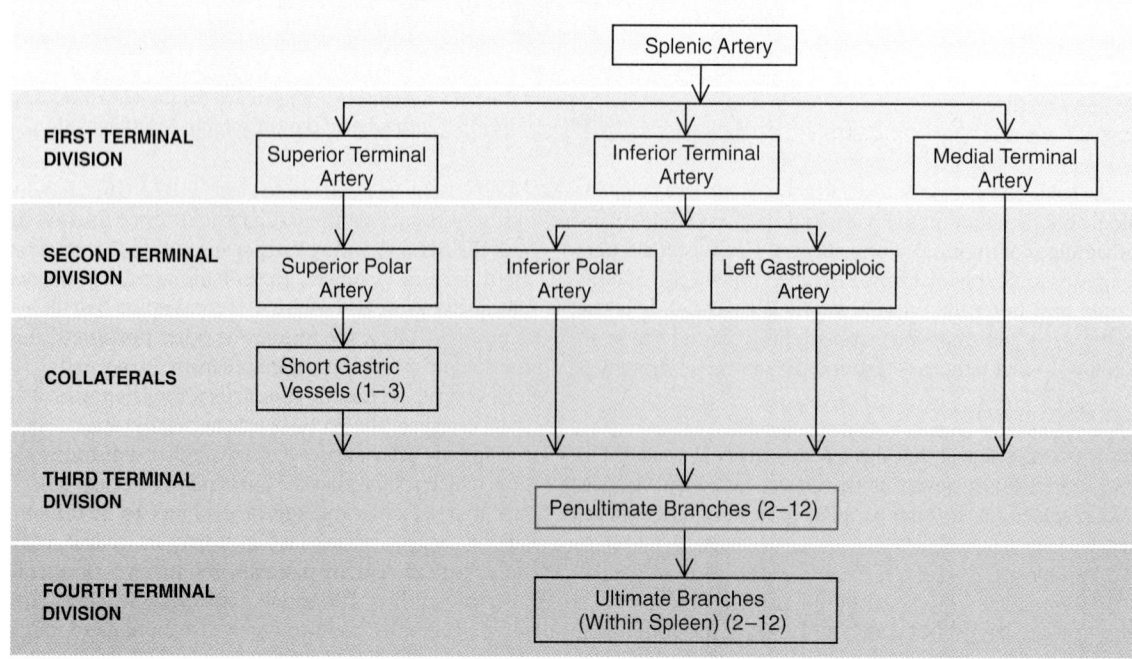

Figure 2   Outlined is a general scheme of the levels of division of the splenic artery branches.

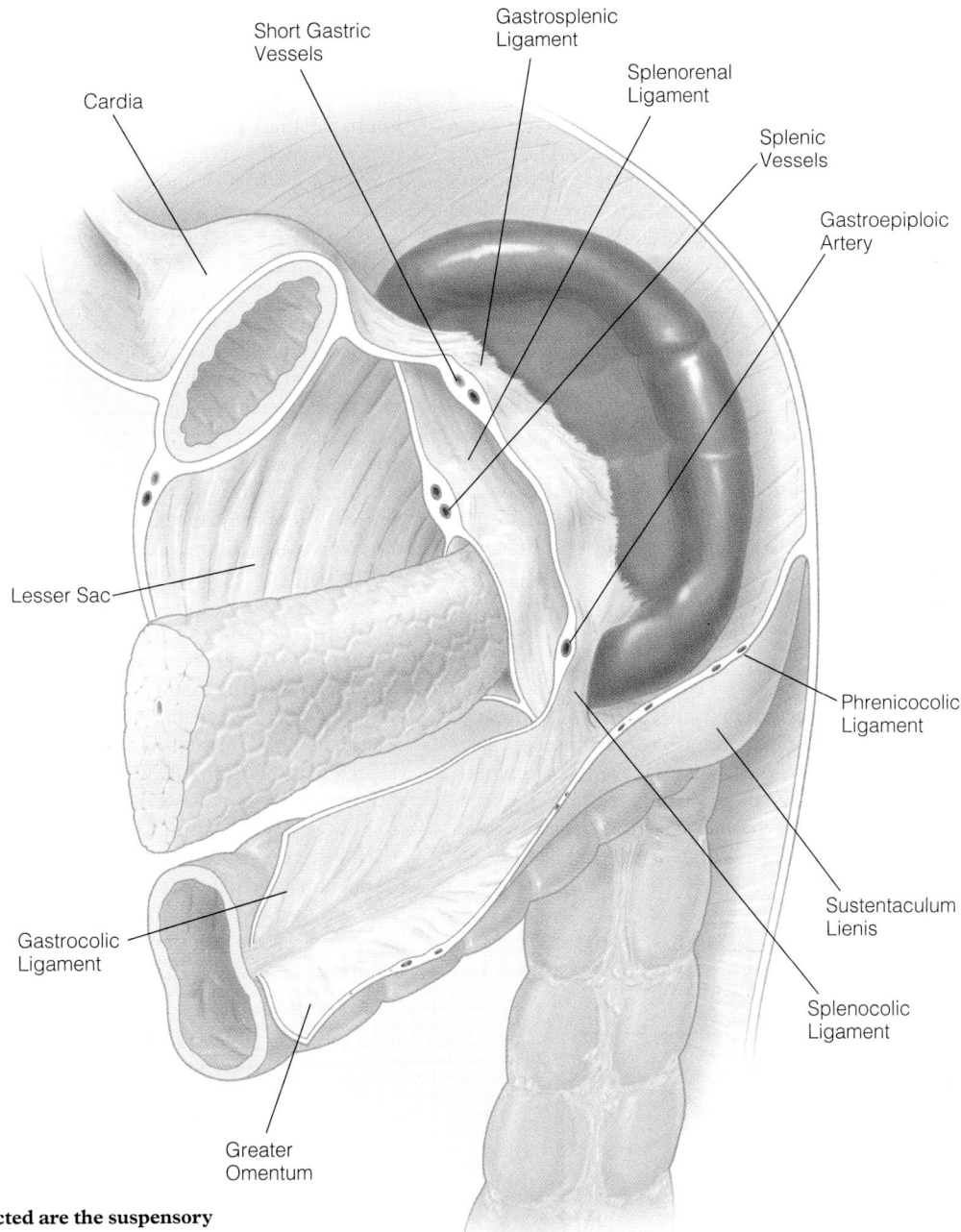

Figure 3 **Depicted are the suspensory ligaments of the spleen.**

splenic trunk, the inferior terminal artery, or, as noted, the left gastroepiploic artery. Inferior polar branches may have multiple origins, and they tend to be of smaller caliber than the superior polar artery.

Left gastroepiploic artery. The most varied of the splenic branches, the left gastroepiploic artery courses along the left side of the greater curvature in the anterior layer of the greater omentum. In 72% of cases, it arises from the splenic trunk several centimeters from its primary terminal division, and in 22% of cases, it originates from the inferior terminal artery or its branches; however, it may also originate from the middle of the splenic trunk or from the superior terminal artery. Characteristically, the left gastroepiploic artery gives off inferior polar arteries, which vary in number (ranging from one to five), size, and length. Typically, these branches are addressed first during laparoscopic splenectomy. When they are small, they can usually be controlled with the electrocautery.

Collaterals *Short gastric arteries.* As many as six short gastric arteries may arise from the fundus of the stomach, but as a rule, only the one to three that open into the superior polar artery must be ligated during laparoscopic splenectomy [*see Figure 1*].

Suspensory Ligaments of Spleen and Tail of Pancreas

Duplications of the peritoneum form the many suspensory ligaments of the spleen [*see Figure 3*]. Medially and posteriorly, the splenorenal ligament contains the tail of the pancreas and the splenic vessels. Anteriorly, the gastrosplenic ligament contains the short gastric and gastroepiploic arteries. In the lateral approach to laparoscopic splenectomy, the splenorenal and gastrosplenic ligaments are easily distinguished, and dissection of the anatomic structures they contain is relatively simple. In the anterior approach, these two ligaments lie on top of each other, and to separate them correctly and safely requires considerable experience with splenic anatomy.

The phrenicocolic ligament courses laterally from the diaphragm to the splenic flexure of the colon; its upper portion is called the phrenicosplenic ligament. The attachment of the lower pole on the internal side is called the splenocolic ligament. Between these two, a horizontal shelf of areolar tissue, known as the sustentaculum lienis, is formed on which the inferior pole of the spleen rests. The sustentaculum lienis is often molded into a sac that opens cephalad and acts as a support for the lower pole. This structure, often overlooked during open procedures, is readily visible through the laparoscope. The phrenicocolic ligament, the splenocolic ligament, and the sustentaculum lienis are usually avascular, except in patients who have portal hypertension or myeloid metaplasia.

A 1937 study found that the tail of the pancreas was in direct contact with the spleen in 30% of cadavers.[16] A subsequent report confirmed this finding and added that in 73% of patients, the distance between the two structures was no more than 1 cm.[17] Care must be exercised to avoid damage with the electrocautery during dissection as well as damage with the linear stapler in the course of en masse ligation of the splenic hilum (a maneuver more easily performed via the lateral approach to laparoscopic splenectomy).

Operative Technique

LATERAL APPROACH

This approach was first described in connection with laparoscopic adrenalectomy and is currently used for most laparoscopic splenectomies.[18] At present, the only indication for the anterior approach to laparoscopic splenectomy is the presence of massive splenomegaly or a megaspleen. Typically, this alternative approach is taken when a spleen reaches or exceeds 23 cm in length or 3 kg in weight.

Step 1: Placement of Trocars

The patient is placed in the right lateral decubitus position, much as he or she would be for a left-side posterolateral thoracotomy. The operating table is flexed and the kidney bolster raised to increase the distance between the lower rib and the iliac crest. Usually, four 12 mm trocars are used around the costal margin so that the camera, the clip applier, and the linear stapler can be interchanged with maximum flexibility [*see Figure 4*]. The trocars must be far enough apart to permit good working angles. Some advantage may be gained from tilting the patient slightly backward; this step gives the operating team more freedom in moving the instruments placed along the left costal margins, especially during lifting movements, when it is easy for instrument handles to touch the operating table. For the same reason, it is also advisable to place the anterior or abdominal side of the patient closer to the edge of the operating table.

A local anesthetic is infiltrated into the skin at the midpoint of the anterior costal margin, and a 12 mm incision is made. The first trocar is inserted under direct vision, and a symmetrical 15 mm Hg pneumoperitoneum is created. The locations of the remaining trocars are determined by considering the anatomic configuration in relation to the size of the spleen to be excised. In most cases, the fourth posterior trocar cannot be inserted until the splenic flexure of the colon has been mobilized. Accordingly, the procedure is usually started with three trocars in place.

Troubleshooting   *Open insertion of first trocar.* After years of using the Veress needle, we now prefer the open method of inserting the first trocar. It is true that use of the Veress needle is for the most part safe; however, the small number of catastrophic complications that occur with blind methods of first trocar insertion are more and more difficult to justify. Admittedly, these complications are infrequent, and thus, it is unlikely that even a large randomized trial would be able to show any significant differences between various methods of first trocar insertion. Nevertheless, even though complications occur with the open method of first trocar insertion as well, they are very uncommon and tend to be limited to trauma to the intestine or the omental blood vessels; they do not have the same serious consequences as the major vessel injury that may arise from blind trocar insertion.

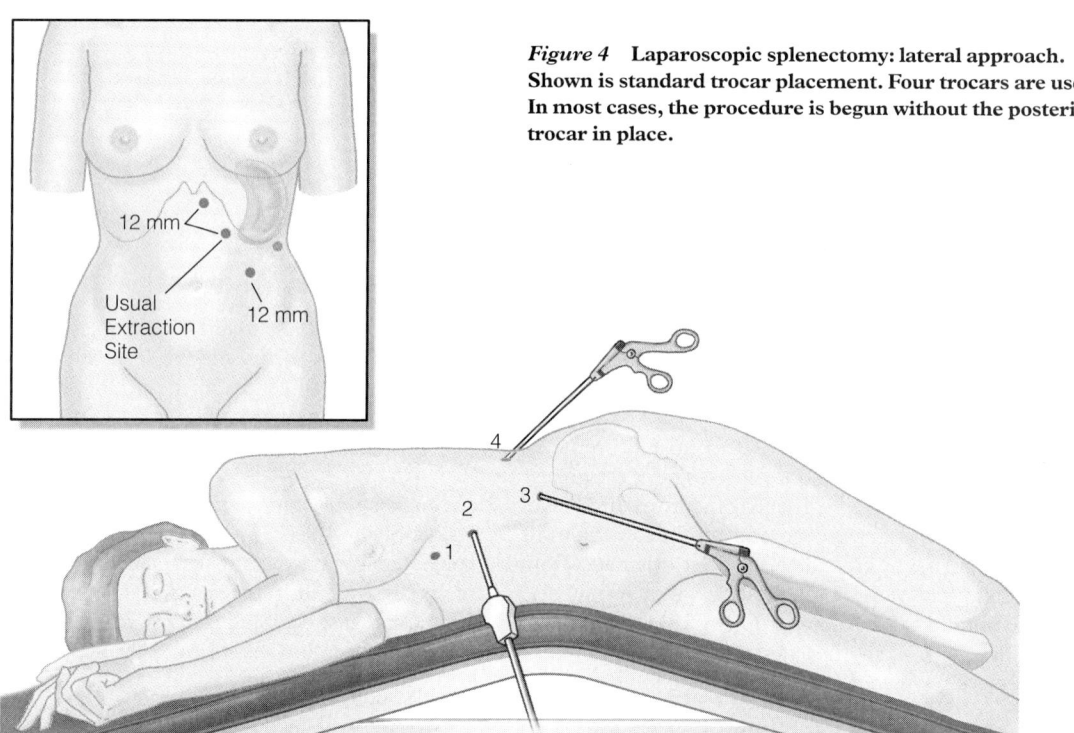

Figure 4   **Laparoscopic splenectomy: lateral approach. Shown is standard trocar placement. Four trocars are used. In most cases, the procedure is begun without the posterior trocar in place.**

Alternative trocar placement. More experienced surgeons (or those simply wishing to make the procedure easier) may choose to replace one or two 12 mm trocars with 5 mm trocars [*see Figure 5a*]. The procedure can also be performed with only three trocars. In leaner patients, one of the trocars can be inserted into the umbilicus to gain a cosmetic advantage. The advent of needlescopic techniques has made it possible to replace some of the 5 and 12 mm trocars with 3 mm trocars. The ultimate (i.e., least invasive) technique, usually reserved for lean patients with ITP and normal-size spleens, involves one 12 mm trocar placed in the umbilicus and two 3 mm trocars placed subcostally [*see Figure 5b*]. This approach requires two different camera-laparoscope setups, so that a 3 mm laparoscope can be interchanged with a 10 mm laparoscope as necessary to permit application of clips or staplers through the umbilical incision once the dissection is completed. The specimen is then retrieved through the umbilicus. Because the use of 3 mm laparoscopes is accompanied by a decrease in available intra-abdominal light and focal width, a meticulously bloodless field and sophisticated surgical judgment are critical for successful performance of needlescopic splenectomy.

Step 2: Search for and Retrieval of Accessory Spleens

The camera is inserted, and the stomach is retracted medially to expose the spleen. Then a fairly standard sequence is followed. A thorough search is then made for accessory spleens. To maximize retrieval, all known locations of accessory spleens should be carefully explored [*see Figure 6*]. Any accessory spleens found should be removed immediately; they are considerably harder to locate once the spleen is removed.

Troubleshooting It is especially important to retrieve accessory spleens from patients with ITP, in whom the presence of overlooked accessory spleens has been associated with recurrence of the disease. Remedial operation for excision of missed accessory spleens has been reported to bring remission of recurrent disease; such operation can be performed laparoscopically. The overall retrieval rate for accessory spleens should fall between 15% and 30%.

Splenic activity has been demonstrated after open and laparoscopic splenectomy for trauma and hematologic disorders[19,20]; accordingly, it is advisable to wash out and recover all splenic fragments resulting from intraoperative trauma at the end of the procedure. This step is particularly important for patients with ITP, in whom intraoperative trauma to the spleen is thought to contribute to postoperative scan-detectable splenic activity. As of this writing, we have recovered accessory spleens in 33% of ITP cases treated laparoscopically.

Step 3: Control of Vessels at Lower Pole, Demonstration of "Splenic Tent," and Incision of Phrenicocolic Ligament

The splenic flexure is partially mobilized by incising the splenocolic ligament, the lower part of the phrenicocolic ligament, and the sustentaculum lienis. The incision is carried slightly into the left side of the gastrocolic ligament. This step affords access to the gastrosplenic ligament, which can then be readily separated from the splenorenal ligament to create what looks like a tent. This maneuver cannot be accomplished in all cases, but when it can be done, it simplifies the procedure considerably. The walls of this so-called splenic tent are made of the gastrosplenic ligament on the left and the splenorenal ligament on the right, and the floor is made up of the stomach. In fact, this maneuver opens the lesser sac in its lateral portion (a point that is better demonstrated with gentle upward retraction of the splenic tip) [*see Figure 7*].

The branches of the left gastroepiploic artery are controlled with the electrocautery or with clips, depending on the size of the branches. The avascular portion of the gastrosplenic ligament, situated between the gastroepiploic artery and the short gastric vessels, is then incised sufficiently to expose the hilar structures in the splenorenal ligament. To accomplish this, the lower pole is gently elevated; in this position, the spleen almost retracts itself as it naturally falls toward the left lobe of the liver. At this point, the surgeon can usually assess the geography of the hilum and determine the degree of difficulty of the operation. The fourth trocar, if needed, is then placed posteriorly under direct vision, with care taken to avoid the left kidney. Caution must also be exercised in placing the trocars situated immediately anterior and posterior to the iliac crest. The iliac crest can impede movement and hinder upward mobilization of structures if the trocars are placed over it rather than in front of or behind it [*see Figure 8*].

Finally, the phrenicocolic ligament is incised all the way to the left crus of the diaphragm, either with a monopolar electrocautery with an L hook or with scissors. A small portion of the ligament is left to keep the spleen suspended and facilitate subsequent bagging. The

a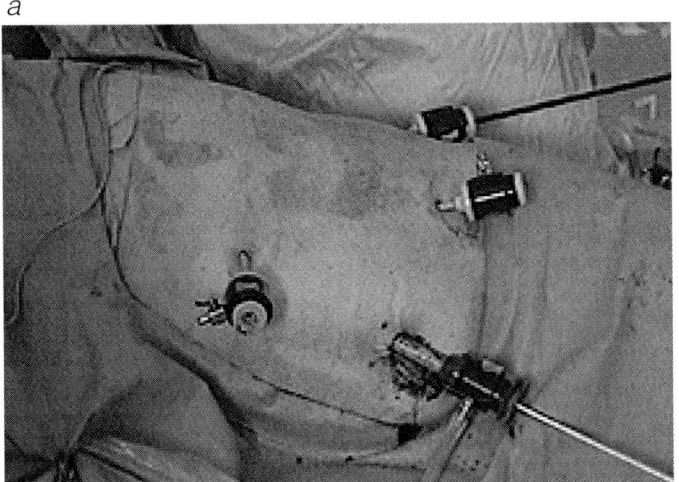

b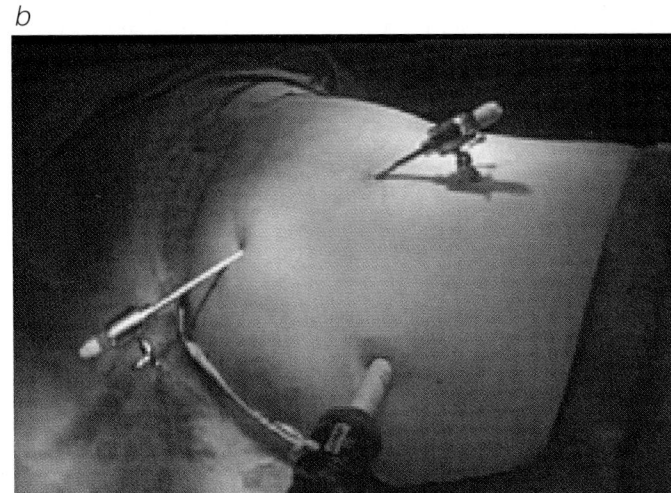

Figure 5 **Laparoscopic splenectomy: lateral approach. Shown are alternative trocar placements. (*a*) In some patients (e.g., thin patients with normal-size spleens), a 12 mm trocar may be placed in the umbilicus to gain a cosmetic advantage, and most of the other trocars may be downsized to 5 mm. (*b*) In the needlescopic approach, only three trocars are placed: a 12 mm trocar in the umbilicus and two 3 mm subcostal trocars. Two camera-laparoscope setups (3 mm and 10 mm) are required.**

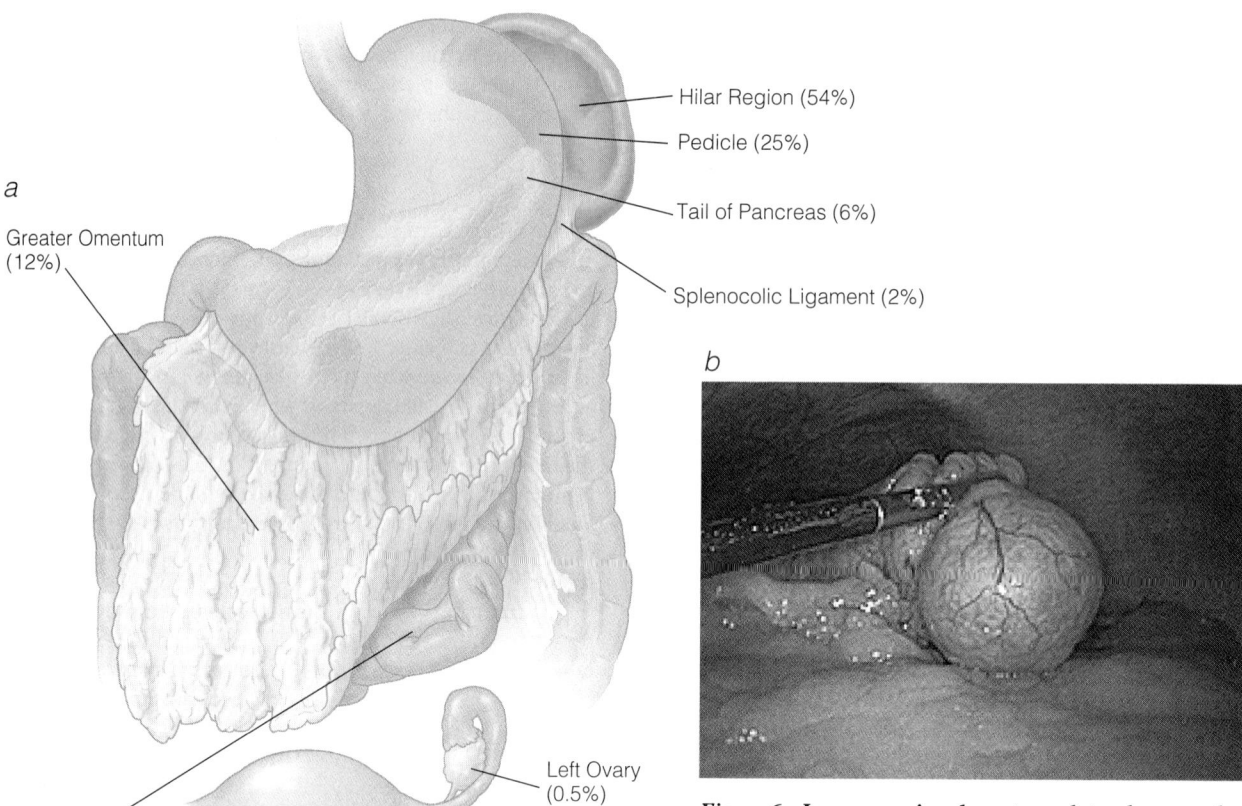

a

Greater Omentum (12%)

Hilar Region (54%)

Pedicle (25%)

Tail of Pancreas (6%)

Splenocolic Ligament (2%)

Mesentery (0.5%)

Left Ovary (0.5%)

b

Figure 6 **Laparoscopic splenectomy: lateral approach. (*a*) Accessory spleens are known to occur at specific sites. (*b*) Shown is an accessory spleen.**

phrenicocolic ligament is avascular except in patients with portal hypertension or myeloproliferative disorders (e.g., myeloid metaplasia). Leaving 1 to 2 cm of ligament all along the spleen side facilitates retraction and handling of the spleen with instruments.

Troubleshooting   Remarkably few instruments are needed for laparoscopic splenectomy [*see Figure 9*]: most of the operation is done with three reusable instruments. A dolphin-nose 5 mm atraumatic grasper is used to elevate and hold the spleen. It is also used to separate tissue planes and vessels with blunt dissection because its atraumatic tip is easily insinuated between tissue planes. A gently curved 5 mm fine-tip dissector (Crile or Maryland) and a 10 mm 90° right-angle dissector are the only other tools required for cost-efficient dissection.

When a powered instrument is called for, we use a monopolar electrocautery with an L hook or a gently curved scissors [*see Figure 9*]. An ultrasonic dissector can also be used.

Step 4: Dealing with Splenic Hilum and Tailoring Operative Strategy to Anatomy

It is advisable to base one's operative strategy on the specific splenic anatomy. If a distributed anatomy is present, the splenic branches are usually dissected and clipped. This is not only the least costly approach but also the simplest, in that the vessels are spread over a wider area of the splenic hilum and are easier to dissect and separate [*see Figure 10*].

A magistral anatomy lends itself more to a single use of the linear stapler, provided that the tail of the pancreas is identified and dissected away when required. When possible, a window is created above the hilar pedicle in the splenorenal ligament so that all structures can

be included within the markings of the linear stapler under direct vision [*see Figure 11*]. The angles provided by the various trocars make this maneuver much easier via the lateral approach than via the anterior approach. Dissection continues with individual dissection and clipping of the short gastric vessels; occasionally, these vessels can also be taken en masse with the linear stapler. So far, we have not used sutures in this setting, except once to control a short gastric vessel that was too short to be clipped safely. This portion of the operation is performed while the spleen is hanging from the upper portion of the phrenicocolic ligament, which has not yet been entirely cut.

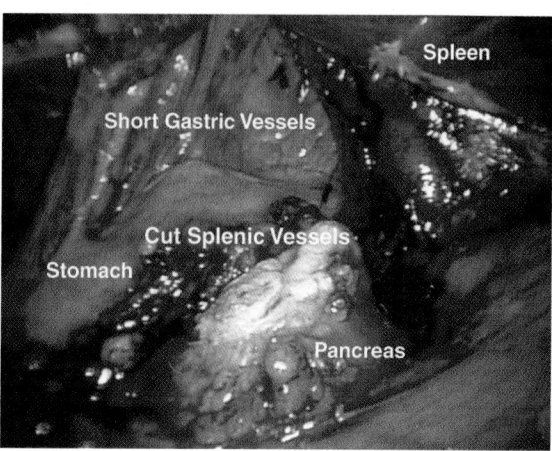

Spleen

Short Gastric Vessels

Cut Splenic Vessels

Stomach

Pancreas

Figure 7 **Laparoscopic splenectomy. The so-called splenic tent is formed by the gastrosplenic and splenorenal ligaments laterally and the stomach below.**

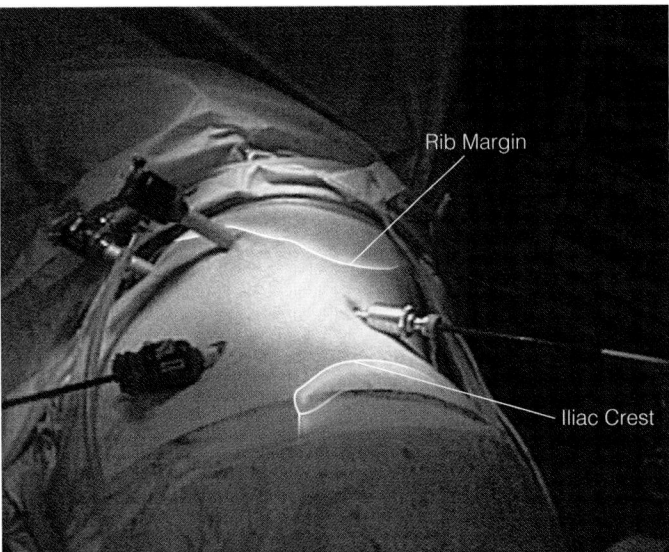

Figure 8 Laparoscopic splenectomy: lateral approach. Shown is the recommended trocar placement around the iliac crest.

Troubleshooting It is at this point in the procedure that experience in designing the operative strategy pays off in reduced operating time. Because of the many variations in size, shape, vascular patterns, and relations to adjacent organs, spleens are almost as individual as fingerprints. Accordingly, an experienced spleen surgeon learns to keep an open mind with regard to operative strategy and must be able to call on a wide range of skills to facilitate the procedure.

The surgeon should start by looking at the internal surface of the spleen. If the splenic vessels cover more than 75% of the internal surface (as is the case in 70% of patients), a distributed anatomy is present, which means that the spleen can be expected to have more vessels spread out over a wider area. The number of splenic branches is also related to the presence of notches on the spleen surface. With a distributed vascular anatomy, the vessels tend to be easier to

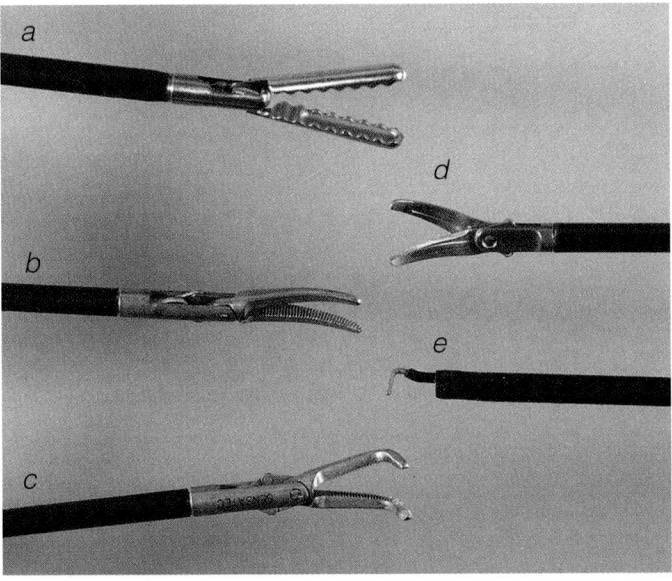

Figure 9 Laparoscopic splenectomy: lateral approach. Laparoscopic splenectomy can be done with a few basic instruments: (*a*) a 5 mm laparoscopic grasper, (*b*) a 5 mm laparoscopic dissector, (*c*) a 10 mm right-angle dissector, (*d*) a curved laparoscopic scissors, and (*e*) a monopolar electrocautery with an L hook.

dissect and isolate and thus can be readily (and cost-effectively) controlled with clips. On the other hand, if the splenic vessels entering the spleen cover only 25% to 35% of the inner surface of the hilum (30% of patients), the pattern is magistral. In such cases, the hilum is more compact and fewer vessels can be expected, especially if the surface of the spleen is smooth and without notches. With a magistral vascular anatomy, the vessels can usually be controlled with a single application of the vascular stapler across the hilum, provided that the tail of the pancreas can be protected.

Step 5: Extraction of Spleen

A medium-size or large heavy-duty plastic freezer bag, of the sort commercially available in grocery stores, is used to bag the spleen. This bag is sterilized and folded, then introduced into the abdominal cavity through one of the 12 mm trocars [*see Figure 12*]. The bag is unfolded and the spleen slipped inside to prevent splenosis during the subsequent manipulations. Grasping forceps are used to hold the two rigid edges of the bag and to effect partial closure. Bagging is facilitated by preserving the upper portion of the phrenicocolic ligament. After final section of the phrenicocolic ligament and any diaphragmatic adhesions present, extraction is performed through one of the anterior port sites. Extraction through a posterior site is more difficult because of the thickness of the muscle mass; usually, the incision must be opened, and more muscle must be fulgurated than is desirable.

The subcostal or umbilical incision through which extraction is to take place is extended slightly. A grasping forceps is inserted through the extraction incision to hold the edges of the bag inside the abdomen. Gentle traction on the bag from outside brings the spleen close to the peritoneal surface of the umbilical incision and then out of the wound [*see Figure 13*]. Specimen retrieval bags have been developed that can accommodate a normal-size spleen and thus make bagging much easier, but they are costly.

A biopsy specimen of a size suitable for pathologic identification is obtained by incising the splenic tip. The spleen is then fragmented with finger fracture, and the resulting blood is suctioned. The remaining stromal tissue of the spleen is then extracted through the small incision, hemostasis is again verified, and all trocars are removed. No drains are used. The incisions are closed with absorbable sutures and paper strips. After verification of hemostasis, the trocar sites are closed with absorbable sutures and paper strips.

Troubleshooting The freezer bags can be more easily introduced into the abdomen if they are pulled in rather than pushed in [*see Figure 12*]. This may be accomplished by bringing out a 5 mm toothed grasper through the introduction trocar from another properly angled trocar, grasping the specimen bag, and pulling the bag back down through the trocar.

Slipping the spleen into a freezer bag is also an acquired skill that takes some time to master. It is an important skill that is useful in many other instances where specimen retrieval is needed (e.g., in procedures involving the gallbladder, the appendix, the adrenal glands, or the colon). In addition, it is highly cost-effective, in that these commercially available bags cost only a few cents each. Admittedly, laparoscopic retrieval bags are easier to use, but their substantially higher cost can become a factor in a busy minimally invasive surgery unit. We recently started to use a powerful suction machine (–70 mm Hg) and a custom-made sharp beveled 10 mm cannula to suction splenic tissue from the plastic retrieval bag [*see Figure 14*].

ANTERIOR APPROACH

The anterior approach is seldom used nowadays; however, it remains the preferable approach in some patients with massive spleno-

a

b

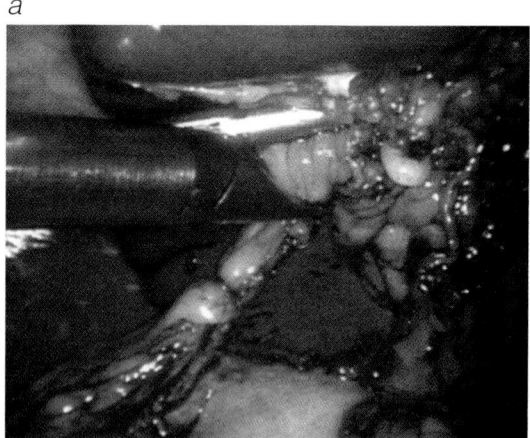
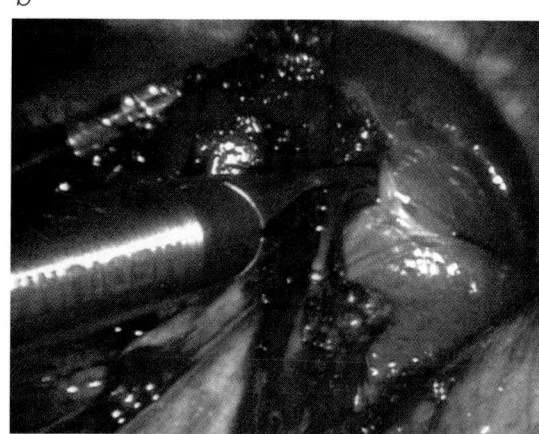

Figure 10 **Laparoscopic splenectomy: lateral approach. (*a, b*) Clipping is well suited to controlling short gastric or gastroepiploic vessels. It is also appropriate for distributed-type splenic vasculatures, in which more splenic vessels are spread over a wider area of the hilum.**

megaly (21 to 30 cm long) and all patients with megaspleens (> 30 cm or > 3 kg). Very large spleens are extremely heavy and difficult to manipulate with laparoscopic instruments, and it is complicated to lift them so as to gain access to the phrenicocolic ligament posteriorly. The anterior approach can also be considered if another procedure (e.g., cholecystectomy) is being contemplated; alternatively, in this situation, the lateral approach can be used, and the patient can be repositioned for the secondary procedure.

Step 1: Placement of Trocars

Under general anesthesia, the patient is placed in a modified lithotomy position to allow the surgeon to operate between the patient's legs and to allow the assistants to stand on each side of the patient. The procedure is performed through five trocars in the upper abdomen [*see Figure 15*], with the patient in a steep Fowler position with left-side elevation. A 12 mm trocar is introduced through an umbilical incision, and a 10 mm laparoscope (0° or 30°) is connected to a video system. A 12 mm trocar is placed in each upper quadrant, and two 5 mm trocars are inserted close to the rib margin on the left and right sides of the abdomen. Alternatively, trocars can be deployed in a semicircle away from the left upper quadrant. Trocar sites are carefully selected to optimize working angles. The 12 mm ports are used to allow introduction of clip appliers, staplers, or the laparoscope from a variety of angles as needed.

Troubleshooting With increasing experience, we find that we prefer to do as many laparoscopic splenectomies as possible via the lateral approach because it is so much easier, even with spleens that are longer than 20 cm and are readily palpable. The decision is arbitrarily made on the basis of estimated available working space. If the spleen comes too close to the iliac crest or the midline, the anterior approach should be taken instead.

Step 2: Isolation of Lower Pole and Control of Blood Supply

The left hepatic lobe is retracted, and the stomach is retracted medially to expose the spleen. Accessory spleens are searched for, and the phrenicocolic ligament, the splenocolic ligament, and the sustentaculum lienis are incised near the lower pole with an electrocautery and a hook probe or with scissors. Vascular adhesions—frequently found on the medial side of the spleen—are cauterized. The gastrocolic ligament is carefully dissected close to the spleen, and the left gastroepiploic vessels are ligated one by one with metallic clips or, if small, simply cauterized. The upper and lower poles of the

spleen are gently lifted with one or both palpators (placed through the 5 mm ports) to expose the splenic hilum and the tail of the pancreas within the splenorenal ligament, thereby facilitating individual dissection and clipping of all the branches of the splenic artery and vein close to the spleen. The short gastric vessels are then identified and ligated with clips or, occasionally, with staples. No sutures are used. Alternatively, the splenic artery itself can be isolated and clipped within the lesser sac before extensive dissection of the lower pole and suspensory ligaments.

When preoperative splenic artery embolization is employed [*see* Preoperative Splenic Artery Embolization, *below*], the dissection plane is situated between the sites of distal embolization of splenic artery branches and the site of proximal embolization of the splenic artery itself. Because of the segmental and terminal distribution of splenic arteries, it is easy to determine the devascularized portions of the spleen: these segments exhibit a characteristic grayish color, whereas the vascularized segments retain a pinkish hue. When the organ is completely isolated, it is left in its natural cavity, and hemostasis is verified.

Troubleshooting If one elects first to clip the splenic artery within the lesser sac, there are a few precautions that must be taken. First, the clipping must be done distal to the pancreatica magna artery to prevent pancreatic injury. Second, one must make sure that the splenic artery proper is clipped, not one of its branches (e.g., the superior terminal branch). This is an easy mistake to commit with the distributed type of splenic vasculature [*see Figure 1*] because the splenic artery itself is short and the branches can take off very early. Third, one must always keep in mind the possibility of an anastomotic branch between the major splenic branches, as described by Testut.[13] Should a major terminal branch be clipped rather than the splenic artery proper, there will be no spleen ischemia if such an anastomosis is present [*see Figure 1*].

Yet another challenge posed by the anterior approach is that if bleeding occurs, the blood tends to pool in the area of the hilum and obscure vision even more, whereas in the lateral approach, the blood tends to flow away from the operative field. One quickly learns that there is a steep price to pay for cutting corners during the dissection. The dissection must be meticulous, especially behind branches of the splenic vein.

Step 3: Extraction of Spleen

Given that the anterior approach is now used only in cases of

a

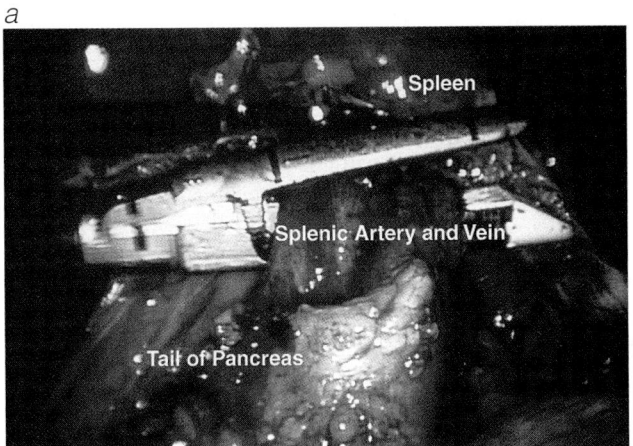

b

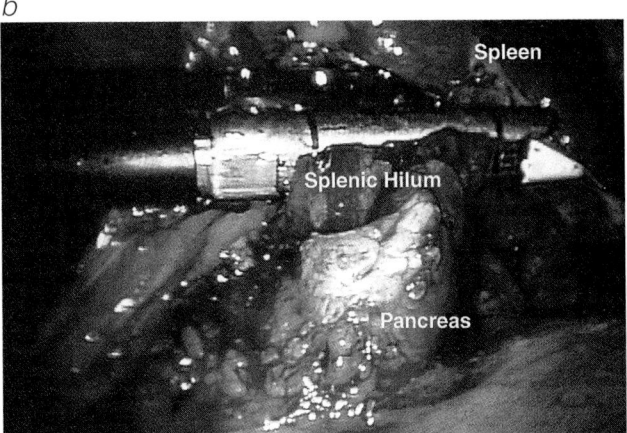

c

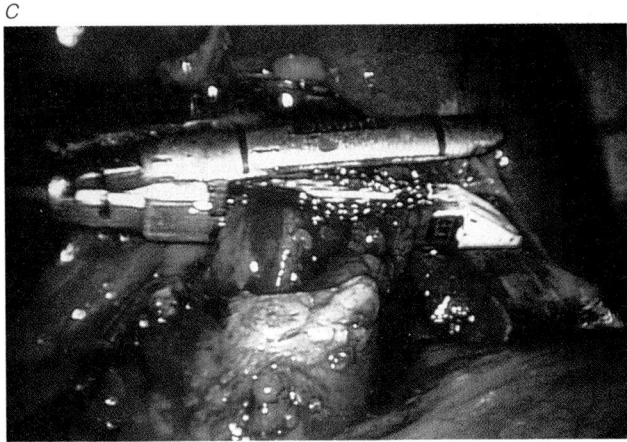

Figure 11 **Laparoscopic splenectomy: lateral approach. (*a through c*) Stapling is particularly well suited to the compact hilum found in the magistral-type distribution of splenic vessels. As shown, all of the vascular structures are within the stapler markers, and the tail of the pancreas is well protected.**

massive splenomegaly or megaspleen, bagging can be problematic. The largest commercially available freezer bag we have seen measures 27 by 28 cm, and the largest spleen we have been able to bag in one of them was 24 cm long. Furthermore, an accessory extraction incision is often required; a Pfannenstiel incision gives better cosmetic results, but a left lower quadrant incision can also be used. A plastic sleeve designed to maintain pneumoperitoneum is also a useful adjunct for vessel dissection and extraction in patients with very large spleens.

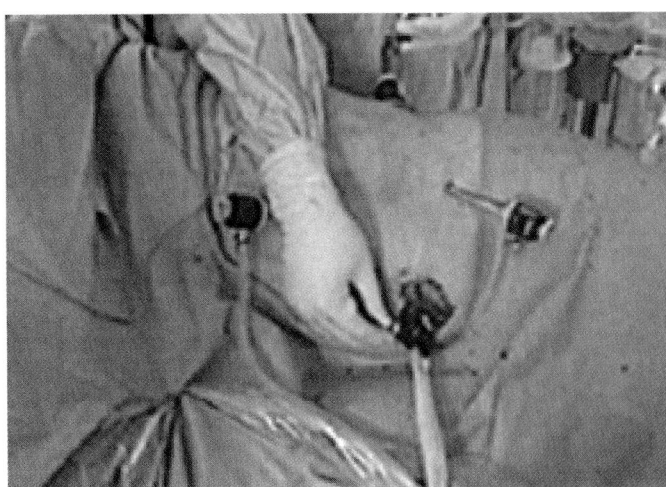

Figure 12 **Laparoscopic splenectomy: lateral approach. Illustrated is the introduction of a sterile freezer bag for specimen extraction via the pull method. A toothed grasper is passed across the abdomen between two trocars and brought out through the 12 mm umbilical trocar site. This grasper is used to pull the extraction bag back into the abdomen.**

If the spleen cannot be bagged, it may be fragmented in the pelvis before extraction, provided that the abdomen is copiously washed and cleaned of any residual spleen fragments before closure to prevent splenosis. Most patients with large spleens have hematologic malignancies; thus, residual splenic activity is not as crucial an issue in these patients as it would be in others.

Troubleshooting Many surgeons advocate the use of pneumatic sleeves as an adjunct to laparoscopic splenectomy. Most such sleeves require at least a 7.5 cm incision for introduction. In our view, use of these sleeves tends to work against the ultimate goal of minimally invasive surgery, which is to produce good surgical outcomes with as little trauma as possible; however, it can be a very helpful aid while one is learning laparoscopic splenectomy as well as in certain special circumstances (e.g., laparoscopic splenectomy for large spleens).

The incision for the pneumatic sleeve may be placed either transversely in the right upper quadrant or vertically in the upper midline. Alternatively, a Pfannenstiel incision may be employed: it has

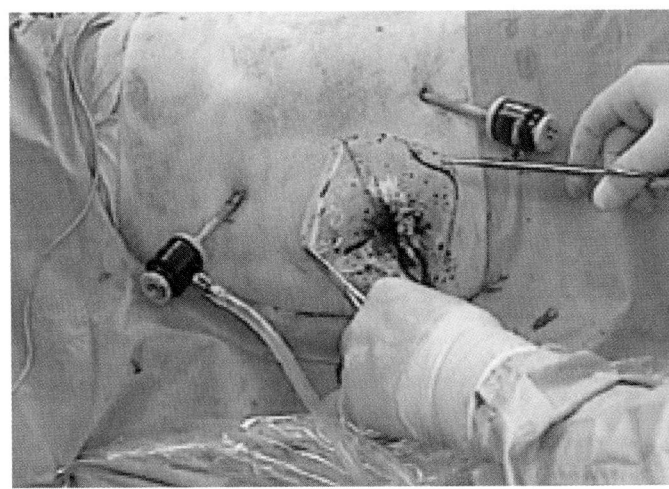

Figure 13 **Laparoscopic splenectomy: lateral approach. Shown is the position of the specimen bag position before finger fragmentation or pulp suction.**

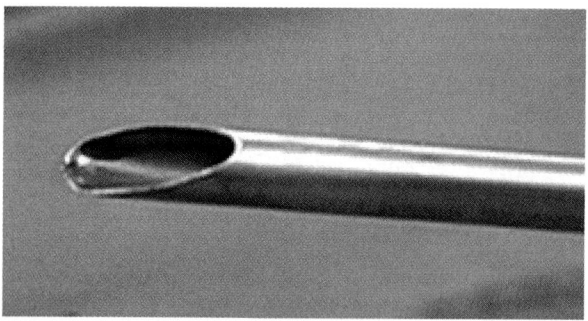

Figure 14 **Laparoscopic splenectomy: lateral approach. A beveled 10 mm suction cannula is used for subcapsular volume reduction in patients with megaspleens. This custom-made suction cannula can also be used to aspirate splenic pulp from the plastic retrieval bag during laparoscopic splenectomy in patients with normal-size or moderately enlarged spleens.**

cosmetic advantages over upper abdominal incisions and may result in fewer pulmonary complications. Use of the pneumatic sleeve may facilitate hilar dissection by improving retraction (especially in the upper pole) and by guiding placement of linear staples or clips. It may also facilitate retraction of enlarged spleens to improve access to all of the suspensory ligaments.

LAPAROSCOPIC PARTIAL SPLENECTOMY

Concern regarding the risk of OPSS has encouraged the practice of preserving splenic tissue and function whenever possible. For this reason, partial splenectomy has occasionally been indicated for treatment of benign tumors of the spleen and for excision of cystic lesions.[21] Its use has been described in connection with the management of type I Gaucher disease, cholesteryl ester storage disease, chronic myelogenous leukemia, and thalassemia major as well as the staging of Hodgkin disease.[22,23] Partial splenectomy has also been an option in the management of splenic trauma when the pa-

tient's condition is stable enough to permit the meticulous dissection required for the operation.[24,25]

Operative Technique

Like standard laparoscopic splenectomy, laparoscopic partial splenectomy is performed with the patient in the right lateral decubitus position. Trocar placement is similar as well. The splenocolic ligament and the lower part of the phrenicocolic ligament are incised to permit mobilization of the lower pole of the spleen. If the lower portion of the spleen is to be excised, branches of the gastroepiploic vessels supplying the lower pole are dissected and clipped close to the parenchyma. An appropriate number of penultimate branches of the inferior polar artery are then taken in such a way as to create a clear line of demarcation between normal spleen and devascularized spleen. This process is continued until the desired number of splenic segments are devascularized. Next, a standard monopolar electrocautery is used to score the splenic capsule circumferentially, with care taken to ensure that a 5 mm rim of devascularized splenic tissue remains in situ; this is the most important technical point for this procedure [see *Figure 16*]. The incision is then carried into the splenic pulp. Atraumatic intestinal graspers are also used to fracture the splenic pulp in a bloodless fashion. The laparoscopic L hook and scissors provide excellent hemostatic control.

Once the spleen has been allowed to demarcate, resection is remarkably bloodless, provided that the 5 mm rim of ischemic tissue is left in place. Complete control of the splenic artery is not required before splenic separation, because division occurs in an ischemic segment of spleen.[9] The feasibility of leaving portions of ischemic spleen in situ has been demonstrated in a large prospective, randomized trial involving partial splenic embolization as primary treatment of hematologic disorders.[26]

If the superior pole is to be removed, the phrenicocolic ligament must be incised almost entirely so that the spleen can be easily mobilized and the proper exposure achieved. The short gastric branch-

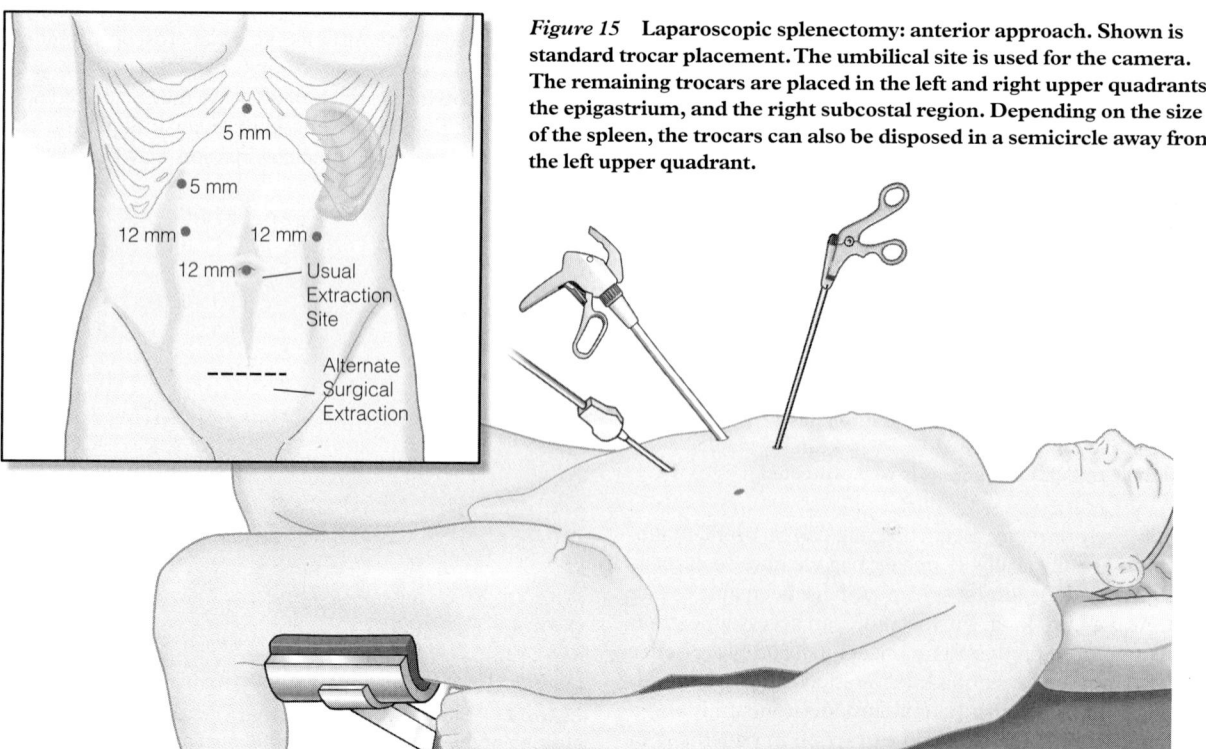

Figure 15 **Laparoscopic splenectomy: anterior approach. Shown is standard trocar placement. The umbilical site is used for the camera. The remaining trocars are placed in the left and right upper quadrants, the epigastrium, and the right subcostal region. Depending on the size of the spleen, the trocars can also be disposed in a semicircle away from the left upper quadrant.**

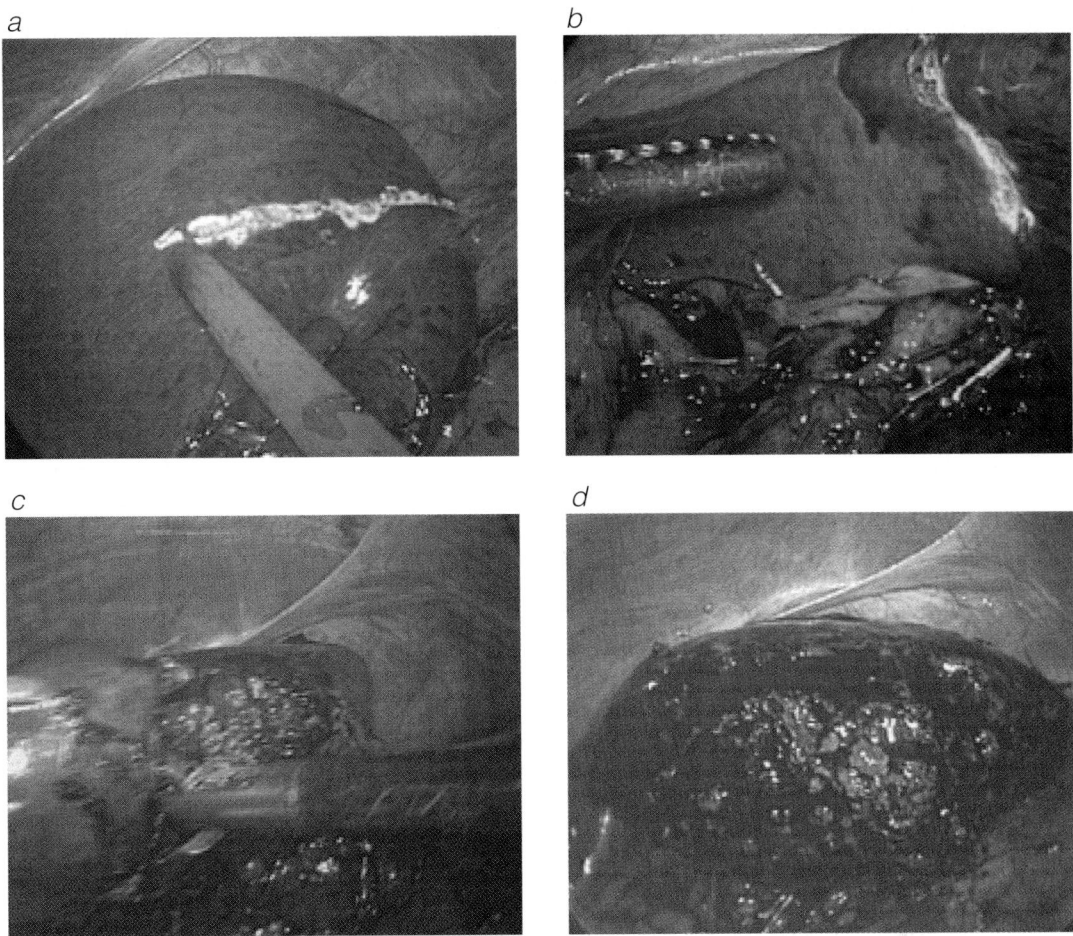

Figure 16 **Laparoscopic splenectomy: partial splenectomy. (*a, b*) The splenic capsule is scored with the monopolar cautery, and a 5 mm margin of devitalized tissue is left. (*c*) The splenic pulp is fractured with an atraumatic grasper. The electrocautery with the L hook is also used to control parenchymal bleeding. (*d*) Shown is the cut surface of the spleen after transection. The operative field remains remarkably dry.**

es are taken first, along with the desired number of superior polar artery branches.

Laparoscopic partial splenectomy can be performed either with or without the aid of selective preoperative arterial embolization. Radiologists are capable of cannulating the desired segmental splenic arterial branch and embolizing the segment that is to be resected. We have removed the superior pole in a patient with a class IV isolated splenic injury sustained while skiing[8]; partial laparoscopic splenectomy was made possible largely by the accuracy of selective arterial embolization, which permitted control of the bleeding and allowed laparoscopy to be performed in unhurried conditions.[27]

PREOPERATIVE SPLENIC ARTERY EMBOLIZATION

Preoperative splenic artery embolization is used as an adjuvant in a few patients to make laparoscopic splenectomy possible and to reduce blood loss. Although it is now infrequently used, it remains a useful tool in the armamentarium of spleen surgeons.

Preoperative splenic artery embolization is usually performed on the morning of operation to reduce the duration of the pain caused by the procedure. Approximately 45% of patients undergoing embolization experience some degree of pain, which is easily controlled by administering narcotics or instituting patient-controlled analgesia. In some patients, thrombosis extends to the venous side of the splenic blood supply when embolization is done on the day before operation. Whether this occurrence translates into any measurable advantage remains to be determined.

Generally speaking, the technique involves embolization of the spleen with coils placed proximally in the splenic artery and absorbable gelatin sponges and small coils placed distally in each splenic arterial branch (the double embolization technique), with care taken to spare vessels supplying the tail of the pancreas [*see Figure 17*]. More specifically, splenic artery embolization is performed through a 5 French catheter (typically a cobra catheter, though sidewinder and various other types are also used) inserted into the right groin with the patient under local anesthesia. The catheter tip is placed in the splenic artery and advanced to the splenic hilum proximal to the left gastroepiploic artery (or the great pancreatic artery) so that distal pancreatic branches of the splenic artery can be observed. At this level, either iohexol 65% or iothalamate 60% is forcefully injected and a digital substraction angiogram done to verify the pattern of the splenic blood supply.

If no pancreatic branches are opacified, there are several techniques that may be used. In particular, 3 to 5 mm microcoils are placed in the hilar branches of the splenic artery; alternatively, absorbable gelatin sponges are used. The catheter is then pulled back 2 to 4 cm, and one or two 5 to 8 mm microcoils are launched into the main trunk of the splenic artery distal to the great pancreatic artery to prevent pancreatitis or pancreatic necrosis. The surgical plane of dissection is therefore situated between the proximal and distal embolization sites.

The procedure is ended when it is estimated radiologically that 80% or more of the splenic tissue has been successfully embolized.

In most cases, successful embolization is achieved with both proximal and distal emboli; in a minority of cases, it is achieved with proximal emboli alone or with distal emboli alone.[28]

Troubleshooting Preoperative splenic artery embolization is safe, provided that two main principles are adhered to. First, embolization must be done distal to the great pancreatic artery to minimize pancreatic damage. Second, neither microspheres nor absorbable gelatin powder should be used, because particles of this small size may migrate to unintended target organ capillaries and cause tissue necrosis; only coils and absorbable gelatin sponge fragments should be used. If these precautions are taken, embolization is safe and remains a useful tool for difficult cases.

Postoperative Care

Postoperative care for patients who have undergone laparoscopic splenectomy is usually simple. The nasogastric tube inserted after induction of general anesthesia is removed either in the recovery room, once stomach emptying has been verified, or the next morning, depending on the duration and the degree of technical difficulty of the procedure. The urinary catheter is usually removed before the patient leaves the recovery room. The patient is allowed to drink clear fluids on the morning after the operation; when clear fluids are well tolerated, the patient is allowed to proceed to a diet of his or her choice.

If the patient has no history of ulcer or dyspepsia, a 100 mg indomethacin suppository is inserted before induction of anesthesia and again every 12 hours for a total of three to five doses. Postoperative pain medication is given on an individualized basis with a view to ensuring complete patient comfort. Meperidine injections (1 mg/kg) are administered during the first night, followed by oral acetaminophen (1 g every 6 hours). If pain is not well controlled, coanalgesia with an NSAID is added; this combination produces the best results. Because of its side effects (i.e., nausea, vomiting, abdominal fullness, and constipation), codeine is currently avoided if at all possible. When indomethacin is used, prophylactic doses of subcutaneous heparin are avoided on empirical grounds, especially if the platelet count is low or platelet function is abnormal.

Patients receiving I.V. cortisone are given oral steroids on postoperative day 1 after an overlap I.V. injection; thereafter, steroids are gradually tapered. Patients are allowed to shower 48 hours after surgery and are advised to keep the paper strips covering the trocar incisions in place for 7 to 10 days. No drains are used. No limitations are imposed on physical activity, and patients are allowed to tailor their activities to their degree of asthenia or discomfort.

Complications

Postoperative complications directly related to splenectomy include intraoperative and postoperative hemorrhage; left lower lobe atelectasis and pneumonia; left pleural effusion; subphrenic collection; iatrogenic pancreatic, gastric, and colonic injury; and venous thrombosis.[24-31]

Successful laparoscopic splenectomy depends to a large extent on proper preparation. Recognition of anatomic elements and their arrangement is paramount. As with other laparoscopic procedures, the keys are avoiding complications and minimizing technical misadventures. Vascular structures should be cleanly isolated and dissected from surrounding fat; they then can usually be controlled with two clips proximally and distally. Staplers should be used with care and should not be applied blindly. The stapler tip should be clearly seen to be free of tissue before it is closed; otherwise, hemorrhage from partial section of a major splenic branch might occur after the instrument is released. Blind application of the stapler may also result in damage to the tail of the pancreas, which often lies in close proximity to the inner surface of the spleen. If both clips and a linear stapler are used, it is vital to prevent interposition of clips in the staple line, which will cause the stapler to misfire and possibly to jam.

Improper use of the electrocautery during the procedure can cause iatrogenic injury to the stomach, the colon, or the pancreas. In a smoke-filled environment, where controlling vessels is difficult and time consuming, blind fulguration of fat in the hilum can lead to bleeding. Structures close to the lower pole in the gastrocolic ligament can be approached more aggressively, but not those in the hilum. To prevent arcing and spot necrosis, which may result in delayed perforation and sepsis, the instrument should be activated only in proximity to the target organ.

The assistants also play an important role in preventing complications. All instruments, including those handled by assistants, should be moved under direct vision. Especially in the anterior approach, retraction of the liver and stomach and elevation of the spleen require constant concentration if lacerations and subsequent hemorrhage or perforation are to be avoided.

Special Considerations

EXTRACTION OF SPECIMENS

Spleens removed via the anterior approach are extracted through the umbilical trocar site after finger fragmentation in a plastic bag. It is rarely necessary to enlarge the umbilical incision to more than 2 or 3 cm. When the lateral approach is used, extraction is more easily performed through one of the ports situated anteriorly. This extraction site also requires little or no enlargement. On occasion, for a spleen longer than 20 cm, a 7.5 to 10 cm Pfannenstiel incision is made, and the operator's forearm is introduced into the abdomen to deliver the spleen into the pelvis for extraction in large fragments under direct vision. Pneumatic sleeves may also be used to facilitate hand-assisted surgery. The abdomen is copiously irrigated before closure.

Special mention should be made of laparoscopic splenectomy in patients with malignant disease. If lymphoma or Hodgkin disease is suspected, neither preoperative splenic artery embolization nor finger fragmentation in a plastic bag should be performed, for fear of

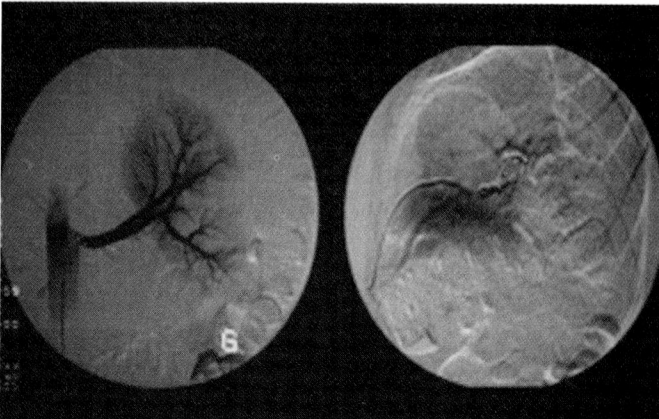

Figure 17 **Laparoscopic splenectomy: splenic artery embolization. Shown are splenic angiograms of a patient with thrombotic thrombocytopenic purpura before (left) and after (right) splenic artery embolization with 3 cm, 5 cm, and 7 cm coils and absorbable gelatin sponge fragments.**

making the histologic diagnosis difficult. Extraction of intact spleens through a small left subcostal or median incision has also been employed when preservation of tissue architecture is required. The various techniques of fragmentation and extraction of splenic tissue during laparoscopic splenectomy should be discussed and agreed on with the pathologist ahead of time to ensure that proper pathologic diagnoses are not compromised by either necrotic tissue (in the case of preoperative splenic artery embolization) or altered tissue architecture (in the case of finger fragmentation), especially if malignancy is suspected but not proven. In practice, however, we have found that the diagnosis is made preoperatively in more than 90% of patients with benign and malignant hematologic disease; hence, the issue rarely arises.

MASSIVE SPLENOMEGALY AND MEGASPLEENS

Massive splenomegaly is defined as the presence of a spleen with an interpole length exceeding 20 cm on ultrasonography or a weight exceeding 1,000 g. Laparoscopic removal of spleens of this size is fraught with problems, mostly related to the size of the organ and its components. Large spleens, besides being heavy and hard to manipulate, carry a high risk of serious hemorrhage. Consequently, preoperative splenic artery embolization is sometimes done beforehand because it helps control arterial flow preoperatively. If embolization is performed long enough before operation, it may even be possible to control the venous side of the blood supply through retrograde thrombosis; that blood clots are occasionally expelled from sections of splenic veins during laparoscopic splenectomy attests to the occurrence of this phenomenon. Finding a sensible way to retrieve the specimen also presents an important challenge.

When a spleen longer than 20 cm is to be removed, some modifications must be made to the technique of laparoscopic splenectomy. Once sectioning of the vessels and the suspensory ligaments is complete, a 7.5 to 10 cm Pfannenstiel incision is made at the pubic hairline. Through this incision, hand revision of the operative site under laparoscopic control can be accomplished, and if necessary, any remaining vessels or ligamentous attachments can be sectioned under video control. Adequate pneumoperitoneum can be maintained with the forearm placed through the lower abdominal incision. Whenever possible, the spleen is placed in a plastic bag; however, to date, we have not been able to bag a spleen longer than 24 cm.

That extraction of a very large specimen requires fragmentation of the spleen in the pelvis and extraction through a Pfannenstiel incision raises the possibility of postoperative splenosis. To minimize this problem, after reconstitution of the pneumoperitoneum, the abdomen is copiously irrigated and reviewed for fragments of spleen and accessory spleens, which can be done very thoroughly with laparoscopy.[32]

For a long time, we had no success with laparoscopic splenectomy for spleens longer than 30 cm (i.e., megaspleens): our conversion rate was 100%. Currently, we use preoperative embolization for these spleens. We also take the anterior approach, using five trocars, and are experimenting with a technique for subcapsular volume reduction with a sharp beveled 10 mm suction cannula connected to a powerful –70 mm Hg aspirator. Megaspleens are next to impossible to move with laparoscopic instruments, and the space constraints make our usual laparoscopic approaches futile. We therefore insert the –70 mm Hg aspirating cannula into the spleen and proceed to reduce the splenic volume so that the spleen can be sectioned into more manageable pieces that can be bagged and extracted in the usual fashion. At present, it is too early to tell whether laparoscopic splenectomy will have a place in the management of megaspleens.

Outcome Evaluation

No randomized, prospective trials comparing open splenectomy with laparoscopic splenectomy have yet been conducted. At present, such trials are unlikely to be held, for a variety of reasons. For one thing, randomization is difficult with procedures that are still in evolution. At one end of the spectrum, laparoscopic splenectomy is done for patients with ITP, who usually are relatively healthy and have normal-size spleens. In many of these patients, needlescopic instruments (< 3 mm) can be used in conjunction with a single 12 mm port site in the umbilicus. This approach permits hospital discharge within 24 hours of operation in a significant number of cases. At the other end of the spectrum, laparoscopic splenectomy is done for patients with myeloid metaplasia and spleens longer than 30 cm. In this setting, a laparoscopic approach poses formidable challenges, and the optimal technique and its justification remain to be determined. The window of opportunity for randomized comparative trials may have been lost.

Large case series and nonrandomized comparative trials, however, have consistently reported better outcomes from laparoscopic splenectomy than from open splenectomy.[33-40] For example, in one set of 528 patients [see Table 2],[35-38] the rate of postoperative pneumonia was 1.1% (6/528), and no subphrenic abscesses occurred as postoperative complications. Many surgeons who have completed the learning curve associated with the procedure feel that there is still room for improvement regarding complication rates and length of stay for pa-

---

Table 2   Clinical Results of Laparoscopic Splenectomy

Authors	N	ITP/Non-ITP	Conversion Rate (%)	OR Time (min)	Morbidity (%)	Mortality (%)	Length of Stay (days)	Accessory Spleen Present (%)
All diagnoses								
Katkhouda et al (1998)[37]	103	67/36	3.9	161	6	0	2.5	16.5
Targarona et al (2000)[35]	122	54/68	7.4	153	18	0	4.0	12
Park et al (2000)[36]	203	129/74	3.0	145	9	0.5	2.7	12.3
Poulin et al (2001)[38]	100	50/50	8.0	180	15	4	3.0	25
ITP								
Trias et al (2000)[39]	48	—	4.2	142	12	N/A	4.0	11
Poulin et al (2001)[38]	51	—	3.9	160	5.9	0	2.0	32
Malignancy								
Schlachta et al (1999)[40]	14	—	21	239	18	9	3.0	—
Trias et al (2000)[39]	28	—	14*	171	28	N/A	5.5	—

*71% required accessory incision because of spleen size.

tients with ITP and other relatively benign conditions necessitating laparoscopic splenectomy. The more serious conditions and the mortality seen in conjunction with the procedure tend to occur in patients with advanced hematologic malignancies or mega-spleens. In such cases, most of the adverse results are related to the disease state rather than to the operation, and it remains to be seen whether laparoscopic splenectomy will have a positive effect on outcome.

One of the great attractions of minimally invasive surgery has been the prospect of significant cost reductions. At this early point in the development of laparoscopic splenectomy, however, we are reluctant to place too much trust in premature cost analyses that do not take into account the "work in progress" nature of minimally invasive surgery. Most surgeons can now perform most cases of laparoscopic splenectomy with simplified trays of reusable instruments. Our basic laparoscopic tray contains a few instruments and two sizes of reusable clip appliers with inexpensive clips. As noted [see Operative Technique, above], clips are used for distributed-type spleens, single-use linear staplers mostly for magistral-type spleens. To reduce costs, ultrasonic dissectors are rarely used. In addition, the use of commercially available freezer bags instead of laparoscopic retrieval bags further reduces the cost of specimen extraction. Finally, even if intraoperative costs are higher with laparoscopic splenectomy, our experience is that the increase is offset by reductions in postoperative stay.

We, like most authorities, believe that as a surgeon gains experience with laparoscopic splenectomy, operating time tends to fall until it approaches that of open splenectomy. We also concur with many authors who have suggested that once laparoscopic splenectomy is mastered, use of blood products tends to decrease substantially.

References

1. Cole F: Is splenectomy harmless? Surg Gynecol Obstet 133:98, 1971
2. Johnston GB: Splenectomy. Ann Surg 48:50, 1908
3. Campos Cristo M: Segmental resections of the spleen: report on the first eight cases operated on. O Hosp (Rio) 62:205, 1962
4. Upadhyaya P, Simpson JS: Splenic trauma in children. Surg Gynecol Obstet 126:781, 1968
5. Delaitre B, Maignien B: Splénectomie par voie laparoscopique, 1 observation. Presse Médicale 20:2263, 1991
6. Carroll BJ, Phillips EH, Semel CJ, et al: Laparoscopic splenectomy. Surg Endosc 6:183, 1992
7. Thibault C, Mamazza J, Létourneau R, et al: Laparoscopic splenectomy: operative technique and preliminary report. Surg Laparosc Endosc 2:248, 1992
8. Poulin EC, Thibault C, DesCôteaux JG, et al: Partial laparoscopic splenectomy for trauma: technique and case report. Surg Laparosc Endosc 5:306, 1995
9. Seshadri PA, Poulin EC, Mamazza J, et al: Technique for laparoscopic partial splenectomy. Surg Laparosc Endosc 10:106, 2000
10. Goerg C, Schwerk WB, Goerg K, et al: Sonographic patterns of the affected spleen in malignant lymphoma. J Clin Ultrasound 18:569, 1990
11. Poulin EC, Thibault C: The anatomical basis for laparoscopic splenectomy. Can J Surg 36:485, 1993
12. Michels NA: The variational anatomy of the spleen and splenic artery. Am J Anat 70:21, 1942
13. Testut L: Traité d'anatomie humaine, 7th ed. Librairie Octave Doin, Paris, 1923, p 942
14. Lipshutz B: A composite study of the coeliac axis artery. Ann Surg 65:159, 1917
15. Henschen C: Die chirurgische Anatomie der Milzgefässe. Schweiz Med Wochenschr 58:164, 1928
16. Ssoson-Jaroschewitsch A: Zür chirurgischen Anatomie des Milzhilus. Zeitsch f. d. ges. Anat I Abt 84:218, 1937
17. Baronofsky ID, Walton W, Noble JF: Occult injury to the pancreas following splenectomy. Surgery 29:852, 1951
18. Gagner M, Lacroix A, Bolte E, et al: Laparoscopic adrenalectomy: the importance of a flank approach in the lateral decubitus position. Surg Endosc 8:135, 1994
19. Gigot JF, Jamar F, Ferrant A, et al: Inadequate detection of accessory spleens and splenosis with laparoscopic approach in hematologic diseases. Surg Endosc 12:101, 1998
20. Nielsen JL, Ellegard J, Marqversen J, et al: Detection of splenosis and ectopic spleens with 99mTc-labeled heat damaged autologous erythrocytes in 90 splenectomized patients. Scand J Haematol 27:51, 1981
21. Pachter HL, Hofstetter SR, Elkowitz A, et al: Traumatic cysts of the spleen: the role of cystectomy and splenic preservation: experience with seven consecutive patients. J Trauma 35:430, 1993
22. Guzetta PC, Ruley EJ, Merrick HFW, et al: Elective subtotal splenectomy: indications and results in 33 patients. Ann Surg 211:34, 1990
23. Hoeckstra HJ, Tamminga RY, Timens W: Partial instead of complete splenectomy in children for the pathological staging of Hodgkin's disease. Ned Tijdschr Geneeskd 137:2491, 1993
24. Sheldon GF, Croom RD, Meyer AA: The spleen. Textbook of Surgery, 14th ed. Sabiston DC, Ed. WB Saunders Co, Philadelphia, 1991, p 1108
25. Jalovec LM, Boe BS, Wyffels PL: The advantages of early operation with splenorrhaphy versus nonoperative management for the blunt splenic trauma patient. Am Surg 59:698, 1993
26. Mozes MF, Spigos DG, Pollak R, et al: Partial splenic embolization, an alternative to splenectomy: results of a prospective randomized study. Surgery 96:694, 1984
27. Poulin E, Thibault C, Mamazza J, et al: Laparoscopic splenectomy: clinical experience and the role of preoperative splenic artery embolization. Surg Laparosc Endosc 3:445, 1993
28. Poulin EC, Mamazza J, Schlachta CM: Splenic artery embolization before laparoscopic splenectomy: an update. Surg Endosc 12:870, 1998
29. Hoeffer RA, Scullin DC, Silver LF, et al: Splenectomy for hematologic disorders: a 20 year experience. J Ky Med Assoc 89:446, 1991
30. Ly B, Albrechtson D: Therapeutic splenectomy in hematologic disorders. Effects and complications in 221 adult patients Acta Med Scand 209:21, 1981
31. Macrae HM, Yakimets WW, Reynolds T: Perioperative complications of splenectomy for hematologic disease. Can J Surg 35:432, 1992
32. Poulin EC, Thibault C: Laparoscopic splenectomy for massive splenomegaly: operative technique and case report. Can J Surg 38:69, 1995
33. Poulin EC, Mamazza J: Laparoscopic splenectomy: lessons from the learning curve. Can J Surg 41:28, 1998
34. Cathode N, Hurwitz MB, Rivera RT, et al: Laparoscopic splenectomy: outcome and efficacy in 103 consecutive patients. Ann Surg 228:568, 1998
35. Targarona EM, Espert JJ, Bombuy E, et al: Complications of laparoscopic splenectomy. Arch Surg 135:1137, 2000
36. Park AE, Birgisson G, Mastrangelo MJ, et al: Laparoscopic splenectomy: outcomes and lessons learned from over 200 cases. Surgery 128:660, 2000
37. Katkhouda N, Hurwitz MB, Rivera RT, et al: Laparoscopic splenectomy: outcome and efficacy in 103 consecutive patients. Ann Surg 228:568, 1998
38. Poulin EC, Schlachta CM, Mamazza J: Unpublished data, February 2001
39. Trias M, Targarona EM, Espert JJ, et al: Impact of hematological diagnosis on early and late outcome after laparoscopic splenectomy: an analysis of 111 cases. Surg Endosc 14:556, 2000
40. Schlachta CM, Poulin EC, Mamazza J: Laparoscopic splenectomy for hematologic malignancies. Surg Endosc 13:865, 1999

Acknowledgment

Figures 1, 3, 4, 6a, and 15   Tom Moore.

20 LAPAROSCOPIC ADRENALECTOMY

Theresa M. Quinn, M.D., F.A.C.S., Francesco Rubino, M.D., and Michel Gagner, M.D., F.A.C.S.

Since the introduction of laparoscopic adrenalectomy in 1992, the minimally invasive approach to the adrenal gland has become the preferred option in a number of settings.[1-18] In particular, the small size of the glands, the superior retroperitoneal location, the benign nature of most adrenal tumors, and the lower morbidity associated with smaller incisions have made laparoscopy a valuable tool in endocrine surgery. Several published series[9,16,19,20] have documented the advantages of laparoscopic adrenalectomy over open adrenalectomy, including decreased operative blood loss, reduced narcotic requirements, and shorter hospital stay and recovery time.

Like its open counterpart, laparoscopic adrenalectomy may be performed via an anterior, a lateral, or a posterior approach. Successful laparoscopic adrenalectomy requires advanced laparoscopic skills, a solid understanding of adrenal anatomy, meticulous hemostasis, and delicate tissue handling. A thorough preoperative evaluation that includes clinical examination, biochemical assessment, diagnostic imaging (computed tomography or magnetic resonance imaging) for localization of the adrenal pathology, and, if necessary, venous sampling or fine-needle aspiration (FNA) cytology is essential.

Indications

Laparoscopic adrenalectomy is now the gold standard for adrenalectomy for selected patients with a variety of conditions [see Table 1], including both functional masses and nonfunctioning tumors. There are also several established contraindications [see Table 1], the most prominent of which is a surgeon's lack of experience with the technique. In addition, patients who are believed to have adrenal carcinoma on the basis of radiographic evaluation or who have a lesion greater than 10 cm in diameter should undergo open adrenalectomy to ensure complete excision of the lesion along with en bloc resection of surrounding organs as necessary. Coagulopathy and portal hypertension, conditions that place the patient at undue risk for perioperative bleeding and limit the exactitude of the laparoscopic procedure, are also contraindications to a minimally invasive approach.

Anatomic Considerations

The two adrenal glands are located in the lateral retroperitoneal area, in front of the 12th rib on the right and in front of the 11th and 12th ribs on the left, and are surrounded by perirenal fascia. They weigh approximately 6 g each, measure $5.0 \times 3.0 \times 0.6$ cm, and are placed like caps on the superomedial poles of the two kidneys. The right adrenal and the left adrenal have very similar relationships to the adjoining anatomy dorsally and laterally but substantially different relationships ventrally and medially. There are also significant right-left differences in adrenal blood supply that have important implications for surgical technique.

DORSAL AND LATERAL RELATIONSHIPS

Because the two adrenal glands have virtually identical dorsal and lateral anatomic relationships, there are no significant differences between posterior and lateral approaches to the right adrenal and posterior and lateral approaches to the left adrenal. Through the pararenal fat and the perirenal fascia, the posterolateral aspect of each adrenal is in contact with the superior part of the posterior abdominal wall. Each gland lies in close proximity to the diaphragmatic crus and to the lateral arcuate ligament. The crus and the arcuate ligament separate the adrenals from the reflection of the pleura, from the 11th and 12th ribs, and from the subcostal, sacrospinalis, and latissimus dorsi muscles.

VENTRAL RELATIONSHIPS

Right Adrenal

The main ventrolateral anatomic relationship of the right adrenal is with the peritoneum between the liver and the kidney. Exposure of the gland is achieved by opening the peritoneum after the right lobe of the liver is mobilized cephalad and medially. The main ventromedial anatomic relationship of the right adrenal is with the inferior vena cava. The right adrenal vein emerges from this aspect of the gland before emptying directly into the inferior vena cava.

Left Adrenal

The main ventrolateral relationships of the left adrenal are with the attachments of the kidney and, occasionally, the splenic flexure of the colon. Mobilization of the splenic flexure and incision of the peritoneal layer overlying Gerota's fascia expose the lateral aspect of the left adrenal. The main ventro-

Table 1 Indications for and Contraindications to Laparoscopic Adrenalectomy

Indications	Functional masses
	Cortisol-secreting adenoma (Cushing syndrome)
	Aldosterone-secreting adenoma (Conn syndrome)
	Adrenocortical hyperplasia (Cushing disease) or other hypercortisolism syndrome
	Pheochromocytoma
	Virilizing/feminizing syndromes
	Nonfunctional tumors
	Incidentaloma (> 3 cm or growing)
	Isolated adrenal metastases
	Symptomatic angiomyolipoma
	Symptomatic adrenal cyst
Contraindications	Surgeon inexperience
	Adrenal carcinoma
	Adrenal mass > 10 cm
	Coagulopathy (uncorrected)
	Portal hypertension

medial relationships of the left adrenal are with the spleen, the pancreas, and the gastric fundus. The splenorenal ligament is divided along the lateral aspect of the spleen to allow medial displacement of the spleen, the tail of the pancreas, and the gastric fundus. The splenic vein can be seen coursing along the posterior margin of the pancreas and the splenic artery along the superior border.

The body of the pancreas separates the adrenal gland from the lesser sac and from the stomach. A second approach to the left adrenal is direct access through the lesser sac after division of the gastrocolic ligament. The adrenal gland can be exposed by means of a peritoneal incision along the inferior or superior border of the pancreatic body. A third approach entails dissection of the transverse mesocolon to provide direct access to the posterior side of the pancreas and the adrenal gland.

BLOOD SUPPLY, LYMPHATIC DRAINAGE, AND INNERVATION

The adrenal glands receive their arterial blood from three sources: a superior adrenal artery arising from the inferior phrenic artery, a middle adrenal artery arising from the abdominal aorta, and an inferior adrenal artery arising from the renal artery.

The arrangement of the adrenal veins is much simpler than that of the adrenal arteries. There is one dominant vein and several smaller accessory veins that follow the arteries. During adrenalectomy for the treatment of a tumor producing excessive amounts of a hormone (especially a pheochromocytoma), the flow of the main adrenal vein is controlled at the beginning of the adrenal dissection.

On the left side, vascular control of the adrenal vein is relatively straightforward because the vein is long (about 30 mm) and empties into either the left inferior phrenic vein or the left renal vein; however, exposure of the left adrenal vein requires more time and more extensive dissection than exposure of the right. Once the inferior pole of the left adrenal has been identified, dissection for 1 to 2 cm along the medial margin of the gland reveals the left adrenal vein. On the right side, vascular control of the adrenal vein is more precarious because the right adrenal vein is much shorter than the left (about 6 mm) and empties directly into the posterior part of the inferior vena cava, an anatomic arrangement that increases the risk of major venous injury. On both sides, numerous accessory adrenal veins follow the arteries and empty into the inferior phrenic vein, the renal vein, or anastomotic branches joining with the azygos system and the posterior gastric veins. These collateral vessels may become significantly enlarged in patients with large adrenal tumors.

Nerves and vessels are ligated simultaneously during adrenalectomy. The nerves are numerous and arise from the sympathetic nervous system. The visceral afferent fibers arise from the celiac ganglia, which is derived from the posterior vagus nerve and the greater and lesser splanchnic nerves. The visceral fibers traverse the cortex to effect direct secretory or indirect vasomotor innervation and finish in the medulla as sympathetic preganglionic fibers.

Preoperative Evaluation

CLINICAL EXAMINATION

The clinical examination should be performed with particular attention to signs and symptoms of aldosterone, catecholamine, or cortisol excess. Nearly all patients with hyperaldosteronism and 60% of patients with pheochromocytoma

have a history of hypertension.[21] About 90% of patients with pheochromocytoma experience nonspecific symptoms, such as headache, diaphoresis, palpitations, abdominal pain, nervousness, nausea, vomiting, chest pain, and weakness. A history of type 2A or 2B multiple endocrine neoplasia can be helpful in diagnosing pheochromocytoma, given that this endocrine tumor ultimately develops in 40% of pheochromocytoma patients. Glucocorticoid-producing adenomas are extremely rare in the absence of the characteristic signs of hypercortisolism (i.e., easy bruising, striae, and myopathy). A functioning adrenocortical carcinoma may be signaled by the abrupt onset of Cushing syndrome or a virilization syndrome, pyrexia, and abdominal pain. Most adrenocortical carcinomas are large (mean diameter, 12.4 cm) and are symptomatic on presentation; only 10% are small and present asymptomatically as incidentalomas.[22]

BIOCHEMICAL ASSESSMENT

Between 0.3% and 5.0% of all abdominal CT scans performed for other reasons reveal incidental adrenal lesions.[23] Determination of hormone levels is important in all such cases because excision of all functioning lesions is recommended. Biochemical evaluation should include measurement of serum potassium concentrations and 24-hour urine collection for determination of metanephrine, vanillylmandelic acid (VMA), 17-hydroxycorticosteroid, and free cortisol levels. A patient with a nonfunctioning adrenal tumor should undergo repeat CT scanning within 6 months so that the evolution of the lesion can be monitored; if the tumor is larger than 4 cm or is found to be growing at the follow-up evaluation, it should be resected.

Hypokalemia in a hypertensive patient suggests primary hyperaldosteronism; an elevated plasma aldosterone level is seen in conjunction with decreased plasma renin activity. Cushing syndrome is caused by excess glucocorticoid secretion; if a glucocorticoid-producing adenoma, an adrenal carcinoma, or macronodular adrenal hyperplasia is noted, resection is indicated. A patient who has a pituitary adenoma or exhibits ectopic production of adrenocorticotropic hormone (ACTH) should undergo bilateral adrenalectomy if pituitary surgery or primary tumor resection fails to control cortisol hypersecretion. Patients with Cushing disease or Cushing syndrome typically have elevated levels of free cortisol and 17-hydroxycorticosteroids. A normal or slightly elevated ACTH level suggests pituitary disease, whereas a markedly elevated level suggests an ectopic source of ACTH. A depressed ACTH level suggests adrenal production of glucocorticosteroids. CT scanning can sometimes differentiate adrenal tumors from macronodular adrenal hyperplasia. Adrenocortical carcinoma is a rare condition but should nonetheless be suspected in patients with large (> 6 cm) adrenal masses, elevated 17-ketosteroid levels, or evidence of local invasion or distant metastasis.

Patients with pheochromocytoma may be normotensive or may have episodic or chronic hypertension. Urinary measurements of metanephrine, VMA, and plasma catecholamine levels allow biochemical confirmation of the diagnosis. CT or MRI is used to localize the tumor. Scintigraphy with 131-metaiodobenzylguanidine may exclude multiple or bilateral tumors or metastasis.[24]

In patients with virilizing syndromes, 24-hour urine collection for 17-ketosteroid, plasma testosterone, and dehydroepiandrosterone levels must be done to confirm the presence of an androgen-producing adrenal tumor.

DIAGNOSTIC IMAGING

Patients with adrenalomas first diagnosed by means of ultrasonography or CT scanning should undergo further evaluation with either helical CT scanning or MRI. In most cases, a thin-cut (3 mm) helical CT scan is capable of localizing the adrenal tumor and determining its size and its relationships with contiguous structures. MRI has the additional advantage of providing T_2-weighted images, which can distinguish various adrenal lesions on the basis of differences in adrenaloma-to-liver signal ratios. For instance, on T_2-weighted images, pheochromocytomas are markedly brighter in relation to the liver than other tumors are.

ADRENAL VENOUS SAMPLING

In selected patients with suspected aldosterone-producing tumors, venous sampling can be used to differentiate an incidentaloma from a cortical adenoma that produces aldosterone.

FNA CYTOLOGY

At present, FNA cytology plays only a limited role in the assessment of adrenal lesions owing to its inability to distinguish an adenoma from a well-differentiated carcinoma. Moreover, a needle biopsy in a patient with a pheochromocytoma can lead to a fatal hypertensive crisis. Consequently, FNA cytology is generally not recommended in this setting.[25]

Operative Planning

PREPARATION FOR OPERATION

Routine bowel preparation and antibiotic prophylaxis are unnecessary. Intermittent pneumatic compression stockings or subcutaneous heparin should be used to prevent thromboembolism.

Preoperative administration of alpha and beta blockers is recommended for patients with pheochromocytoma, who may experience severe hypertension intraoperatively with mild tumor manipulation or hypotension after tumor removal as a consequence of inadequate volume resuscitation before operation.[21] Of the several options available, we prefer phenoxybenzamine, given for at least 1 week preoperatively. The selective alpha-antagonist prazosin is a reasonable alternative. Success has also been reported with the use of either I.V. phentolamine and esmolol[26] or calcium channel blockers starting the day before the procedure.[27] Beta blockers may be given to control intraoperative arrhythmias but should not be started until after alpha blockade has been achieved. In patients with aldosteronomas, potassium deficits should be corrected before operation. Preoperative administration of spironolactone can counteract the aldosterone-producing activity of the tumor.

PATIENT POSITIONING

After placement of intermittent compression stockings and insertion of a Foley catheter, the patient is placed in the lateral decubitus position on a bean bag with the side of the adrenal pathology facing up [see Figure 1a]. An axillary roll (two rolled towels or a 1 L I.V. bag covered with a towel) is used to protect the brachial plexus and a rolled blanket under the flank to facilitate the opposite flank exposure. The flank must be positioned over the table break [see Figure 1b], so that the table can be flexed at this joint to maximize the distance between the costal margin and the iliac crest. Hyperextension of the table is continued until the flank musculature begins to feel taut. The arms are extended over boards and secured, and pressure sites

are padded. The torso and the legs are secured with 2 in. cloth tape. The table is then tested to verify its capability for the reverse Trendelenburg position and for airplaning (i.e., lateral rotation), both of which will be used to facilitate exposure during the operation.

The surgeon and the assistant stand facing the patient's abdomen. To maximize the degree of freedom with which the instruments can be used, the patient's abdomen is moved close to the edge of the table. The area from the umbilicus to the vertebral column and from the nipple to the middle of the iliac crest is prepared and draped. Video monitors are placed on either side of the head of the table.

EQUIPMENT

For adequate vision of the operative field, a 30° laparoscope is recommended. A fan-type liver retractor is useful for liver retraction in a laparoscopic right adrenalectomy.

The surgeon's nondominant hand typically holds an atraumatic bowel grasper. The flat surface of this instrument is used to grasp and retract the tissue adjacent to the adrenal. The surgeon's dominant hand holds an electrocautery scissors, an electrocautery hook, or an ultrasonic scalpel. Because all of these devices can generate thermal energy, care must be taken not to rest their active areas against tissue that is not to be divided. A 5 mm curved ultrasonic endoscopic shears is particularly valuable for dissection around the adrenal. The adrenal vein can be dissected with a right-angle dissector and clipped with either medium or large titanium clips. Arteries can be either ligated with clips and divided with the endoscopic shears or divided directly with the ultrasonic scalpel.

Laparoscopic ultrasonography using a 5 to 7 MHz probe can be useful for localizing the left adrenal gland when large amounts of perirenal and retroperitoneal fat are present.[28] Intraoperative ultrasonography is particularly useful in patients with small tumors when the tumor is not directly visible, the adrenal appears normal, and a paraganglioma is present; it is also helpful in evaluating the venous anatomy and searching for evidence of invasion or metastasis.

A laparoscopic biopsy forceps should be available for biopsy of the adrenal. An impermeable nylon laparoscopic bag is necessary for gland retrieval to prevent seeding of the abdomen or the trocar sites with tumor cells.

Operative Technique

CHOICE OF APPROACH

Two approaches to laparoscopic adrenalectomy—transperitoneal and retroperitoneal—have been described in the literature. We advocate the transperitoneal approach because the anatomy is more familiar to most surgeons, enlarged glands are more easily approached, and the liver can be assessed for metastases. The retroperitoneal approach, much like the open posterior approach, involves creation of a retroperitoneal space. It has often been recommended for patients who have previously undergone abdominal surgery.[19,29,30] Our experience, however, suggests that this approach may not always be superior in this population: more than half of our transperitoneal laparoscopic adrenalectomies have been performed in patients with prior abdominal operations.

The transperitoneal approach may be either anterior or lateral. The anterior transperitoneal approach was the first to be

a

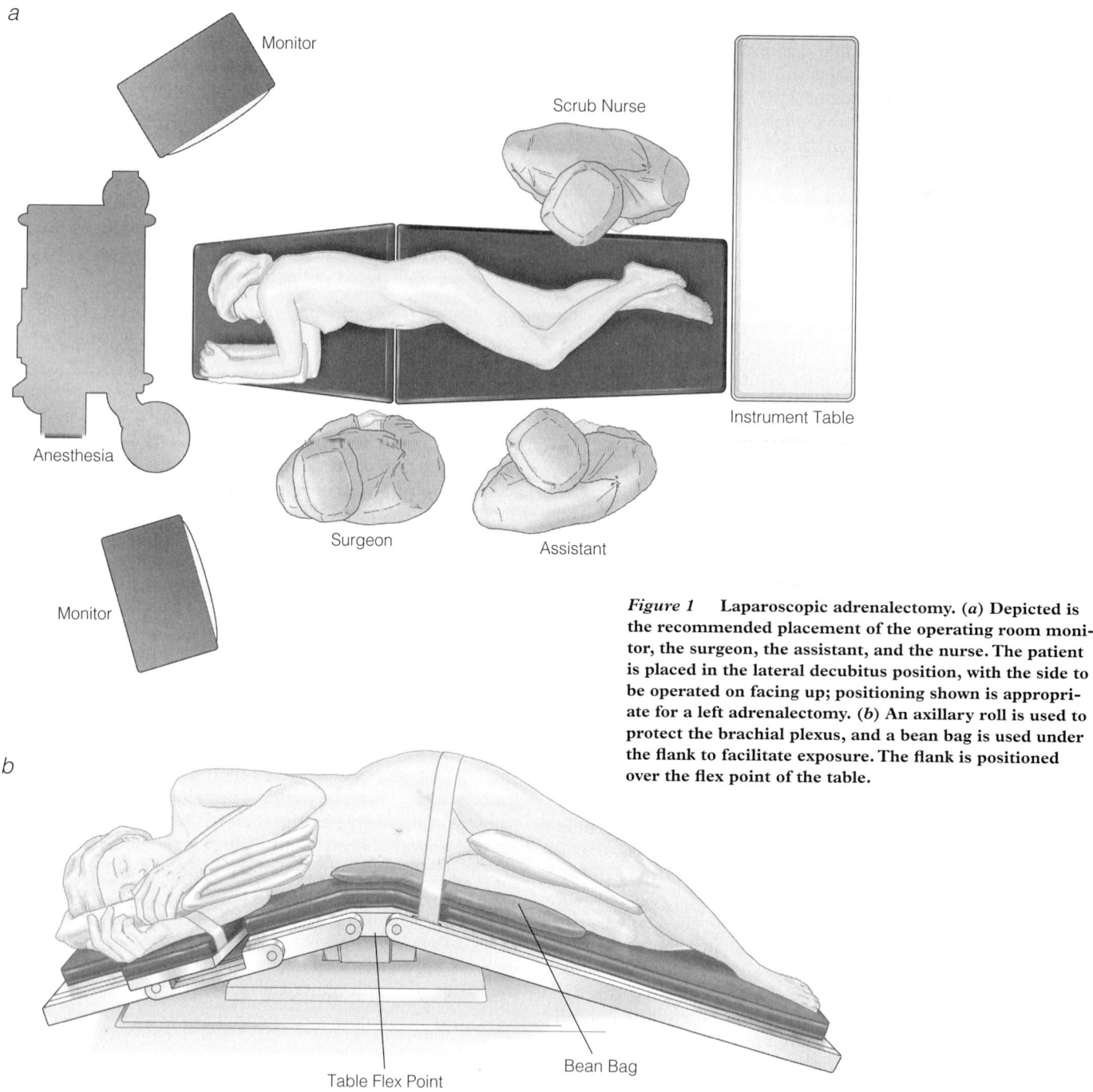

Figure 1 **Laparoscopic adrenalectomy. (*a*) Depicted is the recommended placement of the operating room monitor, the surgeon, the assistant, and the nurse. The patient is placed in the lateral decubitus position, with the side to be operated on facing up; positioning shown is appropriate for a left adrenalectomy. (*b*) An axillary roll is used to protect the brachial plexus, and a bean bag is used under the flank to facilitate exposure. The flank is positioned over the flex point of the table.**

used but was eventually discarded owing to difficulties in exposing the gland, attributable to the supine positioning of the patient. Currently, the lateral transperitoneal approach is the one most commonly used for laparoscopic adrenalectomy. With the patient in the lateral decubitus position, gravity helps to retract anatomic structures, thereby simplifying exposure of the adrenal glands.

We advocate the lateral transperitoneal approach for most cases of adrenal pathology. Accordingly, the bulk of the ensuing technical description is devoted to this technique. The retroperitoneal approach, in our view, is appropriate primarily for tumors less than 6 cm in diameter.

LEFT ADRENALECTOMY: LATERAL TRANSPERITONEAL APPROACH

Step 1: Placement of Trocars

The operation may be performed with either three or four trocars [*see Figure 2*]. In the classic approach, four 10 mm trocars are placed along the subcostal margin. If a 5 mm 30° angled laparoscope is available, the ports can all be 5 mm; if not, a 10 mm 30° angled laparoscope is used and either all three remaining ports are 10 mm as well or the camera port is 10 mm and the other two are 5 mm. The port that is optional is the most posterior one, at the costovertebral angle. This fourth port is sometimes required for retraction of the spleen, but it can generally be dispensed with if the spleen is adequately mobilized and the patient is positioned so that gravity helps pull the spleen down and away from the operative field.

Via either a percutaneous or an open technique, the first port site is created medial to the anterior axillary line, 2 cm below and parallel to the costal margin. Particular care must be taken with the percutaneous technique, because the Veress needle can easily puncture the spleen. CO_2 is insufflated to a pressure of 15 mm Hg, and the initial trocar (5 or 10 mm) is inserted. The abdomen is then visually explored. Under laparoscopic vision, two additional trocars are inserted, one inferior and slightly medial to the tip of the 11th rib and the other more anterior, medial to the initial trocar but lateral to the rectus sheath (approximately a handsbreadth from the midline) so as to avoid the epigastric vessels. The trocars must be placed at least 5 cm—optimally, 10 cm—apart to ensure adequate mobility of the instruments. The most anterior trocar is used for the camera, and the two lateral ports are used for the grasping and cutting instruments.

Step 2: Mobilization of Spleen

With a laparoscopic bowel clamp in the surgeon's left hand and an ultrasonic endoscopic shears in the right, the splenic flexure is mobilized inferiorly and medially to uncover the inferior pole of the splenorenal ligament [see Figure 3]. This ligament is divided along the lateral border of the spleen, from the inferior pole to the superior pole, all the way to the diaphragmatic attachments. When the short gastric vessels are identified, dissection is complete. Once the spleen is fully mobilized, it falls medially, and the retroperitoneum comes into full view. The lateral and anterior portions of the adrenal gland become visible in the perinephric fat, superior and medial to the kidney.

Troubleshooting   Incomplete division of the splenorenal ligament is the most common reason for inadequate exposure

of the left adrenal. The usual solution involves placement of an additional trocar and prolongation of the operation.

Correct patient positioning is key for exposure of the adrenal. The table is tilted to the reverse Trendelenburg position, thereby displacing the surrounding organs and forcing fluids from irrigation or oozing to collect away from the field of dissection. Airplaning the patient toward the surgeon also helps induce the spleen to fall away from the field.

Step 3: Dissection and Removal of Adrenal Gland

The perinephric fat is grasped, and either the lateral and anterior attachments or the medial and inferior attachments are divided with the electrocautery hook or the ultrasonic scalpel to mobilize the adrenal [see Figure 4]. The superior and posterior attachments are left for last: while in place, they act as an anatomic retractor for the gland, thereby facilitating dissection of the adrenal vein. The initial goal of the dissection is to identify and clip the adrenal vein (with two or three clips placed proximally and two distally). The inferior phrenic vein joins the adrenal vein before junction of the adrenal vein with the renal vein. The adrenal vein is clipped above the junction with the inferior phrenic vein, and any branches from the inferior phrenic vein to the adrenal gland are clipped as dissection continues along the medial superior border of the adrenal. The final portion of the dissection of the adrenal gland is performed in the superior and posterior planes. The shaft of a closed instrument can be used to retract the adrenal or elevate it gently during dissection.

The gland is placed in an impermeable nylon bag and removed through the original trocar site, which is widened by gently spreading the abdominal musculature with a clamp. On occasion, the incision may have to be enlarged to permit removal of the specimen.

Troubleshooting   Laparoscopic ultrasonography can be used to identify the adrenal gland or vein in patients who have extensive perinephric fat.[31] If ultrasonography is not available, dissection of the adrenal vein's junction with the renal vein may be necessary to identify the left adrenal.

It is important not to grasp the adrenal gland or the tumor directly. The gland is fragile and prone to tearing. Fracture of the capsule can result in seeding of tumor cells into surrounding tissues, much as sometimes occurs with spleen or parathyroid dissection.

It is not necessary to take the inferior phrenic vein if the adrenal vein is clipped superior to the junction of the two veins and if dissection along the medial superior border of the adrenal stays medial to this vein.

Larger (> 5 cm) adrenal masses may preclude initial access to the adrenal vein. When we encounter a large left adrenal mass, we prefer to dissect laterally and superiorly first, clipping and dividing the inferior phrenic branches to the adrenal. We identify and divide the adrenal vein last.

RIGHT ADRENALECTOMY: LATERAL TRANSPERITONEAL APPROACH

Step 1: Placement of Trocars

In the classic approach to right laparoscopic adrenalectomy, four 10 mm trocars are placed along the subcostal line. If a 5 mm 30° angled laparoscope is available, the ports can all be 5 mm except for the most medial liver retraction port (most liver retractors require a 10 mm trocar). If not, a 10 mm 30° angled laparoscope is used, and either the remaining ports are all 10 mm or the two medial ports (for the camera and the liver retractor) are 10 mm and the remaining one 5 mm.

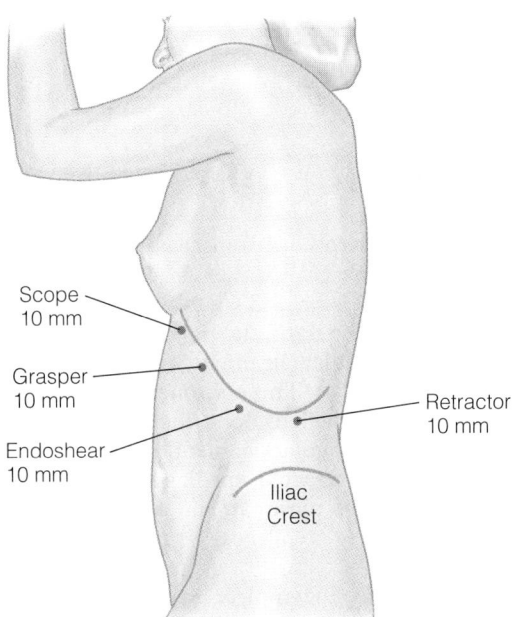

Scope
10 mm

Grasper
10 mm

Endoshear
10 mm

Retractor
10 mm

Iliac
Crest

Figure 2   **Laparoscopic left adrenalectomy: lateral transperitoneal approach. Shown is the recommended trocar placement. The most posterior trocar can often be omitted.**

a

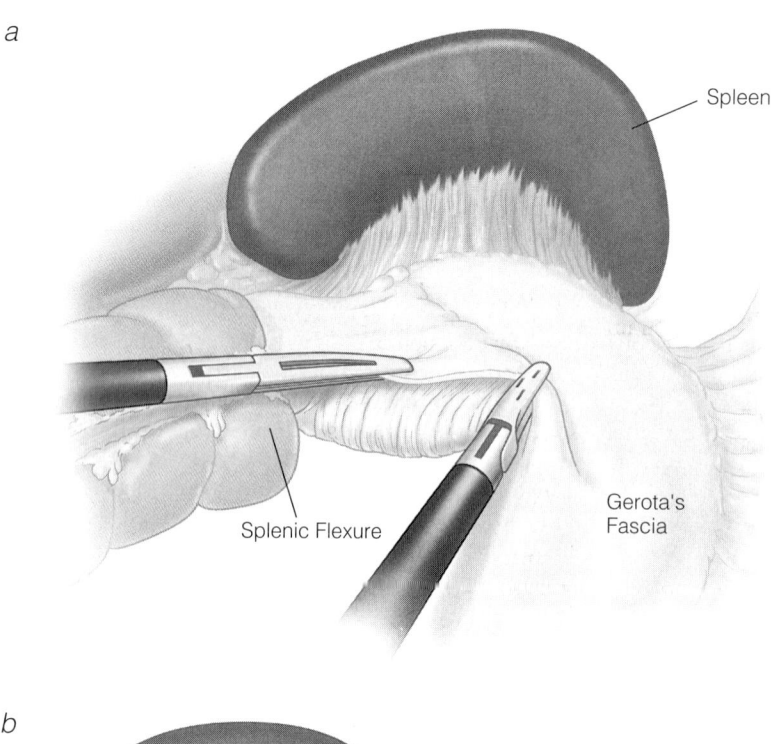

Spleen

Splenic Flexure

Gerota's Fascia

b

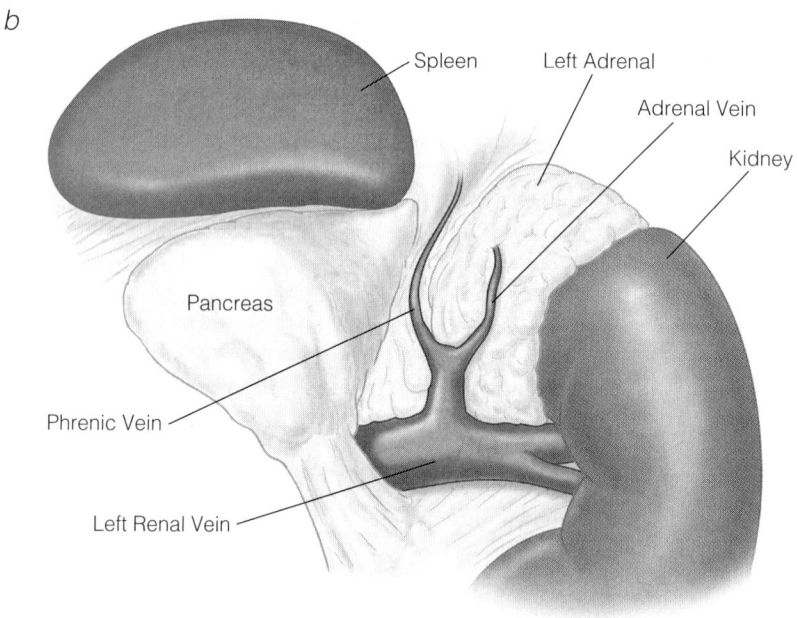

Spleen

Left Adrenal

Adrenal Vein

Kidney

Pancreas

Phrenic Vein

Left Renal Vein

Figure 3 **Laparoscopic left adrenalectomy: lateral transperitoneal approach. Depicted is exposure of the left adrenal. (*a*) The splenorenal ligament is divided and the splenic flexure mobilized, revealing the left adrenal gland. (*b*) After dissection of the lower pole of the adrenal, the adrenal vein and its junctions with the inferior phrenic vein and the left renal vein are revealed.**

Like several other components of a right adrenalectomy, placement of the initial trocar largely mirrors its technical counterpart in a left adrenalectomy (see above), with either percutaneous or open creation of the fascial opening, trocar insertion, insufflation, and visual exploration of the abdomen. The three remaining trocars are then placed under laparoscopic vision at least 5 cm (preferably 10 cm) apart, with one inferior and posterior to the tip of the 11th rib and the other two more anterior and medial. The most medial trocar is placed lateral to the ipsilateral rectus muscle, approximately a handsbreadth from the midline, to avoid the epigastric vessels. The most anterior port is used for the liver retractor, the second port for the camera, and the two lateral ports for the cutting and grasping instruments.

Step 2: Mobilization of Liver

A fan-type liver retractor is inserted through the most anterior port, and the right hepatic lobe is gently reflected medial-

ly. The 30° angled laparoscope is inserted into the second trocar, and liver mobilization is begun. With a laparoscopic curved dissector in the surgeon's left hand and an ultrasonic endoscopic shears in the right, the right lateral hepatic attachments and the triangular ligament are divided along the diaphragm [*see Figure 5a*]. The peritoneum between the liver and the vena cava is divided along the upper border of the renal vein up to the triangular ligament. Once this is done, the liver can readily be retracted medially. At this point, the adrenal gland, the perinephric fat, and the vena cava are generally visible.

Troubleshooting Incomplete division of the right hepatic ligament is the most common reason for inadequate exposure of the right adrenal. As with left adrenalectomy (see above), correct patient positioning is key for exposure of the adrenal.

Step 3: Dissection and Removal of Adrenal Gland

The perinephric fat is grasped, and dissection of the adrenal is begun with the electrocautery hook or the ultrasonic endoscopic shears along the lateral inferior margin of the gland. Dissection continues medially and superiorly until the main adrenal vein coming directly off the vena cava is identified. The adrenal vein is then mobilized with a right-angle clamp and clipped [*see Figure 5b*] with medium or large titanium clips (three on the vena cava side and two on the adrenal side). As dissection progresses superiorly, small veins draining the adrenal gland directly into the inferior phrenic vein or the vena cava may be encountered; these must be clipped. The final portion of the dissection is performed in the superior and posterior planes. The shaft of a closed instrument can be used to retract the adrenal gland or to elevate it gently during dissection.

Finally, the adrenal is placed in an impermeable bag and removed exactly as in a left adrenalectomy.

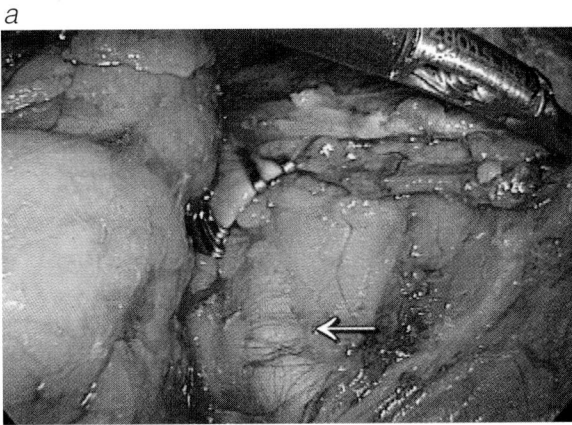

a

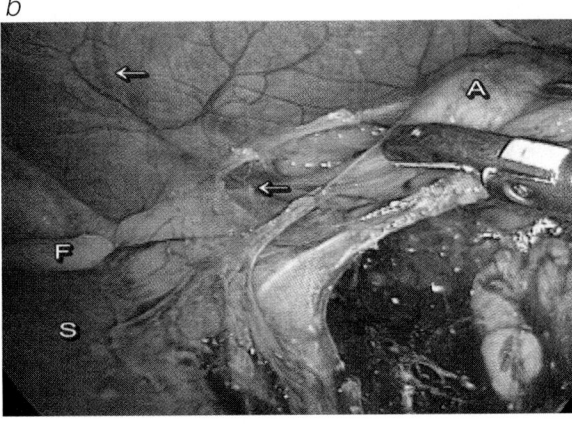

b

Figure 4 **Laparoscopic left adrenalectomy: lateral transperitoneal approach. Depicted is mobilization of the left adrenal gland. (*a*) The lower pole of the adrenal is dissected to reveal the clipped adrenal vein. The pancreas is retracted to the left by gravity, with the splenic vein coursing along its posterior margin. The adrenal is retracted to the right with the laparoscopic instrument. The left renal artery (arrow) is visible. (*b*) The posterior medial attachments of the adrenal are divided with the ultrasonic endoscopic shears. The inferior phrenic vein (arrows) can be seen coursing from the diaphragm along the medial aspect of the adrenal dissection. With sufficient dissection, gravity helps retract the spleen and the gastric fundus from the adrenal.**

Troubleshooting As with a left adrenalectomy, laparoscopic ultrasonography can help define the anatomy; however, it is not needed as often with a right adrenalectomy.

Many problems can be prevented by careful tissue handling. Again, it is important not to grasp the adrenal gland or the tumor directly. In addition, excessive traction during dissection around or clipping of the right adrenal vein can tear the vena cava at the adrenal vein insertion site. Gentle spreading of the right-angle clamp without opening the jaws to their full extent can reduce the likelihood of this complication. The laparoscopic suction tip can also be used for gentle, effective dissection around vessels. If the vein is large, a vascular transverse anastomosis (TA) or gastrointestinal anastomosis (GIA) stapler may be used.

Larger (> 5 cm) adrenal masses may prevent visualization of the adrenal vein and preclude initial dissection and division of the adrenal vein. The solution, again, is to dissect laterally and superiorly first, then continue caudally along the vena cava to reach the adrenal vein. Special care must be taken not to injure the superior pole renal arteries.

BILATERAL ADRENALECTOMY

Most bilateral laparoscopic adrenalectomies are performed to treat Cushing disease or bilateral pheochromocytoma (either benign or malignant). In rare cases, they are performed to treat neoplastic hypercortisolism that cannot be controlled medically or bilateral macronodular hyperplasia associated with Cushing syndrome.

The patient is placed in the lateral decubitus position, with either the left or the right side facing up, depending on which side is to be operated on first. After all wounds have been closed on the first side, the patient is repositioned and redraped to expose the second side. It may be possible to avoid repositioning by making use of an anterior technique, in which trocars are inserted in the anterior subcostal areas on the left and the right, or a posterior technique, in which the patient is prone. Our preference, however, is to start with the left side, with the patient in the lateral decubitus position, then reposition the patient and continue with the right side.

RETROPERITONEAL ADRENALECTOMY

In the retroperitoneal laparoscopic approach to the adrenal gland, first described in 1995,[20,32-35] the patient is placed in the prone position, which enables performance of a bilateral adrenalectomy (if necessary) without repositioning. A retroperitoneal space is created with a balloon dissector. The kidney and the adrenal gland are identified. Dissection is carried out along the inferomedial border of the adrenal, and the renal vein is exposed. The adrenal vein is ligated, and the remainder of the operation proceeds in much the same fashion as with the lateral transperitoneal approach.

The retroperitoneal approach reduces the risk of injury to intra-abdominal organs; however, there are fewer classic anatomic landmarks, the operative field is significantly smaller, and identification of the adrenal glands can be more challenging. In addition, accidental opening of the posterior peritoneal sheath can allow gas to escape into the abdomen, a complication that can further reduce the retroperitoneal space and make dissection even more difficult. A 1997 report that included 111 consecutive retroperitoneal laparoscopic adrenalectomies suggested that this approach is best reserved for management of smaller (< 6 cm) adrenal tumors.[5]

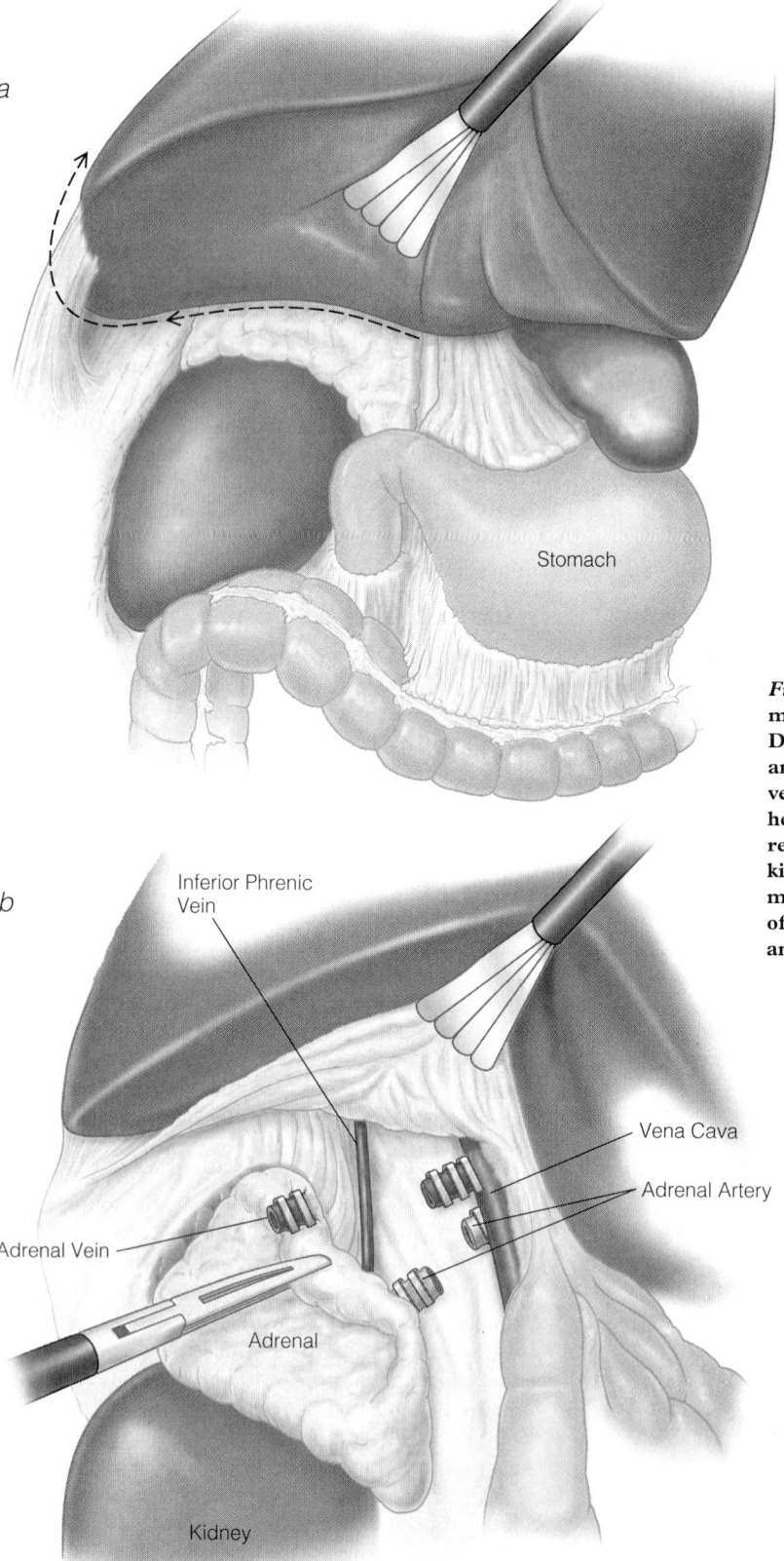

Figure 5 **Laparoscopic right adrenalectomy: lateral transperitoneal approach.
Depicted are exposure of the right adrenal
and dissection and clipping of the adrenal
vein. (*a*) The peritoneal attachments of the
hepatic flexure and the liver are divided to
reveal the right adrenal gland adjacent to the
kidney and the inferior vena cava. (*b*) The
main adrenal vein is clipped, along with one
of the adrenal arteries arising from the aorta
and coursing behind the vena cava.**

Postoperative Care

Oral fluids are started on the day of the operation. Nasogastric
tubes are unnecessary. Most patients need only oral pain medication. The postoperative course is similar to that of laparoscopic cholecystectomy [*see 3:15 Laparoscopic Cholecystectomy*], except
that some endocrine diseases call for hormonal support. Patients
typically are ambulatory on the day of the operation and are discharged on postoperative day 1; however, discharge may be
delayed if perioperative administration of stress-dose steroids or
adjustment of blood pressure medications is required.

Complications

BLEEDING

Operative bleeding can be prevented by meticulous attention to hemostasis. The retroperitoneal fat can be particularly difficult to dissect in male patients: it is extensive and tends to bleed with even gentle manipulation. In this setting, the ultrasonic scalpel is especially useful.

Careful handling of the adrenal vein is crucial. Opening the jaws of a laparocopic dissector can create significant force that the laparoscopic surgeon may fail to appreciate. Gentle spreading, without opening the jaws to their full extent, helps reduce the chances of tearing the vessel. Use of the laparoscopic suction tip also helps reduce the risk of injury to vessels during dissection.

Double or triple clip application to the distal segment of the adrenal vein reduces the chances of clip dislodgment. The clips should be applied at right angles to the tissue. Twisting the clip applier or applying the clips at acute angles can result in scissoring of the clip and division of the vessel. It is of particular importance not to apply clips indiscriminately or blindly if bleeding occurs; to do so puts the renal vein, the vena cava, and other retroperitoneal structures at risk.

The best way of dealing with bleeding during a laparoscopic adrenalectomy is to apply gentle pressure with an instrument or to place an additional trocar to facilitate pressure or exposure. The assistant holding the camera must stay calm and keep the field in view while being careful not to get blood on the lens. Suction devices should be used only under direct vision in the adrenal bed to prevent removal of the clips by the suction.

DAMAGE TO ADJACENT ORGANS

Damage to the pancreas and the spleen (in a left adrenalectomy), to the liver and the vena cava (in a right adrenalectomy), and to the renal arteries (in a left or a right adrenalectomy) can largely be prevented by a thorough knowledge of the anatomy and close attention to key technical details [see Operative Technique, above].

It is not necessary to identify the adrenal vein–left renal vein junction. Tracing the left adrenal vein back to the adrenal gland suffices to confirm its identity. Adequate mobilization of the spleen renders additional retraction of the spleen or pancreas unnecessary. Damage to the pancreas can present either early (as pancreatitis) or late (as a pancreatic pseudocyst). To reduce the risk of such damage, dissection should be kept close to the adrenal and the top of the kidney after division of the splenorenal ligament. Liver lacerations can be controlled with gentle pressure. Bowel lacerations should be closed by means of intracorporeal suture repair.

DEEP VEIN THROMBOSIS

In our series of 100 patients,[2] the incidence of deep vein thrombosis (DVT) was 3%. We routinely use intermittent compression stockings at the beginning of the operation to minimize the occurrence of this complication.

Outcome Evaluation

To date, more than 1,000 cases of laparoscopic adrenalectomy have been reported in the literature. Although no prospective, randomized trials of this new procedure have been published, there is considerable evidence substantiating its effectiveness and safety. A 2000 review examined all English-language studies published between 1995 and 1999 that consisted of more than 20 cases.[18] A total of 1,052 patients underwent 1,082 adrenalectomies (30 of the procedures were bilateral).[18] Patients ranged in age from 17 to 84 years and were equally distributed between males and females. The lesions ranged in size from 0.5 to 14 cm. The lateral transperitoneal approach was followed in 88% of patients, the posterior retroperitoneal approach in 12%. Rates of conversion to open adrenalectomy ranged from 0% to 18%. The most common indications for adrenalectomy were aldosteronoma (42.7%), Cushing syndrome (18.6%), incidentaloma (16.9%), and pheochromocytoma (14.7%); other, less common indications were angiomyolipoma, metastases, small carcinoma, virilizing adenoma, and macronodular hyperplasia.

The retrospective studies comparing laparoscopic adrenalectomy with open adrenalectomy indicated that the average operating time was shorter with open procedures (149 versus 195 minutes). More recently, however, some authors have reported operating times as short as 109 minutes for laparoscopic operations. One of us (M.G.) has now performed more than 200 laparoscopic adrenalectomies.[18] In the first 100, the mean operating time was 123 minutes, the mean blood loss was 70 ml, and the average length of stay was 2.4 days.[2] Currently, the mean operating time is less than 60 minutes for a benign unilateral lesion, and the median length of stay is 1 day.

These retrospective studies also found that laparoscopic adrenalectomy was associated with reduced blood loss (153 versus 355 ml) and a shorter length of stay (2.6 versus 6.5 days).[18] The overall complication rate was lower in the laparoscopic group (7% versus 24%) as well. Laparoscopic adrenalectomy was associated with postoperative hematoma or need for transfusion in approximately 3% of patients and with wound complications, pulmonary complications, or DVT in fewer than 1%. Open adrenalectomy was associated with respiratory problems (e.g., pneumonia or atelectasis) in 6% of patients, with wound infections in 3%, with need for transfusion in 3%, and with splenic injury (sometimes necessitating splenectomy) in 1.5%. Moreover, the open approach was associated with a 54% overall rate of late complications, namely, chronic pain (14%), flank numbness (10%), and muscle laxity (30%). When performed by an experienced laparoscopic surgeon, laparoscopic adrenalectomy can be completed with no mortality, minimal morbidity, and no recurrence of hormonal excess. In the aforementioned experience with more than 200 cases, conversion to an open procedure was required only for removal of invasive or giant (> 15 cm) tumors; in no case was it necessary to manage bleeding.

The retrospective studies comparing the transperitoneal and retroperitoneal approaches to laparoscopic adrenalectomy reported slight differences in operating time and blood loss but no differences in length of stay.[18] As noted [see Operative Technique, Choice of Approach and Retroperitoneal Adrenalectomy, above], the retroperitoneal approach may have advantages in some settings (e.g., the avoidance of intraperitoneal adhesions from previous operations and the elimination of patient repositioning for bilateral procedures), but it also has certain important disadvantages (e.g., the smaller operative field, the greater difficulty of visualizing the adrenal anatomy, and the inability to survey the liver and the peritoneum for metastases). The choice between the lateral transperitoneal approach to laparoscopic adrenalectomy and the retroperitoneal approach is determined primarily by surgeon preference—except in patients with larger tumors, for whom the lateral transperitoneal approach is clearly superior. In general, the retroperitoneal approach is ideal for a surgeon who is experienced with this approach and who is treating a patient with a benign adrenal tumor less than 6 cm in diameter.

References

1. Gagner M, Lacroix A, Bolte E: Laparoscopic adrenalectomy in Cushing's syndrome and pheochromocytoma (letter). N Engl J Med 327:1033, 1992

2. Gagner M, Pomp A, Heniford B, et al: Laparoscopic adrenalectomy: lessons learned from 100 consecutive procedures. Ann Surg 226:238, 1997

3. Gagner M, Breton G, Pharand D, et al: Is laparoscopic adrenalectomy indicated for pheochromocytoma? Surgery 120:1076, 1996

4. Duh QY, Siperstein AE, Clark OH, et al: Laparoscopic adrenalectomy: comparison of the lateral and posterior approaches. Arch Surg 131:870, 1996

5. Bonjer HJ, Lange JF, Kazemeir G: Comparison of three techniques for adrenalectomy. Br J Surg 84:679, 1997

6. Baba S, Miyajima A, Uchida A, et al: A posterior lumbar approach for retroperitoneoscopic adrenalectomy: assessment of surgical efficacy. Urology 50:19, 1997

7. Gagner M, Lacroix A, Prinz RA, et al: Early experience with laparoscopic approach for adrenalectomy. Surgery 114:1120, 1993

8. Chapuis Y, Maignien B, Abboud B: Adrenalectomy under celioscopy: experience of 25 operations. Presse Med 24:845, 1995

9. Brunt LM, Doherty GM, Norton JA, et al: Laparoscopic adrenalectomy compared to open adrenalectomy for benign adrenal neoplasms. J Am Coll Surg 183:1, 1996

10. Fernandez-Cruz L, Saenz A, Benarroch G, et al: Laparoscopic unilateral and bilateral adrenalectomy for Cushing's syndrome: transperitoneal and retroperitoneal approaches. Ann Surg 224:727, 1996

11. de Canniere L, Michel L, Hamoir E, et al: Multicentric experience of the Belgian Group for Endoscopic Surgery (BGES) with endoscopic adrenalectomy. Surg Endosc 11:1065, 1997

12. Jacobs JK, Goldstein RE, Geer RJ, et al: Laparoscopic adrenalectomy: a new standard of care. Ann Surg 225:495, 1997

13. Filipponi S, Guerrieri M, Arnoldi G, et al: Laparoscopic adrenalectomy: a report on 50 operations. Eur J Endocrinol 138:548, 1998

14. Guazzoni G, Montorsi F, Bocciardi A, et al: Transperitoneal laparoscopic versus open adrenalectomy for benign hyperfunctioning adrenal tumors: a comparative study. J Urol 153:1597, 1995

15. Janetschek G, Finkenstedt G, Gasser R, et al: Laparoscopic surgery for pheochromocytoma: adrenalectomy, partial resection, excision of paragangliomas. J Urol 160:330, 1998

16. Winfield HN, Hamilton BD, Bravo EL, et al: Laparoscopic adrenalectomy: the preferred choice? A comparison to open adrenalectomy. J Urol 160:325, 1998

17. Janetschek G, Altarac S, Finkenstedt G, et al: Technique and results of laparoscopic adrenalectomy. Eur Urol 30:475, 1996

18. Jossart G, Burpee SE, Gagner M: Surgery of the adrenal glands. Endocrinol Metab Clin 29.37, 2000

19. Linos D, Stylopoulos N, Boukis M, et al: Anterior, posterior, or laparoscopic approach for the management of adrenal diseases? Am J Surg 173:120, 1997

20. Thompson GB, Grant CS, van Heerden JA, et al: Laparoscopic versus open posterior adrenalectomy: a case-control study of 100 patients. Surgery 122:1132, 1997

21. Grant C: Pheochromocytoma. Textbook of Endocrine Surgery, 1st ed. Clark OH, Duh Q, Eds. WB Saunders Co, Philadelphia, 1997, p 513

22. Icard P, Louvel A, Chapuis Y: Survival rates and prognostic factors in adrenocortical carcinoma. World J Surg 16:453, 1992

23. Herrera MF, Grant CS, van Heerden JA, et al: Incidentally discovered adrenal tumors: an institutional perspective. Surgery 110:1014, 1991

24. Gross MD, McLeod MK, Sanfield JA, et al: Scintigraphic evaluation of clinically silent adrenal masses. J Nucl Med 35:1145, 1994

25. Silverman SG, Mueller PR, Pinkey LP, et al: Predictive value of image-guided adrenal biopsy: analysis of results of 101 biopsies. Radiology 187:715, 1993

26. Pertsemlidis D: Minimal-access versus open adrenalectomy. Surg Endosc 9:384, 1995

27. Proye C, Thevenin D, Cecat P, et al: Exclusive use of calcium channel blockers in preoperative and intraoperative control of pheochromocytomas: hemodynamics and free catecholamine assays in ten consecutive patients. Surgery 106:1149, 1989

28. Miyake O, Yoshimura K, Yoshioka T, et al: Laparoscopic adrenalectomy: comparison of the transperitoneal and retroperitoneal approach. Eur Urol 33:303, 1998

29. Gasman D, Droupy S, Koutani A, et al: Laparoscopic adrenalectomy: the retroperitoneal approach. J Urol 159:1816, 1998

30. Heintz A, Walgenbach S, Junginger T: Results of endoscopic retroperitoneal adrenalectomy. Surg Endosc 10:633, 1996

31. Heniford BT, Iannitti DA, Hale J, et al: The role of intraoperative ultrasonography during laparoscopic adrenalectomy. Surgery 122:1068, 1997

32. Mercan S, Seven R, Ozarmagan S, et al: Endoscopic retroperitoneal adrenalectomy. Surgery 118:1071, 1995

33. Takeda M, Go H, Watanabe R, et al: Retroperitoneal laparoscopic adrenalectomy for functioning adrenal tumors: comparison with conventional transperitoneal laparoscopic adrenalectomy. J Urol 157:19, 1997

34. Terachi T, Matsuda T, Terai A: Transperitoneal laparoscopic adrenalectomy: experience in 100 patients. J Endourol 11:361, 1997

35. Walz MK, Peitgen K, Saller B, et al: Subtotal adrenalectomy by the posterior retroperitoneoscopic approach. World J Surg 22:621, 1998

Acknowledgment

Figures 1 through 3 and 5   Tom Moore.

21 OPEN HERNIA REPAIR

Robert J. Fitzgibbons, Jr., M.D., F.A.C.S., Alan T. Richards, M.D., F.A.C.S., and Thomas H. Quinn, Ph.D.

Herniorrhaphy is one of the most commonly performed operations in all of surgery. Worldwide, some 20 million groin hernia repairs are accomplished each year.[1] In the United States, over 1,000,000 herniorrhaphies are performed each year, of which 750,000 are for inguinal hernias, 166,000 for umbilical hernias, 97,000 for incisional hernias, 25,000 for femoral hernias, and 76,000 for miscellaneous hernias.[2] The significance of these large numbers is that small variations in practice patterns can have huge socioeconomic implications. Operations that might seem unimportant because they account for only a small percentage of herniorrhaphies actually are important in that they account for a large absolute number of procedures. Accordingly, though this chapter is necessarily selective, focusing on the most pertinent of the abdominal wall and groin herniorrhaphies being performed today, it addresses a wide variety of operative approaches to hernia repair.

Epidemiology of Hernia

Approximately 75% of all abdominal wall hernias occur in the groin. Inguinal hernias are more common on the right than on the left and are seven times more likely in males than in females. Indirect inguinal hernias are twice as common as direct hernias. Femoral hernias are much less common than either, accounting for fewer than 10% of all groin hernias; however, 40% of femoral hernias present as emergencies, with incarceration or strangulation, and mortality is higher for emergency repair than for elective repair. Femoral hernias are more common in older patients and in those who have previously undergone inguinal hernia repair. Females are at higher risk than males, by a factor of 4 to 1.[3]

The prevalence of abdominal wall hernias is difficult to determine, as illustrated by the wide range of published figures in the literature. The major reasons for this difficulty are (1) the lack of standardization in how inguinal and ventral hernias are defined, (2) the inconsistency of the data sources used (which include self-reporting by patients, audits of routine physical examinations, and insurance company databases, among others), and (3) the subjectivity of physical examination, even when done by trained surgeons. Prevalence was reported in a United States Health, Education and Welfare study conducted by interview in 1960 for hernia [see Figure 1].[4] Given that a number of persons must have had hernias without knowing it, it can be assumed that these figures underestimate the actual prevalence. Nevertheless, they provide a rough idea of the scope of the hernia problem.

Modern data concerning the risk of major complications from untreated abdominal wall hernias are scarce. Typically, surgeons are taught that all hernias, even if asymptomatic, should be repaired at diagnosis to prevent strangulation or bowel obstruction and that herniorrhaphy becomes more difficult the longer repair is delayed. As a result, it is hard to find a whole patient population in which at least some of the members do not undergo routine hernia repair regardless of symptoms. This state of affairs makes accurate estimates of the natural history of hernia impossible.

Examination of obscure data from the 1800s and some unique data from South America suggests that both the risk of complications from an untreated hernia and the operative mortality

from managing them have been overstated.[5] At the same time, it is becoming clear that abdominal wall herniorrhaphy is associated with a higher morbidity than was previously appreciated. Currently, numerous patients either choose or are counseled by their primary care physicians not to undergo herniorrhaphy if the hernia is not "bothering them too much." A better understanding of the natural history therefore becomes particularly important for identifying patient subgroups who might be at greater risk for complications.

Classification of Hernia Types

Numerous classification schemes for groin hernias have been devised, usually bearing the name of the responsible investigator or investigators (e.g., Casten, Lichtenstein, Gilbert, Robbins and Rutkow, Bendavid, Nyhus, and Schumpelick). The variety of classifications in current use indicates that the perfect system has yet to be developed.[6] The main problem in developing a single classification scheme suitable for wide application is that it is impossible to eliminate subjective measurements and thus impossible to ensure consistency from observer to observer. The advent of laparoscopic herniorrhaphy has further complicated the issue in that some of the measurements needed cannot be obtained via a laparoscopic approach. At present, the Nyhus system enjoys the greatest degree of acceptance [see Table 1].

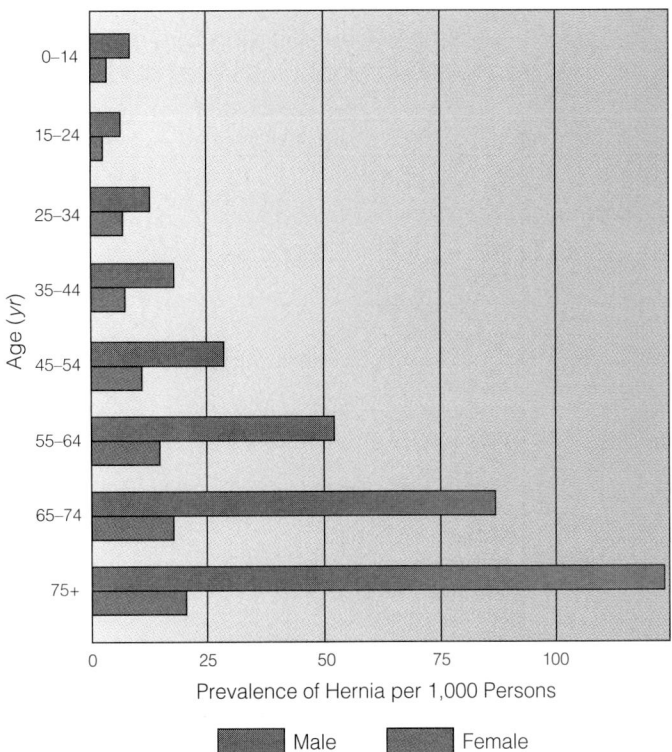

Figure 1 **Illustrated is the prevalence of abdominal wall hernia in the United States per 1,000 population, by age and sex.[4]**

545

Table 1 Nyhus Classification System for Groin Hernias

Type	Description
1	Indirect hernia with normal internal abdominal ring. This type is typically seen in infants, children, and small adults.
2	Indirect hernia in which internal ring is enlarged without impingement on the floor of the inguinal canal. Hernia does not extend to the scrotum.
3A	Direct hernia. Size is not taken into account.
3B	Indirect hernia that has enlarged enough to encroach upon the posterior inguinal wall. Indirect sliding or scrotal hernias are usually placed in this category because they are commonly associated with extension to direct space. This type also includes pantaloon hernias.
3C	Femoral hernia.
4	Recurrent hernia. Modifiers A, B, C, and D are sometimes added to type 4, corresponding to indirect, direct, femoral, and mixed, respectively.

Categorization of ventral abdominal wall hernias is not as critical as categorization of inguinal hernias, because there are so many different types of ventral hernias; however, Zollinger has proposed a classification scheme for these hernias that is frequently used [see Table 2]. Of the ventral hernias, incisional hernias are common enough to warrant their own discrete classification system. The scheme most often used for categorizing incisional hernias [see Table 3] represents the results of a 1998 consensus conference held in conjunction with the European Hernia Society's annual congress.[7] This system is important in that it affords investigators a reliable means of comparing results between one procedure and another or between one center and another.

Table 2 Zollinger Classification System for Ventral Abdominal Wall Hernias

Type	Examples
Congenital	Omphalocele Gastroschisis Umbilical (infant)
Acquired	Midline Diastasis recti Epigastric Umbilical (adult, acquired, paraumbilical) Median Supravesical (anterior, posterior, lateral) Paramedian Spigelian Interparietal
Incisional	Midline Paramedian Transverse Special operative sites
Traumatic	Penetrating, autopenetrating* Blunt Focal, minimal injury Moderate injury Extensive force or shear Destructive

*Penetration from host tissue such as bone.

Abdominal Wall Anatomy

The skin of the lower anterior abdominal wall is innervated by anterior and lateral cutaneous branches of the ventral rami of the seventh through 12th intercostal nerves and by the ventral rami of the first and second lumbar nerves. These nerves course between the lateral flat muscles of the abdominal wall and enter the skin through the subcutaneous tissue.

The first layers encountered beneath the skin are Camper's and Scarpa's fasciae in the subcutaneous tissue. The only significance of these layers is that when sufficiently developed, they can be reapproximated to provide another layer between a repaired inguinal floor and the outside. The major blood vessels of this superficial fatty layer are the superficial inferior and superior epigastric vessels, the intercostal vessels, and the superficial circumflex iliac vessels (which are branches of the femoral vessels).

The external oblique muscle is the most superficial of the great flat muscles of the abdominal wall [see Figure 2]. This muscle arises from the posterior aspects of the lower eight ribs and interdigitates with both the serratus anterior and the latissimus dorsi at its origin. The posterior portion of the external oblique muscle is oriented vertically and inserts on the crest of the ilium. The anterior portion of the muscle courses inferiorly and obliquely toward the midline and the pubis. The muscle fibers themselves are of no interest to the inguinal hernia surgeon until they give way to form its aponeurosis, which occurs well above the inguinal region. The obliquely arranged anterior inferior fibers of the aponeurosis of the external oblique muscle fold back on themselves to form the inguinal ligament, which attaches laterally to the anterior superior iliac spine. In most persons, the medial insertion of the inguinal ligament is dual: one portion of the ligament inserts on the pubic tubercle and the pubic bone, whereas the other portion is fan-shaped and spans the distance between the inguinal ligament proper and the pectineal line of the pubis. This fan-shaped portion of the inguinal ligament is called the lacunar ligament. It blends laterally with Cooper's ligament (or, to be anatomically correct, the pectineal ligament). The more medial fibers of the aponeurosis of the external oblique muscle divide into a medial crus and a lateral crus to form the external or superficial inguinal ring, through which the spermatic cord (or the round ligament) and branches of the ilioinguinal and genitofemoral nerves pass. The rest of the medial fibers insert into the linea alba after contributing to the anterior portion of the rectus sheath.

Beneath the external oblique muscle is the internal abdominal oblique muscle. The fibers of the internal abdominal oblique muscle fan out following the shape of the iliac crest, so that the superior fibers course obliquely upward toward the distal ends of the lower three or four ribs while the lower fibers orient themselves inferomedially toward the pubis to run parallel to the external oblique aponeurotic fibers. These fibers arch over the round ligament or the spermatic cord, forming the superficial part of the internal (deep) inguinal ring.

Beneath the internal oblique muscle is the transversus abdominis. This muscle arises from the inguinal ligament, the inner side of the iliac crest, the endoabdominal fascia, and the lower six costal cartilages and ribs, where it interdigitates with the lateral diaphragmatic fibers. The medial aponeurotic fibers of the transversus abdominis contribute to the rectus sheath and insert on the pecten ossis pubis and the crest of the pubis, forming the falx inguinalis. Infrequently, these fibers are joined by a portion of the internal oblique aponeurosis; only when this occurs is a true conjoined tendon formed.[8]

Aponeurotic fibers of the transversus abdominis also form the structure known as the aponeurotic arch. It is theorized that con-

Table 3 Classification System for Incisional Hernias

Parameter	Categories

Location	Vertical
	  Midline, above or below umbilicus
	  Midline, including umbilicus
	  Paramedian
	Transverse
	  Above or below umbilicus
	  Crosses midline
	Oblique
	  Above or below umbilicus
	  Combined

Size*	< 5 cm 5–10 cm > 10 cm
Recurrence	Primary Multiply recurrent Stratification for type of previous repair

Reducibility	Yes
	  Obstruction
	  No obstruction
	No
	  Obstruction
	  No obstruction

Symptoms	Asymptomatic Symptomatic

*Difficult to measure consistently.

The nerves pass anteriorly in a plane between the internal oblique muscle and the transversus abdominis, eventually piercing the lateral aspect of the rectus sheath to innervate the muscle therein. The external oblique muscle receives branches of the intercostal nerves, which penetrate the internal oblique muscle to reach it. The anterior ends of the nerves form part of the cutaneous innervation of the abdominal wall. The first lumbar nerve divides into the ilioinguinal nerve and the iliohypogastric nerve [*see Figure 3*]. These important nerves lie in the space between the internal oblique muscle and the external oblique aponeurosis. They may divide within the psoas major or between the internal oblique muscle and the transversus abdominis. The ilioinguinal nerve may communicate with the iliohypogastric nerve before innervating the internal oblique muscle. The ilioinguinal nerve then passes through the external inguinal ring to run parallel to the spermatic cord, while the iliohypogastric nerve pierces the external oblique muscle to innervate the skin above the pubis. The cremaster muscle fibers, which are derived from the internal oblique muscle, are innervated by the genitofemoral nerve. There can be considerable variability and overlap.

The blood supply of the lateral muscles of the anterior wall comes primarily from the lower three or four intercostal arteries, the deep circumflex iliac artery, and the lumbar arteries. The rectus abdominis has a complicated blood supply that derives from the superior epigastric artery (a terminal branch of the internal thoracic [internal mammary] artery), the inferior epigastric artery (a branch of the external iliac artery), and the lower intercostal arteries. The lower intercostal arteries enter the sides of the muscle after traveling between the oblique muscles; the superior and

traction of the transversus abdominis causes the arch to move downward toward the inguinal ligament, thereby constituting a form of shutter mechanism that reinforces the weakest area of the groin when intra-abdominal pressure is raised. The area beneath the arch varies. Many authorities believe that a high arch, resulting in a larger area from which the transversus abdominis is by definition absent, is a predisposing factor for a direct inguinal hernia. The transverse aponeurotic arch is also important because the term is used by many authors to describe the medial structure that is sewn to the inguinal ligament in many of the older inguinal hernia repairs.

The rectus abdominis forms the central anchoring muscle mass of the anterior abdomen. It arises from the fifth through seventh costal cartilages and inserts on the pubic symphysis and the pubic crest. It is innervated by the seventh through 12th intercostal nerves, which laterally pierce the aponeurotic sheath of the muscle. The semilunar line is the slight depression in the aponeurotic fibers coursing toward the muscle. In a minority of persons, the small pyramidalis muscle accompanies the rectus abdominis at its insertion. This muscle arises from the pubic symphysis. It lies within the rectus sheath and tapers to attach to the linea alba, which represents the conjunction of the two rectus sheaths and is the major site of insertion for three aponeuroses from all three lateral muscle layers. The line of Douglas (i.e., the arcuate line of the rectus sheath) is formed at a variable distance between the umbilicus and the inguinal space because the fasciae of the large flat muscles of the abdominal wall contribute their aponeuroses to the anterior surface of the muscle, leaving only transversalis (or transverse) fascia to cover the posterior surface of the rectus abdominis.

The innervation of the anterior wall muscles is multifaceted. The seventh through 12th intercostal nerves and the first and second lumbar nerves provide most of the innervation of the lateral muscles, as well as of the rectus abdominis and the overlying skin.

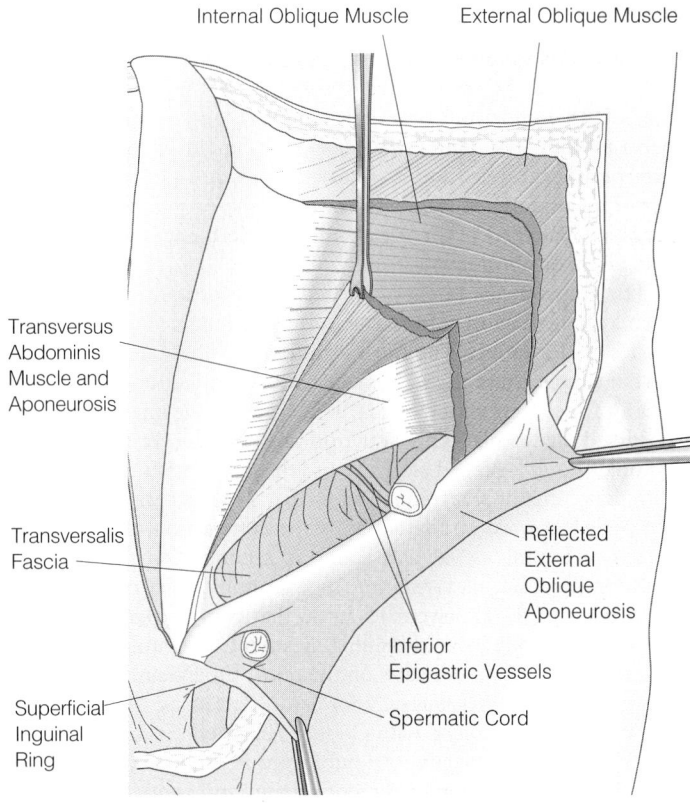

Figure 2 **Depicted is the relationship of the great flat muscles of the abdominal wall to the groin.**

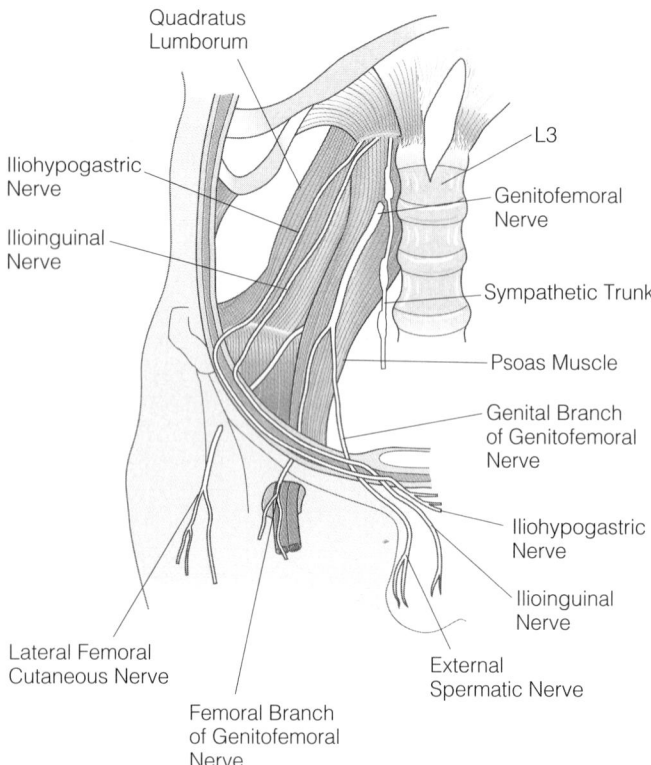

Quadratus
Lumborum

Iliohypogastric
Nerve

Ilioinguinal
Nerve

Lateral Femoral
Cutaneous Nerve

Femoral Branch
of Genitofemoral
Nerve

L3

Genitofemoral
Nerve

Sympathetic Trunk

Psoas Muscle

Genital Branch
of Genitofemoral
Nerve

Iliohypogastric
Nerve

Ilioinguinal
Nerve

External
Spermatic Nerve

Figure 3 **Shown are the important nerves of the lower abdominal wall.**

the inferior epigastric arteries enter the rectus sheath and anastomose near the umbilicus.

The endoabdominal fascia is the deep fascia covering the internal surface of the transversus abdominis, the iliacus, the psoas major and minor, the obturator internus, and portions of the periosteum. It is a continuous sheet that extends throughout the extraperitoneal space and is sometimes referred to as the wallpaper of the abdominal cavity. Commonly, the endoabdominal fascia is subclassified according to the muscle being covered (e.g., iliac fascia or obturator fascia).

The transversalis fascia is particularly important for inguinal hernia repair because it forms anatomic landmarks known as analogues or derivatives. The most significant of these analogues for hernia surgeons are the iliopectineal arch, the iliopubic tract, the crura of the deep inguinal ring, and Cooper's ligament (i.e., the pectineal ligament). The superior and inferior crura form a "monk's hood"–shaped sling around the deep inguinal ring. This sling has functional significance, in that as the crura of the ring are pulled upward and laterally by the contraction of the transversus abdominis, a valvular action is generated that helps preclude indirect hernia formation. The iliopubic tract is the thickened band of the transversalis fascia that courses parallel to the more superficially located inguinal ligament. It is attached to the iliac crest laterally and inserts on the pubic tubercle medially. The insertion curves inferolaterally for 1 to 2 cm along the pectineal line of the pubis to blend with Cooper's ligament, ending at about the midportion of the superior pubic ramus. Cooper's ligament is actually a condensation of the periosteum and is not a true analogue of the transversalis fascia.

Hesselbach's inguinal triangle is the site of direct inguinal hernias. As viewed from the anterior aspect, the inguinal ligament forms the base of the triangle, the edge of the rectus abdominis

forms the medial border, and the inferior epigastric vessels form the superolateral border. (It should be noted, however, that Hesselbach actually described Cooper's ligament as the base.)

Below the iliopubic tract are the critical anatomic elements from which a femoral hernia may develop. The iliopectineal arch separates the vascular compartment that contains the femoral vessels from the neuromuscular compartment that contains the iliopsoas muscle, the femoral nerve, and the lateral femoral cutaneous nerve. The vascular compartment is invested by the femoral sheath, which has three subcompartments: (1) the lateral, containing the femoral artery and the femoral branch of the genitofemoral nerve; (2) the middle, containing the femoral vein; and (3) the medial, which is the cone-shaped cul-de-sac known as the femoral canal. The femoral canal is normally a 1 to 2 cm blind pouch that begins at the femoral ring and extends to the level of the fossa ovalis. The femoral ring is bordered by the superior pubic ramus inferiorly, the femoral vein laterally, and the iliopubic tract (with its curved insertion onto the pubic ramus) anteriorly and medially. The femoral canal normally contains preperitoneal fat, connective tissue, and lymph nodes (including Cloquet's node at the femoral ring), which collectively make up the femoral pad. This pad acts as a cushion for the femoral vein, allowing expansion such as might occur during a Valsalva maneuver, and serves as a plug to prevent abdominal contents from entering the thigh. A femoral hernia exists when the blind end of the femoral canal becomes an opening (the femoral orifice) through which a peritoneal sac can protrude.

Between the transversalis fascia and the peritoneum is the preperitoneal space. In the midline behind the pubis, this space is known as the space of Retzius; laterally, it is referred to as the space of Bogros. The preperitoneal space is of particular importance for surgeons because many of the inguinal hernia repairs (see below) are performed in this area. The inferior epigastric vessels, the deep inferior epigastric vein, the iliopubic vein, the rectusial vein, the retropubic vein, the communicating rectusioepigastric vein, the internal spermatic vessels, and the vas deferens are all encountered in this space.[9]

Inguinal Herniorrhaphy: Choice of Procedure

The major indication for a surgeon to choose any one inguinal hernia repair over another is personal experience with a particular operation. Thus, in theory, any patient can be considered a candidate for any of these procedures. Some general guidelines are useful, however. The overriding consideration should be the need to tailor the operation to the patient's particular hernia. For example, a simple Marcy repair would be completely adequate for a pediatric patient with a Nyhus type 1 hernia but not for an elderly patient who has an indirect hernia in conjunction with extensive destruction of the inguinal floor. The conventional anterior prosthetic repairs are particularly useful in high-risk patients because they can easily be performed with local anesthesia. On the other hand, giant prosthetic reinforcement of the visceral sac (GPRVS), especially when bilateral, necessitates general or regional anesthesia and thus is best for patients with bilateral direct or recurrent hernias or, perhaps, for patients with connective tissue disorders that appear to be associated with their hernia. If surgery has previously been done in either the anterior or the preperitoneal space, the surgeon should choose a procedure that uses the undissected space. If local or systemic infection is present, a nonprosthetic repair is usually considered preferable, though the newer biologic prosthesis now being evaluated may eventually change this view. Uncorrected coagulopathy is a contraindication to elective repair.

Inguinal Herniorrhaphy: Conventional Anterior Nonprosthetic Repairs

ANESTHESIA

Local anesthesia is entirely adequate, especially when combined with I.V. infusion of a rapid-acting, short-lasting, amnesic, and anxiolytic agent such as propofol. This is the approach most commonly employed in specialty hernia clinics. In general practice, general anesthesia is preferred. This approach is reasonable in fit patients but is associated with a higher incidence of postoperative urinary retention.[10] If general anesthesia is used, a local anesthetic should be given at the end of the procedure as an adjuvant to reduce immediate postoperative pain. Spinal or epidural anesthesia can also be used but is less popular.

OPERATIVE TECHNIQUE

The various anterior nonprosthetic herniorrhaphies have a number of initial technical steps in common; they differ primarily with respect to the specific details of the actual repair.

Step 1: Administration of Local Anesthetic

Generally, we use a solution containing 50 ml of 0.5% lidocaine with epinephrine and 50 ml of 0.25% bupivacaine with epinephrine; the epinephrine is optional and may be omitted in patients who have a history of coronary artery disease. In an adult of normal size, 70 ml of this solution is injected before preparation and draping: 10 ml is placed medial to the anterior superior iliac spine to block the ilioinguinal nerve, and the other 60 ml is used as a field block along the orientation of the eventual incision in the subcutaneous and deeper tissues. Care is taken to ensure that some of the material is injected into the areas of the pubic tubercle and Cooper's ligament, which are easily identified by tactile sensation (except in very obese patients). Intradermal injection is unnecessary because by the time the surgeon is scrubbed and the patient draped, anesthesia is complete. The remaining 30 ml is reserved for discretionary use during the procedure. With this technique, endotracheal intubation is avoided and the patient can be aroused from sedation periodically to perform Valsalva maneuvers to test the repair.

Step 2: Initial Incision

Traditionally, the skin is opened by making an oblique incision between the anterior superior iliac spine and the pubic tubercle. For cosmetic reasons, however, many surgeons now prefer a more horizontal skin incision placed in the natural skin lines. In either case, the incision is deepened through Scarpa's and Camper's fasciae and the subcutaneous tissue to expose the external oblique aponeurosis. The external oblique aponeurosis is then opened through the external inguinal ring.

Step 3: Mobilization of Cord Structures

The superior flap of the external oblique fascia is dissected away from the anterior rectus sheath medially and the internal oblique muscle laterally. The iliohypogastric nerve is identified at this time; it can be either left in situ or freed from the surrounding tissue and isolated from the operative field by passing a hemostat under the nerve and grasping the upper flap of the external oblique aponeurosis. Routine division of the iliohypogastric nerve along with the ilioinguinal nerve is practiced by some surgeons but is not advised by most. The cord structures are then bluntly dissected away from the inferior flap of the external oblique aponeurosis to expose the shelving edge of the inguinal ligament and the iliopubic tract. The cord structures are lifted en masse with the fingers of one hand at the pubic tubercle so that the index finger can be passed underneath to meet the ipsilateral thumb or the fingers of the other hand. Mobilization of the cord structures is completed by means of blunt dissection, and a Penrose drain is placed around them so that they can be retracted during the procedure.

Step 4: Division of Cremaster Muscle

Complete division of the cremaster muscle has been common practice, especially with indirect hernias. The purposes of this practice are to facilitate identification of the sac and to lengthen the cord for better visualization of the inguinal floor. Almost always, however, adequate exposure can be obtained by opening the muscle longitudinally, which reduces the chances of damage to the cord and prevents testicular descent. Accordingly, the latter approach should be considered best practice unless there are extenuating circumstances.

Step 5: High Ligation of Sac

The term high ligation of the sac is used frequently in discussing hernia repair; its historical significance has ingrained it in the descriptions of most of the older operations. For our purposes in this chapter, high ligation of the sac should be considered equivalent to reduction of the sac into the preperitoneal space without excision. The two methods work equally well and are highly effective. Some surgeons believe that sac inversion results in less pain (because the richly innervated peritoneum is not incised) and may be less likely to cause adhesive complications. To date, however, no randomized trials have been done to determine whether this is so.[11] Sac eversion in lieu of excision does protect intra-abdominal viscera in cases of unrecognized incarcerated sac contents or sliding hernia.

Step 6: Management of Inguinal Scrotal Hernial Sacs

Some surgeons consider complete excision of all indirect inguinal hernial sacs important. The downside of this practice is that the incidence of ischemic orchitis from excessive trauma to the cord rises substantially. The logical sequela of ischemic orchitis is testicular atrophy, though this presumed relationship has not been conclusively proved. In our view, it is better to divide an indirect inguinal hernial sac in the midportion of the inguinal canal once it is clear that the hernia is not sliding and no abdominal contents are present. The distal sac is not removed, but its anterior wall is opened as far distally as is convenient. Contrary to the opinion commonly voiced in the urologic literature, this approach does not result in excessive postoperative hydrocele formation.

Step 7: Repair of Inguinal Floor

Methods of repairing the inguinal floor differ significantly among the various repairs and thus are described separately [see Details of Specific Repairs, below].

Step 8: Relaxing Incision

A relaxing incision is made through the anterior rectus sheath and down to the rectus abdominis, extending superiorly from the pubic tubercle for a variable distance, as determined by the degree of tension present. Some surgeons prefer to "hockeystick" the incision laterally at the superior end. The posterior rectus sheath is strong enough to prevent future incisional herniation. This relaxing incision works because as the anterior rectus sheath separates, the various components of the abdominal wall are displaced laterally and inferiorly.

Step 9: Closure

Closure of the external oblique fascia serves to reconstruct the superficial (external) ring. The external ring must be loose enough to prevent strangulation of the cord structures yet tight enough to ensure that an inexperienced examiner will not confuse a dilated ring with a recurrence. A dilated external ring is sometimes referred to as an industrial hernia, because over the years it has occasionally been a problem during preemployment physical examinations. Scarpa's fascia and the skin are closed to complete the operation.

Details of Specific Repairs

Marcy repair The Marcy repair is the simplest nonprosthetic repair performed today. Its main indication is for treatment of Nyhus type 1 hernias (i.e., indirect inguinal hernias in which the internal ring is normal). It is appropriate for children and young adults in whom there is concern about the long-term effects of prosthetic material. The essential features of the Marcy repair are high ligation of the sac and narrowing of the internal ring. Displacing the cord structures laterally allows the placement of sutures through the muscular and fascial layers [*see Figure 4*].

Bassini repair Edoardo Bassini (1844–1924) is considered the father of modern inguinal hernia surgery. By combining high ligation of a hernial sac with reconstruction of the inguinal floor and taking advantage of the developing disciplines of antisepsis and anesthesia, he was able to reduce morbidity and mortality substantially. Before Bassini's achievements, elective herniorrhaphy was almost never recommended, because the results were so bad. Bassini's operation, known as the radical cure, became the gold standard for inguinal hernia repair for most of the 20th century.

The initial steps in the procedure are essentially as already described (see above). Bassini felt that the incision in the external oblique aponeurosis should be as superior as possible while still allowing the superficial external ring to be opened,[12] so that the

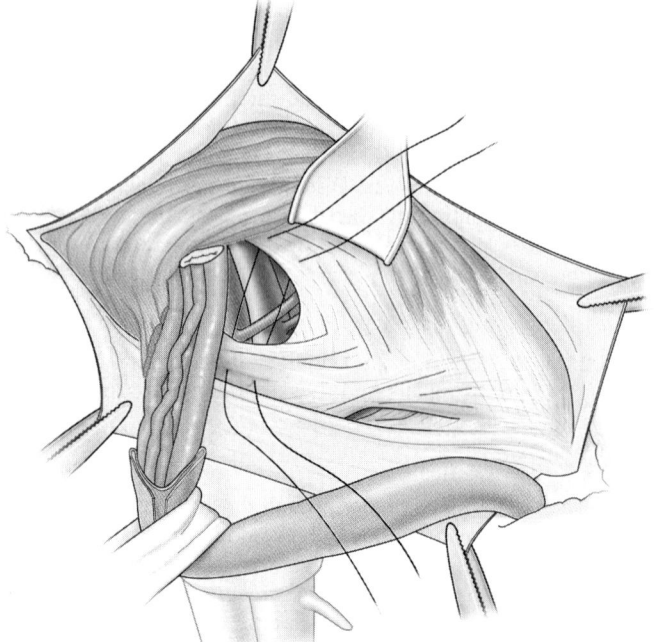

Figure 4 **Inguinal herniorrhaphy: Marcy repair. The deep inguinal ring is narrowed medially with several sutures that approximate the transverse aponeurotic arch to the iliopubic tract.**

reapproximation suture line created later in the operation would not be directly over the suture line of the inguinal floor reconstruction. Whether this technical point is significant is debatable. Bassini also felt that lengthwise division of the cremaster muscle followed by resection was important for ensuring that an indirect hernial sac could not be missed and for achieving adequate exposure of the inguinal floor.

After performing the initial dissection and the reduction or ligation of the sac, Bassini began the reconstruction of the inguinal floor by opening the transversalis fascia from the internal inguinal ring to the pubic tubercle, thereby exposing the preperitoneal fat, which was bluntly dissected away from the undersurface of the superior flap of the transversalis fascia [*see Figure 5a*]. This step allowed him to properly prepare the deepest structure in his famous "triple layer" (comprising the transversalis fascia, the transversus abdominis, and the internal oblique muscle).

The first stitch in Bassini's repair includes the triple layer superiorly and the periosteum of the medial side of the pubic tubercle, along with the rectus sheath. In current practice, however, most surgeons try to avoid the periosteum of the pubic tubercle so as to decrease the incidence of osteitis pubis. The repair is then continued laterally, and the triple layer is secured to the reflected inguinal ligament (Poupart's ligament) with nonabsorbable sutures. The sutures are continued until the internal ring is closed on its medial side [*see Figure 5b*]. A relaxing incision was not part of Bassini's original description but now is commonly added.

Concerns about injuries to neurovascular structures in the preperitoneal space as well as to the bladder led many surgeons, especially in North America, to abandon the opening of the transversalis fascia. The unfortunate consequence of this decision is that the proper development of the triple layer is severely compromised. In lieu of opening the floor, a forceps (e.g., an Allis clamp) is used to grasp tissue blindly in the hope of including the transversalis fascia and the transversus abdominis. The layer is then sutured, along with the internal oblique muscle, to the reflected inguinal ligament as in the classic Bassini repair. The structure grasped in this modified procedure is sometimes referred to as the conjoined tendon, but this is not correct because of the variability in what is actually grasped in the clamp. This imprecise "good stuff to good stuff" approach almost certainly accounts for the inferior results achieved with the Bassini procedure in the United States.

Maloney darn The Maloney darn gets its name from the way in which a long nylon suture is repeatedly passed between the tissues to create a weave that one might consider similar to a mesh. After initial preparation of the groin (see above), a continuous nylon suture is used to oppose the transversus abdominis, the rectus abdominis, the internal oblique muscle, and the transversalis fascia medially to Poupart's ligament laterally. The suture is continued into the muscle around the cord and is woven in and out to form a reinforcement around the cord. On the lateral side of the cord, it is sutured to the inguinal ligament and tied. The darn is a second layer. The sutures are placed either parallel or in a crisscross fashion and are plicated well into the inguinal ligament below. The darn must be carried well over the medial edge of the inguinal canal. Once the darn is complete, the external oblique muscle is closed over the cord structures. The Maloney darn can be considered a forerunner of the mesh repairs, in that the purpose of the darn is to provide a scaffold for tissue ingrowth.[13]

Shouldice repair Steps 1 through 6 are performed essentially as previously described (see above). Particular importance

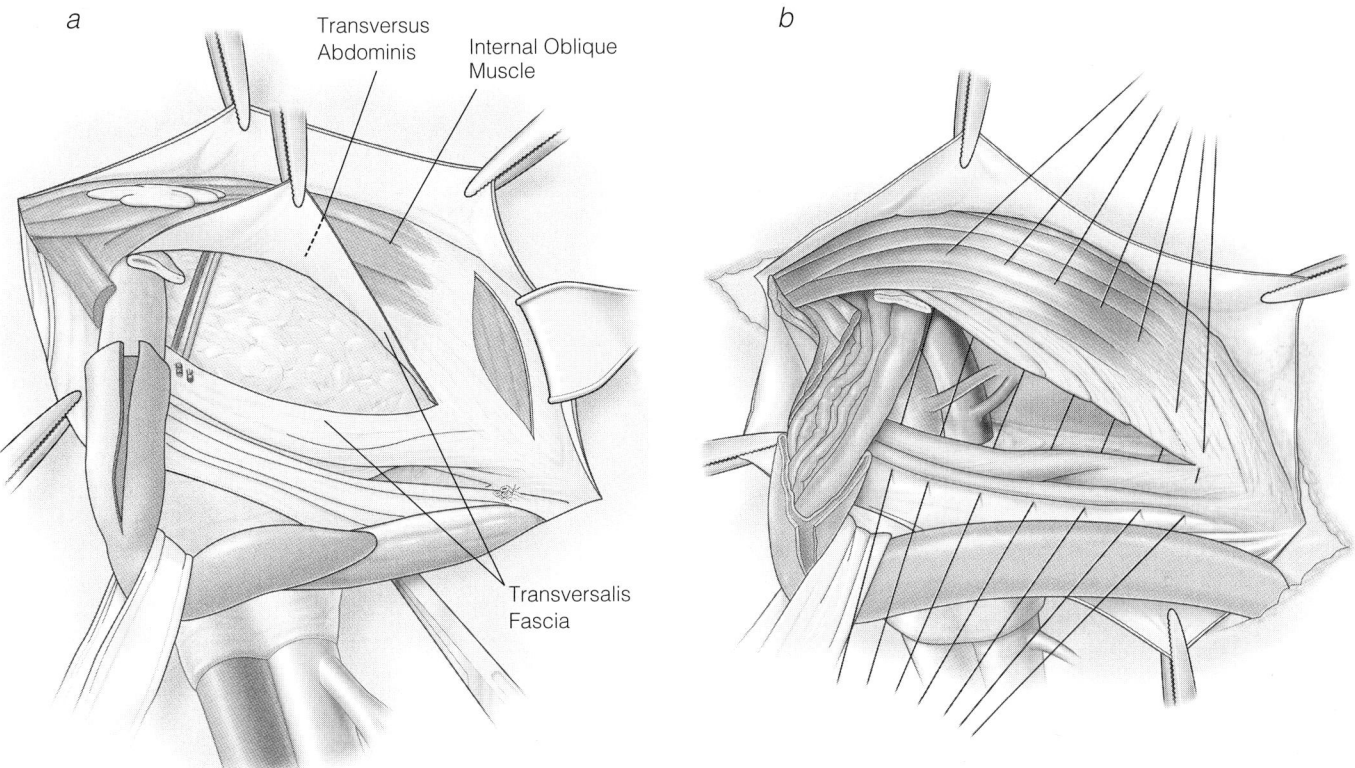

Figure 5   **Inguinal herniorrhaphy: Bassini repair. (*a*) The transversalis fascia has been opened and the preperitoneal fat stripped away to prepare the deepest structure in Bassini's triple layer (comprising the transversalis fascia, the transversus abdominis, and the internal oblique muscle). (*b*) The triple layer superiorly is approximated to the inguinal ligament, beginning medially at the pubic tubercle and extending laterally until the deep inguinal ring is sufficiently narrowed.**

is placed on freeing of the cord from its surrounding adhesions, resection of the cremaster muscle, high dissection of the hernial sac, and division of the transversalis fascia during the initial steps of the procedure.[14] A continuous nonabsorbable suture (typically of monofilament steel wire) is used to repair the floor. The Shouldice surgeons believe that a continuous suture distributes tension evenly and prevents potential defects between interrupted sutures that could lead to recurrence.

The repair is started at the pubic tubercle by approximating the iliopubic tract laterally to the undersurface of the lateral edge of the rectus abdominis [*see Figure 6a*]. The suture is continued laterally, approximating the iliopubic tract to the medial flap, which is made up of the transversalis fascia, the internal oblique muscle, and the transversus abdominis. Eventually, four suture lines are developed from the medial flap. The continuous suture is extended to the internal ring, where the lateral stump of the cremaster muscle is picked up to form a new internal ring. Next, the direction of the suture is reversed back toward the pubic tubercle, approximating the medial edges of the internal oblique muscle and the transversus abdominis to Poupart's ligament, and the wire is tied to itself and then to the first knot [*see Figure 6b*]. Thus, two suture lines are formed by the first suture.

A second wire suture is started near the internal ring, approximating the internal oblique muscle and the transversus abdominis to a band of external oblique aponeurosis superficial and parallel to Poupart's ligament—in effect, creating a second, artificial Poupart's ligament. This third suture line ends at the pubic crest. The suture is then reversed, and a fourth suture line is constructed in a similar manner, superficial to the third line. At the

Shouldice clinic, the cribriform fascia is always incised in the thigh, parallel to the inguinal ligament, to make the inner side of the lower flap of the external oblique aponeurosis available for these multiple layers. In general practice, however, this step is commonly omitted.

The results at the Shouldice clinic have been truly outstanding and continue to be so today. For a time, the Shouldice repair was the gold standard against which all newer procedures were compared. The major criticism of this operation is that it is difficult to teach because surgeons have problems understanding what is really being sewn to what. Unless one is specifically trained at the Shouldice clinic and has the opportunity to work with the surgeons there, one may find it hard to identify the various layers in the medial flap reliably and reproducibly—a step that is crucial for developing the multiple suture lines. To compound the difficulty, modifications developed outside the Shouldice clinic have given rise to different versions of the procedure. For example, some surgeons use three continuous layers instead of four for reconstruction of the inguinal floor.

McVay Cooper's ligament repair   This operation is similar to the Bassini repair, except that it uses Cooper's ligament instead of the inguinal ligament for the medial portion of the repair. Interrupted sutures are placed from the pubic tubercle laterally along Cooper's ligament, progressively narrowing the femoral ring; this constitutes the most common application of the repair—namely, treatment of a femoral hernia [*see Figure 7*]. The last stitch in Cooper's ligament is known as a transition stitch and includes the inguinal ligament. This stitch has two purposes: (1) to com-

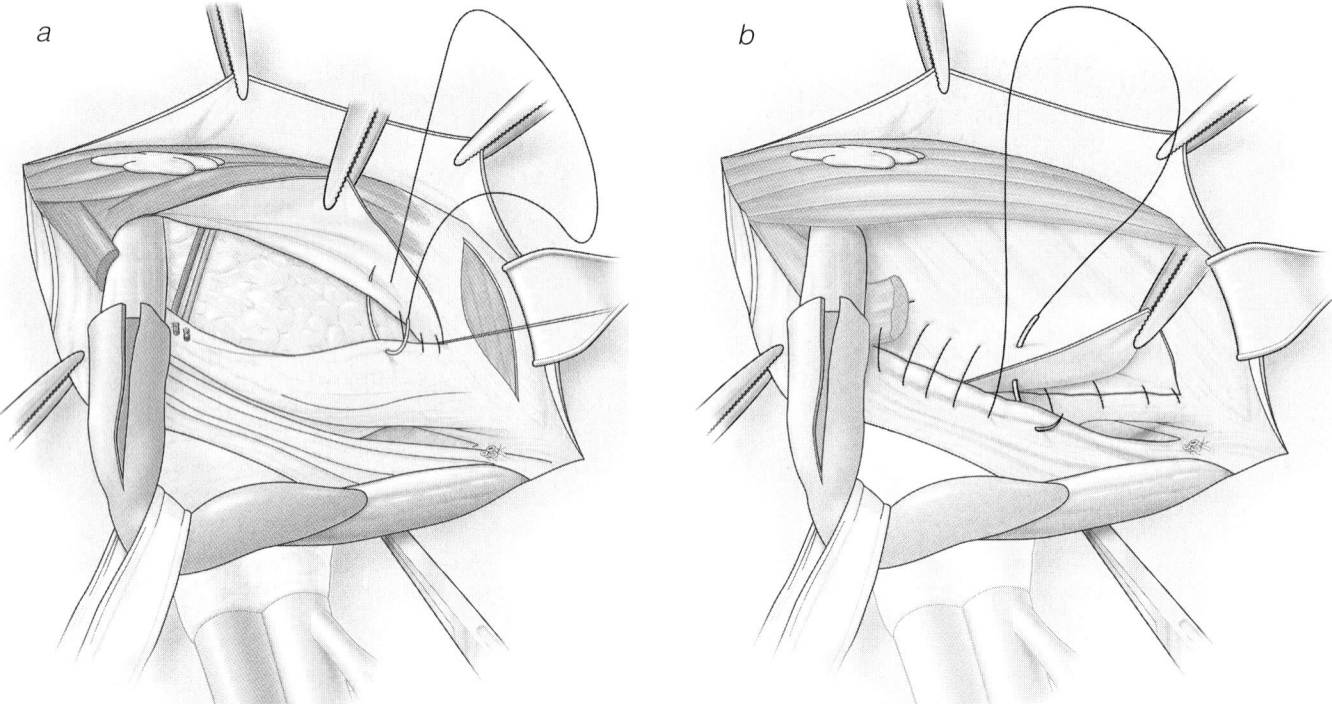

Figure 6 **Inguinal herniorrhaphy: Shouldice repair. (*a*) The first suture line starts at the pubic tubercle by approximating the iliopubic tract laterally to the undersurface of the lateral edge of the rectus abdominis. The suture is continued
laterally, approximating the iliopubic tract to the medial flap (made up of the transversalis fascia, the internal oblique
muscle, and the transversus abdominis). (*b*) The second suture line begins after the stump of the divided cremaster muscle has been picked up. The direction of the suture is reversed back toward the pubic tubercle, approximating the medial
edges of the internal oblique muscle and the transversus abdominis to Poupart's ligament. Two more suture lines will be
constructed by approximating the internal oblique muscle and the transversus abdominis to a band of the inferior flap of
the external oblique aponeurosis superficial and parallel to Poupart's ligament—in effect, creating a second and a third
artificial Poupart's ligament.**

plete the narrowing of the femoral ring by approximating the
inguinal ligament to Cooper's ligament, as well as to the medial
tissue, and (2) to provide a smooth transition to the inguinal ligament over the femoral vessel so that the repair can be continued
laterally (as in a Bassini repair). Given the considerable tension
required to bridge such a large distance, a relaxing incision should
always be used. In the view of many authorities, this tension results
in more pain than is noted with other herniorrhaphies and predisposes to recurrence. For this reason, the McVay repair is rarely
chosen today, except in patients with a femoral hernia or patients
with a specific contraindication to mesh repair.

Subinguinal femoral hernia repair   Femoral hernias in
females can easily be approached via a groin incision with dissection into the fossa ovalis beneath the inguinal ligament without the
external oblique fascia being opened. The defect can be either
closed with sutures or bridged with a mesh plug prosthesis [*see
Figure 8*]. Larger femoral hernias in females and all femoral hernias
in males are better treated with a McVay Cooper's ligament repair.

Pediatric hernia repair   Children and young adults commonly present with an indirect sac only, with no discernible
destruction of the inguinal floor. An extensive repair is not indicated: nearly all such patients are cured with sac ligation or eversion alone. A Marcy repair is the most extensive procedure that
should be considered in this population.

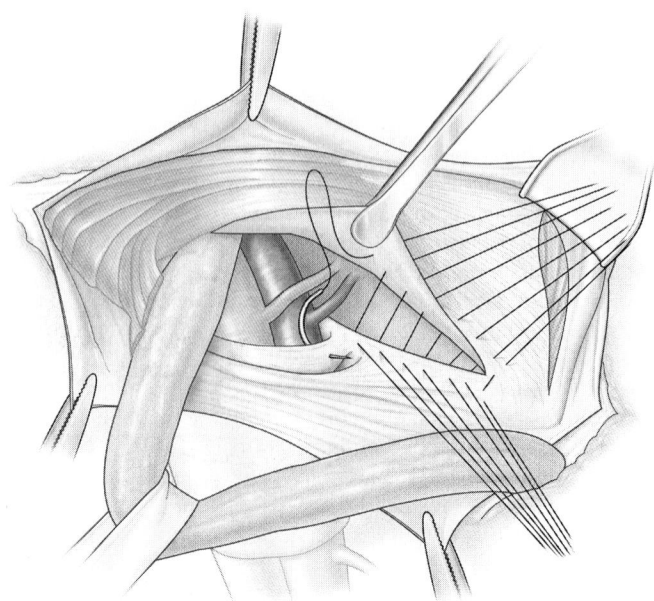

Figure 7 **Inguinal herniorrhaphy: McVay Cooper's ligament
repair. The lateral stitch is the transition stitch to the femoral
sheath and the inguinal ligament.**

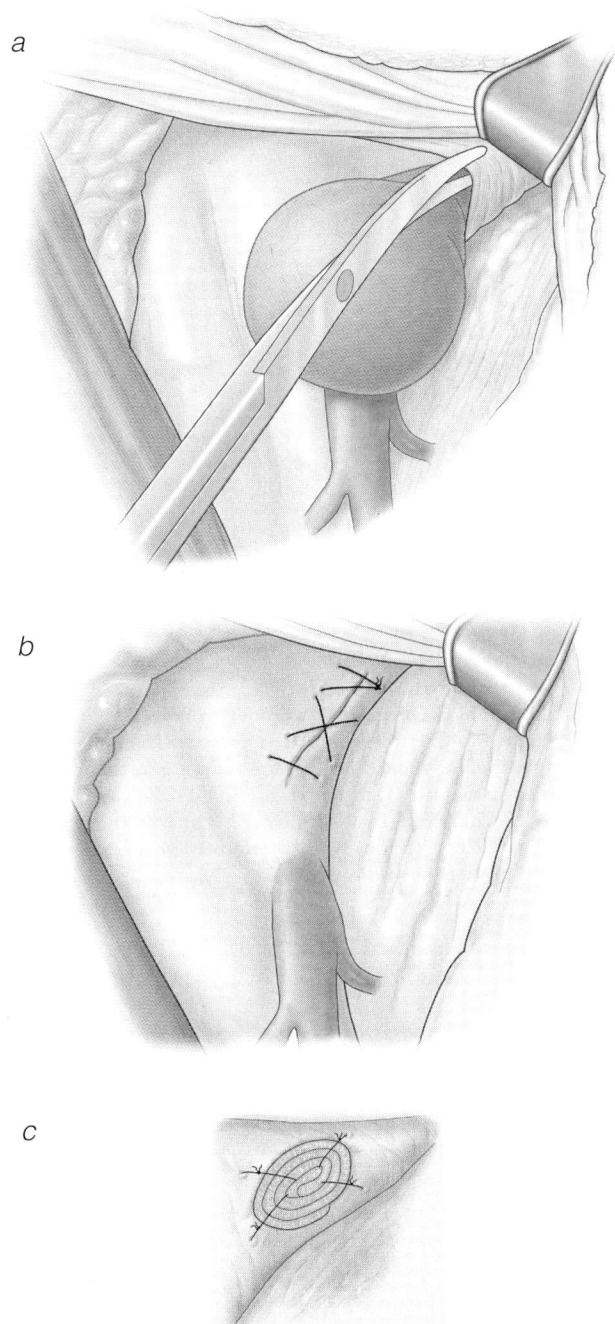

a

b

c

Figure 8 Inguinal herniorrhaphy: femoral hernia repair in females. The femoral canal is opened by dividing the inguinal ligament, the lacunar ligament, or both to facilitate reduction of the contents of the hernia. (*a*) The repair is then accomplished with either a continuous suture (*b*) or a mesh plug (*c*).

Inguinal Herniorrhaphy: Conventional Anterior Prosthetic Repairs

LICHTENSTEIN REPAIR

Steps 1 through 6

The first six steps of a Lichtenstein repair are very similar to the first six steps of a conventional anterior nonprosthetic repair [*see* Inguinal Herniorrhaphy: Conventional Anterior Nonprosthetic Repairs, *above*], but there are certain technical points that are worthy of emphasis. The external oblique aponeurosis is generously freed from the underlying anterior rectus sheath and internal oblique muscle and aponeurosis in an avascular plane from a point at least 2 cm medial to the pubic tubercle to the anterior superior iliac spine laterally. Blunt dissection is continued in this avascular plane from the area lateral to the internal ring to the pubic tubercle along the shelving edge of the inguinal ligament and the iliopubic tract. As a continuation of this same motion, the cord with its cremaster covering is swept off the pubic tubercle and separated from the inguinal floor. Besides mobilizing the cord, these maneuvers create a large space beneath the external oblique aponeurosis that can eventually be used for prosthesis placement. The ilioinguinal nerve, the external spermatic vessels, and the genital branch of the genitofemoral nerve all remain with the cord structures.

For indirect hernias, the cremaster muscle is incised longitudinally, and the sac is dissected free and reduced into the preperitoneal space. Theoretically, this operation could be criticized on the grounds that if the inguinal floor is not opened, an occult femoral hernia might be overlooked. To date, however, an excessive incidence of missed femoral hernias has not been reported. In addition, it is possible to evaluate the femoral ring via the space of Bogros through a small opening in the canal floor.

Direct hernias are separated from the cord and other surrounding structures and reduced back into the preperitoneal space. Dividing the superficial layers of the neck of the sac circumferentially—which, in effect, opens the inguinal floor—usually facilitates reduction and helps maintain it while the prosthesis is being placed. This opening in the inguinal floor also allows the surgeon to palpate for a femoral hernia. Sutures can be used to maintain reduction of the sac, but they have no real strength in this setting; their main purpose is to allow the repair to proceed without being hindered by continual extrusion of the sac into the field, especially when the patient strains.

Step 7: Placement of Prosthesis

A mesh prosthesis is positioned over the inguinal floor. For an adult, the prosthesis should be at least 15 × 8 cm. The medial end is rounded to correspond to the patient's particular anatomy and secured to the anterior rectus sheath at least 2 cm medial to the pubic tubercle. A continuous suture of either nonabsorbable or long-lasting absorbable material should be used. Wide overlap of the pubic tubercle is important to prevent the pubic tubercle recurrences all too commonly seen with other operations. The suture is continued laterally in a locking fashion, securing the prosthesis to either side of the pubic tubercle (not into it) and then to the shelving edge of the inguinal ligament. The suture is tied at the internal ring.

Step 8: Creation of Shutter Valve

A slit is made at the lateral end of the mesh in such a way as to create two tails, a wider one (approximately two thirds of the total width) above and a narrower one below. The tails are positioned around the cord structures and placed beneath the external oblique aponeurosis laterally to about the anterior superior iliac spine, with the upper tail placed on top of the lower. A single interrupted suture is placed to secure the lower edge of the superior tail to the lower edge of the inferior tail—in effect, creating a shutter valve. This step is considered crucial for preventing the indirect recurrences occasionally seen when the tails are simply reapproximated. The same suture incorporates the shelving edge of the inguinal ligament so as to create a domelike buckling effect over the direct space, thereby ensuring that there is no tension, especially when the patient assumes an upright postion. The Lichtenstein group has now developed a customized prosthesis with a built-in domelike configuration, which, in their view, makes suturing the approximated tails to the inguinal ligament unnecessary.

Step 9: Securing of Prosthesis

A few interrupted sutures are placed to attach the superior and medial aspects of the prosthesis to the underlying internal oblique muscle and rectus fascia [see Figure 9]. On occasion, the iliohypogastric nerve, which courses on top of the internal oblique muscle, penetrates the medial flap of the external oblique aponeurosis. In this situation, the prosthesis should be slit to accommodate the nerve. The prosthesis can be trimmed in situ, but care should be taken to maintain enough laxity to allow for the difference between the supine and the upright positions, as well as for possible shrinkage of the mesh.

Step 10: Repair of Femoral Hernia

If a femoral hernia is present, the posterior surface of the mesh is sutured to Cooper's ligament after the inferior edge has been attached to the inguinal ligament, thereby closing the femoral canal.

Step 11: Closure

Closure is accomplished in the same manner as in a conventional anterior nonprosthetic repair.

PLUG-AND-PATCH REPAIR

The mesh plug technique was first developed by Gilbert and subsequently modified by Rutkow and Robbins, Millikan, and others [see Figure 10].[15-17] The groin is entered via a standard

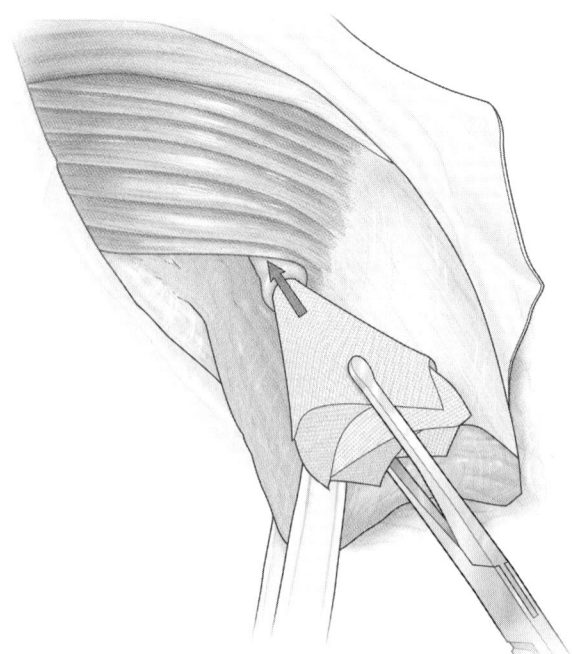

Figure 10 Inguinal herniorrhaphy: Gilbert repair. Depicted is the mesh plug technique for repair of an inguinal hernia. A flat sheet of polypropylene mesh is rolled up like a cigarette or formed into a cone (as shown here), inserted into the defect, and secured to either the internal ring (for an indirect hernia) or the neck of the defect (for a direct hernia) with interrupted sutures. Prefabricated mesh plugs are now available.

anterior approach. The hernial sac is dissected away from surrounding structures and reduced into the preperitoneal space. A flat sheet of polypropylene mesh is rolled up like a cigarette, tied, inserted in the defect, and secured with interrupted sutures to either the internal ring (for an indirect hernia) or the neck of the defect (for a direct hernia).

A prefabricated prosthesis that has the configuration of a flower is commercially available and is recommended by Rutkow and Robbins. This prosthesis is tailored to each patient's particular anatomy by removing some of the "petals" to avoid unnecessary bulk. Many surgeons consider this step important for preventing erosion into surrounding structures (e.g., the bladder); indeed, such complications have been reported, albeit rarely.

Millikan further modified the procedure by recommending that the inside petals be sewn to the ring of the defect. For an indirect hernia, the inside petals are sewn to the internal oblique portion of the internal ring, which forces the outside of the prosthesis underneath the inner side of the defect and makes it act like a preperitoneal underlay. For direct hernias, the inside petals are sewn to Cooper's ligament and the shelving edge of the inguinal ligament is sewn to the conjoined tendon, which, again, forces the outside of the prosthesis to act as an underlay.

The patch portion of the procedure is optional and involves placing a flat piece of polypropylene in the conventional inguinal space so that it widely overlaps the plug, much as in a Lichtenstein repair. The difference with a plug-and-patch repair is that only one or two sutures—or even, perhaps, no sutures—are used to secure the flat prosthesis to the underlying inguinal floor. Some surgeons, however, place so many sutures that they have in effect performed a Lichtenstein operation on top of the plug—a procedure sometimes referred to as a "plugstenstein."

To the credit of its proponents, the plug-and-patch repair, in all

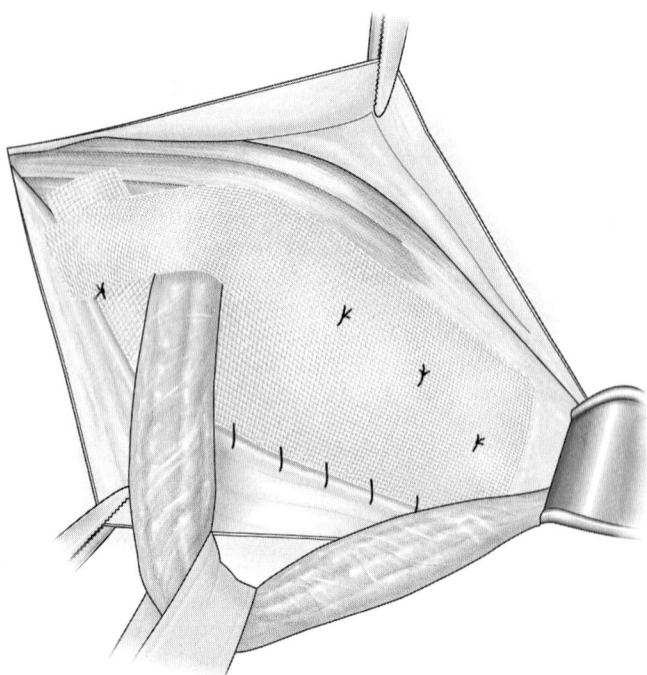

Figure 9 Inguinal herniorrhaphy: Lichtenstein repair. A mesh prosthesis is positioned over the inguinal floor and secured to the rectus sheath with a continuous suture. A slit is made in the mesh to accommodate the cord structures, and the two tails are secured to each other and to the shelving edge of the inguinal ligament with a single interrupted suture. The superior and medial aspects of the prosthesis are secured to the internal oblique muscle and the rectus fascia with a few interrupted sutures.

of its varieties, has been skillfully presented and has rapidly taken a significant share of the overall inguinal hernia market. It is not only fast but also extremely easy to teach, which has made it popular in both private and academic centers.

Inguinal Herniorrhaphy: Preperitoneal Nonprosthetic Repairs

A key technical issue in a preperitoneal hernia repair is how the surgeon chooses to enter the preperitoneal space. In fact, within this general class of repair, the method of entry into this space constitutes the major difference between the various procedures.

Many approaches to the preperitoneal space have been described. For example, the space can be entered either anteriorly or posteriorly. If an anterior technique is to be used, the initial steps of the operation are similar to those of a conventional anterior herniorrhaphy. If a posterior technique is to be used, any of several incisions (lower midline, paramedian, or Pfannenstiel) will allow an extraperitoneal dissection. The preperitoneal space can also be entered transabdominally. This is useful when the patient is undergoing a laparotomy for some other condition and the hernia is to be repaired incidentally. Of course, the transabdominal preperitoneal laparoscopic repairs described elsewhere [see 3:22 Laparoscopic Hernia Repair], by definition, enter the preperitoneal space from the abdomen.

Reed credits Annandale as being the first surgeon to describe the anterior method of gaining access to the preperitoneal space.[18] Bassini's operation, as classically performed, is technically an anterior preperitoneal operation, but it is never discussed in this group, because in the American variant of the procedure, the preperitoneal space is not entered. Cheatle suggested the posterior approach to the preperitoneal space for repair of an inguinal hernia but used a laparotomy to do it.[19] Cheatle and Henry subsequently modified the operation so as to render it entirely extraperitoneal (the so-called Cheatle-Henry approach), which made the procedure more acceptable to surgeons.[20]

The preperitoneal nonprosthetic method remained popular into the second half of the 20th century, championed by proponents such as Nyhus and Condon, who emphasized the importance of the iliopubic tract as the inferior border in primary closures of direct or indirect hernia defects.[21] Today, however, these operations are of little more than historical significance, because it is now universally agreed that better results are obtained in this space when a prosthesis is used. Indeed, after 1975, Nyhus and Condon began routinely placing a 6 × 14 cm piece of polypropylene mesh to buttress the primary repair in all patients with recurrent hernias.[22] When contraindications to a prosthesis are present [see Table 4], most surgeons would opt for a conventional anterior herniorrhaphy (e.g., a Bassini or Shouldice repair) rather than a preperitoneal nonprosthetic herniorrhaphy.

Inguinal Herniorrhaphy: Preperitoneal Prosthetic Repairs

The most important step in any preperitoneal prosthetic repair is the placement of a large prosthesis in the preperitoneal space on the abdominal side of the defect in the transversalis fascia. The theoretical advantage of this measure is that whereas in a conventional repair abdominal pressure might contribute to recurrence, in a preperitoneal repair, the abdominal pressure would actually help fix the mesh material against the abdominal wall, thereby adding strength to the repair. The hernia defect itself may or may not be closed, depending on the preference of the surgeon. The strength of the repair depends on the prosthesis rather

---

Table 4 Contraindications to Use of Prosthesis for Herniorrhaphy

Local infection*[52]	Allergy
Systemic infection	Patient preference

*The newer biological prostheses made of human cadaver skin or of submucosa from porcine small intestine may be acceptable.

---

than on closure of the defect; however, such closure may decrease the seroma formation that inevitably occurs at the site of the undisturbed residual sac. Although these seromas almost always are self-limited and disappear with time, they can be confused with recurrences by both patients and referring physicians. Accordingly, some surgeons prefer to take every step possible to prevent them.

ANTERIOR APPROACH

Read-Rives Repair

The initial part of a Read-Rives repair, including the opening of the inguinal floor, is much like that of a classic Bassini repair. The inferior epigastric vessels are identified and the preperitoneal space completely dissected. The spermatic cord is parietalized by separating the ductus deferens from the spermatic vessels. A 12 × 16 cm piece of mesh is positioned in the preperitoneal space deep to the inferior epigastric vessels and secured with three sutures placed in the pubic tubercle, in Cooper's ligament, and in the psoas muscle laterally. The transversalis fascia is closed over the prosthesis and the cord structures replaced. The rest of the closure is accomplished much as in a conventional anterior prosthetic repair.

POSTERIOR APPROACH

Stoppa-Rignault-Wantz Repair (Giant Prosthetic Reinforcement of Visceral Sac)

GPRVS has its roots in the important contribution that Henri Fruchaud made to herniology. In describing the myopectineal orifice that bears his name [see Figure 11], Fruchaud, who was Stoppa's mentor, popularized a different approach to the etiology of inguinal hernias.[23] Instead of subdividing hernias into direct, indirect, and femoral and then examining their specific causes, he emphasized that the common cause of all inguinal hernias was the failure of the transversalis fascia to retain the peritoneum. This concept led Stoppa to develop GPRVS, which reestablishes the integrity of the peritoneal sac by inserting a large permanent prosthesis that entirely replaces the transversalis fascia over the myopectineal orifice of Fruchaud with wide overlapping of surrounding tissue. With GPRVS, the exact type of hernia present (direct, indirect, or femoral) is unimportant, because the abdominal wall defect is not addressed.

Step 1: skin incision A lower midline, inguinal, or Pfannenstiel incision can be used, depending on the surgeon's preference. The inguinal incision is placed 2 to 3 cm below the level of the anterior superior iliac spine but above the internal ring; it is begun at the midline and extended laterally for 8 to 9 cm.[24]

Step 2: preperitoneal dissection The fascia overlying the space of Retzius is opened without violation of the peritoneum. A combination of blunt and sharp dissection is continued later-

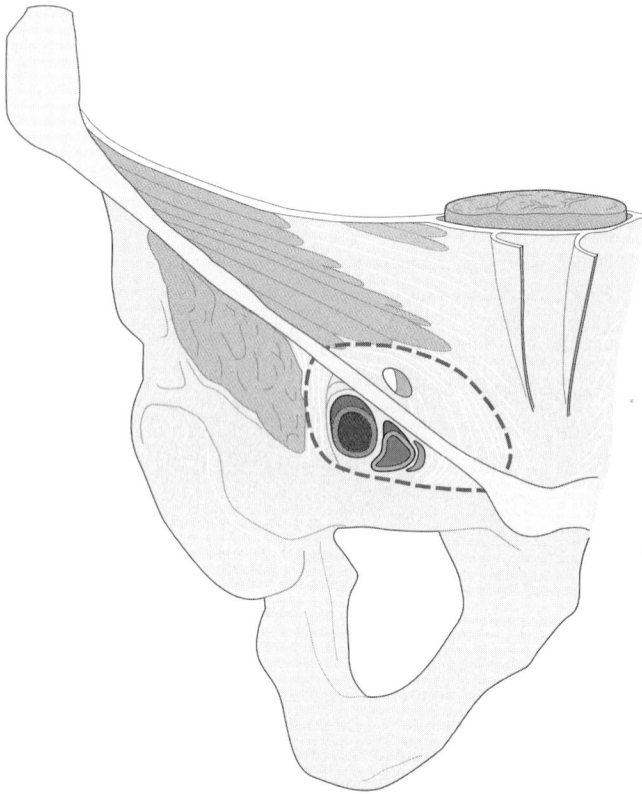

Figure 11 **Inguinal herniorrhaphy. Depicted is the myopectineal orifice of Fruchaud. The area is bounded superiorly by the internal oblique muscle and the transversus abdominis, medially by the rectus muscle and sheath, laterally by the iliopsoas muscle, and inferiorly by Cooper's ligament. Critical anatomic landmarks (e.g., the inguinal ligament, the spermatic cord, and the femoral vessels) are contained within this structure.**

the cord structures and reduced back into the peritoneal cavity. Large sacs may be difficult to mobilize from the cord without undue trauma if an attempt is made to remove the sac in its entirety. Accordingly, large sacs should be divided, with the distal portion left in situ and the proximal portion dissected away from the cord structures. Division of the sac is most easily accomplished by opening the sac on the side opposite the cord structures. A finger is placed in the sac to facilitate its separation from the cord. Downward traction is then placed on the cord structures to reduce any excessive fatty tissue (so-called lipoma of the cord) back into the preperitoneal space. This step prevents the "pseudorecurrences" that may occur if the abnormality palpated during the preoperative physical examination was not a hernia but a lipoma of the cord.

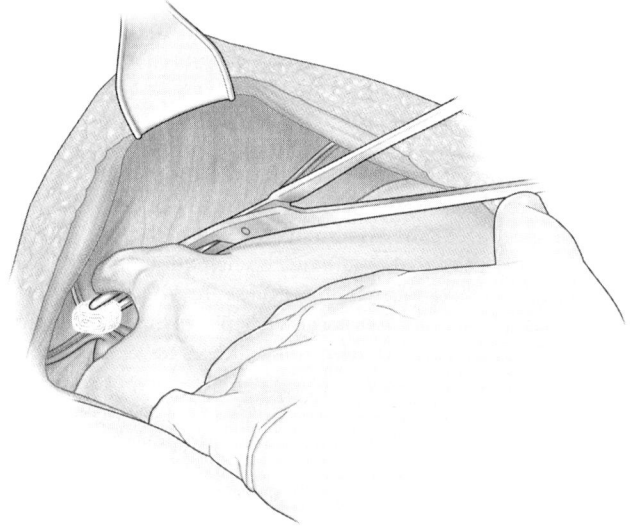

Figure 12 **Inguinal herniorrhaphy: preperitoneal repair. The preperitoneal space is widely dissected from the pubic tubercle to the anterior superior iliac spine. Shown here is isolation of an indirect hernial sac.**

ally posterior to the rectus abdominis and the inferior epigastric vessels. The preperitoneal space is completely dissected to a point lateral to the anterior superior iliac spine [*see Figure 12*]. The symphysis pubis, Cooper's ligament, and the iliopubic tract are identified. Inferiorly, the peritoneum is generously dissected away from the vas deferens and the internal spermatic vessels to create a large pocket, which will eventually accommodate a prosthesis without the possibility of rollup. In the inguinal approach, the anterior rectus sheath and the oblique muscles are incised for the length of the skin incision. The lower flaps of these structures are retracted inferiorly toward the pubis. The transversalis fascia is incised along the lateral edge of the rectus abdominis, and the preperitoneal space is entered; dissection then proceeds as previously indicated.

Step 3: management of hernial sac   Direct hernial sacs are reduced during the course of the preperitoneal dissection. Care must be taken to stay in the plane between the peritoneum and the transversalis fascia, allowing the latter structure to retract into the hernia defect toward the skin. The transversalis fascia can be thin, and if it is inadvertently opened and incorporated with the peritoneal sac during reduction, a needless and bloody dissection of the abdominal wall is the result.

Indirect sacs are more difficult to deal with than direct sacs are, in that they often adhere to the cord structures. Trauma to the cord must be minimized to prevent damage to the vas deferens or the testicular blood supply. Small sacs should be mobilized from

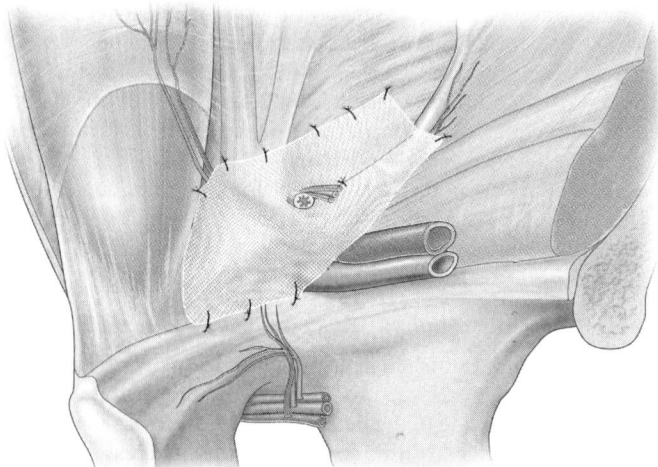

Figure 13 **Inguinal herniorrhaphy: preperitoneal repair. Illustrated is the placement of a mesh prosthesis in the preperitoneal space. The prosthesis is sewn to Cooper's ligament inferiorly and to the transverse fascia well above the hernia defect anteriorly, in the fashion described by Nyhus.**

Step 4: management of abdominal wall defect It is this step that varies most from one author to another. In Nyhus's approach, the defect is formally repaired, and only then is a tailored mesh prosthesis sutured to Cooper's ligament and the transversalis fascia for reinforcement [*see Figure 13*]. In Rignault's approach, the defect is loosely closed to prevent an unsightly early postoperative bulge.[25] In Stoppa's and Wantz's approaches, the defect is usually left alone, but the transversalis fascia in the defect is occasionally plicated by suturing it to Cooper's ligament to prevent the bulge caused by a seroma in the undisturbed sac.

Step 5: parietalization of spermatic cord The term parietalization of the spermatic cord, popularized by Stoppa, refers to a thorough dissection of the cord aimed at providing sufficient length to permit lateral movement of the structure [*see Figure 14*]. In Stoppa's view, this step is essential, in that it allows a prosthesis to be placed without having to be split laterally to accommodate the cord structures; the keyhole defect created when the prosthesis is split has been linked with recurrences. In Rignault's view, on the other hand, creation of a keyhole defect in the mesh to encircle the spermatic cord is preferable, the rationale being that this gives the prosthesis enough security to allow the surgeon to dispense with fixation sutures or tacks. Minimizing fixation in this area is important because of the numerous anatomic elements in the preperitoneal space that can be inadvertently damaged during suture placement.

Step 6: placement of prosthesis Dacron mesh, being more pliable than polypropylene, conforms well to the preperitoneal space and is therefore considered particularly suitable for GPRVS.

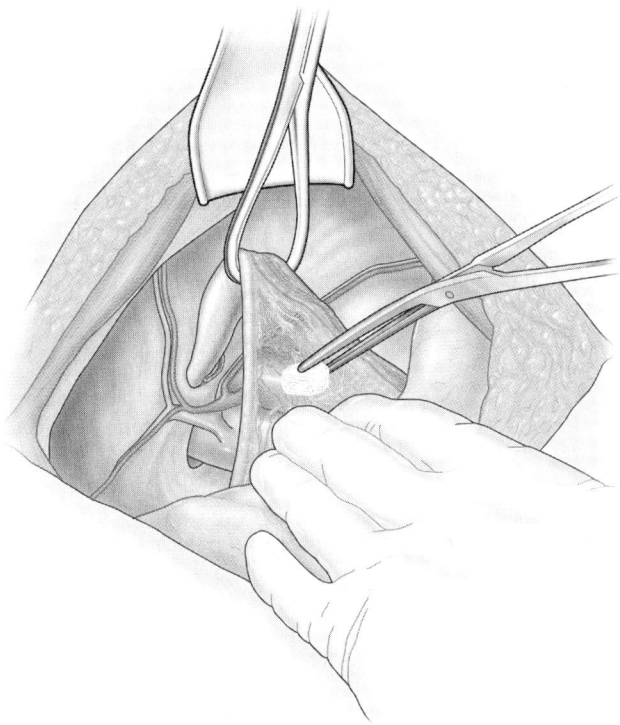

Figure 14 **Inguinal herniorrhaphy: preperitoneal repair. Illustrated is the parietalization of the spermatic cord. The spermatic vessels and the vas deferens are mobilized so that they move laterally. This step is carried out so that the surgeon can place a large prosthesis that widely overlaps the myopectineal orifice without having to slit the prosthesis to accommodate the cord structures.**

Stoppa's technique is most often associated with a single large prosthesis for bilateral hernias. The prosthesis is cut in the shape of a chevron [*see Figure 15a*], and eight clamps are positioned strategically around the prosthesis to facilitate placement into the preperitoneal space [*see Figure 15b*].

Unilateral repairs require a prosthesis that is approximately 15 × 12 cm but is cut so that the bottom edge is wider than the top edge and the lateral side is longer than the medial side. In Wantz's technique, three absorbable sutures are used to attach the superior border of the prosthesis to the anterior abdominal wall well above the defect [*see Figure 16*]. The sutures are placed from medial to lateral near the linea alba, the semilunar line, and the anterior superior iliac spine. A Reverdin suture needle facilitates this task. Three long clamps are then placed on each corner and the middle of the prosthesis of the inferior flap. The medial clamp is placed into the space of Retzius and held by an assistant. The middle clamp is positioned so that the mesh covers the pubic ramus, the obturator fossa, and the iliac vessels and is also held by the assistant. The lateral clamp is placed into the iliac fossa to cover the parietalized cord structures and the iliopsoas muscle. Care must be taken to prevent the prosthesis from rolling up as the clamps are removed.

Step 7: closure of the wound The surgical wound is closed along anatomic guidelines once the surgeon is assured that there has been no displacement or rollup of the prosthesis.

KUGEL AND UGAHARY REPAIRS

The Kugel and Ugahary repairs were developed to compete with laparoscopic repairs. They require only a small (2 to 3 cm) skin incision placed 2 to 3 cm above the internal ring.[26,27] In Kugel's operation, the incision is oriented obliquely, with one third of the incision lateral to a point halfway between the anterior superior iliac spine and the pubic tubercle and the remaining two thirds medial to this point. The incision is deepened through the external oblique fascia, and the internal oblique muscle is bluntly spread apart. The transversalis fascia is opened vertically for a distance of about 3 cm, but the internal ring is not violated. The preperitoneal space is entered and a blunt dissection performed. The inferior epigastric vessels are identified to confirm that the dissection is being done in the correct plane. These vessels should be left adherent to the overlying transversalis fascia and retracted medially and anteriorly. The iliac vessels, Cooper's ligament, the pubic bone, and the hernia defect are identified by palpation. Most hernial sacs are simply reduced; the exceptions are large indirect sacs, which must sometimes be divided, with the distal sac left in situ and the proximal sac closed. To prevent recurrences, the cord structures are thoroughly parietalized to allow adequate posterior dissection.

The key to Kugel's procedure is a specially designed 8 × 12 cm prosthesis made of two pieces of polypropylene with a single extruded monofilament fiber located near its edge. The construction of the prosthesis allows it to be deformed so that it can fit through the small incision; once inserted, it springs open to regain its normal shape, providing a wide overlap of the myopectineal orifice. The prosthesis also has a slit on its anterior surface, through which the surgeon places a finger to facilitate positioning.

Ugahary's operation is similar to Kugel's, but it does not require a special prosthesis. In what is known as the gridiron technique, the preperitoneal space is prepared through a 3 cm incision, much as in a Kugel repair. The space is held open with a narrow Langenbeck retractor and two ribbon retractors. A 10 × 15 cm piece of polypropylene mesh is rolled onto a long forceps

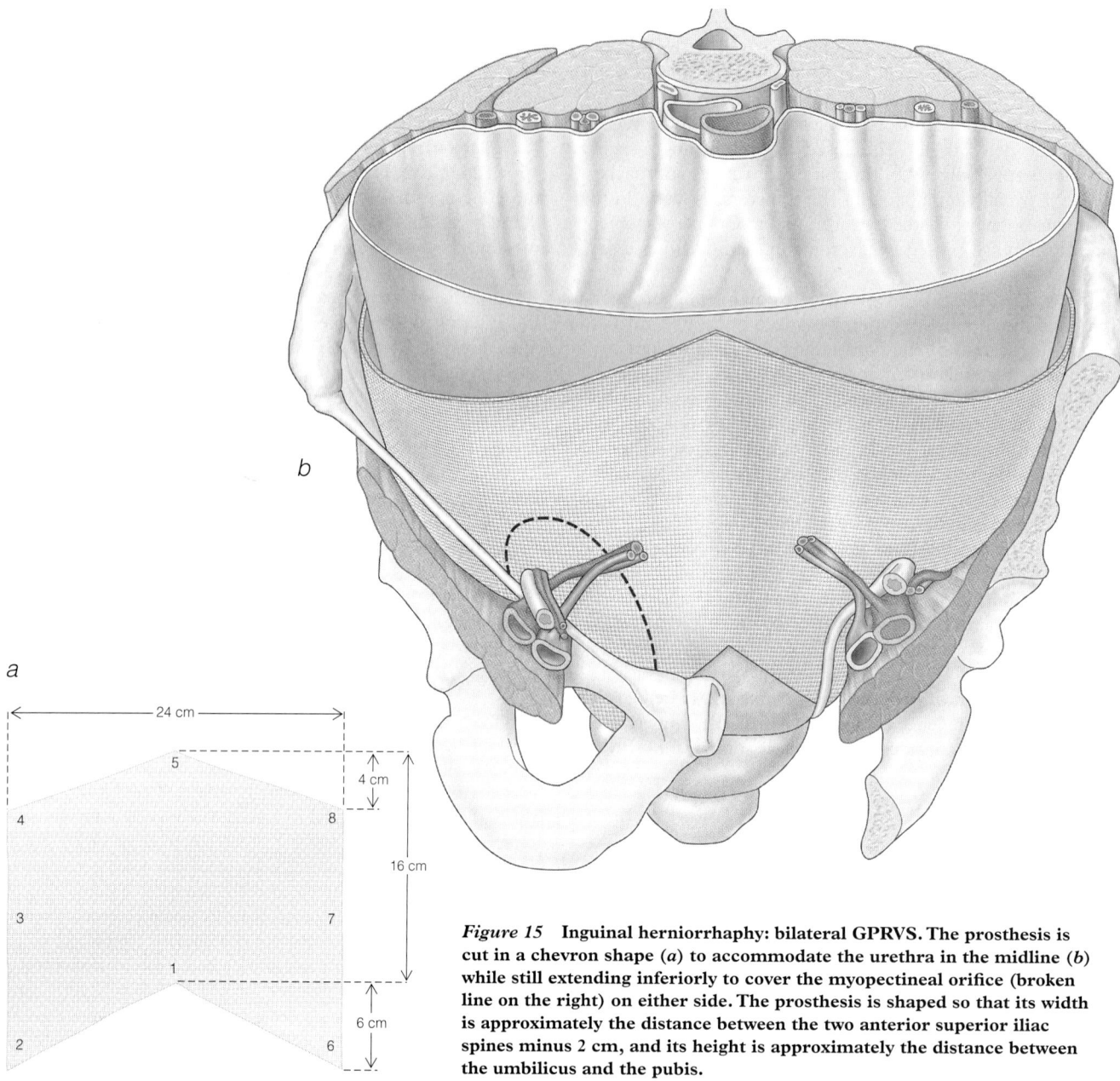

Figure 15 Inguinal herniorrhaphy: bilateral GPRVS. The prosthesis is cut in a chevron shape (*a*) to accommodate the urethra in the midline (*b*) while still extending inferiorly to cover the myopectineal orifice (broken line on the right) on either side. The prosthesis is shaped so that its width is approximately the distance between the two anterior superior iliac spines minus 2 cm, and its height is approximately the distance between the umbilicus and the pubis.

after the edges have been rounded and sutures placed to correspond to various anatomic landmarks. The forceps with the rolled-up mesh on it is introduced into the preperitoneal space, and the mesh is unrolled with the help of clamps and specific movements of the ribbon retractors.

Both operations have been very successful in some hands and have important proponents. However, because they are essentially blind repairs, considerable experience with them is required before the surgeon can be confident in his or her ability to place the patch properly.

COMBINED ANTERIOR-POSTERIOR APPROACH

Bilayer Prosthetic Repair

The bilayer prosthetic repair involves the use of a dumbbell-shaped prosthesis consisting of two flat pieces of polypropylene mesh connected by a cylinder of the same material. The purpose of this design is to allow the surgeon to take advantage of the pre-

sumed benefits of both anterior and posterior approaches by placing prosthetic material in both the preperitoneal space and the extraperitoneal space.

The initial steps are identical to those of a Lichtenstein repair. Once the conventional anterior space has been prepared, the preperitoneal space is entered through the hernia defect. Indirect hernias are reduced, and a gauze sponge is used to develop the preperitoneal space through the internal ring. For direct hernias, the transversalis fascia is opened, and the space between this structure and the peritoneum is developed with a gauze sponge. The deep layer of the prosthesis is deployed in the preperitoneal space, overlapping the direct and indirect spaces and Cooper's ligament. The superficial layer of the device occupies the conventional anterior space, much as in a Lichtenstein repair. It is slit laterally or centrally to accommodate the cord structures and then affixed to the area of the pubic tubercle, the middle of the inguinal ligament, and the internal oblique muscle with three or four interrupted sutures.

Inguinal Herniorrhaphy: Complications

POSTHERNIORRHAPHY GROIN PAIN

It is generally recognized that inguinal herniorrhaphy results in greater morbidity than was previously appreciated. Now that modern hernioplasty techniques have reduced recurrence rates to a minimum, chronic postoperative groin pain syndromes have emerged as the major complication facing inguinal hernia surgeons. In a crit-

ical review of inguinal herniorrhaphy studies between 1987 and 2000, the incidence of some degree of long-term groin pain after surgery was as high as 53% at 1 year (range, 0% to 53%).[28] In the absence of a standard raw database, it was somewhat difficult to extrapolate from these data, but the best estimate was that moderate to severe pain occurred in about 10% of patients and some degree of restriction of activity in about 25%.

Various postherniorrhaphy groin pain syndromes may develop,

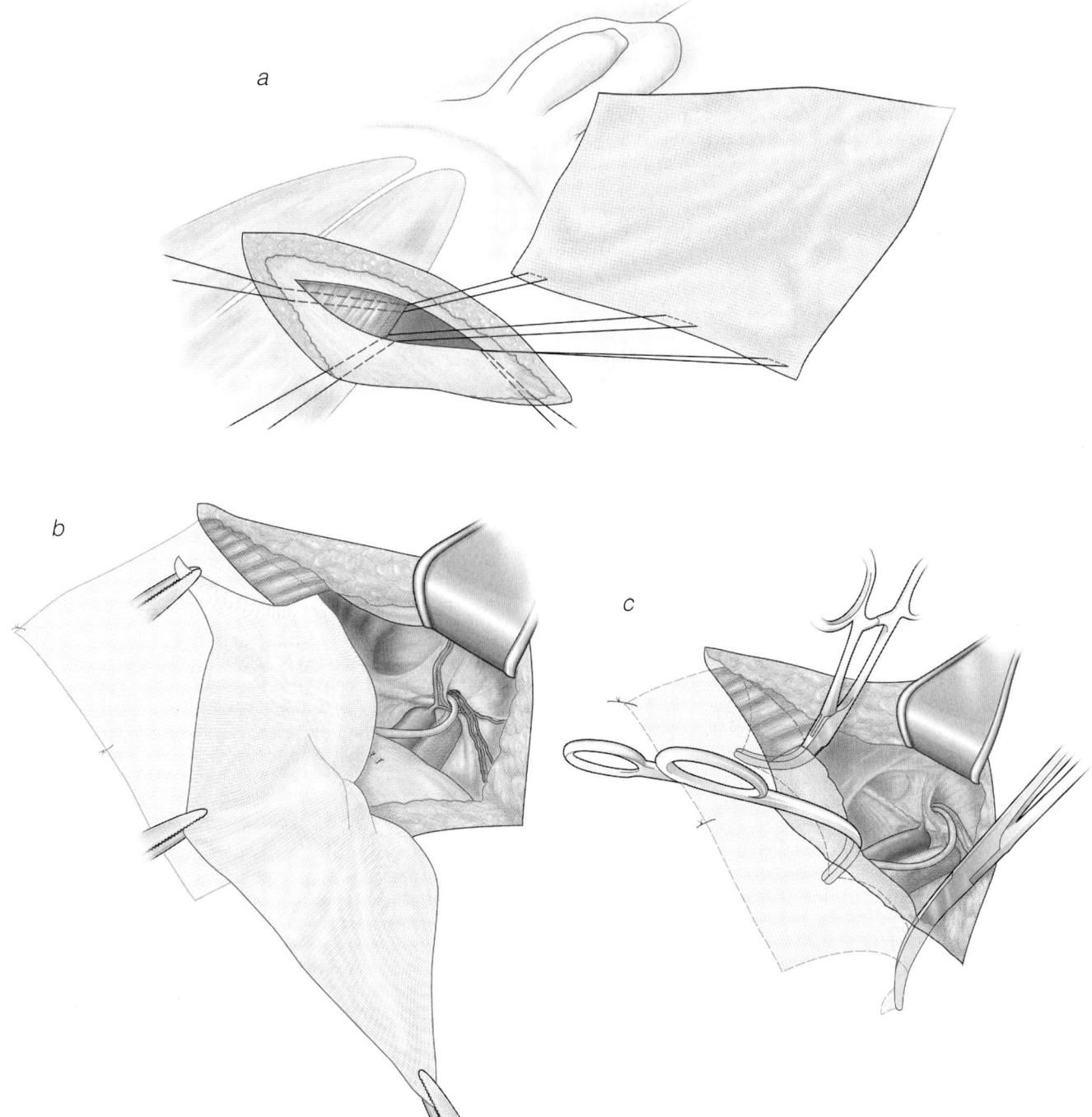

Figure 16   Inguinal herniorrhaphy: unilateral GPRVS (Wantz technique). The prosthesis is cut so that the inferior edge is wider than the superior edge by 2 to 4 cm and the lateral side is longer than the medial side. The width at the superior edge is approximately the distance between the umbilicus and the anterior superior iliac spine minus 1 cm, and the height is approximately 14 cm. Anteriorly, three sutures are placed—near the linea alba, near the semilunar line, and near the anterior superior iliac spine—from medial to lateral to fix the superior border (*a*). Three long clamps on the inferior edge (*b*) are used to implant the prosthesis deep into the preperitoneal space (*c*) with the peritoneal sac retracted cranially.

usually as a consequence of scarring, reaction to prosthetic material, or incorporation of a nerve in staples or suture material during the repair. Chronic postoperative groin pain occurs without regard to the type of repair performed. It can be classified into three general types, as follows:

1. Somatic (nociceptive) pain, the most common form, includes ongoing preoperative pathologic states that were the real causes of patients' pain preoperatively, usually related to ligament or muscle injury; new ligament or muscle injury caused by the operation; scar tissue; osteitis pubis; and reaction to prosthetic material.
2. Neuropathic pain is related to direct nerve damage. Accurate diagnosis is important because if the cause of pain is incorporation of a nerve in staples or sutures, effective surgical treatment is available. The nerves usually involved are the ilioinguinal nerve, the iliohypogastric nerve, the genital and femoral branches of the genitofemoral nerve, and the lateral cutaneous nerve of the thigh. The first two nerves are especially likely to be injured during a conventional herniorrhaphy, whereas the latter two are more likely to be damaged during a preperitoneal herniorrhaphy. Femoral nerve injury, fortunately, is extremely rare and is usually the result of a gross technical misadventure. Neuropathy is generally signaled by pain or paresthesia in the injured nerve's distribution; however, there is significant overlap in the distributions of these nerves, and as a result, it is frequently difficult to determine exactly which nerve is damaged.
3. Visceral pain is related to specific visceral functions; common examples are pain with urination and the dysejaculation syndrome.

Perhaps the most important single issue in dealing with postherniorrhaphy pain is whether the current pain is the same as or different from the pain that brought the hernia to the attention of the physician in the first place. If the latter is the case, efforts must be made to determine which of the numerous potential causative conditions is responsible. Computed tomography, ultrasonography, herniography, laparoscopy, and magnetic resonance imaging all are of diagnostic value in this setting. Of these, MRI has emerged as the most useful because of its ability to differentiate between muscle tears, osteitis pubis, bursitis, and stress fracture. A strain of the adductor muscle complex (comprising the adductor longus, the adductor brevis, the adductor magnus, and the gracilis) is a commonly overlooked cause of pain.

Treatment is difficult and often fails entirely. The difficulty is compounded when workers' compensation issues cloud the picture. The first possibility that must be ruled out is a recurrent hernia. As a rule, all three types of pain are best treated initially with reassurance and conservative treatment (e.g., anti-inflammatory medications and local nerve blocks); frequently, the complaint resolves spontaneously. The only exception to this rule might be the patient who complains of severe pain immediately (i.e., in the recovery room), who might be best treated with immediate reexploration before scar tissue develops. Otherwise, we scrupulously avoid reexploration in the first year after the procedure to allow for the possibility of spontaneous resolution. When groin exploration is required, neurectomy and neuroma excision, adhesiolysis, muscle or tendon repair, and foreign-body removal are all possibilities. The results are often less than satisfying.

ISCHEMIC ORCHITIS AND TESTICULAR ATROPHY

Orchitis or atrophy may result if the testicular blood supply is compromised during herniorrhaphy. Orchitis is defined as postoperative inflammation of the testicle occurring within the first 2

postoperative days. Patients experience painful enlargement and hardening of the testicle, usually associated with a low-grade fever; the pain is severe and may last several weeks. Ischemic orchitis is most likely attributable to thrombosis of the veins draining the testicle, caused by dissection of the spermatic cord. It may progress over a period of months and eventually result in testicular atrophy. This latter development is not inevitable, however. In fact, the occurrence of testicular atrophy is quite unpredictable, in that most patients with this condition have no history of any testicular problems associated with the index herniorrhaphy. Overall, the vast majority of patients who experience testicular problems as an immediate complication of herniorrhaphy go on to recover without atrophy. Bendavid, in a study of the incidence of testicular atrophy at the Shouldice Hospital, found that this complication occurred in only 19 (0.036%) of 52,583 primary inguinal hernia repairs and in only 33 (0.46%) of 7,169 recurrent inguinal hernia repairs.[29]

HEMORRHAGE

Postherniorrhaphy bleeding—usually the result of delayed bleeding from the cremasteric artery, the internal spermatic artery, or branches of the inferior epigastric vessels—can produce a wound or scrotal hematoma. Injuries to the deep circumflex artery, the corona mortis, or the external iliac vessels may result in a large retroperitoneal hematoma.

OSTEITIS PUBIS

Osteitis pubis has diminished in frequency since surgeons began to realize the importance of not placing sutures through the periosteum. In laparoscopic repairs, staples are used to attach the mesh to Cooper's ligament, which may cause osteitis in some cases.

PROSTHESIS-RELATED COMPLICATIONS

The increasingly liberal use of prosthetic material in conventional herniorrhaphy and the routine use of such material in laparoscopic herniorrhaphy make the discussion of complications related directly to foreign material a timely one. Tissue response, which is variable from person to person, can be so intense that the prosthetic material is deformed by contraction. Erosion can result in intestinal obstruction or fistulization, especially if there is physical contact between intestine and prosthesis.[30,31] Erosion into the cord structures has also been reported.[32]

INFECTION

The prostheses used for inguinal herniorrhaphies, unlike those used for ventral herniorrhaphies, rarely become infected. The reasons why the groin is apparently a protected area are unclear. When infections do occur in the groin, they can occasionally be successfully treated with drainage and prolonged antibiotic therapy; more often, however, the prosthesis must be removed. Rejection of the prosthesis because of an allergic response is possible but extremely rare. What patients call rejection in their histories is usually the result of infection.

Incisional Herniorrhaphy

Incisional hernias occur as a complication of previous surgery. They may be caused by poor surgical technique, rough handling of tissues, use of rapidly degraded absorbable suture materials for closing the abdomen, closure of the abdomen under tension, and infection (with or without clinical wound dehiscence).[33] Male sex, advanced age, morbid obesity, abdominal distention, cigarette smoking, pulmonary disease, and hypoalbuminemia have all been incriminated as associated predisposing conditions, but the exact nature of these associations has never been studied in well-controlled trials. Most authorities believe that the best way of preventing incisional hernias is to close abdominal wounds with continuous nonabsorbable monofilament sutures. This is a contentious issue among surgeons, because some feel that the new longer-lasting absorbable sutures are just as good and are less likely to cause suture sinus formation, which is reported in as many as 9% of patients whose abdomens are closed with a nonabsorbable suture.[34]

In 2000, a systematic review and meta-analysis of randomized controlled trials was published that used the MEDLINE and Cochrane Library databases in an effort to determine which suture material and technique best reduced the risk of incisional hernia.[35] The incidence of incisional hernia was significantly lower when nonabsorbable sutures were used in a continuous closure; however, the incidence of suture sinus formation and that of wound pain were significantly higher. The incidence of wound dehiscence or wound infection was not affected by suture material or closure method. Subgroup analyses of individual sutures showed no significant difference in incisional hernia rates between polydioxanone and polypropylene; however, rates were noticeably higher with polyglactin. The authors concluded that surgical practice in this area depended far more on tradition than on high-quality level I scientific evidence.

Continuous suturing is faster, and there has never been convincing evidence that it is inferior to interrupted fascial closure; accordingly, it is favored by most surgeons. In a continuous closure, stitches should be placed 1 cm away from the edge and 1 cm apart from each other. To prevent excessive tension, the length of the suture should be four times the length of the wound.[36] The abdominal wall may be closed with a mass technique, whereby the peritoneum and the anterior and posterior muscle sheaths are fused as a single layer.[37] Alternatively, a multilayered approach may be considered.

The incidence of incisional herniation depends on how the condition is defined. The best definition is any abdominal wall gap, with or without a bulge, that is perceptible on clinical examination or imaging by 1 year after the index operation. If a visible bulge is made part of the definition, the incidence will be underestimated. In the literature, the incidence of incisional herniation after a midline laparotomy ranges from 3% to 20% and doubles if the index operation was associated with infection.

Herniation is most common after midline and transverse incisions but is also well documented after paramedian, subcostal, appendectomy (gridiron), and Pfannenstiel incisions.[38] A 1995 analysis of 11 publications addressing ventral hernia incidence after various types of incisions found the risk to be 10.5%, 7.5%, and 2.5% for midline, transverse, and paramedian incisions, respectively.[34] Upper midline incisions are most likely to lead to ventral hernia formation; transverse and oblique incisions are the least likely. Muscle-splitting incisions probably are associated with a lower incidence of herniation, but they restrict access to the abdominal cavity. Males and females are at roughly equal risk, but early evisceration is more common in males. Most cases are detected within 1 year of surgery, and the basic cause is thought to be separation of aponeurotic edges in the early postoperative period. Incarceration and strangulation occur with significant frequency, and recurrence rates after operative repair approach 50%.

OPERATIVE TECHNIQUE

Simple Nonprosthetic Repair

Simple nonprosthetic repair of an incisional hernia is reserved for only the least complicated defects, because in large series of

unselected patients, the recurrence rate ranges from 25% to 55%.[7] If there is a solitary defect 3 cm or less in diameter, primary closure with nonabsorbable suture material is appropriate. Some surgeons perform a simple edge approximation after flaps are developed on either side of the defect. Others use a Mayo "vest-over-pants" repair. Various advancement and darn procedures have also been described.

A more substantial repair for these defects was popularized by Ramirez.[39] In this operation, known as the component separation technique, fascial planes are incised between muscle groups, so that, in effect, the abdominal wall is lengthened by allowing the muscle to separate on either side of a defect. The hernia can then be repaired primarily with less tension on the repair. This procedure is especially useful at contaminated hernia sites.

A similar procedure is the keel operation of Maingot, which was popular in the middle of the 20th century. The anterior rectus sheath is incised longitudinally, and the medial edge is allowed to rotate behind the rectus abdominis. This, in effect, lengthens the posterior rectus sheath, allowing it to be closed under less tension. The lateral edges of the incised rectus sheath on each side are then approximated to each other.

Onlay Prosthetic Repair

In this technique, a prosthetic onlay is placed over any of a wide variety of simple repairs. Large series of selected patients have documented acceptable results with onlay prosthetic repair, but most surgeons feel that this technique offers little advantage over the simple repair that the prosthesis overlies.[7]

Prosthetic Bridging Repair

Prosthetic bridging repair became popular in the 1990s, in keeping with the tension-free concept for inguinal herniorrhaphy. The basic principle underlying this technique is that for a prosthetic repair to be effective, the defect should be bridged. Although this repair is theoretically attractive, it has not been nearly as successful for incisional hernias as for inguinal hernias. The recurrence rate is especially high in obese patients.

When a hernia defect is bridged with a mesh prosthesis, every attempt should be made to isolate the material from the intra-abdominal viscera to prevent erosion and subsequent fistula formation or adhesive bowel obstruction. This can be accomplished by means of a peritoneal flap constructed from the peritoneal sac or omentum. When contact with intra-abdominal organs cannot be avoided, expanded polytetrafluoroethylene (e-PTFE) should be strongly considered for the prosthesis. Most authorities feel that complications are less likely with e-PTFE, though this has not been unequivocally shown to be the case.

Combined Fascial and Mesh Closure

The issue of contact between the intra-abdominal viscera and the prosthesis has been further addressed by techniques that combine features of the component separation technique with the tension-free concept. The posterior fascia is closed primarily, but the anterior fascia is allowed to remain open, so that there is no tension at all. The anterior fascia is then bridged with a prosthesis.

Sublay Prosthetic Repair

Sublay prosthetic repair, sometimes referred to as the retromuscular approach, is characterized by the placement of a large prosthesis in the space between the abdominal muscles and the peritoneum [*see Figure 17*]. It was popularized by Velamenta, Stoppa, and Wantz and is particularly suitable for large and multiply recurrent hernias when most of the abdominal wall must be

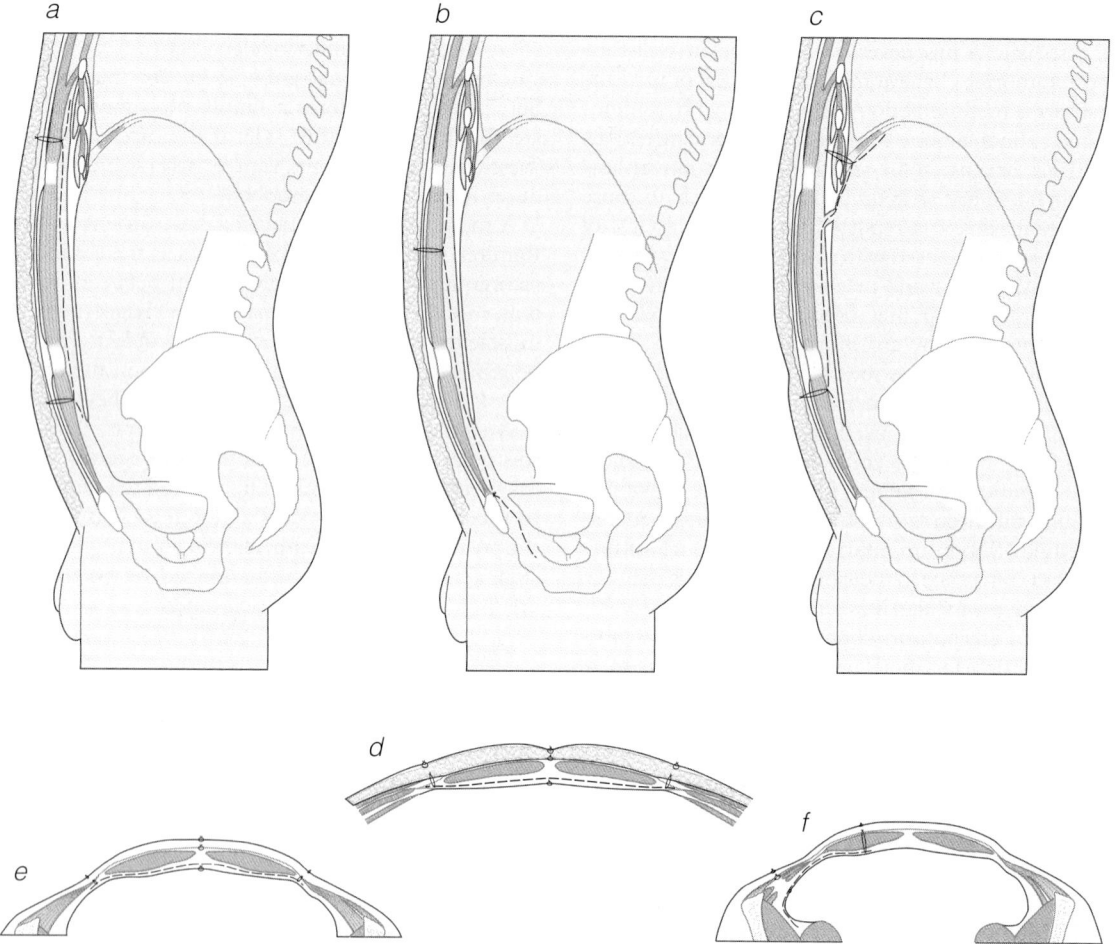

Figure 17 **Incisional herniorrhaphy: sublay prosthetic repair. The lateral views show sites of prosthesis implantation (broken lines) and suture fixation for incisional hernias in (*a*) the upper midline, (*b*) the lower midline, and (*c*) the subcostal region. The cross-sectional views show the same things for incisional hernias in (*d*) the upper midline, (*e*) the lower midline, and (*f*) the right lower quadrant (after appendectomy).**

reconstructed.[40-42] It is considered the most effective conventional incisional hernia repair and therefore the one against which other procedures must be measured.

The posterior rectus sheath is opened on each edge of the hernia defect and dissected away from the undersurface of the recti for a distance of 10 to 15 cm. The posterior rectus sheaths are then approximated to each other primarily. A large mesh prosthesis (composed of e-PTFE if the approximation of the posterior rectus sheath is inadequate) is then placed in this space outside the repaired posterior sheath but beneath the recti. The mesh is secured in this position with several sutures that are placed with a suture passer through small stab incisions at the periphery of the prosthesis and tied in the subcutaneous tissue above the fascia. The laparoscopic incisional herniorrhaphy discussed elsewhere [*see 3:22 Laparoscopic Hernia Repair*] was designed with the principles of this operation in mind.

COMPLICATIONS

Although prosthesis-related infection is rare with prosthetic inguinal herniorrhaphies, it remains a major problem with prosthetic incisional herniorrhaphies. It occurs in about 5% of repairs and can delay healing for prolonged periods. Risk factors for prosthesis infection include preexisting infection or ulceration of the skin overlying the hernia, obesity, incarcerated or obstructed

bowel within the hernia, and perforation of the bowel during hernia repair. Seromas are common, especially when a large prosthesis is required or there has been extensive flap dissection of the subcutaneous layer from the fascia. Untreated seromas commonly become infected secondarily. Suction drains can be useful but are likely to result in prosthesis infection if left in place too long. Strategies for preventing and managing seromas are largely based on empiricism and personal opinion; objective data are virtually nonexistent. It is not always necessary to remove the mesh prosthesis if infection develops. A trial of local wound care after opening the incision and debriding the infected area is warranted. As noted, some authorities believe that e-PTFE is less prone to infection. Nevertheless, once infection is established, e-PTFE prostheses (unlike mesh prostheses) usually have to be removed.

A dilemma arises when a patient has a large incisional hernia and the wound is contaminated either by skin infection or by injury to the bowel during mobilization. In this situation, a nonabsorbable mesh would have a significant chance of becoming infected, and an enterocutaneous fistula could complicate matters further. For these situations, an absorbable mesh made of polyglycolic acid is recommended to prevent evisceration. Granulation tissue forms over the mesh, making skin grafting possible. The mesh itself is absorbed in about 3 weeks, leaving no permanent foreign body to serve as a persistent focus of infection.

Unfortunately, however, recurrence of the incisional hernia is inevitable. The biologic prosthesis now being evaluated for inguinal herniorrhaphy has also been employed in this situation, but the results are as yet unknown.

Several other factors might contribute to the poor results of incisional hernia repair, including preexisting comorbid conditions for which the patient underwent the original operation, cancer-related debilitation, morbid obesity, the use of steroids, and chemotherapy.

Repair of Other Abdominal Wall Hernias

PERIUMBILICAL HERNIA

Gastroschisis

Gastroschisis is seen in fetuses and neonates. The typical presentation is a defect in the abdominal wall to the right of the umbilicus through which the intestines protrude. There is no associated sac. Usually, only the small bowel and the large bowel are eviscerated; however, the stomach, the liver, and the genitourinary system may be involved. Because the bowel is exposed to amniotic fluid, the maternal serum α-fetoprotein (AFP) level tends to be elevated, and the bowel may become thickened and dilated as a result. Bowel complications (e.g., malrotation and segmental atresia) are present in approximately 15% of cases of gastroschisis; however, other anomalies are uncommon. Gastroschisis occurs sporadically and is not associated with chromosome abnormalities, though some familial occurrences are reported.

After the presence of gastroschisis is confirmed, serial ultrasonographic follow-up is indicated for measurement of fetal growth and evaluation of bowel status. Counseling of a couple expecting a baby with gastroschisis should include assessment of the prognosis, description of the surgical and medical support the newborn is likely to need, and discussion with both the neonatologist and the pediatric surgeon.

Omphalocele (Exomphalos)

Omphalocele also is seen in fetuses and neonates. In this condition, a midline defect of the abdominal wall results in herniation of the bowel and intra-abdominal contents into the umbilical cord; the coverings of the hernia are therefore the coverings of the umbilical cord. The defect may be categorized according to whether the liver is present in the omphalocele sac. If the liver is present in the sac, the omphalocele is extracorporeal; if not, the omphalocele is intracorporeal. Omphalocele differs from gastroschisis in that the bowel contents are contained in a membrane, and thus, maternal serum AFP levels generally are not elevated. Often, ascites develops within the omphalocele sac.

Amniocentesis is indicated when an omphalocele is identified in a fetus, because approximately 30% of fetuses with an omphalocele have a chromosome abnormality. The most common such abnormalities are trisomies 18, 13, and 21; Turner syndrome (45, X); and triploidy. Beckwith-Wiedemann syndrome may also be associated with omphalocele. Approximately 67% to 88% of fetuses with an omphalocele have other anomalies as well. These associated anomalies often determine the prognosis.

Umbilical and Paraumbilical Hernia

An umbilical hernia is the result of improper healing of an umbilical scar, which leads to a fascial defect that is covered by skin. If the defect is to one side, it is called a paraumbilical hernia; this variant is more common in adults. The vast majority of umbilical hernias presenting in children are congenital, whereas 90% of those diagnosed in adults are acquired. These hernias are eight times more common in black children than in white ones. The onset of umbilical or paraumbilical hernia in older patients is usually sudden, and the defect tends to be relatively small. In these patients, it is important to look for an underlying cause of increased intra-abdominal pressure (e.g., ascites or an intra-abdominal tumor).

The differential diagnosis of an umbilical hernia should include so-called caput medusae, a condition in which varicosities extend radially from the umbilicus as a consequence of portal hypertension. These varicosities look like varicose veins, exhibit a bluish discoloration, and fill when the patient strains. Another condition to be considered is the so-called Sister Mary Joseph node, which is a metastatic deposit of intra-abdominal cancer at the umbilicus. The cancer cells reach this area via lymphatic vessels in the falciform ligament. A hard nodule is palpable at the umbilicus, and biopsy verifies its cancerous nature. Other periumbilical masses that might be confused with an umbilical hernia are umbilical granulomas, omphalomesenteric duct remnant cysts, and urachal cysts.

Management of umbilical hernias is conservative in children younger than 2 years. A large proportion of these defects heal spontaneously. Consequently, the usual practice is to observe the hernia until the child has reached 2 years of age, by which point about 80% of defects will have healed. Umbilical hernias persisting after the age of 2 years probably will not heal spontaneously and therefore must be treated surgically. The customary recommendation is to repair the hernia by the time the child reaches 5 years of age, so that he or she is not subjected to psychological trauma when participating in normal school sports activities.

In young patients, compression of the hernia with a bandage or a coin is commonly attempted. This practice probably has no real effect but has gained acceptance by parents; the high rate of spontaneous closure fuels the perception (or misperception) of efficacy. In patients who do require surgery—namely, children older than 2 years and adults—the repair used depends on the size of the hernia. Most of the defects are small and can therefore be closed by simple suturing. Alternatively, the Mayo technique may be used. A subumbilical semilunar incision is made, the hernial sac is opened, the contents of the sac are reduced into the abdomen, and the sac is excised. An overlapping or waistcoating technique is then employed, in which the upper edge of the linea alba is placed so as to overlap the lower and fixed in place with a nonabsorbable mattress suture. This technique is controversial: some surgeons argue that the overlapping layers serve only to increase the tension on the repair, thus inviting recurrence.

For larger hernias, particularly those in adults, a popular approach is to dissect the sac away from the undersurface of the skin of the umbilicus and reduce it into the preperitoneal space. The fascial defect is then bridged with a prosthesis without fear of contact with the intra-abdominal viscera. The prosthesis is sutured circumferentially to the defect; alternatively, it can be sutured to the undersurface of the posterior rectus sheath and the linea alba above the peritoneal closure. If the peritoneum cannot be kept intact beneath the defect, omentum should be tacked to the peritoneum circumferentially to isolate the abdominal viscera from the prosthesis at least to some degree.

EPIGASTRIC HERNIA

Epigastric hernias occur through a defect in the linea alba. In most patients with these hernias, as well as those with umbilical hernias, only a single decussation of the fibers of the linea alba is present, as opposed to the triple decussation seen in most persons; this abnormality is the cause of the defect in the midline.

The reported incidence of epigastric hernia ranges from less than 1% to as high as 5%. They are two to three times more common in men than in women, and 20% of them are multiple. Most defects are less than 1 cm long and contain only incarcerated preperitoneal fat, with no peritoneal sac. For this reason, they generally cannot be visualized laparoscopically. The usual complaint is a painful nodule in the upper midline. As a rule, reduction of the preperitoneal fat and simple closure of the defect resolves the complaint. Given the relatively high recurrence rate (up to 10%), however, some surgeons prefer to place a postage stamp–sized piece of prosthetic material in the preperitoneal space to reinforce the repair. Others bridge the defect by suturing the prosthesis circumferentially. Some authorities recommend exposure of the entire linea alba because of the incidence of multicentricity. We believe that this practice leads to unnecessary morbidity. Instead, we make a small incision with the patient under local anesthesia and explain to him or her that additional repairs may be required later.

Left untreated, an epigastric hernia can become large enough to develop a peritoneal sac into which intra-abdominal contents can protrude. Usually, however, the sac is wide, and serious complications are infrequent.

DIASTASIS RECTI

In diastasis recti, the two recti abdominis are separated quite widely, and the linea alba area is stretched and protrudes like a fin. Although the protrusion is easily reducible and almost never produces complications, many patients find it unsightly and request treatment. Surgical therapy would involve removing a strip of the weakened linea alba and reapproximating it; however, this approach could result in tension, which in turn might lead to recurrence. The alternative would be a mesh repair.

PARASTOMAL HERNIA

Parastomal hernia is one of the most common complications of stoma formation. Its incidence is much higher than is generally appreciated. There is good evidence to suggest that more than 50% of patients will eventually be found to have a paracolostomy hernia if followed for longer than 5 years.[43] The rate of herniation with small bowel stomas is also discouraging, though less so than that with colostomies. The results of parastomal hernia repair are particularly dismal, with recurrence being the rule rather than the exception.

Some parastomal hernias can be accounted for by poor site selection or technical errors (e.g., making the fascial opening too large or placing a stoma in an incision), but the overall incidence is too high to be explained by these causes alone. Placement of the stoma lateral to the rectus sheath is widely touted as a cause of parastomal hernia, but this claim is not universally accepted. Obesity, malnutrition, advanced age, collagen abnormalities, postoperative sepsis, abdominal distention, constipation, obstructive uropathy, steroid use, and chronic lung disease are also contributing factors.[44,45]

Newer techniques for stomal construction (e.g., extraperitoneal tunneling) have had little impact on the incidence of parastomal hernia. Fortunately, patients tolerate these hernias well, and life-threatening complications (e.g., bowel obstruction or strangulation) are rare. Routine repair, therefore, is not recommended; repair is appropriate only when there is an absolute or relative indication [see Table 5]. If repair is considered, patients must be informed that there is a significant chance that the hernia will recur.

Three general types of parastomal hernia repairs are currently performed: (1) fascial repair, (2) stomal relocation, and (3) prosthetic repair. Fascial repair involves local exploration around the stoma site, with primary closure of the defect. This approach should be considered of historical interest only because the results are so miserable. Stomal relocation yields much better results and is considered the procedure of choice by many surgeons. This approach is especially appropriate for patients who have other stomal problems (e.g., skin excoriation or suboptimal stomal construction). The use of a prosthesis with stomal relocation is not generally recommended because of the inherent danger of contamination. In the past few years, the popularity of stomal relocation has waned because of the realization that many patients who undergo this procedure ultimately end up with three hernias instead of one: incisional hernias develop in the old stoma site and the laparotomy incision, while a paracolostomy hernia develops at the new site.

Prosthetic repair appears to be the most promising approach, but it is necessary to accept the complications inherent in the placement of a foreign body. The stomal exit site must be isolated from the surgical field to lower the risk of prosthesis-related infection. The prosthesis can be placed extraperitoneally by making a hockey-stick incision around the stoma, taking care to ensure that the incision is outside the periphery of the stomal appliance. Once the subcutaneous tissue is divided, dissection proceeds along the fascia until the sac is identified and removed. The defect is then closed and an overlying prosthesis buttress sutured in place. Alternatively, the fascial defect is bridged with the prosthesis for a "tension-free" repair.

The extraperitoneal prosthetic approach seems logical but can be very technically demanding, in that it is sometimes difficult to define the entire extent of the hernia defect. Moreover, the considerable undermining involved can lead to seroma formation and eventual infection. As an alternative, an intra-abdominal prosthetic approach has also been described that is theoretically attractive because it avoids the local complications of the extraperitoneal operation and incorporates the mechanical advantage gained by placing the prosthesis on the peritoneal side of the abdominal wall.[46,47] Intra-abdominal pressure then serves to fuse the prosthetic material to the abdominal wall rather than being a factor in recurrence. Either e-PTFE or polypropylene mesh can be used. The detractors of the intra-abdominal approach argue that the risk of complications (e.g., adhesive bowel obstruction and fistula formation resulting from the intra-abdominal placement of the prosthesis) outweighs the advantages. The intra-abdominal approach is particularly well suited for laparoscopic repair, and several techniques have been described.[48,49]

SPIGELIAN HERNIA

The Flemish anatomist Adriaan van der Spieghel was the first to describe the semilunar line, which defines the lower limit of the posterior rectus sheath. A spigelian hernia protrudes through an area of weakness just lateral to the rectus sheath and just below this line.[50] The hernia usually is interparietal and rarely penetrates the external oblique fascia; consequently, it can be difficult to appreciate. Spigelian hernias are unusual, with fewer than 750 cases described in the literature to date; however, given that they are so easily diagnosed laparoscopically, it is possible that the incidence will increase. These hernias tend to occur more often in elderly female patients. It is difficult to explain precisely why

Table 5 Indications for Repair of Parastomal Hernia

Absolute indications	Obstruction Incarceration with strangulation
Relative indications	Incarceration Prolapse Stenosis Intractable dermatitis Difficulty with appliance management Large size Cosmesis Pain

spigelian hernias develop; there is no area of weakness in the abdominal wall caused by the passage of blood vessels through the abdominal wall in this position. Undoubtedly, childbirth and various other events that stretch the abdominal wall contribute to their development.

Spigelian hernias are usually small (about 1 to 2 cm in diameter), though large ones (up to 14 cm in diameter) have been described. Omentum, small bowel, or large bowel may enter the sac. Incarceration and strangulation are common complications. The usual clinical presentation is a lower abdominal swelling just lateral to the lateral border of the rectus abdominis. In many cases, however, pain and tenderness are the only signs. Plain x-rays may show a bowel shadow in this area, and of course, CT scanning visualizes the defect and the hernia well.

The standard treatment for a spigelian hernia is operative repair. A transverse incision is centered over the mass. The external oblique aponeurosis is split to reveal the protrusion. If there is a large sac, it is divided and sutured. The aponeurotic defect is triangular, with the base located at or near the lateral border of the rectus abdominis. The defect is closed by joining the separated transversus abdominis and internal oblique muscle layers. Recurrence is uncommon.

SUPRAVESICAL HERNIA

Supravesical hernias develop anterior to the urinary bladder as a consequence of failure of the integrity of the transversus abdominis and the transversalis fascia, both of which insert into Cooper's ligament.[51] The preperitoneal space is continuous with the retropubic space of Retzius, and the hernial sac protrudes into this area. The sac is directed laterally and emerges at the lateral border of the rectus abdominis in the inguinal region, the femoral region, or the obturator region. It also may be associated with an inguinal hernia, a femoral hernia, or an obturator hernia. Treatment of a supravesical hernia involves prompt recognition of the defect at the time of groin exploration and appropriate reinforcement of the area of the defect.

A variant of this hernia, known as an internal supravesical hernia, may also arise. Internal supravesical hernias are classified according to whether they cross in front of, beside, or behind the bladder. Bowel symptoms predominate in patients with these defects, and urinary tract symptoms develop in as many as 30%. Treatment is surgical and is accomplished transperitoneally via a low midline incision. The sac can usually be reduced without difficulty; the neck of the sac should be divided and closed.

INTERPARIETAL HERNIA

With an interparietal hernia, the hernial sac lies between the layers of the abdominal wall. It may be either preperitoneal (between the peritoneum and the transversalis fascia) or interstitial (between the muscle layers of the abdominal wall). Most interparietal hernias are of the latter type and occur in the groin; accordingly, they are designated inguinal interstitial hernias. When the sac passes behind the inguinal ligament in the region of the femoral ring, the resulting defect is known as an inguinocrural hernia.

The cause of interparietal hernias appears to be related to congenital abnormalities (e.g., maldescent of the testis, congenital pouches, absence of the cremaster muscle, and absence of the external abdominal ring). Diagnosis is difficult because there is no obvious swelling of the abdominal wall unless the hernia is large. In many cases, pain is the only symptom; therefore, it is not unusual for patients to present with intestinal obstruction secondary to incarceration. CT, ultrasonography, and laparoscopy can facilitate the diagnosis. Not infrequently, the correct diagnosis is made only at operation. Treatment starts by addressing the intestinal obstruction that is so often the presenting symptom. The defect itself is then repaired in accordance with the same principles followed in inguinal or incisional herniorrhaphy.

RICHTER'S HERNIA

In a Richter's hernia, part of the bowel wall herniates through the defect and may become ischemic and gangrenous, but intestinal obstruction does not occur. The overlying skin may be discolored. The herniated bowel wall is exposed by opening the sac, and the neck of the sac is enlarged to allow delivery of the bowel into the wound. The gangrenous patch is excised and the bowel wall reconstituted. The hernia is then repaired.

LUMBAR HERNIA

The lumbar region is the area bounded inferiorly by the iliac crest, superiorly by the 12th rib, posteriorly by the erector spinae group of muscles, and anteriorly by the posterior border of the external oblique muscle as it extends from the 12th rib to the iliac crest. There are three varieties of lumbar hernia:

1. The superior lumbar hernia of Grynfelt. In this variety, the defect is in a space between the latissimus dorsi, the serratus posterior inferior, and the posterior border of the internal oblique muscle.
2. The inferior lumbar hernia of Petit. Here, the defect is in the space bounded by the latissimus dorsi posteriorly, the iliac crest inferiorly, and the posterior border of the external oblique muscle anteriorly.
3. Secondary lumbar hernia. This hernia develops as a result of trauma—mostly surgical (e.g., renal surgery)—or infection. In the past, it was encountered relatively frequently as a consequence of spinal tuberculosis with paraspinal abscesses; however, it is less common today. Surgical repair is discouraged because the natural history is more consistent with that of a diastasis recti than that of a true hernia. Denervation appears to play a significant role in the pathogenesis. In other words, this "hernia" really reflects a weakness in the abdominal wall more than it does a dangerous hernia defect. Therefore, appropriate repair is commonly followed by gradual eventration, which is perceived by the patient as a recurrence.

Lumbar hernias should be repaired if they are large or symptomatic. A prosthesis or a tissue flap of some kind is usually required for a successful repair. A rotation flap of fascia lata can be used for inferior lumbar hernias.

References

1. Bay-Nielsen M, Kehlet H, Strand L, et al: Quality assessment of 26,304 herniorrhaphies in Denmark: a prospective nationwide study. Lancet 358: 1124, 2001

2. Rutkow IM: Epidemiologic, economic, and sociologic aspects of hernia surgery in the United States in the 1990s. Surg Clin North Am 78:941, 1998

3. McIntosh A, Hutchinson A, Roberts A, et al: Evidence-based management of groin hernia in primary care—a systematic review. Fam Pract 17:442

4. Gaster J: Hernia one day repair. Hafner Publishing Co, Darien, Connecticut, 1970

5. Fitzgibbons RJ, Jonasson O, Gibbs J, et al: The development of a clinical trial to determine if watchful waiting is an acceptable alternative to routine herniorrhaphy for patients with minimal or no hernia symptoms. J Am Coll Surg 196:737, 2003

6. Zollinger RM Jr: Classification of ventral and groin hernias. Nyhus and Condon's Hernia, 5th ed. Fitzgibbons RJ Jr, Greenburg AG, Eds. Lippincott Williams & Wilkins, Philadelphia, 2002, p 71

7. Korenkov M, Paul A, Sauerland S, et al: Classification and surgical treatment of incisional hernia: results of an experts' meeting. Langenbecks. Arch Surg 386:65, 2001

8. Condon RE: The anatomy of the inguinal region and its relation to groin hernia. Hernia. Nyhus LM, Condon RE, Eds. JB Lippincott, Philadelphia, 1995, p 31

9. Bendavid R: The space of Bogros and the deep inguinal venous circulation. Surg Gynecol Obstet 174:355, 1992

10. Kozol RA, Mason K, McGee K: Post-herniorrhaphy urinary retention: a randomized prospective study. J Surg Res 52:111, 1992

11. Smedberg SGG, Broome AEA, Gullmo A: Ligation of the hernia sac? Surg Clin North Am 64:299, 1984

12. Castrini G, Pappalardo G, Trentino P, et al: The original Bassini technique in the surgical treatment of inguinal hernia. Int Surgery 71:141, 1986

13. Lifschutz H: The inguinal darn. Arch Surg 121:717, 1986

14. Bendavid R: The Shouldice technique: a canon in hernia repair. Can J Surg 40:199, 1997

15. Gilbert AI: Sutureless repair of inguinal hernia. Am J Surg 163:331, 1992

16. Millikan KW, Cummings B, Doolas A: The Millikan modified mesh-plug hernioplasty. Arch Surg 138:525, 2003

17. Rutkow IM, Robbins AW: "Tension-free" inguinal herniorrhaphy: a preliminary report on the "mesh plug" technique. Surgery 114:3, 1993

18. Reed RC: Annandale's role in the development of preperitoneal groin herniorrhaphy. Hernia 1:111, 1997

19. Cheatle GL: An operation for the radical cure of inguinal and femoral hernia. Br Med J 2:68, 1920

20. Henry AK: Operation for femoral hernia by a midline extraperitoneal approach, with a preliminary note on the use of this route for reducible inguinal hernia. Lancet 1:531, 1936

21. Condon RE, Nyhus LM: Complications of groin hernia and of hernial repair. Surg Clin North Am 51:1325, 1971

22. Nyhus LM: Iliopubic tract repair of inguinal and femoral hernia: the posterior (preperitoneal) approach. Surg Clin North Am 73:487, 1993

23. Stoppa RE: The midline preperitoneal approach and prosthetic repair of groin hernias. Nyhus and Condon's Hernia, 5th ed. Fitzgibbons RJ Jr, Greenburg AG, Eds. Lippincott Williams & Wilkins, Philadelphia, 2002, p 199

24. Wantz GE, Fischer E: Unilateral giant prosthetic reinforcement of the visceral sac. Nyhus and Condon's Hernia, 5th ed. Fitzgibbons RJ Jr, Greenburg AG, Eds. Lippincott Williams & Wilkins, Philadelphia, 2002, p 219

25. Rignault DP: Properitoneal prosthetic inguinal hernioplasty through a Pfannenstiel approach. Surg Gynecol Obstet 163:465, 1986

26. Kugel RD: Minimally invasive, nonlaparoscopic, preperitoneal, and sutureless, inguinal herniorrhaphy. Am J Surg 178:298, 1999

27. Ugahary F: The gridiron hernioplasty. Hernias of the Abdominal Wall: Principles and Management. Bendavid R, Abrahamson J, Arregui M, et al, Eds. Springer-Verlag, New York, 2001, p 407

28. Poobalan AS, Bruce J, Smith WC, et al: A review of chronic pain after inguinal herniorrhaphy. Clin J Pain 19:48, 2003

29. Bendavid R: Complications of groin hernia surgery. Surg Clin North Am 78:1089, 1998

30. Gray MR, Curtis JM, Elkington JS: Colovesical fistula after laparoscopic inguinal hernia repair. Br J Surg 81:1213, 1994

31. Miller K, Junger W: Ileocutaneous fistula formation following laparoscopic polypropylene mesh hernia repair. Surg Endosc 11:772, 1997

32. Silich RC, McSherry CK: Spermatic granuloma: an uncommon complication of the tension-free hernia repair. Surg Endosc 10:537, 1996

33. Ellis H, Bucknall TE: Abdominal incisions and their closure. Curr Probl Surg 22:41, 1985

34. Carlson MA, Ludwig KA, Condon RE: Ventral hernia and other complications of 1,000 midline incisions. South Med J 88:450, 1995

35. Hodgson NC, Malthaner RA, Ostbye T: The search for an ideal method of abdominal fascial closure: a meta-analysis. Ann Surg 231:436, 2000

36. Israelsson LA, Jonsson T, Knutsson A: Suture technique and wound healing in midline laparotomy incisions. Eur J Surg 162:605, 1996

37. Weiland DE, Bay C, Delsordi S: Choosing the best abdominal closure by meta-analysis. Am J Surg 176:666, 1998

38. Bucknall TE, Cox PJ, Ellis H: Burst abdomen and incisional hernia: a prospective study of 1129 major laparotomies. Br Med J 284:931, 1982

39. Ramirez OM, Girotto JA: Closure of chronic abdominal wall defects: the component separation technique. Hernias of the Abdominal Wall: Principles and Management. Bendavid R, Abrahamson J, Arregui M, et al, Eds. Springer-Verlag, New York, 2001, p 487

40. Temudon T, Saidati M, Sarr MG: Repair of complex giant or recurrent ventral hernias by using tension-free intraparietal prosthetic mesh (Stoppa technique): lessons learned from our initial experience (50 patients). Surgery 120:738, 1996

41. Flament JB, Palot JP, Burde A, et al: Treatment of major incisional hernias. Probl Gen Surg 12:151, 1995

42. Wantz GE: Incisional hernioplasty with Mersilene. Surg Gynecol Obstet 172:129, 1991

43. Rubin MS, Schoetz DJ Jr, Matthews JB: Parastomal hernia. Is stoma relocation superior to fascial repair? Arch Surg 129:413, 1994

44. Sugerman HJ, Kellum JM, Reines HD, et al: Greater risk of incisional hernia with morbidly obese than steroid dependent patients and low recurrence with prefascial polypropylene mesh. Am J Surg 171:80, 1996

45. Pearl RK: Parastomal hernias. World J Surg 13: 569, 1989

46. Byers JM, Steinberg JB, Postier RG: Repair of parastomal hernias using polypropylene mesh. Arch Surg 127:1246, 1992

47. Sugarbaker PH: Peritoneal approach to prosthetic mesh repair of paraostomy hernias. Ann Surg 201: 344, 1985

48. Bickel A, Shinkarevsky E, Eitan A: Laparoscopic repair of paracolostomic hernia. J Laparoendosc Adv Surg Tech A 9:353, 1999

49. Porcheron J, Payan B, Balique JG: Mesh repair of paracolostomy hernia by laparoscopy. Surg Endosc 12:1281, 1998

50. Spangen L: Spigelian hernia. Surg Clin North Am 64:351, 1984

51. Skandalakis JE: Internal and external supravesical hernia. Am Surg 42:142, 1976

52. Franklin ME Jr, Gonzalez JJ Jr, Michaelson RP, et al: Preliminary experience with new bioactive prosthetic material for repair of hernias in infected fields. Hernia 6:171, 2002

Acknowledgments

Supported by a Grant from the United States Agency for Healthcare Research and Quality (5 R01 HS09860-03) and the Department of Veterans Affairs Cooperative Studies Research and Development Program (CSP #456).

Figures 2 through 17 Tom Moore.

22 LAPAROSCOPIC HERNIA REPAIR

Liane S. Feldman, M.D., F.A.C.S., and Marvin J. Wexler, M.D., F.A.C.S.

The introduction of video-assisted minimal access surgery has dramatically altered patient care over the past decade. Certain laparoscopic procedures, including cholecystectomy and antireflux procedures, have shown obvious benefits (e.g., more rapid and less painful recovery) and have been readily and universally adopted. Others, particularly laparoscopic inguinal hernia repair (first described by Ger in 1990[1]), remain controversial. Laparoscopic inguinal herniorrhaphy has shown a great deal of promise; however, concurrently with its development, open anterior herniorrhaphy has evolved into a tension-free, often sutureless mesh repair that is easily performed with the patient under local anesthesia and that is also associated with rapid recovery and low recurrence rates.[2] Thus, to gain acceptance, laparoscopic inguinal hernia repair must be shown to provide a significant advantage over the tension-free open repair now in use.

The two most common techniques for laparoscopic inguinal hernia repair both involve the insertion of mesh into the preperitoneal space; one makes use of a transabdominal preperitoneal (TAPP) approach, the other a totally extraperitoneal (TEP) approach. Both approaches would appear to offer potential advantages, such as reduced postoperative pain, shortened convalescence, quicker and more accurate assessment and repair of bilateral groin hernias simultaneously, and, in the case of recurrent hernia, avoidance of previously dissected and technically difficult scarred areas. In practice, however, these advantages are not invariably realized: a laparoscopic approach is not always minimally invasive, and various disadvantages accrue from the current requirement for general anesthesia, the need to traverse the abdominal cavity in the TAPP technique, and the increase in operating room time and costs.[3]

Meticulous attention to surgical technique is essential. Because surgeons may be unfamiliar with inguinal anatomy as viewed from inside the abdomen and because the potential for complications necessitating laparotomy is increased with the laparoscopic approach, surgeons must be proficient in laparoscopic techniques and must have a precise knowledge of anatomic relations in the region of the groin as seen from the peritoneal surface.

Since the late 1990s, laparoscopic video techniques have also been increasingly applied to the repair of incisional hernias.[4-8] Laparoscopic repair of large incisional hernias resembles open repair in that mesh is inserted to cover the defect in the abdominal wall fascia. A laparoscopic approach is theoretically attractive because an open approach usually necessitates a large incision as well as extensive and tedious wide dissection to expose the abdominal wall defect, resulting in considerable postoperative pain and a risk of wound complications—problems that a laparoscopic approach to the defect from within might minimize.

It may be many more years before we can determine the true safety and efficacy of laparoscopic herniorrhaphy and establish the correct indications for its use. In the meantime, every repair performed should be subjected to careful classification, documentation, and quality-of-life assessment. Surgeons should not perform laparoscopic herniorrhaphy simply because it is novel or potentially economical: they should perform this procedure only when convinced that it is anatomically and physiologically correct and logical.

In what follows, we discuss laparoscopic repair of both inguinal and incisional hernias. In addition to describing current operative techniques, we address inguinal surgical anatomy, preoperative planning, and complications. Finally, we review selected trials measuring the results of laparoscopic repair against those of open repair and comparing the outcomes of TAPP repair with those of TEP repair.

Laparoscopic Inguinal Hernia Repair

LAPAROSCOPIC INGUINAL ANATOMY

To most surgeons, inguinal anatomy as viewed through the laparoscope appears unfamiliar. The surgical perspective on the pelvic anatomy from the intraperitoneal view has been best described by Skandalakis and coworkers[9] and has been elegantly demonstrated in cadaver dissections by Spaw and colleagues,[10] whose work forms the basis of the descriptions we present in this chapter. Excellent descriptions of the preperitoneal space by Wantz[11] and Condon[12] are also worthy of review.

During laparoscopic herniorrhaphy, a number of structures that are usually visible during open herniorrhaphy (e.g., the inguinal ligament, the pubic tubercle, the lacunar ligament, and the ilioinguinal and iliohypogastric nerves) are not seen initially. Conversely, a number of structures that are visible only after significant dissection in the open approach are easily viewed through the laparoscope [*see Figure 1*]. Identification of the iliopubic tract, Cooper's ligament, and the transverse abdominal arch is mandatory to ensure proper coverage and securing of prosthetic material margins. The obliterated umbilical artery, a structure not encountered in the anterior approach to open herniorrhaphy, must be divided or retracted medially to afford visualization and dissection of the pubic tubercle, Cooper's ligament, and often the entire Hesselbach's triangle.

Peritoneum Intact

Four important landmarks should be seen at initial laparoscopic inspection of the inguinal region [*see Figure 2*]: the spermatic vessels, the obliterated umbilical artery (also referred to as the medial umbilical ligament or bladder ligament by various authors), the inferior epigastric vessels (also referred to as the lateral umbilical ligament), and the external iliac vessels.

Spermatic vessels The testicular artery and vein descend from the retroperitoneum, travel directly over and slightly lateral to the external iliac artery, and enter the internal spermatic ring posteriorly. These vessels are covered only by the peritoneum and are usually well visualized as flat structures in the abdominal cavity that assume a cordlike appearance when joined by the vas def-

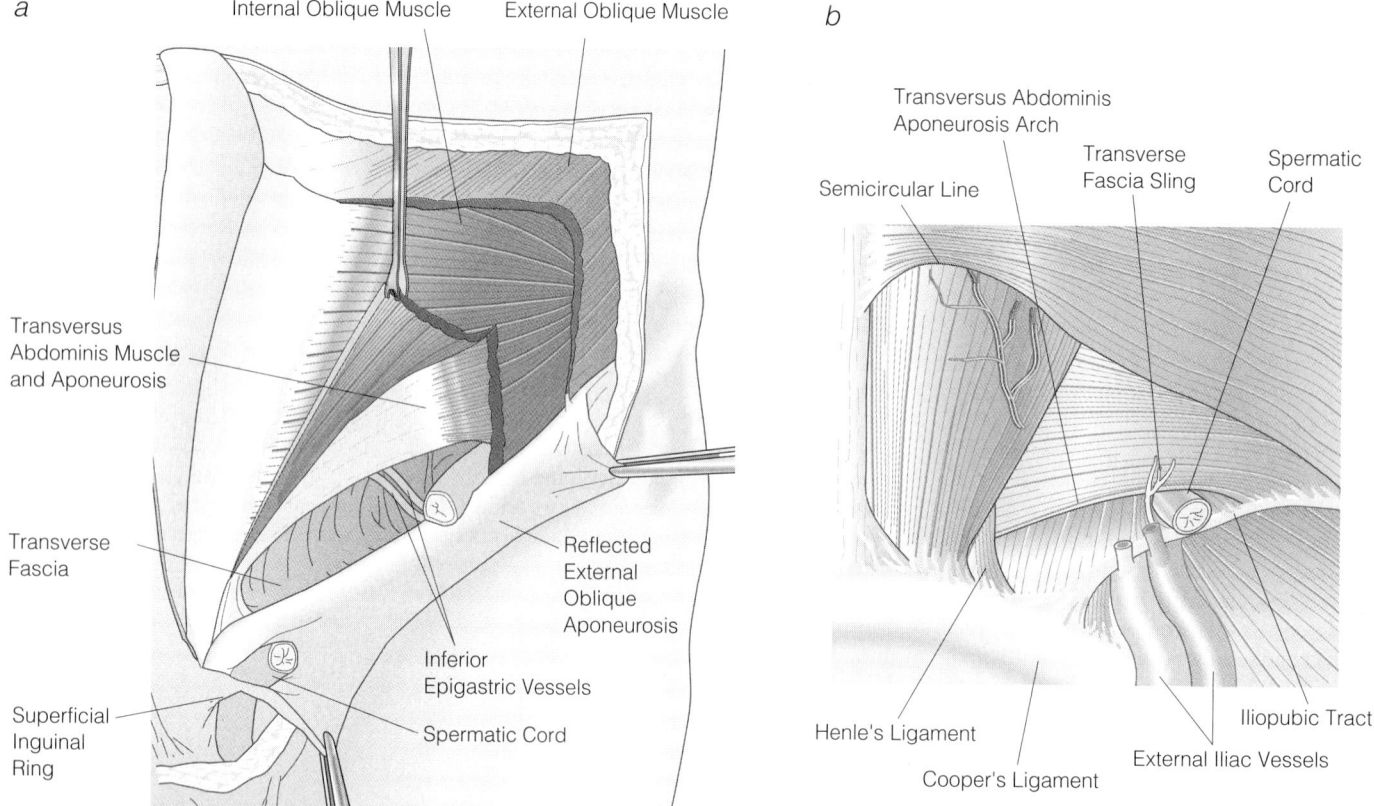

a

Internal Oblique Muscle

External Oblique Muscle

Transversus
Abdominis Muscle
and Aponeurosis

Transverse
Fascia

Superficial
Inguinal
Ring

Reflected
External
Oblique
Aponeurosis

Inferior
Epigastric Vessels

Spermatic Cord

b

Transversus Abdominis
Aponeurosis Arch

Transverse
Fascia Sling

Spermatic
Cord

Semicircular Line

Henle's Ligament

Cooper's Ligament

Iliopubic Tract

External Iliac Vessels

Figure 1 Laparoscopic inguinal hernia repair. Shown are (*a*) the anatomy of the left groin region as seen from the traditional anterior approach to herniorrhaphy and (*b*) the anatomy of the right groin from the posterior, or peritoneal, approach. The inguinal canal floor is covered by transverse fascia alone, and a large space separates the transversus abdominis aponeurosis from the inguinal ligament (*a*). A preperitoneal view of the groin region shows the distance between the transversus abdominis tendon and Cooper's ligament, the iliopubic tract, and the inguinal ligament (*b*).

erens immediately before entering the internal spermatic ring. If no hernia is present, a mere dimple will be seen [*see Figure 2*]. An indirect hernia, if present, will be immediately apparent with an obvious opening [*see Figure 3*]. The vas deferens is best identified where it joins the spermatic vessels. From there, the vas can be traced back medially as it courses over the pelvic brim and falls into the pelvis and behind the bladder. There is a small artery that runs with the vas deferens and is not well seen or known. It is white and cordlike in appearance and can usually be seen just beneath the peritoneum.

Obliterated umbilical artery The obliterated umbilical artery is an unfamiliar but sometimes prominent structure that courses along the anterior abdominal wall toward the umbilicus, often with an apparent mesentery. It is most prominent in the region of the medial inguinal space. This ligament is most readily identified when the umbilical laparoscope is directed toward the pelvic midline, where the ligament's bilateral structure can be best seen directed toward the umbilicus. Medial retraction of this structure is usually necessary for full exposure of the medial aspect of the inguinal canal.

Inferior epigastric vessels The inferior epigastric artery and vein lie in the medial aspect of the internal inguinal ring and ascend the rectus abdominis muscle anteriorly. They are frequently difficult to visualize, particularly in obese patients, and are best identified by locating the internal inguinal ring at the junction of

the vas deferens and the testicular artery and vein. At this location, they exit the medial margin of the internal ring. However, the vessels can quickly fade from view as they travel superiorly and medially along the anterior abdominal wall.

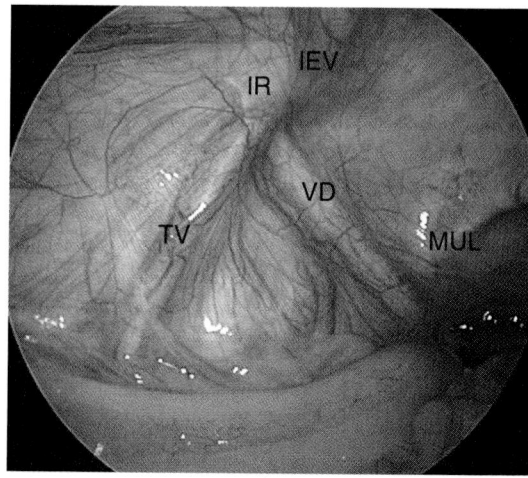

Figure 2 Laparoscopic inguinal hernia repair. Shown is a laparoscopic view of the anatomy of the left groin with the peritoneum intact in a patient without a hernia. (IEV—inferior epigastric vessels; IR—internal ring; MUL—medial umbilical ligament; TV—testicular vessels; VD—vas deferens)

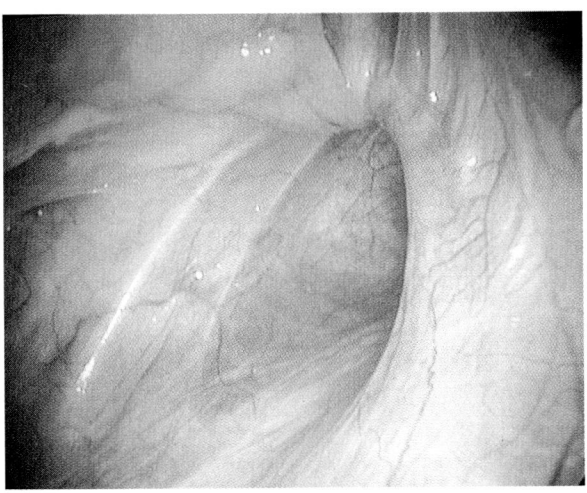

Figure 3 Laparoscopic inguinal hernia repair. Shown is a right indirect inguinal hernia. The vas deferens can be seen below the hernia defect. Omentum is in the hernial sac.

External iliac vessels The lateral spermatic vessels and the medial vas deferens merge at the internal inguinal ring and enter the inguinal canal, where they form the apex of the so-called triangle of doom. Beneath this triangle lie the external iliac artery and the external iliac vein. More laterally, the femoral nerve can be found. The external iliac vessels are often difficult to visualize, though in an elderly patient, a calcified pulsating artery may be prominent. Extreme care must be taken not to dissect within the triangle of doom because such dissection can result in serious bleeding.

Peritoneum Removed

Removal of the peritoneal covering allows access to and visualization of the preperitoneal space and anatomic landmarks critical for repair [see Figure 4].

Internal inguinal ring The internal inguinal ring is normally identified by a slight indentation of the peritoneum at the junction of the vas deferens and the spermatic vessels. When an indirect hernia is present, however, a true ring or opening is easily identified, and by rotating a 30° laparoscope, one can look directly into the hernial sac or insert the laparoscope into the sac, which often allows the external inguinal ring to be identified more medially. An indirect hernial sac lies anterior and lateral to the spermatic cord at this level, as opposed to the familiar medial cord position seen in the classic exterior groin approach to open herniorrhaphy. The medial border of the internal inguinal ring is formed by the transverse fascia and the inferior epigastric vessels. The inferior border is identified by the iliopubic tract, a distinct structure that is the internal counterpart of the inguinal ligament. Anteriorly, the internal inguinal ring is bordered by the transversus abdominis arch (conjoined tendon), which extends medially to insert into the pubic ramus near the pubic tubercle. As the transversus abdominis arch passes laterally over the internal ring, it forms a very well defined visible edge. The layers of the abdominal wall constituting the lateral border of the internal inguinal ring appear the same as when viewed from the exterior approach, and like all margins of the internal inguinal ring, this border is visible only when an indirect hernia is present.

Iliopubic tract The iliopubic tract originates laterally from the anterior superior spine of the ilium and courses medially, forming the inferior margin of the internal inguinal ring and the roof of the femoral canal before inserting medially into the superior pubic ramus. This tract is formed by the condensation of the transverse fascia with the most inferior portion of the transversus abdominis muscle and aponeurosis, and the tract is usually sturdy along its entire course. All inguinal hernial defects lie above the iliopubic tract, either anterior or superior to it. Conversely, femoral hernias occur below the tract, either posterior or inferior to it. Fibers of the iliopubic tract extend into Cooper's ligament medially, where they become the medial margin of the femoral canal. The iliopubic tract is frequently confused with the inguinal ligament, which, though nearby, is part of the superficial muscu-

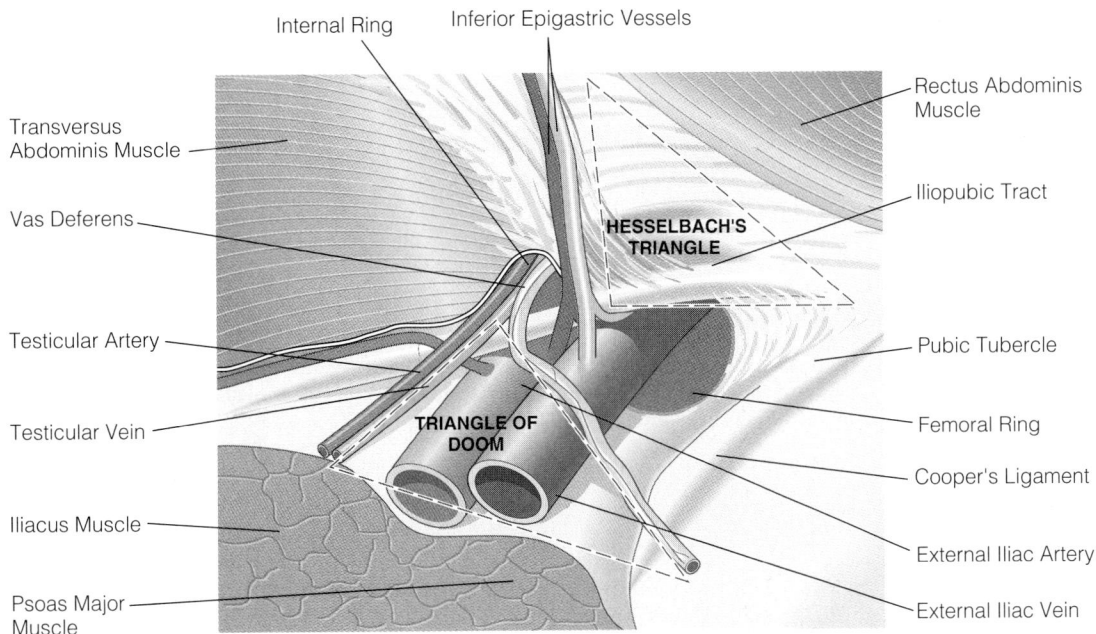

Figure 4 Laparoscopic inguinal hernia repair. Shown is the left inguinal region with the peritoneum removed, as seen during laparoscopic herniorrhaphy.

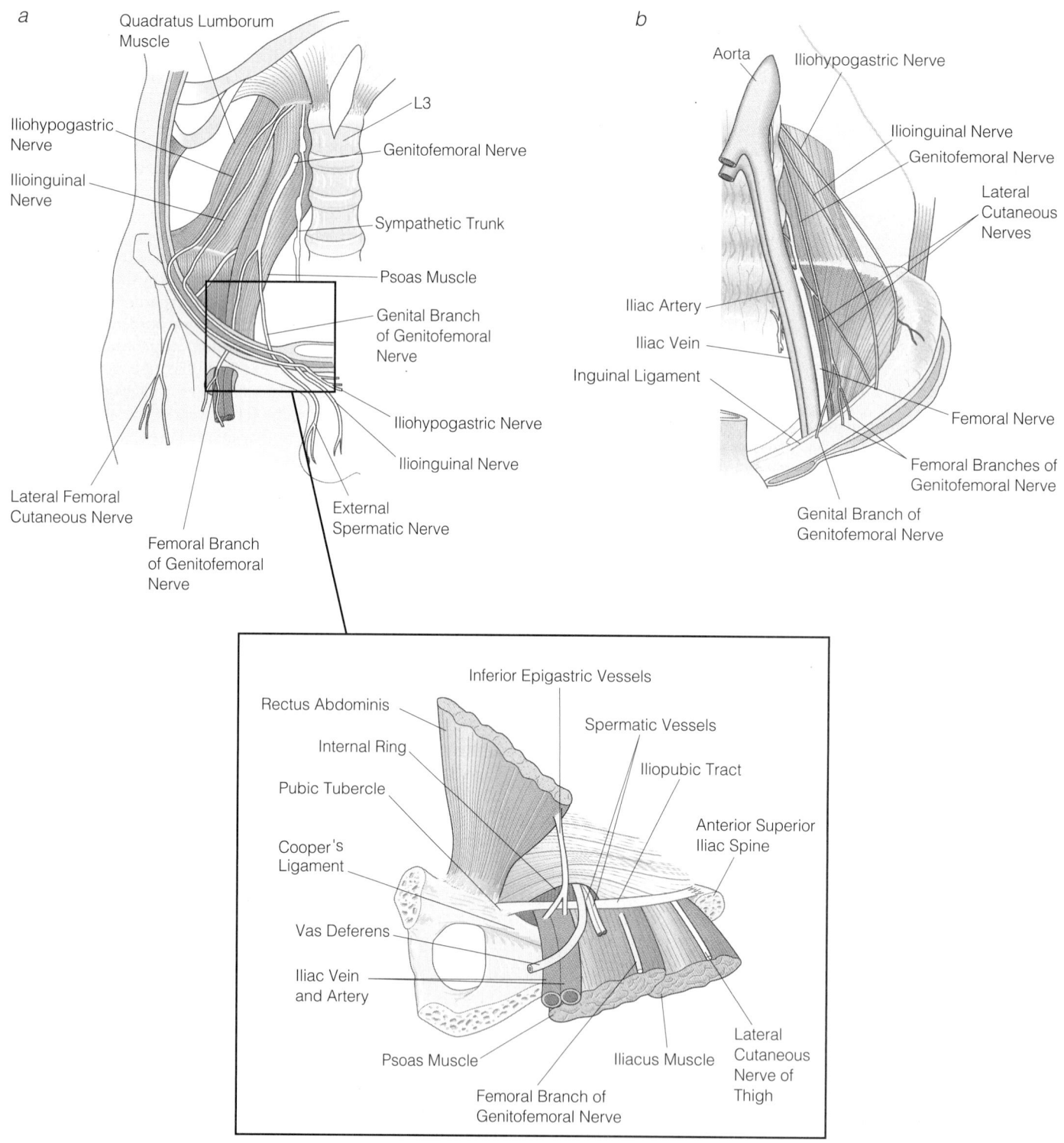

Figure 5 Laparoscopic inguinal hernia repair. Shown are the courses of the genitofemoral and ilioinguinal nerves of the right groin (*a*) and of the left groin (*b*). Inset shows the preperitoneal anatomy of the right groin, as seen by the laparoscopic surgeon.

loaponeurotic layer, which is not seen laparoscopically. The iliopubic tract is part of the deep layer.

Cooper's ligament Cooper's ligament is a condensation of the transverse fascia and the periosteum of the superior pubic ramus lateral to the pubic tubercle. It can be seen only from within the abdominal cavity once the peritoneum is opened and deflected inferiorly, but a considerable amount of preperitoneal

fat must often be cleaned off the ligament before it can be seen. Initially, it is often easier to palpate the ligament than to see it, but once the ligament has been identified and cleaned, its glistening white fibers are apparent. Care must be taken during dissection to avoid the tiny branches of the obturator vein that often run along the ligament's surface. The iliopubic tract inserts into the superior ramus of the pubis just lateral to Cooper's ligament, blending into it.

Femoral canal The femoral canal is seen only in the presence of a femoral hernia in the most medial aspect of the femoral triangle. The anterior and medial borders are bounded by the iliopubic tract, the posterior border is formed by the pectineal fascia, and the lateral border is formed by the femoral sheath and vein.

Trapezoid of disaster. Another area worthy of careful attention is the so-called trapezoid of disaster, containing the genitofemoral, ilioinguinal, iliohypogastric, and lateral cutaneous nerves of the thigh, which innervate the spermatic cord, testicle, scrotum, and upper and lateral thigh, respectively. A detailed knowledge of their anatomic course and careful avoidance of the nerves are essential [*see Figure 5*].

Genitofemoral nerve. The genitofemoral nerve arises from the first and second lumbar nerves; pierces the psoas muscle and fascia at its medial border opposite L3 or L4; descends under the peritoneum, on the psoas major muscle; and divides into a medial genital and a lateral femoral branch. The femoral branch descends lateral to the external iliac artery and the spermatic cord, passing posteroinferior to the iliopubic tract and into the femoral sheath to supply the skin over the femoral triangle. The genital branch crosses the lower end of the external iliac artery and enters the inguinal canal through the internal inguinal ring with the testicular vessels. This branch supplies the coverings of the spermatic cord down to the skin of the scrotum. The genitofemoral nerve is the most visible of the cutaneous nerves and is sometimes confused with the testicular vessels if the latter are not well appreciated in their more medial position.

Ilioinguinal and iliohypogastric nerves. When dissected from the anterior position, the ilioinguinal and iliohypogastric nerves lie between the external oblique and the internal oblique muscles above the internal inguinal ring and descend the spermatic cord. In the abdomen, the ilioinguinal and iliohypogastric nerves arise from the 12th thoracic and first lumbar nerve roots, are more laterally located, and run subperitoneally, emerging from the lateral psoas border to pierce the transversus abdominis muscle near the iliac crest and then pierce and course between the internal oblique and the external oblique muscles close to the internal inguinal ring. Aberrant branches sometimes descend with the genital nerve. The ilioinguinal nerve supplies a small cutaneous area near the external genitals.

Lateral cutaneous nerve of the thigh. Supplying the front and lateral aspect of the thigh, the lateral cutaneous nerve of the thigh arises from the second and third lumbar nerves and emerges at the lateral border of the psoas. There, it descends deep to the peritoneum on the iliac muscle and only comes to lie in a superficial position 3 cm below the anterosuperior iliac spine.

PREOPERATIVE EVALUATION

History and Physical Examination

Preoperative assessment is necessary to determine whether a patient is a suitable candidate for laparoscopic herniorrhaphy. A careful surgical history, including both previous hernia repairs and other procedures (particularly those involving the lower abdomen), should be elicited. A cardiovascular history should also be obtained and risk factors for general anesthesia determined.

Physical examination should confirm the presence of an inguinal hernia. If the patient reports a history of a bulge but no hernia is felt on physical examination, an occult hernia may be presumed. If doubt exists, herniography is indicated. Ultrasonography may be helpful for distinguishing an incarcerated groin hernia from other causes of inguinal swelling (e.g., lymphadenopathy).

Selection of Patients

Indications With the evolution of the open anterior approach to tension-free prosthetic mesh repair, determining which patients will benefit significantly from laparoscopic herniorrhaphy becomes increasingly important. One may choose either (1) to offer laparoscopic repair to all hernia patients in the belief that it is an inherently superior procedure or (2) to reserve laparoscopic repair for specific indications. We prefer the latter choice, believing that these patients are best served when the surgeon has several approaches at his or her command that can be applied to and, if necessary, modified for individual circumstances.

In our opinion, primary unilateral hernias are best treated with an open anterior tension-free repair, preferably with the patient under local or regional anesthesia; possible exceptions include manual laborers and athletes who desire a rapid return to vigorous physical activity and who may benefit from the absence of a sizable incision. We generally reserve laparoscopic inguinal herniorrhaphy for the following clinical situations:

1. Recurrent hernias after previous anterior repair. In such cases, a laparoscopic approach allows one to avoid the scar tissue and distorted anatomy present in the anterior abdominal wall by performing the repair through unviolated tissue, thereby reducing the risk of damage to the vas deferens or the testicular vessels.
2. Bilateral hernias or a unilateral hernia when the presence of a contralateral hernia is strongly suspected. In such cases, a laparoscopic approach allows one to repair both hernias simultaneously and perhaps more rapidly without having to make additional incisions.
3. Repair of an inguinal hernia concurrent with another laparoscopic procedure, provided that there is no contamination of the peritoneal cavity.

Contraindications We do not treat incarcerated hernias laparoscopically. In patients to whom general anesthesia may pose an increased risk, we prefer open anterior repair using local or regional anesthesia. In infants and young children with indirect hernias, for whom repair of the posterior canal wall is unnecessary, we recommend high ligation of the sac via the anterior approach.

Previous lower abdominal surgery, though not an absolute contraindication, may make laparoscopic dissection difficult. In particular, with respect to TEP repair, previous abdominal wall incisions may make it impossible to safely separate the peritoneum from the abdominal parietes for entry into the extraperitoneal plane. Previous surgery in the retropubic space of Retzius, as in prostatic surgery, is a relative contraindication that is associated with an increased risk of bladder injury[13] and other complications.[14]

OPERATIVE PLANNING

Preparation

General anesthesia administered by inhalation is routinely used. Prophylactic antibiotics are unnecessary. The patient is instructed to void before surgery, which means that preoperative bladder catheterization is unnecessary.

Patient Positioning

The patient is placed in the supine position with both arms tucked against the sides. The anesthesia screen is placed as far toward the

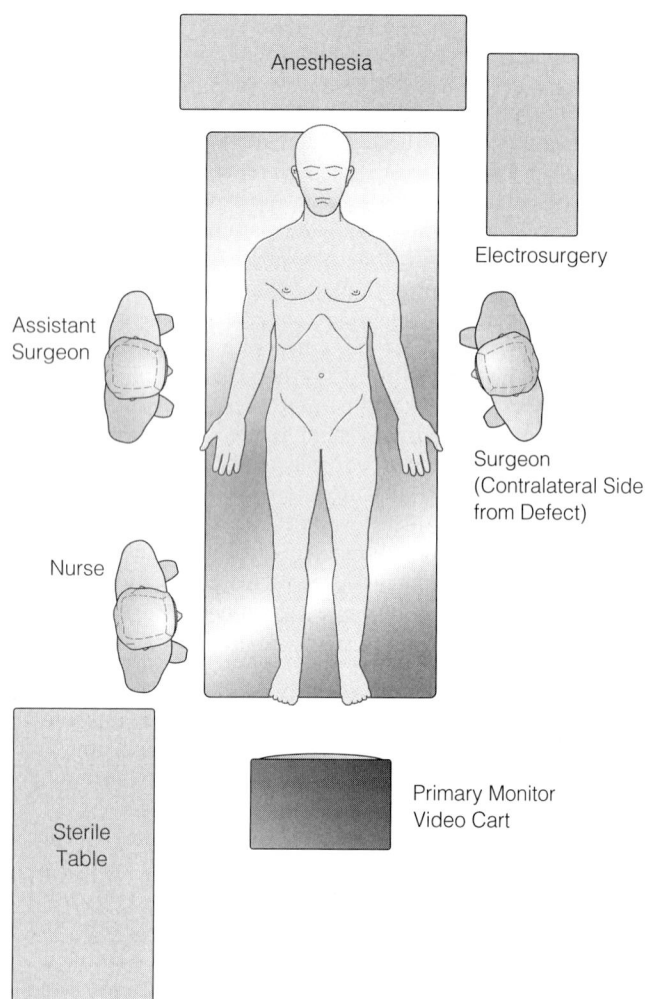

Figure 6 **Laparoscopic inguinal hernia repair. Shown is one of several possible OR setups. The surgeon stands on the side contralateral to the defect, with a nurse on the ipsilateral side. The assistant surgeon stands opposite the surgeon. This positioning may vary, depending on the surgeon's preference and handedness, the visibility of the defect, and the type of defect present, as well as on the prominence of the medial umbilical ligament and the need for its retraction.**

head of the table as possible to allow the surgeon a wide range of mobility with the laparoscope. The skin must be prepared and draped so as to allow exposure of the entire lower abdomen, the genital region, and the upper thighs because manipulation of the hernial sac and the scrotum is frequently necessary. After the laparoscope has been introduced, the patient is placed in a deep Trendelenburg position so that the viscera will fall away from the inguinal areas. Further bowel manipulation is rarely necessary, except to reduce hernial contents. Rotation of the table to elevate the side of the hernia can provide additional exposure, if necessary. A single video monitor is placed at the foot of the bed, directly facing the patient's head.

The surgeon usually begins the repair while standing on the side contralateral to the defect; the assistant surgeon stands opposite the surgeon, and the nurse stands on the ipsilateral side [*see Figure 6*]. Once the key anatomic landmarks and the hernial defect are located and defined, the surgeon should be able to move to either side of the patient, and the surgeon or the assistant should be able to move the camera and the instruments to the ports of preference, the choice of which depends on optimum exposure, angle, right- or left-

handedness, and the designated role of the assistant surgeon as either camera operator or surgical assistant. A two-handed technique provides a distinct technical advantage and also eliminates the need for an additional surgical assistant.

Equipment

Because inguinal hernias occur in the anterior abdominal wall, visualization through the umbilicus requires angling the laparoscope close to the horizontal plane. The view is paralleled anteriorly by the surface of the lower abdominal wall, which may make visualization with a 0° laparoscope difficult. In addition, an indirect hernia is a three-dimensional tubular defect that can be well visualized in its entirety only with an angled lens. For these reasons, we recommend routine use of an oblique, forward-viewing 30° laparoscope. Excellent 30° laparoscopes are currently available in 10 mm, 5 mm, and 3 mm sizes.

A basic set of instruments for laparoscopic hernia repair should include graspers, dissectors, curved scissors, a suction-irrigation device, a hook cautery, and needle drivers. In addition, we use a multifire stapler to fix the mesh and close the peritoneum (though it is certainly possible to use sutures instead). Either a circular tacker or a linear stapler can be employed; both are available in 10 mm and 5 mm sizes. We prefer the linear stapler.

In a TEP repair, besides the equipment needed for a TAPP repair, a blunt trocar is required for gaining access to the preperitoneal space. An operative laparoscope is needed as well. Alternatively, special preperitoneal distention balloon (PDB) systems [*see* Operative Technique, Totally Extraperitoneal Repair, *below*] are also frequently used to develop the preperitoneal space.

OPERATIVE TECHNIQUE

As noted (see above), there are two principal techniques of laparoscopic inguinal hernia repair. The TAPP repair involves insufflating the peritoneal cavity, penetrating the abdomen with trocars, incising the peritoneum overlying the defect, and closing the peritoneum after the repair with a piece of mesh placed in the preperitoneal space. The TEP repair, on the other hand, involves gaining access to the preperitoneal space via trocars placed in a space created between the fascia and the peritoneum, insufflating that space, and placing a piece of mesh between the underside of the anterior abdominal wall and the peritoneum.

We will not describe the intraperitoneal onlay mesh (IPOM) technique, in which polypropylene mesh is fixed directly onto the peritoneum intra-abdominally. This approach has been abandoned by most surgeons out of fear of complications related to adhesions and possible erosion of the mesh into bowel.[3,15]

Transabdominal Preperitoneal Repair

Step 1: placement of trocars Pneumoperitoneum is established through a small vertical infraumbilical incision. Either a closed approach, using a Veress needle, or an open (Hasson) approach, using a 10/12 mm trocar, may be employed. We prefer the open technique, in which the first trocar is inserted into the peritoneal cavity under direct vision. This approach usually prevents injuries to the major blood vessels; although it does not completely prevent bowel injuries, it does facilitate discovery and repair of such injuries.

CO_2 is then insufflated into the abdomen to a pressure of 15 mm Hg. The angled laparoscope is introduced, and both inguinal areas are inspected. Two 10/12 mm accessory ports are then placed at the lateral border of each rectus abdominis muscle at the level of the umbilicus to allow placement of the camera and the instruments [*see Figure 7*]. The 10/12 mm lateral ports can be

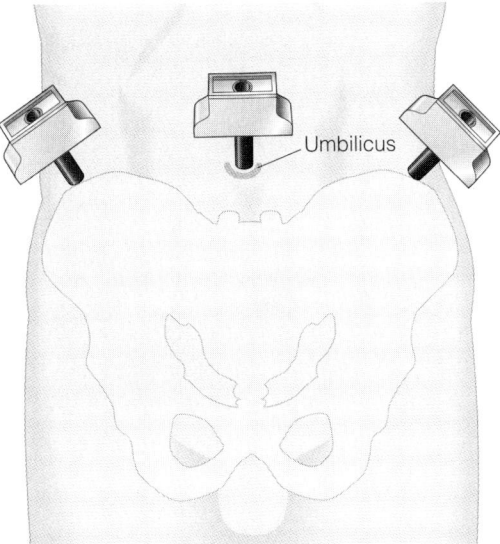

Figure 7 **Laparoscopic inguinal hernia repair: TAPP approach. Shown is standard trocar placement for TAPP repair. Usually, three trocar sites are used. The laparoscope is inserted through the umbilical trocar, and two additional trocars are placed in the right and the left midabdomen. To ensure that the first trocar is not placed too close to the surgical field, the first trocar should be placed either in the umbilicus or immediately above it. The two lateral trocars should be placed lateral to the rectus sheath to prevent bleeding and postoperative muscle spasms. At least one trocar must be 10/12 mm to allow insertion of the mesh.**

replaced with 5 mm ports if 5 mm instruments and a 5 mm laparoscope are available. To facilitate port placement, the abdominal wall is transilluminated with the laparoscope so as to delineate the border of the rectus abdominis muscle, which can be difficult to define in muscular or obese males. Additional care is taken to keep from puncturing the large subcutaneous veins that are frequently present in this region. Failure to transilluminate the abdominal wall can result in placement of the trocar through the rectus muscle, which can cause troublesome bleeding.

Step 2: identification of anatomic landmarks The four key anatomic landmarks mentioned earlier [*see* Laparoscopic In-

guinal Anatomy, Peritoneum Intact, *above*]—the spermatic vessels, the obliterated umbilical artery (medial umbilical ligament), the inferior epigastric vessels (lateral umbilical ligament), and the external iliac vessels—are identified on each side. In the presence of an indirect hernia, the internal inguinal ring is easily identified by the presence of a discrete hole at the junction of the vas deferens and the testicular vessels. Identification of a direct hernia can be more difficult [*see Figure 8*]. A direct hernia sometimes appears as a complete circle or hole and sometimes as a cleft, and at other times it is completely hidden by preperitoneal fat and the bladder and umbilical ligament. Visualization can be particularly difficult in obese patients, who may have considerable lipomatous tissue between the peritoneum and the transversalis fascia, or in patients whose hernia consists of a weakness and bulging of the entire inguinal floor rather than a distinct sac. For adequate definition of this type of hernia and deeper anatomic structures, the peritoneum must be opened, a peritoneal flap developed, and the underlying fatty layer dissected.[16] Direct hernial defects are often situated medial to the ipsilateral umbilical ligament, and retraction or even division of this structure is sometimes necessary. Traction on the ipsilateral testicle can demonstrate the vas deferens when visualization is obscured by overlying fat or pressure from the pneumoperitoneum.

Step 3: creation of peritoneal flap The curved cautery scissors or the hook cautery is used to create a peritoneal flap by making a transverse incision along the peritoneum, beginning just above the upper border of the internal inguinal ring and extending medially above the pubic tubercle and laterally 2 cm beyond the internal inguinal ring [*see Figure 9*]. Extreme care must be taken to avoid the inferior epigastric vessels. Bleeding from the epigastrics can usually be controlled by cauterization, but application of hemostatic clips may be necessary on occasion. Another solution is to pass percutaneously placed sutures above and below the bleeding point while applying pressure to the bleeding vessel so as not to obscure the field of vision.

If the monopolar cautery is used to create the peritoneal flap, the entire uninsulated portion of the instrument must be visible at all times. Unlike laparoscopic cholecystectomy, in which the liver acts as a safe backdrop for scatter and dissection is anterosuperior to the colon, laparoscopic herniorrhaphy may bring bowel loops in contact with instruments, an occurrence that can be particularly dangerous if current is applied to a long-nosed forceps or grasper and a backdrop is lacking. The medial umbilical ligament must be retracted for me-

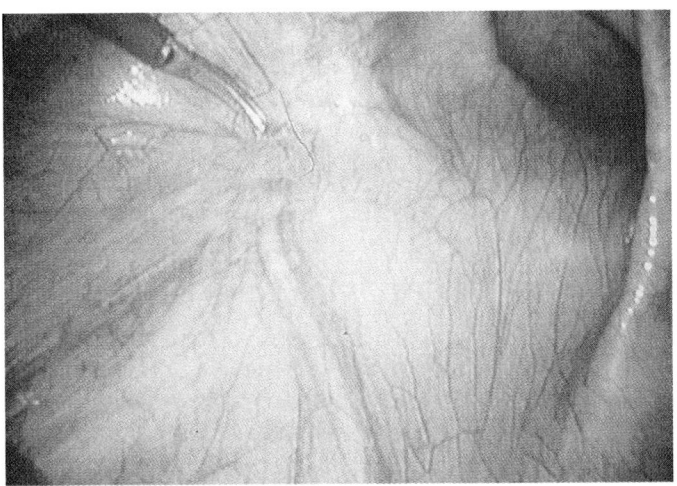

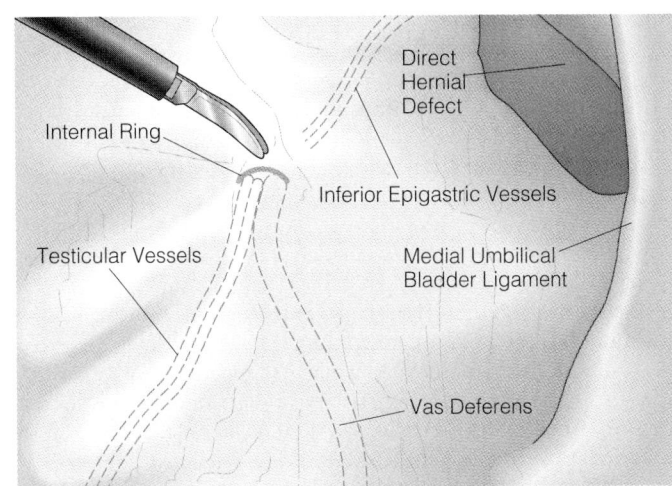

Figure 8 **Laparoscopic inguinal hernia repair: TAPP approach. Shown is a left direct inguinal hernia with the peritoneum intact. The dissector indicates the intact internal ring.**

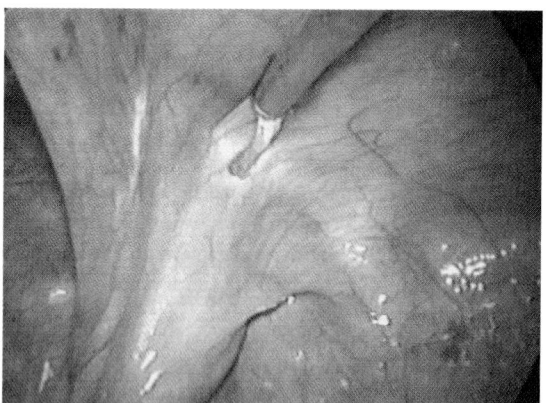

Figure 9 **Laparoscopic inguinal hernia repair: TAPP approach. Shown is dissection of a left direct inguinal hernia. The hernial sac is inverted and the peritoneum incised superior to the sac.**

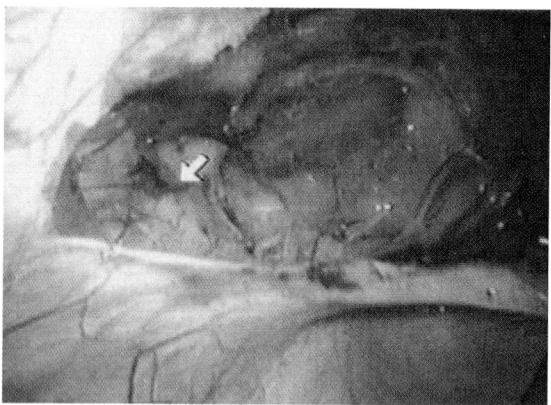

Figure 10 **Laparoscopic inguinal hernia repair: TAPP approach. A flap of peritoneum is dissected downward, revealing a hernial defect and the inferior epigastric vessels (arrow) on the left side.**

dial dissection and may have to be divided. Division of this structure does not have any negative sequelae; however, one should be aware that the obliterated umbilical artery may still be patent and should use the cautery or clips.

The incised peritoneum is grasped along with the attached preperitoneal fat and the peritoneal sac and is dissected caudad with blunt and sharp dissection to create a lower peritoneal flap [*see Figure 10*]. Dissection must stay close to the abdominal wall. A significant amount of preperitoneal fat may be encountered, and this should remain with the peritoneal flap so that the abdominal wall is cleared. When the correct preperitoneal plane is entered, dissection is almost bloodless and easily carried out. A smaller superior peritoneal flap is then created, exposing the posterior rectus muscle and the transversus abdominis arch. Scissors, if used, should always have cautery capability so that bleeding from the multiple small vessels beneath the peritoneum can be prevented.

Step 4: dissection of hernial sac The hernial sac, if present, is removed from Hesselbach's triangle or the spermatic cord and surrounding muscle through inward traction, countertraction, and blunt dissection with progressive inversion of the sac until the musculofascial boundary of the internal inguinal ring and the key deep anatomic structures are identified. An endoscopic Kitner dissector or a 2 × 2 in. piece of gauze on a grasper facilitates blunt dissection of the preperitoneal space. We prefer using a combination of sharp dissection with cautery scissors and a push-and-pull type of dissection in which both hands are used. In most cases, the hernial sac can be slowly drawn away from the transverse fascia or the spermatic cord. The sac is grasped at its apex and pulled inward, thus being reduced by inversion.

Spermatic cord lipomas usually lie posterolaterally and are extensions of preperitoneal fat. In the presence of an indirect defect, such lipomas should be dissected off the cord along with the peritoneal flap to lie cephalad to the internal inguinal ring and the subsequent repair so that prolapse through the ring can be prevented.

A large indirect hernial sac can be divided at the internal ring if it cannot be readily dissected from the cord structures. This step may prevent the cord injury that can result from extensive dissection of a large indirect sac. Division of a large indirect sac is best accomplished by opening the sac on the side opposite the spermatic cord, then completing the division from the inside.[13]

Step 5: reidentification and exposure of landmarks Once the peritoneal flap has been created, the key anatomic landmarks

mentioned earlier [*see* Laparoscopic Inguinal Anatomy, Peritoneum Removed, *above*] must be identified and exposed so that neurovascular structures can be protected from injury and the tissues required for reliable mesh fixation can be located. The pubic tubercle is often more easily felt than seen. Cooper's ligament is initially felt and subsequently seen along the pectineal prominence of the superior pubic ramus as dissection continues laterally and fatty tissue is swept off to expose the glistening white structure. Care must be taken to avoid the numerous small veins that often run on the surface of the ligament as well as to avoid the occasional aberrant obturator artery. The iliopubic tract is initially identified at the inferior margin of the internal inguinal ring, with the spermatic cord above, and is then followed in both a medial and a lateral direction. Minimal dissection is carried out inferior to the iliopubic tract so as not to injure the genitofemoral nerve, the femoral nerve, and the lateral cutaneous nerve of the thigh [*see Figure 11*].

Step 6: placement of mesh A 10 × 6 cm sheet of polypropylene mesh is tapered at its medial end, rolled into a cigarette shape and introduced into the abdomen through the 10/12 mm umbilical trocar. Prolene mesh is preferable to Marlex mesh because it is less dense, conforms more easily to the posterior inguinal wall, and has larger pores, which facilitate visualization and subsequent securing with staples. The inherent elasticity and resiliency of Prolene mesh allow it to unroll easily while maintaining its form. The mesh is used to cover the direct space (Hesselbach's triangle), the indirect space, and the femoral ring areas (i.e., the entire inguinal floor). We do not routinely make a slit in the mesh for the cord, because recurrences through the slits have been noted. An alternative is the double-buttress technique, in which a piece of mesh with a slit and a central opening is placed first and a second, uncut piece is then placed on top of the first for added security and reinforcement.[17]

Although not all surgeons consider fixation of the mesh necessary, it is our practice to staple the mesh to prevent any migration. We use an endoscopic multifire hernia stapler to secure the mesh, beginning at the pubic tubercle and proceeding laterally. The upper margin is tacked first to the rectus muscle and the transversus abdominis fascia and arch, with care taken to stay 1 to 2 cm above the level of the internal inguinal ring and avoid the inferior epigastric vessels, up to a point several centimeters lateral to the internal inguinal ring or the indirect hernial defect. Extending mesh fixation to the anterior iliac spine is neither necessary nor desirable. A

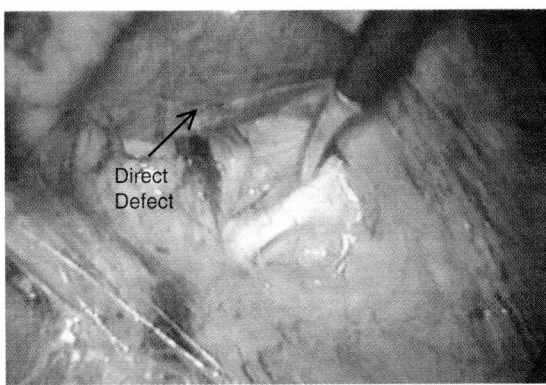

Figure 11 **Laparoscopic inguinal hernia repair: TAPP approach. Dissection of the preperitoneal space on the left side allows identification of the anatomic landmarks. The dissector points to the iliopubic tract inferior to the direct hernial defect.**

two-handed technique is recommended for staple placement: one hand is on the stapler, and the other is on the abdominal wall, applying external pressure to place the wall against the stapler. The stapler itself is frequently pushed against the tissues and used as a spreader and palpator; however, it must not be forced too deeply into the abdominal wall superolateral to the spermatic cord so as not to entrap the sensory nerves inadvertently. The stapler can be moved from the left port to the right port, depending on which position more readily allows placement of the staples perpendicular to the mesh and the abdominal wall.

Once the superior margin is fixed, any excess mesh can be trimmed with scissors; however, this step is rarely necessary with a 10 × 6 cm swatch. Fixation of the inferior margin is then easily accomplished, beginning at the pubic tubercle and moving laterally along Cooper's ligament. The mesh is lifted frequently to ensure adequate visualization of the spermatic cord. Care is taken to avoid the adjacent external iliac vessels, which lie inferiorly. Lateral to the cord structures, all staples are placed superior to the iliopubic tract to prevent subsequent neuralgias involving the lateral cutaneous nerve of the thigh or the branches of the genitofemoral nerve. If the surgeon can palpate the stapler through the abdominal wall with the nondominant hand, the stapler is above the iliopubic tract. When an indirect hernia is present, staples are placed circumferentially to the entire musculoaponeurotic ring of the hernia, which can usually be

visualized through the pores of the polypropylene mesh. The mesh should lie flat at the end of the procedure [*see Figure 12*].

For bilateral repairs, we prefer to make two peritoneal incisions and use two pieces of mesh rather than the single large piece advocated by some authorities; we find that this approach makes the mesh easier to manipulate.

Step 7: closure of peritoneum The peritoneal flap, including the redundant inverted hernial sac, is placed over the mesh, and the peritoneum is reapproximated with the tacker by precocking and partially closing the stapler, then hooking the peritoneum on one side and drawing it to the other side [*see Figure 13*]. Reduction of intra-abdominal pressure and external abdominal wall pressure facilitates a tension-free reapproximation. Alternatively, the peritoneum can be sutured over the mesh, but in most surgeons' hands, this closure takes longer.

Step 8: closure of fascia and skin The peritoneal repair is inspected to ensure that there are no major gaps that might result in exposure of the mesh and subsequent formation of adhesions. The trocars are then removed under direct vision, and the pneumoperitoneum is released. The fascia at the 10/12 mm port sites is closed with 2-0 Prolene sutures to prevent incisional hernias. The skin is closed with 4-0 absorbable subcuticular sutures.

Totally Extraperitoneal Repair

The extra-abdominal preperitoneal approach to laparoscopic hernia repair, developed by McKernan,[18] attempts to duplicate the open preperitoneal repair described by Stoppa[19-21] and Wantz.[11,22] In a TEP repair, the trocars are placed preperitoneally in a space created between the fascia and the peritoneum. An operating laparoscope provides access to the preperitoneal space of the groin, where the mesh repair is effected. Ideally, none of the preliminary exploratory trocars penetrates the peritoneum, and the dissection remains in the extra-abdominal plane at all times.

Patient preparation and positioning are much the same as in a TAPP repair. The surgeon stands on the side opposite the hernia.

Step 1: creation of preperitoneal space With the patient in the Trendelenburg position, the fascia is opened through a 1 cm infraumbilical transverse incision placed slightly toward the side of the hernia, which helps one avoid inadvertently opening the peritoneum. An index finger is inserted on the medial aspect of the exposed rectus muscle and slid over the posterior rectus sheath. A

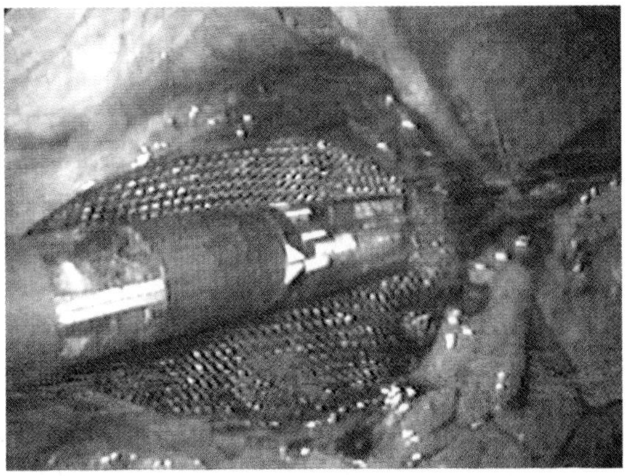

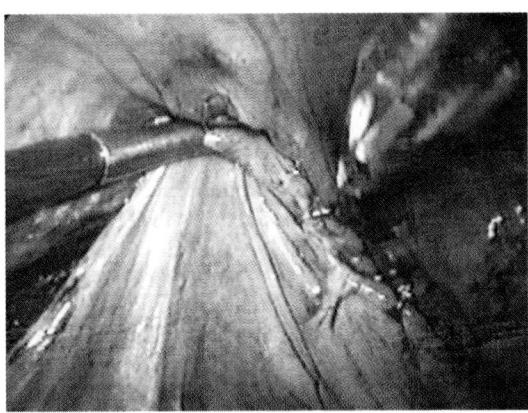

Figure 12 **Laparoscopic inguinal hernia repair: TAPP approach. The mesh is stapled in place.**

Figure 13 **Laparoscopic inguinal hernia repair: TAPP approach. The peritoneum is stapled over the mesh.**

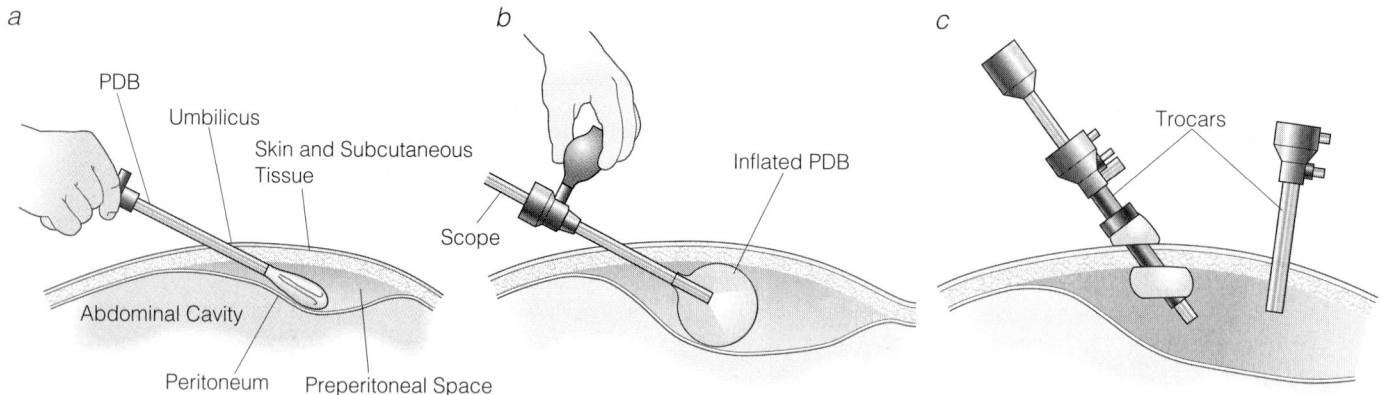

a

PDB
Umbilicus
Skin and Subcutaneous Tissue
Scope
Abdominal Cavity
Peritoneum Preperitoneal Space

b

Inflated PDB

c

Trocars

Figure 14 **Laparoscopic inguinal hernia repair: TEP approach. Shown is the preperitoneal distention balloon (PDB) system. The PDB is introduced into the preperitoneal space (*a*). As it is tunneled inferiorly toward the pubis, the PDB is inflated under laparoscopic vision (*b*). Once the preperitoneal space is created, the PDB is removed and replaced with a blunt-tip trocar. The preperitoneal space is insufflated under low pressure, additional trocars are placed, and the repair is completed (*c*).**

preperitoneal tunnel between the rectus abdominis muscles and the peritoneum is created in the midline with blunt finger dissection. A blunt 10/12 mm trocar is then secured in the preperitoneal space with fascial stay sutures.

An operating laparoscope is inserted through the trocar with a blunt 5 mm probe in the operating channel. Insufflation of the preperitoneal space is begun while the probe depresses the peritoneum and develops the preperitoneal space down to the pubis under direct vision, with the rectus muscles seen anteriorly and the peritoneum posteriorly. Maximum inflation pressure is 8 to 10 mm Hg to prevent disruption of the peritoneum or development of extensive subcutaneous emphysema.

TEP repair can be facilitated by using a preperitoneal distention balloon (PDB) system (Origin Medsystems, Inc., Menlo Park, California). This system consists of a trocar with an inflatable balloon at its tip, which is used to develop the preperitoneal space by atraumatically separating the peritoneum from the abdominal wall. The PDB is inserted into the preperitoneal space below the umbilicus by means of an open Hasson technique and is tunneled inferiorly toward the internal inguinal ring. The preperitoneal working space is developed by gradual inflation of the balloon to a volume of 1 L; the transparency of the balloon permits constant visualization throughout the distention process. Once the working space is created, the PDB is removed and replaced with a blunt sealing trocar. The preperitoneal space is then reinsufflated to a pressure of 8 to 10 mm Hg [*see Figure 14*].

After the peritoneum is dissected away from the rectus muscle, a midline 5 mm trocar is inserted just above the pubis under direct vision, and a 10/12 mm trocar is placed halfway between the pubis and the umbilicus [*see Figure 15*], with care taken not to penetrate the peritoneum. The risk of intraperitoneal entry can be minimized by blunt dissection down to the fascia with a hemostat after the skin incision. If the peritoneum is penetrated, the resulting pneumoperitoneum can reduce the already limited working space. One can try to repair the rent with a suture, but if such repair is unsuccessful, the loss of working space may necessitate conversion to a TAPP approach.

Step 2: dissection of hernial sac The operating laparoscope is replaced by a 45° laparoscope, which facilitates exposure and visualization of this region. Wide dissection of the preperitoneal space is then undertaken with blunt graspers in a two-hand-

ed technique, with the grasper in the left hand depressing the peritoneum. The pubis, Cooper's ligament, and the inferior epigastric vessels are located. If a direct hernia is present, the sac and the preperitoneal contents are carefully dissected away from the fascial defect, with care taken not to enter the peritoneal cavity. The peritoneum is then further dissected cephalad to expose the internal ring and any indirect hernial sac. A small indirect hernial sac is dissected off the spermatic cord and reduced or amputated with an endoscopic ligating loop after reduction of its contents has been ensured. A large indirect hernial sac is transected and closed, with the distal sac left in place and not ligated.

For hernias that are not readily reduced, McKernan[23] suggests making an incision in the groin above the pubis down to the external oblique aponeurosis and severing the adhesions between the sac and the external ring. If this measure does not work, the sac

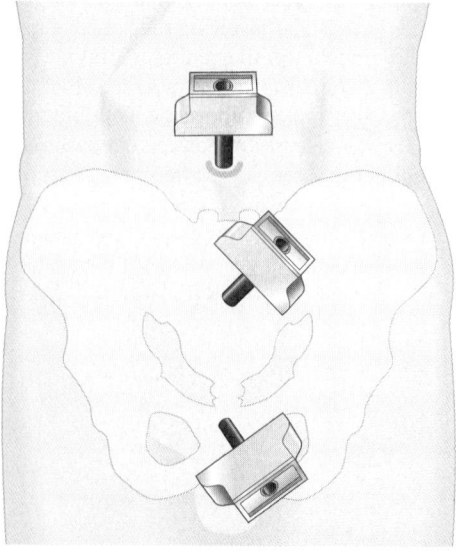

Figure 15 **Laparoscopic inguinal hernia repair: TEP approach. Shown is standard trocar placement for TEP repair. As in TAPP repair, three trocar sites are used. One trocar is placed in the umbilicus; the second is placed in the midline, midway between the umbilicus and the pubis; and the third is placed above the pubic arch. The trocars should not penetrate the peritoneum.**

can be opened through the incision and the adhesions within the sac lysed. If the hernia still cannot be reduced, the TEP repair is abandoned in favor of an anterior approach.

Step 3: placement of mesh A 10×15 cm piece of Prolene mesh is incised vertically, and a 1 cm hole is created centrally for the spermatic cord. The mesh is then folded in half horizontally, with sutures at each corner to maintain the fold, then inserted through the umbilical trocar and drawn behind the cord structures. Once the mesh is well positioned, with the spermatic cord seated in the central hole, the corner sutures are divided, and the mesh is unfolded against the anterior abdominal wall. As in a TAPP repair, the mesh is tacked to key structures, including the pubic tubercle, Cooper's ligament, and the iliopubic tract inferiorly and anteriorly to the posterior aspect of the rectus abdominis muscle. The opening in the mesh is then closed with staples, with great care taken not to compromise cord structures. The mesh must lie flat. No staples are placed inferior to the iliopubic tract lateral to the internal ring. For bilateral hernias, two identical repairs are done, and the two mesh patches are tacked together at the pubis. An additional piece of mesh may be placed cephalad to the pubis for reinforcement.

A major advantage of the TEP approach is avoidance of entry into the peritoneal cavity and thus of the potential risk of adhesions and bowel obstruction. In practice, however, breaches in the peritoneum are common, resulting in decreased operating space and a compromised view of the anatomic structures as pneumoperitoneum ensues. In addition, even when intraperitoneal entry is avoided, the small amount of working space inherent in the nature of the technique can cause the surgeon great difficulty and confusion. For these reasons, considerable experience is required and caution advised before TEP repair is attempted.

Step 4: closure The operative site is inspected for hemostasis. The trocars are removed under direct vision with release of the insufflated CO_2. The fascia at trocar sites larger than 10 mm is closed with 2-0 Prolene sutures, and the skin is closed with subcuticular sutures.

POSTOPERATIVE CARE

Patients are observed in the recovery room until they are able to ambulate unassisted and to void; if they are unable to void at the time of discharge, in-and-out catheterization is performed. Patients are advised to resume their usual activities as they see fit; driving a car is permitted the next day. Outpatient prescriptions for acetaminophen and codeine are given, and follow-up visits in the surgical clinic are scheduled for day 7 after operation. Patients who live alone, who have had an intraoperative complication, who have significant nausea or vomiting, or have unexplained or inordinate pain are admitted overnight.

DISADVANTAGES AND COMPLICATIONS

Disadvantages

Need for general anesthesia The need for pneumoperitoneum and thus for general anesthesia in laparoscopic herniorrhaphy is sometimes considered a major disadvantage. Nausea, dizziness, and headache are more common in the recovery room after TAPP repair than after Lichtenstein repair.[24] It is not necessarily true, however, that local or regional anesthesia is safer than general anesthesia.[25] Anesthesiologic studies critically appraising anesthetic techniques for hernia surgery have shown the choice of general anesthesia over local or regional anesthesia to be safe and, in many cases, advantageous, particularly in patients who are in poor health. Furthermore, TEP repair has been successfully done with patients under epidural[26] and local[27] anesthesia.

Lower cost-effectiveness The costs of laparoscopic repair exceed those of open repair.[24,28-33] For the most part, the differences are accounted for by longer operative time and the use of disposable equipment. Operative time decreases with experience, and disposable trocars and scissors can be replaced with reusable instruments. Suturing the mesh and peritoneum saves the cost of the stapler but requires more operative time.

The higher operative costs of laparoscopic repair notwithstanding, economic impact studies to date have not shown either approach to be clearly more cost-effective. In terms of effectiveness, the laparoscopic approach fares better on most patient-based outcome measures, including pain and convalescence; however, it remains to be seen whether these savings in disability offset the higher operative costs. One randomized study suggested that the total costs of laparoscopic repair were actually lower than those of the Lichtenstein repair when lost workdays were taken into account.[34]

Complications

Most randomized trials comparing laparoscopic repair with open mesh repair have found comparable numbers of total complications in the two groups [*see Table 1*]. Four studies reported fewer overall complications after laparoscopic repair.[24,32,35,36] In general, although intraoperative complications are more common and potentially more serious in the laparoscopic approach, particularly when a TAPP repair is chosen, postoperative complications tend to be less common.

Complications of access to peritoneal cavity A TAPP hernia repair exposes the patient to several potentially serious risks related to the choice of the transabdominal route. Trocar injuries to the bowel, the bladder, and vascular structures can occur during the creation of the initial pneumoperitoneum or the subsequent insertion of the trocars. Use of an open insertion technique to create the pneumoperitoneum should eliminate major vascular injuries as well as make identification and repair of bowel injuries simpler than they would be with the closed technique. Another complication related to trocar sites is incisional hernia, which can lead to postoperative bowel obstruction.[37]

The use of the transabdominal route also exposes the patient to the risk of adhesions and the potential for late bowel obstruction. Fortunately, evidence from study of herniorrhaphy in pigs[38] and from extensive gynecologic application of laparoscopy in humans over many years suggests that adhesions form significantly less often after laparoscopic procedures than after open procedures.

Complications of dissection Injuries occurring during dissection are often linked to inexperience with laparoscopic inguinal anatomy. If serious enough, they can necessitate laparotomy. Conversion of a laparoscopic procedure to an open one, however, is regarded more seriously in herniorrhaphy patients than in cholecystectomy patients. In laparoscopic cholecystectomy, conversion to laparotomy is acceptable and expected in 4% to 5% of cases, and common bile duct injury is a recognized complication of both open and laparoscopic cholecystectomy. In contrast, some of the complications encountered in laparoscopic herniorrhaphy never occur in classic open anterior herniorrhaphy, and conversion to laparotomy to correct a complication arising during laparoscopic herniorrhaphy is not acceptable. Fortunately, such conversion is rare: in more than 800 laparoscopic herniorrhaphies reported by 19 institutions in a multicenter phase II study, only one bladder injury and one bowel perforation requiring laparotomy for repair were documented.[15]

Table 1 Selected English-Language Randomized Controlled Trials
Comparing Laparoscopic with Open Mesh Repairs

Study Authors	Technique Employed	N	OR Time Needed for Unilateral Repairs (min)	Less Early Pain after Laparoscopic Repair?	Complications*	Recovery† (days)	Recurrences (No.)	Cost
Payne et al (1994)	TAPP	48	68	NA	12%	8.9	0	$3,093
	Lichtenstein	52	56		18%	17‡	0	$2,494‡
Wright et al (1996)	TEP	60	58	Yes‡	15	NA	NA	NA
	Lichtenstein	60	45‡		43			
Champault et al (1997)	TEP	51	NA	Yes‡	4%	17	3	NA
	Stoppa	49			30%‡	35‡	1	
Paganini et al (1997)	TAPP	52	67	No	27%	15	2	$1,249
	Lichtenstein	56	48‡		27%	14	0	$306‡
Wellwood et al (1998)	TAPP	200	45	Yes‡	316	5	0	£747
	Lichtenstein	200	45		452‡	8‡	0	£412‡
Zieren et al (1998)	TAPP	80	61	No	19%	3	0	$1,211
	PP	80	36‡		15%	4	0	$124‡
Khoury (1998)	TEP	150	32	Yes‡	13%	8	4	
	PP	142	31		23%‡	15‡	4	
Johansson et al (1999)	TAPP	205	65	Yes‡	66	18	4	5,988 SEK
	Stoppa	204	38		49	24‡	11	350 SEK
MRC (1999)	TAPP/TEP	468	58	NA	30%	10	7	LH £314
	Mixed open§	460	43‡		44%‡	14‡	0‡	more

*Complications are expressed as percentage of patients affected or total number of complications, as reported in the individual studies.
†Definition of recovery varies from study to study..
‡*P* < 0.05.
§Lichtenstein in 94%.
LH—laparoscopic herniorrhaphy   NA—not available   PP—plug-and-patch   TAPP—transabdominal preperitoneal   TEP—totally extraperitoneal

The most common vascular injuries in laparoscopic inguinal herniorrhaphy are those involving the inferior epigastric vessels and the spermatic vessels. The external iliac, circumflex iliac, profunda, and obturator vessels are also at risk. A previous lower abdominal operation is a risk factor.[13] The source of any abnormal bleeding during the procedure must be quickly identified. All vessels in the groin can be ligated except the external iliac vessels, which must be repaired.[13]

Injuries to the urinary tract can also occur. Four bladder injuries requiring repair were documented in a collected series of 762 laparoscopic repairs by different surgical groups.[39] Bladder injuries are most likely to occur when the space of Retzius has been previously dissected (e.g., in a prostatectomy). Renal and ureteral injuries can result from poorly placed trocars. Any urinary tract injuries identified intraoperatively should be repaired immediately. Often, however, these injuries are not apparent until the postoperative period, when they present as lower abdominal pain, renal failure, ascites, dysuria, or hematuria—all of which should be investigated promptly. Although indwelling catheter drainage may constitute sufficient treatment of a missed retroperitoneal bladder injury, intraperitoneal injuries are best treated by direct repair via either laparoscopy or laparotomy.

Complications related to mesh Complications related to the use of mesh include infection, migration, adhesion formation, and erosion into intraperitoneal organs. Such complications usually become apparent weeks to years after the initial repair, presenting as abscess, fistula, or small bowel obstruction.

Mesh infection is very rare. Phillips and colleagues collected information on 2,559 North American patients and found only one patient who required removal of an infected mesh after an IPOM repair.[40] Estour and Mouret reviewed 7,340 patients from 22 European groups and found only seven patients with reported mesh infections.[41] Mesh infection usually responds to conservative treatment with antibiotics and drainage. On rare occasions, the mesh must be removed; this may be accomplished via an external approach. It is noteworthy that removal of the mesh does not always lead to recurrence of the hernia, a finding that may be attributable to the resulting fibrosis.[42]

Mesh migration may lead to hernia recurrence. In a TAPP repair, appropriate stapling of the mesh should reduce this possibility. In a TEP repair, stapling does not appear to be necessary to prevent migration.[43,44]

The risk that adhesions to the mesh will form is substantially augmented if the mesh is left fully exposed to the bowel, as in the case with the IPOM technique. Even with the TAPP approach, the long-term durability and effectiveness of the sometimes flimsy peritoneal coverage have been questioned. Over the past 25 years, however, extensive intraperitoneal use of polypropylene mesh in abdominal wall reconstruction has rarely led to adhesions causing bowel obstruction. Nonetheless, either small bowel[40] or omentum[33] can be incarcerated at a defect in the peritoneal closure site, and reoperation may be required.

Urinary complications Injuries to the urinary tract aside [*see* Complications of Dissection, *above*], urinary retention, urinary tract infection, and hematuria are the most common complications. Avoidance of bladder catheterization reduces the incidence of these complications, but urinary retention still occurs in 1.5% to 2.0% of patients. General anesthesia and the administration of large volumes of I.V. fluids may also predispose to retention.

Vas deferens and testicular complications Wantz[45] believes that the most common cause of postoperative testicular swelling, orchitis, and ischemic atrophy is surgical trauma to the testicular veins (i.e., venous congestion and subsequent thrombosis). Because spermatic cord dissection is minimized with the laparoscopic approach, the risk of groin and testicular complications resulting from injury to cord structures and adjacent nerves should be reduced. When the hernial sac is left undisturbed, there is less trauma to the cord, its vessels, and adjacent nerves.

Most testicular complications, such as swelling, pain, and epididymitis, are self-limited. Testicular pain occurs in about 1% of patients after laparoscopic repair,[34] an incidence comparable to that seen after open repair.[46] A similar number of patients experience testicular atrophy,[32] for which there is no specific treatment.

The risk of injury to the vas deferens appears to be much the same in laparoscopic repair as in open repair.[13] If fertility is an issue, the cut ends should be reapproximated if the injury is recognized intraoperatively.

Postoperative groin and thigh pain Unlike patients who undergo open anterior herniorrhaphy, in whom discomfort or numbness is usually localized to the operative area, patients who undergo laparoscopic repair occasionally describe unusual but specific symptoms of deep discomfort that are usually positional and are often of a transient, shooting nature suggestive of nerve irritation. The pain is frequently incited by stooping, twisting, or movements causing extension of the hip and can be shocklike. Although these symptoms can frequently be elicited in the early postoperative period, they are usually transient. If a neuralgia is present in the recovery room, however, prompt reexploration is the best approach.[13]

Persistent pain and burning sensations in the inguinal region, the upper medial thigh, or the spermatic cord and scrotal skin region occur when the genitofemoral nerve or the ilioinguinal nerve is stimulated, entrapped, or unintentionally injured. When these symptoms persist, they may result in severe morbidity.[47] A more worrisome symptom is lateral or central upper medial thigh numbness, which is reported in 1% to 2% of patients and often lasts several months or longer. Whether this numbness is related to staple entrapment, fibrous adhesions, cicatricial neuroma, or mesh irritation is unknown. Numbness and paresthesia of the lateral thigh are less frequent and are related to the involvement of fibers of the lateral cutaneous nerve. These problems can be prevented by paying careful attention to anatomic detail and technique.[48] After performing 50 cadaveric dissections to determine the relation of the nerves to the internal ring, Rosen and coworkers concluded that both the genitofemoral nerve and the lateral cutaneous nerve of the thigh will be protected in all cases if no staples are placed further than 1.5 cm lateral to the edge of the internal ring.[49]

A great deal of attention has rightly been focused on the risk of nerve injury with laparoscopic hernia repair as well as on ways of preventing it. At the same time, it is important to note that pain and numbness, including thigh numbness, can also occur after open repair and may in fact be more common in that setting than was previously realized. In one study, groin pain lasting longer than 1 month was present in 8% of patients after Lichtenstein repair but in no patients after TAPP.[33] A randomized study of 928 patients found that 1 year after operation, the laparoscopic group had a lower rate of persistent groin pain than the open mesh group (30% versus 37%) and a similar incidence of thigh numbness (14% versus 11%).[32]

Miscellaneous complications Early postoperative examination of patients who have undergone laparoscopic hernia repair frequently reveals groin bogginess, a cough impulse, and deep tenderness over the internal inguinal ring, particularly when the hernia was indirect and when the hernial sac was left in situ.[50] True hydroceles are rare. Well-defined, confined masses 1 to 3 cm in diameter are often palpated at the external inguinal ring or near the pubic tubercle. These typically represent hematomas,[50] which are more common when the sac has been dissected in a TAPP repair. Unlike the diffuse hematomas seen with open repair, these hematomas are very well defined and usually asymptomatic; however, they are very slow to disappear. These findings often mimic those of recurrent hernia and call for careful follow-up. Lipomas of the spermatic cord, if left unreduced in patients with indirect hernias, may produce a persistent groin mass and a cough impulse that mimic recurrence, especially to an uninitiated examiner. These lipomas are always asymptomatic.

OUTCOME EVALUATION

Although there is a large body of literature on laparoscopic inguinal hernia repair—including a variety of randomized controlled trials—the benefits of the laparoscopic approach have not yet been clearly defined or widely accepted. One reason may be that the literature can be difficult to summarize and understand. For example, studies have reported conflicting results: several randomized, controlled trials suggested that the laparoscopic technique offered little benefit,[28,29,34,51,52] but many trials reached the opposite conclusion.[24,30-33,35,36,43,53-57] Furthermore, different trials have compared different operations: TAPP repair, TEP repair, or a mixture of the two, on one hand, against open mesh repair, open sutured repair, or a mixture of the two, on the other hand.

Given the low morbidity and relatively short convalescence already associated with the conventional operation, demonstration of any significant improvements that might be associated with the laparoscopic operation would probably require large study samples. Thus, combining existing studies may be illuminating. In a meta-analysis that included studies performed up to March 1997, Chung and Rowland grouped 18 trials according to the operations compared.[58] In group 1, laparoscopic repair (TAPP, in most cases) was compared with open tension-free repair. In group 2, laparoscopic repair was compared with open sutured repair. In group 3, laparoscopic repair was compared with a mixture of open operations ("at the discretion of the surgeon"). In all comparisons, the laparoscopic operation took longer to perform. Compared with sutured repair, laparoscopic operation yielded significantly less postoperative pain and a significantly shorter recovery. Compared with tension-free repair, however, laparoscopic repair showed no significant advantage with respect to pain but resulted in a slightly shorter recovery (though the reduction was of marginal statistical significance). The results of the meta-analysis suggest that the postoperative course of open tension-free repair is different from that of open sutured repair, with the former clearly resulting in less postoperative pain and a shorter recovery. In that open tension-free repair uses mesh, it resembles laparoscopic repair more closely than open sutured repair does and thus is probably a more relevant comparison procedure. Accordingly, we will briefly review the findings of a number of recent studies that compare laparoscopic inguinal herniorrhaphy with open mesh repair.

Laparoscopic Repair versus Open Mesh Repair

At least 12 prospective, randomized trials comparing laparoscopic repair with open tension-free mesh repair were published in English between 1994 and 1999,[24,28-36,46,59] nine of which are summarized elsewhere [*see Table 1*]. The heterogeneity of the studies' designs (particularly with respect to the different types of repairs done and the different outcome measures assessed) makes direct comparisons difficult. For example, the laparoscopic methods used included TAPP repair alone (eight studies[24,28-31,33,34,59]), TEP repair alone (three studies[35,36,46]), and a combination of TAPP and TEP repair (one study[32]). The open methods used included Lichtenstein repair with local anesthesia (four studies[24,28,33,34]), Lichtenstein repair with general anesthesia (four studies[30,32,46,59]), open Stoppa preperitoneal repair with general anesthesia (two studies[31,35]), plug-and-patch repair with local anesthesia (one study[29]), and plug-and-patch repair with general anesthesia (one study[36]). Most of the studies included bilateral along with unilateral hernias.[24,28,32,33,35,36,46] The considerable differences between these 12 studies notwithstanding, several suggestive patterns do emerge.

Convalescence time The most significant short-term outcome measure after hernia repair is convalescence time, defined as the time required for the patient to return to normal activities. One of the most frequently cited benefits of laparoscopic herniorrhaphy is the patient's rapid return to unrestricted activity, including work. Most of the randomized studies comparing laparoscopic with open mesh repair, including the four largest, report a significantly shorter convalescence time after laparoscopic repair.[24,30-33,35,36] For example, in a study of 400 patients specifically designed to detect differences in convalescence at various defined levels, Wellwood and coworkers found that the self-reported time to return to normal household and social activities was significantly shorter after TAPP repair than after Lichtenstein repair with local anesthesia.[24] In a large multicenter cooperative trial of 928 patients in which TAPP or TEP was compared mainly with tension-free mesh repair, the laparoscopic group returned to normal social activities significantly faster than the open group (10 days versus 14 days).[32]

Convalescence time, particularly time off work, is a complex outcome measure that varies as much with patient expectation, motivation, and disability coverage as it does with surgical morbidity.[33,60] Moreover, measurement of convalescence is subject to bias if the assessor is not blinded to the treatment arm. Finally, the operating surgeon may not assess outcome in the same way as other unbiased observers[61] or the patients themselves would.

Postoperative pain After laparoscopic repair, most patients experience minimal immediate postoperative pain and have little or no need for analgesics after postoperative day 1. In addition, patients are generally able to perform some exercises better after laparoscopic repair than after Lichtenstein repair.[33] That patients experience less postoperative pain after laparoscopic repair than after open mesh repair has been reported in several randomized studies.[24,30,31,35,36,46] A meta-analysis of more than 500 patients in five trials, however, found that postoperative pain, measured on the basis either of analgesic administration or of ratings on a visual analog scale (VAS), was not significantly less after TAPP repair than after open tension-free repair.[58] Zieren and colleagues found no difference in postoperative pain assessed by VAS between 80 patients undergoing TAPP repair and 80 patients undergoing open plug-and-patch repair; however, both groups had significantly lower VAS scores than did 80 patients undergoing Shouldice repair[29]— a finding consistent with almost all of the reports comparing laparoscopic repair with open sutured repair.[43]

Quality of life The studies that have assessed quality of life immediately after hernia repair have tended to favor the laparoscopic approach, albeit marginally. Using the SF-36 (a widely accepted general health–related quality-of-life questionnaire), Wellwood and coworkers found that at 1 month, greater improvements from baseline were apparent in the laparoscopic group in every dimension except general health; however, by 3 months, the differences between the two groups were no longer significant.[24] The MRC group also found no differences in any SF-36 domains at 3 months after operation.[32] Filipi and associates, using the Sickness Impact Profile, found some benefit to the laparoscopic approach.[59]

Bilateral hernias Laparoscopy allows simultaneous exploration of the abdominal cavity and diagnosis and treatment of bilateral groin hernias as well as of coexisting femoral hernias (which are often unrecognized preoperatively), without added risk or disability. Many surgeons avoid performing simultaneous bilateral repair during an open procedure because of the resulting increase in swelling, pain, disability, operative time, and the risk of infection and recurrence. One retrospective study found that simultaneous repair of bilateral hernias via the laparoscopic approach resulted in a shorter convalescence time and a quicker return to work than a modified Shouldice repair.[62] In a prospective, randomized study, Paganini and colleagues found in subgroup analysis that the mean operative time did not differ significantly between bilateral laparoscopic repair and bilateral open mesh repair (85.7 ± 32.2 minutes for TAPP repair versus 75.9 ± 43.3 minutes for open repair).[28] Further prospective, randomized trials designed to compare simultaneous bilateral open tension-free repair with bilateral laparoscopic repair should be undertaken.

Hernia recurrence Open mesh repair has been associated with long-term recurrence rates of 1% or less, even when not performed by hernia specialists.[63,64] If the laparoscopic approach is to be a viable alternative to open repair, it should have comparable results.

In fact, the short-term experience with laparoscopic hernia repair is encouraging. Case series of TAPP and TEP repairs demonstrate recurrence rates ranging from 0% to 2%, with especially low recurrence rates reported after TEP repair.[65] Of the 12 randomized studies of laparoscopic repair versus open mesh repair mentioned earlier (see above), only one found a significant difference in recurrence rates, reporting seven recurrences in 468 laparoscopic patients and no recurrences in 460 open repairs.[32] All seven recurrences occurred in patients who underwent TAPP repair, even though TAPP accounted for only 21% of the laparoscopic repairs.

Most reported recurrences after laparoscopic herniorrhaphy come at an early stage in the surgeon's experience with this procedure and soon after operation.[15] The majority can be attributed to (1) the surgeon's imperfect understanding of the preperitoneal anatomy and the anatomic landmarks for mesh fixation, which leads to inadequate preperitoneal dissection; (2) use of an inadequately sized patch, which fails to provide support for the entire inguinal area, including direct, indirect, and femoral spaces; or (3) staple failure. Secure fascial fixation of the prosthesis is a paramount concern, particularly with TAPP repair; accurate stapling technique, with careful placement of each staple, is vital to prevention of recurrence.

Once a hernia recurs after an initial open repair, laparoscopic repair may be a particularly suitable treatment approach.[66] Normal anatomic and cord structures are not distorted by scar tissue in the preperitoneal space, dissection planes are unmarred, and the risk of causing testicular damage is reduced. The recurrence is usually very well seen and better defined from the peritoneal aspect, and the entire myopectineal inguinal floor can be reinforced and repaired without tension and without the need to use scarred or weakened tissue, which predisposes to further recurrence. Unfortunately, there are few controlled studies that have examined recurrent hernias exclusively. In one randomized study of 79 patients in which TAPP repair of recurrent hernias was compared with open preperitoneal repair, patients experienced less pain and had a shorter convalescence after TAPP repair; however, there were seven recurrences after TAPP repair and only one after open repair.[67]

Transabdominal Preperitoneal Repair versus Totally Extraperitoneal Repair

The TAPP approach is easier to learn and perform than the TEP approach, and even experienced laparoscopic hernia surgeons report more technical difficulties with the latter.[68] Nonetheless, there is a growing body of literature to suggest that TEP repair, by avoiding entry into the peritoneal cavity, provides significant advantages over TAPP repair.[3] In particular, the TEP approach should eliminate trocar site hernias, small bowel injury and obstruction, and intraperitoneal adhesions to the mesh. Kald and colleagues consecutively performed TAPP repairs in 339 patients and TEP repairs in 87 patients, then followed the patients for a mean of 23 and 7 months, respectively.[69] Time off work was shorter after TEP. In the 426 patients studied, 15 major complications were noted, including one death, two bowel obstructions, one severe neuralgia, three trocar site hernias, one epigastric artery hemorrhage, and seven recurrences; all except the epigastric artery hemorrhage occurred in the TAPP group. It is possible, however, that these results can be partly explained by the learning curve, in that the TAPP repairs were all done before the TEP repairs. That six TAPP recurrences occurred in the first 31 cases, whereas only one occurred in the subsequent 395 patients, lends support to this possibility.

In a study comparing 733 TAPP repairs with 382 TEP repairs, 11 major complications occurred in the TAPP group (two recurrences, six trocar hernias, one small bowel obstruction, and two small bowel injuries), whereas only one recurrence and no intraperitoneal complications occurred in the TEP group.[70] Seven TEP procedures were converted to TAPP procedures. Time off work was equal in the two groups but was prolonged in patients receiving compensation. As in the Kald study, the TAPP patients were followed longer than the TEP patients, and the TAPP cases occupied the first part of the learning curve. To avoid this type of selection bias would require a randomized study.

Not all surgeons are convinced that TEP repair is the laparoscopic procedure of choice. Cohen and coworkers compared 108 TAPP repairs with 100 TEP repairs.[68] Although the TEP repairs were done only by surgeons who were already familiar with TAPP repair, many of the surgeons still encountered technical difficulties and problems with landmark identification. Overall, complications did not occur significantly more frequently in either group, but they seemed more severe in the TAPP group: four trocar site hernias, one bladder injury, and six seromas were noted in the TAPP group, compared with one cellulitis and six seromas in the TEP group. The authors concluded that because TAPP repair is easier and does not increase complications significantly, it is an "adequate" procedure. The sample size may have been too small to permit detection of small differences in complication rates.

Laparoscopic Incisional Hernia Repair

Incisional hernias develop in approximately 2% to 11% of patients undergoing laparotomy.[71,72] It has been estimated that 90,000 ventral hernia repairs are carried out in the United States every year.[4] Open incisional hernia repair can be a difficult procedure and may carry a high morbidity. Without prosthetic mesh, repair of large incisional hernias is associated with recurrence rates as high as 50%; in addition, it can be associated with significant complications and a substantial hospital stay.

Laparoscopic repair of incisional hernia was initially described in 1992,[8] and it remains an emerging procedure. Taking a laparoscopic approach allows the surgeon to minimize the abdominal wall incisions, avoid extensive flap dissection and muscle mobilization, and eliminate the need for drains in proximity to the mesh, thereby potentially achieving decreases in pain, recovery time, and duration of hospitalization as well as lower rates of surgical site infections. In addition, the improved visualization of the abdominal wall associated with the laparoscopic view may result in better definition of the defect, the discovery of unrecognized hernia sites, and improved adhesiolysis. If this improved visualization permits more precise and accurate placement and tailoring of the mesh, recurrence rates may also be decreased.

Laparoscopic incisional hernia repair is best suited for repairing large incisional hernias, which may be defined as any incisional hernia in which the smallest diameter is greater than 3 cm. With these large defects, prosthetic material must be used to ensure tension-free repair of the hernia, which reduces the risk of recurrence. Smaller hernias can usually be repaired without mesh, often on an outpatient basis; there is little to be gained by adopting a laparoscopic approach to these defects. Both upper abdominal and lower abdominal incisions are amenable to a laparoscopic approach. The so-called Swiss cheese hernia, which comprises multiple small defects, is particularly well suited to this approach: open repair would necessitate a large incision for access to the multiple fascial defects. Incarcerated hernias can also be approached laparoscopically; however, the suspected presence of compromised bowel is an absolute contraindication. An abdomen that has undergone multiple operations and contains dense adhesions presents a challenge in terms of both access to the abdominal cavity and access to the hernia site. If the surgeon cannot obtain safe access to the peritoneal cavity for insufflation, a laparoscopic approach is contraindicated.

To date, very few comparative trials focusing on laparoscopic incisional herniorrhaphy have been reported. We will therefore concentrate on the technique we currently employ for the repair.

OPERATIVE PLANNING

Preparation

Formal mechanical and antibiotic bowel preparation is administered if it is suspected that there is incarcerated bowel in the hernia. With the patient straining, the edges of the hernia defect are marked on the skin whenever possible. If the defect is in the lower abdomen, a Foley catheter is placed in the bladder. Prophylactic antibiotics are not routinely administered. The procedure is performed with the patient under general anesthesia.

Positioning

The patient is placed in the supine position with the arms extended. If the hernia is in the midline, the surgeon can stand on either side of the patient, with the monitor directly opposite. Initially, the assistant stands on the same side as the surgeon; however, he or she may later have to move to the opposite side to help with dissection and stapling. A second monitor on the opposite side of the table is useful. If the defect is subcostal, the surgeon may prefer to operate from between the patient's legs, with a monitor at the head of the bed.

Equipment

Because laparoscopic incisional hernia repair leaves the mesh exposed to the intraperitoneal cavity, some concern has arisen about the risk of adhesion formation and fistulization if polypropylene mesh is used. A polytetrafluoroethylene (PTFE) prosthesis would have a reduced propensity for adhesion formation and could be more safely placed in an intraperitoneal position, but PTFE is much harder to manipulate laparoscopically than polypropylene and is a less effective scaffold for ingrowth of collagen. We currently use Composix mesh (Bard, Davol Inc., Cranston, Rhode Island), which consists of PTFE on the side facing the peritoneal cavity and two layers of polypropylene mesh on the side facing the abdominal wall. This mesh marries the strength of Marlex with the safety of PTFE.

Additional special equipment used for incisional hernia repair includes 2-0 nonabsorbable sutures, a Keith needle, a 2 mm suture passer, a sterile marking pen, and a stapler (typically, a 12 mm 65° device that uses 4.8 mm staples). Atraumatic bowel instruments are required to reduce incarcerated intestines without injuring them. An ultrasonic scalpel is useful if extensive adhesiolysis is required: it helps expedite the procedure while improving hemostasis.

OPERATIVE TECHNIQUE

In essence, the repair consists of the intraperitoneal placement of a large piece of mesh so that it overlaps the defect in the fascia and the abdominal wall. The defect is not closed. The mesh is anchored with a minimum of four subcutaneously tied transfascial sutures placed at the four corners and is further secured between the sutures with intraperitoneally placed staples.

Step 1: Placement of Trocars

Because of the probability of extensive intra-abdominal adhesions, we begin with open insertion of a blunt 12 mm trocar. This trocar is inserted laterally, at the level of the middle of the hernia, rather than in the midline, even though doing so necessitates dissecting through several layers of muscle.

A 30° scope is then inserted. As in inguinal repair, an angled scope is essential because dissection and repair are done on the undersurface of the anterior abdominal wall, which cannot be adequately visualized with a 0° scope. Laparoscopy is performed and the hernial defect identified. Two additional 5 mm ports are then placed on the same side as the surgeon. These ports are placed superior and inferior to the initial trocar and should be lo-

cated as far laterally as possible, with care taken to ensure that the downward movement of the instruments is not limited by the iliac crest or the thigh. Lateral placement is necessary to optimize exposure of the abdominal wall.

Once all adhesions to the abdominal wall have been dissected sufficiently (see below), a fourth port can be placed on the opposite side to facilitate adhesiolysis and mesh fixation. As noted, some of the ports can be 5 mm, depending on the caliber of the instruments available. Ultimately, port placement depends on the hernia's location, the patient's body habitus, and the surgeon's preference.

Step 2: Exposure of Hernial Defect

The edges of the hernial defect are exposed by reducing the contents of the hernia into the abdominal cavity. All adhesions from bowel or omentum to the abdominal wall in the vicinity of the defect must be transected. This dissection may be performed with cautery scissors or a hook cautery. An ultrasonic scalpel may be useful for optimizing hemostasis if extensive vascularized adhesions are encountered. It is not necessary to excise or reduce the hernial sac itself [see Figure 16].

Step 3: Tailoring of Mesh

The contours of the hernia defect are marked as accurately as possible on the exterior abdominal wall; the edges may be delineated with a combination of palpation and visualization. A rough pictorial representation of the swatch of mesh that will be required is then drawn on the skin around the hernial defect, with care taken to overlap the edges of the defect by at least 2 cm on all sides [see Figure 17]. This template is measured, and the mesh swatch is cut to its dimensions. The four corners of the swatch and those of its representation on the abdominal wall are numbered clockwise from 1 to 4 for later orientation. A mark is made on the inner side of the mesh so that the surgeon can easily determine which side is to face the peritoneum once the mesh is inserted into the peritoneal cavity. A 2-0 Prolene suture is tied in each corner of the mesh swatch, and both ends are left about 15 cm long. Thicker suture material is not easily passed through the abdominal wall.

The mesh swatch is rolled as tightly as possible around a grasping forceps, then introduced into the peritoneal cavity. Small swatches can be inserted through a 12 mm trocar[4]; for larger pieces, we remove a large trocar, enlarge the incision, and insert the mesh directly into the abdomen. The trocar is then repositioned.

a

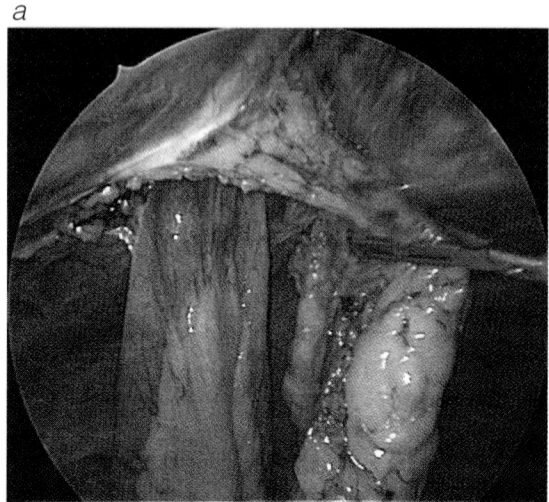

b

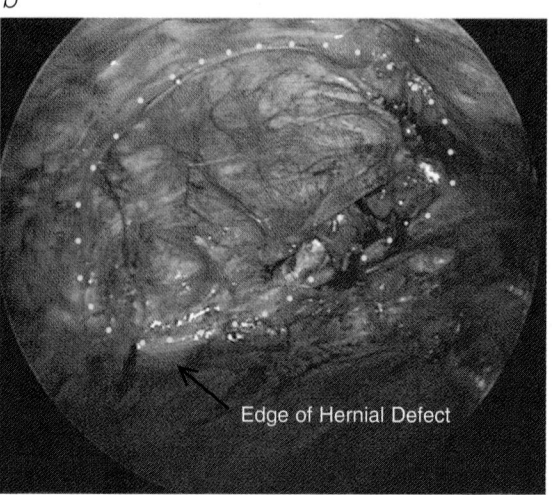

Edge of Hernial Defect

Figure 16 **Laparoscopic incisional hernia repair. (*a*) Shown is dissection of incarcerated small bowel and omentum from an incisional hernia. (*b*) After adhesiolysis, the edges of the defect can be seen.**

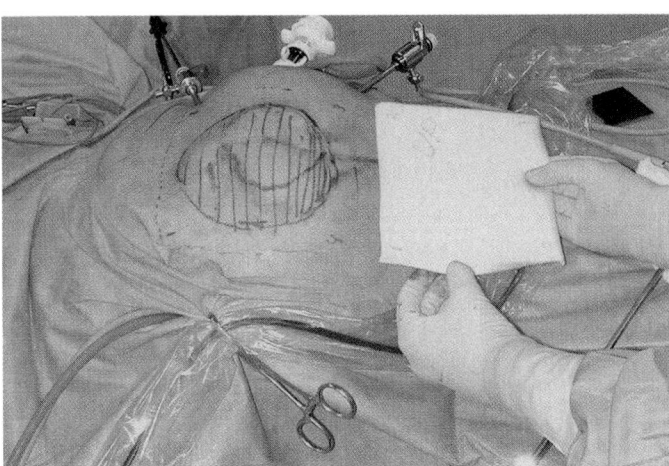

Figure 17 Laparoscopic incisional hernia repair. An outline of the hernial defect is drawn on the abdominal wall, with a 2 cm margin marked around the defect to serve as a template for tailoring the mesh. The four corners of the mesh swatch and of the template are numbered to facilitate orientation of the mesh once it is inside the peritoneal cavity. Patient's head is to the left.

Step 4: Fixation of Mesh

Once the mesh swatch has been introduced into the abdomen, it is unfurled and spread out, with the previously placed corner sutures facing the fascia and oriented so that the four numbered corners are aligned with the numbers marked on the abdominal wall. Small skin incisions are then made in two lateral corners. Through each of these incisions, a suture passer is inserted to grasp one tail of the previously placed 2-0 Prolene suture and pull it out through the abdominal wall, then reintroduced through the incision to pull out the second tail. Each suture is then tied and buried in the subcutaneous tissue so as to anchor the mesh to the fascia and maintain its proper orientation. Once two corners are secured, the mesh is spread out tautly and the other two corners secured in a similar fashion. A stapler is then used to tack the mesh circumferentially at 1 cm intervals [*see Figure 18*].

If multiple defects are present over a large area, we overlap multiple swatches of mesh rather than use a single large swatch, which is cumbersome to manipulate laparoscopically.

Step 5: Closure

The pneumoperitoneum is released. The fascia at any trocar site larger than 10 mm is closed. The skin is then closed with subcuticular sutures.

POSTOPERATIVE CARE

The Foley catheter is removed at the end of the procedure. Patients are admitted to the hospital. Oral intake is begun when bowel sounds are present and there is no abdominal distention; when this state is reached varies according to the extent of adhesiolysis and bowel manipulation required to liberate the contents of the hernial sac. Patients are discharged when a full diet is tolerated. Patients are warned that fluid may accumulate at the hernia site. Any fever or redness should be reported.

OUTCOME EVALUATION

Several series of laparoscopic incisional hernia repairs have been reported. In preparation for a randomized trial, Toy and colleagues described 144 patients at multiple centers who were operated on with a standardized technique and followed prospectively.[4] The mean operating time was about 2 hours. Two enterotomies were made intraoperatively. The most common postoperative complication was wound seroma, which occurred in 23 patients (16%). Surgical site infection occurred in five patients (3%). Two patients required removal of the mesh. One experienced bowel obstruction. Recurrences were observed in eight cases (6%) after a mean follow-up of 222 days. In a study of 122 laparoscopic incisional hernia repairs reported by Franklin and associates, there was one recurrence after a mean follow-up of 30.1 months.[6]

Park and colleagues compared 56 prospective laparoscopic incisional hernia repairs with 49 open incisional hernia repairs assessed through retrospective chart review.[7] The groups were comparable in terms of patient characteristics and hernia size. Although the mean operating time was longer in the laparoscopic group (95.4 minutes versus 78.5 minutes), the postoperative length of stay was significantly shorter after laparoscopic repair than after open repair (3.4 days versus 6.5 days). Overall, there were significantly fewer complications after laparoscopic repair. There were fewer recurrences after laparoscopic repair than after open repair (six versus 17); the mean follow-up time was 24.1 months, but follow-up was significantly longer after open repair, for which the data were collected retrospectively.

Carbajo and colleagues compared 30 laparoscopic incisional hernia repairs with 30 open repairs in a randomized trial.[5] There were no intraoperative complications in the laparoscopic group and two enterotomies in the open group. The mean operating time was significantly shorter in the laparoscopic group (87 minutes versus 111.5 minutes), as was the postoperative length of stay (2.23 days versus 9.06 days). One patient in each group required reoperation for bowel obstruction; in the laparoscopic group, this complication was attributable to incarceration of the bowel between the mesh and the abdominal wall. There were fewer wound complications in the laparoscopic group. After a minimum follow-up of 18 months, no recurrences were noted in the laparoscopic group and two in the open group.

Although the results of other large randomized trials are not available yet, preliminary work suggests that the laparoscopic approach to the repair of large incisional hernias is highly promising. The laparoscopic approach seems to confer the well-known benefits of other video-assisted procedures (e.g., quicker recovery) while comparing favorably to the open operation in terms of complication and recurrence rates.

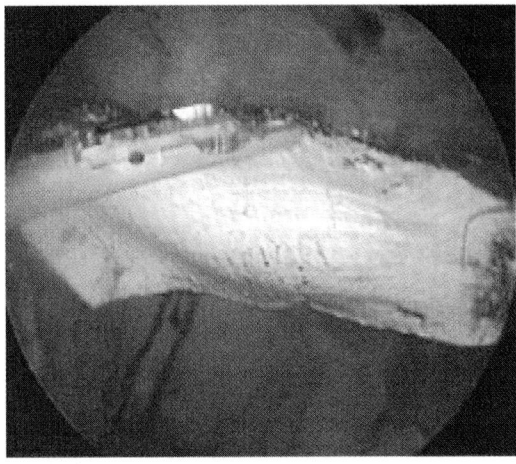

Figure 18 Laparoscopic incisional hernia repair. The mesh is secured to the peritoneum with sutures and staples.

References

1. Ger R, Monroe K, Duvivier R, et al: Management of indirect hernias by laparoscopic closure of the neck of the sac. Am J Surg 159:370, 1990

2. Robbins AW, Rutkow IM: Mesh plug repair and groin hernia surgery. Surg Clin North Am 78:1007, 1998

3. Crawford DL, Phillips EH: Laparoscopic repair and groin hernia surgery. Surg Clin North Am 78:1047, 1998

4. Toy FK, Bailey RW, Carey S, et al: Prospective, multi-center study of laparoscopic ventral hernioplasty: preliminary results. Surg Endosc 12:955, 1998

5. Carbajo MA, Martin del Olmo JC, Blanco JI, et al: Laparoscopic treatment vs open surgery in the solution of major incisional and abdominal wall hernias with mesh. Surg Endosc 13:250, 1999

6. Franklin ME, Dorman JP, Glass JL, et al: Laparoscopic ventral hernia repair. Surg Laparosc Endosc 8:294, 1998

7. Park A, Birch DW, Lovrics P: Laparoscopic and open incisional hernia repair: a comparison study. Surgery 124:816, 1998

8. LeBlanc KA, Booth WV: Laparoscopic repair of incisional abdominal hernias using expanded polytetra-fluorethylene: preliminary findings. Surg Laparosc Endosc 3:39, 1992

9. Skandalakis JE, Gray SW, Skandalakis LJ, et al: Surgical anatomy of the inguinal area. World J Surg 13:490, 1989

10. Spaw AT, Ennis BW, Spaw LP: Laparoscopic hernia repair: the anatomic basis. J Laparoendosc Surg 1:269, 1991

11. Wantz GE: Atlas of Hernia Surgery. Raven Press, New York, 1991

12. Condon RE: The anatomy of the inguinal region and its relation to groin hernia. Hernia, 3rd ed. Nyhus LM, Condon RE, Eds. JB Lippincott Co, Philadelphia, 1989, p 18

13. Memon MA, Fitzgibbons RJ: Laparoscopic inguinal hernia repair: transabdominal (TAPP) and totally extraperitoneal (TEP). The SAGES Manual. Scott-Connor CEH, Ed. Springer, New York, 1999

14. Ramshaw BJ, Tucker JG, Conner T, et al: A comparison of the approaches to laparoscopic herniorrhaphy. Surg Endosc 10:29, 1996

15. Fitzgibbons RJ Jr, Camps J, Cornet DA, et al: Laparoscopic inguinal herniorrhaphy: results of a multicenter trial. Ann Surg 221:3, 1995

16. Arregui ME: Transabdominal retroperitoneal inguinal herniorrhaphy. Operative Laparoscopy and Thoracoscopy. MacFayden BV, Ponsky JL, Eds. Lippincott-Raven, Philadelphia, 1996

17. Felix H, Michas C: Double buttress laparoscopic herniorrhaphy. J Laparoendosc Surg 3:1, 1993

18. McKernan JB, Laws HL: Laparoscopic repair of inguinal hernias using a totally extraperitoneal prosthetic approach. Surg Endosc 7:26, 1993

19. Stoppa R, Warlaumont C, Verhaeghe P, et al: Dacron mesh and surgical therapy of inguinal hernia. Chir Patol Sper 34:15, 1986

20. Stoppa R, Warlaumont CR: The preperitoneal approach and prosthetic repair of groin hernias. Hernia, 3rd ed. Nyhus LM, Condon RE, Eds. JB Lippincott Co, Philadelphia, 1989

21. Stoppa R: The treatment of complicated groin and incisional hernias. World J Surg 13:545, 1989

22. Wantz GE: Giant prosthetic reinforcement of the visceral sac. Surg Gynecol Obstet 169:408, 1989

23. McKernan JB: Extraperitoneal inguinal herniorrhaphy. Operative Laparoscopy and Thoracoscopy. MacFayden BV, Ponsky JL, Eds. Lippincott-Raven, Philadelphia, 1996

24. Wellwood J, Sculpher MJ, Stoker D, et al: Randomized clinical trial of laparoscopic versus open mesh repair for inguinal hernia: outcome and cost. BMJ 317:103, 1998

25. Amado WJ: Anesthesia for hernia surgery. Surg Clin North Am 73:427, 1993

26. Ferzli G, Sayad P, Hallak A, et al: Endoscopic extraperitoneal hernia repair: a 5-year experience. Surg Endosc 12:1311, 1998

27. Ferzli G, Sayad P, Vasisht B: The feasibility of laparoscopic extraperitoneal hernia repair under local anesthesia. Surg Endosc 13:588, 1999

28. Paganini AM, Lezoche E, Carle F, et al: A randomized controlled clinical study of laparoscopic vs. open tension-free inguinal hernia repair. Surg Endosc 12:979, 1998

29. Zieren J, Zieren H, Jacobi CA, et al: Prospective randomized study comparing laparoscopic and open tension-free inguinal hernia repair with Shouldice's operation. Am J Surg 175:330, 1998

30. Heikkinen T, Haukipuro K, Leppälä J, et al: Total costs of laparoscopic and Lichtenstein inguinal hernia repairs: a prospective study. Surg Lap Endosc 7:1, 1997

31. Johansson B, Hallerbäck B, Glise H, et al: Laparoscopic mesh *versus* open preperitoneal mesh *versus* conventional technique for inguinal hernia repair. A randomized multicenter trial (SCUR Hernia Repair Study). Ann Surg 230:225, 1999

32. The MRC Laparoscopic Groin Hernia Trial Group: Laparoscopic versus open repair of groin hernia: a randomised comparison. Lancet 354:185, 1999

33. Payne JH, Grininger LM, Isawa MT, et al: Laparoscopic or open inguinal herniorrhaphy? a randomized prospective trial. Arch Surg 129:973, 1994

34. Heikkinen TJ, Haukipuro K, Hulkko A: A cost and outcome comparison between laparoscopic and Lichtenstein hernia operations in a day-case unit: a randomized prospective study. Surg Endosc 12:1199, 1998

35. Champault GG, Rizk N, Catheline J-M, et al: Inguinal hernia repair. Totally preperitoneal laparoscopic approach versus Stoppa operation: randomized trial of 100 cases. Surg Lap Endosc 7:445, 1997

36. Khoury N: A randomized prospective controlled trial of laparoscopic extraperitoneal hernia repair and mesh-plug hernioplasty: a study of 315 cases. J Laparoendosc Surg 8:367, 1998

37. Phillips EH, Arregui ME, Carroll BJ, et al: Incidence of complications following laparoscopic hernioplasty. Surg Endosc 9:16, 1995

38. Salerno GM, Fitzgibbons RJ Jr, Filipi CJ: Laparoscopic inguinal hernia repair. Surgical Laparoscopy. Zucker KA, Ed. Quality Medical Publishing, St Louis, 1991

39. MacFayden BV Jr, Arregui M, Corbitt J, et al: Complications of laparoscopic herniorrhaphy. Surg Endosc 7:155, 1993

40. Phillips EH, Arregui M, Carroll BJ, et al: Incidence of complications following laparoscopic hernioplasty. Surg Endosc 9:16, 1995

41. Estour E, Mouret PH: Cure laparoscopique des hernies de l'aine. J Coelio Chir 16:15, 1995

42. Avtan L, Avci C, Bulut T, et al: Mesh infections after laparoscopic inguinal hernia repair. Surg Laparosc Endosc 7:192, 1997

43. Leim NSL, Van der Graaf Y, van Steensel CJ, et al: Comparison of conventional anterior surgery and laparoscopic surgery for inguinal hernia repair. N Engl J Med 336:1541, 1997

44. Ferzli GS, Frezza EE, Pecorato AM Jr, et al: Prospective randomized study of stapled versus unstapled mesh in a laparoscopic preperitoneal inguinal hernia repair. J Am Coll Surg 188:461, 1999

45. Wantz GE: Ambulatory surgical treatment of groin hernia: prevention and management of complications. Problems in General Surgery 3:311, 1986

46. Wright DM, Kennedy A, Baxter JN, et al: Early outcome after open versus extraperitoneal endoscopic tension-free hernioplasty: a randomized clinical trial. Surgery 119:552, 1996

47. Starling JR, Harms BA: Diagnosis and treatment of genitofemoral and ilioinguinal neuralgia. World J Surg 13:586, 1989

48. Kraus MA: Nerve injury during laparoscopic inguinal hernia repair. Surg Laparosc Endosc 3:342, 1993

49. Rosen A, Halevy A: Anatomical basis for nerve injury during laparoscopic hernia repair. Surg Laparosc Endosc 7:469, 1997

50. Wexler MJ, Meakins JL, Garzon J: Laparoscopic groin hernia repair: preliminary results from a prospective clinical trial. Can J Surg 36:384, 1993

51. Lawrence K, McWhinnie O, Goodwin, et al: Randomized controlled trial of laparoscopic vs. open repair of inguinal hernia: early results. Br J Surg 311:981, 1995

52. Bassell JR, Baxter P, Riddell F, et al: A randomized controlled trial of laparoscopic extraperitoneal hernia repair as a day surgical procedure. Surg Endosc 10:495, 1996

53. Kald A, Anderberg B, Carisson P, et al: Surgical outcome and cost-minimization analyses of laparoscopic and open hernia repair: a randomised prospective trial with one-year follow up. Eur J Surg 163:505, 1997

54. Kozol R, Lange PN, Kosir N, et al: A prospective randomized study of open vs. laparoscopic inguinal hernia repair. Arch Surg 132:292, 1997

55. Stoker DL, Spiegelhalter DJ, Singh R, et al: Laparoscopic versus open inguinal hernia repair: randomised prospective trial. Lancet 343:1243, 1994

56. Schrenk P, Woisetschlager R, Reiger R, et al: Prospective randomized trial comparing postoperative pain and return to physical activity after transabdominal preperitoneal, total preperitoneal, or Shouldice technique for inguinal hernia repair. Br J Surg 83:1563, 1996

57. Vogt DM, Curet MJ, Pitcher DE, et al: Preliminary results of a prospective randomized trial of laparoscopic onlay versus conventional inguinal herniorrhaphy. Am J Surg 169:84, 1995

58. Chung RS, Rowland DY: Meta-analysis of randomized controlled trials of laparoscopic vs conventional inguinal hernia repairs. Surg Endosc 13:689, 1999

59. Filipi CJ, Gaston-Johansson F, McBride PJ, et al: An assessment of pain and return to normal activity: laparoscopic herniorrhaphy vs open tension-free Lichtenstein repair. Surg Endosc 10:983, 1996

60. Barkun JS, Keyser EJ, Wexler MJ, et al: Short-term outcomes in open vs. laparoscopic herniorrhaphy: confounding impact of worker's compensation on convalescence. J Gastrointest Surg 3:575, 1999

61. Barkun JS, Barkun AN, Sampalis JS, et al: Randomized controlled trial of laparoscopic versus mini cholecystectomy. Lancet 340:1116, 1992

62. Krähenbühl L, Schäfer M, Schilling M, et al: Simultaneous repair of bilateral groin hernias: open or laparoscopic approach? Surg Laparosc Endosc 8:313, 1998

63. Lichtenstein IL, Shulman AG, Amid PK: The cause, prevention, and treatment of recurrent groin hernia. Surg Clin North Am 73:529, 1993

64. Robbins AW, Rutkow IM: Mesh plug repair and groin hernia surgery. Surg Clin North Am 78:1007, 1998

65. Lowham AS, Filipi CJ, Fitzgibbons RJ, et al: Mechanisms of hernia recurrence after preperitoneal mesh repair: traditional and laparoscopic. Ann Surg 225:422, 1997

66. Memon MA, Rice D, Donohue JH: Laparoscop-

ic herniorrhaphy. J Am Coll Surg 184:325, 1997

67. Beets GL, Dirksen CD, Go PM, et al: Open or laparoscopic preperitoneal mesh repair for recurrent inguinal hernia? A randomized controlled trial. Surg Endosc 13:323, 1999

68. Cohen RV, Alvarez G, Roll S, et al: Transabdominal or totally extraperitoneal laparoscopic hernia repair? Surg Laparosc Endosc 8:264, 1998

69. Kald A, Anderberg B, Smedh K, et al: Transperitoneal or totally extraperitoneal approach in laparoscopic hernia repair: results of 491 consecutive herniorrhaphies. Surg Laparosc Endosc 7:86, 1997

70. Felix EL, Michas CA, Gonzalez MH Jr: Laparoscopic hernioplasty: TAPP vs TEP. Surg Endosc 9:984, 1995

71. Hesselink VJ, Luijendik RW, de Wilt JHW, et al: An evaluation of risk factors in incisional hernia recurrence. Surg Gynecol Obstet 176:228, 1993

72. Santora TA, Roslyn JJ: Incisional hernia. Surg Clin North Am 73:557, 1993

Acknowledgment

Figures 1, 4 through 7, 8 (right), 14, and 15   Tom Moore.

Julian Britton, M.S., F.R.C.S.

Intestinal obstruction, peritonitis from a perforated bowel, abdominal trauma, and disease of the bowel are common surgical problems throughout the world. These problems usually must be treated operatively; hence, it is frequently necessary to join two sections of bowel together. Unlike joining two areas of skin, where there is a powerful evolutionary incentive to achieve rapid healing, joining two segments of bowel so as to restore intestinal function without leakage of intestinal contents is not easy. Over time, the basic principles crucial for obtaining successful results have been defined [see Table 1]. Accurate approximation of the bowel without tension and with a good blood supply to both of the structures being joined are obviously fundamental. Surgical technique is equally important: between two given surgeons, rates of anastomotic breakdown can vary by as much as a factor of 60.[1]

Failure of an anastomosis with leakage of intestinal contents is still, regrettably, a common surgical experience. Reported failure rates range from 1.5%[2] to 2.2%,[3] depending on what type of anastomosis was performed and whether the operation was an elective or an emergency procedure. A leaking anastomosis greatly increases the morbidity and mortality associated with the operation: it can double the length of the hospital stay and increase the mortality as much as 10-fold.[4] Dehiscence, when it occurs, has been associated with one fifth to one third of all postoperative deaths in patients who underwent an intestinal anastomosis.[5]

Unfortunately, anastomotic dehiscence can occur even in ideal circumstances. This unwelcome fact has stimulated a great deal of debate regarding the reliability of various methods and approaches. With the aim of clarifying the debate, I will address certain fundamental technical issues in the performance of an intestinal anastomosis and attempt to summarize what is known about how these issues relate to the reliability of the various anastomotic techniques in current use. I will then outline operative approaches to performing three common intestinal anastomoses in somewhat greater detail [see Operative Techniques for Selected Anastomoses, *below*].

Intestinal Anastomotic Healing

Most of the strength of the bowel wall resides in the submucosa[6]; however, for the purpose of suturing bowel segments together, it is important to keep in mind that the serosa (i.e., the visceral peritoneum) holds sutures better than either the longitudinal or the circular muscle layer [see Figure 1]. The absence of a peritoneal layer makes suturing of the thoracic esophagus and the rectum below the peritoneal reflection technically more difficult than suturing the intraperitoneal segments of the intestine. In addition, the stomach and the small bowel possess a richer blood supply than the esophagus and the large bowel and consequently tend to heal more readily.

The process of intestinal anastomotic healing mimics that of wound healing elsewhere in the body in that it can be arbitrarily divided into an acute inflammatory (lag) phase, a proliferative phase, and, finally, a remodeling or maturation phase. The strongest component of the bowel wall, the submucosa, owes most of its strength to the collagenous connective tissue it contains. Collagen is thus the single most important molecule for determining intestinal strength, which makes its metabolism of particular interest for understanding anastomotic healing.

Collagen is secreted from fibroblasts in a monomeric form called tropocollagen; this is a large, stiff molecule that can be visualized by electron microscopy. Collagen itself can be divided into subtypes on the basis of compositional differences (i.e., different combinations of α_1 and α_2 chains). Type I collagen predominates in mature organisms; type II is found primarily in cartilage; and type III is associated with type I in remodeling tissue and in elastic tissues such as the aorta, the esophagus, and the uterus. Synthesis of collagen is an intracellular process that occurs on polysomes. A critical stage in collagen formation is the hydroxylation of proline to produce hydroxyproline; this process is believed to be important for maintaining the three-dimensional triple-helix conformation of mature collagen, which gives the molecule its structural strength. The amount of collagen found in a tissue is indirectly determined by measuring the amount of hydroxyproline, though no significant statistical correlation between hydroxyproline content and objective measurements of anastomotic strength has ever been demonstrated.[7] Vitamin C deficiency results in impaired hydroxylation of proline and the accumulation of proline-rich, hydroxyproline-poor molecules in intracellular vacuoles.

The degree of fiber and fibril cross-linking relates to the maturity of the collagen and is probably important in determining the overall strength of the scar tissue. Of equal importance is the orientation of the fibers and their weave. The bursting pressure of anastomoses has often been used to gauge the strength of the healing process. This pressure has been found to increase rapidly in the early postoperative period, reaching 60% of the strength of the surrounding bowel by 3 to 4 days and 100% by 1 week.[8,9]

Collagen synthesis is a dynamic process that depends on the balance between synthesis and collagenolysis. Degradation of mature collagen begins in the first 24 hours and predominates for

---

Table 1 **Principles of Successful Intestinal Anastomosis**

Well-nourished patient with no systemic illness

No fecal contamination, either within the gut or in the surrounding peritoneal cavity

Adequate exposure and access

Well-vascularized tissues

Absence of tension at the anastomosis

Meticulous technique

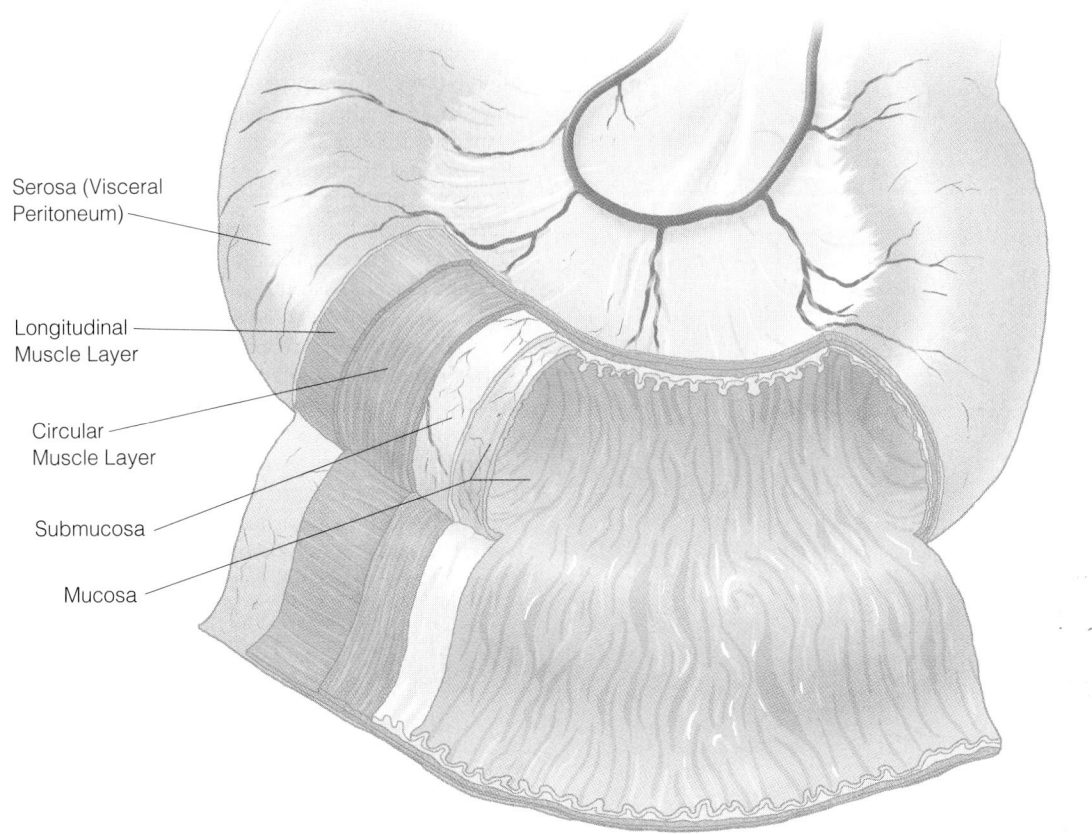

Serosa (Visceral Peritoneum)

Longitudinal Muscle Layer

Circular Muscle Layer

Submucosa

Mucosa

Figure 1 **Shown are the tissue layers of the jejunum. Most of the bowel wall's strength is provided by the submucosa.**

the first 4 days. By 1 week, collagen synthesis is the dominant force, particularly proximal to the anastomosis. After 5 to 6 weeks, there is no significant increase in the amount of collagen in a healing wound or anastomosis, though turnover and thus synthesis are extensive. The strength of the scar continues to increase for many months after injury. Local infection increases collagenase activity and reduces levels of circulating collagenase inhibitors.[10,11]

Collagen synthetic capacity is relatively uniform throughout the large bowel but less so in the small intestine: synthesis is significantly higher in the proximal and distal small intestine than in the midjejunum. Overall collagen synthetic capacity is somewhat less in the small intestine. Although no significant difference has been found between the strength of ileal anastomoses and that of colonic anastomoses at 4 days, colonic collagen formation is much greater in the first 48 hours.[12] It is noteworthy that the synthetic response is not restricted to the anastomotic site but appears to be generalized to a significant extent.[13]

Various attempts have been made to improve the healing of intestinal anastomoses. A 2002 animal study concluded that locally applied charged particles improved the healing of colonic anastomoses.[14]

Technical Options for Fashioning Anastomoses

Sewing bowel segments together with various suture materials, ranging from catgut to stainless steel wire, has been a standard surgical technique for more than 150 years. Staplers, though first developed early in the 20th century, only began to have a significant impact on GI surgery within the past three decades. Staplers certainly

appeal to the technically minded, and most studies suggest that they save a small amount of operating time[15]; however, they remain relatively expensive, and it is still unclear whether the results are any better than can be achieved with suturing. Accordingly, it is worthwhile to examine the technical aspects of the two approaches to bowel anastomosis and to compare their respective merits.

SUTURING: TECHNICAL ISSUES

Choice of Suture Material

Sutures act as foreign bodies in the anastomosis and thus produce an inflammatory reaction.[7] One study that examined the relative efficiency of absorbable and nonabsorbable material concluded that the strength of the anastomosis, expressed as a percentage of normal tissue strength, was essentially the same regardless of the type of suture used. Other studies that examined the amount of inflammation induced at the anastomosis by various types of sutures found that polypropylene (Prolene), catgut, and polyglycolic acid (Dexon) were equivalent in this regard.[16,17] Silk, however, produced a significantly greater cellular reaction at the anastomosis, and the reaction persisted for as long as 6 weeks.[17] A 1975 study reported on a series of 41 patients who underwent low anterior resection involving a primary side-to-end colorectal anastomosis with 5-0 stainless steel wire.[18] The investigators considered this material ideal because of its strength and relative inertness within the tissues, and they supported their claims with a relatively low clinical leakage rate (7.3%).

The ideal suture material—one that causes minimal inflammation and tissue reaction while providing maximum strength during the lag phase of wound healing—is yet to be discovered.

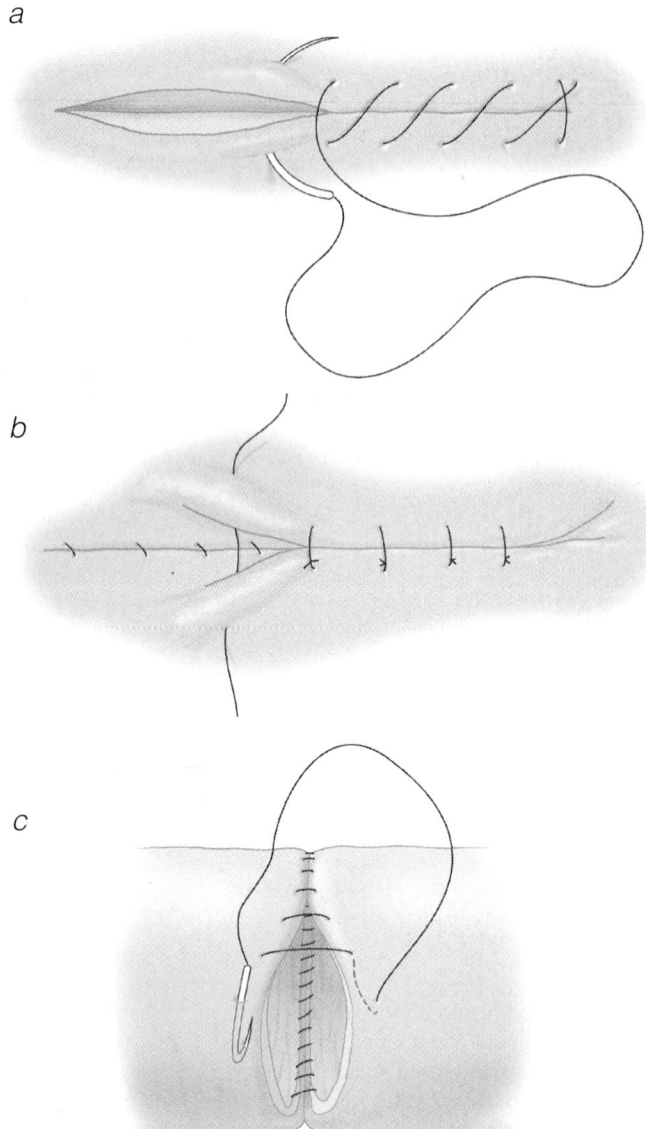

a

b

c

Figure 2 **Shown are stitches commonly used in fashioning intestinal anastomoses: (*a*) the continuous over-and-over suture, (*b*) the interrupted Lembert suture, and (*c*) the Connell suture.**

Clearly, however, monofilament and coated braided sutures represent an advance beyond silk and other multifilament materials.

Continuous versus Interrupted Sutures

Both continuous and interrupted sutures are commonly used in fashioning intestinal anastomoses [*see Figure 2*]. No randomized trials have addressed the question of whether interrupted sutures have a significant advantage over continuous sutures in a single-layer anastomosis; however, retrospective reviews have not revealed any such advantage.[19-21] Animal studies, on the other hand, indicated that perianastomotic tissue oxygen tension was significantly less with continuous sutures than with interrupted sutures.[22] This finding was correlated with an increased anastomotic complication rate and impaired collagen synthesis and healing with continuous sutures in a rat model.[23]

Single-Layer versus Double-Layer Anastomoses

Double-layer anastomoses were described in the literature before single-layer ones. All such anastomoses are of essentially

similar construction, consisting of an inner layer of continuous or interrupted absorbable sutures and an outer layer of interrupted absorbable or nonabsorbable sutures [*see Figure 3*]. Traditionally, double-layer anastomoses have been considered more secure; however, for some time, single-layer anastomoses have been performed in difficult locations (e.g., low in the pelvis or high in the chest) or in difficult circumstances (e.g., in a patient who is unstable or has multiple intra-abdominal injuries) with good results. Moreover, work from the 1980s suggests that the single-layer technique has significant inherent advantages.[23-26]

Double-layer anastomoses were long believed to be essential for safe healing; however, subsequent pathologic analysis of these anastomoses revealed microscopic areas of necrosis and sloughing of the tissues incorporated in the inner layer as a result of strangulation.[27] Animal studies confirmed that single-layer anastomoses take less time to create,[28] cause less narrowing of the intestinal lumen,[24-29] foster more rapid vascularization[23] and mucosal healing, and increase the strength of the anastomosis (as measured by the bursting pressure) in the first few postoperative days.[28] Nonetheless, although clinical studies have fairly consistently demonstrated that single-layer anastomoses are associated with

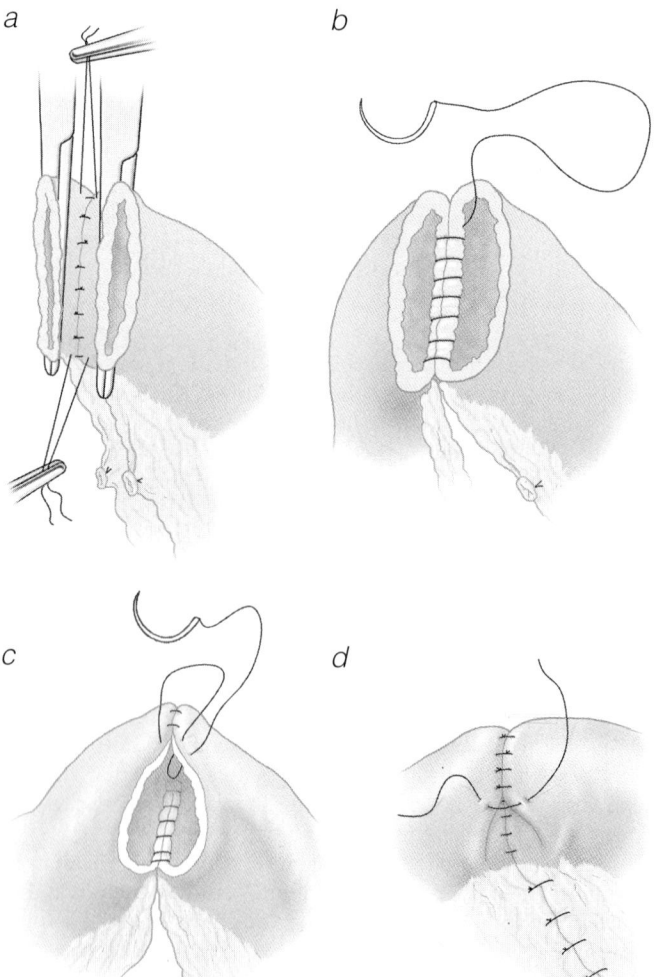

a

b

c

d

Figure 3 **Double-layer end-to-end anastomosis. (*a*) Interrupted Lembert stitches are used to form the posterior outer layer. (*b*) A full-thickness continuous over-and-over stitch is used to form the posterior inner layer. (*c*) A Connell stitch is used to form the anterior inner layer. (*d*) Interrupted Lembert stitches are used to form the anterior outer layer.**

improved postoperative return to normal bowel function (as measured by bowel sounds, passage of flatus, and return to oral intake),[30,31] nonrandomized studies of anastomotic leakage rates have not shown any differences between single- and double-layer anastomoses in this regard.[32-34]

Some authors still favor double-layer anastomoses when the tissues are very edematous or friable, are under minimal tension, or lie in highly vascular areas (e.g., the stomach). There are no data to indicate that this practice yields superior results.

STAPLING: TECHNICAL ISSUES

Choice of Stapler

Surgical stapling devices were first introduced in 1908 by Hültl; however, they did not gain popularity at that time and for some time afterward because the early instruments were cumbersome and unreliable. The development of reliable, disposable instruments over the past 25 years has changed surgical practice dra-

matically. With modern devices, technical failures are rarer, the staple lines are of more consistent quality, and anastomoses in difficult locations are easier to construct.

Three different types of stapler are commonly used for fashioning intestinal anastomoses. The transverse anastomosis (TA) stapler is the simplest of these. This device places two staggered rows of B-shaped staples across the bowel but does not cut it: the bowel must then be divided in a separate step. The gastrointestinal anastomosis (GIA) stapler places two double staggered rows of staples and simultaneously cuts between the double rows. The circular, or end-to-end anastomosis (EEA), stapler places a double row of staples in a circle and then cuts out the tissue within the circle of staples with a built-in cylindrical knife. All of these staplers are available in a range of lengths or diameters. Staplers may be used to create functional or true anatomic end-to-end anastomoses as well as side-to-side anastomoses. The original staplers were all designed for use in open procedures, but there are now a number of instruments (mostly of the GIA type) available for use in laparo-

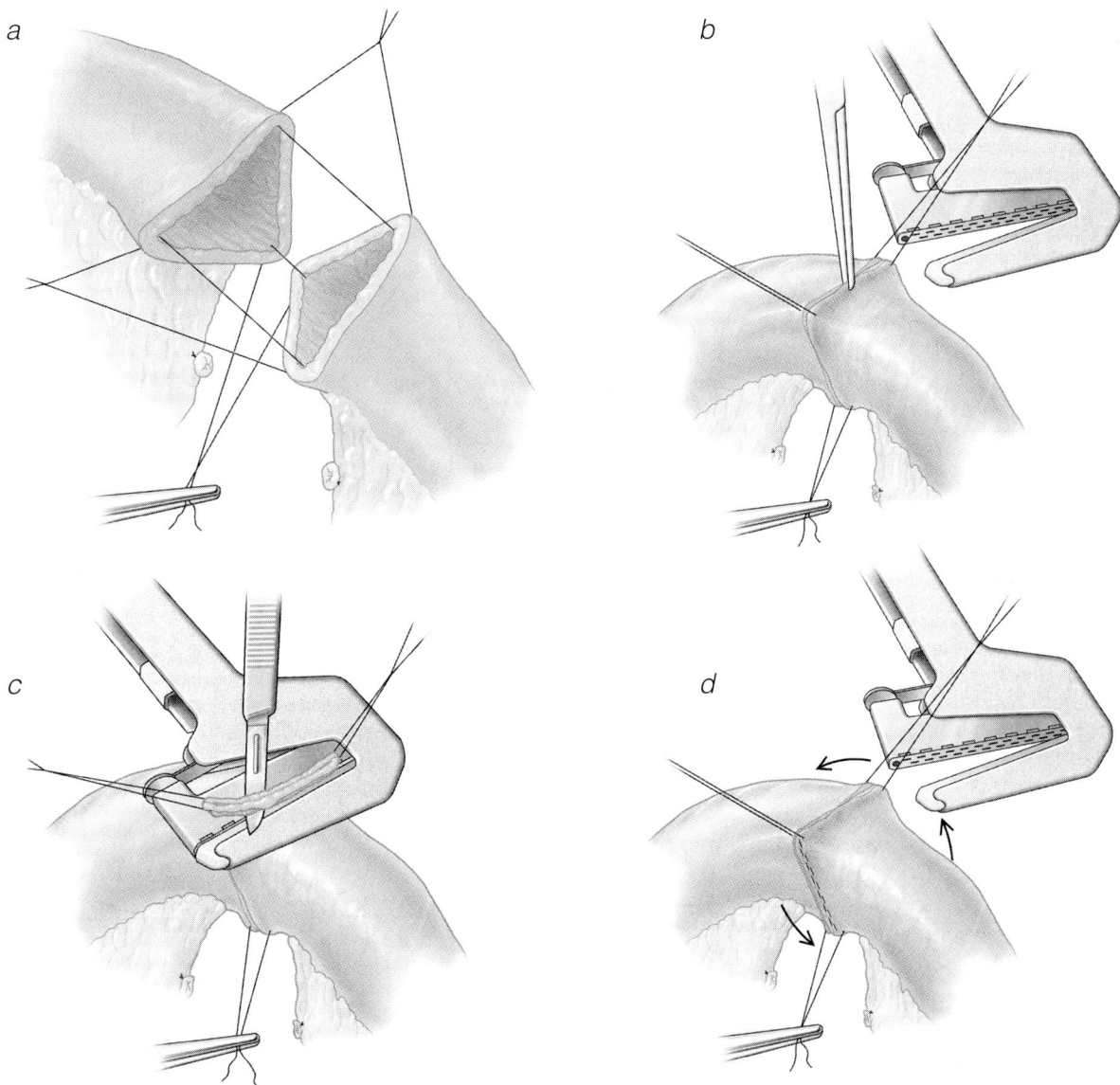

Figure 4 **End-to-end anastomosis with linear noncutting stapler. (a) The bowel ends are triangulated with three traction sutures. (b) A noncutting linear stapler (TA) is placed between two of the sutures. (c) The stapler is closed and the excess tissue excised. (d) The bowel is rotated, and steps b and c are repeated twice more to close the remaining two sides of the triangle.**

scopic procedures. The staples themselves are all made of titanium, which causes little tissue reaction. They are not magnetic and do not cause subsequent difficulties with MRI scanning.

In a functional end-to-end anastomosis, two cut ends of bowel (either open or stapled closed) are placed side by side with their blind ends beside each other. If the bowel ends are closed, an enterotomy must be made in each loop of bowel to allow insertion of the stapler. A cutting linear (GIA) stapler is then used to fuse the two bowel walls into a single septum with two double staggered rows of staples and to create a lumen between the two bowel segments by dividing this septum between the rows. A noncutting linear (TA) stapler is then used to close the defect at the apex of the anastomosis where the GIA stapler was inserted. An alternative, and cheaper, method of closing the defect is to use a continuous suture. The cut and stapled edges of the bowel should be inspected for adequacy of hemostasis before the apex is closed. Some authors suggest cauterizing these edges to ensure hemostasis[35]; however, given that electrical current may be conducted along the metallic staple line to the rest of the bowel, it is probably easier and safer simply to underpin bleeding vessels with a fine absorbable suture. It is also important to offset the two inverted staple lines before closing the apex.[36]

True anatomic end-to-end stapled anastomoses may be fashioned with a linear stapler by triangulating the two cut ends and then firing the stapler three times in intersecting vectors to achieve complete closure [see Figure 4]. The potential drawback of this approach is that the staple lines are all everted. It is often easier to join two cut ends of bowel with an EEA stapler, which creates a directly apposed, inverted, stapled end-to-end anastomosis. However, circular staplers can be more difficult to use at times because of the need to invert a complete circle of full-thickness bowel wall. In addition—at least at locations other than the anus—they typically require closure of an adjacent enterotomy.

Staple Height

TA and GIA staplers are available with a variety of inserts containing several different types of staples. These inserts vary with respect to width, the height (or depth) of the closed staple, and the distance between the staples in the rows. They are designed for use in specific tissues, and it is important to choose the correct stapler insert for a given application. In particular, inserts designed for closing blood vessels should not be used on the bowel, and vice versa. With TA and EEA staplers, it is possible to vary the depth of the closed staples by altering the distance between the staples and the anvil as the instrument is closed. The safe range of closure is usually indicated by a colored or shaded area on the shaft of the instrument. Thus, if full closure would cause excessive crushing of the intervening tissues, the stapler need not be closed to its maximum extent.

A 1987 comparison of anastomotic techniques that used blood flow to the divided tissues as a measure of outcome found that the best blood flow to the healing site was provided by stapled anastomoses in which the staple height was adjusted to the thickness of the bowel wall.[37] The next best blood flow was provided by double-layer stapled and sutured anastomoses, followed by double-layer sutured anastomoses and tightly stapled anastomoses, in that order.

Single-Stapled versus Double-Stapled Anastomoses

To accomplish many of these anastomoses, intersecting staple lines are created. Initially, some concern was expressed about the security of these areas and about the ability of the blade in the cutting staplers to divide a double staggered row of staples. Animal studies, however, demonstrated that even though nearly all (> 90%) of the staple lines that were subsequently transected by a second staple line contained bent or cut staples, the integrity of the anastomosis was not compromised in any way, nor was healing adversely affected.[38,39]

HAND-SEWN VERSUS STAPLED ANASTOMOSES

Stapled anastomoses are said to heal by primary intention, whereas sutured anastomoses are said to heal by secondary intention, though further experimentation is needed to confirm this distinction.[40] Titanium staples are ideal for tissue apposition at anastomotic sites because they provoke only a minimal inflammatory response and provide immediate strength to the cut surfaces during the weakest phase of healing. Initially, tissue eversion at the stapled anastomosis was a major concern, given that everted hand-sewn anastomoses had previously been shown to be inferior to inverted ones; however, the greater support and improved blood supply to the healing tissues associated with stapling tend to counteract the negative effects of eversion. In fact, one study found that bursting strength for canine colonic end-to-end anastomoses was six times greater when the procedure was performed with an EEA stapler than when it was done with interrupted Dacron sutures.[41] Another study demonstrated a significantly reduced radiographic anastomotic leakage rate with staples applied by an EEA stapler as opposed to a double layer of sutures.[42] Various prospective, randomized trials have demonstrated no differences in clinical and subclinical leakage rates, length of hospital stay, or overall morbidity.[15,39,43-46] Even when the anastomosis had to heal under adverse conditions (e.g., carcinomatosis, malnutrition, previous chemotherapy or radiation therapy, bowel obstruction, anemia, or leukopenia), no significant differences were apparent between stapled and hand-sewn anastomoses. Stapling did, however, shorten operating time, especially for low pelvic anastomoses.

Cancer recurrence rates at the site of the anastomosis have been reported to be higher or lower depending on the technique used. Certainly, suture materials engender a more pronounced cellular proliferative response than titanium staples do, particularly with full-thickness sutures as opposed to seromuscular ones,[47] and malignant cells have been shown to adhere to suture materials.[48] Two studies suggested that stapling anastomoses after resection for cancer reduces anastomotic recurrence by 40% and cancer-specific mortality by 50%.[47,49]

UNUSUAL TECHNIQUES

In 1892, Murphy introduced his button, which consisted of a two-part metal stud that was designed to hold the bowel edges in apposition without suturing until adhesion had occurred.[50] Thereafter, the stud was voided via the rectum. Several modifications of this technique have been described since then, primarily focusing on the composition of the rings or stents. In particular, dissolvable polyglycolic acid systems have been developed. These so-called biofragmentable anastomotic rings leave a gap of 1.5, 2.0, or 2.5 mm between the bowel ends to prevent ischemia of the anastomotic line.

The use of adhesive agents such as methyl-2-cyanoacrylate to approximate the divided ends of intestinal segments has been studied as well.[51] There was only a moderate inflammatory response at the wound, which persisted for 2 to 3 weeks. Leakage rates were high, however, and many technical problems remained (e.g., how to stabilize the bowel edges while they underwent adhesion).

Fibrin glues have also been employed in this setting. Although these substances are not strong enough to hold two pieces of bowel in apposition, they have been used to coat a sutured bowel anastomosis in an effort to reduce the risk of anastomotic failure. So far, no controlled clinical trials have confirmed that this approach is worthwhile.

Factors Contributing to Failure of Anastomoses

TYPE AND LOCATION OF ANASTOMOSIS

As a rule, for any given technique, the location of the anastomosis seems not to influence the overall leakage rate. There are two exceptions to this general rule. First, low anterior rectal anastomoses are associated with leakage rates ranging from 4.5% to an incredible 70%.[52,53] Second, esophageal anastomoses are associated with leakage rates of about 5%.[54]

Animal studies demonstrated improved transmission of the intestinal migrating myoelectric complex across hand-sewn end-to-end anastomoses, compared with stapled or sewn side-to-side or end-to-side anastomoses or stapled functional end-to-end anastomoses.[55] This improvement may be significant for patients with diseases affecting small bowel motility, but in ordinary surgical practice, there is no difference between the two methods of anastomosis with respect to return of intestinal function.[56]

PATIENT PREPARATION

Many intestinal anastomoses are constructed in an emergency setting. In this context, careful preoperative preparation, including adequate fluid resuscitation, is important and should be carried out to the extent possible. Elective patients should be as fit as is feasible, and any other active coexisting illnesses should be stabilized or controlled as well as possible. To maximize the chances that the anastomosis will heal uneventfully, patients should be well nourished and not anemic. Adequate preoperative antibiotic prophylaxis has been shown to reduce the risk of postoperative infection in all types of bowel surgery and must be given at the start of the operation [see 1:2 Prevention of Postoperative Infection]. Some patients require additional steroids perioperatively [see 6:11 Endocrine Problems].

For elective operations on the colon, it is traditional to empty the bowel before surgery. Some studies, however, have suggested that mechanical bowel preparation may not be essential for successful healing.[57,58] In one such study, a series of 72 patients underwent elective colonic anastomosis without any mechanical bowel preparation and with a single preoperative dose of I.V. antibiotics.[57] Anastomotic dehiscence was not observed, nor were any differences in wound infection rates (8.3%) or overall mortality (2.7%) noted in comparison with published reports of series of patients who underwent full bowel preparation. On the other hand, a 1989 study reported significantly increased anastomotic bursting pressure and reduced anastomotic dehiscence rates in dogs that underwent mechanical bowel cleansing before low anterior resection.[52] This observation was further supported by a study showing that adding oral erythromycin and kanamycin to bowel preparation led to significantly increased bursting pressure at 7 days after operation.[59] In a number of published clinical series, inadequate bowel preparation increased the incidence of anastomotic complications.[53,60] However, there are also several papers in which mechanical bowel preparation yielded no demonstrable benefit.[61]

Whatever the advantages or disadvantages of preoperative bowel preparation from a postoperative point of view, most surgeons would agree that it is much easier to operate on an empty bowel. Several methods of bowel preparation are in current use, including oral laxatives (e.g., magnesium sulfate and sodium picosulfate), enemas, washouts, and various combinations of these. It is advisable for patients to stop eating solid food 24 hours before the operation. The evidence that adding oral antibiotics is beneficial is inconclusive, but many trials have confirmed the benefits of one, two, or three doses of I.V. antibiotics over the perioperative period. Prophylaxis of thromboembolism [see 4:6 Venous Thromboembolism] is mandatory in all patients scheduled to undergo intestinal anastomosis.

ASSOCIATED DISEASES AND SYSTEMIC FACTORS

Anemia, diabetes mellitus, previous irradiation or chemotherapy, malnutrition with hypoalbuminemia, and vitamin deficiencies are all associated with poor anastomotic healing. Some of these factors can be corrected preoperatively. Malnourished patients benefit from nutritional support delivered enterally or parenterally before and after operation [see 6:23 Nutritional Support]. Well-nourished patients appear not to derive similar benefits from such support.[62]

Resections for Crohn disease appear to carry a significant risk of anastomotic dehiscence (12% in one prospective study) even when macroscopically normal margins are obtained.[3] Strictureplasty has therefore become an attractive alternative to resectional management of Crohn disease even in the presence of moderately long strictures, diseased tissue, or sites of previous anastomoses.

The glucocorticoid response to injury may attenuate physiologic responses to other mediators whose combined effects could be deleterious to the organism.[63] In animal experiments, wound healing, as measured by bursting pressure of an ileal anastomosis 1 week after operation, was optimal at a plasma corticosterone level that maintained maximal nitrogen balance and corresponded to the mean corticosterone level of normal animals.[64] Both supranormal and subnormal cortisol levels resulted in significantly impaired wound healing, probably through different mechanisms. It is believed that slow protein turnover is responsible for delayed anastomotic healing in adrenalectomized animals,[65] whereas negative nitrogen metabolic balance is responsible for increased protein breakdown and delayed healing in animals with excess glucocorticoid activity.[64] Nonsteroidal anti-inflammatory drugs (NSAIDs) may help increase anastomotic bursting pressure by decreasing perianastomotic inflammation,[66,67] but this effect has not been well studied.

Controversial Issues in Intestinal Anastomosis

INVERSION VERSUS EVERSION

The question of the importance of inversion (as described by Lembert in the early 1800s) versus eversion of the anastomotic line has long been a controversial one. It has been argued that the traditional inverting methods ignore the basic principle of accurately opposing clean-cut tissues. In the late 19th century, Halsted proposed an interrupted extramucosal technique, which has since been assessed in retrospective[1] and prospective[3] reviews and found to have a low leakage rate (1.3% to 6.0%) in a wide variety of circumstances. A 1969 study reported greater anastomotic strength, less luminal narrowing, and less edema and inflammation with everted small intestinal anastomoses in dogs.[67] Subsequent laboratory and clinical studies have not confirmed these findings and, in fact, have often yielded quite the opposite results: lower bursting pressure,[68] slower healing,[69] and more severe inflammation[31] have all been associated with an everted suture line. Another argument in favor of inversion is an aesthetic one: an inverted anastomosis always looks neater.

NASOGASTRIC DECOMPRESSION

Routine nasogastric decompression in patients undergoing a procedure involving an intestinal anastomosis remains controversial. In retrospective[70] and prospective,[71] randomized, controlled trials, routine use of a nasogastric tube conferred no significant advantage. In fact, there was a trend toward an increased incidence of respiratory tract infections after routine gastric decompression.[72] Nonetheless, one study found that nearly 20% of patients required insertion of a gastric tube in the early postoperative period.[71] If the choice is made not to place a nasogastric tube routinely, it is important to remain alert to the potential for gastric dilatation, which can develop suddenly and without warning.

ABDOMINAL DRAINS

There has been a great deal of disagreement regarding the ability of abdominal drainage to "protect" an anastomosis. Even before World War I, the old dictum "when in doubt, drain" was called into question by Yates, who wrote that the peritoneal cavity could not be effectively drained because of adhesions and rapid sealing of the drain tract.[73] Six decades later, one study showed a dramatic increase in the incidence of anastomotic dehiscence (from 15% to 55%) after the placement of perianastomotic drains in dogs.[74] This increase was associated with a significant increase in mortality. A 1999 study of pelvic drainage after a rectal or anal anastomosis showed that prophylactic drainage did not improve outcome or reduce complications.[75] Yet another study reported the severe inflammatory reaction caused by drains at anastomoses.[76]

These findings to the contrary, many surgeons elect to place an intra-abdominal drain to the pelvis after an anterior resection or a coloanal anastomosis because of the higher than usual risk that a fluid collection will develop. Drainage is rarely helpful, or indeed easy, after a gastric or small bowel anastomosis. Drains are indicated, however, after emergency operations for peritonitis or trauma in which it was necessary to close or anastomose damaged or inflamed bowel. Rectal tubes are commonly employed after subtotal colectomy for acute colitis and after two-stage pelvic pouch procedures.

Operative Techniques for Selected Anastomoses

In what follows, I outline the essential preliminary steps before a bowel anastomosis and then describe three generic operations involving the small and large bowel. These procedures illustrate many of the general principles previously discussed (see above).

PATIENT POSITIONING AND INCISION

Patients must be positioned on the operating table in a manner that is appropriate for the planned operation. Most abdominal operations are performed through a midline incision of adequate length with the patient supine. For pelvic procedures, the patient is placed in the lithotomy position to allow access to the abdomen and the anus; care must be taken to position the legs and feet in the stirrups correctly, without excessive flexion or abduction and with sufficient padding to prevent pressure ulceration, thrombosis, and neurapraxia. For esophageal procedures, the patient is positioned lying on the appropriate side, and the incision of choice is a lateral thoracotomy [see 3:9 Open Esophageal Procedures]. Occasionally, the patient must be shifted to a different position during the course of an operation.

Gravity can be useful for moving structures out of the way. Accordingly, it is often helpful to alter the axis of the operating table. For example, a 30° head down or Trendelenburg position facilitates pelvic operations.

EXPOSURE, MOBILIZATION, AND DISSECTION

The incision should be held open with a suitable retractor. In addition, sophisticated mechanical systems are available that attach to the operating table and can be positioned to expose the area of the surgeon's attention, thereby reducing the need for surgical assistants. Constructing such systems and adjusting them for specific patients takes some time and skill, but the effort is usually well rewarded. Adequate exposure of the operative field is an essential preliminary to any operation. Given that most intestinal operations are performed inside the body cavity, packing away structures that are not required for the procedure being done is an important skill. In a pelvic operation, for example, the small bowel should be packed into the upper abdomen and retained there with a suitable retractor; in an esophageal resection, the lung should be deflated and held well away.

In the absence of adhesions or tethering caused by disease, the small bowel is usually sufficiently mobile to allow the relevant segment to be brought out of the abdomen. Doing so makes the operation easier and allows the remainder of the bowel to be kept warm and tension free inside the abdominal cavity. Sometimes, the transverse colon and the sigmoid colon are mobile enough to be brought to the surface. More commonly, however, as with the other sections of the large bowel, the peritoneum must be divided along the lateral border of the colon and the retroperitoneal structures reflected posteriorly. Tension is rarely a problem during small bowel anastomosis, but for colonic or esophageal anastomoses, it is absolutely vital that the two ends of bowel to be joined lie together easily. For a large bowel anastomosis, this means that the splenic flexure or the hepatic flexure—or, sometimes, both—must be adequately mobilized.

Classically, the tissues around the bowel are divided with a scissors, whereas the mesentery is divided between clamps and tied with a suitable thread. Recognized tissue planes are separated by means of blunt dissection with either the fingers or a swab. Minor bleeding points are occluded with a coagulating electrocautery, though this approach is often relatively ineffective on mesenteric or omental vessels. The disadvantages of this dissection technique are that oozing from raw surfaces can be a nuisance and that the tissues beyond a tie are often bulky and leave dead tissue within the body that may act as a focus for infection and adhesions. Newer methods of dissection that make use of the ultrasonic scalpel or the bloodless bipolar electrocautery prevent these problems by coagulating a small section of tissue between the jaws of the instrument and simultaneously occluding all blood vessels up to a certain size within the tissues. Consequently, bleeding is reduced, fewer (or no) ties are needed, and only a small quantity of dead tissue results at each point. Becoming skilled in the use of these instruments often takes a little time, but the time is well spent, in that it is now possible to perform an intestinal resection without resort to a single tie.

BOWEL RESECTION

The precise techniques involved in resecting specific bowel segments will not be discussed in great detail here. (Colonic resection, for example, is covered extensively elsewhere [see 3:27 Colorectal Procedures].) The following discussion outlines only the general principles.

Preparation

The segment of bowel to be removed must be isolated with an adequate resection margin. To this end, all surrounding adhesions are divided. Next, the mesentery is divided. The key consideration in this step is to preserve the blood supply to the two remaining ends of bowel while still achieving adequate excision of the diseased bowel. This is more easily accomplished in the small bowel than in the large bowel, thanks to the ample blood supply of the former; even so, transillumination of the mesentery and careful division of the vascular arcade are vital. In the colon, the surrounding fat and the appendices epiploicae should be cleared from the remaining bowel ends so that subsequent suture placement is straightforward.

Care should be taken to avoid two common problems. First, ties placed close to the bowel can bunch tissues excessively and thereby cause angulation or distortion of the free edge of the intestine, which can make the anastomosis difficult and threaten the blood supply. Second, because mesenteric vessels are usually tied very close to their ends, the arteries sometimes slip back beyond the ties. Such slippage results in a hematoma within the leaves of the mesentery, which can itself threaten the viability of the bowel. Generally, the bleeding vessel can be secured with a fine stitch; sometimes, however, a limited further bowel resection is the only safe course of action. Both of these problems can be avoided by using the ultrasonic scalpel or the bipolar coagulating electrocautery.

Division of Bowel

If staplers are not available, the bowel segment to be removed is isolated between noncrushing clamps placed across the intestinal lumen some distance away from the resection margin so as to limit the amount of bowel contents that can escape into the wound. Crushing clamps are then placed on the specimen side of the diseased segment at the point of the resection, and the bowel is divided with a knife just proximal and distal to the clamps. Thus, the lumen of the diseased segment is never open within the abdominal wound. Even so, the contents of the bowel between the open ends and the noncrushing clamps can leak into the wound. To minimize this problem, it is usual to isolate the working area with abdominal packs, which are sometimes soaked in an antiseptic (e.g., povidone-iodine).

One advantage of using staplers for anastomosis is that in most instances, division of the bowel can be accomplished without opening the lumen. A linear cutting stapler (e.g., GIA) transects the bowel and seals the two cut ends simultaneously. Unfortunately, in the pelvis, it is usually necessary to employ an angulated noncutting linear stapler (e.g., TA) so as to obtain as much length as possible distal to the lesion. The proximal rectum is then clamped with a crushing bowel clamp, and a long knife is used to transect the rectum above the staple line. Even so, there remains the potential for leakage of a small amount of fecal material, which must then be suctioned away.

SIMPLE BOWEL CLOSURE

There are many cases in which simple closure of a hole in the bowel is required, as with a perforated duodenal ulcer, a gunshot wound, or the inadvertent perforation of the small bowel during the division of dense peritoneal adhesions. Most surgeons close such holes with two layers of soluble suture material (e.g., 2-0 polyglycolic acid). My own preference is for an inner continuous layer inverted with outer seromuscular interrupted sutures, but there are many perfectly satisfactory alternatives.

Special mention should be made of the technique of stricture-plasty, which is used for a number of benign small bowel strictures (especially those resulting from Crohn disease) as a means of avoiding small bowel resection and anastomoses. In this procedure, the bowel is opened longitudinally and closed transversely with a single layer of 2-0 polyglycolic acid sutures in a Connell stitch. Excellent functional results have been achieved with this technique despite its reputation for fistula formation, which is associated with Crohn disease.

SINGLE-LAYER SUTURED EXTRAMUCOSAL SIDE-TO-SIDE ENTEROENTEROSTOMY

A side-to-side anastomosis [see Figure 5] may be performed when no resection is done, as a bypass procedure (e.g., a gas-

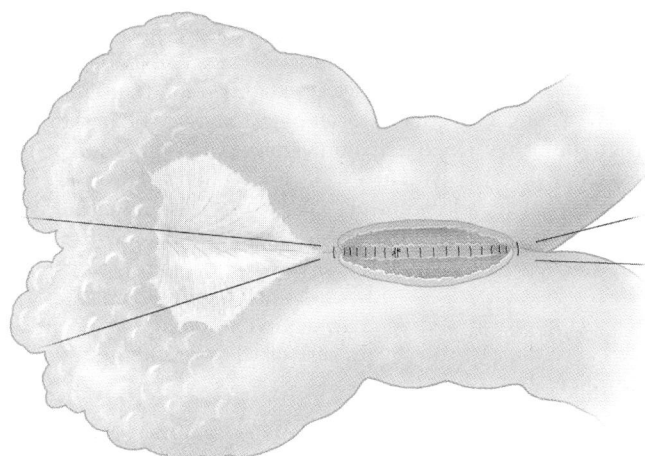

Figure 5 **Single-layer sutured extramucosal side-to-side enteroenterostomy. A full-length suture is started in the back wall and run through the seromuscular and submucosal layers in the direction of the surgeon; the corners of the enterotomy are approximated with a baseball stitch, and a single Connell stitch is used to invert the anterior layer. A second suture is started at the same spot on the posterior wall and run in the opposite direction, again through all layers except the mucosa; the corners of the enterotomies are approximated with a baseball stitch, and the suture is continued in either the Connell stitch or the over-and-over stitch to complete the anterior wall of the anastomosis.**

troenterostomy); after a small bowel resection; when there is a discrepancy in the diameter of the two ends to be anastomosed (e.g., an ileocolic anastomosis after a right hemicolectomy); or when the anatomy is such that the most tension-free position for the anastomosis is with the two bowel segments parallel (as in a Finney strictureplasty).

Two stay sutures of 3-0 polyglycolic acid are placed approximately 8 cm apart on the inner aspect of the antimesenteric border. A 5 cm enterotomy is made on each loop with an electrocautery or a blade on the inner aspect of the antimesenteric border. If electrocautery is used, care must be taken not to injure the mucosa of the posterior wall during this maneuver; placement of a hemostat into the enterotomy to lift the anterior wall usually prevents this problem. Hemostasis of the cut edges is ensured, and the remaining enteric contents are gently suctioned out. A swab soaked in povidone-iodine may be used at this point to cleanse the lumen of the bowel in the perianastomotic region.

A full-length seromuscular and submucosal stitch of 4-0 polyglycolic acid is placed and tied on the inside approximately 5 to 10 mm from the far end of the enterotomies. The stitch is not passed through the mucosa: to do so would add no strength to the anastomosis and would hinder epithelialization by rendering the tissue ischemic. A hemostat is placed on the short end of the tied suture, and the assistant applies continuous gentle tension to the long end of the suture. An over-and-over stitch is started in the direction of the surgeon; small bites are taken, and proper inversion of the suture line is ensured with each pass through tissue. When the proximal ends of the enterostomies are reached, this so-called baseball stitch is continued almost completely around to the anterior wall of the anastomosis. A single Connell stitch may be used to invert this anterior layer.

Another full-length seromuscular and submucosal suture of 4-0 polyglycolic acid is then inserted and tied at the same location in the posterior wall as the first. If the two sutures are placed close enough together, the short ends need not be tied together and may simply be cut off. The remainder of the posterior wall is sewn away from the surgeon in the same manner as the portion already sewn, and the corners are approximated with the baseball stitch. The anterior wall is then completed with this second suture, either with the Connell stitch or with an over-and-over stitch with the assistant inverting the edges before applying tension to the previous stitch.

When the defect is completely closed, the two sutures are tied across the anastomotic line. The stay sutures are removed, and the anastomosis is carefully inspected. Often, there is no mesenteric defect to close in a side-to-side anastomosis, but if there is one, it should be approximated at this point with continuous or interrupted absorbable sutures, with care taken not to injure the vascular supply to the anastomosis.

DOUBLE-LAYER SUTURED END-TO-SIDE ENTEROCOLOSTOMY

In this procedure, the end of the ileum is joined to the side of the transverse colon [see Figure 6]. The distal colon is divided with a cutting stapler so that a blind end is left. Some surgeons underpin or bury this staple line, though this practice is probably unnecessary. The proximal cut end of the intestine is similarly closed either with staples after division with a cutting linear stapler or with a crushing bowel clamp. This proximal end is brought into apposition with the side of the distal bowel segment at a point no farther than 2.5 to 5 cm from the blind end of the distal segment; this proximity to the cut end is important for prevention of the blind loop syndrome.

Stay sutures of 3-0 polyglycolic acid are placed between the serosa of the proximal limb, about 10 to 15 mm from the clamp, and the serosa of the distal limb. Interrupted seromuscular sutures of 3-0 polyglycolic acid are then placed between these stay sutures, spaced about three to six to the centimeter. These stitches

may be tied sequentially or snapped and tied once they are all in place. It is crucial not to apply excessive tension, which could cut the seromuscular layer or render it ischemic. Suction is then readied. The staple line or crushed tissue on the proximal limb is cut off with a coagulating electrocautery or a knife; this maneuver opens the lumen of the proximal limb. All residual intestinal content is gently suctioned.

An enterotomy or colotomy is created on the distal limb opposite the open lumen of the proximal bowel. A full-thickness suture of 3-0 polyglycolic acid is inserted in the posterior wall at a point close to the far end of the enterotomy and run in an over-and-over stitch back toward the surgeon. The corner is rounded with the baseball stitch, and when the anterior wall is reached, the Connell stitch is used. A second full-length 3-0 suture is started at the same point on the posterior wall as the first, and the short ends of the two sutures are tied together and cut. This second suture is then run away from the surgeon to complete the posterior wall, and the anterior wall is completed with the Connell stitch. The two sutures are then tied across the anastomotic line.

A second series of interrupted seromuscular stitches is then placed anteriorly in the same fashion as the seromuscular stitches placed in the posterior wall. It is important not to narrow either lumen excessively by imbricating too much of the bowel wall into this second layer. The lumen of the anastomosis is palpated to confirm patency, and the mesenteric defect is closed if possible with either continuous or interrupted absorbable sutures.

DOUBLE-STAPLED END-TO-END COLOANAL ANASTOMOSIS

Resection of the distal sigmoid colon and the rectum is a common procedure. In the past, it often resulted in a permanent colostomy because of the technical difficulties associated with a hand-sewn

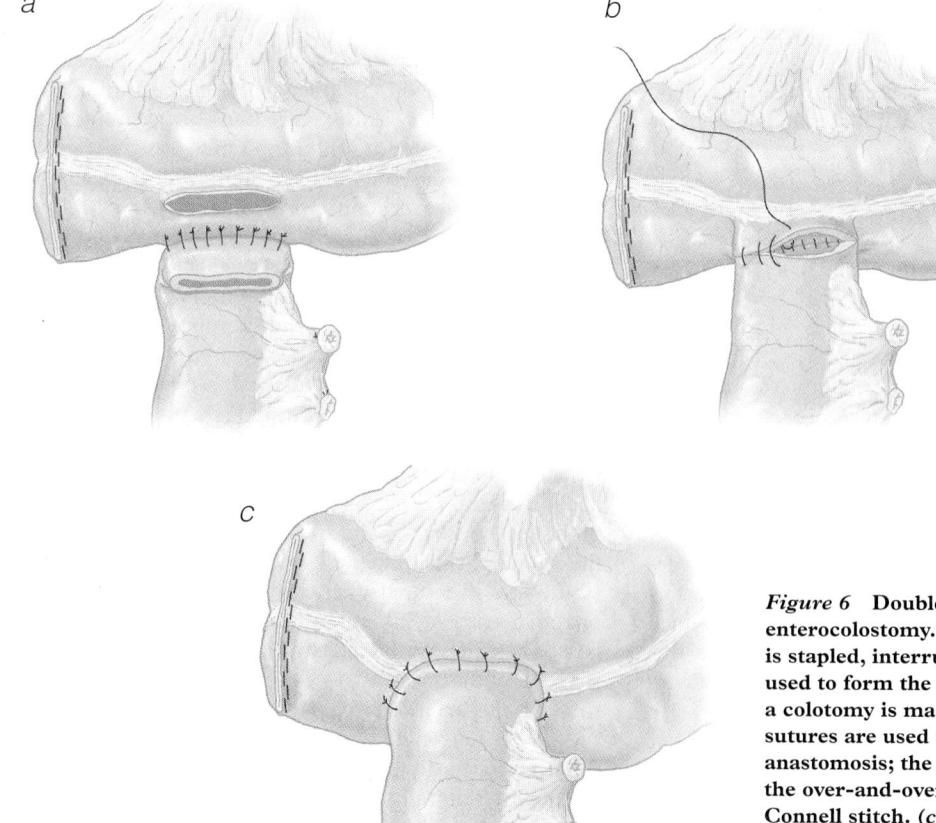

Figure 6 **Double-layer sutured end-to-side enterocolostomy. (*a*) The proximal bowel end is stapled, interrupted Lembert stitches are used to form the posterior outer layer, and a colotomy is made. (*b*) Two continuous sutures are used to form the inner layer of the anastomosis; the posterior portion is done with the over-and-over stitch, the anterior with the Connell stitch. (*c*) Interrupted Lembert stitches are used to form the anterior outer layer.**

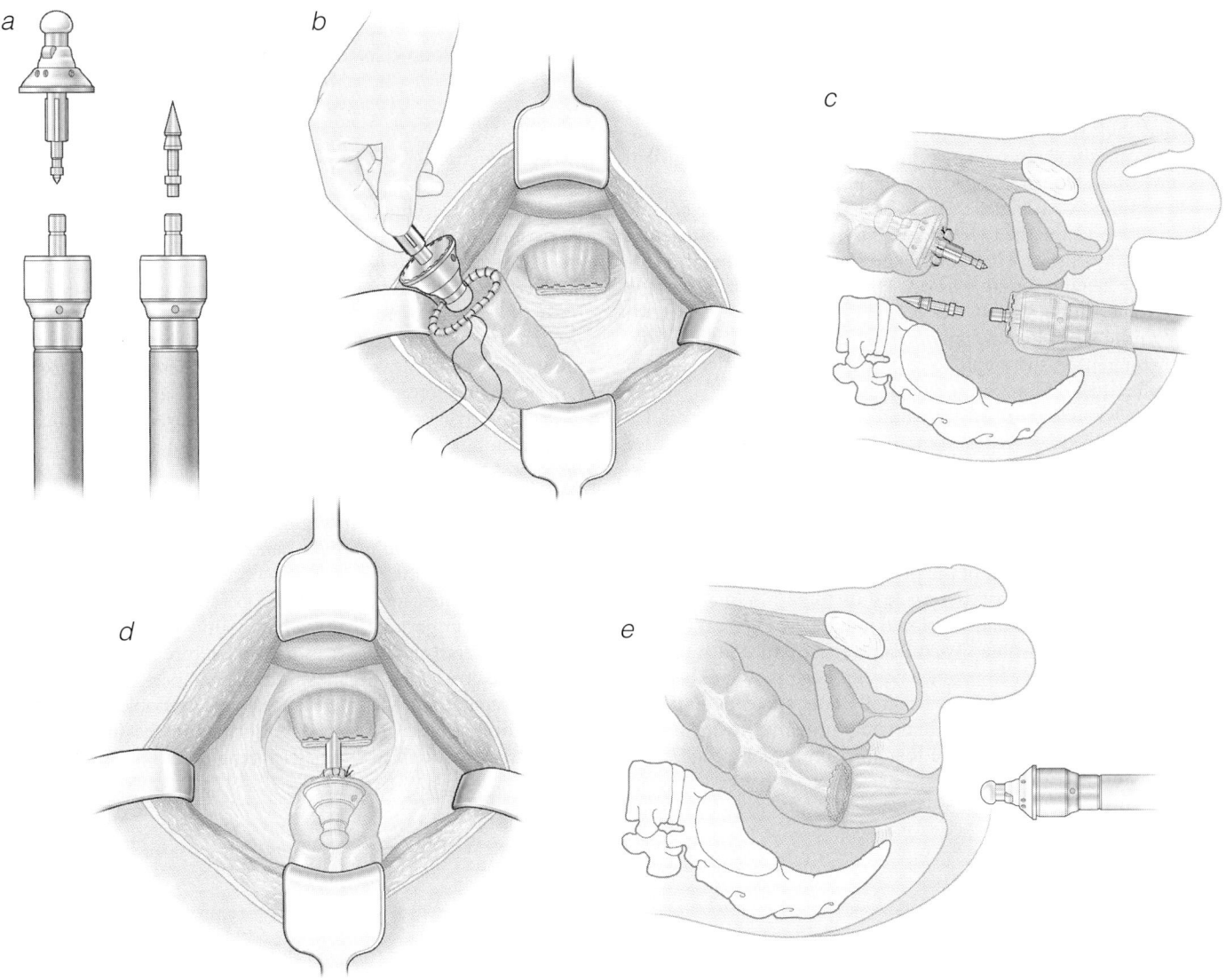

Figure 7   **Double-stapled end-to-end coloanal anstomosis. (*a*) The C-EEA stapler comes with both a standard anvil (left) and a trocar attachment (right). (*b*) The rectal stump is closed with an angled linear noncutting stapler. A purse-string suture is placed around the colotomy, and the anvil of the stapler is placed in the open end and secured. (*c*) The stapler, with the sharp trocar attachment in place, is inserted into the anus, and the trocar is made to pierce the rectal stump at or near the staple line, after which the trocar is removed. (*d*) The anvil in the proximal colon is joined with the stapler in the rectal stump, and the two edges are slowly brought together. (*e*) The stapler is fired and then gently withdrawn.**

anastomosis deep in the pelvis. The development of circular staplers reduced the technical difficulty of the operation and made possible anastomoses as far down as the anus [*see Figure 7*].

Proper preparation of the patient and the bowel is essential before resection of the rectum. The patient is placed in the lithotomy position with the head tilted down, and the small bowel is packed away in the upper abdomen. This positioning gives the surgeon the best access to the pelvis.

The splenic flexure and all of the distal large bowel are fully mobilized along with the rectum. The proximal resection margin is determined and cleared of serosal fat, and the bowel is divided either with a GIA stapler or between crushing bowel clamps. An angled TA stapler is fired across the distal rectal resection margin, and another bowel clamp is placed proximal to it. The rectum is divided with a long-handled knife, with care

taken to avoid plunging the blade into the pelvic sidewall, which could cause significant neurovascular damage. The specimen is removed and the stapler withdrawn. Adequate pelvic hemostasis is ensured.

Once the surgeon is satisfied that the bowel is sufficiently mobilized, a noncrushing bowel clamp is placed on the colon 10 to 15 cm proximal to the margin, and the crushing clamp is removed. At this stage, it is usual to create an 8 to 10 cm colonic J pouch; this measure typically yields a substantially improved functional outcome, especially in the early postoperative period in older patients.[77] A whip-stitch (or purse-string suture) of 2-0 polypropylene is placed around the colotomy, and the anvil from the appropriately sized curved EEA stapler is inserted into the open end and secured in place by tying the suture [*see Figure 7*]. The proximal bowel clamp is removed. The assistant—who may also, if desired, gently wash out the rectal stump with a dilute povidone-iodine solution—performs a digital rectal examination.

The stapler, with its trocar attachment in place, is then inserted into the anus under the careful guidance of the surgeon. The pointed shaft is brought out through or adjacent to the linear staple line, and the sharp point is removed. The peg from the anvil in the proximal colon is snapped into the protruding shaft of the stapler, and the two edges are slowly brought together. The colonic mesentery must not be twisted, and the ends must come together without any tension whatsoever. The stapler is fired, and a distinctive crunching sound is heard. The anvil is then loosened the appropriate amount, and the entire mechanism is withdrawn through the anus. Finally, the proximal and distal rings of tissue, which remain on the stapler, are carefully inspected to confirm circumferential closure of the staple line.

The pelvis is then filled with body-temperature saline, and a Toomey or bladder syringe is used to insufflate the neorectum with air. The surgeon watches for bubbling in the pelvis as a sign of leakage from the anastomosis. If there is a leak, additional soluble sutures must be placed to close the defect and another air test performed. A rectal tube may then be inserted by the assistant or may be placed at the end of the procedure.

When the anastomosis is very low or there is some concern about healing, a drain may be placed in the pelvis behind the staple line; however, as noted [see Controversial Issues in Intestinal Anastomosis, above], this practice has not been shown to be beneficial and may in fact impair healing. Some surgeons prefer to protect the anastomosis with a temporary proximal defunctioning stoma. There is some evidence that such protection reduces the risk of an anastomotic leak, but it is unclear whether a loop ileostomy or a loop colostomy is better for this purpose.[78-82]

Conclusion

A general note about the cosmetic aspect of these procedures is appropriate here. After any of these operations, a close visual inspection of the entire circumference of the anastomosis should be performed. As a rule, if the divided ends appear well apposed, then the anastomosis is probably sound.

Over the past 200 years, our understanding of how the bowel heals and how to perform intestinal anastomoses safely and effectively has improved considerably. This improvement is reflected in lower anastomotic leakage and dehiscence rates, lower operative morbidity, and lower mortality. Some would argue that much of the improved outcome is attributable to improved anesthesia, more potent antibiotics, and better postoperative monitoring and care. No doubt there is a good deal of truth to this argument. There is also no doubt, however, that one of the most significant determinants of outcome after procedures that include intestinal anastomosis is surgical technique. The central importance of meticulous technique means that constant practice and careful attention to detail are essential for all surgeons operating on the GI tract. In addition, it is important that academic surgeons in particular continue to research such issues as the best suture material or stapler for specific operations, the most suitable and best-tolerated type of bowel preparation, the mechanisms and variables involved in wound healing and collagen deposition, and the importance of local and systemic factors in determining overall outcome.

References

1. Smith SRG, Connolly JC, Crane PW: The effect of surgical drainage materials on colonic healing. Br J Surg 69:153, 1982

2. Matheson NA, McIntosh CA, Krukowski ZH: Continuing experience with single layer appositional anastomosis in the large bowel. Br J Surg 72(suppl):S104, 1985

3. Carty NJ, Keating J, Campbell J, et al: Prospective audit of an extramucosal technique for intestinal anastomosis. Br J Surg 78:1439, 1991

4. Debas HT, Thompson FB: A critical review of colectomy with anastomosis. Surg Gynecol Obstet 135:747, 1973

5. Schrock TR, Deveney CW, Dunphy JE: Factors contributing to leakage of colonic anastomoses. Ann Surg 177:513, 1973

6. Halsted W: Circular suture of the intestine—an experimental study. Am J Med Sci 94:436, 1887

7. Hastings JC, Van Winkle W, Barker E, et al: Effects of suture materials on healing of wounds of the stomach and colon. Surg Gynecol Obstet 140:701, 1975

8. Wise L, McAlister W, Stein T, et al: Studies on the healing of anastomoses of small and large intestines. Surg Gynecol Obstet 141:190, 1975

9. Hesp F, Hendriks T, Lubbers E-J, et al: Wound healing in the intestinal wall: a comparison between experimental ileal and colonic anastomoses. Dis Colon Rectum 24:99, 1984

10. Hawley PJ, Hunt TK, Dunphy JE: Aetiology of colonic anastomotic leaks. Proc R Soc Med 63:28, 1970

11. Hawley PJ, Faulk WP: A circulating collagenase inhibitor. Br J Surg 57:900, 1970

12. Martens M, Hendriks T: Postoperative changes in collagen synthesis in intestinal anastomoses of the rat: differences between small and large bowel. Gut 32:1482, 1991

13. Martens M, deMan B, Hendriks T, et al: Collagen synthetic capacity throughout the uninjured and anastomosed intestinal wall. Am J Surg 164:354, 1992

14. Guler M, Kologlu M, Kama NA, et al: Effect of topically applied charged particles on healing of colonic anastomoses. Arch Surg 137:813, 2002

15. Fingerhut A, Hay J-M, Elhadad A, et al: Supraperitoneal colorectal anastomosis: hand-sewn versus circular staples—a controlled clinical trial. Surgery 118:479, 1995

16. Koruda MJ, Rolandelli RH: Experimental studies on the healing of colonic anastomoses. J Surg Res 48:504, 1990

17. Munday C, McGinn FP: A comparison of polyglycolic acid and catgut sutures in rat colonic anastomoses. Br J Surg 63:870, 1976

18. Khubchandani IT: Low end-to-side rectoenteric anastomosis with single-layer wire. Dis Colon Rectum 18:308, 1975

19. Irvin T, Goligher J: Aetiology of disruption of intestinal anastomoses. Br J Surg 60:461, 1973

20. Olsen GB, Letwin E, Williams HTG: Clinical experience with the use of a single-layer intestinal anastomosis. Can J Surg 56:771, 1969

21. Sarin S, Lightwood RG: Continuous single-layer gastrointestinal anastomosis: a prospective audit. Br J Surg 76:493, 1989

22. Shandall A, Lowndes R, Young HL: Colonic anastomotic healing and oxygen tension. Br J Surg 72:606, 1985

23. Jiborn H, Ahonen J, Zederfeldt B: Healing of experimental colonic anastomoses: the effect of suture technique on collagen metabolism in the colonic wall. Am J Surg 139:406, 1980

24. Khoury GA, Waxman BP: Large bowel anastomosis: I. The healing process and sutured anastomoses: a review. Br J Surg 70:61, 1983

25. Abramowitz H: Everting and inverting anastomoses: an experimental study of comparative safety. Rev Surg 28:142, 1971

26. Polglase AL, Hughes ESR, McDermott FT, et al: A comparison of end-to-end staple and suture colorectal anastomosis in the dog. Surg Gynecol Obstet 152:792, 1981

27. O'Neil P, Healey JEJ, Clark RI, et al: Nonsuture intestinal anastomosis. Am J Surg 104:761, 1962

28. Orr NWM: A single layer intestinal anastomosis. Br J Surg 56:77, 1969

29. Templeton JL, McKelvey STD: Low colorectal anastomoses: an experimental assessment of two sutured and two stapled techniques. Dis Colon Rectum 28:38, 1985

30. Goligher J, Morris C, McAdam W: A controlled trial of inverting versus everting intestinal suture in clinical large-bowel surgery. Br J Surg 57:817, 1970

31. Brunius U, Zederfeldt B: Effects of antiinflammatory treatment on wound healing. Acta Chir Scand 129:462, 1965

32. Fielding LP, Stewart Brown S, Blesowsky L, et al: Anastomotic integrity after operations for large bowel cancer: a multicentre study. Br Med J 282:411, 1980

33. Leob MJ: Comparative strength of inverted, everted and endon intestinal anastomoses. Surg Gynecol Obstet 125:301, 1967

34. Undre AR: Enteroplasty: a new concept in the management of benign strictures of the intestine. Int Surg 68:73, 1983

35. Chassin JL, Rifkind KM, Turner JW: Errors and pitfalls in stapled gastrointestinal tract anastomoses. Surg Clin North Am 64:441, 1984

36. Ravitch MM: Intersecting staple lines in intestinal anastomoses. Surgery 97:8, 1985

37. Chung RS: Blood flow in colonic anastomoses: effect of stapling and suturing. Ann Surg 206:335, 1987

38. Julian TB, Ravitch MM: Evaluations of the safety of end-to-end stapling anastomoses across linear stapled closure. Surg Clin North Am 64:567, 1984

39. Brennan SS, Pickford IR, Evans M, et al: Staples or sutures for colonic anastomosis—a controlled clinical trial. Br J Surg 69:722, 1982

40. O'Donnell AF, O'Connell PR, Royston D, et al: Suture technique affects perianastomotic colonic crypt cell production and tumour formation. Br J Surg 78:671, 1991

41. Greenstein A, Rogers P, Moss G: Doubled fourth-day colorectal anastomotic strength with complete retention of intestinal mature wound collagen and accelerated deposition following full enteral nutrition. Surgery Forum 29:78, 1978

42. Bubrick MP: Effects of technique on anastomotic dehiscence. Dis Colon Rectum 24:232, 1981

43. Lafreniere R, Ketcham AS: A single layer open anastomosis for all intestinal structures. Am J Surg 149:797, 1985

44. Beart RW, Kelly KA: Randomized prospective evaluation of the EEA stapler for colorectal anastomoses. Am J Surg 141:143, 1981

45. Kracht M, Hay J-M, Fagniez P-L, et al: Ileocolonic anastomosis after right hemicolectomy for carcinoma: stapled or hand-sewn. Int J Colorect Dis 8:29, 1993

46. Valverde A, Hay JM, Fingerhut A, et al: Manual versus mechanical esophagogastric anastomosis after resection for carcinoma: a controlled trial. French Association for Surgical Research. Surgery 120:476, 1996

47. Akyol AM, McGregor JR, Galloway DJ, et al: Recurrence of colorectal cancer after sutured and stapled large bowel anastomoses. Br J Surg 78:1297, 1991

48. O'Dwyer P, Ravikumar TS, Steele G: Serum dependent variability in the adherence to tumour cells to surgical sutures. Br J Surg 72:466, 1985

49. Everett WG, Friend PJ, Forty J: Comparison of stapling and hand-suture for left-sided large bowel anastomosis. Br J Surg 73:345, 1986

50. Murphy JB: A contribution to abdominal surgery, ideal approximation of abdominal viscera without suture. North American Practitioner 4:481, 1892

51. Ballantyne GH: The experimental basis of intestinal suturing: effect of surgical technique, inflammation and infection on enteric wound healing. Dis Colon Rectum 27:61, 1984

52. O'Dwyer PJ, Conway W, McDermott EWM, et al: Effect of mechanical bowel preparation on anastomotic integrity following low anterior resection in dogs. Br J Surg 76:756, 1989

53. Goligher JC, Graham NG, DeDombal FT: Anastomotic dehiscence after anterior resection of the rectum and sigmoid. Br J Surg 57:109, 1970

54. Fok M, Ah-Chong AK, Cheng SWK, et al: Comparison of a single layer continuous hand-sewn method and circular stapling in 580 esophageal anastomoses. Br J Surg 78:342, 1991

55. Hocking M, Carlson R, Courington K, et al: Altered motility and bacterial flora after functional end-to-end anastomosis. Surgery 108:384, 1990

56. West of Scotland and Highland Anastomosis Study Group: Suturing or stapling in gastrointestinal surgery: a prospective randomized study. Br J Surg 78:337, 1991

57. Irving AD, Scrimgeour D: Mechanical bowel preparation for colonic resection and anastomosis. Br J Surg 74:580, 1987

58. Hughes ESR: Asepsis in large bowel surgery. Ann R Coll Surg Engl 51:347, 1972

59. LeVeen HH, Wapnicks S, Falk D: Effects of prophylactic antibiotics on colonic healing. Am J Surg 131:47, 1976

60. Irvin T, Goligher J, Johnston D: A randomized prospective clinical trial of single-layer and two-layer inverting intestinal anastomoses. Br J Surg 60:457, 1973

61. van Geldere D, Fa-Si-Oen P, Noach LA, et al: Complications after colorectal surgery without mechanical bowel preparation. J Am Coll Surg 194:40, 2002

62. Bozetti F: Perioperative nutrition of patients with gastrointestinal cancer. Br J Surg 89:1201, 2002

63. Munck A, Guyre M, Holbrook N: Physiological functions of glucocorticoids in stress and their relation to pharmacological actions. Endocrinol Rev 5:25, 1984

64. Matsusue S, Walser M: Healing of intestinal anastomoses in adrenalectomized rats given corticosterone. Am J Physiol 263:R164, 1992

65. Quan Z, Walser M: The effect of corticosterone administration at varying levels on leucine oxidation and whole body protein synthesis and breakdown in adrenalectomized rats. Metabolism 40:1263, 1991

66. Gadacz T, Menguy RB: Effects of anti-inflammatory drug oxyphenbutazone on the rate of wound healing and the biochemical composition of wound tissue. Surgery Forum 18:58, 1967

67. Getzen L: Intestinal anastomoses. Curr Probl Surg, August 1969, p 3

68. Kratzer GL, Onsanit T: Single layer steel wire anastomosis of the intestine. Surg Gynecol Obstet 139:93, 1974

69. Ravitch MM, Steichen FM: Techniques of staple suturing in the gastrointestinal tract. Ann Surg 175:815, 1972

70. Burg R, Geigle C, Faso J, et al: Omission of routine gastric decompression. Dis Colon Rectum 21:98, 1978

71. Reasbeck P, Rice M, Herbison G: Nasogastric intubation after intestinal resection. Surg Gynecol Obstet 158:354, 1984

72. Argov S, Goldstein I, Barzilai A: Is routine use of a nasogastric tube justified in upper abdominal surgery? Am J Surg 139:849, 1980

73. Yates JL: An experimental study of the local effects of peritoneal drainage. Surg Gynecol Obstet 1:473, 1905

74. Berliner SD, Burson LC, Lear PE: Use and abuse of intraperitoneal drains in colon surgery. Arch Surg 89:686, 1964

75. Merad F, Hay JM, Fingerhut A, et al: Is prophylactic pelvic drainage useful after elective rectal or anal anastomosis? A multicentre controlled randomized trial. French Association for Surgical Research. Surgery 125:529, 1999

76. Manz CW, LaTendresse C, Sako Y: The detrimental effects of drains on colonic anastomoses. Dis Colon Rectum 13:17, 1970

77. Sailer M, Fuchs K-H, Fein M, et al: Randomized clinical trial comparing quality of life after straight and pouch coloanal reconstruction. Br J Surg 89:1108, 2002

78. Gorfine SR, Gelernt IM, Bauer JJ, et al: Restorative proctocolectomy without diverting ileostomy. Dis Colon Rectum 38:188, 1995

79. Grobler SP, Hosie KB, Keighley MR: Randomized trial of loop ileostomy in restorative proctocolectomy. Br J Surg 79:903, 1992

80. Dehni N, Schlegel RD, Cunningham C, et al: Influence of a defunctioning stoma on leakage rates after low colorectal anastomosis and colonic J pouch-anal anastomosis. Br J Surg 85:1114, 1998

81. Law WL, Chu KW, Choi HK: Randomized clinical trial comparing loop ileostomy and loop transverse colostomy for fecal diversion following total mesorectal excision. Br J Surg 89:704, 2002

82. Edwards DP, Leppington-Clarke A, et al: Stoma-related complications are more frequent after transverse colostomy than loop ileostomy: a randomized prospective clinical trial. Br J Surg 88:360, 2001

Acknowledgments

Figures 1 through 7   Tom Moore.

Portions of this chapter are based on a previous iteration written for *ACS Surgery* by Zane Cohen, M.D., and Barry Sullivan, M.D. The author wishes to thank Drs. Cohen and Sullivan.

24 APPENDECTOMY

Hung S. Ho, M.D., F.A.C.S.

The vermiform appendix was first depicted in anatomic drawings in 1492 by Leonardo da Vinci and was first described as an anatomic structure in 1521 by Jacopo Berengari da Carpi, a professor of human anatomy at Bologna. Appendicitis became recognized as a surgical disease when the Harvard University pathologist Reginald Heber Fitz reported his analysis of 257 cases of perforating inflammation of the appendix and 209 cases of typhlitis or perityphlitis at the 1886 meeting of the Association of American Physicians. In this landmark paper, Fitz correctly pointed out that the frequent abscesses in the right iliac fossa were often due to perforation of the vermiform appendix, and he referred to the condition as appendicitis.[1] Among his classic observations of the disease was his emphasis on the "vital importance of early recognition" and its "eventual treatment by laparotomy." It was not until 1894 that Charles McBurney first described the surgical incision that bears his name and the technique of appendectomy that was to become the gold standard for appendectomy throughout the 20th century and into the 21st.[2]

Although appendectomy has traditionally been done—and largely continues to be done—as an open procedure, there has been increasing interest in laparoscopic appendectomy since the beginning of the 1990s. In what follows, I describe both approaches to the operation and briefly discuss factors affecting the choice between them.

Open Appendectomy

With the patient in the supine position, general anesthesia is induced and the abdomen is prepared and draped in a sterile fashion so as to expose the right lower quadrant. The skin incision is made in an oblique direction, crossing a line drawn between the anterior superior iliac spine and the umbilicus at nearly a right angle at a point about 2 to 3 cm from the iliac spine. This point, McBurney's point, is approximately one third of the way from the iliac spine to the umbilicus [see Figure 1]. The subcutaneous fat and fascia are incised to expose the external oblique aponeurosis. A slightly shorter incision is made in this aponeurosis; first, a scalpel is used, and then, the incision is extended with scissors in the direction of the fibers of the muscle and its tendon in such a way that the fibers are separated but not cut. The fibers of the internal oblique muscle and the transversus abdominis are separated with a blunt instrument at nearly a right angle to the incision on the external oblique aponeurosis. The parietal peritoneum is lifted up, with care taken not to include the underlying viscera, and is opened in a transverse fashion with a scalpel. This incision is then enlarged transversely with scissors. When greater exposure is required, the lateral edge of the rectus sheath is incised and the rectus abdominis retracted medially without being divided [see Figure 2].

A foul smell or the presence of pus on entry into the peritoneum is an indication of advanced appendicitis. The free peritoneal fluid is collected for bacteriologic analysis. The appendix is located by following the cecal taeniae distally. The inflamed appendix usually feels firm and turgid. The appendix, together with the cecum, is delivered into the surgical incision and held with a Babcock tissue forceps. If this step proves difficult, the appendix can sometimes be swept into the field with the surgeon's right index finger as gentle traction is maintained on the cecum with a small, moist gauze pad held in the left hand [see Figure 3]. Care should be taken at this point not to avulse the friable and possibly necrotic appendix. To deliver a retrocecal appendix, it may be necessary to mobilize the ascending colon partially by dividing the peritoneum on its lateral side, starting from the terminal ileum and proceeding toward the hepatic flexure.

The mesoappendix, containing the appendicular artery, is divided between clamps and ligated with 3-0 absorbable sutures [see Figure 4]. The appendix is held up with a Babcock tissue forceps, and its base is crushed with a straight mosquito arterial forceps. The mosquito forceps is then opened, moved up the appendix, and closed again. The base of the appendix is doubly ligated with 2-0 absorbable sutures at the point where it was crushed, so that a cuff of about 3 mm is left between the forceps and the tie. The appendix is divided by running a scalpel along the underside of the forceps. The mucosa of the appendiceal stump is fulgurated with the electrocautery. The stump is not routinely invaginated into the cecum. In those rare cases in which the viability of the appendiceal base is in question, a 2-0 absorbable purse-string suture is placed in the cecum, and the stump is invaginated as the suture is tied; if this is done, palpation for a patent ileocecal valve is indicated. The operative field is then checked for hemostasis. In cases of perforated appendicitis, the right paracolic gutter and pelvis are irrigated and thoroughly aspirated to ensure that any collected pus or particulate material is removed.

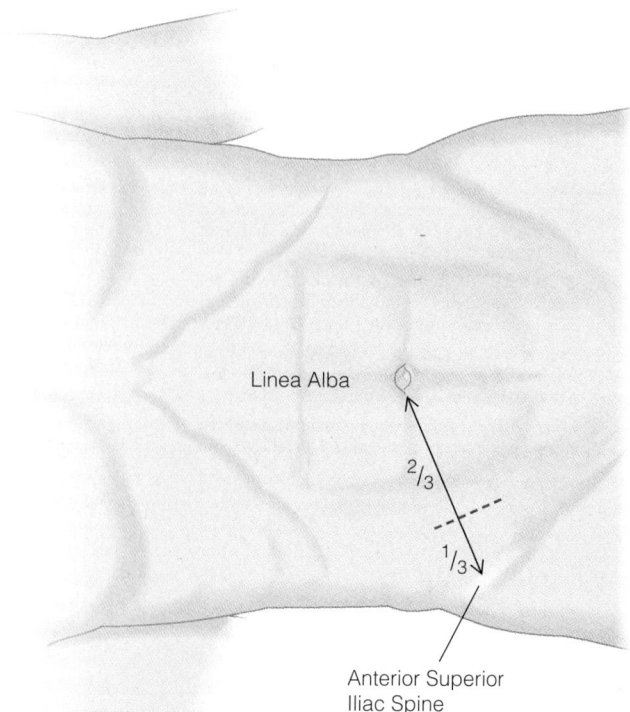

Linea Alba

Anterior Superior
Iliac Spine

Figure 1 **Open appendectomy. Shown are McBurney's point and McBurney's incision.**

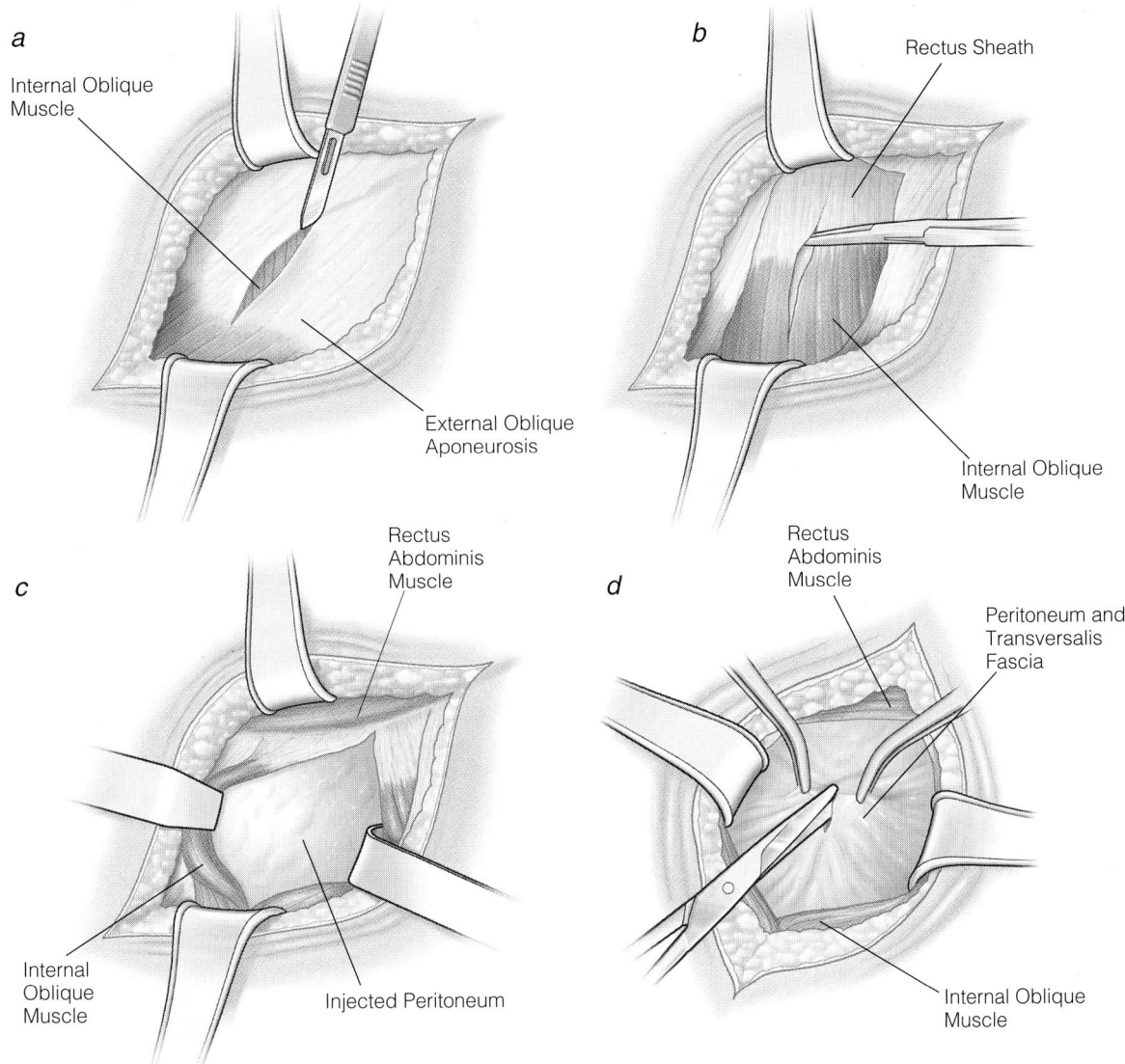

a Internal Oblique Muscle

External Oblique Aponeurosis

b Rectus Sheath

Internal Oblique Muscle

c Rectus Abdominis Muscle

Internal Oblique Muscle

Injected Peritoneum

d Rectus Abdominis Muscle

Peritoneum and Transversalis Fascia

Internal Oblique Muscle

Figure 2 **Open appendectomy. Depicted is exposure of the abdominal cavity. The external oblique aponeurosis is opened (*a*). The fibers of the internal oblique muscle are separated bluntly (*b*). The parietal peritoneum is exposed (*c*) and opened transversely (*d*).**

The peritoneum is then closed with a continuous 3-0 absorbable suture. The fibers of the transversus abdominis and the internal oblique muscle fall together readily, and their closure can be completed with two interrupted 3-0 absorbable ligatures. The external oblique aponeurosis is closed from end to end with a continuous 2-0 absorbable suture. Scarpa's fascia is approximated with interrupted 3-0 absorbable sutures, and the skin is closed with a continuous subcuticular 4-0 absorbable suture and reinforcing tapes (Steri-Strips). If the wound has been grossly contaminated, the fascia and muscles are closed as described, but the skin is loosely approximated with Steri-Strips, which can easily be removed after the procedure if surgical site infection or abscess develops. An alternative approach is to leave the skin and the subcutaneous tissue open but dressed with sterile nonadherent material and then to perform delayed primary closure with Steri-Strips on postoperative day 4 or 5.

Laparoscopic Appendectomy

The patient is placed in the supine position, with both arms tucked along the sides, and general anesthesia is induced.

Decompression with a temporary nasal or orogastric tube should be routine, as should placement of a Foley catheter and use of lower-extremity sequential compression devices. The surgeon should stand on the patient's left side, with the assistant (who operates the camera) near the patient's left shoulder [*see Figure 5*]. The monitors are placed on the opposite side of the operating table, so that both the surgeon and the assistant can view the procedure at all times.

The abdomen is prepared and draped in a sterile fashion so as to expose the entire abdomen. A three-port approach is routinely used [*see Figure 5*]. All skin incisions along the midline are made vertically to allow a more cosmetically acceptable conversion to laparotomy, should this become necessary. The suprapubic port must be large enough to accommodate the laparoscopic stapler (usually 12 mm); the other two ports can be smaller (e.g., 5 or 10 mm). The ports are placed as far away from the operative field as possible to permit the application of a two-handed dissection technique. The use of a 25° or 30° angled scope facilitates operative viewing and dissection. With the patient pharmacologically relaxed and in the Trendelenburg position, a Veress needle is inserted into the peritoneal cavity at

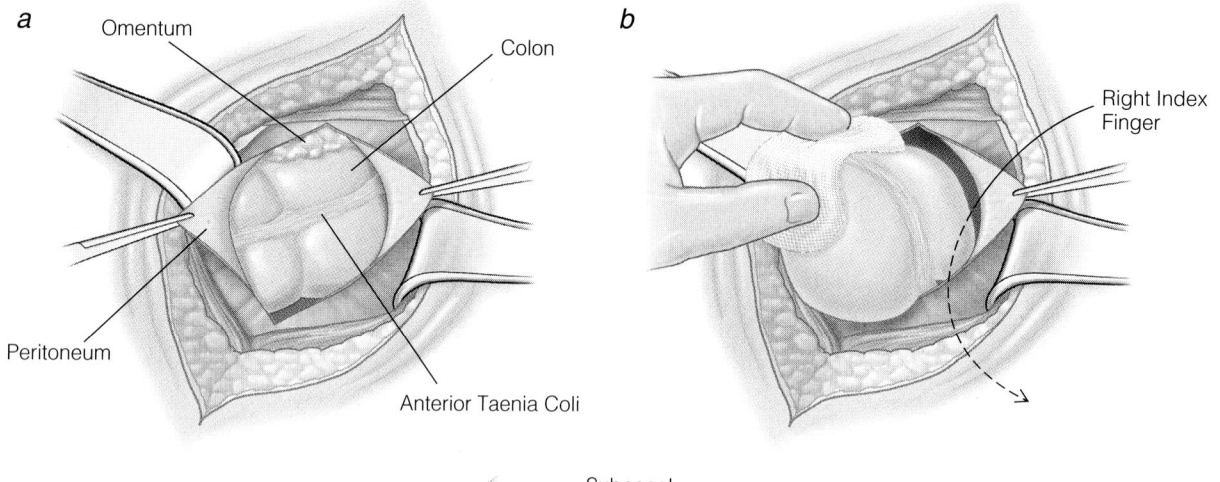

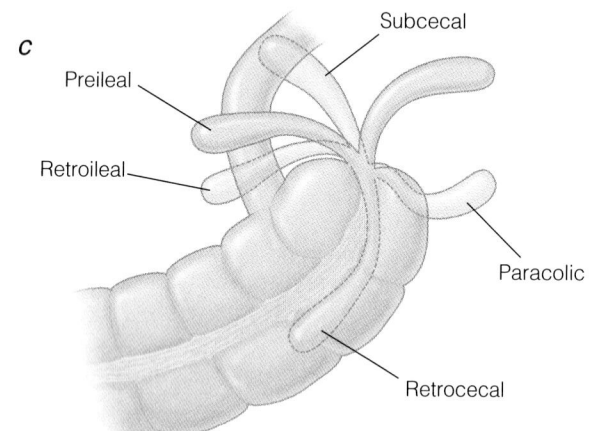

Figure 3 **Open appendectomy. Depicted is the mobilization of the appendix. The ascending colon is identified (*a*). The inflamed appendix and the cecum are delivered into the surgical incision; if this is difficult, the appendix can be swept into the field with the right index finger as traction is maintained on the cecum with a gauze pad (*b*). The appendix may be seen to occupy any of a number of potential locations (*c*).**

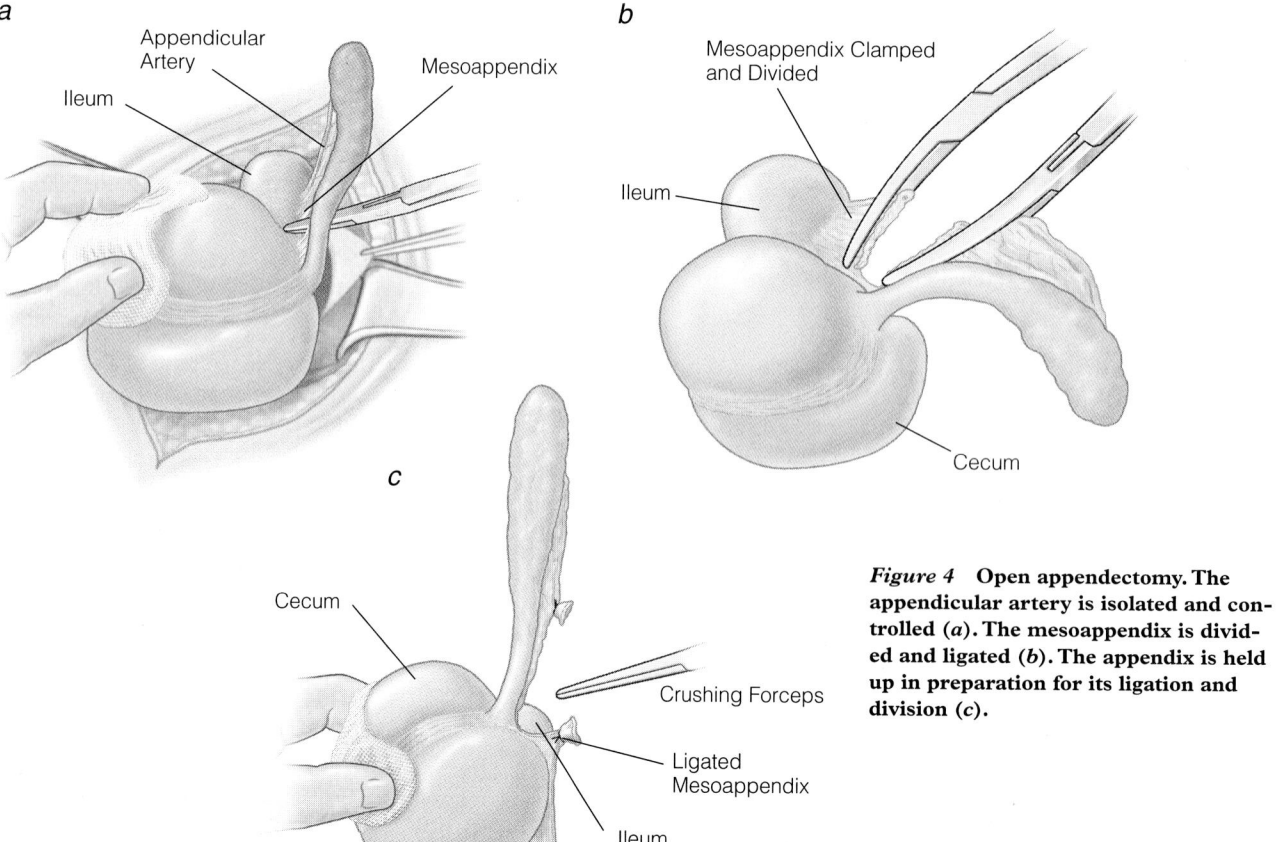

Figure 4 **Open appendectomy. The appendicular artery is isolated and controlled (*a*). The mesoappendix is divided and ligated (*b*). The appendix is held up in preparation for its ligation and division (*c*).**

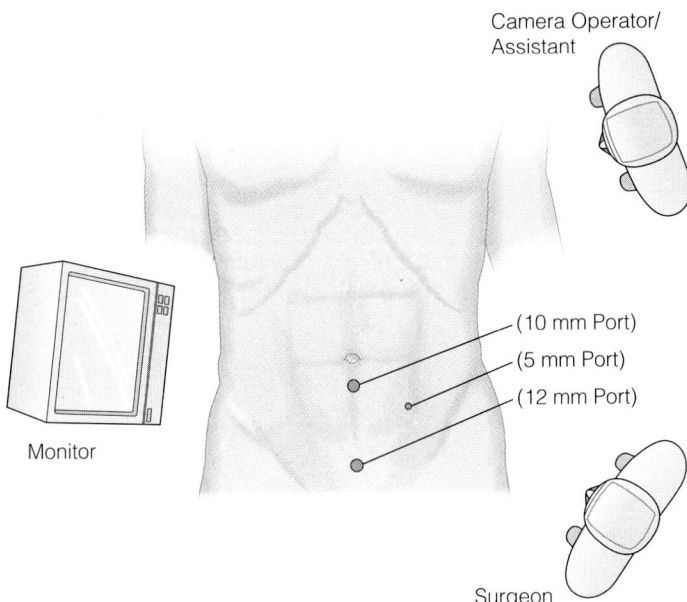

Camera Operator/
Assistant

(10 mm Port)
(5 mm Port)
(12 mm Port)

Monitor

Surgeon

Figure 5 **Laparoscopic appendectomy. Shown are the positioning and placement of the operative ports, as well as the recommended positions for the surgeon, the camera operator, and the video monitor.**

the base of the umbilical ligament. Aspiration and the saline-drop test are performed to ensure that the tip of the needle is correctly positioned. Pneumoperitoneum is established by insufflating CO_2 to an intra-abdominal pressure of 14 mm Hg. The first port is placed at the infraumbilical skin incision, the laparoscope is inserted, and a complete diagnostic laparoscopy is performed. Once the diagnosis of acute appendicitis is confirmed by inspection, the two remaining ports are placed under direct vision. In many cases, however, the diagnosis cannot be confirmed without first placing the second and third ports and exposing the appendix.

The appendix is exposed and traced to its base on the cecum by using an atraumatic retracting forceps. In cases of retrocecal appendix or severe appendiceal inflammation, it is best first to mobilize the cecum completely by taking the lateral reflection of the peritoneum around the terminal ileum and up the ascending colon with an ultrasonic scalpel (e.g., the Harmonic Scalpel, Ethicon Endo-Surgery, Inc.). Surrounding structures, such as the iliac and gonadal vessels and the ureter, should be clearly identified to avoid injury. Dissection of the appendix can then begin. The tip of the appendix is grasped and retracted anteriorly toward the anterior abdominal wall and slightly toward the pelvis; the mesoappendix is thus exposed in a triangular fashion. A window between the base of the appendix and the blood supply is created with a curved dissecting forceps. The mesoappendix is divided either with hemostatic clips and scissors or with a laparoscopic gastrointestinal anastomosis (GIA) stapler loaded with a vascular cartridge [*see Figure* 6]. If a window on the mesoappendix cannot be safely created because of intense inflammation, antegrade dissection of the blood supply is necessary. The ultrasonic scalpel is a handy (albeit expensive) instrument for this purpose. Endoscopic hemostatic clips usually suffice to control the small branches of the appendicular artery during the course of this dissection.

The base of the appendix is then cleared circumferentially of any adipose or connective tissue and is divided with a laparoscopic GIA stapler loaded with an intestinal cartridge [*see Figure*

7]. To ensure an adequate closure away from the inflamed appendiceal wall, a small portion of the cecum may have to be included within the stapler. To ensure proper placement of the stapler and to prevent injury to the right ureter or the adjacent small bowel, the tips of the stapler must be clearly visualized before the instrument is closed. The angled scope and the roticulator laparoscopic GIA stapler will facilitate this maneuver. A noninflamed or minimally inflamed appendix can be ligated with sutures, as described earlier [*see* Open Appendectomy, *above*].

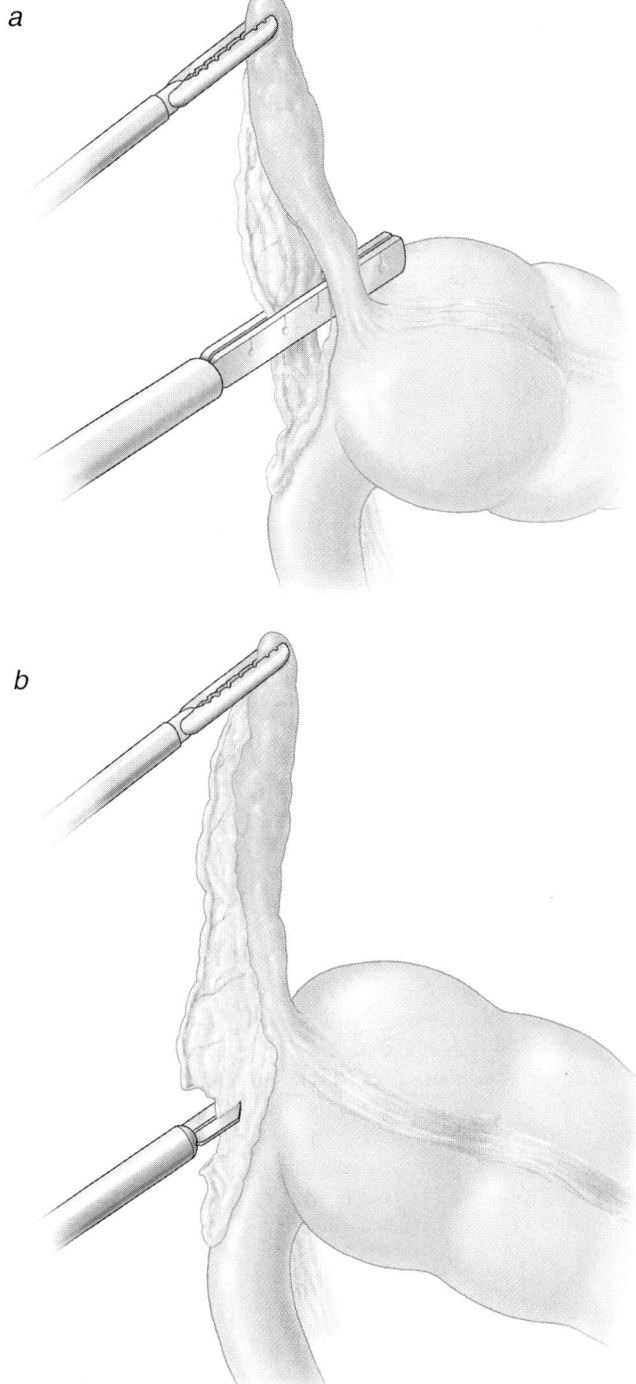

a

b

Figure 6 **Laparoscopic appendectomy. The mesoappendix is divided either with a laparoscopic GIA stapler (*a*) or with hemostatic clips and scissors (*b*).**

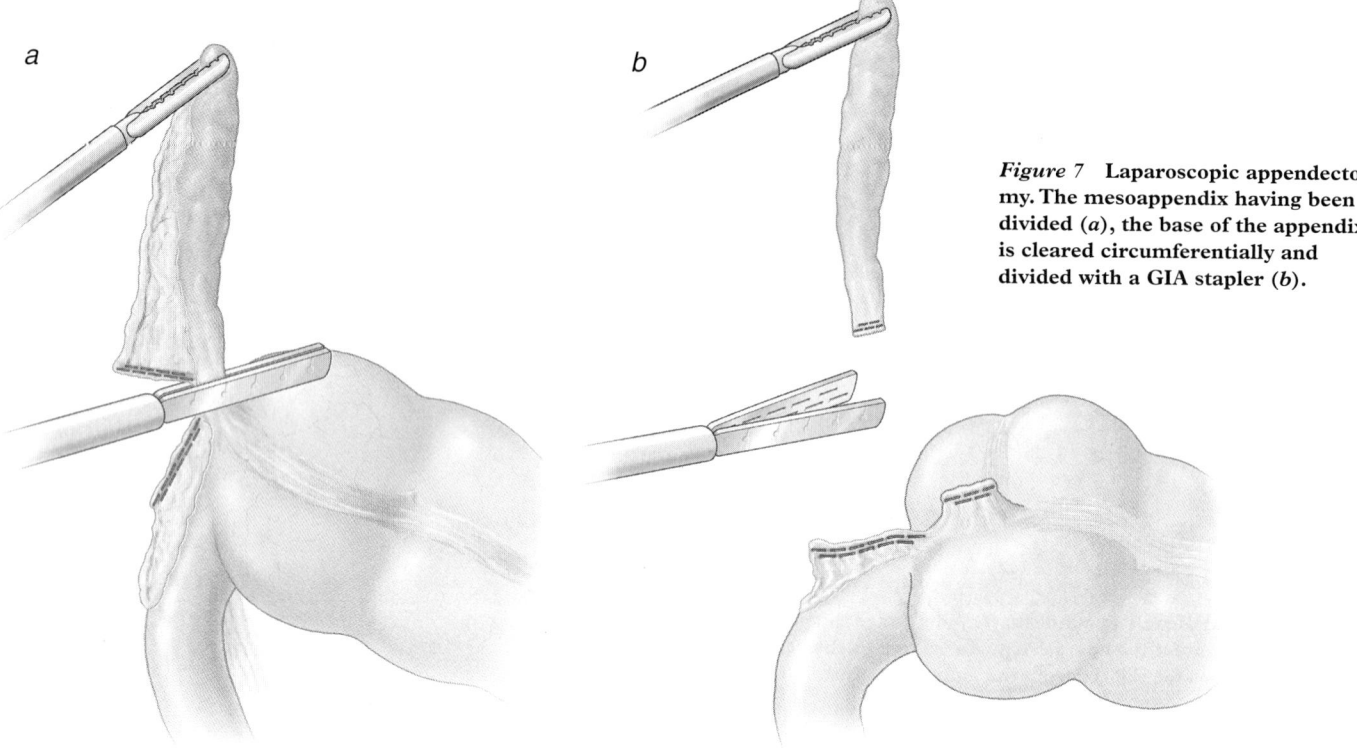

Figure 7 Laparoscopic appendectomy. The mesoappendix having been divided (*a*), the base of the appendix is cleared circumferentially and divided with a GIA stapler (*b*).

The appendix is removed from the abdominal cavity, with care taken to avoid direct contact with the abdominal wall. A mildly inflamed appendix can be delivered through one of the larger ports; a severely inflamed appendix is often too big and hence should be delivered in a specimen retrieval bag [*see Figure 8*].

The operative field is irrigated and aspirated dry. Hemostasis is confirmed, and the cecum is inspected to ensure proper closure of the appendiceal stump. The ports are removed under direct vision, the absence of back-bleeding from the port sites is confirmed, and the abdomen is completely decompressed. All fascial defects larger than 5 mm are closed with 0 absorbable sutures. The skin incisions are reapproximated with a subcuticular 4-0 absorbable suture and reinforcing Steri-Strips.

Choice between Open and Laparoscopic Appendectomy

To date, 27 reports of randomized, controlled trials comparing laparoscopic appendectomy with open appendectomy have been published as full manuscripts in English [*see Table 1*]. These reports involved a total of 3,755 patients, of whom 1,905 underwent laparoscopic appendectomy and 1,850 underwent open appendectomy.[3-29] Similar incidences of histologically normal appendix were found in the two groups (15.9% with laparoscopic appendectomy versus 16.5% with open appendectomy). The conversion rate from laparoscopic appendectomy to open appendectomy was 11% (range, 0% to 23%). Laparoscopic appendectomy was associated with a lower incidence of postoperative wound infection than open appendectomy was (3.4% versus 7%), but it was also associated with a higher incidence of postoperative intra-abdominal abscess (2.4% versus 1%). The length of stay was slightly shorter after laparoscopic appendectomy (1 to 4.9 days; average, 2.7 days) than after open appendectomy (1.2 to 5.3 days; average, 3.2 days). In men with suspected acute appendicitis, laparoscopic appendectomy has no major advan-

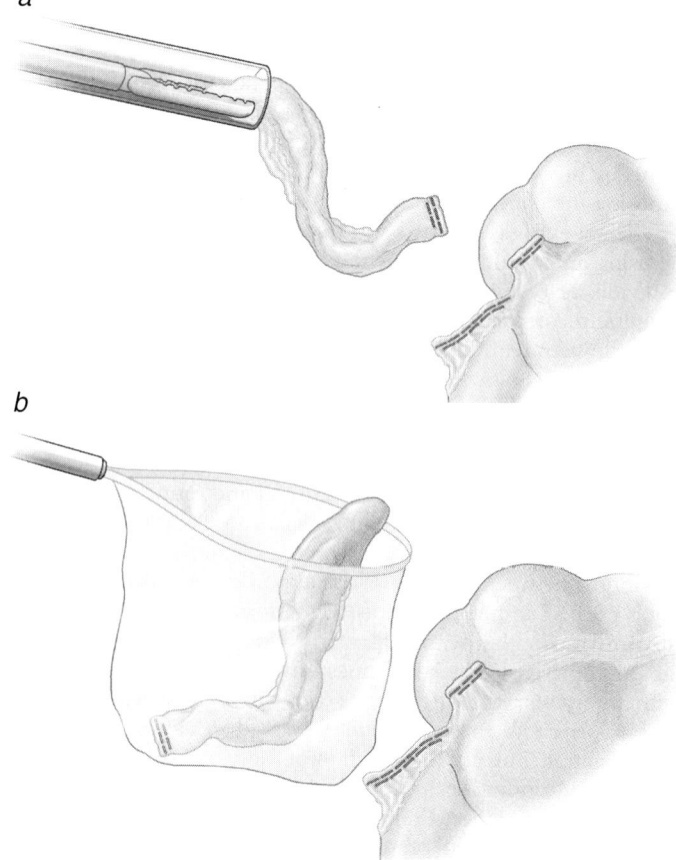

Figure 8 Laparoscopic appendectomy. The specimen is delivered either through one of the larger ports (*a*) or in a specimen retrieval bag (*b*).

Table 1 Results of 27 Prospective, Randomized Trials Comparing Laparoscopic Appendectomy with Open Appendectomy

Variable	Laparoscopic Appendectomy (N=1,905)		Open Appendectomy (N=1,850)	
	No.	Range	No.	Range
Negative appendix	302 (15.9%)	7.7%–36.0%	305 (16.5%)	0%–35.5%
Conversion to open procedure	205 (10.8%)	0%–23.9%	NA	NA
Surgical site infection	64 (3.4%)	0%–18.3%	129 (7%)	0%–17.3%
Intra-abdominal abscess	45 (2.4%)	0%–7.4%	19 (1%)	0%–4.6%
Days in hospital	2.7	1–4.9	3.2	1.2–5.3

tage over open appendectomy.[10,11] In women of childbearing age and in equivocal cases, laparoscopy may be valuable as a diagnostic tool, but the practice of not removing a normal-looking appendix during exploration for right lower quadrant pain is controversial. Laparoscopic appendectomy appears to offer the potential benefit of less postoperative adhesion formation, but the evidence is inconclusive in the light of the short follow-up times reported in these trials, and the higher incidence of intra-abdominal abscess formation remains cause for concern.

At the beginning of the 21st century, as throughout the 20th, the gold standard for surgical treatment of acute appendicitis remains open appendectomy as described by McBurney in 1894. Meta-analyses of prospective, randomized trials showed that although laparoscopic appendectomy is at least as safe as the corresponding open procedure, it is more time-consuming and more costly. Moreover, it remains questionable whether the benefits of laparoscopic appendectomy—reduced postoperative pain, earlier resumption of oral feeding, shortened hospital stay, quicker return to normal preoperative activities, and lower incidence of surgical site infection—outweigh the doubled incidence of postoperative intra-abdominal abscess formation. Further randomized clinical studies focusing on the efficacy of laparoscopic appendectomy as a diagnostic tool and on the incidence of postoperative intra-abdominal abscess and adhesion formation are needed, as are additional cost analyses. At present, the only patients for whom laparoscopic appendectomy appears to offer significant advan-

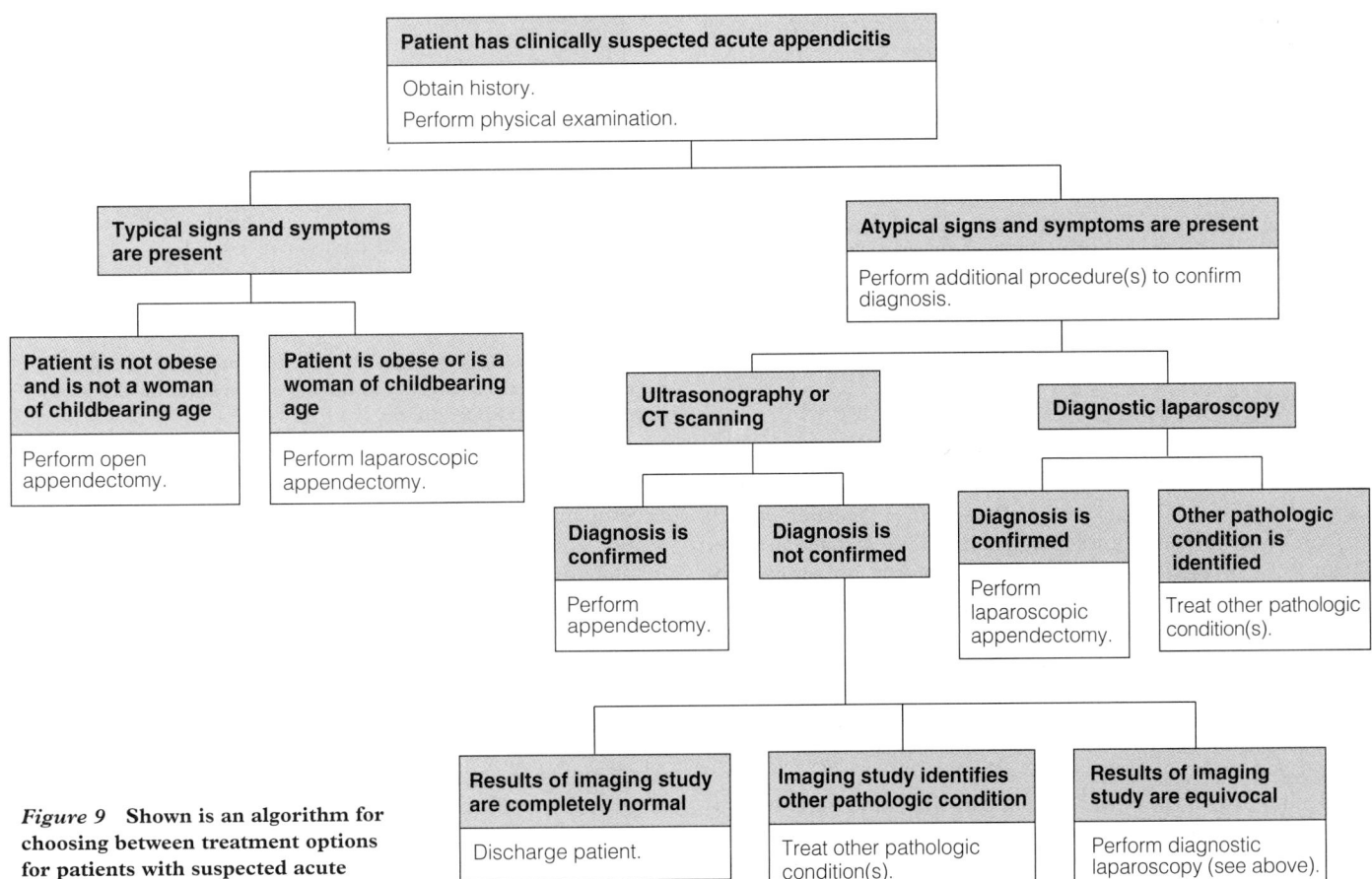

Figure 9 Shown is an algorithm for choosing between treatment options for patients with suspected acute appendicitis.

tages are female patients of childbearing age, obese patients, and patients with an unclear diagnosis [*see Figure 9*].

Special Considerations

THE HISTOLOGICALLY NORMAL APPENDIX

Acute appendicitis is the most common cause of acute surgical abdomen in the United States, and it remains one of the most challenging diagnoses to make in the emergency department. Although the use of advanced diagnostic imaging modalities (e.g., ultrasonography and computed tomography) has led to more accurate diagnosis of acute appendicitis in research settings, it has not been shown to reduce the rate of misdiagnosis of acute appendicitis in the general population.[30]

The incidence of histologically normal appendix in patients with clinical signs and symptoms of acute appendicitis ranges from 8% to 41%.[31-40] Nonetheless, appendectomy relieves symptoms in the vast majority of these patients. When extensive sectioning is done on histologically normal specimens, it often happens that a focus of inflammation is found in only a few serial sections. This condition is known as focal appendicitis—so called because the polymorphonuclear infiltration is confined to a single focus, while the remaining appendix is devoid of any polymorphonuclear cells.[41] It is not clear that all cases of acute appendicitis arise from this focal inflammation; however, such inflammatory foci may be the earliest recognizable manifestations of appendicitis in some so-called negative appendectomies. Furthermore, a substantial proportion of histologically normal appendices removed from patients with clinical signs and symptoms of acute appendicitis exhibit significantly increased expression of tumor necrosis factor–α and interleukin-2 messenger RNA (a sensitive marker of inflammation in appendicitis) in germinal centers, the submucosa, and the lamina propria.[42] Therefore, appendectomy is recommended in patients with clinically suspected acute appendicitis even when the appendix does not appear inflamed during exploration.[43]

As noted [*see* Choice between Open and Laparoscopic Appendectomy, *above*], the results of numerous randomized, controlled trials indicate that laparoscopic appendectomy does not reduce the incidence of negative exploration in patients with clinically suspected acute appendicitis.[3-29] In these 27 English-language reports, the incidence ranged from 7.7% to 36% (average, 15.9%) with laparoscopic appendectomy and from 0% to 35.5% (average, 16.5%) with open appendectomy [*see Table 1*].

APPENDICEAL NEOPLASM

Neoplastic lesions of the appendix are found in as many as 5% of specimens obtained with routine appendectomy for acute appendicitis.[44-47] Most are benign. Preoperative detection of such conditions is rare, and intraoperative diagnosis is made in fewer than 50% of cases. Appendectomy alone may be curative for appendiceal mucocele, localized pseudomyxoma peritonei, most appendiceal carcinoids, and other benign tumors. Definitive management of an appendiceal mass unexpectedly encountered during exploration for clinically suspected acute appendicitis depends on whether the tumor is carcinoid, its size and location, the presence or absence of metastatic disease, and histologic and immunohistochemical findings [*see Figure 10*].

Benign neoplasms of the appendix include mucosal hyperplasia or metaplasia, leiomyomas, neuromas, lipomas, angiomas, and other rare lesions. Appendiceal adenomas tend to be diffuse and to have a predominant villous character. Mucus-producing

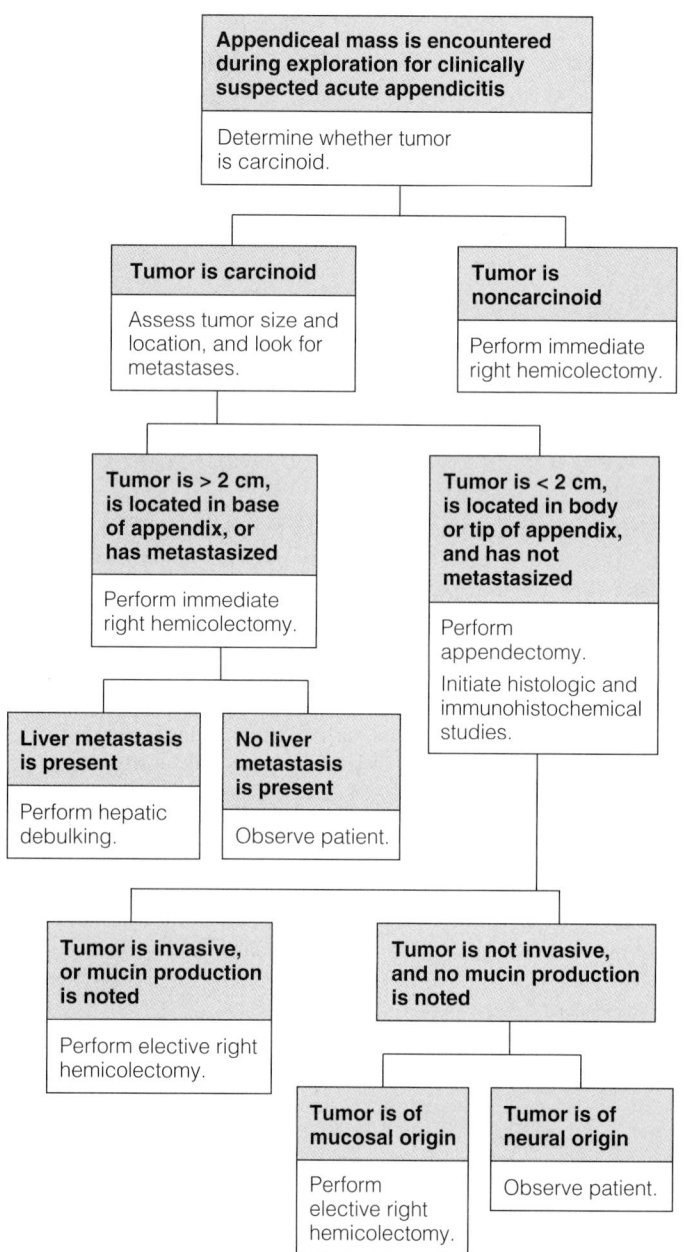

Figure 10 **Shown is an algorithm for the management of an appendiceal mass encountered during exploration for clinically suspected acute appendicitis.**

cystadenomas predispose to appendiceal mucocele, sometimes accompanied by localized pseudomyxoma peritonei. These lesions are rarely symptomatic and are often encountered incidentally during operation; however, they may also be clinically manifested as acute appendicitis, torsion, intussusception, ureteral obstruction, or another acute condition. If the base of the appendix is free of disease, appendectomy alone is sufficient treatment.

Malignant tumors of the appendix primarily consist of carcinoids and adenocarcinomas; altogether, they account for 0.5% of all GI malignancies.[48] The incidence of malignancy in the appendix is 1.35%.[44] Metastasis to the appendix is rare. Carcinoids are substantially more common than adenocarcinomas in the appendix: as many as 80% of all appendiceal masses are carcinoid tumors. Overall, carcinoid tumors are found in 0.5% of all appendiceal specimens, and appendiceal carcinoid tumors account for 18.9% of all carcinoid lesions.[49] These tumors are predominantly of neural cellular origin and have a better prognosis than all other intestinal carcinoid tumors, which typically are of mucosal cellular origin. If the tumor is less than 2 cm in diameter, is located within the body or the tip of the appendix, and has not metastasized, appendectomy is the treatment of choice. If the lesion is at the base of the appendix, is larger than 2 cm in diameter, or has metastasized, right hemicolectomy is indicated. In addition, secondary right hemicolectomy is indicated if the tumor is invasive, if mucin production is noted, or if the tumor is found to be of mucosal cellular origin at final pathologic examination.[50,51] Patients with metastatic appendiceal carcinoid tumors appear to have a far better prognosis than those with other types of metastatic cancers.[50] Therefore, hepatic debulking for symptomatic control is indicated and justified in cases of liver metastasis.

Primary adenocarcinoma of the appendix is rare, and as yet there is no firm consensus regarding prognosis, treatment of choice, and outcome.[52] Currently, the recommended treatment is right hemicolectomy: a 1993 study found that this approach resulted in an overall 5-year survival rate of 68%, compared with 20% when appendectomy alone was performed.[51] The prognosis is determined by the degree of tumor differentiation and by the histologic stage. As many as one third of these patients have a second primary neoplasm, which will be located within the GI tract about half the time.

Finally, nonepithelial appendiceal tumors, though extremely rare, occur as well. Such lesions include malignant and Burkitt lymphomas, smooth muscle tumors, granular cell tumors, ganglioneuromas, and Kaposi sarcoma.

INFLAMMATORY BOWEL DISEASE

The appendix is frequently involved in Crohn disease and ulcerative colitis (25% and 50% of cases, respectively), but isolated Crohn disease of the appendix is rare.[53-56] When a histologically normal appendix is encountered in a patient with active Crohn disease, appendectomy should be performed because of the high risk of recurrent right lower quadrant pain, fever, and tenderness. Although isolated Crohn disease of the appendix may present as acute appendicitis, it is not clear that this condition will necessarily develop into a more extensive form of Crohn disease. Appendectomy is safe in such cases because fistulas almost never develop after appendectomy in patients with isolated involvement of the appendix.

GYNECOLOGIC CONDITIONS

It is clear that the presentation of right lower quadrant pain in a female patient remains a challenge to the treating physician. Frequently, the causes can be identified by means of proper blood work or ultrasonography, but often they can be revealed only through surgical exploration. In such cases, diagnostic laparoscopy provides an excellent view of the pelvic organs, and it offers the potential for easy continuation on to laparoscopic treatment. Ovarian cysts found in premenopausal women include unilocular clear fluid cysts (e.g., follicular cysts and corpus luteum cysts), dermoid cysts, and endometrial cysts. They can be removed by making an incision on the ovary and separating the cyst from the ovarian cortex. Dermoid cysts should be removed in toto to prevent chemical peritonitis. Endometrial cysts are best evaporated with the laser: complete removal is very difficult and sometimes impossible. Torsion of the fallopian tube or the ovary can be reversed by gentle detorsion of the organ with atraumatic forceps. If there is no evidence of ischemia, no further therapy is indicated. If there is gangrene with no indication of recovery, resection is indicated. If the organ shows partial recovery within 10 minutes after the pedicle is untwisted, a second-look laparoscopy is indicated in 24 hours. Pelvic inflammatory disease should be treated on an individualized basis in accordance with the degree of inflammation, the patient's age and desire to have children, and the microbiologic findings.

References

1. Fitz RH: Perforating inflammation of the vermiform appendix with special reference to its early diagnosis and treatment. Trans Assoc Am Physicians 1:107, 1886

2. McBurney C: The incision made in the abdominal wall in cases of appendicitis, with a description of a new method of operating. Ann Surg 20:38, 1894

3. Attwood SEA, Hill ADK, Murphy PG, et al: A prospective randomized trial of laparoscopic versus open appendectomy. Surgery 112:497, 1992

4. Tate JJT, Dawson JW, Chung SCS, et al: Laparoscopic versus open appendectomy: prospective randomised trial. Lancet 342:633, 1993

5. Kum CK, Ngoi SS, Goh PMY, et al: Randomized controlled trial comparing laparoscopic and open appendicectomy. Br J Surg 80:1599, 1993

6. Frazee RC, Roberts JW, Symmonds RE, et al: A prospective randomized trial comparing open versus laparoscopic appendectomy. Ann Surg 219:725, 1994

7. Ortega AE, Hunter JG, Peters JH, et al: A prospective, randomized comparison of laparoscopic appendectomy with open appendectomy. Am J Surg 169:208, 1995

8. Martin LC, Puente I, Sosa JL, et al: Open versus laparoscopic appendectomy: a prospective randomized comparison. Ann Surg 222:256, 1995

9. Hansen JB, Smithers BM, Schache D, et al: Laparoscopic versus open appendectomy: prospective randomized trial. World J Surg 20:17, 1996

10. Mutter D, Vix M, Bui A, et al: Laparoscopy not recommended for routine appendectomy in men: results of a prospective randomized study. Surgery 120:71, 1996

11. Cox MR, McCall JL, Toouli J, et al: Prospective randomized comparison of open versus laparoscopic appendectomy in men. World J Surg 20:263, 1996

12. Lejus C, Dellie L, Plattner V, et al: Randomized, single-blinded trial of laparoscopic versus open appendectomy in children. Anesthesiology 84:801, 1996

13. Williams MD, Collins JN, Wright TF, et al: Laparoscopic versus open appendectomy. South Med J 89:668, 1996

14. Hart R, Rajgopal C, Plewes A, et al: Laparoscopic versus open appendectomy: a prospective randomized trial of 81 patients. Can J Surg 39:457, 1996

15. Reiertsen O, Larsen S, Trondsen E, et al: Randomized controlled trial with sequential design of laparoscopic versus conventional appendicectomy. Br J Surg 84:842, 1997

16. Laine S, Rantala A, Gullichsen R, et al: Laparoscopic appendectomy—is it worthwhile? a prospective, randomized study in young women. Surg Endosc 11:95, 1997

17. Macarulla E, Vallet J, Abad JM, et al: Laparoscopic versus open appendectomy: a prospective randomized trial. Surg Laparosc Endosc 7:335, 1997

18. Kazemier G, de Zeeuw GR, Lange JF, et al: Laparoscopic versus open appendectomy: a randomized clinical trial. Surg Endosc 11:336, 1997

19. Minne L, Varner D, Burnell A, et al: Laparoscopic versus open appendectomy: prospective randomized study of outcomes. Arch Surg 132:708, 1997

20. Hay SA: Laparoscopic versus conventional appendectomy in children. Pediatr Surg Int 13:21, 1998

21. Klinger A, Henle KP, Beller S, et al: Laparoscopic appendectomy does not change the incidence of postoperative infectious complications. Am J Surg 175:232, 1998

22. Hiekkinen TJ, Haukipuro K, Hulkko A: Cost-effective appendectomy: open or laparoscopic? a prospective randomized study. Surg Endosc 12:1204, 1998

23. Hellberg A, Rudberg C, Kullman E, et al: Prospective randomized multicentre study of laparoscopic versus open appendicectomy. Br J Surg 86:48, 1999

24. Ozmen MM, Zulfikaroglu B, Tanik A, et al: Laparoscopic versus open appendectomy: prospective randomized trial. Surg Laparosc Endosc Percutan Tech 9:187, 1999

25. Pedersen AG, Petersen OB, Wara P, et al: Randomized clinical trial of laparoscopic versus open appendicectomy. Br J Surg 88:200, 2001

26. Lavonius MI, Liesjarvi S, Ovaska J, et al: Laparoscopic versus open appendectomy in children: a prospective randomised study. Eur J Pediat Surg 11:235, 2001

27. Long KH, Bannon MP, Zietlow SP, et al: A prospective randomized comparison of laparoscopic appendectomy with open appedectomy: Clinical and economic analyses. Surgery 129:390, 2001

28. Lintula H, Kokki H, Vanamo K: Single-blind randomized clinical trial of laparoscopic versus appendicectomy in children. Br J Surg 88:510, 2001

29. Huang MT, Wei PL, Wu CC, et al: Needlescopic, laparoscopic, and open appendectomy: a comparative study. Surg Laparosc Endosc Percutan Tech 11:306, 2001

30. Flum DR, Morris A, Koepsell T, et al: Has misdiagnosis of appendicitis decreased over time? a population-based analysis. JAMA 286:1748, 2001

31. Chang AR: An analysis of the pathology of 3,003 appendices. Aust NZ J Surg 51:169, 1981

32. Knight PJ, Vassy LE: Specific diseases mimicking appendicitis in childhood. Arch Surg 116:744, 1981

33. Pieper R, Kager L, Nasman P: Acute appendicitis: a clinical study of 1,018 cases of emergency appendectomy. Acta Chir Scand 148:51, 1982

34. Arnbjornsson E, Asp NG, Westin SI: Decreasing incidence of acute appendicitis, with special reference to the consumption of dietary fiber. Acta Chir Scand 148:461, 1982

35. Blind PJ, Dahlgren ST: The continuing challenge of the negative appendix. Acta Chir Scand 152:623, 1986

36. Lau WY: Correlation between gross appeareance of the appendix and histological examination. Ann R Coll Surg Edinb 70:336, 1988

37. Budd JS, Armstrong CP: The correlation between gross appearance at appendix and histological examination. Ann R Coll Surg Edinb 70:395, 1988

38. Blair PM, Bugis PS, Turner LJ, et al: Review of the pathologic diagnosis of 2,216 appendectomy specimens. Am J Surg 165:618, 1993

39. Dahlstom JE, MacArthur EB: *Enterobius vermicularis:* a possible cause of symptoms resembling appendicitis. Aust NZ J Surg 64:692, 1994

40. Pearl RH, Hale DA, Molloy M, et al: Pediatric appendectomy. J Pediatr Surg 30:173, 1995

41. Truji M, Puri P, Reen DJ: Characterization of the local inflammatory response in appendicitis. J Pediatr Gastroenterol Nutr 16:43, 1993

42. Wang Y, Reen DJ, Puri P: Is a histologically normal appendix following emergency appendicectomy always normal? Lancet 347:1076, 1996

43. Grunewald B, Keating J: Should the 'normal' appendix be removed at operation for appendicitis? J R Coll Surg Edinb 38:158, 1993

44. Collins DC: 71,000 human appendix specimens: a final report, summarizing 40 years' study. Am J Proctol 14:265, 1963

45. Chan W, Fu KH: Value of routine histopathological examination of appendices in Hong Kong. J Clin Pathol 40:429, 1987

46. Lenriot JP, Hugier M: Adenocarcinoma of the appendix. Am J Surg 155:470, 1988

47. Gupta SC, Gupta AK, Keswani NK, et al: Pathology of tropical appendicitis. J Clin Pathol 42:1169, 1989

48. Thomas RM, Sobin LH: Gastrointestinal cancer. Cancer 75:154, 1995

49. Modlin IM, Sandor A: An analysis of 8305 cases of carcinoid tumors. Cancer 79:813, 1997

50. Moertel CG, Weiland LH, Nagorney DM, et al: Carcinoid tumor of the appendix: treatment and prognosis. N Engl J Med 317:1699, 1987

51. Gouzi JL, Laigneau P, Delalande JP, et al: Indications for right hemicolectomy in carcinoid tumors of the appendix. Surg Gynecol Obstet 176:543, 1993

52. Nitecki SS, Wolff BG, Schlinkert R, et al: The natural history of surgically treated primary adenocarcinoma of the appendix. Ann Surg 219:51, 1994

53. Yang SS, Gibson P, McCaughey RS, et al: Primary Crohn's disease of the appendix. Ann Surg 189:334, 1979

54. Jahadi MR, Shaw ML: The pathology of the appendix in ulcerative colitis. Dis Colon Rectum 19:345, 1976

55. Ruiz V, Unger SW, Morgan J, et al: Crohn's disease of the appendix. Surgery 107:113, 1990

56. Goldblum JR, Appelman HD: Appendiceal involvement in ulcerative colitis. Mod Pathol 5:607, 1992

Acknowledgments

Figures 1 through 8   Tom Moore.
Figures 9 and 10   Marcia Kammerer.

25 STOMAL CARE

M. Joyce Rosenthal, R.N., M.S., C.E.T.N., and Daniel Rosenthal, M.D., F.A.C.S.

Approach to Perioperative Stomal Care

Preoperative Counseling

Once a surgeon decides that the creation of a stoma is essential to the cure or alleviation of a patient's disease, the next task is to convince the patient that the cure is not worse than the disease. It must be emphasized to the patient that although the stoma will be an inconvenience, the chances are excellent that he or she will 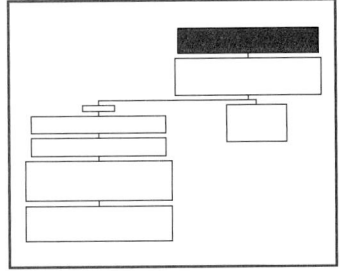 go on to live a fruitful life after recovery from operation. Elderly patients or patients with an advanced stage of cancer may not be as receptive to these words of comfort as a younger or healthier patient would be. In such instances, strong emotional support from the entire health care team and from the patient's family is crucial.

Certain specific topics should always be discussed with the patient preoperatively:

1. The procedure itself. The normal intestinal anatomy, the patient's specific disease process, and the planned rerouting of the bowel should be outlined with the help of simple sketches or preprinted diagrams. Common complications associated with the intended operation should be candidly reviewed. Whether the stoma will be temporary or permanent and whether a pouch will have to be worn at all times should also be discussed. Finally, there should be a brief discussion addressing how long the operation is likely to take; what the postoperative recovery room routine will be; when the patient is likely to be able to return to the hospital room; how the nasogastric tube and the urinary catheter are used and how long they are likely to be needed; how soon after the operation the family will be able to visit the patient; and how soon after the operation the patient will be able to eat. These points have no bearing on the actual procedure, but addressing them instills in the patient and the family some sense of participation in the event and provides some answers they can use when questioned by relatives or friends. Such discussion may seem trivial to the surgeon, but it is of great importance for bolstering patient and family morale.

2. Stoma appliances. The stoma appliances currently available should be described to the patient, with special emphasis placed on their inconspicuousness and ability to contain odor completely. An easy-to-use pouch (probably a one-piece appliance) should be selected and shown to the patient and the family, who should be told that in the postoperative period they will receive detailed instruction in its use. The patient should also be made aware that at some future date, whether because of a change in body habitus or out of a desire to try another type of

appliance more suitable to a particular lifestyle, he or she may switch to another pouch system. If time permits, the pouch may be worn before the procedure to yield a better idea of the suitability of the stoma site.

3. Bathing and showering. Soap and water do not hurt a stoma: ostomates can bathe or shower, with or without their pouch, as often as they wish. If circumstances permit and the patient is physically able, he or she should take a shower in the hospital after the operation with the pouch off, then reapply the pouch just as would be the routine at home. In so doing, the patient gains confidence in his or her ability to return to normal daily activities. Good hygiene is crucial to the care of the peristomal skin. Soaps with creams or oils may prevent the pouch from adhering properly and thus should not be used in the peristomal area. Often, patients want to use strong lye-based or antimicrobial soaps to sterilize the peristomal skin. This practice should be discouraged because such soaps may cause local irritation and alter the normal skin flora. The use of alcohol to clean the peristomal skin should also be discouraged.

4. Employment and physical activities. Once patients have recovered from their operation, they can generally go back to their former occupations with few or no physical limitations; however, heavy lifting or straining should be avoided because the presence of a stoma predisposes to the development of a peristomal hernia.

5. Diet. After the operation, the patient should be fed in the same manner as any other patient who has undergone a major GI operation (whether conventionally or laparoscopically performed), progressing from sips of water to clear liquids to full liquids and then to a soft, low-roughage, low-fat diet. Moving directly to a regular diet after a full-liquid diet often results in premature exposure to high-fat, gas-forming, high-roughage items. Very often, new ostomates cannot tolerate such a diet and may start vomiting or experience ileus.

In our practice, the Dietary Department is involved in coordinating the foods offered after the patient has shown the ability to tolerate a fluid diet. An "ostomy diet" order on the chart alerts the dietitian to the presence of a newly created stoma, which necessitates adjustments to the patient's diet. An ostomy diet should include three small meals supplemented by between-meal snacks. A soft or regular diet should be changed to a low-residue, low-fat, and low-lactose diet for about 2 days. Snacks should be offered at midmorning, midafternoon, and bedtime. Provided that the hospital course has been uneventful, a sample menu for postoperative day 1 might be as follows:

- Breakfast: orange juice, cream of wheat, scrambled egg, white toast, and coffee, tea, or water.

Approach to Perioperative Stomal Care

Stoma with external pouch

In operating room

Mature the stoma and apply disposable pouch, allowing for 3 mm postoperative swelling. If necessary, trim adhesive area to avoid drains or retention sutures. Support loop colostomy with bridge (e.g., segment of No. 16 rubber catheter with ends folded) inside stoma pouch. If opening of digestive stoma is delayed, cover exteriorized bowel segment with petrolatum gauze and sterile dressing.

First postoperative day

Do not change pouch if it is not leaking and stoma color is good. If stoma color cannot be determined, remove pouch, gently wipe off stoma with wet gauze, and inspect. If stoma appears healthy, apply new disposable pouch.

Start involving patient's family in care. If patient is alert, begin teaching process.

Subsequent days

48 hr after operation: Remove entire pouch system, and clean peristomal skin. Select and apply long-term pouch system. Demonstrate working of clamp or spigot, and gradually increase patient involvement.

- Digestive stoma: During next 48 to 72 hr, whenever pouch is one half to two thirds full, remove clamp, empty pouch, and rinse, using water-filled bulb syringe.
- Urinary stoma: Once a day, rinse pouch through spigot with 20 to 30 ml vinegar; reconnect to drainage.

Change pouch system every other day (unless leakage occurs): carefully detach portion adhering to abdomen with help of moist gauze or washcloth, and gently wipe stoma and peristomal skin clean.

Teach patient to fit adhesive wafer snugly around stoma, connect wafer and pouch, and position appliance over stoma and to recognize potential local skin problems.

Consider use of nonadhesive reusable pouch system (VPI).

In preparation for discharge from hospital

If necessary, ensure assistance of relative, friend, or social worker. Advise patient and caretaker of available social and medical support systems.

Patient or caretaker should be familiar with one type of pouch system, including the following:
- Emptying pouch and cleansing closure tail
- Detaching adhesive portion of pouch
- Caring for peristomal skin
- Measuring stoma and cutting hole of correct size in adhesive portion of pouch
- Applying pouch
- Recognizing, preventing, and correcting peristomal skin problems

Early postoperative skin problems include allergic contact dermatitis, folliculitis, and irritant dermatitis; problems that may arise later include radiation reactions, parastomal abscesses and ulcers, pseudoepithelial hyperplasia, and pyoderma gangrenosum.

Do not change pouch as long as wafer is securely fixed to and protecting peristomal skin. Wearing time generally ranges from 3 to 6 days; if patient has problems, consult enterostomal therapist and consider changing systems.

Counsel patient and family preoperatively

Discuss:
- Procedure itself
- Stoma appliances
- Bathing and showering

- Employment and physical activities
- Diet

- Sports and travel
- Sexual activity
- Reproduction and pregnancy

- Availability of home health care and financial support
- Importance of family support system
- Ostomate Bill of Rights

Enlist services of enterostomal therapist and trained ostomy visitor.
For emergency procedures, explain briefly and clearly what a stoma is and why its creation may be unavoidable.

Select and mark stoma site

Site must be visible to the patient and surrounded by a radius of 5 cm of flat, unencumbered skin; flexing thigh, standing, sitting, or lying should not interfere. Avoid iliac crest, costal margins, umbilicus, symphysis pubis, and folds, grooves, or scars in skin.
Proper sites tend to fall in right or left lower quadrant, below beltline, over body of rectus muscle, and 5 cm lateral to and below umbilicus.

Special considerations in site selection:
- Transverse colostomy or continent stoma
- Multiple stomas

- Abdominal shape in obese patient, newborn, or infant; unusual lower abdominal skin folds; abdominal scars

- Handicaps and prostheses
- Anticipated need for or history of radiation therapy
- Laparoscopic creation of a stoma

To mark stoma site, the preferred technique is intradermal injection of methylene blue. Superficial scratch marks are sometimes used.

Continent stoma (Kock pouch)

Intubate with No. 30 Silastic catheter.
Mark correct position of tube with silk tie at stomal level.
Affix tube securely to skin. Leave in place for 10 days, and allow intestinal pouch to empty by gravity.
Irrigate tube with 30 ml normal saline q. 6 hr.

10 days after operation: Teach patient to extubate and intubate intestinal pouch. Do not keep tube out of pouch for > 30 min at a time.

4 wk after operation: Have patient extubate and reintubate stoma at gradually increasing intervals.

609

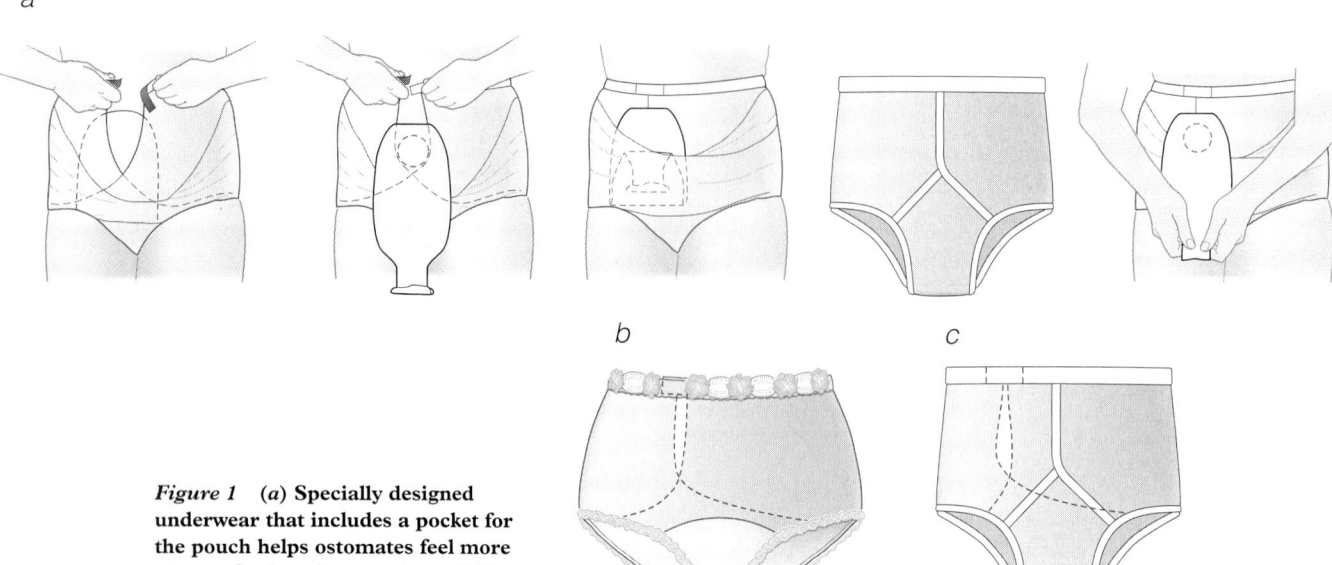

Figure 1 (*a*) **Specially designed underwear that includes a pocket for the pouch helps ostomates feel more at ease. Such underwear is available in female (*b*) and male (*c*) versions.**

• Lunch: baked chicken, mashed potatoes, boiled carrots, roll, and coffee, tea, or water.
• Dinner: turkey, cup of soup, canned fruit, and coffee, tea, or water.
• Snacks: midmorning, crackers and canned fruit; midafternoon, vanilla wafers with juice; and bedtime, low-fat flavored yogurt with tea or coffee.

Specific instructions are needed for the first week or two at home as more roughage and fats are introduced into the diet. Any lactose-intolerance problems should also be taken into account as milk products are slowly reintroduced into the diet. Patients with an ileostomy should have more fluids in their diet to make up for increased stomal water loss. Patients with cardiac or renal disease should be closely monitored by their physicians so that fluid overload may be prevented.

A sample menu plan for week 1 at home might be as follows:

• Breakfast: orange juice, cream of wheat, toast with jam, and milk, coffee, or tea.
• Lunch: pureed soup, turkey sandwich with reduced mayonnaise, canned fruit, and milk, coffee, or tea.
• Dinner: tomato juice; boneless, skinless chicken breast; white rice; cooked carrots; roll with margarine; and coffee or tea.
• Snacks: midmorning, half a banana and four or five graham crackers with water or juice; midafternoon, applesauce and three or four vanilla wafers with water or juice; and bedtime, low-fat flavored yogurt with milk, coffee, or tea.

Beyond the postoperative period, the diet of an ostomate, except for whatever individual modifications are necessary, can be relatively unrestricted. Overall, there is no specific ostomy diet. Any dietary restrictions adhered to are generally voluntary, and their main purpose is the prevention and relief of gas, diarrhea, constipation, or unusual odor. If any of these problems persist for more than 24 hours, the patient should notify a physician. Most difficulties can be averted if patients follow a few simple instructions, which should be emphasized to the patient before discharge:

• Avoid foods that were troublesome preoperatively. (Often, patients know which foods do not agree with them.)
• Chew foods well to break down bulk and fiber. (Failure to chew adequately may lead to stomal obstruction.)
• Eat slowly to minimize swallowing of air. (Eating fast may also result in stomal obstruction.)
• For the first few weeks after operation, avoid high-residue foods, such as fresh fruits and vegetables and whole-grain breads and cereals.
• About 6 weeks after operation, reintroduce high-residue foods into the diet, one at a time. If any food causes problems, try it again at a later date.
• If you have diarrhea, do not restrict fluid intake; instead, drink beverages that contain salt, such as Gatorade or bouillon.
• Keep well hydrated: drink four to six extra glasses of fluid a day.
• If you wish to drink alcoholic beverages, practice moderation.

Some patients with ileostomies tend to pass enteric-coated tablets or time-release capsules before the medication can be absorbed. In such cases, these products should be avoided. If a liquid form of the medication is available, it should be given instead; alternatively, a similar product that is available as a liquid may be substituted.

6. Sports and travel. Contact sports may injure the stoma and should therefore be avoided. Otherwise, ostomates may enjoy a wide range of sports activities, including swimming, as their general state of health allows. They need not avoid Jacuzzis or hot tubs, and they pose no health threat to themselves or to others if they use community pools. Any fears of possible pouch leakage may be allayed by "picture-framing" the stoma appliance with waterproof tape (i.e., placing tape on all four sides of the wafer).

Ostomates should feel free to travel, although they should be careful not to place all of their stoma supplies in their checked luggage when traveling by air. In areas where it is not safe to drink the water, they should use bottled water to irrigate their colostomies.

7. Sexual activity. Sexual activity will be a paramount consideration to some future ostomates, although probably not to all.

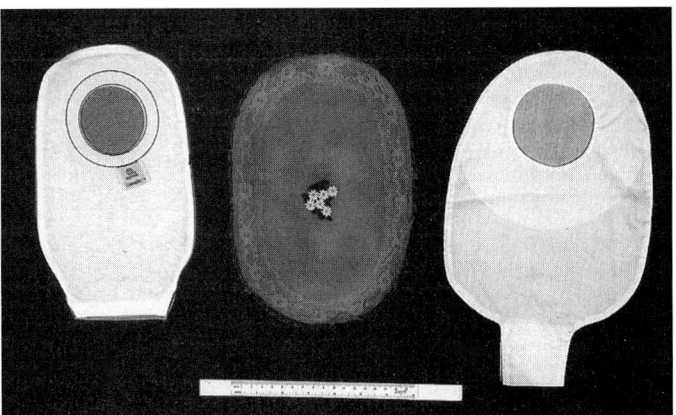

Figure 2 **Shown are three different pouch covers: a commercially available cover (ConvaTec), a lace cover, and a plain handmade cover.**

This matter is of such importance that it should be candidly discussed not only in the preoperative period but during follow-up visits as well. The surgeon should not hesitate to offer any patient the opportunity to voice his or her concerns about this matter. Male patients should be made aware that the amount of erectile or ejaculatory dysfunction that occurs after pelvic surgery or the removal of the rectum is related to the extent of the pelvic dissection necessary to eradicate the disease as well as to the degree of sexual vigor present before operation. Those male patients who are interested in having children may be advised to bank their sperm for future use; a certain number of patients will have permanent ejaculatory dysfunction in spite of the most careful pelvic surgery.[1] Female patients should be told that loss of the rectum and the presence of a stoma do not preclude sexual activity, even though dyspareunia, increased vaginal discharge, and altered orgasmic response are common complications of total rectal excision in women.[2-4] The use of specially designed underwear [*see Figure 1*] or pouch covers [*see Figure 2*] may help patients feel more at ease with their sexuality by enhancing the feeling of normality during intimacy.

8. Reproduction and pregnancy. Women in their reproductive years should be reassured that a stoma is not incompatible with pregnancy and that many female ostomates do in fact become pregnant and undergo normal vaginal delivery. For pregnant women who have an ileal pouch after a proctocolectomy for inflammatory bowel disease, cesarean section may be preferable to vaginal delivery at term, given that anal sphincter damage would be catastrophic in their case. Pregnant women undergoing stoma surgery for Crohn disease should be made aware that recurrent disease and some of the medications required to treat such recurrence may be detrimental to the fetus.[5] As a rule, a pregnant woman undergoing an ostomy procedure should be managed exactly as a nonpregnant woman would be. Major reconstructive procedures, however, should probably be deferred until after delivery. Closer to term, uterine enlargement may preclude even a conventional proctectomy, in which case a staged operation that spares the rectum is appropriate.[6] In our practice, we have seen 11 cases in which pregnant ostomates came to term with normal babies. A few were followed for the entire 9 months of gestation, whereas others were seen only during the last month or two for support and reassurance. We have seen both vaginal deliveries and cesarean sections in patients with ileostomies, colostomies, or ileal conduits; however,

we have not been involved in the care of any pregnant patients with Kock or J ileal pouches. One women who had undergone a total colectomy and an ileostomy for Crohn disease and who had a vaginal fistula became pregnant and gave birth to a normal baby girl via cesarean section. These women are some of the best ostomy visitors we know of—living proof that life goes on despite a stoma.

9. Home health care needs. After an ostomy, some patients may require additional nursing care at home or a period of recuperation in a convalescent center.

10. Financial support. The expense of stoma equipment, along with that of home health care needs, may place a heavy financial burden on patients and their families. Surgeons should anticipate such problems preoperatively and should not hesitate to inquire into patients' insurance coverage. Patients who are 65 years of age or older should be made aware that Medicare covers, to some extent, posthospital nursing care facilities, home health care, and stoma appliance expenses. Because Medicare and Medicaid benefits and deductible expenses tend to vary annually, medical personnel may wish to update their knowledge by obtaining new schedules of Medicare and Medicaid benefits. Handbooks listing Medicare Part B benefits are reviewed annually and are available at Medicare state headquarters; their locations can be obtained by calling 800-442-2620. Pamphlets describing Medicaid benefits can be obtained by calling the individual state's department of human services. The help of a hospital social worker familiar with these problems is frequently invaluable. Retired military personnel and military dependents who are not eligible for Medicare or Medicaid should consult an adviser from the Civilian Help and Medical Program of the Uniformed Services (CHAMPUS) to determine the extent of the benefits available to them.

11. Family support system. It is vital that the surgeon keep a relative or friend of the patient informed of the upcoming operation and its consequences. Well-informed relatives who are involved in the patient's care and demonstrate by words and deeds that they will continue to offer love and concern, regardless of the outcome of the procedure, can exert a positive influence on the patient's recovery.

12. The Ostomate Bill of Rights. According to this manifesto, developed by the United Ostomy Association (UOA), the ostomate shall have the following:

- Preoperative counseling.
- An appropriately positioned stoma site.
- A well-constructed stoma.
- Skilled postoperative nursing care.
- Emotional support.
- Individual instruction.
- Information on the availability of supplies.
- Information on community resources.
- Posthospital follow-up and lifelong supervision.
- Team efforts of health care professionals.

The process of counseling can be greatly aided by the publications for patients available from the UOA [*see Table 1*], 19772 MacArthur Boulevard, Suite 200, Irvine, CA 92612-2405 (800-826-0826; http://www.uoa.org; e-mail uoa@deltanet.com); Crohn's and Colitis Foundation of America, Inc., 386 Park Avenue South, New York, NY 10016-8804 (800-932-2423; http://www.ccfa.org; e-mail info@ccfa.org); and the Wound, Ostomy and Continence Nurses Society, 1550 South Coast Highway, Suite 201, Laguna Beach, CA 92651 (888-224-WOCN [9626]; http://www.wocn.org; e-mail maria@wocn.org).

<table>
<tr><td>

Table 1   Selected Publications for Patients, Available from the United Ostomy Association

The Ostomy Handbook
Colostomies: A Guide
Transverse Colostomies: A Guide
Ileostomy: A Guide
The Continent Ileostomy
Urostomy: A Guide
My Child Has an Ostomy
All about Jimmy and His Friend
Sex and the Female Ostomate
Sex and the Male Ostomate
Sex, Courtship, and the Single Ostomate
Pregnancy and the Woman with an Ostomy
Employment of the Ostomate
Handicapped Ostomate

</td></tr>
</table>

CONSULTING AN ENTEROSTOMAL THERAPIST

Before operation, the surgeon may wish to consult an enterostomal therapy (ET) nurse. (In the United States, most enterostomal therapists are registered nurses; however, there are a few very able ones who are not.) By training and experience, ET nurses are ideally suited to the physical and emotional preparation of ostomy candidates for surgery. Reassurance aimed at dispelling any lingering apprehensions about the upcoming operation often allows the ET nurse to establish a good rapport with the patient and his or her family. To alleviate the patient's fears further, the ET nurse may display a sample pouch, which can even be worn by the candidate if desired. The ET nurse can also explain how one cares for the pouch and how one lives comfortably wearing it, provided that the patient is able and willing to assimilate this information. The patient should be assured that he or she will be taught how to take care of the stoma before leaving the hospital. This point should be reinforced by telling the patient that the ET nurse will be caring for the patient's stoma and the peristomal skin after the operation and will be slowly teaching the patient and any other personal care provider how to provide this care.

If the patient is not opposed, the ET nurse may bring in a well-adjusted ostomate of the same gender as the patient, preferably a trained ostomy visitor. This approach can reassure the patient considerably, especially if the visitor appears self-confident, is well dressed, and is about the same age as the patient. It is helpful, but not necessary, for the visitor to have the same type of stoma as the patient. Ostomy visitors are usually quite eager to help; they can generally be contacted through the local chapters of the UOA or the American Cancer Society. Local telephone directories list numbers for both agencies. In communities where no local chapters are present, the location of the nearest facility can be obtained by calling the national headquarters of either organization. The headquarters of the American Cancer Society is located at 1599 Clifton Road N.E., Atlanta, GA 30329 (800-ACS[227]-2345; http://www.cancer.org).

EMERGENCY COUNSELING

When creation of an intestinal stoma is being planned or considered under emergency conditions, the time available for counseling may be short. This time is best used in briefly but clearly explaining to the patient and the family what a stoma is and why its creation may be unavoidable in this case. Emergency stomas must be constructed according to the same basic principles of stoma construction that govern nonemergency stomas.

Preoperative Selection and Marking of the Stoma Site

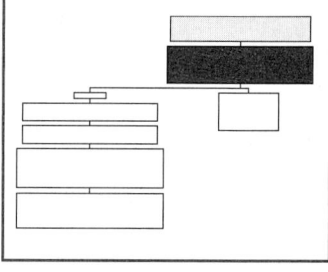

The selection and marking of the stoma site directly affect the likelihood of complications associated with the creation of the stoma.[7,8] Proper location of a stoma can mean the difference between an active, independent life and one of social isolation. Poorly placed stomas are hard to pouch and tend to leak. Accidental pouch leaks are a nuisance and a source of considerable embarrassment to ostomates. Many, in fact, avoid social contacts out of fear of such accidents.

GENERAL CONSIDERATIONS FOR SITE SELECTION

There are several general considerations for site selection that the surgeon must take into account. Proper placement of the stoma may prevent parastomal hernia, prolapse, and leakage (which can lead to skin problems and consequent patient anxiety). Stomas should be placed away from the iliac crest, the costal margins, the umbilicus, the symphysis pubis, and any folds, grooves, or scars in the skin [*see Figure 3*]. There must be a radius of about 5 cm of flat, unencumbered skin around the stoma site if an appliance is to fit well. Flexing the ipsilateral thigh should not interfere with the wearing of the appliance. The stoma site should also be visible to the patient and, ideally, should not interfere with the beltline. If the stoma site is to be placed above the beltline, care should be taken to ensure that pendulous breasts are not hanging over it. In this situation, not only would the patient find it difficult to see the stoma, but the weight of the breast would apply pressure on the appliance wafer, causing it to loosen and thus resulting in leakage.

Because the shape of the abdomen tends to change as an individual stands, sits, or lies down, it is imperative that the stoma site selected be suitable for the wearing of an appliance in all three positions—

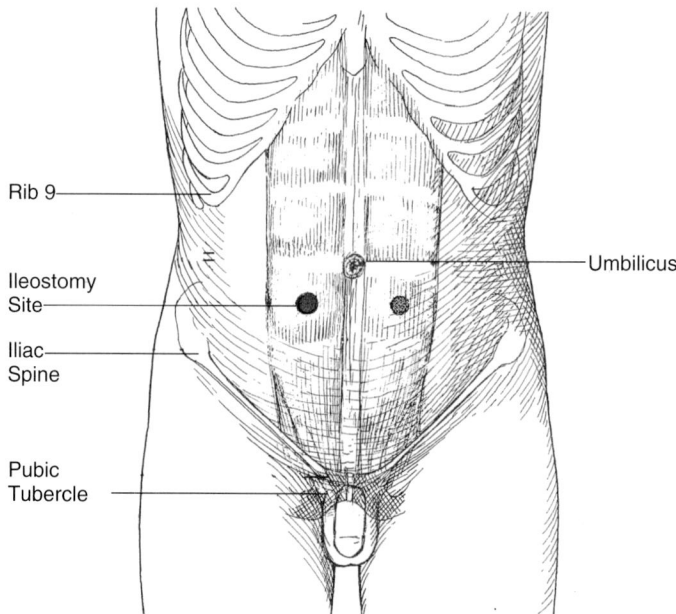

Figure 3   **Shown is a stoma site selected for a conventional ileostomy. A site located in the same spot on the left side of the abdomen would be ideally suited for a sigmoid colostomy.**

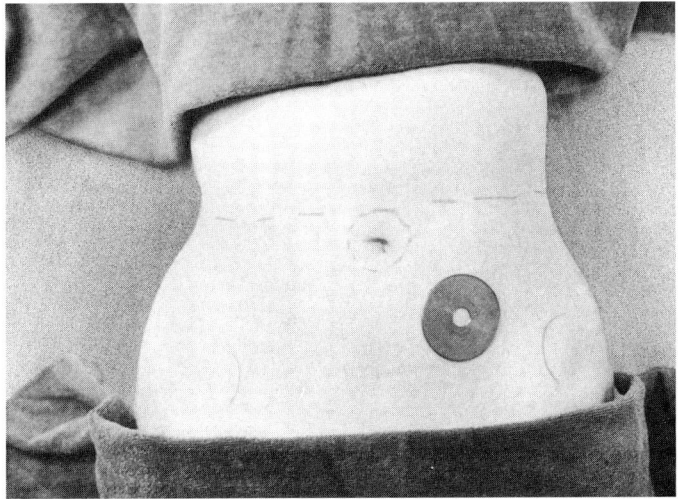

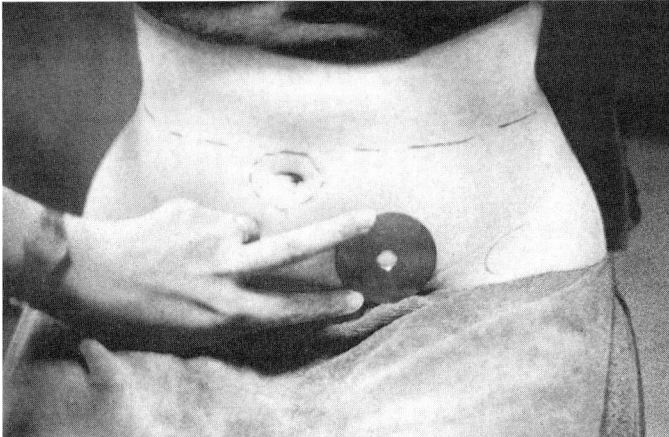

Figure 4 **A 5 cm marking disk is used to select the proper stoma site with the patient lying down (*above*) and sitting up (*below*).**

especially the sitting position, because it is sitting that brings about the greatest changes in abdominal contours. Often, a lower stoma site is selected so that the patient can wear the beltline low; however, a low site may lead to kinks in the appliance when the patient sits, which could result in overfilling of the upper part of the appliance. The use of a skin barrier wafer or a marking disk [*see Figure 4*] is invaluable for determining the adequacy of the stoma site selection.

The right and left lower quadrants of the abdomen are still the most common locations for digestive and urinary stomas. Properly selected stoma sites in these areas tend to fall below the beltline, over the body of the rectus muscle, about 5 cm lateral to and below the umbilicus. In our experience, creation of the stoma through the rectus sheath and muscle is associated with a lower incidence of peristomal hernia.

SPECIAL CONSIDERATIONS FOR SITE SELECTION

Besides these general considerations, the surgeon must also take into account five special considerations: (1) the type of stoma to be created, (2) whether more than one stoma is to be constructed, (3) the shape of the patient's abdomen, (4) whether the patient is handicapped or wears special prosthetic equipment, and (5) whether future radiation therapy to the abdomen is likely to be necessary.

Type of Stoma

In transverse colostomies, the stoma is generally placed in the right

or left upper quadrant of the abdomen, away from the costal margins and the umbilicus. It should also be brought through the rectus sheath and muscle [*see Figure 5*] to minimize the chances of peristomal herniation. Transverse loop colostomies have a tendency to prolapse, particularly if they are created close to the hepatic flexure.

Because with a continent stoma (e.g., Kock pouch or reservoir) there is no need to wear an external pouch, the stoma can be created below the bikini line, in an inconspicuous yet accessible and visible area of the abdomen. A location about 2.5 cm above the pubic hairline over the right rectus sheath area is generally a suitable site.

Multiple Stomas

Unless there is no alternative, two functioning stomas should not be placed on the same side of the abdomen. To do so would greatly reduce the area of peristomal skin available for affixing the appliances and would complicate the emptying of the individual pouches. In addition, the weight of each pouch impinges on the other and makes the wearing of a belt very difficult for the patient. If both a urinary stoma and a digestive stoma are to be created, the stoma that is more likely to necessitate the use of a belt (i.e., the urinary stoma) should be placed somewhat higher than the other. If both stomas were placed at the same level, a belt would interfere with the second one.

Abdominal Shape

A patient must be able to see a stoma to be able to care for it [*see Figure 6*]. As a rule, therefore, a stoma cannot be placed over the lower abdomen in obese patients or patients with unusual lower abdominal skin folds [*see Figure 7*]. The deep skin creases associated with obesity also render the lower abdomen unsuitable for the placement of an appliance. In such patients, the stoma should be placed higher on the abdomen (generally above the belt line), brought through the rectus muscle, and located where it is visible and can easily be pouched [*see Figure 8*]. In a patient with a distended abdomen, the stoma site chosen should be where the stoma is to sit once the abdomen has regained its normal contour.

The general principles of stoma site selection on the abdomen apply to newborns and infants. Because their abdominal walls are more rounded and their hips are usually flexed, however, their abdominal stomas should be placed somewhat higher than is usual in adults. A diaper should not be used instead of a pouch to contain bowel efflux or urine. Many companies make stoma pouches specif-

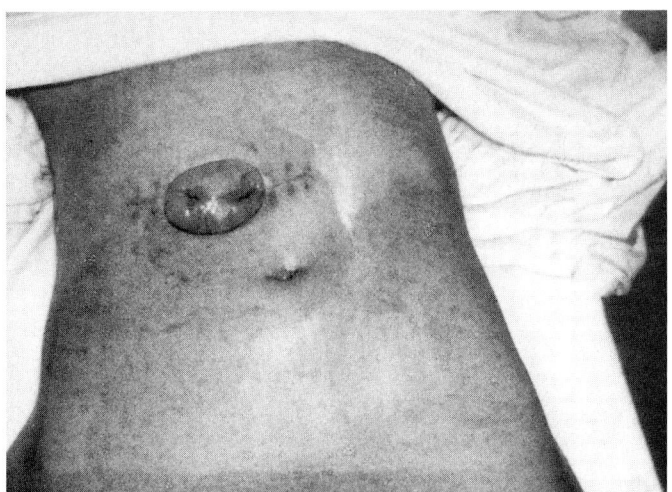

Figure 5 **Shown is a properly placed loop colostomy in the right upper quadrant.**

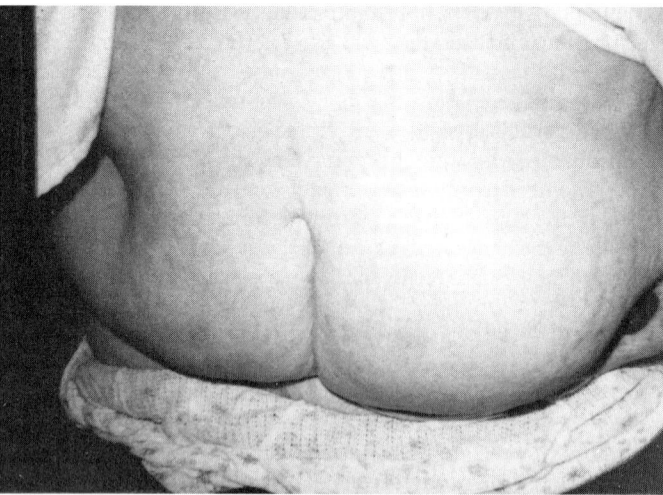

Figure 6 This poorly placed stoma is in a deep skin fold, on top of the iliac crest; it is invisible to the patient.

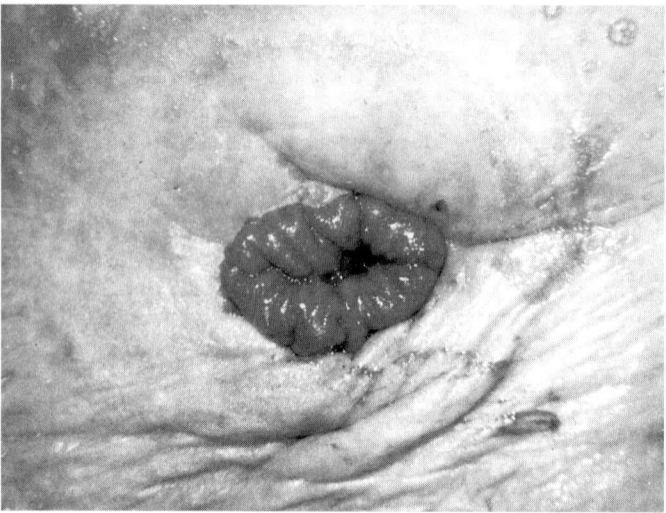

Figure 7 These multiple skin folds make the use of a leakproof pouch system very difficult.

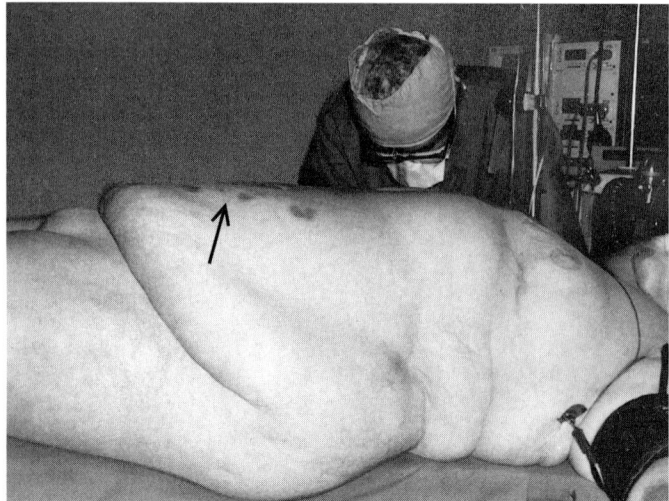

Figure 8 In this massively obese patient about to undergo an abdominoperineal proctectomy, the colostomy site selected (black dot) is above the belt line. The arrow points to the umbilicus.

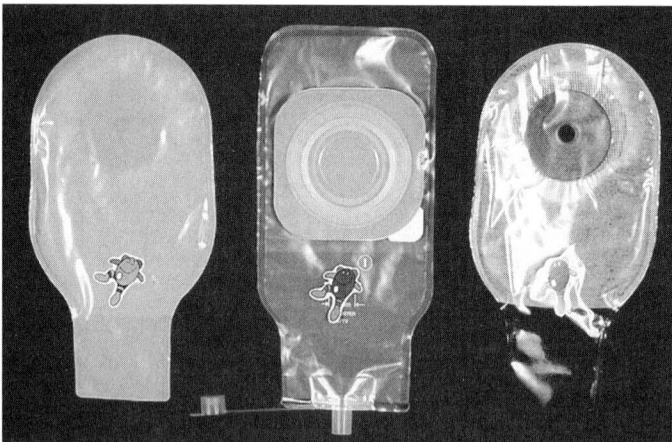

Figure 9 Shown are three pouches that are suitable for infant and newborn ostomates: a one-piece opaque pouch, a two-piece urinary pouch, and a one-piece clear infant pouch (Hollister).

ically for infants and newborns. These pouches not only are smaller but also have skin barriers that are gentler to and safer for newborns' skin [*see Figure 9*].

If the creation of a stoma in the vicinity of a scar is unavoidable, use of easily molded paste or wafers made of pectin, gelatin, and cellulose (e.g., Stomahesive or Hollihesive) can minimize, to some extent, the fitting problems such skin irregularities present.

Stomas for Handicapped Patients

In patients who wear orthopedic braces, are confined to wheelchairs, or are restricted by other handicaps, the stoma may have to be placed in an unconventional location. A surgeon must select a stoma site for such a patient with particular care, taking into consideration both the patient's infirmity and the position in which the patient plans to be when caring for the stoma. Accordingly, it may be advisable to choose the stoma site with the patient sitting in a wheelchair or wearing braces.

Often, with bedridden patients, the surgeon does not select a specific stoma site preoperatively. This is a mistake: when the patient is repositioned, especially into a sitting position, an appliance covering a stoma that was placed in a skin fold or a deep crease, too close to a scar, under a sagging breast, or too close to a feeding tube will tend to loosen and spill its contents. To minimize such problems, the surgeon need only spend a few minutes looking at the patient lying in bed in the usual position and then examine the abdomen for scars, deep folds, feeding tube sites, and other physical features that might impinge on the stoma. This simple step will save the surgeon many calls asking for a revision or a relocation of the stoma.

Stomas and Radiation Therapy

When it is anticipated that radiation therapy through lower abdominal portals will be necessary after operation, the stoma site should be located outside the radiation field, if possible.

When a patient has already undergone irradiation, the stoma should be placed outside the treated area to prevent skin breakdown and delayed healing.

MARKING THE STOMA SITE

It is essential that skin marks placed at the selected stoma site not fade away when the patient showers preoperatively or when his or her abdomen is washed in the operating room. Because truly indelible skin markers are unavailable, the preferred technique for identifying the selected stoma site is intradermal injection of methylene blue. Placement of superficial scratch marks, unless done immediately before operation, can cause local cellulitis that may contribute to postoperative problems with the stoma.

THE LAPAROSCOPICALLY CREATED STOMA

Because the only major difference between laparoscopic and conventional surgery is the access to the operative site,[9] stomal care is, for the most part, the same in patients who have undergone laparoscopic procedures as in those who have undergone open procedures. Creating a stoma laparoscopically involves pulling a segment of intestine through a trocar site and then enlarging the site to deliver the bowel onto the abdomen. Too often, either by necessity or by lack of foresight, the trocar site is not where the stoma site ideally should be. Additional thought must be given to trocar placement when one plans to create a stoma; a good site for the stoma must be selected and marked, even if this means inserting an additional port devoted exclusively to pulling out the stoma. The common practice of enlarging the trocar site by simply incising the adjacent skin is not to be recommended: it causes the stoma to be slit-shaped, with poor projection and a tendency to retract. Instead, the trocar orifice should be enlarged by excising a circular button of skin around the trocar site.

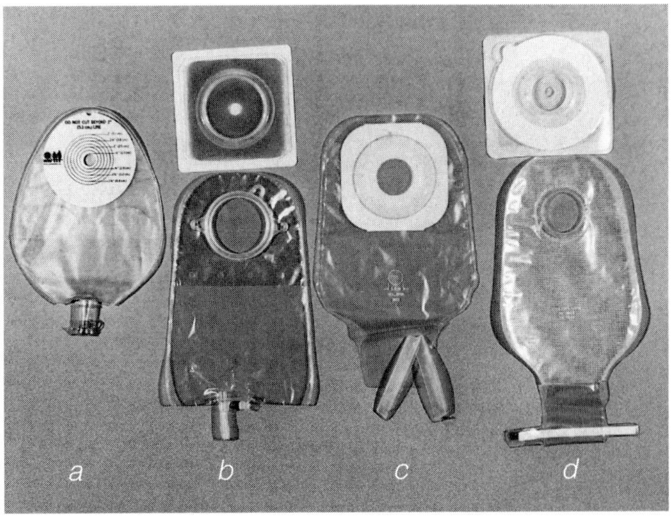

Figure 10 **Four different types of pouch are shown: a one-piece urinary system (United) (*a*), a two-piece urinary system (ConvaTec) (*b*), a one-piece digestive pouch system (Hollister) (*c*), and a two-piece digestive pouch system (Coloplast) (*d*).**

Postoperative Care

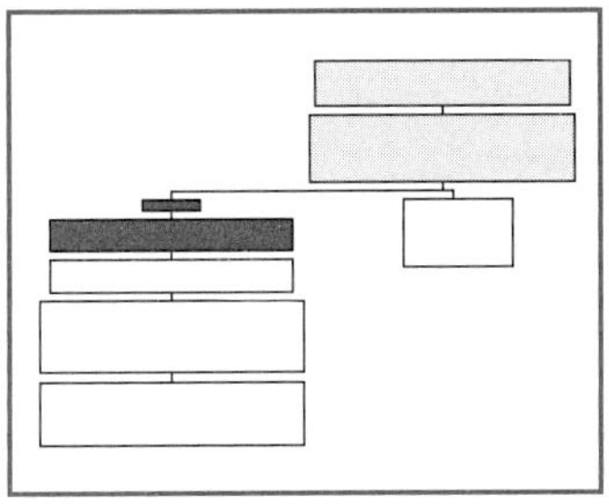

The following discussion is on general principles of stomal care. We do not address care of the various types of stoma separately, because the basic principles governing care are essentially the same for all types, except for some details that will be noted. Care of a continent pouch will be described separately.

IN THE OPERATING ROOM

Provided that the general principles of stoma construction are clearly followed (i.e., that the bowel is brought through the abdominal wall to the skin without tension, is brought through the rectus muscle with a good blood supply, and is everted and sutured primarily to the skin away from the incision, drains, and retention sutures), all electively created stomas, with very few exceptions, are matured and are ready for pouching at the end of the operation. Stomas created under emergency conditions should also be matured. The advantages of maturing the stoma (i.e., the immediate decompression of the bowel and the ease of caring for a matured stoma) far outweigh the disadvantages (i.e., the additional operating time needed to mature the stoma and the theoretical possibility of contaminating the peritoneal cavity with bowel contents). When a surgeon decides to delay the opening of a digestive stoma, the exteriorized bowel segment can simply be covered with a piece of petrolatum gauze and a sterile dressing. The gaseous distention, serositis, and bowel wall edema that eventually develop in such cases often make pouching and caring for these stomas after their opening a challenge.

The pouch used in the operating room should be transparent, drainable, disposable, and of one- or two-piece construction [*see Figure 10*]. A pouch system is available for digestive stomas that is simple and inexpensive yet fully adequate for the purpose. Before applying the pouch, the surgeon should cut a hole in the adhesive backing about 3 mm larger than the stoma to allow for postoperative swelling. Whereas digestive stoma pouches are closed by means of a clamp, urinary stoma pouches are connected to a drainage system.

Once a segment of bowel (i.e., the future stoma) has been exteriorized, the surgeon should exert his or her utmost efforts to avoid impinging on the peristomal skin necessary for securing the appliance. All too often, one sees retention sutures, drains, and feeding catheters placed carelessly in close proximity to a stoma. Such carelessness makes pouching difficult at best and frequently leads to leaks and the attendant skin problems. The problem of insufficient peristomal skin area can be circumvented to some degree by cutting and reshaping the adhesive area; however, this loss of adhesive surface may reduce the stability of the appliance.

Rigid bridges of various designs are available for support of loop colostomies [*see Figure 11*]. These bridges should fit inside the stoma pouch; however, many do not. In addition, if these rigid bridges are sewn to the skin, the pouch opening will not fit adequately around the stoma. The peristomal skin will be bathed by stomal efflux, and the stitch holes create an avenue by which urine or stool can infect the skin. We recommend using a segment of No. 16 rubber catheter with its ends folded [*see Figure 12*]; this will serve the same purpose and can easily be inserted completely into the pouch. If a supporting bridge cannot be accommodated within the pouch, it is difficult

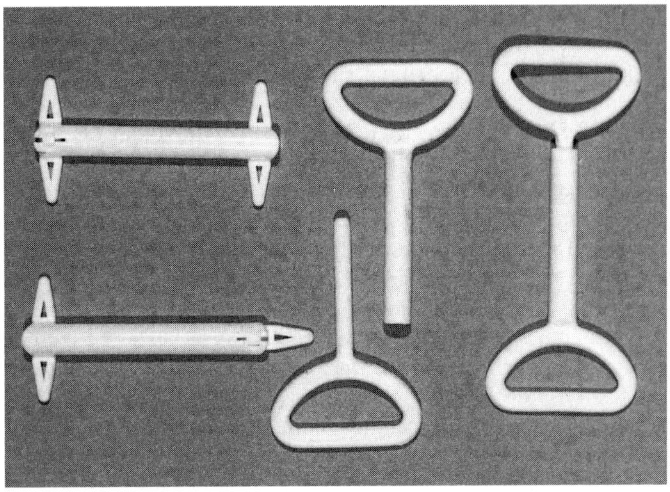

Figure 11 **Rigid colostomy bridges that can fit inside a pouch system are used to support loop colostomies. They come in one- and two-piece forms.**

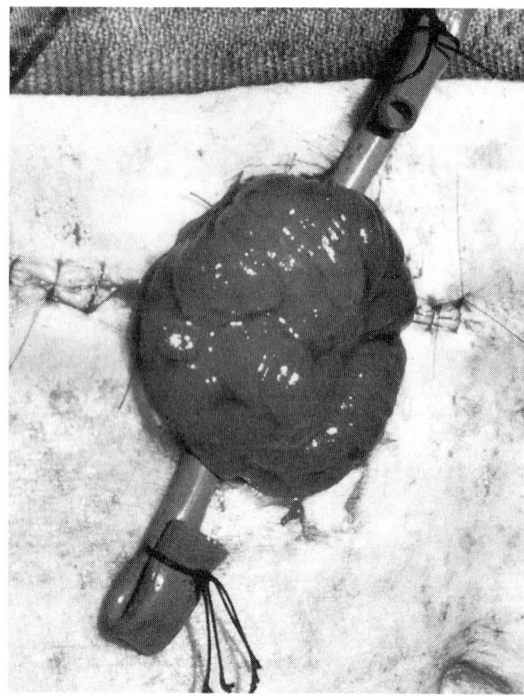
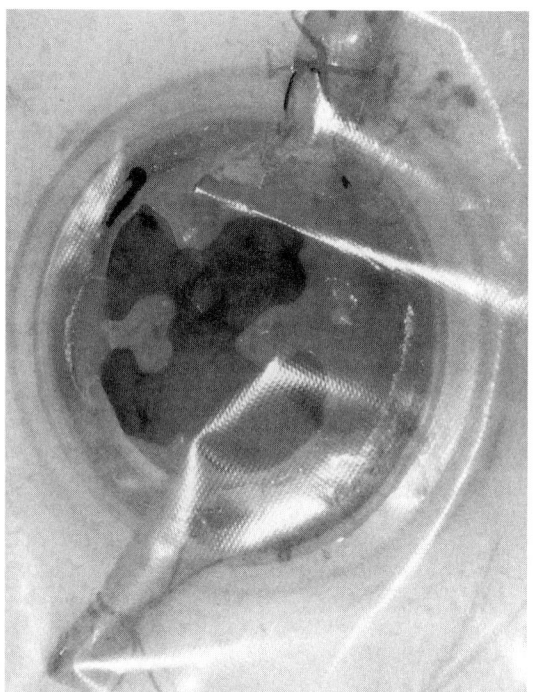

Figure 12 Use of a segment of No. 16 catheter is an easy and practical way to support a loop colostomy (*left*). The rubber bridge shown at left fits into the pouch (*right*).

to make the pouch system leakproof, unless some adhesive paste is used to fill the gap created by the rod between the skin and the adhesive wafer. The bulky plastic rods with rubber tubing that are traditionally used to hold a loop colostomy are out of place in modern stomal care.

FIRST POSTOPERATIVE DAY

If the pouch is not leaking and the stoma color is good, there is little to be gained by changing the pouch. If a stoma is smeared with stool or its color cannot be determined, the pouch should be removed and the stoma gently wiped off with wet gauze and inspected. If the stoma appears to be healthy, a new disposable pouch should be applied; if not, the surgeon should be notified. The patient should be reassured and told that in the next few days he or she will be thoroughly instructed in the care of the stoma. Given the pressure for accelerated discharges imposed by managed care, it is necessary to begin involving the family in the care of the patient on the day after the operation, even if the patient is still somewhat obtunded. If the patient is alert at this time, the ET nurse or the staff nurse can start the postoperative education process by showing the patient how the pouch is changed and doing it for him or her. On the next day, the ET nurse or the staff nurse helps the patient change the pouch, and by the third day (or at least the third teaching session), the patient should be able to change the pouch unassisted under the guidance of the ET nurse or the staff nurse.

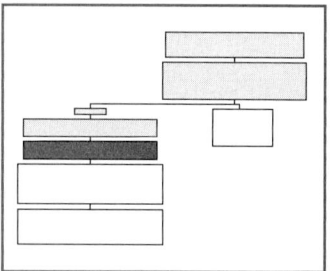

Whereas urinary stomas drain immediately, ileostomies generally begin to function within the first 48 postoperative hours, and colostomies take about twice that long. Stomas created under emergency conditions to relieve bowel obstruction may start to discharge promptly.

SUBSEQUENT DAYS

About 48 hours after operation, the entire pouch system should be removed and the peristomal skin cleaned. If any discoloration, retraction, or mucocutaneous separation is noted or, in a urinary stoma, if any of the stents seem displaced, these problems should be promptly reported to the surgeon. Mucocutaneous separation at the base of the stoma may be caused either by the breaking or untying of the sutures uniting the intestine to the skin or by the sutures having cut through the tissues. If such a separation is noted, one must apply a minimum of pressure at the base of the stoma when pouching to prevent further separation. If the separation is superficial, the area can be covered with a coating of Stomahesive powder. If the separation is wider and deeper, it should be filled with Stomahesive paste to protect the area, keep it moist, and promote granulation. The pouch wafer should cover the filled site to protect the subcutaneous tissue from the stoma efflux.

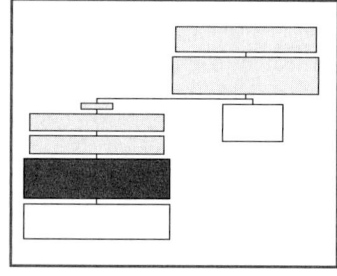

The pouch system with which the patient is to become familiar is then selected. The patient should be shown how the clamp or the spigot at the bottom of the pouch works. If the system is a two-piece one, the pouch and adhesive wafer are connected and then applied over the stoma as a unit, with care taken not to put pressure on the newly created stoma and the sutures fixing it to the skin. The patient should then be invited to place and close the clamp or to connect the spigot to drainage on the newly applied pouch; in this way, he or she is coaxed into looking at the stoma and touching the pouch. Further involvement of the patient in the care of the stoma should progress gradually, under the gentle and patient supervision of a member of the health care team.

During the next 48 to 72 hours, whenever the pouch of a diges-

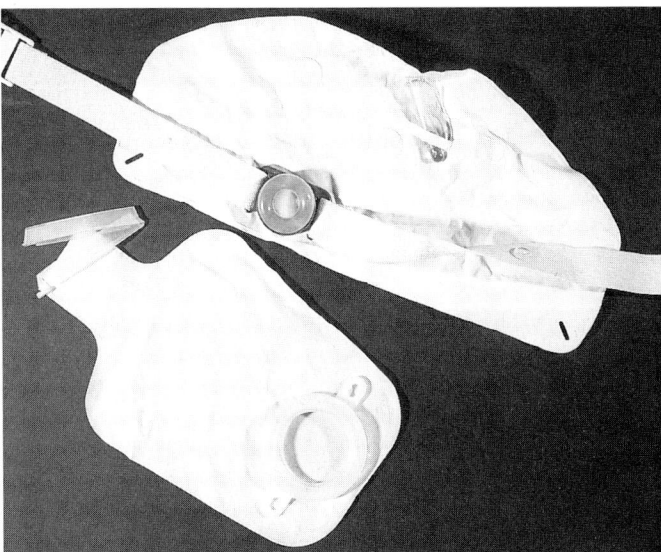

Figure 13 Shown is the VPI nonadhesive pouch system for intestinal and urinary stomas. The urinary appliance is the larger of the two.

tive stoma is one half to two thirds full, the pouch clamp should be removed and the pouch emptied and rinsed out rather than replaced. Rinsing is easily accomplished by means of a bulb syringe filled with tap water. The pouch should not be allowed to fill to the point where its sheer weight pulls it away from the patient's skin.

Once a day, the pouch of a urinary stoma should be rinsed through its spigot with 20 to 30 ml of vinegar to break up mucous plugs and to acidify the pouch wall so as to prevent bacterial proliferation and

the formation of uric acid crystals. The pouch should then be reconnected to drainage.

At this stage, the pouch system should be changed every other day, unless leakage occurs. This schedule allows the staff to teach the patient how to care for the stoma. When the patient's appliance is changed, the portion adhering to the patient's abdomen should be carefully detached with the help of a cloth (either a piece of gauze or a washcloth) moistened with tap water; it should never be pulled off. The stoma and the peristomal skin should then be gently wiped clean with a moist cloth. We do not use permanent appliances that are cemented to the skin in the postoperative period. If such appliances are used, it must be remembered that skin cement solvent rather than water is needed to detach them from the skin. Currently, with the large assortment of disposable pouch systems available, the use of cement and rigid faceplates is seldom, if ever, indicated.

A reusable pouch system (the VPI system) [*see Figure 13*] has been developed that uses no adhesive and consists of a Silastic ring held in place with a belt. This system is favored by patients who have problems with adhesive pouch systems or who wish to change their pouch frequently. In particular, it is attractive to active people and to persons in wheelchairs, who appreciate the large capacity of the pouch and the fact that they can easily and atraumatically change their pouch system frequently. All of the components of the system—the belt, the Silastic ring, and the large-capacity pouch—are reusable and easy to clean and care for.

The patient should learn to measure the stoma with a measuring guide [*see Figure 14*] and cut out a properly sized hole in the appliance wafer so that the edge of the wafer is approximately 3 mm away from the stomal mucosa; this allows for expansion. The wafer and the pouch should be connected and the appliance positioned as one piece over the stoma. The importance of a well-fitting stoma appliance to protect the peristomal skin cannot be overemphasized. The patient should be told about some of the potential local skin problems associated with the type of stoma selected and taught how to recognize them. The instructor must stress that most of these skin problems can be prevented by (1) proper fitting of the pouch system, (2) using the least irritating products at the stoma site, and (3) avoiding physical trauma to the skin in the region around the stoma. When a stoma is being pouched, additional support for the appliance can be provided by use of a belt or by framing the adhesive wafer with adhesive tape. Waterproof Perma Type tape can be used by patients planning to swim.

DISCHARGE OBJECTIVES

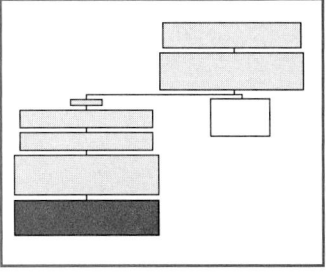

The psychosocial aspects of care discussed earlier [*see* Preoperative Counseling, *above*] should be reemphasized and elaborated on throughout the postoperative period. If the patient did not see or refused to see an ostomy visitor preoperatively, it may be appropriate to ask if he or she wants to see one at this time. If the patient is willing, a relative may learn to help him or her look after the stoma. If infirmity or age prevents a patient from attending to the stoma, a relative or friend must be called in. If relatives and friends are unavailable or are unable or unwilling to help, the services of a social worker must be obtained as soon as possible. In fact, this need for postdischarge assistance should have been anticipated preoperatively, and steps should have been taken to provide the patient with adequate support. Patients and caretakers should be made aware of the social and medical support systems available to them [*see Table 2*]. Either the surgeon or

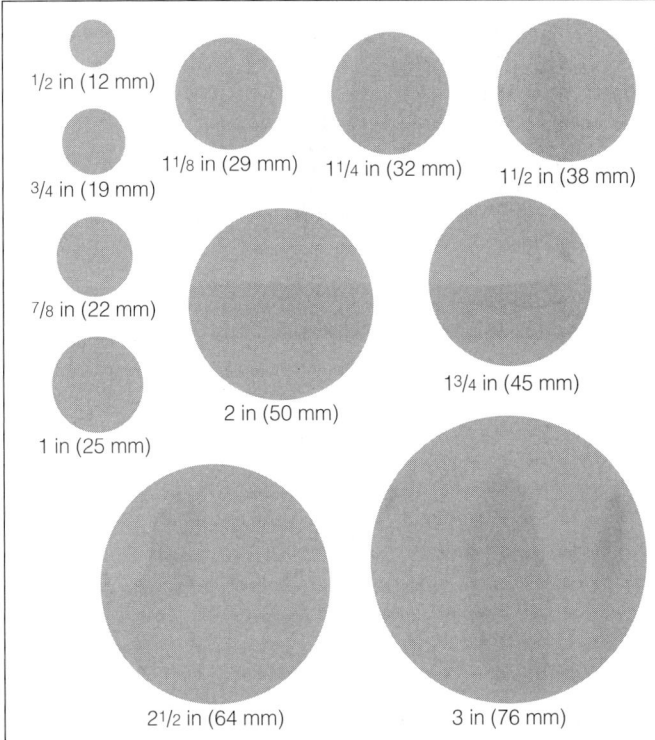

Figure 14 Patients must learn to measure their stomas with the help of measuring guides, such as this one, provided by the manufacturers of stoma appliances.

Table 2 Social and Medical Support Systems Available to Ostomates and Caretakers

Social Resources	Medical Resources
Hospital social worker	Surgeon
Medicare or CHAMPUS advisers	Enterostomal therapy (ET) nurse
Local chapter of the United Ostomy Association	Family physician
United Ostomy Association ostomy visitor	Psychologist
American Cancer Society	Dietitian

the ET nurse should provide the patient with written instructions, supplies, and lists of suppliers (including phone numbers).

Before discharge, a patient or caretaker should be familiar with one type of pouch system. He or she should be able to (1) empty the pouch and cleanse the closure tail [*see Figure 15*], (2) detach the adhesive portion of the pouch system properly, (3) care for the peristomal skin, (4) measure the stoma and cut a hole of the correct size in the adhesive portion of the system, (5) apply the pouch system properly, and (6) be aware of the telltale signs of peristomal skin problems and know how to prevent and correct them.

Peristomal Skin Care

As noted, many skin problems can be prevented by taking a few simple precautions. Fungal infections (most commonly caused by *Candida*) often occur under a wafer because of body heat. These infections respond rapidly to topical antifungal powders such as Mycostatin. Fungal overgrowth can also occur where the warm plastic appliance presses over the abdomen. This problem can often be prevented by using a pouch cover, wearing bikini underpants under the pouch, or wearing specially designed underwear [*see Figure 1*] to keep the plastic away from the skin.

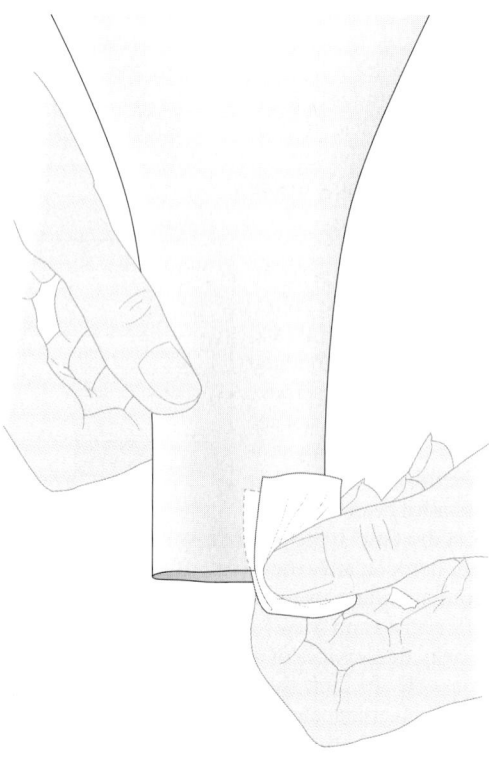

Figure 15 Once an open-end pouch is emptied, the closure tail must be cleansed.

The following three conditions can arise soon after surgery and demand immediate attention if they do:

1. Allergic contact dermatitis. The skin appears erythematous, weepy, or eroded in a pattern exactly corresponding to the shape of the offending product (e.g., tape or a skin barrier). Before a change is made to another skin barrier, a skin-barrier wipe or a transparent dressing should be used on the damaged skin in the interim so that a pouch can be secured. Patch test-

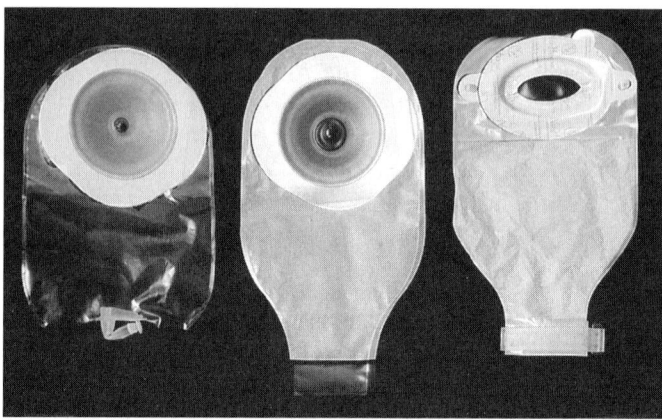

Figure 16 Shown are three convex pouches: a one-piece precut urostomy pouch (ConvaTec), an open-end bowel pouch (ConvaTec), and a one-piece bowel stoma pouch (NuHope).

a

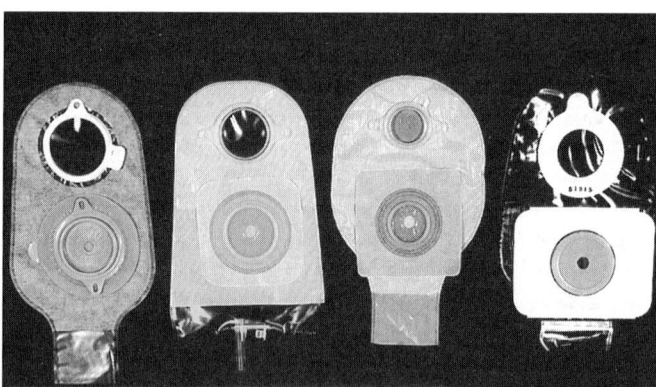

b

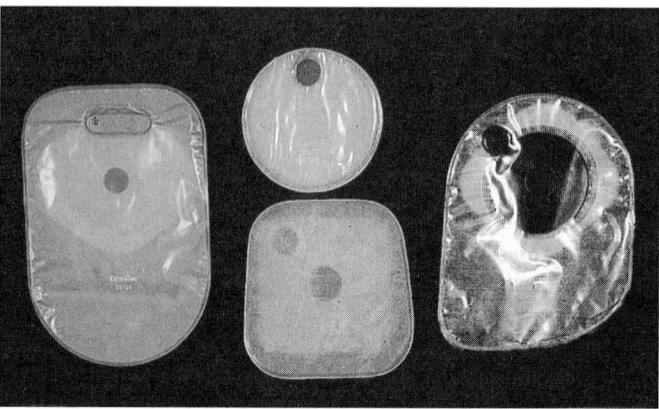

Figure 17 Shown are selected (*a*) two-piece pouches (Coloplast open-end, ConvaTec urinary, and Cymed open-end) and (*b*) closed-end pouches (ConvaTec, Dansac, United, and Hollister).

3. Irritant dermatitis. Either efflux from the stoma or the use of harsh cleansers may cause chemical burns. The skin appears erythematous, weepy, and painful, and the irritation may be restricted to a specific area of leakage. Treatment consists of (1) gently cleansing all of the peristomal skin, (2) dusting with Stomahesive powder, and (3) correcting any pouching problems that may have caused the leak.

Besides these three conditions, all of which may appear in the early postoperative period, there are a number of complications that may arise later, such as radiation reactions, parastomal abscesses, caput medusae, pseudoepithelial hyperplasia, pyoderma gangrenosum, and parastomal ulcers.

The patient should be seen for stomal and pouch evaluation 3 months after the operation and subsequently on an annual basis or as necessary for management of complications. Either weight gain or weight loss may necessitate changing the pouch system. In either event, the use of convex pouches may prove helpful [see Figure 16].

The patient must be aware that as long as the wafer is protecting the peristomal skin and is securely fixed to it, there is no compelling reason to change it. Wearing time generally ranges from 3 to 6 days and depends on both the individual and the pouch system used. If a patient has problems with the appliance, he or she should consult the surgeon or an ET nurse, who may recommend a change in the pouching steps or, if necessary, a change of pouch systems. Improvements are constantly being made in the design and manufacture of stoma equipment; some of the newer systems may fit or be worn more comfortably. There are several makers of high-quality equipment whose products [see Figure 17] we use regularly [see Table 3].

Written Patient Information

Most ostomy patients are under such intense stress after the op-

ing of another pouch system can be done by cutting a small piece of the new barrier wafer and tape and placing them on the opposite side of the patient's abdomen, forearm, or back for 24 hours and checking for any reaction.

2. Folliculitis (i.e., inflammation or infection of hair follicles). This condition usually arises when the abdominal hairs have grown back in the peristomal area and are forcibly pulled out with each pouch change. The patient should be instructed to remove the pouch using a wet piece of gauze or washcloth in a push-pull motion. When the folliculitis has healed, the patient should use an electric razor to shave the area and apply a skin sealant to protect the skin during pouch removal. Safety razors may cause small skin cuts that lead to skin infections. Application of an antimicrobial powder after the skin has been cleaned and dried is also helpful.

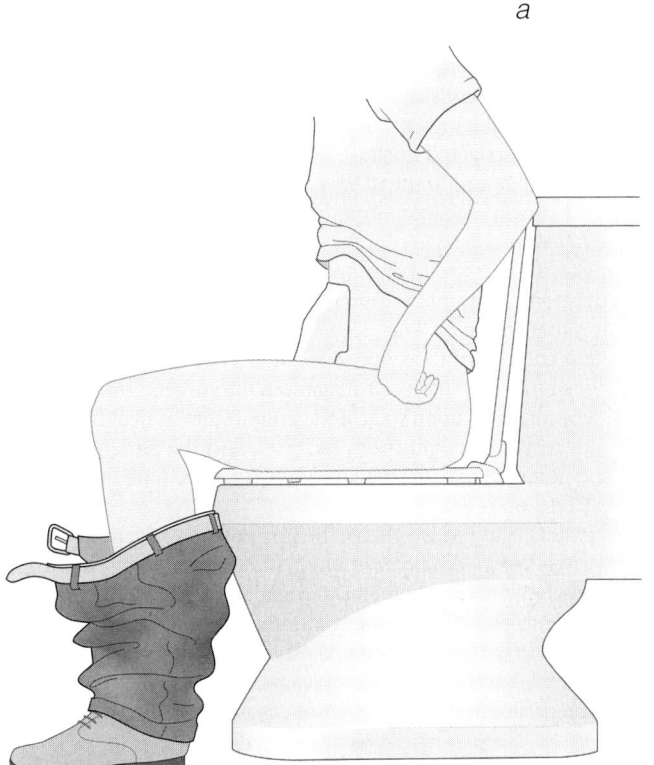

a

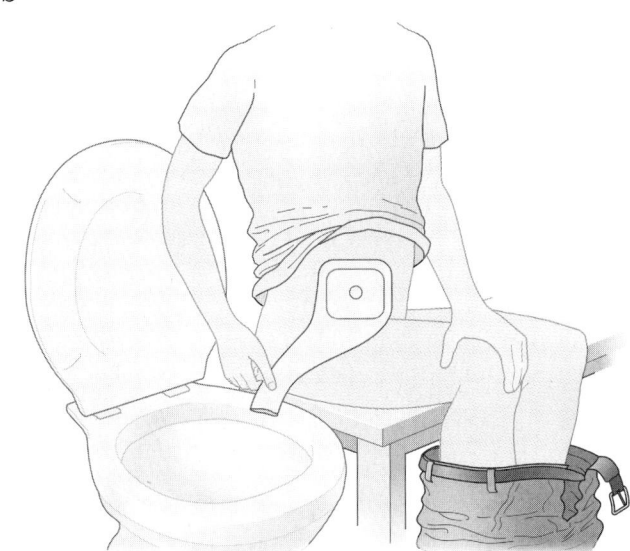

b

Figure 18 Illustrated are (*a*) the standard method of emptying a pouch and (*b*) an alternative emptying method that may be necessary after abdominoperineal resection or extensive rectal surgery. (For patients who have undergone lower GI surgery of this type, sitting beside the commode can be more comfortable than sitting on it, placing less stress on the perineal wound or the suture line.)

Table 4   Selected Companies Selling Stoma Appliances through Mail-Order Catalogues

AOS—American Ostomy Supply Guide, P.O. Box 13396, Milwaukee, WI 53213-9906; 800-858-5858

Edgepark Surgical, Inc., 1810 Summit Commerce Park, Twinsburg, OH 44087-9931; 800-321-0591

MED EXPRESS, P.O. Box 49850, Minneapolis, MN 55449-9908; 877-409-1234

Parthenon Co., 3311 W. 2400 Street, Salt Lake City, UT 84119; 800-453-8898

eration and the creation of the stoma that they cannot absorb all the oral instructions they receive. For this reason, it is important to give them some written information, preferably in a folder; they may or may not read this material while in the hospital, but they will have it at home to use as a reference after discharge. The patient information folder should contain the following components:

1. General stomal care instructions [*see Figure 18*].
2. Specific instructions on caring for their particular type of stoma.
3. Specific directions for applying and caring for their particular pouch system.
4. A list of the steps involved in changing the pouch.
5. Some general dietary instructions, along with explanations of what a stoma blockage is, how to prevent it, and what to do before calling the physician.
6. A guide to recognizing signs of urinary infection (for patients with ileal conduits).
7. A number where the ET can be reached for answers to questions and for discussion of any stoma or pouch problems that may arise, along with the date of the 3-month return visit to the ET for evaluation of the stoma and the pouch system.
8. A referral to local ostomy support group meetings. Ideally, the patient will have seen an ostomy visitor while in the hospital.

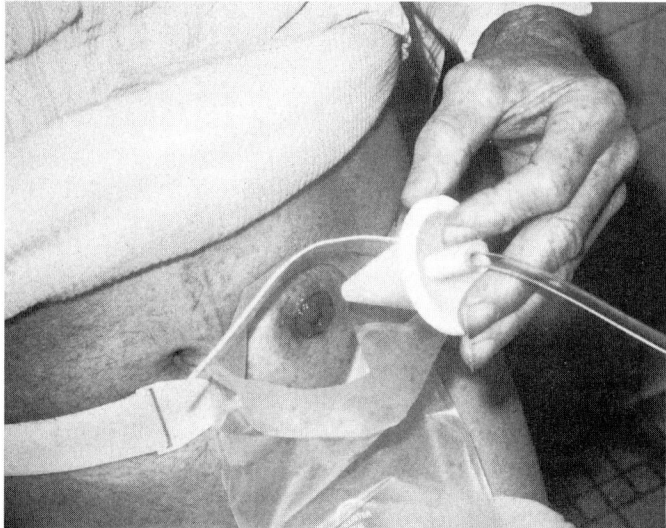

Figure 19   **This patient is about to insert an irrigating cone into his stoma. Note the presence of the irrigation sleeve and the retaining belt.**

9. Information on where and how to obtain stoma appliances and a reminder to check with the insurance company to see whether supplies must be purchased from a specific vendor. A list of local pharmacies or medical suppliers should be included, along with, if needed or desired, a mail-order catalogue [*see Table 4*].

POSTOPERATIVE CARE OF PATIENTS WITH CONTINENT STOMAS

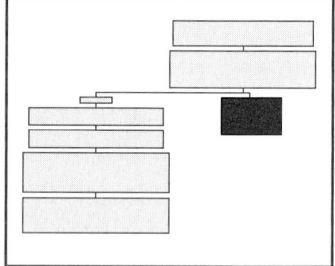

A patient with a continent stoma does not use an external pouch, and hence, certain aspects of his or her care are different. Nevertheless, a patient with a continent stoma also requires the expert planning, counseling, and care that other ostomates require.

After the construction of a continent ileostomy, the surgeon intubates the intestinal pouch with a No. 30 Silastic catheter. A silk tie is placed around the catheter at the level of the stoma to mark the correct position of the tube. The tube is then affixed securely to the skin. It is left in place for about 10 days, and the intestinal pouch is allowed to empty by gravity. The tube must be irrigated with 30 ml of normal saline solution every 6 hours or so to ensure that it remains patent. As soon as the patient expresses interest, he or she may participate in the irrigation of the intestinal pouch and in the washing of the stoma and the surrounding skin. About 10 days after operation, the patient should be taught how to extubate and intubate the intestinal pouch. At this point, the tube should not be kept out of the pouch for more than 30 minutes at a time. Drainage through the catheter is facilitated by saline irrigations.

About 4 weeks after the operation, the patient will extubate and reintubate the stoma at preset times separated by gradually longer intervals, which allows the intestinal pouch to distend progressively.

A similar postoperative approach is required after the creation of a urinary continent pouch, such as the so-called Indiana pouch.[10]

COLOSTOMY IRRIGATION

Colostomy irrigation is not essential to the good functioning of a stoma.[11] It is time consuming and should be performed only for the convenience of the patient. Stomas proximal to the splenic flexure should not be irrigated because of the liquid stools present in that portion of the bowel. In most cases, the teaching of colostomy self-irrigation [*see Sidebar* Recommended Procedures for Irrigation *and Figure 19*] should be deferred for several weeks, until the patient has recuperated from the operation and has gained some familiarity with the stoma. Another reason for deferring instruction in self-irrigation is that the colon may need several weeks to recover from the operation and return to its previous pattern of motility. When deciding who should be taught self-irrigation, the surgeon must take into consideration the patient's age and general state of health, the availability of reasonable bathroom facilities, and the patient's motivation and ability to put up with the inconvenience (and, at times, the variable results) of self-irrigation.

If a patient is to receive chemotherapy postoperatively, instruction in self-irrigation should be postponed. If the patient is already irrigating when placed on chemotherapy, irrigation should be discontinued. All too often, a patient receiving chemotherapy is too tired to perform an adequate irrigation; moreover, the diarrhea that frequently accompanies chemotherapy will render irrigation ineffectual. Irrigation can be resumed, if desired, after chemotherapy is completed.

Recommended Procedures for Irrigation

If irrigation is to be performed, the following instructions for the patient are recommended.

Supplies

Irrigation bag with long tube and cone; sleeve with belt.

Water

Tepid tap water, 1,000–1,500 ml.

Procedure

1. Fill the irrigation bag with tepid water, remove air in the tube by allowing water to run through it and into the sink, close the clamp, hang up the irrigation bag at a height that will allow the bottom of the bag to be at the level of your shoulder when you are seated.

2. Sit on the toilet or a chair beside the toilet (if the perineum is still sore).

3. Remove the colostomy appliance.

4. Center the opening of the irrigation sleeve over the stoma, and place the end of the sleeve in the toilet bowl. To avoid splashing, the sleeve need only be long enough to touch the water. If it is too long, it may be cut. Tighten the irrigation sleeve belt to prevent leakage.

5. Lubricate the end of the cone with water or a water-soluble lubricant. Insert the cone tip gently through the top of the open sleeve and into the stoma, and rotate the cone until the water flows in freely. (If the water does not flow in freely, do not push the cone in further; instead, pull the cone back and rotate it because usually the cause of the limited water flow is that the opening of the cone is against the bowel wall.)

6. Press the cone firmly and gently against the stoma to prevent leakage.

7. The water must flow in slowly. It takes about 5 minutes to instill a quart. Stop the flow of water if you become uncomfortable or experience cramps, but do not remove the cone, because removal would allow the water to return too soon.

8. When all the water has been emptied from the irrigation bag and tube, remove the cone from the stoma. Close the top of the irrigation sleeve with clips or ties.

9. Allow about 15 to 20 minutes for the bowel to empty, with the sleeve end remaining in the toilet.

10. Rinse the sleeve with water, and clamp the end closed. You may leave the bathroom and do what you wish for the next 30 to 45 minutes. During this time, additional water and stool may be expelled.

11. Return to the bathroom, unclamp the sleeve, empty any effluence, and rinse the sleeve. With time, you will know when evacuation is completed. Unsnap the belt, and remove the sleeve.

12. Wash the peristomal skin with warm water, rinse well, pat dry, and replace your appliance.

13. Clean the sleeve with detergent and water, rinse it well, and allow it to air-dry. Let any remaining fluid in the irrigation bag and tubing drain out. Wash, rinse, and dry off the cone.

The entire procedure should take about 1 hour.

General Pointers

1. For the first irrigations you perform, write down the amount of water used, the amount of time for the procedure, and the amount and character of the water and stool expelled. If you record this information for the first few irrigations, you will learn how long to wait for a total evacuation, how much fluid to use, and how often you need to irrigate.

2. Good results are obtained by performing the procedure at about the same time each day. Some individuals need to irrigate only every other day.

3. Because you do not eat the same type or amount of food daily, the amount of elimination will vary from day to day. Persons who are dehydrated may at times need extra irrigation fluid because some of that fluid will be quickly absorbed by the colon.

4. Try to relax when performing irrigation. If you are nervous or upset, often this method will not work for you. If you are ill or experiencing diarrhea, you should temporarily discontinue irrigation.

5. Remember: to irrigate or not to irrigate is your choice.

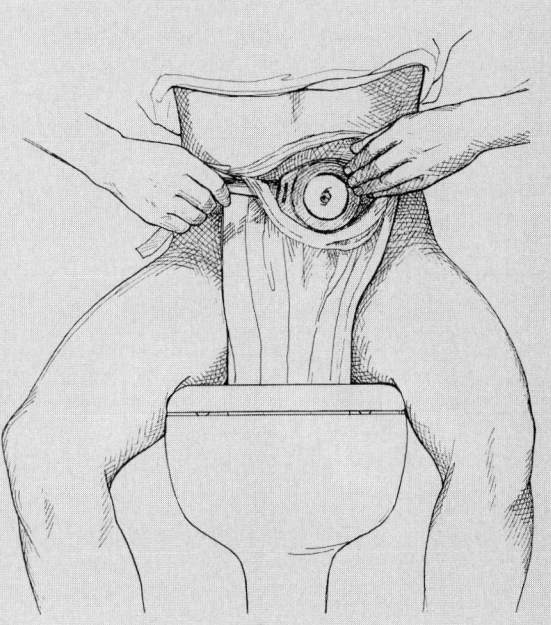
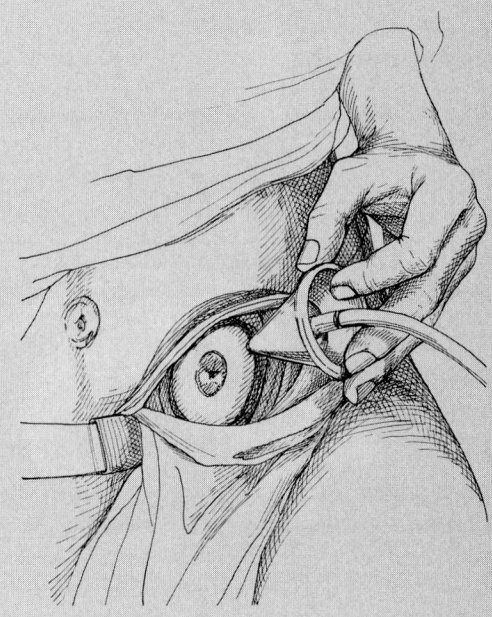

References

1. Rothman CP: Sperm banking. Common Problems in Infertility and Impotence. Rajfer J, Ed. Year Book Medical Publishers, Chicago, 1990, p 200

2. Metcalf AM, Dozois RR, Kelly KA: Sexual function in women after proctocolectomy. Ann Surg 204:624, 1986

3. Emblem R, Stray Pedersen S, Bergan A, et al: Female complaints after proctocolectomy. Proceedings of the Seventh Biennial Congress of the World Council of Enterostomal Therapists. Palex International SA, 1990, p 20

4. Gloeckner MR, Starling JR: Providing sexual information to ostomy patients. Dis Colon Rectum 25:575, 1982

5. Physician's Desk Reference, 51st ed. Medical Economics, Montvale, New Jersey, 1997, pp 1103, 1677, 2588

6. Fazio VW, Erwin-Toth P: Enterostomal therapy. Colon and Rectal Surgery, 4th ed. Corman ML, Ed. Lippincott-Raven, Philadelphia, 1998

7. Ohmura Y: Evaluation of preoperative stoma site marking. Proceedings of the Seventh Biennial Congress of the World Council of Enterostomal Therapists. Palex International SA, 1990, p 27

8. Bass EM, Pino AD, Tan A, et al: Does preoperative stoma marking and education by the enterostomal therapist affect outcome? Dis Colon Rectum 40:440, 1997

9. Milsom JW, Bohm B: Laparoscopic Colorectal Surgery. Springer, New York, 1995

10. Rowland RG, Mitchell ME, Bihrie R, et al: Indiana continent urinary reservoir. J Urol 137:1136, 1986

11. Laucks SS 2nd, Mazier WP, Milsom JW, et al: An assessment of colostomy irrigation. Dis Colon Rectum 31:279, 1988

Reviews

Broadwell DC, Jackson BS: Principles of Ostomy Care. CV Mosby Co, St. Louis, 1982

Celestin LR: Color Atlas of the Surgery and Management of Intestinal Stomas. Year Book Medical Publishers, Chicago, 1987

Dozois R: Alternatives to Conventional Ileostomy. Year Book Medical Publishers, Chicago, 1985

Goldstein BG, Jackson BS: Principles of Ostomy Care. CV Mosby Co, St. Louis, 1982

Gordon PH, Nivatvong S: Colon, Rectum, and Anus. Quality Medical Publishers, St. Louis, 1999

Jeter K: These Special Children: The Ostomy Book for Parents of Children with Colostomies, Ileostomies, and Urostomies. Bull Publishing Co, Palo Alto, 1982

McDougal WS: Use of intestinal segments and urinary diversions. Campbell's Urology, vol 3. Walsh PC, Retik AB, Vaughan ED, et al, Eds. WB Saunders Co, Philadelphia, 1998, p 3121

Smith DB, Johnson DE: Ostomy Care and the Cancer Patient: Surgical and Clinical Considerations. Grune & Stratton, Orlando, Florida, 1986

Acknowledgments

Figures 1, 15, and 18   Tom Moore.

Figure 3 and Sidebar illustrations   Carol Donner.

26 ANAL PROCEDURES

Ira J. Kodner, M.D., F.A.C.S.

Operative Management of Hemorrhoids

In recent years, the frequency of hemorrhoid surgery has diminished significantly. More patients seem to be achieving adequate symptomatic relief by means of bowel control medications and improved diet (e.g., increased intake of fiber, fruit, vegetables, and grain). It is probable that both for these reasons and because more and better patient information is available, fewer patients today have hemorrhoids that progress to a stage advanced enough to necessitate operative treatment for relief of symptoms.

OPERATIVE PLANNING

It is important to distinguish between internal and external hemorrhoids [*see Figure 1*]. Internal hemorrhoids are treated to relieve specific symptoms, including prolapse and bleeding, not simply because hemorrhoidal tissue was seen on routine examinations. Prolapsing tissue occasionally results in maceration of the perianal skin that may not be clearly evident at the time of examination, especially if the patient is in the prone position. External hemorrhoids are treated because they thrombose and cause pain. There are no other symptoms of the anorectum that should be attributed to the presence of hemorrhoids [*see Table 1*]; in particular, difficulties with bowel movements (e.g., straining, the need for digital evacuation of the rectum, and cramping abdominal pain) must not be ascribed to hemorrhoids.

Accordingly, the ability to recognize and diagnose the spectrum of pelvic floor abnormalities (of which rectal prolapse is the most florid manifestation), especially obstructed defecation, is critical to the decision whether to correct hemorrhoids surgically. Attempting to alleviate nonhemorrhoidal symptoms by means of hemorrhoid surgery is likely to yield unsatisfactory

results for both patient and surgeon. It is not uncommon for anal fissure/ulcer disease to coexist with hemorrhoids, in which case the chances of a good operative result can be increased by performing a posterior lateral internal sphincterotomy at the time of hemorrhoid surgery.

Before embarking on the surgical treatment of hemorrhoids, one must always rule out neoplastic disease, compromise of the immune system, and defective clotting mechanisms. Patients with a personal or family history of colorectal cancer and those 50 years of age or older should undergo colonoscopy to eliminate the possibility of polyps or cancer before surgical treatment of hemorrhoids is initiated. The patient's general health status and ability to tolerate pain and an operative procedure should also be taken into account. The postoperative response to anorectal surgery varies enormously among patients. For example, young men tend to strain to have bowel movements after anorectal procedures, and this tendency can lead to bleeding and disruption of postoperative healing. These patients often benefit from the administration of parenteral pain medication for the first 12 to 24 hours after operation, which usually requires hospitalization. Elderly patients, on the other hand, prefer not to be in the hospital. For these patients, single elastic ligation of individual clusters of internal hemorrhoids is performed in the outpatient office.

The next step is to determine the appropriate procedure for the patient. The options include (1) elastic ligation of internal hemorrhoids, (2) excision of thrombosed external hemorrhoids, (3) complete excisional hemorrhoidectomy, and (4) elastic ligation of internal hemorrhoids combined with excision of external hemorrhoids. One should always consider whether complete sigmoidoscopy, rigid or flexible, will be necessary at the time of

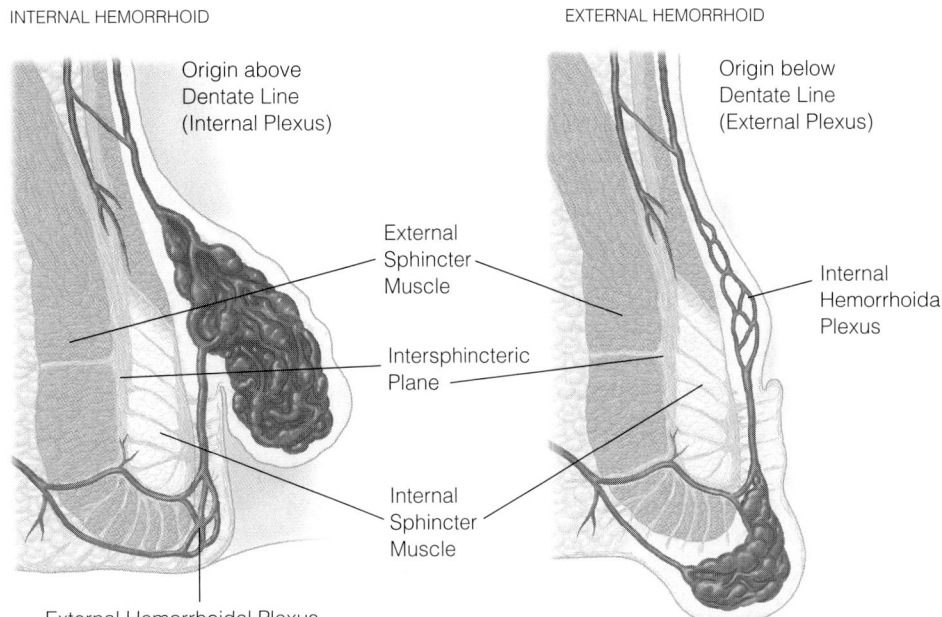

INTERNAL HEMORRHOID

Origin above
Dentate Line
(Internal Plexus)

External
Sphincter
Muscle

Intersphincteric
Plane

Internal
Sphincter
Muscle

External Hemorrhoidal Plexus

EXTERNAL HEMORRHOID

Origin below
Dentate Line
(External Plexus)

Internal
Hemorrhoidal
Plexus

Figure 1 **Operative management of hemorrhoids. A key issue is the differentiation of internal hemorrhoids from external hemorrhoids. Internal hemorrhoids (left) originate from the internal hemorrhoidal plexus, above the dentate line. External hemorrhoids (right) originate from the external hemorrhoidal plexus, below the dentate line.**

Table 1 Anal Symptoms Mistakenly
Attributed to Hemorrhoids

Symptoms	Cause
Pain and bleeding after bowel movement	Ulcer/fissure disease
Forceful straining to have bowel movement	Pelvic floor abnormality (paradoxical contraction of anal sphincter)
Blood mixed with stool	Neoplasm
Drainage of pus during or after bowel movement	Abscess/fistula, inflammatory bowel disease
Constant moisture	Condyloma acuminatum
Mucous drainage and incontinence	Rectal prolapse
Anal pain with no physical findings	*Caution:* possible psychiatric disorder

the procedure and whether anal sphincterotomy will be indicated, especially in young men with a history of straining. This second consideration is important because many patients are treated for hemorrhoids when in fact their primary disease is anal ulcer/fissure disease, the symptoms of which are pain and some bleeding at defecation. These are not symptoms that can be attributed to hemorrhoids. If a patient undergoes hemorrhoid surgery when the primary disease is anal fissure, proper healing will be impeded.

Finally, one should explain the procedure and its attendant risks to the patient in the outpatient office because in most cases, given the restrictions imposed by health care insurers and managed care administrators, one will not see the patient again until the operating room on the day of operation. Specific complications to be discussed preoperatively include urinary retention, bleeding, and infection. In the event that several symptomatic hemorrhoids are present, surgeon and patient should jointly decide between multiple small procedures done in the office and a single larger procedure done in the OR. Individual economic concerns, as well as employment and lifestyle, should be considered.

Special Situations

Acute thrombosed external hemorrhoids This condition is signaled by acute pain and a swelling blood clot within the skin-covered external hemorrhoid. Often, the clot is eroding through the skin, causing bleeding that may be frightening to the patient but is typically insignificant. If I encounter this problem days after its onset, I generally treat it with bowel control and topical medications as the process resolves. If the hemorrhoid is acutely painful or the clot is eroding, the best therapy is surgical excision of the external hemorrhoid, with the anoderm left intact; this is best done with the patient under adequate local anesthesia. Mere evacuation of the clot is rarely appropriate.

Postpartum hemorrhoids The postpartum rosette of acute thrombosed external (and, often, prolapsed internal) hemorrhoidal tissue is appropriately treated with hemorrhoidectomy (see below), carried out as soon after delivery as is convenient. The risk of infection is minimal, and I know of

no good reason to send a new mother home with hemorrhoids in addition to a new baby and a healing episiotomy.

OPERATIVE TECHNIQUE

Step 1: Positioning

Operative treatment of hemorrhoids, like the vast majority of anorectal procedures, should be done with the patient in the prone-flexed position [*see Figure 2*]. The transporting stretcher should be kept in the room. The patient will be given I.V. narcotics to allow painless injection of local anesthetics, and if any respiratory compromise results because of the prone-flexed position, the patient can quickly be returned to the supine position on the stretcher until respiration resumes without difficulty.

Step 2: Intravenous Sedation and Local Anesthesia

Before administering a local anesthetic, I usually give the following drugs for sedation: midazolam, 2 to 5 mg, given in the holding area for sedation and amnesia; alfentanil, 0.5 to 1 mg, or fentanyl, 50 to 100 mg, for analgesia to help alleviate the discomfort of the local anesthetic injection; and propofol, 20 to 50 mg, or methohexital, 20 to 50 mg, to achieve patient cooperation with the injection. Sedation is followed by the injection into perianal tissue of 40 ml of bupivacaine (0.5%) along with a buffer that is added immediately before injection (0.5 ml of 8.4% sodium bicarbonate [1 mEq/ml] added to 50 ml of local anesthetic). If resection is anticipated, epinephrine (1:200,000) is usually included with the local anesthetic. To achieve adequate local anesthesia, 5 ml of bupivacaine is injected into the subcutaneous tissue in each quadrant of the tissue immediately surrounding the anus [*see Figure 3a*]. Next, 10 ml of local anesthetic is injected deep into the sphincter mechanism on each side of the anal canal [*see Figure 3b*].

Step 3: Anoscopy or Sigmoidoscopy

Anoscopy, sigmoidoscopy, or both should be performed at this point if neither procedure was done before the operation.

Step 4: Sphincterotomy

As noted, sphincterotomy should always be considered, especially if a hypertrophic band of the lower third of the internal

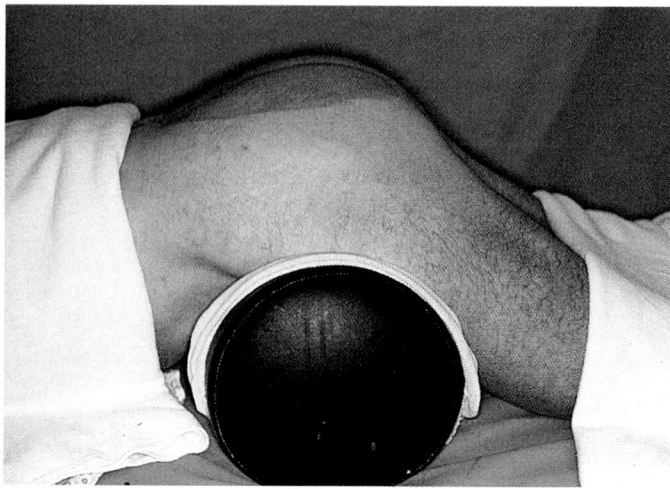

Figure 2 **Operative management of hemorrhoids. The patient is positioned on the operating table in the prone-flexed position, with a soft roll under the hips.**

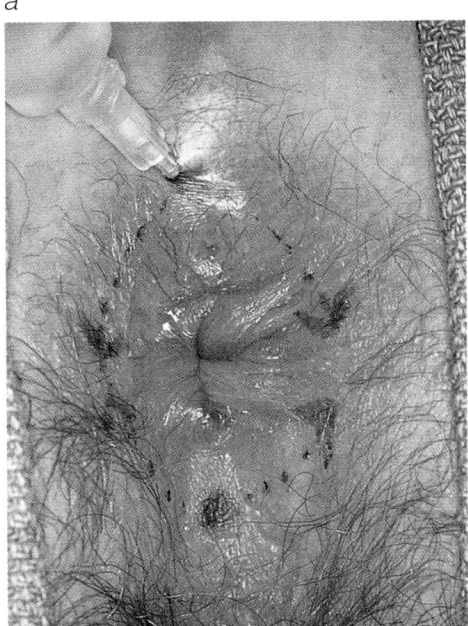

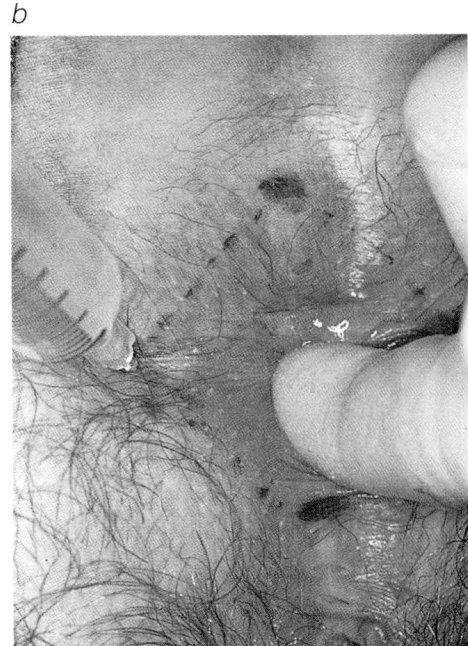

Figure 3 Operative management of hemorrhoids. (*a*) Five milliliters of bupivacaine is injected into subcutaneous tissue. (*b*) Ten milliliters of local anesthetic is injected deep into the sphincter muscle on each side of the anal canal.

sphincter muscle persists after the local anesthetic has been injected and an anoscope has been inserted. It is always best to obtain permission to do this beforehand on the operative consent form.

Step 5: Treatment of Hemorrhoids

Elastic ligation of internal hemorrhoids This is a very safe operation because by the nature of the banding procedure [*see Figure 4*], bridges of normal mucosa are maintained between treated clusters of hemorrhoids. Any clusters of tissue with squamous metaplasia and obviously friable internal hemorrhoids can be treated in this manner. I find that these tissue clusters are not always confined to the three classic positions

identified for hemorrhoids and that in many cases it is necessary to band three or four clusters. If the bands do not stay on, then the tissue probably need not be treated and no further action need be taken.

I use two rubber bands on each cluster. If one of them breaks, bleeding is unlikely to occur, because the tissue rapidly becomes edematous and necrotic. It is important that the placement of the rubber band be proximal to the mucocutaneous junction; if it is not, the procedure will be too painful, given the extensive innervation of the skin. On the other hand, the band should not be placed so proximally as to incorporate the full thickness of the rectal wall; to do so can be risky for patients in whom difficulties with bowel movements indicate the presence of intus-

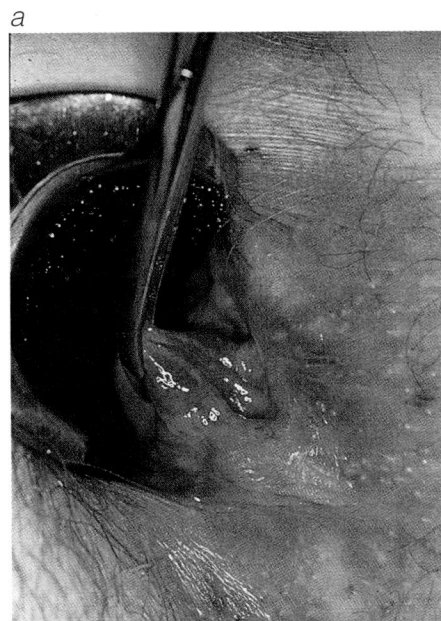

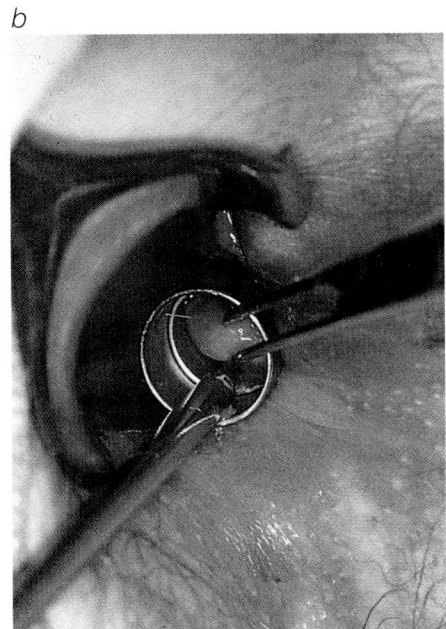

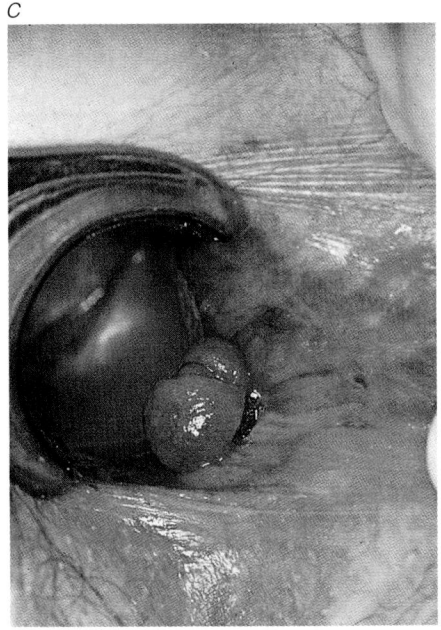

Figure 4 Operative management of hemorrhoids. Shown is the elastic ligation technique for internal hemorrhoids. (*a*) The hemorrhoidal tissue is identified. (*b*) The hemorrhoid is grasped and pulled through the drum. (*c*) The elastic band is applied to the base of the hemorrhoid.

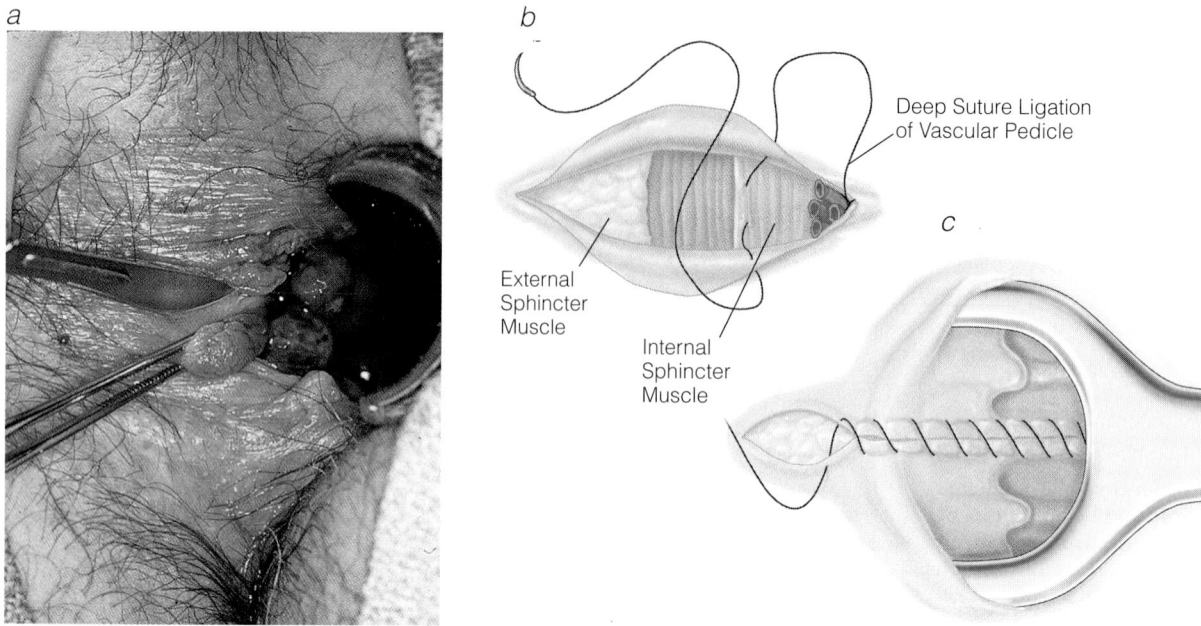

Figure 5 **Operative management of hemorrhoids. Shown is an excisional hemorrhoidectomy. (*a*) An elliptical incision is made in the perianal skin. (*b*) A continuous suture is used in a three-point placement in such a way as to incorporate skin edges and muscle. (*c*) The elliptical defect is closed and the dead space obliterated.**

susception or some other pelvic floor abnormality. Occasionally, the friable tissue gives rise to a suspicion of cancer. If this is the case, rubber bands may be placed at the base, and the tip may be excised for biopsy.

Excision of residual external hemorrhoids Residual external hemorrhoids are rarely treated as a primary problem: true symptoms are few, and the main indication for treatment is maintenance of hygiene. In addition, I find that much of the external tissue is pulled in when the internal hemorrhoids are ligated. Accordingly, I do the internal ligation first and then excise any residual symptomatic external tissue. An elliptical incision is made in the perianal skin, with care taken to protect the underlying sphincter muscle and avoid the previously placed elastic band [*see Figure 5a*]. Although the perianal skin is very forgiving, it is essential to protect the anoderm; this is achieved through careful placement of the rubber band. The elliptical defect is then closed with a continuous absorbable suture in a three-point placement to obliterate the underlying dead space [*see Figures 5b and 5c*]. The suture is tied loosely to allow for swelling. There is no need for separate ligation or coagulation of the small bleeding vessels; this problem is obviated by the continuous suture. It is important not to use slowly absorbable suture material, because it may give rise to infection in this highly susceptible tissue. I prefer to use 3-0 chromic catgut on an exaggeratedly curved needle.

Complete excisional hemorrhoidectomy This procedure is indicated in patients who have large combined internal and external hemorrhoids, patients who are receiving anticoagulants, and patients who have massive edema and thrombosis, as seen in the postpartum rosette of tissue [*see Figure 6*]. I find that even massive edema generally resolves after the local anesthetic is injected and the muscle is allowed to relax. Resolution of edema then permits identification of the specific clusters of hemorrhoids, which can be isolated with a forceps and excised via an elliptical incision. Care must be taken to preserve the underlying muscle, especially in the anterior region in women.

I use 3-0 chromic catgut with a deep stitch at the apex and a continuous three-point suture that is extended on the perianal skin [*see Figure 5b*]. It is important to preserve a bridge of anoderm between the areas of excision. I know of no indications for a radical circumferential procedure (the so-called Whitehead procedure); in fact, I see numerous patients who are seeking a remedy for the stenosis and ectropion that frequently occur after this radical operation [*see Figure 7*].

Currently, a new technique, in which a circumferential band of anorectal mucosa is excised with a special circular stapler, is

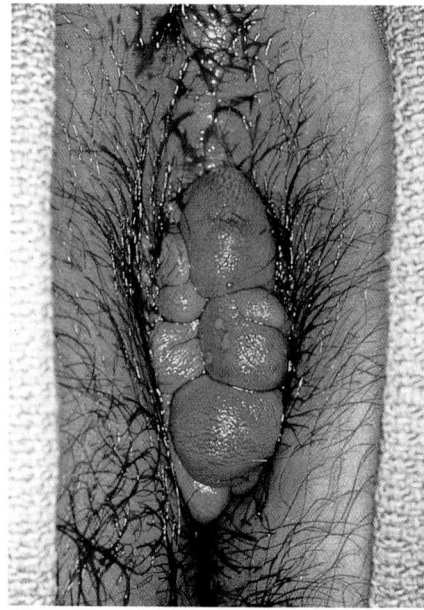

Figure 6 **Operative management of hemorrhoids. Massive edema and thrombosis, as seen in the postpartum rosette of tissue, can be reduced after a local anesthetic is injected and the muscle is allowed to relax.**

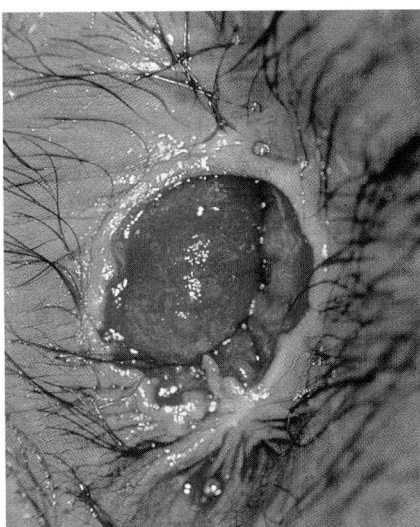

Figure 7 **Operative management of hemorrhoids. Stenosis and ectropion often result from radical circumferential (Whitehead) procedures.**

under investigation. This technique is intended for patients who have profound prolapsing internal hemorrhoids without much of an external component. Its proponents claim that it results in minimum postoperative discomfort; however, special training with the instrument is required. European centers report excellent success rates, and trials are currently under way in the United States.

Step 6: Postoperative Care

Immediately after the procedure—in fact, after any anorectal procedure—antibiotic ointment and a gauze pad are applied. Pressure dressings are unnecessary. Only a very small amount of adhesive tape should be used, so as to prevent traction avulsion of the perianal skin, an event for which we surgeons too often avoid responsibility by ascribing it to a "tape allergy" on the part of the patient.

TROUBLESHOOTING

The most fundamental way of preventing problems is to make an accurate diagnosis. Surgical treatment of hemorrhoids in a patient whose main disease process is Crohn's disease, a pelvic floor abnormality, or ulcer/fissure disease inevitably yields inferior results. It is especially important to recognize the anal pain and spasm of ulcer/fissure disease because in patients with this condition, excision of hemorrhoidal tissue without sphincterotomy leads to increased postoperative pain and poor wound healing.

I prefer to operate with the patient in the prone-flexed position, using local anesthesia supplemented by I.V. medication. I have found over the years that with this approach, patients retain no unpleasant memories of the OR experience, and good pain control is achieved in the immediate postoperative period.

In the postoperative period, efforts must be made to minimize straining on the part of the patient. To accomplish this, pain must be kept at a low level. I prefer to give only parenteral pain medication, in relatively high doses, on the first night. The patient and the nursing staff must be cautioned that the first sensation of pain, especially after elastic ligation of hemorrhoids, is the urge to defecate. This urge is an indication that pain medication should be given. The patient must not sit on the toilet and strain; to do so is likely to result in extrusion of the recently ligated tissue.

At least 20% of patients experience some degree of urinary retention. If this occurs, an indwelling catheter should be placed. In-and-out straight catheterization is contraindicated. No bladder stimulants should be given: such agents encourage straining and increase the risk of complications.

Bulk-forming agents and stool softeners are started in the immediate postoperative period. I encourage patients to take warm soaks, either in a bathtub or in a shower, rather than try to squeeze into the disposable sitz-bath mechanisms provided by the hospitals, which are often too small. I also encourage patients to sit on soft cushions rather than the rubber rings marketed for postoperative care; the rings seem to cause more dependent edema and pain.

COMPLICATIONS

Bleeding

Either immediate or delayed bleeding may occur after hemorrhoid surgery. Bleeding within the first 12 to 24 hours after the operation represents a technical error. The only management is to return the patient to the OR, with good anesthesia and adequate visualization, so that the bleeding site can be suture ligated. Frequently, spinal or epidural anesthesia is necessary because the patient is too uncomfortable, and the tissue perhaps too edematous, to allow local anesthesia. Bleeding within 5 to 10 days after the operation usually results from sloughing of the eschar created by suturing or elastic ligation. This delayed bleeding is usually minimal, and the patient is encouraged to rest and to take stool softeners. If the bleeding is significant, examination with adequate anesthesia is indicated to allow cauterization or suture ligation of the bleeding site.

It is important to discourage patients from taking aspirin-containing compounds in the postoperative period, and it is especially important to follow patients taking systemic anticoagulants closely. I prefer to treat these patients with excisional hemorrhoidectomy so that sutures can be placed; in this way, I avoid the risk that the elastic-ligated tissue will slough after 5 to 10 days.

Infection

Infection is unusual after hemorrhoidectomy because perianal tissue is normally well vascularized and extremely resistant to infection despite constant bombardment by bacteria. When it does occur, it is most likely to be in an immunocompromised patient—that is, one who has a blood dyscrasia, diabetes, or AIDS or has recently undergone chemotherapy. In my view, it is imperative to obtain at least a complete blood count and a chemistry profile before embarking on anorectal procedures; if the results are abnormal, elective hemorrhoid surgery is contraindicated.

Any local focus of infection noted in the postoperative period must be drained. I have seen this complication only when slowly absorbable suture material was used, which is the reason why I have returned to using 3-0 chromic catgut. Postoperative perianal infection can be severe and life-threatening, and it is therefore critically important to be familiar with its symptoms and to treat it intensively. Frequently, such infection is initially manifested by pain that is greater than anticipated, urinary retention, and fever. These symptoms have occasionally been reported after elastic ligation of hemorrhoids. In this event, it is critical that the patient be seen on an emergency basis, the elastic bands removed, the patient hospitalized, and parenteral administration of antibiotics begun. In retrospect, I find that all such patients whom I have

Disease Processes That Cause Anorectal Abscess and Fistula in Ano

Cryptoglandular Abscess and Fistula

This condition results from obstruction of the duct of a gland, the body of which resides in the intersphincteric plane. The orifice of the gland is at the base of the crypt. The disease process has both an acute aspect and a chronic aspect.

Abscess is the acute process of the disease. The anatomy is complex because of the tissue planes in the anorectal-perineal area.[2] Surgical drainage, or at least surgical evaluation, is always necessary. Attempts to manage this condition medically can result in progressive tissue destruction and life-threatening infection. It is also essential always to be alert to the possibility of an immunocompromised state. Normally, the anoperineum is quite resistant to microbial invasion; however, in immunocompromised patients, infection can be life-threatening.

Fistula is the chronic process of the disease. Persistent inflammation results in the formation of tracts from the anal duct to the anoperineal skin or to the inside of the anorectum. These tracts can take extremely complex courses. For this reason and because of the complicated tissue planes of dissection, surgical treatment must be carefully planned: the status of the sphincter mechanism may be jeopardized if inappropriate surgical incisions are employed to open a fistula tract.

Crohn's Disease

Anal and perineal infection is a major factor in the clinical course of one third of all patients who have Crohn's disease. The main pathologic process is full-thickness penetration of Crohn's ulcers, occurring at any location in the anal canal (as opposed to uncomplicated cryptoglandular abscess or fistula, which is usually found posteriorly or anteriorly in the midline). The infection associated with Crohn's disease can be massive but is surprisingly well tolerated by the patient. The infectious process can be progressively destructive to the sphincter and to the surrounding tissue. Patients are at lifelong risk for severe diarrhea and loss of rectal distensibility; accordingly, meticulous preservation of the sphincter mechanism is crucial.

The incisional surgical procedures usually employed for infectious foci in the anal canal may be too hazardous, and excisional procedures are never indicated. Given that Crohn's disease tends to persist and recur, long-term drainage may be necessary. Medical management is useful

and efficacious, but it should be provided in combination with surgical consultation and drainage of abscesses. Because patients with anal Crohn's disease usually exhibit some degree of intestinal involvement as well, it is important to evaluate the remainder of the GI tract, especially the rectum, before embarking on any surgical treatment of the anus.

Hidradenitis Suppurativa

This condition is caused by blockage and disruption of the apocrine sweat glands in the perianal and perineal tissue. It gives rise to destructive infected sinus tracts in the perineal tissue. Although the destruction can be profound, there is no connection with the intestinal tract (either the rectum or the anus). No specific pathologic diagnosis can be made, because all that is left is the destructive fibrotic reaction to the content of the ruptured gland. Hidradenitis suppurativa occurs in persons with seborrheic skin and in those who perspire profusely; it often involves the axillary, suprapubic, and inguinal areas as well as the perineum.

Because the lesions are actually sinus tracts in the skin, therapy involves simply incising the tracts; biopsy is appropriate at some point during the course of management.

Sepsis Resulting from the Immunocompromised State

Anoperineal infection in an immunocompromised patient is a very serious and possibly life-threatening situation. Because this part of the body is so highly contaminated, failure of immune barriers can be disastrous. This condition is seen in patients who have diabetes mellitus, HIV infection, or other forms of blood dyscrasias; in patients undergoing chemotherapy; and in transplant patients requiring long-term immunosuppression. It is diagnosed on the basis of its symptoms: the clinical findings may be obscured by the absence of pus resulting from leukopenia.

Treatment involves aggressive antibiotic therapy, careful examination with the patient under anesthesia, extremely conservative drainage procedures, and biopsy of the tissue (leukemic infiltrates are occasionally found). The potential consequences of failing to recognize and treat this condition are serious enough to warrant evaluation of all patients with perineal infection for an immunocompromised state before any treatment is undertaken or before these patients are discharged from the surgeon's supervision.

seen had preoperative symptoms of a pelvic floor abnormality with difficulty in defecation—not clear symptoms of hemorrhoids.

Urinary Retention

Urinary retention is apparently caused by reflex spasm of the pelvic musculature, which may not become evident until the local anesthesia wears off. Often, a patient still under the influence of local anesthesia seems to be doing exceedingly well for the first few hours after operation, only to go into urinary retention later that night. It may be helpful to reduce the fluid load in the perioperative period. When a patient has trouble urinating, an indwelling urinary catheter should be placed and left in place for at least 12 hours. This, in my view, is one of the major reasons for in-hospital observation after treatment of more than one cluster of hemorrhoids. Placement of the indwelling catheter is of particular importance for the patient's well-being, even if it is not looked on with favor by managed care administrators. Urinary retention is a frightening experience for the patient to undergo at home. What is more, if placement of an indwelling catheter is postponed for 12 to 24 hours, recovery may be delayed. Again, it is important to remember that urinary retention may be an early sign of pelvic infection.

Stricture

Stricture, with or without ectropion, results from circumferential excision of hemorrhoids. I mention this point only to discourage the performance of this procedure.

OUTCOME EVALUATION

Because hemorrhoids are treated only when symptoms—bleeding, prolapse, pain, and difficulty with hygiene—are present, success is determined simply by the extent to which the symptoms are alleviated. If other symptoms were present before operation and persist after the procedure, the primary diagnosis should be called into question. Many elderly patients with a single prolapsing hemorrhoid that causes bleeding or maceration of the perianal skin are well served by outpatient ligation; occasionally, there is a second cluster that requires treatment some months later.

The basic point is that any patient treated surgically for hemorrhoids should experience symptomatic relief. With newer surgical techniques and improved methods of postoperative management, there is no reason for the patient to experience the severe pain described by those who have undergone extensive excisional procedures.

Operative Management of Abscess and Fistula

The conditions that cause suppurative processes in the anoperineum are cryptoglandular abscess and fistula, Crohn's disease, and hidradenitis suppurativa [see Sidebar Disease Processes That Cause Anorectal Abscess and Fistula in Ano]. Accurate diagnosis is essential for proper surgical management. Although these conditions may appear similar at times, each one is managed somewhat differently.

OPERATIVE PLANNING

The most important initial step is to determine the activity and severity of the disease process and the immune status of the patient. For example, a large, fluctuant abscess surrounded by erythema, induration, and superficial necrosis of the skin in an insulin-dependent diabetic is a surgical emergency. On the other hand, a chronic abscess or fistula that drains periodically over a matter of months is not nearly as urgent a problem. Multiple fistula tracts to the perineum in a patient with Crohn's disease require that one perform an adequate study of the intestinal tract and the sphincter mechanism before attempting definitive surgical treatment. It is important to determine the etiology of the process whenever possible. Unfortunately, the determination cannot always be made without examination under anesthesia, during which treatment as well as diagnosis could be accomplished, and this complicates the obtaining of informed consent and the choice of anesthesia.

It is also important to gain as accurate a picture as possible of the complexity of the disease process; this facilitates the planning of the procedure, the choice of anesthesia, and the selection of the information given to patient and family before treatment. For example, in the absence of other significant health problems, a small, well-localized, low intersphincteric abscess often can be easily drained with the patient under local anesthesia if an internal opening can be seen preoperatively on anoscopy, although on occasion even this procedure calls for spinal or epidural anesthesia. (It should be remembered that use of the prone-flexed position [see Figure 2], which is my preference, makes general anesthesia more difficult.) Multiple infected tracts associated with undrained infectious foci in a case of rectal Crohn's disease necessitate examination with the patient under spinal or epidural anesthesia. The treating surgeon should perform careful anoscopy and sigmoidoscopy and conservative temporary drainage procedures until consultation with a specialist can be arranged. Severe destruction and suspected deep tissue necrosis, especially in immunocompromised patients, may necessitate extensive resection of tissue and perhaps a completely diverting colostomy.

Bowel preparation should include mechanical cleansing and antibiotics but may not be possible when the situation is urgent (as is most often the case). Appropriate antibiotic coverage (i.e., agents effective against gram-negative organisms and anaerobes) is indicated for all but the simplest cases, with special consideration given to patients who require prophylaxis because of cardiac disease or the presence of prosthetic material.[1] Usually, a urinary catheter should be inserted before operation, especially if the infectious process is located in the anterior region in a man, where the urethra is at risk for injury.

OPERATIVE TECHNIQUE

Many technical elements are common to all operations for conditions that cause suppurative processes in the perineum. The patient should be in the prone-flexed position, with the buttocks taped apart. Conduction anesthesia (spinal, caudal, or epidural) is usually required. The perineum should be examined carefully with an eye to areas of abscess or external drainage sites. Endoscopic examination of the anus, the rectum, and the vagina should be undertaken to search for primary inflammatory bowel disease, internal openings of the fistula, or vaginal openings of the fistula.

Cryptoglandular Abscess and Fistula

The abscess must be located and characterized because drainage will depend on the location of the abscess, the course of the fistula tract, and any related infectious processes [see Figure 8]. It is important not to create a fistula through the levator plate of the pelvic floor. This means that an abscess with a low origin must be drained low, with care taken to avoid iatrogenic perforation of the rectum, and an abscess with a high origin (e.g., a high intersphincteric abscess) must be drained high by incising the mucosa and the longitudinal (internal sphincter) muscle of the rectal wall (not a procedure for the occasional rectal surgeon). The internal opening—that is, the crypt where the abscess originated—must be sought; this is best done by means of anoscopy, very careful probing, and sigmoidoscopy to rule out a high source (e.g., Crohn's disease). If the internal opening is found,

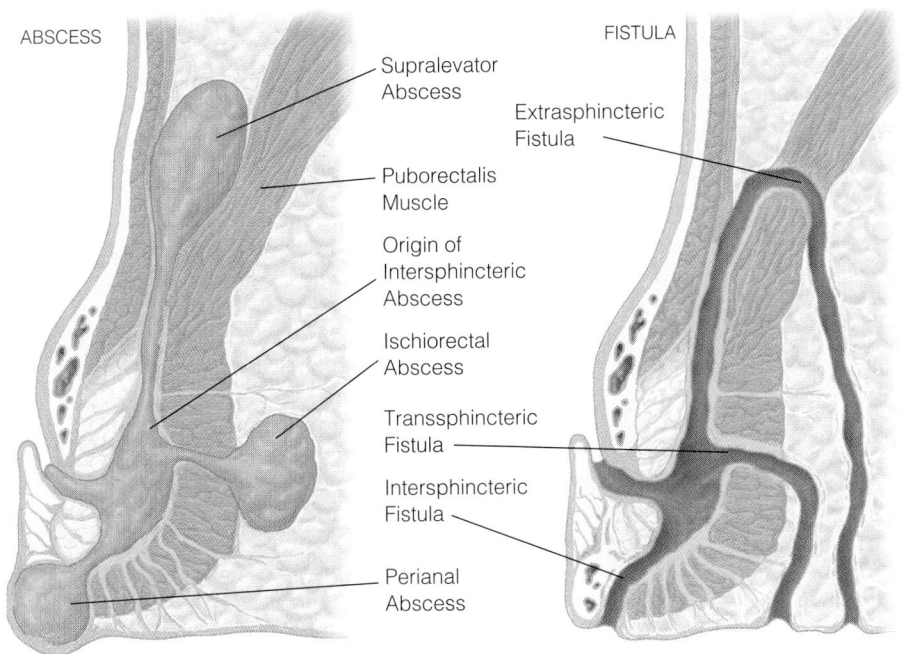

ABSCESS

Supralevator Abscess

Puborectalis Muscle

Origin of Intersphincteric Abscess

Ischiorectal Abscess

Perianal Abscess

FISTULA

Extrasphincteric Fistula

Transsphincteric Fistula

Intersphincteric Fistula

Figure 8 Abscess and fistula are, respectively, the acute aspect and the chronic aspect of a single disease process. Acute inflammation can lead to different types of abscesses (left), depending on the direction in which the inflammation extends. Chronic inflammation leads to communication of the abscess sites with the surface—that is, fistula tracts (right).

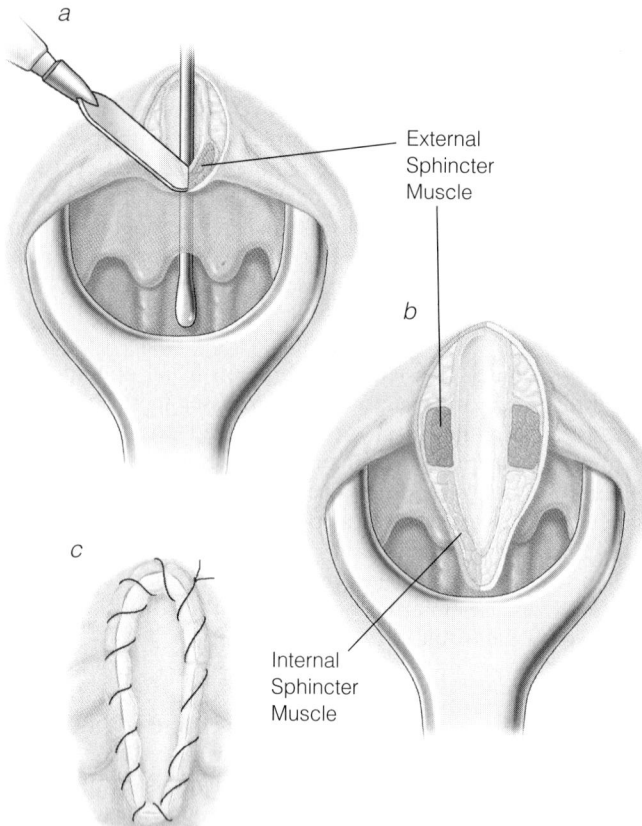

Figure 9 Operative management of abscess and fistula. Shown is a fistulotomy in a patient with cryptoglandular abscess/fistula. (*a*) The fistula tract is carefully probed, a decision is made about which muscle and how much muscle to cut, and the tract is incised. (*b*) Once the tract is open, the involved crypt is excised. (*c*) The defect is marsupialized by sewing skin to the tract.

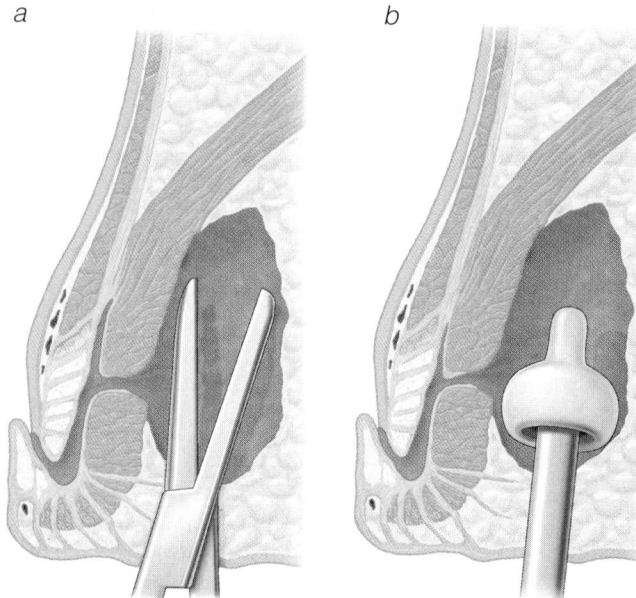

Figure 10 Operative management of abscess and fistula. Shown is drainage of an ischiorectal abscess. Such abscesses may be palpated above the anorectal ring, even though their location is more inferior. (*a*) The abscess is incised. (*b*) A mushroom-tipped catheter is placed.

the abscess can be drained or a fistulotomy can be performed [*see Figure 9*]. With a fistulotomy, determination of safety is a paramount concern. Careful consideration must be given to which muscle—and how much of the muscle—is to be cut. The anterior location in a woman is especially precarious. If the fistula involves a significant amount of muscle, or any muscle in the anterior region in a woman, either a seton should be placed or a drain should be placed without disruption of the muscle, in preparation for advancement flap closure of the internal opening.

If the internal opening is not found, one should not make one by probing. The abscess should be drained with a mushroom-tipped catheter [*see Figure 10*]; this is preferable to unroofing and eliminates painful packing. The catheter can be left in place for an extended period, and it permits subsequent injection of dye or contrast material. Once the mushroom catheter is in place in the OR, the surgeon can inject diluted methylene blue to search again for internal openings, which, if found, allow one to consider fistulotomy. The drain is usually sutured in place. The patient should be seen a few days after the operation to confirm that the abscess is adequately drained.

After 2 weeks, the patient is seen in the office, and povidone-iodine is injected through the drain while the inside of the anal canal is inspected via an anoscope. If an internal opening is seen, then fistulotomy is planned. If no internal opening is seen (as is the case in about 50% of patients), the drain should be removed 1 week later. This allows any irritant effect of the povidone-iodine to resolve and prevents the abscess from recurring.

If the fistula tract is known to have an external opening and fistulotomy is planned, the following approach should be considered. First of all, fistulectomy is never indicated. Fistulotomy is performed rarely and with great caution in the face of Crohn's disease. To perform the fistulotomy, one must first find the internal opening. In this regard, Goodsall's rule is often helpful: external fistula openings anterior to the midanal line are usually connected to internal openings via short, straight tracts, whereas external openings posterior to this line usually follow a curved course to internal openings in the posterior midline. Dilute methylene blue is injected through the external opening, often via a plastic I.V. catheter.

Careful probing, perhaps with a lacrimal duct probe, is then carried out. If the internal opening still cannot be found, a drain is placed so that the surgeon can return at another time to search for the internal opening. If the internal opening is found, a probe is passed and an effort is made to determine how much muscle and which muscle must be transected to accomplish the fistulotomy and how much muscle will remain to maintain continence [*see Figure 11*].

If the surgeon is not sure of the extent of muscle involvement or of how safe a fistulotomy would be, the infectious process should be drained, and either the patient should be referred to a specialist, or plans should be made for an advancement flap procedure to close the internal opening. If a fistulotomy is done, a biopsy specimen should be obtained from the infected tract, and the tract should be marsupialized to prevent premature healing of the superficial aspect.

It is important to keep in mind that the sphincter mechanism is innervated by a branch of the pudendal nerve that enters the sphincter from the posterolateral aspect. Accordingly, extreme caution must be exercised when a deep fistulotomy is required in the posterolateral perianal quadrants.

There is a growing body of evidence suggesting that injection of commercially available fibrin glue is effective for treatment of fistulas in perianal tissue. Longer tracts appear to respond bet-

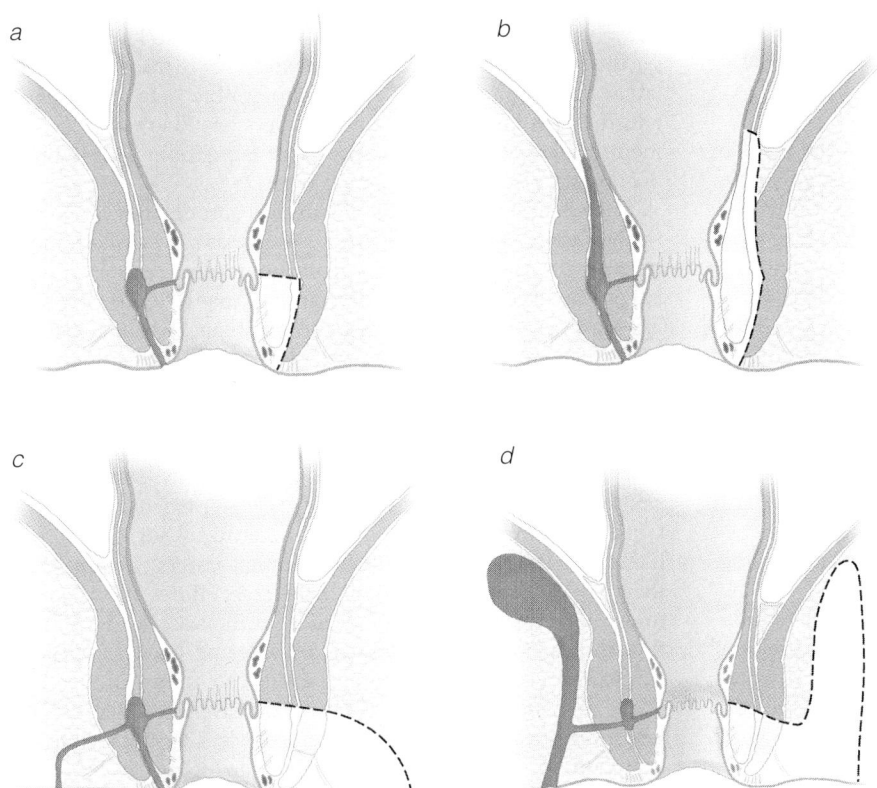

Figure 11 **Operative management of abscess and fistula. Shown are examples of the different types of fistulotomies indicated for some of the many types of fistulas: intersphincteric fistula with a simple low tract (*a*), intersphincteric fistula with a high blind tract (*b*), uncomplicated transsphincteric fistula (*c*), and transsphincteric fistula with a high blind tract (*d*). In each image, the left half of the drawing shows the disease process, and the right half illustrates the recommended operation.**

ter to this modality than shorter tracts do. The long-term efficacy of this approach remains to be proved.

Special problems A cryptoglandular abscess that extends into the posterior anal and posterior rectal spaces is often missed as a source of infection. Diagnosis of such abscesses typically involves bidigital examination, often with the patient under anesthesia; needle aspiration may be required as well. Fistulotomy in this area often necessitates opening large amounts of tissue, including partial transection of the sphincter muscle; the tract

may also have to be marsupialized. If one is unsure of the anatomy or has never done the procedure before, the abscess should be drained as simply as possible and the patient referred to a specialist.

The so-called horseshoe abscess [*see Figure 12*] results from an undiagnosed posterior-space abscess that has dissected laterally and may have been drained several times through the lateral extension into one or both ischiorectal fossae. This condition is cured by opening the posterior space and placing a long-term lateral drain, after which healing proceeds by secondary intention (the so-called Hanley procedure). The drain should not be

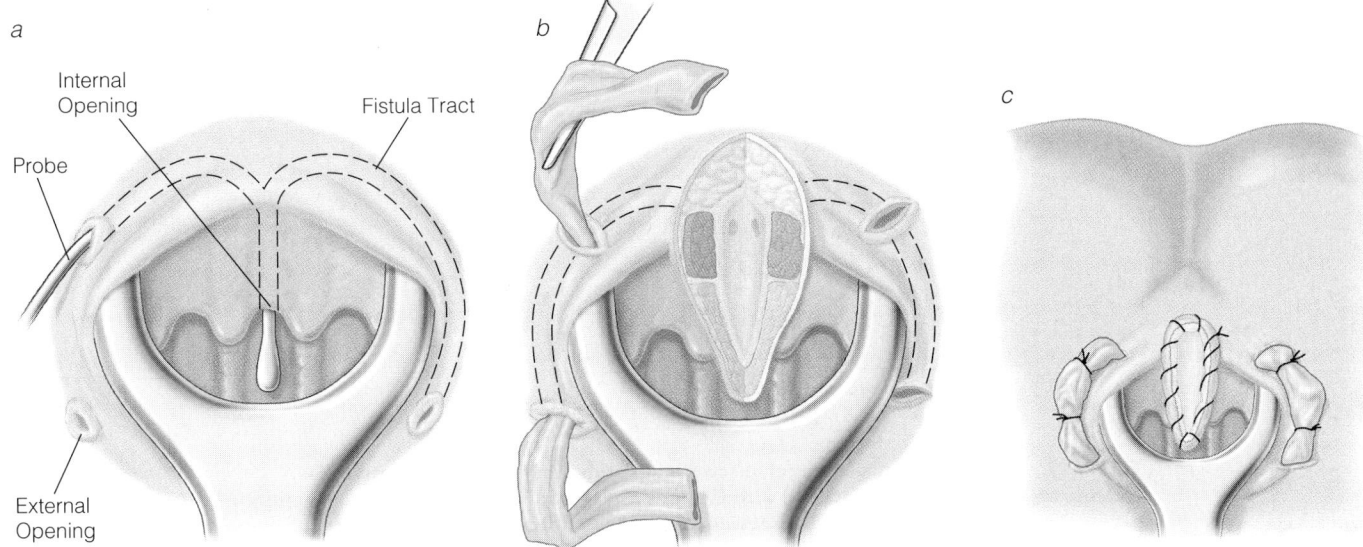

Figure 12 **Operative management of abscess and fistula. Shown is the surgical treatment of a horseshoe fistula. (*a*) The main posterior tract of the fistula is identified by probing. (*b*) The posterior tract is opened, and drains are placed laterally. (*c*) The posterior tract is marsupialized.**

removed until there is solid healing in the posterior midline; this may take weeks or even months.

Abscess and Fistula Associated with Crohn's Disease

The goals of treatment are to drain and control the focus of infection, to preserve sphincter function, to plan and implement a staged approach to preservation of anorectal function, and to make the correct diagnosis. To these ends, careful identification of the location and course of the abscess and any associated fistulas is essential; this is accomplished via endoscopic dye injection, probing, and vaginoscopy.

The safest approach, in my view, is to place mushroom catheters in abscesses and complicated fistula tracts or, in some cases, to use setons to allow drainage of the fistulas (not to cut through the tissue, which is often the intended result of seton placement) [see Figure 13]. For optimal resolution of inflammation at the site of the internal opening in anticipation of a possible advancement flap procedure, perirectal mushroom catheters are preferable to setons placed through the internal opening. Superficial fistula tracts may occasionally be managed with fistulotomy if the Crohn's disease is otherwise inactive. Sphincterotomy is never indicated in a patient with Crohn's disease if severe infection is present or the disease is active. When a patient is known or believed to have Crohn's disease, biopsy of the edematous external skin tags that are often present can be a good way of finding granulomatous tissue to confirm the diagnosis.

The newer forms of medical treatment of Crohn's disease, in which a monoclonal antibody to tumor necrosis factor (infliximab) is given either by itself or in combination with immunosuppressive agents, seem to display some of their most beneficial results in patients with complicated anoperineal fistulas. In my view, a good way of managing abscess and fistula associated with Crohn's disease is for the surgeon to drain and control the suppurative process and for the gastroenterologist then to employ the latest medical regimen to force the disease into remission.

Hidradenitis Suppurativa

Patients with infected fistula tracts or abscesses secondary to hidradenitis suppurativa must be positioned in such a way as to allow visualization of and access to all tracts. This is crucial because some of the tracts may extend into the scrotum, the labia, the inguinal areas, or the suprapubic area. Conduction anesthesia is important in that it covers broad areas of the perineum; adequate local anesthesia is impossible unless one is dealing with very small, isolated tracts.

The definitive therapeutic surgical procedure is incision (rather than excision) of these often extensive inflammatory tracts [see Figure 14]. The surgeon should do as much as possible at one time, with the understanding that it is not unusual to leave a few tracts undrained or to return later to address new areas of dissection. Because the primary disease process does not involve the sphincter, intestinal diversion is rarely indicated. Biopsy is indicated because on rare occasions, these long infected tracts exhibit malignant changes or result from an anal malignancy. The perineal skin can tolerate the extensive incisions necessary to cure the process. Special precautions must be taken not only to preserve the sphincter itself but also to avoid damaging the neurovascular bundle that enters the anus from the posterolateral aspect. In male patients, efforts must be made to avoid the urethra during incision in the anterior midline; to this end, a Foley catheter should always be placed before the surgical procedure is begun. Because so many incised skin edges remain after treatment of extensive hidradenitis, it is imperative to achieve adequate hemostasis. The disposable suction cautery units currently available can be especially helpful for this purpose. The wounds may be either left open or loosely packed until good granulation tissue forms.

Bathing the perineum, especially after a bowel movement, is helpful. Often, showers are better for this purpose than the portable minuscule sitz baths commonly used. For patients who have undergone extensive procedures, twice-daily trips to a whirlpool bath (often located in the physical therapy department) are helpful. Despite the multiple lengthy incisions, there is usually little pain, and most of the postoperative care can be done at home. Adequate follow-up is necessary to treat residual or new areas of disease before the dissection becomes extensive again. Care must be taken, especially in the OR, to search for the infected tracts, which may contain little pus

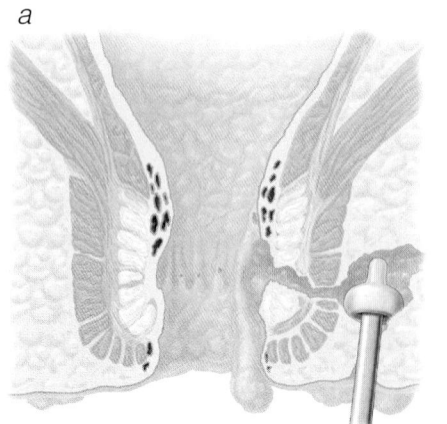 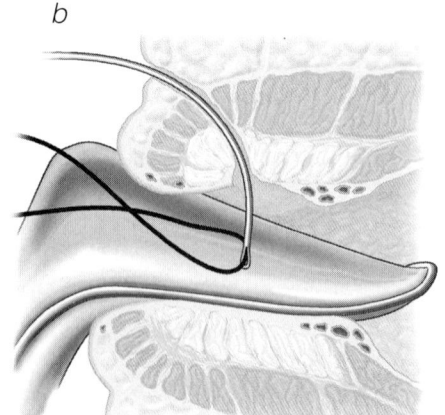

a   b

Figure 13 **Operative management of abscess and fistula. Shown are alternatives for treating abscess or fistula associated with Crohn's disease. In Crohn's disease, multiple perianal and perineal fistulas and abscesses may be seen, often in atypical locations. (a) Abscesses may be drained by placing a small mushroom-tipped catheter as close to the anus as possible. A Malecot catheter should not be used. (b) In some settings, it is appropriate to place a seton between internal and external openings. This seton may then be left in situ for a time for drainage and for prevention of further disease progression.**

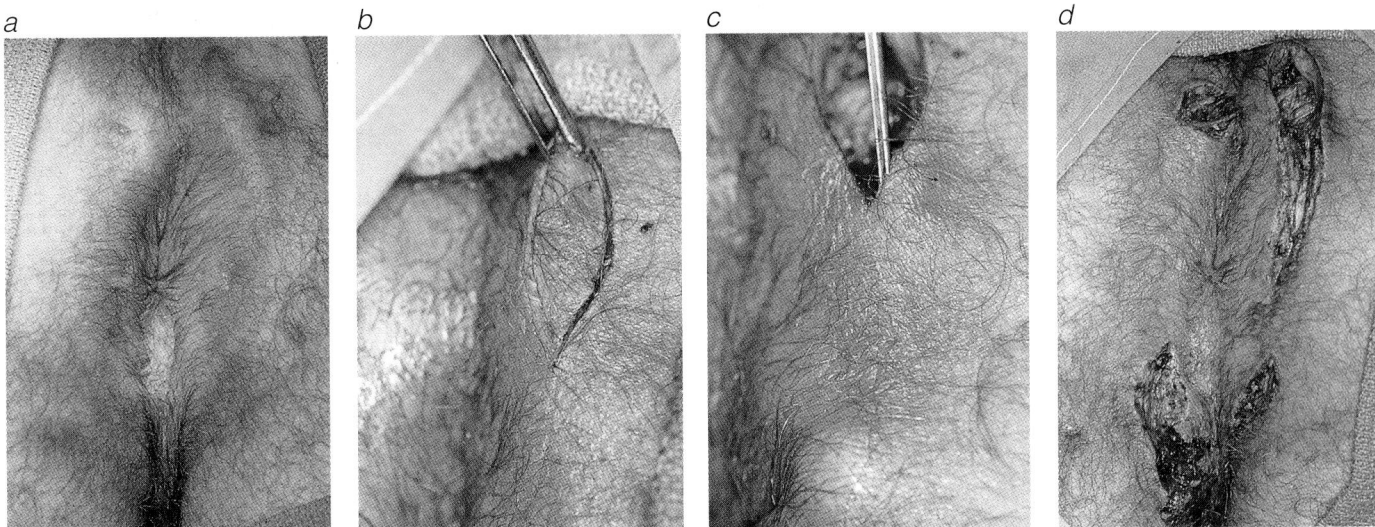

Figure 14 **Operative management of abscess and fistula. In this patient, the causative condition is hidradenitis suppurativa. (*a*) Multiple openings of sinus tracts can be seen and extensive indurated tracts palpated. (*b*) Abscesses are unroofed. (*c*) Indurated tracts are probed. (*d*) All tracts are identified and incised.**

and may be apparent only as indurated cords within the perineal skin.

TROUBLESHOOTING

Most of the important steps for avoiding problems have already been described in the course of addressing preoperative planning and operative technique (see above). The goals in the treatment of all of the processes associated with anorectal abscess and fistula in ano are to preserve sphincter function, to control acute infection, and to eliminate the source of the infection. If it is likely that sphincter function will be compromised at all, a baseline level of sphincter function (including the status of muscles and nerves) must be determined before any surgical procedure is initiated. One should never hesitate to perform an examination with the patient under anesthesia and to inject dilute methylene blue to delineate the extent and location of the infectious process.

Anyone embarking on surgical management of such processes must keep in mind the option of performing an advancement flap procedure to close the internal opening, especially in the anterior region and most particularly in women. If such a procedure is planned, initial drainage should be done external to the rectum with a mushroom catheter rather than through the internal opening with a seton. Simple 3-0 chromic catgut should be used to marsupialize fistula tracts because employing the newer, less quickly absorbable materials may lead to a chronic nidus that gives rise to ongoing infection. Patients should be watched closely in the immediate postoperative period to ensure that all infection is controlled. Not uncommonly, a superficial collection is drained, but a deeper abscess remains that must be sought more aggressively.

One should always take into account the risk of anoperineal infection in immunocompromised patients. Given that the anatomy of the anal tissue planes is complex and can be rendered even more so by multiple surgical procedures, one should not venture beyond one's level of expertise. One should never hesitate to drain an infectious focus with a simple mushroom-tipped catheter and, if appropriate, refer the patient to a colon and rectal surgical specialist who is trained to manage complex anoperineal suppurative processes safely and definitively.

COMPLICATIONS

Complications occur if one or more of the goals just mentioned (see above) have not been achieved. Persistent or recurrent infection is seen with some frequency. In patients with cryptoglandular abscess or fistula, infection usually results from failure to locate the internal opening or to discover a deep posterior midline abscess; such failure is often seen in patients with a horseshoe abscess, in whom repeated lateral drainage procedures may have been undertaken without the primary cavity in the posterior anal or posterior rectal space being discovered and dealt with.

In patients with Crohn's disease, infection can persist if a deeper pocket or extension has gone undiscovered or if the disease has recurred, leading to further penetration and infection in the anoperineum or the perirectal tissue. Extensive examination with the patient under anesthesia, including transrectal ultrasonography or CT scanning, may be required to determine the source and extent of the infection. It is always possible that the infection derives from a superlevator abscess secondary to intestinal disease; consequently, a detailed evaluation of the intestinal tract is indicated in patients with Crohn's disease.

In patients with hidradenitis suppurativa, the most common problems are residual undrained tracts and recurrent disease. Again, examination with the patient under anesthesia and repeated drainage are called for. Because this disease process does not originate in the rectum, care must be taken not to enter the rectum or to cut any of the nerves entering the anus from the posterolateral aspect. It has been reported anecdotally that very chronic or persistent fistula tracts may eventually exhibit malignant changes (squamous cell carcinoma); for this reason, such tracts should be biopsied.

OUTCOME EVALUATION

No sophisticated surveillance is necessary: if drainage persists or some degree of incontinence develops, the patient usually will volunteer the information freely. Either of these complaints could be an indication for a detailed examination, including a sophisticated evaluation of sphincter function.

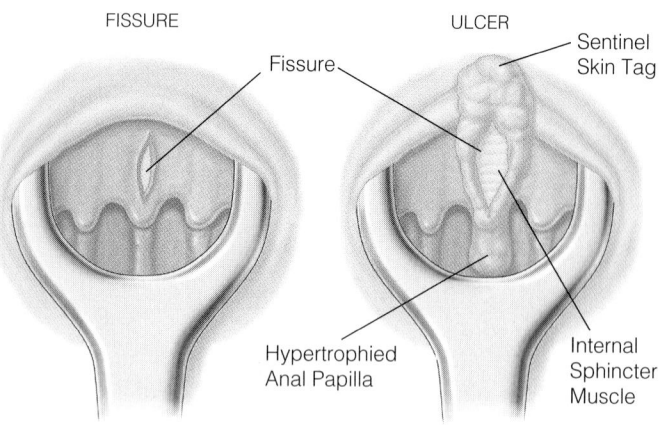

Figure 15 **Operative management of ulcer/fissure disease. Anal fissure (left) and anal ulcer (right) are, respectively, the acute aspect and the chronic aspect of a single disease process.**

FISSURE

Fissure

ULCER

Sentinel Skin Tag

Hypertrophied Anal Papilla

Internal Sphincter Muscle

Operative Management of Ulcer/Fissure Disease

Ulcer and fissure are two aspects of a single anorectal disease process with an unclearly defined pathophysiology [*see Figure 15*]. Accurate diagnosis is crucial [*see Sidebar* Ulcer/Fissure Disease: Diagnosis and Treatment]. Not uncommonly, patients are treated for hemorrhoids when the true primary condition is ulcer/fissure disease.

OPERATIVE PLANNING

Fundamental concerns in planning the operation—besides confirming the diagnosis—are to verify that there are no other conditions that could threaten complete healing of an incision in the anal tissue and to make sure that there is no significant incontinence before the sphincterotomy.

For example, a history of diarrhea compatible with the presence of inflammatory bowel disease indicates the need for further evaluation to eliminate the possibility of Crohn's disease; if Crohn's disease is present, the risk of poor healing is greater, and it will be necessary to preserve all of the available sphincter function of the anus for a long period. As another example, a woman who has borne children by vaginal delivery and has any degree of incontinence should undergo manometry, ultrasonography, and perhaps electromyography to confirm that the sphincter is not compromised by a mechanical or neurologic deficiency. Yet another example is a patient with irritable bowel syndrome or a pelvic floor abnormality who experiences a multitude of difficulties with bowel movements. It is important to recognize such conditions and to advise the patient of the need for special attention to maintain adequate bowel function in the postoperative period.

It is essential to clearly explain the nature of the operative procedure (i.e., the incision of a portion of the internal sphincter mechanism) to the patient and to warn him or her that minor incontinence of flatus may persist for as long as a few months postoperatively. To be fair, significant incontinence is highly unusual: in fact, most patients experience very rapid relief of their often distressing symptoms. One should also advise the patient that any other anal procedures that may be indicated (e.g., elastic ligation of internal hemorrhoids or excision of symptomatic external hemorrhoids) can and should be accomplished at the time of sphincterotomy, with or without excision of the anal ulcer, and that he or she should take 3 to 5 days off from work. The risk of urinary

Ulcer/Fissure Disease: Diagnosis and Treatment

This condition is a very common one; however, the pathophysiology remains unclearly defined. Like abscess and fistula, ulcer/fissure disease has an acute phase and a chronic phase.

A fissure (the acute phase) results from a tear in the tissue at the mucocutaneous junction of the anal canal. The cause is usually a hard bowel movement that stretches the anal opening and tears the tissue. In fact, fissures are also seen in patients with persistent diarrhea. The anal canal has an extremely rich blood supply, and most fissures heal with bowel control (i.e., bulk-forming agents and stool softeners), warm soaks, and mild analgesics. Patients must be assured that although the condition is extremely painful and is associated with some degree of bleeding, it is not a significant health threat.

For reasons that are not clear, perhaps as many as 50% of fissures do not heal spontaneously. As the opening persists, the surrounding tissue becomes hypertrophied and the process extends into the underlying internal sphincter muscle as an ulcer (the chronic phase) with a sentinel hemorrhoidal tag and a hypertrophied anal papilla (the triad of findings typical of an anal ulcer). Spasm and hypertrophy of the lower third of the internal sphincter muscle of the anal canal are always associated with this condition. Many believe, as I do, that spasm of this involuntary muscle results in diminishment of the blood supply to the anal canal and subsequent poor healing of the acute tear. It seems that as the process persists, the ulcer burrows deeper. The condition then becomes more painful, and the muscular spasm evolves into actual hypertrophy. At present, optimal therapy is based on the principle of incising the hypertrophied band of muscle, releasing the spasm, and improving the relative ischemia, thus allowing the injury to heal.

Ulcer/fissure disease can usually be diagnosed on the basis of the typical history of sudden onset of anal pain (often with a tearing sensation) and bleeding. Symptoms are usually exacerbated during bowel movements and may go on for weeks to months with intermit-

tent healing and recrudescence of the process as the ischemia prevents solid, definitive healing. Diagnosis is complicated in that digital rectal examination can be extremely painful, and most physicians do not have the equipment and skills to perform an adequate anoscopic examination. If examination is too painful, local anesthesia may be necessary. Diagnosis can be facilitated by passage of a lubricated cotton swab to look for the typical streak of blood from the ulcer.

Medical treatment is often begun before the specific diagnosis can be verified. I usually try 2 weeks of medical therapy, often including topical antibiotics and anti-inflammatory suppositories or foam preparations. Once the diagnosis is confirmed, it becomes the patient's choice whether or when to undergo surgical treatment. I explain that the reason for the operation is to relieve discomfort, not to cure a life-threatening condition; however, I also point out that once significant spasm and hypertrophy of the sphincter are identified, definitive cure is unlikely unless a sphincterotomy is performed.

Recently, there has been some enthusiasm for alleviating the muscle spasm and hypertrophy and the subsequent ischemia by using medical rather than surgical measures. The most popular medical approaches are (1) topical application of a low-concentration nitroglycerin paste (a much less concentrated preparation than that used to treat cardiac conditions) and (2) local injection of botulinum toxin. The initial enthusiasm for these modalities notwithstanding, it remains to be seen whether they provide any long-term benefit in comparison with anal sphincterotomy. In addition, some reports have described the use of oral diltiazem to reduce sphincter spasm and ischemia. Again, it remains to be seen whether this approach consistently leads to long-term resolution of the pathologic process.

In my own experience, when a fissure is present, resolution can be achieved with any of a number of nonsurgical maneuvers; however, when an ulcer with muscle hypertrophy is present, surgical management ultimately proves necessary for resolution.

retention, pain, and bleeding must also be discussed. In planning the operative procedure and immediate postoperative care, one must take into account the patient's specific needs, idiosyncrasies, and home environment. Some patients are comfortable undergoing the procedure completely on an outpatient basis, whereas others clearly need to be admitted for short-term observation and parenteral administration of pain medication.

When possible, I keep patients on a liquid diet for 24 hours before operation and use small, self-administered enemas to empty the rectum immediately before the procedure. I advise patients to discontinue any aspirin-containing products and any other anticoagulants, if possible, at least 10 days beforehand.

OPERATIVE TECHNIQUE

Operative treatment of ulcer/fissure disease consists of a posterior lateral internal anal sphincterotomy, in which the internal sphincter is divided but the external sphincter, the anoderm, and the longitudinal muscle remain intact. I generally prefer to place the patient in the prone-flexed position with the buttocks taped apart and adequate local anesthesia in place. The operation can then be performed in one of three ways: (1) as a closed procedure involving the use of a No. 11 blade and digital palpation of the muscle [see Figure 16], (2) as an open procedure without direct visualization of the muscle, or (3) as an open procedure with clear identification of the muscle before its transection. The third option is the one I prefer.

An open procedure with visualization of the muscle is done as follows [see Figure 17]. The first step is anoscopy, preferably with a medium Hill-Ferguson instrument. The hypertrophied band of the lower third of the internal sphincter muscle is clearly identified. If this band is not a distinctly identifiable entity, sphincterotomy should not be performed. The ulcer or fissure itself need not be present, because the disease may be in a relatively inactive state at the time of surgery.

Rigid or flexible sigmoidoscopy should then be performed if it was not done in the immediate preoperative period. The primary purpose of this step is to make sure that no features of Crohn's disease are visible in the rectum. When the endoscopic examination is complete, I usually repeat the preparation of the anal opening.

A 1 cm incision is made in the posterior lateral aspect of the perianal skin, hemostasis is obtained, and a delicate dissection is done with a curved hemostat in the intersphincteric plane. The posterior midline is avoided because healing in this position may result in scar tissue that interferes with perfect continence (the so-called keyhole deformity). The white hypertrophied band of muscle is then elevated into the wound with a curved hemostat. If a rent is made in the anal mucosa, it must be repaired with 3-0 chromic catgut. The band of muscle is then incised with the electrocautery, and pressure is maintained for a few minutes to ensure hemostasis. Digital examination confirms adequate transection of the band. The skin is left open.

Attention is then directed to the ulcer, which may be excised sharply in an elliptical fashion so as to incorporate the entire triad of the ulcer (i.e., the ulcer itself, the sentinel hemorrhoidal tag, and the hypertrophied anal papilla) while avoiding additional transection of the underlying muscle. If I excise the ulcer complex, I usually close the wound with a continuous three-point suture of 3-0 chromic catgut to obliterate any dead space and thus to lower the risk of postoperative infection.

Any additional anal surgery required is then completed, the surgical site is covered with antibiotic ointment, and a very light gauze bandage is applied with a minimum of tape and traction on the perianal skin.

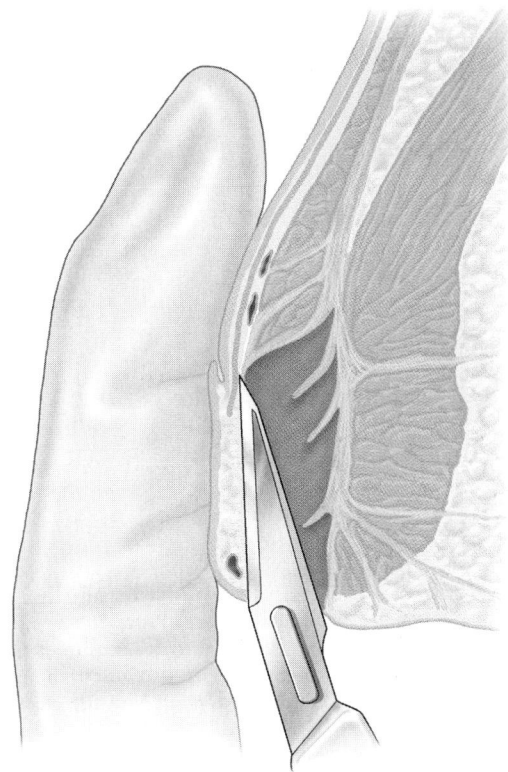

Figure 16 **Operative management of ulcer/fissure disease. Shown is the closed approach to posterior lateral internal sphincterotomy. A No. 11 blade is inserted in the intersphincteric groove and moved upward to the level of the dentate line. Medial movement of the blade divides a portion of the internal sphincter muscle. The anoderm and the other anal muscles are not divided.**

TROUBLESHOOTING

To perform this simple procedure well, one must have a clear understanding of the surgical anatomy of the anal canal and must be able to clearly identify the internal sphincter, the intersphincteric groove, and the external sphincter muscle. The hypertrophied band of muscle must be accurately identified and cleanly transected. No attempt should be made to extend or amplify the procedure by stretching the anal canal and thus bursting the muscle.

Although the procedure and anatomy are simple, the best way of learning the operation is to watch an experienced surgeon perform it. I do not believe this procedure can be learned through reading alone.

COMPLICATIONS

Because the internal sphincter muscle is responsible for resting, involuntary continence, injury to this structure can lead to nocturnal incontinence. Again, special caution is advised with respect to the anterior aspect of the anoperineum in women. On the other hand, incising the posterior midline can also lead to the keyhole deformity, which may cause prolonged anal seepage because of the configuration of the scar tissue; a good analogy is a bent rim on a tubeless tire. It is tempting to close the tiny skin incision at the site of sphincterotomy, but I think it should be left open to reduce the already low risk of infection.

There should be very little postoperative pain. If the patient does complain of significant pain, especially in the presence of fever or urinary hesitancy, one must assume that infection is present in the anoperineum, a structure that is normally highly

a
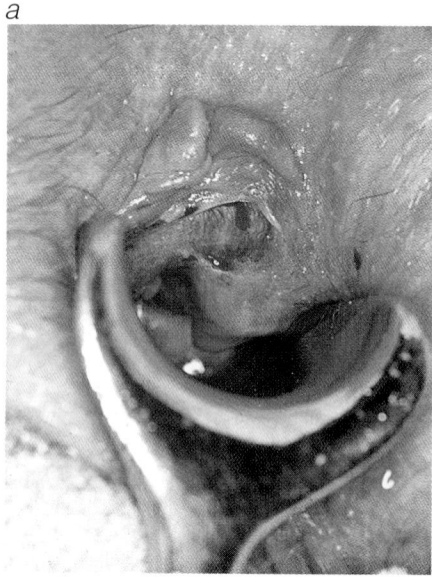

b
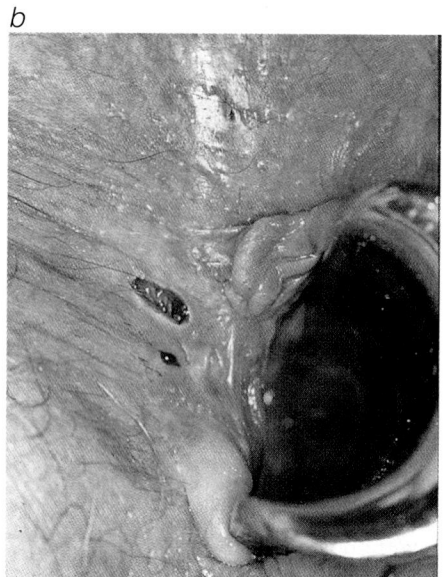

c
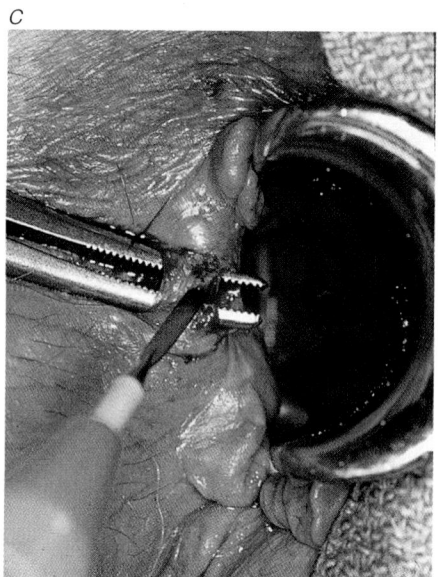

Figure 17 **Operative management of ulcer/fissure disease. Shown is the open approach to posterior lateral internal sphincterotomy. (*a*) The triad of the ulcer complex is visualized. (*b*) Once the hypertrophied band of internal sphincter muscle is identified, a 1 cm incision is made in the posterolateral aspect of the perianal skin. (*c*) The hypertrophied band is elevated into the wound and divided with the electrocautery.**

resistant to microbial invasion. Urgent evaluation, removal of sutures, antibiotic therapy, bowel rest, placement of a urinary catheter, and very close observation in the hospital are indicated.

The major causes of complications are incorrect diagnosis of the disease process (especially overlooking the presence of Crohn's disease) and failure to fully understand the anatomy of the continence mechanism of the anal canal. If too much of the internal sphincter muscle is cut, if this muscle is already compromised, or if the external sphincter muscle is transected by mistake, the patient will be rendered incontinent. On the other hand, if not enough of the internal muscle is transected, the ulcer will not heal and the symptoms will persist.

Overall, the single most common cause of complications that I have observed is the failure even to suspect, much less diagnose, ulcer/fissure disease as the source of a patient's symptoms. I frequently see patients who seem to have failed to heal months after a hemorrhoidectomy. When their symptoms are reviewed and a thorough examination performed, it becomes apparent that the underlying disease process was always ulcer/fissure dis-

ease rather than hemorrhoids and that the hemorrhoidectomy only intensified the anal pain and bleeding. These patients are finally cured when an adequate sphincterotomy is performed.

In very rare instances, drainage continues at the site of the sphincterotomy. If drainage persists for weeks, the patient should be examined under appropriate anesthesia, and the focus of infection should be opened. This is essentially equivalent to a very superficial fistulotomy.

OUTCOME EVALUATION

Again, no sophisticated surveillance is necessary: when the patient returns 2 weeks after the procedure, free of pain and bleeding and able to have bowel movements without difficulty, one may be sure that an acceptable outcome has been achieved. Digital rectal examination should confirm good healing and normal sphincter tone (both while resting and while contracting). For additional confirmation, I have patients continue to take bulk-forming agents and stool softeners and then examine them 1 month later to verify that healing is complete.

References

1. Practice parameters for antibiotic prophylaxis to prevent infective endocarditisor infected prosthesis during colon and rectal endoscopy. Standards Practice Task Force, American Society of Colon and Rectal Surgeons. Dis Colon Rectum 35:277, 1992

2. Kodner IJ, Fry RD, Fleshman JW, et al: Colon, rectum and anus. Principles of Surgery, 6th ed. Schwartz SI, Ed. McGraw-Hill, New York, 1994

Recommended Reading

Corman ML: Colon and Rectal Surgery, 3rd ed. JB Lippincott Co, Philadelphia, 1993

Fry RD, Kodner IJ: Anorectal disorders. Clin Symp 37:6, 1985

Gordon PH, Nivatvongs S: Principles and Practice of Surgery for the Colon, Rectum and Anus. Quality Medical Publishers, St. Louis, 1992

Keighley MRB, Williams NS: Surgery of the Anus, Rectum and Colon, Vols 1 and 2. WB Saunders, London, 1993

Kodner IJ: Differential diagnosis and management of benign anorectal diseases. Gastrointestinal Diseases Today 5:8, 1996

Standards Practice Task Force, American Society of Colon and Rectal Surgeons: Practice parameters for treatment of fistula-in-ano. Dis Colon Rectum 39:1361, 1996

Acknowledgment

Figures 1, 5b, 5c, 8 through 13, 15, 16 Tom Moore. Adapted from original illustrations by John Craig.

27 COLORECTAL PROCEDURES

Theodore R. Schrock, M.D., F.A.C.S.

Total Colectomy with Ileorectal Anastomosis

OPERATIVE PLANNING

Total colectomy involves resection of the entire colon with oversewing of the rectum or construction of an ileorectal anastomosis. Candidates for this operation include certain patients with inflammatory bowel disease, familial adenomatous polyposis, hereditary nonpolyposis colorectal cancer syndromes, chronic constipation, or severe lower gastrointestinal hemorrhage [*see 3:7 Lower Gastrointestinal Bleeding*].[1-5] The operation is performed in two stages in patients with fulminant colitis, severe inflammation of the rectum, pelvic abscess, or severe associated disease. Some surgeons perform total colectomy with ileorectal anastomosis via a laparoscopic or laparoscopic-assisted approach[6] [*see 3:28 Laparoscopic Colectomy*]; however, in what follows, I address only conventional open techniques.

OPERATIVE TECHNIQUE

Step 1: Positioning and Incision

The lithotomy position, with the lower extremities in Lloyd-Davies leg rests or Allen universal stirrups, has the advantage of providing good access to the anus. The rectum can be examined and irrigated with saline before preparation and draping, and intraoperative colonoscopy, stapling maneuvers, and inspection of the anastomosis for integrity can be performed.

The positioning of the surgical team depends on the experience and the anticipated role of the assistants. If the first assistant is able to dissect under the surgeon's guidance, the surgeon should stand on the patient's left side, a position that gives the surgeon control of retraction and exposure of the right colon and the transverse colon. (I assume this arrangement in the description of the procedure.) When working on the left colon, the assistant retracts with one hand and dissects with the other, while the surgeon displays the tissues to be incised laterally. In the teaching environment, positions sometimes shift around the table.

A midline incision is standard, but a transverse incision below the umbilicus is feasible in slender patients and in patients with long-standing inflammatory bowel disease, which often shortens the colon and the mesocolon.

Step 2: Mobilization and Removal of the Colon

The sigmoid colon is occluded with an encircling ligature of heavy material (e.g., umbilical tape) to prevent perineal soilage from distal passage of colonic contents.

Mobilization of the colon usually begins on the right side. The surgeon pinches the peritoneal surfaces together lateral to the cecum to protect the bowel from injury, and the peritoneum is incised very close to the cecal wall. The surgeon inserts the left

index finger into the defect, retracting the cecum and the ascending colon medially while the lateral peritoneum is incised [*see Figure 1*]. The white line of Toldt is ignored on the right side, and the peritoneum is incised as close to the colon as possible. (Incising the peritoneum close to the wall of the right colon makes it unlikely that the surgeon will incise Gerota's fascia and dissect into perinephric fat.) The cecum is pulled laterally, and the medial layer of peritoneum of the distal ileal mesentery is incised proximally as far as necessary. The right ureter is identified.

As the hepatic flexure is approached, the duodenum appears, and the mesocolon is detached from it by dividing filmy tissue containing tiny vessels. In patients with benign disease, separation of the mesocolon from the duodenum up to the pancreas is unnecessary, but it does facilitate division of the mesocolon. In patients with cancer, full mobilization is necessary to ensure that vessels are ligated close to their origin. Hepatic flexure attachments contain vessels of varying size, some of which are large enough to necessitate ligation.

At this point, the surgeon must decide whether to preserve the greater omentum or to remove it. If the omentum is to be preserved, it is detached from the transverse colon; if it is to be removed, the gastrocolic ligament is serially divided and ligated. (I prefer to excise the greater omentum with the colonic specimen because the omentum causes obstruction of the small bowel after total colectomy much more frequently than it does after segmental colectomy.)

The lesser sac is entered to the left of the midline. (One should do this before the hepatic flexure is taken down completely and then work back to the right.) In the lesser sac, adhesions of the stomach to the transverse mesocolon are lysed, the gastrocolic ligament is serially divided and ligated outside the gastroepiploic vessels [*see Figure 2*], and the hepatic flexure is approached from the left. The mesocolon is left intact until it is fully separated from the gastrocolic, duodenal, and pancreatic attachments. The ileocolic, right colic (if present), and middle colic vessels are then divided at a level determined by the pathologic problem being treated [*see Figure 3*]. (Some surgeons preserve the ileocolic vessels in case a pelvic pouch is possible later; however, because I deliberately divide the ileocolic vessels when constructing an ileoanal pouch, I do not preserve them when fashioning an ileorectal anastomosis.) The ileum is divided at the ileocecal valve with a linear cutting stapler or between intestinal clamps.

Once the dissection has reached the distal transverse colon, the sigmoid colon is mobilized so that the splenic flexure can be approached from the left and below. The sigmoid colon and the mesocolon are retracted to the right by the assistant, who remains on the patient's right side. Adhesions of the appendices epiploicae, the colon, and the mesocolon to the parietal peritoneal attachments of the descending colon are incised a little at a time. (If the colonic attachments are divided all the way to the splenic flexure first, one can stray too far laterally and even end up within Gerota's fascia. The surgeon can insert one or two fingers into the space behind the peritoneum to display the next

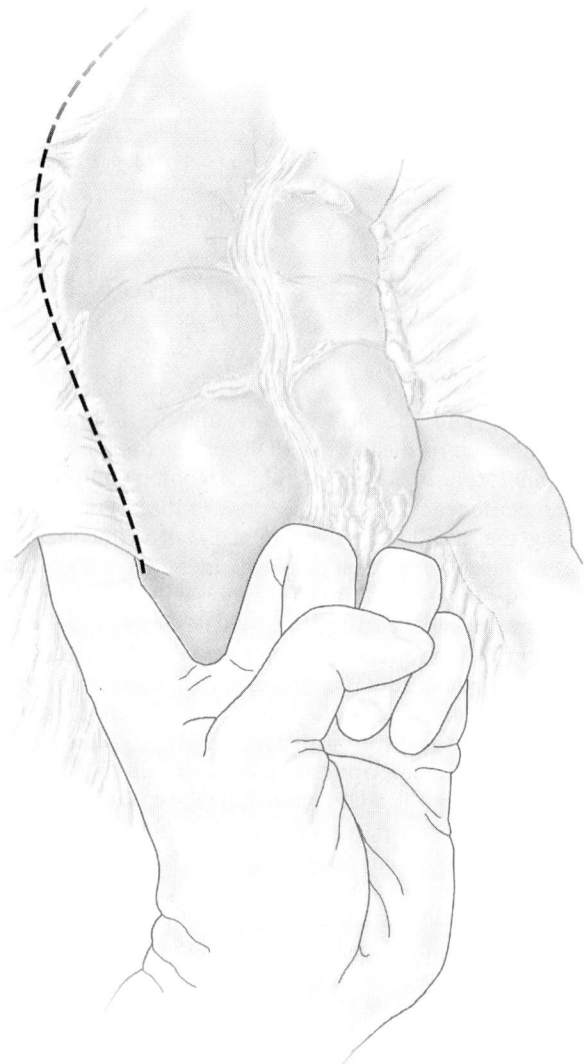

Figure 1 Total colectomy with ileorectal anastomosis. The surgeon inserts the left index finger into the peritoneal defect, retracting the cecum and the ascending colon medially while the lateral peritoneum is incised as close to the colon as possible.[33]

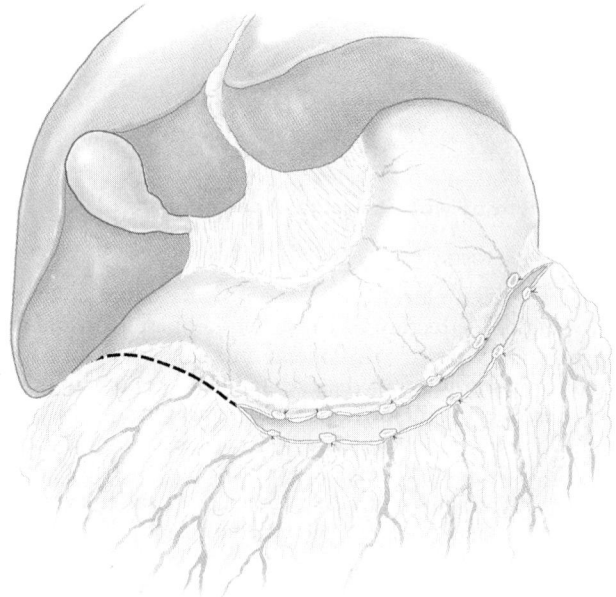

Figure 2 Total colectomy with ileorectal anastomosis. The gastrocolic ligament is serially divided and ligated outside the gastroepiploic vessels, and the hepatic flexure is approached from the left.[33]

toneum are divided. (This must be done in a bloodless plane. No fat should be cut in mobilizing the sigmoid colon. There is no fat in the proper plane; if one is cutting through fat, one is in the wrong plane.)

The sigmoid colon is then pulled farther to the right, and the mesosigmoid is incised at its base. (The incision should be made on the left side, medial to the left ureter. If the ureter is not seen through the intact posterior parietal peritoneum, it should be visible after this incision is made.) The peritoneal incision is extended longitudinally, parallel to the course of the ureter, and the ureter is swept laterally. (Care should be taken to avoid the sympathetic nerves on the surface of the aorta, about 1 cm posterior to the superior hemorrhoidal vessels; injury to these nerves can cause ejaculatory impairment. In men with benign disease, there is no need to risk such impairment. Accordingly, dissection in the vicinity should be minimized once the ureter is seen and protected.)

The splenic flexure is taken down by approaching it from the left, from below, and from behind. The colon and the mesocolon are separated from Gerota's fascia, and the lateral peri-

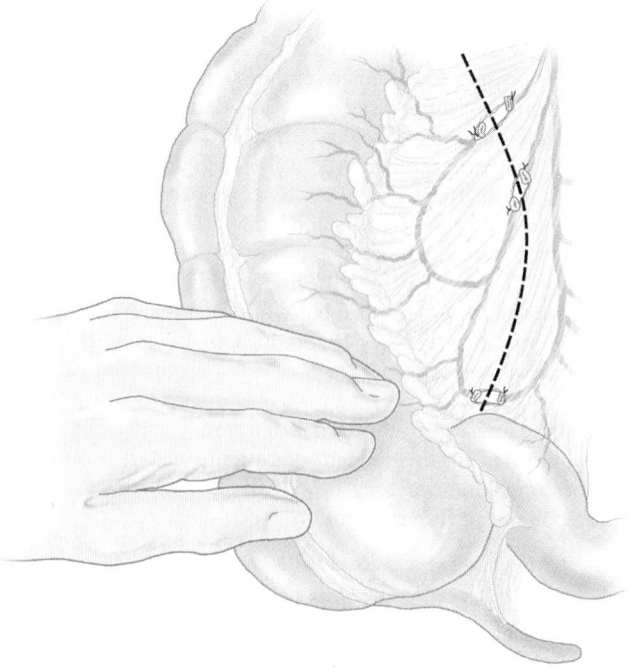

Figure 3 Total colectomy with ileorectal anastomosis. The ileocolic, right colic, and middle colic vessels are ligated and divided at a level called for by the pathologic problem being treated.[33]

portion for incision [*see Figure 4*]. It is important that the path of dissection remain within a few millimeters of the colon as the flexure is taken down. In this way, one follows the plane of attachment of the omentum, which is relatively avascular.) These maneuvers separate the omentum from the colon. If the omentum is to be removed, the remaining portion of the gastrocolic ligament must be divided and ligated so that a connection can be made with the plane established earlier.

The anterior layer of the peritoneum of the transverse mesocolon must be incised to take the splenic flexure down. Behind this thin layer, of course, lie the mesocolic vessels, which must be ligated. In patients with malignant disease, the inferior mesenteric artery and vein are divided and ligated (usually separately) after the left colic vessels are divided. In men with colitis or another benign disease, it is preferable to divide the left colic vessels and then the sigmoidal branches, leaving the inferior mesenteric vessels intact to obviate dissection in the vicinity of the sympathetic nerves. If the inferior mesenteric vessels must be divided, dissection should be carried out as close to them as possible to minimize the risk of nerve injury. The peritoneum on the right side of the base of the mesosigmoid is incised to facilitate vascular division.

The vessels at the rectosigmoid are divided close to the rectal wall in men with benign disease, and the proximal rectum is prepared for transection by division of the mesorectum. (The rectosigmoid is a 4 cm long transitional zone at the sacral promontory, where the taeniae coli merge into a confluent circular muscle coat and the lumen widens.) The rectum is divided between clamps.

Step 3: Ileorectal Anastomosis

Whether an ileorectal anastomosis should be done by hand suturing or by stapling and whether it should be end-to-end or side-to-end are matters of personal preference. My own predilection is for a side-to-end stapled anastomosis, as described here.

A basic problem in ileorectal anastomosis is that the ileal lumen is substantially smaller than the rectal lumen. When performing an end-to-end anastomosis, one can obviate the luminal discrepancy problem by making an antimesenteric slit in the ileum to enlarge it. Another way of obviating the problem is to construct a side-to-end ileorectal anastomosis, either with sutures or with staples (see below). (One caveat is that side-to-end stapling of a very small ileum to a very large rectum seems to bunch up the ileal wall. Although the anastomosis generally heals well and functions satisfactorily, it may not look quite right to the eye. For this reason, I usually hand suture if the luminal discrepancy is very great.)

In a side-to-end stapled ileorectal anastomosis [*see Figure 5*], the stapled end of the ileum is arranged with the cut edge of the mesentery to the patient's right. A 0 polypropylene purse-string suture is placed on the rectal stump. (A finer suture might break when it is tied.) A divot large enough to accommodate the intraluminal stapler is excised from the antimesenteric wall of the ileum. (I generally prefer to use the largest intraluminal stapler available—31 or 33 mm, depending on the manufacturer—but sometimes the next smaller size seems to fit better.) The anastomosis should be about 1 cm from the stapled stump of the ileum. (It should not be so close that the zone between is devascularized.) A 2-0 polypropylene purse-string suture is placed on the ileal defect. The stapler is inserted through the anus and opened, and the distal purse-string suture is tied. (The stapler should have a flat anvil: if the anvil has a protruding knob, it will bump into the opposite wall.) The shaft is separated, and the anvil is secured

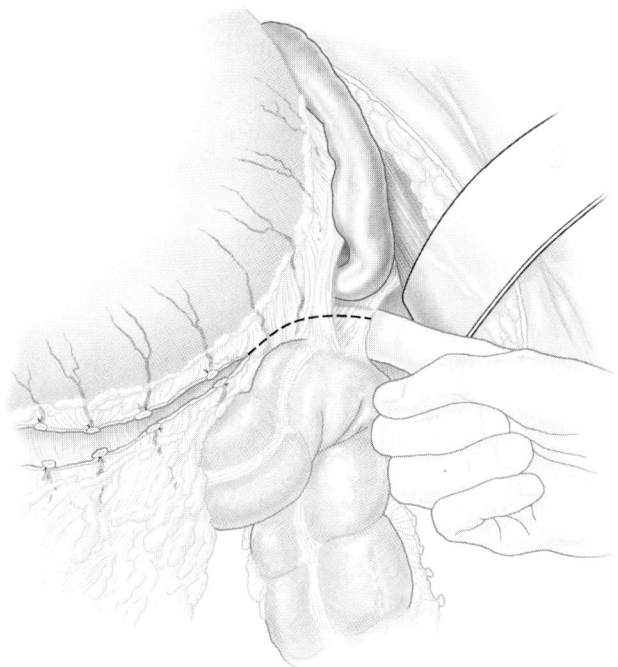

Figure 4 **Total colectomy with ileorectal anastomosis. The surgeon can insert one or two fingers into the space behind the peritoneum to display the next portion for incision.[33] The avascular plane is within a few millimeters of the colon as the flexure is taken down.**

in the ileum by tying the proximal purse-string suture. The stapler is then reassembled and fired. Two intact rings of tissue ("doughnuts") should be obtained. The anastomosis is checked for integrity by inserting a rigid sigmoidoscope through the anus and insufflating air with the pelvis filled with saline.

Step 4: Completion

The edge of the ileal mesentery is sutured to the retroperitoneal surface to eliminate the potential hernial defect. Drains are not required. A diverting loop ileostomy is rarely necessary with this procedure.

COMPLICATIONS

Ileus can be prolonged after total colectomy [*see 3:5 Intestinal Obstruction*]. Obstruction of the small bowel after total colectomy can be minimized by excising the omentum and closing the mesenteric defect. Anastomotic leakage after ileorectal anastomosis is more common in patients with inflammatory bowel disease than in patients with other conditions; in any case, the incidence of this complication should be lower than 4%.[7] Large leaks necessitate reoperation, takedown of the anastomosis, closure of the rectal stump, and end ileostomy until conditions are right for reconnection of the bowel. Small leaks may be managed nonoperatively.

OUTCOME

Return of function depends on the indication for the operation, the presence or absence of rectal disease, the patient's age, and the presence or absence of comorbid factors.[1,2,4,8,9] Once stools begin, diarrhea is the rule, sometimes accompanied by urgency and even minor incontinence. Loperamide is effective against diarrhea. Generally, otherwise healthy persons who undergo total colectomy with ileorectal anastomosis will have from three to five stools a day for the remainder of their lives. This stool pattern does not interfere with physical activities or daily routine. Incontinence should not be a lingering problem once stools slow and thicken, provided that the preoperative assessment of sphincter adequacy was correct.

Total Proctocolectomy with Conventional Ileostomy

OPERATIVE PLANNING

Proctocolectomy with a permanent ileostomy is appropriate for patients with Crohn colitis and for some patients with familial adenomatous polyposis or ulcerative colitis who are not candidates for restorative proctocolectomy because of obesity, advanced age, or the presence of cancer in the distal rectum.[10-13]

Preoperative education of the patient regarding the ileostomy is essential. Either an enterostomal therapist or the surgeon should, if possible, select the site for the stoma with the patient

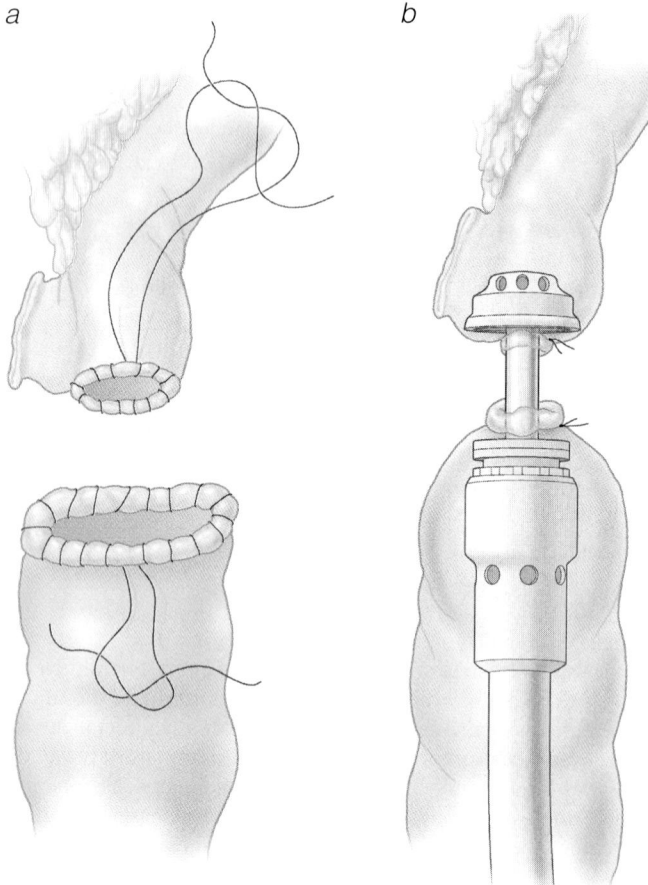

Figure 5 **Total colectomy with ileorectal anastomosis.[33] (*a*) In a side-to-end stapled ileorectal anastomosis, a 0 polypropylene purse-string suture is placed on the rectal stump. A divot is excised from the antimesenteric wall of the ileum, and a 2-0 polypropylene purse-string suture is placed on the ileal defect. (*b*) An end-to-end or intraluminal stapler is inserted through the anus and opened, and the distal purse-string suture is tied. The proximal purse-string suture is tied to secure the anvil in the ileum. The stapler is then reassembled and fired.**

supine, standing, and sitting [*see 3:25 Stomal Care*]. The ileostomy must pass through the rectus sheath and must be located away from depressions and elevations. The ideal site is nearly always in the right lower quadrant.

OPERATIVE TECHNIQUE

Step 1: Positioning

If the operation is to be performed by two teams, the lithotomy position obviously is necessary. If the entire operation is to be performed by a single surgeon, the patient can be repositioned after the abdomen is closed. The anus is closed with a heavy purse-string suture.

Step 2: Creation of Ileostomy Aperture

The first step in creating the ileostomy aperture is to excise a circle of skin about 2.5 cm in diameter.[14] (This aperture should be made before the abdominal incision so as to maintain normal alignment of the layers of the abdominal wall.) My preferred technique is to grasp the skin with a Kocher clamp and elevate it strongly, then to excise a disk of skin with a heavy curved scissors oriented in the longitudinal direction; stress along Langer's lines converts an elliptical aperture on the vertical axis to a circular opening. Dermis that was crushed but not excised is removed with the electrocautery. (Admittedly, this method looks crude, but it nearly always results in a perfect circle.)

The fat is spread with a clamp, not excised. Dead space is not desirable at an ileostomy site. The anterior rectus sheath is incised longitudinally, the rectus is separated with a clamp, and the posterior rectus sheath is exposed. A moist sponge is stuffed into this space, and the aperture is completed after the main abdominal incision is made. (Care should be taken not to injure the inferior epigastric vessels.)

Step 3: Colectomy and Preparation of Ileal Mesentery

Colectomy is carried out as described earlier [*see* Total Colectomy with Ileorectal Anastomosis, *above*]. (It is important to prepare the ileal mesentery in such a way that the bowel projects straight ahead and is not curved by tension on the mesentery. The ileal mesentery is divided in an L fashion so that the blood supply is preserved but the tissue that is to be brought through the abdominal wall is thinned [*see Figure 6*].)

Step 4: Pelvic Dissection

Dissection proceeds close to the rectal wall until well below the sacral promontory. (In this way, one can usually keep from injuring the sympathetic nerves of the superior hypogastric plexus—that is, the presacral nerves. These nerves lie at the level of the aortic bifurcation and divide into the left and right hypogastric nerves, which extend into the pelvis.)

In the classical method of posterior dissection, the presacral connective tissue was incised for a short distance, the surgeon's hand was inserted, and the mesorectum was separated from the endopelvic fascia by blunt dissection; the separation created a characteristic sucking sound. (This technique crudely tears the soft tissues in what the surgeon can only hope is the proper plane, sometimes injuring the presacral veins, the pelvic nerves, or both. Consequently, it should be abandoned except in the most difficult situations, such as in obese men in whom there is limited visibility of the posterior pelvis.) In the method I use, the rectum is pulled forward with a deep pelvic retractor, and the loose areolar tissue between the intact mesorectum and the intact endopelvic fascia is cut with the electrocautery or

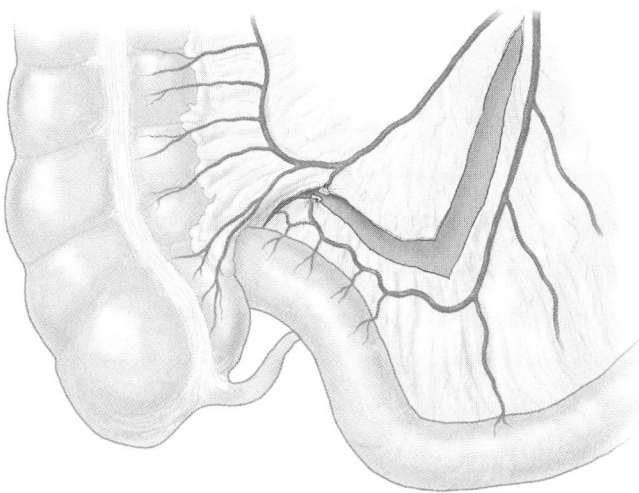

Figure 6 **Total proctocolectomy with conventional ileostomy. The ileal mesentery is divided in an L fashion to thin the tissue that will be brought through the abdominal wall.[14] After the ileocolic vessels are divided and ligated, the mesentery is incised toward the bowel about 1 cm away from the vessels to be preserved; this plane is crossed by no important vessels. The mesenteric incision is then extended at a right angle toward the ileocecal area. Transillumination shows the vessels that must be divided so that the edge of the ileum at the cecum can be reached; there are usually two of these.**

with sharp instruments under direct vision. (This dissection is bloodless or nearly so, and it rarely results in injury to the presacral veins.) Posterior dissection is carried down to the surface of the levator muscles. The pelvic peritoneum is incised bilaterally 1 cm or more medial to the ureters, and the two incisions are connected anteriorly. In men, the rectum is separated from the anterior structures posterior to Denonvilliers' fascia; the seminal vesicles and the prostate are separated from the rectum by blunt dissection or electrocauterization. In women, the rec-

tum is separated from the vagina. If no cancer is present, the lateral dissection should be close to the wall of the rectum. The surgeon's left hand retracts the rectum strongly to the left as the right hand dissects the right side of the pelvis, and the assistant provides the same exposure on the left side. The lateral ligaments are divided completely down to the levators. Either electrocauterization or serial ligation is appropriate.

Step 5: Proctectomy (Perineal Phase)

In patients with benign disease, an intersphincteric proctectomy is performed to minimize the risk of autonomic neurologic sequelae [*see Figure 7*]. In some patients with extensive fistulas, this method is not advantageous or even possible, and an extrasphincteric proctectomy must be done.

For an intersphincteric proctectomy, an elliptical incision is made around the anus over the intersphincteric groove, an easily palpable landmark just at the anal verge. Pennington clamps on the skin edges facilitate retraction. The incision is deepened with the electrocautery or with scissors to display the white fibers of the internal sphincter muscle running circumferentially. (The plane between the internal and external sphincters is fairly obvious laterally and posteriorly because the external sphincter is skeletal muscle and therefore reddish.) Circumferential dissection continues proximally as the longitudinal muscle fibers are cut. Posteriorly, the external sphincter and the puborectalis sling are retracted until the pelvic space is entered by incision through Waldeyer's fascia. The specimen is delivered posteriorly, and the remaining anterior attachments are severed.

Step 6: Closure of Perineal Wound

Sump drains are placed into the pelvic space through the buttocks rather than through the perineal wound itself. The levator muscles are approximated with absorbable sutures, and the soft tissues are closed in layers. The skin is closed with a subcuticular suture. (Primary closure should not be attempted in the presence of anorectal abscesses or complex fistulas.) Closure of the pelvic peritoneum is unnecessary if the perineal wound is sutured primarily.

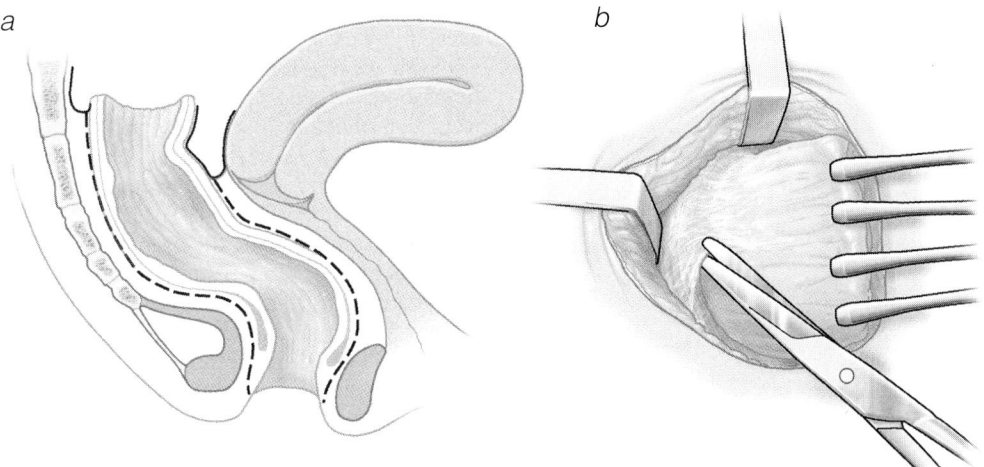

Figure 7 **Total proctocolectomy with conventional ileostomy. The perineal phase usually involves the performance of an intersphincteric proctectomy.[34] (*a*) The pelvic dissection is accomplished from the abdomen, and the perineal dissection preserves the external sphincters and the levators. (*b*) The internal and external sphincters are separated circumferentially by dividing the longitudinal muscle fibers of the gut, which lie in this plane. The specimen is delivered posteriorly (not shown), and the remaining anterior attachments are severed.**

Step 7: Fashioning of Ileostomy

The ileal stump is brought through the aperture so that it projects straight ahead about 5 to 6 cm above the skin.[14] The lateral gutter should be closed to prevent herniation of small bowel around the stoma [*see Figure 8*]. It is unnecessary to suture the bowel to fascia.

A Brooke-type everting ileostomy is fashioned by placing interrupted 4-0 absorbable sutures between the full thickness of the ileal wall and the subcuticular tissue [*see Figure 9*]. One suture in each quadrant also grasps a seromuscular bite of ileum at the skin level. (This facilitates eversion.) The completed stoma should project about 2.5 cm above the skin level. An appliance is placed immediately.

COMPLICATIONS

Early postoperative complications from ileostomy construction include ischemia, paraileostomy abscess, and intestinal obstruction from herniation of small bowel through the gutter.

Perineal wounds may become infected or fail to heal for other reasons. Persistent perineal sinus is a difficult problem that may occur in as many as 50% of patients with Crohn colitis, especially if complex abscesses and fistulas were present at the time of operation.

Postoperative bladder dysfunction is common but is usually transient.

OUTCOME

Operative mortality for proctocolectomy with ileostomy is less than 1% in elective settings; it is higher when the procedure is done on an emergency basis.[8,13] Long-term sequelae include a variety of ileostomy complications, such as retraction, stenosis, prolapse, and paraileostomy hernia. Approximately 90% of patients with a permanent ileostomy are reasonably content, but much depends on the availability of alternatives when the initial operative decision was discussed.[12]

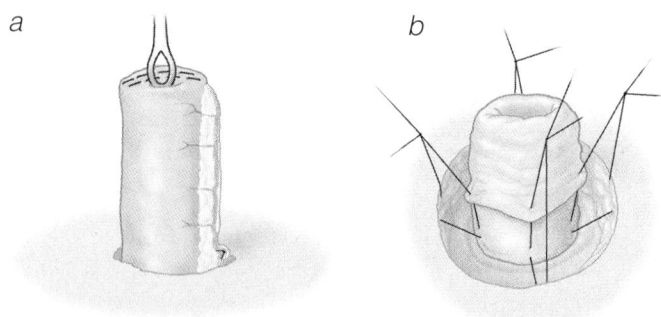

Figure 9 **Total proctocolectomy with conventional ileostomy. A Brooke-type everting ileostomy is fashioned.[14] (*a*) The ileum should project straight ahead for a distance of 5 to 6 cm above the skin. (*b*) One interrupted 4-0 absorbable suture in each quadrant also grasps a seromuscular bite of ileum at the skin level to facilitate eversion. Two additional interrupted sutures (not shown) are placed in each quadrant between the full thickness of the ileal wall and the subcuticular tissue.**

As many as 15% of men who undergo proctocolectomy for benign disease exhibit some postoperative change in sexual function; only about 1% become totally impotent. Some women experience dyspareunia as a result of pelvic fibrosis; others experience sexual dysfunction as a result of altered body image.[15]

Restorative Proctocolectomy with Ileal Pouch–Anal Anastomosis

OPERATIVE PLANNING

Restorative proctocolectomy with ileal pouch–anal anastomosis—complete resection of the colon and rectum and anastomosis of an ileal pouch to the anal canal—is the operation of choice for most patients with ulcerative colitis or familial adenomatous polyposis.[12,15-18] Good anal sphincter function is a requisite. Crohn disease is a contraindication. The operation is difficult but usually possible in obese patients. There is no absolute upper age limit for candidacy for this procedure; however, many elderly, infirm persons may have a better quality of life with an ileostomy. In patients who are acutely ill or malnourished, are receiving huge doses of steroids, or have a significant complication (e.g., perforation), the procedure should be staged.

Whether to perform rectal mucosectomy as part of the procedure is controversial.[19-21] The approach described here involves excising all of the columnar epithelium down to the transitional zone and restoring continuity with a double-stapling technique that renders mucosectomy unnecessary in most patients. The main advantage of this approach is that it minimizes the risk of minor functional impairment resulting from the direct trauma to the sphincters associated with mucosectomy and from the anal dilatation necessary to obtain exposure for mucosectomy. (Insertion of a self-retaining retractor that can be cranked open to improve exposure is risky. Although such devices yield a good view, they can damage the sphincters, often permanently.) The disadvantage of not performing mucosectomy is that one may leave behind some diseased columnar epithelium, which could remain inflamed in patients with ulcerative colitis or become malignant in patients with colitis or polyposis.[21]

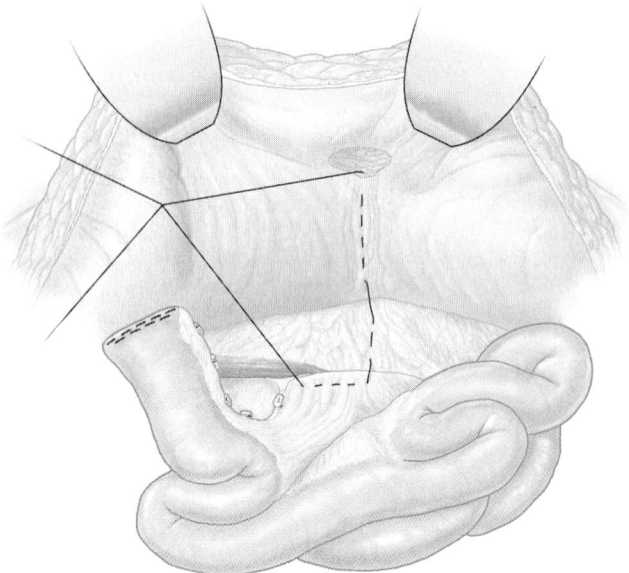

Figure 8 **Total proctocolectomy with conventional ileostomy. One method of closing the gutter uses a purse-string suture passing laterally from the ileostomy aperture to the parietal peritoneum, the retroperitoneal tissue (with care taken to avoid the ureter), and the edge of the mesentery to a point about 8 cm from the ileal stump.[14] The suture is tied and then continued cephalad to the duodenum.**

OPERATIVE TECHNIQUE

Step 1: Positioning

The patient is positioned as for total proctocolectomy with ileostomy.

Step 2: Colectomy and Preparation of Ileal Mesentery

Colectomy is carried out as in total proctocolectomy with ileostomy. (Again, it is important to prepare the ileal mesentery in an L fashion as described for proctocolectomy with ileostomy. Some surgeons preserve the ileocolic vessels, but I do not: if these vessels are divided and the mesentery is prepared properly, the pouch will reach the anus in nearly every instance. It is also important to mobilize the base of the mesocolon and the small bowel mesentery in the hepatic flexure area all the way to the pancreas. Attachments to the duodenum are lysed thoroughly. The peritoneum should be incised on the medial side of the small bowel mesentery all the way up as well.) The ileum is divided with a linear cutting stapler flush with the ileocecal valve.

The ability of the proposed pouch to reach the anus is tested by grasping the ileum about 15 cm proximal to the stapled stump and pulling it to the pubis. If it reaches or extends beyond the lower edge of the pubic bone, there will be no problem; if it does not extend to the lower edge of the pubis, it probably will still reach the anus, but there may be some tension. If additional length is needed, it can be obtained via relaxing incisions through the peritoneum of the mesentery on both sides. (Some surgeons divide mesenteric vessels to gain length, but I have never found this step necessary.) Construction of the pouch is deferred until the colectomy is completed.

Step 3: Proctectomy

The abdominal and pelvic portions of the operation are carried out as described for total proctocolectomy with ileostomy. The rectum is mobilized to the levator muscles circumferentially, but one does not stop at this point: the bowel is dissected from the enveloping puborectal muscles posteriorly and laterally and from urogenital structures anteriorly. (This portion of the large bowel is actually the anal canal. It is lined by columnar epithelium in the upper 1 cm and by transitional epithelium in the lower 1 cm down to the dentate line, though there is anatomic variation in this regard. The pelvic staple line should be in the anal canal rather than the rectum so that diseased mucosa will not be left behind. The surgeon can judge the adequacy of distal mobilization by inserting a finger into the anus from the perineum with the other hand in the pelvis. It is possible to mobilize all the way to the dentate line in most persons, but the intent is to staple across the anal canal 1.0 to 1.5 cm proximal to the dentate line. The end-to-end stapler removes another 1 cm. An assistant can apply pressure to the perineum with a fist, but this is seldom necessary.)

The anal canal is closed off with a right-angle stapler. (I use a 30 mm stapler. If a 30 mm device is too small to close the anal canal across its entire width, one may be certain that mobilization has not been carried far enough distally. The stapler must be aligned so that the distance above the anal verge is uniform.) A crushing intestinal clamp is applied above the stapler, and the bowel is divided and removed. When the stapler is detached, the stump of the anal canal slips within the puborectal muscle.

Step 4: Construction of Ileal Pouch

A J pouch is constructed by approximating two 15 cm limbs measured proximally from the closed end of the ileum [see

Figure 10]. (The J pouch and the W pouch are favored over other types that once were more popular.[17,19,20,22,23] Of the two, I prefer the J pouch because it functions as well as the W pouch and is simpler to construct.) Three or four sutures are placed to align the limbs for side-to-side stapling. A divot is excised from the apex of the J with scissors, and an 80 mm linear cutting stapler is inserted with the anvil in one limb and the cartridge in the other. The stapler is fired and reloaded, and the bowel is bunched up in an accordionlike manner for the second firing. Two applications of the stapler are sufficient to construct a pouch 15 cm long.

A 2-0 polypropylene purse-string suture is placed on the cut edge of the apex of the J pouch, and the anvil of an end-to-end stapler is inserted and secured as the purse-string suture is tied. (I prefer to use the largest stapler available—31 or 33 mm—in the hope that all of the staple line on the anal canal stump will thereby be excised to minimize the possibility of leaving an ischemic corner.)

Step 5: Ileoanal Anastomosis

The end-to-end stapler is inserted into the anus with the spike withdrawn into the cartridge. (It is helpful to insert a sequence of progressively larger stapler sizers into the anus to ensure that the anus can accommodate the stapler and also to show the anal canal stump from the pelvic side. At this point, one must be certain that there is adequate separation from surrounding structures, especially the vagina. I find it essential to insert the stapler into the anus with both hands and then to manipulate it into place with the left hand while palpating the anal canal stump with the right hand in the pelvis. The contamination from this maneuver is a small price to pay for the assurance that the stapler is resting firmly against the stump of the anal canal circumferentially. The entire head of the stapler does not slip into the anal canal above the sphincters, as is normally the case in colorectal anastomoses; instead, the stapler rests within the anal sphincters because the anastomosis is so low. If the stapler is not properly positioned, staples may be fired through empty space rather than through tissue.)

The stapler is opened, and the spike is allowed to penetrate the anal stump adjacent to the staple line. The cut edge of the small bowel mesentery is placed toward the patient's right, and a quick check is done to make sure that the pouch has not been rotated 360°. The stapler is then closed and fired. (Before the stapler is closed, one should be sure that the vagina is adequately cleared away and thus will not be caught in the anastomosis. As the stapler is closed, there is inevitably some rotation of the pouch and its mesentery, but this does not seem to cause any problem.)

Two intact doughnuts should be obtained. The anastomosis is tested by palpation and by direct inspection with a rigid sigmoidoscope inserted into the anus. A noncrushing clamp is placed across the ileum above the pouch, and a pool of saline is placed in the pelvis. Air is insufflated to test for leaks. Leaks can usually be repaired by suturing through the anus (see below). In some patients, a diverting ileostomy may be advisable (see below).

Step 6: Optional Steps

Placement of transanal purse-string suture If, for some reason, one cannot use the stapler or if there has been a mishap in the course of the operation (e.g., entry into the lumen), the procedure can be salvaged by transanal placement of a purse-string suture. (This step can be difficult for surgeons who lack experience with the technique. Exposure is limited, and bleeding can obscure the view. A headlight is essential. Separate instruments should be available for the perineal operator.)

Two Gelpi retractors are placed to evert the anus, and a Hill-Ferguson retractor is inserted to expose the anoderm and the epithelium of the anal canal above the dentate line. The full thickness of the wall of the anal canal is incised with a curved scissors in the posterior midline about 1 cm above the dentate line. This incision should provide entry into the pelvic dissection space if the earlier dissection was extended low enough. The entire circumference of the anal canal is divided, and the purse-string suture is placed through the full thickness of the bowel. (I prefer to start this suture in the posterior midline so that it will be easier to tie with the stapler in place. A curved

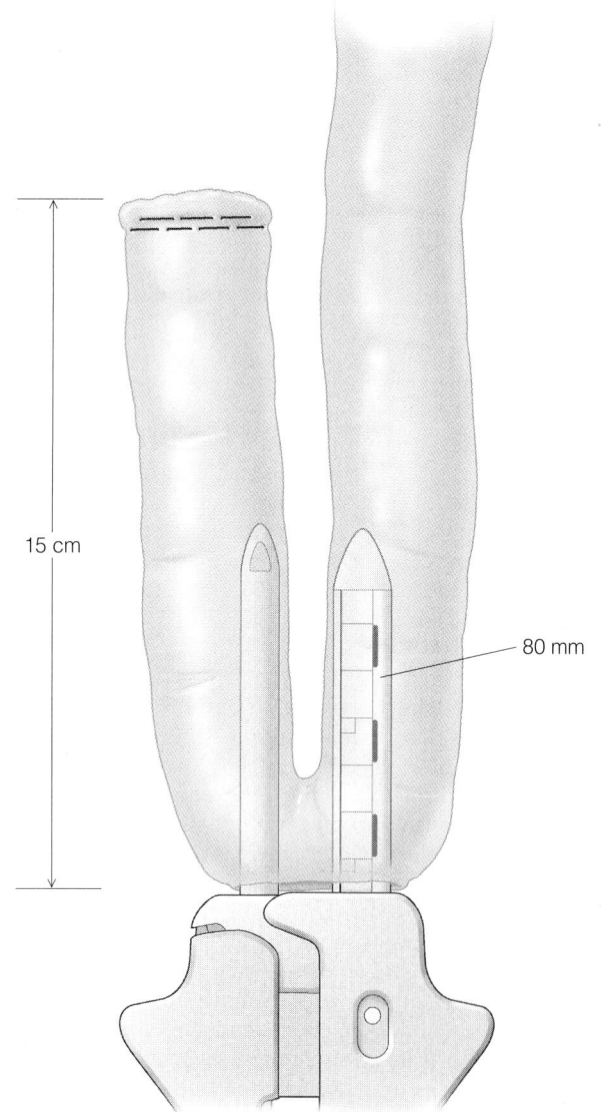

15 cm

80 mm

Figure 10 **Restorative proctocolectomy with ileoanal pouch. Shown is the construction of a J pouch. Two 15 cm limbs, measured proximally from the closed end of the ileum, are aligned; sutures (not shown) may help hold the alignment for stapling. A divot is excised from the apex of the J with scissors. An 80 mm linear cutting stapler is inserted through the resulting opening with the anvil in one limb and the cartridge in the other. Two applications of the stapler are sufficient to construct a 15 cm pouch.**

needle holder is helpful.) The Hill-Ferguson retractor is moved to bring successive portions of the circumference into view. The stapler is inserted and opened, and the shaft is reattached. The distal purse-string suture is tied. The stapler is then closed and fired. (This method is more likely to yield incomplete distal doughnuts.)

Construction of diverting ileostomy If there is concern about anastomotic integrity or the patient's healing capacity, a diverting ileostomy should be constructed. (Diverting loop ileostomy was once routine for all restorative proctocolectomy patients, but I no longer do it in low-risk patients whose anastomosis looks satisfactory and does not leak on testing.[24]) If an ileostomy is constructed, it can be taken down in about 2 months.

Step 7: Completion

Drains are inserted into the pelvis from the abdominal side. The edge of the small bowel mesentery is sutured to the retroperitoneum down to the pelvic brim; it is usually impossible to complete this closure.

COMPLICATIONS

The main complications of this procedure are abscess, anastomotic leakage, and so-called pouchitis. Most abscesses are related to minor anastomotic leaks that are contained in a small area; they tend to be small and easily drained. Large anastomotic or pelvic abscesses or fistulas are uncommon; they may result in failure of the procedure if corrective steps cannot salvage the pouch. So-called cuff abscesses are a complication of mucosectomy in which infected fluid accumulates in the space between the denuded rectal muscle tube and the ileal pouch.

Anastomotic leaks are usually masked by the presence of a diverting ileostomy. They may be revealed by imaging studies before the ileostomy is taken down, or they may remain undetected until the fecal stream is reestablished. If a diverting ileostomy is not performed, leaks become clinically evident in the first few postoperative days. If leakage is significant, laparotomy with ileostomy is the only recourse; however, leakage of this severity is uncommon.[24]

Pouchitis is a late postoperative complication that presumably is related to bacterial overgrowth in the stagnant pouch contents. It is rare in patients with familial adenomatous polyposis and consequently is believed to be related in some way to inflammatory bowel disease.[25] Perhaps 25% of patients with an ileoanal pouch experience pouchitis at some point. The typical manifestations are cramps and diarrhea (sometimes bloody); occasionally, there are systemic symptoms (e.g., fever or arthralgia). The pouch appears inflamed on endoscopy, but this finding is deceptive because some asymptomatic pouches appear red and friable also. Treatment with antibiotics (e.g., metronidazole or a cephalosporin) is usually successful. In a few patients, medical management fails and the pouch must be excised.

OUTCOME

The average patient has about five stools a day after restorative proctocolectomy, but stool frequency may range from two to 10 a day without complications.[15,17-19,22,23] Minor seepage is common in the first weeks after operation, but significant fecal incontinence is uncommon. With the techniques currently in use, infection, pouchitis, incontinence, and other problems lead to failure in about 5% of patients.[20,24]

Low Anterior Resection with Coloproctostomy

OPERATIVE PLANNING

Anterior resection is the procedure of choice for most cancers in or above the midrectum. The goal is to excise the portion of the rectum that contains the tumor and to remove the entire mesorectum as well as pararectal tissue containing lymphatic vessels and lymph nodes. Good technique is critical for minimizing the likelihood of recurrence in the pelvis.[26]

Tumor Assessment

Resection and anastomosis are anatomically impossible when the distal edge of the cancer is lower than about 4 cm above the anal verge (2 cm above the dentate line). In practice, many midrectal cancers that are large, deeply invasive, or poorly differentiated cannot be dealt with by anterior resection either. If the tumor can be moved at all before dissection is begun, it can usually be excised; however, fixity on digital palpation is not a reliable sign that the tumor is unresectable. Computed tomography, magnetic resonance imaging, and endorectal ultrasonography may be helpful. The patient's body habitus and preferences should be taken into account. Sometimes, the final decision regarding sphincter preservation can be made only during the operation. Occasionally, the potential for anastomosis cannot be assessed until the rectum has been mobilized. Extension into the urogenital structures may be apparent, and it should be possible to determine whether the anterior structures (the uterus or the vagina in particular) must be resected en bloc to effect cure.

Excision of the primary tumor is the most effective way of palliating rectal adenocarcinoma. Prevention or relief of tenesmus is a goal worth pursuing, even in patients with distant metastases. Tenesmus is not relieved by fecal diversion, nor is it reliably eliminated by radiation therapy or other forms of local treatment.

OPERATIVE TECHNIQUE

Step 1: Positioning

The patient should be placed in the lithotomy position in Lloyd-Davies leg rests or Allen universal stirrups. Rectal examination is performed to confirm the preoperative assessment of the tumor, and the rectum is irrigated with saline to eliminate any residual stool.

Step 2: Mobilization of Sigmoid and Mesosigmoid

The distal sigmoid is occluded with an encircling umbilical tape to prevent movement of luminal contents from the proximal colon into the rectum and intraluminal migration of malignant cells from the primary rectal cancer into the portion of colon to be retained.

The sigmoid colon and the mesocolon are dissected away from peritoneal attachments, and the left base of the mesosigmoid is incised medial to the ureter as described for total colectomy with ileoanal anastomosis. The splenic flexure is taken down partially or completely, with the redundancy of the sigmoid and the level of the tumor kept in mind. The peritoneum at the base of the mesosigmoid on the right is incised, and the incision is continued cephalad toward the duodenum for a variable distance, depending on the planned level of vessel ligation. (Care should be taken not to injure the preaortic sympathetic nerves during this step. In addition, it is vital that the colon be mobilized in such a way that the proximal end of the bowel will reach the rectal stump with no tension. There must be no compromise on this point.)

Step 3: Ligation of Vessels

There is some controversy regarding the level at which vessels should be ligated during curative resection of rectal cancer. Some surgeons ligate just below the origin of the left colic artery; others ligate at the origin of the inferior mesenteric artery to remove the few nodes that remain with ligation more distally. The data consistently indicate, however, that the level of ligation does not influence survival rates. Today, most surgeons ligate the inferior mesenteric vessels just distal to the origin of the left colic artery.[27]

The mesocolon is divided radially to the point at which the surgeon plans to transect the colon. The colon may be transected either at this time or after the pelvic dissection has been completed.

Step 4: Pelvic Dissection

Dissection is carried out under direct vision.[26] In men, the anterior plane of dissection is anterior to Denonvilliers' fascia if the cancer is nearby; if the lesion is more proximal, dissection can be posterior to Denonvilliers' fascia. In women, the rectum is separated from the vagina, but if there is an anterior lesion invading the vagina, the posterior vaginal wall must be excised. It may be possible to restore colorectal continuity in this situation; however, adjacent suture lines should be avoided, and abdominoperineal resection (see below) may be safer.

The aim of lateral dissection is to leave the pelvis devoid of lateral soft tissue. (To this end, one should remove all of the node-bearing tissue all the way to the pelvic sidewall but not external to the parietal pelvic fascia. One can ligate the middle hemorrhoidal vessels close to the pelvic sidewall and still achieve complete extirpation of soft tissues if this maneuver is conducted under direct vision.) The lateral ligaments are completely divided down to the levator muscles, with the bilobed so-called lipoma of the mesorectum left intact.

Step 5: Removal of Mesorectum

If the tumor is in the midrectum (especially if it is in the distal portion), one should excise the entire mesorectum rather than dissect through it to reach the rectal wall. This approach is referred to as total mesorectal excision.[28] (Residual tumor in the mesorectum is an important cause of local recurrence.) At the levator muscles, the rectal lumen is small, no more than 2.5 to 3.0 cm in diameter; above that point, the rectal lumen enlarges substantially.

Step 6: Anastomosis

Colorectal anastomosis The anastomosis may be done either by hand suturing or by stapling. (Because hand suturing a low anastomosis is tedious, I prefer either the double-staple technique or an open stapled approach.)

In a double-stapled coloproctostomy, the lumen above the planned line of transection is occluded with a right-angled crushing bowel clamp. The distal anorectum is irrigated transanally with dilute povidone-iodine to destroy malignant cells. A 30 mm right-angle stapler (or a device of comparable size) is positioned and fired. (If dissection of the mesorectum is incomplete or if all of the pararectal tissue has not been divided, the 30 mm stapler will not close off the entire rectal stump. One can usually tell when this problem is likely to arise, because the tissue grasped by the stapler will feel unusually bulky. The solution is to remove the stapler without firing it and then to dissect more completely.) The rectum is divided sharply between the stapler and the crushing clamp. A purse-string suture is applied to the colonic stump proximally, and an intraluminal or end-to-end stapler is inserted through the anus. (With a large stapler—31 or 33 mm—one can usually excise the entire original rectal staple line.)

Alternatively, a purse-string suture can be placed distally by hand. (If the rectum is transected deeply in the pelvis, currently available mechanical purse-string appliers do not work well.) The rectum is occluded with a clamp proximal to the proposed site of transection, and the distal portion is irrigated as described for double stapling. The proximal clamp is placed immediately above the planned site of transection so that the bowel can be divided on the distal side flush with the clamp. A beaver blade scalpel with a long handle is used to incise into the rectal lumen in the center, and placement of the purse-string suture is begun with only a portion of the lumen open. (If the rectum is completely divided before the suture is begun, the stump will retract and the mucosa will pout, making the task of suturing unnecessarily difficult.) The rectal transection is completed gradually as the suture is continued.

The anastomosis is tested by digital rectal examination and inspection through a rigid sigmoidoscope as described for ileoanal anastomosis. Drains are placed through a stab wound in the left lower quadrant.

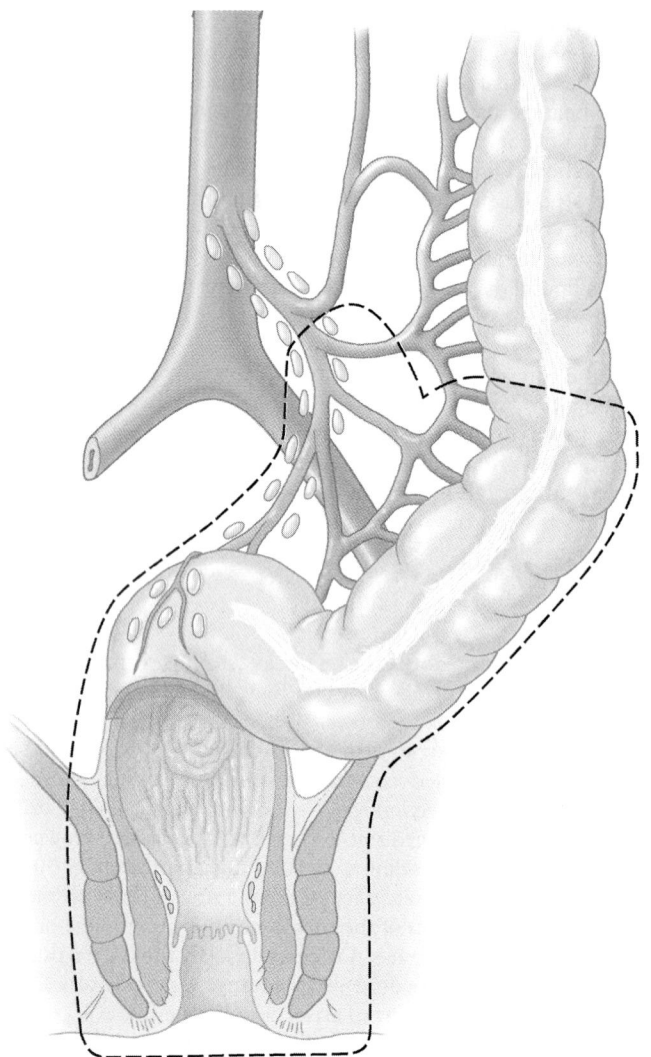

Figure 11 **Abdominoperineal resection. The extent of the resection is outlined.**[35]

Coloanal anastomosis   When a tumor lies in the distal portion of the midrectum but is still high enough for a margin to be obtainable, one may avoid abdominoperineal resection (APR) by performing a coloanal anastomosis. (Coloanal anastomosis is contraindicated in patients with impaired sphincters and persons with infirmities that prevent ready access to bathroom facilities.[29]) Usually, the final decision is made during the operation. This procedure can be performed by means of the double-staple technique or by placing a purse-string suture transanally. Dissection within the levator muscles and the stapling procedure itself are performed as described for restorative proctocolectomy. Postoperative function may be improved by constructing a colonic J pouch and anastomosing the pouch to the anal canal.[30]

COMPLICATIONS

The incidence of clinically significant anastomotic leakage is about 4%.[27] This complication is more common after colorectal anastomoses than after colonic anastomoses, in part because the rectum is devoid of serosa. Tension on the anastomosis is an important—and avoidable—precipitating factor. Infected pelvic fluid can erupt into the lumen and create a leak.

Anastomotic stricture is usually the consequence of a leak, but membranous stenosis can develop in stapled anastomoses. This is rarely a significant problem if large-caliber staplers are used. Digital or sigmoidoscopic stretching of a membranous stenosis usually solves the problem permanently.

OUTCOME

Long-term survival of cancer patients after low anterior resection depends on the tumor stage; it should be no different from survival after APR if patients are selected properly.[31]

The results of very low colorectal or coloanal anastomoses are sometimes functionally unsatisfactory. Mucous leakage is not uncommon. Bowel habits are unpredictable, and patients may experience irregularity and urgency.

Abdominoperineal Resection

OPERATIVE PLANNING

Abdominoperineal resection is the standard procedure for cancers of the distal rectum that are too low to permit preservation of the sphincter [*see Figure 11*].[31,32] Whether APR is appropriate in a given setting depends on the characteristics of the tumor and the general condition of the patient. The tumor is assessed as described for low anterior resection. Ascites is a strong contraindication to APR because ascitic leak through the perineal wound may be troublesome or even fatal if it leads to peritonitis. Palliative APR is worthwhile in many instances.

A colostomy site is selected, and the educational process is begun preoperatively.

OPERATIVE TECHNIQUE

Step 1: Positioning

How the patient is positioned depends on whether APR is to be done in separate stages by a single team or synchronously by two teams. (The synchronous technique is more efficient, but a second experienced surgeon is needed to perform the perineal dissection.) If the two-stage approach is selected, the patient is supine for the abdominal phase and in the lithotomy position or the left lateral decubitus position for the perineal phase. The lateral decubitus position is more cumbersome because the patient must be turned, but it provides superb exposure of the anterior structures. In a difficult patient with an extensive tumor on the anterior wall, the lateral decubitus position is recommended. If the synchronous approach is selected, the patient is in the lithotomy position. If it is certain that APR will be done, the anus is closed with a purse-string suture of heavy material; two sutures should be placed, one within the other. (If there is no doubt about the need for a colostomy, the colostomy aperture is made before the main abdominal incision, as described for total proctocolectomy with ileostomy.)

Step 2: Pelvic Dissection

It is unnecessary to take down the splenic flexure. In men, the anterior pelvic dissection plane is anterior to Denonvilliers' fascia. In women with anterior rectal cancer, the posterior vaginal wall is included with the specimen [*see Figure 12*]. Hysterectomy is usually advisable in this situation.

Step 3: Management of Pelvic Peritoneal Floor

If the operation is done in separate phases, the sigmoid is divided at this point, and the distal stump is covered with a rubber glove secured with an umbilical tape. The specimen is placed in the pelvis, and the pelvic peritoneum is closed. (If the entire specimen does not fit into the pelvic space, the bowel must be divided again, but this must not be done too close to the tumor.) If the synchronous approach is used, the specimen is passed through the posterior aspect of the perineal wound to the perineal operator. (Some surgeons do not close the pelvic peritoneum routinely; in a few patients, it is impossible to close this layer because of previous pelvic surgery or irradiation. With the pelvic peritoneal floor open, the small bowel falls into the pelvis, but this occurrence probably does not increase the incidence of intestinal obstruction. If postoperative radiation therapy is likely, the pelvic peritoneal floor should be closed, and if there is insufficient peritoneum for this purpose, either omentum or polyglycolate mesh can be used to create a floor.)

Step 4: Colostomy

A conventional sigmoid colostomy is made by bringing the colon straight through the rectus muscle. Once this is done, a space is left lateral to the colon through which small bowel can herniate and become obstructed; this space should be closed. Alternatively, the colostomy can be placed extraperitoneally; however, few surgeons favor this approach, because the advantages of extraperitoneal colostomy do not seem to justify the additional time and effort.

Although protrusion above the skin level is essential for an ileostomy, it is not necessary with a colostomy.

Step 5: Perineal Dissection (Perineal Phase)

An elliptical incision encompassing the anus is made with a scalpel or the electrocautery. The incision is extended through the ischiorectal fat in such a way that much—but not all—of this tissue is included with the specimen. Large rake retractors are used to expose the levator muscles.

The anococcygeal raphe is incised just anterior to the coccyx. (Amputation of the coccyx is unnecessary in routine cases.) With the anus retracted forward, the white Waldeyer's fascia is exposed and incised transversely. The pelvic dissection space is thus entered. The surgeon can insert one or two fingers to locate the levator muscles for division with the electrocautery. (Inadequate levator excision seldom leads to local or regional recurrence; unless the tumor is deeply invasive at this level, a

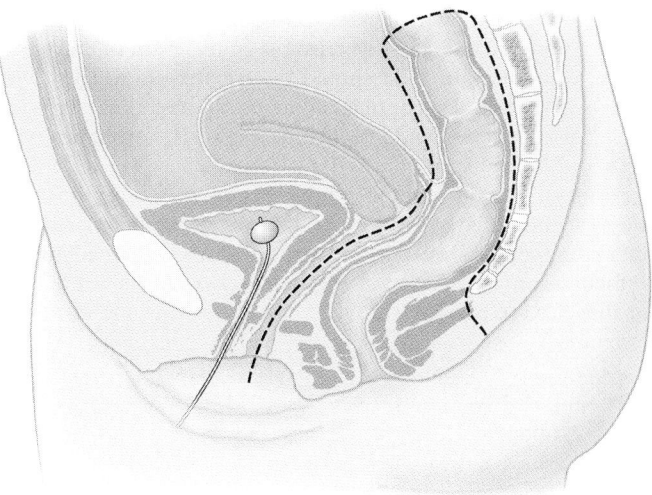

Figure 12 Abdominoperineal resection. In women with anterior rectal cancer, the posterior vaginal wall is included with the specimen.[35] Hysterectomy (not shown) is often done as well.

margin of iliococcygeal muscle can be left laterally to facilitate closure of the perineal wound.)

When the levator muscles have been divided, the specimen is delivered through the posterior part of the perineal wound, with only the anterior attachments left to be severed.

Step 6: Closure of Perineal Wound

If the pelvic peritoneal floor is closed, the perineal wound is sutured in layers with drainage. If bacterial contamination is heavy, the perineal wound is left open or partially closed with drainage.

COMPLICATIONS

The overall complication rate in this predominantly elderly patient population is 35%, but most of the complications—such as atelectasis and postoperative urinary retention—are relatively minor.[31,32] Operative mortality ranges from 0% to 7%; most contemporary series report mortalities of 2% to 3%.[31,32] The majority of deaths are from cardiovascular complications and pulmonary embolism. Surgical complications leading to death are increasingly uncommon in experienced hands.

Intraoperative hemorrhage most commonly arises from injury to the presacral veins. Bulky tumors, previous radiation therapy, a narrow pelvis, and obesity make this complication more likely. If presacral veins are torn, bleeding may stop with pressure. If pressure is ineffective, the bleeding can sometimes be controlled by electrocauterization or ligation with fine sutures; however, if the vessel is torn where it emerges from the bone, these measures may not be effective. (Special metal tacks are manufactured for the purpose of controlling bleeding from these vessels, but I have never found it necessary to use them.) The last resort would be to pack the pelvis and then to return to the operating room later to remove the pack.

Injury to the left ureter must be repaired immediately. The urethra is vulnerable to injury during the anterior perineal dissection; fortunately, such injury is rare. Injury to the urethra should be repaired primarily, and a suprapubic cystostomy tube should be placed.

The rectum can be torn during the posterior pelvic dissection or during the perineal phase. The greatest concern is contamination of the field by malignant cells; bacterial contamination is also problematic but is less worrisome. In the event of entry into the rectal lumen, the field should be irrigated thoroughly with water, a tumoricidal agent (e.g., dilute povidone-iodine), or both.

Colostomy complications include necrosis, retraction, and paracolostomy abscess.

Perineal wound complications occur in about 15% of patients who undergo APR for rectal cancer; the most common such complication is persistent perineal sinus.[23] Perineal hernia is uncommon after APR but is more likely to occur if the levator muscles are excised widely.

OUTCOME

Late colostomy complications are mainly limited to paracolostomy hernia. Prolapse is an uncommon complication of a sigmoid colostomy.

Sexual dysfunction in men after APR is usually neurogenic, but advanced age and psychological factors may play a role as well. Total impotence occurs in 5% to 40% of men after APR.[32] Sexual dysfunction in women may result from psychological problems related to altered body image. Dyspareunia, presumably arising from pelvic fibrosis, is reported by as many as 50% of women after APR.

References

1. Andriesse GI, Gooszen HG, Schipper ME, et al: Functional results and visceral perception after ileo neo-rectal anastomosis in patients: a pilot study. Gut 48:683, 2001

2. Eu KW, Lim SL, Seow-Choen F, et al: Clinical outcome and bowel function following total abdominal colectomy and ileorectal anastomosis in the Oriental population. Dis Colon Rectum 41:215, 1998

3. Mollen RM, Kuijpers HC, Claassen AT: Colectomy for slow-transit constipation: preoperative functional evaluation is important but not a guarantee for a successful outcome. Dis Colon Rectum 44:577, 2001

4. Pastore RL, Wolff BG, Hodge D: Total abdominal colectomy and ileorectal anastomosis for inflammatory bowel disease. Dis Colon Rectum 40:1455, 1997

5. van Duijvendijk P, Slors JFM, Taat CW, et al: Functional outcome after colectomy and ileorectal anastomosis compared with proctocolectomy and ileal pouch-anal anastomosis in familial adenomatous polyposis. Ann Surg 230:648, 1999

6. Milsom JW, Ludwig KA, Church JM, et al: Laparoscopic total abdominal colectomy with ileorectal anastomosis for familial adenomatous polyposis. Dis Colon Rectum 40:675, 1997

7. Nakamura T, Pikarsky AJ, Potenti FM, et al: Are complications of subtotal colectomy with ileorectal anastomosis related to the original disease? Am Surg 67:417, 2001

8. Ko CY, Rusing LC, Schoetz DJ, et al: Does better functional result equate with better quality of life? Implications for surgical treatment in familial adenomatous polyposis. Dis Colon Rectum 43:829, 2000

9. Soravia C, Klein L, Berk T, et al: Comparison of ileal pouch-anal anastomosis and ileorectal anastomosis in patients with familial adenomatous polyposis. Dis Colon Rectum 42:1028, 1999

10. Bernell O, Lapidus A, Hellers G: Recurrence after colectomy in Crohn's colitis. Dis Colon Rectum 44:647, 2001

11. Hulten L: Proctocolectomy and ileostomy to pouch surgery for ulcerative colitis. World J Surg 22:335, 1998

12. Vasen HF, van Duijvendijk P, Buskens E, et al: Decision analysis in the surgical treatment of patients with familial adenomatous polyposis: a Dutch-Scandinavian collaborative study including 659 patients. Gut 49:231, 2001

13. Yamamoto T, Keighley MR: Proctocolectomy is associated with a higher complication rate but carries a lower recurrence rate than total colectomy and ileorectal anastomosis in Crohn colitis. Scand J Gastroenterol 34:1212, 1999

14. Schrock TR: Ileostomy and colostomy. Gastrointestinal Surgery. Fromm D, Ed. Churchill Livingstone, New York, 1985

15. McLeod RS, Baxter NN: Quality of life of patients with inflammatory bowel disease after surgery. World J Surg 22:375, 1998

16. Gorfine SR, Bauer JJ, Harris MT, et al: Dysplasia complicating chronic ulcerative colitis: is immediate colectomy warranted? Dis Colon Rectum 43:1575, 2000

17. Parc YR, Moslein G, Dozois RR, et al: Familial adenomatous polyposis: results after ileal pouch-anal anastomosis in teenagers. Dis Colon Rectum 43:893, 2000

18. Takao Y, Gilliland R, Nogueras JJ, et al: Is age relevant to functional outcome after restorative proctocolectomy for ulcerative colitis? Prospective assessment of 122 cases. Ann Surg 227:187, 1998

19. Karlbom U, Raab Y, Ejerblad S, et al: Factors influencing the functional outcome of restorative proctocolectomy in ulcerative colitis. Br J Surg 87:1401, 2000

20. Regimbeau JM, Panis Y, Pocard M, et al: Handsewn ileal pouch-anal anastomosis on the dentate line after total proctectomy: technique to avoid incomplete mucosectomy and the need for long-term follow-up of the anal transition zone. Dis Colon Rectum 44:43, 2001

21. O'Riordain MG, Fazio VW, Lavery IC, et al: Incidence and natural history of dysplasia of the anal transitional zone after ileal pouch-anal anastomosis: results of a five-year to ten-year follow-up. Dis Colon Rectum 43:1660, 2000

22. Farouk R, Pemberton JH, Wolff BG, et al: Functional outcomes after ileal pouch-anal anastomosis for chronic ulcerative colitis. Ann Surg 231:919, 2000

23. O'Bichere A, Wilkinson K, Rumbles S, et al: Functional outcome after restorative panproctocolectomy for ulcerative colitis decreases an otherwise enhanced quality of life. Br J Surg 87:802, 2000

24. Sugerman HJ, Sugerman EL, Meador JG, et al: Ileal pouch anal anastomosis without ileal diversion. Ann Surg 232:530, 2000

25. Simchuk EJ, Thirlby RC: Risk factors and true incidence of pouchitis in patients after ileal pouch-anal anastomosis. World J Surg 24:851, 2000

26. Polglase AL, McMurrick PJ, Tremayne AB, et al: Local recurrence after curative anterior resection with principally blunt dissection for carcinoma of the rectum and rectosigmoid. Dis Colon Rectum 44:947, 2001

27. Enker WE, Merchant N, Cohen AM, et al: Safety and efficacy of low anterior resection for rectal cancer: consecutive cases from a specialty service. Ann Surg 230:544, 1999

28. Kapiteijn E, Kranenbarg EK, Steup WH, et al: Total mesorectal excision (TME) with or without preoperative radiotherapy in the treatment of primary rectal cancer: prospective randomised trial with standard operative and histopathologic techniques. Dutch ColoRectal Cancer Group. Eur J Surg 165:410, 1999

29. Di Matteo G, Mascagni D, Keri KP, et al: Evaluation of anal function after surgery for rectal cancer. J Surg Oncol 74:11, 2000

30. Lazorthes F, Chiotasso P, Gamagami RA, et al: Late clinical outcome in a randomized prospective comparison of colonic J pouch and straight coloanal anastomosis. Br J Surg 84:1449, 1997

31. Ferulano GP, Dilillo S, La Manna S, et al: Influence of the surgical treatment on local recurrence of rectal cancer: a prospective study (1980–1992). J Surg Oncol 74:153, 2000

32. Enker WE, Havenga K, Polyak T, et al: Abdominoperineal resection via total mesorectal excision and autonomic nerve preservation for low rectal cancer. World J Surg 21:715, 1997

33. Schrock TR: Total colectomy and ileoanal anastomosis. Mastery of Surgery, 3rd ed. Nyhus LM, Baker RJ, Fischer JE, Eds. Little, Brown & Co, Boston, 1997

34. Schrock TR: Inflammatory disease of the colon and rectum. Gastrointestinal Surgery. Fromm D, Ed. Churchill Livingstone, New York, 1985

35. Schrock TR: Abdominoperineal resection—technique and complications. Cancer of the Colon, Rectum, and Anus. Cohen AM, Winawer SJ, Eds. McGraw-Hill, New York, 1995, p 595

Acknowledgment

Figures 1 through 12   Tom Moore.

28 LAPAROSCOPIC COLECTOMY

Babak N. Rad, M.D., and Robert W. Beart, Jr., M.D., F.A.C.S.

The growing emphasis on minimally invasive approaches in modern surgery has forced surgeons to reevaluate traditional approaches to proven procedures. Laparoscopic cholecystectomy, laparoscopic appendectomy, and laparoscopic inguinal and incisional herniorrhaphy all have proved to be viable alternatives to their open counterparts.[1] Their success has led to the application of laparoscopy to bowel surgery in an effort to reduce the morbidity associated with conventional open colon resections. There is now considerable published evidence indicating that laparoscopic colectomy is both safe and effective and has certain advantages over open techniques—namely, decreased operative morbidity, decreased pain, shorter length of stay, more rapid return to work, and improved cosmesis.[1-3]

Laparoscopic bowel surgery does require that surgeons acquire a new set of skills. Thus, it should not be surprising that the natural human tendency to resist change has, to date, limited its utilization. If, however, encouraging study findings are confirmed by subsequent trials, it is likely that laparoscopic colectomy will become the treatment of choice in the future.

Indications

Accepted indications for laparoscopic colectomy include most of the benign colonic diseases (e.g., colorectal polyps, rectal prolapse, diverticular disease, inflammatory bowel disease, intestinal stomas for diversion, cecal or sigmoid volvulus, and symptomatic colonic lipomas).[2] The role of laparoscopic bowel resection in the management of malignant colonic disease, however, remains controversial. Specifically, there are questions about the incidence of port-site recurrence and about long-term survival rates that have not yet been answered.[3-6] These questions have provided the impetus for prospective, randomized studies in several countries. A number of such trials have been initiated, most of which are being conducted at multiple centers. Results from these studies should help resolve these important issues.

Operative Planning

No patient should undergo laparoscopic bowel surgery without a defined diagnosis. Colonoscopy, barium enemas, and computed tomography are all potentially useful in determining the diagnosis before operation; the choice of diagnostic modality should be governed by the patient's initial presenting signs and symptoms. The distance from the tumor to the anal verge is readily measured in the course of colonoscopy, but such measurement does not always result in accurate identification of the corresponding segment of diseased bowel intraoperatively. Furthermore, with the exception of the ileocecal valve (which remains a constant and easily identifiable landmark), the general shape and curves of the colon are indistinct. Therefore, it is recommended that India ink tattooing be used to mark lesions located in segments of the bowel outside the area of the ileocecal valve, thereby facilitating intraoperative localization of the tumor.

Patients who have a history of severe cardiopulmonary disease, hepatic disease, coagulopathy, significant respiratory compromise, or a complex colonic disorder (e.g., obstruction, contained perforation, or colovesical fistula) should not be considered for laparoscopic colectomy, nor should patients who are known to have extensive intra-abdominal adhesions. Patients who have tumors larger than 8 to 10 cm in diameter are also unsuitable candidates for laparoscopic colectomy. Larger specimens inevitably require larger incisions for removal; accordingly, patients with large tumors would benefit from having an appropriately sized incision in place from the beginning of the operation.

Before operation, the surgeon must recognize that the laparoscopic colectomy may have to be converted to an open procedure, and he or she must discuss this possibility with the patient. Standard bowel preparation is provided. An epidural catheter is placed to facilitate postoperative pain control, which is an important consideration for the first 2 days after laparoscopic bowel surgery.

Operative Technique

RIGHT HEMICOLECTOMY

Step 1: Positioning of Patient and Operative Team

The patient is initially placed supine on the operating table. Because the position of the patient is changed several times during the operation, some form of restraining device should be employed to minimize the possibility of a fall; we favor the use of a beanbag that is secured to the table. Pneumatic compression stockings are placed on the patient to minimize the risk of deep vein thrombosis. After induction of general anesthesia, a nasogastric tube and a Foley catheter are placed to decompress the bladder and the stomach so that these organs will not be perforated when the trocars are inserted. The abdomen is then prepared and draped in the usual fashion.

The surgeon and the camera operator stand to the left of the patient, the assistant surgeon and the nurse to the right. The monitors are placed on either side of the patient, adjacent to the shoulders. With this configuration, all members of the operative team can easily view the operative field [*see Figure 1*].

Step 2: Placement of Trocars

We use a standardized trocar placement for all colectomies [*see Figure 2*]. A 12 mm Hasson trocar is inserted through the rectus muscle and into the abdominal cavity via a small left upper quadrant incision placed 3 to 4 cm below the costal margin. The trocar is secured with sutures, and the abdomen is insufflated with CO_2 to achieve pneumoperitoneum. We use a pressure of 10 to 12 mm Hg to minimize the risk of pneumatosis, which can involve the entire body (presumably as a result of dissection through the extraperitoneal tissue planes, which are opened during the operation). After a complete survey of the peritoneal cavity, including the liver, three

649

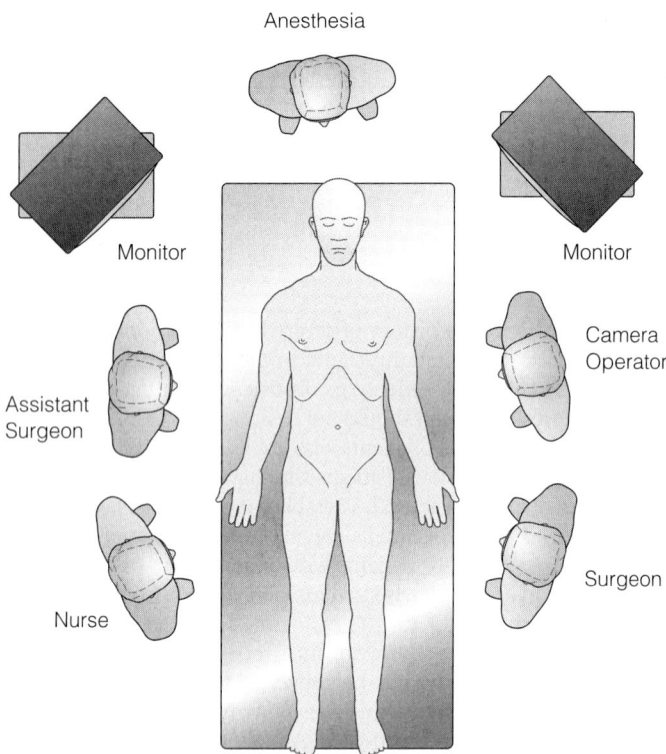

Figure 1 **Laparoscopic colectomy: right hemicolectomy. Shown is the recommended positioning of the operating team.**

additional ports are inserted under direct vision. A 10/12 mm port is placed at the suprapubic location. (Here and at the first site, we recommend the use of 10/12 mm ports to minimize the risk of postoperative port-site herniation.) Two 5 mm ports are placed at sites where stomas could be placed in a conventional procedure. We tend to use a 0° scope for viewing the pelvis, but many surgeons prefer a 30° angled scope. Attempts should be made to close all 10/12 mm ports at the end of the operation.

Step 3: Mobilization of Ascending Colon

The patient is placed in the Trendelenburg position, maximally rotated to the left. This positioning causes the small bowel to fall away from the right colon and allows visualization of the colonic mesentery. Dissecting scissors are inserted through the suprapubic port, and a grasper is inserted through the 5 mm port in the left lower quadrant. The surgeon, standing on the patient's left, operates these two instruments using a two-handed technique. The assistant uses a grasper to retract the peritoneum, taking care not to grasp the bowel but instead to grasp the mesentery or the peritoneum to place the tissues on traction.

The surgeon begins the dissection by incising the peritoneum along the cecum [*see Figure 3*]. The appendiceal and terminal ileal attachments are easily visualized and similarly divided. The bowel is then bluntly reflected from the retroperitoneum. At this point, the ureter can usually be identified in the retroperitoneum. The bowel is further mobilized medially by means of blunt dissection. The dissection is extended upward to the hepatic flexure, and the transverse colon is mobilized as necessary for the diseased bowel segment to be resected. For complete dissection of the transverse colon, it may be necessary to put the patient in the reverse Trendelenburg position. Additional dissection of the colon can also be done under direct vision during the removal of the specimen. The duodenum can usually be visualized during this mobilization.

Step 4: Dissection

The bowel is returned to its normal position, the mesentery is grasped, and the medial aspect of the colon and the ileocolic vessels are placed on traction. With traction placed on the mesentery, the ileocolic vessels are easily visualized. The key technical point here is that on each side of the mesenteric vessels, there exists a clear avascular space, which can be rapidly and readily dissected back into the previously dissected retroperitoneum to create a window [*see Figure 4*]. Once this window is complete, the vessels are isolated and can be controlled with minimal difficulty. The artery and the vein can usually be identified at their origin, separated, and individually clipped. The right colic vessels are then similarly exposed and clipped.

With the dissection of the bowel complete, attention is turned to mobilization and division of the ileocolic and right colic vessels. Once this is accomplished, the bowel is completely mobile and can be retrieved through the abdominal wall. To facilitate creation of the anastomosis, the attachments of the terminal ileum must be completely divided; if this is not done, the surgeon will find it difficult to bring the bowel through the abdominal wall.

Step 5: Anastomosis and Closure

A 5 cm incision is made at the right lower quadrant port site and extended downward through the muscle. Hemostatic techniques must be used: no bleeding should be allowed to occur through this incision. The bowel can then be grasped and brought through the wound with relative ease. Once the bowel is outside the abdomen, any additional mesenteric dissection and ligation that may be needed can be completed under direct vision. Before creating the anastomosis, the surgeon must ensure that the bowel has not been rotated; this can be accomplished by maintaining the orientation of the bowel as it is brought out through the abdominal wall.

The bowel is then divided and reanastomosed either with staples or with sutures. It is not necessary to close the mesenteric defect. The bowel is returned to the peritoneal cavity, and the abdominal wound is closed in layers. The peritoneal cavity is reinsufflated, laparoscopically inspected for hemostasis, and irrigated. The cannulas are removed under direct vision, and the 10/12 mm port sites are closed. Finally, the skin is closed with a subcuticular absorbable suture and Steri-Strips.

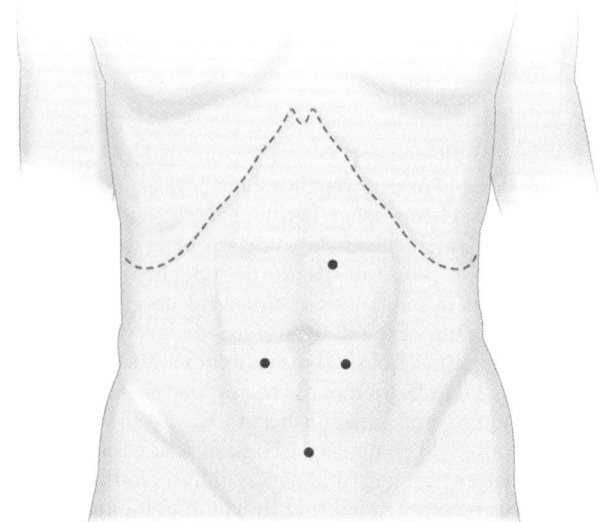

Figure 2 **Laparoscopic colectomy: right hemicolectomy. Standard port placement.**

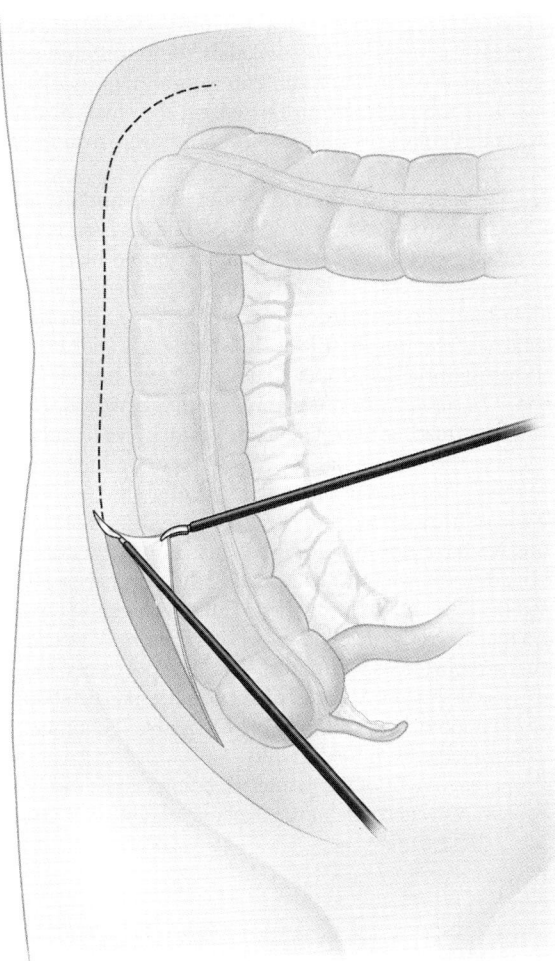

Figure 3 **Laparoscopic colectomy: right hemicolectomy. Right colon mobilization.**

LEFT HEMICOLECTOMY AND SIGMOID RESECTION

Step 1: Positioning of Patient and Operative Team

Initial positioning and preparation of the patient are essentially the same as for a right hemicolectomy (see above). The position of the operative team differs somewhat, in that the surgeon and the nurse stand to the right of the patient, and the camera operator and the assistant stand to the left [*see Figure 5*]. The monitors are placed in the same locations as for a right hemicolectomy.

Step 2: Placement of Trocars

As in a right hemicolectomy, a Hasson trocar is placed in the left upper quadrant via a small incision over the rectus muscle 3 to 4 cm below the costal margin. After pneumoperitoneum is established through this trocar, three additional ports are inserted under direct vision in the same locations used for a right hemicolectomy.

Step 3: Mobilization of Descending Colon

The patient is placed in a steep Trendelenburg position, maximally rotated to the right. For the initial dissection, the laparoscope (either 0° or 30°) is placed in the left upper quadrant port. As the assistant retracts the peritoneal attachments laterally to the left, the surgeon, using the electrified scissors in the suprapubic port and the grasper in the right lower quadrant port, retracts the descending colon cephalad and to the right. The dissection commences along the peritoneal reflection of the sigmoid and descending colon, with

the peritoneum incised along the white line of Toldt. Once the peritoneum has been incised, the colon can be mobilized by blunt reflection off the retroperitoneum.

As in a right hemicolectomy, the ureter must be identified. As a rule, the gonadal vessels appear first, then the ureter. After the ureter is carefully identified and dissected away from the mesentery, the bowel is again laid laterally. To ensure adequate length, the splenic flexure should be mobilized in much the same way as the hepatic flexure.

Step 4: Dissection

After the bowel is returned to its normal anatomic location, the mesentery is grasped and the inferior mesenteric vessels identified. Using the avascular space around the origin of the vessels, the surgeon creates a window that extends laterally to the previously dissected plane. Once the pedicle is isolated, the fat around the vessels can be stripped, and the artery and the vein can be individually controlled and clipped. We use large clips, placing two on the aortic side of the vessels and one on the distal side. In dividing large arteries, it is best to cut partway through the artery and then remove tension from the vessel to make sure that the clips are correctly applied [*see Figure 6*]; alternatively, the pedicle can be divided with a vascular endoscopic stapler. The choice of approach is a matter of individual preference.

Step 5: Anastomosis and Closure

Once the inferior mesenteric artery is ligated, the left colic artery may be divided, depending on which bowel segment is to be removed. A 5 cm incision is then made at the port site in the left lower quadrant. The bowel is grasped and brought up through the incision. The entire bowel can usually be seen, and any additional mesentery can be divided. The bowel is then divided and reanastomosed by means of standard anastomotic techniques. When the anastomosis is complete, the bowel is returned to the abdominal cavity. The fascia is closed in two layers with continuous absorbable sutures, and the skin is closed with a subcuticular absorbable suture.

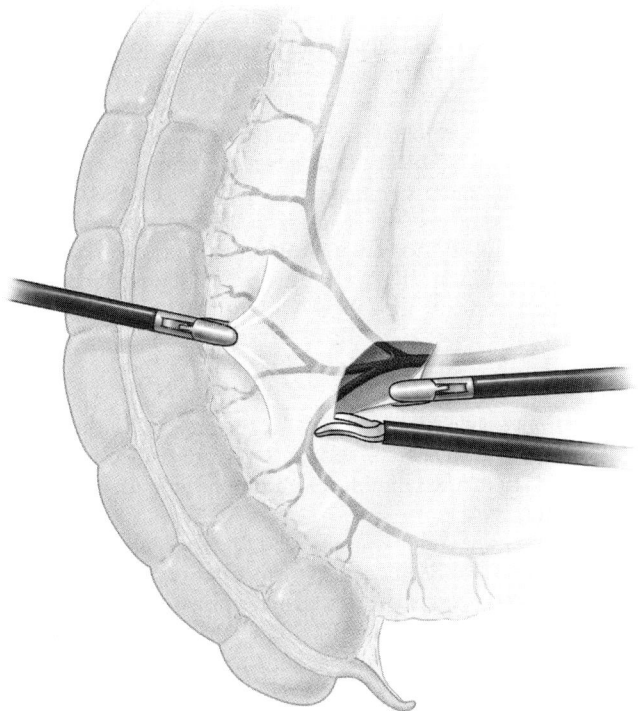

Figure 4 **Laparoscopic colectomy: right hemicolectomy. Right colon mesenteric dissection.**

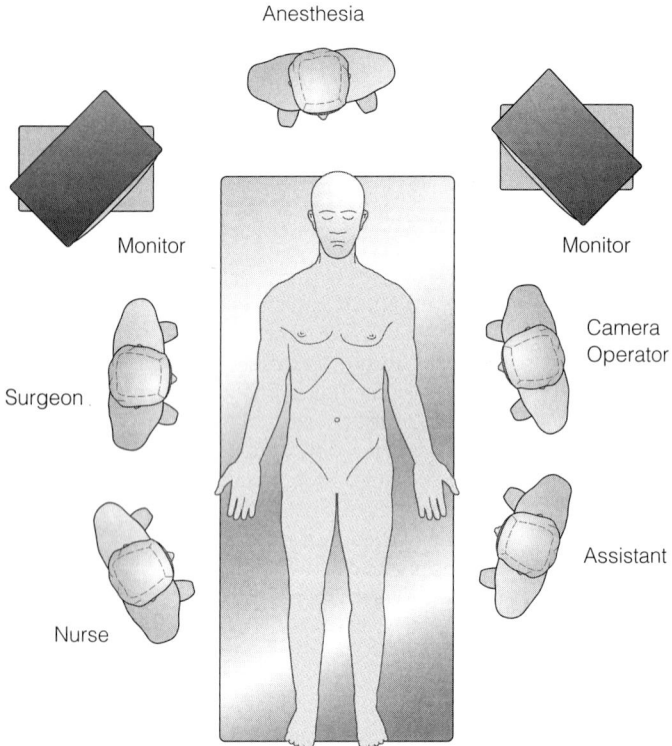

Figure 5 **Laparoscopic colectomy: left hemicolectomy and sigmoid resection. Shown is the recommended positioning of the operating team.**

Postoperative Care

Postoperative care of patients who have undergone laparoscopic colectomy should be similar to that of patients who have undergone open colectomy; however, a shorter recovery period is to be expected with the less invasive procedure. As a rule, patients are started on clear liquids in the evening of the day of surgery and maintained on epidural analgesia until oral intake is adequate. Subsequently, enteral feeding is advanced until patients are on a regular diet, at which point they can be discharged from the hospital. Oral medications are generally adequate for controlling any postoperative pain, and patients are encouraged to pursue desired activities to the extent tolerated. On the whole, it is our impression that patients who have undergone laparoscopic colectomy experience less respiratory and immune dysfunction and can tolerate food more rapidly than those who have undergone open colectomy. They can usually be discharged between postoperative days 3 and 4.

Troubleshooting

A major troubleshooting issue is that of conversion of a laparoscopic bowel resection to an open procedure. Such conversion should not be construed as a failure but rather as the application of sound surgical judgment.

Several findings or conditions may lead to conversion to an open procedure. Inability to identify critical structures (e.g., the ureter or major blood vessels) or concern about appropriate anatomic orientation should encourage the surgeon to open the abdomen. Early in the case, the presence of dense adhesions, which may prolong the procedure excessively, should encourage early conversion to an open procedure. Care and prudence must be exercised during extensive adhesiolysis. In addition, lack of adequate exposure, poor hemostasis, disorientation, inadequate resection or reconstruction,

and the presence of an enterotomy, structure, abscess, or fistula may all prompt early conversion. In particular, we have found it difficult to recognize serosal abrasions and enterotomies, particularly when dissecting over the pelvic brim. Dissecting the small bowel out of the pelvis is difficult. This finding is a common reason for conversion to an open laparotomy.

A key point is that the operation should not be unduly prolonged by troublesome intra-abdominal findings. The decision whether the case can be completed laparoscopically or should be converted to an open laparotomy usually can and should be made rapidly.

Another issue concerns trocar placement. When placing the trocars, we favor a Hasson technique, in which the initial 12 mm port is placed through the left upper quadrant rectus muscle under direct vision. The reason we have come to prefer this location is that in the right upper quadrant, the falciform ligament frequently complicates access to the abdominal cavity. The second, third, and fourth ports are then placed under direct vision. Initial studies reported injuries to major intra-abdominal vessels in the course of port placement, but we have not encountered this problem with our technique.[7] In addition, we favor minimizing the number of 10/12 mm ports used because the larger incisions can be difficult to repair accurately and may be associated with bowel herniation. Bowel herniation has not been reported at 5 mm port sites. The port sizes and instrument sizes necessary for colonic dissection are predictable; thus, a standardized approach, as outlined [*see* Operative Technique, *above*], can be established with little difficulty.

Finally, management of the primary feeding vessels can be an irksome problem. On each side of the ileocolic and inferior mesenteric

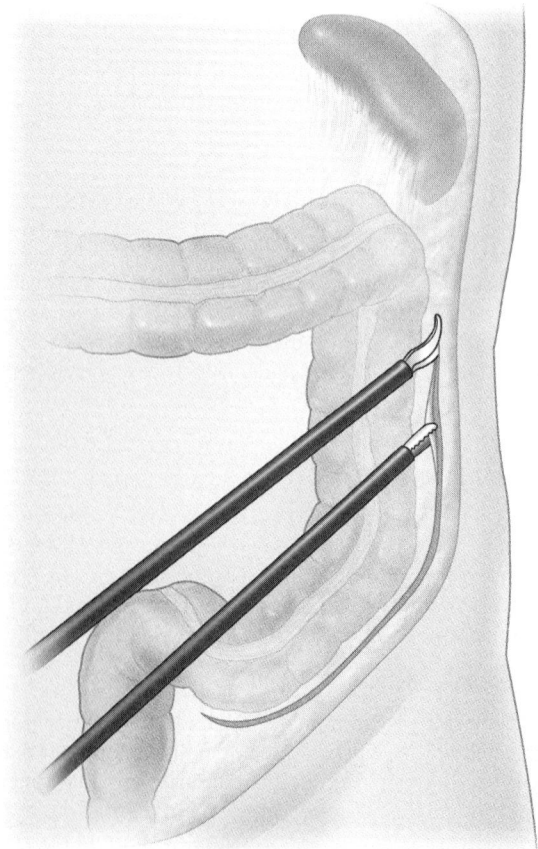

Figure 6 **Laparoscopic colectomy: left hemicolectomy and sigmoid resection. Sigmoid mesentery and pelvic dissection.**

vessels, there is a large avascular window. We take advantage of this predictable anatomic finding and aggressively dissect and isolate these vessels. Our usual practice is to separate the vein from the artery with a right-angle dissecting clamp and clip them separately. Occasionally, a fibrotic sheath prevents this separation, in which case we use an endovascular stapler to occlude and divide the vessels.

Complications

Complications associated with laparoscopic colectomy include major vessel injuries and enterotomies (both recognized and unrecognized). These can generally be minimized and managed through careful troubleshooting (see above).

A potential complication that has given rise to considerable concern is recurrence at port sites after laparoscopic colectomy for cancer. Anecdotal reports of wound and port-site recurrences after laparoscopic colon cancer resection were widely published in the early 1990s. Experience suggests that such recurrences are rare: the average incidence appears to be about 1%, which is comparable to the recurrence rates reported after open procedures.[3-6] Nevertheless, these anecdotal reports led to a resurgence of the theory that tumoricidal agents might prevent such recurrence. One group found that taurolidine combined with heparin decreased tumor cell growth in a rat model.[8] Another showed that 5% pyrrolidone iodine mixed with 0.5% chloramine killed almost all tumor cells in vitro and prevented their growth in vivo.[9] We demonstrated that povidone decreased tumor cell growth in laparoscopic ports in a murine model.[10] If these results can be confirmed by other studies, use of tumoricidal agents to prevent port-site recurrence may well become the standard of care.

The best way of putting the issue of port-site recurrence to rest is to perform a prospective, randomized study comparing laparoscopic colectomy with open colectomy in patients with colon cancer. In 1995, the National Cancer Institute (NCI) initiated a multicenter study designed to address this issue and others having to do with safety, staging, and 5-year survival rates. The results of this study should be available in 2004. The general consensus in the United States is that until the results are in hand, laparoscopic colectomies for cancer should be performed at those centers involved in the study. Data from Barcelona suggest that laparoscopic colectomy may have some advantages over traditional open colectomy. If this observation is confirmed by the NCI study, laparoscopic colectomy may rapidly become the preferred technique for resection of colon cancer.

Outcome Evaluation

To date, laparoscopic approaches have been most successful for right hemicolectomy, sigmoid resection, and stoma formation. Ab-

dominoperineal resection is also easily and safely performed with laparoscopic techniques.

Studies have found that laparoscopic colectomy results in decreased short-term morbidity, decreased abdominal wall trauma, earlier tolerance of food, shortened hospital stays, and reduced pain and narcotic requirements.[11] It has also been reported that surgical blood loss and the need for transfusions are reduced and that postoperative cell-mediated immunity and neutrophil function are improved.[12,13] There appear to be less immunosuppression after laparoscopic colectomy and, therefore, greater resistance to tumor regrowth (theoretically, at least). Because of the overall improvement in function, patients can return to normal activities and work more quickly.

With respect to short-term outcome, laparoscopic colectomy is comparable to open colectomy. No major differences in the number of lymph nodes resected or the length of bowel resected have been found between the two approaches; there is a trend toward greater length of bowel resection in open colectomy, but the difference is not statistically significant.[14,15] No significant cost differences between the two procedures have been documented: the decreased length of stay associated with laparoscopic colectomy is effectively balanced by the increased operating expenses. If, however, the rate of conversion to open colectomy is high (i.e., > 20%), the cost of laparoscopic surgery may be higher than that of open surgery.

At present, there is a great deal of interest in the use of laparoscopy to resect colon cancers and to minimize the short-term morbidity associated with treatment of malignant diseases. There has been sufficient research into and experience with laparoscopic treatment of colorectal cancer to show that it is a feasible modality offering the same advantages as laparoscopic treatment of benign colonic disease. The heart of the current debate surrounding the application of laparoscopy to malignant colonic disease is the question of how a laparoscopic approach might affect long-term patterns of recurrence and survival.[3,5,6]

Concerns regarding the efficacy of laparoscopic colectomy for cancer have centered on the completeness of the bowel and lymph node resections. As noted, multiple studies have shown no differences between laparoscopic colectomy and open colectomy with respect to proximal and distal margins of resection or the adequacy of lymph node dissection. Most of the concerns regarding the incidence and pattern of recurrence after laparoscopic treatment were generated early in surgeons' experience with laparoscopic colectomy, and subsequent studies tended not to find substantial differences. However, further studies that include long-term follow-up to determine the adequacy of resection and the comparability of cure rates are needed to assess any changes in the long-term staging and survival patterns after laparoscopic colectomy.

References

1. Beart RW Jr: Laparoscopic colectomy: status of the art. Dis Colon Rectum 37(suppl):S47, 1994

2. Monson JRT, Hill ADK, Darzi A: Laparoscopic colonic surgery. Br J Surg 82:150, 1995

3. Ramos JM, Gupta S, Anthone GJ, et al: Laparoscopy and colon cancer: is the port site at risk? a preliminary report. Arch Surg 129:897, 1994

4. Paik PS: Abdominal incision tumor implantation following pneumoperitoneum laparoscopic procedure vs. standard open incision in a syngeneic rat model. Dis Colon Rectum 41:419, 1998

5. Wexner SD, Cohen SM: Port site metastases after laparoscopic colorectal surgery for cure of malignancy. Br J Surg 82:295, 1995

6. Lacy AM, Garcia-Valdecasas JC, Pique JM, et al: Short-term outcome analysis of a randomized study comparing laparoscopic vs open colectomy for colon cancer. Surg Endosc 9:1101, 1995

7. Nordestgaard AG, Bodily KC, Osborne RW Jr, et al: Major vascular injuries during laparoscopic procedures. Am J Surg 169:543, 1995

8. Jacobi C, Ordemann J, Bohm B, et al: Inhibition of peritoneal tumor cell growth and implantation in laparoscopic surgery in a rat model. Am J Surg 174:359, 1997

9. Basha G, Penninckx F, Geboes K, et al: Tumoricidal activity of antiseptics with assessment of cell viability in mice with severe combined immunodeficiency. Tumour Biol 18:213, 1997

10. Hoffstetter W, Ortega A, Chiang M, et al: The effects of topical tumoricidals on port-site recurrence of colon cancer: an experimental study in rats. J Laparoendosc Adv Surg Tech A 11:9, 2001

11. Chen HH, Wexner SD, Iroatulam AJN, et al: Laparoscopic colectomy compares favorably with colectomy by laparotomy for reduction of postoperative ileus. Dis Colon Rectum 43:61, 2000

12. Harmon GD, Senganore AJ, Kilbride MJ, et al: Interleukin-6 response to laparoscopic and open colectomy. Dis Colon Rectum 37:754, 1994

13. Kloosterman T, Von Blomberg ME, Borgstein P, et al: Unimpaired immune function after laparoscopic cholecystectomy. Surgery 113:424, 1994

14. Kockerling F: Prospective multicenter study of the quality of oncologic resections in patients undergoing laparoscopic colorectal surgery for cancer. Dis Colon Rectum 41:963, 1998

15. Hida J, Yasutomi M, Maruyama T, et al: The extent of lymph node dissection for colon carcinoma: the potential impact on laparoscopic surgery. Cancer 80: 188, 1997

Recommended Reading

Beart RW Jr: Increased tumor establishment and growth after laparotomy vs laparoscopy in a murine model (invited commentary). Arch Surg 130:653, 1995

Dorrance HR, Oien K, O'Dwyer PJ: Effects of laparoscopy on intraperitoneal tumor growth and distant metastases in an animal model. Surgery 126:35, 1999

Fleshman JW, Wexner SD, Anvari M, et al: Laparoscopic *vs.* open abdominoperineal resection for cancer. Dis Colon Rectum 42:930, 1999

Hewitt PM: Laparoscopic-assisted vs. open surgery for colorectal cancer. Dis Colon Rectum 41:901, 1998

Huguet EL, Earnshaw JJ, Heather BP: Major vascular injury during laparoscopy. Br J Surg 84:1479, 1997

Liberman MA, Phillips EH, Carroll BJ, et al: Laparoscopic colectomy vs traditional colectomy for diverticulitis: outcome and costs. Surg Endosc 10:15, 1996

Schwandner O, Schiedeck THK, Bruch HP: Advanced age—indication or contraindication for laparoscopic colorectal surgery? Dis Colon Rectum 42:356, 1999

Solomon MJ, Egan M, Roberts RA, et al: Incidence of free colorectal cancer cells on the peritoneal surface. Dis Colon Rectum 40:1294, 1997

Wolf JS Jr, Stoller ML: The physiology of laparoscopy: basic principles, complications and other considerations. J Urol 152:294, 1994

Acknowledgment

Figures 1 through 6   Tom Moore.

4 VASCULAR SYSTEM

1 STROKE AND TRANSIENT ISCHEMIC ATTACK

Thomas S. Maldonado, M.D., and Thomas S. Riles, M.D., F.A.C.S.

Assessment and Management of Stroke and TIA

Stroke is defined as any damage to the central nervous system caused by interruption of the blood supply. Ischemic strokes result from the failure of oxygen and nutrients to reach the affected brain. Transient ischemic attacks (TIAs) are defined as transient neurologic deficits lasting no longer than 24 hours; longer-lasting deficits are considered to be indicative of a cerebral infarction ("brain attack").

Infarction from ischemia is typically confined to a vascular territory, at whose center can be found the injured or obstructed artery supplying that parenchyma. The full extent of a stroke may not become apparent until days or weeks later, when the tenuous peripheral watershed zone, or penumbra, either survives or succumbs to cell death. Smaller infarcts, adequate collateral circulation, and prompt intervention and resuscitation are associated with improved outcome.

Hemorrhagic stroke damages the brain by cutting off connecting pathways and causing localized or generalized pressure injury. Brain edema and hydrocephalus after hemorrhagic stroke may also be deleterious. In some cases, hemorrhagic stroke can lead to ischemia as a consequence of vasospasm, as is seen in the setting of subarachnoid hemorrhage (SAH). Likewise, some ischemic strokes can undergo hemorrhagic transformation.

Incidence and Risk Factors

Stroke is the third leading cause of death in the United States: about 168,000 stroke-related deaths are reported each year.[1] Approximately 500,000 first-time strokes are reported annually. In addition, stroke is the leading cause of serious long-term disability in the United States and poses a substantial economic burden. For 2003, U.S. expenditure on stroke-related medical costs and disability payments amounts to roughly $51 billion. Although a sharp decline in stroke incidence and mortality was noted throughout most of the 20th century, the decline leveled off in the early 1990s, and stroke incidence and mortality are now rising for the first time since 1915.[2,3]

Numerous population studies and stroke registries have been designed to examine the incidence, risk factors, and natural history of stroke.[4-10] Some of the independent risk factors that have been identified—such as age (> 55 years), sex (male), race (African American and Asian), and genetic predisposition—cannot be modified and therefore carry a fixed level of stroke risk. The Rochester (Minnesota) population study demonstrated a marked progressive incidence of cerebral infarction with advancing age, as well as nearly 1.5 times greater risk of stroke in males.[4] The Lausanne Stroke Registry data confirmed the overall higher incidence of stroke in males, though it also demonstrated a female preponderance in very young (< 30 years) and very old (> 80 years) patients. These latter findings may be attributable to the high frequency of oral contraceptive use in young women in that

study as well as to the lower life expectancy of men, especially those with vascular risk factors.[9] Race and genetic predisposition are also considered independent risk factors, with African Americans more than twice as likely to die of stroke as whites.[10] The underlying mechanism of stroke appears to vary with race as well: intracranial occlusive disease tends to occur more frequently in African and Asian Americans than in whites or in males as a whole.[11,12] The importance of hereditary risk for stroke has long been recognized. In the Framingham Study, both paternal and maternal histories of stroke were associated with an increased risk of stroke.[10,13]

There are, however, certain risk factors for stroke that are clearly modifiable, including hypertension, smoking, hyperlipidemia, asymptomatic high-grade carotid stenosis, and atrial fibrillation.[14-16] Other purported modifiable risk factors for stroke, such as obesity, diabetes, oral contraceptive use, and alcohol intake, are more controversial.[17-20] Hypertension (systolic as well as diastolic) is perhaps the most prominent modifiable risk factor for stroke and is associated with a substantial risk of atherothrombotic, lacunar, or subarachnoid hemorrhage. The Systolic Hypertension in the Elderly Program (SHEP) study demonstrated that treating systolic hypertension in patients 60 years of age or older can result in a stroke reduction of up to 36%.[21] Prompt diagnosis and intervention for stroke may be critical, but many authorities feel that primary prevention is the true cornerstone of therapy for this lethal disease.

Clinical Evaluation

When assessing patients who present with a neurologic deficit, clinicians must immediately ask themselves the following two questions: (1) what is the mechanism of the deficit (i.e., ischemic or hemorrhagic), and (2) where is the lesion (e.g., cerebral lacunae, the territory around a large vessel, or a watershed region)? A thorough history and physical examination, in conjunction with brain imaging studies, usually suffice to guide initial management. Nonvascular conditions that can mimic stroke (e.g., hypoglycemia, migraine, a postictal state, encephalopathy, trauma, and brain tumors or abscesses) must be excluded. Although these syndromes can all cause focal findings, they usually lack the abrupt onset of symptoms consistently seen with stroke.

Ischemic and hemorrhagic stroke must be differentiated early in the course of an acute stroke because a number of therapeutic interventions that are beneficial for some subtypes of stroke are potentially catastrophic to others. Approximately 71% of all

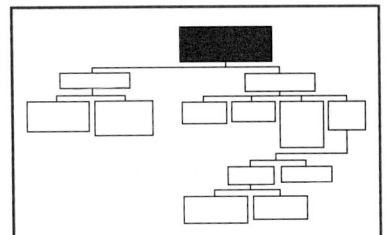

Assessment and Management of Stroke and TIA

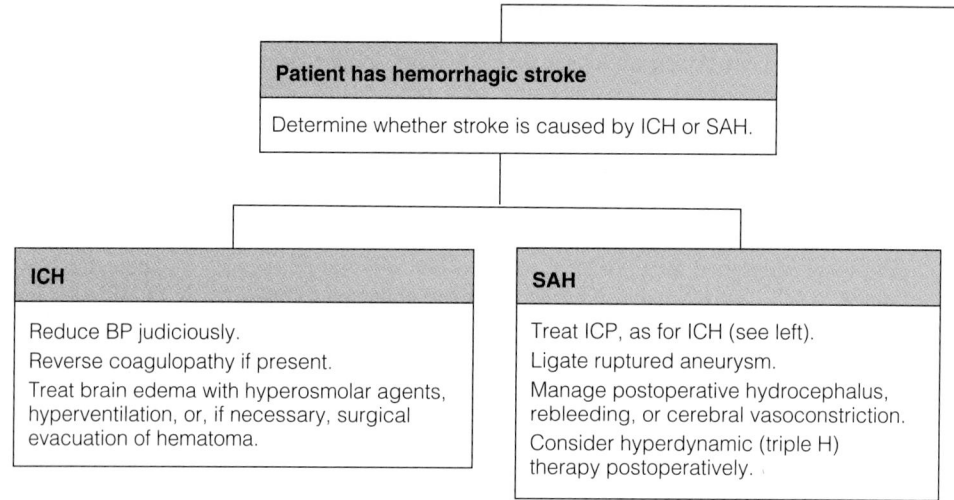

Patient has hemorrhagic stroke

Determine whether stroke is caused by ICH or SAH.

ICH

Reduce BP judiciously.

Reverse coagulopathy if present.

Treat brain edema with hyperosmolar agents, hyperventilation, or, if necessary, surgical evacuation of hematoma.

SAH

Treat ICP, as for ICH (see left).

Ligate ruptured aneurysm.

Manage postoperative hydrocephalus, rebleeding, or cerebral vasoconstriction.

Consider hyperdynamic (triple H) therapy postoperatively.

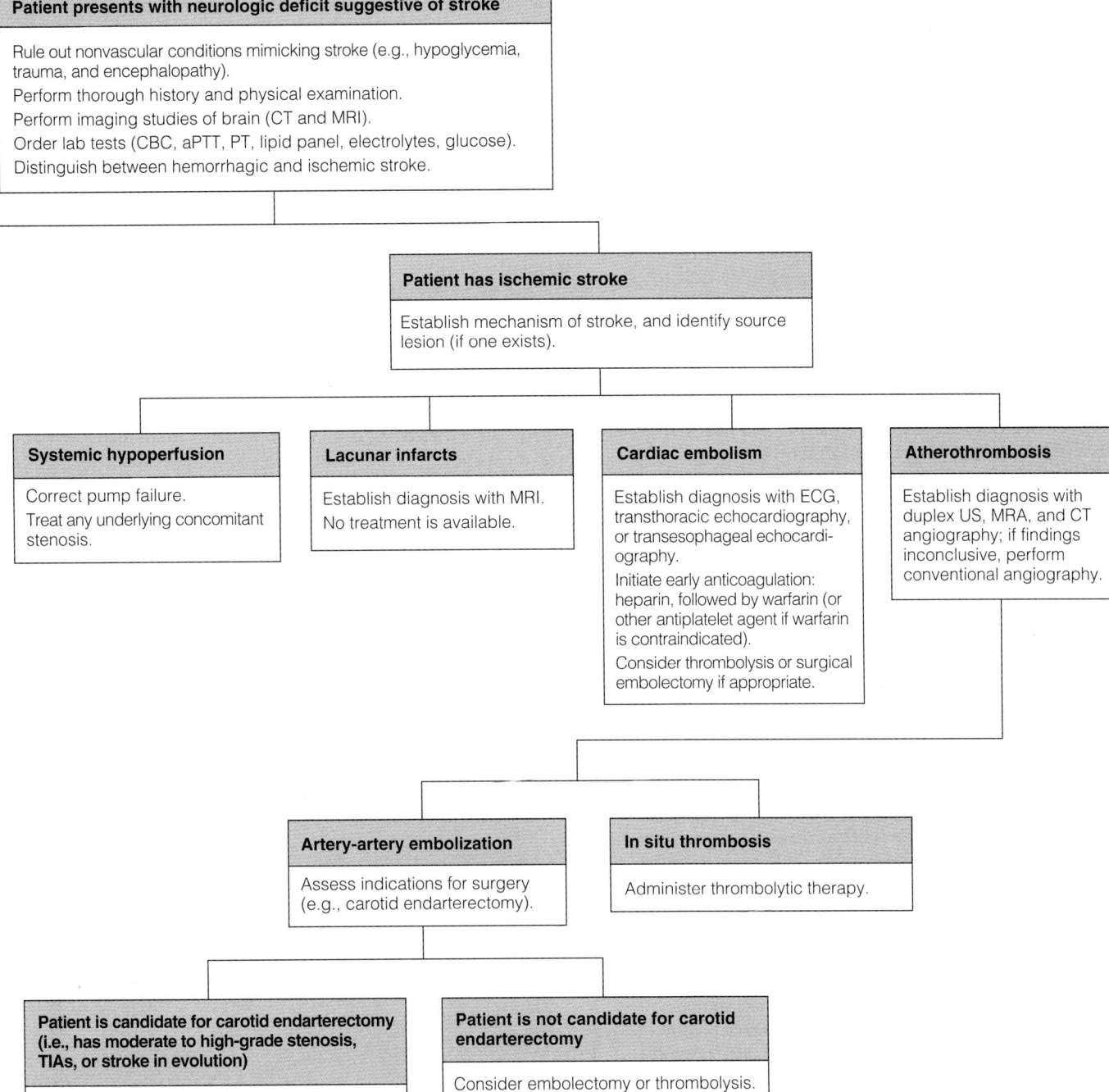

Patient presents with neurologic deficit suggestive of stroke

Rule out nonvascular conditions mimicking stroke (e.g., hypoglycemia, trauma, and encephalopathy).
Perform thorough history and physical examination.
Perform imaging studies of brain (CT and MRI).
Order lab tests (CBC, aPTT, PT, lipid panel, electrolytes, glucose).
Distinguish between hemorrhagic and ischemic stroke.

Patient has ischemic stroke

Establish mechanism of stroke, and identify source lesion (if one exists).

Systemic hypoperfusion

Correct pump failure.
Treat any underlying concomitant stenosis.

Lacunar infarcts

Establish diagnosis with MRI.
No treatment is available.

Cardiac embolism

Establish diagnosis with ECG, transthoracic echocardiography, or transesophageal echocardiography.
Initiate early anticoagulation: heparin, followed by warfarin (or other antiplatelet agent if warfarin is contraindicated).
Consider thrombolysis or surgical embolectomy if appropriate.

Atherothrombosis

Establish diagnosis with duplex US, MRA, and CT angiography; if findings inconclusive, perform conventional angiography.

Artery-artery embolization

Assess indications for surgery (e.g., carotid endarterectomy).

In situ thrombosis

Administer thrombolytic therapy.

Patient is candidate for carotid endarterectomy (i.e., has moderate to high-grade stenosis, TIAs, or stroke in evolution)

Perform carotid endarterectomy.
Administer antiplatelet therapy.

Patient is not candidate for carotid endarterectomy

Consider embolectomy or thrombolysis.
Administer antiplatelet therapy.

Table 1 Causes of Stroke as Recorded in NINCDS Data Bank[22]

Cerebral ischemia	71%
Atherosclerosis	10%
Larger-artery stenosis	6%
Tandem arterial lesions	4%
Lacunae	19%
Cardioembolism	14%
Infarct of undetermined cause	27%
Cerebral hemorrhage	26%
Parenchymatous	13%
Subarachnoid	13%
Other	3%

NINCDS—National Institute of Neurological and Communicative Disorders and Stroke

strokes are ischemic and 26% hemorrhagic; the remaining 3% are of unknown origin [see Table 1].[22] Hemorrhagic strokes result from subarachnoid or intracerebral bleeding, whereas ischemic strokes result from systemic hypoperfusion, cardioembolism, or atherothrombosis. Although various different laboratory and radiographic tests are available and should be performed, the diagnosis of stroke is primarily a clinical one.

HISTORY

A patient who has suffered a stroke typically presents with a history of sudden onset of a focal brain deficit and a clinical syndrome on neurologic examination. A medical history should elicit any of a number of risk factors associated with either ischemic or hemorrhagic stroke. For example, hypertension is often associated with deep infarcts and hemorrhages, whereas cigarette smoking, hyperlipidemia, and hypertension are more commonly associated with ischemic infarcts resulting from atherosclerosis.[9] The presence of atrial fibrillation, a recent myocardial infarction (MI) (< 6 weeks old), or a prosthetic heart valve suggests a possible cardioembolic mechanism.

The onset and course of the neurologic deficit may also be telling. A steady onset is suggestive of hemorrhage, whereas symptoms that progress in a stepwise fashion are more likely to derive from ischemia. Likewise, accompanying signs are frequently useful in differentiating stroke mechanism subtypes. Headache, vomiting, and loss of consciousness constitute the classic picture of hemorrhagic stroke, whereas a focal deficit preceded by TIAs is more suggestive of ischemic stroke.[23] Although the clinical manifestations are generally helpful in differentiating stroke subtypes, it sometimes happens that large infarcts mimic the classic picture of hemorrhage or that lobar or small deep hemorrhages resemble infarction resulting from atherosclerosis. Analysis of 1,000 consecutive patients from the Lausanne Stroke Registry who experienced their first stroke confirmed that the classic hemorrhagic picture (headaches, progressive neuralgic deficits, and decreased level of consciousness) was indeed more common in patients with hemorrhage but found that only one third of patients with hemorrhagic strokes had this clinical triad.[9]

PHYSICAL AND NEUROLOGIC EXAMINATION

A general physical and neurologic examination should detect vascular and cardiac abnormalities as well as localize the process within the CNS. Heart size and sounds, irregular rhythms or dis-crepant pulse exams, and carotid bruits should all be noted. Careful examination of the extremities is essential, in that peripheral vascular disease is highly correlated with the presence of atherosclerosis of the carotid and vertebral arteries.[6,24] An ophthalmologic examination should detect subhyaloid hemorrhages as well as cholesterol emboli (Hollenhorst plaques).

Besides localizing the lesion anatomically, the neurologic examination should be able to identify a probable cause. The absence of major focal neurologic signs is often consistent with SAH; focal deficits localized to the superficial cortex are often attributable to thromboembolism or ischemia. A number of well-described lacunar syndromes also exist; these typically suggest small-vessel disease.

Diagnostic Studies

IMAGING

Imaging is a mandatory and integral part of evaluation for acute stroke and should be performed expeditiously. Computed tomography is the initial test of choice; it is readily available in most hospitals and is well tolerated by critically ill patients.[25] CT can promptly identify nonvascular causative conditions (e.g., masses) and can readily diagnose intracerebral hemorrhage (ICH) [see Figure 1]. Diagnosis of SAH without I.V. contrast can be more difficult, especially if bleeding is minor or occurred more than 1 day before; the accuracy of CT in detecting SAH decreases after 24 hours.[26] SAH should appear as an increased density in the CSF. If SAH is clinically suspected, lumbar puncture may be necessary for definitive diagnosis.

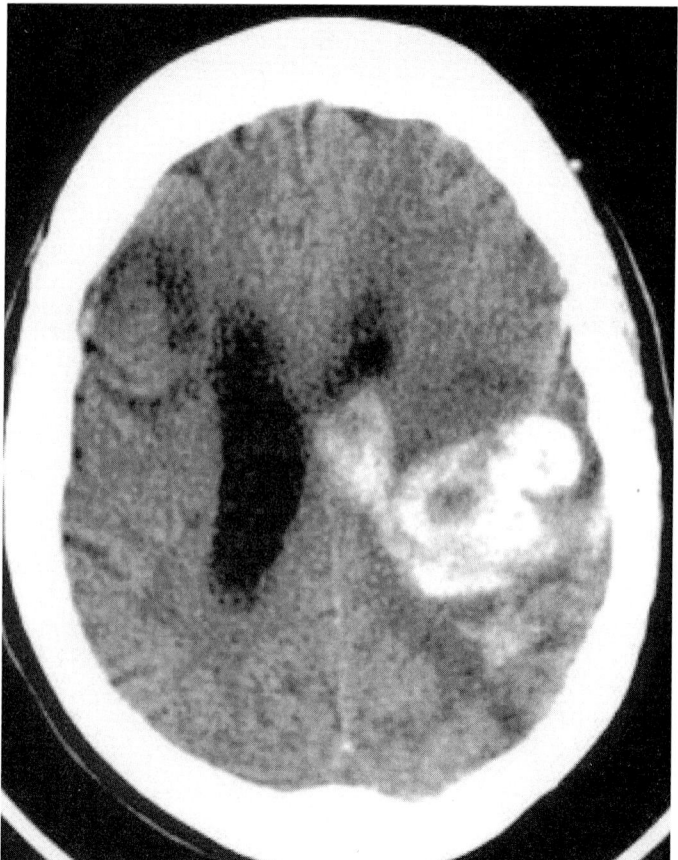

Figure 1 Shown is a CT image of an acute hemorrhagic infarct, with intraparenchymal bleeding apparent.

a   *b*

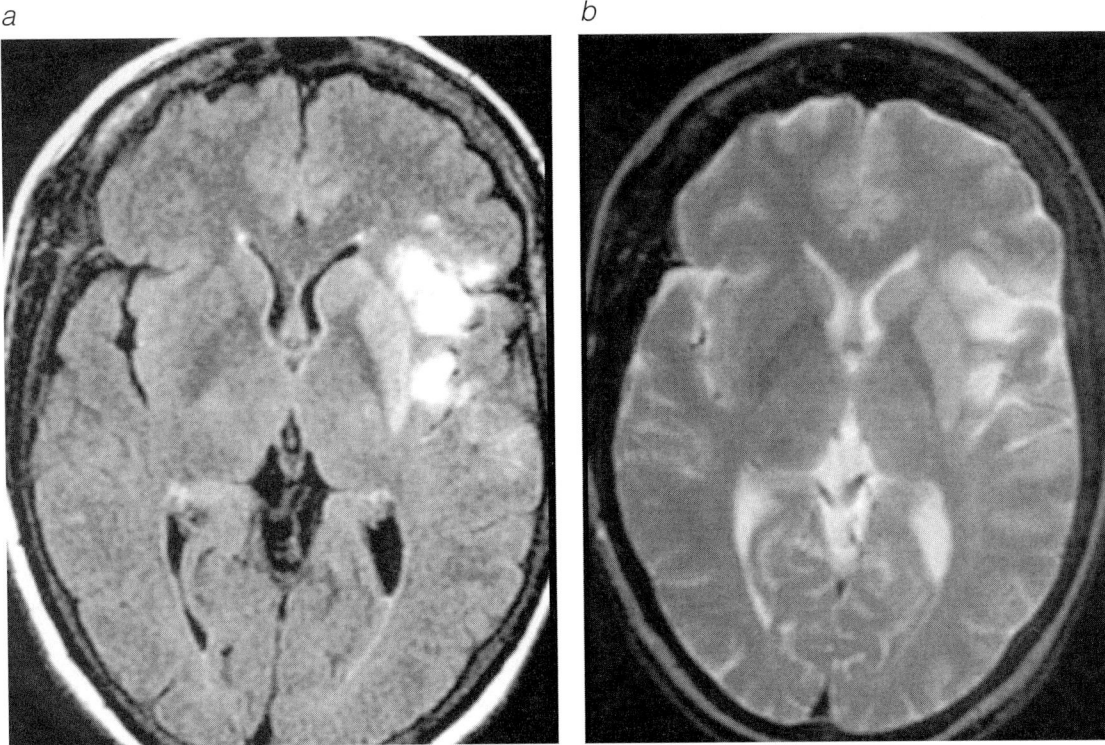

Figure 2   Shown are (*a*) a fluid-attenuated inversion-recovery (FLAIR) MRI image and (*b*) a T$_2$-weighted MRI image of an acute ischemic infarct in the left middle cerebral artery distribution.

In cases of acute ischemic stroke, diagnosis of infarction by means of CT can be more difficult. I.V. contrast CT is of limited value in this setting. Signs of infarction can be absent or subtle in the first few hours after the stroke. A lesion may appear as a slight hypodensity within the infarcted zone or as a loss of definition between gray and white matter.[27] Newer CT scanners may be better at delineating these nuances.[28,29] In the days following an ischemic stroke, an infarct may first appear round or oval and then as a hypodense, dark, or wedge-shaped lesion on CT.

Magnetic resonance imaging is more expensive and time-consuming than CT and is less well tolerated by critically ill patients. Nonetheless, MRI is more sensitive than CT in detecting early ischemic changes after a stroke. It can be used to distinguish an old stroke from a new one and to assess the size and location of a lesion, especially when it is adjacent to bony structures [*see Figure 2*].[30] The size of the infarct as determined by MRI may be of great importance for prognosis. Although lesion size may not correlate with severity of clinical presentation, larger infarcts in the same vascular territory are associated with more severe deficits than smaller infarcts in similar anatomic locations are.

MRI is especially useful for diagnosing lacunar infarcts. In a review of 227 patients with lacunar infarcts, 44% were diagnosed by CT and 78% by MRI.[31] Infarction appears as dark, hypodense areas on T$_1$-weighted sequences and as bright areas on T$_2$-weighted sequences. Edema usually develops around the infarct within the first few days and is readily apparent on MRI as a low-density area surrounding the lesion with mass effect. Sometimes, the infarct is small but is still associated with substantial edema. Such edema may be insignificant in an older patient with an atrophied brain whose cranium is able to accommodate a mass effect but may be life-threatening in a younger patient with little intracranial room to spare.

The high sensitivity of MRI in detecting infarction has been demonstrated in studies evaluating patients experiencing TIAs.

When patients without signs or symptoms of infarction underwent brain imaging after a TIA, 27% were found to have evidence of so-called silent infarcts on CT and 73% on MRI.[32]

Diagnosis of ICH can be a more delicate task with MRI than with CT. Careful scrutiny by an experienced observer using different acquisition techniques is required. The appearance of a lesion on T$_1$- and T$_2$-weighted sequences varies as a cerebral hematoma matures and edema resolves. Acute hematomas are black on T$_1$-weighted images, and chronic hematomas are white on T$_1$- and T$_2$-weighted images.

Normal neuroimaging findings are not uncommon in patients presenting with neurologic deficits suggestive of acute stroke. A patient with a neurologic deficit and a negative CT scan should undergo further cerebral imaging with MRI. The absence of ischemic infarction and hemorrhage on both CT and MRI may suggest transient ischemia or persistent ischemia without infarction. In such cases, one may have to rely on signs and symptoms to localize the ischemic lesion responsible for the stroke. Alternatively, electroencephalography (EEG), positron emission tomography (PET), single-photon emission CT (SPECT), or xenon-enhanced CT (XeCT) may be employed to help localize ischemic foci.[33,34]

LABORATORY TESTS

Blood should be sent to the laboratory as part of the initial assessment of a patient with an acute stroke. Measurement of serum electrolyte and glucose levels is essential to rule out nonvascular conditions mimicking stroke (e.g., hypoglycemia and dehydration). A complete blood count (CBC), an activated partial thromboplastin time (aPTT), a prothrombin time (PT), and a lipid panel are likewise essential components of the initial assessment. Severe anemia has the potential to exacerbate or precipitate cerebral ischemia in stroke; though this is an uncommon occurrence, it should be considered and, if present, corrected.[35]

Additional laboratory blood tests, such as a cardiac injury panel to rule out myocardial infarction or an erythrocyte sedimentation rate to assess the possibility of vasculitis, may be helpful.

Screening should be performed for hematologic disorders that result in hypercoagulable states, including homocystinuria,[36] antiphospholipid antibody syndrome, protein C and S deficiency, antithrombin deficiency, and activated protein C resistance from factor V Leiden mutation [see 4:6 Venous Thromboembolism].[37,38] Hemoglobinopathies (e.g., sickle cell disease and thalassemia) can also lead to altered blood flow, hypercoagulability, and stroke.[39] Finally, hyperviscosity syndromes (e.g., polycythemia vera, thrombocytosis, and myeloproliferative disorders) should be included in the differential diagnosis. If a hyperviscosity syndrome is recognized in the setting of acute stroke, hemodilution therapy may be warranted. Experimental and clinical trials have shown hemodilution to increase blood flow in the ischemic brain; however, other studies have failed to show improvement of neurologic status.[40,41] Hemodilution remains indicated in stroke patients who have a high hematocrit or are in a hyperviscosity state; however, close monitoring is required in patients with heart disease or cerebral edema.

Differentiation of Hemorrhagic from Ischemic Stroke

HEMORRHAGIC STROKE

Hemorrhagic stroke can result from ICH or SAH. The consequences of cerebral bleeding can progress rapidly from neurologic deficit to coma to death in a significant number of patients.

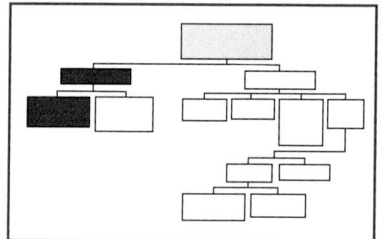

Intracerebral Hemorrhage

ICH accounts for approximately 10% to 15% of all strokes in the United States and Europe.[22,42] Potential causative mechanisms include hypertension, trauma, arteriovenous malformations, cerebral amyloid angiopathy, brain tumors, blood dyscrasias, and medications (e.g., anticoagulants and thrombolytics). Of these, hypertensive arteriopathy is most commonly responsible for nontraumatic ICH.[22,43] Hypertensive brain hemorrhages are usually deep and are typically located in the lateral ganglionic region, the subcortex, the thalamus, the caudate nucleus, the pons, or the cerebellum. As early as the 1870s, Charcot and Bouchard correctly postulated that such events were the result of microaneurysmal disease of arteries and arterioles penetrating deep into the brains of hypertensive patients.[44,45] These discrete hemorrhages go on to compress neighboring capillary networks, causing them to burst and bringing about a rapid enlargement of the intracerebral hematoma. Indeed, such enlargement is not uncommon: one prospective study found that 38% of patients with ICH had a hematoma that was enlarged at 3 hours in comparison with its size on baseline CT after the initial bleeding event.[46]

Patients presenting with sizable ICH often rely on a marked compensatory elevation of blood pressure to maintain a pressure gradient in the setting of acute increases in intracranial pressure (ICP). It is vital to resist the impulse to lower blood pressure aggressively in these patients: a rapid drop in blood pressure may induce brain ischemia. Short-acting antihypertensives should be administered only when the systolic blood pressure is persistently higher than 180 to 200 mm Hg or when there is evidence of active bleeding or an enlarging hematoma. Other medical treatment of hemorrhagic stroke from ICH includes reversal of coagulopathies with transfusions of fresh frozen plasma and platelets when appropriate.

Mortality from ICH has plummeted from 90% before the 1970s to less than 50% in the first years of the 21st century.[2,22,47] This precipitous decline probably reflects improved antihypertensive therapy as well as decreased prevalence of hypertension.[48] Death from ICH most commonly occurs secondary to herniation from the hematoma itself coupled with brain edema, which can develop within the first hours after ICH.[47,49] Thus, treatment of brain edema is the main focus of treatment. Corticosteroids, though indicated for reducing cerebral edema in patients with tumors or abscesses, are contraindicated in patients with ICH because they are not beneficial and may in fact be injurious, predisposing patients to infection and worsening diabetes.[50] Hyperosmolar agents (e.g., mannitol or glycerol solutions) may be more useful for reducing cerebral edema rapidly.[51] Alternatively, in cases of severe brain edema, hyperventilation may reduce ICP by inducing diffuse vasoconstriction in the brain. Any physiologic perturbation that might increase cerebral blood volume (e.g., hypercarbia, hypoxia, or vasodilation) or reduce cerebral perfusion (e.g., hypotension) should be avoided. Finally, surgical evacuation of a hematoma, though controversial, may be employed as a last resort for decompression after ICH.[52]

Subarachnoid Hemorrhage

Rupture of saccular or berry aneurysms with subsequent SAH carries significant morbidity and mortality, depending largely on the patient's age, the extent of the hemorrhage,

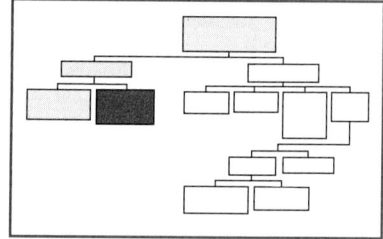

and the presence and severity of rebleeding, cerebral vasospasm, and surgical complications.[53] SAH accounts for 6% to 10% of all strokes and 22% to 25% of all deaths from cerebrovascular accidents.[54] The reported incidence of incidental aneurysms discovered in autopsy studies ranges from 0.8% to 18%.[55-57] SAH tends to occur more often in patients 50 to 60 years of age than in younger or older patients and in women more often than in men (12.3% versus 7.9%).[58] The pathogenesis of saccular aneurysms has not been fully explicated, but the risk factors are well described and include a family history of SAH,[59] hypertension, pregnancy,[60] and black race.[61]

SAH presents with warning signs in as many as 20% of patients within the 3 months preceding a major rupture, presumably because a minor leak develops before the rupture. Such warning signs include a so-called sentinel headache, oculomotor symptoms, nausea and vomiting, and loss of consciousness.[62] The rupture itself is accompanied by sudden severe headache, nuchal rigidity, back pain, nausea, vomiting, photophobia, lethargy, loss of consciouness, and seizure.[60,63]

Medical management of SAH includes tranquil bed rest with the head elevated 30°, stool softeners, antiemetics, and analgesics, as well as deep vein thrombosis (DVT) prophylaxis using pneumatic compression boots. Management of ICP in SAH patients is similar to that in ICH patients (see above). Furthermore, one must be vigilant for signs of hypothalamic dysfunction manifesting as cardiac dysrhythmias or the syndrome of inappropriate antidiuretic hormone secretion (SIADH).

The timing of microsurgical clip ligation of aneurysms after SAH is somewhat controversial. The International Cooperative Study on the Timing of Aneurysm Surgery showed no overall differences in outcome between early surgery (0 to 3 days after SAH) and delayed surgery (11 to 14 days after SAH).[64] Nonetheless, patients who were alert preoperatively did better with early surgery and demonstrated significantly better rates of good recovery.

Three major neurologic complications affect outcome after surgery for SAH: hydrocephalus, rebleeding, and cerebral vasoconstriction. Hydrocephalus may develop acutely as a result of obstruction of CSF outflow. Ventricular drainage can lead to immediate reduction of ICP and improvement in neurologic symptoms. The risk of rebleeding peaks on postoperative day 1; it is as high as 20% in the first 2 weeks and rises to 50% within 6 months if the aneurysm is not treated.[53] Unlike rebleeding, vasospasm manifests itself gradually over hours to days; it may be associated with up to a threefold increase in mortality during the 2 weeks after SAH.[65-67] The diagnosis is initially made via angiography and followed via transcranial Doppler sonography.[68,69] Hyperdynamic, or triple H, therapy consists of keeping patients hyperdynamic (to increase cardiac output), hypervolemic-hypertensive (to augment cerebral perfusion pressure), and hemodiluted (to improve cerebral microcirculation by decreasing viscosity). Because of the risk that the aneurysm will rerupture before operation, triple H therapy is reserved for postoperative patients.[70,71] Calcium blockers may also reduce the incidence of symptoms secondary to vasospasm, though they most likely have little effect on spasm per se.[72]

ISCHEMIC STROKE

If hemorrhagic stroke is ruled out and ischemic stroke is diagnosed, the next step is to establish the mechanism of the stroke and identify the source lesion responsible (if one exists). Systemic hypoperfusion, cardiac embolism, large-artery atherosclerosis, and small-vessel disease should be systematically considered as potential causes.

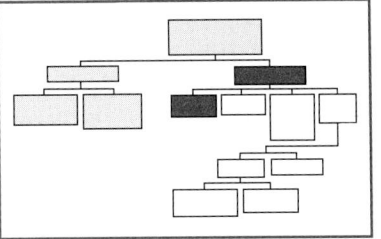

Systemic Hypoperfusion

Only a small fraction of all ischemic strokes are attributable to systemic hypoperfusion. A quick assessment of vital signs and symptoms may provide the first clues that a patient is suffering from cerebral ischemia secondary to systemic hypoperfusion. Patients are characteristically either unconscious on arrival in the emergency department or awake but exhibiting neurologic symptoms resembling near-syncope.[73] Generally, they are pale, diaphoretic, and hypotensive. Neurologic signs and symptoms are varied and are explained by ischemia in the border zone (or watershed) between two or three adjacent arterial territories. Difficulty in reading or identifying visual stimuli (or even frank blindness) may be observed; this may be attributed to ischemia between the middle and posterior cerebral arteries. Bilateral arm weakness or cognitive difficulty may suggest ischemia between the middle and anterior cerebral arteries. Global symptoms usually arise from bilateral border-zone infarcts, which can develop in association with prolonged cardiogenic shock, dysrhythmias, or cardiac arrest.[74,75] Alternatively, symptoms may be asymmetrical if they derive from inadequate perfusion distal to a site of severe stenosis or occlusion of major feeding cerebral vessels. Treatment should focus primarily on correcting the pump failure. Certain patients with concomitant underlying stenosis proximal to border-zone ischemic territories may benefit from treatment of the flow-limiting lesions to eliminate the hemodynamic impairment and thus may do better than patients with systemic hypoperfusion.[76]

Lacunar Infarcts

Neurologic examination of a patient believed to have experienced an acute ischemic stroke should be attentive to the possibility of lacunar infarcts, manifested by pure motor hemi-

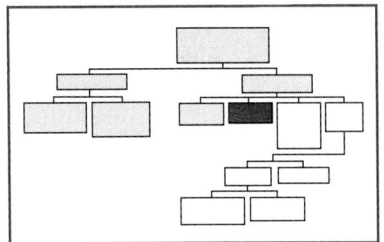

paresis, pure sensory syndrome, sensorimotor syndrome, ataxic hemiparesis, and dysarthria–clumsy hand syndrome.[77,78] Lacunae are small (1 to 2 cm) subcortical lesions that result from small-vessel disease deep in the brain. They can occur either alone or in groups and may be present in as many as 23% of persons over the age of 65 years. Lacunar infarcts, unlike other forms of stroke, do not present with headache and are associated with hypertension and diabetes.[79] Although they are asymptomatic (silent) in as many as 89% of patients, their benignity is currently in some doubt: there is evidence to suggest that they may increase the risk of dementia and cognitive decline.[80,81] Lacunar syndromes are characteristic and highly predictive of the presence of lacunae, but they may be less reliable for excluding other mechanisms of stroke. A review of the Northern Manhattan Stroke Study experience demonstrated that as many as 25% of patients presenting with radiographically confirmed lacunar infarcts were ultimately found to have other mechanisms of ischemic stroke.[82] Thus, MRI should be used to confirm or exclude the presence of lacunar infarcts as well as to screen for nonlacunar mechanisms of stroke.

At present, there is no treatment for lacunar infarcts, but the prognosis is quite good. The survival rate is high, the recurrence rate is low (mean annual stroke rate, 4% to 7%), and patients generally achieve relatively good functional recovery, with as many as 74% experiencing mild or no disability at 1 year.[83-86]

Cardiac Embolism

Embolism of cardiac origin accounts for approximately 14% of ischemic strokes [see Table 1]. Given that many infarcts of undetermined cause are probably of cardioembolic origin, this figure may in fact be an

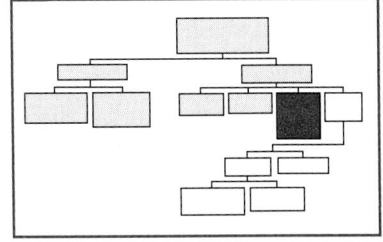

underestimate.[22] Whereas clinical suspicion for cardioembolism may be high in the setting of acute stroke, confirming the diagnosis can be more difficult. In most instances, cardioembolic stroke can be diagnosed on the basis of the history, the physical examination, and electrocardiography. A number of conditions are known to predispose to cardioembolism, including atrial fibrillation or flutter, recent MI (< 6 weeks old), placement of a prosthetic valve, disease of the aortic or mitral valves, and paradoxical emboli (usually from DVT).[87] Key clinical manifestations include sudden onset with rapid progression to maximal deficit, infarcts in different arterial territories, rapid regression of symptoms, and decreased consciousness at onset.[88-90] Headache and seizure activity are not specific for cardioembolic stroke. The rapid regression of symptoms—also known as the spectacular shrinking deficit (SSD)—is thought to result from rapid recanalization or fragmentation and migration of cardioembolus downstream.[91] Ironically, the very mechanism purported to result in rapid regression of symptoms may trigger the hemorrhagic transformation seen in as many as 70% of cardioembolic strokes.[92,93] The vast majority of hemorrhagic transformations are caused by cardioembolism. A 2001 study found that delayed recanalization occurring less than 6 hours after an acute cardioembolic stroke developed in 52.8% of patients and was an independent risk factor for hemorrhagic transformation.[93] Other risk factors for such transformation are severe strokes, decreased alertness, and absence of collateral flow.[94]

Atrial fibrillation (AF) may or may not be detected on ECG, especially if it is paroxysmal; it remains an elusive but increasingly important risk factor for cardioembolic strokes in older patients.[95] Holter monitoring and electrophysiologic testing may be especially useful for diagnosing paroxysmal AF.[96] Likewise, transthoracic echocardiography and transesophageal echocardiography are useful for detecting mural thrombus caused by AF or another cardiomyopathy as well as for detecting valvular diseases, vegetations, tumors, and patent foramina ovalia.

The presence of nonrheumatic AF has been shown to result in a fivefold greater overall incidence of stroke, which rises from 1.5% in persons 50 to 59 years of age to 23.5% in those 80 to 89 years of age.[97] Moreover, data from the International Stroke Trial indicate that mortality is twice as high in patients with AF as in those without AF (17% versus 7.5% at 2 weeks).[98] It is noteworthy that noncardioembolic strokes are estimated to account for about one third of the strokes that occur in AF patients. A 1997 autopsy study of 82 consecutive patients with symptomatic stroke and nonrheumatic AF demonstrated that 29 (35%) of the infarctions in patients with nonrheumatic AF were in fact of noncardioembolic origin.[95]

As a rule, acute ischemic stroke of cardioembolic origin is best treated with early anticoagulation to prevent recurrent brain embolism. Numerous studies have shown that recurrent embolism to the brain occurs within 2 weeks in 6% to 12% of patients after an initial ischemic infarct from a cardioembolic source.[99-101] A 1999 meta-analysis of 16 AF trials indicated that the overall risk of stroke could be reduced by an average of 62% with anticoagulation.[102] Thus, once a hemorrhagic stroke has been ruled out, heparinization and treatment with warfarin are indicated. Patients with ischemic stroke of cardioembolic origin who are at increased risk for hemorrhage or who have a contraindication to warfarin may be treated with aspirin or another antiplatelet agent; however, such agents are less effective than warfarin in secondary prevention of cardioembolic ischemic stroke.[103,104] Finally, despite the clear benefits of early anticoagulation in stroke patients with cardioembolism, such therapy has not been shown to be advantageous in the general stroke population.

For patients who suffer ischemic strokes of noncardioembolic origin, warfarin appears to offer no additional benefit over aspirin in preventing stroke recurrence.[105] Furthermore, most authorities would agree that patients with acute ischemic stroke who present within 48 hours of symptom onset should be given aspirin, 160 to 325 mg/day, to reduce mortality and morbidity from stroke.[106,107]

Atherothrombosis

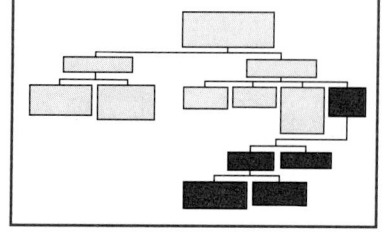

Roughly 10% of acute ischemic strokes are believed to occur secondary to large-vessel atherosclerosis, thrombosis, or artery-to-artery distal embolization.[22] Smoking and age are the most important contributors to the development of carotid atheroma.[108] Unlike cardioembolism, carotid atheroemboli and thrombosis are more likely to be associated with TIAs. Moreover, TIAs of carotid arterial origin tend to occur in the same vascular territory, whereas TIAs of cardioembolic origin are more haphazard in location.[88,90] Once the history, the physical examination, and brain imaging studies are complete, duplex ultrasonography should be performed to search for extracranial atherosclerosis of the carotid arteries. Duplex examination of the carotid arteries may also identify ulceration and assess plaque echolucency, both of which may increase the level of risk.[109,110] Other important diagnostic modalities commonly used to assess extracranial sources for atherothrombotic-embolic mechanisms of stroke are magnetic resonance angiography (MRA) and CT angiography. We routinely use these modalities to corroborate the findings of duplex ultrasonography. In patients with carotid arterial stenosis, conventional angiography is usually limited to cases in which duplex ultrasonography disagrees with MRA or CT angiography; in patients with vertebral arterial stenosis, angiography is mandatory before any attempt is made at reconstruction.

Diagnosis of symptomatic carotid artery lesions in the setting of acute ischemic stroke is critical because this subtype of stroke patient stands to benefit significantly from surgical intervention. The results of three prospective randomized trials from the early 1990s comparing medical with surgical treatment of symptomatic carotid arterial stenosis demonstrated that carotid endarterectomy had a significant advantage over medical treatment (aspirin).[111-113] Perhaps the most convincing of the three studies was the North American Symptomatic Carotid Endarterectomy Trial (NASCET), which was terminated prematurely because of the clear superiority of the results in the surgical arm.[111] In NASCET, the cumulative risk of ipsilateral stroke was 9% with surgical treatment and 26% with medical treatment at 2-year follow-up, for an absolute risk reduction of 17% and a relative risk reduction of 65.4% (P < 0.001). Patients with carotid arterial stenosis of less than 50% did not benefit from carotid endarterectomy. Conversely, studies have shown that patients who have a completely occluded carotid artery in the setting of an acute stroke should not undergo carotid endarterectomy either. Emergency carotid endarterectomy in an acutely occluded artery can result in conversion of an ischemic infarct to a hemorrhagic cerebral infarct, with potentially catastrophic results.[114]

Indications for and Timing of Therapy

CAROTID ENDARTERECTOMY

Carotid endarterectomy [*see 4:8 Carotid Arterial Procedures*] should be performed only when a low (< 5%) morbidity and mortality from stroke can be expected.[111,115] When a symptomatic patient with moderate or high-grade stenosis presents with TIAs or a mild stroke, the decision to perform a carotid endarterectomy is relatively straightforward. Patients who have suffered devastating infarcts, however, usually are not appropriate surgical candidates. Generally speaking, the extent to which neurologic function is spared, the presence and severity of medical comorbidities, and the patient's life expectancy should all be assessed before the decision is made to embark on carotid endarterectomy.

The timing of carotid endarterectomy after acute stroke continues to be the subject of controversy. According to some authorities, the risk that an ischemic infarct will undergo hemorrhagic transformation after urgent carotid endarterectomy is a contraindication to early surgery.[116,117] ICH after endarterectomy is most likely the result of postoperative hyperperfusion. The combination of hypertension (which is common after stroke) and diminished vasomotor regulation in the penumbra may predispose small vessels in this region to hemorrhage. Other authorities, however, argue that delaying surgery exposes the patient to a substantial risk of recurrent stroke or carotid occlusion and that early intervention is therefore warranted.[118] Although it would probably be generally agreed that waiting an obligatory 30 days before surgery is prudent, there are numerous small series in the literature supporting the idea that early carotid endarterectomy following acute ischemic stroke is indeed safe and may be indicated.[119,120] Furthermore, documentation of the location and size of the lesions may help identify infarcts that are at increased risk for hemorrhagic transformation after carotid endarterectomy.[120] Ultimately, the optimal timing of surgery after an acute ischemic stroke must be determined on the basis of prospective, randomized clinical trials.

THROMBOLYSIS

Any patient who presents with an acute ischemic stroke, regardless of subtype, is potentially a candidate for thrombolytic therapy. However, ICH documented on the initial head CT is a clear absolute contraindication to I.V. thrombolysis. Other considerations affecting the decision whether to administer thrombolytic agents include a history of GI or urologic hemorrhage, recent major surgery, and rapidly improving neurologic signs, any of which may constitute a clinical contraindication to treatment. Vigilant monitoring of the aPTT, the PT (or the international normalized ratio [INR]), platelet counts, and fibrinogen levels is essential throughout the course of thrombolytic treatment.

It has been suggested that maximal benefit is derived from I.V. thrombolytic therapy for acute ischemic stroke when it is delivered within a "golden 3-hour window" starting from the onset of symptoms. The National Institute for Neurological Disorders and Stroke (NINDS) trial (parts 1 and 2) randomly assigned 624 patients to receive either recombinant tissue plasminogen activator (rt-PA), 0.9 mg/kg I.V. to a maximum of 90 mg/kg, or placebo.[121] Patients with all types of ischemic stroke were eligible, provided that they could be treated within 3 hours of the onset of symptoms. Outcome at 3 months was better with rt-PA than with placebo on each of the four outcome measures studied. The odds ratio for a favorable outcome in the rt-PA group was 1.7 (95% CI; $P = 0.008$). The overall rate of symptomatic hemorrhage was 6.4% in the rt-PA group and 0.6% in the placebo group ($P < 0.001$).[121] The beneficial effects of rt-PA were similar for all stroke subtypes and persisted for up to 12 months after the stroke.[122] Patients treated with rt-PA were at least 30% more likely to have minimal or no disability at 12 months than patients treated with placebo were. Mortality at 1 year was comparable in the two groups.

Other randomized, double-blind, placebo-controlled trials of rt-PA for treatment of acute ischemic stroke have examined the effect of thrombolytic therapy given within the first 6 hours after the onset of symptoms. The European Cooperative Acute Stroke Study (ECASS) found no significant differences in functional outcome measures at 90 days between placebo and rt-PA in an intention-to-treat analysis.[123] Similarly, the Alteplase ThromboLysis for Acute Noninterventional Therapy in Ischemic Stroke (ATLANTIS) trial reported no benefit in patients treated with rt-PA within 3 to 5 hours of the onset of symptoms. However, patients treated within the golden 3-hour window were more likely to have a favorable outcome at 90 days than patients treated with placebo (60.9% versus 26.3%; odds ratio, 4.4; $P = 0.01$).[124,125]

Unfortunately, most patients are ineligible for I.V. rt-PA because of delays in obtaining treatment. Indeed, studies show that only 1% to 2% of ischemic stroke patients receive I.V. rt-PA.[126,127]

Compared with I.V. thrombolysis, intra-arterial thrombolytic therapy ought, in theory, to be able to deliver a higher local concentration of the agent where it is needed while minimizing the systemic concentration. Proponents of intra-arterial thrombolysis hope that it may lengthen the 3-hour treatment window. The PROACT II trial provided the best evidence to date that intra-arterial thrombolysis can improve patient outcomes.[128] This randomized, open-label, multicenter study with blinded follow-up randomly assigned 180 patients with stroke of less than 6 hours' duration to receive either heparin with recombinant prourokinase (r-proUK), 9 mg intra-arterially, or heparin alone. Intra-arterial thrombolysis resulted in significantly better recanalization rates than heparin alone did (66% versus 18%; $P < 0.001$). In addition, more of the r-proUK group had no neurologic deficit or only a slight deficit at 90 days (40% versus 25%; $P = 0.04$). However, intra-arterial thrombolysis did result in significantly increased rates of ICH (35% versus 13%; $P = 0.003$). Symptomatic ICH with neurologic deterioration within 24 hours occurred in 10% of r-proUK patients and 2% of control patients ($P = 0.06$). Patients who experienced ICH after r-proUK therapy had a high mortality (83%).[129] It is noteworthy that only 2% (180/12,333) of the screened patients in the PROACT II trial were randomized according to inclusion criteria, which suggests that intra-arterial thrombolysis may be of limited applicability. Finally, intra-arterial thrombolyis requires an experienced staff capable of performing cerebral angiography and navigating a microcatheter to the clot. At present, I.V. thrombolysis is certainly more practical than intra-arterial thrombolysis; more important, it can be done earlier in the course of the stroke.

Stroke in Evolution

A patient with neurologic deficits that worsen progressively in a stuttering fashion is considered to have a stroke in evolution. This state is associated with the highest level of risk, whether it is treated medically or surgically.[130] A patient with a stroke in evolution should promptly undergo CT to rule out hemorrhagic stroke, followed immediately by systemic anticoagulation with heparin and urgent operation. In a 1981 study of patients with stroke in evolution or crescendo TIAs that compared medical treatment (N=31) with urgent carotid endarterectomy (N=24), nonoperative management of stroke in evolution yielded a significantly higher mortality than surgical management (15% versus 6%).[131] Furthermore, 70% of the patients who underwent carotid endarterectomy achieved complete or near-complete recovery, compared with 19% of those managed medically.

References

1. Association AS: Stroke Facts 2003: All Americans. CDC/NCHS 2001-2003

2. Broderick JP, Phillips SJ, Whisnant JP, et al: Incidence rates of stroke in the eighties: the end of the decline in stroke? Stroke 20:577, 1989

3. Gillum RF, Sempos CT: The end of the long-term decline in stroke mortality in the United States? Stroke 28:1527, 1997

4. Matsumoto N, Whisnant JP, Kurland LT, et al: Natural history of stroke in Rochester, Minnesota, 1955 through 1969: an extension of a previous study, 1945 through 1954. Stroke 4:20, 1973

5. Sacco RL, Wolf PA, Kannel WB, et al: Survival and recurrence following stroke: the Framingham study. Stroke 13:290, 1982

6. Wolf PA, D'Agostino RB, Belanger AJ, et al: Probability of stroke: a risk profile from the Framingham Study. Stroke 22:312, 1991

7. Sobel E, Alter M, Davanipour Z, et al: Stroke in the Lehigh Valley: combined risk factors for recurrent ischemic stroke. Neurology 39:669, 1989

8. Mohr JP, Caplan LR, Melski JW, et al: The Harvard Cooperative Stroke Registry: a prospective registry. Neurology 28:754, 1978

9. Bogousslavsky J, Van Melle G, Regli F: The Lausanne Stroke Registry: analysis of 1,000 consecutive patients with first stroke. Stroke 19:1083, 1988

10. Sacco RL, Benjamin EJ, Broderick JP, et al: American Heart Association Prevention Conference: IV. Prevention and rehabilitation of stroke. Risk factors. Stroke 28:1507, 1997

11. Wong KS, Huang YN, Gao S, et al: Intracranial stenosis in Chinese patients with acute stroke. Neurology 50:812, 1998

12. Caplan LR, Gorelick PB, Hier DB: Race, sex and occlusive cerebrovascular disease: a review. Stroke 17:648, 1986

13. Kiely DK, Wolf PA, Cupples LA, et al: Familial aggregation of stroke: the Framingham Study. Stroke 24:1366, 1993

14. Amarenco P: Blood pressure and lipid lowering in the prevention of stroke: a note to neurologists. Cerebrovasc Dis 16(suppl 3):33, 2003

15. Leys D, Deplanque D, Mounier-Vehier C, et al: Stroke prevention: management of modifiable vascular risk factors. J Neurol 249:507, 2002

16. Goldstein LB, Adams R, Becker K, et al: Primary prevention of ischemic stroke: a statement for healthcare professionals from the Stroke Council of the American Heart Association. Stroke 32:280, 2001

17. Jorgensen H, Nakayama H, Raaschou HO, et al: Stroke in patients with diabetes. The Copenhagen Stroke Study. Stroke 25:1977, 1994

18. Tegos TJ, Kalodiki E, Daskalopoulou SS, et al: Stroke: epidemiology, clinical picture, and risk factors (part I of III). Angiology 51:793, 2000

19. Stadel BV: Oral contraceptives and cardiovascular disease (first of two parts). N Engl J Med 305:612, 1981

20. Gill JS, Zezulka AV, Shipley MJ, et al: Stroke and alcohol consumption. N Engl J Med 315:1041, 1986

21. Prevention of stroke by antihypertensive drug treatment in older persons with isolated systolic hypertension: final results of the Systolic Hypertension in the Elderly Program (SHEP). SHEP Cooperative Research Group. JAMA 265:3255, 1991

22. Foulkes MA, Wolf PA, Price TR, et al: The Stroke Data Bank: design, methods, and baseline characteristics. Stroke 19:547, 1988

23. Gorelick PB, Hier DB, Caplan LR, et al: Headache in acute cerebrovascular disease. Neurology 36:1445, 1986

24. Kannel WB, McGee DL: Diabetes and cardiovascular disease. The Framingham study. JAMA 241:2035, 1979

25. Welch KM, Levine SR, Ewing JR: Viewing stroke pathophysiology: an analysis of contemporary methods. Stroke 17:1071, 1986

26. Adams HP Jr, Kassell NF, Torner JC, et al: CT and clinical correlations in recent aneurysmal subarachnoid hemorrhage: a preliminary report of the Cooperative Aneurysm Study. Neurology 33:981, 1983

27. von Kummer R, Nolte PN, Schnittger H, et al: Detectability of cerebral hemisphere ischaemic infarcts by CT within 6 h of stroke. Neuroradiology 38:31, 1996

28. Hunter GJ, Hamberg LM, Ponzo JA, et al: Assessment of cerebral perfusion and arterial anatomy in hyperacute stroke with three-dimensional functional CT: early clinical results. AJNR Am J Neuroradiol 19:29, 1998

29. von Kummer R, Allen KL, Holle R, et al: Acute stroke: usefulness of early CT findings before thrombolytic therapy. Radiology 205:327, 1997

30. Maeda M, Abe H, Yamada H, et al: Hyperacute infarction: a comparison of CT and MRI, including diffusion-weighted imaging. Neuroradiology 41:175, 1999

31. Arboix A, Marti-Vilalta JL, Garcia JH: Clinical study of 227 patients with lacunar infarcts. Stroke 21:842, 1990

32. Nicolaides AN PK, Grigg M, et al: Amaurosis Fugax. Springer, New York, 1988

33. Kilpatrick MM, Yonas H, Goldstein S, et al: CT-based assessment of acute stroke: CT, CT angiography, and xenon-enhanced CT cerebral blood flow. Stroke 32:2543, 2001

34. Green JB, Bialy Y, Sora E, et al: High-resolution EEG in poststroke hemiparesis can identify ipsilateral generators during motor tasks. Stroke 30:2659, 1999

35. Kim JS, Kang SY: Bleeding and subsequent anemia: a precipitant for cerebral infarction. Eur Neurol 43:201, 2000

36. Eikelboom JW, Hankey GJ, Anand SS, et al: Association between high homocyst(e)ine and ischemic stroke due to large- and small-artery disease but not other etiologic subtypes of ischemic stroke. Stroke 31:1069, 2000

37. Kenet G, Sadetzki S, Murad H, et al: Factor V Leiden and antiphospholipid antibodies are significant risk factors for ischemic stroke in children. Stroke 31:1283, 2000

38. Madonna P, de Stefano V, Coppola A, et al: Hyperhomocysteinemia and other inherited prothrombotic conditions in young adults with a history of ischemic stroke. Stroke 33:51, 2002

39. Brass LM, Prohovnik I, Pavlakis SG, et al: Middle cerebral artery blood velocity and cerebral blood flow in sickle cell disease. Stroke 22:27, 1991

40. Asplund K: Haemodilution for acute ischaemic stroke. Cochrane Database Syst Rev (4): CD000103, 2002

41. Strand T: Evaluation of long-term outcome and safety after hemodilution therapy in acute ischemic stroke. Stroke 23:657, 1992

42. Sivenius J, Heinonen OP, Pyorala K, et al: The incidence of stroke in the Kuopio area of East Finland. Stroke 16:188, 1985

43. Wityk RJ, Caplan LR: Hypertensive intracerebral hemorrhage: epidemiology and clinical pathology. Neurosurg Clin North Am 3:521, 1992

44. Cole FM, Yates P: Intracerebral microaneurysms and small cerebrovascular lesions. Brain 90:759, 1967

45. Caplan L: Intracerebral hemorrhage revisited. Neurology 38:624, 1988

46. Brott T, Broderick J, Kothari R, et al: Early hemorrhage growth in patients with intracerebral hemorrhage. Stroke 28:1, 1997

47. Schuetz H, Dommer T, Boedeker RH, et al: Changing pattern of brain hemorrhage during 12 years of computed axial tomography. Stroke 23:653, 1992

48. Ueda K, Hasuo Y, Kiyohara Y, et al: Intracerebral hemorrhage in a Japanese community, Hisayama: incidence, changing pattern during long-term follow-up, and related factors. Stroke 19:48, 1988

49. Silver FL, Norris JW, Lewis AJ, et al: Early mortality following stroke: a prospective review. Stroke 15:492, 1984

50. Poungvarin N, Bhoopat W, Viriyavejakul A, et al: Effects of dexamethasone in primary supratentorial intracerebral hemorrhage. N Engl J Med 316:1229, 1987

51. Steiner T, Ringleb P, Hacke W: Treatment options for large hemispheric stroke. Neurology 57(5 suppl 2):S61, 2001

52. Ziai WC, Port JD, Cowan JA, et al: Decompressive craniectomy for intractable cerebral edema: experience of a single center. J Neurosurg Anesthesiol 15:25, 2003

53. Kassell NF, Torner JC, Haley EC Jr, et al: The International Cooperative Study on the Timing of Aneurysm Surgery: part 1. Overall management results. J Neurosurg 73:18, 1990

54. Sacco RL, Wolf PA, Bharucha NE, et al: Subarachnoid and intracerebral hemorrhage: natural history, prognosis, and precursive factors in the Framingham Study. Neurology 34:847, 1984

55. McCormick WF, Acosta-Rua GJ: The size of intracranial saccular aneurysms: an autopsy study. J Neurosurg 33:422, 1970

56. Inagawa T, Hirano A: Autopsy study of unruptured incidental intracranial aneurysms. Surg Neurol 34:361, 1990

57. Dell S: Asymptomatic cerebral aneurysm: assessment of its risk of rupture. Neurosurgery 10:162, 1982

58. Kojima M, Nagasawa S, Lee YE, et al: Asymptomatic familial cerebral aneurysms. Neurosurgery 43:776, 1998

59. Nakagawa T, Hashi K, Kurokawa Y, et al: Family history of subarachnoid hemorrhage and the incidence of asymptomatic, unruptured cerebral aneurysms. J Neurosurg 91:391, 1999

60. Dias MS, Sekhar LN: Intracranial hemorrhage from aneurysms and arteriovenous malformations during pregnancy and the puerperium. Neurosurgery 27:855, 1990

61. Broderick JP, Brott T, Tomsick T, et al: The risk of subarachnoid and intracerebral hemorrhages in blacks as compared with whites. N Engl J Med 326:733, 1992

62. Bassi P, Bandera R, Loiero M, et al: Warning signs in subarachnoid hemorrhage: a cooperative study. Acta Neurol Scand 84:277, 1991

63. Hart RG, Byer JA, Slaughter JR, et al: Occurrence and implications of seizures in subarachnoid hemorrhage due to ruptured intracranial aneurysms. Neurosurgery 8:417, 1981

64. Haley EC Jr, Kassell NF, Torner JC: The International Cooperative Study on the Timing of Aneurysm Surgery: the North American experience. Stroke 23:205, 1992

65. Pasqualin A: Epidemiology and pathophysiology of cerebral vasospasm following subarachnoid hemorrhage. J Neurosurg Sci 42(1 suppl 1):15, 1998

66. Corsten L, Raja A, Guppy K, et al: Contemporary management of subarachnoid hemorrhage and vasospasm: the UIC experience. Surg Neurol 56:140, 2001

67. Torner JC, Kassell NF, Wallace RB, et al: Preoperative prognostic factors for rebleeding and survival in aneurysm patients receiving antifibrinolytic therapy: report of the Cooperative Aneurysm Study. Neurosurgery 9:506, 1981

68. Sloan MA, Burch CM, Wozniak MA, et al: Transcranial Doppler detection of vertebrobasilar vasospasm following subarachnoid hemorrhage. Stroke 25:2187, 1994

69. Newell DW, Winn HR: Transcranial Doppler in cerebral vasospasm. Neurosurg Clin North Am 1:319, 1990

70. Tommasino C, Picozzi P: Physiopathological criteria of vasospasm treatment. J Neurosurg Sci 42(1 suppl 1):23, 1998

71. Treggiari MM, Walder B, Suter PM, et al: Systematic review of the prevention of delayed ischemic neurological deficits with hypertension, hypervolemia, and hemodilution therapy following subarachnoid hemorrhage. J Neurosurg 98:978, 2003

72. Feigin VL, Rinkel GJ, Algra A, et al: Calcium antagonists in patients with aneurysmal subarachnoid hemorrhage: a systematic review. Neurology 50:876, 1998

73. Caplan LR: Diagnosis and treatment of ischemic stroke. JAMA 266:2413, 1991

74. Torvik A: The pathogenesis of watershed infarcts in the brain. Stroke 15:221, 1984

75. Angeloni U, Bozzao L, Fantozzi L, et al: Internal borderzone infarction following acute middle cerebral artery occlusion. Neurology 40:1196, 1990

76. Bogousslavsky J, Regli F: Borderzone infarctions distal to internal carotid artery occlusion: prognostic implications. Ann Neurol 20:346, 1986

77. Mori E, Tabuchi M, Yamadori A: Lacunar syndrome due to intracerebral hemorrhage. Stroke 16:454, 1985

78. Fisher CM: A lacunar stroke: the dysarthria-clumsy hand syndrome. Neurology 17:614, 1967

79. Mast H, Thompson JL, Lee SH, et al: Hypertension and diabetes mellitus as determinants of multiple lacunar infarcts. Stroke 26:30, 1995

80. Longstreth WT Jr, Bernick C, Manolio TA, et al: Lacunar infarcts defined by magnetic resonance imaging of 3660 elderly people: the Cardiovascular Health Study. Arch Neurol 55:1217, 1998

81. Vermeer SE, Prins ND, den Heijer T, et al: Silent brain infarcts and the risk of dementia and cognitive decline. N Engl J Med 348:1215, 2003

82. Gan R, Sacco RL, Kargman DE, et al: Testing the validity of the lacunar hypothesis: the Northern Manhattan Stroke Study experience. Neurology 48:1204, 1997

83. Clavier I, Hommel M, Besson G, et al: Long-term prognosis of symptomatic lacunar infarcts: a hospital-based study. Stroke 25:2005, 1994

84. Salgado AV, Ferro JM, Gouveia-Oliveira A: Long-term prognosis of first-ever lacunar strokes: a hospital-based study. Stroke 27:661, 1996

85. Gandolfo C, Moretti C, Dall'Agata D, et al: Long-term prognosis of patients with lacunar syndromes. Acta Neurol Scand 74:224, 1986

86. Hier DB, Foulkes MA, Swiontoniowski M, et al: Stroke recurrence within 2 years after ischemic infarction. Stroke 22:155, 1991

87. Special report from the National Institute of Neurological Disorders and Stroke. Classification of cerebrovascular diseases III. Stroke 21:637, 1990

88. Arboix A, Oliveres M, Massons J, et al: Early differentiation of cardioembolic from atherothrombotic cerebral infarction: a multivariate analysis. Eur J Neurol 6:677, 1999

89. Timsit SG, Sacco RL, Mohr JP, et al: Brain infarction severity differs according to cardiac or arterial embolic source. Neurology 43:728, 1993

90. Kittner SJ, Sharkness CM, Sloan MA, et al: Infarcts with a cardiac source of embolism in the NINDS Stroke Data Bank: neurologic examination. Neurology 42:299, 1992

91. Minematsu K, Yamaguchi T, Omae T: 'Spectacular shrinking deficit': rapid recovery from a major hemispheric syndrome by migration of an embolus. Neurology 42:157, 1992

92. Hornig CR, Bauer T, Simon C, et al: Hemorrhagic transformation in cardioembolic cerebral infarction. Stroke 24:465, 1993

93. Molina CA, Montaner J, Abilleira S, et al: Timing of spontaneous recanalization and risk of hemorrhagic transformation in acute cardioembolic stroke. Stroke 32:1079, 2001

94. Alexandrov AV, Black SE, Ehrlich LE, et al: Predictors of hemorrhagic transformation occurring spontaneously and on anticoagulants in patients with acute ischemic stroke. Stroke 28:1198, 1997

95. Yamanouchi H, Nagura H, Mizutani T, et al: Embolic brain infarction in nonrheumatic atrial fibrillation: a clinicopathologic study in the elderly.

96. Peters NS, Schilling RJ, Kanagaratnam P, et al: Atrial fibrillation: strategies to control, combat, and cure. Lancet 359:593, 2002

97. Wolf PA, Abbott RD, Kannel WB: Atrial fibrillation as an independent risk factor for stroke: the Framingham Study. Stroke 22:983, 1991

98. Saxena R, Lewis S, Berge E, et al: Risk of early death and recurrent stroke and effect of heparin in 3169 patients with acute ischemic stroke and atrial fibrillation in the International Stroke Trial. Stroke 32:2333, 2001

99. Immediate anticoagulation of embolic stroke: a randomized trial. Cerebral Embolism Study Group. Stroke 14:668, 1983

100. Cardiogenic brain embolism. Cerebral Embolism Task Force. Arch Neurol 43:71, 1986

101. Cardiogenic brain embolism. The second report of the Cerebral Embolism Task Force. Arch Neurol 46:727, 1989

102. Hart RG, Benavente O, McBride R, et al: Antithrombotic therapy to prevent stroke in patients with atrial fibrillation: a meta-analysis. Ann Intern Med 131:492, 1999

103. Warfarin versus aspirin for prevention of thromboembolism in atrial fibrillation: Stroke Prevention in Atrial Fibrillation II Study. Lancet 343:687, 1994

104. Petersen P, Boysen G, Godtfredsen J, et al: Placebo-controlled, randomised trial of warfarin and aspirin for prevention of thromboembolic complications in chronic atrial fibrillation. The Copenhagen AFASAK study. Lancet 1:175, 1989

105. Mohr JP, Thompson JL, Lazar RM, et al: A comparison of warfarin and aspirin for the prevention of recurrent ischemic stroke. N Engl J Med 345:1444, 2001

106. CAST: randomised placebo-controlled trial of early aspirin use in 20,000 patients with acute ischaemic stroke. CAST (Chinese Acute Stroke Trial) Collaborative Group. Lancet 349:1641, 1997

107. The International Stroke Trial (IST): a randomised trial of aspirin, subcutaneous heparin, both, or neither among 19435 patients with acute ischaemic stroke. International Stroke Trial Collaborative Group. Lancet 349:1569, 1997

108. Lees RS: The natural history of carotid artery disease. Stroke 15:603, 1984

109. Kardoulas DG, Katsamouris AN, Gallis PT, et al: Ultrasonographic and histologic characteristics of symptom-free and symptomatic carotid plaque. Cardiovasc Surg 4:580, 1996

110. el-Barghouty N, Nicolaides A, Bahal V, et al: The identification of the high risk carotid plaque. Eur J Vasc Endovasc Surg 11:470, 1996

111. Beneficial effect of carotid endarterectomy in symptomatic patients with high-grade carotid stenosis. North American Symptomatic Carotid Endarterectomy Trial Collaborators. N Engl J Med 325:445, 1991

112. MRC European Carotid Surgery Trial: interim results for symptomatic patients with severe (70-99%) or with mild (0-29%) carotid stenosis. European Carotid Surgery Trialists' Collaborative Group. Lancet 337:1235, 1991

113. Mayberg MR, Wilson SE, Yatsu F, et al: Carotid endarterectomy and prevention of cerebral ischemia in symptomatic carotid stenosis. Veterans Affairs Cooperative Studies Program 309 Trialist Group. JAMA 266:3289, 1991

114. Blaisdell WF, Clauss RH, Galbraith JG, et al: Joint study of extracranial arterial occlusion. IV. A review of surgical considerations. JAMA 209:1889, 1969

115. Easton JD, Sherman DG: Stroke and mortality rate in carotid endarterectomy: 228 consecutive operations. Stroke 8:565, 1977

116. Bruetman M, Fields W, Crawford E, et al: Cerebral hemorrhage in carotid artery surgery. Arch Neurol 9:458, 1963

117. Wylie E, Hein M, Adams J: Intracranial hemorrhage following surgical revascularization for treatment of acute strokes. J Neurosurg 21:212, 1964

118. Dosick SM, Whalen RC, Gale SS, et al: Carotid endarterectomy in the stroke patient: computerized axial tomography to determine timing. J Vasc Surg 2:214, 1985

119. Whittemore AD, Ruby ST, Couch NP, et al: Early carotid endarterectomy in patients with small, fixed neurologic deficits. J Vasc Surg 1:795, 1984

120. Toni D, Fiorelli M, Bastianello S, et al: Hemorrhagic transformation of brain infarct: predictability in the first 5 hours from stroke onset and influence on clinical outcome. Neurology 46:341, 1996

121. Tissue plasminogen activator for acute ischemic stroke. The National Institute of Neurological Disorders and Stroke rt-PA Stroke Study Group. N Engl J Med 333:1581, 1995

122. Kwiatkowski TG, Libman RB, Frankel M, et al: Effects of tissue plasminogen activator for acute ischemic stroke at one year. National Institute of Neurological Disorders and Stroke Recombinant Tissue Plasminogen Activator Stroke Study Group. N Engl J Med 340:1781, 1999

123. Hacke W, Kaste M, Fieschi C, et al: Intravenous thrombolysis with recombinant tissue plasminogen activator for acute hemispheric stroke. The European Cooperative Acute Stroke Study (ECASS). JAMA 274:1017, 1995

124. Clark WM, Albers GW, Madden KP, et al: The rtPA (Alteplase) 0- to 6-hour acute stroke trial, part A (A0276g) : results of a double-blind, placebo-controlled, multicenter study. Thrombolytic Therapy in Acute Ischemic Stroke Study Investigators. Stroke 31:811, 2000

125. Clark WM, Wissman S, Albers GW, et al: Recombinant tissue-type plasminogen activator (Alteplase) for ischemic stroke 3 to 5 hours after symptom onset. The ATLANTIS Study: a randomized controlled trial. Alteplase Thrombolysis for Acute Noninterventional Therapy in Ischemic Stroke. JAMA 282:2019, 1999

126. Hacke W, Brott T, Caplan L, et al: Thrombolysis in acute ischemic stroke: controlled trials and clinical experience. Neurology 53(7 suppl 4):S3, 1999

127. Katzan IL, Furlan AJ, Lloyd LE, et al: Use of tissue-type plasminogen activator for acute ischemic stroke: the Cleveland area experience. JAMA 283:1151, 2000

128. Furlan A, Higashida R, Wechsler L, et al: Intra-arterial prourokinase for acute ischemic stroke. The PROACT II study: a randomized controlled trial. Prolyse in Acute Cerebral Thromboembolism. JAMA 282:2003, 1999

129. Kase CS, Furlan AJ, Wechsler LR, et al: Cerebral hemorrhage after intra-arterial thrombolysis for ischemic stroke: the PROACT II trial. Neurology 57:1603, 2001

130. Moore WS, Mohr JP, Najafi H, et al: Carotid endarterectomy: practice guidelines. Report of the Ad Hoc Committee to the Joint Council of the Society for Vascular Surgery and the North American Chapter of the International Society for Cardiovascular Surgery. J Vasc Surg 15:469, 1992

131. Mentzer RM Jr, Finkelmeier BA, Crosby IK, et al: Emergency carotid endarterectomy for fluctuating neurologic deficits. Surgery 89:60, 1981

2 ASYMPTOMATIC CAROTID BRUIT

*Claudio S. Cinà, M.D., Sp.Chir. (It.), M.Sc., F.R.C.S.(C), Catherine M. Clase, M.B., B.Chir., M.Sc.,
and Aleksandar Radan, M.D., B.Sc., B.F.A.*

Assessment of Asymptomatic Carotid Bruit

The term bruit refers to any noise detected on auscultation in the neck. The conventional method of auscultation is to use the bell of the stethoscope and listen over an area extending from the upper end of the thyroid cartilage to just below the angle of the jaw.[1-3] The principal reason why bruits in the neck are matters of some concern is that they may reflect underlying occlusive carotid artery disease, which carries an increased risk of stroke.

In what follows, we outline a problem-oriented approach to the workup of patients found to have cervical bruits at the time of routine or focused vascular examination.

Clinical Assessment

CAROTID BRUITS VERSUS OTHER CERVICAL SOUNDS

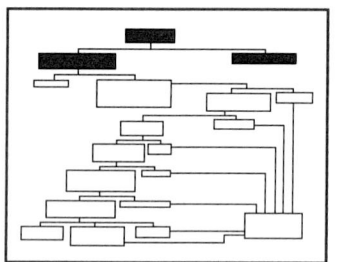

Clinical assessment begins with evaluation of the character of the bruit and examination of the precordium and the cervical structures. Carotid bruits must be distinguished from other sounds heard in the neck. Venous hums are relatively common, being reported in 27% of young adults.[4] They tend to have a diastolic component, are louder when the patient sits or turns the head away from the side of auscultation, and disappear when the patient lies down or when the Valsalva maneuver is performed.[4] Ejection systolic murmurs of cardiac origin may radiate into the neck, but generally, they are bilateral, are louder within the chest, and are less audible distally in the neck[5]; the same is true of bruits arising in other intrathoracic vessels.[6,7] No definitive clinical sign has yet been identified that clearly differentiates bruits from transmitted cardiac murmurs. On occasion, a bruit may be heard over the thyroid gland; however, this finding is extremely rare and is usually accompanied by thyromegaly and other features of autoimmune thyroid disease.[5] In dialysis patients, a bruit may be generated by the increased flow resulting from the creation of an arteriovenous fistula in the forearm.[8]

SYMPTOMATIC VERSUS ASYMPTOMATIC CAROTID BRUITS

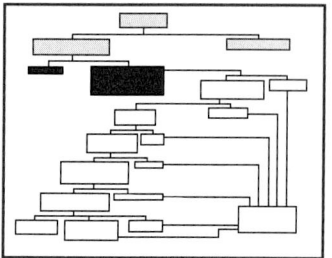

Transient ischemic attacks (TIAs) are defined as brief episodes of focal loss of brain function that can usually be localized to a specific portion of the brain supplied by a single vascular system.[9] By arbitrary convention, such an ischemic episode is considered a TIA if it lasts less than 24 hours; a similar episode, in the absence of evidence of trauma or hemorrhage, is considered an ischemic stroke if it lasts more than 24

hours or causes death.[9] Amaurosis fugax is a transient (< 24 hours) loss of vision in one eye or a portion of the visual field.[9] If a patient with a carotid bruit has a history of any of these conditions in the ipsilateral eye or brain, then the bruit is regarded as neurologically symptomatic, and the relevant question at that point is whether the patient has significant carotid stenosis and may be a candidate for carotid endarterectomy on that basis. Given the substantial differences between the management of patients with symptomatic bruits and those with asymptomatic bruits, the distinction between these two patient groups is crucial.

The history is of critical importance in the diagnosis of TIA because most TIAs last less than 4 hours,[10] which means that patients typically are not seen by physicians during the period of neurologic deficit.[11] Patients should be specifically asked about transient focal problems with vision, language, facial paresis, dysarthria, and arm or leg numbness or weakness. A 1984 study reported good interobserver agreement ($\kappa = 0.65$) [see Table 1] between clinicians diagnosing previous ischemic episodes.[12] Assigning a probable neurologic territory to a TIA or stroke, however, proved more difficult: for TIAs, the interobserver agreement between two independent neurologists asked to distinguish between carotid and vertebrobasilar events was relatively poor ($\kappa = 0.31$).[12] There is some evidence that using a standardized protocol for the diagnosis of previous ischemic episodes might improve this low interobserver agreement (e.g., to $\kappa = 0.65$[12] or $\kappa = 0.77$[13]). Similar difficulties attend diagnosis of stroke by means of history and physical examination.[14]

Many patients with a possible TIA or stroke will have undergone neurologic imaging. Such imaging is unhelpful if it yields negative results; however, in some cases, it reveals the presence of an infarct, thereby confirming the ischemic nature of the event and establish-

Table 1 Quantification of Interobserver Agreement*

$\kappa^\dagger$	Strength of Agreement
≤ 0.2	Poor
$> 0.2, \leq 0.4$	Fair
$> 0.4, \leq 0.6$	Moderate
$> 0.6, \leq 0.8$	Good
$> 0.8, \leq 1$	Very good

*Reliability (how closely an assessment agrees with another similar assessment on a second occasion or by a second observer) and validity (how closely the assessment agrees with another criterion or a gold standard) are the key properties of any assessment. When agreement between two observers is poor, the assessment in question, whether it is a physical finding, a clinical diagnosis, or an interpretation of a diagnostic test, is lacking in reliability; if more reliable methods are available, they should be considered instead. In clinical medicine, however, more reliable methods are not always available. When this is the case, the physician must use a relatively unreliable assessment as the best available alternative, while remaining aware of its limitations.[118]
$^\dagger \kappa$ is a statistical measure used to quantify agreement between two or more observers. It takes a value between 0 and 1, where 0 represents agreement no better than expected by chance alone and 1 represents perfect agreement.[118]

ing its location. For a bruit to be regarded as symptomatic on the basis of imaging studies, at least one infarct must be seen in the appropriate ipsilateral anterior vasculature.

It is evident that distinguishing between symptomatic and asymptomatic bruits on clinical grounds may be difficult; nonetheless, it is worthwhile to make the effort because the risk of stroke in the asymptomatic population is quite different from that in the symptomatic population. For example, whereas the Asymptomatic Carotid Atherosclerosis Study (ACAS), which included patients believed on clinical grounds to be neurologically asymptomatic, reported an overall stroke rate of 6.2% at 2.7 years in its medically managed group,[15] the North American Symptomatic Carotid Endarterectomy Trial (NASCET), which included patients assessed as neurologically symptomatic (i.e., with a history of amaurosis fugax, TIA, or minor stroke), reported a stroke rate of 26% at 3 years in its medically managed group.[16]

In determining whether a unilateral bruit is symptomatic or asymptomatic, the physician should concentrate primarily on ischemic deficits in the ipsilateral hemisphere (i.e., those causing focal contralateral motor or sensory deficits) and ipsilateral amaurosis fugax. However, symptoms referable to the contralateral carotid artery, even if no bruit is heard on that side, might prompt evaluation of the patient for symptomatic carotid stenosis on the contralateral side. The absence of a bruit by no means excludes the diagnosis: carotid bruits are absent in 20% to 35% of patients with high-grade stenosis of the internal carotid artery.[17] In the NASCET subgroup in which the physical finding of a carotid bruit was compared with angiographic imaging of the carotid system, the presence of a focal ipsilateral carotid bruit had a sensitivity of 63% and a specificity of 61% for high-grade (70% to 99%) stenosis; the absence of a bruit did not significantly change the probability of significant stenosis in this population (pretest 52%, posttest 40%).[18]

Workup of patients with symptomatic bruits is beyond the scope of this chapter. Accordingly, the ensuing discussion focuses on assessment of patients with asymptomatic bruits.

VASCULAR RISK ASSESSMENT

Vascular diseases and other vascular risk factors are common in patients with asymptomatic carotid bruits. Hypertension is twice as common in patients who have bruits as in those who do not[19]; smoking, ischemic heart disease, and peripheral vascular disease are also more prevalent.[20,21] Consequently, detection of a bruit should prompt a thorough vascular risk assessment. Standard vascular risk factors—hypertension, hyperlipidemia, diabetes, and smoking—can be integrated into risk profiles for particular patients by using either the New Zealand risk tables (http://www.nzgg.org.nz/library/gl_complete/bloodpressure/appendix.cfm) or the formula and spreadsheets provided by Anderson et al.[22,23] The probability of stroke for various follow-up periods may be quantified by using the Framingham stroke-risk profile.[24] From age, systolic blood pressure, diabetes, smoking, cardiovascular disease, atrial fibrillation, and left ventricular hypertrophy, probability of stroke may be calculated for men and women according to a point system.[24]

Smoking cessation should be recommended to all patients,[25-27] and hypertension should be controlled (BP < 140/90).[28-31] Depending on a patient's individual risk profile, dietary and pharmacologic management of hyperlipidemia may also be warranted.[32-34] Diabetic control should be optimized.[35,36]

Patients should be asked specifically about any concurrent vascular disease—in particular, symptoms suggestive of ischemic heart disease or of claudication or rest pain. In patients with established vascular disease, the risk that future vascular events (e.g., coronary-related death, myocardial infarction [MI], new angina, stroke, TIA, new con-

Table 2 Annual Risk of Stroke

Patient Population	Annual Risk of Stroke
Population without bruits, age > 60 yr[19,43,44]	0.86% (95% CI, 0.8–0.9)
Population with bruits, age > 60 yr[19,20,43]	2.1% (95% CI, 0.6–8.5)
Male population without bruits, age > 60 yr[19,24]	0.9% (95% CI, 0.1–3.0)
Male population with bruits, age > 60 yr[19]	8.0% (95% CI, 0.2–38.0)
Female population without bruits, age > 60 yr[24]	2.0% (95% CI, 0.8–4.2)
Female population with bruits, age > 60 yr[19]	2.4% (95% CI, 0.7–5.5)

gestive heart failure, or peripheral vascular syndrome) will occur in the next 5 years is greater than 20%.[22,37] In such patients, consultation of formulas or tables is unnecessary, and all modifiable risk factors should be aggressively managed (target BP < 140/90; target ratio of total cholesterol to high-density lipoprotein [HDL] cholesterol < 4).[22]

A meta-analysis of randomized, controlled trials showed that aspirin reduced the risk of subsequent stroke, MI, and death from vascular events for patients who had previously experienced a cerebrovascular event, MI, or unstable angina.[38] Other meta-analyses of randomized, controlled trials[39,40] were unable to confirm the effectiveness of aspirin in preventing cerebrovascular events in asymptomatic patients or in patients with TIAs or strokes of noncardiac (and presumably vascular) origin[41]; however, one randomized, controlled trial involving hypertensive patients at modest vascular risk found that aspirin reduced the risk of vascular events, if not the risk of stroke.[42] In the absence of contraindications, we recommend that aspirin be considered for all patients who have established vascular disease elsewhere and for all patients who have a bruit in association with any vascular risk factors.

INDICATIONS FOR SURGICAL INTERVENTION

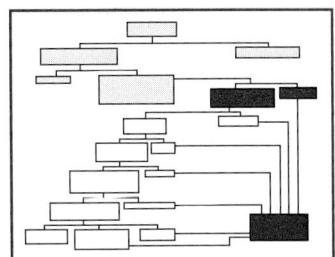

The absolute risk of stroke is increased in the presence of a carotid bruit. In population-based studies, the annual risk of stroke was 2.1% (95% confidence interval [CI], 0.6 to 8.5)[19,20,43,44] for persons who had a carotid bruit and 0.86% (95% CI, 0.8 to 0.9) for those who did not.[19,43,44] These figures represent an absolute risk increase for stroke of 1.24% a year and a relative risk for stroke of 2.4. The mean patient age in these studies was approximately 65 years, and sex distribution and prevalence of risk factors for atherosclerotic disease were similar in patients with bruits and those without bruits. Even after adjustment for age, sex, and the presence of hypertension, the presence of a carotid bruit remained an independently significant variable, with a relative risk of 2.0.[19]

Table 3 Prevalence of Carotid Stenosis in Patients with Bruits and in Healthy Volunteers

Patient Population	Prevalence of Carotid Stenosis
Overall population with cervical bruits	
> 35% stenosis[20,56-58,119]	58% (95% CI, 55–60)
> 60%–75% stenosis[56-58]	21% (95% CI, 18–24)
Healthy volunteers*	
Age > 70 yr[89]	5.1% (95% CI, 2.6–9.0)
Age ≤ 70 yr[89]	1.5% (95% CI, 0.2–5.3)

*In healthy volunteers, the incidence of asymptomatic carotid stenosis is significantly correlated with age (P < 0.01) and with the presence of hypertension (P < 0.005).

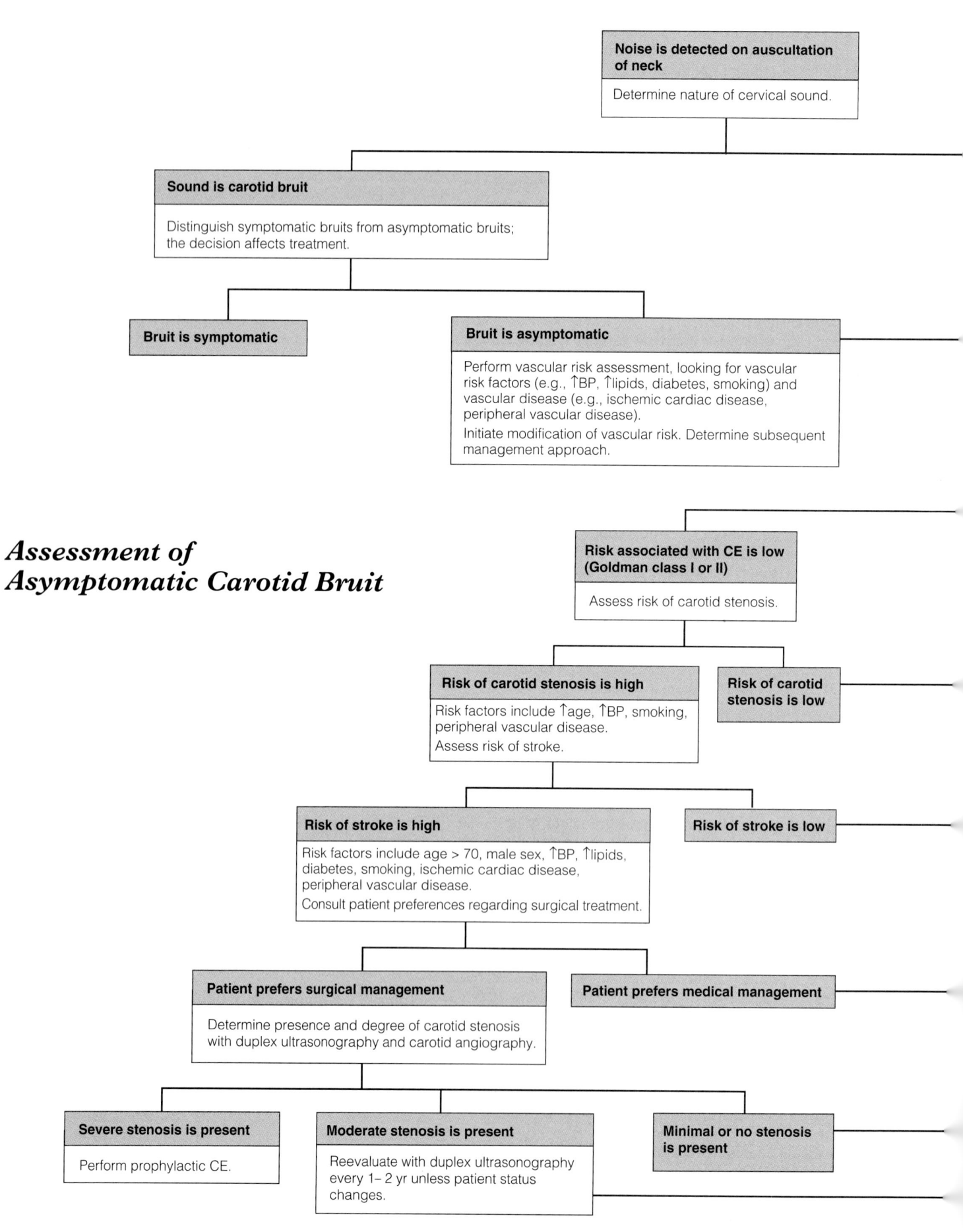

Noise is detected on auscultation of neck

Determine nature of cervical sound.

Sound is carotid bruit

Distinguish symptomatic bruits from asymptomatic bruits; the decision affects treatment.

Bruit is symptomatic

Bruit is asymptomatic

Perform vascular risk assessment, looking for vascular risk factors (e.g., ↑BP, ↑lipids, diabetes, smoking) and vascular disease (e.g., ischemic cardiac disease, peripheral vascular disease).

Initiate modification of vascular risk. Determine subsequent management approach.

Assessment of Asymptomatic Carotid Bruit

Risk associated with CE is low (Goldman class I or II)

Assess risk of carotid stenosis.

Risk of carotid stenosis is high

Risk factors include ↑age, ↑BP, smoking, peripheral vascular disease.

Assess risk of stroke.

Risk of carotid stenosis is low

Risk of stroke is high

Risk factors include age > 70, male sex, ↑BP, ↑lipids, diabetes, smoking, ischemic cardiac disease, peripheral vascular disease.

Consult patient preferences regarding surgical treatment.

Risk of stroke is low

Patient prefers surgical management

Determine presence and degree of carotid stenosis with duplex ultrasonography and carotid angiography.

Patient prefers medical management

Severe stenosis is present

Perform prophylactic CE.

Moderate stenosis is present

Reevaluate with duplex ultrasonography every 1– 2 yr unless patient status changes.

Minimal or no stenosis is present

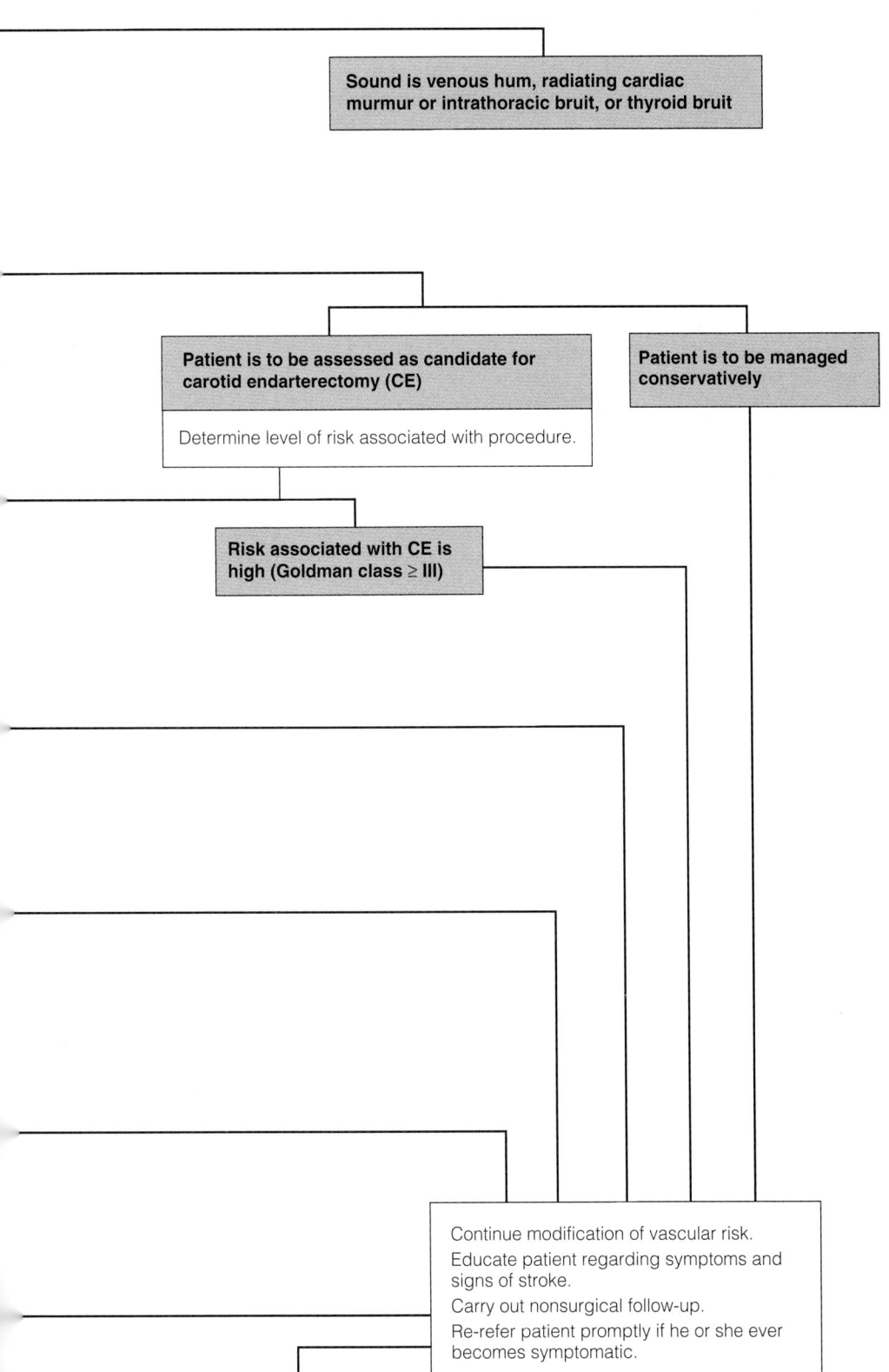

Sound is venous hum, radiating cardiac murmur or intrathoracic bruit, or thyroid bruit

Patient is to be assessed as candidate for carotid endarterectomy (CE)

Determine level of risk associated with procedure.

Patient is to be managed conservatively

Risk associated with CE is high (Goldman class ≥ III)

Continue modification of vascular risk.

Educate patient regarding symptoms and signs of stroke.

Carry out nonsurgical follow-up.

Re-refer patient promptly if he or she ever becomes symptomatic.

Table 4   Necessary Criteria for Offering
an Interventional Approach to Selected
Patients with Carotid Bruits

Center-specific criteria
Either
DUS is documented to have a > 90% PPV for stenosis > 50% on
angiography and is used alone
or
DUS has a lower PPV and is used as a screening test only, and
angiography in patients with cerebrovascular disease has a
documented complication (stroke or death) rate of around 1%
Surgeon-specific criterion
Perioperative rate of stroke or death is < 3% for carotid
endarterectomy

DUS—duplex ultrasonography   PPV—positive predictive value

Given the low absolute risk of stroke in asymptomatic patients with bruits [*see Table 2*], the low prevalence of surgically relevant stenosis in patients with bruits [*see Table 3*], and the small (and only marginally statistically significant) absolute benefit of carotid endarterectomy in patients with asymptomatic stenosis,[45,46] we and others[47-51] do not believe that further investigation with a view to carotid endarterectomy is mandatory in the asymptomatic population. Many surgeons may prefer to manage these patients conservatively, reevaluating them promptly if they become symptomatic [*see* Discussion, *below*]. Other surgeons may wish to pursue a more interventional strategy with selected patients, in which case further evaluation with an eye to surgical treatment depends on the presence of the following key findings in a given patient: (1) low risk associated with carotid endarterectomy, (2) relatively high risk of carotid stenosis, and (3) high risk of stroke if carotid stenosis is documented. In addition, the patient's preferences should be consulted: no patient should be subjected to further evaluation who is not prepared to undergo surgical treatment if such management is recommended. Patients who, on the basis of any of these criteria, are not suitable candidates for intervention will not benefit from imaging studies and should be managed medically.

Finally, surgeons and centers who are contemplating offering prophylactic carotid endarterectomy for asymptomatic stenosis should be able to document that their rates of stroke or perioperative death for this procedure are lower than 3% [*see Table 4*]. When complication rates exceed this threshold, the value of carotid endarterectomy becomes negligible, and surgeons may find themselves doing more harm than good.[45,46]

Low Risk Associated with Carotid Endarterectomy

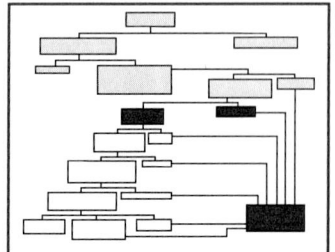

In NASCET and ACAS, patients were excluded if they had coexisting medical disease likely to produce significant mortality and morbidity (e.g., cardiac valvular or rhythm disorders, uncontrolled hypertension or diabetes, unstable angina pectoris, or MI in the previous 4 months)[16]; accordingly, the results of these trials are not generalizable to patients who have such conditions. Further evidence for the impact of operative risk on outcomes is provided by a retrospective review of 562 patients who underwent carotid endarterectomy for symptomatic and asymptomatic disease in a large community hospital.[52] For patients in Goldman class I or II,[53] the overall rate of death or

nonfatal MI was 2% (95% CI, 1.1 to 3.9), whereas for patients in class III or IV, the corresponding figure was 21% (95% CI, 9.2 to 39.9) [*see Table 5*]. Given that 50 prophylactic carotid endarterectomies would have to be performed to prevent one stroke over the subsequent 3-year period (i.e., the number needed to treat [NNT] is 50), it is clearly unacceptable to perform this procedure in a population facing a 21% incidence of MI or death, in which for every 5 patients undergoing the operation, one would experience an MI or die (i.e., the number needed to harm [NNH] is only 5). Further consideration of prophylactic carotid endarterectomy in patients for whom the procedure carries a high risk is not warranted.

High Risk of Carotid Stenosis

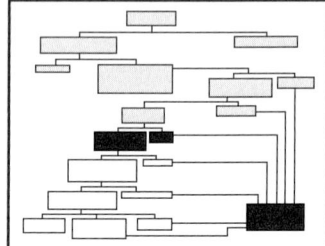

Cohort[45,54-60] and population-based[19,61,62] studies suggest that patients with asymptomatic carotid bruits are more likely to have significant carotid stenosis if they are older, are hypertensive, smoke, or have advanced peripheral vascular disease. In one study, hemodynamically significant stenosis (i.e., > 50%) was found by means of ultrasonography in 32% of patients scheduled to undergo peripheral vascular procedures but in only 6.8% of those scheduled to undergo coronary artery bypass grafting (CABG).[63] (All figures for degree of stenosis in this chapter are determined according to the formula used in NASCET [*see Table 6 and Figure 1*].)

Further consideration of carotid endarterectomy may be warranted in patients with vascular risk factors or known peripheral vascular disease; in the absence of these findings, the risk of significant carotid stenosis is low. Further evaluation is unnecessary for patients who are younger, do not smoke, are not hypertensive or diabetic, and are not known to have peripheral vascular disease.

High Risk of Stroke

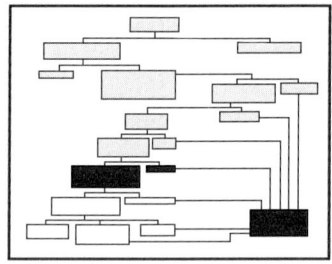

Within the group of patients with asymptomatic carotid stenosis, there is only limited direct evidence for the existence of subgroups of patients at higher risk for stroke. Men seem to be at higher risk for stroke than women are: in the medical arm of ACAS, the incidence of stroke or death at 2.7 years was 7.0% (95% CI, 4.9 to 9.4) for men and 4.9% (95% CI, 2.7 to 8.0) for women. Gender-related differences aside, however, identification of other subgroups at higher risk relies on extrapolation of data from other populations at risk for artery-to-artery embolism. Data from NASCET indicate that for symptomatic patients with greater than 70% carotid stenosis, the presence of a higher number of identifiable clinical risk factors (age > 70 years; male sex; systolic or diastolic hypertension; the occurrence of a cerebrovascular event within the preceding 31 days; the occurrence of a more serious cerebrovascular event, namely, stroke rather than a TIA or amaurosis fugax; smoking; MI; congestive heart failure; diabetes; intermittent claudication; or hyperlipidemia) was associated with a higher annual stroke risk. For patients with zero to three risk factors, the annual stroke risk was 6.6%; for those with four or five, 9.2%; and for those with six or more, 15.8%. Data from the same study indicate that among patients with a contralateral asymptomatic stenosed carotid artery, patients with zero to three risk factors have an annual stroke risk of 1.4% in the territory of the asymptomatic stenosis; those with four or five, 2.8%; and those with six or more, 3.8%.[64]

Obesity is another risk factor for stroke.[49,50] Some 60% of patients who experience a stroke before 65 years of age have a body mass index greater than 24 kg/m[2].[49] This finding, in conjunction with a history of smoking, was found to predict 60% of strokes in men in this age group.[50]

Patients with carotid bruits who do not have significant systemic risk factors or other vascular disease are at low absolute risk for stroke and are unlikely to benefit from carotid endarterectomy; hence, further investigation is not warranted.[5,18,49] Patients with numerous (i.e., six or more) clinical risk factors [see Table 7] are at relatively high risk for stroke, and it is in this population that most of the benefit from carotid endarterectomy is likely to be concentrated.

Patient Preference for Surgical Intervention

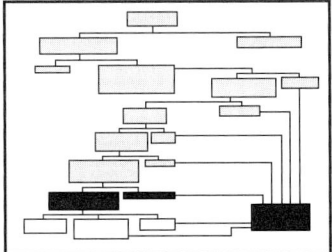

Before pursuing the diagnosis of carotid stenosis with imaging techniques, the surgeon must discuss prophylactic surgical intervention with the patient. The essential question is, if significant stenosis is documented, will the patient wish to undergo carotid endarterectomy? It should be remembered that at this point in the workup, we are considering only those patients (1) for whom the cardiac risk associated with the procedure is acceptably low and (2) who are considered to be at relatively high risk for stroke if carotid stenosis is demonstrated.

Patients should be informed that if they are found to have significant carotid stenosis, their risk of stroke is 6.3% over the ensuing 2.7 years if they do not undergo operation and 4.0% over the same period if they do.[15] They should also be informed that these figures take into account a 3% risk of perioperative stroke or death (2.7% risk of stroke and 0.3% risk of death).[15] The 2.3% absolute risk reduction associated with surgical treatment translates into an NNT of 43, meaning that 43 patients would have to undergo endarterectomy to prevent one stroke over the next 2.7 years.

Given the front-loaded risks of surgery, some patients will prefer a simple risk-modification strategy to a strategy including both risk modification and surgical intervention. In such cases, carotid imaging is not necessary, because knowledge of the degree of stenosis will not affect subsequent management.

Diagnosis of Asymptomatic Carotid Stenosis

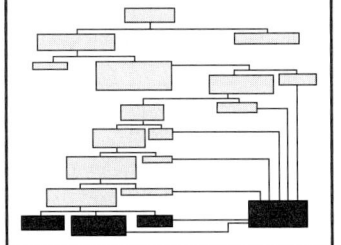

The purpose of investigation of asymptomatic neck bruits is to identify persons with significant carotid stenosis who are at increased risk for cerebrovascular disease[65,66] and who are likely to benefit from carotid endarterectomy. In the absence of other significant findings, cervical bruits are not sufficiently predictive of significant carotid stenosis or ischemic stroke to be useful in selecting candidates for noninvasive imaging.[51] Noninvasive testing is a reasonable step in patients with the characteristics listed above, but routine screening of all patients with asymptomatic carotid bruits is not warranted.[51]

DUPLEX ULTRASONOGRAPHY

Duplex ultrasonography (DUS) should be performed bilaterally. A meta-analysis conducted in 1995 found that for detecting greater

Table 5 Cardiac Risk Assessment*

Parameter	Weighted Score on Cardiac Risk Index		
	Goldman	Detsky	Eagle
Age > 70 yr	5	5	1
MI			1
< 6 mo	10	10	
> 6 mo		5	
Angina			1
Class III		10	
Class IV		20	
Unstable		10	
Diabetes			1
Operation			
Emergency	4	10	
Aortic, abdominal, or thoracic	3		
CHF	11		1
< 1 wk		10	
> 1 wk		5	
ECG			
Rhythm other than sinus	7	5	
> 5 PVCs/min	7	5	
Poor medical status†	3	5	

Risk of Perioperative Cardiac Events

Low	0–12 (class I, II)	0–15	0
Intermediate	13–25 (class III)	16–30	1–2
High	> 25 (class IV)	> 30	≥ 3

*The Goldman cardiac risk index[53] is a multifactorial index of cardiac risk in patients undergoing noncardiac surgery. Modifications have been proposed by Detsky,[121-123] who included angina and institution-specific perioperative cardiac event rates in the model. The Eagle index[124-126] is another risk index based on five clinical variables. Despite the lack of consensus regarding the relative merits of these tools for preoperative cardiac risk assessment, stratification of patients into risk categories is helpful in assessing the risk and benefits of a procedure such as carotid endarterectomy.
†P_aO_2 < 60 mm Hg; P_aCO_2 > 50 mm Hg; K^+ < 3 mmol/L; serum HCO_3 < 20 mmol/L; serum urea > 18 mmol/L; creatinine > 260 μmol/L; abnormal ALT; signs of chronic liver disease; bedridden from cardiac causes.
CHF—congestive heart failure   MI—myocardial infarction   PVC—premature ventricular contraction

than 50% stenosis (determined by means of angiography, the gold standard), DUS had a sensitivity of 91% (95% CI, 89 to 94) and a specificity of 93% (95% CI, 88 to 95).[67] Given a disease prevalence of approximately 41% in patients referred for DUS, these findings translate into a positive predictive value of 90% and an accuracy of 92%.[67] A subsequent prospective study of patients (both symptomatic and asymptomatic) in whom carotid endarterectomy was being considered reported a sensitivity of 100% and a specificity of 98% for greater than 60% stenosis, with a positive predictive value of 99%.[68]

At centers where DUS has been internally validated in comparison with angiography and where this level of performance has been documented, the surgeons may choose to proceed to surgery without angiography.[68-70] At centers where DUS is less reliable, however, it should be regarded as a screening test, and angiography should be performed when DUS suggests greater than 50% stenosis.

CAROTID ANGIOGRAPHY

As an invasive procedure, carotid angiography carries a significant risk of morbidity and mortality. All centers performing carotid angiography for cerebrovascular disease should audit their stroke rates

Table 6 Conversion between Different Methods of Measuring
Degree of Carotid Stenosis

Method	Severity of Disease				
	Minimal	Moderate		Severe	Occlusion
ECST*	24%–57%	58%–69%	70%–81%	82%–99%	100%
NASCET	0%–29%	30%–49%	50%–69%	70%–99%	100%
CC method†	35%–56%	57%–61%	62%–80%	81%–99%	100%

*Conversion from ECST to NASCET was done according to the following formula: ECST % stenosis = 0.6(NASCET % stenosis) + 40.[127]
†The relation of the NASCET method to the CC method is linear, with a ratio of 0.62 between the distal internal carotid diameter and the common carotid diameter.[117]

periodically. Since 1990, four prospective studies[71-74] have addressed the question of the risks associated with angiography in patients with atherosclerotic cerebrovascular disease. When the data from these studies were pooled, the risk of permanent neurologic deficit or death was 1.1% (95% CI, 0.6 to 2.0).[75] In ACAS, the 1.2% of patients in the intervention arm who experienced stroke or died after angiography accounted for 40% of the strokes and deaths attributable to surgical intervention.[15] Angiographic complication rates significantly worse than these will adversely impact the risk-benefit ratio associated with surgical intervention. Centers that consistently record relatively high angiographic complication rates should not offer evaluation for and surgical treatment of asymptomatic carotid disease.

Carotid Endarterectomy

At this point in management, it is reasonable to offer surgical treatment of asymptomatic disease to patients with greater than 50% stenosis. ACAS[15] and two meta-analyses[45,46] that included other trials of surgical therapy for asymptomatic carotid stenosis documented a small and marginally statistically significant benefit from prophylactic carotid endarterectomy in asymptomatic patients with greater than 50% to 60% carotid stenosis. Because the absolute benefit is small, we do not consider it obligatory to pursue the diagnosis or to follow an invasive strategy in patients identified solely on the basis of an asymptomatic bruit; however, patients possessing all the characteristics listed earlier [*see* Indications for Surgical Intervention, *above*] probably constitute a group that is particularly able to benefit from surgical intervention. Patients with higher degrees of stenosis are at higher risk for stroke and are therefore most likely to benefit.[76-79]

The degree of stenosis and the presence or absence of plaque ulceration may modify the final decision for or against operative management [*see* Discussion, Subgroup Analyses for Potential High-Risk Factors, *below*].

Technical details of carotid endarterectomy are discussed elsewhere [*see* 4:8 *Carotid Arterial Procedures*].

Patient Education

All patients with asymptomatic carotid bruits, whether they are undergoing prophylactic endarterectomy or not, should be carefully advised regarding the symptoms and signs of stroke, TIAs, and amaurosis fugax and should be strongly encouraged to seek urgent medical attention if such problems arise. Patients who experience one of these untoward events should undergo full reevaluation for stroke risk factors (e.g., hypertension, hyperlipidemia, diabetes, smoking, and atrial fibrillation); in the absence of atrial fibrillation (which should prompt consideration of prophylactic anticoagulation[80-82]), a change in antiplatelet therapy should be considered. Both ticlopidine[83] and clopidogrel[84,85] are more effective than aspirin in preventing stroke. (Ticlopidine is associated with reversible but severe neu-

tropenia in fewer than 1% of cases; accordingly, monitoring for this complication is indicated.)

If a patient who is a surgical candidate experiences a TIA or stroke as a result of an ischemic event in the carotid region in the absence of atrial fibrillation, he or she must be promptly referred back to the vascular surgeon. This possibility should be clearly explained to patients once the initial evaluation is complete and they have been referred back to their primary care physicians. Patients referred back to a vascular surgeon under these circumstances should then be regarded as having symptomatic carotid disease. A subgroup analysis of patients with symptomatic stenosis reported that carotid endarterectomy performed soon after a nondisabling stroke was not associated with a significantly higher operative complication rate than endarterectomy performed 30 days or longer after a stroke.[75,86] Performing endarterectomy early reduces the risk period for recurrent stroke and may therefore increase the potential benefit of the intervention; the usual approach is to perform the procedure within a week or two of a patient's first neurologic event.[86]

Management of cardiovascular risk factors and concurrent vascular disease should continue. In the absence of concurrent vascular disease, patients may be referred back to the family practitioner, internist, or cardiologist in place of specific surgical follow-up.

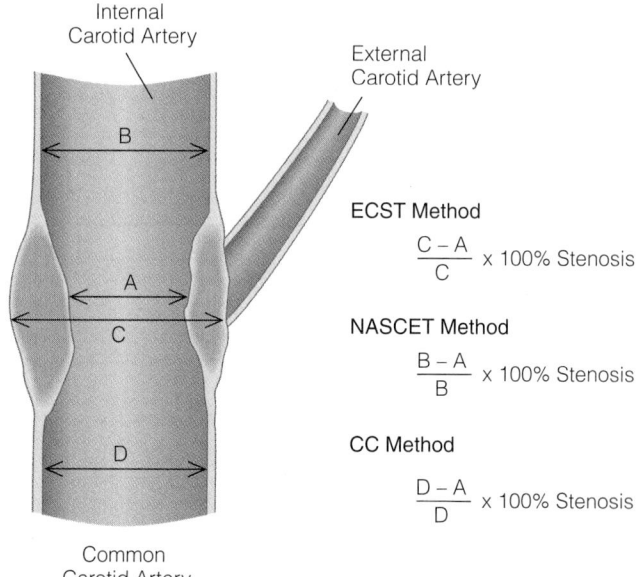

Internal
Carotid Artery

External
Carotid Artery

B

ECST Method

$$\frac{C - A}{C} \times 100\% \text{ Stenosis}$$

A

NASCET Method

C

$$\frac{B - A}{B} \times 100\% \text{ Stenosis}$$

D

CC Method

$$\frac{D - A}{D} \times 100\% \text{ Stenosis}$$

Common
Carotid Artery

Figure 1 **Carotid angiography remains the gold standard for determining the extent of carotid arterial disease. Several methods of reporting angiographically defined stenosis have been described in the literature.[115] The most commonly used methods are those adopted by the NASCET and ECST investigators, though the so-called common carotid (CC) method has its advocates as well.[116,117]**

Table 7 Risk Factors for Stroke[128,129]

Age > 70 yr	Smoking (or history of smoking)
Male sex	> 80% carotid stenosis
Hypertension*	Presence of ulceration
Hyperlipidemia	Ischemic heart disease†
Diabetes	Peripheral vascular disease

*Defined as systolic BP > 160 mm Hg or diastolic BP > 90 mm Hg.
†MI or CHF.

Follow-up of Patients with Lower-Grade Stenosis

Carotid stenosis progresses in about one quarter of patients with asymptomatic carotid stenosis monitored with DUS over a 2-year period.[87] In a population of asymptomatic patients with bruits who were referred to a vascular laboratory, 282 stenotic carotid arteries (average stenosis, 50%) were followed for 38 ± 18 months. Progression of stenosis, defined as an increase in degree of stenosis to 80% or beyond, occurred in 17% of arteries, and 2% became completely occluded. Progression was associated with an increase in stroke risk of 4.9% at 1 year, 16.7% at 3 years, and 26.5% at 5 years. In comparison, the estimated stroke risk in an asymptomatic population of patients with 50% to 79% stenosis was 0.85%, 3.6%, and 5.4% for the same three periods ($P = 0.001$).[76]

Although carotid stenosis, once identified, tends to progress over time,[20,54,76,88] the data are currently insufficient to permit recommendation of routine ultrasonographic or other surveillance for all patients with neck bruits outside a research setting. In our view, reevaluation every 1 to 2 years with noninvasive diagnostic tests is a reasonable approach to patients (1) who are already known to have greater than 50% stenosis, (2) who do not undergo surgery, and (3) who are at high risk for stroke, are surgical candidates, and are not averse to surgery.

Discussion

Epidemiology

In cross-sectional and population-based studies, the overall prevalence of greater than 75% carotid stenosis has been low. A 1992 study reported a 2.3% prevalence in men and a 1.1% prevalence in women; there was a significant ($P < 0.0001$) increase with age with each decade from 65 years to beyond 85 years, but there were no significant differences between men and women.[62] In the Framingham study population, the incidence of greater than 50% stenosis was 8% (95% CI, 6.5 to 9.8).[61] In a study of healthy volunteers, the incidence of greater than 50% stenosis was 5.1% (95% CI, 2.6 to 9.0) in patients 70 years of age or older and 1.5% (95% CI, 0.2 to 5.3) in younger patients.[89]

The pooled risk of greater than 60% to 75% stenosis in patients with carotid bruits referred for noninvasive vascular evaluation at an average age of 65 years is reported to be 21% (95% CI, 18 to 24),[56-58] which is three to four times the prevalence expected on the basis of population-based studies. Thus, five persons with neck bruits must be screened to detect one patient with moderate to severe carotid stenosis. The absolute benefit of surgery is small and of borderline statistical significance. In ACAS, as noted (see above), the relative risk reduction for an ipsilateral major stroke or perioperative death over a 2.7-year period was 36.5% (95% CI, 27.5 to 47.1), the absolute risk reduction was 2.3% (95% CI, 0.2 to 7.0), and the NNT was 43 (95% CI, 14 to 500); the number of patients that would have to be screened with DUS to prevent one stroke over a 3-year follow-up period was 250 (95% CI, 70 to 2,500).

Economic Considerations

A cogent argument in favor of pursuing a surgical strategy in at least some patients was made by a 1997 economic analysis,[90] which demonstrated that although prophylactic endarterectomy in patients with asymptomatic carotid stenosis did not reduce societal costs appreciably, it was nonetheless, at a cost of $8,000/quality-adjusted life year (QALY), within the range of many interventions considered by society to be cost-effective. It should be pointed out, however, that this economic analysis addressed only carotid endarterectomy in patients with identified carotid stenosis, not screening strategies for patients with bruits, and consequently did not consider costs associated with investigation and follow-up to the point of recommendation for or against carotid endarterectomy in the broader group of patients with bruits. These costs would alter the economic analysis substantially, and if they are included, it is far from clear whether the resulting overall cost/QALY would still be acceptable. To date, no trial or economic analysis of a screening strategy has been published.

Screening Issues

For the reasons previously discussed, we do not feel justified in recommending routine screening for patients with asymptomatic carotid bruits. Given the available evidence, we believe that such patients may reasonably be managed in either of two ways. One choice is simply to conclude that screening patients with carotid bruits as possible candidates for carotid endarterectomy has not been proved to be a useful intervention and to concentrate instead on general vascular risk reduction. The other, which is appropriate in centers where noninvasive or invasive diagnostic tests reach acceptable standards with an acceptable degree of risk and where the procedure is done by surgeons whose documented perioperative stroke and death rates are less than 3%, is to take a selective approach that addresses various issues related to stroke risk, cardiac risk, and patient preferences before noninvasive tests are ordered.

Subgroup Analyses for Potential High-Risk Factors

Given the small absolute risk reduction reported by ACAS[15] and by the two meta-analyses of all asymptomatic carotid stenosis trials,[45,46] it would be useful to be able to identify one or more high-risk groups within the broader group of patients identified as having stenosis.

SEX

ACAS included a subgroup analysis addressing the effect of sex on ability to benefit from surgery: the absolute reduction in the risk of perioperative stroke or death or ipsilateral stroke at 2.7 years was 3.6% (95% CI, 1.1 to 9.9) for men and 0.5% (95% CI, 0.01 to 2.7) for women.

DEGREE OF STENOSIS

In asymptomatic patients stratified according to their ultrasonographically determined degree of stenosis, the risk of stroke is low both for patients with less than 30% stenosis (4% cumulative event rate at 3 years) and for those with 30% to 74% stenosis (9% cumulative event rate at 3 years); it is highest for those with greater than 75% stenosis (21% cumulative event rate at 3 years).[20] The European Carotid Surgery Trialists (ECST) study,[47] using angiographic data from the asymptomatic carotid arteries of 2,295 patients, reported that the Kaplan-Meyer estimate of stroke risk at 3 years was only 2% and remained low (< 2%) when patients with less than 79% stenosis were considered; stroke risk increased to 9.8% for patients with 70% to 79% stenosis and to 14.4% for those with 80% to 99% stenosis. In a population of patients referred to a vascular laboratory with asymptomatic carotid stenosis on DUS who were followed for a mean of 38 months, the incidence of stroke was 2.1% in patients with 50% to 79% stenosis and 10.4% in those with greater than 80% stenosis.[76]

In ACAS, there were too few strokes to permit subgroup analysis of the effect of degree of stenosis on ability to benefit from carotid endarterectomy. In both ECST[79] and NASCET,[75,77,78,91] however, higher degrees of stenosis in symptomatic patients were consistently observed to be associated with higher stroke risk as well as with greater ability to benefit from surgical treatment [see Table 8].

PLAQUE ULCERATION AND PLAQUE STRUCTURE

At present, there are no subgroup analyses examining the effect of plaque ulceration on the ability of asymptomatic patients to benefit from surgical treatment. In NASCET, however, when symptomatic patients with 70% to 99% stenosis were considered, those with angiographic evidence of plaque ulceration were at higher risk for stroke than those without ulceration[92] and derived greater benefit from surgery.[75] Angiography had a sensitivity of 46% and a specificity of 74% in the detection of ulcerated plaques, with a positive predictive value of 72%.[93] A 1994 study reported that when ulceration was detected with B-mode imaging in patients with asymptomatic carotid stenosis, the incidence of silent cerebral infarction detected by magnetic resonance imaging was 75%, compared with an incidence of 25% when ulceration was absent.[94]

It has also been suggested that carotid plaques of differing structures may have differing embolic potentials.[95] DUS can distinguish between fibrous plaques (which are highly echogenic) and plaques with high concentrations of lipid and necrotic material (which are echolucent). Echolucent plaques are more frequently associated with neurologic symptoms and computed tomography–proven cerebral infarction.[95-97] Interobserver reliability for plaque echostructure, however, seems to be highly variable, ranging from good (κ = 0.79) for greater than 70% stenosis[95] to average (κ = 0.51) for greater than 40% stenosis[98] to poor (κ = 0.29) for greater than 80% stenosis.[99] A 1994 report found no correlation between the presence or type of symptoms and plaque structure as determined by DUS.[100] The true importance of carotid plaque echomorphology and surface characteristics as predictors of cerebrovascular events remains to be defined.

CONTRALATERAL DISEASE

It has been suggested that the presence of contralateral carotid disease is a risk factor for future cerebrovascular events. In NASCET patients with greater than 70% stenosis,[101] contralateral occlusion significantly increased the benefit of surgery with respect to the incidence of stroke or death, but contralateral high-grade stenosis did not.[75]

ASYMPTOMATIC CEREBRAL INFARCTION

The presence of areas of asymptomatic cerebral infarction ipsilateral to the area of carotid stenosis on head CT may identify patients who would benefit from surgery.[102] In asymptomatic patients with carotid stenosis, the incidence of silent strokes demonstrated by CT has been reported to be 10% in patients with 35% to 50% stenosis on DUS, 17% in those with 50% to 75% stenosis, and 30% in those with greater than 75% stenosis.[103] The incidence of silent cerebral infarctions demonstrated by MRI in the same type of population has been reported to be 42%, increasing to 75% for greater than 50% stenosis.[94] Use of CT and MRI of the brain in risk stratification of patients with asymptomatic carotid stenosis is controversial and currently is not advised.

CONCLUSIONS

Although only limited data on patients with asymptomatic stenosis are available, we believe that consideration of sex, degree of stenosis, and possibly the presence of plaque ulceration may be helpful in making the final decision on whether to offer carotid endarterectomy to these patients; at present, plaque morphology is insufficiently reliable to be a useful guide to clinical management.

Special Situations

RESTENOSIS OR PREVIOUS CAROTID SURGERY

Patients who have previously undergone carotid surgery have been excluded from most studies of asymptomatic patients; when they have been included in trials addressing symptomatic stenosis, they have experienced increased rates of perioperative complications.[16,50] Patients in whom restenosis occurs after an earlier carotid endarterectomy should be advised against surgery while they remain asymptomatic.[15] It is therefore unnecessary to follow patients with ultrasonography after carotid endarterectomy if no symptoms develop.

PREOPERATIVE ASSESSMENT FOR CORONARY ARTERY BYPASS GRAFTING

Some 20% to 30% of patients undergoing assessment for CABG are found to have carotid bruits,[49,104] and 5% to 20% have greater than 50% stenosis on DUS[105-107] or ocular plethysmography.[108] In asymptomatic patients with carotid stenosis who are undergoing CABG, there is no direct evidence favoring prophylactic carotid endarterectomy either before or in conjunction with CABG. Cohort studies including symptomatic and asymptomatic carotid ste-

Table 8 Effectiveness of Surgery by Degree of Stenosis in Patients with Symptomatic Carotid Stenosis[75]

Degree of Stenosis	Relative Risk Reduction or Increase	Absolute Risk Reduction or Increase	Number Needed to Treat or Harm
70%–99%	RRR, 48% (95% CI, 27–63)	ARR, 6.7% (95% CI, 3.2–10)	NNT, 15 (95% CI, 10–31)
50%–69%	RRR, 27% (95% CI, 5–44)	ARR, 4.7% (95% CI, 0.8–8.7)	NNT, 21 (95% CI, 11–125)
≤ 49%	RRI, 20% (95% CI, 0–44)	ARI, 2.2% (95% CI, 0–4.4)	NNH, 45 (95% CI, 22–∞)

ARI—absolute risk increase   ARR—absolute risk reduction   NNH—number needed to harm   NNT—number needed to treat
RRI—relative risk increase   RRR—relative risk reduction

nosis indicate that patients undergoing CABG and carotid endarterectomy in the same operation have a stroke rate of 6% (95% CI, 4.6 to 7.8), an MI rate of 4.6% (95% CI, 3.1 to 6.5), and a mortality of 4.7% (95% CI, 3.4 to 6.4).[109] For cohorts in which carotid endarterectomy was performed before CABG, the stroke rate is 3.2% (95% CI, 2.1 to 4.5), the MI rate is 5.2% (95% CI, 3.6 to 6.9)—a nonsignificant increase—and the mortality is 4.7% (95% CI, 3.4 to 6.4).[109] For cohorts in which CABG was done first and carotid stenosis was treated on its own after the cardiac procedure, the stroke rate is 3.5% (95% CI, 1.0 to 9.0), the MI rate is 2% (95% CI, 0.2 to 6.0), and the mortality is 0.8% (95% CI, 0.02 to 4.8).[110-112]

We recommend against a combined surgical approach in patients with asymptomatic carotid stenosis. Given the equivalent stroke rate and the lower MI rate and mortality, we believe that the preferred strategy in patients with bruits is first to proceed with CABG if indicated and then to determine whether the patient should be further evaluated as a candidate for carotid endarterectomy in the same manner as other elective patients would be.

Effect of Center-Specific Variations on Risk-to-Benefit Ratio

In ACAS, 1.2% of the overall 2.7% perioperative stroke rate was accounted for by strokes occurring after angiography. Centers where ultrasonography has been documented to have high predictive values may avoid this risk by proceeding directly from ultrasonography to surgery. If these complications had been avoided in ACAS, the absolute risk reduction would have been more substantial: 3.43% (95% CI, 1.1 to 9.9), corresponding to an NNT of 29 (95% CI, 1 to 80). The true perioperative combined stroke and death rate achieved in this study was 1.5%, a result that is definitive of excellence in the surgical management of carotid endarterectomy and that constitutes a useful quality assurance measure for centers and individual surgeons.

Issues for the Future

It is possible, perhaps likely, that in the future, magnetic resonance angiography[67] and three-dimensional CT angiography,[113,114] together with DUS, will replace angiography as preferred imaging methods for diagnosing internal carotid artery stenosis. As for surgical treatment and screening, further data on patients with asymptomatic carotid stenosis are necessary before definitive recommendations can be made. The Asymptomatic Carotid Surgery Trial (ACST), a large study currently under way in Europe, will be completed in the next few years; it is to be hoped that this trial will provide these additional data.

References

1. Chambers BR, Norris JW: Clinical significance of asymptomatic neck bruits. Neurology 35:742, 1985
2. Harrison MJ: Cervical bruits and asymptomatic carotid stenosis. Br J Hosp Med 32:80, 1984
3. Ratcheson RA: Clinical diagnosis of atherosclerotic carotid artery disease. Clin Neurosurg 29:464, 1982
4. Jones FL: Frequency, characteristics and importance of the cervical venous hum in adults. N Engl J Med 267:658, 1962
5. Sauve JS, Laupacis A, Ostbye T, et al: Does this patient have a clinically important carotid bruit? JAMA 270:2843, 1993
6. Caplan LR: Carotid artery disease. N Engl J Med 315:886, 1986
7. Thompson JE, Patman RD, Talkington CM: Asymptomatic carotid bruit: long term outcome of patients having endarterectomy compared with unoperated controls. Ann Surg 188:308, 1978
8. Messert B, Marra TR, Zerofsky RA: Supraclavicular and carotid bruits in hemodialysis patients. Ann Neurol 2:535, 1977
9. National Institute of Neurological Disorders and Stroke: Special Report from the National Institute of Neurological Disorders and Stroke. Classification of Cerebrovascular Diseases III. Stroke 21:637, 1990
10. Werdelin L, Juhler M: The course of transient ischemic attacks. Neurology 38:677, 1988
11. Albers GW, Hart RG, Lutsep HL, et al: AHA Scientific Statement. Supplement to the guidelines for the management of transient ischemic attacks: a statement from the Ad Hoc Committee on Guidelines for the Management of Transient Ischemic Attacks, Stroke Council, American Heart Association. Stroke 30:2502, 1999
12. Kraaijeveld CL, van Gijn J, Schouten HJ, et al: Interobserver agreement for the diagnosis of transient ischemic attacks. Stroke 15:723, 1984
13. Koudstaal PJ, van Gijn J, Staal A, et al: Diagnosis of transient ischemic attacks: improvement of interobserver agreement by a check-list in ordinary language. Stroke 17:723, 1986
14. von Arbin M, Britton M, de Faire U, et al: Validation of admission criteria to a stroke unit. J Chronic Dis 33:215, 1980
15. Toole JF, Baker WH, Castaldo JE, et al: Endarterectomy for asymptomatic carotid artery stenosis. JAMA 273:1421, 1995
16. North American Symptomatic Carotid Endarterectomy Trial Collaborators (NASCET): Beneficial effect of carotid endarterectomy in symptomatic patients with high-grade carotid stenosis. N Engl J Med 325:445, 1991
17. Davies KN, Humphrey PRD: Do carotid bruits predict disease of the internal carotid arteries? Postgrad Med J 70:433, 1994
18. Sauve JS, Thorpe KE, Sackett DL, et al: Can bruits distinguish high-grade from moderate symptomatic carotid stenosis? The North American Symptomatic Carotid Endarterectomy Trial. Ann Intern Med 120:633, 1994
19. Heyman A, Wilkinson WE, Heyden S, et al: Risk of stroke in asymptomatic persons with cervical arterial bruits: a population study in Evans County, Georgia. N Engl J Med 302:838, 1980
20. Chambers BR, Norris JW: Outcome in patients with asymptomatic neck bruits. N Engl J Med 315:860, 1986
21. Meissner I, Wiebers DO, Whisnant JP, et al: The natural history of asymptomatic carotid artery occlusive lesions. JAMA 258:2704, 1987
22. Anderson KM, Odell PM, Wilson PW, et al: Cardiovascular disease risk profiles. Am Heart J 121(1 pt 2):293, 1991
23. Anderson KM, Wilson PW, Odell PM, et al: An updated coronary risk profile: a statement for health professionals. Circulation 83:356, 1991
24. Wolf PA, D'Agostino RB, Belanger AJ, et al: Probability of stroke: a risk profile from the Framingham Study. Stroke 22:312, 1991
25. Wolf PA, D'Agostino RB, Kannel WB, et al: Cigarette smoking as a risk factor for stroke. The Framingham Study. JAMA 259:1025, 1988
26. Wannamethee SG, Shaper AG, Whincup PH, et al: Smoking cessation and the risk of stroke in middle-aged men. JAMA 274:155, 1995
27. Shinton R, Beevers G: Meta-analysis of relation between cigarette smoking and stroke. BMJ 298:789, 1989
28. Prevention of stroke by antihypertensive drug treatment in older persons with isolated systolic hypertension: final results of the Systolic Hypertension in the Elderly Program (SHEP). SHEP Cooperative Research Group. JAMA 265:3255, 1991
29. Sutton-Tyrrell K, Alcorn HG, Herzog H, et al: Morbidity, mortality, and antihypertensive treatment effects by extent of atherosclerosis in older adults with isolated systolic hypertension. Stroke 26:1319, 1995
30. Sutton-Tyrrell K, Wolfson SK Jr, Kuller LH: Blood pressure treatment slows the progression of carotid stenosis in patients with isolated systolic hypertension. Stroke 25:44, 1994
31. Collins R, Peto R, MacMahon S, et al: Blood pressure, stroke, and coronary heart disease. Part 2, Short-term reductions in blood pressure: overview of randomised drug trials in their epidemiological context. Lancet 335:827, 1990
32. Randomised trial of cholesterol lowering in 4444 patients with coronary heart disease: the Scandinavian Simvastatin Survival Study (4S). Lancet 344:1383, 1994
33. Furberg CD: Lipid-lowering trials: results and limitations. Am Heart J 128(6 pt 2):1304, 1994
34. Furberg CD, Adams HP Jr, Applegate WB, et al: Effect of lovastatin on early carotid atherosclerosis and cardiovascular events. Asymptomatic Carotid Artery Progression Study (ACAPS) Research Group. Circulation 90:1679, 1994
35. The effect of intensive treatment of diabetes on the development and progression of long-term complications in insulin-dependent diabetes mellitus. The Diabetes Control and Complications Trial Research Group. N Engl J Med 329:977, 1993
36. Intensive blood-glucose control with sulphonyl-ureas or insulin compared with conventional treatment and risk of complications in patients with type 2 diabetes (UKPDS 33). UK Prospective Diabetes Study (UKPDS) Group [published erratum appears in Lancet 354:602, 1999]. Lancet 352:837, 1998

37. Anderson KM, Wilson PW, Odell PM, et al: An updated coronary risk profile: a statement for health professionals. Circulation 83:356, 1991

38. Collaborative overview of randomised trials of antiplatelet therapy—I. Prevention of death, myocardial infarction, and stroke by prolonged antiplatelet therapy in various categories of patients. Antiplatelet Trialists' Collaboration [published erratum appears in BMJ 308:1540, 1994]. BMJ 308:81, 1994

39. Hart RG, Halperin JL, McBride R, et al: Aspirin for the primary prevention of stroke and other major vascular events: meta-analysis and hypotheses. Arch Neurol 57:326, 2000

40. Kronmal RA, Hart RG, Manolio TA, et al: Aspirin use and incident stroke in the cardiovascular health study. CHS Collaborative Research Group. Stroke 29:887, 1998

41. Barnett HJM, Eliasziw M, Meldrum HE: Drugs and surgery in the prevention of ischemic stroke. N Engl J Med 332:238, 1995

42. Hansson L, Zanchetti A, Carruthers SG, et al: Effects of intensive blood-pressure lowering and low-dose aspirin in patients with hypertension: principal results of the Hypertension Optimal Treatment (HOT) randomised trial. HOT Study Group. Lancet 351:1755, 1988

43. Wiebers DO, Whisnant JP, Sandok BA, et al: Prospective comparison of a cohort with asymptomatic carotid bruit and a population-based cohort without carotid bruit. Stroke 21:984, 1990

44. Shorr RI, Johnson KC, Wan JY, et al: The prognostic significance of asymptomatic carotid bruits in the elderly. J Gen Intern Med 13:86, 1998

45. Benavente OR, Moher D, Pham B: Carotid endarterectomy for asymptomatic carotid stenosis: a meta-analysis. BMJ 317:1477, 1998

46. Chambers BR, You RX, Donnan GA: Carotid endarterectomy for asymptomatic carotid stenosis. Cochrane Database Syst Rev (2):CD001923, 2000

47. European Carotid Surgery Trialists' Collaborative Group: Risk of stroke in the distribution of an asymptomatic carotid artery. Lancet 345:209, 1995

48. Gorelick PB: Carotid endarterectomy: where do we draw the line? (editorial) Stroke 30:1745, 1999

49. Gorelick PB, Sacco RL, Smith DB, et al: Prevention of a first stroke: a review of guidelines and a multidisciplinary consensus statement from the National Stroke Association. JAMA 281:1112, 1999

50. Feinberg RW: Primary and secondary stroke prevention. Curr Opin Neurol 9:46, 1996

51. Lee TT, Solomon NA, Heidenreich PA, et al: Cost-effectiveness of screening for carotid stenosis in asymptomatic persons. Ann Intern Med 126:337, 1997

52. Musser DJ, Nicholas GG, Reed JF III: Death and adverse cardiac events after carotid endarterectomy. J Vasc Surg 19:615, 1994

53. Goldman L, Caldera DL, Nussbaum SR, et al: Multifactorial index of cardiac risk in noncardiac surgical procedures. N Engl J Med 297:845, 1977

54. Roederer GO, Langlois YE, Jager KA, et al: The natural history of carotid arterial disease in asymptomatic patients with cervical bruits. Stroke 15:605, 1984

55. Fowl RJ, Marsh JG, Love M, et al: Prevalence of hemodynamically significant stenosis of the carotid artery in an asymptomatic veteran population. Surg Gynecol Obstet 172:13, 1991

56. Zhu CZ, Norris JW: Role of carotid stenosis in ischemic stroke. Stroke 21:1131, 1990

57. AbuRahma AF, Robinson PA: Prospective clinico-pathophysiologic follow-up study of asymptomatic neck bruit. Am Surg 56:108, 1990

58. Lusiani L, Visonà A, Castellani V, et al: Prevalence of atherosclerotic lesions at the carotid bifurcation in patients with asymptomatic bruits: an echo-Doppler (duplex) study. Angiology 36:235, 1985

59. Kartchner MM, McRae LP: Noninvasive evaluation and management of the "asymptomatic" carotid bruit. Surgery 82:840, 1977

60. Clagett GP, Youkey JR, Brigham RA, et al: Asymptomatic cervical bruit and abnormal ocular pneumoplethysmography: a prospective study comparing two approaches to management. Surgery 96:823, 1984

61. Wilson PWF, Hoeg JM, D'Agostino RB, et al: Cumulative effects of high cholesterol levels, high blood pressure, and cigarette smoking on carotid stenosis. N Engl J Med 337:516, 1997

62. O'Leary DH, Polak JF, Kronmal RA, et al: Distribution and correlates of sonographically detected carotid artery disease in the Cardiovascular Health Study. The CHS Collaborative Research Group. Stroke 23:1752, 1992

63. Hennerici M, Aulich A, Sandmann W, et al: Incidence of asymptomatic extracranial arterial disease. Stroke 12:750, 1981

64. Barnett HJ, Eliasziw M, Meldrum HE, et al: Do the facts and figures warrant a 10-fold increase in the performance of carotid endarterectomy on asymptomatic patients? Neurology 46:603, 1996

65. Warlow C: Endarterectomy for asymptomatic carotid stenosis? Lancet 345:1254, 1995

66. Amarenco P, Cohen A, Tzourio C, et al: Atherosclerotic disease of the aortic arch and the risk of ischemic stroke. N Engl J Med 331:1474, 1994

67. Blakeley DD, Oddone EZ, Hasselblad V, et al: Noninvasive carotid artery testing: a meta-analytic review. Ann Intern Med 122:360, 1997

68. Ballotta E, DaGiau G, Abbruzzese E, et al: Carotid endarterectomy without angiography: can clinical evaluation and duplex ultrasonographic scanning alone replace traditional arteriography for carotid surgery workup? A prospective study. Surgery 126:20, 1999

69. Wolf RK, Williams EL II, Kistler PC: Transbrachial balloon catheter tamponade of ruptured abdominal aortic aneurysms without fluoroscopic control. Surg Gynecol Obstet 164:463, 1987

70. Baird RN: Should carotid endarterectomy be purchased? treatment avoids much morbidity. BMJ 310:316, 1995

71. Hankey GJ, Warlow CP, Molyneux AJ: Complications of cerebral angiography for patients with mild carotid territory ischaemia being considered for carotid endarterectomy. J Neurol Neurosurg Psychiatry 53:542, 1990

72. Heiserman JE, Dean BL, Hodak JA, et al: Neurologic complications of cerebral angiography. AJNR Am J Neuroradiol 15:1401, 1994

73. Davies KN, Humphrey PR: Complications of cerebral angiography in patients with symptomatic carotid territory ischaemia screened by carotid ultrasound. J Neurol Neurosurg Psychiatry 56:967, 1993

74. Grzyska J, Freitag J, Zeumer H: Selective cerebral intraarterial DSA: Complication rate and control of risk factors. Neuroradiology 32:296, 1990

75. Cinà CS, Clase CM, Haynes RB: Refining indications for carotid endarterectomy in patients with symptomatic carotid stenosis: a systematic review. J Vasc Surg 30:606, 1999

76. Rockman CB, Riles TS, Lamparello PJ, et al: Natural history and management of the asymptomatic, moderately stenotic internal carotid artery. J Vasc Surg 25:423, 1997

77. Cina CS, Clase CM, Haynes RB: Carotid endarterectomy for symptomatic carotid stenosis. Cochrane Database Syst Rev (2):CD001081, 2000

78. Rothwell PM, Slattery J, Warlow CP: Clinical and angiographic predictors of stroke and death from carotid endarterectomy: systematic review. BMJ 315:1571, 1997

79. European Carotid Surgery Trialists' Collaborative Group: Randomized trial of endarterectomy for recently symptomatic carotid stenosis: final results of the MRC European Carotid Surgery Trial. Lancet 351:1379, 1998

80. Stroke Prevention in Atrial Fibrillation Study: Final results. Circulation 84:527, 1991

81. Warfarin versus aspirin for prevention of thromboembolism in atrial fibrillation: Stroke Prevention in Atrial Fibrillation II Study. Lancet 343:687, 1994

82. Go AS, Hylek EM, Phillips KA, et al: Implications of stroke risk criteria on the anticoagulation decision in nonvalvular atrial fibrillation: the Anticoagulation and Risk Factors in Atrial Fibrillation (ATRIA) study. Circulation 102:11, 2000

83. Hass WK, Easton JD, Adams HP Jr, et al: A randomized trial comparing ticlopidine hydrochloride with aspirin for the prevention of stroke in high-risk patients. Ticlopidine Aspirin Stroke Study Group. N Engl J Med 321:501, 1989

84. Creager MA: Results of the CAPRIE trial: efficacy and safety of clopidogrel. Clopidogrel versus aspirin in patients at risk of ischaemic events. Vasc Med 3:257, 1998

85. A randomised, blinded, trial of clopidogrel versus aspirin in patients at risk of ischaemic events (CAPRIE). CAPRIE Steering Committee. Lancet 348:1329, 1996

86. Gasecki AP, Ferguson GG, Eliasziw M, et al: Early endarterectomy for severe carotid artery stenosis after a nondisabling stroke: results from the North American Symptomatic Carotid Endarterectomy Trial. J Vasc Surg 20:288, 1994

87. Bornstein NM, Chadwick LG, Norris JW: The value of carotid Doppler ultrasound in asymptomatic extracranial arterial disease. Can J Neurol Sci 15:378, 1988

88. Bornstein NM, Norris JW: Management of patients with asymptomatic neck bruits and carotid stenosis. Neurol Clin 10:269, 1992

89. Colgan MP, Strode GR, Sommer JD, et al: Prevalence of asymptomatic carotid disease: results of duplex scanning in 348 unselected volunteers. J Vasc Surg 8:674, 1988

90. Cronenwett JL, Birkmeyer JD, Nackman GB, et al: Cost-effectiveness of carotid endarterectomy in asymptomatic patients. J Vasc Surg 25:298, 1997

91. Barnett HJ, Taylor DW, Eliasziw M, et al: Benefit of carotid endarterectomy in patients with symptomatic moderate or severe stenosis. North American Symptomatic Carotid Endarterectomy Trial Collaborators (NASCET). N Engl J Med 339:1415, 1998

92. Eliasziw M, Streifler JY, Fox AJ, et al: Significance of plaque ulceration in symptomatic patients with high-grade carotid stenosis. North American Symptomatic Carotid Endarterectomy Trial. Stroke 25:304, 1994

93. Streifler JY, Eliasziw M, Fox AJ, et al: Angiographic detection of carotid plaque ulceration. comparison with surgical observations in a multicenter study. North American Symptomatic Carotid Endarterectomy Trial. Stroke 25:1130, 1994

94. Hougaku H, Matsumoto M, Handa N, et al: Asymptomatic carotid lesions and silent cerebral infarction. Stroke 25:566, 1994

95. Sabetai MM, Tegos TJ, Nicolaides AN, et al: Hemispheric symptoms and carotid plaque echomorphology. J Vasc Surg 31(1 pt 1):39, 2000

96. Meairs S, Hennerici M: Four-dimensional ultrasonographic characterization of plaque surface motion in patients with symptomatic and asymptomatic carotid artery stenosis. Stroke 30:1807, 1999

97. Kessler C, von Maravic M, Bruckmann H, et al: Ultrasound for the assessment of the embolic risk of carotid plaques. Acta Neurol Scand 92:231, 1995

98. de Bray JM, Baud JM, Delanoy P, et al: Reproducibility in ultrasonic characterization of carotid plaques. Cerebrovasc Dis 8:273, 1998

99. Albers GW: Expanding the window for thrombolytic therapy in acute stroke: the potential role of acute MRI for patient selection. Stroke 30:2230, 1999

100. Hill SL, Donato AT: Ability of the carotid duplex scan to predict stenosis, symptoms, and plaque structure. Surgery 116:914, 1994

101. Gasecki AP, Eliasziw M, Ferguson GG, et al: Long-term prognosis and effect of endarterectomy in pa-

tients with symptomatic severe carotid stenosis and contralateral carotid stenosis or occlusion: results from nascet. North American Symptomatic Carotid Endarterectomy Trial (NASCET) group. J Neurosurg 83:778, 1995

102. Findlay JM, Tucker WS, Ferguson GG, et al: Guidelines for the use of carotid endarterectomy: current recommendations from the Canadian Neurosurgical Society. Can Med Assoc J 157:653, 1997

103. Norris JW, Zhu CZ: Silent stroke and carotid stenosis. Stroke 23:483, 1992

104. Halliday AW, Thomas D, Mansfield A: The Asymptomatic Carotid Surgery Trial (ACST): rationale and design. Steering Committee. Eur J Vasc Surg 8:703, 1994

105. Ricotta JJ, O'Brien MS, DeWeese JA: Carotid endarterectomy for non-hemispheric ischaemia: long-term follow-up. Cardiovasc Surg 2:561, 1994

106. Faggioli GL, Curl GR, Ricotta JJ: The role of carotid screening before coronary artery bypass. J Vasc Surg 12:724, 1990

107. Courbier R, Jausseran JM, Poyen V: Current status of vascular grafting in supraaortic trunks. Personal experience. Int Surgery 73:210, 1988

108. Pillai L, Gutierrez IZ, Curl GR, et al: Evaluation and treatment of carotid stenosis in open-heart surgery patients. J Surg Res 57:312, 1994

109. Borger MA, Fremes SE, Weisel RD, et al: Coronary bypass and carotid endarterectomy: does a combined approach increase risk? A metaanalysis. Ann Thorac Surg 68:14, 1999

110. Rosenthal D, Caudill DR, Lamis PA, et al: Carotid and coronary arterial disease: a rational approach. Am Surg 50:233, 1984

111. Newman DC, Hicks RG, Horton DA: Coexistent carotid and coronary arterial disease. Outcome in 50 cases and method of management. J Cardiovasc Surg (Torino) 28:599, 1987

112. Ennix CL Jr, Lawrie GM, Morris GC Jr, et al: Improved results of carotid endarterectomy in patients with symptomatic coronary disease: an analysis of 1,546 consecutive carotid operations. Stroke 10:122, 1979

113. Sameshima T, Miyao J, Oda T, et al: [Effects of allopurinol on renal damage following renal ischemia.] Masui—Japan J Anesthesiol 44:349, 1995

114. Cinat ME, Pham H, Vo D, et al: Improved imaging of carotid artery bifurcation using helical computed tomographic angiography. Ann Vasc Surg 13:178, 1999

115. Fox AJ: How to measure carotid stenosis (editorial). Radiology 186:316, 1993

116. Rothwell PM, Gibson RJ, Slattery J, et al: Equivalence of measurements of carotid stenosis: a comparison of three methods on 1001 angiograms. European Carotid Surgery Trialists' collaborative group. Stroke 25:2435, 1994

117. Eliasziw M, Smith RF, Singh N, et al: Further comments on the measurement of carotid stenosis from angiograms. North American Symptomatic Carotid Endarterectomy Trial (NASCET) group. Stroke 25:2445, 1994

118. Landis R, Koch G: The measurement of observer agreement for categorical data. Biometrics 33:159, 1997

119. Floriani M, Giulini SM, Anzola GP, et al: Predictive value of cervical bruit for the detection of obstructive lesions of the internal carotid artery: data from 2000 patients. Ital J Neurol Sci 10:321, 1989

120. Thiele BL, Jones AM, Hobson RW, et al: Standards in noninvasive cerebrovascular testing. Report from the Committee on Standards for Noninvasive Vascular Testing of the Joint Council of the Society for Vascular Surgery and the North American Chapter of the International Society for Cardiovascular Surgery. J Vasc Surg 15:495, 1992

121. Detsky AS, Abrams HB, Forbath N, et al: Cardiac assessment for patients undergoing noncardiac surgery. Arch Intern Med 146:2131, 1986

122. Detsky AS, Abrams HB, McLaughlin JR, et al: Predicting cardiac complications in patients undergoing non-cardiac surgery. J Gen Intern Med 1 (July–August):211, 1986

123. Wong T, Detsky AS: Preoperative cardiac risk assessment for patients having peripheral vascular srugery. Ann Intern Med 116:743, 1992

124. Eagle K, Brundage B, Chaitman B, et al: Guidelines for perioperative cardiovascular evaluation for non-cardiac surgery: report of the American College of Cardiology/American Heart Association Task Force on Practice Guidelines (Committee on Perioperative Cardiovascular Evaluation for Noncardiac Surgery). J Am Coll Cardiol 27:910, 1996

125. Eagle K, Froelich J: Reducing cardiovascular risk in patients undergoing noncardiac surgery (editorial). N Engl J Med 335:1761, 1996

126. Eagle KA, Coley CM, Newell JB, et al: Combining clinical and thallium data optimizes preoperative assessment of cardiac risk before major vascular surgery. Ann Intern Med 110:859, 1989

127. Rothwell PM, Gibson RJ, Slattery J, et al: Prognostic value and reproducibility of measurements of carotid stenosis: a comparison of three methods on 1001 angiograms. European Carotid Surgery Trialists' collaborative group. Stroke 25:2440, 1994

128. NASCET: Clinical alert: benefit of carotid endarterectomy for patients with high-grade stenosis of the internal carotid artery. national institute of neurological disorders and stroke stroke and trauma division. North American Symptomatic Carotid Endarterectomy Trial (NASCET) investigators. Stroke 22:816, 1991

129. NASCET: North American Symptomatic Carotid Endarterectomy Trial. Methods, patient characteristics, and progress. Stroke 22:711, 1991

Acknowledgment

Figure 1 Laurie Grace.

3 PULSATILE ABDOMINAL MASS

Timothy A. Schaub, M.D., and Gilbert R. Upchurch, Jr., M.D., F.A.C.S.

Assessment of a Pulsatile Abdominal Mass

When a pulsatile abdominal mass is found on physical examination, the location of the mass and the symptoms associated with it become essential clinical clues. The underlying condition may range in severity from benign to life threatening. Further evaluation is imperative; in certain clinical settings, immediate transport to the operating room is indicated. Because inappropriate treatment can be catastrophic, it is important to base one's approach to assessment and management of a pulsatile abdominal mass as firmly as possible on the available evidence. In what follows, a clinical approach based on relevant evidence is outlined.

Clinical Evaluation

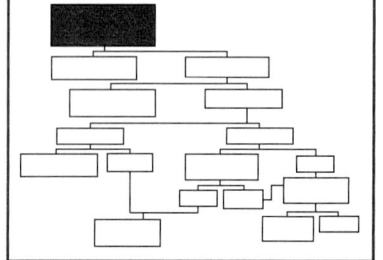

The most feared cause of a pulsatile abdominal mass is an abdominal aortic aneurysm (AAA). In the United States, AAAs are present in 3% to 9% of the population, resulting in more than 15,000 fatalities each year.[1] In 1999, AAAs were the 15th leading cause of death in the United States. These figures, coupled with the overall aging of the U.S. population, indicate that this disease is a major threat to public health.[2]

PRESENTATION

Asymptomatic AAAs are considerably more common than symptomatic AAAs and are often discovered on abdominal or pelvic scans done for other indications (e.g., back pain or renal cysts) rather than on physical examination.[3,4] Plain films of the lumbar region, routinely obtained in patients with back pain, may show a calcified shell of the aorta. In one review of 31 patients with surgically proven ruptured AAAs, 65% had calcification of the aneurysm that was visible on a plain abdominal radiograph.[5] In addition, ultrasonography and computed tomography are nearly 100% sensitive in detecting AAAs.[6] In elderly patients, evaluation of the aorta should be routinely included in abdominal ultrasonography; scanning of the aorta adds, on average, only 43 seconds to the study.[7] If an AAA is unexpectedly found, either the patient is followed or the aneurysm is repaired, depending on the clinical situation and the size of the aneurysm (see below).

Ruptured AAAs, on the other hand, give rise to pronounced symptoms, and the patient's condition may range from hemodynamic stability to class IV shock. When the patient is unstable, further workup is unnecessary and emergency repair is indicated. The situation is less clear when the patient is stable. The traditional presentation of a ruptured AAA is a triad comprising hypotension, back

or abdominal pain, and a pulsatile abdominal mass. Unfortunately, this traditional presentation occurs less than half of the time. In a study of 116 patients with ruptured AAAs, 45% were hypotensive, 72% had pain, and 83% had a pulsatile abdominal mass.[8] Accordingly, it is essential not to be lulled into a false sense of security when evaluating a hemodynamically stable patient with a pulsatile abdominal mass. Although a ruptured AAA is an uncommon event in a patient with a stable blood pressure and no abdominal pain, the absence of these symptoms does not rule out the possibility.

Symptomatic or ruptured aneurysms can mimic many other acute medical conditions and therefore are part of multiple differential diagnoses. The following conditions all may be confused with ruptured AAAs: (1) perforated viscus, (2) mesenteric ischemia, (3) strangulated hernia, (4) ruptured visceral artery aneurysm, (5) acute cholecystitis, (6) acute pancreatitis, (7) ruptured appendix, (8) ruptured necrotic hepatobiliary cancer, (9) lymphoma, and (10) diverticular abscess. Fortunately, misdiagnosis of a ruptured AAA is rare. Moreover, most patients who do undergo an operation for a misdiagnosis either benefit from or at least are not harmed by the operation, which should alleviate some potential concerns about taking an aggressive approach to a suspected ruptured AAA.[9] Conversely, AAAs can mimic other disease processes: in one study, nearly one in five patients with symptomatic AAAs in an emergency department were originally diagnosed as having nephroureterolithiasis.[10] Patients who have urologic symptoms but whose urinalysis is normal may benefit from an AAA workup; radiologic evidence of ureteric involvement is present in as many as 71% of AAAs.[11]

HISTORY

The medical history may be helpful in determining the patient's level of risk for an AAA. Even in the absence of clinical symptoms, knowledge of the risk factors may facilitate earlier diagnosis. The Aneurysm Detection and Management Veterans Affairs Cooperative Study Group trial (commonly referred to as the ADAM trial) found a number of factors to be associated with increased risk for AAA: advanced age, greater height, coronary artery disease (CAD), atherosclerosis, high cholesterol levels, hypertension, and, in particular, smoking.[12] The risk was lower in women, African Americans, and diabetic patients.

AAAs occur almost exclusively in the elderly and are rarely seen in patients younger than 50 years. In a 2001 study, the mean age of patients undergoing repair for AAAs in the United States was 72 years.[13] Male patients outnumber female by a factor of 4 to 6, depending on the study cited.[13-17] Family members of AAA patients are also at significant risk: 12% to 19% of persons undergoing AAA repair have a first-degree relative with an AAA.[18-20] Accordingly,

Table 1 Risk Factors Associated with AAA Development

Factors Positively Associated with Development of AAA	Factors Negatively Associated with Development of AAA
Increased age	Female sex
Increased height	Black race
Coronary artery disease	Presence of diabetes
Any atherosclerosis	
High cholesterol levels	
Hypertension	
Smoking	
Male sex	
Family history (first-degree relative)	

screening is recommended in all first-degree relatives of AAA patients.[21] AAAs are over seven times more likely to develop in smokers than in nonsmokers, with the duration of smoking, rather than total number of cigarettes smoked, being the key variable [see Table 1].[22]

Of particular importance is identification of risk factors for rupture. The United Kingdom Small Aneurysm (UKSA) trial reported 103 AAA ruptures in 2,257 patients over a period of 7 years, with an annual rupture rate of 2.2%.[23] The factors found to be significantly and independently associated with an increased risk of rupture were female sex, a larger initial AAA diameter, a lower forced expiratory volume in 1 second (FEV_1), a current smoking habit, and a higher mean blood pressure.[22,23] Women are two to four times more likely to experience rupture of an AAA than men are.[23,24] AAAs in cardiac and abdominal transplant patients also appear to have high expansion and rupture rates.[25]

The patient's surgical history is also crucial, particularly in that it can shorten the differential diagnosis at presentation by ruling out disease processes (e.g., appendicitis and cholecystitis). In addition, the nature and extent of any previous abdominal procedures may influence the surgeon's operative approach to the AAA repair. When a pulsatile abdominal mass is discovered in a patient who previously underwent open repair of an AAA, it is important to remember that anastomotic pseudoaneurysms[26] or synchronous lesions (e.g., iliac artery aneurysms[27]) can occur at sites remote from the previous repair.

Patients who have undergone endovascular AAA repair may also present with symptoms in the presence [see Figure 1] or absence of an endoleak. In a 2002 review, most ruptures after endovascular AAA repair occurred with type I endoleaks in the tube endograft configuration.[28] This clinical scenario is well described and can present as a pulsatile abdominal mass.[28-30] The risk of rupture after endovascular repair is small,[28] but the long-term outcome of this relatively new approach remains to be determined. Overall mortality after rupture in patients with previous endografts approaches 50%, and the operative mortality is 41%.[28]

PHYSICAL EXAMINATION

Before the advent of modern radiologic tests, the abdominal examination was the key to detecting an AAA. Gray's Anatomy, first published in 1858, noted that AAAs formed "a pulsating tumour, that presents itself in the left hypochondriac or epigastric regions."[31] The abdominal aorta begins at the level of the diaphragm and the 12th thoracic vertebra and runs in the retroperitoneal space just anterior to and slightly to the left of the spine. At approximately the level of the umbilicus and the 4th lumbar vertebra, it bifurcates into the right and left common iliac arteries. In young, thin individuals, the abdominal aorta runs close to the sur-

face of the abdomen and thus can often be palpated during a normal physical examination. Palpation of an AAA is safe and has not been reported to precipitate rupture. A 1997 report found, however, that only 31% of the AAAs studied at a major teaching institution were initially detected by physical examination.[32] Nonaneurysmal common iliac arteries also are often difficult to palpate, even in thin individuals.

There are several methods of conducting a proper physical examination of the abdominal aorta. Our preferred approach resembles that of Lederle and Simel[33]:

1. Have the patient lie supine with the knees raised. Encourage the patient to relax the abdomen. A relaxed abdomen is often obtainable with passive exhalation after a deep inhalation.
2. Beginning a few centimeters cephalad to the umbilicus and just to the left of the midline, palpate deeply for the pulsation of the aorta.
3. To confirm that the aorta is being palpated, place both hands on the abdomen with the palms down in such a way that the pulsation is between the tips of the index fingers. The index fingers should move apart with each heartbeat.
4. Once it is certain that the index fingers are bracketing the aorta, estimate the diameter of the aorta by measuring the distance between the fingertips, taking into account the thickness of the overlying tissue.

Unfortunately, physical examination is not very accurate in detecting AAAs: in one study, approximately 62% of known AAAs were missed.[34] Whether an AAA is detectable on physical examination alone depends primarily on the size of the aneurysm. AAAs more than 5 cm in diameter are detectable on physical examination in 76% of the population, whereas those 3 to 3.9 cm in diameter are detectable in only 29%. Palpation of an AAA 3.0 cm in diameter or larger has a positive predictive value of only 43%.[33] In addition, detection of AAAs is significantly limited by truncal obesity.[35,36] Thus, physical examination is clearly insufficient for ruling out or screening for AAAs.[33,35]

In the past, it was considered important to measure the abdominal aorta accurately by means of physical examination. Several studies have been published comparing ultrasonography, the cur-

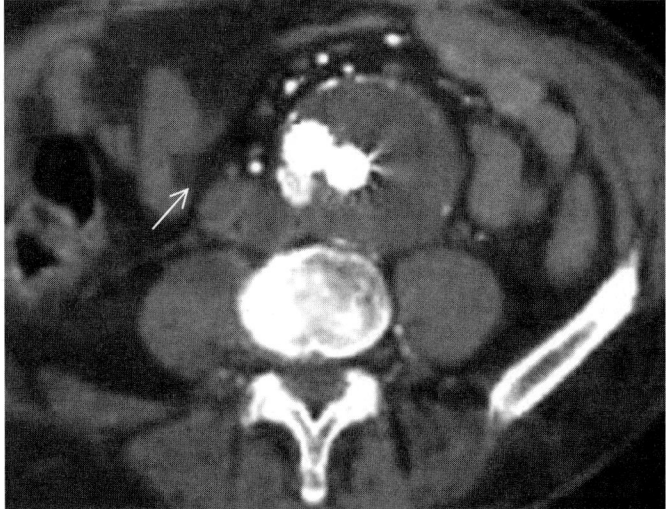

Figure 1 Shown is a CT scan of a patient who presented to the emergency room with increasing back pain 2 years after an endovascular AAA. The patient was found to have a type II endoleak (arrow), which was treated with coil embolization of a lumbar artery.

Patient presents with pulsatile abdominal mass

Perform clinical evaluation.
- *Presenting signs and symptoms:* presence or absence of pain, location, associated symptoms.
- *Medical and surgical history:* risk factors for development or rupture of AAA, previous operations, other surgical disease.
- *Physical examination:* vital signs, abdominal palpation (safe but poor at screening and detection).

Assess stability of patient.

Patient is unstable

Assume ruptured aneurysm until proven otherwise.

Perform emergency repair. Standard of care is open repair, but endovascular repair may be possible in certain circumstances.

No aneurysm is found

Search for other possible causes of complaints.

If aortic diameter is normal and patient > 60 yr, no further screening is indicated.

If aorta is enlarged, rescreen in 5–8 yr or if symptoms develop.

Pain is absent

Base subsequent treatment on aneurysm size.

Aneurysm ≥ 5.5 cm

Risk of rupture in 1 yr is greater than risk of operative repair.

Consider elective AAA repair [*see Figure 4*].

Aneurysm < 5.5 cm

Risk of rupture in 1 yr is less than risk of operative repair.

Optimize medical management.

Perform follow-up US in 6 mo.

If aneurysm grows by > 0.4 cm in 12 mo or becomes symptomatic, offer repair.

Educate patient to signs/symptoms of AAA development and rupture.

Assessment of a
Pulsatile Abdominal Mass

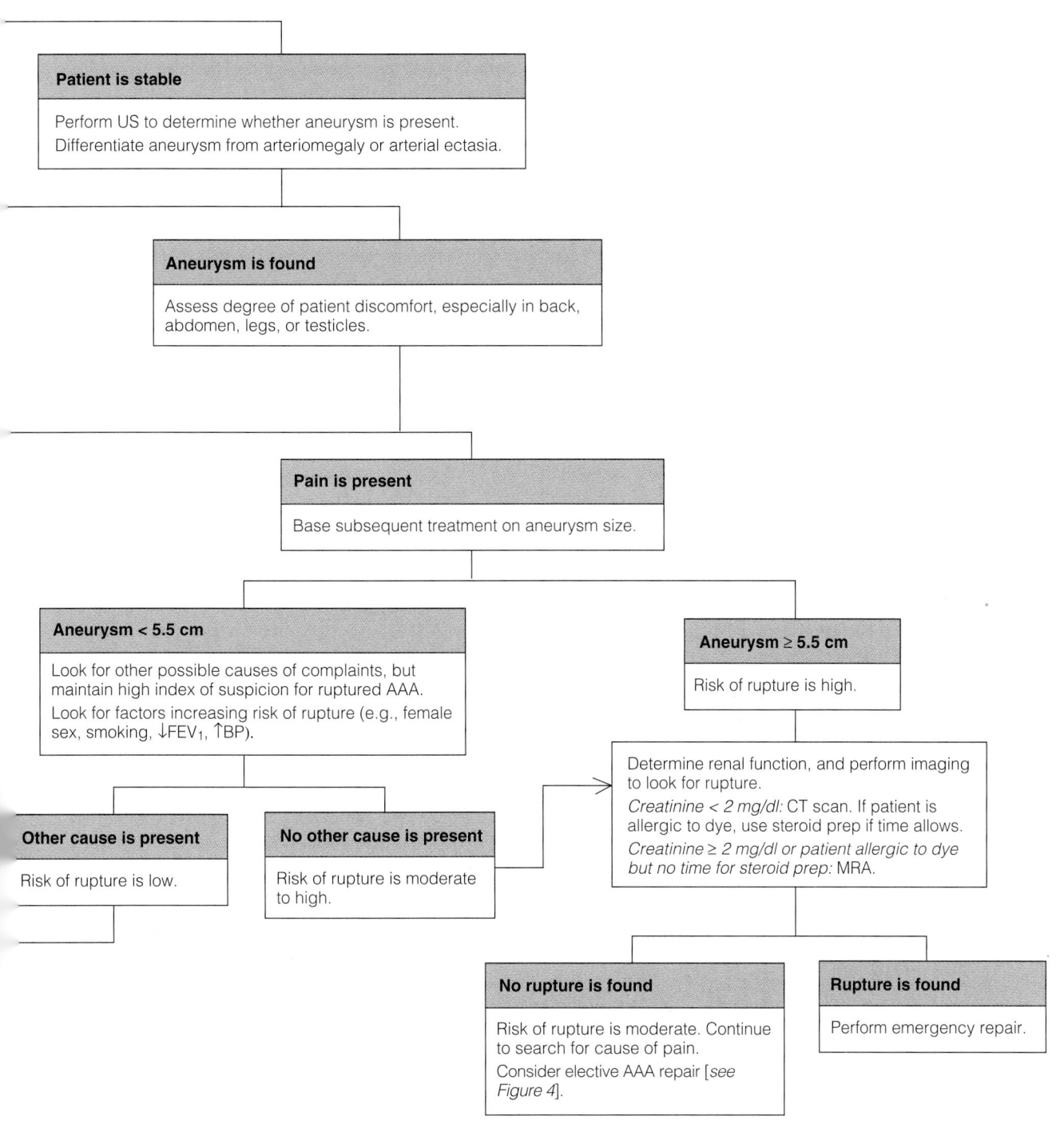

Patient is stable

Perform US to determine whether aneurysm is present.
Differentiate aneurysm from arteriomegaly or arterial ectasia.

Aneurysm is found

Assess degree of patient discomfort, especially in back, abdomen, legs, or testicles.

Pain is present

Base subsequent treatment on aneurysm size.

Aneurysm < 5.5 cm

Look for other possible causes of complaints, but maintain high index of suspicion for ruptured AAA.
Look for factors increasing risk of rupture (e.g., female sex, smoking, ↓FEV$_1$, ↑BP).

Aneurysm ≥ 5.5 cm

Risk of rupture is high.

Determine renal function, and perform imaging to look for rupture.
Creatinine < 2 mg/dl: CT scan. If patient is allergic to dye, use steroid prep if time allows.
Creatinine ≥ 2 mg/dl or patient allergic to dye but no time for steroid prep: MRA.

Other cause is present

Risk of rupture is low.

No other cause is present

Risk of rupture is moderate to high.

No rupture is found

Risk of rupture is moderate. Continue to search for cause of pain.
Consider elective AAA repair [*see Figure 4*].

Rupture is found

Perform emergency repair.

Large Right Common
Iliac Artery Aneurysm

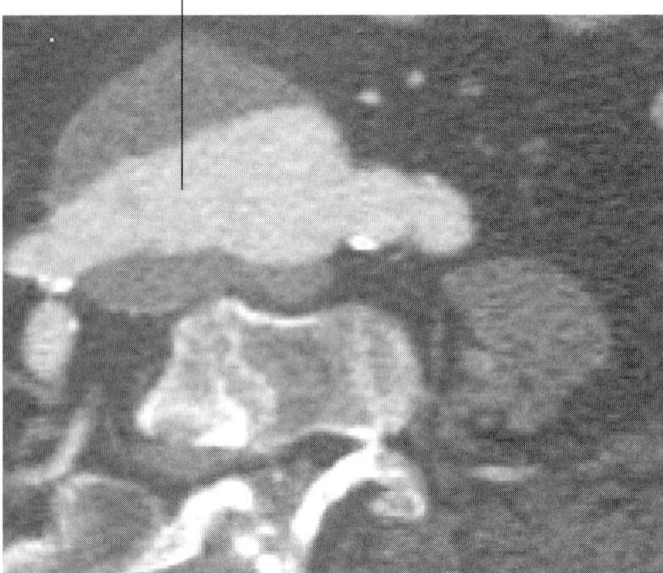

Figure 2 **Shown is a CT scan of a patient presenting with an abdominal mass who, in addition to having a small AAA, was found to have a large right common iliac artery aneurysm, palpable in the right lower quadrant of the abdomen.**

rently preferred screening method, with physical examination.[36,37] One such study found that abdominal palpation had a poor (14.7%) positive predictive value for detecting AAAs greater than 3.5 cm in diameter.[37] At present, with the wide availability of ultrasound screening, physical examination is playing a smaller role in AAA detection.

Although most AAAs appear supraumbilically, not all pulsatile abdominal masses appear there. In some patients, the abdominal aorta becomes more tortuous and elongated with age. As a result, an AAA may appear infraumbilically or to one side of the abdomen or the other. The common iliac arteries may become aneurysmal and palpable in one of the lower abdominal quadrants as well [*see Figure 2*].[38]

Another indication that an AAA may exist is the presence of a femoral or popliteal artery aneurysm on physical examination. A patient with a femoral artery aneurysm has an 85% chance of having a concomitant AAA, and a patient with a popliteal artery aneurysm has a 62% chance.[39,40] Conversely, in a study evaluating 251 patients with documented AAAs, 14% had either a femoral or a popliteal artery aneurysm.[41] There is a significant male predominance, for unknown reasons.[14,41,42]

Patient Is Unstable

If a patient presents with a pulsatile abdominal mass and is medically unstable, no further study or workup is necessary: the diagnosis, until proved otherwise, is a ruptured AAA. The only cure for a ruptured AAA is an emergency operation.

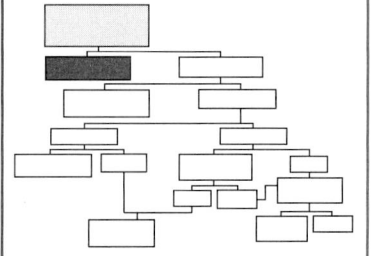

Indeed, when all patients experiencing a ruptured AAA are taken into account, including both those who arrive at the hospital alive

and those who do not, overall mortality is still between 77% and 94%, with over 50% of patients expiring before reaching the hospital.[43,44] Most ruptured AAAs leak into the left retroperitoneum, which may serve to confine the bleeding.[45] However, AAAs that rupture freely into the abdominal cavity usually result in death, either at home or en route to the hospital. Even if the patient makes it to the OR, the expected mortality approaches 50%[46,47] (though values as low as 15% and as high as 90% have been noted[48]). Mortality after a ruptured AAA has declined since the middle of the 20th century by approximately 3.5% per decade; however, the most recent estimate, for the year 2000, is still 41%.[48]

Although some physicians suggest that patients with predictably high morbidity and mortality from a ruptured AAA may not benefit from attempted repair,[49] most would still maintain that even in this population, this presentation necessitates operative intervention.[50] The high cost of repair and the substantial operative mortality notwithstanding, surgical repair of ruptured AAAs appears to be cost-effective in comparison with no intervention.[51] Thus, cost should not be considered in the management of patients with AAAs.

Open repair of ruptured AAAs is the current standard of care [*see 4:9 Repair of Infrarenal Abdominal Aortic Aneurysms*]. There is evidence, however, that endovascular approaches may come to play a more significant role. A 1999 study described endovascular repair of 25 ruptured AAAs and reported a mortality of only 16%.[52]

Patient Is Stable

If a patient with a pulsatile abdominal mass is medically stable, further workup is called for. As noted, ultrasound imaging is significantly more accurate in detecting an AAA than physical examination alone is.[37] Duplex ultrasonography is used extensively as a primary screening tool for evaluating the

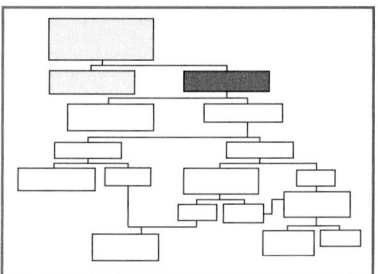

size of an abdominal aorta because of certain advantages it possesses over other, more extensive modalities, such as CT, magnetic resonance angiography (MRA), and conventional angiography. Its main advantages are that (1) it is noninvasive, (2) it is relatively inexpensive, (3) it does not require exposure to radiation, (4) it is portable, and (5) it is as reliable as the other modalities in determining aortic anterior-posterior (AP) diameter. Ultrasound-derived measurements are reproducible to within 3 to 5 mm,[53] and the interobserver variability is less than 5 mm in 84% of AP measurements.[54] In about 75% of cases, ultrasonography underestimates the size of the aorta. Although investigators have not always found ultrasound-derived measurements to correlate closely with CT-derived measurements, it appears that when radiologists take more care with their measurements (e.g., by using magnifying glasses and calipers), the results correlate better.[55]

Ultrasonographic measurement of the infrarenal aorta and the common iliac arteries has been evaluated in patients with no known vascular disease. In one study of patients older than 50 years (the age group in which abdominal aortic and iliac artery aneurysms are most common), the aorta measured 1.68 ± 0.29 cm in men and 1.46 ± 0.19 cm in women ($P < 0.001$).[56] The common iliac arteries measured 1.01 ± 0.20 cm in men and 0.92 ± 0.13 cm in women. An aneurysm is commonly defined as a permanent localized or focal expansion of an artery to 1.5 times its expected diameter.[45] Thus, an infrarenal AAA would be considered to be approximately 3 cm in diameter. It must be remembered, however, that infrarenal aortic di-

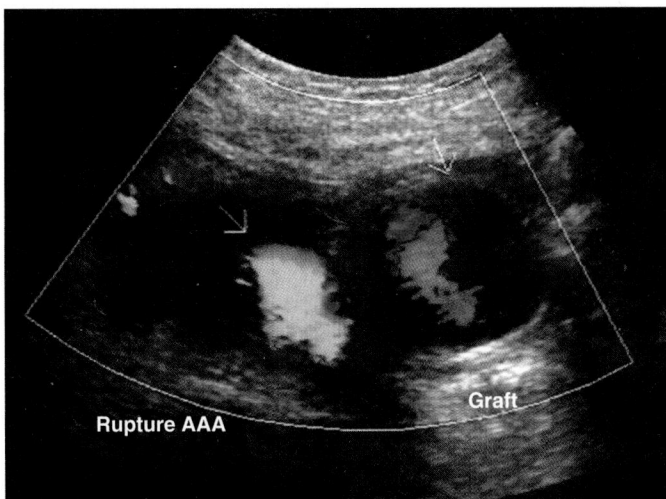

Figure 3 **Depicted is rare ultrasonographic documentation of a ruptured AAA proximal to an old aortic tube graft.**

ameter is affected by height, age, race, body surface area, and sex.[57-59] An aneurysm should be differentiated from arteriomegaly and from arterial or aortic ectasia. Arteriomegaly is a diffuse enlargement of an artery by an amount that is at least 50% of the normal diameter; ectasia is an enlargement of an artery by an amount that is less than 50% of the normal diameter.[60]

The main limitations of ultrasonography are that (1) the results are highly technician dependent and (2) resolution is dependent on body habitus and intestinal gas.[45] Another limitation is that it is unreliable in detecting rupture [*see Figure 3*]. Because ultrasonography does not provide an accurate picture of the aorta proximal to the renal arteries and because it is subject to the limitations already mentioned, it cannot be routinely used to differentiate a ruptured AAA from a symptomatic intact AAA. If ultrasonography is inconclusive in the evaluation of a palpable abdominal mass, then either CT or MRA (see below) is the next step [*see Table 2*].

ANEURYSM IS ABSENT

If ultrasonography indicates that a patient with a pulsatile abdominal mass does not have an aneurysm, the risk of aortic or common iliac artery rupture is very low. Consequently, if symptoms (e.g., abdominal pain) persist, another causative condition must be considered.

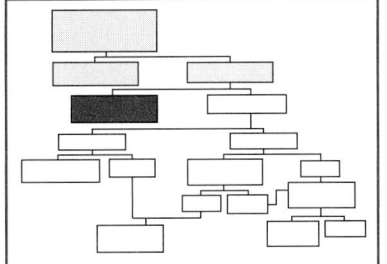

If arteriomegaly is found to be the cause of the pulsatile abdominal mass and there are no symptoms of occlusion, then no specific treatment is required. Routine ultrasonographic follow-up is indicated because the risk of rupture still applies as the aorta continues to expand. In one study, an aneurysm was present in 1.6% of aortas with arteriomegaly.[61] If aortic ectasia (by most standards, an aorta measuring 2.5 to 3 cm) is found to be the cause, follow-up ultrasonography in 5 to 8 years is recommended.[60,62] It has been suggested that for a 65-year-old man with a normal aortic diameter (defined as less than 2.6 cm), the risk that a significantly dilated aneurysm will develop during the remainder of his life is essentially zero.[63] The distinction between a normal and an ectatic aorta remains something of a gray area, and the preferred follow-up period remains controver-

sial. In general, ectatic infrarenal aortas expand slowly and are not associated with rupture.[60]

In the ADAM trial, independent and significant predictors of a new aneurysm on follow-up ultrasonography included (1) current smoking (odds ratio, 3.09), (2) coexisting CAD (1.81), and, in a separate model with composite variables, (3) any atherosclerosis (1.97).[62] Accordingly, when a patient has any of these risk factors, a lower threshold for follow-up ultrasonography and a shorter period between examinations may be practical.

ANEURYSM IS PRESENT

Once the diagnosis of an aneurysm is made in a stable patient, the subsequent course of action is determined by the clinical presentation and the size of the pulsatile abdominal mass. It must be emphasized that if the patient

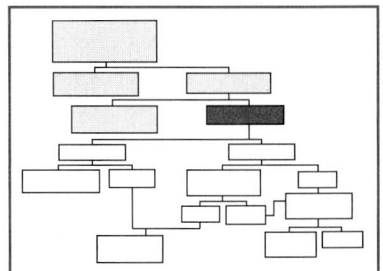

becomes hemodynamically unstable at any point during evaluation, operative intervention is necessary—unless the patient has a terminal condition or has indicated that nothing further should be done to prolong life.

If the patient is experiencing no discomfort and is otherwise stable, the risk of active rupture can be considered extremely low. If, however, the patient is experiencing significant pain or discomfort, especially in the back, the abdomen, the legs, or the testicles, AAA rupture should remain a strong diagnostic possibility.

Pain Is Absent

A patient with a pulsatile abdominal mass who has a known AAA and who is hemodynamically stable without complaints of pain should be further categorized on the basis of the size of the aneurysm. This categorization is traditionally

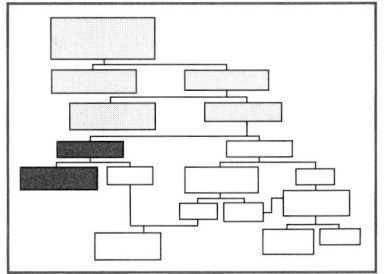

based on the physics of an expanding aneurysm and on the association between increased risk of rupture and increased aneurysm size. The key considerations in these patients are (1) whether the risk associated with AAA repair exceeds the risk of rupture in a given period and (2) what other factors are present that may affect this decision.

Indications for operative intervention The physics of aneurysm expansion and rupture are probably best understood via the law of Laplace,[7] according to which the tangential stress (τ) placed on a cylinder filled with fluid (e.g., a blood vessel) is determined by the equation

$$\tau = Pr/\delta$$

where P is the pressure (dynes/cm²) exerted by the fluid, r is the internal radius (cm) of the cylinder, and δ is the thickness (cm) of the cylinder wall. When the aorta expands, its radius increases while its wall thickness decreases; thus, there is a geometric increase in tangential stress. As an aneurysm grows from 2 cm in diameter to 4 cm, tangential pressure increases not twofold but fourfold. When the increased tangential stress exceeds the elastic capacity of the wall, rupture occurs. Elastic tissue in the abdominal aorta becomes attenuated as a result of age and of certain acquired and genetic factors; thus, a modest degree of expansion

Table 2 Advantages and Disadvantages of Aortic Imaging Techniques

Imaging Modality	Advantages	Disadvantages
Ultrasonography	Noninvasive Relatively inexpensive Does not require radiation exposure Portable Comparable in reliability to other modalities in determining aortic AP diameter	Highly technician dependent Resolution dependent on body habitus and intestinal gas Unreliable in detecting AAA rupture Achieves poor visualization of aorta proximal to renal arteries and of iliac arteries
CT	Yields highly precise measurements Defines proximal and distal extent of AAAs precisely Delineates anatomy of iliac arteries Evaluates AAA wall integrity (notes location and amount of calcification and thrombus) Effective at discovering venous anomalies, retroperitoneal blood, aortic dissection, inflammatory aneurysms, and other intra-abdominal pathology and anomalies	Requires radiation exposure Requires iodinated contrast Expensive
MRA	Comparable to CT in preoperative evaluation Uses nonnephrotoxic contrast agent (gadolinium) Highly sensitive and specific in detecting stenoses of splanchnic, renal, and iliac arteries	Not widely available Very expensive May cause claustrophobia in select patients Requires longer scan time Contraindicated in patients with certain metal foreign bodies
Angiography	Superior in evaluating intraluminal characteristics of aorta Superior in determining visceral branch involvement Superior in delineating variations in vascular anatomy	More expensive than spiral CT Associated with multiple risks (e.g., infection, arterial thrombosis, distal embolization, groin hematoma, local arterial dissection, and risk of renal failure secondary to contrast)

over time is not uncommon. An abnormal rate of expansion is usually considered to be 5 mm/yr or greater. Documentation of an accelerated aneurysm growth rate should cause the surgeon to give serious consideration to operative intervention [*see 4:9 Repair of Infrarenal Abdominal Aortic Aneurysms*].[45]

Multiple studies have examined aneurysm diameter, usually indicated by the greatest AP diameter of the aorta, as a risk factor for rupture; several studies have documented that increased AP diameter is in fact the greatest predictor of rupture. This conclusion has been challenged, however, by studies using three-dimensional CT scanning to evaluate wall stress via a mathematical technique called finite element analysis.[64-66] In these studies, maximal wall stress was a better predictor of rupture than maximal AP diameter was. For example, one patient with a ruptured 4.8 cm aneurysm had a wall stress equivalent to that of a patient with an electively repaired 6.3 cm AAA.[65] Future management of AAAs may be based on actual wall stress in addition to maximum AP diameter.

In a 2001 study addressing open operative repair of intact AAAs, increased mortality was associated with increased patient age, female sex, cerebral vascular occlusive disease, preoperative renal insufficiency, and the presence of more than three comorbid conditions before operation.[13] In the UKSA trial, the 30-day mortality in patients undergoing elective open AAA repair was 5.8%.[67] The point at which the risk of elective repair became acceptable in relation to the risk of rupture with medical management and serial ultrasonographic follow-up was an aneurysm diameter of 5.5 cm. The investigators suggested that in patients with AAAs less than 5.5 cm in diameter, medical management is the best course of action. The operative mortality reported in this study is considered high, in that many single-center series have documented mortalities of 1% to 3% after open repair of intact AAAs.[68-70] The ADAM investigators also found that survival was not improved when AAAs smaller than 5.5 cm were repaired electively, even if a low operative mortality was associated with the procedure.[69]

Hospital volume may have a significant effect on patient outcome after elective AAA repair. A 2002 study found that mortali-ty after this procedure was 56% higher at low-volume hospitals than at high-volume hospitals.[71] Moreover, mortality after repair of an intact AAA exhibited a ninefold variation that could be attributed to hospital volume, sex, and age alone. Thus, when a patient is being evaluated for AAA repair, it is important to take into account not only the size of the aneurysm but also age, sex, comorbidities, and hospital volume.

Given the various possible complicating factors, it is clear that no single aortic diameter can serve as a definitive indication for operative intervention in every patient. It is well known that ruptures can occur unpredictably at aneurysm diameters smaller than 5.5 cm.[72] Therefore, the timing of AAA repair must be individualized, with the 5.5 cm figure serving as a general guideline in the counseling of patients.

Advanced age, terminal conditions, and various end-of-life issues may deter patients from wishing to proceed with operative intervention. In addition, severe coexisting diseases significantly affect the morbidity and mortality associated with AAA repair.[46,73] Accordingly, older patients with multiple comorbidities may be preferentially offered endovascular AAA approach in place of open repair.[29] The surgeon must, however, consider the possibility that any operative intervention will be too risky in this population or that other interventions must be carried out before AAA repair can be attempted. These issues should be addressed via appropriate preoperative evaluation [*see Figure 4*].

Small AAAs (< 5.5 cm): medical management and follow-up When a patient with stable vital signs and no abdominal pain is diagnosed as having a small AAA (i.e. < 5.5 cm), serial ultrasonography and optimization of medical management are

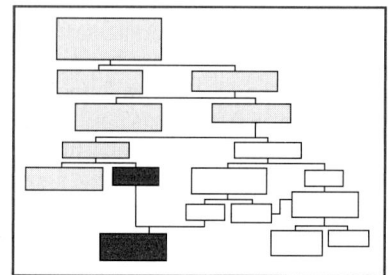

indicated.[74] Small AAAs usually do not rupture.[23,75] Most small AAAs continue to grow, however, typically by 0.2 to 0.4 cm in diameter per year.[69,74,76] Small AAAs can also expand rapidly with unpredictable frequency. A rapidly expanding AAA is at high risk for rupture, regardless of how small it may be.[67,69,76,77]

Many risk factors have been identified that may affect the risk of small aneurysm expansion and rupture. For example, one study suggested that diastolic hypertension and chronic obstructive pulmonary disease (COPD) increased the risk that a small AAA would rupture,[72] whereas another found advanced age, severe cardiac disease, previous stroke, and a history of cigarette smoking to be risk factors for rapid expansion.[76] AAAs smaller than 5.5 cm may rupture more frequently in women than in men. A 2002 study found that in almost one quarter of women with ruptured AAAs, the diameter of the aneurysm was less than 5.5 cm at the time of rupture.[43] Currently, the safest and easiest method of following small AAAs is serial ultrasonography.[10,78] When the diameter of an AAA approaches 5.5 cm, a more detailed study (e.g., CT or MRA) is indicated if repair is being considered.[45]

Over the past several decades, the number of AAAs (especially smaller AAAs) detected has increased.[79] This increase has been attributed to two causes: (1) increased serendipitous detection in the course of scans done for other indications and (2) the "graying" of the population.[45,79] With the potential advent of a screening program for AAA in the near future, thanks to growing evidence that such screening is cost-effective,[80] it is likely that even more AAAs will be detected yearly. This prospect raises an interesting issue, in that at present, the only proven treatment for AAAs is operative; current medical therapy is notably limited. Clearly, there is a need to find medical therapies that can prevent, reduce, or stabilize the growth of AAAs. To that end, a better understanding of how AAAs develop is essential.

Basic science studies have helped elucidate the etiology of AAAs in greater detail. In particular, current research is focusing on (1) evaluating the role various proteolytic enzymes, such as matrix metalloproteinases (MMPs), play in processes involving the structural elements in the aortic wall; (2) investigating the importance of the immune system, specifically the macrophage, in the development of AAAs; (3) determining how hemodynamic and biomechanical stress affects aortic wall remodeling; and (4) identifying molecular genetic variables that contribute to AAA development.[81]

Proteolytic enzymes are currently being evaluated as potential predictors of the course of AAA growth.[82] Doxycycline, which decreases MMPs in animal aneurysm models independently of its antibiotic properties, was evaluated in a prospective, randomized phase II trial published in 2002.[83] Although it did not exert a significant effect on aneurysm growth over the short study period (6 months), doxycycline significantly reduced serum levels of MMP-9, a gelatinase that plays a central role in degrading elastin and collagen in the abdominal aortic wall. Few side effects were noted, and most of them were easily reversible. These findings, though not conclusive, suggest that the use of doxycycline may one day prove to be a viable medical means of slowing AAA growth.

Control of hypertension would seem to be an obvious approach to medical control of aneurysms, in that hypertension is a significant risk factor for both development and rupture of AAAs.[23,72,75,84] To this end, various antihypertensive agents, including beta blockers, calcium channel blockers, and angiotensin-converting enzyme (ACE) inhibitors, have been evaluated in patients with AAAs.[85] The results have been somewhat equivocal.

Beta blockers have been shown to reduce the expansion rate of large AAAs (≥ 5 cm) but not that of smaller AAAs.[86,87] Some of them (e.g., propranolol) may be poorly tolerated at high doses.[87]

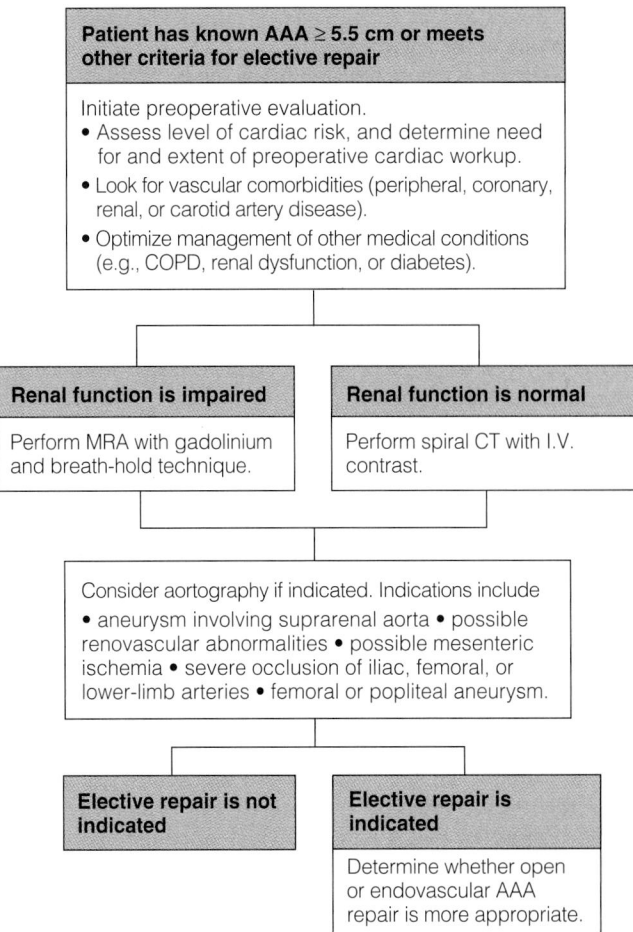

Figure 4 **Shown is an algorithm that may be used to guide the preoperative workup of a patient who is to undergo elective AAA repair.**

In addition, beta blockers are often contraindicated in patients with severe COPD, though as many as 11% of COPD patients have AAAs.[88] A 1999 study suggested that receiving a calcium channel blocker was an independent risk factor for the presence of an AAA (odds ratio, 2.6).[85] The same study also noted, however, that patients receiving calcium channel blockers had stiffer aortic walls. ACE inhibitors, in contrast, were associated with decreased aortic wall stiffness and increased collagen turnover, whereas diuretics and beta blockers had no effect on aortic wall stiffness. None of the medications examined were found to affect the growth rate of AAAs. Aortic stiffness appears to be an important variable: increased aortic wall distensibility is associated with an increased risk of AAA rupture, and it is almost as powerful a predictor of rupture as actual AAA diameter.[89]

A link between COPD and AAAs is suggested by the presence of a common development pathway: both conditions are associated with elastin breakdown and smoking. A 1999 study argued, however, that the strong association between AAAs and COPD was most likely attributable to coexisting cardiovascular disease and medications.[88] In this study, the average annual aortic diameter expansion rate was 4.7 mm in patients who used oral steroids but only 2.6 mm in those who did not. The use of beta-adrenergic agonists was also a positive predictor of aneurysm expansion. Thus, oral steroids and beta agonists must be used cautiously in COPD patients who have AAAs. If an AAA patient must use one of these medications, close follow-up is indicated to monitor the expansion rate of the aneurysm.

Atherosclerosis is associated with AAAs but is currently believed to be a secondary phenomenon, with inflammation and matrix-degrading enzymes being the primary factors in AAA development.[90] Lipoprotein (a) has been found to be an independent risk factor for atherosclerosis and is elevated in patients with AAAs independently of the patients' cardiovascular risk factors or the extent of atherosclerosis.[91] It seems reasonable that lowering lipid levels would decrease the development of atherosclerosis of the abdominal aorta. This is a potentially important effect because patients with small atherosclerotic AAAs often experience thrombotic complications involving the lower extremities.[92] Levels of apolipoprotein-AI and high-density lipoproteins have also been found to be significantly lower in patients with AAAs.[93] Overall, however, lipids appear to play only a minor role in AAA progression.[94] An animal study suggested that regression of plaque by lowering serum lipid levels after atherosclerotic aneurysm formation may result in increased aneurysm dilation in the abdominal aorta.[95] A subsequent study, however, demonstrated that statins reduce the production of MMPs in the wall of AAAs.[96] The role of lipid-lowering medications in the treatment of AAAs remains to be clarified.

Smoking is an independent risk factor for AAA development,[62,84] expansion,[76,94] and rupture.[23] Current smokers are 7.6 times more likely to have an AAA than nonsmokers are, and ex-smokers are three times more likely to have an AAA.[22] The duration of smoking is the key variable[12,22,84]: the relative risk of AAA development is increased by 4% for each year of smoking.[22] The ADAM trial noted that a longer interval since the cessation of smoking was significantly associated with a decreased risk of AAA formation[12]; however, the decline in risk appears to be slow.[22] The UKSA trial showed that former smokers were at lower risk for death from AAA repair than current smokers were.[67] A 2002 study found that there was an independent association between smoking and high-grade tissue inflammation in AAAs,[97] lending support to the idea that smoking is an initiating event in AAA formation.

At present, intriguing possibilities notwithstanding, few definitive recommendations can be made regarding the use of medical therapy to reduce AAA growth. The indications for perioperative beta blockade are primarily cardioprotective. Administration of antihypertensives may be beneficial from a practical perspective, but current level I data supporting this practice are lacking. If an antihypertensive is given, the choice of agent should be based on associated clinical data (e.g., the presence of coexisting medical conditions, such as angina or renal insufficiency, whose management must be optimized). The administration of lipid-lowering drugs to patients with AAAs also requires further study, though the utility of such agents in the presence of CAD, which is found in almost 50% of AAA patients,[98] is well documented. Finally, it is clear that smoking cessation is mandatory.

Pain Is Present

When a patient presenting with a pulsatile abdominal mass is hemodynamically stable but complains of pain in the abdomen, the back, the testicles, or the femoral region, the index of suspicion must be high for a symptomatic or rup-

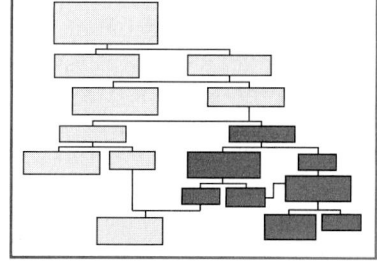

tured AAA. Other possible causes should be considered as well. As noted (see above), many abdominal processes may mimic an AAA; however, it is important that recognition of an AAA not be delayed unduly, because the length of the interval between the onset of symptoms and subsequent diagnosis and operation can have a direct bearing on overall survival. The size of the aneurysm, as determined by ultrasonography, is helpful for identifying patients at highest risk for rupture. Ultrasonography is sometimes able to detect a ruptured aneurysm, but it should not be relied on to rule out rupture. In one study, ultrasonography demonstrated extraluminal blood in only 4% of ruptured AAAs in the emergency department.[99]

In stable patients with AAAs larger than 5.5 cm who are experiencing pain, either CT or MRA may be used to detect AAA rupture; the choice typically depends on the patient's medical history [see Table 2]. After ultrasound evaluation, if an aneurysm smaller than 5.5 cm was found and no associated risk factors for rupture were identified, a search for other possible causes of the pain is reasonable, provided that it is performed expeditiously.

If no other cause for the pain can be found, possible rupture should remain a prime consideration, and the next step in evaluation—namely, spiral CT or MRA—should be implemented. Missing or delaying the diagnosis of a ruptured AAA can be disastrous. If retroperitoneal blood is noted, then the study need not be completed, and the patient should be taken to the OR [see Figure 5]. If the aneurysm is not ruptured, repair should be undertaken urgently (i.e., within the next 24 hours), with the patient's medical condition optimized to the extent possible [see 4:9 Repair of Infrarenal Abdominal Aortic Aneurysms]. Precipitous repairs of nonruptured symptomatic AAAs have an operative mortality five times that of elective repairs,[100] for reasons yet unknown.

Preoperative Evaluation of Nonemergency AAA Repair Candidates

Evaluation of a patient before elective AAA repair begins with assessment of the expected benefit of repair in relation to the estimated risk. If the decision is made to operate, the history and the physical examination should be completed as described earlier [see

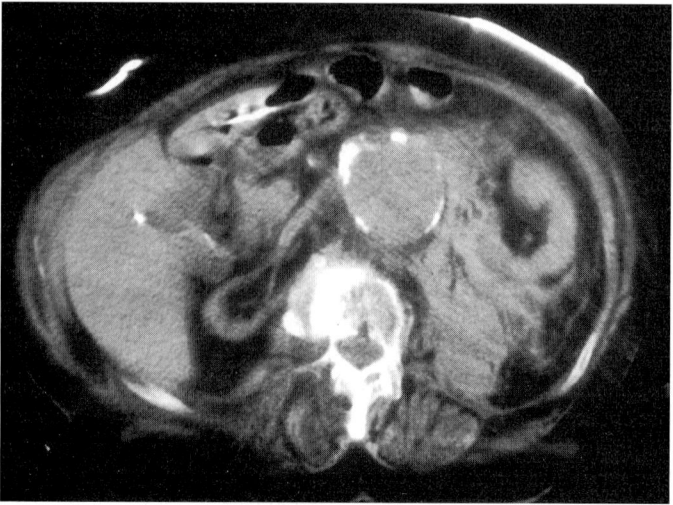

Figure 5 **Shown is a CT scan of a patient presenting with a pulsatile abdominal mass and dull, aching back pain. The scan was obtained before contrast administration and demonstrates free extravasation of blood into the retroperitoneum.**

Clinical Evaluation, *above*]. The clinical findings, in conjunction with ECG and routine laboratory test results, provide most of the information that is needed for evaluating a patient's candidacy for AAA repair.

COMORBID CONDITIONS

CAD is common in patients with AAAs and is the leading cause of early and late mortality after AAA repair.[101] Renal insufficiency, COPD, and diabetes mellitus also may influence morbidity and mortality after AAA repair. Accordingly, when any of these disease entities is present, further evaluation before repair may be beneficial. Optimization of perioperative medications is also important for maximizing risk reduction. Finally, adequate preoperative imaging is essential. The decision regarding which type of repair is most appropriate in an AAA patient should be based on the preoperative evaluation.

Coronary Artery Disease

Before AAA repair, it is important to identify patients who are at high risk for a perioperative cardiac event and who need a preoperative cardiac intervention. It is also important to identify patients who are at low risk, so that they are not subjected to unneeded testing. A report from the American College of Cardiology/American Heart Association (ACC/AHA) Task Force on Practice Guidelines provided useful guidelines for preoperative cardiac evaluation in patients undergoing noncardiac vascular surgery [*see Table 3*], with the express goal of limiting the use of perioperative cardiac procedures in patients at moderate and high risk for complications.[102] Use of these guidelines and permutations thereof has proved both safe and effective at reducing resource use and overall costs.[103-105] According to the ACC/AHA guidelines, patients needing urgent or elective AAA repair are stratified first by whether coronary revascularization was done within the past 5 years. If so, and symptoms have not recurred, the patient is cleared for operation. If the patient never underwent coronary revascularization, underwent revascularization more than 5 years before, or is experiencing recurrent symptoms or signs of cardiac ischemia, further evaluation of clinical predictors is necessary.

Clinical predictors of major perioperative cardiovascular risk—defined as myocardial infarction (MI), congestive heart failure, or death—may be divided into three categories[102]: major, intermediate, and minor. The presence of a major predictor requires that the symptom or disease be managed appropriately before nonemergency surgery. The presence of an intermediate predictor is associated with an increased risk of perioperative cardiac complications and requires that current status be fully investigated. The presence of a minor predictor is indicative of cardiovascular disease but has not been shown to independently increase the risk of perioperative cardiovascular complications.

Once the clinical predictors have been evaluated, additional predictive factors, involving the patient's ability to perform various activities (ranging from minor activities of daily living to strenuous sports) are assessed. The energy required to perform an activity is quantified in terms of metabolic equivalents (METs). The number of METs of which a patient is capable directly correlates with the ability to perform specific tasks [*see Table 4*]. Patients who are unable to attain 4 METs are considered to be at high risk for perioperative cardiac events and long-term complications. Finally, the inherent risk of the procedure to be performed is evaluated. AAA repair is considered high-risk.

The original ACC/AHA recommendations for supplemental preoperative testing were updated in a 2002 statement.[106] Cur-

rently, it is generally agreed that preoperative testing should be limited to patients in whom the results have the potential to alter the current course of management. The following noninvasive tests may be considered.

1. 12-lead ECG. This test is recommended. Certain ECG abnormalities are clinical predictors of perioperative and long-term cardiac risks in patients undergoing high-risk operative procedures [*see Table 5*].
2. Transthoracic echocardiography to evaluate resting left ventricular function. This test is indicated in the presence of heart failure. If it was previously done and demonstrated severe left ventricular dysfunction, repeat evaluation is unnecessary. It may be of benefit in patients with prior heart

Table 3 ACC/AHA Guidelines for Preoperative Cardiac Evaluation in Patients Undergoing Elective High-Risk Vascular Procedures[106]

1. Revascularization in the past 5 years?	If **yes**, without recurrence of signs or symptoms of ischemia, then further cardiac testing is not indicated. Proceed with surgery. If **no**, go to 2.
2. Coronary evaluation in the past 2 years?	If **yes**, findings are favorable on adequate test without onset of new symptoms, or symptoms change, proceed with surgery. If **no** or findings are unfavorable, go to 3.
3. Major clinical predictor of risk present?	Major clinical predictors include Unstable coronary syndromes Decompensated CHF Significant arrhythmias Severe valvular disease Presence of these predictors cancels or delays intervention until they are ameliorated. Implement medical management. Consider coronary angiography. Go to 4.
4. Intermediate clinical predictor of risk present?	Intermediate clinical predictors include Mild angina pectoris Prior MI Compensated or prior CHF Diabetes mellitus Renal insufficiency When these indicators are present, performance of noninvasive testing in AAA repair candidates is indicated, especially if 2 or more are present. If, after noninvasive testing, patient is determined to be low risk, continue with operation. If risk is high, consider coronary angiography. If **no** predictors are present, go to 5.
5. Minor or no clinical predictors present?	Minor clinical predictors include Advanced age Abnormal ECG Nonsinus rhythm Low functional capacity Previous stroke Uncontrolled systemic hypertension If minor or no clinical predictors are present and patient can attain 4 METs or more, proceed with surgery. Consider noninvasive testing when < 4 METs are attained, especially in presence of multiple minor clinical predictors; then go to 6.
6. Risk after noninvasive testing?	Low risk: proceed with operation. High risk: consider coronary angiography.

ACC—American College of Cardiology AHA—American Heart Association
CHF—congestive heart failure MET—metabolic equivalent MI—myocardial infarction

Table 4 Estimated Energy Required for Various Activities[106,131]

Activity Level	METs*	Sample Activities
Mild	1–3	Eating; playing a musical instrument; walking at 2 mph; getting dressed; golfing (with cart)
Moderate	3–5	Calisthenics without weights; climbing a flight of stairs; housework; golfing (without cart); running a short distance
Vigorous	4–12+	Chopping wood; strenuous sports such as football, basketball, singles tennis, karate, or jogging (10 min mile or faster)

*1 MET = 3.5 ml · kg^{-1} · min^{-1} oxygen uptake.

failure and those with dyspnea of unknown etiology. Routine use is not beneficial in the absence of heart failure.

3. Exercise or pharmacologic stress testing. Such testing is useful for diagnosing CAD in patients with an intermediate pretest probability of CAD, but its value is less well established in those with a high or low pretest probability. It is a good prognosticator for patients with suspected or proven CAD who are undergoing initial evaluation, for patients whose clinical disposition has changed significantly, and for those who have experienced an acute coronary syndrome. Stress testing is also recommended for demonstrating the presence of myocardial ischemia before coronary revascularization and for evaluating the efficacy of medical therapy. It may be useful in patients whose subjective assessment of exercise tolerance is unreliable and in whom evaluation in terms of METs is therefore impossible. Less clear are the following indications for stress testing: (1) diagnosis of CAD in patients who have resting ST depression of less than 1 mm, are on digitalis, or show evidence of left ventricular hypertrophy on ECG, and (2) detection of restenosis in high-risk patients who have recently (i.e., within the past few months) undergone percutaneous transluminal coronary angioplasty (PTCA). Exercise stress testing should not be done (1) to diagnose patients with ECG findings that would prevent adequate assessment, (2) in patients with severe comorbidities that would preclude coronary revascularization, (3) for routine screening of asymptomatic patients, or (4) to evaluate young patients with isolated ectopic beats on ECG.

Table 5 ECG Findings as Clinical Predictors of Increased Perioperative Cardiovascular Risk[130]

Major predictors
High-grade atrioventricular block
Symptomatic ventricular arrhythmias in the presence of underlying heart disease
Supraventricular arrhythmias with uncontrolled ventricular rate

Intermediate predictor
Pathologic Q wave indicating previous myocardial infarction

Minor predictors
Left ventricular hypertrophy
Left bundle-branch block
ST-T abnormalities
Rhythm other than sinus (e.g., atrial fibrillation)

Coronary angiography, if indicated, may be performed next. Current indications in patients scheduled to undergo AAA repair include (1) high-risk status after noninvasive testing, (2) continued angina despite adequate medical therapy, (3) unstable angina, and (4) an equivocal result on noninvasive testing in high-risk patients. Coronary angiography may be beneficial in patients with multiple intermediate clinical risk factors. If noninvasive testing reveals moderate-sized to large areas of ischemia in a patient without high-risk criteria and a lower left ventricular ejection fraction, or if testing is nondiagnostic in a patient at intermediate clinical risk, coronary angiography may also be indicated. The indication for coronary angiography is more controversial in patients who have experienced a perioperative MI. Coronary angiography is not indicated in patients who are asymptomatic after coronary revascularization and who are capable of at least 7 METs.

Both coronary artery bypass grafting (CABG) and PTCA have been employed to treat CAD before AAA repair. CABG is usually done in this setting only if it has been decided that the patient needs the intervention regardless of the current status of the abdominal aorta. Such patients have a high-risk coronary anatomy and have a long-term prognosis that may improve if coronary revascularization is performed. The combination of AAA repair and CABG has been evaluated, and there are some data to support its use in highly select patients.[107]

To date, no controlled trials have evaluated the efficacy of PTCA against that of medical therapy before noncardiac aortic surgery. Although some small observational studies have indicated a low cardiac mortality when preoperative PTCA is performed in this setting, complications after PTCA are not infrequent and include the need for emergency CABG. One retrospective review found that patients who underwent prophylactic PTCA before noncardiac surgery were twice as likely to have an adverse cardiac outcome as healthy patients were.[108] This study did not control for CAD severity, medical management, or comorbidities. A later study concluded that both CABG and PTCA offered only modest protection against adverse cardiac events after major arterial surgery (CABG, < 5 years; PTCA, < 2 years).[109] General indications for PTCA use are outlined in the 2001 revision of the 1993 ACC/AHA Guidelines for Percutaneous Coronary Intervention.[110] It is recommended that patients wait at least 2 weeks—preferably, 4 to 6 weeks—after PTCA before undergoing AAA repair; this delay allows the plaque to stabilize after stenting and permits full treatment with antiplatelet agents.

Pulmonary Disease

Between 7% and 11% of patients with COPD have an AAA.[88] Traditionally, when such patients are to undergo AAA repair, room air arterial blood gas values are determined and pulmonary function tests performed to assess the extent of COPD. If COPD is severe, formal pulmonary consultation may be necessary for prediction of short- and long-term prognoses and optimization of treatment. Several studies have reported that COPD is an independent predictor of operative mortality.[13,70,111] A 2001 study of Veterans Affairs (VA) patients, however, found no significant correlation between the presence of COPD and increased operative mortality (though morbidity was notably higher).[112] A 2003 study evaluating morbidity and mortality after AAA repair in patients with COPD showed that the preoperative factors significantly associated with a poor outcome included (1) suboptimal COPD management, as evidenced by fewer inhalers used, (2) a lower preoperative hematocrit, (3) preoperative renal insufficiency, and (4) the presence of CAD.[113] It is noteworthy that abnormal preoperative pulmonary function tests and arterial blood gas values were not predictive of a poor outcome. Thus, COPD by itself is not a contraindication to AAA repair.

Renal Failure

Preoperative renal insufficiency [see 6:7 Renal Failure] is known to be a risk factor for a poor outcome after AAA repair[13,70,112,113] and thus should be evaluated and corrected if possible. In certain patients with AAAs, renal artery stenosis may be contributing to impaired renal function; if so, it may be corrected either noninvasively, before AAA repair, or in the course of the repair.[45]

Diabetes Mellitus

Whether diabetes mellitus is truly an independent risk factor for morbidity or mortality after aortic surgery is controversial. Several studies have shown that the risk of death is not increased in diabetic patients, but the risk of perioperative complications may be.[114-116] Most of these studies had small study groups and thus lacked the statistical power needed to demonstrate that diabetes had a significant influence. A 2002 study of patients at VA medical centers who underwent major vascular procedures found that diabetic patients were indeed at higher risk for death and cardiovascular complications.[117] When examined separately, however, patients undergoing AAA repair did not have higher rates of cardiovascular complications or death than patients undergoing other procedures.

PERIOPERATIVE MEDICATIONS

Multiple studies have addressed optimization of medical management in patients with AAAs. Beta blockers, alpha$_2$-adrenergic agonists, nitrates, and calcium channel blockers have all been evaluated in this setting. Other agents used in the treatment of cardiovascular disease (e.g., aspirin) have not been specifically evaluated in regard to reduction of perioperative cardiac complications in patients undergoing aortic surgery.[118]

A review of the literature supporting perioperative beta blockade was published in 2002.[119] Five randomized, controlled trials were evaluated, and the results suggested that this measure had a beneficial effect on perioperative cardiac morbidity. The number needed to treat to prevent one MI was 2.5 to 6.7 patients; the number needed to treat to produce a significant effect on cardiac or all-cause mortality was 3.2 to 8.3 patients. All but one of the studies reported a significant reduction in postoperative MIs after beta blocker use, with the effect being most obvious in high-risk patients. Thus, it appears that perioperative beta blockade is most likely beneficial for patients at high risk for cardiac events who are to undergo AAA repair, unless it is otherwise contraindicated (e.g., by COPD). The therapeutic goal should be to attain a resting heart rate of 60 beats/min or lower before operation.[118]

Alpha$_2$-adrenergic agonists (e.g., clonidine) have not been shown to reduce MI rates or mortality from cardiac causes. In one study, mivazerol did not exert a significant overall effect in patients undergoing major vascular or orthopedic procedures but was associated with a significant reduction in MI rates and mortality from cardiac causes in patients with known CAD.[120] Therefore, when perioperative beta blockade is contraindicated, administration of alpha$_2$-adrenergic agonists may be of benefit in high-risk patients.

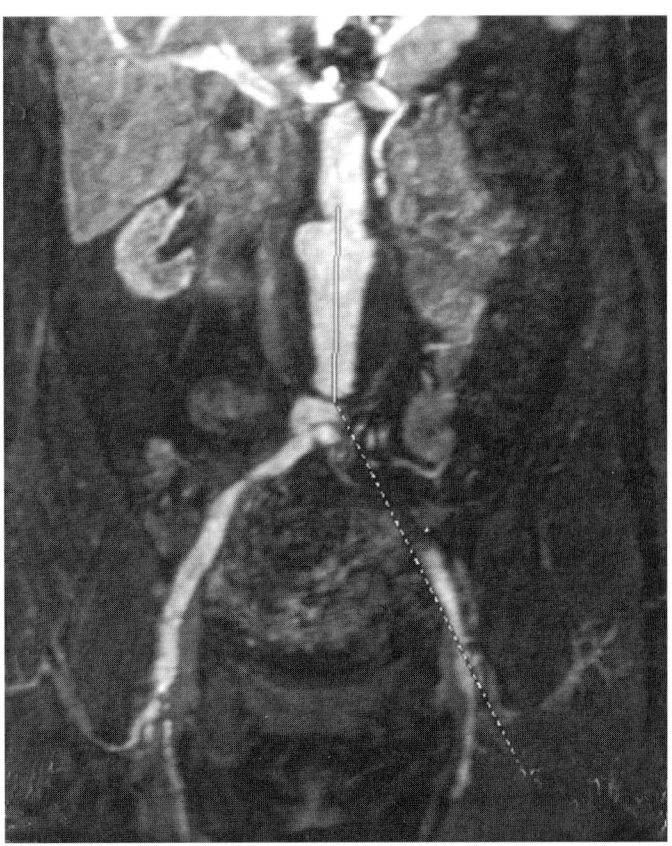

Figure 6 **Shown is an MRA of a patient who had undergone both open infrarenal AAA repair and aortobifemoral bypass off the terminal aorta. The AAA grew between the two previous repairs and was subsequently managed endovascularly.**

To date, studies evaluating the perioperative use of nitroglycerin and diltiazem to lower the risk of cardiac events have not found this practice to be beneficial in this regard. It may be best to reserve these agents for patients who need them for angina or ischemic symptoms and for those who have myocardial ischemia after operation.[118]

It is widely accepted that aspirin is beneficial in reducing the risks associated with CAD.[121] Its continued use throughout the perioperative period is controversial, however, as is the use of clopidogrel, because of the potential complications associated with decreased platelet function. Indications for the use of these antiplatelet agents may be patient dependent.[122] Traditionally, aspirin is discontinued at least 1 week before aortic surgery.

FURTHER IMAGING

The main methods used to evaluate the aortic anatomy before AAA repair are ultrasonography, CT, MRA, and aortography. Which method is employed in a given situation depends largely on the clinical presentation, the history, the comorbid conditions present, and the availability of equipment and expertise. Each has its advantages and disadvantages [see Table 2].

Ultrasonography

Further ultrasonographic evaluation of the aortic anatomy, if indicated, is performed in accordance with the approach described earlier [see Patient Is Stable, above].

CT Scanning

The current standard for preoperative imaging of AAAs is contrast-enhanced CT scanning. This modality is more accurate than aortography at measuring AAA diameter and determining the presence of rupture.[53] With spiral CT, it is possible to obtain a three-dimensional view of the abdominal aorta. CT scanning is highly accurate, with measurements reproducible to within 2 mm. Measurement variations as great as 5 mm are sometimes seen, however, occurring 9% to 17% of the time.[54,55] Such variations may be reduced by standardizing measurements, reducing the number of radiologists reading the images, and using calipers and magnification for greater accuracy.[55]

The advantages of CT over ultrasonography include (1) more precise definition of the proximal and distal extent of AAAs, (2) better delineation of the iliac arterial anatomy, (3) the ability to evaluate AAA wall integrity, noting the location and amount of calcification within vessel walls, and (4) the ability to identify venous anomalies, retroperitoneal blood, aortic dissection, inflammatory aneurysms, and other intra-abdominal pathologic conditions and anomalies (e.g., horseshoe kidney). Therefore, CT is the study of choice for excluding AAA rupture in stable but symptomatic patients.[1,53,123] It is also the current study of choice for evaluating patients before endovascular AAA repair as well as for determining whether an endoleak has occurred after endovascular AAA repair. In the near future, ultrasonography may supplant CT for these applications.

The main drawbacks associated with CT scanning are (1) radiation exposure and (2) the requirement for iodinated contrast material, which cannot be used in patients with dye allergies or renal insufficiency. In addition, spiral CT with three-dimensional reconstruction is relatively expensive at present. Allergic reactions to the contrast agent can usually be prevented by giving a standard steroid-diphenhydramine preparation. Alternatively, CT scanning may be done without contrast to determine whether there is a large retroperitoneal hematoma, which would be indirectly suggestive of a ruptured AAA. If the patient has renal insufficiency, MRA may be more appropriate.

MRA

In patients with renal insufficiency who are scheduled for AAA repair, MRA with gadolinium and the breath-hold technique may be the preoperative study of choice; it is comparable to CT scanning in evaluating elective AAA repair candidates [see Figure 6].[82,124] The main advantages of MRA are that (1) it does not require the use of nephrotoxic agents or radiation and (2) it is highly sensitive and specific in detecting stenoses of the splanchnic, renal, and iliac arteries.[82] Its main drawbacks are that (1) it is not widely available, (2) it is expensive, (3) it may cause claustrophobia in select patients, and (4) it takes longer to perform than CT scanning. MRA is contraindicated in patients with pacemakers, metallic foreign bodies in the eye, cochlear implants, and certain berry aneurysm clips. Over time, however, as MRA becomes faster, more widely available, and less expensive, its advantages may make it a more attractive alternative in the preoperative workup of patients with AAAs.

Aortography

Preoperative digital subtraction aortography is not routinely used for diagnosis but rather as an adjunct to other studies in preparation for AAA repair. Being an invasive test, it carries an added risk over other imaging modalities. Aortography is currently indicated in the preoperative evaluation of an AAA when

(1) the extent of the aneurysm may include the juxtarenal or suprarenal aorta, (2) the clinical history is indicative of lower-extremity arterial occlusive disease (i.e., claudication or rest pain), (3) renovascular disease may be present, as evidenced by uncontrolled hypertension or azotemia, or (4) the patient has previously undergone arterial reconstruction.[78] Aortography is superior at evaluating the intraluminal characteristics of the aorta, determining visceral-branch involvement, and delineating variations in the vascular anatomy.[10]

Aortography has a number of important limitations in comparison with CT or MRA. In particular, it is associated with multiple risks that are not incurred with CT or MRA, such as infection, arterial thrombosis necessitating emergency thrombectomy and repair, distal embolization, groin hematoma, and local arterial dissection.[125] There is also a 10% risk of renal failure in patients with elevated creatinine levels ($\geq$ 2.5 mg/dl)[125]; this can often be prevented with adequate hydration before the study. Finally, the cost of aortography is three to four times that of spiral CT, which gives health care providers an incentive to replace aortography with spiral CT whenever possible.[126]

Complications of AAAs

Rupture of an AAA obviously is often life threatening, but erosion of an aneurysm into adjacent structures may be catastrophic as well. In certain instances, ruptured AAAs may form a continuous luminal connection with a surrounding structure. High-output cardiac failure may result from an arteriovenous shunt between the aorta and the inferior vena cava, which occurs in as many as 2% to 4% of patients with ruptured AAAs.[127,128] AAA patients with intermittent GI bleeding may present with a so-called herald bleed from a primary aortoenteric fistula. Most such fistulas occur in the third or fourth part of the duodenum.[129] Aorta–inferior vena cava shunts and aortoenteric fistulas are medical emergencies that demand immediate operative attention.

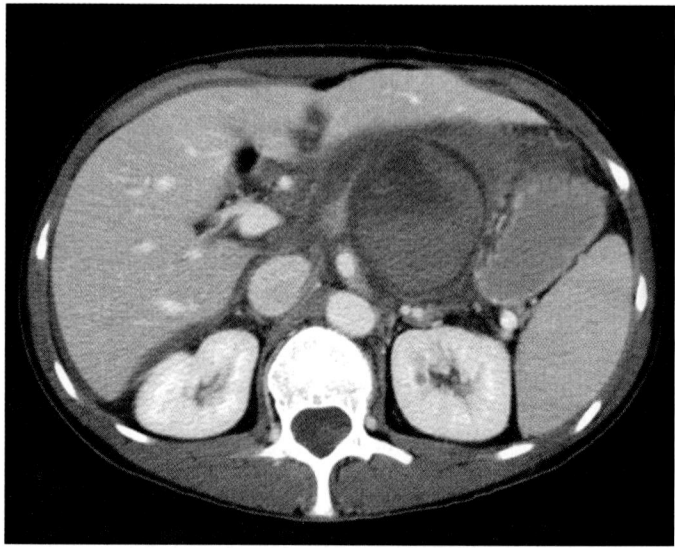

Figure 7 **CT scan of a patient with Marfan syndrome who presented with increasing abdominal pain reveals a large hematoma along the lesser curvature of the stomach. The hematoma was localized via angiography and was found to be consistent with a ruptured left gastric artery aneurysm.**

AAAs may also give rise to distal lower-extremity atheroemboli [see 4:4 Pulseless Extremity and Atheroembolism]. Small AAAs appear to be the most common sources: infrarenal AAAs with mean diameters of 3.5 cm have been linked to lower-extremity atheroemboli.[130] Thrombosis of an AAA also occurs; if it develops acutely, severe ischemia of the entire lower torso may result, manifested by a bilateral lack of femoral pulses, a drop in skin temperature beginning at the level of the upper thigh, and a change in skin color beginning at the level of the knees.[129] Recognizing these symptoms as potential complications of AAAs can facilitate diagnosis.

Rare Causes of Pulsatile Abdominal Mass

Finally, when a patient presents with a pulsatile abdominal mass that is suggestive of aneurysmal disease, the most likely diagnosis is an infrarenal AAA, in that 80% of aortic aneurysms are found in this location. It is important to keep in mind, however, that various less common types of aneurysms may also present as a pulsatile abdominal mass, including (but not limited to) iliac artery aneurysms [see Figure 2], traumatic pseudoaneurysms, and visceral artery aneurysms [see Figure 7].

References

1. Upchurch GR Jr, Wakefield TW, Williams DM, et al: Abdominal aortic aneurysms. Practical Cardiology: Evaluation and Treatment of Common Cardiovascular Disorders. Eagle KA, Baliga RR, Eds. Lippincott Williams & Wilkins, Philadelphia, 2003

2. Hoyert DL, Arias E, Smith BL, et al: National Vital Statistics Reports: Deaths: Final Data for 1999. Division of Vital Statistics, Centers for Disease Control and Prevention. National Center for Health Statistics, vol 49, no 8 (September 21, 2003) http://www.cdc.gov/nchs/data/nvsr49/nvsr49_08.pdf

3. Huber TS, Ozaki CK, Seeger JM: Abdominal aortic aneurysms. Surgery: Scientific Principles and Practice, 3rd ed. Greenfield LJ, Mulholland MW, Oldham KT, et al, Eds. Lippincott Williams & Wilkins, Philadelphia, 2001, p 1803

4. Shames ML, Thompson RW: Abdominal aortic aneurysms: surgical treatment. Cardiol Clin 20:563, 2002

5. Loughran CF: A review of the plain abdominal radiograph in acute rupture of abdominal aortic aneurysms. Clin Radiol 37:383, 1986

6. LaRoy LL, Cormier PJ, Matalon TA, et al: Imaging of abdominal aortic aneurysms. AJR Am J Roentgenol 152:785, 1989

7. Davies AJ, Winter RK, Lewis MH: Prevalence of abdominal aortic aneurysms in urology patients referred for ultrasound. Ann R Coll Surg Engl 81:235, 1999

8. Wakefield TW, Whitehouse WM, Wu S, et al: Abdominal aortic aneurysm rupture: statistical analysis of factors affecting outcome of surgical treatment. Surgery 91:586, 1982

9. Valentine RJ, Barth MJ, Myers SI, et al: Nonvascular emergencies presenting as ruptured abdominal aortic aneurysms. Surgery 113:286, 1993

10. Borrero E, Queral LA: Symptomatic abdominal aortic aneurysms misdiagnosed as nephroureterolithiasis. Ann Vasc Surg 2:145, 1988

11. Hodgson KJ, Webster DJ: Abdominal aortic aneurysm causing duodenal and ureteric obstructions. J Vasc Surg 3:364, 1986

12. Lederle FA, Johnson GR, Wilson SE, et al: Prevalence and associations of abdominal aortic aneurysm detected through screening. Aneurysm Detection and Management (ADAM) Veterans Affairs Cooperative Study Group. Ann Intern Med 126:441, 1997

13. Huber TS, Wang JG, Derrow AE, et al: Experience in the United States with intact abdominal aortic aneurysm repair. J Vasc Surg 33:304, 2001

14. Johnston KW and the Canadian Society for Vascular Surgery Aneurysm Study Group: Influence of sex on the results of abdominal aortic aneurysm repair. J Vasc Surg 20:914, 1994

15. Vardulaki KA, Walker NM, Day NE, et al: Quantifying the risks of hypertension, age, sex and smoking in patients with abdominal aortic aneurysm. Br J Surg 87:195, 2000

16. Singh K, Bonaa KH, Jacobsen BK, et al: Prevalence of and risk factors for abdominal aortic aneurysm in a population-based study: the Tromso Study. Am J Epidemiol 154:236, 2001

17. Steickmeier B: Epidemiology of aortic disease: aneurysm, dissection, occlusion. Radiologe 41:624, 2001

18. Darling RC III, Brewster DC, Darling RC, et al: Are familial aortic aneurysms different? J Vasc Surg 10:39, 1989

19. Johansen K, Kopsell T: Familial tendency for abdominal aortic aneurysm. JAMA 256:1934, 1986

20. van Vlijmen-van Keulen CJ, Pals F, Rauwerda JA: Familial abdominal aortic aneurysm: a systematic review of a genetic background. Eur J Vasc Endovasc Surg 24:105, 2002

21. Dillavou E, Kahn MB: Peripheral vascular disease: diagnosing and treating the 3 most common peripheral vasculopathies. Geriatrics 58:37, 2003

22. Wilming TB, Quick CR, Day NE: The association between cigarette smoking and abdominal aortic aneurysms. J Vasc Surg 30:1099, 1999

23. Brown LC, Powell JT: Risk factors for aneurysm rupture in patients kept under ultrasound surveillance. U.K. Small Aneurysm Trial Participants. Ann Surg 230:289, 1999

24. Brown PM, Zelt DT, Sobolev B: The risk of rupture in untreated aneurysm: the impact of size, gender, and expansion rate. J Vasc Surg 37:280, 2003

25. Englesbe MJ, Wu AH, Clowes AW, et al: The prevalence and natural history of aortic aneurysms in heart and abdominal organ transplant patients. J Vasc Surg 37:27, 2003

26. Hallett JW Jr, Marshall DM, Petterson TM, et al: Graft-related complications after abdominal aortic aneurysm repair: reassurance from a 36-year population-based experience. J Vasc Surg 25:277, 1997

27. Brunkwall J, Hauksson H, Bengtsson H, et al: Solitary aneurysms of the iliac arterial system: an estimate of their frequency of occurrence. J Vasc Surg 10:381, 1989

28. Bernhard VM, Mitchell RS, Matsumura JS, et al: Ruptured abdominal aortic aneurysm after endovascular repair. J Vasc Surg 35:1155, 2002

29. Faries PL, Brener BJ, Connelly TL, et al: A multicenter experience with the Talent endovascular graft for the treatment of abdominal aortic aneurysms. J Vasc Surg 35:1123, 2002

30. Pearce WH: What's new in vascular surgery. J Am Coll Surg 196:253, 2003

31. Gray H: Anatomy: Descriptive and Surgical, 15th ed. Pick TP, Howden R, Eds. Chancellor Press, London, 1994, p 526

32. Kiev J, Eckhardt A, Kerstein MD: Reliability and accuracy of physical examination in detection of abdominal aortic aneurysms. Vasc Surg 31:143, 1997

33. Lederle FA, Simel DL: Does this patient have abdominal aortic aneurysm? JAMA 281:77, 1999

34. Chervu A, Clagett GP, Valentine RJ, et al: Role of physical examination in detection of abdominal aortic aneurysms. Surgery 117:454, 1995

35. Lederle FA, Walker JM, Reinke DB: Selective screening for abdominal aortic aneurysms with physical examination and ultrasound. Arch Intern Med 148:1753, 1988

36. Fink HA, Lederle FA, Roth CS, et al: The accuracy of physical examination to detect abdominal aortic aneurysm. Arch Intern Med 160:833, 2000

37. Beede SD, Ballard DJ, James EM, et al: Positive predictive value of clinical suspicion of abdominal aortic aneurysm: implication for efficient use of abdominal ultrasonography. Arch Intern Med 150:549, 1990

38. Feinberg RL, Trout HH: Isolated iliac artery aneurysm. Current Therapy in Vascular Surgery, 4th ed. Ernst CB, Stanley JC, Eds. Mosby, St Louis, 2001, p 313

39. Graham LM, Zelenock GB, Whitehouse WM Jr, et al: Clinical significance of arteriosclerotic femoral artery aneurysms. Arch Surg 115:502, 1980

40. Whitehouse WM Jr, Wakefield TW, Graham LM, et al: Limb-threatening potential of arteriosclerotic popliteal artery aneurysms. Surgery 83:694, 1983

41. Diwan A, Sarkar R, Stanley JC, et al: Incidence of femoral and popliteal artery aneurysms in patients with abdominal aortic aneurysms. J Vasc Surg 31:863, 2000

42. Lawrence PF, Wallis C, Dobrin PB, et al: Peripheral aneurysms and arteriomegaly: is there a familial pattern? J Vasc Surg 28:599, 1998

43. Heikkinen M, Salenius J-P, Auvinen O: Ruptured abdominal aortic aneurysm in a well-defined geographic area. J Vasc Surg 36:291, 2002

44. Chew HF, You CK, Brown MG, et al: Mortality, morbidity, and costs of ruptured and elective abdominal aortic aneurysm repairs in Nova Scotia, Canada. Ann Vasc Surg 17:171, 2003

45. Ernst CB: Abdominal aortic aneurysm. N Engl J Med 328:1167, 1993

46. Katz DL, Stanley JC, Zelenock GB: Operative mortality rates for intact and ruptured abdominal

aortic aneurysms in Michigan: an eleven-year state-wide experience. J Vasc Surg 19:804, 1993

47. Wakefield TW, Whitehouse WM Jr, Wu SC, et al: Abdominal aortic aneurysm rupture: statistical analysis of factors affecting outcome of surgical treatment. Surgery 91:586, 1982

48. Bown MJ, Sutton AJ, Bell PRF, et al: A meta-analysis of 50 years of ruptured abdominal aortic aneurysm repair. Br J Surg 89:714, 2002

49. Johansen K, Kohler TR, Nicholls SC, et al: Ruptured AAA: the Harborview experience. J Vasc Surg 13:240, 1991

50. Gloviczki P, Pairolero PC, Mucha P Jr, et al: Ruptured abdominal aortic aneurysms: repair should not be denied. J Vasc Surg 15:851, 1992

51. Patel ST, Korn P, Haser PB, et al: The cost-effectiveness of repairing ruptured abdominal aortic aneurysms. J Vasc Surg 32:247, 2000

52. Ohki T, Veith FJ, Sanchez LA, et al: Endovascular graft repair of ruptured aortoiliac aneurysm. J Am Coll Surg 189:102, 1999

53. Nowygod R: Ultrasonography and computed tomography in the evaluation of abdominal aortic aneurysm. Current Therapy in Vascular Surgery, 4th ed. Ernst CB, Stanley JC, Eds. Mosby, St Louis, 2001, p 221

54. Jaakkola P, Hippelainen M, Farin P, et al: Inter-observer variability in measuring the dimensions of the abdominal aorta: comparison of ultrasound and computed tomography. Eur J Vasc Endovasc Surg 12:230, 1996

55. Lederle FA, Wilson SE, Johnson GR, et al: Variability in measurement of abdominal aortic aneurysms. Abdominal Aortic Aneurysm Detection and Management Veterans Administration Cooperative Study Group. J Vasc Surg 21:945, 1995

56. Pedersen OM, Aslaksen A, Vik-Mo H: Ultrasound measurement of the luminal diameter of the abdominal aorta and iliac arteries in patients without vascular disease. J Vasc Surg 17:596, 1993

57. Pearce WH, Slaughter MS, LeMaire S, et al: Aortic diameter as a function of age, gender, and body surface area. Surgery 144:691, 1993

58. Lederle FA, Johnson GR, Wilson SE, et al: Relationship of age, gender, race, and body size to infrarenal aortic diameter. Aneurysm Detection and Management (ADAM) Veterans Administration Cooperative Study Group. J Vasc Surg 26:595, 1997

59. da Silva ES, Rodrigues AJ, Castro de Tolosa EM, et al: Variation of infrarenal aortic diameter: a necropsy study. J Vasc Surg 29:920, 1999

60. d'Audiffret A, Santilli S, Tretinyak A, et al: Fate of the ectatic infrarenal aorta: expansion rates and outcomes. Ann Vasc Surg 16:534, 2002

61. Hollier CH, Stenson AW, Gloviczki P, et al: Arteriomegaly: classification and morbid implications of diffuse aneurismal disease. Surgery 93:700, 1983

62. Lederle FA, Johnson GR, Wilson SE, et al: Yield of repeated screening for abdominal aortic aneurysm after a 4-year interval. Aneurysm Detection and Management Veterans Affairs Cooperative Study Investigation. Arch Intern Med 160:1117, 2000

63. Crow P, Shaw E, Earnshaw JJ, et al: A single normal ultrasonographic scan at age 65 years rules out significant aneurysm disease for life in men. Br J Surg 88:941, 2001

64. Vorp DA, Raghavan ML, Webster MW: Mechanical wall stress in abdominal aortic aneurysm: influence of diameter and asymmetry. J Vasc Surg 27:632, 1998

65. Fillinger MF, Raghavan ML, Marra SP, et al: In vivo analysis of mechanical wall stress and abdominal aortic aneurysm rupture risk. J Vasc Surg 36:589, 2002

66. Fillinger MF, Marra SP, Raghavan ML, et al: Prediction of rupture risk in abdominal aortic aneurysm during observation: wall stress versus diameter. J Vasc Surg 37:724, 2003

67. Brady AR, Brown LC, Fowkes FGR, et al: Long-term outcomes of immediate repair compared with surveillance of small abdominal aortic aneurysms. United Kingdom Small Aneurysm Trial. N Engl J Med 346:1445, 2002

68. Cruz CP, Drouilhet JC, Southern FN, et al: Abdominal aortic aneurysm repair. Vasc Surg 35:335, 2001

69. Lederle FA, Wilson SE, Johnson GR, et al: Immediate repair compared with surveillance of small abdominal aortic aneurysms. Aneurysm Detection and Management Veterans Affairs Cooperative Study Group. N Engl J Med 346:1437, 2002

70. Hertzer NR, Mascha EJ, Karafa MT, et al: Open infrarenal abdominal aortic aneurysm repair: the Cleveland Clinic experience from 1989 to 1998. J Vasc Surg 35:1145, 2002

71. Dimick JB, Stanley JC, Axelrod DA, et al: Variation in death rate after abdominal aortic aneurysmectomy in the United States: impact of hospital volume, gender, and age. Ann Surg 235:579, 2002

72. Cronenwett JL, Murphy TF, Zelenock GB, et al: Actuarial analysis of variables associated with rupture of small abdominal aortic aneurysms. Surgery 98:472, 1985

73. Menard MT, Chew DKW, Chan RK, et al: Outcome in patients at high risk after open surgical repair of abdominal aortic aneurysm. J Vasc Surg 37:285, 2003

74. Biancari F, Mosorin M, Antilla V, et al: Ten-year outcome of patients with very small abdominal aortic aneurysm. Am J Surg 183:53, 2002

75. Santilli SM, Littooy FN, Cambria RA, et al: Expansion rates and outcomes for the 3.0-cm to the 3.9-cm infrarenal abdominal aortic aneurysm. J Vasc Surg 35:666, 2002

76. Chang JB, Stein TA, Liu JP, et al: Risk factors associated with rapid growth of small abdominal aortic aneurysms. Surgery 121:117, 1997

77. Scott RAP, Tisi PV, Ashton HA, et al: Abdominal aortic aneurysm rupture rates: a 7-year follow-up of the entire abdominal aortic aneurysm population detected by screening. J Vasc Surg 28:124, 1998

78. Beebe HG, Kritpracha B: Screening and preoperative imaging of candidates for conventional repair of abdominal aortic aneurysm. Semin Vasc Surg 12:300, 1999

79. Hallett JW Jr: Management of abdominal aortic aneurysms: concise review for clinicians. Mayo Clin Proc 75:395, 2000

80. Multicentre aneurysm screening study (MASS): cost effectiveness analysis of screening for abdominal aortic aneurysms based on four year results from randomized controlled trial. Multicentre Aneurysm Screening Study Group. BMJ 325:1135, 2002

81. Wassef M, Baxter T, Chisholm RL, et al: Pathogenisis of abdominal aortic aneurysms: a multidisciplinary research program supported by the National Heart, Lung, and Blood Institute. J Vasc Surg 34:730, 2001

82. Lindholt JS, Vammen S, Fasting H, et al: The plasma level of matrix metalloproteinase 9 may predict the natural history of small abdominal aortic aneurysms: a preliminary study. Eur J Vasc Endovasc Surg 20:281, 2000

83. Baxter BT, Pearce WH, Waltke EA, et al: Prolonged administration of doxycycline in patients with small asymptomatic abdominal aortic aneurysms: report of a prospective (phase II) multicenter study. J Vasc Surg 36:1, 2002

84. Vardulaki KA, Walker NM, Day NE, et al: Quantifying the risks of hypertension, age, sex and smoking in patients with abdominal aortic aneurysm. Br J Surg 87:195, 2000

85. Wilmink TBM, Quick CRG, Day NE: The association between cigarette smoking and abdominal aortic aneurysms. J Vasc Surg 30:1099, 1999

86. Gadowski GR, Pilcher DB, Ricci MA: Abdominal aortic aneurysm expansion rate: effect of size and beta-adrenergic blockade. J Vasc Surg 19:727, 1994

87. Propranolol for small abdominal aortic aneurysms: results of a randomized trial. Propranolol Aneurysm Trial Investigators. J Vasc Surg 35:72, 2002

88. Brown LC, Powell JT: Risk factors for aneurysm rupture in patients kept under ultrasound surveillance. U.K. Small Aneurysm Trial Participants. Ann Surg 230:289, 1999

89. Wilson KA, Lee AJ, Lee AJ, et al: The relationship between aortic wall distensibility and rupture of infrarenal abdominal aortic aneurysm. J Vasc Surg 37:112, 2003

90. Grange JJ, Davis V, Baxter BT: Pathogenesis of abdominal aortic aneurysm: an update and look toward the future. Cardiovasc Surg 5:256, 1997

91. Schillinger M, Domanovits H, Ignatescu M, et al: Lipoprotein (a) in patients with aortic aneurismal disease. J Vasc Surg 36:25, 2002

92. Keen RR, McCarthy WJ, Shireman PK, et al: Surgical management of atheroembolization. J Vasc Surg 21:773, 1995

93. Simoni G, Gianotti A, Ardia A, et al: Screening study of abdominal aortic aneurysm in a general population: lipid parameters. Cardiovasc Surg 4:445, 1996

94. Lindholt JS, Heegaard NH, Vammen S, et al: Smoking, but not lipids, lipoprotein(a) and antibodies against oxidized LDL, is correlated to the expansion of abdominal aortic aneurysms. Eur J Vasc Endovasc Surg 21:51, 2001

95. Zarins CK, Xu CP, Glasgov S: Aneurysmal enlargement of the aorta during regression of experimental atherosclerosis. J Vasc Surg 15:90, 1992

96. Nagashima H, Aoka Y, Sakomura Y, et al: A 3-hydroxy-3-methylglutaryl coenzyme A reductase inhibitor, cerviastatin, suppresses production of matrix metalloproteinase-9 in human abdominal aortic aneurysm wall. J Vasc Surg 36:158, 2002

97. Rasmussen TE, Hallett JW Jr, Tazelaar HD, et al: Human leukocyte antigen class II immune response genes, female gender, and cigarette smoking as risk and modulating factors in abdominal aortic aneurysms. J Vasc Surg 35:988, 2002

98. Hertzer NR, Beven EG, Young JR, et al: Coronary artery disease in peripheral vascular patients: a classification of 1000 coronary angiograms and results of surgical management. Ann Surg 199:223, 1984

99. Sheeman WP: Suspected leaking AAA: use of sonography in the emergency room. Radiology 168:117, 1988

100. Sullivan CA, Rohrer MJ, Cutler BS: Clinical management of the symptomatic but unruptured AAA. Surgery 113:286, 1993

101. Roger VL, Ballard DJ, Hallett JW, et al: Influence of coronary artery disease on morbidity and mortality after abdominal aortic aneurysmectomy: a population-based study 1971–1987. J Am Coll Cardiol 14:1245, 1989

102. Eagle KA, Brundage BH, Chaitman BR, et al: Guidelines for perioperative cardiovascular evaluation for noncardiac surgery: report of the American College of Cardiology/American Heart Association Task Force on Practice Guidelines (Committee on Perioperative Cardiovascular Evaluation for Noncardiac Surgery). J Am Coll Cardiol 27:910, 1996

103. Froehlich JB, Karavite D, Russman PL, et al: American College of Cardiology/American Heart Association preoperative assessment guidelines reduce resource utilization before aortic surgery. J Vasc Surg 36:758, 2002

104. Samain E, Farah E, Leseche G, et al: Guidelines

for perioperative cardiac evaluation from the American College of Cardiology/American Heart Association task force are effective for stratifying cardiac risk before aortic surgery. J Vasc Surg 31:971, 2000

105. Bartels C, Bechtel JFM, Hossmann V, et al: Cardiac risk stratification for high-risk vascular surgery. Circulation 95:2473, 1997

106. Eagle KA, Berger PB, Hugh C, et al: ACC/AHA guideline update for perioperative cardiovascular evaluation for noncardiac surgery: executive summary: a report of the American College of Cardiology/American Heart Association Task Force on Practice Guidelines (Committee to update the 1996 Guidelines on Perioperative Cardiovascular Evaluation for Noncardiac Surgery). Circulation 105:1257, 2002

107. Falk V, Walther T, Mohr FW: Abdominal aortic aneurysm repair during cardiopulmonary bypass: rationale for a combined approach. Cardiovasc Surg 5:271, 1997

108. Posner KL, Van Norman GA, Chan V, et al: Adverse cardiac outcomes after noncardiac surgery in patients with prior percutaneous transluminal coronary angioplasty. Anesth Analg 89:553, 1999

109. Back MR, Stordahl N, Cuthbertson D, et al: Limitations in the cardiac risk reduction provided by coronary revascularization prior to elective vascular surgery. J Vasc Surg 36:526, 2002

110. Smith SC Jr, Dove JT, Jacobs AK, et al: ACC/AHA guidelines for percutaneous coronary intervention: executive summary and recommendations: a report of the American College of Cardiology/American Heart Association Task Force on Practice Guidelines Committee to Revise the 1993 Guidelines for Percutaneous Transluminal Coronary Angioplasty. J Am Coll Cardiol 37:2215, 2001

111. Johnston KW: Multicenter prospective study of nonruptured abdominal aortic aneurysm: part II.

Variables predicting morbidity and mortality. J Vasc Surg 9:437, 1989

112. Axelrod DA, Henke PK, Wakefield TW, et al: Impact of chronic obstructive pulmonary disease on elective and emergency abdominal aortic aneurysm repair. J Vasc Surg 33:72, 2001

113. Upchurch GR Jr, Proctor MC, Henke PK, et al: Predictors of severe morbidity and death after elective abdominal aortic aneurysmectomy in patients with chronic obstructive pulmonary disease. J Vasc Surg 37:594, 2003

114. Berry AJ, Smith RB III, Wintraub WS, et al: Age versus comorbidities as risk factors for complications after elective abdominal aortic reconstructive surgery. J Vasc Surg 33:345, 2001

115. Dardik A, Lin JW, Gordon TA, et al: Results of elective abdominal aortic aneurysm repair in the 1990's: a population based analysis of 2335 cases. J Vasc Surg 30:985, 1999

116. Treiman GS, Treiman RI, Foran RF, et al: The influence of diabetes mellitus on the risk of abdominal aortic surgery. Am Surg 60:436, 1994

117. Axelrod DA, Upchurch GR Jr, DeMonner S, et al: Perioperative cardiovascular risk stratification of patients with diabetes who undergo elective major vascular surgery. J Vasc Surg 35:894, 2002

118. Fleisher LA, Eagle KA: Lowering cardiac risk in noncardiac surgery. N Engl J Med 345:1677, 2001

119. Auerbach AD, Goldman L: β-Blockers and reduction of cardiac events in noncardiac surgery: scientific review. JAMA 287:1435, 2002

120. Oliver MF, Goldman L, Julian DG, et al: Effect of mivazerol on perioperative cardiac complication during non-cardiac surgery in patients with coronary heart disease: the European Mivazerol Trial (EMIT). Anesthesiology 91:951, 1999

121. Willard JE, Lange RA, Hillis LD: The use of aspirin in ischemic heart disease. N Engl J Med

327:175, 1992

122. Ehlers R, Eagle KA: Lowering cardiac risk in noncardiac surgery (letter). N Engl J Med 346:1096, 2002

123. Cronenwett JL, Krupski WC, Rutherford RB: Abdominal aortic and iliac aneurysms. Vascular Surgery, 5th ed. Rutherford RB, Ed. WB Saunders Co, Philadelphia, 2000, p 1246

124. Petersen MJ, Cambria RP, Kaugman JA, et al: Magenetic resonance angiography in the preoperative evaluation of abdominal aortic aneurysms. J Vasc Surg 21:891, 1995

125. Baker KD, Bandyk DF, Back MR: Arteriography in the evaluation of abdominal aortic aneurysm. Current Therapy in Vascular Surgery, 4th ed. Ernst CB, Stanley JC, Eds. Mosby, St Louis, 2001, p 215

126. Rubin GD, Armerding MD, Dake MD, et al: Cost identification of abdominal aortic aneurysm imaging by using time and motion analyses. Radiology 215:63, 2000

127. Duong C, Atkinson N: Review of aortoiliac aneurysms with spontaneous large vein fistula. Aust N Z J Surg 71:52, 2001

128. Rajmohan B: Spontaneous aortocaval fistula. J Postgrad Med 48:203, 2002

129. Connolly JE, Kwaan JH, McCart PM, et al: Aortoenteric fistula. Ann Surg 194:402, 1981

130. Messina LM, Sarkar R: Peripheral arterial embolism. Surgery: Scientific Principles and Practice, 3rd ed. Greenfield LJ, Mulholland MW, Oldham KT, et al, Eds. Lippincott Williams & Wilkins, Philadelphia, 2001, p 1568

131. Fletcher GF, Baledy G, Froelicher VF, et al: Exercise standards: a statement for healthcare professionals from the American Heart Association. Circulation 91:580, 1995

4 PULSELESS EXTREMITY AND ATHEROEMBOLISM

Vicken N. Pamoukian, M.D., and Cynthia K. Shortell, M.D., F.A.C.S.

Approach to the Acutely Ischemic Limb

Pulseless Extremity

Acute limb ischemia (ALI) is a sudden reduction in limb perfusion that poses a potential threat to the viability of an extremity. The incidence of ALI in the general population is approximately 1.7/10,000 per year.[1] The clinical presentation ranges from subtle to dramatic. Management of ALI is challenging and is complicated by the myriad comorbid conditions typically seen in conjunction with ALI.

In the early 1970s, a study comprising more than 3,000 patients with ALI from 35 centers documented a mortality of 26% and an amputation rate of 37%.[2] Substantial improvements in surgical management approaches, techniques, and instruments have been achieved since then, but morbidity and mortality remain high, with death rates around 15% and amputation rates between 10% and 30%.[3]

Cardiac risk assessment with the Goldman index allows rapid evaluation of the level of physiologic risk patients face. Again, the major cause of morbidity in ALI patients is the associated medical conditions typically present [see Table 1].

Given the general frailty of ALI patients and the multiplicity of available therapeutic options, it is important to take a logical, methodical approach to the treatment of this condition. In particular, the use of algorithms, decision trees, or clinical pathways for patient care helps the clinician visualize and evaluate multiple potential avenues for management and select the path likely to yield the best outcome.

CLINICAL EVALUATION

History

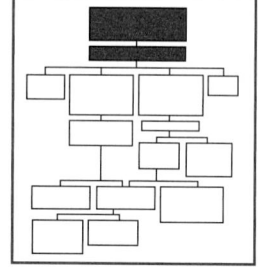

A thorough history should be taken. Generally, the dominant symptoms are related to pain or loss of function. The onset and duration of symptoms should be determined, and the location and the intensity of any changes should be established. The pain of ALI is not well localized and is not affected by gravity. Pain of sudden onset suggests that an embolic cause is likely, whereas long-standing pain before the acute event suggests a thrombotic cause [see Discussion, Etiology of ALI, *below*].

It is imperative to ask whether the patient experienced pain before the current ischemic episode and whether the current episode is the first. It is also important to ask about previous surgical revascularization as well as previous or current cardiac disease (e.g., myocardial infarction [MI], atrial fibrillation, or valvular disease), aneurysmal disease, or vasculitis. Finally, inquiries should be made about previous atherosclerotic disease, current risk factors for atherosclerosis (e.g., hypertension, smoking, diabetes, tobacco abuse, hyperlipidemia, and stroke), and previous clotting episodes.

Physical Examination

The characteristic signs and symptoms of ALI may be summarized as the six Ps: *P*ulselessness, *P*ain, *P*allor, *P*oikilothermia, *P*aresthesia, and *P*aralysis.

- Pulses should be palpated and documented. Any previous documentation should be noted.
- Pain should be documented with regard to severity, area, and progression.
- Pallor may be seen in the early stages, followed by cyanosis.
- Poikilothermia may propagate the ischemic cascade through its vasoconstrictive effects. The level of coolness and pallor is typically one level below the point of occlusion on the arterial tree, and it should correlate with the pulses or signals found. As always, baseline documentation should be done so that the progression or resolution of the process can be tracked.
- Paresthesia is an essential finding. The earliest sign of tissue loss is the loss of light touch, two-point discrimination, vibratory perception, and proprioception, especially in the first dorsal web space of the foot.
- Paralysis, if present, is an indication of advanced limb-threatening ischemia. The extent of paralysis must be determined. The intrinsic muscles of the foot are affected by ischemia of the vessels around the ankle. Dorsiflexion and plantar flexion of the foot are functions of muscles that rely on blood supplied by the popliteal and superficial femoral arteries. Loss of dorsiflexion and plantar flexion indicates that blood flow is cut off at a higher level and signals that more tissue may be at risk.

Peripheral Pulses

Careful assessment of peripheral pulses will help localize the area of arterial obstruction. When clot is fresh, its soft, semiliquid consistency allows the pulse to be translated at the level of obstruction. Only when the thrombus becomes organized and densely compacted is the pulse lost at the site of occlusion. As an example, in a patient with obstruction at the popliteal artery, popliteal pulses remain palpable in the earlier stages of the process, but distal pulses are lost [see Table 2].

Staging of Limb Ischemia

A prime goal of clinical evaluation is to determine the severity of the disease process so that appropriate management can be rapidly instituted. To this end, the key question that must be

Approach to the Acutely Ischemic Limb

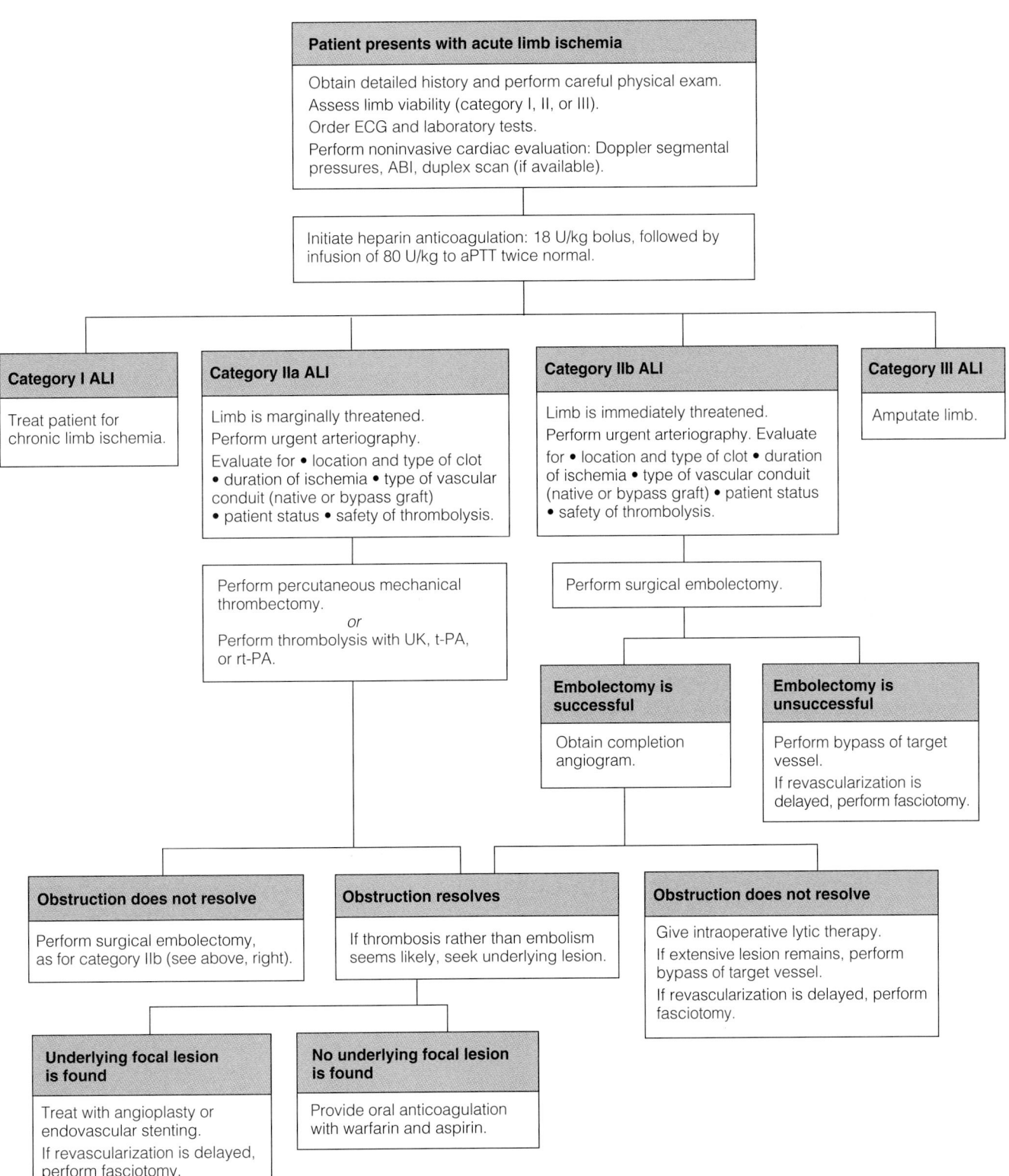

Patient presents with acute limb ischemia

Obtain detailed history and perform careful physical exam.
Assess limb viability (category I, II, or III).
Order ECG and laboratory tests.
Perform noninvasive cardiac evaluation: Doppler segmental pressures, ABI, duplex scan (if available).

Initiate heparin anticoagulation: 18 U/kg bolus, followed by infusion of 80 U/kg to aPTT twice normal.

Category I ALI

Treat patient for chronic limb ischemia.

Category IIa ALI

Limb is marginally threatened.
Perform urgent arteriography.
Evaluate for • location and type of clot • duration of ischemia • type of vascular conduit (native or bypass graft) • patient status • safety of thrombolysis.

Perform percutaneous mechanical thrombectomy.
or
Perform thrombolysis with UK, t-PA, or rt-PA.

Category IIb ALI

Limb is immediately threatened.
Perform urgent arteriography. Evaluate for • location and type of clot • duration of ischemia • type of vascular conduit (native or bypass graft) • patient status • safety of thrombolysis.

Perform surgical embolectomy.

Category III ALI

Amputate limb.

Embolectomy is successful

Obtain completion angiogram.

Embolectomy is unsuccessful

Perform bypass of target vessel.
If revascularization is delayed, perform fasciotomy.

Obstruction does not resolve

Perform surgical embolectomy, as for category IIb (see above, right).

Obstruction resolves

If thrombosis rather than embolism seems likely, seek underlying lesion.

Obstruction does not resolve

Give intraoperative lytic therapy.
If extensive lesion remains, perform bypass of target vessel.
If revascularization is delayed, perform fasciotomy.

Underlying focal lesion is found

Treat with angioplasty or endovascular stenting.
If revascularization is delayed, perform fasciotomy.

No underlying focal lesion is found

Provide oral anticoagulation with warfarin and aspirin.

Table 1   Incidence of Medical Comorbidities in Patients Presenting with ALI[97]

Comorbidity	Incidence (%)			
	Rochester Trial (N = 114)	TOPAS-1 Trial (N = 213)	TOPAS-2 Trial (N = 544)	Total (N = 871)
Cerebrovascular disease	NR	15.4	11.5	11.6
Congestive heart failure	NR	15.5	12.5	13.3
Coronary artery disease	56.1	47.1	42.5	45.4
Diabetes mellitus	28.1	36.7	29.0	30.8
Hypercholesterolemia	31.6	29.6	23.5	26.0
Hypertension	63.2	60.9	69.6	60.3
Malignancy	NR	11.9	11.5	11.6
Tobacco history	51.8	79.3	77.5	74.6

NR—not reported   TOPAS—Thrombolysis Or Peripheral Arterial Surgery

answered is whether the limb is viable or not. In 1997, the Joint Council of the Society for Vascular Surgery and the North American Chapter of the International Society for Cardiovascular Surgery developed reporting standards for ALI and stratified it into three distinct categories on the basis of the severity of the disease process [see Table 3].[4]

In category I ALI, patients present with acute occlusion of an artery that is chronically narrowed. Therefore, abundant collaterals can be found, and the limb is viable. In category II ALI, the ischemic limb is threatened but may be salvaged without the need for an amputation if adequate revascularization can be achieved. This category is further subdivided into categories IIa and IIb. Category IIa includes patients with mild forefoot numbness or any lesion for which prompt revascularization of the limb achieves a good result. Category IIb includes patients with diminished sensation of the entire foot and weakness of calf muscles whose limb is still salvageable but who require immediate revascularization. In category III, ischemia is irreversible and amputation is required. Clinical features include permanent tissue loss, anesthesia, and paralysis of the limb.

DIAGNOSTIC TESTING

In addition to the clinical evaluation, a full battery of diagnostic tests should be performed. An electrocardiogram should be obtained, and if a cardiac source is suspected, a transesophageal echocardiogram should be obtained as well. A full set of laboratory tests, including a complete blood count and a platelet count,

blood chemistries, and coagulation profiles, should be ordered. In addition, chest and abdominal x-rays should be done to look for obvious calcifications. If it appears that a hypercoagulable state may be causing thrombosis, a hypercoagulability profile should be ordered [see 4:6 Venous Thromboembolism].

Evaluation of Arterial Tree

An objective evaluation of the arterial tree should be performed when feasible. If ischemia is particularly severe and long-lasting, a full angiographic evaluation may not be possible; however, noninvasive Doppler studies and, if time permits, angiography should be considered strongly in this setting.

Doppler segmental pressures and ankle-brachial index Examination should begin at the level of the ankle and should include assessment of arterial signals and venous hums. When arterial signals are found, the ankle-brachial index (ABI) should be measured.

The ABI is derived from the ankle systolic pressure and the brachial systolic pressure and is determined as follows. The systolic pressure is measured in each arm, and the higher of the two measurements is taken to be the brachial systolic pressure. A cuff is then placed on each calf, and the examiner listens to signals in the dorsalis pedis and posterior tibial arteries. The cuff is inflated until the signal is no longer heard. At this point, the cuff is slowly released, and the systolic pressure is recorded at the point where the signal is once again audible. Again, the higher of the two systolic measurements is taken to be the ankle systolic pressure. The systolic ankle

Table 2   Localization of Arterial Obstruction through Palpation of Peripheral Pulses[97]

Palpable Pulses			Location of Obstruction	Possible Causes
Femoral	Popliteal	Pedal		
–	–	–	Aortoiliac segment	Aortoiliac atherosclerosis; embolus to common iliac bifurcation
+	–	–	Femoral segment	Thrombosis, femoral atherosclerosis; common femoral embolus
+	++	–	Distal popliteal ± tibials	Popliteal aneurysm with embolization
+	+	–	Distal popliteal ± tibials	Popliteal embolus; popliteal/tibial atherosclerosis, diabetes

Table 3 Clinical Categorization of ALI[4]

Category	Findings			Doppler Signals	
	Description/Prognosis	Sensory Loss	Muscle Weakness	Arterial	Venous
I. Viable	Not immediately threatened	None	None	Audible	Audible
IIa. Marginally threatened	Salvageable if promptly treated	Minimal (toes) or none	None	(Often) inaudible	Audible
IIb. Immediately threatened	Salvageable with immediate revascularization	More than toes, associated with rest pain	Mild, moderate	(Usually) inaudible	Audible
III. Irreversible*	Major tissue loss or permanent nerve damage inevitable	Profound, anesthetic	Profound, paralysis (rigor)	Inaudible	Inaudible

*When presenting early, category IIb and category III may be difficult to differentiate.

pressure is then divided by the brachial systolic pressure to yield the ABI. An ABI in the range of 1 is normal; however, the ABI can be falsely elevated if the distal arteries are not compressible. When the ABI falls below 0.6, there is a significant difference in blood pressure between the proximal arterial tree and the distal extremity, which usually denotes an occlusive process. Next, segmental pressures are obtained by placing cuffs at the ankle, below the knee, above the knee, and on the thigh. Systolic blood pressures are measured at each location, and any pressure drop greater than 15 mm Hg is considered significant.

When the venous Doppler signal or hum is lost in addition to the arterial Doppler signal, the ischemia is severe. In addition, when a Doppler signal is present, intervention may be delayed slightly. However, the absence of signals does not always signify an irreversibly threatened limb.

Duplex ultrasonography Duplex scanning can be valuable for localizing the site of occlusion, especially in bypass grafts. Unfortunately, it is not always a practical option in acute circumstances, both because the machine is often unavailable in the emergency setting and because the results of scanning are highly operator dependent. However, in specialized centers where a duplex ultrasound machine is readily available and personnel are experienced in its use, a quick look at the suspected site may yield helpful information.[5] In stenotic regions, the velocities measured across the lesion are greatly increased.[6,7] In addition, duplex ultrasonography can be used to visualize plaque morphology, stenoses, dissections, and thrombi. In some centers of excellence, duplex ultrasound technology has obviated the need for lengthy arteriograms and has benefited patients by reducing ischemia time.

Arteriography Arteriography remains the gold standard for diagnosis of ALI and may even be a primary tool in its management. It should not, however, be performed if doing so would keep a critically ischemic leg from receiving prompt surgical therapy. Arteriography should be reserved for patients with viable limbs who can tolerate the additional delay before revascularization.

Arteriography should be performed from a site remote from the point of concern. Thus, if lytic therapy is to be administered, entry-site bleeding will be minimized. A complete angiogram that includes the runoff vessels in the foot should be performed to establish the baseline degree of arterial disease and delineate the inflow and outflow anatomy. This information facilitates subsequent planning for revascularization, should this step prove necessary. Digital subtraction angiography is preferred in that it allows a reduced contrast load and lowers the incidence of contrast-associated renal injury.[8,9] If the patient is allergic to the contrast agent

or has renal insufficiency, CO_2- or gadolinium-based angiography may be performed instead. These two modalities have the advantage of possessing minimal to no nephrotoxicity, but they yield poorer suprainguinal arterial visualization than standard contrast angiography does.[10,11]

The arteriogram can provide useful clues for differentiating emboli from thrombi. In a patient with arterial embolism, there is often an identifiable source, there is rarely a history of claudication, contralateral and proximal pulses are normal, cutoff is sharp, atherosclerosis is minimal, a few collateral vessels are present, and a discrete clot is clearly visible on contrast studies. In a patient with arterial thrombosis, the thrombus has no identifiable source, there is a history of claudication with evidence of peripheral vascular disease, diffuse atherosclerotic vessel wall disease is present, cutoff is tapered and irregular, and there is ample collateral circulation.

TREATMENT

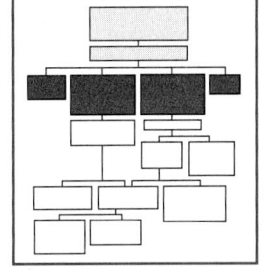

Until the middle of the 20th century, when revascularization techniques were developed, amputation was the only treatment for acute lower-extremity ischemia [*see 4:14 Lower-Extremity Amputation for Ischemia*]. Today, however, the vascular surgeon possesses an immense armamentarium for the treatment of this condition, ranging from emergency bypass to embolectomy to thrombolytic therapy.

The treatment of ALI is an emergency situation. Rapid restoration of flow to the extremity substantially reduces morbidity and mortality. Accordingly, the clinician must be thoroughly familiar with the therapeutic modalities available and capable of making an appropriate choice among them without undue delay. Whichever therapeutic modality is chosen for a given patient, several primary measures should be undertaken to protect and optimize the status of the extremity. Full systemic heparinization should not be delayed. The extremity should be placed in a dependent position, with care taken to avoid extrinsic pressure on the limb. Temperature fluxes should be minimized: cold induces vasoconstriction, and heat increases tissue demand and metabolic and circulatory demands. Finally, tissue oxygenation should be maximized via transfusion, improvement of cardiac function, and restoration of intravascular volume.

Laboratory tests, radiologic studies, and a cardiology evaluation are required. The ABI should be documented. Abnormalities in blood counts, electrolyte concentrations, and coagulation profiles should be corrected. The duration of ischemia should be noted and any comorbid conditions identified so that the examiner can determine the appropriate degree of monitoring required (e.g., arterial line or pulmonary arterial catheter). Proper and timely preoperative preparation is crucial for preventing rapid deterioration of the patient's condition.

Anticoagulation

Heparin administration should be started as soon as the diagnosis of ALI is entertained. Numerous studies have shown that this measure decreases the morbidity and mortality associated with ALI and increases the limb salvage rate. Heparin impedes the propagation of clots and, in the instance of embolism, may help prevent additional events.

Heparin acts at multiple sites in the normal coagulation system, inhibiting reactions that lead to the clotting of blood and the formation of fibrin clots both in vitro and in vivo. Small amounts of heparin, in combination with antithrombin (heparin cofactor), can inhibit thrombosis by inactivating activated factor X and inhibiting the conversion of prothrombin to thrombin.[12] Once active thrombosis has developed, larger amounts of heparin can inhibit further coagulation by inactivating thrombin and preventing the conversion of fibrinogen to fibrin. Heparin also prevents the formation of a stable fibrin clot by inhibiting the activation of fibrin-stabilizing factor.[12-14]

Heparin does not have fibrinolytic activity and therefore does not lyse existing clots. Heparin therapy can be complicated by thrombocytopenia, which has a reported incidence of 0% to 30%.[15] If the thrombocyte count falls below 100,000/mm³ or if recurrent thrombosis develops, heparin should be discontinued.[16,17] Patients receiving heparin may experience new thrombus formation, either early or late, in association with this thrombocytopenic phenomenon as a consequence of irreversible heparin-induced platelet aggregation (the so-called white clot syndrome). This process may lead to severe thromboembolic complications, including skin necrosis, gangrene of the extremities, MI, pulmonary embolism, stroke, and, possibly, death.[16,18,19] Accordingly, if new thrombosis develops in association with thrombocytopenia, heparin should be promptly discontinued.

Periodic platelet counts, hematocrits, and tests for fecal occult blood are recommended during the entire course of heparin therapy, regardless of the route of administration.

Bleeding time is usually unaffected by heparin. Clotting time is prolonged by full therapeutic doses of heparin, but in most cases, it is not measurably affected by low doses.

Thrombolysis

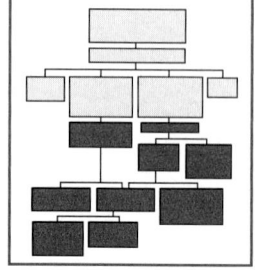

The use of thrombolysis to treat chronic and acute arterial insufficiency dates back to the 1970s, when it was popularized by Dotter.[20] Systemic fibrinolytic therapy has not proved effective and consequently has been supplanted by intra-arterial (catheter-directed) thrombolysis, which yields significantly better results. Still, the role of thrombolytic therapy for ALI is somewhat controversial. In addition, such therapy requires a skilled team with considerable clinical expertise, typically including a vascular surgeon, an interventional radiologist, and a well-trained ancillary staff. The benefits of pharmacologic clot lysis must always be weighed against those of surgical intervention and the risk of bleeding associated with fibrinolysis.

Despite the use of fibrin-specific agents and catheter-directed infusion, thrombolytic agents still exert systemic effects, most of which are dose related. About 10% of patients receiving thrombolytic therapy experience significant bleeding, including bleeding from both puncture and remote sites. Absolute contraindications to the use of lytic agents include recent surgery, recent stroke or brain tumor, pregnancy, a bleeding diathesis, recent trauma, and active bleeding [see Table 4].

Thrombolysis versus surgical treatment   Three prospective, randomized trials—the University of Rochester trial,[21] the Surgery versus Thrombolysis for Ischemia of the Lower Extremity (STILE) trial,[22] and Thrombolysis Or Peripheral Arterial Surgery (TOPAS) trial[23,24]—addressed the differences between thrombolytic therapy and traditional surgery.

Rochester trial. This randomized, controlled single-center trial compared urokinase (UK) with surgery in patients with ischemia of less than 7 days' duration.[21] At the end of 1 year, overall mortality was lower in the thrombolysis group (25%) than in the surgery group (48%). The amputation rates were similar in the two groups. Total hospital charges were comparable as well, which suggests that at initial treatment, thrombolytic therapy is as costly as surgery. Major bleeding was encountered in 11% of patients.

STILE trial. This randomized, controlled multicenter trial compared surgery with recombinant tissue plasminogen activator (rt-PA) and with UK.[22] It was stopped early because of an increase in the number of patients with ongoing ischemia in the thrombolysis groups. An ad hoc committee later determined that the reason for this increase was the inclusion of chronically symptomatic patients in the study. In any case, the study clearly demonstrated that patients with less than 14 days of ischemia had a lower amputation rate when treated with thrombolysis (11% versus 30%; P = 0.02) but that patients with more than 14 days of ischemia had a lower amputation rate when treated with surgery.

TOPAS trial. This randomized, controlled multicenter trial compared surgery with recombinant urokinase (r-UK) thrombolysis in patients with ischemic symptoms of less than 14 days' duration.[23,24] At the end of 1 year, the amputation rates in the two groups were similar. Bleeding complications were seen only in patients undergoing thrombolysis, four of whom had intracranial

---

Table 4   Contraindications to Thrombolytic Therapy[98]

Absolute contraindications
Established cerebrovascular event (including TIAs) within past 2 mo
Active bleeding diathesis
GI bleeding within past 10 days
Neurosurgery (intracranial, spinal) within past 3 mo
Intracranial trauma within past 3 mo

Major relative contraindications
Cardiopulmonary resuscitation within past 10 days
Major nonvascular surgery or trauma within past 10 days
Uncontrolled hypertension: systolic BP > 180 mm Hg, diastolic BP > 110 mm Hg
Puncture of noncompressible vessel
Intracranial tumor
Recent eye surgery

Minor relative contraindications
Hepatic failure, particularly in patients with coagulopathy
Bacterial endocarditis
Pregnancy
Diabetic hemorrhagic retinopathy

TIA—transient ischemic attack

hemorrhage. When additional end points were considered, the thrombolysis group was found to require significantly fewer major interventions at the time of discharge and at 12 months.

A prospective, randomized multicenter trial evaluated local thrombolysis with either rt-PA or urokinase in 234 patients with thrombotic occlusions (223 native femoral or popliteal arteries, 11 bypass grafts).[25] Complete reperfusion occurred in 62% of the patients treated with rt-PA and in 50% of the patients treated with urokinase ($P = 0.18$). However, bleeding was observed in 12.8% of rt-PA–treated patients (including one instance of cerebral hemorrhage) and in 9.1% of UK-treated patients (none of whom experienced cerebral bleeding).

Current data suggest, but do not prove, that thrombolytic therapy is effective as initial therapy for patients with acute arterial and graft occlusions and no sensorimotor deficits. Such an approach, however, is not suitable for patients with common femoral artery emboli, which should be treated surgically, and there are certain patients with sensorimotor deficits (e.g., those without any runoff) for whom the potential benefits of thrombolysis outweigh the risks of delay.

At present, acute thrombotic arterial occlusion in an occluded bypass graft is the area where intra-arterial fibrinolysis may be most useful, permitting better planning of the subsequent operation and resulting in a less extensive procedure. Such therapy, however, does not necessarily yield improvements in major long-term end points. It is important to remember that thrombosis of femoropopliteal or similar bypasses is related to early or late surgical stenosis and atherosclerosis and that restoring flow usually does not suffice to ensure continued patency.

Logistics of thrombolysis In patients with mild or no sensory deficits, angiography is performed first. Depending on the location of the obstruction, the type of clot present, and the level of patient risk, the patient may be offered thrombolysis as initial therapy.

In our practice, the patient is taken from the emergency department to the angiography suite. Informed consent is obtained for diagnostic and therapeutic angiography, including the use of stents, balloon angioplasty, stent grafts and thrombolysis, and finally the requirement for an emergency surgical procedure. A discussion is undertaken with the patient to outline the course of treatment and to explain that indwelling catheters may have to be placed and that a stay in the ICU may be required.

Access to the arterial system is gained via a single-wall puncture technique; the risk of posterior-wall bleeding associated with a double-wall technique is thereby avoided. Access should be obtained from a site as remote from the intervention site as possible. Generally, this is accomplished by starting from the contralateral counterpart of the target artery and going up and over the aortic bifurcation, then back to the ipsilateral artery. By removing the puncture site from the site of catheter-directed thrombolysis, the incidence of bleeding and formation of hematomas or pseudoaneurysms is reduced.

After completion of the angiogram and delineation of the pathology, a guide wire is passed into the occluded area. We use a 0.035 in. hydrophilic guide wire, which has a slippery, wet coating that enables it to cross nonhydrophilic lesions. Once in place, the wire is guided through the clot. A multiple-sidehole catheter is placed through the clot, and a hand-injection angiogram is performed to confirm that the catheter tip is in the true lumen. The guide wire is then left within the catheter to occlude the tip, so that the lytic agent is infused through the sideholes preferentially. This graded "coaxial" infusion technique allows the agent to reach the greatest possible surface area, maximizes the length of infusion, and enables the surgeon to treat some of the longest bypass grafts.

In many cases, mechanical thrombus removal, with or without pulse spray, is employed initially, followed by continuous infusion of a thrombolytic agent. In addition to lytic therapy, administration of heparin is started (200 to 400 units I.V. or via sheath) to prevent pericatheter thrombosis. Serial laboratory evaluation is carried out to verify that the patient is not bleeding and that the fibrinogen level is higher than 100 mg/dl. Serial follow-up arteriograms are performed to monitor progress. It is critically important that successful thrombolysis be followed by treatment, whether endovascular or open, of any lesions uncovered during thrombolysis; if it is not, reocclusion is inevitable. At the conclusion of thrombolysis and before intervention, the patient must be kept on a heparin drip to prevent the formation of a new thrombus. The rate of successful reperfusion is approximately 90% to 95% in most studies.

An important advantage of this selective approach is that it allows simultaneous angiographic definition of the nature of the occlusion (i.e., embolic versus thrombotic) and of any vessel wall abnormalities that would lead to rethrombosis if not corrected by surgery or balloon angioplasty. A major drawback to this approach is that arterial catheterization is required for prolonged periods (20 hours, on average), leading to major bleeding and thromboembolic complications in 6% to 20% of patients. Therefore, the end points of thrombolytic therapy are (1) resolution and reconstitution of flow through the obstruction, (2) absence of change in the occlusion of the vessel on angiography, and (3) bleeding complications. If it is determined that thrombolysis is not progressing, it should be abandoned and surgical intervention undertaken.

Thrombectomy

Percutaneous aspiration thrombectomy This technique uses a large, thin-walled catheter and a large syringe to remove an embolus or thrombus from a vascular conduit, whether native vessel or graft. The catheter is placed as previously described [see Logistics of Thrombolysis, *above*] and is parked immediately by the clot. Aspiration of the clot with the syringe is then attempted. If the clot is new, success is likely, but an old clot that is organized will not be as amenable to removal. Percutaneous aspiration thrombectomy is most effective as an adjunct to catheter-directed thrombolysis.[26,27]

Percutaneous mechanical thrombectomy Percutaneous mechanical thrombectomy (PMT) functions on the basis of a hydrodynamic circulation. The basic concept is that a hydrodynamic vortex is created around the tip of the PMT catheter. Thrombectomy is accomplished with the introduction of a pressurized saline jet stream through the directed orifices in the distal tip of the catheter. The jets generate a localized low-pressure zone via the Bernoulli effect, which entrains and macerates thrombus. The saline and the fragmented thrombus are then sucked back into the exhaust lumen of the catheter and out of the body for disposal.

This technique has proved beneficial when used in appropriate settings and properly selected patients. Its efficiency relies on the age of the clot. Fresh thrombus is readily treated with PMT, but older clots are much less amenable to this technique and may have to be treated with an adjunctive catheter-based modality (e.g., angioplasty, intra-arterial thrombolysis, or atherectomy).[28-31]

Surgical Embolectomy and Revascularization

When a patient has significant sensory and motor deficits related to a profoundly ischemic limb, immediate surgical revascularization is indicated. The decision whether to accomplish this percutaneously or surgically should be made expeditiously. OR availability should be determined, the method of anesthesia should be chosen, and the technical details of the procedure should be planned [see 4:11

Infrainguinal Arterial Procedures]. Heparin administration should be started before the patient enters the OR. General anesthesia is the preferred method of anesthesia.

For lower-extremity emboli, access to the femoral vessels should be obtained rapidly. The common, deep, and superficial femoral arteries are controlled proximally and distally with tape, and the common femoral artery is opened transversely. Catheter embolectomy of the superficial femoral, deep femoral, common femoral, and external iliac arteries is then performed. Differently sized embolectomy catheters are used, depending on the size of each artery. In our experience, a No. 3 catheter is usually suitable for the deep femoral artery, a No. 4 for the superficial femoral artery, and a No. 5 for the common femoral and external iliac arteries. The extracted clot is sent for pathologic evaluation. When the clot is believed to be in the distal vessels of the lower extremity, control of the popliteal artery and its trifurcation is obtained via a popliteal incision. A No. 3 catheter should be adequate at this site.

For upper-extremity emboli, a curvilinear incision is made that starts on the medial aspect of the upper arm, extends transversely across the antecubital fossa, and ends halfway down the middle of the lower arm. This incision allows control of the brachial, radial, and ulnar arteries. A No. 3 embolectomy catheter is typically used here.

Several passes are done in each vessel until no more clot can be seen and there is brisk back-bleeding from the vessel. When no further clot can be retrieved, a completion angiogram is done to visualize the distal vessels and elucidate any anatomic pathology in the native vessels. If distal clot is still present after the completion angiogram, intraoperative thrombolysis can be employed for a brief period to soften the clot. The multiple-sidehole catheter is advanced distally to the location of the clot, the guide wire is passed through the lesion, and the catheter is passed over the wire into the substance of the clot. Infusion of the lytic agent is then started.

Repeat angiograms indicate whether the clot has dissolved or is still present. If the clot is still apparent, repeat embolectomy is attempted. If thrombosis rather than embolism is suspected, an underlying lesion must be sought. In performing the embolectomy, attention should be paid to the tactile sensations felt as the balloon is withdrawn. Such sensations give the operator a sense of the disease process. When several deflations are needed and the withdrawal path of the balloon feels rough, a long-standing process (e.g., an atherosclerotic calcified vessel with anatomic discrepancies) is likely.

If there appears to be no residual clot after embolectomy, then a completion angiogram is sufficient and the artery can be closed primarily. Heparin is continued, and the patient is eventually switched to warfarin, which is continued for at least 6 months postoperatively. Finally, the location from which the embolus originated is sought and appropriately treated. When an underlying lesion is identified, a decision must be made as to whether it can be treated with angioplasty or stenting or whether a formal bypass is required to correct the problem and salvage the limb.

Key to the final management of these patients is assessment of the lower extremities, especially the calves, for compartment syndrome. To minimize the chances that an otherwise successful surgical operation may fail as a consequence of this syndrome, we typically perform intraoperative fasciotomies on the extremity if profound ischemia has been present for several hours.

Cost Considerations

A retrospective study published in 1995 compared thrombolysis with surgical thrombectomy as first-line therapy for ALI.[32] Only the costs of the initial admission were documented. The average charge for the three treatments ranged from $20,000 to $26,000. Economic analysis confirmed that the total economic impact of thrombolysis

approximated that of initial operative therapy. The conclusion of the study was that there was no difference between an endovascular approach and an operative approach with respect to cost. Thus, when acute treatment of ALI is being considered, cost should not be factored into the decision-making process.[32,33]

Atheroembolism

Atheroembolism is a condition in which microscopic cholesterol-laden debris travels from proximal arteries until it reaches the most distal arterial segments, typically in the skin of the lower extremities and in the end-organs.[34-37] This debris usually originates from unstable plaque found at inflection points in the arterial tree, especially in the aorta.[38,39] It may also originate from aneurysmal sacs either in the aorta or in the peripheral arteries.

CLINICAL EVALUATION

Patients with atheroembolism usually present with focal toe ischemia—the so-called blue-toe syndrome—in conjunction with palpable pulses in the distal extremity [*see Figure 1*]. Acute pain of sudden onset is typically noted in the affected area. This pain can often establish the exact timing of embolization. Cyanosis is present either on the toe or over a more extensive area if the atheroemboli were circulated throughout the extremity.[40,41] When both lower extremities are involved, an aortic source of the microemboli is commonly found.

A complete vascular examination should be performed and pulses documented. Although a patent arterial tree is the rule, emboli that are sufficiently small may travel through collateral channels. Palpation should be done to detect any aneurysmal disease. A massive proximal atheroembolic event may affect the entire abdominal wall and both extremities, giving the appearance of livedo reticularis. As the source of the atheroemboli ascends in the arterial tree, more vital organs (e.g., the kidneys and the GI tract) may be damaged.

Previous manipulation of the catheter or clamping or surgical manipulation of the arterial tree can also result in plaque disruption. In these cases, the adverse effects are usually apparent immediately after the procedure.

DIAGNOSTIC TESTING

Doppler examination may visualize unstable ulcerated plaques or aneurysmal disease. Doppler segmental pressures may be used to identify the responsible lesion by localizing a significant drop in pressure and determining where the plaque is. Duplex imaging with noncolor flow can also provide clues to the morphology of a plaque. This is only true, however, in the extremity arteries. When the aorta is the suspected source of the emboli, computed tomography, magnetic resonance imaging, or magnetic resonance angiography is performed; these modalities provide better visualization of intraluminal disease. Arteriography also plays a useful role in identifying intraluminal pathology along the entire vascular tree. In addition, intravascular ultrasonography may be performed with the guide wire in place and may help delineate the extent of the underlying disease.

TREATMENT

If the atheroembolic events are minor and solitary, conservative medical management is recommended. If, however, the emboli are recurrent or massive, a thorough evaluation should be initiated, followed by urgent treatment.

Medical management of atheroembolism consists primarily of antiplatelet therapy. Given that most patients with atheroemboli are already receiving aspirin, addition of clopidogrel or ticlopidine

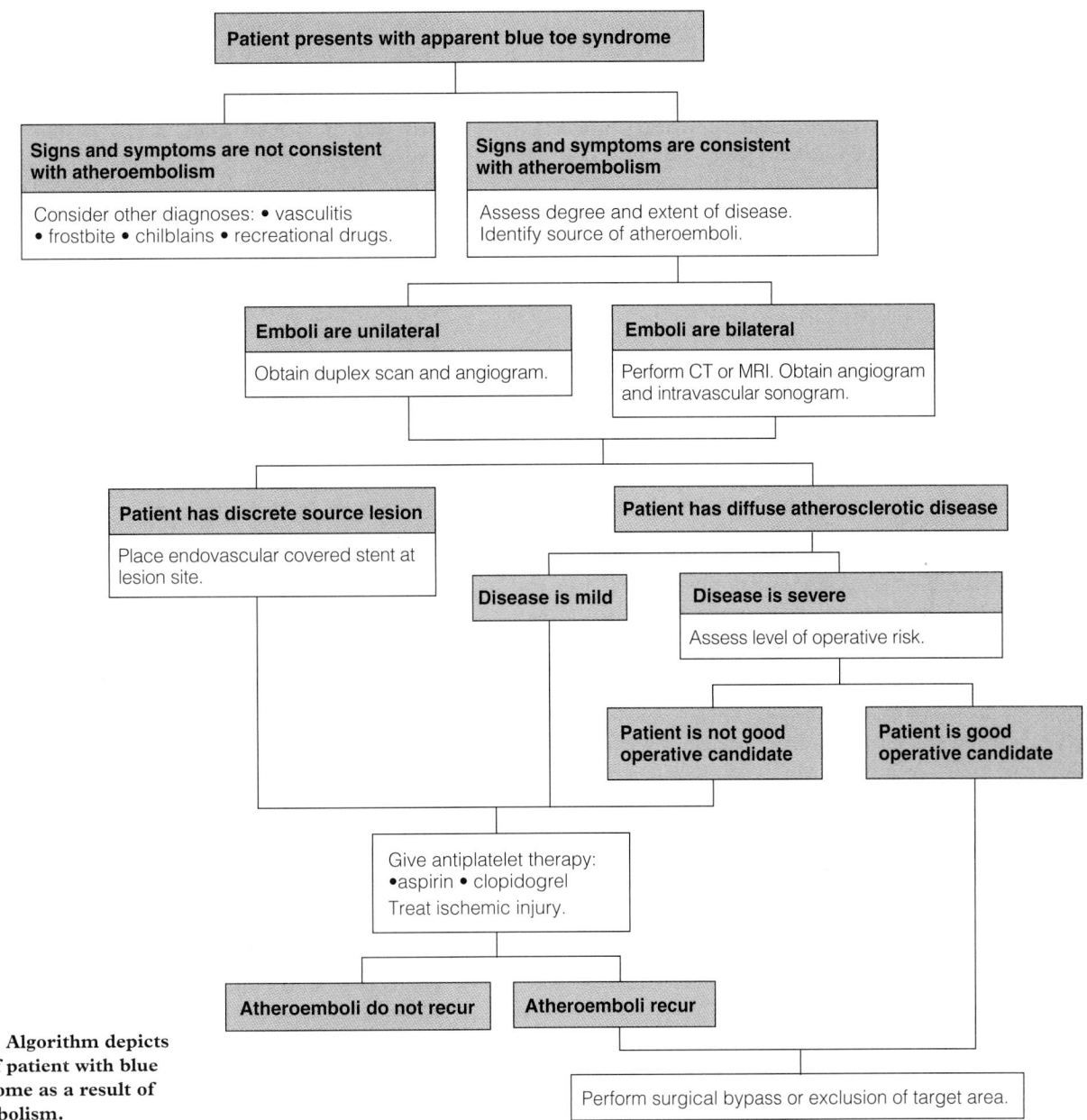

Figure 1 **Algorithm depicts workup of patient with blue toe syndrome as a result of atheroembolism.**

is appropriate. The optimal agents for preventing recurrence of atheroembolism may prove to be lipid-lowering drugs, particularly statins. At present, direct evidence from randomized trials supporting the use of statins to prevent atheroembolism is lacking, but the hypothesis remains under investigation.

The role of warfarin therapy in treating atheroembolic disease has not been established with certainty. Such therapy may even aggravate the disease process by causing intraplaque hemorrhage and increased embolization. The Warfarin Aspirin Recurrent Stroke Study (WARSS), a randomized multicenter study that included 2,206 patients who had recently experienced an ischemic stroke, found no evidence that warfarin is superior to aspirin for preventing recurrent ischemic stroke or death within 2 years.[42] Nor was there a significant difference in bleeding risk between warfarin-treated patients and aspirin-treated patients.

For patients with diffuse atherosclerotic disease, the mainstay of therapy is an antiplatelet regimen. Traditionally, an atheroembolic source has been treated by surgical excision or by exclusion of the disease process with a bypass graft, either of which provides a good

degree of safety from further embolization.[43] With the advent of endovascular surgery, however, the use of covered stents, placed securely and precisely at the site of the offending lesion, appears to be an increasingly effective and popular option [*see Table 5*].[44,45]

Table 5 Surgical Management of Atheroembolism

Source of Emboli	Treatment
Upper extremity	Bypass of subclavian or axillary artery First rib or cervical rib resection
Aorta	Focal disease: covered aortic stent Diffuse disease: aortobifemoral bypass
Iliac artery	Covered iliac stent
Popliteal artery	Ligation and bypass of popliteal artery

Our current approach to treating atheroembolism may be summarized as follows. The source lesion is first identified by means of the modalities already discussed. If embolization is minor, aspirin and clopidrogel are started. If embolization is recurrent or massive, an endovascular approach is attempted, involving the placement of a covered stent over the lesion. This approach is indicated for segments of the arterial tree where there are no collaterals, so that vital blood flow to organs is not hindered. If aneurysmal disease is present, either conventional or endovascular therapeutic approaches may be applied to exclude any source of emboli. In the case of thoracic aortic disease, covered stents may be placed to push the plaque against the wall and prevent further embolization. If suprarenal plaque cannot be treated with a stented graft, aortic ligation with an axillo-bifemoral bypass may be performed [see 4:10 Aortoiliac Reconstruction]. Such treatment does not, however, protect the renal and visceral vessels, and these patients require lifelong strict antiplatelet therapy.

Discussion

Pathophysiology of ALI

The course of ALI usually begins with occlusion of a peripheral artery or bypass graft. It can then develop either slowly, over an extended period, or quickly, over a few hours. A protracted course leading to thrombosis allows collateral vessels to form, and the onset of symptoms is gradual. When occlusion is acute, however, as in embolization or acute thrombosis of a vessel or a bypass graft, signs and symptoms of acute ischemia may become rapidly apparent, including excruciating pain, mottling, cyanosis, and, commonly, sensorimotor changes. Patients typically are seen in an emergency setting within hours after the onset of such symptoms.

With the advent of aggressive surgical management of peripheral vascular disease, more and more patients are being treated with bypass grafts. As a result, graft occlusions now outnumber thromboses of native arteries by a ratio of 1.3 to 1. Thrombotic occlusions outnumber embolic events by a ratio of 6 to 1.

The pathophysiology of limb ischemia is related to the progression of tissue infarction and irreversible cell death. The lower extremity comprises different tissues with different metabolic rates. The extent to which each cell type can tolerate ischemia depends on its metabolic rate. Bone and skin are the most resistant to ischemia, nervous tissue is the least resistant, and muscle is somewhere in between. For muscle and nerve cells, 6 hours is the approximate upper limit of ischemic tolerance; nervous tissue is affected well before this point.[46] Knowledge of the varying degrees of ischemic tolerance helps in determining the viability of the limb.

HYPOPERFUSION-REPERFUSION STATE

Hypoperfusion leads to ischemic infarcts via various mechanisms. During the hypoperfusion state, three major physiologic events occur. First, movement of blood through the vessels is slowed. As a result, the thrombus is able to grow and propagate, occluding collateral vessels and further decreasing blood flow. Second, ischemic cells swell and accumulate water. The resulting increase in pressure within a fixed space between fascial structures creates a compartment syndrome that further decreases flow and exacerbates the injury. Third, the precapillary arteriolar cells swell, narrowing the lumina of distal arterioles, capillaries, and venules and again reducing blood flow.

The reperfusion state that results when flow is restored can be as detrimental to the ischemic extremity as the hypoperfusion state was. During reperfusion, highly active oxygen metabolites are produced by neutrophils.[47] These free radicals destroy cells by attacking the unsaturated bonds of fatty acids within the phospholipid membrane, thereby disrupting the cell membrane, allowing water to enter the cell, and eventually causing cell lysis. Free radical scavengers (e.g., mannitol and superoxide dismutase) have a slight protective effect against reperfusion injury when given before large-scale release of these radicals.[48,49] In addition, myoglobin from injured muscle cells is released into the circulation and is cleared via the renal system. Myoglobin may cause renal failure through its direct toxic effect on the renal tubules and through the accumulation of casts in the tubules.

Creatinine phosphokinase levels may also increase to dramatic levels once perfusion is reestablished. High concentrations of lactic acid, potassium, thromboxane, and cellular enzymes are secreted as a consequence of the rhabdomyolysis; these substances accumulate in the ischemic limb and are released into the systemic circulation upon reperfusion.[50] In one study that measured the venous effluent from a series of patients with limb ischemia, the pH was 7.07 and the mean potassium level 5.7 mEq/L 5 minutes after surgical embolectomy.[51]

Detrimental physiologic changes are seen when toxic oxygen metabolites are released systemically. Depression of myocardial function, an increase in cardiac dysrhythmias, and loss of vascular tone may induce shock and even death.[52]

Etiology of ALI

The etiology of ALI can be divided into two distinct categories: thrombosis and embolism. A thorough evaluation must be performed to elucidate the precise cause of ischemia in each individual patient.

The two categories are each associated with specific symptoms and signs [see Table 6]. Knowledge of these associations helps direct the clinician toward the most appropriate means of accomplishing limb salvage in a given situation.

Thrombosis of a native vessel or bypass graft almost always develops in conjunction with an underlying lesion in the vessel or graft. The lesion usually has been present for some time, and the throm-

Table 6 Differentiation of Embolism from Thrombosis

Variable	Embolism	Thrombosis
Identifiable source	Frequently detected	None
Claudication	Rare	Frequent
Physical findings	Proximal and contralateral pulses normal	Evidence of ipsilateral and contralateral peripheral vascular disease
Angiographic findings	Minimal atherosclerosis; sharp cutoff; few collaterals; multiple occlusions	Diffuse atherosclerotic disease; tapered and irregular cutoff; well-developed collateral circulation

bosis occurs as a result of it. In contrast, embolic events occur in nondiseased vessels that become resting places for emboli.

THROMBOSIS

Native Artery Thrombosis

Native artery thrombosis is usually the end stage of a long-standing disease process of atheromatous plaque formation at specific sites in the arterial tree. Atherosclerotic plaque begins with the slow deposition of lipids in the intima of the vessel and continues with the deposition of calcium, resulting in an atherosclerotic core.[53] This core is a highly thrombogenic surface that encourages platelet aggregation, which results in disturbances of blood flow.[54] The flow disturbances create a zone of separation, stagnation, turbulence, and distorted velocity vectors. These factors cause low shear rates at inflection points in the arterial tree, and endothelial damage ensues. The endothelial damage activates a repair process that results in intimal hyperplasia, which causes further attraction of platelets and eventual thrombus formation. The process by which occlusion develops from an atheromatous plaque may be more important than the degree of stenosis within the lumen. This would explain why acute occlusion occurs in vessels with minimal (< 50%) stenosis: the contact between the atherosclerotic core and the bloodstream leads to platelet aggregation and hence to eventual thrombosis.

Occasionally, thrombosis of a native artery occurs without any obvious underlying pathologic condition. In such cases, a thorough investigation should be initiated into other causes of thrombosis (e.g., hypovolemia, malignancy, hypercoagulable states, and blood dyscrasias).

Bypass Graft Thrombosis

Aggressive management of patients with peripheral vascular disease has led to an increase in bypass graft procedures. As a result, graft thrombosis has become the leading cause of acute lower-extremity ischemia. In patients with native conduits, intimal hyperplasia and valvular hyperplasia are the two leading causes of graft failure.[55] The situation is different in the prosthetic graft population, where the inherent thrombogenicity of the graft material and kinking of the graft from crossing joints are the leading causes. These patients often have graft occlusions without any definable underlying lesion.

EMBOLISM

Peripheral arterial embolization results in the sudden onset of extreme ischemia as the absence of collateral vessels compounds the reduction in flow to the extremity. The heart is by far the predominant source of spontaneous arterial emboli. As the population ages, the number of patients with significant cardiac disease increases and the incidence of embolic phenomena increases. Over the past 20 years or so, the incidence of embolization has doubled, from 23 to 51 per 100,000 admissions. Atherosclerotic heart disease currently accounts for as many as 60% to 70% of all cases of arterial embolism,[56,57] and atrial fibrillation and rheumatic valvular disease account for the remaining 30% to 40%.[56,58]

With respect to peripheral emboli in particular, atrial fibrillation is currently associated with two thirds to three quarters of cases. Transthoracic echocardiography is notoriously insensitive in visualizing atrial clots, especially in the left atrial appendage, which is the most common cardiac source of emboli.[59,60] Transesophageal echocardiography, however, offers significantly better imaging of all four chambers and hence is considered the superior diagnostic test for suspected cardiac embolic sources.[61-64]

MI is the next most important cause of peripheral emboli. A 1986 study of 400 patients found that MI was a causative factor in 20%.[58]

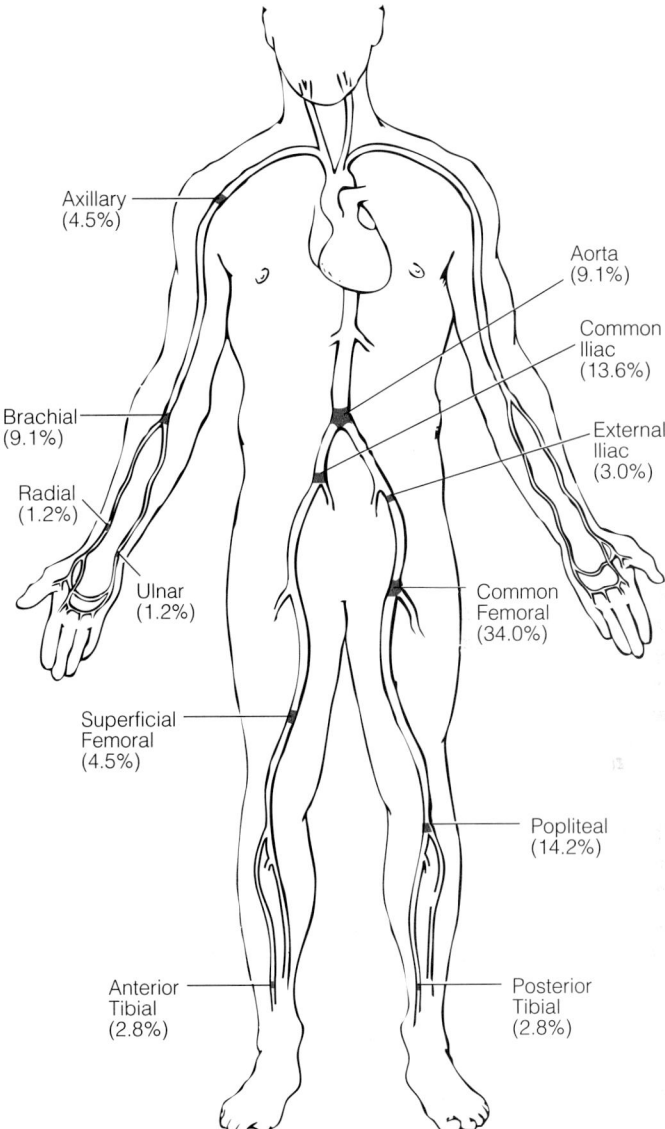

Figure 2 **Depicted are the most common sites of arterial embolic occlusions.**

After an MI, a left ventricular wall thrombus is often seen, with[65] or without[66-68] a left ventricular wall aneurysm; however, only 5% of such thrombi embolize and cause a problem.[66-68] Other studies suggest that the period in which the risk of embolization is highest for an intracardiac thrombus is that between day 3 and day 28.[69]

The ring portions of prosthetic cardiac valves are major intracardiac embolic sources before anticoagulation,[70] as are biologic xenovalves, which do not require anticoagulation.[71] Finally, tumors (e.g., atrial myxomas) are occasional sources of peripheral emboli.[69] Cardiac vegetations from bacterial or fungal endocarditis should be considered as possible sources of peripheral emboli when I.V. drug abuse is suspected in a patient with no previous history of cardiac disease.[72,73]

Noncardiac sources account for 5% to 10% of peripheral emboli. The majority of these involve downstream atherosclerotic arterial disease (e.g., aneurysms or unstable plaques).[74-77] Foreign objects (e.g., missiles[78,79]) and tumors (e.g., melanoma[80,81]) can also embolize if they gain access to the arterial tree. So-called paradoxical embolization occurs when a venous thrombus crosses from right to left via an atrial or ventricular route, gains access to the arterial side, and becomes an arterial embolus.[82-84] About 5% to 10% of emboli remain unidentified despite a thorough diagnostic evaluation[85,86]; some of these are now being attributed to hypercoagulable states.[87]

Incidence

As a consequence of the ongoing growth in the number of endovascular interventions being performed, overall incidence patterns for embolism are shifting yet again, with a greater number of emboli now arising from intravascular handling. A 1996 study found that 45% of all atheroemboli were iatrogenic and that the majority of these originated during manipulation of the abdominal aorta, the iliac artery, or the femoropopliteal artery, with the remainder originating during surgery.[88] Emboli usually lodge at arterial bifurcations and consequently impair blood flow to more than one vessel. Axial limb vessels account for 60% to 80% of clinically significant embolic events,[58,69,89] with the remainder divided between cerebral vessels (20%) and upper-extremity vessels (10% to 20%). The most common site for embolic lodgment is the common femoral bifurcation [see Figure 2]. The aortoiliac region is the next most common site, followed closely by the popliteal artery.[52,57,58,69,90,91]

The presence of normal pulses in the contralateral leg in a patient with an ischemic leg should elicit an aggressive workup to rule out cardiac sources for the emboli and may be a clue that the occlusive event is more likely to be embolic than thrombotic.

Upper-Extremity Emboli

Acute ischemia of the upper extremity is usually caused by embolism, usually deriving from an intracardiac source. Subclavian aneurysms, arteriovenous fistulae, upper-extremity arterial bypasses, and iatrogenic manipulation of the arteries are rare causes.[92] As noted (see above), emboli lodge at inflection points of the arterial tree. In the upper extremity, the bifurcation of the brachial artery into the radial and ulnar arteries is the most common lodgment site, followed by the takeoff of the deep brachial artery. Adequate exposure of all three arteries can be obtained via an elongated S-shaped incision that runs medially to laterally across the elbow joint.

Other Causes

Sepsis and cardiogenic shock bring about a low-flow state that places patients at high risk for thrombosis. Certain vasoconstrictors and recreational drugs are also associated with lower-extremity thrombosis.[93,94] Patients with these conditions usually present with bilateral extremity ischemia. Vasculitides (e.g., Takayasu) may also cause extremity ischemia.[95]

The hypercoagulable states (e.g., antithrombin deficiency, antiphospholipid syndrome, protein C and S deficiencies, factor V Leiden mutation, and hyperprothrombinemia) are the most common disorders associated with acute arterial thrombosis.[96] The consequences are usually devastating.

References

1. Davies B, Braithwaite BD, Birch PA, et al: Acute leg ischaemia in Gloucestershire. Br J Surg 84:504, 1997

2. Blaisdell FW, Steele M, Allen RE: Management of acute lower extremity arterial ischemia due to embolism and thrombosis. Surgery 84:822, 1978

3. Dormandy J, Heeck L, Vig S: Acute limb ischemia. Semin Vasc Surg 12:148, 1999

4. Rutherford RB, Baker JD, Ernst C, et al: Recommended standards for reports dealing with lower extremity ischemia: revised version. J Vasc Surg 26:517, 1997

5. Katzenschlager R, Ahmadi A, Atteneder M, et al: Colour duplex sonography-guided local lysis of occlusions in the femoro-popliteal region. Int Angiol 19:250, 2000

6. Mazzariol F, Ascher E, Hingorani A, et al: Lower-extremity revascularisation without preoperative contrast arteriography in 185 cases: lessons learned with duplex ultrasound arterial mapping. Eur J Vasc Endovasc Surg 19:509, 2000

7. Ascher E, Mazzariol F, Hingorani A, et al: The use of duplex ultrasound arterial mapping as an alternative to conventional arteriography for primary and secondary infrapopliteal bypasses. Am J Surg 178:162, 1999

8. Kim D, Porter DH, Brown R, et al: Renal artery imaging: a prospective comparison of intra-arterial digital subtraction angiography with conventional angiography. Angiology 42:345, 1991

9. Lindholt JS: Radiocontrast induced nephropathy. Eur J Vasc Endovasc Surg 4:296, 2003

10. Kerns SR, Hawkins IFJ, Sabatelli FW: Current status of carbon dioxide angiography. Radiol Clin North Am 33:15, 1995

11. Waver FA, Pentecoast MJ, Yellin AE, et al: Clinical applications of carbon dioxide/digital subtraction arteriography. J Vasc Surg 13:266, 1991

12. Bjork I, Lindahl U: Mechanism of the anticoagulant action of heparin. Mol Cell Biochem 48:161, 1982

13. Hirsh J, Dalen Je, Deykin D, et al: Heparin, mechanism of action, pharmacokinetics, dosing consideration, monitoring, efficacy and safety. Chest 102:337S, 1992

14. Salzman EW, Deykin D, Shapiro RM, et al: Management of heparin therapy: controlled prospective trial. N Engl J Med 292:1046, 1976

15. Walenga JM, Frenkel EP, Bick RL: Heparin-induced thrombocytopenia, paradoxical thromboembolism, and other adverse effects of heparin-type therapy. Hematol Oncol Clin North Am 7:259, 2003

16. Warkentin TE, Bernstein RA: Delayed-onset heparin-induced thrombocytopenia and cerebral thrombosis after a single administration of unfractionated heparin. N Engl J Med 348:1067, 2003

17. Kelton JG: Heparin-induced thrombocytopenia: an overview. Blood Rev 16:77, 2002

18. Rice L, Attisha WK, Drexler A, et al: Delayed-onset heparin-induced thrombocytopenia. Ann Intern Med 136:210, 2002

19. Visentin GP: Heparin-induced thrombocytopenia: molecular pathogenesis. Thromb Haemost 82:448,1999

20. Dotter C: Selective clot lysis with low-dose streptokinase. Radiology 111:31, 1974

21. Ouriel K, Shortell C, DeWeese JA, et al: A comparison of thrombolytic therapy with operative revascularization in the initial treatment of acute peripheral arterial ischemia. J Vasc Surg 19:1021, 1994

22. Weaver FA, Camerota AJ, Youngblood M, et al: Surgical revascularization versus thrombolysis for non-embolic lower extremity native artery occlusions: results of a prospective randomized trial. The STILE investigators: Surgery versus Thrombolysis for Ischemia of the Lower Extremity. J Vasc Surg 24:513, 1996

23. Ouriel K, Veith FJ, Sasahara AA: Thrombolysis or peripheral arterial surgery: phase I results. TOPAS investigators. J Vasc Surg 23:64, 1996

24. A comparison of recombinant urokinase with vascular surgery as initial treatment for acute arterial occlusion of the legs. Thrombolysis or Peripheral Arterial Surgery (TOPAS) investigators. N Engl J Med 338:1105, 1998

25. Mahler F, Schneider E, Hess H: Recombinant tissue plasminogen activator versus urokinase for local thrombolysis of femoropopliteal occlusions: a prospective, randomized multicenter trial. J Endovasc Ther 8:638, 2001

26. Morgan R, Belli AM: Percutaneous thrombectomy: a review. Eur Radiol 12:205, 2002

27. Zehnder T, Birrer M, Do DD, et al: Percutaneous catheter thrombus aspiration for acute or subacute arterial occlusion of the legs: how much thrombolysis is needed? Eur J Vasc Endovasc Surg 20:41, 2000

28. Crain MR: Percutaneous mechanical thrombolysis and thrombectomy. Tech Vasc Interv Radiol 1:235, 1998

29. Demin VV, Zeienin VV, Zheludkov AN, et al: Initial experience of transcutaneous rheolytic thrombectomy for peripheral major arterial lesions. Angiol Vasc Surg 5:1, 1999

30. Dick A, Neuerburg J, Schmitz-Rode T, et al: Declotting of embolized temporary vena cava filter by ultrasound and the AngioJet: comparative experimental in vitro studies. Invest Radiol 33:91, 1998

31. Douek PC, Gandjbakhche A, Leon MB, et al: Functional properties of a 'prototype rheolytic thrombectomy catheter' for percutaneous thrombectomy—in vitro investigations. Invest Radiol 29:547, 1994

32. Ouriel K, Kolassa M, DeWeese JA, et al: Economic implications of thrombolysis or operation as the initial treatment modality in acute peripheral arterial occlusion. Surgery 118:810, 1995

33. Korn P, Khilnani NM, Fellers JC, et al: Thrombolysis for native arterial occlusions of the lower extremities: clinical outcome and cost. J Vasc Surg 33:1148, 2001

34. Carvajal JA, Anderson WR, Weiss L, et al: Atheroembolism: an etiologic factor in renal insufficiency, gastrointestinal hemorrhages, and peripheral vascular diseases. Arch Intern Med 119:593, 1967

35. Karmody AM, Jordan FR, Zaman SM: Left colon gangrene after acute mesenteric artery occlusion. Arch Surg 111:972, 1976

36. Gore L, Collins DP: Spontaneous atheromatous embolization: review of the literature and a report of 16 additional cases. Am J Clin Pathol 33:416, 1960

37. Ramirez G, O'Neill WM, Lambert R, et al: Cholesterol embolization: a complication of angiography. Arch Intern Med 118:534, 1966

38. Williams GM, Harrington D, Burdick J, et al: Mural thrombus of the aorta: an important, frequently neglected cause of large peripheral emboli. Ann Surg 194:737, 1981

39. Khatibzadeh M, Mitusch R, Stierle U, et al: Aortic atherosclerotic plaques as a source of systemic embolization. J Am Coll Cardiol 27:664, 1996

40. Falanga V, Fine MJ, Kapoor WN: The cutaneous manifestations of cholesterol crystal embolization. Arch Dermatol 122:1194, 1986

41. Karmody AM, Powers SR, Monaco VJ, et al: "Blue toe syndrome": an indication for limb salvage surgery. Arch Surg 111:1263, 1976

42. Mohr JP, Thompson JL, Lazar RM, et al: A comparison of warfarin and aspirin for the prevention of recurrent ischemic stroke. N Engl J Med 345:1444, 2001

43. Keen RR, McCarthy WJ, Shireman PK, et al: Surgical management of atheroembolism. J Vasc Surg 21:773, 1995

44. Dougherty MJ, Calligaro KD: Endovascular treatment of embolization of aortic plaque with covered stents. J Vasc Surg 36:727, 2002

45. Kumins NH, Owens EL, Oglevie SB, et al: Early experience using the Wallgraft in the management of distal microembolism from common iliac artery pathology. Ann Vasc Surg 16:181, 2002

46. Blebea J, Kerr JC, Franco CD, et al: Technetium 99m pyrophosphate quantitation of skeletal muscle ischemia and reperfusion injury. J Vasc Surg 8:117, 1998

47. Quinones-Baldrich WJ, Chervu A, Hernandez JJ, et al: Skeletal muscle function after ischemia: "no reflow" versus reperfusion injury. J Surg Res 51:5, 1991

48. Ricci MA, Graham Am, Corbisiero R, et al: Are free radical scavengers beneficial in the treatment of compartment syndrome after acute arterial ischemia? J Vasc Surg 9:244, 1989

49. Ouriel K, Smedira NG, Ricotta JJ: Protection of the kidney after temporary ischemia: free radical scavengers. J Vasc Surg 2:49, 1985

50. Mathieson MA, Dunham BM, Huval WV, et al: Ischemia of the limb stimulates thromboxane production and myocardial depression. Surg Gynecol Obstet 157:500, 1983

51. Fischer R, Fogarty T, Morrow A: A clinical and biochemical observation of the effect of transient femoral artery occlusion in man. Surgery 68:233, 1970

52. Green RM, DeWeese J, Rob CG: Arterial embolectomy before and after the Fogarty catheter. Surgery 77:24, 1975

53. Stary HC, Chandler AB, Dinsmore RE, et al: A definition of advanced types of atherosclerotic lesions and a histological classification of atherosclerosis: a report from the committee on vascular lesions of the council on arteriosclerosis, American Heart Association. Circulation 92:1355, 1995

54. Fernandez-Ortiz A, Badimon JJ, Falk E, et al: Characterization of the relative thrombogenicity of atherosclerotic plaque components: implications for consequences of plaque rupture. J Am Coll Cardiol 23:1562, 1994

55. Ouriel K, Shortell CK, Green RM, et al: Differential mechanisms of failure of autogenous and non-autogenous bypass conduits: an assessment following successful graft thrombolysis. Cardiovasc Surg 3:469, 1995

56. Abbott W, Maloney R, McCabe C et al: Arterial embolism a 44 year perspective. Am J Surg 143:460, 1982

57. Fogarty T, Daily P, Shumway N, et al: Experience with balloon catheter technique for arterial embolectomy. Am J Surg 122:231, 1971

58. Paneta T, Thomson J, Talkington C, et al: Arterial embolectomy: a 34 year experience with 400 cases. Surg Clin North Am 66:339, 1986

59. Shresta N, Moreno F, Narcisco F, et al: Two dimensional echocardiographic diagnosis of left atrial thrombus in rheumatic heart disease: a clinicopathologic study. Circulation 67:341, 1983

60. Schweizer P, Bardos F, Erbel R: Detection of left atrial thrombi by echocardiography. Br Heart J 45:148, 1981

61. Daniel W, Mugge A: Transesophageal echocardiography. N Engl J Med 332:1268, 1995

62. Husain A, Alter M: Transesophageal echocardiography in diagnosing cardioembolic stroke. Clin Cardiol 18:705, 1995

63. Seward J, Khandheria B, Oh J, et al: Transesophageal echocardiography: technique, anatomic correlations, implementation, and clinical applications. Mayo Clin Proc 63:649, 1988

64. Rubin B, Barzilai B, Allen B, et al: Detection of the source of arterial emboli by transesophageal echocardiography: a case report. J Vasc Surg 15:573, 1992

65. Loop F, Effler D, Navia J, et al: Aneurysms of the left ventricle: survival and results of a ten-year surgical experience. Ann Surg 178:399, 1973

66. Hellerstein H, Martin J: Incidence of thromboembolic lesions accompanying myocardial infarction. Am Heart J 33:443, 1947

67. Keely E, Hillis L: Left ventricular mural thrombus after acute myocardial infarction. Clin Cardiol 19:83, 1996

68. Asinger R, Mikell F, Elsperger J: Incidence of left ventricular thrombosis after acute transmural myocardial infarction. N Engl J Med 305:297, 1981

69. Darling R, Austen W, Linton R: Arterial embolism. Surg Gynecol Obstet 124:106, 1967

70. Perier P, Bessou J, Swanson J, et al: Comparative evaluation of aortic valve replacement with Starr, Bjork, and porcine valve prostheses. Circulation 72:140, 1985

71. Pipkin R, Buch W, Fogart T: Evaluation of aortic valve replacement with porcine xenograft without long-term anticoagulation. J Thorac Cardiovasc Surg 71:179, 1976

72. Kitts D, Bongard F, Klein S: Septic embolism complicating infective endocarditis. J Vasc Surg 14:1480, 1991

73. Freischlag J, Asburn H, Sedwitz M, et al: Septic peripheral embolization from bacterial and fungal endocarditis. Ann Vasc Surg 3:318, 1989

74. Lord J Jr, Rossi G, Daliana M, et al: Unsuspected abdominal aortic aneurysm as the cause of peripheral arterial occlusive disease. Ann Surg 177:767, 1973

75. Kempczynski R: Lower extremity emboli from ulcerating atherosclerotic plaque. JAMA 241:807, 1979

76. Kwaan J, Vander Molen R, Stemmer E, et al: Peripheral embolism resulting from unsuspected atheromatous plaques. Surgery 78:583, 1975

77. Machleder H, Takiff H, Lois J, et al: Aortic mural thrombus: an occult source of arterial thromboembolism. J Vasc Surg 4:473, 1986

78. Shannon J, Nghia M, Stanton P Jr, et al: Peripheral arterial missile embolization: a case report and a 22 year review of the literature. J Vasc Surg 5:773, 1987

79. Symbas P, Harlaftis N: Bullet emboli in the pulmonary and systemic arteries. Ann Surg 185:318, 1977

80. Harriss R, Andros G, Dulawa L, et al: Malignant melanoma embolus as a cause of acute aortic occlusion: report of a case. J Vasc Surg 3:550, 1986

81. Prioleau P, Katzenstein A: Major peripheral artery occlusion due to malignant tumor embolism: histologic recognition and surgical management. Cancer 42:2009, 1978

82. Ward R, Jones D, Haponik E: Paradoxical embolism: an underrecognized problem. Chest 108:549, 1995

83. Katz S, Andros G, Kohl R, et al: Arterial emboli of venous orign. Surg Gynecol Obstet 174:17, 1992

84. Gazzaniga A, Dalen J: Paradoxical embolism: its pathophysiology and clinical recognition. Ann Surg 171:137, 1970

85. Hight D, Tilney N, Couch N: Changing clinical trends in patients with peripheral emboli. Surgery 79:172, 1976

86. Thompson J, Sigler L, Raut P, et al: Arterial embolectomy: a 20 year experience. Surgery 67:212, 1970

87. Eason J, Mills J, Beckett W: Hypercoagulable states in arterial thromboembolism. Surg Gynecol Obstet 174:211, 1992

88. Sharma P, Babu P, Shah P, et al: Changing patterns of atheroembolism. Cardiovasc Surg 4:573, 1996

89. Elliott J, Hageman J, Szilagyi D: Arterial embolization: problems of source, multiplicity, recurrence, and delayed treatment. Surgery 88:833, 1980

90. Elliott JP Jr, Hageman J, Szilagyi D, et al: Arterial embolization: problems of source, multiplicity, recurrence and delayed treatment. Surgery 88:883, 1980

91. Dale W: Differential management of acute peripheral ischemia. J Vasc Surg 1:269, 1984

92. Banis JC Jr, Rich N, Whelan TJ Jr: Ischemia of the upper extremity due to noncardiac emboli. Am J Surg 134:131, 1977

93. Balbir-Gurman A, Braun-Moscovici Y, Nahir AM: Cocaine-induced Raynaud's phenomenon and ischaemic finger necrosis. Clin Rheumatol 20:376, 2001

94. Disdier P, Granel B, Serratrice J, et al: Cannabis arteritis revisited—ten new case reports. Angiology 52:1, 2001

95. Ishikawa K: Patterns of symptoms and prognosis in occlusive thromboarthropathy (Takayasu's disease). J Am Coll Cardiol 8:1401, 1986

96. Mira Y, Todoli T, Alonso R, et al: Factor V Leiden and prothrombin G20210A in relation to arterial and/or vein rethrombosis: two cases. Clin Appl Thromb Hemost 7:234, 2001

97. Ouriel K: Acute ischemia and its sequelae. Vascular Surgery, 5th ed. Rutherford RB, Ed. WB Saunders Co, Philadelphia, 2000

98. Thrombolysis in the management of lower limb peripheral arterial occlusion—a consensus document. Working Party on Thrombosis in the Management of Limb Ischemia. Am J Cardiol 81:207, 1998

5 DIABETIC FOOT

Cameron M. Akbari, M.D., F.A.C.S., and Frank W. LoGerfo, M.D., F.A.C.S.

Evaluation and Management of the Diabetic Foot

Surgeons caring for diabetic patients are faced with a diverse spectrum of foot disease.[1,2] The clinical presentation may range from the asymptomatic patient who requires nothing more than preventive foot care to the unstable and critically ill patient in whom both loss of limb and death are imminent threats. This wide range of disease severity, coupled with inappropriate and untimely use of diagnostic testing, contributes to the clinical confusion that often leads to delays in diagnosis and treatment and, ultimately, to limb loss. It is important, therefore, that surgeons caring for diabetic patients develop a simple but comprehensive and orderly approach to diabetic foot problems that (1) can be implemented for any such problem, (2) recognizes the pathogenic roles of neuropathy, ischemia, and infection, and (3) emphasizes the initial clinical assessment at the bedside.[3]

Clinical Evaluation

Evaluation of any diabetic foot problem begins with a complete history and a careful physical examination. Broadly speaking, such evaluation should address the healing potential of the foot, the details of the foot problem (e.g., ulcer, gangrene, infection, or osteomyelitis), the systemic consequences of diabetes, and any immediate threats to life or limb. With this information in hand, the surgeon can usually make an accurate diagnosis and start a comprehensive treatment plan without having to order further diagnostic tests, which are liable to be both costly and time-consuming.

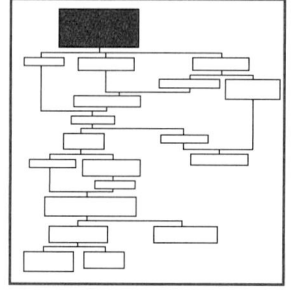

HISTORY

The history of the foot problem can yield valuable insights into the potential for healing, the presence of coexisting infection or arterial occlusive disease, and the need for further treatment. Whenever a patient presents with a foot ulceration or gangrene, possible underlying arterial insufficiency should immediately be suspected, even if neuropathy or infection is present. It is helpful to be aware of the event that incited the foot problem. In a patient with diabetes and arterial insufficiency, the inciting event for a foot ulcer may be a seemingly benign action, such as cutting a toenail, soaking the foot in a warm bath, or applying a heating pad. Unfortunately, because of the broad microneurovascular and macrovascular abnormalities associated with diabetes, these relatively innocuous actions can progress to a nonhealing ulcer and gangrene. Similarly, failure to heal after any podiatric procedure is strongly suggestive of underlying unrecognized arterial insufficiency.

The duration of the ulcer also provides important clues, in that

a long-standing, nonhealing ulcer is strongly suggestive of ischemia. Certainly, an ulcer or gangrenous area that has been present for several months is unlikely to heal without some further treatment, whether it be offloading of weight-bearing areas, treatment of infection, or, most commonly, correction of arterial insufficiency. In some cases, the present ulcer has already healed at least once, and the current episode represents a relapse. A history of intermittent healing followed by relapse raises the possibility of underlying untreated infection (e.g., recurrent osteomyelitis) or an uncorrected architectural abnormality (e.g., a bony pressure point or a varus deformity).

In view of the many vague and unsupported therapies advocated for the diabetic foot, it is helpful to know the type and duration of any treatments the patient has already undergone for the current problem. For example, a patient with an ischemic ulceration may have completed several different courses of antibiotics without success. Thus, if antibiotic therapy is contemplated for a current infection, possible antibiotic resistance must be taken into account in choosing the appropriate agent. It is also helpful to know which treatments were not previously offered to the patient and to look critically at why they were not offered. For example, many diabetic patients with correctable foot ulceration and limb ischemia are told that their only option is limb amputation, usually because of the physician's inherited pessimism or his or her inadequate knowledge of the advances made in limb and foot salvage. No patient should be denied an opportunity for limb salvage on the basis of a previous medical or surgical opinion without a new comprehensive evaluation being performed.

Inquiries should be made about any previous foot and limb problems—for instance, whether the patient had other ulcers on the same foot that healed spontaneously, how long such healing took, and whether foot surgery was ever performed on that side. A history of recent ipsilateral ulceration or foot surgery that healed in a timely and uncomplicated manner suggests, but does not prove, that the arterial supply is adequate. Problems and procedures more remote in time, however, are less useful indicators. A history of previous leg revascularization (including percutaneous therapies) is also an important clue to possible underlying arterial insufficiency. Because of the predilection for mirror image–type atherosclerotic occlusive disease, the contralateral leg must be considered as well: previous revascularization in the opposite leg is often associated with arterial insufficiency on the affected side. Other cardiovascular risk factors, such as cigarette smoking and hyperlipidemia, must also be taken into account: their presence increases the likelihood that ischemia is contributing to the current foot problem.

Although claudication and rest pain have traditionally been associated with vascular disease, they may be obscured by diabetic neuropathy; hence, their absence in the diabetic patient certainly does not rule out ischemia. Because even moderate

a *b*

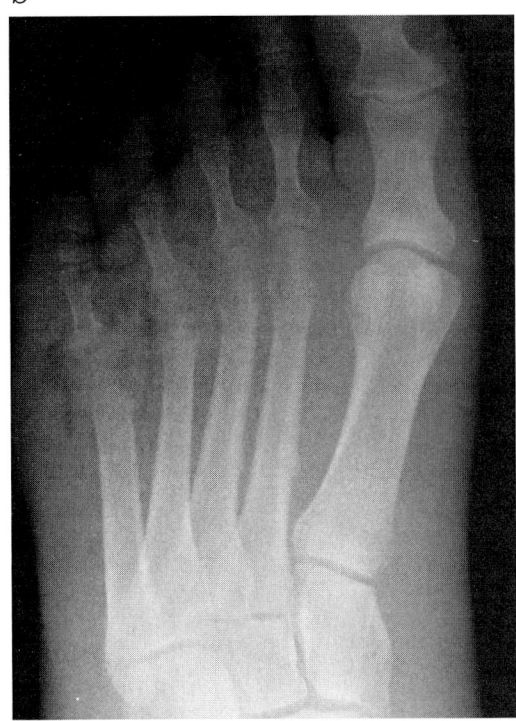

Figure 1 Shown is a benign-appearing gangrenous eschar (*a*) on the foot of a diabetic patient. Plain x-ray (*b*) reveals extensive subcutaneous air in soft tissue, consistent with severe necrotizing fasciitis.

ischemia precludes healing in the diabetic foot, the absence of rest pain is not a reliable indicator of an adequate arterial blood supply; moreover, many patients may not be walking long enough distances for vasculogenic claudication to develop. Conversely, some patients with true ischemic rest pain are dismissed for years as having "painful neuropathy."

Both the systemic effects of the foot problem and the systemic consequences of diabetes itself should be assessed. Because unrecognized infection in the diabetic patient may rapidly progress to a life-threatening condition, attention should be directed toward detecting the subtle manifestations of an infected foot ulcer.

The patient should be asked about worsening hyperglycemia, recent erratic blood glucose control, and higher insulin requirements. As a consequence of the microvascular and neuropathic abnormalities in the diabetic foot, classic symptoms of infection (e.g., chills and pain) are often absent, and hyperglycemia is often the sole presenting symptom of undrained infection. Faced with ongoing infection and hyperglycemia, the surgeon should strongly suspect impending ketoacidosis or nonketotic hyperglycemic hyperosmolar coma, with the attendant symptoms of weakness, confusion, and altered mental status.

Because a patient with a diabetic foot problem often needs some type of operative intervention, the history should also include a comprehensive assessment of overall health status to help stratify perioperative risk. For example, knowledge of previous cardiac events (e.g., myocardial infarction or revascularization) and current cardiac status (e.g., New York Heart Association [NYHA] class or anginal severity) can help determine whether perioperative cardiac monitoring or preoperative cardiac testing is indicated and what form such monitoring or testing should take. Similarly, in a patient with suspected infection and ischemia, a history of worsening renal function or

impending need for hemodialysis can help determine the choice and dosage of antibiotics and may alter plans for standard contrast arteriography. The essential point is that diabetes may affect virtually every organ system, often in an indolent pattern; thus, in the evaluation of any diabetic patient with foot disease, attention must be paid to all of these systems.

Functional status also becomes an important consideration at this point, and the history should carefully determine the patient's ambulatory and rehabilitative potential. Many different methods of quantifying functional status have been suggested. One simple approach is to classify functional status as a point on a continuum. One end of the continuum might be a fully ambulatory patient; almost all surgeons would recognize that such a patient should be offered every attempt at limb salvage. The other end might be a completely bedridden patient with multiple comorbid conditions; most surgeons would adopt a far less aggressive approach to such a patient. In practice, many patients fall somewhere between these two extremes, in which case a more thorough evaluation of functional and social status becomes imperative before any firm decisions can be made regarding limb salvage.

PHYSICAL EXAMINATION

Fever and tachycardia are strongly suggestive of deep or undrained infection, with hypotension being a late manifestation of ongoing sepsis. It is important to remember, however, that these signs may be absent in diabetic patients with impending or progressive infection. A focused cardiopulmonary examination helps confirm the presence or absence of congestive heart failure, valvular abnormalities, or rhythm disturbances, which must be recognized in diabetic patients with poor underlying medical reserve.

Evaluation of the diabetic foot ulcer should include a strong

Evaluation and Management of the Diabetic Foot

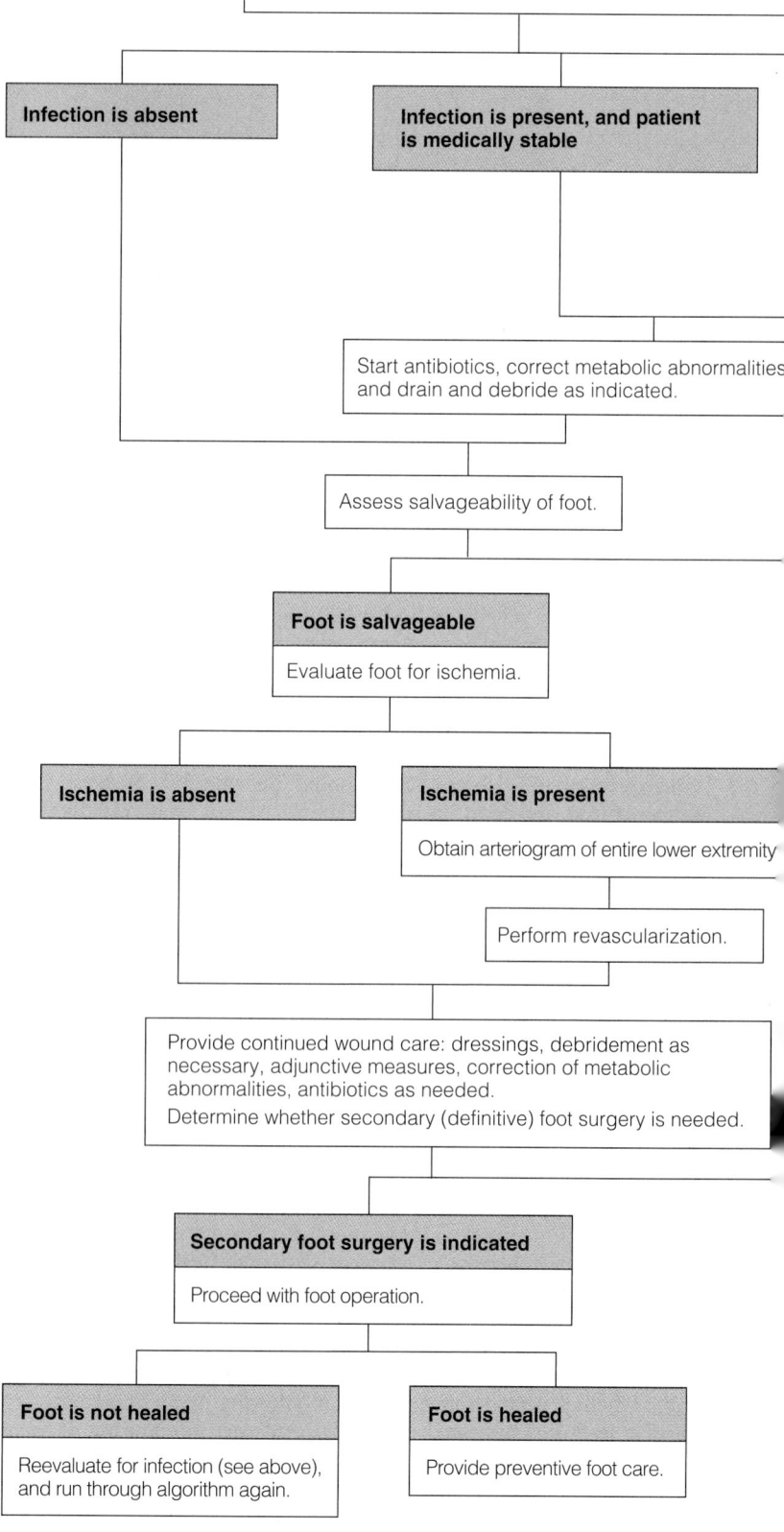

Diabetic patient has foot problem

Obtain history: inciting event, duration, healing, previous treatment (including surgery), vascular disease and risk factors, overall health, functional status.

Perform physical examination: signs of infection, diabetic neuropathy, pulses, arterial perfusion.

Assess clinical findings to determine direction of subsequent workup and treatment.

Infection is absent

Infection is present, and patient is medically stable

Start antibiotics, correct metabolic abnormalities and drain and debride as indicated.

Assess salvageability of foot.

Foot is salvageable

Evaluate foot for ischemia.

Ischemia is absent

Ischemia is present

Obtain arteriogram of entire lower extremity

Perform revascularization.

Provide continued wound care: dressings, debridement as necessary, adjunctive measures, correction of metabolic abnormalities, antibiotics as needed.

Determine whether secondary (definitive) foot surgery is needed.

Secondary foot surgery is indicated

Proceed with foot operation.

Foot is not healed

Reevaluate for infection (see above), and run through algorithm again.

Foot is healed

Provide preventive foot care.

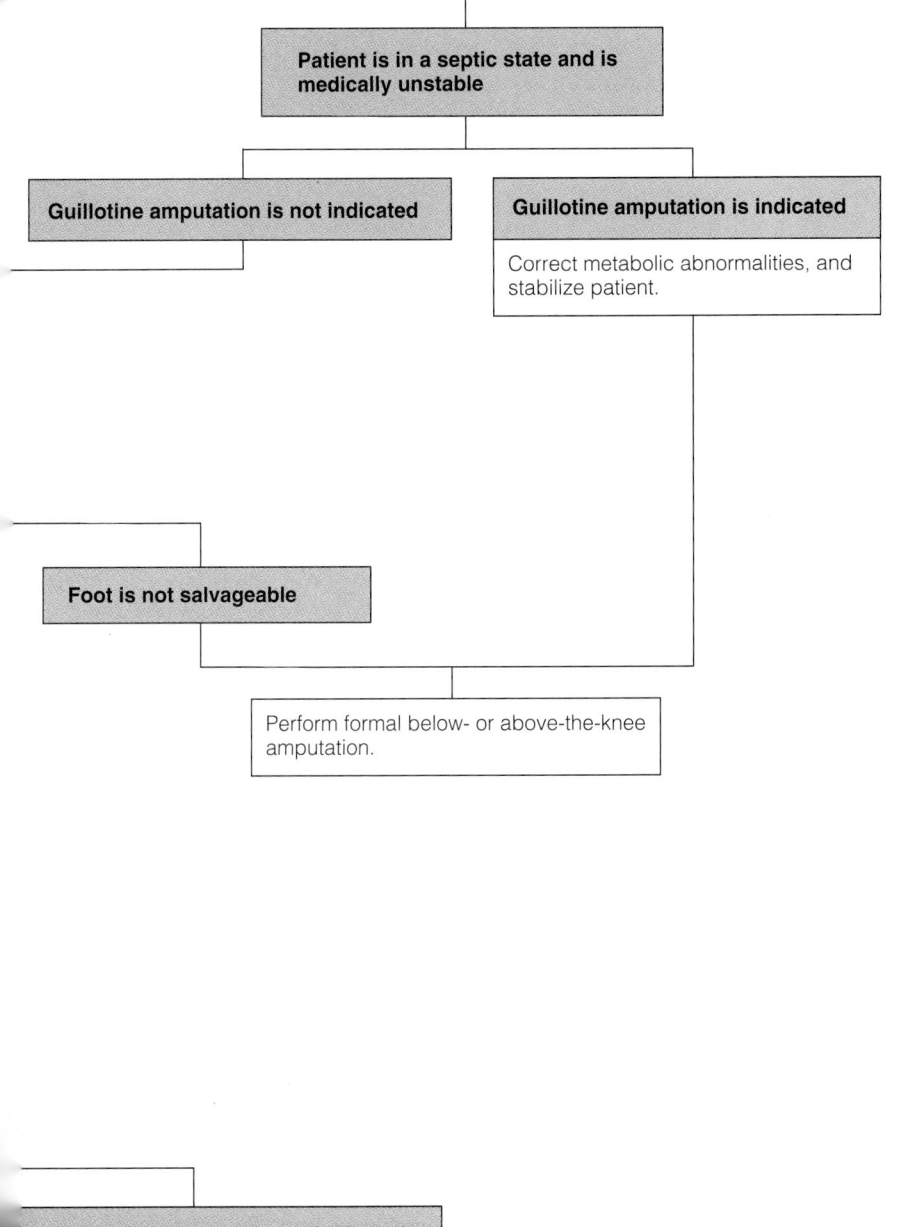

Patient is in a septic state and is medically unstable

Guillotine amputation is not indicated

Guillotine amputation is indicated

Correct metabolic abnormalities, and stabilize patient.

Foot is not salvageable

Perform formal below- or above-the-knee amputation.

Secondary foot surgery is not indicated

Continue wound care.

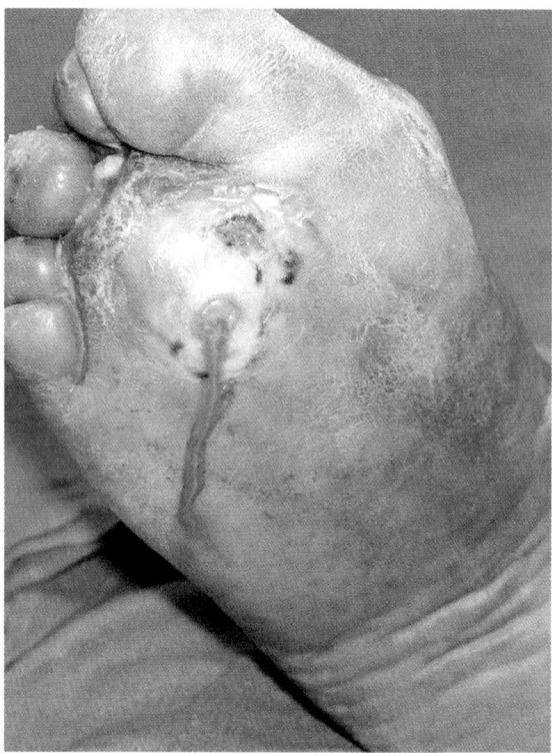

Figure 2 Purulent drainage is seen from a sub-metatarsal ulcer on the plantar surface of the foot of a diabetic patient.

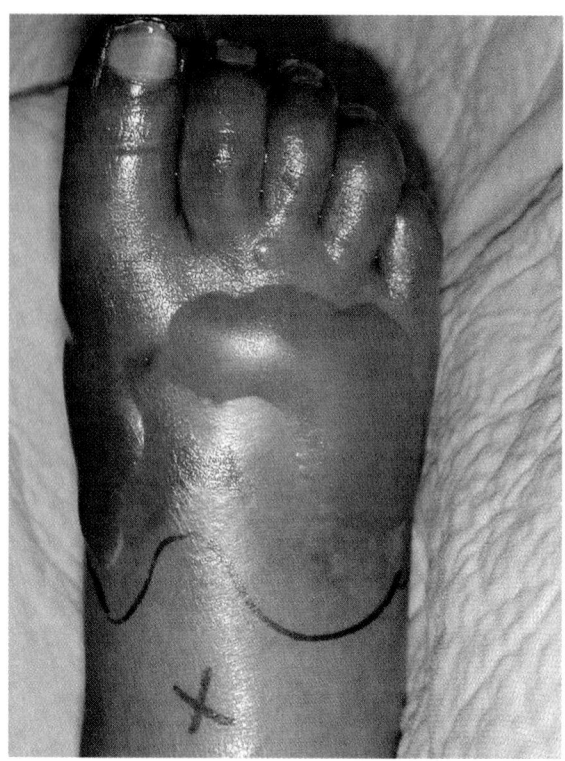

Figure 3 Shown is wet gangrene with edema and undrained severe infection in the foot of a diabetic patient presenting with hyperglycemia and ketoacidosis.

suspicion of infection and a thorough search for it. In a patient with cellulitis, the entire foot, including the web spaces and the nail beds, should be examined for any potential portals of entry, such as a puncture wound or an interdigital ("kissing") ulcer. Encrusted and heavily calloused areas over the ulceration should be unroofed and the wound thoroughly inspected to determine the extent of involvement. A benign-appearing dry gangrenous eschar often hides an undrained infectious collection [*see Figure 1*]. Cultures should be taken from the base of the ulcer; superficial swabs may yield only colonizing organisms.

Findings consistent with infection include purulent drainage, crepitus, tenderness, mild erythema, and sinus formation [*see Figure 2*], though these findings may be entirely absent in the neuropathic foot. With more advanced and deep infection, edema may be present as a result of elevated pressures within one or more of the plantar compartments [*see Figure 3*]. If left untreated, this process may spread proximally along tendon sheaths to involve the ankle or even the calf. Close inspection of the ulcer and the use of a sterile probe may also confirm the presence of osteomyelitis, which occurs commonly even in conjunction with benign-appearing ulcers. If bone is detected with gentle probing, osteomyelitis is presumed present.

Because of its prevalence and its causative role in diabetic foot ulceration and limb loss, neuropathy should be assessed in every diabetic patient, and appropriate preventive measures should be taken to guard against foot ulceration in the high-risk neuropathic foot. Protective sensation may be assessed by pressing a Semmes-Weinstein 5.07 monofilament against the skin; inability to feel the monofilament correlates well with an increased risk of foot ulceration. Advanced sensorimotor neuropathy will lead to the presence of a so-called claw foot (from gradual atrophy of the intrinsic muscles) or to Charcot degeneration with bone and joint

destruction at the midfoot. Both of these conditions give rise to abnormal pressure points on the plantar prominences and the potential for foot ulceration.

Assessment of the arterial perfusion in the diabetic foot is a fundamental consideration, in that the diabetic foot needs maximal perfusion to heal. In the presence of ischemia, all efforts at limb salvage will fail. Therefore, the physical examination must include a systematic approach to the assessment of arterial insufficiency. Simple inspection of the leg and foot, including the ulcer, often provides suggestive clues. For example, distal ulceration (on the tip of a digit), ulceration unassociated with an exostosis or a weight-bearing area, and gangrene are all strongly consistent with underlying ischemia [*see Figure 4*]. Multiple ulcerations or gangrenous areas on the foot, the absence of granulation tissue, and the lack of bleeding with debridement of the ulcer should immediately be taken as signals of possible underlying arterial insufficiency. Other signs suggestive of ischemia are pallor with elevation, fissures (particularly at the heel), and the absence of hair growth. Poor skin condition and hyperkeratosis, though not always good indicators of arterial disease, should be noted because they may help confirm initial clinical impressions.

The pulse examination, including the status of the foot pulses, is the single most important component of the physical examination. In the absence of a palpable pulse, ischemia is always presumed to be present. Although not difficult, an accurate pulse examination of the lower extremities is an acquired skill, and time should be devoted to practicing and perfecting the technique.

The femoral pulse is palpated midway between the superior iliac spine and the pubic tubercle, just below the inguinal ligament. The popliteal pulse is palpated with both hands and with the knee flexed no more than 15°. Palpation of the foot pulses is somewhat more demanding, requiring close attention and a good

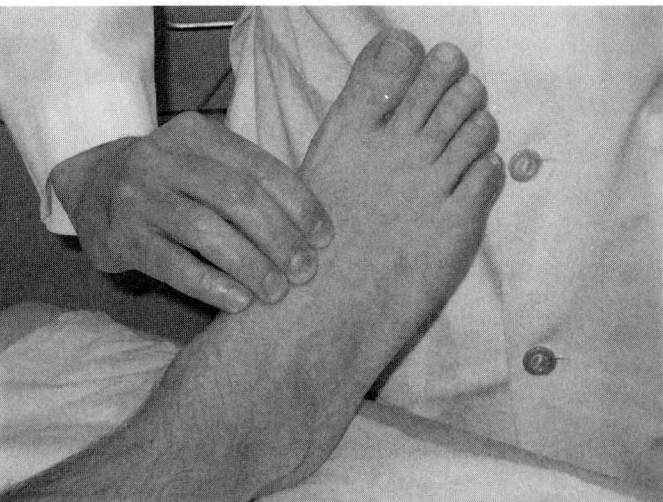

Figure 5 **Illustrated is the correct technique for palpation of the dorsalis pedis pulse.**

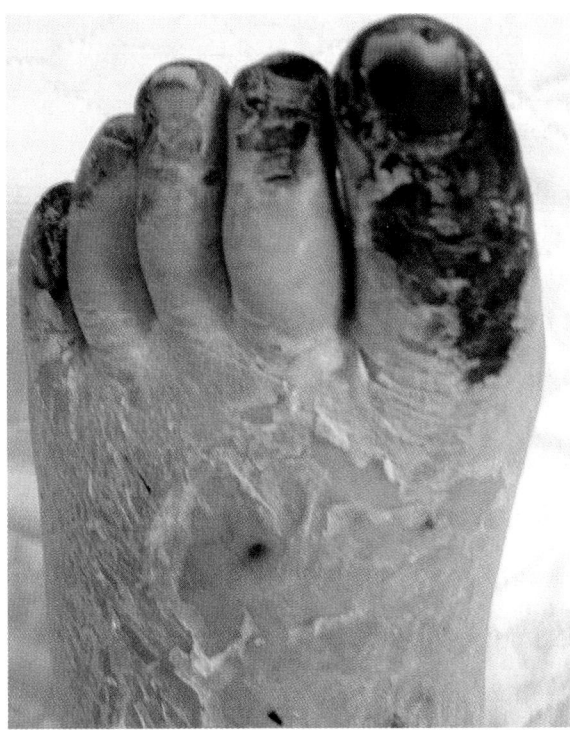

Figure 4 **Shown is dry gangrene of several toes in a diabetic patient with femoropopliteal and tibial arterial occlusive disease.**

knowledge of the usual locations of the native arteries. The dorsalis pedis is located between the first and second metatarsal bones, just lateral to the extensor hallucis longus tendon, and its pulse is palpated with the pads of the fingers as the hand is partially wrapped around the foot [*see Figure 5*]. If the pulse cannot be palpated, the fingers may be moved a few millimeters in each direction; the dorsalis pedis occasionally follows a slightly aberrant course. A common mistake is to place a single finger at one location on the dorsum of the foot. The posterior tibial artery is typically located in the hollow curve just behind the medial malleolus, approximately halfway between the malleolus and the Achilles tendon. The examiner's hand should be contralateral to the examined foot (i.e., the right hand should be used to palpate the left foot, and vice versa), so that the curvature of the hand naturally follows the contours of the ankle [*see Figure 6*].

Assessment of Clinical Findings

Once the clinical evaluation is complete, the next step is to assess the findings from the history and the physical examination so as to determine the course and urgency of the subsequent workup and treatment. This assessment is made at the bedside, focusing on three main concerns: (1) the presence and severity of infection, (2) the salvageability of the limb, and (3) the presence of ischemia.

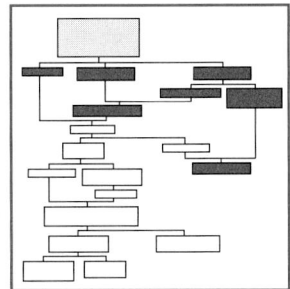

PRESENCE OF INFECTION

Evaluation for and treatment of infection is the first priority in the management of any diabetic foot problem.[4,5] Although radiographic tests may confirm initial clinical suspicions, the deter-

mination of the severity of infection is almost always made on the basis of clinical findings. Infection in the diabetic foot may range from a minimal superficial infection to fulminant sepsis with extensive necrosis and destruction of foot tissue. Accordingly, the treatment plan should address the choice of antibiotic (which requires knowledge of the microbiology), the need for drainage, the option of local or even guillotine amputation, and the patient's overall medical condition.

The microbiology of the diabetic foot varies according to the depth and severity of the infection and the nature of the patient's environment (e.g., hospitalized or outpatient). Certain general assumptions can be made about likely causative organisms. Mild localized and superficial ulcerations, particularly in outpatients, are usually caused by aerobic gram-positive cocci (e.g., *Staphylococcus aureus* and streptococci). In contrast, deeper ulcers and generalized limb-threatening infections are usually polymicrobial. In addition to gram-positive cocci, potential causative organisms include gram-negative bacilli (e.g., *Escherichia coli*, *Klebsiella*, *Enterobacter aerogenes*, *Proteus mirabilis*, and *Pseudomonas aeruginosa*)

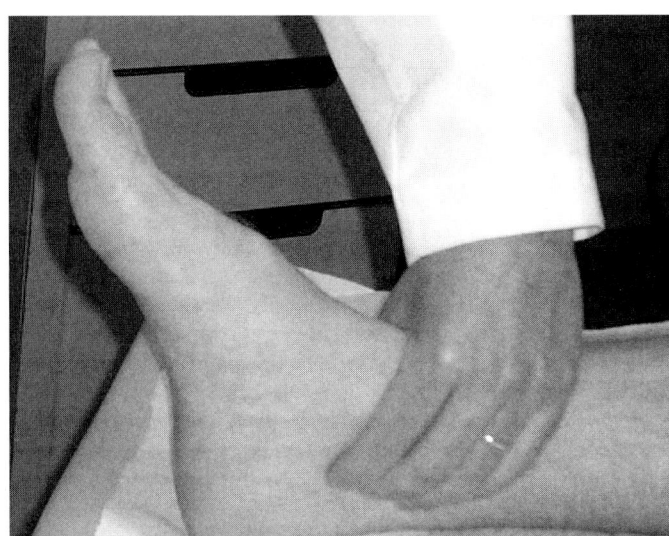

Figure 6 **Illustrated is the correct technique for finding the posterior tibial pulse.**

a

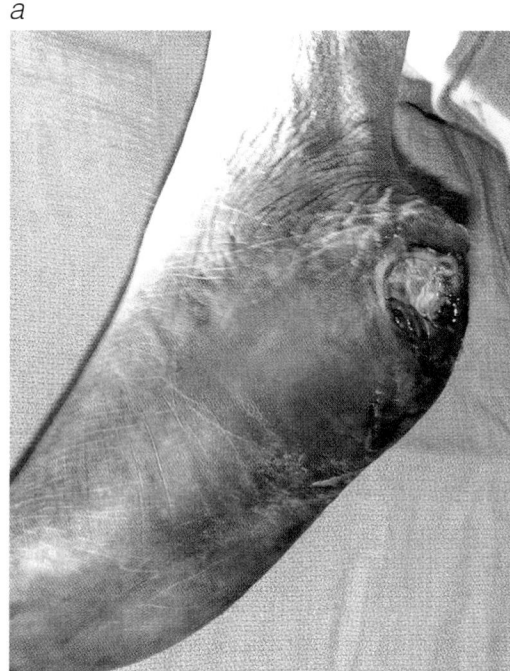

b

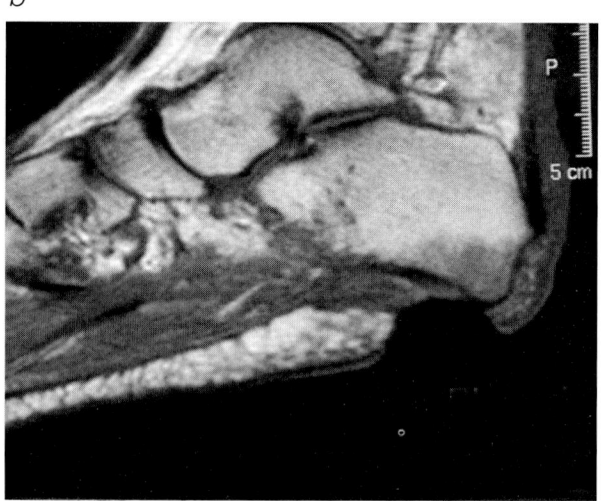

Figure 7 **Shown is heel ulceration with eschar (*a*) in a diabetic patient. MRI findings (*b*) are consistent with calcaneal osteomyelitis.**

and anaerobes (e.g., *Bacteroides fragilis* and peptostreptococci). Enterococci may also be isolated from the wound, notably in hospitalized patients; in the absence of other cultured virulent organisms, they should probably be considered pathogenic. Initially, the choice of antibiotics is made empirically on basis of these general assumptions. When the results of the initial cultures become available, antibiotic coverage may be broadened or narrowed as appropriate.

In the compliant patient with no evidence of deep space involvement or systemic infection, treatment may be delivered on an outpatient basis. An oral antibiotic (pending culture results) is given; a first-generation cephalosporin, with activity against staphylococci and streptococci, is usually adequate. In addition, the patient is instructed to offload weight from the involved extremity and is taught appropriate methods for changing wound dressings. Frequent follow-up is vital, and guidelines should be imparted by which improvement or worsening of the lesion can be determined.

A more common presentation, unfortunately, is the patient with ulceration or gangrene who has a deep infection affecting tendon or bone and possible systemic involvement. For such patients, immediate hospitalization is indicated, including bed rest with elevation of the infected foot, correction of any systemic abnormalities, and broad-spectrum I.V. antibiotic therapy (which may be focused more tightly once culture results are complete). Because the clinical findings of impending sepsis may be subtle, these patients should undergo a complete laboratory workup to detect and correct electrolyte and acid-base imbalances.

The choice of antibiotic agent and the duration of therapy are dependent on the extent of the infection. For non–life-threatening deep or chronic recurrent ulcers, which are typically polymicrobial, appropriate empirical antibiotic options include clindamycin plus a fluoroquinolone, clindamycin plus a third- or fourth-generation cephalosporin, and an antipseudomonal penicillin. Subsequent culture results then dictate further antibiotic coverage, if any. In the absence of osteomyelitis, antibiotics should be continued until the wound appears clean and all surrounding cellulitis has resolved (typically, 10 to 14 days). If osteomyelitis is

present, treatment should include both surgical debridement and a prolonged (4- to 6-week) course of antibiotic therapy (though the course may be abbreviated if the entire infected bone has been removed, as with digital or transmetatarsal amputation). Heel lesions often present with some degree of calcaneal destruction, and determination of osteomyelitis may be made by either clinical examination alone or in conjunction with other radiographic tests (e.g., magnetic resonance imaging) [*see Figure 7*].

In the presence of an abscess or deep space infection, immediate incision and drainage of all infected tissue planes is mandatory. Incisions should be chosen with an eye to the normal anatomy of the foot (including the various compartments) and the need for subsequent secondary (foot salvage) procedures [*see Figure 8*]. Drainage should be complete, with incisions placed to allow for dependent drainage, and all necrotic tissue must be debrided. Repeat cultures (including both aerobes and anaerobes) should be obtained from the deep tissues. Drainage incisions on the dorsum of the foot should be avoided. Abscesses in the medial, central, or lateral compartment should be drained via longitudinal incisions made in the direction of the neurovascular bundle and extending the entire length of the abscess. The medial and central compartments are drained through a medial incision, and the lateral compartment is drained through a lateral incision; both of these incisions are made just above the plantar surface of the forefoot [*see Figure 9*]. Web space infections may be drained similarly through the plantar aspect of the foot. In some instances, open amputation of the foot (e.g., an open toe or transmetatarsal amputation) may be necessary to allow complete drainage and resection of necrotic tissue. Strict adherence to textbook amputations may lead to unnecessary soft tissue removal and possibly to a higher amputation during future closure; therefore, all viable tissue should be conserved.

A patient with an ongoing undrained infection may present with an unsalvageable foot and fulminant sepsis, manifested by hemodynamic instability, bacteremia, and severe acid-base and electrolyte abnormalities. Such patients should undergo prompt open (guillotine) below-the-knee amputation [*see 4:14 Lower-*

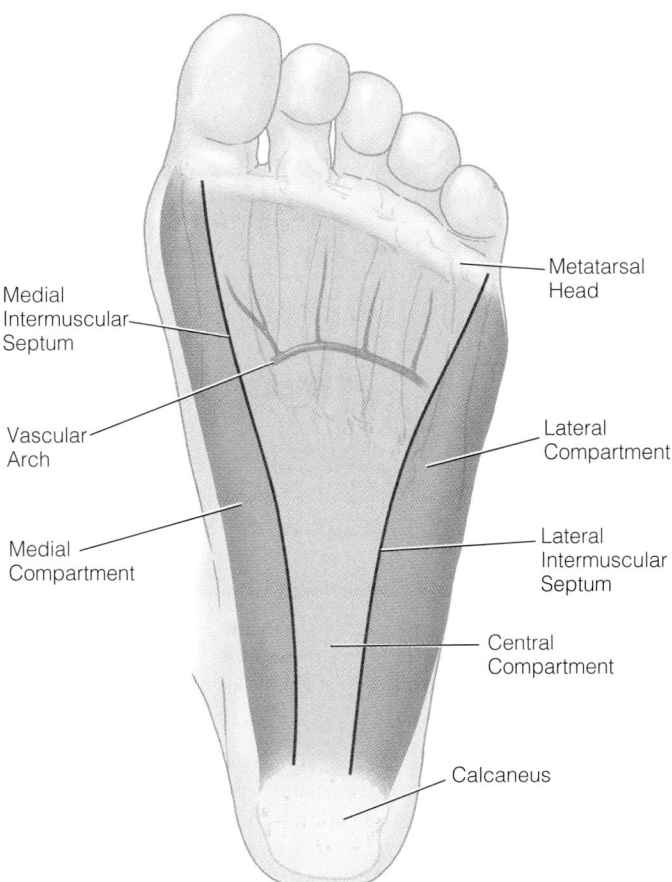

Figure 8 **The foot has three plantar compartments: medial, central, and lateral. The intrinsic muscles of the great toe are in the medial compartment, and those of the fifth toe are in the lateral compartment. The central compartment contains the intrinsic muscles of the second through fourth toes, the extensor flexor tendons of the toes, the plantar nerves, and the plantar vascular structures. The floor of each compartment is the rigid plantar fascia; the roof is composed of the metatarsal bones and interosseous fascia. The medial and central compartments are separated by the medial intermuscular septum, which extends from the medial calcaneal tuberosity to the head of the first metatarsal. The lateral and central compartments are separated by the lateral intermuscular septum, which extends from the calcaneus to the head of the fifth metatarsal.**

Extremity Amputation for Ischemia]. This type of amputation is usually performed at the ankle level, with the aim of removing the septic source while allowing for revision and closure at a later date. Administration of I.V. antibiotics, correction of dehydration and electrolyte abnormalities, and continuous cardiac monitoring are absolutely essential throughout treatment.

Once the infection has been drained and tissues debrided, continued wound inspection and management are essential. Ongoing necrosis should raise the possibility of undrained infection or untreated ischemia, in which case further debridement and treatment may be necessary. Avoidance of weight-bearing should be continued. Neither whirlpool therapy nor soaks are beneficial.

Medical Stabilization

Concomitant with the measures outlined above to control infection, medical stabilization of the diabetic patient must be carried out, and the surgeon must be directly involved in this process. Hyperglycemia is almost always seen when infection is present; it

should be gradually corrected. More advanced hyperglycemia leads to ketotic or nonketotic hyperosmolar states, which carry a 10% to 25% mortality. Serum concentrations of electrolytes, magnesium, and creatinine should be obtained and osmolality determined at frequent intervals; any abnormalities should be corrected [*see 6:8 Disorders of Water and Sodium Balance and 6:9 Disorders of Acid-Base and Potassium Balance*]. Dehydration is common in hyperglycemic patients and should be corrected. A urinary catheter is mandatory to help guide the response to fluid therapy; in unstable patients, a central venous pressure catheter or a pulmonary arterial catheter may be needed [*see 6:4 Cardiopulmonary Monitoring*]. Continuous cardiac monitoring is essential in patients with the hyperglycemic hyperosmolar syndrome or ketoacidosis.

SALVAGEABILITY OF LIMB

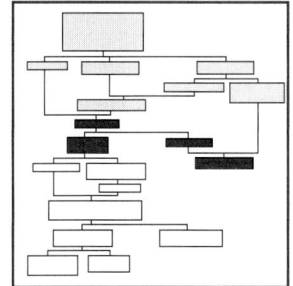

While the infection is being treated and controlled, the surgeon should determine whether limb salvage is feasible. This determination is based largely on the patient's functional status and the degree of foot destruction. For example, primary limb amputation may be considered in a nonambulatory, bedridden patient or in a patient with severe Charcot destruction and degeneration, for whom no further reconstructive foot surgery is possible. Poor medical condition, by itself, is not necessarily an indication for primary limb amputation, given the high perioperative morbidity associated with amputation. Moreover, it is often possible to improve the patient's overall medical status while he or she is being treated for infection and evaluated for ischemia.

Assessment of limb salvageability should be carried out simultaneously with treatment of infection because appropriate drainage and antibiotics can dramatically change the appearance and viability of the foot. If limb salvage is not deemed possible, the patient should undergo formal below-the-knee or above-the-knee amputation [*see 4:14 Lower-Extremity Amputation for Ischemia*].

PRESENCE OF ISCHEMIA

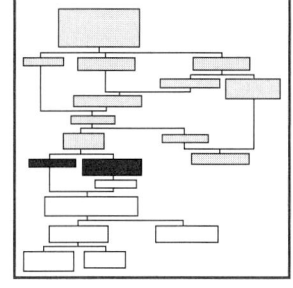

Evaluation of the diabetic foot for ischemia begins with the history and the physical examination. By the conclusion of the clinical evaluation, the surgeon can usually make an accurate assessment of the adequacy of the arterial circulation to the foot. As noted [*see* Clinical Evaluation, Physical Examination, *above*], the absence of a palpable foot pulse strongly suggests ischemia unless proved otherwise.

Noninvasive arterial testing plays only a limited role in the assessment of diabetic patients with foot ulceration and should not be employed in place of the bedside evaluation. Certainly, for patients with poor healing or gangrene and absent foot pulses, noninvasive testing adds little additional useful information to the initial clinical evaluation and typically serves only to further delay vascular reconstruction. For selected patients, however, noninvasive testing, in conjunction with the clinical findings, may be useful. Patients who might benefit from such testing include those with absent foot pulses who have a superficial ulcer with evidence of healing or a previous history of a healed foot ulcer and those without any foot lesions who are scheduled to undergo elective foot surgery.

a
b

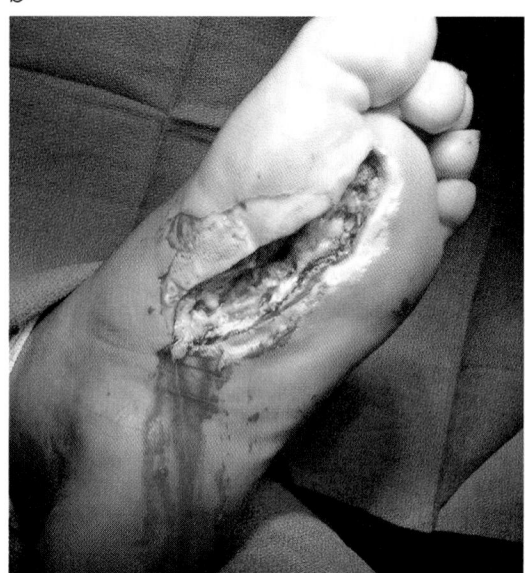

Figure 9 Shown is an infection in the central compartment of the foot from a submetatarsal ulcer that has extended proximally to include the medial compartment (*a*). A plantar incision through the ulcer and both compartments (including the septum) allows complete dependent drainage (*b*).

The presence of diabetes imposes limitations on all of the noninvasive arterial tests currently available. Medial arterial calcinosis occurs frequently and unpredictably in patients with diabetes and can result in noncompressible arteries and artificially elevated segmental systolic pressures and ankle-brachial indices. Because calcification levels tend to be lower in the toe vessels, toe systolic pressures are sometimes obtained, but their value is often limited by the proximity of the foot ulcer to the cuff site. Segmental Doppler waveforms and pulsed volume recordings are unaffected by medial calcification, but evaluation of these waveforms is primarily qualitative rather than quantitative. In addition, the quality of the waveforms is affected by peripheral edema, and cuff placement is commonly affected by the presence of ulceration. Regional transcutaneous oximetry measurements are also unaffected by medial calcinosis, and this modality appears to be reliable for predicting ulcer healing and amputation levels. However, transcutaneous oximetry measurements are actually higher in patients with diabetes and foot ulcers than in nondiabetic patients, possibly because of the effects of arteriovenous shunting. Other limitations, including lack of equipment standardization, user variability, and a large gray area in the interpretation of the measurements, further limit the ability of this test to predict ischemia. Therefore, although these measurements have been used to predict healing in patients without diabetes, high values may not correlate with healing potential in the presence of diabetes.

When a patient presents with absent foot pulses in conjunction with gangrene, nonhealing ulceration, or significant tissue loss, it can be assumed that ischemia is present and must be corrected if the limb is to be salvaged. In such patients, arteriography of the entire lower extremity should be performed. The decision to perform arteriography and vascular reconstruction should be made as soon as infection has started to resolve and signs of systemic toxicity have disappeared; prolonged delays in making this decision may result in further tissue loss and make salvage impossible. For a complete assessment, the arteriogram should include the foot vessels in both lateral and anterior views.

Concern over possible contrast-induced renal failure should not be considered a contraindication to high-quality angiography of the entire lower extremity. The incidence of contrast nephropathy is not higher in diabetic patients without preexisting renal disease, even when ionic contrast agents are employed. Selective use of magnetic resonance angiography (MRA), carbon dioxide angiography, and duplex scanning may help minimize the contrast dye load.

In patients with preexisting renal disease, use of a nonionic contrast agent, in conjunction with appropriate hydration and judicious administration of kidney-protecting agents, should minimize the risk of contrast-induced nephrotoxicity. N-acetylcysteine, 600 mg twice daily, should be started on the day before the arteriogram and continued for 48 hours, and 0.45 N saline should be given I.V. at a rate of 1 mg/kg/hr, beginning 12 hours before the scheduled arteriogram.[6]

Therapy

REVASCULARIZATION

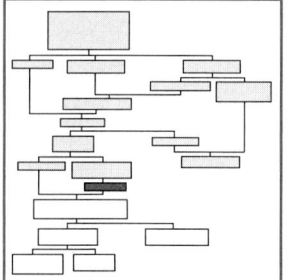

The goals of arterial reconstruction are to restore maximal perfusion to the foot and, ideally, to restore a palpable foot pulse. Possible approaches include endovascular techniques (angioplasty and stenting), bypass grafting (with autogenous or prosthetic grafts), and some combination of the two. Ultimately, the choice of procedure in any given case is based on the individual patient's anatomy, the comorbid conditions present, and the results of the preoperative assessment, with the aim being to provide the most durable procedure with the least risk. For example, in rare patients with isolated iliac artery stenoses, angioplasty may be effective by itself, but in patients with multilevel disease, it may have to be combined with an infrainguinal bypass [*see 4:11 Infrainguinal Arterial Procedures*]. In patients who have previously undergone surgical revascularization, careful consideration should be given to the availability of an autogenous conduit (e.g., an arm vein or the lesser saphenous vein), given the superiority of autogenous vein over prosthetic grafts.

As a rule, arterial bypass grafting is required for restoration of the foot pulse.[7] Proximal bypass to either the popliteal artery or the tibial and peroneal arteries may restore foot pulses, and preference should be given to these vessels if they are in continuity with the foot. Often, however, because of the presence of more distal obstructive disease, bypass grafting to the popliteal or even the tibial artery will not restore the foot pulse. In such cases, restoration of pulsatile flow to the foot may be accomplished with autogenous vein bypass grafts to the paramalleolar or inframalleolar arteries (e.g., the dorsalis pedis). The vein graft can be prepared as an in situ graft, a reversed graft, or a nonreversed graft, without any significant difference in outcome; the choice of approach should be based on the patient's particular vascular anatomy.

As noted (see above), the absence of ipsilateral greater saphenous vein is not a contraindication to pedal bypass: comparable results may be obtained by using arm vein or lesser saphenous vein grafts. Prosthetic material should not be used for dorsalis pedis or other extreme distal bypass grafts. Active infection in the foot is not a contraindication to pedal bypass, provided that the proximal dorsum of the foot is free of infection and that incisions can be placed in clean tissue planes. The foot should be free of cellulitis, lymphangiitis, and edema before any inframalleolar bypass.

CONTINUED WOUND CARE

Once the foot is fully revascularized—or once it is clear that the foot was adequately perfused to begin with—care of the foot wound should be continued. Revascularization of a severely ischemic foot ulcer may result in an immediate paradoxical worsening of the infection, and frequent inspection is mandatory post-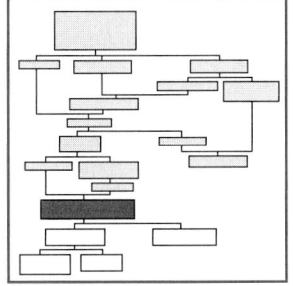operatively. New-onset cellulitis, hyperglycemia, or fever should prompt concern regarding potential worsening of the foot infection. Frequent debridement to healthy, bleeding tissue is required more often than not.

Wounds should be kept moist, with wet-to-dry dressings avoided in favor of normal saline wet-to-wet dressings. Various adjunctive wound treatments are available, including chemical enzymatic debriding agents, growth factors, and hyperbaric oxygen therapy. Some of these may offer a slight additional benefit in terms of improved healing, but they are expensive; blanket use of these costly modalities is therefore discouraged. Failure of wound healing in the diabetic foot is usually attributable to unrecognized ischemia, ongoing infection, or poor conventional wound care—not, as a rule, to the absence of more sophisticated wound therapy.

Hyperglycemia and malnutrition are common in hospitalized diabetic patients with foot ulceration, and both adversely affect wound healing. Correction of these abnormalities should begin early and continue throughout the wound-healing period. Attention should also be directed toward preventing new foot lesions (e.g., decubitus ulcers on the heel from prolonged bed rest). Heel splints, air mattresses, and leg pillows are all valuable in this regard.

SECONDARY FOOT PROCEDURES

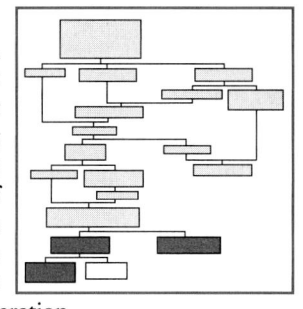

After successful revascularization, secondary procedures on the foot may be performed for maximal foot salvage, with the aim of addressing both the acute problem and the underlying cause. The basic goals of such procedures are (1) to remove infected bone (if present), (2) to restore functional stability, and (3) to reduce the risk of subsequent ulceration.

In the forefoot, digital, single metatarsal (ray), or transmetatarsal amputation [see 4:14 Lower-Extremity Amputation for Ischemia] may be performed, depending on the location of the ulcer. Tissue should be handled gently, forceps should not be used, and incisions should be carefully placed. Care must be taken to prevent dead spaces along tendon sheaths, bone splintering, and areas of residual necrosis, all of which can lead to failure of the procedure. If there is persistent infection or an abscess, the wound should be left open. Every effort, however, should be made to perform a closed amputation so as to avoid the time and cost associated with open wound care. This is a particularly important consideration in the occasional diabetic patient with unreconstructible foot ischemia, because open amputations rarely heal in the presence of ischemia.

Underlying bony structural abnormalities in the diabetic foot are often the cause of ulceration. Such abnormalities may be corrected with hallux arthroplasty, metatarsal head resection, metatarsal osteotomy, or sesamoidectomy; if ulceration is present, these procedures may be combined with ulcer excision. Similarly, ulceration on a previous transmetatarsal amputation may be the result of an equinovarus deformity (from disrupted tendons and a decrease in calcaneal inclination). This problem should be treated with revision of the transmetatarsal amputation (perhaps in conjunction with ulcer excision) and biomechanical correction (e.g., Achilles tendon lengthening or, in more severe cases, posterior tibial tendon release).

Heel lesions are particularly formidable, and there is considerable confusion regarding how best to manage them. Generally, dry eschars with no evidence of deep infection or abscess may be treated with offloading alone so as to allow healing beneath the eschar in the fully revascularized foot. In patients with chronic ulceration or osteomyelitis, partial calcanectomy may be considered. The presence of calcaneal osteomyelitis may be determined by means of probing or adjunctive studies such as MRI [see Figure 7]. Primary closure is occasionally possible, but given the relatively fixed nature of the heel, either secondary healing or some type of flap coverage is usually indicated. Both local and free flaps may be used in the fully revascularized foot.

After any type of surgery of the diabetic foot, frequent postoperative observation of the wound is mandatory. Delays in healing or wound breakdown should immediately raise the possibility of infection or unrecognized ischemia and should trigger the appropriate workup.

PREVENTIVE FOOT CARE

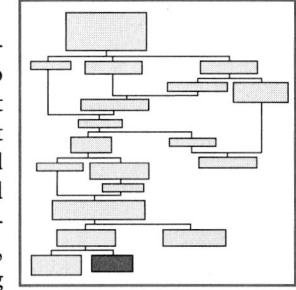

Once the foot has healed, preventive measures should be initiated to prevent future ulceration. Foremost among these measures is patient education, focusing on general hygiene (e.g., daily washing and moisturizer use) and daily inspection of the feet. Walking barefoot, employing heat pads, wearing thong sandals, and using caustic over-the-counter foot medications should all be strongly discouraged.

Neuropathy continues to be the most common cause of diabetic foot ulceration, and its presence is a strong predictor of the likelihood of future ulceration. As noted (see above), inability to feel a Semmes-Weinstein 5.07 monofilament when it is pressed to the skin correlates well with an increased risk of foot ulcera-tion. In addition, abnormal pressure points (secondary to mechanical deformity of the foot and motor neuropathy) can be identified by means of pedobarography, a procedure in which plantar pressure is measured on specialized contour plots as the patient walks on a pressure-sensitive platform. Identification of any high-pressure areas can facilitate the construction of specific, custom-molded orthotics and insoles to help in offloading.

References

1. LoGerfo FW, Coffman JD: Vascular and microvascular disease of the foot in diabetes. N Engl J Med 311:1615, 1984
2. Akbari CM, LoGerfo FW: Diabetes and peripheral vascular disease. J Vasc Surg 30:373, 1999
3. Caputo GM, Cavanagh PR, Ulbrecht JS, et al: Assessment and management of foot disease in patients with diabetes. N Engl J Med 331:854, 1994
4. Fox HR, Karchmer AW: Management of diabetic foot infections, including the use of home intravenous antibiotic therapy. Clin Podiatr Med Surg 13:671, 1996
5. Joshi N, Caputo GM, Weitekamp MR, et al: Infections in patients with diabetes mellitus. N Engl J Med 341:1906, 1999
6. Tepel M, van der Giet M, Schwarzfeld C, et al: Prevention of radiographic-contrast-agent-induced reductions in renal function by acetylcysteine. N Engl J Med 343:180, 2000
7. Akbari CM, LoGerfo FW: Distal bypasses in the diabetic patient. Current Techniques in Vascular Surgery. Yao JST, Pearce WH, Eds. McGraw-Hill, New York, 2001, p 285

Acknowledgment

Figure 8   Tom Moore.

6 VENOUS THROMBOEMBOLISM

John T. Owings, M.D., F.A.C.S.

Deep venous thrombosis (DVT) (deep thrombophlebitis) occurs in approximately 2.5 million people in the United States each year.[1] The incidence of DVT in surgical patients varies widely depending on the method of study: in eight series, the incidence of DVT verified by venography or autopsy ranged from 18% to 90% (average, 42%).[2]

Reviews suggest that pulmonary embolism (PE) occurs in approximately 700,000 people in the United States each year, of whom about 200,000 will die as a result.[3,4] In the absence of prophylaxis, fatal PE occurs in 4% to 7% of hip surgery patients and in 0.1% to 0.8% of general surgery patients.[3,5] In 40% to 60% of patients who die of PE, the diagnosis is not made clinically. PE may be responsible for as many as 5% of postoperative deaths, and it may occur in as many as 25% of patients admitted to the hospital.[6,7] Pulmonary infarction occurs in about 10% of PE patients.[8]

Significant PE is believed, as a rule, to arise from thrombosis of the deep veins of the thigh and the pelvis. Most studies of thromboembolism use DVT as a surrogate end point for PE. The only major study of thromboembolism prophylaxis to date that successfully used death from PE as an end point required more than 5,000 patients to reach statistical significance.[9] Accordingly, the National Institutes of Health has concluded that using DVT as a surrogate for PE is a valid approach.[10]

The optimal treatment of thromboembolism is prevention, particularly in persons at high risk [*see Table 1*].[11,12] Risk factors for venous thromboembolism include increased age (≥ 30 years in some studies),[13] major trauma (Injury Severity Score of 15 or greater or the presence of a pelvic or lower-extremity long bone fracture), morbid obesity, major operation, prolonged immobility, thrombophilia, and previous thromboembolism.

Prophylaxis against Thromboembolism

In evaluating the effectiveness of the methods used to prevent thromboembolic complications, it is important to consider the specific population of patients studied. Within the surgical patient population, there is one reasonable division: between (1) patients who have an ongoing pathologic process that affects coagulation when first encountered and (2) truly elective patients for whom the surgical insult is the inciting risk factor. For the first group, the typical patient is the polytrauma patient; for the second, the patient undergoing elective hip or knee replacement. The key distinction between the two groups lies in whether prophylaxis can be given before the inciting insult (group 2) or must be given after it (group 1). Many prophylactic methods that are effective if started before the inciting insult are completely ineffective if given afterward.

COMPRESSION TECHNIQUES

Elastic stockings have long been used as prophylaxis for thromboembolism. Most commercial stockings, however, do not fit adequately or provide adequate compression and thus probably offer little or no benefit.[4] Low-molecular-weight dextran, which lowers blood viscosity and inhibits platelet aggregation, may be helpful in certain instances, but data showing efficacy against current techniques are lacking.[12]

Pneumatic devices that compress the venous plexuses of the lower extremities are popular because they do not require anticoagulation and thus are not associated with increased bleeding risk. Intermittent pneumatic compression is capable of intermittently increasing venous flow velocities in the femoral and pelvic veins.[14] It has been argued that some of the benefit might derive from the known tourniquet effect of enhancing fibrinolytic activity, attributed both to an increase in tissue plasminogen activator (t-PA) and to a decrease in plasminogen activator inhibitor (PAI). This argument seems to be valid for up to 24 hours of continuous use,[15] but after this point, the effect is exhausted.[14] Intermittent pneumatic compression is a safe, albeit somewhat uncomfortable, method of preventing clots in patients immobilized for prolonged periods. It is particularly useful in critical care units, where other forms of prophylaxis are inapplicable or contraindicated.[11]

Several different pneumatic compression devices have been developed. The first to gain widespread acceptance was the full-length (calf and thigh) sequential compression stocking, which proved effective in a number of settings, including trauma.[16] Because some injured patients were unable to wear the device, various modified compression devices were developed, including a calf-only device and a foot pump designed to compress the plantar venous plexus. Compared with the thigh-high stocking, both the calf-high stocking and the foot pump are associated with higher compliance rates and lower hospital costs. However, substantive data demonstrating that these modified devices reduce PE and DVT are lacking.

Table 1 **Risk Factors for the Development of Venous Thromboembolism**

Hypercoagulability
  Congenital hypercoagulability
  Malignancy
  Oral contraceptives
  Polycythemia
  Thrombocytosis
Venous stasis
  Immobility
  Varicose veins
  Advanced age
  Congestive heart failure
  Obesity
Endothelial injury
  Trauma
  Recent surgery
  Severe infection

PROPHYLACTIC ANTICOAGULATION

A major study of thromboembolic prophylaxis in hip surgery patients found that subcutaneous administration of 5,000 units of heparin two or three times daily before, during, and after the operation substantially reduced thromboembolic complications without increasing bleeding.[5] This low-dose protocol has been criticized as being insufficiently individualized for specific high-risk patients. Low-dose heparin acts by markedly augmenting the antithrombotic effect of antithrombin[17]; therefore, it may be ineffective if antithrombin levels are reduced, and higher doses may be more appropriate in such settings.

Because of these pitfalls, an adjusted-dose technique was devised in the mid-1980s.[18] In this method, heparin is given (either subcutaneously or I.V.) in sufficient doses to elevate the activated partial thromboplastin time (aPTT) by 2 to 5 seconds, thereby compensating for depleted antithrombin levels in high-risk patients. This technique is superior to the low-dose method for preventing venous thromboembolism,[18] and for practical purposes, it should replace the latter as the standard prophylactic dosing technique for unfractionated heparin.[18,19]

In the 1990s, low-molecular-weight heparin (LMWH) appeared on the market. LMWH possesses the same antithrombin-potentiating pentasaccharide chain that unfractionated heparin does. Consequently, it is similarly ineffective if antithrombin levels are depleted. The main advantage of LMWH over unfractionated heparin is that it has a more dependable half-life and bioavailability. Thus, it can be given without monitoring of drug effect or plasma heparin level.

Most of the clinical trials documenting the efficacy of LMWH evaluated patients undergoing elective hip[20,21] or knee operations. A few, however, addressed other patient populations (e.g., trauma patients).[22] In these studies, the incidence of DVT in patients receiving unmonitored LMWH therapy was generally lower than that in patients receiving placebo[20] or low-dose heparin.[21,22] LMWH therapy and adjusted-dose heparin therapy were of roughly equal efficacy.

In the light of these data, it appears that LMWH can be recommended over low-dose unfractionated heparin in elective, emergency, and trauma patients. Whether it is superior to adjusted-dose unfractionated heparin therapy remains uncertain, though it is clearly simpler to manage. Where compliance with monitoring and dose-adjusting protocols is an issue, unmonitored LMWH therapy may well be preferable.

A synthetic form of the specific pentasaccharide that interacts with antithrombin to potentiate its effect has now been introduced. This agent is smaller than the LMWHs and seems to have the same advantages over these substances that they have over unfractionated heparin: increased bioavailability, longer half-life, and more consistent effect. Several studies comparing the pentasaccharide with LMWH reported a decreased incidence of DVT with the pentasaccharide—though at the cost of increased bleeding.[23,24] As the molecular weight of the antithrombin potentiator decreases, the antithrombotic effect focuses more sharply on inhibiting factor X (as opposed to factors II, IX, XII, etc.); this probably explains the improved consistency of action. Given that all of these compounds are used to stop in vivo clotting, it should not be surprising that newer drugs capable of achieving this goal more effectively also cause more bleeding.

In some patients (e.g., those undergoing major gynecologic procedures), warfarin may be used instead of heparin.[12,25] A low-dose regimen (as little as 1 mg/day) may offer some prophylactic benefit.[25] Warfarin anticoagulation must be started 3 or 4 days before the surgical procedure. The international normalized ratio (INR) [see General Principles of Anticoagulation and Lytic Therapy, below] should be kept below 3.0 to prevent excessive bleeding. Warfarin is not as easy to regulate as heparin is. In addition, the therapeutic effect takes several days to be realized and several more days to wear off. Frequently, postoperative patients are unable to resume a normal stable diet. Because warfarin interferes with the clotting factors in the vitamin K pathway, dosage management in the immediate postoperative period is challenging. Because the risk of intracranial bleeding is greater with warfarin than with heparin, great care should be taken in using warfarin for immediate perioperative prophylaxis.

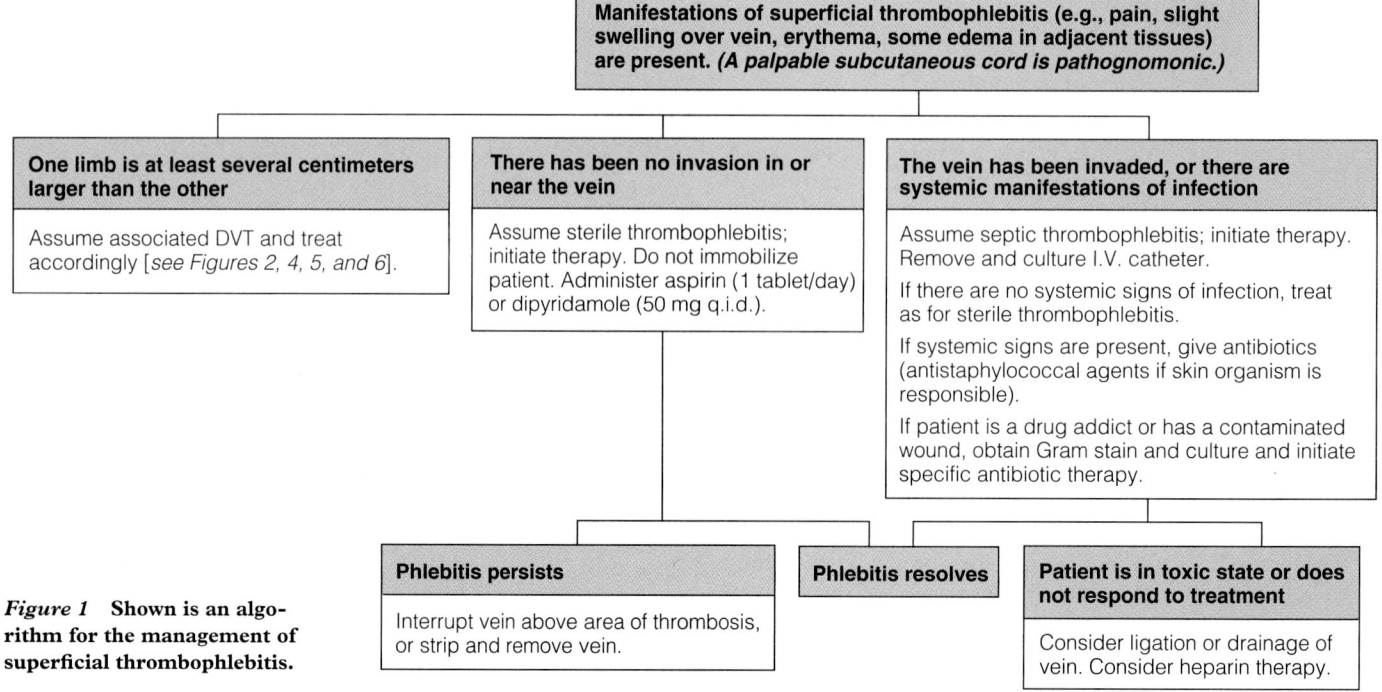

Figure 1 Shown is an algorithm for the management of superficial thrombophlebitis.

PROPHYLACTIC VENA CAVAL INTERRUPTION

Prophylactic vena caval interruption or filter placement provides prophylaxis only against PE, not against DVT, and thus is discussed elsewhere [see Pulmonary Embolism, Minor, Vena Cava Filters, below]. There is evidence that placement of a vena cava filter in fact increases the likelihood of DVT.[26]

Superficial Thrombophlebitis

Characteristic clinical manifestations of superficial thrombophlebitis [see Figure 1] include pain and slight swelling of the extremity, with most of the edema over the course of the involved vein. Unless the patient is obese, a palpable, tender subcutaneous cord is usually found (a pathognomonic finding). Erythema may be present in the overlying skin. The differential diagnosis includes cellulitis and streptococcal lymphangitis. For both conditions, there should be a proximal source (e.g., an open wound). If there is overt limb swelling in a patient who appears to have superficial phlebitis, DVT should be assumed and appropriate treatment [see Deep Venous Thrombosis, below] initiated.

Superficial thrombophlebitis is largely benign but is often overtreated out of fear that infection may be contributing to phlebitis. It is therefore important to differentiate between sterile and septic superficial thrombophlebitis.

STERILE

If there is no invasion in or near the superficial vein involved, sterile thrombophlebitis can be assumed with minimal risk of misdiagnosis. It is best treated simply by giving aspirin (one tablet daily) or dipyridamole (50 mg four times daily).

If superficial phlebitis of the saphenous vein extends to the saphenofemoral junction, interruption of the vein may be appropriate. The choice of treatment is between interrupting the vein above the area of palpable thrombosis and stripping the vein. The second alternative carries a higher morbidity but can be effective when there are associated varicosities. Stripping of the channels above and below the phlebitic process as well as the phlebitic area itself removes the risk of extension and subsequent recurrence. Several authors have explored medical management of patients with above-the-knee superficial thrombophlebitis, using an approach similar to that used for DVT. Therapeutic-dose heparin (unfractionated heparin or LMWH) is given initially, followed by long-term oral anticoagulation. The incidence of extension may be higher than with surgical management, but the operative risks are avoided.[27]

SEPTIC

If there are systemic manifestations of severe infection, septic thrombophlebitis is likely. In addition, the induration, tenderness, and redness over and along the course of the vein are usually more extensive than with sterile thrombophlebitis.

Septic thrombophlebitis associated with an I.V. catheter can be detected by removing the device and culturing the tip [see 6:17 Nosocomial Infection]. Antibiotics should be administered. In most cases, antistaphylococcal drugs are appropriate. If the patient is a drug addict or phlebitis is associated with a contaminated wound, blood samples for culture and Gram staining should be obtained by aspirating the vein. Specific antibiotic therapy directed toward the organisms identified should then be instituted.

If the patient is in a toxic state from presumed septic thrombophlebitis in a subcutaneous vein or is not responding to treatment, it may be appropriate to ligate the vein, to drain it by cutting down on the phlebitic process with the patient under local or general anesthesia and laying the vein open, or to combine ligation with drainage. Moist compresses are then applied, the area is immobilized, and antibiotics are administered. Heparin may occasionally be of value, particularly when the process appears to be extending into the deep venous system.

Deep Venous Thrombosis

DVT can involve either obstructive clots, which affect drainage of venous blood from an extremity, or nonobstructive clots, which are relatively asymptomatic. The latter may be more dangerous because such clots are not circumferentially attached to the vein wall and thus are more likely to embolize. DVT may be divided into three main forms: nonocclusive, occlusive, and phlegmasia cerulea dolens (massive, limb-threatening DVT).

NONOCCLUSIVE

Nonocclusive DVT is common in postoperative and trauma patients but all too often is not suspected until an embolic complication occurs.[28] There may be absolutely no manifestations of clot on clinical examination, or there may be nonspecific swelling in an extremity; rarely is there sufficient pain or tenderness to suggest DVT. Consequently, it is essential to be aware of the major risk factors [see Table 1].

When DVT develops in an outpatient, every effort should be made to determine the cause [see Figure 2]. Apparent spontaneous onset is often the manifestation of an underlying malignancy or even a congenital clotting tendency that will necessitate lifelong treatment [see Hypercoagulability States, below]. Conversely, when risk factors for DVT are identified in a hospitalized patient, it can be assumed that the cause is acquired and that the clotting tendency will be reversed upon recovery.

Before therapy is begun, the diagnosis should be verified. The differential diagnosis includes muscle contusion, plantar or gastrocnemius muscle rupture, ruptured Baker's cyst, popliteal artery aneurysm, arthritis of the knee or the ankle, cellulitis, and myositis. The gold standard for diagnosis of DVT is ascending venography. However, study of the entire lower-extremity venous system often involves injection of dye not only at the foot or ankle level [see Figure 3] but also at the groin level for visualization of the iliac and femoral veins. This approach is uncomfortable and is associated with morbidity; in critically ill ICU patients, it may not be feasible. Accordingly, noninvasive evaluation techniques are favored.

The presence of intravascular clot can be confirmed by detecting D-dimer, a product formed when cross-linked fibrin is broken down by the fibrinolytic system. Both qualitative and quantitative assays are in current use. The various quantitative assays available have differing negative predictive values. The gold standard is the enzyme-linked immunosorbent assay (ELISA) method. Generally, 500 µg/L (in fibrin-equivalent units) or 250 µg/L (in standard units) is an acceptable threshold for a positive result. The latex agglutination test, though inexpensive, has an unacceptably low sensitivity and is the one quantitative method that should not be used. Because some amount of physiologic intravascular clot (e.g., at a wound site) is to be expected in many, if not most, patients at risk for DVT, a positive D-dimer assay is of little diagnostic value. D-dimer assay is therefore unsuitable for screening. In patients suspected of having DVT or PE, however, a negative D-dimer assay can, for the most part, rule out DVT and, by extension, PE.[29-31]

Various forms of plethysmography (e.g., impedance plethysmography) have been used to identify nonocclusive DVT.[32,33] These techniques are accurate only when there is at least 50% obstruction of the lumen of a deep vein. The presence of large col-

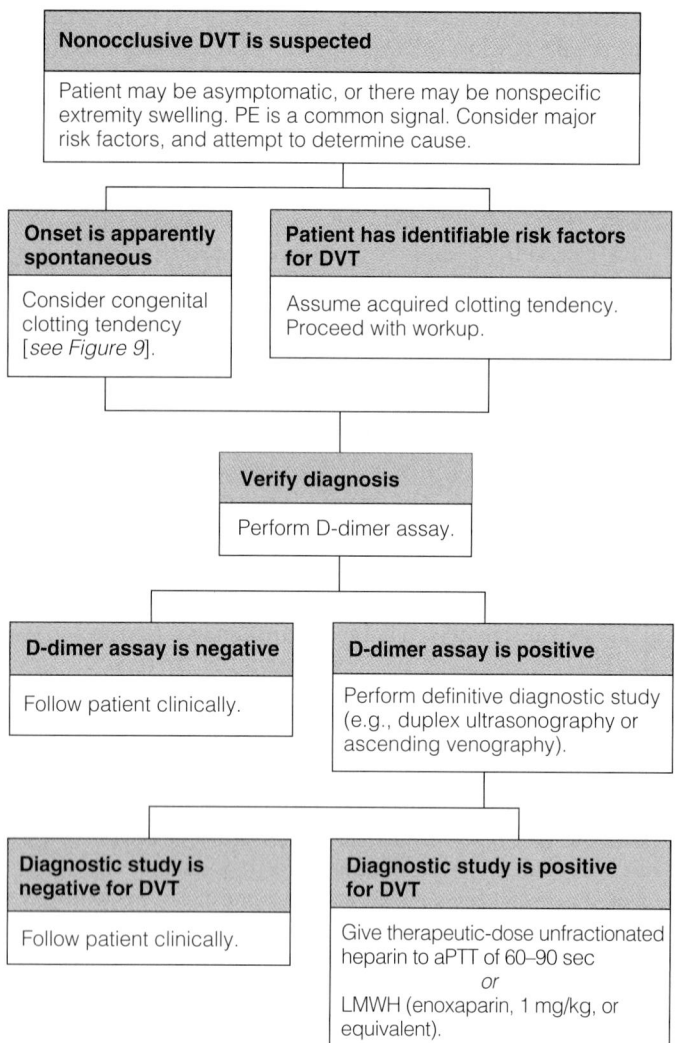

Nonocclusive DVT is suspected

Patient may be asymptomatic, or there may be nonspecific extremity swelling. PE is a common signal. Consider major risk factors, and attempt to determine cause.

Onset is apparently spontaneous

Consider congenital clotting tendency [*see Figure 9*].

Patient has identifiable risk factors for DVT

Assume acquired clotting tendency. Proceed with workup.

Verify diagnosis

Perform D-dimer assay.

D-dimer assay is negative

Follow patient clinically.

D-dimer assay is positive

Perform definitive diagnostic study (e.g., duplex ultrasonography or ascending venography).

Diagnostic study is negative for DVT

Follow patient clinically.

Diagnostic study is positive for DVT

Give therapeutic-dose unfractionated heparin to aPTT of 60–90 sec
or
LMWH (enoxaparin, 1 mg/kg, or equivalent).

Figure 2 **Shown is an algorithm for the management of nonocclusive DVT.**

lateral vessels may result in a false-negative test result as well. Doppler ultrasonography can be performed quickly and easily, though interpretation of the results requires considerable experience. It has essentially the same drawbacks as plethysmography.[32]

Real-time B-mode (duplex) ultrasonography can be valuable in this setting.[32,34,35] It can actually visualize thrombus within a vessel. Inability to obliterate the vein with probe compression is additional evidence of thrombus. Often, experienced users can even differentiate between new and old thrombi on the basis of echogenicity. Duplex ultrasonography is quite sensitive and specific in patients with suspected DVT, and its diagnostic qualities can be further enhanced by the addition of color flow imaging. It has in fact become the noninvasive procedure of choice for assessment of clot in the neck and the extremity vessels. Unfortunately, it is less specific proximal to the axilla and the inguinal ligament, where compression of the vessels is difficult or impossible. Duplex ultrasonography is particularly valuable for detecting associated conditions that may confuse the diagnosis (e.g., muscle hematomas or a Baker's cyst).[35]

Ultimately, ascending venography is the most accurate method of diagnosing DVT.[36,37] If a good contrast study fails to demonstrate the presence of clot, DVT is conclusively ruled out.

Once nonocclusive DVT is diagnosed, the treatment of choice is initial therapeutic-dose heparin therapy followed by warfarin

therapy. If the patient is responsible and reasonably well educated, initial heparin anticoagulation can be done on an outpatient basis with subcutaneous LMWH.[38,39] If this approach is not appropriate, inpatient therapeutic-dose I.V. heparin anticoagulation is employed. After 3 or 4 days, depending on the response, heparin is replaced with warfarin.

OCCLUSIVE

Lower Extremity

Lower-extremity occlusive DVT [*see Figure 4*] is usually associated with swelling; however, if good collateral circulation or duplicate veins are present, especially in the thigh, only local inflammation may be apparent. Typical findings include pain and tenderness over the involved veins as well as swelling in the distal limb (which may be minimal with the patient supine). The differential diagnosis is essentially the same as for nonocclusive DVT. In addition, lower-extremity DVT can be associated with PE: free-floating clot may occur in conjunction with occlusive clot.

If both legs are swollen, the proximal extent of the thrombus is likely in the vena cava. If one entire leg is swollen, the proximal extent must be in the iliac veins. If the swelling is limited to the lower leg below the knee, the thrombus is probably in the superficial femoral vein. If the only manifestations are minimal swelling and calf tenderness, the thrombus is probably limited to the sural vein, the gastrocnemius vein, or both.

If the patient has a history of DVT, is hospitalized, and is at risk for recurrence, heparin therapy may be started before test results are available (provided that there is no contraindication to anticoagulation). If the patient is an outpatient, is hospitalized but lacks risk factors for DVT, or has a contraindication to anticoagulation, a D-dimer assay should be performed. If the assay is negative, an alternative diagnosis should be sought. If it is positive, the diagnostic workup of DVT should proceed. If diagnostic studies yield equivocal results and venography is difficult or impossible, treatment should proceed as if the diagnosis had been confirmed.

The treatment of choice is immobilization in bed, elevation of the limb (with or without elastic compression), and therapeutic-dose heparin (unfractionated heparin or LMWH), followed by 3 to 6 months of warfarin therapy. If the episode is mild, recovery is usually prompt. If pain and swelling do not respond promptly to anticoagulation, either the diagnosis is wrong or anticoagulation is inadequate. Lytic therapy combined with heparin anticoagulation may be superior to heparin anticoagulation alone, leading to better clearance of clot from the valves with improved function and less risk of postphlebitic syndrome.[40]

Upper Extremity

For all practical purposes, upper-extremity DVT [*see Figure 5*] involves only the axillary, the subclavian, or the innominate vein (or a combination thereof). Involvement of the superior vena cava is rare, mainly occurring in chronic conditions (e.g., long-term venous catheterization). Arm thrombophlebitis is characterized by pain and swelling with tenderness over the involved vein. Often, it is relatively asymptomatic: because of the excellent collateral circulation in the arm, thrombosis must be extensive to produce marked swelling.

Spontaneous onset of axillary or subclavian vein thrombosis can occur in association with thoracic compression syndromes (effort thrombosis) or as a complication of so-called Saturday night palsy, in which an alcoholic sleeps with the axilla compressed by the arm of a chair. If a potential mechanical cause is not apparent, other possible causes must be explored. The onset of swelling, tender-

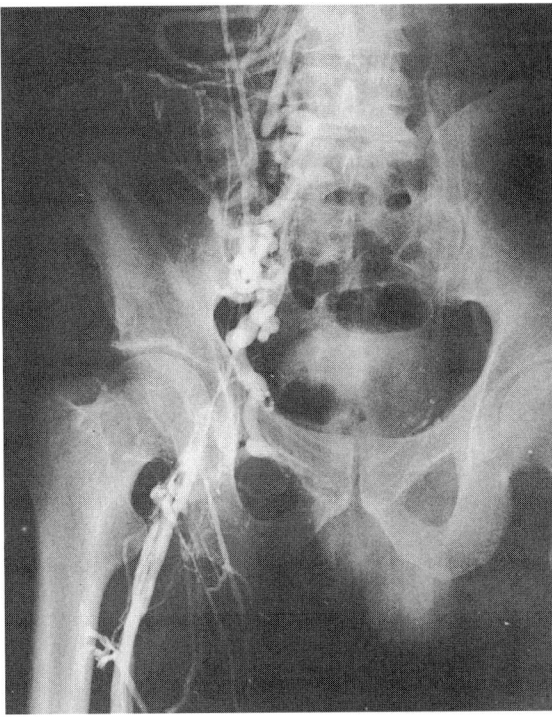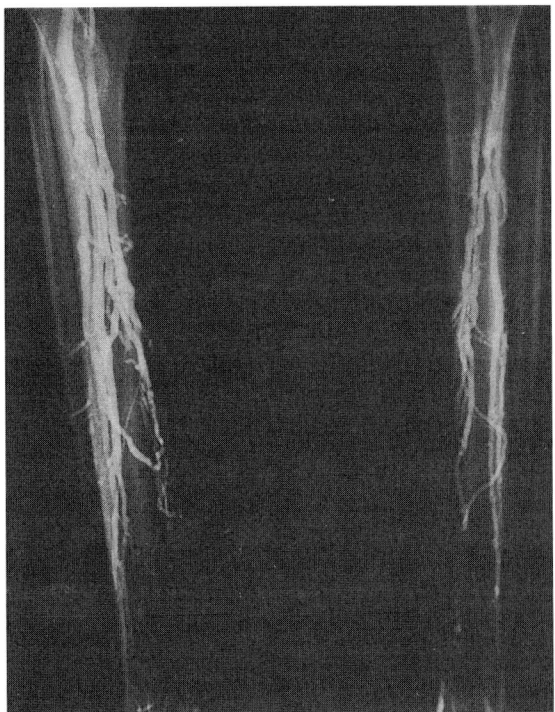

Figure 3 **Injection of dye into dorsal foot veins demonstrates occlusion of iliac veins with excellent pelvic collateral circulation.**

ness, or fever in a patient with a central venous catheter is an indication for removal of the catheter. If there is no bacteremia or fever, if there has been a catheter in the vein, and if the problem developed spontaneously, sterile thrombophlebitis may be assumed. In these cases, once the catheter is removed, anticoagulation is unnecessary.[41]

Subclinical nonocclusive clot is probably of little significance because documented PE from the upper extremity is quite rare. Noninvasive tests [*see* Nonocclusive DVT, *above*] typically yield positive results when the upper extremity is involved.[36] Moreover, distal vein catheterization is easy, and phlebography is relatively uncomplicated. These techniques should be used whenever the diagnosis is in doubt.

The morbidity of occlusive upper-extremity DVT can be quite significant. Thus, if the patient presents with massive swelling of the upper limb, therapeutic-dose heparin anticoagulation should be initiated immediately, and consideration should be given to lytic therapy.[40] If phlebography shows compression of arm veins at the thoracic inlet after lytic therapy or spontaneous recovery from the thrombotic process, resection of rib 1 may be indicated, particularly if positional morbidity is present.[42,43]

Septic DVT is more common in the upper extremity than in the lower, primarily because upper-extremity veins are more frequently catheterized and more often used for injection of illicit drugs. If phlebitis occurs in a catheterized vein with fever and sepsis, the catheter should be removed immediately, the tip cultured, and Gram staining done on any clot present. Broad-spectrum antibiotics should be administered until more specific antibiotic therapy can be instituted. Heparin anticoagulation is the primary treatment unless contraindicated.

Ligation and drainage are not as practical for deep veins as for superficial veins, but either may be indicated on rare occasions if the process does not respond to conventional therapy within 3 or 4 days and marked swelling and fever persist. Drainage is done on

---

Signs of lower-extremity occlusive DVT or PE are present

Determine whether condition is immediately threatening to life or limb.

Condition is immediately life- or limb-threatening

Treat as for phlegmasia cerulea dolens [*see Figure 5*].

Condition is not immediately life- or limb-threatening

Perform D-dimer assay.

D-dimer assay is negative

Follow patient clinically.

D-dimer assay is positive

Perform definitive diagnostic study to confirm DVT or PE.
DVT: duplex ultrasonography or ascending venography.
PE: pulmonary angiography.

Diagnostic study is negative for DVT or PE

Follow patient clinically.

Diagnostic study is positive for DVT of PE

Give therapeutic-dose unfractionated heparin to aPTT of 60–90 sec
or
LMWH (enoxaparin, 1 mg/kg, or equivalent).
Follow with 3–6 mo of warfarin therapy.

Figure 4 **Shown is an algorithm for the management of lower-extremity occlusive DVT.**

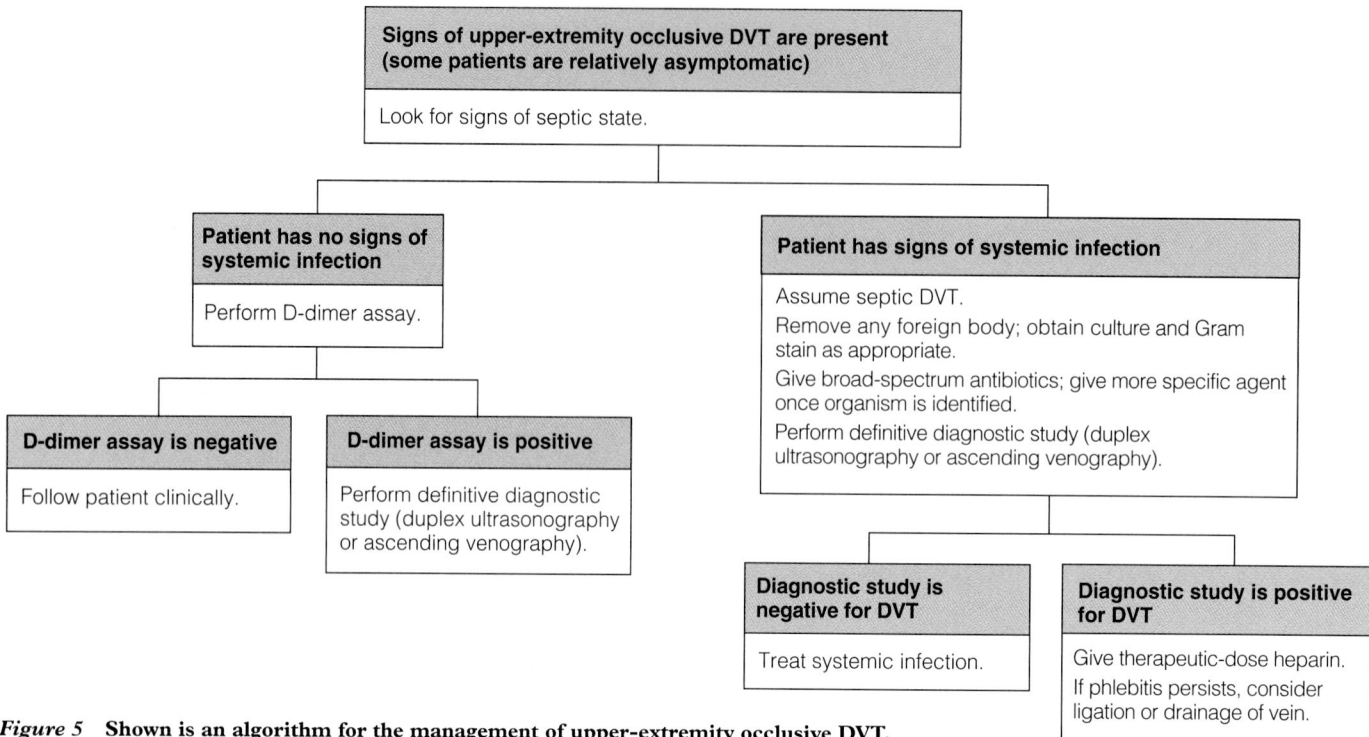

Figure 5 Shown is an algorithm for the management of upper-extremity occlusive DVT.

the most accessible portion of the phlebitic process. For ligation, the proximal end of the process should be identified via surgery or phlebography and the vein then ligated proximally.

MASSIVE (PHLEGMASIA CERULEA DOLENS)

Phlegmasia cerulea dolens [see Figure 6] is most apt to occur in dehydrated, cachectic patients and is usually superimposed on another critical illness. It can involve either the upper or the lower extremity but more commonly affects the lower. In the lower extremity, there is usually simultaneous thrombosis of the iliac, femoral, common femoral, and superficial femoral veins. The limb is massively swollen, bluish, and mottled. Eventually, it becomes nonviable as arterial flow stops because of arterial spasm associated with venous outflow obstruction. The problem is compounded by acute massive fluid loss into the limb, which can result in hypovolemic shock.

Treatment involves rapid and aggressive fluid replacement, elevation of the limb, and aggressive heparin anticoagulation or catheter-directed lytic therapy.[44,45] If the patient does not respond, thrombectomy may be considered, provided that the associated disease does not carry a fatal prognosis.[46] The procedure is best done transfemorally with a limited incision so that anticoagulation can be continued postoperatively. If anticoagulation cannot be continued, thrombophlebitis will recur immediately.

Pulmonary Embolism

It is widely agreed that PE is grossly underdiagnosed.[3,4,47,48] Most episodes (up to 90%) are unsuspected,[49,50] and only a minority (10% to 25%) of fatal episodes are diagnosed before death. Clinical manifestations include dyspnea, hemoptysis, pleurisy, heart failure, and cardiovascular collapse; however, each of these is also associated with other conditions [see Table 2]. Risk factors for PE are similar to those for DVT [see Table 1].

PE should be distinguished from pulmonary infarction. Of the approximately 10% of all pulmonary emboli that are recognized

clinically, only 10% are associated with pulmonary infarction.[8] Because the lung has excellent collateral circulation, obstruction of the larger pulmonary arteries rarely leads to death of lung tissue. When pulmonary infarction does occur, the diagnosis is usually obvious; hemoptysis, pleuritic chest pain, and a wedge-shaped density on chest x-ray are the classic manifestations. In most PE patients (i.e., those without pulmonary infarction), these findings are absent, and the chest x-ray may even be normal.

For the purposes of clinical diagnosis and treatment, PE is best classified as minor (or suspected), moderate, or catastrophic [see Figure 7].

MINOR

Manifestations of minor PE [see Figure 7a] may include transient tachypnea (with perhaps a slight change in blood gas values)

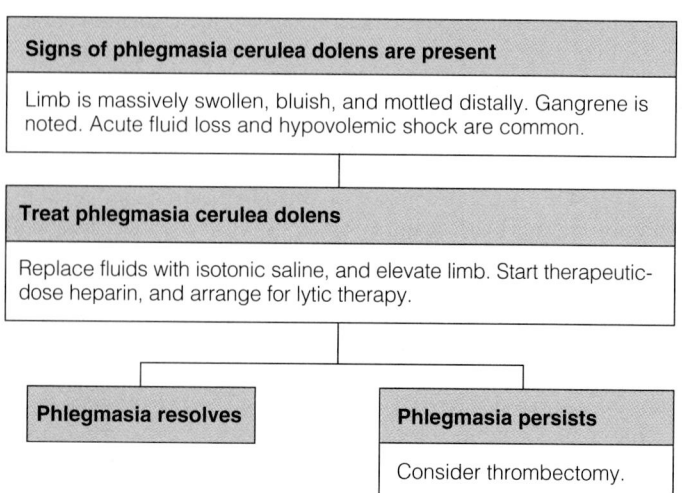

Figure 6 Shown is an algorithm for the management of massive DVT (phlegmasia cerulea dolens).

Table 2 Clinical Features of Pulmonary Embolism: Differential Diagnosis

Clinical Feature	Other Conditions Associated with Feature
Dyspnea	Aspiration Atelectasis Pneumonia Pneumothorax Pulmonary edema Systemic infection
Heart failure	Cardiac tamponade Intracardiac injury Myocardial contusion Myocardial infarction
Hemoptysis	Bronchial injury Pulmonary contusion Tracheal erosion Unsuspected neoplasm
Pleurisy	Chest wall injury Pneumonia Pneumothorax Subphrenic inflammation
Cardiovascular collapse	Air embolism Cardiac tamponade Hypovolemia Myocardial infarction Severe hypoxemia Systemic infection Tension pneumothorax

and cardiac irritability (with frequent premature beats or tachyarrhythmias).[51-53] These changes may resolve in moments, and the patient may then appear perfectly normal. In these circumstances, the embolus probably either is small or is composed of relatively fresh clot that produces only transient obstruction when it enters the pulmonary vascular tree.

It was long believed that after operation, hospitalization, or injury, the earliest PE might occur was 4 to 7 days after the insult. A 1997 study of previously healthy trauma patients, however, found that approximately 25% of the PE episodes occurred in the first 4 days after injury.[54] Accordingly, the presence of clinical signs and symptoms consistent with PE in a patient with risk factors calls for appropriate workup, regardless of how soon after the insult they appear.

The differential diagnosis includes acute respiratory distress syndrome (ARDS), aspiration, atelectasis, heart failure, pneumonia, and systemic infection. If the diagnosis is not obvious but the risk of PE is substantial and there is no contraindication to anticoagulation, heparin therapy (therapeutic-dose unfractionated heparin or LMWH) may be instituted while diagnostic tests are being selected and performed.

If PE is unlikely, the risk from anticoagulation is high, or other serious diagnostic possibilities cannot be ruled out, specific studies (intravascular coagulation, spiral computed tomography, or pulmonary angiography) should be ordered before anticoagulation.

In a stable patient with suspected PE, a blood D-dimer level should be obtained. If the result is negative, PE can be excluded and further diagnostic studies canceled. As with DVT, a positive D-dimer assay does not confirm DVT or PE. The negative predictive value of the assay for DVT and PE is between 90% and 100% when an appropriate assay with an appropriate cutoff value is used.[28-30] If a patient is experiencing a life-threatening respiratory event consistent with PE, the D-dimer assay should be skipped, therapy instituted, and formal diagnostic studies performed.

Noninvasive evaluation of the legs may establish the presence of DVT necessitating anticoagulation. This circuitous way of establishing the diagnosis of PE has severe limitations. When noninvasive assessment aimed at detecting clot in the major leg veins is done before documented PE, it yields positive results in only 33% to 45% of cases.[55] Venography is more sensitive than duplex ultrasonography. When it is used to diagnose venous thrombosis, as many as 30% to 40% of patients with PE are found not to have clot in the major veins of the leg or the abdomen. If the duplex scan or venogram is positive for DVT and there are no contraindications, anticoagulation may be begun. If, on the other hand, a patient is suspected of having PE but is sent for a duplex scan in place of a pulmonary arteriogram, and the duplex scan is negative, workup must continue. It is unacceptable in such cases to assume that the negative result excludes PE.

The initial enthusiasm for the use of lung scans to diagnose or screen for PE has diminished.[56,57] Current thinking about the use of scans for this purpose may be summarized as follows. If a scan is read as high probability, there is roughly an 85% chance that the diagnosis is correct. If a scan is read as normal, there is roughly a 5% chance that the patient had PE. If a scan is read as low or intermediate probability (the most likely scenario), the likelihood that the diagnosis is correct is little better than random chance.

As a result of the dramatic improvements in CT imaging, many have proposed replacing pulmonary angiography with CT. There are several good arguments for this proposal. First, CT scanning is less invasive than pulmonary angiography. Second, it does not require the immediate presence of a radiologist. Third, it is less costly at most institutions. Finally, CT scanning is usually more easily obtained than pulmonary angiography. Initially, the results from CT scanning for PE were quite promising.[58] Subsequently, studies were published in which blinded radiologists from secondary institutions reviewed CT scans and found them to have a sensitivity of 53% to 60% and a specificity of 81% to 97% when compared to pulmonary angiograms.[59] It is generally agreed that the accuracy of the new-generation CT scanners in diagnosing PE is critically dependent on both technique and correct interpretation. Accordingly, physicians working at institutions where CT has replaced pulmonary angiography for diagnosis of PE should be cautious when excluding the diagnosis on the basis of a CT scan.

For critically ill patients, who tolerate diagnostic testing poorly, pulmonary angiography is a more appropriate initial study [see Figure 8].[3,47,60] If the angiogram is obtained immediately after the clinical episode, particularly if the patient is still symptomatic, a negative result rules out PE. However, if the patient improves or recovers before angiography, the angiogram may be falsely negative, implying that the clot was minimal or was disposed of by natural lytic processes. Thus, a negative angiogram in such a patient does not unequivocally rule out PE.[61] The pulmonary angiogram does, however, establish the degree of patency of the pulmonary vasculature, which affects prognosis.

PE can occur even immediately after injury in previously healthy persons.[54] These early emboli are generated from fresh clot and thus are more easily fragmented and broken down. They are much more likely to be found in the periphery.[62] For these reasons, CT is less sensitive in detecting them.[62] Accordingly, patients with suspected PE shortly after injury or operation should undergo pulmonary arteriography.

If all diagnostic tests for PE yield negative results, therapeutic anticoagulation is not indicated; however, if risk factors are present,

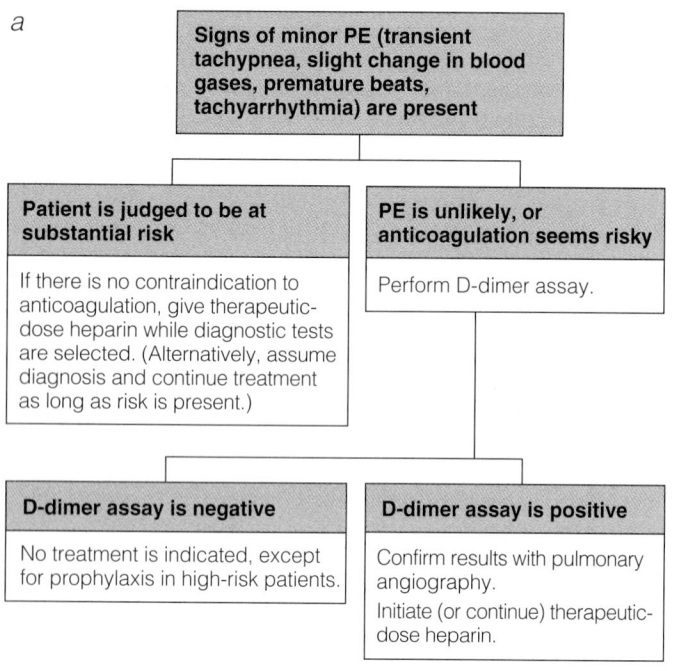

a

Signs of minor PE (transient tachypnea, slight change in blood gases, premature beats, tachyarrhythmia) are present

Patient is judged to be at substantial risk

If there is no contraindication to anticoagulation, give therapeutic-dose heparin while diagnostic tests are selected. (Alternatively, assume diagnosis and continue treatment as long as risk is present.)

PE is unlikely, or anticoagulation seems risky

Perform D-dimer assay.

D-dimer assay is negative

No treatment is indicated, except for prophylaxis in high-risk patients.

D-dimer assay is positive

Confirm results with pulmonary angiography.

Initiate (or continue) therapeutic-dose heparin.

b

Signs of moderate PE (transient hypotension, tachycardia or other arrhythmias, tachypnea, $\downarrow$ Po$_2$ and Pco$_2$, apprehension, symptoms and signs of pulmonary infarction) are present

Perform D-dimer assay.

D-dimer assay is negative

Seek alternative explanation for signs.

D-dimer assay is positive

Assess risk of anticoagulation and likelihood of PE.

PE is likely

Give therapeutic-dose heparin.

Consider lytic therapy for acute episodes.

PE is unlikely, or anticoagulation seems risky

Attempt to make specific diagnosis via pulmonary angiography.

Diagnosis is not confirmed

If patient is at risk for embolism and anticoagulation is not contraindicated, give prophylactic-dose heparin.

Diagnosis is confirmed

If anticoagulation is not contraindicated, give therapeutic-dose heparin. If it is, consider vena caval interruption.

Figure 7 **Shown are algorithms for the management of (*a*) minor, (*b*) moderate, and (*c*) catastrophic PE.**

c

Signs of catastrophic PE (cardiac arrest, circulatory collapse, bradyarrhythmia, severe hypotension, left heart failure) are present

Give 100% O$_2$ by ET tube. Give cardiotonic agents and massive doses of heparin. Consider Trendelenburg's procedure or cardiopulmonary bypass.

Provide further treatment as needed

If patient survives emergency treatment and improves, continue therapeutic-dose heparin and consider lytic therapy or a caval filter.

prophylaxis is indicated. If test results are suggestive or indicative of PE, therapeutic heparin anticoagulation should be continued.

MODERATE

Manifestations of moderate PE [*see Figure 7b*] include transient hypotension, tachycardia or other cardiac dysrrhythmias, tachypnea with a significant fall in arterial oxygen and carbon dioxide tension, apprehension, and symptoms or signs of pulmonary infarction[51,53]; there may be signs of right heart failure as well. Electrocardiography is rarely helpful in the differential diagnosis. Acute right axis deviation, new incomplete right bundle branch block, and changes in S_1, Q_3, or T_3 are thought to characterize this disorder but are found in only a small percentage of patients with proven PE.

If the diagnosis is probable and there are no likely alternatives, heparin therapy should be initiated. Lytic therapy is of debatable utility in these patients: compared with standard heparin therapy, it appears not to reduce mortality or pulmonary dysfunction significantly, yet it carries a higher risk of bleeding.[3,63] Moreover, lytic therapy is often contraindicated because of recent surgery, injury, or vascular punctures.

If there is a relative contraindication to anticoagulation (e.g., an acute surgical wound, a previous bleeding episode, or an allergic reaction to heparin) or alternative diagnoses are likely, specific diagnosis is required, ideally via pulmonary angiography. Peripheral noninvasive venous studies may be helpful because if they show significant venous obstruction, the likelihood of PE increases and the need for therapy is documented. Ventilation-perfusion scanning, again, is valuable only if strongly positive.

If there is no contraindication to heparin therapy and the diagnosis is strongly suspected but not confirmed, therapeutic-dose heparin anticoagulation should be started.[64,65] Treatment is continued if the diagnosis is verified and stopped if the diagnosis is excluded.[66-69]

Vena Cava Filters

Vena caval interruption has often been recommended for patients with documented PE despite apparently adequate sys-

temic anticoagulation, but many authorities now advocate vena caval filter placement even in patients who do not have documented thromboembolism but are at high risk and in whom anticoagulation is contraindicated.[70-72] Supporting data come largely from studies with historic controls. In the one prospective, randomized, controlled trial involving patients with thromboembolic disease, there was no reduction in mortality at any time, nor was there even a reduction in PE at 2 years; however, there was an increased incidence in DVT over that period.[26] These findings suggest that vena cava filters should be reserved for patients with documented DVT, a contraindication to anticoagulation, and a high risk of subsequent PE.

If vena caval interruption is considered necessary, it should be done percutaneously via either the jugular or the femoral route. If it is done by the latter route, phlebography (from the insertion site

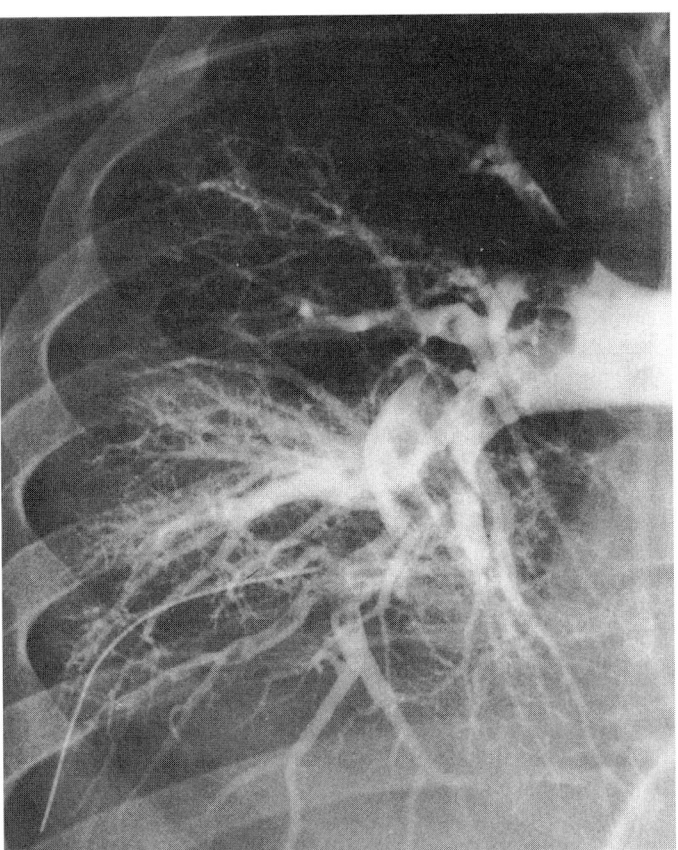

Figure 8 **Pulmonary angiogram shows unequivocal filling defects in multiple arteries.**

through the vena cava) should be performed first to document the absence of clot along the planned route. A number of different vena caval filters are currently on the market. Each is slightly different from the others, but none has demonstrated clear superiority in preventing PE or reducing caval thrombosis. Surgeons should be aware of the advantages and disadvantages of the types available at their institutions. Removable filters have been described in several reports. At present, these are not approved by the Food and Drug Administration (FDA), and no consensus has been reached on the appropriate time, if any, for removal.

CATASTROPHIC

Catastrophic PE [*see Figure 7c*] is most apt to be superimposed on a critical illness or a major operation. The peak incidence is 7 to 10 days after the procedure or the onset of clinical illness, though emboli may occur at any time.[51] The reason for this apparent delay is that for the clot to remain intact after embolization to the pulmonary vasculature, it must mature in the vascular system, a process that takes several days. Fresh clot breaks up readily and dissipates promptly, whereas older clot is resistant to lysis. The manifestation of early embolization of fresh clot to the pulmonary vasculature is ARDS. Embolization of older clot can produce acute pulmonary obstruction and acute right heart failure, making radiologic diagnosis of PE relatively easy.[51] Occlusion of large portions of the vasculature is associated with hemodynamic catastrophe.

Typically, the clinical onset of catastrophic PE comes when a patient, having just been mobilized, performs a vigorous Valsalva maneuver in the course of his or her first postoperative bowel movement. The great abdominal veins distend, and any clot present tends to be stripped loose. If a large clot embolizes, immediate collapse and cardiac arrest may result; in some cases, bradyarrhythmia or severe hypotension precedes the actual arrest. Immediate emergency treatment comprises intubation and administration of 100% oxygen, heparin anticoagulation, and, if cardiac arrest occurs, cardiopulmonary resuscitation. A Swan-Ganz catheter should be inserted as soon as possible so that the effects of therapy can be monitored. Cardiotonic agents (e.g., dopamine, 2.0 to 5.0 µg/min, or dobutamine, 2.5 to 10.0 µg/kg/min) should be administered to strengthen myocardial function. If sudden arrest occurs in circumstances that permit emergency thoracotomy, Trendelenburg's procedure can be performed; however, it is rarely indicated and even more rarely successful. If the patient survives initial emergency treatment and improves, high-dose heparin therapy should be continued and lytic therapy considered.[68,73]

General Principles of Anticoagulation and Lytic Therapy

HEPARIN ANTICOAGULATION

Therapeutic Dose

Heparin therapy may be instituted with either unfractionated heparin or LMWH. In either case, the key is to give enough heparin soon enough to have a beneficial effect. Both types of heparin exert their effect by potentiating antithrombin; thus, if a patient's antithrombin stores are depleted, progressively higher heparin doses will be required to achieve the same degree of anticoagulation.

Unfractionated heparin therapy is also frequently referred to as conventional anticoagulation.[74-76] Before therapy is begun, a clotting battery should be performed, consisting of the aPTT, the INR, the platelet count, and levels of fibrinogen, antithrombin, and D-dimer. High fibrinogen levels and platelet counts are seen in patients with chronic clotting syndromes,[77] probably representing overcompensation for increased utilization. Elevated D-dimer levels suggest intravascular clotting with activation of the fibrinolytic system.

In the average patient, therapeutic-dose heparin anticoagulation begins with administration of 5,000 to 10,000 units, followed by continuous I.V. infusion at a rate sufficient to double or triple the aPTT—typically, 1,000 to 2,000 units/hr. When dosages higher than 2,000 units/hr are required, antithrombin depletion is highly probable.

Tight control of the aPTT change as a result of heparin therapy is not as important as monitoring for evidence of bleeding and platelet depletion. Clinical evidence of bleeding is not necessarily a contraindication to anticoagulation. Minimal amounts of blood may be lost in the urine or through the GI tract; if the patient has a clearly identifiable need for anticoagulation, such minor blood loss should be accepted. Only when transfusion is indicated to maintain the hematocrit should discontinuance of heparin be considered. At that point, if the risks of bleeding seem to outweigh the benefits of anticoagulation, heparin infusion can be stopped or reduced to prophylactic levels. It is important to watch for falls in the hematocrit indicative of significant bleeding. The most common sites for hemorrhagic complications are surgical wounds and the retroperitoneum. Retroperitoneal bleeding is generally asymptomatic until the patient progresses to hemorrhagic hypovolemic shock.

As a rule, the therapeutic dose of LMWH is twice the prophylactic dose. The various LMWHs currently on the market all have slightly different activities and half-lives. Enoxaparin may be taken as prototypical. The accepted prophylactic dose for enoxaparin is 30 mg, given twice daily, and the therapeutic dose is 60 mg (or 1 mg/kg), given twice daily.

A major benefit of using LMWHs to treat DVT and PE is that therapeutic doses can be given subcutaneously.[38,39] As a result, patients may be treated as outpatients both in the acute phase of the disease and in the subacute phase, during the transition to oral anticoagulants. This approach requires that patients be clinically stable and able to follow dosing instructions. Because there are no validated methods of monitoring LMWH therapy, an initial assessment of antithrombin activity is appropriate. If this is low, unfractionated heparin therapy in conjunction with PTT monitoring is probably preferable.

High Dose

High-dose heparin therapy is reserved for patients who are dying of PE or are at risk for immediate limb loss from phlegmasia cerulea dolens. Such therapy consists of administering a large enough dose of heparin to elevate the PTT off scale. The maximum PTT that can be measured by our laboratory is 150 seconds; high-dose heparin treatment should therefore yield a PTT higher than this value. Theoretically, given that a fully anticoagulated patient should not form clot at all, the PTT should be infinite. This method of treatment may be used in patients with immediately life-threatening PE or phlegmasia cerulea dolens when the more conventional technique, catheter-directed thrombolytic therapy, is unavailable.

In most patients, high-dose therapy begins with a 20,000 unit I.V. bolus, followed by infusion of 5,000 units/hr I.V.[78-82] The end point of therapy is clinical evidence of improvement. In patients being treated for PE, pulmonary function should improve.

Because complete anticoagulation is the essential principle of high-dose heparin therapy, there is no need to be concerned about an upper limit for the dosage: if the patient cannot clot, doubling or even tripling the dosage should not increase the risk of bleeding. Moreover, because the incidence of bleeding is very low in the first 2 or 3 days of therapy, regardless of the dosage,[81,82] high initial dosages do not carry an unacceptable bleeding risk. After heparin has been observed to have an effect and a prolonged aPTT documented, the high dosage should be continued for at least 24 hours, then decreased by 500 to 1,000 units/hr over the next 24 hours. If the clinical effect is maintained and improvement continues, the dosage can be decreased by another 500 to 1,000 units/hr over the following 24 hours. In theory, once all clotting stops, natural antithrombin levels should recover, allowing lower dosages of heparin to be effective. After 3 or 4 days of therapy, the dosage may be reduced to more conventional levels [*see* Therapeutic Dose, *above*].

If the initial improvement is lost, the dosage should be restored to its previous high level and maintained there for several days before any attempt is made to reduce it again. The platelet count and the hematocrit should be carefully monitored, the latter at least four times a day. Heparin should be discontinued or the dosage reduced only when the risks of bleeding and transfusion exceed the benefits of anticoagulation. In a monitored environment, patients very rarely die of hemorrhage; rather, they die of the consequences of clotting.

Complications

The most devastating hemorrhagic risk of heparin therapy—fortunately, a rare one—is intracranial bleeding. The risk of major hemorrhage ranges from 4% to 9% and is directly affected by how tightly the INR is controlled.[83] The risk is greatest in elderly patients, particularly women,[75] but it is still small in comparison with the obvious risks posed by the clotting episode. Nevertheless, the existence of this risk makes it appropriate to use high-dose heparin primarily in life-threatening conditions.

A more common complication of full heparin anticoagulation is retroperitoneal bleeding. This problem is accentuated in elderly patients. Because aging is associated with loss of connective tissue elasticity, bleeding into retroperitoneal connective tissue that would normally be insignificant can become life-threatening. Usually, this is not a serious problem if the hematocrit is followed, heparin dosing adjusted, and lost blood replaced. When the perceived risk of bleeding outweighs the thrombotic risk, heparin should be discontinued.

Two forms of acute heparin-induced thrombocytopenia (HIT) have been reported.[84-87] Mild HIT occurs in 2% to 5% of patients 2 to 15 days after the initiation of therapy. The platelet count usually remains at about 100,000/mm³, and treatment can be continued without undue risk of bleeding or thrombosis. Severe HIT is much less frequent. It usually occurs about 7 to 14 days after the initiation of heparin therapy and is reversible once the drug is discontinued. It is not dependent on the heparin dose given. Clinical manifestations include a substantial (at least 50%) drop in the platelet count followed by a thrombotic episode (frequently both arterial and venous). An ELISA directed at the platelet factor 4–heparin complex is generally accepted for laboratory confirmation of the diagnosis. Treatment consists of discontinuance of heparin. If the patient still requires anticoagulation, a different anticoagulant must be used. The most widely accepted agent for this purpose is lepirudin (a direct thrombin inhibitor).[88] Other direct thrombin inhibitors (e.g., argatroban) and heparinoids (e.g., danaproid) have also been successfully used to provide anticoagulation in patients with HIT. None of the LMWHs are acceptable in this setting, and at present, the FDA does not allow use of the pentasaccharide in severe HIT.

Unlike warfarin, heparin does not cross the placenta and has not been associated with fetal malformations; thus, it is preferred for thrombotic complications of pregnancy. Heparin can be administered subcutaneously in an outpatient setting for 3 to 6 months. Long-term administration can lead to osteoporosis and spontaneous vertebral fractures.[89]

Very rarely, heparin therapy can lead to adrenal hemorrhage and consequent adrenal insufficiency [*see 6:11 Endocrine Problems*].[75] If acute adrenal insufficiency is suspected, anticoagulant therapy should be discontinued and high-dose steroid therapy (preferably with hydrocortisone) initiated. Treatment should not await laborato-

---

Table 3 Recommendations for Use of Varying Dosages of Warfarin

The dosage of warfarin is regulated by monitoring the INR. A less intense therapeutic range (INR = 2.0 to 3.0, corresponding to a PT 1.3 to 1.5 times normal with a WHO-designated thromboplastin) is appropriate for the following applications:

1. The prevention of venous thromboembolism in high-risk patients.
2. The treatment of venous thrombosis and PE after an initial course of heparin.
3. The prevention of systemic embolism (a) in patients with tissue heart valves, (b) in selected patients with atrial fibrillation, (c) in patients with acute anterior wall myocardial infarction, and (d) in patients with valvular heart disease.

A more intense therapeutic range (INR = 3.0 to 4.5, corresponding to a PT 1.5 to 2.0 times normal with a WHO-designated thromboplastin) is appropriate for patients with mechanical prosthetic valves and patients with recurrent systemic embolism.

INR—international normalized ratio   PT—prothrombin time   WHO—World Health Organization ry confirmation. CT scanning may be useful. Heparin may suppress aldosterone synthesis, especially with prolonged use.[75]

Reversal of Heparin Effect

The anticoagulant effect of heparin disappears within hours after discontinuance. If the effect must be reversed quickly, the patient should receive protamine sulfate I.V. This agent should be given in the smallest dosages that still evoke the desired result—typically, about 1 mg for every 100 units of heparin remaining in the patient. Protamine sulfate should be administered slowly over 5 to 10 minutes; rapid infusion can cause shortness of breath, flushing, bradycardia, hypotension, or anaphylaxis. On rare occasions, patients previously sensitized to protamine may experience massive platelet aggregation, as manifested by catastrophic arterial thrombosis.

ORAL ANTICOAGULATION

Warfarin is the prototypical oral anticoagulant; the agents in this class have much the same effects, differing primarily with respect to potency and duration of action.[75,76] Warfarin is also available in an I.V. form; however, in view of its mechanism of action, caution should be exercised when it is given parenterally.

Dosage

Historically, warfarin dosage has been regulated by monitoring the prothrombin time (PT), with a PT 1.5 to 2.5 times normal (11 or 12 seconds) generally considered to represent the optimal level. In response to the wide variations in PT reported by different laboratories, the World Health Organization (WHO) has recommended substituting the INR for the PT ratio so that all laboratory assessments will be comparable.[90] An INR of 2.0 to 3.0 corresponds to a PT that is 1.3 to 1.5 times normal (moderate dose); an INR of 3.0 to 4.5 corresponds to a PT that is 1.5 to 2.0 times normal (high dose). Lower INRs are recommended for all but extremely high-risk patients (e.g., those with mechanical heart valves) [see Table 3].[90]

Initially, the daily dose of warfarin required to increase the INR to between 2.0 and 3.0 is estimated and administered. The INR is then checked every morning. If it suddenly overshoots the target range, the warfarin dosage is reduced. If the INR has not reached or surpassed 1.5 after the third dose, the dosage is increased. The maintenance dosage averages about 5 mg/day but may range from 1 to 10 mg/day.

While the maintenance dosage is being determined, the INR should be checked daily. Once the patient stabilizes, the INR can be checked less often: twice weekly for the first few weeks, once weekly for the next several months, and once monthly thereafter if the patient is stable. The patient should be cautioned about drug interactions. If the dosages of other medications are changed, the impact on the INR should be investigated and the warfarin dosage adjusted as appropriate.

Duration

There is no general agreement on how long oral anticoagulant therapy should be continued after a thromboembolic event. Current data suggest that the duration of therapy should be based on the level of underlying risk rather than on the severity of the event. For patients with a limited risk period (e.g., a young patient with a femur fracture and no other risk factors), an 8- to 12-week course is as efficacious as a longer course.[91] For patients with a lifelong risk (e.g., a patient with a congenital hypercoagulability syndrome or cancer), a therapeutic dosage for 3 to 6 months followed by a low dosage for the remainder of the patient's life is indicated.[83] Lengthening the duration of full anticoagulant therapy in

patients with long-term risk factors appears only to delay the recurrence of thromboembolism, not to prevent it.

Drug Interactions

Response to warfarin is affected not only by various bodily factors but also by drug interactions [see Table 4]. Such interactions are most dangerous when drugs administered in parallel are taken intermittently.[75,76] Increased metabolic clearance of the drug can result from administration of barbiturates, rifampin, or phenytoin; long-term use of alcohol; ingestion of large amounts of vitamin K; and rich foods. Elevated levels of coagulation factors during pregnancy also decrease warfarin's effectiveness.

Decreased metabolism or displacement from protein-binding sites caused by phenylbutazone, sulfinpyrazone, metronidazole, disulfiram, allopurinol, cimetidine, amiodarone, or acute intake of ethanol can elevate the INR and increase the risk of hemorrhage. Relative vitamin K deficiency, resulting from inadequate diet or the elimination of the intestinal flora by antimicrobial agents, may have similar effects. For these reasons, warfarin should be used with great caution in patients who are receiving antibiotics or who cannot tolerate a regular diet.

There are some serious interactions that increase the risk of bleeding without altering the INR. These include inhibition of platelet function by drugs such as aspirin and gastritis or gastric ulceration induced by anti-inflammatory drugs. Obviously, when placing a patient on more than one anticoagulant simultaneously, great care must be taken.

Complications

Bleeding is the major complication of oral anticoagulation. Tight control of warfarin therapy is essential for minimizing this complication.[83] Bleeding is rare when the INR is kept below 3.0. When bleeding does occur, a preexisting lesion is likely. If the bleeding is minor, the warfarin dosage should be adjusted; if it is

Table 4 Factors Influencing Response to Warfarin

Factors Leading to Increased Response	Factors Leading to Decreased Response
Drugs	Drugs
Allopurinol	Barbiturates
Amiodarone	Cholestyramine
Aspirin	Diuretics
Cephalosporins	Ethanol (chronic use)
Cimetidine	Phenytoin
Clofibrate	Rifampin
Disulfiram	Vitamin K
Ethanol (acute intoxication)	Foods
Heparin	Green leafy vegetables
Metronidazole	Bodily factors
Sulfinpyrazone	Hereditary resistance
Trimethoprim-sulfamethoxazole	Hypometabolic states
Bodily factors	Pregnancy
Age	Uremia
Congestive heart failure	
Dietary inadequacy	
Hypermetabolic states	
Intestinal flora loss	
Liver disease	

Table 5 Characteristics of Current Thrombolytic Agents

Agent	Abbreviation	Half-life (min)	Fibrin-Specific	Antigenic	FDA-Approved Indication	Comments	Current Trials
Streptokinase	SK	30	No	Yes	AMI, PE, DVT, PAO, AV cannulae	Systemic plasminogen activator	—
Urokinase	UK	15	No	No	AMI, PE, catheter occlusion	Systemic plasminogen activator	—
Alteplase	t-PA	4–8	Yes	No	AMI, acute stroke, PE	Sometimes termed accelerated t-PA	GUSTO TIMI
Reteplase	rt-PA	14–18	Yes	No	AMI	Increased fibrin specificity; increased resistance to PAI-1	ASSENT-II In-Time II
Tenecteplase	TNK-tPA	11–20	Yes	No	AMI	Resistance to plasmin cleavage; increased effectiveness on arterial thrombi	ASSENT-II
Anistreplase	APSAC	40–70	No	No	AMI	Not commonly used, Lys-plasminogen complex with streptokinase	—
Lanoteplase	n-PA	23–37	No	No	—	Increased resistance to PAI-1, less fibrin specificity	In-TIME II
Saruplase	rpro-UK	7–9	No	No	—	Recombinant urokinase-type plasminogen activator without immunogenicity	PROACT III
Staphylokinase	SakSTAR rSak	6	Selectively	Yes	—	Reduction in antigenicity with variants, fibrin-bound is not inhibited by α_2–antiplasmin	CAPTORS II
Pamiteplase	YM866	30–47	No	No	—	Resistance to plasmin cleavage	—
Desmoteplase	Bat-PA b-PA DSPA DSPAα1	t½α:1 t½β:17	Yes	Minimally	—	Vampire bat PA; greater fibrin specificity than tissue plasminogen activator	DEDAS
Monteplase	E6010	23	No	Unlikely	—	—	COMA

AMI—acute myocardial infarction ASSENT— Assessment of the Safety and Efficacy of a New Thrombolytic Agent AV—arteriovenous CAPTORS—Collaborative Angiographic Patency Trial of Recombinant Staphylokinase COMA—Combining Monteplase with Angioplasty DEDAS—Dose Escalation study of Desmoteplase in Acute Ischemic Stroke DVT—deep venous thrombosis In-TIME—Intravenous n-PA for Treatment of Infarcting Myocardium Early PA—plasminogen activator PAI—plasminogen activator inhibitor PAO—peripheral arterial occlusion PE—pulmonary embolism PROACT—Prolyse in Acute Cerebral Thromboembolism

major, the drug may have to be discontinued. The risk of intracerebral or subdural hematoma is greater with warfarin than with heparin, particularly in patients older than 50 years. If there is any sign of hemorrhage, the next anticoagulant dose should be withheld and the INR measured. For continued or serious bleeding, 5 to 10 mg of vitamin K_1 oxide (phytonadione) I.V. is effective. Several hours may pass before hemostasis improves significantly, and 24 hours or longer may be needed for maximal effect. If immediate restoration of hemostatic competence is necessary, levels of vitamin K–dependent coagulation factors can be raised by giving fresh frozen plasma, 10 to 20 ml/kg body weight, or prothrombin complex concentrate.[92]

Administration of warfarin during pregnancy can cause birth defects and abortion and therefore is contraindicated. Warfarin-induced skin necrosis is a rare complication of oral anticoagulant therapy.[86] This syndrome, characterized by the appearance of skin lesions shortly after initiation of treatment , may be the result of a transient hypercoagulable state caused by depletion of the natural anticoagulants (proteins C and S) before the onset of warfarin's effect. To mitigate the initial hypercoagulable state, some advocate starting warfarin therapy only after initial heparinization.

LYTIC THERAPY

A number of lytic agents are currently being studied [see Table 5]. Generally, however, lytic therapy is understood to refer to administration of streptokinase, urokinase, or t-PA,[75,76,93–96] all of which act on the endogenous fibrinolytic system to convert plasminogen to plasmin [see 1:4 Bleeding and Transfusion]. Streptokinase combines with plasminogen to form streptokinase-plasminogen complexes that are converted to streptokinase-plasmin complexes, which then convert residual plasminogen to plasmin.[75,96] Urokinase directly cleaves a peptide bond in the plasminogen molecule to form plasmin. t-PA binds to fibrin via lysine binding sites at the N-terminal.

Lytic therapy is most effective when it can be initiated within hours. It is worth attempting when the clot has been present for less than 1 week, particularly if it has been present for less than 3 days. When lytic therapy is begun, heparin therapy usually is temporarily discontinued because of the theoretical possibility of increased bleeding risk; it may be resumed immediately upon completion of lytic therapy. If, however, the problem is immediately life-threatening (e.g., myocardial infarction or massive PE), anticoagulation should probably be done in parallel with lytic therapy to prevent rethrombosis.

Indications and Contraindications

The indications for lytic therapy are being extended.[92] Urokinase, t-PA, and, to a much lesser degree, streptokinase are being used for venous thrombotic conditions, such as symptomatic obstruction of major upper-extremity veins. The morbidity of axillary vein thrombosis can be considerable; clearance of clot may not only help restore patency but also help identify the underlying cause. In the lower extremities, more thorough clearance of clot should, in theory, help restore valve function and prevent so-called postphlebitic syndrome.[95,97]

Contraindications to lytic therapy include surgery in the previous 10 days, serious GI bleeding in the previous 3 months, a history of hypertension, an active bleeding or hemorrhagic disorder, a previous cerebrovascular accident, and an active intracranial process. As with heparin, the risk of intracranial bleeding is increased in older patients; the risk appears to be higher with t-PA than with streptokinase or urokinase.

Agents

Streptokinase Streptokinase is a 47 kd protein produced by β-hemolytic streptococci. Because it is not endogenous, circulating antibodies to it (from previous streptococcal infections) often are already present in plasma. When streptokinase is infused, a loading dose must be given to overcome these antibodies. Once the antibodies are depleted, the half-life of streptokinase is about 80 minutes. Achievement of the desired therapeutic effects is confirmed by documenting a rise in the thrombin time (TT), a fall in the fibrinogen level, or an abrupt rise in the D-dimer level. Because streptokinase may deplete circulating plasminogen after a few hours, the optimal approach may be to administer it for 6 hours by continuous infusion every 24 hours for 2 or 3 days, then to administer heparin in the intervals between infusions.

Urokinase Urokinase is a 34 kd globulin originally found in human urine and now isolated from cultured human cells. It has a half-life of 15 minutes and is metabolized by the liver. It was removed from the U.S. market for several years as a result of concerns expressed by the FDA, but it subsequently was reintroduced after these concerns were satisfactorily addressed. For catheter clearance, a solution containing 5,000 units/ml should be infused into the obstructed tubing. Urokinase is not fibrin-specific and therefore produces a systemic lytic state. Its primary disadvantage is that it costs far more than streptokinase.

t-PA Tissue plasminogen activator is an enzymatic glycoprotein composed of 527 amino acids that is produced from a human melanoma cell line by means of recombinant DNA technology. Its half-life is approximately 4 minutes; it is metabolized by the liver, and approximately 80% of the dose is excreted in the urine within 18 hours. It is not antigenic and does not promote antibody formation. Theoretically, t-PA should be somewhat more specific for fibrin clot than urokinase or streptokinase. In practice, however, its effects are clinically indistinguishable from those of urokinase. Like urokinase, t-PA is extremely expensive.

Technique of Administration

The traditional method of administering lytic therapy, venous infusion, is widely used to treat coronary artery thrombosis[98]; however, it is only modestly effective against peripheral arterial occlusion and is associated with a high rate of hemorrhagic complications.[99] Current methods focus more closely on the site of occlusion, particularly with the development of intra-arterial infusion techniques.

Lytic therapy for acute PE has attractive theoretical benefits; however, the FDA currently approves this approach only for patients with so-called massive PE (i.e., PE resulting in both shock and heart failure). Clinical trials demonstrated that in patients who were hemodynamically unstable as a result of PE, thrombolysis achieved greater improvements in intermediate end points (e.g., right ventricular function) than heparin alone did, though survival was not improved.[100] Subsequent studies evaluated recombinant t-PA in patients with so-called submassive PE, with similar results.[63]

Monitoring

Although monitoring of lytic therapy is less standardized than monitoring of anticoagulant therapy, several principles should be followed. The effects must be monitored from both a clinical and a laboratory perspective. Clinical monitoring involves following improvements on the angiograms. Laboratory monitoring has three components. First, D-dimer levels should be measured; a marked increase signals that cross-linked fibrin is undergoing breakdown. Second, adequate stores of plasminogen should be documented; without plasminogen, none of the thrombolytic drugs are effective. Third, fibrinogen levels should be followed to prevent exhaustion of native clotting; most authorities recommend that lytic therapy be discontinued once fibrinogen levels fall below 50 mg/dl. Previously, the TT was used for monitoring thrombolysis; today, however, given the recommendation for concurrent use of heparin,[98] the TT is considered to be of little value in this setting.

Complications

The major toxicity of all three major lytic agents is hemorrhage, resulting from (1) lysis of physiologic thrombi occurring at vascular injury sites and (2) a systemic lytic state caused by the systemic formation of plasmin. The incidence of bleeding is many times higher after lytic therapy than after anticoagulant therapy and is dependent on both the dosage and the duration of lytic therapy. Careful administration of lytic agents can keep the incidence of major hemorrhage below 5% and the incidence of intracranial hemorrhage below 1%.[96]

A potential major complication is distal embolism of partially lysed clot. In theory, this possibility should rule out lytic therapy for treating thrombus in the heart or in the cerebrovascular system.[96] Surprisingly, however, dislodgment of intracardiac clot as a result of lytic therapy is rare.

Streptokinase causes several adverse reactions that urokinase and t-PA do not. When first produced, streptokinase was associated with a very high incidence of antigenicity and severe pyrogenic reactions. The current purified formulation is relatively free of pyrogens and has a reduced incidence of allergic side effects, but it is still antigenic and may still cause allergic reactions or, in rare instances, anaphylaxis. Streptokinase may also induce the formation of additional antibodies that make re-treatment impossible. In contrast, retreatment with urokinase may be carried out as often as necessary with minimal risk of allergic reactions.

Hypercoagulability States

Certain patients seem to have a tendency to clot spontaneously. So-called hypercoagulability states were long thought to exist,

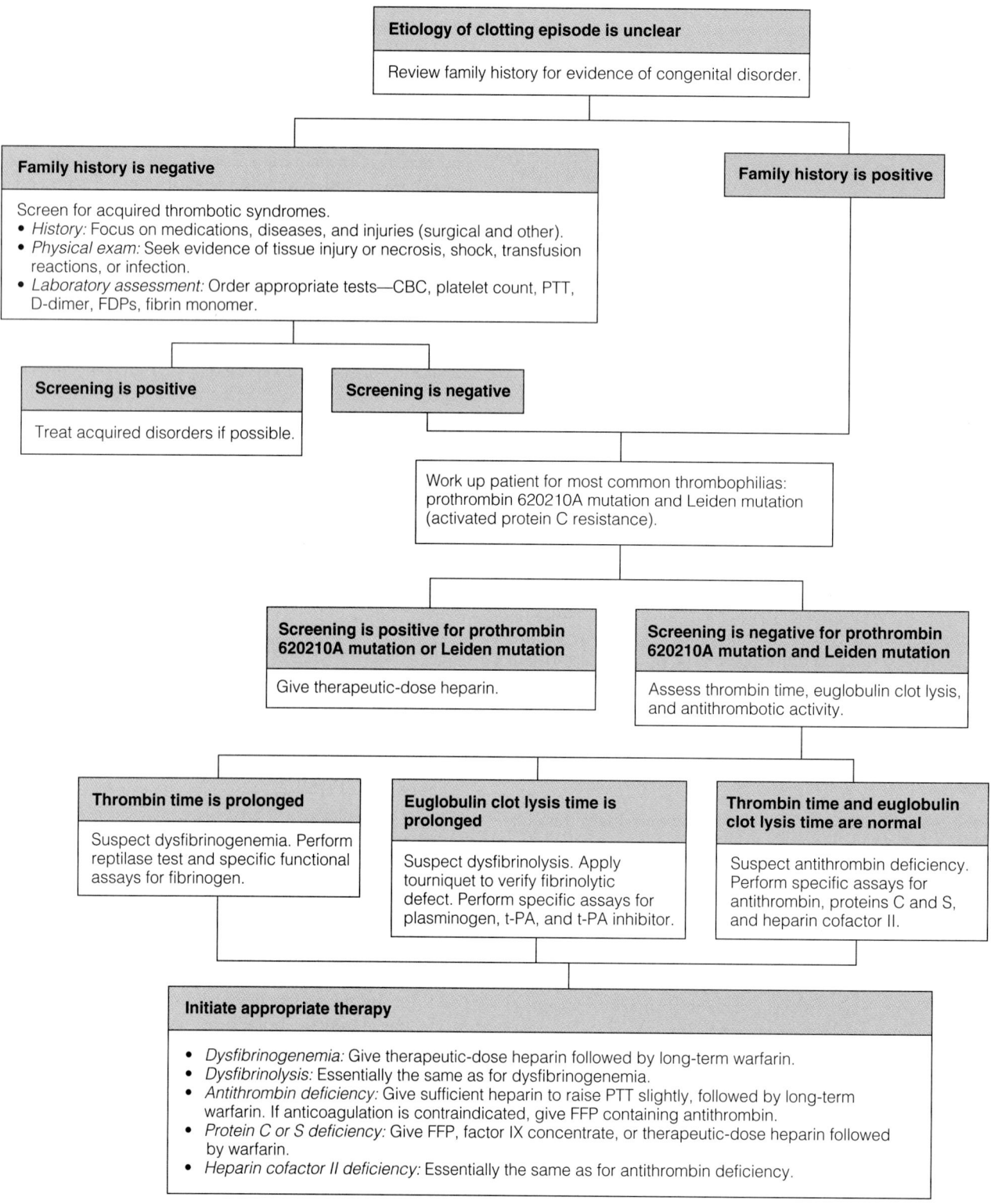

Figure 9 Shown is an algorithm for screening for acquired and congenital thrombotic syndromes.

but they were difficult to document except on clinical grounds. Currently, however, these clotting tendencies are better understood,[101] thanks in large part to recognition of the role of antithrombins. If an antithrombin deficiency exists and clotting goes unchecked, activation of a clotting cascade could theoretically progress to clotting throughout the entire vasculature. Another important development was the recognition that deficiencies of certain natural clot-removing substances in the blood may lead to a clinical thrombotic tendency. Both types of deficiency can be either acquired or congenital.

SCREENING

When the etiology of a clotting episode is unclear, the family history should be reviewed for evidence of a congenital disorder.

Table 6 Etiology of Acquired Hypercoagulability

Tissue and cellular damage
  Shock
  Trauma
  Surgery
  Tissue necrosis
  Transfusion necrosis
Drugs
  Estrogens
  Drug reactions and interactions
  Heparin platelet antibody
  Warfarin

Disease
  Blood dyscrasias
  Cancer
  Diabetes
  Homocystinuria
  Hyperlipidemia
  Presence of lupuslike anticoagulant
  Severe infection
Pregnancy

Even if the history is negative, the patient should be screened for both acquired and congenital disorders [*see Figure 9*].

Acquired Clotting Conditions

Screening for acquired clotting conditions [*see Table 6*] is based on the history, physical examination, and laboratory assessment. The history should include medications, diseases, and surgical procedures or other injuries.[102-104] Examination may disclose causes of hypercoagulability.[105] Soft tissue injury, for example, is a potent activator of the coagulation system. If the injury is severe enough, it may be capable of causing a severe acquired coagulopathy. The problem is usually obvious, but on occasion, detailed study may be necessary to identify tissue damage or ischemic injury to bowel or extremities. Hypovolemia—especially hypovolemic shock—markedly reduces clotting time: blood from a patient in profound shock may clot instantaneously in the syringe as it is being drawn. The breakdown of red cells in a hemolytic transfusion reaction can cause clotting. Severe infection, especially from gram-negative organisms, is a potent activator of coagulation.[106]

Of the acquired hypercoagulability syndromes, Trousseau syndrome is a particularly important condition for surgeons to recognize because it occurs in the surgical population (cancer patients) and must be treated with heparin (it is unresponsive to warfarin). It occurs when an adenocarcinoma secretes a protein recognized by the body as tissue factor, resulting in multiple episodes of venous thromboembolism over time (migratory thrombophlebitis). Simple depletion of vitamin K–dependent factors is ineffective. Patients should receive therapeutic-dose heparin indefinitely or until the cancer is brought into remission.[107]

Laboratory screening may facilitate diagnosis. A complete blood count may document the presence of polycythemia or leukemia. Thrombocythemia may be a manifestation of a hypercoagulable disorder, and thrombocytopenia after the administration of heparin raises the possibility of intravascular platelet aggregation. A prolonged aPTT is suggestive of lupuslike anticoagulant. Increased levels of D-dimers, FDPs, or fibrin monomers in the plasma may reflect low-grade intravascular coagulation.

Congenital Clotting Conditions

Congenital clotting tendencies can result from deficiencies in inhibitors of thrombosis (antithrombin, proteins C and S, and possibly heparin cofactor II), dysfibrinogenemias, or dysfibrinolysis [*see Table 7*]. Most congenital clotting defects are transmitted as an autosomal dominant trait. A negative family history does not

preclude inherited thrombophilia, because the defects have a low penetrance and fresh mutations may have occurred.

INITIAL LABORATORY ASSESSMENT

Initial evaluation of a patient with an unexplained thrombotic episode should be directed at the most common causes of hypercoagulability. Acquired causes of clotting are more commonly seen by surgeons than congenital causes and therefore must be excluded first. If a clotting disorder is determined to be congenital, a laboratory workup should be undertaken. Several of the relevant assays (see below)—specifically, the functional assays—should be performed after the acute phase of the disorder has passed. If they are performed during the acute phase, levels of several antithrombotics (e.g., antithrombin and proteins C and S) will be misleadingly low—not because deficiencies of these substances caused the underlying thrombotic process but because they were consumed in that process.

SPECIFIC CAUSES OF THROMBOTIC TENDENCY

The most common congenital causes of accelerated clotting are mutations of prothrombin (prothrombin G20210A mutation) and factor V (Leiden mutation, or activated protein C resistance).[108-110] The prevalence of each these each ranges from 1% to 5% in the general population and may be much higher in specific ethnic subpopulations.[111] Each mutation may be identified conclusively by means of polymerase chain reaction (PCR) techniques. Detection of these mutations, unlike assays for antithrombin and proteins C and S, is not dependent on the patient's current inflammatory state. It must be remembered that the presence of one of these mutations, especially in the heterozygous form, does not imply that it is the sole cause of thrombosis. In many patients, a second precipitating factor must be present for the pathologic genetic thrombotic potential to be manifested.

Prothrombin G20210A Mutation

The prothrombin G20210A mutation is known to involve a single amino acid substitution in the prothrombin gene, but precisely how this increases the risk of venous thromboembolism is unclear. The one apparent manifestation of the mutation is a 15% to 40% increase in circulating prothrombin. Regardless of the mechanism at work, patients who are at least heterozygous for the trait are at two- to sixfold greater risk for venous thromboembolism than those without the mutation.[112]

Resistance to Activated Protein C (Factor V Leiden)

Resistance of human clotting factors to inactivation by activated protein C is believed to be the most common inherited proco-

---

Table 7 Congenital Clotting Disorders

Prothrombin G20210A mutation
Activated protein C resistance (Leiden V mutation)
Antithrombin deficiency
Proteins C and S deficiency
Dysfibrinogenemias
Dysfibrinolysis
  Hypoplasminogenemia
  Impaired release of t-PA
  High levels of t-PA inhibitor
  Factor XII deficiency

agulant disorder.[108] Normally, activated factor V is degraded by activated protein C in the presence of membrane surface as part of normal regulation of thrombosis. Activated protein C resistance is caused by a single substitution mutation in the factor V gene, which is passed in an autosomal dominant fashion. The mutant factor V that results, termed factor V Leiden, is resistant to inactivation by activated protein C and thus has a greater ability to activate thrombin and accelerate clotting.

Two techniques are commonly used to diagnose this disorder. The first is a functional assay that compares a standard aPTT to one performed in the presence of exogenous activated protein C. If the latter aPTT does not exhibit significant prolongation, the patient is probably resistant to activated protein C. The results of this assay must be interpreted with caution if the patient is still in the acute phase of the illness. The second technique, which is more reliable, involves direct detection of the mutation via PCR analysis of DNA.

Antithrombin Deficiency

Antithrombin (once termed antithrombin III) is a 65 kd protein that decelerates the coagulation system by inactivating activated factors—primarily factor Xa and thrombin but also factors XII, XI, and IX.[113,114] Antithrombin therefore acts as a scavenger of activated clotting factors. Its activity is enhanced 100-fold by the presence of heparans on the endothelial surface and 1,000-fold by administration of exogenous heparin.

Congenital antithrombin deficiency occurs in approximately 0.01% to 0.05% of the general population and 2% to 4% of patients with venous thrombosis.[113] The trait is passed on as an autosomal dominant trait, with the heterozygous genotype being incompatible with life. Antithrombin-deficient patients are at increased risk for thromboembolism when their antithrombin activity falls below 70% of normal.[115]

Patients with congenital antithrombin deficiency frequently present after a stressful event. They usually have DVT but sometimes have PE. If anticoagulation is not contraindicated, the treatment of choice is heparin at a dosage sufficient to raise the aPTT to the desired level, followed by warfarin. If anticoagulation is contraindicated (as it is during the peripartum period), antithrombin concentrate should be given to raise the antithrombin activity to 80% to 120% of normal during the period when anticoagulants cannot be given.

Acquired antithrombin deficiency is a well-recognized entity. In most patients undergoing severe systemic stress, antithrombin levels fall below normal.[116] Patients with classic risk factors for venous thromboembolism tend to have the lowest levels.

Protein C and Protein S Deficiency

Protein C is a 62 kd glycoprotein with a half-life of 6 hours. Because it is vitamin K dependent, a deficiency will develop in the absence of vitamin K. Acquired protein C deficiency is seen in liver disease, malignancy, infection, the postoperative state, and disseminated intravascular coagulation.[46] Protein C deficiency occurs in approximately 4% to 5% of patients younger than 40 to 45 years who present with unexplained venous thrombosis.[117] It is transmitted as an autosomal dominant trait, and the family history is usually positive for a clotting tendency. Protein C levels range from 70% to 164% of normal in patients without a clotting tendency; levels below 70% of normal are associated with a thrombotic tendency. The most appropriate tests for screening are functional assays; there are cases of dysfunctional protein C deficiency in which protein C antigen levels are normal but protein C activity is low, and these would not be detected by the usual immunoassays.

Protein S is a vitamin K–dependent protein that acts as a cofactor for activated protein C by enhancing protein C–induced inactivation of activated factor V. The incidence of protein S deficiency is similar to that of protein C deficiency.[117] It is transmitted as a dominant trait, and the family history is often positive for a thrombotic tendency.

Hyperhomocysteinemia

Although hyperhomocysteinemia is more commonly associated with cardiac disease and arterial thrombosis, it may also be associated with an increased incidence of venous thromboembolism.[118] This association is not as strong as those already discussed (see above). Accordingly, anticoagulation of asymptomatic patients with elevated homocysteine levels is not currently recommended.

Dysfibrinogenemia

More than 100 qualitative abnormalities of fibrinogen (dysfibrinogenemias) have been reported.[119] Dysfibrinogenemias are inherited in an autosomal dominant manner, with most patients being heterozygous. Most patients with dysfibrinogenemia have either no clinical symptoms or symptoms of a bleeding disorder; a minority (about 11%) have clinical features of a recurrent thromboembolic disorder.[120,121] Congenital dysfibrinogenemias associated with thrombosis account for about 1% of cases of unexplained venous thrombosis occurring in young people. The most commonly observed functional defect in such dysfibrinogenemias is abnormal fibrin monomer polymerization combined with resistance to fibrinolysis. Decreased binding of plasminogen and increased resistance to lysis by plasmin have been noted.

In addition to a prolonged TT, patients who have dysfibrinogenemia associated with thromboembolism may have a prolonged INR. The diagnosis is confirmed if the reptilase time is also prolonged. Measured with clotting techniques, fibrinogen levels may be slightly or moderately low; measured immunologically, levels may be normal or even increased.

Dysfibrinolysis

Fibrinolysis can be impaired by inherited deficiencies of plasminogen, defective release of t-PA from the vascular endothelium, and high plasma levels of regulatory proteins (e.g., t-PA inhibitors).[121,122] In addition, factor XII (contact factor) deficiency may induce failure of fibrinolysis activation.

Inherited plasminogen deficiency is probably only rarely responsible for unexplained DVT in young patients. It is transmitted as an autosomal dominant trait. In heterozygous persons with a thrombotic tendency, plasminogen activity is about one half normal (3.9 to 8.4 μmol/ml). The euglobulin clot lysis time is prolonged. Functional assays should be carried out, and there should be full transformation of plasminogen into plasmin activators.

The important role of t-PA inhibitors I and II in the regulation of fibrinolysis is well defined.[122,123] In normal plasma, t-PA inhibitor I is the primary inhibitor for both t-PA and urokinase. Release of t-PA inhibitor I by platelets results in locally increased concentrations where platelets accumulate. The ensuing local inhibition of fibrinolysis may help stabilize the hemostatic plug. t-PA inhibitor II is present in and secreted by monocytes and macrophages.

Factor XII deficiency is a rare cause of impaired fibrinolysis. Initial contact activation of factor XII not only results in activation of the clotting cascade and of the inflammatory response but also leads to plasmin generation. This intrinsic activation of fibrinolysis requires factor XII, prekallikrein, and high-molecular-weight kininogen. Patients with factor XII deficiencies can be identified by a prolonged aPTT in the absence of clinical bleeding.[101,124]

TREATMENT

Treatment of a clinical hypercoagulable state involves both prophylaxis [see Prophylaxis against Thromboembolism, above] and specific treatment.[125] Prophylaxis in postoperative patients consists primarily of maintaining good hydration, ensuring normal cardiac output, and early mobilization. Low-dose heparin, intermittent pneumatic compression, low-molecular-weight dextran, or some combination of these may also be appropriate.

Patients with activated protein C resistance who present with venous thrombosis should be treated with heparin in the standard fashion. They also should receive genetic counseling and refrain from using oral contraceptives.

Treatment of antithrombin deficiency associated with active clotting involves initiating heparin anticoagulation at a dosage sufficient to ensure a significant rise in the aPTT. Warfarin is the drug of choice for long-term prophylaxis and should be given at a dosage sufficient to maintain an INR of 2.0 to 3.0. When anticoagulation is contraindicated, a purified form of antithrombin may be administered directly. Patients with acquired antithrombin deficiency should receive prophylaxis in the form of heparin at a dosage sufficient to raise the aPTT 5 seconds above the upper limit of the normal laboratory value.

Treatment of clotting states related to protein C or protein S deficiency involves administering fresh frozen plasma or factor IX concentrate. Therapeutic-dose heparin followed by warfarin may be appropriate for long-term treatment.

Treatment of thromboembolism associated with dysfibrinogenemia involves therapeutic-dose heparin followed by long-term warfarin. Treatment of thromboembolic disorders associated with dysfibrinolysis is essentially the same as that of dysfibrinogenemia. Some patients with these qualitative plasminogen defects and acute massive thrombotic events may not respond to fibrinolytic treatment with urokinase or streptokinase.

References

1. Dunmire SM: Pulmonary embolism. Emerg Med Clin North Am 7:339, 1989
2. Shackford SR, Moser KM: Deep venous thrombosis and pulmonary embolism in trauma patients. J Intensive Care Med 3:87, 1988
3. Hirsh J, Hull RD: Venous Thromboembolism: Natural History, Diagnosis, and Management. CRC Press, Boca Raton, Florida, 1988
4. Bergqvist D: Postoperative Thromboembolism: Frequency, Etiology, Prophylaxis. Springer-Verlag, New York, 1983
5. Kakkar VV, Stringer MD: Prophylaxis of venous thromboembolism. World J Surg 14:670, 1990
6. Bell WR, Simon TL: Current status of pulmonary thromboembolic disease: pathophysiology, diagnosis, prevention and treatment. Am Heart J 103:239, 1982
7. Sabiston DC Jr: Pathophysiology, diagnosis and management of pulmonary embolism. Am J Surg 138:384, 1979
8. Dalen JE, Haffajee CI, Alpert JS 3rd, et al: Pulmonary embolism, pulmonary hemorrhage and pulmonary infarction. N Engl J Med 296:1431, 1977
9. Kakkar VV, Corrigan TP, Fossard DP, et al: Prevention of Fatal Postoperative pulmonary embolism by low doses of heparin. Reappraisal of results of international multicentre trial. Lancet 1:567, 1977
10. Prevention of venous thrombosis and pulmonary embolism. NIH Consensus Development. JAMA 256:744, 1986
11. Blaisdell FW: Preventing postoperative thromboembolism. West J Med 151:188, 1989
12. Reilly DT: Prophylactic methods against thromboembolism. Acta Chir Scand Suppl 550(suppl):115, 1989
13. Knudson MM, Lewis FR, Clinton A, et al: Prevention of venous thromboembolism in trauma patients. J Trauma 37:480, 1994
14. Christen Y, Wutschert R, Weimer D, et al: Effects of intermittent pneumatic compression on venous haemodynamics and fibrinolytic activity. Blood Coagul Fibrinol 8:185, 1997
15. Comerota AJ, Chouhan V, Harada RN, et al: The fibrinolytic effects of intermittent pneumatic compression: mechanism of enhanced fibrinolysis. Ann Surg 226:306, 1997
16. Elliott CG, Dudney TM, Egger M, et al: Calf-thigh sequential pneumatic compression compared with plantar venous pneumatic compression to prevent deep-vein thrombosis after non-lower extremity trauma. J Trauma 47:25, 1999
17. Rosenberg RD: Action and interactions of antithrombin and heparin. N Engl J Med 292:145, 1975
18. Leyvraz PF, Richard J, Bachmann F, et al: Adjusted versus fixed-dose subcutaneous heparin in the prevention of deep-vein thrombosis after total hip replacement. N Engl J Med 309:954, 1983
19. Owings JT, Blaisdell FW: Low-dose heparin thromboembolism prophylaxis. Arch Surg 131:1069, 1996
20. Turpie AG, Levine MN, Hirsh J, et al: A randomized controlled trial of a low-molecular-weight heparin (enoxaparin) to prevent deep-vein thrombosis in patients undergoing elective hip surgery. N Engl J Med 315:925, 1986
21. Levine MN, Hirsh J, Gent M, et al: Prevention of deep vein thrombosis after elective hip surgery: a randomized trial comparing low molecular weight heparin with standard unfractionated heparin. Ann Intern Med 114:545, 1991
22. Geerts WH, Jay RM, Code KI, et al: A comparison of low-dose heparin with low-molecular-weight heparin as prophylaxis against venous thromboembolism after major trauma. N Engl J Med 335:701, 1996
23. Eriksson BI, Bauer KA, Lassen MR, et al: Steering Committee of the Pentasaccharide in Hip-Fracture Surgery Study: Fondaparinux compared with enoxaparin for the prevention of venous thromboembolism after hip-fracture surgery. N Engl J Med 345:1298, 2001
24. Bauer KA, Eriksson BI, Lassen MR, et al: Steering Committee of the Pentasaccharide in Major Knee Surgery Study: Fondaparinux compared with enoxaparin for the prevention of venous thromboembolism after elective major knee surgery. N Engl J Med 345:1305, 2001
25. MacCallum PK, Thomson JM, Poller L: Effects of fixed minidose warfarin on coagulation and fibrinolysis following major gynaecological surgery. Thromb Haemost 64:511, 1990
26. Decousus H, Leizorovicz, A, Parent F, et al: A clinical trial of vena caval filters in the prevention of pulmonary embolism in patients with proximal deep-vein thrombosis. N Engl J Med 338:409, 1998
27. Belcaro G, Nicolaides AN, Errichi BM, et al: Superficial thrombophlebitis of the legs: a randomized, controlled, follow-up study. Angiology 50:523, 1999
28. Geerts WH, Code KI, Jay RM, et al: A prospective study of venous thromboembolism after major trauma. N Engl J Med 331:1601, 1994
29. Owings JT, Gosselin RC, Battistella FD, et al: Whole blood D-dimer assay: an effective non-invasive method to rule out pulmonary embolism. J Trauma 48:795, 2000
30. Owings JT, Gosselin RC, Anderson JT, et al: Practical utility of the whole blood D-dimer assay for excluding thromboembolism in severely injured trauma patients. J Trauma 51:425, 2001
31. Gosselin RC, Owings JT, Jacoby RC, et al: Evaluation of a new automated quantitative d-dimer, Advanced D-Dimer, in patients suspected of venous thromboembolism. Blood Coag Fibrinol 13:323, 2002
32. Bergqvist D, Bergentz SE: Diagnosis of deep vein thrombosis. World J Surg 14:679, 1990
33. Hirsh J: Reliability of non-invasive tests for the diagnosis of venous thrombosis (editorial). Thromb Haemost 65:221, 1991
34. Krupski WC, Bass A, Dilley RB, et al: Propagation of deep venous thrombosis identified by duplex ultrasonography. J Vasc Surg 12:467, 1990
35. Lensing AW, Prandoni P, Brandjes D: Detection of deep-vein thrombosis by real-time B-mode ultrasonography. N Engl J Med 320:342, 1989
36. Haire WD, Lynch TG, Lund GB: Limitations of magnetic resonance imaging and ultrasound directed (duplex) scanning in the diagnosis of subclavian vein thrombosis. J Vasc Surg 13:391, 1991
37. Barnes RW, Nix ML, Barnes CL: Perioperative asymptomatic venous thrombosis: role of duplex scanning versus venography. J Vasc Surg 9:25, 1989
38. Simonneau G, Sors H, Charbonnier B, et al: A comparison of low-molecular-weight heparin with unfractionated heparin for acute pulmonary embolism. The THESEE Study Group. Tinzaparine ou Heparine Standard: Evaluations dans l'Embolie Pulmonaire. N Engl J Med 337:663, 1997
39. Low-molecular-weight heparin in the treatment of patients with venous thromboembolism. The Columbus Investigators. N Engl J Med 337:657, 1997

40. Hirsh J, Turpie AG: Use of plasminogen activators in venous thrombosis. World J Surg 14:688, 1990

41. Sakakibara Y, Shigeta O, Ishikawa S, et al: Upper extremity vein thrombosis: etiologic categories, precipitating causes, and management. Angiology 50:547, 1999

42. DiFelice GS, Paletta GA Jr, Phillips BB, et al: Effort thrombosis in the elite throwing athlete. Am J Sports Med 30:708, 2002

43. Schmacht DC, Back MR, Novotney ML, et al: Primary axillary-subclavian venous thrombosis: is aggressive surgical intervention justified? Vasc Surg 35:353, 2001

44. Wells PS, Forster AJ: Thrombolysis in deep vein thrombosis: is there still an indication? Thromb Haemost 86:499, 2001

45. Patel NH, Plorde JJ, Meissner M: Catheter-directed thrombolysis in the treatment of phlegmasia cerulea dolens. Ann Vasc Surg 12:471, 1998

46. Lord RS, Chen FC, DeVine TJ, et al: Surgical treatment of acute deep venous thrombosis. World J Surg 14:694, 1990

47. LeClerk JR: Venous Thromboembolic Disorders. Lea & Febiger, Philadelphia, 1991, pp 54, 176

48. Smith GT, Dammin GJ, Dexter L: Postmortem arteriographic studies of the human lung in pulmonary embolization. JAMA 188:143, 1964

49. Goldhaber SZ, Hennekens CH, Evans DA, et al: Factors associated with correct antemortem diagnosis of major pulmonary embolism. Am J Med 73:822, 1982

50. Karwinski B, Svendsen E: Comparison of clinical and postmortem diagnosis of pulmonary embolism. J Clin Pathol 42:135, 1989

51. Moser KM, Hull R, Saltzman HA, et al: Recent advances in diagnosis of pulmonary embolism and deep venous thrombosis. Am Rev Respir Dis 138:1046, 1988

52. Coon WW: Risk factors in pulmonary embolism. Surg Gynecol Obstet 143:385, 1976

53. Boneu B, Bes G, Pelzer H, et al: D-dimers, thrombin antithrombin III complexes and prothrombin fragments 1 + 2 diagnostic value in clinically suspected deep vein thrombosis. Thromb Haemost 65:28, 1991

54. Owings JT, Kraut EJ, Battistella FD, et al: Timing of the occurrence of pulmonary embolism in trauma patients. Arch Surg 132:862, 1997

55. Killewich LA, Nunnelee JD, Auer AI: Value of lower extremity venous duplex examination in the diagnosis of pulmonary embolism. J Vasc Surg 17:934, 1993

56. PIOPED Investigators: Value of ventilation/perfusion scan in acute pulmonary embolism: results of prospective investigation of pulmonary embolism diagnosis (PIOPED). JAMA 263:2753, 1990

57. Hull RD, Hirsh J, Carter CJ, et al: Diagnostic value of ventilation-perfusion lung scanning in patients with suspected pulmonary embolism. Chest 88:819, 1985

58. Remy-Jardin M, Remy J, Deschildre F, et al: Diagnosis of pulmonary embolism with spiral CT: comparison with pulmonary angiography and scintigraphy. Radiology 200:699, 1996

59. Drucker EA, Rivitz SM, Shepard JA, et al: Acute pulmonary embolism: assessment of helical CT for diagnosis. Radiology 209:235, 1998

60. Hull RD, Raskob GE, Hirsh J: The diagnosis of clinically suspected pulmonary embolism: practical approaches. Chest 89:4175, 1986

61. Ferris EJ, Holder JC, Lim WN, et al: Angiography of pulmonary emboli: digital studies and balloon-occlusion cineangiography. Am J Roentgenol 142:369, 1984

62. Anderson JT, Jeng, T, Bain M, et al: Diagnosis of post traumatic pulmonary embolism: is chest computed tomographic angiography acceptable? J Trauma 54:472, 2003

63. Konstantinides S, Geibel A, Heusel G, et al; Management Strategies and Prognosis of Pulmonary Embolism-3 Trial Investigators. Heparin plus alteplase compared with heparin alone in patients with submassive pulmonary embolism. N Engl J Med 347:1143, 2002

64. Atik M, Broghamer WL Jr: The impact of prophylactic measures on fatal pulmonary embolism. Arch Surg 114:366, 1979

65. Collins R, Scrimgeour A, Yusuf S, et al: Reduction in fatal pulmonary embolism and venous thrombosis by perioperative administration of subcutaneous heparin: overview of results of randomized trials in general, orthopedic, and urologic surgery. N Engl J Med 318:1162, 1988

66. Geerts WH: Pulmonary embolism. Conn's Current Therapy 1992. Rakel RE, Ed. WB Saunders Co, Philadelphia, 1992, p 179

67. Moser KM: State of the art: pulmonary embolism. Am Rev Respir Dis 115:829, 1977

68. Thomas DP: Therapeutic role of heparin in acute pulmonary embolism. Curr Ther Res 18:21, 1975

69. Silver D: Pulmonary embolism: prevention, detection and nonoperative management. Surg Clin North Am 54:1089, 1974

70. Rohrer MJ, Scheidler MG, Wheeler HB, et al: Extended indications for placement of an inferior vena cava filter. J Vasc Surg 10:44, 1989

71. Fink JA, Jones BT: The Greenfield filter as the primary means of therapy in venous thromboembolic disease. Surg Gynecol Obstet 172:253, 1991

72. Wells I: Inferior vena cava filters and when to use them. Clin Radiol 40:11, 1989

73. Schmitz-Rode T, Janssens U, Duda SH, et al: Massive pulmonary embolism: percutaneous emergency treatment by pigtail rotation catheter. J Am Coll Cardiol 36:375, 2000

74. Rooke TW: Deep venous thrombosis of the extremities. Conn's Current Therapy 1992. Rakel RE, Ed. WB Saunders Co, Philadelphia, 1992, p 289

75. Majerus PW, Broze GJ Jr, Miletich JP, et al: Anticoagulant, thrombolytic and antiplatelet drugs. Goodman & Gilman's The Pharmacological Basis of Therapeutics. Goodman AG, Rall TW, Nies AS, et al, Eds. Pergamon Press, New York, 1990, p 1311

76. USP DI, Drug Information for the Health Care Professional, vol IB. The United States Pharmacopeial Convention, Inc, Rockville, Maryland, 1992, pp 1505, 2357, 2658

77. Owen CA Jr, Bowie EJ, et al: Chronic intravascular coagulation syndromes: a summary. Mayo Clin Proc 49:673, 1974

78. Blaisdell FW, Graziano CJ, Effeney DJ: In vivo assessment of anticoagulation. Surgery 82:827, 1977

79. Blaisdell FW, Steele M, Allen RE: Management of acute lower extremity arterial ischemia due to embolism and thrombosis. Surgery 84:822, 1978

80. Blaisdell FW, Graziano CJ: Assessment of clotting by the determination of fibrinogen catabolism. Am J Surg 135:436, 1978

81. Conti S, Daschbach M, Blaisdell FW: A comparison of high-dose versus conventional-dose heparin therapy for deep vein thrombosis. Surgery 92:972, 1982

82. Kashtan J, Conti S, Blaisdell FW: Heparin therapy for deep venous thrombosis. Am J Surg 140:836, 1980

83. Ridker PM, Goldhaber SZ, Danielson E, et al, for the PREVENT Investigators: Long-term, low-intensity warfarin therapy for the prevention of recurrent venous thromboembolism. N Engl J Med 348:TK, 2003

84. Silver D, Kapsch DN, Tsoi EK: Heparin induced thrombocytopenia, thrombosis and hemorrhage. Ann Surg 198:301, 1983

85. Becker PS, Miller VT: Heparin-induced thrombocytopenia. Stroke 20:1449, 1989

86. Celoria GM, Steingart RH, Banson B, et al: Coumarin skin necrosis in a patient with heparin-induced thrombocytopenia: a case report. Angiology 39:915, 1988

87. Walker AM, Jick H: Predictors of bleeding during heparin therapy. JAMA 244:1209, 1980

88. Mudaliar JH, Liem TK, Nichols WK, et al: Lepirudin is a safe and effective anticoagulant for patients with heparin-associated antiplatelet antibodies. J Vasc Surg 34:17, 2001

89. Ginsberg JS, Kowalchuk G, Hirsh J, et al: Heparin effect on bone density. Thromb Haemost 64:286, 1990

90. Hirsh J, Poller L, Deykin D, et al: Optimal therapeutic range for oral anticoagulants. Chest 95(2 suppl):5s, 1989

91. Pinede L, Ninet J, Duhaut P, et al; Investigators of the "Duree Optimale du Traitement Anti-Vitamines K" (DOTAVK) Study. Comparison of 3 and 6 months of oral anticoagulant therapy after a first episode of proximal deep vein thrombosis or pulmonary embolism and comparison of 6 and 12 weeks of therapy after isolated calf deep vein thrombosis. Circulation 103:2453, 2001

92. Yasaka M, Minematsu K, Naritomi H, et al: Predisposing factors for enlargement of intracerebral hemorrhage in patients treated with warfarin. Thromb Haemost 89:278, 2003

93. Blaisdell FW: Hemostasis and thrombosis. Vascular Surgery: A Comprehensive Review, 2nd ed. Moore WS, Ed. Grune & Stratton, New York, 1986, p 909

94. Meyerovitz MF, Goldhaber SZ, Reagan K, et al: Recombinant tissue-type plasminogen activator versus urokinase in peripheral arterial and graft occlusions: a randomized trial. Radiology 175:75, 1990

95. Turpie AG: Thrombolytic agents in venous thrombosis. J Vasc Surg 12:196, 1990

96. Marder VJ, Sherry S: Thrombolytic therapy: current status. N Engl J Med 318:1585, 1988

97. Goldhaber SZ, Buring JE, Lipnick RJ, et al: Pooled analyses of randomized trials of streptokinase and heparin in phlebographically documented acute deep venous thrombosis. Am J Med 76:393, 1984

98. The effects of tissue plasminogen activator, streptokinase, or both on coronary-artery patency, ventricular function, and survival after acute myocardial infarction. The GUSTO Angiographic Investigators. N Engl J Med 329:1615, 1993

99. Amery A, Deloof W, Vermylen J, et al: Outcome of recent thromboembolic occlusions of limb arteries treated with streptokinase. Br Med J 4:639, 1970

100. Meyer GJ, Sors H, Charbonnier B, et al: Effects of intravenous urokinase versus alteplase on total pulmonary resistance in acute massive pulmonary embolism: a European multicenter double-blind trial. The European Cooperative Study Group for Pulmonary Embolism. J Am Coll Cardiol 19:239, 1992

101. Schafer AI: The hypercoagulable states. Ann Intern Med 102:814, 1985

102. Baehner RL: Alterations in blood coagulation with trauma. Pediatr Clin North Am 22:289, 1975

103. Jansson IG, Hetland O, Rammer LM, et al: Effects of phospholipase C, a tissue thrombo-

plastin inhibitor, on pulmonary microembolism after missile injury of the limb. J Trauma 28:S222, 1988

104. Effeney DJ, McIntyre KS, Blaisdell FW, et al: Fibrinogen kinetics in major human burns. Surg Forum 29:56, 1978

105. Blaisdell FW: Acquired and congenital clotting syndromes. World J Surg 14:664, 1990

106. Hauptman JG, Hassouna HI, Bell TG, et al: Efficacy of antithrombin III in endotoxin induced disseminated intravascular coagulation. Circ Shock 25:111, 1988

107. Callander N, Rapaport SI: Trousseau's Syndrome. West J Med 158:364, 1993

108. Dahlbäck B, Carlsson M, Svensson PJ: Familial thrombophilia due to a previously unrecognized mechanism characterized by poor anticoagulant response to activated protein C: prediction of a cofactor to activated protein C. Proc Natl Acad Sci USA 90:1004, 1993

109. Bertina RM, Reitsma PH, Rosendaal FR, et al: Resistance to activated protein C and factor V Leiden as risk factors for venous thrombosis. Thromb Haemost 74:449, 1995

110. De Stefano V, Martinelli I, Mannucci PM, et al: The risk of recurrent deep venous thrombosis among heterozygous carriers of both factor V Leiden and the G20210A prothrombin mutation. N Engl J Med 341:801, 1999

111. Hessner MJ, Luhm RA, Pearson SL, et al: Prevalence of prothrombin G20210A, factor V G1691A (Leiden), and methylenetetrahydrofolate reductase (MTHFR) C677T in seven different populations determined by multiplex allele-specific PCR. Thromb Haemost 81:733, 1999

112. Marder VJ, Matei DE: Hereditary and aquired thrombophilic syndromes. Hemostasis and Thrombosis. Colman, Hirsch, Marder, et al, Eds. Lippincott Williams & Wilkins, Philadelphia, 2001

113. Egeberg O: Inherited antithrombin deficiency causing thrombophilia. Thromb Diath Haemorrhag 13:516, 1965

114. High KA: Antithrombin-III, protein-C, and protein-S: naturally occurring anticoagulant proteins. Arch Pathol Lab Med 112:28, 1988

115. Bauer KA, Goodman TL, Kass BL, et al: Elevated factor Xa activity in the blood of asymptomatic patients with congenital antithrombin deficiency. J Clin Invest 76:826, 1985

116. Owings JT, Bagley M, Gosselin R, et al: Effect of critical injury on plasma antithrombin activity: low antithrombin levels are associated with thromboembolic complications. J Trauma 41:396, 1996

117. Gladson CL, Scharrer I, Hach V, et al: The frequency of type I heterozygous protein-S and protein-C deficiency in 141 unrelated young patients with venous thrombosis. Thromb Haemost 59:18, 1988

118. den Heijer M, Koster T, Blom HJ, et al: Hyperhomocysteinemia as a risk factor for deep-vein thrombosis. N Engl J Med 334:759, 1996

119. Rocha E, Paramo JA, Aranda A, et al: Congenital dysfibrinogenemias: a review. Ric Clin Lab 15:205, 1985

120. Liu Y, Lyons RM, McDonagh J: Plasminogen San Antonio: an abnormal plasminogen with a more cathodic migration, decreased activation and associated thrombosis. Thromb Haemost 59:49, 1988

121. Nilsson IM, Ljungner H, Tengborn L: Two different mechanisms in patients with venous thrombosis and defective fibrinolysis: low concentration of plasminogen activator or increased concentration of plasminogen activator inhibitor. Br Med J 290:1453, 1985

122. Kruithof EK, Gudinchet A, Bachmann F: Plasminogen activator inhibitor 1 and plasminogen activator inhibitor 2 in various disease states. Thromb Haemost 59:7, 1988

123. Juhan-Vague I, Roul C, Alessi MC, et al: Increased plasminogen activator inhibitor activity in non insulin dependent diabetic patients—relationship with plasma insulin. Thromb Haemost 61:370, 1989

124. Rodgers GM, Shuman MA: Congenital thrombotic disorders. Am J Hematol 21:419, 1986

125. Blaisdell FW: What's new in clotting and anticoagulation. Progress in Vascular Surgery. Najarian JS, Delaney JP, Eds. Year Book Medical Publishers, Chicago, 1988, p 75

7 FUNDAMENTALS OF ENDOVASCULAR SURGERY

Jon Matsumura, M.D., F.A.C.S., and Joseph Vijungco, M.D.

Endovascular techniques are becoming an important part of vascular surgery. Ongoing technological advances are making it possible to treat a growing number of vascular diseases by minimally invasive means. To perform these new therapeutic techniques, it is necessary to possess certain basic endovascular skills. Accordingly, in what follows, we describe some of the fundamental techniques that a skilled vascular interventionalist must master.

Choice of Vascular Access Site

The initial step in endovascular surgery is selection of the vascular access site. Several choices are available. The ideal access vessel is large, close to the treatment site, free of disease, and only minimally tortuous. Such a vessel is least likely to be associated with complications.[1] For most endovascular interventions, the femoral artery is the preferred choice, though the axillary, brachial, subclavian, common carotid, and iliac arteries may also be used, as may the aorta (by direct puncture).

Before puncture, the vessel undergoes evaluation, including palpation to assess the strength of the pulse in comparison with the opposite side. A weak pulse suggests disease at or proximal to the area, and the vessel should therefore be used with caution. Preoperative assessment also includes noninvasive imaging (e.g., blood flow studies) to check for significant lesions. Finally, with any endovascular procedure, it is helpful to mark the peripheral pulses beforehand to provide reference points for possible subsequent complications.

Puncture of Artery

GENERAL TECHNICAL PRINCIPLES

Once the skin site has been prepared with drapes and towels, 1% lidocaine is infiltrated into the skin and the perivascular tissue. Besides providing anesthesia to the area, lidocaine helps prevent vasospasm.[2] The pain and discomfort from intradermal injection of lidocaine is caused by the low pH of commercially available preparations and can be reduced by adding sodium bicarbonate (1 ml of a 1 mEq/ml $NaHCO_3$ solution in 10 ml of 1% lidocaine).[3] A small nick should be made in the skin about 1 to 2 cm beyond the intended site of arterial entry and the subcutaneous tissue gently dissected with a clamp; this will allow smoother entry of the needle, the guide wire, the sheath, and the catheter.

There are two main methods of cannulating the artery with the needle [*see Figure 1*]: single-wall entry and double-wall entry. Certain principles apply to both methods. The needle is advanced at an angle of 45° to 60°. When it is within the subcutaneous tissue, it should proceed in a straight line: the needle tip is as sharp as a scalpel blade, and side-to-side movement may cause inadvertent laceration of a neurovascular structure. When a needle

must be repositioned, it should first be withdrawn into the subcutaneous tissue superficial to the intended target, then redirected along another course. If the needle becomes dulled as a result of contact with bone or other hard surfaces, it should be discarded and a new one used.

In the single-wall entry method, the needle is slowly moved toward the anterior wall of the vessel. The arterial pulsation can be felt through the shaft of the needle. Gentle pressure is applied, and the needle is advanced through the anterior wall only. It may be helpful to think of the arterial pulse wave as pushing the anterior artery onto the needle. The appearance of pulsatile flow confirms entry into the arterial lumen. The needle may be rotated or deflected slightly to optimize pulsatile back-bleeding. A guide wire can then be passed into the needle, and the needle can be removed.

The double-wall entry method involves a through-and-through puncture of both the anterior wall and the posterior wall of the vessel. A multipart needle is usually required. After the needle is advanced through both walls of the artery, the inner trocar is removed. The needle is then slowly withdrawn until arterial pulsation is noted. The needle is stabilized, and a guide wire is advanced through it into the artery. Once the guide wire is in place, the needle is removed.

Pulsations should be transmitted through the needle in a to-and-fro manner. If the pulsations are localized to one side or the other, the needle is either medial or lateral to the artery.[2] Once the needle is in the vessel, the flow pattern should be observed. A forceful but irregular spraying flow may indicate arterial stenosis in the vicinity of the needle. A barely pulsatile flow may signal occlusive disease, a subintimal location of the needle, or a venous puncture.[2] If the guide wire cannot be passed after access is obtained, the needle tip may be against the wall or against a plaque. Often, the situation can be remedied by making a small change in the needle's insertion angle or by withdrawing the needle slightly.

FEMORAL ARTERY PUNCTURE

As noted, the common femoral artery (CFA) is the vessel most commonly used for arterial access. It is generally quite well suited to this purpose, being readily accessible, fairly large, and easily compressible. CFA puncture facilitates study and treatment of a number of key structures, including the lower-extremity arteries, the abdominal aorta and its branches, the thoracic aorta, the brachiocephalic vessels, the coronary arteries, and the left ventricle. In addition, it is associated with a lower complication rate than puncture of other arteries.[1] The CFA should, however, be avoided when the patient is known to have severe iliofemoral occlusive disease, a local infection, a femoral artery aneurysm, or marked tortuosity of the iliac arteries that would preclude catheter placement or manipulation.

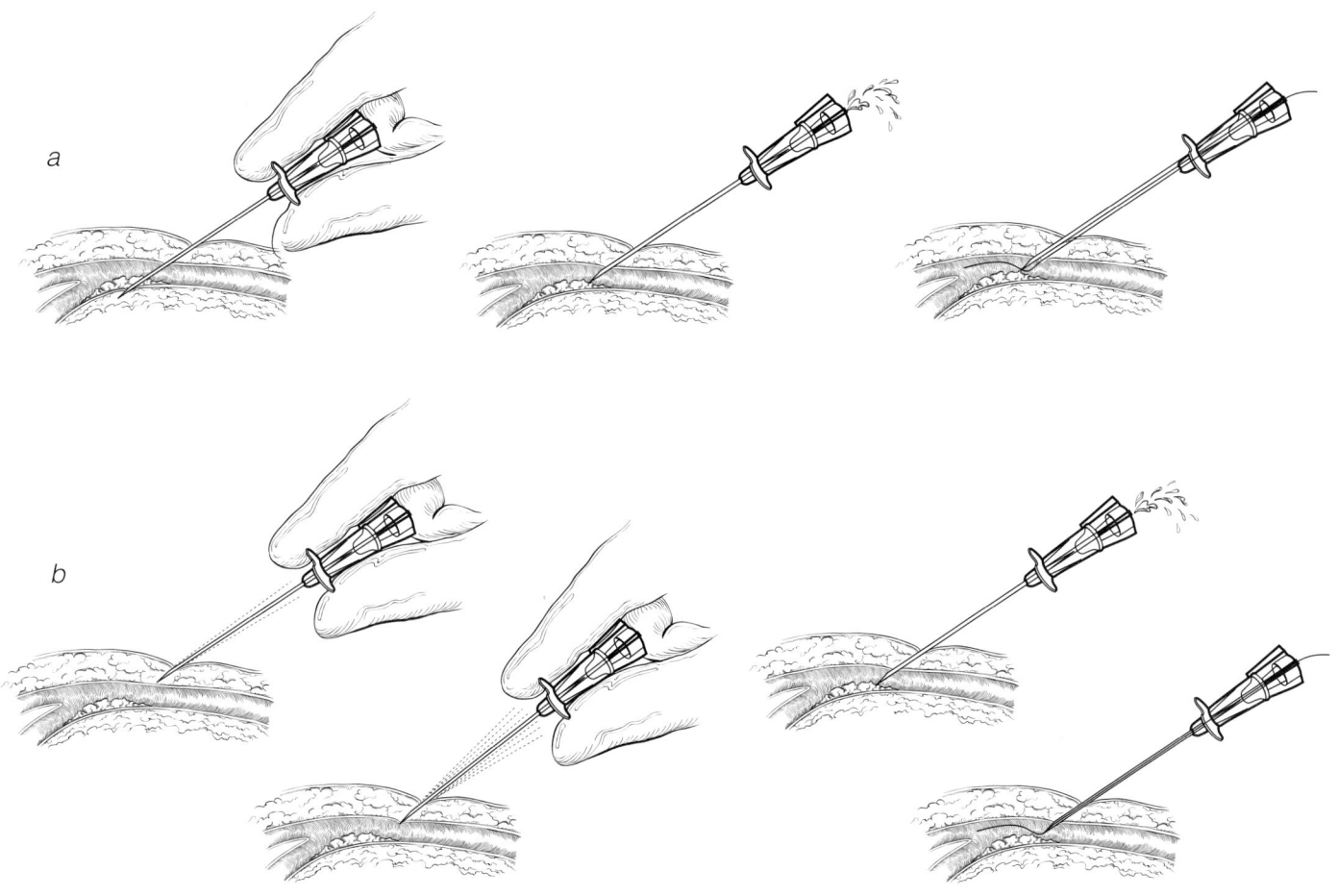

Figure 1 **Shown are the two methods of entry into an artery: (*a*) through-and-through puncture of both walls and (*b*) puncture of the anterior wall only.**

The CFA runs lateral to the common femoral vein and beneath the inguinal ligament. It may be localized by palpation just proximal to its bifurcation into the superficial femoral artery (SFA) and the profunda femoris (PF). The inguinal ligament, which runs from the anterior superior iliac spine to the pubic tubercle, is a convenient landmark for localization of the CFA, but these bony landmarks provide only a rough approximation of the location of the inguinal ligament. The CFA typically lies about two fingerbreadths lateral to the pubic tubercle along the line of the inguinal ligament. The artery should be punctured over the middle of the medial third of the femoral head [*see Figure 2*]. The window available for safe CFA puncture is small—only 3 to 5 cm.

There are several methods that can be used to localize the CFA in patients with difficult anatomy (e.g., those who have previously undergone groin surgery, those who are obese, and those who have a pulseless artery). The bony landmarks are even less reliable guides to the location of the inguinal ligament in these patients. According to a 1993 study, in the majority of cases, the position of the inguinal ligament is about 1 to 2 cm below where palpation would suggest it to be, and the average position of the ligament is approximately 1.5 cm superior to the midfemoral head.[4]

Fluoroscopy may help localize the CFA over the medial third of the femoral head. The chances of hitting the artery are maximized by aiming for the middle (craniocaudal) portion of the medial third of the femoral head. To minimize parallax errors, the femoral head should be centered in the image intensifier. The anatomic relations of the arteries in this area vary little with body habitus, gender, or age. A 1999 anatomic study showed that the CFA bifurcates into the SFA and the PF approximately 2 cm below the femoral head.[5] Occasionally, calcifications in the arteries may serve as landmarks for locating the CFA.

Another localization approach involves palpation of anatomic landmarks; this approach may be especially useful when the artery is pulseless.[6] With a finger placed immediately lateral to the pubic tubercle and inferior to the inguinal ligament, palpation is carried out to locate the point allowing the greatest degree of posterior depression. Anatomically, this point of maximal depression lies between the iliopsoas muscle laterally and the pectincus muscle medially. The common femoral vein lies in the floor of this depression, and the CFA lies 1.5 cm lateral to the depression.[6]

Ultrasonography has also proved useful for finding the CFA. The projection of choice with real-time ultrasonography is the transverse plane. The nonpalpable CFA is identified lateral to the compressible common femoral vein. Occasionally, the artery can be identified on the basis of sonographic shadowing from calcified atheromatous plaques.[7] A second ultrasound technique involves the use of a so-called smart needle, which has an ultrasound probe at its tip. The needle emits a signal as it approaches the artery, thereby giving notice of proximity to the vessel.

Another method of localizing and puncturing a pulseless CFA involves performing a contralateral femoral artery puncture, obtaining a diagnostic angiogram, and passing a guide wire over the aortic bifurcation and then antegrade through the iliac artery into the ipsilateral femoral artery.[8] Under fluoroscopy, the guide wire becomes a visible target for introduction of the needle into the pulseless CFA.

Troubleshooting

Anatomy textbooks typically describe the CFA as being lateral to the common femoral vein; however, one study showed that the CFA overlapped its corresponding vein in the anteroposterior plane 65% of the time.[5] Accordingly, attempts to puncture the CFA sometimes result in puncture of the common femoral vein, signaled by the appearance of dark, nonpulsatile venous blood. If this occurs, one should note the position of the original stick, move the needle 1 to 2 cm laterally, and reinsert the needle. At times, especially when pulse pressure is low, arterial blood may be dark and may resemble venous blood. If it is unclear whether the blood is coming from an artery or a vein, a small amount of contrast agent should be gently injected into the needle by hand so that its location can be confirmed.

If the puncture is done too high—that is, into the external iliac artery—there is an increased risk of potentially life-threatening retroperitoneal bleeding. Such bleeding should be suspected in any patient with an unexplained drop in the hemoglobin concentration or the hematocrit, hypotension, or flank pain. In addition, when the puncture is too high, the tense inguinal ligament and the deep location of the external iliac artery may make complete compression of the vessel impossible. To minimize this problem, the artery should be entered caudal to the inguinal ligament at a site where it can be compressed against the femoral head.[9]

If the puncture is done too low—that is, into the SFA or the PF—there is a greater incidence of hematoma, pseudoaneurysm, arteriovenous fistula, and catheter-related thrombosis.[4,10] The reason for this increased incidence may be that it is harder to compress the SFA and the PF adequately than it is to compress the CFA, which lies for most its length over bone. The CFA is larger in diameter than either the SFA or the PF and thus is better suited for the passage of large catheters and sheaths.

BRACHIAL ARTERY PUNCTURE

The brachial artery is typically the second choice for arterial access after the femoral artery. The brachial artery is located in the lower third of the upper arm, anteromedial to the humerus. The median nerve lies just medial to the artery at this level, and the radial nerve lies posterior to the artery. Even though the brachial artery is best palpated in the lower middle third of the arm, some clinicians prefer to puncture it in the high brachial position because complications may be less frequent with this approach.

The patient's arm is extended and supinated. The upper portion of the brachial artery is entered several fingerbreadths distal to the axillary crease, over the proximal humeral shaft. The middle portion of the brachial artery is entered just above the antecubital fossa. The vessel is very mobile and thus should be fixed between the surgeon's middle and index fingers before puncture.

Troubleshooting

The brachial artery is typically smaller than the CFA and more prone to thrombosis. Accordingly, the needles, guide wires, catheters, and sheaths used for brachial artery puncture must be smaller as well. Occasionally, the median nerve or the radial nerve may be damaged by the puncture. Not uncommonly, the brachial artery goes into spasm after puncture. Intra-arterial injection of papaverine, tolazoline, or nitroglycerin may reduce the risk of spasm.

AXILLARY ARTERY PUNCTURE

The axillary artery is divided into three parts on the basis of its relation to the overlying pectoralis minor. The third portion of the artery lies lateral to the pectoralis minor, and its most distal portion extends beyond the pectoralis major, at which location it is very superficial.[2] The axillary artery is typically used for vascular access when neither the femoral nor the brachial artery is available. This approach is contraindicated in patients who have subclavian artery occlusive disease or aneurysmal disease. A physical examination should be performed before the procedure to look for a blood pressure differential between the two arms, as well as to auscultate for the presence of a supraclavicular bruit. A BP differential greater than 20 mm Hg suggests the presence of hemodynamically significant arterial stenosis in the arm with the lower pressure.

Axillary artery puncture is useful in patients with a steeply downward-coursing mesenteric or renal artery as well as in those who have a history of cholesterol embolization from previous retrograde aortic catheterization.[3] However, access at this site may be problematic, in that the artery is located near the brachial plexus, which may be damaged by direct trauma or compression

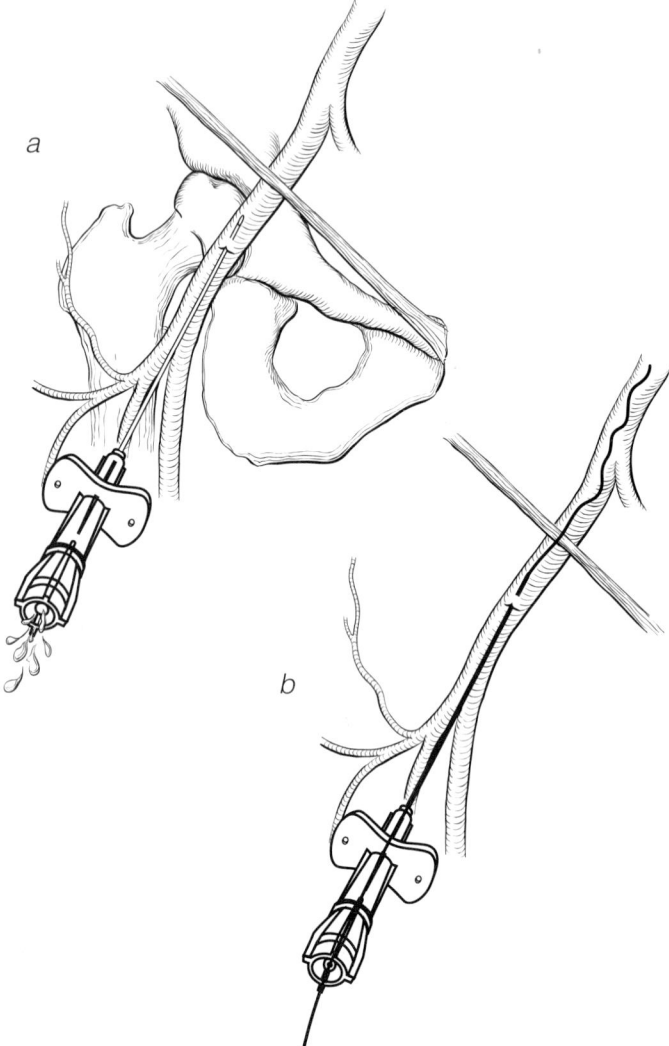

Figure 2 Puncture of the common femoral artery. (*a*) The needle enters the CFA. (*b*) The guide wire is passed through the needle.

from a hematoma. In addition, access via the axillary artery is relatively uncomfortable for both patient and physician. Generally, for access to the descending thoracic aorta, the abdominal aorta, and the lower-extremity vessels, the left axillary artery should be used, whereas for access to the ascending aorta and the coronary vessels, the right axillary artery should be used.

The arm can be placed in either of two positions: (1) abducted 90° or (2) maximally abducted with the patient's hand placed under the head. The second position stretches the artery and fixes it in place. The artery is palpated along the lateral axillary fold over the proximal humerus at the neck so that the underlying bone provides support during compression.[11] The vessel is then entered over the proximal humeral shaft just distal to the axillary fold. Like the brachial artery, the axillary artery is quite mobile. It should be compressed along its length between the index and middle fingers to fix it in place for subsequent puncture.

Troubleshooting

Thrombosis and pseudoaneurysm formation are more common with the axillary artery approach.[3] In addition, the median and ulnar nerves run along with the axillary and proximal brachial arteries in a fascial sheath, so that a small hematoma can cause nerve compression. If a sensory or motor deficit develops, surgical decompression may be required. Cerebral embolization occurs in as many as 4% of cases of axillary artery puncture.[3]

TRANSLUMBAR PUNCTURE

Translumbar puncture of the aorta is indicated when femoral, axillary, and brachial methods are all relatively unsuitable. It is frequently used in patients who have abdominal aneurysms after endovascular repair.

An upper translumbar approach is indicated if visualization of the visceral and renal arteries is required. The patient is placed in a prone position. The 12th thoracic vertebra is located either by palpating the 12th rib or, more accurately, by means of fluoroscopy. The skin is entered 1 to 2 cm below the level of the 12th rib and 8 to 10 cm to the left, lateral to the posterior spinous process of the 12th rib. The needle is aimed ventrally and cephalad toward the level of the middle to lower portion of the body of T12 until the needle strikes the vertebra. Care must be taken to keep the needle below the diaphragm so that it does not hit the lung and the pleura. Particular care must also be taken to avoid the renal arteries inferiorly. After striking T12, the needle is withdrawn several centimeters and aimed laterally and ventrally until the pulsations of the aorta are felt. When the needle hits the aorta, slight resistance will be felt, followed by release of tension and a very slight give or "pop" when the needle enters the aorta. Only the proximal wall should be punctured. The needle is then advanced about 3 to 5 mm to the middle of the lumen [*see Figure 3*].

A lower translumbar approach may be used to access an aortic aneurysm sac after endovascular repair. The puncture site is located via fluoroscopy of radiopaque markers on the device already in place. With the patient in the prone position, the needle is introduced 8 to 10 cm lateral to the spinous process of L2 and directed anterior to the lumbar spine. Often, careful review of the CT images suggests a specific target and tract. As with an upper translumbar puncture, a "pop" can be felt when the needle enters the aneurysm sac; alternatively, the needle can be visualized entering a calcified wall.

Troubleshooting

The high translumbar technique is limited by its inability to deliver the contrast material at the bifurcation of the aorta or to

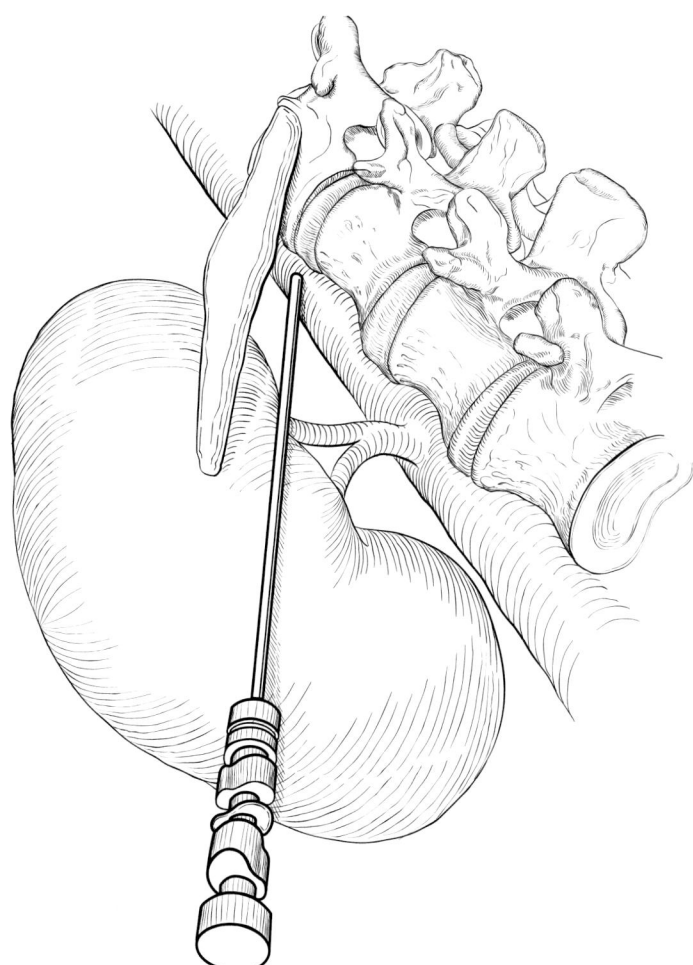

Figure 3 **Translumbar puncture of the aorta. The vessel is approached at the level of T12.**

perform selective catheterization of vessels. Too high a puncture (e.g., at T11) can lead to inadvertent puncture of the lung and cause a hemothorax or a pneumothorax. If the needle moves with the respiratory diaphragmatic movements of the patient, it may be in the thoracic cavity. If the initial needle stick is too medial, only the lateral wall of the aorta is reached. If the needle stick is too lateral, the needle passes between the vertebral body and the aorta. If the needle is advanced at too shallow an angle, it may enter the spinal canal.[2] If resistance is felt when the guide wire is placed, the wire may have entered the renal, celiac, or superior mesenteric artery. Small retroperitoneal hematomas develop in most patients who undergo translumbar puncture, but the incidence of major complications is only 3%.[3] Multiple aortic punctures should be limited to reduce the risk of severe retroperitoneal hemorrhage.

Placement of Guide Wires

Once vascular access has been obtained through arterial puncture, it is maintained through placement of a guide wire. The guide wire consists of a soft tip and a relatively stiff main body. The flexibility of the soft tip allows the surgeon to manipulate the guide wire past lesions or severe stenoses while minimizing the risk of perforation or dissection. For best results, the guide wire must be suitable for the intended procedure in terms of (1) tip configuration, (2) diameter, and (3) length.

Guide wires come in several different tip configurations, including straight, angled, and J-shaped. Straight-tipped wires are used in vessels that are relatively straight and free of disease. J-tipped guide wires are sometimes preferred for atherosclerotic vessels because the shape of the tip reduces the likelihood that the wire will go into the subatheromatous space and consequently loosen plaque.

Guide wires also come in a variety of diameters, typically ranging from 0.014 to 0.052 in. The diameters most commonly used for endovascular procedures are 0.038, 0.035, 0.018, and 0.014 in. Larger guide wires are typically stiffer, which makes it easier to pass sheaths and catheters over them over the wire. Smaller wires are typically used for endovascular work involving the carotid, renal, or infragenicular vessels. In choosing the diameter of the wire, the interventionalist must keep in mind the gauge of the needle that was used to access the vessel. The guide wire should fit the needle yet be large enough to prevent large amounts of blood from flowing back through the cannula of the needle.

The length of the guide wire is an important concern because choosing an appropriate length facilitates exchange of catheters or interventional devices without loss of access across a remote lesion. A general rule for determining optimal guide wire length is as follows[12]:

Optimal guide wire length = Length from outer edge of sheath or insertion site to lesion + length of longest catheter or interventional device + 10 cm

In an average adult, the wire used for selective angiography is typically about 100 to 150 cm long. Longer wires (180 to 300 cm) are used for interchanging vascular catheters. Occasionally, a 450 cm long wire is needed for combined brachial-femoral access.

Once arterial access is obtained, several safety measures should be undertaken. The needle should have its bevel facing upward to optimize conditions for wire advancement. A downward-facing bevel may cause the sharp edge of the needle to damage or even sever the wire. The floppy end of the wire should be used for initial introduction into the needle and the vessel; the stiff end may damage the vessel if used for initial entry. Caution should be exercised in introducing the guide wire if there is unexpectedly poor flow from the needle.

After entry into the lumen, the guide wire is advanced about 15 to 20 cm. The needle is then removed, and a catheter or an introducer sheath is placed over the wire. Further advancement of the wire is done under fluoroscopic guidance. Once placed, the guide wire should be carefully monitored and kept in place (pinned) whenever any other devices are manipulated. As a rule, the guide wire is not removed until the very end of the procedure. The wire should be stored loosely coiled in heparinized saline.

TROUBLESHOOTING

The guide wire should never be forcefully introduced into the vessel. If significant resistance is encountered, the end of the needle may be against the vessel wall or partially within the wall. In this situation, the needle should be repositioned slightly and another attempt made to pass the wire. Occasionally, the guide wire may pass easily for several centimeters before encountering resistance to further advancement. Such resistance may be secondary to stenosis or a tortuous proximal vessel, especially in an atherosclerotic patient. Placement of a different wire with a different tip configuration or insertion of a guide catheter may be necessary to advance the wire past the lesion.

Wiping the guide wire with heparinized saline minimizes thrombus formation on the wire. If thrombus is allowed to build

up, friction will increase during catheter exchange, making the exchange more difficult. Some hydrophilic-coated guide wires require constant wetting to maintain their characteristics. Other guide wire coatings swell after prolonged wetting and thus may inhibit catheter exchanges. Damaged or kinked guide wires should be exchanged for new undamaged wires when this can be done safely.

Placement of Sheaths

Once arterial access is obtained and guide wire access achieved, a sheath is typically placed over the guide wire to maintain a stable pathway for catheter exchange or for placement of a device. Before the sheath is placed, dilators are first passed over the guide wire to create a smooth tract through the soft tissue into the vessel. Sheaths are measured according to their inner circumference (1 mm circumference = 1 French). Dilators, on the other hand, are measured according to their outer circumference. Therefore, for placement of a 5 French sheath, a 6 French dilator is required to create the tract.

Most introducer sheaths have hemostatic valves and side ports. Guide catheters can be effectively converted to sheaths by adding a Touhy-Borst valve apparatus. These valves seal around a smaller catheter and prevent spillage of blood. The side port can be used for continuous infusion of heparinized saline to prevent thrombus formation. The sheath can also be used to straighten tortuous arteries (e.g., the iliac arteries). For example, when a guide wire has been passed through the iliac artery and into the abdominal aorta, the sheath can be advanced over the wire into the abdominal aorta. Passage of a sheath through the tortuous iliac vessel permits easier exchange of catheters and devices.

Once properly placed, sheaths should be secured in position (i.e., pinned or sutured) so that they are not inadvertently advanced without the introducer or accidentally withdrawn.

Insertion of Catheters

Catheters may be categorized in several different ways. They are sized according to their outer diameter (French) and length (cm). In addition, they are classified as either selective or nonselective. Nonselective catheters have multiple side and end holes that allow a large burst of contrast material to be infused over a short period. They are typically used to opacify large vessels. Selective catheters have only a single hole at their distal tip and are typically used to opacify smaller vessels. Generally, opacification of smaller vessels requires a smaller dose of contrast material administered at a slower rate. Finally, catheters are classified on the basis of the shapes of their distal ends [*see Figure 4*] (e.g., straight, cobra, headhunter, angled, shepherd's hook, reverse curve, pigtail, and racquet). Any of the different shapes available may be preferred in a given patient, depending on the specific circumstances present and the specific vessels involved. Generally, within the abdominal aorta, the angle of the primary curve of the catheter tip should be similar to that of the vessel takeoff. A gentle secondary curve in the catheter helps guide the primary curve of the tip deeper into the selected vessel once its origin has been engaged.[2]

Before contrast is injected, the catheter should be aspirated to remove any air bubbles and to verify intraluminal location by means of back-bleeding. A small test injection is useful for checking the catheter's position. If the operation is expected to be long, the patient should receive I.V. heparin at the start of the procedure to reduce the risk of thrombus formation on the outside of the catheter. Periodically, the catheter may be flushed with heparinized saline to prevent thrombus formation within it. When catheters are advanced forward, they are almost always advanced over a pinned guide wire to minimize the risk of intimal injury. In addition, catheters should be removed over a wire, especially if the distal end of the catheter is not straight. This maneuver also lessens the risk that the catheter will scrape the vessel wall.

TROUBLESHOOTING

There are several areas in the handling of catheters where attention to detail and good technique can help optimize results. Two common errors of selective catheterization are (1) looking for a specific artery in the wrong location (e.g., as a consequence of miscounting lumbar vertebral bodies) and (2) failing to recognize when the appropriate vessel has been entered (particularly in patients with anomalous vessels or postoperative changes).[13] Another potential problem is loss of guide wire access, which can be prevented by holding or pinning the guide wire in place while a catheter is being pulled out. Finally, when a sheath is not being used, the subcutaneous tissue can be spread apart with a small clamp, and the catheter can be pushed through the tissue and into the vessel in a rotating motion. There are many other, more advanced catheter and guide wire techniques that are beyond the scope of this discussion.

Use of Balloon Catheters

The purpose of a balloon catheter is to exert a radial force on the luminal surface of a blood vessel to dilate a stenotic lesion. As the balloon inflates, the media and adventitia of the artery stretch, causing a longitudinal fracture of the plaque. A minor arterial dissection is expected with this technique. Thus, the compression of the plaque is not the principal means of increasing the cross-sectional area of the vessel.

Several features are considered in selecting a balloon catheter for a specific intervention, including balloon diameter and length, catheter size and length, trackability, balloon type (e.g., compliant, noncompliant, or coated), and catheter profile [see Figure 5]. Typically, balloons range from 1.5 to 28 mm in diameter and from 1.5 to 10 cm in length. The vessel should be slightly overdistended when the balloon is inflated. Thus, measuring the diameter of the normal vessel distal to the lesion will help determine an appropriate balloon diameter. The shortest balloon length that spans the entire lesion with a slight extension into the normal artery is chosen, with care taken to ensure that the shoulder of the balloon does not dilate the vessel. If the balloon is too short and is not centered, it may be squeezed away from the stenosis during inflation. Catheters typically range from 40 to 150 cm in length. The shortest catheter length that reaches the lesion from the access site without difficulty is chosen; the shorter the catheter, the easier it is to manipulate. The diameter of the catheter depends on the type and size of the balloon but generally is between 3 and 7 French. As a rule, the catheter should be 1 French smaller than the sheath to permit contrast injection when the balloon is in position. Finally, the initial profile of the balloon catheter is the overall diameter of the catheter shaft plus the uninflated balloon. Smaller profiles permit use of smaller guide wires and sheaths.

The balloon catheter is advanced over the guide wire through the sheath to the lesion, and the balloon is centered over the lesion. If it appears possible that the chosen balloon will be too large, it is best to switch to a smaller-diameter balloon and then move up in size as necessary. The balloon is inflated with a dilute contrast solution so that its expansion can be monitored fluoro-

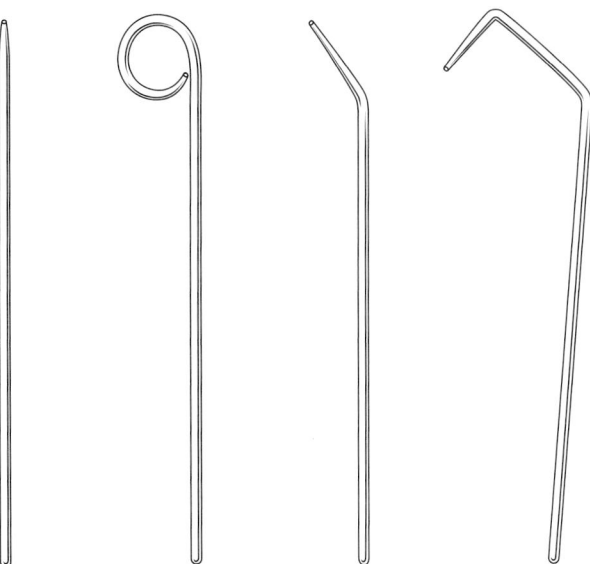

Figure 4 Catheters come with various tip configurations. Shown are straight, pigtail, angled, and double-angled tips (left to right).

scopically. Guidelines for inflation techniques vary with respect to duration of inflation, number of dilatations, and balloon pressure. Typically, the balloon is inflated for 30 to 90 seconds, then deflated. A second dilatation follows, lasting another 30 to 90 seconds. Inflation pressures commonly range from 4 to 10 atm; as a rule, they should not exceed rated burst pressures. After dilatation, the balloon catheter is removed, but the guide wire is kept in place across the lesion. A completion angiogram is obtained for evaluation of the results, including assessment of distal vascular beds.

Dilatation may be considered successful if (1) flow-limiting dissection is absent, (2) residual luminal diameter stenosis is less than 30%, and (3) the systolic pressure gradient is less than 5 to 10 mm Hg. Vasodilators can unmask a significant gradient.

TROUBLESHOOTING

Complications associated with the use of balloon catheters include thrombosis, vessel rupture, embolization, and dissection. The incidence of these complications is influenced by patient selection and by the nature of the lesion being treated. For example, complications may be more likely with treatment of stenoses adjacent to aneurysms, long segments of stenosis, tandem lesions, lesions near major branches, and calcified eccentric plaques. Even though some degree of dissection is expected after balloon angioplasty, larger flow-limiting dissections may call for further management. This problem can often be solved by placing a stent over the dissection.

Most patients feel discomfort and mild pain during balloon inflation. If a patient experiences severe pain even after deflation of the balloon, the possibility of vessel rupture must be considered. If the vessel ruptures, the balloon may be reinflated over the injury to tamponade it. Prolonged balloon inflation often closes the leak, but at the risk of causing thrombosis. If the vessel continues to leak, a covered stent may be placed over the injury, or open vascular repair may be necessary.

If inflation of the balloon fails to dilate the vessel completely, it may be helpful to use a larger-diameter balloon or a higher inflation pressure. Higher inflation pressures may be cautiously attempted, but the vessel may simply recoil after dilatation.[14] A stent is often useful in this scenario.

If the balloon only crosses the lesions partially, it should not be inflated. The position of the guide wire should be checked: the wire may be in a subintimal location. If the stenosis is very tight, the lesion should be predilated with a smaller-profile balloon catheter.

Placement of Vascular Stents

Intravascular stents are commonly used to treat vascular disease, particularly after failed percutaneous transluminal angioplasty (PTA). Placement of an iliac artery stent is indicated when there is significant residual stenosis, flow-limiting dissection, or a persistent pressure gradient. Although PTA is often successful, it may fail when there is elastic recoil of the arterial wall or when the lesion is resistant to dilatation because of heavy calcification. Stenting can often remedy these situations by providing physical support to keep the vessel open. Many physicians now regard primary stenting (i.e., routine use of stents) as a preferred approach for most vascular lesions.

CHOICE OF STENT TYPE

Stents are divided into two categories: balloon expandable stents and self-expanding stents. They may also be described as being covered (with a graft material), coated (with a therapeutic compound), or radioactive. Stent types differ with respect to hoop strength (for resisting arterial recoil), radiopacity, longitudinal flexibility (for crossing tortuous vessels), radial elasticity (for resisting repeated external compression), and profile. Stents come in many different lengths and expanded diameters on a wide variety of deployment catheters.

Balloon Expandable Stents

Balloon expandable stents come either premounted on balloon catheters or unmounted; unmounted stents must be manually crimped onto a balloon to be delivered. With unmounted stents, a smaller inventory can be maintained, and a wider range of stent-balloon combinations is available. Premounted stents, however, tend to be more solidly mounted and less likely to be lost during delivery. Once the stent is at the desired lesion, the balloon is inflated and the stent expanded.

The main advantage balloon expandable stents have over self-expanding stents is that they have greater hoop strength, which

means that they can better resist the recoil of the vessel after full expansion of the stent. In addition, balloon expandable stents may be easier for interventionalists to place with precision. However, greater dilatation may cause some shortening of the stent, which may result in malpositioning of the device. Finally, older balloon expandable stents are less flexible than current models, and navigating such older devices in a tortuous vessel can be difficult.

Self-expanding Stents

Self-expanding stents are placed within a delivery catheter and rely on a self-expansion mechanism for full deployment. A common deployment mechanism involves the use of an outer jacket and a plunger: the jacket is withdrawn while the stent is held in position by the plunger, and the stent then expands to its predetermined diameter. Commonly, a balloon is employed to ensure that the stent is fully expanded and impacted into the plaque.

An advantage of self-expanding stents is that they offer a greater degree of longitudinal flexibility and thus are more easily placed. In addition, they may be delivered by catheters with smaller profiles, which may induce fewer arterial-access complications. Self-expanding stents may also be placed in regions of the body where they are subject to crushing forces (e.g., the carotid artery) because they are capable of recovering from the deformation and maintaining the arterial lumen.[15] As noted, however, self-expanding stents have less hoop strength than the balloon expandable stents.

Covered Stents

Stents may be covered with Dacron, polytetrafluoroethylene, or polyurethane. Covered stents do not yield significantly better long-term results than open mesh stents do. These types of stents are useful for aneurysms, arterial rupture, and arteriovenous fistulas.[15,16]

GENERAL TECHNICAL PRINCIPLES

Stent placement is very similar to transluminal balloon angioplasty, except that the stent is also placed over the lesion [see Figure 6]. Preoperatively, the patient is often given an antiplatelet agent, which may be continued for 4 weeks to 6 months postoperatively to reduce the risk of thrombosis. The diameter of the

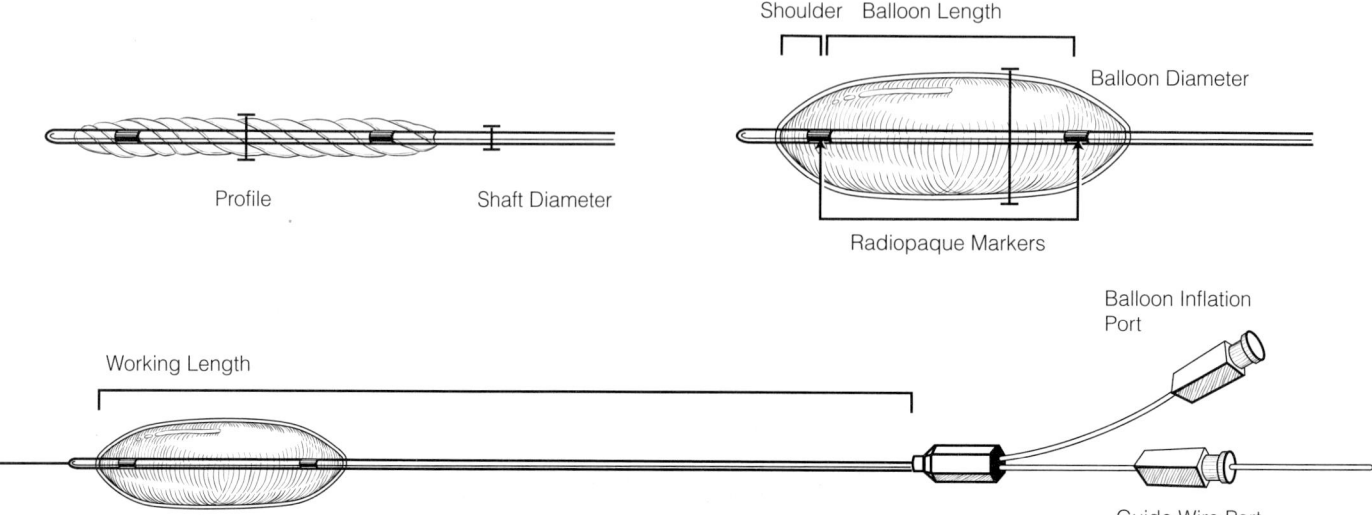

Figure 5 **Shown is a balloon angioplasty catheter.**

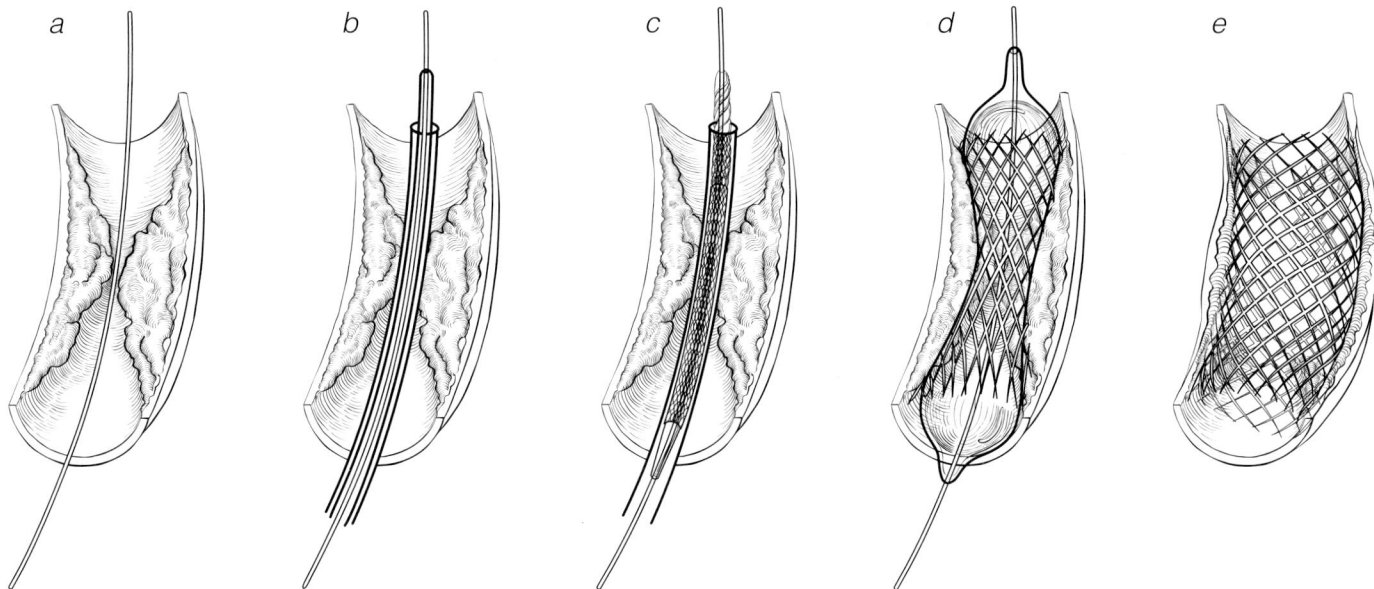

Figure 6 **Deployment of a balloon expandable stent. (*a*) The guide wire is passed across the lesion. (*b*) The sheath-dilator combination is passed over the guide wire across the lesion. (*c*) The dilator is removed and replaced with the balloon-stent combination. (*d*) The sheath is retracted and the balloon inflated. (*e*) The balloon is deflated and withdrawn, leaving the stent fully deployed.**

fully deployed stent should slightly exceed that of the vessel, but by no more than 20%.[11] If occlusion makes the exact diameter of the artery difficult to measure, the vessel's contralateral counterpart can be used as a guide.[16] The stent should also be slightly longer than the lesion to ensure that the entire lesion is covered. In this way, good wall apposition can be achieved and stent migration prevented.

After the guide wire is passed across the lesion, a guide (or a long sheath) is advanced across the stenosis. The vascular stent is passed through the guide and positioned at the lesion. The guide is then withdrawn and the stent deployed. Several stents may be necessary to complete the procedure.

TROUBLESHOOTING

The leading end of a self-expanding stent can be placed slightly beyond the lesion. This permits the stent to be pulled back just before complete deployment, thereby improving deployment accuracy when significant stent foreshortening is present. The struts of the stent can injure the vessel wall if advanced forward. Failure to cover the entire lesion with the stent results in residual disease after the procedure, which can cause subsequent thrombosis. When multiple stents are deployed, there must be no gaps between them. Generally, stents should overlap each other to prevent restenosis. Finally, dilatation of the vessel should be gentle and gradual so as not to cause extensive dissection and vessel rupture.

Postprocedural Management of Arterial Access Site

After any endovascular procedure, the arterial access site must be addressed. External compression is a common method of promoting hemostasis and is effective in most instances. The artery often must be compressed for longer than 20 minutes to prevent bleeding complications. If the patient is receiving anticoagulant therapy, it may be necessary to wait until the coagulation parameters have had time to decrease before pulling out the sheath. This can be done when the patient is out of the OR or interventional suite and in the recovery room or when the patient has been moved onto the hospital floor. After hemostasis has been achieved at the access site, the patient should refrain from walking for about 6 hours to keep from dislodging the clot. In situations involving relatively large devices, use of an arterial closure device may be prudent. Several such closure devices are now commercially available.

Summary: Basic Steps in Endovascular Procedures

1. Before operation, consider prescribing antiplatelet agents.
2. Sedate and monitor the patient as necessary.
3. Prepare and drape the selected arterial access site or sites.
4. Infiltrate a local anesthetic at the selected site.
5. Cannulate the artery with the entry needle.
6. Pass the guide wire into the needle for at least 20 to 25 cm. Use fluoroscopy to follow the guide wire.
7. Remove the needle while pinning the guide wire in place.
8. Use a scalpel to nick the skin where the guide wire exits the skin.
9. Dissect the subcutaneous tissue with a small clamp.
10. Use dilators to create an appropriate tract while pinning the guide wire. After the tract is created, the dilators may be removed.
11. Pass a sheath over the pinned guide wire. Often, the dilator is within the sheath, and the two devices are placed simultaneously. Remove the dilator.
12. Heparinize the patient.
13. Manipulate the guide wire to the appropriate position past the lesion.
14. Pass the catheter over the guide wire and through the sheath. The catheter is manipulated to select the branches for guide wire cannulation.
15. Perform angiography through the catheter or the sheath to clarify the anatomy.
16. Remove the catheter while pinning the guide wire.

17. Pass the balloon catheter over the guide wire. The balloon is advanced across and centered over the lesion.
18. Inflate the balloon.
19. Deflate the balloon.
20. If necessary, remove the balloon catheter while pinning the guide wire.
21. Perform angiography.

22. Pass the vascular stent over the guide wire and advance it across the lesion.
23. Deploy the stent.
24. Perform completion angiography.
25. If the angiogram is satisfactory, remove the guide wire, the catheter, and the sheath.
26. Maintain pressure over the access site.

References

1. Tortorici M: Fundamentals of Angiography. CV Mosby Co, St Louis, 1982

2. Johnsrude I, Jackson D, Dunnick N: A Practical Approach to Angiography, 2nd ed. Little, Brown & Co, Boston, 1987

3. Valji K: Vascular and Interventional Radiology. WB Saunders Co, Philadelphia, 1999

4. Rupp SB, Vogelzang RL, Nemcek AA, et al: Relationship of the inguinal ligament to pelvic radiographic landmarks: anatomic correlation and its role in femoral arteriography. J Vasc Intervent Radiol 4:409, 1993

5. Baum PA, Matsumoto AH, Teitelbaum GP, et al: Anatomic relationship between the common femoral artery and vein: CT evaluation and clinical significance. Cardiovasc Radiol 173:775, 1999

6. Millward SF, Burbride BE, Luna G: Puncturing the pulseless femoral artery: a simple technique that uses palpation of anatomic landmarks. J Vasc Intervent Radiol 4:415, 1993

7. Jaques PF, Mauro MA, Keefe B: US guidance for vascular access: technical note. J Vasc Intervent Radiol 3:427, 1992

8. Khangure MS, Chow KC, Christensen MA: Accurate and safe puncture of a pulseless femoral artery. Radiology 144:927, 1982

9. Spijkerboer AM, Scholten FG, Mali WPTM, et al: Antegrade puncture of the femoral artery: morphologic study. Radiology 176:57, 1990

10. Grier D, Hartnell G: Percutaneous femoral artery puncture: practice and anatomy. Br J Radiol 63: 602, 1990

11. Kandarpa K, Aruny JE: Handbook of Interventional Radiologic Procedures. Lippincott Williams & Wilkins, Philadelphia, 2002

12. Moore WS, Ahn SS: Endovascular Surgery, 3rd ed. WB Saunders Co, Philadelphia, 2001

13. Neiman HL, Yao JST: Angiography of Vascular Disease. Churchill Livingstone, New York, 1985

14. Hood DB, Hodgson KJ: Percutaneous transluminal angioplasty and stenting for iliac artery occlusive disease. Surg Clin North Am 79:575, 1999

15. Nicholson T: Stents: an overview. Hosp Med 60: 571, 1999

16. Henry M, Clonaris C, Amor M, et al: Which stent for which lesion in peripheral interventions? Texas Heart Inst J 27:119, 2000

Acknowledgment

Figures 1 through 6   Alice Y. Chen.

8 CAROTID ARTERIAL PROCEDURES

Wesley S. Moore, M.D., F.A.C.S.

The rationale for operating on patients with carotid artery disease is to prevent stroke. It has been estimated that in 50% to 80% of patients who experience an ischemic stroke, the underlying cause is a lesion in the distribution of the carotid artery, usually in the vicinity of the carotid bifurcation. It would follow, then, that appropriate identification and surgical intervention could significantly reduce the incidence of ischemic stroke.

Carotid endarterectomy for both symptomatic and asymptomatic carotid artery stenosis has been extensively evaluated in prospective, randomized trials. Symptomatic patients have been studied in the North American Symptomatic Carotid Endarterectomy Trial (NASCET),[1] the European Carotid Stenosis Trial (ECST),[2] and the symptomatic carotid stenosis trial from the Veterans Affairs (VA) Cooperative Studies Program.[3] The results of all three trials conclusively demonstrate that symptomatic patients with greater than 50% stenosis on arteriography are at substantially lower risk for stroke after carotid endarterectomy than control subjects receiving medical management alone. Asymptomatic patients with hemodynamically significant stenosis also benefit from surgical treatment: the Asymptomatic Carotid Atherosclerosis Study (ACAS)[4] and the asymptomatic carotid stenosis trial from the VA Cooperative Studies Program[5] show that the risk of both transient ischemic attacks (TIAs) and stroke is markedly lower in patients treated with carotid endarterectomy and best medical management than in control subjects treated with best medical management alone.

Surgical reconstruction of the carotid artery yields the greatest benefits when done by surgeons who can keep complication rates to an absolute minimum. The majority of complications associated with carotid arterial procedures are either technical or judgmental; accordingly, in what follows, I emphasize the procedural details that I consider particularly important for deriving the best short- and long-term results from surgical intervention.

Preoperative Evaluation

PATIENT SELECTION

Indications for carotid artery surgery can be divided into two major categories: (1) asymptomatic critical stenosis and (2) symptomatic hemodynamically significant stenosis.[6]

Asymptomatic Critical Stenosis

ACAS and the VA asymptomatic carotid stenosis study both found that in patients with diameter-reducing stenosis of 60% or greater on angiography, carotid endarterectomy resulted in fewer fatal and nonfatal strokes over a 5-year period than nonoperative treatment with best medical management alone. It is important to keep in mind that there are several different ways of measuring stenosis [*see 4:2 Asymptomatic Carotid Bruit*]. The 60% figure cited by ACAS and the VA study was determined according to the North American method rather than the European method. Moreover, it was determined by means of contrast angiography rather than duplex ultrasonography (DUS) or magnetic resonance imaging. If the decision for carotid endarterectomy is to be based on DUS, some conversion of values is required. A patient who has an 80% to 99% stenosis on DUS can generally be assumed to have a diameter-reducing stenosis of at least 60% on angiography; a stenosis that is less than 80% on DUS may fall short of a 60% diameter-reducing stenosis on angiography.

Symptomatic Hemodynamically Significant Carotid Stenosis

Transient ischemic attacks Both NASCET and ECST found that symptomatic patients with hemodynamically significant stenoses experienced fewer fatal and nonfatal strokes after carotid endarterectomy combined with best medical management than after best medical management alone, provided that the perioperative morbidity and mortality from stroke was 6.0% or less. Thus, patients with monocular or hemispheric TIAs are good candidates for carotid endarterectomy. Global ischemic attacks have also been used as an indication for carotid endarterectomy. This practice has not been evalutated in clinical trials; it is usually justified on the basis of the ACAS data alone.

Prior stroke Patients who have previously experienced a hemispheric stroke but who are not disabled and have made a reasonable recovery are also good candidates for carotid endarterectomy if they have a hemodynamically significant stenosis.

IMAGING

Indications for Carotid Duplex Scanning

Identification of a carotid lesion that can be treated with endarterectomy usually begins with a carotid duplex scan. Indications for carotid duplex scanning fall into three main categories: symptoms, signs, and risk factors. Symptoms include classic TIAs and strokes that give rise to clinical suspicion of carotid bifurcation disease. The primary sign is the presence of a carotid bruit on auscultation. Risk factors include cigarette smoking, hypertension, diabetes mellitus, hypercholesterolemia, peripheral vascular disease, and coronary artery disease. As the number of risk factors present increases, the likelihood of associated carotid bifurcation disease increases exponentially.

Other Considerations in Symptomatic Patients

Patients who present with focal ischemic symptoms are likely to have associated carotid bifurcation disease; however, other pathologic conditions (e.g., emboli of cardiac origin, aortic arch disease, intracranial vascular disease, coagulopathy, and brain tumors) can also be responsible for focal symptoms. Accordingly, a complete workup of a symptomatic patient should include cardiac evaluation as well as intracranial imaging.

Additional Arterial Imaging

The accuracy of carotid duplex scanning is highly dependent on the technician performing it and on the laboratory where it is done. A carefully performed carotid duplex scan is often the most accurate indicator of carotid bifurcation disease; however, a hastily or carelessly performed scan can result in overestimation of the extent of the carotid bifurcation disease. For this reason, additional imaging studies (e.g., MRI, computed tomographic angiography, and, when there is serious doubt, contrast angiography) may be indicated.

Operative Planning

Before operation is scheduled, the general health of the patient must be assessed, with particular attention paid to cardiac and pulmonary status. Given that many patients with carotid artery disease are hypertensive or diabetic, good preoperative control of diabetes mellitus and blood pressure is mandatory. Finally, to reduce the risk of thromboembolic complications, patients should receive antiplatelet drugs (e.g., aspirin) up to and on the day of operation.

ANESTHESIA

Surgery on the cervical portion of the carotid artery may be performed with the patient under either general or cervical block anesthesia. Both techniques have their advocates, their advantages, and their disadvantages.

The advantages of general anesthesia include a quiet operative field, maximal patient comfort, good airway control, and convenient blood gas management. In addition, general anesthesia may lead to improved cerebral blood flow and give better protection against reduced blood flow during carotid clamping. The disadvantages of general anesthesia include blood pressure swings during induction and the inability to monitor the patient's conscious response to carotid clamping. Some reports also suggest that the incidence of cardiac complications is higher during general anesthesia than during cervical block anesthesia.

The main advantage of cervical block anesthesia is the ability to monitor cerebral function during carotid clamping: an awake patient can be engaged in conversation and can be asked to carry out motor activities of the extremities. The disadvantages of cervical block anesthesia include possible patient discomfort, restlessness, and intolerance of the longer operations that are sometimes necessary for technical reasons. Another disadvantage is that on occasion, a patient cannot tolerate carotid clamping and demonstrates an immediate neurologic deficit with clamp application. Such an occurrence heightens the anxiety level of the surgical team, thereby increasing the risk that they will commit technical errors in the rush to place an internal shunt.

Besides considering the inherent advantages and disadvantages of these two anesthetic techniques with respect to the patient, it is important to consider their advantages and disadvantages with respect to individual surgical practice. A given surgeon may well work better and achieve better results with one technique or the other.

Whichever anesthetic approach is used, all patients should have a radial arterial line in place to allow continuous blood pressure monitoring as well as provide access for determining blood gas levels. As a rule, there is no need to place a central venous line or a right heart catheter, except in patients with marginal cardiac function.

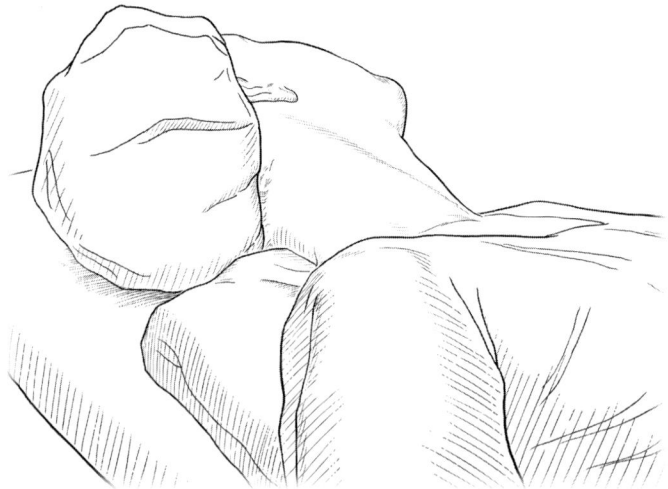

Figure 1 **Carotid arterial procedures. Shown is the recommended patient positioning.**

PATIENT POSITIONING

Proper positioning of the patient is necessary to provide optimal exposure of the neck from the clavicle up to the mastoid process on the side of the proposed operation [*see Figure 1*]. The patient is placed in the supine position with a folded sheet under the shoulders to induce a mild degree of neck extension. Excessive neck extension should be avoided, however, because it places tension on the artery and actually hinders rather than facilitates exposure. This potential problem can be addressed by placing one or more towels under the head to adjust the neck to the optimal degree of extension. The patient's head is then turned away from the side of the operation to improve cervical exposure further. Finally, the table top may be rotated slightly away from the side of the operation so as to provide a flat surgical field. The head of the table may be elevated slightly if the patient's blood pressure is adequate; this step helps

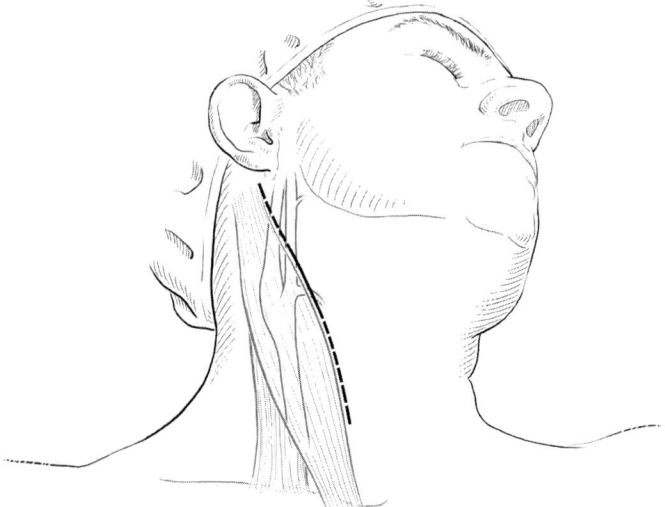

Figure 2 **Carotid arterial procedures. The incision most commonly used to expose the cervical carotid artery is a vertical one placed along the anterior margin of the sternocleidomastoid muscle and centered over the presumed location of the carotid bifurcation. It may be extended proximally or distally, depending on where the carotid bifurcation turns out to be.**

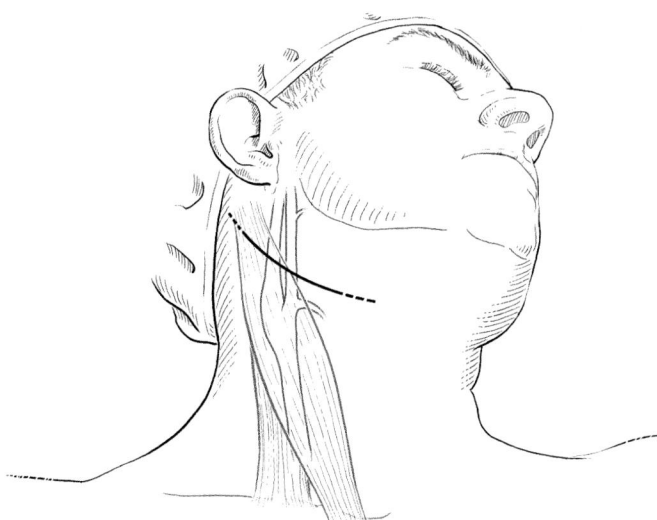

Figure 3 **Carotid arterial procedures. An alternative incision to the vertical incision is a transverse incision along a skin crease in the vicinity of the carotid bifurcation.**

lower venous pressure and reduce venous bleeding during the operation [*see Figure 1*].

Operative Technique

STEP 1: INITIAL INCISION

Either of two incisions may be used for exposure of the cervical carotid artery. The more common choice is a vertical incision placed along an imaginary line that extends from the sternoclavicular junction to the mastoid process, paralleling the anterior margin of the sternocleidomastoid muscle as well as the course of the carotid artery and the contents of the carotid sheath [*see Figure 2*]. The incision is centered over the presumed location of the carotid bifurcation. The advantage of this incision is that it provides optimal exposure of the cervical carotid artery and can readily be extended either proximally or distally along the aforementioned imaginary line to give additional exposure when needed (e.g., when the carotid bifurcation is unusually high). The disadvantage of this incision is that it runs against Langer's lines; thus, if a keloid occurs, it is likely to be in an unsightly position. In most patients, the incision heals to a fine line, and it usually is not noticeable once healing is complete.

The alternative to the vertical incision is a transverse incision that is placed in a skin crease on the anterior portion of the neck and then curved toward the mastoid process posteriorly [*see Figure 3*]. Skin flaps are raised in a subplatysmal layer, and the incision is deepened along the anterior border of the sternocleidomastoid muscle. The advantage of this alternative incision is that it may be more cosmetically acceptable; however, its inferior portion frequently crosses the neck anteriorly, which may make it more visible than an incision confined to the line of the sternocleidomastoid muscle would be. The disadvantage of this incision is that it requires the raising of skin flaps, which takes additional time and may limit the extent of any proximal exposure that may be required.

STEP 2: EXPOSURE OF CAROTID ARTERY

Once the incision through the platysmal layer has been completed, an avascular areolar plane is developed along the anterior border of the sternocleidomastoid muscle for the full length of the incision so as to expose the carotid sheath. The internal jugular vein is usual-

ly the most visible vessel, and the carotid sheath is opened along this vessel's anterior border. The common facial vein, which drains into the internal jugular vein, is a relatively constant landmark. Because the common facial vein is the venous analogue of the external carotid artery, it can generally be used as a guide to the position of the carotid bifurcation [*see Figure 4*]. On occasion, a patient has several accessory facial veins instead of a single common facial vein. The common facial vein or the accessory facial veins are then divided between ligatures so that the jugular vein can be retracted laterally. The common carotid artery and the carotid bifurcation lie immediately beneath the divided facial veins.

At this point, care must be taken to look for the vagus nerve. This nerve is usually located posterior to the common carotid artery, but it is sometimes rotated into a more superficial position. Another important neurologic structure in this area is the ansa cervicalis, which is formed by the junction of fibers from the hypoglossal (12th cranial) nerve and fibers from the first cervical nerve and which continues inferiorly as a single trunk, providing innervation to the strap muscles. This nerve should be spared if possible, but it can be divided without significant sequelae if it interferes with optimal exposure of the carotid bifurcation. One convenient method of separating the nerve from the artery is to divide the fibers running from the first cervical nerve to the ansa cervicalis; when this is done, the nerve is readily mobilized and retracted anteriorly away from the carotid artery.

The perivascular plane of the common carotid artery is then entered, and the common carotid artery is circumferentially mobilized. The common carotid artery is palpated against a right-angle clamp to determine the proximal extent of the atherosclerotic plaque. If possible, the common carotid artery should be mobilized proximal to the plaque until a circumferentially soft portion of that vessel is

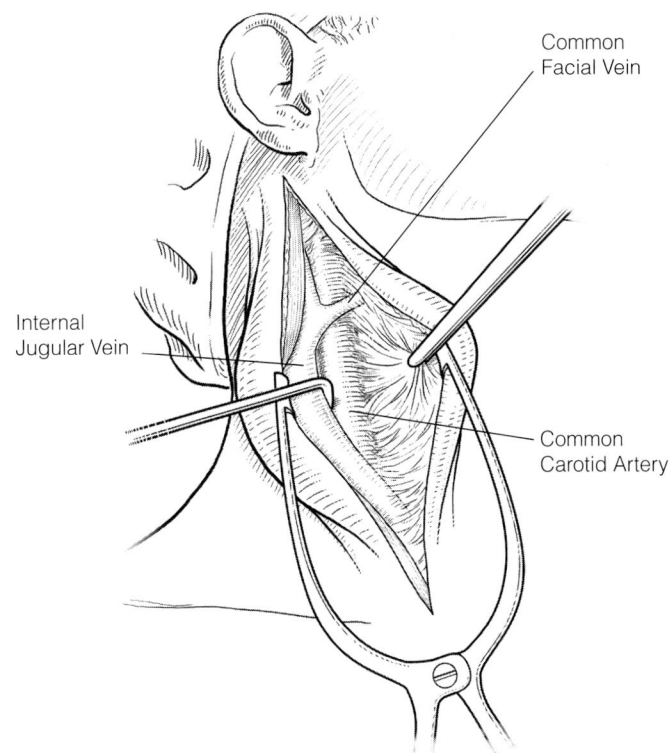

Figure 4 **Carotid arterial procedures. After the sternocleidomastoid muscle is mobilized off the carotid sheath, the jugular vein is identified. The perivascular plane along the jugular vein is opened until the common facial vein is exposed.**

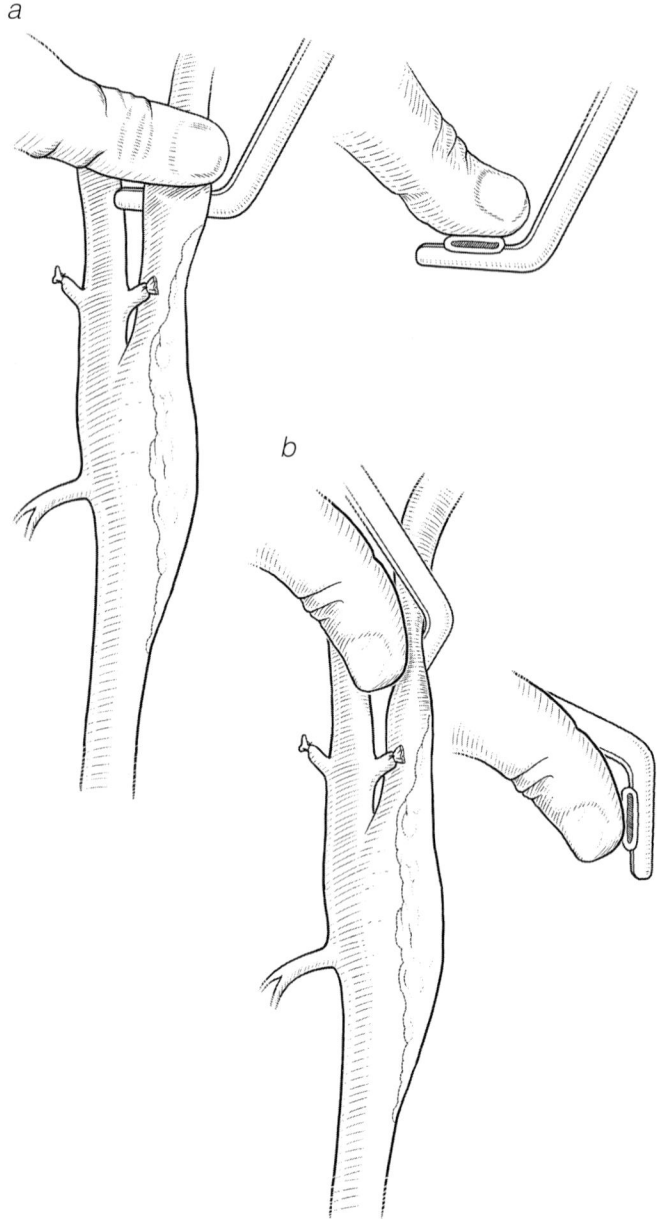

Figure 5 **Carotid arterial procedures. After the common carotid artery and the internal and external carotid arteries have been mobilized, the internal carotid artery is palpated against a right-angle clamp in at least two planes (*a, b*) to confirm that the artery has been freed beyond the end point of the plaque.**

reached. During mobilization, the vagus nerve should be identified in its usual location posterior to the vessel and carefully protected; this nerve sometimes spirals anterior to the carotid artery as the vessel is dissected distally.

Dissection is then extended distally toward the carotid bifurcation and continued along both the internal and external carotid arteries. Excessive manipulation of the area around the carotid bifurcation must be avoided. In particular, it is important to be careful around the bulb of the internal carotid artery: this is where the majority of the plaque will be located, and manipulation can easily dislodge plaque or thromboembolic material. With exposure of the carotid bifurcation, the hypoglossal nerve may come into view. Care should be taken not to injure this nerve, though it may have to be mobilized to permit sufficient distal exposure of the internal carotid artery.

Dissection should then continue distally beyond the bulb of the internal carotid artery to a point where the internal carotid artery is normal. At this point, the relevant portion of the vessel is circumferentially mobilized and palpated against a right-angle clamp in at least two planes to confirm that the atheromatous plaque does not reach up to the level of the proposed clamping [*see Figure 5*]. Once this is accomplished, the external carotid artery is mobilized beyond the end point of plaque extension in a similar manner.

If the patient has a high carotid bifurcation or if the plaque in the internal carotid artery extends further distally than usual, a more extensive exposure of the carotid bifurcation, the internal carotid artery, or both is required. To provide such exposure, the skin incision is extended all the way to the mastoid process. The sternocleidomastoid muscle is fully mobilized up to the mastoid process, with

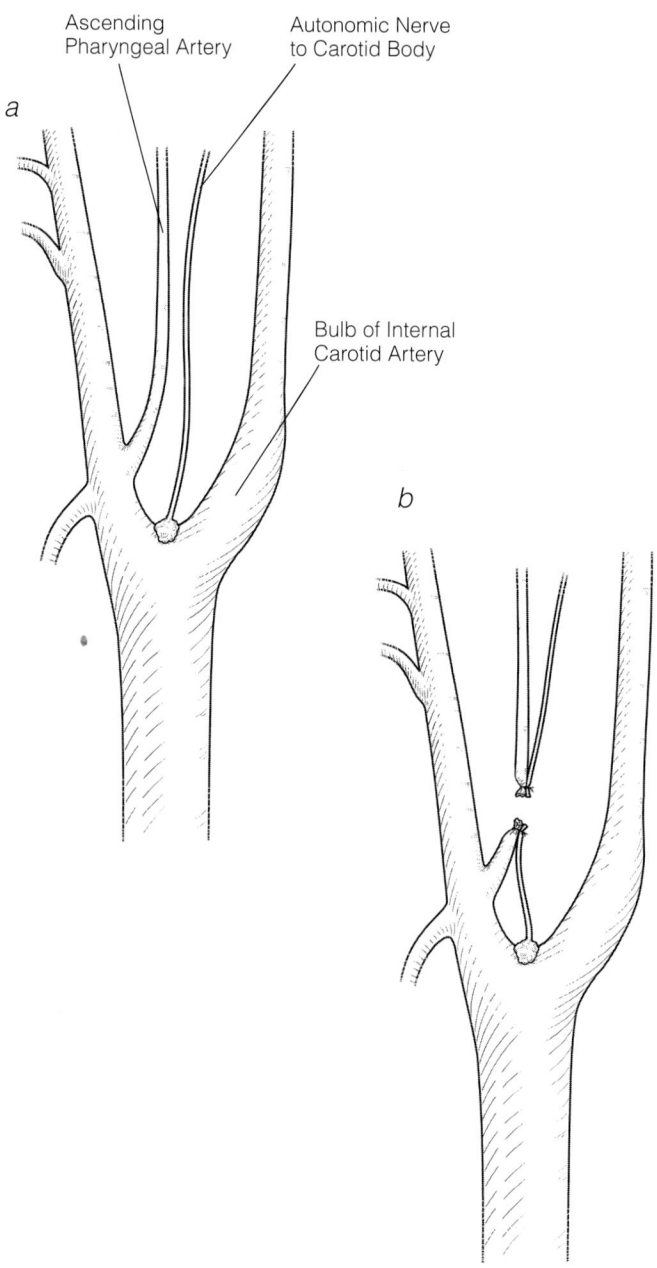

Figure 6 **Carotid arterial procedures. Once the common, internal, and external carotid arteries are fully mobilized, the structures between the internal and external carotid arteries (*a*) are divided (*b*) to allow the carotid bifurcation to drop down.**

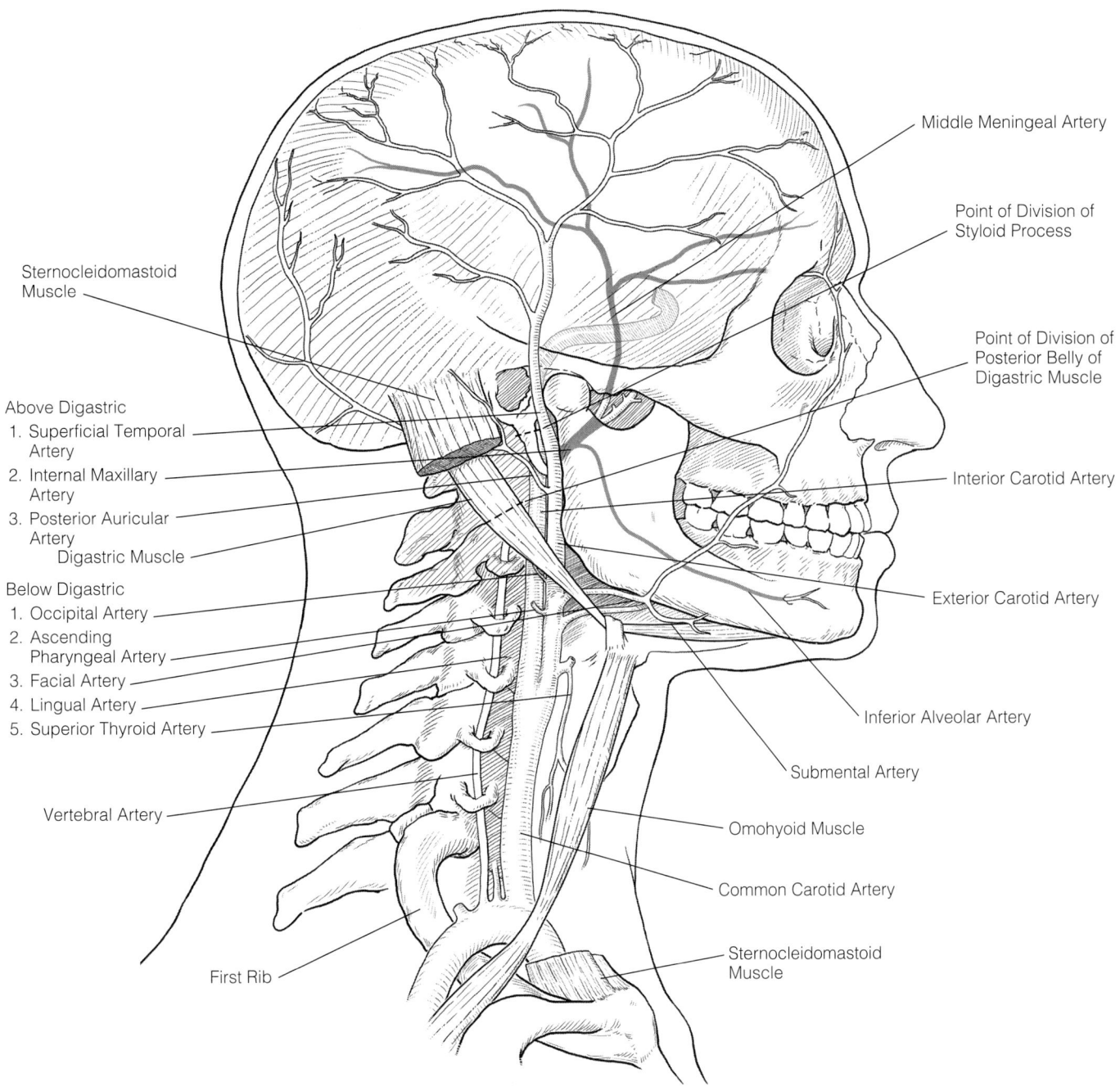

Figure 7 Carotid arterial procedures. Division of the posterior belly of the digastric muscle yields additional exposure of the internal carotid artery. If the internal carotid artery must be mobilized all the way to the base of the skull, further distal exposure is obtained by separating the attachments of the ligaments to the styloid process and dividing the styloid process.

care taken to look for the spinal portion of the accessory (11th cranial) nerve as it enters the sternocleidomastoid muscle on the medial surface. With the sternocleidomastoid muscle fully mobilized and retractors in place, the internal carotid artery can then be further exposed.

The jugular vein is mobilized up toward the base of the skull, with care taken to look for additional accessory facial branches, which must be divided between ligatures so that the jugular vein can be fully mobilized and moved posteriorly. The perivascular plane of the internal carotid artery is carefully defined, and the artery is gently mobilized with a sharp-tipped clamp applied in a spreading motion; in this way, the more distal portion of the inter-

nal carotid artery can be mobilized downward. If the vessel is still insufficiently mobile, then the nerve to the carotid body and the ascending pharyngeal artery within the crotch between the internal and external carotid arteries are mobilized and divided between ligatures. These two structures often serve as a de facto suspensory ligament for the carotid bulb; dividing them allows the carotid bifurcation to drop down and permits further downward traction of the internal carotid artery as the vessel is gently mobilized distally [see Figure 6].

Once the internal carotid artery is further exposed distally and the hypoglossal nerve is mobilized along its vertical portion and moved anteriorly, the posterior belly of the digastric muscle is encountered.

An areolar plane is developed posteriorly and superiorly along the inferior margin of the posterior belly of the digastric muscle, allowing the muscle to be mobilized anteriorly to yield additional exposure of the internal carotid artery. If the resulting exposure is not sufficient, the muscle may be carefully encircled with a right-angle clamp and divided [*see Figure 7*]. In those relatively uncommon cases in which even further distal exposure is required, the styloid process is palpated and the muscular and ligamentous attachments to the styloid process divided, so that the styloid process can be exposed with a periosteal elevator. Once the styloid process has been completely freed of its muscular and ligamentous attachments and the cranial nerves in the vicinity have been identified and carefully protected, the styloid process is cut close to the base of the skull [*see Figure 7*].

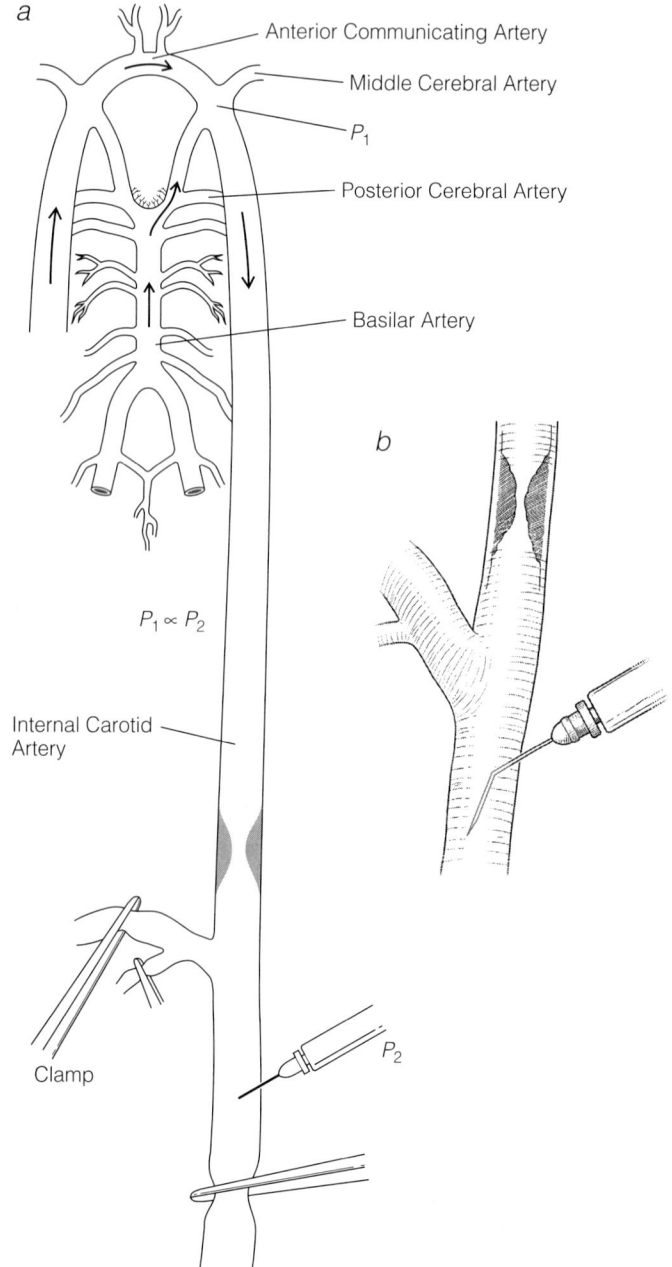

Figure 8 Carotid arterial procedures. (*a*) Shown is a graphic representation of the measurement of internal carotid artery back-pressure. (*b*) The needle is bent at a 45° angle before being inserted into the common carotid artery.

This step yields optimal exposure of the internal carotid artery all the way to the base of the skull.

Additional adjunctive measures for more extensive exposure of the internal carotid artery have been described. These include subluxation or dislocation of the mandible,[7] wiring of the mandible into a subluxed position, and division of the ramus of the mandible with rotation of the mandible away from the base of the skull. In my view, these measures are unnecessary, provided that the sternocleidomastoid muscle and the jugular vein have been adequately mobilized, the plane around the internal carotid artery has been developed, and the carotid bifurcation has been released.

A significant risk associated with extended exposure of the internal carotid artery is possible injury to the vagus nerve, the accessory nerve, or the hypoglossal nerve. Retraction of the vagus nerve may produce either temporary or permanent vocal cord palsy, and extensive retraction of or injury to the hypoglossal nerve causes denervation of the ipsilateral side of the tongue, manifested by tongue deviation to the ipsilateral side on protrusion or difficulty with mastication or swallowing. In addition, posterior exposure of a high carotid bifurcation may result in injury to branches of the glossopharyngeal (ninth cranial) nerve.

A common error in carotid artery mobilization is failure to recognize that the plaque in the internal carotid artery extends beyond the upper limit of the arterial exposure. It is far better to anticipate this problem before clamping and opening the artery than to discover it afterward and be forced to mobilize the vessel after it has been clamped. Once the common carotid and internal carotid arteries have been mobilized sufficiently, they are encircled with umbilical tapes; Rumel tourniquets are used if an internal shunt is required or desired.

STEP 3: CEREBRAL CIRCULATORY SUPPORT

Clamping of the carotid artery necessarily results in interruption of blood flow through the vessel. Patients who have good collateral circulation via the contralateral carotid artery or the vertebral arteries generally (though not always) tolerate the temporary interruption of flow through the clamped artery well.[8] Patients who have inadequate collateral blood flow require cerebral circulatory support, usually in the form of placement of an internal shunt. There are three basic approaches to shunt use: (1) routine use of an internal shunt, (2) selective use of an internal shunt, and (3) routine avoidance of shunting in an attempt to minimize clamp time.

Shunting Options

Routine shunting In approximately 10% of patients undergoing carotid artery surgery, collateral blood flow is inadequate and temporary use of an indwelling shunt is necessary to prevent brain damage; in the remaining 90%, collateral blood flow is adequate and clamping generally well tolerated, and shunting is therefore unnecessary. Clearly, routine use of an internal shunt takes care of the 10% of patients who require shunts. Its disadvantage is that it is an additional procedure that carries its own complications, to which not only the 10% of patients who require shunting but also the 90% who do not are subjected. The potential complications associated with placement of a shunt include intimal injury (including the raising of an intimal flap), atheroma embolization (if atheromatous material is scooped up during shunt placement), and air embolization (if air bubbles are trapped within the shunt and not recognized).

Selective shunting Selective placement of a shunt has an advantage over routine placement in that the procedure and its potential complications are limited to the 10% of patients who actually re-

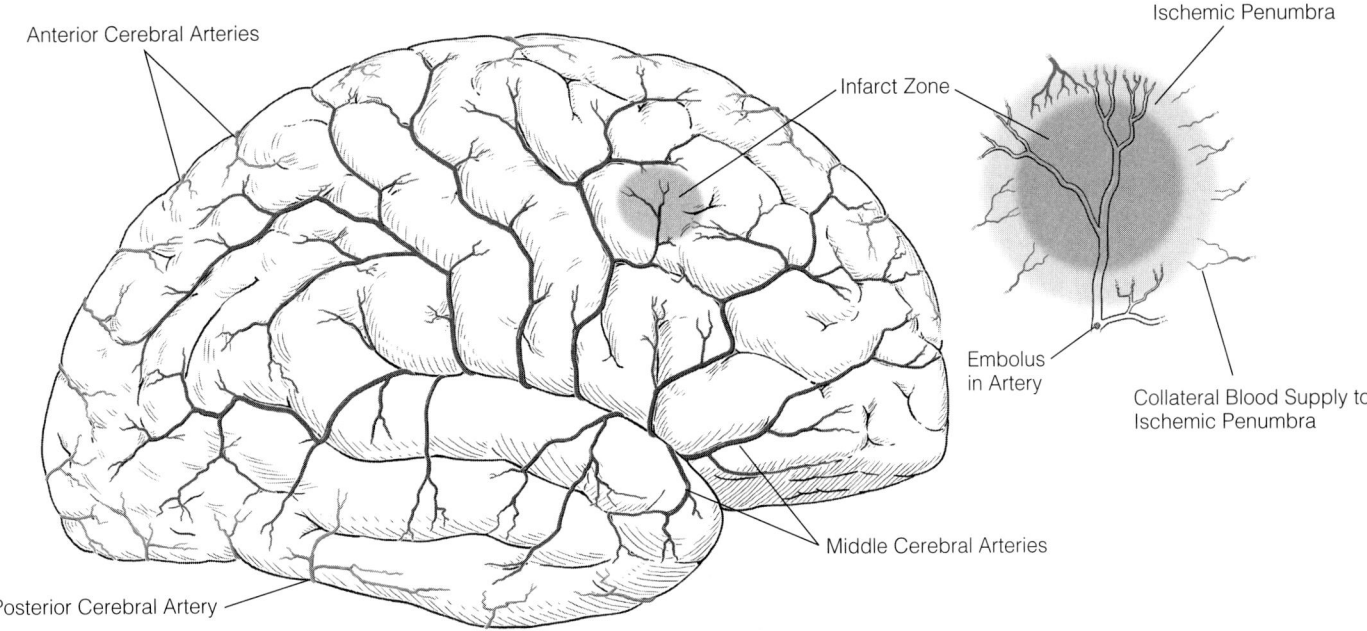

Anterior Cerebral Arteries

Ischemic Penumbra

Infarct Zone

Embolus
in Artery

Collateral Blood Supply to
Ischemic Penumbra

Middle Cerebral Arteries

Posterior Cerebral Artery

Figure 9 **Carotid arterial procedures. When a thromboembolic fragment occludes a cortical arterial branch, a central infarct zone develops, surrounded by an ischemic zone that derives some residual blood supply from collateral vessels. In this zone, known as the ischemic penumbra, the residual blood supply is sufficient to maintain viability.**

quire a shunt. Its main disadvantage is that the methods used to identify patients who require shunting may not be entirely reliable.

Selective identification of patients who require shunting can be accomplished in several ways. The most direct—and perhaps safest—method is to employ local or cervical block anesthesia so that the effect of temporary carotid clamping can be assessed in a conscious patient; if clamping leads to a neurologic deficit, then the patient clearly requires an internal shunt. Other methods of identifying patients who require a shunt make use of techniques such as continuous electroencephalographic monitoring, measurement of somatosensory evoked potential, and monitoring of middle cerebral blood flow with transcranial Doppler ultrasonography.

A useful method of determining the adequacy of collateral cerebral blood flow is measurement of back-pressure in the internal carotid artery.[9] Back-pressure has been shown to be a good index of the adequacy of collateral blood flow, and it correlates well with the safety of temporary clamping and thus with the necessity of placing an internal shunt. Back-pressure is measured by placing into the common carotid artery a needle that is connected to pressure tubing and a pressure transducer. The tip of the needle is bent at a 45° angle. Systemic blood pressure is measured, and clamps are placed on the common carotid artery proximal to the needle and on the external carotid artery. The residual pressure in the common carotid artery, which is in continuity with the internal carotid artery, is then allowed to equilibrate; the resulting pressure reading represents internal carotid artery back-pressure [*see Figure 8*]. It has been determined that patients with back-pressures higher than 25 mm Hg can tolerate temporary clamping without incurring brain damage.

Selective shunting is also appropriate for patients who have previously had strokes, regardless of the degree of neurologic recovery. In these patients, a central area of cerebral infarction is surrounded by a zone of relatively ischemic tissue—the so-called ischemic penumbra. The ischemic penumbra is made up of live and potentially functional brain tissue, but its viability is highly dependent on maximization

of cerebral perfusion pressure through collateral channels. Accordingly, any interruption of carotid circulation, regardless of the degree of collateral circulation present, may threaten the ischemic penumbra and extend the infarct [*see Figure 9*]. In my opinion, all carotid endarterectomy patients with prior strokes should receive shunts on a routine basis.

Routine avoidance of shunting   The advantage of routinely avoiding the use of shunts is that the technical issues and potential complications associated with the additional procedure are avoided entirely. The disadvantage is that unshunted patients with poor collateral blood flow may sustain ischemic brain damage, particularly if the clamp time turns out to be longer than was anticipated.

Technique of Shunt Placement

Internal shunts must be placed with great care if shunt-associated complications are to be avoided. Of the various shunts currently available, I prefer the Javid shunt, which is tapered, has smooth leading edges, and possesses external bulbous circumferential extensions that permit it to be held in place with a circumferential Rumel tourniquet, thereby minimizing the chances of inadvertent dislodgment. Optimal placement of an internal shunt may be achieved by means of the following steps [*see Figure 10*].

After the patient has been adequately heparinized and the artery clamped and opened, the distal portion of the internal shunt is placed into the internal carotid artery. A clamp is placed on the shunt and briefly opened to allow back-bleeding; good back-bleeding confirms that the shunt is lying free in the lumen of the internal carotid artery. The shunt is then secured by tightening a Rumel tourniquet, and the bulbous portion of the shunt is engaged to prevent dislodgment.

Next, the proximal portion of the shunt is placed into the common carotid artery. As this is done, the clamp is removed from the shunt so that backflow from the shunt will dislodge any loose material and air within the common carotid artery. The shunt is then re-

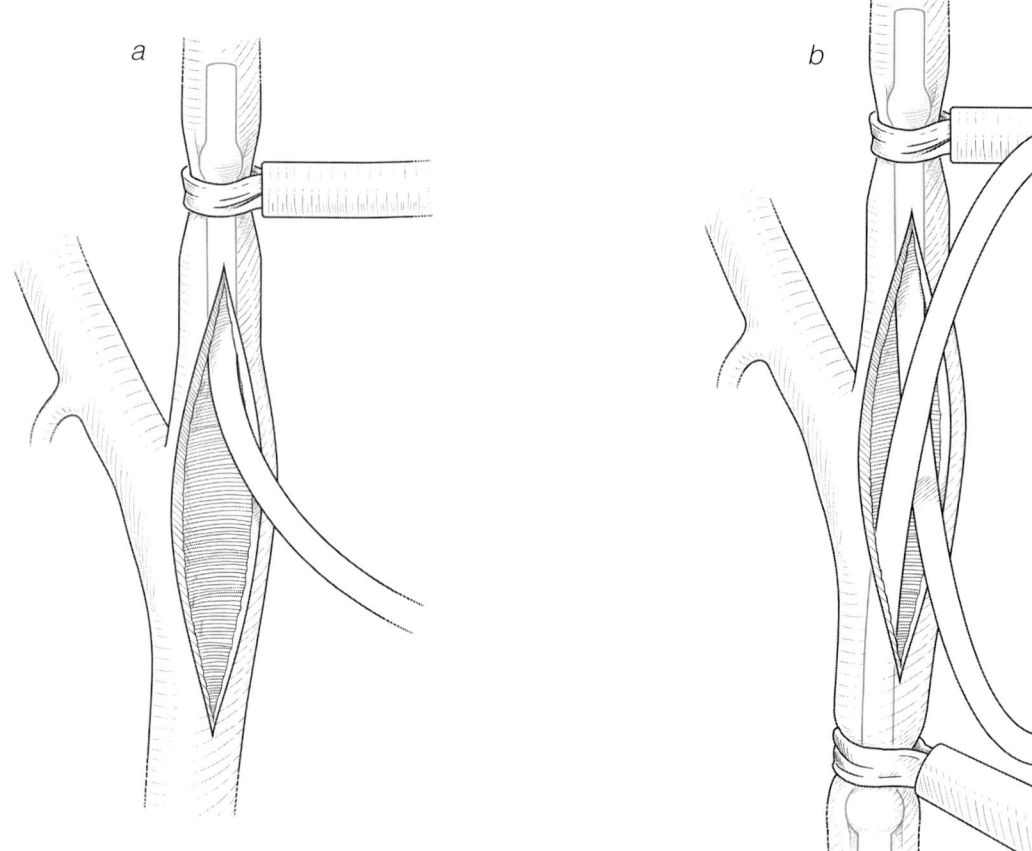

Figure 10 **Carotid arterial procedures. Shown is the technique of shunt placement, first distally (*a*) and then proximally (*b*).**

clamped, and the clamp is removed from the common carotid artery as the proximal portion of the shunt is passed into that vessel.

When the proximal portion of the shunt is in the proper position in the common carotid artery, it is secured by tightening a Rumel tourniquet on the vessel. The clamp on the shunt is then slowly opened so that the surgeon can observe flow through the translucent device and thus verify that no solid particles or air bubbles are passing through it. Because the shunt is relatively long, the surgeon has a reasonable amount of time in which to observe flow. If any particles or air bubbles are identified, the shunt can be quickly clamped, removed from the common carotid artery, and back-bled, and the procedure can then be repeated.

Once the shunt is secured in place and open, its length and redundancy allow it to be easily manipulated medially and laterally; endarterectomy can then be performed without the encumbrance of an inlying shunt.

STEP 4: RECONSTRUCTION OPTIONS

There are four principal reconstructions involving the common carotid artery and the carotid bifurcation: (1) conventional open carotid endarterectomy with either patch angioplasty or primary closure, (2) eversion endarterectomy, (3) reconstruction for proximal lesions of the common carotid artery, and (4) reconstruction for recurrent stenosis with resection of the carotid bifurcation and grafting.

Open Carotid Endarterectomy

Once the carotid bifurcation has been fully mobilized both proximal and distal to the lesion, systemic anticoagulation with heparin is initiated. I generally give 5,000 units, an amount that is sufficient to produce adequate anticoagulation for the duration of carotid clamping but is not large enough to necessitate heparin reversal on completion of the operation. If internal carotid artery back-pressure is to be used to determine whether the patient requires an internal shunt, then it is measured at this time. If cerebral electrical activity is to be the determinant, then the internal, external, and common carotid arteries are clamped and electrical activity is monitored (e.g., via EEG) with the clamps in place. If electrical changes are noted with clamping, an internal shunt is required.

Arteriotomy The common carotid artery and the carotid bifurcation are rotated so as to be positioned for an arteriotomy that begins on the common carotid artery and extends through the bulb of the internal carotid artery to a point 180° opposite the flow divider [*see Figure 11*]. This incision effectively bivalves the carotid bulb, thus making possible a more accurate primary or patch closure. The arteriotomy continues through the plaque and extends well up into the internal carotid artery, beyond the visible end point of the atherosclerotic plaque.

Plaque removal A dissection plane separating the atherosclerotic intima from the media and the adventitia is then developed with a sharp-bladed dissector. As a rule, it is easiest to begin the endarterectomy at the point where the plaque is bulkiest. At this point, the medial fibers are usually gone, but as the dissection continues both proximally and distally, more normal medial tissue may be seen. It is important to develop the dissection plane between the intima and the media if possible because doing so permits the creation of a feathered end point distally as dissection proceeds into a relatively normal portion of the internal carotid artery [*see Figure 12*]. If the dissection plane is between the media and the adventitia, a feathered end point is much harder to achieve. Failure to achieve a feathered end point often results in a sharp shelf at the internal carotid artery level, which increases the risk of subsequent intimal dissection when blood flow is restored.

Once the dissection plane is complete on one side of the arteriotomy at the level of the common carotid artery, a right-angle clamp is gently inserted into the plane and advanced through it to the opposite side of the arteriotomy, thereby separating the plaque from the arterial wall around the entire circumference of the vessel. The clamp is then gently spread and brought downward to complete the circumferential dissection of the plaque proximally. The proximal end point of plaque dissection is obtained by cutting the intima with a No. 15 blade.

With the same depth of dissection now existing on both sides of the open common carotid artery, dissection then continues distally up to the carotid bifurcation. At this point, the plaque within the external carotid artery is carefully separated in a circumferential fash-

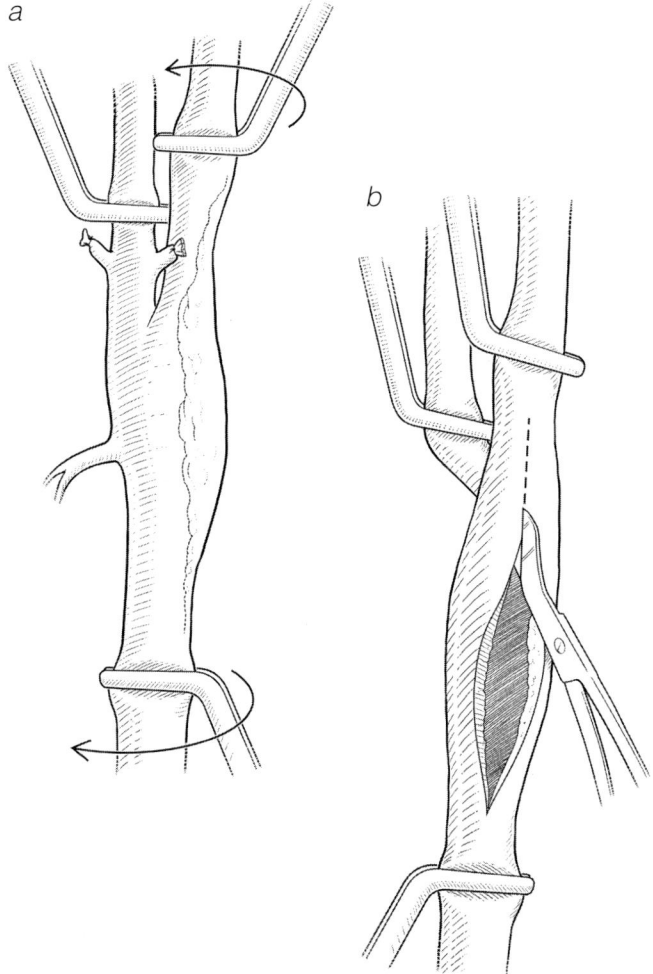

Figure 11 Carotid arterial procedures: open endarterectomy. Clamps are applied to the common, internal, and external carotid arteries, and the structures are rotated (*a*) so that an arteriotomy can be made in the common carotid artery 180° opposite the flow divider (*b*).

ion. This is usually done by using a sharp mosquito clamp until all of the plaque has been separated from the vessel wall and dissection has reached normal intima. The freed plaque is gently grasped with the opened mosquito clamp, traction is applied, and the distal end point of plaque dissection in the external carotid artery is obtained.

Dissection then continues up the internal carotid artery, with care taken to leave normal intima behind. Often, the plaque becomes a relatively narrow tongue of atheroma on the posterior wall of the internal carotid artery. If the edge of the atheromatous plaque is followed to its end, a tapered, feathered end point can be achieved.

Irrigation and clearing of debris   After removal of the specimen, the intimectomized surface is vigorously irrigated with heparinized saline. Any medial debris present is carefully removed. The distal end point is irrigated to determine whether there is a residual flap that might lead to subsequent intimal dissection; if there is a flap, it is carefully removed. If there is a sharp shelf at the distal end point, it is usually an indication that the endarterectomy has not been carried far enough distally. When this is the case, the arteriotomy should be lengthened so that the endarterectomy can be extended to a point where the intima is completely normal. If the patient has a very high carotid bifurcation, very distal plaque, or both and further dissection is impeded by the base of the skull, it may be necessary to secure the distal end point with tacking sutures. Tacking sutures should be used only in exceptional circumstances because their use may lead to healing abnormalities or to the presence of platelet aggregate material that can cause thromboembolic or occlusive complications.

Once the intimectomized surface is completely clear of debris, the lumen of the external carotid artery should be visually inspected to confirm that all overlying dissected intima has been cleared. Any residual dissected intima can be gently teased out with a mosquito clamp. Once the vessel is completely clear, preparation is made for closure of the arteriotomy.

Closure of arteriotomy   If the arteriotomy is relatively short and extends only up to the central portion of the bulb of the internal carotid artery, it can usually be closed primarily with a continuous 6-0 polypropylene suture. Placing very small stitches close together in the internal carotid artery should minimize the risk of vessel narrowing.

If the vessel is relatively small or the arteriotomy was extended well up on the internal carotid artery to ensure a complete endarterectomy, the arteriotomy should be closed with a patch angioplasty. Of the several patch options available, the basic choice is between a prosthetic patch and an autogenous patch composed of a segment of saphenous vein obtained from an extremity. The relative merits of autogenous and prosthetic patches have been extensively debated in the literature, but no definitive conclusions have been reached. One of the disadvantages of an autogenous patch is that surgeons tend to use the entire open portion of the saphenous vein, which then dilates further under arterial pressure, leading to an artery of aneurysmal proportions. Another disadvantage is the potential for patch blowout, which, though rare, has been reported in several series. The main disadvantage of a prosthetic patch is the risk of infection, but this is extremely low.

At present, it would appear that a prosthetic patch is at least as acceptable as an autogenous patch, and the prosthetic patch has an additional advantage in that there is no need to remove a normal saphenous vein segment from an extremity. Prosthetic patches can be composed of either fabric or polytetrafluoroethylene (PTFE). Fabric patches now come impregnated with either collagen or gelatin to make them leakproof; PTFE patches do not leak on the surface, but they are prone to leakage at suture needle puncture sites.

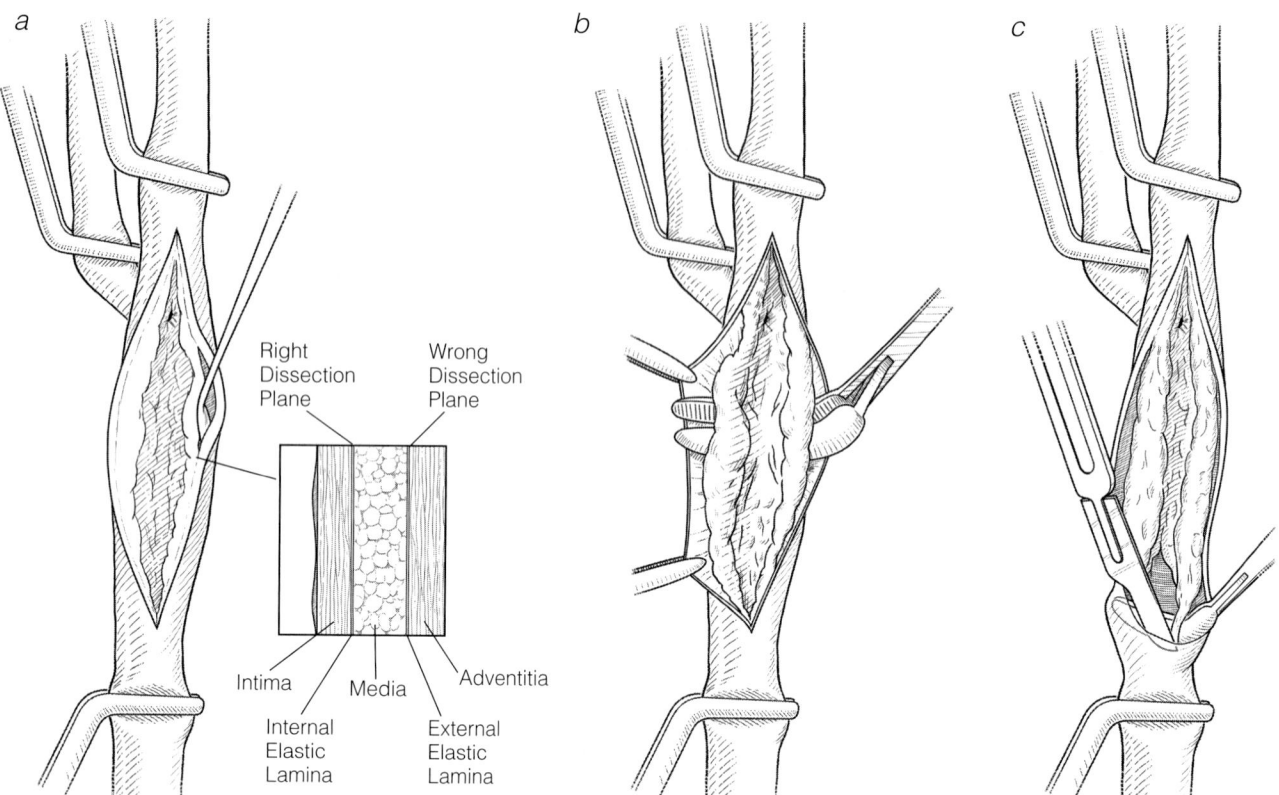

a

b

c

Figure 12 **Carotid arterial procedures: open endarterectomy. (*a*) Dissection is started where plaque is thickest. Often, medial fibers are completely gone here. Dissection proceeds both proximally and distally along one side, and more normal medial tissue may be found. Development of a plane between intima and media, if possible, is valuable for creating a feathered end point distally. (*b*) Once dissection is complete on one side, the same plane is established on the opposite side. (*c*) The end point of proximal dissection is established by sharp division of plaque against the clamp.**

Patch size is a crucial consideration: it is important that the patch be neither too wide nor too narrow. If the patch is too narrow, it will not provide the additional material needed to restore the carotid bifurcation to a normal diameter. If the patch is too wide, it will provide too much additional material and create what virtually amounts to a carotid aneurysm; this would represent a significant disadvantage to the patient in terms of flow dynamics and the risk of producing laminated thrombus in the most dilated portion of the carotid bulb. My preference is to use a 6.0 mm wide collagen-impregnated fabric patch for patch angioplasty.

Whichever patch is selected is cut to length, beveled at each end, and sewn in place with a continuous 6-0 polypropylene suture.

Before completion of the closure, the internal carotid artery and the external carotid artery are back-bled, and the common carotid artery is flushed. The arteriotomy is then completely closed. Removing the clamp on the internal carotid artery allows blood flow to fill the carotid bulb and permits one last internal flush. The origin of the internal carotid artery is then occluded with a vascular forceps, and the clamps are removed first from the external carotid artery and then from the common carotid artery to allow resumption of blood flow. After several heartbeats, the forceps on the origin of the internal carotid artery is removed, and blood flow through the internal carotid artery is restored. There may be some leakage of blood along the suture line, which can usually be controlled with the placement of thrombin-soaked absorbable gelatin sponge. If any obvious defect is noted between sutures, an additional stitch should be placed.

Eversion Endarterectomy

Eversion endarterectomy was designed and developed to eliminate the need for a suture line on the internal carotid artery, in the hope that doing so would reduce the incidence of myointimal hyperplasia and consequent restenosis. There is evidence to suggest that the use of eversion endarterectomy has led to some reduction in the incidence of myointimal hyperplasia, but the data are controversial and certainly are not conclusive. Nonetheless, the technique may well have merit, and it should be a part of the vascular surgeon's armamentarium.

Besides the avoidance of a suture line on the internal carotid artery, the advantages of eversion endarterectomy include the simple end-to-side anastomotic closure and the possibility of managing a redundant internal carotid artery by moving it down the common carotid artery. One disadvantage is the potential difficulty of achieving an end point in cases in which the bifurcation is high or plaque extends well up the internal carotid artery toward the base of the skull. Another disadvantage arises with patients who require an internal shunt, in that it is not possible to keep an internal shunt in place for the entire duration of an eversion endarterectomy. Yet another disadvantage is that the distal end point cannot be viewed as clearly as it can in open endarterectomy. A fourth disadvantage is that eversion endarterectomy is poorly suited to cases in which the internal carotid artery is relatively small and contracted and thus better treated with patch angioplasty.

Eversion and plaque dissection After the carotid bifurcation is fully mobilized, the internal, external, and common carotid arteries are clamped. A circumferential incision is placed in an oblique fashion at the junction of the common carotid artery and the bulb of the internal carotid artery to permit division of the bulbous portion of the internal carotid artery from the common carotid [*see Figure 13*]. The edges of the adventitia of the bulb of the internal carotid artery are grasped, and the outer layers of the vessel wall are gradually everted away from the plaque within the artery. Eversion continues cephalad until it reaches the distal end point of the atherosclerotic lesion, which is marked by the presence of a thin, filmy intima that clearly separates with the specimen, leaving normal vessel behind. The plaque in the common carotid artery and the external carotid artery is then removed in the traditional manner; the opening in the common carotid artery may be extended proximally to facilitate this portion of the endarterectomy.

Reversion and reanastomosis   The internal carotid artery is then reverted to its normal anatomic position, and an anastomosis between the end of the divided bulb of the internal carotid artery and the common carotid artery is fashioned with a continuous 6-0 polypropylene suture. If the internal carotid artery is redundant [*see Special Considerations, below*], the arteriotomy on the common carotid artery is extended proximally and the arteriotomy on the medial aspect of the bulb of the internal carotid artery is extended distally so that the carotid bifurcation may be advanced between the internal and common carotid arteries to eliminate the redundancy.

Reconstruction for Proximal Lesions of Common Carotid Artery

Lesions at the origin of the common carotid artery, either at the level of the aortic arch (in the case of the left common carotid artery) or at the innominate bifurcation (in the case of the right common carotid artery), are relatively rare but do occur. Such lesions may arise

either in isolation or in combination with carotid bifurcation disease. They can be managed by dividing the common carotid artery and transposing it to the adjacent subclavian artery, provided that there is no occlusive disease in the ipsilateral subclavian artery.

Exposure and mobilization   If the lesion at the origin of the common carotid artery is the only one being treated, both the common carotid artery and the subclavian artery should be exposed through a supraclavicular incision that parallels the clavicle. If a carotid bifurcation lesion is present in conjunction with the lesion at the origin of the common carotid artery, the supraclavicular incision is supplemented with a vertical incision along the sternocleidomastoid muscle to permit exposure of the carotid bifurcation. Exposure of the bifurcation has already been addressed (see above); accordingly, I focus here on exposure of the subclavian artery and the proximal common carotid artery.

A supraclavicular incision is placed approximately 1.5 fingerbreadths above the clavicle and centered over the lateral head of the sternocleidomastoid muscle. The lateral head of the sternocleidomastoid muscle is divided, and the scalene triangle is defined. The scalene fat pad is mobilized off the anterior scalene muscle. The phrenic nerve is identified, mobilized off the scalene muscle, and gently retracted. A plane is developed with gentle dissection between the posterior portion of the anterior scalene muscle and the underlying subclavian artery, and the anterior scalene muscle is divided. Division of the muscle exposes the underlying subclavian artery, a sufficient length of which can then be mobilized in the perivascular plane to permit an anastomosis.

The jugular vein is identified at the medial aspect of the incision and mobilized anteriorly and medially to expose the common carot-

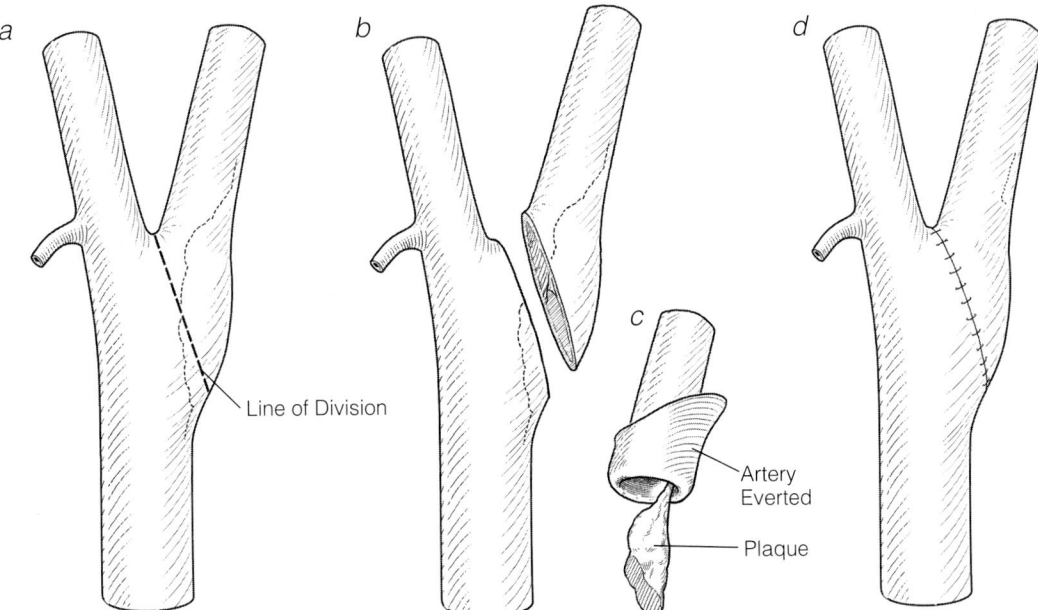

Figure 13   **Carotid arterial procedures: eversion endarterectomy. (*a, b*) The internal carotid artery is divided from the common carotid artery in an oblique line. (*c*) The divided internal carotid artery is everted on itself so that it can be separated from the underlying plaque. Eversion proceeds distally until the plaque end point is encountered, and the plaque is removed from the internal carotid artery. Proximal endarterectomy of the common carotid artery and endarterectomy of the external carotid artery are then carried out. (*d*) Once all of the plaque has been removed, the internal carotid artery is reverted and an end-to-side anastomosis is fashioned between the common carotid artery opening and the internal carotid artery.**

id artery. The vagus nerve is identified and carefully protected. The common carotid artery is then mobilized both proximally and distally; proximal mobilization should extend as far behind the sternoclavicular junction as the surgeon can comfortably manage.

Transection and anastomosis   The common carotid artery is clamped proximally and distally, then divided; the proximal portion of the vessel is oversewn. The transected common carotid artery is brought posterior to the jugular vein in the vicinity of the subclavian artery. The subclavian artery is clamped proximally and distally, a longitudinal arteriotomy is made, and a small ellipse of subclavian arterial tissue is removed. The end of the common carotid artery is then sewn to the side of the subclavian artery with a continuous 6-0 polypropylene suture.

Before completion, the vessels are back-bled and flushed. Once the anastomosis is complete, blood flow is restored, first to the distal subclavian artery and then to the common carotid artery.

Reconstruction for Recurrent Carotid Stenosis

For an initial recurrence of carotid stenosis that primarily results from myointimal hyperplasia, conversion to a patch angioplasty is generally the best treatment. For second or third recurrences or for recurrences that develop in spite of patch angioplasty, resection of the carotid bifurcation with interposition grafting between the common carotid artery and the normal distal internal carotid artery is the best treatment.

Exposure and mobilization   Exposure of a carotid bifurcation for treatment of recurrent carotid stenosis can be challenging. The initial skin incision is reopened, and dissection is carried down through the scar tissue to the common carotid artery. The common carotid artery is sharply dissected from the surrounding scar tissue, with the dissection plane kept close to the adventitia to minimize the risk of injury to the vagus nerve and the hypoglossal nerve. Once the common carotid artery has been adequately mobilized, dissection is carried distally to include the carotid bifurcation and the internal carotid artery. In the course of distal dissection, care must be taken to watch for the hypoglossal nerve, which may be incorporated into the scar tissue; this structure must be carefully dissected away from the artery and protected.

Distal dissection continues beyond the end point of the previous closure of the internal carotid artery. Beyond this end point, it is usually possible to enter a previously undissected plane of the internal carotid artery; from here onward, the artery typically is soft around its circumference and is not involved in the recurrent stenosis. The external carotid artery is then mobilized sufficiently to allow the surgeon to control back-bleeding.

Conversion to patch angioplasty   If the artery was originally closed primarily, an arteriotomy is made through the old suture line and carried distally through the area of stenosis and onto a relatively normal area of the internal carotid artery. Exploration of the luminal surface usually reveals a smooth, glistening neointima, and observation of the cut section of the artery reveals an area where a whitish, firm thickening of the intimal wall has occurred as a result of myointimal hyperplasia. No attempt should be made to reendarterectomize the stenotic area, because the intimal lesion is not, in fact, plaque but scar tissue. If the intima is removed, the cascade of events that led to the myointimal hyperplasia will simply be reinitiated. Accordingly, the healed intimal surface should be carefully protected. A patch angioplasty across the stenotic area, extending from the common carotid artery proximally to a relatively normal portion of the internal carotid artery distally, is usually sufficient to treat the lesion.

Resection of carotid bifurcation with interposition grafting   If the stenosis is recurring for the second or third time or the artery was originally closed with a patch, the surgeon should proceed with resection and interposition grafting. In most cases, it is necessary to sacrifice the external carotid artery and oversew its origin. The internal carotid artery is divided distal to the intimal hyperplastic lesion, the common carotid artery is divided proximally, and the diseased specimen is removed.

I prefer to use 6.0 mm thin-walled PTFE for the interposition graft. The internal carotid artery distally and the common carotid artery proximally are spatulated by making vertical incisions approximately 6.0 mm in length. The PTFE graft is appropriately beveled both proximally and distally, and beveled or spatulated end-to-end anastomoses are performed, first to the internal carotid artery and then to the common carotid artery.

Before completion, the vessels are back-bled and flushed; once the anastomoses are complete, blood flow is reestablished.

Some surgeons may be tempted to use autogenous saphenous vein for the interposition graft. To use such grafts would appear, on the face of it, to be a good idea; in fact, it is a mistake. For reasons not clearly understood, the use of autogenous saphenous vein in the neck has an extremely poor track record, yielding unacceptably high rates of recurrent stenosis and occlusion in comparison with the use of prosthetic grafts.

Special Considerations

Fibromuscular dysplasia of internal carotid artery   Fibromuscular dysplasia of the internal carotid artery is a congenital or acquired lesion that has been subdivided into four pathologic varieties, of which the most common is medial fibroplasia. On contrast angiography, medial fibroplasia has a characteristic appearance, resembling a string of beads in the extracranial portion of the internal carotid artery [*see Figure 14*]. A common initial manifestation is a relatively loud bruit in the neck of a young woman. Fibromuscular dysplasia can cause symptoms of monocular or hemispheric TIAs, or it

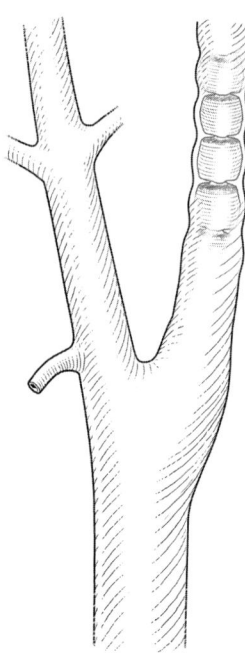

Figure 14   **Carotid arterial procedures: repair of fibromuscular dysplasia. Depicted is the so-called string of beads deformity of the cervical portion of the internal carotid artery, which is characteristic of medial fibroplasia.**

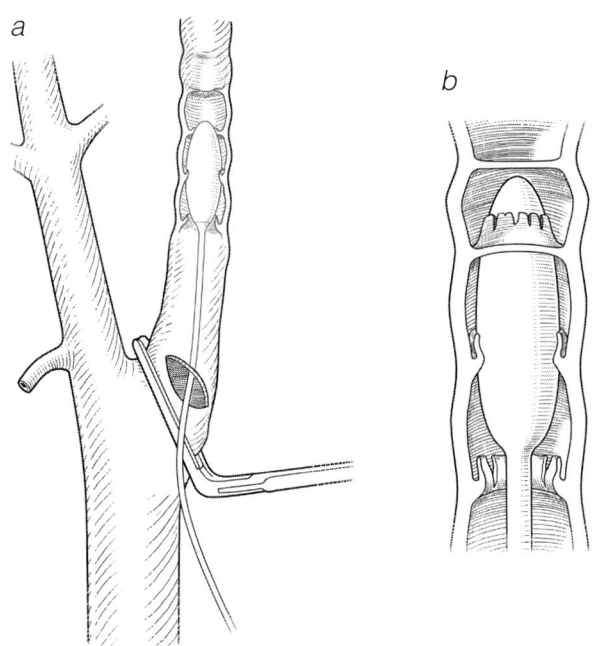

Figure 15 Carotid arterial procedures: repair of fibromuscular dysplasia. (*a*) The proximal portion of the internal carotid bulb is clamped, a transverse arteriotomy is made, and a coronary dilator is passed into the internal carotid artery and advanced up the vessel to the base of the skull. (*b*) The small septa in the internal carotid artery are disrupted by the advancing probe.

may go on to cause a stroke, usually as a consequence of a dissection resulting in thrombotic occlusion. If symptoms develop, they can generally be controlled by means of antiplatelet drugs. Currently, the only indication for surgical intervention is the persistence of symptoms despite antiplatelet therapy.

Treatment of fibromuscular dysplasia has evolved in recent years. The first attempts at surgical repair involved a total resection of the internal carotid artery coupled with interposition of a graft (usually composed of saphenous vein). This technique is now largely abandoned because of the extensive surgical dissection required and the substantial risk of cranial nerve injury; its only remaining application is in cases where there is associated aneurysmal dilatation in the dysplastic segment that calls for resection and graft interposition. At present, the two most popular modes of therapy both involve intraluminal dilatation with disruption of the small septa within the artery. One mode achieves intraluminal dilatation via an open approach, and the other achieves the same end via a percutaneous approach that includes balloon angioplasty. Dilatation and fracturing of the intraluminal septa often result in the release of particles of septal tissue, which in turn can lead to cerebral embolization and infarction. Consequently, open methods, which enable the surgeon to flush out the disrupted segments, are usually favored.

In symptomatic patients with fibromuscular dysplasia, the carotid bifurcation may be exposed in the usual manner. If there is significant redundancy of the internal carotid artery, as documented by preoperative imaging, the artery should be mobilized relatively extensively so that it can be straightened by downward traction before intraluminal dilatation is begun. If, on the other hand, the artery is relatively straight, only minimal mobilization is required. It should be kept in mind that approximately 25% of patients with fibromuscular dysplasia have associated atheromatous disease of the carotid bifurcation that must be dealt with at the time of operation. In addi-

tion, about the same number of patients have associated intracranial aneurysms that should be checked for by means of intracranial imaging studies.

Once the carotid bifurcation has been suitably mobilized and it has been established that no associated atheromatous plaque is present, a small transverse incision is made on the bulb of the internal carotid artery, with flow being maintained between the common and external carotid arteries. Serial intraluminal dilatations are then performed with coronary artery dilators of progressively increasing diameter [*see Figure 15*]. The first dilator (usually 2.5 mm in diameter) is passed up the carotid artery to the base of the skull under digital control. The dilator is then withdrawn, and the artery is back-bled to flush out any fractured segments. The next larger dilator (3.0 mm in diameter) is passed in a similar fashion. Dilatation is repeated with progressively larger dilators (3.5, 4.0, and possibly 4.5 mm in diameter) to complete the procedure.

The transverse arteriotomy is closed with 6-0 polypropylene suture material and flow is reestablished. A completion angiogram verifies that the dysplastic segment is fully restored.

Coiling or kinking of internal carotid artery Redundancy of the internal carotid artery, often resulting in a 360° coil of the high cervical portion of the internal carotid artery, is usually thought to be developmental in origin [*see Figure 16a*]. Elongation of the internal carotid artery, which often results in kinking of the vessel, is believed to be related to the degenerative changes that occur with aging and atherosclerosis [*see Figure 16b*]. Both of these phenomena, in and of themselves, are usually asymptomatic; exceptions occur when an atheromatous plaque develops at the apex of the coil or when kinking of the internal carotid artery is accentuated with changes in head position in a patient who depends on relatively normal blood flow through that vessel. Redundancy of the internal carotid artery often becomes a technical consideration during standard surgical treatment of a carotid bifurcation atheroma. When redundancy occurs, it must be appropriately dealt with to prevent postoperative complications.

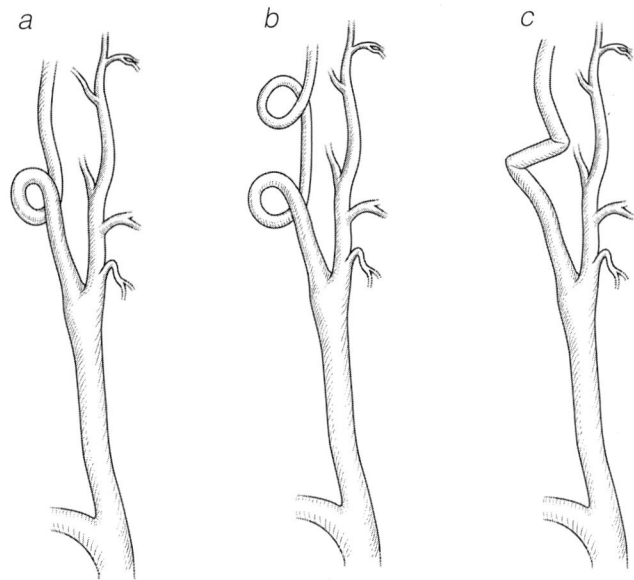

Figure 16 Carotid arterial procedures: repair of coiling or kinking of the internal carotid artery. (*a, b*) Redundancy of the internal carotid artery can result in one or more 360° coils in the vessel. (*c*) Degenerative atheromatous changes of the internal carotid artery can cause elongation with associated kinking or buckling.

Anticipated redundancy of the internal carotid artery at the time of carotid bifurcation endarterectomy can usually be managed with a patch angioplasty. Provided that the arteriotomy extends beyond the apex of the kink, the patch should smooth out the curvature of the redundant vessel and eliminate the kink. If it appears that internal carotid artery redundancy is greater than can be corrected by an elongated patch, then detachment of the internal carotid artery followed by eversion endarterectomy and reimplantation is indicated.

If the arteriotomy has already been closed when it becomes apparent that a kink is present, the problem may be dealt with by mobilizing the external carotid artery sufficiently and then resecting a segment of the common carotid artery and pulling down on the carotid bifurcation with a new end-to-end anastomosis to straighten the redundant internal carotid artery [see Figure 17]. Segmental resection of the internal carotid artery itself combined with end-to-end repair has also been described; this approach is less desirable, being more technically demanding and hence more subject to technical error.

Patients with coiling of the internal carotid artery may present a more difficult problem. If the atheromatous plaque involves only the first portion of the internal carotid artery and the vessel beyond that first portion is relatively normal up to the point where coiling begins, the surgeon can simply avoid the problem by leaving the smooth coil in place and not carrying out an extensive distal dissection. If, on the other hand, it appears that there may be plaque in the coil, then the entire coil must be dissected free, and the patient is left with a very redundant internal carotid artery that must be dealt with. Once again, the best method of managing the problem is to resect the redundant segment of the internal carotid artery, with or without eversion endarterectomy, and to reimplant the internal carotid artery onto the distal common carotid artery at the point of transection.

Upon completion of the reconstruction, a completion angiogram should be obtained to verify that the coiling or kinking has been adequately treated.

STEP 5: COMPLETION IMAGING

Given that the majority of neurologic complications after carotid artery surgery are attributable to technical error, it is imperative that the technical accuracy of the reconstruction be confirmed before the incision is closed and the patient is sent to the recovery room. There are two principal methods of determining the technical quality of the reconstruction: on-table angiography and direct-contact duplex scanning of the carotid artery. To perform either of these techniques routinely in all patients adds relatively little time to the surgical procedure and offers significant advantages to both the patient and the surgeon.[10,11]

My preferred method of confirming the quality of the reconstruction is completion angiography using a C-arm with digital imaging. For this reason, the operation is done on a table that has angiographic capability, and the radiology technician and the equipment are called for at the beginning of the arteriotomy closure. A 10 ml syringe is connected to flexible tubing, and a 20-gauge needle is attached to the end of the tubing and bent at a 45° angle. Air bubbles are carefully evacuated from the tubing and the needle. Placing the needle into the artery or, in the case of a patched artery, into the midportion of the patch in a retrograde fashion will provide good stability for the needle, which lies in the lumen of the artery in an axial position. Once the C-arm is in place and the fluoroscopy unit turned on, the contrast material is injected by hand. The resulting image of the carotid bifurcation can be continuously replayed until maximal radiographic opacity of the carotid bifurcation and the intracranial circulation has been attained. The image is then carefully inspected for defects at the end points in the internal and external carotid arteries.

Intimal defects in the internal carotid artery are unusual, though

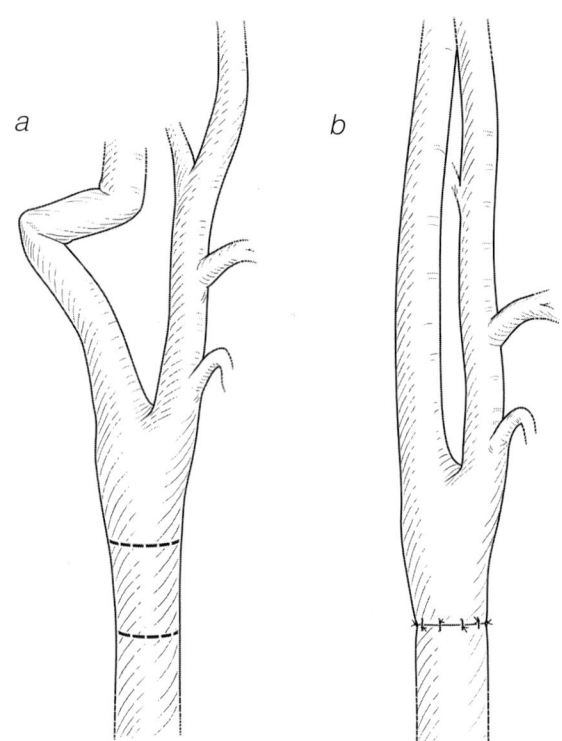

Figure 17 Carotid arterial procedures: repair of coiling or kinking of the internal carotid artery. Kinking or redundancy of the internal carotid artery can be managed by mobilizing the external carotid artery, then resecting a segment of the common carotid artery (a). The surgeon can then draw down the carotid bifurcation for a new primary anastomosis (b).

not unknown. Defects in the external carotid artery are more common because the endarterectomy is essentially done in a blind or closed manner. Defects in the external carotid artery are matters of concern because they may lead to thrombus formation in the external carotid artery; if the thrombus propagates proximally, it may embolize up the internal carotid artery and cause a stroke.[12] For this reason, if a defect is found in the external carotid artery, it is repaired at the time of the operation. To accomplish the repair, clamps are placed on the external carotid artery proximally at its origin and distally beyond the intimal flap. A transverse arteriotomy is made in the external carotid artery to permit identification and removal of the intimal flap. Once the flap has been carefully removed, the transverse arteriotomy is closed with two or three interrupted 6-0 polypropylene sutures and flow is restored.

Completion angiography also has the advantage of permitting the surgeon to image the intracranial circulation. Now that many operations are being performed on the basis of preoperative carotid duplex scanning, intracranial imaging is typically unavailable beforehand, which means that the status of the intracranial circulation with respect to atherosclerotic lesions in the area of the siphon or the middle cerebral artery or with respect to intracranial aneurysms is usually unknown at the start of the procedure. A completion angiogram gives the surgeon the opportunity to rule out these lesions by looking not only at the area around the reconstruction but also at the intracranial circulation.

An alternative to completion angiography is DUS. DUS can be a highly satisfactory way of examining the area of reconstruction, provided that the operating room has duplex scanning capability and that a technologist is available to operate the equipment. Standard B-mode imaging, in conjunction with Doppler ultrasonography, can accurately identify patent or compromised internal and external carotid arteries.

Once the surgeon has confirmed that a good technical reconstruction has been achieved, preparations can be made for closure.

STEP 6: CLOSURE

The dissected area around the reconstructed carotid artery is carefully irrigated with an antibiotic solution, and the wound is meticulously inspected for hemostasis. Even when good hemostasis has been achieved, it is my practice to place a drain overnight—specifically, a 7.0 mm Jackson-Pratt drain brought out through a small separate stab wound. The platysmal layer is closed with a continuous 3-0 absorbable suture, and the skin is closed with a continuous 4-0 subcuticular absorbable suture. A clear adhesive plastic dressing is applied to the skin, and the patient is sent to the recovery room.

Postoperative Management

The main patient variables to be evaluated in the postoperative period are neurologic status, blood pressure, and wound stability.

On awakening from anesthesia, the patient is carefully observed with a view to determining gross cerebral function on the basis of response to commands and movement of extremities. When the patient is fully awake, vagus nerve and hypoglossal nerve function can be tested.

Blood pressure monitoring is of critical importance after carotid endarterectomy. It is essential first to decide on an acceptable blood pressure range for the patient and then to ensure that this pressure is maintained: neither hypertension nor hypotension is acceptable. Patients with severe carotid bifurcation disease who have undergone carotid endarterectomy temporarily lose autoregulation on the side of the operation; therefore, hypertension can result in reperfusion injury to that side of the brain, ranging all the way from simple headache to fatal intracerebral hemorrhage.

The surgical site should be carefully observed for possible wound expansion resulting from hematoma formation. Even when good hemostasis is achieved and a drain is in place, there is still the possibility of delayed bleeding leading to hematoma and airway compromise. If an expanding hematoma is noted, the safest response is to return the patient to the OR so that the hematoma can be evacuated and a bleeding site sought. The earlier this is done, the better.

If the patient is neurologically intact, blood pressure is well controlled, and there is no evidence of an expanding hematoma, then the remaining postoperative care can be provided in a regular hospital room. It is seldom necessary to observe the patient in the intensive care unit, as was once standard practice.

Follow-up

Periodic follow-up examination is essential. There are two major areas of concern: (1) the possibility of recurrent stenosis on the operated side and (2) the possibility of disease developing or progressing in the contralateral carotid artery. It is my practice to see the patient approximately 3 weeks after carotid endarterectomy. In that visit, the patient is examined for quality of wound healing and the presence or absence of carotid bruit on both the operated side and the contralateral side, and a carotid duplex scan is performed. If at this time there are no grounds for concern about the contralateral side, scanning is done only on the side of the operation. The scan serves to establish the new baseline and confirms that the carotid reconstruction is satisfactory. The new baseline is then used as the basis for assessing patient status during subsequent follow-up.

The next patient visit takes place 6 months after operation, at which time a bilateral carotid duplex scan is performed. If the operated side continues to be normal and there are no major problems on the contralateral side, the patient is seen again at the 1-year anniversary of the procedure. If examinations yield satisfactory results at this time, the patient may thereafter be seen at 1-year intervals, with bilateral carotid duplex scanning done at each visit.

Alternatives to Direct Carotid Reconstruction

Angioplasty with stenting has been investigated as a therapeutic alternative to carotid endarterectomy for carotid artery stenosis. In the Wallstent trial (an industry-supported prospective, randomized study), patients with stenosis of 60% to 99%, which was angiographically confirmed according to the North American method of measurement, were randomized into two groups: (1) angioplasty and stenting and (2) carotid endarterectomy.[13] Initially, it was proposed that the study would include 700 patients with symptomatic lesions; however, the trial was stopped by the safety-monitoring committee after 219 patients were randomized. The results were reported at the 26th International Stroke Conference in February 2001.

Of the 219 patients, 107 were randomized to angioplasty and stenting and 112 to carotid endarterectomy. Patients were well matched with respect to age, gender, symptoms, degree of stenosis, and median follow-up. The primary end point was ipsilateral stroke, procedure-related death, or vascular death within 1 year. At approximately 1 year, the primary end-point rate was 12.1% in the angioplasty/stent group and 3.6% in the carotid endarterectomy group ($P = 0.022$). The 30-day stroke morbidity and mortality was 12.1% in the angioplasty/stent group and 4.5% in the carotid endarterectomy group ($P = 0.049$). Upon cessation of the study, the investigators concluded that angioplasty and stenting was not equivalent to carotid endarterectomy for treatment of symptomatic carotid stenosis.

In the SAPPHIRE trial (Stenting and Angioplasty with Protection in Patients at High-Risk for Endarterectomy, which is also an industry-sponsored study), carotid angioplasty and stenting with the use of a cerebral antiembolism device was compared with carotid endarterectomy.[14] Nonrandomized patients were entered into either a stent registry or a surgical registry, but the important part of the study was a randomized, multicenter trial involving 307 patients at 29 investigational sites. Of these 307 patients, 156 were entered into the angioplasty/stent/cerebral protection arm and 151 into the carotid endarterectomy arm. The primary end points were (1) death, any stroke, or nonfatal myocardial infarction (MI) within 30 days after the procedure and (2) 30-day major morbidity plus death and ipsilateral stroke between 31 days and 12 months after the procedure. Secondary end points included (1) patency (defined by restenosis < 50%), (2) disabling stroke between 30 days and 6 months, and (3) a composite of major adverse clinical events at 6 months, 1 year, 2 years, and 3 years.

At 30 days, there were no statistically significant differences between the two study arms when the individual parameters—death, stroke, and nonfatal MI—were considered separately. When these events were viewed in the aggregate, their composite incidence was 5.8% in the angioplasty/stent/cerebral protection group and 12.6% in the carotid endarterectomy group ($P = 0.047$). When death and stroke were considered together, however, the incidence was 4.5% in the angioplasty/stent/cerebral protection group and 6.6% in the carotid endarterectomy group ($P = 0.46$). Thus, it is apparent that the major benefit of angioplasty and stenting over carotid endarterectomy lies in reducing the incidence of nonfatal MI.

References

1. Beneficial effect of carotid endarterectomy in symptomatic patients with high-grade carotid stenosis. North American Symptomatic Carotid Endarterectomy Trial Collaborators. N Engl J Med 325:445, 1991

2. MRC European Carotid Surgery Trial: interim results for symptomatic patients with severe (70-99%) or with mild (0-29%) carotid stenosis. European Carotid Trialists' Collaborative Group. Lancet 337:1235, 1991

3. Mayberg MR, Wilson SE, Yatsu F, et al: Carotid endarterectomy and prevention of cerebral ischemia in symptomatic carotid stenosis. Veterans Affairs Cooperative Studies Program 309 Trialist Group. JAMA 266:3332, 1991

4. Endarterectomy for asymptomatic carotid artery stenosis. Executive Committee for the Asymptomatic Carotid Atherosclerosis Study. JAMA 273:1421, 1995

5. Hobson RW II, Weiss DG, Fields WS, et al: Efficacy of carotid endarterectomy for asymptomatic carotid stenosis. The Veterans Affairs Asymptomatic Cooperative Study Group. N Engl J Med 328:221, 1993

6. Moore WS, Barnett HJM, Beebe HG, et al: Guidelines for carotid endarterectomy—a multidisciplinary consensus statement from the Ad Hoc Committee, American Heart Association. Circulation 91:566, 1995

7. Fisher DF Jr, Clagett GP, Parker JI, et al: Mandibular subluxation for high carotid exposure. J Vasc Surg 1:727, 1984

8. Moore WS, Yee JM, Hall AD: Collateral cerebral blood pressure—an index of tolerance to temporary carotid occlusion. Arch Surg 106:520, 1973

9. Moore WS, Hall AD. Carotid artery back pressure—a test of cerebral tolerance to temporary carotid occlusion. Arch Surg 99:702, 1969

10. Blaisdell FW, Lim R Jr, Hall AD: Technical results of carotid endarterectomy: arteriographic assessment. Am J Surg 114:239, 1967

11. Schwartz RA, Peterson GJ, Noland KA, et al: Intraoperative duplex scanning after carotid reconstruction: a valuable tool. J Vasc Surg 7:260, 1988

12. Moore WS, Martello JY, Quiñones-Baldrich WJ, et al: Etiologic importance of the intimal flap of the external carotid artery in the development of post-carotid endarterectomy stroke. Stroke 21:1497, 1990

13. Alberts MJ: Results of a multicenter prospective randomized trial of carotid artery stenting vs. carotid endarterectomy (abstr). Stroke 32:325d, 2001

14. Yadav J, for the SAPPHIRE Investigators: Stenting and angioplasty with protection in patients at high risk for endarterectomy: the SAPPHIRE study (abstr). Circulation 106:2986a, 2002

Acknowledgment

Figures 1 through 17   Tom Moore.

9 REPAIR OF INFRARENAL ABDOMINAL AORTIC ANEURYSMS

Frank R. Arko, M.D., and Christopher K. Zarins, M.D., F.A.C.S.

An arterial aneurysm is defined as a permanent localized enlargement of an artery to a diameter more than 1.5 times its expected diameter. Aneurysms are classified according to morphology, etiology, and anatomic site. The most common morphology is a fusiform, symmetrical, circumferential enlargement that involves all layers of the arterial wall. A saccular morphology is also seen, in which aneurysmal degeneration affects only part of the arterial circumference.

The most common cause of an arterial aneurysm is atherosclerotic degeneration of the arterial wall. The pathogenesis is a multifactorial process involving genetic predisposition, aging, atherosclerosis, inflammation, and localized activation of proteolytic enzymes. Most aneurysms occur in elderly persons, and the prevalence rises with increasing age. Aneurysms also occur in genetically susceptible individuals with Ehlers-Danlos syndrome or Marfan syndrome. Other causes include tertiary syphilis and localized infection resulting in a mycotic aneurysm.

Aneurysms of the infrarenal aorta are by far the most common arterial aneurysms encountered in clinical practice today: they are three to seven times more common than thoracic aneurysms and affect four times as many men as women.[1] Abdominal aortic aneurysms (AAAs) have a tendency to enlarge and rupture, causing death. In the United States, AAAs result in approximately 15,000 deaths each year and are thus the 13th leading cause of death in the United States.[2,3] The only way to reduce the death rate is to identify and treat aortic aneurysms before they rupture.

The relationship between aneurysm size and risk of rupture is well known. The annual risk of rupture is 1% to 2% for aneurysms less than 5 cm in diameter, 10% for aneurysms 5 to 6 cm in diameter, and 25% or higher for aneurysms greater than 6 cm.[4] Although large aneurysms are much more likely to rupture than small aneurysms, small aneurysms can and do rupture on occasion.

The exact size at which an asymptomatic small AAA should be treated remains unsettled. This issue was the subject of two prospective, randomized clinical trials in the past few years: the United Kingdom Small Aneurysm Trial[5] and the Aneurysm Detection And Management (ADAM) Veterans Affairs (VA) Cooperative Study.[6] Both trials randomly assigned low-risk patients with small (4.0 to 5.4 cm) AAAs to either open surgical repair or ultrasound surveillance. Patients in the surveillance groups were closely monitored with serial ultrasound examinations and underwent open surgical repair if the aneurysm enlarged, became tender to palpation, or became symptomatic. With respect to the primary end point—overall survival—the two trials came to similar conclusions: there was no difference in overall survival between surgery and surveillance groups.[5,6] There was, however, a late survival benefit in the surgery group in the U.K. Small Aneurysm Trial.[7]

Aneurysm rupture rates were low (1%) in both trials, leading many clinicians to conclude that aneurysms smaller than 5.5 cm need not be treated because the risk of rupture is so low. Closer examination of the data, however, reveals that more than 60% of the patients in the surveillance groups underwent open surgical repair during the two trials, with 81% of patients with 5.0 to 5.4 cm aneu-

rysms undergoing surgery in the ADAM trial and almost all patients in the U.K. trial ultimately requiring surgical management. Thus, it is likely that the reason for the low rupture risk in these trials was that surgical treatment of the aneurysm was provided when clinically indicated. This conclusion is supported by data from a prospective study of patients from the VA hospitals involved in the ADAM trial who were not eligible for randomization and did not undergo operative repair. In these patients, the 1-year risk of rupture for slightly larger (5.5 to 5.9 cm) aneurysms was 9.4%.[8] Furthermore, very close surveillance with ultrasound examinations every 3 to 6 months did not prevent aneurysm rupture in 1% of patients. Thus, the decision whether to treat an aneurysm is based on assessment of the risk of aneurysm rupture relative to the risk associated with treatment rather than on an absolute size criterion or a surveillance protocol.

Preoperative Evaluation

IDENTIFICATION OF RISK FACTORS

For successful surgical reconstruction of AAAs, any significant comorbidities that would increase the risk of operative repair must be identified and managed at an early stage. Patients undergoing the procedure usually are elderly and often have coexisting cardiac, pulmonary, cerebrovascular, renal, or peripheral vascular disease. The major anesthetic risk factors for elective resection of AAAs are similar to those for other major intra-abdominal operations; in particular, they include inadequate cardiopulmonary and renal function. Patients with unstable angina or angina at rest, a cardiac ejection fraction of less than 25%, a serum creatinine concentration higher than 3 mg/dl, or pulmonary disease (manifested by oxygen tension < 50 mm Hg, elevated carbon dioxide tension, or both on room air) are considered to be at high risk.[9,10]

Myocardial ischemia is the most common cause of perioperative morbidity and mortality after arterial reconstruction of the aorta. Optimization of preoperative medical management, perioperative invasive monitoring, and long-term risk-factor modification are all facilitated by an accurate preoperative cardiac evaluation. Such evaluation may include transthoracic echocardiography, exercise stress testing, myocardial scintigraphy, stress echocardiography, and coronary angiography; each test has its own merits and limitations with regard to clinical risk assessment. To reduce the mortality associated with resection of AAAs, it is necessary not only to identify high-risk groups but also to institute appropriate preoperative, intraoperative, and postoperative alterations in patient care. Patients who have severe coronary disease (manifested by unstable angina, ischemic congestive heart failure, or recent myocardial infarction [MI]) benefit from invasive cardiac evaluation and possibly from preliminary coronary intervention.

With intensive perioperative monitoring and support in place, resection of AAAs has been successfully performed even in high-risk patients, with operative mortalities of less than 6%.[11-13]

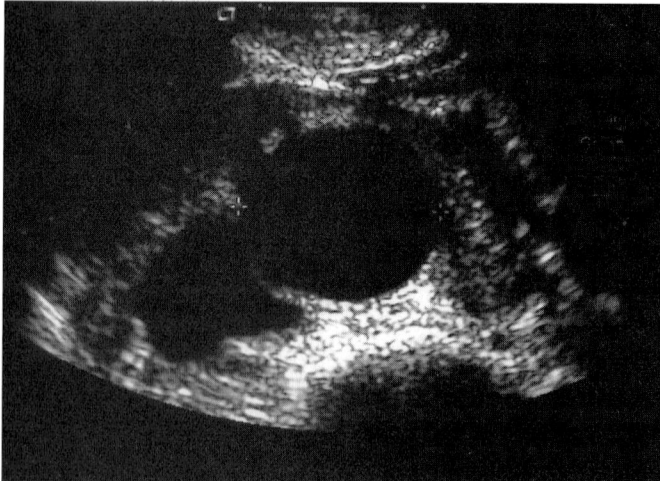

Figure 1 **Duplex ultrasonography may be used as a screening test and to determine the actual size of the aneurysm.**

CONFIRMATION OF DIAGNOSIS AND DETERMINATION
OF ANEURYSM SIZE

Physical examination suffices for detection of most large aneurysms. To determine the exact size of the aneurysm as well as to identify smaller aneurysms, however, more objective methods are available and should be used. Determination of the size of the aneurysm is extremely important because size is the most important determinant of the likelihood of rupture and plays a crucial role in subsequent management decisions. Imaging modalities commonly employed to diagnose and measure aneurysms include duplex ultrasonography (DUS), aortography, computed tomography, and magnetic resonance imaging.

The main advantages of DUS are its ready availability in both inpatient and outpatient settings, its low cost, its safety, and its good performance; many studies have documented the ability of DUS to establish the diagnosis and accurately determine the size of AAAs [see Figure 1].[14–16] The primary limitations of DUS are that imaging of the thoracic and suprarenal aorta is poor, that the quality of the images is considerably lower in the presence of obesity or large amounts of intestinal gas, and that it must be performed by a skilled imaging technician.

Aortography yields excellent images of the contours of the aortic lumen, but it is not a reliable method for determining the diameter of an aneurysm or even for establishing its presence, because the mural thrombus within the aneurysm tends to reduce the lumen to near-normal size. Nonetheless, aortography can be helpful in determining the extent of an aneurysm, especially when there is iliac or suprarenal involvement, defining associated arterial lesions involving the renal and visceral arteries, and detecting lower-extremity occlusive disease. There are risks associated with aortography that place some restrictions on its use. Among these risks are the potential renal toxicity resulting from the use of contrast agents. In addition, manipulation of catheters through the laminated mural thrombus increases the risk of distal embolization. Finally, local arterial complications may arise at the arterial puncture site.

CT provides reliable information about the size of the entire aorta, thereby allowing accurate determination of both the size and the extent of the AAA [see Figure 2]. Spiral CT scanning permits identification of the visceral and renal arteries and their relationship to the aneurysm. The administration of I.V. contrast material allows assessment of the aortic lumen, the amount and location of mural thrombus, and the presence or absence of

retroperitoneal hematoma [see Figure 3]. Overall, spiral CT scanning is currently the most useful imaging method for evaluation of the abdominal aorta.

MRI is also useful in preoperative evaluation of aortic aneurysms.[17,18] It employs radiofrequency energy and a magnetic field to produce images in longitudinal, transverse, and coronal planes. The advantages of MRI over CT are that no ionizing radiation is administered, multiplane images can be obtained, and no nephrotoxic contrast agents are used.

CLASSIFICATION OF PATIENTS FOR ELECTIVE OR URGENT
REPAIR

Patients may usefully be classified into three categories according to how they present for repair: (1) elective patients, (2) symptomatic patients, and (3) patients with ruptured aneurysms.

Elective aneurysm repair is recommended for asymptomatic patients who have aneurysms 5.0 cm in diameter or larger, who have an acceptable level of operative risk, and who have a life expectancy of 1 year or more. Furthermore, elective operation should be considered for patients with aneurysms smaller than 5.0 cm who are not at high operative risk if they are hypertensive or live in a remote area where proper medical care is not readily available. Repair is also appropriate for aneurysms that are between 4.0 and 5.0 cm in diameter and have shown growth of more than 0.5 cm on serial images in less than 6 to 12 months. Peripheral embolization originating from the aneurysm is an indication for repair, regardless of the size of the aneurysm.

Urgent operation is indicated for patients with symptomatic aneurysms, regardless of the size of the aneurysm. Such patients typi-

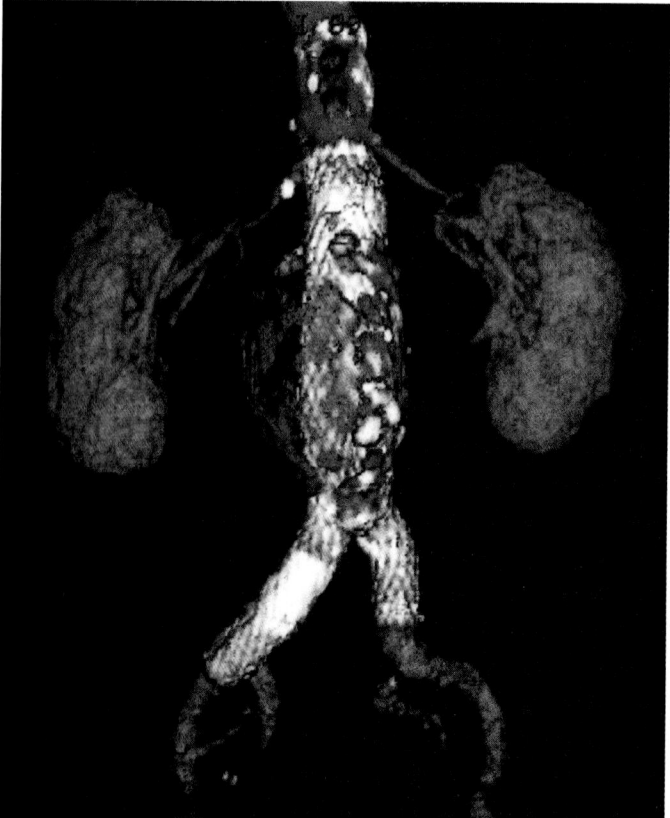

Figure 2 **Shown is a CT angiogram providing a three-dimensional reconstruction of an infrarenal AAA after endovascular repair. Of particular interest is the relation of the graft to the renal arteries and the hypogastric arteries distally.**

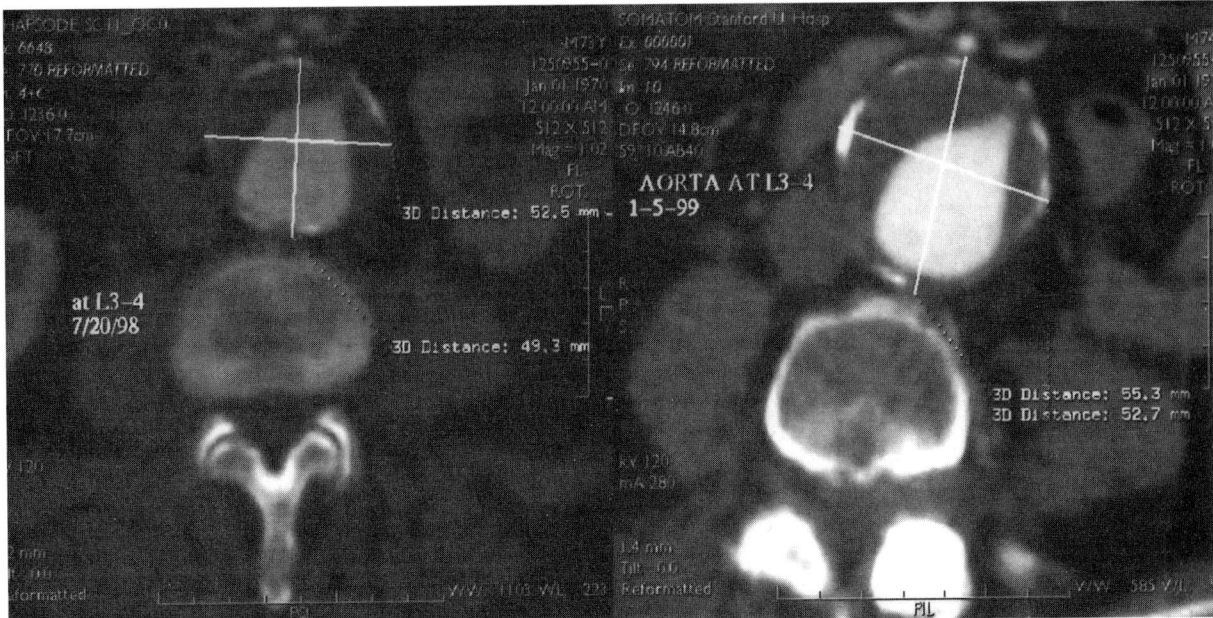

Figure 3 **CT scanning assesses the size of the aneurysm, the amount of mural thrombus present, and the relation of other intra-abdominal structures to the aneurysm.**

cally present with abdominal or back pain. Sometimes, the back pain radiates to the groin, much as in ureteral colic; this pain may be elicited by palpating the aneurysm. In most cases, DUS, CT, and MRI will reliably detect the presence of periaortic blood; however, the absence of this finding should not delay operation, because actual rupture of the aneurysm can occur at any time.

Emergency operation is indicated for almost all patients with known or suspected rupture of an aneurysm.

Operative Planning

Preoperative planning is essential for a successful outcome after repair of an infrarenal AAA. Like the choice between elective and urgent or emergency repair, operative planning is governed by the presentation of the patient. In patients with ruptured aneurysms, diagnosis is immediately followed by operative repair. In patients with symptomatic aneurysms, the amount of preoperative imaging done is balanced against the risk of impending rupture. In patients presenting for elective repair, it is generally possible to perform extensive imaging to determine whether the repair is best done via an endovascular approach or a standard open approach. Current preoperative imaging methods utilizing CT angiography obviate several common pitfalls. The recent introduction of endovascular techniques for excluding an aneurysm should not alter the patient selection criteria for aneurysm repair. Endovascular grafting does introduce certain morphologic criteria into the process of patient selection, in that stent grafting is appropriate only for patients in whom the infrarenal neck and the iliac arteries are suitable.

Given that the long-term outcome of endovascular grafting is currently unknown, younger patients who are at low operative risk and are expected to survive into the long term are typically better served with open surgical repair. In addition, patients who require additional abdominal or pelvic revascularization procedures, who have small or diseased access vessels, or who have short (< 10 mm) or tortuous infrarenal necks are not candidates for endovascular grafting and should undergo open surgical repair instead.

Preoperative preparation to optimize cardiopulmonary function, administration of preoperative antibiotics, and intraopera-

tive hemodynamic monitoring with appropriate fluid management can significantly reduce the risks associated with AAA repair. Before aortic cross-clamping, appropriate volume loading, combined with vasodilatation, is carried out to help prevent declamping hypotension.

Operative Technique

OPEN REPAIR

Step 1: Initial Incision and Choice of Approach

Open surgical repair of infrarenal AAAs is performed through a transperitoneal or retroperitoneal exposure of the aorta with the patient under general endotracheal anesthesia. The aneurysm may be exposed through either a long midline incision (for the transperitoneal approach) or an oblique flank incision (for the retroperitoneal approach) [see Figure 4a]. An upper abdominal transverse incision may also be used for either retroperitoneal or transperitoneal exposure. The results with the two exposures are equivalent. The transperitoneal approach is preferred when exposure of the right renal artery is required and when access to the distal right iliac system or to intra-abdominal organs is necessary. The retroperitoneal exposure offers advantages when extensive peritoneal adhesions, an intestinal stoma, or severe pulmonary disease is present and when there is a need for suprarenal exposure. Use of the retroperitoneal approach has been associated with a shorter duration of postoperative ileus, a lower incidence of pulmonary complications, and a reduction in length of stay in the ICU.

Step 2 (Transperitoneal Approach): Exposure and Control of Aorta and Iliac Arteries

When the transperitoneal approach is used, the small bowel (including the duodenum) is retracted to the right, and the retroperitoneum overlying the aneurysm is divided to the left of the midline [see Figure 4b]. The duodenum is completely mobilized, and the left renal vein is identified and exposed. The normal infrarenal neck, which is just below the left renal vein, is then exposed and encircled

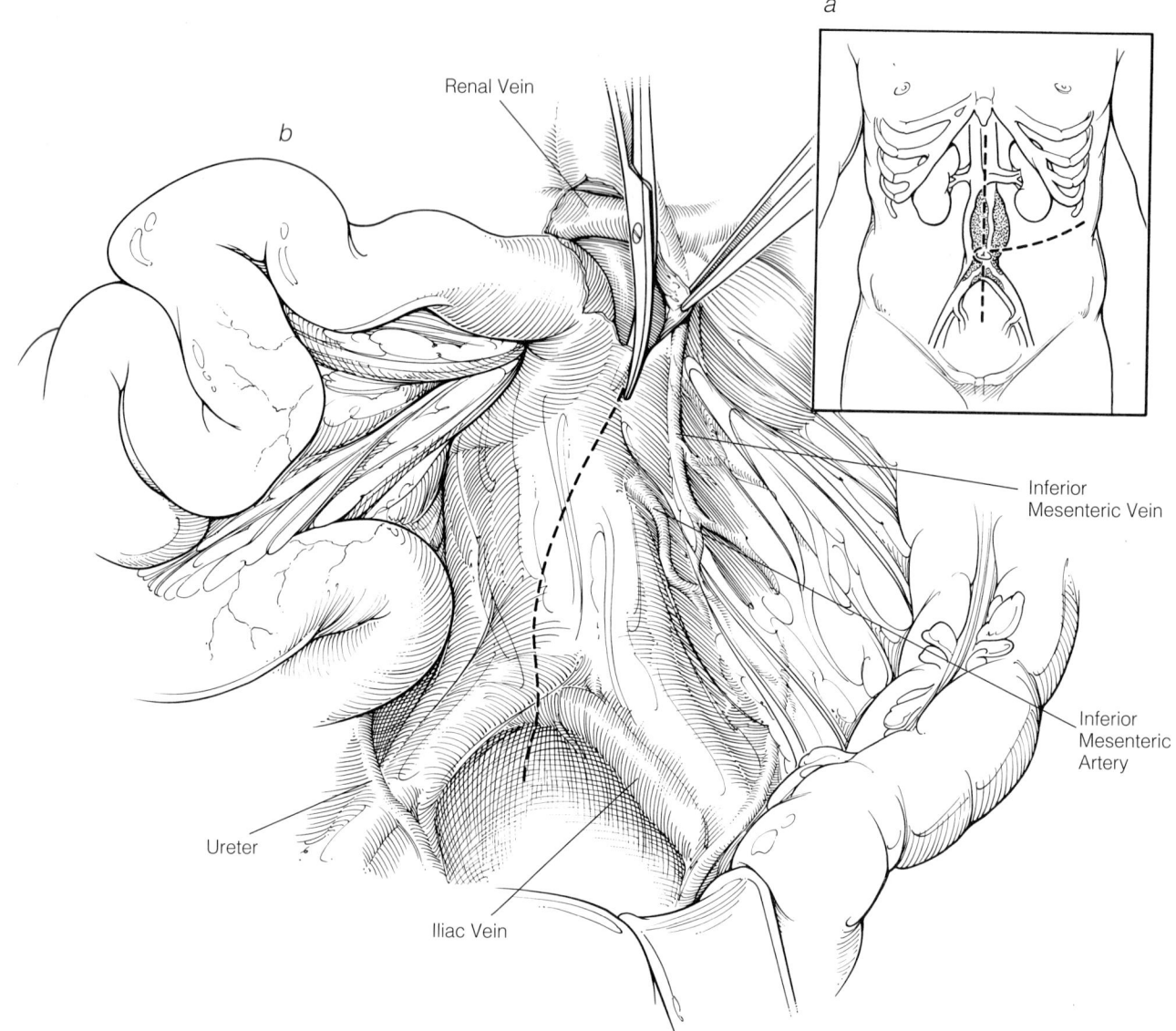

Figure 4 **Open repair of infrarenal AAAs. (*a*) For the transabdominal approach to the abdominal aorta, a midline or transverse incision is appropriate. For the retroperitoneal approach, an oblique flank incision may be used. (*b*) The small intestine (including the duodenum) is retracted laterally after the ligament of Treitz is mobilized, and the retroperitoneum is incised in the midline. The left renal vein is the landmark for the infrarenal neck.**

for proximal control. Both common iliac arteries are then mobilized and controlled, with care taken to avoid the underlying iliac veins and ureters that cross over at the iliac bifurcation [*see Figure 5*]. If the common iliac arteries are aneurysmal, then both the internal and the external iliac arteries are controlled. The inferior mesenteric artery is then dissected out and controlled for possible reimplantation into the graft after the aneurysm has been repaired.

Step 2 (Retroperitoneal Approach): Exposure and Control of Aorta and Iliac Arteries

When the retroperitoneal approach is taken, a transverse left abdominal or flank incision is made, and the peritoneum is reflected anteriorly. The left kidney usually is left in place but may be mobilized anteriorly to expose the posterolateral aorta. Exposure of the right iliac system can be achieved by dividing the inferior mesenteric artery early in the course of dissection. The aorta and the iliac arteries are controlled in essentially the same fashion regardless of the type of incision used.

Step 3: Opening of Aneurysm and Creation of Proximal Anastomosis

Systemic anticoagulation with I.V. heparin is then performed. After sufficient time (3 to 5 minutes) has elapsed to permit adequate circulation, the infrarenal neck and the iliac arteries are clamped. To prevent distal embolization, the distal clamps should be applied before the proximal aortic clamp. The aneurysm is then opened longitudinally, the mural thrombus is removed, and back-bleeding lumbar arteries are oversewn. Depending on its degree of backflow and on the patency of the hypogastric arteries, the inferior mesenteric artery may be either ligated or clamped and left with a rim of aortic wall for subsequent reimplantation [*see Troubleshooting, below*].

The aortic neck is then partially or completely transected, and an appropriately sized tubular or bifurcated graft is sutured to the aorta with a continuous nonabsorbable monofilament suture [*see Figure 6*]. When the proximal aortic neck is very short, suprarenal aortic clamping may be required for performance of the proximal anastomosis. If suprarenal clamping is necessary, the security of the proximal anastomosis should be verified, and the clamp should then be moved onto the graft below the renal arteries as soon as possible to minimize renal ischemia. If the aorta is especially weak or friable, the anastomosis may be supported with Teflon-felt pledgets.

Step 4: Creation of Distal Anastomosis

When the aneurysm is confined to the aorta, the distal anastomosis is performed by suturing a straight tube graft to the aortic bi-furcation [see Figure 7]; straight tube graft reconstructions are used about 30% of the time. Distally, the dissection should avoid the fibroareolar tissue overlying the left common iliac artery because this tissue contains branches of the inferior mesenteric artery and the autonomic nerves that control sexual function in men.

When the aneurysm extends into the common iliac arteries, the distal anastomosis is accomplished by suturing a bifurcated graft to the distal common iliac arteries or, in the case of significant occlusive disease, to the common femoral arteries. In these situations,

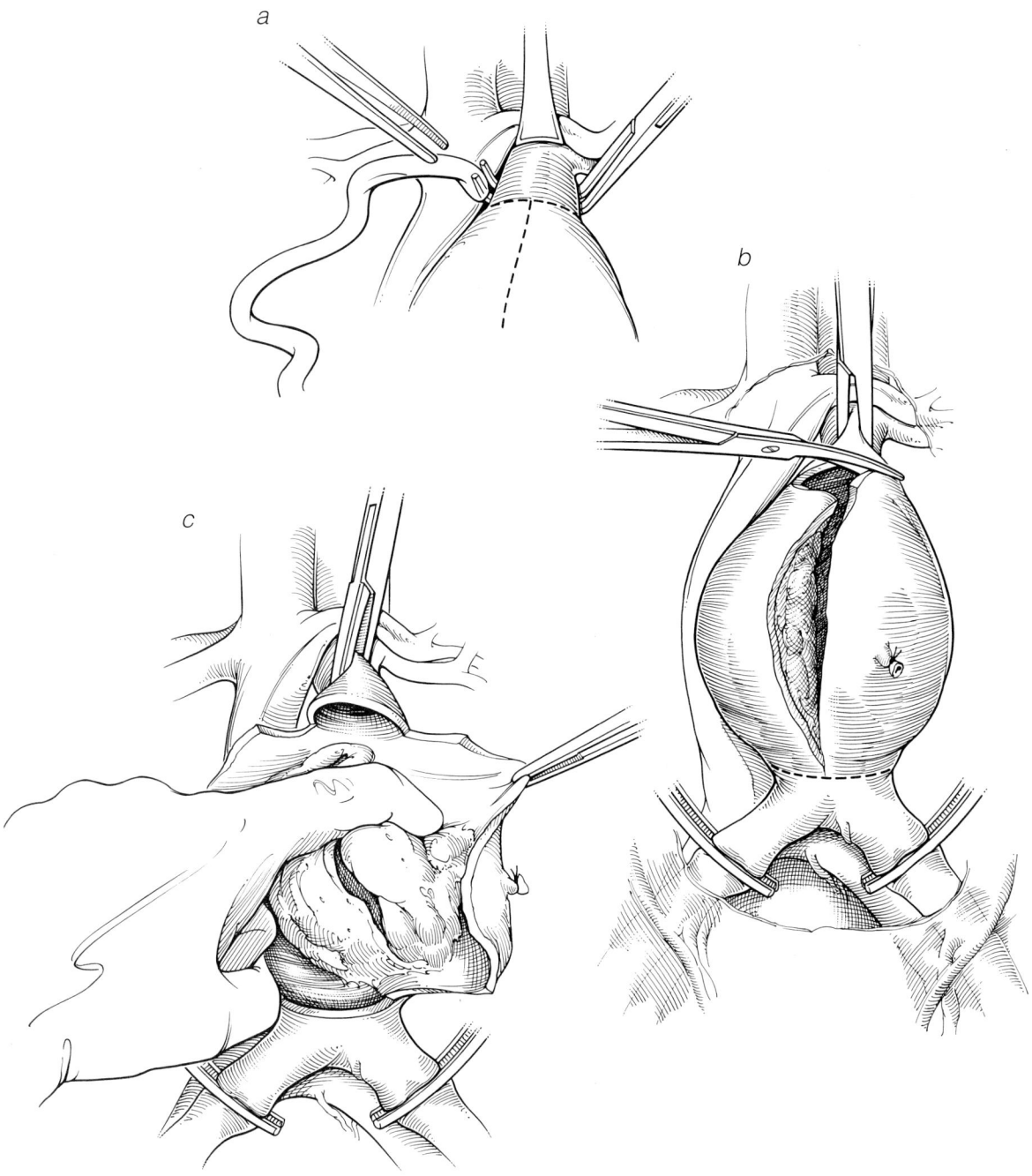

Figure 5   **Open repair of infrarenal AAAs. (*a*) Once the aneurysm is exposed, proximal control is obtained by encircling the proximal neck with an umbilical tape or heavy Silastic. The inferior mesenteric artery is identified and then either clamped or ligated for possible reimplantation at the end of the procedure. (*b*) The iliac arteries are dissected free, systemic heparin anticoagulation is instituted, and distal control is obtained, followed by proximal control to prevent distal embolization. The aneurysm sac is then opened longitudinally. (*c*) All mural thrombus is removed, and the proximal and distal necks of the aorta are incised.**

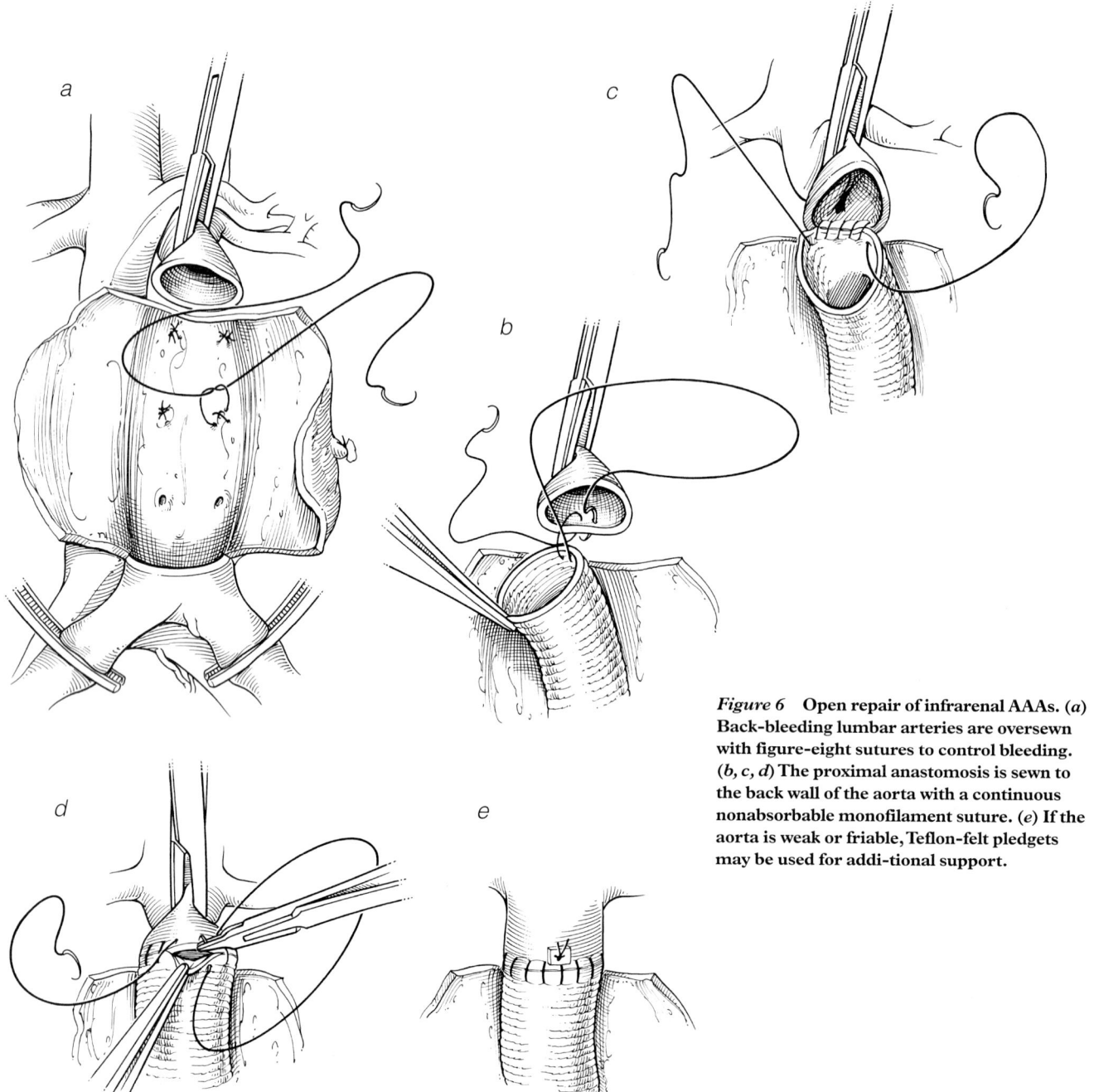

Figure 6 **Open repair of infrarenal AAAs.** (*a*) **Back-bleeding lumbar arteries are oversewn with figure-eight sutures to control bleeding. (*b, c, d*) The proximal anastomosis is sewn to the back wall of the aorta with a continuous nonabsorbable monofilament suture. (*e*) If the aorta is weak or friable, Teflon-felt pledgets may be used for addi-tional support.**

control of the iliac arteries is best achieved by mobilizing the external and internal arteries and clamping them individually [*see Figure 8*]. It is sometimes easier to control iliac artery back-bleeding by using intraluminal balloon catheters and oversewing the common iliac arteries from within the opened aortic or iliac aneurysms. Care must be taken not to injure the accompanying venous structures or the ureters, which cross anterior to the iliac bifurcation. Every effort should be made to ensure perfusion of at least one hypogastric artery to help minimize the risk of postoperative left colon ischemia.

Declamping hypotension may occur after reperfusion of the lower extremities. It is essential to maintain communication with the anesthesiologist so that blood and fluid replacement can be adjusted in anticipation of lower-extremity reperfusion. Even though the graft and vessels are flushed and back-bled before distal flow is reestablished, it is preferable first to establish flow into one of the hypogastric arteries so as to minimize the chances of distal embolization to the legs.

Before the abdomen is closed, adequate perfusion of the lower extremities and the left colon should be ensured via either direct inspection or noninvasive monitoring. The open aneurysm sac is then sutured closed over the aortic graft to separate the graft from the duodenum and the viscera [*see Figure 9*]. This step reduces the risk of aortoenteric fistula.

Troubleshooting

If the inferior mesenteric artery is small and back-bleeding is adequate, it may be ligated [*see Figure 10a*]; however, if the vessel is large or back-bleeding is meager, it should be reimplanted. Reimplantation of the inferior mesenteric artery can be accomplished with relative ease by using the Carrel patch technique. After the graft has been completely sewn to the aorta, a partial occluding clamp is placed on the main body of the graft or on one of the limbs. An opening in the graft is then created, and an end-to-side anastomosis [*see Figure 10b*]—with an interposition graft added if necessary [*see Figure 10c*]—

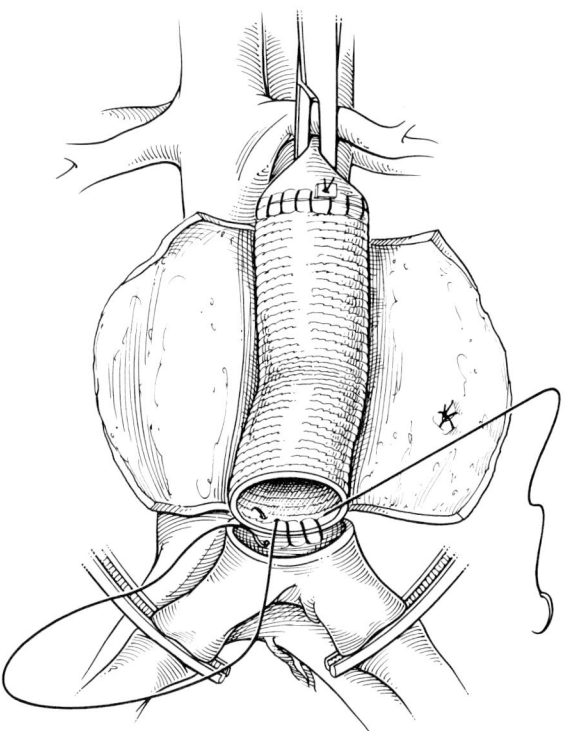

Figure 7 **Open repair of infrarenal AAAs. When the aneurysm does not extend into the iliac arteries, a straight tube graft is used. The distal anastomosis is completed with a continuous suture. Before completion of the anastomosis, the graft is flushed by backbleeding the iliac arteries and flushing the proximal anastomosis.**

is used to reconstruct the inferior mesenteric artery. This anastomosis is created with a continuous monofilament suture.

Special Considerations

CONCURRENT DISEASE PROCESSES

At times, a concurrent disease process complicates repair of an AAA. The most common problems encountered are hepatobiliary, pancreatic, gastrointestinal, gynecologic, and genitourinary disorders. Careful evaluation of the situation is necessary to determine whether to treat the two disease entities concurrently. As a rule, the more life-threatening disorder is treated first.

There are three key points that should be remembered in the management of patients with AAAs and concurrent diseases. First, a careful preoperative diagnostic workup usually detects any concomitant disease processes. Second, in emergency situations such as ruptured or symptomatic aneurysms, the aneurysm always takes priority unless the other condition is life-threatening and the aneurysm is clearly not the cause of the critical symptoms. Finally, many concomitant intra-abdominal problems can be avoided by taking an endovascular approach.

ANATOMIC VARIANTS

Several anatomic variants may be encountered during repair of AAAs, including horseshoe kidney, accessory renal arteries, and venous anomalies.

Horseshoe Kidney

The incidence of horseshoe kidney in the general population is

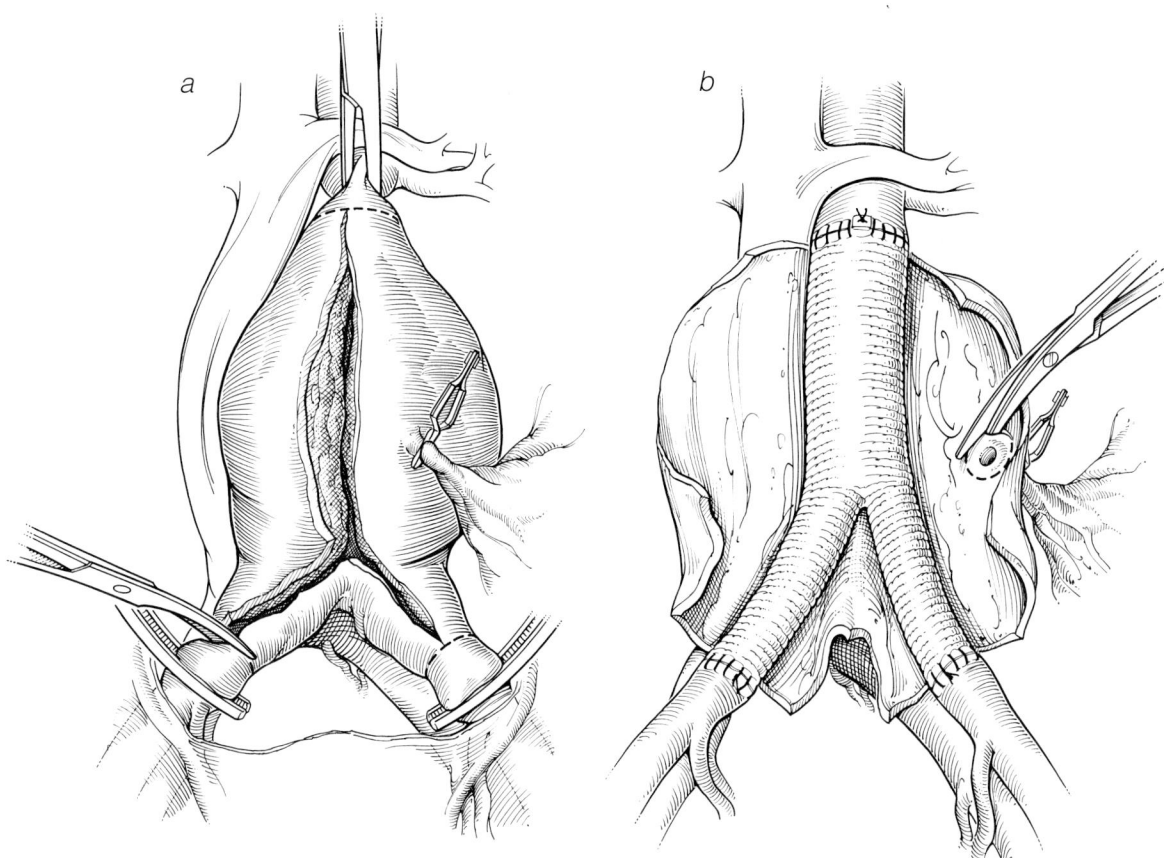

Figure 8 **Open repair of infrarenal AAAs. When the common iliac arteries are aneurysmal, both the internal and the external iliac arteries must be clamped individually (*a*), and a bifurcated graft is sewn to the iliac arteries bilaterally (*b*).**

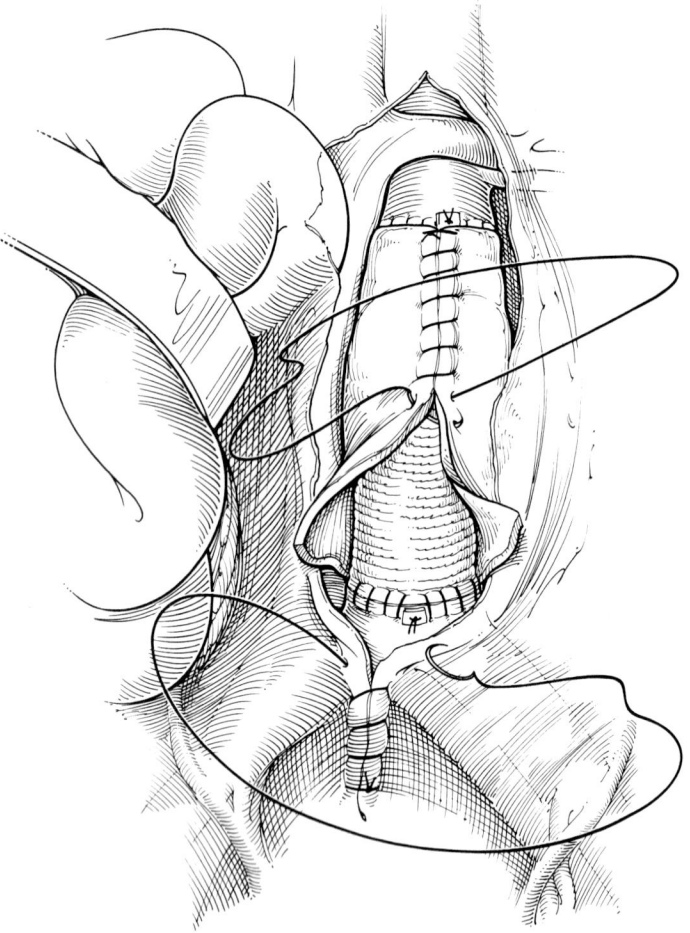

Figure 9 **Open repair of infrarenal AAAs. Once the anastomoses have been completed and adequate flow to the lower extremities and the left colon has been confirmed, the open aneurysm sac is sutured closed over the aortic graft.**

less than 3%. Most patients with horseshoe kidneys have between three and five renal arteries.[19] To preserve renal function, renal arteries arising from the aneurysm should be reimplanted. In patients with horseshoe kidneys who have more than five renal arteries, there often are multiple small accessory arteries, some of which originate from the aneurysm, the iliac arteries, or both.

The presence of a horseshoe kidney may complicate—but does not preclude—an anterior approach to repair of an infrarenal AAA.[20] In such cases, the left retroperitoneal approach provides excellent exposure of the infrarenal aorta. This approach requires that the surgeon dissect the space between the aneurysm and the left portion and isthmus of the kidney; the kidney can then be reflected to the right and the aneurysm fully exposed. The left ureter crosses the iliac arteries from the right in this position, and duplication of ureters may be noted.

Venous Anomalies

A number of different venous anomalies may be observed in the course of AAA repair; however, the overall incidence is quite low. Left renal vein variants, such as retroaortic left renal veins and circumaortic venous rings, are the most commonly seen venous anomalies.[21] Azygous continuation of the inferior vena cava and bilateral inferior vena cava have also been noted. Unnecessary bleeding can be prevented by means of careful dissection and meticulous technique.

INFLAMMATORY ANEURYSM

Approximately 5% of infrarenal AAAs are inflammatory.[22] These AAAs have a dense fibroinflammatory rind that typically adheres to the fourth portion of the duodenum; they may also involve the inferior vena cava, the left renal vein, or the ureters. Patients with inflammatory AAAs typically experience abdominal or flank pain and may present with weight loss. The erythrocyte sedimentation rate is usually elevated as well. Inflammatory aneurysms rarely rupture, because most are symptomatic and consequently are treated before rupture can occur. Repair of inflammatory aneurysms poses technical problems because of the involvement of adjacent structures. A retroperitoneal approach is usually advocated for these aneurysms.

RUPTURED ANEURYSM

Infrarenal AAAs can rupture freely into the peritoneal cavity or into the retroperitoneum. Free rupture into the peritoneal cavity is usually anterior and is typically accompanied by immediate hemodynamic collapse and a very high mortality. Retroperitoneal ruptures are usually posterior and may be contained by the psoas muscle and adjacent periaortic and perivertebral tissue. This type of rupture may occur without significant blood loss initially, and the patient may be hemodynamically stable.

When an aortic aneurysm ruptures, immediate surgical repair is indicated. If the patient is unstable and either an abdominal aortic aneurysm was previously diagnosed or a palpable abdominal mass is present, no further evaluation is necessary and the patient should be taken directly to the OR. If the patient is stable and the diagnosis is questionable, CT scanning may be performed to confirm the presence of an aneurysm and determine its extent, the site of the rupture, and the degree of iliac involvement. Bedside ultrasonography may also be used for quick confirmation of the presence of an AAA.

Surgical repair of ruptured aneurysms is performed via a transperitoneal approach. In cases of contained rupture, supraceliac control should be achieved before infrarenal dissection; once the neck of the aneurysm has been dissected free, the aortic clamp may be moved to the infrarenal level. In cases of free rupture, efforts to obtain vascular control may include compression of the aorta at the hiatus and infrarenal control with a clamp or an intraluminal balloon. Once proximal and distal control have been achieved, the operation is conducted in much the same way as an elective repair.

Outcome Evaluation

The mortality associated with repair of AAAs has been greatly reduced by improvements in preoperative evaluation and perioperative care: leading centers currently report death rates ranging from 0% to 5%.[23] Mortality after repair of inflammatory aneurysms and after emergency repair of symptomatic nonruptured aneurysms continues to be somewhat higher (5% to 10%), primarily as a consequence of less thorough preoperative evaluation.

Overall morbidity after elective aneurysm repair ranges from 10% to 30%. The most common complication is myocardial ischemia, and MI is the most common cause of postoperative death. Mild renal insufficiency is the second most frequent complication, occurring after 6% of elective aneurysm repairs; however, severe renal failure necessitating dialysis is rare in this setting. The third most common complication is pulmonary disease; the incidence of postoperative pneumonia is approximately 5%.

Postoperative bleeding may occur as well. Common sources of such bleeding include the anastomotic suture lines, inadequately recognized venous injuries, and coagulopathies resulting from intra-

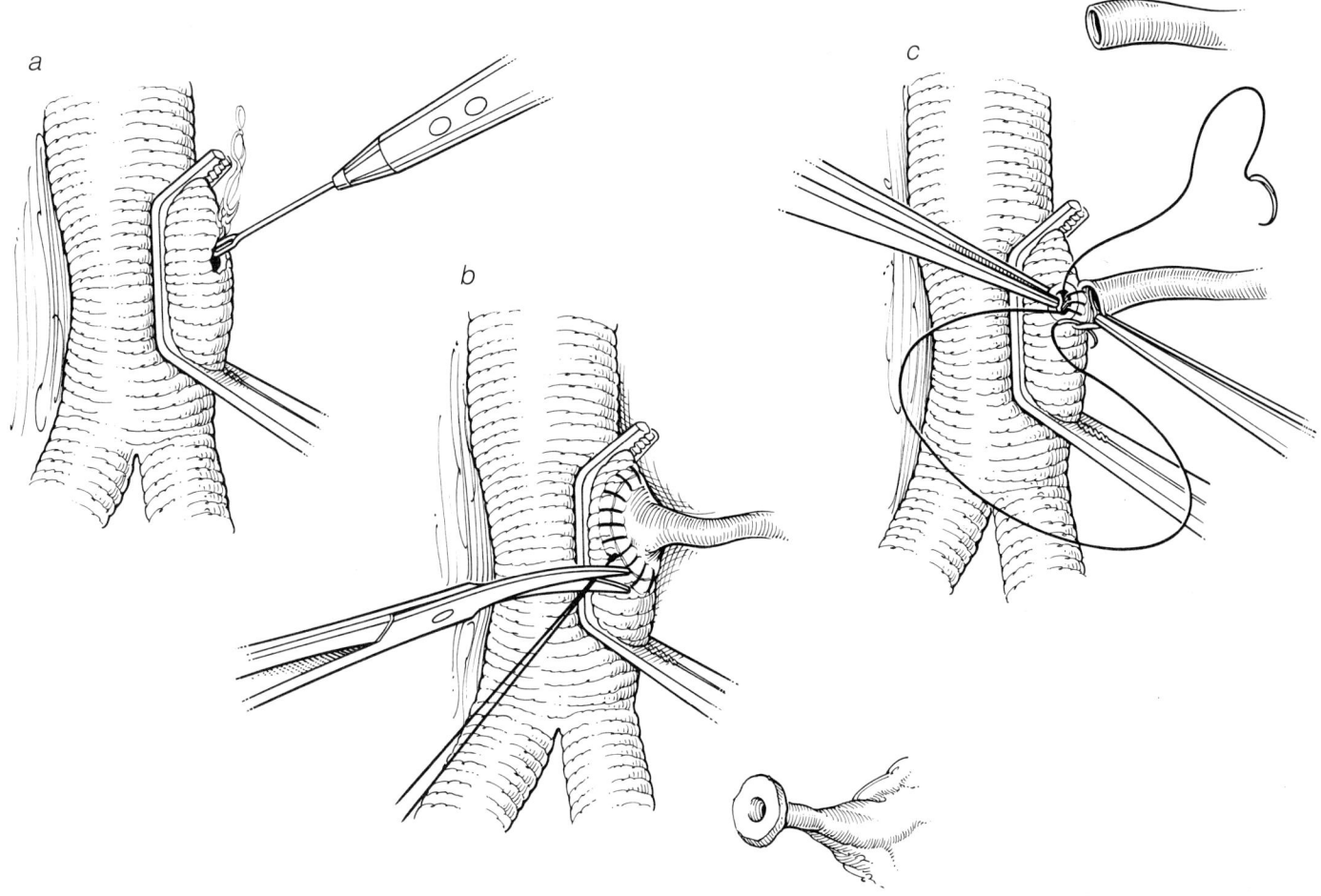

Figure 10 **Open repair of infrarenal AAAs. (*a*) A small, adequately back-bleeding inferior mesenteric artery may be ligated. (*b*) A large or meagerly back-bleeding inferior mesenteric artery should be reimplanted. A side-biting clamp is applied to the graft, and an end-to-side anastomosis is created with a fine monofilament suture. (*c*) If the inferior mesenteric artery is not long enough for a direct anastomosis, an interposition graft—either a segment of a vein or a prosthetic graft—may be used for added length.**

operative hypothermia or excessive blood loss. Any evidence of ongoing bleeding is an indication for early exploration.

Lower-extremity ischemia may occur as a result of either emboli or thrombosis of the graft and may necessitate reoperation and thrombectomy. So-called trash foot may also develop when diffuse microemboli are carried into the distal circulation.

Colon ischemia develops after 1% of elective aneurysm repairs. Patients usually present with bloody diarrhea, abdominal pain, a distended abdomen, and leukocytosis. Diagnosis is confirmed by sigmoidoscopy, which reveals mucosal sloughing. In cases of transmural colonic necrosis, colon resection and exteriorization of stomas are warranted.

Paraplegia is rare after repair of infrarenal AAAs: the incidence is only 0.2%. Most instances of paraplegia occur after repair of a ruptured aneurysm or when the pelvis has been devascularized. The majority of patients recover at least some degree of neurologic function.

Late complications—such as pseudoaneurysms at the suture lines, graft or graft limb thrombosis, and graft infection—may occur but are extremely rare. Graft infection may be associated with graft-enteric fistula and is notoriously difficult to diagnose and treat.

Long-term survival in patients who have undergone successful AAA repair is reduced in comparison with that in the general population. The 5-year survival rate after AAA repair is 67% (range, 49% to 84%), compared with 80% to 85% in age-matched control subjects, and the mean duration of survival after AAA repair is 7.4 years.

Part of the difference in survival can be attributed to associated coronary disease in patients with aneurysms. Late deaths result primarily from cardiac causes.

Endovascular Repair

Endovascular repair was introduced during the 1990s as a less invasive approach to treating infrarenal AAAs. In this approach, a stent-graft is placed endoluminally via bilateral groin incisions; thus, there is no need for a major abdominal incision and aortic clamping. Early results are promising: blood loss is decreased, hospital stay is shortened, and earlier return to function is achieved. Not all patients are candidates for endovascular repair, however. In September 1999, the Food and Drug Administration approved two stent-graft devices for use in surgical management of AAAs: the Ancure device (Guidant, Indianapolis, Indiana), which is a balloon-expandable one-piece bifurcated stent-graft, and the AneuRx device (Medtronic AVE, Santa Rosa, California), which is a self-expanding bifurcated modular device that is fully supported externally by a nitinol stent. Since then, the FDA has approved two more devices for endovascular repair of AAAs: the Excluder Bifurcated Endoprosthesis (W. L. Gore and Associates, Flagstaff, Arizona), in November 2002, and the Zenith AAA Endovascular Graft (Cook Incorporated, Bloomington, Indiana), in May 2003 (premarket approval).

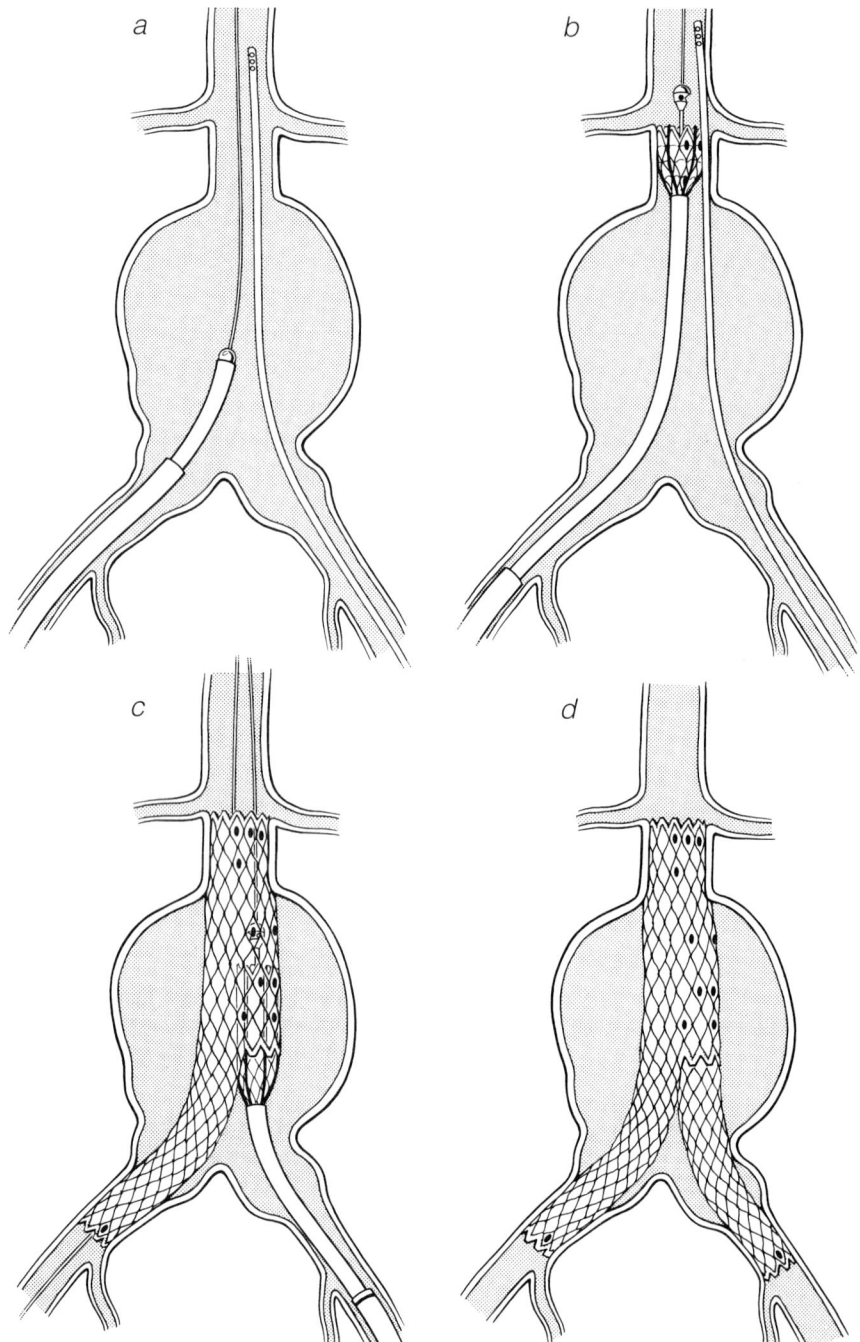

Figure 11 Endovascular repair of infrarenal AAAs. (*a*) The main bifurcated stent-graft is advanced through the aortoiliac system under fluoroscopic guidance. (*b*) The sheath over the stent-graft is retracted under fluoroscopic guidance. Controlled deployment allows the graft to be gradually positioned directly below the renal arteries. (*c*) With the main body of the stent-graft deployed, the contralateral limb is cannulated. Once this is done, the contralateral limb is positioned within the junction gate and the common iliac artery. (*d*) Shown is proper deployment of the stent-graft within the aortoiliac system, with good proximal and distal fixation of the stent to the arterial wall.

PREOPERATIVE PREPARATION

Precise preoperative evaluation that yields accurate measurements will result in proper planning and effective prevention of problems. Both CT angiography and contrast biplane angiography are used for this purpose. Of the two, spiral CT angiography is currently preferred. This imaging modality is capable of obtaining high-quality images of the vascular anatomy and reconfiguring them into detailed three-dimensional images. For optimal evaluation, images should be obtained at 3 mm intervals from the celiac artery to the femoral arteries. Spiral CT angiography accurately defines the proximal and distal characteristics of the AAA, as well as detects any significant renal, visceral, or iliac occlusive disease. It is particularly helpful in defining the infrarenal neck between the renal arteries and the proximal portion of the aneurysm.

Angiography is employed as a complement to spiral CT angiography in this setting. An arteriogram is useful in that it helps define renal, mesenteric, and distal arterial anatomy; helps characterize tortuosity, calcification, and stenoses in access arteries; and helps determine the angles between the aorta, the proximal neck, and the aneurysm.

Proper patient selection is mandatory for successful outcome. The common femoral arteries must be large enough to accept a 22 French sheath. The proximal infrarenal aortic neck must be suitable for device implantation—that is, its diameter must be between 16 and 25 mm, and it must be longer than 10 mm. The common iliac artery implantation should be at least 10 mm above the hypogastric artery, and the iliac artery diameter must be between 8 and 15 mm. In patients with iliac artery aneurysms, it is possible to land the end of the stent in the external iliac artery and thereby exclude one internal iliac artery; however, exclusion of both internal iliac arteries should be avoided so as to prevent ischemic sequelae.

TECHNIQUE

The methods and technical principles we briefly describe here derive from the personal experience one of us (C.K.Z.) has accumulated with more than 150 modular implants. The ensuing technical description is not intended to be exhaustive, nor is it meant as a substitute for the instructions provided by the manufacturer.

The patient is placed under epidural or general anesthesia. Bilateral femoral artery cutdowns are performed through transverse groin incisions to allow exposure of the common femoral artery from the inguinal ligament to the femoral bifurcation. Proximal control of the femoral arteries is obtained with umbilical tapes. Systemic anticoagulation with I.V. heparin is instituted to prolong the activated clotting time (ACT) to greater than 250 seconds. The ACT is monitored and maintained at this level throughout the procedure, and additional heparin is given as needed.

The femoral arteries are cannulated with an 18-gauge needle, and 0.035-in. guide wires are placed bilaterally under fluoroscopic guidance; 10 French sheaths are then placed over the two guide wires and advanced into the aneurysm under fluoroscopic guidance. A superstiff 0.035-in. guide wire 260 cm in length is inserted into the thoracic aorta, usually from the right limb. In the contralateral iliac artery, a pigtail catheter is placed just above the level of the renal arteries, and an initial roadmapping aortogram is obtained. The 10 French sheath in the right femoral artery is exchanged for a 22 French sheath, which is placed over the superstiff guide wire and carefully advanced into the proximal infrarenal aorta under fluoroscopic guidance. The main stent-graft module, which is chosen on the basis of preoperative measurements, is then advanced over the guide wire and through the delivery sheath into the perirenal aorta [see Figure 11a]. A second aortogram is performed to verify the position of the renal arteries. Under fluoroscopic guidance, the stent-graft is then gradually deployed by retracting the outer sheath and allowing the graft to expand, and it is positioned directly below the level of the renal arteries [see Figure 11b].

Once the main bifurcation module has been deployed, the 10 French sheath in the contralateral iliac artery is pulled back, and a 0.035-in. angled hydrophilic wire and a guide catheter are inserted into the contralateral limb of the bifurcation module. The hydrophilic wire is then exchanged for a superstiff guide wire, over which a 16 French sheath is advanced into the contralateral limb under fluoroscopic guidance. The contralateral limb is then advanced through the sheath into the contralateral limb and deployed [see Figure 11c]. A final aortogram is then performed to confirm that a satisfactory technical result has been achieved [see Figure 11d]. Proximal and distal extender cuffs may be placed if necessary. The femoral arteriotomies are repaired, and lower-extremity perfusion is reestablished.

OUTCOME EVALUATION

Endovascular aneurysm repair is significantly less invasive than open surgical repair and consequently is associated with a significant reduction in major procedure-related morbidity. Prospective clinical trials comparing open with endovascular AAA repair have consistently found that patients undergoing endovascular repair experience less intraoperative blood loss, need less postoperative ICU care, have shorter lengths of stay, and regain normal function earlier.[24,25] Procedure-related mortality after endovascular repair is 1% to 2%, which is essentially equivalent to that reported after open repair in prospective clinical trials but lower than the 5% mortality reported after open repair in most multicenter studies.[26,27]

On occasion, endovascular AAA repair fails to exclude blood flow from the aneurysm sac completely. This condition, known as endoleak, may arise from an incomplete seal at the site where the endograft is affixed to the aortic neck or the iliac arteries (type I endoleak), from retrograde flow into the aneurysm from the inferior mesenteric artery or the lumbar arteries (type II endoleak), or from the graft or modular junction site (type III endoleak). Type I and type III endoleaks call for secondary treatment to prevent possible aneurysm rupture. The significance of type II endoleaks is less certain. There is no clear evidence that type II endoleaks lead to aneurysm rupture; however, most such endoleaks are treated if they are associated with aneurysm enlargement.

Numerous studies have shown that endovascular AAA repair results in less morbidity and mortality than open repair,[28-31] but reports describing endograft migration over time, aneurysm enlargement, and occasional aneurysm rupture have raised questions about the long-term durability of the procedure.[32,33] These adverse events, though uncommon, serve as reminders that endovascular repair is still a new technology, one whose long-term outcome is unknown. Accordingly, close patient monitoring and follow-up surveillance are warranted, and secondary treatments may be required (e.g., endovascular procedures or, possibly, open surgical repair). New endovascular devices are currently being designed and evaluated in clinical trials, and endovascular treatment strategies continue to evolve and improve.

Clinical follow-up of patients treated during the initial prospective clinical trials now extends to more than 6 years, with endovascular repair continuing to show favorable results. The largest multicenter endovascular clinical trial to date, involving 1,193 patients followed up for as long as 6 years, found that prevention of aneurysm rupture (the primary objective) was achieved in 99% of patients, whereas procedure-, aneurysm-, or graft-related death was avoided in 97%.[34,35] These results are consistent with the favorable overall outcomes reported from a European registry of endovascular repair using a variety of endovascular devices.[36] Thus, the midterm results of endovascular aneurysm repair are favorable and support the consideration of endovascular repair for most patients who are candidates for the procedure.

References

1. Taylor LM, Porter JM: Basic data related to clinical decision-making in abdominal aortic aneurysms. Ann Vasc Surg 1:502, 1980

2. Bickerstaff LK, Hollier LH, Van Peenen HJ, et al: Abdominal aortic aneurysm: the changing natural history. J Vasc Surg 1:6, 1984

3. Melton L, Bickerstaff L, Hollier LH, et al: Changing incidence of abdominal aortic aneurysms: a population based study. Am J Epidemiol 120:379, 1984

4. Finlayson SRG, Birkeyer JD, Fillinger MF, et al: Should endovascular surgery lower the threshold for abdominal aortic aneurysms? J Vasc Surg 29:973, 1999

5. The UK Small Aneurysm Trial Participants: Mortality results for randomized controlled trial of early elective surgery or ultrasonographic surveillance for small abdominal aortic aneurysms. Lancet 352:1649, 1998

6. Lederle FA, Wilson SE, Johnson GR, et al: Immediate repair compared with surveillance of small abdominal aortic aneurysms. N Engl J Med 346:1437, 2002

7. The United Kingdom Small Aneurysm Trial Participants: Long-term outcomes of immediate repair compared with surveillance of small abdominal aortic aneurysms. N Engl J Med 346:1445, 2002

8. Lederle FA, Johnson GR, Wilson SE, et al: Rupture rate of large abdominal aortic aneurysms in patients refusing or unfit for elective repair. JAMA 287:2968, 2002

9. Darling RC, Messina CR, Brewster DC, et al: Autopsy study of unoperated aortic aneurysms. Circulation 56(suppl 2):161, 1977

10. Thurmond AS, Semler JH: Abdominal aortic aneurysm: incidence in a population at risk. J Cardiovasc Surg 27:457, 1986

11. Whittemore AD, Clowes AW, Hechtman HB, et al: Aortic aneurysm repair reduced operative mortality associated with maintenance of optimal cardiac performance. Ann Surg 120:414, 1980

12. Pairolero PC: Repair of abdominal aortic aneurysms in high-risk patients. Surg Clin North Am 69:755, 1989

13. Stokes J, Butcher HR: Abdominal aortic aneurysms: factors influencing operative mortality and criteria of operability. Arch Surg 107:297, 1973

14. Quill DS, Colgan MP, Summer DS: Ultrasonic screening for the detection of abdominal aortic aneurysms. Surg Clin North Am 69:713, 1989

15. Bluth EI: Ultrasound of the abdominal aorta. Arch Intern Med 144:377, 1994

16. Gomes MN, Choyke PL: Preoperative evaluation of abdominal aortic aneurysms: ultrasound or computed tomography? J Cardiovasc Surg 28:159, 1987

17. Amparo EG, Hoddick WK, Hricak H, et al: Comparison of magnetic resonance imaging and ultrasonography in the evaluation of abdominal aortic aneurysms. Radiology 154:451, 1985

18. Lee JKT, Ling D, Heiken JP, et al: Magnetic resonance imaging of abdominal aneurysms. Am J Roentgenol 143:1197, 1984

19. Papin E: Chirurgie du rein. Anomalies du rein. Paris, G. Doin, 1928, p 205

20. Zarins CK, Gewertz BL: Atlas of Vascular Surgery. New York, Churchill Livingstone, 1988, p 56

21. Trigaux JP, Vandroogenbroek S, De Wispelaere JF, et al: Congenital anomalies of the inferior vena cava and left renal vein: evaluation with spiral CT. J Vasc Interv Radiol 9:339, 1998

22. Crawford JL, Stowe CL, Safi HJ, et al: Inflammatory aneurysms of the aorta. J Vasc Surg 2:133, 1985

23. Crawford ES, Saleh SA, Babb JW 3rd, et al: Infrarenal abdominal aortic aneurysm: factors influencing survival after operation performed over a 25-year period. Ann Surg 193:699, 1981

24. Zarins CK, White RA, Schwarten D, et al: AneuRx stent graft vs. open surgical repair of abdominal aortic aneurysm: multicenter prospective clinical trial. J Vasc Surg 29:292, 1999

25. Makaroun MS: The Ancure endografting system: an update. J Vasc Surg 33:S129, 2001

26. Nonruptured abdominal aortic aneurysm: six-year follow-up results from the multicenter prospective Canadian aneurysm study. Canadian Society for Vascular Surgery Aneurysm Study Group. J Vasc Surg 20:163, 1994

27. Zarins CK, Harris EJ: Operative repair of aortic aneurysms: the gold standard. J Endovasc Surg 4:232, 1997

28. Arko FR, Lee WA, Hill BB, et al: Aneurysm-related death: primary endpoint analysis for comparison of open and endovascular repair. J Vasc Surg 36:297, 2002

29. Moore WS, Kashyap VS, Vescera CL, et al: Abdominal aortic aneurysm: a 6 year comparison of endovascular versus transabdominal repair. Ann Surg 230:298, 1999

30. Adriansen MEAPM, Bosch JL, Halpern EF, et al: Elective endovascular versus open surgical repair of abdominal aortic aneurysms: systematic review of short-term results. Radiology 224:739, 2002

31. Arko FR, Hill BB, Olcott C, et al: Endovascular repair reduces early and late morbidity compared to open surgery for abdominal aortic aneurysm. J Endovasc Ther 9:711, 2002

32. Cao P, Verzini F, Zannetti S, et al: Device migration after endoluminal abdominal aortic aneurysm repair: analysis of 113 cases with a minimum follow-up period of 2 years. J Vasc Surg 35:229, 2002

33. Torsello GB, Klenk E, Kasprzak B, et al: Rupture of abdominal aortic aneurysm previously treated by endovascular stent graft. J Vasc Surg 28:184, 1998

34. Zarins CK, White RA, Moll FL, et al: The AneuRx stent graft: four-year results and worldwide experience 2000. J Vasc Surg 33:S135, 2001

35. The U.S. AneuRx Clinical Trial: 6-year clinical update 2002. AneuRx Clinical Investigators. J Vasc Surg 37:904, 2003

36. Harris PL, Vallabhaneni SR, Desgranges P, et al: Incidence and risk factors of late rupture, conversion, and death after endovascular repair of infrarenal aneurysms: the Eurostar experience. J Vasc Surg 32:739, 2000

Acknowledgment

Figures 4 through 11   Susan Brust, C.M.I.

10 AORTOILIAC RECONSTRUCTION

Mark K. Eskandari, M.D., F.A.C.S.

Symptomatic aortoiliac occlusive disease is the consequence of a diffuse atherosclerotic process that is exacerbated by smoking, hypertension, hypercholesterolemia, and diabetes.[1-4] The resultant narrowing of the aorta and the iliac vessels impairs circulation into the pelvis and the lower extremities, thereby causing myriad patient complaints. Manifestations range from impotence, claudication (in the buttock, the thigh, or the calf), and rest pain (in the forefoot) to ulceration or gangrene.

Hemodynamically significant obstruction of blood flow arising from aortoiliac occlusion may be either segmental or diffuse. Fortunately, there are a number of different vascular reconstructions that can be performed to reestablish sufficient flow to the lower body. The choice of a surgical revascularization approach is based on two factors: (1) anatomic constraints and (2) comorbid conditions. Regardless of which technique is selected, preoperative workup and planning are essentially the same.

Preoperative Evaluation

Once it has been established that a patient's symptoms (e.g., claudication, rest pain, or a nonhealing wound) are attributable to hemodynamically significant aortoiliac occlusive disease, a thorough preoperative evaluation is initiated. Such evaluation typically includes obtaining objective physiologic documentation of the extent of occlusive disease by measuring lower-extremity blood flow with arterial waveforms and ankle-brachial indices. An imaging study is also required to guide revascularization. Percutaneous diagnostic angiography is widely used for this purpose; however, technological advancements may allow magnetic resonance angiography (MRA) to supplant traditional contrast arteriography.[5-7] If an extra-anatomic bypass is anticipated, ancillary tests, including bilateral arm blood pressure measurements and computed tomography scans of the chest, abdomen, or pelvis, may be necessary. A standard cardiac risk assessment is mandatory before any form of revascularization, and the extent of testing is tailored to the level of cardiac risk.

Operative Technique

AORTOILIAC ENDARTERECTOMY

Although localized aortoiliac endarterectomy is less commonly performed today than it once was, it remains useful for a subgroup of patients with focal aortic bifurcation disease. The classic candidate for this procedure has minimal disease of the infrarenal abdominal aorta and the external iliac arteries but a severely diseased and narrowed aortic bifurcation.

Step 1: Incision and Approach

A standard lower midline transperitoneal incision allows rapid, direct access. Usually, the incision can be made below the umbilicus and extended to the pubis.

Step 2: Exposure and Control of Aorta and Iliac Arteries

Upon entry into the abdominal cavity, exposure of the aortic bifurcation is achieved by retracting the small bowel cephalad. A self-retaining retractor, such as an Omni (Omni-Tract Surgical, Minneapolis, Minnesota) or a Bookwalter (Cardinal Health, V. Mueller, McGaw Park, Illinois), is often helpful. The retroperitoneum overlying the aortic bifurcation is then incised in the midline, and the aorta is exposed to the level of the inferior mesenteric artery [see 4:9 Repair of Infrarenal Abdominal Aortic Aneurysms]. Both common iliac arteries are exposed, with care taken not to damage the underlying iliac veins and the overlying ureters, which normally cross at the iliac bifurcation.

Given that this procedure is best suited for treatment of localized disease, exposure beyond the iliac bifurcation is rarely necessary. If it appears that the disease process extends into the external iliac arteries or more proximally in the infrarenal aorta, another form of treatment, such as aortobifemoral bypass (see below), may be indicated.

Step 3: Aortoiliac Endarterectomy

Once the aorta and the iliac vessels are exposed, I.V. heparin is given for systemic anticoagulation. The vessels are then controlled with vascular clamps. As a rule, the iliac vessels should be clamped first to reduce the risk of distal embolization during placement of the aortic cross-clamp. These vessels should be clamped only enough to prevent retrograde bleeding. They must not be repeatedly clamped and unclamped, because they are prone to the development of flow-limiting intimal flaps or fractured atherosclerotic plaques.

Next, the aorta is incised longitudinally from a point just above the bifurcation (where the aorta is soft) down into the common iliac artery in which the disease process extends further. Sometimes, the middle sacral or lower lumbar arteries must be oversewn to control back-bleeding. A dissection plane is developed between the media and the adventitia, and a standard endarterectomy of the infrarenal aorta and the more diseased iliac artery is performed. The endarterectomy of the contralateral iliac artery is performed by means of eversion through the aortotomy [see Figure 1]. If the distal termination points in the iliac vessels are irregular or have a significant step-off, the plaque should be tacked down with two or three 6-0 polypropylene sutures, with the knots tied on the outside of the vessel wall.

Troubleshooting Occasionally, endarterectomy results in a very thin residual wall, or the distal termination points are too steep to fix with tacking sutures alone. In such cases, the best recourse is to replace this section of the aorta and the common iliac vessels with a short standard bifurcated prosthetic interposition graft. Proximally, the graft is sewn to the infrarenal aorta in an end-to-end fashion. Distally, the two limbs are sewn to the two common iliac arteries in the same manner.

Step 4: Repair of Arteriotomy

The arteriotomy can be closed either primarily or with a patch, depending on the size of the aorta and the iliac vessels. Primary closure is preferred, but if it appears that such closure will significantly narrow the aorta or the iliac artery, a patch (either prosthetic or autogenous) should be used instead. Before closure is completed, the vessels should be flushed and back-bled to diminish the risk of distal embolization to the legs upon reestablishment of inline flow. The adequacy of the repair is confirmed pri-

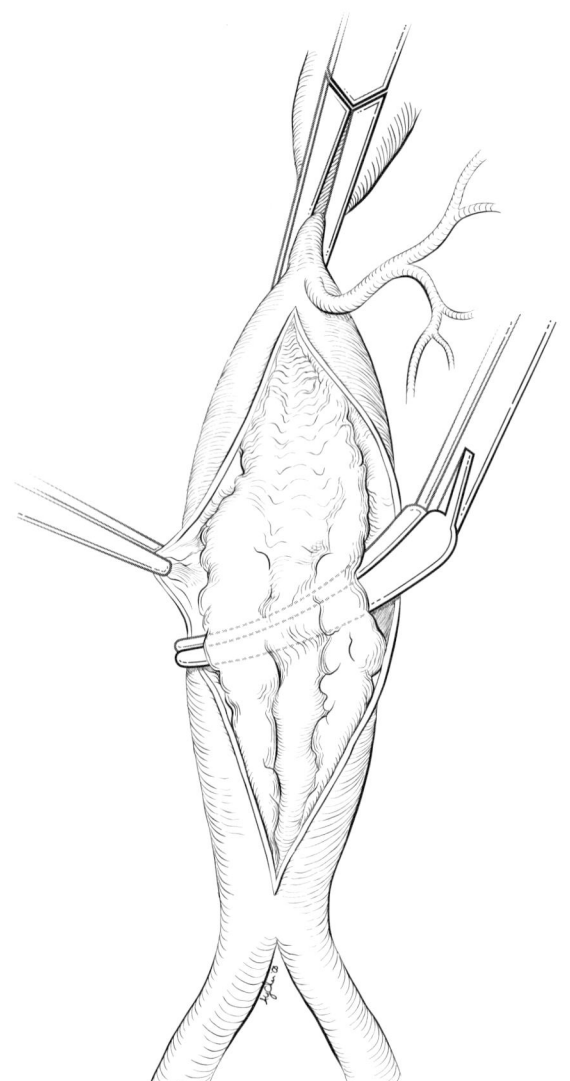

Figure 1 **Aortoiliac endarterectomy. Plaque is removed through a longitudinal aortotomy.**

marily by the palpation of normal femoral pulses in the groins.

Step 5: Closure of Retroperitoneum

Before abdominal closure, the retroperitoneum is closed with an absorbable suture so as to isolate the repair from the GI tract. This step reduces the risk of an aortoenteric fistula.

ILIOFEMORAL BYPASS

Iliofemoral bypass, already an uncommon procedure, has now largely been supplanted by advances in percutaneous endoluminal techniques. Nevertheless, it is still used on occasion and thus is worth knowing. One limitation on the application of iliofemoral bypass is that aortoiliac occlusive disease typically causes diffuse aortic and bilateral iliac artery narrowing. For this operation to be successful, there must be a relatively disease-free common iliac artery that can provide unimpeded inflow. Accordingly, iliofemoral bypass is most suitable for those rare patients who have isolated unilateral external iliac artery disease.

Step 1: Incision and Approach

The patient is placed in the supine position, and two incisions are made [*see Figure 2*]. The common iliac artery is approached

through a lower-quadrant retroperitoneal incision positioned medial to the lateral border of the rectus muscle. The femoral artery is approached through a standard vertical groin incision.

Step 2: Exposure of Iliac and Femoral Arteries

Once the retroperitoneum is entered, the visceral contents and the ureter are bluntly dissected away from the psoas muscle medially. This dissection, which takes place through a mostly bloodless field, yields full exposure of the targeted common iliac artery and its bifurcation into the external and internal iliac arteries. It should proceed far enough to allow control of the arteries with vascular clamps. Care must be taken not to damage the underlying iliac veins. In particular, no attempt should be made to isolate these vessels circumferentially, which can lead to troublesome bleeding.

The vertical incision in the groin permits full exposure of the common femoral artery and its bifurcation into the superficial femoral artery and the profunda femoris. Unlike the iliac arteries, the femoral artery and its branches may be circumferentially dissected.

Step 3: Tunneling of Bypass Graft

Once the inflow and outflow vessels are adequately exposed, the bypass graft is tunneled from the retroperitoneum to the groin, passing beneath the ureter and the inguinal ligament. During tunneling, care must be taken not to avulse the bridging epigastric vein found just cephalad and posterior to the inguinal ligament. Typically, a prosthetic graft 6 to 8 mm in diameter is used; however, autogenous material (e.g., a segment of the greater saphenous vein) may be used if desired.

Step 4: Proximal Anastomosis to Iliac Artery

With the bypass graft in position, the patient undergoes systemic anticoagulation with I.V. heparin. The common, external, and internal iliac arteries are controlled with vascular clamps. The proximal anastomosis is then performed to the selected common iliac artery. If practicable, the anastomosis should be an end-to-side one so as to preserve antegrade flow into the internal iliac artery.

Troubleshooting Occasionally, the common iliac artery is too diseased to clamp or to use as an inflow source. In such cases, the infrarenal aorta may be clamped instead or used as the site of the proximal anastomosis.

Step 5: Distal Anastomosis to Femoral Artery

Vascular clamps are placed on the common femoral artery and its branches, and the distal anastomosis is performed in an end-to-side manner. The configuration of the longitudinal arteriotomy depends on the presence and extent of disease in the femoral arteries. If both the superficial femoral artery and the profunda femoris are relatively free of disease, the arteriotomy should extend from the common femoral artery into the superficial femoral artery. If, however, the superficial femoral artery is occluded or heavily diseased, the arteriotomy should extend down into the profunda femoris [*see Figure 3*]. In either case, an end-to-side anastomosis is fashioned. Before completion of the bypass, the inflow vessel is flushed and the outflow vessel backbled to reduce the risk of distal embolization to the legs.

AORTOFEMORAL BYPASS

Before the application of percutaneous balloon angioplasty and stenting, aortofemoral bypass grafting was the revascularization operation of choice for patients with diffuse aortoiliac occlusive disease. This operation is still favored by many, and it yields excellent long-term patency.

Step 1: Incision and Approach

Typically, the patient is placed in the supine position, and the operation is performed through a midline laparotomy and two longitudinal groin incisions. A self-retaining retractor is recommended to facilitate exposure of the infrarenal aorta.

Alternatively, the infrarenal aorta may be exposed via a left retroperitoneal incision extending obliquely from the lateral border of the rectus muscle, at the level of the umbilicus, to the tip of the 11th rib. For this approach, the patient is placed in a right semilateral decubitus position with the assistance of an inflatable beanbag. The hips are rotated so that they are flat on the bed, providing easy access to the groins.

Step 2: Exposure of Aorta

Upon entry into the abdominal cavity, the fourth portion of the duodenum is dissected free of its retroperitoneal attachments, and the small bowel is retracted to the right of the aorta. The self-retaining retractor may then be placed to facilitate exposure. Next, the retroperitoneum overlying the infrarenal aorta is incised in the midline to expose the vessel, ideally in a location that is not heavily diseased or calcified. Unlike the dissection required in a localized endarterectomy [*see* Aortoiliac

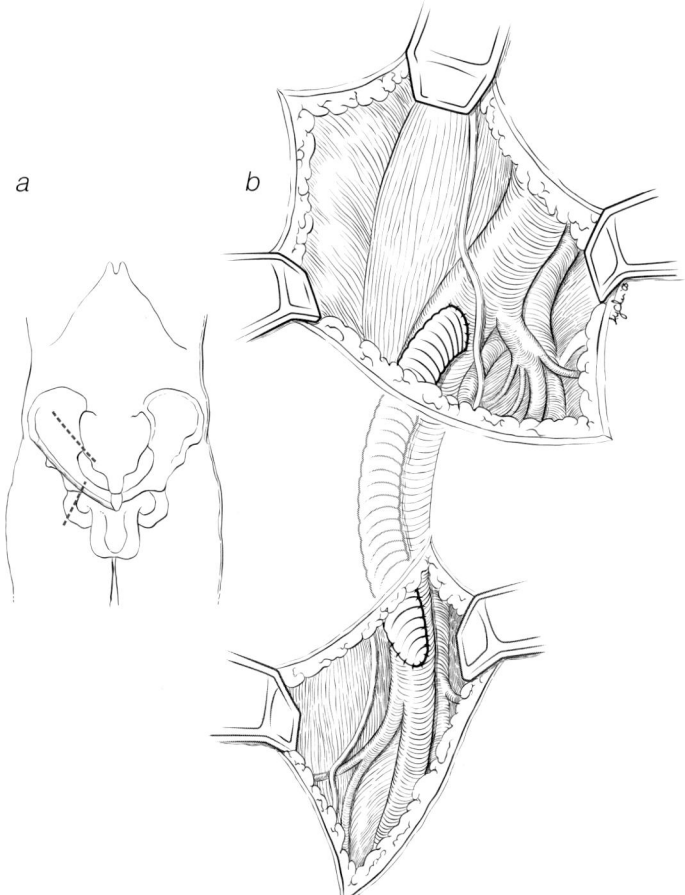

Figure 2 *Iliofemoral bypass. (a)* **A low retroperitoneal incision and an ipsilateral groin incision are made for exposure of the inflow and outflow bypass vessels. (b) The graft is tunneled beneath the ureter and the inguinal ligament.**

Endarterectomy, *above*], this dissection is primarily between the renal arteries and the inferior mesenteric artery. In most cases, the dissection need not be extended downward below the aortic bifurcation into the iliac arteries.

When this operation is performed through a left retroperitoneal incision, the external and internal oblique muscles and the transversus abdominis are divided, and the retroperitoneum is entered. Complete exposure of the infrarenal aorta is obtained by mobilizing the abdominal contents, the left kidney, and the left ureter medially after blunt dissection along the anterior border of the psoas muscle.

Troubleshooting In those cases in which aortofemoral bypass is being done for a patient with complete infrarenal aortic occlusion, the operative approach is modified to allow placement of a vascular clamp above the renal arteries. The dissection is carried cephalad by retracting the small bowel mesentery and the superior mesenteric artery to the right. The left renal vein is found anterior to the aorta at the level of the renal arteries. Generally, this vein need not be divided to expose the suprarenal aorta. Rather, it should be thoroughly dissected and encircled with a vessel loop so that it can be retracted cephalad and caudad. Sometimes, an adrenal or gonadal vein draining into the left renal vein must be ligated and divided to give the renal vein added mobility. With the left renal vein retracted caudad, the suprarenal aorta is dissected.

Step 3: Exposure of Femoral Artery

A vertical groin incision provides full exposure of the common femoral artery and its bifurcation into the superficial femoral artery and the profunda femoris. The femoral artery and its branches should be circumferentially dissected to give the surgeon an unobstructed view for placement of the vascular clamps.

Step 4: Tunneling of Bypass Graft

Once the inflow and outflow vessels are adequately exposed, the bypass graft—typically, a bifurcated prosthetic graft measuring 14×7 mm or 16×8 mm—is tunneled from the abdomen to the groins. Its course should pass beneath the ureter and the inguinal ligament. To create the tunnel, one index finger, oriented so that its dorsum faces the vessel wall, is inserted in the midline incision and advanced caudad down to the groin. Simultaneously, the other index finger, oriented so that its volar aspect faces the common femoral artery, is inserted into a groin incision and advanced cephalad until the two fingers meet. As with an iliofemoral bypass graft, care must be taken not to avulse the bridging epigastric vein found just cephalad and posterior to the inguinal ligament. With one of the two fingers held in place, a Silastic tube or vessel loop is passed through the tunnel. The limbs of the graft are attached to the tube or loop and passed through the tunnel down to the groins.

Step 5: Proximal Anastomosis to Aorta

The proximal aortic anastomosis can be done in either an end-to-end or an end-to-side configuration. An end-to-side beveled anastomosis is preferable for (1) patients with a small (< 1.5 cm) infrarenal aorta and (2) patients with severe occlusive disease of both external iliac arteries in whom it is desirable to preserve flow into the pelvic circulation via the internal iliac arteries. An end-to-end anastomosis is preferable for (1) patients with occlusive iliac disease and a concomitant aortic aneurysm and (2) patients undergoing revascularization for chronic total aortic occlusion. The latter configuration is also less bulky and easier to cover and

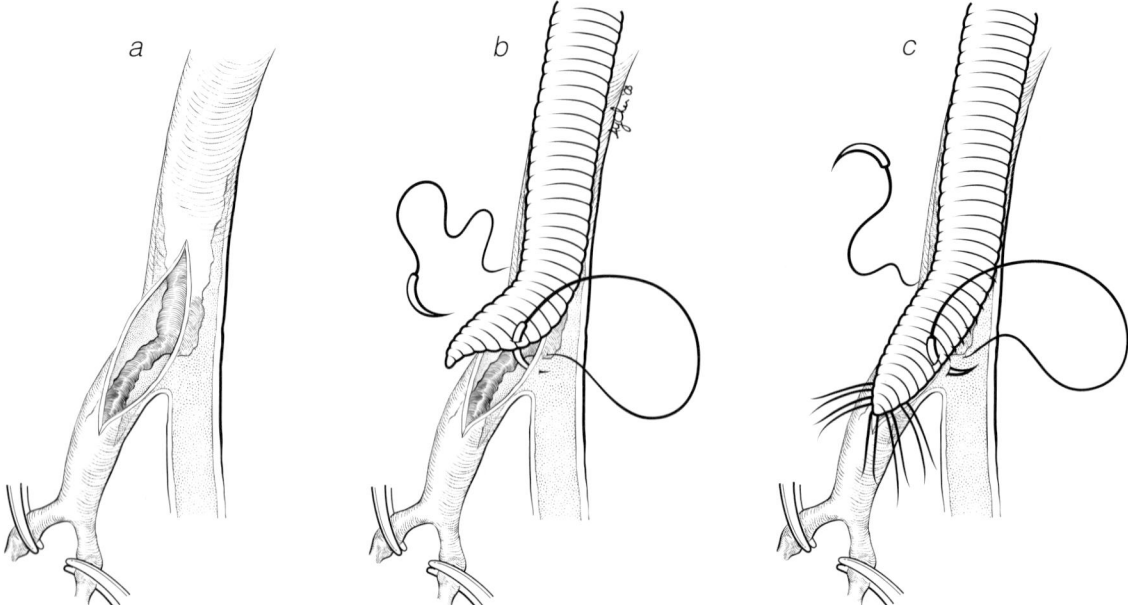

a *b* *c*

Figure 3 **Iliofemoral bypass. (*a*) When concomitatnt superficial femoral artery disease is present, the distal anastomosis is performed to a longitudinal arteriotomy that extends onto the proximal profunda femoris. (*b*) The heel of the hood of the graft is anastomosed to the common femoral artery. (*c*) The tip of the graft is extended down the profunda femoris.**

isolate from the GI tract at the conclusion of the operation.

Once a configuration for the anastomosis has been chosen, I.V. heparin is given for systemic anticoagulation. The graft is trimmed so that its bifurcation lies close to the proximal anastomosis. The infrarenal aorta is controlled, most commonly with vascular clamps above and below the site of the intended anastomosis. Control of the aorta with a partially occluding vascular clamp may be attempted, but the size of the vessel and the coexistence of aortic disease typically make this difficult or impossible to accomplish.

If an end-to-side anastomosis is to be performed, a longitudinal aortotomy is made and the graft sewn in place in a spatulated fashion. The toe of the graft is oriented cephalad [*see Figure 4*]. The anastomosis should be spatulated steeply so that it is not too bulky in the retroperitoneum and can be covered at the end of the procedure. Before completion of the anastomosis, the graft is flushed and back-bled.

If an end-to-end anastomosis is to be performed, a small portion of the aorta is resected to allow the graft to fit neatly into the retroperitoneum. In some cases, back-bleeding lumbar arteries in the region of the resected aorta must be oversewn. The distal stump is oversewn with 2-0 or 3-0 polypropylene in two rows; the first row is done with a continuous suture in a horizontal mattress stitch, the second with a continuous suture in a baseball stitch [*see Figure 5*].

Troubleshooting Vascular control of the aorta is achieved differently when chronic infrarenal aortic occlusion is present. In this setting, placement of a vascular clamp just below the renal arteries may squeeze atherosclerotic debris up into the renal arteries. To prevent this, the vascular clamp should be placed between the superior mesenteric artery and the renal arteries. Once the distal clamp is in place, the aorta is opened below the renal arteries and the atherosclerotic plug removed. The suprarenal clamp can then be moved to just below the renal arteries, and the proximal anastomosis can be fashioned as already described (see above).

A heavily calcified infrarenal aorta encountered at the time of

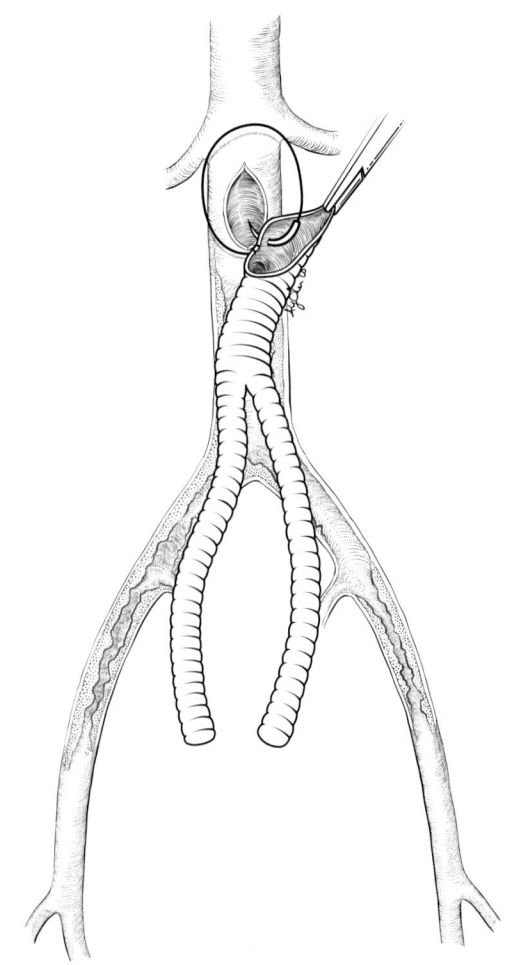

Figure 4 **Aortofemoral bypass. Shown is an end-to-side proximal anastomosis.**

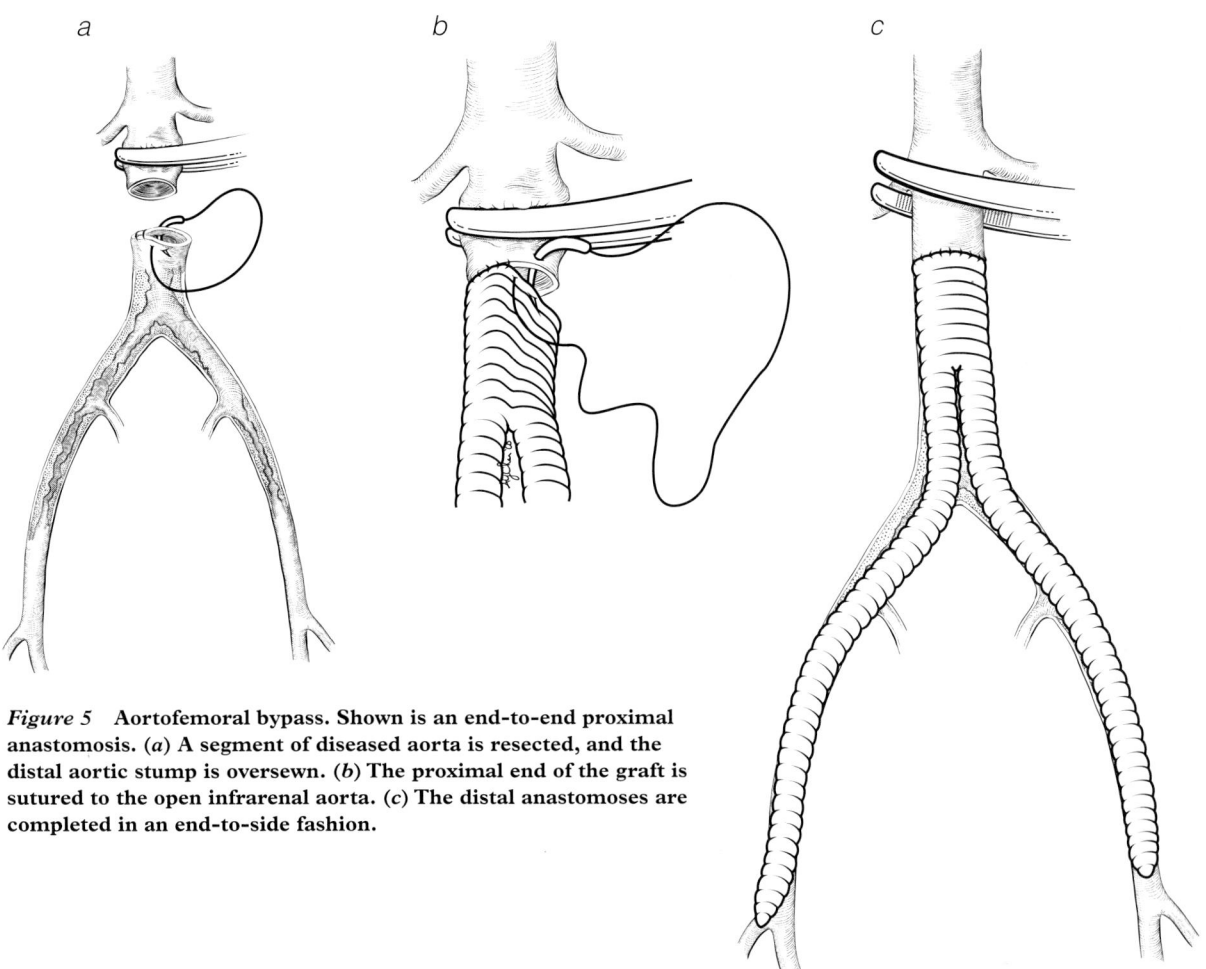

a   *b*   *c*

Figure 5 **Aortofemoral bypass. Shown is an end-to-end proximal anastomosis. (*a*) A segment of diseased aorta is resected, and the distal aortic stump is oversewn. (*b*) The proximal end of the graft is sutured to the open infrarenal aorta. (*c*) The distal anastomoses are completed in an end-to-side fashion.**

operation presents a difficult problem. In most cases, the infrarenal aorta can still be used, but the proximal anastomosis should be performed in an end-to-end configuration. Even in the most calcified aortas, the region 1 to 2 cm below the renal arteries is often soft enough to allow an anastomosis to be fashioned. If this is not the case, there are two alternatives: (1) suprarenal aortic control and endarterectomy of the infrarenal aorta just below the renal ostia before the proximal anastomosis and (2) conversion to a thoracofemoral bypass graft [*see* Thoracofemoral Bypass, *below*].

Step 6: Distal Anastomosis to Femoral Artery

Vascular clamps are placed on the common femoral artery and its branches, and the distal anastomosis is performed. As with an iliofemoral bypass, the configuration of the longitudinal arteriotomy depends on the existence of disease in the femoral arteries. If both the superficial femoral artery and the profunda femoris are relatively free of disease, the arteriotomy should extend from the common femoral artery into the superficial femoral artery. If, however, the superficial femoral artery is occluded or heavily diseased, the arteriotomy should extend downward into the profunda femoris. In either case, an end-to-side anastomosis is indicated. Before completion of the bypass, the inflow vessel is flushed and the outflow vessel back-bled to diminish the risk of distal embolization to the legs.

Step 7: Closure of Retroperitoneum

Before abdominal closure, the retroperitoneum is closed with an absorbable suture to isolate the repair from the GI tract and reduce the risk of an aortoenteric fistula. The ureters should be

visualized and preserved. Careless closure of the retroperitoneum can lead to laceration or entrapment of the ureter, particularly the right ureter. Every attempt should be made to cover the graft. If the retroperitoneum is too thin or the graft too bulky, an omental pedicle flap may be used.

THORACOFEMORAL BYPASS

A thoracofemoral bypass is ideal for a small subgroup of patients, comprising (1) those with an occluded old aortofemoral bypass graft, (2) those with a so-called lead-pipe calcified infrarenal aorta that is unusable as an inflow source, and (3) those with a so-called hostile abdomen (i.e., those with an ileal conduit, an ileostomy or colostomy, or a previous aortic graft infection). Candidates for this procedure must have adequate pulmonary reserve and be able to tolerate a thoracotomy. They must also be informed of and accept the low but real risk of paralysis.

The patient is placed in a right semilateral decubitus position so that the hips are nearly flat on the table and the torso is slightly rotated to the patient's right [*see Figure* 6]. An axillary roll and an inflatable beanbag will help maintain this position. Because single-lung ventilation will be necessary when the proximal anastomosis is done, either a double-lumen endotracheal tube or a bronchial blocker must be used. Placement of an orogastric tube to decompress the stomach helps keep the diaphragm down during exposure of the descending thoracic aorta.

Step 1: Incision and Exposure of Descending Thoracic Aorta

The descending thoracic aorta is approached through a left posterior lateral thoracotomy at the level of the 7th or 8th interspace. Additional exposure can be gained by resecting part of the rib and using a self-retaining table-mounted retractor. With the left lung decompressed, the parietal pleura overlying the descending thoracic aorta is incised. The aorta is cleanly dissected, with care taken not to damage the esophagus, which lies medially. Having an orogastric tube in place is advantageous in this regard: the esophagus can easily be located by palpating the tube. Any intercostal vessels in the region of the anticipated aortotomy can be preserved and controlled at the time of the anastomosis.

Step 2: Exposure of Femoral Artery

Full exposure of the common femoral artery and its bifurcation into the superficial femoral artery and the profunda femoris is obtained via a standard groin incision.

Step 3: Tunneling of Bypass Graft

The tunnel for the prosthetic graft has two components: (1) a left retroperitoneal tunnel and (2) a subcutaneous tunnel over the pubis. Usually, a tube prosthetic graft is sutured to a bifurcated graft before being tunneled through the retroperitoneum. The retroperitoneal tunnel is started in the chest by making a 1 cm hole in the posterior lateral aspect of the left diaphragm. An index finger is inserted through this hole and advanced caudad into the retroperitoneum as far as it can go. The other index finger is inserted through the left groin incision, oriented directly over the external iliac artery, and advanced cephalad into the retroperitoneum [see Figure 7]. Care is taken not to avulse the bridging epigastric vein found posterior and inferior to the inguinal ligament. In most cases, the left retroperitoneal tunnel must then be completed by using a long, hollow metal tunneling device such as the Gore Tunneler (W. L. Gore & Associates, Inc., Tempe, Ariz.). Once this tunnel is completed, the graft is passed through it in such a way that the bifurcated limbs are brought caudad down into the left groin wound.

Next, the subcutaneous tunnel from the left groin to the right groin is bluntly fashioned anterior to the pubis. It should not be oriented superior to the pubis because of the risk of injury to an overdistended bladder. To minimize this risk, an indwelling urinary catheter is advocated. The subcutaneous tunnel is used to pass the right limb of the graft over to the right groin. It is not uncommon for the bifurcation of the prosthetic graft to lie just cephalad to the left groin wound.

Step 4: Proximal Anastomosis to Descending Thoracic Aorta

Once the graft has been tunneled, the patient undergoes systemic anticoagulation with I.V. heparin. The descending thoracic aorta is controlled either with a side-biting clamp or with two completely occluding aortic clamps placed in close proximity to each other. In the latter case, one or two intercostal arteries may have to be temporarily controlled as well. A longitudinal aortotomy is then made along the left lateral aspect of the thoracic aorta, and a beveled end-to-side anastomosis is fashioned. Exposure can be enhanced by ventilating the right lung and attaching the orogastric tube to suction to decompress the stomach. Before completion of the anastomosis, the aorta is flushed and back-bled.

Troubleshooting Partial aortic control with a side-biting vascular clamp is successful in most cases, but it is not recommended when the descending thoracic aorta is heavily diseased and calcified or when preoperative imaging studies show thrombus in this location. If an intercostal artery cannot be temporarily controlled with clamps, it can be oversewn from the inside of the aorta to prevent nuisance back-bleeding.

Step 5: Distal Anastomosis to Femoral Artery

Vascular clamps are placed on the common femoral artery and its branches, and an end-to-side anastomosis is fashioned distally. Again, the configuration of the longitudinal arteriotomy depends on the existence of disease in the femoral arteries. If both the superficial femoral artery and the profunda femoris are relatively free of disease, the arteriotomy should extend from the common femoral artery into the superficial femoral artery. If, however, the superficial femoral artery is occluded or heavily diseased, the arteriotomy should extend downward into the profunda femoris. Before completion of the bypass, the inflow vessel is flushed and the outflow vessel back-bled.

Step 6: Closure of Chest

Once the proximal anastomosis is complete, the left lung is reinflated. At the conclusion of the operation, the chest is closed in a standard fashion over two chest tubes. The proximal anastomosis should be covered with either a prosthetic patch or bovine pericardium to diminish the risk of an aortopulmonary fistula.

AXILLOFEMORAL BYPASS

Axillofemoral bypass is ideally suited to elderly patients who cannot tolerate an aortic operation. The hemodynamic changes occurring during the operation are minimal, and recovery from the three small incisions used is substantially quicker than that from a laparotomy or a thoracotomy.

Because hemodynamically significant occlusive disease is less common in the right innominate artery than in the left subclavian artery, the right axillary is more often used as the inflow vessel than the left axillary artery is. Such occlusion can easily be identified preoperatively by measuring blood pressure in both arms. The sterile field includes both groins, the appropriate side of the chest (usually the right) up to the neck, and the appropriate flank (again, usually the right). It need not include the entire inflow arm; however, the arm should be abducted 90° and positioned on an arm board.

Step 1: Incision and Exposure of Axillary Artery

The patient is placed in the supine position. The axillary artery is approached through a horizontal 6 cm infraclavicular incision placed approximately 2 cm below the inferior border of the clavicle. Dissection is carried through the subcutaneous tissue, the fascia overlying the pectoralis major is incised, and the muscle is bluntly dissected along the length of its fibers. The dissection plane should remain medial to the pectoralis minor.

Next, the axillary vein is encountered and retracted caudad, and the underlying axillary artery is visualized. The axillary artery is cleanly dissected, with care taken not to retract or damage the brachial plexus lying deep and superior to the artery. For full exposure of the axillary artery, the thoracoacromial artery may have to be ligated at its origin. For easier retraction, the axillary artery may be encircled with vessel loops.

Step 2: Exposure of Femoral Artery

The femoral artery and its bifurcation into the superficial femoral and profunda femoris arteries are approached through a standard groin incision.

Step 3: Tunneling of Bypass Graft

Once the inflow and outflow vessels are adequately exposed, a prosthetic graft 80 to 100 cm long and 8 or 10 mm in diameter is tunneled from the axillary incision, beneath the pectoralis

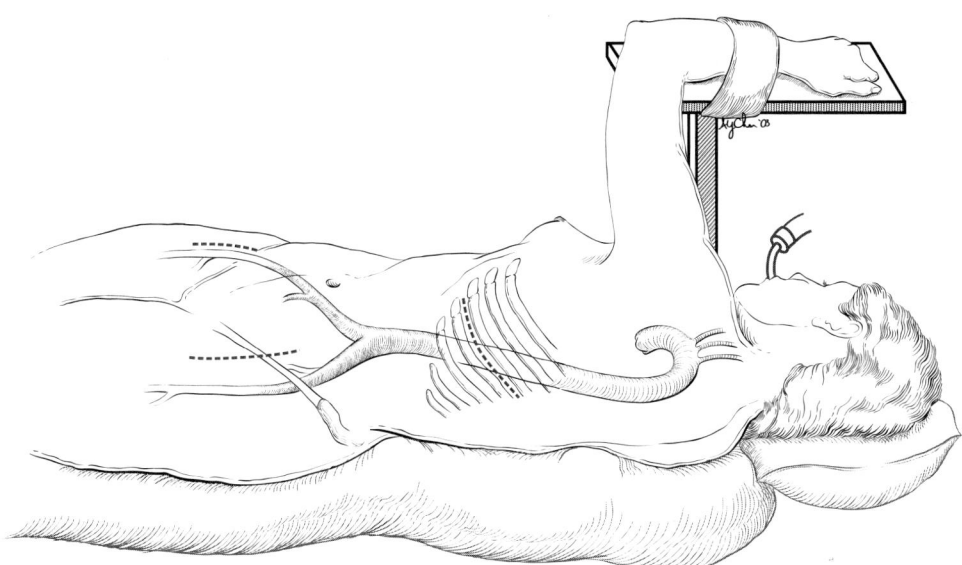

Figure 6 **Thoracofemoral bypass. The patient is positioned so that the hips are flat but the torso is slightly rotated to the patient's right. Three incisions are made: a left postero-lateral thoracotomy and two groin incisions.**

minor, and down to the flank. The use of a long, hollow metal tunneler is recommended at this point. To facilitate tunneling, a single counterincision is made in the midaxillary line over the sixth or seventh intercostal space. From this counterincision, the graft is tunneled along the flank, over the iliac crest, anterior to the anterior superior iliac process, and into the ipsilateral groin wound. Except for the portions in the axilla and the groin, the entire graft should lie in a subcutaneous plane.

Next, a subcutaneous tunnel from the ipsilateral groin to the contralateral groin is bluntly fashioned anterior to the pubis to allow passage of a second prosthetic graft (a short crossover graft 8 mm in diameter). This tunnel should not be oriented superior to the pubis because of the risk of injury to an overdistended bladder.

Step 4: Proximal Anastomosis to Axillary Artery

With the long graft in place, I.V. heparin is given for systemic anticoagulation. The pectoralis minor may be retracted laterally to provide additional exposure. The axillary artery is controlled with vascular clamps, with care taken not to include any part of the brachial plexus lying nearby. A longitudinal arteriotomy is made along the length of the axillary artery. The proximal anastomosis is then fashioned in an end-to-side configuration. The anastomosis must lie medial to the pectoralis minor. This is critical for preventing avulsion of the graft from the axillary artery when the patient fully abducts the arm. Before the anastomosis is completed, it is flushed and back-bled. Once blood flow to the arm is reestablished, the graft should be positioned so that it lies parallel to the axillary artery for a length of 2 to 3 cm before diving deep and caudad.

Step 5: Distal Anastomosis to Femoral Artery

The distal anastomosis to the femoral arteries is performed as described earlier [see Thoracofemoral Bypass, *above*]. There remains some controversy over the formation of the short crossover

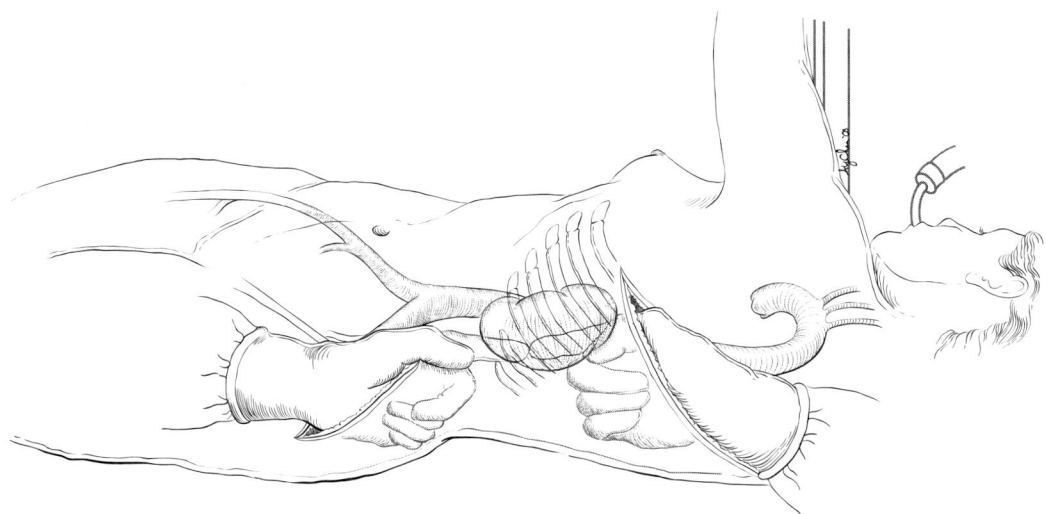

Figure 7 **Thoracofemoral bypass. A left retroperitoneal tunnel is fashioned for passage of the prosthetic graft downward to the groin. (The right arm of the graft is subsequently passed to the right groin via a subcutaneous tunnel anterior to the pubis.)**

graft from the axillary bypass graft to the contralateral femoral artery. My practice is to place the proximal anastomosis of the crossover femorofemoral anastomosis on the hood (or distal anastomosis) of the axillofemoral bypass graft [see Figure 8]. Others prefer to use a commercially available bifurcated axillofemoral prosthetic graft or to place the crossover graft more proximally along the length of the axillofemoral graft.

FEMOROFEMORAL BYPASS

A femorofemoral crossover bypass is well suited to patients who have unilateral complete occlusion or a diffusely diseased iliac system but have a relatively normal contralateral iliac system. It is performed with the patient supine and is conducted in essentially the same fashion as an axillofemoral bypass, but without the axillary anastomosis.

ENDOVASCULAR THERAPY

The use of percutaneous balloon angioplasty and stenting for the treatment of peripheral vascular disease has grown exponentially since its introduction in the 1990s. As regards short-term results, patients clearly experience less pain, recover more quickly, and regain function earlier. Initially, there was some question about the durability of stenting; however, data from longer follow-up periods indicate that this approach is an acceptable alternative for patients with focal aortoiliac occlusive disease.[8-10]

Complications

Certain complications are associated with all of the revascularization procedures discussed, such as bleeding, distal embolization, graft thrombosis, and graft infection. Late graft infection, recurrent disease, and pseudoaneurysm formation are known long-term complications as well. In addition, the following complications are unique to one or more of the procedures but do not arise with the others.

1. Injury to the ureters, resulting from their position overlying the iliac vessels (aortoiliac endarterectomy, iliofemoral bypass, axillofemoral bypass).
2. Impotence, resulting from damage to the autonomic nerve fibers around the origin of the left common iliac artery (aortoiliac endarterectomy, iliofemoral bypass, axillofemoral bypass).
3. Bleeding or deep venous thrombosis, related to trauma to the underlying iliac venous structures (all).
4. Paraplegia, resulting from the sacrifice of intercostal vessels supplying the anterior spinal artery (thoracofemoral bypass).
5. Colonic ischemia or infarction, resulting from hindered primary flow via the inferior mesenteric artery or collateral vessels from the hypogastric arteries (axillofemoral bypass).
6. Buttock claudication, resulting from disruption of inline flow to the pelvic circulation (axillofemoral bypass).
7. Aortoduodenal fistula, resulting from incomplete coverage of an aortic graft (axillofemoral bypass).
8. Renal failure, resulting from acute tubular necrosis or embolization when a suprarenal aortic clamp is used (thoracofemoral bypass, axillofemoral bypass).
9. Arm paralysis, resulting from injury to the deep and superiorly oriented brachial plexus (axillofemoral bypass).
10. Respiratory failure resulting from effusion or hemothorax after a left thoracotomy or from inadvertent pneumothorax

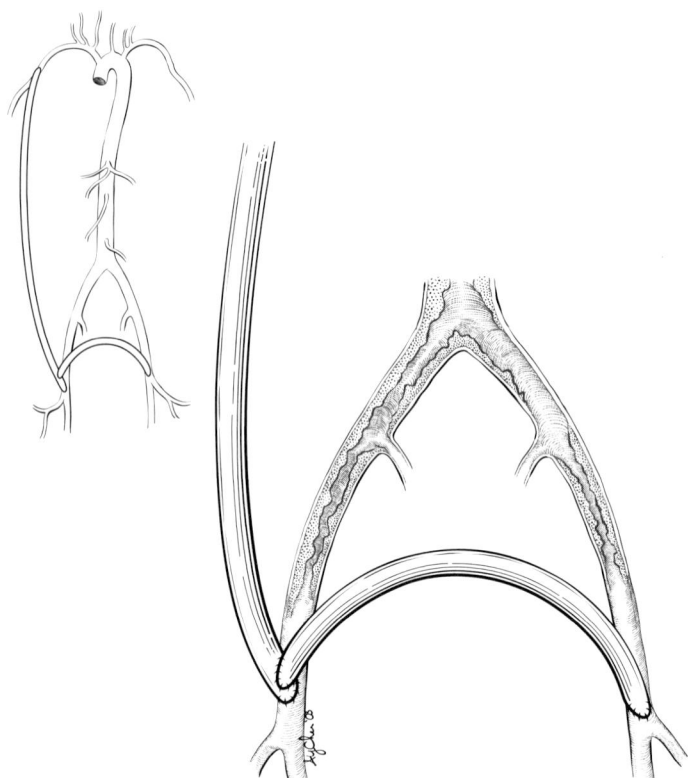

Figure 8 Axillofemoral bypass. Shown is the recommended configuration for the short femorofemoral crossover graft originating from the long axillofemoral graft. The femorofemoral graft originated from the hood of the axillofemoral graft.

during exposure of the axillary artery (thoracofemoral bypass, axillofemoral bypass).

Outcome Evaluation

Regardless of which operation is performed to treat aortoiliac occlusive disease, the subsequent outcome should be immediate relief of presenting symptoms—for example, reduced claudication, resolution of rest pain, or improved distal wound healing. Unfortunately, overall long-term survival in patients with symptomatic aortoiliac occlusive disease is not improved by operative management and is typically 10 to 15 years less than that in a normal age-matched group. Not surprisingly, by far the most significant long-term cause of death in these patients is atherosclerotic cardiac disease, which underscores the importance of a thorough preoperative cardiac evaluation.

In general, direct aortoiliac reconstructions (i.e., endarterectomy, aortofemoral bypass, and thoracofemoral bypass) have an expected patency rate of 85% to 90% at 5 years and 70% to 75% at 10 years.[11-13] When these operations are performed at experienced centers on patients who are considered to be good risk candidates, mortality is typically less than 3%.[14,15] Femorofemoral bypass and axillobifemoral bypass have expected 5-year patency rates of 70% to 75% and 60% to 85%, respectively.[16-19] Coexistent superficial femoral artery disease in the recipient vessels has a detrimental effect on the long-term patency of these bypasses.[20] Long-term anticoagulation may improve the patency for an axillobifemoral bypass graft.

References

1. Witteman JC, Grobbee DE, Valkenburg HA, et al: Cigarette smoking and the development and progression of aortic atherosclerosis: a 9-year population-based follow-up study in women. Circulation 88:2156, 1993

2. McGill HC Jr, McMahan CA, Malcom GT, et al: Effects of serum lipoproteins and smoking on atherosclerosis in young men and women. The PDAY Research Group. Pathobiological determinants of atherosclerosis in youth. Arterioscler Thromb Vasc Biol 17:95, 1997

3. Van Der Meer IM, De Maat MP, Hak AE, et al: C-reactive protein predicts progression of atherosclerosis measured at various sites in the arterial tree: the Rotterdam study. Stroke 33:2750, 2002

4. Faries PL, LoGerfo FW, Hook SC, et al: The impact of diabetes on arterial reconstructions for multilevel arterial occlusive disease. Am J Surg 181:251, 2001

5. Morasch MD, Collins J, Pereles FS, et al: Lower extremity stepping-table magnetic resonance angiography with multilevel contrast timing and segmented contrast infusion. J Vasc Surg 37:62, 2003

6. Loewe C, Schoder M, Rand T, et al: Peripheral vascular occlusive disease: evaluation with contrast-enhanced moving-bed MR angiography versus digital subtraction angiography in 106 patients. AJR Am J Roentgenol 179:1013, 2002

7. Pandharipande PV, Lee VS, Reuss PM, et al: Two-station bolus-chase MR angiography with a stationery table: a simple alternative to automated-table techniques. AJR Am J Roentgenol 179:1583, 2002

8. Back MR, Novotney M, Roth SM, et al: Utility of duplex surveillance following iliac artery angioplasty and primary stenting. J Endovasc Ther 8:629, 2001

9. Sanchez LA, Wain RA, Veith FJ, et al: Endovascular grafting for aortoiliac occlusive disease. Semin Vasc Surg 10:297, 1997

10. Gray BH, Sullivan TM: Aortoiliac occlusive disease: surgical versus interventional therapy. Curr Interv Cardiol Rep 3:109, 2001

11. Kalman PG: Thoracofemoral bypass: proximal exposure and tunneling. Semin Vasc Surg 13:65, 2000

12. Nash T: Aortoiliac occlusive vascular disease: a prospective study of patients treated by endarterectomy and bypass procedures. Aust N Z J Surg 49:223, 1979

13. Brewster DC: Clinical and anatomical considerations for surgery in aortoiliac disease and results of surgical treatment. Circulation 83:I42, 1991

14. de Vries SO, Hunink MG: Results of aortic bifurcation grafts for aortoiliac occlusive disease: a meta-analysis. J Vasc Surg 26:558, 1997

15. Passman MA, Taylor LM, Moneta GL, et al: Comparison of axillofemoral and aortofemoral bypass for aortoiliac occlusive disease. J Vasc Surg 23:263, 1996

16. Martin D, Katz SG: Axillofemoral bypass for aortoiliac occlusive disease. Am J Surg 180:100, 2000

17. Taylor LM Jr, Moneta GL, McConnell D, et al: Axillofemoral grafting with externally supported polytetrafluoroethylene. Arch Surg 129:588, 1994

18. Rutherford RB, Patt A, Pearce WH: Extra-anatomic bypass: a closer view. J Vasc Surg 6:437, 1987

19. Naylor AR, Ah-See AK, Engeset J: Axillofemoral bypass as a limb salvage procedure in high risk patients with aortoiliac disease. Br J Surg 77:659, 1990

20. Criado E, Burnham SJ, Tinsley EA Jr, et al: Femorofemoral bypass graft: analysis of patency and factors influencing long-term outcome. J Vasc Surg 18:495, 1993

Acknowledgments

Figures 1 through 8   Alice Y. Chen.

11 INFRAINGUINAL ARTERIAL PROCEDURES

William D. Suggs, M.D., F.A.C.S., and Frank J. Veith, M.D., F.A.C.S.

Since the early 1980s, there have been enormous advances in the treatment of lower-extremity ischemia secondary to infrainguinal arteriosclerosis. Effective interventional management strategies have been developed for virtually all patterns of arteriosclerosis underlying limb-threatening ischemia.[1,2] Bypasses to the infrainguinal arteries using segments of autologous vein have become routine for limb salvage. As this technique has evolved, the distal limits of revascularization have been extended. Bypasses to arteries near the ankle or in the foot can now be offered to patients who have no patent arteries suitable for more proximal bypasses. In addition, bypasses to distal tibial or tarsal vessels may be performed in some patients whose popliteal arteries are patent but who have three-vessel distal occlusive disease and forefoot gangrene.[3,4] Frequently, patients who require very distal bypasses have already undergone vascular reconstruction; these patients may be candidates for alternative approaches, such as a popliteal-distal bypass or a tibiotibial bypass.[5-7]

Patients with limbs threatened by distal tibial occlusive disease present an ongoing challenge to the vascular surgeon. Provided that careful attention is paid to obtaining high-quality preoperative angiograms and that the surgeon is willing to consider alternative approaches, it is generally possible to achieve good results from limb salvage procedures.

It should be kept in mind that only patients with threatened limbs—manifested by rest pain, frank gangrene, or nonhealing ulcers—should be considered candidates for infrainguinal bypass. Patients who have gangrene that extends into the deeper tarsal region of the foot, who have a severe organic mental syndrome, or who are nonambulatory are not candidates for limb salvage surgery and should be treated with primary amputation instead.[1,2]

Preoperative Evaluation

HISTORY AND PHYSICAL EXAMINATION

A careful history and a thorough physical examination are crucial for accurate assessment of the extent of the patient's atherosclerotic disease. In the course of the history, the examiner should pay particular attention to distinguishing true rest pain from other causes of pain (e.g., arthritis and neuritis). Significant ischemic pain is usually associated not only with decreased pulses but also with other manifestations of ischemia (e.g., atrophy, decreased skin temperature, marked rubor, and pain that is relieved when the foot is dangled). In the course of the physical examination, the examiner should look for and assess the extent of any underlying infection and should closely examine any surgical scars for clues to the nature and extent of any previous vascular operations involving the use of the saphenous vein. In addition, a careful pulse examination should be performed to assess the patient's baseline arterial status; these baseline measure-

ments provide a basis for comparison if the disease subsequently progresses and may help determine the approach to be used to salvage the threatened limb.

NONINVASIVE TESTING

Noninvasive tests are helpful in that they provide semiquantitative assessment of the circulation and help confirm the diagnosis made on the basis of the history and the physical examination. Such test measurements include the ankle-brachial index (ABI) and pulse volume recordings (PVRs).

The ABI is determined by dividing the ankle pressure in each lower limb by the higher of the two brachial pressures. Normal circulation typically yields an ABI of 1.0 to 1.2; claudication, an ABI of 0.40 to 0.95; and limb-threatening ischemia, an ABI of 0 to 0.5. It is vital to remember, however, that lower-extremity pressure measurements are less reliable in patients with heavily calcified vessels (e.g., diabetics and patients with end-stage renal disease). In these patients, ABIs are falsely elevated as a result of the higher cuff pressures required to occlude calcified vessels, which in some cases are not occluded even with pressures higher than 300 mm Hg.

PVRs are obtained by means of calibrated air-cuff plethysmography. Standard blood pressure cuffs are placed at different levels of the lower extremity, and the increases in pressure within the cuffs resulting from the volume increase during systole are recorded as pulse waves. Tracings exhibiting a brisk rise during systole and a dicrotic notch are characterized as normal, those exhibiting loss of the notch and a more prolonged downslope are characterized as moderately abnormal, and those exhibiting a flattened wave are characterized as severely abnormal. Absolute amplitudes on PVRs are not directly comparable between patients; however, serial PVRs from a single patient are highly reproducible and thus are quite useful for following the course of severe peripheral vascular disease in individual cases.[4] One disadvantage of PVRs is that they cannot differentiate proximal femoral disease from iliac occlusive disease.[8]

IMAGING

Duplex Scanning

Duplex scanning is a useful noninvasive method of assessing the aortoiliac and infrainguinal arterial systems. Several studies have evaluated the ability of duplex scanning to predict iliac artery stenosis. A 1987 trial found that duplex scanning was highly sensitive (89%) and specific (90%) in predicting iliac stenosis of 50% or greater.[9] Three subsequent trials corroborated these findings, reporting sensitivities ranging from 81% to 89% and specificities ranging from 88% to 99%.[10-12] This noninvasive modality may be especially useful for improving evaluation of diabetic patients before invasive procedures (e.g., angiography and angioplasty).[10]

Duplex scanning has also been used to allow infrapopliteal bypasses to be performed without preoperative angiography. In one study, a limb salvage rate of 86% was achieved with this approach, and completion arteriography matched the runoff status predicted by duplex scanning in 96% of cases.[13] In a study from our own institution, we were able to perform femoropopliteal bypasses without preoperative arteriography and were able to perform distal bypasses with confirmatory arteriograms at the time of operation.[14]

Magnetic Resonance Angiography

Magnetic resonance angiography (MRA), a noninvasive modality that does not require contrast agents, often yields good arterial images and may, in fact, be more sensitive than angiography in imaging distal lower-extremity runoff vessels.[15,16] More recently, developments such as gadolinium enhancement, multistation examination, and the floating table technique have further improved the resolution of MRA,[17-19] to the point where many institutions that use current forms of MRA no longer routinely obtain preoperative angiograms. MRA, in combination with arterial duplex scanning, has the potential to replace contrast arteriography in the assessment of patients with distal arterial occlusive disease.

Arteriography

Until MRA and duplex scanning become more widely available, contrast angiography will remain the gold standard for the evaluation of patients with distal arterial occlusive disease. A complete evaluation of the existing arterial disease from the aorta to the pedal vessels is necessary for diabetic patients, who frequently have multilevel occlusive disease. Obtaining intra-arterial pressure measurements at the time of angiography significantly improves detection of clinically significant stenosis. The systolic pressure gradient across the lesion should also be measured: gradients greater than 15 mm Hg are considered hemodynamically significant.[20]

In the general population, arteriography has a complication rate of only 1.7% to 3.3%.[21] Elderly patients with severe aortoiliac or infrainguinal disease must be carefully evaluated before the procedure because they are more likely to experience local and systemic complications than patients in the general population are. For the majority of patients, the transfemoral approach is the safest; however, for patients with weak or nonpalpable femoral pulses, other approaches (e.g., translumbar, transbrachial, or transaxillary) may be preferable. These alternative approaches are associated with higher rates of local complications, including hematomas, pseudoaneurysms, dissections, thrombosis, and embolization.

Renal insufficiency is an important complication of angiography: 6.5% to 8.2% of patients who undergo arteriography experience some degree of impairment associated with contrast agents.[22,23] Patients who have preexisting azotemia and whose baseline creatinine concentrations exceed 2.0 mg/dl are at highest risk for renal complications after angiography. Elderly patients typically have lower creatinine clearances for a given serum creatinine level and thus should always be considered at higher risk for nephrotoxicity. All possible precautions should be taken to limit the renal insult. There is some evidence to suggest that the use of low-osmolar contrast agents can decrease the incidence of renal impairment,[24,25] but the data are not unanimous on this point.[26] Adequate hydration and administration of oral acetylcysteine before arteriography are highly effective in diminishing the risk of contrast nephropathy. Administration of mannitol, which has an osmotic diuretic effect, helps prevent contrast toxicity as well. These measures, coupled with judicious use of contrast agents, should minimize renal impairment associated with arteriography.

Femoropopliteal Bypass

Patients whose limbs are clearly threatened and who have undergone arteriographic examination should undergo femoropopliteal bypass when the superficial femoral artery or the popliteal artery is occluded and when arteriography indicates that a patent popliteal artery segment distal to the occlusion has luminal continuity with any of its three terminal branches (even if one or more of these branches ends in an occlusion anywhere in the leg). Even if the popliteal artery segment into which the graft is to be inserted is occluded distally, femoropopliteal bypass to this segment can be considered.[27,28] If the isolated popliteal segment is shorter than 7 cm or if there is extensive gangrene or infection in the foot, a femorodistal artery bypass or a sequential bypass is sometimes performed in one or two stages.

OPERATIVE TECHNIQUE

Femoropopliteal bypass may be carried out either above or below the knee.

Above-the-Knee Bypass

For above-the-knee bypass, the patient is placed in the supine position with the thigh externally rotated and the knee flexed approximately 30°. This position affords easy exposure of the femoral and popliteal arteries as well as of the saphenous vein.

Harvesting of saphenous vein The greater saphenous vein is harvested through intermittent skip incisions starting in the groin and proceeding distally toward the knee [see Figure 1]. Multiple short skin incisions heal better than a single long one and are less likely to result in skin necrosis.

Dissection of the saphenous vein begins at the groin. This proximal incision is also used for exposure of the femoral artery. The saphenofemoral junction is carefully mobilized, and the tributaries are ligated with fine silk close to where they enter the main trunk, with care taken not to impinge on the wall of the trunk. As dissection continues distally, the main trunk of the saphenous vein is progressively elevated, and all tributaries are identified and ligated. The vein is then removed from its bed and

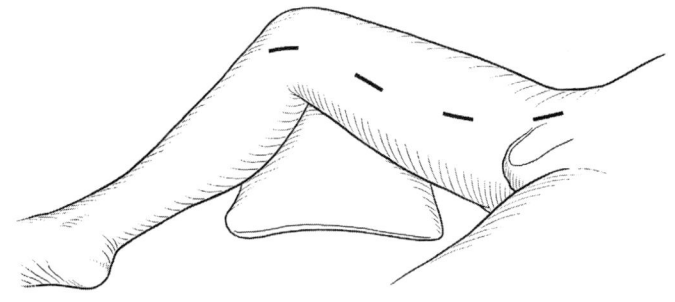

Figure 1 **Femoropopliteal bypass: above knee. Shown is the appropriate position of the leg. Interrupted skin incisions are made in the thigh and upper leg to permit harvesting of the saphenous vein.**

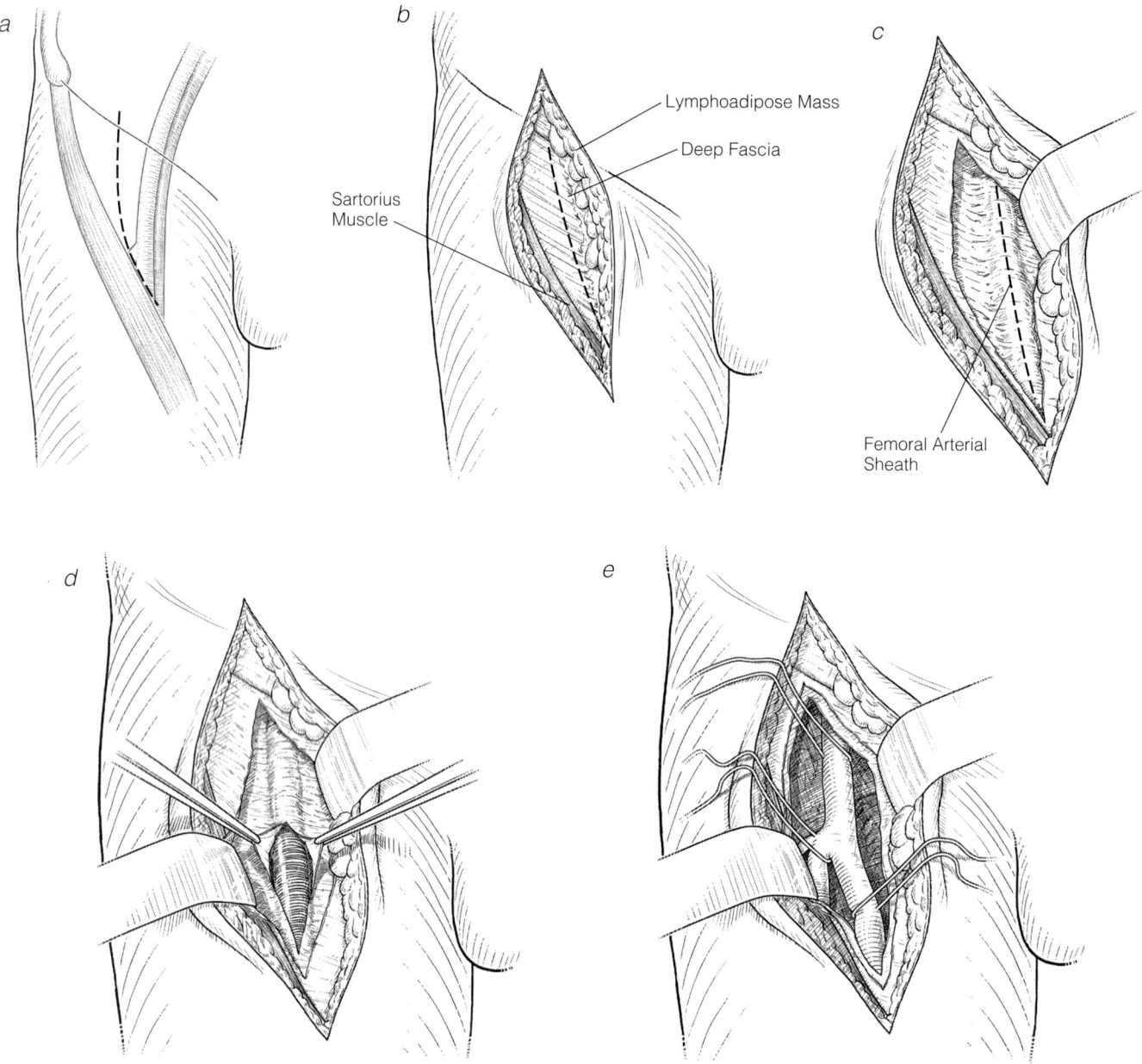

Figure 2 Femoropopliteal bypass: above knee. Depicted is exposure of the femoral artery. (*a*) A curved 4 to 5 in. skin incision is made slightly lateral to the pulsation of the femoral artery. (*b*) Lymphoadipose tissue is retracted to expose the deep fascia overlying the course of the femoral artery. (*c*) The deep fascia is incised, exposing the femoral arterial sheath, which is then opened along its axis (*d*). (*e*) The common and superficial femoral arteries are mobilized and encircled with Silastic vessel loops.

immediately placed into a basin containing heparinized saline (or heparinized whole blood) at a temperature of 4° C or cold Hanks solution. A small cannula is passed through the distal end of the divided vein, and the vessel is irrigated with cold Hanks solution to expel any liquid blood or clot and to locate any leaks. If a leak is found, it is repaired with 6-0 Prolene.

Step 1: exposure of femoral artery A slightly curved skin incision, with the concavity facing the medial aspect, is made starting at a point slightly above the inguinal crease and extending distally for 10 to 12.5 cm [*see Figure 2a*]. The incision should be slightly lateral to the pulsation of the femoral artery so as to avoid the lymphatics as much as possible. Any minor bleeding or

divided lymphatic vessels should be controlled with electrocoagulation or fine ligatures. Self-retaining retractors are placed both proximally and distally in the wound, and the lymphoadipose tissue is gently retracted medially [*see Figure 2b*].

The deep fascia is opened along the femoral artery [*see Figure 2c*], and the sheath of the artery is opened along its axis [*see Figure 2d*]. The common and superficial femoral arteries are mobilized, and Silastic loops are placed around them [*see Figure 2e*]. These vessels are then elevated slightly, and the origin of the deep femoral artery comes into view lateral and posterior to the common femoral artery and just proximal to the superficial femoral artery. Dissection of the origin of the deep femoral artery must be done carefully so as not to injure the collateral

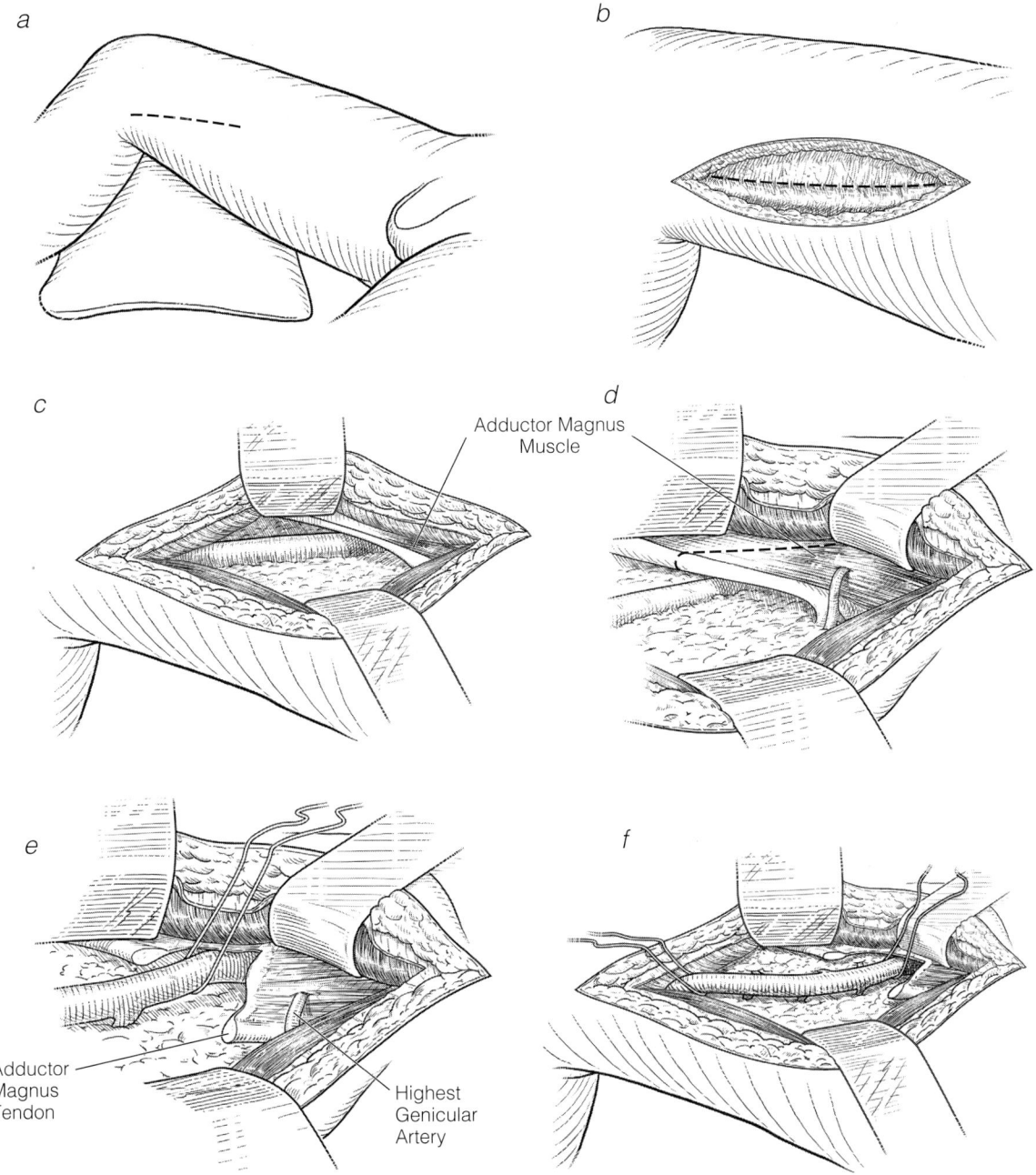

Figure 3 Femoropopliteal bypass: above knee. Depicted is medial exposure of the proximal popliteal artery. (*a*) An incision is made in the lower third of the thigh, anterior to the sartorius muscle. (*b*) The deep fascia is incised, and the sartorius muscle is retracted posteriorly, allowing the popliteal artery to be readily palpated. (*c*) The popliteal arterial sheath is opened, exposing the vessel and its surrounding venules. The adductor magnus tendon may be seen covering the proximal end of the artery (*d*), and it may have to be divided (*e*) to provide better exposure of the artery. (*f*) The popliteal artery, freed of the venous plexus, is mobilized between two vessel loops.

vessels coming off the artery at that level and the one or two branches of the satellite veins that cross the anterior portion of its initial segment. If mobilization of the deep femoral artery proves difficult, the satellite vein branches can be divided and ligated.

Step 2: exposure of proximal popliteal artery   For the approach to the popliteal artery, the surgeon moves to the opposite side of the table. An incision is made in the lower third of the thigh anterior to the sartorius muscle and is extended close to the medial aspect of the knee [*see Figure 3a*]. The deep fascia anterior to the sartorius muscle is opened, and the sartorius

muscle is detached from the vastus medialis muscle and retracted posteriorly. The popliteal artery is identified by palpation; it is the most superficial structure palpable through this exposure [*see Figure 3b*]. The overlying fascia is incised, and the adipose tissue usually present at this level is dissected until the vascular bundle is reached.

The sheath of the artery is opened [*see Figure 3c*]. At this level, there is almost always a network of venules surrounding the artery, which must be carefully dissected away from the arterial wall. Division of the adductor magnus tendon may be required to yield adequate exposure of the proximal portion of the popliteal artery [see Figures 3d and 3e]. The venous network is separated from the arterial adventitia, and the various branches are divided and ligated. The popliteal vein is then separated from the artery—a process that, because of the intimate connection between the two vessels, is sometimes quite difficult. In separating the vein from the artery, care must be taken not to injure any of the genicular branches of the artery. The popliteal artery is freed for a length of approximately 1.5 to 2 in., and vessel loops are placed around it [see Figure 3f].

If the proximal popliteal artery appears markedly sclerotic and unsuitable for anastomosis to the graft, the exposure must be extended to the middle portion of the artery. To achieve this extended exposure, the hamstring muscles and their tendons are mobilized and retracted posteriorly, and the medial head of the gastrocnemius muscle is divided close to the medial condyle of the femur.

Next, the sheath of the popliteal artery is opened farther distally, and the tributaries of the veins surrounding the artery are further dissected away from it. Dissection of the middle portion of the popliteal artery may be facilitated by flexing the knee; this measure relaxes the artery, thereby allowing it to be readily drawn closer to the superficial level of the exposure.

Step 3: creation of tunnel Implantation of the graft may be started in either the popliteal artery or the femoral artery; the former is our usual preference. Before the anastomoses are constructed, a tunnel is created under the sartorius muscle by means of either a tunneler or an aortic clamp with a red rubber catheter attached to it to mark the tunnel.

Step 4: construction of distal anastomosis to popliteal artery Heparin is routinely administered before the vascular clamps are applied. A longitudinal arteriotomy is made in the anterior wall of the artery with a sharp No. 15 knife blade. This arteriotomy is then enlarged with a scalpel or a Potts angled scissors. The length of the opening in the artery should be approximately twice the diameter of the vessel. If the edges of the arteriotomy are calcified and the atheromatous intima overlaps the cut edge, the diseased intima should be excised with arteriotomy scissors.

The saphenous vein segment is then brought into the field. It is reversed so that its proximal end becomes the distal end for the anastomosis. This distal end is then enlarged with a longitudinal incision in its posterior wall, and the right-angle tips of the two sides of the divided posterior wall are cut away. Double-armed sutures are placed through the proximal angle (or heel) of the graft, with the needles going from the outside of the arteriotomy to the inside and then from the inside to the outside. Next, a similar double-armed suture is passed through the distal angle (or toe) of the graft from the outside to the inside and then from the inside to the outside through the end of the arteriotomy.

The edge of the vein is then approximated to that of the arteriotomy with a continuous suture starting at the toe of the graft and proceeding toward the heel [see Figure 4]. When half of the anastomosis has been completed, the edge of the vein graft is separated from the edge of the opposite side of the arteriotomy to permit inspection of the arterial lumen and the completed suture. The other half of the anastomosis is then completed by placing a second continuous suture, starting at the heel and proceeding toward the toe. Finally, the two sutures are tied together midway between the heel and the toe to complete the popliteal anastomosis.

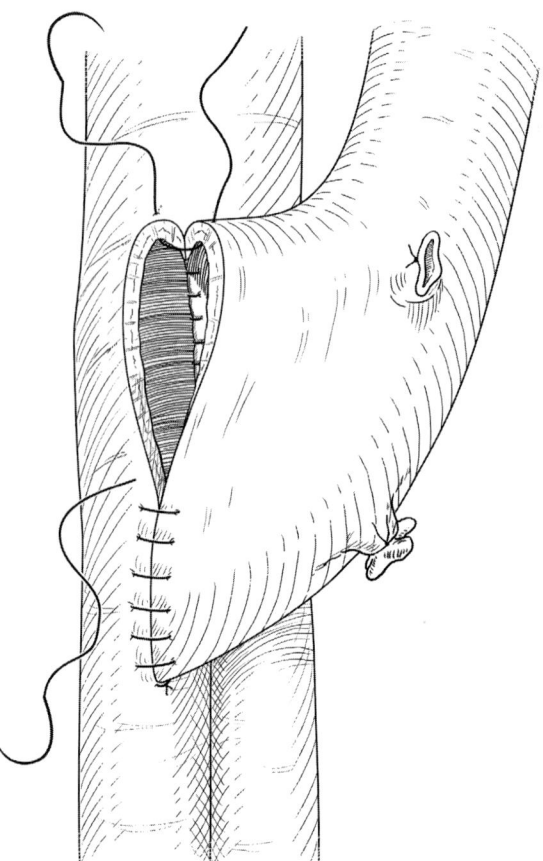

Figure 4 **Femoropopliteal bypass: above knee. Shown are details of the anastomotic suturing, which is begun at the distal end and continued to the middle portion of each side of the anastomosis of the artery and the saphenous vein graft. Equal bites of all layers of each vessel are included in each stitch, all of which are placed under direct vision.**

Step 5: placement of graft in tunnel The graft is distended by injecting heparinized saline solution into it to test for leaks either from the vein segment itself or from the anastomotic site. The graft is then marked to ensure that it does not become twisted when brought through the tunnel. The graft is brought through the tunnel either by using an aortic clamp or by attaching it to the previously placed red rubber catheter.

Step 6: construction of proximal anastomosis to femoral artery Before the proximal anastomosis is begun, the proper length of the graft should be determined to ensure that there is no redundancy. The proximal end of the graft is split and enlarged in the same fashion as the distal end, and the resulting right-angle corners are similarly trimmed. The graft is then anastomosed to the arteriotomy made in the femoral artery (which, like the popliteal arteriotomy, should be at least twice as long as the vessel is wide). The graft is attached by double-armed needles at its proximal angle and then in a similar fashion at its distal angle. The anastomosis is then completed from each end toward the center, just as the popliteal anastomosis was.

Below-the-Knee Bypass

When occlusion or marked stenosis renders the proximal and middle portions of the popliteal artery unsuitable for graft implantation, the lower portion of the vessel, which is often relatively free of atherosclerosis, may be used for the distal anastomosis instead.

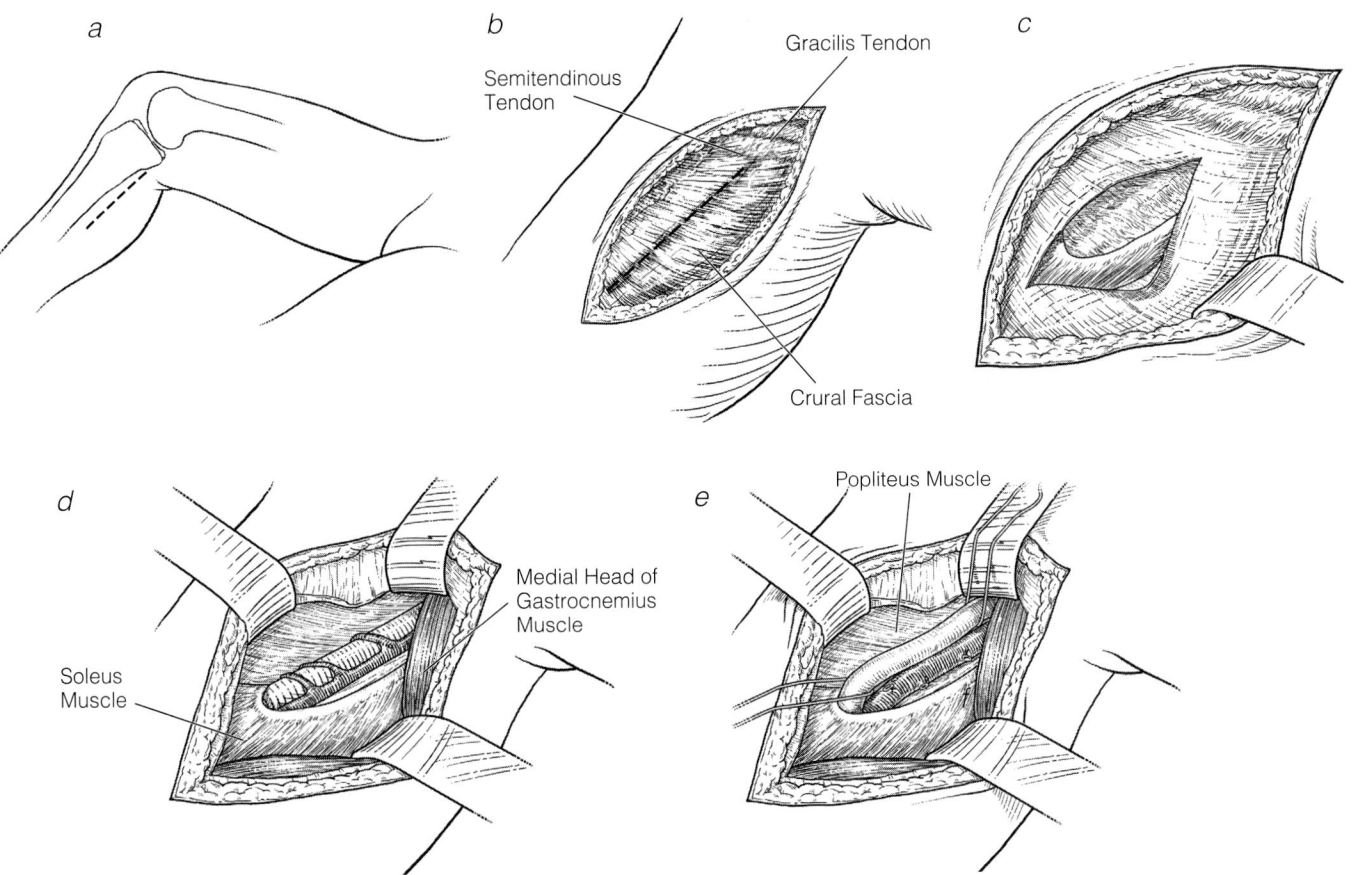

Figure 5 **Femoropopliteal bypass: below knee. Depicted is medial exposure of the distal popliteal artery. (*a*) An incision is made just behind the posteromedial surface of the tibia. (*b*) The crural fascia is exposed. (*c*) The fascia is incised, exposing the vascular bundle. (*d*) The medial head of the gastrocnemius muscle is retracted posteriorly, exposing the distal popliteal vessels and the arcade of the soleus muscle. (*e*) The distal popliteal artery is freed and mobilized between vessel loops.**

Step 1: exposure of popliteal artery   With the knee moderately flexed and supported by a rolled sheet placed under it, a vertical skin incision is made just behind the posteromedial surface of the tibia [*see Figure 5a*], exposing the crural fascia [*see Figure 5b*]. Care must be taken to avoid injury to the greater saphenous vein during the skin incision. When a saphenous vein graft is to be used, the same incision can serve both for harvesting of the vein and for exposure of the artery.

The crural fascia is opened along its fibers [*see Figure 5c*], its distal attachments are separated from the semitendinosus and gracilis tendons, and the two tendons are mobilized proximally and, if necessary, divided. The medial head of the gastrocnemius muscle is retracted posteriorly [*see Figure 5d*] to expose the popliteal artery and vein and the posterior tibial nerve as these structures cross the popliteus muscle posteriorly [*see Figure 5e*].

It should be noted that (1) the distal popliteal artery has few branches below the inferior geniculate arteries, (2) atheromatous plaques are rarely present at this level, and (3) the arterial wall is often more suitable for graft implantation in this portion of the popliteal wall than it is above the knee.

Step 2: exposure of femoral artery   This exposure is accomplished in essentially the same way as it would be in an above-the-knee bypass.

Step 3: creation of tunnel   Tunneling for a below-the-knee femoropopliteal bypass is carried out through Hunter's canal,

through the upper popliteal space, and finally through the region behind the popliteus muscle.

Steps 4 through 6   Steps 4, 5, and 6 of a below-the-knee femoropopliteal bypass—the distal anastomosis of the vein graft to the distal popliteal artery, the placement of the graft in the tunnel, and the proximal anastomosis to the femoral artery—are carried out in much the same way as the corresponding steps in an above-the-knee bypass. A completion angiogram should be obtained to confirm the adequacy of the distal anastomosis and verify the position of the graft in the tunnel [*see Figure 6*].

OUTCOME EVALUATION

Femoropopliteal bypasses performed with segments of the greater saphenous vein are associated with 4-year primary patency rates ranging from 68% to 80% and limb salvage rates ranging from 75% to 80%.[29] Femoropopliteal bypasses performed with polytetrafluoroethylene (PTFE) grafts yield comparable patency and limb salvage rates above the knee but are significantly less successful below the knee.[30]

Newer vein harvesting techniques may help improve outcome further. The use of endoscopic vein harvesting methods has been shown to reduce the incidence of wound complications associated with femoropopliteal bypass.[31] This approach allows above-the-knee bypasses to be performed through two incisions.

Infrapopliteal Bypass

Bypasses to the small arteries beyond the popliteal artery are performed only when femoropopliteal bypass is contraindicated according to accepted criteria [see Femoropopliteal Bypass, above]. Infrapopliteal bypasses are performed to the posterior tibial artery, the anterior tibial artery, or the peroneal artery, in that order of preference. As a rule, a tibial artery is used only if its lumen runs without obstruction into the foot, though bypasses to isolated tibial artery segments and other disadvantaged outflow tracts have been performed and have remained patent for more than 4 years.[2,3] Generally, the peroneal artery is used only if it is continuous with one or two of its terminal branches, which communicate with foot arteries [see Figure 7]. Neither the absence of a plantar arch nor vascular calcification is considered a contraindication to a reconstruction.[2,7] With both femoropopliteal and infrapopliteal bypasses, stenosis of less than 50% of the diameter of the vessel is acceptable at or distal to the site chosen for the distal anastomosis.

OPERATIVE TECHNIQUE

Bypasses to tibial arteries should be performed with autogenous vein grafts, and either the reversed technique (as previously described [see Femoropopliteal Bypass, above]) or the in situ technique [see In Situ Bypass, below] may be used. Placement of a tourniquet above the knee allows the distal anastomosis to be performed without extensive dissection of the tibial vessels or the application of clamps.[32] Exposure of the inflow vessel (i.e., the femoral artery or the popliteal artery) is achieved in the same way as in femoropopliteal bypass. Accordingly, bypasses to tibial and

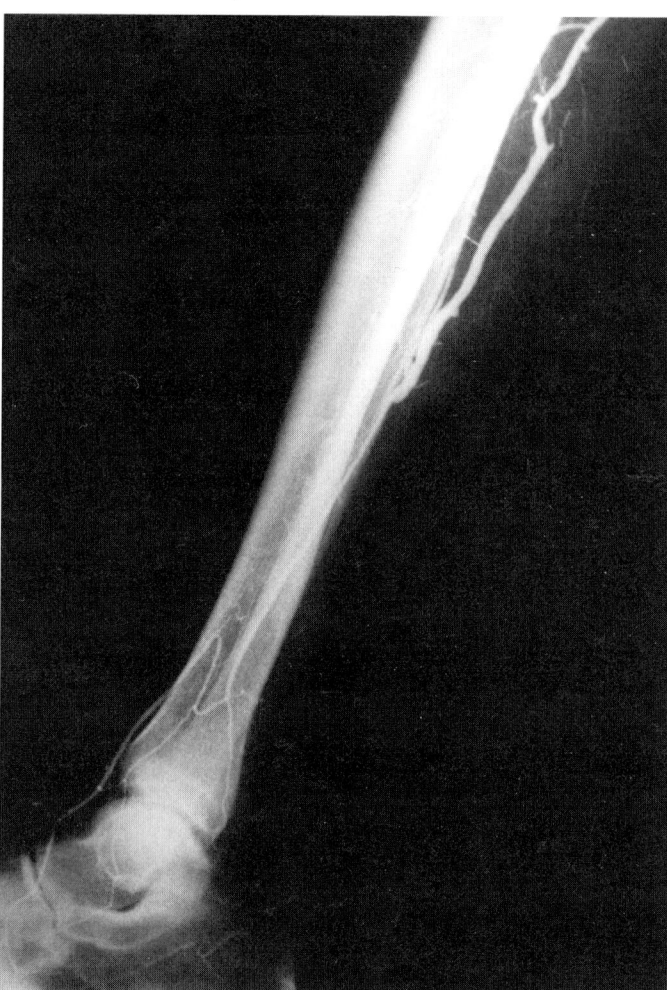

Figure 7 **Infrapopliteal bypass. An arteriogram from a 65-year-old female with rest pain in the right foot who underwent in situ bypass to the middle portion of the peroneal artery shows communication of the peroneal artery with foot arteries and reconstitution of the dorsalis pedis artery.**

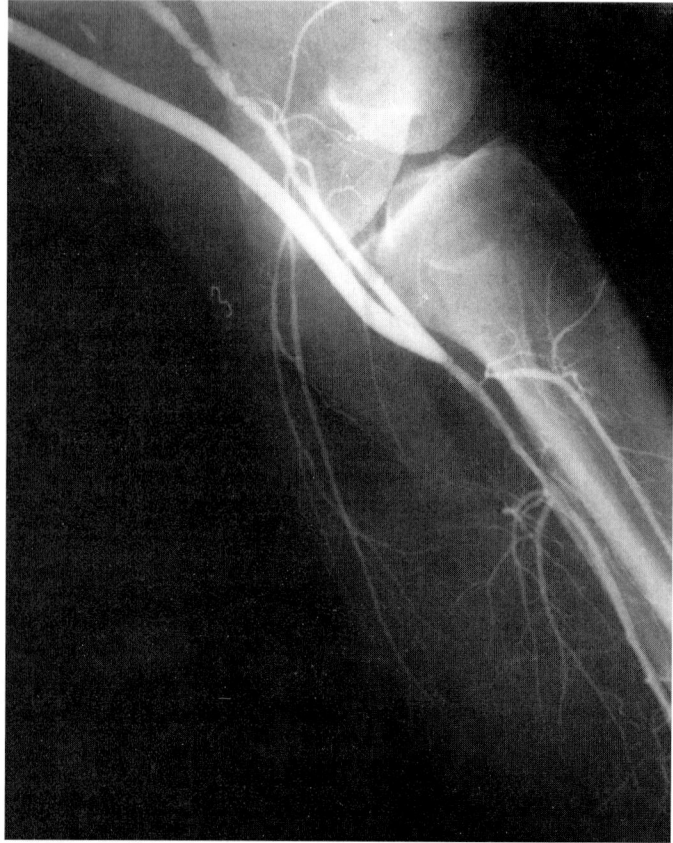

Figure 6 **Femoropopliteal bypass: below knee. A completion arteriogram from a patient who underwent below-the-knee femoropopliteal bypass for a nonhealing toe amputation site shows runoff through all three tibial vessels.**

peroneal arteries are best described in terms of the approaches required for exposure of these vessels and the tunnels required for routing the bypass conduits.

Exposure of Posterior Tibial Artery

The very proximal portion of the posterior tibial artery is aproached via a below-the-knee popliteal incision. The deep fascia is incised, and the popliteal space is entered. The gastrocnemius muscle is retracted posteriorly, and the soleus muscle is separated from the posterior surface of the tibia. The distal portion of the posterior tibial artery is approached via a medial incision along the posterior edge of the tibia [see Figure 8]; deepening this incision along the posterior tibialis muscle and the posterior surface of the tibia allows exposure of the posterior tibial artery. The tunnel from the popliteal fossa to the distal posterior tibial artery is made just below the muscle fascia, ideally with a long, gently curved clamp.

Exposure of Anterior Tibial Artery

To expose the proximal portion of the anterior tibial artery, an anterolateral incision is made in the leg midway between the tibia and the fibula over the appropriate segment of patent artery [see

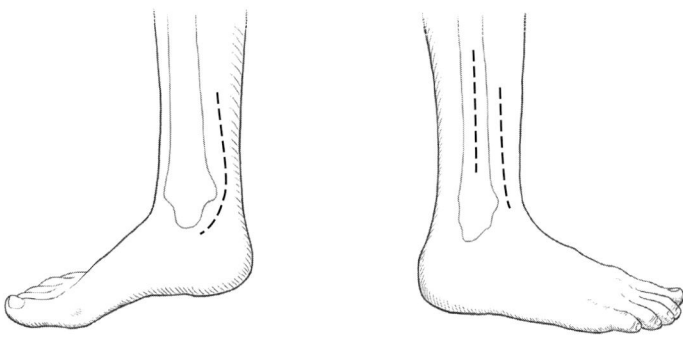

Figure 8 **Infrapopliteal bypass: posterior tibial artery. Shown are incisions for bypasses to the distal regions of the leg.**

Figure 9a]. Additional small medial incisions are also required for tunneling. The anterior incision is carried through the deep fascia, and the fibers of the anterior tibial muscle and the extensor digitorum longus muscle are separated to reveal the neurovascular bundle. The accompanying veins are mobilized and their branches divided to allow visualization of the anterior tibial artery, which can then be carefully mobilized [*see Figure 9b*]. With the artery mobilized, further posterior dissection can be performed, and the interosseous membrane can then be visualized and incised in a cruciate fashion.

Careful blunt finger dissection via the anterior incision and from the popliteal fossa via the medial incision facilitates creation of a tunnel without injury to the numerous veins in the area [*see*

Figure 9c]. Alternatively, the tunnel for the bypass may be placed lateral to the knee in a subcutaneous plane.

The distal anterior tibial artery is approached via an anterior incision placed midway between the tibia and the fibula [*see Figure 8*]. A tunnel is made from the distal popliteal fossa across the interosseous membrane (like the tunnel to the peroneal artery) and beneath the deep fascia to a point 5 to 7 cm above the lateral malleolus. Once the distal anastomosis is complete and the graft has been drawn through the tunnel, any tendons that may be distorting or compressing the graft in its course around the tibia are divided; this measure proves necessary in most low anterior tibial bypasses.

Exposure of Peroneal Artery

The peroneal artery is usually approached via the same incision as the posterior tibial artery [*see* Exposure of the Posterior Tibial Artery, *above*]. The artery is located and isolated just medial to the medial edge of the fibula. In its distal third, however, and in patients with stout calves and ankles, the peroneal artery should be approached via a lateral incision [*see Figure 8*], followed by excision of the fibula.

For lateral exposure of the peroneal artery, a long segment of fibula is freed from its muscle attachments with a combination of blunt and sharp dissection; particular care should be taken in dissecting along the medial edge of the bone because the peroneal vessels run just below this edge and are easily injured by instruments. Next, a finger is passed around the fibula [*see Figure 10a*]; once this is done, the free edge of bone is further developed by

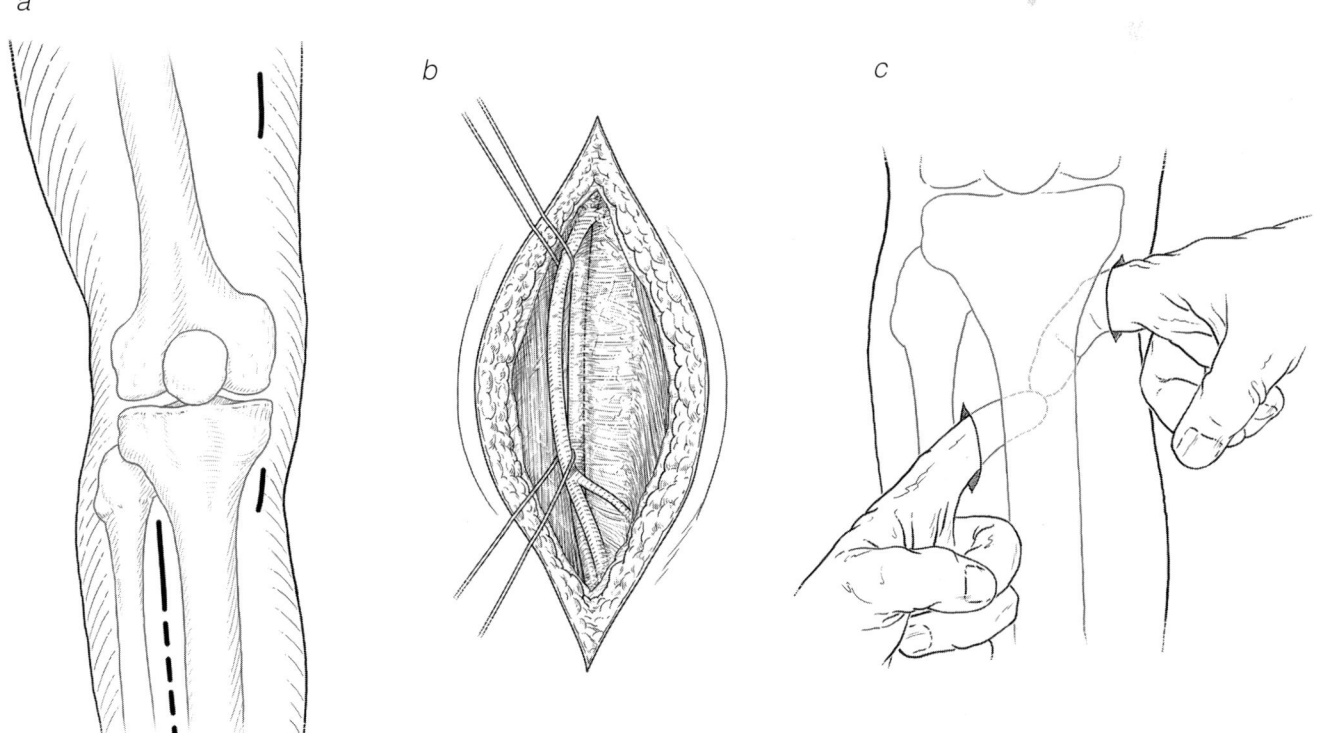

Figure 9 **Infrapopliteal bypass: anterior tibial artery. (*a*) An anterolateral incision is made midway between the tibia and the fibula over the artery; small medial incisions are also made for tunneling. (*b*) The anterior incision is carried through the deep fascia, the anterior tibial and extensor digitorum longus muscles are separated, the accompanying veins are mobilized and divided, and the anterior tibial artery is mobilized. (*c*) A tunnel is created with careful blunt finger dissection.**

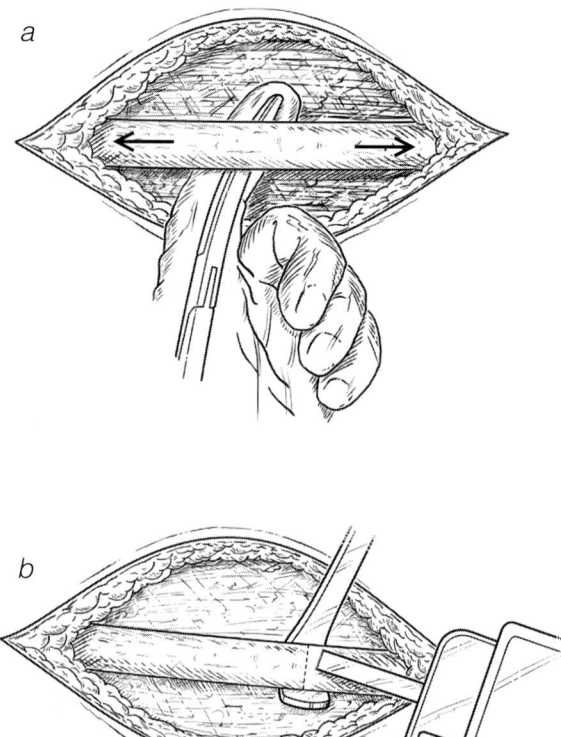

Figure 10 **Infrapopliteal bypass: lateral exposure of peroneal artery. Lateral exposure of the peroneal artery typically requires excision of part of the fibula; this is done by (*a*) passing a finger behind the fibula, developing the free bone edge further with a right-angle clamp, (*b*) passing a right-angle retractor behind the fibula, and dividing the bone with a power saw.**

forcefully pushing a right-angle clamp inferiorly and superiorly [*see Figure 10b*]. A right-angle retractor is passed behind the bone, and the fibula is divided with a power saw. The peroneal artery can then be dissected free from surrounding veins and used in the construction of the distal anastomosis.

Gentle blunt finger dissection is required to develop a tunnel from this lateral wound to the distal popliteal fossa, and great care should be taken to avoid injury to the numerous veins in the area. Because the peroneal artery is the least accessible of the three leg arteries used for infrapopliteal bypasses and normally has the poorest connections with the arteries of the foot, we recommend that it be used as a distal implantation site only when the anterior and posterior tibial arteries are not suitable.

Exposure of Dorsalis Pedis Artery

When no more proximal procedure is possible, a bypass to the ankle region or the foot may be performed. The dorsalis pedis artery is easily approached via a lateral incision on the dorsum of the foot [*see Figure 11a*]. The incision is curved slightly and a flap raised so that the incision will not be directly over the anastomosis [*see Figure 11b*]. If the artery must be approached at the ankle, the extensor retinaculum must be divided. Otherwise, the operation is performed in much the same fashion as a distal anterior tibial bypass [*see Figure 12*]. The posterior tibial artery can be

approached down to a point several centimeters below the medial malleolus.

In Situ Bypass

In situ bypass is an acceptable alternative to reversed vein bypass. Minimally invasive techniques have been developed to reduce the wound complications encountered when in situ bypass is performed with long incisions.

With the help of a side-branch coil occlusion system, in situ bypass can be performed through the two arterial access incisions. The angioscopic coil device is passed through the proximal greater saphenous vein, and the coils are placed into the side branches under angioscopic guidance [*see Figure 13*]. As the device is advanced more distally through the vein, the valves are lysed with a flexible valvulotome.

Another approach to side-branch occlusion involves the use of an endoscopic vein harvesting system. Three skin incisions are made: two incisions for arterial access and one 2 cm incision above the knee for insertion of an endoscopic device to locate and clip the side branches of the saphenous vein. Once the proximal anastomosis is complete, the valves are lysed with a flexible valvulotome passed through the distal end of the vein. Completion cineangiography is then performed to confirm side-branch occlusion and to assess the entire reconstruction.[33]

OUTCOME EVALUATION

Infrapopliteal bypasses should have 5-year primary patency rates ranging from 60% to 67% and limb salvage rates ranging from 70% to 75% whether they are done with the reversed-vein technique or with the in situ technique.[34,35] For all such grafts, close patient follow-up and graft surveillance improve secondary

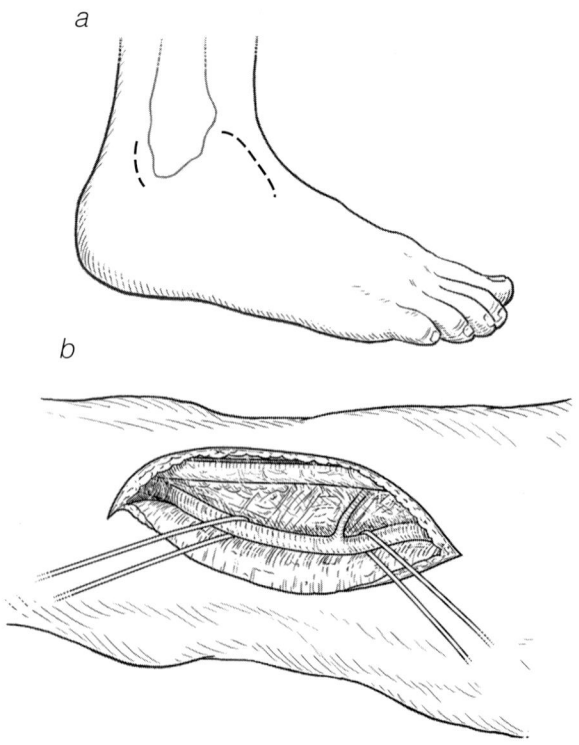

Figure 11 **Infrapopliteal bypass: dorsalis pedis artery. (*a*) The dorsalis pedis artery is approached via an incision on the dorsum of the foot. (*b*) The incision is curved and a flap raised so that the incision is not directly over the anastomosis.**

patency rates. Reduced complications and decreased length of stay have been reported for patients undergoing distal in situ bypasses using either the endoscopic or the coil occulsion approach.[36,37]

Plantar Bypass

Extension of the standard approaches to limb salvage has led to the performance of bypasses to vessels below the ankle joint [*see Figures 14 and 15*]. Such bypasses are indicated when the more proximal tibial vessels are occluded, which frequently occurs secondary to failure of a more proximal bypass. The technique required for performing bypasses to secondary branches in the foot is essentially the same as that required for performing bypasses to major infrapopliteal vessels.

Optimal illumination by means of head lamps is important for achieving technical success with plantar bypass, and loupe magnification is helpful when the vessel is less than 1.5 mm in diameter. In addition, visualization of perimalleolar and inframalleolar arteries requires excellent preoperative imaging studies.

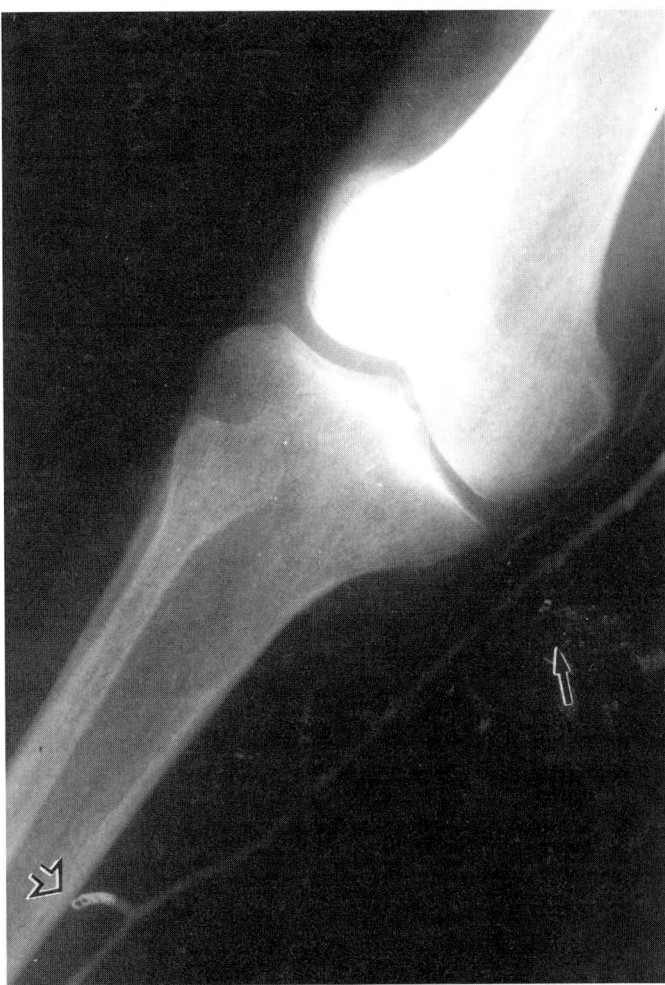

Figure 13 **Infrapopliteal bypass: in situ technique. A completion arteriogram from a patient who underwent an in situ bypass with coil occlusion of the side branches shows the two coils (arrows), which have successfully occluded the side-branch veins.**

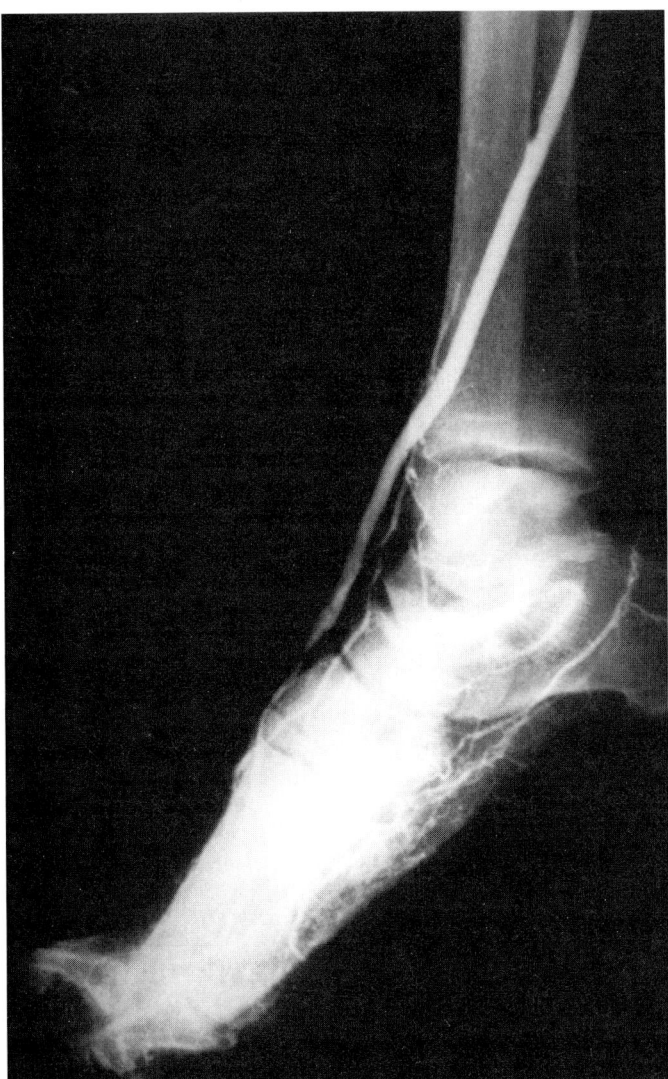

Figure 12 **Infrapopliteal bypass: dorsalis pedis artery. Shown is an arteriogram from a 72-year-old diabetic patient who underwent a popliteal artery–dorsalis pedis artery bypass with a reversed saphenous vein graft for a nonhealing great toe amputation.**

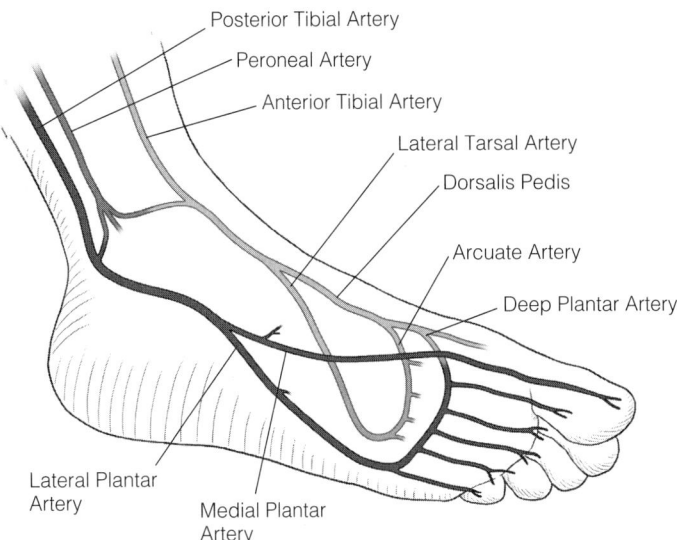

Figure 14 **Plantar bypass. Shown are the major arteries of the foot, including the two major branches of the posterior tibial artery.[3] The lateral plantar artery is usually the larger and ends in the deep plantar arch.**

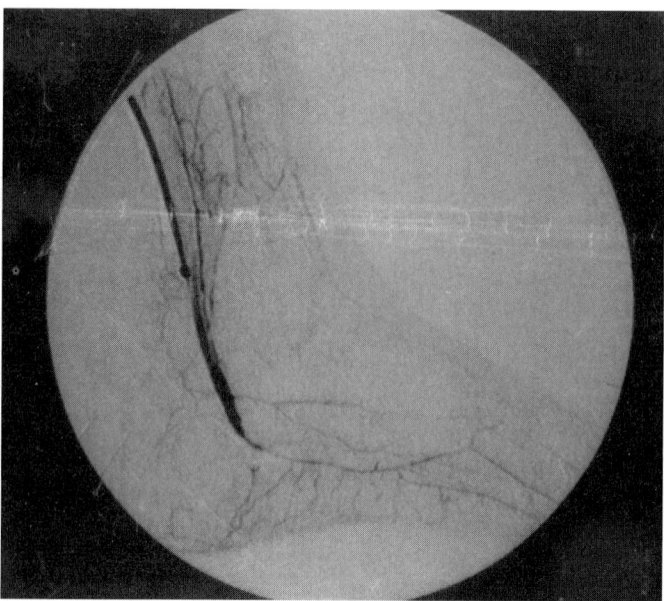

Figure 15 **Plantar bypass. A completion arteriogram from a 62-year-old diabetic with nonhealing toe ulcers who underwent a popliteal artery–medial plantar artery bypass with a reversed saphenous vein graft shows the distal anastomosis, with flow visible through a small but patent medial plantar artery.**

These very distal bypasses offer a viable alternative to a major amputation. Like infrapopliteal bypasses, they are best described in terms of the anatomic approaches to the distal branch vessels. In what follows, we outline exposure of the plantar and tarsal arteries; exposure of the dorsalis pedis artery is outlined elsewhere [*see* Infrapopliteal Bypass, *above*].

OPERATIVE TECHNIQUE

Exposure of Lateral and Medial Plantar Arteries

The lateral and medial plantar branches are the continuation of the posterior tibial artery in the foot [*see Figure 16*]. The lat-

eral plantar artery forms the deep plantar arch and is larger than the medial plantar artery. If the lateral branch is occluded, the medial branch may enlarge and feed the plantar arch through collateral vessels.

The initial incision is made over the termination of the posterior tibial artery below the malleolus. The artery is isolated, and the incision is extended inferiorly and laterally onto the sole. A direct approach to the individual branches is difficult, for several reasons. First, because the skin of the sole is not easily retracted, adequate exposure of the lateral and medial plantar arteries is hard to obtain if the incision does not follow their course exactly. Second, because these arteries are small in diameter and lie deep within the foot, they can be quite difficult to locate. Third, it is sometimes hard to distinguish the lateral plantar artery from the medial plantar artery. Dissection of the termination of the posterior tibial artery can help the surgeon make this distinction. The lateral branch is usually located inferiorly when the foot is externally rotated on the operating table.

Exposure of the proximal 2 to 3 cm of the plantar branches is accomplished by incising the flexor retinaculum and the adductor muscle of the great toe. More distal exposure of these branches can be obtained by dividing the medial border of the plantar aponeurosis and the extensor digitorum brevis muscle.

Exposure of Deep Plantar Artery and Lateral Tarsal Artery

The deep plantar artery and the lateral tarsal artery are branches of the dorsalis pedis artery. The deep plantar artery originates at the metatarsal level, where it descends into a foramen bounded proximally by the dorsal metatarsal ligament, distally by the dorsal interosseous muscle ring, and medially and laterally by the bases of the first and second metatarsal bones. As the deep plantar artery exits from this tunnel, it connects with the lateral plantar artery to form the deep plantar arch [*see Figure 17*].

A slightly curved longitudinal 3 to 4 cm incision is made over the dorsum of the middle portion of the foot, and the dorsalis pedis artery is dissected distally down to its bifurcation into the deep plantar and first dorsal metatarsal branches. The extensor hallucis brevis muscle is retracted laterally—or, if necessary,

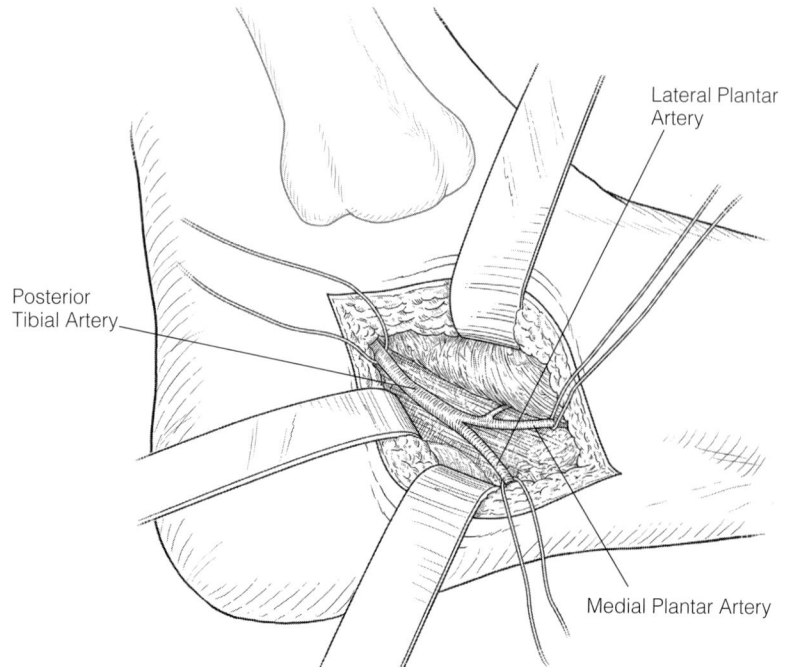

Lateral Plantar
Artery

Posterior
Tibial Artery

Medial Plantar Artery

Figure 16 **Plantar bypass. Depicted is exposure of the distal portion of the posterior tibial artery. The lateral and medial plantar arteries branch from this vessel and lie beneath the flexor retinaculum and the abductor hallucis muscle, which can be incised.**

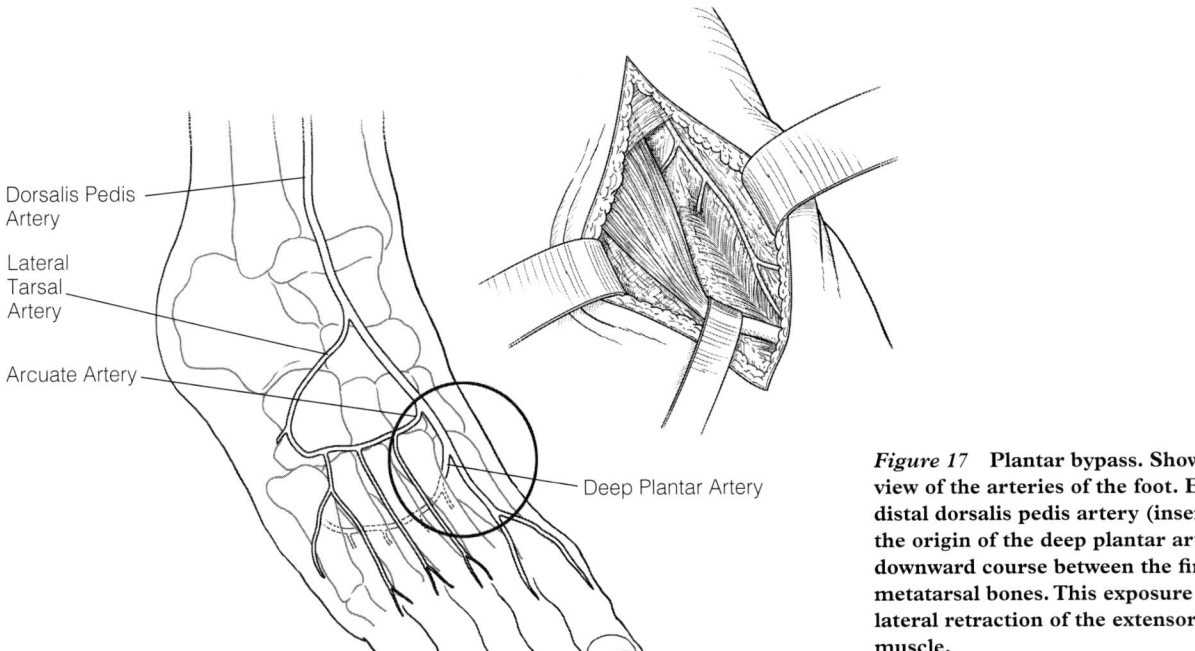

Dorsalis Pedis
Artery

Lateral
Tarsal
Artery

Arcuate Artery

Deep Plantar Artery

Figure 17 **Plantar bypass. Shown is a dorsal view of the arteries of the foot. Exposure of the distal dorsalis pedis artery (insert) highlights the origin of the deep plantar artery and its downward course between the first and second metatarsal bones. This exposure is facilitated by lateral retraction of the extensor hallucis brevis muscle.**

transected—and the dorsal interosseous muscle ring is split to allow better exposure of the proximal portion of the deep plantar artery. The periosteum of the proximal portion of the second metatarsal bone is then incised and elevated. A fine-tipped rongeur is used to excise enough of the metatarsal shaft to permit ample exposure of the deep plantar artery.

OUTCOME EVALUATION

Bypasses to the dorsalis pedis artery and its branches have yielded results comparable to those of bypasses to more proximal tibial vessels, with 3-year primary patency rates ranging from 58% to 60% and limb salvage rates ranging from 75% to 95%.[38-40] In one review, patency rates were higher in patients who had an intact plantar arch than in those who did not; however, failure to visualize the plantar arch on preoperative arteriograms does not preclude the performance of these bypasses for limb salvage. With careful follow-up, the assisted primary patency rates for these grafts have been substantially improved.[41] The available reports emphasize the need to repair failing grafts because their secondary patency was much better than that of failed grafts. In one study, patients who required shorter bypasses or had lower preoperative C-reactive protein levels experienced significantly better outcomes.[42] In some patients, occlusion of the distal tibial vessel necessitates performance of a tibiotibial bypass to achieve wound healing.[7]

Bypasses to plantar or tarsal vessels performed with vein grafts yield 2-year patency rates ranging from 65% to 75% and limb salvage rates higher than 80%.[4,5] In one report, the primary patency rate for these grafts was 74% at 1 year and 67% at 2 years, and the limb salvage rate was 78% at 2 years.[3]

Alternative Bypasses Using More Distal Inflow Vessels

Traditionally, the femoral artery has been the inflow site of choice for infrainguinal bypasses. Since the early 1980s, the superficial femoral, deep femoral, popliteal, and tibial arteries have all been used as inflow sources when these vessels were relatively disease free or when the amount of autologous vein available was lim-

ited. Currently, the superficial femoral artery and the popliteal artery are preferentially used for primary bypasses when they are free of disease.

The strategy of utilizing more distal inflow sources is particularly applicable to inframalleolar bypasses, in which very long vein segments would be required to reach the dorsalis pedis or other pedal arteries from the usual more proximal inflow sites. Two studies from the latter half of the 1980s reported that the patency rates in bypasses originating from the superficial femoral and popliteal arteries were comparable to those in bypasses originating from the common femoral artery.[43,44] In a review of our own experience with popliteal-distal vein graft bypasses,[5] we reported a patency rate of 65% at 4 years—a figure comparable to rates reported for femorodistal bypasses with reversed or in situ vein grafts (67% and 69%, respectively).[34] Given these results, surgeons should not hesitate to employ either the popliteal artery or the superficial femoral artery as an inflow source. Use of these more distal inflow sites results in shorter grafts and allows portions of saphenous vein to be preserved for other purposes.

An increasing number of limb salvage procedures are secondary interventions. These secondary procedures are generally more difficult to perform because the access routes to the arteries have been previously dissected and because there frequently is little good autologous vein left. In some cases, patients present with gangrene developing below a functioning bypass or after a previous failed bypass. Some of these patients need nothing more than a short distal extension of their functioning bypass; others have only enough vein left to make up a short graft. For such patients, a tibiotibial bypass may be an effective alternative revascularization approach.

In 1994, our group reported our 11-year experience with tibiotibial bypasses, comprising 42 procedures in 41 patients.[7] Ten of these bypasses were performed because previous bypasses failed; the remainder were performed because the amount of autologous vein available was limited. Approximately 50% of the bypasses were to pedal or tarsal vessels. At 5 years, the patency rate for these grafts was 65%, and the limb salvage rate was 73%.[7] A subsequent study reported comparable results.[45]

References

1. Veith FJ, Gupta SK, Wengerter KR, et al: Changing arteriosclerotic disease patterns and management strategies in lower-limb–threatening ischemia. Ann Surg 212:402, 1990

2. Veith FJ, Gupta SK, Samson RH, et al: Progress in limb salvage by reconstructive arterial surgery combined with new or improved adjunctive procedures. Ann Surg 194:386, 1981

3. Ascer E, Veith FJV, Gupta SK: Bypasses to plantar arteries and other tibial branches: an extended approach to limb salvage. J Vasc Surg 8:434, 1988

4. Andros G: Bypass grafts to the ankle and foot: a personal perspective. Surg Clin North Am 75:715, 1995

5. Wengerter KR, Yang PM, Veith FJ, et al: A twelve-year experience with the popliteal-to-distal artery bypass: the significance and management of proximal disease. J Vasc Surg 15:143, 1992

6. Veith FJ, Gupta SK, Samson RH, et al: Superficial femoral and popliteal arteries as inflow site for distal bypasses. Surgery 90:980, 1981

7. Lyon RT, Veith FJ, Marsan BU, et al: Eleven-year experience with tibiotibal bypass: an unusual but effective solution to distal tibial artery occlusive disease and limited autologous vein. J Vasc Surg 17:1128, 1994

8. Baker JD, Dix D: Variability of Doppler ankle pressures with arterial occlusive disease: an evaluation of ankle index and brachial-ankle pressure gradient. Surgery 79:134, 1976

9. Kohler TR, Nance DR, Cramer MM, et al: Duplex scanning for diagnosis of aortoiliac and femoropopliteal disease—a prospective study. Circulation 76:1074, 1987

10. Langsfeld M, Nupute J, Hershey FB, et al: The use of deep duplex scanning to predict hemodynamically significant aortoiliac stenosis. J Vasc Surg 7:395, 1988

11. Moneta GL, Yeager RA, Antonovic R, et al: Accuracy of lower extremity arterial duplex mapping. J Vasc Surg 15:275, 1992

12. Legemate DA, Teeuwen C, Hoenveld H, et al: Value of duplex scanning compared with angiography and pressure measurement in the assessment of aortoiliac lesions. Br J Surg 78:1003, 1991

13. Ascer E, Mazzariol F, Hingorani A, et al: The use of duplex ultrasound arterial mapping as an alternative to conventional arteriography for primary and secondary infrapopliteal bypasses. Am J Surg 178:162, 1999

14. Wain RA, Berdejo GL, Delvalle WN, et al: Can duplex scan arterial mapping replace contrast arteriography as the test of choice before infrainguinal revascularization? J Vasc Surg 29:100, 1999

15. Owens RS, Carpenter JP, Baum RA, et al: Magnetic resonance imaging of angiographically occult runoff vessels in peripheral arterial occlusive disease. N Engl J Med 326:1577, 1992

16. Carpenter JP, Owen RS, Baum RA, et al: Magnetic resonance angiography of peripheral runoff vessels. J Vasc Surg 16:807, 1992

17. Earls JP, Patel NH, Smith PA, et al: Gadolinium-enhanced three-dimensional MR angiography of the aorta and peripheral arteries: evaluation of a multistation examination using two gadopentetate dimeglumine infusions. AJR Am J Roentgenol 171:599, 1998

18. Fellner F, Janka R, Fellner C, et al: Post occlusion visualization of peripheral arteries with "floating table" MR angiography. Magn Reson Imaging 17:1235, 1999

19. Fenlon HM, Yucel EK: Advances in abdominal, aortic, and peripheral contrast-enhanced MR angiography. Magn Reson Imaging Clin North Am 7:319, 1999

20. Brewster DC, Waltman AC, O'Hara PJ, et al: Femoral artery pressure measurement during aortography. Circulation 60:120, 1979

21. Hessel SJ, Adams DF, Abrams HL: Complications of angiography. Radiology 138:273, 1981

22. Gomes AS, Baker JD, Martin-Paredero V, et al: Acute renal dysfunction after major arteriography. AJR Am J Roentgenol 145:1249, 1985

23. Martin-Paredero V, Dixon SM, Baker JD, et al: Risk of renal failure after major angiography. Arch Surg 118:1417, 1983

24. Nikonoff T, Skau T, Berglund J, et al: Effects of femoral arteriography and low osmolar contrast agents on renal function. Acta Radiol 34:88, 1993

25. Katholi RE, Taylor GJ, Woods WT, et al: Nephrotoxicity of nonionic low-osmolality versus ionic high osmolality contrast media: a prospective double-blind randomized comparison in human beings. Radiology 186:183, 1993

26. Lautin EM, Freeman NJ, Schoenfeld AH, et al: Radiocontrast-associated renal dysfunction: a comparison of lower-osmolality and conventional high-osmolality contrast media. AJR Am J Roentgenol 157:59, 1991

27. Kram HB, Gupta SK, Veith FJ, et al: Late results of two hundred seventeen femoropopliteal bypasses to isolated popliteal artery segments. J Vasc Surg 14:386, 1991

28. Veith FJ, Gupta SK, Daly V: Femoropopliteal bypass to the isolated popliteal segment: is polytetrafluoroethylene graft acceptable? Surgery 89:296, 1981

29. Taylor LM, Edwards JM, Porter JM: Present status of reversed vein bypass grafting: five-year results of a modern series. J Vasc Surg 11:193, 1990

30. Veith FJ, Gupta SK, Ascer E, et al: Six year prospective multicenter randomized comparison of autologous saphenous vein and expanded polytetrafluoroethylene grafts in infrainguinal arterial reconstructions. J Vasc Surg 3:104, 1986

31. Jordan WD, Voellinger DC, Schroeder PT, et al: Video-assisted saphenous vein harvest: the evaluation of a new technique. J Vasc Surg 26:405, 1997

32. Wagner WH, Treiman RL, Cossman DV, et al: Tourniquet occlusion technique for tibial artery reconstruction. J Vasc Surg 18:637, 1993

33. Suggs WD, Sanchez LA, Woo D, et al: Endoscopically assisted in situ lower extremity bypass: a preliminary report of a new minimally invasive technique. J Vasc Surg 34:668, 2001

34. Bergamini TM, Towne JB, Bandyk DF, et al: Experience with in situ saphenous vein bypasses during 1981 to 1989: determinant factors of long-term patency. J Vasc Surg 13:137, 1991

35. Wengerter KR, Veith FJ, Gupta SK, et al: Prospective randomized multi center comparison of in situ and reversed vein infrapopliteal bypasses. J Vasc Surg 13:189, 1991

36. Rosenthal D, Arous EJ, Friedman SG, et al: Endovascular-assisted versus conventional in situ saphenous vein bypass grafting: cumulative patency, limb salvage, and cost results in a 39-month multi center study. J Vasc Surg 21:60, 2000

37. Piano G, Schwartz LB, Foster L, et al: Assessing outcomes, costs, and benefits of emerging technology for minimally invasive saphenous vein in situ distal arterial bypasses. Arch Surg 133:613, 1998

38. Schneider JR, Walsh DB, McDaniel MD, et al: Pedal bypass versus tibial bypass with autogenous vein: a comparison of outcome and hemodynamic results. J Vasc Surg 17:1029, 1993

39. Harrington EB, Harrington ME, Schanzer H, et al: The dorsalis pedis bypass: moderate success in difficult situations. J Vasc Surg 15:409, 1992

40. Panayiotopoulos YP, Tyrrell MR, Arnold FJ, et al: Results and cost analysis of distal [crural/pedal] arterial revascularization for limb salvage in diabetic and nondiabetic patients. Diabet Med 14:214, 1997

41. Rhodes JM, Gloviczki P, Bower TC, et al: The benefits of secondary interventions in patients with failing or failed pedal bypass grafts. Am J Surg 178:151, 1999

42. Biancari F, Alback A, Kantonen I, et al: Predictive factors for adverse outcome of pedal bypasses. Eur J Vasc Endovasc Surg 18:138, 1999

43. Cantelmo NL, Snow JR, Menzoian JO, et al: Successful vein bypass in patients with an ischemic limb and a palpable popliteal pulse. Arch Surg 121:217, 1986

44. Rosenbloom JS, Walsh JJ, Schuler JJ, et al: Long-term results of infragenicular bypasses with autogenous vein originating from the distal superficial femoral and popliteal arteries. J Vasc Surg 7:691, 1988

45. Plecha EJ, Lee C, Hye RJ: Factors influencing the outcome of paramalleolar bypass grafts. Ann Vasc Surg 10:356, 1996

Acknowledgment

Figures 1 through 17 Tom Moore.

12 SCLEROTHERAPY

William R. Finkelmeier, M.D., F.A.C.S.

Sclerotherapy involves the injection of a caustic solution (a sclerosant) into an abnormal vein so as to cause localized destruction of the venous intima and obliteration of the vessel. It is not a new technique, having been practiced since the early 20th century, but it has evolved significantly over the past 50 years.[1] Improvements in the technology used (e.g., hypodermic syringes, fine needles, sclerosants, compression technique, and duplex ultrasonography) have greatly enhanced the results achievable with sclerotherapy. To ensure optimal results, it is essential to have a thorough knowledge not only of the technique but also of the indications, expected outcomes, and possible complications associated with the procedure.

Sclerotherapy is primarily used to treat small varicose veins, reticular veins, and spider veins. The prevalence of varicose and spider veins is well documented: they affect millions of people in the United States alone.[1] The incidence is two to three times higher in women than in men and increases with age. The precise etiology of varicose veins and spider veins is unknown. Heredity, pregnancy, female sex, obesity, an occupation that requires long periods of standing, and a low-fiber diet all have been implicated as causative factors. The choice of treatment method for varicose veins and spider veins must be individualized for each patient. Although sclerotherapy is only one of a number of techniques available for treatment, it is an important therapeutic tool and a key component of a vascular surgeon's armamentarium.

Preoperative Evaluation

Proper evaluation of the patient before sclerotherapy is the most important step in achieving successful results. Such evaluation should include a thorough clinical arterial and venous examination. Close attention should be paid to the size, location, and distribution of vessels; these variables are critical for determining the appropriate treatment. Any patient who is believed to have axial reflux or whose clinical complaints far exceed the findings from physical examination should undergo venous duplex ultrasonography.

Venous duplex ultrasonography has revolutionized the treatment of varicose and spider veins. It is reproducible and noninvasive, and it can objectively identify areas of reflux in the greater and lesser saphenous systems, as well as detect pathologic conditions in the deep venous system and incompetent perforating vessels. Duplex ultrasonography can also identify the lesser saphenous–popliteal junction and facilitate skin mapping in preparation for surgery.

Patients with duplex-documented axial reflux or reflux from the greater or lesser saphenous junction are best managed by means of surgical correction of the reflux rather than primary treatment with sclerotherapy. In a 1993 randomized study, ligation and stripping were compared with compression sclerotherapy in 164 patients who had symptomatic primary varicose veins.[2] After 5 years, 74% of the patients treated with sclerotherapy were considered to have had treatment failures, compared with only 10% of the patients treated surgically. In a 1991 trial, real-time color duplex ultrasonography was used to evaluate 89 limbs in 55 patients who had previously undergone

sclerotherapy of the greater saphenous vein.[3] Obliteration of the greater saphenous vein was noted in only 20% of the injected limbs and in only 6% of the limbs below a refluxing junction. These poor results from sclerotherapy were confirmed in a subsequent study.[4] The superiority of surgical treatment was also demonstrated in a randomized 10-year study comparing surgery with sclerotherapy alone.[5]

Ultrasound-guided sclerotherapy has also been advocated. The advantages of this approach are that it allows much higher concentrations of the sclerosant solution and that it permits direct visualization of the injections. Reported recurrence rates are still quite high, however: 22.8% at 1 year and 27.2% at 2 years.[6] A number of authors, primarily in the dermatologic literature, have advocated ultrasound-guided foam sclerotherapy for patients with axial reflux.[7,8] The longevity of the results achieved with this technique is still in question, and further studies (including randomized trials) are needed for validation.

Given the available data, my preferred approach in patients with axial reflux is to ligate the greater saphenous vein, strip the vein at least to the knee, and then ligate the lesser saphenous vein before sclerotherapy. Patients who do not have axial reflux and whose vessels are less than 6 mm in diameter can be treated successfully with sclerotherapy alone. Varicose veins more than 6 mm in diameter are best treated surgically by means of phlebectomy, either with a hook or with a transilluminated powered phlebectomy device. The cosmetic results are far better and the recovery time much shorter with the surgical option.

Operative Planning

PATIENT PREPARATION

Before undergoing sclerotherapy, the patient should receive a thorough explanation of the procedure, including the possible risks and complications [*see Table 1*]. He or she should be informed about the expected outcomes and the length of time needed for healing. In particular, it should be emphasized that multiple treatments are usually necessary to eliminate varicosities. Most patients can expect to undergo four or five treatments in a 6-month period. Time and patience are essential for achieving an optimal outcome.

Because sclerotherapy is primarily cosmetic and therefore rarely reimbursable, it is important to have a clear understanding regarding costs. A good-faith estimate of the cost per procedure should be provided to the patient before treatment is initiated. It is advisable to have the patient sign a copy of this estimate so that there is no subsequent misunderstanding about the costs to be incurred during the course of therapy.

To reduce bruising, aspirin and antiplatelet agents should be avoided for 10 days before treatment. On the day of the procedure, the patient should be asked to refrain from applying lotion to the legs so that the tape applied after treatment will adhere better to the skin [*see Table 2*]. The patient should sign and date an informed consent form. Once informed consent is obtained, photographs of the areas

Table 1 Complications of Sclerotherapy

	Complication	Comment
Common	Itching	Usually mild; lasts for 1–2 days
	Hyperpigmentation	Occurs in about 20%–30% of patients treated; usually fades in a couple of weeks but may take several months to a year to resolve totally; lasts longer than 1 yr in 1% of cases
	Telangiectatic matting	Occurs in approximately 10% of patients treated; usually resolves in 3–12 mo if left untreated but in rare cases can be permanent
	Pain	Lasts 1 to, at most, 7 days
	Bruising	May be minimized by avoiding aspirin and ibuprofen for 10 days before and after each treatment session
	Minor allergic reaction	Typically resolves within about 1 hr
Rare	Ulceration at injection site	Can take 4 to 6 wk to heal completely; small scar may result
	Anaphylaxis	Incidence is extremely low
	PE or DVT	Incidence is extremely low

DVT—Deep venous thrombosis   PE—pulmonary embolism

to be treated should be taken. Either a digital camera or a conventional 35 mm camera may be used. Digital photography offers much greater flexibility, in that there is no need to wait for film development. The pictures should be standardized as much as possible with respect to lighting and background. The problem areas are photographed again after treatment, and additional pictures are obtained during subsequent treatments to document progress. The aim is to give patients a reliable means of objectively comparing the legs' appearance before and after sclerotherapy [*see Figures 1 through 3*]. Such photographs often reassure patients that significant cosmetic improvement has been achieved and encourage them to continue treatments.

MATERIALS

Sclerosants cause thrombosis and subsequent fibrosis when injected into a blood vessel. An ideal sclerosant would exert this effect reliably while also being inexpensive, widely available, approved by the Food and Drug Administration (FDA), and nontoxic. In addition, it would be painless on injection and would not cause hyperpigmentation or ulceration with extravasation. Unfortunately, this ideal sclerosant does not exist. All of the solutions currently available have disadvantages.

Sclerosants may be classified into two main categories: osmotic agents and detergents. Hypertonic saline (HS) is the most widely used osmotic agent. FDA-approved as an abortifacient, it is commonly employed to treat superficial telangiectasias. HS in a 23.4% concentration damages the endothelial cells of the vessel walls through hyperosmolarity-induced dehydration. Such damage leads to thrombosis and fibrin deposition. Sodium tetradecyl sulfate (STS) and polidocanol (POL) are the most widely used detergent agents in the United States. These agents form aggregates on endothelial cell surfaces and cause endofibrosis by disrupting the integrity of the cells.

In the United States, HS has been used to treat spider and varicose veins for more than 50 years. Because it is a naturally occurring bodily substance, it does not cause allergic reactions; however, it causes patients much more pain and discomfort than either STS or POL does.[9] Adding lidocaine to HS reduces the pain associated with the injections without significantly decreasing the effectiveness of treatment or increasing the incidence of complications.[10] Even

with the addition of lidocaine, injection of HS is associated with some degree of patient discomfort. Moreover, HS is more viscous than STS and thus more difficult to administer. Extravasation of HS is also associated with a higher risk of skin necrosis.

Table 2 Sample Instructions to Patients after Sclerotherapy

NEXT APPOINTMENT _____ TIME _____

Be sure to keep your follow-up appointment so the physician can monitor your progress.

Please be considerate and give our office at least 72 hours' notice if you are unable to keep an appointment. This will allow us time to call patients who are on the waiting list for an appointment.

Please walk for a few minutes before driving home.
Wear your support hose for 48 continuous hours.
After 48 hours, remove the hose, cotton balls, and tape before getting your legs wet.
After 48 hours, wear your support hose for a minimum of 7 days during the waking hours. Note, you may continue to wear them longer if you prefer.
Do not run, do high-impact aerobics, lift weights with your legs, or do sit-ups for 2 weeks. These activities can increase the venous pressure in your legs.
For 2 weeks, do not take hot baths or showers or sit in a hot tub. The heat can cause vein dilatation. You may take a warm shower or bath after 48 hours.
Avoid aspirin and ibuprofen products for 10 days before and after each treatment. These products may increase the amount of bruising that may develop from the treatment. Acetaminophen is permitted.
For further information regarding sclerotherapy, please refer to the handout "Sclerotherapy Informed Consent and Before and After Treatment Instructions."

Preparation for Your Next Treatment

Bring your support hose.
Do not apply creams, lotions, or powders to your legs the evening before or the morning of your treatment.
Bring a pair of loose shorts to wear during your treatment.
Avoid aspirin and ibuprofen products for 10 days before and after each treatment. These products may increase the amount of bruising that may develop from the treatment. Acetaminophen is permitted.

a

b

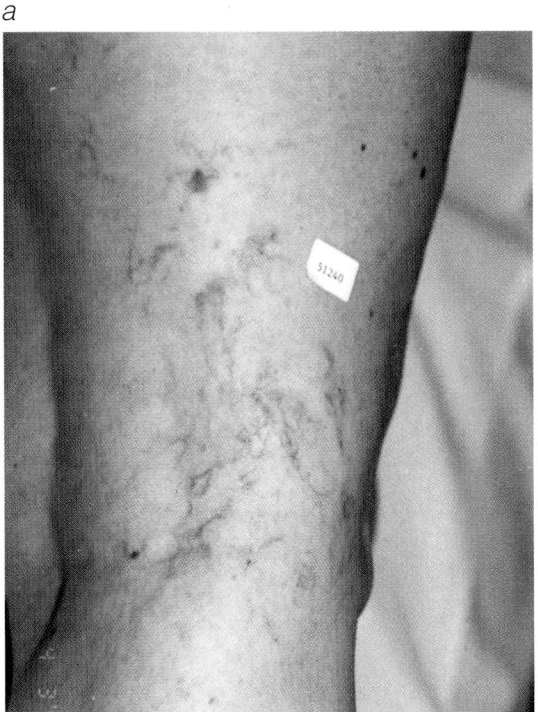
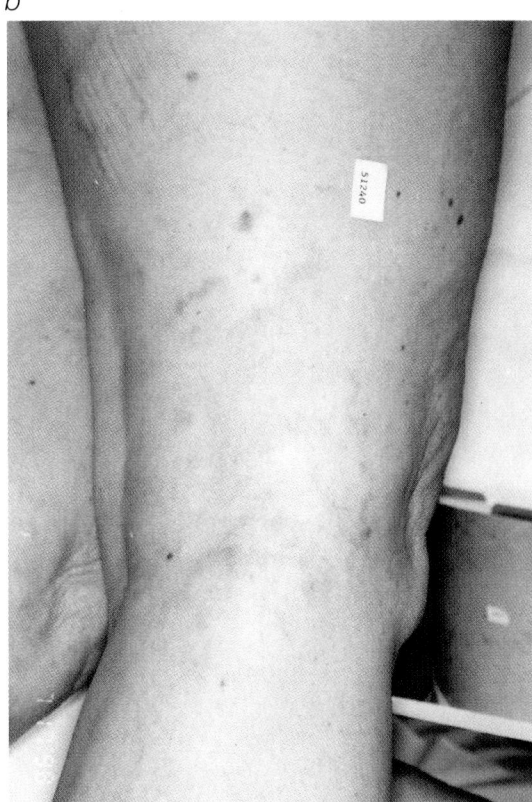

Figure 1 **Sclerotherapy. Shown is a 63-year-old woman (*a*) before and (*b*) after two treatments with 0.2% STS.**

Of the detergent sclerosants, both STS and POL are widely used in the United States, but only STS is FDA approved. FDA approval of POL has been pending for years, and it is unclear why it has not yet been granted. POL appears to be a very good sclerosant, comparable to STS: it is safe, relatively painless, and highly effective in all vein types.[11,12] In a 2002 randomized study comparing STS with POL, both agents were found to be safe and effective, yielding a 70% clinical improvement, and there were no significant differences in adverse effects, aside from a small decrease in ulcerations with POL.[13] Nevertheless, until POL is approved by the FDA, we recommend that it not be used. Two other FDA-approved detergent sclerosants are available: sodium morrhuate (SM) and ethanolamine oleate (EO). However, both SM and EO are associated with an unacceptably high risk of complications, including but not limited to ulceration and anaphylactic reactions, and hence are rarely used. For these reasons, my practice is to use STS for sclerotherapy, and the ensuing technical discussion will focus solely on this agent.

Sclerotherapy is an outpatient procedure performed in the physician's office. Aside from the sclerosant, very few special materials are needed [*see Table 3*]. Because there is a risk of significant allergic reactions (albeit an extremely small risk), a fully stocked resuscitation cart including intubation equipment should be available and checked regularly to confirm that all equipment is up to date and ready for immediate use.

Technique

A variety of sclerotherapy techniques have been developed. Typically, each individual practitioner develops his or her own variation of the procedure.

STEP 1: POSITIONING AND SKIN PREPARATION

Sclerotherapy is best performed with the patient supine. On very rare occasions, it may be necessary to puncture a vein with the patient standing. However, the sclerosant is not injected until the patient has been returned to the supine position, thus allowing the vein to empty.

The skin is wiped with alcohol swabs to increase the visibility of the vessels. The sclerosant is then placed in plastic 3 ml syringes. These syringes fit more easily in the hand than tuberculin syringes do and are less cumbersome to use. In addition, because injection pressure is inversely proportional to the squared radius of the plunger, a 3 ml syringe generates less pressure than a 1 ml syringe does. The endothelial cells in these small vessels are quite fragile, and using a syringe that generates less pressure substantially reduces the risk of vessel disruption.

STEP 2: CHOICE OF SCLEROSANT CONCENTRATION

The solution concentration selected depends on the size of the vessel. I use 0.2% STS for vessels less than 2 mm in diameter and 0.5% for larger vessels. The volume per injection site is generally less than 0.5 ml, but larger volumes may be preferable for reticular or small varicose veins.

At present, there is enthusiasm in the literature for the use of foam sclerotherapy, a technique in which air is repetitively injected into STS to create a foam.[14] This technique is ultimately based on the work of Orbach, who in 1944 advocated expelling blood from the vein by injecting small boluses of air before injecting the sclerosant.[15] The rationale for foam sclerotherapy is that the foam displaces blood in the vessel, resulting in less dilution of the solution. The sclerosant then has more contact with the surface area of the venous endothelium and thus can sclerose the endothelial cells more efficiently at

a   *b*

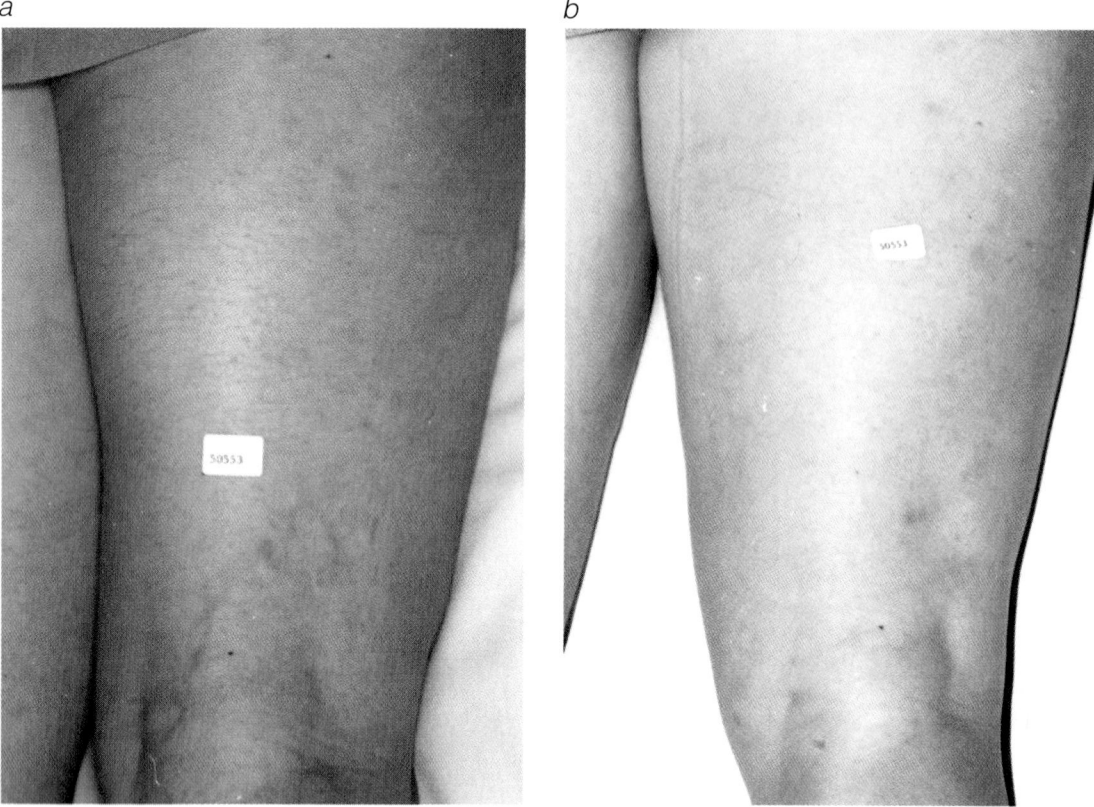

Figure 2 Sclerotherapy. Shown is a 52-year-old woman (*a*) before and (*b*) after two treatments with 0.5% STS.

lower concentrations. Of the various methods of creating a foam sclerosant solution,[16] that described by Tessari and coworkers appears to be the easiest.[17] In this approach, air is injected into the solution via a three-way stopcock and two syringes. Because of the size of the bubbles in a foam solution, foam sclerotherapy is best suited to treatment of reticular and varicose veins. Spider telangiectasias are best treated with standard solutions.

STEP 3: INJECTION OF SCLEROSANT

I use 30-gauge needles for all sclerotherapy treatments; some physicians prefer 27-gauge needles for larger reticular and small varicose veins. The needle is bent at a 45° angle, with the bevel up. Countertraction is applied with the nondominant hand, and the needle is inserted parallel to the vessel and the skin surface [*see Figure 4*]. As the vessel is entered, the sclerosant is gently injected. The slight reduction of pressure that occurs when the vessel is entered becomes increasingly easy to appreciate as the physician accumulates experience with sclerotherapy. Blanching of the vein is another signal of entry into the vessel. If the solution is injected outside the vein, a small superficial wheal will appear, in which case the injection should be discontinued and a new site selected for injection. Such wheals are unlikely to be a problem when STS concentrations lower than 0.25% are used. When more concentrated solutions are used in larger veins, aspiration of blood ensures correct placement of the needle within the vein before injection.

STEP 4: COVERAGE AND COMPRESSION OF INJECTION AREAS

After injection, cotton balls or foam or gauze pads are secured with tape and applied to the injection areas. Compression hose (20 to 30 or 30 to 40 mm Hg) are then applied. Studies have shown that using some type of bandage or pad in addition to support hose is beneficial. The degree of compression achieved with this approach can be as much as 50% greater than that achieved with support hose alone.[18] Gauze pads or cotton balls are more cost-effective than foam pads while providing comparable compressive effects.[19]

Compression approximates the endothelial surfaces of the vein walls after sclerotherapy, thereby reducing thrombus formation and promoting sclerosis of the vessel. It also enhances the calf muscle pump function to help clear any solution that has progressed into the deep venous system. Reduction of thrombus formation after sclerotherapy is important for minimizing hyperpigmentation. In a multicenter randomized trial that evaluated patients who underwent bilateral sclerotherapy but who received compression to only one leg, hyperpigmentation and edema were significantly greater in the uncompressed leg.[20]

Varying recommendations have been made as to how long compression hose should be worn after sclerotherapy. A controlled comparative trial of the effects of compression in patients with reticular and telangiectatic veins found that patients who wore hose for 3 weeks exhibited greater improvement (e.g., less hyperpigmentation) than those who wore no hose.[21] However, the improvement in patients wearing hose for 3 weeks was not appreciably greater than that in patients wearing hose for 1 week. I find that it is difficult to get patients to wear compression hose for several weeks. Therefore, I have adopted the standard practice of instructing the patient first to wear the hose for 48 hours without removing them, then to wear them during waking hours only for the next 7 days.

Once the compression hose are in place, the patient is asked to walk for 15 minutes before leaving the office. This further assists

a

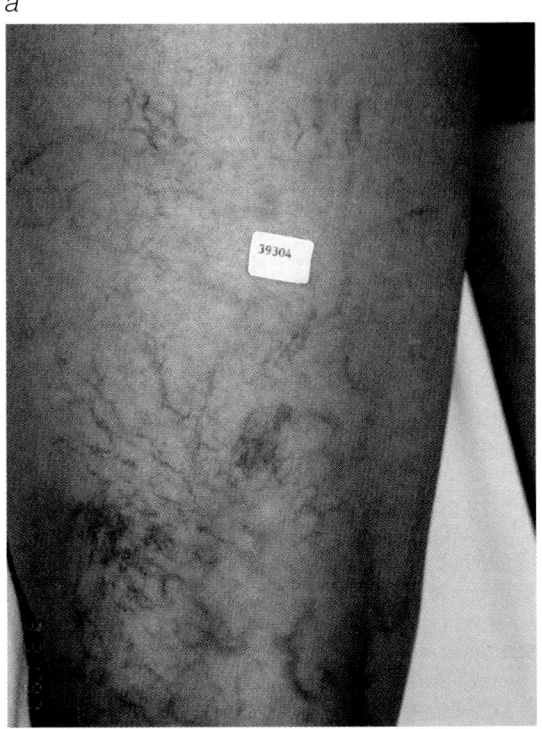

b

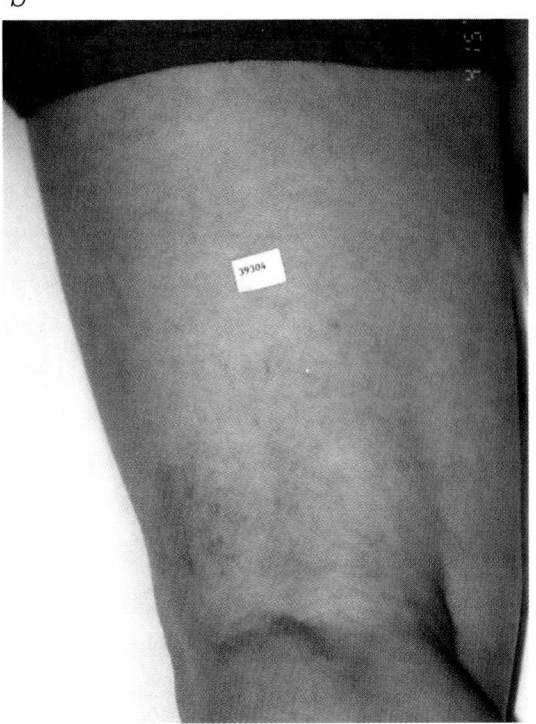

Figure 3 **Sclerotherapy. Shown is a 36-year-old woman (*a*) before and (*b*) after four treatments with a combination of 0.5% and 0.2% STS. Mild hyperpigmentation may be seen on the lateral thigh.**

in clearing any solution that may have progressed into the deep venous system.

STEP 5: SCHEDULING OF RETREATMENT

As noted (see above), multiple treatments are usually required for optimal outcome. Therefore, all patients are instructed to return in 4 to 6 weeks for assessment and possible retreatment. After this interval, vessels requiring further treatment are apparent, and additional injections can be performed. The average patient undergoes four or five treatments.

Complications

Although sclerotherapy is generally quite safe, complications do occur. Physicians must therefore be cognizant of the potential risks and prepared to treat any adverse events that arise. The most significant complications of sclerotherapy are allergic reactions (either minor or major), skin necrosis, hyperpigmentation, deep venous thrombosis (DVT), and telangiectatic matting. Cramping, pain, edema, and blistering from tape or compression may be observed as well.

Minor allergic reactions are quite common. For example, localized urticaria and edema may occur secondary to histamine

release. In the vast majority of cases, such reactions are self-limited, typically resolving in less than 1 hour. Itching often accompanies this response, but it usually resolves by the time the patient leaves the office. Should reactions persist, oral antihistamines or, on rare occasions, steroids may be required.

With the sclerosants used today, anaphylactic reactions are extraordinarily rare but can be life-threatening. The incidence of anaphylaxis with STS is not known with precision but is certainly very low. The reaction is usually mediated by immunoglobulin E and occurs within minutes of exposure. Appropriate emergency

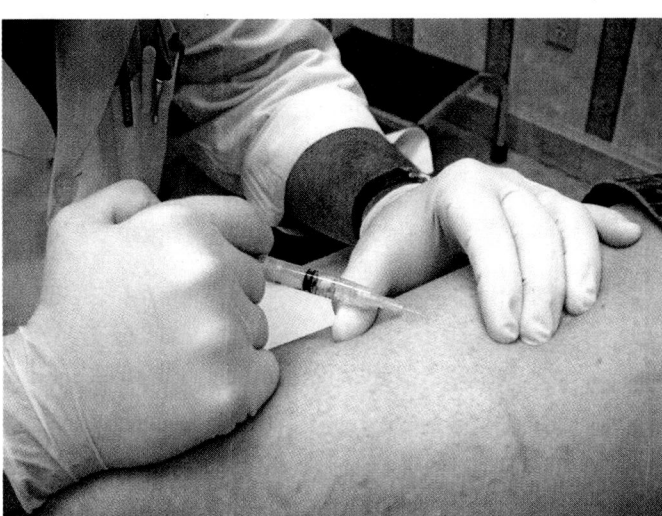

Figure 4 **Sclerotherapy. Illustrated is the standard hand position for sclerotherapy. Countertraction is applied with the nondominant hand.**

Table 3 Materials Needed for Sclerotherapy	
Alcohol swabs	Cotton balls and tape
Protective gloves	18-gauge needles
3 ml syringes	4 × 4 in. gauze pads
30-gauge needles	Adhesive bandages

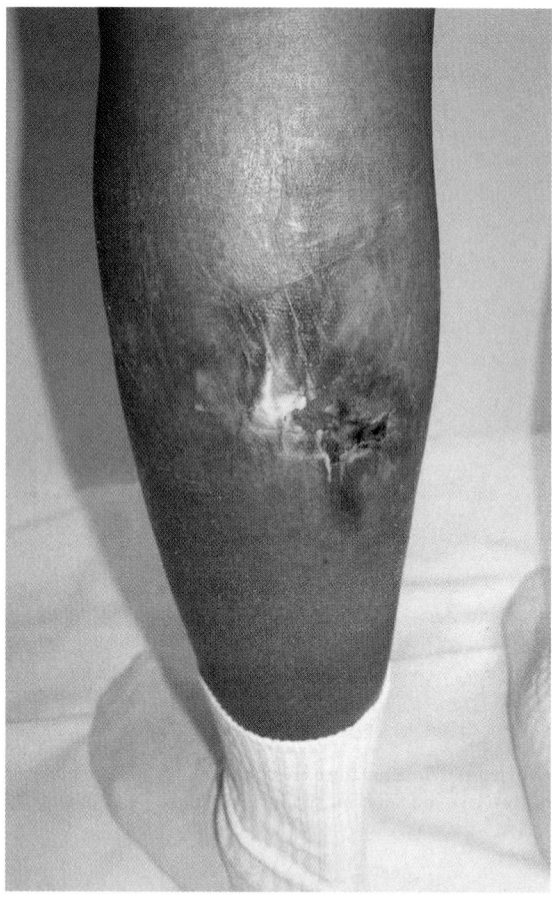

Figure 5 **Sclerotherapy. Shown is skin necrosis on the left posterior calf of a 48-year-old woman after ultrasound-guided sclerotherapy.**

measures must be undertaken immediately, including subcutaneous administration of epinephrine, delivery of supplemental oxygen, and securing of the airway. The patient should then be given antihistamines and transferred to an emergency department for continued evaluation and treatment. As noted (see above), a properly stocked emergency response cart, including endotracheal intubation supplies and medications, is essential in any office where sclerotherapy is performed. Periodic review of procedures with staff and maintenance of the emergency medications and supplies is imperative.

Skin necrosis occurs with 0.2% to 1.2% of sclerotherapy injections.[22] It is a potentially devastating complication and is often unpreventable. Depending on the extent of necrosis, healing may take months. The main causes of necrosis are extravasation of the sclerosant into subcutaneous tissue, inadvertent injection into an arteriole, and vasospasm. Extravasation of the sclerosant can destroy tissue, with the degree of damage determined by the type, concentration, and amount of sclerosant used [*see Figure 5*]. Necrosis is rare when small amounts of dilute (< 0.25%) STS are given, but extensive skin and soft tissue necrosis has been observed when higher concentrations of STS (3%) are administered to treat varicose veins.[23] Inadvertent injections into the arteriole feeding the telangiectasia is impossible to prevent and probably occurs frequently. In a 2001 study, pulsatile Doppler sounds could be detected above spider vein complexes in 72% of cases.[22] Backwash of the solution through arteriovenous shunts may cause occlusion of the arteriole and skin necrosis. Blanching of the skin often occurs with intra-arteriolar injections. Skin massage or, if spasm persists, application of nitroglycerin ointment to the skin may increase microcirculation. Why ulcerations develop in some patients but not others is unknown. The question of whether it is related to injection pressure or injectate volume also remains unanswered.

Hyperpigmentation [*see Figure 6*] is quite common, occurring in a significant percentage of patients, and it may be caused by any of the

a

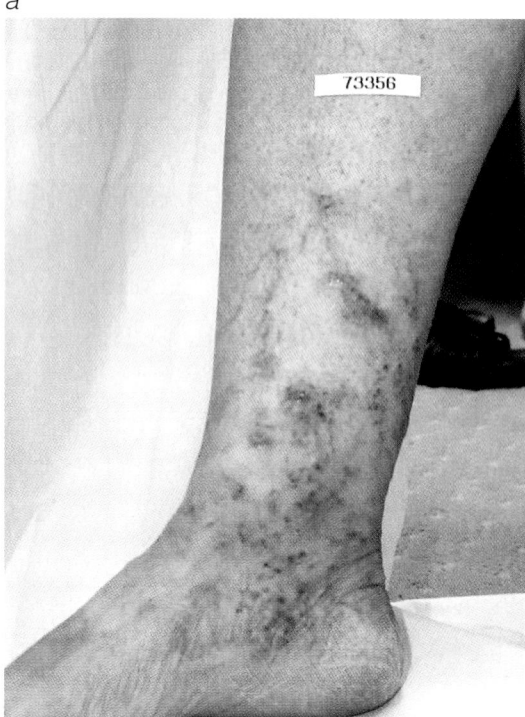

b

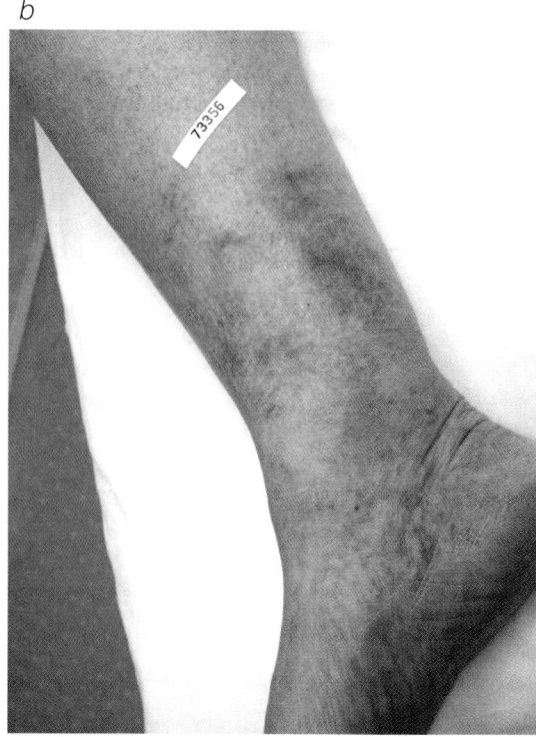

Figure 6 **Sclerotherapy. Shown is residual hyperpigmentation in a 56-year-old woman after treatment with 0.2% STS.**

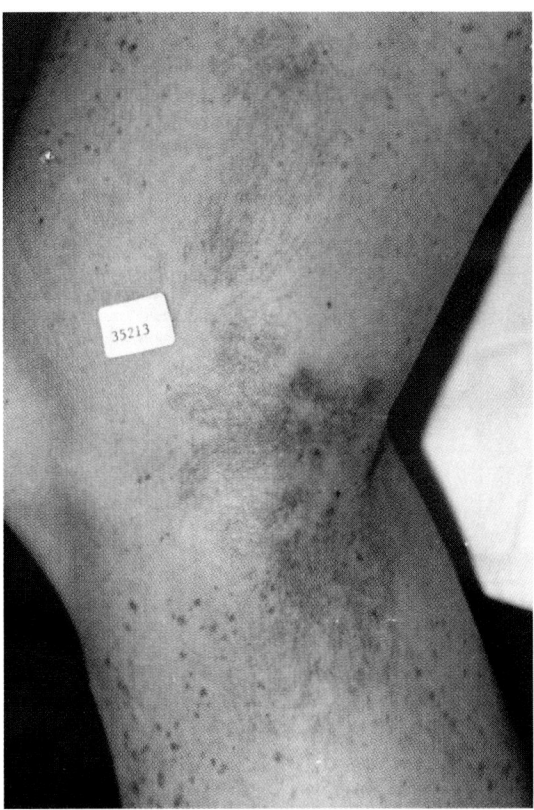

Figure 7 **Sclerotherapy. Shown is telangiectatic matting in a 43-year-old woman after treatment with 0.2% STS.**

sclerosants in current use. It is more common in persons with dark complexions and in those with dark-purple vessels. Fortunately, hyperpigmentation usually resolves with time, but the process can take months. Postsclerotherapy compression lowers the incidence of hyperpigmentation, and removal of any intraluminal thrombi remaining after sclerotherapy reduces the degree of hyperpigmentation present. The latter is accomplished by puncturing the skin with an 18-gauge needle and manually expressing the thrombus. There is no firm consensus on how hyperpigmentation should be treated once it develops. Some authorities recommend the use of fade creams, whereas others advocate laser treatments to lighten the pigmentation. A 2001 study found that 80% depigmentation could be

achieved with weekly subcutaneous injections of the chelating agent deferoxamine mesylate.[24] That various different treatments continue to be recommended suggests that none of them is clearly superior at eliminating hyperpigmentation. The passage of time appears to be the most reliable therapy.

The precise incidence of DVT after sclerotherapy is unknown but appears to be extremely low overall. The risk is somewhat higher when more concentrated solutions are used or larger volumes administered; however, it may be minimized by performing sclerotherapy only for established indications. Treating axial reflux and larger vessels surgically, with sclerotherapy limited to an adjunctive role, will reduce the volume and concentration of solution needed. Ambulation in the physician's office after treatment will help wash away any solution that has progressed into the deep venous system.

The development of tiny new red vessels at an area of previous injection is called telangiectatic matting [*see Figure 7*]. Like ulceration, it is unpredictable. Excessive pressure during injections is thought to play a causative role, but the exact etiology is unknown. Telangiectatic matting is very difficult to treat once it has developed. Occasionally, it resolves spontaneously, but more often, it must be addressed by means of either repeat sclerotherapy with treatment of the feeding reticular vein or laser therapy. Treatment of telangiectatic matting may in fact be the one potential efficacious use for laser-type devices in treating diseased leg veins.

Cost Considerations

I strongly believe that all sclerotherapy, with the exception of that performed for spontaneous hemorrhage, is cosmetic. Accordingly, in the practice to which I belong, patients seeking sclerotherapy for reasons other than hemorrhage are informed well in advance that the procedure is cosmetic and not reimbursable, and they receive a good-faith estimate of expected costs in writing. As noted (see above), venous ligation is the treatment of choice for symptomatic axial reflux and large varicose veins; therefore, sclerotherapy for these conditions is considered medically unnecessary.

Obtaining reimbursement from insurance carriers for sclerotherapy performed to treat small varicose veins or hemorrhage is frustrating at best. Both physicians and patients have contributed to the problem in the past by filing inappropriate claims for reimbursement of cosmetic procedures. This past misuse of insurance coverage has made it difficult to obtain reimbursement even for the one solid medical indication for sclerotherapy, hemorrhage.

References

1. Goldman MP, Bergan JJ: Sclerotherapy: Treatment of Varicose and Telangiectatic Leg Veins, 3rd ed. Mosby–Year Book, Inc, St Louis, 2001, p 1

2. Einarsson E, Eklof B, Neglen P: Sclerotherapy or surgery as treatment for varicose veins: a prospective randomized study. Phlebology 8:22, 1993

3. Bishop C, Fronek H, Fronek A, et al: Real-time color duplex scanning after sclerotherapy of the greater saphenous vein. J Vasc Surg 14:505, 1991

4. Goren G: Real-time color duplex scanning after sclerotherapy of the greater saphenous vein (letter). J Vasc Surg 16:497, 1992

5. Belcaro G, Nicolaides A, Ricci A, et al: Endovascular sclerotherapy, surgery, and surgery plus sclerotherapy in superficial venous incompetence: a randomized, 10-year follow-up trial—final results. Angiology 51:529, 2000

6. Kanter A, Thibault P: Saphenofemoral incompetence treated by ultrasound-guided sclerotherapy. Dermatol Surg 22:648, 1996

7. Cabrera J, Cabrera J Jr, Garcia-Olmedo MA: Treatment of varicose long saphenous veins with sclerosant in microfoam form: long-term outcomes. Phlebology 15:19, 2000

8. McDonagh B, Huntley DE, Rosenfeld R, et al: Efficacy of the comprehensive objective mapping, precise image-guided injection, anti-reflux positioning, and sequential sclerotherapy technique in the management of greater saphenous varicosities with saphenofemoral incompetence. Phlebology 17:19, 2002

9. McCoy S, Evans A, Spurrier N: Sclerotherapy for leg telangiectasia—a blinded comparative trial of polidocanol and hypertonic saline. Dermatol Surg 25:381, 1999

10. Bukhari R, Lohr J, Paget D, et al: Evaluation of lidocaine as an analgesic when added to hypertonic saline for sclerotherapy. J Vasc Surg 29:479, 1999

11. Guex J: Indications for sclerosing agent polidocanol. J Dermatol Surg Oncol 19:959, 1993

12. Conrad P, Malouf GM, Stacey MC: The Austra-

lian polidocanol (aethoxysklerol) study. Dermatol Surg 21:334, 1995

13. Goldman M: Treatment of varicose and telangiectatic leg veins: double-blind prospective comparative trial between aethoxysklerol and sotradecol. Dermatol Surg 28:52, 2002

14. Cavezzi A, Frullini A, Ricci S, et al: Treatment of varicose veins by foam sclerotherapy: two clinical series. Phlebology 17:13, 2002

15. Orbach EJ: Sclerotherapy of varicose veins: utilization of an intravenous air block. Am J Surg 66:362, 1944

16. Frullini A: New technique in producing sclerosing foam in a disposable syringe. Dermatol Surg 26:705, 2000

17. Tessari L, Cavezzi A, Frullini A: Preliminary experience with a new sclerosing foam in the treatment of varicose veins. Dermatol Surg 27:58, 2001

18. Raj TB, Goodard M, Makin GS: How long do compression bandages maintain their pressure during ambulatory treatment of varicose veins? Br J Surg 67:122, 1980

19. Smith SL, Belmont JM, Casparian JM: Analysis of pressure achieved by various materials used for pressure dressings. Dermatol Surg 25:931, 1999

20. Goldman MP, Beaudoing D, Marley W, et al: Compression in the treatment of leg telangiectasia. J Dermatol Surg Oncol 16:322, 1990

21. Weiss RA, Sadick NS, Goldman MP, et al: Post-sclerotherapy compression: controlled comparative study of duration of compression and its effects on clinical outcome. Dermatol Surg 25:105, 1999

22. Bihari I, Magyar E: Reasons for ulceration after injection treatment of telangiectasia. Dermatol Surg 27:133, 2001

23. Bergan JJ, Weiss RA, Goldman MP: Extensive tissue necrosis following high-concentration sclerotherapy for varicose veins. Dermatol Surg 26:535, 2000

24. Lopez L, Dilley R, Henriquez J: Cutaneous hyperpigmentation following venous sclerotherapy treated with deferoxamine mesylate. Dermatol Surg 27:795, 2001

13 VARICOSE VEIN SURGERY

John J. Bergan, M.D., F.A.C.S., *and Luigi Pascarella*, M.D.

Varicose veins are a common problem, accounting for approximately 85% of the venous problems treated surgically. Consequently, a wide variety of operative strategies for dealing with this problem have evolved. From the plethora of procedures in current use, several specific individual techniques have emerged that, when joined together, satisfactorily achieve the objectives of operation.

Indications for Varicose Vein Surgery

The indications for surgical treatment of varicose veins are well established [see Table 1]. Although many physicians believe that varicose veins are nothing more than a cosmetic nuisance, this is in fact true only for some men. Women, for the most part, have specific symptoms (e.g., aching, burning pain, and heaviness) that are related to their varicose veins and are exacerbated by the presence of progesterone. Such symptoms develop with prolonged standing or sitting and reach maximal levels on the first day of the menstrual period, when progesterone levels are at their peak. Men, lacking progesterone, have few such symptoms until the varicose veins progress with aging to the point where they press on somatic nerves. In general, the severity of the symptoms bears no relation to the size of the vessels being treated. Telangiectasias can produce symptoms identical to those of varicose veins, and such symptoms can be relieved by simple sclerotherapy [see 4:12 Sclerotherapy].

Longitudinal studies have shown that large varicose veins can produce venous ulcerations within 15 years. Given that the incidence of venous ulceration is 20% in patients who are first seen with large varicose veins, large varicosities constitute an indication for surgery. Various skin changes characteristic of chronic venous insufficiency precede the development of venous ulceration.

Varicose thrombophlebitis is followed by recurrent varicose thrombophlebitis in nearly every case, at intervals ranging from a few weeks to many months. Nevertheless, the superficial thrombophlebitis, which can be quite disabling, can be prevented by removing varicose vein clusters.

It is true that for many women, the undesirable appearance of varicose veins is a major reason for seeking surgical treatment. When questioned, however, such patients often admit to having symptoms such as pain, heaviness, and fatigue. Typically, they do not relate these symptoms to the varices themselves but instead attribute them to the necessity for prolonged standing during daily work.

Preoperative Evaluation

DUPLEX MAPPING

Over the years, surgical treatises have devoted a great deal of space to clinical examination of the patient with varicose veins. Numerous clinical tests have been described, many of which carry the names of famous persons interested in venous pathophysiology. This august history notwithstanding, the Trendelenburg test, the Schwartz test, the Perthes test, and the Mahorner and Ochsner modifications of the Trendelenburg test are, for the most part, useless in preoperative evaluation of patients today.[1] There is no doubt that clinical evaluation can be improved by using handheld Doppler devices. In our view, however, preoperative evaluation is best performed by means of duplex scanning and physical examination.[2] Although many cite cost considerations as a reason for omitting duplex evaluation, we believe that duplex scanning for venous insufficiency is in fact both simple and cost-effective. Duplex mapping defines individual patient anatomy with considerable precision and provides valuable information that supplements the physician's clinical impression.

A protocol for duplex mapping of incompetent superficial veins has been published.[2] In essence, the examination consists of interrogating specific points of reflux with the patient standing [see Table 2]. Forward flow is produced with muscular compression, and reverse flow is then assessed in the crucial areas that are important to operative planning.

The patient is placed in an upright position so that the leg veins are maximally dilated. No clothing is worn on the lower extremities from the waist down, except for nonconstricting underwear. The patient is instructed to inform the ultrasonographer of any sensation of light-headedness, faintness, dizziness, or nausea. These symptoms seem to be associated with the overall atmosphere of the room and the presence of Doppler velocity signals; they appear to be less likely to occur when the examination itself is performed silently. If a tendency to fainting because of vagovagal reflux is encountered, the examination may have to be modified so that the patient is in a semiupright position instead.

Examination should include both lower extremities, though posttreatment examinations may be targeted to a single extremity or a single area of an extremity. The full length of the axial venous system from ankle to groin is examined. The probe is aligned transversely so that specific named veins can be identified and their relations to other limb structures determined. The veins are scanned by moving the probe up and down along their courses. Double segments, sites of tributary confluence, and large perforating veins (along with their deep venous connections) are identified. (Perforating veins are those that course from the subcutaneous tissue through deep fascia to anastomose with one of the named deep venous structures; communicating veins are those that anastomose with one another within a single anatomic plane.) Varicose veins are often arranged in multiple parallel channels. It is unnecessary to follow reflux into all of the varicose clusters, because these are obvious to the treating physician. Augmentation of flow (distal compression) is done sharply, quickly, and aggressively, and pressure is applied to the calf to activate the gastrocnemius and soleus pump. When a color or pulsed-wave

---

Table 1 Indications for Varicose Vein Surgery

Pain: leg aching, leg heaviness
Patchy burning (venous neuropathy)
Swelling: foot, ankle, leg
Dermatitis: focal, extensive
Lipodermatosclerosis
Ulceration: present or healed
Superficial thrombophlebitis
External hemorrhage
Appearance

Table 2 Interrogation Points in the Venous Reflux Examination

Common femoral vein
Femoral vein
  Upper third
  Distal third
Popliteal vein
Sural veins
Saphenofemoral junction*
Saphenous vein, above the knee
Saphenous vein, below the knee
Saphenopopliteal junction†
Mode of termination, lesser saphenous vein

*Record diameter of refluxing long saphenous vein.
†Record distance from floor.

Doppler device is used, the probe is angled to provide an insonation angle of 60° or less.

For the anterior examination, the patient faces the ultrasonographer with his or her weight borne on the lower extremity that is not being examined. The non–weight-bearing extremity is then evaluated. The common femoral vein and the saphenofemoral junction are assessed with the Valsalva maneuver and with distal compression and release. If reflux is present, the diameter of the refluxing greater saphenous vein is noted for subsequent use in selecting the proper endovenous catheter during saphenous ablation.

The greater saphenous vein is identified on the basis of its relation to the deep and superficial fascia that ensheathe it to form the saphenous compartment. High-resolution B-mode ultrasonographic imaging of the superficial fascia in the transverse plane has shown this structure to be strongly ultrasound reflective, yielding a characteristic image of the saphenous vein known as the saphenous eye [see Figure 1]. The saphenous eye is a constant marker, clearly demonstrable in transverse sections of the medial aspect of the thigh, that serves to differentiate the saphenous vein from varicose tributaries and other superficial veins. Casual examination of the thigh often reveals an elongated, dilated vein that is incorrectly assumed to be the long saphenous vein. This mistaken assumption can be corrected by means of ultrasound scanning using the saphenous eye as an anatomic marker.

Venous reflux can be elicited manually by calf muscle compression and release, by the Valsalva maneuver, or by pneumatic tourniquet release. There is no difference between pneumatic tourniquet release and manual compression and release. Pneumatic tourniquet release is cumbersome and requires two vascular sonographers, which makes the manual compression and release method very attractive by comparison. If saphenofemoral reflux lasting longer than 0.5 second is present, the diameter of the saphenous vein is recorded 2.5 cm distal to the saphenofemoral junction.

The examination continues distally along the greater saphenous vein, with distal augmentation of flow performed at intervals to check for reflux. Reflux frequently ends in the region of the knee. The point at which reflux stops is recorded in terms of distance from the floor in centimeters. The femoral vein (formerly termed the superficial femoral vein) is checked at midthigh for reflux and vein wall irregularities.

The posterior examination is also done on the non–weight-bearing lower extremity, with attention paid to reflux in the popliteal vein, the saphenopopliteal junction, and the sural veins. The Valsalva maneuver may be used to stimulate reflux, as may

distal augmentation and release. Valsalva-induced reflux is halted by competent proximal valves. The lesser saphenous vein is followed from its retromalleolar position on the lateral aspect of the ankle proximally to the saphenopopliteal junction, and augmentation maneuvers are performed every few centimeters.

The termination of the lesser saphenous vein is noted. If the vein terminates proximally in the vein of Giacomini, the femoropopliteal vein, or another vein, a specific check is made for a connection to the popliteal vein. If the lesser saphenous vein is refluxing, the distance from the saphenopopliteal junction to the floor is measured and recorded.

A search for incompetent perforating veins is necessary only in limbs with chronic venous insufficiency (CVI) manifested by hyperpigmentation, atrophie blanche, woody edema, scars from healed ulceration, or actual open ulcers. Incompetent perforating veins in limbs without CVI are associated with varicose veins and can be controlled with varicose phlebectomy. Identification of perforating veins in the lower extremity can be difficult even for the experienced sonographer.

Operative Planning

OBJECTIVES OF SURGICAL TREATMENT

Three principal goals must be kept in mind in planning treatment of varicose veins:

1. The varicosities must be permanently removed and the underlying cause of venous hypertension treated.
2. The repair must be done in as cosmetic a fashion as possible.
3. Complications must be minimized.

To speak of permanent removal of varicosities implies that all potential causes of recurrence have been considered and that surgery has been planned so as to address them. There are four principal causes of recurrence of varicose veins, of which three can be dealt with at the time of the primary operation.

One cause of recurrent varicosities is failure to perform the primary operation in a correct fashion. Common errors include missing a duplicated saphenous vein and mistaking an anterolateral or accessory saphenous vein for the greater saphenous vein. Such errors can be eliminated by careful and thorough groin dissection. Accordingly, failure to do a proper groin dissection has

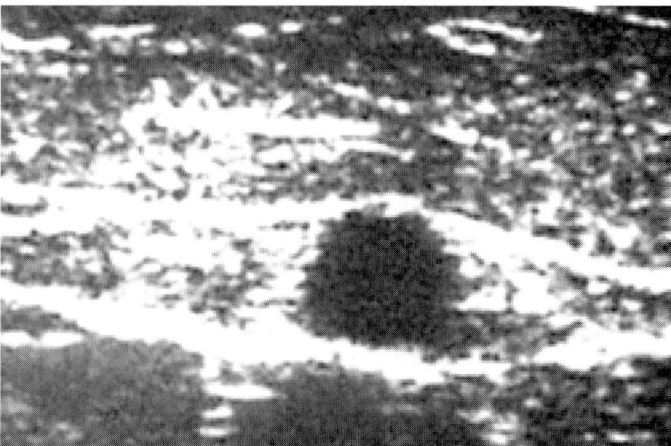

Figure 1 **Shown is an ultrasonographic image of the so-called saphenous eye. Correct identification of this marker is crucial to correct performance of the preoperative ultrasonographic reflux examination.**

Table 3 Options Available for Varicose Vein Surgery

Ankle-to-groin saphenous vein stripping with stab avulsions
Groin-to-knee saphenous vein stripping with stab avulsions
Saphenous vein ligation (high, low, or both)
Saphenous vein ligation and sclerotherapy
Saphenous vein ligation and stab avulsion of varices
Stab avulsion of varices without saphenous vein stripping (ambulatory phlebectomy)
Radiofrequency ablation of saphenous vein
Laser-light ablation of saphenous vein
Foamed sclerosant ablation of saphenous vein and varices

---

long been held to be a second principal cause of recurrent varicose veins. It is now known, however, that such dissection causes neovascularization in the groin, leading to recurrence of varicose veins [*see* Outcome Evaluation, *below*]. A third cause of recurrent varicosities is failure to remove the greater saphenous vein from the circulation. A reason often cited for this failure is the desire to preserve the saphenous vein for subsequent use as an arterial bypass. It is clear, however, that the preserved saphenous vein continues to reflux and continues to elongate and dilate its tributaries, thus producing more varicosities even after primary operation removed what was present at that time. A fourth cause of recurrent varicosities is persistence of venous hypertension through nonsaphenous sources—chiefly, perforating veins with incompetent valves. Muscular contraction generates enormous pressures that are directed against valves in perforating veins. Venous hypertension

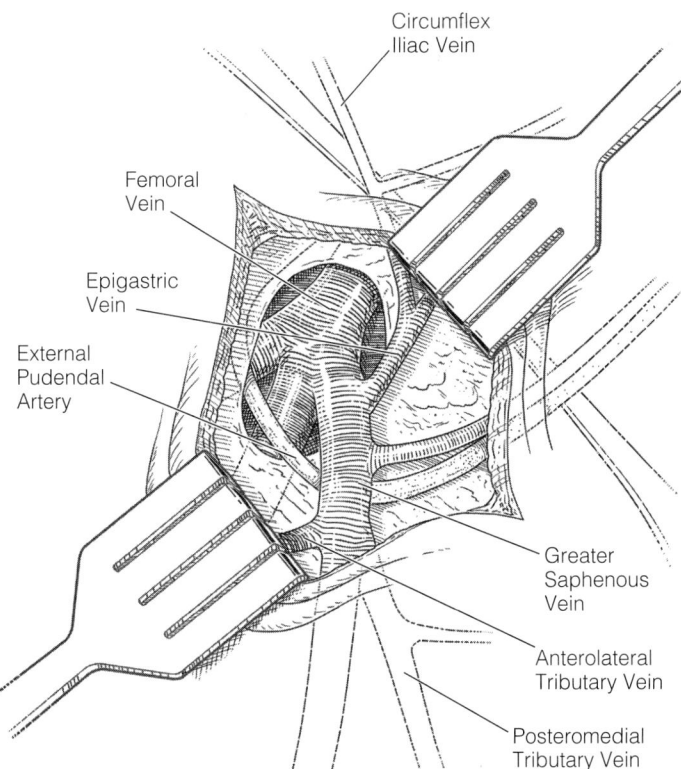

Figure 2 **Shown are a typical saphenofemoral junction and the most important tributary vessels. The classic surgical approach dictates total disconnection of all tributaries at this junction.**

Circumflex Iliac Vein
Femoral Vein
Epigastric Vein
External Pudendal Artery
Greater Saphenous Vein
Anterolateral Tributary Vein
Posteromedial Tributary Vein

induces a leukocyte endothelial reaction, which, in turn, incites an inflammatory response that ultimately destroys the venous valves and weakens the venous wall.[3] The perforating veins most commonly associated with recurrent varicosities are the midthigh perforating vein, the distal thigh perforating vein, the proximal anteromedial calf perforating vein, and the lateral thigh perforating vein, which connects the profunda femoris vein to surface varicosities.

Finally, there is a fifth cause of recurrent varicosities, which is out of control of the operating surgeon—namely, the genetic tendency to form varicosities through development of localized or generalized vein wall weakness, localized blowouts of venous walls, or stretched, elongated, and floppy venous valves.[4,5]

For varicose vein surgery to be successful, two tasks must be accomplished. The first is ablation of reflux from the deep to the superficial veins, including the saphenofemoral junction, the saphenopopliteal junction, and midthigh varices from the Hunterian perforating vein. Accomplishment of this task is guided by careful preoperative duplex ultrasonographic mapping of major superficial venous reflux. The second task is removal or destruction of all varicosities present at the time of the surgical intervention. Accomplishment of this task is guided by meticulous marking of all varicose vein clusters.

SURGICAL OPTIONS

A number of options are available for surgical treatment of varicose veins [*see Table 3*]. Regardless of the specific approach taken, the general technical objectives are the same: (1) ablation of the hydrostatic forces of axial saphenous vein reflux and (2) removal of the hydrodynamic forces of perforator vein outflow. These objectives should be combined with extraction of the varicose vein clusters in as cosmetic fashion as possible.

Ligation of the saphenous vein at the saphenofemoral junction [*see Figure 2*] has been widely practiced in the belief that it would control gravitational reflux while preserving the vein for subsequent arterial bypass. It is true that the saphenous vein is largely preserved after proximal ligation[6]; however, reflux continues and hydrostatic forces are not controlled.[7] Recurrent varicose veins are more frequent after saphenous ligation than after stripping[8] and are more common after saphenous ligation and sclerotherapy than after saphenous stripping and sclerotherapy.[9] A prospective randomized trial comparing proximal saphenous vein ligation and stab avulsion of varices with stripping of the thigh portion of the saphenous vein and stab avulsion of varices showed the latter approach to be superior.[10,11] Routine saphenous vein stripping reduces the rate of varicosity recurrence and the need for reoperation for recurrent saphenofemoral incompetence.

Although there are arguments in favor of retaining the greater saphenous vein for possible arterial bypass grafting, the relatively high reoperation rate (> 20%) makes this strategy undesirable. Almost three quarters of the limbs that have undergone ligation of the saphenous vein alone have an incompetent long saphenous vein on duplex imaging. Until studies show a clear advantage to retaining the long saphenous vein in defined patient populations, stripping should remain a routine part of primary long saphenous vein surgery. In several studies, preservation of patency of the saphenous vein and continuing reflux in this vein were found to be the most frequent elements in recurrence of varicosities.[12-14] In one group of patients undergoing reoperation for relief of recurrent variceal symptoms, two thirds required removal of the saphenous vein as part of the procedure.[12]

Ankle-to-groin stripping of the saphenous vein has been a dominant treatment of varicose veins over the past 100 years.[15-17] One argument against routine stripping of the leg (i.e., ankle-to-knee)

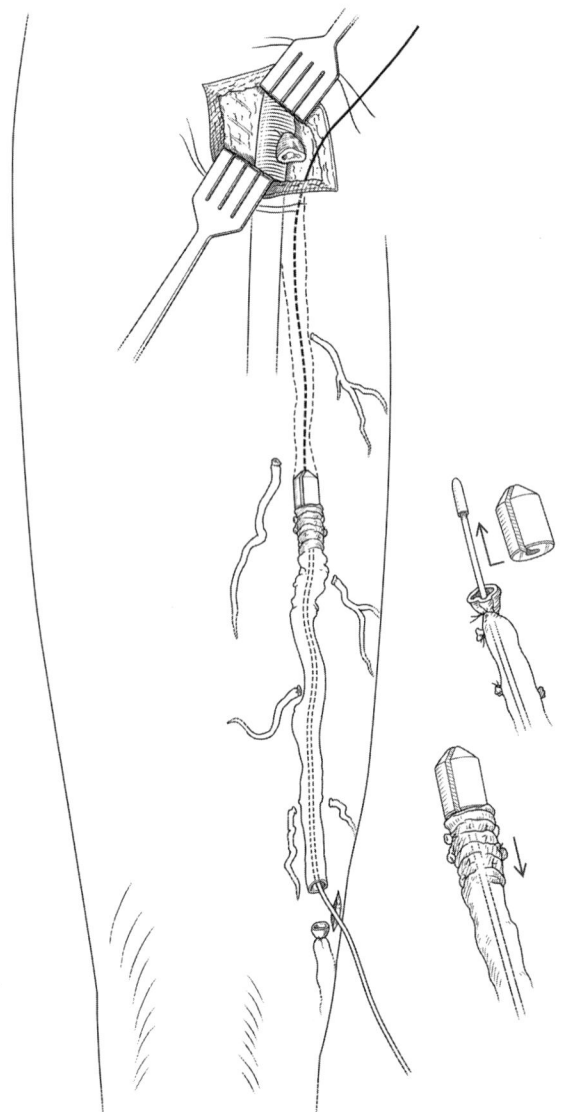

Figure 3 **Illustrated is an early attempt to minimize distal incisions and prevent saphenous nerve injury at the knee. The stripper and its obturator are pulled to knee level, then retrieved through the groin incision. (Note division of perforating and communicating veins.)**

portion of the saphenous vein is the risk of concomitant saphenous nerve injury [*see Figure 3*].[8] Another argument is that whereas the objective of saphenous vein removal is detachment of perforating veins emanating from the saphenous vein, which are seen in the thigh, the perforating veins in the leg are actually part of the posterior arch vein system rather than the saphenous vein system. This latter argument notwithstanding, preoperative ultrasonography frequently shows that the leg portion of the saphenous vein is in fact directly connected to perforating veins. Therefore, removal of the saphenous vein from ankle to knee should be a consideration in every surgical case.

Operative Technique

GREATER SAPHENOUS VEIN STRIPPING

The surgical approach taken must be individually tailored to each patient and each limb. Groin-to-knee stripping of the saphenous vein should be considered in every patient requiring surgical

intervention.[18] In nearly all patients, this measure is supplemented by removal of the varicose vein clusters via stab avulsion or some form of sclerotherapy [*see Table 4*].

Step 1: Placement of Incisions

Preoperative marking, if correctly performed, will have documented the extent of varicose vein clusters and identified the clinical points where control of varices is required. Incisions can then be planned. As a rule, incisions in the groin and at the ankle should be transverse and should be placed within skin lines. In the groin, an oblique variation of the transverse incision may be appropriate. This incision should be placed high enough to permit identification of the saphenofemoral junction [*see Figure 2*]. Generally, throughout the leg and the thigh, the best cosmetic results are obtained with vertical incisions. Transverse incisions are used in the region of the knee, and oblique incisions are appropriate over the patella when the incisions are placed in skin lines.

A major cause of discomfort and occasional permanent skin pigmentation is subcutaneous extravasation of blood during and after saphenous vein stripping. Such extravasation can be minimized by applying a hemostatic tourniquet after Esmarch exsanguination of the limb. The pressure in the hemostatic tourniquet should be between 250 and 300 mm Hg, and the tourniquet should not be in place for longer than 1 hour. If a tourniquet is not used, the entire operation on one limb can be performed with the limb elevated 30° so that the major varicose clusters are higher than the heart. In addition, hemostatic packing can be placed into the saphenous vein tunnel [*see Step 4, below*].

Troubleshooting A common error is to place the groin incision too low. The practice of identifying and carefully dividing each of the tributaries to the saphenofemoral junction has been dominant over the past 50 years. The rationale for this practice has been that it would be inadvisable to leave behind a network of interanastomosing inguinal tributaries. Accordingly, special efforts have been made to draw each of the saphenous tributaries into the groin incision so that when they are placed on traction, their primary and even secondary tributaries can be controlled. The importance of these efforts has been underscored by descriptions of residual inguinal networks as an important cause of varicose vein recurrence.[12] Currently, however, this central principle of varicose vein surgery is under challenge, on the grounds that groin dissection can lead to neovascularization and hence to recurrence of varicosities [*see Outcome Evaluation, below*].

Step 2: Introduction of Stripping Device

Preoperative duplex studies having already demonstrated incompetent valves in the saphenous system, a disposable plastic Codman stripper can be introduced from above downward; alternatively, an Oesch stripper can be employed.[19] Both of these devices can be used to strip the saphenous vein from groin to knee

---

Table 4 Methods of Variceal Ablation

Formal ligation, division, and excision
Stab avulsion
Sclerotherapy
   With liquid sclerosant
   With foamed sclerosant
Sclerotherapy aided by transillumination
Sclerotherapy aided by ultrasound guidance

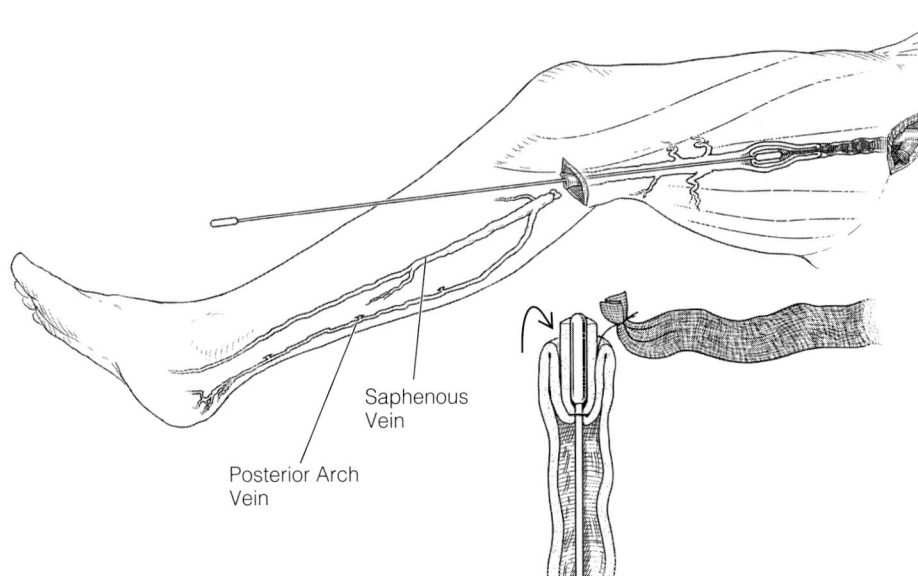

Figure 4 **Greater saphenous vein stripping. Inversion stripping of the saphenous vein decreases soft tissue trauma in the thigh. However, tearing of the vein occurs on occasion. This problem may be largely prevented by attaching a corner of a 2 in. gauze roll soaked in lidocaine-epinephrine solution to the end of the stripper. As the stripper is pulled, the gauze is drawn into the vein, thereby assisting hemostasis. The gauze can then be left in place for 10 to 20 minutes while the stab wounds from the avulsion part of the procedure are being closed.**

via the inversion technique [*see Figure 4*]. This approach has been shown to reduce soft tissue trauma in the thigh.[20]

In the groin, the stripper is inserted proximally into the upper end of the divided internal saphenous vein and passed down the main channel through incompetent valves until it can be felt lying distally approximately 1 cm medial to the medial border of the tibia at a point approximately 4 to 6 cm distal to the level of the tibial tubercle. The saphenous vein is anatomically constant in this location, just as it is in the groin and ankle. If the saphenous vein is removed from the groin to this level, both the midthigh perforating vein, which usually enters the saphenous vein, and the most distal incompetent perforating veins, which are in the distal third of the thigh, will be treated.

A small incision is made over the palpable distal end of the stripper. The saphenous vein will subsequently be divided through this incision, and the stripper and the inverted vein will be delivered through it. In exposing the saphenous vein at knee level, the superficial fascia must be incised because the vein lies between this structure and the deep fascia of the thigh.

If the stripper passes unimpeded to the ankle, it can be exposed there with an exceedingly small skin incision placed in a carefully chosen skin line. Passage of the stripper from above downward to the ankle serves to confirm the absence of functioning valves, and stripping of the vein from above downward is unlikely to cause nerve damage. At the ankle, the vein should be carefully and cleanly dissected to free it from surrounding nerve fibers. If this is not done, saphenous nerve injury will result, and the patient will experience numbness of the foot below the ankle.

Step 3: Stab Avulsion

Stripping of the saphenous vein has been shown to produce profound distal venous hypertension. This occurs in virtually every operation, even when the limb is elevated. Therefore, after the stripper is placed, one should consider performing the stab avulsion portion of the procedure before the actual stripping maneuver. In other words, one should (1) place the stripper correctly, (2) prepare the proximal end of the device for stripping, (3) leave the stripper in place, (4) perform stab avulsions to remove varicosities, and (5) strip the saphenous vein, in that order.

Incisions to remove varicose clusters vary according to the size of the vein, the thickness of the vein wall, and the degree to which the vein is adhering to the perivenous tissues. In general, vertical incisions 1 to 3 mm in length are appropriate, except in areas where skin

lines are obviously horizontal [*see Figure 5*]. Successive incisions are spaced as widely as possible. Varicosities are exteriorized by means of hooks or forceps [*see Figures 6 and 7*]. Particularly useful for this pur-

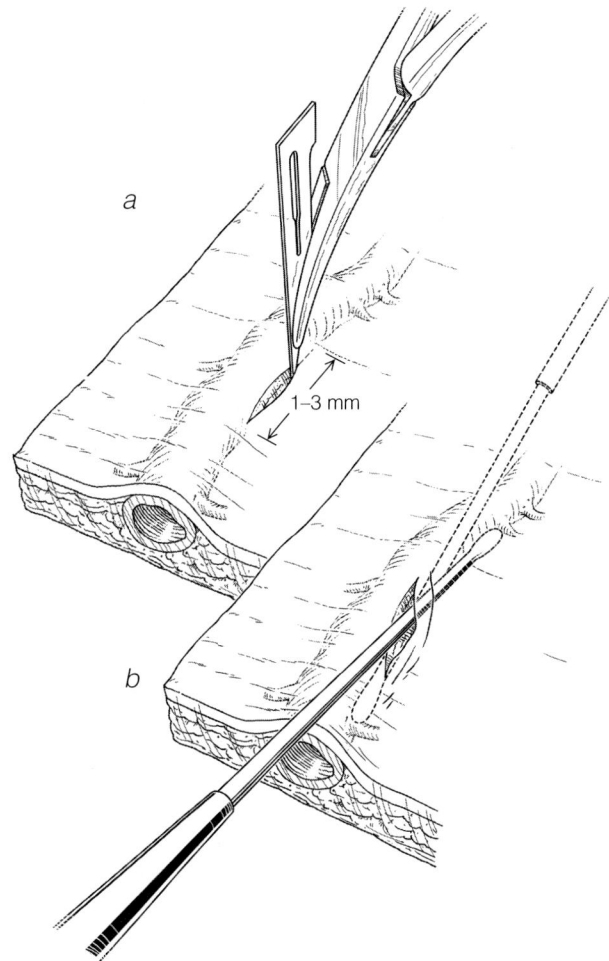

Figure 5 **Greater saphenous vein stripping. Skin incisions for stab avulsion of varicosities are limited with respect to both length and depth (*a*). The dissector blade facilitates mobilization of the vein before removal (*b*).**

pose are the specially designed vein hooks known by such names as the Varady dissector, the Muller hook, and the Oesch hook.[21] These devices efficiently detach perforating veins from their tributary varicose clusters. Dissection of each perforating vein at the fascial level is not required and may in fact be cosmetically undesirable. There is no need to ligate or clip the ends of each vein: the combination of leg elevation, trauma-induced venospasm, and direct pressure ensures adequate hemostasis. Once exteriorized, the varicosity is divided and each end avulsed for as long a length as possible. After avulsion, skin edges are approximated with tape or with a single inverted absorbable monofilament suture.

Phlebectomy techniques for varicose clusters have been markedly refined by experienced workers in Europe.[22]

Step 4: Stripping of Saphenous Vein

Once the stab avulsion portion of the procedure is complete, saphenous vein stripping is performed. The previously placed stripper is pulled distally to remove the saphenous vein. Although plastic disposable vein strippers and their metallic equivalents were designed to be used with various-sized olives to remove the saphenous vein, in fact, a more efficient technique is simply to tie the vein to the stripper below its tip so that the vessel can then be inverted into itself and removed distally, usually at knee level.

To decrease oozing into the tract created by stripping, a 5 cm roller gauze soaked in a 1% lidocaine-epinephrine solution is attached to the stripper by using the ligature fastening the saphenous vein to the device. Thus, inversion stripping is accompanied by hemostatic packing. The hemostatic pack, which lies within the saphenous vein, can be pulled into the tract with minimum tissue trauma; when it is not inverted into the vein itself, it can act as an obturator to facilitate removal of the saphenous vein without tearing. As the vein is removed by inversion, the gauze is left in place in the tract for hemostasis while the remainder of the surgical procedure (i.e., closure of the stab wounds) is being completed.

Complications

Surgical removal of the saphenous vein on an outpatient basis still requires two incisions, one in the groin and the other near the knee. Postoperative compression bandaging is standard, and most patients experience little downtime. Some, however, do experience hematomas, pain, and extensive bruising. These three complications are linked; thus, every effort should be made to prevent oozing. The most feared complication of varicose vein surgery is venous thromboembolism, but the incidence of this complication is quite low (probably about 1%). In countries where postoperative immobilization, hospitalization, and delayed ambulation are employed for patients with varicosities, prophylaxis against venous thromboembolism is common. In the United States, however, this measure is generally considered unnecessary in these patients. The most common complication of varicose vein surgery is recurrence of varicosities, which is experienced by 15% to 30% of patients treated.[23]

Outcome Evaluation

Study of surgical saphenous stripping has shown that when undesirable outcomes occur, they become evident quite early.[10] As noted (see above), it has long been accepted practice to dissect tributary vessels at the saphenofemoral junction very carefully, taking each of the vessels back beyond the primary and even the secondary tributaries if possible.[20] In practice, however, such dissection appears to cause neovascularization in the groin.[24] Duplex

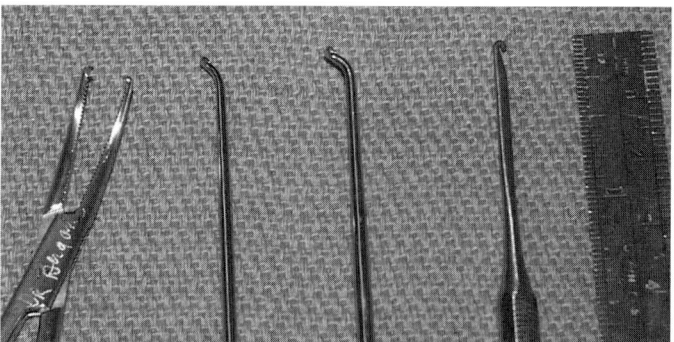

Figure 6 Greater saphenous vein stripping. Shown are tools used for exteriorizing varicosities in the stab avulsion portion of the procedure: a Hartman clamp with its single tooth placed distally, two Muller clamps, and a Varady hook and dissector (left to right).

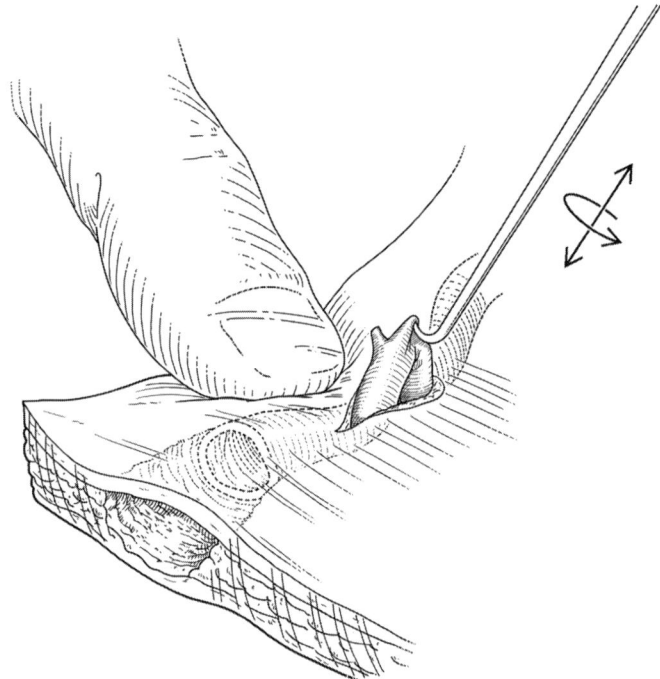

Figure 7 Greater saphenous vein stripping. The varix is exteriorized with a hook, then divided to permit proximal and distal avulsion.

ultrasound surveillance supports this finding.[25] It has now been amply confirmed that neovascularization causes recurrent varicose veins. Clearly, this is a significant disadvantage of standard surgical treatment of varicosities. A number of alternatives to surgical saphenous vein stripping have been developed and are being explored. These alternatives are proving to be effective and may be superior to saphenous stripping, if only because they are not followed by groin neovascularization.

Alternatives to Saphenous Vein Stripping

RADIOFREQUENCY ABLATION OF SAPHENOUS VEIN

In an attempt to minimize postoperative discomfort while maintaining the benefits of saphenous vein ablation, alternating current has been applied to effect rapid thermic electrocoagulation of the vein wall and its valves. Prolonged exposure to such high-frequen-

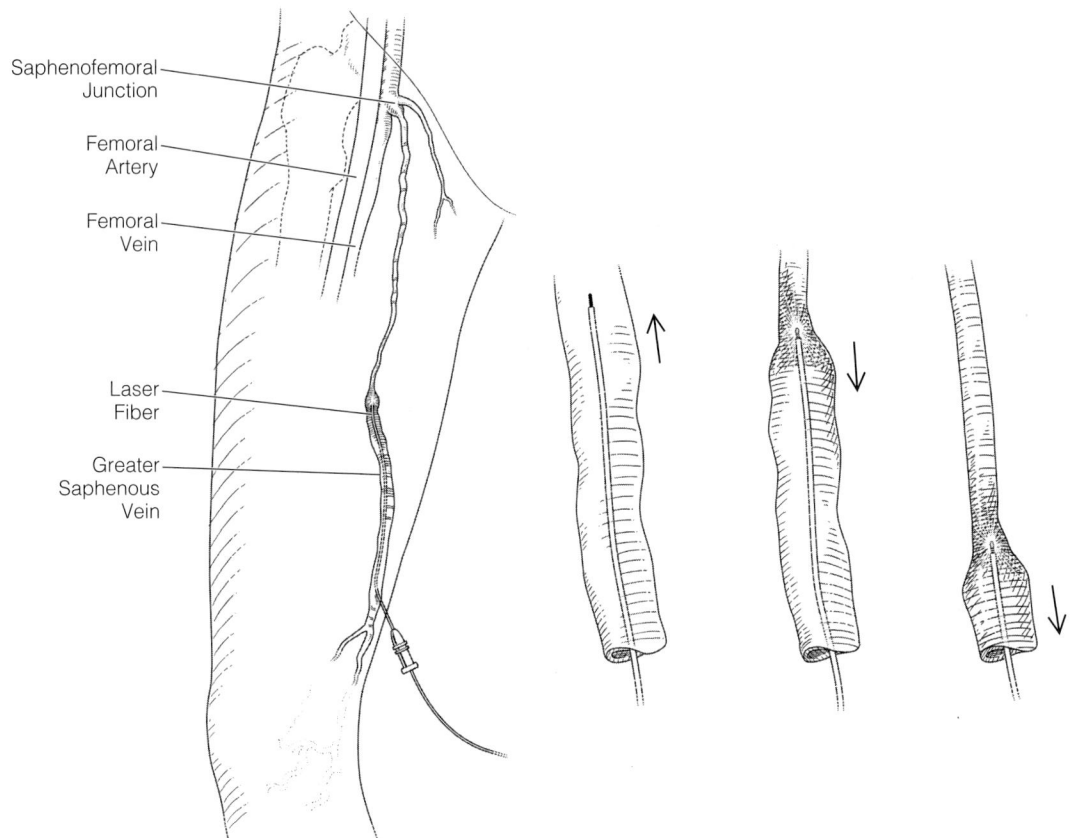

Figure 8 **Ablation of saphenous vein. Shown is percutaneous placement of a quartz fiber for laser ablation of the saphenous vein. In practice, the catheter used for radiofrequency (RF) ablation is placed in a similar fashion. Both laser ablation and RF ablation deliver electromagnetic energy to the vein wall to destroy the vessel and remove it from the circulation.**

cy energy results in total loss of vessel wall architecture, disintegration, and carbonization.[26] There is now level I evidence indicating that such treatment is beneficial.[27] Additional supporting data come from simple registry recording of results.[28] At 1 to 2 years, reported results from ablation of the saphenous vein are as good as those from conventional surgical treatment. Ultrasonography shows treated saphenous veins disappearing after the 2-year point. Clinical observations suggest that patients are much more comfortable after saphenous vein ablation than after stripping.[29]

The issue of varicose vein recurrence after saphenous vein obliteration without saphenofemoral junction tributary disconnection is unsettled at present. It does appear, however, that endovenous radiofrequency (RF) ablation of the saphenous vein—for example, with the Closure procedure (VNUS Medical Technologies, Inc., San Jose, California)—prevents subsequent neovascularization in the groin. Many centers have reported no neovascularization in the absence of a groin incision.

The specific goal of endoluminal treatment of venous reflux is obliteration of the saphenous vein. Follow-up to 3 years shows that RF ablation with the Closure procedure accomplishes this. Laser light energy has also been used to achieve this goal in place of RF energy, but its efficacy has not yet been proved [*see Figure 8*].

One study compared the Closure procedure with endovenous laser treatment (EVLT) for occlusion of the saphenous vein in 100 legs in 50 patients.[30] With each patient, one long saphenous vein was treated with a laser, the other with RF energy [*see Table 5*]. Although this study was not a true randomized trial, bias was prevented by the carefully drawn protocol.

Hemodynamic outcomes were placed into one of three categories: (1) primary occlusion, (2) assisted primary occlusion, and (3) failure of treatment. This categorization is similar to the reporting standards for lower-extremity ischemia, in which the terms primary patency, primary assisted patency, and secondary patency and failure are used. Clear differences between RF ablation and EVLT were observed. RF ablation was more effective than EVLT in achieving primary occlusion (41 versus 28 veins). In addition, there were somewhat fewer treatment failures with RF than with EVLT (4 versus 8 legs), even after ultrasound-guided foam sclerotherapy was carried out for veins in which endovenous treatment had failed.

Ten RF-treated legs showed early recurrent patency. Of these, one closed without further treatment, five closed after ultrasound-guided sclerotherapy, two did not undergo follow-up duplex scans, and two failed to close after repeated sessions of ultrasound-guided sclerotherapy. In these 10 patients, the contralateral leg was treated

Table 5 Comparison of Saphenous Veins Treated with RF Ablation and EVLT[30]

Results (at Last Visit)	RF-Treated Veins	EVLT-Treated Veins	P
Primary occlusion	41	28	< 0.05
Assisted primary occlusion	5	14	< 0.05
Failure of treatment	4	8	< 0.05

EVLT—endovenous laser treatment   RF—radiofrequency

a

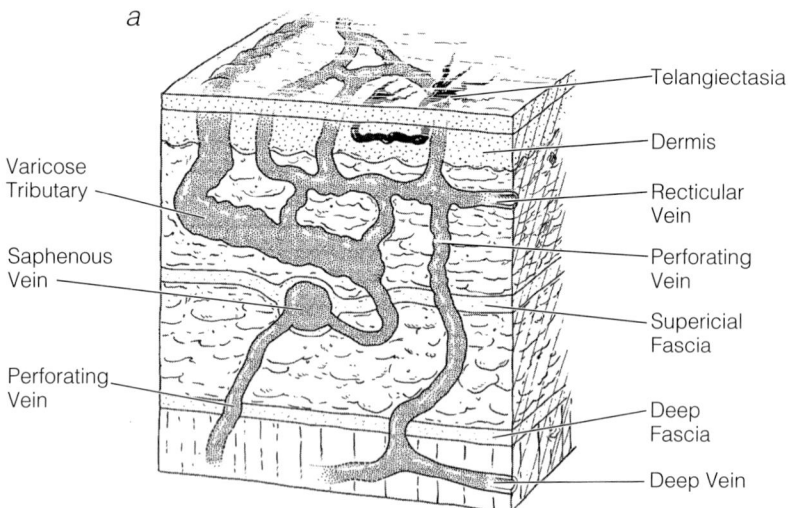

- Telangiectasia
- Dermis
- Recticular Vein
- Perforating Vein
- Supericial Fascia
- Deep Fascia
- Deep Vein

Varicose Tributary

Saphenous Vein

Perforating Vein

b

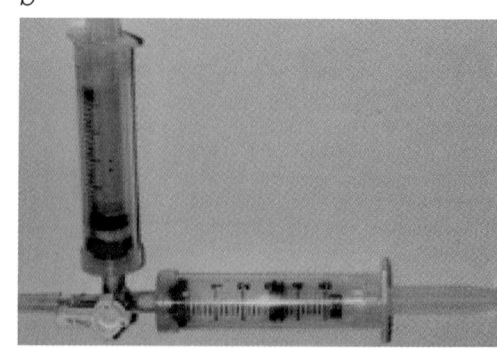

c

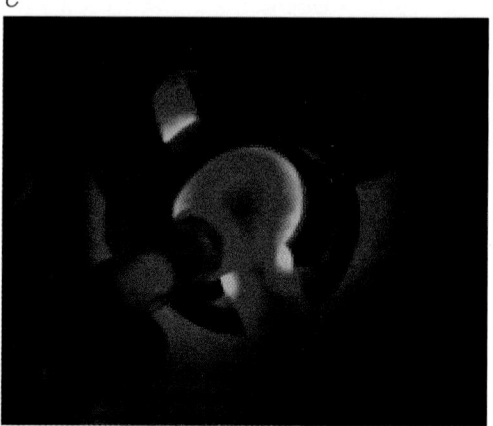

Figure 9 **Microfoam sclerotherapy. (*a*) The relationships among the venous structures in a lower extremity with varicosities explain why microfoam sclerotherapy can succeed. Injections into varices, reticular veins, or perforating veins can place the foam into varicose structures and even into telangiectatic blemishes. (*b*) Sclerosant foam is made by mixing room air with 0.5% sodium tetradecyl sulfate (STS) in a 2-to-1 ratio via a three-way stopcock. The syringes are emptied 35 times to create a foam that lasts about 5 minutes. (*c*) A halogen light (vein light), as used here during a foam injection, is helpful for treating persistent or recurrent varices as well as the saphenous vein in situations where surgery is undesirable.**

with EVLT. In seven of the 10 EVLT-treated legs, the saphenous vein failed to close primarily. Of the 24 EVLT-treated legs that showed recurrent patency and flow, two closed without further intervention, 14 closed after ultrasound-guided sclerotherapy, four did not undergo follow-up duplex scans, and four failed to close after repeated sessions of ultrasound-guided sclerotherapy. The four legs that failed to close with EVLT and ultrasound-guided sclerotherapy were treated with a second ablation procedure, this time with RF. Two of the four closed after the second ablation procedure. For the two legs that showed recurrent patency and flow even after a second ablation procedure, a high ligation of the greater saphenous vein was done in the office with the patient under local anesthesia.

FOAMED SCLEROSANT

The prospect of a rapid, minimally invasive, and durable treatment of varicose veins is an attractive one. It appears as though these objectives may be achieved without operative intervention by using sclerosant microfoam [*see Figure 9*]. In 1944 and 1950, E. J. Orbach introduced the concept of a macrobubble air-block technique to enhance the properties of sclerosants in performing macrosclerotherapy.[31,32] At the time, few clinicians evinced much interest in the subject, and the technique languished.

Half a century later, the work of Juan Cabrera and colleagues in Granada attracted the attention of some phlebologists and reawakened interest in using foam technology for treatment of venous insufficiency.[33] These investigators showed that foam sclerotherapy was technically simple and worked well in small to moderate-sized varicose veins, and they demonstrated that the limitations of liquid sclerotherapy could be erased by using microfoam. Their 5-year report represents the longest observation period reported to date for microfoam sclerotherapy for varicose veins. For most of the patients, a single injection sufficed to treat saphenous veins and varicose tributaries. Extensive vasospasm was seen immediately, but compression was applied after treatment. Complete fibrosis of the saphenous vein was achieved in 81% of cases, and patency with reflux persisted in only 14%. Tributary varicosities disappeared in 96% of cases. Vessels that remained open and were refluxing were successfully closed with retreatment.

If subsequent work continues to confirm these favorable results, it may be that microfoam sclerotherapy will eventually replace all other methods of varicose vein treatment.

References

1. Ballard JL, Bergan, JJ, DeLange M: Venous imaging for reflux using duplex ultrasonography. Noninvasive Vascular Diagnosis. AbuRahma AF, Bergan JJ, Eds. Springer-Verlag, London, 2000, p 329

2. Mekenas LV, Bergan JD: Venous reflux examination: technique using miniaturized ultrasound scanning. J Vasc Technol 26:139, 2002

3. Ono T, Bergan JJ, Schmid-Schönbein GW, et al: Monocyte infiltration into venous valves. J Vasc Surg 27:158, 1998

4. Thulesius O, Ugaily-Thulesius L., Gjores JE, et al: The varicose saphenous vein, functional and ultrastructural studies, with special reference to smooth muscle. Phlebology 3:89, 1988

5. Rose SS, Ahmed A: Some thoughts on the aetiology of varicose veins. J Cardiovasc Surg 27:534, 1986

6. Rutherford RB, Sawyer JD, Jones DN: The fate of residual saphenous vein after partial removal or ligation. J Vasc Surg 12:422, 1990

7. McMullin GM, Coleridge Smith PD, Scurr JH: Objective assessment of high ligation without stripping the long saphenous vein. Br J Surg 78:1139, 1991

8. Munn SR, Morton JB, MacBeth WAAG, et al: To strip or not to strip the long saphenous vein? A varicose veins trial. Br J Surg 68:426, 1981

9. Neglen P: Treatment of varicosities of saphenous origin: comparison of ligation, selective excision, and sclerotherapy. Bergan JJ, Goldman MP, Eds. Varicose Veins and Telangiectasias: Diagnosis and

Management. Quality Medical Publishing, St Louis, 1993, p 148

10. Sarin S, Scurr JH, Coleridge Smith PD: Assessment of stripping the long saphenous vein in the treatment of primary varicose veins. Br J Surg 79:889, 1992

11. Dwerryhouse S, Davies B, Harradine K, et al: Stripping the long saphenous vein reduces the rate of reoperation for recurrent varicose veins; five-year results of a randomized trial. J Vasc Surg 29:589, 1999

12. Stonebridge PA, Chalmers N, Beggs I, et al: Recurrent varicose veins; a varicographic analysis leading to a new practical classification. Br J Surg 82:60, 1995

13. Darke SG: The morphology of recurrent varicose veins. Eur J Vasc Surg 6:512, 1992

14. Conrad P: Groin-to-knee down stripping of the long saphenous vein. Phlebology 7:20, 1992

15. Mayo CH: Treatment of varicose veins. Surg Gynecol Obstet 2:385, 1906

16. Babcock WW: A new operation for extirpation of varicose veins. NY Med J 86:1553, 1907

17. Keller WL: A new method for extirpating the internal saphenous and similar veins in varicose conditions: a preliminary report. NY Med J 82:385, 1905

18. Goren G, Yellin AE: Primary varicose veins: topographic and hemodynamic correlations. J Cardiovasc Surg 31:672, 1990

19. Goren G, Yellin AE: Invaginated axial saphenectomy by a semirigid stripper: perforate-invaginate stripping. J Vasc Surg 20:970, 1994

20. Bergan JJ: Saphenous vein stripping by inversion: current technique. Surg Rounds 23:118, 2000

21. Bergan JJ: Varicose veins: hooks, clamps and suction: application of new techniques to enhance varicose vein surgery. Semin Vasc Surg 15:21, 2002

22. Ricci S, Georgiev M, Goldman MP: Ambulatory Phlebectomy: a Practical Guide for Treating Varicose Veins. Mosby, St Louis, 1995

23. Darke SG: The morphology of recurrent varicose veins. Eur J Vasc Surg 6:512, 1992

24. Jones L, Braithwaite BD, Selwyn D, et al: Neovascularization is the principal cause of varicose vein recurrence: results of a randomized trial of stripping the long saphenous vein. Eur J Vasc Endovasc Surg 12:442, 1996

25. Fischer R, Linde N, Duff C, et al: Late recurrent saphenofemoral junction reflux after ligation and stripping of the greater saphenous vein. J Vasc Surg 34:236, 2001

26. Petrovic S, Chandler JG: Endovenous obliteration: an effective, minimally invasive surrogate for saphenous vein stripping. J Endovasc Surg 7:11, 2000

27. Rautio T, Ohinmaa A, Perala J, et al: Endovenous obliteration versus conventional stripping operation in the treatment of primary varicose veins: a randomized, controlled trial with comparison of the costs. J Vasc Surg 35:958, 2002

28. Kabnick LS, Merchant RF: Twelve- and 24-month followup after endovascular obliteration of saphenous reflux: a report from the multicenter register. J Phlebol 1:17, 2001

29. Goldman MP: Closure of the greater saphenous vein with endoluminal radiofrequency thermal heating of the vein wall in combination with ambulatory phlebectomy: preliminary 6-month followup. Dermatol Surg 26:105, 2000

30. Morrison N, Neuhardt D: Comparative study of radiofrequency versus laser ablation of the greater saphenous vein. J Vasc Surg (in press)

31. Orbach EJ: Sclerotherapy of varicose veins: utilization of intravenous air block. Am J Surg 66:362, 1944

32. Orbach EJ: Contribution to the therapy of the varicose complex. J Intl Coll Surg 13:765, 1950

33. Cabrera J, Cabrera J, Garcia-Olmedo MA: Treatment of varicose long saphenous vein with sclerosant in microfoam form: long term outcomes. Phlebology 15:19, 2000

Acknowledgment

Figures 2 through 9a   Tom Moore.

14 LOWER-EXTREMITY AMPUTATION FOR ISCHEMIA

William C. Pevec, M.D., F.A.C.S.

Patients with infected, painful, or necrotic lower extremities can be restored to a better functional level by means of a properly selected and performed amputation. This procedure should be considered reconstructive and restorative. In what follows, I address amputations across the toe, the forefoot, the leg, and the thigh. Because Symes' amputations and hip disarticulations are seldom appropriate on ischemic limbs, I omit discussion of these procedures.

General Preoperative Planning

Selecting the appropriate level of amputation is of primary importance for healing and preservation of function. For an ambulatory patient who has either a palpable pulse over the dorsal pedal or posterior tibial arteries or a functioning infrainguinal arterial bypass graft, amputation on the foot (either toe amputation or transmetatarsal amputation) is appropriate. For an ambulatory patient who has a palpable femoral pulse and a patent profunda femoral artery, whose skin is warm at least to the level of the ankle, and who has no skin lesions on the proposed amputation flaps, amputation below the knee is appropriate. For a nonambulatory patient who has ischemic rest pain, ulceration, or gangrene, amputation above the knee is appropriate. Arterial reconstruction is not indicated if the extremity is nonfunctional. Below-the-knee amputation does not offer nonambulatory patients any functional advantage; moreover, it is less likely to heal and often results in a flexion contracture at the knee that leads to pressure ulceration of the stump. Above-the-knee amputation depends on pulsatile flow into the ipsilateral internal iliac artery for successful healing. Above-the-knee amputation is also necessary for a patient whose skin is cool at or above the midcalf or who has skin lesions at or proximal to the midcalf.

Several adjunctive measurements (e.g., transcutaneous oxygen tension and segmental arterial pressure) have been used to select the level of amputation but have not proved particularly helpful. Generally, these adjuncts can reliably determine a level of amputation at which healing is virtually assured, but they cannot reliably determine the level at which an amputation will not heal. Consequently, reliance on such measures to select the level of amputation will result in an unnecessarily high percentage of more proximal amputations.

In most cases, definitive amputation can be accomplished in a single stage. Local cellulitis can usually be controlled beforehand with bed rest and systemic administration of antibiotics. Undrained pus or recalcitrant cellulitis, however, must be treated with debridement and drainage in advance of definitive amputation. This can be accomplished with local soft tissue debridement, single-toe amputation, or guillotine amputation across the ankle.

Careful preoperative medical assessment is essential. Lower-extremity amputation for ischemia is associated with a mortality of 4.5% to 16%,[1-5] owing to the poor overall condition of the patient population. Accordingly, optimization of cardiac and pulmonary function and control of systemic infection are mandatory.

Finally, the timing of elective amputation is crucial. Because the loss of a limb is a difficult and frightening thing for a patient to accept, there is a natural tendency to delay amputation for as long as possible. This tendency is understandable but must be weighed against the potential problems associated with delay, such as poor preoperative pain control, which leads to an increased incidence of postamputation phantom limb pain, and extended preoperative immobility, which leads to physical deconditioning and makes prosthetic limb rehabilitation more difficult. A preoperative consultation with a physiatrist can allay some of the patient's anxiety by addressing the expected postoperative course of rehabilitation and thereby removing some of the fear of the unknown.

Toe Amputation

Amputation of the toe can be done either across a phalanx or across a metatarsal bone; the latter procedure is commonly referred

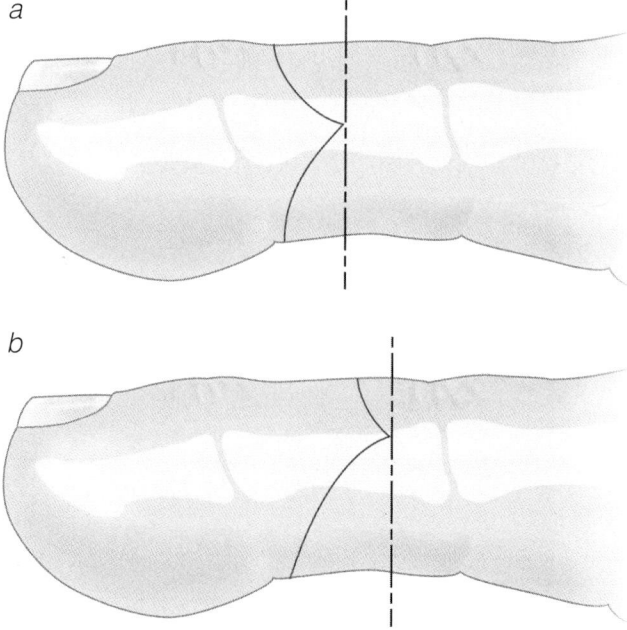

Figure 1 **Toe amputation: transphalangeal amputation. Transphalangeal amputation can be performed either with dorsal and plantar flaps of equal length (*a*) or with a plantar flap that is longer than the dorsal flap (*b*). The phalanx is transected at the level of the apex of the skin flaps (dashed line). The bone is transected through the shaft of the phalanx, never across the joint.**

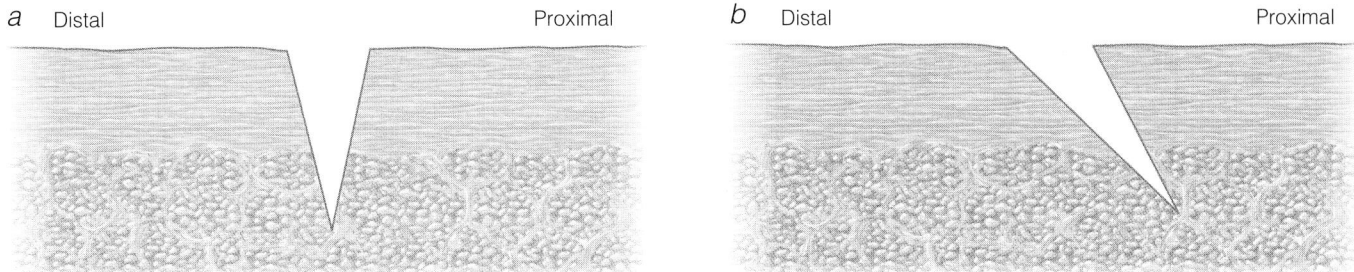

Figure 2 **In a lower-extremity amputation, the skin is always incised perpendicular to its surface (*a*). Given the varying contours encountered during extremity amputation, it can be difficult to maintain the perpendicular orientation of the scalpel; however, an incision that undermines the proximal skin flap (*b*) will devascularize the epidermis and lead to necrosis of the suture line.**

to as a ray amputation. Many of the perioperative issues are essentially similar for the two approaches; however, indications and operative details differ somewhat and thus will be described separately.

OPERATIVE PLANNING

As noted (see above), for a toe amputation to heal properly, there must be either a palpable pulse over the dorsal pedal or posterior tibial artery or a functioning bypass graft to an infrapopliteal artery. If tissue necrosis or infection is confined to the distal or middle phalanx, transphalangeal amputation is appropriate; if tissue loss or necrosis involves the proximal phalanx, ray amputation is indicated. If tissue necrosis or infection extends over the metatarsophalangeal joint, either transmetatarsal amputation of the entire forefoot or below-the-knee amputation is usually necessary (see below).

Multiple transphalangeal amputations are functionally well tolerated. If, however, ray amputation of the great toe or of more than one smaller toe is called for, it is preferable to perform a transmetatarsal amputation of the forefoot. Adequate skin coverage is usually difficult to achieve with a great-toe or multiple-toe ray amputation. In addition, ray amputation of more than one of the middle toes often causes central deviation of the remaining outside toes, which can lead to ulcerations secondary to abnormal pressure points. Finally, loss of the first metatarsal head or of several of the other metatarsal heads results in abnormal weight-bearing on the remaining metatarsal heads, which may give rise to late ulceration.

OPERATIVE TECHNIQUE

Transphalangeal Amputation

Digital block anesthesia is ideal for transphalangeal amputation. A 25-gauge needle is inserted into the skin over the medial aspect of the dorsum of the proximal phalanx and advanced until the bone is encountered. The needle is then withdrawn slightly, and a small amount of fluid is aspirated to confirm that the tip of the needle is not in a blood vessel. Next, 0.5 to 1.0 ml of lidocaine, 0.5% or 1.0% without epinephrine, is slowly injected. The needle is then carefully advanced medial to the bone until the tip can be felt pressing against (but not puncturing) the plantar skin. Again, the needle is withdrawn slightly, fluid is aspirated, and 0.5 to 1.0 ml of lidocaine is injected. The same technique is repeated on the lateral aspect of the proximal phalanx. In this way, all four digital nerve branches are blocked. If multiple toe amputations are required, an ankle block, epidural anesthesia, spinal anesthesia, or general anesthesia can be used.

An incision is made to create dorsal and plantar skin flaps. Typically, these flaps are equal in length [*see Figure 1a*]; however, depending on the location of the skin lesion, either the dorsal flap or the plantar flap can be left longer [*see Figure 1b*]. Care must be tak-

en not to create excessively long flaps, which may lack sufficient perfusion for healing, or to create undermined bevels with the scalpel [*see Figure 2*], which will lead to epidermolysis of the suture line.

The incision is extended down to the phalanx, and the soft tissues are gently separated from the bone with a small periosteal elevator. All tendons and tendon sheaths are debrided because the poor vascularity of these tissues may compromise the healing of the toe. The phalanx is transected at the level of the apices of the skin incisions [*see Figure 1*]. Care must be taken not to leave the remaining bone segment too long: this places undue tension on the skin flaps and is a primary cause of poor healing. The best way of transecting the phalanx is to use a pneumatic oscillating saw. Manual bone cutters can splinter the bone, and manual saws can cause extensive damage to the soft tissues. The bone is always transected across the shaft: because of the poor vascularity of the articular cartilage, disarticulation across a joint typically leads to poor healing.

Hemostasis is achieved with absorbable sutures and limited use of the electrocautery. Excessive tissue manipulation and electrocauterization should be avoided. The skin edges are carefully approximated with simple interrupted nonabsorbable monofilament sutures; perfect apposition is necessary to maximize the potential for primary healing. The sutures must not be placed too close to the skin edges, because the heavily keratinized skin of the foot is easily lacerated. The final step is the application of a soft dressing.

Ray Amputation

For ray amputation, spinal, epidural, or general anesthesia can be employed. A so-called tennis racket incision is made—that is, a straight incision along the dorsal surface of the affected metatarsal bone coupled with a circumferential incision around the base of the toe [*see Figure 3a*]. The goal is to save all available viable skin on the toe; this skin is used to ensure a tension-free closure, and any excess skin can be debrided later, at the time of closure. Again, undermined bevels are avoided. The incision is taken down to the bone, and the soft tissues are separated from the distal metatarsal bone with a periosteal elevator. Dissection must be kept close to the affected metatarsal head to prevent injury to the adjacent metatarsophalangeal joint, which can lead to necrosis of the adjacent toe. The metatarsal bone is transected across the shaft with a pneumatic oscillating saw [*see Figure 3b*]. The tendons and the tendon sheaths are debrided.

Meticulous hemostasis is achieved with absorbable sutures and limited use of the electrocautery. The skin is approximated with simple interrupted nonabsorbable monofilament sutures. If sufficient viable skin was preserved, a flap of plantar skin is rotated dorsally, and the incision is closed in the shape of a Y [*see Figure 4a*]. Alternatively, the medial and lateral edges are shifted, one proximally and the other distally, the corners are trimmed, and the incision is

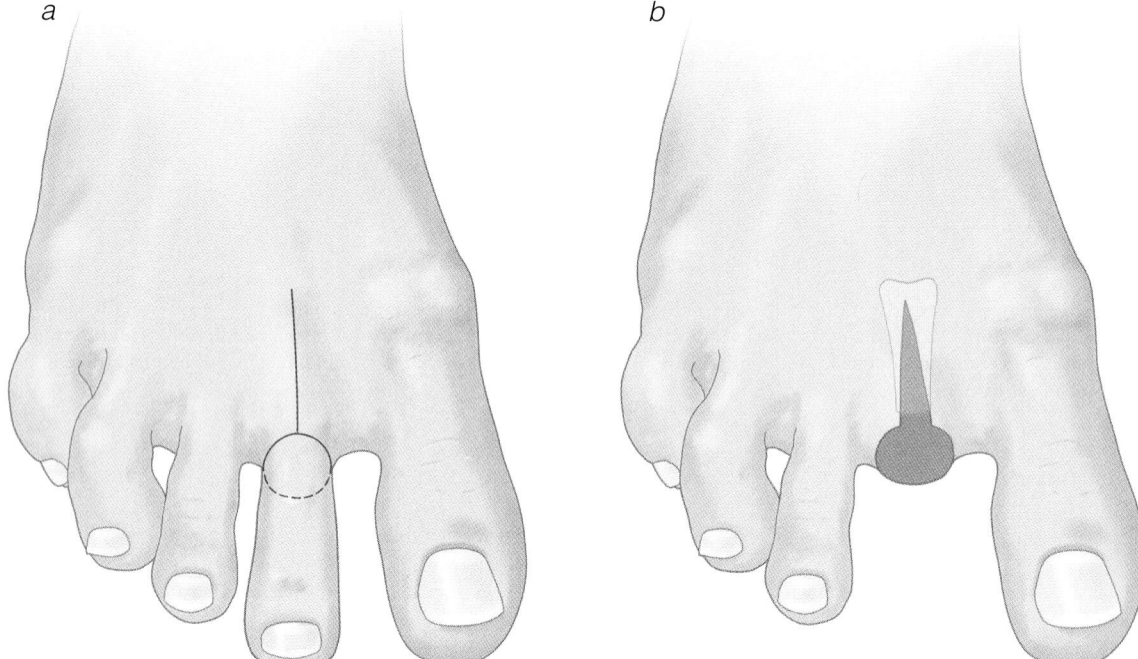

Figure 3 Toe amputation: ray amputation. (*a*) A longitudinal incision is made along the dorsum of the shaft of the metatarsal bone of the affected toe. A circumferential incision is then made around the phalanx. The circumferential incision should be placed as distal on the toe as there is viable skin so that as much skin as possible is retained for closure of the wound. (*b*) The metatarsal bone is transected across its shaft, proximal to the metatarsal head; the joint is never disarticulated.

closed in a linear fashion [*see Figure 4b*]. A soft supportive dressing is applied.

COMPLICATIONS

Complications of toe amputation include bleeding, infection, and failure to heal. Because even a small amount of bleeding under the skin flaps can prevent proper healing, meticulous hemostasis is mandatory. In most cases, infection and failure to heal are attributable to poor patient selection and poor surgical technique; the usual result is a more proximal amputation.

OUTCOME

For optimal healing, there must be an extended period (2 to 3 weeks) during which no weight is borne by the foot that underwent toe amputation. Once healing is complete, the patient should be able to walk normally, with no need for orthotic or assist devices. Beginning ambulation too early can disrupt healing flaps and necessitate more proximal amputation, which lengthens the hospital stay and increases long-term disability. For these reasons, toe amputation in patients with arterial occlusive disease is not an outpatient procedure. Patients are kept on bed rest and instructed in techniques (e.g., use of a wheelchair, a walker, or crutches) that allow them to function without stepping on the foot that was operated on. Hospital discharge is delayed until such techniques are mastered.

Transmetatarsal Amputation

OPERATIVE PLANNING

As noted (see above), transmetatarsal amputation is indicated if there is tissue loss in the forefoot involving the first metatarsal head, two or more of the other metatarsal heads, or the dorsal forefoot. It is contraindicated if there is extensive skin loss on the plantar sur-

face of the foot or on the dorsum proximal to the midshaft of the metatarsal bones. The peroneus longus and peroneus brevis muscles insert on the proximal portions of the fourth and fifth metatarsal bones; if these insertions are sacrificed, inversion of the foot results, eventually leading to chronic skin breakdown from the side of the foot repeatedly striking the ground during ambulation. Transmetatarsal amputation is also contraindicated if there is a preexisting footdrop (peroneal palsy).

OPERATIVE TECHNIQUE

Spinal, epidural, or general anesthesia may be employed. Placement of a tourniquet on the calf is a useful adjunctive measure. This step greatly reduces intraoperative blood loss. More important, the bloodless operative field that results allows more accurate assessment of tissue viability and hence more precise selection of the level of amputation; in a field stained with extravasated blood, it is easy to leave behind nonviable tissue that will doom the amputation. Use of a tourniquet is, however, contraindicated in patients who have a functioning infrapopliteal artery bypass graft.

After sterile preparation and draping, the leg is elevated to help drain the venous blood, and a sterile pneumatic tourniquet is placed around the calf, with care taken to pad the skin under the tourniquet and to position the tourniquet over the calf muscles, where it will not apply pressure over the fibular head (and the common peroneal nerve) or other osseous prominences. The tourniquet is then inflated to a pressure higher than the systolic blood pressure. In patients who do not have diabetes mellitus, a tourniquet inflation pressure of 250 mm Hg is typically employed; in patients who have diabetes mellitus and calcified arteries, a pressure of 350 to 400 mm Hg is preferred.

An incision is made across the dorsum of the foot at the level of the middle of the shafts of the metatarsal bones, extending medially and laterally to the level of the center of the first and fifth metatarsal bones, respectively [*see Figure 5*]. The dorsal incision is curved prox-

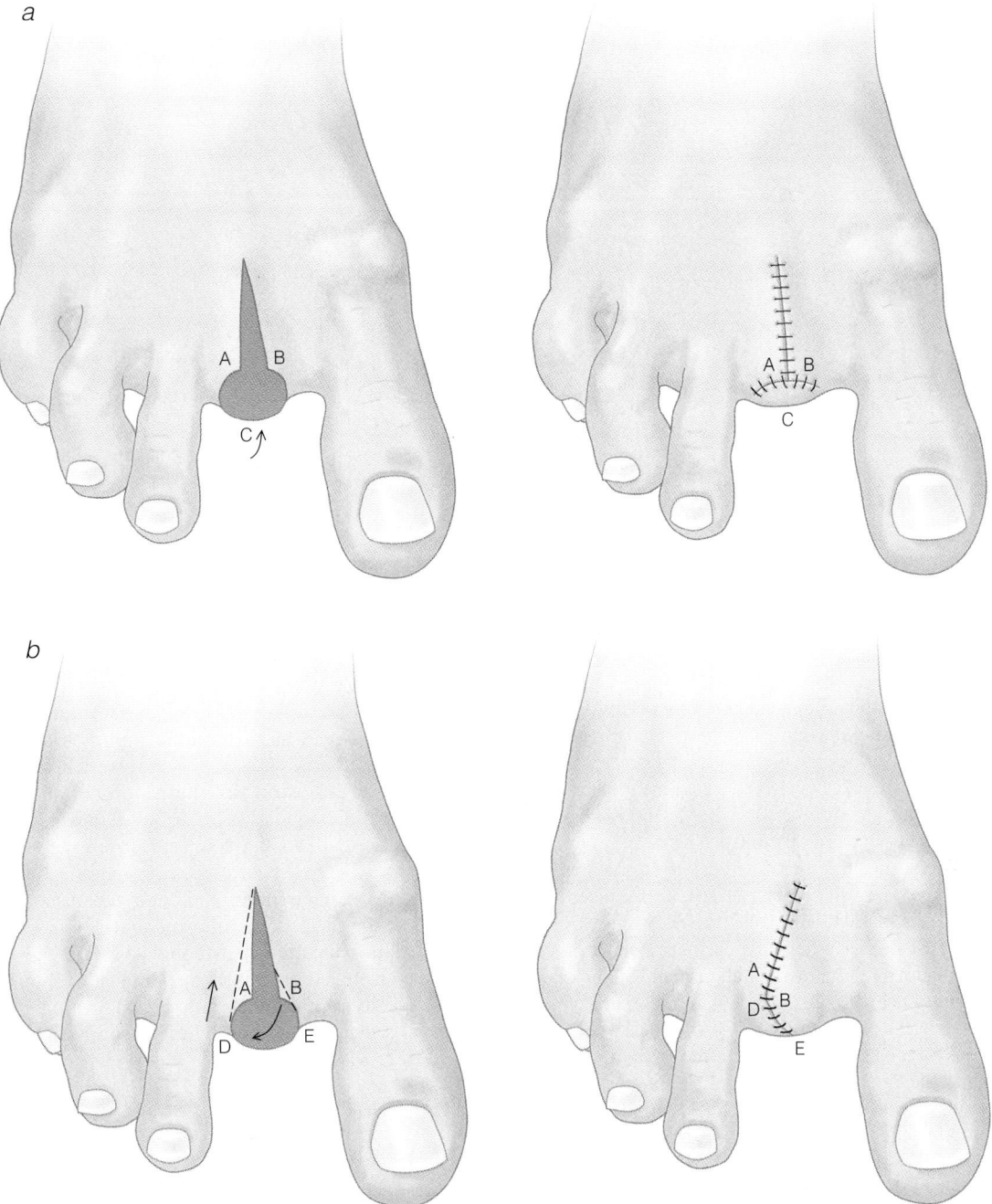

Figure 4   **Toe amputation: ray amputation. (*a*) If adequate skin is available, a plantar flap can be rotated dorsally and the skin closed in a Y configuration. This closure is technically easy to perform; however, there is a risk of skin necrosis at corners A and B. (*b*) Alternatively, the skin can be closed in a linear fashion. Corners A and B are gently trimmed. Corner B is shifted distally toward point D as corner A is shifted proximally. A slight dogear will result at point E; however, it will diminish with time.**

imally at the medial and lateral edges to ensure that no dog-ears remain at the time of closure. The dorsal incision is continued perpendicularly through the soft tissues on the dorsum down to the metatarsal bones. The plantar incision is extended distally to a point just proximal to the toe crease. Care is taken not to bevel the skin incisions.

A plantar flap is created by making an incision with the scalpel adjacent to the metatarsophalangeal joints; the incision is then carried more deeply to the level of the midshafts of the metatarsal bones on their plantar surfaces. The periosteum of the first metatar-

sal bone is scored circumferentially with the scalpel, and the soft tissue is dissected away from the first metatarsal bone with a periosteal elevator to a point about 1 cm proximal to the dorsal skin incision. The first metatarsal bone is then transected perpendicular to its shaft at the level of the dorsal skin incision with a pneumatic oscillating saw. This process is repeated for each individual metatarsal bone, with care taken to follow the normal contour of the forefoot by cutting the lateral metatarsal bones at a level slightly proximal to the level at which the more medial bones are transected. All visible digital arteries are clamped and tied with absorbable ligatures. If a

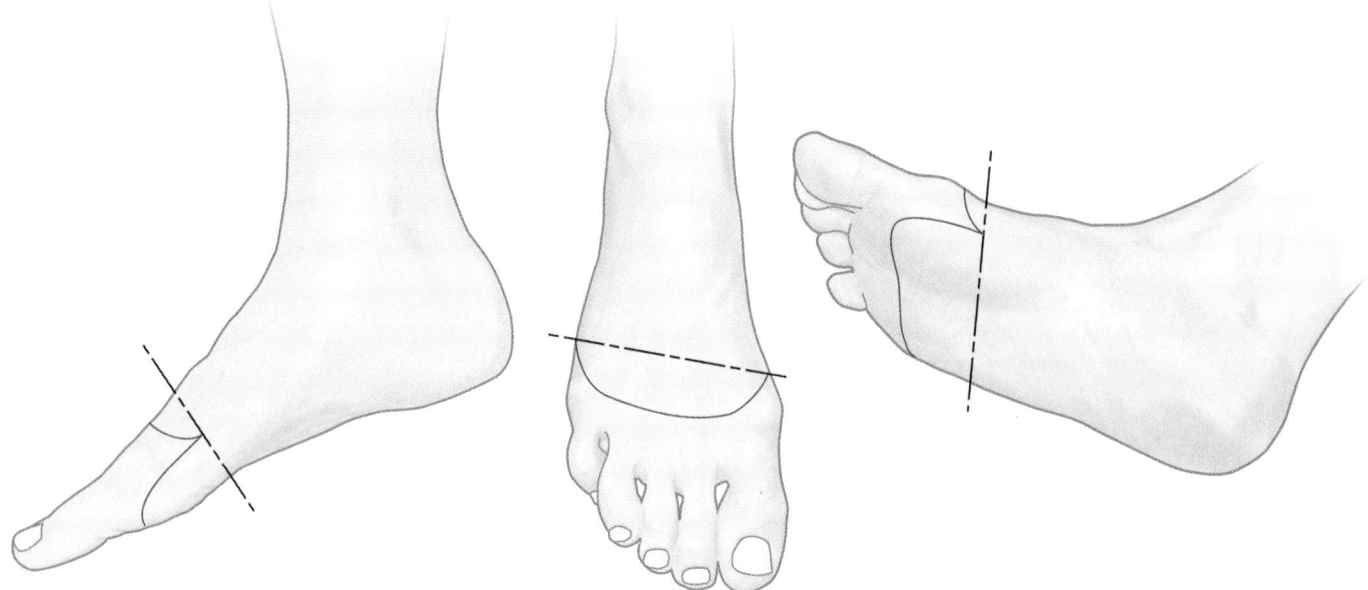

Figure 5 **Transmetatarsal amputation. The skin incisions are shown from various angles. The metatarsal shafts are divided in their midportions (dashed line). The metatarsal bone transection is at the level of the apices of the skin incision, and the lateral metatarsal bones are cut slightly more proximally than the medial metatarsal bones, in a pattern reflecting the normal contour of the forefoot.**

tourniquet was used, it is deflated at this time. All tendons and tendon sheaths are debrided from the wound.

Meticulous hemostasis is achieved with absorbable sutures and limited use of the electrocautery. Any sharp edges on the metatarsal bones are smoothed with a rongeur or a rasp. The wound is irrigated to flush out devitalized tissue and thrombus. The plantar flap is trimmed as needed. The dermis is approximated with simple interrupted absorbable sutures, and the knots are buried. Because the edge of the plantar flap is generally longer than the edge of the dorsal flap, the sutures must be placed slightly farther apart on the plantar flap than on the dorsal flap if perfect alignment is to be obtained. It is imperative to achieve the correct skin alignment with the dermal suture layer. Once this is accomplished, the skin edges are gently and perfectly apposed with interrupted vertical mattress sutures of nonabsorbable monofilament material. Finally, a soft supportive dressing with good padding of the heel is applied; casts and splints are avoided because of the risk of ulceration of the heel or over the malleoli.

COMPLICATIONS

If a tourniquet is not used, intraoperative blood loss can be substantial; the blood pools in the sponges and drapes, often out of the anesthesiologist's field of view. Consequently, good communication between the surgeon and the anesthesiologist is crucial for preventing ischemic complications secondary to hemorrhage.

Postoperative complications include bleeding, infection, and failure to heal, all of which are likely to result in more proximal amputation. They can best be prevented by means of careful patient selection and meticulous surgical technique.

OUTCOME

For proper healing, postoperative edema must be avoided and the plantar flap protected against shear forces. To prevent swelling, the patient is kept on bed rest with the foot elevated for the first 3 to 5 days. This step is particularly important if the transmetatarsal amputation was performed simultaneously with arterial reconstruction, which carries a high risk of reperfusion edema of the foot. After 3 to 5 days, the patient is instructed in techniques for moving in and out of the wheelchair without stepping on the foot. The foot that was operated on should not bear any weight at all for at least 3 weeks; early weight-bearing may disrupt the healing of the plantar flap and necessitate more proximal amputation.

Once healed, patients should be able to walk independently with standard shoes. There is, however, a risk that they may trip over the unsupported toe of the shoe. In addition, the pushoff normally provided by the toes is lost after transmetatarsal amputation, and this change results in a halting, flat-footed gait. These problems can be obviated by using an orthotic shoe with a steel shank (to keep the toe of the shoe from bending and causing tripping) and a rocker bottom (to provide a smooth heel-to-toe motion).

Guillotine Ankle Amputation

OPERATIVE PLANNING

Guillotine amputation across the ankle is indicated when a patient presents with extensive wet gangrene that precludes salvage of a functional foot (e.g., wet gangrene that destroys the heel, the plantar skin of the forefoot, or the dorsal skin of the proximal foot). In such patients, initial guillotine amputation through the ankle is safer than extensive debridement: the operation is shorter, less blood is lost, the risk of bacteremia is reduced, and better control of infection is possible. Guillotine amputation is also indicated in patients with foot infections who have cellulitis extending into the leg. Transection at the ankle, perpendicular to the muscle compartments, tendon sheaths, and lymphatic vessels, allows effective drainage and usually brings about rapid resolution of the cellulitis of the leg, thus permitting salvage of the knee in many cases in which the knee might otherwise be unsalvageable.

OPERATIVE TECHNIQUE

General anesthesia is preferred; regional anesthesia is relatively contraindicated for critically ill patients who are in a septic state. Anesthesia is required for no more than 15 to 20 minutes.

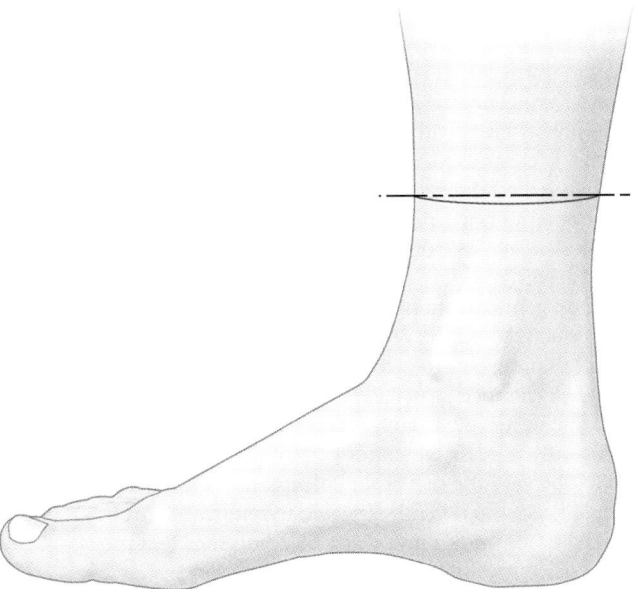

Figure 6 **Guillotine ankle amputation. The skin incision is made circumferentially at the narrowest portion of the ankle. The bones are then transected at the same level (dashed line).**

A circumferential incision is made at the narrowest part of the ankle (i.e., at the proximal malleoli) regardless of the level of the cellulitis [*see Figure 6*]. This placement takes the line of incision across the tendons, thereby preventing bleeding from transected muscle bellies. The incision is then carried through the skin and soft tissues to the bone. If the arteries are patent, the assistant applies circumferential pressure to the distal calf. The distal tibia and fibula are then divided with a Gigli saw. Hemostasis is achieved with suture ligation and electrocauterization. A moist dressing is applied.

OUTCOME

After the procedure, the patient is kept on bed rest and given systemic antibiotics. Formal below-the-knee amputation can be performed when the cellulitis resolves, usually within 3 to 5 days. Routine dressing changes are unnecessary—first, because they are painful, and second, because the decision to proceed with formal below-the-knee amputation is based on the extent of the cellulitis in the calf, not on the appearance of the transected ankle.

Below-the-Knee Amputation

OPERATIVE PLANNING

Below-the-knee amputation is indicated when the lower extremity is functional but the foot cannot be salvaged by arterial reconstruction or by amputation of one or more of the toes or the forefoot. Healing can be expected if there is a palpable femoral pulse with at least a patent deep femoral artery, provided that the skin is warm and free of lesions at the distal calf. Before formal below-the-knee amputation, infection should be controlled with antibiotic therapy, debridement, and, if indicated, guillotine amputation. It is advisable to obtain consent to possible above-the-knee amputation beforehand in case unexpected muscle necrosis is encountered below the knee.

As with any amputation, the surgeon's preoperative interaction with the patient should be as positive as possible. A constructive perspective to convey is that the amputation, though regrettably nec-

sary, is in fact the first step toward rehabilitation. A well-motivated patient whose cardiopulmonary status is not too greatly compromised can generally be expected to walk again, albeit at an increased energy cost. In this regard, a preoperative discussion with a physiatrist can be very helpful, as can a meeting with an amputee who is doing well with a prosthesis. By inculcating a positive attitude in the patient before the procedure, the surgeon can greatly improve the patient's chances of achieving full rehabilitation as well as decrease the time needed for rehabilitation.

OPERATIVE TECHNIQUE

Epidural, spinal, or general anesthesia is appropriate.

The lines of incision should be marked on the skin. The primary level of amputation is determined by measuring a distance of 10 cm from the tibial tuberosity [*see Figure 7*]. The circumference of the leg at this level is then measured by passing a heavy ligature around the leg and cutting the ligature to a length equal to the circumference. The ligature is folded into thirds and cut once more at one of the folds, so that two segments of unequal length remain. The longer segment of the ligature, which is equal in length to two thirds of the leg's circumference 10 cm below the tibial tuberosity, is used to measure the anterior transverse incision; this incision is centered not on the tibial crest but on the gastrocnemius-soleus muscle complex. The shorter segment, which is one third of the leg's circumference at this level, is used to measure the posterior flap; the line of the posterior incision runs parallel with the gastrocnemius-soleus complex. To prevent dog-ears, the medial and lateral ends of the anterior transverse incision are curved cephalad before meeting the posterior incision, and the distal corners of the posterior incision are curved as well [*see Figure 7*].

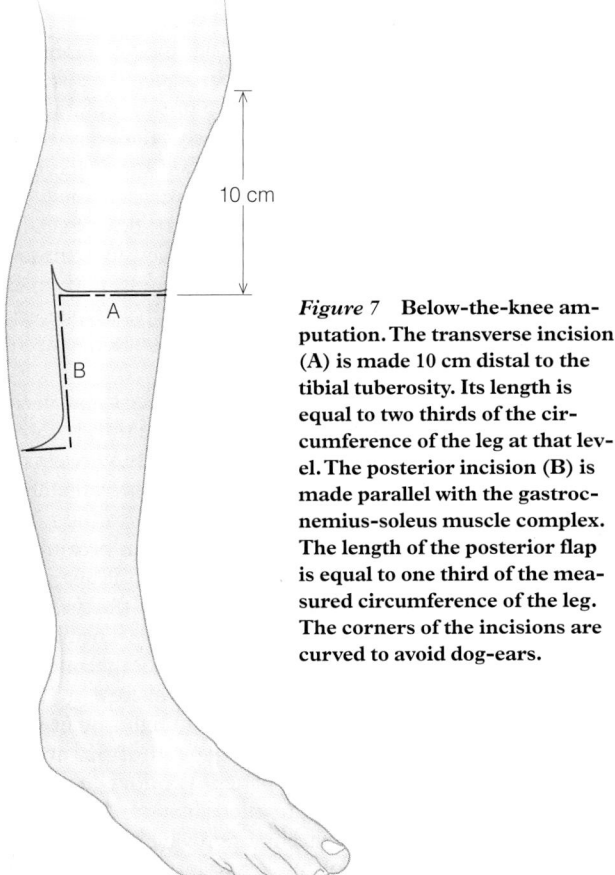

Figure 7 **Below-the-knee amputation. The transverse incision (A) is made 10 cm distal to the tibial tuberosity. Its length is equal to two thirds of the circumference of the leg at that level. The posterior incision (B) is made parallel with the gastrocnemius-soleus muscle complex. The length of the posterior flap is equal to one third of the measured circumference of the leg. The corners of the incisions are curved to avoid dog-ears.**

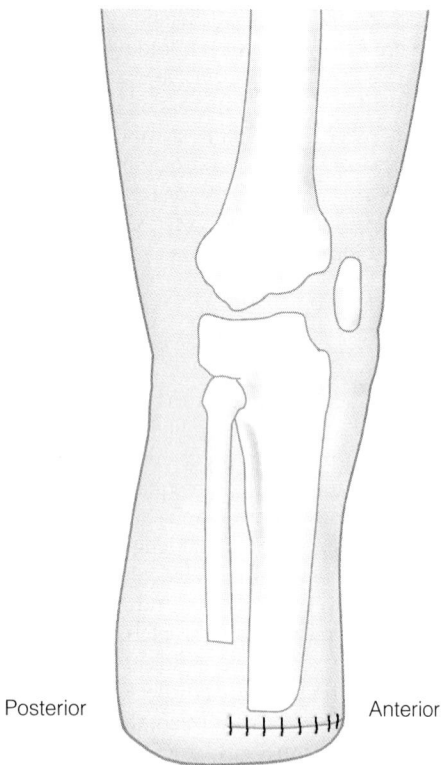

Figure 8 **Below-the-knee amputation. In this lateral view of the right leg, the tibia is beveled anteriorly, and the anterior portion is smoothed with a rasp. The fibula is transected at least 1 cm proximal to the level of transection of the tibia.**

Blood loss can be reduced by using a sterile pneumatic tourniquet. A gauze roll is passed around the distal thigh. The leg is elevated to drain the venous blood, and the tourniquet is applied over the gauze roll. The tourniquet is inflated to a pressure of 250 mm Hg (350 to 400 mm Hg if the patient has heavily calcified arteries). The assistant elevates the leg, and the incision on the posterior flap is made first, followed by the anterior transverse incision; this sequence helps prevent blood from obscuring the field while the incisions are being made. The incisions are carried fully through the dermis, and the skin edges are allowed to separate and expose the subcutaneous fat. Care is taken to keep the scalpel perpendicular to the skin so as not to bevel the incision, which can lead to necrosis of the epidermal edges [*see Figure 2*].

The anterior muscles are transected with the scalpel in a direction parallel to the transverse skin incision. The tibia is scored circumferentially, and a periosteal elevator is used to dissect the soft tissues away from the tibia for a distance of approximately 3 to 4 cm. The tibia is then transected just proximal to the transverse skin incision. Dividing the tibia more than 1 cm proximal to the anterior skin incision will cause the thin skin of the anterior leg to be pulled taut over the cut end of the tibia by the weight of the posterior flap, thereby leading to skin ulceration. The tibia is transected perpendicularly, with a cephalad bevel of the anterior 1 cm to keep from creating a sharp point at the tibial crest [*see Figure 8*]. The tibia can be transected with either a Gigli saw or an oscillating saw; because of the unpleasant sound of the power saw, the Gigli saw is preferred if the patient is under regional anesthesia. Sedation should be augmented in awake patients before division of the tibia. Benzodiazepines provide good sedation and amnesia.

The lateral muscles are divided, and the fibula is scored circumfer-

entially. A periosteal elevator is used to dissect the soft tissues away from the fibula to a point 2 to 3 cm cephalad to the level at which the tibia was transected. The fibula is then transected with a bone cutter at least 1 cm cephalad to the tibial transection level. The distal end of the tibia is lifted with a bone hook, and division of the posterior muscles is completed with an amputation knife. The specimen is then handed off the field.

The anterior tibial, posterior tibial, and peroneal arteries and veins are clamped, and the tourniquet is released. Clamps are placed on all other bleeding vessels. The posterior tibial and sural nerves are placed on gentle traction and clamped proximally. The distal nerves are transected, and the proximal nerves are allowed to retract into the soft tissues so as to prevent painful neuromas at the end of the stump. All clamped structures are then ligated with absorbable ligatures. The nerves are ligated because their nutrient vessels can bleed significantly. The distal anterior tip of the tibia is smoothed with a rasp to decrease the risk of skin ulceration over this osseous prominence. The stump is gently irrigated to remove all thrombus and devitalized tissue and to reveal any bleeding sites that may have been missed. Electrocauterization is rarely necessary.

The deep muscle fascia—not the Achilles tendon—is approximated with simple interrupted absorbable sutures, with care taken to align the posterior flap with the anterior incision. The dermis is approximated as a separate layer with simple interrupted absorbable sutures; if correctly placed, the dermal sutures should take all tension off the skin. The skin edges are then accurately apposed with interrupted vertical mattress sutures composed of monofilament nonabsorbable material. A carefully padded posterior splint or cast is applied to prevent flexion contracture.

COMPLICATIONS

The most common complications after below-the-knee amputation are bleeding, infection, and failure to heal, all of which are likely to result in a more proximal amputation, frequently accompanied by loss of the knee. Prevention of these complications depends on careful patient selection, preoperative control of infection, and meticulous surgical technique.

To walk with a prosthetic leg, the patient must be able to fully extend and lock the knee; thus, flexion contracture at the knee is a major complication. Such contractures are usually attributable either to poor pain control or to noncompliance with knee extension exercises. Good perioperative analgesia is of vital importance because knee flexion is the position of comfort and the patient will be unwilling to extend the knee if doing so proves too painful. To maintain knee extension, the patient should be placed in either a cast or a splint in the early postoperative period. Once postoperative pain has abated, the splint or cast can be removed. At this point, the patient must be taught extension exercises, in which the quadriceps muscles are contracted to maintain the length of the hamstring muscles. If a patient spends all of his or her time in a sitting position with the knee flexed, a flexion contracture will quickly develop. Once this happens, the patient may find it very difficult to regain full knee extension, and without full knee extension, prosthetic limb rehabilitation is impossible.

Phantom sensation is a common complication after below-the-knee amputation but is rarely of any consequence. Phantom pain, on the other hand, can be devastating. Sometimes, phantom pain develops as a consequence of unintentional suggestions made to the patient by medical personnel who fail to distinguish between the two entities. For example, a patient remarks to a medical attendant that he or she can still feel the amputated foot and toes, and the attendant suggests in response that the patient has phantom pain; the patient then focuses on the sensation and exaggerates the severity of

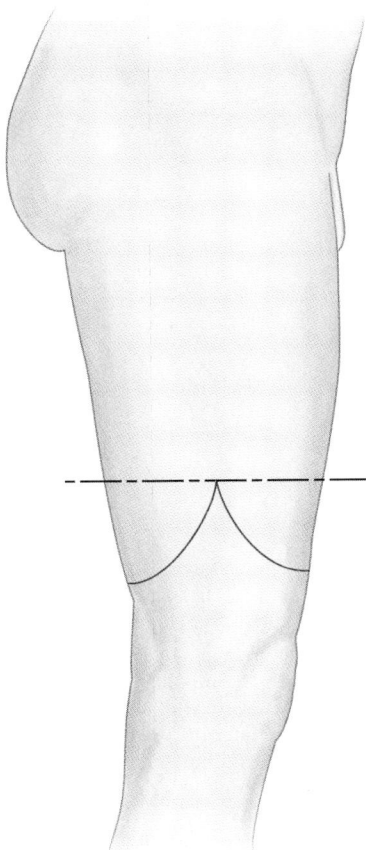

Figure 9   **Above-the-knee amputation. Broadly based anterior and posterior flaps are created. The femur is transected along the dashed line, at the apices of the skin flaps. The skin flaps and the level of transection of the femur can be placed more proximally if clinically indicated.**

the foot and toe discomfort, setting up a cycle of ever-worsening pain. This scenario is even more likely if the patient has had prolonged ischemic rest pain before the amputation. Phantom pain can be prevented by (1) encouraging early amputation in a patient with a hopelessly ischemic foot (while taking into account the patient's need to come to grips with the prospect of amputation), (2) providing good pain control in the early postoperative period, and (3) assuring the patient that phantom sensation after a below-the-knee amputation is common and that any discomfort in the foot immediately after the operation period will vanish once he or she begins walking again with a prosthetic leg.

Ulceration of the skin over the transected anterior portion of the tibia is another serious complication that may preclude successful prosthetic limb fitting. This complication is also best managed through prevention, which depends on meticulous surgical technique. As noted (see above), the anterior tibial crest must be carefully beveled and smoothed at the level of transection, and the tibia must not be transected more than 1 cm proximal to the anterior skin incision.

OUTCOME

Shortly after the amputation, the patient should be encouraged to start working on strengthening the upper body; upper-body strength is critical for making transfers and for using parallel bars, crutches, or a walker. In patients who have preoperative intractable ischemic rest pain, postoperative administration of epidural analgesia can break

the cycle of pain. Once postoperative pain is adequately controlled, patients are taught to transfer in and out of a wheelchair. A compression garment is used on the stump once the sutures have been removed and the stump is fully healed.

Prosthetic rehabilitation begins when the stump achieves a conical shape. Unfortunately, a number of patients who have undergone amputation for ischemia are unable to walk with a prosthetic limb because of comorbid medical conditions and general debility. In many cases, however, even if full ambulation is impossible, patients can maintain relative independence if the knee is salvaged by using a combination of a prosthetic leg and a walker for transfers and movement around the house.

Above-the-Knee Amputation

OPERATIVE PLANNING

Above-the-knee amputation is indicated if the lower extremity is unsalvageable and there is no femoral pulse. The presence of pulsatile flow into a well-developed ipsilateral internal iliac artery usually ensures healing, but even when there is more severe arterial occlusive disease in the pelvis, healing can sometimes be achieved. Above-the-knee amputation is also indicated if there is tissue necrosis or uncontrollable infection extending cephalad to the midleg. Above-the-knee amputation is the procedure of choice in the case of gangrene or ulceration of a completely nonfunctional lower extremity.

OPERATIVE TECHNIQUE

Epidural, spinal, or general anesthesia may be used.

For the best functional results, it is desirable to keep the femur as long as possible. A longer stump improves the prognosis for prosthetic limb rehabilitation and provides better balance for sitting and transfers. Healing potential, however, is lower with a longer stump; therefore, if the pelvic circulation is severely compromised, a shorter stump should be fashioned.

Anterior and posterior flaps of equal length are marked on the skin. The flaps should be wide and long [*see Figure 9*], and their apices should be centered on the line dividing the anterior and posterior muscle compartments. The posterior incision is made first to minimize the presence of blood in the operative field. The anterior incision is made second and carried through the anterior muscles in a plane parallel to the skin incision. The skin incisions are carried through the dermis, and the skin edges are allowed to separate and expose the subcutaneous fat; as in other amputations, they should be perpendicular to the skin surface so as not to undermine the skin.

If the superficial femoral artery is patent, the artery and vein are isolated and clamped after the sartorius muscle is divided but before the remainder of the anterior muscles are divided. The femur is scored circumferentially. The soft tissues are dissected away from the femur to the level of the apices of the flaps, and the femur is divided with an oscillating saw at this level. If the end of the resected femur extends beyond the apices of the flaps, the wound cannot be closed without tension. The posterior flap is completed with an amputation knife, and the specimen is handed off the field.

All bleeding points are clamped and tied with absorbable sutures. The sciatic nerve is placed on gentle traction, clamped, divided, and ligated, and the transected nerve is allowed to retract into the muscles. The deep fascia is approximated with interrupted absorbable sutures, with adjustments made for any discrepancy in length between the two flaps. The dermis is approximated with interrupted absorbable sutures; the dermal sutures should take all tension off

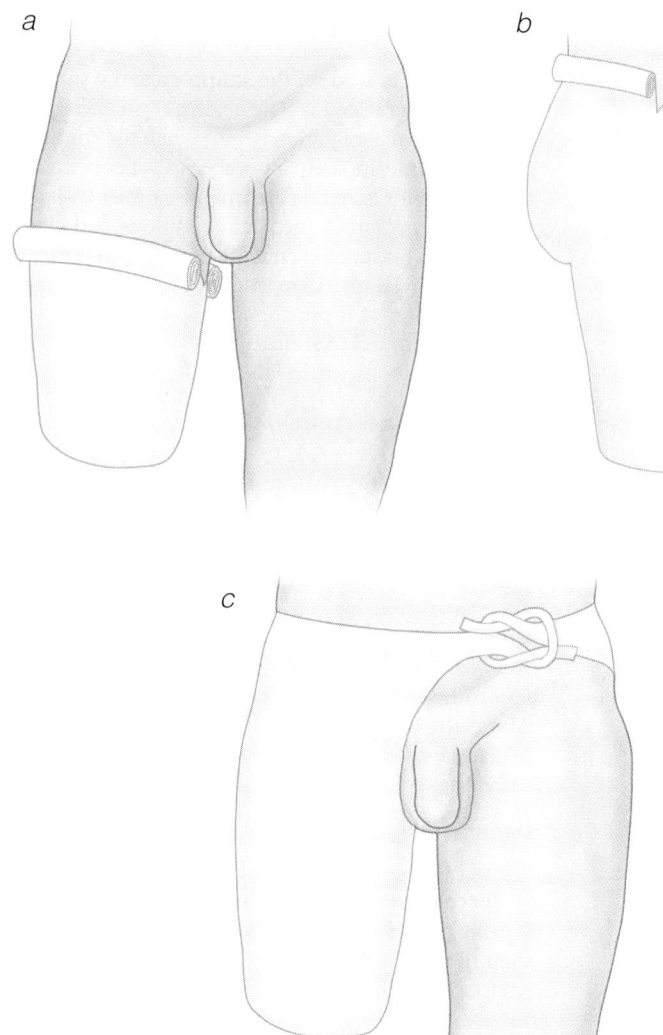

Figure 10 **Above-the-knee amputation. (*a*) After an aerosol tincture of benzoin is applied to the thigh, the hip, and the lower abdomen, a 4 in. wide stockinette is rolled over the amputation stump. The cuff of the stockinette is cut medially at the groin. (*b*) The remainder of the stockinette is then rolled laterally up over the hip, and the cuff is cut on the lateral midline. (*c*) The two resulting strips of cloth are passed around the waist, one anteriorly and one posteriorly, and these strips are tied on the anterior midline to complete the dressing.**

the skin. The skin edges are then carefully apposed with interrupted vertical mattress sutures.

A nonadherent dressing is placed on the suture line and covered with dry, fluffed gauze bandages. An aerosol tincture of benzoin is sprayed on the thigh, the hip, and the lower abdomen. When the benzoin is dry, a cloth stockinette with a diameter of 4 in. is stretched over the stump [*see Figure 10*]. The cuff of the stockinette is cut medially at the groin, and the stockinette is rolled laterally above the hip, where the cuff is then cut on the midaxillary line. This process yields two strips of cloth, one anterior and one posterior, which are passed around the patient's waist and tied on the anterior midline.

If the patient is a candidate for prosthetic limb rehabilitation, a traction rope is passed through a hole cut in the distal end of the stockinette and tied. The traction rope is hung over the end of the bed and tied to a 5 lb weight; this step helps prevent flexion contracture at the hip.

The stockinette need not be removed for the wound to be inspected. A window is cut in the distal end of the stockinette, and the gauze is removed. Once the incision has been inspected, fresh gauze is applied, and the window in the stockinette is closed with safety pins.

COMPLICATIONS

Postoperative complications include bleeding, infection, and fail-

ure to heal, all of which are likely to result in the need for surgical revision of the amputation stump. Control of preoperative infection and meticulous surgical technique and hemostasis are necessary to prevent these complications.

Flexion contracture of the hip is a major complication of above-the-knee amputation. Such contractures preclude successful prosthetic limb rehabilitation. In dealing with this complication, prevention is far more effective than treatment: once a flexion contracture at the hip becomes fixed, it is very difficult to reverse. If a patient is a candidate for prosthetic limb rehabilitation, the traction weight mentioned earlier (see above) can be very helpful. As soon as postoperative pain is controlled, the patient should be taught to spend three periods daily in a prone position to help extend the hip. He or she should then be taught exercises for maintaining range of motion in the hip before prosthetic limb rehabilitation is initiated. Flexion contracture of the hip is less of a problem in nonambulatory patients; however, it can still lead to wound breakdown and chronic skin ulceration.

OUTCOME

Once postoperative pain has abated, patients are mobilized to wheelchair transfers. The prognosis for successful prosthetic limb ambulation in patients undergoing above-the-knee amputation for ischemia is very poor.

References

1. Reichle FA, Rankin KP, Tyson RR, et al: Long-term results of 474 arterial reconstructions for severely ischemic limbs: a fourteen year follow-up. Surgery 85: 93, 1979

2. Maini BS, Mannick JA: Effect of arterial reconstruction on limb salvage. Arch Surg 113:1297, 1978

3. Ellitsgaard N, Andersson AP, Fabrin J, et al: Outcome in 282 lower extremity amputations: knee salvage and survival. Acta Orthop Scand 61:140, 1990

4. Stewart CPU, Jain AS, Ogston SA: Lower limb amputee survival. Prosthet Orthot Int 16:11, 1992

5. Inderbitzi R, Buttiker M, Pfluger D, et al: The fate of bilateral lower limb amputees in end-stage vascular disease. Eur Vasc Surg 6:321, 1992

Acknowledgment

Figures 1 through 10   Tom Moore.

15 VASCULAR AND PERITONEAL ACCESS

Bernard Montreuil, M.D., Laurie Morrison, M.D., Lawrence Rosenberg, M.D., Ph.D., F.A.C.S., and Carl Nohr, M.D., Ph.D., F.A.C.S., F.R.C.S.(C)

Vascular Access via Arteriovenous Fistulas

The number of patients with end-stage renal disease (ESRD) in the United States increased steadily through the 1990s, reaching 300,000 by the end of 1997.[1] Extracorporeal dialysis of blood was introduced in 1943 by Kolff and associates[2]; however, application of this approach was hindered by the requirement for repeated and routine access to the circulation. The full potential of hemodialysis for patient salvage was realized only after the introduction of the external arteriovenous (AV) shunt by Quinton and colleagues in 1960[3] and of the endogenous AV fistula (AVF) by Brescia and coworkers in 1966.[4] The subsequent introduction of synthetic vascular prostheses has permitted continued access in patients who have exhausted peripheral venous sites[5]; however, the long-term performance of such prostheses remains inferior to that of autogenous fistulas. The creation and maintenance of functioning vascular access, along with the associated complications, constitute the most common cause of morbidity, hospitalization, and cost in patients with end-stage renal disease.

The ideal vascular access route permits a flow rate that is adequate for the dialysis prescription ($\geq$ 300 ml/min), can be used for extended periods, and has a low complication rate. The native AVF remains the gold standard. In 1997, the National Kidney Foundation Dialysis Outcome and Quality Initiative (NKF-DOQI)[6] organized multidisciplinary work groups that evaluated all available data on vascular access and concluded that quality of life and overall outcome could be improved significantly for hemodialysis patients if two primary goals were achieved:

1. Increased placement of native AVFs: a minimum of 50% of new dialysis patients should have primary AVFs.
2. Detection of dysfunctional access before thrombosis of the access route occurs.

OPERATIVE PLANNING

At least 4 to 6 weeks—preferably 3 to 4 months—is required for a native AVF to heal and mature before it can be used. Therefore, access planning should be done early in the course of progressive renal failure. Patients should be referred for surgical treatment when creatinine clearance approaches 25 ml/min, the serum creatinine level reaches 4 mg/dl, or dialysis is likely to be necessary within 1 year. Every effort should be made not to puncture forearm veins, particularly the cephalic veins of the nondominant arm; the dorsal hand veins may be used for venipuncture. Subclavian vein catheterization should also be avoided because of the risk of central vein stenosis, which may preclude the use of any part of the ipsilateral arm for vascular access.

Assessment of Venous System

A history of subclavian vein cannulation or transvenous pacemaker placement is associated with a 10% to 40% rate of central vein stenosis or thrombosis.[7] Previous injuries or operative procedures involving the arm, the neck, or the chest, including previous vascular access, also may give rise to significant venous abnormalities. Physical signs of venous outflow obstruction include extremity edema, differences in arm size, and development of collateral veins. All of these historical and physical findings call for investigation by means of phlebography or color flow duplex scanning.[8] Central vein stenosis greater than 50% is a contraindication to creation of an ipsilateral distal AVF: it is a predictor of venous hypertension and edema in the arm and of poor function in the fistula.

Selection of the ideal vein for access is facilitated by distending the veins with a tourniquet around the upper arm. In particular, the cephalic vein is palpated from the region of the anatomic snuffbox to the area above the elbow. Percussion of the vein is performed to confirm that it is patent and to rule out stenosis from previous venipuncture. The fingertips of one hand are positioned over the vein at the elbow, and the vein is gently tapped distally with the other hand. If the vein is patent and of substantial diameter, a fluid wave is felt over the proximal vein.

Assessment of Arterial System

A history of arterial trauma or catheterization, diabetes mellitus, or peripheral arterial disease may be associated with chronic damage to the arterial system. Physical examination involves palpation of the pulses (including both brachial and axillary pulses) and comparison of blood pressure in the arms. A difference of more than 20 mm Hg between the two sides suggests proximal arterial occlusive disease, which may cause the AVF to fail as a result of inadequate inflow. An Allen test is also performed to confirm that the palmar arch is patent, to determine which artery is the dominant vascular supply to the hand, and to ensure that the ulnar artery can support the hand if the radial artery must be divided. Any abnormality on physical examination should be further investigated by means of arterial studies in the vascular laboratory; in select cases, angiography may be indicated.

Noninvasive Preoperative Assessment

Systematic use of noninvasive evaluation in the vascular laboratory permits objective assessment of arterial and venous conduits. If necessary, venous conduits other than the cephalic and basilic veins may be identified,[9] and both arterial and venous segments may be mapped with skin marks to facilitate the operative procedure. The aims are to increase the use of autogenous fistulas and to raise the early and late patency rates by decreasing the use of suboptimal veins and arteries.

Complete noninvasive assessment includes segmental pressure measurements of the upper extremity, arterial waveform recording, and arterial and venous duplex studies. A tourniquet should be placed on the arm, and tapping and stroking maneuvers should be used to distend the vein maximally. Established criteria [see Table 1] are then applied to determine whether venous outflow and arterial inflow are likely to be satisfactory.

Choice of Type of AVF

Multiple varieties of AV fistulas have been used in hemodialysis patients. According to the NKF-DOQI report,[6] the order of preference for AV fistulas in patients requiring long-term hemodialysis is as follows:

1. Wrist (radiocephalic) primary AV fistula.
2. Elbow (brachiocephalic) primary AV fistula.

If neither of these can be constructed, access may be achieved via either of the following:

3. AV graft of synthetic material.
4. Transposed brachiobasilic AV fistula.

All of these fistulas should be established in the nondominant arm, if possible.

The distal radiocephalic AVF remains the gold standard in terms of ease of creation and long-term results. Its advantages considerably outweigh its disadvantages—namely, a higher primary failure rate (10% to 15%) and a long maturation time (1 to 4 months). Radiocephalic AVFs may be constructed either in the anatomic snuff-box or just above the wrist crease. Although the radial artery is smaller in the snuff-box than it is at the classical Brescia-Cimino fistula site, the long-term results at the two sites are comparable if only arteries of adequate diameter are used.[10]

An alternative method of creating an AVF in the forearm that was not mentioned in the NKF-DOQI report is vein transposition.[11] Preoperative duplex ultrasonography often identifies veins that, except for their deep subcutaneous location, are suitable for AVF formation. In addition, the basilic vein in the forearm is often spared and is frequently suitable for AVF formation; however, use of this vein in situ for needle cannulation and hemodialysis may necessitate placing the forearm in an uncomfortable position. In the great majority of cases, such veins can be successfully transposed to a superficial tunnel in the midportion of the volar aspect of the forearm, and the resulting fistula theoretically has the same advantages as a radiocephalic fistula in terms of long-term patency and complication rates. This aggressive approach to autogenous forearm fistula formation also has the advantage of preserving more proximal vessels for future access placement.

If duplex ultrasonography does not identify an adequate forearm vein conduit, a brachiocephalic primary AVF is the next choice. It is easy to create and has the advantage of providing higher blood flow than the wrist fistula. The cephalic vein in the upper arm, because of its position and superficial location, is easy to cannulate and easily covered (a potential cosmetic benefit). The elbow AVF has a theoretical advantage in diabetic patients, in whom medial calcification of the distal radial artery commonly prevents the gradual arterial dilatation required for full maturation of a radiocephalic fistula. In fact, some authors[12] consider an upper-arm autogenous AVF (either a brachiocephalic or a transposed basilic vein fistula) the preferred approach in this particular subgroup of patients. Disadvantages of

brachiocephalic fistulas include higher frequencies of arm swelling and steal syndrome than are seen with forearm fistulas.

If the cephalic vein in the upper arm is unsuitable, the remaining options include a prosthetic graft and transposed basilic vein. An AVF using transposed basilic vein has all the attributes of an autogenous fistula and consequently is preferred to a graft despite being more difficult to create. Its protected, deep subfascial position and large caliber make it a high-quality conduit for hemodialysis access. Its advantages over a prosthetic graft include the avoidance of the distal venous anastomosis (which causes the majority of stenoses in synthetic graft fistulas) and higher primary and secondary patency rates.[13,14] Flow rates are high in basilic vein fistulas because of the large size of the vein, and the infection rate is relatively low. Furthermore, thrombosis of a brachiobasilic fistula does not compromise the integrity of the axillary vein and thus does not preclude subsequent use of a prosthetic conduit at the same site.

If no veins in either upper extremity are suitable for a native AVF, then the use of prosthetic material should be considered. Two options are available. First, if a segment of vein at least 15 cm long is available but is too far from the artery to be used in the creation of a fully native fistula, a jump graft can be constructed between the artery and the vein, and the arterialized vein can be used as the needle conduit for dialysis. Second, the graft itself can be used as the needle conduit for dialysis. The data currently available suggest that extruded polytetrafluoroethylene (ePTFE) is preferable to other biologic and synthetic materials: ePTFE grafts are less likely to disintegrate with infection, they are more widely available, they remain patent longer, and they are easily handled by surgeons. Grafts may be placed in straight, looped, or curved configurations on either the forearm or the upper arm.

OPERATIVE TECHNIQUE

Autogenous AVFs

Radiocephalic fistula The arm is placed on an arm board in 90° of abduction. A tourniquet is applied to the upper arm to distend the cephalic vein, and the vein's course is marked on the skin. The tourniquet is then released.

Local anesthesia using 0.5% or 1% lidocaine without epinephrine is usually adequate for construction of an autogenous AVF at the wrist or the antecubital fossa. General anesthesia may depress cardiac output and thus may, by reducing fistula flow, exert a negative impact on the success of the fistula. Conversely, brachial or supraclavicular regional anesthesia may cause peripheral vasodilatation and thus increase arterial blood flow.

Table 1 **Noninvasive Criteria for Selection of Upper-Extremity Arteries and Veins for Dialysis Access Procedures[9]**

Venous examination

Venous luminal diameter ≥ 2.5 mm for autogenous AVFs, ≥ 4.0 mm for bridge AV grafts

Absence of segmental stenoses or occluded segments

Continuity with the deep venous system in the upper arm

Absence of ipsilateral central vein stenosis or occlusion

Arterial examination

Arterial luminal diameter ≥ 2.0 mm

Absence of pressure differential ≥ 20 mm Hg between arms

Patent palmar arch

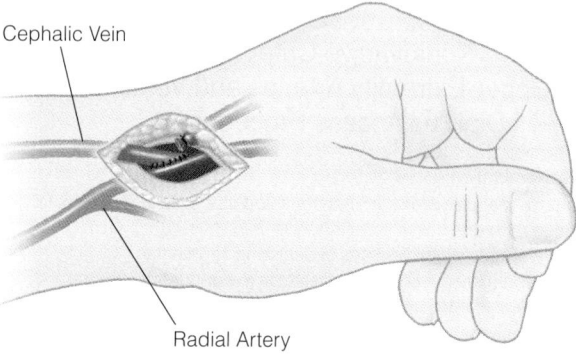

Figure 1 **Vascular access via AVFs: radiocephalic fistula. Shown is the anatomic snuff-box fistula, with the end of the cephalic vein anastomosed to the side of the radial artery.**

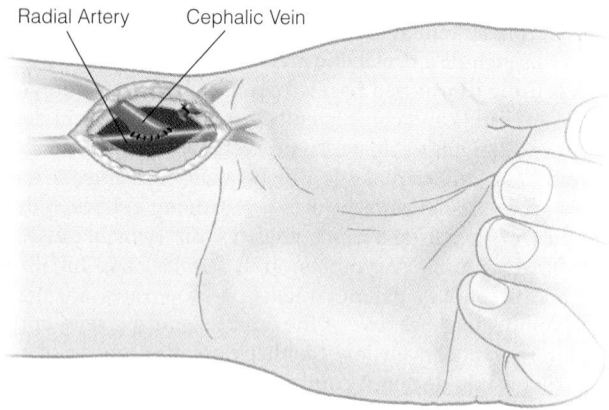

Figure 2 **Vascular access via AVFs: radiocephalic fistula. Shown is the Brescia-Cimino fistula. An incision is made midway between the radial artery and the cephalic vein, and the end of the vein is anastomosed to the side of the artery.**

A longitudinal incision is placed either in the anatomic snuff-box, between the tendons of the extensor pollicis longus and the extensor pollicis brevis [*see Figure 1*], or midway between the cephalic vein and the radial artery, proximal to the wrist skinfold [*see Figure 2*]. In the anatomic snuff-box, the cephalic vein overlies the radial artery, so that minimal mobilization is required to approximate the two vessels. Slightly more mobilization is required to approximate the cephalic vein to the radial artery above the wrist without kinking or twisting. A comparable length of radial artery, found under the deep fascia, is also isolated. Care is taken to preserve the superficial branch of the radial nerve, which lies lateral to the radial artery and is separated from it by the brachioradialis muscle.

Four types of anastomoses can be constructed: side to side, end of vein to side of artery, end to end, and end of artery to side of vein. The side-to-side anastomosis [*see Figure 3a*] yields the highest flow through the fistula but may be associated with venous congestion of the hand. Over time, arterial pressure may render the valves of the distal vein incompetent, resulting in retrograde flow toward the hand and venous hypertension. The end of artery–side of vein anastomosis [*see Figure 3b*] also presents a risk of venous hypertension. This configuration reduces the risk of distal steal by preventing retrograde flow into the fistula, but at the price of lower flow through the fistula. Of the four options, the end of artery–end of vein variation [*see Figure 3c*] produces the least distal arterial steal and venous hypertension but yields the lowest flow.

The preferred configuration of the anastomosis is end of vein to side of artery [*see Figure 3d*]. Dividing the vein reduces the risk of venous congestion in the hand; moreover, by allowing retrograde flow from the distal radial artery and the ulnar artery into the vein, which contributes approximately 30% of the total flow of the fistula, this approach yields maximal blood flow through the fistula. There is a risk of steal syndrome with such fistulas, but this problem is easily corrected by ligating the radial artery distal to the fistula, thereby converting the anastomosis to an end-to-end configuration.

Vascular control is obtained with small vessel loops or Heifets clamps. Heparinization is not needed unless the artery is an end artery. A 1 cm arteriotomy is performed, and the vein is ligated and divided distally and tailored to match the arteriotomy. Coronary dilators are then inserted gently to verify patency and to ensure that the vessel lumina are large enough: the artery should easily admit a 2 mm dilator; the vein, a 3 mm dilator. The vessels are then anastomosed in the desired configuration with a fine continuous monofilament suture (6-0 or 7-0 polypropylene) placed by means of standard techniques. The vessels can be probed with the coronary dilators before the anastomosis is completed, to confirm that the vein is not twisted or to overcome any arterial spasm. Once vascular control is released, a thrill should be easily felt over the fistula and for a moderate distance along the venous conduit. The skin is closed with an absorbable suture.

Vein transposition in the forearm The artery and the vein selected for the primary AVF are identified and mapped preoperatively by means of duplex ultrasonography. Positioning and anesthetic considerations are essentially the same as for a radiocephalic fistula.

A longitudinal incision is made directly over the mapped vein, beginning at its distal end and extending toward the antecubital fossa for a distance of at least 15 cm [*see Figure 4a*]. The vein is gently skeletonized and mobilized by ligating and dividing all side branches. The targeted artery (either the radial or the ulnar) is identified and dissected through a separate incision. A superficial subcutaneous tunnel is made between the two incisions with a blunt tunneling instrument, and the vein is passed through the tunnel [*see Figure 4b*]. The vein should be marked along its length with a marking pen before tunneling; this step provides a usual visual check that allows the surgeon to confirm that the vein is not twisted as it passes through the tunnel. A 1 cm anastomosis is then carried out in the same fashion as for a radiocephalic fistula (see above).

Brachiocephalic fistula After adequate local anesthesia, a transverse incision is made 1.5 cm distal to the antecubital crease[15] to expose the superficial antecubital venous system [*see Figure 5a*]. If the median cubital vein is patent, sufficiently wide, and in continuity with the cephalic vein, it is dissected so that the perforating branch of the antecubital venous system (vena mediana cubiti profunda) can be located. The bicipital aponeurosis is divided, and the perforating branch is followed down to the deep system. In the process, the brachial artery is also exposed, as are the origins of the radial and ulnar arteries.

Once the patient is fully heparinized, the confluence of the brachial vein and the perforating vein is identified, and part of the brachial vein is excised so as to form a venous patch. The perforating vein is gently dilated, so that any valves are rendered incompetent, and the proximal median cubital vein is ligated to prevent diversion of blood flow into the basilic vein. The perforating vein is then anastomosed to the brachial artery in an end-to-side fashion [*see Figure 5b*].[16] To prevent subsequent steal syndrome, the arteriotomy should be no larger than 5 to 6 mm.

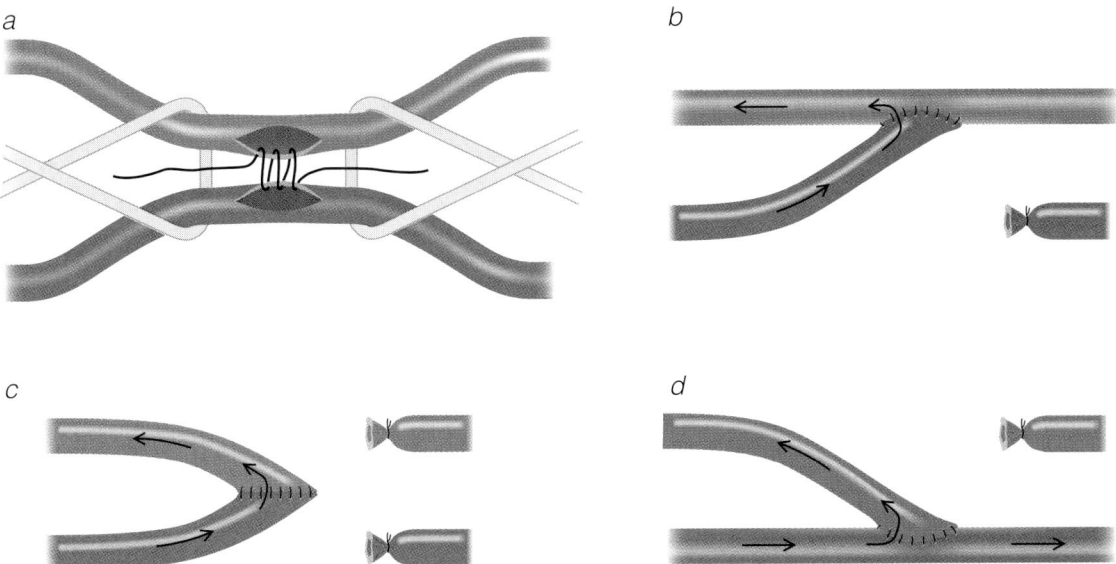

Figure 3 Vascular access via AVFs: radiocephalic fistula. Four anastomotic configurations are possible for an autologenous radiocephalic fistula: (*a*) side of artery to side of vein, (*b*) end of artery to side of vein, (*c*) end of artery to end of vein, and (*d*) end of vein to side of artery (the preferred configuration).

Other techniques may be used if the perforating vein is very large or very small. If the perforating vein is 5 mm or more in diameter, it may be anastomosed directly to the artery without a patch. If the vein is less than 2.5 mm in diameter, it should not be used; instead, the median cubital vein should be ligated and divided and the cephalic end of the vein anastomosed directly to the brachial artery in an end-to-side fashion [*see Figure 5c*]. If the median cubital vein is too small, the incision is extended laterally and proximally to allow mobilization of the cephalic vein. The length of this incision depends on the extent to which the cephalic vein must be mobi-

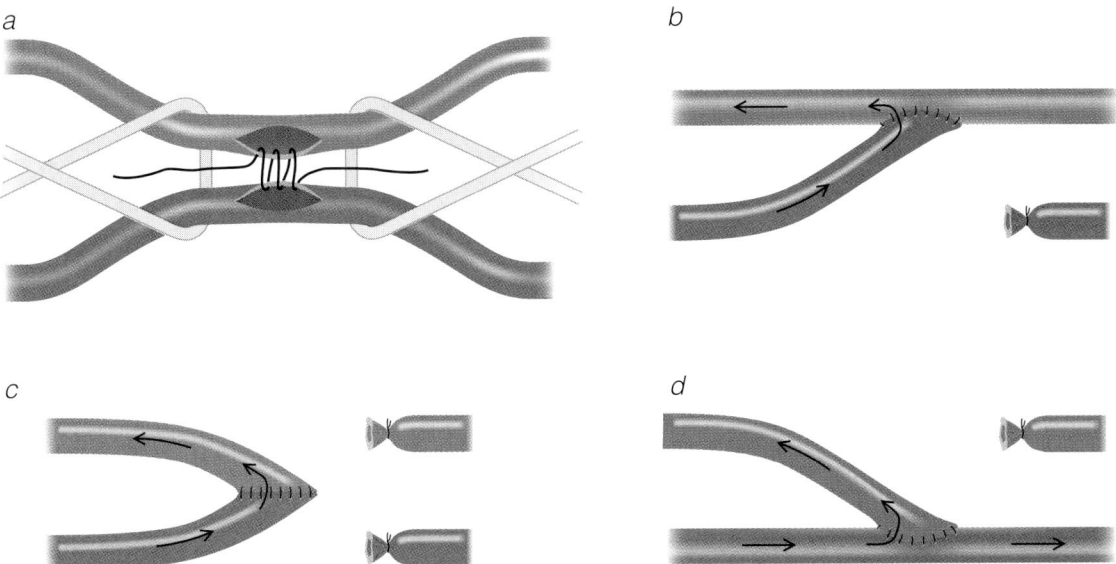

a

b

Radial Artery

Figure 4 **Vascular access via AVFs: vein transposition in the forearm. (*a*) The selected vein, identified by duplex ultrasonography, is completely mobilized. (*b*) The vein is transposed through a superficial tunnel in the midportion of the volar aspect of the forearm and anastomosed to the radial artery in an end-to-side fashion.**

lized to ensure a tension-free end-to-side anastomosis. The accessory cephalic vein, though located far laterally, may also be used.

Repeated venipunctures in the antecubital fossa frequently render the antecubital venous system unsuitable for AVF construction. In such cases, two options are available if the patient has at least 15 cm of good-quality cephalic vein in the upper arm. The first option is to mobilize a sufficient length of the cephalic vein in the distal upper arm through a longitudinal incision, to transpose it medially through a superficial tunnel, and then to anastomose it in an end-to-side fashion to the brachial artery, which has been exposed above the elbow through a separate incision. The second, which avoids extensive dissection of the cephalic vein, is to place two short longitudinal incisions over the brachial artery and the cephalic vein a few centimeters above the elbow crease, to tunnel a short segment of 6 mm ePTFE graft between the two incisions, and to anastomose the ePTFE graft to both the brachial artery and the cephalic vein in an end-to-side fashion [*see Figure 6*].[17] The cephalic vein is used as the needle conduit for this type of bridge AV graft.

Brachiobasilic fistula The technique for constructing a brachiobasilic fistula was described first by Dagher and associates in 1976[18] and then by Logerfo and colleagues in 1978.[19] Local anesthesia can be used, but an axillary block eases the procedure considerably.

An oblique incision overlying the median basilic vein is made in the antecubital fossa, and the vein is mobilized. The brachial artery is exposed as usual by dividing the bicipital aponeurosis. The incision is extended along the medial aspect of the upper arm (the so-called hockey-stick incision), and the basilic vein is mobilized from beneath the fascia, with care taken to preserve the medial cutaneous nerve of the forearm [*see Figure 7a*]. The basilic vein usually pierces the brachial fascia just below the middle of the upper arm, then parallels the course of the brachial artery and vein while remaining superficial to them. At the axillary level, the basilic vein joins the brachial vein to form the axillary vein; this junction constitutes the proximal limit of the dissection.

The distal end of the conduit vein may consist of either the basilic vein or a section of the median cubital vein, which is already exposed. All venous tributaries are ligated and divided. Once this is done, the vein is divided distally, and its anterior surface is

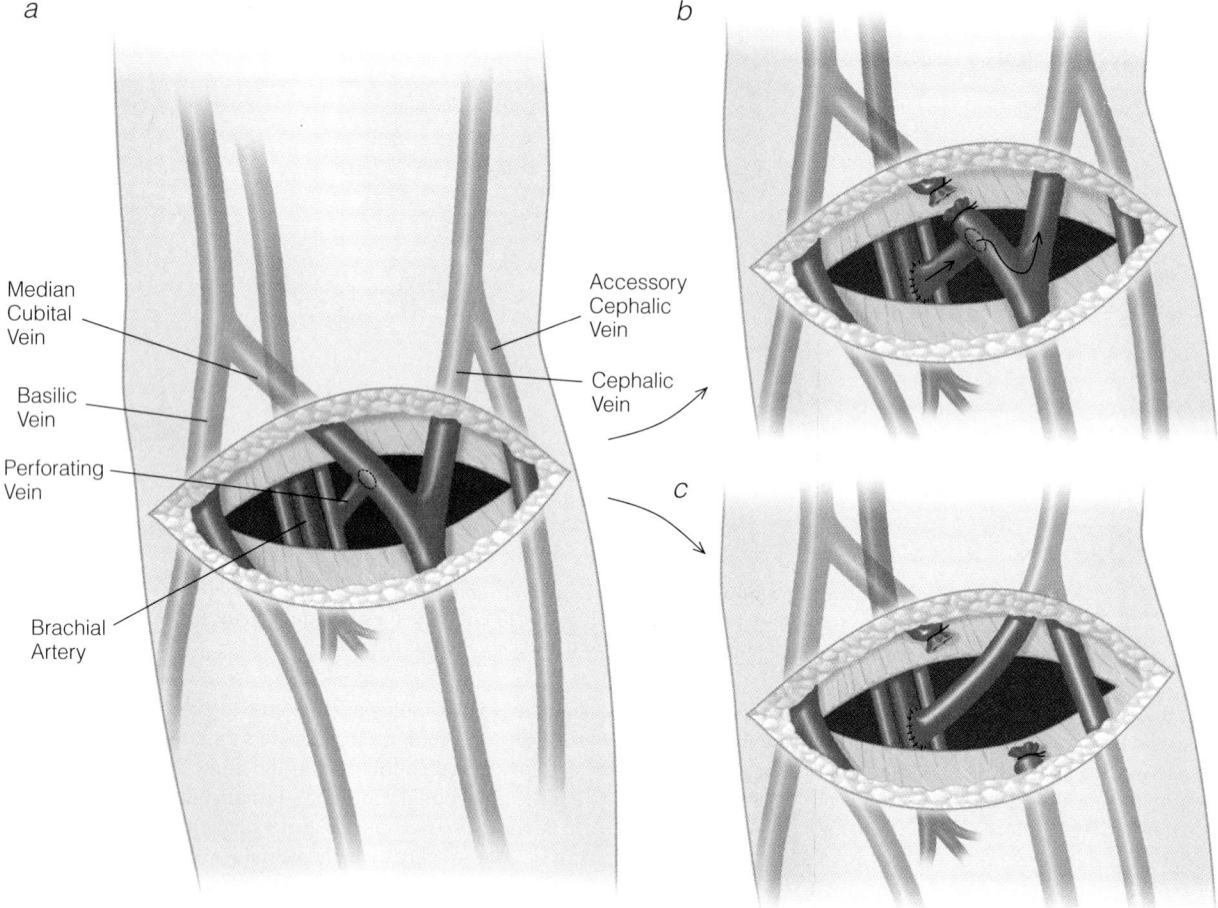

Figure 5 **Vascular access via AVFs: brachiocephalic fistula. (*a*) A transverse incision exposes the antecubital venous system (including the perforating branch) and the brachial artery under the bicipital aponeurosis. (*b*) An end-to-side anastomosis is made between the perforating vein and the brachial artery. (*c*) If the perforating vein is too small, the cephalic vein is mobilized and anastomosed to the brachial artery in an end-to-side fashion.**

marked to help the surgeon avoid axial rotation during transposition. The vein is then passed through a subcutaneous tunnel on the anterior surface of the arm and anastomosed in an end-to-side fashion to the brachial artery in the antecubital fossa with 6-0 or 7-0 polypropylene [*see Figure 7b*]. This transposition places the vein in a more superficial location and positions it anterolaterally on the arm, thereby facilitating cannulation during hemodialysis sessions. Closure involves approximating the fascia and the subcutaneous tissue in two separate layers.

A modification of the procedure just described is the so-called elevated basilic vein arteriovenous fistula.[20] In this variant, the vein is left in situ rather than transposed anterolaterally, but it is elevated by closing the deep fascia and the subcutaneous tissue beneath the vein. The brachial artery anastomosis is created, and the overlying skin is reapproximated with clips or interrupted sutures. Although the vein remains in its medial location, its new superficial position facilitates cannulation for dialysis.

Bridge AV Grafts

Bridge AV graft procedures involve placing an interposition graft between an artery and a vein and using that graft as the needle conduit for dialysis. In the forearm, the most common configurations are loop grafts between the brachial artery and an antecubital vein (including the brachial veins)[21] and straight bridge AV grafts from the radial artery to an antecubital vein. Most studies report superior patency rates with a loop configuration.[22] Adequate results may be obtained with a straight graft in the forearm if the radial artery is at least 2.5 to 3.0 mm in diameter.

Secondary options for bridge AV graft construction include a variety of unusual configurations, including reverse grafts between the axillary artery and the brachial or the antecubital vein and axilloaxillary grafts, which may be looped in the upper arm or may cross the sternum. It is also possible to construct a looped graft between the proximal superficial femoral artery and the proximal saphenous vein or a straight, reversed graft between the distal superficial femoral or popliteal artery and the proximal saphenous or femoral vein [*see Figure 8*]. Such lower-limb AV grafts are associated with an increased risk of potentially life- or limb-threatening infection and thus are used only as a last resort.

Either local anesthesia or axillary block is usually appropriate for upper-extremity bridge AV grafts. A single dose of a cephalosporin should be given before the procedure. Separate longitudinal incisions are placed to expose the artery and the vein—except when the procedure involves the brachial artery and the antecubital venous system, which are better exposed through a single transverse incision. A 6 mm or a tapered 4 to 7 mm ePTFE graft is then passed through a superficial tunnel between the two incisions. Both anastomoses are constructed in an end-to side fashion, beginning with the venous side. Systemic heparinization is used if an end artery is occluded for the arterial anastomosis.

TROUBLESHOOTING

Autogenous AVFs

Although the quality of the AV conduit is assessed preoperatively by means of physical examination and noninvasive studies, it should also be confirmed intraoperatively for optimal results.

Arterial inflow Normally, a strong pulse is felt over the targeted artery; however, dissection may cause spasm, which can render intra-operative assessment difficult. The following three measures will help minimize this problem:

1. Elimination of epinephrine from the anesthetic solution.
2. Gentle dissection and avoidance of direct manipulation of the arterial wall. It may be preferable to use a proximal tourniquet for inflow occlusion so that there is no need to place clamps on small arteries.
3. Local application of a papaverine solution, which relaxes vascular smooth muscle.

If spasm occurs, gentle probing of the artery with coronary dilators may help relieve the spasm and restore full flow.

Stiff, calcified arteries can sometimes be successfully used in the creation of fistulas, but it is difficult to assess flow in such vessels. Quantitative and qualitative analyses of the arterial waveform and the intraluminal diameter by means of duplex scanning can help confirm the adequacy of the vessel. Arteries smaller than 1.5 mm are less likely to provide sufficient flow for a fistula. It is particularly important not to place clamps on calcified arteries; a tourniquet is always preferred in this situation.

Venous outflow A venous diameter of at least 2.5 to 3.0 mm is required for successful maturation of an autogenous fistula. The diameter of the target vein should be known preoperatively from the duplex examination and should be confirmed intraop-

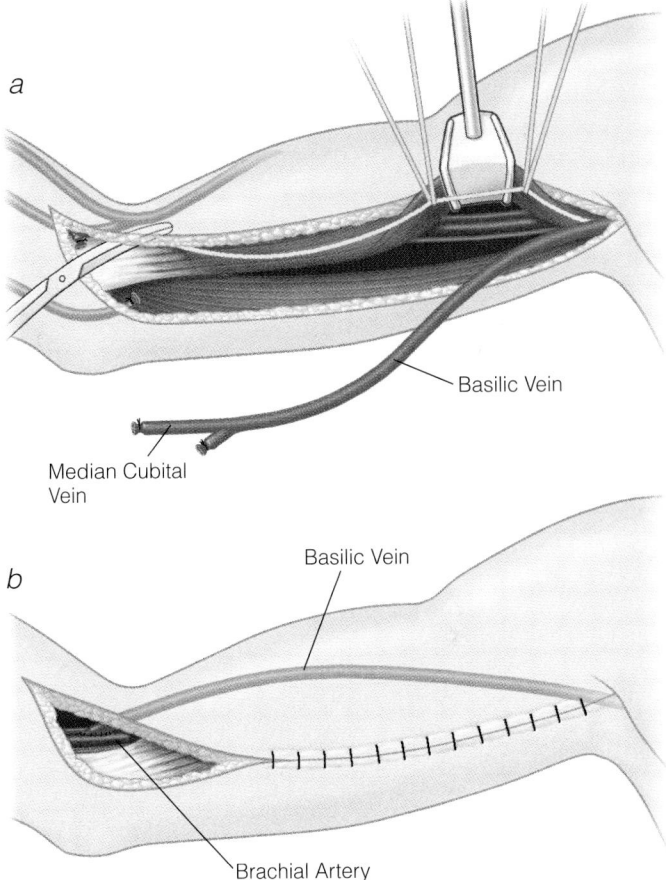

a

Basilic Vein

Median Cubital Vein

b

Basilic Vein

Brachial Artery

Figure 7 **Vascular access via AVFs: brachiobasilic fistula. (*a*) The basilic vein is completely mobilized from underneath the fascia in continuity with a section of the median cubital vein in the antecubital fossa. (*b*) The vein is transposed in a subcutaneous tunnel on the anterior surface of the arm and anastomosed to the brachial artery in an end-to-side fashion.**

eratively by calibration with coronary dilators. No attempt should be made to dilate the vein, however, because endothelial injury may result.

Webs, thickened valve leaflets, and areas of sclerosis from previous phlebitis or punctures are common in upper-extremity veins and may be the cause of poor venous outflow and fistula failure. Passage of the coronary dilator helps to localize such obstructive lesions, which should be corrected when found. The patency of the proximal vein can be demonstrated by free flow of injected heparinized saline or by successful passage of a Fogarty catheter. The evoked thrill is also a useful maneuver: intermittent, pulsatile injection of saline into the vein, mimicking arterial flow, should produce a palpable thrill over the proximal vein.[23] The absence of an evoked thrill suggests the presence of stenosis or areas of thickened, nondistensible vein wall proximally. Intraoperative phlebography is indicated in any doubtful situation.

AV anastomosis Both the artery and the vein should be mobilized sufficiently to ensure that the anastomosis is tension-free once completed. As noted (see above), marking the most superficial aspect of the vein with a sterile pen before mobilization helps ensure that the vein is not rotated when it is approximated to the artery. The ideal anastomosis is constructed by transecting the vein just distal to a bifurcation and using the branch vessel as

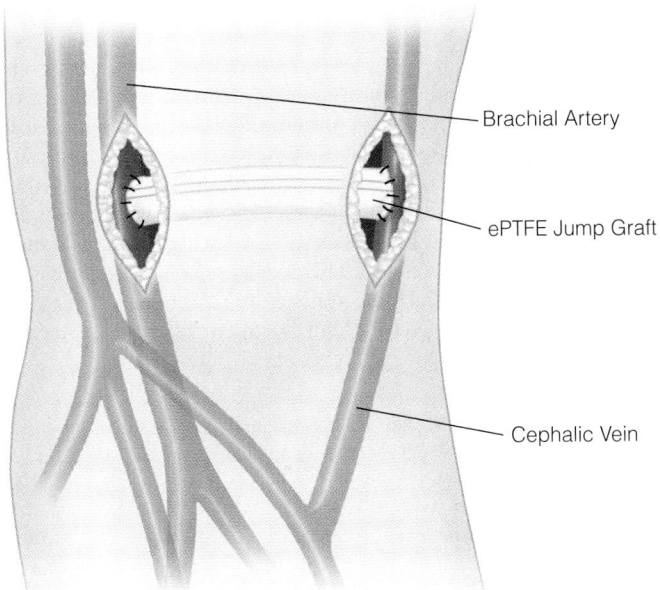

Brachial Artery

ePTFE Jump Graft

Cephalic Vein

Figure 6 **Vascular access via AVFs: brachiocephalic fistula. If the antecubital venous system is unsuitable for AVF construction, one option is to place an ePTFE interposition graft between the brachial artery and the cephalic vein.**

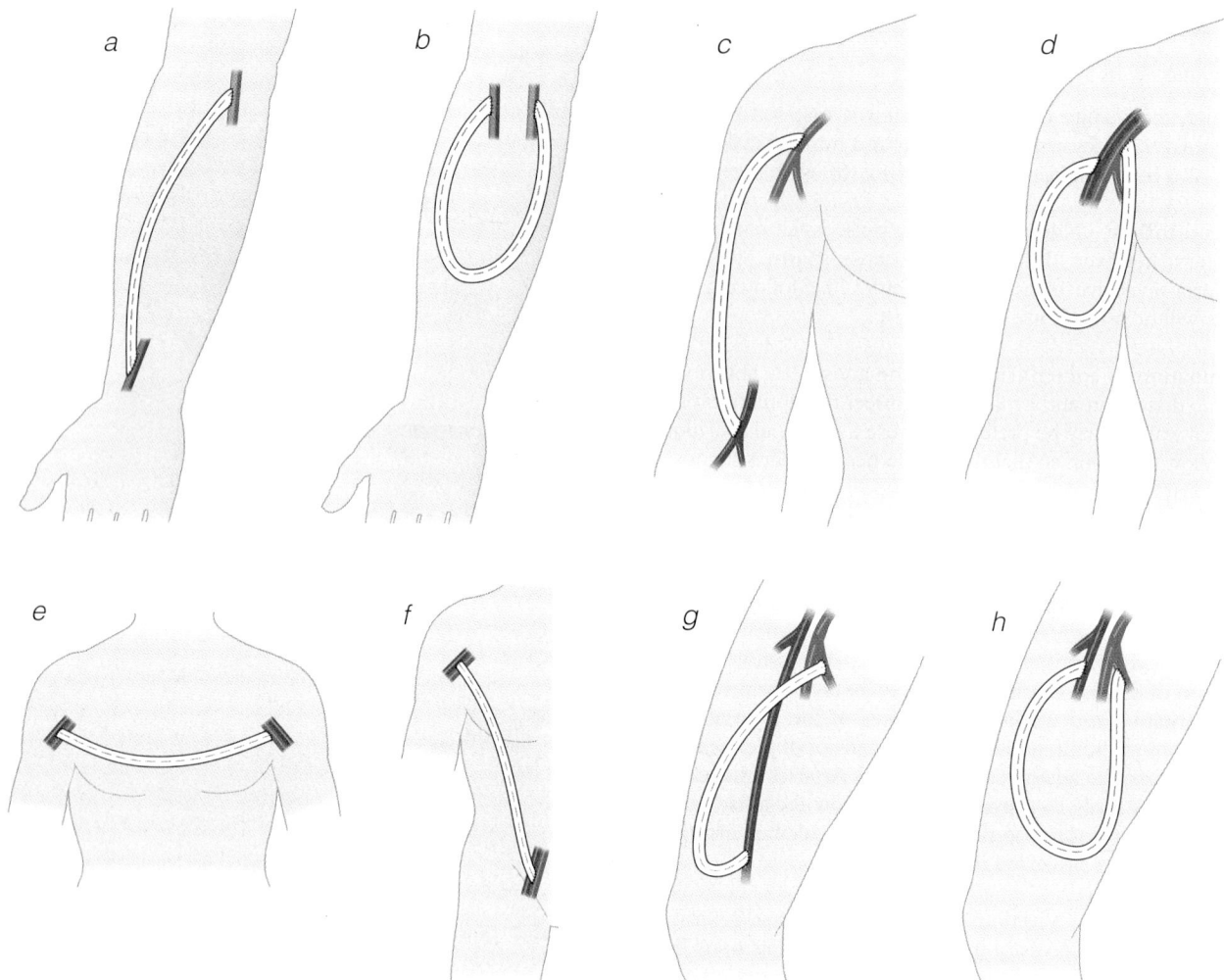

Figure 8 **Vascular access via AVFs: bridge AV grafts. Options for bridge graft construction include (*a*) straight forearm AV graft, (*b*) loop forearm AV graft, (*c*) brachioaxillary AV graft, (*d*) loop axilloaxillary AV graft, (*e*) axillary artery–contralateral axillary vein AV graft, (*f*) axillary artery–iliac vein AV graft, (*g*) distal superficial femoral or popliteal artery–saphenous vein AV graft, and (*h*) proximal superficial femoral artery–saphenous vein loop AV graft.**

a patch. Such a spatulated venous conduit facilitates the anastomosis and minimizes the risk of anastomotic stenosis.

For a distal AVF, the anastomosis should be about 10 mm long to ensure that a gradual increase in flow through the fistula can occur. An anastomosis that is too small may impair the normal dilation of the artery and the vein. For AVFs in the antecubital space and the upper arm, in contrast, the arteriotomy should be limited to 5 to 6 mm to prevent excessive shunting.

The anastomosis can be performed with standard vascular techniques. However, construction of the anastomosis with a single continuous suture may have a purse-string effect; accordingly, the use of two separate running sutures may be preferable for small vessels. Interrupted stitches are preferable for very small vessels. Loupes and microvascular instruments are helpful in this setting.

When the anastomosis is completed, vascular control should be released from the proximal vein and the distal artery first; the resultant back-bleeding will confirm the patency of the palmar arch and reveal any major anastomotic defects. Gentle compression is usually sufficient to obtain hemostasis. Any additional sutures deemed necessary should be placed with great caution because of the risk that they may narrow the anastomosis.

The presence of a pulse rather than a thrill in the arterialized vein indicates inadequate outflow, whereas the absence of either a thrill or a pulse indicates poor inflow. The draining vein should be examined for kinking, twisting, or compression by a fibrous band. If the vein appears to be satisfactory, the anastomosis and the distal vein are inspected and probed with dilators through a venous side branch or a transverse phlebotomy. If no abnormality is identified, the fistula is examined with I.V. contrast studies and fluoroscopy. Focal lesions may be corrected by placement of a vein patch or a short interposition graft or by resection and primary reanastomosis. Alternatively, a short segment of the vein may be excised and the anastomosis repositioned more proximally.

AV Grafts

Skin incisions Incisions should be placed so that neither the graft nor the anastomoses lie directly beneath them. Proper placement reduces the risk of skin erosion, minimizes the risk that the graft will become infected if a surgical site infection occurs, and maximizes the length of conduit available for needle insertion. The subcutaneous tissue and skin should be closed in separate layers to minimize the risk of graft infection in the event of skin dehiscence.

Tunneling The tunnel should be made atraumatically with a Kelly-Wick bidirectional tunneler. It should be superficial to the muscle fascia but no more than 5 mm beneath the skin surface. To decrease the risk of hematoma, there should be a close fit between the diameter of the graft and that of the tunnel, and the graft should be placed before systemic heparinization is initiated.

For a loop configuration, a counterincision at the apex of the tunnel permits the tunnel to be created in two passes of the Kelly-Wick tunneler. This approach gives the tunnel a smooth curve and limits kinking of the graft. In the forearm, this transverse counterincision is usually made 3 to 4 cm proximal to the wrist skinfold [*see Figure 9*]. Careful observation of the stripe on the graft as it is passed through the tunnel helps prevent twisting.

Venous anastomosis   To minimize arterial occlusion time, the venous anastomosis is usually performed first. The vein must be at least 4 mm in diameter; venous diameter and patency are verified by passing coronary dilators or a Fogarty catheter through the vessel and irrigating it with heparinized saline. Before the anastomosis is performed, the vein and all distal branches are ligated to prevent venous hypertension and arm edema.

If no veins of adequate diameter are available, either two adjacent veins or a portion of a transverse communicating vein can be used to construct a venoplasty that will increase the net diameter of the venous outflow tract. Alternatively, the deep brachial or axillary veins can be used for outflow. The latter option is often required when the superficial veins have been exhausted in a patient who has previously had AVFs.

Arterial anastomosis   Systemic heparin is given only if an end artery is occluded for anastomosis. The artery should have a lumen of at least 3 mm, and the arteriotomy should be no more than 6 mm long to prevent distal ischemia. ePTFE sutures are useful for arterial anastomoses: because they have the same diameter as the attached needles, needle-hole bleeding is minimized.

Before the arterial anastomosis is completed, the graft is unclamped and allowed to fill with venous blood; this step prevents air embolism when arterial control is released. When the anastomosis is complete, a thrill should be palpable over the venous outflow tract rather than directly over the graft.

Graft type   The choice between a tapered 4 to 7 mm ePTFE graft and a 6 mm straight graft is a matter of personal preference. The tapered graft was introduced to reduce the incidence of steal syndrome by increasing the resistance to flow through the prosthesis; however, it has not been shown to provide consistent protection from ischemic complications. Both types of graft are also available in either a standard or a thin-wall configuration; the only randomized study published to date reported superior results with the standard configuration.[24] Stretch ePTFE appears to yield better results than the older, nonstretch grafts.[25]

FOLLOW-UP

Upon discharge, the patient is instructed to elevate the arm so as to reduce edema. Regular hand and arm exercise, though not of proven benefit, is nonetheless recommended until the fistula matures.

Physical examination of the fistula, including inspection and palpation for pulse and thrill, should be done on a weekly basis. The patient should also be advised to seek prompt medical attention if the quality of the thrill changes. Normally, a thrill is palpable throughout the cardiac cycle, though it is more intense during systole. Disappearance of the diastolic component of the thrill is generally a consequence of outflow obstruction. Such obstruction (usually from venous or anastomotic stenosis) may also cause intensification of the thrill or bruit. In addition, diminished flow or outflow stenosis may cause the thrill to be converted to a pulse. Any of these abnormal

findings is an indication for a diagnostic procedure: salvage attempts are much more likely to succeed if carried out before thrombosis has occurred.

ePTFE AV grafts should not be used until at least 14 days have passed since placement or until the swelling has subsided enough to allow palpation of the graft. This waiting period allows adhesions to form between the subcutaneous tunnel and the graft, thereby decreasing the risk of hematoma in the graft tunnel, which may ruin the access site. A minimum of 1 month is required before a primary AVF may be cannulated. It is preferable, however, to wait until the fistula matures fully, which may take 3 to 4 months.

COMPLICATIONS

Venous Stenosis

Venous stenosis, either at the anastomosis (particularly with ePTFE grafts) or in the body of the vein, is a common complication of AVF construction. Prophylactic intervention for venous stenoses reduces the rate of thrombosis and graft loss, and stenoses detected before thrombosis occurs are more responsive to therapy than those detected afterward. Intervention is indicated when stenosis of 50% or greater (documented by duplex ultrasonography or fistulography) is accompanied by a hemodynamic, functional, or clinical abnormality (e.g., decreased access blood flow, elevated static or dynamic venous pressure, increased recirculation, reduced delivered dialysis dose, or arm edema). Prophylactic intervention for anatomic stenosis is not warranted when such findings are absent.[26]

Although the question of whether angioplasty or surgical revision is the preferable method of intervention remains controversial, experience to date suggests that surgical revision tends to provide better long-term results. This difference may derive from the elasticity of intimal hyperplastic lesions, whose rapid recoil may limit the efficacy of angioplasty. As a rule, if angioplasty is required more than twice within 3 months, the patient should be referred for surgical revision. Treatment options include patch angioplasty for localized or anastomotic stenoses, bypass for longer stenoses, relocation of the venous anastomosis to a new vein, and resection of the stenotic segment with interposition grafting.

Central venous stenosis   Stenotic or occlusive lesions of the central veins develop in as many as 40% of patients who have previously undergone subclavian hemodialysis catheter placement for temporary vascular access.[7] When a vascular access graft or fistula is placed distal to these lesions, they may become symptomatic,

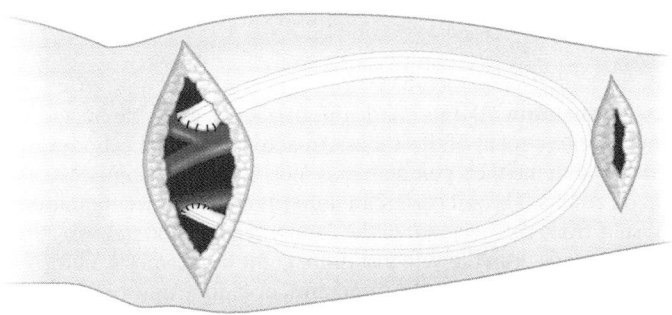

Figure 9   **Vascular access via AVFs: bridge AV grafts. With a loop forearm graft, tunneling of the graft is facilitated by making an incision 1.5 cm distal to the elbow crease to expose the brachial artery and the antecubital venous system, followed by a counterincision at the apex of the tunnel 3 to 4 cm proximal to the wrist skinfold.**

resulting in venous hypertension, arm edema, low access flow, or thrombosis. Percutaneous intervention with transluminal angioplasty is the preferred treatment; the tendency for central venous stenosis to recur soon after treatment[27] may be circumvented by the addition of a stent. Stents are particularly helpful for treating rigid or kinked stenoses, for sealing dissections or circumscribed perforations, and for reestablishing the patency of chronically occluded veins. Surgical repair of central venous obstruction is a major undertaking and is reserved for those occasional cases in which percutaneous procedures have failed in a patient with no alternative access site.

Arterial Stenosis

Arterial stenosis is relatively uncommon. It should be corrected if it is associated with diminished access flow and elevated arterial prepump pressure. Arterial stenosis may be suspected even before dialysis is initiated if a patent vein does not enlarge significantly within several weeks of fistula creation. Angiography provides a definitive diagnosis. Stenosis of the distal artery, the anastomosis, or the distal vein is best treated with reanastomosis proximal to the stenotic area. More proximal stenosis may have to be treated with conventional arterial reconstruction.

Early Thrombosis

Early thrombosis is defined as thrombosis occurring within 3 months of access construction. It is usually the result of technical factors or of inadequate assessment of the arterial or venous conduit. The following are the most common causes of early thrombosis:

1. Inadequate arterial inflow caused by proximal arterial disease.
2. Narrowing of the anastomosis during construction.
3. Kinking or twisting of the vein proximal to the anastomosis or in a subcutaneous tunnel.
4. Undetected occlusion of venous outflow.
5. Compression of the fistula by a hematoma resulting from either inadequate hemostasis during the procedure or early puncture of the fistula with subsequent extravasation of blood.

If early thrombosis is thought to be caused by technical complications and not by the use of marginal vessels, reexploration is worthwhile. Reexploration usually involves takedown of the anastomosis, thrombectomy of the conduit, reevaluation of both arterial inflow and venous outflow, corrective measures as needed, and reanastomosis. Both autogenous AVFs and AV grafts may be profitably reexplored. With an autogenous AVF, reexploration should be done within 24 hours of thrombosis to minimize ischemic endothelial injury.

Late Thrombosis

Autogenous AVFs Little information is available on success rates for treatment of thrombosis in autogenous AVFs; however, it seems that neither percutaneous nor surgical techniques offer good results. Thrombosis of an autogenous AVF most commonly results from an aneurysm of the fistula, hyperplastic stenosis at the anastomosis or in the vein just distal to the anastomosis, fibrosis at an area of repeated needle punctures, or kidney transplantation.

The surgical approach should include exposure of the vein just distal to a clinically apparent or suspected venous stenosis. The vein is opened longitudinally and the thrombus evacuated. Adequacy of venous outflow is assessed with a Fogarty catheter or coronary dilators. If a segment less than 4 mm in diameter is encountered, the problem is corrected with patch angioplasty, vein bypass, or resection and primary anastomosis. (The last of these three approaches is often easy to perform because the tortuosity of the vein allows easy mobilization and length extension.) Central vein stenosis is corrected with intraoperative balloon angioplasty.

When the venous side of the AVF is in satisfactory condition, the thrombus is removed from the arterial limb. Any suspected anastomotic or proximal arterial stenosis should be corrected [see AV Grafts, *below*]. If the thrombosis resulted from a fistula aneurysm containing adherent thrombus, the aneurysm should be repaired to prevent its recurrence.

AV grafts About 85% of AV graft thromboses are caused by stenosis of the venous anastomosis or of the draining vein (as a result of intimal hyperplasia), and most instances of graft loss are attributable to such stenosis. Treatment of a thrombosed graft has only a 10% chance of success if the underlying venous stenosis is not addressed. Although arterial stenoses are less common causes of late thrombosis, they should be sought out and corrected as well. Before treatment is initiated, information about recent graft performance should be obtained. Signs of venous or outflow stenosis include increasing venous resistance and prolonged bleeding from puncture sites. Inadequate flow rates and increased negative pressures during dialysis are associated with stenosis of the arterial inflow. Hypotension or excessive graft compression can explain spontaneous thrombosis in a previously well-functioning graft.

Graft thrombosis may be corrected either with surgical thrombectomy or with pharmacomechanical or mechanical thrombolysis. On the whole, technical success and long-term patency rates are similar for the two approaches, though there is some evidence for a trend toward longer primary patency with surgical management.[28] The choice between these two approaches continues to be controversial, and the decision should generally be based on local expertise. To date, neither surgical treatment nor endovascular management has produced unassisted patency rates higher than 50% at 6 months. If graft thrombosis occurs repeatedly in a given patient, plans for a new access site should be considered.

If surgical treatment is chosen, it should be carried out in an operating suite with the capacity for intraoperative fluoroscopy. Unless preoperative findings indicate that an arterial lesion is present, the incision is made at the venous anastomosis, and an adequate length of graft and outflow vein is mobilized. A transverse graftotomy is made within 1 or 2 mm of the suture line, any clot found on the venous side is removed with suction and a forceps, and the anastomosis is inspected. The anastomosis is calibrated but not dilated: if a 5 mm dilator passes easily through the venous anastomosis, then thrombectomy alone is often sufficient treatment. A 4 French Fogarty catheter is passed proximally into the right atrium and pulled back slowly with the balloon inflated to check for proximal venous stenosis and to evacuate clot. Any abnormality encountered is an indication for operative phlebography. The presence of a venous abnormality does not rule out the possibility of a coexisting arterial defect; both should be corrected if found.

After the venous anastomosis is examined, a 4 French Fogarty catheter is used to evacuate any clot in the graft itself. Thrombectomy at the arterial anastomosis is delayed until any structural problems in the body of the graft are corrected; this delay permits the structural corrections to be carried out in a bloodless field. Narrowing in the body of the graft is usually caused by fibrous material adherent to the wall, which can be removed with the aid of a curette, an endarterectomy instrument, or suction. Once the body of the graft is clear, any thrombus present at the arterial anastomosis is removed. Free passage of the Fogarty balloon catheter suggests that there is no arterial anastomotic stenosis. The arterial anastomosis may be examined under direct vision if necessary to

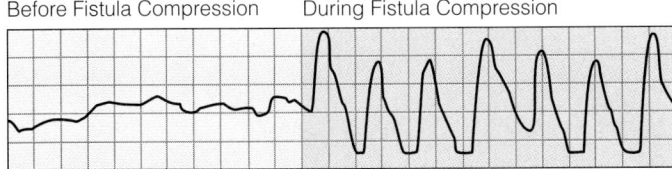

Before Fistula Compression   During Fistula Compression

Figure 10 **Vascular access via AVFs. Shown are digital photo-plethysmographic waveforms on an arm with steal syndrome before and during fistula compression.**

ensure complete removal of the compacted thrombus at the arterial end of the graft.

The graft is filled with heparinized saline before the arterial or the venous anastomosis is repaired. When the arterial side of the graft is involved, a new arterial anastomosis usually suffices to solve the problem. A new arterial site proximal to the old one is selected, and either the graft is moved to the new site or a new free segment is added.

More commonly, the defect is at the venous anastomosis. In this case, the graftotomy is extended longitudinally through the anastomosis. If the stenosis is short, smooth, and hyperplastic, a small patch angioplasty is adequate for repair. If the stenosis is long or if the vein is sclerotic, revision to a new venous outflow site is preferred. The graft can be reanastomosed to another nearby vein, or the stenosis can be bypassed by anastomosing an ePTFE graft of appropriate size to a more proximal segment of the original vein. Joints may be crossed if necessary, in which case an externally supported prosthesis is used.

Steal Syndrome

The incidence of symptomatic steal syndrome has been reported to be approximately 2% for autogenous AVFs and as high as 4% for AV grafts. Ischemic complications result from preferential diversion of arterial flow into the low-pressure venous outflow of the fistula. When collateral arterial flow is inadequate or when proximal or distal occlusive arterial disease is present, distal ischemia occurs. In some cases, the flow into the venous side of the fistula is sufficient to induce reversal of the flow in a portion of the artery distal to the fistula, a phenomenon referred to as steal. Unfortunately, there is no reliable method of predicting the development of symptomatic steal after the construction of an autogenous AVF or AV graft.

The ischemia is usually mild and is characterized by coldness, numbness, and pain during dialysis. In most cases, the problem resolves without treatment within a few weeks. If the patient experiences constant pain, severe numbness, a nonhealing ischemic fissure, digital cyanosis or gangrene, or finger contracture, the ischemia should be corrected. The differential diagnosis of vascular steal syndrome includes the neuropathies of uremia and diabetes as well as secondary hyperparathyroidism. Carpal tunnel syndrome—an uncommon but distinct condition occurring in hemodialysis patients—presents with symptoms similar to those of vascular steal but can be differentiated from steal on the basis of the characteristic electromyographic findings.

A classic indicator of clinically significant steal is that digital pulse waves are absent or markedly diminished on digital photo-plethysmography (PPG) or pulse volume recordings (PVR) but rise to normal amplitude and contour when the fistula is compressed [*see Figure 10*]. Digital pressures lower than 50 mm Hg and a digital-brachial index lower than 0.47 are also indicative of clinically significant distal ischemia.[29] A significant difference in segmental or digital pressure between the two arms with the fistula compressed may be indicative of superimposed arterial disease proximal or distal to the fistula, in which case arteriography is indicated before surgical correction. Identification of reversed flow distal to the fistula on duplex studies is not, in itself, sufficient reason to conclude that clinically significant steal is present: steal is a common phenomenon and is a physiologic consequence of the rheology of the fistula in 73% of autogenous AVFs and 92% of AV grafts.[30]

The goal of treatment is to reduce steal to a level where there is both adequate residual flow volume for dialysis and adequate perfusion to the hand to eliminate ischemic symptoms. Treatment options include the following:

1. Elimination of the fistula. This is the simplest form of treatment and invariably corrects ischemia; however, it raises the vexing problem of reestablishing access in another extremity.
2. Reducing the flow but maintaining patency. Usually, this option involves narrowing a portion of the access to reduce flow. One technique for accomplishing this narrowing is to excise an elliptical portion of the graft or vein just distal to the anastomosis and reapproximate the edges or to plicate the graft or outflow vein with mattress or continuous sutures[31] [*see Figure 11a through c*]. Another technique is to band the fistula or graft with a crossed ePTFE band.[32] The tails of the band are secured with hemostatic clips, and once the appropriate degree of narrowing has been achieved, the clips are held in place with a figure-eight suture of 5-0 polypropylene [*see Figure 11d*]. Both techniques should narrow the outflow over a fairly long distance ($\geq$ 1 cm). A third technique involves interposing a small-diameter (4 mm) ePTFE graft between the artery and the vein or graft[33] [*see Figure 11e*]; however, this technique does not allow progressive calibration of the narrowing to achieve the desired hemodynamic result.
3. Ligation of the source of steal, with distal revascularization when necessary. When steal occurs in a patient who has a radiocephalic fistula at the wrist with flow reversal in the radial artery distal to the fistula (documented by duplex scans) and whose ulnar artery and palmar arch are patent and competent to perfuse the hand, it is easily treated by ligating the radial artery distal to the fistula.[34] The effect of this treatment is easily demonstrated by compressing the radial artery distal to the fistula, which should relieve the ischemia. With a more proximal fistula, in which ligation of a terminal artery would inevitably result in severe distal ischemia, the distal artery is ligated and an arterial bypass established from a point 5 cm proximal to the fistula to a point just distal to the ligation [*see Figure 12*]. This so-called distal revascularization–interval ligation (DRIL) procedure, originally reported by Schanzer and coworkers,[35] is an elegant way of both preserving adequate flow through the fistula and reversing the ischemia. The pathway of steal is eliminated, and antegrade flow into the extremity is restored through the bypass. This technique is particularly helpful when concomitant arterial stenosis proximal or distal to the fistula contributes to the distal ischemic process, because the bypass can be positioned so as to bypass the arterial stenosis as well.

With any of these techniques, intraoperative assessment is required to ensure adequate residual flow volume in the fistula (assessed by intraoperative duplex scanning) and adequate distal perfusion (assessed by evaluation of digital PPG or PVR waveforms). The goal is to achieve a digital pressure of at least 60 mm Hg, a digital-brachial index of 0.6 or greater, and a residual flow of at least 300 ml/min in the fistula (a level of flow that is adequate both for hemodialysis and for maintenance of patency).[36]

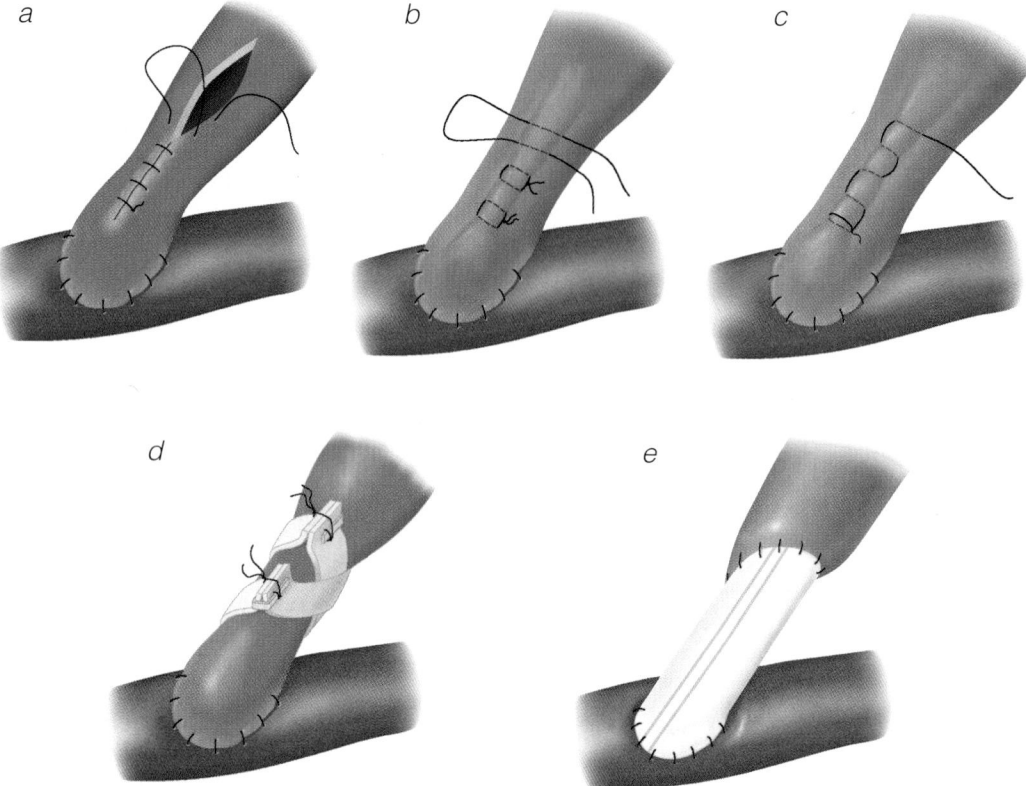

Figure 11 **Vascular access via AVFs. One option for treating steal is to decrease blood flow in the access conduit. Methods that may be used include (*a*) excision of a portion of the vein or graft, (*b*) plication with mattress sutures, (*c*) plication with continuous sutures, (*d*) placement of a crossed ePTFE band with application of hemostatic clips, and (*e*) interposition of a 4 mm ePTFE graft.**

Inadequate Maturation of the Vein

Failure of a fistula to mature may result from either inadequate inflow or venous abnormality. Physical examination combined with Doppler ultrasonography or fistulography should identify the underlying cause. If stenosis is not identified in a nonmaturing radiocephalic fistula, venous side branches may be draining critical flow from the primary vessel; ligation of these branches sometimes leads to successful maturation. Median cubital vein ligation may be attempted, as may temporary banding of the main venous channel in the antecubital fossa. Banding is accomplished by narrowing the vein with a 3-0 Vicryl tie over a 4 mm probe. The Vicryl resorbs in 3 to 4 weeks, during which period it is hoped that the increased resistance to flow will cause dilatation of the vein.[37] If none of these measures succeed, another access site should be sought.

True Aneurysm (Autogenous AVFs)

Aneurysmal dilatation of the vein develops in 5% to 8% of autogenous AVFs as a result of high pressure applied to a vein wall weakened by repeated punctures. Usually, the course of such aneurysms is benign and does not preclude use of the fistula; however, large aneurysms containing mural thrombus have been reported to cause late thrombosis and embolization. On rare occasions, progressive enlargement can compromise circulation to the skin above the aneurysmal vein, leading to incomplete hemostasis when the needle is withdrawn and ultimately to graft rupture. Skin compromise and progressive enlargement are therefore indications for surgical correction. Surgical revision is also recommended if the aneurysm involves the arterial anastomosis or is associated with stenosis of the venous outflow.

Options for revision include total excision of the aneurysm with primary reanastomosis, exclusion of the aneurysm with vein bypass grafting, and partial excision in which part of the vein wall is kept as the arterial conduit. The last option frequently results in early recurrence as the vein wall continues to weaken and dilate with time.

Pseudoaneurysm (AV Grafts)

Pseudoaneurysms occur in prosthetic AV grafts and are usually small and asymptomatic. They can be prevented by allowing sufficient time after graft placement to ensure firm fibrous encapsulation of the graft and by avoiding repeated needle insertion at the same site. On occasion, however, pseudoaneurysms are precipitated by underlying venous stenosis, which should be documented and corrected whenever present. Urgent surgical repair is indicated if the pseudoaneurysm is expanding rapidly or is causing ischemia of the overlying skin. Elective repair is indicated if the diameter of the false aneurysm is more than twice that of the graft.

Infection

Infection is the second most common cause of loss of AV access, occurring in 0% to 3% of autogenous AVFs and 6% to 25% of AV grafts. Infection may be acquired during surgery or cannulation of the conduit and is most often caused by *Staphylococcus aureus.*

Autogenous AVFs Infection of an autogenous AVF should be treated aggressively with 6 weeks of antibiotic therapy, much as subacute bacterial endocarditis would be. Local measures, such as

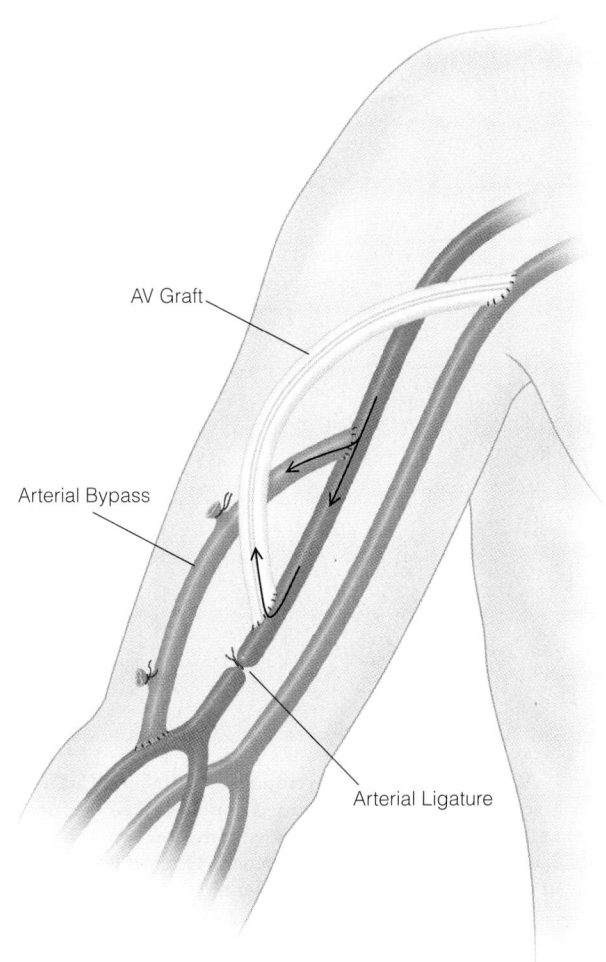

Figure 12 **Vascular access via AVFs. Another option for treating steal is to ligate the source. Shown is the so-called DRIL procedure, which involves arterial ligation distal to the takeoff of the AV graft or the autogenous AVF and arterial bypass from a point 5 cm proximal to the fistula to a point just distal to the ligation.**

drainage of a perifistular abscess, may be necessary. In rare instances, infection-induced anastomotic pseudoaneurysm or septic emboli necessitate takedown of the fistula.

AV grafts Generally, both antibiotic therapy and surgical treatment are necessary for cure. An antibiotic regimen that covers gram-negative organisms, staphylococci, and streptococci should be given until culture results are available. In most cases, complete excision of the prosthetic graft is required,[38] along with vein patch reconstruction of the artery. If the anastomosis is not grossly involved, a small cuff of ePTFE may be left on the arterial side and used to close the arterial defect; this does not seem to alter the prognosis.

In selected cases of well-localized infection, it is possible to resect only the infected portion of the graft and to restore the continuity of the fistula by placing a new conduit in a clean subcutaneous tunnel away from the infected area. A useful approach to managing an infected forearm loop graft is to resect the graft and reconstruct the fistula with an immediate anastomosis between the artery and the arterialized vein remaining after graft excision. Superficial surgical wound infections occurring in the postoperative period can sometimes be treated successfully with aggressive local debridement in combination with systemic administration of antibiotics. Deeper wound infections occurring in the postoperative period must be assumed to involve the entire graft, given that the graft is not yet well incorporated.

OUTCOME EVALUATION

Thrombotic events are the leading cause of access loss. For the most part, they result from venous outflow stenosis that can be detected before thrombosis occurs. An organized monitoring approach that includes regular assessment of the clinical parameters of the access and of the adequacy of the dialysis should be implemented in every dialysis center.[6] Such a proactive approach can be expected to reduce the incidence of thrombosis and increase patency.

Physical examination of the AV graft or autogenous AVF should be performed weekly and should include not only inspection and palpation for changes in the physical characteristics of the pulse or thrill but also a search for indirect signs of graft dysfunction (e.g., arm swelling, prolonged bleeding after needle withdrawal, and aneurysm or pseudoaneurysm). In addition to physical examination, the NKF-DOQI committee recommended routine access monitoring at least monthly with one or more of the following techniques:

1. Intra-access flow assessment using Doppler flow, magnetic resonance imaging, or ultrasound dilution online during dialysis. A trend toward decreasing flow or a flow rate lower than 600 ml/min for an AV graft and lower than 200 to 300 ml/min for an autogenous AVF is predictive of a high likelihood of access stenosis and eventual thrombosis.
2. Static or dynamic venous pressure measurement. Progressively increasing pressures or pressures that exceed the threshold value determined by each center's own protocol are predictive of significant venous outlet stenosis.
3. Urea and nonurea recirculation measurement. Recirculation is defined as the percentage of flow that is recirculated from the venous line into the dialyser inflow by retrograde blood flow through the fistula. A recirculation value exceeding 10% to 20% is significant and usually indicates low arterial blood flow or venous stenosis.
4. Delivered dialysis dose. A decrease is associated with venous outflow stenosis.
5. Arterial prepump pressure. An elevated negative pressure is a sign of inflow insufficiency.

Vascular Access via Percutaneous Catheters

Percutaneous venous catheterization is a useful method of gaining immediate access to the circulation; however, it is associated with significant risks, and the use-life of this type of access is shorter than that of AVFs. Percutaneous catheterization should be reserved for patients with acute renal failure who have an immediate need for dialysis and for patients with chronic renal failure in whom a permanent vascular or peritoneal access route either cannot be established or has not yet matured.

OPERATIVE PLANNING

Patient Assessment

A history is taken, a physical examination is performed, laboratory data are reviewed, and radiologic studies are ordered as for AVFs [*see* Vascular Access via Arteriovenous Fistulas, *above*]. Any finding that might affect the integrity of the central venous system should be noted.

A history or physical signs of previous central venous catheterization, a history of major injury or operation in the area where the catheter is to be inserted, a body mass index greater than 30 or less than 20, and an increasing number of insertion attempts are all known risk factors for perioperative complications from the insertion of venous access devices.[1] If there is any question about the patency of the central venous system, duplex scanning[39] or phlebography is indicated.

On physical examination, the surgeon should note the patient's body type, assess the flexibility of the patient's neck and shoulders, and evaluate the patient's ability to tolerate Trendelenburg's position without dyspnea or discomfort. Chest x-rays are reviewed to verify the patient's pleuropulmonary status and to identify any bony deformities.

The only laboratory study absolutely necessary is a complete blood count (including the platelet count and the differential count); prothrombin and partial thromboplastin times are required if the patient is receiving anticoagulant therapy. The effects of warfarin or heparin should be reversed before the procedure; patients with platelet counts lower than 50,000/mm[3] should undergo platelet transfusion immediately before and during catheter placement.[40]

Choice of Type of Catheter

The catheters best suited for hemodialysis are high-flow, large-diameter (12 French or larger) devices with external ports. Silicone catheters are more flexible, are less likely to give rise to injury or thrombosis, and remain patent longer than polyethylene, polyvinyl chloride, and polytetrafluoroethylene catheters. Silicone catheters are available in both noncuffed (temporary) and cuffed (semipermanent) double-lumen configurations through which flow rates of 250 ml/min or higher can be achieved [see Figure 13]. The venous and arterial orifices are separated by 1 to 2 cm; recirculation is thereby limited to 5%.

Noncuffed (temporary) catheters Noncuffed catheters can be percutaneously inserted into the internal jugular, subclavian, or femoral vein without the need for fluoroscopic guidance. They are suitable for immediate use and provide acceptable flow rates (250 ml/min). Their main disadvantages are their high rates of infection, thrombosis, and venous stenosis and their short use-life (2 to 3 weeks). For these reasons, noncuffed catheters should be reserved for patients in whom access is expected to be needed for less than 3 weeks, and they should be inserted no earlier than required.

Cuffed (semipermanent) catheters Cuffed catheters are placed in a subcutaneous tunnel under fluoroscopic guidance. They are free of some of the shortcomings of noncuffed catheters; in particular, they are associated with lower infection rates and permit higher flow rates. Cuffed catheters are preferred when temporary access is required for longer than 3 weeks, particularly for patients in whom a primary AV fistula is maturing but who require immediate hemodialysis. Semipermanent catheters have been used for as long as 4 years, but long-term follow-up data on large numbers of patients is lacking.[41] Most patients readily accept this approach to dialysis: cuffed catheters allow so-called no-needle dialysis with high flow rates, they eliminate the problem of vascular steal, and they have no effect on cardiac function. In addition, patients appreciate that the access site is hidden from view, does not limit physical activity, and does not require particular care between treatments.

Choice of Insertion Site

The subclavian veins have given way to the right internal jugular (IJ) vein as the preferred site of primary central access. This site

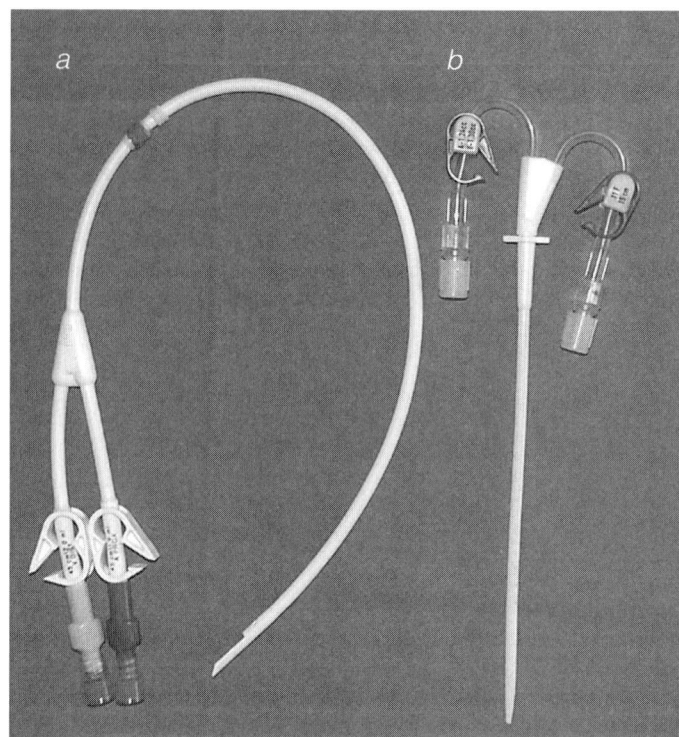

Figure 13 **Vascular access via percutaneous catheters. Catheters used for hemodialysis include (*a*) cuffed double-lumen (semipermanent) catheters, introduced by means of the peelaway sheath technique, and (*b*) noncuffed double-lumen (temporary) catheters, introduced by means of the Seldinger technique.**

has four main advantages: (1) it offers a consistent, predictable anatomic location with palpable landmarks, (2) it provides a short, straight course to the superior vena cava, (3) success rates are high, and (4) the risk of complications is diminished in comparison with other catheter insertion sites.[42] Of particular importance is that the risk of subclavian vein stenosis is decreased; this complication is a major concern for dialysis patients, who may require subsequent construction of an AVF in the ipsilateral arm. The right IJ vein is preferable to the left IJ vein as an access site because the latter calls for longer catheters, which increase the risk of kinking and diminish flow rates. The left IJ approach is also associated with a high rate of stenosis or thrombosis of the left brachiocephalic vein and may hinder subsequent use of the left arm for an AVF. Placement of the catheter in a subclavian vein either via the percutaneous approach or via cutdown on the cephalic vein should be reserved for cases in which neither jugular vein can be used.[6]

The right IJ vein can be catheterized percutaneously, or it can be surgically exposed and catheterized via direct needle puncture or phlebotomy (venous cutdown). The cutdown approach on the internal jugular vein or the external jugular vein allows greater control over the vessel than the percutaneous approach does and is preferred in patients who have a bleeding diathesis, patients whose body habitus or venous anatomy limits percutaneous access, and patients in whom a percutaneous attempt at placement has failed.

A less commonly used approach is femoral vein catheterization. It is technically easy and has few immediate complications, but it necessitates hospitalization (because the patient cannot ambulate) and is associated with high infection rates that limit use of the catheter to 5 days. Alternatively, access to the inferior vena cava can be gained by cannulating the greater saphenous, inferior epigastric, right gonadal, and lumbar veins. It is also possible to cannulate the azygos vein and the right atrium directly via thoracotomy.

OPERATIVE TECHNIQUE

Right Internal Jugular Vein Approach

Step 1: patient preparation Noncuffed catheters may be inserted at the bedside; cuffed catheters should be inserted in a standard OR with facilities for fluoroscopy.

The anatomy is surveyed before preparation and draping. Important anatomic landmarks include the sternal notch, the clavicle, and the sternocleidomastoid (SCM) muscle. The carotid artery should be palpated lateral to the trachea, under the medial (sternal) head of the SCM. The IJ vein lies lateral and slightly anterior to the carotid artery, between the sternal head and the clavicular head of the SCM muscle.

The patient is placed supine in Trendelenburg's position so that the neck veins are distended and the risk of air embolism is minimized. The head is extended and turned slightly to the left to expose the right side of the neck and keep the chin from interfering with the procedure. The neck should not be overextended or overrotated, however, because either of these actions flattens out the vein, making it more difficult to cannulate, and may increase the risk of arterial puncture by causing the internal jugular vein to overlie the carotid artery.

Step 2: cannulation of right IJ vein The jugular vein is located with a 22-gauge finder needle. This needle is left in place and used to guide the subsequent placement of an 18-gauge needle, through which the guide wire is passed. Use of the smaller needle minimizes the consequences of arterial or pleural puncture occurring during blind attempts at venous puncture.

After local anesthesia is administered, the fingers of the left hand are gently positioned on the carotid pulse to provide an anatomic landmark. The right hand locates the IJ vein by applying negative pressure to the 22-gauge finder needle mounted on a 5 ml syringe [*see Figure 14*]. The needle is inserted at the apex of the triangle formed by the two heads of the SCM muscle and directed toward the ipsilateral nipple at an angle of 30° from the plane of the skin. Alternatively, the needle may be inserted under the medial border of the SCM muscle and directed toward the thoracic inlet while the carotid artery is dislocated medially, or it may be inserted under the lateral border of the SCM muscle and directed toward the contralateral nipple.

Once the vein is located, the syringe is disconnected from the finder needle, which is left in place. The vein is then repunctured with an 18-gauge needle oriented parallel to the finder needle. When venous backflow is obtained, the 18-gauge needle is reoriented at a more acute angle to the skin and is advanced 2 to 3 mm. The syringe is disconnected and the needle hub occluded to prevent air embolism. A 0.035-in. guide wire with either a J tip or a flexible straight tip is then inserted through the needle, and the needle is withdrawn over the wire.

Troubleshooting. Because of the predictable anatomic location of the right IJ vein, the first attempt at cannulation is successful in the majority of cases. If the first attempt fails, the finder needle should be withdrawn and its tip reoriented slightly laterally; however, the needle should not be entirely withdrawn from the skin puncture site. An orderly, systematic search performed in this manner often identifies the vein while posing little risk of carotid artery injury as long as the carotid artery remains palpable medially. To avoid lacerating deep structures, the needle orientation should be changed only when the needle is inserted very superficially. If the vein cannot be located after several passes of the needle, the finder needle is withdrawn completely and the anatomy reassessed. Alternative puncture sites can be attempted. In difficult cases, cannulation may be carried out under ultrasound guidance, or a cutdown can be performed on the external or IJ vein through a small transverse incision.

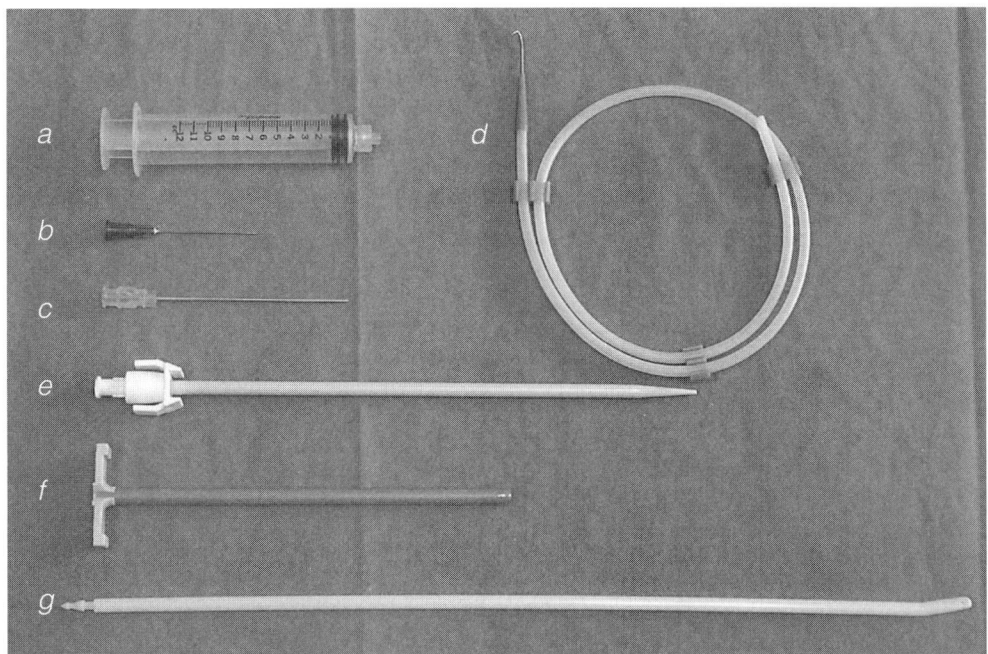

Figure 14 **Vascular access via percutaneous catheters. The equipment used in percutaneous catheter insertion includes (*a*) a 5 ml syringe, (*b*) a 22-gauge finder needle, (*c*) an 18-gauge needle, (*d*) a guide wire, (*e*) a dilator, (*f*) a peelaway sheath, and (*g*) a plastic subcutaneous tunneler.**

When the 18-gauge needle is advanced, the lumen of the jugular vein is often compressed, with the result being that the needle may transfix both front and back walls almost simultaneously. The needle tip should be advanced only slightly beyond the expected depth, then slowly withdrawn, with gentle aspiration maintained on the syringe. Entry into the vein is confirmed by the sudden and easy return of venous blood.

Pulsatile back-bleeding of bright-red blood from the needle usually indicates arterial puncture. If any doubt exists, the aspirated blood can be compared with a simultaneously obtained arterial sample, or the 18-gauge needle can be connected to a pressure transducer. Whenever there is any possibility of arterial puncture, it is preferable to withdraw the needle rather than take the risk of creating a large hole in the artery with a dilator.

The guide wire should be inserted with caution because any forceful movement can result in perforation of the vein wall. The risk is minimized by using a soft-tipped or J-tipped wire. The wire should advance easily into the vein without resistance; if it does not, the guide wire and the needle should be withdrawn together to ensure that the tip of the guide wire is not sheared off and does not embolize.

Step 3 (Seldinger technique): insertion of noncuffed catheter   A small nick is made at the point where the guide wire enters the skin [*see Figure 15*]. The dilator is passed over the wire only far enough to enter the vein; it is then removed, and the catheter is inserted over the wire. The catheter tip should be placed in the superior vena cava, above the right atrial junction. This position is typically 15 to 18 cm from the puncture site if the catheter is placed in the right IJ vein; an additional 3 to 5 cm is required for the left IJ approach. The guide wire is then retrieved, venous blood is aspirated from both ports, and each lumen is flushed with heparinized saline. The catheter is anchored to the skin.

Troubleshooting.   Dilators are relatively inflexible, and their stiffness increases with size. Consequently, they can easily perforate the vein wall if inserted deeper than the point of entry into the vein. Catheters may also cause perforation, though less commonly. The risk of catheter-related perforation is increased with the left IJ approach and the subclavian approach because catheters inserted from the left side must traverse the innominate vein and enter the superior vena cava at an acute angle, and this course increases the possibility that the tip of the catheter will perforate the right lateral wall of the superior vena cava. No resistance should be felt when the catheter is inserted. In addition, the guide wire should move freely within the catheter during insertion; such free movement suggests that the catheter is not compressing the wire against the wall of the vein.

Manual control of the guide wire must be maintained at all times; without such control, pushing a catheter or dilator over the wire can cause the wire to be completely advanced into the vein.

Inadvertent placement of a dilator or catheter into the carotid artery makes a large hole in the vessel wall, thereby creating the potential for substantial bleeding when the device is removed. In such cases, the catheter should be left in the artery, and a vascular surgeon should be consulted.

Step 3 (peelaway sheath technique): insertion of cuffed catheter   A small transverse incision is made at the point where the guide wire enters the skin. Once adequate local anesthesia is achieved, a subcutaneous tunnel is created between the guide-wire entry point and a site on the chest wall at least 10 cm away [*see Figure 16*]. The position of the catheter is estimated by laying the catheter out along its intended tract; the course forms an

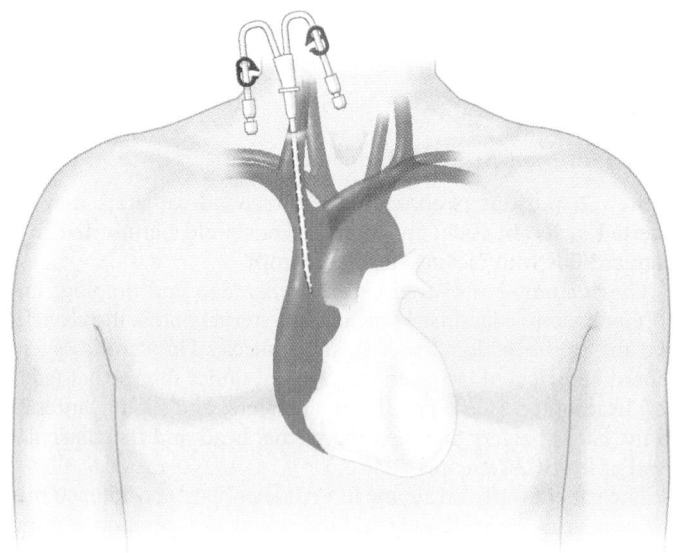

Figure 15   **Vascular access via percutaneous catheters: Seldinger technique. Shown is a noncuffed (temporary) catheter inserted in the right IJ vein.**

inverted U, with the apex at the entry point of the guide wire and the tip of the catheter 5 cm caudad to the angle of Louis (at the second or third intercostal space). The position of the Dacron cuff is noted, and a stab wound is made in such a way that the cuff will be positioned in the subcutaneous tunnel, 2 cm from the wound. This placement simplifies removal of the catheter, prevents the cuff from eroding through the skin, and reduces the incidence of inadvertent catheter dislodgment. The exit wound should be at least 3 to 4 cm from the nipple-areola complex to allow space for the dressing.

A plastic subcutaneous tunneler is attached to the catheter and used to pull the catheter through the tunnel so that the tip emerges adjacent to the guide wire. The venous dilator is then inserted over the wire to effect entry into the vein. Once entry is effected, the dilator is removed and inserted into the peelaway sheath, and sheath and dilator are introduced together into the vein over the guide wire. The guide wire and the dilator are removed, and the open end of the peelaway sheath is occluded with the fingers to prevent air embolism and bleeding. The flushed catheter is then inserted into the peelaway sheath and its position confirmed via fluoroscopy. When the catheter is well positioned, the peelaway sheath is cracked, peeled apart, and removed. Both lumina are tested for easy aspiration of blood and irrigated with heparinized saline. The two incisions are closed with absorbable sutures, and an adequate dressing is applied.

Troubleshooting.   Because the procedure is performed under fluoroscopic guidance, fluoroscopy should be used to confirm that the position of the guide wire is satisfactory before the catheter is inserted. If the guide wire is not satisfactorily positioned, a 14-gauge plastic I.V. catheter is placed over the wire into the vein, and the wire is removed and repositioned through the catheter.

The peelaway sheath must be inserted to its full length, which means that the dilator must be inserted to its full length as well. Bending the dilator and the sheath into a gentle curve that matches the curve of the vein minimizes the risk of venous wall perforation, particularly if the left IJ approach or the subclavian vein approach is used.

If resistance is encountered when the catheter is inserted through the sheath, the usual cause is a kink in the sheath. In most instances, partial withdrawal of the sheath resolves the problem. If this step is taken and the catheter still cannot be advanced, the guide wire and the dilator can be reinserted through the sheath, which is then replaced.

Step 4: evaluation The location of the catheter tip should be documented with a chest x-ray after the procedure. To reduce the risk of complications (e.g., central vein thrombosis or perforation of the right atrium), the tip should be located at the junction of the right atrium and the superior vena cava.[43]

Subclavian Vein Approach

The patient is positioned and prepared in much the same way as for the right IJ approach. The arms should be at the sides, and a small roll should be placed between the shoulder blades to allow full exposure of the infraclavicular area. An insertion site is selected 2 to 3 cm caudad to the midpoint of the clavicle, far enough from its inferior edge to allow the needle to remain parallel to the clavicle as it passes beneath its inferior border. A slightly lateral position is preferred to prevent kinking of the peelaway sheath or compression of the soft silicone catheter between the clavicle and the first rib.

Local anesthesia should include the clavicular periosteum. The 18-gauge needle should be advanced into the space between the clavicle and the first rib in the direction of a finger placed in the suprasternal notch. The needle is oriented as horizontally as possible, and the bevel of the needle is oriented downward to decrease the risk that the guide wire will pass upward into the ipsilateral IJ vein.

Careful technique helps prevent pneumothorax and puncture of the subclavian vein. For example, "walking" the tip of the needle down the clavicle, so that it passes as closely underneath the clavicle as possible, reduces the risk of deep puncture and thus of pneumothorax. The rate of complications is directly related to the number of puncture attempts made; consequently, if the subclavian vein is not punctured on the second or third attempt, one should resist the temptation to make additional needle thrusts.

Once the vein is cannulated, the catheter may be inserted by means of either the Seldinger technique or the peelaway sheath technique as previously described [*see* Right Internal Jugular Vein Approach, *above*].

A chest x-ray will confirm the positioning of the tip of the catheter and the presence or absence of kinking. It will also rule out so-called pinch-off, which is a narrowing or notching of the catheter as it pass-

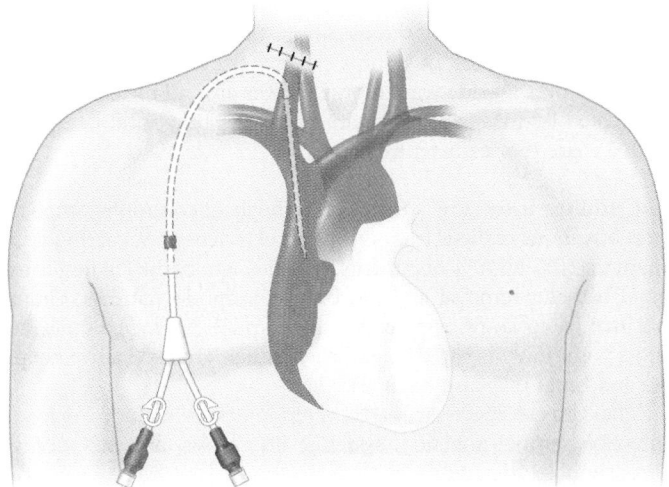

Figure 16 **Vascular access via percutaneous catheters: peelaway sheath technique. Shown is a cuffed (semipermanent) catheter inserted in the right IJ vein and placed in a subcutaneous tunnel.**

es through the tight space between the clavicle and the first rib that may result in transection and embolization of the catheter tip.

Femoral Vein Approach

Femoral venipuncture is performed below the inguinal ligament just medial to the palpated femoral arterial pulse. The catheter is inserted by means of the Seldinger technique. The catheter should be at least 19 cm long to reach the inferior vena cava, thereby minimizing recirculation.

COMPLICATIONS

Early Complications

In more than 5% of catheter insertions, the catheter is improperly positioned. Such malpositioning may cause central venous perforation, venous thrombosis, or device malfunction. The most common positioning error is entry of a subclavian catheter into the ipsilateral IJ vein; less commonly, the catheter tip may inadvertently be placed in an axillary, internal mammary, azygos, or hepatic vein. Placement of the tip within the more cephalad portion of the superior vena cava at an obtuse angle to the venous wall or directly in the heart increases the risk of perforation. Catheter malpositioning is diagnosed by means of fluoroscopy or chest x-ray; management involves immediate repositioning of the catheter with the help of guide wires and fluoroscopy.

Guide-wire embolism can be prevented by being careful not to withdraw the wire through the 18-gauge needle, which can shear off the tip of the wire. Catheter embolism, though rare, may occur when a subclavian venous catheter is inserted too medially and as a consequence is compressed between the costoclavicular ligament, the clavicle, and the first rib. Such compression may lead to biomaterial fatigue, fracture of the catheter, or embolization. Embolized portions of a guide wire or catheter should be removed by means of interventional radiologic techniques to prevent thrombotic complications.

Air embolism occurs when air is inadvertently aspirated into the patient's venous system while the catheter is being inserted, removed, or used. It is easily prevented by using a fingertip to cover all potential communication sites between the venous lumen and the outside air, including the needle hub before guide-wire insertion, the open end of the peelaway sheath just before catheter insertion, and the disconnected external ports of catheters. Patients whose pulmonary status is compromised or who have aspirated large volumes of air may experience respiratory distress. Cardiovascular collapse, caused by obstruction of right ventricular outflow by gas bubbles, can also result. Auscultation may reveal a characteristic millwheel precordial murmur. The patient should be placed in the left lateral decubitus position with the foot of the table elevated so as to trap the air pocket away from the right ventricular outflow tract, and immediate ventilatory support for hypoxemia should be instituted.

Internal hemorrhage may occur at any site, usually as a result of perforation of a central venous or arterial structure during needle puncture or insertion of a guide wire, a dilator, or a catheter. Mediastinal hemorrhage, manifested by mediastinal widening on chest x-ray, occurs in fewer than 1% of all insertions.[44] It is usually self-limited in that the bleeding generally tamponades before hemodynamic compromise occurs.

If both a vascular structure and the parietal pleura are lacerated, hemothorax may result. The chest x-ray will suggest the diagnosis. Treatment includes placement of a thoracostomy tube and early consultation with a thoracic surgeon. Fortunately, the bleeding ceases spontaneously in most cases.

Pericardial tamponade, the most lethal complication of central venous catheterization, may arise as a consequence of perforation into the pericardial space, either through the wall of the vein or through the heart. It can occur immediately, or it can appear hours to days later as a result of delayed perforation by the catheter tip. Proper positioning of the catheter tip is the key to preventing pericardial tamponade. Treatment involves pericardiocentesis, creation of a pericardial window, or median sternotomy, depending on the patient's clinical status.

Cardiac arrhythmias are frequent during catheter insertion: atrial and ventricular arrhythmias occur in as many as 41% and 11% of patients, respectively.[45] These arrhythmias are usually benign; fewer than 1% call for cardioversion.

Pneumothorax occurs in 1% to 4% of attempts at percutaneous catheter placement. The incidence varies according to the experience of the operator and the site selected; in particular, it is higher with the subclavian approach. The presence of pneumothorax may be suggested by air in the syringe during attempts at vein cannulation and may be confirmed by chest x-ray. If the pneumothorax is asymptomatic, with less than 25% lung collapse, it can be treated conservatively; if it is large, symptomatic, or increasing in size, placement of a thoracostomy tube is indicated. Tension pneumothorax is an unusual but important complication that calls for immediate chest tube decompression.

Inadvertent puncture of a lymphatic duct may occur during left subclavian vein or left IJ vein catheterization in patients with hepatic portal hypertension or superior vena caval obstruction. The diagnosis is usually made when clear or milky fluid is aspirated in the syringe during vein cannulation; however, if the duct is punctured at the junction with the vein, the appearance of blood mixed in with the lymphatic fluid may mask the complication. Once lymphatic duct puncture is recognized, the procedure should be abandoned, and pressure should be applied to the site until lymphorrhagia abates. If the complication is recognized late on the basis of spontaneous leakage of lymph around the catheter, either the catheter can be removed or the leak can be stopped with a purse-string suture around the catheter. If persistent fluid drainage, subcutaneous edema, mediastinal enlargement, or chylothorax is noted, the leak is ongoing, and the catheter should be removed.

Late Complications

Central venous thrombosis Catheter-associated central venous thrombosis is more common than was once believed. It is often asymptomatic because of the rich venous collateral circulation in the area. Central venous thrombosis has been estimated to occur in 13% to 35% of catheter insertions[46] and to carry less than a 10% risk of pulmonary embolism and a 19% risk of postphlebitic syndrome. The incidence of catheter-associated thrombosis is correlated with the following factors:

1. Placement site. The incidence of thrombosis or stenosis is as high as 38% with subclavian vein catheters but less than 10% with IJ vein catheters.
2. Site of catheter entry. Surgical cutdown causes less endothelial injury than percutaneous puncture and dilation of the vein and may therefore be less likely to cause thrombosis.
3. Catheter tip position. Catheters placed high in the superior vena cava, near the brachiocephalic vein, are more likely to cause thrombosis.
4. Catheter size. Larger, stiffer catheters are more likely to traumatize the endothelium and to obstruct flow.
5. Catheter material. Silicone is less thrombogenic than other materials.
6. Duration of catheter placement. The incidence of thrombosis increases with the duration of catheter placement.
7. Underlying hypercoagulable state.
8. Associated catheter infection.

The diagnosis is easily made by means of duplex scanning or phlebography. Treatment involves removal of the catheter and administration of anticoagulant therapy. Asymptomatic patients who have no alternative sites for venous access should undergo anticoagulation without removal of the catheter. Thrombolytic therapy through the catheter, though never evaluated in a prospective randomized study, may be useful if the thrombosis is new or symptomatic, is progressing in the face of standard therapy, or is associated with catheter occlusion in a patient with no alternate site of venous access.

Catheter malfunction Catheter malfunction is the most common noninfectious complication of central venous catheterization. Malfunction is defined as either (1) failure to achieve a blood flow rate of at least 300 ml/min on two consecutive occasions or (2) failure to achieve a blood flow rate of 200 ml/min on a single occasion. In addition, partial or complete so-called withdrawal occlusion, in which solutions can be infused but blood cannot be withdrawn, may occur, as may complete occlusion.

Early catheter malfunction is usually caused by improper positioning of the catheter tip proximal to the distal superior vena cava, positioning of the tip against the venous wall, or subcutaneous kinking of the catheter. The precise cause can be determined via chest x-ray and contrast study. Malpositioning of the catheter tip can be corrected by using a tip deflector wire inserted through the lumen of the catheter, by snaring the catheter via the femoral approach and repositioning it, or by replacing the catheter.

Late catheter malfunction is usually caused by intraluminal thrombi; less commonly, it may be caused by extraluminal thrombi (e.g., fibrin tails or sheaths enveloping the distal portion of the catheter) or central venous thrombosis. Most late catheter dysfunction can be successfully managed with thrombolytic therapy. Thrombolysis with urokinase should be attempted first because of its high success rate (up to 90%) and its ease of administration.[47] Multiple protocols have been described. Typically, 5,000 units of urokinase, in a volume sufficient to fill the catheter lumen (usually 1.2 ml), is injected in each port and left in place for 20 to 30 minutes. The urokinase is then withdrawn, and another attempt is made to flush the line. The procedure can be repeated if necessary; the dose and the incubation time may be increased if desired because the urokinase is unlikely to reach the circulation. If catheter function fails to improve, imaging of the catheter with infused contrast material will allow identification and correction of other problems. Residual thrombus in the catheter lumen can be treated by means of intracatheter urokinase infusion (20,000 U/lumen/hr for 6 hours), catheter embolectomy, or catheter exchange over a guide wire. Fibrin sheaths around the catheter can be treated by means of urokinase infusion, fibrin sheath stripping with a snare,[48] or catheter exchange.

Catheter infection Infection is the most common complication of venous catheterization for vascular access, occurring in as many as 30% to 40% of patients. It is also one of the leading causes of catheter removal and morbidity in dialysis patients. Gram-positive bacteria, principally *S. aureus* and *S. epidermidis*, are the most commonly isolated organisms, though gram-negative bacteria and fungi may also be involved.

The clinical spectrum of catheter infection includes exit-site infection, tunnel infection, systemic line sepsis, and suppurative thrombophlebitis.

Exit-site infection. The characteristic signals are localized erythema, induration, tenderness, and exudate at the catheter exit site. Systemic symptoms are absent, and blood cultures are negative.

Treatment involves local wound care and application of topical antibiotics. The catheter need not be removed.

Tunnel infection. If the inflammatory process extends along the entire course of the subcutaneous tunnel, a more extensive cellulitic process, with or without purulent discharge, results. Initially, tunnel infection can be treated with parenteral antibiotics and local measures; however, it usually does not respond to this regimen, and removal of the catheter is often required. If a new catheter is called for, it should use a different tunnel and exit site.

Systemic line sepsis. This condition is manifested by systemic symptoms and signs of bacteremia in a patient who has a central venous catheter in place but exhibits no local evidence of catheter or tunnel infection and has no other identifiable source of infection. It is defined on the basis of the following two criteria: (1) in comparison with peripheral blood, a 10-fold increase in colony-forming units (CFU)/ml blood drawn from the catheter, or (2) in the absence of a positive peripheral blood culture, more than 1,000 CFU from blood drawn through the device. Empirical I.V. antibiotic treatment (including coverage for penicillin-resistant staphylococci) should be administered through the catheter. This measure will eliminate the clinical sepsis syndrome in 70% of patients. Once the antibiotics are discontinued, however, there is a 40% risk of reinfection; for this reason, catheter exchange over a guide wire, using the same tunnel and exit site, is recommended once bactericidal levels have been obtained[49] and the sepsis syndrome has resolved. I.V. antibiotics should be continued for 3 weeks thereafter. If the patient is unstable or still symptomatic after 24 to 36 hours of antibiotic therapy, removal of the catheter is mandatory. The catheter should also be removed if fungemia is suspected or confirmed.

Suppurative thrombophlebitis. When arm edema occurs in addition to systemic sepsis, suppurative thrombophlebitis of a great vein should be suspected. The diagnosis may be confirmed by means of duplex scanning or contrast phlebography. Treatment involves catheter removal, systemic I.V. antibiotic therapy, and heparin anticoagulation and is successful in more than 50% of patients. Vein excision is associated with significant morbidity and consequently is not indicated. Patients who do not respond to treatment can be treated with vena caval filter placement and central vein thrombectomy.

OUTCOME EVALUATION

To improve dialysis outcomes and to maintain or improve quality of care for dialysis patients, percutaneous catheterization should be performed only in selected cases. Given that percutaneous catheterization is associated with higher complication rates, morbidity, and mortality than AV fistulization, the goal should be to use percutaneous catheters in fewer than 10% of hemodialysis patients requiring long-term vascular access. In those cases in which central catheter placement is the best available option, the use of a consistent technique by skilled operators should, according to the NFK-DOQI, reduce the risk of serious complications necessitating intervention to 2% or lower.

Peritoneal Access

OPERATIVE PLANNING

Patient Assessment

For short-term peritoneal access, little formal patient assessment is required. The insertion site should be away from any areas of soft tissue infection and as far from any abdominal scars as is practical.

For long-term peritoneal access, more thorough patient assessment is required. Peritoneal dialysis is absolutely contraindicated in patients who have lost more than 50% of their peritoneal surface area. This degree of loss occurs in some patients who have previously undergone extensive intra-abdominal surgery or have had peritonitis or inflammatory bowel disease. Nonetheless, many patients who have undergone operation have a peritoneal cavity that either is usable for dialysis as is or could be made usable by lysis of adhesions. Patients who have previously undergone intra-abdominal vascular procedures are not candidates for peritoneal dialysis unless the graft is not accessible to the dialysate, so that episodes of peritonitis will not result in graft infection. In addition, adhesions are to be expected in such patients, and preparations to deal with them should be made when catheter insertion is being planned. If active local or distant bacterial infection is present, a permanent catheter should not be inserted until the infection has completely resolved. Advanced age is not a contraindication to peritoneal dialysis, but if the procedure is to be performed in an ambulatory setting, the patient must have sufficient motivation, dexterity, and mental capacity. A prolapsed rectum or uterus is considered a contraindication. Relative contraindications include very large polycystic kidneys, cutaneous stomas, and abdominal hernias. In patients with umbilical or groin hernias, herniorrhaphy may be done either before or at the time of catheter insertion. After herniorrhaphy, it is probably best not to use the catheter for several weeks; a small volume of heparin should be infused every other day while the site of the repair heals.

Choice of Type of Catheter

The catheters used for short-term access to the peritoneal cavity, as in diagnostic peritoneal lavage or short-term peritoneal dialysis, are constructed of rigid plastic and have no Dacron cuff. They may be inserted either percutaneously or under direct vision through small cutdown incisions; the preferred location is the midline.

To obtain long-term access to the peritoneal cavity for chemotherapeutic purposes, the surgeon may elect to place a subcutaneous reservoir to which a catheter is attached in such a way that the unattached end enters the peritoneal cavity. (The same devices are also sometimes used to obtain long-term nondialysis venous access.) The reservoir is accessed with special Huber-point needles; between uses, it is filled with heparinized saline. Alternatively, the surgeon may insert a Dacron-cuffed Silastic catheter [*see* Operative Technique, Step 1: Insertion of Catheter, *below*].

For long-term peritoneal dialysis, transcutaneous catheters made of silicone and equipped with one or two Dacron cuffs are used. These devices are available in a variety of configurations: the intra-abdominal portion may be straight or curved or may have plastic disks attached to it, and the subcutaneous portion may be straight or bent [*see* Figure 17]. The preferred configuration is a pigtail catheter with a preformed bend in the subcutaneous portion.

OPERATIVE TECHNIQUE

General Principles

Long-term peritoneal dialysis catheters may be inserted by means of percutaneous, laparoscopic, or cutdown techniques. Certain general principles apply to all these approaches. The double-cuffed catheter should be placed so that the catheter tip is in the pelvis, the inner cuff is in the rectus abdominis muscle (or adjacent to the linea alba), and the outer cuff is in the subcutaneous tissues. The exit site chosen should permit the patient to see the site to provide local care and should cause minimal interference with clothing. The catheter should exit the skin pointing in a caudal direction;

use of special curved or bent catheter configurations facilitates this. Nearly all patients need only local anesthesia; however, patients who have undergone abdominal operation should be prepared for general anesthesia in case extensive lysis of adhesions is required for satisfactory catheter placement.

What follows is a description of the most commonly used approach to insertion of a long-term peritoneal dialysis catheter, namely, use of a cutdown technique with the patient under local anesthesia [*see Figure 18*].

Step 1: Insertion of Catheter

Catheter insertion and exit sites are chosen so as to avoid old scars, belt lines, and possible future transplantation incisions. Full sterile precautions are taken. A local anesthetic is infiltrated at the catheter insertion site, and an incision is made down to the anterior rectus sheath. This incision is opened longitudinally, the rectus abdominis muscle is split, and the posterior rectus sheath is exposed. A purse-string suture of 2-0 absorbable material is placed in the posterior rectus sheath, and a small incision is made in the peritoneum.

The catheter is inserted into the peritoneal cavity and directed into the pelvis; if a curled catheter is used, it is directed by means of a lubricated straight metal rod. The inner cuff is positioned just outside the posterior rectus sheath, and the purse-string suture is tied. With the ends of the purse-string suture providing traction, the posterior sheath is held up, and a free tie of absorbable material is placed around the tented-up peritoneum and catheter to keep the insertion site watertight. The barrel of a 50 ml syringe full of saline is then attached to the catheter. When the syringe barrel

is held above the abdomen, the fluid should flow freely into the abdomen by gravity alone. Conversely, when the syringe barrel is placed in a dependent position, the fluid should flow rapidly and freely out of the peritoneal cavity and back into the barrel. This test confirms that catheter position is satisfactory.

Troubleshooting The possibilities for error during placement are numerous: the catheter may be misdirected into the upper abdomen, it may be placed in a pocket of adhesions and blocked from reaching the greater peritoneal cavity, or it may be kinked in the abdomen, in muscle, or in the subcutaneous fascia. Plain radiographs sometimes facilitate recognition of incorrect placement. Surgical management—involving reexploration of the catheter insertion site, laparoscopy, or simple removal of the catheter and replacement at another site—is usually necessary if catheter malpositioning is not recognized at the time of the initial insertion.

Step 2: Tunneling of Catheter

The catheter is then tunneled to the exit site. It should emerge from the skin pointing in a caudal direction; this is more easily achieved with a catheter that has a preformed bend. The anterior sheath is closed snugly around the catheter, with the inner felt cuff left in the rectus abdominis muscle. The skin is closed with subcuticular sutures. If the catheter is to be used immediately, dialysis tubing is connected and a dressing is applied. If the catheter is not to be used immediately, 50 ml of saline containing 5,000 units of heparin is placed in the peritoneal cavity and the catheter is capped; this procedure is repeated every other day until dialysis begins.

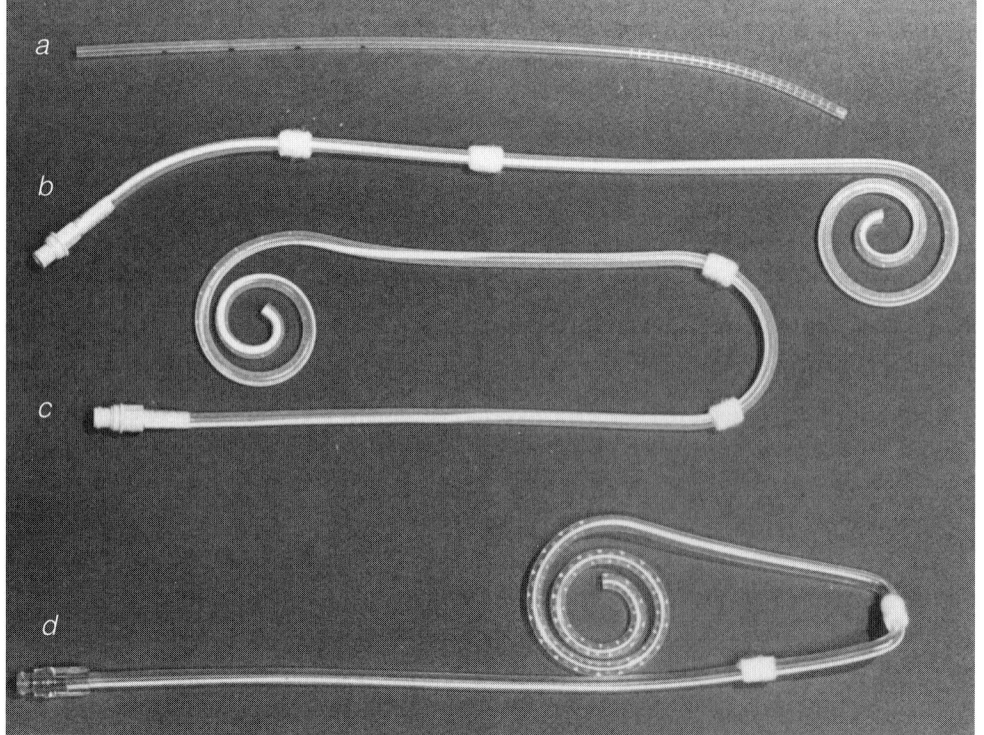

Figure 17 **Peritoneal access. Four types of peritoneal access catheters are shown: (*a*) a rigid catheter without a cuff, designed for temporary use, (*b*) a pigtail silicone catheter with a straight subcutaneous portion, (*c*) a pigtail silicone catheter with a curved subcutaneous portion, and (*d*) a pigtail silicone catheter with a preformed bend in the subcutaneous portion, which is currently the preferred configuration.**

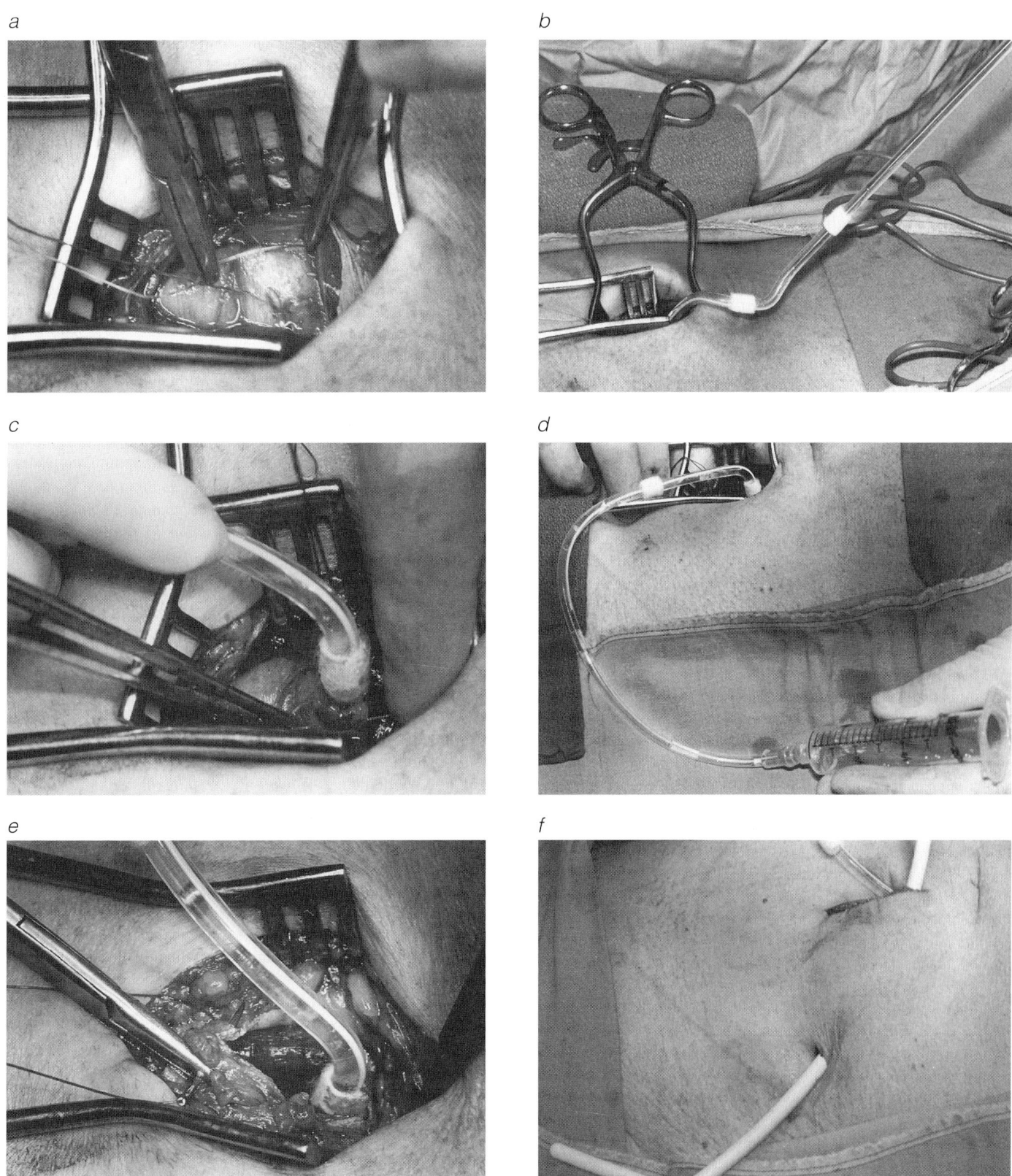

Figure 18 **Peritoneal access. Illustrated is the procedure for inserting a peritoneal dialysis catheter by cutdown with the patient under local anesthesia. (*a*) A local anesthetic is infiltrated, the anterior rectus sheath is opened, the rectus abdominis muscle is split, and a purse-string suture is placed in the posterior rectus sheath. (*b*) With the stylet in place, the catheter is inserted in the direction of the pelvis (left). (*c*) With the inner cuff at the level of the rectus abdominis, the purse-string suture is tied and reinforced with an additional circumferential free tie around the peritoneum, if possible. (*d*) A flow test is performed to confirm satisfactory catheter position. (*e*) The anterior rectus sheath is closed over the inner cuff. (*f*) The catheter is tunneled to the exit site so that it emerges pointing inferiorly (left), with the outer cuff in the subcutis.**

Step 3: Maintenance of Catheter

Maintenance of the catheter involves use of sterile dressings until the skin sites are healed, after which time a routine of skin cleansing and dressing is maintained. Whenever the catheter is disconnected, sterile precautions are taken to limit the possibility of contamination.

Step 4: Removal of Catheter

A Tenckhoff catheter is removed as follows. First, a local anesthetic is infiltrated into the original insertion site, and the inner Dacron cuff is dissected out of the rectus abdominis muscle (or the linea alba) with the electrocautery. Next, the catheter is divided and the abdominal portion removed. The rectus sheath (or the linea alba) is repaired with sutures, and the incision is closed. The subcutaneous cuff is then dissected out from the outside, and the outer portion of the catheter is removed. Finally, the insertion site is debrided, and the small skin opening is left to heal by second intention.

Troubleshooting Infection of the catheter tunnel or the Dacron cuffs necessitates some modification of this technique. If both the inner Dacron cuff and the outer are infected, salvage is impossible and the entire catheter must be removed. Areas of gross infection are treated with drainage and debridement and left open to heal by second intention. If alternative temporary peritoneal access for dialysis is available, a new catheter is not placed until the skin has healed completely. If no alternative temporary access is available, it may be necessary to insert a new catheter simultaneously at another site that is distant from the original infected location.

If only the outer cuff is infected and no other sites are available for subsequent catheter replacement, salvage may be attempted as follows: the outer cuff is dissected out of the subcutaneous tissue, the Dacron is shaved off, and this portion of the catheter is left outside the skin. This approach may allow resolution of the infection; however, it makes the inner cuff the sole barrier to deep infection and thus should not be used when alternative access is possible.

Special Considerations

Peritoneal access in children The technical considerations for peritoneal access in children are much the same as those for peritoneal access in adults. There are, however, some significant differences. If a Tenckhoff catheter is to be used in a child weighing less than 20 kg (44 lb), it should have only one Dacron cuff, which should be placed in the rectus abdominis muscle. The appropriate length for the catheter must be determined; this is done by measuring the size of the child from the point of insertion to the pelvic basin. Leaks should be prevented by ligating the peritoneum underneath the purse-string suture in the posterior rectus sheath [see Step 1: Insertion of Catheter, above]. General anesthesia is usually required. Postoperative dialysis volumes are selected according to patient size.

Alternative technology Laparoscopic techniques have also been developed for placement of peritoneal catheters. These techniques employ the standard 5 to 10 mm diameter trocars commonly used for laparoscopic procedures.[50] The catheter is inserted into the abdomen through a large cannula. One problem with this technique is that it is difficult to confirm that the deep cuff is placed within the musculature until after the cannula is removed. Moreover, despite the excellent visualization of the peritoneal cavity achieved with catheters placed in this manner, there is a high incidence of pericatheter leakage. Alternatively, one may resort to new techniques using specially designed equipment, such as the Y-Tec 2.2 mm–diameter Peritoneoscope, which always positions the deep cuff tightly within the musculature.[51] In fact, randomized, controlled studies have indicated that catheters placed via peritoneoscopy survive approximately twice as long as catheters placed via traditional surgical dissection.[52] Furthermore, such procedures can always be performed at the bedside with local anesthesia or in an outpatient setting.

COMPLICATIONS

The following are the most significant early complications of peritoneal access procedures:

1. Injury to intra-abdominal organs, most commonly the small bowel, the colon, the bladder, and the fallopian tubes. Immediate exploration is necessary.
2. Leakage of peritoneal dialysate soon after catheter placement. This complication is caused by inadequate closure of the peritoneum around the catheter.
3. Incorrect catheter placement, usually manifested by relatively good inflow but poor outflow.
4. Intra-abdominal bleeding, signaled by a bloody dialysate. Although most episodes of intra-abdominal bleeding are minor and self-limited and consequently do not call for transfusion or specific intervention, investigation to determine the underlying cause is warranted.

The following are the most significant late complications of procedures for peritoneal access:

1. Intra-abdominal bleeding. The most common causes of such bleeding are related to menstruation and ovulation.
2. Erosion of the outer cuff of the catheter through the skin. This complication can be treated by dissecting the remaining cuff completely out of the subcutaneous tissues and shaving off the Dacron [see Operative Technique, Step 4: Removal of Catheter, above]. Because this approach, as noted, leaves only the inner cuff as a barrier to infection, it is usually advisable to treat outer-cuff erosion by removing the catheter completely and replacing it at another site.
3. Catheter breakage. If more than 2 cm remains outside the skin, special repair kits may be used to splice a new external catheter piece onto the original catheter.
4. Tunnel infections. Such infections are typically associated with contamination and infection of the outer cuff. The most common causative organisms are *Staphylococcus* species and *Pseudomonas* species.[53] Nasal carriage of *Staphylococcus* is a risk factor for tunnel infections, and pretreatment with rifampin may help decrease the risk.[54] Although many tunnel infections can be controlled with several weeks of antibiotic therapy and some can even be cured, most eventually necessitate removal of the catheter, especially if there is concomitant peritonitis.[55]
5. Catheter malfunction. Late catheter malfunction is uncommon. Complete obstruction of both inflow and outflow is generally attributable to fibrin plugs and can be corrected by infusing streptokinase. Good inflow coupled with poor outflow frequently signals wrapping of the catheter by omentum. This problem can be corrected by performing an omentectomy either laparoscopically or in an open fashion via a low midline incision.

OUTCOME EVALUATION

When peritoneal dialysis catheter function is poor shortly after operative placement, possible causes to be suspected include misdirection into the upper abdomen, kinking, previous abdominal adhesions, and omental obstruction of the catheter. Most of these complications present with satisfactory inflow but poor drainage.

Plain radiographs of the abdomen (or contrast studies if the catheter is not radiopaque) may reveal the problem. Sometimes, the complications respond to enemas (which may alter the location of the catheter) and to persistent attempts to achieve satisfactory exchange. Frequently, however, abdominal exploration via a lower midline incision is required, followed by omentectomy, redirection of the catheter, or catheter replacement. If omental wrapping of the catheter is the problem, the entire omentum should be removed to prevent a recurrence. General anesthesia is often necessary, though in some cases, certain of these procedures can be done with the patient under local anesthesia with sedation or under regional anesthesia. Laparoscopy has also been used to diagnose and treat peritoneal dialysis catheter dysfunction; general anesthesia is usually required.

References

1. US Renal Data System: USRDS 1999 Annual Data Report. The National Institute of Health, National Institute of Diabetes and Digestive and Kidney Disease. Am J Kidney Dis 34(suppl 1):540, 1999

2. Kolff WJ, Berk HT, ter Welle M, et al: The artificial kidney: a dialyzer with a great area. 1944. J Am Soc Nephrol. 8:1959, 1997

3. Quinton WE, Dillard DH, Scribner BH: Cannulation of blood vessels for prolonged hemodialysis. Trans Am Soc Artif Intern Organs 6:104, 1960

4. Brescia MJ, Cimino JE, Appell K, et al: Chronic hemodialysis using venipuncture and surgically created arteriovenous fistula. 1966. J Am Soc Nephrol 10:193, 1999

5. Baker LD, Johnson JM, Goldfarb D: Expanded polytetrafluoroethylene (PTFE) subcutaneous arteriovenous conduit: an improved vascular access for chronic hemodialysis. Trans Am Soc Artif Intern Organs 22:382, 1976

6. National Kidney Foundation DOQI: Clinical Practice Guidelines for Hemodialysis Vascular Access. Am J Kidney Dis 30(suppl 3):S150, 1997

7. Schwab SJ, Quarles LD, Middleton JP, et al: Hemodialysis-associated subclavian vein stenosis. Kidney Int 33:1156, 1988

8. Passman MA, Criado E, Farber MA, et al: Efficacy of color duplex imaging for proximal upper extremity venous outflow obstruction in hemodialysis patients. J Vasc Surg 28:869, 1998

9. Silva MB, Hobson RW, Pappas PJ, et al: A strategy for increasing use of autogenous hemodialysis access procedures: impact of preoperative noninvasive evaluation. J Vasc Surg 27:302, 1998

10. Marx AB, Landmann J, Harder FH: Surgery for vascular access. Curr Probl Surg 28(1):15, 1990

11. Silva MB, Hobson RW, Pappas PJ, et al: Vein transposition in the forearm for autogenous hemodialysis access. J Vasc Surg 26:981, 1997

12. Hakaim AG, Nalbandian M, Scott T: Superior maturation and patency of primary brachiocephalic and transposed basilic vein arteriovenous fistulae in patients with diabetes. J Vasc Surg 27:154, 1998

13. Matsuura JH, Rosenthal D, Clark M, et al: Transposed basilic vein versus polytetrafluoroethylene for brachial-axillary arteriovenous fistulas. Am J Surg 176:219, 1998

14. Coburn MC, Carney WI: Comparison of basilic vein and polytetrafluoroethylene for brachial arteriovenous fistula. J Vasc Surg 20:896, 1994

15. Gracz KC, Ing TS, Soung L, et al: Proximal forearm fistula for maintenance hemodialysis. Kidney Int 11:71, 1977

16. Bender MHM, Bruyninckx CMA, Gerlag PGG: The brachiocephalic elbow fistula: a useful alternative angioaccess for permanent hemodialysis. J Vasc Surg 20:808, 1994

17. Polo JR, Vazquez R, Polo J, et al: Brachiocephalic jump graft fistula: an alternative for dialysis use of elbow crease veins. Am J Kidney Dis 33:904, 1999

18. Dagher FJ, Gelber R, Ramos E, et al: The use of basilic vein and brachial artery as an A-V fistula for long term hemodialysis. J Surg Res 20:373, 1976

19. LoGerfo FW, Menzoian JO, Kumaki DJ, et al: Transposed basilic vein-brachial arteriovenous fistula: a reliable secondary-access procedure. Arch Surg 113:1008, 1978

20. Humphries AL, Colborn GL, Wynn JJ: Elevated basilic vein arteriovenous fistula. Am J Surg 177:489, 1999

21. Benedetti E, Del Pino A, Cintron J, et al: A new method of creating an arteriovenous graft access. Am J Surg 171:369, 1996

22. Santaro TD, Cambria RA: PTFE shunts for hemodialysis access: progressive choice of configuration. Semin Vasc Surg 10:166, 1997

23. Lazarides MK, Staramos DN, Tzilalis VD, et al: Evoked thrill: a simple intraoperative maneuver predicts early patency of arteriovenous fistulas. J Vasc Surg 27:750, 1998

24. Lenz BJ, Veldenz HC, Dennis JW, et al: A three-year follow-up on standard versus thin wall ePTFE grafts for hemodialysis. J Vasc Surg 28:464, 1998

25. Tordoir JH, Hofstra L, Bergmans DC, et al: Stretch versus standard expanded PTFE grafts for hemodialysis access. Vascular Access for Hemodialysis IV. Henry ML, Ferguson RM, Eds. WL Gore & Associates and Precept Press, Chicago, 1995, p 277

26. Lumsden AB, MacDonald MJ, Kikeri D, et al: Prophylactic balloon angioplasty fails to prolong the patency of expanded polytetrafluoroethylene arteriovenous grafts: results of a prospective randomized study. J Vasc Surg 26:382, 1997

27. Shoenfeld R, Hermans H, Novick A, et al: Stenting of proximal venous obstruction to maintain hemodialysis access. J Vasc Surg 19:532, 1994

28. Marston WA, Criado E, Jacques PF, et al: Prospective randomized comparison of surgical versus endovascular management of thrombosed dialysis access grafts. J Vasc Surg 26:373, 1997

29. DeMasi RJ, Gregory RT, Sorrell KA, et al: Intraoperative noninvasive evaluation of arteriovenous fistulae and grafts: "the steal study." J Vasc Tech 18:192, 1994

30. Kwun KB, Schanzer H, Finkler N, et al: Hemodynamic evaluation of angioaccess procedures for hemodialysis. Vasc Surg 13:170, 1979

31. Odland MD, Kelly PH, Ney AL, et al: Management of dialysis-associated steal syndrome complicating upper extremity arteriovenous fistulas: Use of intraoperative digital photoplethysmography. Surgery 110:664, 1991

32. Mattson WJ: Recognition and treatment of vascular steal secondary to hemodialysis prostheses. Am J Surg 154:198, 1987

33. West JC, Evans RD, Kelley SE, et al: Arterial insufficiency in hemodialysis access procedures: reconstruction by an interposition polytetrafluoroethylene graft conduit. Am J Surg 153:300, 1987

34. Bussel JA, Abbott JA, Lim RC: A radial steal syndrome with arteriovenous fistula for hemodialysis. Ann Intern Med 75:1657, 1971

35. Schanzer H, Schwartz M, Harrington E, et al: Treatment of ischemia due to "steal" by arteriovenous fistula with distal artery ligation and revascularization. J Vasc Surg 7:770, 1988

36. Shemesh D, Mabjeesh NJ, Abramowitz HB: Management of dialysis access-associated steal syndrome: use of intraoperative duplex ultrasound scanning for optimal flow reduction. J Vasc Surg 30:193, 1999

37. Beathard GA, Settle SM, Shields MW: Salvage of the nonfunctioning arteriovenous fistula. Am J Kidney Dis 33:910, 1999

38. Zibari GB, Rohr MS, Landreneau MD, et al: Complications from permanent hemodialysis vascular access. Surgery 104:681, 1988

39. Haire WD, Lynch TG, Lieberman RP, et al: Duplex scans before subclavian vein catheterization predict unsuccessful catheter placement. Arch Surg 127:229, 1992

40. Whitman ED: Complications associated with the use of central venous access devices. Curr Probl Surg 33:324, 1996

41. Dunea G, Domenico L, Gunnerson P, et al: A survey of permanent double-lumen catheters in hemodialysis patients. ASAIO Trans 37:M276, 1991

42. Chimochowski GE, Worley E, Rutherford WE, et al: Superiority of the internal jugular over the subclavian access for temporary hemodialysis. Nephron 54:154, 1990

43. The Food and Drug Administration Task Force: Precautions necessary with central venous catheters. FDA Drug Bulletin 15:6, 1989

44. Mansfield PF, Hohn DC, Fornage BD, et al: Complications and failures of subclavian-vein catheterization. N Engl J Med 331:1735, 1994

45. Stuart RK, Shikora SA, Akerman P, et al: Incidence of arrhythmia with central venous catheter insertion and exchange. J Parenter Enteral Nutr 14:152, 1990

46. Horattas MC, Wright DJ, Fenton AH, et al: Changing concepts of deep venous thrombosis of the upper extremity: report of a series and review of the literature. Surgery 104:561, 1988

47. Suchoki P, Conlon P, Knelson M, et al: Silastic cuffed catheters for hemodialysis vascular access: thrombolytic and mechanical correction of HD catheter malfunction. Am J Kidney Dis 28:279, 1996

48. Crain MR, Mewissen MW, Ostrowski GJ, et al: Fibrin sleeve stripping for salvage of failing hemodialysis catheters: techniques and initial results. Radiology 198:41, 1996

49. Schaffer D: Catheter-related sepsis complicating long-term, tunnelled central venous dialysis catheters: management by guidewire exchange. Am J Kidney Dis 25:593, 1995

50. Douglas AF, Deardon DA, Barclay CA, et al: Laparoscopic insertion of CAPD catheters. Proceedings of the 3rd International Congress on Access for Dialysis. Maastricht, 1997

51. Ash SR: Bedside peritoneoscopic peritoneal catheter placement of Tenckoff and newer peritoneal catheters. Adv Peritoneal Dialysis 14:1, 1998

52. Gadallah MF, Pervez A, El-Shahawy M, et al: Peritoneoscopic versus surgical placement of Tenckhoff catheters: a prospective study on outcome. J Am Soc Nephrol 7:A0904, 1996

53. Prevention of peritonitis in CAPD (editorial). Lancet 337:22, 1991

54. Piraino B: A review of *Staphylococcus aureus* exit-site and tunnel infections in peritoneal dialysis patients. Am J Kidney Dis 16:89, 1990

55. Holley JL, Bernardini J, Piraino B: Risk factors for tunnel infections in continuous peritoneal dialysis. Am J Kidney Dis 18:344, 19

Acknowledgments

Figures 1 through 9, 11, 12, 15, and 16   Jean Montreuil, B.Ing, M.Sc. Digitized and adapted by Tom Moore.

5 TRAUMA AND THERMAL INJURY

1 TRAUMA RESUSCITATION

Frederick A. Moore, M.D., F.A.C.S., and Ernest E. Moore, M.D., F.A.C.S.

Initial Approach to the Critically Injured Patient

Salvage of the critically injured is optimized by a coordinated team effort in an organized trauma system. Management of life-threatening injuries must be decided according to physiologic necessity for survival; that is, active efforts to support airway, breathing, and circulation (the ABCs) are usually initiated before specific diagnosis. This chapter presents a systematic approach to severely injured patients within the so-called golden hour. The discussion is divided into prehospital care and emergency department management; the ED component is further divided into (1) primary survey and initial resuscitation, (2) evaluation, with continuation of resuscitation, and (3) secondary survey and definitive diagnosis.

Prehospital Care

Resuscitation and evaluation of trauma patients begin at the injury site. Prehospital care and hospital destination are much different from those of the medical arrest victim. Whereas provision of advanced cardiac life support (ACLS) at the scene clearly improves survival for the medical patient,[1] the goal in trauma is to get the *right patient to the right hospital at the right time.* First responders (typically, firefighters and police) provide rapid basic trauma life support (BTLS) and are followed by paramedics and flight nurses with advanced skills. Medical control is ensured by preestablished field protocols, radio communication with a base hospital physician, and subsequent trip audits. Management priorities of BTLS on the scene are to (1) assess and control the scene for the safety of the patient and the prehospital care provider, (2) tamponade external hemorrhage with direct pressure, (3) protect the spine after blunt trauma, (4) supplement inspired oxygen, (5) extricate the patient, and (6) stabilize long bone fractures. Active airway support is a major asset of advanced trauma life support (ATLS) in prehospital systems, achieved with skilled paramedics under close medical control.[2] However, the value of intravenous fluid administration in such systems remains controversial.[3-5] The heart of the controversy is whether it is preferable (1) to give fluids until a normal blood pressure is reached, thus causing hemodilution and disruption of early hemostatic clots, or (2) to withhold resuscitation, thus prolonging cellular shock, which may become irreversible by the time operative control is accomplished. The compromise between these two approaches is moderate volume loading.[5-8]

Application of the pneumatic antishock garment (PASG) is warranted for active hemorrhage caused by major pelvic fractures and may be appropriate for profound shock if transport time is expected to exceed 30 minutes.[6,9,10] In any situation, implementation of

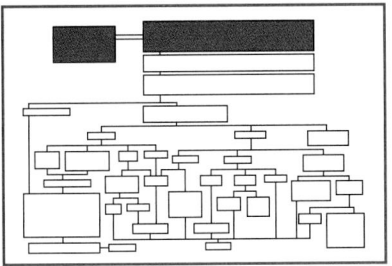

ATLS depends on the expertise of field personnel, the patient's condition, and the distance to the hospital.[11-13]

Prehospital trauma scores have been devised to identify critically injured trauma victims, who represent about 10% to 15% of all injured patients. When it is geographically and logistically feasible, critically injured patients should be taken directly to a designated level I facility (i.e., an Urban Regional Trauma Center) or to a level II facility (i.e., a Rural Regional Trauma Center). The currently available field trauma scores, however, are imperfect for identifying critically injured patients.[14] A 25% over-triage is probably necessary to capture most of the patients with life-threatening injury. Advance transmission of key patient information to the receiving trauma center facilitates organization of the trauma team and ensures availability of ancillary services.

Emergency Department Management

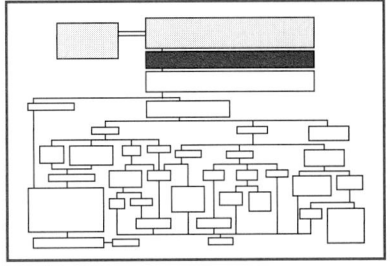

Initial ED management of seriously injured patients requires simultaneous treatment and evaluation. Rapid assessment of vital function is done while an empirical sequence of lifesaving therapeutic and diagnostic procedures is initiated.[15] The ultimate goal is to establish adequate oxygen delivery to the vital organs. This is accomplished by first progressing through the ABCs: airway control with cervical spine precautions—along with assisted breathing, ventilation, and occasional empirical tube thoracostomy to relieve a pneumothorax—maximizes oxygen delivery to the alveoli. Support of circulation (tamponade of external bleeding and fluid administration via large-bore I.V. catheters) is required to restore effective blood volume, thus enhancing myocardial performance and oxygen delivery to the tissues.

PRIMARY SURVEY AND INITIAL RESUSCITATION

Airway/Breathing

After blunt trauma, airway control should proceed on the assumption that an unstable cervical spine fracture exists; thus, hyperextension of the neck must be avoided. Airway management in the seriously injured victim can usually be accomplished with simple techniques, but occasionally, it can be extremely challenging. Evaluation begins by asking the patient a question such as "How are you?" A response given in a normal voice indicates that the airway is not in immediate jeopardy; a breathless, hoarse response or no response at all indicates that the airway may be compromised.

Initial Approach to the Critically Injured Patient

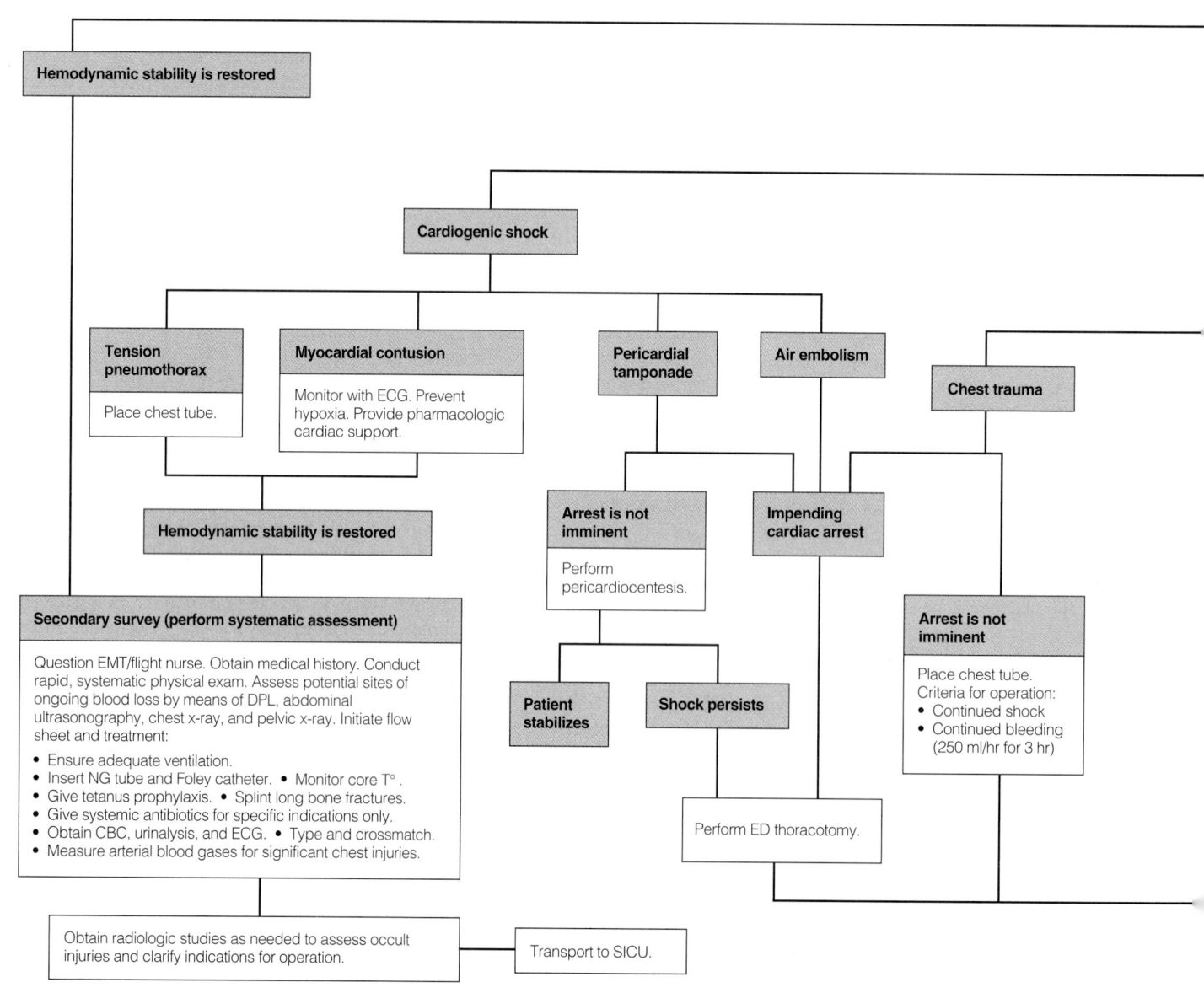

Communicate with base hospital

Field triage: Level I, II, or III facility
Assemble trauma team:
- Trauma surgeon
- ED physician
- Surgical specialist
- Radiology technicians
- Nurses
- Respiratory technicians

Ensure ancillary services:
- OR
- CT scanning
- Blood bank
- Interventional radiology

Hemodynamic stability is restored

Cardiogenic shock

Tension pneumothorax

Place chest tube.

Myocardial contusion

Monitor with ECG. Prevent hypoxia. Provide pharmacologic cardiac support.

Pericardial tamponade

Air embolism

Chest trauma

Hemodynamic stability is restored

Arrest is not imminent

Perform pericardiocentesis.

Impending cardiac arrest

Arrest is not imminent

Place chest tube.
Criteria for operation:
- Continued shock
- Continued bleeding (250 ml/hr for 3 hr)

Secondary survey (perform systematic assessment)

Question EMT/flight nurse. Obtain medical history. Conduct rapid, systematic physical exam. Assess potential sites of ongoing blood loss by means of DPL, abdominal ultrasonography, chest x-ray, and pelvic x-ray. Initiate flow sheet and treatment:

- Ensure adequate ventilation.
- Insert NG tube and Foley catheter. • Monitor core T°.
- Give tetanus prophylaxis. • Splint long bone fractures.
- Give systemic antibiotics for specific indications only.
- Obtain CBC, urinalysis, and ECG. • Type and crossmatch.
- Measure arterial blood gases for significant chest injuries.

Patient stabilizes

Shock persists

Perform ED thoracotomy.

Obtain radiologic studies as needed to assess occult injuries and clarify indications for operation.

Transport to SICU.

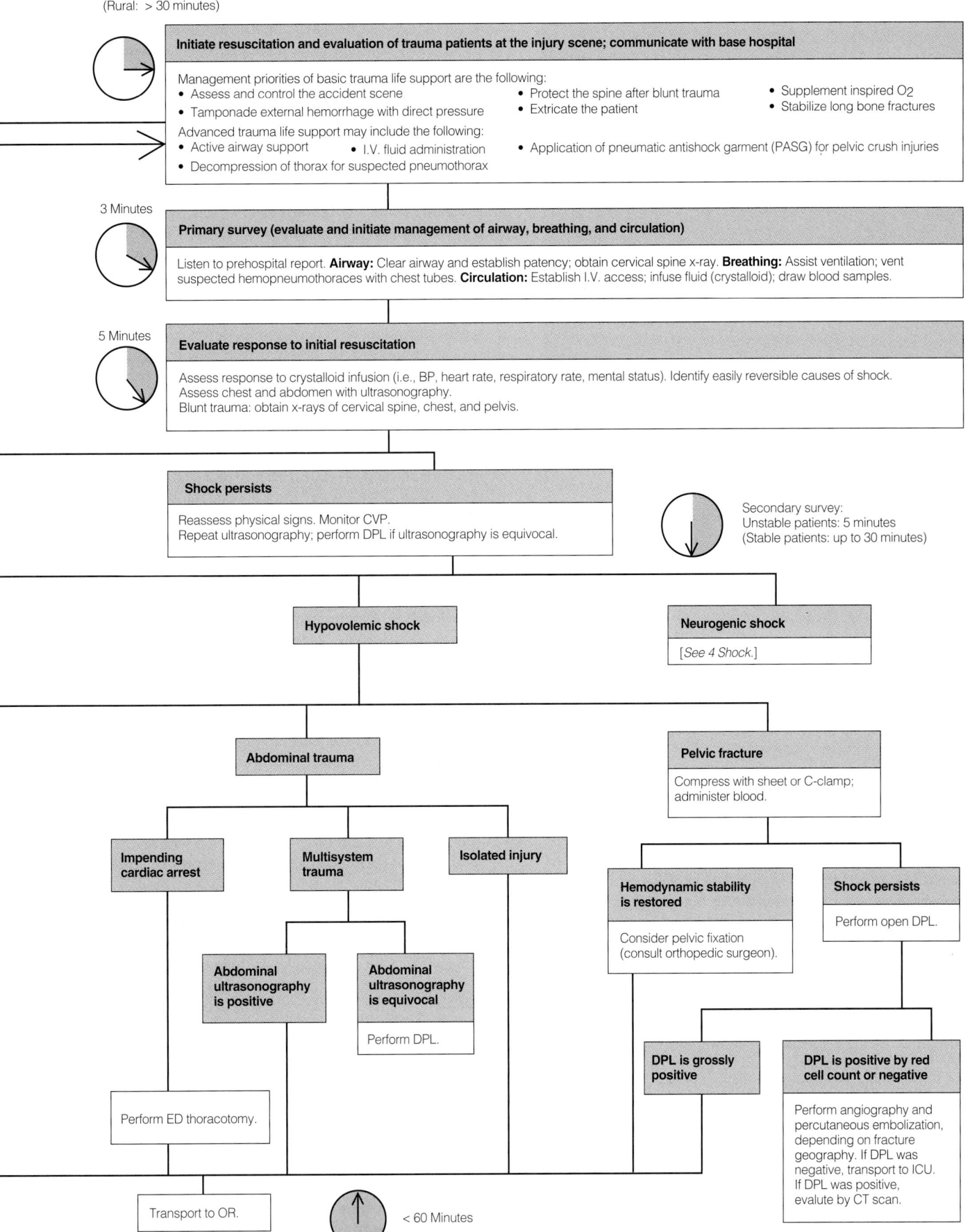

Urban: < 15 minutes
(Rural: > 30 minutes)

Initiate resuscitation and evaluation of trauma patients at the injury scene; communicate with base hospital

Management priorities of basic trauma life support are the following:
- Assess and control the accident scene
- Tamponade external hemorrhage with direct pressure
- Protect the spine after blunt trauma
- Extricate the patient
- Supplement inspired O₂
- Stabilize long bone fractures

Advanced trauma life support may include the following:
- Active airway support
- I.V. fluid administration
- Decompression of thorax for suspected pneumothorax
- Application of pneumatic antishock garment (PASG) for pelvic crush injuries

3 Minutes

Primary survey (evaluate and initiate management of airway, breathing, and circulation)

Listen to prehospital report. **Airway:** Clear airway and establish patency; obtain cervical spine x-ray. **Breathing:** Assist ventilation; vent suspected hemopneumothoraces with chest tubes. **Circulation:** Establish I.V. access; infuse fluid (crystalloid); draw blood samples.

5 Minutes

Evaluate response to initial resuscitation

Assess response to crystalloid infusion (i.e., BP, heart rate, respiratory rate, mental status). Identify easily reversible causes of shock.
Assess chest and abdomen with ultrasonography.
Blunt trauma: obtain x-rays of cervical spine, chest, and pelvis.

Shock persists

Reassess physical signs. Monitor CVP.
Repeat ultrasonography; perform DPL if ultrasonography is equivocal.

Secondary survey:
Unstable patients: 5 minutes
(Stable patients: up to 30 minutes)

Hypovolemic shock

Neurogenic shock

[*See 4 Shock.*]

Abdominal trauma

Pelvic fracture

Compress with sheet or C-clamp; administer blood.

Impending cardiac arrest

Multisystem trauma

Isolated injury

Hemodynamic stability is restored

Consider pelvic fixation (consult orthopedic surgeon).

Shock persists

Perform open DPL.

Abdominal ultrasonography is positive

Abdominal ultrasonography is equivocal

Perform DPL.

Perform ED thoracotomy.

DPL is grossly positive

DPL is positive by red cell count or negative

Perform angiography and percutaneous embolization, depending on fracture geography. If DPL was negative, transport to ICU. If DPL was positive, evalute by CT scan.

Transport to OR.

< 60 Minutes

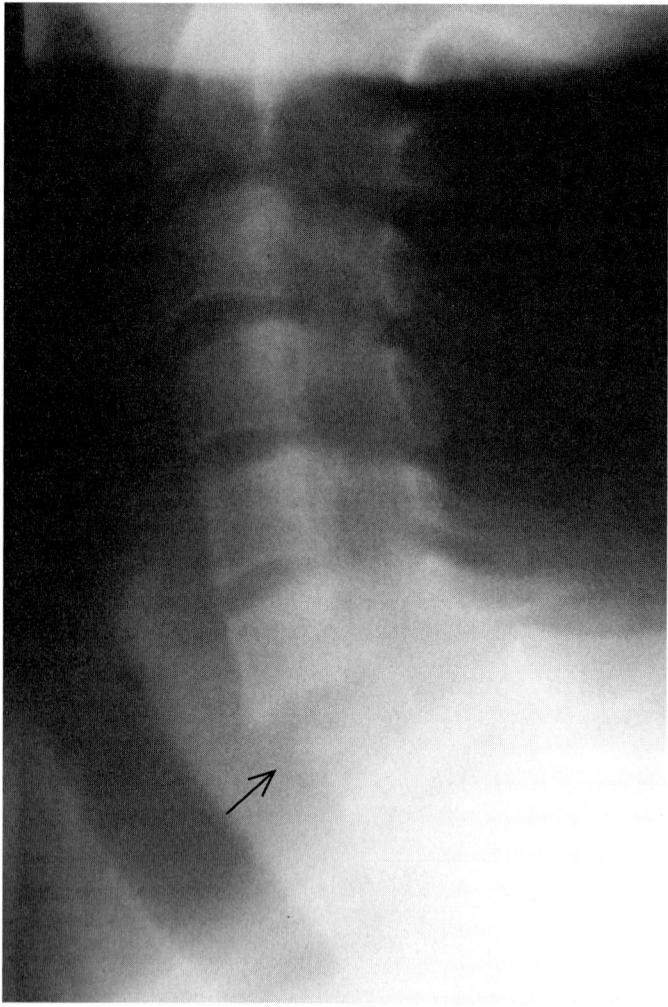

Figure 1 **The cross-table lateral cervical spine x-ray is integral to acute airway management decisions. The most frequent mistake is inadequate visualization of the seventh cervical vertebra (arrow).**

Airway obstruction and hypoventilation are the most likely causes of respiratory failure. The critical decision is whether active airway intervention is needed. The first maneuver is to clear the airway of debris and to suction secretions. In the obtunded patient, this procedure is followed by elevation of the angle of the mandible to alleviate pharyngeal obstruction and placement of an oropharyngeal or nasopharyngeal tube to maintain airway patency. Supplemental oxygen is given via a nasal cannula (6 L/min) or a non-rebreathing oxygen mask (12 L/min). Airway patency does not ensure adequate ventilation. Clinical evidence of hypoventilation includes poor air exchange at the nose and mouth, diminished breath sounds, and decreased chest wall excursion; the most likely causes are head injury, spinal cord transection, hemopneumothorax, flail chest, and profound shock. Suspected hemopneumothoraces should be vented with large-bore chest tubes inserted via the midlateral thorax.

Early cervical spine assessment is integral to airway management. The timing of active airway control is pivotal. The majority of significant spinal injuries in adults arriving alive at the emergency department are at the C5 to C7 levels.[16] In children 8 years old or younger, the most frequent site of spinal injury is between the occiput and C3 level.[17] Moreover, children experience a higher incidence of significant spinal cord injury without radiographic abnormalities (i.e., the SCIWORA syndrome).[18] A fractured cervical spine is usually tender to direct palpation in alert patients, but pain may be masked by distracting injuries.[19] A good-quality cross-table lateral cervical spine (CTLCS) x-ray will delineate 98% of unstable fractures [*see Figure 1*]. In high-risk patients, initial airway management is based on the CTLCS film and clinical judgment,[20] although a cervical collar is left in place until the cervical spine has been radiologically evaluated for bony integrity.

Ideally, after blunt trauma or transcervical gunshot wounds, intubation should be deferred until CTLCS films are available, although neurologic injury from a gunshot wound to the neck is virtually always complete at the time of injury. Bag-mask ventilation is an effective temporizing measure, but it consumes the attention of a skilled trauma team member, it may insufflate air into the stomach, it is resisted by spontaneously breathing patients, and it is ineffective in the presence of severe maxillofacial trauma. The decision for urgent airway control is clinical; there is no time to obtain a confirmatory arterial blood gas (ABG) analysis.[21] Persistent airway obstruction or signs of inadequate ventilation mandate prompt intervention. Patients with expanding neck hematomas, deteriorating vital signs, or severe head trauma are also best managed with an aggressive airway approach. On the other hand, in equivocal situations (e.g., increased P_aCO_2 or base deficit despite a satisfactory S_aO_2), an ABG analysis may be decisive.

The best method of airway control depends on (1) the presence of maxillofacial trauma, (2) suspected cervical spine injury, (3) overall patient condition, and (4) the experience of the physician. Patients in respiratory distress with severe maxillofacial trauma warrant operative intervention. Cricothyrotomy is the preferred approach in adults and has virtually replaced tracheostomy in the ED [*see Figure 2*]; the rare exceptions are in patients with direct laryngeal trauma or complete tracheal disruption. Percutaneous transtracheal ventilation may be safer than both of these surgical procedures for temporary airway management, particularly in children.[22] Nasotracheal intubation is the airway route of choice in nonapneic patients with potential cervical injury in the field but is rarely employed in the ED. The current standard approach is rapid sequence intubation (RSI) of the trachea orally with inline immobilization.[23,24] Our RSI guidelines include nine steps: (1) preparation of equipment and supplies; (2) preoxygenation; (3) sedation to decrease anxiety; (4) premedication to mitigate the negative effects of intubation (e.g., a defasciculating dose of pancuronium or lidocaine for patients with head injuries to prevent increased intracranial pressure); (5) cricoid pressure; (6) paralysis with either succinylcholine, 1.0 to 1.5 mg/kg, or rocuronium, 0.5 to 1.2 mg/kg; (7) intubation with visualization of the vocal cords to permit confident airway access; (8) confirmation of tube position by auscultation and capnography; and (9) securing of the airway. In adults, a large (8 mm internal diameter) cuffed endotracheal tube should be inserted to a distance of 23 cm from the incisors. In children, tube size is gauged to equal the diameter of the little finger or may be estimated by the following formula:

$$\frac{age + 16}{4} = internal\ diameter\ (mm)\ of\ endotracheal\ tube$$

The proper depth (in centimeters) to which the tube should be inserted can be estimated by multiplying the tube's internal diameter (in millimeters) by 3. A chest x-ray should be obtained as soon as possible to rule out the common problem of right mainstem intubation.

Circulation

Once alveolar ventilation is ensured, the next priority is to optimize oxygen delivery by maximizing cardiovascular performance. Hypovolemia is the most likely cause of shock that occurs after the patient receives an injury [*see 6:3 Shock*]; therefore, treatment is

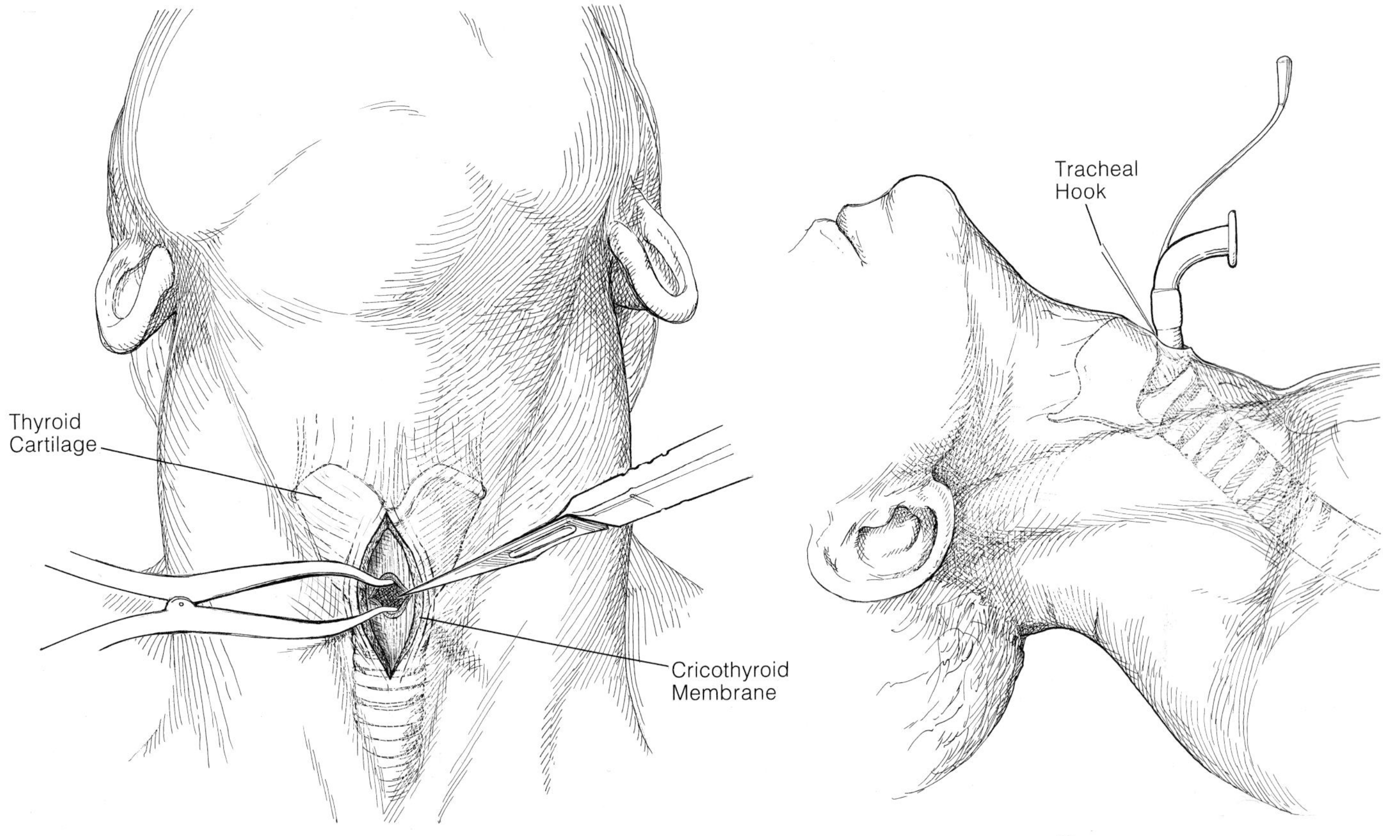

Figure 2 Technique for cricothyrotomy is illustrated here. The larynx is stabilized with one hand, and a 2 cm vertical incision is made over the cricothyroid space. The cricothyroid membrane is palpated and incised horizontally. A Trosseau dilator is inserted and spread vertically for visualization of the subglottic space (left). A tracheal hook is used to retract the inferior border of the thyroid cartilage as a tracheostomy tube with a 6 mm internal diameter is inserted into the trachea (right).

initiated with crystalloid infusion via large-bore I.V. cannulas, and external hemorrhage is controlled by manual compression. If the PASG has been applied in the field, it should not be removed until effective volume restitution has been achieved. Of special concern are cases in which the PASG has been applied to manage otherwise uncontrollable lower-extremity hemorrhage. In such cases, with effective volume loading, bleeding may become profuse. Application of the PASG in the ED should be reserved for the control of bleeding from major pelvic fractures—if used at all. In fact, wrapping the pelvis with a sheet in the ED is now preferred for initial mechanical stabilization of major pelvic fractures.

The size, number, and sites of I.V. catheters depend on the degree of shock and on estimates of the severity of the injury. If the patient arrives in shock or has obvious multiple injuries, a short 14 French catheter should be placed in each antecubital vein. When vascular collapse precludes peripheral percutaneous access, saphenous vein cutdown at the ankle is preferred [*see Figure 3*] because the site is distant from sites of other resuscitative efforts, the vein will easily accept a large catheter, and the only adjacent structure is a trivial branch of the saphenous nerve. An acceptable alternative is intubation of the femoral vein at the groin by means of the Seldinger technique. Intraosseous infusion through a cannula placed in the medullary cavity of a long bone is a safe and efficacious method for emergency vascular access in infants and children 6 years old or younger. This procedure is typically performed in the anteromedial aspect of the tibial plateau in an uninjured extremity; the distal femur, the distal tibia, and the sternum are other potential sites. Intraosseous infusion gen-

erally allows administration of sufficient fluid to facilitate subsequent cannulation of the venous circulation.[25] With establishment of the first intravenous line, blood should be drawn for hematocrit, white blood cell count, amylase level, electrolyte concentrations, blood-group typing, coagulation profile, and toxicology screen as indicated.

EVALUATION AND CONTINUED RESUSCITATION

Systemic blood pressure, heart rate, respiratory rate, and the patient's general appearance are most helpful in judging the degree of acute blood loss and in assessing the response to initial crystalloid resuscitation.

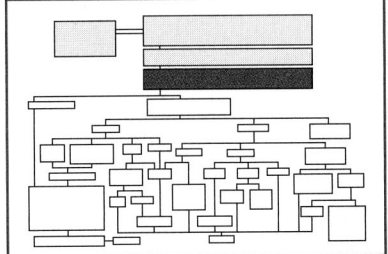

As a general rule, the carotid pulse is palpable at a systolic blood pressure of 60 mm Hg, the femoral pulse at 70 mm Hg, and the radial pulse at 80 mm Hg. In patients with hypovolemic shock, crystalloid loading is initiated with ongoing monitoring of vital signs. Studies from Houston, however, emphasize that in patients with free intraperitoneal or intrathoracic bleeding, overzealous fluid administration before definitive vascular control is achieved may increase blood loss.[3] Consequently, such patients should be promptly transported to the operating room without aggressive efforts to normalize vital signs. It is important to note that acute massive blood loss may paradoxically trigger a vagal-mediated

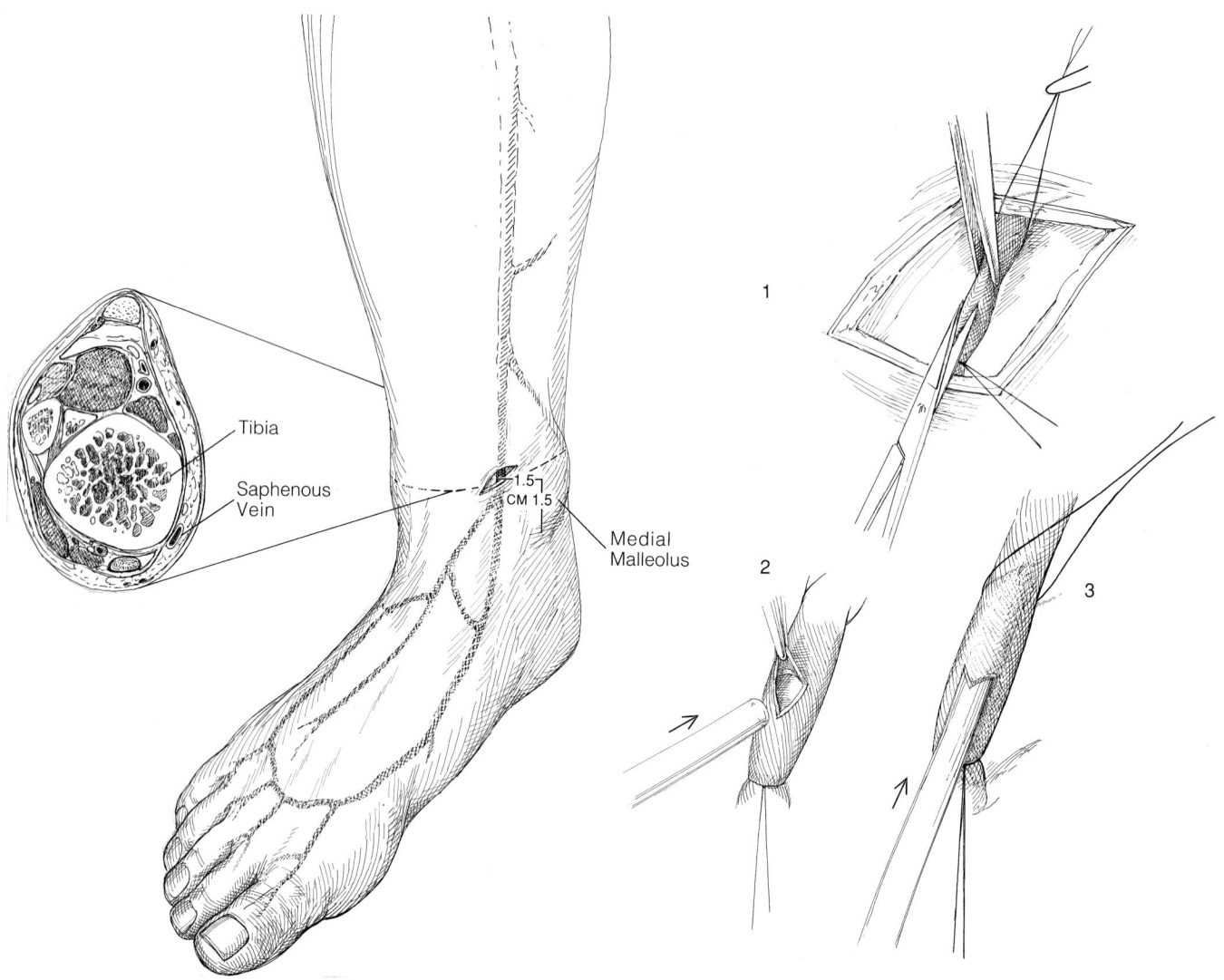

Tibia

Saphenous Vein

1.5
CM 1.5

Medial Malleolus

1

2

3

Figure 3   **Saphenous vein cutdown is indicated when vascular collapse precludes peripheral access. The greater saphenous vein lies superficial to the anterior periosteum at the medial malleolus. A transverse skin incision is made one fingerbreadth superior and anterior to the malleolus. A hemostat is inserted and brought across the anteromedial aspect of the tibia. The only structures that should be included under the hemostat are the saphenous vein and a trivial branch of the saphenous nerve.**

bradycardia, and therefore, the traditional inverse correlation of increasing heart rate and reduced effective blood volume may not occur in the early resuscitation period.[26] When crystalloid infusion exceeds 50 ml/kg, blood should be administered[27]; type-specific whole blood is rarely associated with complications and should be available within 20 minutes. If type-specific blood is not available, reconstituted O-negative packed red blood cells may be used. Micropore filters are not used in blood infusion lines in hemodynamically unstable patients, because they impede infusion capabilities.[28] In the future, hemoglobin-based blood substitutes may become available that would obviate the need for crossmatching and filtration. Electrocardiographic monitoring, serial measurement of vital signs, rapid physical examination, rectal temperature reading, and initiation of a flow sheet complete the initial assessment of the patient.

The next step is to evaluate the response to resuscitation. In patients with persistent shock, chest x-rays [*see Figure 4*], pelvic x-rays, and thoracic and abdominal ultrasonography are performed early in the resuscitation to identify occult sources of hemorrhage.[29,30]

Persistent shock may be hypovolemic, cardiogenic, or neurogenic [*see 6:3 Shock*]. Measurement of central venous pressure (CVP) may aid in differentiating between these types of shock. With hypovolemic shock, the CVP is generally less than 5 mm Hg, whereas in clinically significant cardiogenic shock, the CVP usually exceeds 20 mm Hg. Unfortunately, the CVP may be falsely elevated because of rapid volume infusion, hyperventilation, patient straining, a malfunctioning catheter, or improper location of the catheter tip.

The differential diagnosis of traumatic cardiogenic shock consists basically of (1) tension pneumothorax, (2) pericardial tamponade, (3) myocardial contusion, and (4) air embolism. Except for refractory shock, telltale physical signs are frequently hard to discern in a noisy ED, especially when compounded by persistent hypovolemia. Timely diagnosis requires a high index of suspicion. Tension pneumothorax, the most common etiology, is often confirmed with emergency chest tube placement [*see Figure 5*]. In traumatic pericardial tamponade, the classic signs of tamponade, termed Beck's triad (hypotension, muffled heart sounds, and jugular venous distention), are frequently absent, and pulsus paradoxus is rarely detectable. With

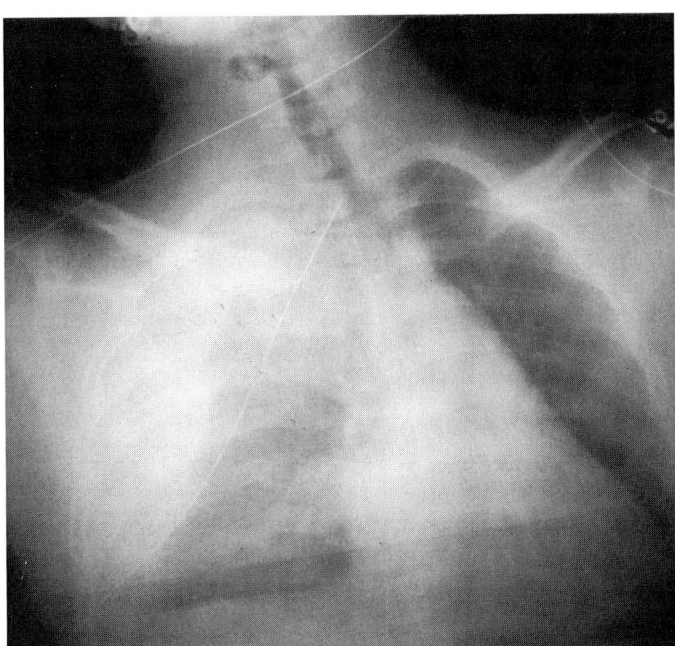

Figure 4 ED chest x-ray shows a massive hemothorax. If the chest tube fails to evacuate the blood, this is a so-called caked hemothorax, which is an indication for emergency thoracostomy in the OR.

the wider use of ultrasonography by trauma surgeons, ED echocardiography should be the first test employed in patients with a high-risk penetrating wound, clinical signs of tamponade, and persistent central venous hypertension.[31,32] With documented pericardial blood on echocardiography and persistent tachycardia, pericardiocentesis should be performed even in the presence of normal systolic blood pressure to relieve any ongoing subendocardial ischemia [*see Figure 6*]. Patients who have persistent signs of pericardial tamponade despite a negative echocardiogram or pericardiocentesis should be transported to the OR for a subxiphoid pericardial window. It is important to remember that results of pericardial aspiration for acute hemopericardium are falsely negative in 15% of patients because the blood in the pericardial sac is clotted and cannot be aspirated. If the patient is in extremis, ED thoracotomy should be performed promptly [*see Figure 7*].[33] Myocardial contusion should be suspected in a patient with unexplained cardiogenic shock or arrhythmia. ECG changes are usually nonspecific.[34,35] Fundamental measures include correction of acidosis, hypoxia, and electrolyte abnormalities; judicious administration of fluid; and pharmacologic suppression of life-threatening arrhythmias. Air embolism into the left atrium from a pulmonary laceration is probably more common than is recognized[36]; typically, hemodynamic instability occurs after positive pressure ventilation is initiated, forcing

Figure 5 In acute trauma, a tube thoracostomy is performed through the fourth or fifth interspace at the midaxillary line, well above the diaphragm (*a*). A short subcutaneous tunnel is fashioned over the superior edge of the rib, and the overlying fascia and intercostal muscle are divided sharply. The pleural space is entered by bluntly perforating the pleura with a Kelly clamp (*b*). A gloved finger is then inserted to confirm penetration of the thoracic cavity and to free up intrapleural adhesions (*c*). A large-bore tube (36 French) is directed posteriorly toward the pleural apex; the proximal port must be well inside the chest (*d*). The tube is then secured to the chest wall with No. 5 braided polyethylene suture and connected to a standard collection apparatus.

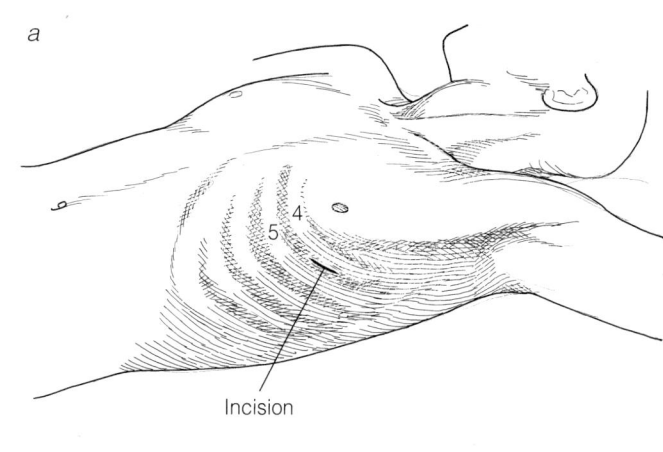

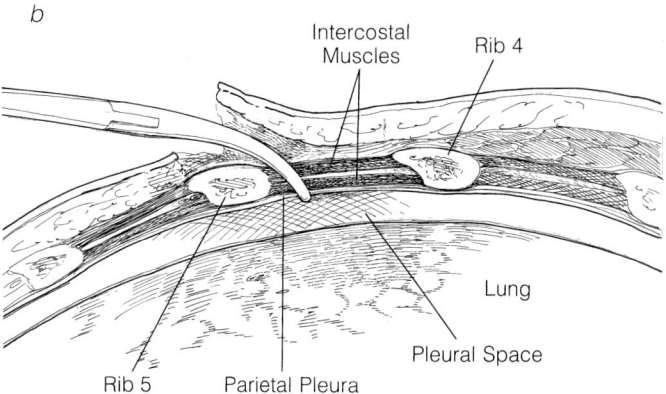

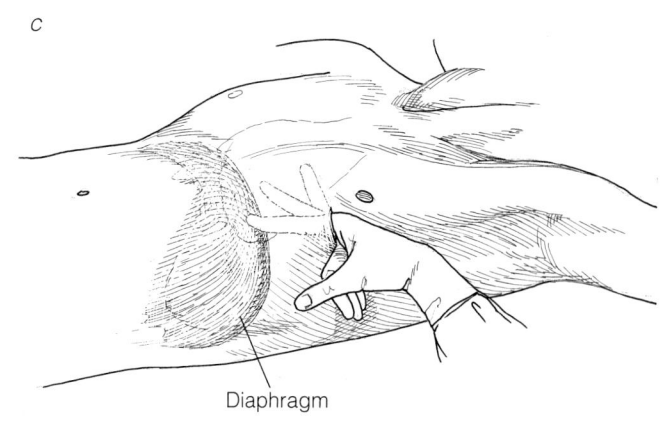

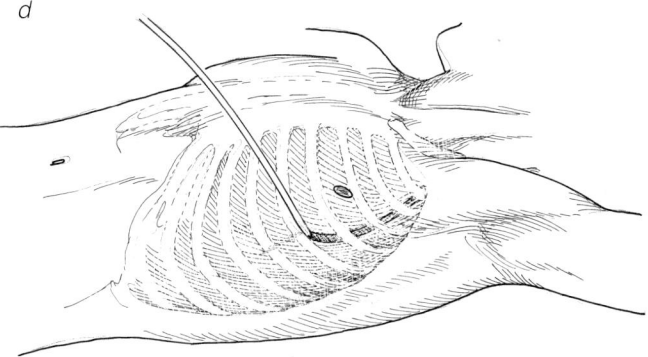

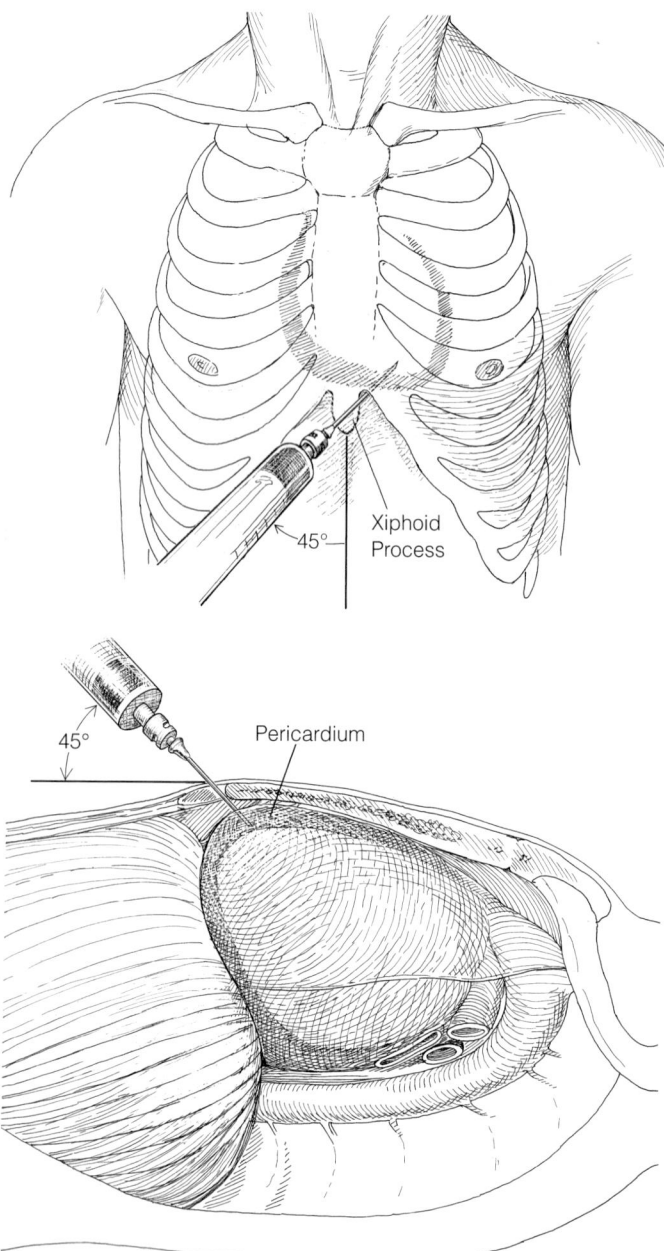

Figure 6 For pericardiocentesis, an 18-gauge spinal needle is inserted at the left xiphoid-costal junction and inserted toward the inferior tip of the left scapula (angled 45° to the patient's right and 45° from the chest wall). The needle is advanced until blood or air is encountered; a "pop" may be appreciated as the needle tip traverses the pericardium. If air is withdrawn, the needle tip should be directed more toward the patient's midline. If blood is withdrawn, 50 ml should be aspirated and injected onto a sheet so that it can be inspected for clots. As a rule, intraventricular blood will clot, whereas defibrinated pericardial blood will not clot.

air from the injured lung into the open pulmonary veins and ultimately into the coronary arteries. ED thoracotomy is essential for pulmonary hilar cross-clamping, air aspiration from the left ventricle, and cardiac massage. The patient is then transferred to the OR for definitive management of the pulmonary lesion before the hilar clamp is released.

ED thoracotomy is an integral part of the initial management of the patient who arrives in extremis and deteriorates to imminent

cardiac arrest [*see Figures 7 and 8*].[33] The physiologic rationale is to minimize the time of profound shock; ED thoracotomy permits (1) release of pericardial tamponade, (2) control of intrathoracic blood loss, (3) internal cardiac massage, and (4) cross-clamping of the descending thoracic aorta to enhance coronary and cerebral perfusion as well as to reduce subdiaphragmatic bleeding. Internal cardiac massage should be done bimanually; otherwise, a forceful thumb may rupture the relatively thin right ventricle as it becomes distended. Simple ventricular lacerations are repaired with pledgeted horizontal mattress sutures, whereas atrial injuries are controlled with a partially occluding vascular clamp and repaired with a running suture [*see Figure 8*].

SECONDARY SURVEY AND DEFINITIVE DIAGNOSIS

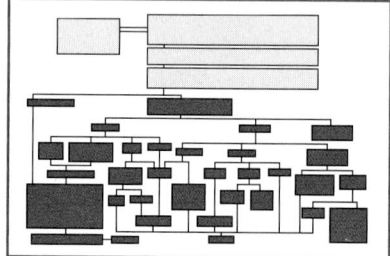

After immediate physiologic demands have been addressed, acutely injured patients can usually be rendered hemodynamically stable, and the secondary survey phase can begin. In this phase, the goal is to complete a systematic assessment to identify all potentially life-threatening injuries. Such assessment is crucial to allow proper triage from the ED to the OR, the CT scanning suite, the interventional suite, or the ICU. Mechanism of injury, severity of shock, and response to resuscitation will dictate the time expended. Details of the patient's medical history as well as those related to the injury are critical. The prehospital emergency medical technicians can provide important details and should be questioned before they leave the ED. A minimal review of the patient's medical history should include preexisting medical illness, current medications and when they were most recently ingested, allergies, tetanus immunization, and time of last meal. A rapid but systematic physical examination is done, literally from head to toe. Patients must be completely disrobed and, once spinal injury is excluded, rolled side to side so that the back and flanks can be inspected. Rectal examination for blood and sphincter tone, inspection of the perineum and axillae, and assessment of neurologic function and peripheral pulses are essential.

A good-quality lateral cervical spine x-ray should be obtained as soon as possible after blunt trauma. Until the x-ray is available and all seven cervical vertebral bodies are clearly visualized, the neck is rigidly immobilized. Splinting of long bone fractures minimizes pain, blood loss, and soft tissue damage. Insertion of a nasogastric tube serves to decompress the stomach and reduce the risk of pulmonary aspiration, but because maxillofacial injury may provide a pathway into the cranial vault,[37] the tube should be placed orally when there are midfacial fractures. Blood in the gastric aspirate may be the only sign of an otherwise occult injury of the stomach and duodenum. A Foley catheter empties the bladder, may disclose hematuria, and permits the physician to monitor urinary output, but it should not be inserted until abdominal ultrasonography is completed. Urine volume is a sensitive index of tissue perfusion. The trauma victim is uniquely susceptible to hypothermia; a rectal temperature probe is therefore essential in patients who have been exposed to a cold environment or who require massive volume replacement. A core temperature reading lower than 32° C (89.6° F) should be confirmed with an esophageal probe, and rewarming measures appropriate for the degree of hypothermia should be initiated.[38-40] Tetanus prophylaxis is routine. Systemic antibiotics should be withheld until a specific indication arises. Minimal laboratory tests for trauma include a complete blood count and urinalysis. An electrocardiogram is obtained after blunt chest trauma, and an ABG analysis is done in select patients to confirm adequate ventilation and metabolic balance. The size of the base deficit can be a useful measure of the depth of hemorrhagic shock.[41] In any patient with evidence of hypovolemia, a blood sample should be sent for blood-group typing.

All potential sites of ongoing blood loss should be evaluated in the hypovolemic patient. A chest x-ray is the most reliable screening test for intrathoracic bleeding; it also confirms the location of endotracheal, nasogastric, and thoracostomy tubes as well as the central venous catheter. Pleural fluid can be difficult to appreciate on a supine chest x-ray; 1 L of blood may produce only a hazy appearance in a hemithorax. Hemothoraces should be drained promptly by tube thoracostomy [see Figure 5]. Continued bleeding must be monitored carefully by means of chest tube output, serial chest films to detect retained intrapleural blood, and vital signs. Abrupt cessation of chest tube output may be deceptive; if hypotension persists or recurs, a second chest tube should be inserted and another chest x-ray should be obtained. The inability to clear the thorax with chest tubes (so-called caked hemothorax [see Figure 4]) is an indication for prompt thoracotomy.

Abdominal examination is notoriously misleading in detecting acute hemoperitoneum.[42] The peritoneal cavity may sequester up to 3,000 ml of blood with only minimal abdominal distention. Laparotomy is clearly indicated for gunshot wounds with violation of the peritoneum[43] or in patients with overt peritonitis after a stab wound or blunt trauma. After blunt trauma, however, head injury or intoxication frequently alters the patient's response to acute injury, and pain from associated fractures may overshadow peritoneal irritation secondary to bleeding. Ultrasonography is the most rapid method of identifying free blood, but it may yield false negative results in as many as 5% to 10% of patients on initial examination. Diagnostic peritoneal lavage (DPL) [see Figure 9] is the most expedient and reliable method of identifying significant intraperitoneal hemorrhage; in patients with life-threatening bleeding, sensitivity approaches 100%. Paradoxically, because of its extreme sensitivity in identifying blood, DPL lacks specificity for determining the need for laparotomy in stable patients.[44,45] A grossly positive aspirate (> 10 ml of blood) mandates emergency laparotomy in cases of penetrating wounds and in cases of blunt trauma with hemodynamic instability. A red blood cell count higher than 100,000/mm³ in a patient with penetrating trauma is an indication for semiemergent celiotomy, whereas a red blood cell count exceeding 50,000/mm³ in a patient with blunt trauma

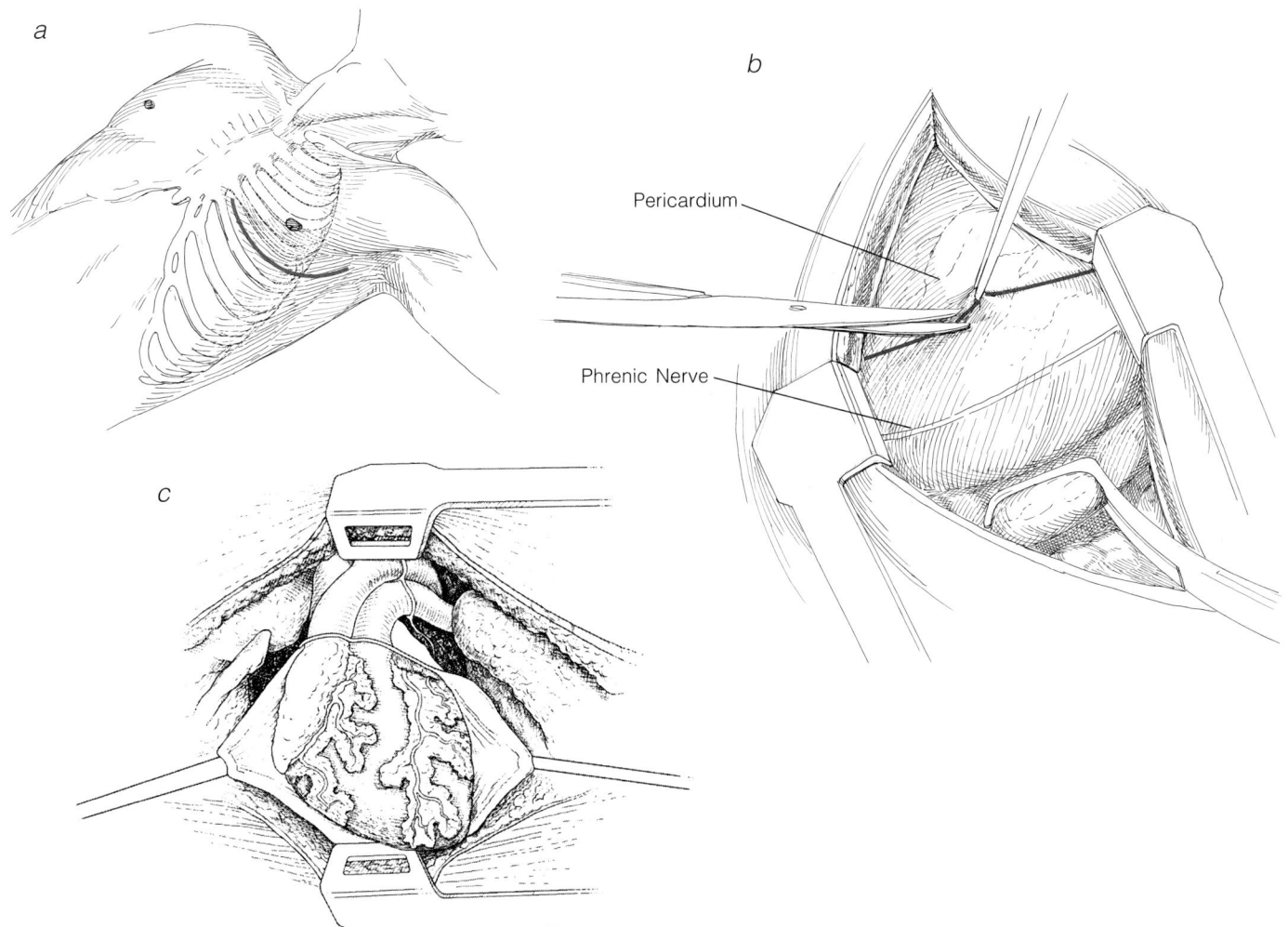

Figure 7 (*a*) A left anterolateral thoracotomy is performed through the fifth intercostal space. (*b*) The lung is reflected superomedially, and a Satinsky vascular clamp is placed on the descending thoracic aorta. A pericardiotomy is performed with scissors anterior to the phrenic nerve. (*c*) A so-called butterfly extension across the sternum creates a bilateral anterolateral thoracotomy, providing access to both thoracic cavities and to the pulmonary hila, heart, and proximal great vessels.

warrants further evaluation by computed tomography of the abdomen. Furthermore, in the setting of both blunt trauma and penetrating trauma, elevation in the peritoneal lavage white blood cell count, the amylase level, and the alkaline phosphatase concentration may identify hollow viscus injury; threshold levels, however, have not been determined.[46-48] In penetrating wounds to the lower chest, the red blood cell count threshold for abdominal exploration is lowered to 10,000/mm³ because isolated diaphragmatic perforations may not bleed.[49] An intermediate red blood cell count of 1,000 to 10,000/mm³ warrants further definitive evaluation by thoracoscopy.[49,50] Because DPL does not sample the retroperitoneum, triple-contrast CT scanning may be of help in cases of high-risk penetrating wounds to the back or the flank.[51,52] Most injuries to retroperitoneal hollow viscera, however, are identified on the basis of extraluminal gas or fluid rather than contrast extravasation.

Assessment of bony stability by physical examination and plain films of the pelvis is crucial for the early identification of major pelvic fractures. Life-threatening hemorrhage occurs most commonly with fracture patterns involving the posterior columns [see Figure 10].[53,54] Appropriate initial management includes vigorous blood volume replacement and mechanical support of the pelvis [see Figure 11]. Most patients can be rendered hemodynamically stable and are potential candidates for external skeletal fixation if the fracture geography is appropriate.[55,56] The unstable patient with a clearly positive ultrasonogram should undergo laparotomy because of a high probability of major hepatic, splenic, or mesenteric bleeding.[57] Conversely, the hemodynamically unstable patient in whom the ultrasonogram is normal and DPL yields confirmatory negative results should undergo prompt pelvic arteriography for selective embolization.[58]

The length of time expended in the ED, the decision for urgent operation, and the need for special radiologic studies are critical triage decisions that must take into account the mechanism of injury, the response to resuscitation, and the availability of a staffed OR. A patient in refractory shock with a central abdominal gunshot wound, for example, should be assigned by triage to the OR in a matter of minutes, whereas a far more complex decision is required in the case of a motor vehicle accident victim with altered mental status, a widened mediastinum on chest x-ray, and a positive ultrasonogram. If the latter patient is hemodynamically unstable, laparotomy should be performed first because intraperitoneal bleeding is the most likely cause of persistent shock. If this patient is hemodynamically stable, however, CT scanning and aortography should be performed first because the results of these procedures facilitate a multiteam approach and allow prioritizing of operative needs.[59,60]

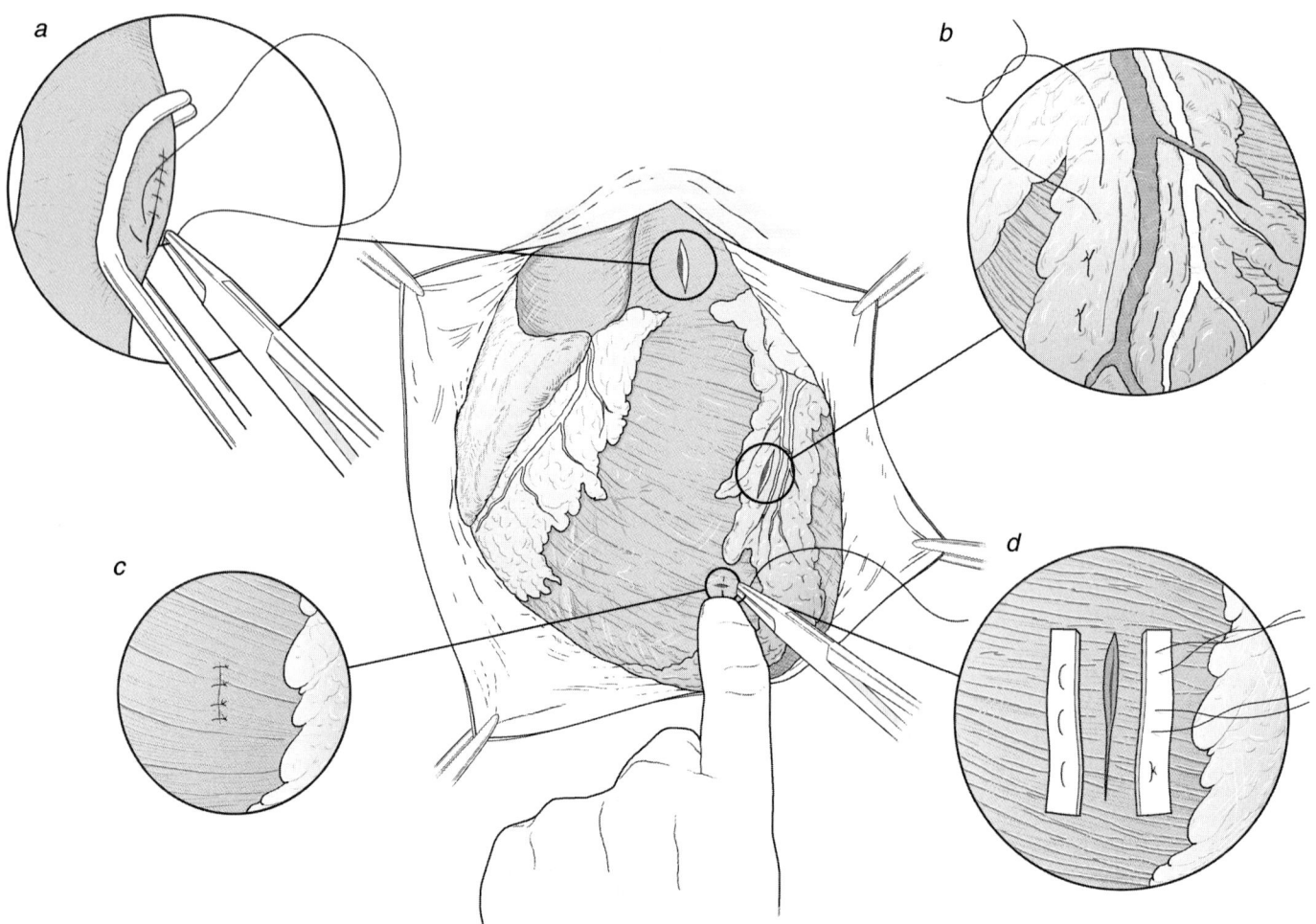

Figure 8 (a) A Satinsky vascular clamp is used to control arterial and major vessel injuries while they are closed with a running suture. (b) For wounds close to coronary arteries, horizontal mattress sutures should be used to exclude the arteries. (c) Small wounds to the thick left ventricle can be closed with interrupted simple sutures. (d) Larger wounds should be closed using pledgets.

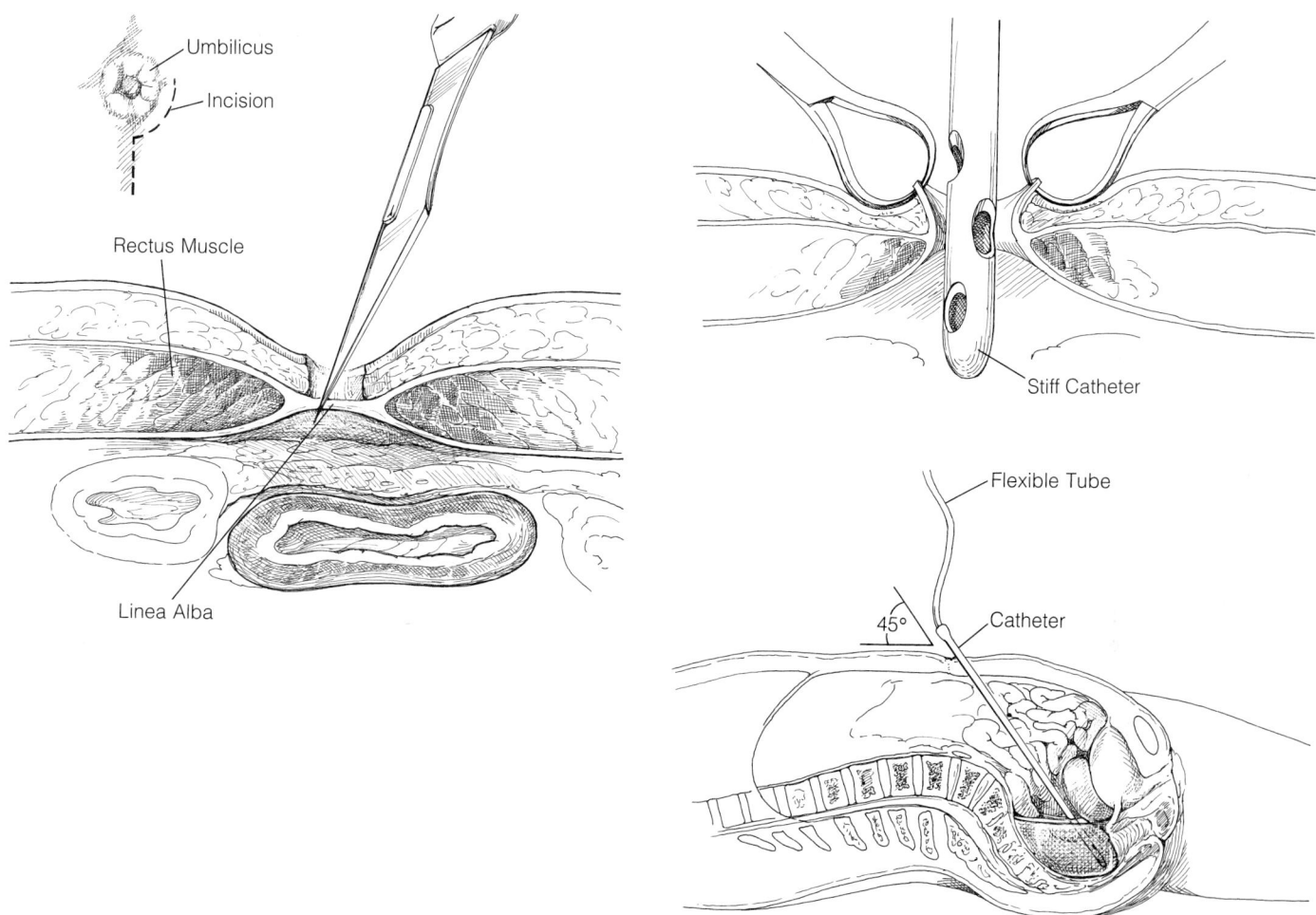

Figure 9 **Illustrated here is the semiopen technique for peritoneal lavage. A 3 to 4 cm incision is made over the infraumbilical ring, and the linea alba is incised vertically for 1 cm. The fascial edges are grasped with towel clips and elevated. A standard peritoneal dialysis catheter is introduced into the peritoneum at a 45° angle and then advanced into the pelvis without use of the trocar. If 10 ml of gross blood is aspirated, the study is considered to be positive. Otherwise, 1 L of normal saline (10 ml/kg for children) is infused. The lavage fluid is retrieved by gravity siphonage; the empty saline bag is dropped to the floor. A 50 ml sample of the fluid is submitted for laboratory analysis.**

Discussion

Prehospital Care

ADVANCED TRAUMA LIFE SUPPORT

The principles of initial assessment and management in ACLS and ATLS are based on the ABCs—airway maintenance, breathing, and circulation. In both settings, upper airway control and assisted ventilation are imperative for optimizing alveolar oxygen tension. With respect to circulation, however, the protocols diverge markedly because of differing pathophysiology.

It is estimated that 60% of deaths caused by coronary artery disease occur within 1 hour of initial symptoms, usually before the patient can receive medical care.[61] Rhythm disturbance is the most frequent cause of death after cardiac arrest; there is only a 6-minute period until irreversible cerebral damage occurs.[62] Temporary artificial circulation in these normovolemic patients can be achieved by closed-chest compression. The technique is simple and effective and requires no special equipment. However, arrhythmias, the most common cause of preventable death, become refractory if pharma-

cologic or electrical treatment is delayed.[63] ECG monitoring and venous access allow the necessary interventions to be initiated effectively in the field, and indeed, ACLS results in a fivefold reduction in the incidence of cardiac arrest en route to the hospital. In contrast, the major reversible threat to life for the severely injured patient is persistent hemorrhage, which requires hospital facilities for effective treatment.

Sophistication of emergency medical services has dramatically expanded the scope of prehospital care. Qualified paramedics using ACLS skills have produced dramatic improvement in survival of acute myocardial infarction by treating arrhythmias in the field.[64] Unquestionably, these efforts also improve trauma resuscitation, but the extent of prehospital ATLS remains a highly controversial issue. Advocates of the so-called scope-and-run philosophy argue that field stabilization is detrimental because it delays definitive care. However, in systems with rigorous medical control, the addition of advanced techniques (e.g., endotracheal intubation, I.V. access, and fluid administration) adds less than 10 minutes to the on-scene time.[2] In the Denver Emergency Medical Service system, para-

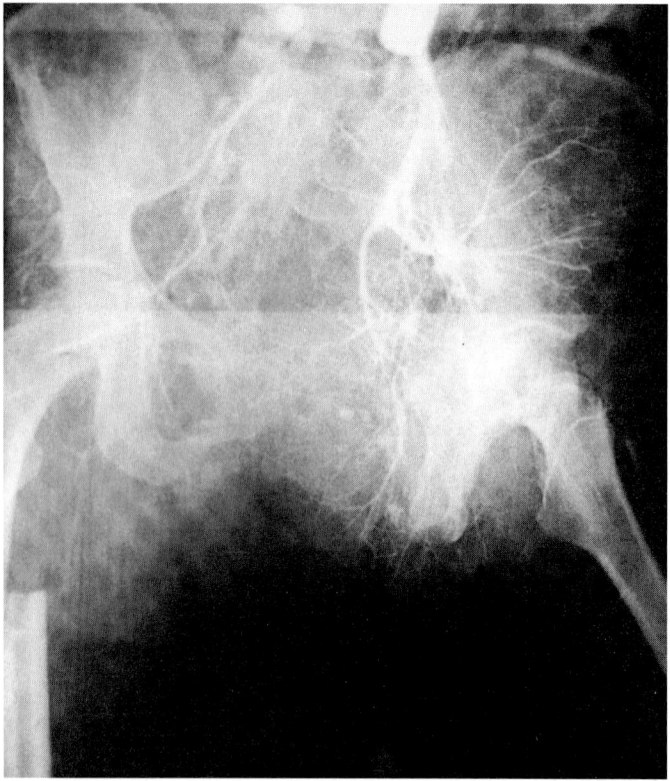

Figure 10 **Pelvic angiography with selective embolization may be an integral component in the early management of a pelvic crush injury.**

medics routinely insert I.V. catheters in critically ill patients within 1.0 to 1.5 minutes.[65] Moreover, the availability of hypertonic saline solution and human polymerized hemoglobin for prehospital fluid resuscitation may provide an undisputed physiologic rationale for establishing I.V. access at the scene.[66-71] Clearly, the relative benefits of paramedic intervention depend on mechanism of injury, patient status, and availability of a trauma center. An efficient prehospital care system should be tailored to the community's needs, providing well-thought-out protocols, appropriate field personnel, and active medical control. Unfortunately, a paradox exists: ATLS skills are needed most in sparsely populated rural areas where transport time exceeds 30 minutes, but the limited volume of trauma precludes the experience necessary to maintain this expertise.

AIRWAY MANAGEMENT

The principles of initial resuscitation are governed by physiologic rationale. The goal is to reestablish adequate oxygen delivery to vital organs. Efforts to improve tissue perfusion will be unproductive unless the oxygen content of the circulating blood is sufficient. Airway patency and maintenance of adequate ventilation are thus the initial priorities. Current policy dictates that emergency airway control after blunt vehicular trauma be performed with the assumption that an unstable cervical spine fracture exists until such injuries are excluded radiologically; however, this policy does not preclude RSI.[72] Cervical neck injury has been documented in 25% of accidental fatalities[73] and in 60% of fatalities in which the patient had sustained head trauma,[74] but the incidence of truly occult unstable cervical fractures in neurologically intact survivors of vehicular trauma is unknown. The current recommendation of orotracheal intubation with in-line manual stabilization of the head and neck has proved safe in clinical series to date. For patients with extensive maxillofacial trauma that precludes oral intubation, the traditional alternative

has been to do a cricothyrotomy, but this surgical procedure has definite risks. The success achieved with percutaneous dilatational tracheostomy in ICU patients[75] suggests that similar approaches with percutaneous cricothyrotomy may be easier and would pose less risk to the patient. Finally, we believe that percutaneous transtracheal ventilation is a viable option in challenging airway problems and that it remains underutilized.[22]

PNEUMATIC ANTISHOCK GARMENT

In the 1970s, the PASG was mandated as essential prehospital equipment for ambulances on the basis of the assumption that inflation produced autotransfusion by redistributing blood from the lower extremities into the central circulation. Subsequent experimental work challenged this concept and showed that the rise in mean arterial pressure is merely the result of an elevated systemic vascular resistance.[76] Randomized prospective evaluations of the PASG in urban prehospital care have failed to demonstrate a benefit and in fact suggest that PASG inflation may be detrimental in cases of thoracic trauma.[6] However, the role of PASGs in the rural setting, in which transport times are longer, has not been studied adequately. In the hospital setting, we consider either wrapping the pelvis or use of the C clamp preferable to the PASG for management of unrelenting bleeding from unstable pelvic fractures.

Emergency Department Management

AIRWAY, BREATHING, AND CIRCULATION

The primary goal of the ABCs is to establish adequate oxygen delivery to vital organs so as to give the physician time to identify and treat immediately life-threatening injuries. Oxygen delivery is the product of cardiac output (CO) and arterial oxygen content (C_aO_2). By convention, CO is generally indexed to body surface area and expressed as cardiac index (CI), which when multiplied by C_aO_2 yields an oxygen delivery index (DO_2). Normal DO_2 is roughly 500 ml/min/m² ; it will increase by as much as 30% in response to injury. C_aO_2 and DO_2 are calculated as follows:

$$C_aO_2 \text{ (ml/dl)} = [Hb] \text{ (g/dl)} \times 1.38 \times S_aO_2 \text{ (\%)} +$$
$$[P_aO_2 \text{ (mm Hg)} \times 0.003]$$
$$DO_2 \text{ (ml/min/m}^2) = CI \text{ (L/min/m)} \times C_aO_2 \text{ (ml/dl)} \times 10$$

where [Hb] is the hemoglobin concentration, S_aO_2 is oxyhemoglobin saturation, P_aO_2 is arterial oxygen tension, and 0.003 is the solubility of O_2 in blood.

Oxyhemoglobin saturation is the first important variable to consider. Given the low solubility of oxygen in plasma, the level of P_aO_2 is only important insofar as it relates to S_aO_2. A review of the oxyhemoglobin dissociation curve makes it clear why pushing P_aO_2 to levels higher than 100 mm Hg will not affect S_aO_2 appreciably and thus will have little impact on DO_2. During initial resuscitation, a high fraction of inspired oxygen (F_IO_2) is administered, and pulse oximetry is used to assess S_aO_2. As a rule, a low S_aO_2 is easily treated by increasing the F_IO_2 further. Intubated patients who do not respond when the F_IO_2 is increased to 100% can be treated with low levels of positive end-expiratory pressure (PEEP) once adequate volume status is ensured.

The second important variable is the hemoglobin concentration. The initial hemoglobin level is notoriously misleading because the patients have not yet been volume loaded and because there has not been sufficient time for substantial flux of interstitial fluid into the intravascular space. The initial hemoglobin level is also problematic because of the lag time before the results come back from the laborato-

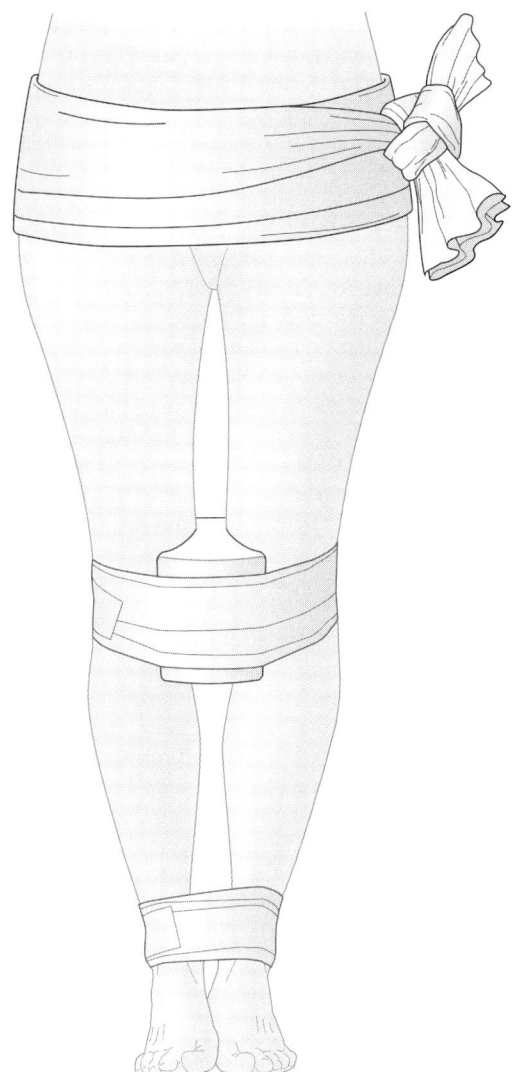

Figure 11 **Shown is the wrapping technique currently used for mechanical support of the pelvis.**

ry. Once recognized, a low hemoglobin level is easily treated with blood transfusion. Given the concerns just mentioned, however, early blood transfusion should be empirically administered in patients who arrive in severe class IV hemorrhagic shock or who have injuries associated with significant bleeding (e.g., vertical shear pelvic fracture or bilateral femur fractures), especially if they are elderly.

CO is the third important variable to consider. Unfortunately, it is difficult to monitor CO in the ED. Decreased preload is by far the most likely problem; consequently, empirical volume loading is recommended. When the patient is unresponsive, a central venous pressure reading can be helpful in differentiating persistent hypovolemia from cardiogenic shock. There is evidence to suggest that noninvasive monitoring of subcutaneous tissue perfusion status may be a valuable adjunct in assessing the adequacy of Do_2.[77]

BLOOD VOLUME RESTITUTION

During profound shock, fluid is lost from the intravascular as well as interstitial space because of sodium flux into the cellular compartment.[78] Crystalloid solutions, which rapidly equilibrate with the total extracellular space, are preferred.[79] Most authorities agree that albumin or artificial plasma expanders are no more effective in restoring tissue perfusion when adequate sodium is provided.[80,81] Moreover, they are costly and may aggravate posttraumatic compli-

cations. The type of crystalloid fluid used for initial volume replacement is of less importance. Lactated Ringer solution is theoretically preferred to normal saline because it provides a better buffer for metabolic acidosis of protracted shock.[82,83] The role of hypertonic saline continues to be investigated. There is some evidence to suggest that hypertonic saline may attenuate neutrophil-mediated injury.[84,85] Acute whole blood loss can be replaced initially with crystalloid because (1) this solution repletes the total extracellular space, (2) hemodilution enhances perfusion by means of reduced blood viscosity, and (3) increased CO and peripheral oxygen extraction provide adequate tissue oxygenation.[86] There is, of course, a limit to these compensatory mechanisms. With massive hemorrhage, the crystalloid replacement for blood may approach a ratio of 8 : 1 because of a progressive fall in plasma oncotic pressure and intracellular sequestration of sodium.[87] In general, blood should be added to fluid resuscitation when crystalloid infusion exceeds 50 ml/kg.[27,88] Diagnosis and management of shock, as well as the pathophysiology of the various shock states, is discussed in detail elsewhere [*see 6:3 Shock*].

Fully crossmatched blood is rarely available for emergency trauma resuscitation. Uncrossmatched type-specific whole blood or packed red blood cells can be safely administered[89,90] and are available in most hospitals within 20 minutes. If type-specific blood is unavailable, reconstituted O-negative packed red blood cells should be used. Type O-negative blood has no cellular antigens; therefore, the risk of major hemolytic reactions caused by patient antibodies attacking donor antigens is minimal. However, O-negative whole blood, the universal donor, is not considered safe, because its plasma contains anti-A and anti-B antibodies.[91] When O-negative packed cells are unavailable, the O-positive packed red blood cells may be used. The patient will become sensitized to the Rh factor, but this is significant only in women of childbearing age.

A 1994 clinical trial found that for hypotensive patients with penetrating torso injuries, survival improved when fluid resuscitation was delayed until surgical intervention had controlled the source of hemorrhage.[3] A subsequent subset analysis revealed that survival was improved only in patients who had sustained cardiac injuries and not in patients who had sustained major vascular, abdominal solid organ, and noncardiac thoracic injuries.[92] Although this clinical trial had some methodologic flaws, it is important for the appropriate emphasis it placed on source control of hemorrhage as an imperative priority. Whether resuscitation should be totally withheld until control of hemorrhage is achieved is doubtful; such an approach is clearly not the current standard of care.[15]

Animal studies using the traditional controlled hemorrhagic shock models have shown that if shock is allowed to persist for several hours, an irreversible shock state occurs from which the animals cannot be resuscitated.[93] On the other hand, more recent animal studies using uncontrolled hemorrhagic shock models with graded resuscitation have found that moderately resuscitated animals survive better than animals who receive either less aggressive or more aggressive resuscitation. A systolic pressure of 90 mm Hg may be acceptable, but the overriding priority must be timely surgical intervention. What this means in blunt trauma is not clear. If a non–head-injured patient arrives in class IV shock with a positive abdominal ultrasonogram, operative control of bleeding is the overriding priority. However, the possibility of a serious associated head injury frequently exists. The surgeon cannot determine whether the low Glasgow Coma Scale score is attributable to cerebral hypoperfusion or to intracranial pathology. If the brain is indeed injured, decreased perfusion pressure can produce secondary brain injury and worsen outcome.[94] Moreover, prehospital extrication and initial ED assessment times are longer with blunt trauma, and definitive con-

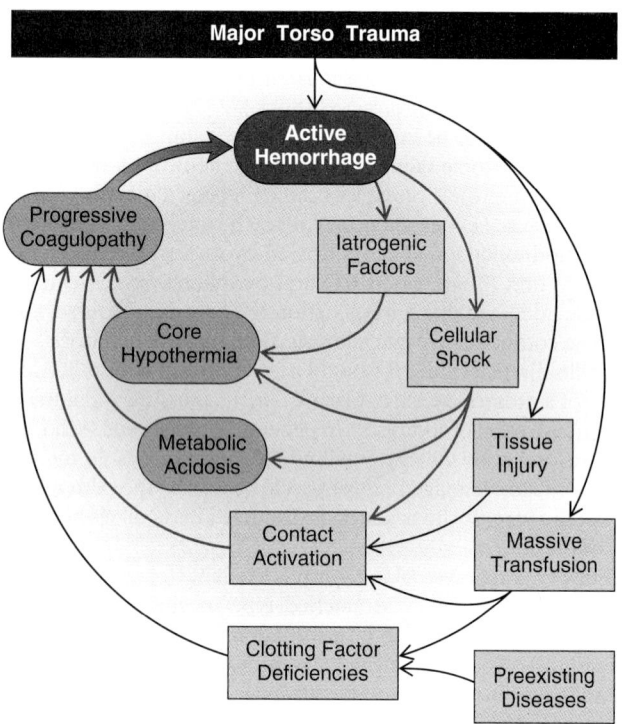

Major Torso Trauma

Active Hemorrhage

Progressive Coagulopathy

Iatrogenic Factors

Core Hypothermia

Cellular Shock

Metabolic Acidosis

Tissue Injury

Contact Activation

Massive Transfusion

Clotting Factor Deficiencies

Preexisting Diseases

Figure 12 **Illustrated is the so-called bloody vicious cycle. This syndrome has a multifactorial pathogenesis, with the usual manifestations including coagulopathy, hypothermia, and metabolic acidosis.**[118]

trol of bleeding may take hours to orchestrate. Finally, for blunt trauma patients who survive early prolonged hypoperfusion, soft tissue injury combined with severe shock contributes to a high incidence of late multiple organ failure.[95]

Diverse clinical experience has substantiated the feasibility of autotransfusion, and in trauma, there has been increasing enthusiasm for its use in the ED as well as in the OR.[96] Autotransfusion clearly eliminates the infectious, allergic, and incompatibility problems of stored blood, an important concern because of the acquired immunodeficiency syndrome (AIDS). However, when large amounts of unprocessed collected blood are reinfused, a consumptive coagulopathy and platelet dysfunction occur.[97] These risks may outweigh the benefits of autotransfusion in the critically injured patient who has multiple potential bleeding sites.

Much attention has been directed toward production of a red blood cell substitute. Fluosol-DA, a perfluorocarbon, appeared promising,[98] but clinical trials failed to demonstrate an advantage over standard lactated Ringer solution, and animal studies clearly established an immunologic penalty.[99] Consequently, Fluosol-DA failed to receive the approval of the Food and Drug Administration. In contrast, progress has been made with hemoglobin-based blood substitutes, although tetrameric hemoglobin has been problematic.[71,100] Experience with human polymerized hemoglobin as a blood substitute after major surgical procedures suggests that this agent may be available for trauma resuscitation in the near future. Transfusion considerations are discussed in detail elsewhere [*see 1:4 Bleeding and Transfusion*].

EMERGENCY DEPARTMENT THORACOTOMY

ED thoracotomy is an integral part of the initial management of trauma patients who arrive in extremis.[33,101] With insufficient blood volume, open cardiac massage is superior to closed-chest compression in maintaining systemic blood flow[102]; coronary and cerebral perfusion is maintained at adequate levels for up to 30 minutes. Adjunctive thoracic aorta occlusion enhances both coronary and cerebral perfusion by maintaining aortic diastolic pressure and by increasing carotid systolic pressure. Aortic cross-clamping also decreases subdiaphragmatic bleeding in the event of associated abdominal injury.[103,104] These benefits are obtained at the expense of increased myocardial oxygen demand and a lack of perfusion to the lower torso. Irreversible cardiovascular collapse and splanchnic dysfunction occur with prolonged cross-clamping times. Clinical experience suggests that 30 minutes is the limit for prevention of serious ischemic sequelae. The possibility of patient salvage is largely determined by the mechanism of injury as well as the patient's condition at the time of thoracotomy. Success approaches 50% in patients arriving with profound shock from a penetrating cardiac wound and 20% for all penetrating wounds. On the other hand, patient outcome is dismal when ED thoracotomy is performed for blunt trauma; it is now considered futile in patients lacking cardiac activity. Adding laparotomy in the ED for definitive control of abdominal hemorrhage has not improved outcome.[105]

PHYSIOLOGIC MONITORING

It is imperative that the critically injured patient undergo early hemodynamic monitoring and assessment of oxygen transport. The adequacy of resuscitation is initially determined by blood pressure, pulse rate, and general patient appearance. Once these factors have stabilized, urine output (> 0.5 ml/kg/hr in adults) is used to gauge additional fluid requirements. All major trauma patients should have continuous ECG and pulse oximetry monitoring. In addition, core temperature should be monitored with a rectal temperature probe capable of recording temperatures lower than 32° C (89.6° F). Atrial and ventricular arrhythmias from cardiac contusion or ischemia may require therapy. A data flow sheet for physiologic indices, laboratory test results, and fluid administration allows quick analysis of trends, but isolated points may be misleading. Measurement of central venous pressure is helpful in differentiating persistent hypovolemia from cardiogenic shock [*see 6:3 Shock*], but several conditions can produce a false elevation of the CVP. Although arterial lines and pulmonary arterial catheters are of limited use in ED trauma management, they are important in the radiology suite, particularly if the patient requires beta blockade for a suspected torn aorta.[60] End-tidal CO_2 monitoring should be available for patients undergoing emergency endotracheal intubation.

COAGULOPATHY

The most devastating complication of massive blood and fluid resuscitation is a bleeding diathesis. Paradoxically, although clotting is accelerated at the capillary level because of shock and tissue damage,[106] the circulating blood becomes hypocoagulable.[107,108] The pathogenesis of bloody vicious cycle is complex [*see Figure 12*]. Factors predictive of a severe coagulopathic state (i.e., prothrombin time [PT] > 2 times normal and partial thromboplastin time [PTT] > 2 times normal) include (1) massive rapid blood transfusion (10 units/4 hr), (2) persistent cellular shock (oxygen consumption index < 110 ml/min/m², lactate concentration > 5 mmol/L), (3) progressive metabolic acidosis (pH < 7.20, base deficit > 14 mEq/L), and (4) refractory core hypothermia (< 34° C).[109] The extent of tissue disruption (as quantitated by the Injury Severity Score) is not a strong independent risk factor; however, it clearly is a facilitating event.

Stored blood is deficient in factors V and VIII and platelets and replete with fibrin split products and vasoactive substances. Timely administration of fresh frozen plasma and platelets will minimize the risk of coagulopathy after massive transfusion [*see 1:4 Bleeding and Transfusion*]. Although blood components are not usually indicated in the early resuscitation phase, they may be appropriate in patients with massive hemorrhage caused by pelvic fracture.

Germane to the initial period of massive blood transfusion are the potential complications of hypocalcemia, acidosis, and hypothermia. Hypocalcemia caused by citrate binding of ionized calcium does not occur until the blood transfusion rate exceeds 100 ml/min (1 U/5 min). Decreased serum levels of ionized calcium depress myocardial function before impairing coagulation.[110,111] Calcium gluconate (10 mg/kg I.V.) should be reserved for cases in which there is ECG evidence of ST interval prolongation or, rarely, for cases of unexplained hypotension during massive transfusion. Moderate hypothermia (< 32° C) causes platelet sequestration and inhibits the release of platelet factors that are important in the intrinsic clotting pathway.[39] In addition, moderate hypothermia has consistently been associated with poor outcome in trauma patients.[112] Core temperature often falls insidiously because of exposure at the scene and in the ED and because of administration of resuscitation fluids stored at ambient temperature. The first step is to prevent further heat loss by covering the body (including the head) and infusing warm blood and fluid. Another simple technique is to heat and aerosolize ventilator gases. Active external rewarming with heating blankets and increased room temperature should also be used. However, it is important to note that the above techniques are not very effective in reversing established hypothermia. In this setting, lavage of the abdominal or chest cavities can increase core temperature at a rate of 1° to 2° C an hour. Recently, Gentilello and others have introduced relatively simple extracorporeal techniques that can increase core temperature at a rate of 2° to 5° C an hour.[113] Whether these rapid rewarming techniques improve patient outcome is currently being investigated.

The use of bicarbonate in the treatment of systemic acidosis remains controversial. Moderate acidosis (pH < 7.20) impairs coagulation,[114] myocardial contractility,[115] and oxidative metabolism.[116] Acidosis in the trauma patient is caused primarily by a rise in lactic acid production secondary to tissue hypoxia and will usually resolve when the volume deficit has been corrected [*see 6:9 Disorders of Acid-Base and Potassium Balance*]. Administration of sodium bicarbonate may cause a leftward shift of the oxyhemoglobin dissociation curve, reducing tissue oxygen extraction, and it may worsen intracellular acidosis caused by carbon dioxide production.[117] Bicarbonate infusion, therefore, should be limited to persons with protracted shock. Patients in shock should be ventilated on 100% oxygen; thus, blood gases obtained from a central venous line are clinically useful in the assessment of acid-base status. Blood gases should be corrected for core body temperature; pH should be increased by 0.15 for every 1° C drop below normal.

References

1. Eisenberg MS, Bergner L, Hallstrom A: Cardiac resuscitation in the community: importance of rapid provision and implications for program planning. JAMA 241:1905, 1979

2. Copass MK, Oreskovich MR, Baldergroen MR, et al: Prehospital cardiopulmonary resuscitation of the critically injured patient. Am J Surg 148:20, 1984

3. Bickell WH, Wall MJ Jr, Pepe PE, et al: Immediate versus delayed fluid resuscitation for hypotensive patients with penetrating torso injuries. N Engl J Med 331:1105, 1994

4. Soucy DM, Rude M, Hsrg WC, et al: The effects of varying fluid volume and rate of resuscitation during uncontrolled hemorrhage. J Trauma 46:209, 1999

5. Burris D, Rhee P, Kaufman C, et al: Controlled resuscitation for uncontrolled hemorrhagic shock. J Trauma 46:216, 1999

6. Mattox KL, Bickell WH, Pepe PE, et al: Prospective randomized evaluation of antishock MAST in post-traumatic hypotension. J Trauma 26:779, 1986

7. Capone AC, Safar P, Stezoski W, et al: Improved outcome with fluid restriction in treatment of uncontrolled hemorrhagic shock. J Am Coll Surg 180:49, 1995

8. Kowalenko T, Stern S, Dronen S, et al: Improved outcome with hypotensive resuscitation of uncontrolled hemorrhagic shock in a swine model. J Trauma 33:349, 1992

9. Cayten CG, Berendt BM, Byrne DW, et al: A study of pneumatic antishock garments in severely hypotensive trauma patients. J Trauma 34:728, 1993

10. Domerer RM, O'Conner, Delbridge TR, et al: National Association of EMS Physicians, Position Paper: Use of the pneumatic anti-shock garment (PASG). Prehosp Emerg Care 1:32, 1997

11. Aprahamian C, Thompson BM, Towne JB, et al: The effects of a paramedic system on mortality of major open intra-abdominal vascular trauma. J Trauma 23:687, 1983

12. Jacobs LM, Sinclair A, Beiser A, et al: Prehospital advanced life support: benefits in trauma. J Trauma 24:8, 1984

13. Pons PT, Honigman B, Moore EE, et al: Prehospital advanced trauma life support for critical penetrating wounds to the thorax and abdomen. J Trauma 25:828, 1985

14. Hoyt DB, Mikulaschek AW, Winchel RJ: Trauma triage and interhospital transfer. Trauma, 4th ed. Mattox KL, Feliciano DV, Moore EE, Eds. McGraw-Hill, New York, 2000

15. Committee on Trauma, American College of Surgeons: Advanced Trauma Life Support Manual. American College of Surgeons, Chicago, 1981

16. Ducker TB, Russo GL, Bellegarrique R, et al: Complete sensorimotor paralysis after cord injury: mortality, recovery, and therapeutic implications. J Trauma 19:837, 1979

17. Bohn D, Armstrong D, Becker L, et al: Cervical spine injuries in children. J Trauma 30:463, 1990

18. Pang D, Pollack IF: Spinal cord injury without radiographic abnormality in children—the SCIWORA syndrome. J Trauma 29:654, 1989

19. Roth BJ, Martin RR: Roentgenographic evaluation of the cervical spine: a selective approach. Arch Surg 129:643, 1994

20. Shaffer MA, Doris PE: Limitation of the cross table lateral view in detecting cervical spine injuries: a retrospective analysis. Ann Emerg Med 10:508, 1981

21. Robinson RJS, Mulder DS: Airway control. Trauma, 4th ed. Mattox KL, Feliciano DV, Moore EE, Eds. McGraw-Hill, New York, 2000

22. Jorden RC, Moore EE, Marx JA, et al: A comparison of PTV and endotracheal ventilation in an acute trauma model. J Trauma 25:978, 1985

23. Norwood S, Myers MB, Butler TJ: The safety of emergency neuromuscular blockade and orotracheal intubation in the acutely injured trauma patient. J Am Coll Surg 179:646, 1994

24. Vijayakumar E, Bosscher H: The use of neuromuscular blocking agents in the Emergency Department to facilitate tracheal intubation in the trauma patient: help or hindrance? J Crit Care 13:1, 1998

25. Sawyer RW, Bodai BI, Blaisdell FW, et al: The current status of intraosseous infusion. J Am Coll Surg 179:353, 1994

26. Vayer JS, Henderson JV, Bellamy RF, et al: Absence of a tachycardic response to shock in penetrating intraperitoneal injury. Ann Emerg Med 17:227, 1988

27. Rush BF Jr, Richardson JD, Bosomworth P, et al: Limitations of blood replacement with electrolyte solutions: a controlled clinical study. Arch Surg 98:49, 1969

28. Durtschi MB, Haisch CE, Reynolds L, et al: Effect of micropore filtration on pulmonary function after massive transfusion. Am J Surg 138:8, 1979

29. Rozycki GS, Ochsner MG, Jaffin JH, et al: Prospective evaluation of surgeon's use of ultrasound in the evaluation of trauma patients. J Trauma 34:516, 1993

30. Rozycki GS, Feliciano DV, Ochsner MG, et al: The role of ultrasound in patients with possible penetrating cardiac wounds: a prospective multicenter study. J Trauma 46:543, 1999

31. Breaux EP, Dupont JB Jr, Albert HM, et al: Cardiac tamponade following penetrating mediastinal injuries: improved survival with early pericardiocentesis. J Trauma 19:361, 1979

32. Plummer D, Brunette D, Asinger R, et al: Emergency department echocardiography improves outcome in penetrating cardiac injury. Ann Emerg Med 21:709, 1992

33. Biffl WL, Moore EE, Harken AH: Emergency department thoracotomy. Trauma, 4th ed. Mattox KL, Feliciano DV, Moore EE, Eds. McGraw-Hill, New York, 2000

34. Biffl WL, Moore FA, Moore EE, et al: Cardiac enzymes are irrelevant in the patient with suspected myocardial contusion. Am J Surg 169:523, 1994

35. Illig KA, Swierzewski MJ, Feliciano DV, et al: A rational screening and treatment strategy based on the electrocardiogram alone for suspected cardiac contusion. Am J Surg 162:537, 1991

36. King MW, Aitchison JM, Nel JP: Fatal air embolism following penetrating lung trauma: an autopsy study. J Trauma 24:753, 1984

37. Fremstad JD, Martin SH: Lethal complication from insertion of nasogastric tube after severe basilar skull fracture. J Trauma 18:820, 1978

38. Gentilello LM: Temperature-associated injuries and syndromes. Trauma, 4th ed. Mattox KL, Feliciano DV, Moore EE, Eds. McGraw-Hill, New York, 2000

39. Patt A, McCroskey BL, Moore EE: Hypothermia induced coagulopathies in trauma. Surg Clin North Am 68:775, 1988

40. Reed RL II, Bracey AW Jr, Hudson JD, et al: Hypothermia and blood coagulation: dissociation between enzyme activity and clotting factor levels. Circ Shock 32:141, 1990

41. Davis JW, Kaups KL: Base deficit in the elderly: a marker of severe injury and death. J Trauma 45:873, 1998

42. Thompson JS, Moore EE, Van Duzer-Moore S, et al: The evolution of abdominal stab wound management. J Trauma 20:478, 1980

43. Moore EE, Moore JB, Van Duzer-Moore S, et al: Mandatory laparotomy for gunshot wounds penetrating the abdomen. Am J Surg 140:847, 1980

44. Marx JA, Moore EE, Jorden RC, et al: Limitations of computed tomography in the evaluation of acute abdominal trauma: a prospective comparison with diagnostic peritoneal lavage. J Trauma 25:933, 1985

45. Fabian TC, Mangiante EC, White TJ, et al: A prospective study of 91 patients undergoing both computed tomography and peritoneal lavage following blunt abdominal trauma. J Trauma 26:602, 1986

46. Feliciano DV, Bitondo-Dyer CG: Vagaries of the lavage white blood cell count in evaluating abdominal stab wounds. Am J Surg 168:680, 1994

47. Jacobs DG, Angus A, Rodriguez A, et al: Peritoneal lavage white count: a reassessment. J Trauma 30:607, 1990

48. McAnena OJ, Marx JA, Moore EE: Peritoneal lavage enzyme determinations following blunt and penetrating abdominal trauma. J Trauma 31:1161, 1991

49. Moore JB, Moore EE, Thompson JS: Abdominal injuries associated with penetrating trauma in the lower chest. Am J Surg 140:724, 1980

50. Uribe RA, Pachon CE, Frame SB, et al: A prospective evaluation of thoracoscopy for the diagnosis of penetrating thoracoabdominal trauma. J Trauma 37:650, 1994

51. McAllister E, Perez M, Albrink MH, et al: Is triple contrast computed tomographic scanning useful in the selective management of stab wounds to the back? J Trauma 37:401, 1994

52. Easter DW, Shackford SR, Mattrey RF: A prospective, randomized comparison of computed tomography with conventional diagnostic methods in the evaluation of penetrating injuries to the back and flank. Arch Surg 126:1115, 1991

53. Burgess AR, Eastridge BJ, Young JWR, et al: Pelvic ring disruptions: effective classification system and treatment protocols. J Trauma 30:848, 1990

54. Cryer HM, Miller FB, Evers BM, et al: Pelvic fracture classification: correlation with hemorrhage. J Trauma 28:973, 1988

55. Latenser BA, Gentilello LM, Tarver AA, et al: Improved outcome with early fixation of skeletally unstable pelvic fractures. J Trauma 31:28, 1991

56. Riemer BL, Butterfield SL, Diamond DL, et al: Acute mortality associated with injuries to the pelvic ring: the role of early patient mobilization and external fixation. J Trauma 35:671, 1993

57. Moreno C, Moore EE, Rosenberger A, et al: Hemorrhage associated with major pelvic fracture: a multispecialty challenge. J Trauma 26:987, 1986

58. Panetta T, Sclafani SJA, Goldstein AS, et al: Percutaneous transcatheter embolization for massive bleeding from pelvic fractures. J Trauma 25:1021, 1985

59. Harris JH, Horowitz DR, Zelitt DL: Unenhanced dynamic mediastinal computed tomography in the selection of patients requiring aortography for detection of acute traumatic aortic injury. Emerg Radiol 2:67, 1995

60. Fabian TC, Davis KA, Gavant ML, et al: Prospective study of blunt aortic injury: helical CT is diagnostic and antihypertensive therapy reduces rupture. Ann Surg 227:666, 1998

61. Lombardi G, Gallagher EJ, Gennis P: Outcome of out-of-hospital cardiac arrest in New York City. JAMA 271:678, 1994

62. Messer JV: Management of emergencies: XIV. Cardiac arrest. N Engl J Med 275:35, 1966

63. Roth R, Stewart RD, Rogers K, et al: Out-of-hospital cardiac arrest: factors associated with survival. Ann Emerg Med 13:237, 1984

64. DeBard ML: Cardiopulmonary resuscitation: analysis of six years' experience and review of the literature. Ann Emerg Med 10:408, 1981

65. Pons PT, Moore EE, Cusick JM, et al: Prehospital venous access in an urban paramedic system: a prospective on-scene analysis. J Trauma 28:1460, 1988

66. Kramer GC, Perron PR, Lindsey DC, et al: Small-volume resuscitation with hypertonic saline dextran solution. Surgery 100:239, 1986

67. Mattox KL, Maningas PA, Moore EE, et al: Prehospital hypertonic saline/dextran infusion for post-traumatic hypotension. Ann Surg 213:482, 1991

68. Younes RN, Aun F, Accioly CQ, et al: Hypertonic solutions in the treatment of hypovolemic shock: a prospective, randomized study in patients admitted to the emergency room. Surgery 111:380, 1992

69. Vassar MJ, Fischer RP, O'Brien PE, et al: A multicenter trial for resuscitation of injured patients with 7.5% sodium chloride. Arch Surg 128:1003, 1993

70. Shackford SR, Schmoker JD, Zhuang J: The effect of hypertonic resuscitation on pial arteriolar tone after brain injury and shock. J Trauma 37:899, 1994

71. Gould SA, Moore EE, Holt D, et al: The first randomized trial of human polymerized hemoglobin as a blood substitute in acute trauma and emergency surgery. J Am Coll Surg 187:113, 1998

72. Aprahamian C, Thompson BM, Finger WA, et al: Experimental cervical spine injury model: evaluation of airway management and splinting techniques. Ann Emerg Med 13:584, 1984

73. Bucholz RW, Burkhead WZ, Graham W, et al: Occult cervical spine injuries in fatal traffic accidents. J Trauma 19:768, 1979

74. Davis D, Bohlman H, Walker AE, et al: The pathological findings in fatal craniospinal injuries. J Neurosurg 34:603, 1971

75. Moore FA, Haenel JB, Moore EE, et al: Percutaneous tracheostomy/gastrostomy in brain-injured patients: a minimally invasive alternative. J Trauma 33:435, 1992

76. Gaffney FA, Thal ER, Taylor WF, et al: Hemodynamic effects of medical anti-shock trousers (MAST garment). J Trauma 21:931, 1981

77. McKinley BA, Marvin RG, Cocanour CS, et al: Tissue hemoglobin O_2 saturation during resuscitation of traumatic shock monitored using near infrared spectometry. J Trauma 48:637, 2000

78. Shires GT, Cunningham JN, Backer CR, et al: Alterations in cellular membrane function during hemorrhagic shock in primates. Ann Surg 176:288, 1972

79. Shires GT, Canizaro PC: Fluid resuscitation in the severely injured. Surg Clin North Am 53:1341, 1973

80. Cochrane Injuries Group Albumin Reviewers: Human albumin administration in critically ill patients: systematic review of randomised controlled trials. BMJ 317:235, 1998

81. Choi PT-L, Yip G, Quinonez LF, et al: Crystalloids vs. colloids in fluid resuscitation: a systematic review. Crit Care Med 27:200, 1999

82. Trinkle JK, Rush BF, Eiseman B: Metabolism of lactate following major blood loss. Surgery 63:782, 1968

83. Healey MA, Davis RE, Liu FC, et al: Lactated Ringer's is superior to normal saline in a model of massive hemorrhage and resuscitation. J Trauma 45:894, 1998

84. Ciesla DJ, Moore EE, Gonzalez R, et al: Hypertonic saline inhibits neutrophil (PMN) priming via attenuation of p38 MAPK signaling. Shock 14:265, 2000

85. Rhee P, Wang D, Ruff P, et al: Human neutrophil activation and increased adhesion by various resuscitation fluids. Crit Care Med 28:74, 2000

86. Moore FD, Dagher FJ, Boyden CM, et al: Hemorrhage in normal man: I. Distribution and dispersal of saline infusions following acute blood loss: clinical kinetics of blood volume support. Ann Surg 163:485, 1966

87. Cervera AL, Moss G: Progressive hypovolemia leading to shock after continuous hemorrhage and 3:1 crystalloid replacement. Am J Surg 129:670, 1975

88. Mann DV, Robinson MK, Rounds JD, et al: Superiority of blood over saline resuscitation from hemorrhagic shock: a ^{31}P magnetic resonance spectroscopy study. Ann Surg 226:653, 1997

89. Blumberg N, Bove JR: Un–cross-matched blood for emergency transfusion: one year's experience in a civilian setting. JAMA 240:2057, 1978

90. Gervin AS, Fischer RP: Resuscitation of trauma patients with type-specific uncrossmatched blood. J Trauma 24:327, 1984

91. Barnes A Jr, Allen TE: Transfusions subsequent to administration of universal donor blood in Vietnam. JAMA 203:695, 1968

92. Wall MJ, Granchi T, Liscum K, et al: Delayed versus immediate resuscitation in patients with penetrating trauma: subgroup analysis. J Trauma 39:173, 1995

93. Wiggers CJ: Physiology of Shock. Commonwealth Publications, New York, 1950

94. Rosner MJ, Daughton S: Cerebral perfusion pressure management in head injury. J Trauma 30:933, 1990

95. Sauaia AJ, Moore FA, Moore EE, et al: Multiple organ failure can be predicted as early as 12 hrs postinjury. J Trauma 45:291, 1998

96. Jurkovich GJ, Moore EE, Medina G: Auto-transfusion in trauma: a pragmatic analysis. Am J Surg 148:782, 1984

97. Silva R, Moore EE, Bar-Or D, et al: The risk:benefit of autotransfusion—comparison to banked blood in a canine model. J Trauma 24:557, 1984

98. Tremper KK, Friedman AE, Levine EM, et al: The preoperative treatment of severely anemic patients with a perfluorochemical oxygen-transport fluid, Fluosol-DA. N Engl J Med 314:1653, 1986

99. Gould SA, Rosen AL, Lakshman RS, et al: Fluosol-DA as a red-cell substitute in acute anemia. N Engl J Med 314:1653, 1986

100. Sloan EP, Koenigsberg M, et al: Diaspirin cross-linked hemoglobin (DCLHb) in the treatment of severe traumatic hemorrhagic shock: a randomized controlled efficacy trial. JAMA 282:1857, 1999

101. Rhee PM, Acosta J, Bridgeman A, et al: Survival after emergency department thoracotomy: review of published data from the past 25 years. J Am Coll Surg 190:288, 2000

102. Sanders AB, Kern KB, Ewy GA, et al: Improved resuscitation from cardiac arrest with open-chest massage. Ann Emerg Med 13:672, 1984

103. Ledgerwood AM, Kazmers M, Lucas CE: The role of thoracic aortic occlusion for massive hemoperitoneum. J Trauma 16:610, 1976

104. Millikan JS, Moore EE: Outcome of resuscitative thoracotomy and descending aortic occlusion performed in the operating room. J Trauma 24:387, 1984

105. Mattox KL, Allen MK, Feliciano DV: Laparotomy in the emergency department. JACEP 8:180, 1979

106. Hardaway RM, Chun B, Rutherford RB: Coagulation in shock in various species including man. Acta Chir Scand 130:157, 1965

107. Collins JA: Problems associated with the massive transfusion of stored blood. Surgery 75:274, 1974

108. Miller RD, Robbins TO, Tong MJ, et al: Coagulation defects associated with massive blood transfusions. Ann Surg 174:794, 1971

109. Cosgriff N, Moore EE, Sauaia A, et al: Predicting life-threatening coagulopathy in the massively transfused trauma patient: hypothermia and acidoses revisited. J Trauma 42:857, 1997

110. Stulz PM, Scheidegger D, Drop LJ, et al: Ventricular pump performance during hypocalcemia: clinical and experimental studies. J Thorac Cardiovasc Surg 78: 185, 1979

111. Trunkey D, Carpenter MA, Holcroft J: Calcium flux during hemorrhagic shock in baboons. J Trauma 16: 633, 1976

112. Jurkovich GJ, Greiser WB, Luterman A, et al: Hypothermia in trauma victims: an ominous predictor of survival. J Trauma 27:1019, 1987

113. Gentilello LM, Jurkovich GJ, Maier R, et al: Is hypothermia in the victim of major trauma protective or harmful? a randomized prospective study. Ann Surg 226:439, 1997

114. Dunn EL, Moore EE, Breslich DJ, et al: Acidosis-induced coagulopathy. Forum on Fundamental Surgical Problems 30:471, 1979

115. Clowes GHA Jr, Sabga GH, Konitaxis A, et al: Effects of acidosis on cardiovascular function in surgical patients. Ann Surg 154:524, 1961

116. Fry DE, Ratcliffe DJ, Yates JR: The effects of acidosis on canine hepatic and renal oxidative phosphorylation. Surgery 88:269, 1980

117. Douglas ME, Downs JB, Mantini EL, et al: Alteration of oxygen tension and oxyhemoglobin saturation: a hazard of sodium bicarbonate administration. Arch Surg 114:326, 1979

118. Moore EE: Thomas G. Orr Memorial Lecture. Staged laparotomy for the hypothermia, acidosis, and coagulopathy syndrome. Am J Surg 172:405, 1996

Acknowledgments

Figures 2 and 6   Carol Donner, revised by Tom Moore.

Figures 3, 5, 7a, 7b, and 9   Carol Donner.

Figures 7c, 8, and 11   Tom Moore.

Figure 12   Seward Hung.

2 INJURIES TO THE CENTRAL NERVOUS SYSTEM

Marike Zwienenberg-Lee, M.D., and J. Paul Muizelaar, M.D., Ph.D.

Approach to Injuries to the Head and Spinal Cord

It is estimated that each year, two million patients present to physicians with a primary or secondary diagnosis of head injury. Of these patients, approximately 400,000 are admitted and 70,000 die, most of traumatic brain injury. Thus, brain injury can be considered epidemic. Neurosurgeons, who number 4,000 in the United States, are probably best trained to manage patients with severe head injuries, but the initial resuscitation and stabilization is usually performed by emergency department physicians, general surgeons, and trauma surgeons. These professionals are the ones who can make a difference for patients: recent insights into the pathophysiology of traumatic brain injury indicate that treatment during the first few hours is critical and often determines outcome.

Nonetheless, the role of surgeons immediately after resuscitation and in the ensuing days is not to be underestimated. Patients with multiple system injuries often receive care in surgical intensive care units under the supervision of a general surgeon. Less than optimal management at an early stage will have a greater impact because of the larger number of patients involved, but less than optimal management at a later stage, even in a mildly injured patient, will have a much more dramatic impact. Initial recovery, followed by relentless decline attributable to insufficient cerebral perfusion, is not an expected outcome. Although we cannot promote healing of the brain with pharmacologic means, we can prevent secondary injury to the brain by ensuring adequate cerebral circulation and oxygenation.

The reported incidence of spinal cord injury in the United States ranges from 29 to 53 per million.[1-3] About 50% of the injuries are related to motor vehicle accidents, 15% to 20% to falls, 15% to 20% to interpersonal violence, and the remaining 15% to 20% to sports and recreational activity. In general, the group at highest risk is between 16 and 30 years of age, not unlike the group at highest risk for head injuries. Most of those injured are males: several studies report that the percentage is approximately 75%.[4] Between 45% and 50% of patients with spinal cord injury have associated injuries that seriously affect their prognosis.[5]

The cervical spine is most often involved in spinal cord injury. The major study of trauma outcome, conducted from 1982 to 1989, revealed that the cervical spinal cord was involved in 55% of cases, the thoracic spinal cord in 30% of cases, and the lumbar spinal cord in 15% of cases of acute injury.[6] In an analysis of 358 patients with spinal cord injury, 78% of the 71 cases of thoracic injury were accompanied by complete neurologic injury; 60% of the 202 cases of cervical injury and 65% of the 85 cases of thoracolumbar injury were accompanied by complete neurologic injury.[7] Average direct costs of spinal cord injury (including hospitalization, rehabilitation, residence modification, and long-term care) are tremendous. In 1992, it was estimated that

lifetime costs (in 1989 dollars) of such injury were $210,379 for a paraplegic and $571,854 for a quadriplegic.[8]

Initial resuscitation and evaluation of injured patients are discussed more fully elsewhere [see 5:1 Trauma Resuscitation]. In this chapter, we outline approaches to the management of severe head injury and acute spinal cord injury. In addition, we address the pathophysiology of such injuries to provide the reader with the understanding required for making appropriate decisions about diagnosis and treatment of injured patients [see Discussion, below].

Head Injury

EMERGENCY DEPARTMENT MANAGEMENT

Because hypoxia and hypotension interfere with cerebral oxygenation, complete and rapid physiologic resuscitation is the first priority for patients with head injuries. A large study from the Traumatic Coma Data Bank demonstrated that a single observation of systolic blood pressure below 90 mm Hg in the field or hypoxia (arterial oxygen tension [P_aO_2] below 60 mm Hg) was a major predictor of poor outcome.[9] A multidisciplinary team should provide the patient with an adequate airway and ventilation (intubation, ventilation, and detection of hemothorax or pneumothorax) and restore and maintain hemodynamic stability (with adequate fluid replacement and detection and treatment of any bleeding), all according to the principles developed by the Advanced Trauma Life Support system.[10] The ABCs of emergency care (airway, breathing, and circulation) take precedence, irrespective of neurologic injuries. The initial neurologic assessment, which does not take more than 10 seconds, consists of rating the patient on the Glasgow Coma Scale (GCS) [see Table 1] and assessing the width and reactivity of the pupils. Although the same assessment is made after resuscitation as a guide for prognosis and therapy, it should also be made (and recorded) before resuscitation to permit evaluation of the effect of resuscitative measures and differentiation between primary and secondary neurologic injury.

Early orotracheal intubation and ventilation, if not performed in the field, is recommended for patients with a GCS score of 8 or lower or a motor score of 4 or lower. Other indications for immediate intubation are loss of protective laryngeal reflexes and ventilatory insufficiency (indicated by measurement of blood gases), including hypoxemia ($P_aO_2 < 60$ mm Hg), hypercarbia (arterial carbon dioxide tension [P_aCO_2] > 45 mm Hg), spontaneous hyperventilation (causing $P_aCO_2 < 26$ mm Hg), and respiratory arrhythmia. Indications for intubation before transport are deteriorating consciousness (even if the patient is not in a coma), bilateral fractured mandible, copious bleeding into the mouth (as occurs with fracture of the base of the skull), and seizures. An intubated patient must also be ventilated ($P_aCO_2 \approx 35$ mm Hg).

Table 1 Glasgow Coma Scale

Test	Response	Score
Eye opening (E)	Spontaneous	4
	To verbal command	3
	To pain	2
	None	1
Best motor response (arm) (M)	Obedience to verbal command	6
	Localization of painful stimulus	5
	Flexion withdrawal response to pain	4
	Abnormal flexion response to pain (decorticate rigidity)	3
	Extension response to pain (decerebrate rigidity)	2
	None	1
Best verbal response (V)	Oriented conversation	5
	Disoriented conversation	4
	Inappropriate words	3
	Incomprehensible sounds	2
	None	1
	Total (E + M + V)	3–15

Fluid replacement should be performed with isotonic solutions such as lactated Ringer's solution, normal saline, or packed red blood cells when appropriate. The patient should be examined rapidly and thoroughly for any concomitant life-threatening injuries.

Patients with spinal cord injury above T5 and vasogenic spinal shock may have severe hypotension, which should be treated vigorously; induction of mild hypertension or application of pneumatic antishock trousers may be necessary. Intracranial hypertension should be suspected if there is rapid neurologic deterioration. Clinical evidence of intracranial hypertension, manifest by signs of herniation, includes unilateral or bilateral dilatation of the pupils, asymmetrical pupillary reactivity, and motor posturing.

Intracranial hypertension should be treated aggressively. Hyperventilation, which does not interfere with volume resuscitation and results in rapid reduction of intracranial pressure (ICP), should be established immediately in cases of pupillary abnormalities. Recent research has shown that unilateral or bilateral pupillary abnormalities do not result from compression of the third cranial nerves, as previously thought, but from compression of the brain stem, with resulting brain stem ischemia.[11] Therefore, administration of mannitol is effective because it not only decreases ICP but also increases cerebral blood flow (CBF) through modulation of viscosity. Because mannitol is not used to dehydrate the body, all fluid losses through diuresis must be replaced immediately or even preventively, especially in patients suffering shock as a result of blood loss. Although arterial hypertension occurring after a severe head injury may reflect intracranial hypertension (Cushing's phenomenon), especially when accompanied by bradycardia, it should not be treated, because it may be the sole mechanism permitting the brain to maintain perfusion despite increasing intracranial pressure.

In the absence of signs of herniation, sedation should be used when indicated for safe and efficient transport of the patient. Transport of the patient should be kept to a minimum because it is often accompanied by secondary insults (e.g., hypoxia or hypotension). Pharmacologic paralysis, which interferes with neurologic examination, should be used only if sedation alone is inadequate for safe and effective transport and resuscitation of the patient. When phar-macologic paralysis is used, short-acting agents are preferred. Prophylactic hyperventilation, which may exacerbate early ischemia, is not recommended for these patients. A guide to the resuscitation and initial treatment of patients with severe head injuries will assist in management [see Figure 1].

Minimal radiologic evaluation consists of a lateral cervical spine film or a swimmer's view [see Spinal Cord Injury, below]. After hemodynamic stability is achieved, unenhanced CT of the head should be used for all patients with persistent impairment of consciousness.

Operative Management

Rapid evacuation of mass lesions decreases intracranial pressure and consequently improves cerebral perfusion pressure (CPP) and CBF. Schroder and colleagues[12] have demonstrated reversal of ischemia soon after removal of a subdural hematoma. Subdural hematomas require emergent evacuation by a neurosurgeon; evacuation performed within 4 hours of injury has been shown to result in a better outcome.

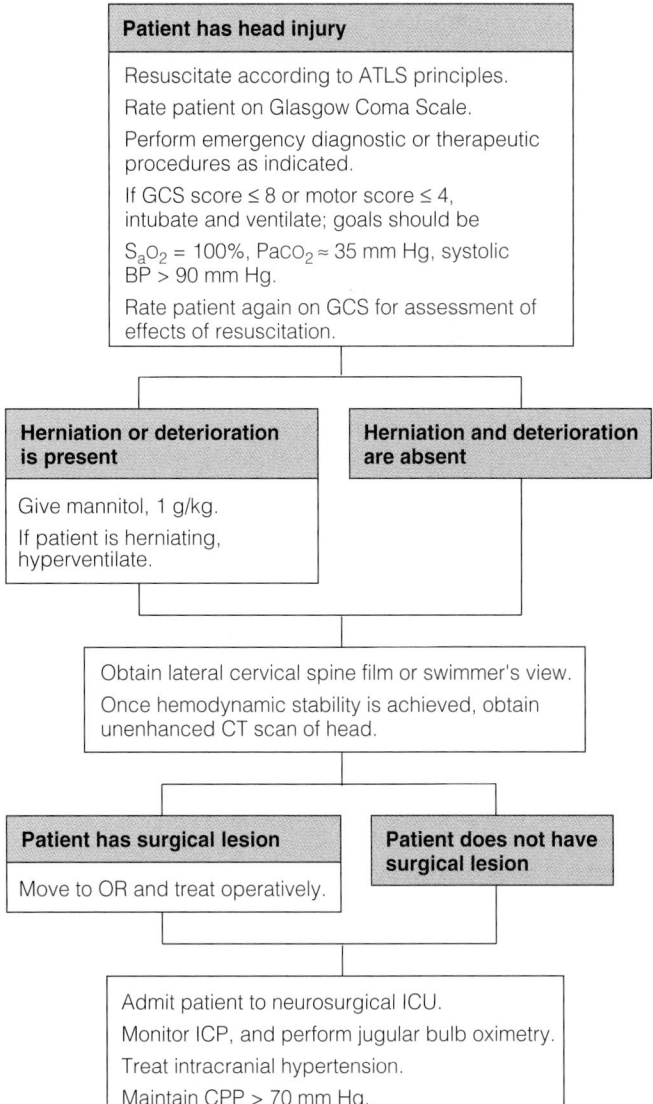

Figure 1 Shown is an algorithm for initial management of the patient with a severe head injury.

An epidural hematoma, which is a life-threatening neurosurgical emergency, should be evacuated urgently. In cases of temporal fracture and rapid clinical deterioration, a temporal craniectomy can be performed. If there is no temporal fracture, an unenhanced CT scan should be obtained to avoid searching for a lesion with multiple bur holes. In cases of progressive deterioration, moderate hyperventilation ($P_aCO_2 \approx 30$) should be initiated and mannitol (1 g/kg) given while the patient is being readied for surgery.

Posterior fossa hematomas, which are rare, also require urgent evacuation, because obstructive hydrocephalus and brain stem compression can result in rapid neurologic deterioration. An intracerebral hematoma causing a midline shift larger than 5 mm is an indication for operative treatment, but surgery can usually be delayed for a few hours.

ICU MANAGEMENT

A GCS score of 8 or lower after resuscitation is an indication for admission to a neurosurgical ICU. Although the focus of ICU management is prevention of secondary injury and maintenance of adequate cerebral oxygenation, admission to an ICU does not eliminate the occurrence of secondary insults.[13] In a series of 124 patients admitted to a neurosurgical ICU, more than one episode of hypotension occurred in 73% of all patients, and more than one episode of hypoxia occurred in 40%.[14] Kirkpatrick and coworkers[15] performed online monitoring of CPP, jugular venous saturation, local CBF, and local tissue oxygenation in 14 patients who had sustained a severe head injury; 37% of the episodes involving decreased CBF, CPP, and saturation were related to clinical and nursing procedures.

Monitoring

A variety of bedside devices are available for monitoring of ICP, local CBF, and local and global cerebral oxygenation.[13,15,16] Aside from monitors for ICP and jugular venous oxygen saturation, most of these devices are experimental.

Intracranial pressure Monitoring of ICP has never been subjected to a prospective, randomized clinical trial designed to assess its efficacy in improving patient outcome. Nevertheless, many clinical studies indicate that ICP monitoring is useful for early detection of intracranial mass lesions; that it allows calculation of CPP, an important clinical indicator of CBF; that it limits the indiscriminate use of potentially harmful therapies for control of ICP; that it helps determine prognosis; and that it may improve outcome. ICP monitoring is indicated in patients with a GCS score of 3 to 7 after resuscitation or a GCS score of 8 to 12 and an abnormal CT scan at the time of admission. In patients with a GCS score of 8 to 9 and a normal CT scan, ICP monitoring is indicated if the patient is older than 40 years, has a systolic BP below 90 mm Hg, and exhibits unilateral or bilateral motor posturing.[16]

Jugular bulb oximetry CBF is an important determinant of neurologic outcome, and the arterial–jugular venous oxygen difference ($A\text{-}VDO_2$) is an important parameter of the adequacy of CBF. Monitoring of therapy by measuring CBF and $A\text{-}VDO_2$ would be ideal, but there is no practical way of doing this directly and continuously.

An estimate of global $A\text{-}VDO_2$ can be obtained from simultaneous monitoring of arterial oxygen saturation (S_aO_2) and jugular venous oxygen saturation ($S_{jv}O_2$). Jugular venous oxygen saturation is monitored by percutaneous retrograde insertion of a fiberoptic catheter in the internal jugular vein, with the tip of the catheter located in the jugular bulb. The catheter is usually inserted into the

jugular vein with the dominant cerebral venous drainage (the right jugular vein in 80% to 90% of the population), but some prefer to insert the catheter at the site of most significant brain damage.

$A\text{-}VDO_2$ is calculated according to the following formula:

$$A\text{-}VDO_2 = (S_aO_2 - S_{jv}O_2) \times 1.34 \times Hb + [(P_aO_2 - P_{jv}O_2) \times 0.0031]$$

The contribution of the variables within the brackets, which is small, is usually ignored for practical purposes. Because calculation of $A\text{-}VDO_2$ requires the drawing of blood samples, it can be done only intermittently.

For continuous monitoring, $S_{jv}O_2$, the result of arterial oxygen input and cerebral extraction, is used. In normal individuals, $S_{jv}O_2$ ranges from 50% to 70%.[17] If $S_{jv}O_2$ values below 50% last for more than 15 minutes, they are considered desaturations, resulting either from insufficient arterial oxygenation (S_aO_2) or oxygen-carrying capacity (Hb concentration) or, when arterial saturation and oxygen-carrying capacity are normal, from inadequate CBF. Gopinath and colleagues[18] [*see Table 2*] described a relation between the occurrence of desaturations and neurologic outcome in patients with severe head injuries. Without desaturation, mortality was 16%; with one documented desaturation, 42%; and with multiple desaturations, 70%. High $S_{jv}O_2$ values indicate low oxygen extraction, which is the case when the cerebral metabolic rate of oxygen ($CMRO_2$) is low.

The limitations of jugular bulb oximetry should be kept in mind when $S_{jv}O_2$ values are interpreted.[19,20] Because $S_{jv}O_2$ represents global oxygenation, regional ischemia may go undetected if the ischemic region is too small to be represented in the total hemispheric $S_{jv}O_2$ value. Ischemia may also occur in a part of the brain being drained by the opposite jugular vein. In addition, extracerebral veins drain into the internal jugular vein approximately 2 cm below the jugular bulb. With low flow values, significant extracerebral contamination may occur, resulting in deceptively high $S_{jv}O_2$ values. Finally, artifactual readings are often encountered as a result of reduced light intensity when the catheter lodges against the vessel wall. With a new type of catheter, however, the number of artifacts appears to be much lower.

Management of Cerebral Perfusion Pressure

The rationale behind CPP therapy is expressed in Poiseuille's law [*see* Discussion, Pathophysiology, *below*]. Although the effect of CPP therapy has not been investigated in a randomized, controlled clinical trial, several studies suggest that a CPP of 70 to 80 mm Hg may be the clinical threshold below which mortality and morbidity increase.[21,22] CPP therapy involves manipulation of both arterial BP and ICP, but its objective is the reduction of ICP. If ICP reduction does not achieve a CPP of 70 mm Hg, arterial

Table 2 Jugular Desaturation* and Outcome in 116 Patients with Severe Head Injuries[18]

Jugular Desaturations (No.)	Outcome		
	Good Recovery/ Moderate Disability (%)	Severe Disability/ Vegetative (%)	Deceased (%)
0	45	39	16
1	26	32	42
>1	10	20	70

*Defined as jugular venous oxygen saturation < 50% for longer than 15 min.

hypertension is instituted. Mean arterial BP should be raised first by achieving good volume status: ample fluids, including albumin (25 to 30 ml/hr), are administered to maintain central venous pressure at 5 to 10 mm Hg. A pulmonary arterial catheter is suggested for patients older than 50 years and for individuals with known cardiac disease, multiple trauma (particularly chest or abdominal injuries), or a need for vasopressors or high-dose barbiturates. Pulmonary arterial wedge pressure (PAWP) should be maintained between 10 and 14 mm Hg. If necessary, an alpha-adrenergic drug (e.g., phenylephrine, 80 mg in 250 or 500 ml of normal saline) can be combined with the fluids.

Management of Intracranial Pressure

Because ICP is a determinant of CPP, treatment of ICP inevitably affects CPP. Because the goal is maintenance or improvement of CBF, measures for treating ICP should be evaluated in the light of their effect on CBF. It is not possible to establish an arbitrary threshold for treatment of elevated ICP that would be applicable in all situations. Any interpretation of ICP must be combined with assessment of clinical features and evaluation of CT scan findings because it is possible to have transtentorial herniation with an ICP of 20 mm Hg in the presence of a mass lesion. Conversely, with diffuse brain swelling, adequate CPP can be maintained despite an ICP as high as 30 mm Hg. As a general rule, ICP values between 20 and 25 mm Hg indicate that therapy should be initiated.

The recommended regimen for treatment of ICP starts with drainage of CSF through a ventriculostomy-ICP catheter and continues with sedation of the patient with morphine sulfate or propofol, administration of mannitol, paralysis of the patient with pancuronium or vecuronium, initiation of hyperventilation, and induction of a coma with pentobarbital or etomidate.

Although drainage of CSF has no documented deleterious side effects, concern is occasionally expressed that it may aggravate brain shift. Therefore, only a minimal amount should be drained to decrease the ICP below 20 mm Hg. Sedation with morphine sulfate, 4 mg I.V., is standard treatment. Muscular paralysis, which is used by many clinicians, has been shown to increase the risk of respiratory complications.

Mannitol is usually administered in I.V. boluses of 0.25 to 1 g/kg over 10 to 15 minutes until ICP is controlled or serum osmolality reaches 320 mOsm/L. Because volume depletion is an important side effect of mannitol therapy, urine losses should be replaced.

As mentioned, hyperventilation reduces ICP (by vasoconstriction) and CBF, which may be at ischemic levels in certain parts of the brain. Therefore, hyperventilation ($P_aCO_2 < 30$) should not be instituted prophylactically. If P_aCO_2 must be reduced to extremely low levels, hyperventilation can be combined with mannitol, improving CBF by reducing blood viscosity. Jugular bulb oximetry is recommended in these situations because it will determine how much the cerebral blood flow can be constricted.

Hemoglobin, Hematocrit, and Blood Viscosity

To ensure optimal cerebral oxygenation, CPP, hemoglobin concentration, and oxygen saturation should be optimized; vessel diameter should be maximized; and viscosity should be in the low range. The hematocrit and viscosity are inversely related, and a balance must be established to ensure optimal oxygenation. If the hematocrit is too high, viscosity increases; if the hematocrit is too low, the oxygen-carrying capacity of blood decreases. Maintaining the hematocrit between 0.30 and 0.35 is recommended: below 0.30, the oxygen-carrying capacity falls without a significant change in viscosity, and above 0.35, the viscosity increases out of proportion to the oxygen-carrying capacity.

Brain Protection

When oxygen delivery cannot be sufficiently improved, the brain can be protected by decreasing $CMRO_2$. Barbiturates appear to protect the brain and lower ICP through several mechanisms, including alteration of vascular tone, suppression of metabolism, and inhibition of free radical lipid peroxidation. The most important effect may involve coupling of CBF to regional metabolic demands, so that the lower the metabolic requirements, the lower the CBF and the related cerebral blood volume (CBV), with subsequent beneficial effects on ICP and global cerebral perfusion. Barbiturate therapy (usually pentobarbital to a blood level of 4 mg/L) is instituted when other measures to control ICP fail. Marshall and associates,[23] in a series of 25 patients with an ICP higher than 40 mm Hg, reported that barbiturates not only controlled ICP but also improved outcome. Of the patients whose ICP was controlled, 50% had a good recovery; in the patients whose ICP was not controlled by barbiturates, 83% died. Prophylactic barbiturate therapy failed to improve neurologic outcome.[24] Of the barbiturate-treated patients, 54% were hypotensive, compared with 7% of the control subjects,[24] but this trial was conducted before the present emphasis on maintaining CPP was recognized.

Etomidate, a rapidly acting agent with hypnotic properties similar to those of barbiturates, has fewer adverse effects on systemic BP or ICP. However, it suppresses adrenocortical function, and its solvent, propylene glycol, can cause renal insufficiency.[25]

Propofol is a sedative hypnotic with a rapid onset and a short duration of action.[26,27] It depresses $CMRO_2$, but not as effectively as barbiturates and etomidate. Studies of patients with head injuries have demonstrated that ICP decreases with administration of propofol, but systemic BP usually decreases as well, resulting in a net decrease in CPP. Blood lactate levels do not increase when propofol is administered, indicating that cerebral oxygenation is adequate. Propofol is being used with increasing frequency in neurosurgical ICUs, mainly because its short half-life allows accurate neurologic examination minutes after discontinuance of its use. If propofol is used, correction of hypovolemia is recommended to prevent hypotension associated with bolus injection. Finally, because of its preservative-free, lipid-base vehicle, there is an increased risk of bacterial or fungal infection, and the high caloric content (1 kcal/ml) may be problematic during a prolonged infusion.

Hypothermia produces a balanced reduction in energy production and utilization, decreasing $CMRO_2$ and CBF proportionally. Current protocols for hypothermia include cooling to 32° to 33° C (89.6° to 91.4° F) within 6 hours of injury and maintenance of this temperature for 24 to 48 hours. Two pilot clinical trials showed improvement in neurologic outcome.[28,29] Hypothermia to 33° C has also been shown to be effective for refractory high intracranial pressure and for improved outcome under those conditions. Side effects of hypothermia are cardiac arrhythmias and coagulation disorders, reported after cooling to 32° to 33° C. Another drawback of hypothermia is that it is difficult to detect infection because of the lack of warning signs (e.g, spiking and elevated temperature). Finally, hypothermia requires specialized equipment (rotor beds with cooling control) as well as personnel to induce and maintain the condition.

Spinal Cord Injury

DIAGNOSIS AND INITIAL MANAGEMENT

In the field, all patients with significant trauma, any trauma patients who lose consciousness, and any patients suffering minor trauma who have complaints referable to the spine or spinal cord should be treated as if they had a spinal cord injury until proven otherwise [*see Figure 2*]. If cardiopulmonary resuscitation is necessary, it takes precedence. The objectives are to maintain adequate oxygenation and maintain blood pressure by administering fluids and vasopressors (avoiding phenylephrine) and placing the patient in military antishock trousers (MAST). The main concerns of management in the field are immobilization before and during extrication from a vehicle (or removal from the scene of another type of accident) and immobilization during transport to prevent active or passive movement of the spine. Subsequently, the patient may require a rigid Philadelphia collar, support from sandbags and straps, a spine board, or a log-roll for turning. A brief motor examination may detect possible deficits.

Patient has apparent spinal cord injury

(In the field, all patients with significant trauma, any trauma patient who loses consciousness, and any patient with minor trauma who has complaints referable to the spine or the spinal cord should be treated as having spinal cord injury until proven otherwise.)

Resuscitate according to ATLS principles.

Immobilize spine, and use spine board, cervical orthosis, sandbags, straps, log-roll, and tape on forehead as necessary.

Perform trauma evaluation.

Perform emergency diagnostic or therapeutic procedures as indicated.

Maintain oxygenation; intubate and ventilate as needed.

Maintain systolic BP > 90 mm Hg with volume replacement (isotonic fluids), MAST, vasopressors (dopamine, 2–10 μg/kg/min) and, if bradycardia (< 45 beats/min) occurs, atropine, 0.5–1.0 mg I.V.

Place NG tube to prevent vomiting and aspiration.

Place Foley catheter to prevent urinary retention.

Normalize T°.

Perform detailed neurologic examination.

Evalute axial skeleton, and obtain x-rays of spine.

Cervical spine: lateral view showing craniocervical and C7–T1 junctions, followed by AP and odontoid views.

Thoracic and lumbosacral spine: AP and lateral views.

Urgent MRI is indicated if (1) there is an incomplete lesion with normal alignment, (2) deterioration occurs, (3) fracture level ≠ deficit level, or (4) a bony injury cannot be identified.

X-rays are clear; patient is alert, neurologically intact, and free of spinal pain or tenderness; and results of neurologic examination are normal

Discontinue immobilization of spine.

X-rays are clear; patient has impaired consciousness, is not neurologically intact, has spinal pain or tenderness, or has abnormal neurologic examination

Continue immobilization of spine.

Obtain specialist evaluation.

X-rays show evidence of fracture/dislocation

Obtain specialist evaluation.

Figure 2 **Shown is an algorithm for management of the patient with an acute spinal cord injury.**

When the patient arrives at the hospital, care should be taken to provide adequate oxygenation, prevent hypotension, and maintain immobilization. Patients with an injury above C4, who may have respiratory paralysis, may need ventilatory assistance. Lesions above T5 may be accompanied by loss of sympathetic tone and consequently by significant venous pooling and arterial hypotension. Because paralytic ileus is common, usually lasting several days, a nasogastric tube should be placed to prevent vomiting and aspiration. Because urinary retention is common, a Foley catheter should be inserted. Vasomotor paralysis may cause poikilothermy (uncontrolled temperature regulation), which should be treated with cooling blankets when necessary.

A detailed neurologic examination should ascertain whether the injury is complete or incomplete and at what level of the spinal cord the injury has occurred. If possible, a history should be taken to determine the mechanism of injury (e.g., hyperflexion, extension, axial loading, or rotation). There exists a protocol for sensory and motor examination of patients with spinal cord injuries, developed by the American Spinal Injury Association, that is precise and relatively easy to follow [*see Figure 3*].

Spinal shock, which occurs during major injury to the spinal cord, consists of loss of motor, sensory, and autonomic function. The motor component may consist of paralysis, flaccidity, and areflexia. The sensory component may involve both spinothalamic and dorsal column sensory function, and the autonomic component may include systemic hypotension, bradycardia, skin hyperemia, and warmth. Although the cause of spinal shock is unknown, it may be related to a disturbance in impulse conduction caused by a reversible imbalance of electrolytes or neurotransmitters. Usually, motor and sensory symptoms of spinal shock last 1 hour or less; longer-lasting deficits should be attributed to pathologic changes in the cord. Autonomic symptoms, however, may persist for days to months.

All patients with possible spine injuries should be examined radiologically. Roentgenography of the cervical spine, while the patient is in a rigid collar, should include a lateral view showing both the craniocervical and the C7-T1 junction. If the lateral view is obtained and the patient is coherent and has no neck tenderness or neurologic deficit, the collar can be removed for anteroposterior and odontoid views. If the lower cervical spine or the cervical-thoracic junction (or both) are not well visualized, a lateral view with caudal traction on the arms, or a swimmer's view, should be obtained. If the spine is still not visualized or if there is neurologic deficit, a CT scan should be obtained through the poorly visualized levels.

Anteroposterior and lateral views of thoracic and lumbosacral vertebrae should be obtained for all trauma patients who were thrown from a vehicle or fell more than 6 ft to the ground, complain of back pain, are unconscious, cannot reliably describe back pain or have altered mental status preventing adequate examination, or have an unknown mechanism of injury or other injuries that suggest the possibility of spinal injury.

Indications for an urgent MRI include the following: an incomplete lesion with normal alignment (to rule out the possibility that soft tissue is compressing the spinal cord); deterioration (worsening deficit or rising level); a fracture level different from the level of deficit; and the inability to identify a bony injury (to rule out the possibilities of soft tissue compression, disk herniation, or hematoma that would necessitate surgery).

In approximately 10% to 15% of adults and 40% of children with injury to the cervical spinal cord, no radiologic abnormalities are evident in plain, flexion, and extension films. Many patients have reversible incomplete cord lesions, but more severe lesions

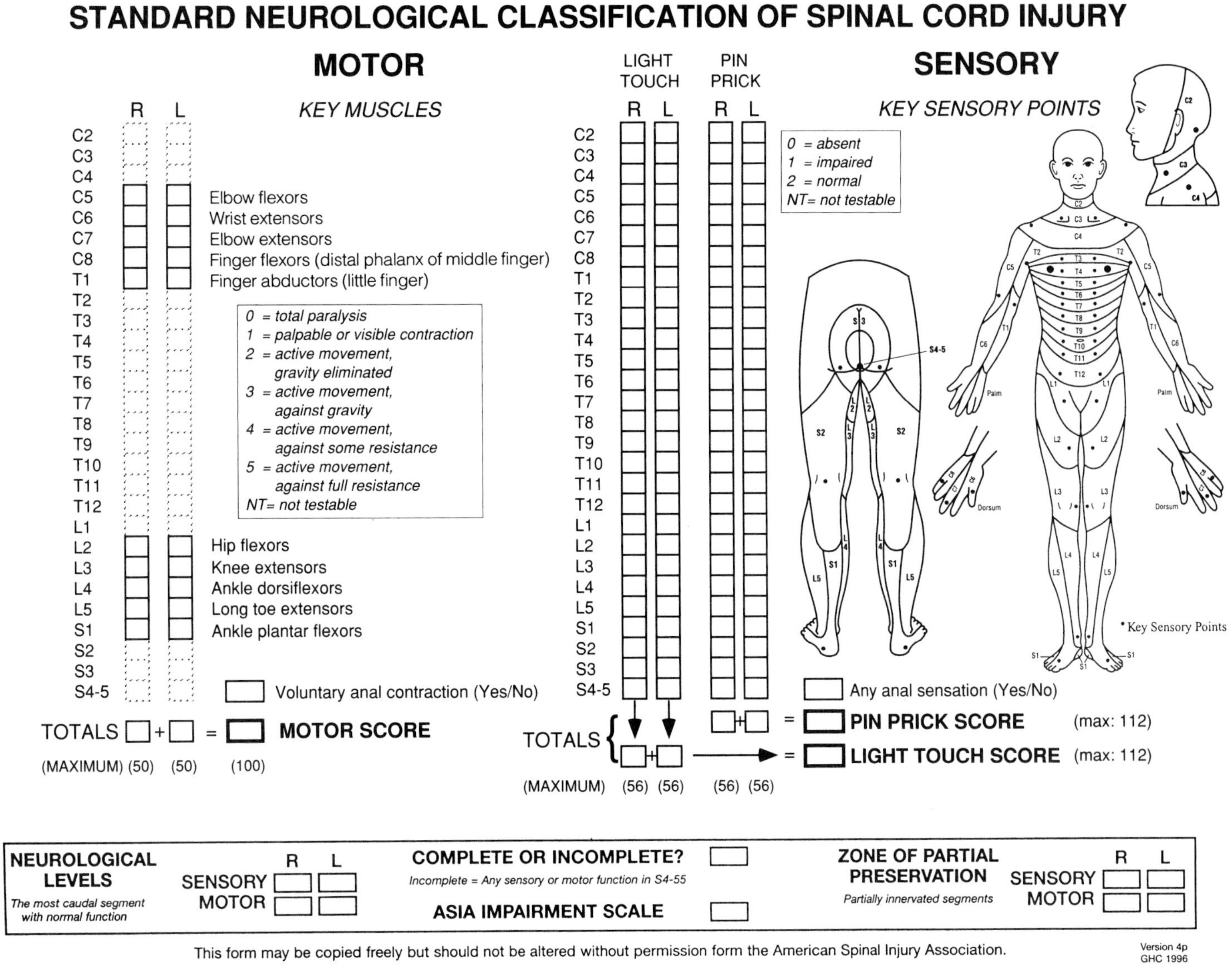

STANDARD NEUROLOGICAL CLASSIFICATION OF SPINAL CORD INJURY

MOTOR

KEY MUSCLES

R L

C2
C3
C4
C5 — Elbow flexors
C6 — Wrist extensors
C7 — Elbow extensors
C8 — Finger flexors (distal phalanx of middle finger)
T1 — Finger abductors (little finger)
T2
T3
T4
T5
T6
T7
T8
T9
T10
T11
T12
L1
L2 — Hip flexors
L3 — Knee extensors
L4 — Ankle dorsiflexors
L5 — Long toe extensors
S1 — Ankle plantar flexors
S2
S3
S4-5

```
0 = total paralysis
1 = palpable or visible contraction
2 = active movement,
      gravity eliminated
3 = active movement,
      against gravity
4 = active movement,
      against some resistance
5 = active movement,
      against full resistance
NT= not testable
```

Voluntary anal contraction (Yes/No)

TOTALS ☐ + ☐ = ☐ **MOTOR SCORE**

(MAXIMUM) (50) (50) (100)

SENSORY

LIGHT TOUCH / PIN PRICK

R L R L

KEY SENSORY POINTS

```
0 = absent
1 = impaired
2 = normal
NT= not testable
```

C2, C3, C4, C5, C6, C7, C8, T1, T2, T3, T4, T5, T6, T7, T8, T9, T10, T11, T12, L1, L2, L3, L4, L5, S1, S2, S3, S4-5

* Key Sensory Points

Any anal sensation (Yes/No)

TOTALS ☐ + ☐ = ☐ **PIN PRICK SCORE** (max: 112)

☐ + ☐ = ☐ **LIGHT TOUCH SCORE** (max: 112)

(MAXIMUM) (56) (56) (56) (56)

NEUROLOGICAL LEVELS
The most caudal segment with normal function

	R	L
SENSORY		
MOTOR		

COMPLETE OR INCOMPLETE? ☐
Incomplete = Any sensory or motor function in S4-S5

ASIA IMPAIRMENT SCALE ☐

ZONE OF PARTIAL PRESERVATION
Partially innervated segments

	R	L
SENSORY		
MOTOR		

This form may be copied freely but should not be altered without permission form the American Spinal Injury Association.

Version 4p
GHC 1996

Figure 3 **Shown is a form developed by the American Spinal Injury Association to record the principal information about motor, sensory, and sphincter function required for accurate neurologic classification of spinal cord injury. For the motor examination, 10 key muscles are tested (left). For the sensory examination, 28 key dermatomes are tested (right).**

---

are observed in elderly people. Explanations for this phenomenon include spontaneous reduction of a subluxation, hyperextension injury, and disk prolapse. With MRI, T_2 (spin-spin)-weighted images may show increased signal within the spinal cord parenchyma.

TREATMENT

Traction

The objectives of craniocervical traction are to reduce fracture-dislocations, to maintain normal alignment or immobility of the cervical spine, to prevent further injury, to decompress the spinal cord and roots, and to facilitate bone healing. A common technique is placement of Gardner-Wells tongs.

Pharmacologic Treatment

A variety of drugs are known to interfere with the processes of secondary injury. The challenge is to identify the most effective treatment or combination of treatments with the fewest severe side effects, a challenge requiring many experiments for each treatment tested. Methylprednisolone, thought to act by scavenging free rad-

icals, has been reported to be neuroprotective in spinal cord injury.[30,31] Patients treated with methylprednisolone within 8 hours of injury exhibited significant improvements in both motor and sensory function compared with patients treated with naloxone or placebo, regardless of whether the injury was complete. After 1 year of follow-up, the advantage was still evident in patients treated with methylprednisolone, but this improvement in outcome was not seen in patients treated more than 8 hours after injury. The regimen studied comprised a 30 mg/kg bolus followed by 5.4 mg/kg/hr for 23 hours. Many centers use methylprednisolone, administered within 8 hours of injury.

The calcium channel blocker nimodipine causes significant increases in blood flow in the spinal cord,[32,33] but the dosage necessary to exert this effect is accompanied by significant systemic hypotension. In a prospective, placebo-controlled, double-blind study, a significant improvement in neurologic outcome was seen in patients treated with GM_1 ganglioside.[34] However, because of the small sample size (34 patients), certain aspects of spinal cord injury or treatment that might have affected outcome were not analyzed in detail. The third National Acute Spinal Cord Injury Study (NASCIS), initiated in 1991, compared methylprednisolone given for either 24 or 48 hours with tirilazad mesylate (an oxygen and lipid radical scavenger).[35] Methylprednisolone was administered in a bolus of 30 mg/kg within 8 hours of injury. Patients receiving methylprednisolone for 48 hours exhibited significant improvement in motor function compared with patients treated with the same agent for 24 hours after injury; however, the patients treated for 48 hours suffered from more severe sepsis and pneumonia. Overall, mortality was identical in the two groups receiving methylprednisolone. Motor function after 6 months in patients treated with tirilazad was similar to that of patients treated with methylprednisolone for 24 hours. On the basis of these findings, the authors suggested that methylprednisolone therapy started within 3 hours of injury should be continued for 24 hours, whereas methylprednisolone treatment started 3 to 8 hours after injury should be continued for 48 hours.

Surgical Treatment

The role of neurosurgery in the treatment of spinal fractures and spinal cord injury is controversial. There is considerable disagreement as to whether surgery should be performed, what type of surgery should be done, and when should it be done. The primary goal of treatment is to restore spinal stability, provide for early mobilization and rehabilitation, and maximize neurologic recovery.

There is general agreement among physicians that early immobilization and early stabilization of fractures and dislocations of the spine are necessary. The single widely accepted indication for early surgical treatment is ongoing neurologic deterioration in the presence of spinal canal compromise from bone and disk fragments, hematoma, or unreduced subluxation. Surgical indications still under debate include incomplete spinal cord injury (with persistent spinal cord deformity) and complete spinal cord injury with the possibility of some neurologic recovery.

Early surgical intervention has been associated with an increased risk of systemic complications (especially pulmonary) and neurologic deterioration. Marshall and coworkers[36] found that one third of all cases of neurologic deterioration could be attributed directly to surgical intervention; 4 of 26 patients who underwent spinal surgery within 5 days deteriorated, while none of the patients treated after 5 days had any neurologic sequelae.

Other studies, however, have not found an increased risk of deterioration with early intervention. Wilberger[37] studied 110 patients with cervical spinal cord injury, of whom 88 underwent surgery for spinal stabilization; in the 39 patients treated within 24 hours, the incidence of systemic complications was reduced by 50% compared with the incidence in the 49 patients treated 24 hours to 3 weeks after injury. In addition, the incidence of neurologic deterioration was 0% in the early-stabilization group versus 2.5% in the late-stabilization group. Data from the NASCIS II study showed improved outcome in patients undergoing surgery within 24 hours of injury compared with patients treated after 200 hours, but the difference was not statistically significant.[38] To date, there is no clear evidence that early surgical intervention improves outcome.

Diagnosis and Treatment of Specific Fractures and Dislocations

Cervical spine Injuries to the cervical spine include atlas fractures, axis fractures, fractures of the lower cervical spine, and atlanto-occipital and atlantoaxial dislocations. Atlanto-occipital dislocations are rare, occurring in approximately 1% of the patients with injury to the cervical spine. Most of these patients die immediately after trauma because of brain stem injury and respiratory arrest. Treatment, which is controversial, consists of either operative fusion or 4 to 6 months of immobilization in a Halo brace. Atlantoaxial dislocations, which are often fatal and there-fore seldom encountered in clinical practice, are usually associated with an odontoid fracture. Because of severe ligamentous injury, these lesions are unstable.

Atlas (Jefferson) fractures, which represent 5% to 10% of all cervical spine fractures, result from axial load. Because of the large diameter of the spinal canal and the tendency of fragments to move outward, these fractures usually are not accompanied by significant neurologic injury, but 40% of patients with an atlas fracture have another cervical fracture (e.g., a fracture through both C1 arches). Treatment requires rigid immobilization in a Halo vest.

Axis fractures account for 10% to 20% of all cervical spine fractures in adults and 70% of cervical fractures in children. Odontoid fractures are the most common (60%). Fractures of the tip of the odontoid process (avulsion fracture, type I) are uncommon and unstable and may require surgical fusion. Fractures of the neck (type II) or at the junction of the odontoid process and the axis (type III) are more common (65% to 80% and 20% to 35%, respectively); they call for Halo-vest immobilization when the dislocation is less than 6 mm and open reduction and internal fixation when the dislocation is greater than 6 mm. Traumatic spondylolisthesis, or hangman's fracture, accounts for approximately 20% of C2 fractures. Injury usually results from axial compression in combination with hyperextension of the occipito-atlanto-axial complex on the lower spine, resulting in bilateral fracture of the pars interarticularis. Fractures affecting the ring of the axis without C2-C3 angulation are stable and can be treated with immobilization in a Philadelphia collar or a sterno-occipito-mandibular immobilizer (SOMI) brace. Halo-vest immobilization is recommended in unreliable patients or patients with both C1 and C2 fractures. The average healing time is 11.5 weeks.

Approximately 80% of all fractures of the lower cervical spine are produced by indirect forces. The vertebra most commonly involved is C5, and dislocations are most frequent at the C5-C6 level. The following injury mechanisms are observed: flexion and distraction (approximately 40% of cases), flexion and compression (22%), vertical compression (8%), extension and compression (24%), extension and distraction (6%), and lateral flexion (3%).

Flexion and distraction injuries usually result from a blow to the occiput from below. The initial disruption is within the posterior ligamentous complex, leading to facet dislocation and abnormally large divergence of the spinous processes. Unilateral facet dislocation and facet interlocking result when a rotatory component is involved. Bilateral facet dislocation with anterior translation of the superior vertebra results from severe hyperflexion. Cord and root involvement vary with the degree of luxation and translation: 50% of patients with unilateral facet dislocation present with moderate cord and root injury, and 90% of patients with bilateral facet dislocation and a full translation of the vertebral body have neurologic deficits, predominantly a complete cord lesion. Teardrop fractures (a bone chip just beyond the anterior inferior edge of the vertebral body) result from severe hyperflexion injury, and the fractured vertebra is usually displaced posteriorly on the vertebra below; these patients are often quadriplegic. Flexion and extension x-rays should be obtained to evaluate ligamentous injury.

Flexion and compression injuries, usually observed at C4-C5 and C5-C6 levels, usually result from a blow to the back of the head. The effect on the anterior vertebral body varies from a moderate rounding or loss of anterior height to a wedge shape with an oblique fracture from the anterior surface to the inferior subchondral plate. Approximately 50% of patients with the latter type of injury have a neurologic deficit. More severe injuries are accompanied by translation of the inferior posterior margin of the vertebral body into the neural canal. About 75% of pa-

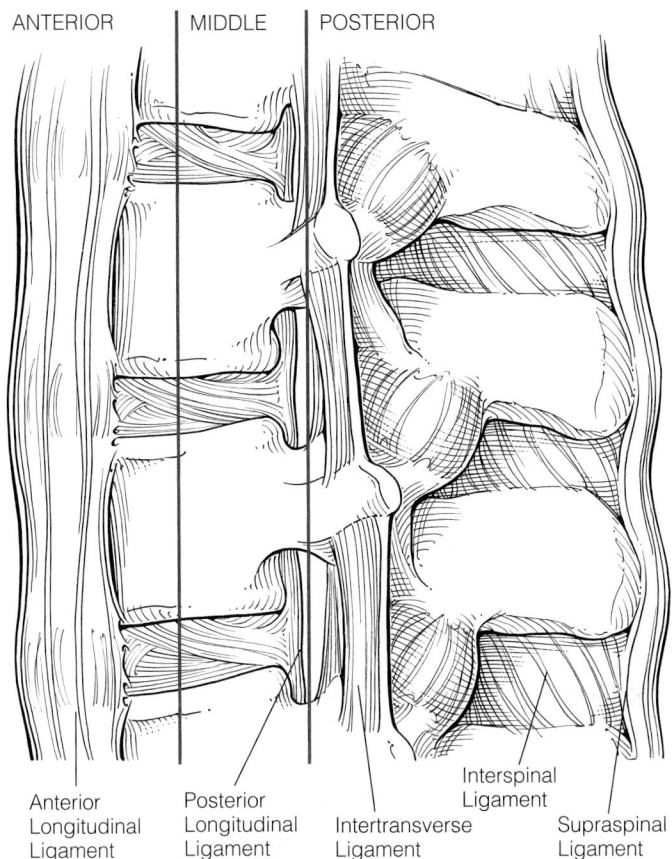

ANTERIOR | MIDDLE | POSTERIOR

Anterior Longitudinal Ligament
Posterior Longitudinal Ligament
Intertransverse Ligament
Interspinal Ligament
Supraspinal Ligament

Figure 4 **Illustrated is the three-column concept for assessment of spinal stability. If two or more columns are destroyed or nonfunctional, instability is likely.**

tients have neurologic involvement. Translations of more than 3 mm result in a complete spinal cord lesion in most cases.

Extension and compression injuries are usually caused by a blow to the forehead and result in fractures of the posterior complex. About 40% of patients with unilateral vertebral arch fractures (articular process, pedicle, or lamina) have a neurologic deficit, predominantly a radiculopathy. Bilaminar fractures are accompanied by a complete cord lesion in 40% of cases. Bilateral vertebral arch fractures with complete anterior translation of the vertebral body present with radiculopathy (30%), central cord syndrome (30%), or incomplete cord lesion (30%). In Allen's series,[39] no complete cord lesions were observed with this type of injury.

Treatment of injuries to the lower cervical spine has not been standardized. As a general rule, severe ligament involvement and severe vertical compression require surgical intervention. Severely comminuted vertebral body fractures may also require surgery because of the high risk of progressive kyphosis. In the series reported by Lind and Nordwall,[40] 87% of patients with distractive flexion injury and 88% of those with compressive flexion injury healed with Halo-vest immobilization.

Thoracolumbar spine Approximately 64% of fractures of the spine occur at the T12-L1 junction, and 70% of these fractures are unaccompanied by immediate neurologic injury. Evaluation according to Denis' three-column principle[41] [*see Figure 4*] is useful for determining whether a fracture is stable, although the precise definition of stability remains controversial. Fractures of the thoracic spine (T1–T10) are more stable because of support from the surrounding rib cage and the strong costovertebral ligaments. When two of the three columns are affected, the fracture is considered unstable and generally requires surgical intervention. If there is no neurologic deficit, surgery can be performed by an orthopedic surgeon or a general surgeon, but if there is a neurologic deficit, a neurosurgeon should perform the operation. In general, the following conditions require surgical intervention: open lesions and dural lacerations, progressive neurologic deficit, marked and progressive angulation, and spinal instability.

The four major types of thoracolumbar spine injuries are compression fractures, burst fractures, seat belt fractures, and fracture-dislocations. These four types of fracture involve the anterior, middle, and posterior columns of the spine in different ways [*see Table 3*].

Minimal to moderate compression fractures with an intact posterior column can be treated with analgesics and bed rest. Ambulation should be started early, and depending on the degree of kyphosis, external immobilization (from a corset or a Boston brace) may or may not be indicated.

Severe compression injuries and seat-belt injuries should be treated with external immobilization in extension. If the loss of anterior height of the vertebral body exceeds 75%, there is an increased risk of progressive kyphosis. Occasionally, surgical intervention is required. An anterior injury is considered unstable if more than three elements in a row, or more than 50% of the height in a single element with angulation, is present.

Burst fractures are considered unstable even if there is no initial neurologic deficit. Early ambulation should be avoided because the axial loading may result in progressive collapse or angulation, with concomitant neurologic damage. Severe burst fractures with neurodeficit should be treated with surgical decompression and stabilization. L5 burst fractures are usually managed conservatively, because it is difficult for spinal instrumentation to maintain alignment at this level; if progressive deformity occurs, L4-S1 fixation is indicated.

Fracture-dislocations require surgical decompression and stabilization.

Table 3   Column Failure in the Four Types of Major Thoracolumbar Spinal Injury[41]

Fracture Type	Anterior Column	Middle Column	Posterior Column
Compression	Compression	Intact	Intact, or distraction if severe
Burst	Compression	Compression	Intact
Seat belt	Intact or mild compression of 10%–20% of anterior vertebral body	Distraction	Distraction
Fracture-dislocation	Compression, rotation, shear	Distraction, rotation, shear	Distraction, rotation, shear

Discussion

Pathophysiology

HEAD INJURY

Cerebral Metabolism

At 1,200 to 1,400 g, the brain accounts for only 2% to 3% of total body weight and does not do any mechanical work; yet it receives 15% to 20% of all cardiac output to meet its high metabolic demands. Of the total energy generated, 50% is used for interneuronal communication and the generation, release, and reuptake of neurotransmitters (synaptic activity), 25% is used for maintenance and restoration of ion gradients across the cell membrane, and the remaining 25% is used for molecular transport, biosynthesis, and other, as yet unidentified, processes.

Cell metabolism involves the consumption of adenosine triphosphate (ATP) during work and the ensuing consumption of metabolic substrates to resynthesize ATP from adenosine diphosphate (ADP). ATP is generated both in the cytosol (via glycolysis) and in the mitochondria (via oxidative phosphorylation). Glucose is the sole energy substrate, unless there is ketosis, and 95% of the energy requirement of the normal brain comes from aerobic conversion of glucose to water and CO_2. ATP generation is highly efficient. Glycolysis and subsequent oxidative phosphorylation result in the generation of 38 molecules of ATP for each molecule of glucose:

$$1 \text{ glucose} + 6 \text{ O}_2 + 38 \text{ ADP} + 38 \text{ P}_i \rightarrow 6 \text{ CO}_2 + 44 \text{ H}_2\text{O} + 38 \text{ ATP}$$

In the absence of oxygen, anaerobic glycolysis can proceed, but energy production is much less efficient. Two molecules of ATP and two molecules of lactate are generated for each molecule of glucose:

$$1 \text{ glucose} + 2 \text{ ADP} + 2 \text{ P}_i \rightarrow 2 \text{ lactate} + 2 \text{ ATP}$$

Regulation of Blood Flow

Because the reserves of glucose and glycogen within the astrocytes of the brain are limited and there is no significant storage capacity for oxygen, the brain depends on blood to supply the oxygen and glucose it requires. More specifically, substrate availability is determined by its concentration in blood, flow volume, and the rate of passage across the blood-brain barrier.

Under normal circumstances and with certain physiologic alterations, an adequate supply of substrates can be maintained by regulation of CBF. CBF increases with vasodilatation and decreases with vasoconstriction. Caliber changes take place mainly in cerebral resistance vessels (i.e., arterioles with a diameter of 300 μm down to 15 μm).[42,43] Control of CBF by influencing vessel caliber is commonly referred to as autoregulation of blood flow.

Metabolic autoregulation CBF is functionally coupled to cerebral metabolism, changing proportionally with increasing or decreasing regional or global metabolic demand. Thus, the brain precisely matches local CBF to local metabolic needs. Because 95% of the energy in the normal brain is generated by oxidative metabolism of glucose, $CMRo_2$ is considered to be a sensitive measure of cerebral metabolism. The relation between CBF and metabolism is expressed in the Fick equation:

$$CMRo_2 = CBF \times A\text{-}VDo_2$$

$CMRo_2$, expressed in milliliters per 100 g of brain tissue, is normally about 3.2 ml/100 g/min in awake adults.[17] The average CBF value for mixed cortical flow is 53 ml/100 g/min in a healthy adult. A-VDo_2, a measure of cerebral oxygen extraction, can be calculated by subtracting the oxygen content of jugular venous blood (6.7 ml/dl) from that of arterial blood (13 ml/dl), resulting in a value of 6.3 ml/dl; this value can then be corrected for hemoglobin content according to the formula discussed earlier [*see* Head Injury, ICU Management, *above*]. Under conditions of increasing metabolic demand (increased $CMRo_2$), such as seizures or fever, CBF increases proportionally, thus keeping A-VDo_2 constant. With decreasing metabolism (anesthesia, deep coma), CBF decreases.

Pressure autoregulation Another important physiologic property of the cerebral circulation is maintenance of a constant supply of substrates at the level set by metabolism. According to Poiseuille's equation,

$$CBF = k \frac{CPP \times d^4}{8 \times 1 \times v}$$

in which k is a constant of proportionality, d is vessel diameter, l is vessel length, and v is blood viscosity, changes in CPP (e.g., arterial hypotension or increases in ICP) are followed by changes in CBF, unless diameter regulation (pressure autoregulation) takes place.[44] In humans, the limits of pressure autoregulation range from 40 to 150 mm Hg of CPP.

Viscosity autoregulation In accordance with Poiseuille's equation, CBF can vary with changes in the viscosity of blood. Blood viscosity changes with variations in hematocrit, γ-globulin, and fibrinogen components of plasma protein. Increased viscosity would increase cerebrovascular resistance ($8 \times 1 \times v/d^4$). By means of diameter adjustment (viscosity autoregulation), cerebrovascular resistance is decreased and CBF can be kept constant.[45]

CO_2 reactivity Vascular caliber and cerebral blood flow are also responsive to changes in arterial P_aco_2. Cerebral blood flow changes 2% to 3% for each mm Hg in P_aco_2 within the range of 20 to 60 mm Hg. Hypercarbia (hypoventilation) results in vasodilatation and higher CBF, and hypocarbia (hyperventilation) results in vasoconstriction and lower CBF. Autoregulation is a compensatory or adaptive response adjusting cerebral blood flow to metabolism; with CO_2 variation, vessel caliber changes and CBF follow passively. The vessels respond not to changes in P_aco_2 but to the pH in the perivascular space. CO_2 can cross the blood-brain barrier freely, thus changing the pH, but over 20 to 24 hours, with a constant new level of P_aco_2, the pH in blood and in the perivascular space returns to baseline, and the diameter of cerebral blood vessels also returns to baseline.[46] With CO_2 reactivity, changes in CBF are compensated for by changes in A-VDo_2, so that a constant supply of substrates is maintained at the level set by metabolism ($CMRo_2$). A constant A-VDo_2 is a common feature of metabolic, pressure, and viscosity autoregulation; because CBF is tuned to metabolism (CBF ≈ $CMRo_2$), A-VDo_2 can be kept constant.

Cerebral Circulation and Metabolism after Severe Head Injury

Arterial hypoxia and hypotension It is known from eyewitness reports of head injury and experimental studies immediately after the impact that arterial hypotension and interruption of normal respiration, sometimes with a period of prolonged apnea, are common findings. In the days after a head injury, there are many occasions and opportunities for hypoxic and hypotensive insults. Studies have identified hypotension (systolic BP below 90 mm Hg) and hypoxia (P_aO_2 below 60 mm Hg) as major determinants of poor outcome.[9,14,47]

The effect of hypotension on the brain depends on the status of autoregulation. If autoregulation is defective, decreased blood pressure leads directly and linearly to a decrease in CBF. If autoregulation is intact, arterial hypotension can lead to a considerable increase in ICP, which interferes with CBF by decreasing perfusion pressure.

Raised intracranial pressure According to the Monro-Kellie doctrine,[48,49] ICP is governed by three factors within the confines of the skull: brain parenchyma plus cytotoxic edema; CSF plus vasogenic edema; and CBV. When the volume in one compartment increases, ICP increases unless there is a compensatory decrease in volume in the other compartments. The relation between intracranial volume and ICP is expressed in the pressure-volume index (PVI).[50] PVI is defined by the volume that must be added to or withdrawn from the craniospinal axis to raise or decrease ICP 10-fold:

$$PVI = \frac{\Delta V}{\log ICP_i / ICP_o}$$

where ΔV represents the change in volume, ICP_o represents ICP before the volume change, and ICP_i represents ICP after the volume change. PVI is thus a measure for the compliance ($\Delta V/\Delta P$) or tightness of the brain. Under normal circumstances, PVI is 26 ± 4 ml; 26 ml of volume will raise ICP from 1 to 10 mm Hg, but the same volume will also raise ICP from 10 to 100 mm Hg. Conversely, a change in volume of only 6.4 ml is necessary to increase intracranial pressure from 10 mm Hg (normal) to the treatment threshold of 20 mm Hg. Thus, small changes in volume have a relatively large effect on ICP.

Apart from mass lesions, intracranial pressure typically increases after severe head injury because of cerebral edema. Initial compensation is by displacement of CSF from the cranium, which is visualized in a CT scan of the head as small ventricles and basal cisterns. Subsequent compensation would be by a decrease in CBV, which can be accomplished by means of vasoconstriction.

Relation between vessel diameter, cerebral blood volume, and intracranial pressure The total diameter of the cerebrovascular bed determines CBV. Cerebral veins contain most of the total blood volume, but their diameter and, thus, their volume are relatively constant. Approximately 20 ml of blood (i.e., one third of total CBV) is located in the cerebral resistance vessels (which range in diameter from 300 μm down to 15 μm).[51] Because most autoregulatory and CO_2-dependent variations in diameter take place in these vessels, cerebral blood volume is determined mainly by their diameter. Typically, the diameter ranges from 80% to 160% of baseline, resulting in volume changes between 64% and 256% of baseline. With a baseline value of 20 ml in the resistance vessels, CBV will range from 13 ml (maximal vasoconstriction) to 51 ml (maximal vasodilatation). Given a pressure-volume index of 26, change from maximal vasoconstriction to maximal vasodilatation will be accompanied by an almost 29-fold change in ICP.

Cerebral blood volume, intracranial pressure, and cerebral blood flow CBF and CBV are governed by vascular di-

ameter. Thus, depending on other parameters influencing CBF (such as mean arterial BP, ICP, and blood viscosity), changes in vascular caliber also affect CBF.

Hypocarbia reduces ICP by means of vasoconstriction, consequently improving CPP. However, net CBF is decreased because in Poiseuille's equation, vessel diameter is carried to the fourth power. A randomized clinical trial has shown that preventive hyperventilation retards clinical improvement after severe head injury, perhaps through reduction of CBF to ischemic levels.[52] However, its rapid effect on ICP is of great advantage in cases of acute neurologic deterioration (e.g., in the presence of an expanding mass lesion before evacuation can take place) and should be reserved for these situations.

There are two methods of reducing ICP by means of vasoconstriction without affecting CBF. The first is to reduce blood viscosity. As can be deduced from Poiseuille's equation, decreasing the blood viscosity will, by itself, lead to vasoconstriction, provided that viscosity autoregulation is intact. With impaired autoregulation, decreased viscosity will result in an increase in CBF but no decrease in ICP. However, this effect can be used to maintain CBF under vasoconstriction with hypocarbia. The effect of mannitol on ICP is thought to be mediated in part by lowering blood viscosity.[53,54]

The second method of reducing ICP without affecting CBF is to increase CPP, which can be done by raising blood pressure. Again, with intact autoregulation, an increase in CPP will lead to vasoconstriction, with net CBF remaining constant. With impaired autoregulation, CBF will follow CPP passively, and maintenance of normal blood pressure may be indicated in these cases. More important, however, is the avoidance of hypotension under these circumstances; the effect of CPP therapy may be attributable in part simply to prevention of hypotension.[21,55]

Cerebral ischemia Cerebral ischemia, defined as CBF that is inadequate to meet the metabolic demands of the brain, is an important mechanism of secondary injury in patients with severe head injury, and the adequacy of CBF has been associated with neurologic outcome. In autopsy findings from patients dying after severe head injury, histologic damage indicative of cerebral ischemia was seen in 80% of cases.[56] Bouma and associates[57] found ischemia (CBF < 18 ml/dl with abnormally high A-VDo$_2$ values) in 20% to 33% of patients with severe head injuries within 4 to 12 hours of injury, and the ischemia was associated with a poor prognosis. Of the intracranial lesions, acute subdural hematoma and diffuse cerebral swelling were most often associated with ischemia.

The relation between cerebral metabolism and CBF is expressed in the Fick equation [see Metabolic Autoregulation, *above*]. The normal brain tends to keep A-VDo$_2$ constant and to react to changes in metabolism with adjustments in blood flow. When CBF decreases in response to metabolism (as with hyperventilation or decreasing CPP with impaired autoregulation), oxygen supply is maintained by increasing oxygen extraction (i.e., A-VDo$_2$ increases). Increasing A-VDo$_2$ is thus a sensitive marker of insufficient cerebral perfusion. However, oxygen extraction is limited, and this limit is reached when A-VDo$_2$ is doubled (13.2 ml/dl). Consequently, any further reduction in CBF results in neuronal dysfunction (i.e., CMRo$_2$ decreases). Because 50% of the energy is used for synaptic activity, a reversible and functional loss is usually observed first. Further decline, however, will result in ion pump failure, loss of membrane integrity, consequent cell swelling (cytotoxic edema), and cell death (irreversible infarction). The occurrence of irreversible infarction depends on both the level and the duration of ischemia. When cerebral blood flow decreases to approximately 18 ml/100 g/min for more than 4 hours, it reaches the threshold for irreversible infarction.[58]

Maintenance or improvement of CBF is thus essential to the treatment of severe head injury, and A-VDO$_2$ is a sensitive marker of the adequacy of therapy. When therapeutic measures fail to sustain CBF, CMRo$_2$ can be decreased to reinstate the match between CBF and metabolism. CNS suppression can be obtained with the administration of hypnotic agents (e.g., barbiturates or propofol) or the induction of hypothermia. Decreasing cell metabolism will result in reduced production of CO$_2$, lactic acid, or both and (with blood vessels almost always remaining responsive to perivascular pH changes) in vasoconstriction accompanied by reductions in both CBF and ICP. The relations between CMRo$_2$, CBF, CBV, CPP, and A-VDo$_2$ are complicated. An overview is available elsewhere[59] [see Table 4].

Altered cerebral metabolism Anaerobic metabolism of glucose to the end product lactate is characteristic of cerebral hypoxia/ischemia.[60] Increased lactate production, hyperglycolysis, and low tissue glucose levels have been observed after severe head injury, suggesting an increased turnover of glucose by the anaerobic glycolytic pathway. Increased lactate levels have also been found in the presence of preserved CBF,[61,62] suggesting impairment not only of oxygen delivery but also of oxidative metabolism (i.e., of mitochondrial function). Recent findings in animals and humans indicate that mitochondrial function is impaired after severe head injury, which may explain poor outcomes despite adequate CBF levels; ATP generation by anaerobic glycolysis is usually insufficient to maintain the metabolic activity of the brain.[63,64] In part, however, such poor outcomes may be attributable to the effects of lactate production (acidosis), because high lactate and hydrogen ion levels interfere with the functional recovery of tissue.

SPINAL CORD INJURY

Spinal cord injury is often viewed as an all-or-nothing event that is irreversible from the moment of injury. By this view, spinal cord injury is classified as either incomplete or complete. This dichotomy is not absolute, however, because some functional recovery occurs even after severe spinal cord injury. The Second National Acute Spinal Cord Injury Study revealed that patients with so-called complete loss of neurologic function recovered on average 8% of the function they had lost, and patients with an incomplete injury recovered 59% of what they had lost.[65] An injury classified as complete does not necessarily involve loss of all connections. Several studies have demonstrated that many patients with a clinically complete lesion show evidence of residual connection.[66] A certain number of intact connections is probably necessary for functional recovery. The determinants of functional outcome are complex, however, and probably include not only the extent of axonal loss but also the level of dysfunction of the surviving axons and the plasticity of the spinal cord.

Animal studies have found that a small number of axons may be sufficient to support functional recovery.[67-69] Animals recover evoked potentials and the ability to walk with as few as 10% of their spinal axons. Nerve sprouting, one of the mechanisms of plasticity, allows a few nerves to carry out the function of many. Finally, animal studies have also shown that many of the axons surviving traumatic injury are dysfunctional and that many of the axons had lost part or all of their myelin sheath, which is the structural component that improves the reliability and speed of conduction. 4-Aminopyridine, an axon-excitatory drug used for the treatment of multiple sclerosis, has significantly improved

Table 4 Changes in CBF, CBV, ICP, and A-VDO$_2$ Associated with Primary Reduction of Selected Variables[59]

Variable Reduced	CBF	CBV (ICP)	A-VDO$_2$
CMRO$_2$	↓	↓	—
CPP (autoregulation intact)	—	↑	—
CPP (autoregulation defective)	↓	↓	↑
Blood viscosity (autoregulation intact)	—	↓	—
Blood viscosity (autoregulation defective)	↑	—	↓
P$_a$CO$_2$	↓	↓	↑
Conductance vessel diameter (vasospasm above ischemia threshold)	↓	↑	↑

A-VDO$_2$—arteriovenous oxygen content difference   CBF—cerebral blood flow CBV—cerebral blood volume   CMRO$_2$—cerebral metabolic rate of oxygen   CPP—cerebral perfusion pressure   ICP—intracranial pressure   P$_a$CO$_2$—arterial carbon dioxide tension

conduction in animals and humans with spinal cord injury.[70-72] Unfortunately, the drug must be given continuously to support axon function, and this is not feasible in humans because of its side effects (seizures, tachycardia, and hyperthermia).

Injury initiates complex responses in the body and the spinal cord. Ischemia is a prominent feature of events occurring after spinal cord injury.[73,74] Within 2 hours of a spinal cord injury, there is a significant reduction in spinal cord blood flow. It is unclear whether this is mechanically or biochemically induced. Like the brain, the spinal cord possesses autoregulatory capacity (pressure autoregulation). When this autoregulation is impaired, blood flow becomes dependent on systemic blood pressure. In a patient with multiple injuries or vasogenic spinal shock (a lesion above T5) complicating the spinal cord injury, severe systemic hypotension may exacerbate the effects of spinal cord injury.

Edema, another prominent feature of spinal cord injury, tends to develop first at the injured site, subsequently spreading to adjacent and sometimes distant segments. The relation between spreading edema and potential worsening of neurologic function is poorly understood. The inflammatory response to injury ideally cleans up cellular debris and repairs tissue. This response is accompanied, however, by the release of toxic substances, which cause further tissue damage, or secondary injury. Processes resulting in secondary injury involve generation of free radicals, excessive calcium influx and excitotoxicity, the release of eicosanoids and cytokines, and programmed cell death.

Conclusion

Mortality has decreased considerably in patients with severe head injury. In the patients we have studied, mortality has decreased from approximately 40% to 45% in the decade between 1975 and 1984 to 25% to 30% at present, with a further downward trend evident. Increased recognition of the mechanism of secondary brain injury as well as avoidance of secondary insults by optimizing cerebral perfusion and oxygenation are probably responsible for most of the improvement in outcome. Pharmacologic brain protection and attempts to intervene in the damaging cascade of biochemical events occurring after injury have shown some beneficial effects in phase II trials, but no compound has clearly shown efficacy when tested in multicenter phase II clinical trials. Targeted strategies or combinations of drugs, based on pathophysiologic concepts, are expected to provide the major breakthrough in research on treatment of head injury.

The results in patients with acute spinal cord injury are not spectacular. Methylprednisolone has provided a modest improvement in outcome, suggesting that pharmacologic intervention can curtail damage from ongoing biochemical cascades in central nervous system injuries. As in research on head injuries, better insight into pathophysiology is a major focus. Early stabilization and multidisciplinary care, which can prevent some of the systemic and neurologic complications of spinal cord injury, can improve outcome.

References

1. Fine P, Kuhlemeier K, DeVivo M, et al: Spinal cord injury: an epidemiological perspective. Paraplegia 17:237, 1979

2. Kalsbeek W, McLaurin R, Harris B, et al: The National Head and Spinal Cord Injury Survey: major findings. J Neurosurg 53:S19, 1982

3. Kraus J, Franti C, Riggins R, et al: Incidence of traumatic spinal cord lesions. J Chron Dis 28:471, 1975

4. Kraus J: Epidemiological aspects of acute spinal cord injury: review of incidence, prevalence, causes and outcome. Central Nervous System Trauma Status Report, 1985. Becker D, Poulishock J, Eds. National Institute of Neurological and Communicative Disorders and Stroke, Bethesda, Maryland, 1985, p 313

5. Factsheet No. 2: Spinal cord injury statistical information. National Spinal Cord Injury Association, Woburn, Massachusetts, 1992

6. Burney R, Maio R, Maynard F, et al: Incidence, characteristics, and outcome of spinal cord injury at trauma centers in North America. Arch Surg 128:596, 1992

7. Tator C: Spine-spinal cord relationships in spinal cord trauma. Clin Neurosurg 30:479, 1983

8. Gibson C: An overview of spinal cord injury. Phys Med Rehab Clin North Am 3:699, 1992

9. Chesnut RM, Marshall SB, Piek J, et al: Early and late systemic hypotension as a frequent and fundamental source of cerebral ischemia following severe brain injury in the Traumatic Coma Data Bank. Acta Neurochir Suppl (Wien) 59:121, 1993

10. American College of Surgeons Committee on Trauma: Advanced Life Support Course for Physicians, Instructor Manual, 2nd ed. American College of Surgeons, Chicago, 1985

11. Ritter AM, Muizelaar J, Barnes T, et al: Brain stem blood flow, pupillary response and outcome in patients with severe head injures. Neurosurgery 44:941, 1999

12. Schroder M, Muizelaar J, Kuta A: Documented reversal of global ischemia immediately after removal of a subdural hematoma: report of two cases. J Neurosurg 80:324, 1994

13. Andrews P, Piper I, Dearden N, et al: Secondary insults during intrahospital transport of head injured patients. Lancet 335:327, 1990

14. Jones P, Andrews P, Midgley S: Measuring the burden of secondary insults in head-injured patients during intensive care. J Neurosurg Anesthesiol 6:4, 1994

15. Kirkpatrick P, Smielewski P, Czosnyka M, et al: Near-infrared spectroscopy use in patients with severe head injury. J Neurosurg 83:963, 1995

16. Kanter M, Narayan R: Management of head injury: intracranial pressure monitoring. Neurosurg Clin North Am 2:257, 1991

17. Gibbs E, Lennox W, Nims L, et al: Arterial and cerebral venous blood: arteriovenous differences in man. J Biol Chem 144:325, 1942

18. Gopinath S, Robertson C, Contant C, et al: Jugular venous desaturation and outcome after severe head injury. J Neurol Neurosurg Psychiatry 57:171, 1994

19. Robertson C, Gopinath SP, Goodman J, et al: $S_{jv}O_2$ monitoring in head-injured patients. J Neurotrauma 12:891, 1995

20. Stochetti N, Paparella A, Bridelli F, et al: Cerebral venous oxygen saturation studied with bilateral samples in the internal jugular veins. Neurosurgery 34:38, 1994

21. Rosner M, Rosner S, Johnson A: Cerebral perfusion pressure: management protocol and clinical results. J Neurosurg 83:949, 1995

22. McGraw C: A cerebral perfusion pressure greater than 80 mm Hg is more beneficial. Springer-Verlag, Berlin, 1989

23. Marshall L, Smith R, Shapiro H: The outcome with aggressive treatment in severe head injuries, part II: acute and chronic barbiturate administration in the management of head injury. J Neurosurg 50:26, 1979

24. Ward J, Becker D, Miller JD, et al: Failure of prophylactic barbiturate coma in the treatment of severe head injury. J Neurosurg 62:383, 1985

25. Levy M, Aranda M, Zelman V, et al: Propylene glycol toxicity following continuous etomidate infusion for the control of refractory cerebral edema. Neurosurgery 37:363, 1995

26. Pinaud M, Lelasque J, Chetanneau A, et al: Effects of Diprivan on cerebral blood flow, intracranial pressure and cerebral metabolism in head-injured patients. Annales Françaises d'Anesthésie et de Réanimation 10:2, 1991

27. Bullock R, Stewart L, Rafferty C, et al: Continuous monitoring of jugular bulb oxygen saturation and the effect of drugs acting on cerebral metabolism. Acta Neurochir (Wien) 59:113, 1993

28. Clifton G, Allen S, Barrodale P, et al: A phase II study of moderate hypothermia in severe brain injury. J Neurotrauma 10:263, 1993

29. Marion D, Obrist W, Carlier P, et al: The use of moderate therapeutic hypothermia for patients with severe head injuries: a preliminary report. J Neurosurg 79:354, 1993

30. Bracken M, Shepard M, Collins W, et al: A randomized controlled trial of methylprednisolone or naloxone in the treatment of acute spinal cord injury. N Engl J Med 322:1405, 1990

31. Bracken M, Shepard M, Collins W, et al: Methylprednisolone or naloxone treatment after acute spinal cord injury: 1-year follow-up data. J Neurosurg 76:23, 1992

32. Guha A, Tator C, Piper I, et al: Increase in rat spinal cord blood flow with the calcium channel blocker nimodipine. J Neurosurg 63:250, 1985

33. Guha A, Tator C, Smith C, et al: Improvement in posttraumatic spinal cord blood flow with a combination of a calcium channel blocker and a vasopressor. J Trauma 29:1440, 1989

34. Geisler F: GM-1 ganglioside and motor recovery following human spinal cord injury. J Emerg Med 11(SII):49, 1993

35. Bracken M, Shepard M, Holford T, et al: Administration of methylprednisolone for 24 or 48 hours or tirilazad mesylate for 48 hours in the treatment of acute spinal cord injury: results of the Third National Acute Spinal Cord Injury Randomized Controlled Trial. National Acute Spinal Cord Injury Study. JAMA 227:1597, 1997

36. Marshall L, Knowlton S, Garfan S, et al: Deterioration following spinal cord injury: a multi-center study. J Neurosurg 66:400, 1987

37. Wilberger J: Advances in the diagnosis and management of spinal cord trauma. J Neurotrauma 8:75, 1992

38. Wilberger J, Duh M: Surgical treatment of spinal cord injury—the NASCIS II experience. Presented at the annual meeting of the AANS, Boston, Massachusetts, April 1993

39. Allen BL Jr: Recognition of injuries to the lower cervical spine. The Cervical Spine, 2nd ed. The Cervical Spine Research Society, Ed. JB Lippincott Co, Philadelphia, 1989, p 286

40. Lind BL, Nordwall A: Halo-vest treatment of unstable traumatic cervical spine injuries. Spine 13:425, 1988

41. Denis F: The three column spine and its significance in the classification of acute thoracolumbar spinal injuries. Spine 8:817, 1983

42. Kontos H, Raper A, Patterson J: Analysis of vasoreactivity of local pH, pCO_2, and bicarbonate on pial vessels. Stroke 8:358, 1977

43. Kontos H, Wei E, Navari R, et al: Responses of cerebral arteries and arterioles to acute hypotension and hypertension. Am J Physiol 234:H371, 1978

44. McHenry LC Jr, West JW, Cooper ES: Cerebral autoregulation in man. Stroke 5:695, 1974

45. Muizelaar J, Wei E, Kontos H, et al: Cerebral blood flow is regulated by changes in blood pressure and in blood viscosity alike. Stroke 17:44, 1986

46. Muizelaar J, Poel H, Li Z, et al: Pial arteriolar vessel diameter and CO_2 reactivity during prolonged hyperventilation in the rabbit. J Neurosurg 69:923, 1988

47. Chesnut R, Marshall L, Klauber MR, et al: The role of secondary brain injury in determining outcome after severe head injury. J Trauma 34:216, 1993

48. Monro A: Observations on the structure and function of the nervous system. Creech and Johnson, Edinburgh, 1783

49. Kellie G: On death from cold, and on congestions of the brain: an account of the appearances observed in the dissection of two of three individuals presumed to have perished in the storm of 3rd November 1821; with some reflections on the pathology of the brain. Trans Med Chir Soc Edinburgh 84-169, 1824

50. Marmarou A, Shulman K, Rosende R: A nonlinear analysis of the cerebral spinal fluid system and intracranial pressure dynamics. J Neurosurg 48:332, 1978

51. Muizelaar JP: Cerebral Blood Flow, Cerebral Blood Volume, and Cerebral Metabolism after Severe Head Injury. WB Saunders Co, Philadelphia, 1989

52. Muizelaar JP, Marmarou A, Ward JD, et al: Adverse effects of prolonged hyperventilation in patients with severe head injury: a randomized clinical trial. J Neurosurg 75:731, 1991

53. Muizelaar JP, Wei EP, Kontos H, et al: Mannitol causes compensatory cerebral vasoconstriction and vasodilation in response to blood viscosity changes. J Neurosurg 59:822, 1983

54. Muizelaar JP, Lutz HI, Becker D: Effect of mannitol on ICP and CBF and correlation with pressure autoregulation in severely head-injured patients. J Neurosurg 61:700, 1984

55. Rosner M, Daughton S: Cerebral perfusion management in head injury. J Trauma 30:933, 1990

56. Adams J, Di G: The Pathology of Blunt Head Injury. Heinemann, London, 1972

57. Bouma G, Muizelaar JP, Choi S, et al: Cerebral circulation and metabolism after severe traumatic brain injury: the elusive role of ischemia. J Neurosurg 75:685, 1991

58. Jones T, Morawetz R, Crowell R, et al: Thresholds of

focal cerebral ischemia in awake monkeys. J Neurosurg 54:773, 1981

59. Muizelaar JP, Schroder M: Overview of monitoring of cerebral blood flow and metabolism after severe head injury. Can J Neurol Sci 21:S6, 1994

60. Hochachka P, Mommsen T: Protons and anaerobiosis. Science 219:1391, 1983

61. Andersen B, Marmarou A: Functional compartmentalization of energy production in neural tissue. Brain Res 585:190, 1992

62. Inao S, Marmarou A, Clarke G, et al: Production and clearance of lactate from brain tissue, CSF and serum following experimental brain injury. J Neurosurg 69:736, 1988

63. Verweij B, Muizelaar J: Mitochondrial dysfunction after experimental and human brain injury and its possible reversal with a selective N-type calcium channel antagonist (SNX-111). Neurol Res 19:334, 1997

64. Xiong Y, Gu Q, Peterson P, et al: Mitochondrial dysfunction and calcium perturbation induced by traumatic brain injury. J Neurotrauma 14:23, 1997

65. Young W, Bracken M: The second National Acute Spinal Cord Injury Study. J Neurotrauma 9:S429, 1992

66. Dimitrijevic M, Dimitrijevic M, Faganel J, et al: Residual Motor Functions in Spinal Cord Injury. Raven Press, New York, 1988

67. Blight A, Young W: Central axons in injured cat spinal cord recover electrophysiological function following remyelination by Schwann cells. J Neurol Sci 91:15, 1989

68. Blight A, Decrescito V: Morphometric analysis of experimental spinal cord injury in the cat: the relation of injury intensity to survival of myelinated axons. Neuroscience 19:321, 1986

69. Blight A, Young W: Axonal morphometric correlates of evoked potentials in experimental spinal cord injury. Humana Press, New York, 1990

70. Blight A, Gruner J: Augmentation by 4-aminopyridine of vestibulospinal free fall responses in chronic phases of traumatic spinal cord injury in dogs: a phase I clinical trial. J Neurol Sci 82:155, 1987

71. Hayes K, Blight A, Potter P, et al: Preclinical trial of 4-aminopyridine in patients with chronic spinal cord injury. Paraplegia 31:216, 1993

72. Hayes K, Potter P, Wolfe D, et al: 4-aminopyridine-sensitive neurologic deficits in patients with spinal cord injury. J Neurotrauma 11:433, 1994

73. Sandler A, Tator C: Review of the effects of spinal trauma on vessels and blood flow in the spinal cord. J Neurosurg 45:638, 1972

74. Young W: Blood flow, metabolic and neurophysiologic mechanisms in spinal cord injury. Central Nervous System Trauma Status Report, 1985. Becker D, Poulishock J, Eds. National Institute of Neurological and Communicative Disorders and Stroke, Bethesda, Maryland, 1985

Acknowledgments

Figure 3   Reprinted courtesy of the American Spinal Injury Association, Chicago, Illinois.
Figure 4   Susan Brust, C.M.I.

3 INJURIES TO THE FACE AND JAW

Seth Thaller, M.D., F.A.C.S., and F. William Blaisdell, M.D., F.A.C.S.

Assessment and Management of Maxillofacial Injuries

Tremendous progress has been made in the management of patients with facial injuries. Reconstructive surgeons are treating an increasing number of challenging facial injuries because of excellent advances in the transportation of trauma victims and the regionalization of care in trauma centers. Although severe facial injuries are often associated with devastating cosmetic and functional defects, reconstructive surgeons are achieving better long-term surgical results and are able to repair certain injuries that were once considered nonreconstructible by employing craniofacial surgical techniques developed through the pioneering efforts of Dr. Paul Tessier, of Paris. These techniques include widespread subperiosteal exposure, rigid internal fixation with miniature plates and screws, and widespread primary bone grafting.

Initial Survey

Maxillofacial injuries are secondary to either blunt or penetrating trauma. Motor vehicle accidents remain the most common cause of facial injuries characterized by bony comminution and distraction. However, penetrating injuries, such as knife wounds, can cause extensive soft tissue injuries to skin and under-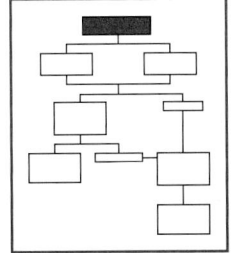lying nerves, blood vessels, parotid structures, and other structures of the upper aerodigestive system. Gunshot wounds can cause devastating injuries that necessitate extensive flap reconstruction to provide satisfactory soft tissue coverage of the underlying bone.

On initial assessment, the physician must always pay special attention to correcting the most life-threatening problems, including an obstructed airway, bleeding, and shock [*see 5:1 Trauma Resuscitation, 6:3 Shock, and 1:4 Bleeding and Transfusion*]. Patients with facial injuries often have multisystem involvement; priorities in the evaluation and treatment of associated significant injuries are discussed elsewhere. After establishing that the patient is stable, the examiner should quickly make note of lacerations and contusions, extensive bony disruptions, loss of vision, malocclusion, trismus, and bleeding.

In the evaluation of facial injuries, a quick analysis of occlusion provides extremely important diagnostic information that serves as the foundation for future fracture repair. Angle's classification of malocclusion, which is more than 100 years old, remains one of the most commonly used systems. The maxillomandibular relation is determined by the position of the mesiobuccal cusp of the maxillary first molar in relation to the buccal groove of the mandibular first molar. Angle's class I, or neutroclusion, exists when the permanent maxillary first molar is ideally positioned—that is, the buccal cusp of the maxillary first molar and the mesiobuccal groove of the mandibular first molar occlude, resulting in a normal anteroposterior relation of the maxillary and mandibular dentition. Angle's class II, or distoclusion, exists when the maxillary first molar is mesial (i.e., toward the midline) to the corresponding mandibular first molar. Angle's class III, or mesioclusion, exists when the mandibular first molar is mesial to the maxillary first molar.

AIRWAY ASSESSMENT

Facial bone fractures, bleeding, loose dentition, debris, and laryngeal injuries can contribute to airway compromise. Accordingly, whenever there is any evidence of maxillofacial injuries, it is essential to monitor the airway status carefully. If the patient is conscious, alert, and breathing at a rate of less than 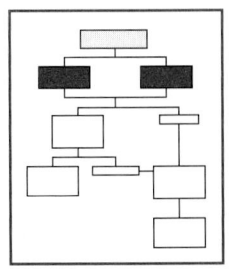20 respirations/min, without excessive airway secretions or excessive hemorrhage, it can be assumed that the patient has an adequate airway.

In a comatose patient with compromised vital reflexes (i.e., gag, cough, and swallow), an endotracheal tube must be inserted immediately to prevent aspiration. In the presence of nasopharyngeal bleeding, major maxillofacial injuries, or cerebrospinal fluid leakage, nasal intubation should be avoided because of the potential for intracranial contamination. If there is a possible fracture of the cribriform plate, either an orotracheal tube should be placed or a cricothyrotomy should be performed. In an agitated or restless patient, only a single attempt should be made at inserting an endotracheal or nasotracheal tube; if the attempt is unsuccessful, an emergency cricothyrotomy should be performed [*see 5:1 Trauma Resuscitation*]. In slightly more elective circumstances, a deliberate tracheotomy may be the optimal means of ensuring an adequate airway. Cricothyrotomy and tracheotomy must never be taken lightly, because they can lead to significant complications. In addition, because newer treatment modalities using rigid fixation decrease the time required for extensive maxillo-

Assessment and Management of Maxillofacial Injuries

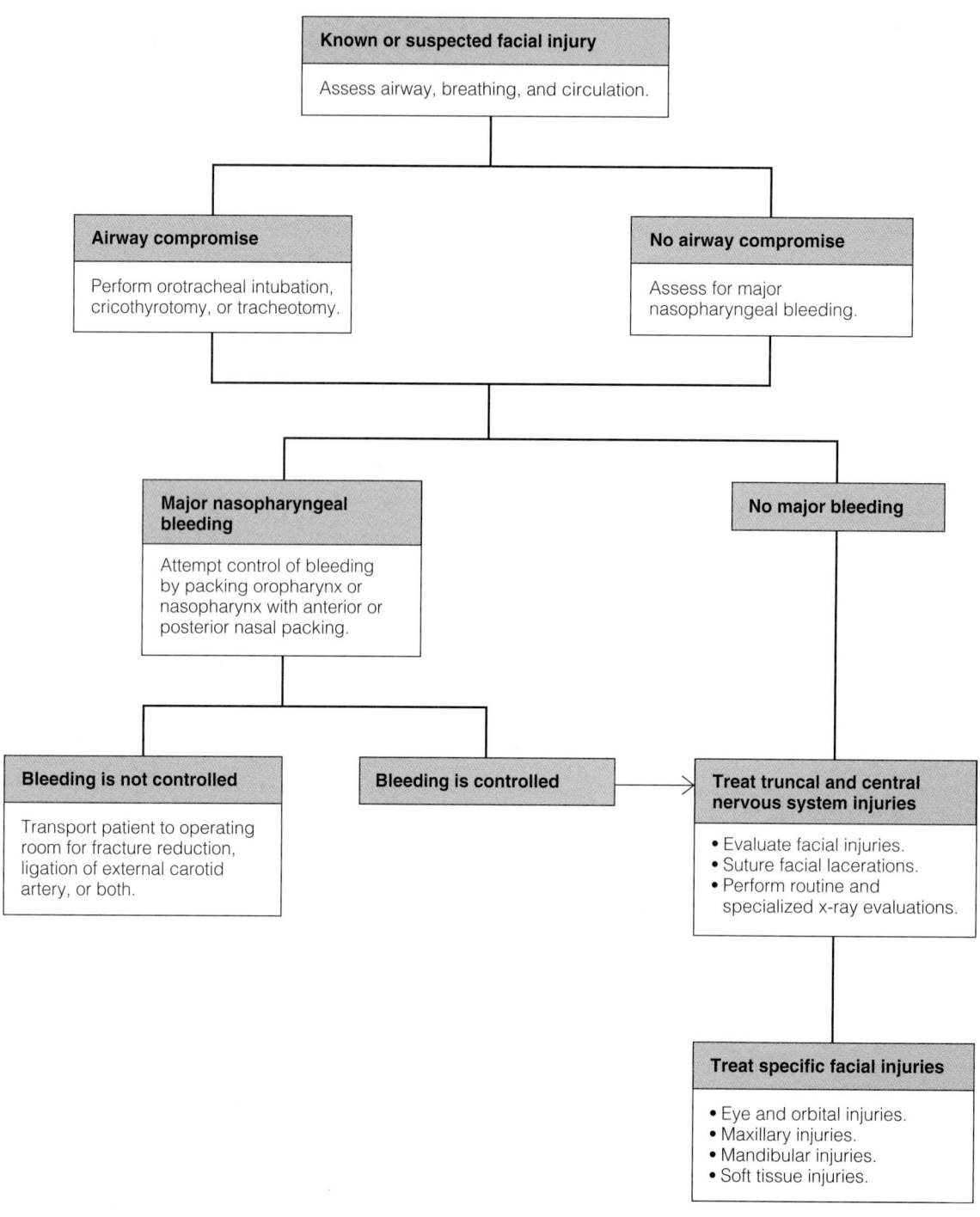

880

mandibular fixation, more conservative methods of airway control are often indicated.

If the respiratory rate is higher than 25/min or if there is evidence that the airway is obstructed or compromised, the patient should be carefully monitored. When the respiratory rate increases to 30/min or higher, an immediate assessment of arterial blood gases should be made under close observation. A respiratory rate higher than 35/min is an indication for both intubation and respiratory support unless the cause of the rapid rate can be identified and immediately reversed.

MAXILLOFACIAL BLEEDING

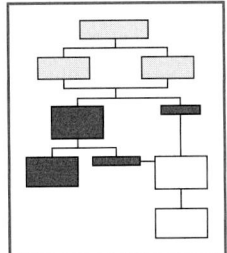

Once the airway has been satisfactorily stabilized, the next priority is to manage maxillofacial bleeding. There is a misconception that patients do not bleed profusely from facial injuries and that facial bleeding can be controlled easily.[1] Unfortunately, this is not necessarily always the case. In addition, because facial injuries themselves can be so striking, associated significant hemorrhage can often be overlooked or underestimated. Firm compression with moist sponges will temporarily stop most arterial and venous bleeding. Careful application of digital pressure or definitive ligation of the bleeding point can often control external bleeding. These procedures are best performed in the operating room, with the patient under general anesthesia.

If the source of hemorrhage is in the depths of a narrow laceration, bleeding can be controlled temporarily by packing. Blind clamping or suture ligation can damage important underlying facial structures, particularly branches of the facial nerve; therefore, such procedures must be avoided. Insertion of an anterior pack moistened with 1:10,000 epinephrine may be used to control nasal bleeding. However, persistent nasopharyngeal hemorrhage will necessitate either placement of a posterior pack or ligation of the internal maxillary artery or the external carotid artery.

In patients with major maxillofacial injuries who are experiencing extensive pharyngeal bleeding, immediate airway access is mandatory, either via an endotracheal tube or by means of cricothyrotomy. Once airway control has been achieved, the patient should be brought to the operating room for reduction of gross bony injuries, which will often stop uncontrollable hemorrhage. In those rare instances when maxillofacial injuries are associated with serious and uncontrollable hemorrhage, it may be necessary to obtain access to the external carotid artery for ligation of the major trunk or a branch if either vessel is the source of bleeding [see 5:4 Injuries to the Neck].

Definitive Evaluation

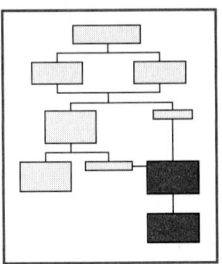

When there is no associated airway compromise, facial injuries are a lower priority than potential thoracic, abdominal, or head injuries [see 5:1 Trauma Resuscitation]. In fact, in the absence of airway compromise and severe hemorrhage, definitive diagnostic evaluation and management of maxillofacial injuries can be delayed until the more life-threatening injuries have been stabilized and treated.

EXAMINATION

Like any other anatomic region, the face must be examined in an orderly fashion, with careful attention paid to gross asymmetry, paralysis, weakness, eye movements, occlusal discrepancies, and ecchymosis. Areas of hypesthesia or anesthesia should be noted. Special attention should be directed toward bimanual palpation of bony prominences within the craniofacial region to look for crepitus, tenderness, irregularities, and step-offs. Palpation should start with the frontal bones and lateral and inferior orbital rims.

The zygomatic arch should be palpated for evidence of depression, and the region of the malar eminence should be evaluated for recession [see Figures 1 through 4]. Fracture of the

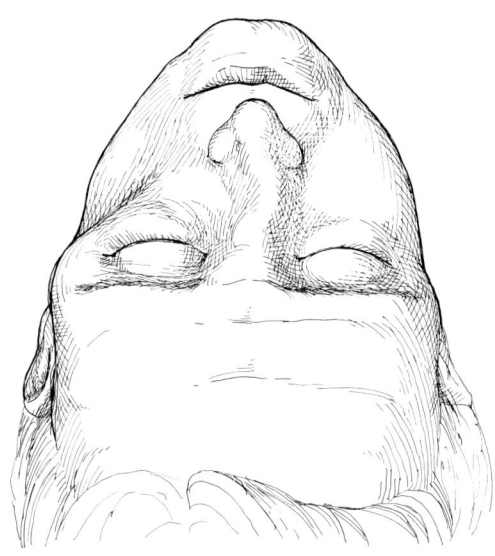

Figure 1 **Broken nose.**

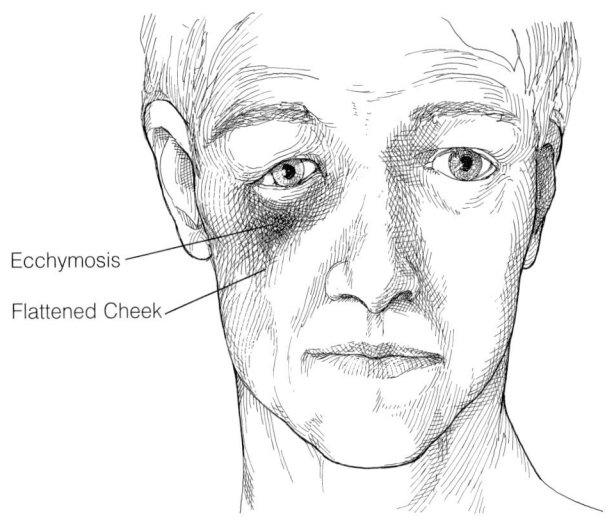

Figure 2 **Fractured zygoma.**

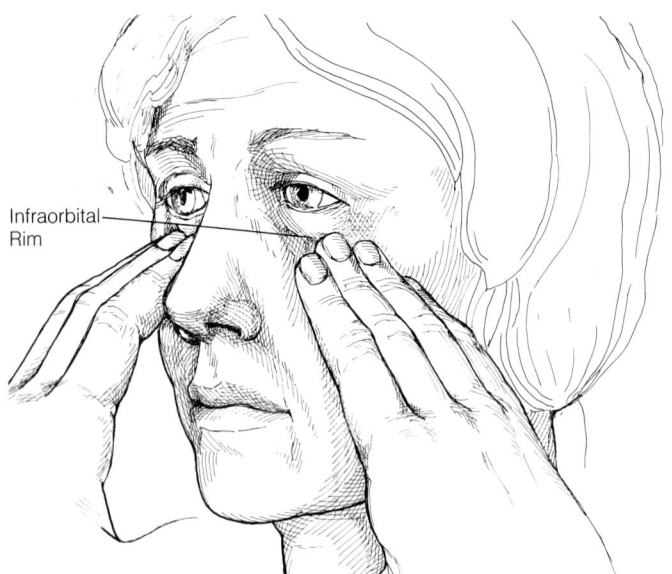

Figure 3 **Infraorbital fracture.**

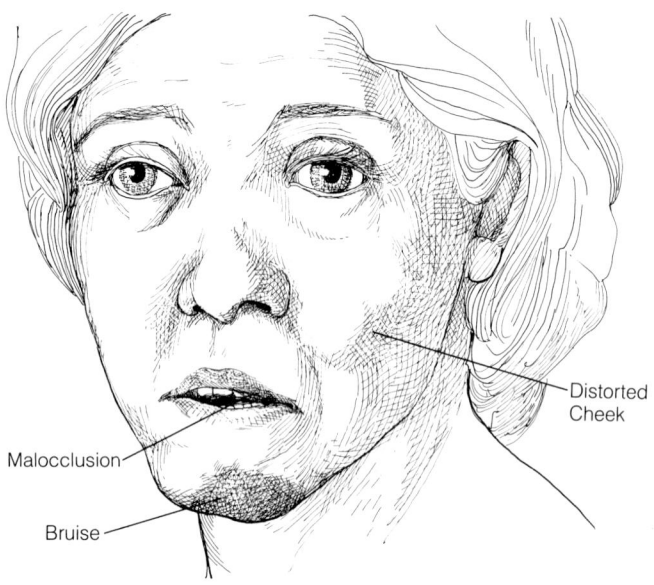

Figure 4 **Fractured mandible.**

zygomatic complex is often identified with an inferiorly displaced lateral canthus, paresthesias of the infraorbital nerve, visual impairment, displacement of the globe, or trismus secondary to impingement of the zygomatic arch on the coronoid process or temporal muscle.

Orbital evaluation is key to the assessment of facial injuries. The nasolacrimal duct should be inspected, and the distance between the medial canthi should be measured for the presence of telecanthus. (The normal intercanthal distance in the average adult is less than 35 mm.) Pupils should be checked for reactivity, and extraocular muscle motion should be assessed. Diplopia secondary to extraocular muscle entrapment should be determined. The position of the globe should also be assessed; orbital floor fractures may cause enophthalmos and severe swelling, and a blow-in type fracture may result in exophthalmos. A visual acuity test must be performed before any surgical intervention for correction of facial fractures. An ophthalmologic consultation is essential if there is any evidence of ocular damage, such as lens displacement, hyphema, retinal detachment, acute visual impairment, or global disruption.

Next, the nose should be gently palpated. Any depression, abnormal motion, or deviation of the nasal bones and cartilages should be noted. The nasal cavity should be examined specifically for the presence of septal deviation, septal hematoma, or leakage of cerebrospinal fluid. A septal hematoma can be ruled out by aspiration with an 18-gauge or 20-gauge needle and syringe; if bleeding is present, an incision and drainage and placement of a drain are necessary. If left untreated, a septal hematoma may lead to the development of a saddle-nose deformity. Flattening of the face, or dish-face deformity, is characteristic of midfacial fractures.

Mobility of the maxilla is determined by placing one hand over the bridge of the nose while the other grasps the palate and upper dentition and moves the maxilla anteriorly and posteriorly, checking for separation of the midfacial structures. The mandible should be palpated carefully with both hands to locate any intraoral mucosal lacerations or lesions. Bimanual palpation of the mandible is accomplished by placing the thumbs over the molar occlusal surfaces and the index fingers externally over the inferior border of the mandible and torquing the bone to check for movement. Any missing or mobile teeth must be recorded. The floor of the mouth should also be examined with bimanual palpation.

The ears should be examined for evidence of lacerations or contusions of the external auditory canal that may be caused by condylar neck fractures. A simple diagnostic method is to insert the fingertip into the external auditory canal on one side; if no movement can be determined with mandibular excursion, a diagnosis of condylar fracture can be made.

FACIAL X-RAYS

A spectrum of available radiologic modalities plays a significant role in the diagnosis and treatment of facial injuries. Appropriate studies are mandatory. In addition, x-rays provide an excellent permanent record for medicolegal purposes. The initial x-rays of patients in the emergency room (the first level for assessment and clarification of maxillofacial injuries) should be performed using conventional films and should consist of a cervical spine series (with all the cervical vertebrae adequately visualized), skull x-rays, and facial x-rays, including the anteroposterior, lateral, Waters, Towne, submentovertex, panorex, and mandibular views. More definitive x-rays can be obtained later for complete evaluation of specific injuries. The Caldwell view defines the orbital walls and the frontal sinus structures. The Waters view is important for determining the bony continuity of the orbit, nose, zygoma, and lateral portion of the maxilla. The lateral skull view is helpful for evaluation of frontal sinus fractures. Oblique views of the orbit are excellent for demonstrating the apex and the medial, lateral, and orbital walls.

The lateral oblique and modified Towne views are used to evaluate the mandible. The lateral oblique is the most common and useful view and provides evaluation of the body, angle of the body, and the ascending ramus. A posteroanterior view is helpful in assessing the symphyseal and body regions as well as the condylar and coronoid processes. Panoramic x-rays are the best screening views for assessing mandibular fractures, especially within the condyles. Associated injuries to the dentition and supporting structures may necessitate dental spot films for more specific information.

OTHER STUDIES

Computed tomographic scanning can be of great value in diagnosing the more complex traumatic injuries, such as craniomaxillofacial injuries and associated central nervous system injuries. Computed tomography is used to evaluate most critically injured patients with craniocerebral trauma, and the studies can easily be extended to include the patient's facial skeleton with little additional risk. Both 3 mm axial and coronal CT cuts of the facial skeleton should be obtained, especially for examination of the orbit. A lateral oblique scan through the midportion of the globe provides additional information regarding the bony architecture of the orbit. This information can be reformatted, and three-dimensional reconstructions can be made for further evaluation. Magnetic resonance imaging is proving to be of benefit in assessing both bony and soft tissue injuries. Arteriography may be needed to evaluate the source of a hemorrhage or to rule out major vascular injuries.

Treatment of Soft Tissue Injuries

Soft tissue injuries are most often the result of penetrating trauma but can also be the result of blunt trauma [see Treatment of Maxillofacial Fractures, below]. Any patients who need general anesthesia, such as a child or a patient with extensive complex lacerations involving deeper structures, should be treated in the operating room after appropriate evaluation of their overall status. Soft tissue injuries can involve nerves, parotid ducts, lacrimal ducts, and other critical facial structures. Abrasions must be thoroughly cleaned, and lacerations should be irrigated with normal saline and conservatively debrided as necessary. With deeply embedded foreign material, debridement and irrigation must be particularly meticulous and extensive to prevent residual cosmetic deformities. Dermabrasion is especially good for large involved areas. Most facial lacerations can be closed primarily with standard suturing procedures [see 1:7 Acute Wound Care]. Antibiotic coverage is left to individual preferences; however, 24 hours of prophylactic perioperative antibiotic coverage with a cephalosporin is strongly recommended. The examiner must always consider the possibility of underlying injuries, and careful palpation and visualization of important underlying structures should be part of the definitive wound evaluation and treatment.

Local anesthetic agents used in the head and neck region should always contain epinephrine for hemostasis. To decrease pain and discomfort, the local anesthetic should be administered through the margins of the wound rather than through the surrounding skin. Regional nerve blocks are preferred for suture closure of lacerations involving the forehead, cheeks, lips, and chin. The forehead can be blocked by local infiltration of the supraorbital nerve, which is located just superior to the eyebrow. The upper lip, side of the nose, and adjacent skin can be blocked by anesthetizing the infraorbital nerve. Injection of the mental nerve, located between the first and second bicuspids, will anesthetize the lower lip and surrounding chin. Regional blocks also provide the advantage of minimizing tis-

sue damage to already traumatized skin and lead to less scar formation.

NERVE INJURIES

The facial nerve is the nerve most vulnerable to maxillofacial trauma, and its function must be thoroughly evaluated before the administration of any local anesthetic. In addition, facial nerve injuries result in the most serious functional disabilities and aesthetic defects. Sensory nerves, such as the infraorbital and supraorbital nerves, can also be involved in traumatic injures; however, the associated hypesthesia causes only minimal long-term disability.

Whenever the posterior half of the parotid gland suffers a deep laceration, it should be assumed that a major branch of the facial nerve has been divided, and the face should be carefully examined. If there is a clean, sharp division of one of the five major trunks or of the proximal main nerve trunk, it can be repaired immediately with microanastomotic techniques. If there is substantial nerve loss, the nerve ends should be identified and appropriately tagged for future nerve grafting. If a nerve laceration occurs anterior to the region of the lateral canthus, nerve repair is generally unnecessary because there is sufficient crossover from the opposite side. Peripheral branch injury is manifest by inability to raise the eyebrow (frontal branch), inability to close the eyelids (malar), smoothness of the cheek (infraorbital), inability to smile (buccal), and inability to frown (marginal mandibular).

PAROTID DUCT INJURIES

The parotid duct is located between the parotid gland and the oral mucosa, opening opposite the second upper molar. Any deep laceration of the anterior parotid gland can damage this duct. If there is a possibility that the parotid duct is injured, the orifice of Stensen's duct should be probed. Should the probe enter the wound, division of the duct is verified. The proximal cut end of the duct can be located by expressing saliva from the gland. A catheter should then be passed through Stensen's duct and through the area of laceration, and the duct should be repaired over the catheter [see Figure 5].

LACRIMAL DUCT INJURIES

Whenever there is a laceration involving the medial canthal region, a lacrimal duct injury should be assumed. Acute reconstruction of the lacrimal duct is controversial. If both ends of the duct can be easily discerned, the severed ends should be realigned, splinted internally, and repaired. This procedure is best accomplished over a fine Silastic rod. Dissection to locate the residual parts of the duct should be delicate and meticulous, because traumatic dissection can aggravate the injury and result in further permanent damage.

SCALP INJURIES

When scalp injuries are repaired, extensive shaving is unnecessary. Scalp injuries can be associated with profuse bleeding because of the scalp's extensive vascular supply. To obtain adequate control of hemorrhage from the wound margins, closure can be achieved in a single layer with a running, locking 3-0 chromic suture on a large cutting needle. Associated underlying skull fractures are always a possibility, and the skull should be palpated and inspected through any full-thickness scalp wound.

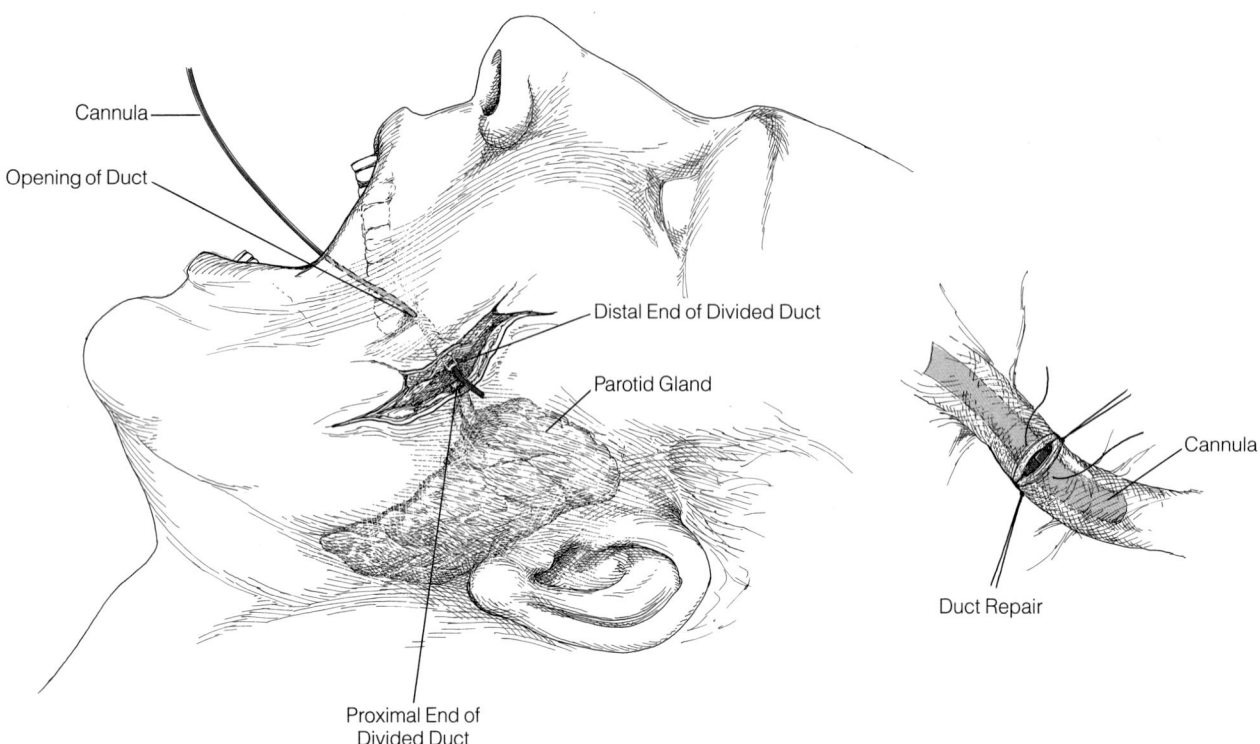

Cannula

Opening of Duct

Distal End of Divided Duct

Parotid Gland

Cannula

Duct Repair

Proximal End of
Divided Duct

Figure 5 **Injuries to the parotid duct are repaired by passing a catheter through Stensen's duct and through the area of laceration and then repairing the parotid duct over the catheter.**

EYELID INJURIES

If the patient reports excessive eye pain, the initial examiner must always first rule out an associated ocular injury. In addition, when faced with through-and-through lid lacerations, the examiner must perform a very careful eye examination. Lacerations of the eyelid should be meticulously repaired by approximation of the margins of the lid defect, followed by closure of the laceration in three layers. The conjunctiva may be left unsutured if good apposition can be obtained by closing the tarsal plate and the pretarsal muscles that occupy the middle layer, which is preferably closed with fine absorbable sutures. Fine nonabsorbable skin sutures are employed to close the final layer. All skin sutures should be removed within 48 hours. When there is extensive tissue loss, it may be necessary to use plastic techniques to mobilize sufficient conjunctiva for closure.

EYEBROW INJURIES

For optimal cosmetic results, the eyebrows should be closed meticulously in layers with careful alignment of the eyebrow margins. Lacerations passing through the eyebrow should not be shaved; leaving them intact facilitates good plastic closure. Because the hairs of the eyebrow run obliquely to the surface of the skin, any incision for debridement should follow the line of the eyebrows to avoid further loss of hair.

EXTERNAL-EAR INJURIES

If avulsions of the ear are properly repaired, the chances are good that they will heal because of the highly vascular pedicle. Circulation is maintained if even a small pedicle is present.

Repair of ear wounds should be done in three layers by using fine nonabsorbable sutures to approximate the cartilage and the skin. If the ear is completely detached, the cartilage should be preserved within a subcutaneous pocket in the mastoid region for future reconstruction.

Hematomas can occur secondary to the shearing of the vascular mucoperichondrium from the underlying cartilage. These must be evacuated early, and a conforming pressure dressing should be placed to maintain the normal ear contour.

NASAL INJURIES

Through-and-through lacerations of the nose and near-avulsion injuries are cosmetic problems. Because the nose is extremely vascular, repair of these injuries should be especially meticulous and done in layers. The cartilage and skin should be aligned with fine nonabsorbable interrupted sutures. Absorbable sutures should be employed for repair of the mucosa. Key cosmetic points (i.e., epidermal-mucosal junctions, nasal fold junctions, or critical angles in jagged lacerations) should be sutured first to ensure that no deformity results.

LIP INJURIES

If the margin of the lip has been divided, the vermilion border should be carefully identified and tattooed, and the first sutures should be placed to approximate this critical margin. A common problem in the treatment of lip injuries is that it may become more difficult to identify landmarks when they are obliterated by local anesthetic injections or associated edema.

Treatment of Maxillofacial Fractures

Management of maxillofacial fractures can be extremely challenging. The common maxillofacial fractures include nasal, mandibular, orbital, zygomatic complex, sinus (e.g., maxillary, sphenoid, ethmoid, and frontal), and maxillary fractures (e.g., Le Fort I, II, or III). Management of these fractures often requires sophisticated specialty treatment involving plastic surgeons, ophthalmologists, neurosurgeons, otolaryngologists, or a combination of these.[2-7]

FRONTAL SINUS FRACTURES

The frontal sinus region is prone to injury because of its prominent location and relatively thin anterior bony wall.[8,9] Injuries to the frontal sinus area require comprehensive treatment, often with a team approach. The key to treatment lies in determining the status of the nasofrontal ducts.[10,11] Patients with such injuries also require careful, regular, long-term follow-up care because potentially life-threatening complications, such as meningitis, osteomyelitis, and mucopyocele, may develop.[12-15]

NASAL AND NASO-ORBITO-ETHMOIDAL FRACTURES

The nasal bone is the most commonly fractured facial bone.[16] Before any treatment is embarked on, it is always helpful to have the patient provide a preinjury photo of himself or herself so that it can be determined whether the nasal deformity is from the acute episode.[17] If a patient is seen almost immediately after injury and the associated swelling and ecchymosis are minimal, closed reduction can be performed at once. Nasal bone fractures can be reduced simply by inserting a scalpel handle or large hemostat into the nostril; the fracture segments can then be elevated and relocated. Usually, the nasal cavity is packed with petroleum jelly gauze to maintain alignment of the fracture and nasal septum, and a malleable splint is taped over the nose to provide counterpressure and assist in maintaining alignment. Packing is removed within 48 hours. However, treatment is generally not urgent and, depending on the individual situation, may be delayed for 7 to 10 days.

Naso-orbito-ethmoidal fractures generally occur secondary to direct force applied over the nasal bridge, resulting in posterior displacement of bony structures and involvement of the medial canthus, lacrimal duct, canaliculi, and sac.[18] Repair of naso-orbito-ethmoidal fractures can be extremely challenging because of the number of important structures involved and their extensive comminution.[19] Satisfactory surgical management should be conducted through a coronal approach, thereby permitting precise three-dimensional reduction and stabilization and extensive primary bone grafting for replacement augmentation.[20] If there is associated CSF rhinorrhea, neurosurgical assistance should be obtained and early fracture reduction done.

ORBITAL FRACTURES

Orbital fractures can occur as isolated events or as a component of more extensive injuries. Orbital fractures, such as lacrimal duct lacerations and injuries to the globe, require highly specialized management with the aid of an ophthalmologist. Naso-orbital fractures with telecanthus should be treated with open reduction and fixation, as should all displaced fractures of the orbital rim and floor.[21,22]

ZYGOMATIC FRACTURES

The zygoma is a tetrapod structure that forms the malar prominence and the inferior and lateral aspects of the orbit. Fractures of the zygomatic complex should be repaired to prevent the development of serious aesthetic and functional deformities. Satisfactory stabilization requires three-point fixation achieved through incisions placed within the regions of the upper and lower lids and the upper buccal sulcus.[23]

MAXILLARY FRACTURES

In 1901, maxillary fractures were classified by René Le Fort into three types.[24] Although the Le Fort classification system remains entrenched in the literature and serves as a basis for both communication and description, it is rare that patients exhibit pure Le Fort fracture patterns. Instead, trauma sur-

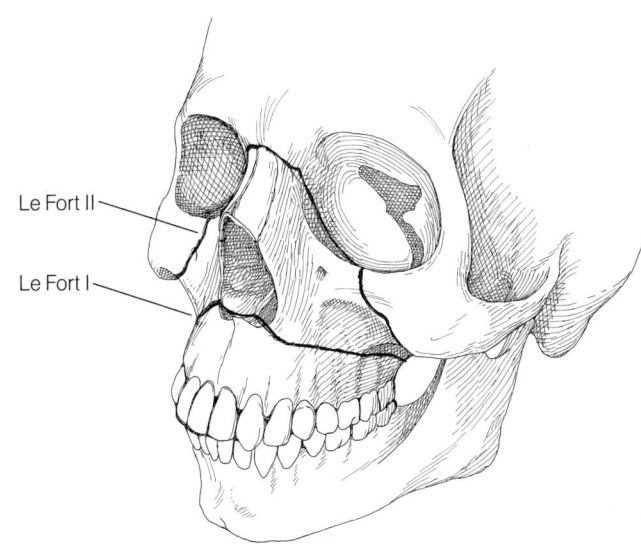

Figure 6 **Le Fort I fractures (black line) affect the upper jaw alone. In Le Fort II fractures (red line), the upper jaw and the central portion of the face are separated from the skull.**

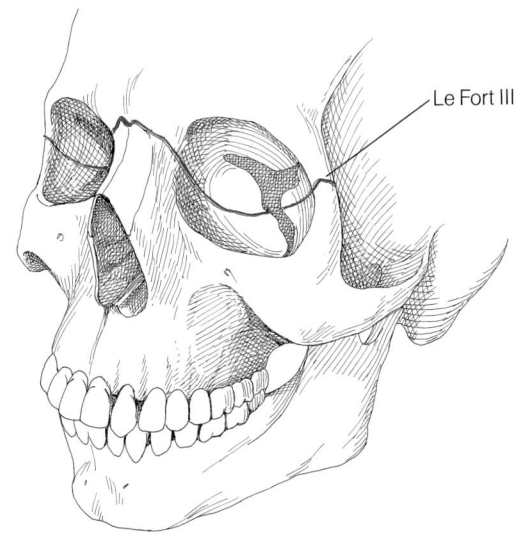

Figure 7 **In Le Fort III fractures, all of the facial bones are separated from the skull.**

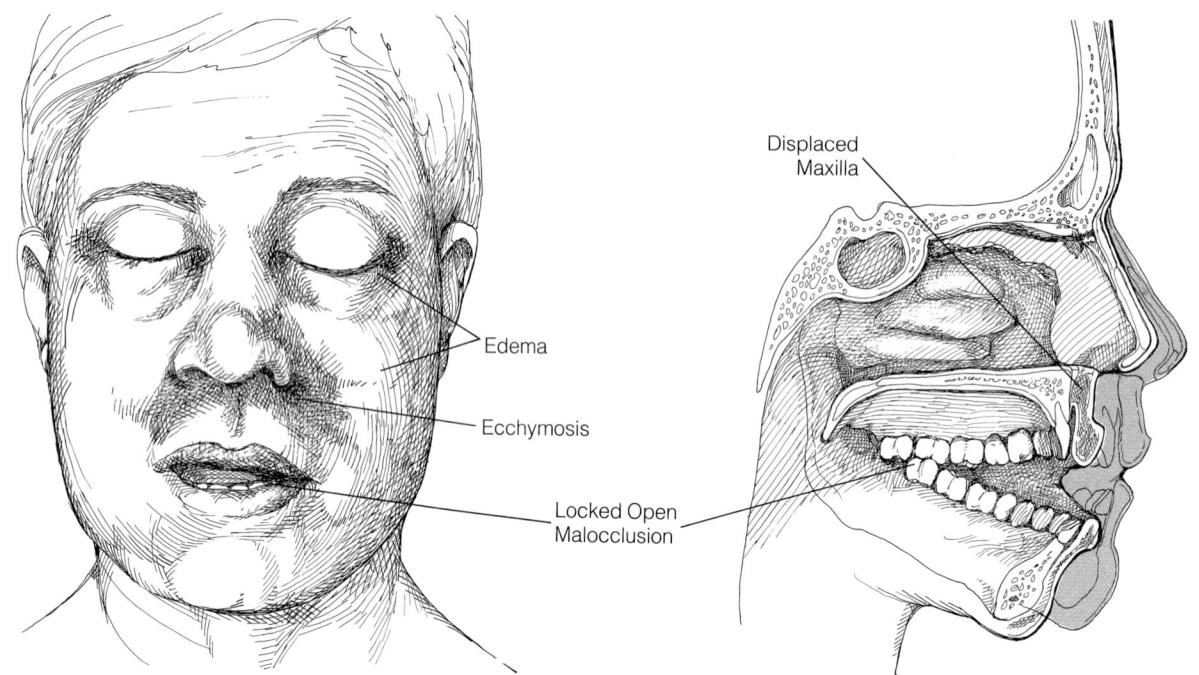

Figure 8 **Findings in patients with Le Fort III maxillary fractures immediately after injury, before obliterative edema develops.**

geons are generally challenged by severe bony comminution and distraction.

Le Fort I, or lower maxillary fractures, are the simplest type of maxillary fracture, consisting of horizontal detachment of the tooth-bearing segment of the maxilla at the level of the nasal floor [*see Figure 6*]. Le Fort II, or central or pyramidal fractures, pass through the central portion of the face, which includes the right and left maxillae, the medial aspect of the antra, the infraorbital rim, the orbital floor, and the nasal bones. Le Fort III, or craniofacial disjunction, is characterized by complete separation of all facial structures from the cranium [*see Figures 7 and 8*]. Le Fort III fractures pass through the upper portions of the orbits as well as through both zygomas.

All Le Fort fractures require highly specialized treatment that involves the use of craniofacial techniques, consisting of exploration and visualization of the entire fracture pattern, precise reduction, and rigid stabilization of bony segments.

MANDIBULAR FRACTURES

Diagnosis of mandibular fractures can usually be made on physical examination. Common findings include malocclusion, intraoral lacerations, and mobility at the fracture site. Radiographs are useful for planning treatment. Fractures of the mandible rarely involve the midline or symphyseal region. Most often, fractures will pass through areas of weakness, including the parasymphyseal region and the angle or neck of the condyle [*see Figure 9*]. The fracture pattern is usually determined by the site and mechanism of injury. Because of the mandible's architectural arrangement, more than one half of mandibular fractures involve multiple sites.

Mandibular fractures are not an emergency, but early defin-

itive treatment results in a decreased number of complications. Preinjury occlusal relations remain the keystone to treatment. Mandibular fractures can be repaired by closed reduction with maxillomandibular fixation or by open reduction and fixation with wire osteosynthesis. However, newer techniques with rigid internal fixation with miniature plates and screws have attained widespread popularity because of increased patient comfort.[25-31] In cooperative patients, a nondisplaced fracture can sometimes be handled conservatively with a dental soft diet and serial x-rays.

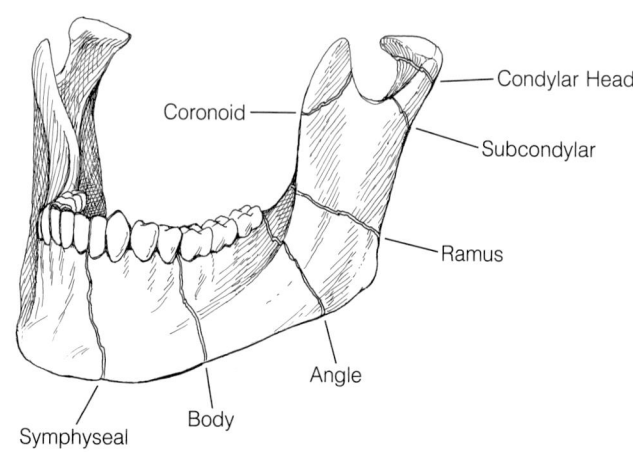

Figure 9 **Mandibular fractures.**

Discussion

Because the face is so thoroughly exposed, it is one of the most frequently injured areas of the body. Facial injuries can occur under a variety of circumstances, such as automobile accidents, altercations, or falls; more specifically, these injuries can be the results of bites, fires, explosions, lacerations, and contact with sharp or blunt objects. In automobile accidents, shards of glass may penetrate the wound, and these shards may not be radiopaque. If abrasions are present, note should be made of the abrading agent, whether it be grease, particles of dirt, gravel from a highway, or other contaminants. Underlying bony injury may or may not be obvious near the wounds. Because such injuries can expose the patient to tetanus or other anaerobic infections, antitetanic agents should be administered as part of the treatment regimen [see 1:7 Acute Wound Care]. If treatment is delayed for any reason, a systemic prophylactic antibiotic should be administered. Minor lacerations of the face caused by domestic assaults or household accidents can be adequately treated in the emergency department under local anesthesia [see 1:7 Acute Wound Care]. Lacerations that are contaminated are often best treated in the operating room with the patient under general anesthesia.

Only as much hair should be removed as is necessary for adequate assessment of the wound or for effective suturing. Eyebrows are best left unshaved to facilitate cosmetic repair. Local anesthesia should be induced, and abrasions should be scrubbed with a stiff brush until every particle of dirt is removed. If the dirt is deeply embedded, some tissue may have to be excised; this step can often be accomplished through the use of a fine curette or the point of a No. 11 blade. If dirt is not removed initially, it may be extremely difficult to remove later, and permanent tattooing may result.

Any dead or devitalized tissue should be excised, but there is no place for radical debridement of facial wounds. Tissue can survive on small pedicles. Full-thickness skin loss can be replaced with a free graft, which provides a better cosmetic match than a split-thickness skin graft [see 2:7 Surface Reconstruction Procedures]. If the wound is so ragged that it cannot be approximated, careful squaring of the edges may be advisable to facilitate a cosmetic closure. Dead or devitalized subcutaneous tissue should be removed conservatively.

Most facial wounds can be closed by simple suturing. Although the deadline for closure of wounds to other sites is usually 6 to 8 hours, facial wounds, unless heavily contaminated, can be closed as long as 24 hours after injury, particularly if meticulous attention is paid to procedural details. Such details include irrigation of the wound, removal of all foreign bodies, excision of devitalized tissue, and accurate approximation of tissue, with minimal dead space and no tension.

If the wound cannot be closed within the first 24 hours, delayed primary closure may be undertaken after 48 hours. In this event, the patient should be given systemic antibiotics, and the wound should be kept moist and protected as much as possible in the interval before closure. For best cosmetic results, the wound should be closed in multiple layers.

Sutures made of fine monofilament nylon, such as 6-0, are ideal for approximating the skin because they are nonreactive. The sutures should be applied loosely so that they do not strangulate tissue.

Key anatomic points should be identified and tattooed, mucosal edges should be approximated, and irregular margins of the skin should be excised and squared to provide the best possible fit. Margins of damaged structures, such as the nose or the ear, should be defined, and the critical margins should be determined and approximated initially. While the wound is being closed, all dead space in the wound should be obliterated and the edges everted. If the needle is passed through the skin at right angles, the edges of the skin will abut and eversion will occur. If, however, the needle is passed through the skin edge obliquely, inversion will result, and healing will be compromised. Subcutaneous or subcuticular sutures should be placed in such a way as to allow the skin edges to be approximated with minimal tension. If this procedure is done, through-and-through sutures can be removed in 3 days, and no marks will be left on the skin.

Any skin defects that require closure should be closed by grafting. No facial wound should be allowed to heal by granulation, because this would lead to excessive scarring. Instead, a temporary cover in the form of a skin graft should be provided to minimize scar formation; any deformity that results from the graft can be repaired at a later date [see 2:7 Surface Reconstruction Procedures].

The more complex of the maxillofacial fractures, such as major maxillary fractures, orbital fractures, malar fractures, and mandibular fractures [see Treatment of Maxillofacial Fractures, above], must be treated with specialty techniques; therefore, corresponding specialty consultation must be sought. However, in treating these fractures and soft tissue injuries [see Treatment of Soft Tissue Injuries, above], the priorities are to ensure adequacy of the airway and to control immediate bleeding. Once these aims have been achieved, none of the defects described, except for facial lacerations, require emergency treatment; they can be repaired days to even months later, if necessary, without jeopardizing a good cosmetic result.

References

1. Thaller S, Beal S: Maxillofacial trauma: a potentially fatal injury. Ann Plast Surg 27:281, 1991
2. Tung TC, Tseng WS, Chen CT, et al: Acute life-threatening injuries in facial fractures: a review of 1025 patients. J Trauma 49:420, 2000
3. Girotto JA, Gamble WB, Robertson B, et al: Blindness after reduction of facial fractures. Plast Reconstr Surg 104:875, 1999
4. Manson PN, Clark N, Robertson B, et al: Subunit principles in midface fractures: the importance of sagittal buttresses, soft tissue reductions, and sequencing treatment of segmental fractures. Plast Reconstr Surg 104:875, 1999
5. Gruss JS, Whelan MF, Rand RP, et al: Lessons learnt from the management of 1500 complex facial fractures. Ann Acad Med Singapore 28:677, 1999
6. McDonald WS, Thaller SR: Priorities in the treatment of facial fractures for the millennium. J Craniofac Surg 11:97, 2000
7. Mauriello JA, Lee HJ, Nguyen L: CT of soft tissue injury and orbital fractures. Radiol Clin North Am 37:241, 1999
8. Stanley R: Management of frontal sinus fractures. Facial Plast Surg 5:231, 1988
9. Stanley R: Fractures of the frontal sinus. Clin Plast Surg 16:115, 1989

10. Wolfe SA, Johnson P: Frontal sinus injuries: primary care and management of late complications. Plast Reconstr Surg 82:781, 1988

11. Luce E: Frontal sinus fractures: guidelines to management. Plast Reconstr Surg 80:500, 1987

12. Wilson B, Davidson B, Corey J, et al: Comparison of complications following frontal sinus fractures managed with exploration with or without obliteration over 10 years. Laryngoscope 98:516, 1988

13. Shockley W, Stucker F, White L, et al: Frontal sinus fractures: some problems and some solutions. Laryngoscope 98:18, 1988

14. Wallis A, Donald P: Frontal sinus fractures: a review of 72 cases. Laryngoscope 98:593, 1988

15. Rohrich R, Hollier L: Management of frontal sinus fractures. Clin Plast Surg 19:219, 1992

16. Spira M, Hardy S: Management of the injured nose. Tex Med 67:72, 1971

17. Rohrich RJ, Adams WP: Nasal fracture management: minimizing secondary nasal deformities. Plast Reconstr Surg 106:266, 2000

18. Gruss J: Naso-ethmoid-orbital fractures: classification and role of primary bone grafting. Plast Reconstr Surg 75:303, 1985

19. Gruss J, Pollock R, Phillips J, et al: Combined injuries of the cranium and face. Br J Plast Surg 42:385, 1989

20. Manson P, Crawley W, Yaremchuk M, et al: Midface fractures: advantages of immediate extended open reduction and bone grafting. Plast Reconstr Surg 76:1, 1985

21. Koutroupas S, Meyerhoff W: Surgical treatment of orbital floor fractures. Arch Otolaryngol 108:184, 1982

22. Antonyshyn O, Gruss J, Galbraith D, et al: Complex orbital fractures: a critical analysis of immediate bone reconstruction. Ann Plast Surg 22:220, 1989

23. Covington DS, Wainwright DJ, Teichgraeber JF, et al: Changing patterns in the epidemiology of treatment of zygoma fractures: 10-year review. J Trauma 37:243, 1994

24. Le Fort R: Etude expérimentale sur les fractures de la mâchoire supérieure. Rev Chir 23:208, 1901

25. Pogrel M: Compression osteosynthesis in mandibular fractures. Int J Oral Maxillofac Surg 15:521, 1986

26. El-Degwi A, Mathog R: Mandible fractures: economic considerations. Otolaryngol Head Neck Surg 108:213, 1993

27. Eid K, Lynch D, Whitaker L: Mandibular fractures: the problem patient. J Trauma 16:658, 1976

28. Thaller S, Reavie D, Daniller A: Rigid internal fixation with miniplates and screws: a cost-effective technique for treating mandible fractures? Ann Plast Surg 24:469, 1990

29. Bayles SW, Abramson PJ, McMahon SJ, et al: Mandibular fracture and associated cervical spine fracture, a rare and predictable injury: protocol for cervical spine evaluation and review of 1382 cases. Arch Otolaryngol Head Neck Surg 123:1304, 1997

30. Chu L, Gussack GS, Muller T: A treatment protocol for mandible fractures. J Trauma 36:48, 1994

31. Troulis MJ, Kaban LB: Endoscopic approach to the ramus/condyle unit: clinical applications. J Oral Maxillofac Surg 59:503, 2001

Acknowledgment

Figures 1 through 9   Carol Donner.

4 INJURIES TO THE NECK

David Wisner, M.D., F.A.C.S., and F. William Blaisdell, M.D., F.A.C.S.

Assessment and Management of Neck Injuries

Injuries to the neck can be secondary to both blunt and penetrating trauma. Most blunt injuries to the neck are managed nonoperatively; the initial diagnosis and treatment of these injuries in the emergency department setting are discussed elsewhere [*see 5:1 Trauma Resuscitation*]. Occasionally, blunt trauma to the neck causes injury to the airway, the carotid artery system, or the vertebral artery system. Blunt airway injuries are sometimes surgical emergencies; the approach to these injuries is similar to that of penetrating injuries [*see* Airway Compromise *and* Isolated Laryngotracheal Injuries, *below*]. Blunt arterial injuries are almost always discovered by angiography and are usually treated nonoperatively. In the rare instance of a patient who undergoes operative treatment for a blunt injury to carotid or vertebral arteries, the operative and postoperative principles for penetrating arterial injuries should be applied [*see* Injuries to the Carotid Arteries, Jugular Veins, Pharynx, and Esophagus, *below*].

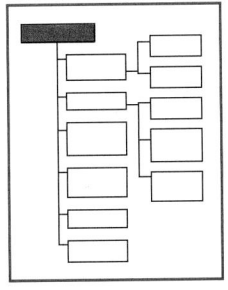

Patients with penetrating wounds of the neck can be loosely categorized into the following six groups according to the location and nature of the wound:

1. Patients with emergency or impending airway compromise.
2. Patients with an isolated injury to the larynx or trachea.
3. Patients with suspected or known injuries to the carotid arteries, jugular veins, pharynx, or esophagus.
4. Patients with wounds at the base of the neck (particularly when intrathoracic injury is suspected).
5. Patients with known injury to the vertebral arteries.
6. Patients with obviously superficial wounds of the neck.

Division of patients into these groups, though somewhat arbitrary, helps in choosing an incision and the initial operative priorities at exploration.

Airway Compromise

Some patients will present with emergency or impending airway compromise. The initial priority should be to ensure an adequate airway. In some patients, this requires orotracheal intubation. In other patients, a surgical airway must be

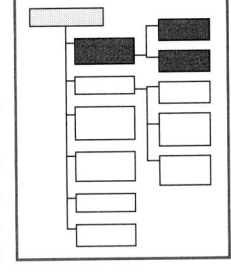

created by means of either cricothyrotomy (in emergency cases) or tracheotomy (in less extreme cases).

CRICOTHYROTOMY

In true emergency situations, a cricothyrotomy should be done. The landmarks of the superior (notched) and inferior borders of the thyroid and the cricoid cartilage should be palpated. For this, it is helpful to stand on the patient's right side (for a right-handed surgeon) and to stabilize the cartilaginous framework by holding the thyroid cartilage in place with the left hand. A transverse incision should be made at the level of the cricothyroid membrane and developed rapidly through the subcutaneous tissue [*see 5:1 Trauma Resuscitation*]. As with any transversely oriented incision of the anterior neck, the anterior jugular veins are at risk for injury. If such injury occurs, the damaged veins are best controlled with suture ligation after an airway is obtained. In true emergency circumstances when the exact site of injury is unknown, a vertical rather than transverse incision should be used to allow access to as much of the anterior surface of the airway as possible and to decrease the chance of injury to the anterior jugular veins.

After the skin and subcutaneous tissue have been divided, an incision should be made through the cricothyroid membrane. This is most rapidly done with a No. 11 knife blade. It is important to avoid pushing the knife blade too far and causing injury to the posterior wall of the airway or to the posteriorly located hypopharynx and esophagus. After the incision has been made, the opening should be enlarged by placing the knife handle in the incision and twisting it 90°. At this point, an indwelling endotracheal airway should be placed and secured. In most adults, a No. 6 airway is the largest that can be inserted; a No. 4 or larger airway is adequate for initial placement. Any incisional bleeding from the anterior jugular vein or other vessels should be controlled. Cricothyrotomies should be converted to tracheotomies within 48 to 72 hours as long as the patient's general condition permits [*see* Discussion, Conversion of Cricothyrotomy to Tracheotomy, *below*].

TRACHEOTOMY

In some instances, airway compromise may not be extreme but a surgical airway may still be necessary for safety or subsequent management of a laryngeal injury. In such circumstances, a tracheotomy rather than a cricothyrotomy should be done, because cricothyrotomy is more likely than tracheotomy to make definitive treatment more difficult.

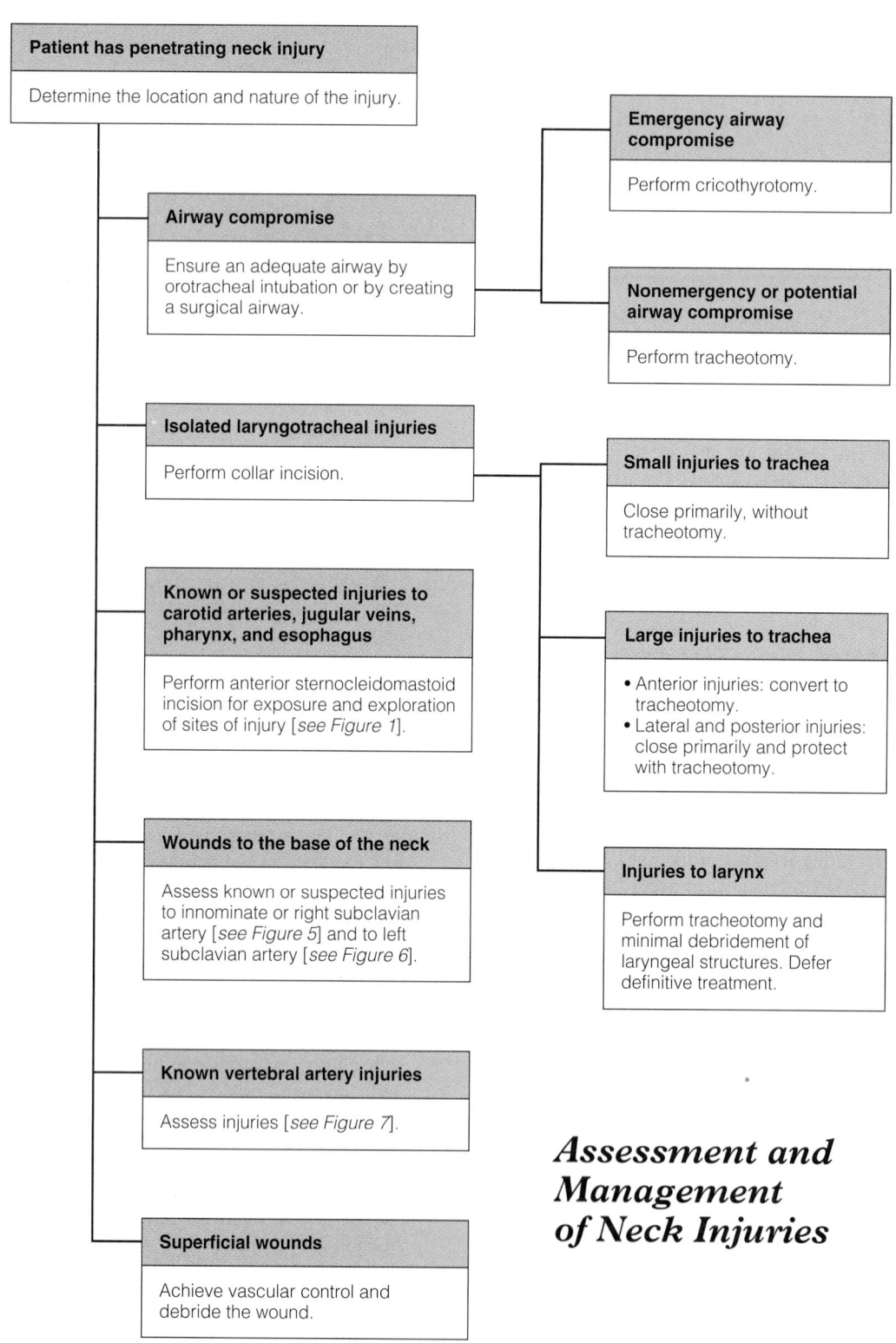

Patient has penetrating neck injury

Determine the location and nature of the injury.

Airway compromise

Ensure an adequate airway by orotracheal intubation or by creating a surgical airway.

Emergency airway compromise

Perform cricothyrotomy.

Nonemergency or potential airway compromise

Perform tracheotomy.

Isolated laryngotracheal injuries

Perform collar incision.

Small injuries to trachea

Close primarily, without tracheotomy.

Known or suspected injuries to carotid arteries, jugular veins, pharynx, and esophagus

Perform anterior sternocleidomastoid incision for exposure and exploration of sites of injury [see Figure 1].

Large injuries to trachea

- Anterior injuries: convert to tracheotomy.
- Lateral and posterior injuries: close primarily and protect with tracheotomy.

Wounds to the base of the neck

Assess known or suspected injuries to innominate or right subclavian artery [see Figure 5] and to left subclavian artery [see Figure 6].

Injuries to larynx

Perform tracheotomy and minimal debridement of laryngeal structures. Defer definitive treatment.

Known vertebral artery injuries

Assess injuries [see Figure 7].

Superficial wounds

Achieve vascular control and debride the wound.

Assessment and Management of Neck Injuries

The initial approach for emergency tracheotomy is similar to that for cricothyrotomy, the difference being that a so-called collar incision is made at a point one to two finger-breadths inferior to the level of the cricothyroid membrane. The incision should be wide enough to provide rapid exposure and should extend as far as the anterior border of the sternocleidomastoid bilaterally. Anteriorly located injuries at the level of the cricoid or trachea may already have a hole in the airway. In such cases, if the need for a surgical airway is immediate, the wound should be enlarged and used as a route of access to the airway.

On rare occasion, the injury is in the distal cervical or proximal intrathoracic trachea. In such circumstances, access to the trachea may not be possible through a cervical incision alone. Median sternotomy and lateral retraction of the innominate artery and left internal carotid artery allow exposure of the anterior surface of the trachea at the thoracic inlet. Right thoracotomy provides access to the more distal intrathoracic trachea.

Isolated Laryngotracheal Injuries

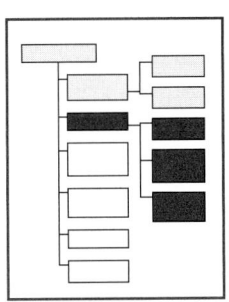

Most commonly, the presence of an isolated laryngotracheal injury is not recognized preoperatively. On occasion, however, isolated injuries to the larynx and trachea are recognized preoperatively on the basis of a suspicious history and the results of diagnostic studies, such as laryngoscopy and bronchoscopy.

Injuries to the larynx should be treated initially with a collar incision for the creation of a surgical airway [see Airway Compromise, Tracheotomy, above]; however, definitive treatment should be deferred. Minimal debridement of laryngeal structures should be carried out during the initial operative procedure. Injuries to the larynx should be handled on a semielective basis by otolaryngologists with expertise in laryngeal repair and reconstruction. Further investigation of the larynx, including laryngeal x-rays, laryngoscopy, and computed tomographic scanning, may be necessary.

Small injuries of the trachea can be repaired primarily without tracheotomy. Absorbable 3-0 or 4-0 sutures should be placed transversely, if possible, and should include tracheal rings above and below the site of injury. Large anterior defects should be converted to a tracheotomy, whereas defects to the lateral or posterior aspects of the trachea should be closed primarily and protected with a tracheotomy. Tension can be relieved from a repair by mobilizing the trachea proximally and distally. During this mobilization, the recurrent laryngeal nerves are subject to injury if the dissection is carried into the tracheoesophageal groove. Laryngotracheal injuries do not require routine drainage unless there is an associated injury to the pharynx or esophagus [see Injuries to the Carotid Arteries, Jugular Veins, Pharynx, and Esophagus, below].

If a large segment of trachea has been destroyed, primary anastomosis can be accomplished for defects up to five or six tracheal rings in length. Anastomosis requires mobilization of the intrathoracic trachea inferiorly and the laryngeal complex superiorly and is best done electively.[1,2]

Patients with laryngeal injuries should be watched carefully in the postoperative period for signs of mediastinitis, which may be from persistent airway leak or a missed pharyngo-esophageal injury. The chest x-ray should also be checked for pneumomediastinum as a sign of continued airway leakage, particularly in patients who remain on positive pressure ventilation.

Injuries to the Carotid Arteries, Jugular Veins, Pharynx, and Esophagus

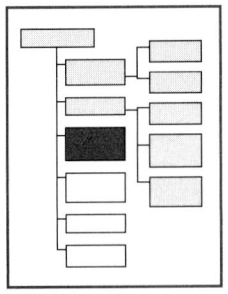

Probably the most common situation in penetrating cervical trauma is the patient with underlying structural injuries, the precise location and nature of which are unknown. Patients with known injuries to the carotid arteries, jugular veins, pharynx, and esophagus are less common. An anterior sternocleidomastoid incision provides good access to these areas and should be employed because of its relative ease and versatility.

STERNOCLEIDOMASTOID INCISION

If the location of underlying neck injuries is either unknown or confirmed by preoperative studies to be in the carotid arteries, the jugular veins, the pharynx, or the esophagus, an incision along the anterior border of the sternocleidomastoid muscle should be used [see Figure 1]. The sternocleidomastoid incision is particularly important in patients with true emergency conditions, such as external bleeding, focal neurologic deficits, coma, and an expanding neck hematoma. When bilateral exploration is necessary, separate sternocleidomastoid incisions should be done.

The use of an incision along the anterior border of the sternocleidomastoid muscle has several important advantages [see Figure 2]. For example, the incision can be lengthened to provide more extensive proximal or distal exposure. If a superior extension to below the earlobe is necessary, the incision should be curved posteriorly to avoid injury to the marginal mandibular branch of the facial nerve. Another advantage of the sternocleidomastoid incision is that it provides exposure of the carotid sheath, the pharynx, and the cervical esophagus.

Operative Technique

The patient should be supine with the head turned away from the side of exploration and the neck extended. In this regard, it is helpful to clear the cervical spine before operation. If both sides of the neck require exploration, the head should be left in the midposition, facing up. The entire neck and the appropriate side of the face and head should be prepped. The anterior chest should also be included in the preparation in case a median sternotomy is necessary for proximal control [see Exploration and Exposure, Arteries and Veins, below]. The patient should be draped in such a way as to leave the lateral neck as the primary field while the chest is kept easily accessible. The lateral chin and tip of the earlobe should also be kept in the field to provide landmarks. If the possibility exists that the injury is to the distal subclavian artery or the axillary artery, the patient's arm should be draped in a way that allows it to be manipulated.

The skin incision should be carried through the dermis and the platysma. After the platysma is divided in the direction of the incision, the investing fascia overlying the anterior border of the sternocleidomastoid muscle is incised, and the muscle is retracted laterally and posteriorly to expose the carotid sheath.

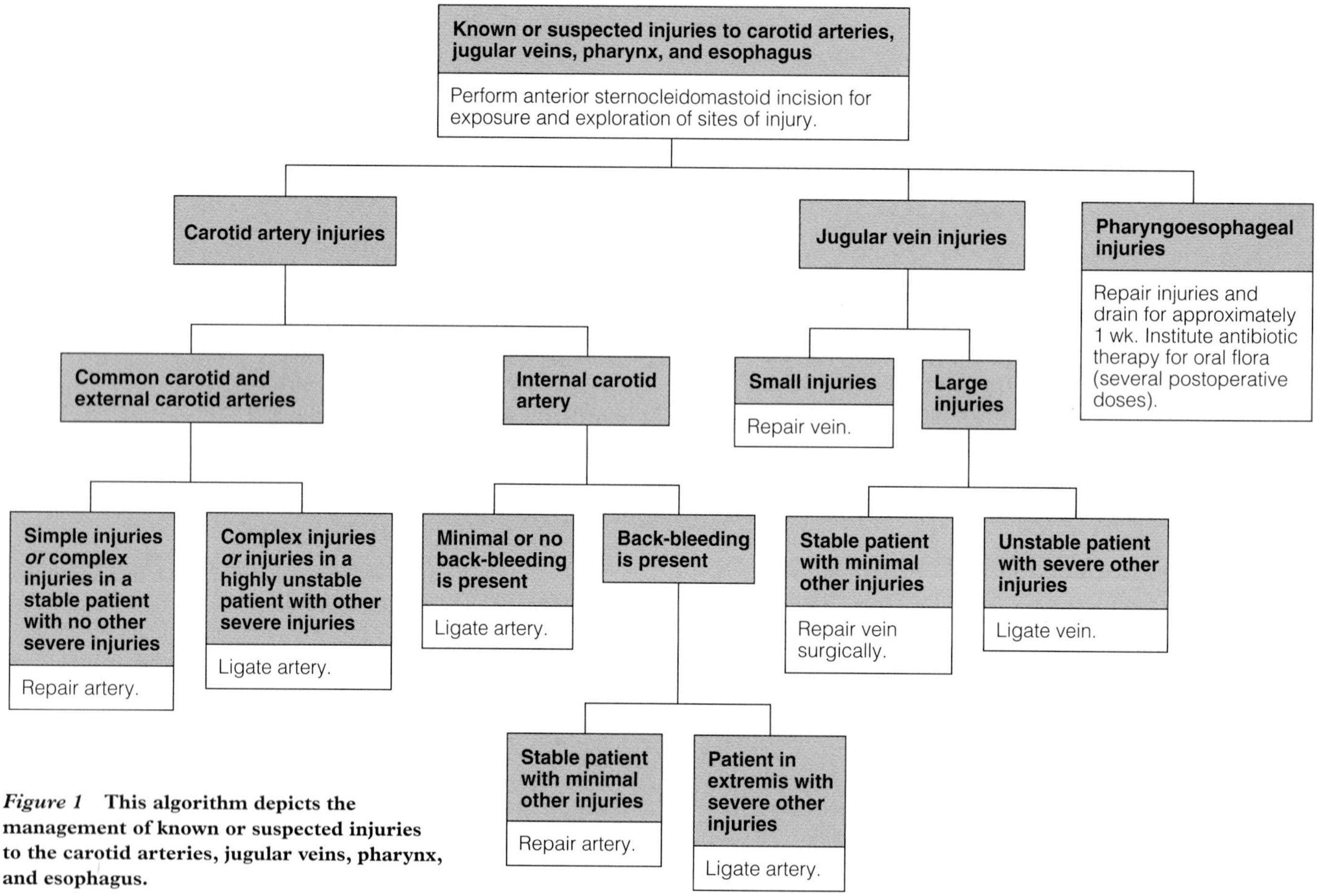

Known or suspected injuries to carotid arteries, jugular veins, pharynx, and esophagus

Perform anterior sternocleidomastoid incision for exposure and exploration of sites of injury.

Carotid artery injuries

Jugular vein injuries

Pharyngoesophageal injuries

Repair injuries and drain for approximately 1 wk. Institute antibiotic therapy for oral flora (several postoperative doses).

Common carotid and external carotid arteries

Internal carotid artery

Small injuries

Repair vein.

Large injuries

Simple injuries *or* complex injuries in a stable patient with no other severe injuries

Repair artery.

Complex injuries *or* injuries in a highly unstable patient with other severe injuries

Ligate artery.

Minimal or no back-bleeding is present

Ligate artery.

Back-bleeding is present

Stable patient with minimal other injuries

Repair vein surgically.

Unstable patient with severe other injuries

Ligate vein.

Stable patient with minimal other injuries

Repair artery.

Patient in extremis with severe other injuries

Ligate artery.

Figure 1 This algorithm depicts the management of known or suspected injuries to the carotid arteries, jugular veins, pharynx, and esophagus.

It is often necessary to divide a venous branch that connects the external jugular vein posterolaterally to the anterior jugular vein anteromedially. This vein lies in a plane immediately deep to the platysma.

Exploration and Exposure

When possible, proximal and distal control should be obtained before exploration of a carotid artery injury. In practice, obtaining proximal control before entering a perivascular hematoma is all that is absolutely necessary. Distal bleeding can be controlled with digital pressure while the dissection of the injured vessel is completed. Although it is often difficult to obtain control before addressing the area of injury, proximal and distal control of the vessel should be obtained at some point before any attempts at definitive repair. For injuries near the carotid bifurcation, it is necessary to control the common, internal, and external carotid arteries as well as the proximal branches of the external carotid artery.

Arteries and veins   The initial exploration should attempt to rule out arterial or venous injury, unless an overt airway injury is present and requires immediate attention [*see* Airway Compromise, *above*]. If the airway is patent, the location of the carotid artery can then be confirmed by the presence of a pulse. It is often necessary to retract the jugular vein posterolaterally to provide adequate arterial exposure [*see* Figure 3]. Jugular vein retraction is facilitated by division of the facial vein, which is superficial to the carotid bifurcation. The

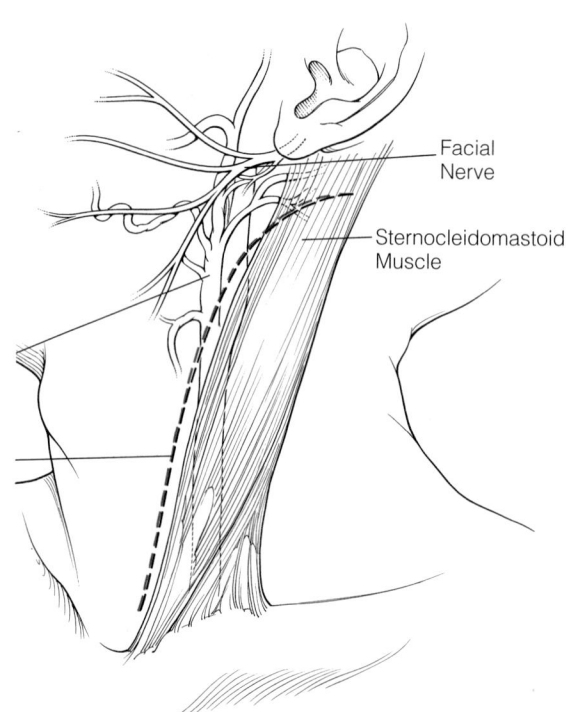

Facial Nerve

Sternocleidomastoid Muscle

Figure 2 In general, exposure of structures in the anterior areas of the neck is best done through an incision oriented along the anterior border of the sternocleidomastoid muscle.

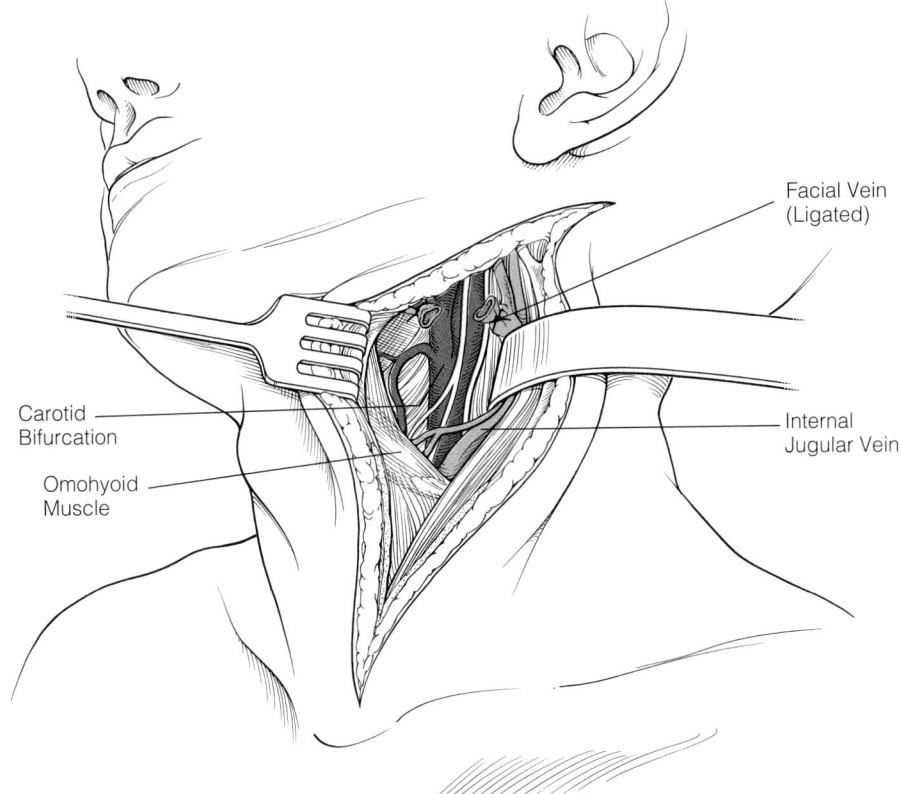

Figure 3 After a plane along the anterior border of the sternocleidomastoid muscle has been developed, dissection is carried down to the level of the carotid sheath. Suture ligation of the facial vein facilitates this dissection. Lateral retraction of the internal jugular vein improves exposure of the carotid bifurcation.

severed ends of the facial vein should be suture-ligated to ensure that the ties will not come off with increased intravenous pressure in the postoperative period—for example, secondary to a cough or a Valsalva maneuver.

Exposure of the proximal common carotid artery at the base of the neck is easier after division of the omohyoid muscle at the point where its superior and inferior bellies are joined. Division of the omohyoid muscle results in minimal functional deficit postoperatively. For proximal control of the common carotid artery, it may be necessary to enter the chest via median sternotomy. To minimize blood loss, the decision to do a sternotomy should be made without undue delay. Control of the proximal right common carotid artery via this route is relatively easy and is accomplished by first obtaining control of the innominate artery and then dissecting distally. Proximal control of the left common carotid artery via median sternotomy is more difficult, because its origin from the aortic arch is more posterior than the origin of the innominate artery.

Exposure of the distal internal carotid artery can be very difficult, particularly if there is an injury in that location. As dissection is carried distally on the internal carotid artery, a number of important structures should be identified and protected [*see Figure 4*]. The hypoglossal nerve is usually encountered within several centimeters of the carotid bifurcation and should be dissected free of the internal carotid and retracted upward. This is facilitated by division of the occipital artery, which crosses superficial to the hypoglossal nerve on its course

from the external carotid artery toward the occiput. It is also helpful to divide the ansa cervicalis branches that run inferiorly from the hypoglossal nerve to supply the muscles of the neck. Injury to the hypoglossal nerve results in impaired motor function of the tongue and can lead to dysarthria and dysphagia. Injury to or sectioning of the ansa cervicalis causes little or no morbidity.

Further distal exposure of the internal carotid artery may require unilateral mandibular subluxation or division of the ascending ramus of the mandible.[3,4] Such maneuvers are somewhat easier when the patient is nasotracheally intubated. They increase the size of the small area immediately behind the condyle and allow for easier division of the stylohyoid ligament and the styloglossus and stylopharyngeus muscles. These three structures can be divided together adjacent to their common origin at the styloid process. If this is done, care should be taken to preserve the facial nerve, which lies superficial to these muscles. The underlying glossopharyngeal nerve, which lies deep to these muscles and superficial to the internal carotid artery, should also be protected. Injury to the facial nerve results in loss of function of the muscles of facial expression. If the glossopharyngeal nerve is injured, loss of motor and sensory supply to parts of the tongue and pharynx increases the risk of aspiration.

Once the muscles originating from the styloid process have been divided, the styloid process itself can be resected to gain a further short distance of distal exposure. In very rare instances, it may prove useful to remove portions of the mastoid bone to provide even more distal exposure of the internal carotid artery as it enters the carotid canal. This can generally be accomplished via a cervical incision. For more distal lesions, it is necessary to place a posterolateral scalp incision, reflect a medially based scalp flap, and divide the ipsilateral external auditory canal. This approach results in better exposure of the mastoid process and allows exposure of the intrapetrous portion of the internal carotid after removal of the overlying bone of the mastoid with a high-speed bone drill.

Pharynx and esophagus The oropharynx, hypopharynx, and cervical esophagus are exposed via the same anterior sternocleidomastoid incision used for arterial and venous injuries. If the patient has a known right-side injury, the incision should be made in the right neck. If the injury is on the patient's left side or if the exact site of injury is unknown, the exposure should be made from the left because the cervical esophagus is located slightly to the left of the midline. After the initial incision, the contents of the carotid sheath should be retracted laterally, exposing the lateral aspect of the pharynx and esophagus. This maneuver is made easier if the anesthesiologist places a large esophageal dilator through the mouth. The dilator makes identification of the otherwise flat esophagus easier, and the colored tubing of the dilator can sometimes be seen through defects in the esophageal wall.[5]

Sometimes, a pharyngoesophageal injury is suspected but cannot be confirmed preoperatively. In such cases—especially when the injury is more than 1 or 2 hours old—salivary amylase may be present in the wound, giving the surgeon's gloves a greasy feel. The presence of salivary amylase can be a valuable clue to the existence of an otherwise unknown occult injury.

CAROTID ARTERY INJURIES

During dissection of the external carotid artery, the branches should be identified. They can be ligated if necessary but should be preserved if possible (this usually depends on whether they can be temporarily occluded with vessel loops, a looped suture, or clips). During dissection around the common and internal carotid arteries, care should be taken to avoid cutting or clamping the posterolaterally located vagus nerve; the recurrent laryngeal nerve runs with the vagus nerve at this level, and damage to the laryngeal nerve can lead to paralysis of the ipsilateral vocal cord.

For wounds of the distal internal carotid artery, distal control may be a problem, particularly in the presence of vigorous ongoing bleeding, in which case a Fogarty balloon catheter (size 3 to 5 French) should be placed through the area of injury or through a proximal arteriotomy. The catheter should be advanced distally, and the balloon should be inflated to provide a dry field for arterial repair. Repair can be done around

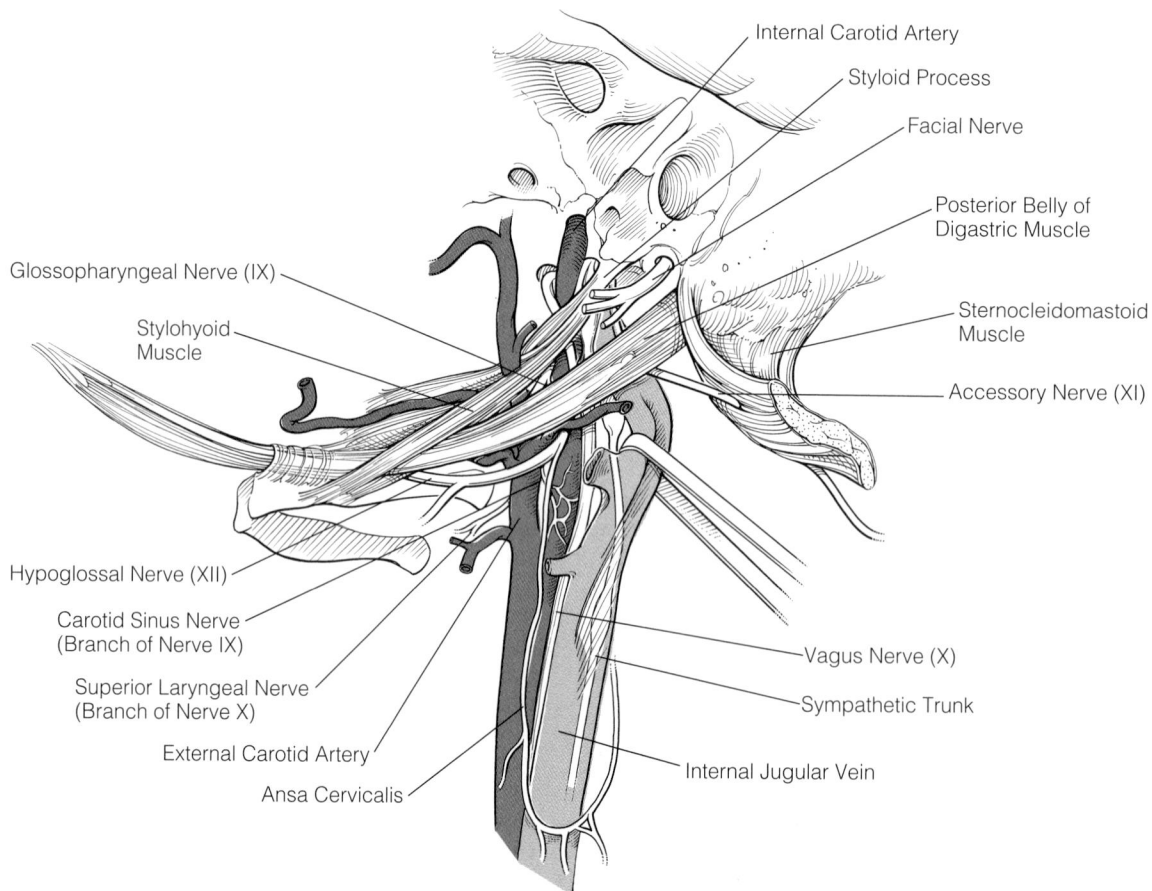

Figure 4 **During distal dissection of the internal and external carotid arteries, a number of important structures are encountered, including the hypoglossal nerve and the occipital artery.**

the catheter; the balloon is deflated near the conclusion of the repair, and the catheter is removed before the final several sutures are tied.

If associated injuries allow, a 5,000 to 10,000 unit bolus of heparin should be given before any of the arteries in the neck are occluded. Because they have no branches, the common and internal carotid arteries can be safely mobilized for some distance from the injury to ensure a tension-free repair.

Management of common or external carotid artery injuries is governed by the extent of injury and the overall status of the patient. Small, simple injuries should be repaired. Complex injuries should be repaired in stable patients and treated with ligation in patients with severe hemodynamic instability or major associated injuries.

Initial management of injuries to the internal carotid artery depends on a determination of the amount of back-bleeding from the artery distal to the site of injury.[6,7] If back-bleeding is minimal or absent, the artery should be ligated. If significant back-bleeding is present, the overall status of the patient and the nature of the associated injuries should be taken into account [see Discussion, Repair versus Ligation of Carotid Arteries, below]. If the patient is hemodynamically stable and has minimal or moderate associated injuries, the internal carotid artery should be repaired. If the patient is hemodynamically unstable or has devastating associated injuries, the internal carotid artery should be ligated even when back-bleeding is present.

If a carotid artery injury involves minimal loss of vascular wall, primary repair is straightforward and can be done with either a running or interrupted technique; interrupted sutures will not purse-string the vessel. In younger patients who are still growing, interrupted sutures should be used to prevent later stenosis. As in elective vascular surgery, nonabsorbable sutures should be used; the carotid arteries generally require a 5-0, 6-0, or 7-0 monofilament suture, depending on the location of the injury and the type of suture material employed.

Defects longer than 1 to 2 cm should not be repaired primarily, because this will place excessive tension on the repair. For large defects limited to one surface of the vessel, a patch repair should be done. Either a venous patch or a synthetic patch can be used; when available, a venous patch is preferred for better long-term patency and to avoid placing a foreign body in a potentially contaminated wound.[8] Saphenous vein from the groin is preferable for patches because of its durability; a saphenous vein from the ankle is easiest to harvest when time is of the essence.[9] Although the jugular vein is in the operative field and can be easily harvested, it is better not to interfere with venous outflow in a neck in which the arterial inflow is to undergo repair; in addition, the jugular vein is very thin and difficult to handle.

For repairs near the carotid bifurcation, an alternative to venous patches and synthetic patches is the use of the proximal external carotid artery. This approach is especially appropriate when the origin of the external carotid artery is itself involved in the area of injury. If the injury is to the proximal internal carotid artery and the origin of the external carotid artery is free of injury, it is better to leave the external carotid artery patent and to use a venous patch or a synthetic patch instead; if the repair fails, the external carotid artery provides collateral distribution to the internal carotid artery via the ophthalmic artery.

Repair of circumferential loss of the common or internal carotid arteries is difficult. In this circumstance, if the defect is too long for primary anastomosis and the patient's general and neurologic condition permits, an interposition graft should be done. As with patch grafts, either venous or synthetic material can be used. As for patch grafts, saphenous vein from the groin is generally the donor material of first choice because of its strength. The saphenous vein from the groin is also well suited for reconstruction of the common carotid artery.

Completion angiography should be done after interposition graft placements and complex repairs of the common or internal carotid arteries. In general, patients with carotid artery injuries should be admitted postoperatively to an intensive care unit. ICU observation need not be prolonged but should be continued for at least 12 to 24 hours postoperatively. In the early postoperative period, the patient should be observed for bleeding or for the development of a neck hematoma; large postoperative hematomas may compromise the airway. If the patient develops a tense hematoma postoperatively, the neck should be reexplored.

Labile blood pressure—particularly in patients with extensive dissection around the carotid bifurcation—is another potential postoperative problem. It is related to manipulation of the carotid body, and control may require pharmacologic intervention. Labile blood pressure is usually self-limiting and disappears over the first 1 to 3 days after operation, but it is another reason why patients with carotid artery repairs should be monitored initially in the ICU.

Antibiotics should be administered to cover common skin flora and should generally be continued only for one or two postoperative doses.

JUGULAR VEIN INJURIES

Any of the veins in the neck can be ligated when necessary. An exception to this rule is the rare instance when both internal jugular veins have been injured, in which case an attempt should be made to repair one of the veins, if possible. However, even in such cases, bilateral internal jugular ligation, if necessary, is usually tolerated. It is particularly important to use suture ligatures rather than simple ligatures on the cut ends of the internal jugular vein.

If the injury to the internal jugular is simple, the vein should be repaired. Large jugular vein injuries should be repaired only if the patient's general condition and associated injuries allow; if the patient is hemodynamically unstable or has severe associated injuries, large jugular vein injuries should be treated with ligation.

It is not always necessary to completely encircle the jugular vein proximal and distal to the site of injury; pressure with a finger or sponge stick will sometimes control bleeding while simple lateral venorrhaphy is done. In the case of more elaborate repairs, it is better either to encircle and occlude the proximal and distal vein or to place a side-biting vascular clamp for control during repair. Nonabsorbable 4-0 or 5-0 sutures should be used.

PHARYNGOESOPHAGEAL INJURIES

Either one-layer or two-layer repair of the pharynx and esophagus is acceptable, for which 3-0 or 4-0 absorbable sutures should be used. Attempts should be made to repair nearly all injuries, even when they are severe or are found on a delayed basis. In extreme cases of very large injuries or very delayed operative intervention, it may be necessary simply to drain the neck widely and turn the injury into a cervical esophagostomy. Esophageal diversion with distal esophageal ligation is rarely necessary in patients with isolated cervical esophageal injuries, except in cases when the injury is very low in the neck or in the thoracic esophagus.

Pharyngoesophageal injuries should be drained; either closed or Penrose drainage can be used. The drains should be left in place for approximately 1 week, at which time a radiographic contrast study should be obtained to determine whether the repair is competent. If the contrast study is negative for extravasation and the patient's general status permits, feeding can begin. If the feedings are well tolerated, the drains can be removed.[10]

Patients with pharyngoesophageal injuries should receive antibiotics appropriate for oral flora for several postoperative doses. If the repair is inadequate or breaks down, the resultant fistula will often heal with nonoperative management, provided that drainage is adequate. A high index of suspicion for mediastinitis should be maintained; the prevertebral space provides a ready route of access from the pharynx and cervical esophagus into the mediastinum. Therefore, missed or inadequately drained injuries may result in profound infection and a septic response.

Wounds at the Base of the Neck

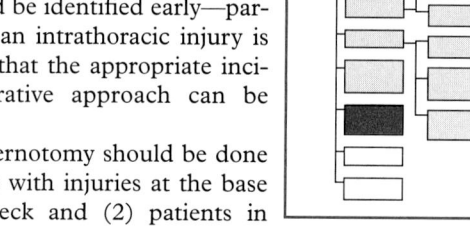

Patients with wounds at the base of the neck should be identified early—particularly when an intrathoracic injury is suspected—so that the appropriate incision and operative approach can be undertaken.

A median sternotomy should be done for (1) patients with injuries at the base of the right neck and (2) patients in whom the superior mediastinum is the most likely site of injury and the most likely arterial injuries are to either the innominate artery or the right subclavian artery[11,12] [see Figure 5]. Exposure of injuries to the proximal left subclavian artery is extremely difficult via sternotomy because of the artery's posterior location; in patients with such injuries, a left thoracotomy is needed [see Figure 6]. If a left thoracotomy is necessary, it is helpful to bump up the patient's left hip and shoulder to position the left chest 20° to 30° anteriorly. The head should be turned to the right, and the left arm should be prepped to the elbow and draped in such a way as to allow it free movement. Moving the arm is helpful in cases in which proximal exposure and control are done through the chest and distal exposure and control are done through a supraclavicular incision. It also allows for improved exposure of the axillary artery if necessary.

In stable patients with angiographically diagnosed injuries to either subclavian artery, a supraclavicular approach alone can be used, thereby eliminating the need for initial entry into the chest. Because proximal control may not be feasible via this limited incision, the patient should still be positioned, prepped, and draped so that sternotomy or thoracotomy is possible. If the injury is on the right side of the neck and proximal control is not possible, a median sternotomy should be done. If the injury is on the left side of the neck and proximal control is not possible, a left thoracotomy should be performed.

If a median sternotomy has been done for exposure of an innominate artery or right subclavian artery injury, it may prove necessary to extend the incision into the right neck to obtain adequate distal control and exposure. Either a right supraclavicular or an anterior sternocleidomastoid extension can be used. Although both are easily accomplished, the anterior sternocleidomastoid extension is the more versatile of the two. If a left thoracotomy is done for proximal control and exposure of the left subclavian artery, the distal subclavian artery should be exposed via a left supraclavicular incision. Improved exposure of the left subclavian artery at the thoracic outlet can be obtained either by resection of the medial one third to one half of the left clavicle or by a so-called trapdoor incision.[13] The trapdoor incision consists of a superior sternotomy and connection of the medial aspects of the thoracotomy and supraclavicular incisions. We find the trapdoor approach somewhat limited and cumbersome and prefer clavicular resection. Medial clavicular resection is accomplished by encircling the midclavicle in the subperiosteal plane via the supraclavicular incision. A Gigli wire saw is then passed around the clavicle, and the clavicle is divided. The medial aspect of the divided bone is then grasped with a bone hook or a Kocher clamp, and the dissection is carried medially in the subperiosteal plane to the sternoclavicular joint, which is disarticulated. If necessary, this dissection and resection can be accomplished in a matter of a few minutes.

After adequate exposure and control of innominate or subclavian artery injuries have been obtained, further management is determined by the nature of the injury and the status of the patient. Small injuries should always be repaired. Large injuries are not often seen, because they are usually incompatible with survival to a point where medical attention is available. Nonetheless, such injuries do occur, and their management is influenced by the status of the patient. Attempts at repair should be made for most such injuries, but in highly unstable patients, the artery should be ligated. However, arterial ligation is sometimes associated with severe morbidity, and it should be avoided if possible.

The wall of the subclavian artery is thin, and extra care should be taken in dissecting around it. Primary repair should be done with either interrupted or running nonabsorbable 4-0 or 5-0 sutures, laterally placed. Because of its location and the large number of branches, the subclavian artery is difficult to mobilize extensively. None of the branches are vital, however, and all can be divided as necessary to gain mobility. The vertebral artery should be preserved if possible, because in rare instances, ligation of the artery can lead to cerebral ischemia. Even with division of arterial branches, only short segments of the artery can be removed without the need for an interposition graft to prevent an anastomosis under tension. Saphenous vein is usually too small to be used as a graft, even when it is harvested from the groin. Accordingly, a synthetic graft is usually the better choice. Infections in this location are rare, even when the graft is placed in a contaminated field.[14]

Complex injuries of the innominate and subclavian veins should be treated with suture ligation, particularly when the patient has severe associated injuries. Simple injuries can be treated with lateral venorrhaphy. Depending on the circumstances, formal control of the proximal and distal vein can first be obtained, or pressure can be applied proximally and distally to provide for a bloodless field during repair. Another alternative for control of bleeding during venous repair is the use of a side-biting vascular clamp.

Some patients with injuries to the subclavian artery or subclavian vein require dissection of the supraclavicular area. The supraclavicular fat pad contains a large number of lymph nodes and lymphatic channels, and dissection of the fat pad can result in considerable weeping of lymphatic fluid; these wounds should therefore be drained. Either a closed or an open drain can be used, and the drain should be brought out through a separate stab wound near the incision. After a left-sided procedure, persistent milky drainage via either drains or the wound suggests injury to the thoracic duct and may necessitate repeat operative intervention if it persists.

Elevation or paralysis of the hemidiaphragm ipsilateral to the side of dissection can indicate injury to the phrenic nerve, which courses in the field of dissection on the anterior surface of the anterior scalene muscle.

Known Vertebral Artery Injuries

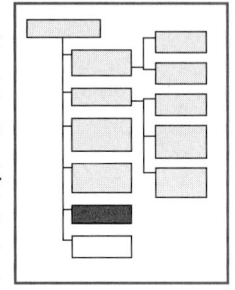

On occasion, patients who present with penetrating cervical wounds and are hemodynamically and neurologically stable are demonstrated on angiographic workup to have an injury to the vertebral artery. In rarer instances, the location of an injury in the posterior triangle of the neck and the presence of ongoing hemorrhage may also indicate the high likelihood of an injury to the distal vertebral artery [see Figure 7].

Most vertebral artery injuries occur in stable patients and are discovered on angiography. Because operative attempts at ligation are associated with blood loss that can be problematic, an alternative approach utilizing angiographic embolization has been developed.[15] In most cases of injury to the distal vertebral artery, the angiographic approach is preferred if available [see Discussion, Angiographic Embolization of Distal

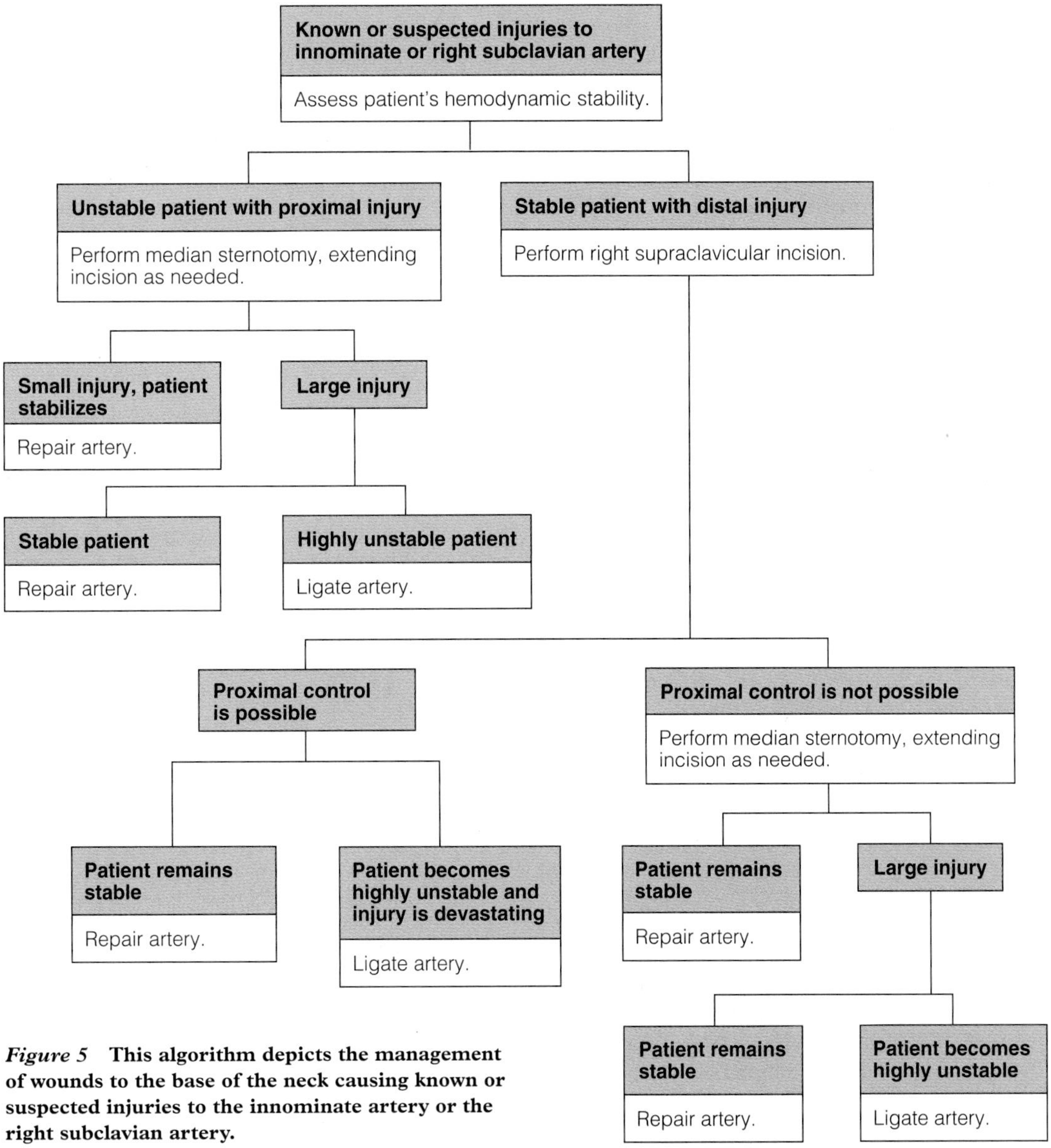

Known or suspected injuries to innominate or right subclavian artery

Assess patient's hemodynamic stability.

Unstable patient with proximal injury

Perform median sternotomy, extending incision as needed.

Stable patient with distal injury

Perform right supraclavicular incision.

Small injury, patient stabilizes

Repair artery.

Large injury

Stable patient

Repair artery.

Highly unstable patient

Ligate artery.

Proximal control is possible

Proximal control is not possible

Perform median sternotomy, extending incision as needed.

Patient remains stable

Repair artery.

Patient becomes highly unstable and injury is devastating

Ligate artery.

Patient remains stable

Repair artery.

Large injury

Patient remains stable

Repair artery.

Patient becomes highly unstable

Ligate artery.

Figure 5 **This algorithm depicts the management of wounds to the base of the neck causing known or suspected injuries to the innominate artery or the right subclavian artery.**

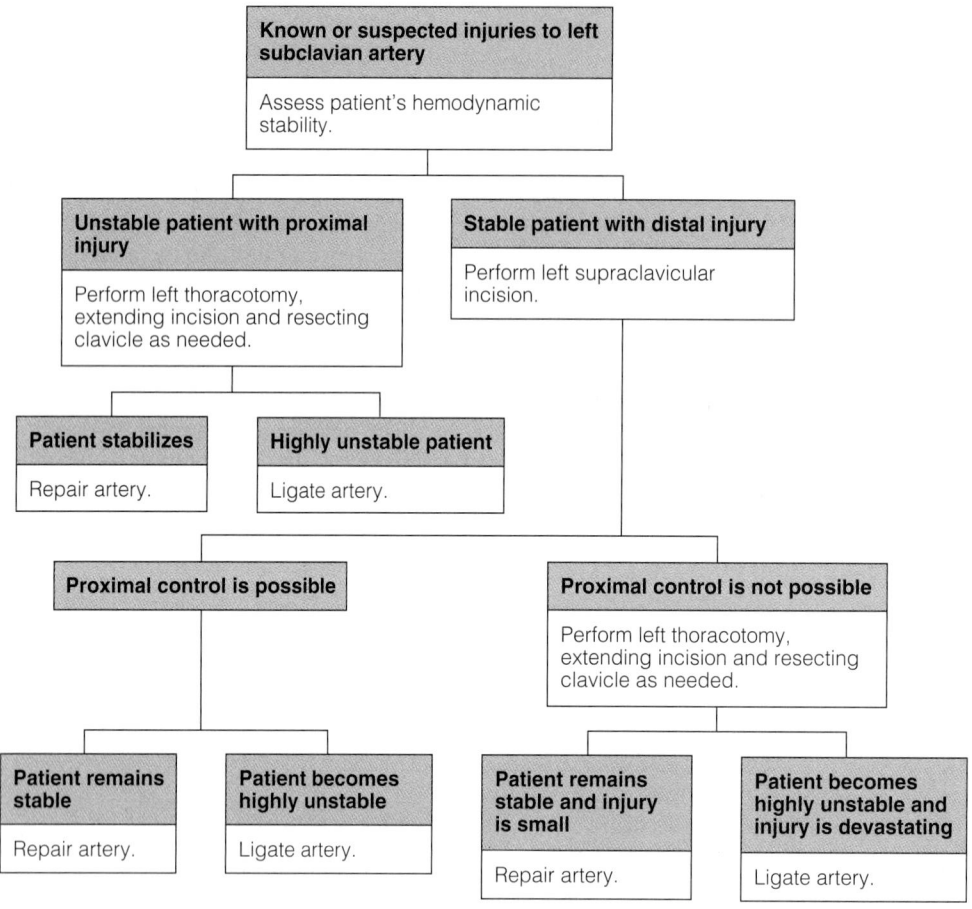

Figure 6 **This algorithm depicts the management of wounds to the base of the neck causing known or suspected injuries to the left subclavian artery.**

Vertebral Artery Injuries, *below*]. If angiographic expertise is not available and the patient is stable enough for transfer, it is preferable to send the patient to a center with angiographic embolization capability if at all possible. In urgent circumstances, an angiographic approach is not practical. In such situations, the direct surgical approach is necessary.[16,17]

EXPOSURE AND EXPLORATION

In the rare case of a patient who presents with active, severe bleeding and in whom the most likely source of bleeding is the distal vertebral artery, exposure of the vertebral artery should be obtained by means of an anterior sternocleidomastoid incision [*see* Injuries to the Carotid Arteries, Jugular Veins, Pharynx, and Esophagus, *above*]. This approach can be used for exposure of both the proximal and the distal vertebral artery. The incision is developed down to the level of the carotid sheath. The lateral margin of the internal jugular vein is developed sharply, and the internal jugular vein and other contents of the sheath are retracted medially. After retraction of the carotid sheath, the plane just superficial to the prevertebral muscles is encountered. The ganglia of the cervical sympathetic chain are located here and should be protected, though this is not always possible in emergency circumstances. The anterior longitudinal ligament is located deep in the medial aspect of the wound and should be incised longitudinally. The ligament, the underlying periosteum, and the overlying longus colli and

longissimus capitis should be mobilized laterally with a periosteal elevator [*see Figure 8*]. The elevation should be carried laterally along the lateral margin of the bodies of the cervical vertebrae and along the anterior aspect of the transverse processes of the cervical vertebrae. To avoid injury to the laterally and posteriorly placed cervical nerve roots, the dissection should not be extended laterally beyond the tips of the transverse processes.

After the anterior aspects of the transverse processes of the cervical vertebrae have been exposed, they can be removed with a small rongeur. This should be done distal to the area of injury only; proximal ligation of the vertebral artery can be done in its more easily exposed proximal portion. Although the vertebral artery is also accessible in the spaces between the transverse processes, there are a number of venous branches in these regions, and it is therefore safer to approach the artery within the confines of the bony foramina.

The third and most distal portion of the vertebral artery can be approached most easily between the atlas and the axis. The segment of the artery between the transverse processes of these two vertebrae is longer and more exposed than the segments between the other cervical vertebrae and is therefore, in theory, somewhat easier to expose. In practice, rapid exposure of this portion of the vertebral artery can be very difficult, particularly in an actively bleeding patient. As with exposures to the second portion of the vertebral artery, lesions requiring this

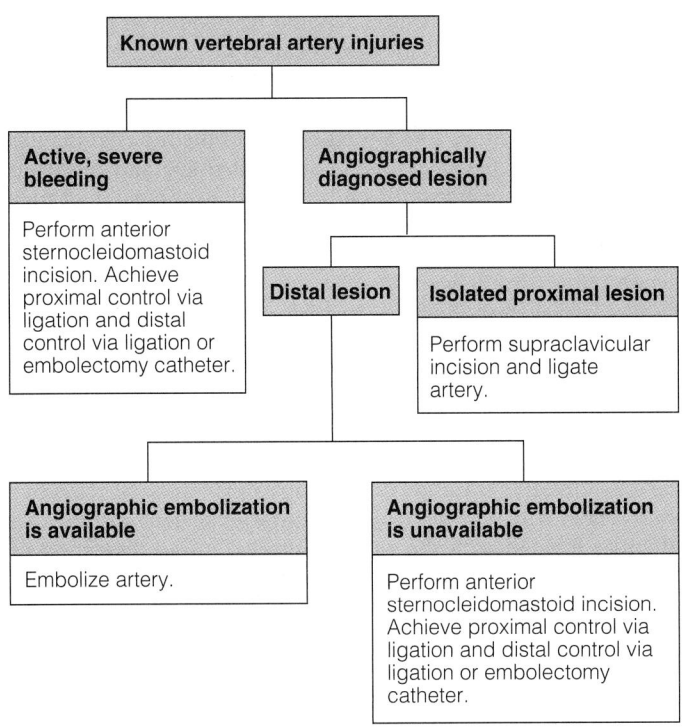

Figure 7 boxes:

Known vertebral artery injuries

Active, severe bleeding

Perform anterior sternocleidomastoid incision. Achieve proximal control via ligation and distal control via ligation or embolectomy catheter.

Angiographically diagnosed lesion

Distal lesion

Isolated proximal lesion

Perform supraclavicular incision and ligate artery.

Angiographic embolization is available

Embolize artery.

Angiographic embolization is unavailable

Perform anterior sternocleidomastoid incision. Achieve proximal control via ligation and distal control via ligation or embolectomy catheter.

Figure 7 **This algorithm depicts the management of known injuries to the vertebral artery, which are most often discovered by angiography.**

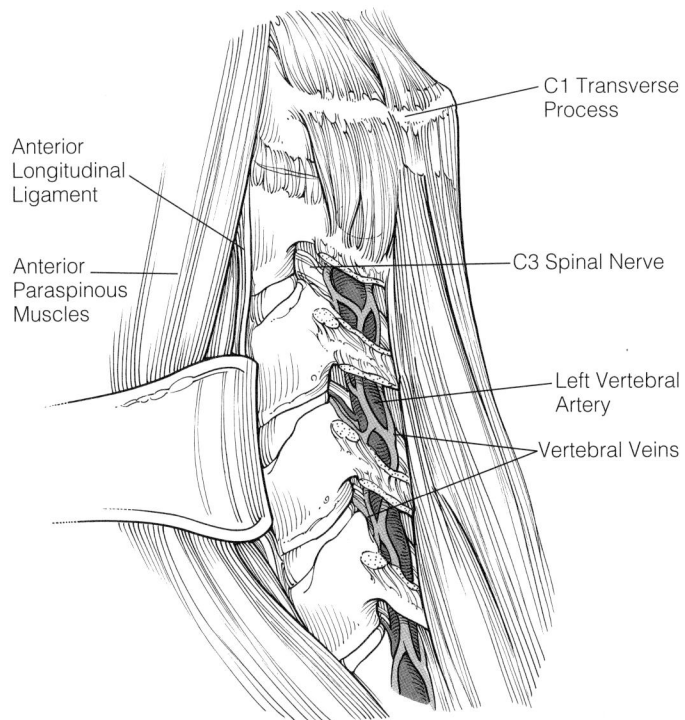

Anterior Longitudinal Ligament

Anterior Paraspinous Muscles

C1 Transverse Process

C3 Spinal Nerve

Left Vertebral Artery

Vertebral Veins

Figure 8 **Throughout most of their course, the vertebral artery and the vertebral veins are surrounded by the transverse processes of the cervical vertebrae. Exposure of this portion of the vertebral artery is best done with lateral mobilization of the longus colli and longissimus capitis.**

exposure are best treated with angiographic embolization if such expertise is available. If angiographic embolization is not an option, however, a surgical approach may be necessary.[18]

The standard anterior sternocleidomastoid incision is used but is carried superiorly with a curved extension to just below the tip of the ear. Once the plane is developed along the anterior border, the sternocleidomastoid muscle should be divided near its origin at the mastoid process. The spinal accessory nerve, which enters the sternocleidomastoid 2 to 3 cm below the tip of the mastoid, should be dissected free of the muscle and mobilized anteriorly. After division of the sternocleidomastoid muscle and anterior retraction of the spinal accessory nerve, the transverse process of the atlas is palpable and the prevertebral fascia is visible in the depths of the wound. The fascia should be incised in a line with the spinal accessory nerve, and the laterally placed levator scapulae and splenius cervicis should be divided as close to the transverse process of the atlas as possible [*see Figure 9*]. The anterior ramus of the nerve root of C2 is closely associated with the anterior edge of the levator scapulae and should be protected. After division of the levator scapulae and splenius cervicis, the distal vertebral artery is visible in the medial aspect of the wound. Venous branches associated with the vertebral artery are most likely to be located near the transverse processes; therefore, ligation should be preferentially directed to the middle of the interspace between the transverse processes.

Exposure of the proximal vertebral artery at the base of the neck can also be achieved via an incision along the anterior border of the sternocleidomastoid muscle. Initial exposure is identical to that used for exposure of the carotid arteries [*see Injuries to the Carotid Arteries, Jugular Veins, Pharynx, and Esophagus, above*]. At the level of the carotid sheath, however, dissection is carried lateral to the internal jugular vein, which is retracted medially to expose the supraclavicular fat pad. The proximal vertebral artery can then be controlled after dissection deep to the fat pad as described for the supraclavicular approach to isolated proximal vertebral artery injuries (see below).

TREATMENT

As opposed to injuries of the carotid arteries, in which either repair or ligation is an option, injuries to the vertebral arteries should always be treated with interruption of flow by surgical or other means. Proximal ligation should usually be done at the origin of the vertebral artery, because the approach to the artery at this point is easier than the approaches to the more distal segments. The artery should be suture-ligated as close to its origin as possible so as not to create a thrombogenic blind pouch off the subclavian artery. Distal ligation can be accomplished by first exposing the artery (see above) and then ligating with ligatures, suture ligatures, or surgical clips. The use of clips minimizes dissection around the artery, which, in turn, decreases the likelihood of further injury to surrounding veins.

In emergency circumstances, a useful technique is to surgically approach the proximal artery at the base of the neck and pass a thrombectomy catheter distally to the site of injury [*see Figure 10*]. First, the proximal vertebral artery is exposed and ligated at its origin. The thrombectomy catheter is then passed distally via an arteriotomy. The catheter balloon is inflated, and the wound is checked to determine whether bleeding has been controlled. If bleeding has been controlled, the distal end of the catheter is left in place, and the proximal end is brought

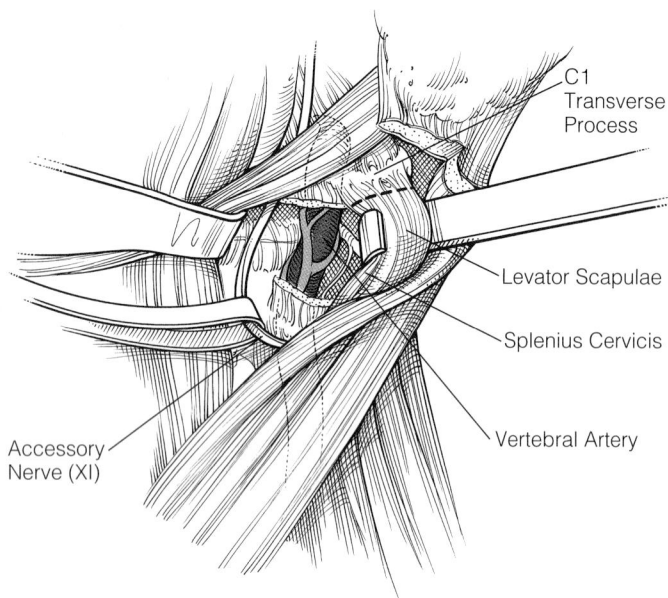

Figure 9 **Exposure of the distal vertebral artery is done via an incision along the anterior border of the sternocleidomastoid muscle. The sternocleidomastoid muscle is then divided near its origin at the mastoid process. The spinal accessory nerve is mobilized anteriorly. The vertebral artery is accessible after division of the levator scapulae and splenius cervicis.**

out through the wound. The catheter is left in situ for approximately 48 hours, at which time the balloon is deflated and the wound is again checked for bleeding. If there is no bleeding for 4 to 6 hours, the catheter can be withdrawn. If the use of a thrombectomy catheter is unsuccessful, a direct surgical approach to the second or third portion of the artery is necessary. However, one of the potential disadvantages of adopting a surgical approach is that proximal ligation of the vertebral artery precludes angiographic embolization except via the contralateral vertebral artery. Embolization via the contralateral vertebral artery is extremely difficult and may result in ischemia or uncontrolled embolization.

If the injury is known by preoperative angiography to be isolated to the first portion of the vertebral artery, both proximal and distal ligation may be possible via a supraclavicular incision [*see Figure 11*]. The patient is positioned with the head turned away from the side of injury, and the chest and ipsilateral neck are prepared and draped. Preparation and draping include the chest so that a left thoracotomy can be done later if necessary for proximal control of the left subclavian artery. In such cases, it is helpful to bump the patient up on the left so that an anterolateral thoracotomy incision can be carried further posteriorly.

The supraclavicular incision should be made approximately one fingerbreadth superior to the clavicle and should extend medially to the midpoint of the sternocleidomastoid insertion and laterally to the juncture of the middle and lateral thirds of the clavicle. The skin, subcutaneous tissue, and platysma should be incised. The external jugular vein, if in the operating field, should be suture-ligated. The clavicular head of the sternocleidomastoid muscle is encountered next, and its lateral aspect should be divided with the electrocautery at its insertion on the clavicle. The muscle is then retracted superiorly and medially. In the plane deep to the sternocleidomastoid

muscle, the omohyoid muscle should be divided in its middle tendinous portion with the electrocautery.

At a level just deep to the sternocleidomastoid and omohyoid muscles, the carotid sheath is encountered in the medial aspect of the wound. The lateral border of the internal jugular vein should be dissected free of adjacent tissue and retracted medially. If the operation is on the left, the thoracic duct may be found in the medial portion of the wound. The thoracic duct is easily injured with retraction and should be divided and ligated if it is in the way.

Just lateral to the internal jugular vein at the same depth is the supraclavicular fat pad, which should be dissected from the supraclavicular fossa in which it lies. Exposure is further enhanced by dissection and division of the laterally located anterior scalene muscle. The phrenic nerve is closely applied to the anterior surface of the anterior scalene muscle and should be dissected free from the underlying muscle and retracted out of the field with a vessel loop. The anterior scalene muscle can then be divided with the electrocautery. During dissection of the supraclavicular fat pad, it may be necessary to divide branches of the thyrocervical and costocervical trunks. The most prominent of these branches is the inferior thyroid artery, which stems from the thyrocervical trunk and courses medially toward the thyroid.

After the supraclavicular fat pad has been dissected, the proximal portion of the vertebral artery is reached. The vertebral vein usually lies slightly superficial and medial to the ver-

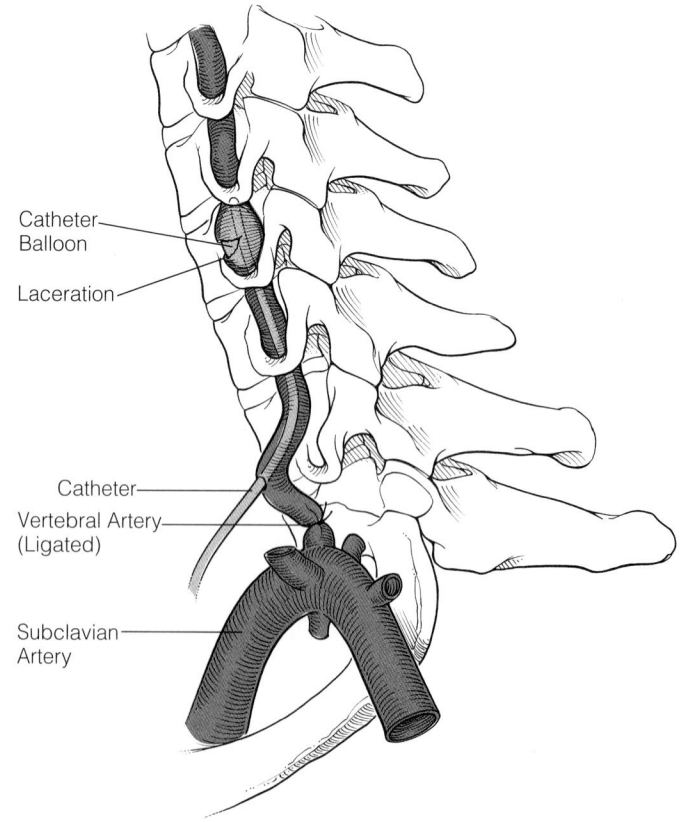

Figure 10 **Bleeding from vertebral artery injuries located within the transverse process of the cervical vertebrae can sometimes be controlled by exposing the proximal vertebral artery at the base of the neck, passing a thrombectomy catheter distally, and inflating the balloon at the site of injury.**

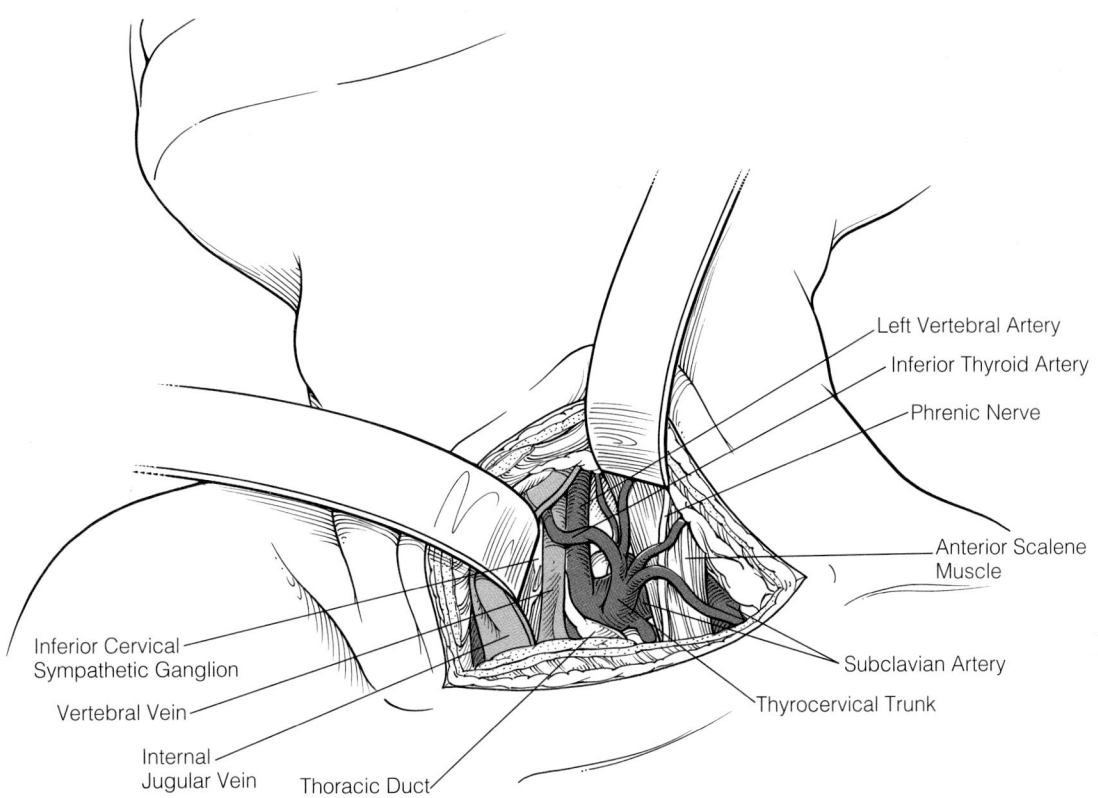

Figure 11 **The proximal vertebral artery can be approached via a supraclavicular incision. Dissection of the supraclavicular fat pad reveals the underlying vertebral artery where it diverges from the subclavian artery. During dissection, care should be taken to avoid injuring the phrenic nerve.**

tebral artery. It should be divided and suture-ligated for better exposure. Care should be taken not to retract too vigorously on the vertebral vein before suture ligation to avoid its avulsion from the subclavian vein. At the depth of the vertebral artery, the white, cordlike elements of the brachial plexus are often visible in the superolateral aspect of the wound. If possible, traction should not be placed on the brachial plexus, and use of the electrocautery around the plexus should be minimized. After exposure, the proximal vertebral artery should be ligated both proximal and distal to the site of injury. No attempts at repair should be made.

Angiographic embolization, the preferred treatment of angiographically diagnosed injuries of the distal vertebral artery, depends on the availability of equipment and expertise with the procedure [*see* Discussion, Angiographic Embolization of Distal Vertebral Artery Injuries, *below*]. Stable patients with angiographically documented injuries to the distal vertebral artery should be transferred to the closest center with cerebral embolization capability. If angiographic embolization is not available, exposure and ligation should be carried out as described above.

In cases where angiographic embolization of the vertebral artery has been employed, a postprocedure angiogram should be done several days to weeks after the procedure to ensure

that the artery remains occluded and that no arteriovenous fistula has developed between the injured vertebral artery and the surrounding venous plexus. Duplex scanning has also been used to a limited extent for follow-up screening. It can be used as an alternative to angiography, but its sensitivity relative to angiography is not yet proved.

Superficial Wounds

Some wounds are obviously superficial on the initial physical examination. Most commonly, these wounds are slash wounds caused by a knife or other sharp object as opposed to being true stab wounds. Rapid exposure and vascular control are sometimes easily accomplished through these wounds. In such circumstances, the surgical procedure 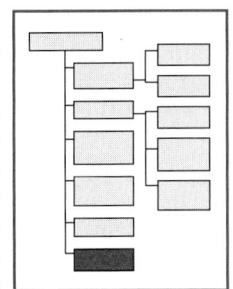 consists of debridement of the neck wound, and deep dissection is not necessary. If greater access and control are needed to rule out further injuries or for definitive repair, a standard anterior sternocleidomastoid incision should be done [*see* Injuries to the Carotid Arteries, Jugular Veins, Pharynx, and Esophagus, *above*].

Discussion

Repair versus Ligation of Carotid Arteries

Simple injuries to the external carotid artery should be repaired, whereas complex injuries should be ligated.

Injuries to the common carotid artery and internal carotid artery are more problematic. If the injury is simple and there is no suggestion that flow in the vessel has been interrupted, repair should always be undertaken. An example of such an injury is a simple stab wound of part of the circumference of the artery with an associated pseudoaneurysm and good distal flow. In this circumstance, lateral repair can be done quickly and easily with a short cross-clamp time. After control of the vessel proximally and distally, a check should be made for back-bleeding. If the back-bleeding from the distal circulation is brisk, as it usually is, repair can be done safely.

If an injury to the common carotid artery or internal carotid artery has interrupted flow in the vessel, repair creates a theoretical disadvantage. Interruption of flow may lead to focal brain ischemia and partial disruption of the blood-brain barrier. Sudden restoration of blood flow may cause hemorrhage in the area of the ischemia and worsen the extent of brain injury; an anemic, or white, infarct of the brain may be converted to a hemorrhagic, or red, infarct. Whether this pathophysiology is important after traumatic injury is unclear and controversial.

Deciding whether to repair or ligate when flow has been interrupted is often difficult.[6,7] One approach is to base the decision on the patient's preoperative neurologic status. If there is no neurologic deficit, it is presumed that there are no areas of brain ischemia and that repair is safe. Conversely, a focal neurologic deficit is presumed to be related to ischemia, and in such cases, the risk of worsening the patient's neurologic status with restoration of blood flow is increased. Even though this approach is rational, it is not applicable in cases in which a detailed neurologic examination before surgery is not possible. Furthermore, this approach may be applicable only to patients in coma or with severe neurologic deficits. There are indications that milder neurologic deficits respond favorably to revascularization.

Yet another approach is to gauge the appropriateness of repair according to the nature of the injury itself. In this approach, large, complicated injuries requiring involved and lengthy procedures for repair should be ligated, whereas simple injuries requiring only simple and quick repairs are repaired. Similarly, repair is not indicated in patients with severe or multiple associated injuries. There is also a difference between the management of injuries of the common carotid artery and management of injuries of the internal carotid artery. Common carotid injuries are more accessible and easier to repair, and repair is generally associated with a good outcome. Continued prograde flow in the internal carotid artery is more likely after injury to the common carotid artery than to the internal carotid artery because of the possibility of collateral flow via the external carotid artery.

A reasonable way to deal with repair dilemmas is to make the decision on the basis of distal back-bleeding. Interruption of blood flow to the brain is tolerated only for a short time, and restoration of flow is unlikely to be accomplished quickly enough to improve outcome. It is therefore logical to base the decision about revascularization on the state of back-bleeding from the internal carotid artery. If back-bleeding is brisk, the patient is presumed to have good collateral flow, and the chances that there is an area of ischemia are low. Repair rather than ligation is safe in such circumstances. If internal carotid artery back-bleeding is minimal or absent, an ischemic infarct is more likely and restitution of arterial inflow is more dangerous. A corollary to this reasoning is that if back-bleeding is poor, a clot distal to the area of injury may be present, and return of flow with repair may dislodge the clot distally.

Nonoperative Management and Stenting of Carotid Artery Injuries

It is now well accepted that certain minimal injuries to the vasculature of the extremities (e.g., small pseudoaneurysms and endothelial injuries) do not always have to be repaired if they do not compromise distal flow and that such injuries usually heal over time without sequelae. It has been hypothesized that minimal injuries to the carotid vasculature can be approached in a similar fashion. The consequences of distal embolization or pseudoaneurysm rupture in the carotid circulation make such an approach somewhat risky; further experience with nonoperative management is necessary before this approach can be accepted for routine use with small carotid artery injuries.[19,20]

Another relatively new approach to carotid artery injuries is intraluminal stenting.[21-23] This approach is now commonly used for aneurysms of the thoracic and abdominal aorta and is also employed for more distal peripheral vascular lesions. On rare occasions, it has also been applied in the management of traumatic injuries to the thoracic aorta and selected injuries to the peripheral and the visceral vasculature. Not surprisingly, stenting has also been used for the management of carotid artery injuries, particularly injuries to the distal internal carotid artery that are not easily approached surgically. At present, however, only limited data on this approach are available, and the long-term results of carotid stenting are not yet known. It is possible that once more experience with intraluminal stenting has been amassed, it will become an accepted part of the armamentarium for managing carotid injuries. Given that most minor injuries seem to heal well with nonoperative management and that major injuries of the proximal carotid system are relatively easy to approach surgically and often call for emergency surgical repair, the most likely niche for carotid stenting after injury is in treating medium to large lesions of the distal internal carotid artery.

Angiographic Embolization of Distal Vertebral Artery Injuries

Most patients with vertebral artery injuries are stable without external bleeding, and the injury is discovered by angiography. A number of series have now been reported in which such lesions have been successfully treated with angiographic embolization. Given the difficulties of surgical exposure, lesions of the distal vertebral artery should be treated angiographically when the patient's general condition permits and when the necessary expertise is available.[15] If the patient is bleeding profusely, such an approach is not possible, and a rapid surgical approach should be done, with ligation of the proximal vertebral artery and an attempt at thrombectomy catheter control or packing of the wound until an angiographic approach can be attempted. If this is unsuccessful, the lesion should be approached directly [see Known Vertebral Artery Injuries, above].

If a patient with a distal vertebral artery lesion is stable—particularly when the lesion is otherwise silent and has been detected angiographically—an attempt should be made at angiographic embolization if the necessary expertise is available. If the patient is stable, transfer to the nearest center with cerebral angiographic embolization capability is appropriate. Embolization is done via the ipsilateral proximal vertebral artery. Detachable balloons or coils can be used.

Conversion of Cricothyrotomy to Tracheotomy

Cricothyrotomy is typically reserved for life-threatening airway compromise when the need for a rapid surgical airway is paramount [see Airway Compromise, above, and 5:1 Trauma Resuscitation]. Tracheotomy is preferred if time and a lesser degree of urgency permit. Similarly, in the postoperative period, tracheotomy is preferred to cricothyrotomy. Traditional thinking, initially promulgated by Chevalier Jackson in 1921, is that cricothyrotomy is more likely than tracheotomy to result in airway stricture or damage to more proximal structures in the larynx. On the basis of this rationale, cricothyrotomies are converted to tracheotomies on a semielective basis within 24 to 48 hours of admission if the patient's general condition permits.[24,25]

Evidence to support a policy of routine conversion is mixed. Several series document a low but increased incidence of complications to the larynx and trachea from prolonged maintenance of cricothyrotomies. Even though incidence is low, the complications can be severe and may require extensive reconstructive procedures. Conversely, studies of cardiac patients undergoing routine cricothyrotomy do not demonstrate a significant increase in the incidence of airway complications. Cricothyrotomy is sometimes favored over tracheotomy in these patients because of concerns about the proximity of tracheotomy wounds to the patient's sternotomy incision. The results of studies of routine cardiac patients may be different from results of studies showing an increase in complications after cricothyrotomy, in that cardiac patients were intubated for shorter periods.

There have been no studies documenting a high incidence of complications in trauma patients who have undergone emergency cricothyrotomy and have remained intubated via the cricothyrotomy for longer than 2 or 3 days. Because complications are potentially so devastating, however, emergency cricothyrotomies should be converted to tracheotomy within 1 to 2 days of admission in stable patients. Assuming a stable patient, the risks of conversion are minimal, and conversion is justified to avoid the possibility of future complications.

References

1. Fuhrman GM, Steig FH III, Buerk CA: Blunt laryngeal trauma: classification and management protocol. J Trauma 30:87, 1990

2. Symbas IN, Hatcher CR Jr, Boehm GAW: Acute penetrating tracheal trauma. Ann Thorac Surg 22:473, 1976

3. Dossa C, Shepard AD, Wolford DG, et al: Distal internal carotid exposure: a simplified technique for temporary mandibular subluxation. J Vasc Surg 12:319, 1990

4. Fisher DF Jr, Clagett GP, Parker JI, et al: Mandibular subluxation for high carotid exposure. J Vasc Surg 1:727, 1984

5. Beal SL, Pottmeyer EW, Spisso JM: Esophageal perforation following external blunt trauma. J Trauma 28:1425, 1988

6. Fabian TC, George SM Jr, Croce MA, et al: Carotid artery trauma: management based on mechanism of injury. J Trauma 30:953, 1990

7. Richardson R, Obeid FN, Richardson JD, et al: Neurologic consequences of cerebrovascular injury. J Trauma 32:755, 1992

8. Feliciano DV, Mattox KL, Graham JM, et al: Five-year experience with PTFE grafts in vascular wounds. J Trauma 25:71, 1985

9. Archie JP Jr, Green JJ Jr: Saphenous vein rupture pressure, rupture stress, and carotid endarterectomy vein patch reconstruction. Surgery 107:389, 1990

10. Winter RP, Weigelt JA: Cervical esophageal trauma: incidence and cause of esophageal fistulas. Arch Surg 125:849, 1990

11. Abouljoud MS, Obeid FN, Horst HM, et al: Arterial injuries of the thoracic outlet: a ten-year experience. Am Surg 59:590, 1993

12. Rich NM, Baugh JH, Hughes CW: Acute arterial injuries in Vietnam: 1,000 cases. J Trauma 10:359, 1970

13. Wood VE: The results of total claviculectomy. Clin Orthop 207:186, 1986

14. McCready RA, Procter CD, Hyde GL: Subclavian-axillary vascular trauma. J Vasc Surg 3:24, 1986

15. Higashida RT, Halbach VV, Tsai FY, et al: Interventional neurovascular treatment of traumatic carotid and vertebral artery lesions: results in 234 cases. AJR Am J Roentgenol 153:577, 1989

16. Hatzitheofilou C, Demetriades D, Melissas J, et al: Surgical approaches to vertebral artery injuries. Br J Surg 75:234, 1988

17. Reid JD, Weigelt JA: Forty-three cases of vertebral artery trauma. J Trauma 28:1007, 1988

18. Blickenstaff KL, Weaver FA, Yellin AE, et al: Trends in the management of traumatic vertebral artery injuries. Am J Surg 158:101, 1989

19. Demetriades D, Asensio JA, Velmahos G, et al: Complex problems in penetrating neck trauma. Surg Clin North Am 76:661, 1996

20. Panetta TF, Sales CM, Marin ML, et al: Natural history, duplex characteristics, and histopathologic correlation of arterial injuries in a canine model. J Vasc Surg 16:867, 1992

21. Gomez CR, May AD, Terry JB, et al: Endovascular therapy of traumatic injuries of the extracranial cerebral arteries. Crit Care Clin 15:789, 1999

22. Kerby JD, May AD, Gomez CR, et al: Treatment of bilateral blunt carotid injury using percutaneous angioplasty and stenting: case report and review of the literature. J Trauma 49:784, 2000

23. Liu AY, Paulsen RD, Marcellus ML, et al: Long-term outcomes after carotid stent placement for treatment of carotid artery dissection. Neurosurgery 45:1368, 1999

24. Esses BA, Jafek BW: Cricothyroidotomy: a decade of experience in Denver. Ann Otol Rhinol Laryngol 96:519, 1987

25. Milner SM, Bennett JDC: Review article: emergency cricothyrotomy. J Laryngol Otol 105:883, 1991

Reviews

Surgical Anatomy, 6th ed. Anson B, McVay CB, Eds. WB Saunders Co, Philadelphia, 1984

Anatomic Exposures in Vascular Surgery. Wind G, Valentine R, Eds. Williams & Wilkins, Baltimore, 1991

Acknowledgments

Figure 1   Marcia Kammerer.
Figures 2 through 4   Susan E. Brust, C.M.I.
Figures 5 through 7   Marcia Kammerer.
Figures 8 through 11   Susan E. Brust, C.M.I.

5 INJURIES TO THE CHEST

Asher Hirshberg, M.D., and Kenneth L. Mattox, M.D., F.A.C.S.

Injuries to the chest account for about one quarter of all trauma deaths in the United States. This high mortality is the result of the malignant interaction between three pathophysiologic mechanisms: bleeding, hypoxia, and direct cardiac injury. Because the chest wall is stiff and noncompliant, the three visceral compartments of the chest (i.e., the two pleural spaces and the mediastinum) are particularly susceptible to pressure elevation resulting from accumulation of undrained air or blood. At least 80% of patients with chest injuries do not require an operative intervention and can be safely managed by means of a tube thoracotomy; however, in approximately one out of every six patients, an urgent thoracotomy will be indicated.

In this chapter, we outline our operative strategy and management tactics for handling penetrating and blunt thoracic injuries, highlight the underlying technical principles of gaining access and repairing traumatic injuries to the thoracic viscera, and describe the pitfalls that await the inexperienced surgeon.

Resuscitative Thoracotomy

A resuscitative thoracotomy is typically performed in the emergency department and occasionally in the OR if the pulse is lost before injuries to other cavities can be addressed. An endotracheal tube is placed, and the left arm is abducted to get it out of the way. An incision is then immediately made beneath the nipple in men or beneath the manually retracted breast in women, beginning at the sternum and extending as far laterally as possible. The incision is rapidly performed with a knife, and heavy scissors are used to cut the intercostal muscles. No time is wasted on skin preparation, wound hemostasis, or identification of the severed internal mammary artery. A chest wall retractor is inserted with the handle away from the sternum and facing the axilla.

Subsequent operative maneuvers depend on the clinical circumstances. If tamponade is suspected, the pericardial sac is opened longitudinally—anterior and parallel to the phrenic nerve—up to the aortic root superiorly and down to the diaphragm inferiorly. The heart is manually delivered into the left hemithorax and carefully examined for injuries. Reliance on external visualization of the intact pericardium is a classic pitfall: such visualization should never be considered sufficient in itself to exclude tamponade. Attempts at definitive repair of cardiac lacerations in the suboptimal technical circumstances of the ED are frequently futile. Evacuation of blood and temporary control of the lacerations by means of digital pressure, a Foley catheter, or a skin stapler will allow transfer of the patient to the OR for definitive repair under optimal conditions.

For clamping of the thoracic aorta or the pulmonary hilum, the inferior pulmonary ligament must be incised to permit mobilization of the lung. The descending thoracic aorta should be clamped to maintain cerebral and coronary perfusion in the agonal patient. Clamping is also an important adjunct to open cardiac massage. This maneuver involves manual upward traction of the left lung after division of the inferior pulmonary ligament,

incision of the mediastinal pleura, and just enough blunt finger dissection around the aorta to accommodate an aortic clamp. Occluding the aorta digitally by simply pinching the flaccid vessel or compressing it against the spine may be a safer and less traumatic alternative when visualization of the area is not optimal. When hemorrhage arises from the pulmonary hilum or parenchyma or when coronary air embolism is suspected, the pulmonary hilum is clamped. This maneuver is performed by placing a Satinsky side-biting clamp across the hilum, with special care taken not to injure the phrenic nerve, which crosses immediately anterior and in close proximity to the hilum. A newer and simpler technique for vascular control of the hilum is the pulmonary hilar twist. After the inferior pulmonary ligament has been divided, the injured lung is simply twisted around the hilum, so that its apex lies against the diaphragm while its base is in the upper chest [*see Figure 1*]. The twist is a rapid and effective temporary control technique that does not require precise anatomic identification of the lung and the hilar structures.

As a general rule, the injured hemithorax is entered first. However, when it becomes apparent that the patient's agonal state cannot be explained by the findings in the open hemithorax, the incision should rapidly be extended across the sternum into the other hemithorax. This is particularly true for a right-side thoracotomy, which does not provide access to the heart and the descending thoracic aorta. Extension of a left thoracotomy to the right hemithorax is done in the third intercostal space (above the nipple) to facilitate access to the innominate artery. The resulting clamshell incision provides excellent access to all thoracic viscera (except the posterior mediastinal structures), albeit at the price of increased morbidity.

The technical keys to resuscitative thoracotomy are (1) speed in entering the chest and (2) avoidance of complex repairs or maneuvers until the patient is in the OR, where definitive repair of the injuries can be safely accomplished. The major pitfalls are (1) iatrogenic injuries to the phrenic nerve or the heart during pericardiotomy and (2) avulsion of an intercostal artery or esophageal perforation during aortic clamping. Care should be taken to avoid laceration of the inferior pulmonary vein during division of the inferior pulmonary ligament. If the resuscitative thoracotomy is successful, the patient regains a pulse and adequate BP, and the transected internal mammary artery begins to bleed. This vessel should then be identified and both its transected ends ligated before closure.

Choice of Incision

It is not possible to gain access to all three thoracic visceral compartments through a single utility incision. Therefore, the correct choice of incision is a key decision that can determine the success or failure of the operation.

The operative approach to thoracic trauma is determined primarily by the hemodynamic stability of the patient. In the unstable patient, an anterolateral thoracotomy is the incision of choice because it allows rapid access to the visceral content of the

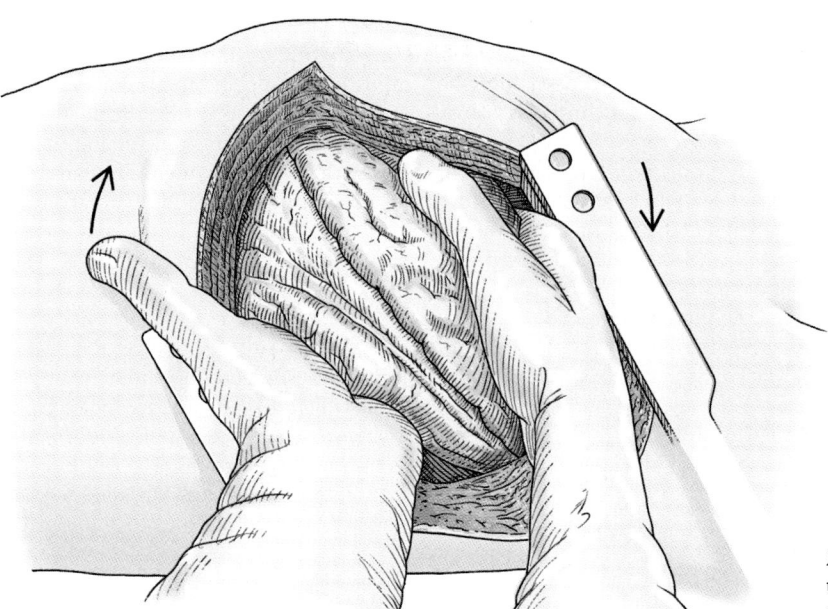

Figure 1 **Temporary vascular control of the hilum can be gained by means of the pulmonary hilar twist.**

hemithorax, requires no special positioning, and does not interfere with access to other visceral compartments. The incision can also be rapidly extended across the sternum to the contralateral hemithorax. In the stable patient, where thoracotomy follows a diagnostic workup with precise delineation of the injury, the incision can be targeted on the injured structure. The choice of thoracotomy incision in stable patients with bleeding into the pleural cavity or the airway is determined by the location of the injury. The heart, the ascending aorta, the arch, and the thoracic inlet vessels are approached via a median sternotomy. A posterolateral thoracotomy is indicated for injuries to the descending aorta, the esophagus, the lung, or the bronchus. In patients with blunt or penetrating trauma to the right lower chest, bleeding is usually from an injured liver, and the initial approach is therefore via a midline laparotomy. The right chest is entered only if laparotomy fails to reveal the source of bleeding. Injuries above the right nipple line and to any part of the left chest are approached through an anterolateral thoracotomy on the injured side.

Penetrating wounds to the base of the neck (i.e., the thoracic inlet) present special access problems. Injuries to the base of the right neck or those bleeding into the right pleural cavity are approached via a median sternotomy. However, the first part of the left subclavian artery is intrapleural and posterior, and the appropriate incision for proximal control of this vessel is a left anterolateral thoracotomy in the third or fourth intercostal space. This incision is used for thoracic inlet injuries bleeding into the left pleura or for presumed left subclavian artery laceration. The more lateral parts of both subclavian arteries are approached through a supraclavicular incision, and exposure can be facilitated by removal of the medial third of the clavicle. An important operative adjunct is the insertion of a Foley balloon catheter into the missile tract, which allows temporary hemostasis to be achieved by inflating the balloon while access and direct control are obtained.

The initial incision chosen for access to an actively bleeding thoracic inlet injury may prove inadequate, in which case it is immediately extended. A median sternotomy can be extended along the border of the sternocleidomastoid muscle or along the clavicle to improve access to the carotid artery and the subclavian artery, respectively. A so-called trapdoor incision is created by extending the median sternotomy into an anterolateral thoracotomy in conjunction with a supraclavicular incision. This incision may be useful for proximal left carotid injuries and for obtaining control of the proximal left subclavian artery if the initial incision was a median sternotomy.

Cardiac Trauma

SIMPLE INJURIES

Repair of simple anterolateral cardiac lacerations is usually straightforward. The major determinants of a successful outcome in these cases are timely diagnosis and a swift thoracotomy. Such lacerations are repaired with either simple or pledgeted monofilament sutures. The most common site of myocardial disruption from blunt trauma is the right atrium, usually at the atriocaval junction. Atrial lacerations can sometimes be controlled with a partially occluding clamp to facilitate the repair.

COMPLEX INJURIES

Several factors may complicate the cardiorrhaphy [*see Figure 2*]. Injuries to the right side of the heart may not be accessible via a left thoracotomy and thus may necessitate transsternal extension. Multiple holes or lacerations may have to be controlled temporarily with digital pressure, an occluding balloon catheter, or a skin stapler. Lacerations involving a coronary artery present a special problem. Ligation of a distal coronary artery is rarely associated with significant arrhythmias or infarction, whereas proximal coronary lacerations should be repaired. When the cardiac perforation is in close proximity to a coronary artery, horizontal mattress sutures passed beneath the artery help prevent inadvertent interruption of the vessel [*see Figure 3*].

Temporary inflow occlusion is a key maneuver in difficult situations, such as posterior lacerations or injuries to the intrapericardial great vessels. Both venae cavae are rapidly clamped, and the heart is allowed to empty. This results in temporary dryness of the operative field, which may last just long enough to permit several quick critical stitches. Large posterior atrial lacerations can sometimes be repaired from within the heart by opening the atrium, occluding cardiac inflow, and performing an intracardiac repair. Cardiopulmonary bypass is always a theoretical possibility but is rarely a practical option in the acute situation.

SPECIAL CONSIDERATIONS

Missile emboli to the heart can be caused by migration of air or particles from a peripheral venous injury site. Almost all such emboli will become embedded within the right ventricular trabeculations. If they are left in place, they can cause arrhythmias, further embolization to pulmonary arteries, endocarditis, and interference with tricuspid valve function. Such emboli have been removed by means of interventional radiologic techniques, cardiopulmonary bypass with a right atriotomy, or a right ventriculotomy without cardiopulmonary bypass.

The diagnosis of coronary air embolism is made intraoperatively when air bubbles are seen in the coronary arteries. This diagnosis calls for immediate hilar clamping of the injured lung in conjunction with venting of air from the left side of the heart

and the ascending aorta via a needle inserted into the most ventral aspect of these structures. Manual occlusion of the aortic root is then accomplished by placing the fingers of the left hand into the transverse sinus and compressing the aorta between the thumb and the forefinger. The heart is massaged for several beats to drive the air through the coronary microcirculation. Once cardiac activity is reestablished, the left chambers are vented again to remove any residual air. The lung injury that allowed air entry into the pulmonary venous circulation must then be addressed.

Aortic Injuries

Traumatic rupture of the descending thoracic aorta creates a contained hematoma, which allows precise angiographic definition of the injury before operative repair [*see Figure 4*]. The descending aorta is approached through a left posterolateral thoracotomy in the fourth intercostal space. The standard repair technique is direct repair using proximal and distal control, with or

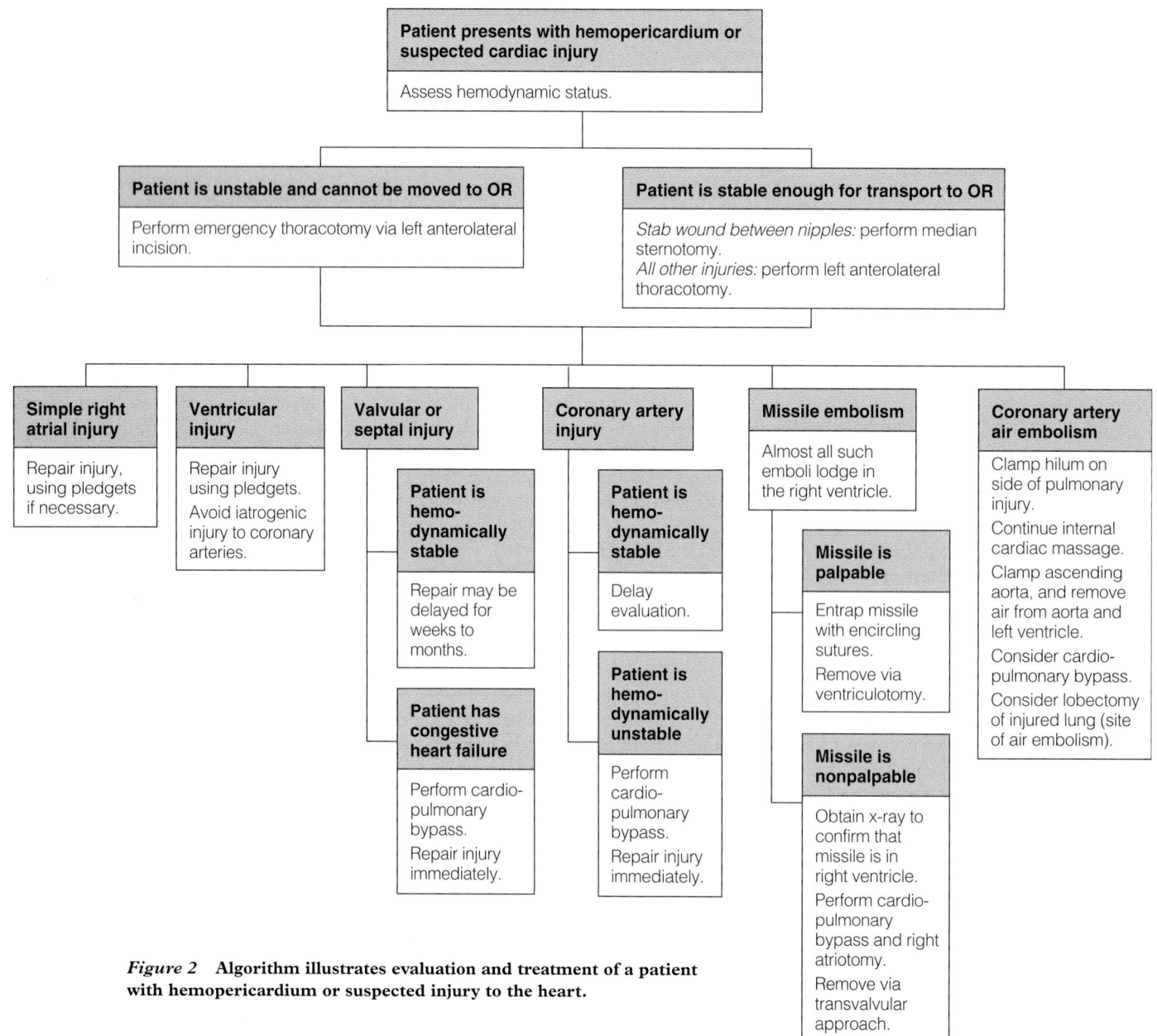

Figure 2 **Algorithm illustrates evaluation and treatment of a patient with hemopericardium or suspected injury to the heart.**

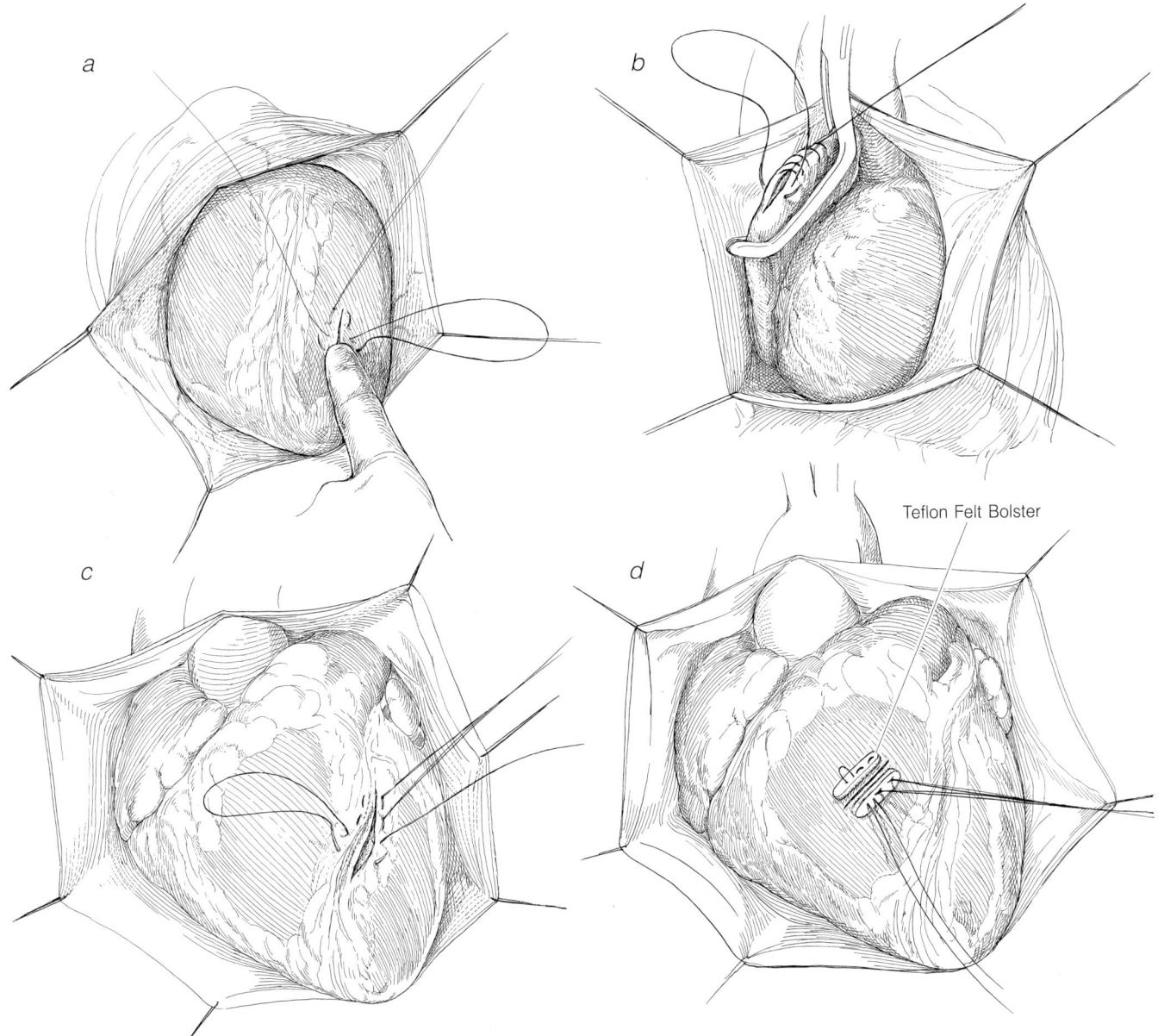

Figure 3 Penetrating injuries to a cardiac chamber can usually be temporarily occluded with the tip of a finger (*a*); a Satinsky clamp can sometimes be used to control an atrial lesion (*b*). If the wound is close to a coronary artery, care must be taken not to obliterate the vessel during repair. Passing horizontal mattress sutures beneath the vasculature will allow closure of the cardiac laceration and avoid ligation of the artery (*c*). Injuries can sometimes be repaired with a simple running suture but are usually best handled with interrupted mattress sutures. Teflon pledgets or strips may be used if there is surrounding contusion or if the injury is to a ventricle (*d*). It is best to use cardiovascular suture material, but absorbable sutures may be used if cardiovascular material is not readily available.

without interposition graft placement. Three commonly used adjuncts to this approach are (1) pharmacologic control of central hypertension during clamping, (2) passive shunting, and (3) pump-assisted left heart bypass. The third adjunct can make use of either a traditional pump system with heparin or a centrifugal pump circuit without heparin [*see Figure 5*]. At present, surgical preference is slowly shifting from clamp repair (proximal and distal control without bypass) to partial cardiopulmonary bypass.

After entry into the left chest, the first operative target is the left subclavian artery, which is encircled by means of careful blunt dissection. Next, the mediastinal pleura overlying the distal descending aorta is incised and the aorta encircled and prepared for clamping, with special care taken not to damage the intercostal vessels. The critical maneuver during dissection is

development of the correct plane around the aortic arch between the subclavian and left carotid arteries in preparation for proximal clamping. The pleura between the vagus and the phrenic nerve is sharply incised, and a plane is developed between the left (or main) pulmonary artery and the undersurface of the aortic arch. The latter is accomplished with a combination of blunt and sharp dissection and may be especially difficult in elderly patients, who often have fibrous periaortic tissue at this location. A large curved clamp is used to encircle the aortic arch, and dissection is limited to the minimum necessary to permit safe passage of an umbilical tape to enable subsequent cross-clamping.

The aortic arch, the subclavian artery, and the distal aorta are then clamped, in this sequence, and the hematoma is entered. The lateral aspect of the aortic wall is carefully incised longitudinally for a distance of no more than 2 cm, a vein retractor is inserted, and the damage to the aortic wall is evaluated. This small incision is subsequently extended as dictated by the operative findings, and a decision is made for primary repair or graft insertion. The aortic incision should be carefully tailored to both the extent of damage and the selected repair technique. Similarly, debridement of the injured wall should be careful and conservative, especially if primary repair seems possible. Direct repair is accomplished with a 4-0 Prolene suture. Graft interposition is accomplished in a standard end-to-end fashion by using a soft woven graft, with care taken not to enter the esophagus with the posterior bites.

After completion of the proximal anastomosis, the clamp should not be moved to the graft. This is particularly true in young adults, whose aortas are relatively friable and thus should not be subjected to excessive tension. Aortic declamping is a critical maneuver that should be accomplished slowly and only after the nitroprusside infusion used to control central hypertension has been discontinued.

Thoracic Outlet Injuries

The second most common blunt thoracic vascular injury is a tear at the origin of the innominate artery off the aortic arch. This injury is repaired in accordance with the bypass and exclusion principle; thus, there is no need for cardiopulmonary bypass, shunts, or heparinization. After precise angiographic definition of the injury, access is obtained via a median sternotomy. The ascending aorta is exposed inside the pericardium. The distal innominate, right subclavian, and right carotid arteries are dissected out and encircled in preparation for clamping, but the hematoma itself is not entered. With a partially occluding (e.g., Satinsky) clamp on the ascending aorta, a 12 mm knitted Dacron graft is sewn to the normal ascending aorta in an end-to-side fashion, away from the injury. Occasionally, the innominate vein is ligated to optimize exposure. A second partially occluding clamp is placed on the aortic arch at the origin of the innominate artery, with special care taken not to occlude the origin of the left carotid artery. The distal innominate artery or its branches are then clamped, and the distal anastomosis is completed. Only then is the hematoma entered and the injury oversewn by placing a row of pledgeted sutures on the aortic arch.

Penetrating injuries to the innominate vessels and proximal carotid arteries produce a mediastinal hematoma, sometimes accompanied by torrential hemorrhage, which can be temporarily controlled either digitally or by placing a Foley balloon catheter in the missile tract before obtaining access. The cardinal technical principle in the management of these injuries is never to enter a contained or partially contained mediastinal hematoma without first obtaining proximal and distal control. Proximal control of

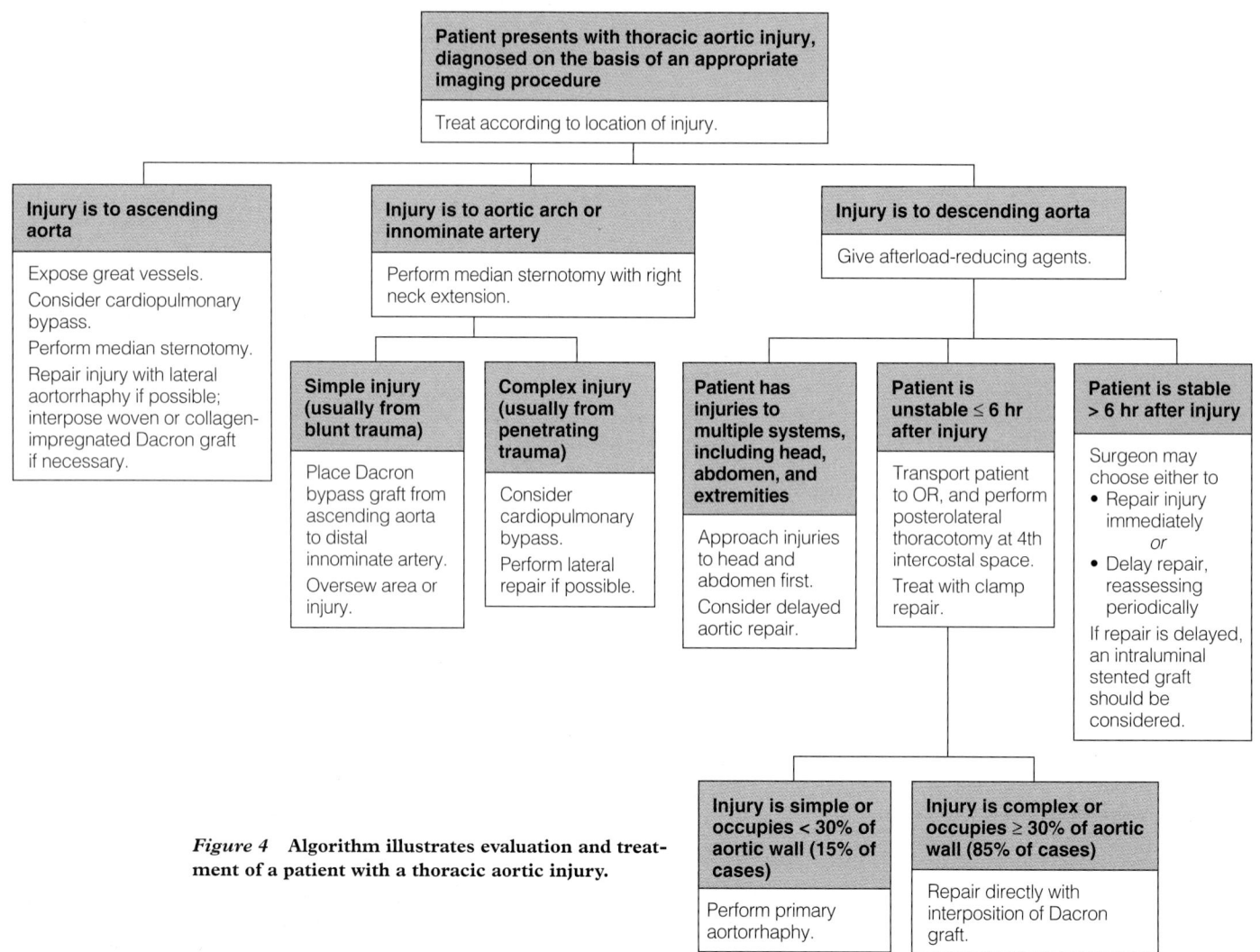

Figure 4 **Algorithm illustrates evaluation and treatment of a patient with a thoracic aortic injury.**

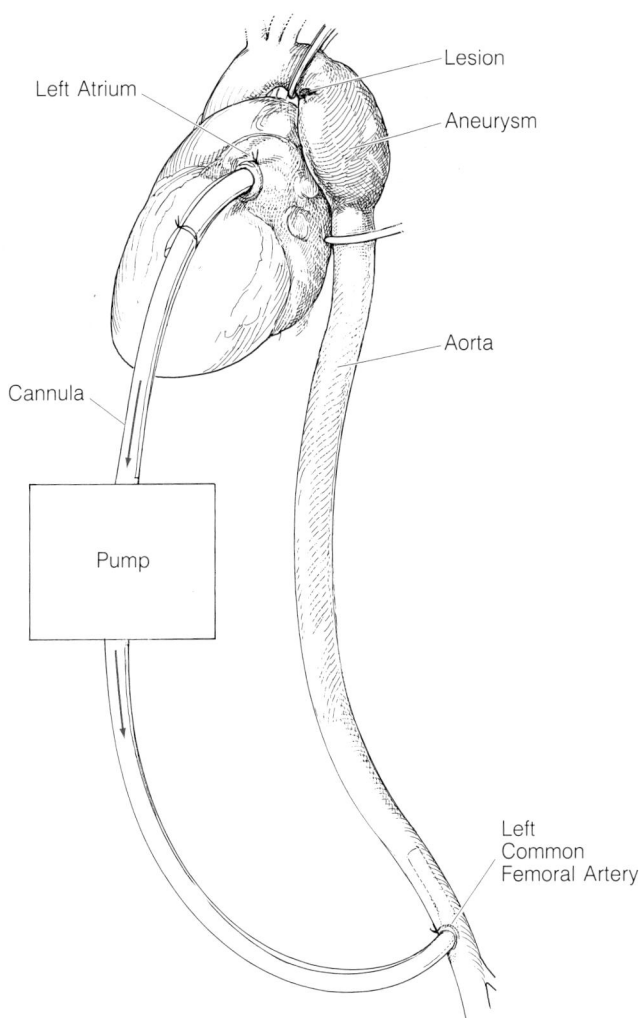

Figure 5 **Illustrated is a bypass from the left atrium to the left common femoral artery during operation for a transected descending thoracic aorta. This maneuver permits decompression of upper body hypertension, complete perfusion of the viscera, and some perfusion of the spinal cord. Once the transected area has been dissected out, the clamps should be placed as close as possible to the damaged area to allow maximal perfusion of the collateral circulation.**

these vessels can be obtained from within the pericardium, where the anatomy is not obscured by the hematoma. During dissection within the hematoma, the technical key is identification of the innominate vein, which may be ligated and divided with impunity if necessary.

Injuries to the distal subclavian vessels can often be approached via a limited supraclavicular incision, but the safest approach, especially in the presence of active bleeding, is via a more extensive incision. The medial third of the clavicle is rapidly resected by performing early subperiosteal division of the bone, grasping it with a towel clip, and lifting it out of its bed. The subclavian artery is a very friable vessel, and limited resection of the injured segment with interposition of a graft (preferably one made of knitted Dacron) is a safer option than extensive mobilization and attempted end-to-end anastomosis.

Major Airway Disruption

The precise location of major airway injury is determined through bronchoscopy, and the operative approach is planned accordingly. Use of a double-lumen endotracheal tube is an important adjunct. The thoracic trachea and the right mainstem bronchus are approached via a right posterolateral thoracotomy, and the left mainstem bronchus is approached through a similar incision on the left. The anterior and left lateral aspects of the mediastinal trachea can also be approached through a median sternotomy. More than 80% of blunt tracheobronchial disruptions occur within 2 cm of the carina [*see Figure 6*].

The technical key to the management of airway injuries is to perform a primary repair with precise mucosa-to-mucosa tension-free apposition of the lacerated edges using interrupted absorbable sutures. Small tracheal wounds with well-opposed edges and no tissue loss can be managed conservatively via tracheal intubation and inflation of the balloon distal to the laceration. Large tracheobronchial wounds are managed by means of conservative debridement and airtight single-layer closure of the defect. Lacerations of the distal airways resulting in a large air leak or bleeding into the airway are managed with resection of the injured lung parenchyma.

Pulmonary Lacerations

Bleeding pulmonary lacerations can be either oversewn or resected [*see Figure 7*]. A continuous over-and-over Prolene suture controls bleeding from small or shallow lacerations; deeper wounds call for resection of the injured parenchyma. As a general rule, parenchymal resections for trauma are not anatomic. Rapid and simple resection of the injured lung tissue is usually accomplished with a wide transverse anastomosis (TA) stapler (e.g., a TA-90), which is positioned just proximal to the injured segment, closed, and fired across the segment. The tissue distal to the stapled line is then amputated, and the stapler is opened. If any residual bleeding or air leakage is noted, the staple line is oversewn with a continuous monofilament suture.

Deep through-and-through injuries to the lung that do not involve hilar structures present a special technical problem because simple closure of the entry and exit wounds does not suffice for management. These injuries can be treated with pulmonary tractotomy using a linear gastrointestinal anastomosis (GIA) stapler or, if an appropriate stapler is not immediately available, a pair of aortic clamps [*see Figure 8*]. The bridge of tissue overlying the bleeding tract is cut by the stapler or divided between the clamps, which allows any bleeding vessels or air leaks inside the tract to be selectively suture-ligated. The tract is carefully inspected to ensure that no major vascular or bronchial injury is present that would necessitate a formal resection. If clamps are used for the tractotomy, the lung tissue held between them is then oversewn with a continuous monofilament suture, and the tractotomy is left open.

Central lung injuries are a source of exsanguinating hemorrhage as well as of air embolism. The key operative maneuver in the management of these injuries is early hilar clamping. The inferior pulmonary ligament is rapidly divided, and the entire hilum is clamped with a large vascular clamp in such a way as to incorporate the pulmonary artery, both pulmonary veins, and the mainstem bronchus. The next step is a meticulous evaluation of the injuries to determine the method of definitive repair (i.e., vascular repair or pulmonary resection). If the vascular injury is immediately below the hilar clamp and the patient's hemodynamic status allows, the pulmonary vessels can be individually isolated and controlled from within the pericardium to facilitate exposure and repair of the injury. In theory, isolated vascular injuries can be repaired, but in practice, these wounds are often

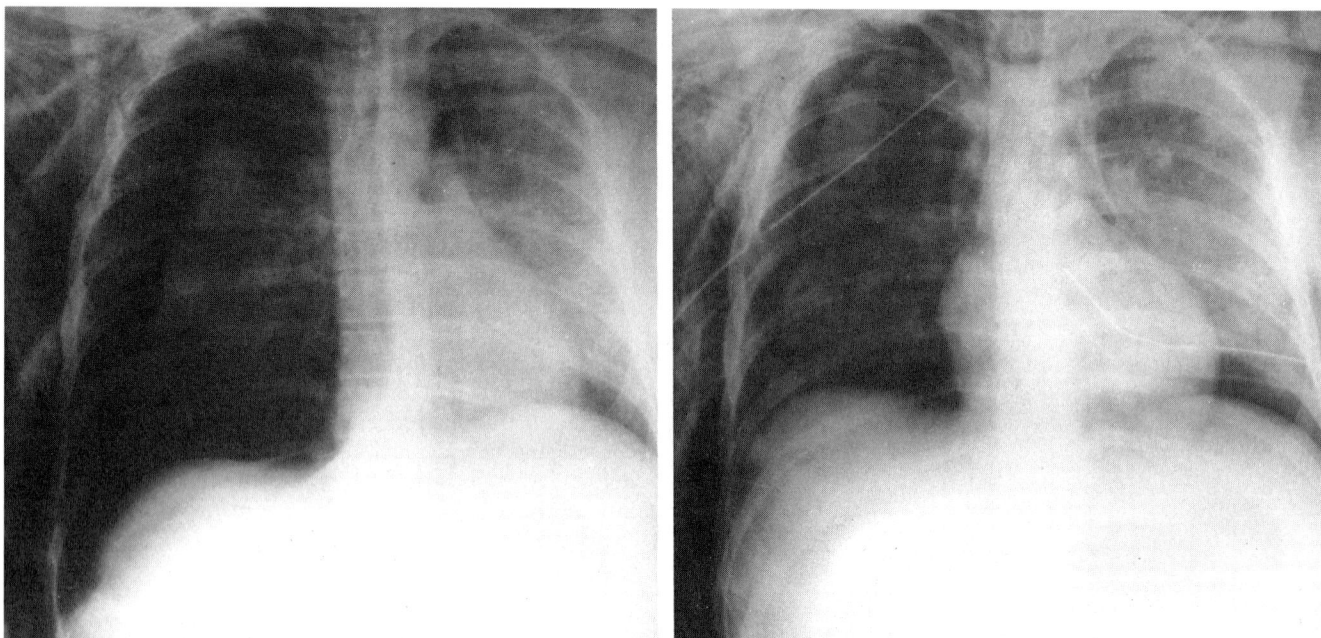

Figure 6   These x-rays are of a patient who was involved in a high-speed motor vehicle accident. His initial blood pressure was 90/60 mm Hg, and he was in respiratory distress. The initial chest x-ray (left) shows a right pneumothorax and a left hemothorax with pulmonary contusion. There is significant subcutaneous and mediastinal air. After bilateral tube thoracostomies, the chest x-ray shows persistent right pneumothorax (right); there was also a significant air leak through the chest tube. Bronchoscopy revealed disruption of the right mainstem bronchus, which was repaired.

associated with extensive parenchymal destruction of the lung and massive blood loss. In these hostile circumstances, rapid resection of the lobe or the entire lung is the only practical option.

Esophageal Injuries

Injuries to the upper thoracic esophagus are approached via a right posterolateral thoracotomy, and similar injuries to the lower esophagus are best approached through the same incision on the left side. Anterolateral thoracotomy provides suboptimal exposure of these injuries, and the thoracic esophagus is totally inaccessible when the chest is entered through a median sternotomy.

The key consideration in esophageal repair is timing. An early perforation (less than 12 to 24 hours old) is associated with minimal spillage into the adjacent mediastinum and is therefore amenable to primary repair. Late perforations are associated with a marked inflammatory response in the esophageal wall and the surrounding mediastinum, which makes primary repair unsafe or technically impossible. In these circumstances, excision and diversion are the only options. Although a 12- to 24-hour delay usually serves as the dividing line between early and late injuries, the final decision depends more on the amount of local inflammation and the feasibility of a sound closure than on arbitrary time limits.

Repair of an esophageal perforation is done in one or two layers, with the aim of obtaining a tension-free, watertight closure. It is important to maintain the suture line in a transverse orientation so as not to narrow the repaired segment. The repair is buttressed with nontraumatized adjacent tissue, such as a small intercostal muscle flap, a tongue of parietal pleura, or the gastric fundus (by means of a Thal patch or a Nissen fundoplication [*see 3:9 Open Esophageal Procedures*]). Wide mediastinal drainage with a large Argyle tube completes the repair.

Delayed operation for esophageal perforation employs the principles of proximal diversion and wide drainage to effectively control an inflamed and friable esophageal wall that will not hold sutures [*see Figure 9*]. The noninflamed intact esophagus above and below the injured segment is mobilized, encircled, and stapled with a linear stapler, and the area is widely drained. This step is then followed by laparotomy with construction of a gastrostomy and a feeding jejunostomy. The final step is the creation of a loop cervical esophagostomy into the left neck. Total exclusion and diversion (see above) will necessitate subsequent

---

Patient presents with penetration or laceration of lung, manifested by air leakage, hemothorax, or pneumothorax
Perform tube thoracostomy. Do not use trocar chest tubes.

Patient's lungs reexpand; air leakage is minimal to moderate; initial hemothorax is ≤ 1,200 ml; chest tube output is ≤ 300 ml/hr	Intubated patient on positive pressure ventilation exhibits sudden CNS and cardiac deterioration	Air leakage is massive; initial hemothorax is > 1,500 ml; chest tube output is > 300 ml/hr
Thoracotomy is unnecessary in 85% of cases.	Perform thoracotomy. Assess patient for air embolism.	Perform lateral thoracotomy and assess injury. Consider pulmonary tractotomy.

Figure 7   Algorithm illustrates evaluation and treatment of a patient with penetrations or lacerations of the lung.

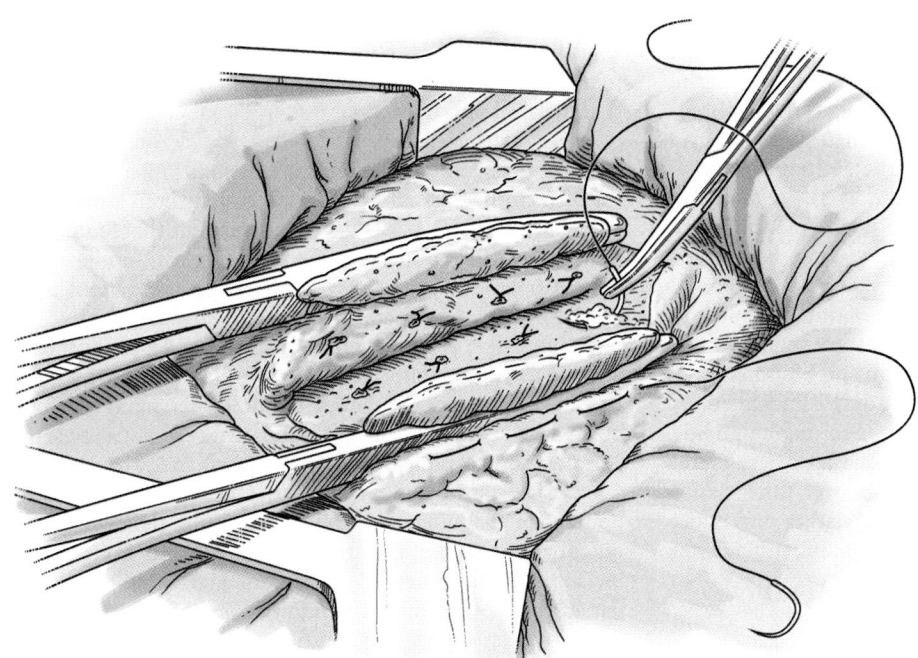

Figure 8 **Deep through-and-through pulmonary injuries that do not involve the hilum can be treated by means of pulmonary tractotomy, either with a linear GIA stapler or, as shown here, between two aortic clamps.**

esophageal resection and reconstruction using colon interposition. Thus, when the local situation allows and repair of the perforation is technically feasible, a less radical technical solution should be considered. The perforation may be repaired and temporarily excluded in continuity by means of Teflon band closure of the esophagogastric junction in conjunction with a lateral cervical esophagostomy. The decision to repair or exclude an esophageal injury is not based solely on the length of delay and the local inflammatory response. Even with early perforations, it is safer to exclude the esophageal injury when it is extensive or when other serious associated injuries are present.

Chest Wall Injuries

The most common source of ongoing bleeding into the pleural cavity is a lacerated intercostal or internal mammary artery. The keys to successful control of bleeding vessels in the chest wall are adequate exposure and ligation of the vessel on both sides of the injury (because each artery has a bidirectional blood supply).

Massive chest wall defects are uncommon and are usually associated with extensive underlying visceral damage. Chest wall reconstruction is a low priority in these circumstances and is therefore postponed until after the patient is stabilized. A myocutaneous flap based on the latissimus dorsi or on the pectoralis major muscle is the surgical solution for these wounds.

Surgical reduction and stabilization of the fractured sternum is indicated only when the fracture interferes with cardiac or pulmonary function or when the fractured segments override, sometimes producing a painful pseudoarthrosis. It is important to remember that a sternal fracture is often a marker of underlying visceral damage, which is the first priority.

Special Operative Considerations

Thoracic injuries involving more than one truncal visceral compartment present unique operative problems. Transmediastinal penetrations are serious injuries for which the diagnostic and operative approaches must be individualized. Whenever a transmediastinal penetration is suspected on the basis of the chest x-ray, the missile trajectory, or the clinical circumstances, injury to all three mediastinal components (i.e., heart, great vessels, and esophagus) must be ruled out. In hemodynamically unstable patients, this is done during operative exploration. However, an esophageal injury cannot be ruled out through a median sternotomy, which means that either a different incision or esophagoscopy is required. Penetrating great vessel injuries cause massive hemorrhage and immediately become the focus of clinical attention. Cardiac wounds, however, do not always present with a dramatic clinical picture and may be missed even during surgical exploration if the pericardium is not opened.

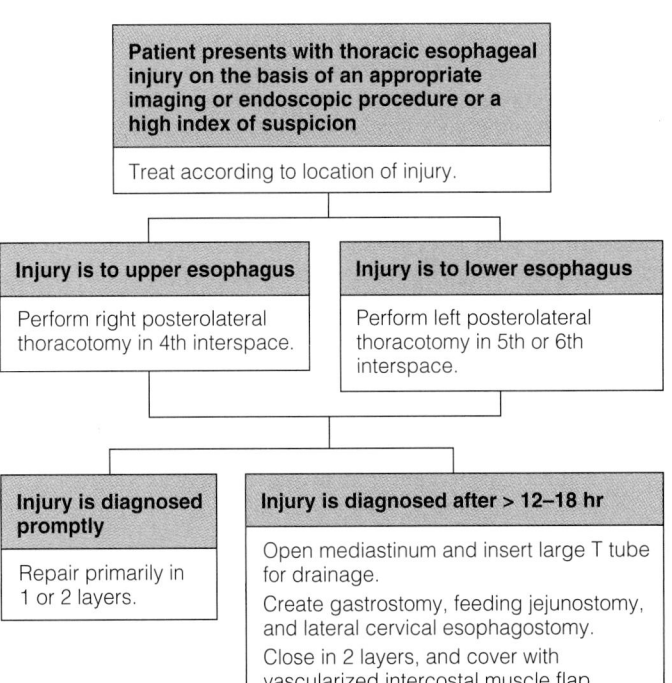

Figure 9 **Algorithm illustrates evaluation and treatment of a patient with thoracic esophageal injury.**

Thoracoabdominal injury is another type of trauma involving more than one truncal visceral compartment. Diaphragmatic lacerations discovered at celiotomy are repaired from within the abdomen after reduction of any herniated viscera. The diaphragmatic injury itself can be repaired from the chest as well, but a laparotomy is required for exploration of the abdominal cavity. Before transabdominal repair, the diaphragmatic laceration can be enlarged to permit limited visualization of the pleural space and lung on the injured side. The presence of blood in the pericardial space can be ruled out by performing a transabdominal subxiphoid pericardiotomy. However, the limited exposure yielded by this incision does not allow any further interventions if blood is found in the pericardial cavity; thus, if blood is present, an immediate left anterolateral thoracotomy is indicated.

Reduction and repair of a chronic traumatic diaphragmatic hernia are undertaken from the chest through a posterolateral thoracotomy. This route is preferred because over time, dense adhesions surround the herniated abdominal viscera and make transabdominal reduction and repair technically difficult or even impossible.

Damage Control Tactics

Rapid emergency surgical techniques are employed to abbreviate the operative procedure in critically injured patients who are rapidly approaching their physiologic limits. Hypothermic and coagulopathic patients are poor candidates for lengthy formal procedures, and temporary or unorthodox technical solutions to control bleeding, air leakage, and spillage are often employed in these patients. Formal anatomic repair either is postponed until after restitution of physiologic reserves postoperatively or is not performed at all.

Stapled nonanatomic lobectomy and pneumonectomy provide a rapid technical solution to exsanguinating hemorrhage from central lung injuries. The technique involves firing a wide linear stapler across the entire bronchovascular pedicle and subsequently oversewing any residual bleeding from the stump with a continuous Prolene suture. Pulmonary tractotomy and selective ligation (see above) are also useful for damage control. Under emergency conditions, the subclavian and innominate arteries are sometimes ligated and not reconstructed. Coagulopathic bleeding from soft tissue damage to the chest wall is packed, and the perforated esophagus is excluded by ligating the esophagus above and below the injured segment with cotton tapes. In extreme circumstances, formal closure of the chest is time-consuming and unnecessary; instead, only the skin is closed with a continuous heavy monofilament suture.

Postoperative Management

PRIMARY CONCERNS

The three major concerns in the immediate postoperative management of thoracic trauma are oxygenation, hypothermia, and bleeding.

The combination of pulmonary trauma, massive bleeding, and aggressive preoperative and intraoperative fluid administration translates into compromised oxygen delivery. Early insertion of a pulmonary arterial catheter is the key to maintaining adequate oxygenation in these circumstances. The physiologic insight provided by the pulmonary arterial catheter allows tailored support of preload, cardiac contractility, and afterload, as well as optimization of positive end-expiratory pressure (PEEP)

and fraction of inspired oxygen ($F_{I}O_2$). Every attempt is made to avoid fluid overload: because the posttraumatic lung exhibits a marked degree of capillary leakage, fluid overload is immediately translated into interstitial pulmonary congestion and adversely affects oxygenation.

All critically injured patients are hypothermic, and rapid reversal of hypothermia is therefore an urgent concern. Heat loss is especially severe in patients who underwent thoracotomy in conjunction with laparotomy and in patients who underwent a prolonged operative procedure. In the ICU, the patient is meticulously protected from additional conductive heat loss and undergoes aggressive active external rewarming. All intravenous fluids and blood components are warmed before they are administered. In selected patients with severe hypothermia, rapid correction can be achieved by means of continuous arteriovenous rewarming via percutaneous cannulation of the femoral artery and vein.

Massive transfusion and hypothermia contribute to the development of coagulopathy, which is clinically signaled by continuous oozing of blood into the chest tubes and from the surgical incisions. This coagulopathy is managed by rewarming the patient and by empirical administration of fresh frozen plasma and platelets; coagulation studies are unreliable in hypothermic patients. Continuous bleeding from the hemithorax that was operated on raises the question of reoperation. As a general rule, the first priority is always to correct hypothermia and coagulopathy first, leaving reoperation to be considered later if necessary.

A specific consideration in the postoperative chest trauma patient is that the cause of a sudden deterioration in oxygenation or hemodynamic collapse can often be found in the hemithorax that was operated on. Tension pneumothorax, cardiac tamponade, and systemic air embolism are three mechanisms of sudden cardiovascular collapse that call for immediate surgical action. If the patient also underwent a laparotomy and exhibits a sudden deterioration in oxygenation coupled with excessive inspiratory pressures, decreasing urinary output, and increased intra-abdominal pressure, the surgeon should suspect the abdominal compartment syndrome, and immediate decompression should be performed.

Misleading chest tube output is a major pitfall in the postoperative patient. Chest tubes often become clogged, are misplaced, or are incorrectly connected to the underwater seal and suction system. Whenever the chest tube output becomes a cause for concern, the tube and its connections should be examined closely for evidence of clogging, kinking, and misplacement. A chest x-ray should be obtained and the tube exchanged if it is felt that the tube is not functioning properly. A chest tube should always be removed when it is no longer functioning for the purpose of its insertion. In a patient undergoing mechanical ventilation after operation, a functioning chest tube is retained until the patient is weaned from positive-pressure ventilation.

The possibility of a missed injury should be considered whenever there is a deviation from the expected course of postoperative recovery. Unexplained bleeding and unexpected sepsis are the two most common manifestations that should prompt a diligent search for a missed injury. The two most common sites for missed thoracic injuries are the chest wall vessels (i.e., the intercostal and internal mammary arteries) and the heart. Missed injuries at either site call for urgent reoperation. Missed esophageal perforations are uncommon but devastating. They are managed with proximal diversion, drainage of the perforation, distal drainage of GI contents via a large tube gastrostomy, and creation of a feeding tube jejunostomy; total esophageal diversion is no longer considered an option.

Reoperation for thoracic trauma may be either planned or unplanned. Planned reoperation is performed in patients who underwent a damage control procedure and subsequent stabilization in the ICU. The aim of this reoperation is to perform definitive repairs and formal chest closure. It is undertaken only after correction of hypothermia and coagulopathy and after oxygen delivery has been optimized. Unplanned procedures are usually performed for bleeding and may have to be undertaken in the surgical ICU if the patient's condition is deteriorating rapidly. There are no firm quantitative guidelines for urgent reoperation, but generally speaking, reoperation should be considered in any patient whose postoperative bleeding markedly exceeds the surgeon's expectations. This decision should always be made by the surgeon who performed the initial thoracotomy.

SPECIFIC COMPLICATIONS

Pulmonary Complications

Persistent air leakage Patients on sustained PEEP or with elevated ventilatory pressures may exhibit persistent and at times high-volume air leaks. Often, increasing the negative pressure on the pleural space produces parietal and visceral pleura apposition that decreases the leakage. Sometimes, however, increased negative pressure actually increases leakage and leads to hypoxemia. On rare occasions, operative repair of a large torn lung or of a missed injury to a major bronchus is required. Operative repair should be undertaken only after the patient is off PEEP and has normal ventilatory pressures.

Retained clotted hemothorax and empyema Unevacuated or retained clotted hemothorax is an indication for early evacuation, often via thoracoscopy or thoracotomy. The minimally invasive option of video-assisted thoracoscopy [*see 3:11 Video-Assisted Thoracic Surgery*] is growing in popularity, but this option may be technically difficult or impossible when the clotted hemothorax is large or long-standing, in which case decortication through a formal thoracotomy is the safest course of action for the patient.

Effusion and empyema may occur because of undrained pleural fluid, undetected esophageal or pulmonary leakage, or sympathetic reaction to subdiaphragmatic conditions. Management of these conditions consists of early detection and drainage.

Systemic air embolism Systemic air embolism can occur with pulmonary parenchymal injury and increased intrabronchial pressure, creating a bronchopulmonary venous fistula. Sudden cerebral or cardiac insufficiency may be the initial sentinel clue that air has embolized to the coronary or cerebral vessels. Immediate prevention of further air embolism with possible removal of the intravascular air is a therapeutic goal. The mortality associated with this complication is high.

Cardiac Complications

Intracardiac shunts Left-to-right intracardiac shunts, which are manifested by continuous murmurs, are often found postoperatively. Detection may be aided by color Doppler imaging. Depending on the size of the fistula, closure of the fistula by means of operative or transvascular interventional techniques may be required.

Cardiac herniation Cardiac herniation can occur postoperatively in patients with a pericardium that has been only partially incised or incompletely repaired. It usually occurs when a patient is lying on the left side, and it is manifested by sudden hypotension and distended neck veins. Cardiac herniation is often reversible if the patient lies with the right side down. Management involves either pericardiorrhaphy or wider pericardectomy.

Pericardial effusion Pericardial effusion is a rare but important entity that arises after pericardiotomy or cardiorrhaphy. Such effusion may be sympathetic, chylous, reactive, or infectious. Diagnosis is made via echocardiography or a pericardial window. Such effusion may be part of a postpericardiotomy syndrome in some patients.

Complications of Great Vessel Repair

Paraplegia Paraplegia, the dreaded complication of thoracic aortic surgery, is the result of spinal cord ischemia, and there is currently no universally recognized preventive measure to reduce its incidence. Although ischemic myelopathy is most often apparent immediately after operation, it may occur as long as 5 days after surgery, suggesting other possible causes, such as spinal compartment syndrome and reperfusion injury.

False aneurysms False aneurysms occur at the site of undetected arterial injury or at vascular anastomotic sites. Some surgeons have recommended postoperative arteriograms in thoracic vascular reconstructions to establish a baseline study, whereas others obtain vascular images only when routine radiographs or symptoms suggest a posttraumatic false aneurysm. Delayed thoracic posttraumatic aneurysms frequently appear weeks or months after the injury rather than in the ICU. Depending on the location of the aneurysm, direct surgical repair is indicated. Stenting of both arteriovenous fistulas and traumatic false aneurysms with intraluminal stents is a modern therapeutic option.

Arteriovenous fistula Arteriovenous fistulas can occur in many thoracic locations (e.g., from one intercostal vessel to another, from the aorta to a pulmonary artery, or from a pulmonary artery to a pulmonary vein). The location of the last fistula listed may be the pulmonary parenchyma. Diagnosis is accomplished by means of arteriography, and treatment involves vascular reconstruction, occasionally after pulmonary resection.

Esophageal, Tracheal, and Diaphragmatic Complications

Breakdown of esophageal repair Penetrating injury to the thoracic esophagus repaired via an anterior thoracic incision has a 50% breakdown rate. Accordingly, it is recommended that a contrast esophagogram be performed before resumption of oral food intake in every patient who underwent an esophageal repair. When esophageal injury is discovered, it is best repaired via a posterior approach. Late esophageal leaks are handled as outlined earlier (see above).

Stenosis Tracheal or bronchial stenosis can occur from a missed injury, a constricted repair, or a buildup of granulation tissue around suture material at the site of a bronchial or tracheal repair. Suture-line granuloma is less common when absorbable suture material is used. When braided or polypropylene suture materials are used, the externally placed knots are often discovered to be intraluminal upon subsequent bronchoscopy.

Diaphragmatic hernia Acute diaphragmatic herniation is rare: the appearance of this condition is usually delayed for months or years. Diagnosis is aided by gastric or colonic contrast studies. Posttraumatic diaphragmatic hernias are repaired via a thoracic incision, whereas acute herniations are approached via an abdominal incision.

Chest Wall Complications

Chylothorax An uncommon but worrisome occurrence, chylothorax usually becomes manifest on postinjury days 3 to 7. Conservative therapy involves either intravenous alimentation or enteral feedings with medium-chain triglycerides. To assist in the localization of persistent chylous leaks, olive oil can be administered into the GI tract before or during operation.

Causalgia Posttraumatic causalgia, or reflex sympathetic dystrophy, may be caused by a partial injury to a peripheral nerve. Causalgia is also common after a so-called trap-door thoracotomy and is occasionally seen when a median sternotomy is opened very widely. Management is conservative and is based on the patient's response to physical therapy and stellate ganglion blocks. Occasionally, dorsal sympathectomy is required.

Intercostal pain Intercostal radicular pain is common after a lateral thoracotomy. Such pain can frequently be controlled by means of analgesics and intercostal nerve blocks initially, but it can be disabling if it becomes chronic. Use of permanent suture material for pericostal sutures during rib reapproximation contributes to radicular pain as the intercostal nerve becomes entrapped. Symptoms may be lessened by permanent intercostal nerve ablation.

Chondritis Thoracoabdominal incisions across the chondral border in trauma patients often give rise to chronic chondritis. This painful condition may be due to devascularization of the cartilaginous structures as a result of necrosis or infection. It is best treated by placing a muscle flap into the area after adequate debridement.

Recommended Reading

RESUSCITATIVE THORACOTOMY

Champion HR, Sykes L: Emergency room thoracotomy. Trauma Surgery, Part 1, 4th ed. Champion HR, Robbs JV, Trunkey DD, Eds. Butterworth & Co, London, 1989, p 70

Feliciano DV, Bitondo CG, Cruse PA, et al: Liberal use of emergency center thoracotomy. Am J Surg 152:654, 1986

Shannon FL, Moore EE, Moore JB: Emergency department thoracotomy. Trauma. Mattox KL, Moore EE, Feliciano DV, Eds. Appleton & Lange, Norwalk, Connecticut, 1988, p 175

CHOICE OF INCISION

Mattox KL: Indications for thoracotomy: deciding to operate. Surg Clin North Am 69:47, 1989

Mattox KL: Thoracic injury requiring surgery. World J Surg 7:47, 1982

Pickard LR, Mattox KL: Thoracic trauma and indications for thoracotomy. Trauma. Mattox KL, Moore EE, Feliciano DV, Eds. Appleton & Lange, Norwalk, Connecticut, 1988, p 315

CARDIAC INJURIES

Mattox KL, Beal AC Jr, Jordan GL Jr, et al: Cardiorrhaphy in the emergency center. J Thorac Cardiovasc Surg 68:886, 1974

Mitchell ME, Muakkassa FF, Poole GV, et al: Surgical approach of choice for penetrating cardiac wounds. J Trauma 34:17, 1993

Symbas PN: Cardiothoracic Trauma. WB Saunders Co, Philadelphia, 1989, p 300

AORTIC INJURIES

Mattox KL: Red River Anthology. J Trauma 42:353, 1997

Mattox KL, Holzman M, Pickard LR, et al: Clamp-repair: a safe technique for treatment of blunt injury to the descending thoracic aorta. Ann Thorac Surg 40:456, 1985

Mattox KL, Wall MJ Jr, Hirshberg A: Traumatic aneurysm of the thoracic aorta. Aneurysms—New Findings and Treatments. Yao JST, Pearce WH, Eds. Appleton & Lange, Norwalk, Connecticut, 1994, p 207

von Oppell UO, Dunne TT, De Groot MK, et al: Traumatic aortic rupture: twenty-year metaanalysis of mortality and risk of paraplegia. Ann Thorac Surg 58:585, 1994

THE EXTRAPERICARDIAL VESSELS

Brawley RK, Murray GF, Crisler C, et al: Management of wounds of the innominate, subclavian and axillary blood vessels. Surg Gynecol Obstet 148:1130, 1970

Graham JM, Feliciano DV, Mattox KL: Management of subclavian vascular injuries. J Trauma 20:537, 1980

Johnston RH, Wall MJ Jr, Mattox KL: Innominate artery trauma: a thirty year experience. J Vasc Surg 17:134, 1993

MAJOR AIRWAY DISRUPTION

Symbas PN: Cardiothoracic trauma. Curr Probl Surg 28:747, 1991

Urschel HC, Razzuk MA: Management of acute traumatic injuries of tracheobronchial tree. Surg Gynecol Obstet 136:113, 1973

PULMONARY LACERATIONS

Wall MJ Jr, Hirshberg A, Mattox KL: Pulmonary tractotomy with selective vascular ligation for penetrating injuries to the lung. Am J Surg 168:665, 1994

Weincek RG Jr, Wilson RF: Central lung injuries: a need for early vascular control. J Trauma 28:1418, 1988

ESOPHAGEAL INJURIES

Cheadle W, Richardson JD: Options in management of trauma to the esophagus. Surg Gynecol Obstet 155:380, 1982

Defore WW Jr, Mattox KL, Hansen HA, et al: Surgical management of penetrating injuries of the esophagus. Am J Surg 134:734, 1977

CHEST WALL INJURIES

Pate JW: Chest wall injuries. Surg Clin North Am 69:59, 1989

DAMAGE CONTROL TACTICS

Hirshberg A, Wall MJ Jr, Mattox KL: Planned reoperation for trauma: a two year experience with 124 consecutive patients. J Trauma 37:365, 1994

POSTOPERATIVE MANAGEMENT

Hirshberg A, Wall MJ Jr, Ramchandani MK, et al: Reoperation for bleeding in trauma. Arch Surg 128:1163, 1993

Acknowledgments

Figures 1 and 8 Tom Moore. Adapted from original illustrations provided by the Baylor College of Medicine.

Figures 2, 4, 7, and 9 Marcia Kammerer.

Figures 3 and 5 Carol Donner.

6 INJURIES TO THE LIVER, BILIARY TRACT, SPLEEN, AND DIAPHRAGM

Jon M. Burch, M.D., F.A.C.S., and Ernest E. Moore, M.D., F.A.C.S.

Assessment and Management of Injuries to the Liver, Biliary Tract, Spleen, and Diaphragm

Injuries to the Liver

ASSESSMENT

The initial step in the management of penetrating abdominal injuries and of blunt abdominal injuries in cases when nonoperative treatment is contraindicated or has failed is exploratory laparotomy [*see 5:8 Operative Exposure of Abdominal Injuries and Closure of the Abdomen*].

Visualization of the right lobe of the liver is hindered by the lobe's posterior attachments and by the right lower costal margin. Exposure of the right lobe is facilitated by elevating the right costal margin with a large Richardson retractor. Further exposure can be achieved with mobilization, which requires division of the right triangular and coronary ligaments. In dividing the superior coronary ligament, care must be taken not to injure the lateral wall of the right hepatic vein; in dividing the inferior coronary ligament, care must be taken not to injure the right adrenal gland (which is vulnerable because it lies directly beneath the peritoneal reflection) or the retrohepatic vena cava. When the ligaments have been divided, the right lobe of the liver can be rotated medially into the surgical field. Mobilization of the left lobe poses no unusual problems other than the risk of injury to the left hepatic vein, the left inferior phrenic vein, and the retrohepatic vena cava.

If optimal exposure of the junction of the hepatic veins and the retrohepatic vena cava is necessary, the midline abdominal incision can be extended by means of a median sternotomy. The pericardium and the diaphragm can then be divided toward the center of the inferior vena cava. This combination of incisions provides superb exposure of the hepatic veins and the retrohepatic vena cava while avoiding injury to the phrenic nerves.

The American Association for the Surgery of Trauma's Committee on Organ Injury Scaling has developed a grading system for classifying injuries to the liver [*see Table 1 and Figure 1*].[1] Hepatic injuries are graded on a scale of I to VI, with I representing superficial lacerations and small subcapsular hematomas and VI representing avulsion of the liver from the vena cava. Isolated injuries that are not extensive (grades I to III) often require little or no treatment; however, extensive parenchymal injuries and those involving the juxtahepatic veins (grades IV and V) may require complex maneuvers for successful treatment, and hepatic avulsion (grade VI) is lethal.

Clamping of the hepatic pedicle—the Pringle maneuver—is a helpful technique for evaluating grade IV and V hepatic injuries

[*see Figure 2*]. This maneuver allows one to distinguish between hemorrhage from branches of the hepatic artery or the portal vein, which ceases when the clamp is applied, and hemorrhage from the hepatic veins or the retrohepatic vena cava, which does not. When performing the Pringle maneuver, we prefer to tear the lesser omentum manually and place the clamp from the left side while guiding the posterior blade of the clamp through the foramen of Winslow with the aid of the left index finger. The advantages of this approach are the avoidance of injury to the structures within the hepatic pedicle, the assurance that the clamp will be properly placed the first time, and the inclusion of a replacing or accessory left hepatic artery between the blades of the clamp.

MANAGEMENT OF INJURIES

Techniques for Temporary Control of Hemorrhage

Temporary control of hemorrhage is essential for two reasons. First, during treatment of a major hepatic injury, ongoing hemorrhage may pose an immediate threat to the patient's life, and temporary control gives the anesthesiologist time to restore the circulating volume before further blood loss occurs. Second, multiple bleeding sites are common with both blunt and penetrating trauma, and if the liver is not the highest priority, temporary control of hepatic bleeding allows repair of other injuries without unnecessary blood loss. The most useful techniques for the temporary control of hepatic hemorrhage are manual compression, perihepatic packing, and the Pringle maneuver.

Periodic manual compression with the addition of laparotomy pads is useful in the treatment of complex hepatic injuries to provide time for resuscitation [*see Figure 3*].[2-4]

Perihepatic packing with carefully placed laparotomy pads is capable of controlling hemorrhage from almost all hepatic injuries.[5-9] The right costal margin is elevated, and the pads are strategically placed over and around the bleeding site [*see Figure 4*]. Additional pads may be placed between the liver and the diaphragm and between the liver and the anterior chest wall until the bleeding has been controlled. Ten to 15 pads may be required to control the hemorrhage from an extensive right lobar injury. Packing is not as effective for injuries of the left lobe, because with the abdomen open, there is insufficient abdominal and thoracic wall anterior to the left lobe to provide adequate compression. Fortunately, hemorrhage from the left lobe can be controlled by dividing the left triangular and coronary ligaments and compress-

Table 1 AAST Organ Injury Scales for Liver, Biliary Tract, Diaphragm, and Spleen

Injured Structure	AAST Grade	Characteristics of Injury	AIS-90 Score
Liver*	I	Hematoma: subcapsular, nonexpanding, < 10% surface area	2
		Laceration: capsular tear, nonbleeding, < 1 cm parenchymal depth	2
	II	Hematoma: subcapsular, nonexpanding, 10%–50% surface area; intraparenchymal, nonexpanding, < 10 cm in diameter	2
		Laceration: capsular tear, active bleeding, 1–3 cm parenchymal depth, < 10 cm in length	2
	III	Hematoma: subcapsular, > 50% surface area, expanding; ruptured subcapsular hematoma with active bleeding; intraparenchymal, > 10 cm or expanding	3
		Laceration: > 3 cm parenchymal depth	3
	IV	Hematoma: ruptured intraparenchymal hematoma with active bleeding	4
		Laceration: parenchymal disruption involving 25%–75% of hepatic lobe or 1–3 Couinaud's segments within a single lobe	4
	V	Laceration: parenchymal disruption involving > 75% of hepatic lobe or > 3 Couinaud's segments within a single lobe	5
		Vascular: juxtahepatic venous injuries (i.e., injuries to retrohepatic vena cava or central major hepatic veins)	5
	VI	Vascular: hepatic avulsion	5
Extrahepatic biliary tree*	I	Gallbladder contusion/hematoma	2
		Portal triad contusion	2
	II	Partial gallbladder avulsion from liver bed; cystic duct intact	2
		Laceration or perforation of gallbladder	2
	III	Complete gallbladder avulsion from liver bed	3
		Cystic duct laceration	3
	IV	Partial or complete right or left hepatic duct laceration	3
		Partial common hepatic duct or common bile duct laceration (< 50%)	3
	V	> 50% transection of common hepatic duct or common bile duct	3–4
		Combined right and left hepatic duct injuries	3–4
		Intraduodenal or intrapancreatic bile duct injuries	3–4
Diaphragm†	I	Contusion	2
	II	Laceration < 2 cm	3
	III	Laceration 2–10 cm	3
	IV	Laceration > 10 cm, with tissue loss < 25 cm²	3
	V	Laceration with tissue loss > 25 cm²	3
Spleen*	I	Hematoma: subcapsular, nonexpanding, < 10% surface area	2
		Laceration: capsular tear, nonbleeding, < 1 cm parenchymal depth	2
	II	Hematoma: subcapsular, nonexpanding, 10%–50% surface area; intraparenchymal, nonexpanding, < 5 cm in diameter	2
		Laceration: capsular tear, active bleeding, 1–3 cm parenchymal depth, not involving a trabecular vessel	2
	III	Hematoma: subcapsular, > 50% surface area or expanding; ruptured subcapsular hematoma with active bleeding; intraparenchymal, > 5 cm or expanding	3
		Laceration: > 3 cm parenchymal depth or involving trabecular vessels	3
	IV	Hematoma: ruptured intraparenchymal hematoma with active bleeding	4
		Laceration: laceration involving segmental or hilar vessels producing major devascularization (> 25% of spleen)	4
	V	Laceration: completely shattered spleen	5
		Vascular: hilar vascular injury that devascularizes spleen	5

*Advance one grade for multiple injuries, up to grade III.
†Advance one grade for bilateral injuries, up to grade III.
AAST—American Association for the Surgery of Trauma

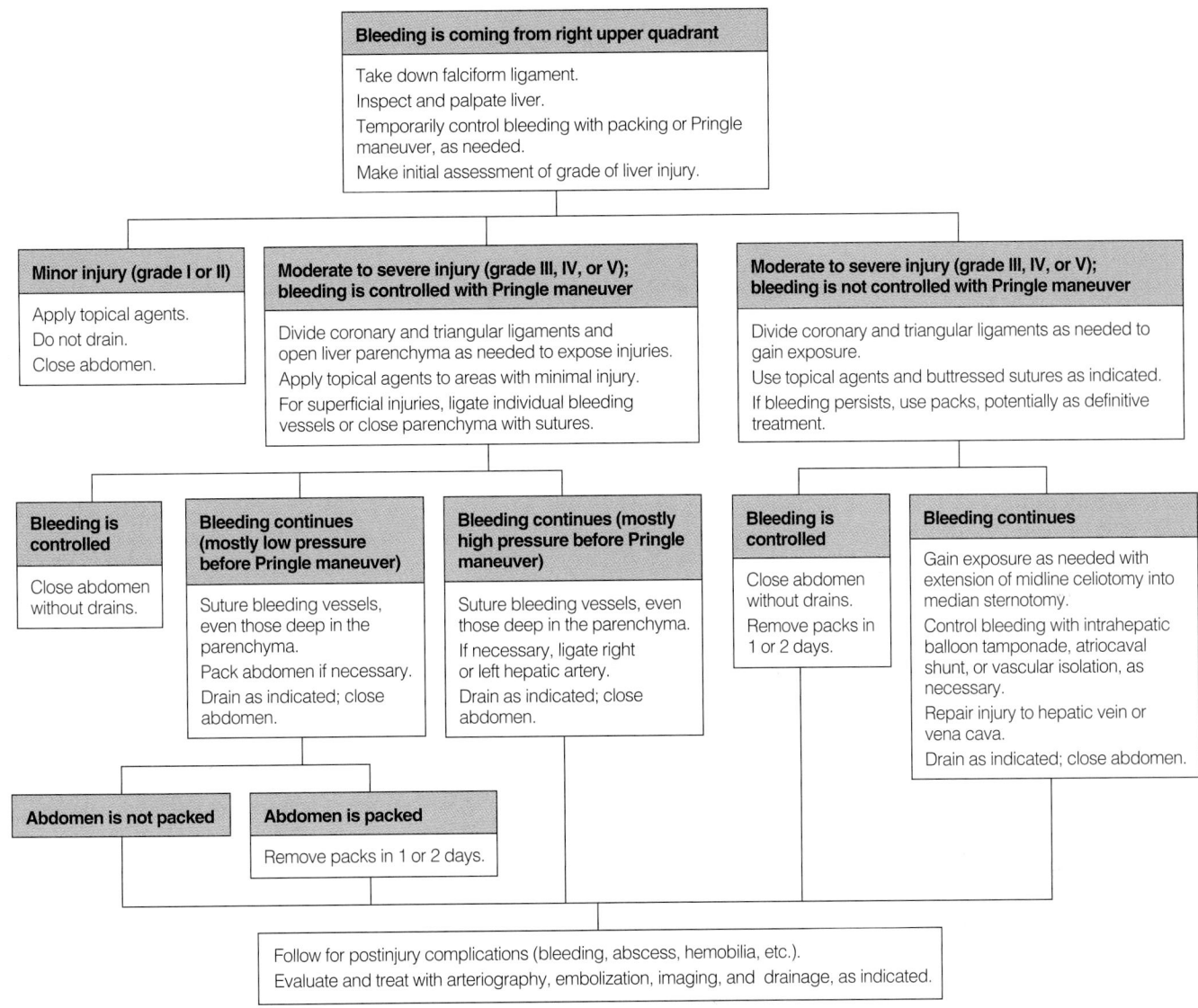

Figure 1 **Shown is an algorithm for the treatment of hepatic injuries.**

ing the lobe between the hands. Two complications may be encountered with the packing of hepatic injuries. First, tight packing compresses the inferior vena cava, decreases venous return, and reduces left ventricular filling; hypovolemic patients may not tolerate the resultant decrease in cardiac output. Second, perihepatic packing forces the right diaphragm superiorly and impairs its motion; this may lead to increased airway pressures and decreased tidal volume. Careful consideration of the patient's condition is necessary to determine whether the risk of these complications outweighs the risk of additional blood loss.

The Pringle maneuver is often used as an adjunct to packing for the temporary control of hemorrhage.[3] Over the years, the length of time for which surgeons believe a Pringle maneuver can be maintained without causing irreversible ischemic damage to the liver has increased. Several authors have documented the maintenance of a Pringle maneuver for longer than 1 hour in patients with complex injuries, without appreciable hepatic damage.[4,10] When a life-threatening hepatic injury is encountered on entry into the abdomen, the Pringle maneuver should be performed immediately and perihepatic packs placed. This combination of techniques should eliminate all hepatopetal blood flow and control retrograde venous bleeding.

Another technique for temporary control of hepatic hemorrhage is the application of a tourniquet or a liver clamp.[11] Once the bleeding lobe is mobilized, a 2.5 cm Penrose drain is wrapped around the liver near the anatomic division between the left lobe and the right. The drain is stretched until hemorrhage ceases, and tension is maintained by clamping the drain. Unfortunately, tourniquets are difficult to use: they tend to slip off or tear through the parenchyma if placed over an injured area. An alternative is the use of a liver clamp; however, the application of such devices is hindered by the variability in the size and shape of the liver.

Juxtahepatic venous injuries are technically challenging and often lethal. Complex procedures may be required for temporary control of these large veins. Of these procedures, the most important are hepatic vascular isolation with clamps, placement of the atriocaval shunt, and use of the Moore-Pilcher balloon.

Hepatic vascular isolation is accomplished by executing a Pringle maneuver, clamping the aorta at the diaphragm, and clamping the suprarenal and suprahepatic vena cava.[12] In patients scheduled for elective procedures, this technique has enjoyed nearly uniform success, but in trauma patients, the results have been disappointing. The relative ineffectiveness of hepatic vascular isolation with clamps in this setting is presumably due to the inability of a patient

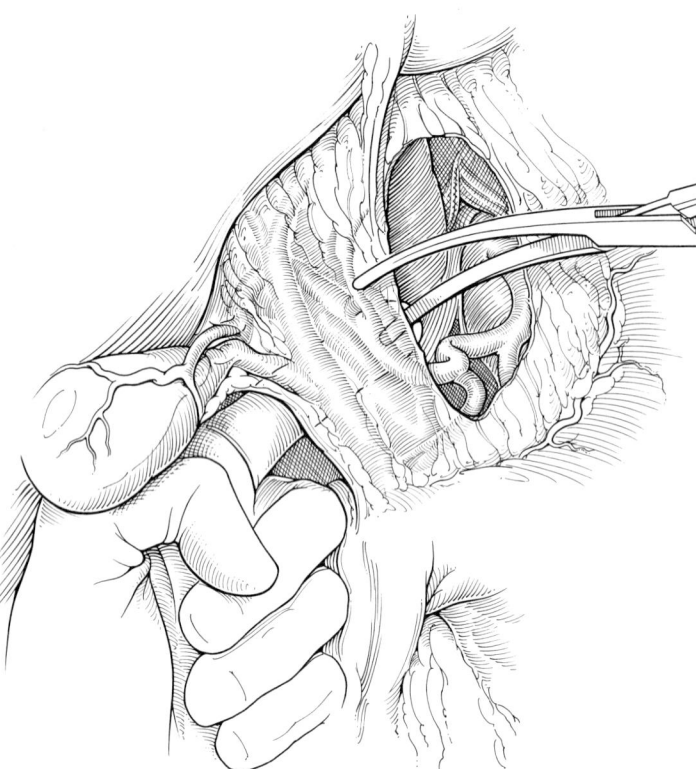

Figure 2 **The Pringle maneuver controls arterial and portal vein hemorrhage from the liver. Any hemorrhage that continues must come from the hepatic veins.**

in shock to tolerate an acute reduction in left ventricular filling pressure; on occasion, sudden death has occurred on placement of the venous clamps.[13] If, however, a trauma patient requiring hepatic vascular isolation has been maintained in a relatively normal physiologic condition, it is reasonable to consider this method.

A new approach to exposure of complex injuries to the retrohepatic vena cava and the hepatic veins has recently been developed.[14] Vascular isolation of the liver is achieved by means of the clamping technique, and the suprahepatic vena cava is divided between vascular clamps. The liver and the suprahepatic vena cava are then rotated anteriorly to provide direct access to the posterior aspect of the retrohepatic vena cava. Anterior injuries of the large veins are repaired through an incision in the posterior aspect of the retrohepatic vena cava.

The atriocaval shunt was designed to achieve hepatic vascular isolation while still permitting some venous blood from below the diaphragm to flow through the shunt into the right atrium.[4] After a few early successes, the initial enthusiasm for the atriocaval shunt declined as high mortalities associated with its use began to be reported.[15-20] Surgeons' lack of familiarity with the technique; manipulation of a cold, acidotic heart; and poor patient selection have all contributed to the poor overall results.[13] A variation on the original atriocaval shunt has been described in which a 9 mm endotracheal tube is substituted for the usual large chest tube [see *Figure 5*].[21] The balloon of the endotracheal tube makes it unnecessary to surround the suprarenal vena cava with an umbilical tape. This minor change eliminates one of the most difficult maneuvers required for the original shunt procedure: because hemorrhage must be controlled by posterior pressure on the liver during the insertion of the shunt, access to the suprarenal vena cava is severely restricted, and thus, surrounding this vessel with an umbilical tape is almost impossible. A side hole must be cut in the

tube to allow blood to enter the right atrium. Care must be taken to avoid damage to the integral inflation channel for the balloon.

An alternative to the atriocaval shunt is the Moore-Pilcher balloon.[22] This device is inserted through the femoral vein and advanced into the retrohepatic vena cava. When the balloon is properly positioned and inflated, it occludes the hepatic veins and the vena cava, thus achieving vascular isolation. The catheter itself is hollow, and appropriately placed holes below the balloon permit blood to flow into the right atrium, in much the same way as the atriocaval shunt. At present, the survival rate for patients with juxtahepatic venous injuries who are treated with this device is similar to that for patients treated with the atriocaval shunt.[18]

Surgeons who attempt hepatic vascular isolation should be aware that none of these techniques provide complete hemostasis. Drainage from the right adrenal vein and the inferior phrenic veins and persistent hepatopetal flow resulting from unrecognized replacing or accessory left hepatic arteries contribute to this problem. The relatively small volume of blood that continues to flow after vascular isolation is readily removed by means of suction.

An adjunct to vascular isolation with clamps is venovenous bypass. This technique provides vascular decompression for the small bowel and maintains high cardiac filling pressures, which are often necessary. Venovenous bypass is accomplished by placing catheters in the inferior vena cava via the femoral vein and in the superior mesenteric vein via the inferior mesenteric vein. A centrifugal pump withdraws blood from these veins and pumps it into the superior vena cava through a third catheter placed in the jugular vein.

Techniques for Definitive Management of Injuries

Techniques available for the definitive management of hepatic injuries range from manual compression to hepatic transplantation. Grade I or II lacerations of the hepatic parenchyma can generally be controlled with manual compression. If these injuries do not respond to manual compression, they can often be controlled with topical hemostatic measures.

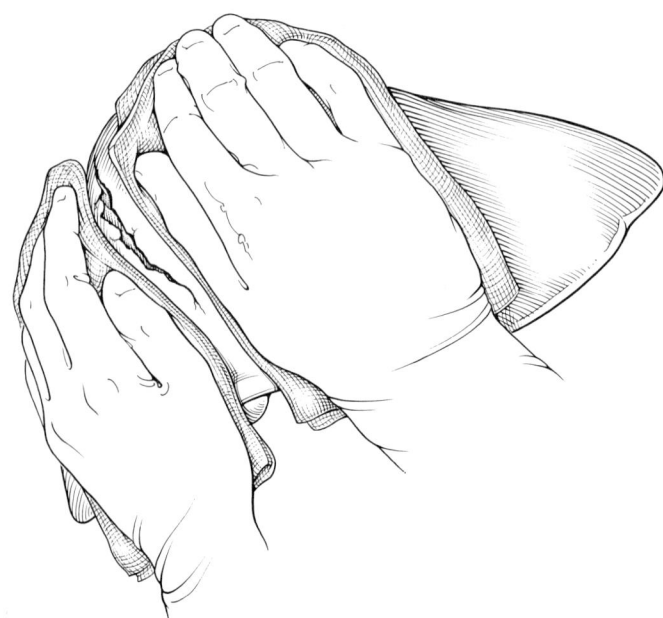

Figure 3 **Manual compression of large hepatic injuries temporarily controls blood loss in hypovolemic patients until the circulating blood volume can be restored.**

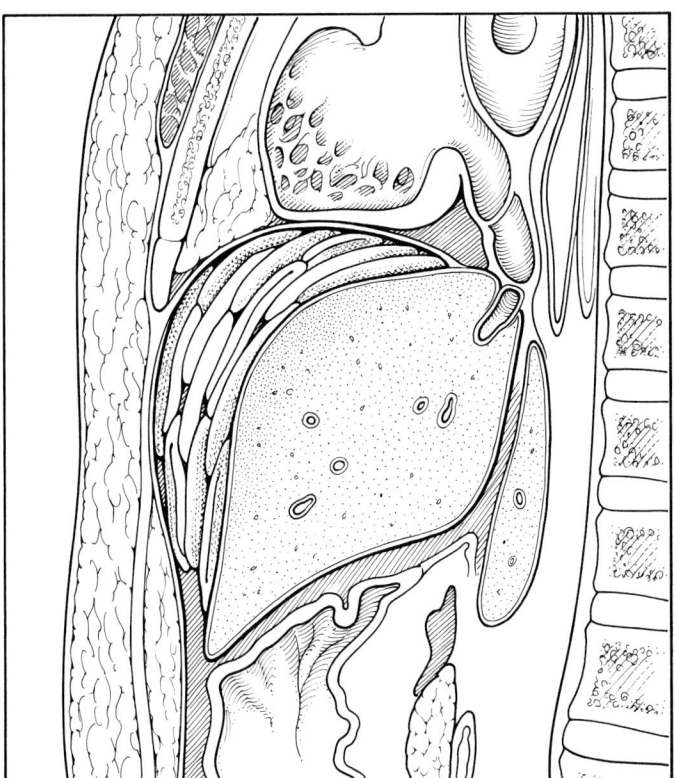

Figure 4 **Perihepatic packing is often effective in managing extensive parenchymal injuries. It has also been successfully employed for grade V juxtahepatic venous injuries.**

The simplest of these measures is electrocauterization, which can often control small bleeding vessels near the surface of the liver (though the machine's power output may have to be increased). Bleeding from raw surfaces of the liver that does not respond to the electrocautery may respond to the argon beam coagulator. This device imparts less heat to the surrounding hepatic tissue and creates a more consistent eschar, which enhances hemostasis. Also useful in similar situations is microcrystalline collagen in the powdered form. The powder is placed on a clean 10 × 10 cm sponge and applied directly to the oozing surface, with pressure maintained on the sponge for 5 to 10 minutes. Thrombin can also be applied topically to minor bleeding injuries by saturating either a gelatin foam sponge or a microcrystalline collagen pad and pressing it to the bleeding site.

Fibrin glue has been used in treating both superficial and deep lacerations and appears to be the most effective topical agent. It can also be injected deep into bleeding gunshot and stab wound tracts to prevent extensive dissection and blood loss. Fibrin glue is made by mixing concentrated human fibrinogen (cryoprecipitate) with a solution containing bovine thrombin and calcium. Because a coagulum forms quickly, the fibrinogen and the thrombin-calcium solution are placed in separate syringes joined with a Y connector, so that they are not mixed until immediately before application. Spray-on applicators have also been used. Topical hemostasis with fibrin glue became very popular after the publication of reports of large series of patients with serious hepatic injuries that were successfully managed with this material.[2,23,24] The initial enthusiasm, however, was tempered by subsequent reports of fatal anaphylactic reactions and hypotension temporally related to the application of fibrin glue.[25,26] The current role of this agent in the treatment of hepatic injuries remains to be defined.[27]

Although some grade III and IV lacerations respond to topical measures, many do not. In these instances, one option is to suture the hepatic parenchyma. Although this hemostatic technique has been maligned as a cause of hepatic necrosis, it still is frequently used.[3,4,10,17,28,29] Suturing of the hepatic parenchyma is often employed to control persistently bleeding lacerations less than 3 cm in depth; it is also an appropriate alternative for deeper lacerations if the patient cannot tolerate the further hemorrhage associated with hepatotomy and selective ligation. If, however, the capsule of the liver has been stripped away by the injury, this technique is far less effective.

The preferred suture material is 0 or 2-0 chromic catgut attached to a large, blunt-tipped, curved needle; the large diameter prevents the suture from pulling through Glisson's capsule. For shallow lacerations, a simple continuous suture may be used to approximate the edges of the laceration. For deeper lacerations, interrupted horizontal mattress sutures may be placed parallel to the edges. When tying sutures, one may be sure that adequate tension has been achieved when hemorrhage ceases or the liver blanches around the suture.

Most sources of venous hemorrhage can be managed with parenchymal sutures. Even injuries to the retrohepatic vena cava and the hepatic veins have been successfully tamponaded by

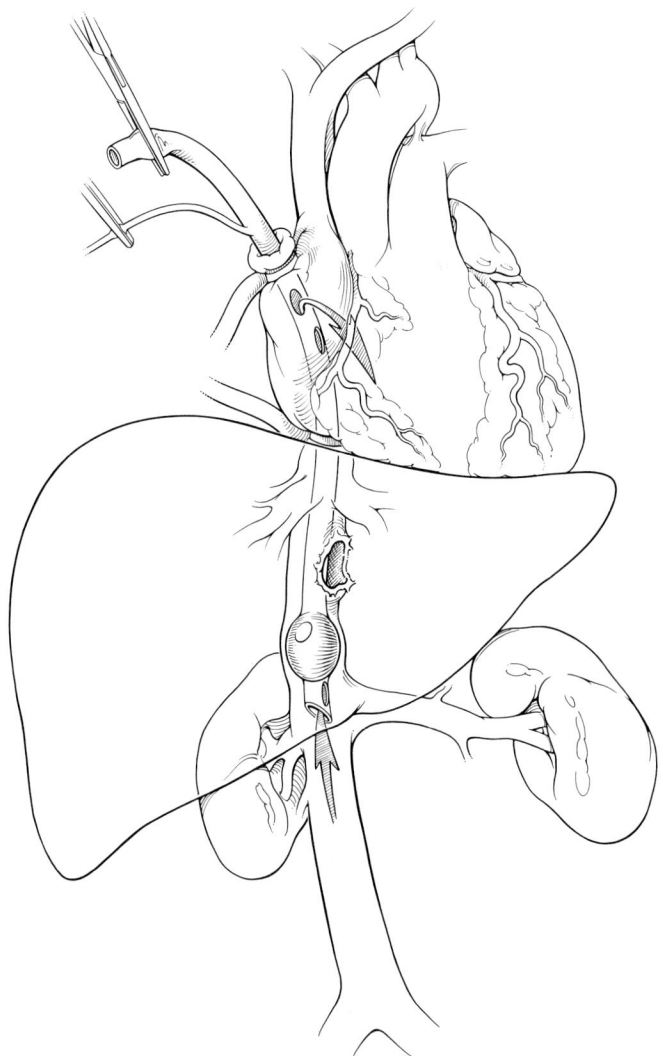

Figure 5 **Shown is a method of achieving hepatic vascular isolation with a 9 mm endotracheal tube.**

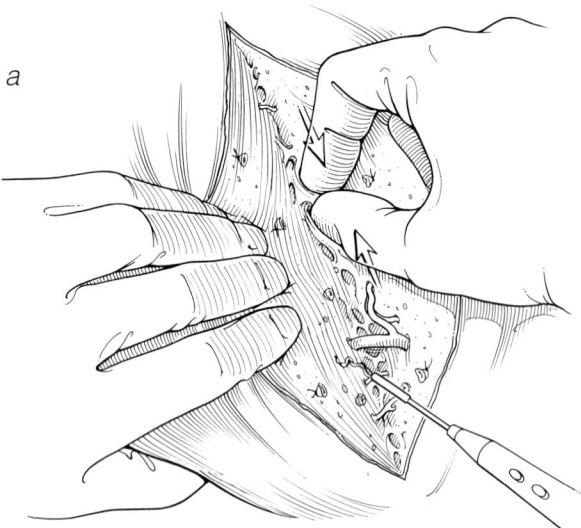

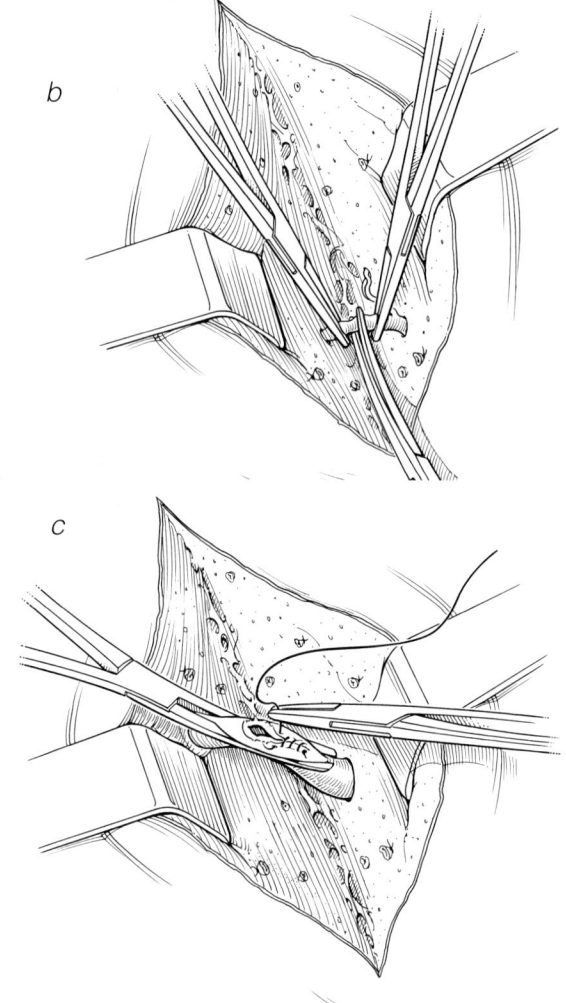

Figure 6 **Hepatotomy with selective ligation is an important technique for controlling hemorrhage from deep (usually penetrating) lacerations. This technique includes finger fracture to extend the length and depth of the wound (*a*), division of vessels or ducts encountered (*b*), and repair of any injuries to major veins (*c*).**

closing the hepatic parenchyma over the bleeding vessels.[13,30] Venous hemorrhage caused by penetrating wounds traversing the central portion of the liver may be managed by closing the entrance and exit wounds with interrupted horizontal mattress sutures. Although this measure may lead to the formation of intrahepatic hematomas that may then become infected, the risk is reasonable compared with the risks posed by an intracaval shunt or a deep hepatotomy. Still, suturing of the hepatic parenchyma is not always successful in controlling hemorrhage, particularly hemorrhage from the larger branches of the hepatic artery. If it fails, one must acknowledge the failure promptly and remove the sutures so that the wound can be explored.

Hepatotomy with selective ligation of bleeding vessels is an important technique that is usually reserved for deep or transhepatic penetrating wounds. Most authorities prefer it to parenchymal suturing[3,4,10,31,32]; some even favor it over placement of an atriocaval shunt for exposure and repair of juxtahepatic venous injuries.[20] The finger-fracture technique is used to extend the length and depth of a laceration or a missile tract until the bleeding vessels can be identified and controlled [*see Figure 6*]. It should be remembered that considerable blood loss may be incurred with the division of viable hepatic tissue in the pursuit of bleeding from deep penetrating wounds.

An adjunct to parenchymal suturing or hepatotomy is the use of the omentum to fill large defects in the liver and to buttress hepatic sutures. The rationale for this use of the omentum is that it provides an excellent source for macrophages and fills a potential dead space with viable tissue.[33] In addition, the omentum can provide a little extra support for parenchymal sutures, often enough to prevent them from cutting through Glisson's capsule.

Hepatic arterial ligation may be appropriate for patients with arterial hemorrhage from deep within the liver[34]; however, it plays only a limited role in the overall treatment of hepatic injuries, because it does not stop hemorrhage from the portal and hepatic venous systems.[35] Its primary role is in the management of deep lobar injuries when application of the Pringle maneuver results in the cessation of arterial hemorrhage. If the bleeding from the wound stops once the left or right hepatic artery is isolated and clamped, hepatic arterial ligation is a reasonable alternative to deep hepatotomy. Generally, ligation of the right or left hepatic artery is well tolerated; however, ligation of the proper hepatic artery (distal to the origin of the gastroduodenal artery) may produce hepatic necrosis.[36]

An alternative to suturing the entrance and exit wounds of a transhepatic penetrating injury or to performing an extensive hepatotomy is the use of an intrahepatic balloon.[37] These devices are hand-crafted by the surgeon in the OR. One method of fashioning such a device is to tie a 2.5 cm Penrose drain to a hollow catheter [*see Figure 7*]. The balloon is then inserted into the bleeding wound and inflated with a soluble contrast agent. If the hemorrhage is controlled, a stopcock or clamp is used to occlude the catheter and maintain the inflation. (It should be noted that the balloon catheter may not be able to generate sufficient intraparenchymal pressure to tamponade major arterial hemorrhage.) The balloon is left in the abdomen and removed at a subsequent operation after 24 to 48 hours. The hemorrhage may recur when the balloon is deflated.

Resectional debridement is indicated for peripheral portions of nonviable hepatic parenchyma. Except in rare circumstances, the amount of tissue removed should not exceed 25% of the liver. Resectional debridement is performed by means of the finger-fracture technique and is appropriate for selected patients with grade III to grade V lacerations. Because additional blood loss occurs during removal of nonviable tissue, this procedure should be reserved for patients who are in sound physiologic condition and can tolerate additional blood loss.

Perihepatic packing is the most significant advance in the treatment of hepatic injuries to occur in the past 20 years. The practice of packing hepatic injuries is not a new one, but the concepts and techniques associated with it have changed. In the past, liver lacerations were packed with yards of gauze, and one end of the gauze strip was brought out of the abdomen through a separate stab wound[38]; the remainder of the gauze was then teased out of the wound over a period of days. Unfortunately, this approach often led to abdominal infection and failed to control the hemorrhage, and as a result, it eventually fell from favor. The current approach is not to place packing material in the laceration itself but rather to place it over and around the injury to compress the wound by compressing the liver between the anterior chest wall, the diaphragm, and the retroperitoneum.[5-9] The abdomen is closed, and the patient is taken to the SICU for resuscitation and correction of metabolic derangements. Within 24 hours, the patient is returned to the OR for removal of the packs. Perihepatic packing is indicated for grade IV and V lacerations and for less severe injuries in patients who have a coagulopathy caused by associated injuries.

A technique that may be attempted if packing fails is to wrap the injured portion of the liver with a fine porous material (e.g., polyglycolic acid mesh) after the injured lobe has been mobilized.[39,40] Using a continuous suture or a linear stapler, the surgeon constructs a tight-fitting stocking that encloses the injured lobe. Blood clots beneath the mesh, which results in tamponade of the hepatic injury. Although this technique is intuitively attractive, to date it has achieved only limited success.

The final alternative for patients with extensive unilobar injuries is anatomic hepatic resection. In elective circumstances, anatomic lobectomies can be performed with excellent results; however, in the setting of trauma, the mortality associated with this procedure exceeds 50% in most series.[28,29,31,41-43] Consequently, hepatic resection is rarely performed in trauma patients, having been largely replaced by perihepatic packing, resectional debridement, and hepatotomy with selective ligation. Nonetheless, there are two circumstances in which anatomic resection may still be a reasonable choice. The first is prompt resection in patients with extensive injuries of the lateral segment of the left lobe; because hemorrhage from the left lobe is easily controlled with bimanual compression, the risk of uncontrolled blood loss is not as high as with left or right anatomic lobectomies. The second is delayed anatomic lobectomy in patients whose hemorrhage has been controlled but whose left or right lobe is nonviable as a result of ligation or thrombosis of essential blood vessels. Because of the large mass of necrotic liver tissue, there is a high risk of subsequent infection or persistent hyperinflammation, setting the stage for the multiple organ dysfunction syndrome (MODS). The necrotic lobe should be removed as soon as the patient's condition permits.

Hepatic transplantation has been successful in several trauma patients with devastating hepatic injuries who required total hepatectomy.[44-47] In each of these five patients, the mean anhepatic period was approximately 24 hours. All five survived the transplantation, though two died of disseminated viral infections within two months of the procedure. Two others were alive and well 16 and 17 months after the procedure; no follow-up was reported for the fifth patient. Hepatic transplantation represents the ultimate expression of aggressive trauma care. All other injuries must be well delineated (particularly injuries to the CNS), and the patient must have an excellent chance of survival aside from the hepatic injury. High cost and limited availability

of donors restrict the performance of hepatic transplantation for trauma, but it seems probable that this procedure will continue to be performed in extraordinary circumstances.

Subcapsular Hematoma

An uncommon but troublesome hepatic injury is subcapsular hematoma, which arises when the parenchyma of the liver is disrupted by blunt trauma but Glisson's capsule remains intact. Subcapsular hematomas range in severity from minor blisters on the surface of the liver to ruptured central hematomas accompanied by severe hemorrhage [see Table 1]. They may be recognized either at the time of the operation or in the course of CT scanning.

Regardless of how the lesion is diagnosed, subsequent decision making is often difficult. If a grade I or II subcapsular hematoma—that is, a hematoma involving less than 50% of the surface of the liver that is not expanding and is not ruptured— is discovered during an exploratory laparotomy, it should be left alone. If the hematoma is explored, hepatotomy with selective ligation may be required to control bleeding vessels. Even if hepatotomy with ligation is effective, one must still contend with diffuse hemorrhage from the large denuded surface, and packing may also be required. A hematoma that is expanding during operation (grade III) may have to be explored. Such lesions are often the result of uncontrolled arterial hemorrhage, and packing alone may not be successful. An alternative strategy is to pack the liver to control venous hemorrhage, close the abdomen, and transport the patient to the interventional radiology suite for hepatic arteriography and embolization of the bleeding vessels. Ruptured grades III and IV hematomas are treated with exploration and selective ligation, with or without packing.

Perihepatic Drainage

For years, all hepatic injuries were drained via Penrose drains brought out laterally or through the bed of the resected 12th rib;

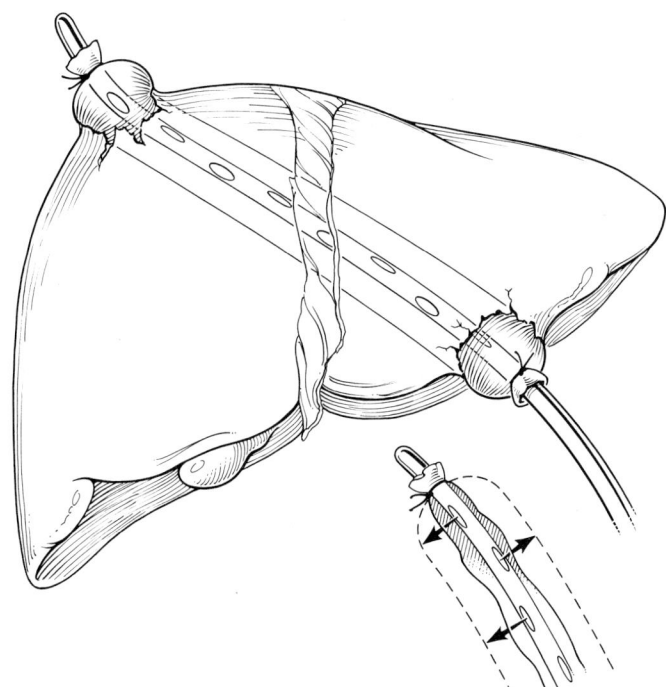

Figure 7 **A hand-made balloon from a Robinson catheter and a Penrose drain may effectively control hemorrhage from a transhepatic penetrating wound.**

recently, the use of large sump drains and closed suction drains has become increasingly popular. Several prospective and retrospective studies have demonstrated that the use of either Penrose or sump drains carries a higher risk of intra-abdominal infection than the use of either closed suction drains or no drains at all.[48-51] It is clear that if drains are to be used, closed suction devices are preferred. What is not clear, however, is whether closed suction drains are better or worse than no drains, particularly in view of the advent of percutaneous catheter drainage. Patients who are initially treated with perihepatic packing may also require drainage; however, drainage is not indicated at the initial procedure, given that the patient will be returned to the OR within the next 48 hours.

MORTALITY AND COMPLICATIONS

Overall mortality for patients with hepatic injuries is approximately 10%. The most common cause of death is exsanguination, followed by MODS and intracranial injury. Three generalizations may be made regarding the risk of death and complications: (1) both increase in proportion to the injury grade and to the complexity of repair; (2) hepatic injuries caused by blunt trauma carry a higher mortality than those caused by penetrating trauma; and (3) infectious complications occur more often with penetrating trauma.

Postoperative hemorrhage occurs in a small percentage of patients with hepatic injuries. The source may be either a coagulopathy or a missed vascular injury (usually to an artery). In most instances of persistent postoperative hemorrhage, the patient is best served by being returned to the OR. Arteriography with embolization may be considered in selected patients. If coagulation studies indicate that a coagulopathy is the likely cause of postoperative hemorrhage, there is little to be gained by reoperation until the coagulopathy is corrected.

Perihepatic infections occur in fewer than 5% of patients with significant hepatic injuries. They develop more often in patients with penetrating injuries than in patients with blunt injuries, presumably because of the greater frequency of enteric contamination. An elevated temperature and a higher than normal white blood cell count after postoperative day 3 or 4 should prompt a search for intra-abdominal infection. In the absence of pneumonia, an infected line, or urinary tract infection, an abdominal CT scan with intravenous and upper gastrointestinal contrast should be obtained. Many perihepatic infections can be treated with CT-guided drainage; however, infected hematomas and infected necrotic liver tissue cannot be expected to respond to percutaneous drainage. Right 12th rib resection remains an excellent approach for posterior infections and provides superior drainage in refractory cases.

Bilomas are loculated collections of bile that may or may not be infected. If a biloma is infected, it is essentially an abscess and should be treated as such; if it is sterile, it will eventually be resorbed. Biliary ascites is caused by disruption of a major bile duct. Reoperation after the establishment of appropriate drainage is the prudent course. Even if the source of the leaking bile can be identified, primary repair of the injured duct is unlikely to be successful. It is best to wait until a firm fistulous communication is established with adequate drainage.

Biliary fistulas occur in approximately 3% of patients with major hepatic injuries.[42] They are usually of little consequence and generally close without specific treatment. In rare instances, a fistulous communication with intrathoracic structures forms in patients with associated diaphragmatic injuries, resulting in a bronchobiliary or pleurobiliary fistula. Because of the pressure differential between the biliary tract and the thoracic cavity, most

of these fistulas must be closed operatively; however, we know of one pleurobiliary fistula that closed spontaneously after endoscopic sphincterotomy and stent placement.

Hemorrhage from hepatic injuries is often treated without identifying and controlling each bleeding vessel individually, and arterial pseudoaneurysms may develop as a consequence. As the pseudoaneurysm enlarges, it may rupture into the parenchyma of the liver, into a bile duct, or into an adjacent branch of the portal vein. Rupture into a bile duct results in hemobilia, which is characterized by intermittent episodes of right upper quadrant pain, upper gastrointestinal hemorrhage, and jaundice; rupture into a portal vein may result in portal vein hypertension with bleeding varices. Both of these complications are exceedingly rare and are best managed with hepatic arteriography and embolization.

Injuries to the Bile Ducts and Gallbladder

Injuries to the extrahepatic bile ducts [see Table 1] can be caused by either penetrating or blunt trauma; however, they are rare in either case.[52-55] The diagnosis is usually made by noting the accumulation of bile in the upper quadrant during laparotomy for treatment of associated injuries. Treatment of common bile duct (CBD) injuries after external trauma is complicated by the small size and thin wall of the normal duct, which render primary repair almost impossible except when the laceration is small and there is no tissue loss. When there is tissue loss or the laceration is larger than 25% to 50% of the diameter of the duct, the best treatment option is a Roux-en-Y choledochojejunostomy [see 3:16 Biliary Tract Procedures].[56,57] Treatment of injuries to the left or right hepatic duct is even more difficult—so much so that we question whether repair should even be attempted under emergency conditions. If only one hepatic duct is injured, a reasonable approach is to ligate it and deal with any infections or atrophy of the lobe rather than to attempt repair.[58] If both ducts are injured, each should be intubated with a small catheter brought through the abdominal wall. Once the patient has recovered sufficiently, delayed repair is performed under elective conditions. Injuries to the intrapancreatic portion of the CBD are treated by dividing the duct at the superior border of the pancreas, ligating the distal portion, and performing a Roux-en-Y choledochojejunostomy.

The Roux-en-Y choledochojejunostomy is done in a single layer with interrupted 5-0 absorbable monofilament sutures. To prevent ischemia and possible stricture, no circumferential dissection of the duct is performed. A round patch of approximately the same diameter as the CBD is removed from the seromuscular layer of the small bowel, but the mucosa and submucosa are only perforated, not resected. The posterior row of sutures is placed first, with full-thickness bites taken through both the duct and the small bowel. The anterior row is then completed. Finally, three or four 3-0 polypropylene sutures are placed to secure the small bowel around the anastomosis to the connective tissue of the porta hepatis. The only purpose for these sutures is to spare the fragile anastomosis any potential tension. No T tubes or stents are employed. Closed suction drainage is added in the case of injuries to the intrapancreatic portion of the duct or at the surgeon's discretion.

Injuries to the gallbladder [see Table 1] are treated by means of either lateral repair with absorbable sutures or cholecystectomy; the decision between the two approaches depends on which is easier in a given situation. Cholecystostomy is rarely, if ever, indicated.

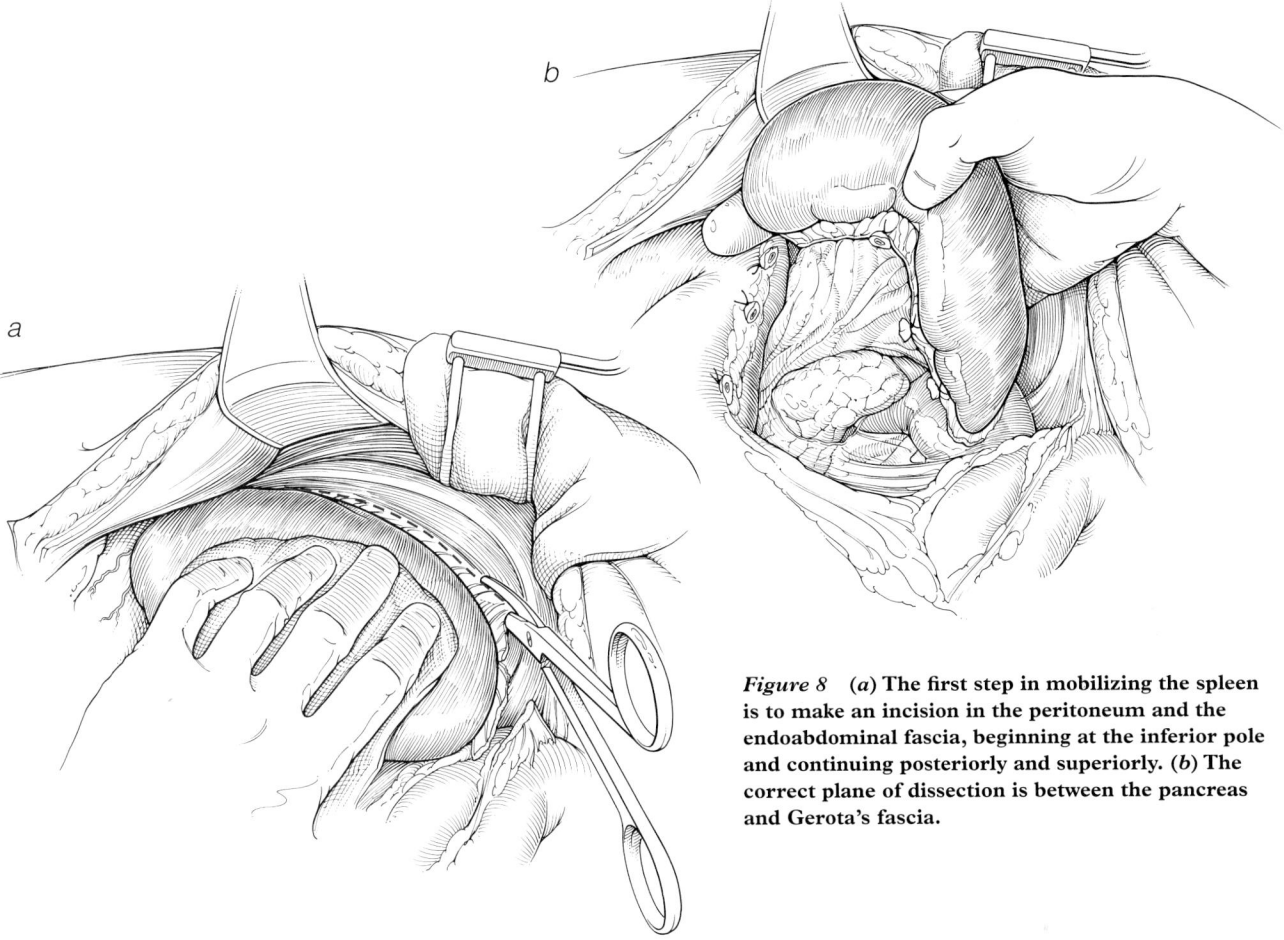

Figure 8 (*a*) **The first step in mobilizing the spleen is to make an incision in the peritoneum and the endoabdominal fascia, beginning at the inferior pole and continuing posteriorly and superiorly. (*b*) The correct plane of dissection is between the pancreas and Gerota's fascia.**

Injuries to the Spleen

Splenic injuries [*see Table 1*] are treated operatively by means of splenic repair (splenorrhaphy), partial splenectomy, or resection, depending on the extent of the injury and the condition of the patient.[59-63] Currently, there is considerable enthusiasm for splenic salvage as a consequence of the evolving trend toward nonoperative management of solid organ injuries and the growing concern about the rare but often fatal complication known as overwhelming postsplenectomy infection (OPSI). OPSI is caused by encapsulated bacteria (e.g., *Streptococcus pneumoniae, Haemophilus influenzae,* and *Neisseria meningitidis*) and is very resistant to treatment: mortality may exceed 50%.[59] OPSI occurs most often in young children and immunocompromised adults and is uncommon in otherwise healthy adults. For this reason, splenic salvage is attempted more vigorously in pediatric patients than in adult ones.

To ensure safe removal or repair, the spleen should be mobilized to the point where it can be brought to the surface of the abdominal wall without tension. To this end, the soft tissue attachments between the spleen and the splenic flexure of the colon must be divided. Next, an incision is made in the peritoneum and the endoabdominal fascia, beginning at the inferior pole, 1 to 2 cm lateral to the posterior peritoneal reflection of the spleen, and continuing posteriorly and superiorly until the esophagus is encountered [*see Figure 8a*]. Care must be taken not to pull on the spleen, so that it will not tear at the posterior peritoneal reflection, causing significant hemorrhage. Instead, the spleen should be rotated counterclockwise, with posterior pres-

sure applied to expose the peritoneal reflection. It is often helpful to rotate the operating table 20° to the patient's right so that the weight of the abdominal viscera facilitates their retraction. A plane is thus established between the spleen and pancreas and Gerota's fascia that can be extended to the aorta [*see Figure 8b*]. With this step, mobilization is complete, and the spleen can be repaired or removed without any need to struggle to achieve adequate exposure.

Splenectomy is the usual treatment for hilar injuries or a pulverized splenic parenchyma. It is also indicated for lesser splenic injuries in patients who have multiple abdominal injuries and a coagulopathy, and it is frequently necessary in patients in whom splenic salvage attempts have failed. Partial splenectomy is suitable for patients in whom only a portion of the spleen (usually the superior or inferior half) has been destroyed. Once the damaged portion has been removed, the same methods used to control hemorrhage from hepatic parenchyma can be used to control hemorrhage from splenic parenchyma [*see Figure 9*]. When horizontal mattress sutures are placed across a raw edge, gentle compression of the parenchyma by an assistant facilitates hemostasis; when the sutures are tied and compression is released, the spleen will expand slightly and tighten the sutures further. Drains are never used after completion of the repair or resection.

If splenectomy is performed, vaccines effective against the encapsulated bacteria are administered. The pneumococcal vaccine is routinely given, and vaccines effective against *H. influenzae* and *N. meningitidis* should also be given if available.

Injuries to the Diaphragm

In cases of blunt trauma to the diaphragm, the injury is on the left side 75% of the time, presumably because the liver diffuses some of the energy on the right side. With both blunt and penetrating injuries [see Table 1], the diagnosis is suggested by an abnormality of the diaphragmatic shadow on chest x-ray. Many of these abnormalities are subtle, particularly with penetrating injuries, and further diagnostic evaluation may be warranted. The typical injury from blunt trauma is a tear in the central tendon; often, the tear is quite large. Regardless of the cause, acute injuries are repaired through an abdominal incision. Because of the concave shape of the diaphragm and the overlying anterior ribs, anterior diaphragmatic injuries may be difficult to suture. Repair is greatly facilitated by using a long Allis clamp to grasp part of the injury and evert the diaphragm. Lacerations are repaired with continuous No. 1 monofilament nonabsorbable sutures. Occasionally, with large avulsions or gunshot wounds accompanied by extensive tissue loss, polypropylene mesh is required to bridge the defect.

The explosive growth of laparoscopic procedures has led to the application of this technology for both diagnostic and therapeutic purposes in trauma patients. In a number of patients with low anterior thoracic stab wounds who otherwise were not candidates for a laparotomy, small diaphragmatic lacerations have been identified and repaired with laparoscopy and stapling.

Discussion

Nonoperative Treatment of Blunt Hepatic and Splenic Injury

Only a few years ago, blunt and penetrating hepatic and splenic injuries were managed in a similar fashion on the basis of a positive diagnostic peritoneal lavage or the probability of peritoneal penetration: a laparotomy was performed, and the injured organs were identified and treated. Currently, although penetrating abdominal injuries are still treated in the same way, nearly all children and 50% to 80% of adults with blunt hepatic and splenic injuries are treated without laparotomy.[64-76] This remarkable change was made possible by the development of the high-speed helical CT scanner, the replacement of diagnostic peritoneal lavage by ultrasonography, and the growth of interventional radiology.

The diagnosis of blunt abdominal trauma is suspected on the basis of the mechanism of injury and the presence of associated injuries (e.g., right or left lower rib fractures). In contemporary urban trauma centers, ultrasonographic examination of the abdomen may reveal a fluid stripe in Morrison's pouch, the left upper quadrant, or the pelvis, which suggests a hemoperitoneum. This observation prompts a CT scan of the abdomen, which delineates injuries of the liver or spleen. CT scanning is a less than optimal means of grading hepatic and splenic injuries; however, patients may be observed either in the SICU or on the ward, depending on the apparent severity of the parenchymal injury on the CT scan and the presence and extent of any associated injuries.[77,78]

The primary requirement for nonoperative therapy is hemodynamic stability.[63-72] To confirm stability, frequent assessment of vital signs and monitoring of the hematocrit are necessary. Continued hemorrhage occurs in 1% to 4% of patients.[65,66,68-73] Hypotension may develop, usually within the first 24 hours after hepatic injury but sometimes several days later, especially when splenic injury is present.[79,80] It is often an indication that operative intervention is necessary. A persistently falling hematocrit should be treated with packed red blood cell (PRBC) transfusions. If the hematocrit continues to fall after two or three units of PRBCs, embolization in the interventional radiology suite should be considered.[74] Overall, nonoperative treatment obviates laparotomy in more than 95% of cases.[65,66,68-73]

Out of concern over the risk of delayed hemorrhage or other complications, follow-up CT scans have often been recommended; unfortunately, there is no consensus as to when or even whether they should be obtained. Given that patients with grade I or II hepatic or splenic injuries rarely show progression of the lesion or other complications on routine follow-up CT scans, it is reasonable to omit such scans if patients' hematocrits remain stable and they are otherwise well. Patients with more extensive injuries often have a less predictable course, and CT scanning may be necessary to evaluate possible complications. Routine scanning before discharge, however, is unwarranted. On the other hand, patients who participate in vigorous or contact sports should have CT documentation of virtually complete healing before resuming those activities.

A more convenient and less expensive alternative to follow-up CT scanning is to monitor lesions ultrasonographically. Ultrasonographic monitoring is particularly useful for following up splenic injuries; however, it may not be useful for following up hepatic injuries, because the technology currently available is incapable of reliably imaging the entire liver.

Other complications of nonoperative therapy for blunt hepatic and splenic injuries occur in 2% to 5% of patients; these include missed abdominal injuries, parenchymal infarction,

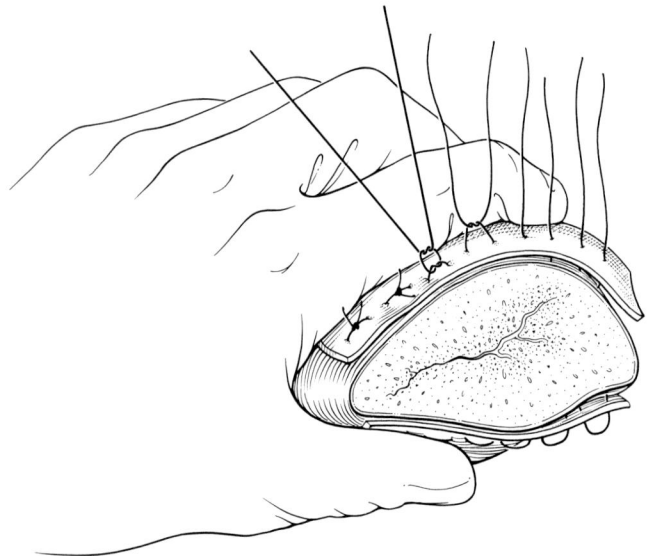

Figure 9 **Methods for controlling hemorrhage from the splenic parenchyma are similar to those for controlling hemorrhage from the hepatic parenchyma. Shown are interrupted mattress sutures across a raw edge of the spleen.**

infection, and bile leakage (a complication associated solely with hepatic injuries).[65,68-71] Aseptic infarcts, infected hematomas, and bile collections are suspected on the basis of a clinical picture suggestive of infection and confirmed by CT-guided aspiration. Aseptic infarction usually does not necessitate operative intervention. Fluid collections are drained, with the method depending on the viscosity of the fluid: CT-guided drainage may be effective in treating thin collections, but operative intervention is required for thicker collections, those with solid components, and those for which percutaneous drainage was attempted without success. Extrahepatic bile collections should be drained percutaneously under CT guidance. Most biliary fistulas close spontaneously; endoscopic stent placement may hasten closure in recalcitrant cases.[81] Intrahepatic collections of blood and bile are managed expectantly. Complete absorption of large intrahepatic collections may take several months. If a collection becomes infected, CT-guided aspiration is performed and drainage obtained as described above.

Missed enteric and retroperitoneal injuries are another cause of failed nonoperative treatment. Such injuries are present in 1% to 4% of patients in whom nonoperative treatment is attempted.[65,68-71] High-quality images and expert interpretation minimize the number of missed injuries on CT scans but cannot eliminate them entirely. Therefore, patients must be watched carefully for the development of peritoneal irritation and other signs of intra-abdominal pathology.

References

1. Moore EE, Cogbill TH, Jurkovich GJ, et al: Organ injury scaling: spleen and liver (1994 revision). J Trauma 38:323, 1995
2. Hepatic trauma revisited. Feliciano DV, Pachter HL, Eds. Curr Probl Surg 26, 1986
3. Moore EE: Critical decisions in the management of hepatic trauma. Am J Surg 148:712, 1984
4. Feliciano DV, Mattox KL, Jordan GL, et al: Management of 1000 consecutive cases of hepatic trauma (1979–1984). Ann Surg 204:438, 1986
5. Feliciano DV, Mattox KL, Burch JM, et al: Packing for control of hepatic hemorrhage. J Trauma 26:738, 1986
6. Ivantury RR, Nallathambi M, Gunduz Y, et al: Liver packing for uncontrolled hemorrhage: a reappraisal. J Trauma 26:744, 1986
7. Carmona RH, Peck DZ, Lim RC: The role of packing and planned reoperation in severe hepatic trauma. J Trauma 24:779, 1984
8. Cue JI, Cryer HG, Miller FB, et al: Packing and planned reexploration for hepatic and retroperitoneal hemorrhage: critical refinements of a useful technique. J Trauma 30:1007, 1990
9. Beal SL: Fatal hepatic hemorrhage: an unresolved problem in the management of complex liver injuries. J Trauma 30:163, 1990
10. Pachter HL, Spencer FC, Hofstetter SR, et al: Significant trends in the treatment of hepatic trauma: experience with 411 injuries. Ann Surg 215:492, 1992
11. Murray DH Jr, Borge JD, Pouteau GG: Tourniquet control of liver bleeding. J Trauma 18:771, 1978
12. Heaney JP, Stanton WR, Halbert DS, et al: An improved technic for vascular isolation of the liver. Ann Surg 163:237, 1966
13. Burch JM, Feliciano DV, Mattox KL: The atriocaval shunt: facts and fiction. Ann Surg 207:555, 1988
14. Buechter KJ, Gomez GA, Zeppa R: A new technique for exposure of injuries at the confluence of the retrohepatic veins and the retrohepatic vena cava. J Trauma 30:328, 1990
15. Schrock T, Blaisdell FW, Matthewson C Jr: Management of blunt trauma to the liver and hepatic veins. Arch Surg 96:698, 1968
16. Bricker DL, Morton JR, Okies JE, et al: Surgical management of injuries to the vena cava: changing patterns of injury and newer techniques of repair. J Trauma 11:725, 1971
17. Yellin AE, Chaffee CB, Donovan AJ: Vascular isolation in treatment of juxtahepatic venous injuries. Arch Surg 102:566, 1971
18. Walt AJ: The mythology of hepatic trauma: or Babel revisited. Am J Surg 125:12, 1978
19. Millikan JS, Moore EE, Cogbill TH, et al: Inferior vena cava injuries: a continuing challenge. J Trauma 23:207, 1983
20. Pachter HL, Spencer FC, Hofstetter SR, et al: The management of juxtahepatic venous injuries without an atriocaval shunt. Surgery 99:569, 1986
21. Rovito PF: Atrial caval shunting in blunt hepatic vascular injury. Ann Surg 205:318, 1987
22. Pilcher DB, Harman PK, Moore EE: Retrohepatic vena cava balloon shunt introduced via the sapheno-femoral junction. J Trauma 17:837, 1977
23. Kram HB, Reuben BI, Flemming AW: Use of fibrin glue in hepatic trauma. J Trauma 28:1195, 1988
24. Kram HB, Nathan RC, Stafford FJ, et al: Fibrin glue achieves hemostasis in patients with coagulation disorders. Arch Surg 124:385, 1989
25. Berguer R, Staerkel RL, Moore EE, et al: Warning: fatal reaction to the use of fibrin glue in deep hepatic wounds: case reports. J Trauma 31:408, 1991
26. Ochsner MG, Maniscalco-Theberge ME, Champion HR: Fibrin glue as a hemostatic agent in hepatic and splenic trauma. J Trauma 30:884, 1990
27. Feliciano DV: Continuing evolution in the approach to severe liver trauma (editorial). Ann Surg 216:521, 1992
28. Trunkey DD, Shires GT, McClelland R: Management of liver trauma in 811 consecutive patients. Ann Surg 179:722, 1974
29. Levin A, Gover P, Nance FC: Surgical restraint in the management of hepatic injury: a review of Charity Hospital experience. J Trauma 18:399, 1978
30. Lucas CE, Ledgerwood AM: Prospective evaluation of hemostatic techniques for liver injuries. J Trauma 16:442, 1976
31. Camona RH, Lim RC Jr, Clark GC: Morbidity and mortality in hepatic trauma: a 5 year study. Am J Surg 144:88, 1982
32. Moore FA, Moore EE, Seagrave A: Nonresectional management of major hepatic trauma: an evolving concept. Am J Surg 150:725, 1985
33. Stone HH, Lamb JM: Use of pedicled omentum as an autogenous pack for control of hemorrhage in major injuries of the liver. Surg Gynecol Obstet 141:92, 1975
34. Mays ET: Lobar dearterialization for exsanguinating wounds of the liver. J Trauma 12:397, 1972
35. Flint LM, Polk HC: Selective hepatic artery ligation: limitations and failures. J Trauma 19:319, 1979
36. Lucas CE: Discussion of: Flint LM, Polk HC. Selective hepatic artery ligation: limitations and failures. J Trauma 19:319, 1979
37. Poggetti RS, Moore EE, Moore FA, et al: Balloon tamponade for bilobar transfixing hepatic gunshot wounds. J Trauma 33:694, 1992
38. Madding GF, Lawrence KB, Kennedy PA: War wounds of the liver. Tex State J Med 42:267, 1946
39. Reed RL, Merrell RC, Meyers WC, et al: Continuing evolution in the approach to severe liver trauma. Ann Surg 216:524, 1992
40. Jacobson LE, Kirton OC, Gomez GA: The use of an absorbable mesh wrap in the management of major liver injuries. Surgery 111:455, 1992
41. Lim RC Jr, Knudson J, Steele M: Liver trauma: current method of management. Arch Surg 104:544, 1972
42. Donovan AJ, Michaelian MJ, Yellin AE: Anatomical hepatic lobectomy in trauma to the liver. Surgery 73:833, 1973
43. Defore WW, Mattox KL, Jordan GL, et al: Management of 1590 consecutive cases of liver trauma. Arch Surg 111:493, 1976
44. Esquivel CO, Bernardos A, Makowka L, et al: Liver replacement after massive hepatic trauma. J Trauma 27:800, 1987
45. Angstadt J, Jarrell B, Moritz M, et al: Surgical management of severe liver trauma: a role for liver transplantation. J Trauma 29:606, 1989
46. Ringe B, Pichlmayr R, Ziegler H, et al: Management of severe hepatic trauma by two-stage total hepatectomy and subsequent liver transplantation. Surgery 109:792, 1991
47. Jeng LB, Hsu C, Wang C, et al: Emergent liver transplantation to salvage a hepatic avulsion injury with a disrupted suprahepatic vena cava. Arch Surg 128:1075, 1993
48. Fischer RP, O'Farrell KA, Perry JF Jr: The value of peritoneal drains in the treatment of liver injuries. J Trauma 18:393, 1978
49. Gillmore D, McSwain NE, Browder IW: Hepatic trauma: to drain or not to drain? J Trauma 27:989, 1987
50. Noyes LD, Doyle DJ, McSwain NE: Septic complications associated with the use of peritoneal drains in liver trauma. J Trauma 28:337, 1988
51. Fabian TC, Croce MA, Stanford GG, et al: Factors affecting morbidity after hepatic trauma. Ann Surg 213:540, 1991
52. Posner MC, Moore EE: Extrahepatic biliary tract injury: operative management plan. J Trauma 25:833, 1985
53. Ivatury RR, Rohman M, Nallathami M, et al: The

morbidity of injuries of the extra-hepatic biliary system. J Trauma 25:967, 1985

54. Sheldon GF, Lim RC, Yee ES, et al: Management of injuries to the porta hepatis. Ann Surg 202:539, 1985

55. Feliciano DV, Bitondo CG, Burch JM, et al: Management of traumatic injuries to the extra-hepatic biliary ducts. Am J Surg 150:705, 1985

56. Bade PG, Thomson SR, Hirshberg A, et al: Surgical options in traumatic injury to the extra-hepatic biliary tract. Br J Surg 76:256, 1989

57. Csendes A, Diaz JC, Burdiles P, et al: Late results of immediate primary end to end repair in accidental section of the common bile duct. Surg Gynecol Obstet 168:125, 1989

58. Howdieshell TR, Hawkins ML, Osler TM, et al: Management of blunt hepatic duct transection by ligation. South Med J 83:579, 1990

59. Sherman R: Perspective in management of trauma to the spleen: 1979 presidential address, American Association for the Surgery of Trauma. J Trauma 20:1, 1980

60. Barrett J, Sheaff C, Abuabara S, et al: Splenic preservation in adults after blunt and penetrating trauma. Am J Surg 145:313, 1983

61. Delany HM, Rudavsky AZ, Lan S: Preliminary clinical experience with the use of absorbable mesh splenorrhaphy. J Trauma 25:909, 1985

62. Beal SL, Spisso JM: The risk of splenorrhaphy. Arch Surg 123:1158, 1988

63. Feliciano DV, Spjut-Patrinely V, Burch JM, et al: Splenorrhaphy: the alternative. Ann Surg 211:569 1990

64. Schiffman MA: Nonoperative management of blunt abdominal trauma in pediatrics. Emerg Med Clin North Am 7:519, 1989

65. Cogbill TH, Moore EE, Jurkovich JJ, et al: Nonoperative management of blunt septic trauma: a multicenter experience. J Trauma 29:1312, 1989

66. Meredith JW, Young JS, Bowling J, et al: Nonoperative management of blunt hepatic trauma: the exception or the rule? J Trauma 36:529, 1994

67. Morrell DG, Chang FC, Helmer SD: Changing trends in the management of splenic injury. Am J Surg 170:686, 1995

68. Pachter HL, Hofstetter ST: The current status of nonoperative management of adult blunt hepatic injuries. Am J Surg 169:442, 1995

69. Croce MA, Fabian TC, Menke PG, et al: Nonoperative management of blunt hepatic trauma is the treatment of choice for hemodynamically stable patients. Ann Surg 221:744, 1995

70. Boone DC, Federle M, Billiar TR, et al: Evolution of management of major hepatic trauma: identification of patterns of injury. J Trauma 39:344, 1995

71. Pachter HL, Knudson MM, Esrig B, et al: Status of nonoperative management of blunt hepatic injuries in 1995: a multicenter experience with 404 patients. J Trauma 40:31, 1996

72. Smith JS, Cooney RN, Mucha P: Nonoperative management of the ruptured spleen: a revalidation of criteria. Surgery 120:745, 1996

73. Powell M, Courcoulas A, Gardner M, et al: Management of blunt splenic trauma: significant differences between adults and children. Surgery 122:654, 1997

74. Sclafani SJA, Shaftan GW, Scalea TM, et al: Nonoperative salvage of computed tomography–diagnosed splenic injuries: utilization of angiography for triage and embolization for hemostasis. J Trauma 39:818, 1995

75. Malhotra AK, Fabian TC, Crou MA, et al: Blunt hepatic injury: a paradigm shift from operative to nonoperative management in the 1990's. Ann Surg 231:804, 2000

76. Richardson JD, Franklin GA, Lukan JK, et al: Evolution in the management of hepatic trauma: a 25-year perspective. Ann Surg 232:324, 2000

77. Sutyak JP, Chiu WC, D'Amelio LF, et al: Computed tomography is inaccurate in estimating the severity of adult splenic injury. J Trauma 39:514, 1995

78. Croce MA, Fabian TC, Kudsk KA, et al: AAST organ injury scale: correlation of CT-graded liver injuries and operative findings. J Trauma 31:806, 1991

79. Gates JD: Delayed hemorrhage with free rupture complicating the nonsurgical management of blunt hepatic trauma: a case report and review of the literature. J Trauma 36:572, 1994

80. MacGillivray DC, Valentine RJ: Nonoperative management of blunt pediatric liver injury—late complications: case report. J Trauma 29:251, 1989

81. Sugimoto K, Asari Y, Sakaguchi T, et al: Endoscopic retrograde cholangiography in the nonsurgical management of blunt liver injury. J Trauma 35:192, 1993

Acknowledgments

Figure 1   Marcia Kammerer.
Figures 2 through 9   Susan Brust, C.M.I.

7 INJURIES TO THE STOMACH, DUODENUM, PANCREAS, SMALL BOWEL, COLON, AND RECTUM

Charles E. Lucas, M.D., F.A.C.S., and Anna M. Ledgerwood, M.D., F.A.C.S.

Injuries to the stomach, duodenum, pancreas, small bowel, colon, and rectum present a broad spectrum of challenges necessitating widely different solutions. The first priorities are recognizing injury and making the decision to operate.

Initial evaluation of injured patients is addressed more fully elsewhere [see 5:1 Trauma Resuscitation]. In what follows, we assume that the patient has been stabilized and that injuries to one or more of the organs just mentioned have been recognized. The need for operation varies according to whether the patient has sustained a stab wound, a gunshot wound, or a blunt injury.

Determination of Need for Operation

STAB WOUNDS

It is universally agreed that patients with symptomatic stab wounds (as evidenced by hypotension, peritonitis, or both) should undergo operation immediately.[1] Likewise, most surgeons agree that mentally competent patients with asymptomatic stab wounds are best treated by observation, even if the wounding object has penetrated the peritoneal cavity.[1] For patients who fall into neither of these categories, however, as when there are no signs of injury but the patient is in a compromised state (e.g., as a result of alcohol, drugs, or mental retardation), the diagnostic and therapeutic approach may take a number of different directions. Options include (1) observation with reexaminations until the patient is sober, (2) local wound exploration, (3) diagnostic peritoneal lavage (DPL), (4) laparoscopy, (5) abdominal ultrasonography in the form of the FAST (Focused Assessment for the Sonographic examination of the Trauma patient [see 3:12 Ultrasonography: Surgical Applications]), or (6) contrast abdominal computed tomography. Of these, we prefer immediate FAST, which, if yielding positive results, is followed by DPL. A positive DPL result is defined as the presence of more than 20,000 red blood cells (RBCs) or more than 500 white blood cells (WBCs) per high-power field. When a stab wound to the lower thorax causes hemothorax, pneumothorax, or both, any return of blood on DPL suggests perforation of the diaphragm, for which the recommended treatment is laparotomy and repair.[1]

GUNSHOT WOUNDS

Early operation is indicated for symptomatic patients with gunshot wounds to the abdomen. More than 90% of patients with penetrating gunshot wounds have intra-abdominal

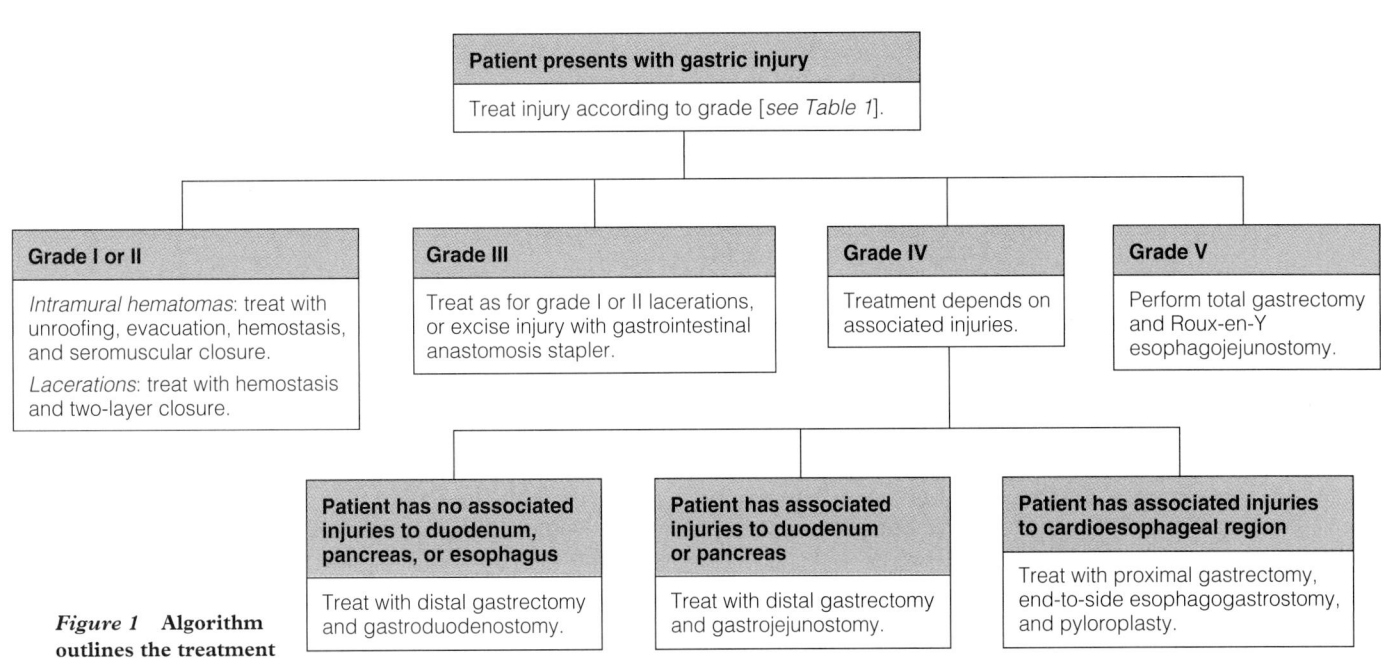

Figure 1 Algorithm outlines the treatment of gastric injury.

Table 1 AAST Organ Injury Scales for GI Tract and Pancreas

Injured Structure	AAST Grade*	Characteristics of Injury	AIS-90 Score
Stomach	I	Intramural hematoma < 3 cm; partial-thickness laceration	2
	II	Intramural hematoma ≥ 3 cm; small (< 3 cm) laceration	2
	III	Large (> 3 cm) laceration	3
	IV	Large laceration involving vessels on greater or lesser curvature	3
	V	Extensive (> 50%) rupture; stomach devascularized	4
Duodenum	I	Single-segment hematoma; partial-thickness laceration	2; 3
	II	Multiple-segment hematoma; small (< 50% of circumference) laceration	2; 4
	III	Large laceration (50%–75% of circumference of segment D2 or 50%–100% of circumference of segment D1, D3, or D4)	4
	IV	Very large (75%–100%) laceration of segment D2; rupture of ampullary or distal bile duct	5
	V	Massive duodenopancreatic injury; devascularization	5
Pancreas	I	Small hematoma without duct injury; superficial laceration without duct injury	2
	II	Large hematoma without duct injury or tissue loss; major laceration without duct injury or tissue loss	2; 3
	III	Distal transection or parenchymal laceration with duct injury	4
	IV	Proximal transection or parenchymal laceration involving ampulla	4
	V	Massive disruption of pancreatic head	5
Small bowel	I	Contusion or hematoma without devascularization; partial-thickness laceration	2
	II	Small (< 50% of circumference) laceration	3
	III	Large (≥ 50% of circumference) laceration without transection	3
	IV	Transection	4
	V	Transection with segmental tissue loss; devascularized segment	4
Colon	I	Contusion or hematoma; partial-thickness laceration	2
	II	Small (< 50% of circumference) laceration	3
	III	Large (≥ 50% of circumference) laceration	3
	IV	Transection	4
	V	Transection with tissue loss; devascularized segment	4
Rectosigmoid and rectum	I	Contusion or hematoma; partial-thickness laceration	2
	II	Small (< 50% of circumference) laceration	3
	III	Large (≥ 50% of circumference) laceration	4
	IV	Full-thickness laceration with perineal extension	5
	V	Devascularized segment	5

*Advance one grade for multiple injuries, up to grade III.
AIS-90—Abbreviated Injury Score, 1990 version   AAST—American Association for the Surgery of Trauma

injuries. If there is any question of possible peritoneal penetration with an anterior or anterolateral wound, diagnostic DPL should be performed; a clear return rules out penetration.[1] Triple-contrast CT helps confirm or rule out penetration in patients with lateral or posterior wounds.

BLUNT TRAUMA

Clinical assessment of stable blunt trauma patients often leads to false positive or false negative conclusions,[1] and the error rate rises in patients whose mental function is compromised. The resultant delay in diagnosis and operative intervention is potentially hazardous. For this reason, FAST and DPL, with or without CT scanning, are essential in mentally compromised patients. When stable patients with no abnormal findings on abdominal examination require operative intervention for nonabdominal injuries, DPL can help identify unsuspected intraperitoneal injuries, and double-contrast CT can help identify unsuspected pancreatic and duodenal injuries.

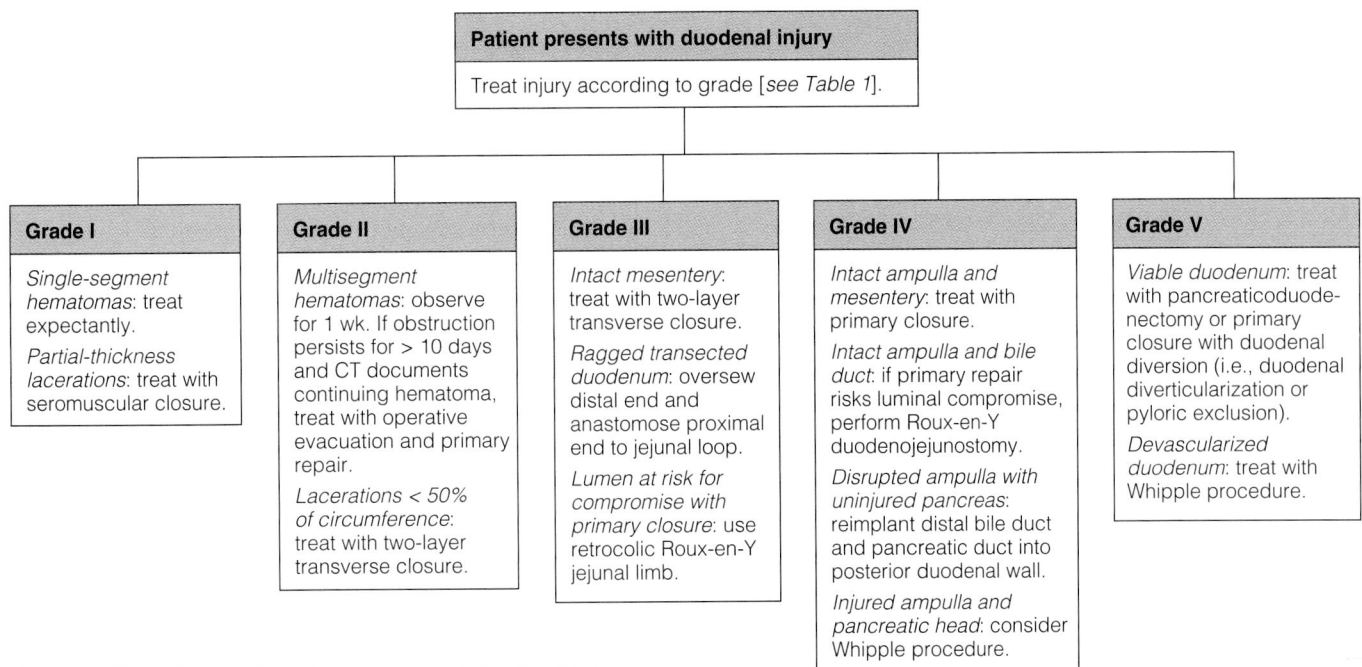

Figure 2 Algorithm outlines the treatment of duodenal injury.

Patient presents with duodenal injury
Treat injury according to grade [*see Table 1*].

Grade I

Single-segment hematomas: treat expectantly.

Partial-thickness lacerations: treat with seromuscular closure.

Grade II

Multisegment hematomas: observe for 1 wk. If obstruction persists for > 10 days and CT documents continuing hematoma, treat with operative evacuation and primary repair.

Lacerations < 50% of circumference: treat with two-layer transverse closure.

Grade III

Intact mesentery: treat with two-layer transverse closure.

Ragged transected duodenum: oversew distal end and anastomose proximal end to jejunal loop.

Lumen at risk for compromise with primary closure: use retrocolic Roux-en-Y jejunal limb.

Grade IV

Intact ampulla and mesentery: treat with primary closure.

Intact ampulla and bile duct: if primary repair risks luminal compromise, perform Roux-en-Y duodenojejunostomy.

Disrupted ampulla with uninjured pancreas: reimplant distal bile duct and pancreatic duct into posterior duodenal wall.

Injured ampulla and pancreatic head: consider Whipple procedure.

Grade V

Viable duodenum: treat with pancreaticoduodenectomy or primary closure with duodenal diversion (i.e., duodenal diverticularization or pyloric exclusion).

Devascularized duodenum: treat with Whipple procedure.

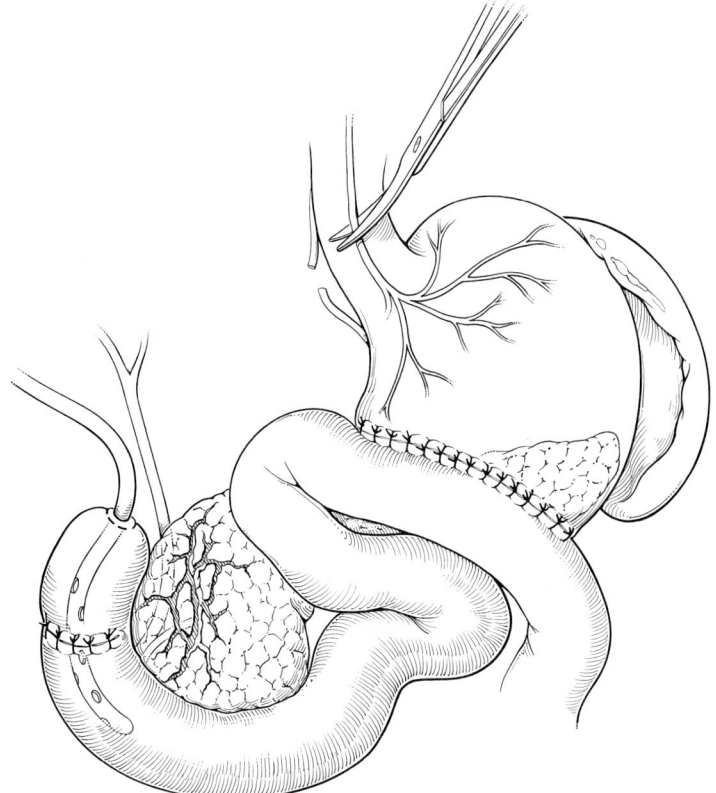

Figure 3 Shown is a grade IV stellate crack to pancreatic head with a grade III (60%) transection of the duodenum (D2). After hemostasis is established, it is possible to perform the so-called duodenal diverticularization, consisting of antrectomy with gastrojejunostomy, tube duodenostomy, vagotomy, and peripancreatic drainage. H_2-receptor blockade precludes the need for vagotomy.

When DPL is positive for amylase, particulate matter, WBCs, or bowel contents, hollow viscus injury is likely and laparotomy is therefore mandatory.

Injuries to the Stomach

The treatment of gastric injuries varies according to their severity [*see Figure 1 and Table 1*]. Most intramural hematomas (grades I and II) are treated by careful evacuation, hemostasis, and seromuscular closure. Perforations from stabs and bullets are usually small (grade I or II) and can be closed primarily in two layers.[1,2] Because the stomach is quite vascular, even small perforations may bleed profusely, especially along the greater curvature. Consequently, the recommended closure is an inner layer of locked hemostatic sutures followed by an outer inverting layer of sutures.

Large (grade III) injuries near the greater curvature can be closed by the same technique or by excising the injury with a long gastrointestinal anastomosis (GIA) stapler. Careful hemostasis and inversion of the staple line provide extra security when the lumen is not compromised. Extensive (grade IV) injuries may necessitate proximal or distal gastrectomy. The type of resection depends on the presence of associated injuries to the duodenum, the pancreas, or the esophagus. Patients with associated duodenal injuries or pancreatic injuries, or both, are best treated with gastrojejunal reconstruction after distal gastrectomy. In patients who survive extensive injury to the cardioesophageal region, an end-to-side esophagogastrostomy can be performed after proximal gastrectomy; a pyloroplasty is added. When total gastrectomy is done for grade V injury, Roux-en-Y esophagojejunostomy is advocated [*see 3:13 Gastroduodenal Procedures*].

Injuries to the Duodenum

The diagnosis of penetrating duodenal injury is usually made during laparotomy performed for hypotension or peritoneal irritation. The decision to explore for isolated blunt duodenal injury is based on the physical examination and roentgeno-

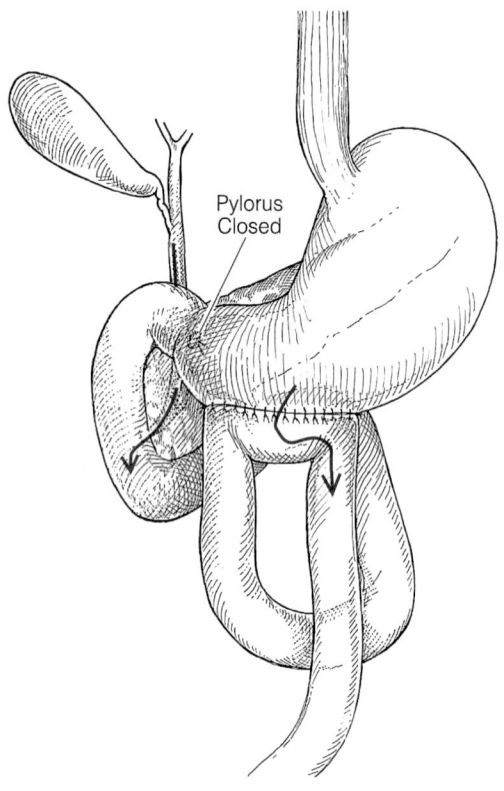

Figure 4 **Duodenal exclusion consists of closure of the pylorus from within the stomach, followed by gastrojejunostomy. The procedure eliminates discharge of gastric acid into the duodenum, thus minimizing the stimulation of pancreatic secretion and reducing morbidity if there is breakdown of a repair.**

graphic findings. Duodenal injury may be present despite negative findings from DPL, and the symptoms of duodenal injury are often slow to evolve.[3] Roentgenograms made within 2 hours of injury typically show scoliosis and partial obliteration of the right psoas shadow. Retroperitoneal gas along the right psoas margin, over the right pole of the kidney, or in the lower mediastinum is seen within 6 hours in most patients. Contrast CT generally identifies the site of perforation.

Treatment varies according to the location (segments D1 through D4) and severity of injury [*see Figure 2 and Table 1*].[4,5] Single-segment (grade I) intramural hematoma usually occurs in segment D1 or D2, seldom leads to obstruction, and can be treated expectantly. Partial-thickness (grade I) lacerations are best treated by simple seromuscular closure. Multisegment hematomas (grade II) often require operative evacuation, especially when the obstruction lasts for more than 10 days and there is CT documentation that the hematoma persists. A generous longitudinal serosal incision along the antimesenteric border permits gentle evacuation without accidental injury to the underlying muscular and mucosal layers. The serosa with attached muscle is carefully reapproximated. Drainage is not necessary. Perforations involving less than 50% of the circumference of the duodenum, whether caused by penetrating wounds or blunt injury, are best treated by simple two-layer closure, preferably in a transverse manner.

Larger perforations that involve more than 50% of the circumference (grade III) require careful suture placement along the mesentery border to prevent unintentional vascular compromise.[6] Near D3 and D4 injuries, careful suture placement and gentle duodenal mobilization help prevent iatrogenic injury to the superior mesenteric vessels. If a transected duodenum is ragged, the distal end may be oversewn and the proximal end anastomosed to a jejunal loop.[7] Alternatively, if primary closure would compromise lumen patency, a retrocolic Roux-en-Y jejunal limb can be used to close large defects.

Large D2 injuries (grade IV) can be closed primarily if the adjacent ampulla and mesentery are spared.[8] If the condition of the distal bile duct is unknown, choledochography through the gallbladder or the proximal bile duct will confirm continuity. When the ampulla and the bile duct are intact but primary repair would cause excessive luminal compromise, a Roux-en-Y duodenojejunostomy is preferred. If the ampulla is disrupted but the pancreas is not injured, primary reimplantation of the distal bile duct and the pancreatic duct into the posterior duodenal wall is preferred. When both the ampulla and the pancreatic head are injured, a Whipple procedure may be needed [*see 3:18 Pancreatic Procedures*].

Duodenopancreatic crunch (grade V) is associated with high morbidity and mortality. This injury can sometimes be treated by pancreaticoduodenectomy or by primary closure done in

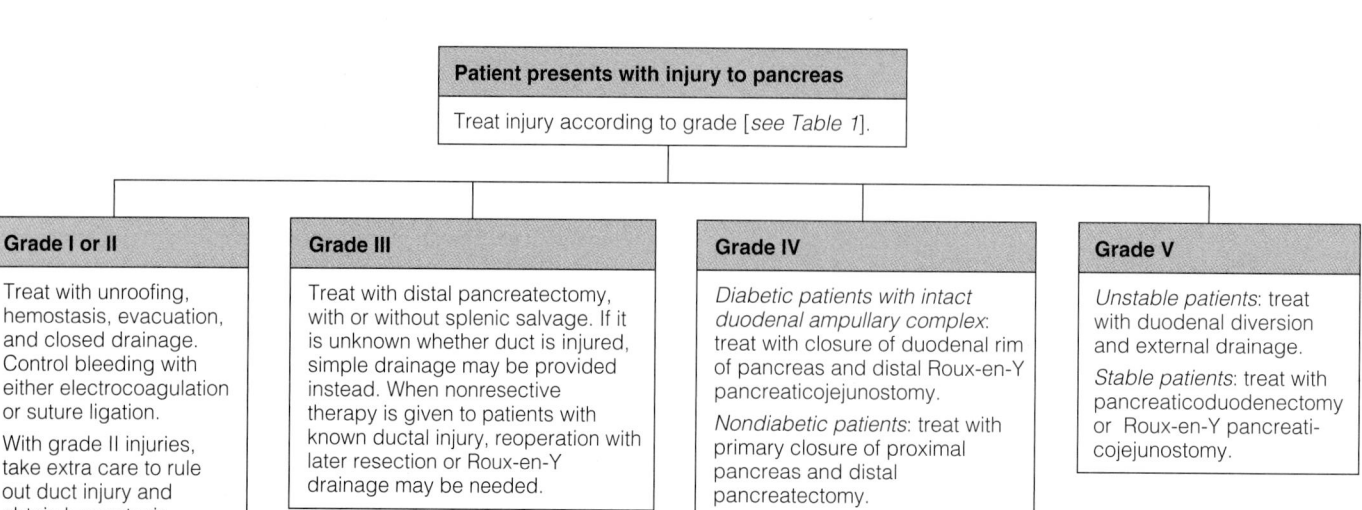

Patient presents with injury to pancreas
Treat injury according to grade [*see Table 1*].

Grade I or II	Grade III	Grade IV	Grade V
Treat with unroofing, hemostasis, evacuation, and closed drainage. Control bleeding with either electrocoagulation or suture ligation. With grade II injuries, take extra care to rule out duct injury and obtain hemostasis.	Treat with distal pancreatectomy, with or without splenic salvage. If it is unknown whether duct is injured, simple drainage may be provided instead. When nonresective therapy is given to patients with known ductal injury, reoperation with later resection or Roux-en-Y drainage may be needed.	*Diabetic patients with intact duodenal ampullary complex:* treat with closure of duodenal rim of pancreas and distal Roux-en-Y pancreaticojejunostomy. *Nondiabetic patients:* treat with primary closure of proximal pancreas and distal pancreatectomy.	*Unstable patients:* treat with duodenal diversion and external drainage. *Stable patients:* treat with pancreaticoduodenectomy or Roux-en-Y pancreaticojejunostomy.

Figure 5 **Algorithm outlines the treatment of pancreatic injury.**

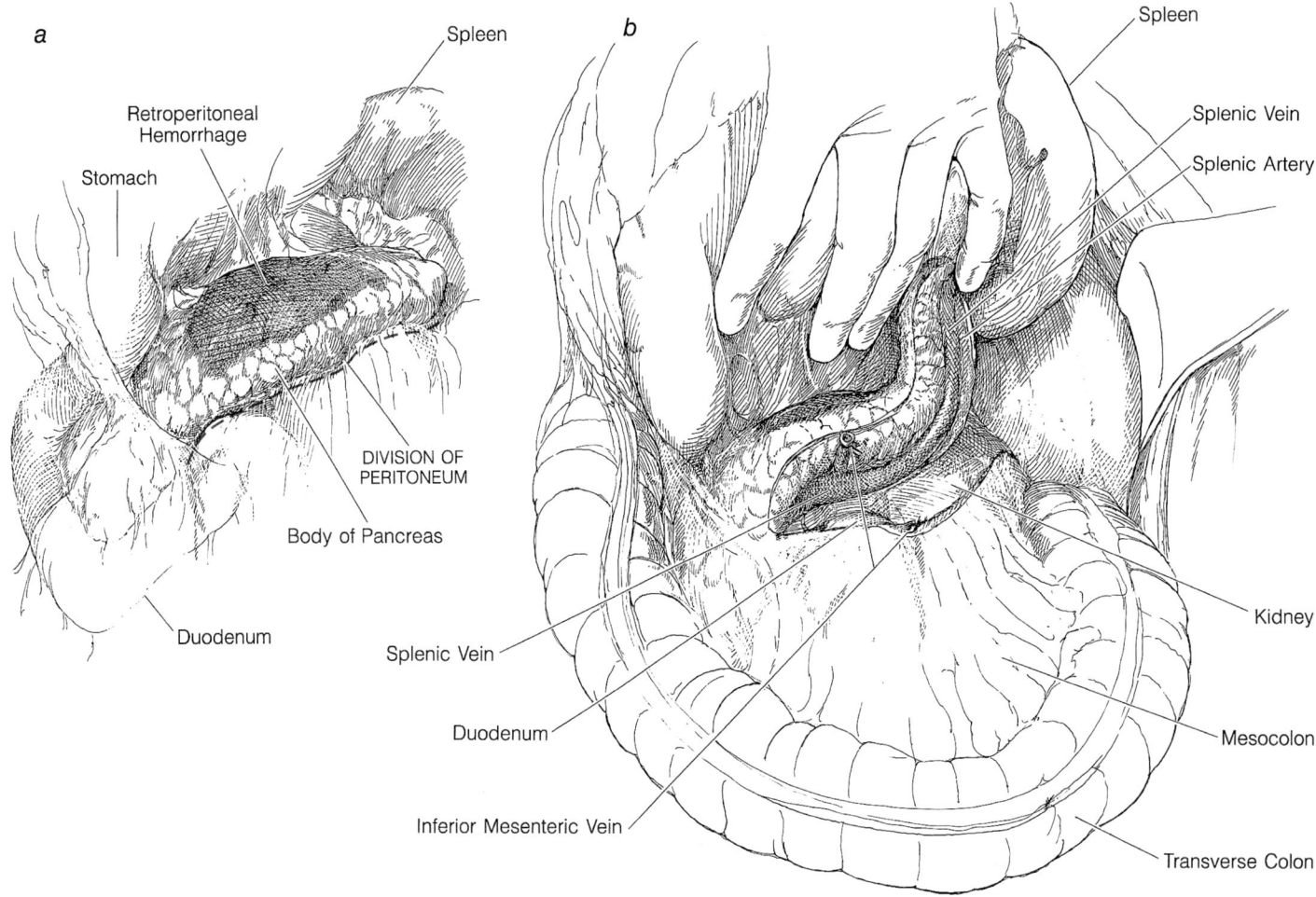

Figure 6 **Illustrated is the appearance of a contusion to the body of the pancreas overlying the vertebral column, as seen from the lesser sac (*a*). Such a contusion necessitates mobilization of the pancreas to determine whether a fracture is present and to assess the likelihood of a duct injury. This exposure is best accomplished by dissecting along the inferior border of the gland, dividing the inferior mesenteric vein if necessary, and reflecting the pancreas superiorly (*b*).**

conjunction with some type of duodenal diversion. When the injury causes devascularization, resection is mandated. Duodenal bypass is performed by either duodenal diverticularization [*see Figure 3*] or pyloric exclusion [*see Figure 4*]; we prefer the former. Duodenal diverticularization includes antrectomy with gastrojejunostomy, tube duodenostomy, and drainage of the associated pancreatic injury.[6] Tube choledochostomy is added only for overt extrahepatic biliary injury. Duodenal exclusion includes pyloric occlusion by sutures or staples, a side-to-side gastrojejunostomy, and appropriate drainage.[9,10]

Injuries to the Pancreas

The treatment of pancreatic injury depends on its grade and extent [*see Figure 5 and Table 1*].[5] The pancreas is best exposed by dividing the greater omentum just outside the arcades of the gastroepiploic vessels. Assessment of the posterior surface may require mobilization of the inferior border or complete relocation of the spleen and pancreatic tail anteriorly [*see Figure 6*]. A small hematoma (grade I) is best treated by unroofing, hemostasis, evacuation, and drainage. Minor bleed-

ing from unnamed vessels is controlled by either electrocoagulation or ligature with fine sutures.

Gentle tension-free tying helps avert iatrogenic injury to the soft pancreatic parenchyma. Careful inspection after hemostasis will confirm the presence of a grade I injury, which does not involve a major duct. The site of the unroofed hematoma is left open and drained externally. Closed-suction drainage permits the exit of pancreatic juices. All small pancreatic lesions without duct injury (grade I) are treated essentially the same way, whether caused by stabs, gunshots, or blunt trauma. If the fluid drained has a high amylase content, skin will not be digested unless the effluent contains enteric juices that activate pancreatic peptidase.[11]

During one 5-year period extending from 1990 through 1994, the surgical services at Detroit Receiving Hospital treated 37 patients with grade I pancreatic injury. All 37 were treated with hemostasis, minimal debridement (if tiny fragments of loose pancreatic tissue were seen), and external drainage. All of the patients survived. Pancreatitis, defined on the basis of an elevated serum amylase level lasting more than 5 days, developed in two patients, and a pancreaticocutaneous fistula developed in two patients whose pancreatic drainage lasted more than 14 days. All of the complications resolved with nonoperative supportive care, including parenteral nutrition.

Treatment of larger hematomas or lacerations without duct injury (grade II injuries) is similar. Extra care is taken to rule out duct injury and to obtain hemostasis. Once hemostasis has been achieved, the injury is left open and drained. This practice helps prevent the development of a pseudocyst, which may occur if tiny ductules leak pancreatic juices within a closed injury.[12,13]

Although the incidence of postoperative pancreatitis (10%) or persistent pancreatic drainage (20%) seen after grade II injury exceeds that seen after grade I injury, few patients (3%) have refractory drainage lasting more than 30 days. When the external drainage system plugs, percutaneous drainage or reoperation may be needed to reestablish drainage. When reoperation is deemed essential for a peripancreatic abscess, dependent drainage through the bed of the 12th rib helps avoid the extensive contamination that occurs when laparotomy is performed through the anterior approach.[13]

Grade III lacerations or transections thought to involve the main duct to the left of the superior mesenteric vein are best treated by distal pancreatectomy, with or without splenic salvage [*see Figure 7 and 3:18 Pancreatic Procedures*].[11,13] If it is not known whether there is injury to the main pancreatic duct, simple drainage may be provided even though it may result in formation of a pancreaticocutaneous fistula. This approach is more expedient than pancreatic resection in unstable patients, especially those with multiple associated injuries requiring multiple transfusions. Total parenteral nutrition permits such patients to recover from the total insult with minimal morbidity.[11] When nonresective therapy is used for patients known to have a duct injury, reoperation with later resection or Roux-en-Y drainage is often needed.[14]

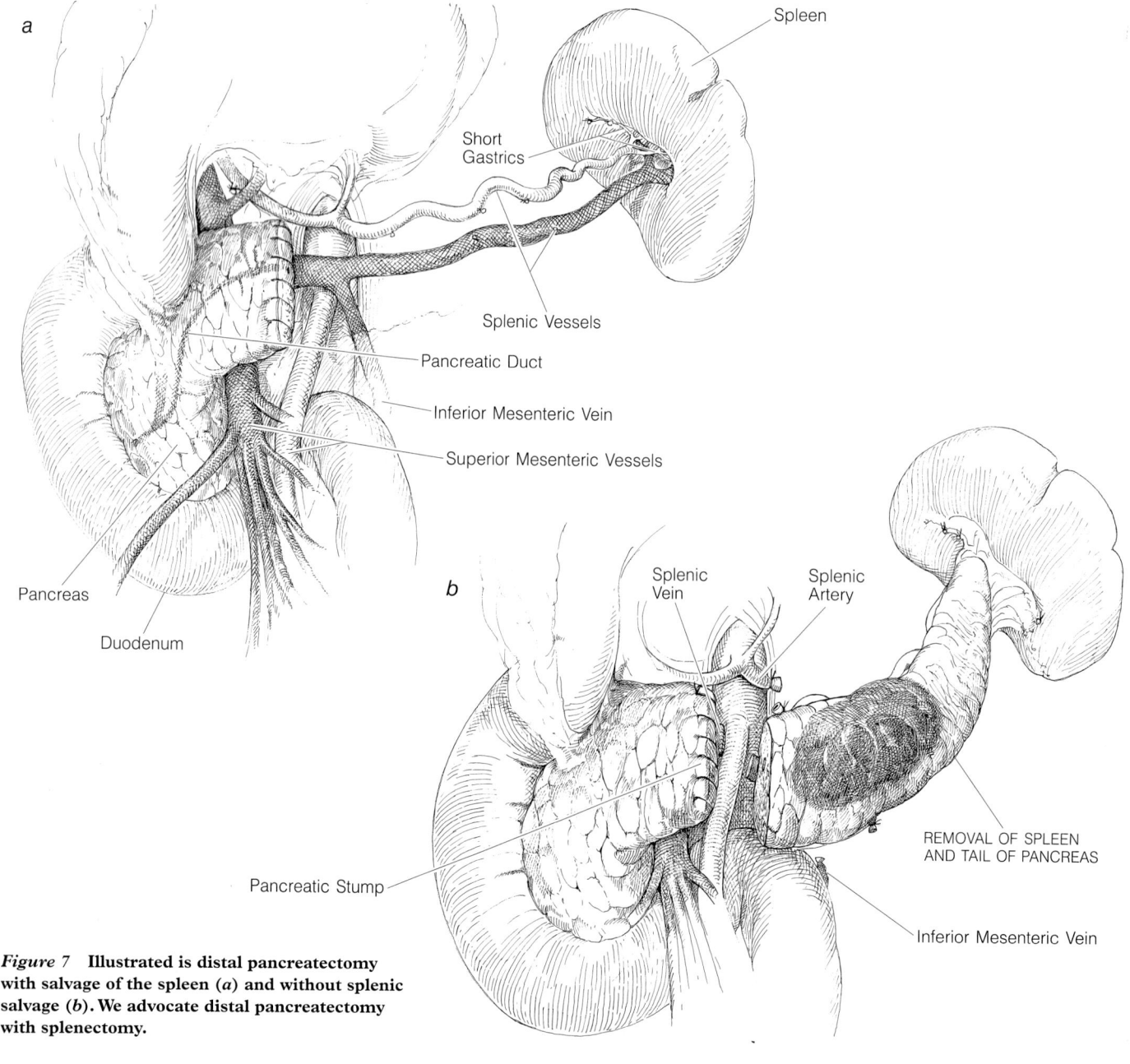

Figure 7 Illustrated is distal pancreatectomy with salvage of the spleen (*a*) and without splenic salvage (*b*). We advocate distal pancreatectomy with splenectomy.

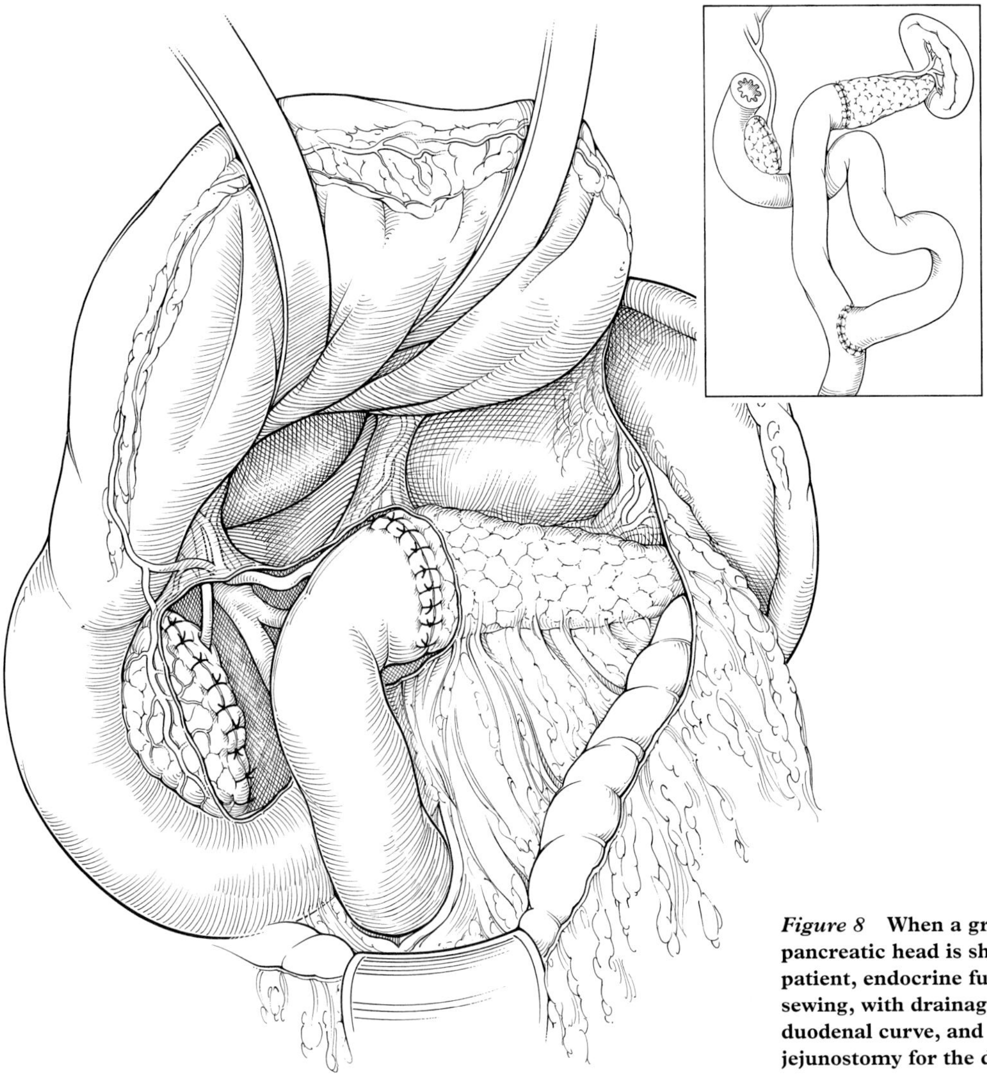

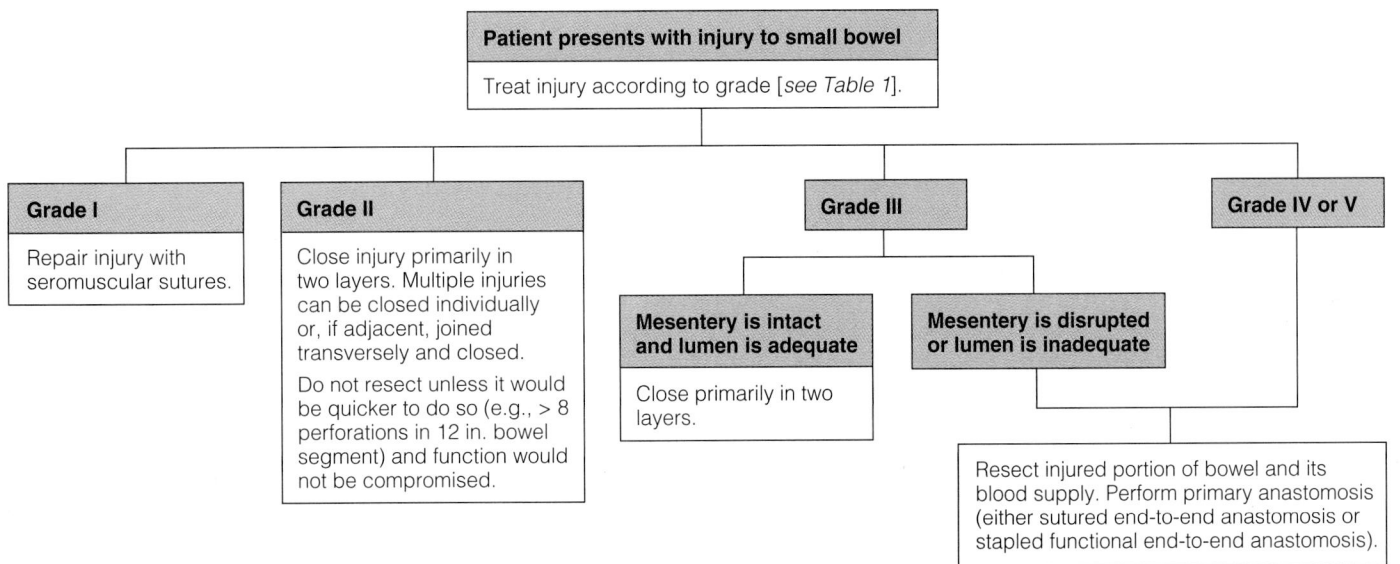

Figure 8 When a grade IV pancreatic injury to the pancreatic head is sharply demarcated in a diabetic patient, endocrine function can be preserved by over-sewing, with drainage of the pancreas along the duodenal curve, and a Roux-en-Y pancreatico-jejunostomy for the distal pancreas.

Patient presents with injury to small bowel

Treat injury according to grade [*see Table 1*].

Grade I

Repair injury with seromuscular sutures.

Grade II

Close injury primarily in two layers. Multiple injuries can be closed individually or, if adjacent, joined transversely and closed.

Do not resect unless it would be quicker to do so (e.g., > 8 perforations in 12 in. bowel segment) and function would not be compromised.

Grade III

Mesentery is intact and lumen is adequate

Close primarily in two layers.

Mesentery is disrupted or lumen is inadequate

Grade IV or V

Resect injured portion of bowel and its blood supply. Perform primary anastomosis (either sutured end-to-end anastomosis or stapled functional end-to-end anastomosis).

Figure 9 Algorithm outlines the treatment of small bowel injury.

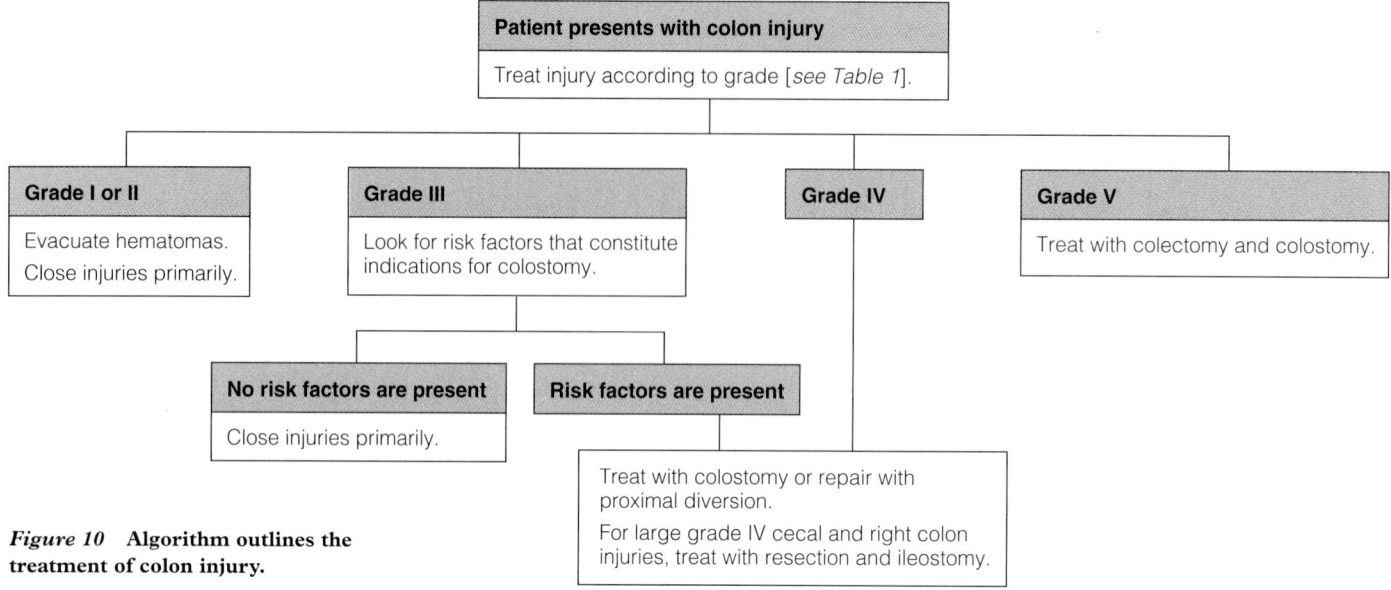

Figure 10 Algorithm outlines the treatment of colon injury.

After distal pancreatectomy with primary closure of the pancreatic stump, about 20% of patients have drainage lasting longer than 2 weeks. In most cases, nonoperative supportive therapy leads to resolution. A left upper quadrant abscess may occur, especially in patients with associated colon injury. On rare occasions, a patient with a left upper quadrant abscess experiences bleeding from the pancreatic stump that necessitates reoperation with more proximal ligation of the splenic vessels and better drainage of the left upper quadrant.

A major pancreatic transection or extensive parenchymal disruption near the ampulla (grade IV) presents special challenges. These injuries to the right of the superior mesenteric vein are often lethal when associated with vascular injury. The first priority is hemostasis, which may be accomplished by primary vascular repair or suture ligature of exposed vessels. Gentle retraction helps prevent accidental injury to the supe-

rior mesenteric vein or to unnamed veins draining the uncinate process. When a clean transection is present, a Roux-en-Y pancreaticojejunostomy allows appropriate drainage of the distal pancreas. Simple oversewing of the proximal stump reduces the likelihood that a pancreatic fistula will develop from the transected proximal pancreas [*see Figure 8*]. When the pancreatic head has a stellate laceration that does not extend posteriorly, one should attempt to establish hemostasis and provide for abundant external drainage. Two or more drains are recommended. Although pancreaticoduodenectomy may be used for grade IV injury, the magnitude of this operation in the midst of pancreatic bleeding argues that it should be performed only by the most experienced trauma surgeons.[13,15] Short-term treatment with well-placed drains often permits the patient to recover from the total insult; if a pancreaticocutaneous fistula persists, reoper-

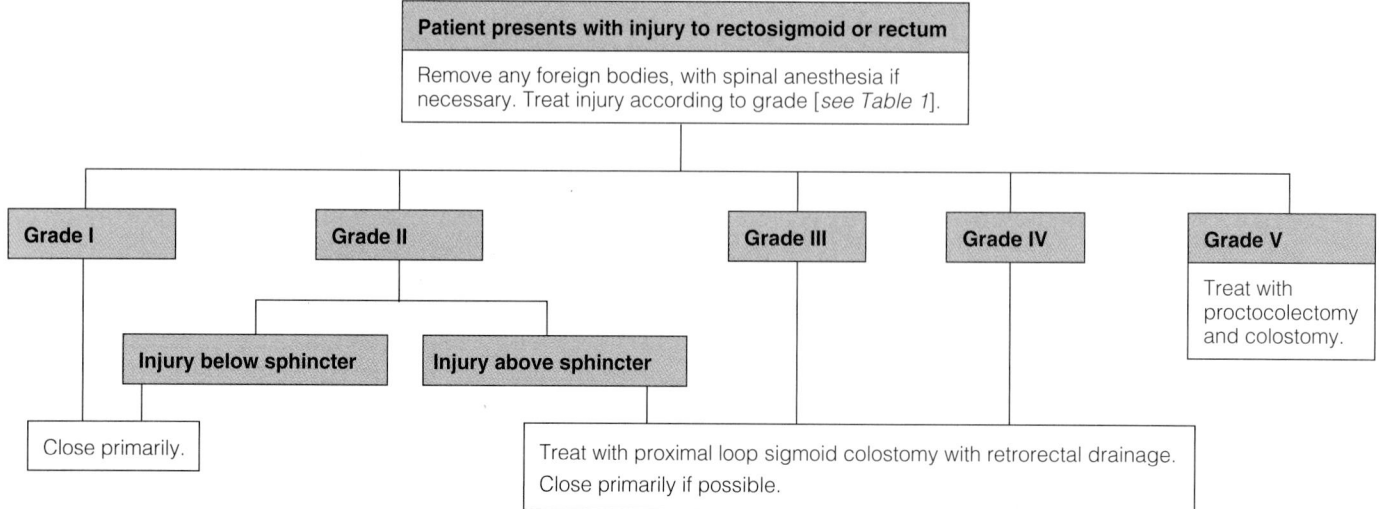

Figure 11 Algorithm outlines the treatment of rectosigmoid or rectal injury.

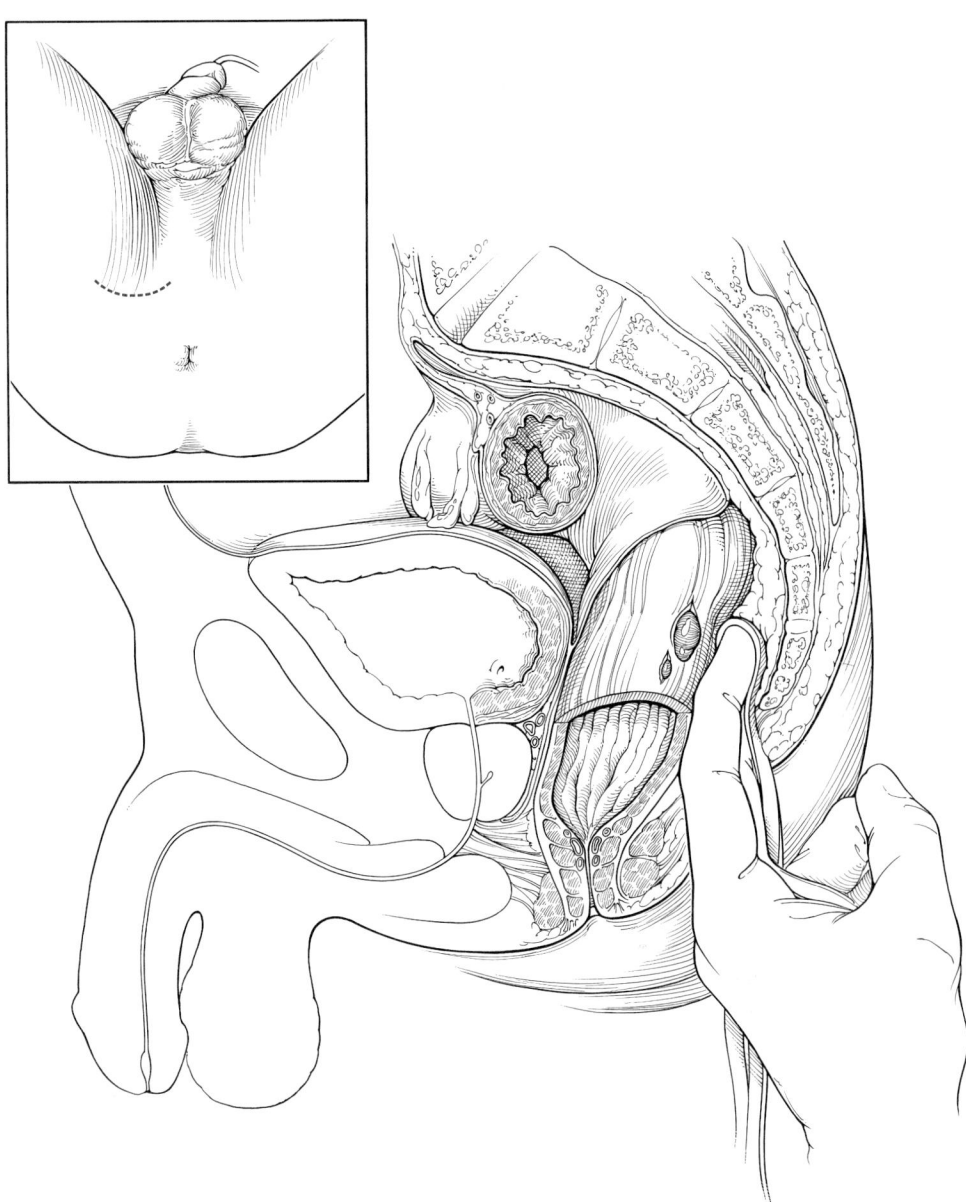

Figure 12 **Presacral drainage is
provided through a curved incision
midway between the anus and the tip
of the coccyx. With blunt dissection,
two fingers are inserted between the
rectum and the hollow of the sacrum.
Penrose drains are inserted and
sutured to the skin.**

ation can provide definitive intraluminal drainage. When a
grade IV pancreatic injury coexists with a duodenal injury,
duodenal diverticularization or duodenal exclusion is recommended; we prefer the former.

Grade V pancreatic injuries with massive disruption of the
pancreatic head (with or without associated duodenal injury)
have the highest morbidity and mortality.[13,15] When these injuries result from gunshot or stab wounds, the high incidence
of injury to the superior mesenteric vein, the superior mesenteric artery, the inferior vena cava, or the aorta often results
in death in the operating room. Once hemostasis has been
obtained, the treatment of choice for grade V injuries is either
simple external drainage of the pancreas (for unstable
patients) or pancreaticoduodenectomy or Roux-en-Y pancreaticojejunostomy (for stable patients).

Between 1990 and 1994, the surgical services at Detroit
Receiving Hospital treated 18 patients with grade V pancreatic injury. The treatment regimens varied but included duodenal diverticularization, segmental resection of the duode-

num with wide drainage of the pancreatic injury, pyloric
exclusion, Roux-en-Y pancreaticojejunostomy, and 95%
pancreatectomy with external drainage of the remaining pancreas. All patients who survived the hemorrhagic shock survived the procedures. Hospitalization was prolonged, however, and many of these patients required long-term total parenteral nutrition and additional operations for drainage of
abscesses.

Injuries to the Small Bowel

The severity of small bowel injury directs the type of treatment [*see Figure 9 and Table 1*].[5] A small intramural hematoma
(grade I) can be safely inverted with seromuscular 4-0 silk
sutures. Partial-thickness tears are gently reapproximated, with
4-0 silk sutures used to invert the torn seromuscular tissue. A
full-thickness tear (grade II) involving less than 50% of the circumference is treated by primary closure, with a continuous
absorbable suture used for the internal layer and interrupted

nonabsorbable sutures used for the outer layer.[2] Multiple grade II injuries from penetrating wounds can usually be closed individually in two layers. Adjacent through-and-through wounds are joined transversely and closed in a similar manner.[16,17] Small bowel resection for multiple injuries is not recommended unless (1) resection and anastomosis would take less time than individual closure of the multiple perforations and (2) the amount of tissue sacrificed does not compromise function. If more than eight perforations exist in a 12 in. segment of bowel, resection with primary anastomosis is more expedient than multiple primary closures.

Full-thickness small bowel perforations involving at least 50% of the circumference (grade III) can usually be closed primarily in two layers, provided that adjacent blood vessels are protected and an adequate lumen (greater than 30% of the circumference) is maintained.[18] A transverse closure helps protect lumen patency.

Complete transection (grade IV) is treated by resection of the injured portion and its adjacent blood supply, followed by prima-

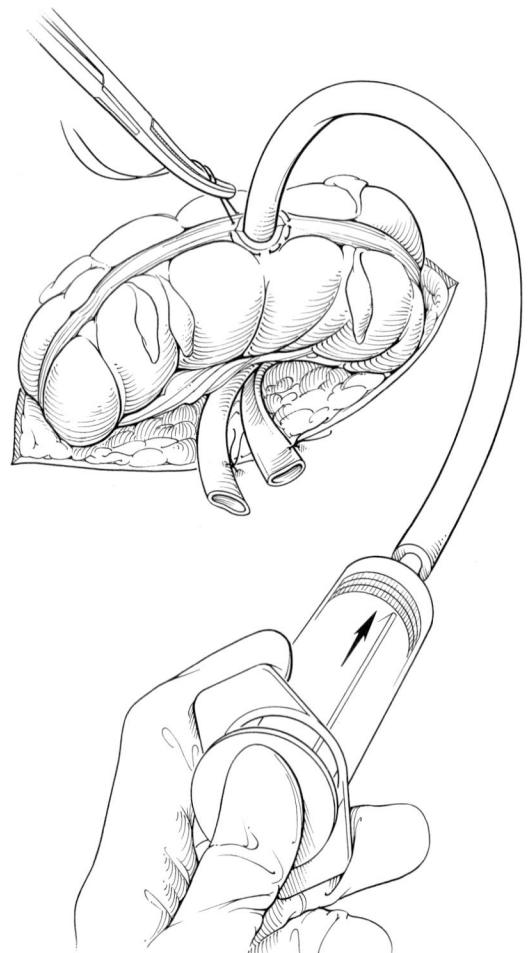

Figure 13 Irrigation of the distal sigmoid colon and rectum reduces soilage of the retrorectal space through unclosed perforations of the rectum as peristalsis returns. At the completion of the operative procedure, a purse-string suture is placed in the sigmoid colostomy and a large Foley catheter passed into the distal limb. The distal limb is irrigated with saline as the anus is held open. The catheter is then removed, and the colostomy is opened and matured.

ry anastomosis.[19,20] This can be accomplished by the hand-sewn end-to-end technique or by fashioning a stapled functional (as opposed to anatomic) end-to-end anastomosis [see 3:23 Intestinal Anastomosis]. Stapled small bowel anastomoses may be associated with higher complication rates in injured patients than hand-sewn anastomoses are. A 1999 study[21] found stapled anastomoses to be more prone to leakage, and a 2000 study[22] reported a higher incidence of intra-abdominal abscesses after stapled anastomoses. Neither group of investigators inverted the staple line of the anastomosis. Inversion of all exposed staple lines with 4-0 silk sutures provides added safety.

Extensive destruction of the small bowel or its mesentery (grade V) necessitates resection and reconstruction using the same techniques recommended for grade III and grade IV bowel injuries.[2,17] Treatment of an isolated mesenteric tear without bowel rupture depends on the vascularity of the bowel. If the bowel is necrotic and devascularized, resection is required; if the bowel remains pink and peristalsis is normal, careful closure of the mesenteric tear is sufficient. If vascularity is marginal, simple closure of the mesentery without resection of the bowel may lead to stenosis; thus, resection with primary reconstruction is recommended.

Injuries to the Colon

As with injuries to other organs, the treatment of colon injury depends on its severity [see Figure 10 and Table 1].[5] Because the ascending, descending, and retrosigmoid segments of the colon are located retroperitoneally, they may still have penetrating injuries even when DPL yields negative results.[23] Such injuries may be seen with contrast CT, but the importance of sequential physical examination to an early diagnosis cannot be overemphasized. Blunt injury is uncommon; when present, it is usually located in the cecum or the sigmoid colon.[23,24] Because these injuries seldom cause pneumoperitoneum, early diagnosis depends on careful sequential physical examination.

Most minor injuries (grades I and II) can be treated with primary repair [see Figure 10]. For small hematomas or partial-thickness lacerations, simple closure with inversion is sufficient. Similarly, a partial-thickness contusion should be inverted to preclude subsequent full-thickness necrosis with perforation.[23,25] Grade II hematomas should be evacuated carefully to prevent full-thickness injury and should be closed primarily. Through-and-through injuries with little or no spill and a minimum of associated injuries can be closed primarily throughout the colon.[25,26]

Because the colon has an increased bacterial level, ranging from 10^6 in the cecum to 10^{13} in the rectum, primary closure of colon injuries is associated with a much greater risk of leakage than primary closure of small bowel perforations. Accordingly, many patients are candidates for colostomy; however, primary closure is preferred for most minor injuries. In a prospective, randomized study of primary closure versus colostomy, Stone and Fabian reported that morbidity was much higher in the colostomy patients.[3] On the basis of these and other studies, primary closure appears to be the preferred technique in patients with the following clinical characteristics: (1) injuries with minimal spill; (2) fewer than three associated injuries; (3) no hypotension; (4) minimal blood loss; (5) a short interval between injury and operation; (6) good colonic vascularity; (7) injury involving no more than 50% of the circumference; and (8) an intact abdominal wall.

ROLE OF COLOSTOMY

Colostomy is preferred in patients with one or more of the following clinical characteristics[3,5,23]: (1) a wound involving more than 50% of the circumference (grade III); (2) extensive free peritoneal fecal spill; (3) associated hypotension; (4) a need for multiple transfusions; (5) three or more associated injuries; (6) colonic devascularization (grade V); (7) a delay of more than 6 hours between injury and operative intervention; (8) an extensive retroperitoneal hematoma from pelvic fractures; (9) an associated abdominal wall defect; and (10) an associated rectal injury.

Specific methods include exteriorization of the segment of injured colon as a loop colostomy; closure of the injured colon, which is then protected by a proximal colostomy; and resection of the injured colon with a proximal end colostomy and a distal mucous fistula (or the Hartmann closure). Simple exteriorization of the injured colon as a loop colostomy is most effective for serious grade III injuries to the right, transverse, left, or sigmoid colon. After the abdomen has been closed, the ostomy is matured primarily to facilitate early fitting with a properly sized appliance. Because exteriorization of the distal sigmoid colon usually is not feasible, such injuries are treated by primary closure with a proximal colostomy (grade III) or by resection of the injury with proximal end colostomy and a distal Hartmann procedure (grades IV and V). For a grade V injury to the distal sigmoid colon with associated devascularization, resection of the injured segment is essential. This type of injury necessitates a proximal end colostomy in conjunction with a Hartmann procedure.

RIGHT COLON INJURY

If the cecum or the first 6 cm of the ascending colon has suffered extensive injury, it may be technically difficult to exteriorize the injured segment as a colostomy.[27] The redundant cecum, including its inferior cul-de-sac, may fill the appliance bag and inconvenience the patient. When large grade IV or V cecal injuries are present, resection with end ileostomy and a distal mucous fistula is safe and effective.

For large cecal and right colon injuries, right hemicolectomy with primary ileotransverse colon anastomosis has been advocated.[23,26] Despite the excellent results reported with right hemicolectomy and primary anastomosis, we recommend that whenever right colon wounds are so extensive that primary closure cannot be done safely, resection with ileostomy should be performed instead. Most patients can tolerate a properly constructed Brooke ileostomy with intraoperative fitting of the appliance [see 3:27 Colorectal Procedures].

The so-called closed-loop exteriorization, in which the colon injury is closed primarily and the injured segment then brought out as a temporary exteriorization for 7 to 10 days, is no longer performed. Patients who healed after this procedure probably would have done as well after primary closure. We recommend that whenever there is doubt about the safety of a primary closure, the patient should be treated with a colostomy.

COLOSTOMY CLOSURE

The optimal time for colostomy closure depends on the underlying insult, postoperative morbidity, and the patient's general condition. A patient is ready for a colostomy closure when general health has been restored, appetite has returned, lost weight has been regained, and all wounds have healed. When these criteria are met, mortality associated with colosto-my closure should approach zero.[28] Although some colostomies may be closed within days or weeks after injury, those associated with extensive peritonitis and enterocutaneous fistulas are best closed 6 to 12 months after injury.

The safest way of closing loop colostomies involves resection of the exteriorized loop through an oval-shaped incision around the loop, followed by closure with an end-to-end colocolostomy. Sutures are preferred to the staples in this setting because they allow closure of the ostomy through this pericolostomy incision with less mobilization of the proximal and distal ends. When end colostomies are closed, full laparotomy with lysis of all adhesions is required to provide tension-free end-to-end anastomosis and reapproximation of the mesentery. On the whole, we prefer hand-sewn anastomoses for colonic reconstruction.[28]

Injuries to the Rectosigmoid and Rectum

Rectosigmoid and rectal injuries also vary in severity [see Figure 11 and Table 1].[5,29] The agents of injury include knives, bullets, cars, and rectal obturators such as enema tips, thermometers, and sexual toys. The rectosigmoid colon begins near the sacral promontory and extends to the retrovesical fold, where only the anterior bowel wall is covered with peritoneum. Posterior injuries in this 3 to 5 cm zone are retroperitoneal; below this point, the rectum is completely retroperitoneal.

Small, clean, easily accessible rectosigmoid wounds (grades I and II) can be closed primarily if conditions are favorable. Larger wounds require that this segment of bowel be exteriorized or diverted by a proximal colostomy. This can often be accomplished by a proximal sigmoid loop colostomy with primary closure of the rectosigmoid wound.[27,29,30] Massive wounds (grades IV and V) in the rectosigmoid junctional zone require excision, with proximal colostomy and a distal Hartmann procedure.

Penetrating rectal injuries can be diagnosed by means of proctoscopic examination. During laparotomy, the retroperitoneal hematoma associated with rectal injuries often interferes with safe dissection and clear identification of the perforation. Small wounds (grades I and II) can be closed primarily if a proximal colostomy is performed in conjunction with retrorectal drainage. The skin incision for retrorectal drainage is placed between the anus and the coccyx [see Figure 12]. The drain should extend proximal to the perforation. When examination shows that the rectum is filled with stool, the colostomy is opened at the time of operation to facilitate disimpaction and copious distal irrigation with balanced electrolyte solution [see Figure 13]. The anus is kept open only during this irrigation, to facilitate passage of saline and associated stool into an adjacent bucket and to decrease the likelihood that stool will be pushed through the site of injury into retroperitoneal tissues.[28,30] Grade III and grade IV rectal injuries are often more difficult to close primarily; they are usually treated with a proximal colostomy and retrorectal drainage. Massive devascularized grade V rectal injuries are rare; they are treated with resection followed by a proximal end colostomy.

Foreign bodies may produce rectal injuries. Although a thermometer is the most common offending agent in pediatric patients, a larger obturator inserted for pleasure is the usual agent in adults. Such obturators include cans, soft drink bottles, light bulbs, vibrators, and other firm objects. When the offending agent is difficult to remove, spinal anesthesia may be helpful. Once the foreign body has been removed, careful endoscopic examination helps rule out intrinsic injury to the upper rectum or the rectosigmoid. When transanal extraction is impossible, full laparotomy and gentle pushing of the offending agent from above usually permit safe removal. Repair of full-thickness injuries from these obturators follows the guidelines for other types of penetrating injuries.[28]

Extensive grade V rectal injuries associated with close-range shotgun wounds often cause devascularization and intrusion of the bony pelvis. These wounds may require extensive resection of the rectum as well as proximal diversion. Occasionally, these injuries are severe enough to preclude subsequent rectal repair. In rare cases, an industrial accident may result in the same type of extensive injury that is associated with pelvic fractures. For such patients, delayed reconstruction of the rectum may be impossible because of extensive damage to the rectum and the adjacent sacral plexus. Permanent colostomy will be needed in such cases.

References

1. Lucas CE: Splenic trauma: choice of management. Ann Surg 213:98, 1991

2. Wisner DH, Blaisdell FW: Visceral injuries. Arch Surg 127:687, 1992

3. Stone HH, Fabian TC: Management of duodenal wounds. J Trauma 19:334, 1979

4. Kline G, Lucas CE, Ledgerwood AM, et al: Duodenal organ injury severity (OIS) and outcome. Am Surg 60:500, 1994

5. Moore EE, Cogbill TH, Malangoni MA, et al: Organ injury scaling: II. Pancreas, duodenum, small bowel, colon, and rectum. J Trauma 30:1427, 1990

6. Berne CJ, Donovan AJ, White EJ, et al: Duodenal diverticulation for duodenal and pancreatic injury. Am J Surg 127:503, 1974

7. Shorr RM, Greaney GC, Donovan AJ: Injuries of the duodenum. Am J Surg 154:93, 1987

8. Cogbill TH, Moore EE, Feliciano DV, et al: Conservative management of duodenal trauma: a multicenter perspective. J Trauma 30:1469, 1990

9. Degiannis E, Krawczykowski D, Velmahos GC, et al: Pyloric exclusion in severe penetrating injuries of the duodenum. World J Surg 17:751, 1993

10. Vaughan GD 3rd, Frazier OH, Graham DY, et al: The use of pyloric exclusion in the management of severe duodenal injuries. Am J Surg 134:785, 1977

11. Pederzoli P, Bassi C, Falconi M, et al: Conservative treatment of external pancreatic fistulas with parenteral nutrition alone or in combination with continuous intravenous infusion of somatostatin, glucagon, or calcitonin. Surg Gynecol Obstet 163:428, 1986

12. Sugawa C, Lucas CE: The role of endoscopic retrograde cholangiopancreatography in surgery of the pancreas and biliary ducts. Endoscopic Retrograde Cholangiopancreatography. Silvis SE, Rohrmann CA, Ansel HJ, Eds. Igaku-Shoin, New York, 1994, p 3

13. Feliciano DV, Martin TD, Cruse PA, et al: Management of combined pancreatoduodenal injuries. Ann Surg 205:673, 1987

14. Stone A, Sugawa C, Lucas C, et al: The role of endoscopic retrograde pancreatography (ERP) in blunt abdominal trauma. Am Surg 56:715, 1990

15. McKone TK, Bursch LR, Scholten DJ: Pancreaticoduodenectomy for trauma: a life-saving procedure. Am Surg 54:361, 1988

16. Flint LM, Cryer HM, Howard DA, et al: Approaches to the management of shotgun injuries. J Trauma 24:415, 1984

17. Schenk WG 3rd, Lonchyna V, Moylan JA: Perforation of the jejunum from blunt abdominal trauma. J Trauma 23:54, 1983

18. Wisner DH, Chun Y, Blaisdell FW: Blunt intestinal injury: keys to diagnosis and management. Arch Surg 125:1319, 1990

19. Coleman EJ, Dietz PA: Small bowel injuries following blunt abdominal trauma: early recognition and management. NY State J Med 90:446, 1990

20. Sherck J, Shatney C, Sensaki K, et al: The accuracy of computed tomography in the diagnosis of blunt small-bowel perforation. Am J Surg 168:670, 1994

21. Brundage SI, Jurkovich GJ, Grossman DC, et al: Stapled versus sutured gastrointestinal anastomoses in the trauma patient. J Trauma 47:500, 1999

22. Witzke JD, Kraatz JJ, Marken JM, et al: Stapled versus hand-sewn anastomoses in patients with small bowel injury: a changing perspective. J Trauma 49:660, 2000

23. Lucas C, Ledgerwood A: Management of the injured colon. Current Surgery 43:190, 1986

24. Ross SE, Cobean RA, Hoyt DB, et al: Blunt colonic injury—a multicenter review. J Trauma 33:379, 1992

25. George SM Jr, Fabian TC, Voeller GR, et al: Primary repair of colon wounds: a prospective trial in nonselected patients. Ann Surg 209:728, 1989

26. Ivatury RR, Licata J, Gunduz Y, et al: Management options in penetrating rectal injuries. Am Surg 57:50, 1991

27. Strada G, Raad L, Belloni G, et al: Large bowel perforations in war surgery: one-stage treatment in a field hospital. Int J Colorectal Dis 8:213, 1993

28. Ledgerwood AM, Lucas CE: Management of colon injuries. Principles and Practice of Trauma Care. Worth MH, Ed. Williams & Wilkins, Baltimore, 1982, p 117

29. Nelken N, Lewis F: The influence of injury severity on complication rates after primary closure or colostomy for penetrating colon trauma. Ann Surg 209:439, 1989

30. Burch JM, Feliciano DV, Mattox KL: Colostomy and drainage for civilian rectal injuries: is that all? Ann Surg 209:600, 1989

Acknowledgments

Supported by the Interstitial Fluid Fund, Account 4-44966.

Figures 1, 2, 5, 9 through 11   Marcia Kammerer.

Figures 3, 8, 12, 13   Susan Brust, C.M.I.

Figures 4, 6, 7   Carol Donner.

8 OPERATIVE EXPOSURE OF ABDOMINAL INJURIES AND CLOSURE OF THE ABDOMEN

Erwin R. Thal, M.D., F.A.C.S., Brian J. Eastridge, M.D., F.A.C.S., and Rusty Milhoan, M.D., F.A.C.S.

Management of abdominal trauma has changed significantly since the beginning of the 1990s. In part, the change is attributable to improvements in the available diagnostic studies and to the advent of nonoperative therapeutic approaches. Those patients who require operative intervention for treatment of abdominal injuries often present a major challenge to the surgical team. Although each such patient is unique, we believe that the application of a standard operative approach is nonetheless necessary to optimize patient care and to minimize the risk of missing injuries. The primary objective of this operative approach is the expeditious prioritization and treatment of injuries. To this end, all surgeons treating injured patients should have a general routine to follow and should be familiar with a variety of exposures and techniques that may be used to carry out this routine. Adequate exposure, rapid assessment, and sound clinical judgment are essential ingredients of the care of patients with abdominal injuries.

Patient Preparation

Before the celiotomy is begun, the patient must be adequately prepared. All contingencies must be planned for in advance. A nasogastric tube and a Foley catheter should be inserted, and a single dose of a broad-spectrum antibiotic should be given before the initial incision is made. With the patient positioned on the operating table, skin preparation is performed in such a way as to include the anterior chest as well as the abdomen; one thus has virtually immediate access to the chest in the event that a thoracic injury is discovered or thoracic vascular control is required. In addition, skin preparation should be extended over the anterior thighs in case distal vascular control is warranted or a vascular reconstruction conduit is needed. All exposed areas of the body that were not prepared must be covered to optimize thermoregulation. Drapes should be placed widely to allow easy access to all potential injuries.

Resuscitation, including the use of blood and blood products, should be continued as the patient is prepared. Both rapid volume infusion systems and cell saver systems are useful adjuncts in this setting. Room temperature must be controlled to minimize loss of heat from the patient during the operation.

Incision and Initial Exploration

CHOICE OF INCISION

A midline incision is the most expedient choice for opening the abdomen. It has several key advantages: it allows the abdominal cavity to be accessed easily and quickly, it provides good exposure (including exposure of the pelvis), and it can be extended into a median sternotomy or into either thoracic cavity if necessary. Its main disadvantage is the occasional difficulty that may be encountered in exploring the deep recesses of the upper quadrants.

Patients who have had previous midline incisions may be more challenging to operate on, depending on the extent to which intraperitoneal adhesions are present. Accordingly, alternative incisions may be considered. For example, a chevron incision or a transverse incision might allow better visualization of viscera adhering to a previous midline wound and thus might tend to protect them better from iatrogenic injury; however, these incisions are associated with certain disadvantages, in particular the need to divide the large rectus abdominis muscle, the restricted exposure provided, the additional time needed to close the incision, and the inherent limitations on extension of the incision if the need arises. Consequently, chevron and transverse incisions are rarely used and seldom recommended in this setting.

There are additional alternative incisions, such as paramedian, subcostal, retroperitoneal, and flank incisions, but they are not recommended, because they generally do not provide adequate exposure for assessment and treatment of abdominal injuries.

INITIAL EXPLORATION

Once the peritoneal cavity has been entered, initial exploration should proceed in an orderly manner so as to minimize hemorrhage and contamination and facilitate the identification of injuries. There may be an incipient drop in blood pressure when the abdomen is opened. The abdominal organs are eviscerated, and any gross blood, clotted or nonclotted, is evacuated. Laparotomy pads are then used for rapid packing of all four quadrants of the abdomen. When bleeding is under control, anesthesia is allowed to catch up with the resuscitation efforts before abdominal exploration is continued.

Once hemodynamic stability has been achieved, the peritoneal portion of the initial exploration is begun. If there is no discrete site of hemorrhage, the temporary packs are carefully removed, except for those around the solid viscera. The enteric viscera are inspected in an orderly fashion. The anterior aspect of the stomach is inspected from the esophagogastric junction to the pylorus. If there is a high index of suspicion, on the basis of the mechanism of injury or the presence of hematoma or soilage in the lesser sac, the gastrocolic omentum is opened to permit inspection of the posterior aspect of the stomach; this exposure also facilitates examination of the body of the pancreas. Exploration then continues distally. If duodenal or pancreatic injury is suspected, the Kocher maneuver is performed to mobilize the duodenum and the head of the pancreas fully. Once the duodenum has been visualized, the small bowel is inspected from the ligament of Treitz to the ileocecal valve. Careful consideration should be given to the possibility of mesenteric vascular injury, which is often manifested as a mesenteric hematoma. Next, the colon is inspected from the cecum to the peritoneal reflection over the rectum. If there are injuries or missile tracts in proximity to a portion of the ascending or descending colon, the colon must be mobilized by incising the peritoneal reflection (the white line of Toldt) so as to permit inspection of the posterior wall of the bowel as well. Finally, attention is turned toward evaluation of the solid viscera. The laparotomy pads are removed, and the liver and the spleen are visualized to ascertain whether any injury is present.

Once the peritoneal survey has been completed, the retroperitoneum is inspected for potential injury. Retroperitoneal hematomas are classified according to their location: zone 1 is the central portion of the retroperitoneum, zone 2 comprises the two lateral portions, and zone 3 is the pelvic portion [*see Figure 1*]. The decision whether to explore a retroperitoneal hematoma is based on its location and on the mechanism of injury [*see Priorities in Management, Repair of Retroperitoneal Injuries, below*]. The retroperitoneum is also evaluated with an eye to identifying any occult injuries to organs such as the pancreas, the duodenum, the posterior colon, the kidneys, and vascular structures. The initial exploration concludes with a brief pelvic survey undertaken to exclude injury to the rectum or the distal genitourinary tract (including the urinary bladder).

Operative Exposure

In what follows, we focus on exposure of specific organs and vessels in patients with abdominal injuries. Definitive repair of such injuries is addressed in more detail elsewhere [*see 5:6 In-*

juries to the Liver, Biliary Tract, Spleen, and Diaphragm; 5:7 Injuries to the Stomach, Duodenum, Pancreas, Small Bowel, Colon, and Rectum; and 5:9 Injuries to the Great Vessels of the Abdomen].

AORTA

Control of the aorta can be achieved at several different levels, depending on the site of injury. The supraceliac aorta can be exposed by incising the gastrohepatic ligament, retracting the left lobe of the liver cephalad, and retracting the stomach caudad. The esophagus and the periesophageal soft tissue are then mobilized laterally to permit identification of the abdominal aorta at the diaphragmatic hiatus, at which point the vessel can be clamped or compressed. The exposure this method gives is limited with respect to vascular access for definitive repair. Better exposure of the supraceliac aorta can be obtained by means of left medial visceral rotation [*see Figure 2*]. To reflect the left-sided viscera, the splenorenal ligament is mobilized with a combination of blunt and sharp dissection. The peritoneal reflection is incised, and the incision is extended down the left paracolic gutter to the level of the distal sigmoid colon. With the aid of blunt dissection, the left-sided viscera are gently mobilized to the right in a plane anterior to Gerota's fascia. This technique permits exploration of the entire length of the abdominal aorta as well as the origin of the celiac axis, the origin of the superior mesenteric artery, the left iliac system, and the origin of the right common iliac artery. In addition, it facilitates control of the left renal pedicle before exploration of a left-sided hematoma within Gerota's fascia.

If only distal access to the aorta is necessary, the vessel can be approached transperitoneally. The small bowel is retracted to the right, the transverse colon is retracted cephalad, and the descending colon is retracted to the left. The peritoneum is incised over the aorta, and the third and fourth portions of the duodenum are mobilized cephalad. The proximal limit of this dissection extends to the level of the left renal vein, which can, if necessary, be divided to provide access to the suprarenal aorta. If the left renal vein is ligated, care should be taken to place the ligature close to the vena cava so as to spare important venous collaterals. A somewhat more limited dissection may suffice to expose the distal infrarenal aorta; the exposure can subsequently be extended distally to expose both iliac vessels.

VENA CAVA

Access to the suprahepatic vena cava can be gained by incising the central tendon of the diaphragm or by performing a median sternotomy and opening the pericardium. The infrahepatic inferior vena cava can be exposed by means of right medial visceral rotation [*see Figure 3*] in much the same way as the aorta is exposed by means of left medial visceral rotation [*see Aorta, above*]. The right colon is mobilized by taking down the hepatic flexure and incising the peritoneal reflection within the right paracolic gutter. The colon, again, is reflected medially toward the aorta in a plane anterior to Gerota's fascia with the aid of blunt dissection. If additional exposure is necessary, the inferior margin of the peritoneal incision can be extended to the root of the mesentery and even beyond by sacrificing the inferior mesenteric vein. This exposure allows visualization of both the aorta below the origin of the superior mesenteric artery and the vena cava below the third portion of the duodenum. The portion of the inferior vena cava immediately below the liver can be exposed by performing the Kocher maneuver [*see Figure 4*] with subsequent medial mobilization of the duodenum and head of the pancreas.

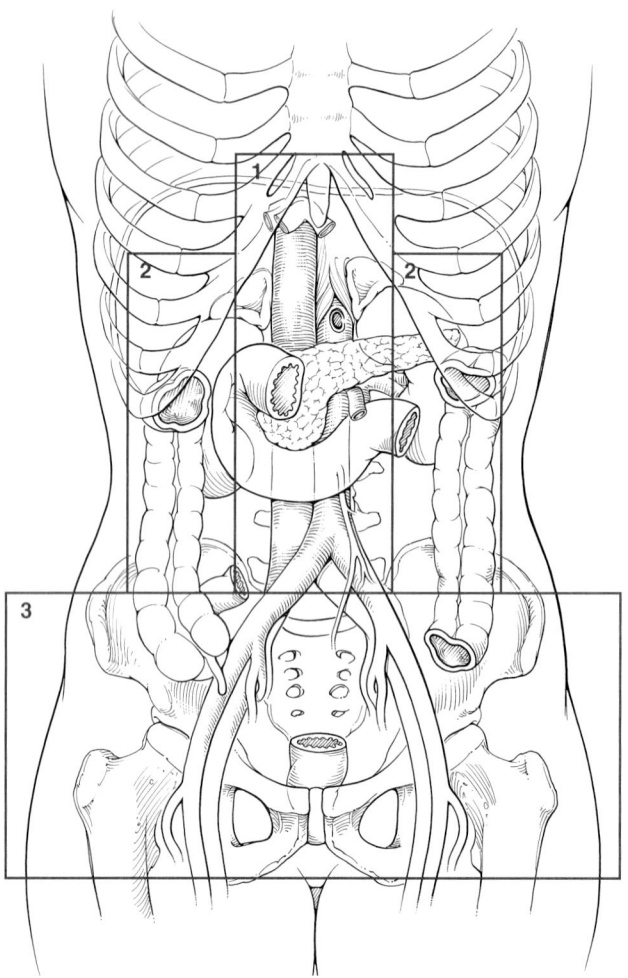

Figure 1 **Shown are the anatomic zones of the retroperitoneum: zone 1 (central), zone 2 (flank), and zone 3 (pelvic).**

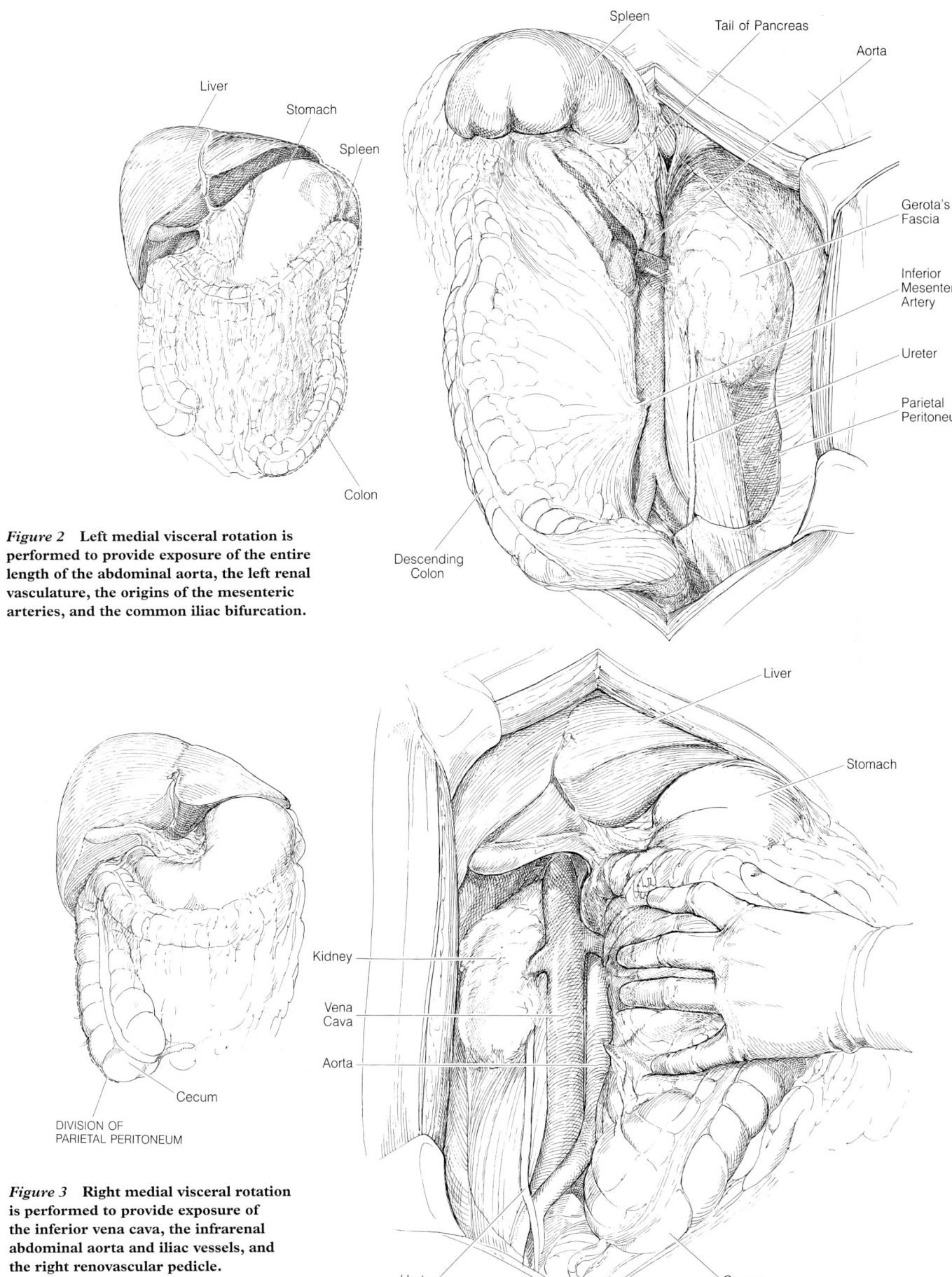

Figure 2 **Left medial visceral rotation is performed to provide exposure of the entire length of the abdominal aorta, the left renal vasculature, the origins of the mesenteric arteries, and the common iliac bifurcation.**

Figure 3 **Right medial visceral rotation is performed to provide exposure of the inferior vena cava, the infrarenal abdominal aorta and iliac vessels, and the right renovascular pedicle.**

This right medial visceral exposure facilitates identification of the right renovascular pedicle for control before exploration of a right-sided perinephric hematoma.

PANCREAS

Intraoperative evidence of a central hematoma, peripancreatic edema, or bile staining in the retroperitoneum or the lesser sac raises the possibility of pancreatic injury. The contents of the lesser sac can be seen through the gastrohepatic ligament by direct inspection or by division of the ligament, or they can be visualized by dividing and ligating two or three gastroepiploic arcades of the gastrocolic ligament. If it proves necessary to explore the pancreas, the stomach is separated from the transverse colon by completing the division of the gastrocolic ligament. A Kocher maneuver is performed to reflect the second, third, and fourth portions of the duodenum medially, along with the head of the pancreas. This exposure allows inspection of the anterior and posterior surfaces of the head of the pancreas as well as the uncinate process. If injury to the body or tail of the pancreas is suspected, the splenorenal and splenocolic ligaments are incised. At this point, the spleen and, subsequently, the pancreas can be mobilized medially to a position near the level of the superior mesenteric vessels, and the anterior and posterior aspects of the body and tail can be examined.

DUODENUM AND BILIARY TRACT

The pancreatic head and the duodenum can be adequately exposed by means of the Kocher maneuver (see above). This technique is also used when injury to the distal extrahepatic biliary system is suspected. The proximal extrahepatic biliary tree is visualized by using the Kocher maneuver in combination with local exploration of the porta hepatis.

Priorities in Management

HEMORRHAGE CONTROL

If the patient remains hemodynamically unstable as a result of persistent hemorrhage, the initial and primary focus of the exploration becomes control of bleeding. There are several techniques by which hemostasis may be established. One is repeat packing of the specific bleeding site with laparotomy pads. The importance of adequate packing to the control of hemorrhage cannot be overestimated. Packing is effective as a temporizing measure until more definitive vascular control can be achieved or until a coagulopathy has been corrected.

If persistent hemorrhage is anticipated, proximal and distal control of the injured vessel is obtained by means of the exposure techniques already discussed [see Operative Exposure, above]. Given the potential for exsanguinating hemorrhage, one must be ready to gain control over aortic inflow at the diaphragmatic hiatus or to control the descending aorta in the chest via a left lateral thoracotomy. Effective aortic control may be obtained through digital compression of the vessel at the hiatus; subsequently, a padded Richardson retractor or an aortic compressor may be used to occlude the vessel. If prolonged occlusion of arterial inflow is necessary, an atraumatic vascular clamp may be applied at the hiatus. Injuries to the proximal abdominal aorta often necessitate control of the vessel within the chest.

In patients with parenchymal injury to the solid viscera, control of vascular inflow is crucial as both a diagnostic and a therapeutic maneuver. Control of the splenic hilum effectively stops

splenic hemorrhage. Likewise, use of the Pringle maneuver [see 5:6 Injuries to the Liver, Biliary Tract, Spleen, and Diaphragm] to control the vessels in the porta hepatis (the hepatic artery and the portal vein) is useful for determining the source of perihepatic hemorrhage. The Pringle maneuver is performed by compressing the portal structures digitally. If bleeding is diminished as a result, control of portal inflow can be maintained by means of an atraumatic vascular clamp or a Rumel tourniquet; however, if significant hemorrhage persists, one must consider the possibility of an injury to the retrohepatic vena cava.

In patients who have a retrohepatic vena caval injury, hepatic exclusion may be necessary for vascular control before definitive repair. This is accomplished by first gaining control of the inferior vena cava both above and below the liver. Control of the inferior vena cava above the liver is obtained by performing a median sternotomy and a pericardiotomy and occluding the vessel within the pericardium. Control of the inferior vena cava below the liver is accomplished by means of right medial visceral rotation in conjunction with the Kocher maneuver. Rumel tourniquets are applied to the vena cava above and below the liver. A monofilament purse-string suture is placed in the right atrial appendage. Extra side holes are cut in the middle portion of a 36 French chest tube. The right atrial appendage is opened, and the chest tube is passed down through the inferior vena cava and positioned so that all of the distal shunt holes are inferior to the Rumel tourniquet below the liver and the proximal shunt holes are superior to the Rumel tourniquet above the liver [see Figure 5]. The tourniquets are then secured around the tube. As an alternative, an endotracheal tube with extra proximal side holes may be used as a shunt. Control of venous inflow below the liver is obtained by inflating the balloon. It is important not to transect the insufflation channel while cutting the side holes. When this type of system is employed, adapters can be used to infuse fluid and blood directly into the right atrium.

Another technique for controlling retrohepatic hemorrhage is occlusion of the inferior vena cava both above and below the liver. This technique often results in significant hemodynamic instability, especially in volume-depleted patients; however, it may be tolerated by patients whose volume status is good. Complete hepatic exclusion involves both atriocaval shunting or clamping of the inferior vena cava and control of hepatic arterial and portal venous inflow.

CONTROL OF CONTAMINATION

Once hemorrhage has been controlled, the next priority is control of contamination. Small enterotomies may be temporarily closed with Babcock clamps while awaiting definitive repair; alternatively, they may be temporarily closed with a continuous suture to prevent ongoing spillage. When multiple enterotomies are present, suture closure is probably preferable to obviate the placement of multiple clamps within the operative field. If the patient has several holes in the bowel that are all in close proximity, the best way of containing the luminal contents is to apply atraumatic clamps at both the proximal end and the distal end of the injury site. If placing bowel clamps is not feasible or the clamps get in the way, a stapling device can be used to control an enteric leak. Once the spillage is controlled, all gross foreign material should be removed from the peritoneal cavity.

VASCULAR REPAIR

After the patient has been stabilized and hemorrhage and bowel contamination have been controlled, attention is directed to defini-

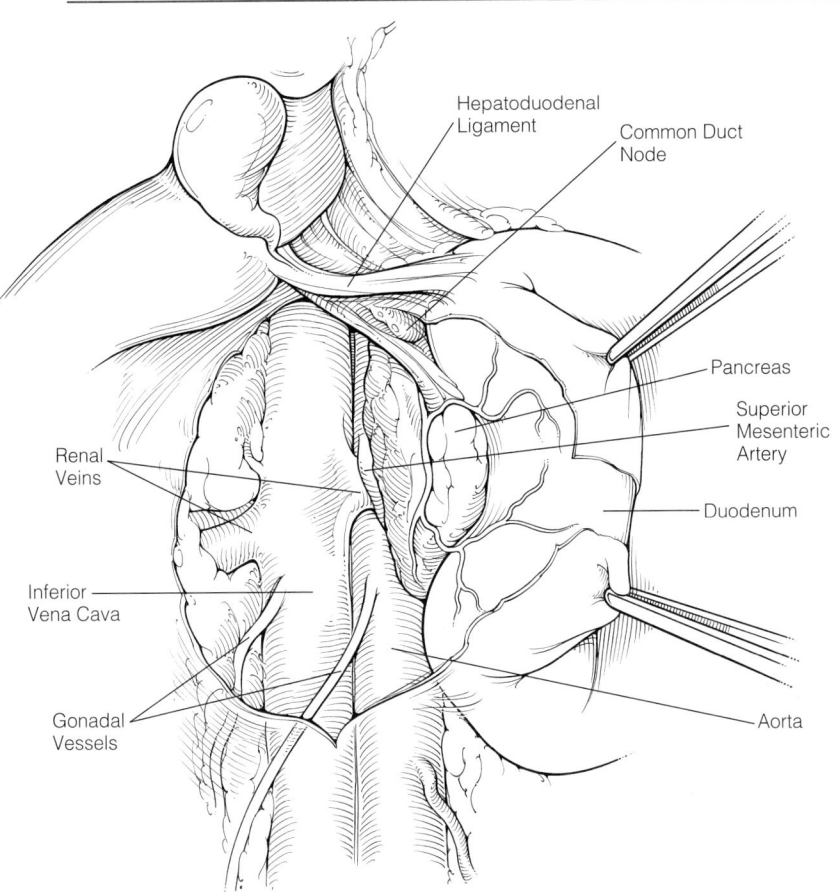

Figure 4 **The Kocher maneuver reflects the duodenum and the pancreatic head from the retroperitoneum, allowing access to the infrahepatic inferior vena cava as well as to the distal common bile duct, the duodenum, and the pancreatic head.**

tive vascular repair. Control of the injured vessel, both proximally and distally, is obtained if this has not already been done. The vascular injury is identified and adequately debrided, and continuity is re-established. If the vascular injury is not amenable to ligation or primary repair, autogenous tissue is procured and used as either a patch or an interposition graft. If no suitable autogenous tissue is available, synthetic material must be considered for use as a vascular conduit. In cases of aortic or iliac arterial injury, primary ligation with subsequent extra-anatomic bypass is an acceptable alternative.

REPAIR OF DAMAGED OR DEVITALIZED BOWEL

The next priority is repair of enteric injuries. Because of the large size of the stomach and its rich vascularity, most gastric wounds can be repaired primarily. In general, small-bowel injuries that involve less than 50% of the circumference after debridement can be repaired primarily with either a one-layer or a two-layer closure. As a rule, single-layer closure is preferred because it is less likely to compromise the lumen of the bowel. If multiple enterotomies or large areas of devitalized tissue in close proximity are present, segmental enterectomy with primary anastomosis is a more prudent option. The entero-enterostomy can be performed as either a hand-sewn or a stapled anastomosis; the latter tends to be more expeditious. Solitary injuries to the colon that do not have to be resected and are not associated with shock, massive blood transfusion, or significant contamination can be repaired primarily. Large or multiple injuries located in the right colon are best managed with a right hemicolectomy followed by primary ileocolic anastomosis. Multiple or large injuries in the left colon are best treated with resection followed by proximal diversion and distal limb exteriorization. If distal diversion is impossible because of inadequate

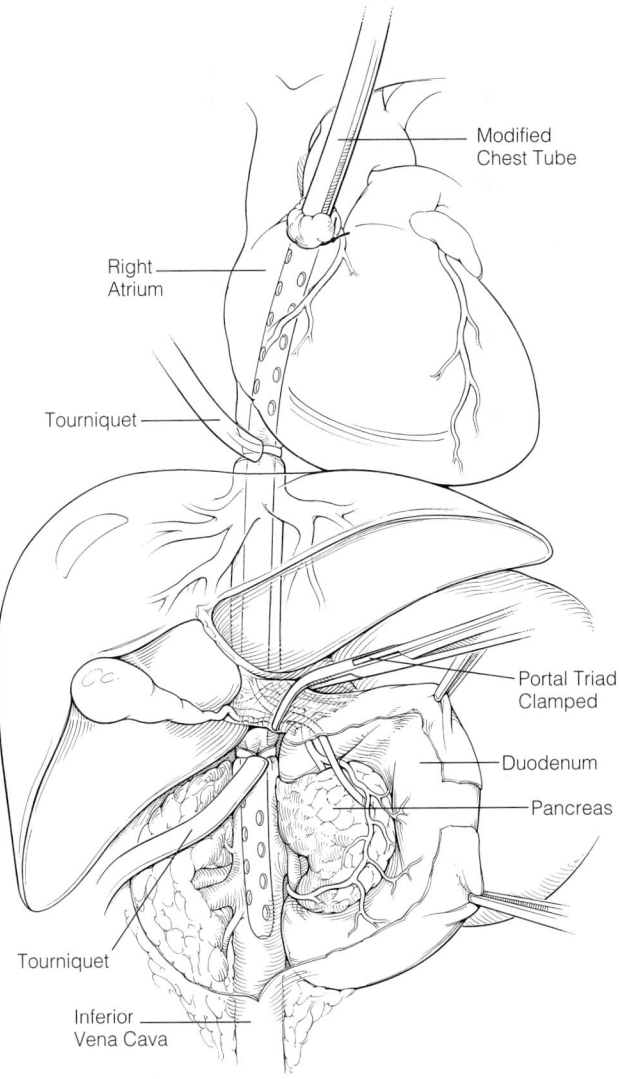

Figure 5 **Control of a retrohepatic vena caval injury is facilitated by the atriocaval shunt technique, in which a chest tube or an endotracheal tube with extra side holes cut in it is passed caudad through the right atrial appendage beyond the level of the inferior vena caval injury. Tourniquets are placed on the inferior vena cava above and below the liver, and the portal triad is clamped.**

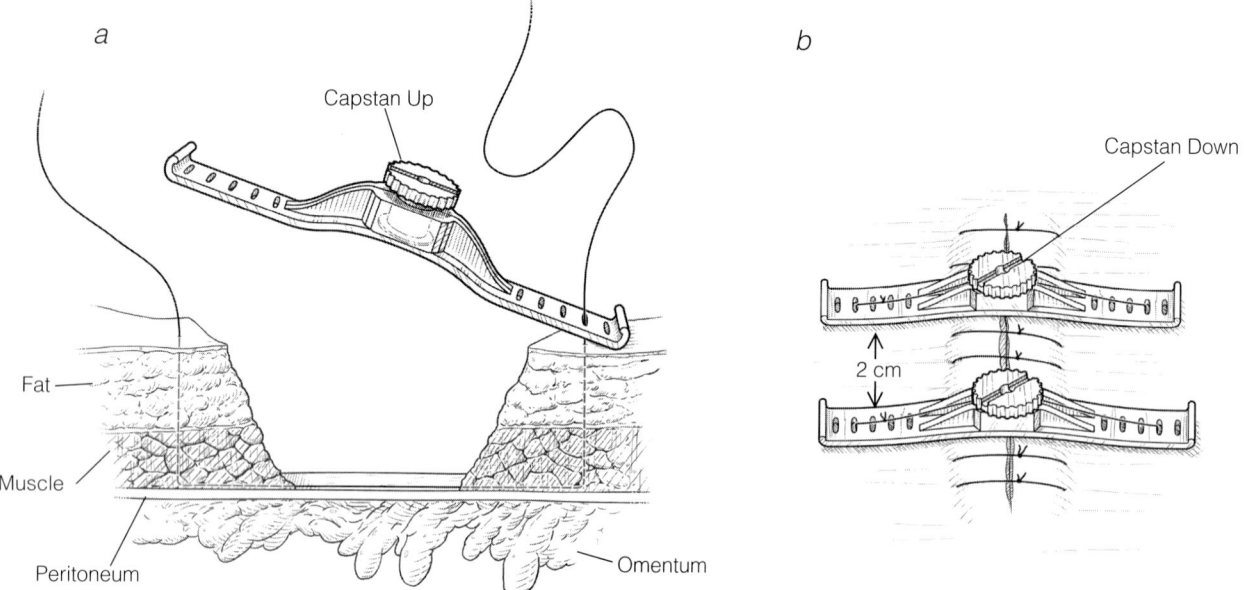

Figure 6   **Retention sutures may be used to bolster fascial closure in wounds at high risk for breakdown. (*a*) Sutures are placed in the subfascial plane. (*b*) The defect is approximated, and the sutures are tied over skin bridges.**

length, a Hartmann procedure can be performed. When significant left colon injury occurs in association with shock or gross contamination, proximal diversion should be considered.

REPAIR OF RETROPERITONEAL INJURIES

Once injuries within the peritoneal cavity have been addressed, the retroperitoneum should be inspected again, with particular attention paid to the possibility of hematoma expansion. Zonal distribution and mechanism of injury are the two important

determinants governing the decision whether to explore a retroperitoneal hematoma. All zone 1 hematomas should be explored regardless of the mechanism: they signal possible aortic, vena caval, duodenal, or pancreatic injury. Zone 2 and 3 hematomas should be explored if the patient sustained a penetrating injury. Generally, except for expanding zone 2 hematomas, zone 2 and 3 hematomas need not be explored in cases of blunt trauma. Even in blunt trauma patients with pelvic fractures, zone 3 hematomas are not explored if one is certain that there is no injury to the dis-

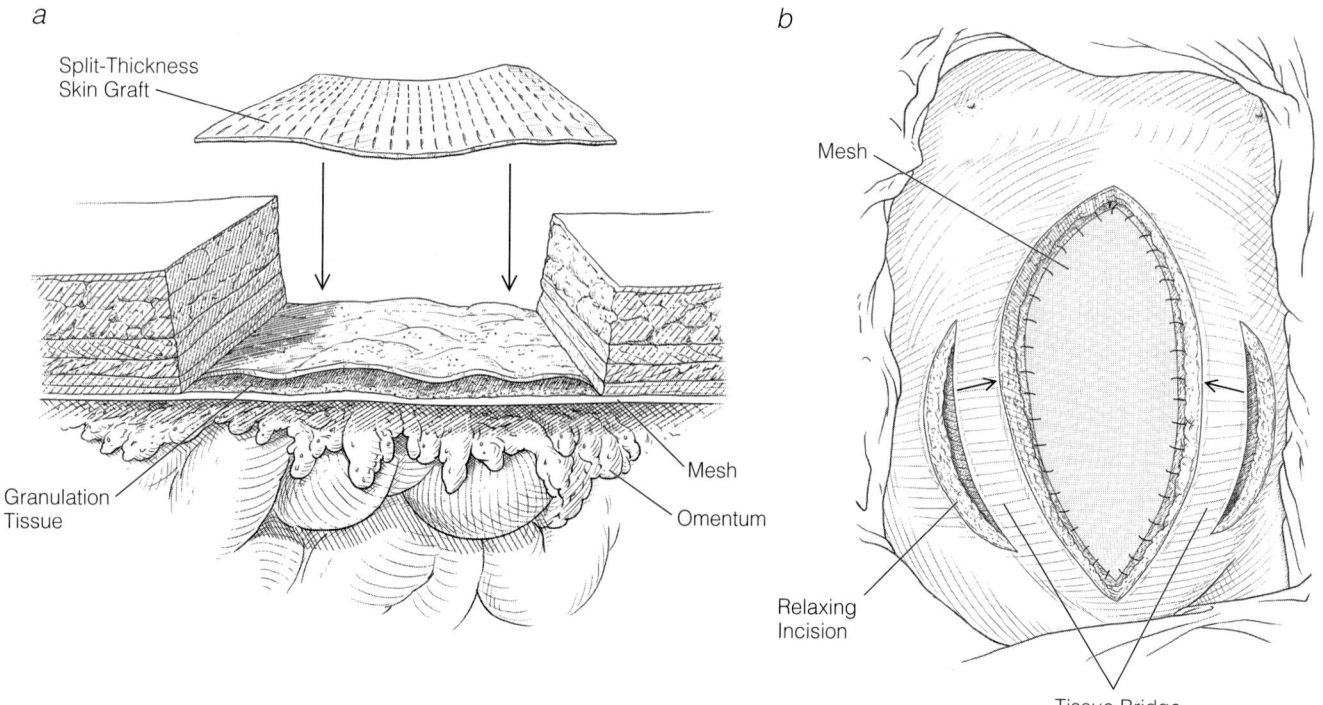

Figure 7   **Mesh may be used for temporary or permanent abdominal closure in patients at risk for increased abdominal pressure. (*a*) Mesh is sutured into the fascial plane. (*b*) The abdominal defect is closed with mesh.**

tal aorta or the iliac vessels. Before exploration of retroperitoneal hematomas, it is important to gain proximal vascular control to minimize hemorrhage once the retroperitoneal tamponade effect is lost. Vascular injuries discovered at this juncture should be repaired as discussed earlier (see above). Injuries to retroperitoneal organs (e.g., kidneys, pancreas, or adrenals) may be treated with debridement or resection with drainage as indicated.

Closure

GENERAL TECHNIQUE

Once the abdominal exploration has been completed, the abdomen should be copiously irrigated with a balanced salt solution. Generally, the optimal closure technique is chosen on the basis of five main considerations: the amount of blood lost, the volume of fluid received, the degree of contamination present, the patient's nutritional status, and the patient's overall stability. In some cases, the speed with which a closure can be performed may be the determining factor. Every effort should be made to close the fascia primarily. There are several methods that can be used to accomplish this. The most commonly used technique involves placement of a continuous monofilament suture. The major benefit of this type of closure is that it can be done relatively quickly. Alternatively, the fascia can be closed with interrupted sutures. There is no difference between the two techniques with respect to the rate of fascial dehiscence; however, the extent of the dehiscence is generally more limited with the interrupted suture method. Whichever method is used, the most important technical point is the necessity of avoiding excessive tension on the tissue.

Large monofilament sutures placed at intervals within the standard closure can serve as retention sutures [see Figure 6]. These sutures are used to support standard closure methods in patients who are at increased risk for fascial dehiscence and wound breakdown. They can be tied over bolsters fashioned from a red rubber catheter or tied over plastic skin bridges. When time is of the essence, the abdomen can be rapidly closed with four or five retention sutures of this type that are placed through and through all layers of the abdominal wall. These sutures should be checked daily and loosened if edema creates tension on the wound.

SKIN CLOSURE

The skin is closed primarily in patients who have minimal injuries and show no evidence of enteric contamination. Either a stapled closure or a sewn closure is acceptable. A degree of clinical judgment is required in dealing with clean-contaminated wounds. In some cases, the skin may be closed primarily; however, one should stand ready to open the wound again without undue delay if subsequent infection is suspected. Alternatively, the wound may be left open for three to five days and then loosely approximated with Steri-Strips if there is no evidence of contamination or infection. When gross intraperitoneal contamination was noted at the time of celiotomy, the patient is best served by leaving the wound open to heal by either secondary intention or delayed primary closure.

OPEN FASCIAL CLOSURE

On occasion, a multiply injured patient must undergo a protracted procedure or must receive massive volume resuscitation to maintain hemodynamic stability. Extensive interstitial edema may occur, precluding primary fascial closure. Closure of the abdomen in these circumstances may result in compromise of respiratory function or increased intra-abdominal pressure and its attendant se-

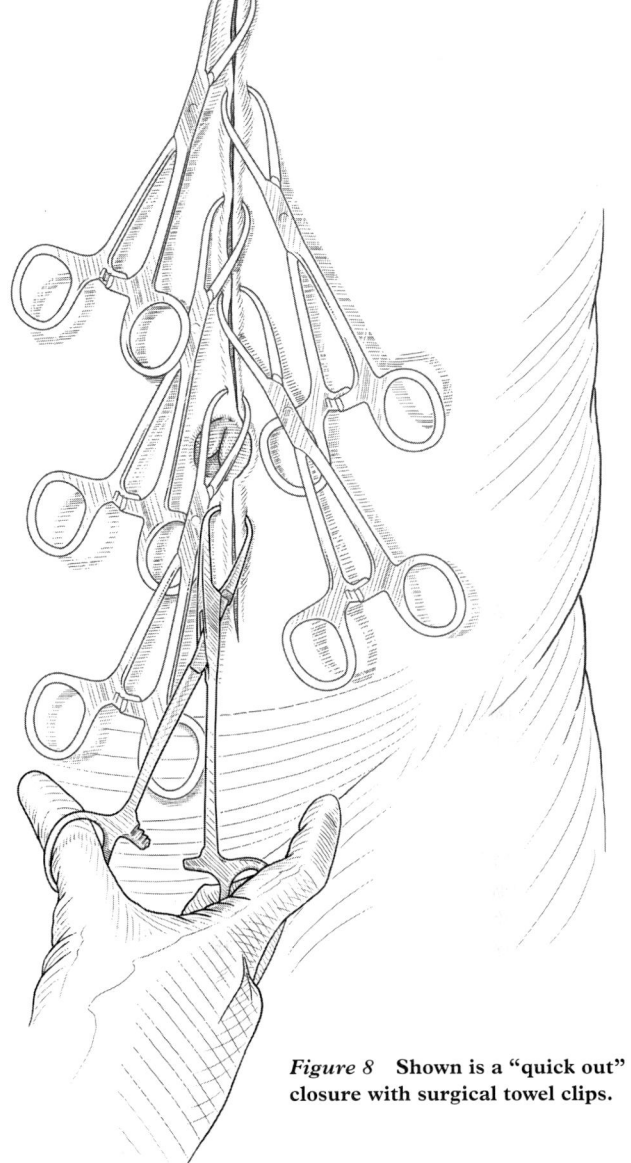

Figure 8 Shown is a "quick out" closure with surgical towel clips.

quelae. Consequently, a number of materials have been developed for use in both temporary and permanent abdominal closure in such conditions. Several absorbable meshes are available [see Figure 7]. Their main advantages are their inherent porosity and their ability to be easily incorporated into tissue. Subsequent abdominal wounds can be left open to heal by secondary intention; ventral hernias may be expected to form at a later date. Abdominal fascial defects may also be closed with sheets of nonincorporable synthetics, such as Gore-Tex. The advantages of these nonabsorbable materials are their innate lack of reactivity with tissue and the decreased rate of complications (e.g., enterocutaneous fistula). On the other hand, they are expensive and must ultimately be removed unless the skin is closed over them to protect the graft from contamination. If a temporary closure that lasts only a few days is all that is needed, then materials such as sterile I.V. bags can be used to close the fascial defect.

"QUICK OUTS" AND DAMAGE CONTROL

In grossly unstable or coagulopathic patients in whom surgical bleeding and contamination have been controlled, rapid abdominal closure may be necessary with the proviso that further exploration will be required. The basic objectives of the closure techniques used in these situations are control of peritoneal contamination and maintenance of intra-abdominal tamponade. One example of such a "quick out" is the use of towel clips to approximate skin [*see Figure 8*] in conjunction with a biooclusive dressing for control of contamination. Another technique involves placement of a sterile plastic barrier within the fascial defect, followed by insertion of several closed suction drains over which open laparotomy pads are placed. Subsequently, an adherent biooclusive sheet is draped over the abdominal wall to minimize thermal and insensible water losses.

Recommended Reading

Blaisdell FW, Trunkey DD: Abdominal Trauma. Thieme Medical Publishers, New York, 1993

Donovan AJ: Trauma Surgery. Mosby–Year Book Co, St Louis, 1994

Greenfield LJ: Complications in Surgery and Trauma. JB Lippincott Co, Grand Rapids, Michigan, 1990

Ivatury RR, Cayten CG: The Textbook of Penetrating Trauma. Williams & Wilkins, Baltimore, 1996

Mattox KL: Complications of Trauma. Churchill Livingstone, New York, 1994

Mattox KL, Feliciano DV, Moore EE: Trauma, 4th ed. Appleton & Lange, Stamford, Connecticut, 1998

Maull KI, Rodriguez A, Wiles CE: Complications in Trauma and Critical Care. WB Saunders Co, Philadelphia, 1996

Thal ER, Weigelt JA, Carrico CJ: Operative Trauma Management: An Atlas, 2nd ed. McGraw-Hill, New York, 2002

Acknowledgments

Figures 1, 4, and 5   Susan Brust, C.M.I.

Figures 2 and 3   Carol Donner.

Figures 6 through 8   Tom Moore. Adapted from *Operative Trauma Management: An Atlas,* by C. J. Carrico, E. R. Thal, and J. A. Weigelt. Appleton & Lange, Stamford, Connecticut, 1998.

9 INJURIES TO THE GREAT VESSELS OF THE ABDOMEN

David V. Feliciano, M.D., F.A.C.S.

In patients who have injuries to the great vessels of the abdomen, the findings on physical examination generally depend on whether a contained hematoma or active hemorrhage is present. In the case of contained hematomas around the vascular injury in the retroperitoneum, the base of the mesentery, or the hepatoduodenal ligament, the patient often has only modest hypotension in transit or on arrival at the emergency center; the hypotension can be temporarily reversed by the infusion of fluids and may not recur until the hematoma is opened at the time of laparotomy. This is usually the situation when an abdominal venous injury is present. In the case of active intraperitoneal hemorrhage, the patient typically has significant hypotension and may have a distended abdomen on arrival. Another physical finding that is occasionally noted in association with an injury to the common or external iliac artery is intermittent or complete loss of a pulse in the ipsilateral femoral artery; this finding in a patient with a transpelvic gunshot wound is pathognomonic of an injury to the iliac artery.

Injuries to the great vessels of the abdomen are caused by penetrating wounds in 90% to 95% of cases; accordingly, they are often accompanied by injuries to multiple intra-abdominal organs, including those in the gastrointestinal tract. The general principles governing the sequencing of repairs of injuries to the great vessels and the GI tract are outlined elsewhere [*see 5:8 Operative Exposure of Abdominal Injuries and Closure of the Abdomen*].

A hematoma [*see Figures 1 and 2*] or hemorrhage associated with an injury to a great vessel of the abdomen occurs in one of the three zones of the retroperitoneum or in the portal-retrohepatic area of the right upper quadrant [*see 5:8 Operative Exposure of Abdominal Injuries and Closure of the Abdomen*]. The magnitude of injury is usually described according to the Abdominal Vascular Organ Injury Scale, devised in 1992 by the American Association for the Surgery of Trauma [*see Table 1*].

Injuries in Zone 1

SUPRAMESOCOLIC

It is helpful to divide midline retroperitoneal hematomas into those that are supramesocolic and those that are inframesocolic. Hematoma or hemorrhage in the midline supramesocolic area of zone 1 is cause to suspect the presence of an injury to the suprarenal aorta, the celiac axis, the proximal superior mesenteric artery, or the proximal renal artery.

When a hematoma is present in the midline supramesocolic area, one usually has time to perform left medial visceral rotation [*see Figure 3 and 5:8 Operative Exposure of Abdominal Injuries and Closure of the Abdomen*]. The advantage of this technique is that it allows visualization of the entire abdominal aorta, from the aortic hiatus of the

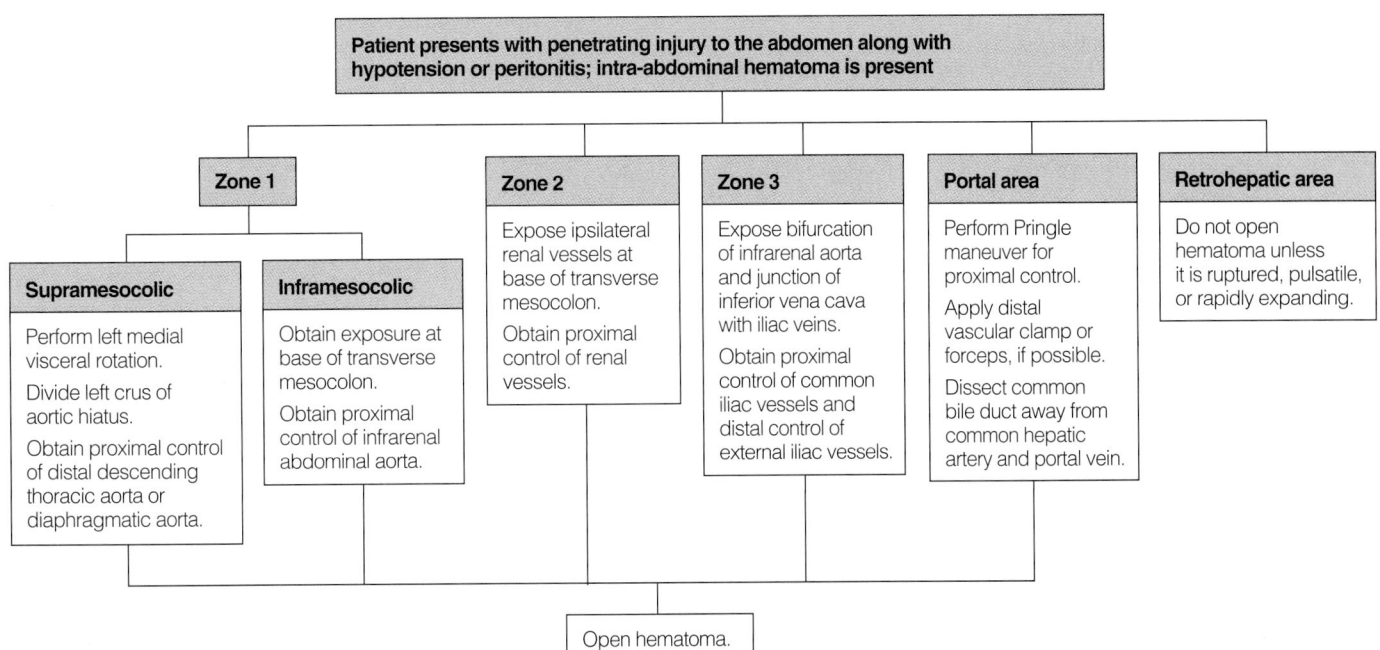

Figure 1 Algorithm illustrates management of intra-abdominal hematoma found at operation after penetrating trauma.

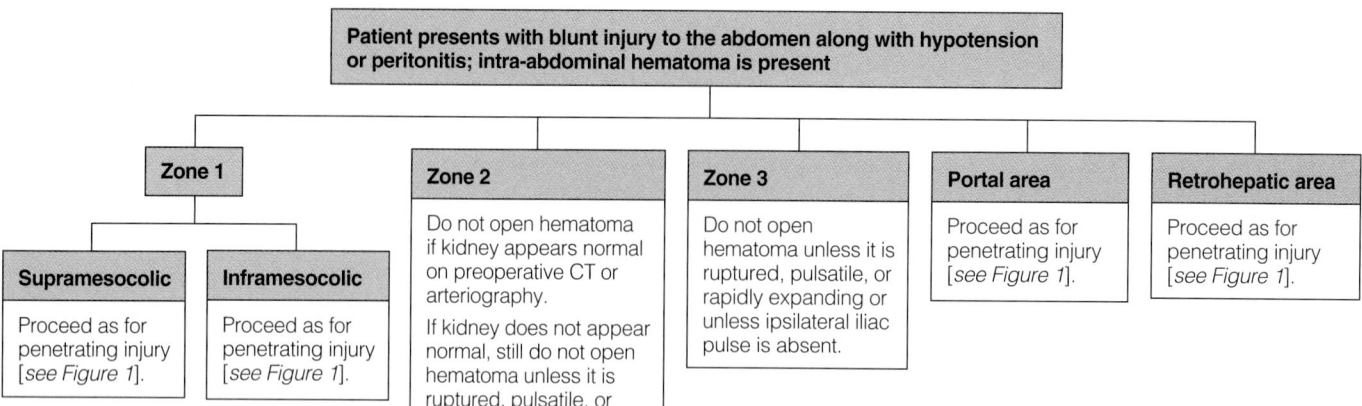

Figure 2 Algorithm illustrates management of intra-abdominal hematoma found at operation after blunt trauma.

diaphragm to the common iliac arteries [*see Figure 4*]. Obvious disadvantages include the 4 to 5 minutes required to complete the maneuver when the surgeon is inexperienced; the risk of damage to the spleen, the left kidney, or the posterior left renal artery as the maneuver is performed; and the anatomic distortion that results when the left kidney and the left renal artery are rotated anteriorly. When the hematoma is near the aortic hiatus of the diaphragm, it may be

advisable to leave the left kidney in its fossa, thereby eliminating potential damage to the structure as well as the distortion resulting from rotation. Because of the density of the celiac plexus and the lymphatic vessels surrounding the upper abdominal aorta, this portion of the aorta is difficult to visualize even when left medial visceral rotation has been performed. It is frequently helpful to transect the left crus of the aortic hiatus in the diaphragm at the 2 o'clock

Table 1   AAST Abdominal Vascular Organ Injury Scale

Grade	Characteristics of Injury	OIS Grade	ICD-9	AIS-90
I	Unnamed superior mesenteric artery or superior mesenteric vein branches	I	902.20/902.39	NS
	Unnamed inferior mesenteric artery or inferior mesenteric vein branches	I	902.27/902.32	NS
	Phrenic artery or vein	I	902.89	NS
	Lumbar artery or vein	I	902.89	NS
	Gonadal artery or vein	I	902.89	NS
	Ovarian artery or vein	I	902.81/902.82	NS
	Other unnamed small arterial or venous structures requiring ligation	I	902.90	NS
II	Right, left, or common hepatic artery	II	902.22	3
	Splenic artery or vein	II	902.23/902.34	3
	Right or left gastric arteries	II	902.21	3
	Gastroduodenal artery	II	902.24	3
	Inferior mesenteric artery, trunk, or inferior mesenteric vein, trunk	II	902.27/902.32	3
	Primary named branches of mesenteric artery (e.g., ileocolic artery) or mesenteric vein	II	902.26/902.31	3
	Other named abdominal vessels requiring ligation or repair	II	902.89	3
III*	Superior mesenteric vein, trunk	III	902.31	3
	Renal artery or vein	III	902.41/902.42	3
	Iliac artery or vein	III	902.53/902.54	3
	Hypogastric artery or vein	III	902.51/902.52	3
	Vena cava, infrarenal	III	902.10	3
IV*†	Superior mesenteric artery, trunk	IV	902.25	3
	Celiac axis, proper	IV	902.24	3
	Vena cava, suprarenal and infrahepatic	IV	902.10	3
	Aorta, infrarenal	IV	902.00	4
V†	Portal vein	V	902.33	3
	Extraparenchymal hepatic vein	V	902.11	3 (hepatic vein) 5 (liver + veins)
	Vena cava, retrohepatic or suprahepatic	V	902.19	5
	Aorta, suprarenal and subdiaphragmatic	V	902.00	4

Note: This classification is applicable to extraparenchymal vascular injuries. If the vessel injury is within 2 cm of the parenchyma of a specific organ, one should refer to the injury scale for that organ.

*Increase grade by I if there are multiple injuries involving > 50% of vessel circumference.

†Reduce grade by I if laceration is < 25% of vessel circumference.

AAST—American Association for the Surgery of Trauma   AIS—Abbreviated Injury Scale   ICD—International Classification of Diseases

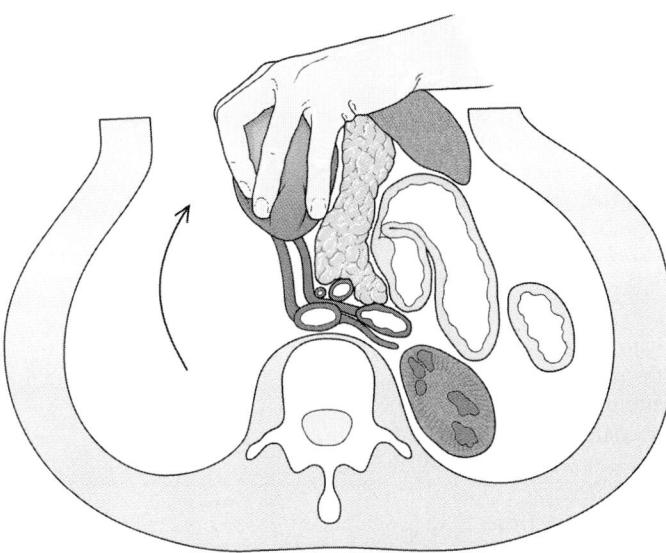

Figure 3 **Left medial visceral rotation is performed by means of sharp and blunt dissection with elevation of the left colon, the left kidney, the spleen, the tail of the pancreas, and the gastric fundus.**

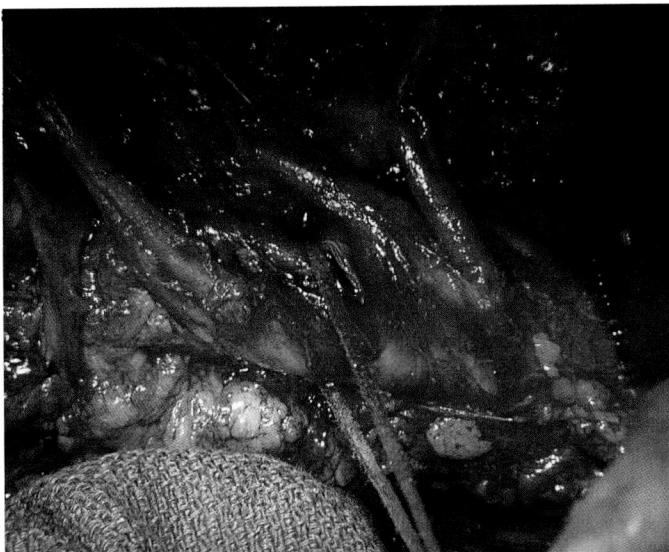

Figure 4 **Shown is an autopsy view of the supraceliac aorta and the celiac axis, the proximal superior mesenteric artery, and the medially rotated left renal artery after removal of lymphatic and nerve tissue.**

position to allow exposure of the distal descending thoracic aorta above the hiatus. Visualization of this portion of the vessel is much easier to achieve than visualization of the diaphragmatic or visceral abdominal aorta below, and an aortic cross-clamp can be applied much more quickly at this level.

Active hemorrhage from the midline supramesocolic area is controlled temporarily by packing with laparotomy pads or using an aortic compression device [*see Figure 5*]. The definitive approach is to divide the lesser omentum manually, retract the stomach and esophagus to the left, and manually dissect in the area just below the aortic hiatus to obtain rapid exposure of the supraceliac abdominal aorta; an aortic cross-clamp can then be applied. Distal control of the upper abdominal aorta is difficult to obtain because of the presence of the anteriorly located celiac axis and superior mesen-

teric artery. In young trauma patients who are otherwise healthy, ligation and division of the celiac axis allow easier application of the distal aortic clamp and better exposure of the supraceliac area for subsequent vascular repair.

Small penetrating wounds to the supraceliac abdominal aorta are repaired with a continuous 3-0 or 4-0 polypropylene suture. If two small perforations are adjacent to each other, they can be connected and the defect closed in a transverse fashion. If closure of a perforation would result in significant narrowing of the aorta or if a portion of the aortic wall is missing, patch aortoplasty with polytetrafluoroethylene (PTFE) is indicated. On rare occasions, in patients with extensive injuries to the diaphragmatic or supraceliac aorta, resection of the area of injury and insertion of a vascular conduit are indicated. Even though many of these patients have associated gastric, enteric, or colonic injuries, the most appropriate prosthesis with such a life-threatening injury is a 12 mm or 14 mm Dacron or PTFE graft [*see Figure 6*]. Provided that vigorous intraoperative irrigation is performed after repair of GI tract perforations, that proper graft coverage is ensured, and that perioperative antibiotics are appropriately employed, it is extraordinarily rare for a prosthesis inserted in the healthy aorta of a young trauma patient to become infected.

The aortic prosthesis is sewn in place with a continuous 3-0 or 4-0 polypropylene suture. Both ends of the aorta are flushed before the distal anastomosis is completed, and the distal aortic cross-clamp is removed before the final knot is tied to eliminate air from the system. The proximal aortic cross-clamp is removed very slowly as the

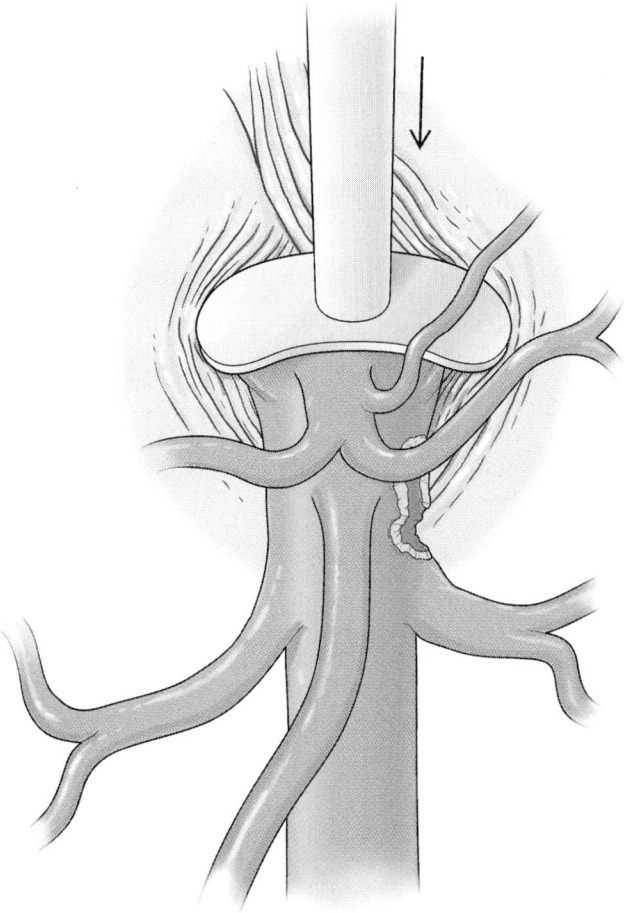

Figure 5 **An aortic compression device is used to control hemorrhage from the visceral portion of the abdominal aorta.**

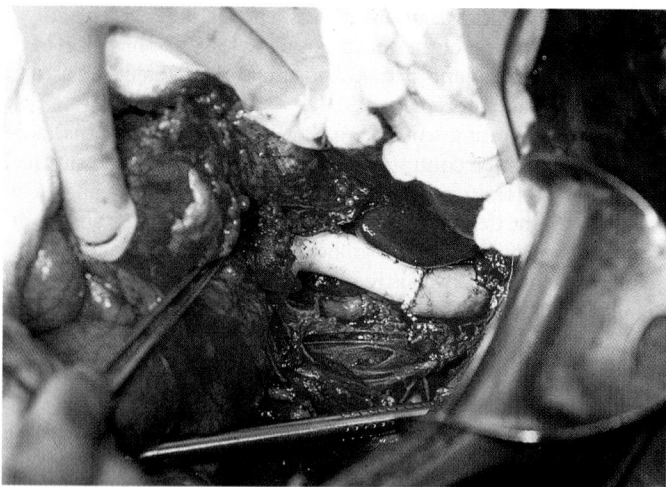

Figure 6 **A 22-year-old man with a gunshot wound to the right upper quadrant had injuries to the prepyloric area of the stomach and to the supraceliac abdominal aorta. The aortic injury was managed by means of segmental resection and replacement with a 16 mm polytetrafluoroethylene (PTFE) graft. The patient went home 46 days after injury.**

sive collateral flow to the liver from the midgut. When the entire celiac axis is injured, it is best to ligate all three vessels and forgo any attempt at repair.

Injuries to the superior mesenteric artery are managed according to the anatomic level of the perforation or thrombosis. On rare occasions, in patients with injuries beneath the neck of the pancreas, one may have to transect the pancreas to obtain proximal control. Another option is to perform left medial visceral rotation (see above) and apply a clamp directly to the origin of the superior mesenteric artery. Injuries to the superior mesenteric artery in this area or just beyond the base of the mesocolon are often associated with injuries to the pancreas. The potential for a postoperative leak from the injured pancreas near the arterial repair has led numerous authors to suggest that any extensive injury to the artery at this location should be ligated [*see Figure 7*].

Because of the intense vasoconstriction of the distal superior mesenteric artery in patients who have sustained exsanguinating hemorrhage from more proximal injuries treated with ligation, the collateral flow from the foregut and hindgut is often inadequate to maintain the viability of the organs in the distal midgut, especially the cecum and the ascending colon. Therefore, it is safest to place a saphenous vein or PTFE graft on the distal infrarenal aorta, away from the pancreatic injury and any other upper abdominal injuries. Such a graft can be tailored to reach the side or the anterior aspect of the superior mesenteric artery, or it can be attached to the transected distal superior mesenteric artery in an end-to-end fashion without significant tension [*see Figure 8*]. Soft tissue must be approximated over the aortic suture line of the graft to prevent the development of an aortoenteric fistula in the postoperative period.

In patients with severe shock from exsanguination caused by a complex injury to the superior mesenteric artery, damage control laparotomy is indicated: the injured area should be resected and a temporary intraluminal Argyle, Javid, or Pruitt-Inahara shunt inserted to maintain flow to the midgut during resuscitation in the surgical intensive care unit. When ligation is indicated for more distal injuries to the superior mesenteric artery, segments of the ileum or even the right colon may have to be resected because of ischemia.

The survival rate in patients with penetrating injuries to the superior mesenteric artery is approximately 50% to 55% overall [*see Table 2*] but only 20% to 25% when any form of repair more complex than lateral arteriorrhaphy is necessary.[1-3]

An injury to the proximal renal artery may also be present under a supramesocolic hematoma or bleeding area. When active hemor-

anesthesiologist rapidly infuses fluids and intravenous bicarbonate to reverse so-called washout acidosis from the previously ischemic lower extremities. The retroperitoneum is then irrigated with an antibiotic solution and closed over the graft in a watertight fashion with an absorbable suture.

The survival rate in patients with injuries to the suprarenal abdominal aorta had been 30% to 35% but was lower than 10% in one 2001 review.[1]

Injuries to branches of the celiac axis are often difficult to repair because of the amount of dissection required to remove the dense neural and lymphatic tissue in this area. Because most patients have excellent collateral flow in the upper abdomen, major injuries to either the left gastric or the proximal splenic artery generally should be ligated. Because the common hepatic artery may have a larger diameter than either of these two arteries, an injury to this vessel can occasionally be repaired by means of lateral arteriorrhaphy, an end-to-end anastomosis, or the insertion of a saphenous vein graft. One should not worry about ligating the common hepatic artery proximal to the origin of the gastroduodenal artery: there is exten-

Table 2 Survival after Injuries to Arteries in the Abdomen

Injured Artery	Asensio et al[2] (2000)		Davis et al[3] (2001)*	Tyburski et al[1] (2001)
	Isolated Injury	With Other Arterial Injury		
Abdominal aorta as a whole	21.7% (10/46)	17.6% (3/17)	39.1% (25/64)	21.1% (15/71)
Pararenal to diaphragm	—	—	—	8.3% (3/36)
Infrarenal	—	—	—	34.2% (12/35)
Superior mesenteric artery	52.4% (11/21)	28.6% (2/7)	53.3% (8/15)	48.8% (20/41)
Renal artery	62.5% (5/8)	33.3% (2/6)	56.2% (9/16)	73.7% (14/19)
Iliac artery				
Common	—	—	55.5% (5/9)	44.7% (17/38)
External	—	—	65.2% (30/46)	62.5% (20/32)

*Excludes patients who exsanguinated before repair or ligation.

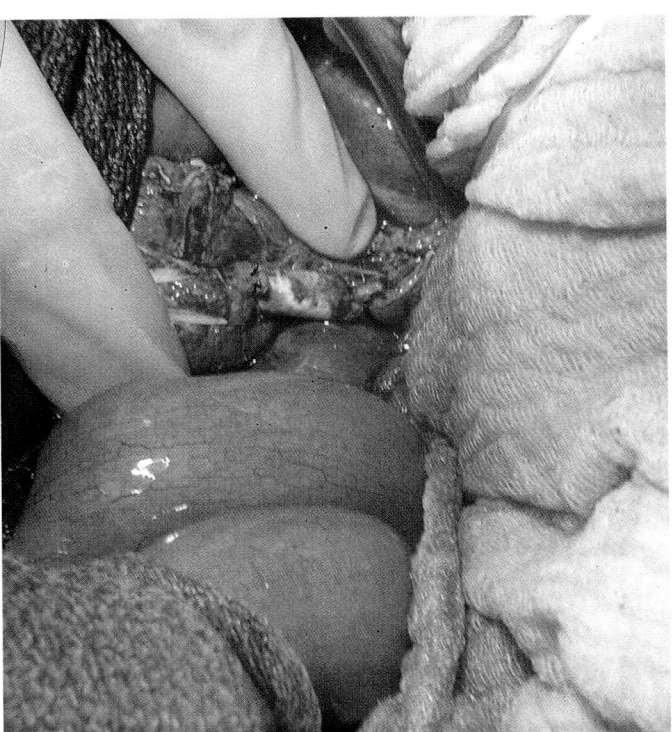

Figure 7 An 18-year-old man experienced a gunshot wound to the head of the pancreas and the proximal superior mesenteric artery. A Whipple procedure was performed, and a 6 mm PTFE graft was placed in the artery. The artery-graft suture line dehisced secondary to a pancreatic leak on day 30 after injury, and the patient died on day 42.

rhage is present, control of the supraceliac abdominal aorta in or just below the aortic hiatus must be obtained. When only a hematoma or a known thrombosis of the proximal renal artery is present, proximal vascular control can be obtained by elevating the transverse mesocolon and dissecting the vessel from the lateral aspect of the abdominal aorta. Options for repair of either the proximal or the distal renal artery are described elsewhere [see Injuries in Zone 2, below].

The superior mesenteric vein is the other great vessel of the abdomen that may be injured in the supramesocolic or retromesocolic area of the midline retroperitoneum. Because of the overlying pancreas, the proximity of the uncinate process, and the close association of this vessel with the superior mesenteric artery, repair of the superior mesenteric vein is quite difficult. As with injuries to the superior mesenteric artery (see above), one may have to transect the neck of the pancreas between noncrushing vascular or intestinal clamps to gain access to a perforation of the superior mesenteric vein. An injury to this vein below the inferior border of the pancreas can be managed by compressing it manually between one's fingers as an assistant places a continuous 5-0 polypropylene suture to complete the repair. When a penetrating injury to the vein has a posterior component, one must ligate multiple collateral vessels entering the vein in this area to achieve proper visualization.

There is now excellent evidence that young trauma patients tolerate ligation of the superior mesenteric vein well when vigorous postoperative fluid resuscitation is performed to reverse the peripheral hypovolemia that results from splanchnic hypervolemia. Typically, ligation is followed almost immediately by swelling of the midgut and discoloration suggestive of impending ischemia. In such cases, temporary coverage of the midgut with a silo, followed by ear-

ly reoperation, may be necessary to reassure the operating surgeon that the ischemia has not become permanent.

The survival rate in patients with injuries to the superior mesenteric vein has ranged from 36% to 71%, depending on whether other vascular injuries are present [see Table 3].[1-3]

INFRAMESOCOLIC

The lower area of the midline retroperitoneum in zone 1 is known as the midline inframesocolic area. Injuries to either the infrarenal abdominal aorta or the inferior vena cava occur in this area.

The infrarenal abdominal aorta is exposed by pulling the transverse mesocolon up toward the patient's head, eviscerating the small bowel to the right side of the abdomen, and opening the midline retroperitoneum until the left renal vein is exposed. A proximal aortic cross-clamp is then placed immediately inferior to this vessel [see Figure 9]. When there is active hemorrhage from this area, rapid proximal control is obtained in the same fashion or, if necessary, by dividing the lesser omentum and applying the cross-clamp just below the aortic hiatus of the diaphragm. Distal control of the infrarenal abdominal aorta is obtained by dividing the midline retroperitoneum down to the aortic bifurcation, taking care to avoid the left-sided origin of the inferior mesenteric artery.

Injuries to the infrarenal aorta are repaired by means of lateral aortorrhaphy, patch aortoplasty, an end-to-end anastomosis, or insertion of a Dacron or PTFE graft. Much as with injuries to the suprarenal abdominal aorta in young trauma patients, it is rarely possible to place a tube graft larger than 12 or 14 mm. Because the retroperitoneal tissue is often thin at this location in young patients, an appropriate option after the aortic repair is to mobilize the gastrocolic omentum, flip it into the lesser sac superiorly, and then bring it down over the infrarenal aortic graft through a hole in the transverse mesocolon. Another option is to mobilize the gastrocolic omentum away from the right side of the colon and then swing the mobilized tissue into the left lateral gutter just below the ligament of Treitz to cover the graft.

The survival rate in patients with injuries to the infrarenal abdominal aorta had been approximately 45% but was 34% in a 2001 review [see Table 2].[1]

Injury to the inferior vena cava below the liver should be suspected when the aorta is found to be intact underneath an inframesocolic hematoma, when such a hematoma appears to be more extensive on the right side of the abdomen than on the left, or when there is active hemorrhage coming through the base of the mesentery of the ascending colon or the hepatic flexure. It is certainly possible to visualize the inferior vena cava through the midline retroperitoneal exposure just described (see above); however, most surgeons are more comfortable with visualizing the vessel by mobilizing the right half of the colon and the C loop of the duodenum [see 5:8 Operative Exposure of Abdominal Injuries and Closure of the Abdomen]. With this right medial visceral rotation maneuver, the right kidney is left in situ unless there is an associated injury to the posterior aspect of the right renal vein, to the suprarenal vena cava, or to the right kidney itself. Right medial visceral rotation, in conjunction with the Kocher maneuver, permits visualization of the entire vena caval system from the confluence of the iliac veins to the suprarenal vena cava below the liver.

For proper exposure of a hole in a large vein such as the inferior vena cava, the loose retroperitoneal fatty tissue must be dissected away from the wall of the vessel. Active hemorrhage coming from the anterior surface of the inferior vena cava is best controlled by applying a Satinsky vascular clamp. If it is difficult to apply this clamp, one should try grasping the area of the perforation with a pair of vascular forceps or several Judd-Allis clamps; this step may

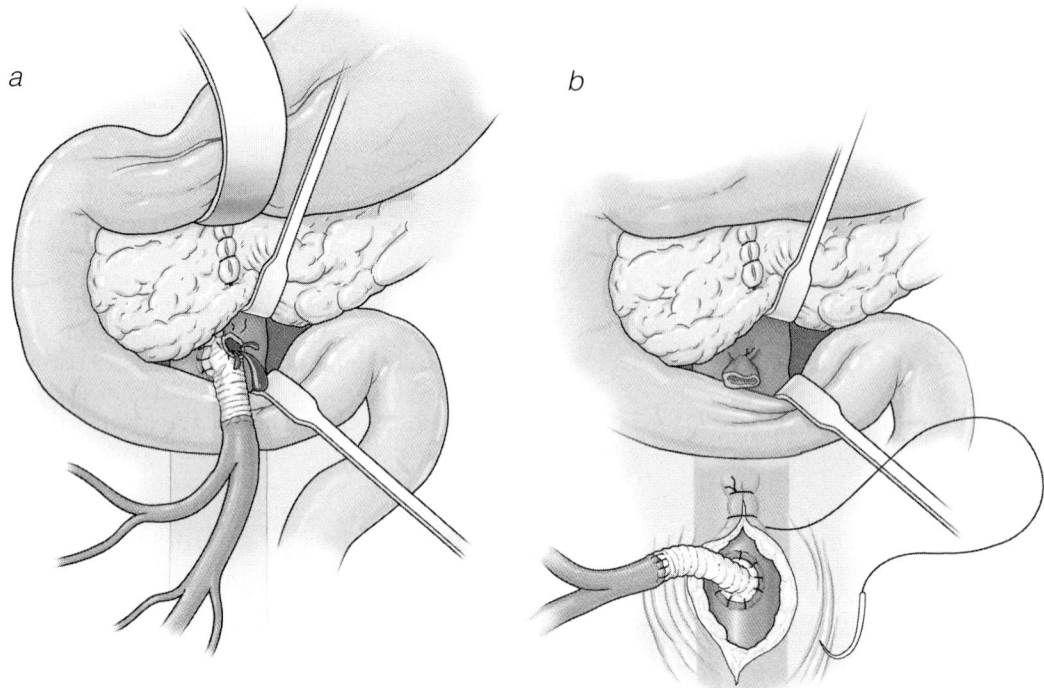

Figure 8 (*a*) **When complex grafting procedures to the superior mesenteric artery are necessary, it may be dangerous to place the proximal suture line near an associated pancreatic injury. (*b*) The proximal suture line should be on the lower aorta, away from the upper abdominal injuries, and should be covered with retroperitoneal tissue.**

facilitate safe application of the Satinsky clamp. When the perforation in the inferior vena cava is more lateral or posterior, it is often helpful to compress the vessel proximally and distally around the perforation, using gauze sponges placed in straight sponge sticks. On occasion, an extensive injury to the inferior vena cava can be controlled only by completely occluding the entire inferior vena cava with large DeBakey aortic cross-clamps. This maneuver interrupts much of the venous return to the right side of the heart and is poorly tolerated by hypotensive patients unless the infrarenal abdominal aorta is cross-clamped simultaneously.

There are two anatomic areas in which vascular control of an injury to the inferior vena cava below the liver is difficult to obtain: (1) the confluence of the common iliac veins and (2) the junction of the renal veins with the inferior vena cava. One interesting approach to an injury to the inferior vena cava at the confluence of the iliac veins is temporary division of the overlying right common iliac artery, coupled with mobilization of the aortic bifurcation to the patient's left. This approach yields a better view of the common iliac veins and the proximal inferior vena cava and makes repair considerably easier than it would be if the aortic bifurcation were left in place. Once the vein is repaired, the right common iliac artery is reconstituted via an end-to-end anastomosis. The usual approach to injuries to the inferior vena cava at its junction with the renal veins involves clamp or sponge-stick compression of the infrarenal and suprarenal vena cava as well as control of both renal veins with Silastic loops to facilitate the direct application of angled

Table 3 Survival after Injuries to Veins in the Abdomen

Injured Vein	Asensio et al[2] (2000)		Davis et al[3] (2001)*	Tyburski et al[1] (2001)
	Isolated Injury	With Other Venous Injury		
Inferior vena cava as a whole	29.3% (12/41)†	22.2% (8/36)†	56% (47/84)	43% (61/142)
Pararenal to diaphragm	—	—	—	40.3% (31/77)
Infrarenal	—	—	—	46.2% (30/65)
Superior mesenteric vein	47.4% (9/19)	35.7% (5/14)	71.4% (15/21)	56.3% (18/32)
Renal vein	—	44.1% (15/34)	70% (21/30)	68.8% (22/32)
Iliac vein (all)	62.2% (23/37)	33.3% (5/15)	—	—
Common	—	—	81% (17/21)	49% (24/49)
External	—	—	74.5% (41/55)	66.7% (16/24)

*Excludes patients who exsanguinated before repair or ligation.
†Excludes retrohepatic vena cava.

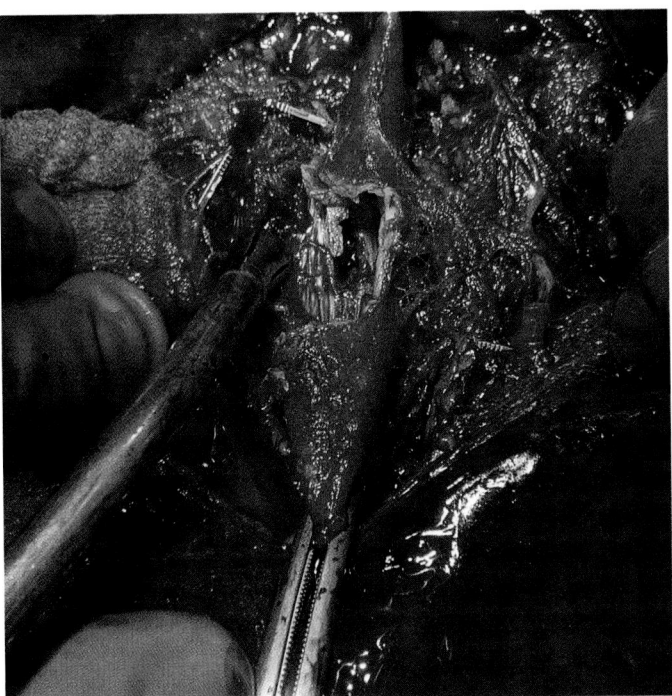

Figure 9 Shown is a gunshot wound to the infrarenal abdominal aorta viewed through standard inframesocolic exposure.

vascular clamps. As noted, medial mobilization of the right kidney may permit the application of a partial occlusion clamp across the inferior vena cava at its junction with the right renal vein as an alternative approach to an injury in this area. Another useful technique for controlling hemorrhage from the inferior vena cava at any location is to insert a 5 ml or 30 ml Foley balloon catheter into the caval laceration and then inflate it in the lumen. Once the bleeding is controlled, vascular clamps are positioned around the perforation, and the balloon catheter is removed before repair of the vessel.

Anterior perforations of the inferior vena cava are managed by means of transverse repair with a continuous 4-0 or 5-0 polypropylene suture. Much has been written about visualizing posterior perforations by extending anterior perforations, but in my experience, opportunities to apply this approach have been rare. It is often easier to roll the vena cava to one side to complete a continuous suture repair of a posterior perforation. When both anterior and posterior perforations have been repaired, there is usually a significant degree of narrowing of the inferior vena cava, which may lead to slow postoperative occlusion. If the patient's condition is unstable and a coagulopathy has developed, no further attempt should be made to revise the repair. If the patient is stable, there may be some justification for applying a large PTFE patch to prevent this postoperative occlusion [*see Figure 10*].

Ligation of the infrarenal inferior vena cava is appropriate for young patients who are exsanguinating and in whom a complex repair of the vessel would be necessary. Such patients require vigorous resuscitation with crystalloid solutions in the postoperative period; in addition, both lower extremities should be wrapped with elastic compression wraps and elevated for 5 to 7 days after operation. Patients who have some residual edema during the later stages of hospitalization despite the elastic compression wraps should be fitted with full-length custom-made support hose. Ligation of the suprarenal inferior vena cava is occasionally necessary when the patient has an extensive injury at this location and appears to be in an irreversible shock state during operation. If the patient's condition improves during a brief period of resuscitation in the SICU, reoperation and reconstruction with an externally supported PTFE graft are necessary to prevent renal failure.

The survival rate in patients with injuries to the inferior vena cava depends on the location of the injury; in the past, it ranged from 60% for the suprarenal vena cava to 78% for the infrarenal vena cava but decreased to approximately 33% to 56% if injuries to the retrohepatic vena cava were included. Current studies indicate survival rates of 22% to 56% for inferior vena cava injuries taken as a whole.[2,3] A 2001 review reported survival rates of 46.1% for the infrarenal inferior vena cava and 40.3% for more superior injuries.[1]

Injuries in Zone 2

Hematoma or hemorrhage in zone 2 is cause to suspect the presence of injury to the renal artery, the renal vein, or the kidney.

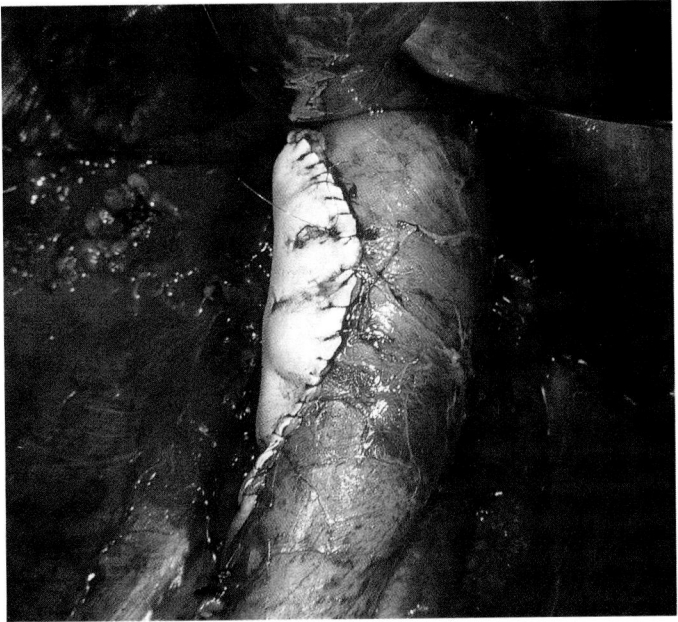

Figure 10 Shown is PTFE patch repair of an injury to the infrarenal inferior vena cava.

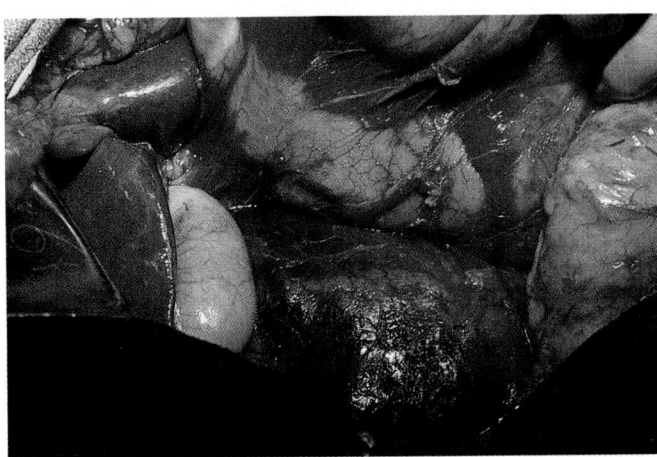

Figure 11 A right perirenal hematoma was not opened at operation, because preoperative abdominal CT documented a reasonably intact kidney.

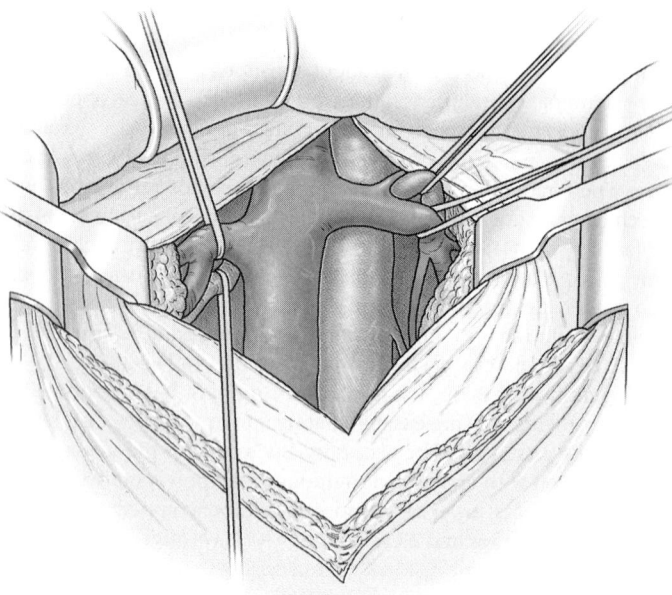

Figure 12   **Midline looping of respective renal vessels is performed before entry into any perirenal hematoma.**

In patients who have sustained blunt abdominal trauma but in whom preoperative intravenous pyelography, renal arteriography, or CT of the kidneys yields normal findings, there is no justification for opening a perirenal hematoma if one is found at a subsequent operation [*see Figure 11*].

In highly selected stable patients with penetrating wounds to the flank, there are some data to justify performing preoperative CT. On occasion, documentation of an isolated minor renal injury in the absence of peritoneal findings on physical examination makes it possible to manage such patients nonoperatively. In all other patients with penetrating wounds, when a perirenal hematoma is found dur-

ing initial exploration, the hematoma should be unroofed and the wound tract explored. If the hematoma is not rapidly expanding and there is no active hemorrhage from the perirenal area, one may control the ipsilateral renal artery with a Silastic loop in the midline of the retroperitoneum at the base of the mesocolon [*see Figure 12*]. Control of the left renal vein can be obtained at the same location; however, control of the proximal right renal vein requires mobilization of the C loop of the duodenum and dissection of the vena cava at its junction with this vessel.

If there is active hemorrhage from the kidney through Gerota's fascia or from the retroperitoneum overlying the renal vessels, no central renal vascular control is necessary. In such a situation, the retroperitoneum lateral to the injured kidney should be opened, and the kidney should be manually elevated directly into the abdominal incision. A large vascular clamp should then be applied directly to the hilar vessels of the elevated kidney to control any further bleeding until a decision is reached on repair versus nephrectomy.

Occasionally, a small perforation of the renal artery can be repaired by lateral arteriorrhaphy or resection with an end-to-end anastomosis. Interposition grafting and replacement of the renal artery with either the hepatic artery (on the right) or the splenic artery (on the left) have been used on rare occasions, but such approaches ordinarily are not indicated unless the injured kidney is the only one the patient has. In patients who have sustained multiple intra-abdominal injuries from penetrating wounds or have undergone a long period of ischemia while other injuries were being repaired, nephrectomy is the appropriate choice for a major renovascular injury, provided that intraoperative palpation has confirmed the presence of a normal contralateral kidney.

The role of renal revascularization in patients who have intimal tears in the renal arteries as a result of deceleration-type trauma remains controversial. If a circumferential intimal tear is noted on preoperative arteriography but flow to the kidney is preserved, the decision whether to repair the artery depends on whether laparotomy is necessary for other injuries and whether the opportunity for anticoagulation is available. If there are no other significant injuries and

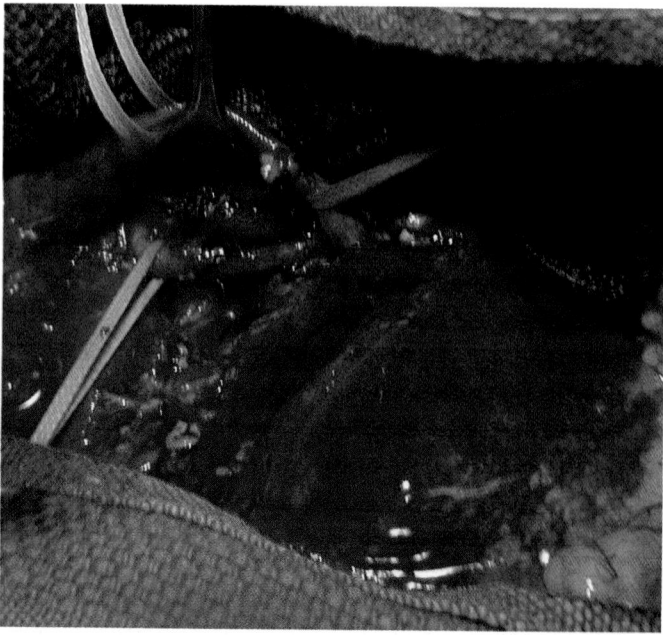

Figure 13   **With the left renal vein elevated, a hematoma ring may be noted overlying a blunt intimal tear in an occluded left renal artery.**

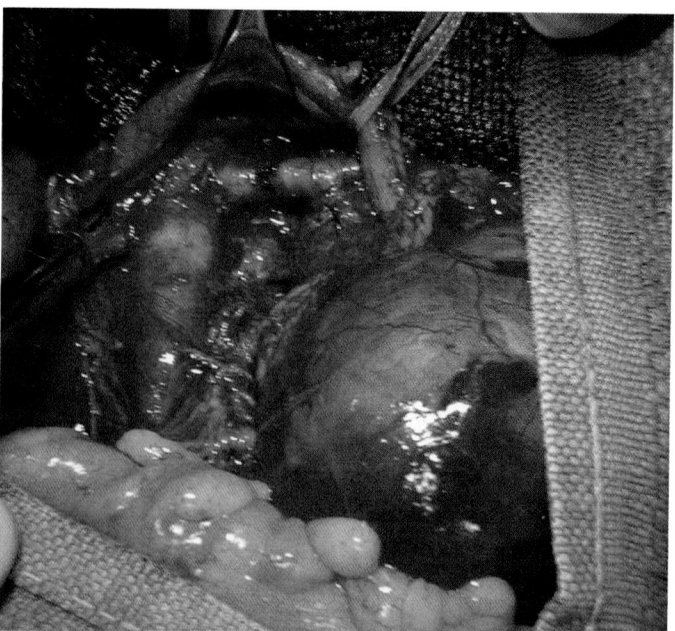

Figure 14   **In the same patient as in Figure 13, the intimal tear in the left renal artery was resected, an end-to-end anastomosis was performed, and blood flow to the left kidney was restored.**

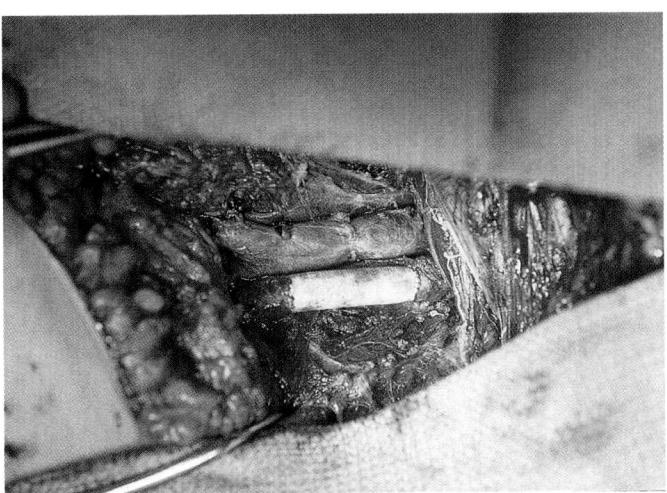

Figure 15 A 24-year-old man experienced a gunshot wound to the left external iliac artery and vein. The arterial injury was repaired with segmental resection and insertion of an 8 mm PTFE graft; the venous injury was repaired with segmental resection and an end-to-end anastomosis.

flow to the kidney is preserved despite the presence of an intimal tear, anticoagulation and a repeat isotope renogram within the first several days may be justified. If occlusion of the proximal renal artery from blunt deceleration-type trauma is documented, the critical factor for renal salvage is the time from occlusion to revascularization. Renal artery occlusion from deceleration-type trauma that is detected within 6 hours of injury is best treated with immediate operation, resection of the area of intimal damage, and an end-to-end anastomosis performed by an experienced vascular trauma team [*see Figures 13 and 14*]. Given proper exposure and medial mobilization of the kidney, this operation is not technically difficult in a young trauma patient whose renal artery is otherwise normal. In a 1998 review,[4] fewer than 20% of kidneys revascularized in this manner regained any significant degree of function. Hypertension develops in 40% to 45% of patients who undergo observation only after thrombosis is detected.

The survival rate in patients with isolated injuries to the renal arteries ranges from 56% to 74% [*see Table 2*].[1,3]

Many patients with penetrating wounds to the renal veins are quite stable as a result of the retroperitoneal tamponade described earlier (see above). Once vascular control is obtained with the direct application of clamps, lateral venorrhaphy is the preferred technique of repair. Nephrectomy should be performed if ligation of the right renal vein is necessary to control hemorrhage, whereas the medial left renal vein may be ligated as long as the left adrenal and gonadal veins are intact. It should be noted, however, that in some series, more postoperative renal complications were noted when this maneuver was used on the left side.

The survival rate in patients with isolated injuries to the renal veins is approximately 70% [*see Table 3*].[1,3]

Injuries in Zone 3

Hematoma or hemorrhage in either lateral pelvic area is suggestive of injury to the iliac artery or the iliac vein.

When lateral pelvic hematoma or hemorrhage is noted after penetrating trauma, compression with a laparotomy pad or the fingers should be maintained as proximal and distal vascular control is obtained. The proximal common iliac arteries are exposed by eviscerating the small bowel to the right and dividing the midline retroperi-

toneum over the aortic bifurcation. In young trauma patients, the common iliac artery usually is not adherent to the common iliac vein, and Silastic loops can be passed rapidly around these vessels to provide proximal vascular control. Distal vascular control is most easily obtained where the external iliac artery and vein come out of the pelvis proximal to the inguinal ligament. Even with proximal and distal control of the common or the external iliac artery and vein, there is often continued back-bleeding from the internal iliac artery. Such bleeding is controlled by elevating the Silastic loops on the proximal and distal iliac artery and then either clamping or looping the internal iliac artery, which is the only major branch vessel that descends into the pelvis.

For transpelvic bilateral iliac vascular injuries resulting from a penetrating wound, a technique of total pelvic vascular isolation has been described. Proximally, the abdominal aorta and the inferior vena cava are cross-clamped just above their bifurcations, and distally, both the external iliac artery and the external iliac vein are cross-clamped, with one clamp on each side of the distal pelvis. Back-bleeding from the internal iliac vessels is minimal with this approach.

Ligation of either the common or the external iliac artery in a hypotensive trauma patient leads to a 40% to 50% amputation rate in the postoperative period; consequently, injuries to these vessels should be repaired if at all possible. The standard options for repair—lateral arteriorrhaphy, completion of a partial transection with an end-to-end anastomosis, and resection of the injured area with insertion of a conduit—are feasible in most situations [*see Figure 15*]. On rare occasions, it may be preferable either to mobilize the ipsilateral internal iliac artery to serve as a replacement for the external iliac artery or to transpose one iliac artery to the side of the contralateral iliac artery. When a patient is in severe shock from exsanguination caused by a complex injury to the common or the external iliac artery, damage control laparotomy [*see* Damage Control Laparotomy, *below*] is indicated. The injured area should be resected and a temporary intraluminal Argyle, Javid, or Pruitt-Inahara shunt inserted to maintain flow to the ipsilateral lower extremity during resuscitation in the SICU.

One unique problem associated with repair of the common or the external iliac artery is the choice of technique when significant enteric or fecal contamination is present in the pelvis. In such cases, there is a substantial risk of postoperative pelvic cellulitis, a pelvic abscess, or both, which may lead to blowout of any type of repair. When extensive contamination is present, it is appropriate to divide the common or external iliac artery above the level of injury, close the injury with a double row of continuous 4-0 or 5-0 polypropylene sutures, and bury the stump underneath uninjured retroperitoneum. If a stable patient has obvious ischemia of the ipsilateral lower extremity at the completion of this proximal ligation, one may perform an extra-anatomic femorofemoral crossover graft to restore arterial flow to the extremity. If the patient is unstable, one should take several minutes to perform an ipsilateral four-compartment below-knee fasciotomy; this step will counteract the ischemic edema that inevitably leads to a compartment syndrome and compromises the early survival of the leg. After adequate resuscitation in the SICU, the patient should be returned to the OR for the femorofemoral graft within 4 to 6 hours.

Injuries to the internal iliac arteries are usually ligated even if they occur bilaterally, because young trauma patients typically have extensive collateral flow through the pelvis.

The survival rate in patients with isolated injuries to the external iliac artery exceeds 80% when tamponade is present. If the injury is large and free bleeding has occurred preoperatively, however, the survival rate is only 45%. Current studies report overall survival rates of approximately 45% to 55% for injuries to the common iliac

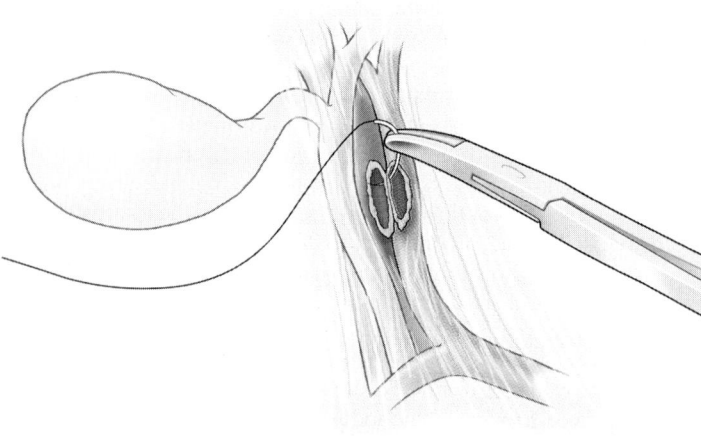

Figure 16 **Failure to properly dissect out the structures in the porta hepatis after a penetrating wound led to the creation of an iatrogenic hepatic artery–portal vein fistula, which was corrected after the arrival of the attending surgeon.**

artery and 62% to 65% for injuries to the external iliac artery [*see Table 2*].[1,3]

Hemorrhage from injuries to the iliac veins can usually be controlled by means of compression with either sponge sticks or the fingers. As noted, division of the right common iliac artery may be necessary for proper visualization of an injury to the right common iliac vein. Similarly, ligation and division of the internal iliac artery on the side of the pelvis yield improved exposure of an injury to an ipsilateral internal iliac vein.

Injuries to the common or the external iliac vein are best treated by means of lateral venorrhaphy with continuous 4-0 or 5-0 polypropylene sutures. Significant narrowing often results, and a number of reports have demonstrated occlusion on postoperative venography. For patients with narrowing or occlusion, as well as for those in whom ligation was necessary to control exsanguinating hemorrhage, the use of elastic compression wraps and elevation for the first 5 to 7 days after operation is mandatory.

The survival rate in patients with injuries to the iliac veins ranges from 33% to 81%, depending on whether associated vascular injuries are present [*see Table 3*].[1-3]

Injuries in the Porta Hepatis or Retrohepatic Area

PORTA HEPATIS

Hematoma or hemorrhage in the area of the portal triad in the right upper quadrant is cause to suspect the presence of injury to the portal vein or the hepatic artery or of vascular injury combined with an injury to the common bile duct.

If a hematoma is present, the proximal hepatoduodenal ligament should be occluded with a vascular clamp (the Pringle maneuver [*see 5:6 Injuries to the Liver, Biliary Tract, Spleen, and Diaphragm*]) before the hematoma is entered. If the hematoma is centrally located in the porta, one may also be able to apply an angled vascular clamp to the distal end of the portal structures at their entrance into the liver.

If hemorrhage is occurring, compression of the bleeding vessels with the fingers should suffice until the vascular clamp is in place. Once proximal and distal vascular control is obtained, the three structures in the hepatoduodenal ligament must be dissected out very carefully because of the danger of blindly placing sutures in proximity to the common bile duct [*see Figure 16*].

Injuries to the hepatic artery in this location are occasionally amenable to lateral repair, though ligation without reconstruction is ordinarily well tolerated because of the extensive collateral arterial flow to the liver. If an associated hepatic injury calls for extensive suturing or debridement, ligation of the common hepatic artery will certainly lead to increased postoperative necrosis of the hepatic repair. Moreover, ligation of the common hepatic artery, the right or left hepatic artery supplying the injured lobe, and the portal vein branch to that lobe will lead to necrosis of the lobe and will necessitate hepatectomy. Finally, ligation of the right hepatic artery to control hemorrhage should be followed by cholecystectomy.

Because of the large size of the portal vein and its posterior position in the hepatoduodenal ligament, injuries to this vessel are particularly lethal. Once the Pringle maneuver has been performed, mobilization of the common bile duct to the left and of the cystic duct superiorly, coupled with an extensive Kocher maneuver, allows excellent visualization of any injury to this vein above the superior border of the pancreas. When the perforation extends underneath the neck of the pancreas, it may be necessary to have an assistant compress the superior mesenteric vein below the pancreas and then to divide the pancreas between noncrushing intestinal clamps to obtain exposure of the junction of the superior mesenteric vein and the splenic vein.

The preferred technique for repairing an injury to the portal vein is lateral venorrhaphy with continuous 4-0 or 5-0 polypropylene sutures. Complex repairs that have been successful on rare occasions include end-to-end anastomosis, interposition grafting with externally supported PTFE, transposition of the splenic vein, and a venovenous shunt from the superior mesenteric vein to the distal portal vein or the inferior vena cava. Such vigorous attempts at restoration of blood flow are not justified in patients who are in severe hypovolemic shock, for whom ligation of the portal vein is more appropriate. In addition, if a portosystemic shunt is performed in such a patient, hepatic encephalopathy will result because hepatofugal flow will be present in the rerouted or bypassed portal vein. As with ligation of the superior mesenteric vein, it is necessary to infuse tremendous amounts of crystalloids to reverse the transient peripheral hypovolemia that occurs secondary to the splanchnic hypervolemia resulting from ligation of the portal vein.

Since the early 1980s, the survival rate in patients with injuries to the portal vein has been approximately 50%.

RETROHEPATIC AREA

Retrohepatic hematoma or hemorrhage is cause to suspect the presence of injury to the retrohepatic vena cava, a hepatic vein, or a right renal blood vessel. In addition, hemorrhage in this area may signal injury to the overlying liver [*see 5:6 Injuries to the Liver, Biliary Tract, Spleen, and Diaphragm*].

If there is a hematoma that is not expanding or ruptured and clearly has no association with the right perirenal area, a tamponaded injury to the retrohepatic vena cava or a hepatic vein is present. Perihepatic packing around the right lobe of the liver for 24 to 48 hours has been shown to prevent further expansion and should be considered.

If hemorrhage is occurring that does not appear to be coming from the overlying liver, the right lobe of the liver should be compressed posteriorly to tamponade the caval perforation. The Pringle maneuver is then applied, and the surgical and nursing team, the anesthesiologist, and the blood blank are notified. Once the proper instruments and banked blood are in the OR, the overlying injured hepatic lobe is mobilized by dividing the triangular and anterior coronary ligaments and then lifted out of the subdiaphragmatic area. On occasion, an obvious perforation of the retrohepatic or suprahepatic vena cava or an obvious area where a hepatic vein was avulsed from the vena cava may be grasped with a forceps or a Judd-Allis clamp; a Satinsky clamp may then be applied. Because of the copious bleeding that occurs as the liver is lifted and the hole in the vena cava sought, the anesthesiologist should start blood transfusions as the lobe is being mobilized.

If the hemorrhage is not controlled after one or two attempts, another technique must be tried. The most common choice is the insertion of a 36 French chest tube or a 9 mm endotracheal tube as an atriocaval shunt [see 5:8 Operative Exposure of Abdominal Injuries and Closure of the Abdomen and 5:6 Injuries to the Liver, Biliary Tract, Spleen, and Diaphragm]. The shunt can reduce bleeding by 40% to 60%, but vigorous hemorrhage persists until full control of the perforation is obtained with clamps or sutures. An alternative approach is to isolate the liver and the vena cava by cross-clamping the supraceliac aorta, the porta hepatis, the suprarenal inferior vena cava, and the intrapericardial inferior vena cava. Because profoundly hypovolemic patients usually cannot tolerate cross-clamping of the inferior vena cava, this approach is rarely used.

The retrohepatic vena cava is repaired with continuous 4-0 or 5-0 polypropylene sutures. When the atriocaval shunt is removed from the heart after the vessel has been repaired, the right atrial appendage is ligated with a 2-0 silk tie.

The survival rate in patients undergoing atriocaval shunting and repair of the retrohepatic vena cava who are not in cardiac arrest has ranged from 33% to 50%.

Damage Control Laparotomy

Patients with injuries to the great vessels of the abdomen are ideal candidates for damage control laparotomy: they are uniformly hypothermic, acidotic, and coagulopathic on completion of the vascular repair, and a prolonged operation would lead to their demise. In such patients, packing of minor or moderate injuries to solid organs, packing of the retroperitoneum, stapling and rapid resection of multiple injuries to the GI tract, consideration of diffuse intra-abdominal packing, and towel-clip closure of the skin are all appropriate. If a towel-clip closure cannot be completed because of distention of the midgut (such as may be seen in association with profound shock or after ligation of the superior mesenteric or portal vein), a temporary silo made from a urologic irrigation bag can be used. The silo can be sewn to the skin edges with a continuous 2-0 polypropylene or nylon suture.

The patient is then rapidly moved to the SICU for further resuscitation. Priorities in the SICU include rapid restoration of normal body temperature, reversal of shock, infusion of intravenous bicarbonate to correct a persistent pH lower than 7.2, and administration of fresh frozen plasma, platelets, and cryoprecipitate when indicated. It is usually possible to return the patient to the OR for removal of clot and packs, reconstruction of the GI tract, irrigation, and reapplication of a towel-clip or silo closure within 48 to 72 hours.

When massive distention of the midgut persists after 7 days of intensive care, the safest approach is to convert the patient to an open abdomen (i.e., without closure of the midline incision) and cover the midgut with a double-thickness layer of absorbable mesh. With proper nutritional support and occasional use of Dakin solution to minimize bacterial contamination of the absorbable mesh, most patients are ready for the application of a split-thickness skin graft to the eviscerated midgut within 3 to 4 weeks of the original operation for an injury to a great vessel.

Complications

Besides those already mentioned, major complications associated with repair of injuries to the great vessels in the abdomen include thrombosis, dehiscence of the suture line, and infection. Because of the risk of occlusion of repairs in small vasoconstricted vessels (e.g., the superior mesenteric artery), it may be worthwhile to perform a second-look operation within 12 to 24 hours if the patient's metabolic state suggests that ischemia of the midgut is present. Early correction of an arterial thrombosis in the superior mesenteric artery may permit salvage of the midgut.

As noted [see Injuries in Zone 1, above], dehiscence of an end-to-end anastomosis or a vascular conduit inserted in the proximal superior mesenteric artery when there is an injury to the adjacent pancreas may be prevented by inserting a distal aorta–superior mesenteric artery bypass graft. To prevent adjacent loops of small bowel from adhering to the vascular suture lines, both lines should be covered with soft tissue (retroperitoneal tissue for the aortic suture line and mesenteric tissue for the superior mesenteric arterial suture line). Also as noted [see Injuries in Zone 3, above], when an extensive injury to either the common or the external iliac artery occurs in the presence of significant enteric or fecal contamination in the pelvis, ligation and extra-anatomic bypass may be necessary.

On occasion, vascular-enteric fistulas occur after repair of the anterior aorta or the insertion of grafts in either the abdominal aorta or the superior mesenteric artery. In my experience, such fistulas all occur at suture lines; hence, once again, proper coverage of suture lines with soft tissue should eliminate this complication.

References

1. Tyburski JG, Wilson RF, Dente C, et al: Factors affecting mortality rates in patients with abdominal vascular injuries. J Trauma 50:1020, 2001
2. Asensio JA, Chahwan S, Hanpeter D, et al: Operative management and outcome of 302 abdominal vascular injuries. Am J Surg 180:528, 2000
3. Davis TP, Feliciano DV, Rozycki GS, et al: Results with abdominal vascular trauma in the modern era. Am Surg 67:565, 2001
4. Hass CA, Dinchman KH, Nasrallah PH, et al: Traumatic renal artery occlusion: a 15-year review. J Trauma 45:557, 1998

Recommended Reading

Asensio JA, Britt LD, Borzotta A, et al: Multiinstitutional experience with the management of superior mesenteric artery injuries. J Am Coll Surg 193:354, 2001

Feliciano DV, Burch JM, Graham JM: Abdominal vascular injury. Trauma, 4th ed. Mattox KL, Feliciano DV, Moore EE, Eds. McGraw-Hill, New York, 2000

Wilson RF, Dulchavsky S: Abdominal vascular trauma. Management of Trauma: Pitfalls and Practice. Wilson RF, Walt AJ, Eds. Williams & Wilkins, Baltimore, 1996

Acknowledgments

Figures 1 and 2 Marcia Kammerer.

Figures 3, 5, 8, 12, and 16 Tom Moore.

Figures 4 and 9 From "Abdominal Vascular Injury," by D. V. Feliciano, J. M. Burch, and J. M. Graham, in Trauma, 3rd ed., edited by D. V. Feliciano, E. E. Moore, and K. L. Mattox. Appleton & Lange, Stamford, Connecticut, 1996. Reproduced by permission.

10 INJURIES TO THE UROGENITAL TRACT

Hunter Wessells, M.D., F.A.C.S., and Jack W. McAninch, M.D., F.A.C.S.

Hematuria is the hallmark of injury to the urogenital system. Location of the injury and identification of its cause help determine which urologic organs are most likely to have been injured by a particular traumatic event. In penetrating trauma to the abdomen, hematuria signals the need to evaluate the kidneys, ureters, and bladder. Urethral and genital injuries are suspected only with wounds to the pelvis, perineum, and buttocks. When hematuria occurs in association with blunt injuries and pelvic fracture, the entire genitourinary system should be evaluated.

This chapter includes a separate algorithm for each of the major urogenital organs. Injury to both the upper and the lower urinary tract is rare, but a high index of suspicion must be maintained for detection of such an injury. Injury to the female reproductive organs requires special expertise in evaluation and management, particularly if the patient is pregnant or the victim of a sexual assault.

Injuries to the Kidneys

INITIAL EVALUATION

The most reliable sign of injury to the kidney is hematuria, whether microscopic or gross. However, the degree of hematuria is not correlated with the severity of injury, and patients with serious injuries may have no blood in their urine.[1] The same staging system is used to classify blunt injuries and penetrating injuries [see Figure 1 and Table 1], and the only significant difference in their management is in the initial evaluation [see Figure 2]. For patients with blunt trauma, we recommend the following criteria for radiographic evaluation of injuries to the kidney[2]: adults with microscopic hematuria and systolic blood pressure of at least 90 mm Hg do not require imaging unless serious associated injuries suggest a deceleration injury; all pediatric trauma patients, patients with gross hematuria, and patients with microscopic hematuria and systolic BP lower than 90 mm Hg require radiographic evaluation. Computed tomography is the first-line imaging modality for all cases of suspected blunt renal trauma. We recommend performance of a delayed CT scan 10 minutes after initial imaging to detect any urinary extravasation or injury to the collecting system.[3]

All penetrating injuries of the kidney require exploration unless a complete radiographic evaluation demonstrates that an injury can be managed nonoperatively. CT, which is ideal for study of penetrating injuries, should be the first radiographic method used in hemodynamically stable patients.[4]

Intravenous urography is adequate for the evaluation of trauma only if it includes tomography and does not demonstrate poor visualization, an irregular contour, or extravasation, which should prompt further studies or exploration.[5]

All grade I and II renal injuries, regardless of the mechanism of injury, can be managed without operation. The absolute indications for renal exploration include pulsatile and expanding hematomas and hemodynamic instability resulting from renal injury.[6] In stable patients with adequate staging, grade III and nonvascular grade IV injuries (including devitalized fragments and urinary extravasation) can be observed.[7] In patients requiring laparotomy for associated injuries, we perform renal exploration and reconstruction to reduce the likelihood of delayed complications.[8,9] Shattered kidneys (grade V) and vascular injuries (grades IV and V) require immediate renal exploration. An exception is thrombosis of the renal artery or its branches, which may be treated expectantly if revascularization is not performed expediently in a patient with no associated injuries.

A significant number of patients with a penetrating injury and a minority of those with blunt trauma require immediate laparotomy before they can be evaluated radiographically.[10] Hematuria is the key clinical sign, alerting the surgeon to the possibility of renal injury in inadequately staged patients. The presence of a retroperitoneal hematoma should prompt further evaluation. We obtain a single-shot intravenous pyelogram (IVP) 10 minutes after bolus injection of 150 ml of iodinated contrast material, ensuring the presence of a functioning contralateral unit before exploration. If the injured kidney is imaged adequately and found to be normal, exploration may be omitted.[11] In patients with blunt injuries and gross hematuria or with microscopic hematuria in the presence of shock, intraoperative imaging is required, even in the absence of a retroperitoneal hematoma. If the kidney is not adequately imaged, the possibility of renal artery thrombosis should be considered.

OPERATIVE MANAGEMENT

A midline transabdominal incision permits exploration of the kidneys and abdomen. After areas of bleeding have been packed with laparotomy sponges, the first step is isolation of the renal vasculature before opening Gerota's fascia. This technique, which has reduced our nephrectomy rate, allows rapid control of bleeding from serious injuries.[12] In all renal explorations, regardless of the degree of injury, we begin with isolation of the renal vessels, which is best performed by opening the posterior peritoneum overlying the aorta, preventing premature entry of the retroperitoneal hematoma. Even in the presence of large hematomas, the inferior mesenteric vein serves as a landmark for location of the aorta. Working cephalad along the aorta, the surgeon encounters the left renal vein first and subsequently both renal arteries. The best way to find the right renal artery is to dissect between the aorta and the vena cava; dissection lateral to the vena cava may lead to inadvertent isolation of a seg-

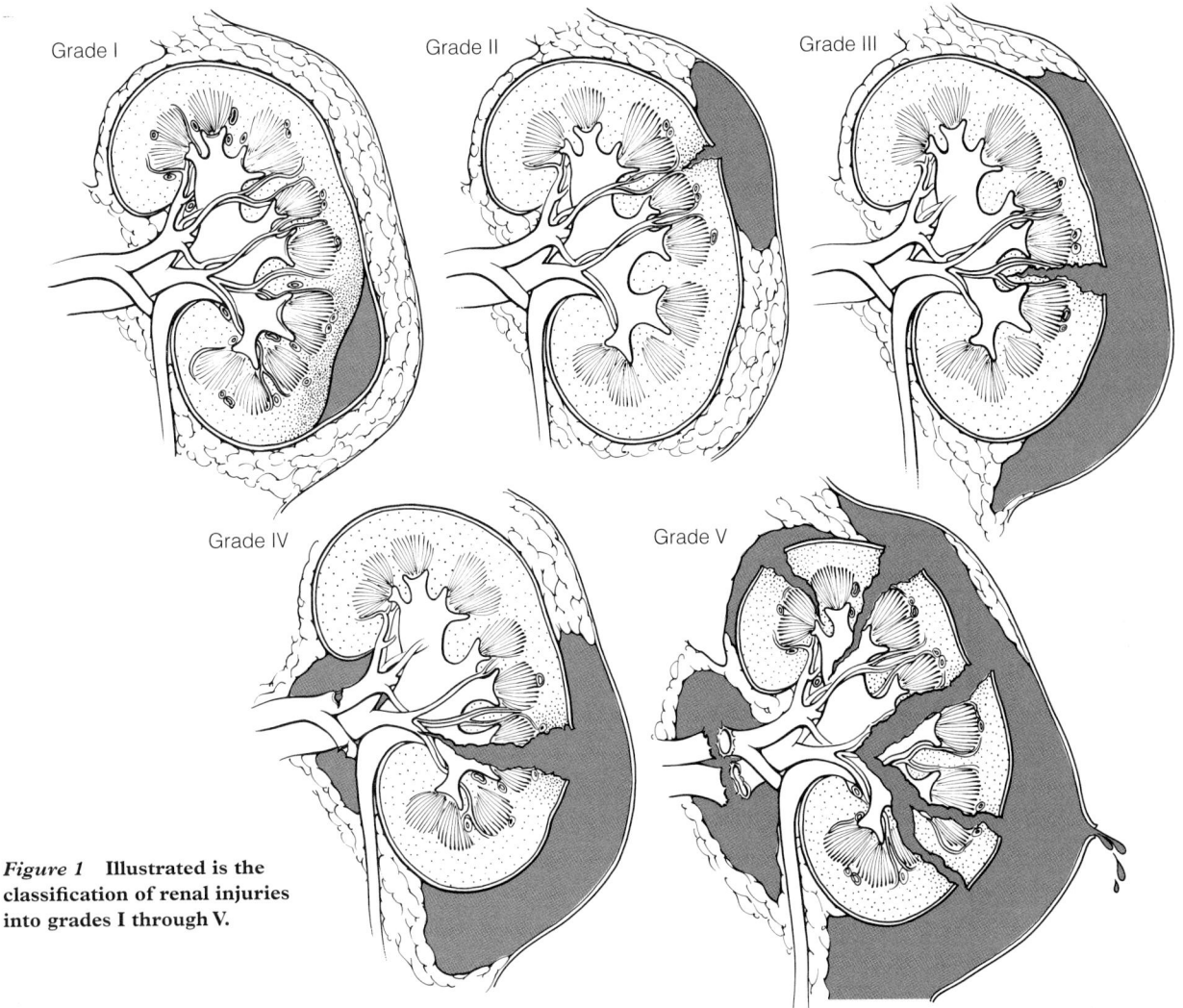

Grade I   Grade II   Grade III

Grade IV   Grade V

Figure 1 Illustrated is the classification of renal injuries into grades I through V.

mental branch of the renal artery. Isolation of the right renal vein may be easier after reflection of the right colon and duodenum. We place vessel loops around the artery and the vein, thus ensuring rapid access to the vessels if significant bleeding occurs. The renal vessels can also be approached laterally if the duodenum or left colon has been mobilized.

Gerota's fascia is opened only after vascular isolation. If release of the tamponade effect causes bleeding, we use Rumel tourniquets or vascular clamps to occlude the renal artery and the renal vein. Clamping of the renal artery alone usually controls bleeding. If it does not, the surgeon should suspect a venous injury and occlude the vein. It is not routine to cool the surface of the kidney after clamping of the renal artery, because patients with trauma are often hypothermic and coagulopathic. Clamp time should be limited to less than 30 minutes, if possible.

Total exposure of the kidney, by means of sharp and blunt dissection, is necessary to rule out injury to the parenchyma, the renal pedicle, and the collecting system. The renal capsule can easily be pulled off the parenchyma if dissection is not meticulous. Once the kidney has been delivered into the field, the extent of injury can be assessed and reconstruction can be planned. Renal reconstruction includes debridement of all devitalized tissue, hemostasis, closure of the collecting system, defect coverage, and drainage [see Figure 3]. With these techniques, renal salvage should be possible in close to 90% of kid-

ney explorations.[5] Nephrectomy should be reserved for destroyed kidneys that cannot be reconstructed or for serious renal injury associated with other life-threatening injuries, such as vascular or hepatic trauma.

Debridement of devitalized tissue permits reconstruction with healthy tissue and prevents delayed bleeding and urinary extravasation. If the renal capsule is present at the margins of the wound, it should be peeled back and preserved for subsequent closure. A scalpel is used to remove the devitalized renal parenchyma until bleeding occurs at the margin. Polar injuries can be debrided by guillotine amputation of the parenchyma.

Manual compression usually controls bleeding during the ligation of small vessels. Ligation of individual vessels with absorbable monofilament suture material, such as 4-0 chromic catgut, achieves hemostasis. Temporary release of renal artery occlusion for the assessment of hemostasis is not recommended. Ligation of venous bleeding points generally controls adjacent arterial sources.

Once hemostasis is satisfactory, the collecting system should be scrutinized for evidence of injury. If the extent is unclear, 2 to 3 ml of methylene blue can be injected directly into the renal pelvis, while the ureter is occluded, to identify any openings in the collecting system. Open calyxes or infundibula can be closed with a continuous 4-0 absorbable suture. For injuries to the renal pelvis, interrupted closure is more reliable.

The renal capsule can often be used to cover exposed renal parenchyma. The defect in the parenchyma is filled with folded absorbable gelatin sponges or other hemostatic agents; and with interrupted sutures through the capsule but not the parenchyma, the capsule is closed over the bolsters. If the capsule is not available, options include an omental or perinephric fat flap tacked down over the defect, a patch of Dexon or peritoneum, or an entire sac of Dexon wrapped around the kidney, with the parenchymal edges kept well apposed.[6,13]

At the end of the procedure, the kidney should be returned to its location within Gerota's fascia. Drainage of the renal region is recommended, and either a closed-suction or a Penrose drain is acceptable. If there are significant injuries to the collecting system, a Penrose drain is preferable because it does not exert negative pressure on the repair site. Internalized drains and double J stents generally are not necessary for renal injuries. However, major injuries to the renal pelvis or the ureteropelvic junction (UPJ) should be drained with an internalized stent as well as a retroperitoneal drain.

POSTOPERATIVE CARE

Management of patients after operative or nonoperative intervention for renal trauma depends to a large extent on associated injuries. Bed rest is prescribed until the urine becomes grossly clear, usually within 24 to 48 hours. Ambulation is allowed unless gross hematuria recurs. Drainage of the bladder with a Foley catheter is necessary only until the patient is ambulatory and the urine clear. Nasogastric suction

Table 1 AAST Organ Injury Scales for Urinary Tract

Injured Structure	AAST Grade	Characteristics of Injury	AIS-90 Score
Kidney*	I	Contusion with microscopic or gross hematuria, urologic studies normal; nonexpanding subcapsular hematoma without parenchymal laceration	2; 2
	II	Nonexpanding perirenal hematoma confined to renal retroperitoneum; laceration < 1.0 cm parenchymal depth of renal cortex without urinary extravasation	2; 2
	III	Laceration > 1.0 cm parenchymal depth of renal cortex without collecting system rupture or urinary extravasation	3
	IV	Parenchymal laceration extending through renal cortex, medulla, and collecting system; injury to main renal artery or vein with contained hemorrhage	4; 4
	V	Completely shattered kidney; avulsion of renal hilum that devascularizes kidney	5; 5
Ureter*	I	Contusion or hematoma without devascularization	2
	II	< 50% transection	2
	III	≥ 50% transection	3
	IV	Complete transection with < 2 cm devascularization	3
	V	Avulsion with > 2 cm devascularization	3
Bladder†	I	Contusion, intramural hematoma; partial-thickness laceration	2; 3
	II	Extraperitoneal bladder wall laceration < 2 cm	4
	III	Extraperitoneal bladder wall laceration > 2 cm or intraperitoneal bladder wall laceration < 2 cm	4
	IV	Intraperitoneal bladder wall laceration > 2 cm	4
	V	Intraperitoneal or extraperitoneal bladder wall laceration extending into bladder neck or ureteral orifice (trigone)	4
Urethra*	I	Contusion with blood at urethral meatus and normal urethrography	2
	II	Stretch injury with elongation of urethra but without extravasation of urethrography contrast material	2
	III	Partial disruption with extravasation of urethrography contrast material at injury site with visualization in the bladder	2
	IV	Complete disruption with < 2 cm urethral separation and extravasation of urethrography contrast material at injury site without visualization in the bladder	3
	V	Complete transection with ≥ 2 cm urethral separation or extension into the prostate or vagina	4

*Advance one grade for bilateral injuries, up to grade III.
†Advance one grade for multiple injuries, up to grade III.
AAST—American Association for the Surgery of Trauma AIS-90—Abbreviated Injury Score, 1990 version

should be continued until peristalsis returns. Retroperitoneal drains should be removed within 48 hours unless the output is significant. Often, peritoneal fluid continues to drain. Comparison of the creatinine level in the fluid with the creatinine level in serum can distinguish urinary leakage from serous fluid. If serous fluid is draining, we remove the retroperitoneal drains regardless of output.

Persistent urinary leakage is best evaluated with CT. Evidence of distal ureteral obstruction should be sought and the obstruction alleviated. Many urinomas without concurrent infection resolve without intervention. If the collection is large, the collecting system should be drained with a double J stent or a percutaneously placed nephrostomy tube. With appropriate drainage, uninfected urinomas and extravasation usually resolve.

Infectious complications after renal reconstruction include urinoma formation and perinephric abscesses. Percutaneous drainage of urinomas and abscesses is preferred. Reexploration may force the surgeon to perform a nephrectomy if there is not enough healthy tissue for a trustworthy repair. The renal collecting system should be drained and the collection studied at intervals until the leak has resolved.

Delayed bleeding is a rare but serious complication of renal reconstruction or nonoperative management of major lacerations. Gross hematuria usually, but not invariably, accompanies the bleeding. If there is evidence of significant bleeding (i.e., hypotension or a decreasing hematocrit), the combination of renal angiography and selective embolization is an effective option that should be attempted before reexploration.[14]

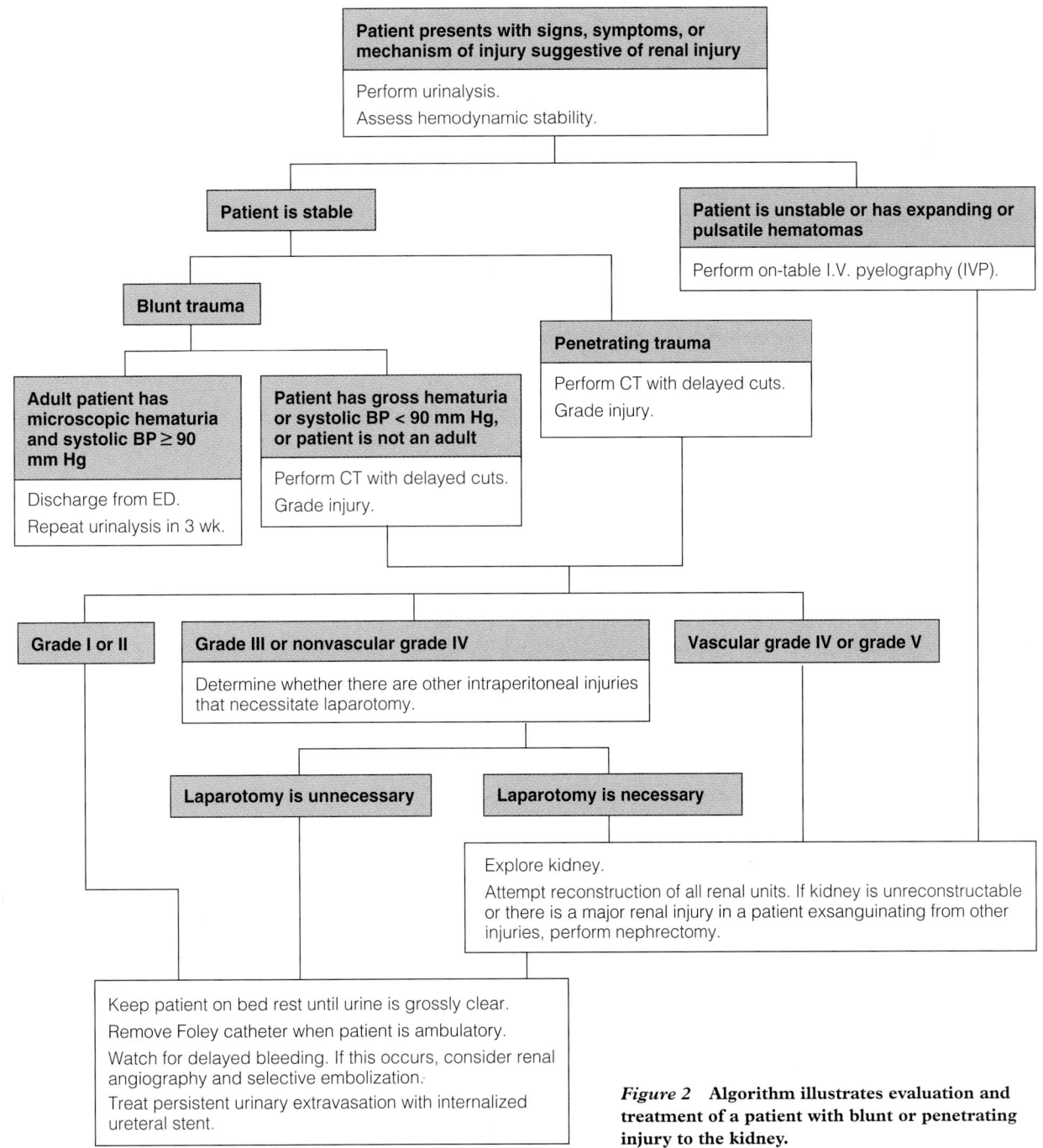

Figure 2 **Algorithm illustrates evaluation and treatment of a patient with blunt or penetrating injury to the kidney.**

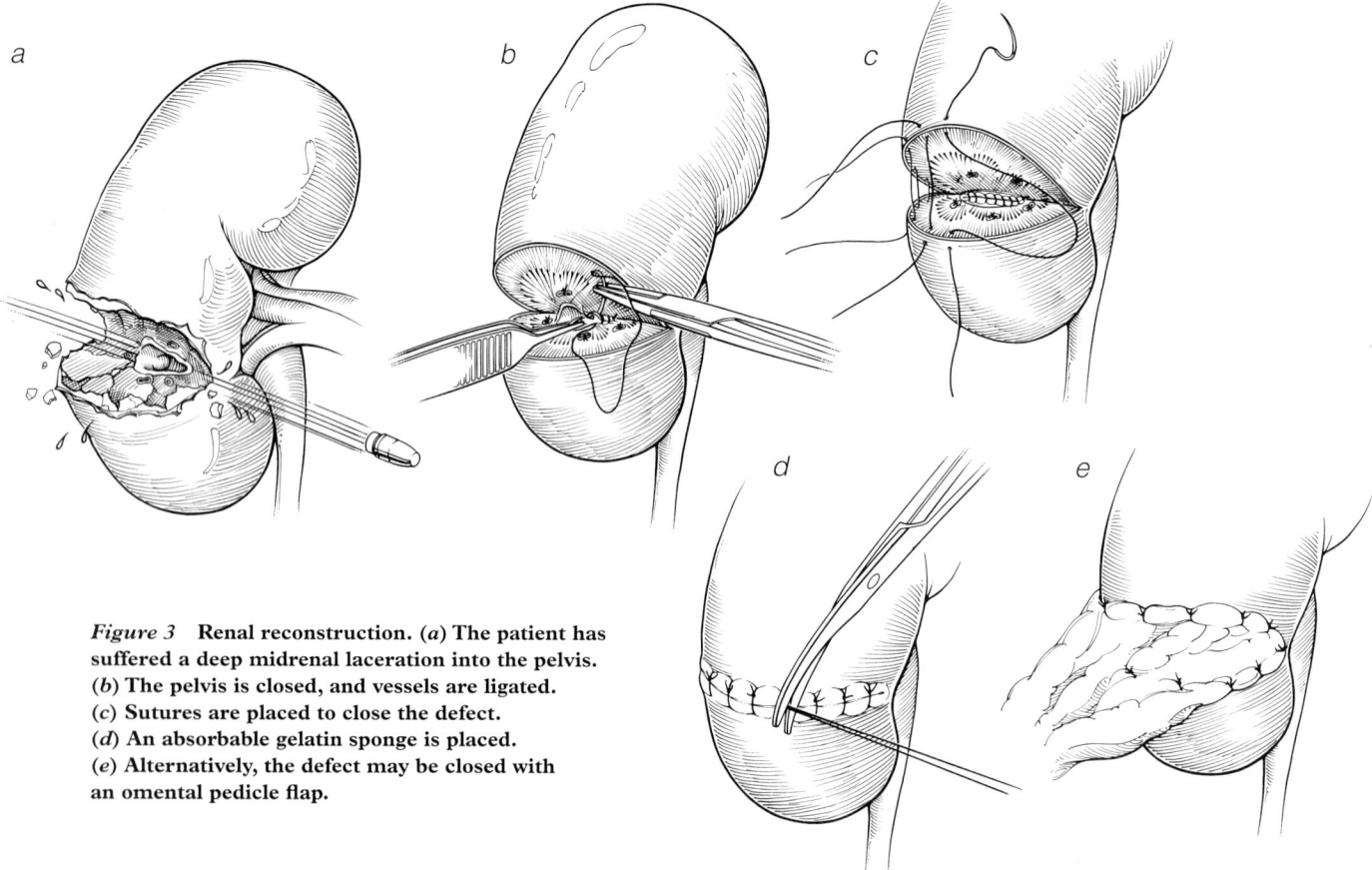

Figure 3 Renal reconstruction. (*a*) The patient has suffered a deep midrenal laceration into the pelvis. (*b*) The pelvis is closed, and vessels are ligated. (*c*) Sutures are placed to close the defect. (*d*) An absorbable gelatin sponge is placed. (*e*) Alternatively, the defect may be closed with an omental pedicle flap.

Postoperative imaging is recommended to evaluate renal function and to rule out the development of hydronephrosis or stones. The optimal follow-up is intravenous urography or radionuclide scanning at 3 months and 1 year. If significant injury to the collecting system was repaired, the imaging study should be performed before discharge from the hospital. Hypertension is a rare late complication of renal reconstruction, usually renin-mediated from an ischemic segment of renal parenchyma. Occasionally, angiography delineates the ischemic segment of the kidney, and excision of the nonperfused segment or nephrectomy may be required.

Injuries to the Ureters

INITIAL EVALUATION

Ureteral injury [*see Table 1*] is rare, accounting for fewer than 1% of genitourinary injuries. Although ureteral injury can be repaired successfully [*see Figure 4*], it may have serious consequences, including loss of renal function and death,[15] if unrecognized. The absence of physical signs of injury makes diagnosis difficult, and a delayed presentation is not uncommon. Up to half of all ureteral injuries resulting from blunt trauma are not recognized immediately, and a high index of suspicion is necessary to prevent the late complications of urinoma, sepsis, and nephrectomy.[16]

A penetrating wound is the predominant cause of ureteral injury, gunshot wounds being the most common cause and stab wounds the second most common. Deceleration injuries may result in UPJ disruption, especially in children. The pediatric ureter is prone to injury because hyperextensibility of the

spine can result in avulsion of the ureter at the UPJ.[17] The patient's history and the physical examination provide little information about ureteral injuries. Signs and symptoms related to associated injuries predominate. In three series, gross or microscopic hematuria was present in only 30% to 70% of ureteral injuries, making vigilance necessary for diagnosis.[15,16,18]

CT with delayed cuts should be performed whenever ureteral injury is suspected. Intravenous urography is of variable usefulness in the detection of ureteral injuries, but extravasation of the contrast agent is diagnostic.[19]

Ureteral injury may not be suspected until the time of laparotomy, when a hematoma is found near the kidney or ureter. If an on-table IVP is not diagnostic, direct inspection of the ureter for injury, contusion, and peristalsis is mandatory. Injection of indigo carmine directly into the collecting system may identify extravasation. All injuries to the ureter should be repaired surgically, unless a delay in diagnosis results in an abscess or a urinoma. For either abscess or urinoma, drainage by percutaneous nephrostomy and ureteral stenting may allow the inflamed ureter to heal, whereas an operative approach may result in nephrectomy.

OPERATIVE MANAGEMENT

Once ureteral injury has been recognized, reconstruction should proceed. Depending on the type of injury and its location, the reconstructive techniques may include debridement of devitalized tissue, a spatulated tension-free anastomosis, watertight mucosal approximation, ureteral stenting, coverage of the repair with vascularized tissue, and appropriate drainage.[15] Stab wounds generally require less tissue debridement

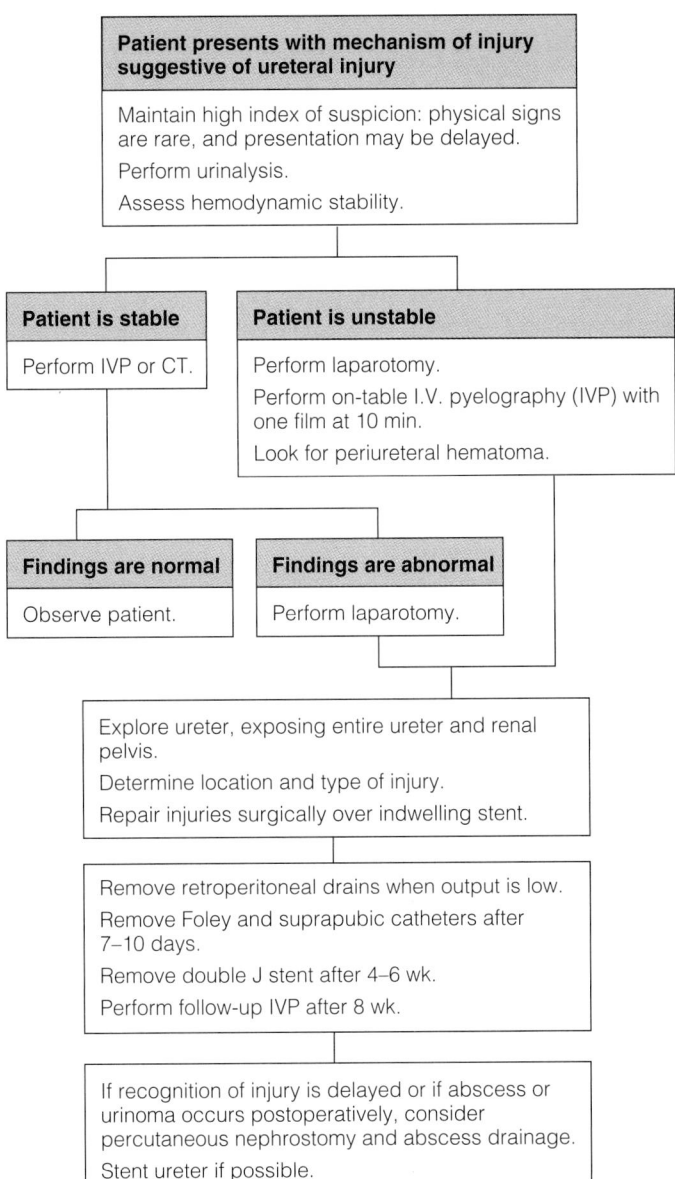

Patient presents with mechanism of injury suggestive of ureteral injury

Maintain high index of suspicion: physical signs are rare, and presentation may be delayed.
Perform urinalysis.
Assess hemodynamic stability.

Patient is stable

Perform IVP or CT.

Patient is unstable

Perform laparotomy.
Perform on-table I.V. pyelography (IVP) with one film at 10 min.
Look for periureteral hematoma.

Findings are normal

Observe patient.

Findings are abnormal

Perform laparotomy.

Explore ureter, exposing entire ureter and renal pelvis.
Determine location and type of injury.
Repair injuries surgically over indwelling stent.

Remove retroperitoneal drains when output is low.
Remove Foley and suprapubic catheters after 7–10 days.
Remove double J stent after 4–6 wk.
Perform follow-up IVP after 8 wk.

If recognition of injury is delayed or if abscess or urinoma occurs postoperatively, consider percutaneous nephrostomy and abscess drainage.
Stent ureter if possible.

Figure 4   **Algorithm illustrates evaluation and treatment of a patient with ureteral injury.**

than gunshot wounds, and partial transections may be closed primarily.

Disruption or transection of the UPJ is repaired by debridement and primary anastomosis of the renal pelvis and ureter. Penetrating low-velocity injuries require minimal or no debridement. Mobilization of the ureter should be limited to avoid compromising the blood supply. Interrupted 5-0 or 6-0 Vicryl sutures are preferred, and a double J ureteral stent or a nephrostomy tube must be inserted before closure of the anastomosis.

Injuries to the abdominal ureter between the UPJ and the pelvic brim are repaired by ureteroureterostomy [*see Figure 5*]. After debridement, the ends are spatulated on opposite sides, and an interrupted approximation is completed over a double J stent. In cases of overlying colonic, duodenal, or pancreatic injury, the anastomosis may be covered with omentum. Large defects in the abdominal ureter may require transuretero-ureterostomy, in which the injured ureter is passed behind the

mesocolon to the contralateral side. Anastomosis of the injured ureter to a 1 to 2 cm opening in the medial normal ureter can be achieved without tension. With transureteroureterostomy, a stent (usually a 5 French pediatric feeding tube) should cross the anastomosis and be brought out through the normal lower ureter or bladder.

Ureteral injuries below the pelvic brim should be debrided and reimplanted into the bladder. The distal stump is ligated, and after the anterior bladder wall is opened, the proximal end of the ureter is brought through a new hiatus on the back wall of the bladder. The ureter is then spatulated and approximated to the bladder mucosa with interrupted chromic sutures. One 3-0 anchoring stitch should bring the distal apex of the ureter to the muscle and mucosa; the rest of the sutures are 4-0 only, approximating mucosa. A nonrefluxing reimplantation is acceptable in adults. Large defects can be bridged by performing a vesico-psoas hitch, in which the bladder dome is mobilized to bridge the ureteral defect and sewn to the central

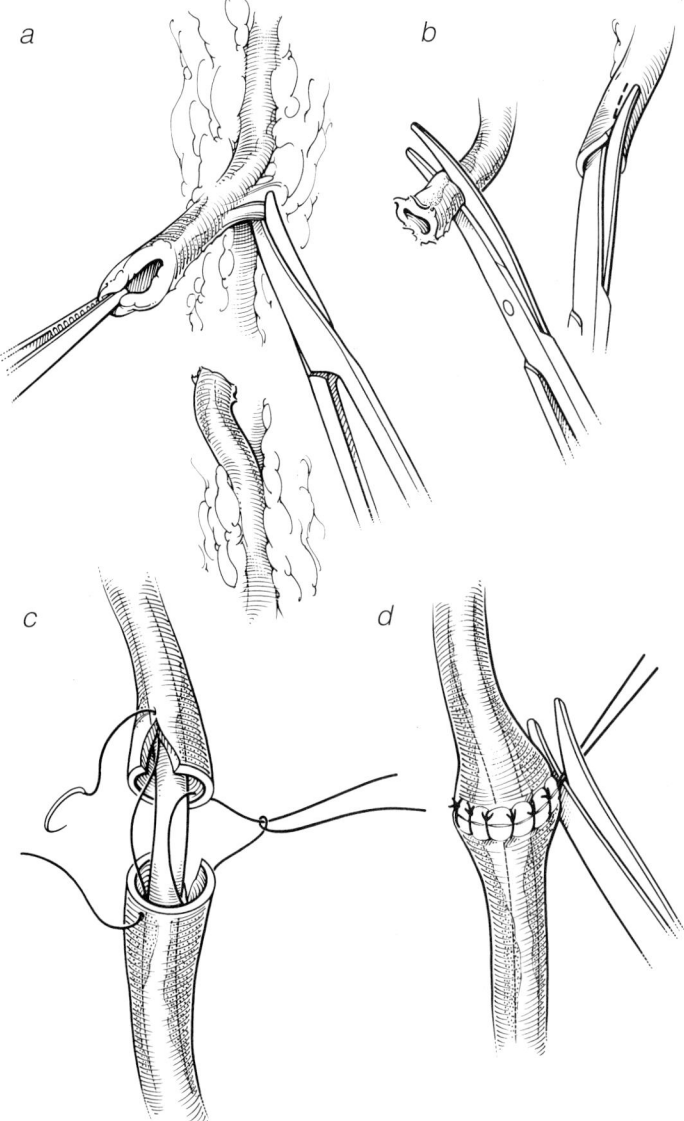

Figure 5   **Ureteroureterostomy. (*a*) The injured ureter is dissected free. (*b*) The ends are spatulated. (*c*) The ends are approximated over a double J stent. (*d*) The anastomosis is completed with interrupted sutures.**

tendon of the psoas muscle. Three interrupted sutures that enter the detrusor muscle but not the bladder lumen should anchor the dome above the iliac vessels. The dome is mobilized by dividing the obliterated umbilical arteries bilaterally and, if necessary, dividing the contralateral superior vesical artery. Significant bladder or vascular damage may make transureterouterostomy a more attractive option to avoid further dissection in the injured area. A ureteral stent should be used in all ureteral reimplantations. The bladder is closed in two layers with a continuous 2-0 Vicryl suture, and a drain is placed in the Retzius space.

A retroperitoneal drain is essential in all ureteral reconstructions. A large-bore Foley catheter is sufficient for bladder drainage unless there is coexistent bladder injury or prolonged catheterization is expected. In either of these cases, a suprapubic catheter allows better drainage of clots and, in males, has fewer long-term complications.[20]

POSTOPERATIVE CARE

Postoperative care of ureteral trauma relates mainly to the manipulation of drains and management of complications. Retroperitoneal drains may have significant output for several days but are removed once the output is minimal. With severe injuries or persistent output from drains, CT or IVP before discharge from the hospital may help rule out the possibility of extravasation. Bladder catheterization is necessary for 7 days after ureteral reimplantation. In combined bladder and ureteral reconstructions, contrast cystography is indicated before catheter removal. Cystoscopic removal of the double J stent is usually performed with local anesthesia 4 to 6 weeks after operation. Intravenous urography 3 months after removal of the stent rules out the possibility of asymptomatic obstruction.

Fistula formation, usually the result of distal obstruction or necrosis of the ureter, should be managed by antegrade or retrograde drainage of the collecting system using percutaneous or endoscopic techniques. Drainage of periureteral collection may also be necessary. If recognition of an injury or complication is delayed, reconstruction should not be undertaken for at least 3 months, to allow resolution of the inflammatory phase of wound healing. Because hydronephrosis may develop as a result of stricture, retroperitoneal fibrosis, or a urinoma, repeat imaging is appropriate 1 year after injury.

Injuries to the Bladder

INITIAL EVALUATION

Bladder injury [see Table 1] occurs in fewer than 1% of trauma patients.[21] Bladder rupture is most often caused by blunt injuries, including injuries resulting from motor vehicle accidents, falls, and direct blows to the abdomen, and is associated with pelvic fracture in 89% of cases. Overall, 9% of patients with a pelvic fracture have an associated injury to the bladder.[22] Penetrating wounds of the bladder may be caused by gunshot, stabs, or pelvic surgery.

The signs and symptoms of bladder injury are nonspecific [see Figure 6]. Patients may complain of suprapubic pain, dysuria, or an inability to void.[23] Physical examination may reveal tenderness in the suprapubic region, ileus, or an acute abdomen. Bladder rupture is associated with gross hematuria in 95% of cases; in a 1989 report, 3% of patients had no hematuria.[24] Laboratory studies are usually inconclusive unless significant reabsorption of urine causes elevated serum creatinine levels.

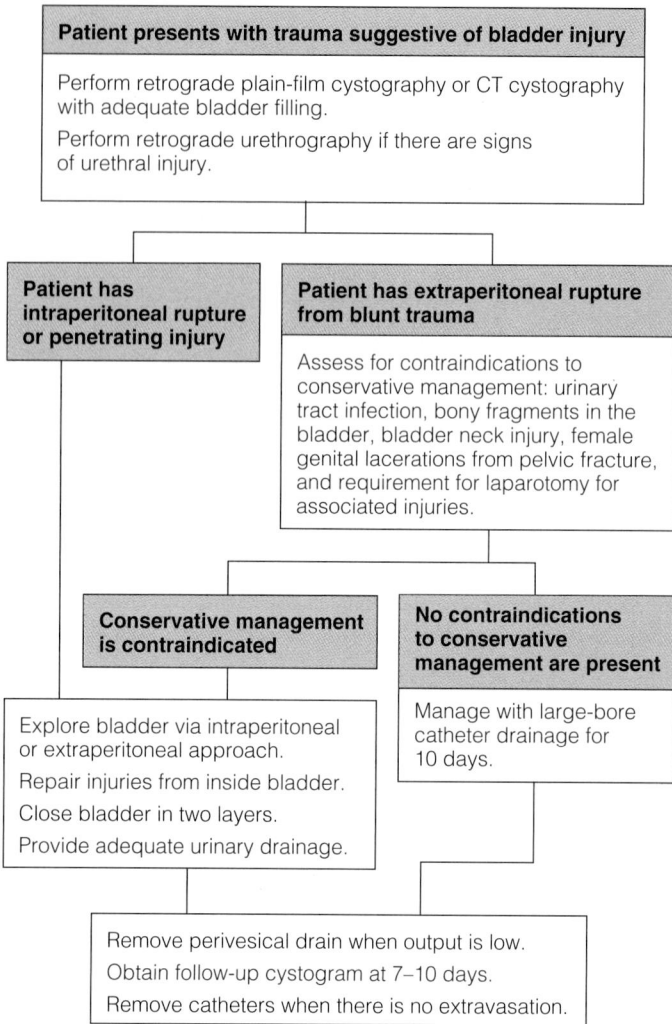

Figure 6 **Algorithm illustrates evaluation and treatment of a patient with bladder injury.**

Bladder rupture can be accurately diagnosed with CT cystography or plain-film cystography. Insufficient instillation of the contrast agent, however, yields false negative results. Standard CT is inadequate for the diagnosis of bladder rupture, because the bladder is not sufficiently distended in most patients. CT cystography involves three sets of images: (1) initial fill images obtained after retrograde instillation of 100 ml of contrast material, (2) complete fill images obtained after instillation of 350 ml, and (3) images obtained after drainage.[25]

A plain-film cystogram is obtained after an initial scout film by instilling 300 to 400 ml of 25% to 30% iodinated contrast through a urethral catheter. An anteroposterior view should be taken with the bladder full and after evacuation. In cases of intraperitoneal bladder injury, extravasation of contrast outlines the bowel loops and may track along the lateral gutters [see Figure 7a]. Extraperitoneal injuries demonstrate flame-shaped extravasation in the pelvis, which may track down into the obturator region, the scrotum, or the thigh [see Figure 7b]. Blunt injuries can cause extraperitoneal, intraperitoneal, or combined rupture. The amount of extravasation has no correlation with the degree of injury and should not influence management.[20]

a

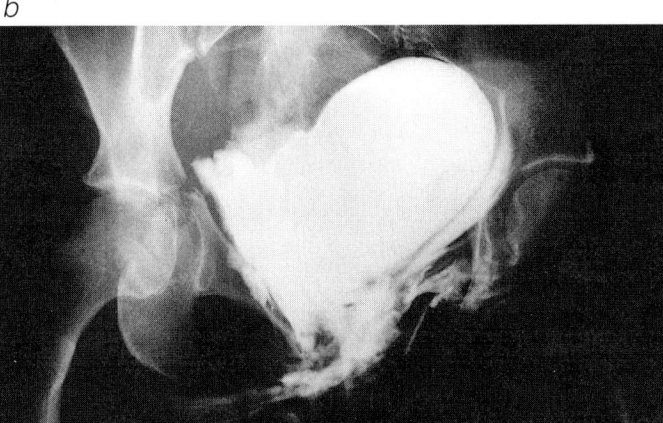

b

Figure 7 X-rays show intraperitoneal (*a*) and extraperitoneal (*b*) bladder rupture.

OPERATIVE MANAGEMENT

Extraperitoneal bladder injuries caused by blunt trauma can be managed with catheter drainage for 10 days, unless contraindications exist.[20] After 10 days, plain-film cystography should be used to document healing and allow removal of the catheter. If extravasation persists, cystography should be repeated weekly until healing occurs. Contraindications to nonoperative management include urinary infection; the presence of bony fragments in the bladder; bladder neck injury, which may compromise continence; and female genital lacerations associated with pelvic fracture.

If the patient requires laparotomy for associated injuries and is not critically ill, repair of extraperitoneal bladder injuries is recommended to decrease the possibility of infecting the pelvic hematoma. If the bladder injury is associated with a pelvic fracture in a male patient, the possibility of a urethral injury is

10% to 29% and must be excluded.[24] A successfully placed Foley catheter rules out a complete urethral disruption.

All penetrating injuries and all intraperitoneal ruptures of the bladder are managed by bladder exploration and repair. Bladder exploration can be performed via an intraperitoneal approach. In addition to repair of the bladder, exploration makes it possible to rule out associated injuries, ensure the integrity of the ureters by direct visualization, and, in the case of pelvic fracture, avoid entering the pelvic hematoma. In cases involving early orthopedic reconstruction of the pelvis, we approach the bladder extraperitoneally through the incision used to expose the pubis. Intraperitoneal injuries generally cause a stellate rupture of the dome of the bladder. By enlarging this opening, one can inspect the interior of the bladder to exclude concomitant extraperitoneal injuries, which occur in 8% of cases.[23]

Penetrating injuries and extraperitoneal ruptures are approached by opening the bladder with the electrocautery, vertically at the dome or along the anterior surface, and identifying the sites of rupture intravesically. These lacerations are then debrided (rarely necessary) and closed with interrupted 3-0 chromic catgut or Vicryl sutures, which approximate detrusor muscle and mucosa in one layer and provide hemostasis. In patients with gunshot wounds, entrance and exit sites must be identified. The cystotomy is then closed with two layers of continuous 2-0 or 3-0 Vicryl sutures, the first layer consisting of mucosa and detrusor muscle and the second consisting of detrusor and serosa.

Adequate urinary drainage is essential to successful healing of the repaired bladder. Large-bore (22 French or larger) Foley catheter drainage is sufficient if bladder injuries are not extensive and hemostasis is excellent. Extensive injuries and coagulopathy warrant additional drainage with a suprapubic tube, which allows irrigation of clots and proper decompression of the bladder. If suprapubic cystostomy is chosen, a 24 French Malecot catheter placed through a separate site into the bladder is preferred. In addition, a closed-suction or a Penrose drain near the bladder closure, but not overlying the suture line, is recommended. Like the suprapubic tube, the drain should exit through a separate site in the skin.

POSTOPERATIVE CARE

In the majority of patients with a bladder repair, 7 days of catheter drainage is sufficient to allow healing. Cystography may be indicated in cases of severe bladder injury or persistent output from drains. The perivesical drain can be removed after the output has decreased to an acceptable rate. Because bladder repair is reliable, complications of bladder injury are related to a delay in diagnosis rather than to postoperative morbidity. Azotemia, ascites, and sepsis may result from an intraperitoneal injury that was overlooked. Because an infected pelvic hematoma can have disastrous effects, nonoperative management of extraperitoneal rupture must be undertaken with caution. Bladder neck injury, if unrecognized, may lead to scarring and incompetence of the proximal sphincter mechanism, with resultant incontinence, especially in females.

Injuries to the Urethra

INITIAL EVALUATION

Almost all injuries to the male urethra [*see Table 1*] are caused by blunt trauma. Posterior urethral (prostatic and membranous urethral) injuries in males occur in 5% of pelvic

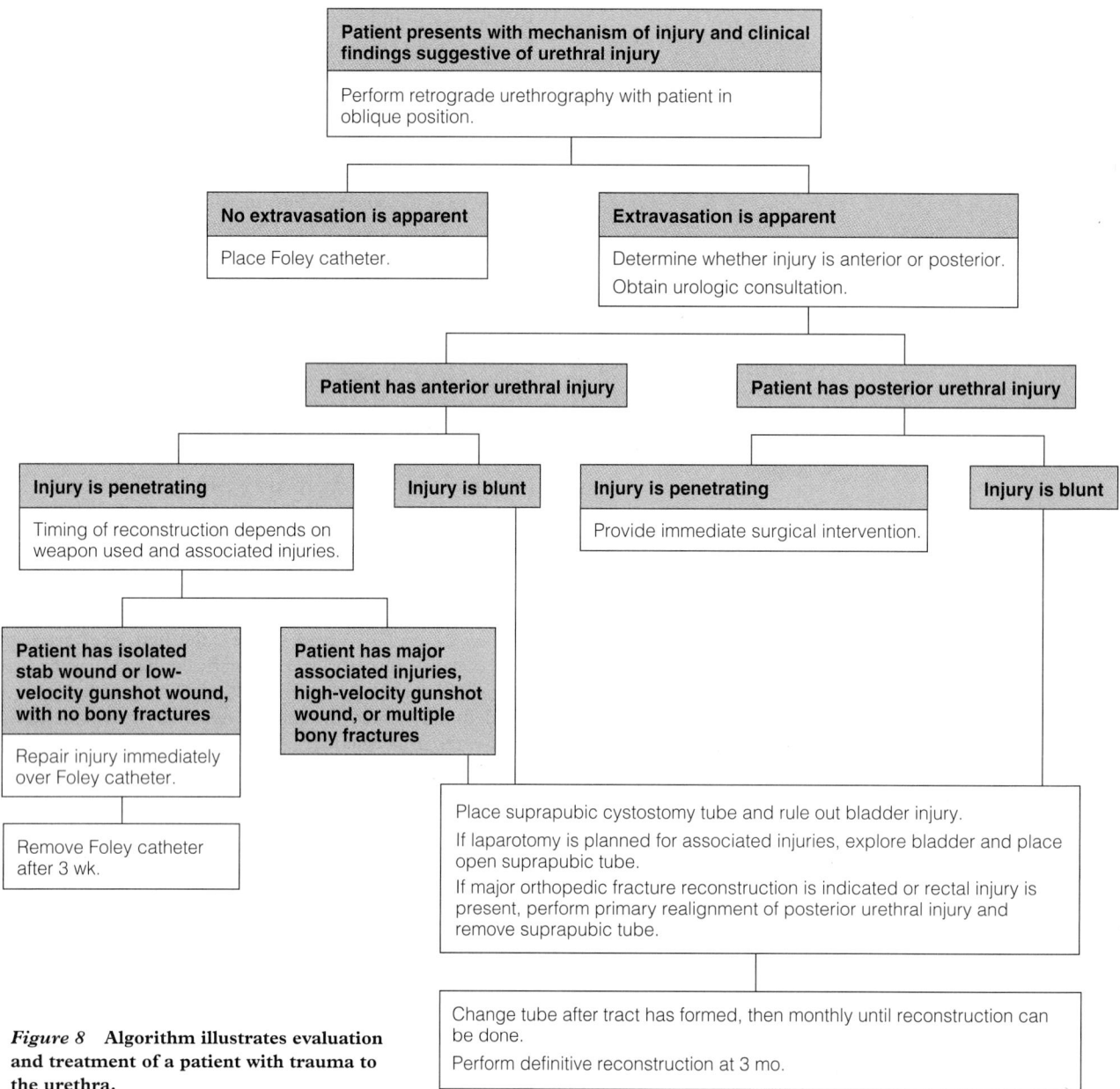

Figure 8 **Algorithm illustrates evaluation and treatment of a patient with trauma to the urethra.**

fractures, which is the most common cause of posterior urethral injury.[26] Anterior urethral (penile and bulbar urethral) injuries are commonly caused by straddle injury but may be the result of penile fracture or penetrating injuries to the genitalia. Penetrating injury to the posterior urethra often leaves the urethral continuity intact. The female urethra is rarely injured, but when it is, it is invariably associated with bladder injury and pelvic fracture.

Blood at the urethral meatus, the classic sign of injury to the male urethra, indicates that urethrography should be performed immediately. Attempts at catheter placement, which may convert incomplete injuries to complete disruptions,[26] are to be condemned in any case of suspected urethral injury. Because signs of urethral injury are variable, urethrography is the essential diagnostic test.

Retrograde urethrography can document the location and nature of urethral injury. Injection of the contrast agent may be accomplished with a Foley catheter placed in the fossa navicularis, a Brodney clamp, or a catheter tip syringe. The patient is placed in the oblique position, with the penis stretched to delineate the anterior urethra. Extravasation of the contrast agent is evidence of urethral injury. In the absence of extravasation, a Foley catheter may be passed. If a catheter has been placed but its position is unclear, contrast injection will confirm its placement in the bladder. In such cases, the catheter should be left in place until a pericatheter contrast study can document the absence of injury. In cases of pelvic fracture and penetrating posterior urethral injury, bladder injury must be excluded via suprapubic tube cystography or open bladder exploration when the suprapubic tube is placed.

OPERATIVE MANAGEMENT

Management of penetrating injuries to the urethra, which are rare, differs considerably from management of blunt trauma [*see Figure 8*]. Traumatic urethral injuries are usually managed by suprapubic cystostomy, with reconstruction delayed for 3 to 6 months. Straddle injuries to the bulbar urethra should always be managed by urinary diversion and delayed repair because the appearance of the crushed tissue makes it difficult to delineate a healthy margin. The majority of prostatomembranous urethral injuries can be managed with suprapubic cystostomy. Immediate surgical intervention is reserved for the following urethral injuries: selected penetrating anterior urethral injuries without major associated injuries; penetrating posterior urethral injuries; blunt posterior urethral rupture with associated rectal injury, bladder neck injury, or an extremely wide separation of bladder and urethra; and urethral injury associated with penile fracture.[27]

Suprapubic cystostomy allows urinary diversion until all associated injuries and bony fractures have healed. The vast majority of blunt anterior and posterior urethral injuries are managed with this approach. If laparotomy is not indicated for other injuries, the suprapubic tube may be placed percutaneously under fluoroscopic guidance. A cystogram can then be performed via the suprapubic tube to rule out associated bladder injury. A patient with urethral injury should not be allowed to void (voiding causes urinary extravasation). If open placement of the suprapubic tube is elected, the bladder can be inspected to rule out simultaneous injury, and a cystogram is not necessary.

Use of a lower abdominal incision and an intraperitoneal approach avoids the pelvic hematoma and allows an anterior vertical incision of the bladder. We lead the suprapubic tube (24 French Malecot or Foley catheter) out the superior aspect of the bladder closure and the inferior aspect of the skin wound in the midline, facilitating subsequent tube changes and reconstructive procedures. The bladder is closed in two layers [*see* Injuries to the Bladder, Operative Management, *above*]. In 3 to 6 months, a repeat cystogram and a retrograde urethrogram will delineate the residual stricture or rupture defect, which will require repair.

Suprapubic cystostomy should be used for management of penetrating injuries to the anterior urethra if they were caused by high-velocity weapons, leading to extensive tissue loss; if they are associated with serious injuries; or if bony fractures prevent use of the lithotomy position. For stab wounds or isolated low-velocity gunshot wounds, the favored approach is primary repair, which is associated with a lower stricture rate.[28]

Penile urethral injuries are approached by making a circumferential distal penile incision and degloving the penis to expose the urethra. Bulbar injuries are approached through a midline perineal incision. In each case, mobilization of the proximal and distal urethra with debridement of devitalized tissue should allow a spatulated end-to-end anastomosis. We use interrupted 6-0 monofilament absorbable suture over a 16 French Foley catheter. Additional drains are usually not necessary, and the wounds can be closed primarily because of the excellent blood supply of the perineum.

Penetrating injuries to the posterior urethra are rare. The prostate acts as a scaffold, preventing total disruption of the prostatic urethra. If contrast agent used during urethrography reaches the bladder, one can assume an incomplete injury. Endoscopic realignment and placement of a Foley catheter may be sufficient treatment of injury to the posterior urethra. A cystoscope or fluoroscopic guidance is used to place a wire into the bladder, beyond the injury, and a Foley catheter is then advanced over the wire. Positioning is confirmed by contrast instillation. After a month of catheter drainage, a voiding cystourethrogram will document healing.

In cases of prostatomembranous urethral disruption caused by blunt injury, immediate surgical intervention is required in only rare and specific instances. In cases of vascular, rectal, and bladder neck injuries or wide separation of the bladder from the urethra, some authors recommend immediate primary surgical realignment of the urethra.[27] If pelvic exploration is performed for major vascular or orthopedic repair, the urethra can be realigned, and a secondary procedure may not be required.[22] Primary realignment is preferred in such cases because the risk of hardware contamination is considerably lower with a urethral catheter than with a suprapubic cystostomy. Because of the risk of infection to the pelvic hematoma, simultaneous rectal injury should prompt evacuation of the pelvic hematoma, irrigation, placement of drains, and primary realignment of the urethra. Bladder neck injuries, which may compromise the continence mechanism of the proximal sphincter, require reconstruction in patients with posterior urethral rupture (whose external sphincter has been compromised by the injury). At the time of bladder neck repair, primary realignment should be performed. Finally,

Patient presents with evidence of gynecologic injury or sexual assault

Examine external genitalia and, by speculum, internal organs.
Notify support services if there is evidence of sexual trauma.

Patient has perineal injury

Look for associated rectal and urinary tract injuries.
Small hematomas: treat conservatively.
Large hematomas: treat with incision, drainage, and ligation of vessels.
Lacerations: treat with irrigation, debridement, and primary closure.

Patient has cervical or vaginal injury

Differentiate between simple and complex injuries.

Patient has pelvic genital organ injury

(Such injury is usually found at laparotomy rather than on examination, and there is a high incidence of associated injuries.)
Close ovarian lacerations primarily; if injury is severe, consider salpingo-oophorectomy.
Repair uterus in two layers.
If bleeding is uncontrolled or uterine artery is avulsed, consider hysterectomy.

Patient has simple vaginal or cervical lacerations

Place antibiotic-soaked vaginal pack and leave for 24 hr.
Give perioperative broad-spectrum antibiotics.
Minor lacerations: close primarily.
Major lacerations: examine via speculum with patient under anesthesia, and repair injury.
Large hematomas: evacuate and drain.

Patient has complex vaginal or perineal lacerations

Evaluate vaginal injuries with patient under anesthesia.
Perform contrast cystography and rigid proctoscopy.
Close vaginal injuries primarily.
Give I.V. antibiotics.
Consider urinary and fecal diversion.

Figure 9 **Algorithm illustrates evaluation and treatment of a female patient with trauma to reproductive organs.**

when the bladder and prostate are completely avulsed from the urethra and are pushed far up into the abdomen, early intervention makes later reconstruction more successful.

Primary realignment is accomplished through a lower midline abdominal incision. In contrast with suprapubic cystostomy, it is necessary to enter the Retzius space anterior to the bladder, thus disturbing the pelvic hematoma.[29] The bladder is opened along its anterior surface, and catheters are passed from the bladder and the urethral meatus into the pelvic hematoma. The ends of the two catheters are located in the midline anterior to the bladder neck. The two ends are brought up into the wound and attached with a suture, which allows the urethral catheter to be guided into the bladder and reestablishes alignment of the urethra. No traction is necessary, because neither mucosal approximation nor direct anastomosis is the goal. Suprapubic catheter drainage is recommended, and a perivesical drain should be used for 48 hours.[29] Either flexible cystoscopy (from the urethra and via a suprapubic approach)[30] or placement of magnetic urethral catheters[31] may be used for endoscopic realignment of membranous urethral disruption, but not all urologists in the community are familiar with these techniques.

POSTOPERATIVE CARE

The ambulatory patient who has been treated for all injuries may be discharged. In patients with a pelvic fracture, prolonged hospitalization and rehabilitation often postpone definitive care of urethral injuries. Delayed reconstruction of prostatomembranous urethral disruption requires an exaggerated lithotomy position, which may not be possible for months after long-bone or pelvic fractures.

Catheter care is of great importance after urethral reconstruction or suprapubic cystostomy. Urethral catheters should be secured to the abdominal wall in the early postoperative period. After immediate urethral repair or realignment, the Foley catheter should remain in place for 3 to 6 weeks, depending on the nature of the repair. Contrast voiding cystourethrography should be obtained at the time of catheter removal. If extravasation is present, the catheter should be replaced for 1 week and the study repeated. When a suprapubic catheter has been used in addition to a Foley catheter, radiographic studies can be performed via the suprapubic tube.

Patients managed initially with a suprapubic tube alone should have the tube changed after a tract has formed, usually in 4 weeks, and then monthly until reconstruction can be performed. Stricture formation or complete obliteration of the urethra may be the final result after initial management. Subsequent radiographic studies can indicate whether secondary endoscopic or open procedures are needed. Voiding dysfunction may occur after pelvic fracture and sacral nerve root injury.

Injuries to the Vagina, Uterus, and Ovaries

INITIAL EVALUATION

Injuries to the female genitalia [see Table 2] must be regarded as especially morbid because of their association with sexual assault as well as the potential complications of infection and bleeding. Perineal and vaginal injuries, usually the result of blunt trauma, straddle injury, and pelvic fracture, are much more common than cervical and uterine trauma [see Figure 9].[32,33] Enlargement of a reproductive organ predisposes that

organ to injury.[34] Penetrating injuries account for almost all injuries to the fallopian tubes, ovaries, and nongravid uterus.[35]

A history of sexual trauma must be sought and, if elicited, appropriate police and support services notified.[32] In addition, if sexual assault has occurred, informed consent for the rest of the patient assessment must be obtained. This assessment includes a history, physical examination, collection of evidence and laboratory specimens, and treatment, as outlined by the American College of Obstetricians and Gynecologists.[36]

All female patients with evidence of genital injury require examination of the external genitalia as well as a speculum examination of internal organs. The presence of blood implies vaginal laceration. In the presence of pelvic fracture or impalement injury, vaginal laceration warrants complete evaluation (using cystourethrography, proctoscopy, and laparotomy, as indicated) to rule out associated urinary tract and gastrointestinal injuries. Failure to identify vaginal injury associated with pelvic fracture may lead to abscess formation, sepsis, and death.

OPERATIVE MANAGEMENT

Perineal lacerations in the absence of associated urinary tract and rectal injury can be managed in the emergency department. Only large hematomas must be incised and drained, with ligation of vessels. Lacerations of the vulva may be closed primarily after irrigation and debridement. Interrupted absorbable sutures allow any accumulated fluid to drain and eliminate the need for suture removal. Drains are used if there is a large cavity; if hemostasis is suboptimal, the wound may be left open and packed.[32]

Vaginal and cervical lacerations, the result of either blunt or penetrating injury, may bleed extensively if pudendal vessels are injured.[32] If bleeding is not severe, examination and repair under local anesthesia is possible in the ED. If large lacerations are associated with bleeding and hematoma, speculum examination under anesthesia permits more complete assessment and repair of injuries. Vaginal lacerations should be closed with continuous or interrupted absorbable sutures that include mucosal and muscular layers. Antibiotic-soaked vaginal packing should be left in place for 24 hours. Perioperative administration of broad-spectrum antibiotics is sufficient, unless injuries are more complex.

Complex vaginal and perineal lacerations associated with pelvic fracture require much more aggressive management to prevent the morbidity and mortality of open fractures.[32] Evaluation of vaginal injuries under anesthesia, contrast cystography, and rigid proctoscopy are mandatory. The vaginal laceration should be closed with absorbable sutures. Even in the absence of injury to the bladder or rectum, diversion of the urinary and fecal streams should be considered to facilitate care of the wounds.[37] Extraperitoneal bladder rupture associated with vaginal lacerations requires operative repair to prevent infection of pelvic hematoma or the formation of a vesicovaginal fistula. Antibiotic therapy is more prolonged, as appropriate for open fractures.[32] Urologic, gynecologic, and orthopedic consultations are necessary for care of associated injuries.

Injury to the pelvic genital organs is rare in a nongravid patient. Penetrating trauma is the most common cause, and the majority of patients have associated injuries necessitating laparotomy.[34] Blunt injury of the nongravid uterus and pelvic organs occurs in the face of preexisting abnormalities; diagnostic peritoneal lavage demonstrates hemoperitoneum in these instances.[35] The uterus, most commonly injured, is

Table 2 AAST Organ Injury Scales for Female Reproductive Tract

Injured Structure	AAST Grade	Characteristics of Injury	AIS-90 Score
Vagina*	I	Contusion or hematoma	1
	II	Superficial laceration (mucosa only)	1
	III	Deep laceration (into fat or muscle)	2
	IV	Complex laceration (into cervix or peritoneum)	3
	V	Injury to adjacent organs (anus, rectum, urethra, bladder)	3
Vulva*	I	Contusion or hematoma	1
	II	Superficial laceration (skin only)	1
	III	Deep laceration (into fat or muscle)	2
	IV	Avulsion (skin, fat, or muscle)	3
	V	Injury to adjacent organs (anus, rectum, urethra, bladder)	3
Nongravid uterus*	I	Contusion or hematoma	2
	II	Superficial laceration (< 1 cm)	2
	III	Deep laceration (≥ 1 cm)	3
	IV	Laceration involving uterine artery	3
	V	Avulsion or devascularization	3
Fallopian tube†	I	Hematoma or contusion	2
	II	Laceration < 50% of circumference	2
	III	Laceration ≥ 50% of circumference	2
	IV	Transection	2
	V	Vascular injury or devascularized segment	2
Ovary†	I	Contusion or hematoma	1
	II	Superficial laceration (depth < 0.5 cm)	2
	III	Deep laceration (depth ≥ 0.5 cm)	3
	IV	Partial disruption of blood supply	3
	V	Avulsion or complete parenchymal destruction	3
Gravid uterus*	I	Contusion or hematoma (without placental abruption)	2
	II	Superficial laceration (< 1 cm) or partial placental abruption (< 25%)	3
	III	Deep laceration (≥ 1 cm) in second trimester or placental abruption > 25% but < 50%; deep laceration in third trimester	3; 4
	IV	Laceration involving uterine artery; deep laceration (≥ 1 cm) with > 50% placental abruption	4; 4
	V	Uterine rupture in second trimester; uterine rupture in third trimester; complete placental abruption	4; 5; 4–5

*Advance one grade for multiple injuries, up to grade III.
†Advance one grade for bilateral injuries, up to grade III.

repaired with figure-eight sutures or a two-layer closure using Vicryl or chromic catgut sutures.[34] Avulsion of the uterine artery or extensive blast destruction of the uterus may necessitate hysterectomy.[32] When hysterectomy is necessary for trauma, the vaginal cuff may be left open to allow drainage of the operative bed.[38] Lacerations to the ovary or the fallopian tube may be managed by primary closure or salpingo-oophorectomy if contralateral structures are normal.

POSTOPERATIVE CARE

Postoperative care should be dictated by the management of associated injuries. After hysterectomy or repair of vaginal lacerations, a vaginal pack should remain in place for 24 hours. Hemorrhage caused by uterine injury has been treated with oxytocin, which increases uterine tone and controls bleeding.[34] Complex lacerations of the perineum may necessitate bowel rest or colostomy to prevent soilage. Fertility after injury to the

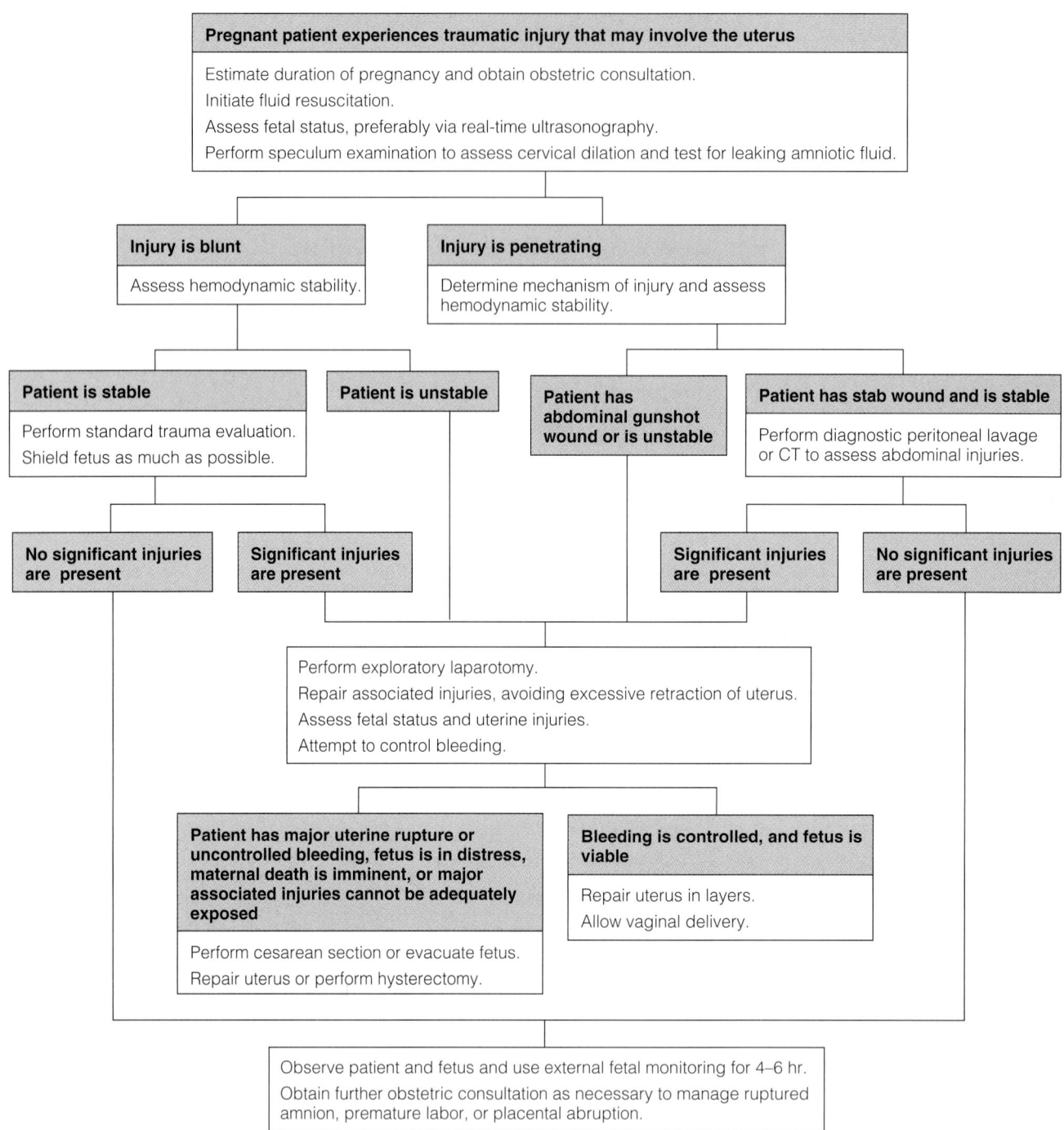

Figure 10 Algorithm illustrates evaluation and treatment of a pregnant female with blunt or penetrating injury to the uterus.

female reproductive organs is not well documented, but patients must be counseled about the possible adverse consequences of uterine and adnexal trauma.

Injuries to the Gravid Uterus

INITIAL EVALUATION

As a result of the increasing incidence of motor vehicle accidents, 6% to 7% of pregnancies are complicated by trauma.[39] Trauma is a leading cause of maternal death, but it more fre-

quently causes death of the fetus.[40-42] Although penetrating injuries are not common, those that do occur are likely to cause uterine injury [see Table 2] and fetal injury because of the size of the uterus.[43] Because of physiologic changes during pregnancy, few signs of injury may be present at initial evaluation, but fetal compromise can easily occur. Conversely, life-threatening hemorrhagic shock may occur with uterine rupture.[38] Maternal survival must remain the first priority, both in initial resuscitation and in the operating room; fetal viability and needs can be managed once the mother's condition has been stabilized.

Table 3 AAST Organ Injury Scales for Male Genitalia

Injured Structure	AAST Grade	Characteristics of Injury	AIS-90 Score
Scrotum	I	Contusion	1
	II	Laceration < 25% of scrotal diameter	1
	III	Laceration ≥ 25% of scrotal diameter	2
	IV	Avulsion < 50%	2
	V	Avulsion ≥ 50%	2
Testis*	I	Contusion or hematoma	1
	II	Subclinical laceration of tunica albuginea	1
	III	Laceration of tunica albuginea with < 50% parenchymal loss	2
	IV	Major laceration of tunica albuginea with ≥ 50% parenchymal loss	2
	V	Total testicular destruction or avulsion	2
Penis†	I	Cutaneous laceration or contusion	1
	II	Laceration of Buck's fascia (cavernosum) without tissue loss	1
	III	Cutaneous avulsion, laceration through glans or meatus, or cavernosal or urethral defect < 2 cm	3
	IV	Partial penectomy or cavernosal or urethral defect ≥ 2 cm	3
	V	Total penectomy	3

*Advance one grade for bilateral injuries, up to grade III.
†Advance one grade for multiple injuries, up to grade III.

All pregnant patients suffering traumatic injury require evaluation [see Figure 10]. Ejection from an automobile, presentation in shock, or pelvic fracture increases the likelihood of uterine injury. Estimation of the gestational age is essential for accurate examination of the gravid uterus. Physical signs outlined in the algorithm generally are not useful in determining the status of the fetus. A sterile speculum examination is necessary to evaluate dilation of the cervix and to test for the presence of amniotic fluid.[43] Resuscitation begins by placing the patient in the left lateral decubitus position to minimize obstruction of venous return by the gravid uterus. Once initial evaluation of the mother has been performed, evaluation with external fetal monitoring and real-time ultrasonography provides information on fetal distress, placental abruption, and the general state of the fetus. Most authors agree that real-time ultrasonography gives the most information about the condition of the fetus.[39,44] Kleihauer-Betke testing for fetomaternal hemorrhage has not been predictive of obstetric complications, whereas the maternal Injury Severity Score is correlated with the likelihood of fetal survival.[39,44,45]

Blunt injury and stab wounds to the gravid uterus in a hemodynamically stable female patient should be evaluated by standard methods, with the fetus being shielded as much as possible during radiographic studies but with all available modalities being used, including limited CT if indicated.[43] In the absence of significant injuries, the patient and fetus should be observed and evaluated with external fetal monitoring for at least 4 to 6 hours. In two studies, all complications developed within this time frame.[39,46] Ruptured amniotic membranes, premature labor, or placental abruption should be managed by the obstetric service.

OPERATIVE MANAGEMENT

Pregnant females who experience significant injuries should undergo laparotomy in the following instances: after a gunshot wound to the abdomen; after a defined associated injury necessitating surgery; after a blunt injury or stab wound causes hemodynamic instability; if fetal parts are palpable; and in cases of fetal distress.[43] A midline incision is always selected, and the obstetric consultant should be on hand. Repair of associated injuries can usually be performed by moving the uterus out of the way, permitting subsequent vaginal delivery. Major vascular or rectal injuries may necessitate a cesarean section to provide adequate exposure. Fetal distress or imminent maternal death necessitates an immediate cesarean section. A nonviable fetus, which must be evacuated, is best managed by induced labor at a later date; uterine salvage may be more likely, possibly maintaining reproductive function.[47]

Uterine injuries during pregnancy cause extensive bleeding, but multilayered closure with absorbable sutures should achieve hemostasis. Serious bleeding may be controlled by ligating the hypogastric arteries.[47] In the absence of fetal distress, the abdomen may be closed to allow spontaneous vaginal delivery, even in the perioperative period.[43] If the uterus cannot be salvaged because of bleeding or extensive uterine destruction, a cesarean section and hysterectomy are indicated.

POSTOPERATIVE CARE

External fetal monitoring should be offered when the estimated gestational age is greater than 20 weeks and there is no indication for cesarean section. Monitoring should continue for at least 6 hours after blunt trauma and according to the obstetric recommendations for fetal monitoring after a penetrating injury or laparotomy. $Rh_0(D)$ immune globulin (RhoGAM) should be administered within 72 hours to all Rh-negative mothers, regardless of Kleihauer-Betke test results.[39,40]

Injuries to the Scrotum

INITIAL EVALUATION

Scrotal trauma may result in testicular injury or genital skin loss [see Table 3]. Because blunt injuries to the testicle may be difficult to recognize, high-resolution ultrasonography has become a key element in the evaluation of scrotal trauma [see Figure 11]. When a straddle injury or penetrating mechanism suggests the possibility of urethral injuries, retrograde urethrography is indicated.

Penetrating scrotal injuries commonly involve not only the testis but also the corpora cavernosa, urethra, and spermatic cord. Because of the excellent blood supply of the scrotal skin, most penetrating injuries may be debrided and closed. Exceptions to this general rule include human and animal bites, which are treated with antibiotics and local wound care (or debridement in cases of severe soft tissue infection).[48]

Rupture of the testicle is often immediately painful, with rapid onset of swelling. Falls, straddle injuries, and direct blows are common mechanisms of injury.[49] However, seemingly minor degrees of trauma may be associated with delayed onset of pain, swelling, and ecchymosis; in this scenario, testicular torsion must be included in the differential diagnosis. Physical signs of rupture include scrotal swelling, tenderness, and ecchymosis. Injury to the scrotal wall or tunica vaginalis may cause significant swelling without rupture of the tunica albuginea of the testis; pelvic hematoma caused by fracture may extend down, resulting in massive scrotal swelling. For these reasons, blunt injury to the scrotum should be evaluated by ultrasonography unless findings of the physical examination are normal.

The ultrasonographic characteristics of testicular rupture include loss of normal homogeneity of the testicular parenchyma, loss of continuity of the tunica albuginea, and intraparenchymal hematoma.[50] A discrete break in the tunica is relatively rare. In cases of pelvic fracture with massive scrotal edema, ultrasonography can document the integrity of the testis and allow conservative management of the swelling. If rupture is not documented, conservative treatment with ice packs, analgesics, and elevation allows resolution of swelling.

OPERATIVE MANAGEMENT

Exploration of the scrotum through a vertical incision allows inspection of the scrotal contents and, when spermatic cord injury is discovered, extension of the incision into the groin. The goal is preservation of testicular parenchyma for endocrine and cosmetic purposes; normal sperm production and transport are not expected after repair of rupture. Clots and extruded seminiferous tubules are debrided with scissors to allow closure of the tunica albuginea over the edematous parenchyma. A continuous absorbable suture (3-0 Vicryl) is preferred to prevent palpable knots. When spermatic cord injury is detected, the first priority is determination of the viability of the testis. If this is in doubt, a small incision into the tunica albuginea should cause some bleeding; if the testis is cyanotic and does not bleed when cut, orchiectomy should be performed. If only the vas deferens or spermatic vessels are injured, the testis may

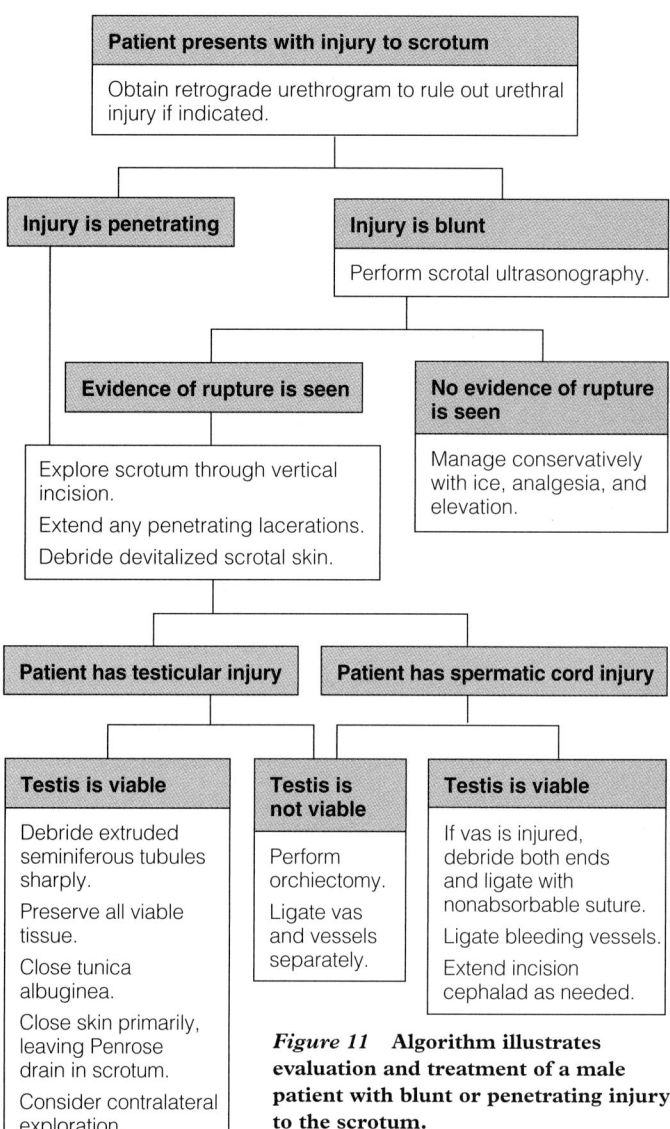

Figure 11 Algorithm illustrates evaluation and treatment of a male patient with blunt or penetrating injury to the scrotum.

remain viable. Ligation of the spermatic vessels is performed in the standard fashion; if vasal ligation is necessary, nonabsorbable suture with long tails is preferable, aiding in later identification for reconstruction if infertility ensues.

Because scrotal skin is well vascularized, it can be closed primarily in almost all instances. Exceptions arise if there is a prolonged delay between injury and definitive care or if grossly contaminated wounds are associated with rectal injuries. Hemostasis should be meticulous because the scrotum will expand massively if bleeding occurs; to prevent such complications, we recommend interrupted suture closure of the tunica dartos and skin in two layers, with a Penrose drain brought out through a separate dependent stab wound. Fluffed gauze should be used for dressing, and a scrotal supporter should be used to keep the scrotum elevated. The Penrose drain is removed on postoperative day 1. There are no major restrictions to activity after scrotal surgery, and patients can be discharged once they have recovered from associated injuries.

Scrotal skin loss caused by burns or electrical or mechanical injury usually spares the testis, which has a separate blood supply. Conservative debridement is possible if there is no infection, but the demarcation between viable and nonviable tissue should be identified before extensive debridement.[51] Management depends on the amount of skin remaining. Options include primary closure, immediate coverage with meshed split-thickness skin grafts, or placement of the testes in subcutaneous pouches in the thigh.

References

1. Bright TC, White K, Peters PC: Significance of hematuria after trauma. J Urol 120:455, 1978

2. Miller KS, McAninch JW: Radiographic assessment of renal trauma: our 15 year experience. J Urol 154:352, 1995

3. Brown SL, Hoffman DM, Spirnak JP: Limitations of routine spiral computerized tomography in the evaluation of blunt renal trauma. J Urol 160:1979, 1998

4. Bretan PN, McAninch JW, Federle MP, et al: Computerized tomographic staging of renal trauma: 85 consecutive cases. J Urol 136:561, 1986

5. Pollack HM: Renal trauma: imaging and intervention. Problems in Urology 8:199, 1994

6. McAninch JW, Carroll PR, Klosterman PW, et al: Renal reconstruction after injury. J Urol 145:932, 1991

7. Matthews LA, Smith EM, Spirnak JP: Nonoperative treatment of major blunt renal lacerations with urinary extravasation. J Urol 157:2056, 1997

8. Cheng DL, Lazan D, Stone N: Conservative management of type III renal trauma. J Trauma 36:491, 1994

9. Husmann DA, Gilling PJ, Perry MO, et al: Major renal lacerations with a devitalized fragment following blunt abdominal trauma: comparison between nonoperative (expectant) versus surgical management. J Urol 150:1774, 1993

10. Sagalowsky AI, McConnel JD, Peters PC: Renal trauma requiring surgery: an analysis of 185 cases. J Trauma 23:128, 1983

11. Morey AF, McAninch JW, Tiller BK, et al: Single shot intraoperative excretory urography for the immediate evaluation of renal trauma. J Urol 161:1088, 1999

12. McAninch JW, Carroll PC: Renal trauma: kidney preservation through improved vascular control, a refined technique. J Trauma 22:285, 1982

13. Corriere JN Jr, McAndrew JD, Benson GS: Intraoperative decision-making in renal trauma. J Trauma 31:1390, 1991

14. Uflacker R, Paolini RM, Lima S: Management of traumatic hematuria by selective renal artery embolization. J Urol 132:662, 1984

15. Presti JC, Carroll PR, McAninch JW: Ureteral and renal pelvic injuries from external trauma: diagnosis and management. J Trauma 29:370, 1989

16. Boone TB, Gilling PJ, Husmann DA: Ureteropelvic junction disruption following blunt abdominal trauma. J Urol 150:33, 1993

17. Corriere JN Jr: Ureteral injuries. Adult and Pediatric Urology, 3rd ed. Gillenwater JY, Grayhack JT, Howards SS, et al, Eds. Mosby–Year Book, St. Louis, 1991

18. Brandes SB, Chelsky MJ, Buckman RF, et al: Ureteral injuries from penetrating trauma. J Trauma 36:766, 1994

19. Medina D, Lavery R, Ross SE, et al: Ureteral trauma: preoperative studies neither predict injury nor prevent missed injuries. J Am Coll Surg 186:641, 1998

20. Corriere JN Jr, Sandler CM: Management of extraperitoneal bladder rupture. Urol Clin North Am 16:275, 1989

21. Fried FA, Rutledge R: A statewide population-based analysis of the frequency and outcome of genitourinary injury in a series of 215,220 trauma patients. J Urol 153:314A, 1995

22. Corriere JN Jr: Trauma to the lower urinary tract. Adult and Pediatric Urology, 3rd ed. Gillenwater JY, Grayhack JT, Howards SS, et al, Eds. Mosby–Year Book, St. Louis, 1991

23. Peters PC: Intraperitoneal rupture of the bladder. Urol Clin North Am 16:279, 1989

24. Cass AS: Diagnostic studies in bladder rupture: indications and techniques. Urol Clin North Am 16:267, 1989

25. Deck AJ, Shaves S, Talner L, et al: Computerized tomography cystography for the diagnosis of traumatic bladder rupture. J Urol 164:43, 2000

26. Sandler CM, Corriere JN Jr: Urethrography in the diagnosis of acute urethral injuries. Urol Clin North Am 16:283, 1989

27. Webster GD: Perineal repair of membranous urethral stricture. Urol Clin North Am 16:303, 1989

28. Husmann DA, Boone TB, Wilson WT: Management of low velocity gunshot wounds to the anterior urethra: the role of primary repair versus urinary diversion alone. J Urol 150:70, 1993

29. Devine CJ Jr, Jordan GH, Devine PC: Primary urethral realignment. Urol Clin North Am 16:291, 1989

30. Guille F, Cipolla B, Leveque S, et al: Early endoscopic realignment of complete traumatic rupture of the posterior urethra. Br J Urol 68:178, 1991

31. Porter JR, Takayama TK, Defalco AJ: Traumatic posterior urethral injury and early realignment using magnetic urethral catheters. J Urol 158:425, 1997

32. Knudson MM, Crombleholme WR: Female genital trauma and sexual assault. Abdominal Trauma. Blaisdell FW, Trunkey DD, Eds. Thieme Medical Publishers, New York, 1993, p 311

33. Mandell J, Cromie WJ, Caldamone AA: Sports-related genitourinary injuries in children. Clin Sports Med 1:483, 1982

34. Quast DC, Jordan GL: Traumatic wounds of the female reproductive organs. J Trauma 4:839, 1964

35. Maull KI, Rozycki GS, Pedigo RE: Injury to the female reproductive system. Trauma, 4th ed. Mattox KL, Moore EE, Feliciano DV, Eds. Appleton-Lange, San Mateo, California, 2000

36. ACOG educational bulletin. Sexual assault. Number 242, November 1997 (replaces No. 172, September 1992). American College of Obstetricians and Gynecologists. Int J Gynaecol Obstet 60:297, 1998

37. Niemi TA, Norton LW: Vaginal injuries in patients with pelvic fracture. J Trauma 25:547, 1985

38. Shires GT: Trauma. Principles of Surgery, 4th ed. Schwartz SI, Shires GT, Spencer FC, et al, Eds. McGraw-Hill, New York, 1984, p 199

39. Towery R, English TP, Wisner D: Evaluation of pregnant women after blunt injury. J Trauma 35:731, 1993

40. Pearlman MD, Tintinalli JE, Lorenz RP: Blunt trauma during pregnancy. N Engl J Med 323:1609, 1990

41. Fildes J, Reed L, Jones N, et al: Trauma: the leading cause of maternal death. J Trauma 32:643, 1992

42. Esposito TJ, Gens DR, Smith LG, et al: Trauma during pregnancy: a review of 79 cases. Arch Surg 126:1073, 1991

43. ACOG educational bulletin. Obstetric aspects of trauma management. Number 251, September 1998 (replaces Number 151, January 1991, and Number 161, November 1991). American College of Obstetricians and Gynecologists. Int J Gynaecol Obstet 64:87, 1999

44. Drost TF, Rosemurgy AS, Sherman HF, et al: Major trauma in pregnant women: maternal/fetal outcome. J Trauma 30:574, 1990

45. Kissinger DP, Rozycki GS, Morris JA, et al: Trauma in pregnancy: predicting pregnancy outcome. Arch Surg 126:1079, 1991

46. Pearlman MD, Tintinalli JE, Lorenz RP: A prospective controlled study of outcome after trauma during pregnancy. Am J Obstet Gynecol 162:1502, 1990

47. Baker DP: Trauma in the pregnant patient. Surg Clin North Am 62:275, 1982

48. Wolf JS, Gomez R, McAninch JW: Human bites to the penis. J Urol 147:1265, 1992

49. Gomez R: Genital injuries. Problems in Urology 8:279, 1994

50. Fournier GR, Laing FC, McAninch JW: Scrotal ultrasonography and the management of testicular trauma. Urol Clin North Am 16:377, 1989

51. McAninch JW: Management of genital skin loss. Urol Clin North Am 16:387, 1989

Acknowledgments

Figures 1, 3, 5 Susan Brust, C.M.I. Adapted from originals by P. Stempen.

Figures 2, 4, 6, 8 through 11 Marcia Kammerer.

11 INJURIES TO THE EXTREMITIES

John T. Owings, M.D., F.A.C.S., James P. Kennedy, M.D., and F. William Blaisdell, M.D., F.A.C.S.

Assessment and Management of Extremity Injuries

Trauma to the extremities falls into two basic categories, penetrating and blunt. After penetrating trauma, the primary problem is vascular or neurologic injury. After blunt traumatic injury, the most common problem is fractures and the soft tissue injuries that accompany them. Nonetheless, high-velocity missile injuries can cause complex bone and soft tissue injuries, and blunt trauma can also cause neurologic and vascular injuries.

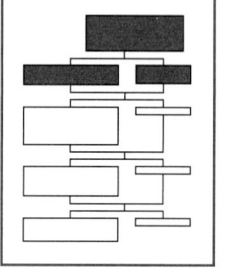

Unless active bleeding is present, injuries to the extremities are less urgent than injuries to the trunk, the head, or the neck: most extremity injuries are not immediately life-threatening and thus can be treated more deliberately. If massive hemorrhage occurs, particularly from a proximal extremity, it can usually be controlled by the application of direct pressure over the bleeding area or, if the conformation of the wound permits, by the introduction of a gloved finger for direct control of the bleeding. In either case, the patient should be directly transferred to the operating room.

Initial Assessment, Temporizing of Fracture-Dislocations, and Secondary Evaluation

Assessment of an injured extremity starts with a history, which can be obtained in parallel with the examination. Failure to elicit the patient's bleeding history at the scene from those transporting the patient may result in failure to recognize the presence of a major vascular injury. The mechanism of injury should also be ascertained.

The initial examination should first be directed toward the circulation. Blood pressure and temperature in both the injured limb and its contralateral counterpart should be determined. Distal pulses should be sought; if they are present and bounding, major vascular injury is unlikely. Injured extremities should be compared with their uninjured counterparts because pulse assessment may be difficult in the face of shock resulting from systemic or torso injuries. If the pulses in one extremity differ significantly from those in the other, vascular injury may be present.

If pulses are absent and a joint dislocation or fracture-dislocation is present, then gentle reduction of the dislocation should be carried out without delay. Frequently, a pulseless extremity with a dislocation regains pulses once the fracture or dislocation is reduced. If pulses return after reduction of the dislocation, assessment may continue on to the next priority. If pulses do not return, vascular injury is assumed, and treatment of such injury becomes the immediate priority.

The circulatory examination should be followed first by a quick neurologic examination aimed at assessing motor function in the hands and feet and ascertaining the presence or absence of sensation and later by a proximal examination of sensory and motor function. Gross deformity is pathognomonic of fracture or dislocation, and appropriate x-rays should be obtained that include portions of the joint above and below the area of suspected injury. Before x-rays are obtained, any gross deformities should be gently reduced to yield a more anatomic alignment of the extremity and splinted to relieve any possible compromise of neural or vascular structures. Finally, soft tissue defects should be noted. If considerable oozing is present, particularly in critical areas such as the hand, proximal application of a tourniquet for a few minutes may facilitate examination, permit definitive control of the bleeding point, and help determine whether significant nerve, muscle, or tendon injury has occurred.

Once the patient's condition has fully stabilized and other injuries have been evaluated, a secondary evaluation of the extremities is appropriate after blunt trauma. The shock, pain, and discomfort associated with more severe truncal injuries may mask the presence of significant extremity injuries. Passive motion of the extremity that results in localized discomfort or crepitation is a signal that x-rays are needed. In the absence of fracture or dislocation, specialized films (e.g., motion or stress studies) may be required if major ligamentous disruption is suspected. Any open wound in the extremity that is associated with a fracture is by definition an open fracture and usually must be explored surgically, ideally within 6 hours of wounding to ensure the removal of any contamination that may have resulted when the bone penetrated the skin.[1] Traumatic penetration of a joint (traumatic arthrotomy) similarly must be expeditiously addressed with prompt irrigation of the joint.

Temporary splinting is in order when definitive treatment of extensive soft tissue injuries, major strains or sprains, or fractures will be delayed. Splints applied in the emergency department must immobilize the injured extremity and prevent movement of the joint above and below the injured area: for example, with a tibial fracture, the leg should be splinted from the toes up to the proximal thigh. Temporary stabilization makes the patient more comfortable and facilitates transfer to the radiology department, the OR, or elsewhere. Immobilization of long bone fractures also helps prevent further soft tissue damage and decrease wound complications. Because most plaster splints obscure radiographic detail, they are best applied after x-rays have been taken. Cardboard splints can be used to stabilize grossly unstable fractures.

Splints vary in width and thickness according to what is appropriate for the extremity. Generally, 15 layers of plaster are applied for arm splints to prevent breakage at the elbow. This thickness is also appropriate for short leg splints; however, 20 to 25 layers may be required for long leg splints. Before being

Assessment and Management of Extremity Injuries

Patient presents with injury to extremity

Management of life-threatening injuries takes priority.

Elicit history (including bleeding history), and ascertain mechanism of injury.

Compare BP, distal pulses, and T° in injured limb and uninjured counterpart.

Check for paralysis or discomfort on motion.

Apply splints or dressing if treatment of fractures or soft tissue injuries must be delayed.

Fracture-dislocation is present, and extremity is pulseless

Reduce fracture-dislocation.

If pulses return, treat as orthopedic injury. If not, assume vascular injury.

No fracture-dislocation is present, and pulses are relatively normal

Major vascular injury is unlikely.

Signs of vascular injury are present

Pulseless extremity from blunt trauma: perform on-table arteriogram.

Pulseless extremity from penetrating trauma: explore or, if location of injury is uncertain, perform on-table arteriogram.

Extremity with pulses but at high risk for vascular injury: perform duplex Doppler evaluation or arteriogram electively.

Repair injuries identified, ideally via primary repair if ≤ 2 cm is resected. If more must be resected, use autogenous vein or a prosthetic graft.

No signs of vascular injury are present

Neurologic injury is present

Penetrating trauma: treat with early debridement and repair unless wound is heavily contaminated or was caused by a gunshot, in which case repair should be delayed.

Blunt trauma: delay repair to allow for possible return of function; these injuries are often contusions rather than lacerations.

No neurologic injuries are present

Orthopedic injuries are present

Open fractures: debride within 6–8 hr of injury, irrigate with saline, and stabilize. Begin antibiotics in ER [*see Figure 3*].

Closed fractures: stabilize.

No orthopedic injuries are present

applied, the splint should be well padded, especially at its edges and at bony prominences, to prevent abrasions, pressure sores, and burns from the exothermic reactions that occur as fiberglass or plaster hardens. Once it has been applied, the splint should be wrapped in such a way as to prevent constriction and held in place with bias-cut stockinette or a similar material.

The ankle should be placed in as close to a neutral position as possible to prevent an equinus deformity. A neutral position can be achieved with a posterior splint bent at 90° or with sugar tong splints applied to the leg medially and laterally. For long leg splints, the knee should be gently flexed. Upper extremity splints should be applied with the limb in the resting position, the wrist extended 20°, and the phalangeal joints gently flexed. An easy way to remember this position is to imagine the hand holding a glass in a drinking position.

The Robert Jones dressing is a very useful all-purpose compressive dressing that immobilizes the injured extremity, helps control swelling, and prevents circulatory compromise. First, a single layer of cast padding is applied to the skin to prevent irritation. Next, one or two layers of thick cotton batting are applied circumferentially or longitudinally and held in place with a roll of cotton bandage. Finally, a splint is applied and kept in place with an elastic bandage or stockinette.

Injuries to Blood Vessels

ARTERIES

Arterial injuries in an upper extremity are generally a less demanding problem than corresponding injuries in a lower extremity. The main reasons are, first, that upper extremity vessels have much better collateral flow and, second, that even ischemic upper extremities tend to 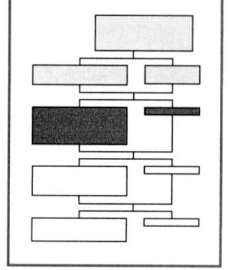 remain viable except when extensive soft tissue damage is present. Moreover, because arteries and veins are smaller in the upper extremities, life-threatening hemorrhages are less common; exceptions are injuries to the subclavian or axillary arteries, which can cause unexpected exsanguination into the chest or present as intrathoracic bleeding.

Blunt and penetrating trauma usually produce different types of injuries. Injuries from blunt trauma usually result in thrombosis of a vessel. Such injuries are primarily stretch injuries rather than transections [see Figure 1]; as the vessel stretches, the tunica intima and the tunica media are disrupted first, leaving the highly thrombogenic tunica externa to maintain temporary vessel continuity. Penetrating injuries that completely divide the vessel may be manifested by thrombosis rather than hemorrhage. If the vessel is only partially divided, however, it contracts and thus will continue to bleed. Accordingly, partial transections are far more dangerous than complete ones.

Bleeding from injured extremity vessels may be ongoing or, if the patient becomes hypotensive, may stop temporarily, only to resume when resuscitation has been initiated. The urgency with which one approaches this type of hemorrhage is governed by whether there is any ongoing limb-threatening ischemia. If limb-threatening ischemia is present, especially in conjunction with anesthesia and paralysis, the extremity is likely to be nonviable: unless vascular repair can be accomplished within 6 hours, normal function is unlikely to return. Moreover, attempts at late repair may be associated with reperfusion injury, the consequences of which also can be life-threatening. If, however, the

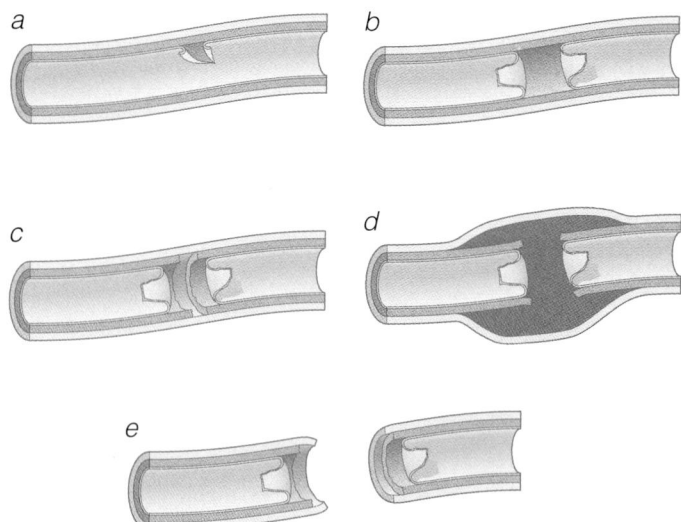

Figure 1 Shown is an avulsion injury, in which the artery is stretched, resulting either in partial (*a*) or complete (*b*) intimal disruption or in complete intimal or medial disruption (*c*), with or without pseudoaneurysm formation (*d*) and complete separation of all layers of the vessel wall (*e*).

limb is viable (as indicated by normal or modestly delayed capillary refill, normal sensation, and normal muscle function), then management of other injuries may justifiably assume priority.

Penetrating Trauma

Penetrating vascular injuries generally declare themselves readily. As a rule, the location of a presumed vascular injury can be relatively easily determined by simply noting the path of the penetrating object. If there is evidence of thrombosis or ongoing bleeding, a prompt trip to the OR and an incision placed so as to ensure proximal and distal control are appropriate. If the location of the penetrating injury is obscure or if multiple injuries may exist, angiographic or ultrasonographic evaluation may be appropriate. If the extremity is nonviable, arteriography in the OR is usually preferable to waiting for specific examination in the radiology department. Extremity arteriography in the OR can be performed by injection into the axillary artery (for upper extremity injuries) or the common femoral artery (for lower extremity injuries). Exposure of the x-ray plate immediately after injection of 15 to 20 ml of full-strength contrast material usually results in visualization of the injured area. If it does not, additional films should be obtained; these may be timed according to the progress of the contrast material as estimated from the initial x-ray.

There is considerable controversy regarding whether exploration or angiography is needed when a penetrating injury passes in proximity to a major blood vessel. If the limb appears viable, a duplex Doppler examination may be the best choice: it will identify significant injuries while causing minimal morbidity.[2,3]

Blunt Trauma

Blunt arterial injuries are more difficult to evaluate than penetrating arterial injuries. With blunt trauma, an artery may be completely disrupted, yet pulses may still be present if sufficient collateral blood flow remains. The injured extremity should be compared with its uninjured counterpart; if there are no major differences, it is unlikely that an arterial injury is present. Because the location of an arterial injury is more difficult to discern in cases of blunt trauma, duplex Doppler evaluation or angiography may be indicated when an injury is suspected. If the limb is viable, the definitive diagnostic study can be done electively. If it is not viable, intraoperative angiography should be performed in the OR. Certain injuries, by their very nature, dictate a diagnostic study of the vasculature even in the presence of normal pulses. One example is dislocations of the knee. These injuries usually cause severe stretching of the popliteal artery. Initially, the disruption may constitute only a minor intimal tear, and examination may reveal no evidence of injury [*see Figure 2*]; however, these internal tears are thrombogenic and result in delayed thrombosis many hours after the initial injury. Because lower extremities are usually splinted to stabilize the extremity, subsequent thrombosis either may not be recognized or may be recognized too late to permit salvage of the limb. Dislocation of the knee with missed popliteal thrombosis is the injury that most often results in subsequent amputation; accordingly, patients with knee dislocations (with a few exceptions) should undergo screening arteriography or duplex Doppler evaluation before any definitive orthopedic treatment of the limb.[4]

VEINS

In the absence of an associated arterial injury, most venous injuries probably go unrecognized. On the whole, the venous system has excellent collateral circulation, and major secondary hemorrhage is rare. Silent venous thrombosis may be responsible for valve damage or may set the stage for subsequent occlusive thrombosis resulting in limb swelling or thromboembolic problems. In the absence of other indications for exploration of the limb, asymptomatic venous injuries need not be repaired; howev-

er, adjusted-dose heparin should be used whenever venous injury is suspected or documented, unless contraindications exist. If there is an associated arterial injury that calls for exposure and operative treatment, the venous injury should be treated simultaneously if the repair is simple. Alternatively, clean ligation may be done; this gives rise to fewer complications than simply ignoring the injury or performing an ill-advised repair of a complex injury. With certain venous injuries, particularly those about the popliteal space or those associated with extensive soft tissue injury, the venous collateral circulation may be inadequate, in which case repair is indicated.

Injuries to Nerves

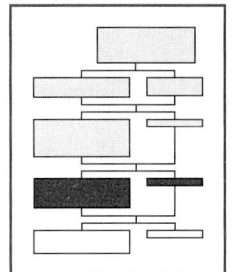

Nerve injury has always been the most challenging aspect of managing trauma to the extremities. It is the principal factor that accounts for limb loss and permanent disability.[5] Some nerve injuries, such as brachial plexus injuries and nerve root injuries, preclude repair.

Because the upper extremities have less muscle and bone mass and more neurologic structures than the lower extremities do, upper extremity injuries are twice as likely to result in nerve damage as lower extremity injuries are. Furthermore, because of the proximity of the upper extremity nerves to arteries, nerve injuries are more common in patients with upper extremity vascular injuries than in patients with lower extremity vascular injuries.

Penetrating injuries from cuts or stab wounds that result in a clean laceration of a nerve are amenable to early intervention and repair. Blunt injuries and penetrating injuries from gunshot wounds are more difficult to assess and manage. When such injuries are explored, one often finds that the nerve is not completely divided, and it is difficult to identify functional injuries—as opposed to anatomic injuries—through visual inspection. Functional loss does not preclude complete recovery without intervention. If exploration reveals complete division of a nerve, it is difficult to determine how much nerve resection may be required to ensure anastomosis of healthy tissue.

CLASSIFICATION

The most practical guide to classification of nerve injuries is that of Sunderland,[6] which comprises five degrees of nerve injury [*see Table 1*].

First-degree nerve injury results from either concussion or compression of the nerve; electrical conductivity distal to the lesion is preserved. Surgical repair is not necessary. Recovery is spontaneous and rapid, occurring within days or weeks. Because it does not depend on regeneration of any neural element, recovery is usually complete.

Second-degree nerve injury occurs when the anatomic continuity of the nerve and the Schwann sheath is preserved but the axons are interrupted and must recover by means of axonal regeneration. It is characterized by complete motor, sensory, and autonomic paralysis and progressive muscle atrophy. Surgical repair is not necessary. Recovery from secondary injuries is typically complete unless the injury is so proximal that motor end-plate and sensory receptors atrophy before the axon can grow back. The usual rate of axonal regeneration is approximately 1 mm/day or 25 mm/month.

Third-degree nerve injuries involve disruption of endoneural sheaths as well as axons. Thus, when the axons regenerate,

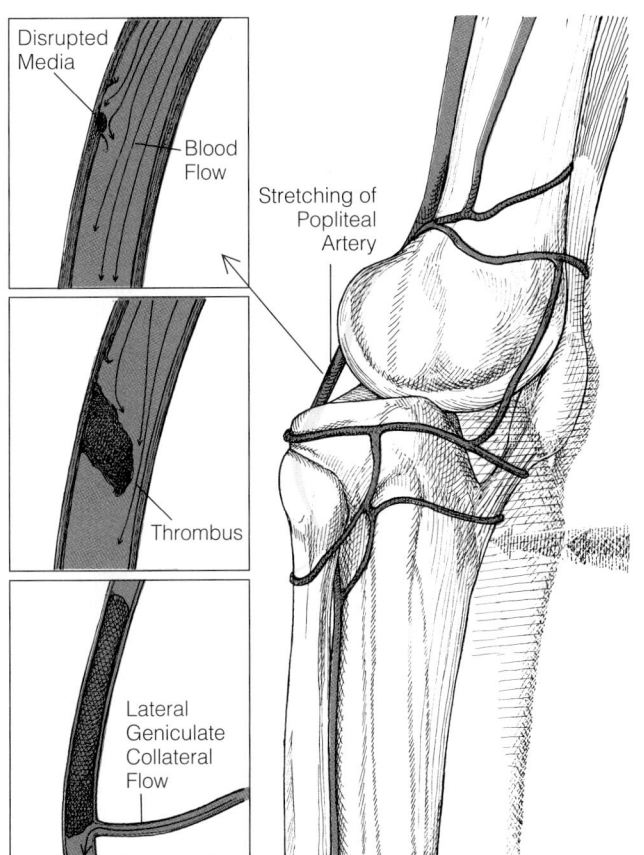

Figure 2   **Knee dislocation is a common mechanism of popliteal artery injury.**

Disrupted Media

Blood Flow

Stretching of Popliteal Artery

Thrombus

Lateral Geniculate Collateral Flow

Table 1 Sunderland's Classification
of Injuries to Nerves[6]

Degree of Injury	Anatomic Disruption
First	Conduction loss only, without anatomic disruption
Second	Axonal disruption, without loss of the neurilemmal sheath
Third	Loss of axons and nerve sheaths
Fourth	Fascicular disruption
Fifth	Nerve transection

they may enter the nerve sheaths of other axons, resulting in aberrant regeneration. The loss of the sheath leads to increased intraneural fibrosis, which makes it more difficult for the regenerating axons to penetrate the site of injury. The time needed for functional improvement depends on the distance between the injury site and the end organ.

Fourth-degree injuries involve disruption of nerve fasciculi and cause a greater degree of intraneural scarring. To regain function, axons must grow through the scar and reenter the endoneural sheaths. When fourth-degree injuries are minimal, partial resection with meticulous anastomosis of the fasciculi improves outcome.

Fifth-degree nerve injuries involve transection of the entire peripheral nerve. Invariably, there is considerable epineural and perineural hemorrhage and subsequent scarring. Recovery of neural function is impossible without surgical intervention. Fifth-degree injuries may be limited to a very short section of nerve (as with sharp transection) or may affect a very long segment (as with gunshot injury); they may also be associated with stretch injury or compartment syndrome.

How quickly and successfully the nerves regenerate depends on several factors. One such factor is age: the younger the patient, the faster and more complete the recovery. Another is the type of nerve involved: a pure motor or sensory nerve recovers better than a nerve containing both motor and sensory fibers. Thus, the radial and musculocutaneous nerves, which are primarily motor nerves, recover better than the mixed medial nerves, and the tibial division of the sciatic nerve fares better than the peroneal division. A third factor is the level of nerve injury and the duration of denervation. If regenerating axons take more than 12 months to reach denervated muscle, a significant degree of muscle atrophy will have occurred, and the muscle may remain dysfunctional despite some degree of reinnervation. Even when this is the case, it may still be possible to restore some sensation. For example, repair of a divided ulnar nerve near the axilla or the peroneal nerve above midthigh is unlikely to improve motor function; however, median nerve repair near the axilla or tibial nerve at about midthigh may allow the return of at least some protective sensation.

TREATMENT

Whenever an extremity is injured, careful assessment of motor and sensory function is essential. If other life-threatening cranial or truncal injuries are present, evaluation and treatment of nerve injuries may be deferred until these more urgent problems are dealt with. Before any orthopedic manipulation or treatment of vascular injury, an examination must be conducted to assess the integrity of the nerves.

For lacerating nerve injuries, surgical exploration is often indicated. Generally, if the wound is clean or minimally con-

taminated, the feasibility of nerve repair can be considered after the more immediate problems (e.g., vascular injuries) are corrected. If the nerve ends appear to have been sharply divided and there is minimal hemorrhage or contusion, immediate repair is appropriate; identification and approximation of nerve fasciculi are more easily accomplished before extraneural scarring obscures nerve anatomy. If, however, the penetrating object is relatively blunt (e.g., a missile), if the injury is dirty, if there is significant soft tissue damage, if associated fractures are present, or if the vascular repair is particularly tenuous, nerve repair should be delayed. In such circumstances, one should clean and debride the wound, identify the nerve ends if they are divided, and fix them in proximity so that they do not retract; the need for subsequent mobilization at the time of repair will thereby be reduced. After the wound has healed, reexploration is indicated for definitive repair about 3 to 4 weeks after the injury.

A progressing neurologic deficit is another indication for urgent surgical exploration. Such a deficit may result from a false aneurysm associated with vascular injury or from compartment syndrome attributable to hemorrhage and swelling in a fascial compartment. Emergency nerve decompression for a worsening neurologic deficit involves opening any skin, fascia, or muscle constricting the nerve. The decompressed nerve should be covered with some soft tissue, although delayed skin closure may be necessary if the fascia cannot be closed. In cases of compartment syndrome, fascial closure should not be attempted.

In all instances of blunt trauma, delayed repair (usually 2 to 3 months after the injury) is recommended. With neurapraxic lesions, this allows time for recovery, and with axonotmesis lesions, it allows time for possible axonal regrowth through the area of injury. When exploration is delayed, nerve action potential should be recorded intraoperatively to determine whether axonal regeneration has crossed the lesion in continuity. Intraoperative recording of nerve action potentials is much superior to waiting for electromyographic evidence of motor recovery, which requires an average waiting period of 6 months. If no action potentials are recorded crossing the injury, the nerve is resected proximal and distal to the injury until a normal fascicular pattern is obtained. If possible, the nerve is then primarily reapproximated, the epineurium is sutured, or cable nerve grafts are employed.

Open Fractures and Dislocations

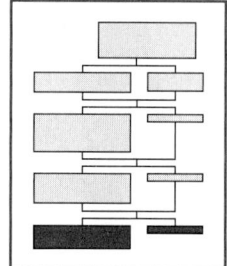

The prognosis after an open fracture is very different from that after a closed fracture; treatment of open fractures is much more complex than treatment of simple fractures or traumatic wounds. The existence of an open fracture means that a great deal of energy has been delivered to the bone to produce soft tissue disruption. Accordingly, it can be inferred that there has been considerable stripping of muscle, periosteum, and ligament from the bone, resulting in relative devascularization, and that varying degrees of contusion, crushing, and devascularization of the associated soft tissues have occurred. All of these events greatly influence the rate of healing, the incidence of nonunion, and the risk of infection.

The basic principles of management for open fractures are aggressive debridement, open wound treatment, soft tissue and bone stabilization, and systemic administration of antibiotics. These principles have reduced the formerly high mortality associated with open fractures to very acceptable levels.

A simple classification for open fractures exists that is well accepted[7] [*see Table 2*]. High-velocity gunshot wounds and open fractures must be approached somewhat differently from closed fractures because of the force imparted to the soft tissues. A fracture that looks like a grade I injury because of a small skin wound may behave as a grade III injury because of soft tissue injury. Any open fracture associated with bone loss is treated as a grade III injury, as is any grade I or grade II soft tissue wound that is associated with severe tissue contusion and periosteal stripping. In addition, any fracture associated with gross contamination (e.g., a farmyard injury with vegetable matter or soil within the wound) is treated as a grade III injury because of the risk of clostridial infection and clostridial myonecrosis.

EVALUATION

The injured extremity should undergo orthopedic examination, with particular attention paid to evaluation of neural and vascular status. Compartment syndrome [*see Compartment Syndrome, below*] should be ruled out in patients at risk; as many as 10% of open tibial fractures are associated with this syndrome as a result of severe soft tissue injury.

The patient's medical condition before the injury, the time elapsed since the injury, the mechanism of injury, and the presence or absence of associated injuries should be noted. If foreign material that is easily removable can be seen, it should be removed promptly, and a quick saline dump (i.e., pouring 1 to 2 L of saline into the wound to help wash out gross contamination and prevent tissue desiccation) is indicated. If the limb is malaligned, gentle gross reduction should be done to relieve any vascular compromise. A sterile dressing moistened with saline or povidone-iodine should then be applied to the wound, and a few minutes should be spent on securing the wound. Ideally, once the wound is assessed and the dressing applied, the dressing should not be removed until the patient is in the OR and preparation for operation is initiated. Once a secure dressing has been applied, a temporary splint should be applied to the limb so that the patient can be transported for x-rays if necessary. Cardboard splints are convenient, inexpensive, and disposable and do not interfere with x-rays.

TREATMENT

When a severe open extremity fracture is accompanied by vascular or neurologic injury, the limb may not be salvageable; such an injury may be essentially a traumatic amputation in which the parts remain connected by a bridge of skin. Although some severely injured limbs can be salvaged, those with both neurologic and vascular injury have a high complication rate and a late amputation rate of 78%. Often, the best treatment in such cases is immediate amputation.

Every open fracture calls for emergency surgical treatment [*see Figure 3*]. Ideally, treatment should begin within 6 hours of injury: the incidence of infection is directly related to delay in initiating treatment. The factors most helpful in reducing infection (the most severe preventable complication) are antibiotic therapy, timely and aggressive surgical debridement, fracture stabilization, and proper treatment of wounds. Tetanus prophylaxis should be given as needed. Cultures should be obtained in the course of debridement because the results may influence subsequent antibiotic therapy. Patients with grade I or grade II injuries should receive cefazolin in a dosage of 1 g every 4 hours while in the OR and 1 g every 8 hours afterward. Patients with grade III fractures

Table 2 Gradation of Open Fractures[7]

Grade	Wound Size	Extent of Soft Tissue Damage
I	< 1 cm	No or minimal tissue damage
II	> 1 cm	Moderate tissue damage
III	Any size	Major tissue damage; soft tissue loss; bone loss; gross contamination
IIIa		Bone can be covered
IIIb		Bone cannot be covered
IIIc		Vascular injury

or grossly contaminated grade I or II fractures should receive penicillin and gentamicin as well.

WOUND CARE

For all open fractures, irrigation and debridement in the sterile, controlled environment of the OR are required [*see Figure 3*]. Even apparently minor injures, such as minimal grade I injuries, benefit from thorough examination. The traumatic wound should be extended in such a way as to be compatible with any fracture fixation that may be necessary, and all devitalized or contused soft tissue should be aggressively debrided back to normal, clean, bleeding tissue. It may be a good idea to have a tourniquet in place, but it should be inflated only long enough to control acute hemorrhage; prolonged inflation leads to further tissue ischemia and eliminates muscle contractility, the best indication of muscle viability. If uncontrollable bleeding is encountered, the tourniquet may be inflated for a few minutes until the bleeding point is located and secured. The fracture ends should be delivered into the wound to facilitate inspection and allow adequate irrigation. Any devitalized, stripped, loose bone fragments that are not crucial to reduction or stabilization should be removed, devascularized bone should be debrided, and bleeding fragments should be carefully handled so as to maintain their attachments to the bone and preserve their vascularity.

A pulsatile lavage system should then be used to irrigate the wound and the bone ends with 8 to 10 L of normal saline. At this point, tissue specimens should be obtained and sent for culture. Irrigation is completed by adding another 2 L of fluid containing 100,000 units of bacitracin. Any surgically created wound extensions may then be closed; however, the traumatic wound itself should be left widely open. If the wound is small, a portion of the surgical extension should be left open to allow adequate drainage and to prevent the traumatic wound from sealing off prematurely. Every attempt should be made to cover bone, joint surfaces, implants, and sensitive structures (e.g., tendons, nerves, and blood vessels) with available local soft tissue, but this must be done without tension. Some surgeons are currently investigating wound coverage with primary closure of the primary wound itself. The value of this approach is controversial; however, the need for early and aggressive management of all open fractures is not.[8]

After the initial debridement, the antibiotic regimen is continued for 24 to 48 hours. At this point, if the postdebridement cultures are positive, the regimen is changed to include agents that are appropriate for the infecting organism. If the cultures are negative, the antibiotic regimen may be stopped if the wound appears clean. Any patient who has a grade III fracture or a grade I or II fracture with a positive culture should be returned to the OR every 48 hours for repeat irrigation and debridement until the wound appears healthy and clean. Each

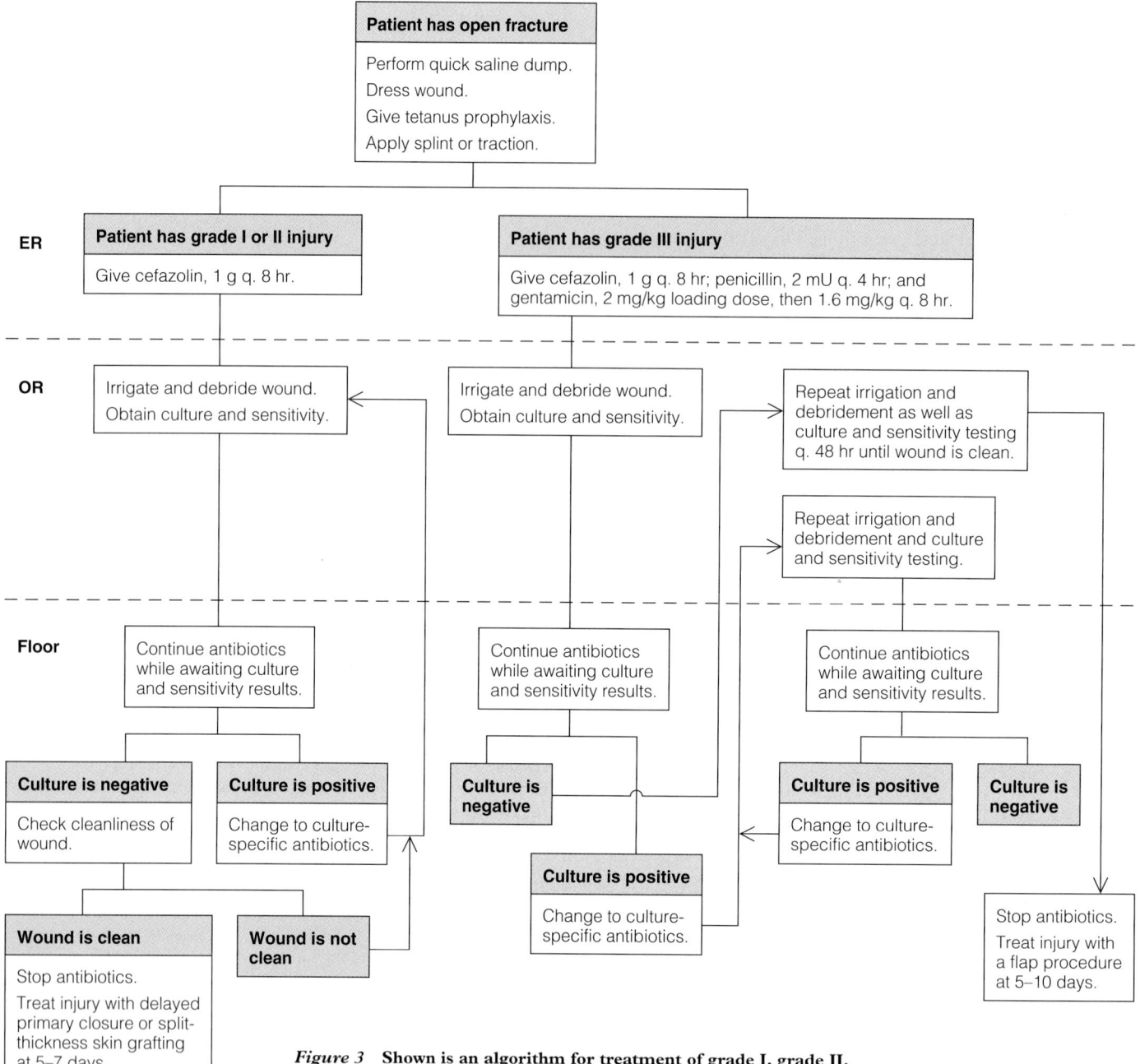

Figure 3 Shown is an algorithm for treatment of grade I, grade II, and grade III open fractures.[7]

time the patient is returned to the OR, new tissue cultures are taken and antibiotics restarted. If the bacterial counts on quantitative culture are higher than 10,000/g tissue, wound infection is probable; lower counts tend to reflect colonization rather than infection. In the case of a grade I or II injury in which the initial culture is negative, the wound may be allowed to close by granulation and secondary intention, or the patient may be returned to the OR in 5 to 7 days for delayed primary closure. For larger wounds, split-thickness skin grafts are often required. For grade III wounds, some type of flap is often required for soft tissue coverage. The flap procedure should be done early, 5 to 10 days after the injury, provided that tissue cultures are negative at this time.

The same protocol used for open fractures is also followed for open dislocations; in addition, the articular surfaces must be kept moist. Cartilage that has been damaged by the force of impact may not be able to tolerate any further insult. Once the

dislocation has been reduced with the patient under anesthesia, the joint should be thoroughly irrigated and debrided as required. The capsule of the reduced joint is closed over a suction drain, and the remaining traumatic wound is left open. In patients who have large grade III injuries associated with soft tissue loss, coverage for the articular surface may not be available, and immediate reconstruction with local or distal flaps may have to be done to keep articular cartilage viable. In these instances, only the joint cartilage should be covered; the remaining portion of the wound must be left open.

FRACTURE STABILIZATION

Operative fixation of open fractures is an extremely complex issue. Many options are open to the orthopedist, and these options change yearly. For open intra-articular fractures, internal fixation is indicated for better healing of cartilage. This is accomplished via anatomic reduction and lag screw fixation, which allow early performance of range-of-motion exercises to minimize permanent loss of range of motion. In addition, any open fractures that are associated with massively traumatized limbs, that occur in patients with multiple injuries to multiple systems, or that are associated with vascular injury should be managed with internal fixation if at all possible.

Generally, it is desirable to stabilize the open fracture during the initial operative procedure. Restoring the anatomy through reduction and stabilization improves circulation; promotes healing of bone and soft tissue; reduces inflammation, bleeding, and dead space; and increases revascularization of devitalized tissue. It also results in earlier mobilization of multiply injured trauma patients and improves their overall status.

Isolated grade I open fractures that are treated promptly can usually be handled with the same techniques as their closed counterparts, with the exception of open tibial fractures. Grade II injuries that occur in ideal circumstances in certain favorable areas (e.g., metaphyseal bone in the forearm and the foot, the humerus, and the femur) can also be treated with the same internal fixation techniques used for closed fractures. Early internal fixation is the optimal method of stabilization for intra-articular fractures.

In other situations, such as those involving open tibial fractures and grade III fractures, the safer approach is conservative treatment with either modified internal fixation techniques or immobilization with external fixators.

Closed Fractures

Of the closed fractures, it is those of the lower extremities with which the trauma surgeon should be most concerned: the prognosis for closed upper extremity fractures is excellent, and these fractures are much less likely to have life-threatening complications than fractures of the lower extremities.

UPPER EXTREMITY FRACTURES

On the whole, fractures of the scapula and the clavicle are relatively benign: they usually heal well, and they typically respond to both conservative and open treatment. Fractures of the neck of the humerus, the shaft, or the condyles (particularly the last) may be associated with vascular complications and may call for immediate fixation. Fractures of the forearm, the wrist, and the hand generally respond to conservative measures and have little or no impact on outcome.

LOWER EXTREMITY FRACTURES

The closed fractures that are of greatest concern for the trauma surgeon and that have the greatest potential effect on outcome are fractures of the femur that involve the acetabulum (with or without hip dislocation), standard hip fractures, and fractures of the shaft of the femur. Other, somewhat less worrisome closed fractures of the lower extremities are fractures that involve the tibial plateau in the knee, fractures that involve the tibia or the fibula, and pilon fractures. Fractures and dislocations of the ankle and the foot, though having the potential to affect long-term morbidity when the ankle joint is involved, generally are not of concern in the immediate overall management of the trauma victim.

Acetabular Fracture and Hip Dislocation

Fractures of the acetabulum and hip dislocations have a common mechanism: they are usually the result of accidents in which a blow is directed down the axis of the femur with the hip and the knee flexed. The telltale sign of soft tissue injury to the knee in an auto accident victim suggests the possibility of hip injury as well. The converse is also true, in that as many as 25% of auto accident victims with posterior hip dislocation also have significant knee injuries. Dislocated hips constitute a pressing orthopedic emergency. Treatment consists of immediate reduction with the patient under general anesthesia to release neurologic compression, restore joint congruency, and reduce any compromise of the femoral head vasculature that may result in aseptic necrosis. This is one situation in which the orthopedist always takes priority over the general surgeon except in the case of impending cardiac arrest. It takes only a few minutes after the induction of anesthesia for the dislocation to be reduced, at which point the case can be turned back over to the general surgeon for definitive treatment of life-threatening emergencies.

Acetabular fractures are of two types. The first type is a fracture associated with hip dislocation; there may be associated cartilage compression with ensuing damage to the joint. The second type results from direct application of force against the pelvis; essentially, it is a pelvic fracture that happens to be intra-articular. The goals of treatment are to obtain anatomic reduction of the articular surfaces and a concentric stable hip joint, to remove intra-articular loose bodies, and to achieve early motion so as to optimize cartilaginous healing. In assessing an acetabular fracture, the most important step is the neurovascular examination, which determines whether any nerve injury has occurred. It is not uncommon to find the nerve entrapped within the sharp edges of a fracture or draped over a displaced fracture under great tension. If a nerve palsy is observed, rapid reduction and stabilization of the fracture are indicated to improve the chances of neurologic recovery. Unless there is an associated hip dislocation, no deformity is noted on examination, but the patient usually complains of deep-seated hip or groin pain. A routine pelvic film usually documents the presence of a fracture; oblique views and computed tomographic scanning permit further localization of the fragments (if necessary) and help determine whether the joint is congruent and the fracture stable.

Although some acetabular fractures (in particular, small chip fractures that have no significant articular component) can be treated with benign neglect, open fixation is usually required if the fracture is displaced or involves the weight-bearing dome of the acetabulum. Fixation may also be necessary for fractures that do not involve the weight-bearing dome if stability is required to prevent recurrent dislocation of the hip. Usually, if an acetabular fracture in a multiply injured patient is displaced severely enough to require internal fixation, intra-articular debris and other indications for open treatment are present. In most situations involving multiple injuries, the best time to fix acetabular injuries is at presentation: at no subsequent point in the early postinjury period will the patient's condition be more favorable and operative fixation easier. If the patient's condition is too unstable to allow immediate fixation, the injury should be treated operatively within 5 to 7 days, before fibrosis and healing begin; once healing has started, mobilization and reduction of the fragments are more difficult. With unstable, displaced fractures, a tibial or femoral traction pin should be inserted if the patient cannot be operated on at presentation or must be stabilized medically before being transferred to a facility that is equipped for operative management of such injuries. In many instances, good reduction can be obtained by using 10 to 15 kg of skeletal traction.

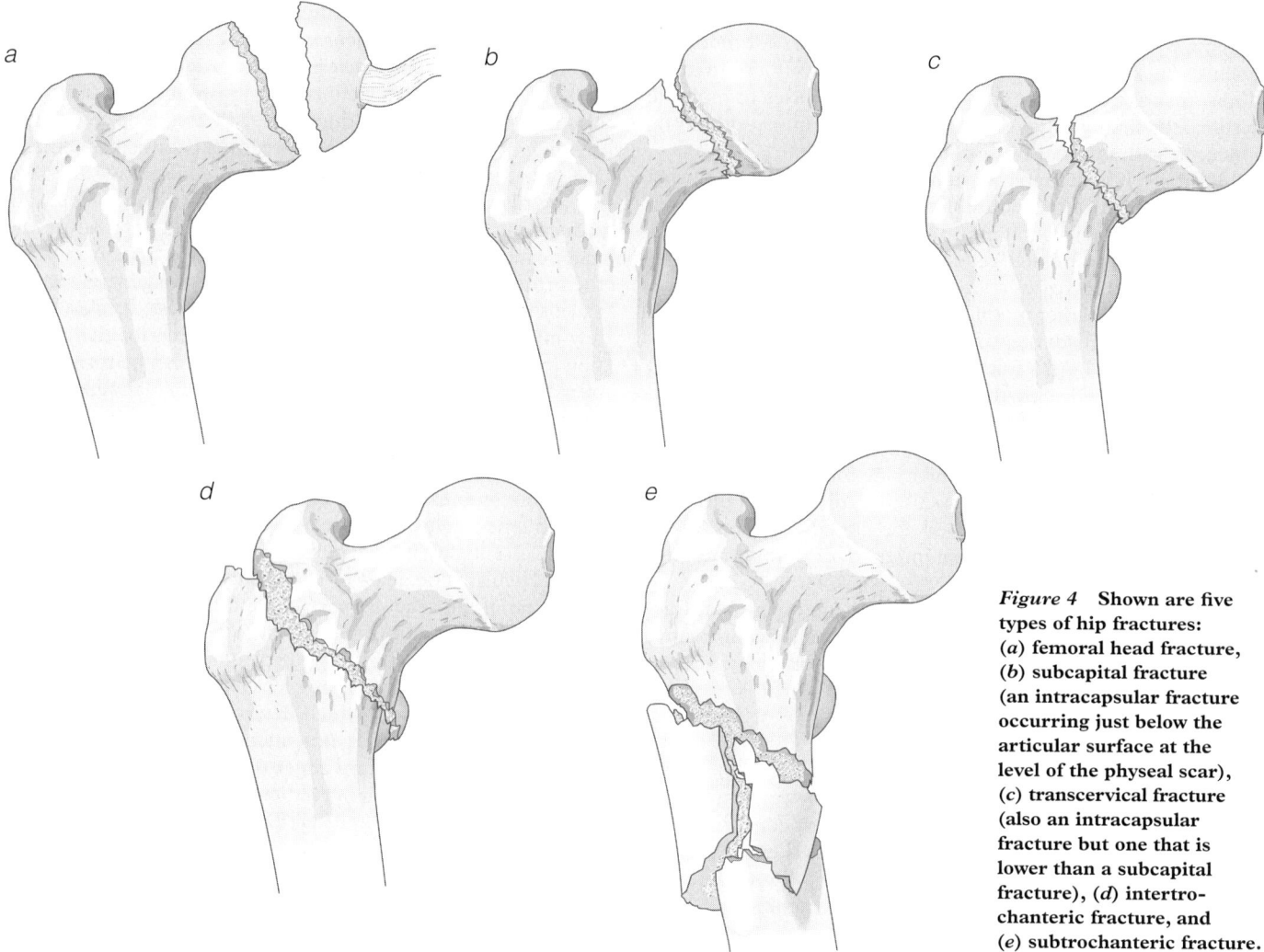

Figure 4 Shown are five types of hip fractures: (*a*) femoral head fracture, (*b*) subcapital fracture (an intracapsular fracture occurring just below the articular surface at the level of the physeal scar), (*c*) transcervical fracture (also an intracapsular fracture but one that is lower than a subcapital fracture), (*d*) intertrochanteric fracture, and (*e*) subtrochanteric fracture.

As soon as the patient's level of discomfort has decreased sufficiently, gentle range-of-motion exercise should be started to help mold the cartilage and facilitate its healing. If the patient cannot cooperate with these efforts because of other injuries, continuous passive motion exercise can be started by using a mechanical device with an electric motor.

Hip Fracture

Fracture of the hip is one of the most common conditions seen by orthopedists. A substantial force is required to fracture a hip in a young, healthy accident victim, whereas a minor trauma or fall may be sufficient to do so in an elderly osteoporotic female. Hip fractures may be classified according to their anatomic site: (1) femoral head fractures, (2) intracapsular fractures (including subcapital and transcervical femoral neck fractures), (3) intertrochanteric fractures, and (4) subtrochanteric fractures [*see Figure 4*]. Treatment differs slightly from one type to the next; the primary influence on the choice of treatment is whether the all-important blood supply to the femoral head is preserved or disrupted. With intracapsular fractures, there is a significant risk of disrupting the tenuous blood supply to the joint involved. Such disruption leads to nonunion or avascular necrosis, which can be compounded in the hip by collapse of the femoral head.

Fractures of the femoral head are the most devastating of hip injuries and must be handled as surgical emergencies.[9]

Once a femoral head fracture is recognized, it must be treated operatively within 24 hours of the injury to achieve optimal results. Closed treatment of such injuries yields uniformly poor results. Although operative treatment is usually necessary to provide the best chance of recovery, the initial trauma often is so great as to preclude good results; at best, good results can be obtained in only 50% of cases.[9]

Impaction fractures of the femoral head, however, may be treated in closed fashion with early range-of-motion exercise, particularly if they do not involve a major weight-bearing surface. Internal fixation of these injuries is technically very difficult. Small fracture fragments in the non–weight-bearing inferior portion of the head are probably best excised; large fragments or those involving a significant portion of the weight-bearing dome are best treated with operative fixation. At present, no one form of treatment yields consistently good results. In some patients, particularly physiologically older patients with significant fractures, it may be best to insert a hip prosthesis primarily.

Intracapsular femoral neck fractures carry a high risk of nonunion and avascular necrosis and should be treated on an emergency basis with operative fixation within 12 hours of injury. Even with early optimal surgical treatment, the incidence of avascular necrosis is 20%; if near-anatomic reduction is not obtained, the incidence approaches 50%.[10] The deformity associated with these fractures is not as great as that associated with extracapsular or intertrochanteric fractures. A typical patient with an intracapsular fracture presents with a shortened, externally rotated, and abducted lower extremity. Traction reduces the pain and, more importantly, may allow increased blood flow across the neck by decreasing the external rotation and thus relieving vascular occlusion resulting from compression of a tight, twisted capsule. Treatment consists of early anatomic reduction with fixation to eliminate the risk of displacement and permit rapid mobilization. Closed reduction of displaced fractures should be attempted with the patient under general anesthesia, and it must be gentle to prevent further vascular damage. If closed reduction does not achieve acceptable anatomic results, open reduction is required, with care taken to minimize soft tissue stripping and preserve the blood vessels encountered in the approach. Once anatomic reduction has been accomplished, internal fixation with any of the several types of fixation devices available (e.g., sliding hip screw devices, blade plates, and multiple pins or screws) is indicated. When the patient is physiologically older than 70 years, a primary hip prosthesis is often indicated instead of internal fixation.

Intertrochanteric and subtrochanteric fractures do not threaten the blood supply to the femoral head, because they occur below the extracapsular ring of vessels. As a rule, operative fixation within 24 hours of injury yields optimal results, permitting rapid mobilization and preventing systemic complications as well. A typical patient with an intertrochanteric femoral neck fracture presents with a limb that appears to be markedly shortened and externally rotated. Traction should be used if a delay of more than 12 hours is expected before operation. Almost all patients with these fractures are candidates for internal fixation; the exception is an elderly patient who had significant arthritis of the hip before the fracture, in whom a hip prosthesis may be the best choice. A sliding hip screw

device is most commonly used for fixation [see Figure 5]. Operative fixation of subtrochanteric fractures, which are located between the lesser trochanter and a point 5 cm distally, can be more difficult because high bending forces in the region (resulting from the angular shape of the proximal femur) often lead to implant failure before union. Possible management approaches include cross-locking, intramedullary nailing, and the use of plates and screws.

Femoral Shaft Fracture

Fractures of the femoral shaft, like intertrochanteric femoral neck fractures, are associated with significant blood loss. Because of the shape of the thigh, more than 1 L may be lost into this space with little or no external indication. Accordingly, the trauma surgeon must anticipate the blood loss from the fractured femur when formulating the initial management strategy.

The advent of intramedullary nailing has revolutionized the treatment of femoral shaft fractures. With stable femoral shaft fractures that undergo nailing, full weight bearing without crutches is possible within a few days of the operation. Reapproximation of the fracture fragments with nailing also dramatically reduces bleeding into the thigh. Femoral shaft fractures are often associated with injuries to knee ligaments, which are difficult to assess in the presence of the femoral fracture. It is important that, when the patient is under anesthesia for treatment of the fracture, the stability of the knee be assessed as well.

Neurovascular injuries are relatively uncommon with femoral shaft fractures; however, when the fracture is in the distal third of the femur, there is the possibility of injury to either the superficial femoral artery or the popliteal artery as a consequence of the tethering of these vessels against the shaft at the level of the adductor canal [see Figure 6]. The most popular method of immobilizing a femoral fracture for transport is the use of a Hare or Thomas splint. These convenient devices consist of a frame buttressed against the ischial tuberosity, along with a nonwound endstrap about the foot for traction. They effectively immobilize the extremity and lessen patient discomfort, and they need not be removed for x-rays to be taken. These splints do, however, exert some pressure on the foot; therefore, the patient should be placed in skeletal traction to maintain the benefits if immediate operation is not feasible. The skeletal traction pin should be placed in the tibia so that the femur is not contaminated by the pin wound. Its placement in the tibia should be distal to the anterior tubercle so that the entire thigh, including the knee joint, can be prepared for operation without the pin site being included.

Very few tenets in orthopedics are held with such absolute conviction as the tenet that femoral fractures are best treated with intramedullary nailing. Nailing lowers the incidence of respiratory distress syndrome, blood loss, and tissue trauma and reduces the patient's need for narcotics. In a multiply injured patient with a fractured femur, nailing should be done immediately to help control hemorrhage to the fracture site and help stabilize the patient hemodynamically. In one study,[11] multiply injured patients with an injury severity score of 18 or higher who underwent nailing more than 48 hours after the injury had a four times greater incidence of pulmonary complications than a similar group of patients who underwent nailing within 24 hours of injury; in addition, they had a longer average stay in the ICU (7.6 days as opposed to 2.8 days). In a patient who does not have multiple injuries, the timing is not crucial, but nailing is

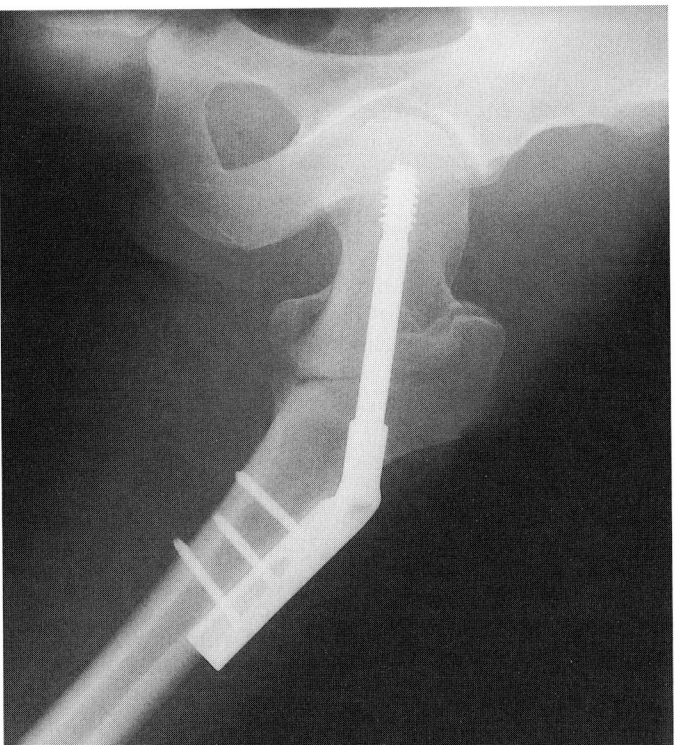

Figure 5 Hip x-ray shows an intertrochanteric fracture stabilized with a sliding hip screw device.

easier to perform if it is done within the first 6 to 12 hours, because after this period, hemorrhage and swelling make reduction more difficult. Although virtually all open femoral fractures are best treated with intramedullary nailing, a plate or an external fixator may be indicated as well in isolated instances.

Femoral fractures were once associated with significant morbidity and mortality but now are among the musculoskeletal injuries with the most predictable results after treatment. Most complications are secondary to technical problems at the time of nailing and therefore can be prevented by paying attention to the technical details.

Fracture and Dislocation of the Knee and the Patella

Knee injuries are common in multiply injured patients, partly because of the vulnerability of this joint to dashboard injuries in motor vehicle accidents and to direct trauma in motorcycle accidents.

Intra-articular knee fracture Fractures about the knee that affect the tibial or femoral condyles are as much an injury to the articular surface of the knee joint as they are a fracture of the periarticular bone. Consequently, even if successful bony union has been achieved, the issues of joint alignment, stability, stiffness, and posttraumatic arthritis must still be taken into account to ensure that the clinical result is not compromised. Knee fractures are characterized by local pain, swelling, and crepitation. A hemarthrosis forms when an intra-articular fracture is present. Such a fracture may be suspected when marrow fat globules are present in the hemarthrosis. With any injury about the knee, ligamentous stressing should not be performed until after x-rays confirm that no fracture is present. If the x-rays show a femoral supracondylar or tibial plateau fracture, x-rays of the entire length of the fractured bone should be obtained to rule out the presence of other fractures.

Unstable intra-articular knee fractures should be treated by means of anatomic reduction, rigid fixation, and early motion. Aspiration of a tense hemarthrosis is sometimes required to decompress the joint and relieve pain. The best results are achieved by means of immediate stabilization through rigid internal fixation; however, if treatment must be delayed for a few days after the injury, acceptable results usually can still be achieved. If delayed fixation is to be done, the extremity should be splinted or placed in balanced traction. Femoral condylar fractures, even when they initially are not displaced, should be treated with rigid fixation to minimize the risk of subsequent displacement from muscle forces or knee motion. Rigid fixation allows early motion to facilitate cartilage healing. Unstable or displaced tibial plateau fractures likewise should be treated with rigid fixation and early motion. Tibial plateau compression fractures are the result of an axial load and are displaced by definition. For active individuals, anatomic reduction and fixation allow early motion and yield the best long-term results. Often, bone grafting is required to maintain elevation of the articular surface.

After rigid stabilization of these fractures, the ligamentous structures about the knee should be evaluated via examination or stress films as warranted: as many as 25% of plateau fractures are associated with ligamentous injuries.[12] Late knee instability may compromise treatment of tibial plateau fractures and is a major cause of unacceptable results.

Patellar fracture The most common injury to the patella in trauma patients is a stellate comminuted fracture result-

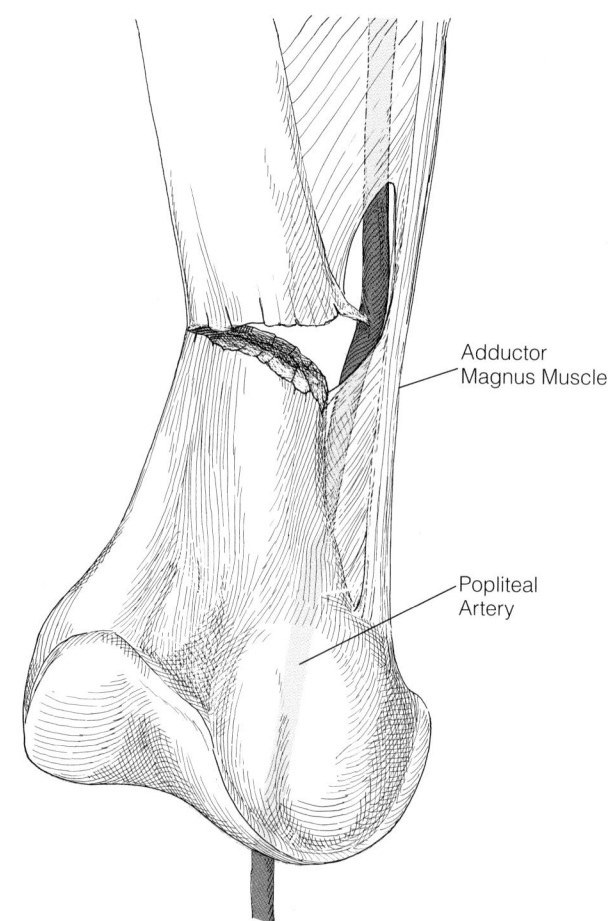

Figure 6 **Vascular injuries resulting from blunt trauma to an extremity are usually associated with fracture. Illustrated here is the mechanism of arterial injury in femoral fracture.**

Adductor Magnus Muscle

Popliteal Artery

ing from a direct blow; the second most common is an avulsion fracture that is a rupture of the extensor mechanism. A patient with a fractured patella exhibits soft tissue swelling about the knee as well as hemarthrosis, which may be tense. Patellar fractures are commonly associated with laceration over the patella; when this is the case, a traumatic arthrotomy must be ruled out. Other injuries, such as cruciate ligament failure and femoral fracture, may be present as well. The most important task in the examination is to make sure that the extensor mechanism is intact. Stellate fractures usually are not associated with extensor ruptures, and the extensor retinaculum keeps many of these fractures from displacing. Avulsion fractures, on the other hand, are associated with tears of the extensor tendon; the patient cannot extend the knee without a lag or perform a straight leg raise against gravity. It may be necessary to infiltrate the joint with local anesthesia so that the patient can attempt the maneuver.

For tensile avulsion fractures, exploration and repair of the fracture are appropriate. Nondisplaced fractures may be treated with a knee immobilizer or a cylindrical cast. Stellate direct blow fractures may be treated initially with simpler immobilization and later with protected motion until the fracture is healed. If the fragments for the joint surface are offset by more than 1 mm, anatomic reduction of the joint surface is necessary to prevent posttraumatic arthritis. Severely comminuted patellar fractures may be irreparable; in such instances, a partial or total patellectomy may be required.

Tibial Fracture, Fibular Fracture, and Pilon Fracture

Tibial fracture Fractures of the tibia are among the most difficult fractures that orthopedic surgeons are called on to treat. The subcutaneous location of the tibia offers little protection from direct violence, and high-energy fractures are associated with an increased healing time in 50% of cases.[13] Tibial fractures are often fraught with complications, such as compartment syndrome, nonunion, delayed union, malunion, and infection. In their severest manifestations, they often end in amputation.

Tibial shaft fracture is the most common shaft fracture affecting the long bones. Minor fractures take 10 to 16 weeks to heal, with a 2% delayed union rate, and severe fractures take an average of 23 weeks to heal, with a 60% delayed union rate. The reason for the slow healing is that the blood supply to the tibia is notoriously poor; furthermore, because most of the bone is located subcutaneously, a good soft tissue envelope is present only posteriorly and, to a lesser extent, laterally, which means that relatively few areas are available where blood vessels can enter the tibia through muscular attachments. Tibial shaft fractures are easily diagnosed clinically in the emergency room. Whenever such an injury is present, the patient's calf should be palpated for evidence of firmness, which would suggest a possible compartment syndrome. The patient's neurovascular status should then be assessed. If the fracture is grossly angulated or malaligned, gentle restoration of axial alignment helps relieve vascular kinking and compromise. The extremity should be splinted and then x-rayed for full assessment of the fracture. After the x-rays, the tibia should be temporarily stabilized by means of a Robert Jones dressing and a splint or by means of skeletal traction through a calcaneal pin.

For unstable tibial fractures—including long spiral fractures, fractures with butterfly fragments or significant comminution, segmental fractures, and tibial and fibular fractures occurring at the same level—operative fixation is the treatment of choice. For isolated stable tibial fractures in which the fracture line is transverse and there is at least 50% bony apposition, long leg casts with weight bearing may be highly successful. If the patient is comatose or has head injuries, operative fixation should be considered, particularly if the patient is agitated or uncooperative.

The standard treatment for tibial shaft fractures—closed, reamed, intramedullary nailing—has a high success rate and a low complication rate. Although the closed technique helps preserve the extraosseous blood supply, the reaming and nailing lead to loss of the intraosseous vasculature that supplies the inner two thirds of the bone. For rotational or axially unstable fractures, interlocking screws may be required. In those unusual circumstances in which the fracture pattern does not permit insertion of an intramedullary rod, a plate or screws may be used; unfortunately, this form of management is associated with a high rate of nonunion. For open fractures with complex wounds, the standard treatment has been external fixation, which permits stabilization of the fracture, allows access to large open wounds, and facilitates nursing care. Currently, however, nonreamed nailing appears be superior to external fixation in this situation: with proper early treatment and aggressive irrigation and debridement, the infection rates are no higher, the complication rate is lower, and the functional end results are better.

Fibular fracture Generally, fibular shaft fractures may be ignored; they heal readily, sometimes so readily that they interfere with the union of associated tibial fractures. Isolated midshaft fibular fractures that do not involve the ankle joint may be treated symptomatically, often without a cast. In some instances, plating the fibular fracture stabilizes an unstable tibial shaft fracture; however, rendering the fibula stable may diminish the cyclic compression that occurs with weight bearing at the site of the tibial fracture and may delay healing. For this reason, in most cases of combined tibial and fibular fracture, the fibula is not stabilized.

Fractures at the distal end of the fibula can be a serious problem if the ankle joint is disrupted. In these circumstances, anatomic reduction (usually with internal fixation) is required to prevent chronic pain or late arthritis from altered joint mechanics. The most common problem associated with proximal fibular head injuries is a peroneal nerve palsy, which usually resolves. If the nerve has been lacerated, however, regeneration may take quite a long time.

Pilon fracture Pilon fracture results from forceful axial compression across the ankle joint, which drives the talus up into the tibial plafond, resulting in a severe intra-articular fracture. It is commonly seen in falls from a height and is usually accompanied by a fracture of the distal fibular diaphysis. Some pilon fractures are so comminuted and severe that reconstruction is technically impossible and primary ankle fusion may be necessary. With severe open fractures, amputation may be required.

Pilon fractures are associated with massive swelling resulting from soft tissue edema and bleeding. Fracture blisters are common. Reconstruction must be done within a few hours of injury; the earlier, the better. If it cannot be done in this period, it must be delayed for 5 to 7 days or longer, until the swelling has decreased. Even with immediate fixation, the swelling can be so great that by the end of the operation, the skin cannot be closed and must be either left open or closed with a skin graft.

The goals of treatment are restoration of ankle joint integrity, congruency and stability, achievement of bony union, and functional painless motion. These are best achieved by means of open reduction and internal fixation, but only if the fracture is amenable to reconstruction. For certain complex fractures, closed treatment may be the only choice.

At best, good surgical technique results in a 50% to 75% return to full function. Accordingly, meticulous attention to detail is essential in performing the procedure. The fibula is usually fixed first through a lateral incision, and the tibia is then fixed via an anterior or medial approach. Dissection should be minimized to prevent further soft tissue injury. Any debris present in the joint should be removed. Plates and screws are necessary for stabilization of the fracture. Bone grafting is often required to fill bony defects and voids. If the tibial fracture is not amenable to reconstruction, the fibula may be plated to help bring the tibia out to length, maintain alignment, and afford some stability. If the fracture cannot be immediately fixed, calcaneal pin traction should be used to bring the limb out to length and permit elevation of the leg to decrease swelling. If posttraumatic arthritic pain is severe, delayed ankle fusion may be required.

Compartment Syndrome

Compartment syndrome is defined as high-pressure swelling within a fascial compartment. The forearm and the lower leg are the classic locations for compartment syndrome—any physician who treats trauma patients will encounter compartment syndromes at these sites—but the syndrome may also occur in the hand or the foot or, less commonly, in the shoulder, the upper arm, the buttock, or the thigh. The reason why compartment syndrome is more common in the forearm and the lower leg than in the less classic sites is that the compartments in these anatomic areas have tighter, better-defined fascial boundaries. Many physicians still believe, incorrectly, that compartment syndrome cannot develop in conjunction with an open fracture because the open nature of the injury provides decompression. This is a dangerous assumption: extensive soft tissue injury is in fact a very common accompaniment to an open fracture, and as many as 10% of open tibial fractures, for example, are associated with compartment syndrome. Alertness to symptoms and physical findings in patients with open fractures is the key to recognizing compartment syndrome.

Compartment syndrome can have any of several causes. The most common cause is hemorrhage and edema in the damaged soft tissue that accompanies a fracture. A dressing or a cast that is too tight can cause external pressure, as can the eschar from a circumferential burn. Massive soft tissue swelling and edema can occur secondary to various toxins found in venomous snakes, spiders, and scorpions. Unintentional infusion of intravenous fluid outside the vascular space can also cause compartment syndrome. A rarer situation is an iatrogenic compartment syndrome induced by the military antishock trousers; several cases have been reported after ill-advised, prolonged occlusion of the extremity with this garment. Disruption of the venous drainage of a limb may also result in edema and high compartment pressures, as may venous thrombosis.

The classic concept of the etiology of compartment syndrome is that as pressure increases within the compartment, it ultimately reaches that of the venous capillary. At this point, complete venous obstruction occurs, which, if arterial flow should continue, would result in continued escalation of compartment pressure. Inevitably, extensive venous obstruction gives rise to reflex spasm of the accompanying arteries, at which point tissues begin to become ischemic. Muscle can tolerate complete ischemia for 3 or 4 hours; after this period, it dies, and limb function is permanently compromised. In advanced ischemia, the microvasculature loses its integrity, with the result that severely ischemic and dead muscle swells and compartment pressure increases. Theoretically, in these circumstances, opening the skin envelope and exposing the dead muscle through fasciotomy would render the tissue vulnerable to infection. With late fasciotomy, when muscle is already necrotic, limb loss occurs primarily as a consequence of loss of skin covering; this consideration should be weighed when fasciotomy is being considered. This issue represents the only significant controversy regarding fasciotomy, which is the treatment of choice for compartment syndrome in all other contexts.

DIAGNOSIS

The key to diagnosis of compartment syndrome is continuous assessment of any extremity injury where there is a chance that the syndrome might develop—for example, fractures of the tibia or the forearm, fractures of the thigh or the upper arm (less likely), and, for that matter, all comminuted fractures associated with severe soft tissue injury. The diagnosis of compartment syndrome is a clinical one: although compartment pressures may be measured, there is no agreement on what constitutes the critical pressure. In fact, it has been shown that there is no specific compartment pressure at which the compartment syndrome occurs. The problem appears to be related more to the difference between the mean arterial pressure and the compartment pres-

sure. As this pressure difference decreases, perfusion of the soft tissues decreases as well, and compartment syndrome occurs. The syndrome is frequently seen when the difference between the mean arterial pressure and the pressure in the involved compartment is less than 40 mm Hg.[14]

The hallmark of the compartment syndrome is the presence of the four Ps: *p*ressure, *p*ain, *p*aresthesia, and intact *p*ulses. On palpation, the compartment will be tense or even boardlike, and this tenseness is usually the critical factor in deciding whether to treat the problem surgically. Pain that is out of proportion to what would be expected for the patient's level of injury and pain that is aggravated by passive stretching of the muscles are also manifestations of compartment syndrome. Muscles are more sensitive to anoxia than nerves are; thus, muscle pain and paralysis occur before paresthesia and anesthesia are noted.

When a patient at risk begins to complain of undue pain, the first step is to remove all circumferential bandages and then split them down to skin to relieve any pressure. If a plaster cast is present, it should be split, spread, or removed; if necessary, maintenance of reduction should be sacrificed. If the clinical picture does not improve after these measures are taken, then a decompressive fasciotomy is indicated.

OPERATIVE TREATMENT

Acute compartment syndrome is treated with wide decompression fasciotomy. To decompress the forearm, two incisions are made, one volar and one dorsal [see Figure 7]. A longitudinal dorsal incision provides access to the extensor compartment and the mobile wad. The fascia overlying these compartments must be widely opened. A curvilinear volar incision allows access to

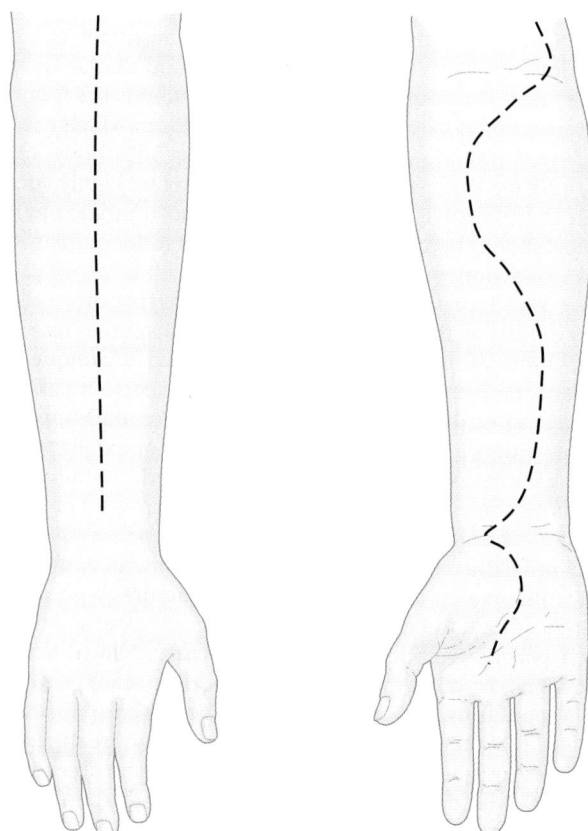

Figure 7 **Shown are incisions for forearm decompression in compartment syndrome.**

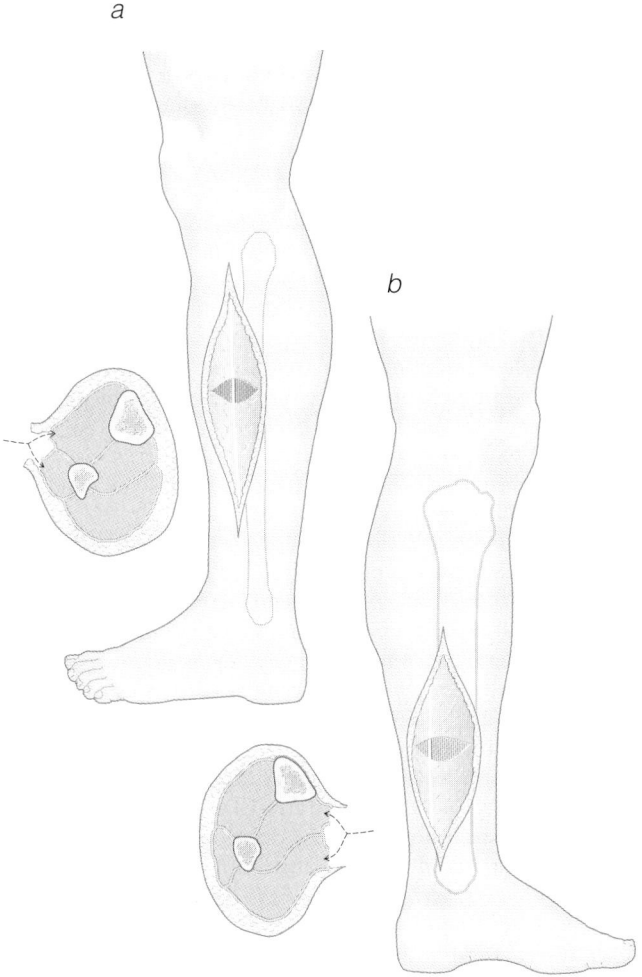

Figure 8 **Illustrated is the two-incision technique for lower leg decompression in compartment syndrome. Short transverse incisions are made in the fascia to locate (*a*) the lateral intermuscular membrane dividing the anterior and lateral compartments and (*b*) the posterior membrane dividing the superficial and deep posterior compartments. Fasciotomies are then performed in all four compartments along the dashed lines.**

the flexor compartment from a point proximal to the antecubital fossa to the midpalm. Here, too, it is imperative that fascia be widely opened. In severe cases, the deep intramuscular fascia enveloping the flexor digitorum superficialis, the flexor digitorum profundus, and the flexor pollicis longus may have to be opened as well. The thick transcarpal ligament is divided distally to perform a carpal tunnel release. The proximal end of the incision should release the lacertus fibrosus so as to decompress the median nerve at the elbow.

To decompress the lower leg, again, two incisions are usually made. A lateral incision between the tibial crest and the fibula provides access to the anterior and the lateral compartment. A short transverse incision is then made through the leg fascia to locate the lateral intramuscular membrane. The superficial peroneal nerve lies posterior to this septum in the lateral compartment and must be avoided. The fascia enveloping the two compartments is then widely opened longitudinally with blunt scissors until the muscles are soft and all pressure is dissipated. Next, a medial incision is made 2 cm posterior to the posterior crest of the tibia to provide access to the posterior compartments, with care taken to avoid the saphenous nerve and the saphenous vein. Again, a short

transverse incision is made through the enveloping fascia to identify the septum between the deep compartment and the superficial compartment [*see Figure 8*].

After fasciotomy, both fascia and skin are left widely open. The skin defects may be closed with skin grafts, provided that this is done without tension or pressure. Alternatively, the patient may be returned to the OR after the swelling resolves for delayed closure of the skin (again, with fascia left open) or split-thickness skin grafting, as indicated.

Injuries to Soft Tissue

The main types of soft tissue injuries encountered in patients who have experienced trauma to an extremity are abrasions, contusions, lacerations (including avulsion injuries), hemarthrosis, and sprains and strains. All such injuries should be examined with the goal of determining their nature and severity and ruling out underlying injuries to tendons, arteries, or nerves. Local or systemic analgesia or anesthesia may be required for appropriate examination of injuries. The entire area around the wound should then be prepared with an antiseptic solution and thoroughly inspected, palpated, and, if necessary, probed to ascertain the probable depth and direction of the wound. The position the extremity was in when wounded should be kept in mind; it may be critical for identifying injuries to underlying structures.

When examination reveals that a break in the skin has occurred, tetanus prophylaxis should be given in accordance with the patient's immunization history. For minor, clean lacerations that are not associated with other injuries, prompt debridement and irrigation are indicated. Simple wounds and lacerations that are seen and managed within 6 to 8 hours can usually be closed.

Abrasions are generally minor injuries. Typically, there is some ground-in foreign material, which may give rise to subsequent infection and complicate other injuries. Sometimes, abrasions may be treated in the ED by anesthetizing the injured area and cleaning it with an antiseptic solution and a soft brush to remove any grit and dirt. For abrasions that are more than 10 cm in diameter and are overtly dirty, however, anesthesia and treatment in the OR may be required. Once the abraded area is clean, an occlusive, nonadherent dressing should be applied to ease the pain of dressing changes and promote healing.

Contusion is the result of disruption of and hemorrhage into subcutaneous tissue or muscle as a consequence of blunt trauma. Large contusions that contain expanding hematomas may have to be treated with operative debridement and hemostasis; smaller contusions are usually treated with supportive dressings, with or without counterpressure.

Lacerations range in severity from simple full-thickness skin injuries to complex undermining lacerations and flap avulsions. As noted, simple lacerations can generally be treated in the ED with irrigation, debridement, and closure. Contaminated wounds more than 6 to 8 hours old call for a more conservative approach: once the wound is clean, it should be left open for 3 to 4 days and then closed by secondary intention. The deeper lacerations seen in avulsion injuries usually call for operative exploration, irrigation, and debridement to ensure removal of devitalized tissue and to minimize the risk of retaining foreign material. In some instances, the wound may have to be extended to permit proper inspection of its depth and to ensure adequate cleaning. Copious irrigation with a pulsatile lavage system dilutes the bacterial load and flushes foreign material from the wound. Because muscle takes sutures poorly, no attempt should be made to close muscles unless major tendinous avulsions have occurred. Once the wound has been cleaned and debrided, closure of the overlying fascia results in close approximation of the muscle ends, particularly if closure is accompanied by suction drainage. In the case of avulsion injuries, the likelihood that the flap will slough is high, particularly if the intact portion of the flap is distally based (that is, if the flap derives its blood supply distally). This problem can be dealt with by removing and defatting the skin, converting it to a full-thickness skin graft, and reapplying it to the injured area (provided that the wound is sufficiently clean).

Any laceration in the vicinity of a joint raises the possibility of traumatic arthrotomy. A long knife blade, a shard of glass, or a jagged piece of metal can travel some distance under the skin and can penetrate a joint. Probing the wound often confirms joint penetration, but it does not necessarily rule it out. Air seen in the joint on x-rays confirms penetration. For other wounds in proximity to synovial joints, an arthrogram should be performed. Saline or dilute methylene blue may be injected into the joint; oozing from the wound confirms arthrotomy. Once arthrotomy is confirmed, irrigation of the wound and the joint should be performed on a timely basis in the OR.

An acute joint effusion that occurs within 6 to 8 hours of injury is usually the result of bleeding. The presence of hemarthrosis can be confirmed by joint aspiration, which is also the treatment of choice. After reoperation, hemarthrosis should be treated with bulky, compressive dressings, ice, elevation, and rest until it resolves.

Sprained ligaments and strained muscles of the extremities rarely necessitate urgent surgical treatment. The diagnosis may not even be apparent until the patient has recovered sufficiently from other injuries to note local discomfort when attempting to bear weight on the extremity. Severe sprains and strains in which gross instability of the joint is apparent may be associated with joint dislocation. As a rule, these more extensive injuries need not undergo urgent surgical repair; repair is usually best done later, on an elective basis. Dislocations asso-ciated with vascular injury (most commonly, knee dislocations) may necessitate emergency revascularization procedures. In these situations, joint stabilization or reconstruction may be required to protect the vascular repair.

The Mangled Extremity

One of the more difficult decisions for a trauma surgeon is whether to amputate an extremity with multiple severe injuries. A number of scoring systems have been devised to facilitate this decision; however, most are cumbersome and hence too impractical to be used in the very patients most likely to need them—namely, unstable, multiply injured trauma patients. Although the ultimate usefulness of an extremity is related to the presence of intact neurologic function, the decision on when to amputate versus when to attempt complex repair of the mangled extremity is more appropriately based on the patient's overall condition and the vascular supply to the extremity.

In severely injured patients, dead or devitalized tissue can help precipitate the onset of disseminated intravascular coagulation. It is not uncommon for patients with mangled extremities to manifest the systemic inflammatory response syndrome until the extremity is removed, at which point they recover promptly. For this reason, if a mangled extremity is not an acute threat to the patient during the initial resuscitation, it may be best treated with irrigation and debridement (as described with respect to open fractures) and some form of stabilization. If, however, the extremity has no palpable pulses or does not appear viable, then the decision whether to amputate should be based on the functional prognosis of the extremity, which in turn is based on the presence or absence of nerve injury and the orthopedist's judgment of whether long-term bony stabilization is likely to be achievable.

If the decision is made to attempt salvage of the limb, regular rechecking of both the extremity and the patient's overall condition is essential. If the patient's condition deteriorates significantly or the previous prognostic estimate changes for the worse, amputation should be promptly performed within the first 24 hours.[15]

References

1. Allgöwer M, Border JR: Management of open fractures in the multiple trauma patient. World J Surg 7:88, 1983

2. Knudson MM, Lewis FR, Atkinson K, et al: The role of duplex ultrasound arterial imaging in patients with penetrating extremity trauma. Arch Surg 128:1033, 1993

3. Dennis JW, Frykberg ER, Veldenz HC, et al: Validation of nonoperative management of occult vascular injuries and accuracy of physical examination alone in penetrating extremity trauma: 5- to 10-year follow-up. J Trauma 43:196, 1997

4. Wagner WH, Calkins ER, Weaver FA, et al: Blunt popliteal artery trauma: one hundred consecutive injuries. J Vasc Surg 7:736, 1988

5. Visser PA, Hermreck AS, Pierce GE, et al: Prognosis of nerve injuries incurred during acute trauma to peripheral arteries. Am J Surg 140:596, 1980

6. Sunderland S: Nerves and Nerve Injuries. Churchill Livingstone, Edinburgh, 1978, p 127

7. Chapman MW: Operative Orthopaedics. JB Lippincott, Philadelphia, 1988

8. DeLong WG Jr, Born CT, Wei SY, et al: Aggressive treatment of 119 open fracture wounds. J Trauma 46:1049, 1999

9. Epstein HC, Wiss DA, Cozen L: Posterior fracture dislocation of the hip with fractures of the femoral head. Clin Orthop 201:9, 1985

10. Swiontkowski MF, Winquist RA, Hansen ST Jr: Fractures of the femoral neck in patients between the ages of twelve and forty-nine years. J Bone Joint Surg [Am] 66:837, 1984

11. Bone LB, Johnson KD, Weigelt J, et al: Early versus delayed stabilization of femoral fractures: a prospective randomized study. J Bone Joint Surg [Am] 71: 336, 1989

12. Delamarter RB, Hohl M, Hopp E Jr: Ligament injuries associated with tibial plateau fractures. Clin Orthop 250:226, 1990

13. Hoaglund FT, States JD: Factors influencing the rate of healing in tibial shaft fractures. Surg Gynecol Obstet 124:71, 1967

14. Heppenstall RB, Sapega AA, Izanty T, et al: Compartment syndrome: a quantitative study of high-energy phosphorus compounds using ^{31}P-magnetic resonance spectroscopy. J Trauma 29:1113, 1989

15. Roessler MS, Wisner DH, Holcroft JW: The mangled extremity: when to amputate? Arch Surg 126:1243, 1991

Acknowledgments

Figures 1, 4, 7, and 8   Tom Moore.
Figures 2 and 6   Carol Donner.
Figure 3   Marcia Kammerer.

12 BURN CARE IN THE IMMEDIATE RESUSCITATION PERIOD

Robert H. Demling, M.D., F.A.C.S.

Approach to the Burn Patient in the First 24 Hours

Neutralization of the Source of the Burn

CLOTHING

The first objective is to stop the burning process because the deeper the burn, the greater the potential for mortality and

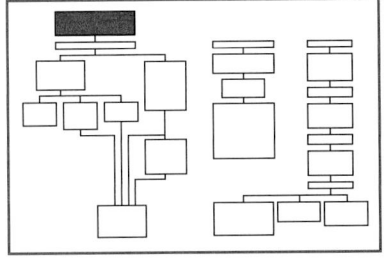

morbidity. With chemical burns, chemicals can remain in fabric and on skin for long periods. With a flame or scald burn, clothing can retain heat for a considerable time. Rapid removal of clothing is thus essential. Clothes are often still smoldering when the patient arrives at the emergency room. If clothing is burned or melted into the tissues, the surrounding fabric can be cut off. Adherent clothing can be removed after admission, when further wound cleaning and debridement are performed.

CHEMICAL BURNS

Removal of the chemical is urgent. Acid burns should be irrigated for up to 60 minutes with warm tap water. For burns resulting from alkali contact, lavage for at least 60 minutes may be beneficial [*see Table 1*]. If necessary, particles of corrosive powders should be surgically removed before the wound is irrigated. The skin burn itself is not the only concern, because the absorption of certain chemicals can lead to systemic toxicities such as neurologic dysfunction, red cell hemolysis, and liver and kidney failure.

It is important to avoid severe hypothermia during irrigation because hypothermia results in significant morbidity. Therefore, once the burn source is removed, the patient should be covered with clean, dry dressings or sheets.

Establishment of Airway and Adequate Ventilation

DIAGNOSIS AND TREATMENT OF CARBON MONOXIDE TOXICITY

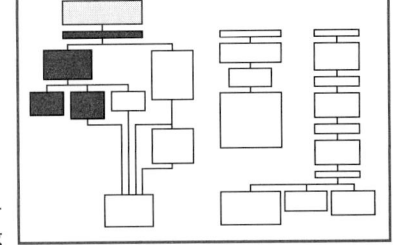

Carbon monoxide toxicity is one of the leading causes of death associated with fires. As oxygen is being consumed in the process of combustion, CO is being released. Carbon

monoxide is rapidly transported across the alveolar membrane and preferentially binds to hemoglobin in place of oxygen to form carboxyhemoglobin (COHb). In addition, CO causes the oxyhemoglobin dissociation curve to shift to the left, thereby impairing oxygen unloading at the tissue level; this shift results in a substantial reduction in oxygen delivery, given that 98% of the oxygen supplied to the tissues comes bound to hemoglobin. With prolonged exposure, CO can saturate the cell, binding to cytochrome oxidase and thereby further impairing mitochondrial function and adenosine triphosphate (ATP) production.

Patients who were injured in a closed space or who have inhalation injuries should be suspected of inhaling CO [*see Table 2*]. CO toxicity is determined by a high index of suspicion and by measuring the COHb level. Persistent metabolic acidosis in a patient with adequate volume resuscitation and adequate cardiac output indicates persistent impairment of oxygen utilization and delivery by CO or hydrocyanide. The chemical alteration of hemoglobin or of the cytochrome system by CO will not affect the amount of oxygen dissolved in plasma, and arterial oxygen tension (P_aO_2) will thus remain relatively normal. However, the measured oxygen saturation of hemoglobin will be markedly decreased relative to the oxygen tension.

Treatment of CO toxicity consists of promptly displacing CO from hemoglobin by administering 90% to 100% oxygen until the COHb level is less than 7%. If 20% oxygen is administered, the half-life of COHb is about 90 minutes; if concentrated high-flow oxygen is administered, the half-life is 20 to 30 minutes. The concentration of COHb is thus reduced by approximately 50% every 20 to 30 minutes if an oxygen concentration of 90% to 100% is used. Hyperbaric oxygen (2 to 3 atm) yields even more rapid displacement, particularly from the cell cytochrome system, and can be used to treat severe CO toxicity (i.e., a CO level > 50% or an elevated CO level that does not respond to standard oxygen therapy).

DIAGNOSIS AND TREATMENT OF CYANIDE TOXICITY

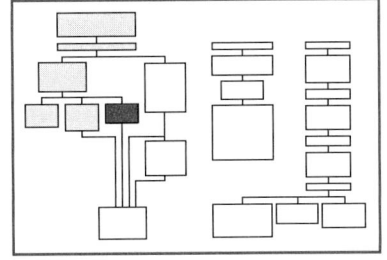

Hydrocyanide, the gaseous form of cyanide, is a well-recognized cause of fire-associated morbidity and mortality, particularly when synthetics such as

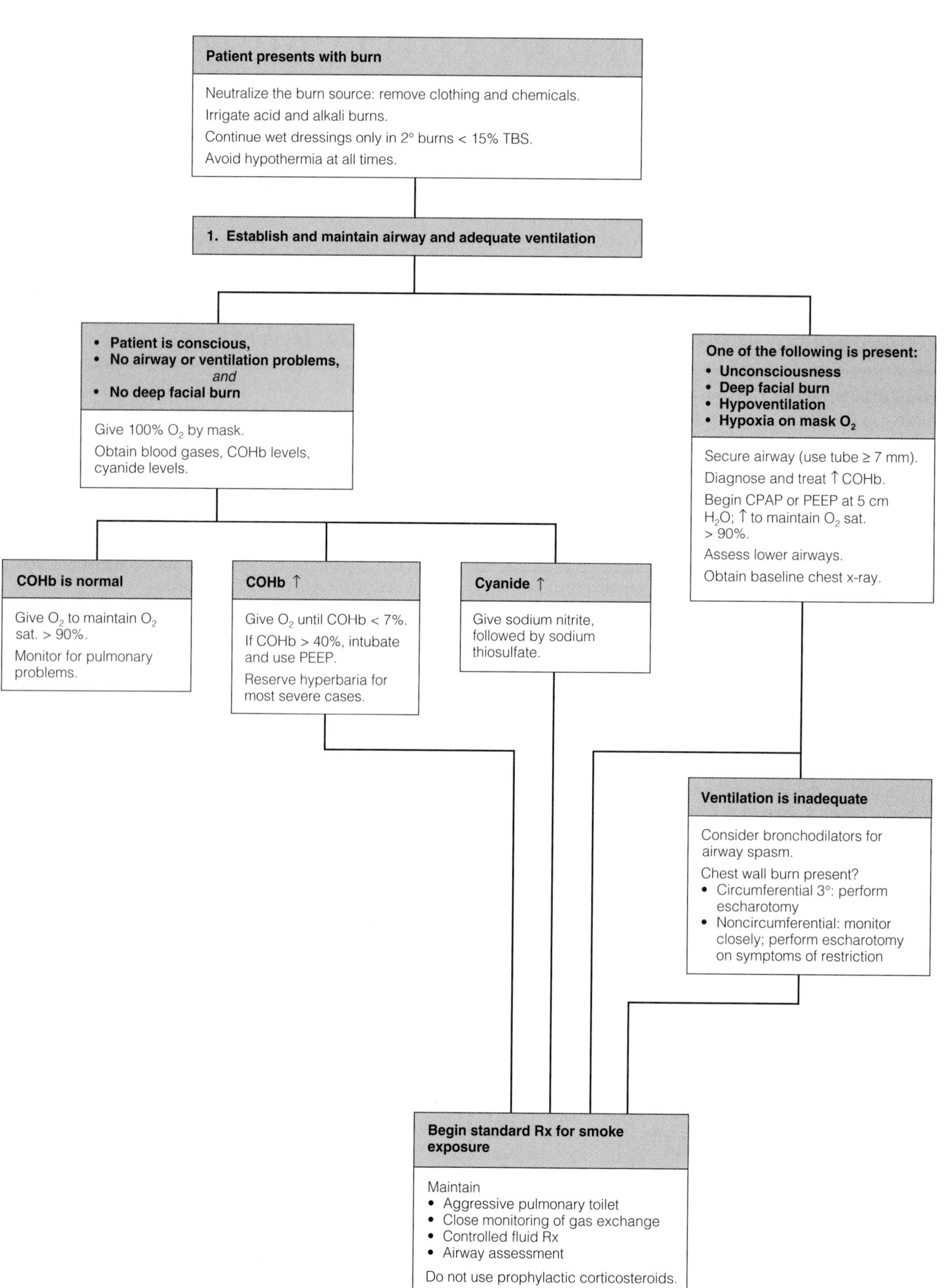

Patient presents with burn

Neutralize the burn source: remove clothing and chemicals.
Irrigate acid and alkali burns.
Continue wet dressings only in 2° burns < 15% TBS.
Avoid hypothermia at all times.

1. Establish and maintain airway and adequate ventilation

- **Patient is conscious,**
- **No airway or ventilation problems,**
  and
- **No deep facial burn**

Give 100% O₂ by mask.
Obtain blood gases, COHb levels, cyanide levels.

One of the following is present:
- **Unconsciousness**
- **Deep facial burn**
- **Hypoventilation**
- **Hypoxia on mask O₂**

Secure airway (use tube ≥ 7 mm).
Diagnose and treat ↑COHb.
Begin CPAP or PEEP at 5 cm H₂O; ↑ to maintain O₂ sat. > 90%.
Assess lower airways.
Obtain baseline chest x-ray.

COHb is normal

Give O₂ to maintain O₂ sat. > 90%.
Monitor for pulmonary problems.

COHb ↑

Give O₂ until COHb < 7%.
If COHb > 40%, intubate and use PEEP.
Reserve hyperbaria for most severe cases.

Cyanide ↑

Give sodium nitrite, followed by sodium thiosulfate.

Ventilation is inadequate

Consider bronchodilators for airway spasm.
Chest wall burn present?
- Circumferential 3°: perform escharotomy
- Noncircumferential: monitor closely; perform escharotomy on symptoms of restriction

Begin standard Rx for smoke exposure

Maintain
- Aggressive pulmonary toilet
- Close monitoring of gas exchange
- Controlled fluid Rx
- Airway assessment

Do not use prophylactic corticosteroids.

Approach to the Burn Patient in the First 24 Hours

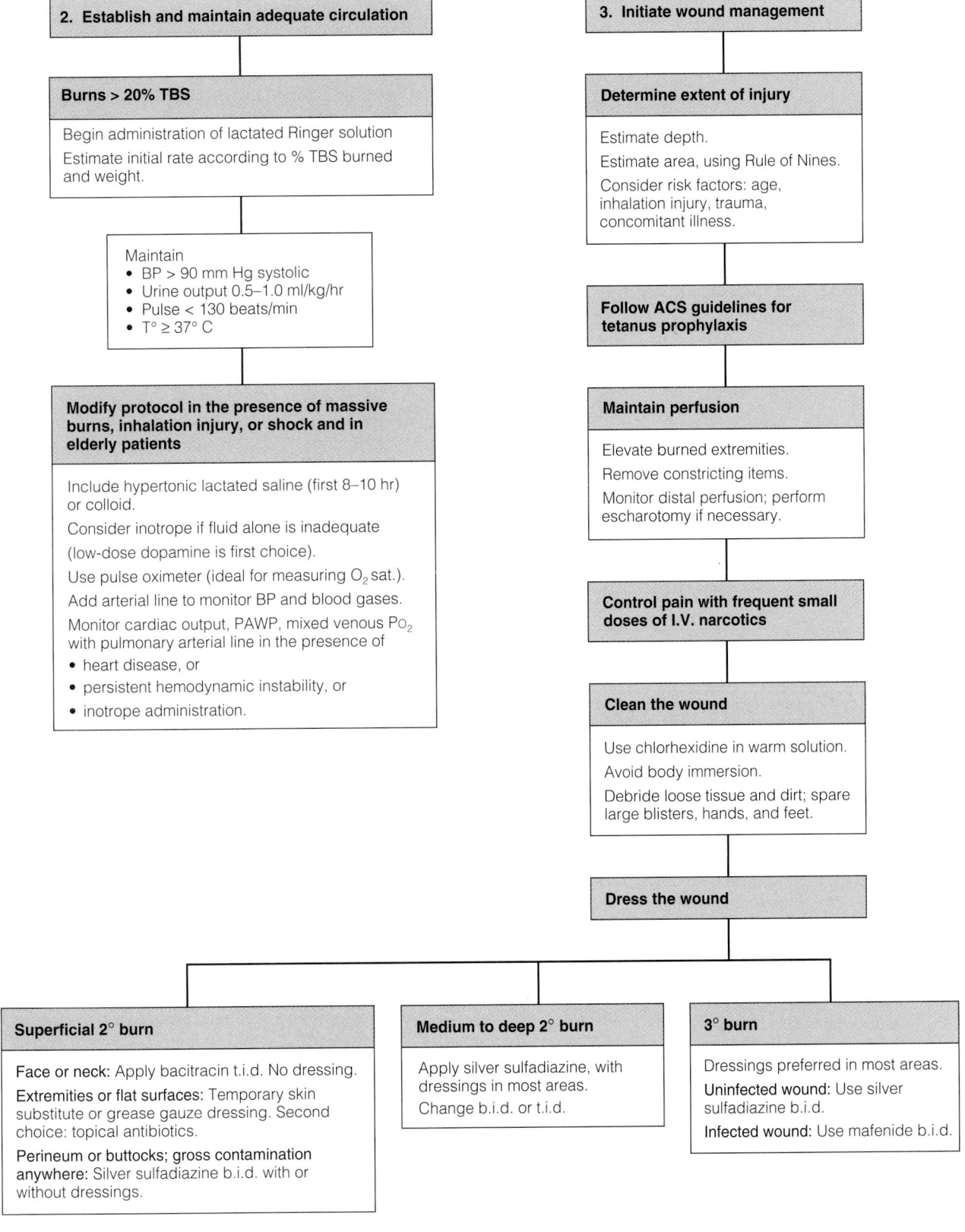

2. Establish and maintain adequate circulation

Burns > 20% TBS

Begin administration of lactated Ringer solution
Estimate initial rate according to % TBS burned and weight.

Maintain
- BP > 90 mm Hg systolic
- Urine output 0.5–1.0 ml/kg/hr
- Pulse < 130 beats/min
- T° ≥ 37° C

Modify protocol in the presence of massive burns, inhalation injury, or shock and in elderly patients

Include hypertonic lactated saline (first 8–10 hr) or colloid.

Consider inotrope if fluid alone is inadequate (low-dose dopamine is first choice).

Use pulse oximeter (ideal for measuring O_2 sat.).

Add arterial line to monitor BP and blood gases.

Monitor cardiac output, PAWP, mixed venous Po_2 with pulmonary arterial line in the presence of
- heart disease, or
- persistent hemodynamic instability, or
- inotrope administration.

3. Initiate wound management

Determine extent of injury

Estimate depth.
Estimate area, using Rule of Nines.
Consider risk factors: age, inhalation injury, trauma, concomitant illness.

Follow ACS guidelines for tetanus prophylaxis

Maintain perfusion

Elevate burned extremities.
Remove constricting items.
Monitor distal perfusion; perform escharotomy if necessary.

Control pain with frequent small doses of I.V. narcotics

Clean the wound

Use chlorhexidine in warm solution.
Avoid body immersion.
Debride loose tissue and dirt; spare large blisters, hands, and feet.

Dress the wound

Superficial 2° burn

Face or neck: Apply bacitracin t.i.d. No dressing.

Extremities or flat surfaces: Temporary skin substitute or grease gauze dressing. Second choice: topical antibiotics.

Perineum or buttocks; gross contamination anywhere: Silver sulfadiazine b.i.d. with or without dressings.

Medium to deep 2° burn

Apply silver sulfadiazine, with dressings in most areas.
Change b.i.d. or t.i.d.

3° burn

Dressings preferred in most areas.
Uninfected wound: Use silver sulfadiazine b.i.d.
Infected wound: Use mafenide b.i.d.

polyurethane are burned. Although cyanide can be absorbed through the GI tract or through skin, it is most dangerous when aerosolized and inhaled because it is absorbed especially rapidly through the respiratory tract. Once absorbed, cyanide binds to the cytochrome system, thereby inhibiting cell metabolism and ATP production. All cells, and hepatocytes in particular, have a detoxifying system in which the enzyme rhodenase converts hydrocyanide to thiocyanate, which is then excreted in the urine. If, however, a large amount of cyanide is absorbed, this protective system can be overwhelmed, especially in the face of hypovolemia, which hinders metabolism and clearance of cyanide.

The diagnosis of cyanide toxicity is made on the basis of the history and a high index of suspicion and is confirmed by the presence of elevated blood cyanide levels (normal, < 0.1 mg/L; values higher than 1 mg/L are usually lethal). Treatment begins with volume replenishment. From 10 to 20 ml of a 3% sodium nitrite solution is then given over a period of 10 minutes; methemoglobin is produced as the cyanide is detoxified. Finally, 50 ml of a 25% solution of sodium thiosulfate is given; this converts the cyanide to sodium thiocyanate, which is excreted in the urine.

DIAGNOSIS OF THE PRESENCE AND EXTENT OF INHALATION INJURY

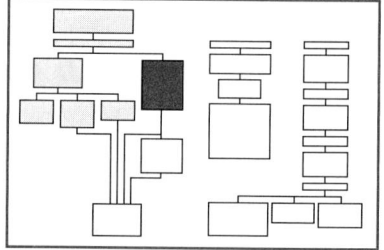

Inhalation injury, a complex and deadly disease process, occurs when the heat and toxins in smoke make contact with airway mucosa and alveoli. The degree of injury depends on the composition of the smoke, which varies according to its source. Heat affects primarily the supraglottic area and causes edema and upper airway obstruction, whereas the gas and particle components of the smoke affect primarily the airway mucosa and cause the actual chemical burn. The initial smoke injury occurs shortly after exposure, but the ensuing intense inflammatory reaction evolves over a period of hours to days [see Figure 1]. The degree of mucosal damage can range from simple erythema and irritation to complete mucosal sloughing that leads to distal airway obstruction and subsequently to atelectasis and increased shunting. Alveolar instability can also occur as a result of direct surfactant denaturation. Alveolar edema is a late finding.

Table 1 Chemical Burns

Agent	Pathophysiology	Treatment
Acids	Acids cause deep skin burns through tissue desiccation and protein denaturation; with concentrated acids, injury may extend well below skin. Acids such as H_2SO_4, HCl, and HNO_3 cause local damage. Burned area is tan to gray in appearance; extreme pain is a common finding. *Hydrofluoric acid:* Hydrofluoric acid causes a deep skin burn that may be extensive. It also exerts systemic effects, which are attributable to hypocalcemia resulting from the formation of a Ca^{2+}-F^- complex.	Perform vigorous water lavage for as long as 60 min after injury; use warm water with extensive exposure to prevent hypothermia. Assume that the burn will be much deeper than initial appearance indicates. Apply standard fluid resuscitation principles. *Hydrofluoric acid:* Perform vigorous water lavage. Inject calcium gluconate locally, and apply 2.5% calcium gluconate gel topically; end point of calcium gluconate administration is relief of pain. Monitor plasma calcium levels, and replace calcium deficits if necessary.
Alkalies	Alkalies cause deep skin burns through tissue desiccation and protein denaturation resulting from chemical reaction with hydrated tissue. Alkali burns tend to be worse than acid burns, but alkalies tend not to be absorbed systemically and thus rarely exert systemic effects. The burned area is tan to gray; extreme pain is a characteristic finding.	Perform vigorous water lavage for at least 60 min after injury—longer for lye burns—and take pains to prevent hypothermia. Assume that the burn will increase in depth. Apply standard fluid resuscitation principles.
Gasoline	Gasoline immersion produces both superficial skin injury and systemic injury (resulting from absorption of hydrocarbons). The systemic injury comprises the following: *Renal injury:* lipid degenerative changes to proximal tubules *Pulmonary injury:* surfactant denaturation, atelectasis, lipoid pneumonia *CNS injury:* edema producing seizures or coma *Hepatic injury:* lipid degenerative changes, hepatitis Burned area is erythematous in appearance.	Immerse injured area in water. Aggressively maintain hydration and pulmonary support, and provide general critical care support.
Phenol	Phenol produces both a partial-thickness burn and systemic injury (resulting from absorption), which is directly proportional to amount of skin exposed. The systemic injury comprises the following: *Renal injury:* direct glomerular and tubular damage as well as indirect damage from precipitated hemoglobin *Hematologic injury:* red cell hemolysis *CNS injury:* seizures or coma *Hepatic injury:* centrolobular necrosis Burned area is dull tan to gray in appearance.	Spray or pour large amounts of water on burned surface. Do not swab or use small amounts of water; these actions serve only to increase surface area of exposure. After lavage, quickly wipe skin with polyethylene or propylene glycol. To minimize hemoglobin precipitation, keep urine alkaline by administering bicarbonate. Maintain optimal hydration and blood volume to support injured kidney and any other injured organs.
Tar	Hot tar causes a superficial to deep skin burn, depending on the temperature of the tar when it contacts the skin. As a rule, there is no systemic absorption.	Remove tar to allow burn wound management. Bacitracin ointment and Neosporin (polymyxin B–bacitracin–neomycin) ointment contain the emulsifier Tween-80, which is very useful for dissolving tar. Apply the ointment and wash it off several times a day until tar is removed. Avoid hydrocarbon solvents. Perform general mechanical debridement if desired.

Table 2 Symptoms of
Carbon Monoxide Intoxication

Carboxyhemoglobin Level (%)	Symptoms
0–15	None
15–20	Headache, confusion
20–40	Disorientation, fatigue, nausea, visual impairment
40–60	Hallucination, combativeness, coma, shock
60+	Death

Inhalation injury should be suspected in (1) individuals who were injured in a closed space; (2) patients with extensive burns or with burns of the face; (3) patients who were unconscious at the time of injury; (4) patients with singed nasal hairs, hoarseness, or wheezing; and (5) patients who are coughing up carbonaceous sputum.

Pulmonary injury is known to result in substantially increased late burn mortality and morbidity as well as increased early fluid requirements and metabolic demands. Early intubation and positive pressure ventilation have been reported to improve outcome. The mode of ventilation used depends on the specific physiologic problem present; different modes may become necessary as the disease changes over time.

Pulmonary changes can be classified according to cause: thermal injury (heat) or chemical injury (incomplete products of combustion).

Thermal Injury

A number of techniques have been used to assess the degree of supraglottic injury and to determine the need for endotracheal intubation. Fiberoptic bronchoscopy or laryngoscopy will reveal physical evidence of mucosal injury. Spirometry detects early

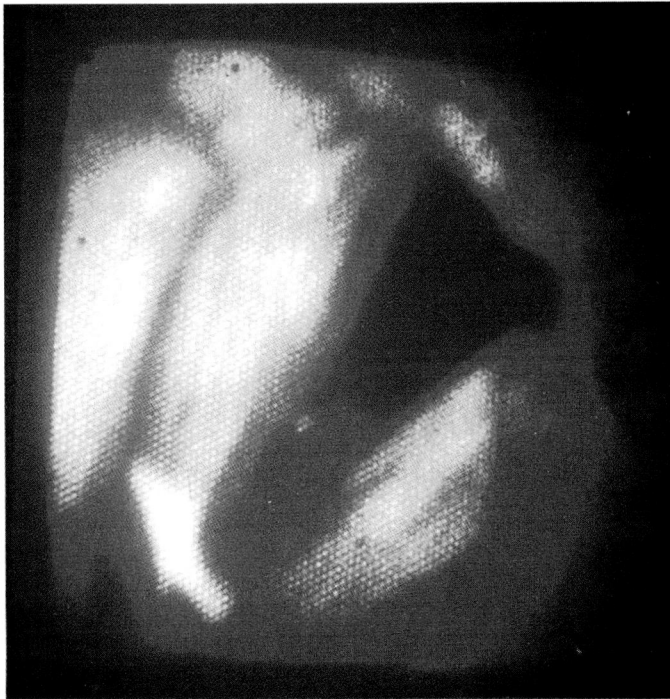

Figure 1 **The view through a fiberoptic bronchoscope shows erythema and edema of the larynx 18 hours after a burn.**

obstructive patterns in the airways, but reliable data can be obtained only in a cooperative patient without severe facial burns. Because the injury process is progressive during the first 18 to 24 hours, none of these tests accurately predicts the severity of subsequent airway compromise; serial studies must be performed.

Chemical Injury

Diagnosis of chemical injury is complicated by the fact that facial burns or other signs evident in heat injury may be absent; indeed, the patient may not have been exposed to heat. Fiberoptic bronchoscopy detects the reddened, sometimes ulcerated mucosa that indicates the presence—but not the severity—of chemical injury. Ventilation-perfusion lung scans using xenon-133 reportedly detect early changes in the small airways, as do analyses of flow-volume curves and a simple 1-second forced expiratory volume (FEV_1). Preexisting lung disease, however, will alter the interpretation of findings. Measurement of lung water is of minimal benefit because major changes in water content usually occur only in an alveolar injury in which early respiratory failure is prominent. Initial chest x-ray, blood gas levels, and physical examination results are frequently normal.

INTUBATION

Endotracheal intubation is indicated for (1) deep facial burns—especially of the lips, the mouth, the neck, or the oropharynx—because subsequent edema will impair airway patency; (2) cases of smoke inhalation in which heat or chemical burns to the airway have been demonstrated by laryngoscopy or bronchoscopy; and (3) massive body burns, especially in the presence of circumferential chest burns, because ventilatory support is needed.

With deep burns of the face, the mouth, or the neck, the airway can be compromised by anatomic distortion and compression from the burn-edema process. Edema-induced distortion peaks at 18 to 24 hours after a burn; both airway patency and the ability to clear secretions are impaired. As edema increases, it becomes much more difficult to secure an airway. Endotracheal intubation is thus preferably performed on admission, before severe edema develops. A patient with inhalation injury can be closely monitored for upper airway obstruction without a tube, preferably with the head elevated at 30°, only if intubation will be technically possible later. However, if anatomic distortion from face and neck burns is increasing to a point where safe intubation might soon be precluded, the procedure is carried out immediately. Tracheostomy through burned tissue is contraindicated because the risk of infection, both in the wound and in the airway, is substantially increased.

Heat injury usually heals in a matter of a few days to a week, as the mucosal edema resolves and the relatively superficial mucosal injury heals.

Positive end-expiratory pressure (PEEP) is frequently necessary to keep the edematous airways open and to maintain an adequate functional residual capacity; it is also often used in the early management of severe CO toxicity (COHb > 40%). Prophylactic endotracheal intubation and PEEP have been reported to decrease deaths from early pulmonary complications after severe burns and smoke inhalation. A large enough tube (i.e., approximately 7.5 mm internal diameter in adults) should be used because very thick secretions develop as the lung injury becomes manifest, and changing tubes in the presence of edema is very dangerous. Therefore, although the nasotracheal route may be more comfortable for the patient, the choice of a route of placement must be based on the tube size required.

INITIATION OF AGGRESSIVE PULMONARY SUPPORT

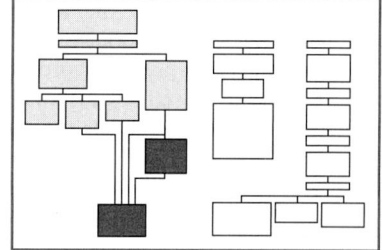

Continuous administration of humidified oxygen is indicated to maintain adequate oxygen delivery as well as to assist in the clearance of secretions. If the patient's hemodynamic condition will tolerate it, elevation of the head and chest by 20° to 30° is helpful in reducing neck and chest wall edema. The early addition of bronchodilators, usually by aerosol, is especially advantageous in managing the bronchospasm seen after chemical injury. The beta$_2$-adrenergic agent metaproterenol (via nebulizer) is an effective bronchodilator. Intravenous aminophylline, although helpful, is frequently limited in its use because of the tachycardia seen in the early postburn period. Intravenous steroids have not been found to decrease the degree of injury; however, aerosolized steroid preparations identical to those used in asthma patients can decrease airway hyperreactivity, which is often a major problem in patients with smoke inhalation injury and which may not be responsive to aerosolized beta agonists. On the other hand, intravenous steroids have been successful in attenuating obliterative bronchiolitis, an uncommon but uniformly fatal late complication of severe smoke inhalation injury. Prophylactic antibiotics are not indicated to prevent a lung infection after smoke injury.

Close monitoring of the adequacy of gas exchange by serial blood gas determination is necessary, particularly during the early evolution of complications from the inhalation injury. An indwelling arterial line is indicated in the presence of severe injuries. When placement of such a line is not possible, a pulse oximeter is very useful if an unburned finger or earlobe is available. The pulse oximeter reads arterial oxygen saturation by means of a photosensor, which detects the color of the blood flowing beneath the probe.

Chest Wall Escharotomy

A full-thickness burn of the anterior and lateral chest wall can lead to severe restriction of chest wall motion as edema develops beneath the nonviable tissue (eschar), even in the absence of a completely circumferential burn. Chest wall escharotomy is required to relieve the restriction; the incision must penetrate completely through the eschar so that the subeschar space can expand and decrease tissue pressure. In a full-thickness burn, nerve endings are destroyed along with the entire epidermis and dermis. Analgesics are thus usually not necessary for escharotomy. The escharotomy incisions are placed along the anterior axillary lines, with bilateral incisions connected by a subcostal incision [see Figure 2 and Initiation of Wound Management, Subeschar Edema

in Extremities, below]. Occasionally, another incision from the suprasternal notch to the xiphoid process is needed. Bleeding can usually be managed by pressure and occasional use of the electrocautery unit.

Restoration and Maintenance of Hemodynamic Stability

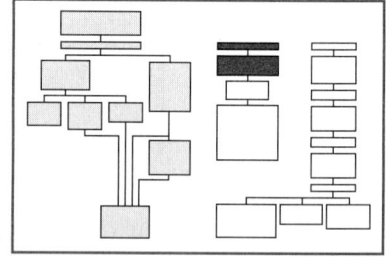

ESTIMATION OF BURN SIZE

Fluid requirements depend on the size of the burn. A simple determination of the burn surface area can be made using the Rule of Nines: each arm is considered to be 9% of total body surface (TBS), each leg 18%, the anterior trunk 18%, the posterior trunk 18%, and the head 9% [see Figure 3]. In small children, the determination must be modified because the head approaches 18% of TBS.

INTRAVENOUS ACCESS

A peripheral venous catheter through unburned tissue is the preferred route for fluid administration. A central venous line or pulmonary arterial line is only occasionally needed to monitor the patient during the initial resuscitation period and is removed as soon as it is no longer needed. These lines are usually required only in elderly patients or in patients who have severe heart disease. An extremely high complication rate reportedly accompanies the use of central catheters in burn patients because of infection and embolic episodes related to a hypercoagulable state. Because of the high infection rate, an intravenous catheter should not be placed through burn tissue unless every other possible route has been ruled out. A line that is dedicated to total parenteral nutrition should be completely isolated from the burn wound and cared for by covering the entrance site with an occlusive dressing [see 5:14 Burn Care after the First Postburn Week].

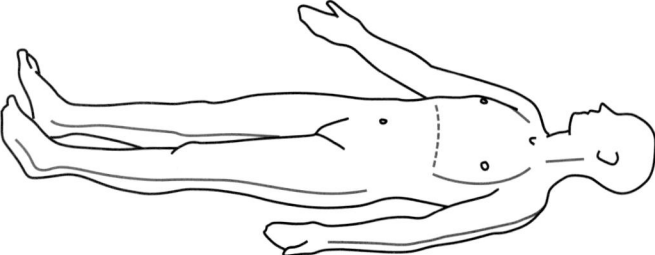

Figure 2 The red lines on the illustrated human figure represent guidelines for the placement of escharotomy incisions.

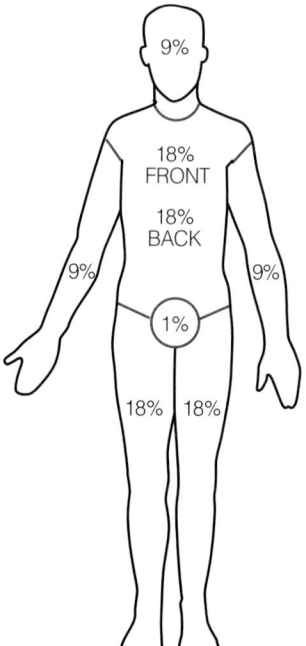

Figure 3 The size of a burn can be estimated by means of the Rule of Nines, which assigns percentages of total body surface to the head, the extremities, and the front and back of the torso.

RESUSCITATION FLUIDS

In general, fluids containing salt in quantities at least isotonic with plasma are appropriate for use in resuscitation after burn injury if given in sufficient amounts. These fluids should be free of glucose because burn patients exhibit early glucose intolerance as a result of the early release of catecholamines and other stress hormones. The oral route can be used in the case of smaller burns, but intestinal ileus frequently occurs after deep burns in excess of 20% of total body surface. A number of intravenous fluids, including colloids, are used to decrease edema in unburned tissues and to maintain a higher blood volume.

Crystalloid

Crystalloid—in particular, lactated Ringer solution, with a sodium concentration of 130 mEq/L—is the most popular resuscitation fluid in the United States. The loss of large quantities of sodium and water from the vascular space into the burn wound is well described. Isotonic crystalloid, if given in sufficient amounts, can restore cardiac output toward normal in most patients, the exceptions being patients who are extremely young or extremely old, those whose burns are massive, and those with superimposed inhalation injury. Lactated Ringer solution is preferred to normal saline because of its physiologic pH of 6.5 versus saline's pH of 5.0. Because isotonic salt solutions generate no differential in osmotic pressure between plasma and interstitial spaces, the entire extracellular space must be expanded to replace intravascular losses.

The amount of isotonic crystalloid required in the first 24 hours is based primarily on the calculated deficit of sodium from the extracellular space. This amount has been estimated to be 0.5 to 0.6 mEq sodium/kg/% TBS burned, which is equal to 4 ml/kg/% TBS burned of lactated Ringer solution. The quantity of crystalloid needed is also determined by measuring the parameters used to monitor resuscitation. In most burn centers, a urine output of 0.5 ml/kg/hr is considered an indication of adequate perfusion. The patient will require about 3 to 5 ml/kg/% TBS burned in the first 24 hours; about half of this amount is given in the first 8 hours [see Table 3].

Sodium is apparently the key element in crystalloid infusion; water is primarily the solvent. Solutions with increased sodium concentration therefore have a theoretical advantage because less water is infused. The hypertonic salt solutions used clinically have an osmolarity of 400 to 600 mOsm/L (isotonic solutions have an osmolarity of 280 to 300 mOsm/L); these solutions thereby transiently generate potential osmotic pressures of several thousand mm Hg relative to the normal isosmolar state. Hypertonic salt solutions have been known for many years to be effective in treating shock states, including burns. Essentially, they induce the body to borrow intracellular water to fill the extracellular space deficit. Infusion of hypertonic solutions thereby limits edema, compared with treatment by infusion of isotonic solutions.

Hypertonic solutions have also been reported to increase myocardial contractility, produce precapillary dilatation, and decrease vascular resistance by exerting a direct effect on the capillary smooth muscle. Current practice is to use a solution with a sodium concentration of approximately 240 mEq/L, which is prepared by adding two ampules of sodium lactate to each liter of normal saline. It is recommended that serum sodium levels not be allowed to exceed 160 mEq/L during infusion of the solution. Complications of hypertonic saline administration relate primarily to hyperosmolarity. A more isotonic solution should be given if an excessive hyperosmolar state develops. Free water cannot be given during infusion, because such action will simply lead to a more isotonic solution and in turn no decrease

---

Table 3 Calculations to Determine Resuscitation Requirements in a Young Patient without an Inhalation Injury

The patient is a 35-year-old male. His weight is 70 kg. His burns cover 50% TBS, most of which are second degree.

Recommendations:

3–4 ml lactated Ringer solution/kg body weight/% TBS burned Administer 1/2 the required volume in the first 8 hr after the burn. Administer 1/2 the required volume during the next 16 hr.

Calculation:

4 ml × 70 kg × 50% TBS burned = 14,000 ml/24 hr

Give

7,000 ml during the first 8 hr (875 ml/hr)
7,000 ml during the next 16 hr (435 ml/hr)

Monitor

Blood pressure (systolic > 90 mm Hg; mean > 80 mm Hg)
Pulse (< 120 beats/min)
Urine output (30–50 ml/hr)
Arterial blood gases (PO_2 > 90 mm Hg)
pH (> 7.35)

Adjust fluid administration in response to circulatory requirements:

Diminish fluid administration if hemodynamic stability is achieved at these infusion rates

or

Add colloid if adequate hemodynamic stability is not achieved at 4 ml/kg/% TBS burned.

---

in total administered fluid. Increased water retention is likely to occur with the institution of hypotonic solutions beginning on postburn day 2, at least until isotonicity results.

Colloids

Unburned tissue appears to regain normal permeability very soon after injury. Because hypoproteinemia may accentuate edema in uninjured tissues, protein restoration should begin 8 to 12 hours after a burn if nonburn edema and total fluid requirements are to be minimized. This method is particularly advantageous in patients who have massive burns and in elderly patients.

The amount of protein to be infused remains undefined. Many investigators have arbitrarily used between 0.5 and 1.0 ml/kg/% TBS burned during the first 24 hours. The amount depends on the magnitude of the injury and on the degree of hemodynamic instability. The protein should be infused at a constant rate [see Adjustment of Infusion Rate, *below*]; pulsed infusion will transiently increase pressure and increase the rate of edema formation.

If early administration of colloids is required because hemodynamic instability persists despite the infusion of large quantities of crystalloid (about 4 ml/kg/% TBS burned), nonprotein colloids are more economical. Although the weight of dextran 70 (70 kd) is almost identical to that of albumin, dextran's molecular size is considerably larger because of its branched configuration. A standard 6% solution of dextran 70 exerts an oncotic pressure more than twice that generated by a 6% albumin solution. This property makes the compound advantageous as a volume expander. Dextran 40 (40 kd) in a 10% solution, infused at about 2 ml/kg/hr, is an even more potent volume expander because it generates a colloid osmotic pressure six to eight times that of a protein of comparable weight. To prevent platelet deficits, the total dose of dextran 70 during any 24-hour period should not exceed 33 ml/kg; the total dose of dextran 40 should not exceed 15 ml/kg during any 24-hour period. Therefore, these preparations are usually used in the early resuscitation period and are replaced by protein in the later resuscitation period. The use of the hapten PROMIT—a 1 kd dextran—before the administration of the dextran solution essentially precludes allergic reactions to the dextran molecule.

Hetastarch, a 6% starch solution, has colloid properties very similar to those of a 6% protein solution and generates a comparable oncotic pressure. Hetastarch molecules are much larger than those of most dextrans, and vascular clearance is therefore much slower. This solution is being used with increasing frequency as a volume expander.

Blood

Because there is no actual early red cell deficit with a burn alone, blood replacement is usually not needed during this period unless severe hemolysis occurs. Occasionally, however, blood can be a very useful volume expander to restore cardiac output if perfusion is not adequately maintained by other resuscitation fluids.

ADJUSTMENT OF INFUSION RATE

Fluids should be infused at a constant rate because rapid fluid challenge transiently increases pressure above the level required for adequate perfusion and contributes to edema formation. Fluid requirements in the first 6 to 8 hours after a burn will clearly exceed those in the subsequent 18 hours because the largest fluid shifts occur early. Approximately half of the total amount of fluid required in the first 24 hours will be given in the first 8 hours. During those first 8 hours, once a fluid infusion rate is reached at which adequate perfusion is maintained, only minor changes should be made so as to avoid large hemodynamic fluctuations. Beginning 8 to 10 hours after a burn, when fluid requirements begin to diminish, an attempt should be made to decrease the infusion rate gradually and to determine the smallest amount of fluid or fluids necessary to maintain adequate perfusion. The rate required in the 12- to 24-hour period must usually deliver around 50% to 60% of the initial requirements. Fluid requirements during the first 24 hours usually range from 3 to 4 ml/kg/% TBS burned, depending on the type of fluid, the patient's age, and the presence of other injuries [*see Table 3*].

HEMODYNAMIC PARAMETERS TO MONITOR

Perfusion-Related Parameters

The adequacy of perfusion is difficult to assess after major burns. Burn in-

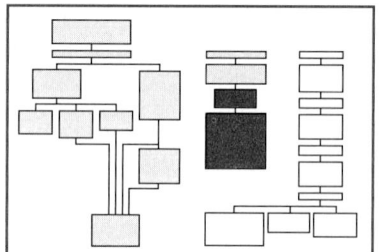

jury leads to increased tissue demand for oxygen, but at the same time, the body's ability to increase oxygen delivery is impaired by capillary leakage into the burn. Inhalation injury places additional fluid requirements and metabolic demands on burn patients. The increased hemodynamic instability seen in burn patients is probably attributable to activation of systemic inflammation by the burn as well as to airway injury. Infusion of larger amounts of resuscitation fluid may be necessary; however, this may lead to additional edema, which also results in complications. The best approach is to rely on repeated clinical assessments based on sound physiologic principles. Monitoring the following parameters can facilitate the assessment and improvement of perfusion.

Mean arterial pressure The increased sympathetic tone characteristic of the early postburn period makes arterial pressure an insensitive measure of volume status; however, minimal perfusion pressure (mean, > 90 mm Hg) must be maintained, which means that blood pressure must be monitored. In each patient, however, the precise blood pressure required to maintain adequate organ perfusion and tissue oxygenation becomes evident only in the process of observing the patient's response to fluid infusion.

If the patient is hemodynamically unstable, if the extremities are burned to such an extent that a sphygmomanometer cannot be used, or if frequent measurement of not only P_aO_2 but also pH and arterial carbon dioxide tension (P_aCO_2) is required, insertion of an arterial catheter may be necessary. The catheter should be placed through unburned skin and should be removed as soon as possible. A pulse oximeter can provide continuous readings of oxygen saturation and has the additional benefit of being noninvasive.

Pulse rate Tachycardia is inevitable in the early postburn period, given the development of hypovolemia and the release of catecholamines as a result of tissue trauma and pain. The degree of tachycardia can be a useful indicator of the adequacy of volume replacement, except in elderly patients or in patients with preexisting heart disease, whose heart rate cannot increase in proportion to the stimulus. In most patients, a pulse rate lower than 120 beats/min usually indicates adequate volume, whereas a pulse rate higher than 130 beats/min usually indicates that more fluid is needed. This guideline assumes that the pulse rate response corresponds to the other monitors of perfusion being used. Sometimes, the pulse rate does not follow the other indicators of impaired perfusion, in which case it becomes less useful for monitoring purposes. A case in point is a burn patient who is taking a beta blocker.

Pulmonary arterial wedge pressure In most young patients, even those with massive burns, it is not necessary to measure pulmonary arterial wedge pressure (PAWP) in the course of initial resuscitation: the risks associated with inserting a pulmonary arterial catheter may well exceed any benefits to be gained with respect to assessing adequacy of perfusion. Like central venous pressure, PAWP is usually normal to low (6 to 10 mm Hg) in the early postburn period, even when perfusion is adequate. Hypoperfusion is almost always attributable to hypovolemia; other well-recognized causes are (1) impaired left ventricular function resulting from impaired left ventricular filling (as with high mean airway pressure or pneumothorax) and (2) a marked increase in afterload resulting from high levels of circulating vasoconstrictors. There are three main patient groups in whom measurement of PAWP may be beneficial: (1) elderly patients who have deep burns covering more than 30% of TBS or who have suffered substantial smoke inhalation injury, (2) patients with preexisting heart disease who have massive burns or substantial smoke inhalation injury, and (3) young patients with massive burns who are not maintaining adequate perfusion despite fluid intake well in excess of predicted requirements.

Cardiac output and mixed venous oxygen tension The primary objective of fluid management is maintenance of adequate delivery of oxygen to tissues. Direct measurement of cardiac output (usually expressed as cardiac index) facilitates this task. In an uninjured person, a cardiac index of 2.5 L/min/m² or higher would be considered normal. In an injured person, however, such a value would not necessarily be indicative of adequate oxygen delivery, because injured tissue requires more oxygen than normal tissue does. Monitoring of mixed venous oxygen tension ($P_{mv}O_2$) can be of great assistance in this situation. A $P_{mv}O_2$ higher than 35 mm Hg indicates that oxygen delivery is adequate, a $P_{mv}O_2$ between 30 and 35 mm Hg indicates that oxygen delivery is marginal, and a $P_{mv}O_2$ lower than 30 mm Hg indicates that oxygen delivery is inadequate.

Arterial blood gas values Whether P_aO_2 and P_aCO_2 must be monitored depends on the percentage of TBS burned and on the risk of respiratory abnormalities (particularly in patients with a history of smoke exposure). Pulse oximetry is useful for measuring P_aO_2. Measurement of pH and evaluation of acid-base balance are also extremely useful in the assessment of tissue oxygenation. A base deficit during the early postburn phase usually reflects impaired tissue oxygenation caused by hypovolemia or by carbon monoxide or hydrocyanide toxicity [*see 6:9 Disorders of Acid-Base and Potassium Balance*].

Blood lactate concentration A normal blood lactate concentration does not indicate that perfusion is optimal; it only indicates that anaerobic metabolism is not taking place. A high lactate concentration, on the other hand, reflects severe hypoperfusion.

Urine output Urine output via a Foley catheter is a valuable indicator of adequate renal blood flow if the urine is nonglycosuric and if output has not been increased by administration of solutes (e.g., mannitol or dextran). An output of 0.5 ml/kg/hr in adults or 1.0 ml/kg/hr in children is adequate. Antidiuretic hormone and aldosterone are automatically released in response to the burn stress; therefore, a urine output greater than 0.5 to 1.0 ml/kg/hr may necessitate a rate of fluid infusion far higher than that necessary to maintain perfusion, and excess edema will result.

Other Parameters

Serum creatinine and blood urea nitrogen concentration Baseline values for serum creatinine and blood urea nitrogen may help rule out intrinsic renal disease, which impairs the reliability of urine output as an index of perfusion.

Body weight and temperature Obtaining a baseline body weight as early as possible after the burn will facilitate assessment of fluid balance. The preburn weight should be used to determine nutrition needs and drug dosages.

Body temperature should be obtained as well. Hypothermia is a major complication of burns; it is controlled by warming the environment. Hyperthermia can also occur as a result of early pyrogen release and can alter vital signs to be misleadingly suggestive of profound hypovolemia; it should be treated with antipyrogens.

Electrocardiographic status Arrhythmias are not common in young patients with burns as long as oxygenation is adequate, but they become a major concern in patients older than 45 years as a result of the stress response to the burn. Because arrhythmias may be the first clues to the presence of hypoxia and electrolyte or acid-base abnormalities, continuous electrocardiographic monitoring is required during the early postburn period.

Intake and output What goes in and what comes out should be carefully tabulated. Intake will far exceed output during the early postburn period as edema develops.

Hematocrit and hemoglobin concentration Although it is helpful to monitor the hematocrit and the hemoglobin concentration, changes in these values may not accurately reflect changes in blood volume. The rate of plasma loss often exceeds the rate of whole blood loss, which means that the hematocrit may be normal even in the face of severe volume depletion; consequently, blood loss (e.g., from escharotomies, line placement, internal bleeding, or fractures) can easily be underestimated. If, however, the hematocrit declines in the absence of hemolysis, this is a clear indication that there is a significant source of blood loss somewhere. After large burns, normalization of blood volume is almost impossible until 24 to 48 hours after the burn.

White blood cell count The initial white blood cell count may be high, normal, or low, depending on the magnitude of the stress response and the degree of white cell sequestration into the burn. The absolute value is not a particularly useful parameter during the early postburn period.

Blood glucose level The increased release of catecholamines in burn patients often leads to hyperglycemia. In elderly and diabetic patients, insulin may be required; some glucose should be infused at this time as well. Infants are prone to hypoglycemia as a result of decreased glucose stores.

Electrolyte status Because most of the fluid lost initially is plasma rather than whole blood, concentrations of sodium, chloride, and potassium remain relatively constant despite hypovolemia; variations in these values are mainly a function of the type of resuscitation fluid used. The potassium concentration will rise if severe hemolysis has occurred or if renal impairment is present. The HCO_3^- concentration varies according to perfusion status and acid-base balance.

Plasma protein and myoglobin levels A marked decrease in the plasma protein level occurs soon after a burn, with the greater part of the decrease coming in the first 4 to 6 hours. Not much can be done about this change until about 10 to 12 hours after the burn, given the rapid fluid and protein shifts. The plasma albumin level should be maintained above 2.5 g/dl.

In patients with very deep burns, especially if the burns are electrical in origin, the plasma myoglobin level should be measured. Myoglobin released from deeply injured muscles will affect renal function. This problem can be largely prevented by maintaining a higher than normal urine output.

Prothrombin time, partial thromboplastin time, and platelet count Initial values for prothrombin time and partial thromboplastin time and an initial platelet count are useful for determining whether administration of coagulation factors will be necessary. In the first 36 hours after the burn, coagulation factors and platelets are rarely needed unless a prolonged shock state has initiated disseminated intravascular coagulation or unless the patient has preexisting hepatic or hematologic disease.

INOTROPIC SUPPORT

Inotropic support in the first 24 hours is indicated if inadequate perfusion persists despite vigorous fluid resuscitation. This situation is most common in the elderly burn patient. If improved renal blood flow is the major goal, low-dose dopamine (1 to 4 µg/kg/min) is preferred. Moderate-dose dopamine (5 to 10 µg/kg/min) or dobutamine will increase contractility and improve cardiac output. Dobutamine results in less tachycardia. Digoxin is not recommended in the immediate postburn period, because the rapid fluid shifts during this period can lead to digitalis toxicity; in addition, digoxin is generally a less potent inotropic agent than dopamine or dobutamine.

DIURETICS

Diuretics are rarely indicated in the first 24 hours of resuscitation. The exceptions are when hemoglobinuria or myoglobinuria is present, as may occur after electrical injuries.

Initiation of Wound Management

COOLING THE WOUND

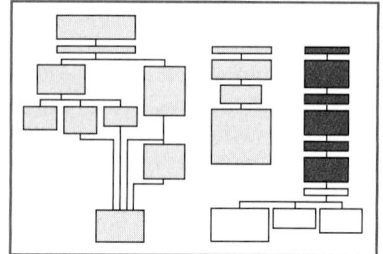

Cooling will increase heat loss, and neutralizing the heat source is a primary goal of initial management. Immediate cooling of the burn also decreases edema, apparently by stabilizing skin mast cells and thereby preventing histamine release. This effect, however, is short-lived. After the first 30 minutes, the benefit of cooling with water at a temperature of approximately 20° C is principally that of pain relief in superficially burned tissues. Prolonged cooling for pain relief is indicated only in second-degree burns covering less than 15% of TBS. Ice should never be used directly on the skin, because a freezing injury can result.

After a deep burn, the normal protective mechanism of skin vasoconstriction is absent. The barrier to water loss by evaporation—and hence the barrier to heat loss—is markedly impaired, an extremely important problem to recognize in the resuscitation period. Body heat is lost 25 times more quickly in water (wet dressings or hydrotherapy) than in air because of increased heat conductivity in water. Once hypothermia develops, rewarming is extremely slow, and decreased body temperature may affect cardiac output and perfusion of vital organs.

ASSESSMENT OF BURN DEPTH

At this point, more precise assessments of burn size and depth are needed to determine the manner of burn care and the need for transfer to a burn facility [see Figure 4 and Table 4]. The size of second- and third-degree burns must be determined in relation to total body surface [see Figure 3].

Burn depth is classified by degree of injury. Unfortunately, clinical assessment of the depth of anything more serious than a superficial second-degree burn is difficult at admission. Moreover, deeper burns tend to increase in depth over a period of hours to days as the injured but viable tissue eventually becomes nonviable, usually as a result of a low-flow state (initially) or inflammation (in the later stages). A number of techniques for clinical determination of burn depth have been employed; all have met with some success, but none have been widely adopted.

First-Degree Burns

A first-degree burn involves only the thinner outer epidermis layer and is characterized by erythema and mild discomfort. Tissue damage is minimal, and protective functions of the skin are intact. Pain, the chief symptom, usually resolves in 48 to 72 hours, and healing takes place uneventfully. The pain is probably caused by local vasodilator prostaglandin production. In 5 to 10 days, the damaged epithelium peels off in small scales, leaving no residual

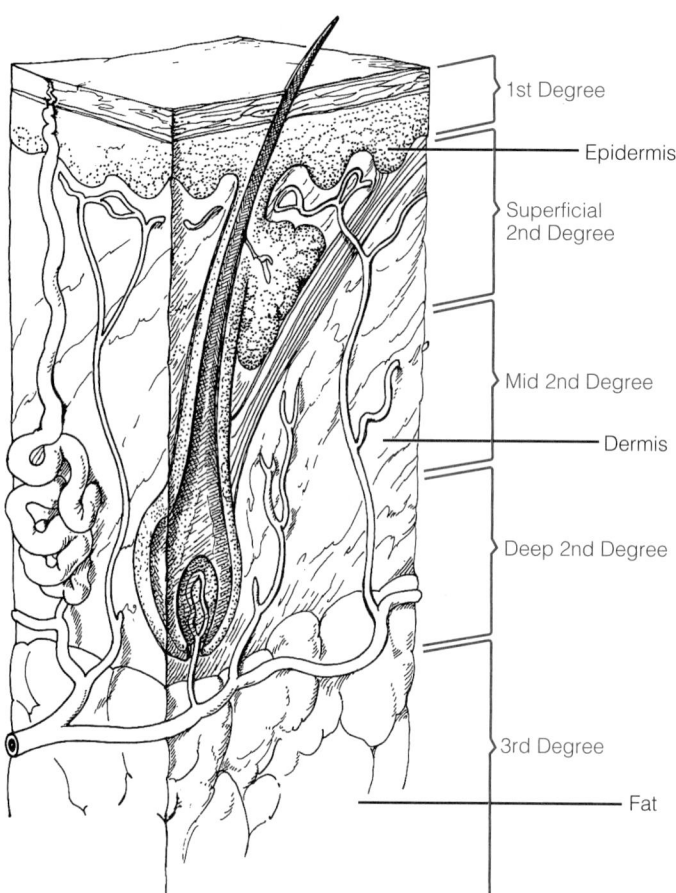

Figure 4 **Illustrated here are the depths to which skin damage extends with burns of varying degrees.**

scarring. The most common causes of first-degree burns are overexposure to sunlight and brief scalding by hot liquids.

Second-Degree Burns

Second-degree burns [see Figure 5] are those in which the entire epidermis and variable portions of the dermis have been destroyed by heat. A superficial second-degree burn involves heat injury to the upper third of the dermis. The microvessels perfusing this area are injured, and permeability is increased, with the result that large amounts of plasma leak into the interstitium. This fluid in turn lifts the thin, heat-destroyed epidermis, forming blisters. Despite the

Table 4 Physical Characteristics of Burns

Cause	Appearance	Depth	Pain
Hot liquids			
Short exposure	Wet; pink; blisters	2°	Severe
Long exposure	Wet; dark red	2°–3°	Minimal
Flames			
Flash exposure	Wet; pink; blisters	2°	Severe
Direct contact	Dry, white, and waxy; leathery brown or black	3°	Minimal
Chemicals			
Acid, alkalies	Light brown to light gray	2° (converts to 3°)	Severe

loss of the entire basal layer of the epidermis, a superficial second-degree burn will heal in 7 to 14 days owing to repopulation by the epithelial cells that line the hair follicles, sweat glands, and other skin appendages anchored deep in the dermis. Minimal scarring occurs because the wound closes rapidly; consequently, inflammation, which stimulates excessive collagen deposition, is short-lived. A deep dermal second-degree burn extends well into the dermal layer; fewer viable epidermal cells remain. Epithelialization is extremely slow, sometimes requiring months. Blister formation is not characteristically seen: because the layer of dead tissue is thick and adherent to underlying dermal collagen, it cannot be readily lifted off the surface. Exceptions occur in very young or very old patients, who have a very thin dermis. The surface of the wound is usually red, with some evidence of plasma leakage from remaining intact blood vessels. Blood supply to the burned tissue is marginal; thus, there is a high probability that tissue damage will deepen with time. Pain is present but to a lesser degree than in more superficial burns. Fluid losses and the metabolic effects of deep dermal burns are basically the same as those seen with third-degree burns. Dense scarring usually results if skin grafts are not performed.

Third-Degree Burns

In a full or third-degree burn [see Figure 6], the entire epidermis and dermis are destroyed; no residual epidermal cells remain to repopulate or epithelialize. Areas of the wound not closed by wound contraction will require skin grafting. Characteristically, avascular burned tissue has the waxy white color typical of any avascular tissue. If the burn extends into the fat or if contact with a flame source has been prolonged, the leathery brown or black color typical of charred tissue is seen. The most common cause of third-degree burns is a short exposure to a very high temperature, such as direct contact with a flame. However, prolonged contact with only moderately hot liquids (e.g., water at 125° F), as seen with intentional scalding, can result in a third-degree burn. Prolonged contact with hot liquid that leads to a third-degree burn will also lead to red cell hemolysis and release of myoglobin from underlying muscle, resulting in a red pigment deposition in the wound. The red-pigmented wound can be mistaken for viable dermis; the same appearance in a flame burn would represent only a deep second-degree injury. Therefore, a dark-red appearance in a scald burn may actually represent a full-thickness injury. The microvessels are not immediately thrombosed in second-degree injury and therefore continue to leak plasma for days. In full-thickness flame burns, however, injured capillaries are usually immediately occluded by thrombosis. The absence of pain sensation in full-thickness burns is the result of heat destruction of nerve endings. This sensory deficit distinguishes a third-degree burn from a partial-thickness injury.

Full-thickness chemical burns are light gray to brown in appearance. Pain is usually extreme because retained chemicals prolong the burning process; these retained chemicals commonly convert partial burns to full-thickness burns.

In the early postburn period (24 to 72 hours after the burn), a zone of ischemia is usually present below the dead tissue and above the deeper living tissue. The vasculature to this area has been injured. Some vessels are thrombosed; others are patent but have endothelial cell damage. The marginally viable tissue can readily convert to eschar if blood flow is further decreased because of local mediator release or infection. A deep second-degree burn—in which healing is still possible—can therefore progress to a third-degree burn. Wound conversion is prevented or minimized with prompt, adequate resuscitation.

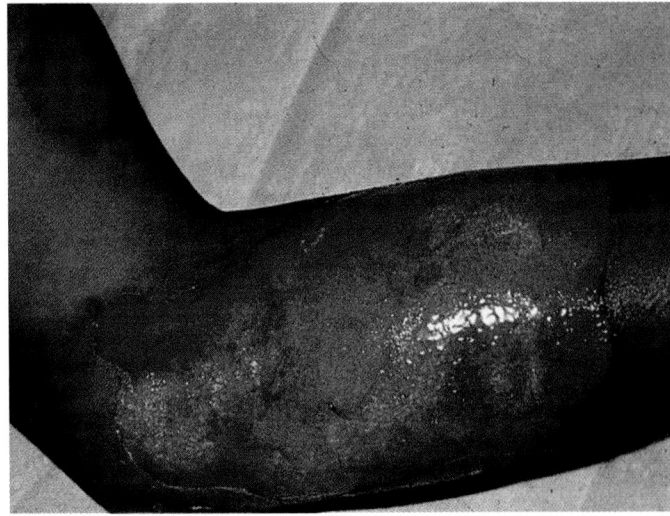

Figure 5 Immediately after injury, a second-degree burn typically has a wet, reddish appearance.

PAIN MEDICATION

Pain medication is necessary for partial-thickness burns, particularly when the wounds are cleaned. Pain control should be initiated before aggressive wound manipulation because it is important to minimize the subsequent stress response. With minor burns, oral or intramuscular narcotics may be adequate if given about 30 minutes before wound care. For major burns [see Table 5], intravenous narcotics in small doses are appropriate; erratic absorption from the gastrointestinal tract, skin, and muscles makes these routes of administration both ineffective and dangerous.

REMOVAL OF FOREIGN BODIES AND LOOSE NONVIABLE TISSUE

When a patent airway, breathing, and circulation are ensured, the wound can be debrided and cleaned. Soot and dirt are best removed with a mild dilute detergent such as a chlorhexidine product. Gross debris, loose sloughed skin, or skin overlying broken blisters should be gently removed with forceps and scissors. Rough scrubbing should be avoided to prevent further harm to the injured tissues. Ground-in dirt will gradually work its way to the surface with daily dressing changes. The surrounding skin should be

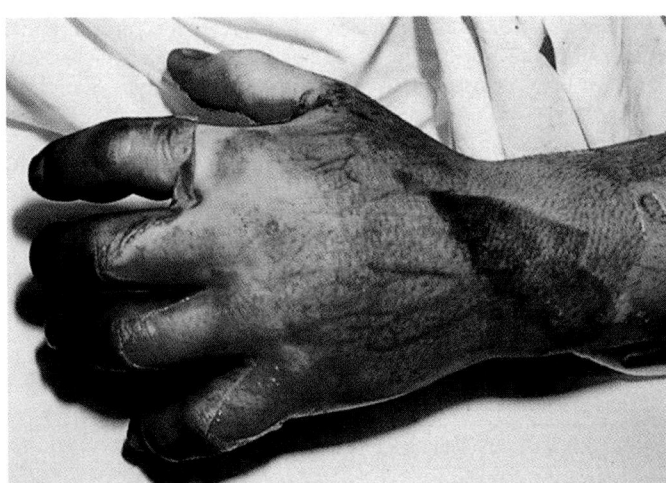

Figure 6 Shown is a full-thickness burn of the hand that actually extends below the dermis into subdermal tissue.

Table 5 Classification of Severity of Burn Injury

Critical burns

2° burns involving > 30% TBS

3° burns involving > 10% TBS

Any burns complicated by respiratory tract injury, fractures, or involvement of critical areas (i.e., face, hands, feet, perineum)

High-voltage electrical burns

Lesser burns in patients with significant preexisting disease

Moderate burns

2° burns involving 15%–20% TBS (if critical areas are not involved)

3° burns involving 2%–10% TBS (if critical areas are not involved)

Minor burns

2° burns involving < 15% TBS (if critical areas are not involved)

3° burns involving < 2% TBS (if critical areas are not involved)

---

shaved to facilitate local wound care. Large intact blisters can be left in place for 48 hours, reducing discomfort and the risk of underlying dermal desiccation.

If a hydrotherapy tank is to be used at this time for wound cleaning, the patient must be hemodynamically stable because good hemodynamic monitoring will be impossible during the procedure. Sequential cleaning of the various burned areas at bedside allows continuous monitoring and minimizes hypothermia and is thus a safer approach. A warm environment during burn care, preferably 30° to 35° C (86° to 95° F), is necessary to avoid heat loss.

Tar burns present unique problems. Tar removal is particularly difficult because the heat of the tar (150° to 200° C) usually results in a deep burn, and the rapid cooling leads to adherence to the skin. Tar can be gently removed without further tissue damage by means of repeated applications of petroleum-based ointments (such as Neosporin), which also contain surface-active emulsifying agents that dissolve the tar and make it easier to remove.

TETANUS PROPHYLAXIS

As with any large wound, the risk of tetanus must be minimized by using standard measures [see 1:7 Acute Wound Care].

PROPHYLACTIC ANTIBIOTICS

Numerous studies have demonstrated that prophylactic systemic antibiotics do not decrease wound infection rates in either minor or major burns. The blood supply to the relatively avascular deep burn is insufficient to provide adequate tissue antibiotic levels. In addition, any open wound will become colonized with bacteria. The only exception to the dictum against prophylactic systemic antibiotics would be prophylaxis against β-hemolytic streptococcus with low-dose penicillin, particularly if the patient is at high risk for infection with this organism (i.e., if the patient is a carrier or was recently exposed).

EARLY INFECTION
CONTROL: TOPICAL
ANTIBIOTICS
AND SKIN SUBSTITUTES

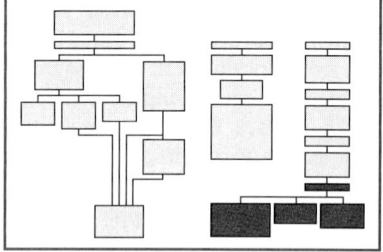

Topical Antibiotics

Because topical antibiotics decrease the rate of wound healing (in particular, the rate of epithelialization) as compared with biologic dressings or other forms of temporary skin substitutes, these agents are most useful for deep burns with eschar present and are less useful for most superficial burns or clean, healing burns. Topical agents are applied to the wound, which is then covered with dressings or left open to the environment. Both techniques are used, but the closed dressing technique is employed more because pain, heat, and fluid loss are decreased if dressings are applied. In addition, residual dermis is less likely to desiccate under a dressing.

The deep burn must be protected from early bacterial invasion, which can rapidly convert the wound to a still deeper injury. Topical antibiotics that are sufficiently water soluble to penetrate the burn eschar will temporarily control bacterial growth in the wound [see Table 6]. The half-life of the currently available topical agents is only a few hours; therefore, the agent must be applied at least twice daily to achieve a reasonable level of antibacterial protection.

Silver sulfadiazine (Silvadene) is the most commonly used topical agent because it has good antibacterial properties and because fewer complications are associated with its use. This agent, however, penetrates thick eschar less readily than some other agents and is therefore better used to prevent infection than to treat an established infection. Antibacterial properties are primarily directed against gram-negative organisms, with some antifungal effects. The primary complication of silver sulfadiazine is leukopenia as a result of transient bone marrow suppression. A white blood cell count of 2,000 to 3,000/mm³ can be seen after application is begun. The effect is transient; the white cell count returns toward normal after several days, even if the agent is continued.

Mafenide (Sulfamylon) is the most effective agent in its ability to penetrate burn eschar. It also has the most potent antibacterial

Table 6 Topical Antibiotic Agents

Agent	Antimicrobial Spectrum	Eschar Penetration	Local Tissue Toxicity	Systemic Toxicity	Pain on Application	Occlusive Dressings
10% Mafenide (Sulfamylon)	Broad*	Excellent	Moderate	Acidosis; carbonic anhydrase inhibition	Yes	Unnecessary
1% Silver sulfadiazine (Silvadene)	Broad	Good	Low	Transient leukopenia	Minimal	Preferred
0.1% Gentamicin sulfate ointment	Broad†	Fair	Low	? Renal toxicity; ? ototoxicity	Minimal	Preferred
0.5% Povidone-iodine (Betadine)	Broad	Fair	Low	Renal, CNS, and iodine toxicity	Yes	Preferred
Bacitracin ointment	Gram-positive organisms	Surface only	Low	Renal toxicity	No	Optional

*Most potent of the topical agents. †Has no antifungal properties.

properties and is particularly effective against gram-negative organisms. The agent has some antifungal properties as well. However, mafenide, as a carbonic anhydrase inhibitor, can potentiate pulmonary insufficiency and metabolic acidosis; hence, it also produces the most significant complications. In addition, application is painful in many cases. This agent is used primarily as a second line of defense or as a primary treatment for small, infected wounds.

Povidone-iodine (Betadine) ointment is usually used only on relatively thin eschar because its tissue penetration is not very good. The active agent is iodine, which is quite effective against both bacteria and fungi. Agents such as gentamicin and bacitracin can be used for more selective infections [*see Table 6*], but systemic toxicity can occur if these agents are used over large open wounds. Bacitracin is reasonably effective against wound colonization with gram-positive organisms. Bacitracin and gentamicin, however, have no antifungal properties, and prolonged use on an open wound can precipitate fungal growth.

Temporary Skin Substitutes

A number of temporary skin substitutes have been developed to improve healing of partial-thickness wounds as well as to protect clean, excised wounds when autografts are not performed immediately. Skin substitutes allow excision of burned tissue even if insufficient skin is available for autograft, permitting more rapid removal of devitalized tissue. The properties required of a temporary skin substitute have been well defined. Most important, it must adhere to the wound to maximize the epithelialization rate and minimize inflammation and fibrosis.

There are two types of temporary skin: biologic and synthetic. Biologic dressings are from previously living tissue, including amniotic membranes, xenografts, and allografts (or cadaver skin), although the last is only of limited availability and is used primarily to cover excised wounds. A number of synthetic skin substitutes have been developed that have the advantages of ready availability, long shelf life, and minimal risk of disease transmission.

SUBESCHAR EDEMA IN EXTREMITIES

The increased pressure that accompanies the development of subeschar edema is of particular concern in extremities with circumferential burns. In such cases, if the increasing pressure cannot be dissipated, a decrease in venous outflow results; this effect speeds the rate of edema formation and further elevates tissue pressure until there is marked impairment of arterial blood flow to the tissues distal to the obstruction.

Immediate elevation of the burned extremity decreases the magnitude of tissue edema. Perfusion is best monitored by the Doppler flowmeter or by assessment of capillary refill. Immediate escharotomy is indicated [*see Figure 2*] if there is a decrease in pulsatile flow beyond the burn.

Transfer to Specialized Burn Facility

Patients whose burns are critical [*see Table 5*] should be transferred to specialized burn facilities as early as possible after their injury, once the initial assessment and resuscitation have begun. Moderate burns necessitate hospitalization but may be manageable outside a burn facility if a local surgeon with an interest or expertise in burns will accept responsibility for the patient's care. Minor burns may be manageable on an outpatient basis.

A major reason for the impressive progress made in the field of burn therapy has been the expansion of the concept of specialized centers for burns. There are now more than 150 burn units in the United States as compared with a mere dozen a few decades ago. About 21,000 burn patients—approximately one third of all hospitalized burn patients—are treated yearly in these 1,700 specialized burn care beds. The centralization of patients has made possible not only improved care but also multidisciplinary research.

Recommended Reading

Barillo D, Goode R, Esch V: Cyanide poisoning in victims of fire: analysis of 364 cases and review of the literature. J Burn Care Rehabil 15:46, 1994

Crapo R: Causes of respiratory injury. Respiratory Injury: Smoke Inhalation and Burns. Haponik E, Munster A, Eds. McGraw-Hill Book Co, New York, 1990, p 47

Crum RL: Cardiovascular and neurohumoral responses following burn injury. Arch Surg 125:1065, 1990

Deitch E: The management of burns. N Engl J Med 323:1249, 1990

Demling R: Fluid resuscitation. The Art and Science of Burn Care. Boswick J, Ed. Aspen, Rockville, Maryland, 1982, p 189

Demling R: Smoke inhalation injury. New Horizons in Critical Care. Demling R, Ed. Williams & Wilkins, Baltimore, 1993, p 422

Demling R, Knox J, Youn Y, et al: Oxygen consumption early post burn becomes oxygen dependent with the addition of smoke inhalation injury. J Trauma 32:593, 1992

Fitzpatrick J, Cioffi W: Diagnosis and treatment of inhalation injury. Total Burn Care. Herndon D, Ed. WB Saunders Co, Philadelphia, 1996, p 174

Fratianno R, Brandt C: Improved survival of adults with extensive burns. J Burn Care Rehabil 18:347, 1997

Heimbach D: Burn depth. World J Surg 16:10, 1992

Jeng J, Lee K, Jordan M: Serum lactate and base deficit suggest inadequate resuscitation of patients with burn injury. J Burn Care Rehabil 18:402, 1997

Masanes M, Legendre C: Fiberoptic bronchoscopy for the early diagnosis of subglottal inhalation injury: comparative value in the assessment of prognosis. J Trauma 36:59, 1994

Pruitt B: The evolutionary development of biologic dressings and skin substitutes. J Burn Care Rehabil 18:52, 1997

Scheulen JJ, Munster AM: The Parkland formula in patients with burns and inhalation injury. J Trauma 22:869, 1982

Silverman S, Purdue G, Hunt J, et al: Cyanide toxicity in burned patients. J Trauma 28:171, 1988

Vinus B, Matsuda T, Coprizo JB, et al: Prophylactic intubation and continuous positive airway pressure in the management of inhalation injury in burn victims. Crit Care Med 9:519, 1981

Youn Y, LaLonde C, Demling R: Oxidants and pathophysiology of burn and smoke inhalation injury. Free Radic Biol Med 12:409, 1992

Acknowledgment

Figures 2 through 4   Carol Donner.

13 BURN CARE IN THE EARLY POSTRESUSCITATION PERIOD

Robert H. Demling, M.D., F.A.C.S.

Approach to the Burn Patient during the Second to Fifth Days after the Burn

Beginning about 36 hours after injury, major physiologic and biochemical changes occur that differ from earlier alterations [*see 5:12 Burn Care in the Immediate Resuscitation Period*]. The interval after resuscitation and before the onset of inflammation is generally the most stable period for burn patients. One exception is the patient with a severe inhalation injury, symptoms of which usually become most severe several days after the injury.

Maintenance of Pulmonary Function

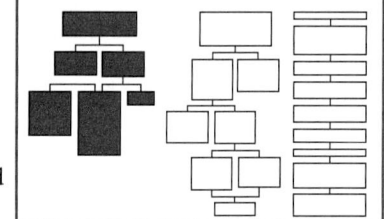

ENDOTRACHEAL INTUBATION

Intubation is required for the three Ps:

1. Maintenance of a *patent* airway.
2. *Pulmonary* toilet.
3. *Positive pressure* ventilation.

If edema threatens to compromise airway patency by distortion and compression, intubation is mandatory and should be continued until the upper airway edema begins to resolve, usually between postburn days 2 and 4; elevating the patient's head 30° to 40° allows faster resolution of edema. Oral and facial edema from the burn begins to resolve at this time as well. In the presence of a full-thickness neck burn, tissue edema—including mucosal edema—resolves much more slowly. Positive end-expiratory pressure during this period will help prevent small airway collapse. The injured mucosa is very prone to superinfection because mucosal irritation and increased mucus production persist for several days, whereas clearance is decreased because of the damaged ciliary action of the mucosa. Aggressive mouth care to prevent mucosal infection (particularly with anaerobes) is necessary because aspiration of infected saliva leads to airway infection.

The decision when to extubate is a difficult one because no test of airway patency is foolproof. Laryngoscopy is helpful in that it can determine whether cord edema is present; however, edema of the false cords or the oropharynx, as well as external compression from a neck burn, can impair airway patency even if minimal cord edema is present. As a rule, therefore, extubation should not be performed unless reintubation is technically feasible. If the patient

clearly has a severe inhalation injury or a large burn that will necessitate airway protection or ventilatory assistance, a tracheostomy through an unburned or an excised and grafted area of the neck should be done at an early stage (e.g., the first excision and grafting procedure). Percutaneous tracheostomy through unburned skin is an effective approach.

VENTILATION

In the patient without an inhalation injury, lung function during this period is usually surprisingly good if blood volume is not excessively increased. Although massive soft tissue edema is present, lung water measurements are consistently normal or only minimally elevated in both animal and human studies. However, in the presence of inelastic burned tissue and subeschar edema, chest wall compliance may remain significantly decreased. Because the work of breathing is increased, the decreased compliance may result in a diffuse microatelectasis if it is not recognized and aggressively treated.

When initial energy stores are depleted, mechanical ventilatory support may be needed to assist with the increased work load that results from the impaired chest wall function. Although parenchymal pulmonary function may be adequate, it is also important to consider work load and caloric demand before removing ventilatory support. Maintaining the patient in a semierect position improves diaphragmatic function. Oxygen administration to maintain adequate blood oxygen content and tissue oxygen tension is frequently required, for several days at least, after any large burn. Arterial oxygen saturation should be maintained at 90% or greater, preferably with a fraction of inspired oxygen (F_IO_2) of 0.5 or less. In addition, the sequential surgical excisions and wound closure initiated around postburn day 2 or 3 frequently make ventilatory assistance necessary for longer periods because general anesthesia is used every 2 to 3 days and narcotic usage is increased to control postoperative pain, particularly in donor sites. Fluid overload should be carefully avoided to minimize lung dysfunction.

MANAGEMENT OF PULMONARY INJURY

The clearance of soot, mucopurulent exudate, and sloughed mucosa is a major problem during this period, particularly if mucociliary action is impaired by smoke damage. An aggressive surgical approach to the burn wound cannot be undertaken, however, in the absence of good lung function. Airway collapse and atelectasis will result in an increasing shunt and an increasing risk of bronchopneumonia. Bronchodilators, in particular those delivered by aerosol, are very helpful, along with chest physical therapy and frequent repositioning of the patient. Mechanical ventilatory assistance may be necessary in severe cases.

The clinical magnitude of a chemical injury to the smaller airways becomes much more evident during this period. At the very least, mucosal irritation will persist for several days, causing bronchorrhea, increased coughing, and mucus production. Impairment of the ciliary function of the airway lining leads to a high risk of infection, manifested first (in the next 3 to 4 days) by bacterial tracheobronchitis and subsequently by bronchopneumonia. Bacterial colonization is inevitable. When the injury is severe, the damaged mucosa typically becomes necrotic 3 to 4 days after injury and begins to slough. Increased viscous secretions can lead to distal airway obstruction and atelectasis and can place the patient at high risk for rapidly developing bronchopneumonia.

If the chemical burn to the lung occurs in combination with a body burn, the morbidity and mortality of both processes are substantially higher than they would be otherwise.

Diagnosis

In the first several days after injury, soot continues to be present in the airway secretions. Diffuse rhonchi are usually present once inflammation develops. Wheezing often persists as a result of continued bronchospasm and (more frequently) bronchial edema. Continued coughing, as well as the residual airway edema and bronchospasm, increases the work of breathing, which can lead to fatigue and hypoventilation. Secretions then become tenacious and more difficult to clear. In the most severe airway injuries, rales compatible with edema are noted, especially when concomitant volume overload is present. Bacterial tracheobronchitis is common and is followed by bronchopneumonia in a substantial number of patients; the primary pathogen is usually *Staphylococcus aureus*. The symptom complex includes the following: (1) sputum changing from loose to mucopurulent, (2) evidence of necrotic tissue in sputum, (3) increased work of breathing, (4) altered gas exchange, and (5) infiltrates on radiographs (a late finding). The initial presentation is not necessarily an accurate guide to the magnitude of injury: lung function may be deceptively good on day 2, only to deteriorate rapidly on day 3 or 4.

In general, chest radiographs obtained during this period do not reveal the full severity of the lung damage, because the injury usually is initially confined to the airways. Clinical evidence of continued respiratory compromise—dyspnea, tachypnea, diffuse wheezing, and rhonchi—precedes any radiographic changes. The first radiographic indication of lung damage is usually diffuse atelectasis, pulmonary edema, or bronchopneumonia. Parenchymal changes are late findings.

Treatment

Endotracheal intubation may be necessary if clearance of secretions is inadequate. Ventilatory assistance may also be necessary if the patient is fatigued and if gas exchange is deteriorating. Bronchodilators, particularly those delivered by aerosol [*see 5:12 Burn Care in the Immediate Resuscitation Period*], are also helpful, as are frequent changes in position to facilitate postural drainage. Continuously rotating beds are ideal for patients with inhalation injury and large body burns, who often find it difficult to move from side to side because of pain and stiffness from tissue edema; the constant postural drainage helps to remove airway plugs.

Infection surveillance is crucial during this early period so that bacterial bronchitis can be detected before pneumonia develops.

Sputum smears should be obtained, and the character of the sputum should be monitored. Systemic antibiotics are not given prophylactically but are administered when a bacterial process becomes evident; it is important not to wait for obvious radiographic evidence of bronchopneumonia, because the process, once well established, is difficult to reverse. Broad-spectrum antibiotics can be used until susceptibility test results become available and a more specific antibiotic regimen can be instituted.

Maintenance of Hemodynamic Stability

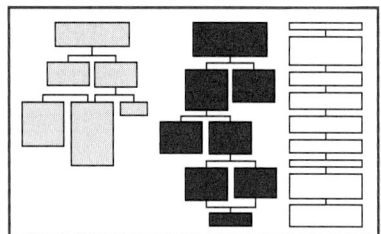

RESTORATION OF BLOOD VOLUME

Although cardiac output may be restored toward normal by fluid resuscitation during the first 24 hours after a burn, blood volume frequently decreases, particularly in the large burn, because of the substantial loss of fluid from the plasma to the interstitial space; edema is maximal at 24 to 36 hours after a burn. Restoration of blood volume is more feasible during the early postresuscitation period. Adequate perfusion pressure must be maintained (i.e., systolic blood pressure greater than 90 mm Hg and urine output 0.5 to 1.0 ml/kg/hr). In the presence of hypovolemia and severe hypoproteinemia (0.5% of normal), plasma protein levels should be restored toward normal to decrease crystalloid needs and to improve gastrointestinal function. Improved gastrointestinal function will be of considerable importance for nutritional support. Protein solutions should be given to replace volume loss [*see 5:12 Burn Care in the Immediate Resuscitation Period*]; such solutions should not be administered to patients who are normovolemic or hypervolemic, because volume overload and its complications may result, especially during the fluid mobilization period.

Red blood cells are injured during the burning process and again as a result of the mediator release from burned tissue. Red cell lipid peroxidation is characteristically seen after a burn. The increased fragility leads to a decreased half-life. Red cell hematopoiesis is also markedly impaired. The combination of these processes leads to anemia, beginning during the early postresuscitation period. Red cells should be provided if necessary to maintain a hematocrit of at least 30%, given the increasing oxygen demands in burn patients during this period and the chronic nature of the impaired production.

MAINTENANCE OF FLUID AND ELECTROLYTE BALANCE

A measurable increase in protein permeability in burned tissue vessels persists for days to weeks. The rate of fluid and protein loss into the burned interstitium lessens considerably after the first two postburn days; however, protein loss from the surface of a partial-thickness burn can still be substantial.

After postburn day 2, evaporation from the surface of deep burns becomes a major source of water loss that persists until the wound is closed. Losses are comparable to those expected from an open pan of water with the same surface area. It is possible to calculate a reasonable estimate of water loss from the surface of deep burns [*see Table 1*].

During the early postresuscitation period, however, intravascular fluid is gained from the resorption of edema fluid. Therefore, continued replacement of free water lost from evaporation and of protein lost into burned tissue and from the burned surface must be balanced against these intravascular fluid gains.

Approach to the Burn Patient during the Second to Fifth Days after the Burn

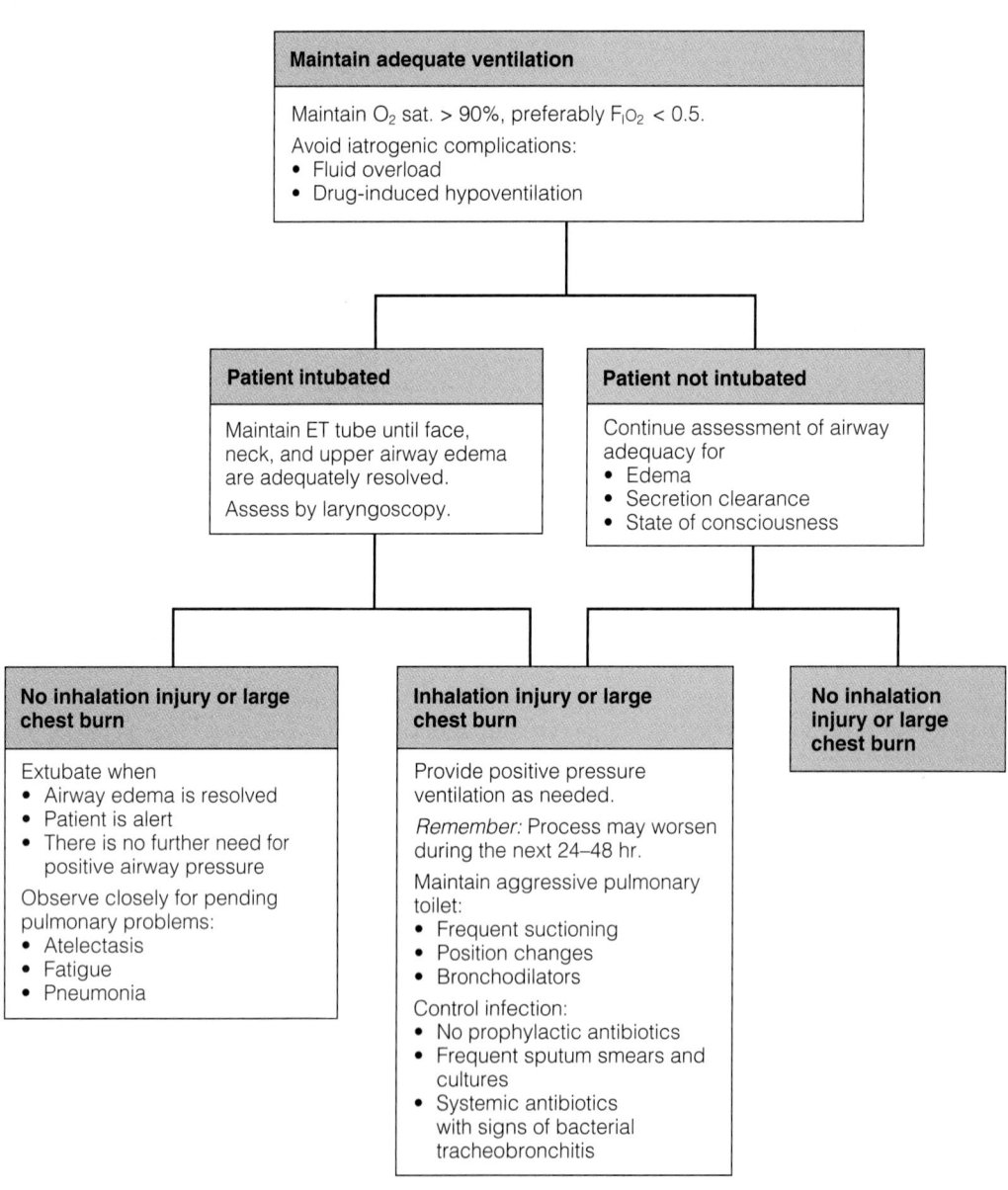

Maintain adequate ventilation

Maintain O_2 sat. > 90%, preferably F_iO_2 < 0.5.

Avoid iatrogenic complications:
- Fluid overload
- Drug-induced hypoventilation

Patient intubated

Maintain ET tube until face, neck, and upper airway edema are adequately resolved.

Assess by laryngoscopy.

Patient not intubated

Continue assessment of airway adequacy for
- Edema
- Secretion clearance
- State of consciousness

No inhalation injury or large chest burn

Extubate when
- Airway edema is resolved
- Patient is alert
- There is no further need for positive airway pressure

Observe closely for pending pulmonary problems:
- Atelectasis
- Fatigue
- Pneumonia

Inhalation injury or large chest burn

Provide positive pressure ventilation as needed.

Remember: Process may worsen during the next 24–48 hr.

Maintain aggressive pulmonary toilet:
- Frequent suctioning
- Position changes
- Bronchodilators

Control infection:
- No prophylactic antibiotics
- Frequent sputum smears and cultures
- Systemic antibiotics with signs of bacterial tracheobronchitis

No inhalation injury or large chest burn

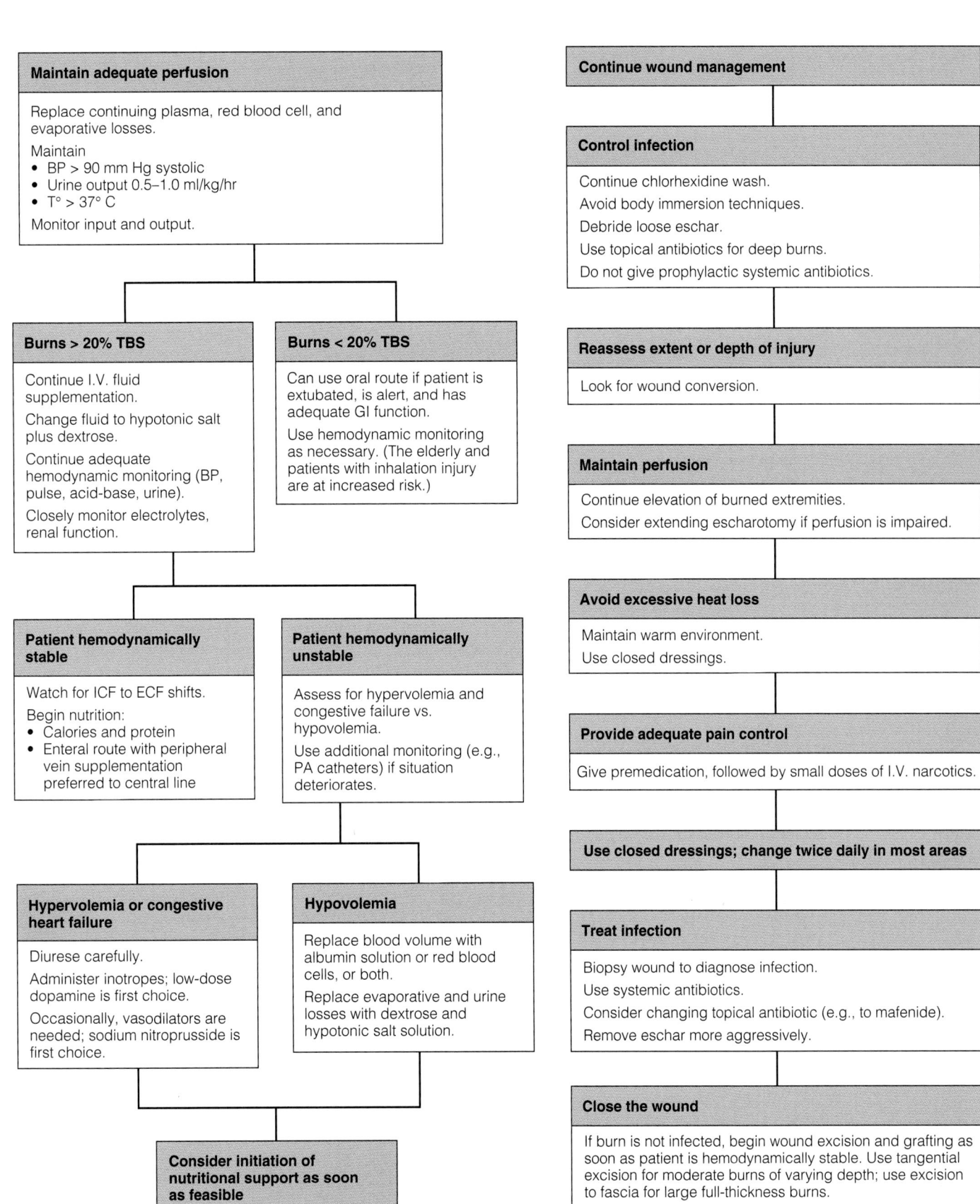

Maintain adequate perfusion

Replace continuing plasma, red blood cell, and evaporative losses.

Maintain
- BP > 90 mm Hg systolic
- Urine output 0.5–1.0 ml/kg/hr
- T° > 37° C

Monitor input and output.

Burns > 20% TBS

Continue I.V. fluid supplementation.

Change fluid to hypotonic salt plus dextrose.

Continue adequate hemodynamic monitoring (BP, pulse, acid-base, urine).

Closely monitor electrolytes, renal function.

Burns < 20% TBS

Can use oral route if patient is extubated, is alert, and has adequate GI function.

Use hemodynamic monitoring as necessary. (The elderly and patients with inhalation injury are at increased risk.)

Patient hemodynamically stable

Watch for ICF to ECF shifts.

Begin nutrition:
- Calories and protein
- Enteral route with peripheral vein supplementation preferred to central line

Patient hemodynamically unstable

Assess for hypervolemia and congestive failure vs. hypovolemia.

Use additional monitoring (e.g., PA catheters) if situation deteriorates.

Hypervolemia or congestive heart failure

Diurese carefully.

Administer inotropes; low-dose dopamine is first choice.

Occasionally, vasodilators are needed; sodium nitroprusside is first choice.

Hypovolemia

Replace blood volume with albumin solution or red blood cells, or both.

Replace evaporative and urine losses with dextrose and hypotonic salt solution.

Consider initiation of nutritional support as soon as feasible

Continue wound management

Control infection

Continue chlorhexidine wash.

Avoid body immersion techniques.

Debride loose eschar.

Use topical antibiotics for deep burns.

Do not give prophylactic systemic antibiotics.

Reassess extent or depth of injury

Look for wound conversion.

Maintain perfusion

Continue elevation of burned extremities.

Consider extending escharotomy if perfusion is impaired.

Avoid excessive heat loss

Maintain warm environment.

Use closed dressings.

Provide adequate pain control

Give premedication, followed by small doses of I.V. narcotics.

Use closed dressings; change twice daily in most areas

Treat infection

Biopsy wound to diagnose infection.

Use systemic antibiotics.

Consider changing topical antibiotic (e.g., to mafenide).

Remove eschar more aggressively.

Close the wound

If burn is not infected, begin wound excision and grafting as soon as patient is hemodynamically stable. Use tangential excision for moderate burns of varying depth; use excision to fascia for large full-thickness burns.

1005

Table 1 Calculation of Evaporative Water Loss and Required Fluid

The patient is a 70 kg male whose burns cover 50% of TBS. His body surface area is 1.7 m².

The patient's output during the previous 24 hours:
Urine: 2,000 ml
Nasogastric tube: pulled

Evaporative water loss (ml/hr) = (25 + % TBS burned) × TBS

In this patient: (25 + 50) × 1.7 = 125 ml/hr
125 ml/hr × 24 hr/day = 3,000 ml/day

Fluid required = evaporative loss + other losses

In this patient: 3,000 ml evaporative loss/day
       + 2,000 ml urine/day
Fluid required = 5,000 ml/day

Give as 5% dextrose in 0.2% normal saline at ~ 200 ml/hr.

The rate of edema absorption depends on the burn depth and subsequent lymphatic damage. It is rapid in superficial burns, beginning at about day 2 or 3 when lymphatics are intact, but much slower after full-thickness injury.

Sodium requirements are usually minimal because of initial sodium loading and because water loss from evaporation is extensive. Therefore, the preferred crystalloid after the resuscitation period is hypotonic salt plus dextrose. Glucose administration is necessary at this point, however, because glycogen stores are totally depleted. Once glucose is administered and tissue utilization improves, large amounts of potassium must be given as well. Potassium administration will be particularly important once nutritional support is initiated because wound healing and new cell formation will increase potassium utilization. Enteral nutrition should begin as soon as the gastric ileus resolves. Nutrition can be supplemented with central or peripheral vein alimentation until the enteral route becomes totally functional [*see 5:14 Burn Care after the First Postburn Week*].

Restoration of blood flow to the burned tissue after resuscitation will result in the resorption of a large load of osmotically active particles made up of solutes from disrupted cells and fragments of denatured proteins. The increased osmotic load is very evident in second-degree burn blisters, which increase dramatically in size and pressure over a period of days. The increased solute load frequently results in an obligate solute diuresis that is manifested by increased output of high–specific gravity urine. It is important that such an increase in urinary output not be mistaken for hypervolemia; therefore, fluids should not be decreased or diuretics initiated. In the diuretic response to hypervolemia, the urine specific gravity is, of course, characteristically low.

TRANSITION FROM HYPOMETABOLISM TO HYPERMETABOLISM

As the hypermetabolic state evolves (beginning at about day 3 or 4), the response of the cardiovascular system changes. Cardiac output begins to increase and exceeds normal values as a hyperdynamic state develops. Mild to modest tachycardia is usually present, partly because of persistently elevated catecholamine levels, which may be even further potentiated by hypothermia, hypoxia, or pain. The tachycardia, however, is usually much less than that seen during the first 24 hours after the burn [*see 5:12 Burn Care in the Immediate Resuscitation Period*]. The early increased systemic vascular resistance (SVR) begins to be replaced by SVR that is lower than normal.

It is important to recognize this transition during the post-resuscitation period. The hyperdynamic state is characterized by (1) a 50% to 100% increase in oxygen consumption, (2) a 1° to 2° F rise in body temperature, (3) increased gluconeogenesis, (4) increased secretion of anti-insulin hormones (decreased glucose tolerance), and (5) increased catabolism (increased ureagenesis). The increase in oxygen consumption usually peaks 5 to 10 days after the burn. Body temperature tends to increase further as pyrogen is released from the burn wound. The characteristic rise in body temperature makes it more difficult to diagnose the presence of infection.

The increasing oxygen consumption necessitates increasing oxygen delivery by ensuring adequate blood volume, hematocrit, and oxygen saturation (i.e., lung function and cardiac output must be maintained). Lactic acidosis indicates inadequate oxygen delivery, even if P_aO_2 or oxygen saturation is normal. Oxygen demands are twice normal (100 to 140 ml/min/m² when 50% or more of the total body surface (TBS) has been burned).

Control of Burn Infection

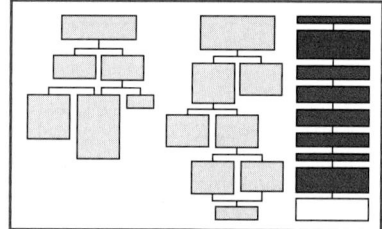

The burn wound is a major site of infection for three reasons: (1) loss of the skin barrier, (2) the presence of dead tissue, and (3) systemic immunosuppression. The stratum corneum is a relatively impermeable barrier to bacterial invasion through the skin. Loss of this barrier as a result of burn injury permits bacteria to populate the underlying tissues. Most of these early colonizing bacteria are endogenous, deriving from heat-injured skin (especially hair follicles, sweat glands, and sebaceous glands), the nares and the oropharynx, the perineum, or stool [*see Tables 2 through 4*]. The bacteria migrate to the wound by way of wet dressings, immersion in water, hand contact, and, to a lesser extent, aerosolization. The reduced blood flow to the surface of the burn impairs local immune defenses (white blood cells need oxygen to kill bacteria); it also decreases the ability of phagocytes and opsonins to reach the wound. In addition, the wound itself releases a number of immunosuppressive substances that impair both cell-mediated and humoral immunity.

DAILY BURN CARE AND INFECTION CONTROL METHODS

In general, significant bacterial colonization of the burn wound does not occur for several days after injury unless the wound initially is heavily contaminated or inadequately cleaned and treated. The eschar remains intact. Surgical excision of the deep burn is most appropriate during this period because the wound is not yet infected or revascularized [*see Wound Closure, below*].

Wound conversion is common during this period as injured tissue becomes nonviable. Frequent reassessment of the wound is

Table 2 Organisms Most Commonly Recovered from Burn Wounds in First Week

Organism	% of Patients
Staphylococcus aureus	85
β-Hemolytic streptococcus	5
Pseudomonas aeruginosa	25
Escherichia coli	40
Enterococcus	55
Candida albicans	40

Table 3 Findings Distinguishing Colonization
of Burn Wound from Invasive Infection

Findings	Colonization	Invasive Infection
Systemic changes	Variable body temperature	Increased body temperature
	WBC count increased, with mild left shift	WBC count either high or low, with pronounced left shift
	Wound may appear either purulent or benign	Wound may appear purulent, or wound surface may appear dry and pale
Bacterial characteristics	Surface bacterial content ranging from trace to large	Surface bacterial content variable
	Usually < 10^5 bacteria/g tissue on biopsy	Usually > 10^5 bacteria/g tissue on biopsy
	No invasion of normal tissue	Invasion of normal tissue

necessary. In addition, continued edema can still lead to excessive increases in tissue pressure, necessitating additional escharotomies. During this period, burned extremities should remain elevated and active and passive range-of-motion exercises should begin.

Evidence of tissue necrolysis remains absent until neutrophils, bacteria, or both proliferate in the eschar, leading to liberation of proteases and breakdown of tissue. Topical antibiotic therapy rehydrates and softens the eschar more rapidly, thereby allowing inflammatory cells to migrate into the subeschar space. Increased bacterial proliferation is then possible if the amount of topical antibiotic is not sufficient.

The epidemiology of burn wound infection seems to indicate that—in the first week, at least—the primary bacteria present are cutaneous organisms and, to a lesser extent, pulmonary and enteric organisms. This predominance of endogenous bacteria is reflected in the early colonization of the wound by gram-positive bacteria, primarily *S. aureus*, followed in several days by the beginning of gram-negative colonization.

Exogenous bacteria are certainly present in any standard critical care unit; these ordinarily resistant organisms become significant pathogens after the normal flora has been altered by the use of systemic antibiotics. The principal mode of cross-contamination with more resistant strains appears to be direct contact; air is a less significant vehicle. Compulsive hand washing between patient contacts is crucial to minimize this problem. Changes of cap, gown, and mask are also very helpful. Sophisticated isolation techniques (e.g., isolators) are not routinely necessary.

Wound Care

In wounds not amenable to early surgical closure or closure with temporary skin substitutes, daily removal of devitalized tissue, wound exudate, and inactive topical agents is important. A number of approaches are used; the primary objective is to maximize wound cleaning while minimizing patient stress. Hydrotherapy is one approach. Adequate pain control [*see* Stress Control, Analgesia and Sedation, *below*] and adequate safeguards against hypothermia are necessary. It has also become clear that immersion in a hydrotherapy tank can result in significant cross-contamination from perineum to wound or from one burned area to another. Therefore, it is recommended that the patient's head be up on a slanted board or that showers be used so that water runs off the wounds, maximizing mechanical debridement and minimizing stagnation. Another approach, which is very effective, is bedside wound care: each portion of the body is cleaned and rewrapped independently, both to minimize pain and to minimize bacterial cross-contamination. When early excision has been performed, bedside wound care is particularly useful to avoid contamination of clean, grafted wounds and donor sites. In addition, vascular catheters can be protected. A warm environment during burn care, preferably 30° to 35° C (86° to 95° F), is necessary to prevent excessive heat loss when the wound is open. Pyrogen release as a result of wound manipulation can be anticipated. Use of antipyretics before wound care is initiated can significantly attenuate this response.

Topical Antibiotics

Topical antibiotics that are sufficiently water soluble to penetrate the burn eschar will temporarily control bacterial growth in the wound [*see 5:12 Burn Care in the Immediate Resuscitation Period*]. Superficial burns do not require topical antibiotics unless they are heavily contaminated—for example, with ground-in dirt. If the burn is extremely deep (i.e., extending into fat or muscle) or clearly infected, mafenide (Sulfamylon) will be more effective in controlling bacterial growth.

Systemic Antibiotics

Systemic antibiotics are used to treat established infection and are not for prophylaxis. Prophylactic antibiotics for small burns

Table 4 Characteristics of Invasive Burn Wound Infection
with Specific Etiologic Organisms

Variable	Infecting Organism		
	S. aureus	*P. aeruginosa*	*C. albicans*
Wound appearance	Loss of wound granulation	Surface necrosis; patchy black	Minimal exudate
Clinical course	Slow onset (days)	Rapid onset (hours)	Slow onset (days)
CNS symptoms	Disorientation	Modest changes	Often no change
Temperature	Marked increase	High or low	Modest changes
WBC count	Marked increase	High or low	Modest changes
Blood pressure	Modest decrease	Often severe decrease	Minimal change
Mortality	5%	20% to 30%	30% to 50%

treated on an outpatient basis have also not been shown to be effective in preventing infection. There are only two exceptions. Low-dose penicillin is indicated during the first 24 to 48 hours if the patient is at particular risk for β-hemolytic streptococcus infection; however, this complication is quite uncommon. Systemic antibiotics are also indicated in the 24 to 48 hours before and after burn wound excision to protect against the effects of a transient bacteremia. The agent is selected on the basis of data from the wound culture. The administration of a dose before surgical wound manipulation, followed by continued doses for 24 hours afterward, is common practice.

Systemic antibiotics play no role in treating wound colonization, simply because the agents are incapable of penetrating the nonviable eschar from beneath in sufficient concentration to control bacterial growth. However, if sufficient bacteria ($\geq 10^5$/g eschar) are present in the wound to cause an invasion of underlying viable tissue by breakdown of tissue defense mechanisms, systemic antibiotics are indicated. Values lower than 10^5/g indicate wound colonization that does not require systemic treatment [*see* Table 3]. Diagnosis of infection is difficult to make by wound inspection alone. Full-thickness biopsies of the burn wound with determination of quantitative bacteriology are used to detect infection. However, there is considerable variability in results with this method, particularly if only a superficial biopsy is obtained. Inclusion of viable subeschar tissue is necessary to limit the inaccuracies [*see Sidebar* Technique for Wound Biopsy]. Histologic inspection of the biopsy is a more accurate method for determining tissue invasion.

Wound Closure

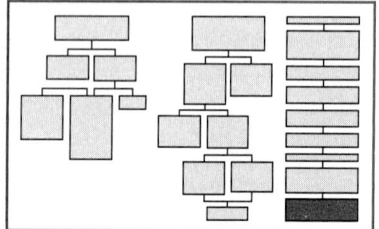

Surgical approaches to the management of large surface burns vary. At one extreme is immediate, complete wound excision to fascia and closure with a combination of autografts and skin substitutes within the first week after the burn. Another method is to initiate sequential excision and graftings, beginning about 2 to 4 days after the burn and continuing every 4 to 5 days until wound closure. The latter appears to be the safer and more common approach.

EARLY EXCISION AND GRAFTING

Risk Assessment

Before the decision is made to proceed with wound excision and grafting, two key judgments must be made:

1. Are the patient's cardiopulmonary status and the operative risk such that the potential benefits of the procedure outweigh the risks?

2. What morbidity may be expected if the wound is not rapidly closed? (This judgment takes into consideration the depth of the wound, the extent of loss of function, and the potential effects of wound inflammation on the host [*see* Table 5].)

General Principles

Four general principles apply to all methods of burn wound excision and grafting.

First, the patient must be hemodynamically stable before excision can be considered. Some degree of pulmonary dysfunction may be expected, but it should not be so severe that the patient cannot be safely moved to the operating room and back.

Second, the potential for significant blood loss must be recognized, and adequate amounts of red cells, plasma, and platelets, if indicated, must be available before treatment is begun. The potential for infection must also be recognized: at this stage, the burn is considered a clean-contaminated wound. Preoperative planning should also include perioperative administration of systemic antibiotics. Given that the initial organisms of concern are gram positive, the drug of choice is usually one of the first-generation cephalosporins.

Third, hypothermia must be avoided. Severe hypothermia is a major hazard in burn patients—particularly if coagulation is crucial, as it is when excision is being done. The operating room temperature should be maintained between 75° and 85° F.

Fourth, the stress induced by anesthesia and the operation must be kept at or below a level that the patient can safely tolerate. Because patients with major burns are potentially highly unstable, the time spent in the operating room should be carefully controlled. A reasonable operating time limit, including anesthesia, is 2 hours—less for elderly or compromised patients. It is better to perform several operations of moderate length at intervals of 1 or 2 days than to perform a single lengthy procedure. Blood loss should be carefully controlled to prevent the development of a coagulopathy: no more than 60% of estimated total blood volume should be lost in the course of any one operation. It is usually possible to stay within this limit, given good timing and careful attention to hemostasis (see below). For large excisions, two operating teams, working simultaneously,

---

Table 5 Factors Affecting Burn Wound Morbidity

Infants and the elderly tolerate burn inflammation and infection poorly.

Burns in infants and the elderly are usually deep.

Pulmonary dysfunction from smoke inhalation will be accentuated by burn-induced hypermetabolism, inflammation, and infection.

Burns tend to get deeper over the first several days as a result of necrosis of ischemic areas.

Burns caused by direct contact with flames, hot grease, chemicals, or electricity are invariably deeper than first appearances would suggest.

Burns on the lower back, the scalp, the palms, and the soles usually have sufficient remaining dermis to allow primary healing in 3 to 5 wk.

Small burns—even if they are deep dermal 2° or 3° burns—are not life threatening; therefore, the timing of operation can be much more flexible, depending on the risks to the patient.

Large 3° burns are life threatening until closed.

are required: one is responsible for obtaining the skin grafts and maintaining hemostasis from the donor site, and the other is responsible for excising the wound, maintaining hemostasis, and closing the wound. Any blood lost should be replaced with blood products rather than with crystalloid.

Other issues that must be considered in planning burn wound excision include timing of operation and recovery. Appropriate timing of excision in relation to the changes occurring in the wound itself is crucial for minimizing associated risks. There is a marked increase in blood flow to the burn wound, beginning several days after injury and peaking between days 5 and 14. This increase, which parallels the development of wound inflammation, occurs in the viable tissue beneath the eschar. Excision performed after day 5 or 6 should therefore be expected to cause significantly more blood loss than earlier excision. Any clotting abnormalities present at this stage can thus cause major problems. In addition, the wound undergoes colonization by bacteria during the first week, and manipulation of the wound after this period carries an increased risk of bacteremia.

Types of Surgical Excision

There are two types of surgical procedures for removing eschar: tangential excision and excision to fascia. Each type has advantages and disadvantages [see Table 6]. There are also several types of grafts and dressing techniques [see Grafting, below].

Tangential (sequential) excision In tangential excision, the wound is excised in thin layers with a blade held at a very acute angle to the skin surface [see Figure 1]. The objective is to remove only nonviable tissue while sparing as much viable tissue as possible. This is particularly true with patients who have deep dermal burns, in whom every effort should be made to preserve viable dermis. The dermis is responsible for the elasticity of skin, and it provides an excellent base for grafts. Fat is a less suitable base for skin grafts because of its lesser vascularity and because of the difficulty of determining viable fat on inspection.

Excision is performed with a handheld dermatome to which guards of variable thickness (0.008 to 0.020 in) may be attached. Either a Goulian knife [see Figure 1] or a Watson knife is used, depending on the area being excised: the Watson knife, being larger, is used on large, flat surfaces, whereas the Goulian knife is used on curvilinear regions (e.g., bony prominences, fingers, toes, the neck, and, occasionally, the face). Excision over bony surfaces can be facilitated by injecting saline beneath the eschar to flatten the wound and push it away from the bone. For the actual cutting, a back-and-forth motion is used, with very little forward force applied. The depth of the excision is controlled by choosing a guard of the appropriate thickness and by maintaining the blade

at the proper angle to the surface. A sharp blade is needed for this procedure, and frequent blade changes are required.

The end point of excision is brisk punctate bleeding and a completely viable wound base [see Figure 2]. Viable dermis is white and shiny; however, one or two large bleeding vessels can make the entire wound look red, which means that careful inspection and considerable experience are needed to assess the adequacy of the wound bed. Nonviable dermis is also white, but punctate bleeding is absent. Nonviable fat is more difficult to recognize because fat often appears to be in better condition than it really is. Healthy fat is light yellow and shiny; any fat that is dark yellow-brown should be removed. It is easy either to underexcise, leaving a poor base for the graft, or to overexcise, thereby removing potentially viable dermis. There is a significant risk of major blood loss, and the procedure must be approached with this risk in mind. Measures must therefore be taken to prepare for the possibility of massive bleeding, and the timing of the procedure must be carefully considered with a view to minimizing this risk [see General Principles, above].

Excision to fascia Excision of the burn wound to fascia is appropriate for patients who have very large full-thickness burns or small deep burns that extend well into fat or underlying tissue. This approach is used when the burn is large but only a limited amount of skin is available for grafting. There are three reasons why excision to fascia is suitable for these settings. First, the end point of excision to fascia is well defined, and graft take is always excellent; therefore, less experience is required to define an adequately excised wound surface. Second, wide-mesh grafts can be used because the fascia appears to be less vulnerable to desiccation than fat or dermis is when covered with a skin substitute. Third, when the procedure is performed early, large amounts of most body areas (except for the face and the perineum) can be excised with only modest blood loss. In the case of the small deep wounds, excision to the depth of the fascia or deeper is required because of the extent of the injury itself.

Excision to fascia involves a combination of sharp dissection, constant tension, and electrocauterization; instruments such as those used for tangential excision are not required. The vessels encountered at the fascial plane are less plentiful and larger than those encountered closer to the skin surface and are much easier to control with the electrocautery and ligatures. If the procedure is performed in the first several days after the burn, when the edema fluid separates fascia from overlying subcutaneous tissue, it is actually very easy. Most of the bleeding derives from the wound edge; often, such bleeding can be controlled and exposure of fat on the wound edge minimized if the skin edge is sutured to the fascia. This form of marsupialization may also decrease the total size of the wound as the edges are pulled

Table 6 Advantages and Disadvantages of Tangential Excision and Excision to Fascia

	Advantages	Disadvantages
Tangential excision	Can be performed rapidly Optimal functional and cosmetic results	Substantial blood loss End point of excision difficult to define Greater risk of underexcision or overexcision Greater need for donor skin for coverage
Excision to fascia	Can be performed rapidly, with relatively little loss of blood End point of excision well defined Tourniquets can be used Wide-mesh grafts can be used Excised areas easily covered with skin substitute	Risk of nerve injury Risk of exacerbating distal edema Risk of exposing joints or tendons Potential cosmetic defect

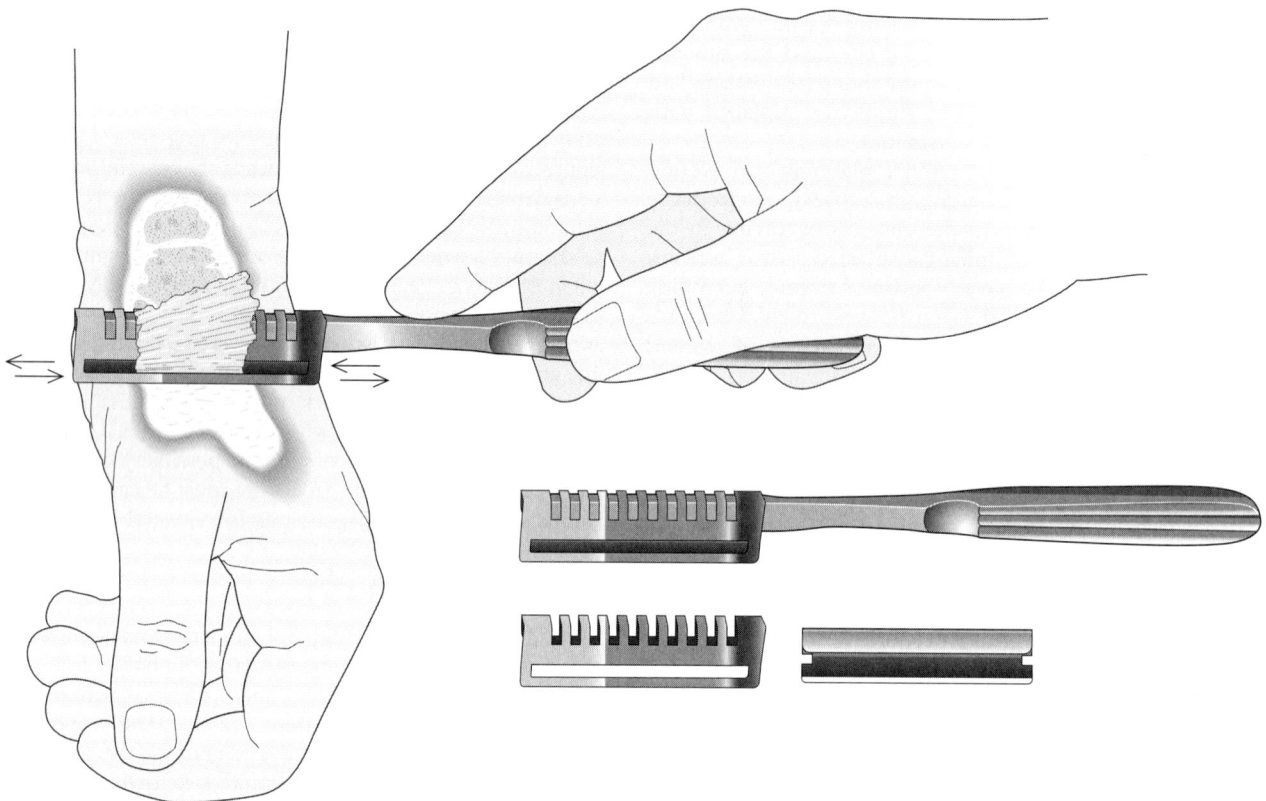

Figure 1 **In tangential excision, nonviable tissue is removed in thin layers with a handheld dermatome. Shown at lower right are the components of a Goulian dermatome.**

toward the middle. As much as 18% of TBS can be excised with only a 10% to 20% blood loss. Total excision per operation should be limited to 18% to 20% of TBS. Tourniquets may be used when an extremity is being excised to fascia (especially if excision is delayed for several days) because the end point is an anatomic one rather than punctate bleeding (as in tangential excision).

There are a number of disadvantages to this approach that must be carefully weighed against the advantages. The major disadvantage is potential impairment of long-term function of the excised and grafted areas, especially extremities. Removal of superficial veins and lymphatics may result in distal edema; however, in many burn patients, these vessels have already been destroyed by heat. Furthermore, removal of cutaneous nerves leads to impaired sensation in addition to the reduced sensation characteristic of any skin graft in comparison with normal skin, and there is a significant risk of injury to other superficial nerves that have motor function.

The second main disadvantage of fascial excision is cosmetic. A rim of tissue remains at the border between excised and nonexcised tissue and produces a balloonlike effect, especially on the extremities; tapering of the excision at its end points helps minimize this problem. Because fat normally does not regenerate between fascia and skin grafts, the cosmetic defect is persistent, particularly in obese patients. Frequently, fascial excision is combined with tangential excision to maximize the benefits of early wound closure and minimize the complications.

In patients with massive burns, these two disadvantages are outweighed by the excellent graft take and the reliability of the excision end point.

Grafting

Tangential excision Once the wound is excised, the wound bed must be closed. Usually, skin grafts are applied immediately. Meshed skin grafts allow the escape of blood and plasma that would lift a sheet graft off the wound bed. The width of the mesh (e.g., 1.5 to 1 or 3 to 1) depends on the availability of donor skin. Sheet grafts (i.e., nonmeshed grafts) are preferred for the face and

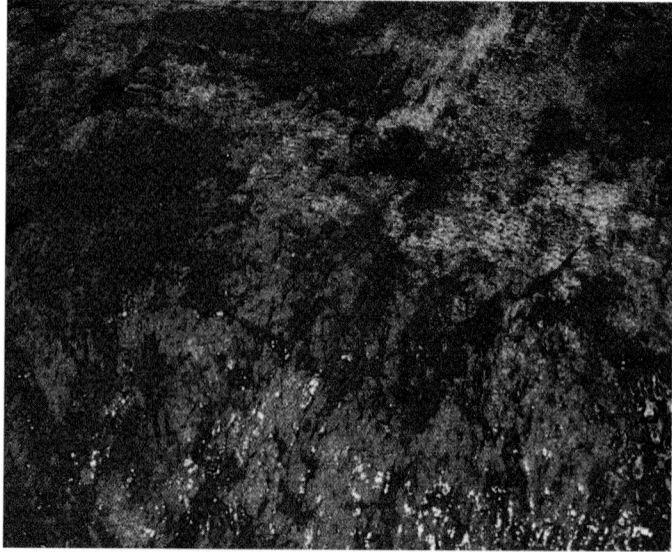

Figure 2 **After appropriate tangential excision, brisk punctate bleeding is observed over a completely viable wound base; this is the end point for the procedure.**

the hands; however, a 1.5 to 1 mesh opened just slightly for drainage can often be used with excellent cosmetic results. The mesh used for grafting after tangential excision is usually no wider than 1.5 to 1 to prevent excessive exposure of viable tissue (especially fat) so that it does not desiccate and form new eschar [*see Figure 3*].

Excision to fascia Once excised, the fascial surface must be covered. Given that donor sites are usually limited unless the wound is small, 3 to 1 meshed grafts can be used. Skin substitutes (Biobrane, pigskin, or cadaver skin) are very effective in occluding the fascial wound until the mesh fills in (between days 7 and 10) or until rehealing makes new donor sites available (between days 10 and 14).

Stress Control

The burn itself initiates the stress response to injury, which includes the development of a marked hypermetabolic state. Hypovolemia or tissue hypoxia leads to additional tissue damage, thereby amplifying the host response. Several factors (e.g., pain, anxiety, psychosis, and hypothermia), most of which are largely controllable, further amplify the stress response, exacerbating both physiologic and metabolic abnormalities. All of these factors increase secretion of stress hormones, catecholamines in particular. Psychosis and resulting sleep deprivation also lead to excessive motor activity, further increasing tissue oxygen demand and the risk of oxygen debt.

HEAT LOSS

The loss of the skin barrier increases the rate of heat loss [*see 5:12 Burn Care in the Immediate Resuscitation Period*]. Decreased body temperature is a potent stimulus for catecholamine release. In addition, a core body temperature that falls below what the hypothalamus regards as normal constitutes a strong stimulus for increased heat production (primarily via increased muscle activity).

Heat loss can be controlled by maintaining a warm (30° to 35° C [86° to 95° F]) external environment (e.g., by using radiant overhead heaters), by using occlusive dressings to prevent further convection losses, by minimizing exposure to a wet environment, and by providing adequate oxygen and nutrients. If muscle paralysis proves necessary, the ambient temperature should be further increased, and efforts should be made to achieve additional reduction of heat loss from the wound surface.

HYPERTHERMIA

Severe hyperthermia accentuates the stress response. For every 1° increase in body temperature, oxygen consumption rises by about 5% to 10%. Evaporative water loss increases as well, particularly in patients with large burn wounds. Fluid administration should be stepped up to replace lost water. Nonsteroidal antiinflammatory drugs may be given; these agents have proved to be very effective in countering hyperthermia in burn patients.

ANALGESIA AND SEDATION

Burn patients experience continuous pain simply from the presence of an open wound. The pain is stimulated by movement and is intensified during dressing changes, debridement, physical therapy, and other burn care–related procedures. Pain increases the stress response and the release of catecholamines, thereby amplifying the hypermetabolic state. The pain-induced increase in sympathetic nervous system activity results in decreased blood flow to skin and soft tissue, which can impair wound healing. Excessive pain also leads to increased release of endogenous

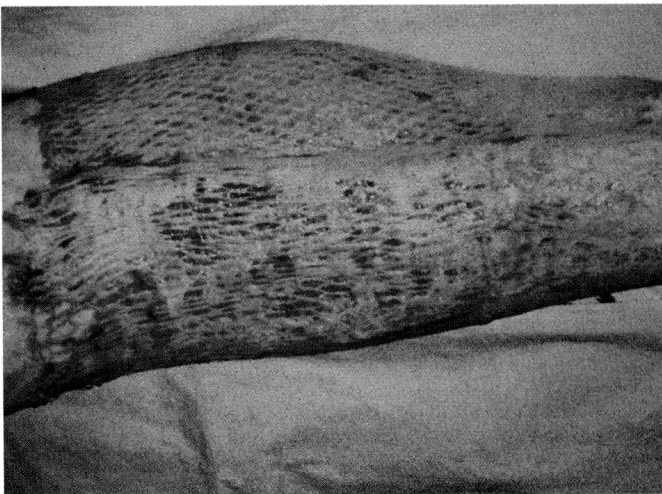

Figure 3 A 1.5 to 1 meshed skin graft has been applied to a tangentially excised wound. Blood and fluid can escape through the interstices of the mesh.

endorphins, which is known to produce both hemodynamic instability and immunosuppression.

Anxiety is also a major problem. Patients suffer from anxiety related to uncertainties about the short- and long-term consequences of their injuries. In addition, many patients experience severe anxiety related to the combination of the stress response and the effects of the ICU environment. There is evidence indicating that the stress response, like pain, leads to increased endorphin release, and it has been well documented that several elements of the ICU environment (e.g., noise, sensory deprivation, and lack of day-to-night cycles) have a major impact on the stress response. Frequent disturbances of sleep patterns may lead to disorientation, greater anxiety, and, eventually, a syndrome loosely described as ICU psychosis. Characteristically, patients with ICU psychosis exhibit a marked increase in muscle activity, which further amplifies the stress response and the hypermetabolic state.

Attempts to control pain and anxiety [*see Table 7*] are required, as well as increased support during the described maneuvers. Relaxation techniques and hypnosis have advantages over narcotics, which suppress gastrointestinal motility and cause other significant side effects.

For severe burns, I.V. narcotics administered by continuous low-dose infusions or on demand can be quite useful. In addition, sedatives such as diazepam and haloperidol are useful for treating anxiety or psychological aberrations. The addition of sedatives to pain medication or hypnosis, biofeedback, or relaxation techniques is also very useful. For chronic burn pain, give narcotics orally, intramuscularly, or intravenously (either intermittently or via low-dose continuous infusion). In addition, administer sedatives to decrease anxiety.

Table 7 Measures for Controlling Pain and Anxiety in Burn Patients

Patient-controlled analgesia

Continuous regional or intravenous infusion

Early use of benzodiazepines for anxiety and of neuroleptics for ICU psychosis

Avoidance of ICU sensory overload

NUTRITIONAL SUPPORT

Hypermetabolism and nutritional support are discussed in more detail elsewhere [*see 5:14 Burn Care after the First Postburn Week and 6:23 Nutritional Support*]. There is, however, one aspect of nutritional management that should be mentioned here—namely, early enteral feeding. Several clinical studies have indicated that initiating enteral feeding soon after the injury (i.e., in the first 48 hours) appears to reduce the degree of subsequent injury-induced hypermetabolism, possibly by preventing early bacterial migration through the gut wall (so-called gut leak). Although the data are not conclusive, it is certainly possible at this point to state that early enteral nutrition is advantageous and that feedings should be started as soon as possible, preferably in the first 48 hours.

GASTRIC pH

Gastrointestinal bleeding from burn stress (i.e., Curling ulcer) was once a major cause of morbidity, but aggressive nutritional support and wound control have decreased this problem. In burn patients as well as in critical care patients in general, maintenance of a gastric pH above 3 has been found to diminish the risk of significant ulceration and bleeding. Scheduled administration of antacids, H_2 receptor blockers, or both can be used to control pH. Continuous tube feeding—or frequent meals, in the absence of a nasogastric tube—is also very effective at decreasing ulceration and maintaining gastric pH at nonulcerogenic levels.

Physical Therapy and Splinting

It is important to maintain as much joint and muscle function as possible during the period of wound closure. If muscle function is not maintained, contraction of the wound by infiltration with myofibroblasts produces permanent impairment of joint motion or a disability requiring extensive reconstructive surgery. Joints must be maintained in the position of function during rest and moved through the limitations of extension, flexion, abduction, and adduction several times a day. Splints are fitted beginning 48 to 72 hours after the burn and refitted as edema resolves.

Recommended Reading

Alexander J: Mechanism of immunologic suppression in burn injury. J Trauma 30:70, 1990

Demling R: Effect of early burn excision and grafting on pulmonary function. J Trauma 24:830, 1984

Desai M, Herdon D, et al: Early burn wound excision significantly reduces blood loss. Ann Surg 211:756, 1990

Dimick P, Heimbach D, Mansen J, et al: Anesthesia assisted procedures in a burn intensive care unit procedure room: benefits and complications. J Burn Care Rehabil 14:446, 1993

Dobke MK, Simoni J, Ninnemann JL, et al: Endotoxemia after burn injury: effect of early excision on circulating endotoxin levels. J Burn Care Rehabil 10:107, 1989

Engrav L, Heimbach D, Reas J, et al: Early excision and grafting vs nonoperative treatment of burns of indeterminate depth. J Trauma 23:1001, 1983

Fuller F, Parrish M, Nance F: A review of dosimetry of silver sulfadiazine cream in burn wound treatment. J Burn Care Rehabil 15:213, 1994

Housinzer T, Lang D, Warden G: A prospective study of blood loss with excisional therapy in pediatric burn patients. J Trauma 34:262, 1993

Hunt J: Is tracheostomy warranted in the burn patient? Indications and complications. J Burn Care Rehabil 7:492, 1986

Lanke K, Liljedahl S: Evaporative water loss from burns, grafts, and donor sites. Scand J Plastic Reconstr Surg 5:17, 1971

Matsumura N, Sugumata A: Aggressive wound closure for elderly patients with burns. J Burn Care Rehabil 15:18, 1994

McDonald W, Deitch E: Immediate enteral feeding in burn patients is safe and effective. Ann Surg 213:177, 1991

Monafo W, Bessey P: Benefits and limitations of burn wound excision. World J Surg 16:37, 1992

Shankowsky H, Callioux L: North American survey of hydrotherapy in modern burn care. J Burn Care Rehabil 15:193, 1994

Acknowledgment

Figure 1   Tom Moore.

14 BURN CARE AFTER THE FIRST POSTBURN WEEK

Robert H. Demling, M.D., F.A.C.S.

Management of the Burn Patient from 7 Days after the Burn until Complete Wound Closure

Beginning at about postburn day 7, dramatic physiologic and biochemical changes occur, related primarily to the onset of burn wound inflammation. Local and systemic infections also become major factors. The patient with a large burn who was stable during the preceding period frequently becomes unstable again, but the pathophysiologic alterations are much different from those seen during the first postburn week.

Maintenance of Adequate Lung Function

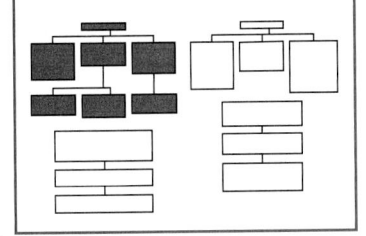

As during the early postresuscitation period, maintenance of pulmonary function is of major importance. There are two reasons for this: first, oxygen demands and carbon dioxide production are increased, and second, infection risks persist from the immunosuppressed state and from any superimposed smoke damage.

MAINTENANCE OF ADEQUATE ARTERIAL OXYGEN SATURATION

Because oxygen demands nearly double during this period in the patient with a major burn, an arterial oxygen saturation of 95% or greater is preferred, especially if it can be maintained with the fraction of inspired oxygen (F_IO_2) below 0.5, to minimize oxygen toxicity. The shunt fraction therefore must be minimized by maintaining both adequate lung volume and adequate blood volume. Atelectasis from hypoventilation or from secretion-induced obstruction of the small airways must be kept to a minimum.

MAINTENANCE OF ADEQUATE TISSUE OXYGENATION

In burn patients, blood volume, cardiac output, and hemoglobin count must be maintained at levels that optimize oxygen delivery to provide for the increased requirements. Oxygen consumption ($\dot{V}O_2$) increases from the normal value of 125 ml/min/m² to values approaching 300 ml/min/m² in burns exceeding 50% of total body surface (TBS). Pulse rate and cardiac output increase, paralleling the increase in $\dot{V}O_2$. Systemic hypertension is relatively common, as is heart failure, in patients with preexisting cardiac disease, especially the elderly. An obligate urine output of 1 to 2 ml/kg/hr is necessary to remove the increased solute load caused by the hypermetabolic state. Inadequate oxygen delivery is reflect-

ed in persistent lactic acidosis or in evidence of early organ failure (in particular, liver dysfunction).

MAINTENANCE OF ADEQUATE MINUTE VENTILATION

The increased carbon dioxide production characteristic of the postburn hypermetabolic state requires a large increase in minute ventilation ($\dot{V}_E$), sometimes twofold or threefold. The increase in $\dot{V}_E$ will depend on how large a portion of the $\dot{V}_E$ is increased dead space ventilation. If excision or grafting is to be performed, the anesthesiologist must be aware that increased ventilation is required to prevent severe hypercapnia.

MECHANICAL VENTILATORY SUPPORT

Frequently, the increased work of breathing necessitates some ventilatory assistance, particularly in the presence of a chest wall burn. Decreased chest wall compliance (in both open and grafted wounds) markedly increases the work necessary to clear the excess carbon dioxide produced. Because oxygen demands are high during this period, mechanical ventilation must be used carefully to allow adequate gas exchange without impeding oxygen delivery. Intermittent mandatory ventilation or, better yet, spontaneous ventilation is preferred to diminish wasted ventilation, provided that adequate energy is available to support the increased work of breathing. In addition, some use of positive end-expiratory pressure (PEEP) may be required to minimize atelectasis. The optimal situation, of course, is adequate spontaneous ventilation, as long as the necessary pulmonary function can be maintained. Any factor that increases carbon dioxide production (e.g., pain, excessive work, or excessive intake of carbohydrate calories) must be controlled.

PULMONARY TOILET

Pneumonia is a major problem during this period, and aggressive maintenance of pulmonary toilet is essential. Among patients in whom the airway mucosal barrier has been injured or actually denuded, pneumonia is particularly frequent and in fact is the major cause of death. The pneumonic process is accentuated by the immunodeficiency state that exists in the presence of the inflamed or infected burn wound.

Careful monitoring of sputum quantity and quality aids in detection of early infection and remains important in preventing the development of a life-threatening pneumonia. In addition, aggressive chest physiotherapy, ambulation, and cough and deep-breathing exercises must be continued until wound closure.

Management of the Burn Patient from 7 Days after the Burn until Complete Wound Closure

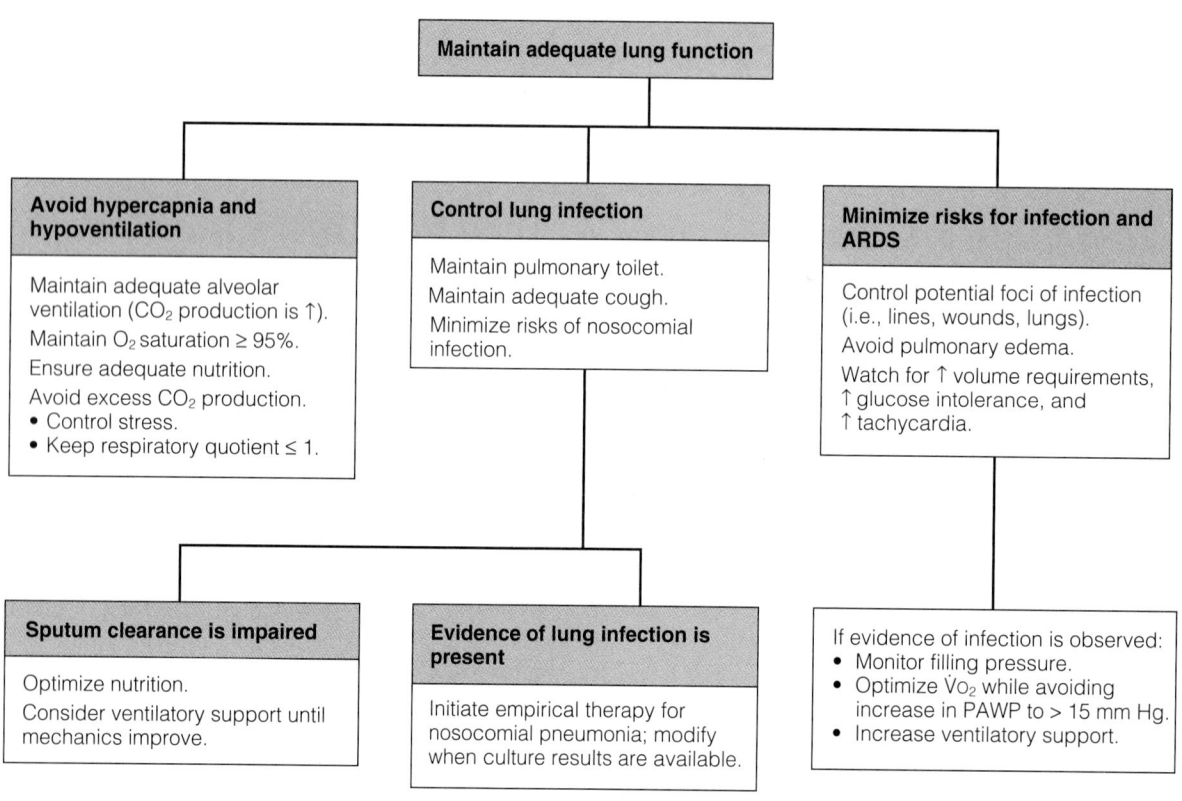

Maintain adequate lung function

Avoid hypercapnia and hypoventilation

Maintain adequate alveolar ventilation (CO_2 production is ↑).
Maintain O_2 saturation ≥ 95%.
Ensure adequate nutrition.
Avoid excess CO_2 production.
• Control stress.
• Keep respiratory quotient ≤ 1.

Control lung infection

Maintain pulmonary toilet.
Maintain adequate cough.
Minimize risks of nosocomial infection.

Minimize risks for infection and ARDS

Control potential foci of infection (i.e., lines, wounds, lungs).
Avoid pulmonary edema.
Watch for ↑ volume requirements, ↑ glucose intolerance, and ↑ tachycardia.

Sputum clearance is impaired

Optimize nutrition.
Consider ventilatory support until mechanics improve.

Evidence of lung infection is present

Initiate empirical therapy for nosocomial pneumonia; modify when culture results are available.

If evidence of infection is observed:
• Monitor filling pressure.
• Optimize $\dot{V}O_2$ while avoiding increase in PAWP to > 15 mm Hg.
• Increase ventilatory support.

Maintain adequate nutritional support

Determine total calories required:
• For burn 20%–40% TBS, 30–35 cal/kg/day.
• For burn ≥ 50% TBS, 35–45 cal/kg/day.
Determine protein requirements:
• Establish calorie-to-nitrogen ratio between 100:1 and 150:1.
Replace lost vitamins and trace elements (e.g., vitamin A, vitamin C, and zinc).

Establish appropriate nutrient mix

Of nonprotein calories, give 70% as carbohydrate.
Of final diet, give 55%–60% as carbohydrate, 20%–25% as fat, 20% as protein.

Select appropriate route

Enteral route is preferred, supplemented by parenteral route as needed.
Consider peripheral vein alimentation with increased water needs.

Maintain hemodynamic stability

Replace lost fluids and electrolytes

Estimate evaporative losses (monitor body weight, urine specific gravity, serum osmolarity, and clinical signs of hydration status).

Replenish evaporative losses: ml/hr = (25 + %TBS burn) × m².

Replace lost RBCs and protein.

Monitor electrolyte levels (particularly with nutritional support).

Maintain tissue perfusion

O_2 consumption is 1.5–2 times normal.

Maintain cardiac output at 1.5–2 times normal.

Maintain hematocrit $\geq$ 30.

Avoid lactic acidosis.

Control stress response

Control the three components of the stress response: (1) systemic inflammation (afferent arc), (2) release of stress hormones (efferent arc), and (3) CNS stimuli such as pain and anxiety (CNS modulation).

Avoid hypothermia:
- Maintain ambient T° $\geq$ 85° F.
- Minimize heat loss from wound exposure or wet dressings.

Sufficient pain control is essential.

Ensure sufficient sedation to allow for adequate rest.

Burn wound care

Gently debride wound daily.

Graft on clean granulation tissue, if wound is heavily colonized.

Excision should be done cautiously during this period because of increased risks of infection and blood loss.

Control wound infection

Control wound surface bacteria with topical antibiotics.

Treat wound infection with systemic antibiotics.

Monitor plasma levels of antibiotics.

Initiate rehabilitation

Begin and continue joint motion early.

Maintain aggressive muscle-strengthening efforts.

Mobilization should be early and continued.

Apply pressure garments (25 mm Hg) to healed wound.

Use skin moisturizers liberally.

TRACHEOSTOMY

Burn patients are at high risk for lung dysfunction, much of which can be prevented if direct access to excessive secretions can be obtained, the risk of aspirating infected oral secretions can be decreased, and patients can be intermittently rested with partial mechanical support so that the cough reflex can be maintained. A good way of achieving these objectives—given that the time course for correction of a large burn wound or a severe smoke inhalation injury is weeks rather than days—is to perform a tracheostomy. The timing of tracheostomy remains somewhat controversial; however, a tracheostomy through unburned or grafted skin should be considered appropriate if the patient is expected to require an artificial airway for several weeks. Improved pulmonary toilet, enhanced patient comfort, and the elimination of the need for frequent reintubation are all assets. If the high-risk period is short, the burn relatively small, and the patient relatively young, then weaning and extubation are appropriate.

MANAGEMENT OF PULMONARY DYSFUNCTION

Pulmonary problems remain a major cause of morbidity and mortality after the first postburn week. In fact, pulmonary failure and pulmonary infection exceed burn wound infection as causes of death in burn patients. Three major processes occur during this period: (1) nosocomial pneumonia, (2) hypermetabolism-induced respiratory fatigue (power failure), and (3) acute respiratory distress syndrome (ARDS), including low-pressure pulmonary edema. These three processes are closely interrelated. Burn patients are highly vulnerable to infection, particularly after inhalation injury. The hypermetabolic state produces a marked elevation in oxygen requirements and carbon dioxide production; the increased demands placed on the lung as a result may exceed pulmonary functional capacity. ARDS is a severe complication of the septic response; it is very difficult to reverse in burn patients.

Nosocomial Pneumonia

The term nosocomial pneumonia refers to a pneumonia that develops in the hospital in a patient who showed no evidence of lung infection on admission (i.e., to a hospital-acquired pneumonia). Although wound infection, another form of hospital-acquired infection, is more common than nosocomial infection, the latter carries a much higher mortality. Burn patients who have both inhalation injury and a major body burn are at highest risk for nosocomial pneumonia, with the incidence in this population exceeding 50%. This high incidence is attributable to the presence of virulent organisms in the hospital environment and to the immunosuppressed state of burn patients. Once pneumonia is established in a burn patient, it is very difficult to eradicate; consequently, prevention is of primary importance. Preventive measures fall into four main categories: (1) improving systemic host defenses, (2) improving local pulmonary defenses, (3) minimizing oropharyngeal colonization, and (4) minimizing tracheobronchial aspiration.

Hypermetabolism-Induced Respiratory Fatigue (Power Failure)

Several processes may impair oxygenation during this period. The severe catabolism initiated by the inflammatory response can lead not only to extremity weakness but also to chest wall muscle weakness. Chronic pain and anxiety can lead to sleep deprivation and fatigue. Heart failure can lead to lung edema, and growing fatigue can lead to hypoventilation-induced atelectasis. As a rule, however, the major problem during this period is not hypoxemia but hypercapnia. Removal of carbon dioxide is directly dependent on alveolar minute ventilation: if carbon dioxide production doubles, alveolar ventilation must also double to maintain normal arterial oxygen tension (P_aO_2). Increased ventilation means increased work of breathing, especially if compliance is decreased or dead space is increased. Large tidal volumes are necessary to maintain adequate alveolar ventilation because small tidal volumes ventilate little more than dead space. Larger tidal volumes call for greater inspiratory force, and the increased work of breathing must be sustained 24 hours a day. Fatigue may then result in impaired clearance of secretions, which can lead to nosocomial pneumonia (see above) as well as hypercapnia.

Serial measurements of tidal volume, vital capacity, and inspiratory force allow one to detect early deterioration of pulmonary function. Measurement of carbon dioxide production allows one to determine whether production exceeds the value predicted on the basis of the burn size alone. Oxygen consumption can also be measured directly by means of either spirometry or the Fick method, and the respiratory quotient can then be calculated directly [see 6:6 Use of the Mechanical Ventilator].

Acute Respiratory Distress Syndrome

ARDS is the name given to the clinical manifestations of a number of indirect lung injury states that are characterized by dyspnea, severe hypoxemia, and decreased lung compliance accompanied by radiographic evidence of diffuse bilateral pulmonary infiltrates. Alveolar consolidation with fluid, protein, and inflammatory cells in the presence of normal pulmonary arterial wedge pressure (PAWP) (i.e., low-pressure pulmonary edema) is also a characteristic finding. Altered permeability results in rapid movement of fluid from plasma to the interstitial space without any increase in PAWP.

ARDS caused by burn inflammation and infection carries an extremely high mortality. The major reason why this is so is that the condition will not resolve until the initiating process is removed. Unfortunately, at this point in the postburn period, burn wounds—especially large ones—cannot be readily excised and closed, because of the increased vascularity of the wound, the presence of colonization or infection, and the further debilitation of the patient. Consequently, efforts must be made to prevent ARDS through early removal of as much of the burn wound (which is a potential source of a systemic inflammatory response) as is feasible.

Maintenance of Hemodynamic Stability

MAINTENANCE OF ADEQUATE HYDRATION

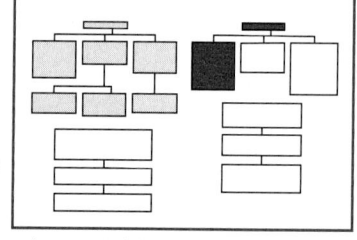

Evaporative loss is greatest from granulation tissue (with its increased blood supply) and least from a third-degree burn (with its thick eschar). Unhealed donor sites must also be considered in the estimation of evaporative loss. In addition, the increased body temperature characteristic of this period increases evaporative loss. Grafted skin restores much of the barrier, but losses may still be greater than evaporation across normal skin until the graft matures. Estimation of these losses depends on close monitoring of body weight, urine specific gravity, serum osmolarity, and clinical signs of hydration status [see 5:13 Burn Care in the Early Postresuscitation Period]. Serum sodium is a helpful indicator of the state of hydration. If the value is elevated, more water should be given.

RESTORATION AND MAINTENANCE OF PERFUSION

The Hyperdynamic State

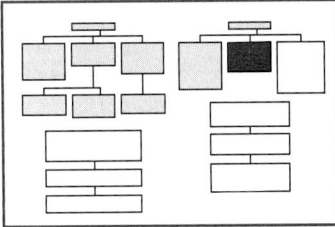

A hyperdynamic state evolves in the postresuscitation period as part of the response to burn injury, peaking about the end of the first postburn week. The degree of hyperdynamism appears to correlate with the degree of initial tissue injury as well as with the degree of initial damage to organs (especially the lungs). The hyperdynamic state is the result of systemic inflammation and the altered hormonal environment: the tissue injury and the secondary inflammatory response it evokes result in increased oxygen demands. Generally, patients remain hemodynamically stable in the postresuscitation period unless volume replenishment is inadequate; however, varying degrees of instability may occur. Physiologic responses range from normal to grossly abnormal or, more specifically, from simple hyperdynamism to the systemic inflammatory response syndrome (SIRS) to septic shock to, finally, the multiple organ dysfunction syndrome (MODS).

It is clear that burn patients who can spontaneously generate a hyperdynamic state in response to injury are capable of supplying enough oxygen to keep up with the increased metabolic demands reflected in increased oxygen consumption. It is also clear that mortality is lower in these patients than in patients who have an oxygen debt. It remains unclear, however, whether patients who cannot spontaneously generate a hyperdynamic response should be artificially maintained in a hyperdynamic state with volume expansion and inotropes, which patients should be so maintained, and what degree of artificial hyperdynamism would be appropriate.

Unfortunately, because of certain direct cellular metabolic changes, lactate concentration is a less sensitive indicator of impaired perfusion in this period than it was in the initial postburn period. Increased quantities of pyruvate are present as a result of the increased glucose utilization. Increased lactate may simply reflect decreased pyruvate utilization. A more reliable indicator of excessive lactate is the lactate-pyruvate ratio. An increase in this ratio would indicate excessive lactate and impaired perfusion. Mixed (or central) venous oxygen saturation may be a less useful monitoring parameter because of inflammation-induced maldistribution of blood flow, which lowers the extraction ratio. Logically, it would appear that maintaining high values for certain physiologic variables might help prevent MODS [see Table 1]; however, this approach has not yet been unequivocally shown to decrease the incidence of MODS during the early stress response.

When bacteria or their by-products are present, a further amplification of the hyperdynamic state occurs, accompanied by increased inflammation; clinical infection may or may not be present. This symptom complex has traditionally been referred to as

Table 2   Unstable Hyperdynamism: Systemic Inflammatory Response Syndrome

Clinical and laboratory findings
Increased temperature, chills
Warm, dry skin
Tachycardia, tachypnea
Blood pressure: usually decreased
Mental changes
Urine changes: variable

Laboratory findings
White blood cell count: increased
Metabolic acidosis
Lactate concentration: 1.5–2.0 mmol/L

Physiologic changes
Increased O_2 consumption, CO_2 production
Arterial-venous oxygen difference: normal to low
PAWP: normal to low
Cardiac output: increased
Systemic vascular resistance: decreased
Local microvascular damage

sepsis but currently is often referred to as SIRS [see Table 2]. The hyperdynamic state persists, but a degree of hemodynamic instability is now present, necessitating both increased fluid infusion and the administration of inotropes to maintain adequate oxygen delivery and perfusion pressure. Cardiac output remains 1.5 to 2.0 times normal, but vascular pressures decrease gradually as a result of a marked downregulation of both alpha and beta agonists by inflammatory mediators, which leads to hypotension and impaired cardiac function.

A modest lactic acidosis may also be present. If the impairment of blood flow is not corrected, the decreased perfusion leads to damage to vital organs. Neurologic changes (usually increased lethargy or confusion attributable to by-products of the metabolic changes) are also evident. As the hemodynamic changes progress, the hyperdynamic state can actually develop into a hypodynamic state.

Methods for Restoring and Maintaining Perfusion

If the patient is incapable of spontaneously increasing oxygen delivery to meet the increased oxygen demands, one may attempt to improve perfusion using the following approaches.

Volume expansion   Volume expansion is the initial treatment of choice for restoring perfusion in the hypermetabolic burn patient. This primarily involves raising filling pressure to increase cardiac output as well as to reopen underperfused microcirculatory beds. The specific role of colloids in restoring volume remains unclear; however, it seems reasonable to use them to supplement crystalloids. Albumin has a number of important properties in addition to its ability to maintain plasma colloid oncotic pressure, including antioxidant activity and the ability to bind free fatty acids, oxidants, and endotoxin.

Administration of inotropes   Because renal and splanchnic perfusion are often decreased even when overall perfusion appears to be adequate, low-dose dopamine (1 to 3 µg/kg/min) is appropriate for maintaining urine output. Medium-dose dopamine (≥ 4 µg/kg/min) is appropriate for raising the cardiac index when PAWP is normal (14 to 16 mm Hg), and dobutamine

Table 1   Physiologic Values to Be Maintained during the Stress Response to Major Burn Injury

Cardiac index > 4 L/min/m²
PAWP 12–16 mm Hg (may have to be as high as 18 mm Hg)
Oxygen delivery 1.5 times normal
Oxygen consumption approximately 1.5 times normal
Normal anion gap (8–12 mEq/L)

(usually 5 to 10 μg/kg/min), a nearly pure beta agonist, is used when PAWP is elevated (> 16 mm Hg).

Blood transfusion The ideal hemoglobin concentration for restoring perfusion in the hypermetabolic burn patient remains undefined. It is certain that in previously healthy young patients whose condition is stable, 8 g/dl is adequate. In severely burned patients who have MODS to any degree, on the other hand, a value of 10 g/dl is probably a more appropriate goal, especially in view of the impaired ability of critically ill patients to make new red blood cells.

Patients with Established MODS

In patients with established MODS, it is difficult to improve metabolic function simply by increasing oxygen delivery; inotropes are also often ineffective in these individuals. To date, it has not been documented that maintaining a hyperdynamic state by itself has any beneficial effect on survival once secondary MODS is established; it appears that the stress response–induced metabolic abnormalities must also be minimized for outcome to be improved.

CONTROL OF THE SYS-
TEMIC STRESS RESPONSE

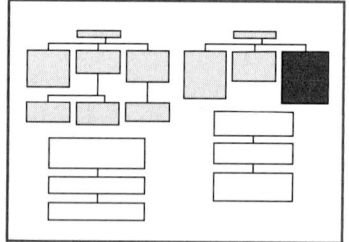

The initial burn insult provokes a reaction on the part of the host. This reaction may be considered a protective mechanism; however, it can in fact produce more injury than the initial insult itself. The components of the stress response are (1) an afferent arc, that is, the inflammatory response; (2) an efferent arc, that is, the release of so-called stress hormones; and (3) a CNS modulation that accentuates the efferent arc, that is, the generation of stimuli such as pain, anxiety, and stress-induced psychosis. The patient's natural response to injury is inflammation, both local and systemic.

Although the physiologic manifestations of the stress response are most evident several days after the injury, cellular biochemical changes caused by activation of this response can be seen very early after injury [*see Figure 1*].

The Afferent Arc: The Inflammatory Response

It has long been known that local inflammation occurs in burn-injured tissue within minutes to hours after injury; it has now also been documented that generalized inflammation also occurs. It is becoming increasingly clear that any severe local tissue trauma can give rise to a massive systemic inflammatory response. Large amounts of cytokines are released soon after major trauma, and inflammatory cells can be found sequestered in the microcirculation in virtually all organs immediately after severe trauma or burn injury. This generalized response appears to be attributable to the systemic activation of a number of inflammatory cascades, including intravascular complement activation. Animal and human studies have found evidence of early tissue oxidant changes, as reflected in elevated levels of circulating lipid peroxides and increased tissue lipid peroxidation.

The inflammatory cell sequestration and adherence to endothelial cells observed initially do not necessarily lead to injury if the inflammatory cells are only primed and not activated. Neutrophils often undergo systemic activation if ischemic or devitalized tissue is not removed or if there is a second insult. Although inflammation begins immediately after injury, physiologic evidence of the systemic response usually is not apparent for several days. The continued presence of devitalized tissue primes the host for a subsequent insult. In addition, the response to any subsequent insult (e.g., endotoxin, vascular catheter bacteremia, or pancreatitis) is amplified, leading to far more tissue damage and hemodynamic instability than would have been expected to result from the same insult in the absence of previous injury or infection.

The observation of this exaggerated response to even modest infection or ischemia on the part of the injured patient has given rise to the so-called two-hit theory of MODS [*see Figure 2*]. The

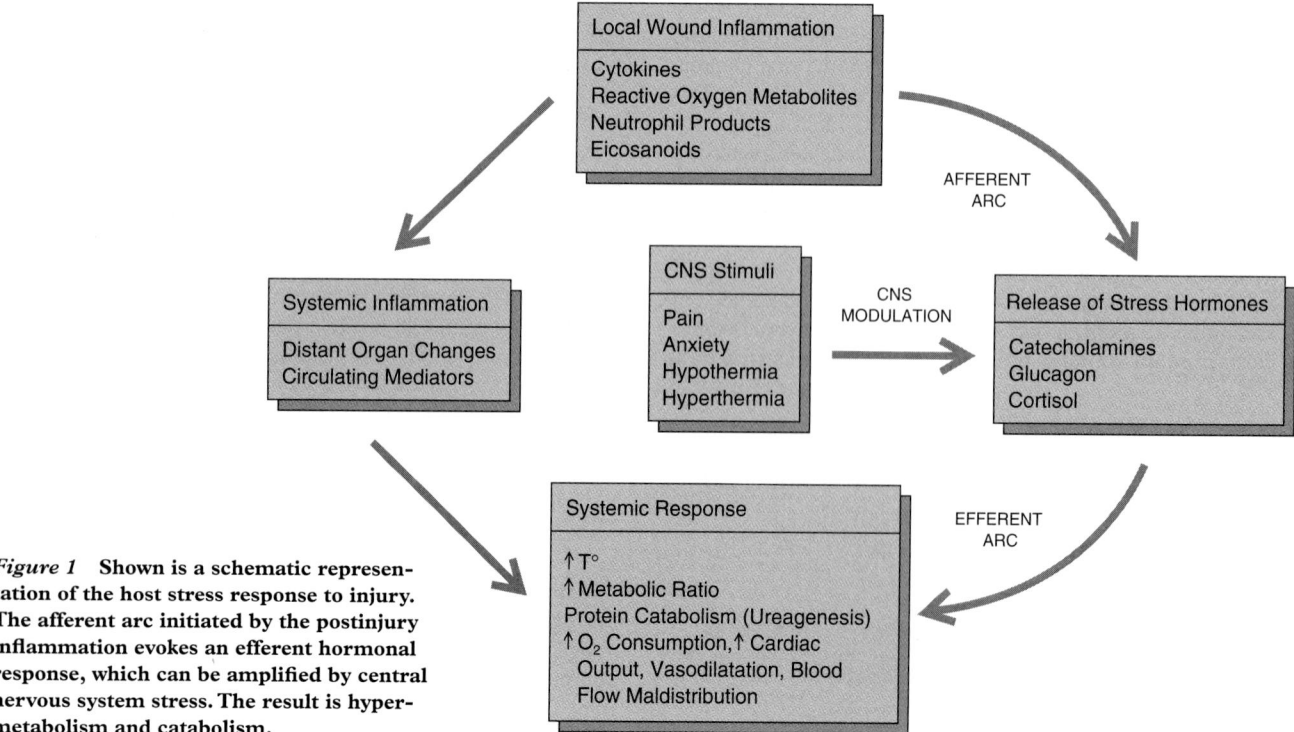

Figure 1 **Shown is a schematic representation of the host stress response to injury. The afferent arc initiated by the postinjury inflammation evokes an efferent hormonal response, which can be amplified by central nervous system stress. The result is hypermetabolism and catabolism.**

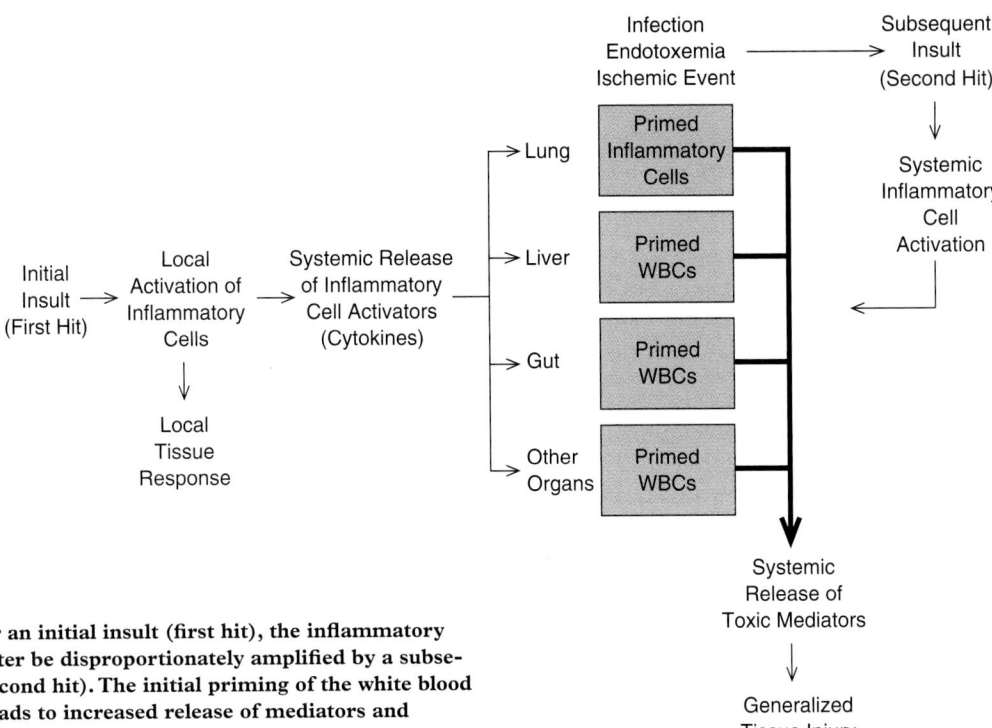

Figure 2 **After an initial insult (first hit), the inflammatory response can later be disproportionately amplified by a subsequent insult (second hit). The initial priming of the white blood cells (WBCs) leads to increased release of mediators and systemic activation.**

initial burn or smoke inhalation injury—the first hit—induces the inflammatory cells to turn on their metabolic machinery; this process usually is not clinically apparent. A subsequent insult—the second hit—causes the mediator factories to synthesize and release larger quantities of toxic compounds than the degree of the second insult would normally call for; these mediators then produce hemodynamic instability and tissue injury. The most prominent mediators of the stress response are the cytokines. These agents activate the inflammatory process and trigger the release of counterregulatory hormones and other potent vasoactive and cytotoxic mediators.

Cytokines are involved in a number of major responses to injury and infection, including hemodynamic changes, tissue inflammation, wound healing, immune defenses, hypermetabolism, and catabolism. Sustained increases in the activity of some of these agents—tumor necrosis factor (TNF) in particular—are thought to be responsible for the organ dysfunction associated with a persistent, progressive inflammatory response. The major cytokines that play a role in the inflammatory response to injury and infection are TNF, interleukin-1 (IL-1), IL-2, IL-6, and interferon gamma.

Endotoxin Endotoxin is a well-known initiator of inflammation and inflammation-induced disease. It activates the release of a number of mediators, including eicosanoids, oxidants, and cytokines (especially TNF). It also leads to generalized immunosuppression, although the mechanism by which it does so remains undefined.

Endotoxemia is considered to play a major role in the postinjury stress response, even when no obvious source of infection is present. In the absence of clinical infection, endotoxin may be absorbed into the circulation from a colonized wound surface or from a leaky GI tract.

Reactive oxygen metabolites Oxygen radicals are unstable metabolites of oxygen that have an unpaired electron in their outer shell and consequently are potent oxidizing agents; two examples are the superoxide anion ($O_2^{\cdot}$) and the hydroxyl anion ($OH\cdot$). There are other toxic oxygen metabolites that, though not true free radicals, are nonetheless potent oxidants; one example is hydrogen peroxide (H_2O_2). Oxidants are now considered to be involved in several aspects of the response to burn injury and inflammation [*see Table 3*]. Studies have shown that the systemic inflammatory response seen after severe burns is attributable to systemic activation of complement by $OH\cdot$. Toxic oxygen metabolites also cause lipid peroxidation in the lungs, liver, kidneys, and other tissues in the early postburn period. Elevated circulating levels of lipid peroxides have been documented in patients who are injured or infected. This early postinjury lipid peroxidation may not result in immediate organ dysfunction, but it may help amplify the response to a second insult by causing the release of more inflammatory cytokines. Tissues injured by oxidants and proteases are much more vulnerable to further injury by a subsequent insult. The degree of oxidant damage is closely correlated with the adequacy of antioxidant defenses. After the process of inflammation and infection is under way, oxygen metabolites are again involved in tissue injury; during this phase, the primary oxidant source is activated white blood cells, with endotoxin playing a major role in the release of these substances.

Table 3 **Effects of Reactive Oxygen Metabolites**

Alteration of vascular permeability
Lipid peroxidation, altering function
Initiation and perpetuation of local and systemic inflammation
Disruption of interstitial matrix
Impairment of macrophage phagocytosis
Alteration of cellular DNA
Initiation of arachidonic acid metabolism
Red blood cell hemolysis

At present, a number of antioxidants normally present in tissues (e.g., vitamin C, vitamin E, catalase, superoxide dismutase, and glutathione or its substrate, glutamine) are available for clinical use. Other oxidants (e.g., xanthine oxidase inhibitors, iron chelators, and 21-aminosteroids, a new class of agents with iron chelating and antioxidant properties) are also being developed for use in humans.

Eicosanoids Arachidonic acid metabolites play a role in both the early and the late response to burn injury. Arachidonic acid is released from the cell membrane in response to injury or infection. It is metabolized via two enzymatic pathways: (1) the cyclooxygenase pathway, which yields prostaglandins and thromboxanes, and (2) the lipoxygenase pathway, which yields leukotrienes.

After a burn, both the vasodilator prostaglandin I_2 (PGI_2), or prostacyclin, and the vasoconstrictor thromboxane A_2 (TXA_2) are released in great quantities. Prostacyclin increases local blood flow, thereby accentuating mediator-induced vascular leakage. The local increase in TXA_2 increases platelet aggregation and neutrophil margination in the wound microcirculation, thereby also potentiating tissue ischemia.

CNS production of prostaglandin E is thought to be the cause of the fever associated with the stress response. The characteristic maldistribution of blood flow observed in marked systemic inflammation appears to be related to excessive production of TXA_2 or PGI_2 in various vascular beds.

The Efferent Arc: Release of Stress Hormones

Certain characteristic hormonal alterations take place during the stress response to burn injury. There is an early increase in circulating catecholamine levels, and this increase produces the peripheral vasoconstriction, anxiety, and tachycardia observed in the early postburn period. Catecholamine levels appear to correlate directly with the degree of injury. The sympathetic adrenal response—namely, increased alpha$_1$- and beta$_1$-receptor activity— appears to correlate with the degree of subsequent hypermetabolism and increased oxygen demands. Beta-receptor activity predominates in the hyperdynamic state. The increased sympathetic activity generally persists throughout the period of critical illness.

Cortisol and glucagon levels are also increased during critical illness. Both of these agents are considered anti-insulin hormones because they promote gluconeogenesis and glycogenolysis. Cortisol also promotes catabolism.

Insulin not only increases glycogen production and is essential for glucose utilization at the cell level but also is a potent anabolic hormone that facilitates the incorporation of amino acids into protein. Insulin administration improves both glucose utilization and protein synthesis.

Human growth hormone is the most potent anabolic hormone. It induces marked increases in protein synthesis and gluconeogenesis; in addition, unlike insulin, it causes lipolysis and increased utilization of ketone bodies for fuel, sparing skeletal muscle and decreasing the catabolic response to stress. Growth hormone levels typically are lower than normal in the catabolic phase of severe injury.

Metabolic alterations Significant alterations in normal metabolic activity are observed in patients with SIRS [see Table 4]. In addition to increases in circulating levels of inflammatory mediators (particularly macrophage-derived products), there are large, sustained increases in levels of anti-insulin hormones and catabolic hormones (e.g., catecholamines, cortisol, and glucagon). Although insulin levels are increased as well, insulin activity appears to be outweighed by the anti-insulin

activity of the catabolic hormones. In hypermetabolic patients, calorie requirements are 50% to 100% higher than normal. Because of the altered metabolism, the compensatory mechanisms normally triggered by starvation are absent, and nutrient utilization is substantially affected.

Acute-phase protein production Hepatic protein synthesis is reprioritized. Production of acute-phase proteins is increased, and production of albumin synthetase is decreased. Acute-phase proteins, which have immunoprotective properties, are released from the liver in response to burn injury, severe smoke inhalation injury, or systemic infection; the specific stimulus appears to be the elevated levels of cytokines (IL-6 and IL-1).

Each acute-phase protein has a characteristic function and duration of action. The downregulation of albumin production results in a hypoalbuminemic state that persists throughout the stress response.

CNS Modulation

The CNS significantly affects the efferent response to a burn. Increased CNS stimulation deriving from pain, anxiety, hypothermia, or hyperthermia amplifies the release of catecholamines, thereby accentuating the hypermetabolic state. Occasionally, patients manifest a stress-induced psychosis, which leads to sleep deprivation and excessive motor activity, thereby further increasing oxygen and nutrient consumption.

Methods for Controlling the Stress Response

Removing the inflammatory focus It is critical to remove deep burned tissue as soon as possible. The objective is to remove a potential inflammatory focus before the host stress response takes hold. Once the hyperdynamic state is clinically present, inflammation is already well established. According to current protocols for preventing secondary MODS, devitalized tissue should be removed even if the patient still appears to be stable.

Modulating release of stress hormones It is essential to minimize the likelihood of further stimuli that will amplify the release of stress hormones, especially catecholamines. Infection must of course be controlled, and further ischemic insults must be avoided (see below). Hypothermia usually is readily controlled. To prevent excessive heat loss during care of the burn wounds, the ambient temperature must be maintained at 30° to 35° C (86° to 95° F). Mild hyperthermia generally is not a major problem, but if body temperature exceeds 103° F, deleterious side effects can result.

Pain control helps prevent excessive release of catecholamines in patients at risk for organ dysfunction. Optimum pain control usually cannot be achieved during initial resuscitation, while patients are still hypovolemic; it is possible only when hemodynamic

---

Table 4 **Major Metabolic Abnormalities with Response to Injury**

Sustained increase in body temperature

Marked increase in glucose demand and therefore strong stimulation of liver gluconeogenesis

Rapid skeletal muscle breakdown caused by demand for amino acid substrate for use as a direct energy source, for gluconeogenesis, and for hepatic acute-phase protein production

Stimulation of the liver to produce large quantities of acute-phase proteins

Absence of ketosis, indicating that fat is not the major calorie source

Unresponsiveness of the rate of gluconeogenesis and catabolism to substrate stability is restored. Patients require larger and more frequent doses of pain medication after the first postburn week because during this period, they experience increasing tolerance to analgesic agents as a result of long-term use and the increasing pain of the debriding wound [*see 5:12 Burn Care in the Immediate Resuscitation Period and 5:13 Burn Care in the Early Postresuscitation Period*]. Self-administration has been found to be quite useful because the patient's perception of the pain is more accurate than that of the care providers. During the postresuscitation period, high-risk patients should receive continuous epidural analgesia or continuous low-dose narcotic infusion to minimize stress.

Anxiety control is crucial. Close attention must be paid to supporting the neuropsychological status of the patient, especially in the presence of organ dysfunction and SIRS. Adequate sleep periods and the avoidance of sensory overload are essential, especially in the ICU. Administration of benzodiazepines, either intermittently or by continuous infusion, can effectively attenuate anxiety-induced stress. The ICU psychosis syndrome [*see 5:13 Burn Care in the Early Postresuscitation Period*] usually must be treated by means of a neuroleptic agent, such as chlorpromazine or haloperidol.

Counteracting or augmenting stress hormone activity
Excessive production of catecholamines occurs in patients with major burns in the later postresuscitation period. This response increases metabolic demands and is responsible for cardiomyopathy, characterized by focal myofiber necrosis. Rapid pulse rate and hypertension are commonly observed. In moderate doses, beta antagonists can reduce the amount of work the heart must perform and actually decrease metabolic demands, especially in patients with head injuries. Oxygen delivery must not be decreased to the point where it fails to meet oxygen demands.

Recent studies suggest that exogenous administration of human growth hormone may be highly beneficial in patients with massive burns. Human growth hormone, 1 to 2 mg/day, has been shown to improve nitrogen balance in normal elderly men. Levels of endogenous human growth hormone are lower than normal in burn patients. When given to such patients in dosages of 5 to 10 mg/day, human growth hormone markedly improved nitrogen retention and increased the rate of wound healing. Exogenous human growth hormone causes more endogenous fat to be used for fuel and reduces protein catabolism. Its use is associated with some complications, namely, a modest (5% to 10%) increase in oxygen consumption, modest hyperglycemia, and positive salt and water retention, especially during the first several days. Efforts are being made to determine how, when, and to which burn patients human growth hormone should be given.

Preventing a second insult As noted (see above), the addition of a second insult to an already primed system evokes an amplified host stress response. To prevent such an occurrence, extreme vigilance and aggressive institution of preventive measures are required in patients who are at high risk for secondary MODS.

Decreasing leakage from the gut Efforts should be made to minimize bacterial translocation and leakage of endotoxin across the impaired gut barrier. A lack of enteral nutrients rapidly leads to mucosal atrophy, especially during the stress response; early enteral nutrition is considered effective in maintaining the mucosal barrier. Several clinical trials have demonstrated that early enteral nutrition—as compared with early parenteral nutrition or delayed enteral nutrition—decreases secondary MODS in burn patients. Placement of a postpyloric feeding tube is becoming an increasingly common practice.

Table 5 Substances with Antioxidant Effects That May Be Given in Nutritional Solutions

Oxidant scavengers
  Vitamin C: 1–2 g/day
  Vitamin E: 400 mg/day
  β-Carotene: 25,000 IU/day
Antioxidant substrate
  Glutamine: 20–30 g/day (required for glutathione synthesis)
Required cofactors
  Selenium: 40 mg/day (cofactor glutathione peroxidase-reductase)
  Zinc: 20 mg/day parenterally (cofactor superoxide dismutase); alternatively, zinc sulfate, 220 mg t.i.d., p.o.

Administering glutamine The amino acid glutamine is the major fuel for the rapidly dividing enterocytes. Injury is often followed by glutamine deficiency as a result of both increased endogenous utilization and decreased exogenous intake. Glutamine is typically absent from central hyperalimentation solutions and standard tube feedings; however, glutamine-enriched enteral and parenteral solutions are now available. The current recommended daily dose of glutamine for adults is 20 to 30 g or 0.5 g/kg.

Using exogenous inhibitors of inflammation Nonsteroidal anti-inflammatory drugs (NSAIDs), particularly ibuprofen, have been shown to attenuate the response to inflammation and endotoxin in humans. Ibuprofen inhibits cyclooxygenase activity, thereby decreasing eicosanoid production. In addition, NSAIDs have antioxidant, anticytokine, and neutrophil-stabilizing properties. Although it is clear that these agents have significant beneficial potential, it has not been determined whether and to what extent they can actually attenuate the stress response and prevent MODS. The use of NSAIDs during the stress response has not led to an increased incidence of renal complications.

Given the deleterious effects of oxidants, the use of agents that prevent or minimize oxidant activity in some fashion is likely to be beneficial [*see Table 5*]. A host of antioxidants and agents that prevent oxidant release or remove oxidants already released (e.g., vitamin C, vitamin E, and β-carotene) are being used clinically. Optimizing cellular defenses against oxidant activity, particularly by nutritional means, has received considerable attention as a method of preventing inflammation. Marked deficiencies in endogenous antioxidants, resulting from both increased turnover and decreased substrate intake, are known to exacerbate the cellular injury caused by the ongoing inflammatory response. Glutamine, besides being fuel for enterocytes (see above), is also an essential substrate for the endogenous antioxidant glutathione. During critical illness and oxidant stress, tissue glutathione levels decrease.

Nutrition

Adequate nutrition must be provided to meet increased tissue demands by postburn day 7 because early delivery of necessary calories and proteins becomes essential for rapid wound closure and to minimize complications from pulmonary dysfunction and infection. Nutritional support should have begun between postburn days 2 and 5. Increased metabolic activity usually peaks between postburn days 7 and 10, and by then, demands should be completely met.

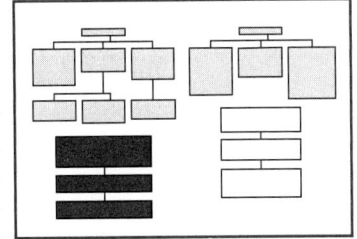

First, energy requirements must be estimated; second, plans for nutrient delivery must be individually tailored according to each patient's requirement for carbohydrate, protein, and fat.

ENERGY REQUIREMENTS

The goal of nutritional support is to provide the necessary calories to meet energy needs. These needs depend on energy expenditure, measurements of which are based on three components: basal metabolic rate (BMR), muscle activity, and stress-induced energy needs.

Basal metabolic rate describes the energy required to maintain cell integrity at the resting state and at thermoneutrality, which for the burn patient is 28° to 30° C ambient (80° to 88° F). Under these environmental conditions, heat loss is minimized and the need to produce additional metabolic heat to maintain body temperature is absent or greatly attenuated. In normal individuals, environmental temperature below thermoneutrality markedly increases sympathetic activity and caloric requirements. The BMR for humans of various ages has been determined and is widely available in chart form. Body size is the principal factor influencing metabolic rate. Other variables include the age and, to a lesser extent, the sex of the patient.

Muscle activity level is a measure of the average amount of energy used by muscles for daily activity. For patients in an ICU, muscle activity is usually quite limited, and the energy cost is usually considered to be no more than 25% above the BMR. The stress of daily exercise, sitting in a chair, and walking all contribute to the additional energy cost. Energy expenditure in bedridden patients can be markedly increased by excessive muscle activity (e.g., in patients who fight the ventilator, who must work excessively hard to breathe, or who are in a combative, disoriented state). Sedation or, if necessary, muscle paralysis will decrease this component of energy expenditure to almost zero. Prolonged muscle paralysis is not desirable, because muscle tone is necessary to maintain strength and positive nitrogen balance; the latter is particularly important for the muscles of respiration.

The third component on which energy requirements are based is stress-induced energy need. A so-called stress factor defines the hypermetabolism that is induced by the burn. The stress factor is a multiple of the basal metabolic rate (normalized to 1.0); its value takes into consideration the size of the burn injury and the average metabolic response that is seen with this size injury [see Table 6].

Oxygen consumption, carbon dioxide production, or both can be measured directly and the metabolic rate calculated. Direct measurement of calorie requirements with an indirect calorimeter (which essentially involves converting oxygen consumption to calorie expenditure) appears to be more accurate than using a formula to estimate calorie requirements; however, formulas can be very useful as guidelines [see Figure 3].

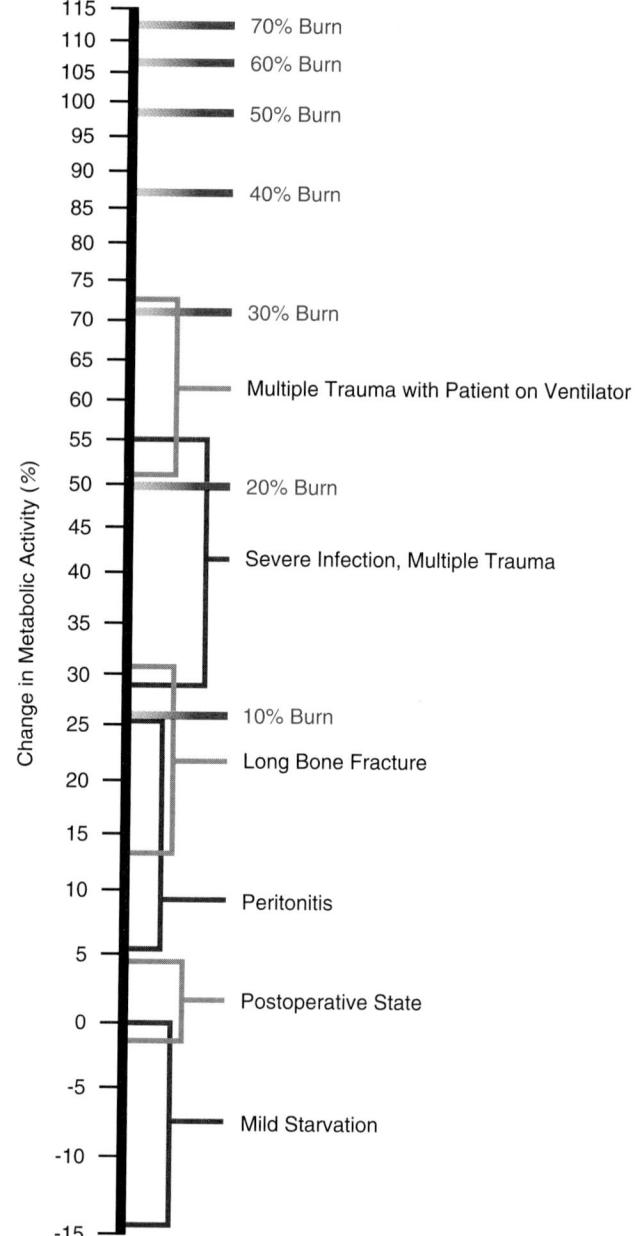

Figure 3 Depicted is the relation between selected injuries and various degrees of change in metabolic activity resulting from these injuries. Major burns cause the largest increases in metabolic rate.

NUTRIENT REQUIREMENTS (CARBOHYDRATE, FAT, AND PROTEIN)

Approximately 70% of estimated nonprotein calorie requirements must be given as glucose to spare nitrogen effectively. If lipid infusions are given, triglyceride levels must be monitored to avoid hypertriglyceridemia. In most burn patients, lipid clearance is not impaired and may in fact be increased. Increasing the proportion of omega-3 fatty acids and decreasing the proportion of omega-6 fatty acids in the infusion may be helpful. Lipids, because of their immunosuppressive effects, should make up no more than 25% of total calories.

When carbohydrates are administered, a large portion is oxidized to carbon dioxide and excreted via the lungs. As the quantity of glucose administered increases, carbon dioxide production

Table 6 Stress Factors

Burn Size (% TBS)	Stress Factor
10	1.25
20	1.50
30	1.70
40	1.85
50	2.00
60–100	2.10

rises and the respiratory quotient shifts from 0.7 (reflecting fat oxidation) toward 1.0 (reflecting carbohydrate oxidation). Excess carbohydrate—that is, more than can be primarily oxidized—is converted to fat. When this conversion occurs, the respiratory quotient exceeds 1.0, and the result may be an increased ventilatory load for the patient.

Protein requirements are also calculated in a number of ways. An estimate of 1.5 to 2.0 g of protein per kilogram of body weight can be used for all major burns. A more specific quantitative estimate can be based on a calorie-nitrogen ratio. (The nitrogen content of protein is determined by dividing the amount of protein by 6.25.) A 150:1 ratio is usually used to calculate protein requirements, but some investigators are now proposing that a 100:1 ratio is preferable. Thus, the final diet provides approximately 20% protein, 55% to 60% carbohydrate, and 20% to 25% fat.

VITAMIN AND TRACE-ELEMENT REQUIREMENTS

The burn patient loses a number of vitamins in increased quantities. Vitamins A and C are of particular concern because they are essential for healing. Vitamin A must usually be replaced in a daily dose of 10,000 to 15,000 units and vitamin C in a daily dose of 1 to 2 g. Zinc, a trace element required for healing, is also lost in increased amounts. Replacement is usually 220 mg of zinc sulfate, given orally three times a day. Administering microminerals in the form of a high-potency vitamin-mineral pill or elixir is necessary to provide trace elements.

ADMINISTRATION OF NUTRITION

Nutritional support is best managed during this period by the enteral route, usually with a combination of balanced tube feeding and voluntary intake. Parenteral supplementation through a peripheral vein may be necessary in the patient with a very large burn (i.e., a burn exceeding 50% of TBS). Central venous feedings are occasionally required if the GI tract is not functioning adequately, as sometimes occurs in patients receiving ventilatory assistance or in patients with SIRS.

For patients with large burns (in whom obligate fluid requirements are high), most of the required calories and protein can be infused through a peripheral vein. Enteral feeding via a nasogastric or postpyloric tube can usually be initiated within 2 to 3 days after a burn. As emphasized elsewhere [see 5:13 Burn Care in the Early Postresuscitation Period], the sooner enteral nutrition can be instituted the better [see 6:23 Nutritional Support]. Ideally, it should begin on postburn day 1 or 2, with a small feeding tube placed through the duodenum.

Burn Wound Care

DIAGNOSIS AND TREATMENT OF BURN WOUND INFECTION

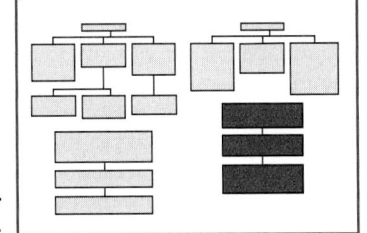

The primary indication for systemic antibiotics in the treatment of the burn wound is (1) evidence of increased bacterial content (i.e., > 10^5 organism/g tissue or histologic evidence of invasion) or (2) cellulitis or other evidence that the wound is increasing in depth or invading adjacent, noninfected tissue. In addition, systemic antibiotics are indicated in the perioperative period (24 to 48 hours) preceding and following debridement and skin grafting [see 5:13 Burn Care in the Early Postresuscitation Period]. The initial topical agent is usually silver sulfadiazine. Mafenide, povidone-iodine, gentamicin, and bacitracin are commonly used topical agents when the wound becomes infected or when bacterial overgrowth retards wound healing.

CHANGES IN THE BURN WOUND

By the second postburn week, the burn wound has changed considerably from its state during the first several days. Superficial burns are healing rapidly by this point. Deep second-degree burns are beginning to debride and are becoming much more uncomfortable and prone to infection. Full-thickness burns are now colonized and revascularized, and the eschar is beginning to separate. Deep burns, being now inflamed, hyperemic, and colonized (or infected) with bacteria, must be managed much more gently than in earlier phases. Any vigorous wound manipulation can lead to bacteremia and endotoxemia. Antibiotic-resistant organisms also become more common.

During the first 6 days after the burn, wound inflammation begins and the various components of healing are initiated [see 5:13 Burn Care in the Early Postresuscitation Period]. In superficial burns, epidermal regeneration is relatively rapid if the wound environment is optimized; this is achieved by providing sufficient amounts of oxygen, nutrients, and wound-healing factors (e.g., vitamin A and vitamin C), by keeping the wound surface from drying out, and by taking steps to prevent infection. The injured dermal elements are usually covered by new epithelium within 2 weeks. The hyperplasia of dermal fibroblasts then begins to resolve, and healing is complete with only modest amounts of collagen deposited. The wound usually becomes relatively pliable with time, and wound contraction is minimal. Superficial second-degree burns typically result in little or no long-term scarring.

The histology of the wound, however, changes dramatically if it has not been closed by 2 weeks after the burn, as would be the case with nongrafted deep dermal or full-thickness burns. Fibroblasts and macrophages become the predominant cells. Large numbers of myofibroblasts—modified fibroblasts that have some of the contractile properties of smooth muscle—also enter the wound. Microfilament bundles can be seen in their cytoplasm, lined parallel to each other and to the direction of contraction. Cells are linked together via extracellular extensions that allow transmission of the contractile forces. This results in a synchronized contractile process similar to that in smooth muscle. More than 75% of the cells in granulating wounds are myofibroblasts; in hypertrophic scars, the number of myofibroblasts present correlates with the rate of wound contraction. Besides leading to contraction, myofibroblasts continue to deposit large quantities of collagen and glycosaminoglycans.

Closure of the wound by reepithelialization or grafting does not eliminate the stimulus for ongoing scar formation. Angiogenesis continues, as does production of mucopolysaccharides and collagen. A marked increase in the proteoglycan content of chondroitin sulfate A can be seen as well. Chondroitin sulfate A, which is usually found in firm tissues such as cartilage, produces a harder, less pliable wound. As myofibroblasts contract, thereby shortening the scar, the deposition of the mucopolysaccharides and ground substances results in the fusion of the collagen fibers in the contracted site. The process of wound contraction leads to joint contractures.

Collagenase is also released by inflammatory cells. Synthesis of new collagen and lysis of old collagen are ongoing processes: any exaggeration of lysis or retardation of synthesis results in the dissolution of the new tissue.

CHANGES IN WOUND CARE

A marked pyrogen release resulting from manipulation of the wound causes a rise in body temperature, which accentuates the stress response and increases oxygen requirements. Use of antipyretics just before burn care begins attenuates the subsequent pyrogen response; the best agent for this purpose appears to be ibuprofen. Quantitative biopsies of the eschar are useful for diagnosing invasive infection and determining whether systemic antibiotics should be added or the topical antibiotic should be changed. Any pockets of suspected purulence below the eschar should be unroofed. Loose eschar should be removed from the wound to lower the bacterial content and to reduce surface exudation and inflammation, which can injure the new tissue being formed. Sharp dissection should not be continued into viable tissue beneath the eschar; if it is continued, substantial blood loss and bacteremia may result. Hypertrophic granulation tissue continues to be formed until the wound is surgically closed. Wound contraction reduces the surface area of the wound somewhat, but at the cost of mobility and function.

SURGICAL MANAGEMENT

As during the early postresuscitation period, surgical management of the burn wound is complicated by both anesthesia-related and wound-related problems.

Anesthesia

After the first postburn week, patients are highly hypermetabolic, and maintenance of anesthesia can be quite complex. The following are the essential components of anesthesia management in burn patients:

1. Airway maintenance and intubation.
2. Provision for increased ventilatory needs.
3. Choice of anesthetic agent.
4. Monitoring.
5. Maintenance of temperature and hemodynamic stability.

It is well known that the skeletal muscle neuromuscular receptors begin to be more sensitive to depolarizing muscle relaxants about 4 or 5 days after a burn injury and that this change results in the release of large amounts of K^+ and potentially fatal hyperkalemia during muscle fasciculations. Depolarizing agents are therefore contraindicated; a nondepolarizing agent is used when paralysis is indicated.

Adequate cardiopulmonary monitoring is extremely important in patients with major burns, who are potentially highly unstable. The relative lack of sites for invasive monitoring—and even for noninvasive monitoring—in these patients calls for considerable ingenuity on the part of the anesthesiologist. Some of the access problems can be avoided by using needle electrocardiographic electrodes, pulse oximetry, and end-tidal carbon dioxide concentrations (obtained from air expired from the ventilator). Advance knowledge of the patient's ventilatory and hemodynamic status and maintenance of preoperative values are essential.

Accurate assessment of blood loss depends on frequent communication between the surgeon and the anesthesiologist. Any blood lost should be replaced with blood products; crystalloid should be given to replace evaporative losses, not blood losses. Blood and blood products should be present in the room before management of a major case begins. The operating room must be warm (at least 80° F), and heating blankets, warm fluids, and similar adjuvants should be available. The operating time should be limited to two hours in patients who have large burns, especially if any significant cardiopulmonary instability is present.

Surgical Procedures

Surgical procedures done in burn patients during the inflammation period should be performed according to the same guidelines that are applicable in the first postburn week [see 5:13 Burn Care in the Early Postresuscitation Period]: the duration of the operation must be limited, blood loss must be minimized, and the grafted area must be carefully immobilized. The patient must be hemodynamically stable before the operation. Perioperative antibiotics are indicated. The choice of an agent is governed by the results of the preoperative wound culture: if no specific organism predominates, a first-generation cephalosporin is usually preferred because it provides reasonable coverage of Staphylococcus aureus and the more common gram-negative bacteria. S. aureus is the most common organism affecting the skin graft and the donor site.

The wound is colonized with bacteria during this period; thus, the potential for producing significant bacteremia also increases. Certainly, endotoxemia develops and inflammatory mediators are released; SIRS results postoperatively. Perioperative antibiotics help combat the bacteremia but do not block the absorption of endotoxins and pyrogens already present in the wound. If the wound infection cannot be controlled by nonoperative management, limited sequential excision can be lifesaving. The primary caution is to avoid large or long procedures that might have been easily tolerated in the first week but that are not as well tolerated during this period.

Wound Remodeling and Scar Formation

HYPERTROPHIC SCARRING

Pressure is the standard means of controlling hypertrophic scarring and accelerating the maturation process. When dressings are still required, pressure is provided by Ace wraps. Form-fitted pressure garments are used later. The pressure is expected to exceed surface vessel capillary pressure and should reach 25 mm Hg or higher. Pressure immediately reduces hyperemia and wound edema, which in turn prevents blister formation. Over a period of several weeks, a decrease in the chrondroitin sulfate content becomes evident, as does a decline in mast cells and myofibroblasts. One theory is that by impeding blood flow to scars, pressure decreases fibroblast and inflammatory cell numbers by means of surface ischemia and thereby decreases overall excess collagen synthesis. In addition, because the water content is decreased, ground substance production is also decreased. The pressure must be continuous to be effective (i.e., about 23 hours every day for up to a year). Therapy with pressure garments is continued until the scar demonstrates complete maturation. Muscle activity and joint motion have been found to be significantly improved when this approach is employed.

It is during this period that permanent skin substitutes are used. There are two types that are commonly used clinically: (1) cultured autologous keratinocytes and (2) bilayer skin with generic dermis covered with the patient's own dermis.

Cultured keratinocytes are used as follows. In the first several days after the burn, the decision is made that cultured keratinocytes will be required to help cover a large burn surface. Full-thickness skin biopsies are then taken for cell preparation, the wound is excised and covered (preferably with cadaver skin), the cells are grown in tissue media for 3 weeks, the skin substitute is removed, the cultured cells are applied, and the area is immobilized. Graft take ranges from 20% to 80%; the best results are obtained with flat surfaces that can be immobilized.

Bilayer skin consists of a dermis, which is absorbed and replaced by the host, and an artificial epidermis in the form of a Silastic sheet, which is eventually replaced by the patient's own epidermis. Bilayer skin, despite its greater potential for providing a dermis and its superior flexibility, is at present less commonly used than cultured keratinocytes, primarily because it is still undergoing developmental changes.

There are a number of experimental skin substitutes in various stages of development. It is likely that before long, skin substitutes will be available that can replace both layers in a predictable fashion.

SKIN LUBRICATION

Because the burn patient's sebaceous glands have been impaired or destroyed, natural skin lubrication is absent; drying, pain, and markedly impaired pliability result. Skin moisturizers will be necessary for months to years to maintain optimal skin function.

Recommended Reading

Alexander W: The role of infections in the burn patient. The Art and Science of Burn Care. Boswick J, Ed. Aspen Publishers, Rockville, Maryland, 1982, p 103

Beeker W: Fungal burn wound infection, a 10 year experience. Arch Surg 126:44, 1991

Bingham H, Gallagher T, Powell R: Early bronchoscopy as a predictor of ventilatory support for burned patients. J Trauma 27:1286, 1987

Bone R, Balk R, Cerra F, et al: Definitions for sepsis and organ failure and guidelines for the use of innovative therapies in sepsis. Chest 101:1644, 1992

Boukoms A: Pain relief in the intensive care unit. J Intens Care Med 3:32, 1988

DeBandt S, Chollet M, Lowry S, et al: Cytokine response to burn injury: relationship with protein metabolism. J Trauma 36:624, 1994

DeBiasse M, Wilmore D: What is optimum nutritional support? New Horizons. Zalaga G, Ed. Society for Critical Care Medicine, Fullerton, California, 1994, p 122

Deitch E: Intestinal permeability is increased in burn patients shortly after injury. Surgery 167:411, 1990

Demling R: Effect of early burn excision and grafting on pulmonary function. J Trauma 24:830, 1984

Demling R: Fluid replacement in burned patients. Surg Clin North Am 67:15, 1987

Demling R, Orgill D: Current concepts and approaches to wound healing. Crit Care Med 16:899, 1988

Demling R, Pomposelli J: Burn wound infection. Surgical Infections: Diagnosis and Treatment. Meakins JL, Ed. Scientific American, Inc, New York, 1994, p 369

Dobke M, Deitch E, Baxter C: Oxidant activity of polymorphonuclear leukocytes after thermal injury. Arch Surg 124:856, 1989

Dong Y, Abdullah K, Yan T, et al: Effect of thermal injury and sepsis on neutrophil function. J Trauma 34:417, 1993

Fong Y, Moldawer L, Shires T, et al: The biologic characteristics of cytokines and their implications in surgical injury. Surg Gynecol Obstet 170:363, 1990

Gatzen C, Scheltinga M, Kimbrough T, et al: Growth hormone attenuates the abnormal distribution of body water in critically ill surgical patients. Surgery 112:181, 1992

Goodwin C, Wilmore D: Surgery and burns. Clinical Nutrition. Paige D, Ed. CV Mosby Co, St Louis, 1988, p 372

Gore D, Honeycutt D, Jahoor F, et al: Effect of exogenous growth hormone on whole body and isolated limb protein kinetics in burned patients. Arch Surg 126:38, 1990

Gottleich M, Warden G: Vitamin supplementation in the patient with burns. J Burn Care Rehabil 11:375, 1990

Hirsch C, Kaemerek R, Stanek K: Work of breathing during CPAP and PSV imposed by the new generation mechanical ventilators. Respir Care 36:815, 1991

Jahoor F, Shangraw RE, Miyoshi H, et al: Role of insulin and glucose oxidation in mediating the protein catabolism of burns and sepsis. Am J Physiol 257:E323, 1989

Jeevandra M, Ramias L, Shamos R, et al: Decreased growth hormone levels in the catabolic phase of severe injury. Surgery 111:495, 1992

Law E, Blecher K, Still J: Enterococcal infections as a cause of mortality and morbidity in patients with burns. J Burn Care Rehabil 15:236, 1994

Machin L, Bendich A: Free radical tissue damage: protective role of antioxidant nutrients. FASEB J 1:441, 1990

Moore E, Jones T: Benefits of immediate jejunostomy feeding after major abdominal trauma: a prospective randomized study. J Trauma 26:874, 1986

Moore F, Haenel J, Moore E, et al: Incommensurate oxygen consumption in response to maximal oxygen availability products post injury multiple organ failure. J Trauma 33:58, 1992

Munster A: Cultured epidermal autograft in the management of burn patients. J Burn Care Rehabil 13:121, 1992

Paxton J, Williamson J: Nutrient substrate: making choices in the 1990s. J Burn Care Rehabil 12:198, 1991

Pinsky M, Matuschak G: A unifying hypothesis of multiple system organ failure: failure of host defense homeostasis. J Crit Care 5:108, 1990

Pruitt B: Infection and the burn patient. Br J Surg 77:1081, 1990

Rodriguez J, Miller C, Till G, et al: Correlation of the local and systemic cytokine response with clinical outcome following thermal injury. J Trauma 34:684, 1993

Servent R, Hansbrough J: Cytotoxicity to human leukocytes by topical antimicrobial agents used for burn care. J Burn Care Rehabil 14:132, 1993

Taddonio T, Thomson P: A survey of wound monitoring and topical antimicrobial therapy practices in the treatment of burn injury. J Burn Care Rehabil 11:423, 1990

Tobin M: Respiratory monitoring. JAMA 264:244, 1990

Wallace B, Caldwell F, Cone J: Ibuprofen lowers body temperature and metabolic rate of humans with burn injury. J Trauma 32:159, 1992

Ward P, Warren J, Johnson K: Oxygen radical inflammation and tissue injury. Free Rad Biol Med 5:403, 1988

Waymack JP, Herndon DN: Nutritional support of the burned patient. World J Surg 16:80, 1992

Wilmore D: Metabolic changes after thermal injury. The Art and Science of Burn Care. Boswick J, Ed. Aspen Publishers, Rockville, Maryland, 1987, p 137

Winchurch R, Thupari J, Munster A: Endotoxemia in burn patients, levels of circulating endotoxins are related to burn size. Surgery 102:808, 1987

Woolf P: Hormonal responses to trauma. Crit Care Med 20:216, 1992

Xia Z, Coolbaugh M, He F, et al: The effects of burn injury on the acute phase response. J Trauma 32:245, 1992

Youn Y, Demling R: The role of mediators in the response to thermal injury. World J Surg 16:30, 1992

Acknowledgments

Figures 1 through 3   Talar Agasyan.

Table 1   Adapted from *Metabolic Management of the Critically Ill*, by D. W. Wilmore. Plenum Publishing Corporation, New York, 1977, p 22.

15 MISCELLANEOUS BURNS AND COLD INJURIES

David Heimbach, M.D., F.A.C.S., and Nicole Gibran, M.D., F.A.C.S.

Electrical Injury

Three forms of electrical injury exist: low-voltage burns (i.e., burns resulting from contact with circuits of less than 440 volts), high-voltage burns (i.e., burns resulting from circuits of greater than 1,000 volts), and super–high-voltage burns (caused by lightning). A poorly defined "intermediate-voltage" burn includes those caused by contact with industrial circuits of 440 to 800 volts; these burns have characteristics of both high-voltage and low-voltage burns, depending on the circumstances.

A common "electrical," though noncontact, injury is an intense flash burn resulting from the short-circuiting of an industrial circuit by an electrician with a metal tool. Such a short-circuiting causes the metal part of the tool to vaporize, as if it were an uncontrolled arc welder; this vaporization results in a very high temperature flash that causes deep burns to the hand holding the tool and less deep burns to the upper body and face. Clothing can catch fire, compounding the problem. These burns are not, however, associated with the problems of contact electrical burns, and they should be treated in a manner similar to other thermal burns.

An electrical burn is managed in essentially the same way as any other burn except that a higher urinary output is necessary in the presence of myoglobinuria. In addition to the potentially devastating tissue destruction seen with high-voltage injury, electrical injuries can lead to nonsurgical, chronic, debilitating conditions that must be addressed.

LOW-VOLTAGE INJURIES

The human body is three to four times as sensitive to alternating current as it is to direct current. Alternating current has generally replaced direct current for all commercial power applications because it is cheaper to transmit and can be more easily transformed to any required voltage. The amount of 60-cycle alternating current that can just be perceived in the hand is about 1.1 milliamperes (mA), which produces a tingling sensation. Skin resistance, however, varies according to the thickness of the epidermal keratin layer, as well as the cleanliness and dryness of the skin. The calloused hand may provide resistance of as much as 1,000,000 ohms/in² while dry; normal skin provides resistance of 5,000 ohms/in²; and wet skin provides resistance of only 1,000 ohms/in². With currents higher than 2 to 4 mA, the tingling gives way to muscle contractions, which get stronger as the current increases. The "let go" current is reached at approximately 15 mA, above which the victim cannot release the grasp of the conductor. Above 20 mA, there is sustained spasm of the respiratory muscles. If the passage of current lasts less than 4 minutes, respiration will resume; however, if it lasts longer than 4 minutes, asphyxiation may occur, and mouth to mouth resuscitation may be required. At levels above 30 to 40 mA, ventricular fibrillation (VF) may be induced. As the current is increased, the heart's susceptibility to fibrillation first increases and then decreases. At 1 to 5 amps, the heart goes into sustained contraction, and the likelihood of VF

becomes negligible. When the high current is terminated, the heart usually reverts back to sinus rhythm, just as happens in cardiac defibrillation, when such high currents are deliberately applied to the chest to depolarize the entire heart.

In the event that the victim of electric shock is unconscious, the initial responder should remove the source of the current (taking care not to himself or herself become a victim of shock) and then provide cardiopulmonary resuscitation (CPR); paramedics may then begin defibrillation. If a sinus rhythm has not been established on arrival at the ER, the physician should treat the patient as he or she would any other dysrhythmia patient. If sinus rhythm has been established, the patient should be treated as a sudden death victim, with evaluation for anoxic damage and cardiac monitoring.

Many patients come to the ER after receiving an electric shock from household current. If the electrocardiogram and rhythm strip are normal, the patient should be reassured and discharged without hospital admission. Muscle soreness will resolve spontaneously in 24 to 48 hours and may be treated with analgesics, such as nonsteroidal anti-inflammatory drugs (NSAIDs).

Cutaneous burns with significant tissue necrosis rarely result from contact with low-voltage current. Usually, the area of contact is large enough to dissipate the heat of the current, and underlying tissue destruction is minimal.

Mouth Burns in Children

The exception to this rule is a child who may chew on the end of a live electric extension cord. The child's saliva completes the circuit between the positive and neutral leads; the resulting electrical short may cause significant tissue destruction of the lips, tongue, or both [see Figure 1]. These burns should be evaluated and treated by a plastic surgeon or a burn surgeon. The patient is often admitted to ensure he or she receives proper nourishment and that the parent is comfortable with pain management and wound cleansing. The parent should be forewarned that the eschar might separate in a few days, resulting in bleeding from the labial branch of the facial artery. Emergently, this can be easily treated by pinching the lip between thumb and forefinger while the child is brought to the ER for suture ligation.

There are two plans for definitive care.[1-3] Long-term results appear to be about equal for nonoperative and operative acute management. If nonoperative management is chosen, splinting is usually recommended to keep the mouth stretched to prevent contracture, but patient and parent compliance with splint use is not always successful. Immediate coverage with flaps hastens the healing but leaves a permanent scar and may result in the sacrifice of some normal tissue.

HIGH-VOLTAGE INJURIES

Current in wires containing 1,000 volts or more may cause massive tissue destruction. The tissue destruction results from electrical energy being converted to heat as it meets resistance in the tissues. The smaller the size of the body part through which the electricity passes, the more intense the heat and the less the heat is dissipated. Fingers, hands, forearms, feet, and lower legs are frequently totally destroyed; areas of larger volume, such as the trunk, usually dissipate enough current to prevent extensive damage to viscera unless the contact wound is on the abdomen or chest. As current passes through the body, arc burns, as well as the usual contact wounds, are common. These deep wounds, which are often as destructive as contact wounds, occur when current takes a direct path, often between joints in close apposition to one another at the time of injury. Burns of the volar aspect of the wrist, the antecubital fossa when the elbow is flexed at the time of injury, and the axilla are most common. Such injuries should always be seen immediately by a surgeon with a special interest in burns. The immediate evaluation of the patient with a major electrical burn is similar to that of any severely injured patient and includes evaluation of airway, breathing, and circulation.

In addition to burns, which may be obvious, the patient may have other associated injuries from falls, or the patient may have broken bones from the tetanic spasms of major muscle groups. Common potential fractures include those of the lumbar spine and hip.

RESUSCITATION

Flash and flame burns without electrical contact injuries are treated in the same manner as are all thermal burns. For patients with electrical contact injuries, fluid requirements are considerably more than are predicted by the various formulae used for thermal burn victims; the reason is that the cutaneous injury is usually only the "tip of the iceberg," and underlying deep tissue damage may be extensive. A good general starting point is to administer lactated Ringer solution at two to three times the quantity specified by the Baxter (Parkland) burn formula. This would initially require providing 8 to 10 ml/kg/% total body surface area that is burned. Fluid administration should be adjusted, based on correction of metabolic acidosis, normalization of vital signs, and attainment of a urinary output of approximately 100 ml/hr in adults, especially in the presence of myoglobinuria. With significant myonecrosis, rhabdomyolysis results in increased levels of circulating myoglobin and hemoglobin, as well as cell fragments, which can plug the renal tubules and cause acute tubular necrosis. Myoglobin precipitation is accentuated by acidic urine and decreased by alkaline urine. There has never been a report of a correlation between exact myoglobin levels in the urine or the blood and development of renal failure.[4,5] Because myoglobin levels in the urine can be significantly elevated even when the urine is clear, the clinical relevance of quantitative levels of myoglobin in urine is unclear. However, gross myoglobin in the urine should be treated with aggressive fluid hydration. If the urine is red or reddish black, urinary flow of at least 1 ml/kg/hr is indicated until the pigment clears, and acidosis should be corrected. An osmotic diuretic such as mannitol (25 g bolus, followed by 12.5 g every 2 to 4 hours) may be necessary to maintain adequate urinary output. Use of sodium bicarbonate to maintain urinary pH above 7 without raising blood pH above 7.5 theoretically may minimize protein precipitation in the urine.

SURGICAL CONSIDERATIONS

There are two reasons for early operation in a patient with a high-voltage electrical burn. If the burn is making the patient sick (e.g., myoglobin will not clear or acidosis will not resolve), the wound should be explored and all grossly necrotic tissue

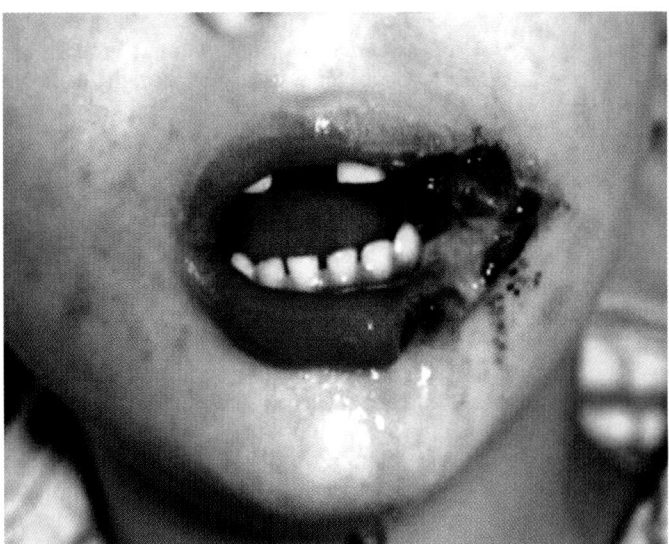

Figure 1 **Shown is an electrical burn caused by a 110-volt household current. The injury resulted from the patient's sucking on an extension plug. The burn was treated conservatively with a mouth splint, which resulted in a nearly normal-appearing mouth with good function.**

removed. If the burn is making an extremity sick (e.g., there are signs of a compartment syndrome), early escharotomy, fasciotomy, or both should be performed. Otherwise, a delay in surgical exploration of a few days can often allow definitive debridement and wound closure through a single operation.[6,7]

Escharotomy and Fasciotomy

In general, an escharotomy is indicated for a circumferential deep burn when there is evidence of impaired distal perfusion. Fasciotomy is indicated for concomitant electrical injury to underlying muscle when there is evidence of increased compartment pressure, myoglobinuria, tense muscle compartments, or nerve or vessel compression. Careful monitoring, including measurement of compartment pressures, is mandatory, and escharotomies and fasciotomies should be performed at the slightest suggestion of progression. Routine compartment pressure measurements may be helpful, but any of the signs of impending compartment syndrome (i.e., increased pain, pallor, absence of pulse, decreased sensation, and tense swelling) mandate prompt compartment release in the operating theater. One unique injury that must be considered in patients with electrical injuries to the hand is a carpal tunnel injury.[7] With the associated swelling, relatively small electrical injuries can lead to swelling in the carpal tunnel that manifests as increasing paresthesias and numbness in the distribution of the median nerve. If the injury is sufficiently devastating to create a mummified hand, carpal tunnel release probably has no role in the treatment plan.

CONTACT SITES

Because most electrical injuries result from alternating current, entrance and exit sites are better referred to as contact points. These are thermal burns resulting from heat generation, but unlike flame burns, they are often associated with significant injury to the deep tissues. The amount of heat generated depends on the resistance to current flow. A dry hand or foot in contact with high voltage may generate heat in excess of 1,000° C, leading to mummification at the contact site [*see Figure 2*].

With passage of a large current, multiple contact sites may be seen along the route of the current, resulting in injuries that suggest the effects of an explosion. Sites of current arcing (described above) should be treated in the same manner as primary contact sites, because underlying damage can be just as severe.

WOUND MANAGEMENT

In general, if there are large amounts of necrotic muscle as a result of high-voltage electrical contact, aggressive surgical debridement to decrease myoglobinemia is indicated. This intervention may minimize subsequent organ dysfunction. If gross myoglobinuria does not resolve after several hours of aggressive hydration, diuresis, and compartment release, the presence of a large amount of dead muscle is a virtual certainty. Muscle of indeterminate viability should be spared, but guillotine amputation may be appropriate and lifesaving on obviously nonsalvageable limbs. The goal of subsequent surgical procedures is to conserve viable tissue while removing neighboring dead tissue. The uneven nature of the injuries makes this approach difficult and time-consuming. If they are not exposed, small, scattered areas of injured muscle will be replaced by fibrous tissue. A high fever and tachycardia, however, may be physiologic evidence that remaining nonviable muscle has become infected. Because bone resists current and becomes very hot, nonviable necrotic muscle tissue along the bone may require debridement. It is not uncommon for superficial forearm muscles to appear viable, while necrotic muscle surrounds the radius and ulna. Use of vascular grafts to replace clotted arteries is sometimes an option. However, such grafts may actually increase morbidity and prolong recovery; better function may result through use of one of the newer prostheses following amputation than would be available in a hand or foot that has poor sensation and motor function.

In accordance with the principles used for thermal burns, devitalized tissue below the skin at the contact sites should be debrid-

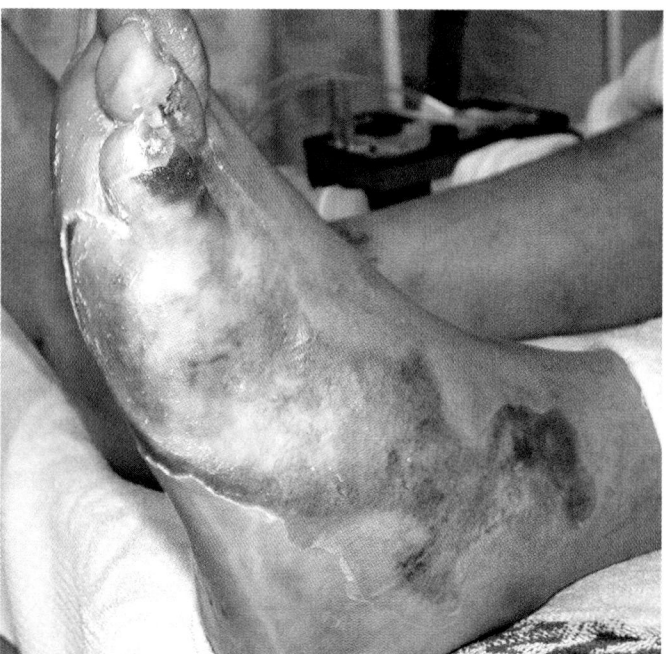

Figure 2 Shown is a contact-point injury caused by a 15,000-volt current, seen on day 1. Although the injury looks relatively simple, a similar injury to this patient's right foot led to a below-the-knee amputation. Careful monitoring for compartment syndrome in the leg is mandatory in such injuries.

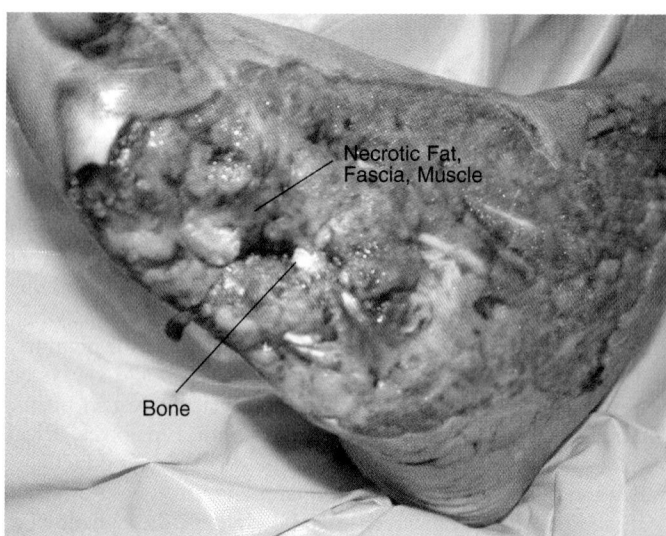

Figure 3 Shown is the same injury seen in Figure 2 just before a second debridement on day 7. Because this patient's right leg was amputated, every attempt was made to salvage as much of the left foot as possible. At initial debridement, it is difficult to tell precisely how much of the foot is possibly viable; note that there is still considerable nonviable soft tissue under the metatarsals and that the metatarsals are considerably exposed. After the second debridement, the foot was treated in a Wound Vac to stimulate vascularization.

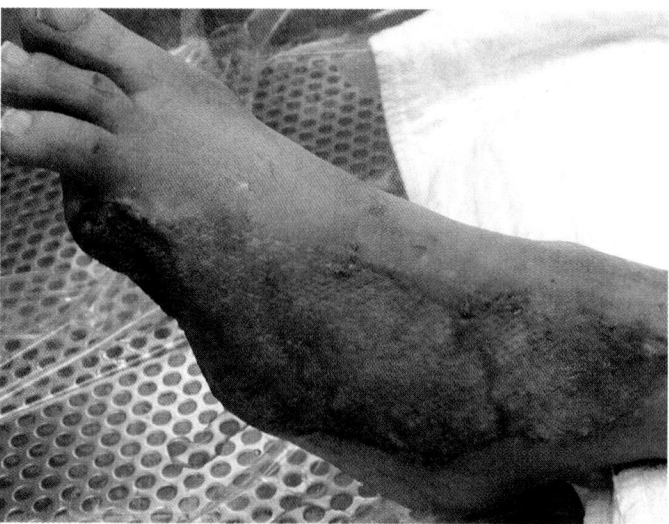

Figure 4 Shown is the same foot as in Figures 2 and 3 at the time of discharge (day 21 after injury). Two toes and the fifth metatarsal were removed, leaving a stable, sensate foot with satisfactory cover.

ed within 7 days after injury [*see Figure 3*]. Sequential debridement of residual necrotic tissue may be necessary over the ensuing 3 to 5 days. Early aggressive debridement, followed immediately by reconstructive surgery with tissue transfer by rotation or free flaps to cover remaining viable tissue, nerves, vessels, and bone, may facilitate early recovery [*see Figure 4*].

To help determine timing and results of operation, Mann reviewed the charts of 62 patients who underwent treatment for high-voltage electrical burns of the upper extremities.[6] A total of 100 upper extremities were treated. Of these, 22% underwent decompression within 24 hours because of progressive nerve dysfunction, clinical compartment syndrome, or failure of resuscitation. This group required a mean of 4.2 operations; the amputation rate was 45%, which was similar to that reported in other series. For 35% of the burned extremities, the first operative procedure was delayed until resuscitation was complete. This group required a mean of 2.1 operations and required no amputations. Forty-three percent of the extremities did not require operations to achieve healing. Overall results showed a 10% amputation rate and a mean hospital stay of 27 days; these results were better than the results reported by others.

Nonsurgical Problems Related to Electrical Injury

CARDIAC INJURIES

Immediate cardiac arrest is the most common cause of death from electrical injury. Low-voltage exposure is likely to induce ventricular fibrillation, whereas high-voltage exposure is more likely to produce cardiac standstill. Cardiac standstill and respiratory arrest may revert spontaneously if CPR prevents anoxia; VF is more likely to require defibrillation. Conventional wisdom states that patients who have sustained high-voltage injuries should be admitted for 24-hour telemetry monitoring; in addition, cardiac isoenzymes should be followed. Studies have shown that if the ECG is normal on admission, subsequent cardiac dysrhythmias are rare and intensive monitoring is probably not necessary.[8,9] A transient interest in isoenzyme and troponin levels has waned, and their assessment has not been useful in predicting cardiac damage.[8,10,11]

Myocardial infarction is uncommon, but it has been reported in a small percentage of cases in each series. In one patient at our burn center, a papillary muscle ruptured within 24 hours; this led to immediate, fatal congestive heart failure.

NEUROLOGIC COMPLICATIONS

Neurologic complications are common sequelae of high-voltage electrical injuries and can affect the brain, spinal cord, and peripheral nerves. Immediate but frequently transient symptoms include varying levels of unconsciousness, respiratory paralysis, and motor paralysis. Permanent changes include cortical encephalopathy, caused by the electrical injury itself or resulting from hypoxia at the time of the accident. Spinal cord injuries are rare but may present as progressive muscular atrophy, amyotrophic lateral sclerosis, or transverse myelitis. These may occur days to months after the injury and progress slowly.[12,13]

A study of 90 patients (82 males and 8 females) with electrical burns was conducted at the University of Washington Burn Center to determine neurologic consequences.[14] There were four deaths. Twenty-two patients sustained low-voltage injury. Of these 22 patients, 11 had immediate neurologic symptoms; these symptoms resolved in nine of the 11 patients. Sixty-four patients sustained high-voltage injury; of these, two thirds had immediate central or peripheral neurologic symptoms, or both. Loss of consciousness accounted for the largest percentage of central nervous system sequelae in the high-voltage group (45%). Twenty-three patients (79%) recovered consciousness before arrival at the hospital. Six patients remained comatose, three died, and three awoke but had neurologic sequelae. One third of patients in the high-voltage group had one or more acute peripheral neuropathies. Of these neuropathies, 64% resolved or improved. Five patients had transient initial paralysis, but there were no delayed spinal cord symptoms. Eleven patients experienced one or more delayed peripheral neuropathies. Half of these delayed neuropathies resolved or improved.

Peripheral neuropathies are relatively common in burned extremities, either from direct nerve injury or fibrosis occurring around the nerves. Reflex sympathetic dystrophy is not uncommon. Many patients suffer aches, headaches, chronic pain, and various nonanatomic neurologic complaints for some months after injury

CATARACTS

The incidence of premature cataract development may be as high as 5% to 10% following electrical injury.[15-17] Surprisingly, they occur equally in patients who do and do not have obvious contact points on the face or head. The latent period may range from weeks to years, with the average being 6 months.[17] Therefore, complete ophthalmologic examination for cataracts at the time of hospitalization and, subsequently, with any subjective decrease in visual acuity is warranted. For workers' compensation claims, an eye examination shortly after the injury is indicated to document normal lens transparency in case cataracts occur as an injury-related disease and not from preexisting problems.

PSYCHOLOGICAL EFFECTS

Posttraumatic stress syndrome is more common after electrical burns than after thermal burns.[18]

Lightning Injury

A lightning strike is an extraordinarily high-voltage discharge of brief duration. The current generated may reach 300,000 amps and 100,000,000 volts. Fortunately, the current often flows around the surface of, rather than through, the body; this "flashover" permits an overall survival rate of 65% or more.[19,20] The most common immediate potentially fatal complications are paralysis of the respiratory center and cardiac standstill. Cardiac activity will usually resume spontaneously, but apnea may be present for 15 minutes or longer—long enough to cause anoxic brain injury in the absence of pulmonary resuscitation. A rare but fascinating complication is keraunoparalysis, which is a transient paralysis associated with extreme vasoconstriction and sensory disturbances of one or more extremities. It usually lasts only an hour (in rare instances, as long as 24 hours); a lifeless appearance should not result in the patient's being treated as a victim of sudden death.[21] Cardiac and neurologic complications are frequent and are generally similar to those resulting from man-made high-voltage injuries.[22] Dendritic superficial skin burns, known as Lichtenberg's flowers or fractals,[23] are sometimes seen. These superficial burns heal rapidly without sequelae. Ruptured tympanic membranes and vertigo are common accompaniments.[24,25] Treatment of systemic effects is generally supportive; tissue injuries are treated in the same manner as other high-voltage injuries.

Chemical Burns

GENERAL EMERGENCY CARE

Immediate treatment of chemical burns involves the immediate removal of affected clothing; the burns should then be thoroughly flushed with copious amounts of water at the scene of the accident. The only exception to this is for chemical burns involving dry powder; for such burns, the powder should be brushed from clothing and skin. Chemicals will continue to burn until removed;

washing for at least 15 minutes under a stream of running water may limit the overall severity of the burn. No thought should be given to searching for a specific neutralizing agent. Delay results in deepening of the burn, and neutralizing agents may cause burns themselves; they frequently generate heat while neutralizing the offending agent, adding a thermal burn to the already potentially serious chemical burn.

Chemical burns, usually caused by strong acids or alkalis, are most often the result of industrial accidents, assaults, or the improper use of harsh solvents and drain cleaners. In contrast to a thermal burn, chemical burns cause progressive damage until the chemicals are inactivated by reaction with the tissue or are diluted by being flushed with water. Individual circumstances vary, but acid burns may be more self-limiting than alkali burns. Acid tends to tan the skin, creating an impermeable barrier that limits further penetration of the acid. Alkalis combine with cutaneous lipids to create soap and thereby continue dissolving the skin until they are neutralized. A full-thickness chemical burn may appear deceptively superficial, seeming to cause only a mild brownish discoloration of the skin. The skin may appear to remain intact during the first few days postburn and only then begin to slough spontaneously. Chemical burns should be considered deep dermal or full-thickness until proved otherwise. In general, definitive treatment of these burns is the same as for thermal injuries—shallow burns heal with infection prevention; deep burns are excised and grafted as soon as their depth is determined.

Some chemicals, such as phenol, cause severe systemic effects; others, such as hydrofluoric acid, may cause death from hypocalcemia even after moderate exposure. Unless the characteristics of the chemical are well known, the treating physician is advised to call the local poison control bureau for specifics on treatment.

ALKALIS

Lime (calcium oxide/hydroxide) and sodium or potassium hydroxide are examples of common alkalis used in industry and around the home.

Sodium or potassium hydroxide (drain cleaner) is ingested by children accidentally and by adults attempting suicide. Mouth burns are the tip of the iceberg. Treatment should be emergently directed to the oropharynx and the upper gastrointestinal tract; description of such treatment is beyond the scope of this chapter. Sodium or potassium hydroxide is also used in assaults, especially in areas where people cannot afford handguns.[26] Teen hoodlums sometimes fill water pistols with sodium hydroxide and squirt sleeping homeless people. Contact of concentrated sodium hydroxide with the cornea results in prompt and permanent corneal destruction and blindness. Drain and oven cleaners are also favorite substances of patients who deliberately and repeatedly inflict injury on themselves (Munchausen syndrome).[27-29] The unwitting homeowner or novice construction worker who does not protect the skin when working with concrete cement (calcium hydroxide) is often surprised at day's end with painful red contact areas on the hands, feet, knees, and forearms. By bedtime, these injuries have become excruciating and require emergency treatment and, frequently, excision and grafting.[30,31]

Strong alkali burns are invariably deep, although at onset they may seem deceptively shallow.

ANHYDROUS AMMONIA

Anhydrous ammonia is a colorless, pungent gas that is stored and transported under pressure in liquid form. Ammonia injury is uncommon, but it is associated with high morbidity and mortality. Particularly devastating is severe acute respiratory distress syn-

drome and long-term restrictive disease with bronchiectasis. Most of the literature consists of case reports, but all emphasize the severity and long-term sequelae of the respiratory and ocular problems.[32-36]

ACIDS

As noted (see above), burns tend to denature (tan) the skin. Although these burns may be full thickness, destruction of deeper tissues is often limited as a result of the formation of an impervious carapace of the dermis.

Hydrochloric and Nitric Acids

Hydrochloric and nitric acids are strong acids that denature proteins but usually do not result in systemic poisoning unless inhaled or ingested.

Chromic Acid

Some acids, such as chromic acid and dichromate, cause both systemic and cutaneous problems. Chromium poisoning is characterized by complete anuria, hepatic damage, and progressive anemia. It can occur from the cutaneous absorption of chromium from chromic acid burns that are as small as 1% of the total body surface area. Aggressive surgical excision and prompt hemodialysis may be lifesaving.[37-40]

Formic Acid

Similarly, formic acid causes metabolic acidosis, intravascular hemolysis, and hemoglobinuria when ingested or when concentrated solutions contact the skin.[41,42]

Carbolic Acid

Phenol (carbolic acid) is used as a hospital, industrial, and home disinfectant. Exposure may lead to rapid CNS depression, vomiting, coughing, stridor, and, in rare instances, seizures.[43] The cutaneous burns are usually first degree.

Hydrofluoric Acid

Hydrofluoric acid burns are unique in presentation and current treatment. Hydrofluoric acid is used in industrial cleaners and rust removers. It is used in concentrated form in the etching of circuit boards and in dilute form as a glass cleaner and to clean milk cans. Hydrofluoric acid is a very strong acid that coagulates skin and allows entry of fluoride ions, which then chelate calcium and magnesium in tissue and plasma. Local cell death results; with severe exposure, severe systemic hypocalcemia and hypomagnesemia can result in fatal cardiac dysrhythmias.[44,45] Fluoride, as the most electronegative element, tightly binds many cations essential to hemostasis, inhibiting normal blood coagulation. As a metabolic poison, it stimulates some enzymes, such as adenylate cyclase, and severely inhibits others, such as Na^+,K^+-ATPase and the enzymes of carbohydrate metabolism.[46] Treatment of severe poisoning requires careful monitoring in an ICU, replacement of magnesium and calcium, and consideration of dialysis.

More commonly, industrial exposure is limited to the hand. Exposure to concentrated solution will cause immediate symptoms, but the more common dilute solutions may not cause symptoms for hours. Often, the worker will go home and experience increasingly severe pain, which will prevent sleep and lead to a nighttime visit to the ER. The worker will likely be unaware of the cause of his pain; the emergency physician should question the patient about solvents used that day.

Conventional treatment of burns to the hand and digits has been local application of calcium liquids and gels. Direct injection of calcium gluconate into the injury site is somewhat effective but risks pressure necrosis of fingers that are already swollen. A much better, almost magical, treatment is direct infusion of a dilute calcium gluconate solution intra-arterially through the radial or brachial artery. The sooner the infusion is started after onset of pain, the better the result. Pain is immediately mitigated if not cured, and tissue destruction is often minimal.[47,48] This has become the treatment of choice in our burn center and has yielded good results with no complications to date. However, therapy needs to be started within the first 24 hours, because tissue damage is permanent by that time. An alternative is intravenous calcium gluconate using the Bier block technique (i.e., a venous tourniquet applied proximal to the infusion site),[49-51] but this can increase swelling in the extremity.

War and Chemicals of Mass Destruction

NAPALM

Napalm is jellied gasoline that is generally ignited and sprayed on material and combatants in wartime. It causes devastating burns, because the gasoline sticks to clothing and skin while it is burning. Injuries are usually fourth-degree thermal burns, which are treated in the same manner as other very deep thermal burns.

WHITE PHOSPHORUS

White phosphorus is used in many types of military munitions, as well as in fireworks and in industrial and agricultural products. In the presence of oxygen, it ignites spontaneously; when in contact with skin, it causes deep thermal injuries. It may also cause multiorgan failure because of its toxic effects on erythrocytes, the liver, the kidneys, and the heart. Treatment of the injured patient is difficult. The particles must be debrided to prevent continued burning and systemic poisoning. Conventional wisdom was to use a solution of copper sulfate to convert the elemental phosphorus into copper phosphate. However, this approach has fallen into disfavor because copper poisoning may result, the effects of which are as bad as those of the phosphorus.[52,53] During debridement in the operating theater, exposure of the particles to air will cause flare-up and endanger the environment and the operating team.

MUSTARD GAS, LEWISITE, AND PHOSGENE

Sulfur mustard is a vesicant that alkylates DNA. In liquid or gas form, its main targets are skin and lungs. Its clinical effects are similar to those of burns, with loss of immunity, respiratory failure, and ophthalmic, gastrointestinal, and hematologic signs. In the Iraq-Iran war (1981–1989), extensive use of chemical weapons such as mustard gas caused injuries with high mortality and morbidity, as well as chronic side effects in vital organs, especially the respiratory tract. Bijani studied the long-term effects in 220 survivors who were exposed to mustard gas. Nearly all the victims complained of cough, dyspnea, and suffocation. Hemoptysis was found in six victims. In four patients, respiratory distress with use of accessory muscles was observed. Two thirds of the subjects had wheezing and coarse rales. Most had obstructive patterns on pulmonary function testing.[54] Cutaneous exposure is manifested by a delayed erythema of skin occurring after about 4 hours, followed by blistering in 12 to 48 hours. The blisters rupture, leaving shallow, painful ulcers. Other vesicants are more corrosive: lewisite (arsine) and phosgene are both more potent; symptoms appear sooner with these agents than with mustard gas.[55]

Rescuers should be protected with suitable clothing, respirators, gloves, and boots. The victim's clothing is removed, and extensive water lavage is provided, along with copious isotonic eye irrigation. Once decontamination has been completed, there is no danger to attendants; blister fluid does not contain chemicals.[56] Burns are usually of partial thickness and can be treated in the same manner as other partial-thickness burns.

Cold Injury

Cold injuries limited to digits, extremities, or exposed surfaces are the result of either direct tissue freezing (frostbite) or more chronic exposure to an environment just above freezing (chilblain or pernio; trench foot). Cold injury has been a major cause of morbidity during war, and it is described as being the single major injury sustained by British soldiers in the Falklands expedition. Cold injury resulted in over 7 million soldier fighting days lost by Allied forces in World War II.[57]

CHILBLAIN, PERNIO, AND TRENCH FOOT

Chilblain and pernio are descriptive terms for a form of local cold injury characterized by red-purple, pruritic skin lesions (papules, macules, plaques, or nodules) often associated with edema or blistering; the lesions are caused by a chronic vasculitis of the dermis. This pathology appears to be provoked by repeated exposure to cold, though not freezing, temperatures. This injury typically occurs on the face, the anterior tibial surface, or the dorsum of the hands and feet—areas poorly protected or subject to long-term exposure to the environment. With continued exposure, ulcerative or hemorrhagic lesions may appear and progress to scarring, fibrosis, and atrophy. Treatment consists of sheltering the patient, elevating the affected part on sheepskin, and allowing gradual rewarming at room temperature. Rubbing or massage is contraindicated, because further damage and secondary infection may result.[58-60]

Trench foot or cold immersion foot (or hand) describes a nonfreezing injury of the hands or feet, typically sustained by sailors, fishermen, or soldiers, as a consequence of long-term exposure to wet conditions (e.g., water or mud) and temperatures just above freezing.[61-65] Alternating arterial vasospasm and vasodilatation appear to occur, with the affected tissue first cold and anesthetic and then progressing to hyperemia after 24 to 48 hours of exposure. With the hyperemia comes an intense, painful burning and dysesthesia, as well as tissue damage characterized by edema, blistering, redness, ecchymosis, and ulceration. Complications consisting of local infection and cellulitis, lymphangitis, and gangrene may occur. After 2 to 6 weeks, a posthyperemic phase ensues, resulting in tissue cyanosis with increased sensitivity to cold. Treatment is best started during or before the reactive hyperemia state; it consists of immediate removal of the extremity from the cold, wet environment and exposure of the extremity to warm, dry air. The limb is elevated to minimize edema; pressure spots are protected, and local and systemic measures to combat infection are undertaken. Massage, soaking of the feet, and rapid rewarming are not indicated.

FROSTBITE

Frostbite is a common, severe form of cold injury that involves local freezing of tissues. Frostbite is classified into four grades of severity:

1. First-degree injury involves the freezing of tissue, with hyperemia and edema but without blistering.
2. Second-degree frostbite involves the freezing of tissue, with hyperemia, edema, and characteristic large, clear blisters.

3. Third-degree frostbite involves the freezing of tissue, with death of subcutaneous tissues and skin, resulting in hemorrhagic vesicles that are generally smaller than is seen in second-degree frostbite.

4. Fourth-degree frostbite is notable for tissue necrosis, gangrene, and, eventually, full-thickness tissue loss.

The degree of severity of frostbite is often not apparent for several days. For all forms of frostbite, the initial presentation is pain or discomfort, as well as pruritus if the injury is mild. With more severe injury, there is a progressive decrease in range of motion, and edema becomes prominent. The injury progresses to numbness and eventual loss of all sensation in the affected tissue. The involved area appears white or blue-white and is firm or even hard (frozen) to the touch. The tissue is cold and insensate. Although the initial symptoms may be mild and may be overlooked by the patient, with rewarming, severe pain, burning, edema, and even necrosis and gangrene may appear.

Weather conditions, altitude, degree of protective clothing, duration of exposure, and degree of tissue wetness are all contributing external factors to the development of frostbite. Acclimation to cold may be protective, whereas a previous history of frostbite probably does predispose an individual to another cold tissue injury. Smoking and a history of arterial disease also are contributing factors. In urban environments, over 50% of frostbite injuries are alcohol related, and a significant portion (16%) of patients have an underlying psychiatric illness.[66,67]

Current evidence suggests that frostbite injury may in fact have two components: the initial freeze injury, and a reperfusion injury that occurs during rewarming.[68-70] The initial response to tissue cooling is vasoconstriction and arteriovenous shunting, intermittently relieved (every 5 to 7 minutes) by vasodilatation. With prolonged exposure, this response fails, and the temperature of the freezing tissue will approximate ambient temperature until a temperature of $-2°$ C is reached. At this point, extracellular ice crystals form; as these crystals enlarge, the osmotic pressure of the interstitium increases, resulting in the movement of intracellular water into the interstitium. Cells begin to shrink and become hyperosmolar, disrupting cellular enzyme function. If freezing is rapid (faster than $10°$ C/min), intracellular ice crystal formation will occur, resulting in immediate cell death. Intravascularly, endothelial cell disruption and red cell sludging result in cessation of circulation.[71-74]

During rewarming, red cell, platelet, and leukocyte aggregation is known to occur; this results in patchy thrombosis of the microcirculation.[75] These accumulated blood elements are thought to release, among other products, the toxic oxygen free radicals and the arachidonic acid metabolites prostaglandin F_2 and thromboxane A_2, which further aggravate vasoconstriction and platelet and leukocyte aggregation. However, the exact mechanism of tissue destruction and death following freeze injury remains poorly defined. Animal studies suggest that vascular injury in the form of endothelial cell damage and subsequent interstitial edema, but not vessel thrombosis, predominate as initial events in rewarming injury. Mileski has demonstrated a marked amelioration of the frostbite injury in a rabbit ear model by treating the animals (after cold injury and before rewarming) with a monoclonal antibody to the neutrophil CD18 glycoprotein complex.[76] The implication of this observation is that neutrophil adherence to the endothelium of frostbitten tissue during rewarming (reperfusion) is at least partially responsible for the subsequent tissue injury. Clinical application of these experimental observations remains untested.

TREATMENT

Prehospital or field care of the victim of cold injury should focus on removing the patient from the hostile environment and protecting the injured body part from further damage. Rubbing or exercising the affected tissue does not augment blood flow and risks further cold injury or mechanical trauma. Because repeated bouts of freezing and thawing worsen the injury, it is preferable for the patient with frostbite of the hands or feet to immediately seek definitive shelter and care rather than to rewarm the tissue in the field and risk refreezing. Once rewarming has begun, weight bearing should be avoided.

The ER treatment of a frostbite victim should first focus on the basic ABCs of trauma resuscitation and on identifying and correcting systemic hypothermia. Frostbitten tissue should be immersed in a large water bath of 40° to 42° C (104° to 108° F). The bath should be large enough to prevent rapid loss of heat, and the water temperature should be maintained. This method of rapid rewarming may significantly decrease tissue necrosis caused by full-thickness frostbite.[71,73,74] Dry heat is not advocated, because it is difficult to regulate and places the patient at risk for a burn injury. The rewarming process should take about 30 to 45 minutes for digits. The affected area appears flushed when rewarming is complete and good circulation has been reestablished. Narcotics are required, because the rewarming process may be quite painful.

The skin should be gently but meticulously cleansed and air-dried, and the affected area should be elevated to minimize edema. A tetanus toxoid booster should be administered as indicated by immunization history. Sterile cotton should be placed between toes or fingers to prevent skin maceration, and extreme care should be taken to prevent infection and to avoid even the slightest abrasion. Prophylactic antibiotics and dermal blister debridement are both controversial; most clinicians debride blisters and reserve antibiotics for identified infections.

After rewarming, the treatment goals are to prevent further injury while awaiting the demarcation of irreversible tissue destruction. All patients with second- and third-degree frostbite should be hospitalized. The affected tissue should be gently cleansed in a warm (38° C) whirlpool bath once or twice a day; some clinicians add an antiseptic such as chlorhexidine or an iodophor to the bath. On the basis of findings of arachidonic acid metabolites in the blisters of frostbite victims, some authors advocate the use of topical aloe vera (a thromboxane inhibitor) and systemic ibuprofen or aspirin. After resolution of edema, digits should be exercised during the whirlpool bath, and physical therapy should begin. Tobacco, nicotine, and other vasoconstrictive agents must be withheld.

Numerous adjuvants have been suggested and tried in an effort to restore blood supply to frostbitten areas. Because of the intense vasoconstrictive effect of cold injury, attention has been focused for many years on increased sympathetic tone. Sympathetic blockade and even surgical sympathectomy have been advocated as early therapy, under the theoretical suspicion that sympathetic blockade will release the vasospasm that may precipitate thrombosis in the affected tissue. Unfortunately, this method of treatment has produced inconsistent results in experimental studies and is difficult to evaluate clinically.[72,77] Experience with intra-arterial vasodilating drugs such as reserpine and tolazoline have also failed to verify this hypothesis. In a controlled clinical study, immediate (mean, 3 hours) ipsilateral intra-arterial reserpine infusion coupled with early (mean, 3 days) ipsilateral operative sympathectomy failed to alter the natural history of acute frostbite injury when compared with the contralateral.[72] Sympathectomy may, however, mollify the chronic pain, hyperhidrosis, and vasospasm of cold injuries; some clinicians also suggest that it reduces the risk of subsequent cold injury. Heparin, low-molecular-weight dextran, thrombolytic agents, and hyperbaric oxygen have failed to demonstrate any substantial treatment benefit.

The difficulty in determining the depth of tissue destruction in cold injury has led to a conservative approach to the care of frostbite injuries. As a general rule, amputation and surgical debridement are delayed for 2 to 3 months unless severe infection with sepsis occurs. The natural history of a full-thickness frostbite injury leads to the gradual demarcation of the injured area; dry gangrene or mummification clearly delineate nonviable tissue. Often, the permanent tissue loss is much less than originally suspected. In Urschel's review, only 39% of urban frostbite victims required debridement and skin grating or amputation.[67] Emergency surgery is unusual, but during the rewarming phase, vigilance should be maintained to detect the development of a compartment syndrome requiring fasciotomy. Open amputations are indicated in patients with persistent infection and sepsis that is refractory to debridement and antibiotics.

Frostbitten tissues seldom recover completely. Some degree of cold insensitivity invariably remains. Hyperhidrosis (occurring in up to 72% of patients), neuropathy, decreased nail and hair growth, and persistent Raynaud phenomenon in the affected part are frequent sequelae to cold injury.[78] The affected tissue remains at risk for reinjury and should be carefully protected during any cold exposure. Treatment with antiadrenergics (prazosin hydrochloride, 1 to 2 mg/day) or calcium channel blockers (nifedipine, 30 to 60 mg/day) and careful protection from further exposure is often helpful. However, there is little that appears to afford significant relief to the chronic symptoms following tissue freeze injury; sympathectomy, beta- and alpha-adrenergic blocking agents, calcium channel blockers, topical and systemic steroids, and a host of home remedies have been tried, all with occasional individual success.[78]

Toxic Epidermal Necrolysis

Toxic epidermal necrolysis (TEN) is a devastating, though (fortunately) rare, exfoliative disease of the skin and mucous membranes that results in full-thickness epidermal necrosis. The first published report of adult TEN appeared in 1956, when Lyell, in Lyon, France, compared four cases to scald burns.[79] Some authors describe a similar skin slough but with lesser involvement, termed the Stevens-Johnson syndrome; in reality, the two diseases are exactly the same. Thirty-four years before Lyell's report was published, Stevens and Johnson described the same pathology in two children in South Africa.[80] Dermatologists have long known the disease as erythema multiforma major exudativum. Thus, even though only one disease process is involved, various names continue to be used: Europeans refer to this condition as Lyell's disease, pediatricians call it the Stevens-Johnson syndrome, dermatologists refer to it as erythema multiforme majus, and American surgeons and internists call it TEN.

TEN can be precipitated by the administration of medications, most commonly sulfonamides, antibiotics, and anticonvulsants. It can also be caused by immunizations, systemic diseases, and viral illnesses; some cases have no known precipitating etiology.

The molecular etiology of TEN is still unclear. One theory suggests certain offending drugs that should be metabolized are instead deposited in the epidermis, leading to an immune response, which causes the body to reject the skin. In 1998, Viard pointed out that keratinocytes normally express the death receptor Fas (CD95); keratinocytes from TEN patients were found to express lytically active Fas ligand (FasL). Antibodies present in pooled human intravenous immunoglobulins (IVIg) blocked Fas-mediated keratinocyte death in vitro. In a pilot study, 10 consecutive individuals with clinically and histologically confirmed TEN were treated with IVIg; disease progression was rapidly reversed, and the outcome was favorable in all cases. Thus, Fas-FasL interactions appear to be directly involved in the epidermal necrolysis of TEN, and IVIg may be an effective treatment.[81] This report sparked numerous small clinical series that have, at best, been inconclusive.[82-86] There may be a role for γ-globulin, but current data show that it is no miracle cure.

TEN should be distinguished from a somewhat similar disease, staphylococcal scalded skin syndrome (SSSS). This entity is caused by a bacterial exotoxin, which splits the epidermis above the dermal-epidermal junction. Although patients with SSSS develop severe erythema, the skin exfoliates rather than blisters. SSSS does not involve mucosa, and the patients are septic from the underlying staphylococcal infection. SSSS usually affects newborns and becomes much less common as people get older. Treatment of this unusual disease is with antibiotics directed against *Staphylococcus*.[87]

The TEN-induced denuded areas are comparable to those affected by a very shallow second-degree burn. Oropharyngeal, esophageal, anal, urethral, and vaginal[88,89] mucosal sloughing are also characteristic of TEN. The disease attacks squamous epithelium, so the remainder of the GI tract is usually spared. There is only one case report of intestinal epithelial sloughing.[90] Complications such as infection, malnutrition, negative nitrogen balance, severe wound pain, and multiple organ dysfunction syndrome are identical to those seen in patients with major burns. The most common cause of death in patients suffering from TEN is systemic infection and pneumonia. The potential mortality from TEN is high, but it is reduced by treatments and protocols common in burn centers, such as wound coverage with biologic dressings. There is good evidence that patients affected with TEN should be referred early for management in a burn center.[91-93] The role of the dermatologist is to define the diagnosis and determine the potential etiology.

CLINICAL MANIFESTATIONS

A prodrome of TEN usually consists of fever, sore throat, and malaise; 1 to 2 days after these symptoms appear, the skin of the face and extremities usually becomes tender and erythematous. Lesions appear either as large areas of red skin or as target lesions that are about 2 cm in diameter and consist of concentric rings of erythema. At the same time, ulcerations in the lips and mouth appear, making oral intake painful.

In 24 to 96 hours, the involved skin begins to form both small blisters and bullae. Moderate traction of the erythematous skin results in separation of the epidermis from the dermis—a positive Nikolsky sign.[94] When the bullae rupture, large denuded areas of skin become apparent. Fingernails, toenails, and the skin of the palms and soles may also slough.

One hallmark of this disease is severe inflammation of the mouth. Blisters develop on the oral mucosa, leaving a very raw, red surface. The lips quickly become swollen and crusted with clotted blood. The oral lesions may be confined to the oral cavity or may extend to the larynx or even to the trachea and the esophagus. The patient is usually unable to eat. The eyelids swell as conjunctival inflammation develops. Conjunctival infection, usually caused by *S. aureus*, may lead to scarring and permanent blindness.[95] The nasal and urethral mucosa may also become inflamed, and erosions can develop on the genital and perianal skin.

Renal failure can occur as a result of hypovolemia, the septic response, or membranous glomerulonephritis. In up to 50% of cases, there are abnormalities in liver enzymes, including modest increases in aspartate aminotransferase (AST) and alanine aminotransferase (ALT). Bilirubin levels often show modest to severe increases.[96] The mechanism of these increases, which appear to be a part of the toxic component of TEN, is unknown.

TREATMENT

The initial focus of treatment is on restoration and maintenance of cardiopulmonary stability. TEN does not induce the intense cytokine reaction that is associated with similar-sized burns, and thus massive anasarca is unusual; resuscitation need not procceed in the manner recommended for burns. Maintenance of normal vital signs and adequate urinary output (0.5 ml/kg) is satisfactory. Because of the high incidence of line sepsis in the absence of epidermis, use of Swan-Ganz catheters is usually avoided when possible.[97]

Treatment involves aggressive wound management, similar to that of a massive second-degree burn, in which the emphasis is on optimizing healing and controlling infection. A crucial feature of TEN is an intact and uninjured dermis, which, if protected, rapidly reepithelializes from sweat glands and hair follicles, which appear to remain intact. Treatment must, therefore, protect the dermis from desiccation and infection. Routine use of ointments and salves not only creates intense pain but also increases the risk of the formation of a "pseudo eschar" of crusts and devitalized dermis that impairs wound healing.

Biologic or manufactured covers have formed an important role in wound treatment.[92,98,99] Emergency operative wound cleansing and application of commercially available pigskin (porcine xenograft) has been the standard of care at the University of Washington Burn Center in over 100 cases. The pigskin is stapled in place, the patient treated for several days in a fluidized bed, and the pigskin removed as the denuded areas heal. The pigskin is relatively inexpensive, adheres well, is nontoxic, and probably provides some growth factors to hasten healing. With this management plan and meticulous systemic care, mortality at the University of Washington has been below 20% for the past 15 years. Alternative covers include Acticoat[100] and Biobrane,[101-104] which follow the same principle of dermal protection to permit uninfected healing.

In addition, associated physiologic and psychological care must be meticulous. Lung function is often impaired as a result of the aspiration of secretions from involved oral mucosa and a reduction in the clearance of secretions as a result of oral pain and overall weakness. Pain control and aggressive pulmonary toilet to assist the patient's cough are the first line of defense. Suctioning can lead to significant bleeding and should be used either sparingly or only after an endotracheal tube is in place. The patient should be intubated if lung function is progressively impaired. Partial ventilatory assistance is often required if the patient is intubated, because chest wall pain, systemic toxicity, and weakness can severely impair spontaneous ventilatory efforts.

Cardiovascular function is initially impaired as a result of hypovolemia caused by plasma leaking from the blisters, increased skin evaporative losses, and decreased oral intake. Controlling the febrile response will also help decrease fluid losses, vasodilatation, and the resulting hyperadrenergic response. Adequate pain control is essential. Methadone is effective for long-acting pain control, and morphine is a good choice for procedural pain.

Aggressive oral care is critical because of the high risk of local mouth infection and consequent wound and lung infection. Early and continued assessment and aggressive management of corneal involvement are required. Administration of ophthalmic antibiotic ointments and gentle breaking of adhesions between conjunctiva and eyelids with a small glass rod are the standard treatment.[105]

OPTIMIZING NUTRITION

Nutrition is a major component of care, and it often cannot be delivered orally because of oral lesions. A small gastric feeding tube is preferred, as the GI tract between stomach and anus is usually intact and is normally functional.[106] In general, standard tube-feeding formulas for an individual under moderate stress are sufficient, because the full ravages of postburn hypermetabolism are probably not present. When sepsis is avoided, it is very unusual for the gut to fail and for intravenous parenteral nutrition to be needed.

The role of corticosteroids in the treatment of TEN remains unclear. Although some patients who are on steroids before developing TEN still get severe disease,[107] some dermatologists feel that the administration of steroids when the disease process is just beginning, before skin sloughing occurs, can attenuate the process and result in less sloughing. However, once vesicles have formed and the separation has occurred, corticosteroids no longer effectively attenuate skin sloughing; in fact, they retard the rate of healing. In one study, the complication rate was found to be higher in patients who received steroids.[108] This study, however, did not take into account the patients whose disease might have been sufficiently limited by steroid use to make burn center treatment unnecessary.

FOLLOW-UP CARE

Fortunately, when treatment is successful, the disease usually resolves without hypertrophic scarring, but there may be some mismatching of epidermal pigmentation. Nails may remain deformed, and eyes are usually dry, requiring periodic lubrication. Obviously, patients must not again contact the medication that caused the disease; for common medications, a Medic Alert bracelet is useful.

Ionizing Radiation Burns

The burn surgeon may encounter ionizing radiation injuries in three settings. Of these, by far the most common involves deliberate exposure to radiation (i.e., radiation used in treatment) or accidental radiation in a hospital, a laboratory, or an industrial complex. In such settings, a single individual is likely to be injured. The second scenario involves failure of a nuclear energy plant, such as occurred at Chernobyl; in this scenario, dozens to hundreds of exposures may occur. The third setting is that resulting from a nuclear explosion through military or terrorist action. In such a scenario, thousands of casualties will immediately overwhelm all resources.

LOCALIZED INJURY

A Gray (Gy) is the current unit of radiation, defined as 1 joule of energy deposited in a kilogram of tissue; 1 Gy is the equivalent of 100 rads.

Localized injury is produced by local radiation to a small area; in localized injuries there are no systemic effects. As with thermal burns, the degree of injury is dependent on the type of radiation, the dose of radiation, and the susceptibility of the tissue. An initial erythema appears within minutes or hours of exposure and subsides over 2 to 3 days. Secondary erythema occurs 1 to 3 weeks after exposure and is associated with hair loss and desquamation of the epidermis. At about 3 weeks, blisters may occur after doses of about 20 Gy; ulcerations occur after doses in excess of 25 Gy. Ulcerations occur within a few weeks to months after injury. Blood vessels become telangiectatic, and deeper vessels become occluded, leading to fibrosis, atrophy, and necrosis.[109]

Wounds are generally treated in a manner similar to the treatment of thermal burns, with the additional caveat that radiation sickness is accompanied by immunosuppression, and that endarteritis obliterans will markedly diminish the blood supply. Infection is common, and the optimal timing of excision and grafting of deep ulcers is not known.

A detailed description of whole-body radiation and its treatment are beyond the scope of this chapter. Radiation sickness, also known as the acute radiation syndrome, may begin within hours of exposure. It is initially characterized by nausea, vomiting, diarrhea, and lethargy; this is followed by the hematopoietic syndrome (neutropenia and thrombocytopenia) and the gastrointestinal syndrome (severe diarrhea, bowel ischemia, bacterial translocation, and sepsis).[110] Treatment is mainly supportive.

In a nuclear explosion, there occurs a supersonic blast with a fireball extending miles from the epicenter and immense amounts of ionizing radiation. All three of these interact, causing severe mechanical injury, flash and flame burns as a result of the igniting of clothing, and, of course, severe radiation exposure.[111] The flash has been described as being so intense that the side of a victim facing the flash will be charred to bone while the opposite side is unburned. Doctors in Hiroshima after the atomic bombing there observed that thermal burns appeared to heal for a time, but in the second and third week the wounds broke down and infection set in as the acute radiation syndrome became manifest.

References

1. Milano M: Oral electrical and thermal burns in children: review and report of case. ASDC J Dent Child 66:116, 1999

2. Canady JW, Thompson SA, Bardach J: Oral commissure burns in children. Plast Reconstr Surg 97:738, 745, 1996

3. Thomas SS: Electrical burns of the mouth: still searching for an answer. Burns 22:137, 1996

4. Gupta KL, Kumar R, Sekhar MS, et al: Myoglobinuric acute renal failure following electrical injury. Ren Fail 13:23, 1991

5. Rosen CL, Adler JN, Rabban JT, et al: Early predictors of myoglobinuria and acute renal failure following electrical injury. J Emerg Med 17:783, 1999

6. Mann R, Gibran N, Engrav L, et al: Is immediate decompression of high voltage electrical injuries to the upper extremity always necessary? J Trauma 40:584, 587, 1996

7. Engrav L, Gottlieb J, Walkinshaw M, et al: Outcome and treatment of electrical injury with immediate median and ulnar nerve palsy at the wrist: a retrospective review and a survey of members of the American Burn Association. Ann Plast Surg 25:166, 1990

8. Purdue GF, Hunt JL: Electrocardiographic monitoring after electrical injury: necessity or luxury. J Trauma 26:166, 1986

9. Bailey B, Gaudreault P, Thivierge RL: Experience with guidelines for cardiac monitoring after electrical injury in children. Am J Emerg Med 18:671, 2000

10. Hammond J, Ward CG: Myocardial damage and electrical injuries: significance of early elevation of CPK-MB isoenzymes. South Med J 79:414, 1986

11. Murphy JT, Horton JW, Purdue GF, Hunt JL: Evaluation of troponin-I as an indicator of cardiac dysfunction after thermal injury. J Trauma 45:700, 1998

12. Ratnayake B, Emmanuel ER, Walker CC: Neurological sequelae following a high voltage electrical burn. Burns 22:578, 1996

13. Kanitkar S, Roberts AH: Paraplegia in an electrical burn: a case report. Burns Incl Therm Inj 14:49, 1988

14. Grube B, Heimbach D, Engrav L, et al: Neurologic consequences of electrical burns. J Trauma 30:254, 1990

15. Reddy SC: Electric cataract: a case report and review of the literature. Eur J Ophthalmol 9:134, 1999

16. Boozalis GT, Purdue GF, Hunt JL, et al: Ocular changes from electrical burn injuries: a literature review and report of cases. J Burn Care Rehabil 12:458, 1991

17. Saffle JR, Crandall A, Warden GD: Cataracts: a long-term complication of electrical injury. J Trauma 25:17, 1985

18. Mancusi-Ungaro HR Jr, Tarbox AR, Wainwright DJ: Posttraumatic stress disorder in electric burn patients. J Burn Care Rehabil 7:521, 1986

19. Milzman DP, Moskowitz L, Hardel M: Lightning strikes at a mass gathering. South Med J 92:708, 1999

20. Graber J, Ummenhofer W, Herion H: Lightning accident with eight victims: case report and brief review of the literature. J Trauma 40:288, 1996

21. ten Duis HJ, Klasen HJ, Reenalda PE: Kerauno-paralysis, a 'specific' lightning injury. Burns Incl Therm Inj 12:54, 1985

22. Muehlberger T, Vogt PM, Munster AM: The long-term consequences of lightning injuries. Burns 27:829, 2001

23. ten Duis HJ, Klasen HJ, Nijsten MW, et al: Superficial lightning injuries: their "fractal" shape and origin. Burns Incl Therm Inj 13:141, 1987

24. Ogren FP, Edmunds AL: Neuro-otologic findings in the lightning-injured patient. Semin Neurol 15:256, 1995

25. Jones D, Ogren F, Roh L, et al: Lightning and its effects on the auditory system. Laryngoscope 101:830, 1991

26. Branday J, Arscott GD, Smoot EC, et al: Chemical burns as assault injuries in Jamaica. Burns 22:154, 1996

27. Barocas D, Difede J, Viederman M, et al: A case of chronic factitious disorder presenting as repeated, self-inflicted burns [letter]. Psychosomatics 3:79, 1998

28. Lutzow-Holm C: [Psycho-cutaneous disorders in practice: self-inflicted skin diseases of psychological origin.] Tidsskr Nor Laegeforen 117:3241, 1997

29. Wiechman SA, Ehde DM, Wilson BL, et al: The management of self-inflicted burn injuries and disruptive behavior for patients with borderline personality disorder. J Burn Care Rehabil 21:310, 2000

30. Buckley D: Skin burns due to wet cement. Contact Derm 8:407, 1982

31. Early S, Simpson R: Caustic burns from contact with wet cement. JAMA 254:528, 1985

32. George A, Bang RL, Lari AR, et al: Liquid ammonia injury. Burns 26:409, 2000

33. Close L, Catlin F, Cohn A: Acute and chronic effects of ammonia burns of the respiratory tract. Arch Otolaryngol 106:151, 1980

34. Leduc D, Gris P, Lheureux P, et al: Acute and long term respiratory damage following inhalation of ammonia. Thorax 47:755, 1992

35. Kerstein MD, Schaffzin DM, Hughes WB, et al: Acute management of exposure to liquid ammonia. Mil Med 166:913, 166, 2001

36. Flury K, Dines D, Rodarte J, et al: Airway obstruction due to inhalation of ammonia. Mayo Clin Proc 58:389, 1983

37. Laitung J, Earley M: The role of surgery in chromic acid burns: our experience with two patients. Burns Incl Therm Inj 10:378, 1984

38. Matey P, Allison KP, Sheehan TM, et al: Chromic acid burns: early aggressive excision is the best method to prevent systemic toxicity. J Burn Care Rehabil 21:241, 2000

39. Schiffl H, Weidmann P, Weiss M, et al: Dialysis treatment of acute chromium intoxication and comparative efficacy of peritoneal versus hemodialysis in chromium removal. Miner Electrolyte Metab 7:28, 1982

40. Terrill P, Gowar J: Chromic acid burns: beware, be aggressive, be watchful. Br J Plast Surg 43:699, 1990

41. Sigurdsson J, Bjornsson A, Gudmundsson ST: Formic acid burn: local and systemic effects: report of a case. Burns Incl Therm Inj 9:358, 1983

42. Chan TC, Williams SR, Clark RF: Formic acid skin burns resulting in systemic toxicity. Ann Emerg Med 26:383, 1995

43. Spiller HA, Quadrani KDA, Cleveland P: A five year evaluation of acute exposures to phenol disinfectant (26%). J Toxicol Clin Toxicol 31:307, 1993

44. Sanz-Gallen P, Nogue S, Munne P, et al: Hypocalcaemia and hypomagnesaemia due to hydrofluoric acid. Occup Med (Lond) 51:294, 2001

45. Mayer T, Gross P: Fatal systemic fluorosis due to hydrofluoric acid burns. Ann Emerg Med 14:149, 1985

46. McIvor M: Acute fluoride toxicity: pathophysiology and management. Drug Saf 5:79, 1990

47. Siegel DC, Heard JM: Intra-arterial calcium infusion for hydrofluoric acid burns. Aviat Space Environ Med 63:206, 1992

48. Lin TM, Tsai CC, Lin SD, et al: Continuous intra-arterial infusion therapy in hydrofluoric acid burns. J Occup Environ Med 42:892, 2000

49. Gupta R: Intravenous calcium gluconate in the treatment of hydrofluoric acid burns. Ann Emerg Med 37:734, 2001

50. Ryan JM, McCarthy GM, Plunkett PK: Regional intravenous calcium: an effective method of treating hydrofluoric acid burns to limb peripheries. J Accid Emerg Med 14:401, 1997

51. Graudins A, Burns MJ, Aaron CK: Regional intravenous infusion of calcium gluconate for hydrofluoric acid burns of the upper extremity. Ann Emerg Med 30:604, 1997

52. Eldad A, Wisoki M, Cohen H, et al: Phosphorous burns: evaluation of various modalities for primary treatment. J Burn Care Rehabil 16:49, 1995

53. Eldad A, Simon GA: The phosphorous burn: a preliminary comparative experimental study of various forms of treatment. Burns 17:198, 1991

54. Bijani K, Moghadamnia AA: Long-term effects of chemical weapons on respiratory tract in Iraq-Iran war victims living in Babol (north of Iran). Ecotoxicol Environ Saf 53:422, 2002

55. Devereaux A, Amundson DE, Parrish JS, et al: Vesicants and nerve agents in chemical warfare: decontamination and treatment strategies for a changed world. Postgrad Med 112:90, 2002

56. Mellor SG, Rice P, Cooper GJ: Vesicant burns. Br J Plast Surg 44:434, 1991

57. DeGroot DW, Castellani JW, Williams JO, et al: Epidemiology of U.S. Army cold weather injuries, 1980–1999. Aviat Space Environ Med 74:564, 2003

58. White AD: Chilblains. Med J Aust 154:406, 1991

59. Goette DK: Chilblains (perniosis). J Am Acad Dermatol 23(2 pt 1):257, 1990

60. Cribier B, Djeridi N, Peltre B, et al: A histologic and immunohistochemical study of chilblains. J Am Acad Dermatol 45:924, 2001

61. Irwin MS, Sanders R, Green CJ, et al: Neuropathy in non-freezing cold injury (trench foot). J R Soc Med 90:433, 1997

62. Irwin MS: Nature and mechanism of peripheral nerve damage in an experimental model of non-freezing cold injury. Ann R Coll Surg Engl 78:372, 1996

63. Mills WJ Jr, Mills WJ 3rd: Peripheral non-freezing cold injury: immersion injury. Alaska Med 35:117, 1993

64. Wrenn K: Immersion foot: a problem of the homeless in the 1990s. Arch Intern Med 151:785, 1991

65. Kyosola K: Clinical experiences in the management of cold injuries: a study of 110 cases. J Trauma 14:32, 1974

66. Urschel JD, Urschel JW, Mackenzie WC: The role of alcohol in frostbite injury. Scand J Soc Med 18:273, 1990

67. Urschel JD: Frostbite: predisposing factors and predictors of poor outcome. J Trauma 30:340, 1990

68. Murphy JV, Banwell PE, Roberts AH, et al: Frostbite: pathogenesis and treatment. J Trauma 48:171, 2000

69. Zook N, Hussmann J, Brown R, et al: Microcirculatory studies of frostbite injury. Ann Plast Surg 40:246, 254, 1998

70. Manson PN, Jesudass R, Marzella L, et al: Evidence for an early free radical-mediated reperfusion injury in frostbite. Free Radic Biol Med 10:7, 1991

71. Greenwald D, Cooper B, Gottlieb L: An algorithm for early aggressive treatment of frostbite with limb salvage directed by triple-phase scanning. Plast Reconstr Surg 102:1069, 1998

72. Bouwman DL, Morrison S, Lucas CE, et al: Early sympathetic blockade for frostbite: is it of value? J Trauma 20:744, 1980

73. Valnicek SM, Chasmar LR, Clapson JB: Frostbite in the prairies: a 12-year review. Plast Reconstr Surg 92:633, 1993

74. Reamy BV: Frostbite: review and current concepts. J Am Board Fam Pract 11:34, 1998

75. Marzella L, Jesudass RR, Manson PN, et al: Morphologic characterization of acute injury to vascular endothelium of skin after frostbite. Plast Reconstr Surg 83:67, 1989

76. Mileski WJ, Raymond JF, Winn RK, et al: Inhibition of leukocyte adherence and aggregation for treatment of severe cold injury in rabbits. J Appl Physiol 74:1432, 1993

77. Porter JM, Wesche DH, Rosch J, et al: Intra-arterial sympathetic blockade in the treatment of clinical frostbite. Am J Surg 132:625, 1976

78. Purdue GF, Hunt JL: Cold injury: a collective review. J Burn Care Rehabil 7:331, 1986

79. Lyell A: Toxic epidermal necrolysis: an eruption resembling scalding of the skin. Br J Dermatol 68:355, 1956

80. Stevens A, Johnson F: A new eruptive fever associated with stomatitis and opthalmia. Am J Dis Child 24:526, 1922

81. Viard I, Wehrli P, Bullani R, et al: Inhibition of toxic epidermal necrolysis by blockade of CD95 with human intravenous immunoglobulin. Science 282:490, 1998

82. Abe R, Shimizu T, Shibaki A, et al: Toxic epidermal necrolysis and Stevens-Johnson syndrome are induced by soluble fas ligand. Am J Pathol 162:1515, 2003

83. French LE, Tschopp J: Protein-based therapeutic approaches targeting death receptors. Cell Death Differ 10:117, 2003

84. Bachot N, Revuz J, Roujeau JC: Intravenous immunoglobulin treatment for Stevens-Johnson syndrome and toxic epidermal necrolysis: a prospective noncomparative study showing no benefit on mortality or progression. Arch Dermatol 139:33, 2003

85. Stella M, Cassano P, Bollero D, et al: Toxic epidermal necrolysis treated with intravenous high-dose immunoglobulins: our experience. Dermatology 203:45, 2001

86. Paquet P, Jacob E, Damas P, et al: Treatment of drug-induced toxic epidermal necrolysis (Lyell's syndrome) with intravenous human immunoglobulins. Burns 27:652, 2001

87. Patel GK, Finlay AY: Staphylococcal scalded skin syndrome: diagnosis and management. Am J Clin Dermatol 4:165, 2003

88. Meneux E, Paniel BJ, Pouget F, et al: Vulvovaginal sequelae in toxic epidermal necrolysis. J Reprod Med 42:153, 1997

89. Meneux E, Wolkenstein P, Haddad B, et al: Vulvovaginal involvement in toxic epidermal necrolysis: a retrospective study of 40 cases. Obstet Gynecol 91:283, 1998

90. Sugimoto Y, Mizutani H, Sato T, et al: Toxic epidermal necrolysis with severe gastrointestinal mucosal cell death: a patient who excreted long tubes of dead intestinal epithelium. J Dermatol 25:533, 1998

91. Kelemen JJ 3rd, Cioffi WG, McManus WF, et al: Burn center care for patients with toxic epidermal necrolysis. J Am Coll Surg 180:273, 1995

92. Heimbach DM, Engrav LH, Marvin JA, et al: Toxic epidermal necrolysis: a step forward in treatment. JAMA 257:2171, 1987

93. Honari S, Gibran NS, Heimbach DM, et al: Toxic epidermal necrolysis (TEN) in elderly patients. J Burn Care Rehabil 22:132, 2001

94. Salopek TG: Nikolsky's sign: is it 'dry' or is it 'wet'? Br J Dermatol 136:762, 1997

95. de Felice GP, Caroli R, Autelitano A: Long-term complications of toxic epidermal necrolysis (Lyell's disease): clinical and histopathologic study. Ophthalmologica 195:1, 1987

96. Masia M, Gutierrez F, Jimeno A, et al: Fulminant hepatitis and fatal toxic epidermal necrolysis (Lyell disease) coincident with clarithromycin administration in an alcoholic patient receiving disulfiram therapy. Arch Intern Med 162:474, 2002

97. Heimbach DM, Engrav LH, Marvin JA, et al: Toxic epidermal necrolysis: a step forward in treatment [published erratum appears in JAMA 258:1894, 1987]. JAMA 257:2171, 1987

98. Sheridan RL, Weber JM, Schulz JT, et al: Management of severe toxic epidermal necrolysis in children. J Burn Care Rehabil 20:497, 1999

99. Yarbrough DR 3rd: Treatment of toxic epidermal necrolysis in a burn center. J S C Med Assoc 93:347, 1997

100. Clennett S, Hosking G: Management of toxic epidermal necrolysis in a 15-year-old girl. J Wound Care 12:151, 2003

101. Arevalo JM, Lorente JA: Skin coverage with Biobrane biomaterial for the treatment of patients with toxic epidermal necrolysis. J Burn Care Rehabil 20:406, 1999

102. Al-Qattan MM: Toxic epidermal necrolysis: a review and report of the successful use of Biobrane for early wound coverage. Ann Plast Surg 36:224, 1996

103. Bradley T, Brown RE, Kucan JO, et al: Toxic epidermal necrolysis: a review and report of the successful use of Biobrane for early wound coverage. Ann Plast Surg 35:124, 1995

104. Kucan JO: Use of Biobrane in the treatment of toxic epidermal necrolysis. J Burn Care Rehabil 16(3 pt 1):324, 327, 1995

105. Power WJ, Ghoraishi M, Merayo-Lloves J, et al: Analysis of the acute ophthalmic manifestations of the erythema multiforme/Stevens-Johnson syndrome/toxic epidermal necrolysis disease spectrum. Ophthalmology 102:1669, 1995

106. Palmieri TL, Greenhalgh DG, Saffle JR, et al: A multicenter review of toxic epidermal necrolysis treated in U.S. burn centers at the end of the twentieth century. J Burn Care Rehabil 23:87, 2002

107. Rzany B, Schmitt H, Schopf E: Toxic epidermal necrolysis in patients receiving glucocorticosteroids. Acta Derm Venereol 71:171, 1991

108. Halebian PH, Corder VJ, Madden MR, et al: Improved burn center survival of patients with toxic epidermal necrolysis managed without corticosteroids. Ann Surg 204:503, 1986

109. Nenot JC: Medical and surgical management for localized radiation injuries. Int J Radiat Biol 57:783, 1990

110. Gus'kova AK, Baranov AE, Barabanova AV, et al: [The diagnosis, clinical picture and treatment of acute radiation sickness in the victims of the Chernobyl Atomic Electric Power Station. II. Non-bone marrow syndromes of radiation lesions and their treatment]. Ter Arkh 61:99, 1989

111. Iijima S: Pathology of atomic bomb casualties. Acta Pathol Jpn 32(suppl 2):237, 1982

6 CRITICAL CARE

1 CARDIAC RESUSCITATION

Terry J. Mengert, M.D.

Sudden cardiac arrest outside the hospital is expected to claim the lives of at least 300,000 persons in the United States in 2003, making it the single leading cause of death.[1-4] In fact, approximately 50% of all cardiac deaths are sudden deaths. In hospitals, a minimum of 370,000 patients will also suffer a cardiac arrest, followed by an attempted, but only sometimes successful, resuscitation.[5] Although most victims of sudden death have underlying coronary artery disease (70% to 80%), sudden death is the first manifestation of the disease in half of these persons.[2] Other causes and contributing factors to sudden death include abnormalities of the myocardium (i.e., chronic heart failure or hypertrophy from any other cause), electrophysiologic abnormalities, valvular heart disease, congenital heart disease, and miscellaneous inflammatory and infiltrative disease processes (e.g., myocarditis, sarcoidosis, and hemochromatosis).[6,7]

The pathophysiology that culminates in a sudden cardiac death is complex and poorly understood. It likely represents a mix of electrical abnormalities combined with acute functional triggers, such as myocardial ischemia, central and autonomic nervous system effects, electrolyte abnormalities, and even pharmacologic influences.[1] Classically, most sudden deaths that occur in adults in the community are thought to be secondary to ventricular tachycardia (VT) that degenerates into ventricular fibrillation (VF). During the past 10 years in the Seattle area, the different arrhythmias found in prehospital cardiac arrest patients presumed to have underlying cardiovascular disease were VF (45%), asystole (31%), pulseless electrical activity (PEA; 10%), VT (1%), and other miscellaneous arrhythmias (14%).[3]

The Chain of Survival

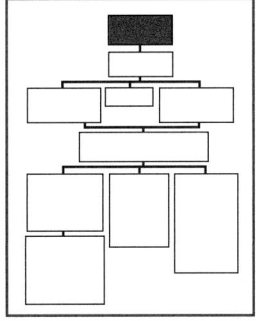

The resuscitation of an adult victim of sudden cardiac arrest should follow an orderly sequence, no matter where the patient's collapse occurs. This sequence is called the chain of survival.[8] It comprises four elements, all of which must be instituted as rapidly as possible: activation of the emergency medical service network, cardiopulmonary resuscitation (CPR), defibrillation, and provision of advanced care.

ACTIVATION OF EMERGENCY MEDICAL SERVICES

A person in cardiac arrest will be unresponsive and pulseless, but agonal respirations may last for minutes. Unresponsiveness should be confirmed by speaking loudly to and shaking the patient. If the patient is unresponsive, help should immediately be sought through activation of the emergency medical service in the community (in most locales, this means calling 911); if the patient is already in the hospital, a code should be called (e.g., code blue, code 199). If an automated external defibrillator (AED) is available, it should be brought to the resuscitation scene; AEDs are easily used and can be lifesaving.[9-12]

INITIATION OF CPR

While awaiting the arrival of a defibrillator and advanced help, the rescuer should assess the patient's airway, breathing, and cir-

culation [*see* The Primary Survey, *below*], and CPR should be initiated [*see Table 1*]. When CPR is started within 4 minutes of collapse, the likelihood of patient survival at least doubles.[13,14]

INITIATION OF DEFIBRILLATION

When the AED or monitor-defibrillator arrives, the device should be appropriately attached to the patient and the rhythm should be analyzed; if the patient is in pulseless VT or VF, a defibrillatory shock should be rapidly applied [*see Tables 2 and 3*]. If required, two additional shocks may be administered sequentially. The importance of rapid access to defibrillation cannot be overemphasized. In a patient who is dying from a shockable rhythm, the chance of survival declines by 7% to 10% for every minute that defibrillation is delayed.[15]

INITIATION OF ADVANCED CARE

If the patient remains pulseless despite the steps described above, CPR should be continued; a definitive airway should be secured; intravenous access should be established; and appropriate medications should be administered, as determined by the rhythm and the arrest circumstances. If the patient is in pulseless VT or VF, repeated attempts at defibrillation are interspersed with delivery of vasoactive and antiarrhythmic medication [*see Table 4*].

RESUSCITATION OUTCOME

When every link in this described chain is quickly and sequentially available, the patient is provided an optimal opportunity for return of spontaneous circulation.[15-18] In the United States, individual communities report survival rates of 4% to 33% or more in cases of sudden cardiac death.[19-22] Prehospital victims of VF have had survival rates to hospital discharge of greater than 50% when an AED

Table 1 **Initial Resuscitation Steps in the Unresponsive Patient**

Confirm unresponsiveness
Activate the emergency medical system
   In the community, call 911 in most locales
   In the hospital, activate the appropriate code response
Call for an automatic external defibrillator (AED)
Begin basic life support (CPR)
   Open airway
   Check breathing; if not breathing, deliver two initial breaths
   Check for a carotid pulse; if pulseless, do the following:
      Begin chest compressions at the rate of 100 compressions/min, depressing the sternum 4–5 cm per compression in patients older than 8 yr
      Intersperse ventilations with chest compressions: in nonintubated patients, deliver 15 compressions, pause for two breaths, then repeat; in intubated patients, deliver one breath every 5 sec, with no pause in compressions
Reassess for return of spontaneous circulation every 1–3 min
When defibrillator arrives, immediately analyze and treat arrhythmia
   Attach patient to AED [*see Table 2*] or the monitor-defibrillator [*see Table 3*]
   Analyze arrhythmia and treat as appropriate

Approach to Cardiovascular Resuscitation

Patient is in cardiac arrest

Confirm unresponsiveness.
If out of hospital, call EMS.
If in hospital, activate appropriate code.
Call for a defibrillator.

Primary survey

Assess ABCs.
Begin CPR; when defibrillator arrives,
   attach to patient and briefly withhold CPR.
Assess rhythm.

Pulseless VT or VF

Immediately administer shock, first at 200 J,
then 200–300 J, then 360 J; if patient is already
attached to a monitor-defibrillator, begin
resuscitation with immediate defibrillation.
Resume CPR.

Pulseless electrical activity

Resume CPR.

Asystole

Resume CPR and confirm asystole.
Ensure that patient is appropriately attached to
monitor-defibrillator, that ECG gain control on
the defibrillator is at maximum, and that the
rhythm is assessed in several leads.

Secondary survey

Endotracheally intubate, confirm tube placement, secure tube, establish I.V. access.
Concomitantly with preceding steps, identify and correct technical difficulties
hampering resuscitation [*see Table 6*]; initiate emergency therapy for conditions
contributing to cardiac arrest [*see Table 7*].

Pulseless VT or VF

Subsequent steps assume continuing VT or VF
despite interventions; do not interrupt CPR
except as required for rapid performance of
lifesaving procedures.
Administer vasoactive drugs with ongoing CPR:
   Epinephrine, 1 mg I.V. push, repeated every
   3–5 min throughout CPR
      or
   Vasopressin, 40 U I.V. push in a single dose;
   if no response after 10 min, administer
   epinephrine as described above.

Administer antiarrhythmic drugs with ongoing CPR:
   Amiodarone, 300 mg I.V. push; if a second dose is
   needed, 150 mg after 5 min
      or
   Lidocaine, 1.0–1.5 mg/kg I.V. push; if a second
   dose is needed, repeat initial dose in 3–5 min.
Hypomagnesemia or torsade de pointes is suspected:
   Magnesium sulfate, 1–2 g I.V. push
*Intermittent or recurrent VT/VF after an initial
response to shocks:*
   Procainamide, 20–50 mg/min I.V. infusion to a
   total dose of 17 mg/kg.
Follow medication delivery with a 20 ml saline
bolus; elevate extremity with I.V. line, and continue
CPR for 30–60 sec to circulate medication; then
administer shock (360 J for up to three shocks).

Pulseless electrical activity

Subsequent steps assume continuing
PEA despite interventions; do not
interrupt CPR except as required for
rapid performance of lifesaving
procedures.
Administer epinephrine, 1 mg I.V. push,
with ongoing CPR; repeat every 3–5
min as long as CPR is required.
If heart rate as shown on monitor is
slow, administer atropine, 1 mg I.V.
push, with ongoing CPR; may repeat
every 3–5 min to a total dose of 3 mg.
Follow medication delivery with a 20 ml
saline bolus and elevation of the
extremity containing the I.V. line.

Asystole

Subsequent steps assume continuing
asystole despite interventions; do not
interrupt CPR except as required for rapid
performance of lifesaving procedures.
Attempt transcutaneous pacing, if
available (may be initiated simultaneously
with above steps).
Administer medications with ongoing CPR:
   Epinephrine, 1 mg I.V. push; repeat
   every 3–5 min for as long as patient
   requires CPR
      and
   Atropine, 1 mg I.V. push; repeat every
   3–5 min to a total dose of 3 mg
Follow medication delivery with a 20 ml
saline bolus and elevation of the
extremity containing the I.V. line.
End resuscitation attempt if patient remains
in confirmed asystole for > 10 min and
there is no technical problem preventing
resuscitation, no imminently treatable
cause, and no extenuating circumstance.

Table 2 Using an Automatic External Defibrillator

Automatic external defibrillator (AED) arrives (CPR is in progress)
　Place AED beside patient.
　Turn on the AED.
　Attach the electrodes to the AED (they may be preattached).
　Attach the electrode pads to the patient (as diagrammed on the pads).
AED analyzes patient's rhythm
　Stop CPR (and ensure no one is touching the patient).
　Press the Analyze button on the AED (some devices analyze the rhythm automatically as soon as the pads are placed on the patient).
AED instructs rescuers (via an audible voice prompt and/or on-screen instructions)
　Shock is indicated: clear the patient (ensure no one is touching the patient) and push the Shock button.
　After delivering shock, press the Analyze button again; the sequence of analysis followed by shock (if so indicated) may be performed a total of three times.
or
　Shock not indicated: reassess the patient for signs of circulation; if present, assess the adequacy of breathing; if there are no signs of circulation, resume CPR for 1–2 min. After 1 min of CPR, assess the patient again for signs of circulation; if present, assess the adequacy of breathing. If the patient is still pulseless, repeat analysis, followed (if indicated) by shock steps.

was expeditiously used.[23] Many other factors also influence patient survival, however; these include whether the patient's collapse was witnessed, the rhythm associated with the cardiac arrest, and underlying comorbidities.[24,25] With inpatient cardiac arrest, for example, overall survival rates vary from 9% to 32%,[26-32] but in one study, survival to hospital discharge was 30% for patients with primary heart disease, 15% for patients with infectious diseases, and only 8% for patients with other end-stage diseases (e.g., cancer, lung disease, liver failure, or renal failure).[33]

Such statistics underline the importance of using cardiac resuscitation appropriately and with discrimination. Cardiac resuscitation provides rescuers with powerful tools that save the lives of thousands of people every year. These techniques are capable of returning patients who would otherwise die to productive and meaningful lives. However, cardiac resuscitation should not be employed to reverse timely and natural death. Under those circumstances, it has the potential to lengthen the dying process and to increase human suffering. All practitioners are well advised to remember that "death is not the opposite of life, death is the opposite of birth. Both are aspects of life."[34] It is untimely death that requires immediate intervention and a well-conducted cardiac resuscitation.

The Primary and Secondary Surveys of Cardiac Resuscitation

A cardiac resuscitation is a stressful event for everyone involved. Too often, clinic and inpatient cardiac arrests and their management are episodes of chaos in the busy lives of resident and attending physicians. Yet, it has been eloquently stated that a good resuscitation team should function like a fine symphony orchestra.[35] Such skill levels require dedicated individual and team practice and careful code team organization. Mastery in cardiac resuscitation is in fact a lifelong pursuit that requires training and retraining in advanced cardiac life support (ACLS); regular practice and review; and leadership and team skill development. Its key elements include not only the resuscitation itself but the response to the announcement of a code, postresuscitation stabilization of the patient, notification of the family and primary care provider, and code critique

and debriefing. To help practitioners learn and apply some of the most essential techniques used in cardiac resuscitation more easily and effectively, the American Heart Association (AHA) has developed the concepts of primary and secondary surveys of a patient in atraumatic cardiac arrest.[36]

THE PRIMARY SURVEY

The primary survey for the victim of sudden cardiac arrest consists of the appropriate assessment of the patient's airway (A), breathing (B), and circulation (C) and the simultaneous application of expert CPR until defibrillation (D) becomes possible (assuming the patient is in pulseless VT or VF). Thus, the primary survey includes the second and third links in the chain of survival (see above). In 1958, Kouwenhoven noted that when 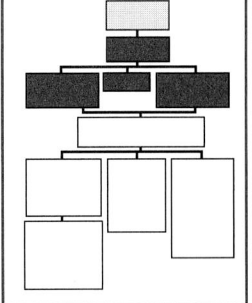 his research fellow forcefully applied external defibrillating electrodes on a dog's chest in the laboratory, an arterial pressure wave

---

Table 3 Using a Manual Defibrillator[45,71]

Defibrillator arrives (CPR is in progress)
　Place defibrillator beside patient.
　Turn defibrillator on (initial energy level setting is typically 200 J).*
　Set Lead Select switch to Paddles. Alternatively, if patient is already attached to monitor leads, set Lead Select switch to lead I, II, or III; ensure all three leads are correctly attached to the patient and the defibrillator: white to right shoulder, black to left shoulder, red to ribs on left side.
　Apply gel to paddles or place conductor pads on patient's chest. Some devices use disposable electrode patches that are prepasted with a conducting gel. In either case, the appropriate positions of the paddles with applied gel, conductor pads, or disposable paddles are as follows: sternal paddle is placed to the right of the sternum, just below the right clavicle; apex paddle is placed to the left of the left breast, centered in the left midaxillary line at the fifth intercostal space.
Analyze rhythm
Briefly withhold CPR
　If using paddles to assess rhythm, apply paddles as described with firm pressure (25 lb of pressure to each paddle) and visually assess rhythm on monitor (if using leads, briefly withhold CPR and assess rhythm in leads I, II, or III). If rhythm is either pulseless VT or VF, proceed as follows:
Defibrillate, then reassess
　Announce to resuscitation team, "Charging defibrillator, stand clear!" and press Charge button on either paddles or defibrillator (initial energy, 200 J, not synchronized).*
　Warn resuscitation team that a defibrillatory shock is coming: "I am going to shock on three! ONE, I'm clear; TWO, you're clear; THREE, everybody's CLEAR!" Simultaneously with these statements, visually ensure that no resuscitation team member is in contact with patient.
　Press the Discharge buttons on both paddles simultaneously to deliver a defibrillatory shock.
　Reassess rhythm on monitor; if patient is still in VT or VF, recharge defibrillator (now 300 J)* and repeat process of loudly informing team members by giving the warning statements as above, and then apply defibrillatory shock.
　Reassess rhythm on monitor; if patient is still in VT or VF, recharge defibrillator (now 360 J)* and repeat process of loudly informing team members by giving the warning statements as above, and then apply defibrillatory shock.
　Reassess rhythm on monitor; if patient is still in VT or VF, resume CPR and continue with resuscitation sequence .

*Note: if using a biphasic defibrillator, a lower initial defibrillatory energy level (< 200 J) without energy escalation on subsequent shocks is acceptable.
VF—ventricular fibrillation　VT—ventricular tachycardia

Table 4 Drugs Useful in Cardiac Arrest[3,72]

Category	Drug and Doses Supplied	Indications in Cardiac Arrest	Adult Dosage	Comments
Vasopressors	Epinephrine, 1 mg in 10 ml emergency syringe; 1 mg/ml (1 ml and 30 ml vials)	Pulseless VT or VF unresponsive to initial defibrillatory shocks; PEA; asystole	1 mg I.V. push; may repeat every 3–5 min for as long as patient is pulseless; can also be given via the endotracheal route: 2–2.5 mg diluted with normal saline (NS) to 10 ml total volume	I.V. boluses of epinephrine (1 mg) are appropriate only in pulseless cardiac arrest patients; if continued epinephrine is required after resuscitation, a continuous infusion should be started (1–10 µg/min). High-dose epinephrine (up to 0.2 mg/kg IV per dose) does not improve survival to hospital discharge in cardiac arrest patients and is no longer recommended in adults.
	Vasopressin, 20 IU/ml (1 ml vial)	Pulseless VT or VF unresponsive to initial defibrillatory shocks	40 IU I.V. push, single dose only; can also be given via endotracheal tube: same dose, diluted with NS to 10 ml total volume	If no response after 10 min of continued resuscitation, administer epinephrine, as above.
Antiarrhythmics	Amiodarone, 50 mg/ml (3 ml vial)	Pulseless VT or VF unresponsive to initial defibrillatory shocks and epinephrine plus shock(s)	VT/VF: 300 mg diluted in 20–30 ml; NS or D5W rapid I.V. push; a repeat dose of 150 mg may be given if required in 5 min; maximum dose in 24 hr should not exceed 2,200 mg	Side effects may include hypotension and bradycardia in the postresuscitation phase.
	Lidocaine, 50 mg or 100 mg in 5 ml emergency syringes; premixed bag, 1 g/250 ml or 2 g/250 ml	Pulseless VT or VF unresponsive to initial defibrillatory shocks and epinephrine plus shock(s)	Initial dose: 1–1.5 mg/kg I.V.; for refractory VF or unstable VT, may repeat 1–1.5 mg/kg I.V. in 3–5 min; maximum dose, 3 mg/kg May also be given endotracheally: 2–4 mg/kg diluted with NS to 10 ml total volume	If lidocaine is effective, initiate continuous I.V. infusion at 2–4 mg/min when patient has return of a perfusing rhythm (but do not use if this rhythm is an idioventricular rhythm or third-degree heart block with an idioventricular escape rhythm). Continuous infusion should begin at 1 mg/min in congestive heart failure or chronic liver disease or in elderly patients.
	Magnesium sulfate, 500 mg/ml (2 ml and 10 ml vials), or 10 ml emergency syringe	Pulseless VT or VF unresponsive to initial defibrillatory shocks and epinephrine plus shock(s) if suspected hypomagnesemic state	Administer 1–2 g diluted in 100 ml D5W I.V. over 1–2 min Total body magnesium deficits should be replaced gradually after initial therapy has stabilized the emergency: administer 0.5–1 g/hr for 3–6 hr, then reassess continued need	Measured magnesium levels correlate only approximately with the actual level of deficiency. Patients with renal insufficiency are at risk for dangerous hypermagnesemia; use appropriate caution. Side effects may include bradycardia, hypotension, generalized weakness, and temporary loss of reflexes.
	Procainamide, 100 mg/ml (10 ml injection); 500 mg/ml (2 ml vial)	Recurrent or intermittent pulseless VT or VF	20–30 mg/min I.V. (up to 50 mg/min if situation is critical); maximum dose is 17 mg/kg over time (but maximum dose is reduced to 12 mg/kg in setting of cardiac or renal dysfunction) Maintenance infusion is 1–4 mg/min	Administer procainamide during a perfusing rhythm. Stop procainamide administration when arrhythmia is adequately suppressed, hypotension occurs, QRS widens to > 50% of original duration, or maximum dose is administered.
Anticholinergic	Atropine, 1 mg in 10 ml emergency syringe	Asystole or PEA (if rate of rhythm is slow)	For asystole or PEA: 1 mg I.V. every 3–5 min up to 3 mg May be given via ET tube: 2–3 mg diluted with NS to 10 ml	Minimal adult dose is 0.5 mg. Avoid use in type II second-degree heart block or third-degree heart block.
Miscellaneous	Bicarbonate, 50 mEq in 50 ml emergency syringe	Significant hyperkalemia Significant metabolic acidosis unresponsive to optimal CPR, oxygenation, and ventilation Certain drug overdoses, including tricyclic antidepressants and aspirin	Hyperkalemia therapy: 50 mEq I.V. Metabolic acidosis: 1 mEq/kg slow I.V. push; may repeat half initial dose in 10 min; ideally, ABGs should help guide further therapy Use in overdose: discuss with toxicologist	In non–dialysis-dependent hyperkalemic patients, bicarbonate is most useful if metabolic acidosis is also present; bicarbonate is less effective in dialysis dependent renal failure patients. The use of bicarbonate in metabolic acidosis management in cardiac arrest patients is controversial. Side effects may include sodium overload, hypokalemia, and metabolic alkalosis.
	Calcium chloride, 100 mg/ml in 10 ml prefilled syringe	Significant hyperkalemia Calcium channel blocker drug overdose Profound hypocalcemia of other causes	In hyperkalemia: 5–10 ml slow I.V. push; may repeat if required In calcium channel blocker overdose: discuss with toxicologist	Do not use if cause of hyperkalemia is suspected acute digoxin poisoning. Do not combine in same I.V. with sodium bicarbonate. Calcium chloride is not a routine medication in cardiac arrest.

Note: All medications used during cardiac arrest, when given via a peripheral venous site in an extremity, should be followed by a 20 ml I.V. saline bolus and elevation of the extremity for 10 to 20 sec.
ABG—arterial blood gases   D5W—5% dextrose in water   ET—endotracheal   PEA—pulseless electrical activity   VF—ventricular fibrillation   VT—ventricular tachycardia

occurred.[37] Further study and refinements led to the technique of closed chest CPR, the careful description of which was published in 1960.[38] The first report of the use of this technique in patients was in 1961.[39] Since those early days, the fundamentals of closed-chest CPR have remained relatively unchanged. Mouth-to-mouth, mouth-to-mask, or bag-valve-mask ventilation oxygenates the blood. Chest compressions produce forward blood flow. This flow appears to result from a combination of direct compression of the heart and intrathoracic pressure changes.[40,41]

CPR in isolation does not defibrillate the heart. Its main benefit is to extend patient viability until a defibrillator and advanced interventions become available and, one hopes, succeed in restoring spontaneous circulation in the patient. CPR is not nearly as effective as a contracting heart; systolic arterial pressure peaks of 60 to 80 mm Hg may be generated, but diastolic blood pressure remains low, and a cardiac output of only 25% to 30% of normal can be achieved.[42] Still, effective CPR is critical to keeping the patient alive. It is worth remembering that the most important rescuers at a cardiac resuscitation are those who are performing expert CPR, because it is only through their efforts that the patient's heart and brain are kept viable until defibrillation and other advanced interventions can restore spontaneous circulation.

After unresponsiveness is confirmed, the emergency medical system is activated, and an AED is called for, the primary survey (A, B, C, and D) proceeds as described below.

Optimization of the Airway

The patient's mouth should be opened and the airway optimized by use of the head-tilt and chin-lift maneuver. A jaw-thrust maneuver should be used instead of the head-tilt technique if cervical spine injury is suspected. It should be remembered that in patients with suspected spine injury, proper spine alignment must be maintained throughout all phases of the resuscitation. In such circumstances, as equipment becomes available, the patient's spine should be immobilized with a padded backboard, hard cervical collar, appropriate bolstering around the patient's head to prevent movement, and strapping of the patient to the backboard.[43]

Assessment of Breathing

To assess breathing, the rescuer should place his or her cheek close to the patient's mouth and look, listen, and feel for the patient's breath. If the respirations are agonal or the patient is apneic, the rescuer should deliver two initial breaths. Each breath should be delivered over 1.5 to 2.0 seconds. The patient's chest should rise with each delivered breath, and exhalation should be allowed for between breaths. Breaths may be delivered using mouth-to-mouth technique with appropriate barrier precautions (the patient's nose should be pinched if the mouth-to-mouth technique is used) or mouth-to-mask technique. The ideal device, if available, is a bag-valve mask device attached to high-flow oxygen; this allows the delivery of a substantially higher oxygen concentration to the patient. If the patient cannot be ventilated, the airway should be repositioned and the technique attempted again. If the airway is still obstructed, up to five abdominal thrusts should be delivered, followed by a finger sweep of the oropharynx, then ventilation attempts repeated. Definitive intervention for an obstructed airway in the hospital setting may involve laryngoscopic visualization of the cause of obstruction and foreign-body removal. If an adequate airway cannot be established by less invasive means, cricothyrotomy may be required.

Initiation of CPR

A check should be made for the carotid pulse, but no more than 10 seconds should be spent doing this. (The AHA no longer recommends pulse checks for rescuers who are not health care providers.[44] Instead, lay rescuers should initiate chest compressions if the patient is not breathing, coughing, or moving after the initial two breaths.) If the patient has no carotid pulse, chest compressions should be initiated. The patient should be on a firm surface, and the heel of the rescuer's hand should be in the center of the inferior half of the patient's sternum (but cephalad to the xiphoid process). The rescuer's other hand is placed on top of the lower hand, with the fingers interlocked.

The rescuer's arms should be straight, and the force of each compression should come from the rescuer's trunk. In patients older than 8 years, the sternum should be smoothly compressed by 4 to 5 cm, then released. The duration of the compression-release cycle should be divided equally between compression and release. The rate of chest compression should be 100 compressions/min. The chest should be allowed to rebound to its precompression dimen-

sions between compressions, but the resuscitator's palm closest to the patient should remain in contact with the sternum.

In nonintubated patients, chest compressions are regularly interrupted for the delivery of ventilations. The sequence is the same, regardless of whether one-rescuer or two-rescuer CPR is being performed: the rescuer delivers 15 compressions, pauses for two breaths (each given over 1.5 to 2 seconds), then resumes compressions. In endotracheally intubated patients, chest compression and ventilation are not synchronized; every 5 seconds, one ventilation is delivered over a period of 2 seconds, while compressions continue without pause.[14]

Good technique is critical throughout CPR delivery. There should be carotid pulses with chest compressions and appropriate breath sounds and chest movement with ventilations. Interestingly, femoral pulsations with CPR do not necessarily indicate effective CPR; frequently, these pulsations are venous rather than arterial. Quantitative end-tidal carbon dioxide levels can be monitored, if practicable. Higher levels correlate with more effective CPR and improved survival of cardiac arrest.[45] The patient should be reassessed for return of spontaneous circulation every 1 to 3 minutes [see Table 1].

Initiation of Defibrillation

When the monitor-defibrillator or AED arrives, it should be attached to the patient; the rhythm should be analyzed, and, if the patient is in pulseless VT or VF, defibrillation should be given [see Tables 2 and 3].

Defibrillation works by simultaneously depolarizing a sufficient mass of cardiac myocytes to make the cardiac tissue ahead of the VT or VF wave fronts refractory to electrical conduction. Subsequently, the sinus node or another appropriate pacemaker region of the heart with inherent automaticity can resume orderly depolarization-repolarization, with return of a perfusing rhythm.[12,46] The sooner defibrillation occurs, the higher the likelihood of resuscitation. When provided immediately after the onset of VF, the success of defibrillation is extremely high.[47] In a study of sudden cardiac arrest patients in Nevada gambling casinos, the survival rate to hospital discharge was 74% for patients who received their first defibrillation no later than 3 minutes after a witnessed collapse.[23] In this study, defibrillation was delivered via an AED operated by casino security officers.

Early defibrillation is so critical that if a defibrillator is immediately available, its use takes precedence over CPR for patients in pulseless VT or VF. If CPR is already in progress, it should of course halt while defibrillation takes place. Newer defibrillators can compensate for thoracic impedance, ensuring that the selected energy level is in fact the energy that is delivered to the myocardial tissue. In addition, defibrillators that deliver biphasic defibrillation waveforms instead of the standard monophasic damped sinusoidal waveforms allow effective defibrillation at lower energy levels (< 200 joules) and without the need for escalating energy levels during subsequent shocks.[12,48-51] In the Optimized Response to Cardiac Arrest (ORCA) study, which involved 115 patients with prehospital VF, the 150-joule biphasic-shock AED was more effective than the traditional high-energy monophasic-shock AED in four respects: it produced successful defibrillation with the first shock (96% versus 59%); it led to a higher rate of ultimate success with defibrillation (100% versus 84%); it had a better rate of return of spontaneous circulation (76% versus 54%); and its use was associated with a higher rate of ultimate good cerebral performance in the survivors (87% versus 53%).[52] There were no differences, however, in terms of survival to hospital admission or discharge. Current AHA guidelines state that lower energy biphasic waveform defibrillators are safe and have equivalent or higher effica-

Table 5 Confirmation of Endotracheal
Tube Placement

Intubation process
  Vocal cords are visualized by intubator
  Tip of ET tube is seen passing between the cords
  Cuff of ET tube also passes cords by 1 cm
Postintubation checks
  Esophageal detector device or end-tidal CO_2 detector confirms ET tube placement in trachea
  Breath sounds are symmetrical (auscultate over lateral anterior chest and in midaxillary line bilaterally)
  No gurgling with auscultation over epigastrium
  Patient's chest rises and falls appropriately with ventilation
  ET tube depth is appropriate: 21 cm at the corner of the mouth in adult women, 23 cm in adult men
Secure the ET tube to prevent dislodgment
Reassess the adequacy of oxygenation and ventilation throughout the resuscitation (bedside patient assessment; also obtain ABGs when feasible)
After resuscitation, obtain a portable chest radiograph

ABG—arterial blood gas ET—endotracheal

cy for termination of VF, as compared with the standard monophasic wave-form defibrillator.[12,44]

THE SECONDARY SURVEY

The secondary survey for a victim of persistent cardiac arrest takes place after completion of the primary survey. Like the primary survey, the secondary survey follows an ABCD format, which in this case consists of advanced airway interventions (A); optimized oxygenation and ventilation by confirmation of endotracheal (ET) tube placement and repeated reassessment of the adequacy of delivered

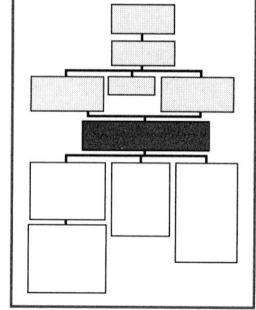

breaths (B); intravenous access and appropriate medication delivery to the patient's circulation (C); and definitive therapy (D), based on a differential diagnosis that considers the specific disease processes thought to be responsible for, or contributing to, the cardiac arrest. The secondary survey includes the fourth link in the chain of survival, rapid advanced care (see above).

Placement of an Advanced Airway

Patients who remain in cardiac arrest after completion of the primary survey require placement of an advanced airway. Depending on the setting and the experience of the rescuers, this advanced airway may be a laryngeal mask airway, an esophageal-tracheal Combitube (a tracheal tube bonded side by side with an esophageal obturator), or an ET tube.[36,53,54] The laryngeal mask airway and the Combitube can be placed by personnel with less training than that required for endotracheal intubation, and they do not require special equipment or visualization of the vocal cords. Nevertheless, endotracheal intubation is generally the preferred advanced airway technique for cardiac resuscitation, both in the hospital setting and in many paramedic systems throughout the United States. Endotracheal intubation isolates the airway, maintains airway patency, helps protect the trachea from the ever-present risk of aspiration, helps permit optimal oxygenation and ventilation of the patient, allows for tracheal suctioning, and even provides a route for delivery of some medications to the systemic circulation (via the pulmonary circulation) if intravenous access is unobtainable or lost.[53]

Optimization of Breathing and Ventilation

When a cardiac arrest patient undergoes endotracheal intubation, correct positioning of the tube must be immediately confirmed and regularly reconfirmed during and after the resuscitation [*see Table 5*]. Routine use of an esophageal detector device or end-tidal CO_2 detector is recommended, along with careful patient examination. Caution is necessary with qualitative colorimetric end-tidal CO_2 detectors, because both false positive and false negative results have been documented during cardiac arrests.[55] Breath sounds should be present during auscultation over the anterior and lateral chest walls, and the patient's chest should rise and fall with delivered ventilations. No gurgling should be heard when the epigastrium is auscultated. The ET tube should be inserted to the appropriate depth marking: 21 cm at the corner of the mouth in the average adult woman, 23 cm in the average adult man. The patient's skin color should be reasonable (i.e., not dusky or cyanotic), provided the patient's pigmentation allows such assessment.

Once correct positioning is confirmed, the ET tube should be appropriately secured to prevent its dislodgment. When feasible, an arterial blood gas (ABG) measurement should be obtained to confirm the adequacy of oxygenation and ventilation as the resuscitation proceeds.

Establishment of Circulation Access

Access to the patient's venous circulation is mandatory; such access may be achieved by a code team member or members simultaneously while other resuscitators pursue steps A and B of the secondary survey. Ideally, a large intravenous cannula should be placed in a prominent upper-extremity vein or external jugular vein to optimize delivery of needed medications. If a peripheral line is not achievable, additional possibilities include central line placement via the internal jugular, subclavian (via the supraclavicular approach) or, less ideally, femoral vein; even intraosseous access is possible (intraosseous access is a common emergency vascular access site in pediatric patients, but it is an unusual route of access in adults). It is useful to remember, as already noted, that some important resuscitation medications can be delivered via the ET tube in cases of failed intravenous access; such medications include naloxone, atropine, vasopressin, epinephrine, and lidocaine (a mnemonic for these agents is NAVEL).

The commonly used medications in cardiac resuscitation may be grouped into the following general categories: vasopressors (epinephrine or vasopressin), antiarrhythmics (amiodarone, lidocaine, magnesium, and procainamide), anticholinergic agents (atropine, if the arrest arrhythmia is asystole or PEA is slow), and miscellaneous drugs used to treat specific problems contributing to the arrest state, such as sodium bicarbonate (for severe metabolic acidosis, hyperkalemia, and certain drug overdoses), and calcium chloride (for hyperkalemia, calcium channel blocker drug overdose, or severe hypocalcemia) [*see Table 4*].

Persons in cardiac arrest (which can result from pulseless VT or VF, PEA, or asystole) should receive 1 mg of epinephrine intravenously every 3 to 5 minutes for as long as they are pulseless. Epinephrine stimulates adrenergic receptors, which leads to vasoconstriction and optimization of CPR-generated blood flow to the heart and brain. In patients with pulseless VT or VF, vasopressin (40 units I.V. once only) is a reasonable alternative to epinephrine, at least initially. Vasopressin in the recommended dose is a potent vasoconstrictor. It also has the theoretical advantage over epinephrine of not increasing myocardial oxygen consumption or lactate production in the arrested heart.[56] Despite its potential advantages, however, a recent study of 200 inpatient cardiac arrest patients found no differences in survival between those given vasopressin and those given epinephrine.[57]

Table 6   Technical Problems That May Prevent a Successful Resuscitation

Problem	Patients at Risk	Recommendations
Ineffective CPR	All cardiac arrest patients	Ensure technically perfect CPR. Confirm carotid pulses with CPR. If arterial line was in place before cardiac arrest, confirm adequate arterial waveform with CPR on arterial line monitor. Monitor end-tidal CO_2 if available (higher levels correlate with better CPR and improved patient survival). Confirm adequate oxygenation with an ABG when feasible.
Inadequate oxygenation and ventilation	All cardiac arrest patients	Ensure optimal airway positioning and control. Have suction immediately available to manage pharyngeal and airway secretions. Ensure use of properly fitting, tightly sealed face mask for bag-valve mask (BVM) ventilation until a definitive airway is established. Apply cricoid pressure to prevent gastric distention during BVM ventilation until a definitive airway is established. Ensure that supplemental oxygen is flowing to BVM at 15 L/min. Deliver an appropriate tidal volume per breath (6–7 ml/kg if oxygen is available) at the rate of 12–15 breaths/min. Confirm bilateral and equal breath sounds with ventilation. Confirm that patient's chest rises with each ventilation. Allow adequate time for exhalation between breaths. Confirm optimal oxygenation and ventilation with an ABG when feasible.
ET tube difficulties	All patients intubated with ET tube	Allow ≤ 20–30 sec/intubation attempt. Intubator should see tip of ET tube and cuff pass between vocal cords at time of intubation. After intubation, immediately confirm correct ET tube placement; regularly reconfirm ET tube placement throughout resuscitation. Confirm adequacy of oxygenation and ventilation with an ABG. After intubation, consider nasogastric tube placement to decompress stomach and optimize diaphragmatic excursions with ventilation.
Intravenous line difficulties	All cardiac arrest patients	Place one or more 18-gauge or larger I.V. cannulas in an antecubital or external jugular vein site. Check for I.V. infiltration regularly throughout the resuscitation. Follow all medications administered through a peripheral I.V. site with a 20 ml saline bolus and elevation of the extremity containing the I.V. for 10–15 sec (if possible). Consider central line placement if the resuscitation is prolonged. Be aware of all I.V. infusions the patient is receiving. Stop all nonessential medications that had been started before the cardiac arrest. During the resuscitation, the only infusions the patient should receive are normal saline, blood products (if clinically indicated), and pertinent medications necessary to assist with return of spontaneous circulation. Pulmonary artery catheters and central lines occasionally act as an arrhythmogenic focus within the right ventricle. If applicable, deflate all relevant balloons on the catheter and withdraw the catheter to a superior vena cava position. Make sure Synchronization Mode button is in the off position when defibrillating patients in pulseless VT or VF. Make sure electricity is not arcing over the patient's chest because of perspiration or smeared conducting gel; dry patient's chest with a towel except for areas directly beneath pads or paddles. Do not administer shock through nitroglycerin paste or patches. If the patient has an internal cardioverter-defibrillator (ICD) or a pacemaker, the patient may still be manually defibrillated, but do not shock directly over the internal device. Under these circumstances, place the pads or paddles at least 2.5 cm away from the patient's internal device. If the ICD is intermittently firing but not defibrillating the patient and if the ICD is thought to be compromising the resuscitation, turn the device off with a magnet so that manual defibrillation may take place without interference. Maximize the gain or electrocardiography "size" and check the rhythm in several leads (or change the axes of the paddles if reading the rhythm in Paddles mode) to confirm asystole when the initial rhythm appears to be asystole.

ABG—arterial blood gas   ET—endotracheal   VF—ventricular fibrillation   VT—ventricular tachycardia

During resuscitation with ongoing CPR, medication delivery through an intravenous cannula should be followed by a 20 ml saline bolus; if the cannula is in a peripheral vein, the extremity containing the cannula should then be elevated for 10 to 15 seconds to augment delivery of the medication to the central circulation. This is especially important because of the low-flow circulatory state with closed-chest CPR.

Differential Diagnosis and Definitive Care

The most challenging part of the secondary survey, and of cardiac resuscitation management in general, is the problem-solving required when spontaneous circulation does not return despite appropriate interventions. This situation poses a critical question to the resuscitators: Why is this patient dying right now? The intellectual challenge of that question, which the resuscitators must try to answer expeditiously and at the bedside, is compounded by the emo-

tional intensity that pervades most cardiac resuscitations.

The solvable problems that can interfere with resuscitation can be grouped into three broad categories: technical [see Table 6], physiologic, and anatomic [see Table 7]. Technical problems consist of difficulties with the resuscitators' equipment or skills; such difficulties include ineffective CPR, inadequate oxygenation and ventilation, ET tube complications, intravenous access difficulties, and monitor-defibrillator malfunction or misuse. The physiologic and anatomic problems consist of life-threatening but potentially treatable conditions that may have led to the cardiac arrest in the first place. This differentiation between physiology and anatomy is admittedly artificial, given that physiology is always involved in a cardiac arrest, but it has some usefulness as a teaching and problem-solving tool. Physiologic problems classically include hypoxia, acidosis, hyperkalemia, severe hypokalemia, hypothermia, and drug overdose. Anatomic problems are hypovolemia/hemorrhage, tension pneumothorax, cardiac tam-

Table 7 Potentially Treatable Conditions That May Cause or Contribute to Cardiac Arrest[3]

Condition	Clinical Setting	Diagnostic and Corrective Actions
Acidosis	Preexisting acidosis, diabetes, diarrhea, drugs, toxins, prolonged resuscitation, renal disease, shock	Obtain stat ABG. Reassess technical quality of CPR, oxygenation, and ventilation. Confirm correct endotracheal tube placement. Hyperventilate patient (P_aCO_2 of 30–35 mm Hg) to partially compensate for metabolic acidosis. If pH < 7.20 despite above interventions, consider I.V. sodium bicarbonate, 1 mEq/kg I.V. slow push.
Cardiac tamponade	Hemorrhagic diathesis, malignancy, pericarditis, postcardiac surgery, postmyocardial infarction, trauma	Initiate large-volume I.V. crystalloid resuscitation. Confirm diagnosis with emergent bedside echocardiogram, if available. Perform pericardiocentesis. Immediate surgical intervention is appropriate if pericardiocentesis is unhelpful but cardiac tamponade is known or highly suspected clinically.
Hypoglycemia	Adrenal insufficiency, alcohol abuse, aspirin overdose, diabetes, drugs, toxins, liver disease, renal disease, sepsis, certain tumors	Consider clinical setting and obtain finger-stick glucose or stat blood glucose measurements (may be obtained on ABG specimen). If glucose < 60 mg/dl, treat: 50 ml = 25 g of D50W I.V. Follow glucose levels closely posttreatment.*
Hypomagnesemia	Alcohol abuse, burns, diabetic ketoacidosis, severe diarrhea, diuretics, drugs (e.g., cisplatin, cyclosporine, pentamidine), malabsorption, poor intake, thyrotoxicosis	Obtain stat serum magnesium level. Treat: 1–2 g magnesium sulfate I.V. over 2 min. Follow magnesium levels over time, because blood levels correlate poorly with total body deficit.
Hypothermia	Alcohol abuse, burns, central nervous system disease, debilitated and elderly patients, drowning, drugs, toxins, endocrine disease, exposure history, homelessness, poverty, extensive skin disease, spinal cord disease, trauma	Obtain core body temperature. If severe hypothermia (< 30° C), limit initial shocks for pulseless VT/VF to three, initiate active internal rewarming and cardiopulmonary support, and hold further resuscitation medications or shocks until core temperature > 30° C† If moderate hypothermia (30°–34° C), proceed with resuscitation (space medications at intervals greater than usual), passively rewarm, and actively rewarm truncal body areas.
Hypovolemia, hemorrhage, anemia	Major burns, diabetes, gastrointestinal losses, hemorrhage, hemorrhagic diathesis, malignancy, pregnancy, shock, trauma	Initiate large-volume I.V. crystalloid resuscitation. Obtain stat hemoglobin level on ABG specimen. Emergently transfuse packed red blood cells (O negative if type-specific blood not available) if hemorrhage or profound anemia is contributing to arrest. Emergently consult necessary specialty for definitive care. Emergent thoracotomy with open cardiac massage is a consideration if experienced providers are available for the patient with penetrating trauma and cardiac arrest.
Hypoxia	All cardiac arrest patients are at risk	Reassess technical quality of CPR, oxygenation, and ventilation. Confirm correct ET tube placement. Obtain stat ABG to confirm adequate oxygenation and ventilation.
Myocardial infarction	Consider in all cardiac arrest patients, especially those with risk factors for coronary artery disease, a history of ischemic heart disease, or prearrest picture consistent with an acute coronary syndrome	Review prearrest clinical presentation and ECG. Continue resuscitation algorithm; proceed with definitive care as appropriate for the immediate circumstances (e.g., thrombolytic therapy, cardiac catheterization/coronary artery reperfusion, circulatory assist device, emergent cardiopulmonary bypass).

ponade, myocardial infarction, and pulmonary embolism.[36]

Whenever possible, the patient's medical and surgical history and the circumstances and symptoms immediately before the cardiac arrest should be sought from family members, bystanders, or hospital staff as the resuscitation proceeds. This information may contain important clues to the principal arrest problem and how it may be expeditiously treated. For example, a patient who presents to an emergency department with chest pain and then suffers a VF cardiac arrest is probably dying of a massive myocardial infarction, pulmonary embolism, or aortic dissection. A tension pneumothorax or cardiac tamponade is also a possibility.

Specific questions to consider include the following: Does the patient have risk factors for heart disease, pulmonary embolism, or aortic disease? What was the quality of the patient's pain and its radiation before the cardiac arrest? What were the prearrest vital signs and physical examination findings? What did the prearrest ECG show (if available)? Can any of this information be used now, at the bedside, to dictate the needed resuscitation interventions during the

D phase of the secondary survey? For example, if the prearrest ECG showed prominent ST-segment elevation in leads V1 through V4 consistent with a large anterior myocardial infarction, if the patient's resuscitation is failing despite appropriate interventions, and if there appear to be no technical problems hampering the resuscitation, then a working diagnosis of massive myocardial infarction can be made; intravenous thrombolytic therapy may be a reasonable part of the resuscitation in such a setting.[58]

Thoughtful consideration of the possible reasons that resuscitation is failing will regularly push the code captain's and the resuscitation team's expertise and clinical skills to the limits. Nevertheless, the failure to consider these formidable issues will deprive the patient of an optimal opportunity to survive the cardiac arrest.

Cardiac Resuscitation Based on Rhythm Findings

When a monitor-defibrillator arrives at the scene of a cardiac arrest, the patient's rhythm is immediately analyzed (the beginning part

Table 7   (continued)

Condition	Clinical Setting	Diagnostic and Corrective Actions
Poisoning	Alcohol abuse, bizarre or puzzling behavioral or metabolic presentation, classic toxic syndrome, occupational or industrial exposures, history of ingestion, polysubstance abuse, psychiatric disease	Consider clinical setting and presentation; provide meticulous supportive care. Emergently consult toxicologist (through regional poison center) for resuscitative and definitive care advice, including appropriate antidote use. Prolonged resuscitation efforts are appropriate. If available, immediate cardiopulmonary bypass should be considered.
Hyperkalemia	Metabolic acidosis, excessive administration, drugs and toxins, vigorous exercise, hemolysis, renal disease, rhabdomyolysis, tumor lysis syndrome, significant tissue injury	Obtain stat serum potassium level on ABG specimen. Treatment: calcium chloride 10% (5–10 ml I.V. slow push [do not use if hyperkalemia is secondary to digitalis poisoning]), followed by glucose and insulin (50 ml of D50W and 10 U regular insulin I.V.); sodium bicarbonate (50 mEq I.V.); albuterol (15–20 mg nebulized or 0.5 mg I.V. infusion).‡
Hypokalemia	Alcohol abuse, diabetes, diuretic use, drugs and toxins, profound gastrointestinal losses, hypomagnesemia, excess mineralocorticoid states, metabolic alkalosis	Obtain stat serum potassium level on ABG specimen. If profound hypokalemia (K+ < 2–2.5 mEq/L) is contributing to cardiac arrest, initiate urgent I.V. replacement (2 mEq/min I.V. for 10–15 mEq) then reassess.§
Pulmonary embolism	Hospitalized patients, recent surgical procedure, peripartum, known risk factors for venous thromboembolism (VTE), history of VTE, prearrest presentation consistent with acute pulmonary embolism	Review prearrest clinical presentation; initiate appropriate volume resuscitation with I.V. crystalloid and augment with vasopressors as necessary. Attempt emergent confirmation of diagnosis, depending on availability and clinical circumstances; consider emergent cardiopulmonary bypass to maintain patient viability. Continue resuscitation algorithm; proceed with definitive care (thrombolytic therapy, embolectomy via interventional radiology, or surgical thrombectomy) as appropriate for immediate circumstances and availability.
Tension pneumothorax	Postcentral line placement, mechanical ventilation, pulmonary disease (including asthma, COPD, necrotizing pneumonia), postthoracentesis, trauma	Consider risks and clinical presentation (prearrest history, breath sounds, neck veins, tracheal deviation). Proceed with emergent needle decompression, followed by chest tube insertion.

*Unrecognized hypoglycemia can cause significant neurologic injury and can be life threatening, but caution with I.V. glucose is appropriate in the setting of cardiac arrest. Available evidence indicates that hyperglycemia may contribute to impaired neurologic recovery in cardiac arrest survivors.

†Active internal or core rewarming includes warm (42°–46° C) humidified oxygen delivered through the endotracheal tube; warm I.V. fluids; peritoneal lavage; esophageal rewarming tubes; bladder lavage; and extracorporeal rewarming if immediately available. Active external rewarming includes warming beds, hot-water bottles, heating pads, and radiant heat sources applied externally to the patient.

‡Glucose is not necessary initially if patient is already hyperglycemic, but glucose levels should be followed closely after administration of I.V. insulin because of the risk of hypoglycemia (especially in patients with renal failure, because of the long duration of action of I.V. insulin in such patients). Sodium bicarbonate is most helpful in patients with concomitant metabolic acidosis; it is less effective in lowering serum potassium in dialysis-dependent renal failure patients. High-dose nebulized albuterol should lower serum potassium by 0.5 to 1.5 mEq/L within 30 to 60 min, but administration during cardiac arrest may be difficult.

§In a non–cardiac arrest situation, usual I.V. potassium replacement guidelines for patients requiring parenteral therapy are generally 10 to 20 mEq/hr with continuous electrocardiographic monitoring. If profound hypokalemia is contributing to cardiac arrest, however, these usual replacement rates are not timely enough, given the critical nature of the situation. Under these circumstances, potassium chloride, 2 mEq/min I.V. for 10 to 15 mEq, is reasonable, but reassessment and careful attention to changing levels, redistribution, and ongoing clinical circumstances are essential to prevent life-threatening hyperkalemia from developing.

ABG—arterial blood gas   COPD—chronic obstructive pulmonary disease   D50W—50% dextrose in water   ET—endotracheal   VF—ventricular fibrillation   VT—ventricular tachycardia

of step D in the primary survey). There are four rhythm possibilities [see Figure 1]: (1) pulseless VT, (2) pulseless VF, (3) organized or semiorganized electrical activity despite the absence of a palpable carotid pulse, which defines PEA, and (4) asystole. The detailed management of these different cardiac resuscitation scenarios is based on the recommendations of the AHA[44] and the International Liaison Committee on Resuscitation.[59]

PULSELESS VENTRICULAR TACHYCARDIA OR VENTRICULAR FIBRILLATION

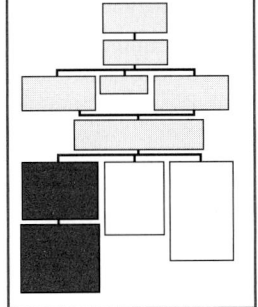

The appearance of either pulseless VT or VF on the rhythm monitor in a patient with ongoing CPR is a relatively favorable finding, because there is reasonable hope for a successful outcome with these rhythms. In addition, the interventions and medications sequentially used in the resuscitation are plainly delineated, and the initial course of action is clear. Pulseless VT or VF is managed identically.

Initiation of Defibrillation

Defibrillation with 200 joules should be attempted immediately; if the VT or VF persists, subsequent attempts should be made with 200 to 300 joules and then 360 joules, successively. A lower, nonescalating equivalent biphasic energy level is acceptable, if the defibrillator offers this option. It is no longer recommended that the patient's carotid pulse be manually checked between shocks, but the displayed rhythm on the monitor must be carefully assessed after each defibrillation attempt. If there are any doubts concerning the rhythm or if there is suspicion of a dysfunctional lead or paddle cable, then a manual pulse check would be appropriate. If pulseless VT or VF persists, CPR should be resumed, the patient should be intubated, correct ET tube placement should be confirmed, and the tube should be secured. Simultaneously, intravenous access should be established.

Initiation of Drug Therapy

A parenteral drug should then be administered, after which further attempts at defibrillation should be made. The first medication given is a vasoconstrictor (either epinephrine or vasopressin) [see Table 4]. If there is no intravenous access, this drug can be given endotracheally. After each intravenous dose, a 20 ml saline bolus should be administered, and the extremity that contains the intravenous line should be elevated. The rescuers should continue CPR for 30 to 60 seconds to allow the drug to reach the heart, after which defibrillation should again be attempted with one to three shocks at 360 joules each. As long as the patient remains pulseless, epinephrine should be repeatedly administered every 3 to 5 minutes, with each dose followed by one to three attempts at defibrillation. When vasopressin is the chosen initial drug, only a single dose is given; if the resuscitation continues 10 minutes or longer after vasopressin is administered, epinephrine should be substituted for vasopressin for the remainder of the code. If pulseless VT or VF persists despite the

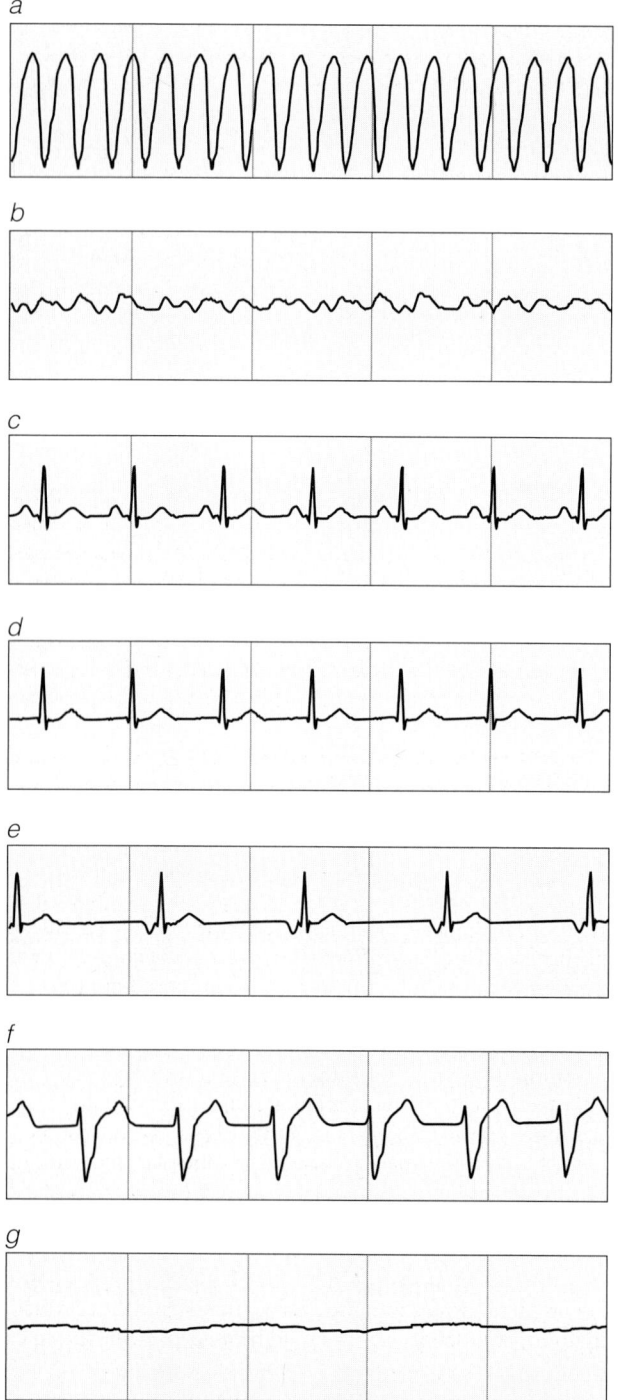

Figure 1 **The sudden cardiac arrest arrhythmias. (*a*) Ventricular tachycardia. (*b*) Ventricular fibrillation. Pulseless electrical activity encompasses any of several forms of organized electrical activity in the pulseless patient; these include (*c*) normal sinus rhythm, (*d*) junctional rhythm, (*e*) bradycardic junctional rhythm, and (*f*) idioventricular rhythm. (*g*) Asystole.**

initial administration of a vasoconstrictor and repeated defibrillation attempts, antiarrhythmic drug therapy is added; amiodarone or lidocaine is an appropriate agent [*see* Choice of Antiarrhythmic Drugs, *below*]. Throughout all of these steps, the code team leader should actively look for technical and physiologic/anatomic problems that may be preventing a successful resuscitation and should correct any problems that are found [*see Table 6*].

Emergency Laboratory Tests

If spontaneous circulation does not return after the first round of antiarrhythmic drug therapy, the resuscitation team must also endeavor to identify and treat the clinically relevant conditions causing or contributing to the cardiac arrest [*see Table 7*]. In theory, the interventions conducted to this point should have resulted in a perfusing rhythm. The code team must ask why this has not occurred, and it must attempt to answer this question as the resuscitation continues. Emergency laboratory studies that may prove helpful include a stat ABG measurement and measurements of hemoglobin, potassium, magnesium, and blood glucose levels (most of which can be obtained from the ABG specimen).

Choice of Antiarrhythmic Drugs

There are four antiarrhythmic drugs used in cardiac resuscitation: amiodarone, lidocaine, magnesium (if the patient is thought or proven to be hypomagnesemic), and procainamide (for intermittent or recurrent VT or VF that initially responds to defibrillation).[60] It is not known which one of these drugs or which combination of them will optimize the chances of patient survival to hospital discharge. Despite many years of routine use, there are no controlled studies demonstrating a survival benefit from lidocaine versus placebo in the management of pulseless VT or VF. Two recent studies in patients with shock-refractory prehospital VF showed that survival to hospital admission was better with amiodarone than with placebo (44% versus 34%; *P* = 0.03)[61] or with lidocaine (22.8% versus 12.0%; *P* = 0.009).[62] Neither of these studies demonstrated an improved survival to hospital discharge in the amiodarone groups, but neither study had the statistical power to demonstrate such a difference. The optimal role and exact benefit of antiarrhythmic medications in cardiac resuscitation has yet to be fully elucidated. According to AHA guidelines, either amiodarone or lidocaine is an acceptable initial antiarrhythmic drug for the treatment of patients with pulseless VT or VF that is unresponsive to initial shocks, CPR, airway management, and administration of epinephrine or vasopressin plus shocks. On the basis of available evidence, however, amiodarone appears to be the antiarrhythmic agent of first choice in the setting of prehospital refractory VF.[60-62]

PULSELESS ELECTRICAL ACTIVITY

Community ACLS providers are encountering nonventricular arrhythmias (i.e., PEA and asystole) with increasing frequency. Classically, the prognosis for PEA has been poor, with outpatient survival rates generally reported as 0% to 7%.[63,64] The sequence of resuscitation steps in the management of PEA is as follows: activation of the emergency medical or code response, primary survey (CPR and rhythm evaluation), and secondary survey (intubation and confirmation of correct ET tube placement, optimal oxygenation and ventilation, establishment of I.V. access, epinephrine administration, and, finally, problem solving for technical difficulties and establishment of cause of cardiac arrest). The two core drugs

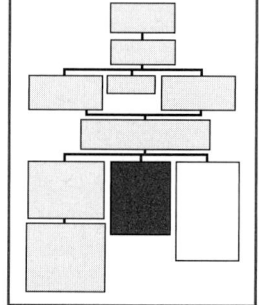

for PEA management are epinephrine (repeated every 3 to 5 minutes for as long as the patient is pulseless) and atropine (up to 3 mg over time if the PEA rhythm on the monitor is inappropriately slow). The best hope for a successful resuscitation is to find and treat the cause of PEA; therein lies the exceptionally challenging aspect of PEA resuscitation management [*see Tables 6 and 7*]. Because coronary artery thrombosis and pulmonary thromboembolism are common causes of cardiac arrest, a recent trial evaluated the efficacy of tissue plasminogen activator (t-PA) in the setting of PEA of unknown or presumed cardiovascular cause in 233 patients in prehospital and emergency department settings.[65] No benefit was found with thrombolytic therapy for PEA in this study; the proportion of patients with return of spontaneous circulation was 21.4% in the t-PA group and 23.3% in the placebo group.

ASYSTOLE

The prognosis for asystole is generally regarded as dismal unless the patient is hypothermic or there are other extenuating but treatable circumstances. The sequence of resuscitation steps in the management of asystole is as follows: activation of the emergency medical or code response, primary survey (CPR, rhythm evaluation, and asystole confirmation), and secondary survey (intubation 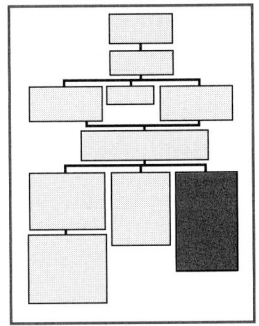 and confirmation of correct ET tube placement, optimal oxygenation and ventilation, I.V. access with epinephrine and atropine administration, immediate transcutaneous pacing if available, and problem solving for technical difficulties and establishment of cause of cardiac arrest). The two core drugs for asystole management are epinephrine (repeated every 3 to 5 minutes for as long as the patient is pulseless) and atropine (up to 3 mg over time). Potentially treatable causes of asystole have traditionally included hypoxia, acidosis, hypothermia, hypokalemia, hyperkalemia, and drug overdose. Resuscitation efforts should stop if asystole persists for longer than 10 minutes despite optimal CPR, oxygenation and ventilation, and epinephrine/atropine administration; if extenuating circumstances (e.g., hypothermia, cold-water submersion, or drug overdose) are not present; and if no other readily treatable condition is identified.

Immediate Postresuscitation Care

Even when the resuscitation is successful, the patient's situation remains tenuous and continued meticulous patient care is essential. When the cardiac monitor indicates what should be a perfusing rhythm, one should immediately confirm the presence of a palpable pulse in the patient. If there is a pulse, the patient's blood pressure should be obtained. Simultaneously, resuscitation team members should quickly reassess the adequacy of the patient's airway, the ET tube position, oxygenation and ventilation, and the patient's level of consciousness.

If the patient is hypotensive, appropriate blood pressure management depends on the presence or absence of fluid overload, as judged at the bedside. If the patient is clinically volume overloaded or in frank pulmonary edema, dopamine should be started at inotropic doses (5 μg/kg/min I.V.) and titrated to a target systolic blood pressure of 90 to 100 mm Hg. If the patient's clinical status suggests normovolemia or hypovolemia, intravenous crystalloid boluses (in 250 to 500 ml increments) should be administered instead of dopamine to support adequate tissue perfusion. If the patient is regaining consciousness, the level of comfort should be carefully as-

sessed and analgesia and sedation administered, as indicated.

If the arrest rhythm was either VT or VF, the parenteral antiarrhythmic drug used immediately before the return of spontaneous circulation is continued as a maintenance infusion (amiodarone, 1 mg/min for 6 hr, then 0.5 mg/min for 18 hr as blood pressure allows; lidocaine, 2 to 4 mg/min). If an antiarrhythmic drug has not yet been administered, it is usually started at this point to prevent the recurrence of pulseless VT or VF. There are important exceptions to this guideline, however. If the perfusing postarrest arrhythmia is an idioventricular rhythm or third-degree heart block accompanied by an idioventricular escape rhythm, an antiarrhythmic medication should not be started at this time, because the antiarrhythmic agent could eliminate the ventricular perfusing focus and return the patient to pulselessness.

Initial postresuscitation studies usually include ECG, portable chest radiography, ABG measurement, serum electrolyte panel, fingerstick or blood glucose measurement, measurement of serum magnesium and cardiac enzyme levels, and measurement of hemoglobin and hematocrit. The resuscitated patient requires urgent transfer to the optimal site for continued definitive care. Depending on the circumstances, this may be either the cardiac catheterization laboratory or the intensive care unit.

Ending a Resuscitation Attempt

Throughout the resuscitation, the team leader should speak with calmness and authority; the leader should orchestrate the resuscitation with clarity and finesse and should make clinical decisions without directly performing specific procedures (if that is possible). All cardiac arrests are emotionally charged, but the leader must insist on a composed, orderly, and technically sound resuscitation. It is appropriate to invite suggestions from team members and to ensure that all members are comfortable with the decision to stop the resuscitation, should that time arrive.

The decision to stop a cardiac resuscitation is burdensome. Clearly, the circumstances of the event, patient comorbidities, the nature of the lethal arrhythmia, and the resuscitation team's ability to correctly identify and treat potential contributing causes to the arrest are all important considerations. Resuscitation efforts beyond 30 minutes without a return of spontaneous circulation are usually futile unless the cardiac arrest is confounded by intermittent or recurrent VT or VF, hypothermia, cold-water submersion, drug overdose, or other identified and readily treated conditions.[66,67]

In the prehospital setting (assuming proper equipment and medications are available and no extenuating circumstances suggest otherwise), full resuscitation efforts should take place at the scene of a nontraumatic cardiac arrest in preference to rapid transport to an emergency department. A prehospital resuscitation that has been appropriately conducted but has not resulted in at least temporary return of spontaneous circulation to the patient may be discontinued. It is important that certain criteria are adhered to, however, including the following: high-quality CPR was provided, an adequate airway was successfully placed, appropriate oxygenation and ventilation occurred, intravenous access was established, appropriate medications specific to the arrest scenario were administered, resuscitation was attempted for at least 10 minutes, the patient is not in persistent VF, and there are no extenuating circumstances that mandate in-hospital continuation of the resuscitation (e.g., hypothermia, drug overdose). The decision to cease resuscitation efforts in the field is enhanced by direct discussion with EMS physicians. It is also essential that services be available to provide immediate assistance and support to the family and loved ones of the patient who has now died.

Discontinuing in-hospital resuscitations is advisable if the arrest was unwitnessed, the initial rhythm was other than VT or VF, and spontaneous circulation does not return after 10 minutes of ongoing resuscitation.[68] In a study of this decision rule, only 1.1% of patients (3 out of 269) who met these three parameters survived to hospital discharge, and none of these survivors were capable of independent living.[69] In a recent study of 445 prospectively recorded resuscitation attempts in hospitalized patients, no patient survived who suffered a cardiac arrest between 12 A.M. and 6 A.M. if the arrest was unwitnessed and if it occurred in an unmonitored bed.[33]

A resuscitation attempt in a persistently asystolic patient should not last longer than 10 minutes, assuming all of the following conditions apply: asystole is confirmed through proper rhythm monitoring and assessment, high-quality CPR is taking place, ET intubation was correctly performed and confirmed, adequate oxygenation and ventilation have occurred, intravenous access is present, appropriate medications (epinephrine and atropine) have been administered, and the patient is not the victim of hypothermia, cold-water submersion, drug overdose, or other readily identified and reversible cause.

After all resuscitation attempts, the code leader should debrief the team so that all may learn from the experience. Finally, marked empathy and skill are needed to carefully and compassionately inform family members about the outcome of the resuscitation.[70]

References

1. Callans DJ: Management of the patient who has been resuscitated from sudden cardiac death. Circulation 105:2704, 2002

2. Zipes DP, Wellens HJ: Sudden cardiac death. Circulation 98:2334, 1998

3. Eisenberg MS, Mengert TJ: Cardiac resuscitation. N Engl J Med 344:1304, 2001

4. 1999 Heart and Stroke Statistical Update. American Heart Association, Dallas, 1998

5. Ballew KA, Philbrick JT: Causes of variation in reported in-hospital CPR survival: a critical review. Resuscitation 30:203, 1995

6. Myerburg RJ, Castellanos A: Cardiac arrest and sudden cardiac death. Heart Disease: A Textbook of Cardiovascular Medicine. Braunwald E, Ed. WB Saunders Co, Philadelphia, 1997, p 742

7. Osborn LA: Etiology of sudden death. Cardiac Arrest: The Science and Practice of Resuscitation Medicine. Paradis NA, Halperin HR, Nowak RM, Eds. Williams & Wilkins, Philadelphia, 1996, p 243

8. Cummins RO, Ornato JP, Thies W, et al: Improving survival from cardiac arrest: the chain of survival concept: a statement for health professionals from the Advanced Cardiac Life Support Subcommittee and the Emergency Cardiac Care Committee, American Heart Association. Circulation 83:1832, 1991

9. Capussi A, Aschieri D, Piepoli MF, et al: Tripling survival from sudden cardiac arrest via early defibrillation without traditional education in cardiopulmonary resuscitation. Circulation 106:1065, 2002

10. Callaham M, Madsen CD: Relationship of timeliness of paramedic advanced life support interventions to outcome in out-of-hospital cardiac arrest treated by first responders with defibrillators. Ann Emerg Med 27:638, 1996

11. Marenco JP, Wang PJ, Link MS, et al: Improving survival from sudden cardiac arrest: the role of the automated external defibrillator. JAMA 285:1193, 2001

12. Peberdy MA: Defibrillation. Cardiol Clin 20:13, 2002

13. Cummins RO, Eisenberg MS: Prehospital cardiopulmonary resuscitation: is it effective? JAMA 253:2408, 1985

14. Stapleton ER: Basic life support cardiopulmonary resuscitation. Cardiol Clin 20:12, 2002

15. Valenzuela TD, Roe DJ, Cretin S, et al: Estimating effectiveness of cardiac arrest interventions: a logistic regression survival model. Circulation 96:3308, 1997

16. Eisenberg MS, Bergner L, Hallstrom A: Cardiac resuscitation in the community: the importance of rapid delivery of care and implications for program planning. JAMA 241:1905, 1979

17. Weaver WD, Cobb LA, Hallstrom AP, et al: Considerations for improving survival from out-of-hospital cardiac arrest. Ann Emerg Med 15:1181, 1986

18. Larsen MP, Eisenberg MS, Cummins RO, et al: Predicting survival from out-of-hospital cardiac arrest: a graphic model. Ann Emerg Med 270:1211, 1993

19. Eisenberg MS, Horwood BT, Cummins RO, et al: Cardiac arrest and resuscitation: a tale of 29 cities. Ann Emerg Med 19:179, 1990

20. Lombardi G, Gallagher J, Gennis P: Outcome of out-of-hospital cardiac arrest in New York City: the Pre-Hospital Arrest Survival Evaluation (PHASE) study. JAMA 271:678, 1994

21. Becker LB, Ostrander MP, Barrett J, et al: Outcome of CPR in a large metropolitan area: where are the survivors? Ann Emerg Med 20:355, 1991

22. Killien SY, Geyman JP, Gossom JB, et al: Out-of-hospital cardiac arrest in a rural area: a 16-year experience with lessons learned and national comparisons. Ann Emerg Med 28:294, 1996

23. Valenzuela TD, Roe DJ, Nichol G, et al: Outcomes of rapid defibrillation by security officers after cardiac arrest in casinos. N Engl J Med 343:1206, 2000

24. Eisenberg M, Bergner L, Hallstrom A: Sudden Cardiac Death in the Community. Praeger, Philadelphia, 1984

25. Becker L: The epidemiology of sudden death. Cardiac Arrest: The Science and Practice of Resuscitation Medicine. Paradis NA, Halperin HR, Nowak RM, Eds. Williams & Wilkins, Philadelphia, 1996, p 28

26. Jastremski MS: In-hospital cardiac arrest. Ann Emerg Med 22:113, 1993

27. Rosenberg M, Wang C, Hoffman-Wilde S, et al: Results of cardiopulmonary resuscitation failure to predict survival in two community hospitals. Arch Intern Med 153:1370, 1993

28. Ballew KA, Philbrick JT, Caven DE, et al: Predictors of survival following in-hospital cardiopulmonary resuscitation: a moving target. Arch Intern Med 154:2426, 1994

29. De Vos R, Koster RW, deHaan RJ, et al: In-hospital cardiopulmonary resuscitation: prearrest morbidity and outcome. Arch Intern Med 159:845, 1999

30. Goodlin SJ, Zhong Z, Lynn J, et al: Factors associated with use of cardiopulmonary resuscitation in seriously ill hospitalized adults. JAMA 282:2333, 1999

31. Van Walraven C, Forster AJ, Stiell IG: Derivation of a clinical decision rule for the discontinuation of in-hospital cardiac arrest resuscitations. Arch Intern Med 159:129, 1999

32. Zoch TW, Desbiens NA, DeStefano F, et al: Short- and long-term survival after cardiopulmonary resuscitation. Arch Intern Med 160:1969, 2000

33. Dumot JA, Burval DJ, Sprung J, et al: Outcome of adult cardiopulmonary resuscitations at a tertiary referral center including results of "limited" resuscitations. Arch Intern Med 161:1751, 2001

34. Meade M: Men and the Water of Life. Harper, San Francisco, 1993, p 442

35. Burkle FM Jr, Rice MM: Code organization. Am J Emerg Med 5:235, 1987

36. ACLS Provider Manual. American Heart Association, Dallas, 2001

37. Safar P: On the history of modern resuscitation. Anesthesiol Clin North Am 13:751, 1995

38. Kouwenhoven WB, Jude JR, Knickerbocker GG: Closed-chest cardiac massage. JAMA 173:1064, 1960

39. Jude JR, Kouwenhoven WB, Knickerbocker GG: Cardiac arrest: report of application of external cardiac massage on 118 patients. JAMA 178:1063, 1961

40. Halperin HR: Mechanisms of forward flow during external chest compression. Cardiac Arrest: The Science and Practice of Resuscitation Medicine. Paradis NA, Halperin HR, Nowak RM, Eds. Williams & Wilkins, Philadelphia, 1996, p 252

41. Ornato JP, Peberdy MA: Cardiopulmonary resuscitation. Textbook of Cardiovascular Medicine. Topol EJ, Ed. Lippincott-Raven, Philadelphia, 1998, p 1779

42. Paradis NA, Martin GB, Goetting MG, et al: Simultaneous aortic, jugular bulb, and right atrial pressures during cardiopulmonary resuscitation in humans: insights into mechanisms. Circulation 80:361, 1989

43. Daya MR, Mariani RJ: Out-of-hospital splinting. Clinical Procedures in Emergency Medicine, 3rd ed. Roberts JR, Hedges JR, Eds. WB Saunders Co, Philadelphia 1998, p 1297

44. Guidelines 2000 for cardiopulmonary resuscitation and emergency cardiovascular care: international consensus on science. Circulation 102(suppl I):1, 2000

45. Levine RL, Wayne MA, Miller CC: End-tidal carbon dioxide and outcome of out-of-hospital cardiac arrest. N Engl J Med 337:301, 1997

46. Hedges JR, Greenberg MI: Defibrillation. Clinical Procedures in Emergency Medicine, 3rd ed. Roberts JR, Hedges JR, Eds. WB Saunders Co, Philadelphia, 1998, p 1297

47. Hossack KF, Hartwig R: Cardiac arrest associated with supervised cardiac rehabilitation. J Cardiac Rehab 2:402, 1982

48. Bardy GH, Marchlinski FE, Sharma AD, et al: Multicenter comparison of truncated biphasic shocks and standard damped sine wave monophasic shocks for transthoracic ventricular defibrillation. Circulation 94:2507, 1996

49. Gliner BE, White RD: Electrocardiographic evaluation of defibrillation shocks delivered to out-of-hospital sudden cardiac arrest patients. Resuscitation 41:129, 1999

50. Gliner BE, Jorgenson DB, Poole JE, et al: Treatment of out-of-hospital cardiac arrest with a low-energy impedance-compensating biphasic waveform automatic external defibrillator. Biomed Instrum Technol 32:631, 1998

51. Poole JE, White RD, Kanz KG, et al: Low-energy impedance-compensating biphasic waveforms terminate ventricular fibrillation at high rates in victims of out-of-hospital cardiac arrest. J Cardiovasc Electrophysiol 8:1373, 1997

52. Schneider T, Martens PR, Paschen H, et al: Multicenter, randomized, controlled trial of 150-J biphasic shocks compared with 200- to 360-J monophasic shocks in the resuscitation of out-of-hospital cardiac arrest victims. Circulation 102:1780, 2000

53. Aehlert B: ACLS: Quick Review Study Guide, 2nd ed. CV Mosby, St Louis, 2001

54. Rumball CJ, MacDonald D: The PTL, Combitube, laryngeal mask, and oral airway: a randomized prehospital comparative study of ventilatory device effectiveness and cost-effectiveness in 470 cases of cardiorespiratory arrest. Prehosp Emerg Care 1:1, 1997

55. Garnett AR, Ornato JP, Gonzales ER, et al: End-tidal carbon dioxide monitoring during cardiopulmonary resuscitation. JAMA 257:512, 1987

56. Paradis NA, Wenzel V, Southall J: Pressor drugs in the treatment of cardiac arrest. Cardiol Clin 20:61, 2002

57. Stiell IG, Hebert PC, Wells GA, et al: Vasopressin versus epinephrine for inhospital cardiac arrest: a randomized controlled trial. Lancet 358:105, 2001

58. Tiffany PA, Schultz M, Stueven H: Bolus thrombolytic infusions during CPR for patients with refractory arrest rhythms: outcome of a case series. Ann Emerg Med 31:124, 1998

59. Cummins RO, Chamberlain DA: Advisory statements of the International Liaison Committee on Resuscitation. Circulation 95:2172, 1997

60. Kudenchuk PJ: Advanced cardiac life support antiarrhythmic drugs. Cardiol Clin 20:79, 2002

61. Kudenchuk PJ, Cobb LA, Copass MK, et al: Amiodarone for resuscitation after out-of-hospital cardiac arrest due to ventricular fibrillation. N Engl J Med 341:871, 1999

62. Dorian P, Cass D, Schwartz B, et al: Amiodarone as compared with lidocaine for shock-resistant ventricular fibrillation. N Engl J Med 346:884, 2002

63. Myerburg RJ, Conde CA, Sung RJ, et al: Clinical, electrophysiologic, and hemodynamic profile of patients resuscitated from prehospital cardiac arrest. Am J Med 68:568, 1980

64. Stratton SJ, Niemann JT: Outcome from out-of-hospital cardiac arrest caused by nonventricular arrhythmias: contribution of successful resuscitation to overall survivorship supports the current practice of initiating out-of-hospital ACLS. Ann Emerg Med 32:448, 1998

65. Abu-Laban RB, Christenson JM, Innes GD, et al: Tissue plasminogen activator in cardiac arrest with pulseless electrical activity. N Engl J Med 346:1522, 2002

66. Bonnin MJ, Pepe PE, Kimball KT, et al: Distinct criteria for termination of resuscitation in the out-of-hospital setting. JAMA 270:1457, 1993

67. Kellermann AL, Hackman BB, Somes G: Predicting the outcome of unsuccessful prehospital advanced cardiac life support. JAMA 270:1433, 1993

68. Van Walraven C, Forster AJ, Stiell IG: Derivation of a clinical decision rule for the discontinuation of in-hospital cardiac arrest resuscitations. Arch Intern Med 159:129, 1999

69. Van Walraven C, Forster AJ, Parish DC, et al: Validation of a clinical decision aid to discontinue in-hospital cardiac arrest resuscitations. JAMA 285:1602, 2001

70. Iserson K: Grave Words: Notifying Survivors about Sudden, Unexpected Deaths. Galen Press, Tucson, Arizona, 1999

71. Cummins RO, Field JM, Hazinski MF, et al: ACLS Provider Manual. American Heart Association, Dallas, 2001, p 36

72. Part 1: introduction to the international guidelines 2000 for CPR and ECC: a consensus on science. Circulation 102(8 suppl):I1, 2000

Acknowledgment

Adapted from Mengert TJ: III Cardiac Resuscitation. 8 Interdisciplinary Medicine. WebMD Scientific American® Medicine Online. Dale DC, Federman DD, Eds. WebMD Inc., New York, 2003. http://www.samed.com/. (April 2003)

2 ACUTE CARDIAC DYSRHYTHMIA

Caesar Ursic, M.D., and Alden H. Harken, M.D., F.A.C.S.

Management of Acute Dysrhythmias

After successful cardiopulmonary resuscitation (CPR) or any myocardial ischemic event, the most common source of hemodynamic instability is an abnormal heart rhythm. This chapter outlines the approach to a patient with an apparent acute cardiac dysrhythmia.

The purpose of the heart's electrical activity is to induce mechanical activity. Abnormal electrical activity that occurs in the absence of hemodynamic compromise should be examined but treated with forbearance because therapy itself poses some hazards: all antidysrhythmic agents, except oxygen, are negatively inotropic. In the evaluation of a patient who appears to exhibit an acute cardiac dysrhythmia, four questions should be asked:

1. Does the patient actually have a cardiac dysrhythmia?
2. Does the patient require any therapy (i.e., is the patient sufficiently stable that treatment is NOT indicated)?
3. How soon should therapy be started (i.e., how unstable is the patient)?
4. Which therapy is the safest and most effective?

Patient Is Hemodynamically Unstable

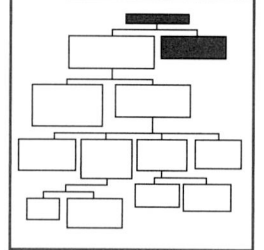

The choice of therapy is determined by the stability of the patient and the origin of the dysrhythmia. An electrocardiogram is helpful but not required. Patients with asystole require CPR [*see 6:1 Cardiac Resuscitation*]. All hemodynamically unstable patients who have a dysrhythmia other than asystole should be treated immediately by cardioversion. Actually, cardioversion of asystole will do no harm; it just will not help, because there is no underlying rhythm to reorganize. If in doubt, therefore, one should proceed with cardioversion.

The two primary goals in the management of an acute dysrhythmia are to control the ventricular rate and to maintain a normal sinus rhythm. It is important to note that hemodynamic instability in a patient who has a ventricular rate between 60 and 100 beats/min is almost certainly not the result of a cardiac rhythm disturbance. Furthermore, heart rates in excess of 100 beats/min do not necessarily require therapy. Most patients can remain hemodynamically stable—and, in fact, increase their cardiac output—while raising their heart rate to 220 beats/min minus their age. In addition, it is not critical to reestablish normal sinus rhythm in all cases.[1] In a young, healthy patient with a nor-

mal heart, the so-called atrial kick adds almost nothing to cardiac output.[2] If normal sinus rhythm is abolished and atrial fibrillation is electrically induced in a young healthy patient, the ventricles and the rest of the cardiovascular system compensate almost immediately to prevent a fall in cardiac output.[3] On the other hand, loss of synchronous atrial activity in patients with end-stage cardiac decompensation may decrease cardiac output by as much as 40%[4]; fortunately, such a degree of end-stage cardiac compromise is rare.

CARDIOVERSION

Cardioversion delivers sufficient electrical energy to the precordium (or directly to the heart) to depolarize cells, even those in a relatively refractory state. Cardioversion imposes electrical reorganization on the heart. In theory, after this massive depolarization, all the myocardial cells will repolarize simultaneously and then reinstitute a synchronous beat [*see Sidebar* The Intracardiac Cardioverter Defibrillator].

Certain precautions are necessary with cardioversion. The procedure is of no use in patients who are in asystole or who have fine ventricular fibrillation (VF), because these patients have no cardiac activity to organize—though, again, cardioversion does no harm in such cases (as it is said, "you cannot fall off the floor"). Supraventricular dysrhythmias such as atrial flutter can be converted with extremely low energy levels (e.g., ≤ 5 joules), but such low levels should not be employed in emergency situations. For a hemodynamically unstable patient, the initial cardioversion should be with 100 joules; if the dysrhythmia is not abolished, the voltage should be increased rapidly (to a maximum of 360 joules).

Patient Is Hemodynamically Stable

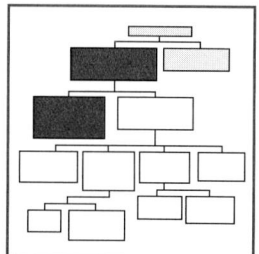

VENTRICULAR RATE IS SLOW

If the patient is bradycardic before or after cardioversion, atropine should be administered in a 0.5 mg I.V. push. This dose may be repeated at 2-minute intervals. Because the effects of atropine are transient, a temporary internal or external pacemaker should be used to maintain the heart rate. Insertion of an internal pacemaker consistently takes longer than predicted; an external pacemaker is a very effective temporizing maneuver [*see Sidebar* Troubleshooting a Pacemaker].

Management of Acute Dysrhythmias

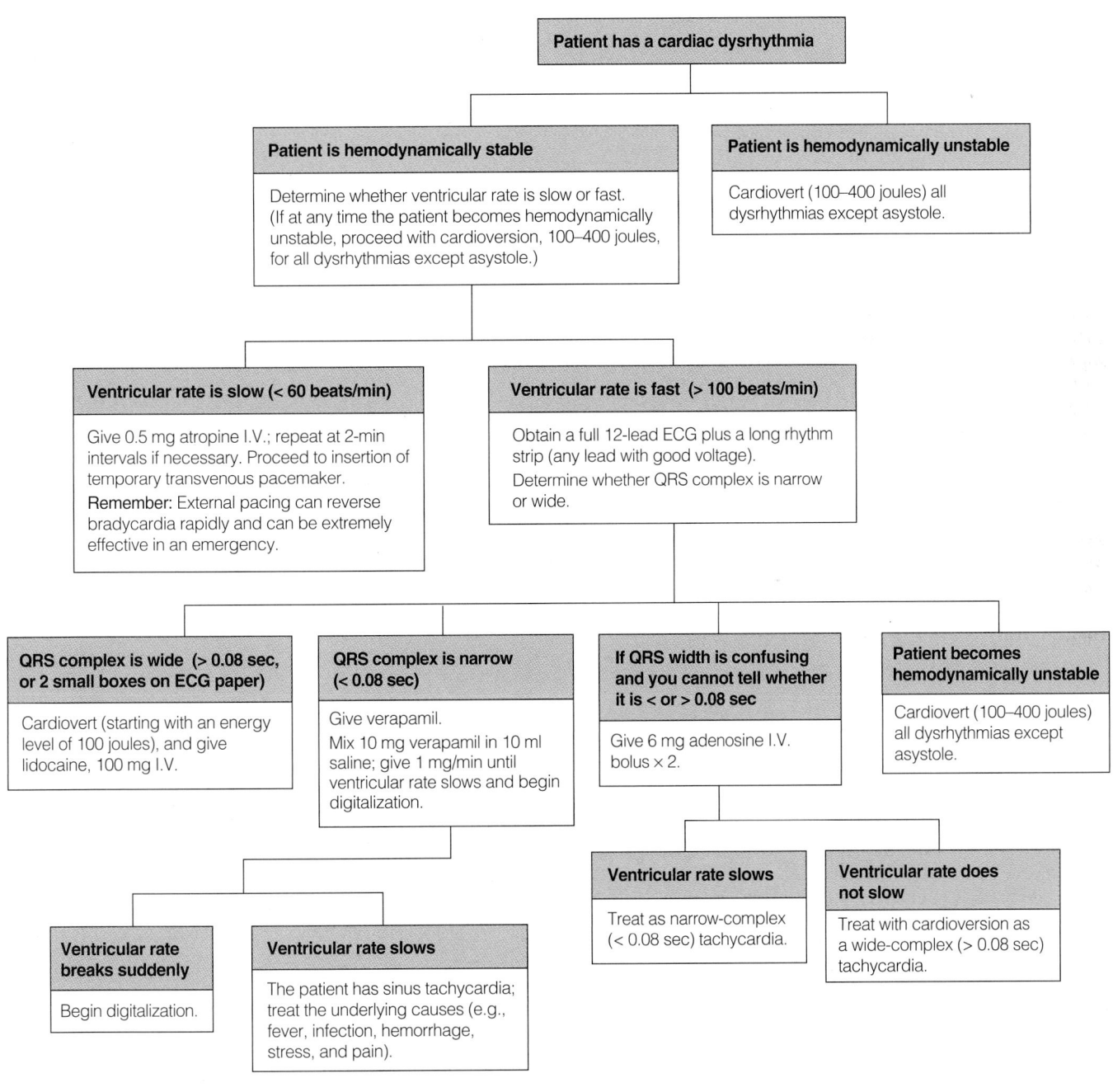

Patient has a cardiac dysrhythmia

Patient is hemodynamically stable

Determine whether ventricular rate is slow or fast.
(If at any time the patient becomes hemodynamically unstable, proceed with cardioversion, 100–400 joules, for all dysrhythmias except asystole.)

Patient is hemodynamically unstable

Cardiovert (100–400 joules) all dysrhythmias except asystole.

Ventricular rate is slow (< 60 beats/min)

Give 0.5 mg atropine I.V.; repeat at 2-min intervals if necessary. Proceed to insertion of temporary transvenous pacemaker.
Remember: External pacing can reverse bradycardia rapidly and can be extremely effective in an emergency.

Ventricular rate is fast (> 100 beats/min)

Obtain a full 12-lead ECG plus a long rhythm strip (any lead with good voltage).
Determine whether QRS complex is narrow or wide.

QRS complex is wide (> 0.08 sec, or 2 small boxes on ECG paper)

Cardiovert (starting with an energy level of 100 joules), and give lidocaine, 100 mg I.V.

QRS complex is narrow (< 0.08 sec)

Give verapamil.
Mix 10 mg verapamil in 10 ml saline; give 1 mg/min until ventricular rate slows and begin digitalization.

If QRS width is confusing and you cannot tell whether it is < or > 0.08 sec

Give 6 mg adenosine I.V. bolus × 2.

Patient becomes hemodynamically unstable

Cardiovert (100–400 joules) all dysrhythmias except asystole.

Ventricular rate breaks suddenly

Begin digitalization.

Ventricular rate slows

The patient has sinus tachycardia; treat the underlying causes (e.g., fever, infection, hemorrhage, stress, and pain).

Ventricular rate slows

Treat as narrow-complex (< 0.08 sec) tachycardia.

Ventricular rate does not slow

Treat with cardioversion as a wide-complex (> 0.08 sec) tachycardia.

The Intracardiac Cardioverter Defibrillator

Over 30 years ago, Michel Mirowski developed the first automatic intracardiac cardioverter defibrillator (ICD), a device that detects dangerous tachyarrhythmias and delivers a cardioverting shock.[55] In the intervening time, it has become abundantly clear that some of the 400,000 Americans who die "suddenly" of tachyarrhythmias each year could have been identified as high risk, although they could not have been saved by pharmacologic or surgical treatment. For these patients, an ICD can be lifesaving.[56]

The ICD identifies dangerous rhythm patterns by means of two algorithms. The first of these algorithms analyzes the patient's heart rate. The patient's maximum attainable sinus rate must be determined by exercise testing before the device is implanted; the ICD is then programmed to detect heart rates above this value. (The ICD can be externally programmed to detect rates between 155 and 200 beats/min.[57])

Using rate criteria alone, however, the ICD cannot discriminate between sinus tachycardia and ventricular or supraventricular tachycardia. Inappropriate shocks are the Achilles heel of the ICD: almost one third of patients experience at least one inappropriate shock annually, when the device detects an episode of sinus tachycardia in which the rate exceeds the threshold programmed earlier. The ICD misinterprets the event as ventricular tachycardia and delivers a shock to the hemodynamically stable patient.[58] Patients liken this to being punched hard in the chest. Although rarely of electrophysiologic significance, an inappropriate shock can be psychologically crippling.[59]

Although computer circuitry is facile and rapid, an ICD recognizes patterns poorly. Fine (or even coarse) VF may not exhibit enough positive spikes to be recognized as a tachyarrhythmia by the ICD. A second algorithm (the probability density function algorithm) was developed to analyze electrophysiologic data and improve the specificity of the ICD's sensing circuitry. A unique feature of ventricular fibrillation is the virtual absence of isoelectric time. Conversely, during sinus tachycardia and supraventricular tachycardia, the ECG is at the isoelectric baseline much of the time. The probability density function algorithm enables the ICD to determine the proportion of time that the ECG is spending at the isoelectric baseline and thereby to detect ventricular fibrillation.

The ICD typically requires more than 5 seconds to appreciate ventricular tachycardia or fibrillation. It then charges its energy storage capacitors for 15 seconds and delivers a 30-joule cardioverting shock. If necessary, the device will deliver a second, third, fourth, and fifth countershock. If the rhythm disorder persists after the fifth countershock, the device will not recycle.

ICD systems are not complex. The device consists of a battery, which is heavy (though newer batteries are becoming lighter), and circuitry, which is light, with a total weight of less than 100 g. Most implanted defibrillators are currently placed without a thoracotomy. A sensing and defibrillating lead system (14 French) is inserted percutaneously via the subclavian vein into right ventricular–right atrial position. The distal electrode tip senses ventricular fibrillation and tachycardia. The cardioverting energy is then discharged between a coil electrode on the diaphragmatic surface of the right ventricle and another coil electrode positioned in the superior vena cava.

It is now clear that ICDs really do work and are capable of extending life. The most effective predictor of outcome in patients with ICDs is the severity of heart failure.[60] The ICD does not prevent malignant arrhythmias: it is, in essence, a safety net that cardioverts ventricular tachycardia or VF when it occurs. Therefore, it must still be used in conjunction with antidysrhythmic drugs.[61,62]

It is easy for a surgeon to become spooked by an ICD. The most effective strategy for managing a patient with an ICD is simply to ignore the ICD. If such a patient is being transported to the OR, however, the device should be inactivated before the electrocautery is used: the ICD will misinterpret the cautery current as VF and respond by delivering a shock to the patient.

The aura of mystery surrounding the ICD may be instantly eliminated by turning off the device (see below). Once the ICD is inactivated, the patient can be treated as any other patient would be. If external cardioversion is indicated, the ICD can be disregarded; external cardioversion will not harm or activate it.

How to Turn the ICD Off

1. If you can find the industry representative to program the device to remain off, do so. Then treat the patient exactly as you would if the ICD were not present.
2. If you cannot find the representative or the situation is urgent:
   a. Palpate the ICD generator, which is typically implanted in the left subcostal region.
   b. Place a heavy pacemaker (or, better yet, an ICD magnet) over the upper corner of the device, toward the patient's left shoulder. Older devices used to emit a soft beep (synchronous with the heartbeat) in response to a magnet when they were active. Unfortunately, that feature has since been engineered out, and newer ICDs are silent.
   c. Tape the magnet in place over the upper border of the device. As long as the magnet is in place, the ICD is off and the electrocautery can be used safely.

VENTRICULAR RATE IS FAST

If a patient is hemodynamically stable, a full 12-lead electrocardiogram is helpful; a long rhythm strip should be obtained as well. The best ECG lead to use for evaluating acute dysrhythmias is one that has good-voltage QRS complexes and maximal P waves, if the latter are present at all.

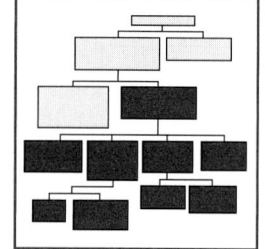

Electrocardiography

A cardiac impulse produces a positive, or upward, deflection on the monitor or oscilloscope as it approaches an ECG electrode and a negative, or downward, deflection as it moves away from the electrode. The important factor in dysrhythmia recognition, however, is not the direction of the impulse but its duration and location. Normal conduction velocity is fast: an impulse is transmitted by healthy Purkinje fibers at a rate of 2 to 3 m/sec.[3] Hence, when an impulse that arises in the atrium (supraventricular) is transmitted via the atrioventricular (AV) node to the high-velocity Purkinje system, the entire ventricle is electrically activated in 0.08 second (80 milliseconds; or two small boxes on ECG paper). An impulse that is generated at an ectopic ventricular site, however, cannot access the high-velocity Purkinje fibers as rapidly as a normal impulse, and ventricular activation is delayed. The QRS complex arising from an ectopic ventricular locus is therefore wider, signifying aberrant ventricular conduction [see Figure 1].

Because dysrhythmias of supraventricular origin typically display a narrow QRS complex, the width of the QRS can generally be used to distinguish dysrhythmias of ventricular origin from those of supraventricular origin [see Figure 2]. A wide QRS, however, may also be produced by an impulse that originates in the atrium and is aberrantly conducted to or through the ventricles (supraventricular rhythm with aberrancy). Such rhythms are relatively uncommon, constituting approximately 10% of all wide-complex tachycardias; more important, these patients will not suffer if their dysrhythmias are treated as though they were of ventricular origin.

When the ventricular rate is fast and the QRS is narrow, the 12-lead ECG should be searched for P waves, which indicate the presence of atrial activity. If P waves are absent and the QRS complexes occur at irregular intervals [see Figure 3], the patient probably has atrial fibrillation. It is not crucial to know this, however; the focus should be on the width of the QRS complex. A calcium channel blocker (verapamil or diltiazem) should be administered to control the ventricular rate. For verapamil, 10 mg is

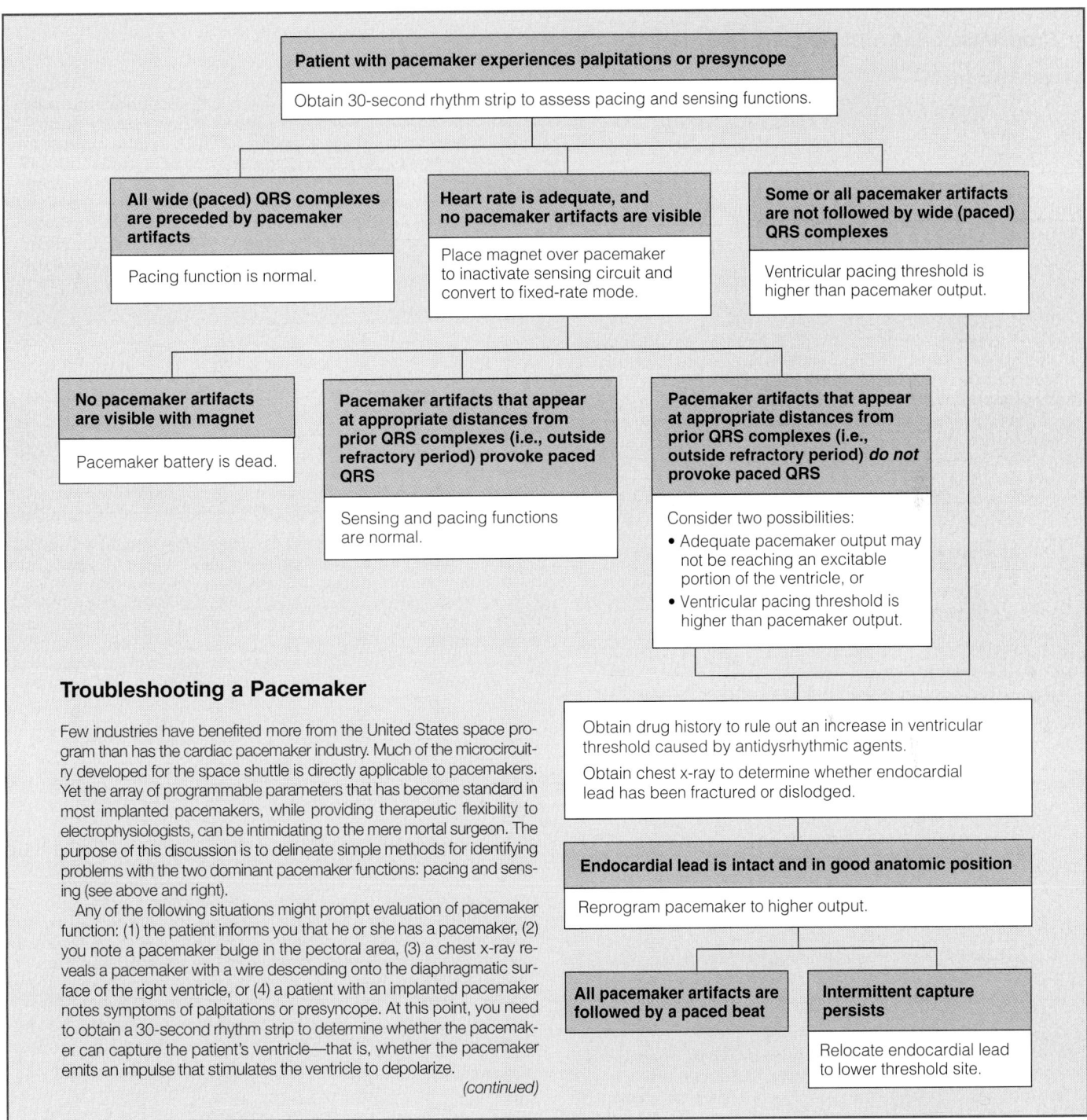

Patient with pacemaker experiences palpitations or presyncope

Obtain 30-second rhythm strip to assess pacing and sensing functions.

All wide (paced) QRS complexes are preceded by pacemaker artifacts

Pacing function is normal.

Heart rate is adequate, and no pacemaker artifacts are visible

Place magnet over pacemaker to inactivate sensing circuit and convert to fixed-rate mode.

Some or all pacemaker artifacts are not followed by wide (paced) QRS complexes

Ventricular pacing threshold is higher than pacemaker output.

No pacemaker artifacts are visible with magnet

Pacemaker battery is dead.

Pacemaker artifacts that appear at appropriate distances from prior QRS complexes (i.e., outside refractory period) provoke paced QRS

Sensing and pacing functions are normal.

Pacemaker artifacts that appear at appropriate distances from prior QRS complexes (i.e., outside refractory period) *do not* provoke paced QRS

Consider two possibilities:
- Adequate pacemaker output may not be reaching an excitable portion of the ventricle, or
- Ventricular pacing threshold is higher than pacemaker output.

Troubleshooting a Pacemaker

Few industries have benefited more from the United States space program than has the cardiac pacemaker industry. Much of the microcircuitry developed for the space shuttle is directly applicable to pacemakers. Yet the array of programmable parameters that has become standard in most implanted pacemakers, while providing therapeutic flexibility to electrophysiologists, can be intimidating to the mere mortal surgeon. The purpose of this discussion is to delineate simple methods for identifying problems with the two dominant pacemaker functions: pacing and sensing (see above and right).

Any of the following situations might prompt evaluation of pacemaker function: (1) the patient informs you that he or she has a pacemaker, (2) you note a pacemaker bulge in the pectoral area, (3) a chest x-ray reveals a pacemaker with a wire descending onto the diaphragmatic surface of the right ventricle, or (4) a patient with an implanted pacemaker notes symptoms of palpitations or presyncope. At this point, you need to obtain a 30-second rhythm strip to determine whether the pacemaker can capture the patient's ventricle—that is, whether the pacemaker emits an impulse that stimulates the ventricle to depolarize.

(continued)

Obtain drug history to rule out an increase in ventricular threshold caused by antidysrhythmic agents.

Obtain chest x-ray to determine whether endocardial lead has been fractured or dislodged.

Endocardial lead is intact and in good anatomic position

Reprogram pacemaker to higher output.

All pacemaker artifacts are followed by a paced beat

Intermittent capture persists

Relocate endocardial lead to lower threshold site.

---

mixed into 10 ml of saline, and 1 mg/min is given until the ventricular rate slows. For diltiazem, 0.25 mg/kg—15 to 20 mg is a reasonable dose for the average patient—is given over 2 minutes; the dose can be repeated in 15 minutes at 20 to 25 mg (0.35 mg/kg) over 2 minutes. A patient with a wide-complex tachycardia—or any patient who is hemodynamically unstable—is treated by cardioversion (see above), commonly followed by administration of lidocaine, 100 mg I.V., whereas a patient with a narrow-complex tachycardia should be treated with verapamil[3,5] or diltiazem to retard impulse conduction through the AV node. Therefore, it is not necessary to identify the specific type of dysrhythmia in order to treat it effectively.

Verapamil and diltiazem act by producing profound AV nodal blockade (see below); however, they are also peripheral vasodilators.[6] Moderate to profound systemic hypotension can be anticipated until the patient converts to sinus rhythm.

Much has been written about the risks of using calcium channel blockers in patients who are already receiving beta blockers. Abrupt and complete AV block rarely occurs, however, and in the vast majority of patients, persistent supraventricular tachycardia poses a greater risk than the possibility of third-degree heart block. Therefore, previous beta blockade should not be considered a contraindication to the use of a calcium channel blocker. Some clinicians may prefer to use adenosine.

Troubleshooting a Pacemaker (continued)

Ventricular Capture

a

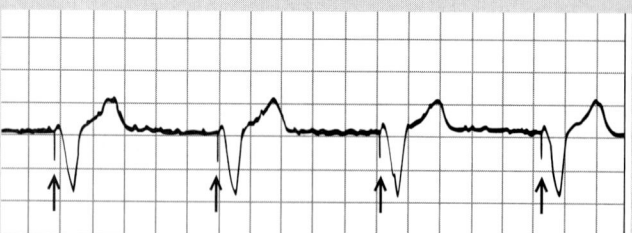

Note the pacemaker artifact (↑) that precedes each wide QRS complex in rhythm strip *a*, above. The QRS complex is wide because ventricular activation does not originate from the AV node, and ventricular conduction is therefore aberrant. At this point, you know that your patient is pacing, and you can determine the pacing rate. You do not, however, know the pacing threshold (i.e., the minimum voltage required for ventricular capture) or the safety margin between pacemaker output and pacing threshold. At this moment (and presumably yesterday and tomorrow), this pacemaker is appropriately discharging its most important function—pacing the heart and maintaining an adequate rate.

Ventricular Sensing

b

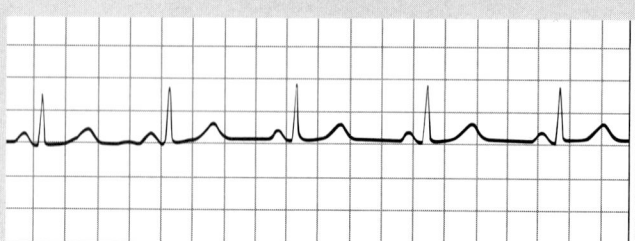

In rhythm strip *b*, above, normal P waves are followed by regular QRS complexes, and no pacemaker artifacts are evident. It is most likely that this patient's pacemaker has been programmed to fire at a paced rate that is slower than this patient's intrinsic heart rate, and the pacemaker is thus appropriately sensing each QRS complex. It is unlikely but possible, however, that the pacemaker is not sensing appropriately. Instead, one of the following problems may be occurring: (1) the pacemaker battery is dead, which is unlikely unless the battery was implanted more than 5 years ago, (2) the intracardiac electrode has been fractured, which is also unlikely, because current leads are remarkably durable, (3) the intracardiac electrode has been dislodged (this is an uncommon late problem that typically results in pacemaker artifacts unrelated to each QRS complex), or (4) the patient is taking an antidysrhythmic drug that has profoundly depressed ventricular excitability below threshold level for capture (this problem is very rare and can be excluded by taking a drug history). It is overwhelmingly likely, therefore, that rhythm strip *b* simply demonstrates that the pacemaker is sensing appropriately.

Assessing Ventricular Capture When the Spontaneous Heart Rate Is High

Typically, by the time you see the syncopal patient in the emergency department or recovery room, the patient is sufficiently excited that his or her

heart rate has recovered, and the rhythm strip will look like rhythm strip *b*. In a patient in whom heart rate is adequate and no pacemaker artifacts are visible, it is necessary to override the pacemaker's sensing circuit to determine whether the pacemaker is capable of emitting a pacing impulse that will capture the ventricle. The pacemaker's sensing circuit may be inactivated by placing a magnet over the pacemaker. Alternatively, the pacemaker may be reprogrammed to a paced rate that is faster than the patient's intrinsic heart rate. In this fashion, capture may easily be assessed. (Unfortunately, the programmers are expensive and are therefore often locked in some inaccessible closet. Programmers have great theoretical value but very little practical value to the surgeon.)

c

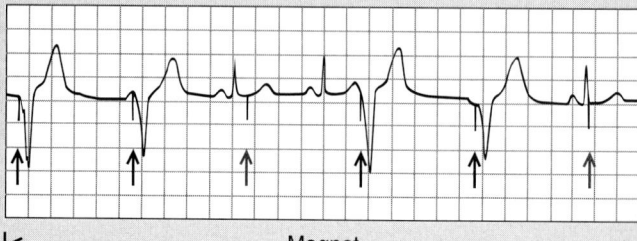

|←——————————————— Magnet ———————————————→|

In rhythm strip *c*, above, a magnet has converted the patient's pacemaker from the demand mode to the fixed-rate mode. The pacemaker artifacts that precede the wide (paced) QRS complexes in this rhythm strip (black arrows) show that the pacing function of this pacemaker is intact. Occasionally, a pacemaker artifact occurs during the electrical refractory period that immediately follows the QRS complex (red arrows). Pacing during the refractory period will not result in ventricular capture. Pacing during the refractory period should not result in ventricular capture and must not be interpreted as intermittent capture. In a patient whose pacemaker seems to be sensing appropriately (as in rhythm strip *b*), the magnet permits assessment of ventricular capture. Rhythm strip *c* demonstrates normal ventricular capture in the presence of a magnet.

Some or All Pacemaker Artifacts Are Not Followed by Wide QRS Complexes

If a pacemaker impulse that occurs outside the refractory period is not followed by a wide QRS complex, two possibilities should be considered. First, an adequate pacemaker impulse may not be reaching an excitable portion of the ventricle because of fracture or dislodgment of the endocardial lead. This problem can usually be identified by a chest x-ray. Second, if the chest x-ray shows that the lead is intact and in good anatomic position, the pacemaker output is not sufficient to reach the pacing threshold. Occasionally, this problem is caused by fibrosis at the endocardial electrode tip. If the pacemaker can be reprogrammed to a higher output, the capture problem should resolve. Otherwise, the lead must be repositioned to a site at which the pacing threshold is lower.

Occasional Pacemaker Artifacts Closely Follow a Spontaneous QRS Complex

If the patient's rhythm strip looks like rhythm strip *c, in the absence of a magnet*, the pacemaker is not sensing properly. In the demand mode, most pacemakers require at least a 2.5 mV signal to suppress output. Thus, if the pacemaker emits stimuli in spite of a normal spontaneous heart rate, an adequate QRS signal either is not being sensed (the lead tip may be lodged at the site of a prior myocardial infarction or scar) or is not being transmitted to the pacemaker (because of lead fracture or dislodgment).

Adenosine (see below) produces conduction delay in the AV node and deserves recognition as a second very good option (albeit only a transiently effective one) for treatment of paroxysmal narrow-complex tachycardia or for diagnosis of supraventricular tachycardia with aberrancy (including Wolff-Parkinson-White syndrome). Adenosine is given in a 6 mg I.V. push, followed 2 minutes later by a 12 mg I.V. push and then, after another 2 min-

utes, by a final 12 mg I.V. push over 2 seconds.[2,7]

Patients receiving adenosine complain of a frightening feeling of breathlessness and pressure that is not angina or dyspnea. This feeling typically resolves within 30 seconds. Facial flushing is also common. Unlike verapamil, adenosine is associated with hypotension in fewer than 1% of patients. Transient atrial or ventricular ectopy, with varying degrees of AV block, occurs in more

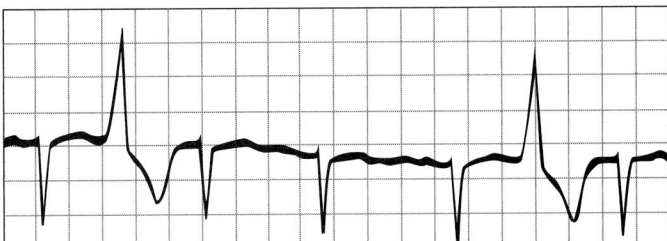

Figure 1 **This tracing depicts frequent ventricular ectopic depolarizations interspersed among depolarizations from a supraventricular source. Note that the QRS depolarizations of supraventricular origin are narrow, whereas the QRS complexes of ectopic ventricular origin are wide.**

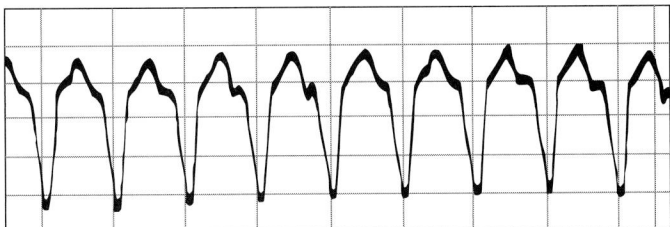

Figure 2 **In a wide-complex tachycardia, each impulse is conducted aberrantly through the ventricles. The QRS complex is therefore prolonged to more than 0.08 second and occupies more than two small boxes on the ECG tracing.**

than half of patients. None of the side effects of adenosine necessitate therapy.

Compared with calcium channel blockers, adenosine has certain advantages. Because of its rapid onset and short duration of action, and because its side effects are trivial and self-limited, adenosine can be used diagnostically. If, as is often the case, the QRS width is confusing and it is therefore uncertain whether the rhythm disorder is supraventricular (QRS < 0.08 second) or ventricular (QRS > 0.08 second), a 6 mg I.V. bolus of adenosine may be infused, and repeated if necessary. If the dysrhythmia slows or breaks, it was supraventricular. If it does not break, proceed to cardioversion (see above). On the other hand, even if a dysrhythmia responds to adenosine, the profound neuroendocrine and electrolyte perturbations that provoked the dysrhythmias in the first place—perturbations that are very common in the surgical intensive care unit—are likely to persist, and the dysrhythmia disorder typically recurs. Continuous (therapeutic) infusion of adenosine (150 to 300 µg/kg/min) is rational from a physiologic standpoint but is frighteningly expensive. Therefore, if adenosine works transiently, it is appropriate to follow with one of the longer-acting calcium channel blockers.

Calcium Channel Blockers

Both the sinoatrial (SA) node and the AV node are activated by the movement of calcium through the so-called slow calcium channels.[8] Calcium channel blockers are the most powerful agents currently available for blocking the transmission of impulses across the AV node. A supraventricular dysrhythmia produces an acceleration in the ventricular rate because impulses generated by an ectopic source above the AV node are transmitted too rapidly to the ventricle [see Figure 4]. Calcium channel blockers produce a pharmacologic blockade of the AV node, reducing the number of impulses reaching the ventricles and thereby controlling the ventricular rate (Remember, keeping the

ventricular rate between 60 and 100 beats/min is the ultimate goal of antidysrhythmia therapy).

Adenosine

Adenosine is an endogenous nucleoside that has differential antidysrhythmic effects in both supraventricular and ventricular tissue. The appeal of adenosine as a therapeutic and diagnostic tool is that it depresses automaticity and conduction within the SA and AV nodes.[9] Two clinically relevant types of adenosine receptors are present in cardiac tissue: (1) A_1 receptors, which are present on AV nodal tissue and cardiomyocytes and which thus mediate AV block and even bradycardia; and (2) A_2 receptors, which reside on vascular endothelial and smooth muscle cells and mediate coronary vasodilatation.[10] A_3 receptors are present in the myocardium, and selective activation of these has a cardioprotective (cardiac preconditioning) effect; however, these receptors are not relevant in antidysrhythmic therapy.[11]

Adenosine and acetylcholine exhibit identical cardiac effects and share similar receptor-effector coupling systems. Adenosine and acetylcholine provide an opposing balance to the sympathetic neurotransmitters norepinephrine and epinephrine. Thus, predictably, the adenosine antagonists caffeine, theophylline, and aminophylline provoke tachycardia and ectopy.

Because of the rapid intravascular metabolism of adenosine (half-life, 6 seconds), an intravenous bolus of adenosine (6 mg or 100 µg/kg) produces a negligible effect on systemic blood pressure, as confirmed by multiple clinical studies. Thus, adenosine is safe, but its effects are transient.

Adenosine is useful in blocking AV nodal conduction. Intracardiac recordings exhibit prolongation of the A-H interval with no alteration in conduction distal to the His bundle and on into the ventricular myocardium (the His-Purkinje system is unaffected).

In more than 90% of cases, adenosine is effective in terminating supraventricular tachycardia. Interestingly, adenosine has proved as effective at terminating atrioventricular reentry (85%) as at terminating atrioventricular node reentry (86%).[9] Because of adenosine's short half-life, however, the supraventricular dysrhythmia is likely to recur within minutes in up to one third of patients. For that reason, adenosine is often used diagnostically, to discriminate supraventricular from ventricular dysrhythmias (see above).

Several clinical studies have compared adenosine with verapamil for therapeutic AV nodal blockade, with predictable results. Both agents block the AV node and control the ventricular rate: cumulative efficacy with either agent is more than 90%. Postconversion dysrhythmias in the two groups were similar. Spontaneous reinitiation of supraventricular dysrhythmias occurs more frequently with adenosine, whereas systemic hypotension is more commonly associated with verapamil (at least until the dysrhythmia breaks). Thus, for help in seconds (approximately 20 seconds), use adenosine (6 mg I.V. bolus, may be repeated); for help in minutes (3 to 5 minutes), use verapamil (1 mg/min I.V. up

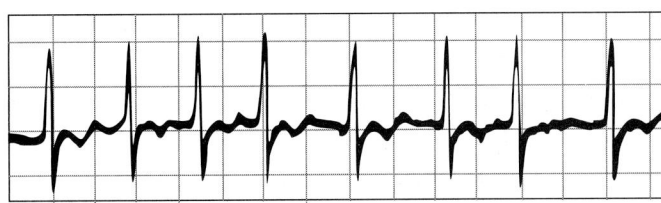

Figure 3 **P waves are absent and the QRS complexes are narrow and irregular in this ECG tracing from a patient with atrial fibrillation.**

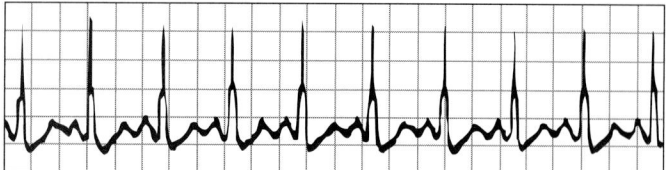

Figure 4 In a narrow-complex tachycardia, the entire ventricle is activated in less than 0.08 second. Presumably, the impulse originated at a supraventricular source and accessed the ventricle via the high-velocity Purkinje system.

to 10 mg); and for help in hours, infuse digoxin, 0.5 mg I.V. Although digitalis effectively blocks the AV node, it should be remembered that digitalis actually increases automaticity and excitability in both the atrium and the ventricle. The calcium channel blockers are superior to digoxin in controlling the ventricular rate.[8]

The adverse effects of adenosine, like the beneficial effects, are transient.[9] Facial flushing, chest pressure (adenosine has been implicated in the sensation of angina), and transient third-degree heart block are very common. Significant side effects are rare. Nebulized adenosine can cause bronchoconstriction, especially in asthmatic patients. Bronchoconstriction has not been reported after intravenous administration of adenosine.

Magnesium

Magnesium is the second most abundant cation in humans. It is involved in many enzymatic reactions that influence the production and utilization of cellular energy. Abnormalities in electrolyte homeostasis (potassium and calcium in particular) are associated with a robust increase in cardiac myocellular excitability and automaticity, especially when these abnormalities are concurrent with myocardial ischemia.[12] Multiple clinical studies confirm the efficacy of intravenous magnesium infusion even when the measured serum values are normal. The mechanism is unknown. When confronted with a patient exhibiting either supraventricular or ventricular ectopy, it is safe (and often effective) to administer magnesium chloride at a dosage of 7 g or 100 mg/kg I.V. over 1 to 3 hours. It is not necessary to measure the serum magnesium concentration first; the serum value will not influence therapy.

Amiodarone

Amiodarone is a class III antiarrhythmic drug that exerts its primary effect by prolongation of the myocardial action potential and refractory period and by delay of both SA node function and AV conduction. Amiodarone is also unique among these compounds by virtue of exhibiting, to varying degrees, the pharmacologic traits of all four classes of antiarrhythmic drugs [see Discussion, Antidysrhythmic Agents, below].[13] Among these is its ability to inhibit alpha- and beta-adrenergic stimulation without the classic side effects associated with beta receptor blockade. It also reduces transmural proarrhythmic heterogeneity (which predisposes to arrhythmias) in the human heart [see Discussion, Pathophysiology of Cardiac Dysrhythmias, Reentrant Dysrhythmias, below].[14]

Intravenous amiodarone was approved in the United States for use against malignant ventricular tachyarrhythmias in 1995. Rates of effective suppression for ventricular arrhythmias have been reported to be as high as 91% in uncontrolled trials.[15] Intravenous amiodarone has also proved effective against refractory ventricular tachycardia and VF. In one double-blind, randomized, placebo-controlled trial, amiodarone significantly improved survival in patients suffering out-of-hospital cardiac arrest.[16] Amiodarone also proved superior to lidocaine (78% versus 27%) for termination of ventricular tachycardia in a randomized, prospective study of 29 patients with ventricular tachycardia refractory to external shock therapy.[17]

Another prospective, double-blind study comparing amiodarone with ibutilide (another class III antiarrhythmic agent) showed the drugs to be equally efficacious in the conversion of atrial fibrillation to sinus rhythm and in the subsequent maintenance of sinus rhythm.[18] Although two patients (10%) in the amiodarone group experienced hypotension during treatment, long-term maintenance therapy using the oral form of amiodarone may make it the drug of choice for this purpose, given ibutilide's lack of oral bioavailablity. Amiodarone was also found superior to both sotalol and propafenone in preventing the recurrence of atrial fibrillation in a randomized, prospective multicenter study of 403 patients with a mean follow-up period of 16 months.[19]

Although gratifyingly effective, amiodarone has significant side effects.[20] In trials of low-dose amiodarone (200 mg/day), thyroid, neurologic, cutaneous, ocular, bradycardic, and hypotensive problems were statistically more frequent; interestingly, pulmonary fibrosis was not.[21]

For the first 24 hours, the recommended dosages for adults are a loading dose of 150 mg I.V. over the first 10 minutes (15 mg/min) followed by 360 mg I.V. over the next 6 hours (1 mg/min); a maintenance infusion of 540 mg (0.5 mg/min) is given over the remaining 18 hours. The maintenance infusion may be continued for up to 3 weeks, at the rate of 0.5 mg/min, or the patient may be converted to oral dosing at 400 to 1,600 mg daily, depending on the duration of the preceding I.V. infusion.

Cardiac Dysrhythmias during Pregnancy

Fortunately, cardiac dysrhythmias are not frequent in young women of childbearing age. When rhythm problems do occur, they tend not to be hemodynamically destabilizing. The most commonly used obstetric drug with electrophysiologic side effects is magnesium sulfate.[22] When magnesium is infused intravenously into the mother, the fetus may exhibit a dose-dependent bradycardia and a progressive decrease in healthy heart rate variability.[23,24] Antidysrhythmic (indeed, any) drugs should be avoided during the first trimester of pregnancy, although most antidysrhythmic agents carry relatively little risk.[22] Quinidine, procainamide, lidocaine, digoxin, adenosine, and beta blockers all have a long record of safety during pregnancy. Flecainide has proved to be effective in treating fetal supraventricular tachycardia complicated by hydrops. Phenytoin and amiodarone have been associated with congenital abnormalities.[22]

The important point is that if the mother is hemodynamically unstable and exhibits a dysrhythmia, direct current cardioversion is safe and effective.

Proarrhythmia with Antidysrhythmic Drugs

Proarrhythmic manifestations of ostensibly antiarrhythmic drugs have been linked primarily to agents that prolong repolarization. Early afterdepolarizations associated with agents that retard repolarization or an increase in spatial and temporal dispersion of repolarization are the putative mechanisms of drug-induced or drug-enhanced arrhythmias.[25,26]

The class III antidysrhythmic agents have traditionally been the agents most likely to cause dysrhythmias.[26] The best way of preventing dysrhythmias, however, is to follow the general policy of not using drugs at all if they are not needed.[27]

Discussion

Antidysrhythmic Agents

Verapamil (or another calcium channel blocker), lidocaine, and adenosine are the only drugs essential for the acute treatment of cardiac dysrhythmias. Because patients may already be taking oral agents for chronic dysrhythmias, however, it is important to be aware of the actions and side effects of these drugs when treating an individual with an acute dysrhythmia. Antidysrhythmic drugs have been classified on the basis of their dominant electrophysiologic effect[28]; this classification has been reviewed and placed in a clinical context.[5] Adenosine has a unique receptor that modulates cyclic adenosine monophosphate (cAMP), resulting in cholinergic activity. It is not similar to other antidysrhythmic agents and is therefore unclassified.

CLASS I AGENTS (MEMBRANE ACTIVE)

Class I agents are fast sodium channel blockers. All class I agents—which include lidocaine, procainamide, quinidine, and disopyramide—are local anesthetics. These agents block the fast inward sodium current and thereby decrease both the amplitude of the action potential, or phase 0 depolarization (see below), and conduction velocity. These agents also depress the rate of spontaneous phase 4 depolarization, or automaticity, and thus are useful for abolishing premature ventricular contractions (PVCs); class I agents are sometimes termed PVC killers. Because these agents slow the conduction velocity, they can actually increase the likelihood of reentrant cardiac dysrhythmias in some patients.[25,27]

CLASS II AGENTS (BETA BLOCKERS)

Class II agents are beta blockers and include such drugs as propranolol. Sympathetic hyperactivity, marked by increased release of catecholamines, is one of the major causes of cardiac dysrhythmias that result from increased automaticity (hyperexcitability).[25,27,29] Beta-adrenergic blockade has produced a decrease in such automatic dysrhythmias under both clinical and experimental conditions.[29]

CLASS III AGENTS (TO PROLONG REPOLARIZATION)

Class III agents, such as bretylium, act directly on the myocardial cell membrane to delay phases 2 and 3 of repolarization and thereby prolong refractoriness. Bretylium is effective in terminating reentrant dysrhythmias because it prolongs the refractory period of the ectopic focus to beyond the point at which an impulse reenters the circuit.[1,2] Bretylium apparently has no effect on either automaticity or conduction velocity.[30]

CLASS IV AGENTS (CALCIUM CHANNEL BLOCKERS)

Class IV agents, of which verapamil and diltiazem are the most effective, block the movement of calcium across the slow calcium channels but have virtually no effect on the so-called fast sodium channels.[28] Because both the SA node and the AV node are composed of slow-response fibers that are activated by the movement of calcium ions across the slow channels, the class IV agents are particularly effective in preventing unwanted supraventricular impulses from reaching the ventricles. These agents decrease the conduction velocity through the AV node and increase the refractory period of the AV node.

CLASS V AGENTS (UNCLASSIFIED)

The vagus nerve innervates the SA node, the atria, and the AV node, but it has almost no influence over the His-Purkinje system or ventricular muscle. At therapeutic levels, digitalis has an antidysrhythmic action that is mediated almost exclusively via the vagus nerve. Toxic doses of digitalis, however, may produce an increased automaticity characterized by multifocal premature ventricular depolarizations [see Pathophysiology of Cardiac Dysrhythmias, below]. Caution must be observed in digitalizing a patient who is prone to atrial dysrhythmias, because digitalis increases atrial excitability and hence increases the risk of atrial ectopy. Because digitalis also induces AV nodal blockade mediated by the vagus nerve, however, any atrial dysrhythmias produced by digitalization will be less clinically significant.[31,32]

Cellular Electrophysiology

Electromechanical activity of all muscle, including the heart, is determined by the concentration and flow of ions, particularly calcium, potassium, and sodium. Knowledge of cardiac electrophysiology can serve as a conceptual framework on which to build a rational therapeutic program. Direct observation of cellular electrical activity using a glass microelectrode reveals that the cell membrane is semipermeable: it permits easy passage of cations such as sodium, potassium, and calcium but provides a barrier to anions and proteins. Negatively charged intracellular proteins that cannot cross the cell membrane create a transmembrane potential in which the interior of the cell is negatively charged relative to the exterior. The membrane potential of a cell, E_K, is proportional to the difference between the logarithms of the intracellular potassium concentration, $[K]_i$, and the extracellular potassium concentration, $[K]_o$:

$$E_K = c(\log [K]_i - \log [K]_o)$$

The proportionality constant, c, varies with temperature, but at 37° C it is –60 mV. Thus, under physiologic conditions,

$$E_K = -60 \text{ mV} \times \log [K]_i / [K]_o$$

This relation, termed the Nernst equation, can be used to calculate the myocardial cell membrane potential if the potassium concentrations are known. For example, if the potassium concentration is normal—that is, 150 mEq/L intracellularly and 3.8 mEq/L extracellularly—then the membrane potential is

$$E_K = -60 \text{ mV} \times \log 150 / 3.8$$
$$E_K = -90 \text{ mV}$$

If, however, the serum potassium concentration rises to 6.0 mEq/L, then the membrane potential also changes:

$$E_K = -60 \text{ mV} \times \log 150 / 6.0$$
$$E_K = -80 \text{ mV}$$

Thus, the resting membrane potential is determined primarily by the concentration gradient for potassium across the cell membrane. The transmembrane potential can be calculated if the transmembrane potassium concentrations are measured with a glass microelectrode. Under clinical conditions, however, only the serum potassium level can be measured. This value does not provide an adequate guide to the transmembrane electrical voltage, because many physiologic factors are capable of altering the intracellular potassium concentration.[13] Such factors include electrolyte and acid-base balance, the level of osmotic and metabolic activity, and the serum levels of glucose and insulin.

Any factor that causes osmotic movement of water into the cell

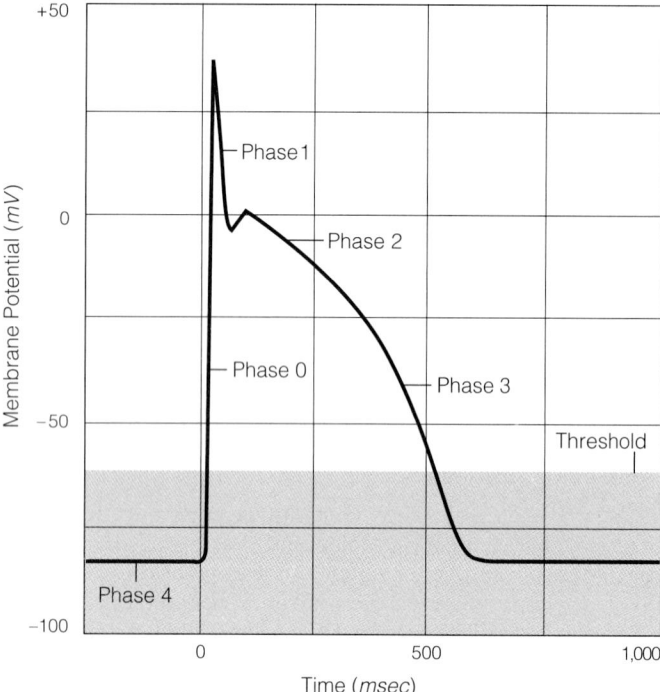

Figure 5 **The standard Purkinje (or ventricular muscle) action potential has five distinct phases: phase 0, rapid depolarization; phase 1, early repolarization; phase 2, plateau; phase 3, rapid repolarization; and phase 4, diastole.**

will dilute and thus decrease the intracellular potassium concentration. The transmembrane gradients of sodium and calcium are maintained by energy-requiring pumps in the cell membrane. When these pumps are inactivated, as during myocardial ischemia,[12] sodium and calcium can leak into the cell. If, as often occurs, sodium leaks into the cell faster than potassium leaks out, water will be drawn in, producing myocardial edema. Tissue acidosis can also alter the transmembrane potassium gradient. In acidosis, hydrogen ions can leak into the cell in exchange for potassium, thereby decreasing the intracellular potassium concentration and increasing the membrane potential. Variations in glucose transport can also affect the potassium gradient. Under the influence of insulin and epinephrine, glucose may move across the membrane into the myocardial cell, drawing in water by osmosis. The decline in intracellular potassium concentration stimulates the sodium pump to exchange extracellular potassium for intracellular sodium. Concurrent administration of glucose and insulin is the standard method for treating hyperkalemia because it shifts potassium from the extracellular fluid back into the cells.

ACTION POTENTIAL GENERATION

Stimulation of either cardiac muscle or skeletal muscle produces an action potential. Unlike a skeletal muscle action potential, which lasts only several milliseconds, a cardiac action potential may persist for as long as several hundred milliseconds.[33] The standard Purkinje, or ventricular muscle, action potential has five discernible phases [*see Figure 5*].

Phase 4

In phase 4, the resting membrane potential, or diastolic potential, of the cell is generated by active metabolic processes that produce substantial transmembrane potassium and sodium gradi-

ents. An energy-dependent (ATP-dependent) sodium-potassium pump counteracts a significant influx of sodium and efflux of potassium in the resting cell to maintain this resting membrane potential. As noted, when the extracellular potassium concentration rises from a typical value of 3.8 mEq/L to 6.0 mEq/L, the resting membrane potential increases from −90 mV to −80 mV. This effect would tend to increase automaticity, but it is superseded by the effect of hyperkalemia on the sodium current. A rise in the extracellular potassium level progressively impairs the flux of sodium through sodium-specific channels, leading to an overall decrease in myocardial excitability.[34]

Phase 0

During phase 0, an electrical stimulus causes the sodium-specific fast channels and the calcium-specific slow channels to open, usually for no longer than 1 msec. As positive ions rush in, depolarization occurs as the membrane potential rises to threshold, or −60 mV, and an action potential is generated [*see Figure 5*]. Under normal physiologic conditions, the stimulus that produces an action potential is electrical, but any stimulus—electrical, physical (such as a precordial thump), or chemical—that depolarizes a membrane up to threshold (again, −60mV) can generate an action potential. There are various abnormalities that can cause the resting membrane potential to move toward threshold. For example, conditions that produce a decrease in energy supply (or, alternatively, an increase in energy demand) will have this effect because energy is required to maintain the potassium and sodium gradients across the resting membrane. Under such conditions, automaticity is enhanced because lesser stimuli can achieve the threshold potential, and the cardiac muscle is said to be hyperexcitable, or irritable.

Phases 1 and 2

Phase 1 is characterized by repolarization to the plateau phase, or phase 2. During phase 2, the slow calcium channels as well as the fast sodium channels are activated, and the membrane potential remains relatively constant for as long as 100 msec.[35] The long duration of this plateau phase is the most dramatic difference between an action potential in cardiac muscle and one in skeletal muscle. During this interval, termed the effective refractory period, the myocardium is relatively resistant to further excitation.

Phase 3

During phase 3, potassium channels reopen to promote efflux of potassium from the cell. Rapid repolarization ensues, and the resting membrane potential is reestablished at −90 mV.

Spontaneous Phase 4 Depolarization

Unlike ordinary atrial and ventricular muscle, the Purkinje fibers do not have a stable phase 4 diastolic potential [*see Figure 6*]. Instead, these fibers undergo continuous depolarization during diastole as a result of deactivation of the potassium efflux current.[35,36] If the Purkinje fibers reach the threshold voltage, they will fire an action potential. Under normal conditions, however, the SA and AV nodes exhibit faster diastolic depolarization and reach threshold sooner than the Purkinje fibers. Because the cells in the SA node normally reach threshold first—winning the race, so to speak—the SA node typically assumes the pacemaker function of the heart. Premature ventricular contractions develop when a hyperexcitable cell or fiber in ventricular myocardium undergoes rapid diastolic depolarization and reaches threshold before the cells in the SA node. This cell or fiber then assumes the pacemaker function of the heart for that beat. The PVCs (or,

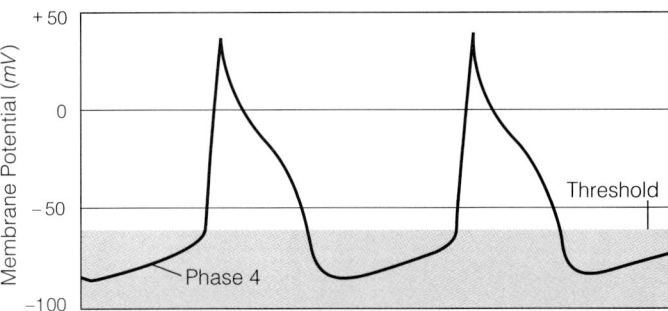

Figure 6 In normal cardiac Purkinje fibers, the membrane potential does not remain flat during phase 4 but instead rises gradually. This spontaneous phase 4 depolarization is the result of a resting potassium current.

more accurately, premature ventricular depolarizations) that result from such ventricular ectopy can be abolished by overdrive pacing. In this situation, a mechanical pacemaker is used to pace the heart at a rate faster than that of the PVC (i.e., the R–R interval is shorter). The artificial device thereby wins the race; it assumes the pacemaker function and regularizes the heart rate, producing a beneficial cosmetic effect on the ECG without altering the hyperexcitability of the diseased cell.

Pathophysiology of Cardiac Dysrhythmias

All dysrhythmias are caused by enhanced automaticity, reentry, or a combination of these two mechanisms.

AUTOMATIC DYSRHYTHMIAS

Any area of myocardial tissue that independently depolarizes, reaches threshold, and fires is termed automatic, and the electrical impulse that activates the adjacent myocardium generates an automatic rhythm. Acute dysrhythmias tend to be automatic; such automatic dysrhythmias are frequently seen in patients in emergency departments and coronary care units and in patients undergoing surgery. Five common clinical phenomena that tend to increase automaticity have been identified: local myocardial hypoxia, hypokalemia, hypercalcemia, increased catecholamine levels, and drugs (most commonly digitalis).

Local Myocardial Hypoxia

Energy-dependent cell membrane pumps maintain the resting membrane potential, and when oxygen supply to myocardial tissue is inadequate because of ischemia, the pumps fail to function properly. Consequently, the potassium gradient declines, and the membrane potential drifts closer toward threshold. Small membrane potential fluctuations or stimuli of less than normal magnitude are then sufficient to bump the membrane potential up to threshold and initiate an action potential. Ventricular muscle cells, not only those cells in specialized conduction tissue, can spontaneously generate electrical fluctuations, or oscillations, in membrane potential [*see* Slow Afterdepolarizations, *below*]. If the resting membrane potential is initially closer to normal because of local myocardial hypoxia, then these spontaneous oscillations are more likely to achieve threshold and fire an action potential.[37]

Hypokalemia

Extracellular hypokalemia increases the resting membrane potential, drawing it further away from threshold and producing hyperpolarization. This effect tends to decrease tissue excitability,

or automaticity.[37,38] Hypokalemia also increases the size of the sodium channels, however, thereby promoting more rapid influx of sodium during phase 0. Because the net result of hypokalemia is increased automaticity, the effect of hypokalemia on sodium influx appears to override its effect on membrane hyperpolarization. Hypokalemia is one of the most easily treated (and overtreated) forms of hyperexcitability.

Hypercalcemia

Calcium is a potent inotropic agent, mediating the interaction between actin and myosin that produces muscle contraction.[35] High extracellular calcium levels may cause myocardial work to exceed the energy supply and thus impair the function of the membrane pump. As a result, the resting membrane potential drifts up toward threshold, enhancing automaticity. Excess calcium also appears to promote spontaneous oscillations in membrane potential [*see* Slow Afterdepolarizations, *below*].[39] Because of calcium's inotropic effect, such oscillations are accompanied by muscle activity.

Elevated Catecholamine Levels

Increased catecholamine levels also appear to predispose to automaticity, as evidenced by an increase in the incidence of multiple PVCs reported in patients who have been infused with high doses of catecholamines, such as epinephrine or dopamine. Catecholamines increase both heart rate and contractility. As with hypercalcemia, elevated catecholamine levels may increase cardiac work beyond the limits of energy supply and cause the membrane potential to move closer to threshold. This effect on the energy-dependent membrane pumps has been observed in isolated preparations of Purkinje muscle fibers. The addition of catecholamines to preparations of Purkinje muscle fibers has decreased the outward potassium current to the point that the resting membrane potential was shifted as much as 25 mV toward depolarization, enhancing automaticity.[36,37] In addition to affecting the operation of the membrane pumps, catecholamines can produce large spontaneous oscillations in membrane voltage.[36,40] Catecholamines are elaborated endogenously; a patient who is in pain, for example, may be releasing large amounts of epinephrine into the circulation. In such cases, morphine can be used effectively as an antidysrhythmic agent.[40]

Drugs

Digitalis is the prototypical cardiac stimulant. Typically, any

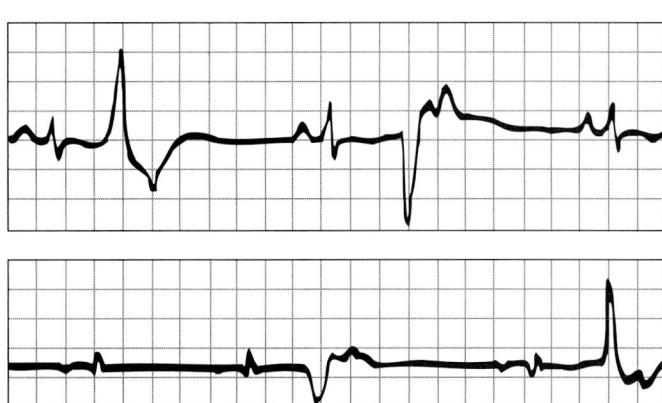

Figure 7 ECG demonstrates multifocal PVCs, indicating a diffuse hyperexcitability of the ventricles. Such hyperexcitability may arise from a metabolic abnormality such as hypokalemia or a pharmacologic cause such as digitalis toxicity.

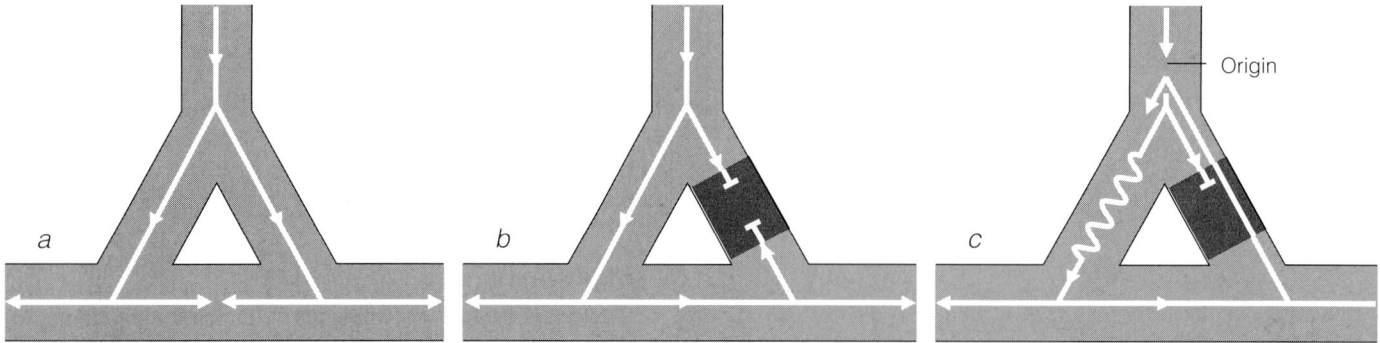

Figure 8   **Schematic diagram portrays a conceptual framework for understanding the generation of reentrant dysrhythmias. In normal conduction (*a*), as in sinus rhythm or ventricular pacing, an impulse is propagated along two different anatomic pathways and is extinguished at the bottom. In (*b*), one pathway has a region of slow conduction (red area), which results in a rate-dependent block. In (*c*), the impulse is also blocked in the right limb (red area), but it travels over the alternative pathway sufficiently slowly (zigzag line) for the origin to be able to repolarize before the initial impulse returns; the conducted impulse then depolarizes the origin and reenters the circuit.**

agent other than oxygen that causes the heart to pump harder and faster also increases cardiac excitability. Digitalis toxicity can produce diffuse myocardial hyperexcitability, manifested by so-called automatic ventricular ectopy. In this condition, the cardiac impulse originates from multiple sites in the ventricle. In patients with ventricular ectopy caused by digitalis intoxication, the whole myocardium becomes hyperexcitable and spontaneous depolarizations derive from multiple different sites. When the QRS complex originates at multiple loci, the ECG will exhibit multiple morphologies, and multifocal PVCs are apparent on the ECG— the classic multifocal ectopy of digitalis toxicity [*see Figure 7*].[41-43]

REENTRANT DYSRHYTHMIAS

In the normally functioning heart, the rich cell-cell conduction pathways promote uniform activation of the atria or ventricles in waves. Because activation occurs by means of large electrical wave fronts and because all cardiac tissue has a long refractory period, it is highly unlikely that any cells will remain excitable at the completion of each beat. However, disorders such as myocardial ischemia, fibrosis, and necrosis slow electrical conduction and also produce nonconductive areas that interrupt the normal electrical wavefront.[44] These conditions set up one of the requirements for reentry: areas of differential myocardial repolarization.[45]

A circuit whose length exceeds the duration of the reentrant impulse circuit is required for the initiation of reentry (i.e., in order to sustain continuous conduction); such a circuit may develop because of anatomic or physiologic heterogeneity in myocardial tissue.[44,45] Slow conduction, a shortened refractory period, and anatomic heterogeneity all favor reentry [*see Figure 8*]. The circuit wavelength of an impulse is the product of the conduction velocity and the duration of the longest refractory period in the circuit.[46] For example, for normal myocardium, the

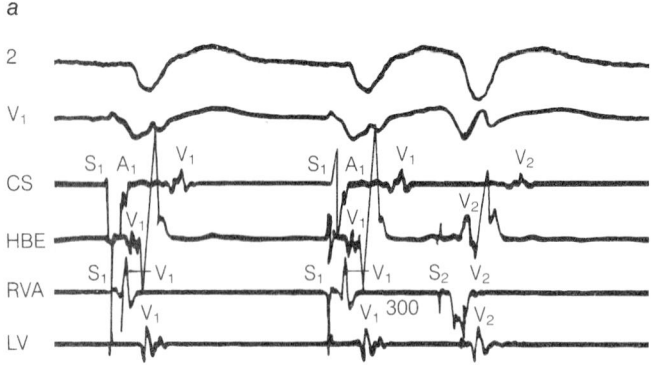

a

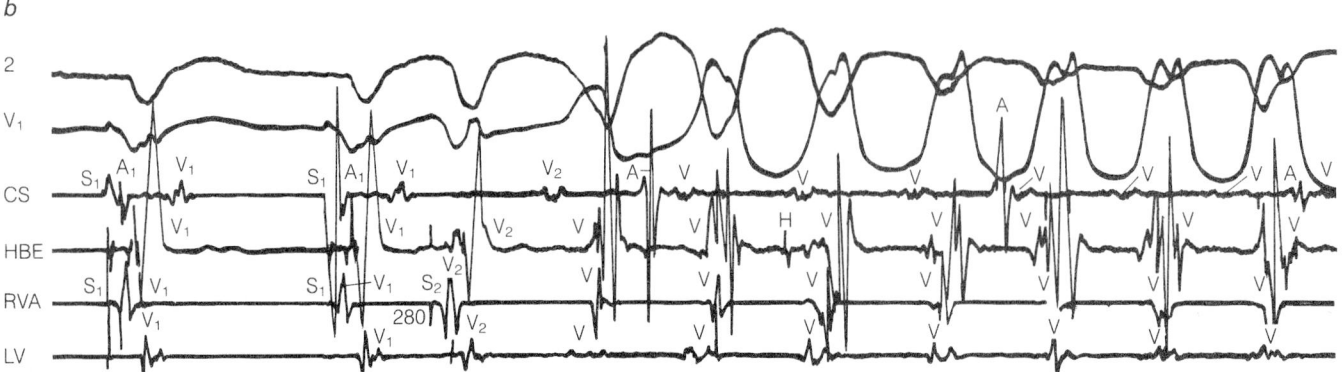

b

Figure 9   **In electrophysiologic testing, the electrical complexes are spread out to facilitate the recognition of ventricular electrical morphology. In (*a*), critically timed paced stimuli capture one ventricle, but when pacing is stopped, the rhythm reverts to sinus rhythm. In (*b*), critically timed paced stimuli achieve rate-dependent block in one arm of a reentrant circuit. When the activation wave front returns to the origin, this tissue is no longer refractory and undergoes depolarization. With reexcitation, the conditions for reentry are met, and the impulse continues after pacing stops.**

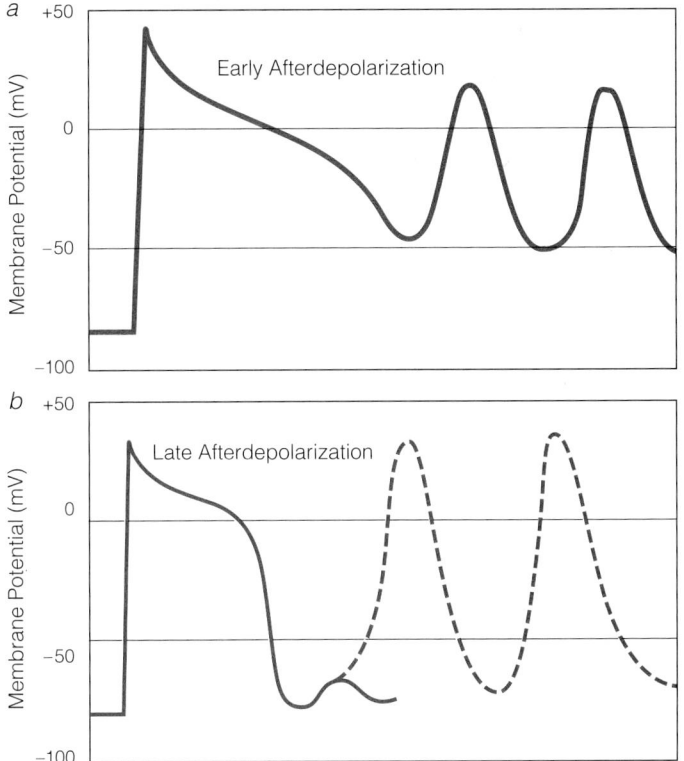

Figure 10 **Membrane oscillatory instability may be manifested by either (*a*) early afterdepolarizations or (*b*) late afterdepolarizations. If the late afterdepolarizations achieve the threshold voltage, they can fire an action potential (dotted lines).**

conduction velocity is 200 cm/sec and the refractory period is 0.4 second; therefore, the circuit length for a normally conducted myocardial impulse would have to be 80 cm. Because the reentrant circuit would have to be extraordinarily tortuous to encompass 80 cm, it would appear that concomitant slow conduction is essentially mandatory to shorten the circuit wavelength and permit initiation of a reentrant dysrhythmia. Regions such as the AV and SA nodes normally exhibit slow conduction, and therefore, any disturbance that produces minor additional slowing in these areas predisposes to reentry. It has also been suggested that extreme anatomic heterogeneity might permit microreentry.[45] For example, a tortuous path over stunned, slowly conducting ventricular muscle in an individual with heterogeneous myocardial infarction might achieve the prerequisites for reentry.

In vitro studies have investigated physiologic factors that might produce changes in conduction and excitability that predispose to reentrant dysrhythmias. For example, abnormal conduction has been observed in a Purkinje network subjected to local changes in potassium concentration.[33,40] The decrease in conduction velocity can vary in different areas of the Purkinje network, leading to functional conduction block.[37,38] In T- or X-shaped Purkinje preparations, the impulses either summate electrically or, conversely, inhibit each other when they arrive at the same junction simultaneously. It is difficult to study the cardiac microenvironment in living animals or humans, but in these studies,[47] electrical instability results when the Purkinje network is subjected to potassium fluctuations (which certainly occur with induced cardioplegia during cardiac surgery, and probably occur in myocardial ischemia).

Electrophysiologic testing with programmed stimulation in a

patient with a history of cardiac dysrhythmias can reveal whether latent substrates of reentry are present. Because organized ventricular reentry does not occur in normal myocardium, all reentrant dysrhythmias, whether they are induced or spontaneous, are pathologic. Rapidly paced stimuli may provoke a decrease in action potential duration and shorten refractoriness in myocardium in which the conduction velocity has already been reduced. Critically timed premature paced stimuli may then penetrate selective zones of myocardium, leading to a reentrant dysrhythmia [*see Figure 9*].[48] A ventricular tachydysrhythmia that can be induced by programmed stimulation carries an ominous prognosis unless it can be abolished by pharmacotherapy or surgery.[48]

SLOW AFTERDEPOLARIZATIONS

Damaged atrial and ventricular muscle exhibits resting membrane potential instability.[49] The oscillations in membrane potential may at times be large enough to raise the membrane voltage to threshold level and cause the cell to fire. The phenomenon of oscillatory instability, which was first recognized in the 1940s,[50] is now thought to play an important role in the genesis of cardiac dysrhythmias. Injury,[49] elevated calcium levels,[33] digitalis,[41,42] and catecholamines all promote membrane oscillatory instability, which may be manifested as either early or late afterdepolarizations. Both phenomena occur after an action potential; however, an early afterdepolarization occurs before repolarization of the cell, whereas a late afterdepolarization occurs after repolarization [*see Figure 10*]. Both early and late afterdepolarizations may be followed by extreme membrane oscillatory instability that leads to slow-response action potentials [*see Figure 11*]. If any of these slow potentials reach threshold, they may result in either organized electrical activity (premature ventricular depolarization) or disorganized electrical activity (fibrillation).

The recognition of slow potentials, depressed fast responses, and very slow conduction was originally based on in vitro studies of cardiac tissue.[51] For example, bathing superfused Purkinje fibers in a solution with a high potassium concentration inactivates the fast sodium channels and markedly alters normal phase 0 depolarization. Under such circumstances, slow potentials that are less than 80 mV in amplitude, that depolarize at a rate of 1 to

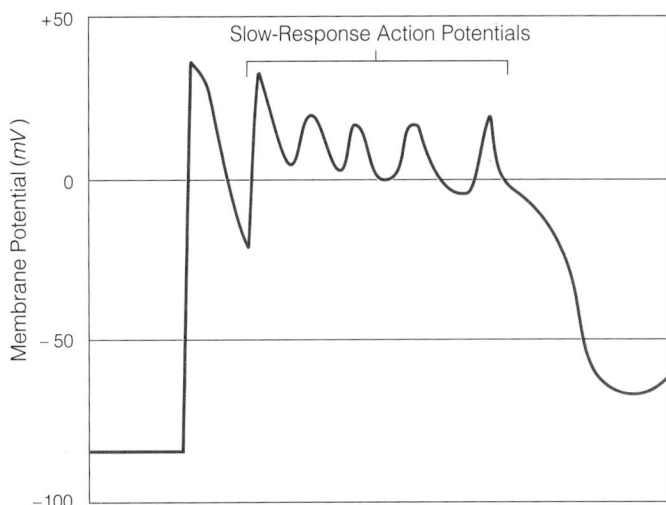

Figure 11 **Early afterdepolarizations may lead to slow-response action potentials. If any of these potentials reach threshold, they may lead to either organized electrical activity (premature ventricular depolarization) or disorganized electrical activity (fibrillation).**

2 V/sec, and that last for up to 1 second are frequently documented.[40,51] The amplitude and the overshoot of these slow potentials can be magnified by increasing the extracellular calcium concentration and can be abolished by adding manganese, an agent that blocks the slow calcium channels. These results suggest that the slow potentials are mediated by the slow calcium channels rather than by the fast sodium channels responsible for routine phase 0 depolarization. Although extraordinary nonphysiologic conditions are employed to induce such slow potentials in the laboratory, the myocardial microenvironment during the peri-infarction and postinfarction periods as well as after cardioplegia may well be similarly bizarre and equally nonphysiologic.

For example, even after extensive myocardial infarction, there are often healthy Purkinje fibers overlying areas of damaged, ischemic myocardium.[52] Slow conduction and slow potentials are characteristic of stunned myocardium.[53,54]

Slow potentials have been incriminated in the generation of reentrant dysrhythmias for three reasons: (1) because they are caused by an active calcium influx that produces 40 to 80 mV depolarizations, they may be conducted long distances; (2) because the conduction velocity may be 1,000 times slower than normal, the circuit wavelength is reduced accordingly; and (3) because slow potentials leave a long refractory wake, they set up zones of functional conduction block.[53,54]

References

1. Saxonhouse SJ, Curtis AB: Risks and Benefits of rate control versus maintenance of sinus rhythm. Am J Cardiol 91:27D, 2003

2. Reiffel JA: Selecting an antiarrhythmic agent for atrial fibrillation should be a patient-specific, data-driven decision. Am J Cardiol 82:72N, 1998

3. Naccarelli GV, Wolbrette DL, Khan M, et al: Old and new antiarrhythmic drugs for converting and maintaining sinus rhythm in atrial fibrillation: comparative efficacy and results of trials. Am J Cardiol 91:15D, 2003

4. Raichlen JS, Campbell FW, Edie RN, et al: Effect of the site of placement of temporary epicardial pacemakers on ventricular function in patients undergoing cardiac surgery. Circulation 70:I, 1984

5. Sarubbi B, Ducceschi V, D'Andrea A, et al: Atrial fibrillation: what are the effects of drug therapy on the effectiveness and complications of electrical cardioversion? Can J Cardiol 14:1267, 1998

6. Bertaglia E, D'Este D, Zerbo F, et al: Effects of verapamil and metoprolol on recovery from atrial electrical remodeling after cardioversion of long-lasting atrial fibrillation. Int J Cardiol 87:167, 2003

7. Bigger JT Jr: Epidemiological and mechanistic studies of atrial fibrillation as a basis for treatment strategies. Circulation 98:943, 1998

8. Botto GL, Bonini W, Broffoni T: Modulation of ventricular rate in permanent atrial fibrillation: randomized, crossover study of the effects of slow-release formulations of gallopamil, diltiazem, or verapamil. Clin Cardiol 11:837, 1998

9. Glatter KA, Cheng J, Dorostkar P, et al: Electrophysiologic effects of adenosine in patients with supraventricular tachycardia. Circulation 99:1034, 1999

10. Hayes A: Adenosine receptors and cardiovascular disease: the adenosine-1 Receptor (A(1)) and A(1) selective ligands. Cardiovasc Toxicol 3:71, 2003

11. Tracey WR, Magee W, Masamune H, et al: Selective activation of adenosine A3 receptors with N6-(3-chlorobenzyl)-5'-N-methylcarboxamidoadenosine (CB-MECA) provides cardioprotection via KATP channel activation. Cardiovasc Res 40:138, 1998

12. Zumino AP, Baiardi G, Schanne OF, et al: Differential electrophysiologic effects of global and regional ischemia and reperfusion in perfused rat hearts. Effects of Mg2+ concentration. Mol Cell Biochem 186:79, 1998

13. Letelier LM, Udol K, Ena J, et al: Effectiveness of amiodarone for conversion of atrial fibrillation to sinus rhythm: a meta-analysis. Arch Intern Med 163:777, 2003

14. Drouin E, Lande G, Charpentier F: Amiodarone reduces transmural heterogeneity of repolarization in the human heart. J Am Coll Cardiol 32:1063, 1998

15. Kowey PR, Marinchak RA, Rials SJ, et al: Intravenous amiodarone. J Am Coll Cardiol 29:1190, 1997

16. Kudenchuk PJ, Cobb LA, Copass MK, et al: Amiodarone for resuscitation after out-of-hospital cardiac arrest due to ventricular fibrillation. N Engl J Med 341:871, 1999

17. Somberg JC, Bailin SJ, Haffajee CI, et al: Intravenous lidocaine versus intravenous amiodarone (in a new aqueous formulation) for incessant ventricular tachycardia. Am J Cardiol 90:853, 2002

18. Bernard EO, Schmid ER, Schmidlin D, et al: Ibutilide versus amiodarone in atrial fibrillation: a double-blinded, randomized study. Crit Care Med 31:1031, 2003

19. Roy D, Talajic M, Dorian P, Connolly S, et al: Amiodarone to prevent recurrence of atrial fibrillation. N Engl J Med 342:913, 2000

20. Using oral amiodarone safely. Drug Therapy Bull 41:9, 2003

21. Vorperian VR, Havighurst TC, Miller S, et al: Adverse effects of low-dose amiodarone: a meta-analysis. J Am Coll Cardiol 30:791, 1997

22. Gowda RM, Khan IA, Mehta NJ, et al: Cardiac arrhythmias in pregnancy: clinical and therapeutic considerations. Int J Cardiol 88:129, 2003

23. Cardosi RJ, Chez RA: Magnesium sulfate, maternal hypothermia, and fetal bradycardia with loss of heart rate variability. Obstet Gynecol 92:691, 1998

24. Hamersley SL, Landy HJ, O'Sullivan MJ: Fetal bradycardia secondary to magnesium sulfate therapy for preterm labor: a case report. J Reprod Med 43:206, 1998

25. Hohnloser SH: Proarrhythmia with class III antiarrhythmic drugs: types, risks, and management. Am J Cardiol 80:82G, 1997

26. Wolbrette DL: Risk of proarrhythmia with class III antiarrhythmic agents: sex-based differences and other issues. Am J Cardiol 91:39D, 2003

27. Sager PT: New advances in class III antiarrhythmic drug therapy. Curr Opin Cardiol 14:15, 1999

28. The Sicilian gambit: a new approach to the classification of antiarrhythmic drugs based on their actions on arrhythmogenic mechanisms. Task Force of the Working Group on Arrhythmias of the European Society of Cardiology. Circulation 84:1831, 1991

29. Brodsky MA, Orlov MV, Allen BJ, et al: Clinical assessment of adrenergic tone and responsiveness to beta-blocker therapy in patients with

30. Kowey PR, Marinchak RA, Rials SJ, et al: Pharmacologic and pharmacokinetic profile of class III antiarrhythmic drugs. Am J Cardiol 80:16G, 1997

31. Stafford RS, Robson DC, Misra B, et al: Rate controls and sinus rhythm maintenance in atrial fibrillation: national trends in medication use, 1980-1996. Arch Intern Med 158:2144, 1998

32. Van Gelder IC, Brugemann J, Crijns HJ: Current treatment recommendations in antiarrhythmic therapy. Drugs 55:331, 1998

33. Uchida T, Yashima M, Gotoh M, et al: Mechanism of acceleration of functional reentry in the ventricle: effects of ATP-sensitive potassium channel opener. Circulation 99:704, 1999

34. Light PE, Wallace CH, Dyck JR: Constitutively active adenosine monophosphate-activated protein kinase regulates voltage-gated sodium channels in ventricular myocytes. Circulation 107:1962, 2003

35. Meldrum DR, Cleveland JC Jr, Rowland RT, et al: Cardiac surgical implications of calcium dyshomeostasis in the heart. Ann Thorac Surg 61:1273, 1996

36. Cleveland JC Jr, Meldrum DR, Rowland RT, et al: Optimal myocardial preservation: cooling, cardioplegia, and conditioning. Ann Thorac Surg 61:760, 1996

37. Janse MJ: Why does atrial fibrillation occur? Eur Heart J 18(suppl C):C12, 1997

38. Yue L, Feng J, Gaspo R, et al: Ionic remodeling underlying action potential changes in a canine model of atrial fibrillation. Circ Res 81:512, 1997

39. Priebe L, Beuckelmann DJ: Simulation study of cellular electric properties in heart failure. Circ Res 82:1206, 1998

40. Levi AJ, Dalton GR, Hancox JC, et al: Role of intracellular sodium overload in the genesis of cardiac arrhythmias. J Cardiovasc Electrophysiol 8:700, 1997

41. Riaz K, Forker AD: Digoxin use in congestive heart failure: current status. Drugs 55:747, 1998

42. Reddy S, Benatar D, Gheorghiade M: Update on digoxin and other oral positive inotropic agents for chronic heart failure. Curr Opin Cardiol 12:233, 1997

43. Umans VA, Cornel JH, Hic C: Digoxin in patients with heart failure. N Engl J Med 337:129, 1997

44. Patterson E, Kalcich M, Scherlag BJ: Phase 1B ventricular arrhythmia in the dog: localized reentry with the mid-myocardium. J Interv Card Electrophysiol 2:145, 1998

symptomatic ventricular tachycardia and no apparent structural heart disease. Am Heart J 131:51, 1996

45. Boineau JP, Cox JL: Slow ventricular activation in acute myocardial infarction: source of reentrant premature ventricular contractions. Circulation 48:702, 1973

46. Swynghedaauw B: Molecular mechanisms of myocardial remodeling. Physiol Rev 79:215, 1999

47. Koning MMG, Gho BCG, Klaarwater EV, et al: Rapid ventricular pacing produces myocardial protection by nonischemic activation of K+-ATP channels. Circulation 93:178, 1996

48. Kastor JA, Horowitz LN, Harken AH, et al: Clinical electrophysiology of ventricular tachycardia. N Engl J Med 304:1004, 1981

49. Burashnikov A, Antzelevitch C: Reinduction of atrial fibrillation immediately after termination of the arrhythmia is mediated by late phase 3 early afterdepolarization-induced triggered activity. Circulation 107:2355, 2003

50. Bozler E: The initiation of the cardiac impulse. Am J Physiol 138:273, 1943

51. Carmeliet EE, Vereecke J: Adrenaline and the plateau phase of the cardiac action potential. Pflugers Arch 313:303, 1969

52. Friedman P, Stewarts J, Fenoglio J: Survival of subendocardial Purkinje fibers after extensive myocardial infarction in dogs. Circ Res 33:597, 1973

53. Masui A, Tamura K, Tarumi N, et al: Resolution of late potentials with improvement of left ventricular systolic pressure in patients with first myocardial infarction. Clin Cardiol 20:466, 1997

54. Ferrari R, Pepi P, Ferrari F, et al: Metabolic derangement in ischemic heart disease and its therapeutic control. Am J Cardiol 82:2K, 1998

55. Pires LA, Lehmann MH, Steinman RT, et al: Sudden death in implantable cardioverter-defibrillator recipients: clinical context, arrhythmic events and device responses. J Am Coll Cardiol 33:24, 1999

56. Yee R, Connolly SJ, Gillis AM: Appropriate use of the implantable cardioverter defibrillator: a Canadian perspective. Canadian Working Group on Cardiac Pacing. Pacing Clin Electrophysiol 22:1, 1999

57. Swygman CA, Homoud MK, Link MS, et al: Technologic advances in implantable cardioverter defibrillators. Curr Opin Cardiol 14:9, 1999

58. Grimm W, Menz V, Hoffmann J, et al: Complications of third generation implantable cardioverter defibrillator therapy. Pacing Clin Electrophysiol 22:201, 1999

59. Pauli P, Wiedemann G, Dengler W, et al: Anxiety in patients with an automatic implantable cardioverter defibrillator: what differentiates them from panic patients? Psychosom Med 61:69, 1999

60. Anvari A, Gottsauner-Wolf M, Turel Z, et al: Predictors of outcome in patients with implantable cardioverter defibrillators. Cardiology 90:180, 1998

61. Movsowitz C, Marchlinski FE: Interactions between implantable cardioverter-defibrillators and class III agents. Am J Cardiol 82:41I, 1998

62. Dorian P, Newman D, Greene M: Implantable defibrillators and/or amiodarone: alternatives or complementary therapies. Int J Clin Pract 52:425, 1998

3 SHOCK

James W. Holcroft, M.D., F.A.C.S.

Approach to the Treatment of Shock

Classification of Shock

Shock may be defined as a state in which either (1) the cardiovascular system lacks adequate power for perfusion of the peripheral tissues or (2) there is adequate power for perfusion, but only at the cost of excessive and inefficient use of oxygen by the heart, which renders the heart vulnerable to ischemia. The first type of shock is commonly termed decompensated shock; the second, compensated shock.

Shock, whether decompensated or compensated, can be classified into five categories according to the physiologic derangement that is the primary cause of the shock state: (1) extracardiac compressive/obstructive shock, (2) hypovolemic shock, (3) inflammatory shock, (4) neurogenic shock, and (5) cardiogenic shock [*see Tables 1 and 2*]. Frequently, this classification is a nonexclusive one—that is, a given clinical condition (e.g., tension pneumothorax) might cause shock by several mechanisms. Nonetheless, a physiologic classification of shock that emphasizes a single primary cause is frequently helpful in the initial stages of treatment.

In extracardiac compressive shock, forces external to the heart compress the thin-walled chambers of the heart (the atria and right ventricle) and the great veins (both systemic and pulmonary) as they enter the heart, thus decreasing ventricular end-diastolic volumes. In extracardiac obstructive shock, the heart fails because it encounters excessive hindrance during contraction or because the extrapericardial veins returning blood to the heart become compressed. Many of the conditions associated with excessive hindrance to contraction also compress the great systemic and pulmonary veins.

In hypovolemic shock, small ventricular end-diastolic volumes lead to inefficient or inadequate cardiac production of power.

Inflammatory shock arises from the release of inflammatory and coagulatory mediators. It can be caused by ischemia-reperfusion injuries, trauma, or infection (in which case it is sometimes referred to as septic shock). Inflammatory shock is also known as distributive shock because the abnormalities in some cases derive partly from increased blood flow to the skin or stagnation of blood in dilated peripheral venules and small veins.

Inflammatory and coagulatory mediators cause inflammatory shock via three main mechanisms: (1) disruption of the microvascular endothelium, both at the inflammatory site and distally, (2) dilation of the microvasculature, both locally and distally, and (3) depression of the myocardium. The result is plasma loss into the interstitium, which produces a hypovolemic state, distant organ failure, and cardiac insufficiency or inadequacy. If the predominant feature of the shock state is loss of plasma volume into the interstitium through a permeable microvasculature, the patient's skin will be cool and clammy (hence the terms cold septic shock and cold inflammatory shock). If blood volume has been restored or the predominant feature of the shock state is cutaneous vasodilatation, the skin will be flushed and warm (hence the term warm inflammatory shock).

The causes of inflammatory shock are all associated with the presence of large amounts of infected or traumatized tissue in prox-imity to a robust blood supply and drainage. An avascular infection (e.g., a contained abscess) will not cause inflammatory shock, because the inflammatory mediators do not have access to the circulation; however, an uncontained abscess (e.g., a ruptured appendiceal abscess or a surgically drained subphrenic abscess) can cause inflammatory shock because the mediators that spill out of the abscess are picked up by the vasculature in the surrounding tissue. In like manner, dry gangrene, because of its poor vascular supply, will not cause inflammatory shock, whereas wet gangrene can.

Neurogenic shock arises from loss of autonomic innervation of the vasculature and, in some cases, of the heart. Causes include spinal cord injury, regional anesthesia, administration of drugs that block the adrenergic nervous system (including some systemically administered anesthetic agents), certain neurologic disorders, and fainting. Loss of arteriolar tone leads to hypotension; loss of venular and small venous tone leads to pooling of blood in the denervated parts of the body. If the blockade is generalized or at a high enough level, the denervation can also decrease myocardial contractility and heart rate.

In cardiogenic shock, the heart itself, through an intrinsic abnormality, is incapable of efficiently pushing its contained blood into the vasculature with adequate power.

Recognition of Shock

The presence of a shock state is typically signaled by one or more characteristic clinical markers [*see Table 3*].

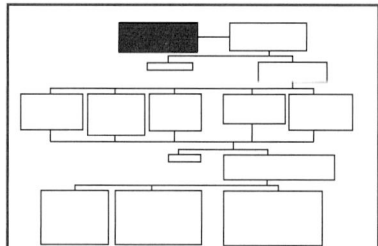

HYPOTENSION

A low blood pressure is a specific sign of shock but not a sensitive one. A very low blood pressure (≤ 89 mm Hg) almost always indicates some form of shock. Postural falls in blood pressure can also be a helpful signal: a sustained (> 30 seconds) systolic pressure drop greater than 10 mm Hg in a patient who has arisen from a supine position to an upright one is abnormal and frequently is an indication of underlying shock.

The absence of hypotension does not, however, rule out shock. Adrenergic discharge and the release of circulating and locally produced vasoconstrictors during shock often sustain blood pressure despite volume depletion or depressed myocardial contractility. Furthermore, how hypotension should be defined in a particular case depends on the patient's usual blood pressure, which may not be known to the physician. For instance, in a patient with severe preexisting hypertension, a systolic pressure of 120 mm Hg might reflect shock. Thus, hypotension—either supine or postural—can strongly suggest the diagnosis of shock, but normotension in a patient suspected of being in shock means nothing.

Table 1   Pathophysiologic Classification of Shock

Type of Shock	Abnormality	Causes
Extracardiac Compressive	Compression of the thin-walled chambers of the heart—the atria and the right ventricle—and compression of the great veins entering the heart	Pericardial tamponade, elevated diaphragm from pregnancy or abdominal bleeding or intestinal distention or ascites, ruptured diaphragm, tension pneumothorax, positive pressure ventilation with large tidal volumes
Obstructive	Excessive hindrance to ventricular emptying imposed by cardiac valvular stenosis or excessive vascular stiffness or resistance	Pulmonary embolism, air embolism, systemic hypertension, tension pneumothorax, hemothorax, ruptured diaphragm, positive pressure ventilation, aortic or pulmonary valvular stenosis
Hypovolemic	Depletion of vascular volume	Bleeding, protracted vomiting or diarrhea, fluid sequestration in obstructed gut or injured tissue, excessive use of diuretics, adrenal insufficiency, diabetes insipidus, dehydration, anaphylaxis
Inflammatory (formerly known as septic or traumatic shock)	Complex response associated with the systemic inflammatory and coagulative reaction to infected or injured tissues	Pneumonia, peritonitis, cholangitis, pyelonephritis, soft tissue infection, meningitis, mediastinitis, crush injuries, major fractures, high-velocity penetrating wounds, major burns, retained necrotic tissue, pancreatitis, anaphylaxis
Neurogenic	Pooling of blood in autonomically denervated venules and small veins; hypotension arising from denervated arterioles and sometimes from a denervated heart	Spinal cord injury, regional anesthetic, administration of drugs that produce autonomic blockade
Cardiogenic	Decreased myocardial contractility	Bradyarrhythmias, tachyarrhythmias, cardiac valvular insufficiency, papillary muscle rupture, myocardiopathy, myocarditis, myocardial ischemia, myocardial contusion (rare), septal defects

Table 2   Clinical Features of Compensated and Decompensated Shock

Parameter	Hypovolemic Shock		Inflammatory Shock		Neurogenic Shock		Left-Sided Cardiogenic Shock	
	Compensated	Decompensated	Compensated	Decompensated	Compensated	Decompensated	Compensated	Decompensated
Cardiovascular								
Heart rate	Increased	Variable	Increased	Increased	Increased	Decreased	Normal	Normal
BP	Normal	Decreased	Decreased	Decreased	Decreased	Decreased	Normal	Decreased
Cardiac output	Normal	Decreased	Increased	Normal	Increased	Decreased	Normal	Decreased
Power	Normal	Decreased	Normal	Decreased	Normal	Decreased	Normal	Decreased
Cardiac efficiency*	Decreased	Decreased	Decreased	Decreased	Decreased	Decreased	Decreased	Decreased
Metabolic								
Acid-base status	Normal	Metabolic acidemia	Metabolic acidemia	Metabolic acidemia	Normal	Metabolic acidemia	Normal	Metabolic acidemia
O_2 consumption	Normal	Decreased	Normal	Decreased	Normal	Decreased	Normal	Decreased
Glucose concentration	Moderately increased	Moderately increased	Increased	Variable	Normal	Normal	Normal	Normal
Clinical								
Temperature	Normal	Normal to decreased	Increased	Variable	Normal	Normal to decreased	Normal	Normal
Respiratory rate	Increased	Increased	Increased	Increased	Normal	Variable	Normal	Increased
Skin	Pale, cool	Pale, cool, clammy	Pink, warm	Pale, cool, clammy	Pink, warm in denervated areas	Pink, warm in denervated areas	Normal	Pale, cool, clammy
Neurologic state	Anxious	Anxious, confused, combative, obtunded	Anxious	Obtunded	Anxious; lower body paralyzed	Anxious; upper and lower body paralyzed	Normal	Anxious
Urine output	Decreased	Minimal	Decreased	Minimal	Decreased	Minimal	Decreased	Minimal

*Cardiovascular power divided by myocardial O_2 requirements.

Patient shows signs of possible shock

Characteristic signs include
- Hypotension
- Tachycardia or bradycardia
- Tachypnea
- Cutaneous hypoperfusion
- Mental abnormalities
- Oliguria
- Myocardial ischemia
- Metabolic acidemia
- Hypoxemia

Approach to the Treatment of Shock

Shock resolves

Extracardiac compressive/obstructive shock

Compression or obstruction of the heart or great vessels, as an immediately life-threatening condition (see above), should already have been treated. However, periodic reassessment during workup is appropriate because this type of shock can develop secondary to another process.

Hypovolemic shock

Control bleeding.

Obtain vascular access, and infuse NS or lactated Ringer solution (to 60 ml/kg or more).

If [Hb] ≤ 9 g/dl, consider giving RBCs. [Hb] should be ≥ 7 g/dl in young healthy patients with controlled bleeding, up to ≥ 11 g/dl in other patients.

Treat pain, hypothermia, acidemia, and coagulopathy.

Inflammatory shock

Obtain vascular access, and infuse fluids as necessary to replenish volume.

Give RBCs as for hypovolemic shock.

Treat pain, hypothermia, and acidemia.

Once resuscitation is well under way, search for and treat underlying inflammatory cause of shock.

Shock resolves

Periphery is priority

Goals: SV 60–100 ml, MAP 90 mm Hg, HR 60–100/min, filling pressures in midteens.

Treatment measures:
- Infuse fluids to ensure generous end-diastolic volumes.
- Increase contractility as needed with dobutamine (5–15 μg/kg/min) and milrinone (50 μg, then 0.375–0.75 μg/kg/min).
- If absolutely necessary to increase BP, give a vasoconstrictor—dopamine (2–20 μg/kg/min) if HR ≤ 90/min, norepinephrine (4–12 μg/kg/min) if HR > 90/min.

Periphery and heart are equal priorities

Goals: SV 55–85 ml, MAP 80 mm Hg, HR 60–90/min, filling pressures in low teens.

Treatment measures:
- Give fluids or initiate diuresis so that the smaller of the two end-diastolic volumes is slightly greater than normal.
- Cautiously increase contractility as necessary with dobutamine (5–15 μg/kg/min) and milrinone (50 μg, then 0.375–0.75 μg/kg/min).
- If absolutely necessary, give a vasoconstrictor—dopamine (2–20 μg/kg/min) if HR ≤ 70/min, norepinephrine (4–12 μg/kg/min) if HR > 70/min.
- For HR ≥ 110/min, initiate beta blockade with esmolol (500 μg/kg, then 50 μg/kg/min), followed by metoprolol (5–10 mg q. 6 hr).

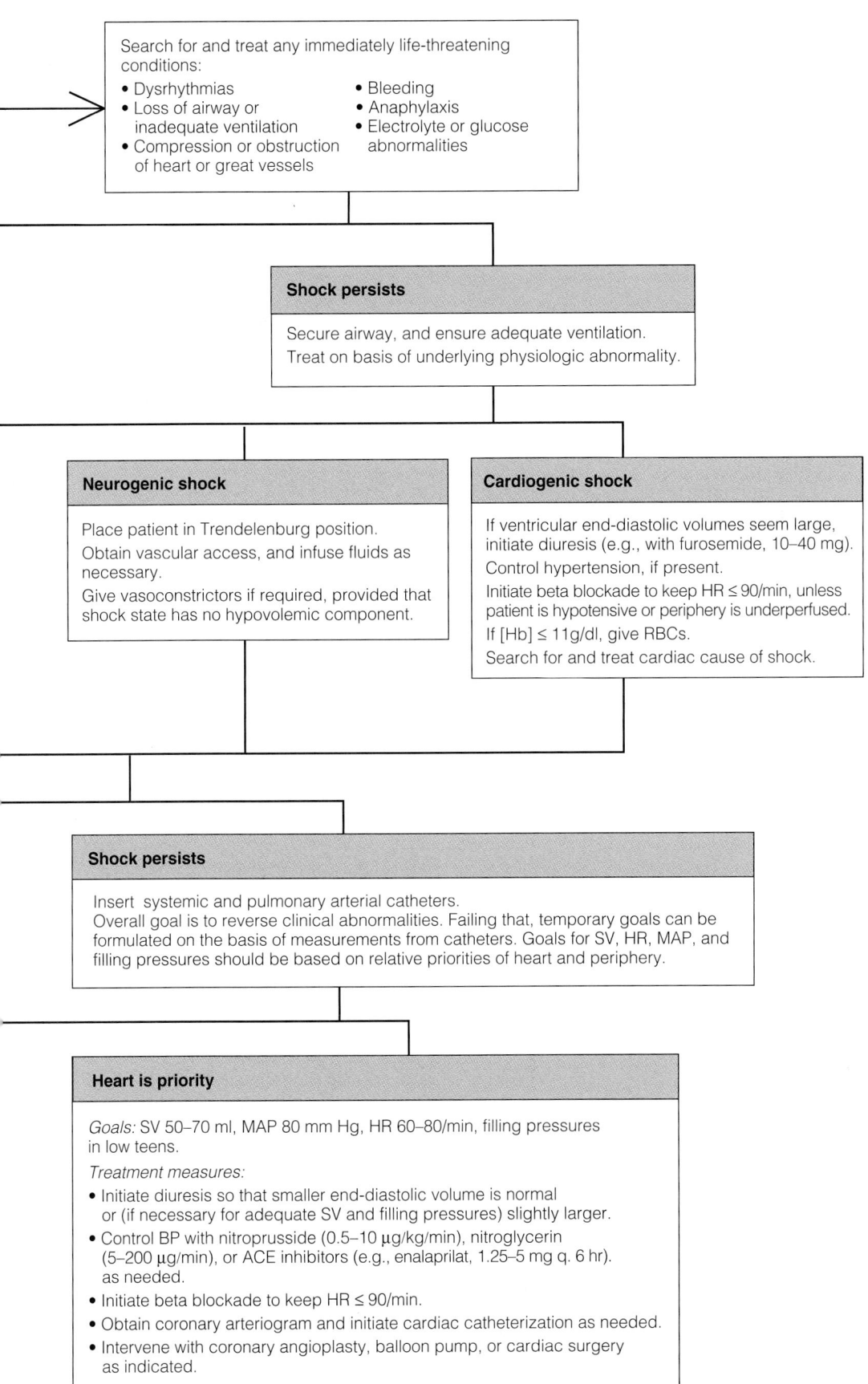

Search for and treat any immediately life-threatening conditions:

- Dysrhythmias
- Loss of airway or inadequate ventilation
- Compression or obstruction of heart or great vessels
- Bleeding
- Anaphylaxis
- Electrolyte or glucose abnormalities

Shock persists

Secure airway, and ensure adequate ventilation.
Treat on basis of underlying physiologic abnormality.

Neurogenic shock

Place patient in Trendelenburg position.
Obtain vascular access, and infuse fluids as necessary.
Give vasoconstrictors if required, provided that shock state has no hypovolemic component.

Cardiogenic shock

If ventricular end-diastolic volumes seem large, initiate diuresis (e.g., with furosemide, 10–40 mg).
Control hypertension, if present.
Initiate beta blockade to keep HR ≤ 90/min, unless patient is hypotensive or periphery is underperfused.
If [Hb] ≤ 11g/dl, give RBCs.
Search for and treat cardiac cause of shock.

Shock persists

Insert systemic and pulmonary arterial catheters.
Overall goal is to reverse clinical abnormalities. Failing that, temporary goals can be formulated on the basis of measurements from catheters. Goals for SV, HR, MAP, and filling pressures should be based on relative priorities of heart and periphery.

Heart is priority

Goals: SV 50–70 ml, MAP 80 mm Hg, HR 60–80/min, filling pressures in low teens.

Treatment measures:

- Initiate diuresis so that smaller end-diastolic volume is normal or (if necessary for adequate SV and filling pressures) slightly larger.
- Control BP with nitroprusside (0.5–10 µg/kg/min), nitroglycerin (5–200 µg/min), or ACE inhibitors (e.g., enalaprilat, 1.25–5 mg q. 6 hr). as needed.
- Initiate beta blockade to keep HR ≤ 90/min.
- Obtain coronary arteriogram and initiate cardiac catheterization as needed.
- Intervene with coronary angioplasty, balloon pump, or cardiac surgery as indicated.

TACHYCARDIA OR BRADYCARDIA

The pulse rate—perhaps the most evident of all the physical findings in clinical medicine—can increase in shock; such an increase is frequently cited as a cardinal feature of shock. When tachycardia is present, the possibility of shock should be considered; however, the absence of tachycardia should not be taken as a sign that the patient is not in shock. In extreme cases of shock, the pulse rate eventually falls to 0/min. Even in less extreme cases, the pulse rate may slow down, presumably to allow added time both for ventricular filling and for coronary perfusion of the myocardium as well as to reduce myocardial oxygen requirements. Thus, a normal or even a slow heart rate does not rule out shock and may even be an indication of a decompensated shock state.[1-3]

TACHYPNEA

A rapid respiratory rate may be a response to a metabolic acidemia, which is a typical finding with decompensated shock of any cause.

CUTANEOUS HYPOPERFUSION

Poor skin perfusion is often the first sign of shock. In all types of shock other than warm inflammatory shock and neurogenic shock, adrenergic discharge and the release of vasopressin and angiotensin II constrict the arterioles, venules, and small veins throughout the body. This constriction compensates for what otherwise could be profound hypotension. Cutaneous vasoconstriction produces the most sensitive sign of shock: the pale, cool, and clammy skin of someone exhibiting the fight-or-flight reaction. This sign is not specific for shock—it can also be the result of hypothermia, for example—but when it is seen in conjunction with collapsed and constricted subcutaneous veins in a patient with suspected hypovolemic or decompensated inflammatory shock, it establishes the diagnosis.

MENTAL ABNORMALITIES

Patients in severe decompensated shock frequently exhibit mental abnormalities, which can range from anxiousness to agitation to indifference to obtundation. These findings are not sensitive—indeed, they develop only in the late stages of shock—nor are they specific. They are, however, a strong warning to the physician that something must be done quickly. The body protects the brain at all costs; if blood supply to the brain is becoming inadequate, there usually is little time left.

OLIGURIA

Whenever the diagnosis of shock is being entertained, a Foley catheter should be placed. In many cases of compensated shock and in all cases of decompensated shock (except those in which shock results from inappropriate diuresis involving either a previously administered drug or ingestion of ethanol), urine output falls off. Oliguria is one of the most sensitive and specific of all the signs of shock.

MYOCARDIAL ISCHEMIA

An electrocardiogram, which should be obtained promptly whenever a patient is suspected of being in shock, may show signs of ischemia. The ischemia may be caused either by a primary myocardial problem or by a secondary extracardiac problem (e.g., hypotension resulting from hemorrhage or excess hindrance to ventricular contraction resulting from pulmonary embolism). In either case, the presence of myocardial ischemia, like the presence of mental abnormalities, should prompt quick action.

METABOLIC ACIDEMIA

Metabolic acidemia, as a sign of shock, may be manifested by an increased respiratory rate, but analysis of blood gases is usually re-

Table 3 Clinical Markers of Possible Shock State

Clinical Marker	Value or Findings Indicative of Shock
Systolic blood pressure Adult Schoolchild Preschool child Infant	 ≤ 110 mm Hg ≤ 100 mm Hg ≤ 90 mm Hg ≤ 80 mm Hg
Sinus tachycardia Adult Schoolchild Preschool child Infant	 ≥ 90 beats/min ≥ 120 beats/min ≥ 140 beats/min ≥ 160 beats/min
Cutaneous vasoconstriction	Pale, cool, clammy skin with constricted subcutaneous veins
Mental changes	Anxiousness, agitation, indifference, lethargy, obtundation
Urine output Adult Child Infant	 ≤ 0.5 ml·kg^{-1}·hr^{-1} ≤ 1.0 ml·kg^{-1}·hr^{-1} ≤ 2.0 ml·kg^{-1}·hr^{-1}
Myocardial ischemia or failure	Chest pain, third heart sound, pulmonary edema, abnormal ECG
Metabolic acidemia	$[HCO_3^-] \leq 21$ mEq/L Base deficit ≥ 3 mEq/L
Hypoxemia (on room air) 0–50 yr 51–70 yr ≥ 71 yr	 ≤ 90 mm Hg ≤ 80 mm Hg ≤ 70 mm Hg

quired for confirmation. The acidemia may take the form of either a low calculated bicarbonate level or a base deficit.[4] Some patients in the early stages of shock—even severe shock—are not acidemic. If flow is sufficiently reduced, the anaerobic products of metabolism will be confined to the periphery; they may not be washed into the central circulation until some degree of resuscitation has taken place. Systemic arterial acidemia may become evident only after the diagnosis has been made and treatment initiated.

HYPOXEMIA

Systemic arterial hypoxemia is a common sign of shock. Low flow results in marked desaturation of blood leaving the metabolizing peripheral tissues and entering the pulmonary artery. If pulmonary function is compromised to any significant degree, as is often the case with shock, the markedly desaturated pulmonary arterial blood becomes only partially saturated as it passes through the lungs.

Identification and Treatment of Immediately Life-Threatening Conditions

If the patient shows signs of possible shock, the next step is to search for and treat any conditions that could

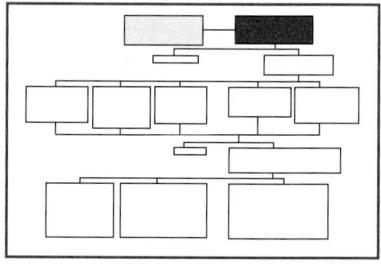

kill the patient immediately. Such conditions include dysrhythmias, loss of airway or inadequate ventilation, extracardiac compression of the heart or obstruction of the vasculature, bleeding, and certain life-threatening medical conditions (e.g., anaphylaxis and highly abnormal electrolyte concentrations).

DYSRHYTHMIAS

Given that an electrocardiogram should be obtained promptly in any patient suspected of being in shock, any dysrhythmias present will usually be recognized at an early point. An agonal patient with a dysrhythmia should undergo cardioversion, ideally even before the airway is secured and before I.V. access is obtained. Cardioversion, when successful, can restore a moribund patient with ventricular fibrillation, ventricular tachycardia, or atrial fibrillation to life with full neurologic recovery. It is of no value for a patient in asystole; however, the possibility of fully resuscitating a patient in ventricular standstill is so remote that it usually makes little difference what mode of therapy is attempted or whether therapy is attempted at all.

A nonagonal patient should be treated in accordance with standard resuscitation routines [see 6:1 Cardiac Resuscitation and 6:2 Acute Cardiac Dysrhythmia].

LOSS OF AIRWAY OR INADEQUATE VENTILATION

If a patient can talk in a full voice without undue effort, the airway can be assumed to be intact; if not, the possibility of airway compromise must be considered. Airway compromise has a number of possible causes, ranging from loss of protective reflexes to mechanical obstruction. Sometimes, a jaw thrust is all that is needed for the physician to make the diagnosis and treat the problem.[5] In cases of profound shock, however, a definitive airway, such as that gained by inserting an oral endotracheal tube, becomes necessary. A definitive airway allows the physician to proceed with other lifesaving measures. If, after initial resuscitation, shock resolves and the patient regains consciousness and begins to struggle against intubation, the tube may be removed.

Of all the conditions that can render ventilation inadequate, tension pneumothorax is the most deadly. The most common causes of tension pneumothorax are trauma and therapeutic interventions by medical personnel (e.g., central venous punctures and positive pressure ventilation). Characteristic signs include decreased or absent breath sounds on the involved side, a hyperresonant hemithorax, and, if the patient is normovolemic, distended neck veins. (A tracheal shift—a commonly described feature in patients with tension pneumothoraces—is hard to detect and, in my experience, rarely helpful in making the diagnosis.) Treatment consists of needle decompression or tube thoracostomy.

Institution of mechanical ventilation does not guarantee that the patient will be adequately ventilated. The ventilator may malfunction, or the endotracheal tube may be misplaced or obstructed. If the chest wall does not rise with inspiration, mechanical ventilation should be promptly discontinued, and ventilation with an Ambu bag should be initiated at an inspired oxygen fraction (F_IO_2) of 1.0. If increasing abdominal distention is apparent, the possibility of esophageal intubation or displacement of the endotracheal tube into the hypopharynx should be considered. Treatment consists of reintubation. If breath sounds are absent on the left, right mainstem bronchial intubation should be considered. Treatment consists of partial withdrawal of the tube. Endotracheal tubes can become obstructed with clotted blood or inspissated secretions. Treatment consists of suctioning. Bleeding in the tracheobronchial tree (from injuries or from friable bronchial mucosa or tumor tissue) can eliminate ventilation from the lung segment supplied by the injured or obstructed bronchus and flood the initially uninjured lung with blood. If the bleeding is thought to be coming from the left lung, the endotracheal tube should be advanced into the right mainstem bronchus. Bleeding from the right lung can be more problematic because selective left mainstem intubation may be impossible. Prompt control of bleeding can sometimes be obtained via endobronchial or open surgical intervention; both interventions also may be needed either for acute control or for definitive management of bleeding from the left lung.

Massive hemothoraces with collapse and compression of the lung should be treated with tube thoracostomy and, if necessary, surgical intervention. A massive left-side air leak from trauma or a ruptured bleb can be treated by advancing the endotracheal tube into the right mainstem bronchus. A massive right-side air leak usually necessitates surgical intervention, as does any leak that does not close quickly.

COMPRESSION OR OBSTRUCTION OF THE HEART OR THE GREAT VESSELS

Acute pericardial tamponade is usually manifested by muffled heart tones and occasionally by an exaggerated (> 10 mm Hg) decrease in systolic blood pressure on spontaneous breathing. If the patient is not hypovolemic, the neck veins are typically distended. Treatment consists of needle decompression or surgical creation of a pericardial window. Chronic tamponade can also produce shock but often does not give rise to the findings characteristic of acute tamponade; it is treated in the same way.

Diaphragmatic rupture and the ensuing intrusion of abdominal viscera into the chest can compress the heart, the great veins, and the extracardiac pulmonary vasculature, as can an intact but elevated diaphragm. Such compression can become a major problem if the patient is also hypovolemic. Treatment of a ruptured hemidiaphragm consists of operative reduction and repair; treatment of gut distention, decompression; treatment of bleeding, vascular control; and treatment of ascites, paracentesis of small amounts of fluid (just enough to lower intra-abdominal pressure).[6] Late-term pregnant women should be turned onto the left side so as to relieve compression of the right common iliac vein and the inferior vena cava.

Positive pressure ventilation can compress the heart, the great veins, and the vasculature in the pulmonary parenchyma.[7-11] In cases of suspected shock, tidal volumes should be kept small (≤ 7 ml/kg ideal body weight); inspiratory times should be short (≤ 1 second); end-expiratory pressure should be set at 0; and the initial respiratory rate should be kept low to minimize the total time spent in inspiration. Oxygenation can be maintained by using a high F_IO_2 (initially, 1.0). When blood gas analysis becomes available, the respiratory rate should be adjusted to prevent respiratory acidemia, and the inspired oxygen concentration should be decreased, provided that arterial saturation remains above 95%. When the patient is more stable, arterial saturation can be kept at a slightly lower level (≥ 92%); however, in the acute setting, it should be kept higher to buffer unanticipated decreases in oxygenation.

Besides compromising ventilation, tension pneumothoraces can compress the heart, the great systemic and pulmonary veins as they enter the atria, and the extracardiac pulmonary vasculature. Massive hemothoraces can exert similar effects. These conditions are treated as previously described [see Loss of Airway or Inadequate Ventilation, above].

Intravascular obstruction from a pulmonary thromboembolism or air embolism can kill quickly. Treatment of massive thromboembolism consists of prompt administration of fibrinolytics or heparin [see 4:6 Venous Thromboembolism], followed, in many cases, by pulmonary arteriography and further lytic therapy. Right-side air embolism can arise from penetrating injuries to large veins in the upper part of the body or from a percutaneous puncture with a large-bore needle if air is allowed access to the venous system while the patient takes a deep breath, especially if the patient is upright. Right-side air embolism can also arise as a complication of insufflation of gas into the peritoneal cavity during laparoscopy. Initial treatment consists of elimination of the source of air. Air that forms an air trap in the outflow tract of the right ventricle can sometimes be translocated to the apex of the ventricle by placing the patient in the Trendelenburg position with the left side down. Treatment consists of administration of 100% oxygen to wash out any residual nitrogen, followed by attempts to aspirate the air with a long central venous catheter. Coronary air embolism can occur whenever a patient with a penetrating injury to the lung parenchyma, either from trauma or from a needle puncture, is placed on positive pressure ventilation. The positive airway pressure can push air from an injured bronchus into an adjacent injured pulmonary vein, thereby allowing the air access to the left ventricle, the coronary arteries, and the brain. The diagnosis is usually made when a patient at risk goes into arrest shortly after initiation of positive pressure ventilation. Coronary air embolism is treated by giving 100% oxygen, opening the chest on the side with the suspected pulmonary penetration, and cross-clamping the hilum of the lung. The heart is then massaged while the descending thoracic aorta is compressed, and vasoconstrictors are administered.

BLEEDING

Bleeding should be controlled by any means necessary. Bleeding from an easily accessible site in an extremity, for instance, may be readily controlled with compression, whereas bleeding from an injury to the suprarenal aorta calls for meticulous exposure and control. Fracture-dislocations should be reduced if possible or, if not immediately reduced, immobilized.

ACUTE MEDICAL CONDITIONS

Anaphylaxis and life-threatening abnormalities in electrolyte or glucose concentrations usually are not recognized in the initial stages of shock management, but once they come to light, they should be treated promptly.

Treatment of Shock on the Basis of the Underlying Physiologic Abnormality

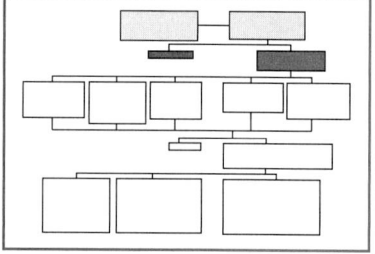

If shock persists after immediately life-threatening conditions have been treated, the next step in management is to categorize the shock state on the basis of the underlying physiologic abnormality and to initiate treatment accordingly.

As a rule, all that is needed to make this preliminary classification is the history, the physical examination, a chest x-ray, an electrocardiogram, and, in some cases, a complete blood count, electrolyte concentrations, a glucose level, and an arterial blood gas analysis. The classification is seldom neat: more than one cause of cardiovascular inadequacy is usually present, as when a patient with a myocardial infarction (MI) requires ventilation or when a patient with a ruptured abdominal aortic aneurysm has a distended abdomen. Nevertheless, such categorization is useful, in that it focuses the physician's attention on the primary problem, the cause of the persistent shock state.

First, the airway should be secured (if it has not been secured al-

ready), and supplemental oxygen should be given via a mask or a nasal cannula. The patient should be intubated, and ventilatory support should be provided if needed. The F_IO_2 should be 1.0 initially. Tidal volumes should be kept small (approximately 7 ml/kg ideal body weight) to minimize overdistention of alveoli and compression of the pulmonary vasculature and the heart. No end-expiratory pressure should be used initially. Inspiratory times should be kept short ($\leq$ 1 second), and the respiratory rate should be kept as slow as possible. These measures will minimize ventilation-induced obstruction of the pulmonary vasculature and compression of the vena cavae and the heart—hemodynamic consequences that can be fatal, especially when superimposed on preexisting shock.

EXTRACARDIAC COMPRESSIVE/OBSTRUCTIVE SHOCK

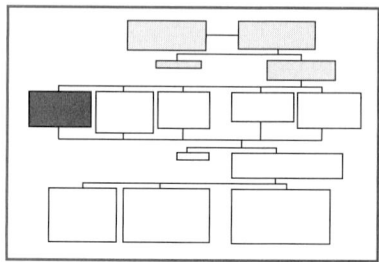

As a condition that can kill quickly, extracardiac compressive/obstructive shock should already have been treated [see Compression or Obstruction of the Heart or the Great Vessels, above]. It is wise, however, to keep these two causes of shock in mind as workup proceeds: they often develop secondarily, as when tension pneumothorax develops in a mechanically ventilated patient who is being worked up or treated for some nonpulmonary problem.

HYPOVOLEMIC SHOCK

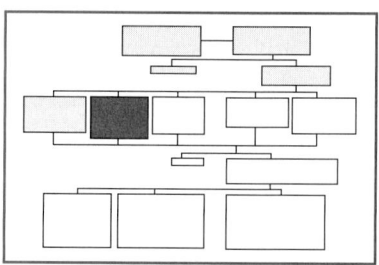

Treatment of Underlying Cause

At first glance, it might seem obvious that treatment of the underlying causes of shock should have the highest of priorities. This is indeed the case for hypovolemic shock caused by hemorrhage: it makes no sense to pour fluid and blood into a patient while controllable bleeding continues unchecked. For other types of shock, however, it is better to postpone treatment of the underlying causes until after the patient has been adequately resuscitated [see Inflammatory Shock, below].

Vascular Access

Simultaneously with efforts to control the underlying cause of hypovolemic shock, vascular access should be obtained, if it has not been already. If possible, superficial veins in the upper extremities should be cannulated with two large-bore catheters. If this is impossible, cutdowns may be performed on an antecubital or a basilic vein in the upper extremity, a cephalic vein at the shoulder, an external jugular vein at the base of the neck, or a saphenous vein at the ankle or in the groin.

Cutdowns in the upper extremity cause little morbidity but can take time to perform because upper-extremity veins are most likely to be thrombosed from earlier use. Morbidity is also low with the cephalic veins and the external jugular veins; however, exposure is sometimes difficult because of either the overlying fascia (in the case of the cephalic veins) or the overlying muscle (in the case of the external jugular veins). The saphenous vein at the ankle is readily exposed, large, and easy to cannulate. It cannot be used if there is extensive trauma to the extremity: if the cannula is left in place at the ankle for more than 24 hours, it is likely to cause superficial thrombophlebitis. The saphenous vein in the groin is harder to expose, but it too is large and easy to cannulate. If the cannula is left in place in the groin for more than 24 hours, there is a substantial chance that it will cause iliofemoral thrombophlebitis, which can lead to massive and possibly disabling edema in the involved extremity. Therapeutic anticoagulation is required in patients who may be at high risk for bleeding.

Percutaneous cannulation of the internal jugular vein provides not only access for infusion of fluids and drugs but also a port for central venous monitoring. In hypovolemic patients, this vein is usually collapsed, and puncture of the adjacent common carotid artery becomes a possibility; if puncture does occur, it may be difficult to recognize. The pulsatility of blood drawn from an arterial catheter may not be apparent; desaturated arterial blood may take on the appearance of a venous aspirate.

Percutaneous puncture of the subclavian vein provides large-bore access and monitoring capability; however, it may be difficult to accomplish in a hypovolemic patient. Pneumothorax may result, but it is usually easy to treat if recognized early. Puncture of the subclavian artery with decompression into the pleural cavity (a nontamponading space) can be fatal, especially in a patient made vulnerable by coexisting shock.

Percutaneous puncture of the common femoral vein is among the easiest of all techniques for venous access and provides large-bore monitoring capability. Because the femoral artery is immediately adjacent to the vein, unintentional puncture of the artery is common under urgent conditions. If the patient is in extremis, the artery should be cannulated. Intra-arterial infusion of fluids is as effective as I.V. infusion. Great care must be taken to ensure that no air gains entry to the system, and the catheter should be removed as soon as other access is gained. A femoral venous catheter should be removed as soon as possible as well. Percutaneous puncture of the common femoral vein is usually a fallback approach. If it is used in the resuscitation of a hypercoagulable shock patient (the usual scenario) and if the catheter is left in place for more than even a few hours, there is a substantial risk of iliofemoral deep vein thrombosis or even septic deep vein thrombosis—a potentially fatal complication in a critically ill patient.

In pediatric patients, intraosseous access has become a useful means of gaining vascular access under difficult conditions. On rare occasions, this approach may be used in young adults.[12,13]

The first attempts at obtaining vascular access should be made in the upper extremities with a percutaneous technique. If these attempts fail, the physician should fall back on a technique with which he or she is comfortable. There is no single best approach.

Fluid Administration

Once vascular access is obtained, a 20 ml/kg bolus of normal saline should be infused. If the patient is in profound shock, the fluid bolus should be given within 5 minutes if possible; if the situation is less urgent, it may be given over a period of 15 minutes or so. If shock does not resolve, two more boluses should be given.

I consider normal saline the fluid of choice for initial resuscitation in most patients. Its sodium concentration (154 mmol/L) is close to that of normal serum. Its chloride concentration (also 154 mmol/L) can induce hyperchloremic metabolic acidemia, but this state seems not to be harmful to the patient; if it is not severe, it may even augment myocardial contractility. The slight hyperosmolality of the solution may yield a modest increase in contractility as well. If the patient has severe metabolic acidemia with a chloride concentration exceeding 115 mmol/L, lactated or acetated Ringer solution is used. Both the lactate and the acetate accept a proton to form an organic acid, which is converted in the liver to carbon dioxide and water. As long

as hepatic function and pulmonary function are adequate, which is usually the case, the result of this process is buffering of the acidemia that can accompany the shock state. Both of these solutions, however, are hyponatremic and hypoosmotic; the latter is a potential problem in patients at risk for increased intracranial pressure.

Solutions containing glucose should not be used in the initial resuscitation of a patient in shock unless the patient is known to be hypoglycemic. Most patients in shock, in fact, are hyperglycemic as a result of high plasma levels of epinephrine and cortisol.[14] Excessively high plasma glucose concentrations can induce an inappropriate diuresis.

Hypertonic saline solutions containing up to 7.5% sodium chloride (compared with 0.9% for normal saline) show promise for resuscitating patients in situations where large-volume resuscitation with isotonic solutions is impossible (e.g., battle, events involving mass casualties, and prehospital trauma care). Hypertonic solutions provide far more blood volume expansion than isotonic solutions do. They also have advantages in treating hypotensive patients with head injuries. These solutions are approved for use and are commercially available in Brazil (the country where the idea originated), Chile, Argentina, and Europe; they are not currently approved for use in the United States.[15-21]

Albumin-containing solutions should not be given in the acute phase of shock resuscitation except perhaps in unusual circumstances—for example, when only small amounts of resuscitative fluids can be given because of logistical problems, such as those encountered with mass casualties or under battlefield conditions. Initially, protein- or colloid-containing solutions achieve greater plasma volume expansion than crystalloid solutions, but the data from randomized trials with albumin convincingly demonstrate that long-term survival is no better and possibly worse if albumin is used in a setting where large-volume crystalloid can be given instead.[22] The reasons for the poorer survival rates are not entirely clear, but it may be that administration of albumin under conditions of increased microvascular permeability results in accumulation of excessive amounts of albumin in the interstitium. Once in the interstitium, albumin, unlike water and other smaller molecules, can regain access to the plasma space only via lymphatic drainage. If lymphatic drainage capacity is exceeded, persistent postoperative edema may result.

Blood should be given to ensure that the hemoglobin concentration is at least 7 g/dl, if not substantially higher. Certain patients require higher concentrations, as reflected in the following guidelines:

1. A hemoglobin concentration of 7 g/dl is adequate in a young patient who has good coronary arteries and whose bleeding is known to be completely under control.[23]
2. A hemoglobin concentration of 8 g/dl is adequate in a young patient who is at slight risk for further bleeding.
3. A hemoglobin concentration of 9 g/dl is required if the risk of bleeding is substantial.
4. A hemoglobin concentration of 10 g/dl should be the goal if there is any possibility of coronary artery disease, even in the absence of ongoing myocardial ischemia. (The heart is a working muscle, even when the body is at rest, and uses much of the oxygen delivered to it by the coronary arteries. Obstruction of the arteries proximal to the working muscle can lead to usage of all the oxygen carried in the blood. Accordingly, it is crucial to maintain an adequate hemoglobin concentration in this setting. Provided that the arteries are not obstructed, the other organs in the resting body are not susceptible, because they use only a fraction of the oxygen delivered to them.)
5. A hemoglobin concentration of 11 g/dl should be maintained if the heart shows any signs of ongoing myocardial ischemia.

In an emergency, O-negative red blood cells reconstituted with normal saline may be given. If the patient can wait a few more minutes, type-specific blood may be given so as to conserve the blood bank's supply of O-negative blood. Whole blood can be administered more quickly than packed red blood cells, but use of packed cells has the advantage of conserving the blood bank's supply of fresh frozen plasma. Filtering reduces the amount of particulate material administered with the blood but may also reduce the rate at which blood can be administered.

The use of blood substitutes for resuscitation is an attractive option from a conceptual perspective. To date, however, clinical trials using these agents in this setting have yielded disappointing results.[24,25]

Treatment of Pain, Hypothermia, Acidemia, and Coagulopathy

Once blood volume has been at least partially replenished, pain may be treated with small I.V. doses of narcotics. Pain relief can decrease the stress response associated with shock and perhaps diminish the severity of its late sequelae; however, narcotics can also decrease tone in the venules and small veins, thereby exacerbating the shock state. Accordingly, it is vital to keep doses small, to titrate the dosage carefully, and to be ready to reverse the effect with a narcotic antagonist if necessary. Sometimes, a drop in blood pressure after administration of a narcotic can even be a good thing if it alerts the physician to an underlying hypovolemia that should be treated more aggressively.

If hypothermia is present initially, it should be corrected; if it is not present initially, it should not be allowed to develop. Hypothermia slows metabolic processes. In some situations (e.g., cold-water drowning), this may be beneficial to a degree. In the majority of cases, however, it is better for the patient to have a normal body temperature, normal myocardial contractility, and intact coagulatory and immune function. The patient must be unclothed during the initial evaluation, but after that, he or she should be covered, especially the head (a potential source of major heat loss). The room should be kept warm, and any fluids administered should be prewarmed either in an oven or with heating devices.

A low arterial pH should be brought up to a 7.20 by means of either modest degrees of hyperventilation or administration of bicarbonate. Attempts to achieve higher values, at least in the initial shock setting, are probably counterproductive. As noted [see Fluid Administration, above], moderate acidemia may enhance myocardial contractility and immune function. Ideally, acidemia is corrected by treating the underlying cause of shock. Administration of bicarbonate should be kept to a minimum.

Coagulopathy should be treated with fresh frozen plasma and platelets [see 1:4 Bleeding and Transfusion]. The decision to use these components should be based on observation of bleeding and clotting in the patient, not on laboratory measurements of coagulation or platelet counts, which can be normal even during exsanguination.

INFLAMMATORY SHOCK

For the most part, initial treatment of inflammatory shock is similar to that of hypovolemic shock because the most pronounced feature of inflammatory shock is loss of plasma into the interstitium through a permeable microvasculature, leading to depletion of vascular volume. The main difference between treatment of hypovolemic shock and treatment of inflammatory shock has to do with when the underlying cause of the shock state should be treated. With hemorrhagic shock, the first priority is control of bleeding. With inflammatory shock, the

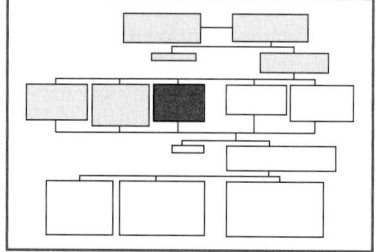

first priority is replenishment of vascular volume, and definitive treatment (e.g., debridement of dead tissue, drainage of pus, or diversion of the GI tract) should be postponed until the patient is at least partially resuscitated. Such definitive procedures can impose a major physiologic burden on the patient; thus, it is usually best to wait until the patient can withstand the operative insult.

Other potential differences between treatment of inflammatory shock and treatment of hypovolemic shock have to do with the replenishment of depleted compensatory factors and with the use of blockers of inflammatory mediators. A 2001 study suggested that infusion of activated protein C might well be lifesaving for some patients with the septic response.[26] To date, however, studies using blockers of inflammatory mediators to treat inflammatory shock have yielded disappointing results.[27,28]

NEUROGENIC SHOCK

Initial management of neurogenic shock is similar to that of hypovolemic shock, with two exceptions. First, patients in neurogenic shock often benefit from being placed in the Trendelenburg position. Autonomic

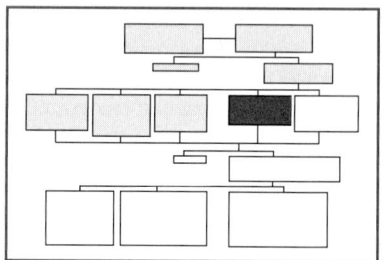

denervation of the systemic venules and small veins leads to pooling of blood in these capacitance vessels. The Trendelenburg position causes this blood to be translocated to the vascular structures in the chest, including the heart, thereby helping to restore ventricular end-diastolic volumes. Patients with other forms of shock, however, derive no benefit from the Trendelenburg position. In hypovolemic shock, for example, the systemic venules and small veins are already depleted of their blood, as a consequence of both volume loss and adrenergic constriction of the vessel walls. Thus, no blood can be translocated. Furthermore, the left ventricle must pump its blood uphill to perfuse the abdominal viscera and the lower extremities, and the increased work can exhaust an overworked heart.[29]

Second, patients in neurogenic shock often benefit from the use of vasoconstrictors. Vasoconstrictors play no role in the initial management of hypovolemic or inflammatory shock. In these forms of shock, fluid replenishment is a crucial initial measure, and constrictors can be deadly in these settings because they can shut off residual flow to organs already rendered ischemic by depletion of the vascular volume. In neurogenic shock, however, the arterioles are fully dilated in the denervated parts of the body, and this dilatation can lead to central hypotension and inadequate perfusion of the brain and heart. Vasoconstrictors constrict the denervated arterioles, thereby helping to restore central pressures. They also constrict denervated systemic venules and small veins, thereby helping to restore ventricular end-diastolic volumes.

If the heart rate is slow, as it may be if denervation extends high enough to block the sympathetic nerves going to the heart, dopamine (2 to 20 μg/kg/min) may be used. If the heart rate is rapid, norepinephrine or phenylephrine is a good choice. Norepinephrine is given by continuous infusion at a dosage of 4 to 12 μg/min; phenylephrine is initially given at a dosage of 100 to 180 μg/min, which is then decreased to 40 to 60 μg/min.

The danger in giving a vasoconstrictor to a patient in neurogenic shock is that the underlying cause of shock may also have caused occult bleeding. Thus, the vasoconstrictor may maintain the blood pressure, reassuring the physician while the patient bleeds to death. Vasoconstrictors should be used in patients in neurogenic shock only after it has been established that the shock state has no hypovolemic component.

CARDIOGENIC SHOCK

In most cases of cardiogenic shock, management begins with diuresis rather than fluid administration. Furosemide (10 to 40 mg I.V. over a period of 2 to 5 minutes) is a good first choice. If the patient

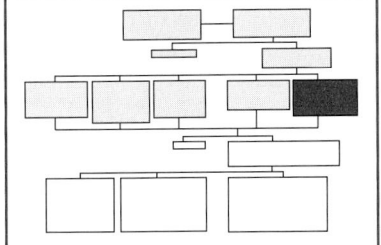

has been receiving furosemide for an extended period, high dosages may be necessary, or spironolactone (25 to 200 mg orally) may have to be added.

Hypertension, if present, may be treated in several ways, depending on the conditions observed. Morphine sulfate (1 to 6 mg I.V. every 1 to 4 hours) is a good first choice if the patient is in pain from an MI and if the physical examination and the chest x-ray indicate pulmonary edema. Nitroglycerine is a good choice if the patient is experiencing angina. It should initially be given I.V. at a dosage of 5 µg/min, which may then be raised in increments of 5 µg/min every 5 minutes. When the dosage reaches 20 µg/min, it may then be raised in increments of 10 µg/min to a maximum dosage of 200 µg/min. Nitroprusside is effective under any conditions. It should initially be given at a dosage of 0.5 µg/kg/min, which may then be raised in increments of 0.5 µg/kg/min to a maximum dosage of 3 µg/kg/min. An angiotensin-converting enzyme (ACE) inhibitor (e.g., enalaprilat, 1.25 to 5.0 mg every 6 hours) is a good choice if the patient's renal function is not compromised and if time is not critical. Sometimes, all of these drugs can be used.

As a rule, hydralazine should not be used; it can increase the heart rate and can markedly increase myocardial oxygen requirements. Calcium channel blockers should be given only after other approaches have failed; they can reduce myocardial oxygen requirements but at the cost of a substantially decreased cardiac output. Nitroprusside and ACE inhibitors generally do not reduce cardiac output, nor, in patients with large ventricular end-diastolic volumes, do morphine and nitroglycerine.

Beta blockade can be extremely effective in controlling blood pressure in a hypertensive patient and heart rate in any patient. Esmolol, a short-acting agent, is the best first choice. A loading dose of 500 µg/kg is given, followed by infusion at a rate of 50 µg/kg/min. If it proves necessary to increase the dosage, another 500 µg/kg loading dose is given, and the infusion rate is raised to 100 µg/kg/min. If the patient responds well to this regimen, he or she should be switched from esmolol to the long-acting agent metoprolol (5 to 15 mg every 6 hours).

Beta blockers can reduce cardiac output, but they also markedly reduce myocardial oxygen requirements by decreasing heart rate, blood pressure, stroke volume, and myocardial contractility. These agents should not be given to patients who are hypotensive or show signs of marked peripheral hypoperfusion, but they should be given to all other patients in whom myocardial ischemia is a possibility.

In many patients with acute myocardial ischemia and shock, all of the aforementioned treatments should be employed, with the addition of heparin anticoagulation and emergency coronary angiography. The mortality associated with cardiogenic shock in a patient with an acute MI is extremely high. Accordingly, every effort should be made to find a correctable lesion and treat it with coronary angioplasty, stenting, or surgical revascularization. If necessary, an intra-aortic balloon pump may be placed once angiography, angioplasty, and stenting have been completed or in preparation for surgical correction of ischemia.

The hemoglobin concentration in patients with cardiogenic shock should be maintained at a generous level (i.e., about 11 g/dl).

Treatment of Shock That Persists Despite Initial Management

INVASIVE MONITORING

In most cases of shock, regardless of category, the initial approach just described leads to resolution

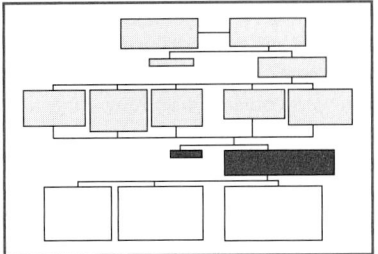

of all the clinical abnormalities. Some patients, however, do not respond to these treatment measures. In my view, invasive monitoring is warranted for these unresponsive patients.

Invasive monitoring permits direct assessment of patients' thermodynamic needs, thus allowing the physician to deal with the most difficult problem in managing unresponsive shock patients—namely, how to balance the metabolic needs of the noncardiac tissues against the demands made on a potentially ischemic myocardium. Almost all interventions that increase perfusion of the peripheral tissues also increase myocardial oxygen requirements, and almost all interventions that decrease myocardial oxygen requirements also decrease perfusion of noncardiac tissues [see Sidebar Thermodynamic Concepts of Clinical Relevance to Shock].[30,31]

GOALS OF RESUSCITATION

The primary goal of shock management is to correct the clinical abnormalities that led to the diagnosis in the first place. The secondary goal is to enable the patient to generate adequate blood pressure and cardiac output—that is, adequate power [see Table 4]—for perfusion of the tissues without overburdening the heart.

Determining what constitutes adequate blood pressure can be difficult at times. The pressure must be, at the very least, high enough to perfuse the brain, an organ that has a very active metabolic rate and very little vascular tone. Drops in blood pressure put the brain at risk because, unlike all the other organs in the body, it is unable to vasodilate in response to falling perfusion pressure. In an alert patient, determining adequate blood pressure is not difficult. In an obtunded patient, an arbitrary value must be assigned; a reasonable systolic pressure might be 90 mm Hg in a younger patient and somewhat higher in an older patient. Carotid stenosis necessitates a higher pressure, and stenoses in any of the arteries supplying actively metabolizing organs call for higher central pressures.

Although, under ordinary circumstances, all noncerebral organs have some tonic contracture of the arterioles that allows vasodilatation if pressure falls, the arterioles in an organ made ischemic by proximal obstruction and active metabolism are maximally dilated; the organ therefore becomes vulnerable to hypotension. The classic example of this phenomenon is the heart in a patient with coronary disease, but the same mechanism comes into play in the gut in a patient with mesenteric arterial occlusive disease, in the kidney in a patient with renal artery stenosis, in the spinal cord in a patient with obstructed intercostal arteries, and in the extremities in a patient with peripheral arterial disease.

In sum, the only way of setting the goal for adequate blood pressure is to combine clinical judgment with assessment of the patient's response to treatment. If a given blood pressure is associated with an altered level of consciousness, myocardial ischemia, oliguria, or any other sign suggesting inadequate flow, it must be increased.

Although there is general agreement on how to set goals for adequate blood pressure, there is little agreement on how to set goals for optimum cardiac output. One approach is to attempt to determine whether the patient's oxygen consumption (measured with a pulmonary arterial catheter and based in part on measurements of cardiac output) is dependent on oxygen delivery (the product of cardiac output, hemoglobin concentration, and arterial oxygen saturation). At very low levels of oxygen delivery, there is no question that oxygen consumption must decrease.[32] At excessively high levels, however, oxygen consumption may continue to rise if oxygen delivery is increased by the administration of inotropes. These agents usually have beta-adrenergic effects and can increase peripheral oxygen metabolism; they also increase myocardial oxygen requirements. Thus, the act of increasing delivery can increase peripheral consumption.

Another approach is to maintain all patients at very high levels of oxygen delivery without making any attempt to see if there is a correlation between delivery and peripheral consumption. This proposed approach was examined in randomized trials in critically ill patients, which found that maintaining supranormal levels of oxygen delivery was of no benefit.[33-36]

A third approach is to use mixed venous oxygen saturation (also measured with a pulmonary arterial catheter) as a primary end point in resuscitation. This approach has the advantage of simplicity and is certainly useful with some forms of shock (e.g., hypovolemic

---

Table 4 Different Forms of Power Generated in the Cardiovascular System

Form of Power	Formula
Power delivered into aortic root each minute	SV·HR·LVESP
Power generated by left atrium	SV·HR·LAP
Power generated by left ventricle	SV·HR·(LVESP-LAP)
Mean power delivered into aortic root	SV·HR·MAP
Oscillatory power delivered into aortic root	SV·HR·(LVESP-MAP)
Power used to perfuse peripheral tissues	SV·HR·(MAP-RAP)
Power used to fill right atrium	SV·HR·RAP

Note: see 6:4 Cardiopulmonary Monitoring.
HR—heart rate   LAP— mean left atrial pressure   LVESP—left ventricular end-systolic pressure   MAP—mean arterial pressure (equivalent to mean aortic root pressure)   RAP—mean right atrial pressure   SV—stroke volume

---

shock). Many patients in inflammatory shock, however, have quite high mixed venous oxygen saturations, partly because of peripheral shunting through the cutaneous vasculature and partly because of functional shunting by cells that cannot metabolize the oxygen presented to them. In these patients, a high mixed venous oxygen saturation might even indicate a severe metabolic derangement rather than resolution of shock.[34]

Yet another resuscitation approach is to avoid using any direct measurement of cardiovascular adequacy and to use other end points of resuscitation instead. Perhaps the most attractive such end point is gastric mucosal pH. In many forms of shock, the gut is quickly made ischemic; conceivably, if the gut mucosa can be shown to be well perfused, one can assume that the rest of the body is also well perfused. Further trials are necessary to ascertain whether gastric mucosal pH can be used in lieu of detailed measurements of cardiac performance.[37]

Thermodynamic principles may also be employed to set resuscitation end points. Such an approach implies that cardiac output itself should be used in conjunction with blood pressure to assess adequacy of resuscitation. Recent work by Chang and associates suggests that a normal cardiac output is probably an adequate one.[38,39] One might wish to aim for slightly supranormal values in patients with major injuries or overwhelming infections, but excessively high values should rarely be necessary.

To define what a normal cardiac output is, one must take some account of patient size, expressed in terms either of body weight (ideal, current, or premorbid) or of body surface area (which in turn is calculated in part on the basis of weight). I prefer to use ideal body weight in the calculations rather than current body weight or premorbid weight. Ideal body weight is calculated on the basis of the patient's height, with adjustments made for age, on the assumption that ideal weight in an unconditioned older individual decreases by 10% each decade after 50 years of age. The age adjustment can have a substantial effect on the calculation. For example, a patient who is 80 years old—not an uncommon age for an ICU patient today—might have had an ideal body weight of 70 kg at age 50. At 80 years of age, if the patient is not in good condition, ideal body weight will have fallen to 51 kg. This makes a significant difference in terms of target cardiac output: whereas a cardiac output of 7 L/min might have been required when the patient was 50 years old, an output of 5 L/min is probably more than adequate 30 years later. Finally, the choice of a goal for cardiac output is sometimes facilitated by trial and error. For example, if a supranormal cardiac output causes an abnormality (e.g., metabolic acidemia) to resolve when a normal output did not, then an effort should be made to keep the output high for a while.

Thermodynamic Concepts of Clinical Relevance to Shock

In my view, treatment of shock is best approached with an eye to the thermodynamics of cardiovascular function. Thermodynamics is the scientific discipline developed in the 19th century to explain the generation and transfer of energy, including power and heat, between systems. For the purposes of this chapter, an exhaustive familiarity with thermodynamic principles is unnecessary; however, there are a few thermodynamic concepts of direct clinical relevance that are worth outlining here. These concepts become increasingly pertinent as one moves from easily managed patients to more challenging ones.

A key concept is that of power. Power, in thermodynamic terms, is flow multiplied by pressure [see Table 4]. In the case of the heart, the power generated by the left atrium and the left ventricle (and consequently the power delivered into the aortic root) is approximately equal to cardiac output multiplied by left ventricular end-systolic pressure (LVESP):

Power into aortic root = SV·HR·LVESP

where cardiac output is expressed as the product of stroke volume (SV) and heart rate (HR).

The main challenge in treating the patient in shock is to balance the needs of the peripheral circulation against the demands made on the heart. Left ventricular oxygen requirements are directly proportional to left ventricular power: doubling power doubles oxygen requirements. The significance of this relation in the management of shock will be apparent from an examination of the formulas for left ventricular power and power for peripheral tissue perfusion:

Left ventricular power = SV·HR·(LVESP-LAP)

Power for peripheral perfusion = SV·HR·(MAP-RAP)

where LAP is mean left atrial pressure, MAP is mean arterial pressure (which is equivalent to mean aortic root pressure), and RAP is mean right atrial pressure.

From these formulas, it is clear that any therapy that increases SV or HR will increase both power for peripheral perfusion and left ventricular power (and thus left ventricular oxygen requirements). Any therapy that increases MAP will increase power for peripheral perfusion and usually will increase ventricular oxygen requirements because LVESP generally rises when MAP rises. Finally, any therapy that decreases RAP will increase power for peripheral perfusion and usually will increase left ventricular oxygen requirements because LAP generally falls when RAP falls. Thus, in increasing power for perfusion of the peripheral tissues, one almost always increases left ventricular oxygen requirements as well. In other words, there is no thermodynamic free lunch.

Thus, the end points of shock management are for the most part clinical end points—namely, reversal of cutaneous signs of shock, hypotension, mental abnormalities, myocardial ischemia, metabolic acidemia, hypoxemia, and heart rate abnormalities. If these end points cannot be reached initially, the goal should then be to reach thermodynamic end points—that is, adequate pressures and adequate flow (power [*see Table 4*])—while trying to minimize myocardial oxygen requirements. This is the main challenge in resuscitating a patient from shock. As a rule, increasing the heart rate, end-diastolic volumes, contractility, and the hindrance against which the ventricles contract (up to a limit) all increase the power output of the heart; they also all increase myocardiac oxygen requirements. Incorporating a thermodynamic perspective into management brings this problem into the open.

Depending on the resuscitative priorities in a given patient, one of the following three hemodynamic goals is generally appropriate:

1. Increased provision of nutrients to noncardiac tissues along with robust amounts of energy, even though production of that energy by the heart puts a strain on the myocardium.
2. Decreased demands on the heart, even though, as a consequence, less energy will be available for perfusion of noncardiac tissues.
3. A balance between (1) and (2), aimed at achieving the most efficient possible production of energy by the heart while admitting the possibility that a compromise between the two might end up achieving neither.

An example of a patient for whom the first goal might be appropriate is a young trauma patient with a robust myocardium but extensive noncardiac injuries. The second goal might be appropriate for a patient with an uncomplicated MI. The third goal might be appropriate for a patient with known coronary artery disease who has just undergone resection of a ruptured abdominal aortic aneurysm.

ASSESSMENT OF RELATIVE PRIORITIES OF PERIPHERY AND HEART

The next task in the management of unresponsive shock states is to determine whether priority should be given to the needs of the periphery or to those of the heart. The difficulty here is that many of the patients who have reached this stage of treatment—that is, in whom initial therapeutic measures have been unsuccessful—have both cardiac and noncardiac problems. Management of these patients is a challenge.

Periphery Is Priority

Fluid administration and assessment of ventricular end-diastolic volumes If priority is given to the periphery, the patient will probably require fluids. As a starting point, the goal should be to achieve a pul- 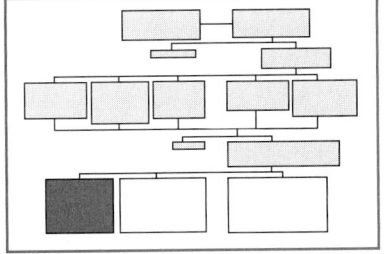 monary arterial wedge pressure in the midteens (assuming that the patient is being mechanically ventilated). As therapy progresses and as more measurements are made, this goal may have to be modified. The ultimate goal, however, is not to produce any specific wedge pressure but rather to produce generous right and left ventricular end-diastolic volumes.[40] To estimate these volumes, it is necessary to synthesize several pieces of information.

Intracavitary right atrial pressure (a commonly measured value obtained via the proximal port of a pulmonary arterial catheter)

yields a good estimate of intracavitary right ventricular end-diastolic pressure. Pulmonary arterial wedge pressure is equivalent to intracavitary left atrial pressure (which, in the absence of mitral valvular stenosis, is the same as left ventricular end-diastolic pressure) if there is an open column of blood when the balloon is inflated between the end of the catheter and the left atrium. This open communication between the catheter tip and the atrium is usually present because the catheter, once inserted, is directed by flow into the well-perfused parts of the pulmonary vasculature. On occasion, however, the catheter ends up in a poorly perfused part of the lung (zone I), in which case it measures intra-alveolar pressure instead of left atrial pressure. This malpositioning is usually signaled by excessive swings in wedge pressure that coincide with the cycling of the ventilator. In theory, inaccuracies can creep into pressure measurements if there is robust collateral flow around the vasculature occluded by the balloon, as with the bronchial circulation. In practice, however, this is seldom a problem.

Given acceptably accurate intracavitary end-diastolic pressure values, the challenge is to extrapolate from these values to reasonably good estimates of ventricular end-diastolic volume. There is not a simple proportional correspondence between pressure and volume, because volume depends not only on pressure but also on the stiffness of the ventricle during diastole and on the stiffness of the structures surrounding the heart.[41-43]

In a patient breathing spontaneously, a right atrial pressure of 2 to 5 mm Hg measured with respect to atmosphere with the transducer zeroed at the midaxillary line is generally sufficient to generate an adequate right ventricular end-diastolic volume. For the left ventricle, a wedge pressure of 5 to 8 mm Hg usually suffices. In a patient with compression of the heart as a result of inflation of the lungs by positive pressure ventilation, an intracavitary right atrial (or right ventricular end-diastolic) pressure of 9 to 12 mm Hg is usually necessary for a normal right ventricular end-diastolic volume; a wedge pressure of 12 to 15 mm Hg is usually necessary for a normal left ventricular end-diastolic volume.

These values work for patients with essentially normal lungs; however, most patients on mechanical ventilators do not have normal lungs. In such patients, the lungs can form a stiff compartment around the heart that does not give when the heart is pushed into the compartment by an elevated diaphragm. To complicate matters further, the diastolic stiffness of the ventricular musculature is increased in many critically ill patients, and the intracavitary pressures must overcome this added stiffness as well. On occasion, right and left intracavitary ventricular end-diastolic pressures exceeding 20 mm Hg are necessary to produce normal end-diastolic volumes.

The estimates of end-diastolic pressure can sometimes be confirmed by increasing the filling pressures of the heart with a fluid bolus and assessing the cardiovascular response. Increases in stroke volume, especially if associated with increases in pulmonary and systemic arterial pressures, suggest that the initial end-diastolic volumes were too small and that more fluid is needed. In other cases, initial end-diastolic volumes might have been unnecessarily large. If so, a diuretic can be given. If stroke volumes and blood pressures do not decrease, further diuresis is indicated.

Right ventricular end-diastolic volume can be measured directly by means of a pulmonary arterial catheter equipped with a fast-response thermistor. These catheters are more expensive than those not so equipped, but they can be helpful in complicated cases.[44] Left ventricular end-diastolic volume can be measured directly with transesophageal echocardiography in difficult cases (e.g., a patient with an elevated diaphragm).

If measurements are available from only one ventricle, the physician can cautiously use this information to estimate the corresponding values from the other, keeping in mind that in many critically ill patients, there is a marked discrepancy between right and left ventricular end-diastolic volumes. The general finding from studies comparing right ventricular end-diastolic volumes (measured with a fast thermistor) and left ventricular end-diastolic volumes (measured with transesophageal echocardiography) is that right ventricular values are frequently larger than left ventricular values in patients in inflammatory shock, sometimes by a factor of 3.[45] In patients with left-sided congestive heart failure, however, left ventricular end-diastolic volumes can be substantially larger than right. Thus, knowing the volume of one chamber does not necessarily mean that one knows the volume of the other, but the clinical scenario can provide some guidance.

Inotropes   Inotropes such as dobutamine (5 to 15 µg/kg/min) and milrinone (50 µg, then 0.375 to 0.75 µg/kg/min) can be given freely. They will increase myocardial oxygen requirements, but this is not a problem in a patient with a strong heart. The only limitation on use of the inotropes is the development of a tachycardia. If the heart rate begins to exceed 100 beats/min, the dosage should be reduced.

Vasoconstrictors   There are only three indications for administration of vasoconstrictors to patients in whom the primary concern is perfusion of the periphery: (1) profound hypotension in a patient who is in neurogenic shock; (2) hypotension so severe that cerebral or spinal cord perfusion is thought to be inadequate on the basis of either neurologic symptoms (if the patient is neurologically intact) or cerebral perfusion pressure (if the patient is not neurologically intact); and (3) hypotension in a patient who has critical stenosis in the cerebral, coronary, mesenteric, or renal arteries or in the arteries supplying the spinal cord or who has a severely ischemic extremity. For virtually all other patients whose main problem is inadequate perfusion of the periphery, fluids and, occasionally, inotropes are enough.

If a vasoconstrictor is indicated, dopamine may be given if the initial heart rate is 90 beats/min or slower. The heart rate should not be driven above 100 beat/min. Norepinephrine may be given if the initial heart rate exceeds 90 beats/min.

Periphery and Heart Are Equal Priorities

Fluid management in patients who have both inadequate peripheral perfusion and marginal myocardial reserve must be finely tuned. Every effort should be made to estimate the ventricular

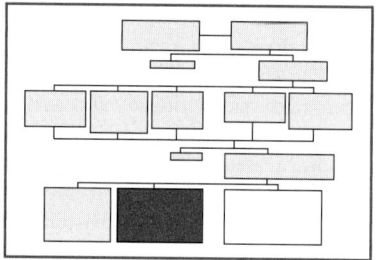

end-diastolic volumes accurately. Excessively large end-diastolic volumes will increase myocardial oxygen requirements unnecessarily, and inadequate end-diastolic volumes will make it impossible for the ventricles to produce adequate pressure and stroke volumes. In some patients, diuresis is indicated; in others, administration of fluids. Frequently, trial and error will be necessary.

If pressures and stroke volumes are still inadequate after fluids have been replenished, inotropes should be tried. These agents must be used with some caution because they will increase myocardial oxygen requirements.

Vasoconstrictors should be used only as previously discussed [*see* Periphery Is Priority, *above*]. Dopamine may be given if the initial heart rate is 70 beats/min or slower. The heart rate should not be driven above 90 beats/min. Norepinephrine may be given if the heart rate exceeds 70 beats/min.

Beta blockade is frequently necessary when the heart rate exceeds 90 beats/min. Maintenance of a slow heart rate is the single most important factor in minimizing myocardial oxygen requirements, but it usually can be achieved only at the cost of decreasing pressures and stroke volumes. Esmolol is a good first choice because it is quickly reversible; metoprolol may be given later if it is clear that beta blockade was needed and the patient is stable.

Heart Is Priority

If the priority is the heart and there is comparatively little reason for concern about noncardiac tissues, treatment is usually straightforward, though the results may be less than might be hoped for. The treatment approach should be patterned on that for cardiogenic shock (see

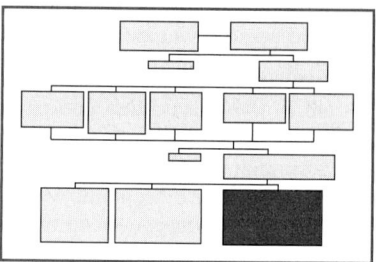

above). Invasive monitoring allows precise measurements that can be useful, particularly during diuresis. The goal of diuresis is to produce normal ventricular end-diastolic volumes so as to minimize myocardial oxygen requirements. Often, this proves impossible. Larger end-diastolic volumes are necessary to make up for poor contractility. Invasive monitoring helps the physician strike the necessary balance. Vasoconstrictors and inotropes should not be used, because they will increase myocardial oxygen requirements. If blood pressure or stroke volumes become inadequate, the therapeutic approach should be changed to take the needs of the periphery into account as described earlier [*see* Periphery and Heart Are Equal Priorities, *above*].

References

1. Demetriades D, Chan LS, Bhasin P, et al: Relative bradycardia in patients with traumatic hypotension. J Trauma 45:534, 1998

2. Little RA: 1988 Fitts Lecture: heart rate changes after haemorrhage and injury—a reappraisal. J Trauma 29:903, 1989

3. Shenkin HA, Cheney RH, Govons SR, et al: On the diagnosis of hemorrhage in man: a study of volunteers bled large amounts. Am J Med Sci 208:421, 1944

4. Gore DC, Ferrando A, Barnett J, et al: Influence of glucose kinetics on plasma lactate concentration and energy expenditure in severely burned patients. J Trauma 49:673, 2000

5. Gausche M, Lewis RJ, Stratton SJ, et al: Effect of out-of-hospital pediatric endotracheal intubation on survival and neurological outcome: a controlled clinical trial. JAMA 283:783, 2000

6. Chang MC, Miller PR, D'Agostino R, et al: Effects of abdominal decompression on cardiopulmonary function and visceral perfusion in patients with intra-abdominal hypertension. J Trauma 44:440, 1998

7. Ventilation with lower tidal volumes as compared with traditional tidal volumes for acute lung injury and the acute respiratory distress syndrome. Acute Respiratory Distress Syndrome Network. N Engl J Med 342:1301, 2000

8. Amato MBP, Barbas CSV, Medeiros DM, et al: Effect of a protective-ventilation strategy on mortality in the acute respiratory distress syndrome. N Engl J Med 338:347, 1998

9. Bulger EM, Jurkovich GJ, Gentilello LM, et al: Current clinical options for the treatment and management of acute respiratory distress syndrome. J Trauma 48:562, 2000

10. Ranieri VM, Suter PM, Tortorella C, et al: Effect of mechanical ventilation on inflammatory mediators in patients with acute respiratory distress syndrome: a randomized controlled trial. JAMA 282:54, 1999

11. Rankin JS, Olsen CO, Arentzen CE, et al: The effects

of airway pressure on cardiac function in intact dogs and man. Circulation 66:108, 1982

12. Sawyer RW, Bodai BI, Blaisdell FW, et al: The current status of intraosseous infusion. J Am Coll Surg 179: 353, 1994

13. Waisman M, Waisman D: Bone marrow infusion in adults. J Trauma 42:288, 1997

14. Wilmore DW: Metabolic response to severe surgical illness: overview. World J Surg 24:705, 2000

15. Angle N, Hoyt DB, Coimbra R, et al: Hypertonic saline resuscitation diminishes lung injury by suppressing neutrophil activation after hemorrhagic shock. Shock 9:164, 1998

16. Ciesla DJ, Moore EE, Zallen G, et al: Hypertonic saline attenuation of polymorphonuclear neutrophil cytotoxicity: timing is everything. J Trauma 48:388, 2000

17. Ho HS, Liu H, Cala PM, et al: Hypertonic perfusion inhibits intracellular Na and Ca accumulation in hypoxic myocardium. Am J Physiol Cell Physiol 278: C953, 2000

18. Rotstein OD: Novel strategies for immunomodulation after trauma: revisiting hypertonic saline as a resuscitation strategy for hemorrhagic shock. J Trauma 49:580, 2000

19. Vassar MJ, Fischer RP, O'Brien PE, et al: A multicenter trial for resuscitation of injured patients with 7.5% sodium chloride. Arch Surg 128:1003, 1993

20. Velasco IT, Pontieri V, Rocha e Silva M, et al: Hyperosmotic NaCl and severe hemorrhagic shock. Am J Physiol 239:H664, 1980

21. Wade CE, Grady JJ, Kramer GC, et al: Individual patient cohort analysis of the efficacy of hypertonic saline/dextran in patients with traumatic brain injury and hypotension. J Trauma 42:S61, 1997

22. Human albumin administration in critically ill patients: systematic review of randomised controlled trials. Cochrane Injuries Group Albumin Reviewers. BMJ 317:235, 1998

23. Hébert PC, Wells G, Blajchman MA, et al: A multicenter, randomized, controlled clinical trial of transfusion requirements in critical care. N Engl J Med 340: 409, 1999

24. Cohn SM: Surgical research review: blood substitutes in surgery. Surgery 127:599, 2000

25. Sloan EP, Koenigsberg M, Gens D, et al: Diaspirin cross-linked hemoglobin (DCLHb) in the treatment of severe traumatic hemorrhagic shock: a randomized controlled efficacy trial. JAMA 282:1857, 1999

26. Bernard GR, Vincent JL, Laterre PF, et al: Efficacy and safety of recombinant human activated protein C for severe sepsis. N Engl J Med 344:699, 2001

27. Angus DC, Birmingham MC, Balk RA, et al: E5 murine monoclonal antiendotoxin antibody in gram-negative sepsis: a randomized controlled trial. JAMA 283:1723, 2000

28. Ketoconazole for early treatment of acute lung injury and acute respiratory distress syndrome: a randomized controlled trial. ARDS Network Authors. JAMA 283: 1995, 2000

29. Sibbald WJ, Paterson NAM, Holliday RL, et al: The Trendelenburg position: hemodynamic effects in hypotensive and normotensive patients. Crit Care Med 7:218, 1979

30. McDonald's Blood Flow in Arteries: Theoretical, Experimental and Clinical Principles, 4th ed. Nichols WW, O'Rourke MF, Eds. Arnold and Oxford University Press, London and New York, 1998

31. Suga H: Ventricular energetics. Physiol Rev 70:247, 1990

32. Cain SM: Oxygen delivery and uptake in dogs during anemic and hypoxic hypoxia. J Appl Physiol 42:228, 1977

33. Durham RM, Neunaber K, Mazuski JE, et al: The use of oxygen consumption and delivery as endpoints for resuscitation in critically ill patients. J Trauma 41:32, 1996

34. Gattinoni L, Brazzi L, Pelosi P, et al: A trial of goal-oriented hemodynamic therapy in critically ill patients. N Engl J Med 333:1025, 1995

35. Hayes MA, Timmins AC, Yau EHS, et al: Elevation of systemic oxygen delivery in the treatment of critically ill patients. N Engl J Med 330:1717, 1994

36. Velmahos GC, Demetriades D, Shoemaker WC, et al: Endpoints of resuscitation of critically injured patients: normal or supranormal? A prospective randomized trial. Ann Surg 232:409, 2000

37. Ivatury RR, Simon RJ, Islam S, et al: A prospective randomized study of end points of resuscitation after major trauma: global oxygen transport indices versus organ-specific gastric mucosal pH. J Am Coll Surg 183:145, 1996

38. Chang MC, Meredith JW, Kincaid EH, et al: Maintaining survivors' values of left ventricular power output during shock resuscitation: a prospective pilot study. J Trauma 49:26, 2000

39. Chang MC, Mondy JS, Meredith JW, et al: Redefining cardiovascular performance during resuscitation: ventricular stroke work, power, and the pressure-volume diagram. J Trauma 45:470, 1998

40. Miller PR, Meredith JW, Chang MC: Randomized, prospective comparison of increased preload versus inotropes in the resuscitation of trauma patients: effects on cardiopulmonary function and visceral perfusion. J Trauma 44:107, 1998

41. Grossman W: Diastolic dysfunction in congestive heart failure. N Engl J Med 325:1557, 1991

42. Hess OM, Osakada G, Lavelle JF, et al: Diastolic myocardial wall stiffness and ventricular relaxation during partial and complete coronary occlusions in the conscious dog. Circ Res 52:387, 1983

43. Isoyama S, Apstein CS, Wexler LF, et al: Acute decrease in left ventricular diastolic chamber distensibility during simulated angina in isolated hearts. Circ Res 61:925, 1987

44. Chang MC, Blinman TA, Rutherford EJ, et al: Preload assessment in trauma patients during large volume shock resuscitation. Arch Surg 131:728, 1996

45. Kraut EJ, Owings JT, Anderson JT, et al: Right ventricular volumes overestimate left ventricular preload in critically ill patients. J Trauma 42:839, 1997

46. Perdue PW, Balser JR, Lipsett PA, et al: "Renal dose" dopamine in surgical patients: dogma or science? Ann Surg 227:470, 1998

4 CARDIOPULMONARY MONITORING

James W. Holcroft, M.D., F.A.C.S., and John T. Anderson, M.D., F.A.C.S.

Making and interpreting measurements of cardiopulmonary function in critically ill patients can be a challenge, for a number of reasons. Invasive monitoring, which is still necessary for many of the measurements, can give rise to complications. Differences among the ICU personnel who make the measurements can raise concerns about accuracy. The patient care decisions that are based on the measurements often must be made quickly, with little time available for on-the-spot cogitation. Finally, the measurements, and the descriptors of cardiopulmonary function derived from them, often are quite abstract and must be interpreted mathematically. Moreover, the measurements are frequently indirect, involving surrogate variables. Extrapolating from the surrogate measurement back to the primary parameter of interest can be a very involved process.

All of these problems can contribute to misinterpretation of the measurements. Incorrect interpretations can lead to incorrect conclusions; incorrect conclusions can lead to death. Our aim in what follows is to describe the technology and reasoning behind measurements of cardiopulmonary function in critically ill surgical patients and to outline ways of interpreting these measurements more accurately and using them more effectively.

Systemic Arterial Pressures

Systemic arterial pressures can be measured in the aortic root via an indwelling central arterial catheter, but this approach is risky. Extremity arteries are used instead. The radial artery is usually accessible, and the risk of cannulation and maintenance of an indwelling catheter in this vessel is acceptable.[1,2] Other arteries (e.g., the brachial artery and the major leg arteries) lend themselves well to measurement of pressure with a cuff.

NONINVASIVE MEASUREMENT TECHNIQUES

In the cuff technique, a blood pressure cuff is applied around the extremity and artery of interest, and a reference point is selected for the pressure measurement. The point is arbitrary, but most physicians use the right atrium. If the patient is supine, the point is taken as the midaxillary line; if upright, the point is taken as the fifth intercostal space in the midaxillary line.[3] The cuff is inflated to a pressure that eliminates flow in the underlying artery (e.g., as determined by obliteration of a distal palpable pulse), then gradually deflated while one listens with a stethoscope over the artery at the distal edge of the cuff. When cuff pressure falls below systolic pressure, blood begins to flow again through the artery. Because the artery is still partially compressed, arterial blood flow is turbulent and thus creates sound that is audible through the stethoscope. The pressure in the cuff at the point where this sound first becomes audible is taken to be the peak systolic pressure in the artery encompassed by the cuff.[4,5]

As deflation continues and the pressure in the cuff falls to levels between the peak systolic pressure and the nadir of the diastolic pressure, the artery becomes less compressed, but some compression remains. Thus, some degree of turbulence and sound remain as well, though their characteristics change. When the pressure in the cuff falls below the nadir of the diastolic pressure in the artery, the vessel becomes widely patent, and turbulence and sound vanish. The pressure in the cuff at the point where sound disappears is taken to be the nadir of the diastolic pressure in the artery.[4]

Various techniques can be used with the cuff technique to detect distal flow. The pressure in the cuff at the point where flow begins to appear distally is taken to be the systolic pressure in the artery. A distal artery can be interrogated with a Doppler device, which picks up movement of individual red blood cells in the vessel; the absence of such movement implies no arterial flow. Arterial flow can also be detected by assessing pulsatility of perfusion in the tip of a digit and can be evaluated by means of photoplethysmography.[6] One can even measure volume changes in the distal portion of the extremity as the heart beats: the limb will expand during systole, as blood is forced into the arteries and veins, and shrink during diastole, as blood runs out of the vessels. This concept can be used to measure arterial pressure waveforms in the finger. Pressure in a cuff around the finger is regulated to maintain a constant blood volume in the finger; the pressure waveform required to accomplish this reflects the finger arterial pressure waveform.[7]

Sphygmomanometry poses no risk to the patient, and pressures are usually easy to obtain.[8] Measured pressures can be misleading, however, in that the technique relies on the assumption that the pressures in the cuff are the same as those in the encompassed artery. This condition is usually met, except in diabetic patients with calcified arteries and obese patients, in whom the pressure in the cuff will be higher than the pressure in the artery. An additional problem arises when diastolic pressures are measured with a cuff and a stethoscope: the sounds are frequently quite soft, and in a noisy ICU, it is often hard to tell exactly when they vanish. Measurement of diastolic pressure is also difficult if the patient is in shock: flow through the brachial artery can be so minimal that very little turbulence is created and very little sound generated. Finally, only a stethoscope can be used to measure diastolic pressure. Audible Doppler signals in a distal artery change little as a proximal artery goes from partial obstruction to full patency; changes are also minimal if oximetry or sphygmomanometry is used.

Other devices that facilitate the measurement of blood pressure by cuff suffer from similar limitations. Some have Doppler probes incorporated into the cuff apparatus. These can automatically record systolic pressures but have the same limitations as handheld Doppler devices. Other automatic devices use an oscillometric method that senses pulsatility in the volume of the extremity enclosed by the cuff. The point where pulsation amplitudes are maximal corresponds to the mean arterial pressure; various algorithms are used to determine systolic and diastolic arterial pressures.[9-11] Oscillometric methods can work well in euvolemic patients but frequently fail in the presence of hypovolemia.

Thus, all of these noninvasive methods for measuring pressure have limitations: the inability to measure any pressures accurately in patients who are obese or have calcified arteries, the uncertainty associated with diastolic pressure measurements in all patients, and the difficulty of making measurements in patients in shock.

MONITORING VIA INTRA-ARTERIAL CATHETER

The limitations of noninvasive measurement techniques can be overcome by using an intra-arterial catheter. Such devices provide ready access to systemic arterial blood, though not without a degree of risk.[1,2] Catheter-related infection can occur, albeit infrequently [*see 6:15 Blood Cultures and Infection in the Patient with the Septic Response and 6:17 Nosocomial Infection*].[12] Thrombosis associated with insertion and maintenance of indwelling arterial catheters can lead to ischemia and even necrosis distal to the insertion site. Catheters should be inserted in arteries with abundant collateral circulation. The radial artery is safer to use than the brachial artery, and the dorsalis pedis artery is safer than the femoral artery. To reduce the risk of

thrombosis, we continuously infuse an isotonic solution through the catheter.[13,14] If the patient is at high risk for thrombosis, we use a dilute heparin solution for flushing, accepting a slight risk of heparin-induced thrombocytopenia; if not, we use normal saline. Flushing must be done carefully, either as a slow continuous infusion or with boluses no larger than 2 ml. Rapid infusion of large amounts of any solution can lead to retrograde flow. In the case of the radial artery, retrograde flushing can lead to embolization of platelet aggregates or air through the vertebral artery to the brain stem.

The decision to use intra-arterial monitoring rests on the potential risks and benefits. We insert arterial catheters if it appears that blood gases will have to be measured more often than three times daily. We also use them in patients who might bleed suddenly (e.g., those undergoing a major operation), patients whose blood pressure is labile (e.g., those who are in a septic state or require titration of vasoactive or cardiotonic drugs), and patients in whom management of one failing organ system might precipitate failure in another.

Once the decision is made to use intra-arterial monitoring, the artery is cannulated. A pressure transducer is calibrated, then opened to the atmosphere and zeroed at the level of the right atrium.[3] The transducer is connected to the cannula. The pressure waveform from the transducer is displayed on a monitor, along with digital readouts of the running averages (means) of the sys-

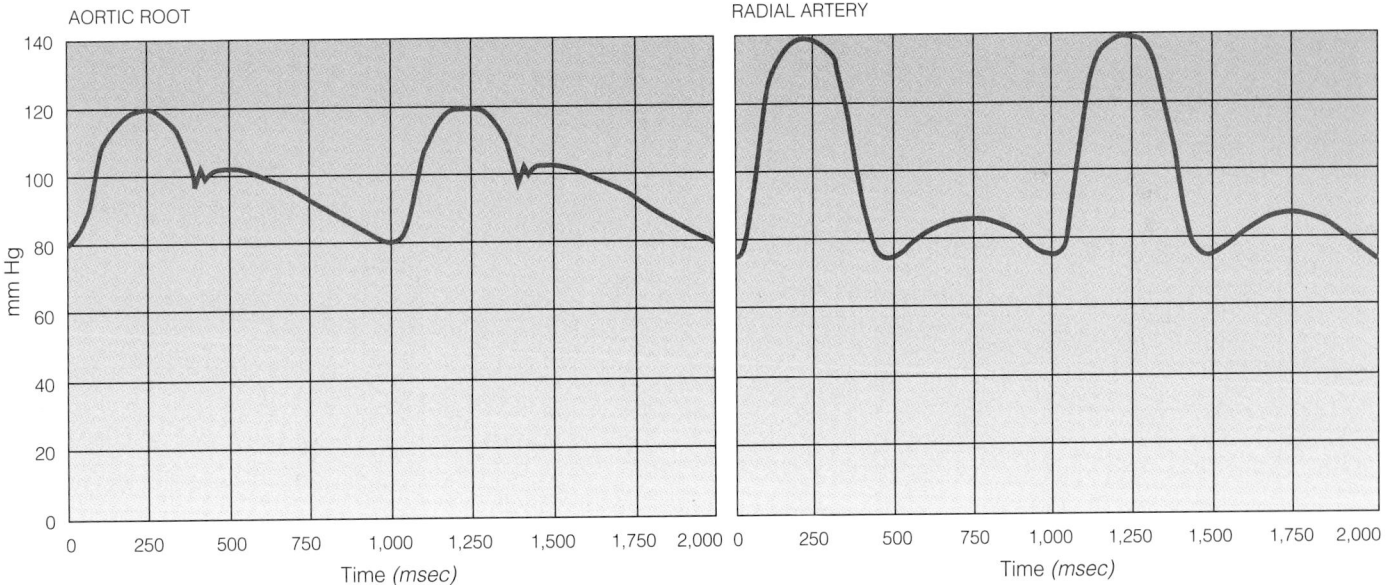

Figure 1 The mean pressure is defined as the area under a pressure tracing divided by the time needed to produce the tracing. A pressure wave in the ascending aorta with a blood pressure of 120/80 mm Hg will have the same mean pressure as a pressure wave in the radial artery of the same patient, even though the radial artery pressure might be 140/75 mm Hg. The systolic pressure in the radial artery is usually inscribed more rapidly. Therefore, even though the peak pressure in the radial artery is greater than that in the aorta, the areas under the tracings from the radial artery and the aorta will be the same. A useful but not infallible approximation of the mean pressure is to take the diastolic pressure plus one third of the difference between the systolic and diastolic pressures. In these examples, this formula would not work. The mean aortic pressure would be approximated at 93 mm Hg, whereas the mean radial artery pressure would be approximated at 97 mm Hg. Such results would be impossible: if the mean pressure in the radial artery were greater than the mean pressure in the aorta, blood would flow backward. This confusion is avoided by measuring the area under the curve and calculating the mean pressure exactly, which can be done with computer circuits that are available in all modern pressure-monitoring systems. The means of the pressures during diastole and systole can be calculated by using analogous formulae. The means of the peak systolic and nadirs of the diastolic pressures over a number of heart beats can be calculated by summing the individual values and dividing the summed values by the number of beats.

Note, in addition, that the systolic pressure in the radial artery is some 20 mm Hg higher than the systolic pressure in the aortic root.

a

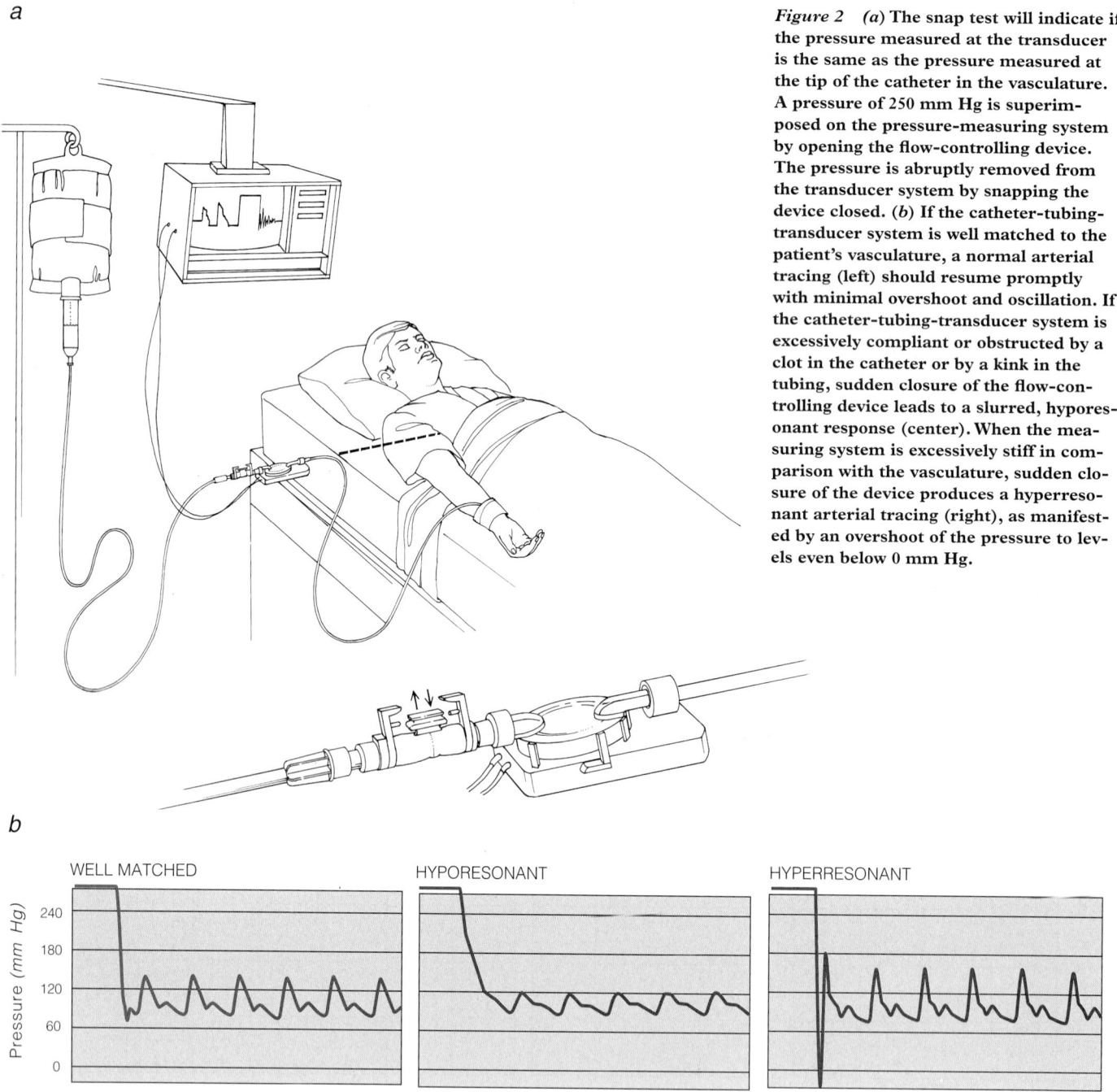

Figure 2 (*a*) The snap test will indicate if the pressure measured at the transducer is the same as the pressure measured at the tip of the catheter in the vasculature. A pressure of 250 mm Hg is superimposed on the pressure-measuring system by opening the flow-controlling device. The pressure is abruptly removed from the transducer system by snapping the device closed. (*b*) If the catheter-tubing-transducer system is well matched to the patient's vasculature, a normal arterial tracing (left) should resume promptly with minimal overshoot and oscillation. If the catheter-tubing-transducer system is excessively compliant or obstructed by a clot in the catheter or by a kink in the tubing, sudden closure of the flow-controlling device leads to a slurred, hyporesonant response (center). When the measuring system is excessively stiff in comparison with the vasculature, sudden closure of the device produces a hyperresonant arterial tracing (right), as manifested by an overshoot of the pressure to levels even below 0 mm Hg.

b

WELL MATCHED   HYPORESONANT   HYPERRESONANT

tolic and diastolic pressures. These running averages are calculated by computer circuitry in the transducer equipment. To calculate peak systolic pressure, for example, the computer might be programmed to sample 10 consecutive heart beats. It would then detect the peak systolic pressure for each of the 10, add the values, and divide the sum by 10. For the next sampling, it might take the last five values, add these to the next five, and divide the sum by 10. A similar logic is followed for diastolic pressures. The number of sampled beats is large enough that pressure variations introduced by ventilation are averaged out. The displayed pressure tracing is also accompanied by a digital readout of the mean pressure. This pressure is calculated as the area under the tracing divided by the time over which the tracing is sampled (typically, about 10 beats), and a running average is obtained in the same manner as the running averages of systolic and diastolic pressure [*see Figure 1*].

The pressures measured in the transducer are very accurate, and the computer's calculation of the running averages is very sophisticated. A problem remains, however: the displayed pressures represent the pressures in the transducer, not the actual pressures in the cannulated artery. This is not a major concern with mean pressure. Because there is no net transfer of energy between the catheterized artery and the transducer, the mean pressure in the transducer is the same as that in the artery, as long as the catheter and the tubing are unobstructed. Nor is diastolic pressure a significant problem as a rule. In both the transducer and the artery, mean pressure largely determines diastolic pressure. Because the mean pressures are the same, the diastolic pressures are usually fairly close together.

The peak systolic pressure in the transducer, however, is sometimes substantially different from that in the cannulated

Snap Test for Detection of Mismatch between Artery and Measuring System

Clinically, arterial pressures are measured with low-fidelity disposable fluid-filled catheter-tubing-transducer systems. The response of these systems can be characterized by two variables: a damped natural frequency and a damping coefficient.[15,16] The natural frequency reflects how rapidly the system oscillates in response to a pressure impulse; the damping coefficient reflects how rapidly the system comes to rest after a pressure impulse.

An arterial pressure waveform is made up of various individual harmonic components. The baseline component depends on the heart rate. For example, at a heart rate of 60 beats/min, the first harmonic component is at a frequency of 1 Hz. Adequate representation of an arterial pressure waveform can be obtained from the first several harmonic components. As the frequency of the arterial pressure waveform approaches the natural frequency of the catheter-tubing-transducer system, there will be resonance and amplification of the signal. The measured systolic pressure will be higher than the input arterial pressure, and the measured diastolic pressure will be lower. For an adequate representation of the arterial pressure waveform, the damped natural frequency of the system should be as large as possible—ideally, at least 7.5 to 8 Hz.

In addition, adequate characterization of the arterial pressure waveform requires a certain degree of damping (quantified by the damping coefficient). A completely undamped system will oscillate continuously in response to a pressure input. At the other extreme, an excessively damped system will respond sluggishly to changes in arterial pressures. Ideally, just enough damping should be present to allow minimal overshooting (i.e., a small amount of oscillatory motion).[15] This optimal damping represents a balance between responsiveness and instability.

Measurement of the damped natural frequency and the damping coefficient is readily accomplished by means of the snap test [see Figure 2].[15,69] This test results in transmission of a square wave impulse to the catheter-tubing-transducer system. Through trial and error, this impulse can be timed to a portion of the arterial waveform that is relatively flat, thereby facilitating evaluation. An arterial pressure waveform strip can generally be printed from a central monitor station. The damped natural frequency is calculated as the inverse of the period of one oscillation. As an approximation, at a standard rate of 25 mm/sec, one oscillatory period should be no longer than three small boxes (0.12 second, corresponding to a frequency of 8.3 Hz). The damping coefficient is reflected by the ratio between the amplitudes of successive oscillations. As the natural frequency of the catheter-tubing-transducer system increases, the range of acceptable damping coefficient values increases as well, while still allowing adequate representation of the arterial pressure waveform. A natural frequency requires a damping coefficient that results in a ratio of roughly 0.15 between successive oscillation amplitudes. Thus, a natural frequency of 10 Hz requires a ratio of 0.1 to 0.25. As the frequency increases to 20 Hz, a ratio ranging from 0.01 to 0.5 would be acceptable.[15]

artery. This difference arises because of (1) mismatching between the physical characteristics of the measuring system and those of the artery[15,16] and (2) catheter whip (or fling).

If the catheter-tubing-transducer system is excessively stiff compared with the vasculature, systolic pressure will be much higher and diastolic pressure somewhat lower in the transducer than in the artery. Conversely, if the measuring system is more compliant than the vasculature, if the vascular catheter is obstructed by a blood clot, or if the tube is too narrow or too long or has a kink, damping at the transducer will be introduced. When such damping occurs, systolic pressure will be lower and diastolic pressure somewhat higher in the transducer than in the artery.

Maintenance of an arterial catheter's patency requires a continuous infusion of fluid, usually from a high-pressure reservoir. A valve inserted in the circuit between the reservoir and the artery limits the amount of fluid infused. One can take advantage of this arrangement by using the so-called snap test to determine whether the systolic and diastolic pressures in the transducer accurately reflect those in the artery [see Figure 2]. In this test, a square pressure wave is introduced into the catheter-tubing-transducer system by pulling on the tab that allows fluid to flow from the high-pressure bag into the transducer and the artery. The tab is then snapped shut, and the pressure in the system returns abruptly to baseline levels [see Sidebar Snap Test for Detection of Mismatch between Artery and Measuring System]. If the system is adequately matched to the vasculature, the pressures in the transducer will abruptly return to baseline with minimal oscillation. If the measuring system is too stiff, the snap test will result in hyperresonance, evidenced by prolonged and exaggerated oscillation. If the measuring system is too compliant or if the catheter or tubing is obstructed, the snap test will lead to a slow and slurred descent toward baseline.

The primary goal in setting up the catheter-tubing-transducer system is accurate representation of the arterial pressure waveform. The system should be set up with the stiffest available tubing, which should be kept as short as is consonant with patient care and should be kept free of compression or clogging. Care should be taken to remove any air bubbles in the tubing or the transducer. Furthermore, the system should be as simple as possible; extraneous connectors and three-way valves should be removed.

If the system ends up with good matching, all of the measured pressures in the transducer can be accepted as accurate reflections of the pressures in the cannulated artery. If the system is hyperresonant, one should make a note of it and keep in mind that systolic and, to a lesser extent, diastolic pressures are not to be trusted. Mean pressures will still be accurate, and in many patients, these are all that is needed. If there is a need to know the systolic and diastolic pressures, any of several commercially available damping devices can be inserted in the transducer-tubing system. If the system is or becomes hyporesonant, an attempt should be made to clear the catheter, both to make the measurements from the catheter more accurate and to prevent propagation of thrombus into the artery from the catheter. If the system continues to be severely damped, it should be replaced and a new catheter inserted, if practicable. None of the measurements from a severely damped system are of any value. In the extreme case of occlusion of the catheter or the tubing, even the mean pressure in the transducer will bear no relation to the mean pressure in the artery.

Catheter whip—movement of the intravascular catheter in the vascular lumen as the heart beats [see Figure 3]—renders systolic and, to a lesser extent, diastolic pressures unreliable.[17] It is usually not a problem in the radial artery, where the catheter cannot move around very much, but it can cause difficulties in the femoral artery or the pulmonary artery, where the catheter has ample room for free movement in the lumen. Catheter whip can introduce errors of 20 mm Hg or more in measurements of femoral and pulmonary arterial pressures. Often, distortion introduced by a hyperresonant measuring system looks very much like catheter whip, and the two cannot be distinguished. When this is the case, a device can be added to the catheter-tubing-transducer system to eliminate hyperresonance; any remaining distortion must be the result of catheter whip. Usually, however, it is sufficient just to make a note of possible catheter whip and then not use the systolic or diastolic values in patient management; mean pressures will not be greatly affected and will remain usable.

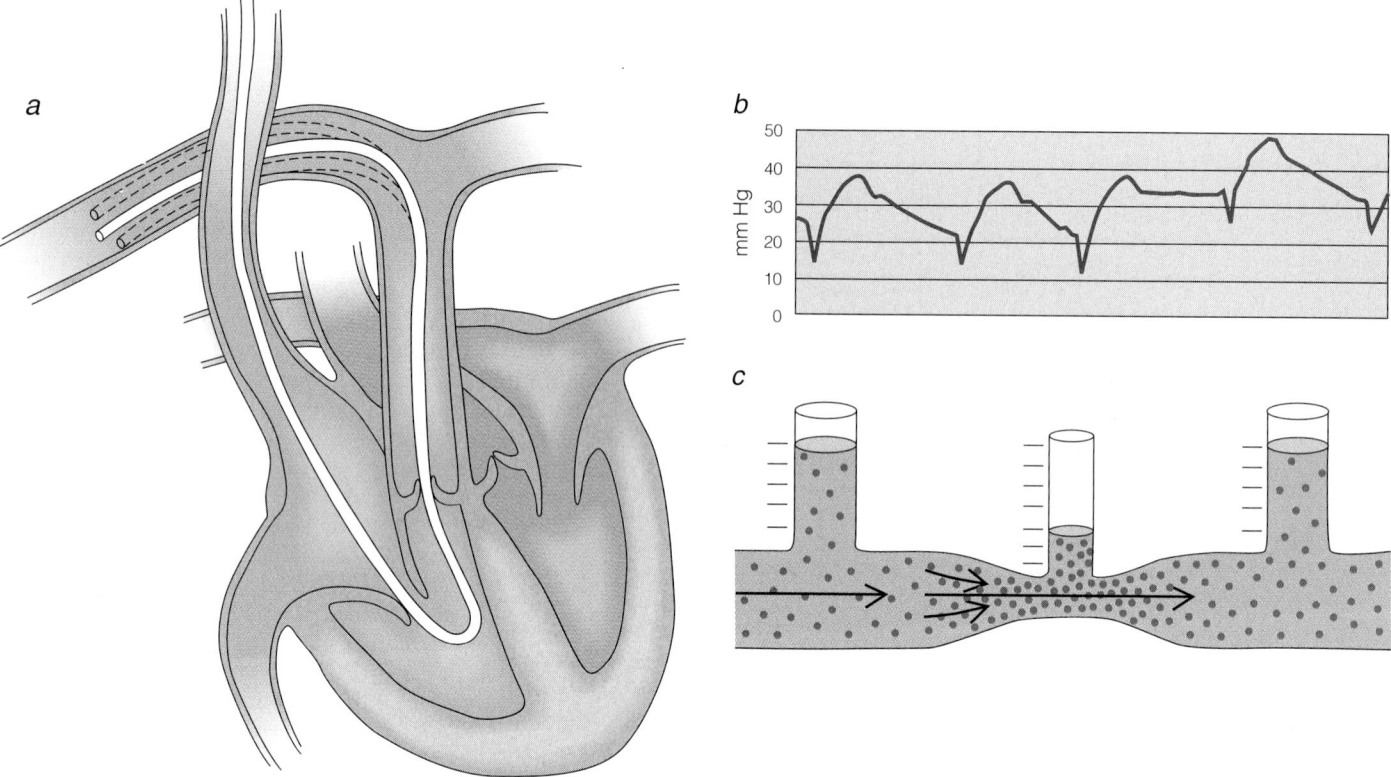

Figure 3 Catheter whip (or fling) results from movement of a catheter within the vasculature (*a*) that produces hydrostatic pressure changes at the tip of the catheter that are independent of any changes in hydrostatic pressure within the vessel itself. Pressure drops during diastole that are the result of catheter whip could be falsely interpreted as true vascular diastolic pressure. In the pressure tracing shown (*b*), the true diastolic pressure in the pulmonary artery is 24 mm Hg; catheter fling produces the lower pressure of 12 mm Hg at the tip of the catheter.

The total energy in a hydraulic system, such as the vasculature, is the sum of hydrostatic pressure and kinetic energy. The kinetic energy depends on the square of the velocity of the fluid. Because the velocity—and thus the kinetic energy—is greater the narrower the system (*c*), and because the total energy measured at any point in the system is constant, the hydrostatic pressure must be less in the narrow portion of the tube, where the velocity of flow is higher.

If a femoral or pulmonary arterial catheter moves within the vasculature as the heart beats, the velocity of blood across its orifice will increase; as the velocity increases and the kinetic energy increases, the hydrostatic pressure as measured at the tip will fall. This transient decrease in hydrostatic pressure at the tip of the catheter (as seen in the tracing) does not reflect the true hydrostatic pressure in the artery.

The radial artery catheter is best for determining the total energy in the blood flow. The catheter will not whip, because the artery is small and the catheter has no room to move about, and there will be no kinetic energy component in the blood, because the radial artery catheter is end-on (i.e., it faces into the direction of the flow), and thus, the velocity of the blood as it runs into the end of the catheter is zero. Therefore, the hydrostatic pressure will represent the total energy of the blood at that point of the vasculature. A catheter placed in the ascending aorta will be buffeted by the rapidly accelerating blood in the aorta, and catheter whip will be introduced. A pulmonary arterial catheter potentially has both the problem of catheter whip and the problem that it measures pressure in the direction of flow rather than end-on.

Once the pressure in the peripheral artery has been determined as accurately as possible, the next step is to extrapolate from this pressure to the aortic root pressure.[18] As a rule, the pressure in the radial artery is of little significance in itself (unless one is concerned about perfusion to the hand); the important concerns are perfusion to the entire body, including the heart, and the metabolic demands made on the heart to provide that perfusion. To address these concerns, one must know the pressures in the aortic root.

The central pressures are the most important of all the systemic arterial pressures. The peak systolic pressure in the aortic root can be used to estimate left ventricular end-systolic pressure—the most important of the left-side pressures for estimating ventricular stroke work and myocardial oxygen requirements.[19,20] In addition, when interpreted in the light of stroke volume, left ventricular end-systolic pressure is the key indicator of the hin-

drance that the ventricle faces when it contracts against the blood in the aortic root.[21] The mean diastolic pressure in the aortic root, defined as the integral of the pressure during diastole divided by the time spent in diastole, is the critical determinant of coronary perfusion. The mean pressure in the aortic root for the entire cardiac cycle, defined as the integral of the pressure over the cycle divided by the time of the cycle, is a critical determinant of the perfusion of noncardiac tissues.

Use of the mean pressure in a peripheral artery as a surrogate for the central aortic mean pressure is rarely a problem. Mean pressure is nearly uniform throughout the arterial system.[22] There is some mean energy loss as the blood flows through the arteries, but the loss is minimal unless the patient has proximal atherosclerotic occlusive disease or shock so severe that the arteries between the aortic root and the site of measurement go into spasm. In the great majority of patients, the mean pressure in any

Propagation of Energy and Generation of Pressures and Volumes in the Arterial System

Each left ventricular contraction pushes a bolus of blood with a high energy content into the aortic root, where it encounters a residual stagnant column of blood left over from the previous contraction. The collision of the two bodies of blood creates an energy impulse that propagates as a wave throughout the arteries to the arterioles. The energy that reaches the arterioles is then either transported through or reflected off them. Most of the energy is transferred through the arterioles without reflection. Much of that energy is used to perfuse the tissues and is dissipated as heat as it travels through them. The energy that remains after passage through the tissues is used to fill the right side of the heart—the atrium during systole and both the atrium and the ventricle during diastole. The energy that is reflected off the arterioles creates a retrograde wave that travels back to the aortic root, where it is attenuated and dies out before the ventricle contracts again.

The summation of the antegrade and retrograde energy waves at any given point in the arterial system creates a specific pressure and volume at that point. This composite wave depends primarily on ventricular contraction and on the characteristics of the arteries and arterioles into which and against which that energy is delivered. (It depends secondarily on the stiffness of the atrium and ventricle into which the blood flows, but this is relatively unimportant for present purposes.) Three characteristics of the vasculature must be considered: (1) the degree of constriction of the arterioles distal to the measurement site; (2) the spatial distribution of these arterioles, including the distance from the measurement site; and (3) the stiffness of the arteries transmitting the energy to the arterioles.

Distal arteriolar constriction increases the amplitude of the reflected wave; dilation decreases it. Symmetrical spatial distribution of arterioles results in uniform reflection of waves that coalesce in phase with one another; the summated reflected wave is compact with sharp contours and is short in duration. Asymmetrical arteriolar distribution results in reflection of waves that are out of phase with one another; the summated reflected wave is slurred and spread out. Arterioles that are distant from the measurement site create a composite reflected wave that comes back late; arterioles that are close create a wave that returns quickly. Stiff arteries result in increased velocities of wave propagation, both outgoing and returning, and thus early return to the measurement site; compliant arteries result in late return.

Systolic pressures in the peripheral arteries increase and diastolic pressures decrease slightly if the arterioles distal to the measurement site are constricted, symmetrically distributed, or nearby or if the conducting arteries are stiff. In this case, the amplitude of the reflected wave will be large (constricted arterioles), its components will be in phase (symmetrical arteriolar distribution), and the retrograde wave will return quickly (stiff arteries). If the measurement site is close to the arterioles, the reflected wave will return very quickly and will pass through the antegrade wave before diastole begins. The duration of systole will be short. The pressure contour created by the superposition of the antegrade and retrograde waves will be sharp, with a rapid upswing and downswing. The systolic pressure will be increased, sometimes substantially, and the diastolic pressure will be slightly decreased.

The opposite occurs if the distal arterioles are dilated, asymmetrically distributed, or distant or if the conducting arteries are compliant. In this case, the amplitude of the reflected wave will be small, its components will be out of phase, and the retrograde wave will be delayed. Unless the measuring site is very close to the arterioles, the wave will return during both systole and diastole. The duration of systole will be lengthened, and the upswing and downswing of the waveform will be smoothed out. The systolic pressure will be minimized, sometimes substantially, and the diastolic pressure will be slightly augmented.

These general characteristics of the arterial vasculature have specific implications for the pressures in the aortic root and the radial artery. In the aortic root, the typical pressure waveform is blunted (damped) and is characterized by lower systolic pressures and higher diastolic pressures than the distal waveforms. The arterioles in the heart, brain, liver, and kidneys are chronically dilated, diminishing the amplitudes of the reflected waves. The arterioles supplied by the aorta are asymmetrically distributed: those in the upper part of the body are close to the aortic root, whereas those in the lower extremities are distant. Thus, the reflected waves return to the aortic root at varying times, with the result that some of their pressure oscillations cancel one another out. Finally, the arteries that come off the aorta have varying degrees of stiffness. Those arteries supplying the upper body are compliant (slow wave propagation velocities and late return), whereas those supplying the lower body are stiff (high propagation velocities but delayed return because of the long distances the waves must travel). This contour of pressure in the aortic root enhances cardiovascular efficiency: the low systolic pressure results in minimal hindrance to ventricular emptying, and the high diastolic pressure results in maximal perfusion of the coronary vasculature [see Figure 1].

In the radial artery, systolic pressures are almost always higher and diastolic pressures usually somewhat lower than in the aortic root [see Figure 1]. The duration of systole is shorter, with a sharper upswing and more precipitous downswing. The arterioles in the hand are usually constricted, symmetrically distributed, and close to the measurement site. The artery is compliant, which decreases the velocity of wave propagation, but its compliance is outweighed by the closeness of the arterioles. Thus, waves return quickly.

The spiked pressure waveform in the peripheral arteries has no adverse effect on distal perfusion. It is the mean pressure in the periphery that is important for perfusion, and that pressure is independent of the reflected pulsatile energy wave. The exaggerated peripheral arterial waveform does, however, make it difficult to extrapolate from distally measured systolic pressures back to the central aortic pressures. Such extrapolation must rest on certain assumptions. For example, in a patient with normally constricted arteries in the hand, the peak systolic pressure in the radial artery is approximately 10 mm Hg higher than that in the brachial artery, which is approximately 10 mm Hg higher than that in the aortic root. If the arterioles in the hand are constricted more than the arterioles in the central portions of the body, the peak systolic pressure in the radial artery can be much higher than that in the aortic root. If the arterioles in the hand are dilated with respect to the central arterioles, the peak systolic pressures in the radial artery and aortic root come closer together.

Thus, if a patient is in moderately severe hemorrhagic shock, with constricted arterioles in the skin of the hand, peak systolic pressures in the radial artery should be substantially higher than those in the aortic root, because of reflected waves with large amplitudes. On the other hand, severe shock might constrict the arteries between the aorta and the hand enough to decrease mean pressure distally, and probably systolic and diastolic pressure as well. In this case, the radial systolic pressure might come to be close to the aortic systolic pressure. If the patient is in warm inflammatory shock, one would expect a close correlation between the systolic pressures in the radial artery and those in the aortic root. A warm hand means dilated cutaneous arterioles; accordingly, the reflected waves will have minimal amplitudes.

peripheral artery can, for practical purposes, be considered equivalent to the mean central aortic pressure.

The diastolic pressure in the periphery is usually somewhat less than that in the aortic root, but this too is rarely a problem.[22] The nadir of the diastolic pressure in the periphery is usually close to the mean diastolic pressure. Mean diastolic pressure is closely related to mean pressure, which is usually the same distally and proximally. The mean pressure in the aortic root is closely related to the mean diastolic pressure in the aortic root. Thus, the nadir of the diastolic pressure in the radial artery is usually close to the mean diastolic pressure in the aortic root. Typically, therefore, the nadir of the diastolic pressure in the periphery can be taken to be the pressure available for perfusion of the coronary arteries.

On the other hand, use of the systolic pressure in the periphery as a surrogate for the systolic pressure in the aorta can be a

Table 1 Effects of Position and Exercise on Cardiovascular Pressures in a Young, Well-Conditioned 60 kg Woman[67,78-95]

Pressures	Supine (Resting)	Upright (Resting)	Upright (Exercising)
Aortic root pressures (mm Hg)			
Peak systolic	110	110	160
End-diastolic	80	80	85
Mean	90	90	110
Brachial artery pressures (mm Hg)			
Peak systolic	120	120	170
End-diastolic	80	80	85
Mean	90	90	110
Radial artery pressures (mm Hg)			
Peak systolic	130	130	180
End-diastolic	80	80	85
Mean	90	90	110
Mean right arterial pressure (mm Hg)	5	5	5
Right ventricular pressures (mm Hg)			
End-diastolic	5	5	5
Peak systolic	25	25	40
End-systolic	22.5	22.5	35
Pulmonary arterial pressures (mm Hg)			
Peak systolic	25	25	40
End-diastolic	10	10	10
Mean	15	15	20
Mean pulmonary arterial wedge pressure (mm Hg)	8	8	8
Left ventricular pressures (mm Hg)			
End-diastolic	8	8	8
Peak systolic	110	110	160
End-systolic	100	100	145

major problem. The systolic pressure in a peripheral artery is almost always larger than its counterpart in the aortic root, sometimes substantially so [*see Figure 1*].[18,22] This difference can be understood by considering that the heart is a pulsatile energy source and that the energy it generates travels to the periphery through a vascular network with complex physical characteristics [*see Sidebar* Propagation of Energy and Generation of Pressures and Volumes in the Arterial System].[22] Understanding why these pressures are different allows one to make better estimates of central pressures from measurements of peripheral pressures, just as understanding why the systolic pressures in a transducer are frequently different from those in the artery to which the transducer is connected allows one to make better estimates of the actual intra-arterial pressures.

Typical values for pressures in the systemic arteries, measured by techniques that avoid all of the potential pitfalls, have been determined [*see Table 1*]. Although these measurements are made in a highly sophisticated manner, they still must be used with some reservations. There is probably no such thing as a normal blood pressure or a normal cardiac output—or, for that matter, a normal value for any cardiopulmonary parameter. That the values given are typical is not to say that they are necessarily desirable or associated with good health or longevity or that they should be the target values in a critically ill patient. Any of these values, in fact, could easily be 25% higher or lower. They can also be affected by the stresses associated with different positions and with exercise. Going from a supine to an upright position requires some cardiopulmonary adjustments; going from a rest-

ing to an all-out exercising state requires extreme adjustments. Gaining a sense of what the heart and lungs can do in different circumstances can give the clinician a valuable perspective on what to expect from a critically ill patient. This is the real relevance of these "typical" values.

Central Venous Pressure

Central venous pressure is very close to right atrial pressure, which is a critical determinant in the formation of peripheral edema. Right atrial pressure, in turn, is very close to right ventricular end-diastolic pressure (in the absence of tricuspid valvular disease), and end-diastolic pressure gives an idea of end-diastolic volume. Right ventricular end-diastolic volume is a critical determinant of right ventricular stroke volume, end-systolic pressure, and stroke work, which, in turn, are critical determinants of right ventricular oxygen requirements.[19] Thus, central venous pressure can give the clinician substantial insight into the functioning of the right side of the heart.

Quantitative measurement of central venous pressure requires insertion of either a central venous catheter or a pulmonary arterial catheter. Access is usually achieved through either a jugular or a subclavian approach. Certain risks are associated with puncture of these large central veins.[23] Penetration of the parietal pleura can produce a pneumothorax. Puncture of the subclavian artery can lead to exsanguination into the pleural cavity. Intrapleural infusion of fluids can occur with improper catheter placement. Puncture of one of the major trunks or divisions of the brachial plexus lying near the large veins can permanently impair the extremity. Puncture of the trachea, the esophagus, or the lung can lead to subcutaneous emphysema and mediastinitis. Puncture of the internal jugular vein on the left side can damage the thoracic duct and lead to a chylothorax. Improper use of the introducing needle can result in shearing of the catheter and catheter emboli. No matter how experienced the person performing the procedure, these complications will occur occasionally; the goal is to keep their incidence to a minimum. The alternative to direct puncture of a central vein is to cannulate a peripheral vein and pass the catheter centrally. This technique, however, carries a very high risk of thrombophlebitis.[24] On balance, it is better to gain direct access to a central vein if this can be accomplished safely.

The central pressures obtained vary with the respiratory cycle. Intracardiac pressures fall during spontaneous inspiration, as the lungs pull away from the great veins and cardiac chambers, and rise during mechanical ventilation, as insufflation of the lungs compresses the cardiac chambers. With pressure control or pressure support ventilation, end-expiratory pressures will be close to those that would result from spontaneous breathing. Intermittent mandatory ventilation, however, can create a confusing picture, producing both augmented vascular pressures when the ventilator gives a mechanical breath but lowered intracardiac pressures when the patient takes a spontaneous breath [*see Figure 4*].

Substantial pressures can be generated during inspiration with these different modes of ventilation. The intracardiac pressure variations induced by mechanical ventilation can exceed 20 mm Hg. To deal with this problem, some clinicians use end-expiratory values, which can be read from the pressure tracings on the monitor screen. The disadvantage of this approach is that even the most experienced physicians and nurses sometimes find end-expiratory pressure tracings difficult to read.[25,26] Another approach is to take the patient off the ventilator while making the measurements. This approach does make it easier to interpret the

SPONTANEOUS VENTILATION

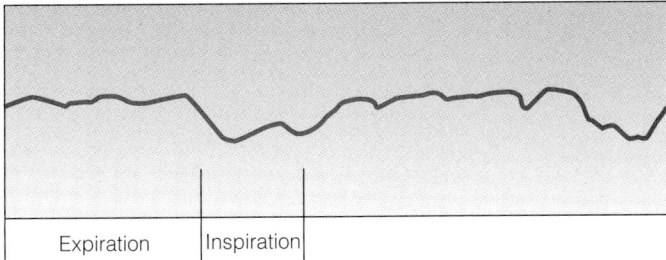

MECHANICAL VENTILATION

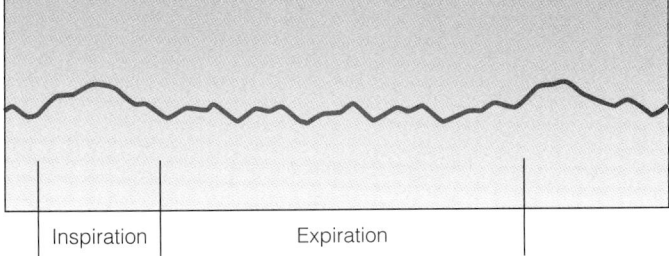

INTERMITTENT MANDATORY VENTILATION

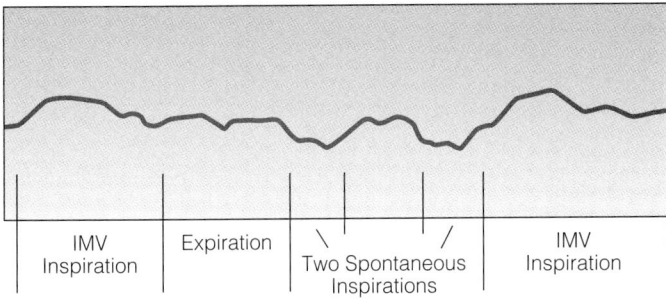

Figure 4 **Ventilation can have marked effects on all of the pressures on the right side of the circulation. For example, in a patient breathing spontaneously (top), central venous pressure (or, equivalently, right atrial pressure) falls as the lungs pull away from the intrathoracic great veins and the right atrium. In these patients, the end-expiratory pressure is the highest pressure measured during the ventilatory cycle. During mechanical ventilation (middle), the lungs are pushed against the outside of the heart and the great veins; intracavitary and intravascular pressures are thereby increased during inspiration, and the end-expiratory pressure is the lowest pressure measured during the ventilatory cycle. If intermittent ventilation is used, the problem is made even more complicated (bottom). The machine-generated breaths produce increases in the atrial pressure and spontaneous breaths produce decreases; the end-expiratory pressure is the plateau pressure between the two extremes. The same considerations come into play with measurement of pulmonary arterial and pulmonary arterial wedge pressures. One way to avoid these problems is to take the reading for all of these right-sided pressures from the digital display of the monitoring equipment. These values are the running means of the various pressures, taken over a number of breaths.**

pressures. Its disadvantage is that the most significant pressures are the ones prevailing while the patient is being ventilated. Removing the patient from the ventilator produces a condition that no longer represents his or her physiologic status.

Currently, most physicians rely on the mean pressure over the entire ventilatory cycle, as obtained from digital readouts [*see*

Systemic Arterial Pressures, *above*]. This approach has two advantages: (1) the readings are independent of the person making the measurement, and (2) the measurements reflect the actual conditions to which the patient is exposed. We also use the running means for pulmonary arterial and pulmonary arterial wedge pressures (see below).

Pulmonary Arterial Pressures

Monitoring of the pressures in the pulmonary artery of an ICU patient can only be accomplished by means of a Swan-Ganz catheter.[27] These pressures, along with other values obtainable from the modern catheter (e.g., cardiac output, right ventricular end-diastolic volume, and mixed venous oxygen levels) can give the clinician an enormous amount of information about a patient's cardiac status.

Pulmonary arterial peak systolic pressure is the same as right ventricular peak systolic pressure. From the latter, right ventricular end-systolic pressure can be approximated, and this value, along with right ventricular end-diastolic volume, is a critical determinant of right ventricular stroke volume, stroke work, and oxygen requirements.[19] It is also useful, along with stroke volume, for estimating the hindrance against which the ventricle contracts. Mean pulmonary arterial pressure is the most important of the pressures for assessing perfusion of the pulmonary microvasculature, filling of the left atrium during systole, and filling of the left atrium and ventricle during diastole.

Pulmonary arterial wedge pressure can also be measured with a Swan-Ganz catheter. Because there are no valves between the pulmonary arteries and the left atrium, the pressure obtained with occlusion of proximal flow will be the same as the pressure in the left atrium [*see Figure 5*], provided that there is no significant bronchial blood flow.[28-30] In the absence of mitral valvular disease, left atrial pressure will be the same as left ventricular end-diastolic pressure.

Knowledge of the pulmonary arterial wedge pressure can help management in two ways. First, it alerts one to possible formation of pulmonary edema. The pulmonary microvascular pressure must lie between mean pulmonary arterial pressure and left atrial (or wedge) pressure. If wedge pressure is high, pulmonary microvascular pressure must be high as well. A high wedge pressure (≥ 25 mm Hg) is always associated with microvascular pressures that generate at least some interstitial pulmonary edema, even if the microvascular endothelium is intact.[31] If the endothelium is disrupted, as in sepsis, pulmonary edema can be produced even with wedge pressures in the midteens.

Second, knowledge of the wedge pressure can facilitate estimation of left ventricular end-diastolic volume, which is one of the prime factors determining left ventricular end-systolic pressure, stroke volume, stroke work, and myocardial oxygen consumption.[19] As noted (see above), pulmonary arterial wedge pressure, in the absence of mitral valvular disease, is essentially equal to ventricular end-diastolic pressure. End-diastolic pressure can then be extrapolated to derive end-diastolic volume.

A caveat is in order here, however. To make this extrapolation, one must take into account ventricular end-diastolic compliance, which can decrease in the face of myocardial ischemia or hypertrophy or scarring of the ventricular wall.[32] One must also consider the possibility of external forces that are compressing the heart. A high end-diastolic pressure in a compliant ventricle that is not compressed from the outside will be associated with a large end-diastolic volume; a similarly high pressure in a ventricle that is stiff or compressed will be associated with a small volume.

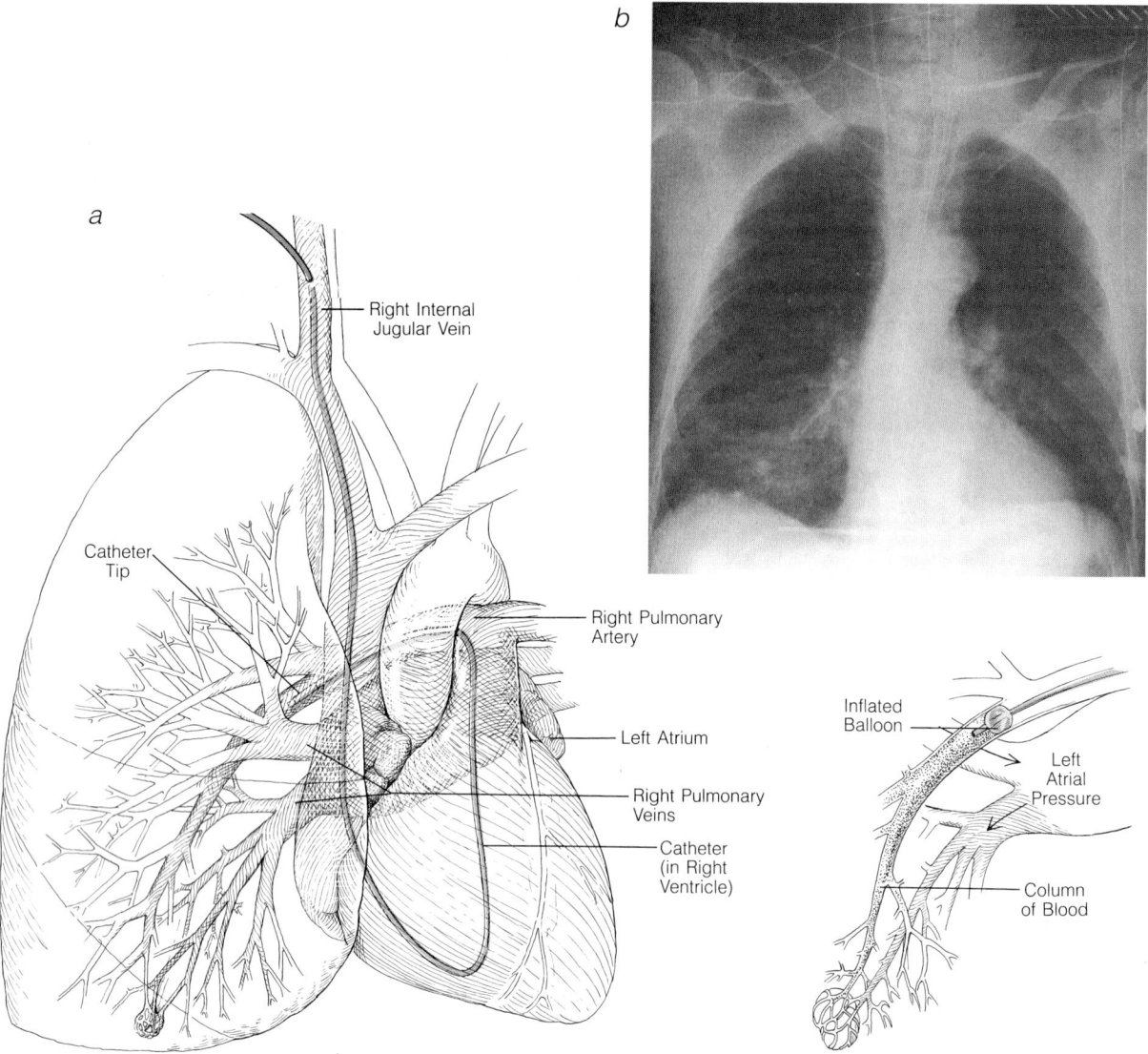

Figure 5 (*a*) The pulmonary arterial catheter measures pressure in the pulmonary artery when the balloon is deflated. Because flow in the vascular system generates a pressure drop as the blood passes through the microvasculature, the pressure from the pulmonary artery to the left atrium gradually falls. When the balloon is inflated, flow in the vasculature distal to the tip is eliminated; therefore, there is no pressure drop. Because there is no pressure drop and because there are no valves between the left atrium and the pulmonary artery, the pressure in the pulmonary artery distal to the point of occlusion must equal the pressure in the left atrium, provided that there is an open column of blood between the end of the catheter and the left atrium. That is, pulmonary arterial wedge pressure will equal left atrial pressure as long as the catheter is in a dependent portion of the lung with a vasculature that remains open during ventilation. Because the catheter is flow directed, it usually will end up in such a dependent, well-perfused area. This is not a certainty, however. If inflated alveoli occlude the microvasculature, wedge pressure will equal alveolar pressure. This inaccuracy might not be easily detected. (*b*) Verification that the catheter is in the dependent portion of the lung requires a cross-table lateral chest x-ray. We do not routinely obtain these x-rays unless the wedge pressures are absolutely critical for treatment and unless the reliability of the wedge pressure tracing is suspect. Suspicion usually arises when excessively wide pressure swings are evident as the lungs are inflated and deflated.

Frequently, the factors affecting end-diastolic compliance and the pressure applied to the outside of the ventricle can only be roughly estimated. In some patients (e.g., a spontaneously breathing patient with no indications of myocardial ischemia), it can be assumed that the end-diastolic volume will be acceptable even with a fairly low end-diastolic (and wedge) pressure. In others (e.g., a patient on a mechanical ventilator with abdominal or retroperitoneal hemorrhage and an elevated diaphragm), the wedge pressure can be completely misleading.[33,34] Extrapolation

from ventricular end-diastolic pressure to end-diastolic volume in such patients becomes very imprecise. The wedge pressure might be in the high teens and still not be associated with an acceptable end-diastolic volume.

There are other potential pitfalls in interpreting measurements from a Swan-Ganz catheter. As with intra-arterial monitoring of systemic arterial pressures, the pressure in the transducer must be extrapolated to the pressure in the artery. The mean pressures are the same, and the diastolic pressures are nearly the same, but again, the systolic pressures can be misleading because of mismatching and catheter whip. These concerns can be dealt with in the same way as in systemic arterial monitoring.

In contrast with measurement of peripheral systemic arterial pressures and extrapolation back to aortic root pressures, measurement of the pressures at the outflow of the ventricle with the Swan-Ganz catheter is not problematic. The lumen of the catheter used for measuing pulmonary arterial pressure is placed far enough proximally that it gives a direct measurement of the pressure to which the right ventricle is exposed.

Typical pulmonary arterial, left atrial, and left ventricular end-diastolic pressures have been determined [see Table 1]. Like the typical systemic arterial pressures, these values are not necessarily either ideal or desirable: they merely give an idea of what the cardiovascular system can do when demands are placed on it.

PROBLEMS ASSOCIATED WITH SWAN-GANZ CATHETERS

In addition to the problems arising from interpretation of measurements made with a Swan-Ganz catheter, there are general problems associated with gaining access to a central vein [see Central Venous Pressure, above] and specific problems associated with passage and maintenance of a pulmonary arterial catheter.[35]

Ventricular dysrhythmias are common during passage of the catheter, particularly in patients who have suffered recent myocardial infarctions or who have an irritable myocardium as indicated by a preexisting arrhythmia or conduction defect. For some of these patients, prophylactic administration of lidocaine is indicated. In rare instances, aggressive treatment of such dysrhythmias may be required. Usually, the dysrhythmia subsides when the end of the catheter finally passes through the ventricle and enters the pulmonary artery; sometimes, however, it can be ablated only by complete removal of the catheter. The balloon on the end of the catheter should be kept inflated during passage to cushion the tip and minimize myocardial irritability.

Passing a Swan-Ganz catheter in a patient with left bundle branch block can be particularly hazardous. The catheter can eliminate conduction through the right ventricle, producing complete heart block. If this condition does not resolve upon prompt withdrawal of the catheter, insertion of a transvenous pacemaker or the use of external pacing may be necessary. The time required to establish a rhythm, however, can be so long that the patient may die first. Therefore, Swan-Ganz catheters should be placed in patients with left bundle branch block only when absolutely necessary.

Lodging of the catheter tip in the trabeculae of the right ventricle is a common problem during catheter passage. On rare occasions, the end of the catheter may puncture the right ventricular wall. The puncture site may not be immediately obvious and may in fact seal by itself; however, it is far more likely to lead to pericardial tamponade and, possibly, death. Measurements from the Swan-Ganz catheter will indicate pericardial tamponade, which mandates emergency operation.

Passage of the catheter through the tricuspid and pulmonic valves can damage them, especially if the device is roughly pulled back through the valves with the balloon inflated. In addition, if the catheter is left in place for more than a few days, valvular damage may result. Besides minimizing long-term use of the catheter, little can be done to prevent this problem.

A problem unique to the Swan-Ganz catheter is intracardiac knotting, which is most likely to develop during placement. The knot can occasionally be untied by manipulating the catheter under fluoroscopic guidance. Passage of a J-wire into the right side of the heart from the groin can also be effective. If these approach-

es do not work, the catheter must be withdrawn to the site of entry and then removed, usually under direct surgical control.

Swan-Ganz catheters left in place for more than a few days can migrate distally and cut off the blood supply to the pulmonary parenchyma, resulting in pulmonary infarction. This situation is best prevented by continuous monitoring of the pulmonary arterial waveform. Development of a permanently wedged wave pattern is an indication that the catheter should immediately be withdrawn far enough to reestablish a normal pulmonary arterial tracing.

On rare occasions, the catheter can perforate the pulmonary artery. This event typically presents with hemoptysis but may present with acute cardiopulmonary collapse during or immediately after measurement of wedge pressure. Risk factors include advanced age, pulmonary arterial hypertension, warfarin anticoagulation, clotting deficiencies, distal migration of the catheter into the pulmonary vasculature, and balloon overinflation. Patients with tumors surrounding the pulmonary artery are also at increased risk. The balloon itself may disrupt the pulmonary artery directly, or inflation of the balloon may force the tip of the catheter through the vessel wall. Prevention consists of continuous monitoring of pulmonary arterial pressure tracings. The catheter location should be confirmed by chest x-ray at least once daily. Wedge pressures should be measured only when needed. The degree of balloon inflation necessary to obtain a wedge tracing should be noted and overinflation avoided. The balloon inflation port should be identified so that infusions are not misdirected into the balloon. The catheter should never be left in the wedge position. Rupture associated with mild hemoptysis can be treated by removing the catheter; rupture associated with cardiovascular collapse calls for lobectomy or pneumonectomy, which occasionally permits patient salvage.

Given the limitations of interpreting measurements from the Swan-Ganz catheter and the risks associated with its use, some have asked if the potential benefits (i.e., increased knowledge of the state of the cardiovascular system) are enough to justify its use. Two groups of investigators have suggested that the risks of Swan-Ganz catheterization outweigh the benefits.[36,37] We disagree, for reasons spelled out more fully elsewhere [see Sidebar Arguments for and against Swan-Ganz Catheterization]. In our view, the question of whether and when to use a Swan-Ganz catheter is still unresolved. A study with a high capture rate of eligible patients with a death rate confirming severe preexisting illness is still needed. We believe that use of the Swan-Ganz catheter is still appropriate in selected patients, provided that the information obtained thereby is employed intelligently and that the associated risks are kept to a minimum.

For example, it would seem reasonable to use a Swan-Ganz catheter when myocardial function is severely compromised. The catheter can provide crucial information on the efficacy of pharmacologic support and can aid in the diagnosis of abnormalities such as pericardial tamponade and acute mitral regurgitation. Another reasonable indication would be hypovolemic shock that does not respond readily to volume administration. The catheter may reveal abnormalities of myocardial function or of the pulmonary or systemic vasculature that require specific interventions in addition to volume loading. Pulmonary arterial monitoring would also seem reasonable in patients with sepsis who have inadequate urine output or who are hypotensive. The catheter can provide valuable information about the adequacy of oxygen consumption and pharmacologic support. Pulmonary disorders, especially those that carry a high probability of associated myocardial dysfunction, might constitute another reasonable

Arguments for and against Swan-Ganz Catheterization

The authors of two observational cohort reviews found that ICU patients who underwent Swan-Ganz catheterization had higher death rates than those who did not.[36,37] They addressed the possibility that the patients in the first group were more seriously ill than those in the second by using statistical tools that relied on numerical descriptors of the patient's condition on admission to the hospital or the ICU. These descriptors consisted of measurements of such indicators of illness as temperature, electrolyte concentrations, and blood gas values (including arterial pH) as well as many other, mostly laboratory, determinations. The authors concluded, in effect, that use of the Swan-Ganz catheter kills patients.

We argue that the evidence currently available does not support this conclusion. Most of the life-threatening complications of Swan-Ganz catheterization (e.g., puncture of the subclavian artery and creation of a tension pneumothorax) are associated with insertion of the catheter and are technical in nature; various others result from maintenance of the catheter. In the hands of a technically proficient person who works in an institution where the catheters are used well, such complications ought to be infrequent. There is no reason why insertion and use of a Swan-Ganz catheter should cause very many fatalities,[23] and the information obtained from the catheter, if used intelligently,[70,71] can only be beneficial.[72-74] In neither of the above-mentioned reviews did the authors indicate how the information obtained with the catheters was used in patient management, nor did they report on the types or frequencies of complications in their institutions.

Furthermore, we believe that given the statistical tools currently available, it is impossible to take into account the preexisting degree of illness in the patients. No scoring system yet developed can match the assessment made by an experienced clinician. Thus, even though the authors of these studies tried to account for severity of illness in their analyses, there is still a very good chance that the ill patients were more likely to have Swan-Ganz catheters inserted than the relatively well patients. One does not institute invasive measures if one thinks that the patient's prognosis is good with current management; one does become more aggressive if one thinks that the patient is going to die.

A randomized prospective trial—the only one in this area to date, to our knowledge—was subsequently published that partially confirmed our reservations.[75] The authors enrolled patients who came to have moderately, but not excessively, high death rates. In-hospital death rates in both patients who were managed with a pulmonary arterial catheter and those who were not so managed were quite low, considering the diagnoses involved, and were essentially identical, at 7.8% and 7.7%. Furthermore, the authors reported on the complications noted with use of the catheter. There were, in fact, very few of these, with the exception of a higher incidence of pulmonary embolism in patients who underwent Swan-Ganz catheterization. Given that the death rates in the two groups were the same, one could reasonably assume either that use of the catheters must have had some offsetting advantage or that the embolisms were clinically inconsequential.

Admittedly, the authors did not detect any significant benefit from Swan-Ganz catheterization either. We think, however, that this lack of benefit could easily be explained by patient selection. The authors enrolled 52% of the patients eligible for the study but were unable to enroll the remaining 48%. A capture rate of 52% is admirable in a study of this nature, but the 48% enrollment failure rate raises questions about the extent to which the study's conclusions about absence of benefit can be generalized to the entire cohort of eligible patients. We suspect that some of the physicians who were taking care of the eligible but excluded patients might have been particularly concerned about those patients and consequently might have wanted to retain the option of using the catheter if they thought it necessary. In other words, it may be that the unenrolled patients included some, perhaps even many, who might have benefited most from use of the catheter.

---

indication. Pulmonary arterial catheters might also be useful in patients with good cardiopulmonary function who are undergoing procedures associated with large volume requirements and fluid shifts as well as in patients with severe preexisting myocardial or pulmonary disease who are undergoing elective procedures. Finally, pulmonary arterial catheterization might be indicated if the patient is experiencing failure of two organs with competing priorities.

Cardiac Output

Modern pulmonary arterial catheters are equipped to obtain a number of other measurements besides pulmonary arterial pressures. Thermistor-tipped catheters can measure cardiac output by means of thermodilution.[38] Typically, this value is obtained by injecting a known quantity of a cool solution in the right atrium and analyzing the temperature drop in the pulmonary artery as the cooled blood flows past the thermistor. Commercially available computers calculate the cardiac output on the basis of indicator dilution theory [see Figure 6]. The calculation takes into account the temperature of the injectate, its volume, its specific heat and gravity, the cold capacity of the blood, and the area inscribed under the thermodilution curve. Adjustments can be made for different amounts and temperatures of injectates. The computer finds the area under the thermodilution curve and gives a digital readout of the cardiac output, usually in L/min.

Although either a room-temperature or an ice-cold solution may be used as the thermal indicator, cold injectates are used more often at present. The advantages of room-temperature injections are simplicity and relative invariability of injectate temperature. Ice-cold injections generate a large signal-to-noise ratio because the magnitude of the changes in the pulmonary arterial temperature increases as the temperature of the injectate decreases. Whichever type of injectate is used, the key is to know its exact temperature, because this value is necessary for accurate calculation of output.

Ventilation affects flow into and out of the right ventricle, and pulmonary arterial temperature changes as a function of insufflation of the lungs. To account for these variations, three injections are usually made for each determination of cardiac output. They are usually given at a consistent point in the ventilatory cycle—typically at end-expiration—though some clinicians make an effort to give them at different points in the ventilatory cycle.[39] The three values should be within 15% of one another; if they are not, the series is repeated.

Pulmonary arterial catheters equipped with heating elements are now available for determination of cardiac output.[40,41] Their main advantage is that the precise amount of heat they generate is known. The temperature pulses are generated randomly so that the values obtained are a mean over several breaths. No injectate is needed, and there is no limit to how many measurements can be made, even in patients in whom fluid administration must be restricted. However, catheters with heating elements seem to be stiffer than catheters without such elements. This added stiffness may make passage of the catheter into the pulmonary artery more difficult and may predispose to tricuspid insufficiency.

Methods of measuring cardiac output have also been developed that do not involve placement of pulmonary arterial catheters. The direct Fick method is best used in awake, alert patients.[42] Transthoracic electrical impedance measurement requires placement of electrodes, which may interfere with surgical procedures.[43] Doppler ultrasonography probes have been placed at the suprasternal notch and the esophagus for measure-

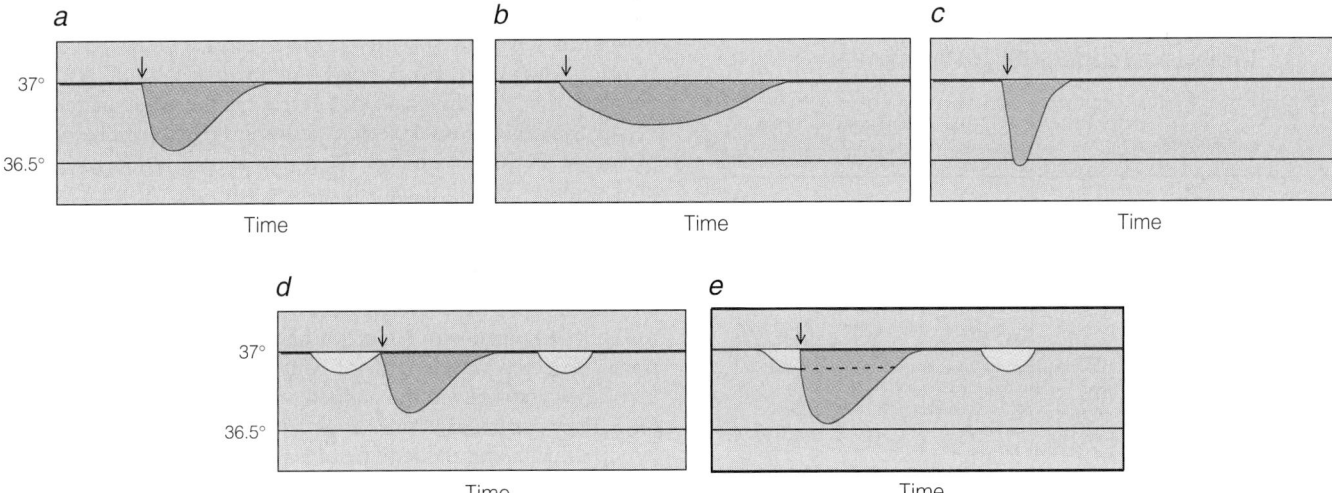

Figure 6 In the normal thermodilution curve shown here (*a*), the baseline pulmonary arterial temperature is 37° C; when a cold solution is injected to measure cardiac output (arrow), the temperature may fall to a low of 36.6° C as the cooled blood flows past the thermistor. When cardiac output is low (*b*), the cooled blood flows sluggishly past the end of the thermistor. The temperature drop in the blood might be to 36.7° C, but the cooled blood stagnates near the thermistor, and the blood at that portion of the pulmonary artery remains cool for a long time. Because the cardiac output is calculated as the inverse of the area, the output is recorded as a smaller number. By contrast, a supranormal cardiac output (*c*) pushes the pulse of cool blood rapidly past the thermistor. The result is a transiently low pulmonary arterial temperature. The area under the curve, however, is smaller than normal because the fall in temperature is brief; this small area leads to a calculation of a high cardiac output. These examples assume a stable temperature for pulmonary arterial blood, however, which is usually not the case. Pulmonary arterial blood temperature can vary during the ventilatory cycle by as much as several hundredths of a degree (represented by the lightly shaded areas in *d* and *e*.) During inspiration, elastic recoil in the venules and small veins of the nonsplanchnic part of the body pushes the cool blood from the extremities back to the right atrium; relatively little blood returns from the hepatic veins as the diaphragm pushes down on the liver and kinks those vessels. During expiration, the diaphragm and liver rise, and the accumulated warm blood in the liver is discharged into the inferior vena cava as the hepatic veins open up and the liver reassumes its normal anatomic position. This cyclic return of blood to the right atrium leads to temperature changes in the blood in that chamber. This fact becomes important in the timing of the three injections for cardiac output determinations. If an injection is superimposed onto the baseline high temperature (*d*), the computer will detect a relatively small area under the curve. If an injection is superimposed onto a dip in the pulmonary arterial temperature (*e*), however, the computer will detect a larger area because it will be using the temperature of 37° C for its baseline. (The excess area is that above the broken line.) The only way to eliminate this variability is to make each of the three injections at the same point in the ventilatory cycle. We make all of our injections at end-expiration. Another option is to systematically spread the injections throughout the ventilatory cycle. Each ICU should establish its own protocol.

ment of blood flow velocity and calculation of continuous cardiac output in the ascending aorta, distal to the coronary ostia, and in the descending thoracic aorta, distal to the origin of the left subclavian artery.[44,45] Suprasternal notch probes require estimation of the diameter of the ascending aorta; esophageal probes require estimation of the diameter of the descending aorta. Expired gas analysis, with rebreathing techniques, has also been used to obtain cardiac output.[46-48] These methods are currently under clinical evaluation.

Typical cardiac output values for a well-conditioned person vary under conditions of rest and strenuous exertion [*see Table 2*]. Once again, these typical values are to be used as indicators of what the heart can do, not as target values for every critically ill patient.

Right Ventricular End-Diastolic Volume

The introduction of fast-response thermistors has allowed development of thermodilution pulmonary arterial catheters that can measure right ventricular end-diastolic volume directly.[49] The measurements are accurate as long as the patient has a regular rhythm and a heart rate lower than 140 beats/min.

Right ventricular end-diastolic volume varies with cardiovascular condition, total blood volume, positioning, exercise, ventricular compliance during diastole, pressures applied to the outside of the ventricle, hindrances against which the ventricles contract, and other factors. The right ventricular end-diastolic volume in a resting, supine, well-conditioned 60 kg person is approximately 150 ml. With assumption of an erect position, some of the blood in the thoracic portions of the cardiovascular system pools in the capacitance vessels of the abdominal viscera and the lower extremities. Ventricular end-diastolic volume decreases by perhaps one eighth, to 133 ml. With exercise, muscular contraction in the lower extremities and the abdomen squeezes the capacitance vessels. Blood is redistributed back to the heart and the pulmonary vasculature, raising the end-diastolic volume to perhaps 145 ml.

Hemoglobin Concentration

Hemoglobin concentration and hematocrit can be measured by a variety of techniques. There is no consensus as to what these values should be in critically ill patients. Both hemoglobin levels and hematocrit are lower in women than in men, for no obvious

Table 2 Effects of Position and Exercise on Cardiopulmonary Variables in a Young, Well-Conditioned 60 kg Woman[67,78-95]

Variables	Supine (Resting)	Upright (Resting)	Upright (Exercising)
Heart rate (beats/min)	60	60	200
Stroke volume (ml)	100	83	110
Cardiac output (L/min)	6	5	22
Ventricular end-diastolic volumes (ml)	150	133	145
Respiratory rate (breaths/min)	14	14	42
Tidal volume (ml)	420	420	2,220
Minute ventilation (L/min)	5.9	5.9	93.2
Hemoglobin concentration (g/dl)	11.4	11.4	12.7
Systemic arterial O_2 tension (mm Hg)	97	97	65
Systemic arterial O_2 saturation	97%	97%	92%
Systemic arterial O_2 content (ml/dl)	15.7	15.7	16
Systemic arterial CO_2 tension (mm Hg)	40	40	30
Systemic arterial pH	7.40	7.40	7.30
Mixed venous O_2 tension (mm Hg)	41	37	14
Mixed venous O_2 saturation (%)	76%	71.6%	11%
Mixed venous O_2 content (ml/dl)	12.2	11.5	2.0
O_2 consumption (ml/min)	210	210	3,180
CO_2 production (ml/min)	170	170	3,180
Respiratory quotient	0.8	0.8	1.0

reason. The relative anemia has no apparent ill effect, and it may even have some survival advantages. The value for a desirable hematocrit depends on many variables [see 6:3 Shock].[50] Physical conditioning in a warm environment typically leads to a substantial increase in plasma volume, by a factor of 1.5 or more, and a less substantial increase in red cell volume. Pregnancy induces changes identical to those induced by hard physical conditioning. The result is a lower hemoglobin concentration. At the end of a vigorous session of exercise, the hemoglobin level increases as a consequence of dehydration [see Table 2]. Living at altitude results in high hemoglobin levels and high hematocrits.

Levels of Oxygen and Carbon Dioxide

SYSTEMIC ARTERIAL BLOOD

The term oxygen saturation (S_{O_2}) refers to the fraction of hemoglobin occupied by oxygen. Oxygen content (C_{O_2}), or con-

Table 3 Conversion of pH to Hydrogen Ion Concentration*

pH	Conversion	Hydrogen Ion Concentration (nmol/L)
7.0	—	100
7.1	100×0.8	80
7.2	80×0.8	64
7.3	63×0.8	50
7.4	50×0.8	40
7.5	40×0.8	32
7.6	32×0.8	25

*Values not indicated in the table can be derived by interpolation. For example, a pH of 7.35 corresponds to a hydrogen concentration of approximately 45 nmol/L.

centration, is the amount of oxygen contained in a given volume of blood. In the United States, it is typically expressed as ml of oxygen dissolved in 100 ml (1 dl) of blood. The partial pressure (tension) of oxygen (P_{O_2}) or carbon dioxide (P_{CO_2}) in blood is the pressure that the dissolved gas exerts on the walls of the blood vessel. Systemic arterial oxygen saturation ($S_{a}O_2$) can be obtained by means of pulse oximetry. Measurement of blood gases, however, requires blood, usually obtained from indwelling catheters.

Pulse oximeters have proved extremely useful for monitoring $S_{a}O_2$ in the ICU, in that they are noninvasive and easy to use and require minimal calibration. The basic principle is that oxygenated and reduced hemoglobin have different absorption properties for light of known wavelengths. Pulse oximeters measure absorption of selected wavelengths of light from pulsatile (i.e., arterial) blood flow, typically in the nailbed on a finger or toe or in the earlobe. They can be used only in patients who have good perfusion: hypoperfusion and inadequate pulsation of blood in the arterioles make it impossible for the oximeter to distinguish between arteriolar and venular blood.

Oxygen saturations may not give enough information, however. For a more complete clinical assessment, it may be necessary to measure arterial oxygen tension ($P_{a}O_2$), arterial CO_2 tension ($P_{a}CO_2$), and pH. Saturation can be approximated from these three measurements along with temperature. These calculations are typically made by computer in the blood gas laboratory, and the approximated saturation value is returned by the laboratory along with the measured $P_{a}O_2$, $P_{a}CO_2$, and pH. Oxygen saturation can also be measured directly on a blood specimen by means of a co-oximeter. This simple and inexpensive device gives a more accurate value because it measures saturation directly. It does require another several milliliters of blood, however, thereby adding to the amount of blood required of the patient.

The greatest significance of $S_{a}O_2$, whether obtained via pulse oximetry or via direct measurement, lies in its role in yielding values for arterial oxygen content ($C_{a}O_2$), which is the value that usually counts most. $C_{a}O_2$ is a measure of all the oxygen in the blood, including that attached to hemoglobin and that dissolved in plasma, and may be approximated as follows:

$$C_{a}O_2 = 1.39 \times [Hb] \times S_{a}O_2 + 0.0031 \times P_{a}O_2$$

[Hb], the hemoglobin concentration in blood, is expressed in g/dl; $S_{a}O_2$ is expressed as a percentage; 0.0031 is the so-called Bunsen coefficient; and $P_{a}O_2$ is expressed in mm Hg.

The amount of oxygen dissolved in plasma is small compared with the amount bound to hemoglobin. As long as $P_{a}O_2$ is less than about 100 mm Hg, the contribution of the oxygen in the plasma to the total oxygen content need not be considered, provided that the hemoglobin concentration is at least 7 g/dl. If the oxygen dissolved in plasma is left out, calculation of $C_{a}O_2$ is even simpler:

$$C_{a}O_2 = 1.39 \times [Hb] \times S_{a}O_2$$

Thus, if the hemoglobin concentration is 11.4 g/dl and $S_{a}O_2$ is 97%, the oxygen content of the blood (excluding that dissolved in plasma) is 15.4 ml/dl. If the oxygen dissolved in plasma is added back in, $C_{a}O_2$ is 15.7 ml/dl, assuming a $P_{a}O_2$ of 97 mm Hg. This is a normal value for a woman who is in good cardiovascular condition or in the late stages of pregnancy, with a hematocrit of 34% [see Table 2].

Although 1.39 is probably the most accurate figure for the purposes of this calculation, other values—some as low as 1.33—have also been reported. Accordingly, the calculation can be simplified yet further by using a value of 4/3 instead of 1.39.

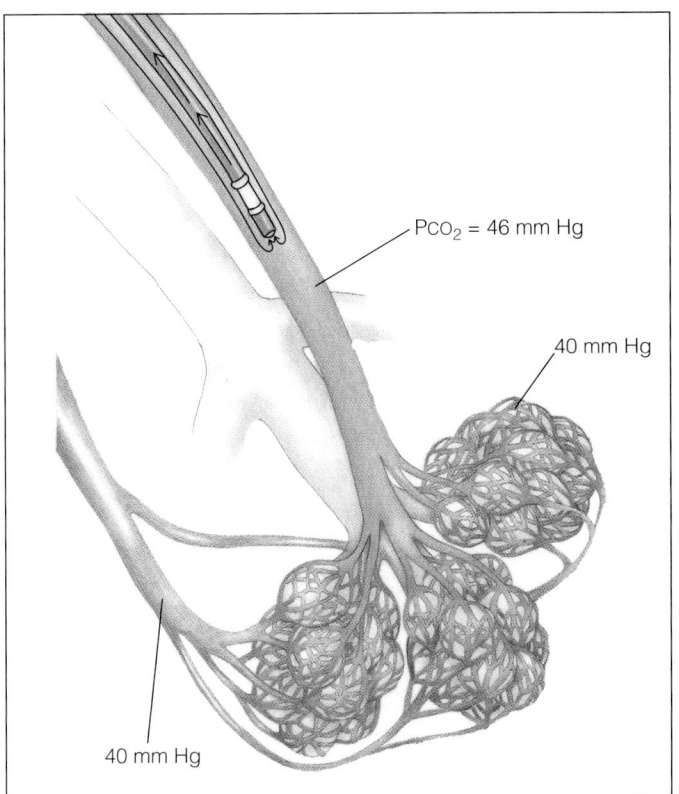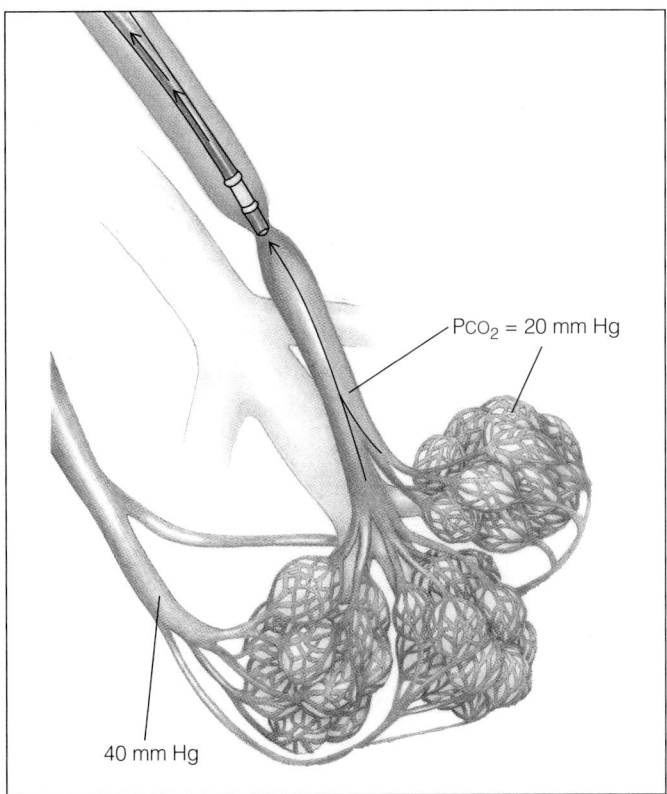

Figure 7 **The Swan-Ganz catheter allows collection of mixed venous blood for measurement of $S_{mv}O_2$ and $C_{mv}O_2$ (left). If blood from the pulmonary artery is withdrawn through the catheter too forcefully, however, arterial walls can collapse around the tip of the catheter (right). The sample will in that case consist of blood from the distal pulmonary vasculature that has been pulled back past ventilated alveoli. To determine whether this has happened, the P_{CO_2} in the sample should be checked. $P_{mv}CO_2$ is typically about 5 mm Hg greater than P_aCO_2. If the arterial walls have collapsed around the catheter, the sample will consist of blood from which much of the CO_2 will already have been excreted into the ventilated alveoli, and the $P_{mv}CO_2$ in the recovered blood may be as much as 20 mm Hg lower than a simultaneously obtained P_aCO_2. Specimens of this sort should be discarded and new specimens obtained. Taking care in obtaining true mixed venous blood is equally important when using a catheter with an oximeter mounted on its tip. Calibration of the oximeter requires direct measurement of $S_{mv}O_2$ in a correctly obtained specimen.**

The blood obtained for direct measurement of P_aO_2 and S_aO_2 can also be used for measurement of P_aCO_2 and pH. P_aCO_2 is a measure of the amount of CO_2 dissolved in the plasma. Arterial carbon dioxide content (C_aCO_2) can be calculated, but it seldom is because within physiologic ranges of P_aCO_2, CO_2 content is almost linearly related to partial pressure. Hydrogen ion concentration is usually expressed as pH and is obtained by direct measurement with ion-sensitive electrodes. It can also be expressed in nmol/L [*see Table 3*].

Blood drawn for blood gas determinations should be placed on ice immediately to inhibit oxygen consumption by neutrophils. Before being measured in the blood gas apparatus, it is rewarmed to 37° C by a heating element in the cuvette, and P_aO_2, P_aCO_2, and pH are then determined with the blood at this temperature. The patient's blood, however, may be either warmer or colder than 37° C. If, for example, the patient's blood is 35° C when it is drawn, some of the oxygen and CO_2 will come out of solution when it is warmed to 37° C. Consequently, the partial pressures measured by the apparatus will be higher than the actual pressures in the blood when it was circulating in the patient.

The physician and nurse caring for the patient need not make this temperature correction themselves: the blood gas laboratory typically reports temperature-corrected values for the partial pressures and pH if the patient's temperature is supplied to the laboratory along with the specimen.[51]

An increasing number of clinicians, however, no longer make temperature corrections for blood gases and manage hypothermic and hyperthermic patients with the so-called alpha-stat method.[52] Treatment based on this method is thought to induce fewer abnormalities in acid-base balance when the patient's temperature returns to normal [*see 6:9 Disorders of Acid-Base and Potassium Balance*].

MIXED VENOUS BLOOD

Mixed venous blood, by definition, represents a mixture of all blood returned from all organs. Venous blood from the heart is returned to the right atrium through the coronary sinus. This blood is markedly desaturated. Thus, blood in the right ventricle or in the pulmonary artery is truly mixed venous blood because it includes the blood from the heart as well as that from the rest of the body. Blood from the superior vena cava, however, is not, because it does not include the blood from the heart. Accordingly, blood gas measurements from vena caval blood may be falsely elevated. Measurements of gases in blood obtained from the right atrium may be falsely low if the catheter tip is placed near the coronary sinus.

Two errors in obtaining pulmonary arterial blood can lead to misleading measurements. The first, contamination of the specimen with residual fluid in the lumen of the catheter, is easily avoided by discarding the initial 3 ml of blood drawn through the catheter. The second error is harder to avoid. It arises if the blood sample is withdrawn too forcefully through the catheter. The pulmonary artery may collapse around the end of the catheter, causing the blood to be drawn in a retrograde manner past ventilated alveoli [*see Figure 7*]. This results in a specimen with very high oxygen levels, which does not accurately reflect desaturated pulmonary arterial blood. The possibility that blood was drawn in a retrograde fashion can be checked by measuring the P_{CO_2} in the specimen. CO_2 tension in true pulmonary arterial blood ($P_{mv}CO_2$) is typically 5 mm Hg higher than that in simultaneously drawn systemic arterial blood.[53] Blood drawn back past ventilated alveoli will have a very low $P_{mv}CO_2$. If the CO_2 tension in the specimen is equal to or less than that in systemic arterial blood, the specimen should be discarded and another specimen obtained by drawing back on the syringe more slowly. One should rely on the oxygen saturation of the specimen (measured by co-oximetry) rather than on the oxygen tension. Mixed venous partial pressure of oxygen ($P_{mv}O_2$) and oxygen saturation ($S_{mv}O_2$) lie on the steep portion of the oxyhemoglobin dissociation curve. A minor error in measurement of the former can result in a major error in calculation of the latter [*see 6:9 Disorders of Acid-Base and Potassium Balance*].

It is frequently worthwhile to monitor $S_{mv}O_2$ continuously with a specially equipped pulmonary arterial catheter that has an oximeter attached to the tip. Calibration of the oximeter requires occasional cross-checking with measurement of $S_{mv}O_2$ in a correctly obtained sample of pulmonary arterial blood. A fall in the $S_{mv}O_2$ can arise from a decline in the cardiac output, a decrease in the hemoglobin concentration, a fall in the S_aO_2, or an increase in oxygen consumption (including an increase in myocardial oxygen consumption).

It must be kept in mind, however, that even though a falling $S_{mv}O_2$ may be a warning signal, a normal or high value does not guarantee that cardiopulmonary status is satisfactory or that there is adequate oxygen for metabolic demands. In patients with low-output septic shock, for example, well-oxygenated blood is returned to the heart because blood is functionally shunted away from the tissues. The high $S_{mv}O_2$ in these patients does not indicate that their metabolic needs are being met; rather, it is the result of deranged peripheral metabolic processes characterized by futile metabolic cycling. In patients with high-output septic shock, $S_{mv}O_2$ may be high because large amounts of blood are shunted to the skin so as to attenuate hyperthermia. Because the skin is metabolically inactive, the blood returning from it will have a high oxygen saturation. Similarly, in cirrhotic patients, who have functional arteriovenous shunts, a high $S_{mv}O_2$ is generated in the presence of inadequate metabolic activity.

Mixed venous oxygen content ($C_{mv}O_2$) is easily calculated in the same manner as C_aO_2. In normal persons, $S_{mv}O_2$ is about 76%. Therefore, if oxygen dissolved in plasma is excluded, $C_{mv}O_2$ is $1.39 \times 11.4 \times 76\%$, or 12.0 ml/dl. If the oxygen in the plasma is added back in, $C_{mv}O_2$ becomes 12.2 ml/dl, on the assumption that $P_{mv}O_2$ is 41 mm Hg.

Minute Ventilation and Tidal Volume

Modern mechanical ventilators have flow meters built into both the inspiratory and expiratory limbs of their tubing. Integration of the flows by computers in the ventilator gives values for inspiratory and expiratory tidal volumes, and multiplying these values by respiratory rate yields inspiratory and expiratory minute ventilation [*see Table 2*]. The inspiratory values are usually ever so slightly larger than the expiratory values. Oxygen consumption per minute is slightly greater than CO_2 production (for a respiratory quotient < 1). Large discrepancies between the two may indicate a leak in the ventilator circuitry.

Cardiopulmonary Descriptors Derived from Primary Measurements

The primary measurements already described can be used to calculate certain derived values that are useful descriptors of specific aspects of the cardiopulmonary system. Although a few of these derived descriptors are simple—such as stroke volume, which is cardiac output divided by heart rate—most are fairly complex and require the use of relatively complicated formulas. Some (e.g., ventricular end-systolic unstressed volumes) can be calculated only from measurements obtained via cardiac catheterization. All of these descriptors, being derived values, are only as accurate and useful as the measurements on which they are based. With that caveat in mind, they can be quite valuable in helping one form a sophisticated overall assessment of cardiopulmonary status. They can also help one make effective choices among therapeutic alternatives.

LEFT AND RIGHT VENTRICULAR END-SYSTOLIC PRESSURE

Left ventricular end-systolic pressure can be precisely measured during cardiac catheterization, but it can only be estimated in the ICU. From measurements during catheterization, it is known that left ventricular end-systolic pressure is approximately 90% of left ventricular peak systolic pressure, which is the same as aortic root peak systolic pressure. In SICU patients, left ventricular end-systolic pressure can be approximated by multiplying aortic root systolic pressure by 0.9.[54] In patients younger than 50 years, aortic root systolic pressure can be estimated by subtracting 20 mm Hg from radial artery systolic pressure; in patients 50 years of age or older, it can be estimated by subtracting 20 mm Hg from radial artery systolic pressure.[55] Left ventricular end-systolic pressure is a useful value to know, but one must keep in mind the limitations of the measurements it is based on.

Right ventricular end-systolic pressure can be calculated by multiplying pulmonary arterial peak systolic pressure by 0.9. This measurement is usually quite reliable, provided that the catheter-tubing-transducer system is well matched to the vasculature.

AORTIC ROOT AND PULMONARY ARTERIAL END-SYSTOLIC PRESSURE-VOLUME RELATIONS

The aortic root end-systolic pressure-volume relation can be calculated by dividing left ventricular end-systolic pressure by stroke volume; the pulmonary arterial end-systolic pressure-volume relation can be determined by dividing right ventricular end-systolic pressure by stroke volume. These relations give a good approximation of the total hindrances or input impedances facing the ventricles when they inject their blood into their respective vasculatures.[21,56] These impedances depend on the same factors that apply in the systemic arteries [*see Sidebar* Propagation of Energy and Generation of Pressures and Volumes in the Arterial System]: the stiffness of the arteries, the degree of constriction of the arterioles, the spatial distribution of the arterioles, and the stiffness of the contralateral heart during filling. The input impedances are a major determinant of myocardial oxygen requirements. Pumping blood into a vasculature with a high impedance requires a great deal of oxygen; pumping blood into a vasculature with a low impedance requires little.[22,57,58]

For purposes of treatment, input impedance can be regarded as having three components: the stiffness of the arteries, the resistance of the arterioles, and the stiffness of the contralateral heart. If the arteries seem excessively stiff, one has several potential options. Diuresis can decrease arterial blood volume and decrease arterial stiffness. Nitroprusside and nitroglycerine can act directly on arterial walls to reduce stiffness. Positive pressure ventilation can increase the stiffness of the pulmonary arteries; adjusting the ventilator can decrease stiffness. Use of aortic balloon counterpulsation can directly decrease aortic input impedance. If arteriolar resistance seems excessively high, as determined by calculation of vascular resistance (see below), a vasodilator may be given. If the contralateral ventricle is thought to be excessively stiff, a diuretic can be administered. If positive pressure appears to be increasing stiffness, the problem may be resolved by adjusting the ventilator.

In resting normal persons, aortic root and pulmonary arterial end-systolic pressure-volume relations are approximately 1.0 and 0.2 mm Hg/ml, respectively.[59] The values can increase enormously (up to four times baseline) in a hypertensive crisis or in compensated hemorrhagic shock. They can plunge to levels 50% of normal in inflammatory shock.

The calculated aortic root end-systolic pressure-volume relation is usually reliable, the main potential problem being the extrapolation from a distal arterial systolic pressure to a central aortic systolic pressure. The calculated pulmonary arterial end-systolic pressure-volume relation is usually very accurate as well, provided that the Swan-Ganz catheter's measuring system is well matched to the vasculature.

SYSTEMIC AND PULMONARY VASCULAR RESISTANCE

Pressure across a resistance equals flow across the resistance multiplied by the resistance itself. Resistance, therefore, equals pressure divided by flow. To calculate systemic vascular resistance, the difference between mean aortic pressure and right atrial pressure is divided by cardiac output. To calculate pulmonary vascular resistance, the difference between mean pulmonary arterial pressure and pulmonary arterial wedge pressure is divided by cardiac output.[35]

Of the two resistances, pulmonary vascular resistance is more difficult to measure and more likely to change under different conditions. Because pulmonary vascular resistance depends on the difference between two relatively small pressures, a slight error in the measurement of either one can result in a large error in the calculation of resistance. The mode of ventilation can substantially affect the calculation as well. Hyperinflation with mechanical ventilation can compress the intra-alveolar vasculature and increase pulmonary vascular resistance[60]; spontaneous ventilation can decrease it. In contrast, systemic vascular resistance depends on the difference between a large pressure and a small one. Hence, a slight error in the measurement of either pressure has little effect on the calculation of resistance.

For these reasons, pulmonary vascular resistance is not, in our view, a reliable descriptor. Systemic vascular resistance can be helpful, however, if considered in the context of clinical condition and input impedance. Patients with a low systemic vascular resistance almost always have warm, well-perfused skin and a high cardiac output. Those with a high resistance usually have constricted cutaneous vessels and a low cardiac output. If input impedance is high and resistance is normal (or, possibly, low), the problem must lie in the stiffness of the arteries or the heart. Treatment should therefore be directed toward these areas, not the arterioles.

The units used to express vascular resistances vary from hospital to hospital. It is simplest, and also perfectly acceptable scientifically, to use arbitrary units. We prefer mm Hg · L^{-1} · min— that is, we use the number obtained through the simple calculation described without making any further corrections. A normal systemic arterial resistance is about 14 mm Hg · L^{-1} · min in a supine, resting 60 kg person. Some multiply this raw number by 80 to convert the resistances to units in the centimeter-gram-second (CGS) system.

LEFT VENTRICULAR END-DIASTOLIC VOLUME

Direct measurement of left ventricular end-diastolic volume requires transesophageal echocardiography. This modality is available in most ORs, but it requires the attendance of a physician, usually an anesthesiologist or a cardiologist. This level of physician involvement is not routinely available in most ICUs. Transthoracic imaging can be used for this purpose, but results are frequently misleading in critically ill surgical patients because of bandaging, chest wall edema, and movement of mediastinal structures with mechanical ventilation.

Left ventricular end-diastolic volume can be estimated by measuring pulmonary arterial wedge pressure and taking into account the factors discussed in relation to pressures in the pulmonary artery [see Pulmonary Arterial Pressures, above]. To improve the precision of the estimate, composite right ventricular end-diastolic compliance can be assessed by comparing directly measured right ventricular end-diastolic volume with right atrial pressure. This value is taken as the volume divided by the difference between intracardiac pressure and atmospheric pressure, zeroed at the level of the atrium.

Given that the pressures applied to the outside of the right ventricle are usually about the same as those applied to the outside of the left, a compliant right ventricle suggests a compliant left ventricle. Thus, if a low right atrial pressure generates a satisfactory right-ventricular end-diastolic volume, one can tentatively assume that a low wedge pressure is probably generating a satisfactory left-ventricular end-diastolic volume. This sort of assumptive reasoning, however, is fraught with danger, for many reasons. Measurements made during cardiac catheterization suggest that left and right ventricular end-diastolic volumes are nearly the same in spontaneously breathing normal persons. In critically ill surgical patients, however, there can be enormous disparities between the two, depending in part on varying pressures applied to the outside of the heart and in part on the different hindrances the ventricles face when they contract.[61] Accordingly, a noninvasive and accurate means of determining left ventricular end-diastolic volume would be extremely useful in managing critically ill patients. Unfortunately, the technology is not yet available.

In a supine, well-conditioned, spontaneously breathing normal person, left ventricular end-diastolic volume is approximately 150 ml. In the upright position, it decreases by perhaps one eighth; with exercise, it returns to close to 150 ml.

LEFT AND RIGHT VENTRICULAR END-SYSTOLIC VOLUME

End-systolic volumes can be obtained by subtracting stroke volume from end-diastolic volumes. In a 60 kg subject with ventricular end-diastolic volumes of 150 ml and a stroke volume of 100 ml, end-systolic volumes are 50 ml.

Ventricular End-Systolic Unstressed Volume

The term end-systolic unstressed volume refers to the volume that a ventricle would assume if all of its blood were removed with the ventricle in a fully contracted state. Unstressed volumes cannot be measured routinely in the ICU, but they can be measured during cardiac catheterization. In most patients, unstressed volumes are quite small (~ 6 ml). In those with severe congestive heart failure, however, they can be as large as 50 ml.

LEFT AND RIGHT VENTRICULAR END-SYSTOLIC PRESSURE-VOLUME RELATIONS

The left ventricular end-systolic pressure-volume relation can be determined by subtracting left ventricular end-systolic unstressed volume from left ventricular end-systolic volume and dividing the difference into the left ventricular end-systolic pressure.[62] The right ventricular end-systolic pressure-volume relation can be determined similarly. These relations give a good indication of the contractile state of the ventricles. For the left ventricle, a typical value in an unstressed person is 2.3 mm Hg/ml; for the right, 0.5 mm Hg/ml. Values can be doubled by exercise or adrenergic stimulation and cut in half by congestive heart failure. Knowledge of these pressure-volume relations can help direct therapy toward contractility,[22] though, as with most interventions in the critically ill patient, it is not clear that doing so is necessarily beneficial.

Calculation of these values requires knowledge of ventricular end-systolic pressure and ventricular end-diastolic volume. In the case of the right ventricle, these estimates are quite good and the calculation of the end-systolic pressure-volume relation quite accurate. In the case of the left ventricle, estimates are less precise and the calculation less dependable.

POWER

Power calculations are a useful way of quantifying the energy available for delivery of nutrients to tissues and delivery of energy to the contralateral heart. The total power delivered into the aorta can be calculated by multiplying left ventricular end-systolic pressure by cardiac output.[59] Steady-flow aortic power is mean arterial pressure multiplied by cardiac output. Oscillatory power is the difference between total power and steady-flow power. Most of the steady-flow power is dissipated as heat in the microvasculature; the amount of heat dissipated can be calculated by subtracting central venous pressure from mean arterial pressure and multiplying the difference by cardiac output. The remaining steady-flow power fills the right atrium and ventricle during diastole and the right atrium during systole; this value can be calculated by multiplying central venous pressure by cardiac output. The power delivered by the right side of the heart into the pulmonary vasculature can be calculated similarly.

OXYGEN TRANSPORT

Oxygen transport—the amount of oxygen delivered to the tissues—is calculated by multiplying cardiac output by C_aO_2. The calculation is simple, though care must be taken to obtain the correct units. Cardiac output is typically expressed in L/min, C_aO_2 in ml/dl. In multiplying the two, it is necessary to introduce a factor of 10 (to convert the liters of blood in cardiac output to the deciliters of blood in C_aO_2). Thus, in a patient with a normal cardiac output of 6 L/min, a normal hemoglobin concentration of 11.4 g/dl, a normal S_aO_2 of 97%, and a normal P_aO_2 of 97 mm Hg, a normal oxygen transport is approximately 940 ml/min:

$$O_2 \text{ transport} = \text{Cardiac output} \times C_aO_2$$
$$= 60 \text{ dl/min} \times 15.7 \text{ ml/dl}$$
$$= 940 \text{ ml/min}$$

A reduction in cardiac output, hemoglobin concentration, or S_aO_2 decreases oxygen transport.

OXYGEN RETURN

The amount of oxygen returned to the heart can be calculated by multiplying cardiac output by $C_{mv}O_2$. For a normal cardiac output of 6 L/min and a $C_{mv}O_2$ of 12.2 ml/dl, oxygen return is approximately 730 ml/min.

OXYGEN CONSUMPTION

Oxygen consumption is the difference between oxygen transport and oxygen return. It is therefore calculated by multiplying cardiac output by the difference between oxygen content in systemic arterial blood and that in mixed venous blood:

$$\text{Oxygen consumption} = \text{Cardiac output} \times (C_aO_2 - C_{mv}O_2)$$

Normal oxygen consumption in a resting, supine, well-conditioned woman is 210 ml/min.

Oxygen consumption seems to have even more normal variability than the other parameters already discussed (see above), and it covers a range of values. It is probably easiest to memorize a single normal value, however, rather than a range. As long as the physician recognizes that, for example, an oxygen consumption of 180 ml/min in a 60 kg patient is close to the average of 210, no harm will be done. An oxygen consumption of 150 ml/min, however, would clearly be abnormally low and should prompt investigation to correct a low cardiac output, a low hemoglobin concentration, or a low S_aO_2.

BICARBONATE CONCENTRATION

The calculated value for bicarbonate concentration is obtained from measurements of P_{CO_2} and hydrogen ion concentration by using the Henderson-Hasselbalch equation [see 6:9 Disorders of Acid-Base and Potassium Balance]. The advantage of this equation is its familiarity; the disadvantage is that it involves the use of logarithms. It is possible, however, to estimate bicarbonate concentration without using logarithms, as follows:

$$[HCO_3^-] = (24 \times P_{CO_2}) \div [H^+]$$

This formula yields a value for bicarbonate concentration in mmol/L. P_{CO_2} should be expressed as mm Hg; however, the hydrogen ion concentration must be expressed as nmol/L rather than pH [see Table 3]. Thus, if P_{CO_2} is 40 mm Hg and hydrogen ion concentration is 80 nmol/L, the bicarbonate concentration is 12 mmol/L.

The bicarbonate concentration closely approximates the actual concentration of bicarbonate in the blood. The value obtained from the clinical laboratories for a peripheral venous blood specimen includes all of the compounds involved with dissociation of carbonic acid, including carbonic acid itself, bicarbonate, and carbon dioxide. In contrast, calculation of the bicarbonate concentration from blood gas values gives a value for a specific compound and therefore tends to be more useful than laboratory values for such specimens.

Noninvasive Summary Measurements

Three main goals can be identified for cardiopulmonary monitoring as technology advances. The first is to make as many measurements as possible noninvasively so as to eliminate the risks now associated with monitoring. The second is to find a single measurement that summarizes overall patient status. If this parameter indicates that a patient is doing well, current therapy can be continued; if not, therapy can be reassessed. The third goal—which contradicts the second to some degree but is nonetheless desirable—is to know the status of the individual organs. If a

Table 4   Effects of Position and Exercise on Organ Blood Flow and Oxygen Consumption in a Young, Well-Conditioned 60 kg Woman[67,78-95]

Variables	Supine (Resting)	Upright (Resting)	Exercising (Upright)
Whole body			
Blood flow	6.0	5.0	22.0
Venous O_2 saturation	76%	71.6%	11%
O_2 consumption	210	210	3,180
Splanchnic viscera			
Blood flow (% of total)	1.50 (25%)	1.25 (25%)	0.30 (1%)
Venous O_2 saturation	77%	73%	18%
O_2 consumption	50	50	40
Kidneys			
Blood flow (% of total)	1.20 (20%)	1.00 (20%)	0.25 (1%)
Venous O_2 saturation	91%	90%	65%
O_2 consumption	12	12	12
Brain			
Blood flow (% of total)	0.90 (15%)	0.75 (15%)	0.75 (3%)
Venous O_2 saturation	67%	60%	59%
O_2 consumption	45	45	45
Heart			
Blood flow (% of total)	0.24 (4%)	0.20 (4%)	0.80 (4%)
Venous O_2 saturation	46%	35%	1%
O_2 consumption	20	20	130
Skeletal muscle			
Blood flow (% of total)	1.20 (20%)	1.00 (20%)	19.5 (89%)
Venous O_2 saturation	61%	54%	8%
O_2 consumption	70	70	2,940
Skin			
Blood flow (% of total)	0.30 (5%)	0.25 (5%)	0.30 (1%)
Venous O_2 saturation	93%	91%	88%
O_2 consumption	2	2	2
Other organs			
Blood flow (% of total)	0.66 (11%)	0.55 (11%)	0.10 (0%)
Venous O_2 saturation	87%	85%	31%
O_2 consumption	11	11	11

patient is not doing well, one would like to know where to direct therapeutic efforts. Ideally, one could identify the organ at greatest risk, keeping in mind that treating one organ usually comes at the expense of another. If one could monitor the state of all organs at once, this problem would be close to being solved. Having a feeling for flows and metabolic activities of individual organ systems, in baseline and stressful conditions [*see Table 4*], is a start toward these goals. This knowledge can provide a useful perspective on the measurements available now.

Skin temperature can be monitored on the toe or the thumb with noninvasive devices. It is directly correlated with cutaneous blood flow and can be a sensitive indicator of overall perfusion.[63] A gradient of less than 2° C between skin temperature and ambient temperature indicates critically low perfusion. A gradient exceeding 2° C suggests that the heart is capable of generating a fairly robust output. Accurate measurements, however, are difficult to obtain unless there is good control of ambient temperatures.

Oxygen tension in soft tissues, which can also be a good indicator of overall perfusion, can be determined by monitoring conjunctival or cutaneous tissues. Conjunctival oxygen tension is measured with a small oxygen sensor placed directly on the conjunctiva. The device is safe, and it does reflect changes in oxygen delivery to the tissue, but it is not commonly used, perhaps because of the potential for damage to the eye. Transcutaneous

oxygen tension can be determined by placing a polarographic surface oxygen electrode directly on heated skin; tissue oxygen tension is measured beneath this surface electrode. This value correlates well with P_aO_2 if local tissue perfusion is good.

Urine output is a good indicator of overall status. It is determined primarily by plasma levels of antidiuretic hormone and aldosterone. Stress increases these levels and thereby reduces output. Blood flow to the kidneys is of secondary importance, but it too can contribute to oliguria. The kidneys, however, are rarely at risk solely because of decreased blood flow. In strenuous exercise, for example, blood flow drops to very low levels, but the kidneys fare well. Their metabolic needs are easily met by increased extraction of oxygen from renal arterial blood [*see Table 4*]. Although a low urine output usually reflects stress and perhaps decreased blood flow to the kidneys, an adequate or even high urine output does not necessarily mean that stress is absent or blood flow is more than adequate. For unclear reasons, some patients in inflammatory and even hypovolemic shock continue to produce apparently adequate urine output. Thus, although oliguria can be a warning sign of patient distress, normal urine production is not a guarantee that all is well.

Blood flow to the gastric mucosa can be assessed by means of gastric tonometry.[64] Low values suggest shock; normal values suggest adequate cardiovascular function. Blood flow to the gut mucosa and mucosal oxygen consumption can be influenced by many factors. Consumption of a large meal increases blood flow to the small intestine and metabolic activity of the gut mucosa, slightly increasing cardiac output and overall oxygen consumption. Oxygen consumption of the gut mucosa typically increases from 50 ml/min to more than 100 ml/min. With stress, blood flow can fall to very low levels. Metabolic activity decreases less dramatically, as the mucosa extracts more oxygen from the perfusing blood [*see Table 4*].

Continuous measurement of end-expiratory carbon dioxide tension gives information about P_aCO_2. The monitoring devices are typically inserted into the ventilator circuit between the end of the endotracheal tube and the Y connector to the ventilator. Credible readings must show a smooth CO_2 tension curve that begins at zero during inspiration and then rises exponentially to a plateau at end-expiration. A long plateau indicates that the alveoli are probably emptying at a regular rate, in which case the value can be used to detect trends in P_aCO_2. Values obtained at end-expiration depend not only on P_aCO_2 but also on dead-space ventilation.[65] Thus, the devices are best used for detecting trends rather than for determining the absolute value for arterial CO_2.

Influence of Age, Body Size, and Other Variables on Cardiopulmonary Descriptors

The typical values for cardiopulmonary descriptors given earlier [*see Tables 1, 2, and 4*] can be affected by several variables, including age, cardiovascular condition, positioning, consumption of a large meal, mechanical ventilation, and thermal stress.

Age does not affect resting heart rate, but it does decrease resting stroke volume and cardiac output, depending on how the values are indexed to body size.[66] As a rule, in an older person who has not maintained good aerobic conditioning and who has not continued to work out against resistance, cardiac output decreases by approximately 10% per decade, starting at age 50. This decline can be mitigated by physical activity, but it cannot be eliminated.

Good cardiovascular conditioning results in a larger blood volume, a slower resting heart rate, larger ventricular end-diastolic volumes, and a larger stroke volume.[50] Conditioning does not influence resting cardiac output or, in otherwise normal persons, resting blood pressures.

Assumption of an upright position does not affect resting heart rate, but it does reduce ventricular end-diastolic volumes, stroke volume, and cardiac output to levels approximately one eighth lower than supine values [see Table 2].

Institution of mechanical ventilation can decrease oxygen consumption by approximately 10%. The effects of mechanical ventilation on the other parameters vary depending on the patient's intravascular volume status. As a rule, mechanical ventilation with tidal volumes of 10 ml/kg decreases ventricular end-diastolic volumes, stroke volume, and cardiac output. These effects can be partially reversed by infusing fluid to return ventricular end-diastolic volumes toward normal values. With the current trend toward using smaller tidal volumes, some, but not all, of these adverse effects of mechanical ventilation can be minimized.

Any environment that places a thermal stress on the patient can influence the values obtained. If the environment is cold enough to produce shivering, oxygen consumption and cardiac output can rise to levels several times higher than those of a person in a thermoneutral environment. Hypothermia in the absence of shivering decreases oxygen consumption and cardiac output. Extreme hypothermia can reduce these values to levels as low as one fourth of normothermic values. Hyperthermia or systemic inflammation can increase oxygen consumption and cardiac output to values as high as twice those of a normothermic

Table 5 Approximate Desirable Weights and Cardiac Outputs in Young, Resting, Supine Persons

Height (ft, in)	Desirable Weight (kg)	Cardiac Output (L/min)
5'0"	50	5.0
5'6"	60	6.0
6'0"	70	7.0
6'6"	80	8.0

Table 6 Effects of Age on Metabolically Active Weight and Cardiac Output in Older, Resting, Supine Persons 5'6" in Height

Age (years)	Weight (kg)	Cardiac Output (L/min)
50	60	6.0
60	54	5.4
70	49	4.9
80	44	4.4
90	39	3.9

Methods of Indexing Cardiopulmonary Variables to Body Size

In the late 1800s, body surface area was used to index for metabolic rate. The rationale was that an increased metabolic rate was known to be associated with increased heat production and that loss of heat from the body to the environment, to maintain an acceptable body temperature, had to occur between the surface of the body and its surroundings. In the 1920s, when it became possible to measure cardiac output as part of metabolic studies, many investigators began to express cardiac output, as well as metabolic rate, in terms of body surface area, on the grounds that the two quantities had to be related. Although it was recognized that the relation was not necessarily a linear one, this approach to indexing worked, in the sense that it minimized some of the inherent variability observed in nonindexed cardiac outputs. Body surface area became the most commonly used measurement of body size for indexing both metabolic rate and cardiac output.

In the 1930s, however, Max Kleiber made the empirical observation that the metabolic rates, and presumably the cardiac outputs, of members of one species of animals could best be compared with those of another species by indexing to body weight raised to the three-fourths power.[76] Such indexing seemed to reduce variability even more effectively than indexing to body surface area, though it was difficult to explain why. Over the ensuing six decades, more and more accumulated evidence came to support Kleiber's contention, but only in the past 10 years have his observations been satisfactorily explained. It now seems established that the Kleiber hypothesis can be explained by relating metabolism and flow with a model that accounts for the fractal geometry of the cardiovascular system and the thermodynamics of metabolism and temperature regulation.[77]

The question of indexing within a species (as opposed to between different species), however, remains unsettled. Many clinicians, particularly those with a primary interest in the cardiovascular system, continue to favor use of body surface area for indexing metabolic rates and cardiac outputs; others, particularly those with a primary interest in the respiratory system, favor use of body weight. A few favor use of body weight raised to the three-fourths power. Still others choose not to index at all.

or uninjured or noninfected person, but no higher [see 6:22 Metabolic Response to Critical Illness]. Blood flow to the skin, during strenuous but not exhausting exercise in a warm environment, can increase from a baseline of 300 ml/min to as much as 6 L/min in an effort to offload heat and keep body temperature within acceptable limits.[67] During extreme exercise, cutaneous flow falls back to baseline as the body redirects flow away from the skin and to the muscles [see Table 4]. The result is hyperthermia. To the best of our knowledge, accurate measurements of skin blood flow have not been obtained in an ICU setting, but it is not unreasonable to speculate that skin blood flow in a patient in warm inflammatory shock could be on the order of 3 L/min.

Some cardiopulmonary variables (e.g., blood pressures and blood gases) are independent of body size; others (e.g., cardiac output and minute ventilation) are not. Many techniques have been used to deal with the problem of indexing these latter variables [see Sidebar Methods of Indexing Cardiopulmonary Variables to Body Size].

Our current practice is to index both cardiovascular and pulmonary variables to desirable body weight—by which we mean the weight associated with a long and healthy life—with adjustments made only for age. We disregard all other variables, including gender. We take a body mass index of 21 as the most desirable value.[68] In practice, we use the patient's height to determine what the weight would be if he or she had a body mass index of 21. We do not use the patient's actual weight when the measurement is made. That weight can be inflated by fluid resuscitation, the hardware used for fracture fixation, or bedclothes, and it can be deflated by malnutrition. It can also be difficult to measure accurately in critically ill patients, who frequently cannot be easily moved to a bedside scale. Nor do we use the patient's weight at admission, which can be unduly influenced by a large mass of metabolically inactive fat.

Approximate desirable weights can easily be calculated for

persons of different heights [*see Table 5*]. We find that height can be approximated to the nearest half foot and the numbers rounded off without affecting how the patient is eventually treated. For example, for a person 5 feet 4 inches tall, we take the desirable weight as 60 kg and the baseline output as 6 L/min.

As noted, we do adjust the calculated desirable weight for age, on the assumption that metabolically active mass decreases by an average of about 10% per decade, starting at age 50 [*see Table 6*].

This adjustment seems to make a difference, especially for persons in their 80s and 90s. An expected cardiac output of 6 L/min at age 50 falls to 4.4 L/min at age 80.

We use the indexing technique described for all of the cardiopulmonary values discussed in this chapter. At key points, we also give heights and weights, so that the values can be adjusted in relation to body surface area or other potential indices. We recognize that there is no unanimity on how best to index these variables.

References

1. Mandel MA, Dauchot PJ: Radial artery cannulation in 1,000 patients: precautions and complications. J Hand Surg [Am] 2:482, 1977

2. Slogoff S, Keats AS, Arlund C: On the safety of radial artery cannulation. Anesthesiology 59:42, 1983

3. Gardner RM, Hollingsworth KW: Optimizing the electrocardiogram and pressure monitoring. Crit Care Med 14:651, 1986

4. Arabidze GG, Petrov VV, Staessen JA: Blood pressure by Korotkoff's auscultatory method: end of an era or bright future? Blood Press Monit 1:321, 1996

5. Geddes LA: Handbook of Blood Pressure Measurement. Humana Press, Clifton, New Jersey, 1991

6. Talke P, Nichols RJ Jr, Traber DL: Does measurement of systolic blood pressure with a pulse oximeter correlate with conventional methods? J Clin Monit 6:5, 1990

7. Penaz J: Photoelectric measurement of blood pressure, volume and flow in the finger. Digest of the 10th International Conference on Medical and Biological Engineering. Albert A, Vogt W, Heilbig W, Eds. International Federation for Medical and Biological Engineering, Dresden, 1973, p 104

8. Jones DW, Appel LJ, Sheps SG, et al: Measuring blood pressure accurately: new and persistent challenges. JAMA 289:1027, 2003

9. Brinton TJ, Walls ED, Chio SS: Validation of pulse dynamic blood pressure measurement by auscultation. Blood Press Monit 3:121, 1998

10. Bur A, Herkner H, Vlcek M, et al: Factors influencing the accuracy of oscillometric blood pressure measurement in critically ill patients. Crit Care Med 31:793, 2003

11. Geddes LA, Voelz M, Combs C, et al: Characterization of the oscillometric method for measuring indirect blood pressure. Ann Biomed Eng 10:271, 1982

12. Band JD, Maki DG: Infections caused by arterial catheters used for hemodynamic monitoring. Am J Med 67:735, 1979

13. Kulkarni M, Elsner C, Ouellet D, et al: Heparinized saline versus normal saline in maintaining patency of the radial artery catheter. Can J Surg 37:37, 1994

14. Randolph AG, Cook DJ, Gonzales CA, et al: Benefit of heparin in peripheral venous and arterial catheters: systematic review and meta-analysis of randomised controlled trials. BMJ 316:969, 1998

15. Gardner RM: Direct blood pressure measurement—dynamic response requirements. Anesthesiology 54:227, 1981

16. Kleinman B: Understanding natural frequency and damping and how they relate to the measurement of blood pressure. J Clin Monit 5:137, 1989

17. Kofke WA, Levy JH: Postoperative Critical Care Procedures of the Massachusetts General Hospital. Little, Brown & Co, Boston, 1986

18. Karamanoglu M, O'Rourke MF, Avolio AP, et al: An analysis of the relationship between central aortic and peripheral upper limb pressure waves in man. Eur Heart J 14:160, 1993

19. Suga H: Ventricular energetics. Physiol Rev 70: 247, 1990

20. Suga H: Total mechanical energy of a ventricle model and cardiac oxygen consumption. Am J Physiol 236:H498, 1979

21. Kelly RP, Ting CT, Yang TM, et al: Effective arterial elastance as index of arterial vascular load in humans. Circulation 86:513, 1992

22. Nichols WW, O'Rourke MF, Hartley C, et al: McDonald's Blood Flow in Arteries: Theoretic, Experimental, and Clinical Principles, 4th ed. Oxford University Press, London, 1998

23. McGee DC, Gould MK: Preventing complications of central venous catheterization. N Engl J Med 348:1123, 2003

24. Merrer J, De Jonghe B, Golliot F, et al: Complications of femoral and subclavian venous catheterization in critically ill patients: a randomized controlled trial. JAMA 286:700, 2001

25. Komadina KH, Schenk DA, LaVeau P, et al: Interobserver variability in the interpretation of pulmonary artery catheter pressure tracings. Chest 100:1647, 1991

26. Morris AH, Chapman RH, Gardner RM: Frequency of wedge pressure errors in the ICU. Crit Care Med 13:705, 1985

27. Swan HJ, Ganz W, Forrester J, et al: Catheterization of the heart in man with use of a flow-directed balloon-tipped catheter. N Engl J Med 283:447, 1970

28. Marini JJ: Obtaining meaningful data from the Swan-Ganz catheter. Respir Care 30:572, 1985

29. O'Quin R, Marini JJ: Pulmonary artery occlusion pressure: clinical physiology, measurement, and interpretation. Am Rev Respir Dis 128:319, 1983

30. Raper R, Sibbald WJ: Misled by the wedge? The Swan-Ganz catheter and left ventricular preload. Chest 89:427, 1986

31. Sibbald WJ, Driedger AA, Moffat JD, et al: Pulmonary microvascular clearance of radiotracers in human cardiac and noncardiac pulmonary edema. J Appl Physiol 50:1337, 1981

32. Grossman W: Diastolic dysfunction in congestive heart failure. N Engl J Med 325:1557, 1991

33. Guazzi M, Polese A, Magrini F, et al: Negative influences of ascites on the cardiac function of cirrhotic patients. Am J Med 59:165, 1975

34. Jardin F, Farcot JC, Boisante L, et al: Influence of positive end-expiratory pressure on left ventricular performance. N Engl J Med 304:387, 1981

35. Civetta JM, Taylor RW, Kirby RR: Critical Care, 3rd ed. Lippincott-Raven, Philadelphia, 1997

36. Connors AF Jr, Speroff T, Dawson NV, et al: The effectiveness of right heart catheterization in the initial care of critically ill patients. SUPPORT Investigators. JAMA 276:889, 1996

37. Polanczyk CA, Rohde LE, Goldman L, et al: Right heart catheterization and cardiac complications in patients undergoing noncardiac surgery: an observational study. JAMA 286:309, 2001

38. Hosie KF: Thermal dilution technics. Circ Res 10:491, 1962

39. Stevens JH, Raffin TA, Mihm FG, et al: Thermodilution cardiac output measurement: effects of the respiratory cycle on its reproducibility. JAMA 253:2240, 1985

40. Yelderman M: Continuous measurement of cardiac output with the use of stochastic system identification techniques. J Clin Monit 6:322, 1990

41. Yelderman ML, Ramsay MA, Quinn MD, et al: Continuous thermodilution cardiac output measurement in intensive care unit patients. J Cardiothorac Vasc Anesth 6:270, 1992

42. Selzer A, Sudrann RB: Reliability of the determination of cardiac output in man by means of the Fick principle. Circ Res 6:485, 1958

43. Porter JM, Swain ID: Measurement of cardiac output by electrical impedance plethysmography. J Biomed Eng 9:222, 1987

44. Huntsman LL, Stewart DK, Barnes SR, et al: Noninvasive Doppler determination of cardiac output in man: clinical validation. Circulation 67:593, 1983

45. Singer M, Clarke J, Bennett ED: Continuous hemodynamic monitoring by esophageal Doppler. Crit Care Med 17:447, 1989

46. Homer LD, Denysyk B: Estimation of cardiac output by analysis of respiratory gas exchange. J Appl Physiol 39:159, 1975

47. Gedeon A, Forslund L, Hedenstierna G, et al: A new method for noninvasive bedside determination of pulmonary blood flow. Med Biol Eng Comput 18:411, 1980

48. de Abreu MG, Quintel M, Ragaller M, et al: Partial carbon dioxide rebreathing: a reliable technique for noninvasive measurement of nonshunted pulmonary capillary blood flow. Crit Care Med 25:675, 1997

49. Dhainaut JF, Brunet F, Monsallier JF, et al: Bedside evaluation of right ventricular performance using a rapid computerized thermodilution method. Crit Care Med 15:148, 1987

50. Åstrand P-O, Rodahl K: Textbook of Work Physiology: Physiological Bases of Exercise, 3rd ed. McGraw-Hill, New York, 1986

51. Andritsch RF, Muravchick S, Gold MI: Temperature correction of arterial blood-gas parame-

ters: a comparative review of methodology. Anesthesiology 55:311, 1981

52. Swain JA: Hypothermia and blood pH: a review. Arch Intern Med 148:1643, 1988

53. Klocke RA: Carbon dioxide transport. Handbook of Physiology, Sect 3, Vol 4. American Physiological Society, Bethesda, Maryland, 1987, p 173

54. Kelly R, Fitchett D: Noninvasive determination of aortic input impedance and external left ventricular power output: a validation and repeatability study of a new technique. J Am Coll Cardiol 20:952, 1992

55. Kelly R, Hayward C, Avolio A, et al: Noninvasive determination of age-related changes in the human arterial pulse. Circulation 80:1652, 1989

56. Piene H: Pulmonary arterial impedance and right ventricular function. Physiol Rev 66:606, 1986

57. O'Rourke MF: Vascular impedance in studies of arterial and cardiac function. Physiol Rev 62:570, 1982

58. O'Rourke MF, Kelly RP, Avolio AP: The Arterial Pulse. Lea & Febiger, Philadelphia, 1992

59. Asanoi H, Sasayama S, Kameyama T: Ventriculoarterial coupling in normal and failing heart in humans. Circ Res 65:483, 1989

60. Rankin JS, Olsen CO, Arentzen CE, et al: The effects of airway pressure on cardiac function in intact dogs and man. Circulation 66:108, 1982

61. Kraut EJ, Owings JT, Anderson JT, et al: Right ventricular volumes overestimate left ventricular preload in critically ill patients. J Trauma 42:839, 1997

62. Sagawa K: The end-systolic pressure-volume relation of the ventricle: definition, modifications and clinical use. Circulation 63:1223, 1981

63. Kaplan LJ, McPartland K, Santora TA, et al: Start with a subjective assessment of skin temperature to identify hypoperfusion in intensive care unit patients. J Trauma 50:620, 2001

64. Ivatury RR, Simon RJ, Islam S, et al: A prospective randomized study of end points of resuscitation after major trauma: global oxygen transport indices versus organ-specific gastric mucosal pH. J Am Coll Surg 183:145, 1996

65. Hoffman RA, Krieger BP, Kramer MR, et al: End-tidal carbon dioxide in critically ill patients during changes in mechanical ventilation. Am Rev Respir Dis 140:1265, 1989

66. Slotwiner DJ, Devereux RB, Schwartz JE, et al: Relation of age to left ventricular function in clinically normal adults. Am J Cardiol 82:621, 1998

67. Rowell LB: Cardiovascular adjustments to thermal stress. Handbook of Physiology, Sect 2, Vol 3. Geiger SR, Shepherd JT, Abboud FM, Eds. Waverly Press, Baltimore, 1983, p 967

68. Willett WC, Dietz WH, Colditz GA: Guidelines for healthy weight. N Engl J Med 341:427, 1999

69. Kleinman B, Powell S, Gardner RM: Equivalence of fast flush and square wave testing of blood pressure monitoring systems. J Clin Monit 12:149, 1996

70. Gnaegi A, Feihl F, Perret C: Intensive care physicians' insufficient knowledge of right-heart catheterization at the bedside: time to act? Crit Care Med 25:213, 1997

71. Iberti TJ, Fischer EP, Leibowitz AB, et al: A multicenter study of physicians' knowledge of the pulmonary artery catheter. Pulmonary Artery Catheter Study Group. JAMA 264:2928, 1990

72. Celoria G, Steingrub JS, Vickers-Lahti M, et al: Clinical assessment of hemodynamic values in two surgical intensive care units: effects on therapy. Arch Surg 125:1036, 1990

73. Eisenberg PR, Jaffe AS, Schuster DP: Clinical evaluation compared to pulmonary artery catheterization in the hemodynamic assessment of critically ill patients. Crit Care Med 12:549, 1984

74. Mimoz O, Rauss A, Rekik N, et al: Pulmonary artery catheterization in critically ill patients: a prospective analysis of outcome changes associated with catheter-prompted changes in therapy. Crit Care Med 22:573, 1994

75. Sandham JD, Hull RD, Brant RF, et al: A randomized, controlled trial of the use of pulmonary-artery catheters in high-risk surgical patients. N Engl J Med 348:5, 2003

76. Kleiber M: Body size and metabolic rate. Physiol Rev 27:511, 1947

77. West GB, Brown JH, Enquist BJ: A general model for the origin of allometric scaling laws in biology. Science 276:122, 1997

78. Astrand P, Cuddy TE, Saltin B, et al: Cardiac output during submaximal and maximal work. J Appl Physiol 19:268, 1964

79. Bevegard S, Holmgren A, Jonsson B: Circulatory studies in well trained athletes at rest and during heavy exercise, with special reference to stroke volume and the influence of body position. Acta Physiol Scand 57:26, 1963

80. Donald DE: Splanchnic circulation. Handbook of Physiology, Sect 2, Vol 3. Geiger SR, Shepherd JT, Abbound FM, Eds. Waverly Press, Baltimore, 1983, p 219

81. Ekblom B, Hermansen L: Cardiac output in athletes. J Appl Physiol 25:619, 1968

82. Heath GW, Hagberg JM, Ehsani AA, et al: A physiological comparison of young and older endurance athletes. J Appl Physiol 51:634, 1981

83. Heistad DD, Kontos HA: Cerebral circulation. Handbook of Physiology, Sect 2, Vol 3. Geiger SR, Shepard JT, Abbound FM, Eds. Waverly Press, Baltimore, 1983, p 137

84. Holmberg S, Serzysko W, Varnauskas E: Coronary circulation during heavy exercise in control subjects and patients with coronary heart disease. Acta Med Scand 190:465, 1971

85. Janicki JS, Sheriff DD, Robotham JL, et al: Cardiac output during exercise: contribution of the cardiac, circulatory and respiratory systems. Handbook of Physiology, Sect 12. Rowell LB, Shephard JT, Eds. Oxford University Press, New York, 1996, p 649

86. Kitamura K, Jorgensen CR, Gobel FL, et al: Hemodynamic correlates of myocardial oxygen consumption during upright exercise. J Appl Physiol 32:516, 1972

87. Knox FG, Spielman WS: Renal circulation. Handbook of Physiology, Sect 2, Vol 3. Geiger SR, Shepherd JT, Abboud FM, Eds. Waverly Press, Baltimore, 1983, p 183

88. Laughlin MH, Korthuis RJ, Duncker DJ, et al: Control of blood flow to cardiac and skeletal muscle during exercise. Handbook of Physiology, Sect 12. Rowell LB, Shepherd JT, Eds. Oxford University Press, New York, 1996, p 705

89. Messer JV, Wagman RJ, Levine HJ: Patterns of human myocardial oxygen extraction during rest and exercise. J Clin Invest 41:725, 1962

90. Milnor WR: Cardiovascular Physiology. Oxford University Press, New York, 1990

91. Pollock ML, Foster C, Knapp D, et al: Effect of age and training on aerobic capacity and body composition of master athletes. J Appl Physiol 62:725, 1987

92. Roddie IC: Circulation to skin and adipose tissue. Handbook of Physiology, Sect 2, Vol 3. Geiger SR, Shepherd JT, Abboud FM, Eds. Waverly Press, Baltimore, 1983, p 285

93. Rowell LB, O'Leary DS, Kellogg DL Jr: Integration of cardiovascular control systems in dynamic exercise. Handbook of Physiology, Sect 12. Rowell LB, Shepherd JT, Eds. Oxford University Press, 1996, p 770

94. Shepherd JT: Circulation to skeletal muscle. Handbook of Physiology, Sect 2, Vol 3. Geiger SR, Shepherd JT, Abboud FM, Eds. Waverly Press, Baltimore, 1983, p 319

95. Wade OL, Bishop JM: The distribution of the cardiac output in normal subjects during exercise. Cardiac Output and Regional Blood Flow. Blackwell Scientific Publications, Oxford, 1962, p 95

Acknowledgments

Figures 1, 4, and 6   Albert Miller.
Figure 2   Top, Dana Burns-Pizer; bottom, Albert Miller.
Figure 3   Top and bottom, Dana Burns-Pizer; center, Albert Miller.
Figure 5   Carol Donner.
Figure 7   Dana Burns-Pizer.

5 PULMONARY INSUFFICIENCY

Robert H. Bartlett, M.D., F.A.C.S., and Preston B. Rich, M.D.

Approach to Pulmonary Insufficiency

Pulmonary insufficiency is the most common complication after surgical procedures. It ranges in incidence from 5% to 50% and in severity from minor atelectasis to lethal acute respiratory distress syndrome (ARDS). The reason why the lung is so vulnerable in the postoperative period is that both of the essential components of lung function—ventilation (anatomy and physiology of breathing) and pulmonary circulation (anatomy and physiology of the pulmonary endothelium and interstitium)—are affected by all the events surrounding tissue injury, anesthesia, and tissue dissection.[1] Abnormal ventilation leads to alveolar collapse, decreased functional residual capacity (FRC), and atelectasis. Abnormal capillary homeostasis leads to lung edema. Bacterial pneumonitis can initiate these events or can be a secondary complication. The term ARDS refers to a combination of atelectasis and edema, with edema predominating; it will be used sparingly in this chapter, primarily to describe the occurrence of pulmonary edema caused by increased capillary permeability.

In what follows, we discuss the care of patients at risk for pulmonary complications, including clinical presentation, pathogenesis, recognition, prevention, and treatment of pulmonary insufficiency. Atelectasis and lung edema are considered as separate events, though it is obvious that both abnormalities can and do occur simultaneously after operation. The emphasis is on disorders of the pulmonary parenchyma as opposed to pulmonary insufficiency secondary to cardiac disease, thromboembolism, CNS depression, and other conditions. The discussion is limited to mild to moderate pulmonary insufficiency because major insufficiency is discussed more fully elsewhere [*see 6:6 Use of the Mechanical Ventilator*]. Perioperative problems related to operations for primary pulmonary disease also are not addressed in this chapter.

Preoperative Pulmonary Function Testing

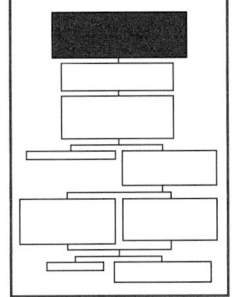

Given that identification of the high-risk patient can reduce the incidence of pulmonary complications, preoperative assessment of respiratory status is clearly important. The history is the most valuable step. Factors indicating a need for more detailed study of pulmonary function include exercise intolerance, dyspnea on exertion, wheezing, cigarette smoking, cough, and sputum production.

Physical examination should include auscultation and percussion of the lung bases during tidal breathing and maximal inspiration to detect hypoventilation in weak or debilitated patients and hyperinflation in patients with chronic airway disease. Wheezing, rales, or rhonchi should trigger further examination. Cardiac insufficiency, obesity, clubbing, tobacco stains, and poor oral hygiene are all relative indications for more detailed pulmonary function testing. Chest x-ray should be considered part of the routine physical examination for any patient with an abnormality detected from the history or physical examination, any patient scheduled to undergo a thoracotomy, and any patient older than 40 years. As part of the physical examination, the patient should be instructed to inhale to the maximum, then to perform a vigorous forced expiration. By observing the patient's chest and the sound of forced expiration, one can make a good guess at the volume of inspiration (which should be at least 1 L/50 kg), forced expiratory volume (which should be at least 2 L/50 kg), and expiratory flow (most of the exhaled volume should come out in the first second without wheezing). Forced expiratory volume—or vital capacity (the two are different names for the same thing)—and maximum voluntary ventilation (MVV) can be directly measured with a handheld turbine spirometer.

The ability to climb one or two flights of stairs at a steady pace without dyspnea provides information about the patient that is not available in any other way short of treadmill or exercise testing. A patient who cannot do this simple exercise may have respiratory, cardiac, or joint disease or may be too obese, too weak, too sedentary, or too debilitated to manage mild exertion. Whatever the cause, an elective operation should be delayed if the patient cannot do the exercise.

Simple spirometry should be done whenever the history, the physical examination, or bedside tests yield findings indicating abnormal pulmonary function. Tidal volume, inspiratory capacity, vital capacity (total and timed intervals), and MVV are measured, and the results are compared with tables for normal persons of the same age, sex, and size and then reported as percentages of predicted normal values. Results between 80% and 120% of predicted values are considered normal. If these tests of lung volume and flow are within the normal range, the risk of pulmonary complications is small (though the tests do not address endurance). Abnormally high values are not important; however, abnormal values below 70% of predicted levels indicate small airway or obstructive lung disease (if the expiratory flow rate is low), loss of lung volume (if vital capacity is low), or localized or generalized muscle weakness. If expiratory flow is abnormally low, spirometry should be repeated after the administration of aerosolized bronchodilators. Low expiratory flow that improves after bronchodilation indicates bronchospasm, which will require special management during and after operation. The test result that correlates best with the incidence of postoperative pulmonary complications is an MVV value below 50% of the

1101

Assess pulmonary function preoperatively

Review history; perform physical exam. Evaluate for wheezing, rales, and rhonchi; cough and sputum production; cardiac insufficiency; and obesity. Estimate volume of inspiration, forced expiration, and expiratory flow.

Obtain chest x-ray if abnormality is detected, thoracotomy is planned, or patient is > 40 years.

If pulmonary dysfunction is suspected:
- Measure tidal volume, inspiratory capacity, vital capacity, and maximum voluntary ventilation.
- Obtain baseline blood gas measurements.
- In special circumstances: Measure FRC. Assess for chronic fibrotic disease. Obtain ventilation-perfusion lung scan if pulmonary resection is contemplated.

Correct abnormalities, and prepare patient before operation

Teach breathing maneuvers, and exercise patient's respiratory muscles.
Reduce risk factors (e.g., smoking, LV failure).
Assess effects of bronchodilators in patients with bronchospasm.
Provide adequate nutrition.

Follow pulmonary prophylaxis regimen during and after operation

Inflate all alveoli regularly:
- Use breathing exercise with incentive spirometer. Use IPPB if necessary.
- Use mechanical ventilation in high-risk patients.
- Use bronchodilators for bronchospasm.

Maintain normal body fluid volume and composition:
- Give blood and fluids as needed, but not excessively.
- If fluid overload is unavoidable, diurese when stable.

Minimize the risk of venous thrombosis and pulmonary embolism.

Postoperative pulmonary insufficiency does not develop

Approach to Pulmonary Insufficiency

Postoperative pulmonary insufficiency develops (e.g., dyspnea, tachypnea, tachycardia, confusion, cyanosis, abnormal x-ray)

Rule out mechanical limitation of breathing, bronchospasm, pulmonary embolism, congestive heart failure, and hypovolemia.
Evaluate for atelectasis or pulmonary edema.
General support: Give O_2 during preliminary investigations (10 L/min by cannula or mask).

Treat atelectasis

Establish large-volume inflation via deep breathing exercises. If unsuccessful, try IPPB without intubation.
Initiate chest physiotherapy and postural drainage. Administer hydration, nebulized bronchodilators, and mucolytic drugs via airway. Perform bronchoscopy or tracheal suctioning as indicated.
If ventilation is still inadequate: Intubate and initiate mechanical ventilation. Provide nutritional support. Treat coexisting lung edema and lung infection. Maintain $F_IO_2 < 60\%$ and airway pressure < 40 cm H_2O.

Treat increased lung water

Decrease pulmonary hydrostatic pressure by improving LV function pharmacologically. (Monitor changes in cardiac output.)
Reduce total extracellular fluid volume by forced diuresis, dialysis, or hemofiltration.
Increase plasma oncotic pressure by administering colloids during diuresis.
Establish and maintain normal pulmonary microvascular integrity by treating any extrapulmonary site of infection or inflammation.

Pulmonary insufficiency resolves

Pulmonary insufficiency progresses to ARDS or pneumonia

Provide specific treatment for respiratory failure or postoperative pneumonia as indicated.

predicted level. MVV may be abnormally low for many reasons, both pulmonary and nonpulmonary.

Arterial blood gas values are obtained only if major pulmonary dysfunction is suspected, and they serve primarily as a baseline for postoperative comparison and for decisions about postoperative ventilation rather than as a screening test for adequacy of pulmonary function. Arterial carbon dioxide tension (P_aCO_2) greater than 45 mm Hg at rest indicates significant alveolar hypoventilation. If the cause is muscle weakness, bronchospasm, or chronic bronchitis, it should be treated before any elective operation is undertaken. If the arterial oxygen tension (P_aO_2) is greater than 70 mm Hg, the patient has significant right-to-left shunting, diffusion block, or ventilation-perfusion mismatch—usually the last, though two or all three of these may occur together. These three causes of hypoxemia can be further identified by the response to breathing 100% oxygen, but this evaluation requires special equipment (a face mask or nasal catheter is not satisfactory), and the information gained is generally not worth the effort for the purposes of preoperative pulmonary assessment.

More detailed tests of pulmonary function are needed only in special situations. The most useful of these is measurement of FRC, which is done in association with simple spirometry using helium dilution or nitrogen washout. FRC is the most difficult lung volume to measure but also the most important: following the FRC is the most specific way of determining when the patient is in optimal pulmonary condition. An abnormally high FRC indicates air trapping from small airway disease or bronchospasm, which should be treated before any elective operation. An abnormally low FRC indicates loss of lung volume that may result from atelectasis, pneumonia, pleural effusion, or congestive heart failure, all of which should be treated until the FRC is normal. Measurement of diffusing capacity by carbon monoxide inhalation is not helpful. Measurement of P_aO_2 during carefully monitored breathing of 100% oxygen is more useful when chronic fibrotic lung disease is suspected. Oxygen consumption, CO_2 production, and respiratory quotient are measures of systemic metabolism rather than of pulmonary function; accordingly, whereas they may be helpful in preoperative screening for the purposes of detecting sepsis or planning nutritional therapy, they generally are not useful guides to pulmonary functional status. Ventilation-perfusion scanning should be added to the regimen of routine preoperative testing in any patient with evidence of compromised pulmonary function in whom resection of pulmonary tissue is contemplated.

In summary, the history, the physical examination, and chest x-ray constitute sufficient preoperative pulmonary assessment in almost all cases. Patients at risk for pulmonary complications, as identified by history or examination, should undergo simple spirometry to identify abnormalities that can be corrected before elective operations. Arterial blood gases should be measured preoperatively in patients with major respiratory dysfunction to serve as a baseline for postoperative management.

Preoperative Measures to Prevent Pulmonary Insufficiency

PREVENTION OF ATELECTASIS AND EDEMA

Given an understanding of how pulmonary insufficiency arises and how patients at high risk for this complication can be detected, one can identify the appropriate steps in prevention. First, measures must be adopted to prevent atelecta-

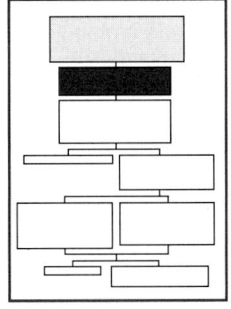

Table 1   Prevention of Atelectasis during and after Operation

Ensure frequent inflation to total lung capacity
    Deep breathing exercises facilitated by incentive spirometer
    Mechanical ventilation after major operations until alert and awake
    Positive pressure breathing for patients who cannot take deep breaths
Minimize respiratory depression
    Adequate, but not excessive, narcotic dosage
    Local and regional anesthesia
Minimize absorption atelectasis from increased F_IO_2
    Add nitrogen (lowest F_IO_2 to keep $S_aO_2 > 90\%$)
    Use PEEP if $F_IO_2 > 50\%$
Avoid pulmonary edema
Clear pleural space of air and fluid
Use abdominal viscera to increase lung volume
    Sitting or standing position
    Avoidance of supine position and high abdominal pressure

F_IO_2—fraction of inspired oxygen   PEEP—positive end-expiratory pressure
S_aO_2—arterial oxygen saturation

sis [*see Table 1*]. The most important of these is to maintain a normal pattern of breathing with regular maximal lung inflation. The patient can usually do this voluntarily and spontaneously, taking deep forced inspiratory breaths at least 10 times each hour. The incentive spirometer may be used to encourage the patient's efforts and to measure the volume of inspiration. If the patient cannot take deep breaths spontaneously, mechanical assistance should be employed—usually on an intermittent basis with a mechanical ventilator and mouthpiece (intermittent positive pressure breathing, or IPPB). In high-risk patients who have undergone major operations, postoperative prophylactic intubation and mechanical ventilation are appropriate preventive measures and should be continued until the patient can sustain a normal breathing pattern. Keeping the airway clear with humidification and postural drainage is important in patients with chronic bronchitis. Coughing is not useful for preventing postoperative pulmonary complications.

Second, measures must be adopted to prevent lung edema [*see Table 2*]. Advising the surgeon to avoid cardiac failure, endotoxemia, and shock is an oversimplified platitude, but it is important to remember that pulmonary insufficiency may be the presenting symptom of these conditions. If preoperative and intraoperative resuscitation has resulted in major fluid overload, diuresis should be instituted when the patient is hemodynamically stable to minimize the potential for symptomatic lung edema and to raise plasma oncotic pressure.

CORRECTION OF ABNORMALITIES

If a patient is scheduled for an elective operation, as much time as is necessary should be spent measuring lung function, correcting abnormalities where present, and changing conditions that may predispose to pulmonary complications. This is particularly true in patients with preexisting cardiopulmonary disease. Patients should be advised to train for a major operation as they would for an athletic event. The respiratory muscles should be exercised and specific breathing maneuvers learned.

Correction of factors that may decrease the efficiency of ventilation includes cessation of smoking, elective weight loss in gross-

---

Table 2   Prevention of Pulmonary
Edema during and after Operation

Avoid extracellular fluid overload
  Routine intraoperative fluids limited to 3% of body weight
  Low threshold for blood or colloid during resuscitation or blood loss
Treat or prevent left ventricular failure
  Optimization of cardiac output with inotropes when filling pressures
  are elevated
Restore or maintain colloid osmotic pressure
  Diuresis to concentrate proteins
  Administration of 25% albumin or plasma if pulmonary edema is
  symptomatic
Minimize pulmonary capillary leakage
  Drainage of pus and excision of dead tissue

---

ly obese patients, and treatment of existing bacterial infection (chronic bronchitis) with culture-specific antibiotics where indicated. Patients with a known tendency for bronchospasm should become accustomed to undergoing bronchodilator treatment preoperatively, and the effect of bronchodilators on pulmonary mechanics should be directly measured, particularly in patients with known bronchospastic disorders (e.g., asthma).

Patients with preexisting lung disease require special consideration beyond the preparation related to bronchospasm or chronic bronchitis (see above). Patients with acute pulmonary insufficiency, increased lung water levels, and atelectasis secondary to an acute disorder such as pancreatitis or sepsis often show improvement during the operation and postoperative mechanical ventilation.

The condition of a patient with severe, chronic obstructive lung disease should be improved as much as possible by means of bronchodilators, treatment of chronic bronchitis (if present), nutritional support, and training in deep breathing. If the pulmonary disorder is very severe (i.e., if P_aO_2 is less than 50 mm Hg on room air or if CO_2 retention is evident), prolonged postoperative intubation and mechanical ventilation should be anticipated and the patient advised accordingly.

Intraoperative Measures to Prevent Pulmonary Complications

Intraoperatively, several factors may minimize the risk of postoperative pulmonary complications. The operation may directly improve pulmonary function (e.g., by repairing a mitral valve or a large abdominal wall hernia) or may mitigate or eliminate factors that of themselves are causing pulmonary insufficiency (e.g., by draining an empyema, removing a foreign body, or resecting dead tissue).

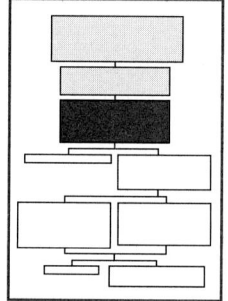

The operative procedure should be planned so as to simultaneously treat the patient and avoid any factors that may cause postoperative complications. With regard to the pulmonary system, planning includes various components, as follows.

Abdominal incisions should be planned to minimize postoperative pain and to maintain the strength of the abdominal wall for forced inspiration. Transverse incisions should be used whenever possible, particularly in patients with chronic heavy sputum production who will have to cough excessively after operation.

Gastrostomy should be considered to avoid prolonged nasogastric intubation. Bone fragments should be manipulated as gently as possible to prevent possible marrow embolism. Veins under negative pressure (e.g., those in the brain) must be managed carefully to prevent air embolism. If the patient has a history of pulmonary embolism or existing deep vein thrombosis (DVT) in the legs, prophylaxis for these conditions is particularly important.

Ventilation with 100% O_2 before intubation is standard practice, and a fraction of inspired oxygen (F_IO_2) higher than 90% is commonly used during operation. However, elimination of inert nitrogen in the alveoli leads to absorption atelectasis very rapidly. Accordingly, restoring normal alveolar nitrogen levels and volume through sustained inspiratory pressure with air before extubation is a valuable maneuver.[2] By the same token, however, maintaining a high F_IO_2 throughout the operation and during the early postoperative period significantly decreases the risk of a surgical site infection.[3]

Much of the intraoperative prevention of pulmonary complications is carried out by the anesthesiologist. Maintaining large tidal volume ventilation (10 to 15 ml/kg) at a low respiratory rate during operation helps maintain alveolar inflation. Particularly during long procedures, alveoli begin to collapse unless regularly hyperinflated at least every hour. The anesthesiologist contributes greatly toward preventing pulmonary complications by avoiding crystalloid fluid overload during operation. Blood and protein losses can be replaced intraoperatively with lactated Ringer solution. Generally, blood or plasma lost during operation should be replaced with blood or plasma. Moderate amounts of saline-type solutions are permissible, but caution should be observed.

Mechanical ventilation should be continued postoperatively until adequate spontaneous ventilation has been clearly established. The action of paralytic drugs should be reversed completely, and a voluntary vital capacity at least twice the tidal volume should be documented before extubation.

Postoperative Measures to Prevent Pulmonary Insufficiency

ROUTINE MEASURES

In the recovery room, the endotracheal tube should be maintained in place as long as is necessary. Patients with preexisting pulmonary dysfunction or those at high risk for pulmonary complications may need to remain intubated and be maintained on mechanical ventilation for hours or days after operation.

Abundant evidence suggests that well-ventilated alveoli are less susceptible to humoral capillary damage than atelectatic alveoli are. Elderly, debilitated patients, patients who have undergone major cardiac procedures, and patients with extensive injuries, multiple fractures, pancreatitis, dead tissue, or severe peritonitis are commonly left intubated and maintained on mechanical ventilation for 12 hours or longer after operation. When the patient is fully alert and awake, when perfusion and cardiac status are stable, and when blood and extracellular fluid volumes are demonstrated to be normal, then the patient is ready for spontaneous ventilation and extubation.

Deep breathing exercises, clearing of sputum and mucus, and avoidance of prolonged periods in the supine position must begin in the recovery room. Profound hypoventilation, ventilation-perfusion imbalance, and resultant hypoxemia are the rule in patients awakening from anesthesia. For this reason, it is common practice to administer moderate amounts (5 to 10 L/min) of supplemental oxygen to all patients in the recovery room. This is a wise precaution for the first hour or two after anesthesia, but it is really prophylactic only against hypoxic arrhythmias, and it may actually impair lung function by suppressing whatever deep breathing may result from moderate hypoxemia. Consequently, supplemental oxygen should not be administered for more than a few hours unless serial blood gas analyses so dictate.

Airway cleaning, suctioning, expectorant drugs, mist inhalation, and mucolytic agents are all useful in patients with preexisting chronic bronchitis or thick, tenacious tracheobronchial secretions. However, these maneuvers and agents may not be necessary in patients who can inflate their lungs adequately by means of inspiratory maneuvers. In the past, a compulsion to force patients to cough dominated much of the thinking on postoperative pulmonary care. Currently, it is generally recognized that coughing maneuvers are painful in thoracotomy or laparotomy patients and should not be necessary if the lung remains well ventilated.

Breathing maneuvers and devices designed to encourage those maneuvers are important adjuncts to postoperative care. Because shallow breathing, the lack of spontaneous deep breaths, and alveolar collapse are the steps that lead to postoperative pulmonary complications, respiratory maneuvers must emphasize maximal lung inflation. Emphasis on breathing out (i.e., with coughing, tracheal stimulation, or so-called blow bottles) does nothing to accomplish alveolar inflation, aside from the preparatory inspiration the patient may take beforehand. The greater the emphasis placed on inhaled volume and inspiratory pressure, the more effective the maneuver will be.

Routine IPPB is not particularly effective in preventing pulmonary complications.[4] This does not mean that IPPB is not a useful treatment method. On the contrary, it is quite useful for patients who are severely obtunded, those who are too weak to carry out spontaneous breathing maneuvers, and those with already established atelectasis. In such circumstances, however, the device should be used frequently (preferably each hour) and monitored by direct measurement of exhaled volumes, with maximum volume inflation attempted with each breath.

Deep inspiratory maneuvers can be done spontaneously or with the aid of a nurse or physical therapist but are better done with the aid of the incentive spirometer. This device allows the patient to see the inspired volume with each breath, thereby assuring the physician, the nurse, the respiratory therapist, and the patient that the maneuver is being done correctly and frequently enough to maintain alveolar inflation. Regular performance of deep breathing exercises using an incentive spirometer can decrease the incidence of pulmonary complications from about 30% to about 10%.[5]

Another method of preventing postoperative atelectasis is the application of continuous positive airway pressure (CPAP) or bilevel positive airway pressure (BiPAP) with a tight-fitting face mask. The potential complications of mask CPAP—gastric distention, vomiting and aspiration, and patient discomfort—are rare but remain a cause for concern. This technique, perhaps combined with mask IPPB, may prove useful in patients who are extubated but cannot or will not breathe deeply.

Whatever method is used to accomplish maximal inflation after operation must be carefully taught to the patient before the procedure: most patients cannot learn breathing exercises in a painful, narcotized, postoperative state.

For patients requiring care in an ICU, keeping the head of the bed elevated at least 30° significantly decreases the risk of developing ventilator-associated pneumonia.[6-8] Accordingly, unless there is a contraindication (e.g., spinal fracture), semirecumbent positioning should be employed routinely. Frequent change of position and early ambulation will minimize fluid collection in the dependent portions of the lung. Postoperative nutrition should be maintained [see 6:23 Nutritional Support]. If the patient must go without oral intake for more than 4 or 5 days, total parenteral nutrition is advisable for several reasons, not the least of which is to maintain the strength of the respiratory effort. Fluids must be managed carefully to avoid overloading the extracellular space and diluting the serum proteins.

Pulmonary thromboembolism from the deep veins of the leg or the pelvis is a constant threat after operation [see 4:6 Venous Thromboembolism]. Patients older than 40 years and patients with cancer are at particularly high risk. Several methods are used to prevent DVT, including anticoagulation, pharmacologic inhibition of platelet function, and application of pressure to the legs with plastic wraps or stockings. Regular muscle exercise is the easiest preventive maneuver, has the fewest complications, and is advised for all postoperative patients.

MEASURES IN PATIENTS WITH PREEXISTING LUNG DISEASE

Patients with chronic disease of the airways or the pulmonary parenchyma have less pulmonary reserve; consequently, in these patients, acute respiratory failure may develop after a minimal insult to the lung. The patient with emphysema or asthma presents an interesting problem. Because of the primary disease, residual volume and FRC are abnormally expanded. The patient is protected to some extent against alveolar collapse secondary to shallow breathing; however, the involved alveoli are difficult to ventilate, even with maximal effort. The dead space is abnormally large, so that the minute ventilation must be higher than normal just to achieve normal CO_2 excretion. In addition, alveolar destruction, fibrosis, or bullae may be present, decreasing oxygenation as well as CO_2 excretion. The effect of shallow breathing in such a patient will not be atelectasis, as would occur with a normal lung, but rather CO_2 retention and hypoxemia. Supplemental oxygen may reverse the hypoxemia, but CO_2 narcosis may result, particularly if the patient is also sedated with narcotics or anesthetics.

Chronic bronchitis (daily production of purulent sputum) narrows the small airways, increasing susceptibility to inadequate inflation and alveolar collapse. Heavy cigarette smoking has the same effect. In these conditions, treating the airways before elective operation (with antibiotics or cessation of smoking) is advisable. Severe restrictive disease from pulmonary fibrosis, pleural thickening, fibrosis, or chest wall deformities predisposes to atelectasis.

Patients with acute respiratory failure may require operation; in fact, the respiratory failure may exist because of the indication for operation (e.g., abscess, ischemic tissue, or long bone fractures). Such patients come to operation with a decreased FRC and increased pulmonary water, following the pathogenetic sequence of acute respiratory failure [see Discussion, Pathogenesis of Postoperative Pulmonary Insufficiency, below]. The pulmonary problem may be mitigated or eliminated by the operation itself (e.g., when pus is drained or a fracture immobilized), but even if pulmonary function does not improve, these patients cannot afford any worsening of alveolar collapse or pulmonary edema. In such patients, further deterioration of pulmonary function must be prevented by means of prolonged postoperative intubation and mechanical ventilation and fine-tuning of hydrostatic pressure and colloid osmotic pressure in relation to cardiac output and blood volume.

Clinical Presentation of Postoperative Pulmonary Insufficiency

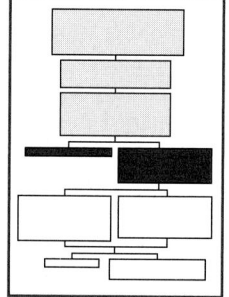

At any time during the first week after a major operation, a patient may manifest dyspnea, tachypnea, tachycardia, confusion, and cyanosis—the syndrome of pulmonary insufficiency. Although the most likely causes of this syndrome are atelectasis and edema, the first step in evaluation is to rule out mechanical limitation of breathing, acute bronchospasm (asthma), pulmonary thromboembolism, congestive heart failure, and hypovolemia.

Mechanical limitation of breathing may be caused by gastric or intestinal distention, ascites, pneumothorax, hydrothorax, or splinting of the chest wall to treat pain or rib fractures. It is diagnosed by physical examination and chest x-ray and treated by removing the limitation.

Bronchospasm occurs in patients with a history of asthma. The diagnosis is made by finding wheezes on physical examination and hyperinflation on x-ray. Treatment consists of bronchodilators.

Pulmonary embolism is the first consideration when the onset of pulmonary insufficiency is sudden, but it is the least common cause. Small (lobar) pulmonary emboli rarely cause symptoms. A patient who is symptomatic from embolism has had a major embolus (or a series of minor emboli) occluding more than 50% of the pulmonary circulation. It is usually easy to differentiate pulmonary embolism from atelectasis on the basis of clinical examination and blood gas measurements [see Table 3].

Congestive heart failure in the postoperative period may be either an exacerbation of a chronic condition or acute cardiac failure secondary to myocardial infarction. In either case, the diagnosis is made by physical and x-ray examination of the chest. In the patient who is fluid overloaded, the use of a pulmonary arterial catheter may be required to differentiate cardiogenic from capillary-injury pulmonary edema. The initial steps in management are the same, however, for the acutely ill patient: diuresis, supplemental oxygen, review of body weight and fluid balance records, and transfer to the ICU for more invasive monitoring.

Hypovolemia is often first manifested by dyspnea associated with metabolic acidosis, and postoperative shortness of breath should always raise the possibility of occult bleeding or third-space sequestration. Clinical examination elicits findings typical of hypovolemia. The chest x-ray is usually clear, and blood gases demonstrate normal oxygenation and CO_2 clearance with metabolic acidosis.

In postoperative pulmonary insufficiency caused by atelectasis and edema, physical examination shows diminished breath sounds over one or both lung bases. Rales and rhonchi may be heard in the middle and lower lung fields. Although tidal volume is normal, vital capacity (judged or actually measured) is abnormally small. Chest x-ray demonstrates incomplete lung inflation, usually with overt collapse or consolidation apparent in the lower lobes. If lung edema is the predominant cause of pulmonary insufficiency, a diffuse increase in lung density is seen, which, when combined with irregular inflation, is often described as diffuse fluffy infiltrates. This radiographic finding will usually differentiate this state from cardiogenic pulmonary edema, which is typically more apparent in the lower and middle lung fields when the x-ray is taken with the patient sitting or standing. Measurement of arterial blood gas values while the patient is breathing air demonstrate hypoxemia, hypocarbia, and respiratory alkalosis.

Supplemental high-flow oxygen (10 L/min) supplied by nasal catheter or face mask supplies approximately 40% inspired oxygen (regardless of the settings on the equipment). Supplemental oxygen substantially mitigates the hypoxemia resulting from ventilation-perfusion mismatch, pulmonary embolism, or cardiogenic pulmonary edema, typically resulting in a P_aO_2 greater than 150 mm Hg. In contrast, supplemental oxygen has a minor effect on hypoxemia caused by atelectasis, yielding a P_aO_2 typically rising from the 40s to the 80s. Fever and mild leukocytosis often accompany atelectasis, and the differential diagnosis between atelectasis and pneumonia is based primarily on con-

Table 3 Differential Diagnosis of Postoperative Dyspnea

	Atelectasis/ Edema	Pulmonary Embolism	Bronchospasm	Congestive Heart Failure
Lung bases	Not aerated	Clear	Wheezes	Rales
Chest x-ray	Consolidation, general edema	Clear ↑ Diameter of main pulmonary artery	Hyperinflated	Hydrostatic edema ↑ Diameter of main pulmonary artery
Central venous pressure	Normal	Elevated	Normal	Elevated
Pulmonary arterial wedge pressure	Normal	Normal or low	Normal or high	High
Arterial P_{O_2} (breathing air) (mm Hg)	40–60	40–80	70–90	40–60
Arterial P_{O_2} (breathing O_2) (mm Hg)	50–100	100–300	200–300	100–300
Arterial P_{CO_2}	Low	Normal or low	High	Normal or high
Lung scan	Regional ischemia	Regional ischemia	± Normal	± Normal
Pulmonary angiogram	Normal	Diagnostic	Normal	Normal

tinuing signs of infection without another obvious source, combined with pathogenic organisms on sputum culture. Thickened or copious bronchial secretions may be present in any patient after operation, particularly if the patient underwent endotracheal intubation, general anesthesia, or both during the procedure. Bronchial secretions are neither the cause nor the result of atelectasis. However, sputum samples for a Gram stain and culture should be acquired from every patient with pulmonary complications.

Treatment of Postoperative Pulmonary Insufficiency Caused by Atelectasis or Edema

GENERAL SUPPORT

Beginning during the preliminary clinical and laboratory examinations and the differential diagnosis, supplemental oxygen should be supplied by nasal catheter or face mask at a rate of 10 L/min. If the patient has a history of severe pulmonary disease with hypoxemia and hypercarbia, preoperative supplemental oxygen may correct the hypoxemia but diminish the respiratory drive and result in CO_2 narcosis; accordingly, special precautions should be taken. The patient should be positioned so as to maximize diaphragmatic excursion—that is, sitting but not hunched forward, with care taken to ensure that the stomach and the abdomen are not distended.

TREATMENT OF ATELECTASIS

The cornerstone of treatment aimed at alveolar inflation [*see Figure 1*] is to establish large-volume inflation by instituting deep breathing exercises. The patient should be taught to carry out a sustained maximal inspiration (basically a yawn maneuver); as noted, an incentive spirometer will encourage and quantitate the patient's efforts. If adequate volumes cannot be generated in this manner, 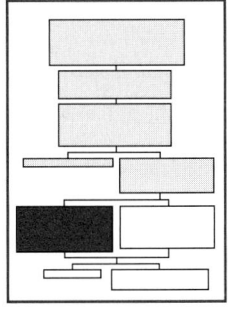 mechanical assistance is necessary—initially with IPPB with a mechanical ventilator, without intubation. This step must be done with direct measurement of exhaled volume, and it often requires high pressures (30 to 40 cm H_2O) with the IPPB device. All of the inflation techniques of mechanical ventilation (positive end-expiratory pressure [PEEP], sighs, inspiratory hold, CPAP) can be used in nonintubated patients. Again, coughing is not a treatment for pulmonary insufficiency: forced expiration collapses alveoli, does not clear small airways, and is painful and ineffective in the postoperative patient.

When an area of lung is not ventilated, mucus secreted in the bronchi draining from that lung segment may become thickened and impacted, hindering efforts at reexpansion. Chest physical therapy (percussion) and postural drainage should clear this mucus. Hydration and nebulized bronchodilator and mucolytic drugs may be used as well. Although coughing is not effective in preventing atelectasis, it is necessary for expelling mucus from airways that have been inflated distally. Coughing will not dislodge mucus from airways leading to nonventilated areas of lung. In this situation, mucus must be removed directly with tracheal suction or bronchoscopy, preferably the latter.

Tracheal suctioning exacerbates hypoxia if not done properly. The catheter is inserted through the nose, passed through the larynx (with passage confirmed by a change in voice), and connected to oxygen administered at 5 L/min. Then, 5 ml of saline

is injected, and the oxygen is reconnected for several coughing breaths. Suction is applied for no longer than 10 seconds, after which oxygen is resumed. This process is repeated until the suction return is clear (1 to 5 minutes). Electrocardiographic monitoring should be done during and after suctioning. Atropine is given for bradycardia. In adults, the primary value of this technique is the stimulation of deep breathing associated with the vigorous coughing that it induces. However, deep breathing can be easily accomplished by other means without the potential vagal complications associated with tracheal suctioning. Thus, routine tracheal suctioning has no rational place in the care of postoperative adult patients. In infants, who have much narrower airways, even a very small amount of mucus may suffice to cause major tracheal or bronchial occlusion. Infants breathe rapidly, with large ventilation of the dead space; thus, their tracheal secretions tend to dry out, and they may have difficulty coughing material from the lower trachea or from the bronchi. Consequently, endotracheal suctioning can be valuable for infants who have undergone operations on the thorax or the upper abdomen.

ALVEOLAR COLLAPSE

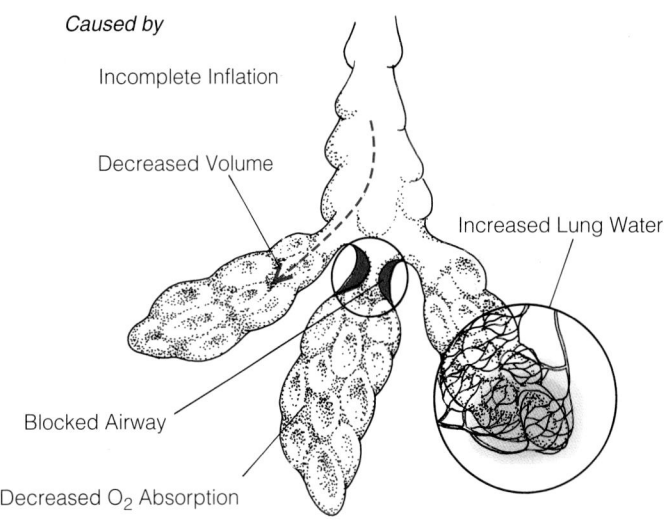

Caused by
Incomplete Inflation
Decreased Volume
Increased Lung Water
Blocked Airway
Decreased O_2 Absorption

Leads to	Ventilation-Perfusion Imbalance
	Hypoxemia
	Decreased FRC
	Decreased Compliance
	Increased Work

Treatment:	Maximum Inflation
	Yawn, Mechanical Ventilator, IPPB, CPAP
	Maintain Lowest Possible F_IO_2
	Decrease Lung Water
	Treat Infection
	Optimize Nutrition

Figure 1 **Illustrated are causes and effects of alveolar collapse in postoperative pulmonary insufficiency.**

Flexible fiberoptic bronchoscopy is preferable to blind tracheal suctioning in the management of atelectasis. Bronchoscopy is performed to examine the airways and clear mucus from the atelectatic area. Use of the endotracheal tube facilitates repeated removal and reinsertion of the bronchoscope, which may be necessary if mucus is too thick to be aspirated through the small suction lumen.

If adequate ventilation cannot be established with these methods, respiratory support is warranted. In many cases, endotracheal intubation can be avoided by using noninvasive mechanical ventilation.[9-11] Mechanical ventilation is indicated if the respiratory rate is consistently higher than 30 breaths/min or if the patient is severely hypoxemic (oxygen saturation < 92% despite supplemental oxygen via nasal cannula or face mask). If either of these indications cannot be reversed by the measures described, intubation and mechanical ventilation are carried out. Intubation with spontaneous breathing and CPAP (5 to 10 cm H_2O) without mechanical ventilation are standard therapy for the respiratory distress syndrome of the newborn and are commonly employed when that syndrome is complicated by a surgical procedure. CPAP may be useful in some adults with respiratory insufficiency associated with absence of surfactant. Generally, if the patient requires intubation, mechanical ventilation is also indicated.

If supplemental oxygen has been instituted as general support, the amount of oxygen should be kept as low as possible to avoid displacing nitrogen from alveoli and causing absorption atelectasis. Nutritional support should be instituted to achieve a positive nitrogen balance so as to maintain respiratory muscle strength and optimize host defenses. To prevent overfeeding, the amount of nutrients given should be based on measured energy expenditure. Overfeeding with carbohydrate causes an excess CO_2 load that may exacerbate pulmonary insufficiency.

TREATMENT OF EDEMA

The amount of lung water can be reduced by decreasing the entire extracellular fluid space, decreasing the hydrostatic pressure in the pulmonary capillary bed, and increasing plasma oncotic pressure without increasing oncotic pressure in the interstitial fluid of the lung [see Figure 2]. Mechanical positive pressure ventilation is not a means of decreasing lung water. In fact, positive pressure ventilation with PEEP actually increases lung water slightly, probably by stretching the pulmonary tissue.[12] Mechanical ventilation improves gas exchange in patients with pulmonary edema by overcoming the ventilation-perfusion mismatch associated with bronchodilators or alveolar thickening, but it does not decrease lung water itself.

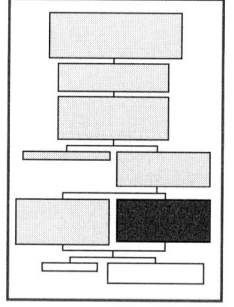

Patients with simple atelectasis need no treatment for increased lung water other than avoidance of fluid overload and cardiac failure. Increased lung water warrants treatment when diffuse interstitial fluid collection is evident from x-rays and the hospital course. For example, patients who have had an episode of severe systemic infection, disseminated intravascular coagulation, or fat embolism; those with peritonitis; those experiencing revascularization of ischemic tissue; and those who received 4 L of lactated Ringer solution during a 3-hour operation are likely to have increased lung water in association with other pulmonary problems.

Total extracellular fluid volume is reduced by forced diuresis (or, if the patient is in renal failure, by dialysis or hemofiltra-tion). Diuresis is induced with a potent agent such as furosemide. The course of diuresis is followed with careful daily measurement of body weight and hourly measurement of fluid intake and output. Usually, a patient with postoperative pulmonary insufficiency is 4 to 5 kg overloaded, primarily with extracellular fluid.

Adequate treatment of increased lung water must include removing excess extravascular fluid (i.e., returning the patient to baseline weight). Diuresis is continued until the patient is close to dry weight and is maintained in this condition. The major decrease in total extracellular fluid volume is accompanied by a minor decrease in pulmonary extracellular fluid volume, but this change is usually enough to improve pulmonary function greatly. Diuretic drugs remove water, sodium, and potassium at differing rates; thus, all of these must be monitored carefully and frequently. Usually, more water is removed than electrolytes, so that extreme forced diuresis leads to a hypernatremic, hyperosmotic state. Serum sodium concentrations should be monitored closely: when they are between 145 and 150 mEq/L, diuresis has reached its limit.

Diuresis concentrates serum proteins, increasing oncotic pressure. It should be combined with colloid loading to further increase plasma oncotic pressure transiently, thereby forcing

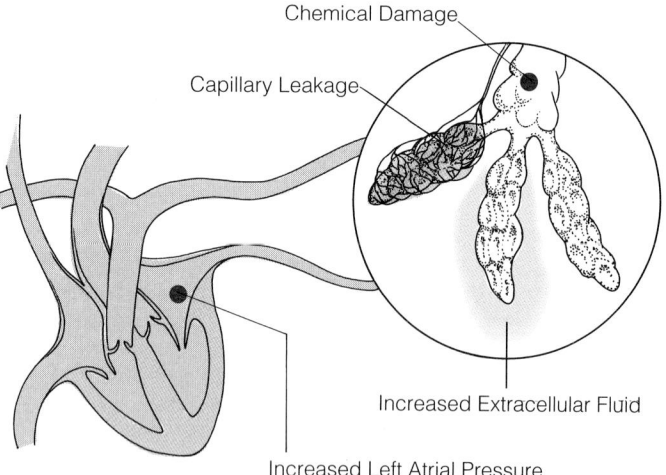

INCREASED LUNG WATER

Caused by

Chemical Damage

Capillary Leakage

Increased Extracellular Fluid

Increased Left Atrial Pressure

Leads to	Increased Pulmonary Vascular Resistance Decreased FRC Ventilation-Perfusion Imbalance Infection
Treatment:	Decrease Extracellular Fluid through Diuresis and Decreased Intake Increase Plasma Oncotic Pressure Treat Capillaries Decrease Hydrostatic Pressure

Figure 2 Illustrated are causes and effects of increased lung water in postoperative pulmonary insufficiency.

fluid to move from the extravascular to the intravascular space. Diuresis and colloid loading should be done concomitantly because most agents used for colloid loading (e.g., albumin) have a molecular weight between 50 and 100 kd and will gradually find their way into the extracellular space within 4 to 12 hours of infusion. The advantages of colloid loading come during the first hour or two after infusion and before the colloid load joins the lymphatic system and is metabolized. Although some studies suggest a deleterious effect from albumin loading in this setting, treatment of individuals with colloid loading (and diuresis) is usually highly successful.[13,14] The technique should be used when capillary integrity has been restored, as determined by response to small initial doses.

Decreasing pulmonary hydrostatic pressure by improving left ventricular function is accomplished pharmacologically; it can and should be done in all patients with major pulmonary insufficiency. A short-acting inotrope (e.g., dopamine) is preferred. The effectiveness of this treatment can be determined only through direct measurement of cardiac output and left atrial (or pulmonary capillary wedge) pressure, for which insertion of a pulmonary arterial catheter is required. Pulmonary arterial pressure monitoring and mixed venous blood sampling are as important as direct arterial blood gas sampling in managing patients with pulmonary insufficiency who have a major increase in lung water. The exact position of the catheter must be carefully determined and the pressure tracings properly interpreted; continuous display on an oscilloscope and careful selection of the end-expiratory point for pressure readings are required.

An effort should be made to establish and maintain normal pulmonary capillary permeability. The most common cause of pulmonary capillary leakage or ARDS is infection or inflammation at a site distant from the lungs. Any postoperative pulmonary insufficiency should trigger a search for wound infection, deep abscess, pancreatitis, and septic phlebitis. Drugs that inhibit the inflammatory response, block mediators of capillary injury, or prevent fibrosis have been investigated for the prevention or treatment of ARDS. Corticosteroids definitely diminish the inflammatory response and appear to be effective against some disorders (e.g., fat embolism), but they have not been confirmed as effective in randomized trials.[15] Drugs such as cyclooxygenase inhibitors, which block production of inflammatory mediators more specifically than steroids do, have been studied.[16] Drugs that inhibit the action of specific mediators—such as antihistamines, superoxide dismutase,[17] catalase, and ketoconazole[18]—have been investigated, but none have proved effective in clinical trials.

Progression to Pneumonia, Intubation, or ARDS

Bacterial infection often complicates atelectasis and edema, and it may occur as a primary event after operation. The progression from atelectasis to pneumonia can be difficult to identify because pulmonary infiltration and consolidation, fever, leukocytosis, and sputum production occur in both conditions. This differential diagnosis is one of the most difficult in postoperative

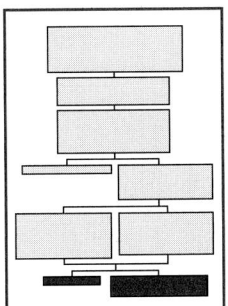

Table 4 Empirical Antibiotic Regimens for Postoperative Pneumonia

Patient Status	Likely Organisms	Empirical Antibiotics
Normal postoperative patients	Pharyngeal organisms; staphylococci; enterococci	Core combination (quinolone plus aminoglycoside)
Postoperative patients with aspirated gastric contents in association with operation	Pharyngeal organisms plus gram-negative organisms and *Candida*	Core combination plus fluconazole
Immunocompromised patients	Pharyngeal organisms plus *Candida* and methicillin-resistant staphylococci	Core combination plus vancomycin or fluconazole
Patients with chronic pulmonary infection	Gram-negative organisms (especially *Pseudomonas* and *Klebsiella*)	Aminoglycoside plus antipseudomonal agent

care; decisions must be based on repeated examination of the patient and the sputum or bronchoalveolar lavage fluid.

In patients with no preexisting lung disease, the organisms that most commonly cause early (first 3 days) postoperative bacterial pneumonia come from the pharynx during the operation: staphylococci, enterococci, or gram-negative bacteria. The same organisms invariably invade the lower airway in chronically intubated ICU patients. Rarely, streptococcal pneumonia occurs in the postoperative period if the pharynx was colonized at the time of the operation. *Candida* is commonly found in the pharynx but rarely causes pneumonia except in immunosuppressed hosts. Treatment for presumed early postoperative pneumonia includes vigorously treating the edema and atelectasis and giving empirical antibiotics. A Gram stain of the sputum will show the common pharyngeal flora but occasionally identifies one predominant organism, the presence of which guides selection of antibiotics while cultures are pending. Usually, however, the Gram stain is not definitive, and antibiotic treatment is therefore selected to cover the most common bacteria.

In patients with preexisting lung disease (emphysema) or lung infection (bronchitis, cystic fibrosis), pneumonia is usually caused by overgrowth of the bacteria already present in the lower airway. Gram-negative organisms predominate. In this circumstance, it is wise to culture a tracheal aspirate sample at the time of operation and to give culture-specific antibiotics if pneumonia occurs. Several choices for empirical antibiotic coverage for postoperative pneumonia are available [see Table 4].

The combination of atelectasis, edema, and pneumonia may necessitate intubation and mechanical ventilation. The subjective findings of dyspnea and confusion, combined with the objective findings of tachypnea and cyanosis, usually trigger ICU transfer, careful monitoring, and intubation. More precise indicators of the need for intubation and ventilation include (1) respiratory rate higher than 30/min; (2) arterial oxygen saturation (S_aO_2) lower than 92% on supplemental O_2; (3) P_aCO_2 higher than 45 mm Hg; (4) inspiratory force less than 20 cm H_2O; and (5) vital capacity less than twice tidal volume. Management of severe respiratory failure is discussed more fully elsewhere [see 6:6 Use of the Mechanical Ventilator].

Discussion

Normal Pulmonary Physiology

VENTILATION AND PULMONARY MECHANICS

The term pulmonary mechanics refers to the gas volumes in the chest and the gas flow rates during forced inspiration and exhalation. These values are depicted in a normal spirogram [*see Figure 3*]. As noted, FRC is approximately 2 L in a normal adult. During tidal breathing, the patient inhales about 500 ml, then exhales back to FRC. During a maximal inspiratory maneuver, the patient inhales to total lung capacity (typically twice the FRC). During pulmonary function testing to measure gas flow and volume, the patient inhales to total lung capacity, then breathes out as hard and fast as possible. The volume that the patient exhales is referred to as the forced expiratory volume or vital capacity. The rate at which the gas is exhaled is measured as the timed vital capacity, or the maximal midexpiratory flow rate. The volume of tidal breaths multiplied by the respiratory rate yields the minute ventilation (typically 8 L/min in a normal adult). Approximately one third of this ventilation passes through the conducting airways (dead space), and two thirds reaches the alveoli, where gas exchange takes place. Inspiration occurs when the diaphragm contracts, generating an intrapleural pressure that is negative relative to the atmosphere and resulting in the influx of air through the airway into the alveoli. Exhalation is largely a passive event, involving relaxation of the diaphragm and the accessory muscles of inspiration. Forced expiration requires the exertion of effort by the abdominal muscles.

The relation between gas volume and alveolar inflating pressure is referred to as pulmonary compliance [*see Figure 4*]. During diaphragmatic contraction, beginning at FRC, an intrapleural pressure of –10 cm H_2O is generated, which results in inspiration. During normal breathing, an inspiratory pressure of –5 to –10 cm H_2O results in inhalation of 500 to 1,000 ml. During forced inhalation against an open airway, intrathoracic pressures of –40 to –50 cm H_2O can be generated, resulting in inhalation to total lung capacity. Exhalation back to atmospheric pressure returns gas volume in the chest to FRC. An inspiratory pressure greater than –40 cm H_2O during spontaneous breathing (or greater than 40 cm

H_2O during mechanical ventilation) causes overdistention of alveoli, stretching of alveolar capillaries, interstitial and pulmonary edema, and potentially severe lung injury.

Compliance relationships obviously depend on the size of the patient [*see Figure 4*]. The actual volumes for FRC, tidal volume, and total lung capacity related to inflating pressure are low for infants, children, and small adults and relatively high for normal large adults. Patients with alveolar collapse, atelectasis, or interstitial pneumonia have an abnormally small FRC; consequently, their compliance characteristics tend to resemble those of a child. Under these circumstances, if a normal inflating tidal volume is used for such adult patients, high pressures are reached, overstretching occurs, and lung injury results.[19]

Minute ventilation (rate and depth of breathing) is controlled by the respiratory center in the brain stem to maintain P_aCO_2 at 40 mm Hg. By definition and in practice, hypoventilation results in a P_aCO_2 higher than 40 mm Hg and hyperventilation in a P_aCO_2 lower than 40 mm Hg. If a patient is hypermetabolic because of exercise or fever, excess CO_2 is produced, and minute ventilation increases proportionately to keep the P_aCO_2 at 40 mm Hg.

GAS EXCHANGE

Although O_2 exchange and CO_2 exchange occur simultaneously and at the same place in the lung, it is worthwhile to consider CO_2 clearance and O_2 uptake as if they were separate physiologic events. CO_2, being highly soluble in water and very diffusible, is readily eliminated from the pulmonary capillary blood to the alveolar gas space, even though the driving gradient is only about 45 mm Hg. The amount of CO_2 removed depends on the amount of alveolar ventilation [*see Figure 5*]. Minute ventilation (and hence alveolar ventilation) is regulated to remove all metabolically produced CO_2 each minute. Dissolved CO_2 combines with water to become carbonic acid (H_2CO_3), which is in equilibrium with the bicarbonate (HCO_3^-) in blood at a definite ratio. As long as this ratio is 1:20, the pH will be 7.4 (the Henderson-Hasselbalch equation). In postoperative patients, hypoventilation can be caused by respiratory depressing drugs (e.g., narcotics and anesthetics), paralysis or

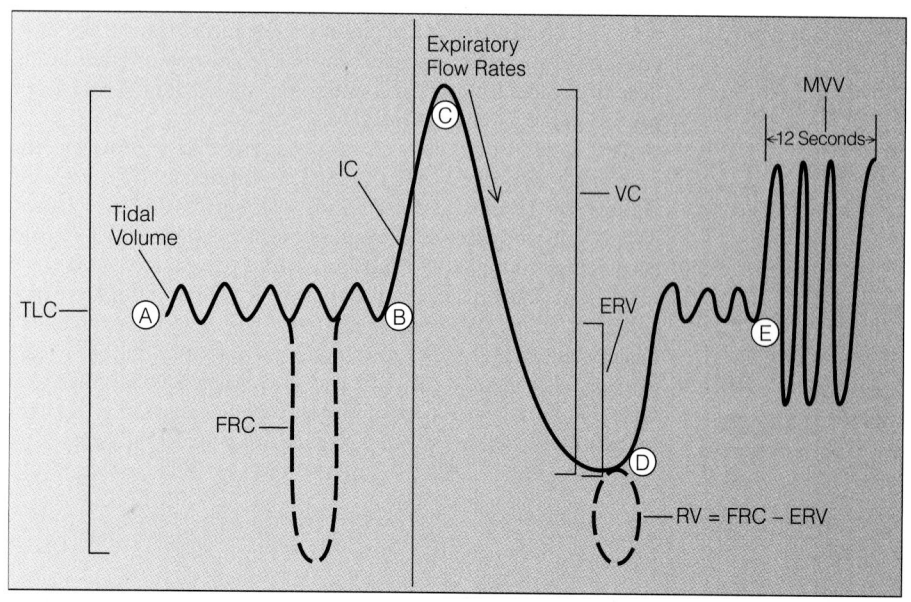

Figure 3 Depicted are gas volume and flow as demonstrated by spirometry. The subject is instructed to (**A**) breathe normally, (**B**) inhale as much as possible, (**C**) blow out as hard and fast as possible, (**D**) breathe normally, and (**E**) breathe as hard and fast as possible for 12 seconds. FRC is measured by a separate test, and residual volume (RV) is determined by subtracting expiratory reserve volume (ERV) from FRC.[1] (TLC—total lung capacity; IC—inspiratory capacity; VC—vital capacity)

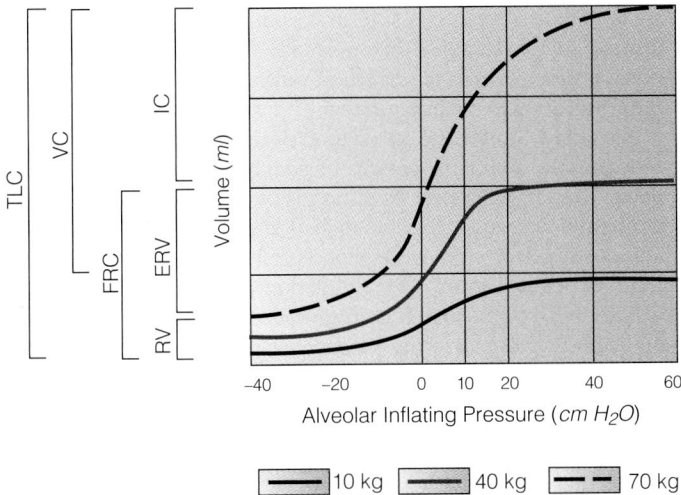

Figure 4 **Shown are volume-pressure curves for three subjects. Compliance is quantified as volume per inflating pressure normalized to body size (80 ml/cm H_2O/kg). Regardless of subject size, total lung capacity is reached at 40 cm H_2O.**[1]

weakness, obesity, and gastric distention, all of which result in CO_2 retention and respiratory acidosis.

Oxygenation of the blood depends more on matching of perfused alveoli to inflated alveoli than on minute ventilation. Under normal conditions, as long as inhaled alveolar gas contains at least 20% oxygen, red blood cells are fully oxygenated and exit the pulmonary capillaries at 100% saturation. During hypoventilation, the concentration of inspired oxygen in the alveoli does not reach 20% unless supplemental oxygen is given at the upper airway. In the recovery room, it is common practice to give supplemental oxygen; thus, a patient may be severely hypoventilated but remain fully oxygenated. The gradient for oxygen transfer from alveolar gas to red blood cells is much higher than that for CO_2 clearance. In a patient breathing room air, the oxygen tension (Po_2) in inhaled gas is approximately 150 mm Hg, and Po_2 in pulmonary capillary blood is approximately 40 mm Hg. Hence, the red cells are oxygenated during a single pass through the pulmonary capillary network. Oxygen in the blood is commonly measured in terms of either saturation (So_2) or Po_2, but the most useful measure is actually oxygen content (Co_2) because that is the major determinant of oxygen delivery at the tissue level. It is noteworthy that when Co_2 is plotted against So_2 and Po_2 at different levels of hemoglobin concentration [*see Figure 6*], blood that is severely hypoxic because of anemia still exhibits normal So_2 and Po_2.

Factors that impair oxygen delivery to blood include hypoventilation causing ventilation-perfusion mismatch, diffusion block caused by chronic lung disease with fibrosis in the interstitial space, and complete atelectasis resulting in transpulmonary shunting of blood from the pulmonary arterial circulation to the venous circulation without participating in gas exchange. The first two generic causes of hypoxemia can be completely corrected by supplemental oxygen breathing, but supplemental oxygen has very little effect on oxygenation when the problem is caused by a transpulmonary shunt.

Pathogenesis of Postoperative Pulmonary Insufficiency

CHANGES IN LUNG FUNCTION

After any major operation, changes occur in lung function. These changes occur in all patients but are not detected on routine exam-

ination. Aside from shallow tidal ventilation and some decreased breath sounds at the lung bases, the patient shows no signs of respiratory abnormality. On direct measurement, lung volumes are decreased (particularly residual volume, expiratory reserve volume, FRC, and vital capacity). Compliance is decreased because of the decrease in FRC. The work of breathing is increased for the same reason: more pressure is required to inhale a given volume into the decreased lung air space. Further evidence that alveoli are not being ventilated is absolute or relative arterial hypoxemia, which occurs with the patient breathing room air or 100% oxygen, indicating that nonventilated alveoli are being perfused (transpulmonary shunting).

These changes in lung function are present immediately after operation, progress slowly over 1 to 2 days, and then return to normal in most patients [*see Figure 7*]. The extent and duration of abnormality are related to the site of operation, the duration of operation and anesthesia, the quality of postoperative care, and preexisting pulmonary status.

The extent and duration of postoperative pulmonary abnormalities are greatest for operations on the thorax and upper abdomen and progressively decrease as the site of operation moves more distally and more superficially on the body structures. These changes may occur after only 1 to 2 hours of general anesthesia if careful attention is not paid to maximal lung inflation during anesthesia. They are superimposed on the patient's preexisting lung status. If, for example, the patient requires operation for complication of pancreatitis 2 weeks after the onset of disease, he or she may already have pleural effusions, increased pulmonary capillary permeability, and existing transpulmonary shunting and thus may be unable to tolerate any further deterioration of lung function. Likewise, if the patient has preexisting chronic obstructive lung disease with high airway resistance, maximal work of breathing, and minimal functional lung tissue before operation, CO_2 retention may develop if the work of breathing is even slightly increased after the procedure. Advanced age per se does not cause lung dysfunction, but elderly patients may have chronic lung disease or cardiac disease and thus be at higher risk for pulmonary failure. More important, elderly patients may be weak, and weak respiratory muscles predispose to alveolar collapse.

Several factors contribute to these changes in pulmonary function, but shallow breathing with incomplete alveolar inflation is the common denominator. If spontaneous deep breaths to maximal

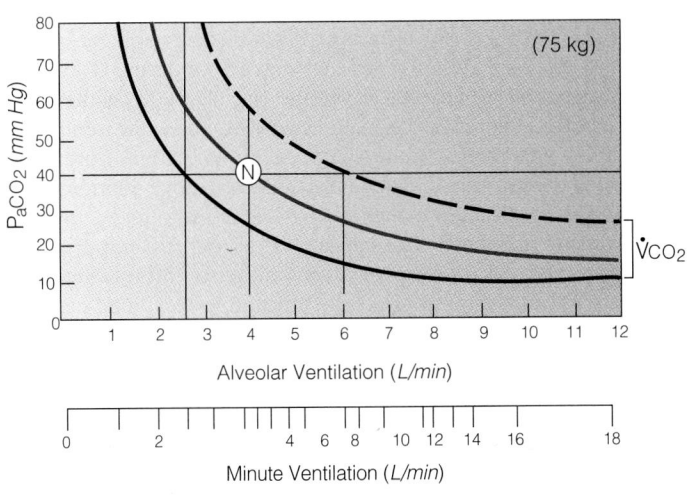

Figure 5 **Illustrated is CO_2 excretion ($\dot{V}CO_2$) related to ventilation for a typical 75 kg adult subject (N = normal).**[1]

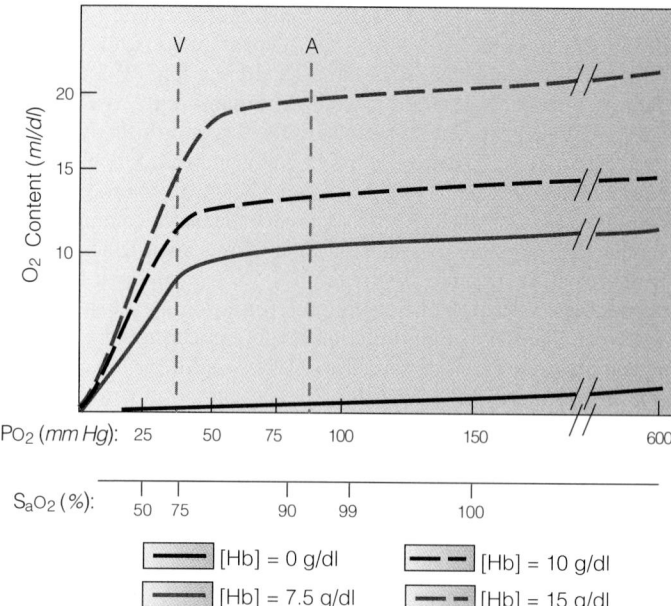

Figure 6 Shown is measurement of oxygen content in blood at four levels of hemoglobin (Hb) concentration. Dotted lines show values for arterial (A) and venous (V) blood. There is much more oxygen in normal venous blood with a Po₂ of 40 mm Hg than there is in anemic arterial blood with a Po₂ of 150 mm Hg.[1]

lung inflation are eliminated from the pattern of breathing, alveolar collapse begins within 1 hour and progresses rapidly to produce significant transpulmonary shunting. Several studies have shown that because of severe pain, anesthetics, or narcotic drugs, postoperative patients often lack the normal pattern of spontaneous deep breaths.[4,20] This finding is further supported by the observation that the postoperative changes in lung function can be returned toward normal by instituting maximal-inflation deep breathing exercises at regular intervals.[5] Excessive tracheobronchial secretions, aspiration of oral or gastric contents, and intraoperative fluid overload or blood transfusion may also contribute to postoperative changes in lung function.

The effects of an increased F$_I$O₂ and nitrogen washout are important to consider. The higher the concentration of oxygen in the alveoli, the lower the concentration of nitrogen. Nitrogen accounts for 80% of alveolar gas. Because nitrogen is inert, it merely occupies space, holding alveoli open as O₂ and CO₂ are rapidly exchanged during each breath. When nitrogen is washed out during O₂ breathing, alveoli tend to decrease in volume or collapse altogether with each breath. Major atelectasis can occur with just a few minutes of 100% O₂ breathing. In one study,[2] chest CT scans during O₂ breathing demonstrated major atelectasis occurring within minutes [*see Figure 8*]. Because a high F$_I$O₂ is commonly (and correctly) used during anesthesia with inhalational agents, it is important to minimize the risk of postoperative atelectasis through frequent recruitment of collapsed alveoli by inflation to total lung capacity and restoration of alveolar nitrogen at the end of the operation.

If the pattern of decreased lung volume and shunting is progressing rather than returning to normal, this development becomes clinically evident within 2 to 4 days after operation [*see Figure 7*]. Decreased lung volume is detectable as decreased breath sounds on physical examination, and atelectatic areas may be visible on chest x-ray. Shunt-produced hypoxemia leads to an increased ventilatory rate and the sensation of dyspnea.

Severe hypoxemia may cause cyanosis. Atelectasis causes fever and pooling of mucus secretions in nonventilated areas, leading to

an apparent increase in sputum production. Against the background of the changes that normally accompany major operations, a more complete picture of pulmonary pathophysiology in the surgical patient can be drawn.

As noted, abnormal ventilation leads to altered pulmonary function; the abnormal pattern of tidal breathing without spontaneous deep breaths after operation is a good example of this phenomenon. A patient supine in bed preferentially ventilates the anterior superior lobes while blood preferentially flows to the posterior dependent lobes. This ventilation-perfusion imbalance itself will result in hypoxemia. If it progresses over time, lower-lobe alveoli begin to collapse in the pathogenetic pathway described earlier. Alveolar collapse will occur in any patient who remains in one position for a prolonged period and in whom the pattern of breathing is that of shallow tidal ventilation. It should be emphasized that 600 ml breaths delivered with a mechanical ventilator will lead to alveolar collapse, just as shallow spontaneous breathing will, if regular maximal inflations are not carried out.

Obesity as a Risk Factor

Obesity is a common risk factor for postoperative pulmonary insufficiency. In the morbidly obese patient, the effort required to lift the chest wall and push the abdominal viscera and omentum aside during inspiration may be more than diaphragmatic contraction can handle. This condition is exacerbated after operation, when the patient may still be partially paralyzed, sedated from anesthetics or narcotics, and lying in the supine position (which allows the abdominal weight to push up on the diaphragm). In addition, obesity narrows the posterior pharyngeal space by the simple accumulation of fat in the submucosal tissues. This combination of factors makes hypoventilation a common problem in the obese patient [*see 3:3 Morbid Obesity*]. The hypoventilation can be profound but may be masked because the patients are receiving supplemental oxygen, so that P$_a$O₂ remains normal while P$_a$CO₂ may exceed 100 mm Hg. Moving the obese patient into a sitting position can minimize hypoventilation.

EDEMA AND THE PULMONARY INTERSTITIUM

Increased pulmonary hydrostatic pressure, decreased plasma oncotic pressure, and increased capillary permeability may all occur in the surgical patient. All of these states will cause increased pulmonary extravascular water and deterioration of lung function.

Fluid flux is a net function of the hydrostatic pressure that tends to force fluid out of the vascular space, on one hand, and the oncotic pressure that tends to pull fluid in, on the other hand. High hydrostatic pressure or low plasma oncotic pressure results in accumulation of fluid in the extravascular space. If the pulmonary endothelium is damaged, fluid may leak into the extracellular space at normal hydrostatic or oncotic pressures (as in ARDS) [*see Figure 2*]. Pulmonary vascular resistance increases because of periarteriolar cuffing. Ventilation-perfusion imbalance is created by peribronchiolar and alveolar compression. Shunting occurs if the alveoli become completely collapsed or filled with fluid. Finally, boggy atelectatic areas of lung are ideal breeding grounds for bacterial pulmonary infection.

Well-intentioned therapy in the normal course of treatment or resuscitation may cause increased lung water. An example is replacement of lost blood or plasma with crystalloid, which must equilibrate into the entire extracellular space, including that in the lung. Excess exogenous fluid combines with increased endogenous production of the water of metabolism during hypermetabolic states to yield increased total body extracellular fluid—the

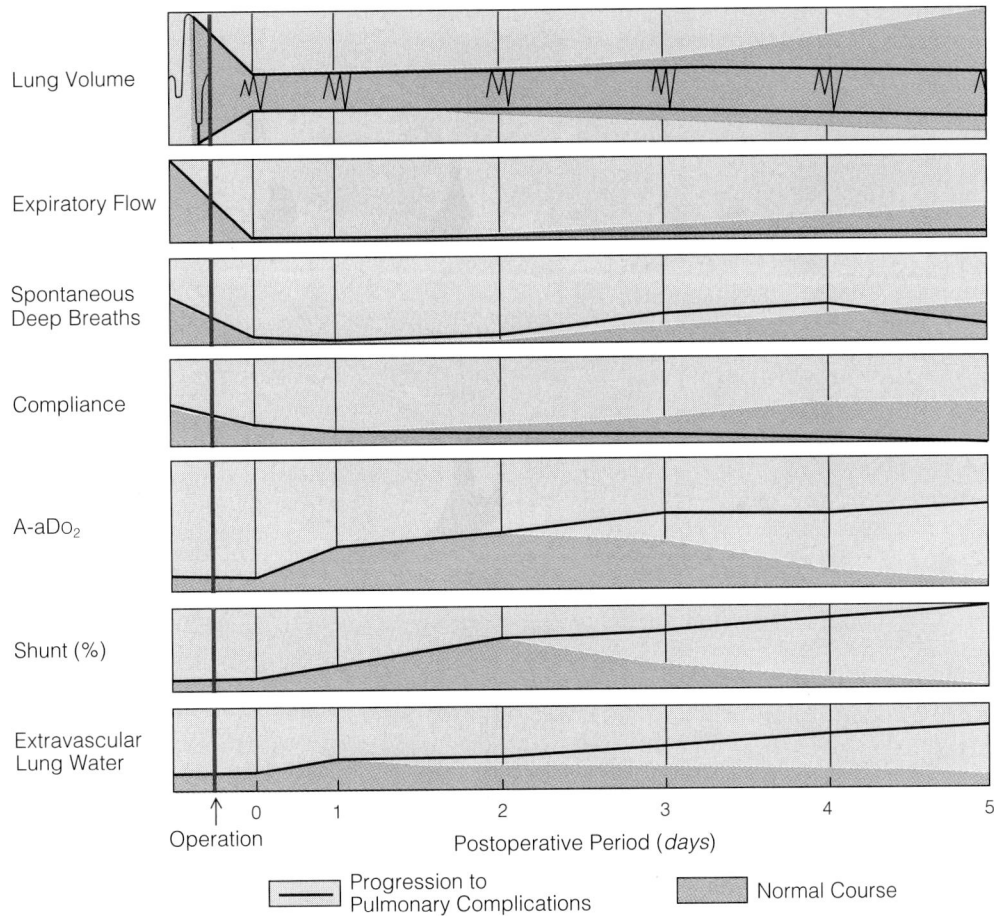

Lung Volume

Expiratory Flow

Spontaneous Deep Breaths

Compliance

A-aDo$_2$

Shunt (%)

Extravascular Lung Water

↑
Operation 0 1 2 3 4 5

Postoperative Period (*days*)

Progression to Pulmonary Complications   Normal Course

Figure 7   **Shaded areas represent normal changes in pulmonary function after an operation. Solid lines represent progression to pulmonary insufficiency. (A-aDo$_2$—alveolar-arterial difference in oxygen)**

major cause of pulmonary extravascular water collection. The effect is compounded by the decreased oncotic pressure that results when protein is lost or replaced with non–colloid-containing fluids. When plasma proteins are diluted in this way, lung interstitial proteins are also diluted; thus, the oncotic gradients stay unchanged, whereas the entire extracellular space expands.

The pulmonary capillary endothelium is the first major vascular bed to be exposed to any toxic substances arising from peripheral organ metabolism or perfusion of ischemic or infected tissue. The venous effluent from underperfused tissue (whether localized to a single organ, as in arterial embolism, or pervading the entire body, as in any type of shock) arrives directly at the lung, where pulmonary capillary damage occurs. Humoral substances (e.g., lysosomal enzymes and bacterial endotoxin) or particulate materials (e.g., microemboli, major thromboemboli, platelet aggregates, and fat particles) may lodge in the pulmonary capillary bed. As these materials are cleared, leaky pulmonary capillaries are left behind, with the resultant accumulation of extravascular water. If the material trapped in pulmonary capillaries includes large amounts of platelets, secondary effects caused by platelet breakdown products (notably serotonin and thromboxane) are also seen. In major thromboembolism, for example, hypoxemia occurs because of ventilation-perfusion imbalance owing to bronchial spasm, presumably secondary to serotonin released from platelets.

The pulmonary effects of materials released into the venous blood in shock entrain a particularly vicious circle.[21] Increased

pulmonary vascular resistance and hypoxia resulting from the capillary damage lead to decreased cardiac output and peripheral oxygen delivery, exacerbating the shock state and perpetuating the pulmonary lesion.

Left ventricular failure with increased left atrial pressure results in pulmonary transcapillary transudation, which may be subtle or grossly obvious, as in congestive heart failure with overt pulmonary edema. Left ventricular pressures may waver at the point of high left atrial pressure for short periods—even minutes—resulting in a transient increase in lung water, then return to a balanced state. This situation in itself may not lead to severe pulmonary edema, but it probably makes the lung more vulnerable when minor capillary damage coexists.

The pulmonary interstitium is particularly vulnerable to the events surrounding an operation. Saltwater infusion usually greatly exceeds fluid losses and thus expands the extracellular space. Bleeding and compression of veins by retractors may cause hypotension and necessitate infusion of blood or fluid. Mediators from sterile tissue injury or bacterial invasion may injure pulmonary capillary endothelium. Transient myocardial depression may cause hydrostatic pulmonary edema. With all of these factors, it is remarkable that there is no primary change in lung water volume after uncomplicated operations, even operations including cardiopulmonary bypass. Nonetheless, it should be remembered that the patient usually leaves the OR overloaded with fluid and primed for the development of lung edema.

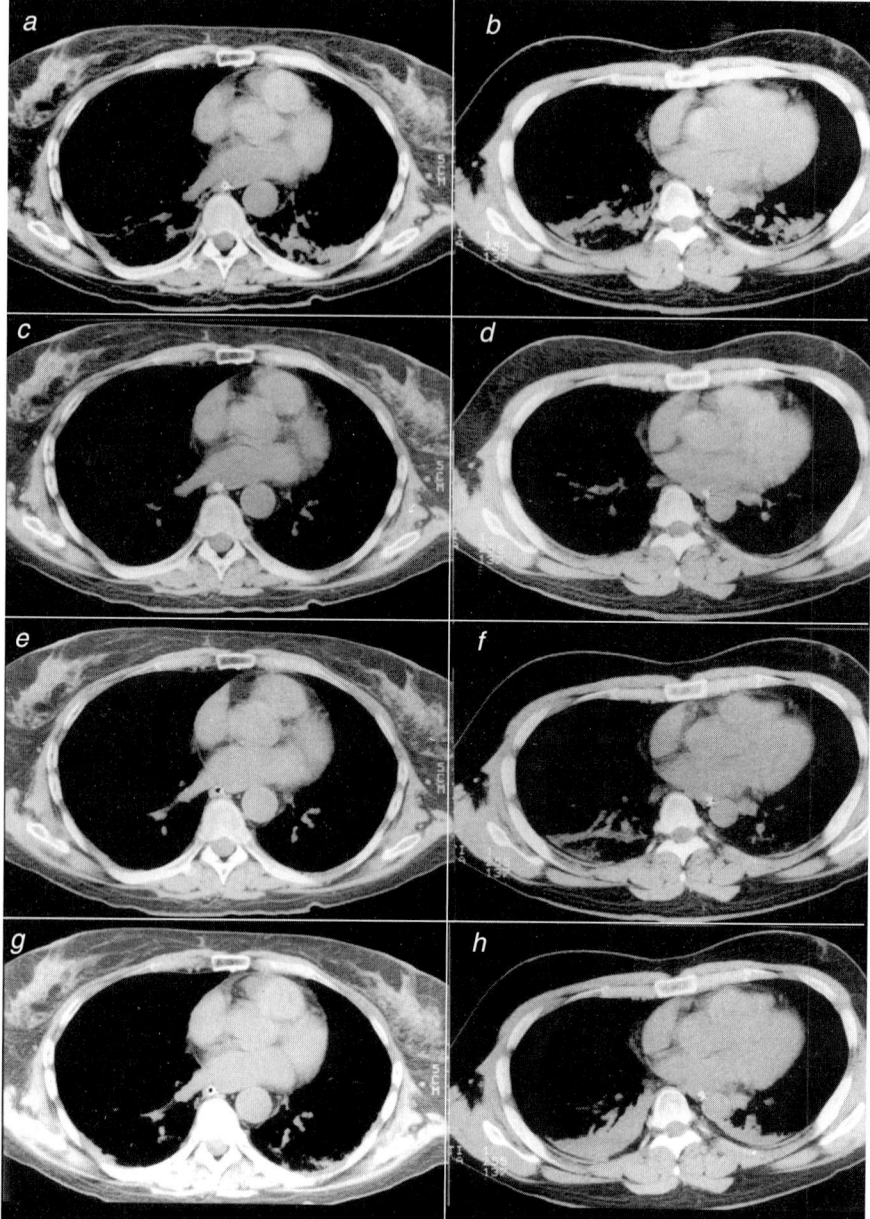

Figure 8   The subject on the left (*a, c, e, g*) is ventilated with 40% O_2; the subject on the right (*b, d, f, h*), with 100% O_2. Atelectasis occurs (posteriorly, of course) after induction and several minutes of tidal breathing (*a, b*) and is completely reversed by inflation to total lung capacity (plateau pressure 40 cm H_2O; *c, d*). Inflation was sustained for 5 and 40 minutes while the patient was breathing 60% nitrogen (*e, g*), but atelectasis recurred by absorption while the patient was breathing 0% nitrogen (*f, h*). Used with permission.[2]

CONDITIONS AND EVENTS ASSOCIATED WITH PULMONARY INSUFFICIENCY

Fat Embolism

In a small percentage of patients with extensive fractures, the clinical syndrome of fat embolism develops. This syndrome results from pulmonary embolization of neutral fat globules from the marrow cavity and is often associated with embolization of megakaryocytes and other marrow cells. Hypoxemia and bilateral patchy pulmonary infiltrates, beginning 12 to 36 hours after an injury or a bone operation, are typical of this lesion. Associated findings include a falling hematocrit, hemolysis, high fever, cerebral symptoms, petechiae (particularly in the anterior axillary folds, the sclerae, and the eyelids), and possibly fat globules in urine, blood, or sputum. Pulmonary capillary damage occurs, apparently as a consequence of sterile inflammation from fatty acids released as the triglyceride particles break down in the lung parenchyma. Steroids have been shown to reduce the inflammation and hence the mortality from the pulmonary lesion, though they must be given early and in large doses to be effective. Intubation and mechanical ventilation are indicated as soon as the syndrome has been diagnosed. Care must be taken to keep the patient's fluid balance as dry as possible because the pulmonary capillaries leak even at normal hydrostatic pressures. This is often difficult in patients with multiple injuries, who may have active bleeding or oliguria concomitantly with the developing pulmonary lesion.

Smoke Inhalation

Several investigators have demonstrated a generalized permeability increase in capillaries (including pulmonary capillaries) after a small burn; the more extensive the burn, the greater the capillary leakage.[22] The pulmonary capillary bed shows signs of increased capillary permeability first, in the form of increased lung water. This phenomenon has confused clinicians caring for patients with smoke inhalation syndrome for many years. However, it has now been clarified by work showing that smoke inhalation injury is a relatively mild pulmonary insult in itself but is a major insult when combined with a body surface burn, as is often the case in humans.[23]

Toxic components of smoke include carbon monoxide, heat, various aldehydes and other organic materials, and a wide range of vaporized compounds. Materials that are totally combustible (e.g., natural gas and gasoline) burn to yield CO_2 and water, producing few toxic organic compounds and causing minimal lung damage when inhaled in smoke. On the other hand, materials that burn incompletely (e.g., wood, paint, and upholstery), yield a number of toxic vapors in addition to the usual products of combustion, and these vapors damage the respiratory epithelium and the alveoli. The heat carried in smoke is a relatively minor cause of lung damage because air is such a poor heat conductor. Deep lung damage from heat is unusual unless the thermal injury is conveyed by hot steam.

Carbon monoxide is the major toxic material in smoke. It does not damage the lungs but renders the brain hypoxic by associating with hemoglobin, thereby inducing potentially lethal brain damage. Patients with smoke inhalation injury who do not have a body surface burn usually pass through a period of mild pulmonary insufficiency and recover completely unless they have suffered irreversible brain damage or metabolic acidosis as a result of carboxyhemoglobinemia. Patients with the same degree of smoke inhalation injury who also have a moderate body surface burn are subject to serious pulmonary insufficiency with combined atelectasis and increased lung water; intubation, mechanical ventilation, and efforts to reduce lung water usually prove necessary.

Chest Trauma

Direct injury to the chest may cause damage to the chest wall, the lung parenchyma, the diaphragm, the airway, and other intrathoracic structures (e.g., the heart and the great vessels) [see 5:5 Injuries to the Chest]. These injuries are usually associated with hemothorax or pneumothorax. Life-threatening hypoventilation may result from injuries to the chest wall or from alveolar collapse caused by fluid or blood in the pleural space. Emergency treatment includes placement of a large chest tube to empty the pleur-

al space and reexpand the lung along with mechanical ventilation if spontaneous breathing is inadequate.

With blunt trauma, fracture of the ribs or sternum may create a segment of the chest wall that moves inward in response to the negative pressure created during spontaneous inspiration (so-called paradoxical motion); this floating segment is referred to as a flail segment, or flail chest. A small amount of paradoxical motion with no physiologic side effects does not warrant specific treatment. If flail chest is associated with hypoxemia or CO_2 retention, then lung contusion is probable and intubation and ventilation are indicated.

If air or fluid is detected in the pleural space, a large chest tube should be placed. If a patient with minor chest injuries requires immediate operation for other problems (e.g., ruptured spleen or head injury), prophylactic chest tubes should be replaced on both sides to eliminate the possibility of a tension pneumothorax or hemothorax developing during anesthesia. Mechanical ventilation is required for patients with major flail segments and lung contusion of chest injury complicating other serious injuries.

Penetrating trauma may result in a sucking chest injury, in which air is inhaled into the pleural space during inspiration, filling the pleural space, eliminating the pressure gradient that would normally cause the lung to inflate, and resulting in atelectasis. If the injury allows air to be inhaled into the pleural space but prevents it from exiting, a tension pneumothorax results, with hypoventilation and blockage of venous return; bleeding into the pleural space from the chest wall or the lung complicates this problem. Placing a chest tube to drain accumulated air and blood, along with appropriate replacement of lost blood, usually returns cardiac output and respiration to normal quite promptly. Because the lung vasculature is a low-pressure system, bleeding from the lung itself usually subsides relatively quickly. Air leaks from the lung usually seal within 1 or 2 days. Prolonged major air leaks suggest the presence of an injury to a large bronchus, the trachea, or the esophagus that requires operative repair.

Thoracotomy and Pulmonary Resection

On the whole, patients experiencing pulmonary problems after thoracic operations are managed in much the same way as those with pulmonary insufficiency from other causes. Special attention should, however, be given to patients who have undergone resection of part or all of a lung as treatment for infection, cancer, congenital abnormalities, or, rarely, trauma. If the remaining lung is normal, removal of lung tissue does not cause a major physiologic deficit. Nevertheless, pulmonary resection does give rise to certain unique concerns. In particular, the empty space formerly occupied by the lung tissue must be managed very carefully, or poor healing and infection may result. If pleural space infection, leakage from the closed bronchus, or pulmonary failure occurs after pulmonary resection, challenging ventilatory problems ensue.

References

1. Bartlett RH: Critical Care Physiology. JB Lippincott Co, Philadelphia, 1996

2. Routhen H, Sporre B, Engberg G, et al: Influence of gas composition on recurrence of atelectasis after a reexpansion maneuver during general anesthesia. Anesthesiology 82:832, 1995

3. Greif R, Akca O, Horn EP, et al: Supplemental perioperative oxygen to reduce the incidence of surgical-wound infection. Outcomes Research Group. N Engl J Med 342:161, 2000

4. Bartlett RH, Gazzaniga AB, Geraghty TR: Respiratory maneuvers to prevent postoperative pulmonary complications: a critical review. JAMA 224:1017, 1973

5. Bartlett RH: Respiratory therapy to prevent postoperative pulmonary complications. Respiratory Intensive Care. Pierson DJ, Ed. Daedalus Enterprises, Dallas, 1986, p 369

6. Drakulovic MB, Torres A, Bauer TT, et al: Supine body position as a risk factor for nosocomial pneumonia in mechanically ventilated patients: a randomised trial. Lancet 354:1851, 1999

7. Orozco-Levi M, Torres A, Ferrer M, et al: Semirecumbent position protects from pulmonary aspiration but not completely from gastroesophageal reflux in mechanically ventilated patients. Am J Respir Crit Care Med 152:1387, 1995

8. Torres A, Serra-Batlles J, Ros E, et al: Pulmonary aspiration of gastric contents in patients receiving mechanical ventilation: the effect of body position. Ann Intern Med 116:540, 1992

9. Antonelli M, Conti G, Rocco M, et al: A comparison of noninvasive positive-pressure ventilation and conventional mechanical ventilation in patients with acute respiratory failure: pressure support ventilation in COPD patients with postextubation hypercapnic respiratory insufficiency. N Engl J Med 339:429, 1998

10. Girou E, Schortgen F, Delclaux C, et al: Association of noninvasive ventilation with nosocomial infections and survival in critically ill patients. JAMA 284:2361, 2000

11. Brochard L, Mancebo J, Wysocki M, et al: Noninvasive ventilation for acute exacerbations of chronic obstructive pulmonary disease. N Engl J Med 333:817, 1995

12. Demling R, Staub N, Edmunds LH: Effect of end expiratory pressure on accumulation of extravascular lung water. J Appl Physiol 38:907, 1975

13. Hauser CJ, Shoemaker W, et al: Hemodynamic and oxygen transport responses to body shifts produced by colloids and crystalloids in critically ill patients. Surg Gynecol Obstet 150:811, 1980

14. Shoemaker W, Hauser CJ: Critique of crystalloid versus colloidal therapy in shock and shock lung. Crit Care Med 7:117, 1979

15. Bernard GR, Luce JM, Sprung CL, et al: High-dose corticosteroids in patients with the adult respiratory distress syndrome. N Engl J Med 317:1565, 1987

16. Johnson A, Malik AB: Pulmonary transvascular fluid and protein exchange after thrombin-induced microembolism: differential effects of cyclooxygenase inhibitors. Am Rev Respir Dis 132:70, 1985

17. Flick MR, Hoeffel JM, Staub NC: Superoxide dismutase with heparin prevents increased lung vascular permeability during air emboli in sheep. J Appl Physiol 55:1284, 1983

18. Yu M, Tomasa G: A double blind prospective randomized trial of ketoconazole, a thromboxane synthase inhibitor, in the prophylaxis of the adult respiratory distress syndrome. Crit Care Med 21:1635, 1993

19. Kolobow T, Moretti MP, Fumagalli R, et al: Severe impairment in lung function induced by high peak airway pressure during mechanical ventilation. Am Rev Respir Dis 135:312, 1987

20. Okinaka AJ: The pattern of breathing after operation. Surg Gynecol Obstet 125:785, 1967

21. Demling R: The pathogenesis of respiratory failure after trauma and sepsis. Surg Clin North Am 60:1373, 1980

22. Staub N: Pulmonary edema: physiologic approaches to management. Chest 74:559, 1978

23. Alpard SK, Zwischenberger JB, Tao W, et al: New clinically relevant sheep model of severe respiratory failure secondary to combined smoke inhalation/cutaneous flame burn injury. Crit Care Med 28:1469, 2000

6 USE OF THE MECHANICAL VENTILATOR

Robert H. Bartlett, M.D., F.A.C.S.

Approach to Mechanical Ventilation

An essential concept in mechanical ventilation is the distinction between two key processes, ventilation and oxygenation. The primary purpose of ventilation is to excrete carbon dioxide. The minute ventilation ($\dot{V}_E$) is the total amount of gas exhaled per minute, computed as the product of the rate and the tidal volume (V_T). Approximately two thirds of the minute ventilation reaches the alveoli and promotes gas exchange (alveolar ventilation, or $\dot{V}_A$); the remaining third moves in and out of the conducting airways and nonperfused alveoli (the dead space ventilation, or $\dot{V}_D$). Thus, the ratio of dead space to tidal volume (V_D/V_T) is normally 0.33. The efficiency of carbon dioxide excretion is directly related to the amount of alveolar ventilation. During spontaneous breathing, the minute ventilation is regulated by the respiratory center; during mechanical ventilation, the operator uses a mechanical ventilator to excrete enough CO_2 to maintain the partial arterial pressure of CO_2 (P_aCO_2) at 40 mm Hg. Ventilation is monitored by measuring P_aCO_2.

Oxygenation, on the other hand, refers to the equilibrium of oxygen in the pulmonary capillary blood and oxygen in inflated alveoli. The partial pressure of oxygen (PO_2) gradient between alveolus and capillary favors transfer of oxygen into blood because alveolar PO_2 is maintained by ventilation or by provision of supplemental oxygen to the airway. Hence, oxygenation depends less on good alveolar ventilation than on the appropriate matching of pulmonary blood flow to well-inflated alveoli, a process that can be affected by patient position, altered airway pressure, pulmonary parenchymal disease, or small airway disease. The efficiency of this ventilation-perfusion matching, and therefore of oxygenation, can be evaluated by measuring the PO_2 in arterial blood (P_aO_2) at a known value for the fraction, or concentration, of inspired oxygen (F_IO_2).

Mechanical ventilators are designed to provide ventilation by regulating tidal volume, rate, and inspiratory flow, thereby controlling CO_2 excretion. Because they can also regulate airway pressure and F_IO_2, they offer some control over oxygenation as well. In either case, proper use of a mechanical ventilator necessitates a solid understanding of normal and abnormal pulmonary mechanics, gas exchange, and the relation between systemic oxygen delivery and consumption. Most mechanical ventilators allow the operator to monitor at least some of these variables. In practice, a mechanical ventilator is employed differently depending on whether the main goal is adequate ventilation or adequate oxygenation. Therefore, these two aspects of ventilator use will be discussed separately.

Basic Mechanical Ventilation

VENTILATION

For basic mechanical ventilation, the rate should initially be set at 10/min and the tidal volume at 10 ml/kg, provided that the inspiratory plateau pressure (P_{plat}) is

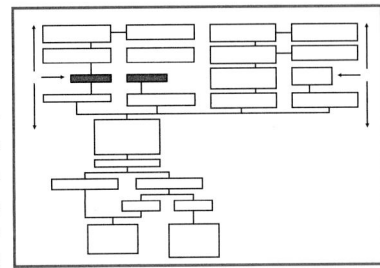

less than 30 cm H_2O; if P_{plat} is higher than 30 cm H_2O, smaller tidal volumes, such as 6 ml/kg, are appropriate. This setting will yield a minute ventilation of 100 ml/kg/min. If the V_D/V_T ratio is nearly normal, the alveolar ventilation produced (approximately 4 L/min) will be sufficient to eliminate all the metabolically produced CO_2 and to maintain the P_aCO_2 at about 40 mm Hg. If the patient's brain stem function is normal, the mechanical ventilator should be set on the assist mode, which allows the patient to adjust his or her own respiratory rate to keep the P_aCO_2 within normal limits. As a safeguard, a controlled backup rate is set below the patient's assist rate in case spontaneous effort ceases.

OXYGENATION

For basic oxygenation, the F_IO_2 should initially be set at 0.5. This level is not damaging to the alveoli and does not deplete nitrogen levels from the alveoli. If the pulmonary parenchyma and ventilation-perfusion relations are normal, P_aO_2 will

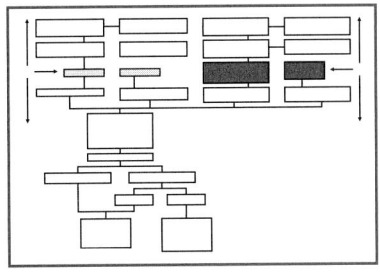

be unnecessarily elevated, and the F_IO_2 should be turned down until the saturation and PO_2 are in the normal range. The positive end-expiratory pressure (PEEP) should be set at +5 cm H_2O. This value is high enough to maintain inflation of some alveoli that would close at end expiration at lower pressures yet low enough not to induce any deleterious effects. The peak inspiratory pressure (PIP), which is always measured after a short inspiratory hold or plateau, is determined by the tidal volume, inspiratory gas flow, and compliance of the lung. If the compliance is relatively normal, the ventilator settings described will lead to a P_{plat} of 20 cm H_2O. The high airway pressure cutoff and alarm should be set at 40 cm H_2O. These settings will result in a mean airway pressure of between 5 and 10 cm H_2O, with the exact lev-

CO₂

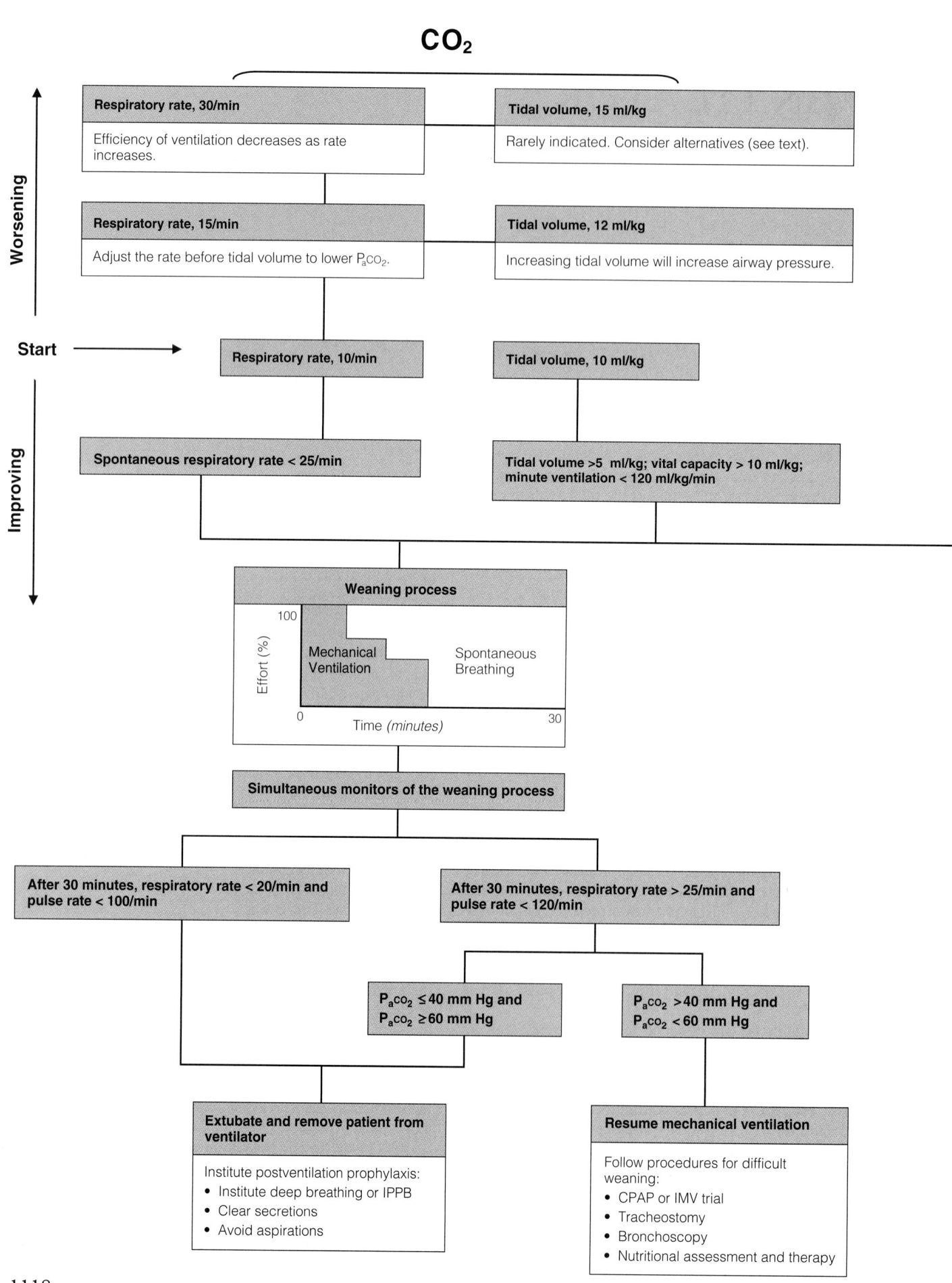

Worsening ↑

Respiratory rate, 30/min	Tidal volume, 15 ml/kg
Efficiency of ventilation decreases as rate increases.	Rarely indicated. Consider alternatives (see text).

Respiratory rate, 15/min	Tidal volume, 12 ml/kg
Adjust the rate before tidal volume to lower P_aCO_2.	Increasing tidal volume will increase airway pressure.

Start →

Respiratory rate, 10/min

Tidal volume, 10 ml/kg

Improving ↓

Spontaneous respiratory rate < 25/min

Tidal volume >5 ml/kg; vital capacity > 10 ml/kg; minute ventilation < 120 ml/kg/min

Weaning process

Effort (%)

100

Mechanical Ventilation

Spontaneous Breathing

0   Time (minutes)   30

Simultaneous monitors of the weaning process

After 30 minutes, respiratory rate < 20/min and pulse rate < 100/min

After 30 minutes, respiratory rate > 25/min and pulse rate < 120/min

P_aCO_2 ≤ 40 mm Hg and P_aCO_2 ≥ 60 mm Hg

P_aCO_2 > 40 mm Hg and P_aCO_2 < 60 mm Hg

Extubate and remove patient from ventilator

Institute postventilation prophylaxis:
- Institute deep breathing or IPPB
- Clear secretions
- Avoid aspirations

Resume mechanical ventilation

Follow procedures for difficult weaning:
- CPAP or IMV trial
- Tracheostomy
- Bronchoscopy
- Nutritional assessment and therapy

O₂

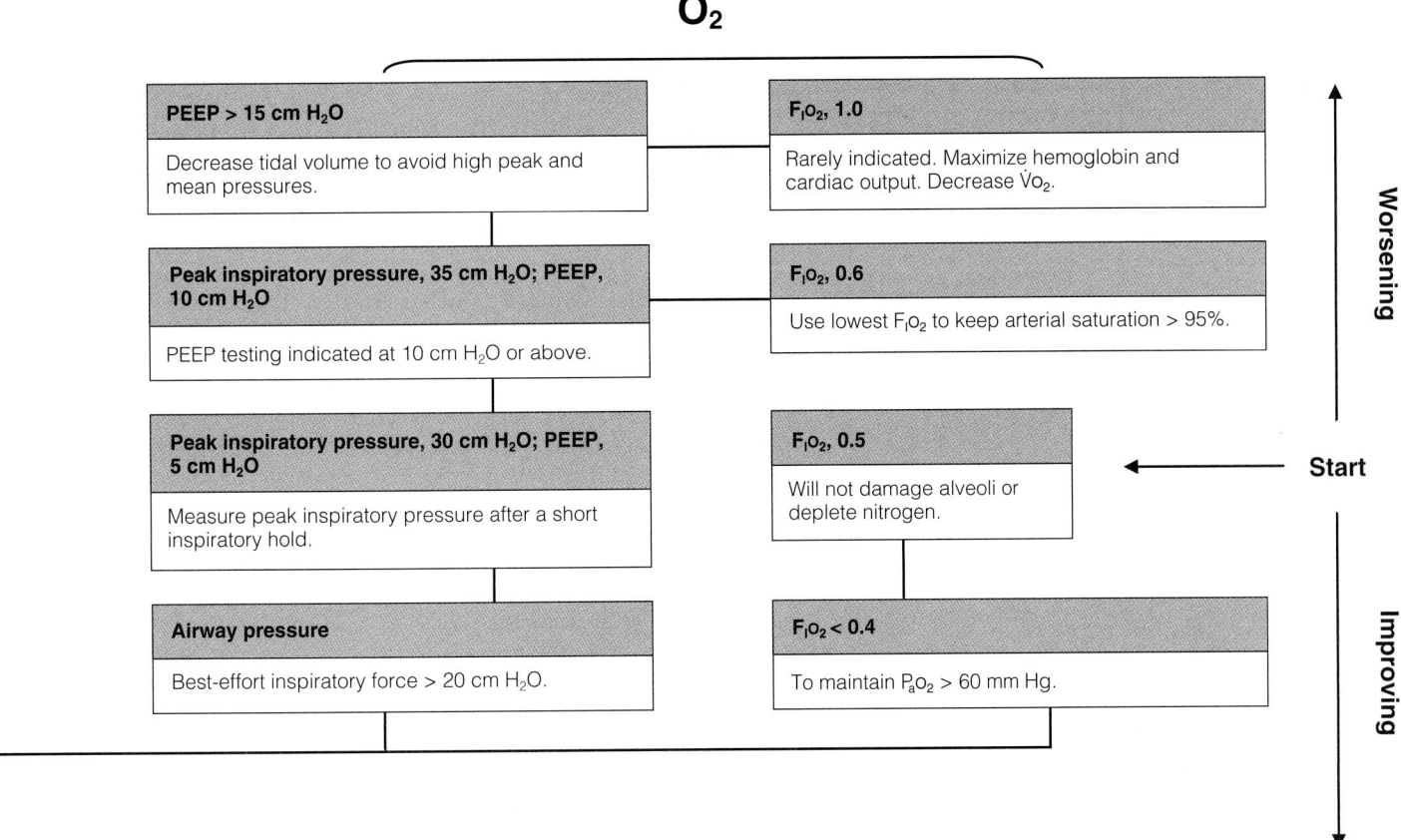

PEEP > 15 cm H₂O	**F₁O₂, 1.0**
Decrease tidal volume to avoid high peak and mean pressures.	Rarely indicated. Maximize hemoglobin and cardiac output. Decrease V̇O₂.
Peak inspiratory pressure, 35 cm H₂O; PEEP, 10 cm H₂O	**F₁O₂, 0.6**
PEEP testing indicated at 10 cm H₂O or above.	Use lowest F₁O₂ to keep arterial saturation > 95%.
Peak inspiratory pressure, 30 cm H₂O; PEEP, 5 cm H₂O	**F₁O₂, 0.5**
Measure peak inspiratory pressure after a short inspiratory hold.	Will not damage alveoli or deplete nitrogen.
Airway pressure	**F₁O₂ < 0.4**
Best-effort inspiratory force > 20 cm H₂O.	To maintain P_aO₂ > 60 mm Hg.

Worsening

Start

Improving

Approach to Mechanical Ventilation

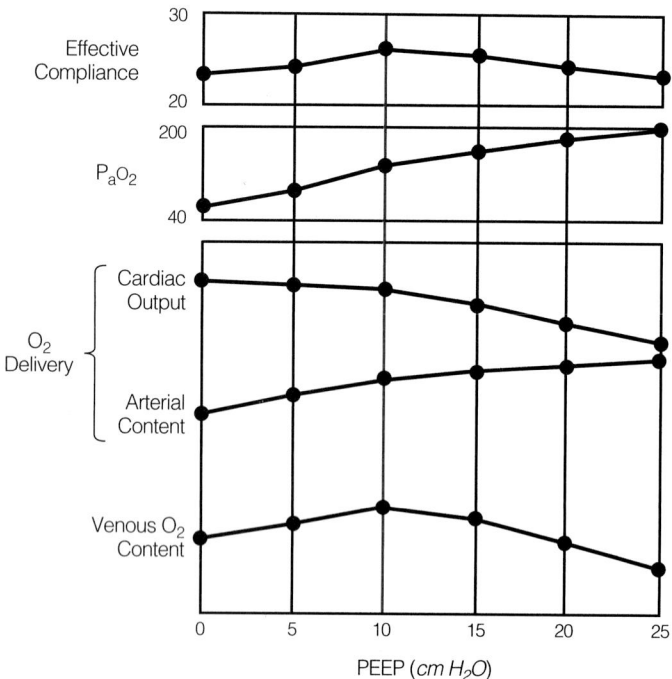

Figure 1 Shown are measurements for determining the optimal PEEP. The objective is to maximize the oxygen delivery:oxygen consumption ratio, which is measured by mixed venous saturation. Here, the best PEEP is 10 cm H_2O, even though the P_aO_2 and the arterial oxygen content are higher at higher levels of PEEP.

el depending on the respiratory rate, the inspiratory gas flow rate, and the amount of spontaneous inspiratory effort generated by the patient. The patient's inspiratory effort will appear as negative pressure measured at the airway, but such effort is beneficial rather than deleterious.

After the patient has been started on a course of mechanical ventilation, ventilation and oxygenation must be assessed, usually by measuring P_aCO_2 and P_aO_2. Adjustments are then made on the basis of this assessment [*see Figure 1*]. If P_aCO_2 and P_aO_2 are normal and if the patient is to remain on mechanical ventilation for pulmonary prophylaxis or because of CNS depression, these settings are maintained until it is time to wean the patient from ventilation [*see* Weaning from Mechanical Ventilation, *below*]. If the settings do not provide adequate gas exchange or if the patient's condition worsens, further adjustments are required.

Worsening Respiratory Status

VENTILATION

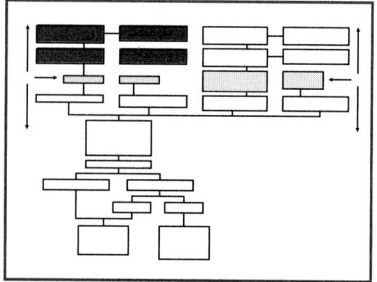

If the P_aCO_2 is elevated despite a minute ventilation of 100 ml/kg/ min, either the metabolically produced carbon dioxide is inappropriately high or the alveolar ventilation is an inappropriately low percentage of the tidal volume, or both. To increase ventilation, the first step should be to increase the respiratory rate (stepwise) to 20/min. (Increasing the respiratory rate raises the mean airway pressure and may necessitate administration of fluid volume to maintain hemodynamic stability; however, because increasing the tidal volume elevates the P_{plat}, possibly lead-

ing to barotrauma, the respiratory rate must be changed first.) The volume of CO_2 excreted is easily measured by collecting and analyzing exhaled gas. If it is greater than normal (130 ml/m²/min), CO_2 production can be decreased by reducing muscular activity or seizures, controlling hypermetabolic states (if possible), and minimizing the exogenous carbohydrate load.

If the P_aCO_2 has still not returned to normal after these measures have been taken, the respiratory rate can be increased to 25/min or higher, although it should be kept in mind that the efficiency of ventilation decreases as the respiratory rate increases (i.e., the percentage of minute ventilation that becomes alveolar ventilation decreases as the respiratory rate increases because there may be inadequate time for alveolar emptying during expiration and because the dead space remains unchanged). A tidal volume greater than 15 ml/kg is rarely necessary unless there is a major air leak. A minute ventilation higher than 300 ml/kg/min indicates major metabolic or respiratory dysfunction. The pressures required to generate this amount of ventilation are harmful to the lungs and adversely affect hemodynamic status. If the P_aCO_2 is higher than 40 mm Hg despite a respiratory rate of 20 to 25/min, a P_{plat} of 35 cm H_2O, and a minute ventilation of 250 to 300 ml/kg/min, alternatives should be seriously considered, such as allowing the patient to equilibrate at an abnormally high P_aCO_2, inducing paralysis to decrease muscular activity and CO_2 production, or instituting extracorporeal circulation through a membrane oxygenator to remove CO_2 [*see* Fighting the Ventilator, Permissive Hypercapnia, *and* Extracorporeal Life Support, *below*].

OXYGENATION

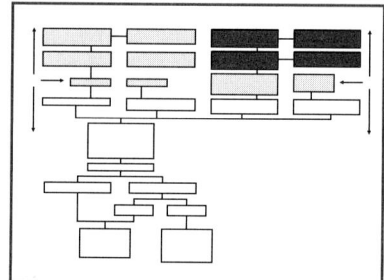

If the initial ventilator settings are not adequate to oxygenate the patient's arterial blood, then some areas in the lung are perfused but not inflated (i.e., right-to-left shunting). To enhance oxygenation, the first step is to raise the PEEP to 10 cm H_2O, in the hope of maintaining or improving alveolar inflation. It is wise to decrease tidal volume and to increase the respiratory rate at the same time, to avoid raising the P_{plat}. The P_{plat} should not exceed 45 cm H_2O. Even with these changes in ventilation, the mean airway pressure may increase to the point at which it interferes with venous return. Whenever the PEEP is raised above 5 cm H_2O, the balance between systemic oxygen delivery and oxygen consumption should be evaluated because increasing the mean airway pressure may raise the P_{O_2} but may actually decrease systemic oxygen delivery by decreasing cardiac output.

Several measurements are necessary for determining the optimal PEEP level [*see Figure 1*]. Effective lung compliance is the simplest measurement, but optimal lung compliance does not always correlate with optimal oxygen delivery. The best measurement is that of venous oxygen content, which is approximated as mixed venous oxyhemoglobin saturation. This measurement requires samples of blood from the pulmonary artery or, better yet, a continuous indwelling catheter to monitor venous saturation. Obviously, therefore, a pulmonary arterial catheter should be inserted whenever PEEP levels higher than 5 cm H_2O are necessary for ensuring adequate oxygenation. Venous saturation measures the ratio of systemic oxygen delivery to oxygen consumption. This ratio is normally 4, which corresponds to a mixed venous saturation of 75%, when arterial saturation is near 100%. (That is, normally 25% of the oxygen delivered to tissues is extracted and utilized.) Consequently, PEEP testing is best done by gradually increasing the

PEEP level until either oxygenation is sufficient to saturate arterial blood or mixed venous saturation drops below 70%, whichever comes first.

PEEP does not cause inflation of collapsed alveoli but only holds open alveolar units that would collapse at a lower airway pressure. Inflation can be facilitated by prolonging inspiration, which can be achieved by using a slower inspiratory flow rate, an inspiratory hold or plateau (0.5 to 1.0 second), or a designated pressure for a specific time (pressure-controlled ventilation). All of these maneuvers will increase the mean airway pressure and the inspiration-expiration ratio (I/E), which may limit venous return, thereby interfering with oxygen delivery. Venous saturation monitoring is the best way to titrate inspiratory pressure maneuvers.

AVOIDING LUNG INJURY

Positive airway pressure and oxygen are lifesaving when delivered in moderation but can damage the lungs when delivered in excess. An F_IO_2 of 0.6 and a peak airway pressure of 30 cm H_2O can be used for days or weeks if necessary without deleterious effects. Because oxygen and pressure are delivered only to inflated alveoli, the most normal area of the lung is subjected to injury when higher levels are used. Thus, excessive positive pressure and oxygen can contribute to the pathogenesis of progressive pulmonary failure in ventilated patients. Moreover, pressure above 40 cm H_2O simply causes overdistention of the inflated alveoli and decreases the efficiency of ventilation [see Discussion, below]. An F_IO_2 above 0.6 has a minimal effect on oxygenation when the major problem is transpulmonary shunt. For these reasons, before P_{plat} is raised above 40 cm H_2O or F_IO_2 is raised above 0.6, all other variables of systemic oxygen delivery should be considered [see Table 1].

If oxygenation remains inadequate at these higher airway pressures, then F_IO_2 can be increased to 0.6 or higher, although it should be noted that if the problem is a major transpulmonary shunt, major increases in F_IO_2 will have little effect on P_aO_2. High concentrations of oxygen in the airway should generally be avoided, primarily because of the resultant depletion of nitrogen, which helps maintain inflation of the alveoli. Only very rarely is it necessary to raise F_IO_2 above 0.6; usually, it is preferable to increase the PEEP instead while progressively decreasing tidal volume and supporting blood volume. PEEP is used to improve ventilation-perfusion matching; prone positioning and diuresis may be even more effective [see Discussion, below].

The goal in severe respiratory failure is to optimize oxygen delivery, not P_aO_2. Measures to be taken include administering red blood cells until a normal hemoglobin concentration (13 to 15 g/dl) is reached, increasing cardiac output by means of volume loading, decreasing systemic oxygen consumption by means of sedation or paralysis, and treating the cause of hypermetabolism (usually infection). The relation between systemic oxygen delivery and oxygen consumption can be monitored by measuring mixed venous saturation. If it is considered necessary to use high airway pressure and 100% oxygen, the variables of oxygen delivery should be set as just described. The F_IO_2 should then be decreased until venous saturation falls to 65% to 70%. If arterial saturation is less than 90% despite an F_IO_2 of 1.0, PEEP of more than 10 cm H_2O, and a hemoglobin of more than 13 g/dl, the next measures to be taken should be (1) to induce paralysis to decrease oxygen consumption, (2) to allow the patient to equilibrate at an abnormally low arterial oxygen saturation (S_aO_2), or (3) to institute extracorporeal circulation through a membrane oxygenator to deliver oxygen.

Improving Respiratory Status

VENTILATION

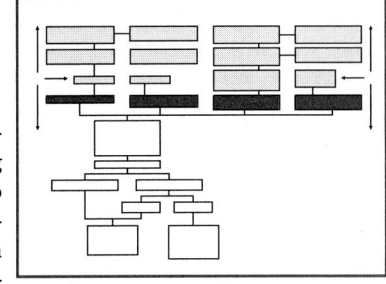

Patients whose respiratory status is improving should be alert enough to regulate their own respiratory rate with the ventilator in the assist mode. Tidal volume is maintained at 10 ml/kg until the patient is ready for weaning. (As noted, if P_{plat} is greater than 30 cm H_2O, a smaller tidal volume is appropriate.) When respiratory status is improving, the ventilator should remain in the assist mode rather than in the controlled mechanical ventilation (CMV) mode because the patient can adjust his or her respiratory rate to maintain a normal P_aCO_2.

Table 1 Interventions to Optimize the Ratio of Oxygen Delivery to Oxygen Consumption in Patients with Impaired Oxygenation

Intervention	Benefits	Risk
Increase O_2 content ↑ F_IO_2 to above 0.6	0.3 ml O_2/dl for each 100 mm Hg P_aO_2 after full saturation	O_2 toxicity to lung Less nitrogen in alveoli
↑ Hemoglobin (Hb) to normal	1.36 ml O_2/dl for each g HbO_2/dl	Transfusion risk (viral infection)
Increase cardiac output ↑ Blood volume to pulmonary capillary wedge pressure of 15–20 mm Hg	200 ml $\dot{D}O_2$ increase for each L/min increase in cardiac output*	Transfusion risk ↑ Pulmonary hydrostatic pressure
Administer inotropic drugs to achieve $S_{\bar{v}}O_2$ 75%–80%	200 ml $\dot{D}O_2$ increase for each L/min increase in cardiac output*	Increased $\dot{V}O_2$ and $\dot{V}CO_2$ with catecholamines Tachycardia
Administer vasodilator drugs to achieve $S_{\bar{v}}O_2$ 75%–80%	200 ml $\dot{D}O_2$ increase for each L/min increase in cardiac output*	Hypotension Variable regional blood flow
Decrease O_2 consumption Drain and treat infection	Eliminate stimulus to metabolism	None
Patient paralysis	10%–15% decrease in $\dot{V}O_2$ and $\dot{V}CO_2$	Weakness, atrophy, need for positional changes, difficult patient examination
↓ Body temperature	7% decrease in $\dot{V}O_2$ and $\dot{V}CO_2$ for each 1° C increase in body temperature	Requires patient paralysis, coagulopathy

*Hb = 15 g/dl; S_aO_2 = 100%.

OXYGENATION

The F_IO_2 should be decreased to a concentration (0.4 or 0.3) that ensures an arterial saturation higher than 90% (equivalent to a P_aO_2 higher than 60 mm Hg). Keeping the F_IO_2 in this range will lead to increased arterial oxygenation, which serves as a slight safety buffer during suctioning or disconnection. The PEEP can be reduced to 0, although there is a theoretical advantage to maintaining a low level of PEEP as long as the patient is intubated.

WEANING PARAMETERS

When the patient can maintain satisfactory gas exchange at the ventilator settings just given, the next step is to determine whether the patient is ready for extubation. Accordingly, the patient's ability to ventilate is measured during spontaneous breathing a few minutes after the removal of mechanical support. The findings that generally indicate that weaning and extubation can be carried out successfully are (1) a spontaneous respiratory rate lower than 25/min, (2) a tidal volume greater than 5 ml/kg, (3) a vital capacity greater than 10 ml/kg, (4) a minute ventilation less than 120 ml/kg/min, and (5) an inspiratory pressure that is more negative than –20 cm H_2O. If the patient meets these parameters and if arterial oxygenation is satisfactory at an F_IO_2 of 0.4 or less, then pulmonary mechanics and gas exchange are probably close enough to normal to permit extubation and spontaneous breathing. It should be kept in mind that these measurements are made while the patient is breathing through a long, narrow endotracheal or tracheostomy tube, which causes significant resistance and increases the work of breathing. Therefore, the results will be even better when the patient is extubated and breathing through his or her own airway. If metabolic alkalosis is present, it should be corrected before weaning is attempted. The one variable that cannot be measured with this amount of testing is the endurance of the patient's respiratory efforts. Measurement of endurance is, in essence, the weaning process.

Weaning from Mechanical Ventilation

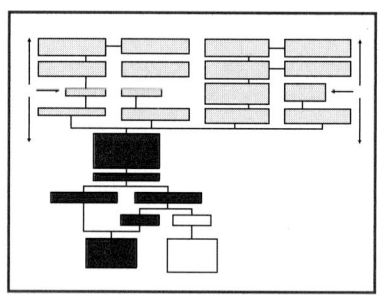

In the weaning process, the work of breathing that had been the task of the mechanical ventilator is reassumed by the respiratory muscles of the patient. When the results of respiratory testing indicate that the patient can be weaned from the ventilator, a trial of spontaneous breathing is indicated. During this trial, supplemental humidified oxygen is supplied by way of the endotracheal tube. The balloon is deflated to allow some breathing around the tube and to minimize airway resistance. The patient should be sitting upright. The transition from mechanical support to spontaneous breathing should be swift: the mechanical ventilator should be either turned down rapidly or simply disconnected [see Figure 2]. In addition, the gas supply to the endotracheal tube must be free-flowing; at no point in the trial should the patient have to trigger a demand valve on the ventilator. Most ventilators do not supply a free flow of gas in the continuous positive airway pressure (CPAP) or intermittent mandatory ventilation (IMV) mode but require patient effort to trigger gas flow. The purpose of the spontaneous breathing trial is to determine the endurance of the patient. If it is obvious that the patient can make a strong respiratory effort and is fully alert and awake, he or she can be extubated without further testing after a few minutes of spontaneous breathing.

The simplest way to monitor a spontaneous breathing trial is to watch respiratory rate and pulse rate. If, after 5 to 30 minutes of spontaneous breathing, the respiratory rate is lower than 25/min, the patient will probably be able to sustain an adequate minute ventilation when extubated. If the pulse rate is less than 120/min, the work of breathing is probably not excessive. If the respiratory rate is lower than 20/min and the pulse rate less than 100/min, the patient can be extubated without any further measurements being made. If, however, the pulse rate and respiratory rate are moderately elevated, the P_aCO_2 and P_aO_2 should be measured; if the P_aCO_2 is 40 mm Hg or lower and the P_aO_2 is 60 mm Hg or higher, the patient may be extubated. Postventilation prophylactic maneuvers, to be discussed later [see Postventilation Prophylaxis, below], are indicated. If the results of these four measurements indicate that the trial of spontaneous breathing has failed, mechanical ventilation is resumed to improve the patient's respiratory status before weaning is tried again.

The weaning process should never take more than an hour. If the indicators for weaning are present, the trial of spontaneous breathing is usually successful, and the patient should be extubated. If the indicators are not present, mechanical support should not be gradually decreased—for example, over a period of hours or days—except under strictly controlled conditions.

Difficult Weaning

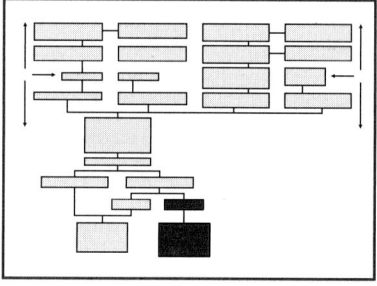

There are a number of reasons why patients may remain ventilator dependent. If the patient has chronic lung disease that predated the acute event, it may be necessary to wean from the ventilator at a level of P_aCO_2 corresponding to compensated respiratory acidosis. If chronic bronchitis, acute resolving pneumonitis, or injury to the respiratory epithelium is present, bronchoscopy is indicated to examine the airway and clear any inspissated secretions. If the patient has lower-lobe infiltrates (as is commonly the case following a prolonged period of ventilation and supine position), vigorous chest physical therapy and postural drainage are indicated.

VENTILATION

Hypoventilation with gradual CO_2 accumulation is the most common finding in patients who are difficult to wean from mechanical ventilation. Hypermetabolism with increased CO_2 load is a common cause of this problem. Patients who have barely enough respiratory endurance to excrete a normal amount of carbon dioxide cannot maintain the extra ventilation necessary for sustained hyperventilation. Often, muscular weakness is the problem, particularly when compliance is decreased by the acute lung disease that requires extra work with every breath.

In addition to the general measures listed (see above), the first step in a patient in whom attempts at weaning have failed is to do a tracheostomy. This procedure not only minimizes the rebreathing space but also eliminates the urgency and potential risk of extubation, thereby greatly facilitating the weaning process. When the tracheostomy is in place and all the general measures have been carried out, progressive breathing exercises are begun. The type of progressive breathing exercise depends to some extent on the type of mechanical ventilator available. The tidal volume should remain greater than 5 ml/kg while the inspiratory work gradually shifts from the ventilator to the patient. The pressure-support mode on newer ventilators is ideal for this purpose, or a pressure-controlled mode can be

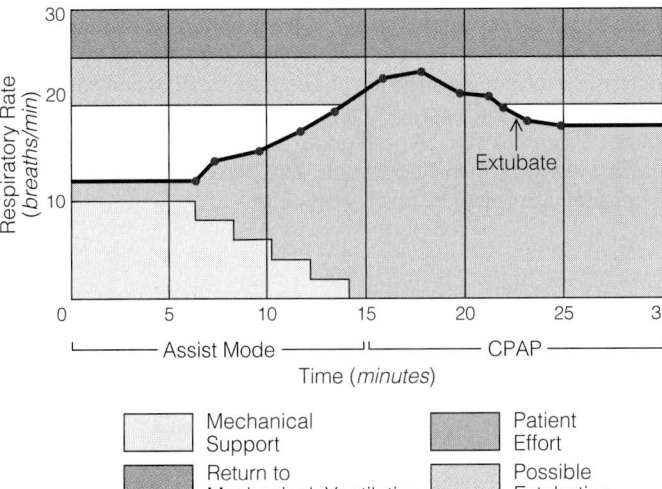

Figure 2   **For most patients, ventilator weaning consists of a brief trial of spontaneous breathing in which pulse and respiratory rates are measured. Mechanical support is decreased until the patient can breathe spontaneously (with or without continuous positive airway pressure [CPAP]), and the respiratory rate is measured every few minutes to determine whether the patient can be extubated. If the respiratory rate is consistently below 20/min and the pulse rate is less than 100/min, the patient can be extubated without the need for further measurements; if it is consistently above 30/min, the patient must be returned to the ventilator; and if it is between 25/min and 30/min, measure PCO_2 and PO_2 to determine whether another trial of mechanical ventilation is needed.**

used. In pressure-controlled or pressure-support ventilation, the peak airway pressure is decreased (typically, 2 cm H_2O/15 min) as long as the respiratory rate is lower than 25/min and the tidal volume is adequate. When the peak airway pressure is 5 to 10 cm H_2O for several hours, the patient can be extubated or can be managed with only humidified air to the tracheostomy [*see Table 2*].

Some volume ventilators do not allow pressure-controlled weaning and instead decrease the rate of volume-controlled breaths. The patient is expected to sustain normal minute ventilation by spontaneous nonassisted breaths. This so-called intermittent mandatory ventilation weaning technique often leads to rapid, shallow breathing and exhaustion in patients [*see Table 2*]. Periods of totally spontaneous breathing should be alternated with assist-mode volume ventilation if pressure-controlled weaning is not possible.

OXYGENATION

Oxygenation is rarely a problem with the hard-to-wean patient because supplemental inspired oxygen (30% to 40%) can counter the hypoventilation that makes weaning difficult. As mentioned earlier [*see* Worsening Respiratory Status, Oxygenation, *above*], other components of the oxygen delivery system (hemoglobin and cardiac output) should be optimized because the patient may have to be weaned at a lower than normal P_aO_2.

NUTRITION AND METABOLISM

A common cause of weaning failure is hypermetabolism caused by occult infection, which manifests itself as increased oxygen consumption ($\dot{V}O_2$) and CO_2 production ($\dot{V}CO_2$). The underlying cause should be treated before weaning is attempted again. Good nutrition is essential for respiratory muscle strength and endurance [*see 6:23 Nutritional Support*]. If a patient is chronically nutritionally depleted, enteral or parenteral feeding to improve muscular strength may be necessary before the patient can be weaned from the ventilator. On the other hand, if carbohydrates are given in amounts exceeding energy expenditure, lipogenesis occurs, which leads to excess CO_2 production. The appropriate nutritional manipulations to avoid this problem depend on direct measurement of $\dot{V}O_2$ and $\dot{V}CO_2$ and calculation of the respiratory quotient. As mentioned earlier [*see* Improving Respiratory Status, Weaning Parameters, *above*], it is important to correct metabolic alkalosis.

Postventilation Prophylaxis

The recently extubated patient is at risk for respiratory failure and consequently should be watched carefully. Airway secretions, stimulated by the chronic indwelling tube, may be thick and difficult to clear. The airway should be carefully lavaged and suctioned before the tube is removed. Direct endotracheal suctioning should be avoided in the period just after removal of the tube because of the risk of hypoxia, vagal stimulation, and vocal cord edema. Postural drainage combined with appropriate airway humidification is a better way of draining airway secretions. The patient should be encouraged to do deep breathing exercises hourly for a few days after extubation, aided, if desired, by an incentive spirometer. If the patient cannot or will not take spontaneous deep breaths, a mechanical ventilator fitted with a mouthpiece should be used every hour or two to ensure periodic maximal inflation (a procedure known as intermittent positive pressure breathing, or IPPB). During IPPB, the ventilator should be used as described in this

Table 2   Methods of Progressive Breathing Exercise in Patients Who Are Difficult to Wean from Mechanical Ventilation

Method	Benefit	Risk
Intermittent mandatory ventilation (IMV)	Commonly available Assisted breath V_T not dependent on compliance	Rapid, shallow breaths may be exhausting Unassisted breaths may require demand valve trigger
Pressure-controlled ventilation	Commonly available V_T supported during each breath	V_T varies with compliance
Pressure support (flow-controlled)	Best support of V_T during each breath	V_T varies with compliance Not commonly available
Pressure support with IMV	V_T supported during each breath IMV not dependent on compliance	IMV may slow the weaning process Not commonly available
Spontaneous-breathing trials	Easy to quantitate status and progress Not dependent on demand valve trigger Universally available	Rapid, shallow breaths may be exhausting

chapter, except that periodic maximal inflation (to a PIP of 30 to 40 cm H₂O) is used to ensure maximal alveolar filling. Even if only a few assisted deep breaths are taken every few hours, inflation will be sufficient to prevent atelectasis. Another option is the use of continuous positive airway pressure by mask or nasal catheter.

The vocal cords will be edematous and may be chronically damaged or dislocated. Aerosolized racemic epinephrine helps to mini-mize upper airway edema. If the voice is abnormal or there is any sign of upper airway obstruction, laryngoscopy should be done to determine the condition of the glottis. Aspiration of oral contents is common in the early postextubation period, particularly if an endo-tracheal tube has been in position for several days. Thick liquids are easier to swallow than clear liquids. The patient should be observed very carefully during the first few feedings.

Discussion

Pulmonary Physiology and Mechanical Ventilation

PULMONARY MECHANICS

The interrelations of gas volumes and pressures that are an inte-gral part of ventilation are collectively referred to as pulmonary mechanics and are more fully described elsewhere [*see 6:5 Pulmon-ary Insufficiency*]. The use of a mechanical ventilator is an exercise in pulmonary mechanics, which may be illustrated by comparing the compliance curve for a normal lung with that for an atelectatic or edematous lung [*see Figure 3*]. The standard compliance, or vol-ume-pressure, curve is obtained by measuring volume and pressure at stages of lung deflation after total inflation. Total lung compli-ance, normalized for patient size, is approximately 1 ml/cm H₂O/ kg. A comparison of volume-pressure curves for normal lungs from three different patients shows the effect of patient size [*see Figure 3, left*]. In fact, the curves would be the same if normalized for patient size. If the lung volume is decreased by half (as a result of pneu-monectomy or main bronchus occlusion, for example), the com-

pliance is decreased by half (to 0.5 ml/cm H₂O/kg). Although the lung is said to be stiffer, it is actually only smaller [*see Figure 3, right*]. Volume, pressure, and flow are related in time [*see Figure 4*]. During a normal volume-controlled mechanical breath, the venti-lator generates gas flow until the desired volume is reached. The pressure is then simply measured. In this example [*see Figure 4*], a short 1-second inspiratory hold is applied to show the difference between plateau pressure, which is equilibrated with alveoli, and peak inspiratory pressure, which is slightly higher because of airflow resistance in the tubing.

In acute respiratory failure, the cause of decreased compliance is almost always associated with a decrease in the functional residual capacity (FRC). In the example cited earlier [*see Figure 3, right*], nor-mal tidal breathing from volume A to volume B would result with 10 cm of inflating pressure. During atelectasis, the decreased FRC (point C) represents the lost alveoli that are either collapsed or filled with fluid but are still perfused with blood. Tidal breathing (to vol-ume D) requires higher pressure. Because the compliance curve is

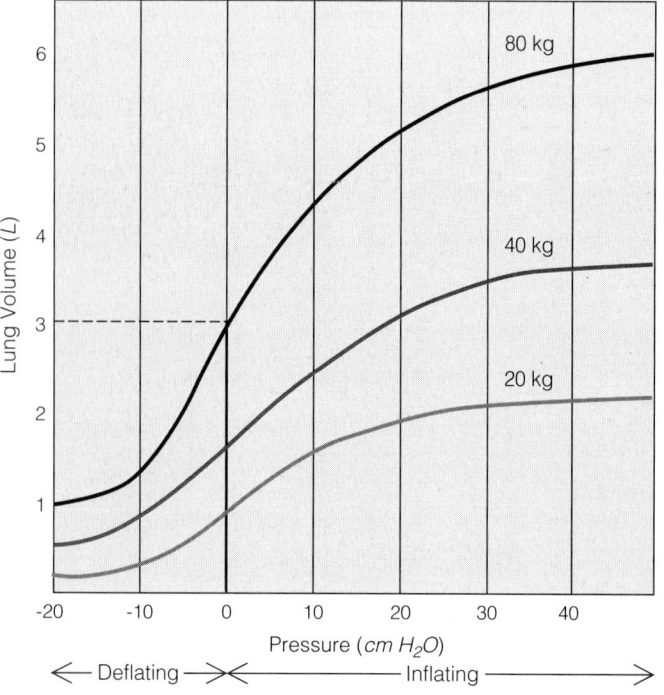

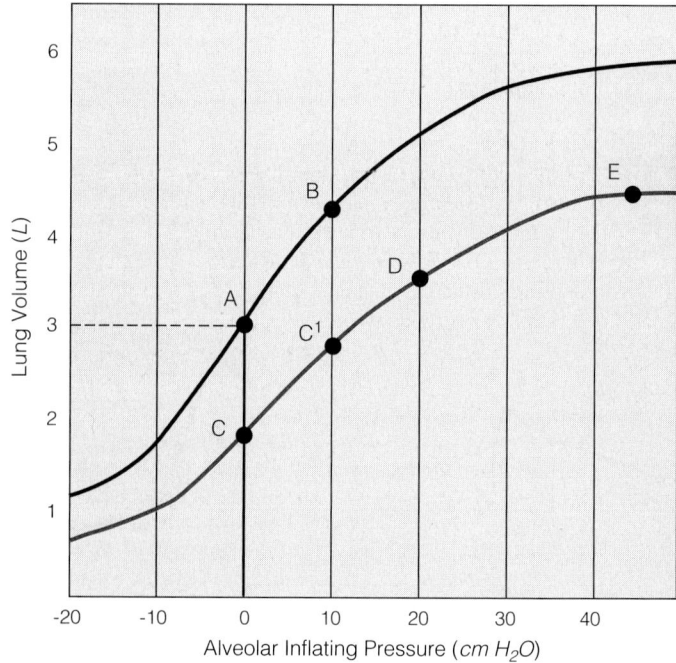

Figure 3 Depicted are pulmonary mechanics involved in mechanical ventilation. At left are compliance curves for a child weighing 20 kg, an adult weighing 40 kg, and an adult weighing 80 kg, all with normal lungs. The dotted line identifies FRC for the person weighing 80 kg. Functional residual capacity (FRC), total lung capacity, and compliance, which are proportional to patient size, must be normalized to patient weight to permit comparisons with other normal persons and between patients. At right are compliance curves for a patient weighing 80 kg who has normal lungs (upper curve) (compliance, 1 ml/cm H₂O/kg) and the same patient with major atelectasis (lower curve). The mechanics are altered in atelectasis because a smaller lung volume is available for inflation.

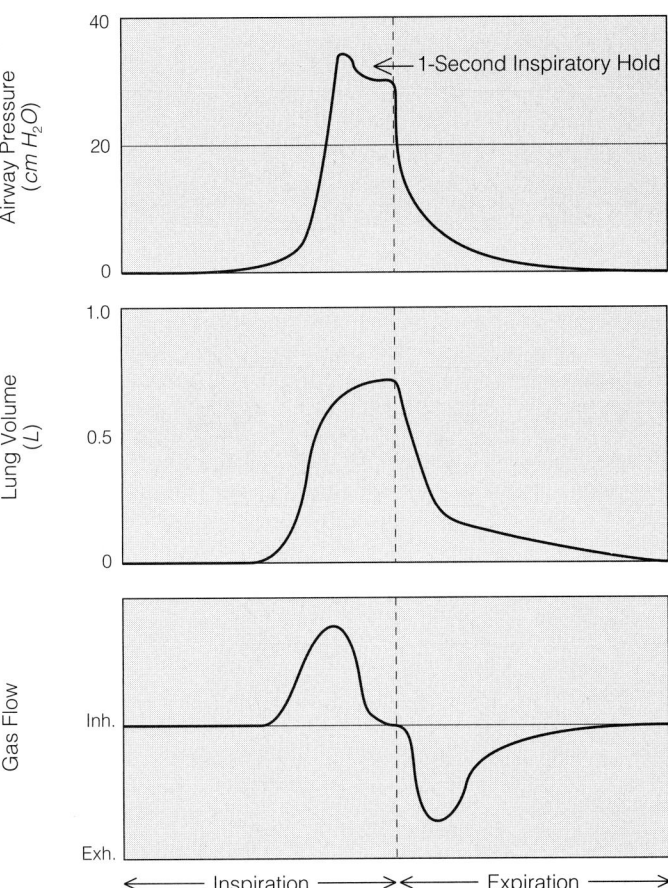

Figure 4 Shown are airway pressure, lung volume, and gas flow during a normal volume-controlled mechanical breath. The ventilator generates gas flow until the desired lung volume is reached, and the airway pressure is simply measured. A 1-second inspiratory hold shows the difference between peak inspiratory and plateau pressures. Dotted line separates inspiration from expiration.

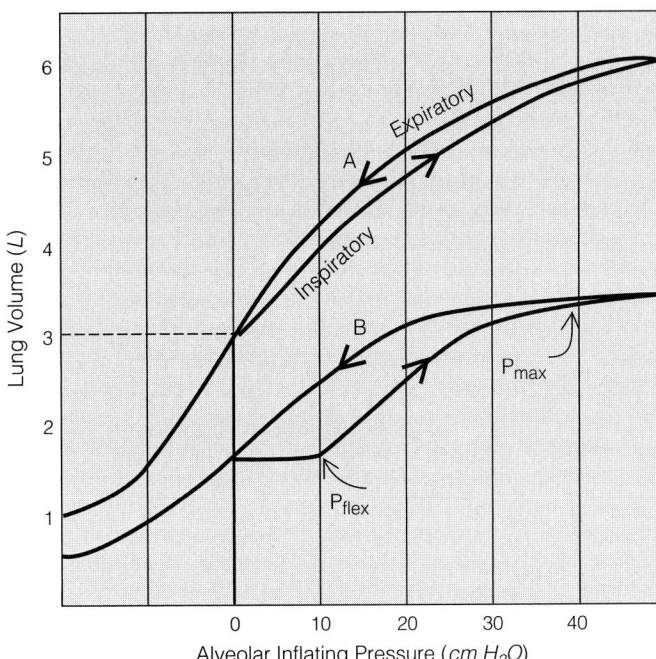

Figure 5 In a patient with normal lungs (black line), the inspiratory volume/pressure curve is very close to the expiratory curve. In a patient with severe parenchymal disease (red line), the inspiratory volume/pressure curve may be nearly flat until enough pressure is exerted to open edematous and collapsed airways and alveoli. As illustrated here, this event (identified as P_{flex}) occurs at 10 cm H_2O. The functional lung is fully inflated at 40 cm H_2O (the curve becomes flat at P_{max}). There is a substantial gap between the deflation curve and the inflation curve.

shifted to the right, much higher pressures are required to achieve the same level of inflation. To inflate the lung to point E, for example, a pressure of 40 cm H_2O would be necessary.

The best way of managing ventilation in these circumstances is to maintain positive end-expiratory pressure at 10 cm H_2O (point C^1 in Figure 3, right) and ventilate to point D with tidal breathing. The PEEP is set at this level to maintain the inflation of alveoli that might close at lower end-expiratory pressures; the volume of pressure used for tidal ventilation is safe and adequate for normal gas exchange.

In normal lungs, the inspiratory limb of the volume/pressure curve is almost the same as the expiratory limb. In severe respiratory failure, variable inspiratory inflation of the lung results in a significant difference between the inflation and deflation limbs, which can be useful in ventilation management [*see Figure 5*]. Collapsed small airways "pop" open at a critical inflating pressure, resulting in an inflation point early in inhalation (P_{flex}). The volume plateaus when all available alveoli are inflated (P_{max}). The P_{flex} and P_{max} are not always well defined, but when they are, it is reasonable to set PEEP above P_{flex} and to set P_{plat} at P_{max}.

Several measurements must be taken to determine whether positive airway pressure is recruiting collapsed alveoli or simply distending normal alveoli [*see Figure 6*]. The signs that collapsed alveoli are being reinflated are (1) improved normalized compliance, (2) decreased dead space ventilation, (3) unaffected cardiac output, and (4) improved oxygenation and decreased shunt at the same ventila-

tor settings. These signs must be kept in mind during management of a patient on a mechanical ventilator.

The effect of the abdominal viscera on pulmonary mechanics is significant. Most data on patients and normal subjects were obtained from individuals in the sitting position, yet most patients on mechanical ventilation are in the supine position. Even in normal subjects, the functional residual capacity is decreased by 25% when measured with the subjects in the supine position. This effect is exaggerated in

Distention	Positive Airway Pressure	Recruitment
↓ Compliance		↑ Compliance
↑ V_D/V_T		↓ V_D/V_T
↓ Cardiac Output		→ Cardiac Output
→ Shunt		↓↓ Shunt
↑ Air Leak		→ Air Leak

Figure 6 The results of serial measurements of compliance, dead space ventilation, cardiac output, oxygenation, shunting, and air-leak risks indicate whether positive airway pressure is recruiting collapsed alveoli or simply distending normal alveoli.

patients with ascites or abdominal distention and is exacerbated by a weak inspiratory effort. The reason is that the weight of the viscera literally pulls down on the diaphragm when patients are in the upright position, creates slight negative (inflating) pressure in the pleural space, and facilitates inspiration. These beneficial effects on lung inflation are even greater in the prone position, if the abdomen is free to expand. When patients are in the supine position, the weight of the viscera pushes against the diaphragm, which decreases alveolar volume and makes inspiration more difficult.[1]

These principles apply to mechanical ventilation as well as spontaneous breathing. Unless unstable hemodynamics make the supine position necessary, patients who are on ventilators (or are being weaned from ventilators) should be placed in a sitting position most of the time. This positioning is particularly important during spontaneous-breathing trials.

Because high airway pressure can cause lung damage, overdistention [see Figure 6] is not merely inefficient but actually detrimental.[2-4] Even in diffuse pulmonary disease, some areas of lung are not inflated and some are nearly normal.[5] The most normal areas of lung have the best compliance and therefore are the areas most vulnerable to overdistention, which may contribute to the steady progression of lung dysfunction in ventilated patients.[6]

The deleterious effects of alveolar overdistention on the lung itself have been demonstrated in many laboratory studies.[2,4] It has been suggested that the resulting lung injury can trigger the multiple organ dysfunction syndrome. Recent prospective randomized clinical studies by Amato and associates[7] and the Acute Respiratory Distress Syndrome Network of the National Institutes of Health[8] confirm the risks of overdistention injury; moreover, these studies report improved survival and decreased organ failure when overdistention is avoided during either pressure-limited[7] or volume-limited[8] modes of mechanical ventilation. The point at which inflation becomes overdistention has not been precisely determined; however, using end-inspiratory P_{plat} as an indicator of alveolar distention, one would be wise to keep P_{plat} below 40 cm H_2O (some would say 30 cm H_2O) during any mode of mechanical ventilation.[9] In patients with decreased FRC and diminished compliance, limiting P_{plat} in this fashion will result in hypoventilation, which in turn will result in hypercapnia. The physiologic risks of respiratory acidosis are minimal in comparison with the risks of alveolar overdistention. Therefore, it is safer to avoid overdistention injury and tolerate respiratory acidosis (so-called permissive hypercapnia[10]).

OXYGEN KINETICS

Oxygen consumption ($\dot{V}O_2$) is normally 3 ml/kg/min (120 ml/m²/min) at rest and is moderately elevated (as high as 6 ml/kg/min) by catecholamines or sepsis. $\dot{V}O_2$, the measure of metabolic rate, is converted to resting energy expenditure expressed in calories through the arithmetic of indirect calorimetry (5 cal for each liter of $\dot{V}O_2$). $\dot{V}O_2$ at rest stays constant from hour to hour, even in critically ill patients. Oxygen delivery ($\dot{D}O_2$) is normally 12 to 15 ml/kg/min (480 to 600 ml/m²/min) at rest. $\dot{D}O_2$ is measured as cardiac output in deciliters per minute times oxygen content (milliliters of oxygen per deciliter). Oxygen content is a function of the saturation and amount of hemoglobin; each gram of fully saturated hemoglobin carries 1.36 ml of oxygen. A very small amount of oxygen is dissolved in plasma, which is measured as P_aO_2.

In patients on a mechanical ventilator, F_IO_2 and pressure are manipulated to optimize oxygen content and delivery without causing injury to the lung. When $\dot{V}O_2$ is increased, as in sepsis or hypermetabolism, $\dot{D}O_2$ increases through an automatic increase in cardiac output until the ratio between $\dot{D}O_2$ and $\dot{V}O_2$ ($\dot{D}O_2/\dot{V}O_2$) is reestablished at 5:1 [see Figure 7]. A compensatory increase in cardiac out-

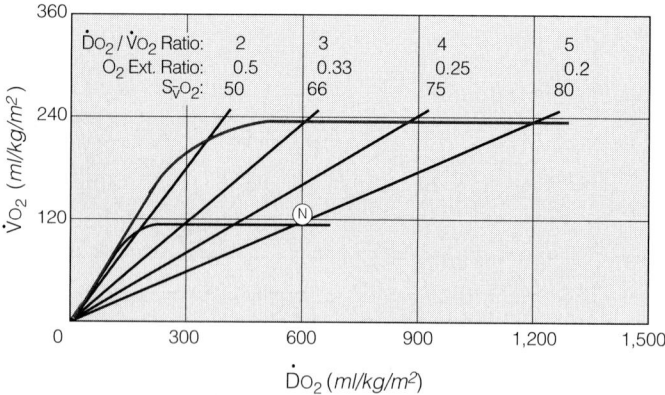

Figure 7 **In mechanical ventilation, F_IO_2 and airway pressure are manipulated to optimize oxygen content and $\dot{D}O_2$ so that the lung is not injured. $\dot{D}O_2$ is normally five times greater than $\dot{V}O_2$. Shown are the relationships between the $\dot{D}O_2/\dot{V}O_2$ ratio, the O_2 extraction (Ext.) ratio, and the $S_{\bar{v}}O_2$ when arterial blood is 100% saturated. Gas volumes are standard temperature (O° C) and pressure (760 mm Hg), dry. N indicates values in a normal person at rest; the red line represents hypermetabolism.**

put also occurs during anemia or hypoxia to maintain a normal $\dot{D}O_2/\dot{V}O_2$. When $\dot{D}O_2$ changes, no corresponding change in $\dot{V}O_2$ occurs unless $\dot{D}O_2/\dot{V}O_2$ is severely decreased to less than 2:1. When $\dot{D}O_2$ is less than twice $\dot{V}O_2$, anaerobic metabolism occurs, $\dot{V}O_2$ falls, and hemodynamic instability results. These changes occur at both normal and elevated metabolic rates [see Figure 7].[11,12] Although it has been reported that pathologic supply dependency occurs in patients with the acute respiratory distress syndrome,[13,14] this is an artifact,[15] and normal oxygen kinetics exist, even in hypermetabolic conditions.[16] $\dot{D}O_2$ is optimal when it is four to five times greater than $\dot{V}O_2$. Although this point could be determined by repeated measurements of $\dot{V}O_2$, oxygen content, and cardiac output, a simpler way exists.

When arterial blood is nearly 100% saturated, the mixed venous oxygen saturation ($S_{\bar{v}}O_2$) directly reflects $\dot{D}O_2/\dot{V}O_2$, regardless of the metabolic rate. For example, if $\dot{D}O_2$ is three times $\dot{V}O_2$, the $S_{\bar{v}}O_2$ will be 66% [see Figure 7]. This variable can be measured in samples of pulmonary arterial blood or by continuous use of a fiberoptic catheter.[17,18] When $\dot{D}O_2$ is adequate, $\dot{V}O_2$ at rest stays constant. Thus, any change in $S_{\bar{v}}O_2$ over minutes or hours directly reflects changes in $\dot{D}O_2$. This phenomenon is used to adjust F_IO_2, PEEP, I/E, and mean airway pressure, in addition to inotropic drug dosages, blood volume, and blood transfusion. The ventilator should be set at the lowest settings that maintain $S_{\bar{v}}O_2$ above 70%.

$S_{\bar{v}}O_2$ does not show the cause of a problem, only whether $\dot{D}O_2/\dot{V}O_2$ is abnormal. If $S_{\bar{v}}O_2$ is abnormally high, the delivery may be higher than necessary (e.g., as in the case of arteriovenous shunt), or the $\dot{V}O_2$ may be decreased at the cellular level (e.g., as in the case of endotoxin affecting cellular enzymes). If $S_{\bar{v}}O_2$ is abnormally low, the delivery might be lower than necessary (e.g., low cardiac output), or the $\dot{V}O_2$ might be elevated above the level at which delivery can compensate (e.g., exercise in a patient with a fixed-rate pacemaker). All of these factors must be taken into account when using $S_{\bar{v}}O_2$ to regulate the mechanical ventilator. The principles of the physiology of oxygen kinetics become particularly important in patients with severe respiratory failure when their pressure and F_IO_2 requirements approach the limits of safety. When $\dot{D}O_2/\dot{V}O_2$ is low, it is better to raise oxygen content by transfusion or decrease $\dot{V}O_2$ by sedation than to use 100% oxygen or very high pressure [see Table 1].

VENTILATION-PERFUSION MATCHING

In surgical patients with pulmonary failure, the lung is usually characterized by areas of congestion and atelectasis (low ventilation-perfusion matching [$\dot{V}/\dot{Q}$], or a shuntlike effect) and areas of normal inflation (high $\dot{V}/\dot{Q}$). When blood shunts through lung areas with low $\dot{V}/\dot{Q}$, arterial hypoxemia and hypercapnia result. Hyperventilation of lung areas with high $\dot{V}/\dot{Q}$ will normalize P_aCO_2 but will not improve oxygenation. Improving oxygenation depends on matching blood flow to inflated ventilated alveoli. This matching can be done in three ways: (1) reinflating alveoli by positive airway pressure, (2) reinflating alveoli by decreasing pulmonary interstitial edema, or (3) diverting blood flow to lung areas with high $\dot{V}/\dot{Q}$. The role of peak inspiratory pressure in opening alveoli and of PEEP in holding alveoli open has been discussed [see Pulmonary Mechanics, above]. Decreasing lung extravascular water is accomplished by diuresis, reduction of left atrial pressure, and postural drainage. The edematous lung is heavy, and dependent alveoli are compressed by the weight of the lung, which is why consolidation occurs in dependent areas in acute respiratory distress syndrome.[19] Decreasing edema minimizes compression, which results in improved lung function[20] and improved survival in patients with the acute respiratory distress syndrome.[21]

Turning the patient so that lung areas with high $\dot{V}/\dot{Q}$ are dependent (usually the prone position) usually improves oxygenation immediately by diverting blood flow to the inflated lung areas and decreasing the blood flow in the consolidated lung areas.[22] When patients are in the prone position for several hours, the effects of lung weight are reversed, so that consolidated areas of the lung may become reinflated, resulting in improved oxygenation even when the patient is returned to the supine position.[23] Of these three maneuvers, diuresis and positioning are usually safer and more effective than airway pressure manipulation.

Types and Features of Mechanical Ventilators

At least 20 makes and models of mechanical ventilators are used in North America today. Almost all the ventilators used in operating rooms, recovery rooms, and intensive care units are volume-controlled ventilators. With a device of this type, the operator sets the tidal volume, the respiratory rate, and the inspiratory gas flow, and the ventilator will keep delivering the set volume of gas regardless of the airway pressure (unless a pressure cutoff is set). In a pressure-controlled ventilator, however, the operator selects the respiratory rate, the inspiratory gas flow, and the peak airway pressure, and the ventilator delivers inspired gas until the desired pressure is reached. The tidal volume is measured. Most ICU ventilators can be used in the volume- or pressure-controlled mode or in combinations of the two.

Ventilators come with an extensive array of knobs, gauges, controls, electronic microprocessors, digital displays, and instruction books. Although the features and accoutrements of mechanical ventilators can be intimidating, the functions and controls are actually quite simple. All ventilators have certain basic controls and monitors [see Table 3]. They all are capable of delivering gas of known composition and volume at a given flow rate and of measuring and controlling the pressure at various phases of the respiratory cycle.

Different ventilators accomplish gas delivery in different ways, such as by employing a motor-driven piston, by metering in a quantity of gas supplied to the ventilator under very high pressure, or by keeping a constant reservoir of gas under moderate pressure. Measurement of airway pressure, gas volume, inspiratory effort, F_IO_2, and other parameters is also accomplished in a variety of different ways. A surgeon caring for ventilator patients should know what ventilator is used in his or her hospital and how these variables are controlled in that specific ventilator. Circuit diagrams and descriptions of how

each make and model of ventilator functions are available from the hospital respiratory therapy department, from the manufacturer, and in the literature. Extensive and excellent descriptions of specific mechanical ventilators have been published by Mushin and Rendell-Baker,[24] Kirby and colleagues,[25] and Burton and associates.[26] Surgeons should familiarize themselves with the available documentation and descriptions so that they can better understand the limitations of the equipment they use as well as alert themselves and others to possible malfunctions.

The primary controls for tidal volume, rate, and F_IO_2 are straightforward. The end-expiratory airway pressure control, or PEEP control, provides graduated occlusion of the expiratory system, thereby regulating positive end-expiratory pressure. There is also a primary control for maximum inspiratory pressure, which is set by the operator. If this pressure is reached, an alarm sounds and inflation stops, so that the preset volume is not reached. These simple primary controls allow regulation of all the components of routine mechanical ventilation.

There is also a set of secondary controls for fine-tuning the mechanical ventilator. These controls vary the flow (and therefore the pressure) during the inflation phase of the ventilator. The most important of them is the inspiratory flow rate control. If the tidal volume is delivered at a low flow rate, the time of inspiration will be long, the pressure accumulation will be gradual and minimal, and ventilation will be smoother, but the patient may feel dyspneic. If the flow rate of gas is high, however, the inspiratory time will be short, the peak inspiratory pressure will be reached abruptly, the mean airway pressure will be increased, the high-pressure cutoff will be reached more often, and the blast of ventilating gas may stimulate coughing. Because the respiratory rate is set per minute, a higher inspiratory flow rate will shorten inspiration and result in a lower I/E. A short inspiratory phase with a low I/E favors expiration and CO_2

Table 3 Controls and Monitors
on a Volume-Controlled Ventilator

Controls	Monitors and Alarms
Primary controls	
F_IO_2	
Tidal volume (minute volume)	Tidal volume
Respiratory rate	Respiratory rate
Positive end-expiratory pressure (PEEP)	PEEP
Maximum inspiratory pressure	PIP
	Mean airway pressure
	Apnea or disconnect
Secondary controls	
Inspiratory flow rate	Inspiratory time, I/E
Inspiratory flow wave pattern	
Inspiratory hold	
Sigh rate, volume, and maximum pressure	Sigh PIP
Trigger sensitivity for assist and IMV models	

Modes of Ventilation
Controlled mechanical ventilation (CMV)
Assist control (AC)
Intermittent mandatory ventilation (IMV)
Synchronized IMV
Continuous positive airway pressure (CPAP)
Pressure-controlled ventilation (PCV)
Pressure-controlled inverse-ratio ventilation (PC-IRV)
Pressure support (PS)

excretion, whereas a long inspiration with a high I/E favors inflation and oxygenation. When a patient with normal lungs is undergoing mechanical ventilation, the inspiratory flow rate should be adjusted so that the patient is comfortable and I/E is close to normal (1:3). This is best done by examining the patient while adjusting the inspiratory flow rate. Often, high mean airway pressures can be decreased significantly simply by decreasing the inspiratory flow rate. When a patient with poor oxygenation is undergoing mechanical ventilation, the time spent during inflation should be increased. I/E can be increased until CO_2 excretion is inadequate. This unusual pattern of breathing is uncomfortable and often requires sedation.

Most ventilators provide an inspiratory flow wave pattern control, which varies the pattern of gas flow from sine wave to square wave to various combinations of waves. The normal inspiratory flow pattern is essentially a sine wave, which is usually the best pattern for mechanical ventilation. Most modern ventilators also provide a control for timed inspiratory hold, or plateau pressure. This setting occludes the expiratory circuit for 1 or 2 seconds. There are two reasons for using the inspiratory hold control: (1) to allow pressures throughout the system to equilibrate so that effective compliance (exhaled volume divided by plateau pressure as measured on the ventilator gauge) can be measured and (2) to simulate a forced sustained inspiration to reinflate collapsed alveoli (a procedure to be distinguished from an automatic sigh [see Modes of Ventilation, below]). As a rule, ventilators deliver gas only during the inflation phase of the respiratory cycle,

but some provide continuous gas flow, which is a significant advantage in the CPAP and IMV modes of ventilation.

Humidification is an essential part of mechanical ventilation. The inspired gas is usually humidified by passing it over water warmed to 37° C. A chamber for nebulizing drugs may be included in the inspiratory circuit; it is powered by a gas line separate from the ventilator.

Modes of Ventilation

Ventilators always have at least two and sometimes as many as six modes of ventilation. Each mode of ventilation is characterized by what starts the gas flow (time- or effort-triggered) and what stops the gas flow (volume-controlled, pressure-time–controlled, or flow-controlled; or volume-limited, pressure-time–limited, or flow-limited) [see Figure 8]. In the controlled mechanical ventilation mode, the ventilator is time-triggered and either volume-limited or pressure-limited, and it functions exactly as determined by the primary controls, regardless of what the patient does. This mode is appropriate for a patient who is under anesthesia, paralyzed, heavily sedated, or suffering from brain stem injury.

In the assist-control mode, the ventilator is effort-triggered and either volume-controlled or pressure-controlled and delivers the V_T and F_IO_2 determined by the primary controls whenever the patient initiates a spontaneous breath. A control or backup rate is specified so that the ventilator will automatically deliver the tidal volume if the pa-

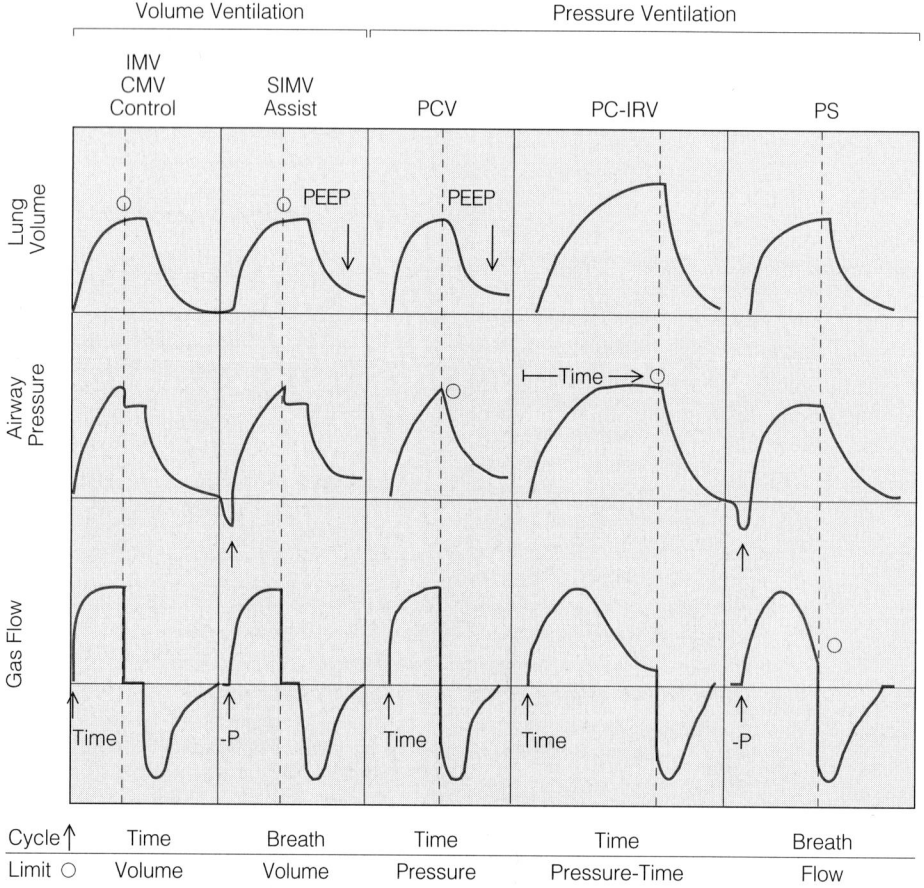

Figure 8 Shown are lung volume, airway pressure, gas flow, and the inspiration-expiration ratio (I/E) during commonly used modes of mechanical ventilation. The event that starts the gas flow is the cycle (↑), and the event that stops the gas flow is the limiting factor (○). The cessation of gas flow is shown by the dotted lines. Time and negative pressure (-P) may be responsible for cycling or limiting gas flow, as indicated. PEEP is shown in two modes of ventilation as examples of the effect of that maneuver.

tient does not initiate a spontaneous breath within an appropriate period. The control rate is usually set at approximately half the spontaneous rate. The ventilator is triggered to deliver an assisted breath when the pressure in the airway is decreased by the pa ent's inspiratory effort. When the assist-control mode is used, the sensitivity of this trigger mechanism should be adjusted. If the setting is too sensitive, a ventilator inflation may be triggered simply by the pressure drop during expiration. If the adjustment is not sensitive enough, the patient may be unable to generate enough pressure to trigger the ventilator.

Because of the relatively poor pressure transmission through the gas in the system, the negative deflection on the ventilator pressure gauge is not nearly as great as the negative pressure actually generated in the pleural space by inspiratory effort. Whenever possible, therefore, the patient's inspiratory pressure should be measured at the airway. The sensitivity control should be adjusted so that the mechanical breath is delivered with the minimum of effort by the patient. It must be readjusted whenever the PEEP level is changed. The assist mode greatly simplifies the monitoring and management of mechanical ventilation. It is the preferred mode in any patient with a normally functioning brain stem and respiratory center.

In the intermittent mandatory ventilation mode, time-triggered controlled mechanical ventilation occurs at the rate and volume determined by the primary controls (time-triggered and either volume-limited or pressure-limited), and additional inspired gas is made available if the patient generates a spontaneous inspiration. (The latter feature distinguishes IMV from CMV, in which no gas flows if the patient makes an inspiratory effort.) The volume of gas provided during the spontaneous effort is proportional to the patient's effort and is usually small. IMV was originally designed to be used with a continuous high-volume gas flow and PEEP (requiring minimal effort by the patient for spontaneous breaths) supplemented by intermittent mechanical breaths at a rate and volume sufficient to maintain CO_2 clearance.[27] The Emerson ventilator functions in this fashion, but most other mechanical ventilators have a type of pseudo-IMV, in which gas is delivered only when a demand valve is activated by the inspiratory effort. This method requires considerable work by the patient[28] and can lead to progressive exhaustion of respiratory muscles rather than the mild exercise desired. Synchronized IMV (SIMV) is simply a modification of IMV in which the controlled ventilation V_T is delivered at the time of spontaneous inspiratory effort (i.e., effort-triggered).

In the continuous positive airway pressure mode, breathing is entirely spontaneous, with expiratory pressure controlled by the PEEP control [see Figure 9]. This mode corresponds to the period of spontaneous breathing with IMV as described earlier and is subject to the same variables and criticisms. The CPAP mode should be used in conjunction with a continuous-flow and reservoir system. Because in most ventilators the CPAP mode requires the patient to trigger a demand valve during inspiration rather than supplying continuous flow of gas, this mode may at times be more exhausting than helpful. A variation of CPAP is so-called pressure-release ventilation, in which CPAP is applied and then released to a controlled PEEP level at intervals.

Pressure support is a time- or effort-triggered, flow-limited mode of ventilation.[29] Rapid gas flow is initiated by effort or a timer and continues until a preset pressure is reached. Gas flow continues at a slower rate, and pressure is maintained until the flow rate is only a fraction of the initial flow rate (typically 25%). This has the effect of an inspiratory hold but continues to supply gas during the inspiratory hold, which results in a relatively large tidal volume at moderate pressure. If the patient generates inspiratory effort during the pressure-support breath, an even higher tidal volume will result, making pressure support a valuable method of weaning. The same principle applies to the pressure-limited mode, without the inspiratory hold.

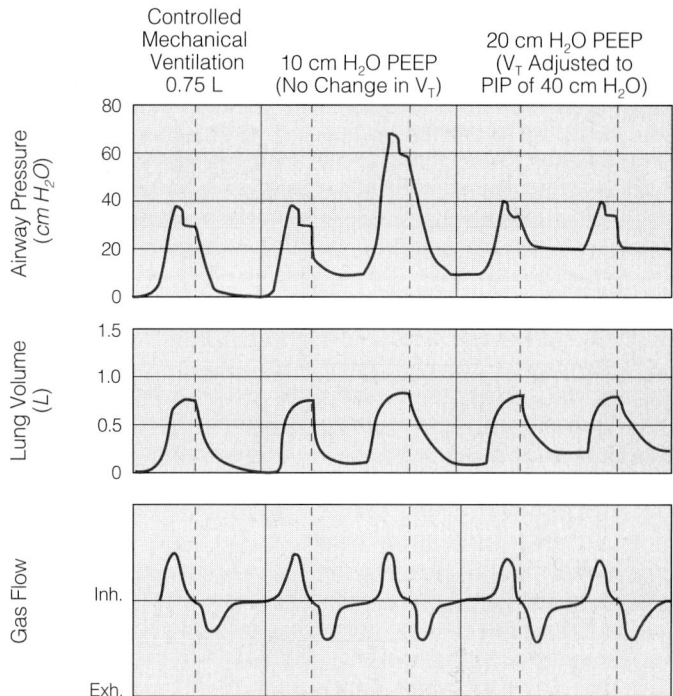

Figure 9   Shown is the effect of positive end-expiratory pressure (PEEP) during five breaths. PEEP is added after the second breath, so the third breath, with the same lung volume, results in unacceptably high peak inspiratory pressure (PIP). The lung volume is decreased until PIP is 40 cm H_2O, as shown in breaths four and five. The dotted vertical line separates inspiration from expiration.

Most ventilators have a control for automatic sighs. (It would be more accurate to call these automatic yawns because sighs are expiratory maneuvers.) In the sigh mode, the ventilator delivers a large V_T (typically 15 to 25 ml/kg) at regular intervals (usually several times each hour). This setting ensures regular maximal inflation, thereby simulating the normal physiologic pattern of breathing, in which total lung capacity is reached six times each hour. A separate high-pressure limit and alarm is provided for the sighs. Although the amount of gas contained in a sigh is considerably larger than the normal V_T, it is delivered at the same inspiratory flow rate; consequently, the inspiratory time will be two or three times longer than normal. This system is a more effective means of achieving maximal alveolar inflation than the inspiratory hold described earlier [see Types and Features of Mechanical Ventilators, *above*], in which a normal-sized tidal volume is simply held at pressure for a second or two. When PEEP is maintained above 5 cm H_2O and P_{plat} is close to 30 cm H_2O, the sigh mechanism is not necessary and may even lead to dangerously high airway pressures; however, when PEEP is 5 cm H_2O or lower and the tidal volume is controlled in the normal range, periodic sighs should be used to maintain alveolar inflation. Overdistention may be avoided by limiting P_{plat} to 40 cm H_2O or lower.

Monitors and Alarms

Most ventilators are equipped with a device to measure exhaled volume, usually by integrating a measurement of flow with time. The exhaled volume can be displayed either breath by breath or as minute ventilation. It should correspond to the preset inspired volume; if it does not, an air leak exists, and the volume of the leak can be calculated by simple subtraction. It should be remembered that a considerable part of the exhaled volume is gas that was compressed in the tubing and in the patient's lungs and that therefore did not enter into the alveolar ventilation. This compression volume in the ventilator and tubing can be measured by capping the airway and measuring the volume exhaled over a range of pressures. In some ventilators, the tubing compression volume is automatically subtracted in the final volume display. This compressed gas will appear as V_D when V_D/V_T is calculated from arterial and mixed expired CO_2. The appearance of compression volume as $\dot{V}_D$ makes it seem as if a patient with poor compliance has a large anatomic or physiologic dead space, but it is nothing more than a measurement artifact.

The apnea or disconnect alarm on most ventilators is triggered by an abnormally low expired volume measurement. Pressure limits and alarms can be set for PIP in all ventilators, PEEP in some, and mean airway pressure in others. The PIP and the PEEP can be displayed either on a gauge or on a digital readout in all ventilators. Some ventilators can display the mean airway pressure as well—a desirable feature because the mean airway pressure affects venous return. The F_IO_2 is displayed on most ventilators, but this display usually reflects the setting made by the operator rather than the actual F_IO_2 value. There can be considerable variation between the desired and the actual F_IO_2, so some device must be used to measure F_IO_2 if the ventilator cannot measure it.

In the process of adjusting the respiratory rate, tidal volume, and inspiratory flow rate, it is possible to arrive at unreasonable settings. Most ventilators have an alarm system to notify the operator. Usually, this alarm system will be triggered if I/E exceeds 2:1.

Some of the newer ventilators can calculate and display effective compliance, flow-volume loops, or volume-pressure curves. In the near future, mechanical ventilators will include apparatus to measure oxygen consumption, CO_2 production, respiratory quotient, and work of breathing. These measurements, combined with measurements of arterial and venous oxyhemoglobin saturation, will allow ventilators to display oxygen delivery-consumption ratios, cardiac output, and other hemodynamic variables, as well as energy expenditure expressed in calories. The same generation of ventilators will be able to regulate minute ventilation on the basis of CO_2 load and to regulate airway pressure and F_IO_2 on the basis of oxygenation. These devices will appear to be even more complex than today's ventilators, but they will have the same basic functions and features.

In addition to monitors built into the ventilator, some other patient monitors are used to manage mechanical ventilation. The use of the pulmonary arterial catheter and mixed venous oximetry has already been discussed [see Worsening Respiratory Status, Oxygenation, above]. An arterial catheter is helpful because of the frequency of arterial blood gas measurement. Pulse oximeters measure arterial saturation in capillary blood by ignoring the nonpulsatile venous phase. These instruments have become invaluable for both safety and management monitoring. Transcutaneous, corneal, and tissue gas sensors have not gained general acceptance, because they drift and require frequent recalibration. End-tidal CO_2 monitoring at the airway generally corresponds to P_aCO_2. End-tidal CO_2 is the same as P_aCO_2 when lung function is normal, and it is less than P_aCO_2 when real or apparent dead space (compression volume) is elevated. End-tidal CO_2 is particularly helpful during weaning.

Learning to Use a Mechanical Ventilator

Every surgeon who is responsible for ventilator patients should understand the mechanical ventilators at his or her hospital and should be able to set all the controls and make any necessary adjustments, even if such tasks are traditionally done by nurses or respiratory therapists. The best way for a surgeon to learn to use a mechan-

ical ventilator is first to regulate the primary control settings by using a rubber-bag test lung, then to regulate the secondary controls and select the modes of ventilation while acting as the patient (easily accomplished by attaching a mouthpiece to the ventilator tubing and applying a noseclip). Whenever a new ventilator is introduced into the ICU, each surgeon who will use the ventilator should go through a detailed self-instruction routine [see Table 4]. It is well worth the cost of an extra set of sterile ventilator tubing.

Writing Ventilator Orders

Mechanical ventilators are generally operated by nurses and respiratory therapists under a set of orders from the responsible physician [see Table 5]. These orders may range from very specific directions to broad guidelines, depending on the experience and ability of the ICU personnel; however, the orders should always include a statement of the goals of mechanical ventilation and specify the system to be used to determine how well those goals have been achieved. For example, in an ICU in which ventilators are routinely used, it may be sufficient merely to say: "Measure arterial saturation and P_aCO_2 every 4 hours. Maintain P_aCO_2 between 35 and 45 mm Hg with rate and tidal volume, and maintain arterial saturation of more than 95% by using F_IO_2 less than 0.6 and PEEP less than 6." Conversely, if mechanical ventilators are not used routinely, or if a nurse or respiratory therapist on a given shift is not comfortable with such responsibility, it is advisable to specify the exact mode, the primary control and secondary control settings, and the monitoring alarm systems that are to be used.

Related Topics

FIGHTING THE VENTILATOR

Fighting the ventilator means that the patient is dyspneic and trying to breathe out while the ventilator is inflating. Usually, this situation can be handled by placing the ventilator in the assist mode

---

Table 4   Self-Instruction Routine for Ventilator Training

1. Set: F_IO_2, V_T, rate, PEEP, PIP.
2. Set mode: CMV.
3. Set ranges for alarms: V_T, rate, PIP, PEEP.
4. Attach test lung (rubber bag), and ventilate.
5. Measure: V_T, rate, minute volume, PIP, PEEP, effective compliance.
6. Limit the bag to simulate poor compliance. Readjust ventilator, and repeat measurements.
7. Set primary controls to ventilate yourself. Rate = 16/min.
8. With a mouthpiece and a noseclip, ventilate yourself. Relax until you are on controlled ventilation. Then, adjust V_T (5–20 ml/kg) and PEEP (0–10 cm H_2O) to get the feel, and observe the measurements. Try the sigh mode.
9. At baseline settings, resist inspiration, cough, and try to hyperventilate. How does it feel? Do the monitors and alarms work?
10. At baseline settings, turn to the AC mode. Rate = 0/min. Adjust the sensitivity from low to high.
11. In the AC mode, adjust the inspiratory flow rate and pattern. Which I/E feels comfortable?
12. Reset mode to IMV, then CPAP. How much work does it take to initiate a breath?
13. Repeat steps 10–12, but using an endotracheal tube instead of a mouthpiece in your mouth. What are the effects of the added resistance?

Table 5 Sample Orders for Ventilator Patients

1. Objectives (range of acceptable values)
   A. Arterial blood oxygenation
      Hemoglobin saturation _____ to _____
      or
      P_aO_2 _____ to _____
   B. Arterial carbon dioxide (P_aCO_2) _____ to _____
2. Standard respiratory care for all ventilator patients
   A. Alternating lateral and sitting positions, never supine.
   B. 100% airway humidity at 35°–37° C.
   C. Airway irrigation and suctioning every 8 hours, more frequently as required.
   D. Percussion and chest physical therapy every 8 hours, more frequently as required.
   E. Deflation of cuffed tubes every 8 hours (before suctioning) and reinflation with the minimum volume necessary to achieve the required peak inspiratory pressure.
   F. Continuous monitoring of V_T and airway pressure.
   G. Mouth care every other hour (for patients with endotracheal tubes).
   H. Tracheal stoma care every other hour for patients with tracheostomy tubes.
3. Ventilator settings: Mode _____
   F_IO_2 _____
   V_T or PIP _____ Rate _____ PEEP _____
   Alarm limits: V_T _____ Rate _____ P_{plat} _____
   Other: _____
4. Monitoring frequency
   Arterial blood gases _____
   Venous blood gases _____
   Compliance _____
   Weaning parameters _____
   Chest x-ray _____

---

and increasing the inspiratory flow and tidal volume until respiratory alkalosis occurs and breathing slows, and then backing off to more comfortable settings. Mild sedation of the patient may be necessary, particularly if he or she is disoriented or extremely anxious. Almost never is it necessary or indicated to paralyze a patient to achieve mechanical ventilation. (There are, however, some specific indications for paralysis, such as tetanus, seizures, delirium tremens, and major ventilatory failure [see Worsening Respiratory Status, above].)

VENTILATION OF INFANTS AND CHILDREN

Although this discussion has been concerned solely with mechanical ventilation for adults, the principles underlying pulmonary mechanics, gas exchange, monitoring and alarms, and modes of ventilation all apply to pediatric patients as well. In children older than 2 years, volume-controlled ventilators can be used according to the guidelines given here for adults. Pressure-limited continuous-flow ventilators are generally preferred in infants. Techniques for neonatal ventilation are well described in standard texts.[30,31]

INTERMITTENT POSITIVE PRESSURE BREATHING

Intermittent positive pressure breathing is nothing more than mechanical ventilation through a mouthpiece rather than through direct tracheal access. All of the relevant variables can be monitored and controlled when a mouthpiece rather than an endotracheal tube is used, and any of the modes can be selected. Intermittent positive pressure breathing is a useful technique in patients who have borderline pulmonary function or minimal reserve.[32] When it is employed,

the ventilator is placed at the bedside and set in the assist mode with a backup rate of zero, and all the primary and secondary controls are adjusted to the appropriate settings. The patient is taught to use the ventilator and is allowed to pick up the mouthpiece for mechanical assistance at will. He or she is encouraged to use the ventilator at least every hour while awake, to prevent or treat atelectasis.[33] This variety of mechanical ventilation differs considerably from intermittent positive pressure breathing provided by a nurse or respiratory therapist every 6 or 8 hours, which is useful for delivering nebulized drugs and for encouraging the patient to think about deep breathing but is usually ineffective unless the mechanical support is provided more frequently.

BRONCHOSCOPY

Bronchoscopy with flexible fiberoptic instruments is an essential adjunct to the management of mechanical ventilation. Introducing the instrument through a sphincter adapter allows bronchoscopy to be performed during ventilation but increases the resistance to gas flow through the airway. Therefore, ventilator adjustments are necessary to maintain adequate gas exchange. The inspiratory flow rate and peak inspiratory pressure must be increased significantly to maintain inspired tidal volume. This clinical setting is the one exception to the PIP limit of 40 cm H_2O; an inspiratory pressure of 50 to 80 cm H_2O may be required. This pressure level, required to overcome airway resistance, is not injurious to the lung. Distal pressure is low, and overdistention will not occur. Expiration is also limited by the increased resistance. More time will be required for exhalation, and PEEP should be decreased. Without these changes, exhalation of each breath will be incomplete, resulting in auto-PEEP [see Auto-PEEP, below] and CO_2 retention. Obviously, ventilator settings must be adjusted carefully to facilitate bronchoscopy.

Conversely, bronchoscopy is used to facilitate mechanical ventilation. Airway placement and positioning, evaluation of tracheal injury and bronchial patency, identification of sources of bleeding and mucus production, tissue level diagnoses, and selective lobar study and treatment all require bronchoscopy. A surgeon who is managing mechanical ventilation should be proficient in performing this procedure.[34]

AUTO-PEEP

When exhalation is incomplete, the functional residual capacity is increased, airway pressure increases, and alveoli are more inflated than they would be if exhalation continued to the point of equilibration with atmospheric pressure. This phenomenon can be exploited by using PEEP to limit exhalation and maintain alveolar inflation. If bronchial or prosthetic airway resistance is increased or if the time for exhalation is short, incomplete exhalation can occur regardless of externally regulated PEEP. If this process continues during many breaths, alveolar volume increases in association with increased alveolar pressure; this process has been referred to as auto-PEEP.[35] This phenomenon also occurs in asthma, with the same physiologic consequences of CO_2 retention and capillary obstruction. Auto-PEEP occurs during mechanical ventilation as a result of the ventilator settings, sometimes combined with bronchospasm. It can be measured by placement of a catheter-transducer system into the trachea or esophagus. Auto-PEEP should be suspected if CO_2 clearance is impaired and is paradoxically worsened by increasing respiratory rate (i.e., shortening exhalation time). If auto-PEEP is suspected, the respiratory rate or tidal volume, or both, should be decreased. If CO_2 clearance is enhanced by this maneuver, ventilator settings are readjusted to permit full exhalation or to control exhalation solely by the external PEEP valve.

Special Techniques for Patients with Severe Respiratory Failure

When the principles outlined above are used, most surgical patients can be managed without difficulty. However, a small percentage of patients with pneumonitis, aspiration, contusion, or the acute respiratory distress syndrome will develop such a large shunt, air leak, or alveolar damage that conventional mechanical ventilation is inadequate. The mortality associated with severe respiratory failure, defined as a shunt persistently over 30% despite and after all appropriate therapy, is 60% to 90%.[36-39] The following innovative approaches have been recommended for these patients.

NONVENTILATORY TREATMENT

Oxygenation can often be improved by placing the patient in the full lateral or prone position.[40] This positioning diverts blood flow to the anterior lung, which is usually the most inflated part of the lung, and promotes reinflation of the posterior lung. Oxygen delivery should be optimized by use of transfusion to achieve a normal hematocrit[41] and administration of inotropes (with the caveat that catecholamines increase $\dot{V}O_2$ and $\dot{V}CO_2$).[42] When the hematocrit and cardiac output are normal, an arterial saturation of 80% to 90% is well tolerated.

PERMISSIVE HYPERCAPNIA

Even in patients with severe lung disease, a normal P_aCO_2 can be maintained at 40 mm Hg by hyperventilation. Indeed, in patients with atelectasis and consolidation, a small portion of the lung is hyperventilated to maintain normocapnia while hypoxia is treated with attempted reinflation. However, because this intervention causes overdistention and induced tissue alkalosis in the most normal and compliant area of the lung, it can damage the lung in a very short time.[43] The risk of hypercapnia is minimal, particularly when it is compared with the risk of hyperventilation-induced lung damage. Therefore, ventilation should be limited to safe levels (plateau pressure below 40 cm) to avoid lung injury. This limitation may result in a P_aCO_2 as high as 80 mm Hg, but the resulting acidosis can be buffered with bicarbonate or TRIS buffer and no deleterious effects result. This approach has been used for many years in the management of asthma[44] and neonatal respiratory failure[45] but has rarely been used in acute adult respiratory failure. Recommendations to strictly limit peak airway pressure[46,47] were generally ignored in favor of normocapnia. In the early 1990s, this approach, named permissive hypercapnia, was advocated in patients with adult respiratory failure.[10] Critical care practitioners recognized the dangers of hyperventilation and began regulating mechanical ventilator peak pressure. Although transient hypercapnia may result, that is a small price to pay for ultimate lung recovery.

PRESSURE-LIMITATION (LOW-STRETCH) VENTILATION

The rationale for limiting overdistention (high pressure, high volume, or high stretch) was defined by Gattinoni and colleagues[5] and demonstrated by Hickling and coworkers.[6,10] Several recent prospective, randomized studies have shown a significant survival advantage to so-called low-stretch modes of ventilation.[7,8] Other studies have shown no advantage,[48] but the differences can be explained by the number of patients in the various treatment groups who were actually ventilated with damaging pressure. Ranieri and colleagues demonstrated that high-stretch ventilation was associated with increased plasma levels of inflammatory cytokines.[49] Amato and coworkers[7] advocate that the high-stretch limit be combined with PEEP adjustment based on P_{flex} (the so-called open-lung approach), a combination providing survival advantage.

HIGH-FREQUENCY OR OSCILLATION VENTILATION

High-frequency ventilation (HFV) is an intriguing technique in which oxygenation is achieved by continuous positive airway pressure with supplemental oxygen, and ventilation is achieved by shaking the airway—that is, by supplying a very small tidal volume (≤ 100 ml) at a very rapid rate (200 to 2,000/min) by means of a jet of gas, a piston, or a loudspeaker. This unusual airway pressure manipulation enhances CO_2 diffusion and induces excretion of a normal metabolic load of CO_2 without conventional tidal ventilation. Reports on HFV in adults indicate that the mean airway pressure is lower than with CMV and that barotrauma and air leaks are less frequent, but the duration of ventilation and the outcome in ventilated patients are about the same.[50,51] There are, however, anecdotal cases of spectacular recovery with HFV despite the apparent failure of conventional mechanical ventilation, suggesting that the development of this technique should be watched carefully.

PRESSURE-CONTROLLED INVERSE-RATIO VENTILATION

If one objective of mechanical ventilation is to inflate collapsed alveoli, inspiration can be prolonged until I/E (normally 1:3 or 1:4) reaches or, in certain cases, exceeds 1:1 (inverse). As long as there is adequate time during expiration for CO_2 clearance and as long as the effects of elevated mean airway pressure are taken into account, pressure-controlled inverse-ratio ventilation is an effective mode of mechanical ventilation. Because it requires total control of the breathing patterns, the patient must be heavily sedated. Pressure-controlled ventilation and pressure-controlled inverse-ratio ventilation are standard techniques in neonatal ventilation.

TRACHEAL INSUFFLATION

During mechanical ventilation, the major bronchi, trachea, and endotracheal airway make up the anatomic dead space. At the end of exhalation, this dead space is filled with alveolar gas that contains carbon dioxide. Under normal conditions, this CO_2 is rapidly diluted with fresh air, which creates a suitable gradient for CO_2 excretion. However, when V_D/V_T is more than 50%, reequilibration at a higher level of blood CO_2 may ultimately occur. This effect is not necessarily deleterious [see Permissive Hypercapnia, above]. However, preferably, a normal P_aCO_2 should be maintained as long as hyperventilation is avoided. CO_2 clearance can be facilitated by the insufflation of ventilating gas near the level of the carina through a small catheter. This maneuver, known as tracheal insufflation, removes CO_2 from the major airway. This removal lowers V_D/V_T and allows CO_2 clearance without overdistention and hyperventilation. When the gas flow is mechanically directed out of the airway, a Bernoulli effect results, which facilitates CO_2 clearance from the distal airways and alveoli.[52] This technique has been studied in detail by Kolobow, who refers to it as intratracheal pulmonary ventilation. This technique can be used in conjunction with conventional mechanical ventilation or as the sole source of ventilating gas. Of course, intratracheal pulmonary ventilation holds the greatest promise for patients whose conducting airways constitute a large fraction of the tidal volume, specifically newborn infants.[53]

EXTRACORPOREAL LIFE SUPPORT

Extracorporeal membrane oxygenation (ECMO) is the use of a modified heart-lung machine for days or weeks to support gas exchange while resting the diseased lung.[54] This technique has the advantage of avoiding the oxygen toxicity and barotrauma that may accompany mechanical ventilation in patients experiencing severe respiratory failure. It has become standard treatment in the management of severe respiratory failure in newborn infants.[55] In patients with adult respiratory failure who are considered moribund, 50% survival with extracorporeal life support (ECLS) has been reported from several centers.[56,57] In adult patients, venovenous blood access is generally used for patients with adequate cardiovascular function; venoarterial access is used when cardiac failure coexists.

ECLS might be considered when the risk of mortality with continuing conventional ventilation is more than 90% and the primary process is reversible. Thus, the specific indications in most ECMO centers are a transpulmonary shunt over 30% and compliance less than 0.5 ml/cm H_2O/kg after and despite optimal therapy. The contraindications to ECLS are advanced age, malignancy or brain damage, and mechanical ventilation longer than 5 to 7 days. ECLS can play a significant role in the management of severe respiratory failure in adults.[58] However, ECLS is complex and requires a well-trained team.

Summary

Management of mechanical ventilation is an exercise in applied pulmonary mechanics, just as the management of respiratory failure is an exercise in the full spectrum of applied pulmonary physiology. CO_2 clearance and oxygenation should be considered and managed as distinctly separate processes, although they are obviously interrelated. CO_2 clearance is the result of breathing and is thus the goal in mechanical ventilation. Although it is almost always possible to maintain normal P_aCO_2 by hyperventilation, a peak airway pressure greater than 40 cm H_2O injures the lung and should be avoided. Maintaining and improving oxygenation is a process of matching pulmonary blood flow to inflated alveoli, which should be done by positioning, diuresis, and optimization of hemoglobin concentration and cardiac output. Although oxygenation can be facilitated by increased F_IO_2 and PEEP, these methods of treatment, like hyperventilation, do more harm than good when applied in excess. The goal of mechanical ventilation is to provide adequate gas exchange without damaging the lung.

References

1. Agostoni E, Mead J: Statics of the respiratory system. Handbook of Physiology, Vol 1. American Physiological Society, Washington, DC, 1964, Sect 3, p 387

2. Kolobow T, Moretti MP, Fumagalli R, et al: Severe impairment in lung function induced by high peak airway pressure during mechanical ventilation. Am Rev Respir Dis 135:312, 1987

3. Bowton DL, Kong DL: High tidal volume ventilation produces increased lung water in oleic acid–injured rabbit lungs. Crit Care Med 17:908, 1989

4. Dreyfuss D, Soler P, Basset G, et al: High inflation pressure pulmonary edema: respective effects of high airway pressure, high tidal volume, and positive end-expiratory pressure. Am Rev Respir Dis 137:1159, 1988

5. Gattinoni L, Pesenti A, Torresin A, et al: Adult respiratory distress syndrome profiles by computed tomography. J Thorac Imaging 1:25, 1986

6. Hickling KG: Ventilatory management of ARDS: can it affect the outcome? Intensive Care Med 16:219, 1990

7. Amato MB, Barbas CS, Medeiros DM, et al: Effect of a protective-ventilation strategy on mortality in the acute respiratory distress syndrome. N Engl J Med 338:347, 1998

8. Ventilation with lower tidal volumes as compared with traditional tidal volumes for acute lung injury and the acute respiratory distress syndrome. The Acute Respiratory Distress Syndrome Network. N Engl J Med 342:1301, 2000

9. Lee PC, Helsmoortel CM, Cohn SM, et al: Are low tidal volumes safe? Chest 97:430, 1990

10. Hickling KG, Henderson SJ, Jackson R: Low mortality associated with low volume pressure limited ventilation with permissive hypercapnia in severe adult respiratory distress syndrome. Intensive Care Med 16:372, 1990

11. Cilley RE, Polley TZ Jr, Zwischenberger JB, et al: Independent measurement of oxygen consumption and oxygen delivery. J Surg Res 47:242, 1989

12. Hirschl RB, Heiss KF, Cilley RE, et al: Oxygen kinetics in experimental sepsis. Surgery 112:37, 1992

13. Danek SJ, Lynch JP, Weg JG, et al: The dependence of oxygen uptake on oxygen delivery in the adult respiratory distress syndrome. Am Rev Respir Dis 122:387, 1980

14. Gutierrez G, Pohil RJ: Oxygen consumption is linearly related to O_2 supply in critically ill patients. J Crit Care 1:45, 1986

15. Bartlett RH, Dechert RE: Oxygen kinetics: pitfalls in clinical research (editorial). J Crit Care 5:77, 1990

16. Vermeij CG, Feenstra BW, Bruining HA: Oxygen delivery and oxygen uptake in postoperative and septic patients. Chest 98:415, 1990

17. Zwischenberger JB, Cilley RE, Kirsh MM, et al: Does continuous monitoring of mixed venous oxygen saturation accurately reflect oxygen delivery and oxygen consumption following coronary artery bypass grafting? Surg Forum 37:66, 1986

18. Rashkin MC, Bosken C, Baughman RP: Oxygen delivery in critically ill patients: relationship to blood lactate and survival. Chest 87:580, 1985

19. Gattinoni L, Mascheroni D, Turresin A, et al: Morphological response to positive end expiratory pressure in acute respiratory failure: computerized tomography study. Intensive Care Med 12:137, 1986

20. Ali J, Duke K: Colloid osmotic pressure in pulmonary edema clearance with furosemide. Chest 92:540, 1987

21. Simmons RS, Berdine GG, Seidenfeld JJ, et al: Fluid balance and the adult respiratory distress syndrome. Am Rev Respir Dis 135:924, 1987

22. Langer M, Mascheroni D, Marcolin R, et al: The prone position in ARDS patients. Chest 94:103, 1988

23. Gattinoni L, Presenti A: Computed tomography scanning in acute respiratory failure. Adult Respiratory Distress Syndrome. Zapol WM, Lemaire F, Eds. Marcel Dekker, New York, 1991, p 199

24. Mushin WW, Rendell-Baker L, Thompson DW, et al: Automatic Ventilation of the Lungs. Blackwell Scientific Publishers, Oxford, 1980

25. Kirby RR, Smith RA, Desautels DA: Mechanical Ventilation. Churchill Livingstone, New York, 1985

26. Burton GG, Hodgkin JE, Ward JJ: Respiratory Care, 3rd ed. JB Lippincott Co, Philadelphia, 1991

27. Downs JB, Mitchell LA: Intermittent mandatory ventilation following cardiopulmonary bypass (abstr). Crit Care Med 2:39, 1974

28. Marini JJ, Rodriguez RM, Lamb V: The inspiratory workload of patient-initiated mechanical ventilation. Am Rev Respir Dis 134:902, 1986

29. MacIntyre N, Nishimura M, Usada Y, et al: The Nagoya conference on system design and patient-ventilator interactions during pressure support ventilation. Chest 97:1463, 1990

30. Gille JP: Neonatal and Adult Respiratory Failure. Elsevier, Paris, 1989

31. Levin DL, Moriss FC: Essentials of Pediatric Intensive Care. Quality Medical Publishing, St. Louis, 1990

32. Anderson HL III, Bartlett RH: Respiratory Care of the Surgical Patient. Respiratory Care, 3rd ed. JB Lippincott Co, Philadelphia, 1991, p 821

33. Bartlett RH: Respiratory therapy to prevent postoperative pulmonary complications. Respiratory Intensive Care. Pierson DJ, Ed. Daedalus Enterprises, Dallas, 1986, p 369

34. Bartlett RH: Bronchoscopy in surgical patients. Surgical Endoscopy. Dent TL, Strodel WE, Turcotte JG, Eds. Year Book Medical Publishers, Inc, Chicago, 1985

35. Blanch L, Fernandez R, Artigas A: The effect of auto-positive end-expiratory pressure on the arterial end-tidal carbon dioxide pressure gradient and expired carbon dioxide slope in critically ill patients during total ventilatory support. J Crit Care 6:202, 1991

36. Zapol WM, Snider MT, Hill JD, et al: Extracorporeal membrane oxygenation in severe acute respiratory failure: a randomized prospective study. JAMA 242:2193, 1979

37. Bartlett RH, Morris AH, Fairley HB, et al: A prospective study of acute hypoxic respiratory failure. Chest 89:684, 1986

38. Gillespie DJ, Marsh HMM, Divertie MB, et al: Clinical outcome of respiratory failure in patients requiring prolonged (> 24 hours) mechanical ventilation. Chest 90:364, 1986

39. Zapol WM, Frikker MJ, Pontoppidan H, et al: The adult respiratory distress syndrome at Massachusetts General Hospital. Adult Respiratory Distress Syndrome. Zapol WM, Lemaire F, Eds. Marcel Dekker, New York, 1991

40. Maunder RJ, Shuman UP, McHugh JW, et al: Preservation of normal lung regions in the adult respiratory distress syndrome: analysis by computed tomography. JAMA 255:2463, 1986

41. Bryan-Brown CW, Gutierrez G: O_2 transport and tissue oxygenation in the critically ill. Clinical Aspects of O_2 Transport and Tissue Oxygenation. Rinhart K, Eyrich K, Eds. Springer-Verlag, Berlin, 1989

42. Ruttimann Y, Chiolero R, Jequier E, et al: Effects of dopamine on total oxygen consumption and oxygen delivery in healthy men. Am J Physiol 257:E541, 1989

43. Gattinoni L, Mascheroni D, Basilico E, et al: Volume/pressure curve of total respiratory system in paralyzed

patients: artefacts and correction factors. Intensive Care Med 13:19, 1987

44. Williams TJ, Tuxen DV, Scheinkestel CD, et al: Risk factors for morbidity in mechanically ventilated patients with acute severe asthma. Am Rev Respir Dis 146:607, 1992

45. Wung JT, James LS, Kilchevsky E, et al: Management of infants with severe respiratory failure and persistence of the fetal circulation, without hyperventilation. Pediatrics 76:488, 1985

46. Eriksen J, Andersen J, Rasmussen JP, et al: Effects of ventilation with large tidal volumes or positive end-expiratory pressure on cardiorespiratory function in anesthetized obese patients. Acta Anaesthesiol Scand 22:241, 1978

47. Bendixen HH, Hedley-White J, Laver MB: Impaired oxygenation in surgical patients during general anesthesia with controlled ventilation. N Engl J Med 269:991, 1963

48. Stewart TE, Meade MO, Cook DJ, et al: Evaluation of a ventilation strategy to prevent barotrauma in patients at high risk for acute respiratory distress syndrome. N Engl J Med 338:355, 1998

49. Ranieri VM, Suter PM, Tortorella C, et al: Effect of mechanical ventilation on inflammatory mediators in patients with acute respiratory distress syndrome: a randomized controlled trial. JAMA 282:54, 1999

50. Hurst JM, Branson RD, Davis K Jr, et al: Comparison of conventional mechanical ventilation and high-frequency ventilation: a prospective, randomized trial in patients with respiratory failure. Ann Surg 211:486, 1990

51. Carlon GC, Guy Y, Groeger JS, et al: Early prediction of outcome of respiratory failure: comparison of high-frequency jet ventilation and volume-cycled ventilation. Chest 86:194, 1984

52. Lehnert BE, Oberdorster G, Slutsky AS: Constant-flow ventilation of apneic dogs. J Appl Physiol 53:483, 1982

53. Wilson JM, Thompson JR, Schnitzer JJ, et al: Intratracheal pulmonary ventilation: human case report. Presented at 3rd Annual Extracorporeal Life Support Organization Meeting, Ann Arbor, Michigan, September 1991

54. Gattinoni L, Pesenti A, Mascheroni D, et al: Low-frequency positive-pressure ventilation with extracorporeal CO_2 removal in severe acute respiratory failure. JAMA 256:881, 1986

55. Stolar CJ, Snedecor SM, Bartlett RH: Extracorporeal membrane oxygenation and neonatal respiratory failure: experience from the extracorporeal life support organization. J Pediatr Surg 26:563, 1991

56. Kolla S, Awad SA, Rich PB, et al: Extracorporeal life support for 100 adult patients with severe respiratory failure. Ann Surg 226:544, 1997

57. Lewandowski K, Lewandowski M, Pappert D, et al: Outcome and follow-up of adults following extracorporeal life support. ECMO: Extracorporeal Cardiopulmonary Support in Critical Care. Zwischenberger JB, Bartlett RH, Eds. ELSO, Ann Arbor, Michigan, 1995

58. Bartlett RH: Management of ECLS in adult respiratory failure. ECMO: Extracorporeal Cardiopulmonary Support in Critical Care. Zwischenberger JB, Bartlett RH, Eds. ELSO, Ann Arbor, Michigan, 1995

Acknowledgments

Figure 1   Albert Miller.

Figures 2, 4, and 7 through 9   Talar Agasyan.

Figures 3 and 5   Marcia Kammerer.

Figure 6   Dana Burns-Pizer.

7 RENAL FAILURE

Renae E. Stafford, M.D., Bruce A. Cairns, M.D., F.A.C.S., and Anthony A. Meyer, M.D., Ph.D., F.A.C.S.

Approach to the Patient with Renal Failure

Normal renal function provides a mechanism for eliminating toxic metabolites and maintaining homeostasis of fluid and electrolytes. Loss of normal function results in alterations in volume and electrolyte homeostasis and inadequate excretion of metabolic wastes. Acute renal failure (ARF) has been defined as a sudden and sustained decline in glomerular filtration rate (GFR) that is usually associated with azotemia and a fall in urine output.[1] This presents clinically as oliguria or anuria and results in a rise in serum creatinine and blood urea nitrogen (BUN). Fortunately, most patients in whom acute renal dysfunction develops do not progress to acute renal failure. However, ARF remains a complex problem associated with a high mortality in surgical patients. Most of the renal failure encountered in contemporary surgical care is not single-organ failure; rather, it occurs in the context of the simultaneous dysfunction or failure of several organ systems.

The annual incidence of ARF is approximately 50 to 100 cases per million population. Among hospitalized patients, ARF is particularly prevalent in the intensive care unit.[2] Risk factors for the development of ARF include hypotension and shock; sepsis and the systemic inflammatory response syndrome; trauma[3]; nephrotoxic agents such as ionic contrast agents,[4,5] aminoglycosides, vancomycin, and cyclosporine; atheroembolic events[6]; abdominal compartment syndrome[7]; and preexisting renal insufficiency. Those factors tend to have an additive effect, particularly in patients whose renal function is already compromised. The mortality of ARF is greater than 50%.[8] Hence, prevention and early recognition of acute renal dysfunction are of paramount importance.

Recognition of Acute Renal Dysfunction

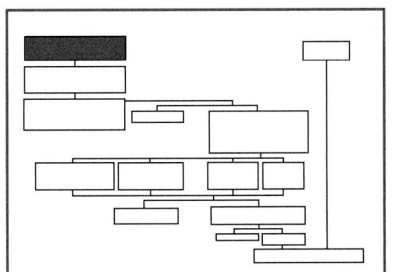

Acute renal dysfunction is approached clinically from the presenting problems of oliguria or rising serum creatinine levels. Evaluation of renal dysfunction generally takes into account prerenal, renal parenchymal, and postrenal mechanisms of dysfunction [see Table 1]. In some patients, more than one cause of renal dysfunction may be present, and it is important to consider all possible mechanisms. The goals in management of ARF are prevention and early diagnosis to limit renal damage and to maintain adequate residual function.

The clinical manifestations of renal dysfunction vary. Patients with acutely deteriorating renal function become symptomatic earlier than those with acute-on-chronic renal failure.[9] In the early stages, patients may be asymptomatic. As the renal dysfunction progresses, they may become oliguric or anuric and develop edema or cardiopulmonary compromise as a result of volume overload. Patients with uremia (creatinine clearance < 10 ml/min) may present with nausea, pruritus, malaise, weakness, and mental status changes.[10-12] Laboratory manifestations include a rising creatinine level and a fall in the serum bicarbonate level. BUN levels usually rise, but they may be normal. Although laboratory values are useful adjuncts for recognizing acute renal dysfunction, they cannot be used to predict outcome in ARF [see Discussion, Perspective on Acute Renal Failure, *below*].

ACUTE OLIGURIA

Acute renal dysfunction may be signaled by the acute onset of oliguria. This is defined as a urine output of less than 0.5 ml/kg/hr or 400 ml/24 hr in an adult and less than 1.0 ml/kg/hr in a child weighing less than 10 kg.[13-16] Patients may progress to or even present with anuria, defined as a urine output of less than 100 ml/24 hr. Acutely decreased urine output most often is the result of a fall in renal perfusion from diminished circulating blood volume [see Initial Clinical Assessment, *below*]. A Foley catheter should be placed in acutely oliguric patients to follow urine output closely and to evaluate the effects of treatment. Efforts should be made to determine the cause of the oliguria and to reestablish adequate urine output. Oliguria has many causes, and most patients who present with oliguria do not have ARF.

INCREASED SERUM CREATININE

Creatinine, a product of amino acid metabolism, is cleared by the kidneys. This is done principally by glomerular filtration, although a limited amount of creatinine is secreted into the tubular fluid.[17] A serum creatinine level of 1.2 mg/dl or less is considered normal. The rate of creatinine production is relatively constant and depends primarily on muscle mass. Among patients with renal dysfunction, therefore, smaller rises in creatinine may be seen in small women than in large, muscular men. In addition, GFR decreases with age, as do creatinine production and muscle mass.[18] Therefore, a normal creatinine level in an elderly patient does not represent the same GFR as the same creatinine level would in a younger patient. A rising serum creatinine level implies decreased renal clearance; an increase of 1 mg/dl over normal or baseline levels indicates a 50% decrease in the GFR. The serum creatinine level can rise acutely even with normal urine output, such as with aminoglycoside-induced acute tubular necrosis (ATN)[19] and thus is another marker of acute renal dysfunction. Not all elevated creatinine levels represent renal insufficiency, however. The presence of ketones[20] or some cephalosporins[21] may produce a factitiously elevated creatinine level by interfering with its assay. Other drugs, such as trimethoprim-sulfamethoxazole[22] and

Patient presents with signs of acute renal dysfunction

- *Oliguria:* urine output < 0.5 ml/kg/hr or < 1.0 ml/kg/hr in child < 10 kg.
- *Rising creatinine level:* ≥ 1.0 mg/dl increase.
- *Worsening of preexisting renal insufficiency.*
  Note: these manifestations may have nonrenal causes, which should be excluded.

Clinical assessment

Perform physical examination to look for signs of hypovolemia, CHF, poor perfusion, and urinary tract obstruction.

- Estimate intravascular volume and peripheral perfusion, and consider possible causes of impaired renal perfusion (cardiac disease, renovascular disease, renal artery injury, abdominal compartment syndrome). If renal artery is injured, consider renal perfusion scan.
- Identify and treat any urinary tract obstruction.

Initial treatment measures

Administer I.V. fluid challenge (~10% of circulating volume, more in hypovolemic patients), preferably isotonic crystalloid bolus. Give blood if patient has acute blood loss or is anemic. Do not administer fluid challenge to patients who have CHF or other primary cardiorespiratory conditions until more extensive evaluation of cause of renal dysfunction has been done. Maintain urine volume. Consider diuresis with mannitol or loop diuretic only in selected cases.

Renal dysfunction resolves

Continue monitoring. Avoid hypovolemia and use of nephrotoxic agents.

Prerenal dysfunction (U_{Na} < 20 mEq/L or FE_{Na} < 1)

Expand intravascular volume if necessary. Improve renal blood flow; if intravascular volume is adequate, consider dopamine, 2–5 μg/kg/min. Monitor CVP, PAWP, or RVEDVI. Decompress abdomen if abdominal compartment pressure remains elevated. If acute renal arterial problems are present, emergency operation and revascularization may be necessary.

Renal parenchymal dysfunction (no obstruction; U_{Na} > 40 mEq/L or FE_{Na} > 3)

Stop nephrotoxic drugs if possible. Avoid using contrast agents if possible. Maintain renal perfusion. Assess tubular function. Consider loop diuretics or mannitol. Evaluate for SIADH and hepatorenal syndrome.

Renal function returns to normal

Continue monitoring. Avoid hypovolemia and use of nephrotoxic agents.

Approach to the Patient with Renal Failure

Patient has chronic renal failure

Evaluate renal function.
Assess patient for symptoms
[*see Table 4*].

Renal dysfunction does not resolve

Initiate more extensive evaluation of renal function. Attempt to identify potentially reversible prerenal, renal parenchymal, and postrenal causes.

Evaluate
- Intravascular volume (CVP, PAWP).
- Perfusion (cardiac output, mixed venous O_2 saturation).
- Tubular function (urine and plasma electrolytes, urinalysis). Calculate FE_{Na}.
- Collecting system (US, IVP).

Review medications. Stop nephrotoxic drugs if possible, and adjust all dosages as necessary.

Consider miscellaneous causes (e.g., abdominal compartment syndrome and damage to renal artery).

Mixed prerenal and renal parenchymal dysfunction (U_{Na} > 20 mEq/L but < 40 mEq/L and FE_{Na} > 1 but < 3)

Expand intravascular volume. Stop nephrotoxic drugs if possible. Monitor CVP, PAWP, RVEDVI, and urine electrolyte concentrations.

Postrenal dysfunction (obstruction of urinary system)

Drain obstructed area.
- *Bladder:* use Foley catheter or suprapubic tube.
- *Ureter:* use nephrostomy tube or stent.

Renal dysfunction continues or progresses

Monitor and adjust medications and fluids. Maintain general supportive care. Provide renal replacement therapy via CVVHD/CAVHD, intermittent hemodialysis, peritoneal dialysis, or hemofiltration.

Renal deterioration stops or slows

Chronic renal failure ensues

Continue renal replacement therapy.

Measure and correct fluid, electrolyte, and metabolic abnormalities as needed. Monitor patient for other chronic complications of renal failure, including hypertension, anemia, and platelet dysfunction. Monitor and adjust medications.

1137

Table 1 Classification of Acute Renal Failure

Prerenal (50%–90% of Total Cases)

Volume depletion

    Dehydration (i.e., from cutaneous or gastrointestinal losses or renal losses in adrenal insufficiency)

    Hemorrhage (i.e., from trauma, surgery, childbirth, or GI lesions)

    Fluid redistribution (e.g., from trauma, crush injury, burns, pancreatitis, peritonitis, sepsis, or hypoalbuminemia)

Cardiac failure

    Myocardial or valvular dysfunction, arrhythmia, or tamponade

Systemic vasodilatation

    Sepsis, anaphylaxis, neurogenic shock, anesthesia, or antihypertensive medications

Renovascular obstructive disease

    Arterial (e.g., arteriosclerosis, embolism, dissection, fibromuscular dysplasia, vasculitis, or disease related to aortic or any retroperitoneal operation)

    Venous (e.g., renal vein thrombosis)

Renal Parenchymal (10%–30% of Total Cases)

Acute tubular necrosis

    Ischemia

    Nephrotoxins

      Endogenous: pigments (myoglobin and hemoglobin), crystals (uric acid, calcium phosphate, and oxalate), or tumors (tumor lysis syndrome and myeloma)

      Exogenous: antibiotics (aminoglycosides, cephalosporins, sulfonamides, and amphotericin B), anesthetics (methoxyflurane and enflurane), chemotherapeutic and immunosuppressive agents (e.g., cisplatin and cyclosporine), contrast media, organic solvents (heavy metals, poisons, or other chemicals), and dextran

Glomerulonephritis

    Postinfectious (e.g., associated with streptococcal, pneumococcal, viral, and shunt infections and abdominal abscesses)

    Membranoproliferative

    Rapidly progressive (e.g., associated with lupus erythematosus, Goodpasture syndrome, polyarteritis nodosa, Wegener granulomatosis, Schönlein-Henoch purpura)

    Serum sickness

    Thrombotic microangiopathy (e.g., hemolytic-uremic syndrome or thrombotic-thrombocytopenic purpura) and other microvascular diseases (e.g., scleroderma, malignant hypertension, radiation, and disseminated intravascular coagulation)

Vasculitides

    Polyarteritis nodosa, hypersensitivity angiitides, scleroderma, hemolytic-uremic syndrome, coagulopathy, radiation, diffuse intravascular coagulation, eclampsia, malignant hypertension, or thrombotic-thrombocytopenic purpura

Interstitial nephritis

    Drugs (e.g., penicillin, cephalosporins, sulfonamides, rifampin, nonsteroidal anti-inflammatory drugs, thiazides, cimetidine, and interferon)

    Infection

      Direct invasion (e.g., by *Staphylococcus,* viruses, or fungi)

      Indirect effects (e.g., of streptococcal or pneumococcal infection, typhoid, or diphtheria)

    Infiltration (lymphoma, leukemia, or sarcoidosis)

    Idiopathic

Papillary necrosis (e.g., associated with analgesics, infection, obstruction, or diabetes)

Acute cortical necrosis (e.g., profound shock, often associated with complicated pregnancy or septic abortion)

Atheroembolic syndrome (renal failure with lower extremity ischemia)

SIADH

Intrarenal shunting

    Systemic infection, SIRS, hepatorenal syndrome

Postrenal (1%–15% of Total Cases)

Obstructive uropathy

    Renal pelvis and ureters (i.e., from calculus, tumor, clot, papillae, infection, trauma, or retroperitoneal fibrosis)

Bladder and urethra (i.e., from calculus, bladder or prostatic tumor, clot, trauma, benign prostatic hypertrophy, neuropathic bladder, obstructed bladder catheter, or phimosis)

Extravasation (i.e., from trauma)

---

cimetidine,[23] inhibit the tubular secretion of creatinine and may cause an elevated serum creatinine level in a patient with normal renal function.

As with oliguria, most patients who present with a rising serum creatinine level do not have acute renal failure. However, an increase of more than 1 mg/dl above normal or baseline levels should be investigated and appropriate preventive and therapeutic measures taken. An increase of more than 2 mg/dl/day, even in the presence of anuria, suggests a rapid rate of protein breakdown, such as might occur in the presence of ischemic muscle or a resolving hematoma.[24] Furthermore, a BUN-to-creatinine ratio higher than 40:1 suggests that volume depletion is the cause of the rising creatinine.[25]

INCREASED BLOOD UREA NITROGEN

The BUN measurement depends on many variables, which include GFR and rates of urea production and tubular reabsorption. In addition, extrarenal factors such as blood in the GI tract, a high-protein diet, the administration of glucocorticoid hormones, protein catabolism, and sepsis can increase BUN.[25] Therefore, a high BUN cannot be equated with a low GFR.

Initial Clinical Assessment

The first step in evaluating acute renal dysfunction, as manifested by acute oliguria or a rising serum creatinine, is physical examination. Laboratory tests and imaging procedures

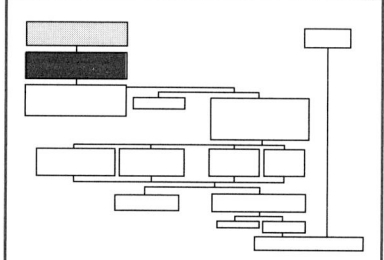

should not be used as surrogates. A clinical examination is necessary to assess the patient's perfusion status and to rule out urinary tract obstruction as a cause of renal dysfunction. Signs of hypovolemia, congestive heart failure, poor peripheral perfusion, and urinary tract obstruction should be sought.

Decreased renal perfusion is the most common cause of acute renal dysfunction in surgical patients[25-28] and is usually the result of decreased intravascular volume, as signaled by flat neck veins, tachycardia, diminished jugular pulse, and other signs of hypovolemia [see 6:3 Shock]. Perfusion can be estimated clinically on the basis of skin color, temperature, and capillary refill. It is important to remember, however, that although patients who have systemic infections, exhibit the systemic inflammatory response syndrome (SIRS), have been burned, or have recently undergone a major surgical procedure or sustained a serious injury may have liters of excess body fluid, their intravascular volume may still be depleted. These patients may have associated systemic vasodilatation that contributes to the poor perfusion. In such patients, tissue edema and weight change may be of limited help in estimating intravascular volume.

Another cause of acute renal dysfunction is diminished peripheral perfusion secondary to poor myocardial function. This should be considered if the patient has a history of cardiac disease or evidence of acute myocardial ischemia.

Obstructive renovascular disease and acute renal artery injury also lead to diminished renal perfusion. The patient with obstructive renovascular disease and acute renal dysfunction may be oliguric and tachycardic but will be hypertensive. Patients who have sustained trauma or have undergone retroperitoneal or invasive vascular procedures may have a renal artery injury. If such injury is thought to be present, a renal perfusion scan should be considered.

Impaired renal perfusion and subsequent ARF have been documented in patients with abdominal compartment syndrome.[7,29] If the abdomen is extremely rigid, abdominal pressure can be measured through a Foley catheter. If the pressure is higher than 30 to 40 cm H_2O and there is a decrease in urine output that cannot be attributed to other causes, decompression should be considered, although this is not without risk.

A similar mechanism accounts for the decreased urine output that is sometimes seen after laparoscopic surgery. Insufflation of the abdominal cavity with gas during laparoscopy causes an increase in intra-abdominal pressure, which can decrease renal function and urine output. The decrease is transient and resolves after release of the pneumoperitoneum.[30]

Urinary tract obstruction causes up to 10% of ARF. Bladder outlet obstruction from prostatic enlargement or a plugged Foley catheter may be missed without a physical examination. Placement of a Foley catheter, or irrigation of the catheter if one is already present, will help eliminate outlet obstruction as a cause of acute renal dysfunction. Obstruction of the upper collecting system is generally unilateral and rarely accounts for acute renal dysfunction. However, patients who experience acute renal dysfunction after surgical procedures in which the ureters could potentially be injured or ligated should be evaluated for ureteral obstruction or injury. Acute dysfunction that is caused solely by obstruction of the upper or lower collecting system should resolve when the obstruction is corrected.[31]

Assessment of the patient with acute renal dysfunction is not a one-time event. Reevaluating the patient after tests and monitoring the patient's response to treatment with measures such as daily weights, total fluid input and output, and hourly urine output are essential to minimize renal injury and prevent progression to frank renal failure.

Initial Treatment Measures

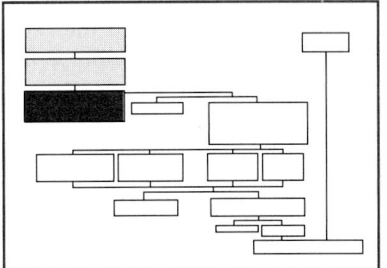

I.V. FLUID CHALLENGE

Because acute oliguria or increased serum creatinine levels in surgical patients are usually the result of decreased renal perfusion, treatment should begin with administration of an intravenous fluid bolus to expand intravascular volume. The bolus should be approximately 10% of the estimated circulating volume if it is to produce a significant increase in perfusion. Under the assumption that blood makes up 7% of body weight, a bolus for an 80 kg patient should be calculated as follows:

$$80 \text{ kg} \times 0.07 \text{ L/kg} = 5.6 \text{ L}$$
$$5.6 \text{ L} \times 0.10 = 560 \text{ ml}$$

An even larger bolus may be appropriate if severe hypovolemia is present. If the patient has suffered acute blood loss or is significantly anemic, blood will be required to expand vascular volume effectively. Otherwise, isotonic salt-containing crystalloid solutions, such as normal saline or lactated Ringer solution, are the most effective volume expanders. Colloid solutions may be used in some patients, such as those with significant burns or liver disease, but they have not been proved to be more effective than crystalloid solutions. In fact, they may be detrimental.[32] Use of hypertonic saline may produce dramatic physiologic effects, but these solutions are not routinely given for management of acute renal dysfunction. The intravenous fluid bolus should improve hypovolemia and should at least partially correct acute renal dysfunction.

Volume infusion should also benefit patients in whom decreased renal perfusion is caused by myocardial dysfunction. Increasing preload will usually improve left ventricular performance. Although in rare cases an intravenous fluid bolus may be harmful to such patients, the renal injury may be worsened if fluid therapy is withheld to prevent the unlikely possibility of congestive heart failure. Patients who are normovolemic will not suffer cardiorespiratory complications as the result of such a fluid challenge, because 65% to 75% of infused fluid leaves the vascular compartment within 30 minutes.

Patients with congestive heart failure or other primary cardiorespiratory conditions, on the other hand, should not receive a fluid bolus until a more extensive evaluation of the cause of their renal dysfunction has been performed [see Evaluation to Determine Cause of Renal Failure, below].

MAINTENANCE OF URINE OUTPUT

Maintenance of urine output during a period of renal injury may have a significant influence on survival. Oliguric renal failure has been shown to have a mortality twice as high as that for nonoliguric failure and has higher morbidity.[33] Prompt fluid therapy may be all that is necessary to handle the problem. Diuretics or osmotic agents have not been shown to prevent or reverse ARF[34] or to decrease mortality from renal failure. However, if prerenal and postrenal causes of oliguria have been corrected, a trial of mannitol[35] or a loop diuretic[33,36] may convert oliguric to nonoliguric renal failure.[19,33] Diuretics may be appropriate in patients with high intravascular volume or who have been taking diuretics for long periods of time and are dependent on them. Critically ill patients who are refractory to intermittent dosing of loop diuretics or have severe fluid overload may have improved diuresis with continuous infusion.[37] This type of dosing is more commonly used in patients with heart failure and in kidney transplant recipients. Mannitol may be used in patients who can tolerate the osmotic load and may be particularly helpful for renal dysfunction caused by rhabdomyolysis.[3] In general, loop and osmotic diuretics should be avoided because their administration will abrogate the use of urine volume and electrolyte levels as useful tests of renal function for approximately 24 hours. In addition, diuretic agents may cause further renal injury in patients who are intravascularly depleted.[38]

Evaluation to Determine Cause of Renal Failure

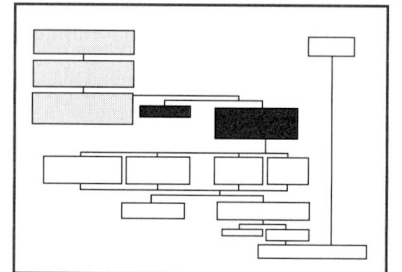

Patients who fail to respond to a fluid challenge or to correction of urinary obstruction, those who require repeat fluid boluses, and those with complicating and severe acute and chronic medical problems require more extensive evaluation to determine the cause or causes of their renal failure before appropriate treatment can be initiated. Potentially reversible prerenal, renal parenchymal, and postrenal causes must be considered. Prerenal causes involve decreased perfusion of the kidney; renal parenchymal causes include ischemia and toxic injury; and postrenal causes involve obstruction of the ureters, bladder, or urethra. Acute renal dysfunction from renal parenchymal causes is usually diagnosed by excluding prerenal and postrenal causes, rather than by specific diagnosis.

In the critically ill patient, maintenance of urine output is an inadequate indicator of renal perfusion.[39] Instead, specific measurements can be made that will help determine the cause of renal dysfunction [see Table 2]. Hemodynamic monitoring will allow assessment of intravascular volume as well as cardiac function. Intravascular volume can be estimated clinically on the basis of the jugular pulse and physiologically on the basis of the central venous pressure (CVP) or the pulmonary arterial wedge pressure (PAWP). Physiologic measures of perfusion are usually derived from measurement of cardiac output by means of a thermodilution pulmonary arterial catheter or measurement of mixed venous oxygen saturation by means of a Swan-Ganz catheter, though other methods of measuring cardiac performance and perfusion can also be used [see 6:4 Cardiopulmonary Monitoring]. These measurements are useful in diagnosing prerenal causes of renal failure (e.g., hypovolemia and decreased perfusion), but they do not reflect renal function itself.

Water and solute dynamics are good measures of renal function. Prerenal causes of renal failure can be distinguished from renal parenchymal or postrenal causes through measurement of the urine sodium level (U_{Na}) on a spot urine sample: a urine sodium level lower than 20 mEq/L indicates a prerenal cause, whereas a level higher than 40 mEq/L indicates a renal parenchymal or postrenal cause. The levels of sodium and creatinine in the urine or plasma (P) can be used to calculate the fractional excretion of sodium (FE_{Na}),[40-42] which represents the fraction of the sodium filtered by the glomeruli that is excreted in the urine. FE_{Na} is expressed as a percentage:

$$FE_{Na} = [(U_{Na} / P_{Na})/(U_{Cr} / P_{Cr})] \times 100$$

An FE_{Na} lower than 1 indicates that the cause of dysfunction is prerenal, whereas an FE_{Na} higher than 3 suggests a renal parenchymal or postrenal cause. Urine sodium measurements of 20 to 40 mEq/L and an FE_{Na} between 1 and 3 have been shown to be nonspecific.[43]

It is essential to review all present and recent medications and treatments, looking for nephrotoxic agents that may be responsible for the acute renal dysfunction or failure. Nonsteroidal anti-inflammatory drugs, cyclosporine and tacrolimus, and the combination of angiotensin-converting enzyme (ACE) inhibitors with diuretics may all precipitate prerenal azotemia.[44] The administration of any such agents that are not absolutely necessary should be limited or stopped. Even if these agents are not the cause of the renal dysfunction, they can exacerbate it substantially. Patients who are to receive nephrotoxic agents, such as intravenous contrast dye, aminoglycosides, or antineoplastic agents, should be adequately hydrated beforehand in an attempt to prevent renal dysfunction or worsening of preexisting renal dysfunction.[5,45] A new dopaminergic agonist, fenoldopam, may prove useful in the prevention of renal toxicity associated with intravenous contrast agents.[46,47] The antioxidant acetylcysteine has been shown to prevent radio-

Table 2 Findings in Acute Renal Dysfunction

Assessment	Findings			
	Prerenal	Renal Parenchymal	Mixed Prerenal and Renal Parenchymal	Postrenal
Intravascular volume (measure central venous pressure or pulmonary arterial occlusion pressure)	Decreased	Normal	Decreased	Normal
Perfusion (measure cardiac output or mixed venous O_2 saturation)	Decreased	Normal	Decreased	Normal
Urine sodium	< 20 mEq/L	> 40 mEq/L	> 20 but < 40 mEq/L	Usually > 40 mEq/L
Fractional excretion of sodium (FE_{Na})	< 1	> 3	> 1 but < 3	Usually > 3
Collecting system (perform sonography or intravenous pyelography)	Normal	Normal	Normal	Dilated
Tubular function (measure urine and plasma electrolytes; perform urinalysis)	Specific gravity > 1.020, pH < 6	Red cell and white cell casts, tubular cells	Red cell and white cell casts, tubular cells	Specific gravity < 1.015, pH > 6

graphic contrast–induced decreases in renal function in patients with chronic renal insufficiency.[48] In addition, dosages of all medications should be adjusted as necessary.

Diagnosis of urinary outlet obstruction in patients with renal dysfunction can usually be made by means of ultrasonography or intravenous pyelography. Ultrasonography can be performed on critically ill patients in the ICU without jeopardizing them by transport to x-ray facilities and can identify urinary tract obstruction in the kidneys or in the bladder. A dilated collecting system indicates a postrenal cause of renal dysfunction. In the acute setting, this may be relieved by percutaneous nephrostomy or retrograde cystoscopy.

Urinalysis can identify urine of high specific gravity and low pH; both findings indicate a prerenal cause. Microscopic urine examination may reveal tubular casts indicative of renal parenchymal dysfunction; hemoglobinuria as a result of transfusion reaction, parenchymal injury, rhabdomyolysis, or vasculitic disease; eosinophilia associated with interstitial nephritis; or myoglobinuria from muscle ischemia or crush injury.[3,49] Relatively benign urinary sediments are often seen in hepatorenal syndrome.

These assessments and measurements can help distinguish the causes of acute renal dysfunction and failure but are of somewhat limited use in elderly patients and in those with preexisting renal disease. They are of little or no use in patients who have received diuretics or osmotic agents in the previous 24 hours. In some patients, results may be difficult to interpret and clinical and laboratory evidence will have to be used to determine the most likely cause. If the specific cause remains uncertain, the condition may have several causes. Further workup and management will depend on whether the problem has a prerenal, renal parenchymal, or postrenal origin. In addition, although urinalysis and determination of urine sodium concentration and the fractional excretion of sodium can help identify the cause of acute renal failure, they do not indicate its severity. These studies can be supplemented by periodic measurements of creatinine clearance, which can be used to estimate the severity of acute renal failure and to assess the patient's clinical course. Normal creatinine clearance is greater than 100 ml/min; however, this value decreases by nearly half by 70 years of age.

Management

ACUTE DYSFUNCTION FROM PRERENAL CAUSES

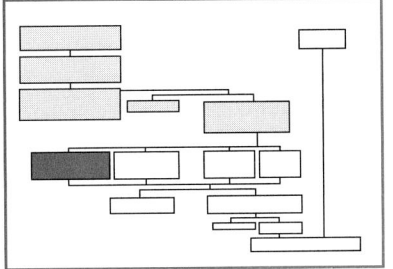

Prerenal causes of acute renal dysfunction include those that diminish blood flow; hence, management is designed to improve renal blood flow. Prerenal azotemia is reversed with treatment of the underlying cause. Intravascular volume is expanded to guarantee adequate preload. CVP, PAWP, or right ventricular end-diastolic volume index (RVEDVI) should be monitored to avoid excess fluid administration. In addition, blood pressure should be controlled adequately, because severe hypertension may worsen preexisting disease. In patients with renovascular disease, however, overcorrection of hypertension may decrease renal blood flow and worsen renal dysfunction.[19,50]

If cardiac dysfunction is present, inotropic support may be useful. It is important not to use agents with alpha-adrenergic activity. Although these agents increase blood pressure, when they are used in high doses their vasoconstrictive effect on

renal arteries leads to reduced renal blood flow.[51,52] Selective renal artery dilation and subsequent diuresis can be achieved with low dosages of dopamine (2 to 5 µg/kg/min).[51,53,54] The contribution of this effect may be trivial or very significant, depending on the patient and coexisting problems. It may also be arrhythmogenic. Administration of dopamine can be useful adjunctive therapy, however, and may be tried in patients who do not respond to simple fluid boluses [see Discussion, Treatment of Developing Acute Renal Failure, below].

If acute renal arterial problems are present, emergency operation and revascularization may be required. Renal artery disease should also be evaluated in the patient undergoing abdominal aortic aneurysm repair, because reimplantation, endarterectomy, or both may be indicated.[55] In cases of documented abdominal compartment syndrome, the abdomen may have to be reapproximated with a prosthetic patch in the fascia to reduce the transmission of external pressure to the kidneys.

Even if prerenal mechanisms do not appear to be the cause of acute renal dysfunction, it is nevertheless important to maintain adequate renal blood flow to minimize injury and facilitate recovery.

ACUTE DYSFUNCTION FROM RENAL PARENCHYMAL CAUSES

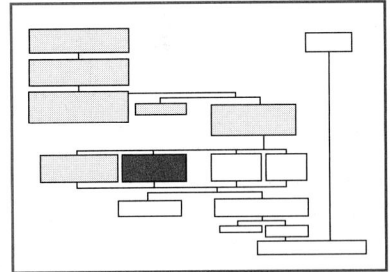

Renal parenchyma can be affected or damaged by many substances and mechanisms. Initial attention in patients with renal parenchymal disorders should be directed at stopping the injury. The most common cause of ARF in surgical patients is ATN from systemic infection, ischemia, or exposure to nephrotoxins.[56] Nephrotoxic drugs, such as aminoglycosides, other antibiotics, and nonsteroidal anti-inflammatory drugs, should be discontinued and nonnephrotoxic drugs substituted where possible. The use of radiographic contrast agents should be avoided. Radiologic studies that do not require intravenous contrast, such as magnetic resonance and carbon dioxide imaging, should be selected where possible. If this is not possible, a nonionic agent should be used. It is also important to limit the amount of contrast medium given, because multiple doses have been associated with an increased risk of contrast-induced nephropathy, and to ensure that the patient's intravascular volume is adequate before administration begins.[5] Clearance of circulating myoglobin and hemoglobin should be increased by encouraging diuresis with crystalloid solution infusion. Osmotic agents and urine alkalinization have been used to treat myoglobinuria,[3,57] but they are no substitute for diuresis of at least 100 ml/hr until the urine is clear. Again, maintenance of renal perfusion is essential.

In patients whose serum creatinine level is normal but whose urine sodium level is greater than 40 mEq/L and whose serum sodium level is normal or low, oliguria may reflect the syndrome of inappropriate antidiuretic hormone secretion (SIADH). SIADH is treated by water restriction and, if necessary, administration of diuretics. In patients who have a history of chronic or acute liver disorders, the combination of persistent oliguria, rising serum creatinine levels, low urine sodium levels, low serum sodium levels, and normal intravascular volume should suggest the hepatorenal syndrome [see 6:10 Hepatic Failure]. There are two findings by which this syndrome can be distinguished from prerenal causes of renal failure: (1) urine output does not increase in response to fluid challenge and (2) the ratio of urine creatinine to plasma creatinine is higher than 30:1 (this ratio is lower than 30:1 when prerenal causes are present).[58] There is no proven treatment for hepatorenal syndrome. Peritoneovenous shunts have been used but are of unproven efficacy. Liver transplantation is sometimes lifesaving.[58] Many patients require dialysis until transplantation or resolution of renal dysfunction.[59]

Renal dysfunction from parenchymal causes often takes longer to resolve and has a less predictable course than renal dysfunction from prerenal or postrenal causes.[6] Identification of the specific injurious agent may not be possible. Any patient who is receiving nephrotoxic substances or who has been exposed to such substances should be monitored closely to limit damage. Daily measurement of serum levels of nephrotoxic drugs and adjustment of dosage are indicated in patients in whom these drugs cannot be substituted.

ACUTE DYSFUNCTION FROM A MIXTURE OF PRERENAL AND RENAL PARENCHYMAL CAUSES

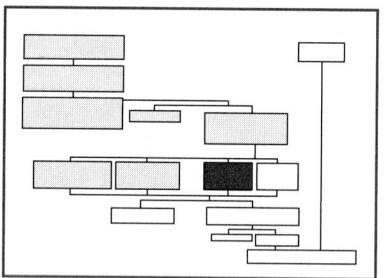

Some patients exhibit a mixed pattern of renal dysfunction, in which the mechanism is not obviously prerenal or renal parenchymal. Such patients typically have oliguria or an elevated serum creatinine concentration. The urine sodium concentration is usually between 20 and 40 mEq/L, and the FE_{Na} is usually between 1 and 3. Several potential causes of dysfunction may be present, including diminished renal perfusion and exposure to nephrotoxic agents. These may be superimposed on some degree of baseline renal dysfunction. The administration of diuretics or osmotic agents in this situation may also lead to this mixed pattern through their effects on renal electrolytes.

Treatment of renal dysfunction of mixed origin is generally based on increasing intravascular volume. Unless the patient is known to have intravascular fluid overload, a fluid bolus should be given, and the I.V. fluid infusion rate should be increased. Edema in itself is not a sufficient reason to withhold further fluid challenge: it may be extravascular, rendering the patient paradoxically hypovolemic. Again, all nephrotoxic drugs should be discontinued to prevent any further injury to the renal parenchyma. The patient's CVP, PAWP, or RVEDVI should be monitored to ensure that intravascular volume is not pushed to a high level. Continued monitoring of urine electrolyte concentrations should be undertaken to detect any further deterioration of renal function.

ACUTE DYSFUNCTION FROM POSTRENAL CAUES

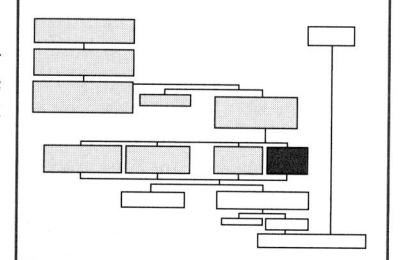

Treatment of obstructive lesions that produce acute renal dysfunction is relatively straightforward. Decompression of the obstructed area will usually correct the problem and permit return of all or some degree of renal function. Obstructing lesions that are

complicated by urosepsis may be associated with more prolonged renal dysfunction. These patients often have prerenal dysfunction as a result of the sepsis, and a Swan-Ganz catheter may be necessary to guide therapy. Similar assessment of cardiac output, using a somewhat less invasive method than pulmonary artery catheterization, may be accomplished by the use of continuous cardiac output arterial thermodilution calibrated pulse contour analysis.[60]

The bladder can be drained by means of a Foley or suprapubic catheter. Continued monitoring of urine output is then possible. If ureteral obstruction is present, ureteral stents or nephrostomy tubes can be placed to relieve the obstruction.

Return to Normal Renal Function

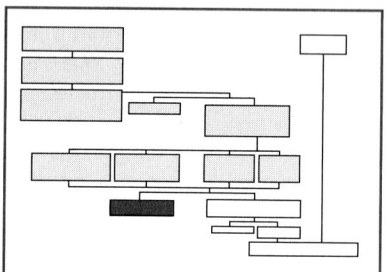

Successful management of acute renal dysfunction will correct oliguria and serum creatinine levels. However, monitoring of renal function must be continued until there appears to be no further risk, particularly if other medical problems necessitate ongoing treatment. Documentation of the acute renal dysfunction is important because it may help prevent recurrent problems in the future. Drug selection should be carefully reviewed with an eye to avoiding nephrotoxic agents, if possible. If nephrotoxic drugs must be used, the serum levels of the drugs and parameters of renal function, such as serum creatinine, must be followed closely.

Progressive Renal Dysfunction

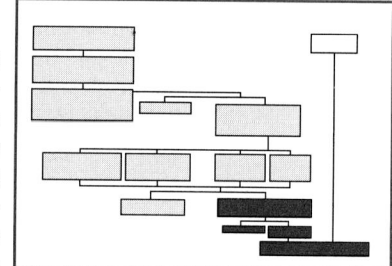

Attempts to maintain renal blood flow and preserve urine output are important even in the presence of advancing renal failure.[61] Nonoliguric renal failure has a better prognosis than oliguric or anuric renal failure.[33] Adequate hydration remains the principal method for sustaining urine output. Inotropic agents may have a positive influence in some patients but are not recommended as routine treatment. Attempts to preserve urine output and convert oliguric to nonoliguric renal failure by administering diuretics[62,63] have been largely unsuccessful; these attempts appear only to identify patients with the least severe renal dysfunction (i.e., those with enough residual renal function to respond to the diuretics).[33] Furthermore, diuretics confer no long-term benefit in the treatment of ARF.

If renal function deteriorates, medication doses and dosing intervals must be adjusted. Adjustments for drugs should be based on product information from the manufacturer or on the recommendations of a pharmacologist. The principles to be considered in adjustment of drug dosage in patients with renal failure are (1) the desired concentration, (2) the volume of distribution of the drug, and (3) the mechanism and rate of metabolism or excretion. Drug levels should be checked frequently as renal function changes; fluid and electrolyte therapy should also be adjusted. Drug dosages should be adjusted downward in elderly patients because of their age-related decline in renal function.[64]

Comorbid conditions also require attention. Urinary tract infections should be aggressively treated to prevent further deterioration of renal function. Uncontrolled hypertension should be treated.[65]

Adequate nutrition appears to be important for recovery from renal failure,[66,67] but nutritional support in the patient with ARF can be complicated.[68] Patients who are critically ill are hypercatabolic, with an increased energy expenditure and increased protein turnover with negative nitrogen balance. They often have comorbid disease processes that impair their nutritional status. Although renal failure decreases energy expenditure, dialysis may increase energy expenditure, so it would seem appropriate to increase protein and caloric intake in these patients. However, in some patients, decreasing the dietary protein intake will decrease glomerular hyperfiltration and may slow the progression of renal failure.[69,70] Measurement of nitrogen balance, along with more sophisticated techniques such as metabolic cart measurements, will help guide nutritional support.

RENAL REPLACEMENT THERAPY

Patients who have symptomatic fluid overload associated with congestive heart failure, encephalopathy, or acid-base and electrolyte disorders may require some degree of artificial renal support. Dialysis is necessary to correct encephalopathy or severe metabolic disorders. Other criteria for initiating renal replacement therapy (RRT) in the critically ill ICU patient have been proposed: these include azotemia, uremic pericarditis, neuropathy and myopathy, acute respiratory distress syndrome, and sepsis.[71,72] Elevated absolute values of BUN and creatinine are not indicators for dialysis.

If dialysis is indicated, it should be initiated promptly. Early dialysis in ARF is associated with improved survival.[14,73,74]

There are many options for providing RRT in the hospital setting, and each has advantages and disadvantages [see Table 3]. RRT can be done with an intermittent or a continuous technique.[75] Standard intermittent techniques include peritoneal dialysis and intermittent hemodialysis. These are typically used in patients with established renal failure who are already receiving some form of RRT and are undergoing an elective procedure. Continuous therapy is most commonly employed in critically ill ICU patients.

Along with the clinical setting, the indications for replacement therapy guide the selection of the appropriate method of RRT. Therapy may be required to remove fluid, metabolic wastes, or both. These management decisions are made in conjunction with nephrologists to provide optimal care to the patient requiring RRT.

Acute continuous hemodiafiltration is an excellent option in critically ill patients, who often are too hemodynamically labile to tolerate standard hemodialysis.[76-79] The most commonly employed method is continuous venovenohemodialysis (CVVHD). This method of dialysis is usually performed via a temporary double-lumen central venous dialysis catheter, which is placed percutaneously in the subclavian, internal jugular, or femoral vein. Blood is pumped by a peristaltic pump through a filter against the flow of peritoneal dialysate, which is pumped into the nonblood portion of the filter in the opposite direction. The machine is programmed and various concentrations of dialysate are chosen to effect the desired removal

Table 3 Comparison of Renal Replacement Therapy Options[147]

	Advantages	Disadvantages
Intermittent hemodialysis	Efficient fluid, filtrate, and solute removal	Hemodynamic instability; resource and personnel intensive
Continuous renal replacement therapy (CVVH/D, CAVH/D, hemofiltration)	Hemodynamic stability; multiple filtration options; relative ease of use	Inefficient fluid and filtrate removal; requires immobilization and continuous anticoagulation
Peritoneal dialysis	No vascular access, hemodynamic stability, minimal equipment	Contraindicated in abdominal surgery patients; peritonitis

of fluid and wastes.[2,79] Continous arteriovenous hemodiafiltration (CAVHD) is performed in the same way but requires large-bore arterial access or a Scribner shunt in addition to venous access. This method allows for slow but continuous removal of fluid and clearance of toxic wastes. Compared with intermittent hemodialysis, continuous RRT provides better hemodynamic stability, maintenance of cerebral perfusion, and control of fluid balance. It is therefore indicated in patients with renal failure and critical illness and may be the treatment of choice for ARF in this patient population.[2,72,80]

Patients who have fluid overload as evidenced by cardiopulmonary congestive failure but no other need for dialysis can be treated with continuous hemofiltration, which permits clearance of fluid and plasma solutes.[2,81,82] Continuous hemofiltration can be performed in patients who are hemodynamically unstable and can be done using the same machine and vascular access as that used for CVVHD. This process may be particularly useful in patients with severe cardiac failure and sepsis, in whom the ability to remove proinflammatory mediators may improve the clinical course.[2]

Treatment of patients requiring dialysis or other RRT should be directed at returning renal function to normal levels, or at least to levels that eliminate the need for renal support. Free water clearance or creatinine clearance should be monitored. Improvement in these urinary clearance measurements may signal a return to normal or baseline renal function. It is important to remember that baseline renal function in the elderly is usually less than normal.

For patients who do progress to renal failure, recovery depends on age, cause of renal failure, and urine output during the time of renal dysfunction. Young patients and those who maintain adequate urine output despite ARF have a significantly better prognosis.[33,83] Mortality in patients with severe ARF has remained unchanged despite improved dialysis and other advances[8]; it ranges from 30% to 80% and varies with comorbid factors. It is highest in patients with multiorgan failure from infection or SIRS. Of patients who survive ARF, most can discontinue dialysis after recovery of renal function.[84]

Death related to renal failure is most often caused by infectious complications. Pneumonia is the most common fatal infection, although peritonitis and urinary infection may lead to sepsis and death. Bleeding complications may occur as a result of platelet dysfunction caused by uremia and heparin anticoagulation during dialysis; this may also contribute to death in these patients.[85-87]

Chronic Renal Failure

Chronic renal failure (CRF), which is irreversible, may be caused by a number of factors. Diabetes mellitus, hypertension, glomerular diseases, obstructive disease with chronic pyelonephritis, congenital hypoplasia or aplasia, tubulointerstitial diseases, and polycystic disease are the most common causes of CRF.[88] These patients will have varying degrees of renal insufficiency, and as in patients with acute renal failure, a good history and physical examination are critical in their evaluation in the perioperative period [see Table 4]. Particular attention should be paid to the baseline status of the patient whenever possible. This includes attention to baseline blood pressure and cardiac function; urine output; medications that may affect blood pressure, renal blood flow, and cardiac output; and any history of preexisting renal disease or signs and symptoms of obstruction and urinary tract infection.

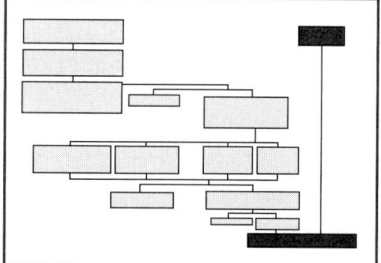

Perioperative Management of Patients with Renal Failure

Elective and emergency operations can be performed safely in patients with renal failure. Many patients will experience some complication. The most common complication is hyperkalemia; others include volume overload, bleeding, and infection.[89] However, most of these complications can be prevented or managed with both preoperative and postoperative dialysis, judicious use of appropriate perioperative antibiotics, choice of anesthetic agents, and meticulous surgical technique and hemostasis. Attention should be paid to maintaining blood pressure and volume homeostasis before, during, and after surgery. In addition, attention to operative planning, exposure, blood loss, and the use of renal protective measures where possible becomes important.[46,55] In patients with a hemodialysis access graft, hospital staff should also be cautioned to avoid measurement of blood pressures and placement of I.V. access in the arm with the graft.

The patient with stable renal failure requires standard preoperative evaluation before elective surgery. Particular attention is paid to fluid and electrolyte status. In patients on chronic dialysis who are stable, dialysis is usually performed the day before and the day after the procedure, and more often as necessary.[9] Patients on peritoneal dialysis who are to have an intra-abdominal procedure will require vascular access for hemodialysis. In the patient with acute or acute-on-chronic renal failure who has volume overload or severe metabolic imbalance, dialysis should be performed early and should be aggressive.[11,90] Patients with hepatorenal syndrome may be dialyzed throughout liver transplantation surgery to deal with the large fluid volumes often required for the procedure.

Patients who require emergency surgery and cannot be dialyzed may become hyperkalemic and require medical management. Calcium (e.g., 5 to 10 ml of 10% calcium chloride solution I.V. over 2 minutes) will stabilize cardiac membranes. Subsequently, the intravenous administration of sodium bicarbonate (44 mEq over 5 minutes) and insulin (e.g., 10 to 25 U over 30 minutes) will drive potassium into the cells; those are given along with glucose (e.g., 250 ml of 20% dextrose) to counterbalance the hypoglycemic effects of the insulin. Sodium polystyrene sulfonate (Kayexalate), an orally or rectally administered exchange resin, will bind potassium. However, this agent takes hours to work.

The actions of some neuromuscular blockers and anticholinesterases are affected by renal failure.[91,92] Their use can potentiate acidosis and hyperkalemia. In particular, the use of succinylcholine, which causes a transient hyperkalemia in normal persons, is controversial in the anesthetic management of the patient with renal failure.[93]

Intraoperative hypotension should be avoided. This is particularly true in patients with chronic renal insufficiency but without end-stage disease requiring dialysis, who are at greatest risk for ARF and for the development of toxic nephropathies in the postoperative period.[94] In addition, hypotension may lead to dialysis graft thrombosis.

Postoperatively, patients with renal failure should be managed as any other patient. However, special consideration must be given to fluid and electrolyte management and acid-base balance. Dialysis should be instituted early to prevent complications.[9] Wound healing may be delayed in renal failure patients.[94] In addition, these patients may be protein malnourished, which will also affect wound healing.[68] Appropriate nutritional support is essential in these patients (see above). Nutritional support should be provided as early as possible postoperatively, and the enteral route is preferred.[66] Drug dosages should be modified for those drugs that are excreted renally or are dialyzable.[95]

Patients who have prolonged bleeding times as a result of renal failure are managed with dialysis. Those with clinically evident bleeding may require cryoprecipitate, vasopressin (DDAVP), and conjugated estrogens to correct bleeding disorders.[96]

Table 4 Findings Suggestive of Chronic Rather Than Acute Renal Failure

History
- Symptoms of uremia (e.g., nausea, pruritus, malaise, weakness, mental status changes, weight loss, edema)
- Hypertension
- Hematuria or proteinuria
- Abnormal blood chemistry values (elevated urea nitrogen or creatinine levels)

Physical examination
- Debility
- Alopecia
- Excoriations and yellow pallor of skin
- Peripheral neuropathy
- Conjunctival calcification
- Band keratopathy
- Gynecomastia, testicular atrophy, or both

Laboratory examination*
- Anemia on presentation (only if there is no history of acute blood loss)
- Low urinary sodium level or high urine osmolarity (either suggests prerenal azotemia)

X-rays or ultrasonography
- Bilateral small kidneys
- Other evidence of long-standing renal dysfunction (e.g., chronic obstruction, pyelonephritis, or polycystic kidney disease)
- Bone changes of secondary hyperparathyroidism (e.g., osteitis fibrosa cystica, osteomalacia, or osteosclerosis)

*Serum chemistry values are not helpful, because they may be altered in both acute and chronic renal failure.

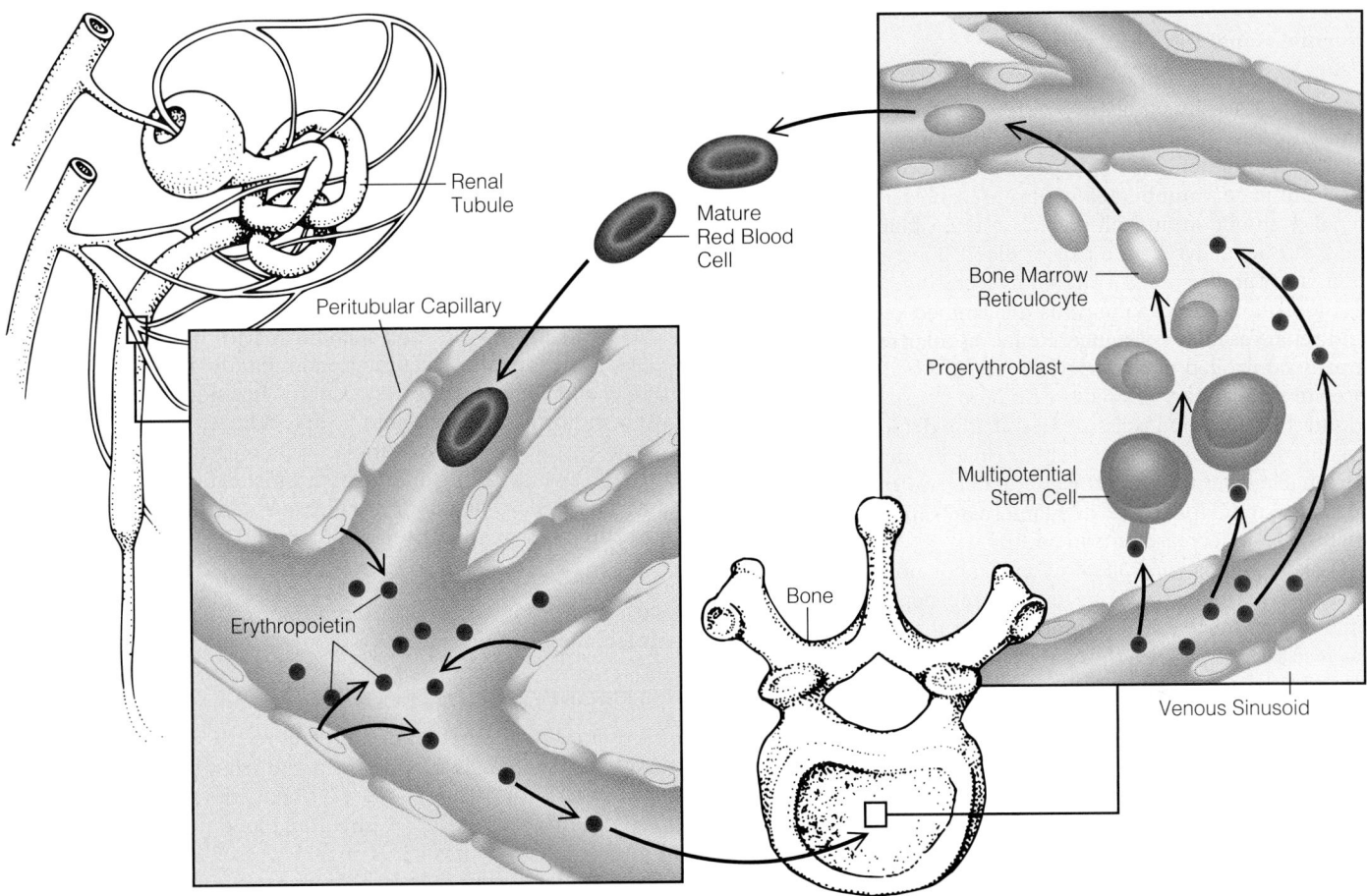

Figure 1 **The rate of red cell production in the marrow is determined by erythropoietin elaboration in the kidneys. In normal kidneys, as shown here, endothelial cells in the tubules or peritubular capillaries are thought to produce most of the renal erythropoietin. Synthesis is stimulated by renal hypoxemia. (The hypoxemia would not necessarily be caused by anemia. It could, for example, be the result of dwelling at high altitudes.) In the marrow, the erythropoietin binds to erythroid progenitors, stimulating their differentiation and proliferation. In patients with renal failure, decreased production of erythropoietin by the diseased kidneys impairs erythropoiesis in the marrow. Red cell morphology is unaffected, however.**

Many patients on chronic hemodialysis are anemic because of decreased endogenous erythropoietin levels [*see Figure 1*] and blood losses during dialysis, as well as depletion of iron stores. Blood transfusions were commonly used to treat anemia in these patients until the 1990s, when recombinant erythropoietin became available. This agent has largely eliminated the need for transfusions and their associated morbidity; it also corrects clotting abnormalities associated with decreased platelet function and improves quality of life.[97-101] Blood transfusion remains necessary, however, in the setting of acute blood loss with hemodynamic compromise.

Discussion

Perspective on Acute Renal Failure

The incidence of ARF has decreased since the mid-1940s; however, mortality among patients who have renal failure severe enough to necessitate dialysis has not been improved.[8,44] This lack of improvement appears to be related to the increasing percentage of patients who experience acute renal failure as one manifestation of multiorgan failure. Mortality from ARF without multiorgan dysfunction is 8% to 30%, whereas mortality from renal failure that is associated with sepsis or multiorgan failure is 70% to 80%.[8,39,44]

Groups of patients at risk for acute renal failure can be identified, but the specific degree of risk for an individual patient cannot be calculated. Patients with burns, severe injury, prolonged periods of hypoperfusion, or cardiopulmonary bypass are at significantly higher risk for ARF than routine surgical patients.[25,102-104] Other than relative amount of injury or ischemia, the variables that correlate with renal failure are older age and a history of limited renal function.[44] Tests to predict renal failure and outcome of renal failure have proved elusive.[42,105]

It is well accepted that the fundamental goal in the management of ARF is prevention, or at least limitation of its severity. Attention to the cause or causes of acute renal dysfunction and to the mechanisms involved often permits correction of the problem before progression to actual renal failure occurs. If acute renal dysfunction and failure are to be managed by prevention, early diagnosis, and correction, it is necessary to understand renal pathophysiology.

Normal Renal Physiology

Understanding of both normal and altered renal physiology is greatly aided by familiarity with the anatomy of the nephron and with the sites of action of the hormones essential to normal renal function [see Figure 2]. Anatomic or functional injury to a sufficient number of nephrons can lead to measurable renal dysfunction and ultimately to renal failure. Renal function can be analyzed in terms of blood flow, glomerular filtration, and tubular reabsorption and secretion.

Blood flow to the kidneys is determined by cardiac output and renal vascular resistance. Renal vascular resistance is principally controlled at the arteriolar level. When renal perfusion pressure falls, the efferent arterioles constrict to maintain glomerular filtration pressure despite the decreased flow. If the systemic systolic pressure drops below 70 mm Hg, however, this mechanism fails and the afferent arterioles constrict, leading to a rapid decrease in glomerular filtration and consequently to a decrease in urine output.

This system is controlled by several hormonal and mediator systems that act at various sites in the nephron. The renin-angiotensin mechanism is important for the control of arteriolar resistance.[106,107] When renal perfusion pressure falls, secretion of renin by the juxtaglomerular apparatus increases. This leads to increased production of angiotensin I, which is converted to angiotensin II. Angiotensin II is a powerful vasoconstrictor that increases peripheral vascular resistance.

Nitric oxide and prostaglandins have been found to be important mediators of blood flow to different areas of the kidney[1,108] and may exert some control over renin release through a feedback mechanism. Catecholamines, ATP-$MgCl_2$, and calcium[109,110] have also been found to participate in the control of renal blood flow. Adequate blood flow largely controls glomerular filtration and is essential for normal renal function.

Glomerular filtration is determined by the hydrostatic pressure in the afferent arteriole and by the filtration coefficient, K_f. The glomerular filtration rate is an important variable but is not easily measured[111]; it is usually approximated by calculations based on creatinine clearance (C_{Cr}) or free water clearance (C_{H_2O}). These clearance values (expressed in ml/min) can be calculated by the following formulas:

$$C_{Cr} = V \times (U_{Cr}/P_{Cr})$$
$$C_{H_2O} = V - C_{osm} = V - [V \times (U_{osm}/P_{osm})]$$

in which V is urine volume (ml/min), C_{osm} is osmolar clearance, U_{osm} is urine osmolality (mOsm/L), and P_{osm} is plasma osmolality (mOsm/L).

These calculations are usually indexed to a standard patient size (1.73 m^2 body surface area) by multiplying each calculated clearance by 1.73/patient's estimated body surface area. The creatinine clearance provides a good estimate of the glomerular filtration rate. A positive C_{H_2O} measures net water excretion; a negative C_{H_2O} measures water retention. A change in free water clearance into the range of ± 0.15 ml/min precedes a rise in creatinine by 24 to 48 hours. Free water clearance is not routinely measured, however, and does not usually establish the diagnosis of renal dysfunction. Rather, renal dysfunction is signaled clinically by the onset of oliguria or a rising serum creatinine level.

Most physicians use the serum creatinine level as an indicator of GFR because it is the simplest to determine. However, a small fraction of creatinine is secreted into the renal tubular fluid. The serum creatinine level becomes a less accurate measure of GFR as the relative component of creatinine clearance from GFR decreases.[112] Furthermore, medications such as cimetidine and the cephalosporin antibiotics can be measured as creatinine in laboratory tests and thus can give a falsely decreased measure of GFR.[20-23] Despite its limitations, however, measurement of serum creatinine levels continues to be the mainstay of the initial assessment of GFR and renal clearance.

The principal functions of the renal tubules are reabsorption of sodium and water.[113] Sodium reabsorption occurs in the distal tubule and is controlled primarily by aldosterone.[114] Water reabsorption occurs predominantly in the collecting tubule and is regulated by antidiuretic hormone (ADH), which is also known as vasopressin.[115] In addition, atrial natriuretic factor appears to affect tubular cells and the renal vasculature.[116] Hypovolemia and hypotension cause increased production of these hormones, which act to increase tubular reabsorption in an attempt to maintain intravascular volume.

Pathophysiology of Acute Renal Failure: Cellular and Molecular Changes

PRERENAL PATHOPHYSIOLOGY

Prerenal causes of acute renal failure are principally associated with inadequate blood flow and altered hemodynamics[117] and account for 50% to 90% of ARF, with the exact distribution somewhat varied.[118,119] Impaired blood flow to the kidneys is the result of hypovolemia in most cases and of depressed myocardial function in a small percentage of patients with an acute cardiac insult or chronic cardiac dysfunction. Renal injury from inadequate perfusion can be exacerbated if low arterial oxygen saturation further impairs oxygen delivery.[120]

The decreased arterial and arteriolar pressures associated with hypovolemia cause production of ADH and aldosterone to increase; the reabsorption of sodium and water is thereby increased as well. If the systemic systolic pressure falls below 70 mm Hg, afferent arterioles constrict, decreasing the GFR further.[121] This decrease in glomerular filtration leads to increased sodium reabsorption and concentrated urine, eventually resulting in the urine characteristics associated with a prerenal cause of renal dysfunction—namely, low urine sodium levels, low fractional excretion of sodium, and high urine specific gravity.

Renal blood flow can also be impaired by high intra-abdominal pressure, which seems to decrease renal blood flow.[7,30,122,123] Prompt reduction of increased intra-abdominal pressure appears to correct developing renal failure, possibly because of improved renal blood flow.

RENAL PARENCHYMAL PATHOPHYSIOLOGY

Redistribution of blood flow inside the kidneys can occur as a result of systemic infection, SIRS, or the hepatorenal syndrome,[58,59] causing glomerular filtration to decrease. The changes in small renal vessel impedance that mediate intrarenal blood flow distribution are probably controlled by local release of prostaglandins and nitric oxide.[108,124] The use of prostaglandin inhibitors or inhibitors of inducible nitric oxide synthase, however, has not been shown to alter function or outcome in patients with systemic infection, SIRS, or the hepatorenal syndrome.

Pathophysiologic changes associated with parenchymal injury depend on the specific cause of renal injury. Several such changes

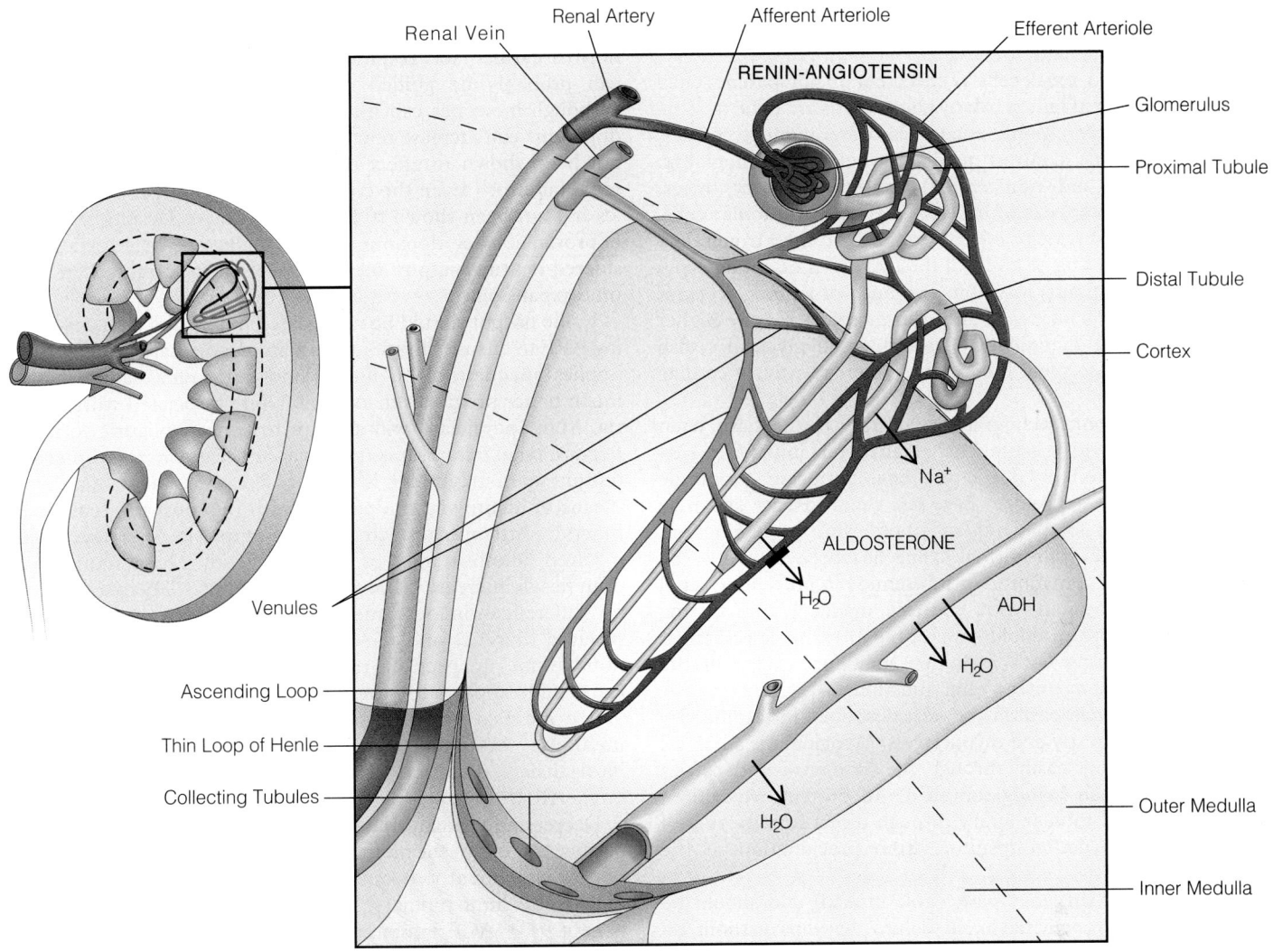

RENIN-ANGIOTENSIN

Renal Vein · Renal Artery · Afferent Arteriole · Efferent Arteriole

Glomerulus

Proximal Tubule

Distal Tubule

Cortex

Na⁺

ALDOSTERONE

H_2O

ADH

H_2O

Venules

Ascending Loop

Thin Loop of Henle

Collecting Tubules

H_2O

Outer Medulla

Inner Medulla

Figure 2 **Depicted are the major anatomic features of a juxtamedullary nephron, its blood supply, and the sites of action of the renin-angiotensin system, aldosterone, and ADH. The renin-angiotensin system controls resistance in the renal arterioles, primarily the efferent arteriole. By constricting the efferent arteriole, angiotensin can increase the glomerular pressure, thereby helping to maintain a relatively constant glomerular filtration rate even in the face of low arterial pressure. Aldosterone affects sodium reabsorption in the late distal tubule and the collecting duct. When aldosterone is present in large amounts, virtually all of the sodium is reabsorbed, and almost none is excreted. In the absence of aldosterone, however, substantial quantities of sodium are not reabsorbed and are excreted in the urine. ADH affects the permeability of the epithelium of the collecting duct. When ADH is absent, the collecting duct is almost totally impermeable to water. When it is present in substantial concentrations, however, the collecting duct becomes highly permeable to water; this increased permeability, coupled with the hyperosmolality of the medullary interstitial fluid, results in rapid reabsorption of water from the collecting duct.**

may occur concomitantly. Impairment of tubular function by ischemia, toxic substances, or increased intraluminal pressure may alter the normal polarity between the luminal and basal surfaces of the cell membranes of the tubular cells. This loss of polarity alters membrane function, disrupts the microfilaments in the cells, and causes intercellular tight junctions to open, thereby affecting transport of sodium and potassium and inducing fluid shifts.[125] Progression of tubular functional impairment eventually leads to alterations in ultrafiltrate flow by several mechanisms. Swelling of tubular cells or increased back pressure from distal obstruction raises tubular luminal pressure, thereby decreasing glomerular filtration. Simultaneously, the loss of integrity of the tubular cell junctions leads to back-leakage of fluid into the renal interstitium.[126,127] Tubular glomerular feedback may also occur, in which the relatively high sodium concentration at the distal tubule near the macula densa leads to reflex vasoconstriction of the afferent arterioles and consequently a further decrease in glomerular filtration.[128] Renal blood flow may be further affected by the shunting of blood from the cortex to the medulla, probably in association with increased nitric oxide production.

There are two major parenchymal causes of ARF. The first is ischemia, which is a common cause of tubular injury. The medullary thick ascending limb of the loop of Henle and the pars recta of the proximal tubule are the segments of the nephron most sensitive to ischemia.[129] Tubular cells can be identified in the urine of patients with this form of renal injury, which is sometimes called acute tubular necrosis. The term is not an accurate pathologic description of this form of renal injury but continues to be used, frequently to describe any renal parenchymal cause of ARF.

Toxic injury to renal cells is the other major parenchymal cause of acute renal failure. Many compounds are toxic to renal tissue; the most commonly encountered are aminoglycosides, ionic radiographic contrast media, myoglobin, hemoglobin, cyclosporine,[130] and nonsteroidal anti-inflammatory drugs. Aminoglycosides appear to have toxic effects on tubular cells, with the extent of toxicity related primarily to their trough levels. Close monitoring of levels of these drugs is essential, especially in burn patients, in whom clearance of aminoglycosides and other drugs is increased and who therefore require higher doses to achieve therapeutic levels.[131] Aminoglycosides also appear to decrease renal blood flow independently of cardiac output.[132]

Intravenous ionic radiographic contrast media have been demonstrated to cause acute renal parenchymal injury. The toxicity is potentiated by decreased renal perfusion. Nonionic contrast material appears to have less renal toxicity and may be an alternative for patients with borderline renal function. Pretreatment with half-normal saline has been shown to be more effective than mannitol or furosemide in preventing renal dysfunction associated with contrast media.[63] Use of the dopaminergic agonist fenoldopam or the nitric oxide scavenger acetylcysteine along with hydration may further lesson the effects of contrast agents on renal function.[47,48]

ARF from myoglobinuria was first described in trauma victims with crush injury and myonecrosis. Myoglobin is an 18 kd protein that filters easily through the glomeruli and causes more damage than hemoglobin, a 67 kd protein. Myoglobin appears to cause tubular injury through direct toxicity as well as through obstruction resulting from precipitation in the tubule.[3]

Many other toxins may play a role in ARF and should be considered if parenchymal renal failure develops without an apparent cause.[126]

Inflammatory and vasculitic causes of ARF are uncommon in surgical patients. These disease processes usually present as medical problems associated with autoimmune or postinfectious states. Still, appropriate workup is required to rule out other contributing causes or processes. Identification of red cell or white cell casts and proteinuria is useful in diagnosing inflammation.

SYNDROME OF INAPPROPRIATE ANTIDIURETIC HORMONE SECRETION

The diagnosis of SIADH is made by excluding other causes of oliguria. Patients with SIADH have low urine output, high urine sodium levels, and low serum sodium levels. Furthermore, serum creatinine levels do not usually rise in these patients, despite prolonged borderline oliguria. Treatment consists of water restriction, although some patients require diuretics.[133] Hypertonic saline is infused only if the patient appears to be symptomatic from hyponatremia. SIADH usually resolves spontaneously with no injurious consequences to the kidneys.

Treatment of Developing Acute Renal Failure

If prevention fails, treatment of developing acute renal failure is directed at preserving remaining renal function and limiting further damage by increasing blood flow and urine output and decreasing tubular cell injury. Adequate renal blood flow is essential in treating renal injury from all causes and is usual-

ly successfully achieved by volume infusion. In patients with normal cardiac and respiratory function, fluid administration can probably be guided with only a central venous line. Although inotropes can increase cardiac output and low-dose dopamine can increase renal blood flow, use of these agents has not been shown to affect the incidence or outcome of acute renal failure.[134] Even the combination of inotropes and diuretics has not been shown to have any effect.[135] Despite this lack of proven efficacy, dopamine (2 to 5 mg/kg/min) should be considered if urine output does not respond to intravascular volume expansion.

Urine output should be maintained in patients with developing ARF to ensure filtration; in addition, adequate urine output implies adequate blood flow. Nonoliguric renal failure has a much better prognosis than renal failure associated with oliguria. Many physicians will attempt to convert oliguric to nonoliguric renal failure. It is unclear whether the increase in urine output upon treatment is an actual conversion or simply a means of identifying the patients with the most residual renal function. Attempts to increase urine output in ARF have often involved administration of diuretics. Studies have found that diuretics do increase GFR and urine output.[33] There have been no differences in outcome, however, between patients who received diuretics and those who did not; this result is most notable in prospective, randomized trials.[136] Response to furosemide appears to have only prognostic value in ARF.[33,136] There are also potential problems with high-dose diuretics, including ototoxicity, arrhythmias, and hypokalemia.[37] Nevertheless, diuretics still are commonly used to treat developing ARF.[37,38,44]

Decreasing tubular injury is an attractive concept. Mannitol has been found to shrink tubular cells, but like diuretics, it does not affect patient outcome.[137] The use of calcium channel blockers to limit tubular cell damage may have some clinical benefit.[138-140] ACE inhibitors may limit injury in patients with diabetic renal disease because of the drugs' ability to decrease arteriolar and glomerular capillary pressures.[141] The use of agents that modify nitric oxide production may provide a means of treating evolving renal failure. Other molecular therapies for renal failure, including the use of epidermal growth factor, are under investigation.[141] Elimination of nephrotoxic substances and maintenance of perfusion are currently the only effective methods for decreasing tubular injury.

Differential Diagnosis of Acute Renal Failure

Because prevention and limitation of renal injury are the goals in the management of ARF, early diagnosis is essential. However, determination of which patients with oliguria or elevated serum creatinine levels will progress to ARF and differentiation among the causes of their renal dysfunction remain difficult.

A measurable change in free water clearance into the range of ± 0.17 ml/min/1.73 m² body surface area or a creatinine clearance of 30 ml/min/1.73 m² body surface area indicates ARF.[41] These calculated clearances do not identify the cause of ARF, however. Identification of the cause is best accomplished through physical examination, review of the history and treatment, urinalysis, and measurement of urine and plasma sodium and creatinine levels. The most reliable means of differentiating prerenal from other causes of ARF are measurement of urine sodium levels and calculation of the fractional excretion of sodium.[43] The renal failure index (RFI) is another means of distinguishing prerenal causes and is defined as follows:

$$RFI = [U_{Na}/(U_{Cr}/P_{Cr})] \times 100$$

This formula is similar to that for the fractional excretion of sodium:

$$FE_{Na} = [(U_{Na}/P_{Na})/(U_{Cr}/P_{Cr})] \times 100$$

Although the RFI is used by some nephrologists, it is not superior to FE_{Na} in discriminating between prerenal and renal parenchymal causes of ARF.[119] The usefulness of FE_{Na} for diagnosing ARF has been challenged in some reports[142,143]; however, these reports failed to measure FE_{Na} at the same period in the course of acute renal failure.[144] Furthermore, complaints that FE_{Na} is not predictive are not well founded, because the calculation is not intended to be a predictor but rather a tool for distinguishing prerenal from renal parenchymal causes of ARF.[14,40,145,146]

Other tests to distinguish the causes of ARF are of limited value, except in identifying possible parenchymal disorders. The presence of red cell and white cell casts may indicate vasculitic or inflammatory causes. Identification of tubular cells in the urine, either microscopically or by detection of surface antigen, suggests a postischemic cause, but these markers are not specific.

Measurement of urine electrolyte concentrations (e.g., chloride and bicarbonate), measurement of the products of inflammation (e.g., complement components), and renal biopsy are useful in assessing chronic renal problems; however, these determinations add little to the diagnosis and treatment of ARF.

References

1. Nissenson AR: Acute renal failure: Definition and pathogenesis. Kidney Int 53 (suppl 66):S-7, 1998

2. Ronco C, Barbacini S, Digito A, et al: Achievements and new directions in continuous renal replacement therapies. New Horizons 3:708, 1995

3. Slater MS, Mullins RJ: Rhabdomyolysis and myoglobinuric renal failure in trauma and surgical patients: a review. J Am Coll Surg 186:695, 1998

4. Quader MA, Sawmiller C, Sumpio BA: Contrast-induced nephropathy: review of incidence and pathophysiology. Ann Vasc Surg 12:612, 1998

5. Tublin ME, Murphy ME, Tessler FN: Current concepts in contrast media induced nephropathy. AJR Am J Roentgenol 171:933, 1998

6. Thadani RI, Camargo CA, Xavier RJ, et al: Atheroembolic renal failure after invasive procedures. Natural history based on 52 histologically proven cases. Medicine (Baltimore) 74:350, 1995

7. Tan IK, Kua JS: Abdominal compartment syndrome and acute anuria. Nephrol Dial Transplant 13:2651, 1998

8. Alkhunaizi AM, Schrier RW: Management of acute renal failure: new perspectives. Am J Kidney Dis 28:315, 1996

9. Lazarus JM, Morgan AP, Tilney NL: Patients with chronic renal failure: general management and acute surgical illness. Surgical Care of the Patient with Renal Failure. Tilney NL, Lazarus JM, Eds. WB Saunders Co, Philadelphia, 1982, p 1

10. Vincent F: Preoperative and postoperative care: renal disease. Handbook of Surgery. Schrock TR, Ed. Jones Medical Publications, Greenbrae, California, 1985, p 47

11. Bellomo R, Parkin G, Love J, et al: A prospective comparative study of continuous arteriovenous hemodiafiltration and continuous venovenous hemodiafiltration in critically ill patients. Am J Kidney Dis 21:400, 1993

12. Rosen T: Uremic pruritus: a review. Cutis 23:790, 1979

13. Engle WD: Evaluation of renal function and acute renal failure in the neonate. Pediatr Clin North Am 33:129, 1986

14. Tilney NL, Lazarus JM: Acute renal failure in surgical patients: causes, clinical patterns, and care. Surg Clin North Am 63:357, 1983

15. Narayanan S: Renal biochemistry and physiology: pathophysiology and analytical perspectives. Adv Clin Chem 29:121, 1992

16. Espinel CH: Diagnosis of acute and chronic renal failure. Clin Lab Med 13:89, 1993

17. Bjornsson TD: Use of serum creatinine concentrations to determine renal function. Clin Pharmacokinet 4:200, 1979

18. Rowe JW: Clinical research on aging: strategies and directions. N Engl J Med 297:1332, 1977

19. Lieberthal W, Levinsky NG: Treatment of acute tubular necrosis. Semin Nephrol 10:571, 1990

20. Nanji AA, Campbell DJ: Falsely elevated serum creatinine values in diabetic ketoacidosis: clinical implications. Clin Biochem 14:91, 1981

21. Guay DR, Meatherall RC, Macauley PA: Interference of selected second and third generation cephalosporins with creatinine determination. Am J Hosp Pharm 40:435, 1983

22. Shouval D, Ligumsky M, Ben-Ishay D: Effects of co-trimoxazole on normal creatinine clearance. Lancet 1:244, 1978

23. Larsson R, Bodemar G, Kagedal B, et al: The effects of cimetidine (Tagamet) on renal function in patients with renal failure. Acta Med Scand 208:27, 1980

24. Baek SM, Makabali GG, Shoemaker WC: Clinical determinants of survival from postoperative renal failure. Surg Gynecol Obstet 140:685, 1975

25. Kellerman PS: Perioperative care of the renal patient. Arch Intern Med 154:1674, 1994

26. Finn WF, Arendshorst WJ, Gottschalk CW: Pathogenesis of oliguria in acute renal failure. Circ Res 36:675, 1975

27. Burnier M, Schrier RW: Pathogenesis of acute renal failure. Adv Exp Med Biol 212:3, 1987

28. Fishchereder M, Trick W, Nath KA: Therapeutic strategies in the prevention of acute renal failure. Semin Nephrol 14:41, 1994

29. Sugrue M: Prospective study of intra-abdominal hypertension and renal function after laparotomy. Br J Surg 82:235, 1995

30. Dunn MD, McDougall EM: Renal physiology. Laparoscopic considerations. Urol Clin North Am 27:609, 2000

31. Link D, Leff RG, Hildel J, et al: The use of percutaneous nephrostomy in 42 patients. J Urol 122:9, 1979

32. Bunn F, Lefebvre C, Li Wan Po A, et al: Human albumin solution for resuscitation and volume expansion in critically ill patients. The Cochrane Database of Systematic Reviews 2:CD 001208, 2000

33. Anderson RJ, Linas SL, Berns AS, et al: Nonoliguric acute renal failure. N Engl J Med 296:1134, 1977

34. Aurora RN: Preventing renal failure in critically ill patients. Crit Care Med 27:2044, 1999

35. Bonventre JV, Weinberg JM: Kidney preservation ex vivo for transplantation. Annu Rev Med 43:523, 1992

36. Cantarovich F, Galli C, Benedetti L, et al: High dose frusemide in established acute renal failure. Br Med J 4:449, 1973

37. Martin SJ, Danziger LH: Continuous infusion of loop diuretics in the critically ill: a review of the literature. Crit Care Med 22:1323, 1994

38. Kellum JA: Use of diuretics in the acute care setting. Kidney Int 53(suppl 66):S67, 1998

39. DuBose TD, Warnock DG, Mehta R, et al: Acute renal failure in the 21st century: recommendations for management and outcomes assessment. Am J Kidney Dis 29:793, 1997.

40. Farber MD, Kupin WL, Krishna GG, et al: The differential diagnosis of acute renal failure. Acute Renal Failure, 3rd ed. Lazarus JM, Brenner BM, Eds. WB Saunders Co, Philadelphia, 1993, p 133

41. Brown R, Babcock R, Talbert J, et al: Renal function in critically ill postoperative patients: sequential assessment of creatinine osmolar and free water clearance. Crit Care Med 8:68, 1980

42. Kellen M, Aronson S, Roizen MF, et al: Predictive and diagnostic tests of renal failure: a review. Anesth Analg 78:134, 1994

43. Miller TR, Anderson RJ, Linas SL: Urinary diagnostic indices in acute renal failure: a prospective study. Ann Intern Med 89:47, 1978

44. Thadani R, Pascual M, Bonventre JV: Acute renal failure. N Engl J Med 334:1448, 1996

45. Belzberg H, Cornwell EE, Berne TV: The critical care of the severely injured patient: pulmonary and renal support. Surg Clin North Am 76:971, 1996

46. Garwood S: New pharmacologic options for renal preservation. Anesth Clin North Am 18:753, 2000

47. Mathur VS, Swan SK, Lambrecht LJ, et al: The effects of fenoldopam, a selective dopamine receptor agonist, on systemic and renal hemodynamics in normotensive subjects. Crit Care Med 27:1832, 1999

48. Tepel M, Van der Giet M, Schwarzfeld C, et al: Prevention of radiographic-contrast induced reductions in renal function by acetylcysteine. N Engl J Med 343:180, 2000

49. Flamenbaum W, Gehr M, Gross M, et al: Acute renal failure associated with myoglobinemia and hemoglobinemia. Acute Renal Failure. Brenner BM, Lazarus JM, Eds. WB Saunders Co, Philadelphia, 1983, p 269

50. Mattern WD, Sommers SC, Kassirer JP: Oliguric acute renal failure in malignant hypertension. Am J Med 52:187, 1972

51. Goldberg LI: Cardiovascular and renal actions of dopamine: potential clinical applications. Pharmacol Rev 24:1, 1972

52. Bellomo R, Cole L, Ronco C: Hemodynamic support and the role of dopamine. Kidney Int 53:(suppl 66):S71, 1998

53. Davis RF, Lappas DG, Kirklin JK, et al: Acute oliguria after cardiopulmonary bypass: renal functional improvement with low-dose dopamine infu-

sion. Crit Care Med 10:852, 1982

54. Pavoni V, Verri M, Volta CA, et al: Plasma dopamine concentration and effects of low dopamine doses on urinary output after major vascular surgery. Kidney Int 53(suppl 66):S75, 1998

55. Allen BT, Anderson CB, Rubin BG, et al: Preservation of renal function in juxtarenal and suprarenal abdominal aortic aneurysm repair. J Vasc Surg 17:948, 1993

56. Pascual J, Liano F, Ortuno J: The elderly patient with acute renal failure. J Am Soc Nephrol 6:144, 1995

57. Braun SR, Weiss FR, Keller AI, et al: Evaluation of the renal toxicity of heme proteins and their derivatives: a role in the genesis of acute tubular necrosis. J Exp Med 131:443, 1970

58. Laffi G, LaVilla G, Gentilini P: Pathogenesis and management of the hepatorenal syndrome. Semin Liver Dis 14:71, 1994

59. Keller F, Heinze H, Jochimsen F, et al: Risk factors and outcome of 107 patients with decompensated liver disease and acute renal failure: the role of hemodialysis. Renal Failure 17:135, 1995

60. Goedje O, Koeke K, Lichtwarck-Aschoff M, et al: Continuous cardiac output by femoral arterial thermodilution calibrated pulse contour analysis: comparison with pulmonary arterial thermodilution. Crit Care Med 27:2407, 1999

61. Finn WF: Enhanced recovery from postischemic acute renal failure: micropuncture studies in the rat. Circ Res 46:440, 1980

62. Russo D, Memoli B, Andreucci VE: The place of loop diuretics in the treatment of acute and chronic renal failure. Clin Nephrol 28(suppl 1):S69, 1992

63. Solomon R, Werner C, Mann D, et al: Effects of saline, mannitol and furosemide on acute decreases in renal function induced by radiocontrast agents. N Engl J Med 331:1416, 1994

64. Rowe JW, Andres R, Tobin JD, et al: The effect of age on creatinine clearance in men: a cross sectional and longitudinal study. J Gerontol 31:155, 1976

65. Shimamura T, Morrison AB: A progressive glomerulosclerosis occurring in partial five-sixths nephrectomized rats. Am J Pathol 79:95, 1975

66. Compher C, Mullen JL, Barker CF: Nutritional support in renal failure. Surg Clin North Am 71:597, 1991

67. Abel RM: Nutritional support in the patient with acute renal failure. J Am Coll Nutr 2:33, 1983

68. Leverve X, Barnoud D: Stress metabolism and nutritional support in acute renal failure. Kidney Int 53(suppl 66):S62, 1998

69. Maschio G, Oldrizzi L, Tessitore N, et al: Effects of dietary protein and phosphorus restriction on the progression of early renal failure. Kidney Int 22:371, 1982

70. Abel RM, Beck CH Jr, Abbott WM, et al: Improved survival from acute renal failure after treatment with intravenous essential L-amino acids and glucose: results of a prospective double blind study. N Engl J Med 288:695, 1973

71. Bellomo R, Ronco C: Indications and criteria for initiating renal replacement therapy in the intensive care unit. Kidney Int 53(suppl 66):S106, 1998

72. Schetz MR: Classical and alternative indications for continuous renal replacement therapy. Kidney Int 53:(suppl 66):S129, 1998

73. Conger JD: Management of acute renal failure. Principles and Practice of Nephrology. Jacobson HR, Striker GE, Klahr S, Eds. BC Decker, Philadelphia, 1991, p 666

74. Gettings LG, Reynolds HN, Scalea T: Outcome in post-traumatic acute renal failure when continuous renal replacement therapy is applied

early vs. late. Intensive Care Med 25:805, 1999

75. Bellomo R, Ronco C: Continuous versus intermittent renal replacement therapy in the intensive care unit. Kidney Int 53(suppl 66):S125, 1998

76. Bellomo R, Boyce N: Acute continuous hemodiafiltration: a prospective study of 110 patients and a review of the literature. Am J Kidney Dis 21:508, 1993

77. Kierdorf H: Continuous versus intermittent treatment: clinical results in acute renal failure. Contrib Nephrol 93:1, 1991

78. Ronco C: Continuous renal replacement therapies for the treatment of acute renal failure in intensive care patients. Clin Nephrol 40:187, 1993

79. Bellomo R, Farmer M, Boyce N: The outcome of critically ill elderly patients with severe acute renal failure treated by continuous hemodiafiltration. Int J Artif Organs 17:466, 1994

80. Silvester W: Outcome studies of continuous renal replacement therapy in the intensive care unit. Kidney Int 53(suppl 66):S138, 1998

81. Reichow W, Koehler H, Dietrich K, et al: Continuous arterio-venous hemofiltration for the treatment of acute renal failure in septic shock. Prog Clin Biol Res 236B:235, 1987

82. Golper TA: Continuous arteriovenous hemofiltration in acute renal failure. Am J Kidney Dis 6:373, 1985

83. Cioffi WG, Ashikaga T, Gamelli RL: Probability of surviving postoperative acute renal failure: development of a prognostic index. Ann Surg 200:205, 1984

84. Briglia A: Acute renal failure in the intensive care unit. Clin Chest Med 20:347, 1999

85. Guild WR, Bray G, Merrill JP: Hemopericardium with cardiac tamponade in chronic uremia. N Engl J Med 257:230, 1957

86. Talalla A, Halbrook H, Barbour BH, et al: Subdural hematoma associated with long-term hemodialysis for chronic renal disease. JAMA 212:1847, 1970

87. Galen MA, Steinberg SM, Lowrie EG, et al: Hemorrhagic pleural effusion in patients undergoing chronic hemodialysis. Ann Intern Med 82:359, 1975

88. Wineman RJ: Endstage renal disease. Dial Transplant 7:1034, 1978

89. Schreiber SS, Korzets A, Powsner E, et al: Surgery in chronic dialysis patients. Isr J Med Sci 31:479, 1995

90. Gillum DM, Dixon BS, Yanover MJ, et al: The role of intensive dialysis in acute renal failure. Clin Nephrol 25:249, 1986

91. Booij LH: Neuromuscular transmission and its pharmacological blockade. Pharm World Science 19:35, 1997

92. Williams AR, Bailey M, Joye T, et al: Marked prolongation of the succinylcholine effect two hours after neostigmine reversal of neuromuscular blockade in a patient with renal insufficiency. South Med J 92:77, 1999

93. Thapa S, Sorin J: Succinylcholine–induced hyperkalemia in patients with renal failure: an old question revisited. Anesth Analg 91:237, 2000

94. Nayman J: Effect of renal failure on wound healing in dogs: response to hemodialysis following uremia induced by uranium nitrate. Ann Surg 164:227, 1966

95. Bennett WM: Altering drug dosage in patients with diseases of the kidney and liver. Clinical Uses of Drugs in Patients with Kidney and Liver Disease. Anderson RJ, Schrier RW, Eds. WB Saunders Co, Philadelphia, 1981, p 16

96. Schetz MR: Coagulation disorders in acute renal failure. Kidney Int 53(suppl 66):S96, 1998

97. Eschbach JW: The anemia of chronic renal fail-

ure: pathophysiology and the effects of recombinant erythropoietin. Kidney Int 35:134, 1989

98. Lim VS, DeGowin RL, Zavala D, et al: Recombinant human erythropoietin treatment in predialysis patients: a double-blind placebo-controlled trial. Ann Intern Med 110:108, 1989

99. Tang WW, Stead RA, Goodkin DA: Effects of epoetin alfa on hemostasis in chronic renal failure. Am J Nephrol 18:263, 1998

100. Macdougall IC: Quality of life and anemia: the nephrology experience. Semin Oncol 25(suppl 7):39, 1998

101. McMahon LP, McKenna MJ, Sangkabutra T, et al: Physical performance and associated electrolyte changes after haemoglobin normalization: a comparative study in haemodialysis patients. Nephrol Dial Transplant 14:1182, 1999

102. Tilney NL, Bailey GL, Morgan AP: Sequential system failure after rupture of abdominal aortic aneurysms: an unsolved problem in postoperative care. Ann Surg 178:117, 1973

103. Abel RM, Buckley MJ, Austen WG, et al: Etiology, incidence, and prognosis of renal failure following cardiac operations: results of a prospective analysis of 500 consecutive patients. J Thorac Cardiovasc Surg 71:323, 1976

104. Kron IL, Joob AW, Van Meter C: Acute renal failure in the cardiovascular surgical patient. Ann Thorac Surg 39:590, 1985

105. Durakovic Z, Durakovic A, Durakovic S, et al: The lack of clinical value of laboratory parameters in predicting outcome in acute renal failure. Ren Fail 11:213, 1989

106. Wilkes BM, Mailloux LU: Acute renal failure: pathogenesis and prevention. Am J Med 80:1129, 1986

107. Henrich WL, Anderson RJ, Berns AS, et al: The role of renal nerves and prostaglandins in control of renal hemodynamics and plasma renin activity during hypotensive hemorrhage in the dog. J Clin Invest 61:744, 1978

108. Garrison RN, Wilson MA, Matheson PJ, et al: Nitric oxide mediates redistribution of intrarenal blood flow during bacteremia. J Trauma 39:90, 1995

109. Humes HD: Role of calcium in pathogenesis of acute renal failure. Am J Physiol 250:F579, 1986

110. Rasmussen H, Kojima I, Apfeldorf W, et al: Cellular mechanism of hormone action in the kidney: messenger function of calcium and cyclic AMP. Kidney Int 29:90, 1986

111. Gates GF: Glomerular filtration rate: estimation from fractional renal accumulation of 99mTc-DTPA (stannous). AJR Am J Roentgenol 138:565, 1982

112. Carrie BJ, Golbetz HV, Michaels AS, et al: Creatinine: an inadequate filtration marker in glomerular diseases. Am J Med 69:177, 1980

113. Cronin RE, de Torrente A, Miller PD, et al: Pathogenic mechanisms in early norepinephrine-induced acute renal failure: functional and histological correlates of protection. Kidney Int 14:115, 1978

114. Morel F, Doucet A: Hormonal control of kidney functions at the cell level. Physiol Rev 66:377, 1986

115. Jard S, Butlen D, Cantau B, et al: The mechanisms of action of antidiuretic hormone. Adv Nephrol 13:163, 1984

116. Capasso G, Anastasio P, Giordano D, et al: Atrial natriuretic factor increases glomerular filtration rate in the experimental acute renal failure induced by cisplatin. Adv Exp Med Biol 212:285, 1987

117. Myers BD, Moran SM: Hemodynamically mediated acute renal failure. N Engl J Med 314:97, 1986

118. Levinsky NG: Pathophysiology of acute renal

failure. N Engl J Med 296:1453, 1977

119. Oken DE: On the differential diagnosis of acute renal failure. Am J Med 71:916, 1981

120. Jones DP: Renal metabolism during normoxia, hypoxia, and ischemic injury. Annu Rev Physiol 48:33, 1986

121. Adams PL, Adams FF, Bell PD, et al: Impaired renal blood flow autoregulation in ischemic acute renal failure. Kidney Int 18:68, 1980

122. Harman PK, Kron IL, McLachlan HD, et al: Elevated intra-abdominal pressure and renal function. Ann Surg 196:594, 1982

123. Kron IL, Harman PK, Nolan SP: The measurement of intra-abdominal pressure as a criterion for abdominal re-exploration. Ann Surg 199:28, 1984

124. Epstein M, Lifschitz M, Ramachandran M, et al: Characterization of renal prostaglandin E responsiveness in decompensated cirrhosis: implications for renal sodium handling. Clin Sci 63:555, 1982

125. Molitoris BA: New insights into the cell biology of ischemic acute renal failure. J Am Soc Nephrol 1:1263, 1991

126. Stein JH: Acute renal failure: lessons from pathophysiology. West J Med 156:176, 1992

127. Hohenfellner M, Thuroff JW, Thurau K: Cellular changes in acute renal failure: functional and therapeutic consequences. Eur Urol 22:265, 1992

128. Braam B, Mitchell KD, Koomans HA, et al: Relevance of the tubuloglomerular feedback mechanism in pathophysiology. J Am Soc Nephrol 4:1257, 1993

129. Brezis M, Rosen S, Silva P, et al: Renal ischemia: a new perspective. Kidney Int 26:375, 1984

130. Myers BD: Cyclosporine nephrotoxicity. Kidney Int 30:964, 1986

131. Loirat P, Rohan J, Baillet A, et al: Increased glomerular filtration rate in patients with major burns and its effect on the pharmacokinetics of tobramycin. N Engl J Med 299:915, 1978

132. Bayliss C: The mechanism of the decline in glomerular filtration rate in agent induced acute renal failure in the rat. J Antimicrob Chemother 6:381, 1980

133. Rose BD: Syndrome of inappropriate ADH (SIADH). Clinical Physiology of Acid-Base and Electrolyte Disorders, 2nd ed. McGraw-Hill Book Co, New York, 1984

134. Duke GJ, Bensten AD: Dopamine and renal salvage in the critically ill patient. Anaesth Intensive Care 20:277, 1992

135. Graziani G, Cantaluppi A, Casati S, et al: Dopamine and frusemide in oliguric acute renal failure. Nephron 37:39, 1984

136. Brown CB, Ogg CS, Cameron JS: High dose frusemide in acute renal failure: a controlled clinical trial. Clin Nephrol 15:90, 1981

137. Warren SE, Blantz RC: Mannitol. Arch Intern Med 141:493, 1981

138. Schrier RW: Role of calcium channel blockers in protection against experimental renal injury. Am J Med 90:21S, 1991

139. Wetzels JF, Burker JF, Schrier RW: Calcium channel blockers: protective effects in ischemic acute renal failure. Renal Failure 14:327, 1992

140. Conger JD: Interventions in clinical acute renal failure: what are the data? Am J Kidney Dis 26:565, 1995

141. Humes HD: Potential molecular therapy for acute renal failure. Cleve Clin J Med 60:166, 1993

142. Pru C, Kjellstrand CM: The FENa test is of no value in acute renal failure. Nephron 36:20, 1984

143. Saha H, Mustonen J, Helin H, et al: Limited value of the fractional excretion of sodium test in the diagnosis of acute renal failure. Nephrol Dial Transplant 2:79, 1987

144. Brosius FC, Lau K: Fractional excretion of sodium in acute renal failure: role of timing of the test and ischemia. Am J Nephrol 6:450, 1986

145. Danielson RA: Differential diagnosis and treatment of oliguria in post-traumatic and post-operative patients. Surg Clin North Am 55:697, 1975

146. Lucas CE: The renal response to acute injury and sepsis. Surg Clin North Am 56:953, 1976

147. Schetz M: Renal replacement therapy in patients with chronic renal failure and acute illness in ESRD. Critical Care Nephrology. Ronco C, Bellomo R, Eds. Kluwer, Dordrecht, Netherlands, 1998, p 1139

Acknowledgment

The authors would like to acknowledge the work of Drs. Nicholas L. Tilney, Julian L. Seifter, and Robert J. Rizzo in a chapter entitled "Renal Dysfunction," which appeared in previous versions of *ACS Surgery: Principles & Practice*. Some of their work was incorporated into this chapter.

Figure 2 Dana Burns.

8 DISORDERS OF WATER AND SODIUM BALANCE

Richard H. Sterns, M.D.

Overview of Body Fluid Homeostasis

Life takes place in an aqueous solution. Cells, the blood bringing nutrients and oxygen to them, and the interstitial fluid bathing them are all mostly water. Each day, water and salt are lost and replaced. To maintain stability of the internal milieu, body fluids are processed by the kidney, guided by intricate physiologic control systems that regulate fluid volume and composition.

DISTRIBUTION AND COMPOSITION OF BODY WATER

Water accounts for approximately half of an adult human's body weight. Because fat contains little water, individuals with more body fat have less body water. On average, total body water constitutes 60% of lean body weight in young men, 50% in young women and older men, and 45% in older women. Two thirds of body water is intracellular and the remainder is contained in the extracellular fluid compartment, which includes intravascular (plasma) and interstitial fluid. Small amounts of water are also contained in bone, dense connective tissue, digestive secretions, and cerebrospinal fluid.[1]

Extracellular solutes are predominantly sodium salts (primarily a mixture of NaCl and NaHCO$_3$). Thus, extracellular fluid can be thought of as saltwater. Except for protein (present at a higher concentration in plasma [approximately 1 mmol/L] than in interstitial fluid), the compositions of the intravascular and interstitial subdivisions of the extracellular fluid compartment are similar.

The sodium-potassium adenosine triphosphatase (Na$^+$,K$^+$-ATPase) pump on cell membranes keeps intracellular sodium at low levels. Potassium, the dominant intracellular cation, is electrically balanced, in large part, by anionic charges on impermeant macromolecules. Stability in the number of intracellular anionic charges makes the total solute content of cells much less variable than that of the extracellular fluid.

Osmolality

Extracellular and intracellular fluids contain different types of solutes, but the concentrations of solutes inside and outside of cells are equal. Concentration differences exist only transiently because they create an extremely strong force for water movement across cell membranes. Osmotic pressure moves water rapidly to the fluid compartment with the higher solute concentration until concentrations once again become equal. The osmotic pressure responsible for water movement across cell membranes depends on the total number of solute particles (osmoles) dissolved in solution, a property known as osmolality.[2] Osmolality is usually expressed as milliosmoles of solute per kilogram of solvent (mOsm/kg), but it can be thought of more simply as the number of millimoles of solute particles per liter of solution. A solute particle's contribution to osmolality is independent of its charge and molecular size. Ionic substances such as sodium chloride that dissociate in solution contribute more than one osmotically active particle. Sodium salts, glucose, and urea, commonly measured as blood urea nitrogen (BUN), are responsible for most of the solute particles normally present in extracellular fluid. Plasma osmolality can be measured directly with an osmometer or can be esti-

mated with reasonable accuracy from the concentrations of the major extracellular solutes, as follows:

$$P_{osm} \cong 2 \times \text{plasma [Na+]} + \frac{[\text{Glucose}]}{18} + \frac{\text{BUN}}{2.8}$$

The multiple of 2 reflects the anions accompanying sodium ions, and 18 and 2.8 are the corrections required to convert glucose and urea nitrogen concentration from mg/dl (the units used by most laboratories in the United States) to mmol/L. Exogenous solutes (e.g., ethanol, methanol, ethylene glycol, glycine, mannitol) are measured by osmometers but are not included in the formula shown above. A discrepancy between the measured and the calculated plasma osmolality values (an osmolar gap) is useful clinically as a way to recognize the presence of an exogenous solute.[2]

Fluid Movement between Body Fluid Compartments

The intravascular and interstitial subdivisions of the extracellular fluid compartment are separated by capillary walls that are freely permeable to small extracellular solutes but relatively impermeable to plasma proteins. Protein-free saltwater continuously moves across the capillary endothelial barrier by filtration, driven by a hydrostatic pressure gradient (generated by contractions of the heart), which forces fluid from the capillary into the interstitium, and an oncotic pressure gradient (the consequence of the osmotic force created by intravascular protein), which draws interstitial fluid into capillaries [see Figure 1]. These so-called Starling forces, which regulate the disposition of fluid within the extracellular compartment, determine how much extracellular saltwater is contained in intravascular plasma and how much is in interstitial fluid [see Disorder of Saltwater Excess: Edematous States, below]. Sodium salts, urea, glucose, and other small extracellular solutes freely cross the capillary wall, achieving similar concentrations in the interstitial fluid and plasma. Thus, changes in plasma osmolality do not influence water movement between the intravascular and interstitial fluid compartments.

Fluid movement between the extracellular and the intracellular fluid compartments is unaffected by Starling forces. Rather, transcellular water movement is driven by osmotic forces, a function of the concentration of solutes in the extracellular fluid. A decrease in extracellular solute concentration (hypotonicity) drives water into cells, causing cell swelling; an increase in the concentration of exclusively extracellular solutes (hypertonicity) draws fluid out of cells, dehydrating them.

Not all solutes contribute to the tonicity of extracellular fluid.[2] Permeant solutes such as urea and ethanol readily cross cell membranes, achieving equal concentrations in the extracellular and intracellular fluid compartments without driving transcellular water movement and without affecting cell volume. Such solutes, which increase plasma osmolality without altering plasma tonicity, are sometimes called ineffective osmoles. Impermeant solutes are excluded from cell water either by active transport (e.g., sodium ions) or because the cell membrane is impermeable to them (e.g., mannitol).

1152

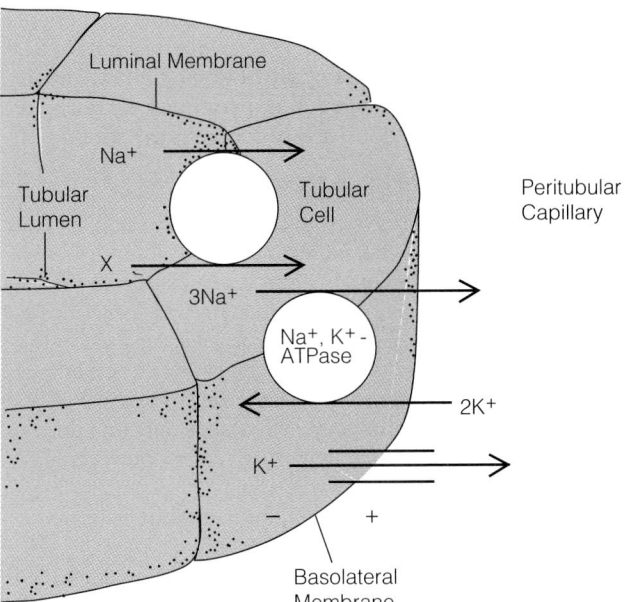

Figure 1 Sodium reabsorption by the renal tubules is driven by the Na⁺, K⁺-ATPase pump in the basolateral (blood side) membrane, which maintains a low sodium concentration within the tubular cell. Filtered sodium in the tubular lumen enters the cell down its concentration gradient via a transmembrane carrier (which may also transport another solute, X) or via a channel in the luminal membrane [*see Figure 2*].

Such solutes, which cause both hyperosmolality and hypertonicity, are sometimes called effective osmoles.

Body Fluid Tonicity and the Plasma Sodium Concentration

Normally, sodium salts are the major effective osmoles in extracellular fluid, and potassium salts are the major effective osmoles in cells. Given that effective osmolality is equal in all fluid compartments, body fluid tonicity can be described by the following equation:

$$\text{Tonicity} \cong$$
$$2 \times \text{Plasma [Na}^+] \cong \frac{2 \,(\text{Exchangeable Na}^+ + \text{Exchangeable K}^+)}{\text{Total body water}}$$

therefore,

$$\text{Plasma [Na}^+] \cong \frac{\text{Exchangeable Na}^+ + \text{Exchangeable K}^+}{\text{Total body water}}$$

(Only the exchangeable fractions of sodium and potassium are included in the equation, because one third of overall body sodi-

um is bound to bone and is therefore osmotically inactive.)

Thus, the plasma sodium concentration is, in effect, a measure of the concentration of tonicity of all body fluids.[3] In the absence of an osmolar gap, the plasma sodium concentration is a more valid measure of body fluid tonicity than plasma osmolality (which includes the ineffective osmole, urea). With a few exceptions, most notably hyperglycemia, a low plasma sodium concentration indicates hypotonicity and cell swelling, whereas a high plasma sodium concentration indicates hypertonicity and cellular dehydration.

RENAL PROCESSING OF BODY FLUIDS

Glomerular Filtration

Approximately 170 L of extracellular saltwater containing over 25,000 mmol of sodium are filtered by the glomerulus each day. Although glomerular hydrostatic pressure is considerably higher than the pressure of other capillary beds, the Starling forces that control fluid movement between intravascular and interstitial fluid also drive glomerular filtration. The glomerular filtrate contains the same concentrations of sodium and other solutes as interstitial fluid and is nearly protein free.

Tubular Reabsorption

On a conventional diet, all but 2 L of filtered fluid and all but 175 mmol of filtered sodium is reabsorbed by the renal tubules. Regulation of tubular reabsorption of salt and water is the key to renal regulation of body fluid balance.[4]

At the end of the proximal tubule, the remaining filtrate has the same sodium concentration as plasma has; as the filtrate passes through downstream tubular segments, it undergoes major changes in composition. In these more distal segments, sodium and water reabsorption are uncoupled; salt can be reabsorbed without water, and water can be reabsorbed without salt. Thus, depending on conditions, the sodium concentration of the final urine can vary from less than 1 mEq/L to nearly 300 mEq/L, and urine osmolality can vary from one sixth (50 mOsm/kg) to four times (1,200 mOsm/kg) that of plasma.

The process of sodium reabsorption is mediated by carriers or channels embedded in the tubular cell's luminal and basolateral (blood side) membranes. In each nephron segment, sodium reabsorption is powered by the so-called sodium pump, Na⁺,K⁺-ATPase, which is located on the blood side of the tubular cell [*see Figure 1*]. This sodium pump exports sodium from the cell, lowering the intracellular sodium concentration. The lowered concentration of cellular sodium creates an electrochemical gradient driving sodium from the tubular lumen into the cell. Tubular segments at various regions of the nephron utilize different luminal mechanisms for sodium reabsorption [*see Table 1 and Figure 2*]. Luminal ex-

Table 1 Sodium Transport in Different Nephron Segments

Nephron Segment	Glomerular Filtrate Reabsorbed	Mechanism of Luminal Sodium Entry	Physiologic Regulation	Diuretic Site of Action
Proximal tubule	60%–70%	Na⁺-H⁺ exchange; cotransport with glucose and other organic solutes	Angiotensin II; renal nerves; peritubular Starling forces	Carbonic anhydrase inhibitors (e.g., acetazolamide)
Loop of Henle	20%–25%	Na⁺-K⁺-2Cl⁻ cotransport	Flow dependent; peritubular Starling forces	Loop diuretics (e.g., furosemide, bumetanide, ethacrynic acid)
Distal tubule	5%	Na⁺-Cl⁻ cotransport	Flow dependent	Thiazide diuretics
Collecting tubule	4%	Na⁺ channels	Aldosterone; atrial natriuretic factor	Potassium-sparing diuretics (e.g., amiloride, triamterene, spironolactone)

changers, cotransporters, and ion channels along the nephron are subject to physiologic control, and they can be inhibited pharmacologically by specific diuretic agents.[5] Mutations in these transport proteins are responsible for well-defined clinical disorders.[6]

The luminal membrane of the collecting duct is impermeable to water in the absence of arginine vasopressin, an antidiuretic hormone (ADH). Thus, when plasma ADH levels are low, this segment progressively reduces the osmolality and sodium concentration of the final urine and permits the excretion of large volumes (as much as 20 L daily) of dilute urine. In the presence of ADH, water chan-

nels—called aquaporins—are inserted in the luminal membrane of the distal tubule and collecting duct.[7,8] When plasma levels of ADH are high, water is attracted osmotically from the tubular lumen to the hypertonic medullary interstitium, permitting excretion of a small volume (as little as 0.5 L daily) of concentrated urine.

REGULATION OF BODY FLUID VOLUMES

Saltwater (isotonic saline) is confined to the extracellular space. Accumulation of saltwater expands extracellular volume; loss of saltwater causes volume depletion. In either case, changes in saltwater balance do not alter the plasma sodium concentration or cell volume. By contrast, so-called electrolyte-free water, or pure water, is distributed throughout body fluids, affecting both extracellular and intracellular fluid compartments. Because only one third of body water is extracellular, electrolyte-free water has only one third the impact on extracellular volume that saltwater has; however, unlike saltwater balance, electrolyte-free water balance has a major impact on the plasma sodium concentration, body fluid tonicity, and cell volume.

Extracellular and intracellular fluid volumes are maintained by separate but interacting control systems [see Table 2]; the extracellular system primarily regulates urinary sodium excretion, whereas the intracellular system regulates the intake and excretion of water. Extracellular fluid volume maintains a proper degree of vascular fullness, a variable that is sensed by atrial stretch receptors and arterial baroreceptors. Intracellular volume is regulated by hypothalamic osmoreceptor cells that swell or shrink in response to changes in plasma tonicity.

Control of Extracellular Fluid Volume

In a healthy person, the amount of sodium in the extracellular space can vary considerably, depending on dietary salt intake. On the other hand, under normal conditions, the extracellular sodium concentration remains almost constant because of physiologic control systems that tightly regulate water intake and excretion. In healthy persons, more salt in the extracellular space means an expanded extracellular fluid volume; less salt means a smaller extracellular volume. In either case, the extracellular sodium concentration does not change.

Sodium balance and intravascular volume are affected by numerous hormonal and nonhormonal mediators; in addition to aldosterone and angiotensin—the best known mediators of sodium excretion—the sympathetic nervous system, natriuretic peptides, and changes in the renal circulation all play important regulatory roles [see Table 2].[9] Because of redundancy and overlap in the control system, failure of a single factor does not cause major, sustained abnormalities in intravascular volume. The relative importance of the various mediators that affect urinary sodium excretion are incompletely understood, and it is likely that some sodium regulatory factors remain undiscovered.

Control of Intracellular Fluid Volume

Water balance and cell volume are controlled by a single hormonal mediator, arginine vasopressin [see Tubular Reabsorption, *above*], which is released into the systemic circulation by the neurohypophysis [see Table 2 and Figure 3]. The hormone activates V_2 receptors on the basolateral membrane of principal cells in the renal collecting duct, initiating a cyclic adenosine monophosphate–dependent process that culminates in the insertion of water channels (aquaporins) into the cells' luminal membranes.[7,8] Modulation of the number of water channels controls urine osmolality and the rate of water excretion by the kidney. Vasopressin's short half-life in the circulation and continuous shuttling of

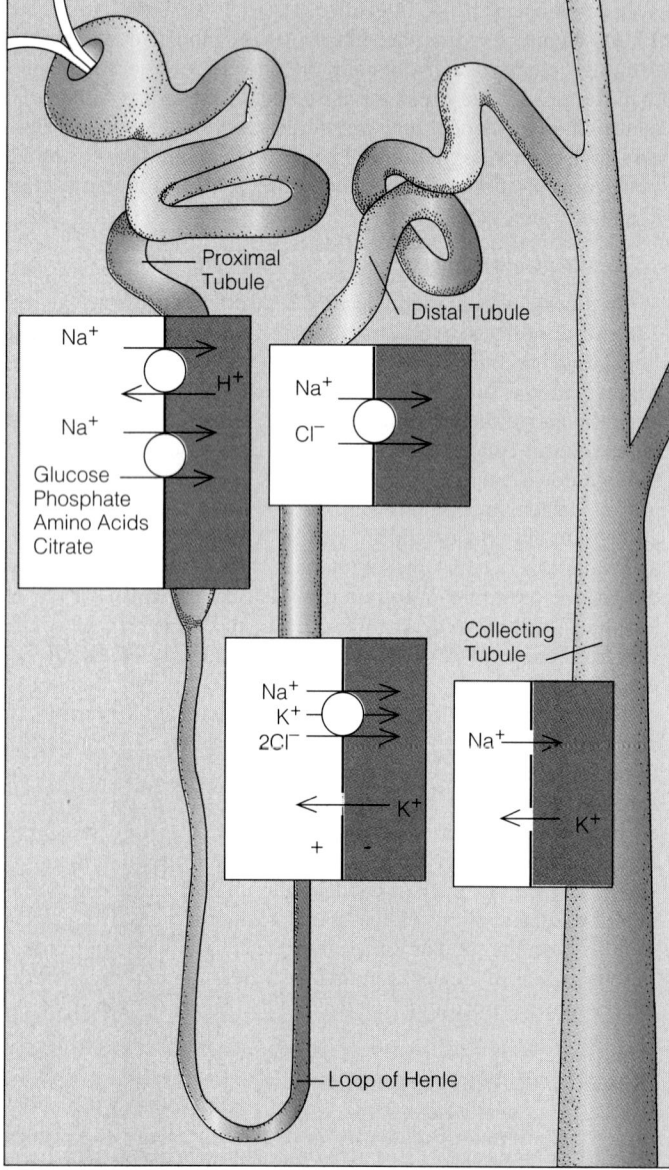

Figure 2 In each tubular segment, sodium enters the tubular cell passively, down the favorable electrochemical gradient created by the Na^+, K^+-ATPase pump. Luminal sodium enters by a different mechanism in each of the nephron segments. The proximal tubule reabsorbs filtered bicarbonate and other solutes, such as glucose, phosphate, amino acids, and citrate. An Na^+, K^+, $2Cl^-$ transporter mediates Na^+ entry into the ascending limb of the loop of Henle. The distal tubule has an Na^+, Cl^- cotransporter. Na^+ enters the principal cells of the cortical collecting tubules through Na^+ channels in the luminal membrane.

Table 2 Control of Body Fluid Volumes

	Saltwater Balance	Electrolyte-Free Water Balance	
		Day to Day	Emergency Backup
Regulated variable	Extracellular volume Vascular fullness	Cell volume	Arterial filling
Clinical indicator	Blood pressure Edema	Plasma sodium concentration	Blood pressure Edema
Sensors	Baroreceptors, atrial volume receptors	Hypothalamic osmoreceptors	Baroreceptors, atrial volume receptors
Mediators	Renin-angiotensin-aldosterone system Sympathetic nervous system Atrial natriuretic peptide Starling forces in peritubular capillaries	Antidiuretic hormone (arginine vasopressin) Thirst	Antidiuretic hormone (arginine vasopressin) Thirst
Affected variable	Urinary sodium excretion	Urine osmolality Water intake	Urine osmolality Water intake

aquaporins between the collecting duct's cell membrane and cytosol ensure that urinary water excretion responds rapidly to changes in body fluid tonicity.

Vasopressin levels are normally unmeasurable when the plasma sodium concentration falls to 135 mEq/L or lower [*see Figure 3*]. Low levels of the hormone result in the excretion of large volumes of a maximally dilute urine (50 mOsm/kg). Above a sodium level of 135 mEq/L, plasma vasopressin levels are linearly related to the plasma sodium concentration and increase measurably in response to changes in the plasma sodium concentration of as little as 1 mEq/L. Once the plasma sodium concentration reaches approximately 142 mEq/L, plasma vasopressin levels are high enough to promote the excretion of maximally concentrated urine (1,200 mOsm/kg). A rising plasma sodium concentration also causes hypothalamic cell volume receptors to relay signals to nearby thirst centers. Mediated by thirst and changes in vasopressin secretion, the plasma sodium concentration is normally prevented from rising above 142 mEq/L or falling below 135 mEq/L.

Under day-to-day conditions, water intake, vasopressin secretion, and urinary free water excretion primarily respond to changes in the plasma sodium concentration created by variations in electrolyte-free water balance. Unlike sodium excretion, which is affected only by changes in intravascular volume, free water excretion can be affected by two types of stimuli—intravascular volume and tonicity. Under pathologic conditions, osmotic control of vasopressin secretion and thirst can be overridden by hemodynamic stimuli. The hypothalamic neurons that secrete vasopressin receive neural input from baroreceptors in the great vessels and volume receptors in the atria. When these receptors are stimulated by hypotension or by a major reduction in plasma volume, impulses are carried via cranial nerves IX and X.[8] Vasopressin and thirst responses to hypovolemia and hypotension can be regarded as back-up systems that serve to maintain arterial blood volume under emergency conditions, sacrificing tonicity to tissue perfusion.

CELL VOLUME REGULATION IN HYPOTONICITY AND HYPERTONICITY

Cell volume is determined by the amount and concentration of intracellular solute. Because intracellular and extracellular solute concentrations must be equal, the relation between cell water and extracellular osmolality can be described by the following equation:

$$\text{Cell volume} = \frac{\text{Cell water}}{\text{Extracellular osmolality}}$$

Normally, water intake and excretion are modulated to maintain body fluid tonicity within a narrow physiologic range. However, under pathologic conditions, body cells can be exposed to a hypotonic or hypertonic milieu.[10] The first response to osmotic stress is a compensatory adjustment to intracellular electrolytes: loss of potassium in hypotonicity and accumulation of sodium and potassium in hypertonicity. With time, changes in organic solutes dominate the response.

Most cells maintain relatively high concentrations of small, osmotically active organic molecules known as organic osmolytes. Or-

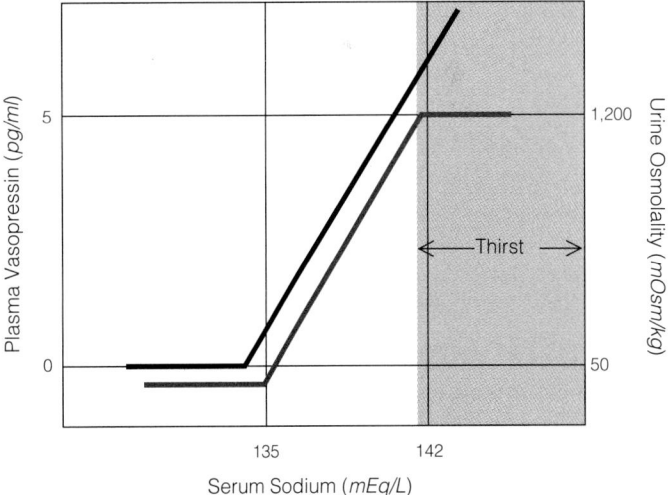

Figure 3 Graph depicts the normal relation between plasma vasopressin levels and urine osmolality (black line) and the plasma sodium concentration (red line). Plasma vasopressin levels change within minutes in response to changes in plasma sodium, and urine osmolality changes within minutes in response to changes in vasopressin levels. When hydration reduces the plasma sodium level below 135 mEq/L, plasma vasopressin becomes undetectable and the urine becomes maximally dilute (osmolality, 50 mOsm/kg). Between sodium concentrations of 135 and 142 mEq/L, vasopressin levels are linearly related to the plasma sodium, causing nearly a 100 mOsm/kg increase in urine osmolality for every 0.5 mEq/L increase in sodium concentration. Above a plasma sodium concentration of 142 mEq/L, the urine is maximally concentrated; increased water intake, mediated by thirst, then becomes the major defense against progressive hypernatremia.

ganic osmolytes are nonperturbing solutes; unlike sodium and potassium, their intracellular concentrations may vary widely without affecting tertiary protein structure. Cells accumulate organic osmolytes under hypertonic conditions and lose them when confronted with hypotonicity.

The need for cell volume regulation is most imperative in the brain, where the rigid calvaria places sharp limits on the degree of tissue expansion or contraction that can be tolerated.[10-13] An increase in brain water content of more than about 5% to 10% is incompatible with life. Variations in the intracellular concentration of organic osmolytes provide the brain with an astonishing ability to adapt to chronic osmotic disturbances. However, because changes in the osmolyte content of brain cells require a few days to develop fully, the brain is imperiled by rapid osmotic changes. Thus, acute hyponatremia or hypernatremia may be fatal at plasma sodium concentrations that are well tolerated chronically.

With sustained osmotic disturbances, adaptations that protect against brain swelling and shrinkage also predispose to injury when the osmotic disturbance is suddenly corrected. In chronic hyponatremia, cellular solutes lost in the adaptive phase must be recovered when the plasma sodium concentration returns to normal—a process that may require several days. Unless solute recovery keeps pace with the rising extracellular osmolality, brain cells will become dehydrated.[11,12] This phenomenon may cause clinical complications [see Disorder of Water Excess: Hyponatremia, Chronic Hyponatremia, Complications of Therapy: Myelinolysis and Osmotic Demyelination Syndrome, below]. Similarly, in chronic hypernatremia, accumulated solutes must be shed during correction of the electrolyte disturbance.[10,13] Cells that have become acclimated to a hypertonic environment lose organic osmolytes slowly because of slow turnover of the efflux mechanism, slow downregulation of hypertonically stimulated uptake pathways, or both. Thus, when chronic hypernatremia is corrected rapidly, brain cells swell to a greater than normal volume.

Disorder of Water Excess: Hyponatremia

Hyponatremia simply means a low plasma sodium concentration. In most cases, hyponatremia is associated with a low plasma osmolality level and body fluids that are too dilute (hypotonic hyponatremia). However, there are exceptions to this rule [see Differential Diagnosis for Hyponatremia, below].

PATHOGENESIS OF HYPONATREMIA

Hypotonic hyponatremia results from two basic mechanisms individually or together: (1) massive water intake, exceeding the capacity to excrete electrolyte-free water, or (2) impaired water excretion. Normally, the capacity for water excretion is rather large. In the absence of vasopressin, urine osmolality falls to approximately 50 mOsm/kg. A typical American diet provides 600 to 900 mOsm of electrolytes and urea that must be excreted each day. At this rate of solute excretion, the volume of maximally dilute urine equals 12 to 18 L. Water intake can occasionally exceed the normal excretory capacity, primarily in psychotic patients who frantically ingest gallons of water over a few hours[14] and in very heavy beer drinkers who ingest large volumes of fluid but take in small amounts of salt and protein.[15] More commonly, hyponatremia occurs in patients with a diminished ability to excrete free water.[8,12]

Impaired Water Excretion

Water excretion is obviously compromised in severe renal failure; oliguric patients become hyponatremic if they are given too much water. However, most cases of hyponatremia occur in patients whose normal kidneys are unable to excrete maximally dilute urine. A pathologically low plasma sodium concentration occurs when water is taken in at a time when renal diluting mechanisms are not functioning maximally because either (1) diuretics or tubular transport defects are blocking sodium reabsorption in the renal diluting segments or (2) antidiuretic hormone levels are elevated.

Nonosmotic Release of Vasopressin

Vasopressin is a water-retaining hormone that is released when water is needed. Because hypotonic hyponatremia normally inhibits vasopressin secretion, detectable vasopressin in a patient who is hyponatremic indicates that a nonosmotic stimulus for vasopressin release must be present. Vasopressin action increases the urine osmolality, which can be thought of as a bioassay for the hormone.

Hemodynamic stimuli for vasopressin Hypovolemia, heart failure, and cirrhosis are the most common nonosmotic stimuli for antidiuretic hormone secretion.[16-18] The hemodynamic abnormalities that stimulate vasopressin release also promote sodium reabsorption by the renal tubules; thus, these conditions result in both sodium and water retention.

Inappropriate antidiuretic hormone secretion Nonosmotic release of vasopressin without a hemodynamic stimulus to account for it is considered "inappropriate." Patients with the syndrome of inappropriate antidiuretic hormone secretion (SIADH) retain water because of nonosmotic release of vasopressin but have no abnormality in sodium balance, evidence of volume depletion, or tendency to form edema; in the steady state, sodium excretion matches intake.[8,12,19] Because of water retention, SIADH causes mild, subclinical volume expansion. Any additional volume expansion is met by a brisk increase in urinary sodium excretion.

Reset osmostat Reset osmostat is a variant of SIADH, commonly seen in patients with chronic, debilitating illness; it is also a characteristic of normal pregnancy. Patients with this condition are able to dilute their urine normally but at a lower set-point than in normal individuals. Such patients are thus mildly hyponatremic, but unlike other patients with SIADH, they are not predisposed to progressive water retention and do not require dietary water restriction or other measures used to treat chronic hyponatremia.[11] Reset osmostat can, however, be seen in malignancies, and like other causes of SIADH, it requires a diagnostic evaluation to determine its cause.

Urinary Electrolyte Losses: Desalination and Hyponatremia

If the urine is concentrated, urinary sodium and potassium losses can contribute to the pathogenesis of hyponatremia. The plasma sodium concentration can be reduced either by loss of sodium or potassium or by water gain. However, to lower the plasma sodium concentration, electrolytes must be lost in urine that has a higher electrolyte concentration than plasma. The combination of high vasopressin levels (which concentrate the urine) and a high rate of sodium and potassium excretion can yield hypertonic urine capable of generating free water, which in essence desalinates the plasma.[20]

DIFFERENTIAL DIAGNOSIS FOR HYPONATREMIA

Several conditions can lower the plasma sodium concentration without causing hypotonicity and are referred to as nonhypotonic hyponatremia [see Table 3]. The diagnostic and therapeutic approach to these conditions differs fundamentally from the approach to hypotonic hyponatremia. Thus, it is important that nonhypotonic hyponatremia be excluded whenever a low plasma sodium concentration is encountered.

Table 3 Causes of Nonhypotonic Hyponatremia

Condition	Plasma Osmolality	Pathogenesis	Therapeutic Implications
Hyperglycemia	High	Extracellular glucose osmotically draws water into the ECF, diluting extracellular sodium	During treatment of hyperglycemia, anticipate 3 mEq/L increase in serum sodium for every 200 mg/dl reduction in blood sugar
Intravenous hypertonic mannitol therapy	High	Water shift from ICF to ECF as with hyperglycemia	Mannitol is rapidly excreted when renal function is normal
Intravenous γ-globulin therapy	High	Maltose present in solution acts like mannitol	Measure plasma osmolality when hyponatremia is suspected
Irrigant absorption (prostatectomy or intrauterine surgery)	Normal or low (when hypoosmolar irrigants are used)	Absorbed solute—mannitol, sorbitol, or glycine (most common)—initially confined to ECF, causing severe hyponatremia but little change in plasma osmolality	Mannitol is rapidly excreted; sorbitol is metabolized, causing late-onset hypotonic hyponatremia; glycine is neurotoxic and causes transient blindness and is metabolized to ammonia, causing encephalopathy; consider hemodialysis
Pseudohyponatremia (severe hyperlipidemia, multiple myeloma, macroglobulinemia)	Normal	Laboratory artifact; plasma water constitutes a smaller fraction of the plasma sample, causing a more serious underestimate of the true sodium concentration	Suspect when serum is lactescent; compare measured plasma osmolality with calculated osmolality or measure plasma sodium with direct-reading sodium electrode

ECF—extracellular fluid   ICF—intracellular fluid

Hyperglycemic Hyponatremia

Hyperglycemia lowers the plasma sodium concentration; in the absence of insulin, glucose is an effective osmole that attracts water from cells and thereby dilutes extracellular sodium. Therefore, the blood glucose level should always be examined when a low plasma sodium concentration is being evaluated. The plasma sodium concentration falls by approximately 3 mEq for every 200 mg/dl (10 mmol) increase in blood glucose and will increase by this amount when hyperglycemia is corrected with insulin. To evaluate hyponatremia in the presence of hyperglycemia, the serum sodium concentration must be "corrected" for the osmotic effect of glucose. In effect, the clinician must ask the question, What would the serum sodium concentration be if the excess glucose were no longer present? The correction factor most commonly used today is a 1.6 mEq/L decrease in serum sodium concentration for every 100 mg/dl increase in blood glucose. A small study has suggested that the true correction factor is approximately 2.4 mEq/L for every 100 mg/dl increase in blood glucose.[21] A precise correction factor is probably unobtainable because in practice, hyperglycemia develops, in part, from the ingestion of glucose with water and resolves, in part, from the urinary excretion of glucose with water.[22]

Exogenous solutes such as mannitol and maltose (a sugar contained in intravenous immunoglobulin preparations) are confined to the extracellular space and have an effect on the plasma sodium concentration similar to that of hyperglycemia. When the clinical setting suggests that these solutes might be responsible for hyponatremia, their presence can be confirmed by measuring the plasma osmolality and comparing it with the calculated value to identify an osmolar gap [*see* Overview of Body Fluid Homeostasis, Distribution and Composition of Body Water, Osmolality, *above*].[2,11]

Postprostatectomy Syndrome and Hysteroscopic Hyponatremia

Irrigants containing mannitol, sorbitol, or glycine are used for endoscopic transurethral and intrauterine procedures [*see Table 3*].[2,23] Occasionally, several liters of irrigant may be absorbed systemically, reducing the plasma sodium in a matter of minutes. Immediately after surgery, the serum sodium concentration is much lower than would be anticipated, because the electrolyte-free solution is initially confined to the extracellular space. Glycine, the most commonly used irrigant in the United States, is metabolized to ammonia and eventually to urea and glucose. Hyperammonemia may be responsible for most of the symptomatology, and glycine itself has direct neuroinhibitory effects and may cause hypotension, bradycardia, and visual disturbances.

Pseudohyponatremia

High plasma concentrations of lipid or protein cause mild nonhypotonic hyponatremia because of an artifact of laboratory measurement [*see Table 3*].[2,11] With extremely high concentrations of lipid (enough to cause lactescent serum) or protein (from multiple myeloma or Waldenstrom macroglobulinemia), plasma water may constitute a smaller fraction of the plasma sample than normal, which can result in an underestimate of the "true" sodium concentration. The plasma osmolality and the sodium concentration in plasma water (as measured by a sodium-sensitive electrode) are unaffected. There are no symptoms, and no therapy is required.

ACUTE HYPONATREMIA (WATER INTOXICATION)

The term water intoxication was coined in the early 1920s to describe a neurologic syndrome that develops when large volumes of water are retained within a relatively short period of time (< 48 hours). The syndrome is often called acute hyponatremia.[12,24]

Etiology

Acute hyponatremia develops when water intake is large and electrolyte-free water excretion is impaired. Potentially, hyponatremia can develop rapidly in any patient predisposed to water retention who takes in a large volume of water in a short period of time. However, this is likely to occur in a limited number of settings [*see Table 4*], and such instances account for most cases of severe symptomatic hyponatremia and for most of the recorded fatalities.

Postoperative hyponatremia   Vasopressin is released immediately after surgical procedures in what appears to be a stress response [*see Table 4*].[20,25] Particularly during the first 24 hours, the concentration of urinary cations (sodium plus potassium) may greatly exceed the plasma sodium concentration. As a result, even isotonic fluids may be "desalinated" and can lower the plasma sodium concentration.[20] Thus, all hypotonic fluids and excessive amounts of isotonic fluids should be avoided after surgery. As discussed earlier, endoscopic prostatectomy and intrauterine proce-

Table 4 Causes and Treatment of Acute Hyponatremia

Causes	Pathogenesis	Effect of Treatment	Recommendations
Postoperative stress*	Vasopressin is secreted in response to surgical stress for 2 or more days; free water from hypotonic I.V. fluids is retained and sodium and potassium are excreted in urine at high concentrations	Normal saline ineffective for correction—administered sodium excreted in concentrated urine, "desalinating" isotonic fluid and causing water retention	Avoid hypotonic fluid (e.g., D5W, 0.45% saline) and excessive volumes of isotonic fluid (lactated Ringer solution or 0.9% saline) after surgery; treat symptomatic hyponatremia with 3% saline and furosemide
Oxytocin	Used in obstetrics to induce labor; direct antidiuretic effect of drug mimics SIADH; free water from I.V. fluids retained	Urine becomes dilute when oxytocin is discontinued	Avoid administration of oxytocin in or with hypotonic fluids; treat hyponatremia by discontinuing drug
Cyclophosphamide	Drug has antidiuretic effect that persists for as long as 12 hours; patients are encouraged to drink large volumes of water to prevent chemically induced cystitis	Normal saline ineffective for correction as in other causes of persistent SIADH	Treat symptomatic hyponatremia with 3% saline and furosemide
Psychotic self-induced water intoxication	Extreme polydipsia (> 1 L/hr) common among patients with severe psychosis; retained water causes hyponatremia by late afternoon or evening, and water diuresis restores normonatremia by morning	Normal ability to dilute urine in most patients so hyponatremia self-corrects when water intake stops; some patients have vasopressin release (often transient) from stress, smoking, or medications (e.g., carbamazepine)	Monitor diurnal weight in institutionalized patients for early detection; avoid antidiuretic medications; treat hyponatremia with water restriction; use hypertonic saline and furosemide for occasional patient with SIADH
Marathon running	Extracellular volume depletion caused by saltwater losses from sweating and possibly stress are nonosmotic stimuli for vasopressin secretion; large volumes of sugar water consumed during race are retained	Isotonic saline restores ability to dilute urine	3% saline without furosemide for seizures; isotonic saline and water restriction for more moderate symptoms
Ecstasy (MDMA) use	Excessive fluid intake and inappropriate antidiuretic hormone secretion, induced by MDMA, is implicated	Isotonic saline ineffective; self-correction typical but may be delayed	Hypertonic saline for severe symptoms

*Excluding irrigant absorption syndromes [see Table 3].
D5W—5% dextrose in water   MDMA—methylenedioxymethamphetamine   SIADH—syndrome of inappropriate antidiuretic hormone

dures can cause hyponatremia if irrigant used in the procedures is absorbed systemically. The management of irrigant absorption syndromes differs from that of other causes of postoperative hyponatremia [see Postprostatectomy Syndrome and Hysteroscopic Hyponatremia, above].[25]

Oxytocin infusions Oxytocin, which is used in obstetrics to induce labor, has a direct antidiuretic effect. If the drug is administered in 5% dextrose in water (formerly a common practice), symptomatic hyponatremia may emerge after the infusion of less than 3 L of fluid [see Table 4].[11] Termination of the infusion permits a water diuresis and correction of hyponatremia; however, the syndrome is best avoided by using isotonic saline as a vehicle for the drug.

Cyclophosphamide infusion Intravenous cyclophosphamide impairs water excretion by an unknown mechanism.[26] The antidiuretic effect of the drug begins 4 to 12 hours after injection and persists for as long as 12 hours. Patients receiving cyclophosphamide are particularly susceptible to hyponatremia, because they are encouraged to drink large volumes of water to prevent chemically induced cystitis [see Table 4].

Psychotic self-induced water intoxication Extreme polydipsia is relatively common in patients with psychiatric illnesses, particularly schizophrenia, and it may lead to symptomatic hyponatremia [see Table 4].[14] Daily intake of 10 to 15 L has been documented, and much of the intake may take place over a few hours. Many patients become hyponatremic in the late afternoon and

evening; however, water diuresis typically restores normonatremia by the following morning. Occasionally, individuals drink enough water to produce seizures. By monitoring diurnal changes in body weight, water intoxication can be recognized before the onset of severe neurologic symptoms. Transient release of vasopressin (most commonly provoked by nausea and vomiting) may contribute to water retention. There is little evidence that any of the major tranquilizers has a significant antidiuretic effect; however, carbamazepine, an anticonvulsant, enhances sensitivity to vasopressin.

Water intoxication during exercise During a race, runners sweat profusely, losing large volumes of saltwater. Extracellular volume contraction and possibly the stress of exertion cause the release of vasopressin. When saltwater losses are replaced by the intake of sugar water, water retention and symptomatic hyponatremia may occur.[27,28] Most severe cases have been reported after marathons or ultramarathons. However, symptomatic hyponatremia may occur after recreational running and military fitness training.

Water intoxication from "ecstasy" During the 1990s, 3,4-methylenedioxymethamphetamine (MDMA, or ecstasy) gained widespread popularity as a recreational drug taken at dances.[29] When malignant hyperthermia was recognized as a complication associated with this drug, MDMA users were advised in underground magazines and the lay press to drink plenty of fluids. Subsequently, acute water intoxication emerged as a potentially lethal complication of the drug [see Table 4]. Excessive fluid intake and inappropriate ADH secretion, induced by MDMA, have been implicated.[29]

Diagnosis

Symptoms of water intoxication include headaches, weakness, nervousness, and vomiting, progressing to disorientation, delirium, tremulousness, and ultimately convulsions and coma.[12,24] The pupils are often dilated, and bilateral Babinski signs may be present. On occasion, patients may present with hemiparesis, mimicking a cerebrovascular accident. The syndrome reflects cerebral edema, which can lead to herniation of the brain and death. Clinical findings may emerge explosively. Complaints of headache and mild confusion may be followed within hours by respiratory arrest and, in some cases, neurogenic pulmonary edema. For reasons that remain obscure, almost all reported fatalities from acute postoperative hyponatremia have been in women (usually of childbearing age) and young children. Fatal cases of acute hyponatremia from other etiologies have been recorded in men and women.

Acute hyponatremia should be suspected in any patient who has unexplained neurologic symptoms, especially in psychiatric patients, marathon runners, users of ecstasy, and patients receiving hypotonic fluids intravenously (e.g., after surgery). Serum electrolytes should be obtained immediately. In the proper setting, a tentative diagnosis of water intoxication is advisable when symptoms develop in a patient whose serum sodium concentration is lower than 130 mEq/L (provided that causes of nonhypotonic hyponatremia have been excluded). Although severe neurologic symptoms do not usually appear until the sodium level has fallen below 120 mEq/L, some patients may be unusually susceptible to brain edema when they become acutely hyponatremic; rare fatalities have been reported at plasma sodium concentrations between 120 and 128 mEq/L.[20,25]

Computed axial tomography demonstrates cerebral edema in severe cases of water intoxication, and it rules out other potential explanations for neurologic findings. However, when symptoms are severe, therapy should not be delayed while imaging studies are being obtained.

Treatment

Free-water intake should be stopped immediately whenever water intoxication is suspected. Hypertonic saline is the treatment of choice for water-intoxicated patients who cannot autocorrect their electrolyte disturbance.[24,25] Each 1 ml of 3% saline contains 0.5 mEq of sodium. Because there are approximately 0.5 L of body water for every 1 kg of body weight, 1 ml of 3% saline per 1 kg of body weight can be expected to increase the plasma sodium concentration by 1 mEq/L. For patients with severe neurologic symptoms, an infusion of 3% saline at 1 to 2 ml/kg/hr will increase the plasma sodium concentration by approximately 1 to 2 mEq/L/hr, a rate that is considered appropriate for initial therapy. Hypertonic saline is best infused in 100 ml containers to avoid inadvertently giving an excessive dose. Except when volume depletion is suspected (as in marathon runners), concurrent administration of a loop diuretic (furosemide, bumetanide, or torsemide) is advisable. The diuretic prevents volume overload and, by blocking sodium reabsorption in the loop of Henle, impedes the formation of concentrated urine.

The goal of therapy in acute hyponatremia is to decrease the severity of cerebral edema and to stop seizures. A 4 to 6 mEq/L increase in plasma sodium concentration is usually sufficient to accomplish these goals. Thus, the plasma sodium concentration should be monitored frequently during therapy and emergency treatment with hypertonic saline should be stopped after 2 to 3 hours. Once initial therapy with high-dose hypertonic saline has been completed, more conservative measures should be substituted

Table 5 Causes of the Syndrome of Inappropriate Antidiuretic Hormone

Tumors	Bronchogenic (small cell) Pancreatic Duodenal Urethral Nasopharyngeal Leukemia Hodgkin disease Thymoma
Neurologic disorders	Psychosis Trauma Neoplasms (primary and metastatic) Vascular (hemorrhage, infarction, and vasculitis) Infection (meningitis, brain abscess, and encephalitis) Miscellaneous (Guillain-Barré syndrome, multiple sclerosis, hydrocephalus, Shy-Drager syndrome)
Pulmonary disorders	Infectious (bacterial, viral, and fungal pneumonia and tuberculosis) Functional (asthma, acute respiratory failure, and mechanical ventilation)
Endocrine diseases	Glucocorticoid deficiency (hypopituitarism) Hypothyroidism
Drugs	Antidiuretic hormones (vasopressin, DDAVP, and oxytocin) Psychotropic agents (tricyclic antidepressants, serotonin reuptake inhibitors, monoamine oxidase inhibitors, and carbamazepine) Ecstasy (MDMA) Antineoplastic agents (cyclophosphamide, vincristine, and vinblastine) Nonsteroidal anti-inflammatory drugs Diabetic agents (chlorpropamide and tolbutamide) Miscellaneous (bromocriptine and nicotine)
Other causes	Postoperative stress Alcohol withdrawal AIDS Nausea

DDAVP—1-desamino-8-D-arginine vasopressin MDMA—methylenedioxymethamphetamine

to gradually return the plasma sodium concentration to normal. To avoid complications from excessive correction of hyponatremia, the plasma sodium concentration should not be intentionally increased by more than 12 mEq/L during the first day of therapy or by more than 6 mEq/L/day thereafter.

CHRONIC HYPONATREMIA

The distinction between acute and chronic hyponatremia is somewhat arbitrary. We consider hyponatremia to be chronic when it has evolved over the course of 48 hours or more.[11,12,24] Although the precise duration of an electrolyte disturbance cannot be known when it develops outside the hospital (except for psychotic water drinkers, marathon runners, and users of ecstasy) outpatients can be assumed to have chronic hyponatremia.[30] Prolonged hyponatremia cannot occur unless there is a sustained defect in water excretion. Except for patients with renal failure, virtually all chronically hyponatremic patients have some abnormality in vasopressin secretion.

Etiology

Advanced renal failure A low glomerular filtration rate limits the ability to excrete electrolyte-free water. Many patients with advanced renal failure excrete urine that has the same osmolality as plasma regardless of physiologic conditions (fixed isosthenuria). In acute oliguric renal failure, the ability to excrete free water is virtually nil; administration of hypotonic fluids must be scrupulously avoided to avoid hyponatremia.

Diuretics Thiazide diuretics are commonly the sole cause or a major contributing factor of hyponatremia requiring hospital admission.[30,31] For unknown reasons, severe hyponatremia caused by thiazides affects elderly women much more often than other groups. By blocking the reabsorption of sodium and chloride in the distal tubule, thiazides and metolazone prevent the generation of maximally dilute urine.[32] Because sodium reabsorption in the ascending limb of the loop of Henle is left unaffected by these agents, they permit excretion of maximally concentrated, hypertonic urine and can lead to simultaneous retention of water and depletion of sodium and potassium. Extraordinarily severe hyponatremia can result from thiazides, with plasma sodium levels as low as 100 mEq/L. Vasopressin levels are usually elevated in patients who present with thiazide-induced hyponatremia, sometimes because of diuretic-induced volume depletion but more often because of the stress of minor intercurrent illnesses. Patients with thiazide-induced hyponatremia do not usually appear clinically volume depleted, presumably because retained water partially sustains extracellular fluid volume. Patients who have become hyponatremic on thiazides should not be given these agents again; recurrent episodes of severe hyponatremia are common.

Hypovolemia Hypovolemic hyponatremia is most often associated with gastrointestinal fluid losses caused by vomiting, diarrhea, or laxative abuse. Surprisingly, particularly in alcoholics, patients who continue to drink while vomiting repeatedly can still absorb enough ingested water to become hyponatremic. Electrolyte losses in the vomitus, combined with urinary sodium and potassium losses that result from metabolic alkalosis, lower the plasma sodium concentration.

Beer potomania Patients who subsist on beer (a practice known as beer potomania) are susceptible to hyponatremia because of their low rates of solute excretion (beer contains little protein or electrolyte). Nonosmotic stimuli to vasopressin secretion caused by nausea or gastrointestinal fluid losses or by treatment with thiazide diuretics are often contributing factors.[15]

Edematous conditions Any disease that can cause edema also predisposes to water retention and hyponatremia. The same hemodynamic factors that promote sodium retention are nonosmotic stimuli for vasopressin release.[8,16-18] Elevated vasopressin levels have been reported in hyponatremic patients with congestive heart failure, cirrhosis, and nephrotic syndrome. In heart failure, hyponatremia is associated with a low cardiac output and a poor prognosis.

SIADH Nonosmotic release of vasopressin that has no hemodynamic explanation is termed inappropriate [see Table 5].[12,19] A number of tumors (most commonly small cell carcinoma of the lung) ectopically synthesize and secrete vasopressin.[33] Unexplained, persistent hyponatremia should be considered a marker for an underlying malignancy.

SIADH may also complicate the course of a wide variety of conditions in which there is damage to or inflammation of the central nervous system.[8,12] In patients with subarachnoid hemorrhage, natriuretic peptides released by the brain may directly promote urinary sodium loss, regardless of extracellular volume (cerebral salt wasting).[34,35] Urinary salt losses combined with vasopressin-induced water retention are responsible for hyponatremia. SIADH is a common complication of chest infection. Antidiuretic activity has been demonstrated by bioassay in patients with tuberculous lung tissue, and tuberculosis causes SIADH.[11] In pneumonia, vasopressin levels are increased during the acute phase of the disease and return to baseline within a few days. Isolated glucocorticoid deficiency caused by anterior pituitary dysfunction also causes hyponatremia; patients with hypopituitarism develop inappropriate ADH secretion, but unlike patients with Addison disease, they have normal levels of mineralocorticoid and do not become hypovolemic or hyperkalemic. Hyponatremia caused by glucocorticoid deficiency promptly resolves when cortisol is replaced. Hypothyroidism also causes inappropriate ADH secretion; hyponatremia gradually resolves when thyroid hormone is replaced.[36] A number of therapeutic agents can induce SIADH.[12,37] Nonsteroidal anti-inflammatory drugs (NSAIDs) decrease water excretion because they inhibit formation of prostaglandin E_2, which modulates vasopressin action.[8] Rare cases of hyponatremia solely attributable to NSAIDs have been reported, but these commonly used agents may exacerbate other causes of hyponatremia.

Hyponatremia in AIDS Hyponatremia is an extremely common finding in AIDS.[38] Many AIDS patients have features of SIADH associated with opportunistic infections that cause pneumonia and meningitis. Others have clinical signs of volume depletion without low urine sodium values, a finding that may indicate coexistent renal disease or adrenal insufficiency.[39] Hyponatremia often occurs when antibiotics are administered in hypotonic intravenous solutions.

Diagnosis

Hyponatremia should be approached in a systematic fashion. First, the various disorders that can lower the plasma sodium concentration without causing hypotonicity should be excluded [see Differential Diagnosis for Hyponatremia, *above*]. Once it has been established that hypotonic hyponatremia is present, the mechanism for impaired water excretion is identified (hypovolemia versus an edematous condition versus SIADH), and the differential diagnosis that applies to that mechanism is considered. The most challenging goals of the diagnostic process are to determine whether chronic SIADH is present and, if it is, to define the specific disease responsible for the syndrome.

Clinical manifestations Because cerebral edema is usually not severe, the symptoms of chronic hyponatremia are much more subtle, vague, and nonspecific than those of acute water intoxication.[12,24] The electrolyte disturbance is often asymptomatic at sodium levels that may be lethal to a patient with acute water intoxication. As the plasma sodium concentration falls below 115 to 120 mEq/L, patients often experience anorexia, nausea, vomiting, muscle weakness, and muscle cramps. They may be irritable and show personality changes, becoming uncooperative, confused, hostile, or simply slow to respond. At plasma sodium concentrations below 110 mEq/L, gait disturbances, falling, stupor, tremulousness, and, more rarely, seizures may occur.

Chronic hyponatremia itself is rarely, if ever, fatal. However, because hyponatremia can be a marker for severe underlying illness, hospitalized patients with hyponatremia often have a high mortality rate, dying with but not of chronic hyponatremia. There is little evidence that chronic hyponatremia itself leads to permanent sequelae, even when the plasma sodium concentration falls below 105 mEq/L.[30,40] However, patients with prolonged severe hyponatremia are susceptible to iatrogenic injury if their electrolyte disturbance is corrected too rapidly [see Treatment, *below*].

History and physical examination The history of patients with chronic hyponatremia should include information about diet, fluid intake, gastrointestinal fluid losses, and use of diuretics, antidepressants, or other antidiuretic drugs. During the physical examination, physicians should look for clinical signs of volume depletion or an edematous condition. Evidence of volume depletion may not always be definitive, however. For example, vomiting may be a symptom rather than the cause of hyponatremia; extreme hyponatremia may occasionally impair baroreceptor reflexes causing postural hypotension and a false impression of volume depletion; and retained water may mask underlying volume depletion. When the distinction between hyponatremia caused by hypovolemia and hyponatremia caused by inappropriate antidiuretic hormone secretion is not obvious, laboratory clues may helpful.

Laboratory tests Measurement of the urinary sodium, chloride concentration, or both is often the most helpful test.[41] Water retention caused by hypovolemia or by an edematous condition is usually associated with a urinary sodium concentration lower than 20 mEq/L. Hypovolemia caused by upper gastrointestinal fluid losses is an important exception. Loss of gastric fluid causes a metabolic alkalosis that may increase urinary sodium excretion despite volume depletion; the diagnosis can be made by measuring the urine chloride concentration, which is reduced in this condition. In SIADH, urinary sodium matches intake; as the urine is usually concentrated, the urinary sodium concentration exceeds 40 mEq/L unless dietary sodium intake is very low. Measurements of the BUN and serum uric acid complement these measurements. When a hemodynamic abnormality is responsible for hyponatremia, the kidney is underperfused, urea and uric acid clearances are diminished, and the BUN and serum uric acid levels are usually elevated. Conversely, SIADH is a volume-expanded state, and BUN and uric acid levels are usually low. Uric acid is a more reliable indicator of volume status than the BUN, because the latter value is affected by dietary protein intake as well as renal clearance. Assessment of acid-base and potassium balance may provide helpful clues to the diagnosis. The serum potassium and bicarbonate levels are normal in SIADH. Hypokalemia and metabolic alkalosis suggest diuretic therapy or vomiting, which can be surreptitious. Hyperkalemia and metabolic acidosis suggest the possibility of adrenal insufficiency. Hypokalemia and acidosis are found in diarrhea and raise the possibility of surreptitious laxative abuse.

Withdrawal of hyponatremic drugs When a patient is taking a drug that can cause hyponatremia, it is important to exclude another underlying cause for hyponatremia before attributing the electrolyte disturbance to the medication. For example, thiazide diuretics can exacerbate hyponatremia caused by SIADH. The best way to make a diagnosis of drug-induced hyponatremia is to eliminate the offending agent and be sure that water excretion returns to normal when the patient is off the drug. Full resolution of hyponatremia and full recovery of diluting function may be delayed for a week or two in patients with thiazide-induced hyponatremia. During repair of sodium and potassium deficits, transient resetting of the osmostat is common and should not necessarily prompt an extensive search for an underlying cause.

Response to therapy On occasion, evidence regarding the cause of hyponatremia can be equivocal. In such cases, the patient's response to isotonic saline (or a generous oral salt intake and the passage of time) is the best clue to the diagnosis. Patients with subclinical edematous conditions will retain the administered sodi-um, developing clinically obvious edema. Volume-depleted patients initially retain the administered sodium, but as soon as hypovolemia is corrected, the urine becomes dilute, the rate of urinary sodium excretion increases to match intake, and hyponatremia improves as water is excreted in the urine. Urinary sodium excretion promptly increases in patients with SIADH, but the urine remains concentrated and hyponatremia persists. Isotonic saline should be given with extreme caution to patients with very low plasma sodium concentrations; in SIADH, saline can exacerbate hyponatremia, whereas in volume depletion, hyponatremia may correct too rapidly.

Identifying a specific cause for SIADH SIADH is a mechanism for developing hyponatremia, not a diagnosis. In all patients with SIADH, a specific etiology for inappropriate vasopressin secretion should be sought. When hyponatremia develops in the hospital, the cause is sometimes obvious (e.g., pneumonia, meningitis, acute respiratory failure) and no further testing is indicated. In a patient with clinical features of SIADH but no obvious cause for it, a more extensive evaluation is indicated. The workup should include a careful search for malignancy and central nervous system pathology and an endocrine evaluation to exclude hypothyroidism and hypocortisolism. Sometimes, no cause for SIADH is found, especially in elderly patients and patients with psychiatric disorders, mental retardation, or alcoholism.[42] Careful follow-up is important, because malignancies may become clinically apparent after several years in so-called idiopathic SIADH.

Treatment

Patients with very low plasma sodium concentrations usually have some neurologic symptoms, and they are at risk of injuries from falls. However, unlike acute water intoxication, there is little risk of an explosive onset of seizures or a fatal outcome in chronic hyponatremia. On the other hand, patients with chronic hyponatremia are at considerable risk of neurologic injury caused by overaggressive correction. Thus, there are four major goals in managing chronic hyponatremia: (1) prevention of a progressive decrease in plasma sodium concentration; (2) amelioration of symptoms caused by hyponatremia; (3) avoidance of excessive correction; and (4) gradual restoration and maintenance of a normal plasma sodium concentration.

Free-water restriction should be instituted in all patients until the plasma sodium concentration has begun to increase. Intravenous fluids should be at least isotonic, and oral fluid intake should be limited to 500 to 1,000 ml/day, depending on the severity of the electrolyte disturbance. In patients with reversible defects in water excretion, limitations on free-water intake should be lifted once the plasma sodium concentration has begun to increase.

Attempts to calculate the dose of sodium chloride needed to correct hyponatremia are doomed to failure. The increase in plasma sodium concentration depends on the amounts of administered sodium and potassium that have been retained without being excreted, as well as on the amount of electrolyte-free water that is eliminated in the urine. Indeed, in some cases, the plasma sodium concentration will return to normal solely because of a water diuresis, with no sodium given. The measures required to increase the plasma sodium concentration, along with the likelihood of inadvertent rapid correction, vary depending on the cause of hyponatremia. For therapeutic purposes, the causes can be divided into reversible and persistent defects in water excretion.

Reversible defects in water excretion Hyponatremia corrects easily when the cause for defective water excretion can be eliminated by volume expansion, by withdrawal of a therapeutic agent, or by treatment of an underlying illness [see Table 4]. In patients with reversible defects in water excretion, prevention of excessive correction may become a major challenge.

Hypovolemic hyponatremia responds readily to 0.9% sodium chloride because the sodium concentration of isotonic saline is higher than the cation concentration of the excreted urine. Once the volume deficit is repaired and the hemodynamic stimulus to vasopressin secretion is removed, the urine becomes dilute and a water diuresis may rapidly return the plasma sodium concentration to normal. Similarly, patients with diuretic-induced hyponatremia are extremely susceptible to rapid correction; restoration of the renal diluting mechanism when the diuretic is discontinued and replacement of sodium and potassium deficits contribute to the increase in plasma sodium concentration.

Intravenous saline should be discontinued once clinically apparent hypovolemia has been corrected and the plasma sodium concentration has begun to increase. Saline should be given cautiously, if at all, to hypokalemic patients who require potassium replacement. During repair of a potassium deficit, potassium enters cells, displacing sodium, which then returns to the extracellular fluid; administered potassium is therefore as effective as sodium in raising the plasma sodium concentration. Diuretic-induced hyponatremia does not usually necessitate use of intravenous saline; for most patients, an adequate diet, replacement of potassium deficits, and discontinuance of thiazide diuretics are sufficient. In severely hyponatremic patients, the plasma sodium concentration should be monitored every 6 to 8 hours for the first 2 to 3 days of therapy. If it appears that a water diuresis is going to increase the plasma sodium by more than the desired amount, replacement of fluid losses with oral water or 5% dextrose in water may become necessary.

Persistent defects in water excretion: SIADH   Patients with SIADH tend to be resistant to rapid changes in plasma sodium concentration (unless the cause of SIADH is short-lived). Water restriction is the cornerstone of therapy, but if used alone, water restriction often leads to an extremely slow resolution of hyponatremia. Isotonic saline is ineffective and may even be counterproductive. Furosemide and loop diuretics are often useful therapeutic adjuncts because by blocking sodium reabsorption in the ascending limb of the loop of Henle, they interfere with the renal-concentrating mechanism, partially blocking the effect of vasopressin. Loop diuretics can be combined with oral salt or a slow infusion (approximately 15 ml/hr) of 3% saline. Oral and intravenous urea have been used extensively to treat SIADH in some parts of Europe, but experience with this agent in the United States is very limited. Demeclocycline, a tetracycline that blocks the effect of vasopressin on the collecting duct, is another therapeutic option in chronic SIADH; however, its expense and long duration of action limit its effectiveness. Several orally active vasopressin receptor blockers have been developed and are currently in clinical trials.[43,44]

Persistent defects in water excretion: edematous conditions and renal failure   Saline should rarely, if ever, be given to correct hyponatremia in edematous patients or patients with renal failure (except for those with prerenal azotemia). Because it has no effect on water excretion, 1 L of 0.9% saline will increase the plasma sodium concentration by only 1 mEq/L.[12] In addition, saline exacerbates edema and ascites in patients with cirrhosis and may cause pulmonary edema in patients with congestive heart failure or renal failure.

Although thiazide diuretics are contraindicated, loop diuretics

are the mainstay of treatment of hyponatremia for patients with edematous conditions because they increase free-water excretion and improve hyponatremia, particularly when dietary salt intake is increased. There is a natural inclination to discontinue loop diuretics when severely edematous patients develop hyponatremia. The usual problem, however, is oliguria and diuretic resistance rather than overdiuresis; the proper response is to increase the dose of loop diuretics and restrict water intake. The combination of a loop diuretic and an angiotensin converting enzyme (ACE) inhibitor is particularly effective in patients with congestive heart failure. The beneficial effect of an ACE inhibitor can be explained by reduced thirst and vasopressin secretion attributable to angiotensin II and by a direct effect on the hydro-osmotic effect of vasopressin, mediated by prostaglandins.[11]

Hyponatremia in edematous conditions is mediated by vasopressin. Clinical trials have shown that vasopressin receptor antagonists can be effective in managing patients with hyponatremia and edema.[43,44]

Treatment of hyponatremic seizures   A small percentage of chronically hyponatremic patients with very low plasma sodium concentrations present with seizures. Regardless of the suspected duration or cause of the electrolyte disturbance, active seizures may be resistant to anticonvulsants alone and should be treated with hypertonic saline. The therapeutic approach is similar to that used for patients with acute water intoxication, except that even more vigilance is required to prevent an excessive increase in plasma sodium concentration once emergency measures have been discontinued.[12,24]

Complications of Therapy: Myelinolysis and Osmotic Demyelination Syndrome

Excessive correction of chronic hyponatremia may be complicated by neurologic injury.[40,45] Typically, the patient's hyponatremic symptoms improve as the plasma sodium concentration increases, but after a delay of one to several days, new findings emerge. The patient may become confused and may exhibit psychotic or catatonic behavior, pathologic crying, or a movement disorder. Swallowing dysfunction, progressive unresponsiveness, and a spastic quadriparesis may develop. In severe cases, locked-in syndrome occurs—that is, the patient is awake but unable to move or respond. The stereotypical pattern of delayed neurologic deterioration after rapid correction of hyponatremia has been named the osmotic demyelination syndrome,[45] because these clinical features are associated with brain lesions (myelinolysis) characterized by disruption of myelin and sparing of neurons and axons.[46,47] Lesions, which are best identified by magnetic resonance imaging, are typically found in the center of the basal pons (central pontine myelinolysis [CPM]), but histologically similar lesions may also occur in a symmetrical distribution in extrapontine areas of the brain where there is a close admixture of gray and white matter. The osmotic demyelination syndrome has been reproduced in animal studies[46]; these experiments have shown that the disorder is a complication of rapid correction of hyponatremia rather than the electrolyte disturbance itself. Observational studies in severely hyponatremic patients suggest that this therapeutic complication can be avoided if rates of correction are maintained below 10 to 12 mEq/L/day and 18 mEq/L/48 hr. Because large increases in the serum sodium concentration are seldom required to relieve hyponatremic symptoms and because unintentional excessive correction is common, the goal of therapy should be to increase serum sodium concentration by 8 mEq/L/day or less.[12]

Disorder of Water Deficiency: Hypernatremia

PATHOGENESIS

Persistent hypernatremia results from one of two basic mechanisms: water is lost and not adequately replaced or, less commonly, too much salt is taken in without enough water [see Table 6].[13,48-50] In either case, electrolyte-free water is needed to return the plasma sodium concentration to normal. Because thirst is the primary defense against hypertonicity, persistent hypernatre-mia means there is a defect in water intake. A maximally concentrated urine minimizes but does not prevent water losses. Insensible water losses from the skin and lungs are unavoidable and urea excretion obligates some urinary losses. Maintenance of a normal serum sodium concentration (135 to 142 mEq/L) requires that daily water losses be replaced.

Most hypernatremic patients are too sick, too young, or too old to obtain water themselves or ask for it.[13,48] Sometimes, the thirst sensation itself is impaired, so that the patient has no desire to drink when the plasma sodium concentration increases above the normal range. Inadequate water intake by itself will lead to hypernatremia. When impaired intake is coupled with excessive water losses, severe hypernatremia results.

ETIOLOGY

Electrolyte-free water can be lost as pure water, with no accompanying electrolyte, or it can be lost in hypotonic fluids, which have lower electrolyte concentrations than plasma. Hypotonic losses can be thought of as mixtures of isotonic fluid and free water. Pure-water and hypotonic fluid losses, the most common causes of hypernatremia, are typically associated with a contracted extracellular fluid volume.[13] However, this is not always the case. When hypernatremia is caused by a rapid intake of salt (acute salt poisoning), the extracellular volume expands because of water drawn from the intracellular space.[48] In critically ill patients, extracellular volume expansion with edema often coexists with hypernatremia[49,51]; the finding reflects free-water losses in patients who become edematous after fluid resuscitation for shock or underlying conditions such as congestive heart failure, renal disease, and hepatic cirrhosis.

Pure-Water Losses

If pure-water losses are responsible for hypernatremia, each body-fluid compartment loses an equal percentage of its volume.[13,48] Plasma constitutes only one twelfth of total body water (one quarter of extracellular fluid volume), and plasma volume is defended by oncotic pressure, which increases with water loss. Thus, plasma volume contracts by less than 83 ml for each 1 L of water lost; clinical signs of hypovolemia are unusual unless the water deficit is extremely large.

Insensible water losses Water is constantly lost by evaporation from the skin and lungs and must be replaced to avoid dehydration. Daily insensible water losses, normally about 0.5 L, can be increased severalfold by high environmental temperature, fever, or hypermetabolic states such as thyrotoxicosis.

Increased urea excretion Although urea is an ineffective osmole that freely crosses most cell membranes, urinary urea excretion can play an important role in water balance. High rates of urea excretion caused by protein-rich diets, catabolism, or recovery from renal failure obligate increased rates of water loss. When the urine solute is composed almost exclusively of urea, the urine becomes an electrolyte-free water solution, regardless of its osmolality.

Table 6 Causes of Hypernatremia

Electrolyte-free water losses	Extrarenal
	  Insensible loss (skin and lungs)
	Renal
	  Neurogenic (central) diabetes insipidus
	  Nephrogenic diabetes insipidus
	    Congenital
	      X-linked (V_2 vasopressin receptor defect)
	      Recessive (aquaporin defects)
	    Acquired
	      Electrolyte abnormalities: hypokalemia, hypercalcemia
	      Drugs: lithium, demeclocycline, methoxyflurane
	      Pregnancy (vasopressinase)
	  Excess urea excretion

Hypotonic losses	Extrarenal
	  Sweat
	  Upper GI tract
	  Osmotic cathartics
	Renal
	  Glycosuria, mannitol, glycerol, diuretics

Salt poisoning	Oral
	Parenteral
	  $NaHCO_3$, 3% or 5% I.V. saline, therapeutic abortion (inadvertent 29% I.V. saline)
	  Hemodialysis with hypertonic dialysate

Diabetes insipidus Because sodium excretion is unaffected in diabetes insipidus (see below), the excess fluid lost in the urine is pure water. As long as water is available and the patient is able to drink, hypernatremia does not occur. Without water replacement, however, hypernatremia develops within a few hours

Hypotonic Losses

Hypernatremia caused by hypotonic fluid loss is associated with extracellular volume depletion.

Sweat Sweat is a hypotonic solution containing water, sodium, potassium, and chloride. Sweat glands respond to aldosterone by lowering the sodium concentration and increasing the potassium concentration of their secretions.

Gastric fluid losses Fluid lost by vomiting or nasogastric suction is hypotonic to plasma. Without adequate water replacement, large gastric fluid losses can cause hypernatremia.

Osmotic cathartics Fecal losses of water contain electrolytes at a concentration comparable to that of plasma, except when osmotic cathartics such as sorbitol or lactulose are given. These cathartic agents osmotically attract electrolyte-free water to the intestinal lumen, leading to hypotonic fluid losses. Oral sorbitol is a nonabsorbable solute, given with sodium polystyrene sulfonate (Kayexalate) to treat hyperkalemia or with charcoal to treat poisoning; the sugar osmotically attracts electrolyte-free water into the intestinal lumen, where it is eliminated in the stool. Similarly, lactulose, which is used to treat hepatic encephalopathy, can promote large electrolyte-free water losses, causing a high incidence of hypernatremia unless the lost water is replaced.

Osmotic diuretics and glycosuria Glucose in the extracellular fluid acts as an effective osmole that attracts water to the extracellular fluid, dehydrating cells and lowering the plasma sodium concentration.[22,48] Excretion of glucose in the urine acts as an osmotic diuretic that can provoke the loss of several liters of hypotonic fluid. Electrolyte-free water losses induced by glycosuria raise the plasma sodium concentration, offsetting the hyponatremic effect of the high blood glucose levels. Intravenous hyertonic mannitol has a similar effect on body fluids.

Acute Salt Poisoning

Water losses increase the serum sodium concentration over hours or days. The oral ingestion of large amounts of salt without water—1 tbsp of salt contains nearly 350 mEq of NaCl, enough to increase the plasma sodium concentration by 8 mEq/L—or the intravenous infusion of hypertonic salt solutions can increase the plasma sodium concentration much more rapidly (i.e., cause acute salt poisoning).[13,48]

DIAGNOSIS

Clinical Manifestations

An acute onset of hypernatremia (seen virtually exclusively in acute salt poisoning) causes the brain to shrink, leading to vascular injury and intracranial bleeding. Patients present with seizures, coma, hyperventilation, hyperreflexia, hypertonia, and high fever. Acutely hypernatremic patients with plasma sodium levels above 170 mEq/L often die.[13,48]

Given time to adapt, brain cells protect their volume by accumulating organic osmolytes, preventing the hemorrhages caused by acute hypernatremia. Thus, the clinical manifestations of chronic hypernatremia are less dramatic than those seen in acute salt poisoning, ranging from lethargy to coma, depending on the severity of the electrolyte disturbance.[13,48,50]

The clinical signs of pure-water loss and acute salt poisoning are primarily neurologic. Hypotonic fluid losses may be associated with signs and symptoms of extracellular fluid volume depletion in addition to symptoms related to hypernatremia.

Recognition of Water Deficit

The plasma or serum sodium concentration can be used to determine how much water is needed to restore normotonicity; it seriously underestimates the magnitude of the water deficit in diabetic patients with hyperglycemic dehydration [see Treatment, Diabetic Dehydration, below]. In patients without severe hyperglycemia, the percentage increase in the serum sodium concentration approximates the percentage decrease in total body water, as stated more precisely in the following:

Water deficit = Normal body water $(1 - \text{serum } [Na^+]/140)$

The value for body water is based on the patient's usual body weight (often an estimate), age, and sex.

The calculated water deficit is the amount of water that will return the serum sodium concentration to normal. It reveals nothing about the volume status of the extracellular fluid. Extracellular fluid volume deficits (or surfeits) must be estimated from the history and physical examination, not from the serum sodium concentration.

TREATMENT

Correction of severe extracellular volume depletion takes precedence over correction of hypernatremia. When the patient is hypotensive, initial therapy should include a rapid infusion of isotonic saline to quickly achieve hemodynamic stability. In hemodynamically stable patients, pure-water losses should be replaced with pure water, and isotonic saline is not required. Edematous patients with hy-

pernatremia can be given diuretics along with electrolyte-free water to replace urinary electrolyte-free water losses; the net effect is reduction of the extracellular volume surfeit and restoration of normotonicity and cell volume.

Electrolyte-free water can be given intravenously in a 5% dextrose solution (D5W) to patients who are unable to drink. Dextrose solutions cannot be infused more rapidly than approximately 500 ml/hr. More-rapid infusions provide more glucose than can be metabolized and therefore cause hyperglycemia, glycosuria, and urinary water losses, which are counterproductive to the correction of hypertonicity. Water replacement should not be based on formulas alone; the serum sodium concentration and urine output should be monitored frequently so that the fluid prescription can be adjusted appropriately.

Rate of Correction

In the vast majority of cases, the onset of hypertonicity is slow enough for brain adaptations to minimize cerebral dehydration. Organic osmolytes that accumulate in the adaptation to hypernatremia are slow to leave the cell during rehydration. If hypernatremia is corrected too rapidly, cerebral edema results.[13,48] To be safe, the serum sodium concentration should be reduced by no more than 10 to 12 mEq/L/day. To achieve the desired rate of correction, electrolyte-free water intake should exceed free-water losses by no more than 2 L daily.

Acute salt poisoning causes devastating brain injury that is largely irreversible. In rare cases when acute salt poisoning can be rapidly diagnosed (e.g., in a case of inadvertent intravenous infusion of hypertonic saline during therapeutic abortion), an effort to prevent a neurologic catastrophe can be made with rapid infusions of electrolyte-free water along with a loop diuretic before the results of the serum electrolyte measurements are known.

Diabetic Dehydration

Hypertonicity associated with diabetes mellitus is a complex disorder.[22] The osmotic diuresis induced by glycosuria results in both saltwater and electrolyte-free water losses; the accumulation of glucose in the extracellular fluid adds impermeant solute, which contributes to hypertonicity and neurologic symptoms. Severely dehydrated hyperglycemic patients may not appear hypovolemic at first, because the high glucose concentration in the extracellular fluid osmotically attracts water from cells, masking the loss of saltwater. With correction of hyperglycemia, marked hypovolemia may emerge. Initial treatment should include 1 to 2 L of isotonic saline in anticipation of this complication, even in patients who are initially normotensive. With volume expansion, excess glucose will be excreted in the urine, creating an ongoing requirement for both saline and electrolyte-free water. An infusion of 0.45% saline at a rate that exceeds urine output by approximately 250 ml/hr will serve to replace the electrolyte-free water deficit and remaining saltwater deficits. The serum sodium concentration, blood glucose level, and urine output should be monitored carefully so that fluid replacement can be tailored to the patient's needs. Rapid correction of hypertonicity should be avoided because of the risk of cerebral edema.

Patients with oliguric renal failure do not become dehydrated when they become severely hyperglycemic. Such patients often experience hypertension or congestive heart failure because of fluid shifts from cells to the extracellular fluid. Even after adjusting for the effect of hyperglycemia, the serum sodium concentration is often low. Insulin is the only required treatment; neither isotonic saline nor 0.45% saline is indicated.

Disorder of Water Conservation: Diabetes Insipidus

PATHOGENESIS

Neurogenic diabetes insipidus (DI) is caused by deficient secretion of vasopressin[8,52,53]; nephrogenic DI results from the kidney's unresponsiveness to normally secreted hormone.[54] Both disorders present with polyuria (loosely defined as the passage of excessive volumes of urine—generally more than 3 to 4 L daily) and polydipsia (excessive thirst). Most patients with polyuria do not become hypernatremic, because thirst maintains electrolyte-free water balance.

Defective responsiveness to vasopressin (nephrogenic DI) may be inherited as an X-linked trait, caused by a mutation in the gene encoding for the V_2 vasopressin receptor or as an autosomal recessive trait caused by a mutation in the gene encoding for the vasopressin-responsive water channel (aquaporin 2). Acquired nephrogenic DI may be caused by lithium or demeclocycline therapy, hypokalemia, or hypercalcemia; or it may complicate a number of renal diseases [see Table 6]. Vasopressin-resistant DI may emerge during the late stage of pregnancy as a result of vasopressinase released by the placenta; many affected patients have underlying, subclinical partial neurogenic or nephrogenic DI that has been exacerbated by increased catabolism of circulating vasopressin.

DIAGNOSIS

Clinical Manifestations

Patients with DI complain of polyuria, nocturia (the need to urinate during the night), and polydipsia. The only significant physical findings or laboratory abnormalities are those of the underlying cause.

Laboratory Tests

A diagnosis of DI can be made if the urine osmolality is less than 250 mOsm/kg despite hypernatremia.[8] When the disease is suspected in a polyuric patient whose serum sodium concentration is normal or borderline, the urine osmolality level can be monitored while the patient is deprived of water, allowing the serum sodium level to increase to higher than 143 mEq/L. Exogenous vasopressin increases urine osmolality by more than 150 mOsm/kg in patients with neurogenic, but not nephrogenic, DI. It is possible to misdiagnose DI in patients who actually have a primary thirst disorder. Excessive water intake suppresses vasopressin secretion and causes polyuria with dilute urine. Because patients with primary polydipsia secrete vasopressin normally, they do not become hypernatremic during diagnostic water deprivation. Correlation with plasma vasopressin levels is often necessary in borderline cases. Polyuric patients whose urine osmolality equals or exceeds plasma osmolality should be distinguished from patients with DI; polyuria in such cases is usually caused by excessive excretion of salt, urea, or glucose or by an osmotic diuretic (solute diuresis).

Magnetic resonance imaging of the brain can be helpful in the evaluation of patients with suspected DI.[8,53] In 85% to 90% of healthy adults and children, the posterior pituitary emits a hyperintense signal, or so-called bright spot, on T_1-weighted magnetic resonance images, apparently related to the vasopressin release of the gland. This bright spot is also normal in 85% to 90% of patients with primary polydipsia, but it is almost always absent or greatly diminished in patients with pituitary DI.

TREATMENT

When access to water is limited, patients with DI are more susceptible to dehydration than normal persons. Thus, water losses must be carefully replaced during superimposed illnesses. Neurogenic DI is best treated with a synthetic antidiuretic hormone, 1-desamino-8-D-arginine vasopressin (DDAVP), which can be given parenterally or intranasally.[8,53] Chlorpropamide or carbamazepine, both of which enhance vasopressin action, or thiazide diuretics, which limit the ability to maximally dilute the urine, can be used in patients with mild disease. Limiting dietary salt and protein intake is also helpful. Nephrogenic diabetes can also be treated with dietary measures or with thiazides and indomethacin (which helps concentrate the urine by inhibiting prostaglandin synthesis). Lithium-induced nephrogenic DI may be improved by amiloride, which blocks lithium entry into the collecting duct cell.

Disorder of Saltwater Excess: Edematous States

Edema, a swelling of the soft tissues that can be indented or pitted by the examiner's fingers, is the clinical manifestation of an expanded interstitial fluid volume. To be detected clinically, interstitial volume must increase by at least 2.5 to 3 L, nearly equaling the total amount of fluid in the intravascular space. Thus, generalized edema requires an increase in the total amount of saltwater in the extracellular space, and it implies retention of dietary or infused sodium, with an impaired ability to excrete saltwater.

PATHOGENESIS

Excess fluid collects in the interstitial space in response to Starling forces, which govern the movement of extracellular fluid into and out of the vasculature. Edema occurs when there is increased capillary blood pressure, decreased plasma oncotic pressure, increased capillary permeability to protein, or obstruction to lymph flow.

When fluid overflows from an overfilled vascular space into the interstitium, impaired sodium excretion is clearly implicated. However, even when edema formation results from decreased oncotic pressure or increased capillary permeablity, renal sodium retention is required to replace the saltwater that has been lost from the vasculature.

ETIOLOGY

Primary Renal Sodium Retention: Edema Caused by Renal Disease

Nephrotic syndrome The nephrotic syndrome is characterized by heavy urinary protein losses (in excess of 3 g/day), hypoalbuminemia, and edema.[55] The syndrome, which can be seen in a variety of glomerular diseases, is caused by increased permeability of the glomerular capillary to protein. Traditionally, edema in the nephrotic syndrome has been ascribed to decreased plasma oncotic pressure. This no longer appears to be the sole explanation. Correction of hypoalbuminemia by infusing albumin does not consistently improve the edema, and resolution of edema in steroid-responsive cases may precede improvement of hypoalbuminemia. Thus, in most patients, primary sodium retention by the kidney, independent of an underfilled vasculature, plays a major contributing role.

Nephritic edema Glomerular diseases characterized by proliferation of mesangial cells (e.g., diffuse proliferative glomerulonephritis and membranoproliferative glomerulonephritis) often cause primary sodium retention that is not associated with heavy proteinuria or hypoalbuminemia (the nephritic syndrome). Patients with nephritic edema are typically hypertensive and may present with congestive heart failure because of an overexpanded vascular volume.

Secondary Renal Sodium Retention: Edema Caused by Extrarenal Disease

In congestive heart failure and hepatic cirrhosis, the body responds as if it were volume depleted. Despite an expanded interstitial fluid volume, as well as increased total body sodium content, the kidney avidly retains salt and water. The normal renal response to a high salt intake is lost, and progressive salt retention occurs. In these conditions, volume regulatory mechanisms are responding to reduced fullness of the arterial portion of the vascular system, which normally contains about 15% of the total blood volume.

Congestive heart failure Advanced stages of the many disorders that affect the pericardium, myocardium, or heart valves can produce congestive heart failure, a disorder characterized by renal sodium retention and interstitial edema in systemic or pulmonary capillary beds.[16,17] Arterial receptors are activated when cardiac output falls (low-output congestive failure) or when cardiac output is not high enough to compensate for decreased peripheral resistance (high-output failure).

Cirrhosis Patients with severe liver disease may exhibit profound salt retention, often excreting less than 10 mEq of sodium in the urine each day. Scarring of the hepatic parenchyma increases resistance to blood flow in the postsinusoidal venules, resulting in high sinusoidal pressures and venous hypertension throughout the portal system. Portal hypertension and hypoalbuminemia promote the formation of ascites. In addition, the cirrhotic patient is vasodilated because of endotoxins, vasodilatory prostaglandins, nitric oxide, various gut hormones, and other mediators. The combined effects of blood pooling in the splanchnic circulation (caused by portal hypertension) and systemic vasodilatation lead to underfilling of the arterial circulation and subsequent activation of sodium-retaining factors.[56]

Idiopathic edema Idiopathic edema is a benign disorder of young, menstruating women who have no cardiac, hepatic, or renal disease.[57] Fluid retention often begins premenstrually and then becomes persistent. Depression and neurotic symptoms are commonly present, and affected patients are often weight conscious and markedly concerned about even minor degrees of edema. Some patients episodically fast for days at a time and then accumulate edema on refeeding. In many others, diuretics play an important role in the pathogenesis of idiopathic edema. Long-term diuretic or cathartic use leads to persistent hypovolemia and chronic activation of sodium-retaining mechanisms, which include hypertrophy of the nephron segments distal to the site of action of the diuretic. When the diuretic is stopped, marked sodium retention occurs because the sodium-retaining forces cannot be shut off rapidly. The patient thus becomes convinced of the need for diuretics, and the cycle continues.

DIAGNOSIS

The symptoms and laboratory findings associated with edematous conditions depend on the underlying cause. Dyspnea on exertion and orthopnea provoked by pulmonary interstitial edema are prominent features in patients with left ventricular failure or nephritic edema, but these symptoms are usually absent when edema is caused by right heart failure, nephrotic syndrome, or cirrhosis. Mild peripheral edema collects in the dependent portions of the anatomy and is usually asymptomatic. Although more severe edema, which can extend to the thighs and buttocks, may be uncomfortable, it is usually harmless. A large volume of ascites not only causes discomfort but also may elevate the diaphragm, causing shortness of breath; promote reflux of gastric fluid, causing bleeding from esophageal varices; or become infected spontaneously.

The diagnosis of edema should be approached systematically, looking for evidence of heart, renal, or liver disease. A diagnosis can usually be made from the history and physical examination, urinalysis, liver function tests, and chest x-ray. More puzzling cases may require echocardiography or, rarely, right heart catheterization. Plasma levels of B-type natriuretic peptide (BNP) are increased in patients with heart failure. Used in conjunction with other clinical information, rapid-measurement BNP is useful in establishing or excluding the diagnosis of congestive heart failure in patients who present with acute dyspnea.[58]

TREATMENT

Dietary salt restriction is important for patients with edema, but this measure alone is impractical or insufficient when urinary sodium excretion is reduced to very low levels. Thus, most edematous patients whose underlying condition cannot be reversed require treatment with diuretics.[5,59] Salt restriction and diuretics are adjunctive treatments for heart failure. Therapy is also directed at improving cardiac performance by using digoxin and vasodilators to reduce afterload. Recombinant human BNP (nesiritide) has become available for the treatment of acute decompensated heart failure. The agent reduces pulmonary capillary wedge pressure and systemic vascular resistance, improves cardiac performance, and has a diuretic effect, in part because of its effect on sodium reabsorption in the distal nephron.[60]

Ascitic fluid is a separate compartment of the extracellular fluid compartment that is much more difficult to mobilize than peripheral edema. Thus, cirrhotic patients who have ascites but no peripheral edema are susceptible to intravascular volume depletion when they are treated with diuretics; weight loss should thus be limited to 0.5 kg daily. Repeated large-volume paracenteses combined with intravenous albumin is a safe and effective alternative to diuretics that avoids intravascular volume depletion.[61] The subsequent administration of diuretics prevents reaccumulation of ascitic fluid.

Use of Diuretics

Diuretics increase saltwater excretion by impairing tubular reabsorption of the sodium filtered by the glomerulus. The diuretic effect is dose-dependent; the maximum response is determined by the diuretic's site of action within the nephron, the filtered load of sodium, and the amount of sodium reabsorbed by nephron segments unaffected by the diuretic.

Mechanism of action All diuretics except spironolactone are specific inhibitors of luminal transporters and must gain access to the tubular fluid to block sodium reabsorption.[5,59] Because diuretic agents are highly protein bound, they are not readily filtered at the glomerulus; instead, they are actively transported into the urine by the organic acid (e.g., acetazolamide, thiazide, and loop diuretic) or organic base (e.g., amiloride and triamterene) secretory pumps in the proximal tubule. A dose-response curve links the amount of drug reaching the urine to the amount of sodium excretion that is elicited [*see Figure 4*]. Spironolactone binds to the cytosolic receptor for aldosterone, and its diuretic action, unlike that of other diuretics, does not depend on secretion into the tubular lumen.

The most potent agents are those that block sodium transport in the loop of Henle. At high doses, loop diuretics almost totally block sodium reabsorption in this nephron segment, causing about 20% of the filtered load of sodium to be excreted in the urine; at low glomerular filtration rates, the same percentage of filtered sodium is excreted, but the total amount is reduced. Conditions such as volume depletion, heart failure, and cirrhosis, which cause avid sodium reabsorption in the proximal and distal tubules, blunt the maximum response to the diuretic.

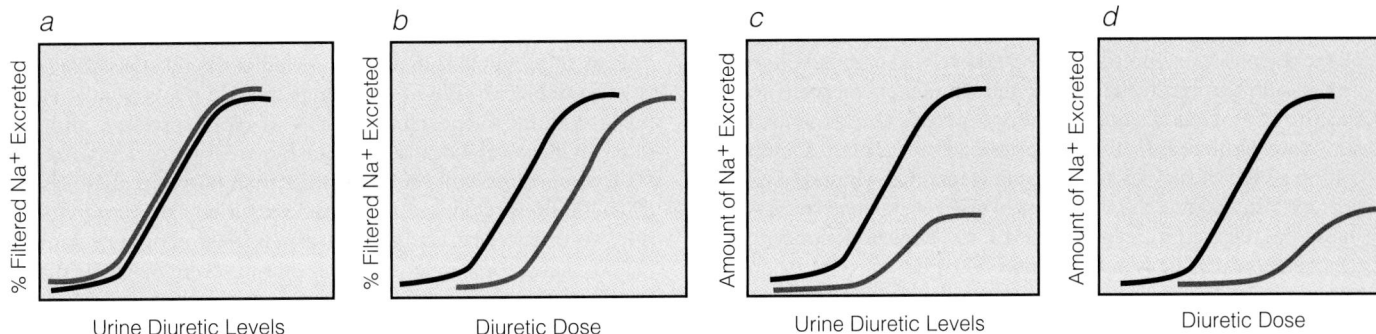

Figure 4 **Dose-response curves for a loop diuretic in patients with normal (black line) and reduced (red line) renal function. Urinary sodium excretion responds to diuretic levels in the tubular lumen (as reflected by urinary drug levels). The diuretic effect reaches a maximum at approximately 20% of the filtered load of sodium regardless of renal function (*a*). Secretion of the diuretic into the tubular lumen is reduced in renal failure; thus, higher doses are required in azotemic patients to achieve the same urinary drug levels found in patients with normal renal function (*b*). Because the filtered load of sodium is reduced in patients with renal failure, absolute sodium excretion is also reduced, even at high doses (*c* and *d*).**

Because gastrointestinal absorption of diuretics is often delayed in edematous conditions (presumably because of bowel edema), higher oral doses must be used to achieve adequate blood levels. In renal disease and cirrhosis, organic anions such as hippurate and bile acids compete with the diuretic for secretion into the proximal tubule; thus, higher plasma levels may be required to achieve adequate drug levels in the urine. Similarly, severe hypoalbuminemia can diminish drug secretion into the tubular lumen, because albumin binding of most diuretics maximizes the rate of diuretic delivery to the organic anion secretory pump in the proximal tubule. Reduced renal blood flow also limits delivery of drug to the tubular lumen. Some patients with advanced cirrhosis who are resistant to furosemide respond to spironolactone, a generally weak diuretic whose effectiveness does not depend on tubular secretion.

Agents that act in the proximal tubule, loop of Henle, or distal tubule cause potassium wasting and hypokalemia because they increase delivery of tubular fluid to the cortical collecting tubule, where potassium secretion is flow dependent. Potassium-sparing diuretics, which act in the cortical collecting tubule, cause hyperkalemia because sodium reabsorption at this site favors potassium secretion. The carbonic anhydrase inhibitor, acetazolamide, causes metabolic acidosis, as do the potassium-sparing diuretics. Thiazides and loop diuretics cause metabolic alkalosis because of increased distal delivery of sodium to sites where sodium reabsorption stimulates hydrogen ion secretion.

Clinical use   Diuretic doses should be adjusted to achieve explicit therapeutic goals. Outpatient therapy is usually designed to produce a gradual loss of fluid, increasing the dose until a desired target weight is reached. The patient should be instructed to keep a daily log that records weight and diuretic dose. Patients are instructed to stop the diuretic if their weight falls too low, resuming at a lower dose when enough saltwater has been retained to restore the target weight.

Inpatient diuretic management should also employ the target-weight concept, but dose adjustments can be made more often and more aggressively, particularly at the start of therapy. It is important to rapidly define the dose that can deliver enough drug to the tubular lumen to reach the steep portion of the dose-response curve. Once an effective dose is defined, larger doses of diuretic provide little benefit. If a greater response is needed, the effective dose should be repeated several times during the day, or alternatively, a continuous infusion can be given to maintain effective urinary drug levels. Continuous infusion of loop diuretics induces a slightly larger natri-

uretic response than does bolus administration and is associated with a shorter hospital stay in patients with advanced heart failure.[62]

Diuretic resistance   Resistance to high doses of loop diuretics may be overcome by administering loop diuretics in combination with thiazide or metolazone. Acetazolamide may be used along with or in place of a thiazide or metolazone. This strategy blocks sodium reabsorption at several sites along the nephron, avoiding resistance caused by increased sodium reabsoption proximal or distal to the loop of Henle. Careful monitoring is extremely important, because these combinations can be extremely potent, causing large potassium and sodium losses.

Diuretic complications   All diuretic agents may cause volume depletion and azotemia, but these complications are most likely to occur with loop diuretics.[4] Hypokalemic alkalosis, hyperglycemia, and hyperuricemia (sometimes with clinical gout) are common dose-dependent complications of both thiazides and loop diuretics. Thiazides decrease calcium excretion and may cause hypercalcemia in patients with underlying conditions that increase gastrointestinal calcium absorption (e.g., sarcoidosis) or bone reabsorption (e.g., hyperparathyroidism). Thiazides are also much more likely to cause hyponatremia than other agents and should be avoided in patients who habitually drink large amounts of fluid. Potassium-sparing agents (e.g., triamterene, amiloride, and spironolactone) may cause hyperkalemia; these agents should generally not be given with potassium supplements, and they should be used with caution in patients with renal insufficiency (particularly diabetic nephropathy) and patients receiving ACE inhibitors or angiotensin II blocking agents. Loop diuretics can predispose to hearing loss, particularly when high doses are administered by bolus injection to patients receiving other ototoxic drugs.[32] Hearing loss from ethacrynic acid is more likely to be permanent.

Disorder of Saltwater Deficiency: Volume Depletion

PATHOGENESIS OF VOLUME DEPLETION

Volume depletion occurs when saltwater is lost from the extracellular fluid at a rate that exceeds intake. Saltwater can be lost from the gastrointestinal tract, kidney, or skin, or it can result from extravascular sequestration (third-space losses) in the abdominal cavity or in traumatized tissues.

Underfilling of the arterial circulation triggers a cascade of physiologic responses that preserve blood flow to vital organs. Volume receptors and baroreceptors activate the sympathetic nervous system and the renin-angiotensin-aldosterone system. Except when renal salt wasting is the cause, these responses reduce urinary sodium excretion so that nearly all ingested salt is retained. Volume-depleted persons also become thirsty; ingested water is retained because vasopressin, released in response to volume depletion, concentrates the urine, decreasing water excretion. The plasma sodium concentration can be high, normal, or low in volume-depleted persons, depending on electrolyte-free water intake and excretion. Vasoconstriction maintains the systemic blood pressure and also reduces renal blood flow. Initially, efferent arteriolar resistance, mediated by angiotensin II, predominates, sustaining intraglomerular pressure and the glomerular filtration rate; in more severe hypovolemia, renal blood flow is further reduced and glomerular filtration falls.

ETIOLOGY

Because renal sodium conservation can reduce urinary sodium losses to less than 10 mmol/day, volume depletion is unlikely to occur from decreased intake alone. The small bowel and colon are the most common sources of isotonic fluid loss. Spectacular amounts of isotonic saltwater can be lost in diarrhea. For example, rice-water stool losses in cholera can reach 20 L/day, causing death within a few hours without fluid replacement. Small bowel obstruction causes pooling of several liters of saltwater within the bowel lumen. Fluid may also be sequestrated in the abdominal cavity in patients with pancreatitis or peritonitis. Sequestration of fluid in the soft tissues may also complicate crush injuries with rhabdomyolysis or burns.

Renal salt wasting can cause volume depletion, but only a few disorders can cause enough renal salt loss to be clinically apparent. Diuretics and osmotic diuresis caused by glycosuria are the most frequent causes of renal salt wasting. Transient renal salt wasting may occur in the recovery phases of acute tubular necrosis or obstructive uropathy, and it can also occur in toxic nephropathies. Renal salt wasting also occurs in adrenal insufficiency.

DIAGNOSIS

Clinical Manifestations

Minor degrees of volume depletion (less than 10% of plasma volume, equivalent to the loss of one unit of blood) cause an increase in heart rate and may also be associated with complaints of fatigue, thirst, or muscle cramps. With modest hypovolemia, arteriolar vasoconstriction is sufficient to maintain the blood pressure when the patient is recumbent. However, dizziness and hypotension emerge on standing or during physical exertion. Severe fluid losses cause hypotension in recumbency and, ultimately, signs of tissue ischemia and shock (e.g., cool, clammy extremities, decreased urine output, lethargy, and confusion). Irreversible tissue injury may occur if this condition is allowed to continue.

Loss of weight within a short period is the most reliable sign of volume depletion. Physical findings include a low jugular venous pulse rate and orthostatic changes in blood pressure and heart rate.[63,64] However, because postural hypotension can occur in up to 30% of normovolemic persons older than 65 years, these changes must be interpreted with caution. Decreased skin turgor and dry mucous membranes are generally unreliable findings in volume-depleted adults; these signs can be absent in severe hypovolemia, and they can be present (particularly in mouth breathers and the elderly) when the patient is actually volume overloaded. The presence of edema makes true volume depletion unlikely.

Laboratory Tests

Laboratory findings are related to the decreased volume of intravascular saltwater and to decreased renal perfusion. Hematocrit increases in proportion to the contraction of plasma volume, and the serum albumin may be increased as well. Urinary sodium is usually less than 20 mEq/L except in metabolic alkalosis (in which the urine chloride is low) or when renal sodium wasting is the cause of the condition.[41,65] Renal blood flow is reduced, but unless the patient is frankly hypotensive, the glomerular filtration rate is maintained by vasoconstriction of the efferent glomerular arteriole. Thus, except in severe volume depletion, the serum creatinine changes very little. Unlike creatinine, urea is reabsorbed from the glomerular filtrate. Thus, in volume depletion (prerenal azotemia), the BUN is increased disproportionately to the increase in creatinine.[65] Azotemia may be blunted in patients with a poor dietary-protein intake and may be exacerbated in patients who are catabolic, bleeding, or receiving steroid therapy.

TREATMENT

Patients with mild volume depletion can be treated by increasing their dietary intake of salt, relying on normal thirst mechanisms to provide the appropriate amount of water. For most patients, the familiar (but misguided) order to drink fluids should be replaced with an order to salt one's food. Even severe volume depletion can be treated with oral solutions containing electrolytes, sugar, and amino acids.[66] Glucose and amino acids promote intestinal absorption of sodium through cotransport mechanisms similar to those found in the proximal tubule of the kidney. Rice-based oral replacement solutions have been a major advance in the treatment of diarrhea in developing countries.

Intravenous fluids are necessary when fluids cannot be taken orally. If the patient is hypotensive, isotonic saline should be given as rapidly as possible until tissue perfusion is adequate. Colloid-containing solutions have no proven advantage over crystalloids.[67] There is no accurate way to estimate the total fluid deficit in hypovolemia other than continued clinical observation of the patient's response to therapy.

References

1. Edelman IS, Leibman J: Anatomy of body water and electrolytes. Am J Med 27:256, 1959

2. Oster JR, Singer I: Hyponatremia, hyposmolality, and hypotonicity: tables and fables. Arch Intern Med 159:333, 1999

3. Mange K, Matsuura D, Cizman B, et al: Language guiding therapy: the case of dehydration versus volume depletion. Ann Intern Med 127:848, 1997

4. Greger R: Physiology of renal sodium transport. Am J Med Sci 319:51, 2000

5. Rasool A, Palevsky PM: Treatment of edematous disorders with diuretics. Am J Med Sci 319:25, 2000

6. Scheinman SJ, Guay-Woodford LM, Thakker RV, et al: Genetic disorders of renal electrolyte transport. N Engl J Med 340:1177, 1999

7. Kozono D, Yasui M, King LS, et al: Aquaporin water channels: atomic structure molecular dynamics meet clinical medicine. J Clin Invest 109:1395, 2002

8. Robertson G: Antidiuretic hormone: normal and disordered functions. Endocrinol Metab Clin North Am 30:671, 2001

9. Levin ER, Gardner DG, Samson WK: Natriuretic peptides. N Engl J Med 339:321, 1998

10. McManus ML, Churchwell KB, Strange K: Regulation of cell volume in health and disease. N Engl J Med 333:1260, 1995

11. Sterns RH, Silver SM, Spital A: Hyponatremia. The Kidney: Physiology and Pathophysiology.

Seldin DW, Giebisch G, Eds. Lippincott Williams & Wilkins, Philadelphia, 2000, p 1217

12. Adrogue HJ, Madias NE: Hyponatremia. N Engl J Med 342:1581, 2000

13. Adrogue HJ, Madias NE: Hypernatremia. N Engl J Med 342:1493, 2000

14. Kawai N, Baba A, Suzuki T, et al: Roles of arginine vasopressin and atrial natriuretic peptide in poly-dipsia-hyponatremia of schizophrenic patients. Psychiatry Res 101:39, 2001

15. Fenves AZ, Thomas S, Knochel JP: Beer poto-mania: two cases and review of the literature. Clin Nephrol 45:61, 1996

16. Cadnapaphornchai MA, Gurevich AK, Wein-berger HD, et al: Pathophysiology of sodium and water retention in heart failure. Cardiology 96:122, 2001

17. Schrier RW, Abraham WT: Hormones and hemodynamics in heart failure. N Engl J Med 341:577, 1999

18. Cardenas A, Gines P: Pathogenesis and treat-ment of fluid and electrolyte imbalance in cir-rhosis. Semin Nephrol 21:308, 2001

19. Schwartz WB, Bennett W, Curelop S, et al: A syndrome of renal sodium loss and hyponatrem-ia probably resulting from inappropriate secre-tion of antidiuretic hormone. 1957. J Am Soc Nephrol 12:2860, 2001

20. Steele A, Gowrishankar M, Abrahamson S, et al: Postoperative hyponatremia despite near-isoton-ic saline infusion: a phenomenon of desalination. Ann Intern Med 126:20, 1997

21. Hillier TA, Abbott RD, Barrett EJ: Hyponatremia: evaluating the correction factor for hyper-glycemia. Am J Med 106:399, 1999

22. Davids MR, Edoute Y, Stock S, et al: Severe degree of hyperglycaemia: insights from integra-tive physiology. QJM 95:113, 2002

23. Istre O, Jellum E, Skajaa K, et al: Changes in amino acids, ammonium, and coagulation factors after transcervical resection of the endometrium with a glycine solution used for uterine irrigation. Am J Obstet Gynecol 172:939, 1995

24. Verbalis JG: Adaptation to acute and chronic hyponatremia: implications for symptomatology, diagnosis, and therapy. Semin Nephrol 18:3, 1998

25. Gowrishankar M, Lin SH, Mallie JP, et al: Acute hyponatremia in the perioperative period: insights into its pathophysiology and recommendations for management. Clin Nephrol 50:352, 1998

26. Spital A, Ristow S: Cyclophosphamide induced water intoxication in a woman with Sjögren's syndrome. J Rheumatol 24:2473, 1997

27. Montain SJ, Sawka MN, Wenger CB: Hyponatremia associated with exercise: risk fac-tors and pathogenesis. Exerc Sports Sci Rev 29:113, 2001

28. Ayus JC, Varon J, Arieff AI: Hyponatremia, cere-bral edema, and noncardiogenic pulmonary edema in marathon runners. Ann Intern Med 132:711, 2000

29. Hartung TK, Schofield E, Short AI, et al: Hyponatraemic states following 3,4-methylene-dioxymethamphetamine (MDMA, 'ecstasy') ingestion. QJM 95:431, 2002

30. Sterns RH: Severe symptomatic hyponatremia: treatment and outcome: a study of 64 cases. Ann Intern Med 107:656, 1987

31. Sonnenblick M, Friedlander Y, Rosin AJ: Diuretic-induced severe hyponatremia: review and analysis of 129 reported patients. Chest 103:601, 1993

32. Akalin E, Chandrakantan A, Keane J, et al: Normouricemia in the syndrome of inappropri-ate antidiuretic hormone secretion. Am J Kidney Dis 37:E8, 2001

33. Sorensen JB, Andersen MK, Hansen HH: Syndrome of inappropriate secretion of antidi-uretic hormone (SIADH) in malignant disease. J Intern Med 238:97, 1995

34. Diringer MN, Wu KC, Verbalis JG, et al: Hypervolemic therapy prevents volume contrac-tion but not hyponatremia following subarach-noid hemorrhage. Ann Neurol 31:543, 1992

35. Maesaka JK, Gupta S, Fishbane S: Cerebral salt-wasting syndrome: does it exist? Nephron 82:100, 1999

36. Hanna FW, Scanlon MF: Hyponatraemia, hypothyroidism, and role of arginine-vaso-pressin. Lancet 350:755, 1997

37. Wilkinson TJ, Begg EJ, Sainsbury R. Incidence and risk factors for hyponatremia following treatment with fluoxetine or paroxetine in elder-ly people. Br J Clin Pharmacol 47:211, 1999

38. Vitting KE, Gardenswartz MH, Zabetakis PM, et al: Frequency of hyponatremia and nonosmo-lar vasopressin release in the acquired immuno-deficiency syndrome. JAMA 263:973, 1990

39. Gebers AL, Gulberg V, Gines P, et al: Therapy of hyponatremia in cirrhosis with a vasopressin receptor antagonist: a randomized double-blind multicenter trial. Gastroenterology 124:933, 2003

40. Sterns RH, Cappuccio JD, Silver SM, et al: Neurologic sequelae after treatment of severe hyponatremia: a multicenter perspective. J Am Soc Nephrol 4:1522, 1994

41. Narins RG, Jones ER, Stom MC, et al: Diagnostic strategies in disorders of fluid, elec-trolyte and acid-base homeostasis. Am J Med 72:496, 1982

42. Anpalahan M: Chronic idiopathic hyponatremia in older people due to the syndrome of inappro-priate antidiuretic hormone secretion (SIADH) possibly related to aging. J Am Geriatr Soc 49:788, 2001

43. Greenberg A: Diuretic complications. Am J Med Sci 319:10, 2000

44. Shimizu K: Combined effects of vasopressin V2 receptor antagonist and loop diuretics in humans. 59:164, 2003

45. Sterns RH, Riggs JE, Schochet SS Jr: Osmotic demyelination syndrome following correction of hyponatremia. N Engl J Med 314:1535, 1986

46. Laureno R, Karp BI: Myelinolysis after correc-tion of hyponatremia. Ann Intern Med 126:57, 1997

47. Brown WD: Osmotic demyelination disorders: central pontine and extrapontine myelinolysis. Curr Opin Neurol 13:691, 2000

48. Feig PU, McCurdy DK: The hypertonic state. N Engl J Med 297:1444, 1977

49. Kahn T: Hypernatremia with edema. Arch Intern Med 159:93, 1999

50. Palevsky PM, Bhagrath R, Greenberg A: Hypernatremia in hospitalized patients. Ann Intern Med 124:197, 1996

51. Sterns RH: Hypernatremia in the intensive care unit: instant quality—just add water. Crit Care Med 27:1041, 1999

52. Maghnie M, Cosi G, Genovese E, et al: Central diabetes insipidus in children and young adults. N Engl J Med 343:998, 2000

53. Singer I, Oster JR, Fishman LM: The manage-ment of diabetes insipidus in adults. Arch Intern Med 157:1293, 1997

54. Bichet DG: Nephrogenic diabetes insipidus. Am J Med 105:431, 1998

55. De Santo NG, Pollastro RM, Saviano C, et al: Nephrotic edema. Semin Nephrol 21:262, 2001

56. Martin PY, Gines P, Schrier RW: Nitric oxide as a mediator of hemodynamic abnormalities and sodium and water retention in cirrhosis. N Engl J Med 339:533, 1998

57. Kay A, Davis CL: Idiopathic edema. Am J Kidney Dis 34:405, 1999

58. Maisel AS, Krishnaswamy P, Nowak RM, et al: Rapid measurement of B-type natriuretic pep-tide in the emergency diagnosis of heart failure. Breathing Not Properly Multinational Study Investigators. N Engl J Med 347:161, 2002

59. Brater DC: Diuretic therapy. N Engl J Med 339:387, 1998

60. Colucci WS, Elkayam U, Horton DP, et al: Intravenous nesiritide, a natriuretic peptide, in the treatment of decompensated congestive heart failure. Nesiritide Study Group. N Engl J Med 343:246, 2000

61. Peltekian KM, Wong F, Liu PP, et al: Cardio-vascular, renal, and neurohumoral responses to single large-volume paracentesis in patients with cirrhosis and diuretic-resistant ascites. Am J Gastroenterol 92:394, 1997

62. Howard PA, Dunn MI: Aggressive diuresis for severe heart failure in the elderly. Chest 119:807, 2001

63. Carlson JE: Assessment of orthostatic blood pressure: measurement technique and clinical applications. South Med J 92:167, 1999

64. McGee S, Abernethy WB 3rd, Simel DL: The rational clinical examination. Is this patient hypovolemic? JAMA 281:1022, 1999

65. Klahr S, Miller SB: Acute oliguria. N Engl J Med 338:671, 1998

66. Farthing MJ: Oral rehydration: an evolving solu-tion. J Pediatr Gastroenterol Nutr 34:S64, 2002

67. Schierhout G, Roberts I: Fluid resuscitation with colloid or crystalloid solutions in critically ill patients: a systematic review of randomised tri-als. BMJ 316:961, 1998

Acknowledgment

Figures 3 and 4   Marcia Kammerer.

9 DISORDERS OF ACID-BASE AND POTASSIUM BALANCE

Robert M. Black, M.D.

Acid-Base Disorders

The blood pH is normally maintained at 7.38 to 7.42. Any deviation from this range indicates a change in the hydrogen ion concentration ($[H^+]$) because blood pH is the negative logarithm of $[H^+]$, as expressed by the following equation:

$$pH = -\log_{10}[H^+]$$

The $[H^+]$ at a physiologic blood pH of 7.40 is 40 nEq/L [*see Figure 1*]. An increase in the $[H^+]$—fall in the blood pH—is termed acidemia. A decrease in the $[H^+]$—a rise in the blood pH—is termed alkalemia. The disorders that cause these changes in the blood pH are acidosis and alkalosis, respectively. Because abnormalities of acid-base metabolism are often associated with potassium imbalance, clinical approaches to hypokalemia and hyperkalemia are also discussed in this subsection.

NORMAL ACID-BASE PHYSIOLOGY

The normal adult diet contains an excess 70 to 100 mEq of acid that must be eliminated every day. Failure to do so results in a persistent fall in the blood pH resulting from a rise in the plasma H^+ ion concentration. The balance of acid-base homeostasis is maintained in part by the relation between the arterial carbon dioxide tension (P_aCO_2) and plasma bicarbonate concentration ($[HCO_3^-]$), as noted in the following equation, a nonlogarithmic expression of the Henderson-Hasselbalch formula[1]:

$$[H^+] = 24 \times P_aCO_2/[HCO_3^-]$$

Similarly, a fall in plasma $[HCO_3^-]$ caused by either gastrointestinal or renal bicarbonate losses also increases the $[H^+]$ and lowers blood pH.

Renal Reabsorption of Bicarbonate

The plasma $[HCO_3^-]$ is normally maintained at approximately 25 mEq/L. If the daily filtered bicarbonate load (about 4,500 mEq) were not reabsorbed, the plasma $[HCO_3^-]$ would fall, as would the blood pH. Thus, maintenance of a normal plasma $[HCO_3^-]$ requires reabsorption of essentially all of the bicarbonate filtered across the glomerular capillaries each day.

Most bicarbonate reabsorption (almost 90%) occurs in the proximal convoluted tubule [*see Figure 2*]; in contrast, the distal nephron reclaims very little bicarbonate. The difference is a result of the greater quantity of carbonic anhydrase in the lumen of the proximal tubule.

Renal Excretion of Acid

In addition to reabsorbing essentially all filtered bicarbonate, the kidneys excrete the daily acid load, derived mainly from sulfur-containing amino acids. The hydrogen ions that are excreted in the final urine are secreted mainly in the collecting tubules [*see Figure 3*]. This secretory process is facilitated by aldosterone.

The daily acid load is excreted into the collecting tubules by the H^+-ATPase pumps located in the luminal membrane of the intercalated cells. This secretory process is inhibited by a trivial quantity of free hydrogen ions that lower the urine pH below the critical level of

4.0 to 4.5. This limitation is normally overcome by the presence of urinary buffers that combine with free hydrogen ions, thus permitting continued secretion of acid. There are several urinary buffers, the most important of which is ammonia because it is the only buffer that can increase substantially in the presence of an acid load. Limitation of the capacity to generate adequate urinary ammonia, as occurs in renal insufficiency, usually leads to acidosis.

The major site of ammonia production in the kidney is the proximal tubule [*see Figure 4*]; ammonia moves from the proximal tubule to the collecting tubule, where it is eliminated [*see Figure 5*]. The quantity of ammonia produced is stimulated both by acidemia and by hypokalemia. Conversely, alkalemia and hyperkalemia inhibit renal tubular ammonia production.

METABOLIC ACIDOSIS

Metabolic acidosis results whenever a primary decrease in the plasma $[HCO_3^-]$ occurs. Such a decrease may be caused by several factors: exogenous acid administration, endogenous acid production, impaired renal hydrogen secretion, and bicarbonate losses from the kidney or in gastrointestinal secretions. Calculation of the plasma anion gap is particularly useful in identifying the specific cause of metabolic acidosis and in narrowing the differential diagnosis.

Anion Gap in Metabolic Acidosis

The anion gap (measured in mEq/L) refers to the difference between the plasma concentrations of the major measured cation

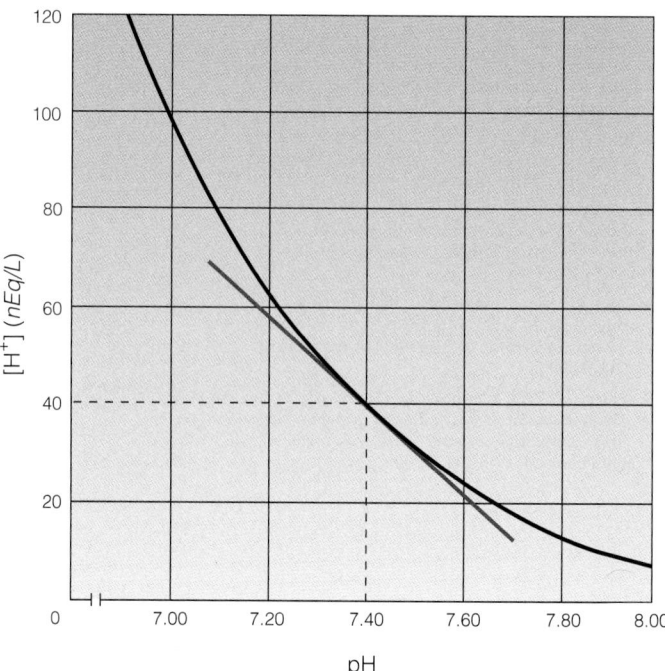

Figure 1 **The relation between the plasma hydrogen ion concentration ($[H^+]$) and the pH of the blood (pH = $-\log_{10}[H^+]$).**

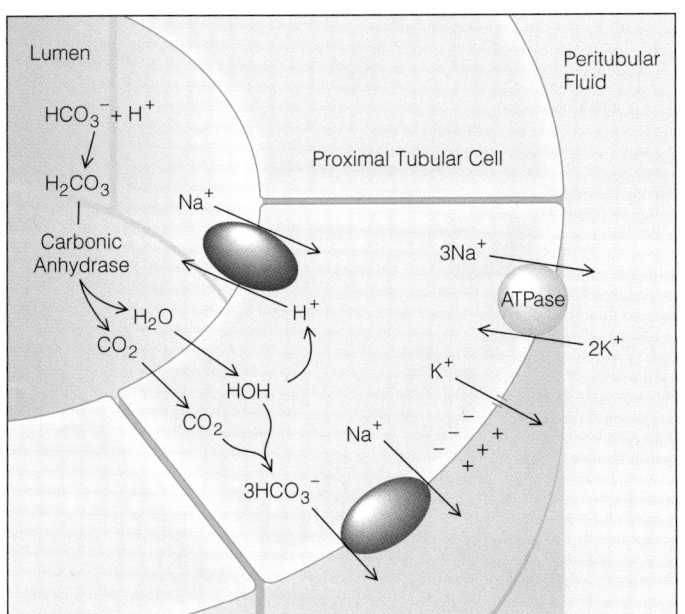

Figure 2 Proximal tubular bicarbonate reabsorption is activated by the Na^+,K^+-ATPase pump in the peritubular cell membrane. Exchanging peritubular K^+ for intracellular Na^+ keeps the intracellular sodium concentration low, allowing Na^+ to move down its concentration gradient from the tubular lumen through the Na^+- H^+ antiporter to the cell interior. HCO_3^- filtered across the glomerular capillaries combines with secreted H^+ to form H_2CO_3. Rapid dissociation of H_2CO_3 to CO_2 and H_2O in the presence of luminal carbonic anhydrase permits movement into the cell, where redissociation occurs. Ultimately, the reabsorbed H^+ is resecreted in exchange for Na^+, and HCO_3^- moves down an electrical gradient from the cell interior to the peritubular space, where it is reabsorbed into the systemic circulation.

(sodium) and the major measured anions (chloride and bicarbonate), as described by the following equation:

$$Anion\ gap = [Na^+] - ([HCO_3^-] + [Cl^-])$$

The normal anion gap ranges from 3 to 13 mEq/L, with a mean of about 7 to 10 mEq/L.[2] It is composed mainly of plasma proteins (primarily albumin) that carry a negative charge. In the setting of hypoalbuminemia, therefore, the baseline anion gap may be less than 3 mEq/L.

The most important clinical use of the anion gap is to identify the etiology of metabolic acidosis.[3] The disorders that cause metabolic acidosis fall into two categories: (1) those that cause a fall in the plasma [HCO_3^-] while concomitantly raising the anion gap and (2) those that cause a fall in the plasma [HCO_3^-] without affecting the anion gap. In the latter setting, the plasma chloride concentration increases to replace the depleted bicarbonate.

Causes of Metabolic Acidosis with a High Anion Gap

Several disorders, as well as the ingestion of toxins, can cause metabolic acidosis with an increased anion gap [see Table 1].

Renal failure Advanced renal failure is the most common cause of metabolic acidosis with an increased anion gap in the outpatient setting. The retention of hydrogen ions leads to a fall in the plasma [HCO_3^-]. Because sulfate and phosphate (which are the accompanying anions) are excreted in the urine while chloride is retained to maintain electroneutrality, the anion gap remains nor-

mal during the early course of renal failure. As renal failure progresses (creatinine > 3.0 mg/dl), these ingested anions and metabolic waste products can no longer be excreted normally. At this point, the anion gap increases. There is, however, no linear correlation between the degree of acidemia (or hypobicarbonatemia) and the level of the anion gap. In uncomplicated renal failure, the plasma [HCO_3^-] rarely decreases to less than 12 mEq/L, and the anion gap characteristically remains less than 20 mEq/L.

Lactic acidosis Lactic acidosis is the most common cause of high-anion-gap metabolic acidosis observed in hospitalized patients. Lactic acid production usually increases as a result of hypotension or sepsis, both of which cause true or relative tissue ischemia. The oxidative pathways of pyruvate metabolism become markedly impaired in states of mitochondrial dysfunction, such as those induced by tissue hypoxemia. This setting enhances the conversion of pyruvate to lactate. The liver and, to a lesser degree, the kidneys are the

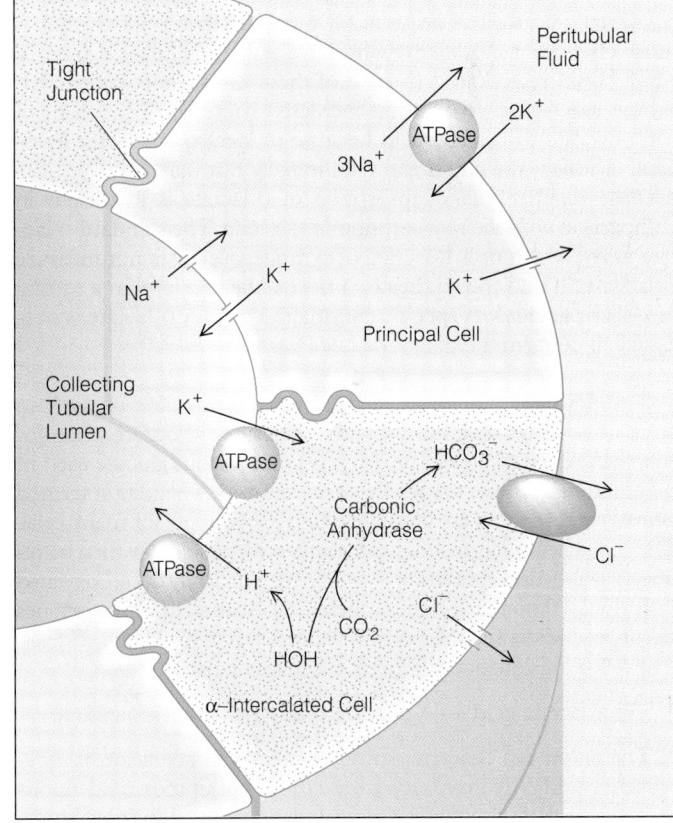

Figure 3 Secretion of H^+ from the cortical collecting tubule is indirectly linked to Na^+ reabsorption. Intracellular potassium is exchanged for sodium in the principal cells, whereas H^+ is actively transported by an ATPase pump from the α-intercalated cells. Aldosterone stimulates H^+ secretion by entering the principal cell, where it opens Na^+ channels in the luminal membrane and increases Na^+, K^+-ATPase activity. The movement of cationic Na^+ into the principal cells then creates a negative charge within the tubular lumen. K^+ moves from the principal cells and H^+ from the α-intercalated cells down this electrochemical gradient and into the lumen. (When K^+ is depleted, principal cell K^+ secretion is reduced, and K reabsorption via an ATPase pump in the α-intercalated cell is stimulated.) Aldosterone apparently also stimulates the H^+-ATPase directly in the intercalated cell, further enhancing H^+ secretion. HCO_3 is returned to the blood across the peritubular membrane in exchange for Cl^-, thus maintaining electroneutrality.

major organs that remove lactate from the circulation. In both organs, lactate is converted back to pyruvate and then to carbon dioxide and water via the tricarboxylic acid cycle. When normal tissue perfusion is restored, metabolism of lactate ($CH_3CHOHCOO^-$) in these organs rapidly regenerates the bicarbonate used initially to buffer the acid load, a process that is largely independent of renal acid excretion and that is summarized by the following equation:

$$CH_3CHOHCOO^- + 3O_2 \rightarrow 2CO_2 + 2H_2O + HCO_3^-$$

The normal rate of lactate production can reach 320 mEq/hr (e.g., during exercise), a rate that is usually greater than the rate of lactate production in lactic acidosis. These findings indicate that for lactic acid to accumulate, lactate metabolism must also be impaired. In shock, for example, the marked reduction in hepatic perfusion slows lactate clearance.

The anion gap is almost always elevated above baseline in lactic acidosis. Because the renal excretory threshold for lactate is 6 to 8 mEq/L and the normal lactate level is less than 1 mEq/L, excess lactate accumulates in the blood, rather than being eliminated in the urine, thus contributing to the increased anion gap.

D-Lactic acidosis is an unusual form of lactic acidosis that is most often seen in patients who have undergone ileal bypass or small bowel resection.[2,4] In each of these cases, short bowel syndrome can occur, resulting in increased bacterial metabolism of carbohydrate to D-lactic acid because of local overgrowth. In D-lactic acidosis, the anion gap rises initially but may fall over time because renal tubular reabsorption of D-lactate is inefficient in comparison with the reabsorption of L-lactate. The standard L-lactate assay, which uses L-lactate dehydrogenase, does not measure D-lactic acid and thus indicates a normal lactate level in a setting of D-lactic acidosis. A specific enzymatic assay for D-lactate is necessary to confirm the diagnosis [see Diagnosis, below].

Ketoacidosis Acidosis caused by overproduction of the keto acids acetoacetic acid and β-hydroxybutyric acid occurs when insulin deficiency, fasting, or insulin resistance impairs glucose use.[5] In these settings, ketone bodies are overproduced (a condition termed ketosis) and serve as an alternative source of energy for many cells. The initial ketone formed is acetoacetic acid, which may then be reduced to β-hydroxybutyric acid or nonenzymatically decarboxylated to acetone. Although acetone is chemically neutral, the other ketones are organic acids, and their accumulation leads to metabolic acidosis. The following equation summarizes the reactions:

Acetoacetic acid ⟷ β-hydroxybutyric acid ⟶ acetone

The anion gap characteristically increases in ketoacidosis. Acetoacetate and β-hydroxybutyrate are the major unmeasured anions that accumulate, although a concomitant lactic acidosis may be observed in some patients. The plasma [HCO_3^-] may be markedly depressed in diabetic ketoacidosis; in contrast, the acidemia is generally mild and the plasma bicarbonate rarely less than 18 mEq/L in starvation, or fasting, ketosis.

In patients with ketoacidosis, isotonic fluid replacement leads to ketonuria. Although the anion gap initially increases, it begins to fall as the rate of urinary excretion of acetoacetate and β-hydroxybutyrate exceeds the rate of production. Ultimately, normalization of the anion gap results, with chloride replacing the lost ketone anions. Because loss of urinary ketones does not regenerate bicarbonate, the plasma [HCO_3^-] remains depressed.

The trend toward normal-anion-gap metabolic acidosis during recovery from ketoacidosis has an important effect on the rate at which acidemia can be corrected. As long as ketones are circulating and insulin is available, acetoacetate and β-hydroxybutyrate can be rapidly

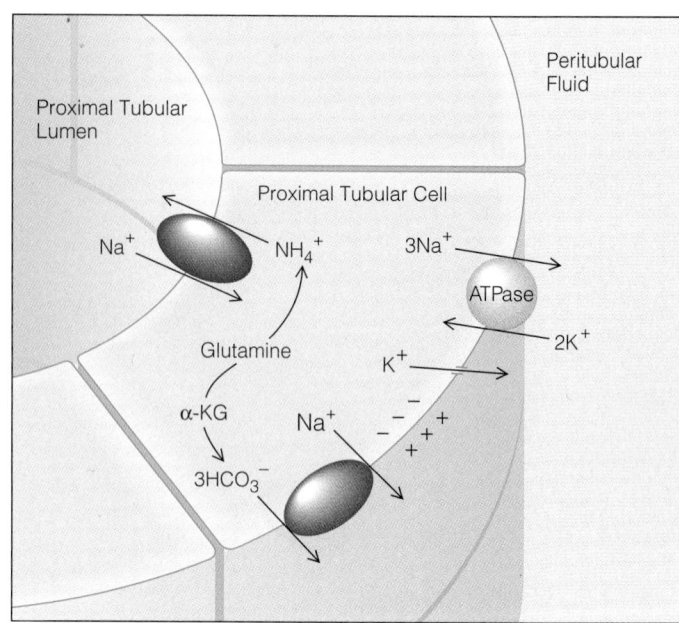

Figure 4 All of the ammonia used to buffer urinary H^+ in the collecting tubule is synthesized in the proximal convoluted tubule, and glutamine is assumed to be the main source of this ammonia. As glutamine is metabolized, α-ketoglutarate (α-KG) is formed, which ultimately breaks down to bicarbonate that is then secreted into the peritubular fluid at an Na^+-HCO_3^- cotransporter.

metabolized to bicarbonate in nonhepatic tissues, such as muscle. Once these anions have been completely eliminated by urinary losses, however, regeneration of bicarbonate requires renal excretion of retained hydrogen ions. This process, which depends on increased ammonia production, requires at least 2 to 3 days to become fully functional. Consequently, resolution of acidemia occurs more rapidly in patients who have a higher anion gap (and higher circulating acetoacetate and β-hydroxybutyrate levels) when treatment with insulin begins.

Any dose of insulin that lowers the blood glucose level will reduce ketone production, because the concentration of insulin that inhibits lipolysis by adipose tissue is much lower than the concentration required for glucose utilization. Although metabolism of the remaining circulating keto acids occurs rapidly, the elimination of acetone, which occurs partly through the lungs, proceeds more slowly. Thus, positive blood and urinary ketone levels that persist for longer than 24 hours do not necessarily indicate ongoing ketogenesis.

Rhabdomyolysis Massive muscle breakdown is an important cause of metabolic acidosis.[6] The retention of metabolic acids and such inorganic anions as phosphate appear to contribute to the increased anion gap. Metabolic acidosis is more likely to develop when concomitant renal failure is present.

Ingested agents and toxins Salicylates and the alcohols ethylene glycol (a component of antifreeze and solvents) and methanol, or wood alcohol (a component of shellac, varnish, deicing solutions, and other commercial preparations), are the most frequent causes of metabolic acidosis among ingested agents and toxins. Ethyl alcohol ingestion is not associated with a high-anion-gap acidosis unless accompanied by either lactic acidosis or ketoacidosis.

The most common acid-base abnormality observed with salicylate intoxication in adults is respiratory alkalosis caused by direct

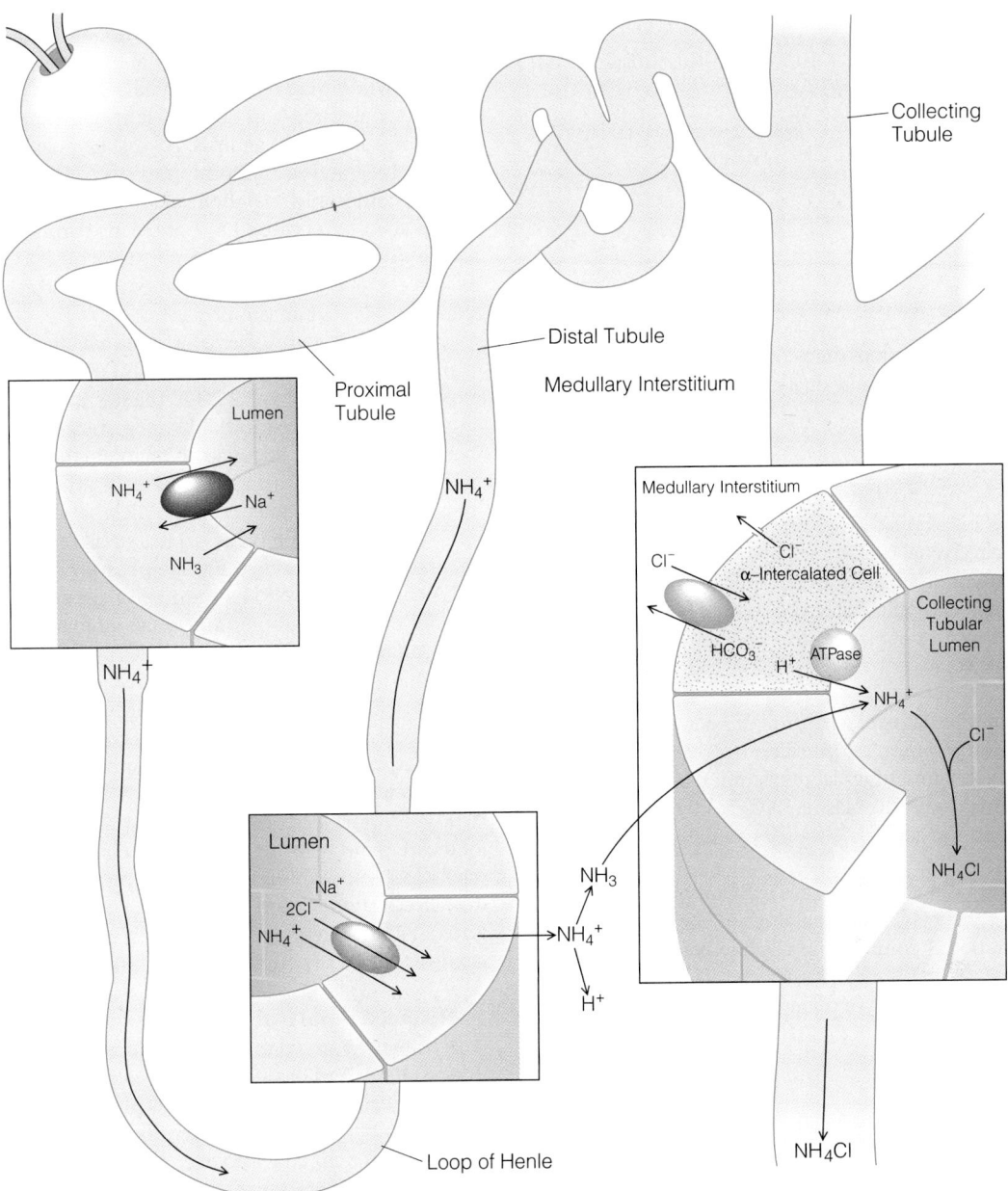

Figure 5 **The ammonia used to buffer urinary hydrogen ions is synthesized in the proximal convoluted tubule. It then diffuses into the proximal tubular lumen or can become acidified within the cell, forming ammonium, which can enter the tubular lumen by substituting for hydrogen ions on the Na^+- H^+ antiporter. Ammonium flows through the thick ascending limb of the loop of Henle, where it is transported from the tubule into the medullary interstitium by replacing potassium on an Na^+-K^+-$2Cl^-$ transporter. In the interstitium, ammonium dissociates to ammonia, which diffuses down its concentration gradient into the lumen of the collecting tubule. Here, ammonia combines with secreted H^+ to form ammonium; NH_4^+ is then excreted as NH_4Cl to maintain electroneutrality. A bicarbonate molecule is regenerated for each H^+ eliminated in the urine.**

stimulation of the medullary respiratory center [*see* Respiratory Acidosis and Alkalosis, *below*]. In adults, the presence of respiratory alkalosis appears to be a prerequisite for the development of metabolic acidosis, because an isolated metabolic acidosis is rare. Moderate to severe salicylate intoxication, on the other hand, leads to a mixed respiratory alkalosis and a high-anion-gap metabolic acidosis. Other clinical findings that may be seen with severe salicylate intoxication include tinnitus, hyperpyrexia, vasodilatation leading to shock, and peripheral or pulmonary edema.

The alcohols methanol and ethylene glycol can produce fatal intoxication. Both can cause a plasma osmolal gap, which refers to the difference between the plasma osmolality (P_{osm}) measured by the laboratory and that calculated by the following formula:

$$\text{Calculated } P_{osm} = (2 \times \text{plasma } [Na^+])$$
$$+ (\text{glucose concentration}/18) + (\text{blood urea nitrogen}/2.8)$$

A high plasma osmolal gap (with the measured level at least 10 mOsm/kg higher than the calculated value) can be detected only when the P_{osm} is measured by freezing-point depression. In contrast, the osmotic contribution of volatile alcohols is not included when a vapor-pressure osmometer, which assumes that only water is in the vapor phase, is used.[7] Furthermore, the presence of an osmolal gap

Table 1 Causes of High-Anion-Gap Metabolic Acidosis

Renal failure*	Ingested agents and toxins
Lactic acidosis	Salicylates
Ketoacidosis*	Ethylene glycol
Rhabdomyolysis	Methanol
	Toluene*

*May also be associated with a normal-anion-gap acidosis.

is not specific for these ingestions, and confirmation of the diagnosis requires plasma assays for the individual drugs [see Diagnosis, below].

Causes of Metabolic Acidosis with a Normal Anion Gap

A normal anion gap in metabolic acidosis can arise from several causes, including administration of inorganic acids such as hydrochloric acid, loss of bicarbonate from the gastrointestinal tract or the kidneys, and impaired renal excretion of hydrogen ions [see Table 2].

In the resultant conditions, electroneutrality is maintained by a decrease in plasma bicarbonate and replacement by chloride. Consequently, these disorders are sometimes collectively referred to as the hyperchloremic acidoses.

Acid and chloride administration The infusion of amino acid solutions during parenteral nutrition supplies abundant hydrochloric acid. In certain settings, administration of a sodium chloride solution also may lower the plasma $[HCO_3^-]$ by dilution (a condition termed expansion acidosis), leading to a fall in blood pH.[8]

Bicarbonate or other alkali losses Bicarbonate can be lost from the body via the gastrointestinal tract or the kidneys. Compared with blood, bowel contents are alkaline because pancreatic and biliary secretions add bicarbonate, which is later exchanged for chloride in the ileum and colon to maintain a normal acid-base sta-

Table 2 Causes of Metabolic Acidosis with a Normal Anion Gap

Acid and chloride administration
 Hyperalimentation*
 NH₄Cl, HCl for treatment of severe metabolic acidosis*

Bicarbonate (or other alkali) losses
 Gastrointestinal alkali loss†
  Diarrhea, pancreatic-intestinal-biliary fistulas, pancreatic transplantation with drainage into the urinary bladder
 Ureteral diversions†
  Ureterosigmoidostomy, ileal bladder (if obstructed)
 Type 2 RTA†
 Recovery from ketoacidosis†
 Posthypocapnia†

Reduced renal and hydrogen excretion
 Renal insufficiency*
 Type 1 RTA
  Hypokalemic forms*
  Hyperkalemic forms†
 Type 4 RTA*

*Normal or increased plasma K⁺.
†Normal or decreased plasma K⁺.
RTA—renal tubular acidosis

tus. Gastrointestinal losses of bicarbonate (or bicarbonate precursors such as lactate and acetate) are most commonly observed in patients with severe diarrhea. The diagnosis of diarrhea as the cause of a normal-anion-gap acidosis is usually apparent from the patient's history [see Diagnosis, below]. Hypokalemia resulting from stool potassium losses also supports the diagnosis.

Less commonly, metabolic acidosis resulting from gastrointestinal alkali losses is caused by pancreatic fistulas, biliary drainage, or urinary diversions to the colon or small bowel.[9] It also occurs after pancreatic transplantation in patients who lose bicarbonate via the pancreas-bladder anastomosis.[10]

Renal bicarbonate losses cause the acidemia observed in type 2, or proximal, renal tubular acidosis (RTA) and in patients who are posthypocapnic. In type 2 RTA, the normal threshold for bicarbonate reabsorption is reduced. Therefore, bicarbonate can no longer be reabsorbed at a rate adequate to maintain the normal plasma level of about 25 mEq/L. During this phase, bicarbonaturia occurs, leading to a urine pH of greater than 5.3. Bicarbonate wasting ceases, however, once the plasma $[HCO_3^-]$ has stabilized at the new, lower concentration; at this time, the urine pH may be less than 5. Proximal RTA can be observed in a number of circumstances, including the administration of carbonic anhydrase inhibitors and in some patients with multiple myeloma. In multiple myeloma, toxic damage to the proximal tubular cells by the filtered myeloma light chains often leads to a generalized reduction in proximal reabsorption (including glucose and phosphate) in addition to bicarbonate. This group of maladies, caused by proximal tubular dysfunction, is called the Fanconi syndrome.[11]

Hypocapnia leads to a fall in the proximal tubular reabsorption of bicarbonate. After 1 to 3 days, the plasma level of bicarbonate decreases. Because this renal adaptive process requires the same time to cease, a sudden increase in the P_aCO_2 does not immediately alter proximal bicarbonate reabsorption. This posthypocapnic metabolic acidosis resolves spontaneously within 24 to 72 hours.

Reduced renal hydrogen ion excretion Reduced renal acid excretion is observed in three conditions: renal insufficiency, type 1 (distal) RTA, and type 4 RTA (hypoaldosteronism) [see Tables 3 and 4].[12] The acidosis of renal failure is primarily caused by a reduction in the number of nephrons. In contrast, type 1 RTA is characterized by a reduction in renal acid excretion by each nephron. Because the total quantity of ammonia that can be synthesized is also reduced in renal failure, the urine pH is lower than 5.3 in most patients.

Type 1 RTA, which may be congenital or may be acquired in association with a number of immune disorders, such as Sjögren syndrome, occurs most commonly when hydrogen ions cannot be pumped out of the α-intercalated cells into the collecting tubular lumen [see Figure 3]. As a result, the urine cannot be maximally acidified, and the urine pH is always higher than 5.3. Furthermore, hypokalemia is characteristically present, in part because of enhanced distal nephron Na⁺-K⁺ exchange, a process that is necessary to maintain sodium balance because hydrogen ions cannot be secreted in response to sodium reabsorption. A hyperkalemic form of type 1 RTA also has been described; it occurs most often in patients with urinary tract obstruction. In contrast to type 4 RTA, this disorder results in an inability to acidify urine maximally (urine pH > 5.3).

The most important clinical complication of hypokalemic type 1 RTA is the formation and deposition of calcium phosphate salts that can cause calculi throughout the kidney (nephrocalcinosis). A major factor contributing to crystal formation is hypocitraturia, which results from metabolic acidosis that leads to an increase in proximal tubular citrate reabsorption; in addition, hypokalemia promotes hypocitraturia. Because calcium citrate is significantly more

Table 3 Causes of Type 1 RTA

Hypokalemic Forms	Hyperkalemic Forms
Primary	Urinary tract obstruction
Idiopathic	Sickle cell anemia
Genetic	Systemic lupus erythematosus
Familial	Renal transplant rejection
Marfan syndrome	
Ehlers-Danlos syndrome	
Nephrocalcinosis	
Chronic hypercalcemia	
Medullary sponge kidney	
Hypergammaglobulinemic states	
Amyloidosis*	
Cryoglobulinemia	
Cirrhosis	
Drugs and toxins	
Amphotericin B	
Lithium carbonate	
Toluene†	
Autoimmune diseases	
Sjögren syndrome*	
Thyroiditis	
Chronic active hepatitis	
Primary biliary cirrhosis	

*May also cause type 2 RTA [see Table 5].
†May also cause metabolic acidosis with an elevated anion gap [see Table 1].

soluble than calcium phosphate, a decrease in urinary citrate facilitates the precipitation of calcium phosphate crystals in the collecting tubular lumen.

Type 4 RTA may be caused by a number of medications, including nonsteroidal anti-inflammatory drugs (NSAIDs), angiotensin-converting enzyme (ACE) inhibitors, angiotensin II blockers, cyclo-

Table 4 Causes of Type 4 RTA and Aldosterone Resistance

Disorder	Cause

Type 4 RTA	Reduced activity of the renin-angiotensin system
	  Hyporeninemic type 4 RTA (diabetes most common)
	  Nonsteroidal anti-inflammatory drugs (with the possible exception of sulindac)
	  Angiotensin-converting enzyme inhibitors
	  Cyclosporine
	  AIDS*
	Reduced aldosterone synthesis
	  Low cortisol levels
	    Primary adrenal insufficiency
	    Enzymatic deficiencies (primarily adrenal hyperplasia)
	  Normal cortisol levels
	    Heparin
	    Immediately after removal of adrenal adenoma in primary aldosteronism
	    Enzymatic deficiencies

Aldosterone resistance (normal or increased aldosterone levels)	Potassium-sparing diuretics, trimethoprim Pseudohypoaldosteronism (hereditary or acquired) Hyperkalemic type 1 RTA†

*Adrenalitis causing type 4 RTA may also occur in persons who are seropositive for HIV.
†In this setting, the urine is alkaline (pH > 5.3).

sporine, and heparin. However, it is most often observed in patients with diabetes mellitus [see Hyperkalemia, below].

The most common electrolyte disturbance in type 4 RTA is hyperkalemia (plasma [K+] > 5.0 mEq/L), which is caused by impaired luminal reabsorption of sodium ions and, thus, reduced potassium ion secretion by the principal cells of the collecting tubule [see Figure 3]. This defect is caused by a reduction in aldosterone production or action. In contrast to hypokalemia, high plasma potassium levels impair renal ammonia production. Insufficient urinary buffer in the form of ammonia limits hydrogen ion secretion in the collecting tubule. Despite this reduced ability to excrete hydrogen ions, the final urine is usually acidified (pH < 5.3). This apparently paradoxical finding occurs because the limited urinary buffer permits the free urine [H+] to exceed the secretory capacity of the α-intercalated cells, thus limiting further hydrogen ion transport from the cells and into the collecting tubular lumen. In contrast to patients with type 1 RTA, patients with type 4 RTA can excrete some acid, albeit in inadequate quantities; consequently, the urine pH is typically lower than 5.3 in patients with this disorder.

Potassium Imbalance in Metabolic Acidosis

Hyperkalemia is frequently observed in patients with metabolic acidosis; in respiratory acidosis, the shift of potassium from cells to plasma is smaller. A fall in the plasma [HCO₃⁻] leads to an exchange of extracellular hydrogen ions for intracellular potassium ions. This defense mechanism permits intracellular buffering of hydrogen ions; the H+-K+ exchange maintains electroneutrality. Therefore, the patient who has diarrhea with a normal-anion-gap metabolic acidosis and a low plasma [K+] has significantly greater potassium depletion than the patient with the same plasma [K+] and a normal blood pH.

In contrast to what occurs in patients with a normal-anion-gap metabolic acidosis, potassium shifts caused by acidemia are less pronounced in patients with endogenous organic acidoses (e.g., lactic acidosis and ketoacidosis).[13] This difference does not imply that hyperkalemia is uncommon in patients who present with these disorders. In lactic acidosis, for example, cellular catabolism permits leakage of potassium from cells. In ketoacidosis, insulin deficiency limits potassium entry into cells, and hyperglycemia promotes potassium exit from cells. In both conditions, the plasma [K+] may be elevated on presentation, although hyperkalemia does not normally correlate with the degree of acidemia.

Diagnosis

Clinical manifestations Kussmaul respirations suggest the presence of metabolic acidosis. The increase in tidal volume rather than respiratory rate that characterizes these ventilatory changes results from stimulation of the brain stem respiratory system by the low blood pH. As acidemia increases, either nausea and vomiting or changes in mental status, including coma, may be seen.

Secondary hypotension also may be observed in severely acidemic persons. In this setting, the reduced blood pressure results from depressed myocardial contractility and arterial vasodilatation, which are induced by the decreased blood pH. Initially, elevated levels of circulating catecholamines counter the cardiovascular effects of acidemia; however, at a blood pH below 7.15 to 7.20, the effects of acidemia may predominate.[14] Reentrant arrhythmias and a reduction in the threshold for ventricular fibrillation can occur, whereas the defibrillation threshold remains unaltered.

The symptoms and signs of lactic acidosis are characteristically those of the underlying disturbance causing the disorder [see Lactic

Table 5 Causes of Type 2 RTA

Hereditary Disorders	Acquired Disorders
Cystinosis	Multiple myeloma
Tyrosinemia	Vitamin D deficiency/hyperparathyroidism
Wilson disease	Amyloidosis*
Glycogen storage disease type I	Renal transplant rejection*
Pyruvate carboxylase deficiency	Sjögren syndrome*
Galactosemia	Toxins and drugs
	Carbonic anhydrase inhibitors
	Lead
	Cadmium
	Mercury
	Uranium
	Copper
	Outdated tetracycline
	Streptozocin

*Is usually associated with classic or hyperkalemic type 1 RTA [see Table 3].

Acidosis, above]. Most commonly, patients exhibit evidence of hypoperfusion, such as low blood pressure and cool or mottled extremities. Less commonly, a medication (such as metformin) may be the cause.

Symptoms of acidosis caused by ingestion of methanol or ethylene glycol [see Ingested Agents and Toxins, above] may develop 12 to 36 hours after ingestion. In addition to acid-base changes, the initial symptoms that occur after ingestion of methanol include weakness, nausea, headache, and decreased vision, which can progress to blindness, coma, and death. Fundoscopic examination may reveal a retinal sheen caused by retinal edema. After ethylene glycol is ingested, the earliest findings are neurologic abnormalities that range from drunkenness to coma. If the patient is not treated, these changes may be followed first by cardiopulmonary symptoms (tachypnea and pulmonary edema) and then by flank pain and renal failure caused by calcium oxalate crystal deposition, which may be seen in the urine sediment.

Several disorders are associated with type 2 RTA [see Table 5]. As discussed earlier, most adults with this disorder also exhibit other abnormalities of proximal tubular reabsorption, such as glucosuria, aminoaciduria, and phosphaturia, together known as Fanconi syndrome. In contrast, the administration of a carbonic anhydrase inhibitor, such as acetazolamide, is associated with bicarbonaturia alone.

Laboratory tests The diagnosis of metabolic acidosis is made relatively easily in the presence of a low blood pH and a low plasma $[HCO_3^-]$. The anion gap can then be used to identify a specific cause. The finding of concomitant hypokalemia or hyperkalemia may also be useful.

Once the presence or absence of a high serum anion gap is determined, the respiratory defense against acidemia can be evaluated. The respiratory response begins immediately, although it may not be maximal for 12 to 24 hours. The appropriate respiratory compensation can be calculated by using the Winter[15] formula:

$$\text{Expected } P_{CO_2} = 1.5\,[HCO_3^-] + 8 \pm 2$$

The respiratory compensation is inadequate when the measured $P_{a}CO_2$ is higher than the expected value and is excessive when the $P_{a}CO_2$ is lower than the expected value. When these inadequate or excessive responses occur, a superimposed respiratory acidosis or respiratory alkalosis, respectively, is present [see Respiratory Acidosis and Alkalosis, below]. For example, if the serum bicarbonate concentration were 16 mEq/L in a patient with a low blood pH (meta-

bolic acidosis), the expected P_{CO_2} would be approximately $32[(1.5 \times 16) + 8]$ mm Hg. A P_{CO_2} below this value indicates a superimposed respiratory alkalosis.

Another laboratory calculation, the urinary anion gap, may be useful in defining the cause of metabolic acidosis when the serum anion gap is normal. For example, although the diagnosis of diarrhea is usually apparent from the patient's history and the presence of hypokalemia, a profile of plasma electrolytes similar to that in persons with diarrhea may be observed in patients with type 1 RTA. These disorders can usually be distinguished by the urine pH; the urine tends to be acidic (pH < 5.3) in patients with diarrhea and tends to be alkaline (pH > 5.3) in patients with type 1 RTA. In some patients with diarrhea, however, the urine may be alkaline, presumably because ammonia production (induced by hypokalemia) increases to such an extent that urinary buffer is produced in excess of hydrogen ion secretion. Calculation of the urinary anion gap, as shown in the following equation, may be quite useful in this setting:

$$\text{Urinary anion gap} = (\text{urinary }[Na^+] + \text{urinary }[K^+]) - \text{urinary }[Cl^-]$$

Whenever secreted hydrogen ions are excreted as ammonium chloride, an increase in urinary chloride excretion results. The increase in urinary chloride excretion decreases the urinary anion gap, leading to a negative value in most patients with diarrhea. By comparison, in type 1 RTA, the urinary anion gap is positive. As an example, a patient with a normal anion gap metabolic acidosis (e.g., $[HCO_3^-] = 10$ mEq/L), a low potassium level (hypokalemia), and an alkaline urine pH (6.0) could have diarrhea or type 1 (distal) renal tubular acidosis. If the urine $[Na^+]$ were 50 mEq/L, the urine $[K^+]$ were 28 mEq/L, and the urine $[Cl^-]$ were 55 mEq/L, the urinary anion gap would be +23, supporting a diagnosis of renal tubular acidosis.

Treatment

Treatment of metabolic acidosis is aimed at correcting both acidemia and the underlying disorder. The likelihood that alkali administration is needed and that it will be effective depends on the blood pH, the compensatory mechanisms, and the underlying condition.

Until the arterial blood pH falls below 7.15 to 7.20, the adverse effects of acidemia are usually compensated for by elevated plasma catecholamines [see Diagnosis, above]. To maintain adequate buffer reserves, alkali therapy should usually be used to keep $[HCO_3^-]$ higher than 10 to 12 mEq/L. Alkali administration is usually unnecessary, however, if the acidosis is likely to resolve spontaneously (as in lactic acidosis after a grand mal seizure). Important issues dealing with specific causes of metabolic acidosis are discussed below.

Chronic renal failure Of interest is the finding that the acidemia tends to be more severe in nondiabetic patients with chronic renal failure than in diabetic patients with similar degrees of renal insufficiency.[16] This difference may be the result of more efficient extrarenal bicarbonate generation in diabetic patients.

As long as the metabolic acidosis is mild, most adults with renal failure are not treated with alkali replacement, partly because of a concern that sodium bicarbonate will exacerbate the volume expansion and hypertension that are commonly present.

Some studies, however, have suggested several reasons for the use of alkali replacement therapy in patients with renal failure.[17] Among the reasons are the likelihood that acidemia can enhance the breakdown of skeletal muscle, reduce albumin synthesis, and (by activating the complement system) contribute to tubulointerstitial injury and that bone buffering of hydrogen ions can lead to bone resorption.[18] These findings have led some physicians to advocate the early use of alkali therapy to maintain plasma [HCO_3^-] above 22 mEq/L. Definitive studies are still needed, however, to ascertain the benefit of such treatment.

Physicians should be aware that electrolyte studies in hemodialysis patients who use non–hospital-based dialysis units may be performed in central laboratories several hundred miles away. Compared with results of samples obtained locally, samples tested at the central laboratories appear to show consistent and clinically important decreases in serum bicarbonate concentration.[19] This in vitro enhancement of metabolic acidosis should be confirmed before treatment is initiated.

Lactic acidosis Correcting the underlying disorder is the primary therapy for lactic acidosis. Reversal of circulatory failure, hypoxemia, or sepsis reduces the rate of lactate production and enhances its removal.

As in chronic renal failure, the use of alkali therapy in lactic acidosis is controversial.[20,21] The principal rationale for bicarbonate administration is the potential maintenance of normal cardiovascular homeostasis. This possible advantage must be weighed against deleterious side effects, such as volume overload, hypernatremia, and alkalosis (when excessive bicarbonate is administered).

Clinical studies[22] also suggest that sodium bicarbonate therapy may not improve either the blood pH or the survival of patients with lactic acidosis. The administration of sodium bicarbonate also has been observed to reduce cardiac performance in patients with cardiac disease, congestive heart failure, or acute myocardial infarction. This lack of efficacy possibly results from an associated increase in net lactic acid production, although hyperosmolality of the administered alkali solution also may be important. The finding that dichloroacetate (which promotes the conversion of pyruvate into the Krebs cycle instead of permitting its conversion to lactate) can lower lactate levels and raise the blood pH in patients with lactic acidosis without seeming to improve survival lends further support to the concept that treating the underlying cause of lactic acidosis is more important than treating the acidemia.

In view of these observations, a reasonable approach may be to administer bicarbonate to maintain the arterial blood pH at higher than 7.15 and the plasma bicarbonate at higher than 10 mEq/L. If one of the complications of bicarbonate therapy ensues, the benefit of continuing alkali therapy should be reevaluated.

THAM (*tris*-hydroxymethyl aminomethane) is an alcohol of low toxicity that buffers carbon dioxide and acids. In vivo, THAM supplements the buffering capacity of the blood bicarbonate system by accepting a proton and generating a bicarbonate molecule. Its buffering capacity does not require pulmonary excretion of generated CO_2, because the protonated THAM is excreted in the urine. Although there is less sodium load with this agent than with sodium bicarbonate, its efficacy and safety in lactic acidosis remain uncertain.[23]

Ketoacidosis A maximal rate of 500 ml of fluid an hour appears to be effective replacement therapy for patients with ketoacidosis. Once intravascular volume has been restored, the advantages of intensive fluid administration may be limited because volume expansion then leads to the excretion of acetoacetate and β-hydroxybutyrate in the urine.

Significantly higher rates of fluid administration can result in a decreased anion gap without an increase in the plasma [HCO_3^-]. When this process occurs, correction of the acidosis requires regeneration of bicarbonate by the kidney, a process that may take 3 or more days. In contrast, a rapid increase in the plasma [HCO_3^-] can be achieved when ketones are metabolized to bicarbonate in extrahepatic tis-

Table 6 Causes of Metabolic Alkalosis

Disorder	Cause

Hydrogen loss	Gastrointestinal losses
	  Removal of gastric secretions (vomiting or nasogastric suction)*
	  Chloride-losing diarrheal states
	Renal losses
	  Loop or thiazide diuretics*
	  Mineralocorticoid excess
	  After rapid correction of chronic hypercapnia
	  Hypercalcemia (including milk-alkali syndrome)
	  High-dose intravenous penicillin derivatives
	  Bartter syndrome

Hydrogen movement into cells	Hypokalemia
Bicarbonate retention	Administration of alkali (as either a bicarbonate or a bicarbonate precursor with massive blood transfusions or with absorbable antacids)†
Contraction alkalosis	Diuretics* Loss of gastrointestinal secretions having high [Cl⁻] and low [HCO_3^-] when compared with plasma (usually with vomiting)*

*These are the most common causes.
†For alkalosis to be maintained, renal bicarbonate excretion also must be impaired by either reduced filtration or enhanced reabsorption by the proximal tubule.

sues.[24] As a result, vigorous fluid administration may delay recovery from acidosis, and the rate of administration should be slowed after intravascular volume compromise—manifested by reduced blood pressure or increased plasma creatinine and urea nitrogen concentrations—has been corrected.

Although exceptions occur, the administration of sodium bicarbonate is not usually necessary in ketoacidosis, because there appears to be no difference in mortality between patients treated with sodium bicarbonate and control subjects. When severe hyperkalemia is present, however, administration of sodium bicarbonate may be beneficial because bicarbonate drives potassium into cells, thereby lowering the plasma potassium concentration. By comparison, bicarbonate therapy may be a risk factor for the subsequent development of cerebral edema in this setting.[25]

Salicylate, ethylene glycol, and methanol intoxication Salicylate removal is enhanced by urinary alkalinization (to maintain the blood pH between 7.45 and 7.5, which increases urinary excretion even in the setting of dialysis.[26] The usual treatment of ethylene glycol or methanol intoxication is to administer an agent that will reduce conversion of the nontoxic alcohol to its toxic metabolic byproducts (ethanol or a new drug) and to use dialysis in the presence of tissue damage or acidemia. Although ethyl alcohol has been administered historically, fomepizole (4-methylpyrazole) is the only potent inhibitor of alcohol dehydrogenase that has been studied prospectively and that has been approved by the Food and Drug Administration for this condition.[27]

Type 1 renal tubular acidosis The acidemia in type 1 RTA can be corrected with bicarbonate or with a bicarbonate precursor, such as citrate. The usual requirement is 1 to 3 mEq/kg/day. Correcting the acidemia reduces tubular citrate reabsorption, which leads to an increase in urinary excretion and a decrease in the tendency toward nephrolithiasis and nephrocalcinosis. Usually, a potassium salt, such as potassium citrate, is administered because it corrects the potassium deficit as well.

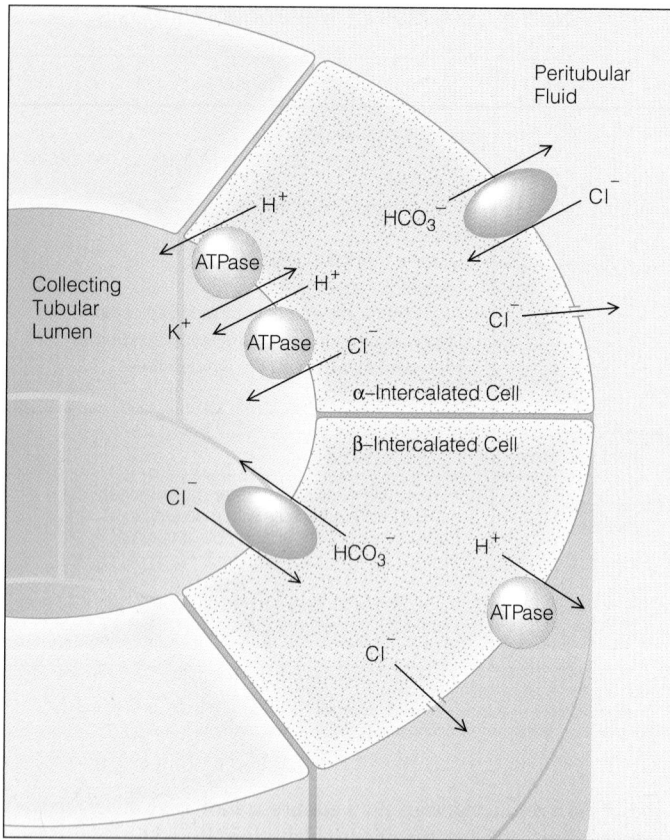

Figure 6 In metabolic alkalosis, the high ratio of α-intercalated to β-intercalated cells decreases. Unlike α-intercalated cells, which regenerate bicarbonate and add it to the venous blood, β-intercalated cells promote urinary HCO_3^- excretion by exchanging HCO_3^- for Cl^- in the glomerular filtrate. As a result, chloride administration serves an important function in the treatment of most persons with metabolic alkalosis.

METABOLIC ALKALOSIS

Primary metabolic alkalosis is characterized by an elevated plasma $[HCO_3^-]$ and an arterial pH greater than 7.42. When there is concomitant metabolic acidosis, however, the blood pH may be increased, decreased, or normal. Furthermore, hyperbicarbonatemia alone is not diagnostic of primary metabolic alkalosis, because it may also represent the appropriate physiologic response to chronic respiratory acidosis. These conditions can usually be easily distinguished by measuring the arterial blood pH, which is reduced in respiratory acidosis.

Causes of Metabolic Alkalosis

Metabolic alkalosis is a relatively common clinical problem that is most often induced by diuretic therapy or the loss of gastric secretions as a result of vomiting or nasogastric suction.[28] Two abnormalities must be present for metabolic alkalosis to develop and to be sustained. First, there must be an initial increase in the plasma $[HCO_3^-]$ caused by hydrogen loss in gastrointestinal secretions or in the urine, hydrogen movement into cells, alkali administration, or contraction alkalosis [*see Table 6*]. Second, one of four factors (in the absence of advanced renal failure) must be present to sustain the high plasma $[HCO_3^-]$ once the initiating event has been terminated: effective circulating volume depletion, chloride depletion and hypochloremia, hypokalemia, or hypercapnia.

Gastrointestinal hydrogen loss Loss of hydrogen ions can occur in gastrointestinal secretions or in the urine. Each 1 mEq of hydrogen lost generates 1 mEq of bicarbonate. Gastric juice contains a high concentration of hydrochloric acid and a lesser amount of potassium chloride. In normal persons, gastric hydrogen secretion does not lead to metabolic alkalosis, because it is matched by pancreatic bicarbonate secretion that is stimulated as the acid enters the duodenum. There is no stimulus to bicarbonate secretion, however, when vomiting or nasogastric tube drainage prevents the hydrogen ions from reaching the duodenum. Vomiting can be surreptitious in some cases, such as in patients with eating disorders.

Renal hydrogen loss An inappropriate increase in renal acid loss may occur when there is an increase in hydrogen ion secretion by the distal nephrons. Aldosterone acts here both by directly stimulating the secretory H^+-ATPase pump and by making the tubular lumen more electronegative through the stimulation of sodium reabsorption [*see Figure 6*]. Distal potassium secretion is also enhanced in this setting and results in concurrent hypokalemia.

Primary hypersecretion of aldosterone can lead to metabolic alkalosis, generally accompanied by hypertension and hypokalemia. In contrast, untreated patients with secondary aldosteronism caused by congestive heart failure or cirrhosis usually do not present with metabolic alkalosis or hypokalemia. In those cases, the effect of aldosterone is counteracted by decreased distal sodium delivery (unless diuretics are administered) and reduced urine volume; these factors limit the quantity of acid and potassium secreted into, and excreted in, the final urine. If, however, a nonreabsorbable anion (such as high-dose ticarcillin) is administered, potassium, sodium, or hydrogen ion losses are required to maintain electroneutrality. This condition leads to a hypokalemic metabolic alkalosis.

When patients are treated with either thiazide or loop diuretics, both adequate distal delivery of sodium chloride and increased secretion of aldosterone occur. The increase in distal hydrogen ion secretion and volume contraction, if the diuresis has been large, contribute to the development of metabolic alkalosis. The laboratory findings are similar to those observed with diuretic use in patients with Bartter and Gitelman syndromes [*see Diagnosis, below*].

Chronic respiratory acidosis brings about an appropriate increase in hydrogen secretion, as the rise in the plasma $[HCO_3^-]$ raises the pH toward normal. Rapid lowering of the P_aCO_2, usually by mechanical ventilation, leads to metabolic alkalosis, as the patient is left with an elevated plasma $[HCO_3^-]$. This abnormality is called a posthypercapnic metabolic alkalosis.

Hypercalcemia Hypercalcemia increases renal tubular bicarbonate reabsorption. Significant metabolic alkalosis in hypercalcemic patients, however, is more commonly seen in those with milk-alkali syndrome. In milk-alkali syndrome, an increased alkaline load (caused by the ingestion of calcium carbonate) and hypercalcemia-induced renal failure both enhance bicarbonate production and diminish bicarbonate excretion.[29]

Intracellular hydrogen shift Hypokalemia is a frequent finding in patients with metabolic alkalosis. Both vomiting and diuretic therapy directly induce potassium and hydrogen loss. Hypokalemia produces a transcellular shift in which potassium leaves cells to replete extracellular stores; to maintain electroneutrality, hydrogen enters the cells. This shift not only raises the extracellular pH but also decreases the intracellular pH; the latter promotes proximal tubular bicarbonate reabsorption and distal hydrogen ion secretion.

Alkali administration   The administration of sodium bicarbonate at a dosage as high as 1,000 mEq/day does not induce metabolic alkalosis in normal persons, because the excess bicarbonate is rapidly excreted in the urine. If the ability to excrete bicarbonate is impaired, however, metabolic alkalosis can occur when a very large quantity of bicarbonate or a bicarbonate precursor (e.g., lactate, citrate, or acetate) is administered, as occurs with citrate in large-volume blood transfusions.

Contraction alkalosis   Contraction alkalosis develops when loss of relatively large volumes of bicarbonate-free fluid occurs. In this setting, the plasma [HCO_3^-] rises because the extracellular volume contracts around a relatively constant quantity of extracellular bicarbonate.

The most common cause of contraction alkalosis is administration of a loop diuretic to induce rapid fluid removal in a patient with marked edema. Similarly, contraction alkalosis occurs under other conditions in which fluid with a high chloride concentration and a low [HCO_3^-] is lost. Among these causes are receipt of thiazide diuretics; loss of gastric secretions (even in patients with achlorhydria); sweat losses in patients with cystic fibrosis; and diarrhea in some patients with villous adenomas or congenital chloridorrhea, a rare disorder characterized by a specific defect in intestinal chloride reabsorption and bicarbonate secretion.[30]

Effective volume depletion   Both the fall in the glomerular filtration rate (GFR) and the associated sodium avidity seen with hypovolemia limit the excretion of sodium bicarbonate. Most bicarbonate is reabsorbed in the proximal tubule [*see Figure 2*]. An important stimulus for enhanced reabsorption in this nephron segment is increased activity of the Na^+- H^+ antiporter in the tubular cell membranes. Volume contraction promotes Na^+- H^+ exchange in this nephron segment, in part through the release of angiotensin II. The hydrogen ions secreted into the lumen combine with filtered bicarbonate, ultimately leading to a higher rate of transport back into the tubular cells. An even higher rate of bicarbonate is returned to the venous blood at the level of the collecting tubules, partly under the influence of secondary aldosteronism.

Chloride depletion   Vomiting and diuretic therapy are associated with loss of both hydrogen and chloride. Chloride depletion can both promote bicarbonate regeneration and decrease distal bicarbonate secretion. Bicarbonate generation in the α-intercalated cells in the cortical collecting tubule is mediated by hydrogen ion secretion via H^+-ATPase pumps in the luminal membrane [*see Figure 6*]. Passive cosecretion of chloride is required to maintain electroneutrality when intracellular bicarbonate is returned to the systemic circulation.

In contrast, the β-intercalated cells in the cortical collecting tubule (which increase in number when metabolic alkalosis develops) are able to secrete bicarbonate directly by reversing the location of the transporters [*see Figure 6*]. Thus, the Cl^--HCO_3^- exchangers are located in the luminal membrane, leading to bicarbonate secretion into the tubular lumen; the H^+-ATPase pumps are located in the basolateral membrane. Although the activity of these cells is appropriately enhanced by alkalemia in an attempt to excrete the excess bicarbonate, the associated fall in the tubular fluid chloride concentration diminishes the favorable inward gradient for chloride, thereby reducing bicarbonate secretion.

Hypokalemia   Hypokalemia directly increases bicarbonate reabsorption by at least two different mechanisms. First, the fall in plasma [K^+] shifts potassium from and hydrogen into cells. The ensuing intracellular acidosis stimulates hydrogen secretion and bicarbonate reabsorption in the proximal and collecting tubules. Second, distal hydrogen and potassium secretion is mediated in exchange for luminal sodium [*see Figure 6*]. In states of potassium depletion, the rate of hydrogen secretion in exchange for sodium increases. As a result, hypokalemia and hyperaldosteronism, which stimulate hydrogen ion secretion, can have a potentiating effect on the development and maintenance of metabolic alkalosis.

Diagnosis

Clinical manifestations   The clinical manifestations of metabolic alkalosis—namely, an elevated plasma [HCO_3^-] and an arterial pH greater than 7.42—are usually a result of volume depletion, hypokalemia, or concomitant hypocalcemia and hypomagnesemia. It is unclear why some individuals have severe cramping, paresthesias, or even tetany but others with similar electrolyte levels do not. Other clinical findings are the result of the underlying etiology (e.g., hypertension with primary hyperaldosteronism).

The diagnosis of metabolic alkalosis is usually evident from the patient's history of vomiting or receipt of diuretic therapy. In some cases, however, no cause for the metabolic alkalosis is apparent. In such a setting, the most likely diagnosis is surreptitious vomiting caused by an eating disorder, use of diuretics, or one of the causes of mineralocorticoid excess (e.g., primary aldosteronism). The first two factors induce effective volume depletion, whereas aldosteronism is usually associated with mild volume expansion as a result of the stimulatory effect of aldosterone on renal sodium reabsorption.

Laboratory tests   Measurement of the sodium concentration in a random urine specimen (U_{Na}) is used in many conditions to distinguish between volume depletion (U_{Na} usually < 20 mEq/L) and euvolemia (U_{Na} > 40 mEq/L). However, metabolic alkalosis is one of the conditions in which volume depletion may not lead to a low U_{Na}. In such cases, a urine [Cl^-] test is more useful. The capacity to retain sodium in this setting may be antagonized by the need to excrete bicarbonate (as the sodium salt) in an attempt to correct the alkalosis.

Sodium wasting is most likely to occur during the first few days of vomiting, when the plasma [HCO_3^-] and thus the filtered bicarbonate load are increased. Early in the course of vomiting, the ability to enhance bicarbonate reabsorption has not yet occurred. The net effects are a high U_{Na} and urinary potassium concentration and a urine pH of greater than 7.0 caused by bicarbonaturia.

As a result, the U_{Na} is not necessarily an accurate reflection of the patient's volume status in metabolic alkalosis. The presence of underlying hypovolemia can be detected more accurately by the finding of a urinary chloride concentration below 25 mEq/L. The appropriate chloride conservation is caused both by volume depletion and by hypochloremia induced by chloride losses in gastric secretions. The urinary chloride concentration may be inappropriately elevated, however, if a defect in chloride reabsorption is present. Such a defect most commonly occurs in patients who receive diuretic therapy and is transient, as chloride is appropriately conserved once the drug effect wears off. Thus, in patients with metabolic alkalosis caused by vomiting, the urinary chloride concentration is typically low; it is higher when diuretics are administered. In both circumstances, the U_{Na} may be elevated.

Bartter syndrome and Gitelman syndrome   The Bartter syndrome and Gitelman syndrome are disorders of sodium chloride reabsorption in the loop of Henle and the distal tubule, respectively.[31] Bartter syndrome is a rare disorder that causes hypokalemic metabolic alkalosis. Because the U_{Na} and urinary chloride concentrations are usually higher than 25 mEq/L, surreptitious diuretic use is the major disorder to be considered in the differential diagnosis. Classic Bartter syndrome generally presents in early life and may be associated with delayed growth and mental retardation. The spectrum of findings, including hypercalciuria, is most compatible with a primary defect in sodium chloride reabsorption in the medullary thick ascending limb of the loop of Henle.

Gitelman syndrome is a more benign condition that may be inherited but that may not be diagnosed until late childhood or even adulthood. In contrast to patients with Bartter syndrome, who have a defect in urinary concentrating ability (normal function of the loop of Henle is needed to generate a high interstitial osmotic gradient), patients with Gitelman syndrome can demonstrate normal urinary concentrating ability and have hypocalciuria. This finding suggests that the defect resides in the distal tubule. Bartter syndrome and Gitelman syndrome are diagnosed only after diuretic use—the other, much more common, cause of these findings—has been excluded.

Treatment

In patients with true volume depletion caused by vomiting, nasogastric suction, villous adenomas, or diuretic therapy, metabolic alkalosis can be corrected by the administration of sodium chloride.[32] The ensuing increase in sodium bicarbonate excretion is primarily caused by two events occurring in the collecting tubules—decreased bicarbonate generation and increased bicarbonate secretion—as well as by a fall in bicarbonate reabsorption in the proximal tubule. The administration of potassium chloride to patients with concurrent hypokalemia also contributes to correction of the alkalemia.

Edematous states Therapy is different for patients who have edema caused by heart failure, cor pulmonale, or advanced liver disease. In these disorders, sodium chloride is contraindicated because it increases the degree of edema. Administration of the carbonic anhydrase inhibitor acetazolamide (beginning with 250 mg p.o., q.d. or b.i.d., or 125 mg I.V., q.d. or b.i.d.), however, may be particularly effective. This drug preferentially inhibits proximal tubular reabsorption of sodium bicarbonate, thereby correcting both the alkalosis and the fluid overload.

A potential side effect of therapy with a carbonic anhydrase inhibitor is the development or worsening of hypokalemia. Although hypokalemia can be treated with potassium supplements, an alternative approach to therapy is to administer a potassium-sparing diuretic (e.g., spironolactone) instead of a carbonic anhydrase inhibitor. Potassium-sparing diuretics impair sodium reabsorption in the collecting tubules and, as a result, limit further potassium and hydrogen secretion [see Figure 6]. In patients with advanced liver disease, spironolactone may be the most effective diuretic.

On extremely rare occasions, metabolic alkalosis may be so severe that administration of hydrochloric acid is required to correct the problem. The standard 0.1N (decinormal) hydrochloric acid solution contains 100 mEq H^+/L. The amount of hydrochloric acid needed to reduce the serum [HCO_3^-] can be estimated from the product of the volume distribution of bicarbonate (approximately 50% of lean body weight) and the bicarbonate deficit per liter. Thus, the equation for lowering the serum [HCO_3^-] from 45 mEq/L to 35 mEq/L in a 70 kg man is as follows:

$$\text{Bicarbonate excess} = 0.5 \times 70 \times (45 - 35) = 350 \text{ mEq}$$

The required amount of 0.1N hydrochloric acid solution would be 3.5 L. Because of the risk of errors in calculation and the cor-

rosive nature of hydrochloric acid solution, this technique should be used only when other measures to correct metabolic alkalosis have failed, and the hydrochloric acid solution must always be administered into a central vein.

Bartter syndrome and Gitelman syndrome The tubular defect in patients with Bartter syndrome or Gitelman syndrome cannot be corrected. As a result, treatment is directed at minimizing the electrolyte and metabolic abnormalities. The combination of an NSAID, including cyclooxygenase-2 inhibitors (because prostaglandin levels are secondarily increased) and a potassium-sparing diuretic, can raise the plasma [K^+] toward normal and largely reverse the metabolic alkalosis.[33] Most patients, however, require continued oral potassium and magnesium supplements because drug therapy is rarely completely effective.

RESPIRATORY ACIDOSIS AND ALKALOSIS

Alveolar ventilation provides the oxygen necessary for oxidative metabolism and eliminates the carbon dioxide produced by these metabolic processes. It is therefore appropriate that the main physiologic stimuli to respiration are a reduced arterial oxygen tension (P_aO_2), termed hypoxemia, and an elevated P_aCO_2. Carbon dioxide stimulates ventilation primarily in chemosensitive areas in the respiratory center in the medulla that respond to carbon dioxide–induced changes in the cerebral interstitial pH. In contrast, the initial hypoxemic enhancement of ventilation is mostly mediated by chemoreceptors in the carotid bodies, which are located near the bifurcation of the carotid arteries. A number of disorders can be responsible for acute and chronic respiratory acidosis and alkalosis [see Tables 7 and 8].

Diagnosis

Clinical manifestations Severe respiratory acidosis can produce a variety of neurologic abnormalities. Initial symptoms include headache, blurred vision, restlessness, and anxiety, which can progress to tremors, asterixis, delirium, and a somnolence termed carbon dioxide narcosis. Some of these signs, including papilledema, appear to be caused by the acidemia-induced increase in cerebral blood flow. Overall, these signs seem to result from the fall in cerebrospinal fluid pH and not from the changes in the arterial pH or P_aCO_2.

The symptoms produced by respiratory alkalosis are related to increased irritability of the central and peripheral nervous systems and include light-headedness, altered consciousness, paresthesias of the extremities and circumoral area, cramps, carpopedal spasm (indistinguishable from that caused by hypocalcemia), and syncope. In critically ill patients, a variety of arrhythmias may also occur. These abnormalities are thought to relate to the ability of alkalosis to reduce cerebral blood flow and to increase membrane excitability; a decrease in ionized calcium or magnesium also contributes to heightened membrane excitability.

Laboratory tests Primary respiratory alkalosis can be diagnosed when the blood pH is greater than 7.42 in the presence of a reduced P_{CO_2}. It can also be identified by use of the Winter formula in patients with metabolic acidosis [see Metabolic Acidosis, above].

Treatment

Usually, respiratory failure causes acute respiratory acidosis. As a result, treatment is normally indicated, and the patient may require mechanical ventilation [see 6:6 Use of the Mechanical Ventilator]. In contrast, treatment of respiratory alkalosis is generally not necessary; evaluation should be aimed at diagnosing and correcting the underlying disorder.

Table 7 Causes of Respiratory Acidosis

Disorder	Cause
Suppression of the medullary respiratory center	Sedative medications Oxygen administration in chronic lung disease Sleep apnea (also caused by extreme obesity) Central nervous system lesions (uncommon) Cardiopulmonary arrest

Reduced respiratory muscle function	Acute
	   Muscle weakness or paralysis (myasthenia gravis, periodic paralysis, intraperitoneal aminoglycosides, Guillain-Barré syndrome, botulism, severe hypokalemia, severe hypophosphatemia)
	Chronic
	   Muscle weakness: poliomyelitis, amyotrophic lateral sclerosis, myxedema
	   Kyphoscoliosis

Upper airway obstruction	Aspiration of a foreign body or vomitus Obstruction in sleep apnea Laryngospasm

Disorders affecting pulmonary gas exchange	Acute
	   Acute respiratory distress syndrome
	   Acute cardiac pulmonary edema
	   Severe asthma or pneumonia
	   Pneumothorax or hemothorax
	Chronic
	   Obstructive pulmonary diseases

Inadequate mechanical ventilation	—

Plasma Potassium Disorders

Potassium is the major intracellular cation, with much higher concentrations inside cells (123 to 140 mEq/L) than in the extracellular space (3.5 to 5.0 mEq/L). This concentration difference is preserved by the Na^+,K^+-ATPase pump, which actively transports sodium ions out of most cells and potassium ions into most cells. The difference between potassium concentration inside and outside the cell is the major determinant of membrane excitability. Thus, despite the comparatively small quantity of extracellular potassium, slight changes can have dramatic effects on muscle contraction and nerve conduction.

POTASSIUM HOMEOSTASIS

In the United States, the daily dietary potassium intake varies from 40 to 120 mEq. Under normal conditions, about 90% of dietary potassium is excreted in the urine; most of the remainder is eliminated in the stool. Gastrointestinal potassium losses increase in patients with renal failure, but the significance of this adaptation is uncertain.

Only about 50% of an oral or intravenous potassium load appears in the urine during the first 4 hours after administration. Marked and potentially life-threatening hyperkalemia can occur if the remaining potassium is confined to the extracellular fluid; this volume is only about 14 L in a 70 kg male. Transport of most of this potassium into cells before excretion in the urine minimizes the rise in the plasma $[K^+]$.

The most important factors in the transport of dietary potassium into cells are the influences of insulin and beta$_2$-adrenergic receptors. Insulin stimulates the Na^+,K^+-ATPase pump, leading to a more rapid rate of potassium entry. Similarly, activation of beta$_2$-adrenergic receptors also promotes potassium movement into cells. Aldosterone is the most important hormone involved in potassium secretion by epithelial surfaces, including epithelial cells of the renal tubule. Aldosterone appears to be less important to the transport of potassium into other cells.

Renal Regulation of Potassium Secretion

Potassium is freely filtered at the glomerulus. The concentration of potassium ions entering the early proximal tubule is approximately 4 mEq/L, identical to the plasma $[K^+]$. By the time the glomerular filtrate reaches the distal tubule, 90% of the filtered potassium has been reabsorbed. Thus, renal potassium excretion occurs almost exclusively by secretion in the collecting tubule.

Potassium secretion into the collecting tubule takes place in the principal cells [see Figure 3]. Movement of potassium ions from the tubular cells into the lumen is controlled by the rates of (1) dietary potassium intake; (2) aldosterone-driven sodium reabsorption, which generates a negative electrical gradient that allows potassium to move down the lumen; and (3) distal urine flow, which maintains a high gradient of tubular cell to tubular lumen concentration by washing away secreted potassium.

Aldosterone produced in the adrenal glands enters the principal cells from the antiluminal, or capillary, surface. Once inside, aldosterone binds to receptors that increase the number of open sodium channels on the luminal cell membrane. The number and activity of Na^+,K^+-ATPase pumps in the cell membrane also increase. The ensuing rise in cellular potassium leads to secretion into the collecting tubular lumen down the favorable concentration and electrochemical gradient.

In states of potassium depletion, secretion of potassium ions by the principal cells is reduced (provided the kidney is not the source of potassium wasting) and potassium reabsorption is stimulated. This process occurs in the adjacent intercalated cells [see Figure 3].

HYPOKALEMIA

Causes of Hypokalemia

Hypokalemia, which can be defined as a plasma $[K^+]$ lower than 3.5 mEq/L, may be caused by low potassium intake, a shift of potassium into cells, or potassium losses from the body [see Table 9]. In

Table 8 Causes of Respiratory Alkalosis

Disorder	Cause
Hypoxemia	Pulmonary disease: pneumonia, emboli, edema, interstitial fibrosis Congestive heart failure Severe anemia High-altitude exposure
Direct stimulation of the medullary respiratory center	Hyperventilation syndrome Hepatic encephalopathy Gram-negative sepsis Salicylate intoxication* After rapid correction of metabolic acidosis Pregnancy (i.e., increased progesterone) Neurologic disorders (cerebrovascular accidents, pontine tumors)
Excessive mechanical ventilation	—

*Respiratory alkalosis is the initial disorder observed, although metabolic acidosis develops later if intoxication is severe.

most persons, potassium losses occur from the gastrointestinal tract, skin, or kidneys.

Low potassium intake   Inadequate potassium intake is uncommon in developed nations because potassium is abundant in most foods. Furthermore, if intake is diminished, urinary and intestinal losses can be reduced to less than 15 mEq/day.

In some rural areas of the United States, however, potassium intake may be only about 25 mEq/day, in part because potassium-containing foods are relatively expensive. Also, the practice of clay ingestion, common in parts of the rural southeastern United States, can result in clay binding to potassium in the bowel, thereby limiting its absorption.

Altered potassium distribution   Even in the presence of normal potassium stores in the body, several conditions can cause transport of potassium into cells and hence reduce the plasma [K$^+$].

Metabolic and, to a much lesser degree, acute respiratory alkalosis may be associated with hypokalemia. The principal mechanism in this setting is the transfer of hydrogen ions out of cells as part of the buffering response that minimizes the rise in the extracellular pH; electroneutrality is maintained in part by potassium entry into cells. The relation between the degree of hypokalemia and the increase in blood pH varies greatly. Potassium loss from the body also plays an important role in the hypokalemia observed with the metabolic alkalosis caused by vomiting or diuretic use.

A catecholamine surge, which occurs during an acute myocardial infarction or delirium tremens, can result in an acute intracellular shift of potassium caused by stimulation of beta$_2$-adrenergic receptors. This phenomenon, in which epinephrine can convert mild hypokalemia to severe hypokalemia, may contribute to the apparent increase in coronary mortality observed in studies of patients with left ventricular hypertrophy and mild hypertension who have been treated with moderate- to high-dose thiazide diuretics. Beta-adrenergic stimulation with terbutaline used in preterm labor can also reduce the plasma [K$^+$] to below normal.[34]

The plasma [K$^+$] typically falls during insulin administration in patients with diabetic ketoacidosis, despite a normal or increased level on presentation. This decrease results in part from insulin-stimulated transfer of potassium into cells. A similar problem can occur when intravenous dextrose is given to nondiabetic patients; for example, 5% dextrose in water can temporarily worsen hypokalemia and possibly lead to cardiac arrhythmias.

Rare causes of redistribution-induced hypokalemia include folic acid or vitamin B$_{12}$ administration in the treatment of megaloblastic anemias (in which the rapid production of new cells results in the uptake of potassium from the extracellular fluid) and poisoning with barium salts (which block cell membrane channels that normally allow potassium to leave the cells). Patients undergoing gastrointestinal radiographic procedures are not at risk for poisoning with barium salts, because barium sulfate, which is used in gastrointestinal studies, is not absorbed into systemic circulation. Severe theophylline overdoses also may cause hypokalemia resulting from catecholamine-induced potassium shifts or glucose-induced insulin release. A similar finding has been reported after chloroquine intoxication.[35]

Hypokalemic periodic paralysis is a rare disorder of uncertain cause that is characterized by potentially fatal episodes of muscle weakness or paralysis resulting from the sudden movement of potassium into cells. Acute attacks are often precipitated by rest after exercise, stress, or a carbohydrate meal, events that are often associated with increased release of epinephrine or insulin.

The disorder may be familial, and the abnormal gene in most patients seems to code for the part of the calcium channel in skeletal muscle that is blocked by dihydropyridine calcium channel blockers (e.g., nifedipine). In contrast, some patients with hyperthyroidism, particularly Asian males, acquire the disease.[36] In these patients, excess thyroid hormone may predispose to paralytic episodes by increasing Na$^+$,K$^+$-ATPase activity in cells [see Treatment, below].

Potassium losses from the body   The gastrointestinal tract can be an important site of potassium wasting, particularly in patients with vomiting or diarrhea. However, the [K$^+$] in gastric secretions (5 to 10 mEq/L) is much lower than that in intestinal secretions, where it can reach 75 mEq/L. As a result, the loss of large volumes of gastric secretions would be required to produce substantial potassium depletion. The decreased [K$^+$] that is seen with vomiting results primarily from increased urinary, rather than gastric, losses.

Two conditions can cause cutaneous potassium losses resulting in hypokalemia: exercise in a hot, humid environment and severe burns. Persons who undergo intense physical exercise may lose more than 10 L of sweat a day. This loss can lead to significant potassium depletion even though the [K$^+$] in sweat is only about 5 mEq/L. In comparison, the [K$^+$] in fluid lost through the skin after extensive

***Table 9* Causes of Hypokalemia**

Disorder	Cause
Inadequate potassium intake	Low dietary content Clay ingestion
Cellular translocation of potassium	Metabolic and, to a lesser degree, acute respiratory alkalosis Beta$_2$-adrenergic stimulation (myocardial infarction, delirium tremens) Insulin administration (or glucose administration in nondiabetics) Increased cell proliferation during the treatment of megaloblastic anemia Hypokalemic periodic paralysis Hypothermia Barium poisoning Theophylline toxicity (may be caused by catecholamine or insulin-induced shifts)

Losses of potassium from the body	Extrarenal losses
	  Gastrointestinal (i.e., diarrhea)
	Skin losses
	  Profuse sweating
	  Extensive burns
	Renal losses
	  Normotensive
	    Diuretics
	    Vomiting or nasogastric suction*
	    Hypomagnesemia
	    Nonreabsorbable anions (high-dose penicillins)
	    Levodopa
	    Tubular disorders: classic type 1 RTA, Bartter syndrome, drugs (cisplatin, aminoglycosides, amphotericin B), and lysozymuria (in leukemia)
	  Hypertensive with high mineralocorticoid activity
	    Low plasma renin activity: primary aldosteronism and licorice ingestion
	    Normal or high plasma renin activity: renal artery stenosis, malignant hypertension, and Cushing syndrome

*Gastric losses of potassium also contribute but are minor.

burns may greatly exceed the plasma level because of local tissue breakdown, which leads to the release of intracellular potassium.

Potassium losses in the urine occur most commonly in patients who are either vomiting or receiving diuretic therapy. Extracellular volume depletion promotes aldosterone release, leading to enhanced Na^+-K^+ exchange in the collecting tubule [see Figure 3]. Aldosteronism alone is insufficient to permit increased potassium excretion, however, because distal urine flow must be maintained for secreted potassium to be excreted. Distal urine flow is maintained in the presence of vomiting or diuretic therapy because sodium and water escape reabsorption. Diuretics inhibit reabsorption of water and sodium in either the loop of Henle or the distal tubule. The increased tubular bicarbonate load present during vomiting allows sodium and water to escape reabsorption in the proximal tubule. The latter mechanism also explains the hypokalemia seen with high-dose penicillins, because these drugs, like bicarbonate, are nonreabsorbable anions. Direct inhibition of potassium reabsorption also contributes to the hypokalemia observed with the use of loop diuretics.

As many as 40% of hypokalemic persons also have hypomagnesemia. At times, the cause of potassium wasting, such as diuretic or cisplatin treatment, is also responsible for impaired magnesium reabsorption. However, potassium depletion usually cannot be corrected without restoring magnesium balance. This connection may exist because magnesium can act as a potassium channel blocker. In the loop of Henle, for example, potassium may leak through the cell membrane into the tubular lumen when magnesium levels are low, thereby contributing to ongoing urinary losses.

Several less common causes of tubular dysfunction can also lead to urinary potassium losses. These causes include classic type 1 RTA; drugs (e.g., cisplatin, amphotericin B, and the aminoglycosides); both acute and, less commonly, chronic leukemia; and levodopa administration. Reduced sodium reabsorption, leading to volume depletion, stimulates aldosterone secretion and plays a role in many of these disorders. Primary aldosteronism should be considered, however, whenever unprovoked potassium wasting is detected in a hypertensive person.

Diagnosis

Clinical manifestations In most circumstances, mild hypokalemia (plasma $[K^+]$ 3.0 to 3.5 mEq/L) causes no symptoms. The major disturbances seen with more severe potassium deficiency result from changes in cardiovascular, neuromuscular, and renal function. Cardiac toxicity may be manifested by serious arrhythmias, which occur because hyperpolarization of the myocardial cell membrane leads to a prolonged refractory period and increased susceptibility to reentrant arrhythmias. Other electrocardiographic changes of hypokalemia include T wave depression and prominent U waves [see Figure 7].

Hyperpolarization also slows nerve conduction and muscle contraction, which may contribute to muscle weakness, cramps, and paresthesias, although these symptoms are usually not observed until the plasma $[K^+]$ is lower than 2.5 mEq/L. When hypokalemia is severe, it can impair respiratory muscle function, leading to hypoventilation. Because potassium normally permits vasodilatation in response to muscle contraction, severe hypokalemia also may cause rhabdomyolysis.

The primary renal manifestations of hypokalemia are polyuria resulting from stimulated thirst and resistance to antidiuretic hormone action. The latter condition is termed nephrogenic diabetes insipidus. Increased thirst is an appropriate response to polyuria, but it is also caused by direct stimulation of the hypothalamic thirst center by hypokalemia. The resistance to antidiuretic hormone is

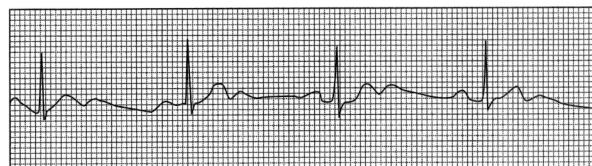

a

II

b

V1

c

V1

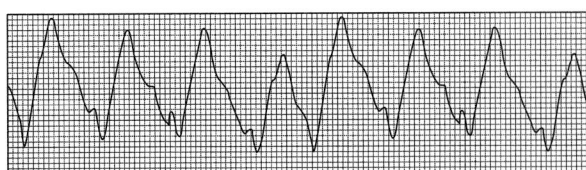

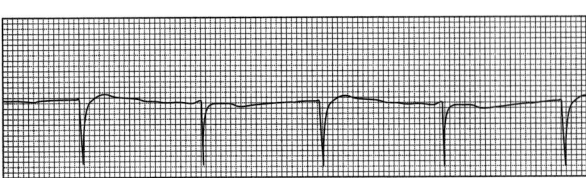

Figure 7 **Both hypokalemia and hyperkalemia can cause changes in the patient's electrocardiogram. (*a*) The ECG from a patient with moderate hypokalemia shows prominent U waves. (*b*) Marked hyperkalemia results in peaked T waves and widened QRS complexes in this ECG. Ten minutes after the patient receives intravenous calcium, however, all ECG manifestations of hyperkalemia have resolved (*c*).**

caused by a hypokalemia-induced fall in the number of collecting tubular water channels.[37] Chronic hypokalemia can lead to chronic interstitial nephritis and a decline in glomerular filtration.

When hypokalemia is severe (plasma $[K^+]$ < 2 mEq/L), the ability of the renal tubules to reabsorb sodium and chloride may be impaired. This condition can lead to volume depletion and to the loss of urinary sodium and chloride, even in states of reduced renal perfusion. The mechanism may involve suppressed activity of tubular chloride transporters, many of which also facilitate sodium reabsorption.

Physiologic tests The history and physical examination usually suggest the diagnosis in the hypokalemic patient. Excretion of more than 30 mEq of potassium a day indicates some renal potassium wasting. Patients with extrarenal potassium losses excrete less potassium daily, as do patients who have discontinued diuretic therapy. Once urinary potassium excretion is measured, the following diagnostic possibilities should be considered in the patient with hypokalemia of uncertain origin:

1. In an asymptomatic patient, metabolic acidosis with a low rate of urinary potassium excretion suggests lower-gastrointestinal losses because of diarrhea, laxative abuse, or villous adenomas.
2. Metabolic acidosis with renal potassium wasting is most often caused by diabetic ketoacidosis or type 1 RTA.
3. Metabolic alkalosis with a low rate of urinary potassium excretion is usually caused by surreptitious vomiting (late phase) or diuretic use (in which the urine sample is obtained after the effect of the diuretic has worn off).
4. Metabolic alkalosis with potassium wasting and a normal blood pressure is most often caused by surreptitious vomiting (early phase), diuretic use, or Bartter syndrome. In this setting, mea-

surement of the urinary chloride concentration is often helpful. It is low in patients who have been vomiting, whereas the U_{Na} and urinary potassium excretion may be relatively high. This diagnosis can be determined at the bedside from the urine pH, which should be 7.0 or higher if significant bicarbonaturia is present.

5. Metabolic alkalosis with potassium wasting and hypertension suggests surreptitious diuretic use by a patient with underlying hypertension, renovascular hypertension, malignant hypertension, or primary aldosteronism.

Treatment

Normalizing the plasma $[K^+]$ is indicated in most cases, although the means of normalization and the quantity and route of potassium administration vary greatly. In the absence of factors that cause transcellular shifts of potassium, a fairly predictable relation exists between the degree of hypokalemia and the extent of total body potassium depletion. For each 1 mEq/L fall in the plasma $[K^+]$, potassium stores fall by 200 to 400 mEq, until the plasma $[K^+]$ drops below 2.0 mEq/L. At that point, the total deficit may exceed 1,000 mEq. With both oral and parenteral replacement, potassium enters the plasma before it is transferred into cells. Consequently, potassium supplementation, particularly when given intravenously, carries the risk of hyperkalemia if the dose is too large or if it is administered too rapidly. Therefore, potassium should be administered orally whenever possible.

Potassium replacement using potassium-rich foods can be effective when metabolic acidosis or renal failure is present. However, dietary potassium is not effective in correcting the potassium deficit that occurs with metabolic alkalosis. In most foods, potassium is bound to poorly reabsorbable anions such as phosphate.[38] Therefore, chloride salts (e.g., potassium chloride, which is used when metabolic alkalosis is caused by diuretics) are usually required to restore potassium losses.

Potassium can be administered intravenously into a peripheral vein in concentrations as high as 40 mEq/L; higher concentrations can cause phlebitis and thus should be infused only into a large vein. Except in unusual settings, the rate of administration should probably not exceed 20 to 40 mEq/hr, although dosages as high as 100 mEq/hr have been infused in selected patients with paralysis or life-threatening arrhythmias.[39] Glucose-containing solutions should be avoided because insulin stimulation can drive potassium into cells, thereby exacerbating the hypokalemia.

For patients taking diuretics for high blood pressure, several alternatives are available to correct hypokalemia without use of potassium chloride supplementation. Because patient compliance decreases as the number of medications (including potassium supplements) increases, reducing the diuretic dose (e.g., to 12.5 mg of hydrochlorothiazide) or substituting an alternative agent should be tried first.

Edematous individuals or patients with primary aldosteronism who also experience hypokalemia can be treated with potassium-sparing diuretics (amiloride or spironolactone) until more definitive therapy can be performed (e.g., the surgical removal of an adrenal adenoma in primary aldosteronism).

In patients with hypokalemic periodic paralysis [see Altered Potassium Distribution, above], administration of potassium chloride can abort acute attacks within minutes. Hyperthyroidism should be treated when present, and the administration of a nonselective beta-adrenergic blocker (e.g., propranolol) may prevent episodes in patients with the familial form of the disorder.

HYPERKALEMIA

Hyperkalemia is a common electrolyte disorder. Because a variety of frequently used medications can interfere with normal potas-

Table 10 Causes of Hyperkalemia

Disorder	Cause
Pseudohyperkalemia	Traumatic hemolysis during blood drawing Thrombocytosis Marked leukocytosis
Increased intake of potassium*	Increased dietary potassium Increased intake of potassium-containing medications Increased release of endogenous potassium (as occurs during rhabdomyolysis)

Increased release from cells	Insulin deficiency
	Beta$_2$-adrenergic blockade
	Acute metabolic acidosis
	Cell breakdown
	  Rhabdomyolysis
	  Trauma or infection with abscess formation
	  Tumor lysis syndrome after chemotherapy
	Marked exercise (transient; resolves with rest)
	Massive cardiac glycoside intoxication (e.g., digoxin)
	Succinylcholine
	Arginine infusion
	Hyperkalemic periodic paralysis

Impaired renal potassium excretion	Oligoanuric renal failure Marked volume depletion (prerenal diseases) Type 4 RTA Hyperkalemic type 1 RTA [see Table 3]

*Sustained hyperkalemia associated with increased intake is always accompanied by impaired renal excretion.

sium homeostasis, hyperkalemia is often iatrogenic and therefore preventable. Severe hyperkalemia is associated with altered neuromuscular or cardiac function.

Causes of Hyperkalemia

Hyperkalemia can be caused by excessive potassium intake, increased potassium release from cells, or reduced renal excretion of potassium [see Table 10].

Increased potassium intake The elevation in plasma $[K^+]$ that occurs after an acute oral or intravenous potassium load depends on four factors: (1) the quantity of potassium administered, (2) the ability of some of the excess potassium to enter cells, (3) urinary potassium excretion, and (4) the preceding level of potassium intake—a process called adaptation. The rise in plasma $[K^+]$ is minimized if potassium intake has increased slowly. During a slow increase, renal excretion and, perhaps, cellular entry become more efficient. Enhanced aldosterone and increased Na^+,K^+-ATPase activity in the cortical collecting tubule play important roles in this process. Even in the absence of adaptation, the kidney ultimately excretes the excess potassium, although more slowly. Thus, hyperkalemia resulting from an acute load is transient unless renal potassium excretion is concomitantly reduced.

Increased potassium release from cells Both insulin deficiency and beta$_2$-adrenergic blockade can increase the plasma $[K^+]$. In patients with end-stage renal disease who are on hemodialysis, for example, propranolol or labetalol, but not the selective beta$_1$-adrenergic blocker atenolol, can raise the plasma $[K^+]$ level by about 1 mEq/L.[40]

At higher doses of atenolol, however, this selectivity may be lost.

An elevation in plasma osmolality results in osmotic water movement from the cells into the extracellular fluid. This event is accompanied by the movement of potassium from cells via two mechanisms. First, the increased cellular potassium concentration caused by the loss of water creates a favorable gradient for passive exit of potassium through the potassium channels in the cell membrane. Second, friction forces between solvent (water) and solute carry potassium along with water through the water pores in the cell membrane.

Acute acidemia can also increase the plasma $[K^+]$ by shifting potassium from cells to plasma. This shift is likely to occur when bicarbonate is lost because of diarrhea and during the infusion of acids; when arginine hydrochloride is infused, for instance, potassium is exchanged for cationic arginine entering the cells. This shift, however, appears to be important in inorganic acidoses only. In comparison, hyperkalemia in lactic acidosis is caused primarily by cell breakdown, and hyperkalemia in ketoacidosis results from insulin deficiency and hyperglycemia.

Massive cell breakdown that occurs during rhabdomyolysis, during abscess formation, with cell necrosis (e.g., bowel infarction), or after chemotherapy for leukemia or lymphoma releases potassium into the plasma. Less common causes of an increased plasma $[K^+]$ include cardiac glycoside intoxication, a result of partial inhibition of the Na^+,K^+-ATPase pump; succinylcholine administration, which depolarizes the cell membrane and thus permits potassium to leave the cells; and the rare form of hyperkalemic periodic paralysis.

Impaired renal excretion of potassium The kidney, the major site of potassium excretion, has the distinct ability to increase the excretion rate as the plasma $[K^+]$ rises. Thus, sustained hyperkalemia is virtually always associated with some impairment of renal potassium elimination. Distal nephron hydrogen ion secretion is frequently impaired as well, leading to a normal-anion-gap metabolic acidosis, because the collecting tubule is the site of both potassium and hydrogen ion secretion. Renal potassium excretion can be impaired by oligoanuric renal failure, reduced effective arterial volume, type 4 RTA, and hyperkalemic type 1 RTA.

Oligoanuric renal failure impairs, but does not halt, potassium excretion. Although renal failure predisposes to potassium retention, excretion of dietary potassium usually continues in chronic renal disease until the GFR is less than 5 to 10 ml/min. Although less efficient in oligoanuric renal failure, renal excretion can still occur because most urinary potassium is derived from tubular secretion, not glomerular filtration.

When the effective arterial volume is reduced, delivery of sodium and water to the collecting tubule is also diminished. Adequate distal delivery of sodium and water is essential to normal potassium excretion. Distal delivery is characteristically reduced, for example, in patients with advanced congestive heart failure or cirrhosis. Both a fall in GFR and a rise in proximal sodium and water reabsorption, mediated in part by angiotensin II, play a role in the reduction of potassium excretion in this setting. Although aldosterone enhances sodium reabsorption and potassium secretion in these conditions, the increase is limited because less sodium is available for reabsorption. Furthermore, secreted potassium may not be eliminated completely if urine flow is markedly decreased.

Aldosterone deficiency or resistance (i.e., type 4 RTA) is responsible for the hyperkalemia in more than 75% to 85% of those cases in which patients have persistent hyperkalemia in the absence of any apparent cause, such as advanced renal failure, an offending drug, or a potassium load.

Type 4 RTA is also associated with diminished hydrogen ion secretion, which is caused in part by impaired ammoniagenesis in the proximal tubule, a possible result of hyperkalemia-induced intracel-

Table 11 Evaluation of the Renal Defect in Hyperkalemia

Disorder	Urine pH	U_{Na} (mEq/L)	Plasma Aldosterone Level
Renal failure	< 5.3	> 20	Normal or increased
Marked volume depletion	Variable	< 20	Increased
Type 4 RTA	< 5.3	> 20	Low*
Hyperkalemic type 1 RTA	> 5.3	> 20	Normal or increased

*Aldosterone level may be normal or increased in states of aldosterone resistance.
U_{Na}—urinary sodium concentration

lular alkalosis. The result is a diminished supply of ammonia in the more distal nephron segments. Consequently, insufficient buffer in the urine plays an important role in the limited hydrogen ion secretion and explains why the urine pH is characteristically acidified (< 5.3) in this disorder.

Several conditions cause type 4 RTA [see Table 4]. Hyporeninemic type 4 RTA is the most common form of the disorder and occurs most often in patients with mild renal insufficiency. Diabetic nephropathy or chronic interstitial nephritis is often present. Medications such as NSAIDs can also contribute to this disorder.

The pathophysiology of type 4 RTA in hyporeninemic patients is incompletely understood. Decreased angiotensin II production is clearly important because potassium and angiotensin II are the major physiologic stimuli for aldosterone release. However, at least some patients must also have a concurrent adrenal defect because observations indicate that the normal adrenal gland can release angiotensin II. It has also been suggested that in some patients, the reduced renin may be secondary. For example, volume expansion, which increases atrial natriuretic peptide, inhibits both renin and aldosterone release.

In other cases of type 4 RTA, the defect in aldosterone synthesis and release seems confined to the adrenal glands. Heparin (or perhaps its preservative, chlorbutol) is a potent inhibitor of aldosterone production, even when given subcutaneously in low doses.[33] Heparin use is not widely associated with hyperkalemia, however, because moderate aldosterone deficiency is not sufficient to cause significant potassium retention in the great majority of patients who still have normal renal function. Hyperkalemia can occur, however, if renal disease is present or if agents that impair the renin-angiotensin-aldosterone system, such as NSAIDs or ACE inhibitors, are concomitantly administered.

The possibility of panadrenal insufficiency (i.e., a deficiency of both aldosterone and cortisol, also termed Addison disease) should be assessed before the diagnosis of selective aldosterone deficiency is made. When panadrenal insufficiency is present, hypoadrenocorticism often impairs water excretion, leading to hyponatremia in addition to the hyperkalemia resulting from aldosterone deficiency.

Although classic type 1 RTA is associated with hypokalemia, some patients with impaired hydrogen ion secretion by the collecting tubule also cannot secrete potassium normally. This condition, hyperkalemic type 1 RTA, is most often seen with urinary tract obstruction but can also be caused by tubulointerstitial damage from such disorders as sickle cell nephropathy, lupus nephritis, or transplant rejection. The hyperkalemia and metabolic acidosis are caused by damage to both the potassium-secreting principal cells and the acid-secreting intercalated cells. Hyperkalemic type 1 RTA can be distinguished from type 4 RTA by the persistently alkaline urine (pH > 5.3) and by a normal or increased plasma aldosterone level [see Table 11].

Finally, it is important to remember the effects of medications that can limit potassium secretion directly.[41] Obvious agents are the potassium-sparing diuretics: amiloride, triamterene, and spironolactone. Another, less common agent is trimethoprim-sulfamethoxazole. Trimethoprim in this combination or alone can impair potassium secretion by blocking sodium transport from the tubular lumen into the collecting tubule cell, in a mechanism similar to that of amiloride.

Diagnosis

Clinical manifestations The symptoms of hyperkalemia are related to impaired neuromuscular transmission. However, the neuromuscular manifestations are not specific. The earliest findings are paresthesias and weakness, which can progress to paralysis affecting respiratory muscles. These symptoms are similar to those seen with hypokalemia; cranial nerve function, however, characteristically remains unaffected.

The ease of generating an action potential (called membrane excitability) is related both to the magnitude of the resting membrane potential and to the activation state of membrane sodium channels. The opening up of these sodium channels, leading to the passive diffusion of extracellular sodium into the cells, is the primary step in this process.

According to the Nernst equation, the resting membrane potential is related to the ratio of the intracellular potassium concentration to the extracellular potassium concentration. An elevation in the (extracellular) plasma [K^+] decreases this ratio and therefore partly depolarizes the cell membrane (i.e., it makes the resting membrane potential less electronegative). This change initially increases membrane excitability because less of a depolarizing stimulus is required to generate an action potential. However, persistent depolarization inactivates sodium channels in the cell membrane, thereby producing a net decrease in membrane excitability that may be manifested clinically by impaired cardiac conduction, muscle weakness, or paralysis.

In general, severe symptoms of hyperkalemia do not occur until the plasma [K^+] is higher than 7.5 mEq/L. There is substantial variability among patients, however, because factors such as concomitant hypocalcemia, metabolic acidosis, and the rate at which hyperkalemia develops can increase the toxicity of excess potassium.[42]

Physiologic tests Careful monitoring of the electrocardiogram and muscle strength is necessary to assess the functional consequences of hyperkalemia. At a plasma [K^+] higher than 7.5 to 8.0 mEq/L, severe muscle weakness or marked ECG changes are potentially life threatening and require immediate treatment with almost all of the available modalities [*see* Treatment, *below*].

The earliest ECG abnormality is symmetrical peaking of T waves, which is followed by reduced P wave voltage and widening of the QRS complexes [*see Figure 7*]. If left untreated, severe hyper-

kalemia may ultimately cause a sinusoidal ECG pattern, with one oscillation representing a wide QRS complex and the complementary oscillation representing an abnormal T wave. ECG changes do not usually occur until the plasma [K^+] exceeds 6.5 mEq/L, and they are more likely to develop when the rise in potassium occurs rapidly. However, there is no absolutely predictive relation between the severity of the electrolyte disturbance and the ECG pattern. In rare cases, the ECG pattern can remain unchanged even in patients with a plasma [K^+] above 9.0 mEq/L.

When hyperkalemia is sustained, reduced renal elimination is usually the cause [*see Table 10*]. When type 4 RTA is documented, the plasma cortisol concentration should be measured to determine whether complete adrenal insufficiency is present.

Differential Diagnosis

Pseudohyperkalemia should be considered when there is evidence of hemolysis in the sample or when the platelet or white blood cell (WBC) count is markedly increased. In contrast to true hyperkalemia, which is associated with altered neuromuscular or cardiac function, pseudohyperkalemia does not put patients at risk.

In this condition, the plasma [K^+] measured by the clinical laboratory is increased because potassium is released during clotting that occurs after the blood specimen has been obtained. This condition is most frequently caused by hemolysis resulting from traumatic blood drawing but is also seen with marked thrombocytosis (platelet count > 1,000,000/μl) or leukocytosis (WBC > 100,000/μl). It can also be observed as familial pseudohyperkalemia, in which potassium leaks out of cells at room temperature after clotting, without overt hemolysis.[43]

The diagnosis of pseudohyperkalemia is made by demonstrating that the [K^+] is normal in a nonhemolyzed plasma sample; such a sample is collected by drawing the blood into a heparinized tube, thus preventing clotting. In cases where no cause for hyperkalemia can be determined (e.g., normal renal function) and when the serum [K^+] is over 1 mEq/L higher than the plasma level, drawing the blood without a tourniquet and finding a normal serum potassium level identifies the cause of hyperkalemia as an in vitro phenomenon.[44] Treatment of pseudohyperkalemia is not indicated, because the in vivo (i.e., plasma) [K^+] is normal.

Treatment

In true hyperkalemia, particularly when it is severe (plasma [K^+] > 6.0 mEq/L), discontinuance of all medications that adversely affect potassium balance is mandatory.[45] These medications include nonselective beta blockers, ACE inhibitors, potassium-sparing diuretics, NSAIDs, and trimethoprim. Salt substitutes, which contain potassium chloride, should also be avoided. Persons with mild hyperkalemia (plasma [K^+] < 6.0 mEq/L) can usually be treated conservatively with reduction of daily intake to less than 2 g and, if indicated, with the addition of a loop diuretic.

Active treatment to lower the plasma [K^+] or to antagonize its effects on the cell membrane should be started if the plasma [K^+] has risen acutely to 6.0 mEq/L or higher, particularly if ECG manifestations of hyperkalemia are present; several therapeutic options are available [*see Table 12*].

An infusion of calcium rapidly normalizes the ECG. An increase in the [Ca^+] raises the threshold potential, thereby returning membrane excitability to normal. Calcium should be administered, however, in the presence of only those ECG manifestations of hyperkalemia that may precede ventricular fibrillation. Because calcium can exacerbate or precipitate glycoside-induced cardiac arrhythmias, it should be used only when necessary and with great care in patients receiving digoxin or other digitalis preparations.

Table 12 Treatment of Hyperkalemia

Agent	Result
Calcium	Antagonism of hyperkalemic membrane effects
Glucose infusion (with insulin in diabetics) Sodium bicarbonate Beta₂-adrenergic agonists	Potassium movement into cells
Loop or thiazide diuretics Cation exchange resins Hemodialysis or peritoneal dialysis	Potassium removal from the body

Calcium is administered intravenously as the gluconate or chloride salt (10 ml of 10% calcium gluconate over 2 to 3 minutes, with ECG monitoring). Normalization of the ECG may persist for less than 60 minutes; furthermore, this treatment does not alter the plasma [K$^+$] or total potassium body stores. Consequently, measures that will lower the plasma level and remove potassium from the body should be initiated simultaneously.

Sodium bicarbonate, glucose (with or without insulin), and beta$_2$-adrenergic receptor stimulation lower the plasma [K$^+$] by promoting the entry of potassium from the extracellular fluid into cells. Bicarbonate appears to be less effective than glucose and insulin, particularly in patients who have severe renal failure. Furthermore, bicarbonate does not appear to potentiate the hypokalemic action of beta$_2$-adrenergic agonists or glucose and insulin, both of which are more effective in this setting.[46]

Beta$_2$-adrenergic agonists can also transiently lower the serum potassium level. Albuterol can be administered as 10 to 20 mg in 4 ml of saline by nasal inhalation over 10 minutes or by a 0.5 mg I.V. infusion. The blood potassium level usually falls by 0.5 to 1.5 mEq/L within 30 minutes after the I.V. infusion, but more than 1 hour is required for a peak effect when albuterol is inhaled.

The hypokalemic effect of insulin is observed within 30 to 60 minutes, and it can be achieved by simply administering 25 g of glucose intravenously, because a glucose infusion rapidly stimulates insulin release. Alternatively, 6 to 8 units of insulin can be given intravenously with this glucose load to patients with diabetes, although this regimen can cause hypoglycemia in normal persons. Regardless of the method, care must be taken to avoid producing severe hyperglycemia by the glucose infusion, because a high plasma glucose concentration can exacerbate hyperkalemia by causing water, which contains potassium, to shift from the intracellular compartment into the plasma.

Like the administration of calcium, the administration of glucose and insulin, bicarbonate, and beta$_2$-adrenergic agonists is a temporary measure because total body potassium stores are not reduced. Therefore, additional measures are required to ensure that the plasma [K$^+$] does not return to pretreatment levels. Furthermore, in some patients, lowering the plasma [K$^+$] with these agents shortly before dialysis can lead to reduced dialytic potassium removal, possibly resulting in rebound hyperkalemia after the dialysis treatment has been completed.[47]

Increasing urine flow with diuretics is sometimes useful, but renal insufficiency frequently limits their effectiveness. However, the Na$^+$-K$^+$ cation exchange resin, sodium polystyrene sulfonate (Kayexalate), can be administered in sorbitol (to promote diarrhea) orally or as a retention enema and is almost always effective. In asymptomatic hyperkalemia, sodium polystyrene sulfonate can be used as the sole therapy, although it requires at least 2 to 4 hours before the plasma [K$^+$] begins to fall. In rare circumstances, the resin has been associated with intestinal necrosis. This serious complication tends to occur in the early postoperative period in surgical patients, although its mechanism is uncertain. The hypertonic nature of the solution possibly damages the intestinal mucosa.

Dialysis should be considered in severe or refractory cases of hyperkalemia, particularly when there is advanced renal failure. When available, hemodialysis is preferable in the acute setting because it removes potassium much more quickly than does peritoneal dialysis.

If aldosterone deficiency has been documented in cases of chronic hyperkalemia that are inadequately controlled by diet or diuretics, aldosterone replacement may be useful. However, because its onset of action may take several days or longer, this therapy is not sufficiently effective to be used alone in the treatment of acute, life-threatening hyperkalemia.

References

1. Kraut JA, Madias NE: Approach to patients with acid-base disorders. Respir Care 46:392, 2001
2. Vella A, Farrugia G: D-lactic acidosis: pathologic consequence of saprophytism. Mayo Clin Proc 73:451, 1998
3. Lolekha PH, Vanavanan S, Lolekha S: Update on value of the anion gap in clinical diagnosis and laboratory evaluation. Clin Chim Acta 307:33, 2001
4. Uribarri J, Oh MS, Carroll HJ: D-lactic acidosis: A review of clinical presentation, biochemical features, and pathophysiologic mechanisms. Medicine (Baltimore) 77:73, 1998
5. Kamel SK, Lin SH, Cheema-Dhadli S, et al: Prolonged total fasting: a feast for the integrative physiologist. Kidney Int 53:531, 1998
6. Vanholder R, Sever MS, Erek E, et al: Rhabdomyolysis. J Am Soc Nephrol 11:1553, 2000
7. Sweeney T, Beuchat C: Limitation of methods of osmometry: measuring the osmolality of biological flluid (editorial). Am J Physiol 264:R469, 1993
8. Jaber BL, Madias NE: Marked dilutional acidosis complicating management of right ventricular myocardial infarction. Am J Kidney Dis 30:561, 1997
9. Cruz DN, Huot SJ: Metabolic complications of urinary diversions: an overview. Am J Med 102:477, 1997
10. Newell KA, Bruce DS, Cronin DC, et al: Comparison of pancreas transplantation with portal venous and enteric exocrine drainage to the standard technique utilizing bladder drainage of exocrine secretions. Transplantation 62:1353, 1996
11. Messiaen T, Deret S, Mougenot B, et al: Adult Fanconi syndrome secondary to light chain gammopathy: clinicopathologic heterogeneity and unusual features in 11 patients. Medicine (Baltimore) 79:135, 2000

12. Gluck SL: Acid-Base. Lancet 352:474, 1998
13. Graber M: A model of hyperkalemia produced by metabolic acidosis. Am J Kidney Dis 22:436, 1993
14. Adrogue HJ, Madias N: Management of life-threatening acid-base disorders: fiirst of two parts. N Engl J Me 338:26, 1998
15. Winter SD, Pearson R, Gabow PA, et al: The fall of the serum anion gap. Arch Intern Med 150:311, 1990
16. Caravaca F, Arrobas M, Pizarro JL, et al: Metabolic acidosis in advanced renal failure: differences between diabetic and nondiabetic patients. Am J Kidney Dis 33:892, 1999
17. Movilli E, Zani R, Carli O, et al: Correction of metabolic acidosis increases serum albumin concentrations and decreases kinetically evaluated protein intake in haemodialysis patients: a prospective study. Nephrol Dial Transplant 13:1719, 1998
18. Boirie Y, Broyer M, Gagnadoux MF, et al: Alterations of protein metabolism by metabolic acidosis in children with chronic renal failure. Kidney Int 58:236, 2000
19. Kirschbaum B: Spurious metabolic acidosis in hemodialysis patients. Am J Kidney Dis 35:1068, 2000
20. Forsythe SM, Schmidt GA: Sodium bicarbonate for the treatment of lactic acidosis. Chest 117:260, 2000
21. Luft FC: Lactosis acidosis update for critical care clinicians. J Am Soc Nephrol 12(suppl 17):S15, 2001
22. Stacpoole PW, Wright EC, Baumgartner TG, et al: A controlled clinical trial of dichloroacetate for treatment of lactic acidosis in adults. N Engl J Med 327:1564, 1992
23. Nahas GG, Sutin KM, Fermon C, et al: Guidelines for the treatment of acidaemia with THAM. Drugs 55:191, 1998
24. Okuda Y, Adrogue HJ, Field JB, et al: Counterproductive

effects of sodium bicarbonate in ketoacidosis. J Clin Endocrinol Metab 81:314, 1996
25. Glaser N, Barnett P, McCaslin I, et al: Risk factors for cerebral edema in children with diabetic acidosis. N Engl J Med 344:264, 2001
26. Higgins RM, Connolly JO, Hendry BM: Alkalinization and hemodialysis in severe salicylate poisoning: comparison of elimination techniques in the same patient. Clin Nephrol 50:178, 1998
27. Barceloux DG, Krenzelok EP, Olson K, et al: American Academy of Clinical Toxicology Practice Guidelines on the Treatment of Ethylene Glycol Poisoning. Ad Hoc Committee. J Toxicol Clin Toxicol 37:537, 1999
28. Galla JH: Metabolic alkalosis. J Am Soc Nephrol 11:369, 2000
29. Beall DP, Scofiield RH: Milk-alkali syndrome associate with calcium carbonate consumption. Medicine (Baltimore) 74:89, 1995
30. Aichbichler BW, Zerr CH, Santa Ana CA, et al: Proton-pump inhibition of gastric chloride secretion in congenital chloridorrhea. N Engl J Med 336:106, 1997
31. Kurtz I: Molecular pathogenesis of Bartter's and Gitelman's syndromes. Kidney Int 54:1396, 1998
32. Adrogue HJ, Madias NE: Management of life-threatening acid-base disorders: second of two parts. N Engl J Med 338:107, 1998
33. Oster JR, Singer I, Fishman LM: Heparin-induced aldosterone suppression and hyperkalemia. Am J Med 98:575, 1995
34. Braden GL, von Oeyen PT, Germain MJ, et al: Ritodrine- and terbutaline-induced hypokalemia in preterm labor: mechanisms and consequences. Kidney Int 51:1867, 1997

35. Clemessy JL, Favier C, Borron SW, et al: Hypokalaemia related to acute chloroquine ingestion. Lancet 346:877, 1995

36. Manoukian MA, Foote JA, Crapo LM: Clinical and metabolic features of thyrotoxic periodic paralysis in 24 episodes. Arch Intern Med 159:601, 1999

37. Marples D, Frokiaer J, Dorup J, et al: Hypokalemia-induced downregulation of aquaporin-2 water channel expression in rat kidney medulla and cortex. J Clin Invest 97:1960, 1996

38. Gennari FJ: Hypokalemia. N Engl J Med 339:451, 1998

39. Kruse J, Carlson R: Rapid correction of hypokalemia using concentrated intravenous potassium chloride infusions. Arch Intern Med 150:613, 1990

40. Allon M: Hyperkalemia in end-stage renal disease: mechanisms and management. J Am Soc Nephrol 6:1134, 1995

41. Perazella MA: Drug-induced hyperkalemia: old culprits and new offenders. Am J Med 109:307, 2000

42. Charytan D, Goldfarb DS: Indications for hospitalization of patients with hyperkalemia. Arch Intern Med 160:1605, 2000

43. Iolascon A, Stewart GW, Ajetunmobi JF, et al: Familial pseudohyperkalemia maps to the same locus as dehydrated hereditary stomatocytosis (hereditary xerocytosis). Blood 93:3120, 1999

44. Wiederkehr MR, Moe OW: Factitious hyperkalemia. Am J Kidney Dis 36:1049, 2000

45. Weiner ID, Wingo CS: Hyperkalemia: a potential silent killer. J Am Soc Nephrol 9:1535, 1998

46. Allon M, Shanklin N: Effect of bicarbonate administration on plasma potassium in dialysis patients: interactions with insulin and albuterol. Am J Kidney Dis 28:508, 1996

47. Allon M, Shanklin N: Effect of albuterol treatment on subsequent dialytic potassium removal. Am J Kidney Dis 26:607, 1995

Acknowledgments

Adapted from Black RM: II Disorders of Acid-Base and Potassium Balance. 10 Nephrology. WebMD Scientifiic American® Medicine Online. Dale DC, Federman DD, Eds. WebMD Inc., New York, 2001. http://www.samed.com/. (June 2003)

Figure 1 Janet Betries.

Figures 2 through 6 Tom Moore.

Figure 7 Electrocardiograms kindly provided by Dr. David Spodick, Professor of Medicine at the University of Massachusetts Medical School, Worcester.

The author thanks Kristin Wilmarth for her assistance in the preparation of this manuscript.

10 HEPATIC FAILURE

Walid S. Arnaout, M.D., F.A.C.S., and Achilles A. Demetriou, M.D., Ph.D. F.A.C.S.

Approach to the Patient with Liver Failure

Hepatic failure and cirrhosis continue to be major causes of morbidity and mortality among critically ill patients. Since the beginning of the 1980s, several advances have been made in the management of hepatic failure. Newer diagnostic techniques and therapeutic modalities have been introduced that have led to significantly better overall outcomes. In addition to improved medical therapy, liver transplantation has proved to be effective in treating end-stage liver disease and liver failure, regardless of etiology.

In what follows, we outline general management guidelines for hepatic failure and its complications. We also discuss the role of artificial liver support and its potential use in managing hepatic failure.

Patient Evaluation

RISK FACTORS AND WORKUP

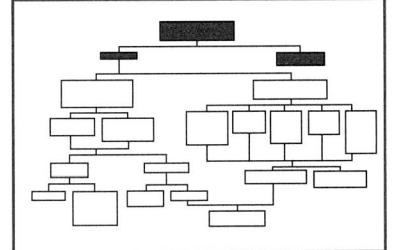

Liver disease is usually suspected on the basis of several risk factors, including a history of alcohol or I.V. drug abuse. Receipt of a blood transfusion before 1992 raises the index of suspicion for viral hepatitis, hepatitis C virus (HCV) infection in particular.[1-3] Other risk factors for liver disease are tattoos, sexual promiscuity, and snorting cocaine. Rare risk factors include a family history of certain liver diseases and exposure to various toxins and chemicals (e.g., aflatoxin and carbon tetrachloride).

Evaluation of patients with suspected liver disease is often complex and typically requires an extensive workup—including a detailed history and physical examination as well as various diagnostic studies—to establish the diagnosis and confirm the underlying cause. The laboratory data usually required include a complete blood count, a platelet count, liver function tests, a prothrombin time (PT), and serum albumin and cholesterol levels. In addition, imaging studies (e.g., abdominal ultrasonography, computed tomography, or magnetic resonance imaging) may be indicated. These studies usually demonstrate anatomic and structural abnormalities in the liver parenchyma, the biliary tree, or the vascular system. Occasionally, a liver biopsy is required to establish or confirm the diagnosis of liver disease.

Liver disease commonly gives rise to several manifestations that are easily recognized by most health care workers: jaundice [see 3:4 Jaundice], muscle wasting, malnutrition, ascites, lower-extremity edema, and varying degrees of hepatic encephalopathy. Common findings on physical examination of patients with liver disease in-clude bitemporal muscle wasting, vascular spiders, abdominal wall collaterals, caput medusae, palmar erythema, and clubbing. Umbilical and inguinal hernias are frequently noted in patients with tense ascites. Bilateral gynecomastia and testicular atrophy are often seen in male patients.

PRIMARY VERSUS SECONDARY HEPATIC FAILURE

Hepatic failure is generally classified as either primary or secondary, depending on the underlying cause. Primary hepatic failure derives from underlying liver disease, whereas secondary hepatic failure is caused by various underlying conditions unrelated to the liver. Most patients with primary hepatic failure have a history of preexisting liver disease and possibly of cirrhosis, generally presenting with one or more complications of chronic liver disease (e.g., GI bleeding, hepatic encephalopathy, spontaneous bacterial peritonitis, or renal failure). A subgroup of patients, however, exhibit hepatic failure secondary to acute exacerbation of the preexisting liver disease (e.g., acute reactivation of hepatitis B, acute decompensated Wilson disease, or autoimmune hepatitis). In another subgroup, primary hepatic failure develops acutely among patients who have no preexisting liver disease and no known risk factors (so-called acute or fulminant hepatic failure). These patients present with massive liver necrosis, jaundice, and profound coagulopathy and often go on to experience deep coma and cerebral edema, which may lead to irreversible brain damage and death. Acute liver failure can be associated with severe multisystem organ involvement, as in the acute respiratory distress syndrome (ARDS) or the multiple organ dysfunction syndrome (MODS), which makes diagnosis difficult. (This may also be the case with chronic liver disease, but to a lesser degree.)

Secondary liver failure is seen among critically ill patients admitted to the ICU for management of a non–liver-related illness. It is usually manifested by cholestatic jaundice, impaired synthetic activity, varying degrees of hepatocellular damage, and altered mental status. Hepatic insufficiency is common in patients with life-threatening injuries, severe systemic infection, or ARDS. These patients usually have no preexisting liver disease: their liver dysfunction is simply a reflection of their overall critical condition. The extent of the liver dysfunction in such cases usually depends on the severity of the underlying nonhepatic disease; in general, it tends to lessen as the causative problem is controlled or resolved. Failure to control the primary underlying condition leads to progressive MODS and death.

Management of secondary hepatic failure typically involves treating underlying nonhepatic disorders. Accordingly, we focus here on management of acute and chronic primary hepatic failure, which by definition involves treating hepatic disease and its associated complications.

Approach to the Patient with Liver Failure

Patient has signs of liver disease or known risk factors

Perform extensive workup: history, physical examination, laboratory tests, and imaging studies as needed. Liver biopsy is occasionally required.

Distinguish primary from secondary hepatic failure.

Primary hepatic failure

Acute liver failure

Determine etiology—viral, drug-induced, toxin-induced, or other—and treat accordingly.

Begin medical management of complications.

Concurrently, assess prognosis by means of King's College criteria.

Cerebral edema

Initiate invasive ICP monitoring.

Manage elevated ICP.

Extrahepatic complications

Treat fluid, electrolyte, and nutritional abnormalities; renal failure; pulmonary complications; infectious complications; and coagulopathy and bleeding.

Good prognosis with medical management

Continue medical therapy.

Poor prognosis with medical management

Medical management succeeds

Medical management fails

Consider emergency OLT if not contraindicated.

Treat toxic liver syndrome with total hepatectomy and end-to-side portacaval shunt, followed by OLT.

Consider use of BAL support system.

Transplantation is contraindicated

Manage medically.

No contraindications to transplantation are present

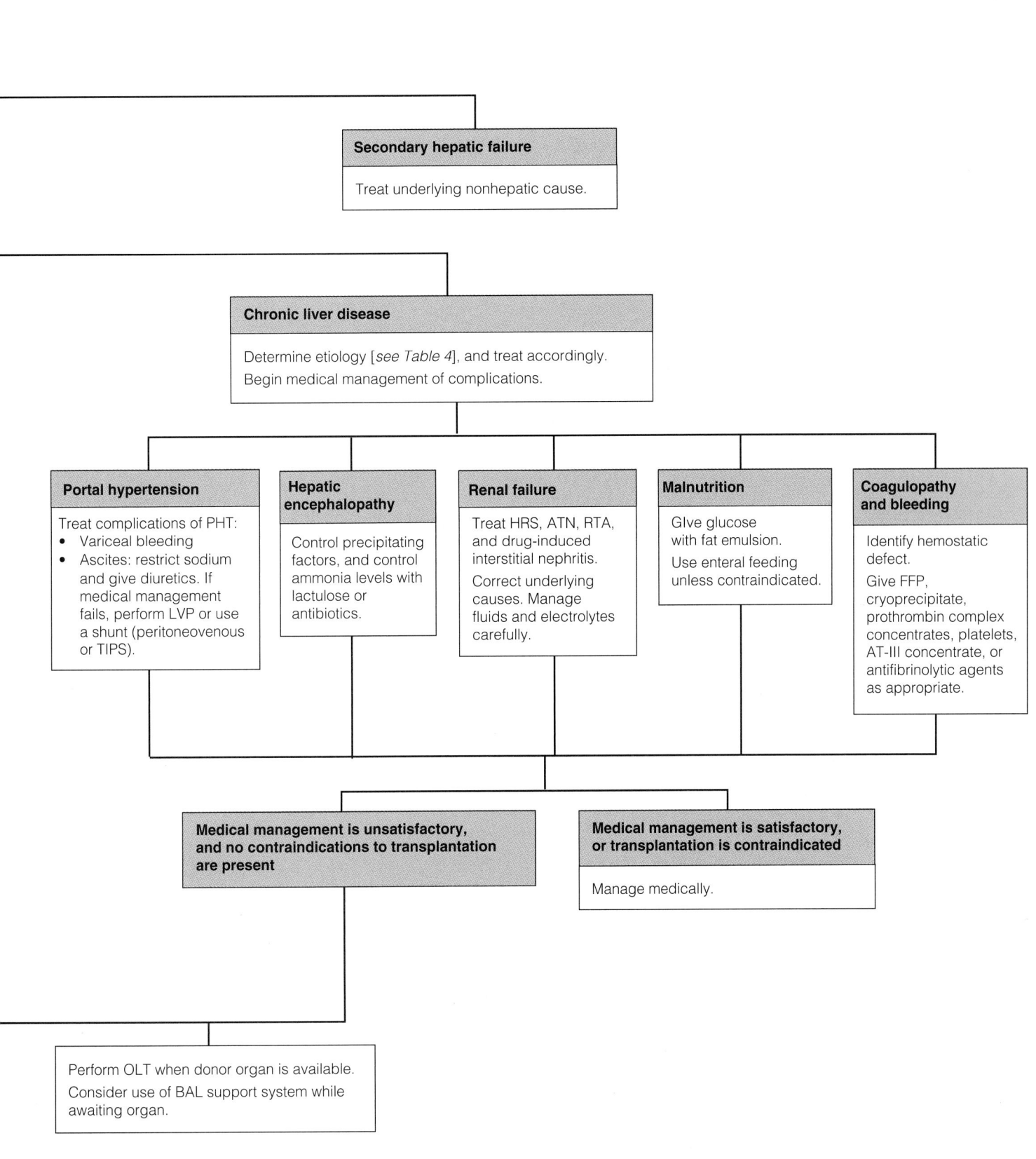

Secondary hepatic failure

Treat underlying nonhepatic cause.

Chronic liver disease

Determine etiology [*see Table 4*], and treat accordingly.
Begin medical management of complications.

Portal hypertension

Treat complications of PHT:
- Variceal bleeding
- Ascites: restrict sodium and give diuretics. If medical management fails, perform LVP or use a shunt (peritoneovenous or TIPS).

Hepatic encephalopathy

Control precipitating factors, and control ammonia levels with lactulose or antibiotics.

Renal failure

Treat HRS, ATN, RTA, and drug-induced interstitial nephritis.
Correct underlying causes. Manage fluids and electrolytes carefully.

Malnutrition

GIve glucose with fat emulsion.
Use enteral feeding unless contraindicated.

Coagulopathy and bleeding

Identify hemostatic defect.
Give FFP, cryoprecipitate, prothrombin complex concentrates, platelets, AT-III concentrate, or antifibrinolytic agents as appropriate.

Medical management is unsatisfactory, and no contraindications to transplantation are present

Medical management is satisfactory, or transplantation is contraindicated

Manage medically.

Perform OLT when donor organ is available.
Consider use of BAL support system while awaiting organ.

Acute Liver Failure

In the United States, acute liver failure (ALF) affects approximately 5,000 persons each year. The definition of ALF depends on the temporal relation between the initial onset of illness and the manifestation 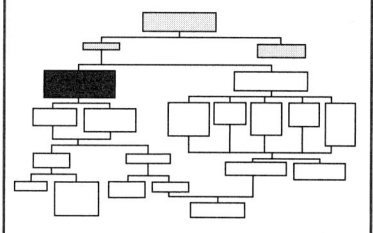 of jaundice, encephalopathy, and coagulopathy. The classic definition of Trey and Davidson is based on massive liver necrosis associated with encephalopathy developing within 8 weeks of the onset of illness.[4] In most cases, however, it is difficult to determine the precise time of onset of the disease process and thus the exact time elapsed before the establishment of hepatic failure. Recognizing that clinical findings and prognosis varied depending on the interval between onset of jaundice and encephalopathy, Bernuau and coworkers defined fulminant hepatic failure (FHF) as ALF complicated by encephalopathy developing within 2 weeks of the onset of jaundice and defined subfulminant hepatic failure (SFHF) as ALF complicated by encephalopathy developing 2 to 12 weeks after onset of jaundice.[5]

Differences in nomenclature and classification notwithstanding, the defining characteristic of ALF is the absence of known preexisting liver disease. We use the term FHF more or less interchangeably with ALF as defined by Trey and Davidson.

ETIOLOGY

The causes of FHF may be classified into four major groups: viral, drug-induced, toxin-induced, and miscellaneous. In one multicenter study, acetaminophen-induced FHF toxicity was found to be the most common variety (20%), followed by FHF of indeterminate etiology (15%).[6]

Viral Hepatitis

Hepatitis A The incidence of FHF and SFHF in hepatitis A virus (HAV) infection is very low (< 0.01%).[5] Young patients with HAV infection rarely manifest FHF, and their chances of survival with medical therapy are relatively good (40% to 60%). About 10% of patients experience relapses, usually within 2 to 3 months after an initial clinical improvement. Relapse is signaled by an increase in serum transaminase and bilirubin levels and the reappearance of virus in the stool. If encephalopathy occurs during this period, the outcome is poor.[7]

Hepatitis B ALF related to hepatitis B virus (HBV) accounts for fewer than 1% of HBV infections but is the most common form of viral-induced FHF.[6,8] Like HAV infection, HBV infection leads to FHF more often than to SFHF. Hepatitis B surface antigen (HBsAg) and HBV DNA may be absent in some cases of FHF secondary to HBV infection.[9] These findings indicate that in certain FHF patients, an enhanced immune response prevents further HBV replication and results in more rapid clearance of HBsAg. The survival rate for patients who are HBsAg-positive on presentation (17%) is much lower than that for patients who are HBsAg-negative (47%).[5] Clearance of HBsAg and HBV DNA results in better survival rates as well as lower recurrence rates after emergency liver transplantation.[10]

Hepatitis D Hepatitis D virus (HDV, also referred to as the delta agent) is a defective virus that uses HBsAg as its envelope protein. HDV RNA is detected in only 10% of patients with fulminant hepatitis D.[11] HDV infection can be either a coinfection, in conjunction with HBV infection, or a superinfection in patients with previous HBV infection [see 6:20 Viral Infection].[12] Among patients with FHF,

HDV coinfection is more common than superinfection; however, HDV superinfection is associated with a higher mortality than HDV coinfection (72% versus 52%) and more often predisposes to chronic liver disease (54% versus 31%).[13]

Hepatitis C and hepatitis of indeterminate etiology Previously, FHF of indeterminate etiology was attributed to non-A, non-B viral hepatitis. It is now clear that some such cases are caused by hepatitis C virus (HCV) infection, though the precise extent to which HCV infection contributes to this indeterminate group is unclear. Unlike HAV and HBV infection, HCV infection is more likely to cause SFHF than FHF. Despite the availability of advanced serologic testing, there are still many cases of FHF and SFHF whose cause cannot be determined.[14,15] These patients are placed into a non-A, non-B, non-C (NANBNC) category, implying a viral etiology. A more accurate designation for this category would be "of indeterminate etiology," in that the true cause is unknown and may not, in fact, be undiagnosed viral hepatitis.

Drugs

Drug toxicity accounts for 35% of all cases of FHF and SFHF and usually runs a subfulminant course.[6] Drug ingestion causes hepatic injury in fewer than 1% of patients, about 20% of whom manifest FHF or SFHF. Increasing the total drug dose, simultaneously ingesting other drugs that induce or inhibit hepatic enzymes, and continuing drug administration after the onset of liver disease all increase the risk of hepatic failure.[5] Acetaminophen toxicity is the most common cause of drug-induced hepatic failure. The prognosis for FHF caused by acetaminophen is usually better than that for FHF caused by other drugs (e.g., isoniazid, psychotropic drugs, antihistamines, and nonsteroidal anti-inflammatory drugs [NSAIDs]).[16] Halothane-induced FHF occurs within 2 weeks of general anesthesia and carries a high mortality.[17]

Toxins

Most cases of toxin-induced FHF involve mushroom poisoning or exposure to industrial hydrocarbons. In mushroom poisoning, the active agents are heat-stable and are not destroyed by cooking. Liver damage from mushroom toxins is delayed and is usually preceded by several days of vomiting and diarrhea. Mortality is high: up to 22% in one series.[18] Emergency liver transplantation is sometimes successful.[19]

Industrial hydrocarbons (e.g., carbon tetrachloride and trichloroethylene) are rare causes of FHF. In developing nations, aflatoxin and herbal medicines have been implicated as causes of FHF.

Miscellaneous Conditions

Wilson disease may present as FHF or SFHF with intravascular hemolysis and renal failure.[20,21] A family history of hepatic and neurologic disease, the presence of Kayser-Fleischer rings, and low serum ceruloplasmin levels help establish the diagnosis. Acute decompensated Wilson disease carries a high mortality and is therefore an indication for emergency liver transplantation.[22]

Acute fatty liver of pregnancy is a rare cause of FHF that carries a high mortality for both mother and infant. Delivery of the fetus results in regression of the microvesicular steatosis and abnormal liver test results for the mother. The risk of FHF is increased with misdiagnosis and continuation of pregnancy. Liver transplantation has been successfully performed.[23]

Several other conditions and disease processes are known to cause ALF in both adults and children [see Table 1].

ASSESSMENT OF PROGNOSIS

Several prognostic criteria and indicators have been proposed for

Table 1 Etiology of Acute Liver Failure

Infectious
  Viral: hepatitis A, B, C, D, and E and hepatitis of indeterminate etiology; infection by herpes simplex virus, cytomegalovirus, Epstein-Barr virus, or adenovirus
  Bacterial: Q fever
  Parasitic: amebiasis

Drugs

Toxins
  Mushrooms: *Amanita phalloides, verna,* and *virosa; Lepiota* species
  Bacillus cereus
  Hydrocarbons: carbon tetrachloride, trichloroethylene, 2-nitropropane, chloroform
  Copper
  Aflatoxin
  Yellow phosphorus

Miscellaneous conditions
  Wilson disease
  Acute fatty liver of pregnancy
  Reye syndrome
  Hypoxic liver cell necrosis
  Hypothermia or hyperthermia
  Budd-Chiari syndrome
  Veno-occlusive disease of the liver
  Autoimmune hepatitis
  Massive malignant infiltration of the liver
  Partial hepatectomy
  Liver transplantation
  Postjejunoileal bypass
  Galactosemia
  Hereditary fructose intolerance
  Tyrosinemia
  Erythropoietic protoporphyria
  Irradiation
  α_1-Antitrypsin deficiency
  Niemann-Pick disease
  Neonatal hemochromatosis
  Cardiac tamponade
  Right ventricular failure
  Circulatory shock
  Tuberculosis

predicting outcome after optimal medical management of FHF. The two main factors determining the likelihood of survival are (1) the extent of liver necrosis and (2) the potential for hepatocyte regeneration. In a 1989 study, investigators at King's College Hospital in London compiled a set of indicators for predicting a poor outcome after medical therapy and hence the need for emergency liver transplantation.[24] Underlying etiology was the single most important predictive variable. Therefore, patients were divided into two groups, one comprising all cases of acetaminophen-induced FHF and the other all cases of FHF from other causes. Age, degree of encephalopathy, serum pH, PT, interval to onset of encephalopathy, and admission serum creatinine and bilirubin levels also proved to be significant variables [see Table 2]. Patients who met the criteria in either group had a 95% chance of dying with medical therapy alone and were identified as candidates for emergency liver transplantation.

The major strength of the King's College study is that it based patient assessment on parameters that are easily obtained within a few hours of admission to the emergency department. This approach to assessment facilitates early referral of patients with a poor prognosis to a specialized liver unit for evaluation for transplanta-

tion. In another study, plasma factor V level and age were found to be independent predictors of survival.[25] The criteria for liver transplantation were the presence of hepatic encephalopathy (stage III or IV) and a factor V level either less than 20% of normal in patients younger than 30 years or less than 30% of normal in patients older than 30 years.

In addition to biochemical and synthetic activities, assessment of the residual functional reserve of the liver has been studied as an indicator of prognosis. The ratio of acetoacetate to β-hydroxybutyrate in an arterial blood sample (also known as the arterial ketone body ratio [AKBR]) is thought to reflect hepatic energy status.[26] Galactose clearance reflects both residual liver mass and hepatic blood flow.[27] This test has long been considered a standard test of liver functional reserve, and newer tests are routinely compared to it. At present, functional assessment tools are not routinely used in patient assessment.

The wide variety of potential prognostic indicators for FHF notwithstanding, the King's College criteria are still the most widely used. These criteria have been validated in several large series and are currently considered the gold standard for predicting outcome in FHF patients undergoing medical management.

At our center, we apply the King's College criteria at admission to predict the likely outcome with medical therapy. Once the initial assessment is completed, the decision for or against emergency evaluation for liver transplantation is made. Evaluation, if indicated, is usually completed within 12 to 24 hours. The evaluation is similar to that of patients with chronic liver disease [see Chronic Liver Disease, below], with a few exceptions. In particular, patients with FHF usually do not have preexisting liver disease; thus, it is vital that the evaluation [see Table 3] reveal the probable cause of liver failure. Unlike chronic liver disease, FHF is associated with cerebral edema and elevated intracranial pressure (ICP), which is the leading cause of death among these patients. Therefore, an extensive neurologic evaluation should be completed before a patient is listed for transplantation. Serial neurologic assessment is necessary to rule out irreversible brain damage and brain-stem herniation; however, previous sedation often makes this step very difficult.

Table 2 King's College Hospital Prognostic Criteria Predicting Poor Outcome for Patients with FHF

Acetaminophen-induced FHF	pH < 7.30 (irrespective of grade of encephalopathy)
	or
	All of the following:
	PT > 100 sec (INR > 6.5)
	Serum creatinine > 3.4 g/dl
	Stage III or IV hepatic encephalopathy
Non–acetaminophen-induced FHF	PT > 100 sec (INR > 6.5) (irrespective of grade of encephalopathy)
	or
	Any three of the following (irrespective of grade of encephalopathy):
	Age < 10 or > 40 yr
	Etiology: non-A, non-B hepatitis, halothane hepatitis, drug toxicity
	Duration of jaundice to encephalopathy > 7 days
	PT 50 sec (INR > 3.5)
	Serum bilirubin > 17.5 g/dl

FHF—fulminant hepatic failure   INR—international normalized ratio
PT—prothrombin time

TREATMENT
OF COMPLICATIONS

Cerebral Edema

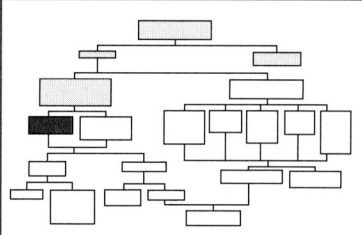

Cerebral edema is one of the hallmarks of FHF, and its presence significantly influences management and outcome. Autopsy studies indicate that cerebral edema is present in 80% of patients who die of FHF.[28,29] It occurs in advanced stages of FHF and can be recognized by clinical, radiologic, or invasive means. Clinical findings include decerebrate posturing, myoclonus, spastic rigidity, seizure activity, systemic hypertension, bradycardia, hyperventilation, and mydriasis with diminished pupillary response. These findings initially are paroxysmal but later become persistent. Papilledema is a late finding and often does not occur at all, even in the advanced stages of the disease.[30] Noninvasive diagnostic modalities (e.g., CT scanning, electroencephalographic monitoring, and transcranial Doppler flow measurement) have not proved helpful for early detection and management of cerebral edema.[31,32] CT scanning of the brain is not a sensitive test for detecting early cerebral edema: 25% to 30% of patients with high ICP exhibit no radiographic changes.[33] It is, however, useful for ruling out intracranial bleeding.

Currently, ICP monitoring is the best means of monitoring intracranial hypertension and is recommended for guiding treatment in patients with stage III or IV encephalopathy. ICP can be measured by using epidural, subdural, or intraventricular catheters. Although epidural catheters are slightly less sensitive to ICP changes, they have the lowest complication rate (3.8%) and lowest rate of fatal hemorrhage (1%).[34] Despite a slightly higher complication rate, we prefer subdural catheters: in our view, they offer more reliable ICP monitoring. Institution of ICP monitoring necessitates aggressive treatment of any concomitant coagulopathy. Fresh frozen plasma (FFP) infusions are given to bring the PT below 25 seconds, and platelet transfusions are indicated if the patient has severe thrombocytopenia (platelet count < 50,000/mm³). Once ICP monitoring is established, bolus administration of FFP is repeated as needed to keep the prothrombin time low (international normalized ratio [INR] ≤ 5) so as to reduce the risk of intracranial bleeding.

The goal of invasive monitoring is to keep ICP below 15 mm Hg while keeping cerebral perfusion pressure (CPP), which is a better predictor of outcome, above 50 mm Hg. CPP is calculated by subtracting ICP from mean arterial pressure (MAP) [see *6:12 Coma, Seizures, Cognitive Impairment, and Brain Death*]. ICP monitoring allows early detection of cerebral edema and hence early introduction of aggressive management. To date, no randomized, controlled trials have addressed the effect of either high ICP or low CPP on outcome after liver transplantation; however, it appears that the persistence of either an ICP higher than 25 mm Hg or a CPP lower than 40 mm Hg for more than 2 hours is associated with an increased risk of irreversible brain damage and a poor outcome.[35,36]

Management of elevated ICP involves hyperventilation, minimization of external stimuli, deep sedation, elevation of the head, maintenance of hemodynamic stability, and infusion of mannitol. Patients are usually sedated with a short-acting agent (e.g., fentanyl) in small boluses before operation, nasotracheal suction, venipuncture, or line placement. Mechanical hyperventilation lowers ICP by lowering arterial carbon dioxide tension (P_aCO_2) to 25 to 30 mm Hg, thereby maximizing cerebral vascular constriction and reducing blood flow. This vascular effect diminishes progressively after 6 hours of therapy, though a clinical response is apparent for days. As many as 80% of patients without renal failure respond to mannitol infusions.[37] Serum

Table 3 Liver Transplant Evaluation and Workup for FHF Patients

Laboratory workup
  CBC and differential count
  Chemistry panel
  Coagulation profile
  24-hr creatinine clearance
  Urinalysis
  Arterial blood gases
  ANA, AMA, ceruloplasmin, urinary copper, α_1-antitrypsin
  AFP
  RPR
  Thyroid function tests
  Alcohol and drug toxicology screen
Viral serologies
  Hepatitis A virus (IgM, IgG)
  Hepatitis B virus (HBsAg, HBcAb, HBeAg, HBV DNA)
  Hepatitis C virus (HCV antibody, HCV RNA-PCR)
  Cytomegalovirus
  Epstein-Barr virus
  HIV
Cultures
  Bacterial, fungal, and viral cultures
  Blood
  Sputum
  Urine
  Ascites
12-lead ECG
Chest x-ray
Pulmonary function tests
Abdominal Doppler ultrasonography
CT scans of head

AFP—α-fetoprotein   AMA—antimitochondrial antibody   ANA—antinuclear antibody   RPR—rapid plasma reagent

osmolality should be measured frequently and maintained at 300 to 320 mOsm/L. Mannitol should be withheld if osmolality reaches or exceeds 320 mOsm/L, if renal failure occurs, or if oliguria and rising serum osmolality develop simultaneously. Repeated administration of mannitol may reverse the osmotic gradient. Mannitol should be discontinued if ICP does not respond after the first few boluses.

Patients who do not respond to conventional therapy may be placed in a barbiturate coma. Thiopental infusion decreases cerebral metabolic activity, lowers CNS oxygen demand, and protects the brain from ischemic injury secondary to decreased cerebral blood flow. In one retrospective, nonrandomized study, it lowered ICP and reduced mortality from FHF.[38] In our experience, however, the effect of thiopental infusion on ICP is transient and unpredictable.

Other Complications

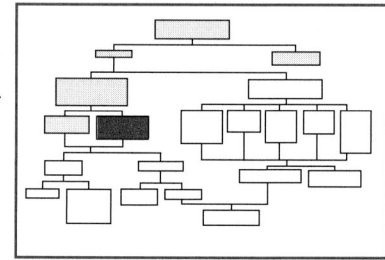

In addition to cerebral edema and increased ICP, MODS and a variety of life-threatening complications are associated with FHF. Most of these complications are similar to those seen in chronic liver disease [see Chronic Liver Disease, Treatment of Complications, *below*]; however, the following complications are seen with particular frequency in FHF.

Fluid, electrolyte, and nutritional abnormalities Euvolemia must be maintained to prevent fluid overload, pulmonary edema, and dehydration; extreme fluid shifts should be avoided. The presence of cerebral edema and intracranial hypertension calls for careful fluid administration so as not to expand the intravascular space or exacerbate the edema. Electrolyte and acid-base imbalances are frequent in FHF patients and should be managed appropriately. Hyperkalemia may be multifactorial; usually, it is secondary to liver necrosis, massive transfusion, acid-base imbalance, or renal failure. Acidosis results from increased lactic acid production and decreased handling of lactate by the failing liver. Compensatory respiratory alkalosis develops initially, but if encephalopathy progresses, respiratory acidosis may result. Sodium or potassium bicarbonate infusions should be administered in cases of severe acidosis. Acetate provides twice the bicarbonate load and is metabolized outside the liver; thus, if sodium and potassium intake is severely restricted, continuous infusion of acetate salts may be useful.

Initially, amino acids should be withheld to prevent excessive nitrogen loading; later, limited nitrogen supplementation (70 to 80 g protein/day) may be provided. Most patients present with severe hypoglycemia, which can be fatal and warrants aggressive therapy. Hypoglycemia should be corrected rapidly by infusion of a 50% dextrose solution, followed by continuous infusion of a more dilute solution at a rate of 4 mg/kg/min. A 10% solution is usually adequate; however, higher concentrations should be considered in patients whose hypoglycemia persists or whose fluid intake is restricted. Caloric supplementation has not been extensively studied in FHF.

Renal failure Renal failure occurs in as many as 55% of FHF patients. Functional renal failure is the most common cause of renal failure in this population. However, acute tubular necrosis is more common in these patients than in those with chronic liver disease and cirrhosis.[39] This is especially true in patients who have not been resuscitated adequately, who have experienced prolonged hypotension, or who have ingested hepatotoxins that are also nephrotoxic (e.g., acetaminophen).

Adequate urine volume can be maintained by means of judicious volume expansion, administration of loop diuretics, or both, along with infusion of renal doses of dopamine. Depleted intravascular volume may be managed by giving blood products, volume expanders, or both. Because the plasma albumin level is invariably low, salt-poor albumin solutions may be preferable to carbohydrate-based volume expanders. If oliguria is present—especially if mannitol is administered to treat ICP—hemodialysis or hemofiltration may be needed to maintain optimal fluid volume.

Pulmonary complications Pulmonary complications—especially pulmonary edema, aspiration pneumonia, and ARDS—are common in FHF patients.[40] Pulmonary edema is seen in as many as 40% of cases. Supplemental oxygen and mechanical ventilation are always indicated. Sedative and paralytic agents may be required to ensure tolerance of ventilation; however, they should be used sparingly because they may hinder neurologic evaluation. Aspiration pneumonia should be treated aggressively because it is a potential contraindication to transplantation.

Infectious complications Infection poses a serious threat to FHF patients both by placing them at risk for sepsis and by constituting a contraindication to liver transplantation. Immunologic defects observed in this setting include impaired opsonization, impaired chemotaxis, impaired neutrophil and Kupffer cell function, and complement deficiency.[41,42] Bacterial infection, usually deriving from the respiratory or urinary tract or from a central venous catheter, occurs in more than 80% of cases. In one study, bacteremia was documented in

25% of patients, with staphylococci, streptococci, and gram-negative rods the most common pathogens.[43] Because most FHF patients have percutaneous lines and indwelling catheters in place, iatrogenic sources must always be considered. Fungal infection is less common than bacterial infection in this setting; however, one series found a significant incidence of fungal infections, with *Candida albicans* cultured in 33% of the patients studied.[44] The majority of these patients had renal failure and had been treated with antibiotics for longer than 5 days.

The high prevalence of infection notwithstanding, we do not advocate antibiotic prophylaxis in this population unless there is a strong suspicion of active infection or an ICP monitor is in place. However, our decision threshold for starting antibiotics is low, given that the usual clinical presentations (e.g., fever and leukocytosis) may be absent in as many as 30% of FHF patients.[43] Surveillance cultures for bacteria and fungi must be obtained at frequent intervals from blood (peripheral and central lines), urine, sputum, and open wounds. If ascites is present, the ascitic fluid should be cultured. In addition, chest x-rays should be obtained to identify developing infiltrates. Administration of broad-spectrum antibiotics should be initiated at the first sign of infection; as soon as an organism is identified, coverage may be focused more narrowly. Initiation of antifungal therapy with either amphotericin B or another agent should be considered either if fungal culture is positive or if fever persists beyond 5 days while the patient is receiving antibiotics—especially if renal failure is present. The duration of antimicrobial therapy should be individualized for each patient. Follow-up cultures are recommended if a specific organism is isolated.

Coagulopathy and bleeding Bleeding is a frequent complication of FHF, typically resulting from massive liver necrosis, impaired hepatic synthesis of clotting factors, and platelet dysfunction. All clotting factors synthesized by the liver (i.e., factors II, V, VII, IX, and X) exhibit depressed plasma activity in FHF. Factor II, with a half-life of 2 hours, is the first to be depleted with hepatocellular dysfunction and also the first to be repleted with hepatocellular recovery. The PT is invariably prolonged, reflecting a generalized clotting factor deficiency; it is used as one of the criteria for determining the chances of spontaneous recovery. At some centers, FFP transfusion is withheld and the PT is followed carefully to determine upward or downward trends in the course of the disease and hence the likelihood of spontaneous recovery or need for transplantation (unless the PT > 25 seconds or the INR > 5, especially if an ICP monitor is in place). Intracranial bleeding and its neurologic sequelae are the most devastating complications of coagulopathy in FHF patients.

Thrombocytopenia and abnormalities of platelet function are also common in FHF. Acute splenomegaly, consumptive coagulopathy, and bone marrow suppression all contribute to the development of thrombocytopenia. Conversely, clearance of older platelets from the blood by the reticuloendothelial system is hindered, which results in an older, less effective platelet pool. In one study, a mean platelet count of 50,000/mm³ was associated with a higher incidence of GI hemorrhage.[45] Our current practice is to give platelets to patients who either are thrombocytopenic (platelet count < 50,000/mm³) or are actively bleeding.

OUTCOME OF MEDICAL THERAPY

Because of the complexity of the underlying disease, medical management of FHF requires a multidisciplinary approach. Hemodynamic and respiratory support and prevention and

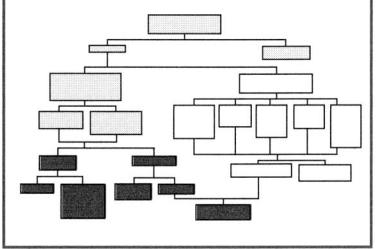

treatment of cerebral edema are major goals. Complications of liver failure must be treated aggressively to prevent sepsis, ARDS, and MODS, which is the second most common cause of death in these patients if they survive the first few days. As noted [*see* Assessment of Prognosis, *above*], liver transplant evaluation must be carried out simultaneously with aggressive ICU care, and the patient's chances of spontaneous recovery must be assessed. In addition to determining the King's College prognostic score at admission, we follow the general trend in the clinical course with respect to the development of encephalopathy, ICP elevation, coagulopathy, metabolic acidosis, and renal failure. The decision whether to continue with medical therapy or to perform liver transplantation must be made whenever a donor liver becomes available. In general, patients who appear to be deteriorating rapidly and who have no contraindications to liver transplantation should undergo emergency liver transplantation. Similarly, patients whose synthetic function does not improve within the first 48 to 72 hours should be considered for liver transplantation: the risk of complications and death from MODS if transplantation is not done outweighs the risk attendant on the procedure.

Toxic Liver Syndrome

Even with a multidisciplinary, comprehensive approach to therapy, a few patients with FHF go on to manifest the so-called toxic liver syndrome, characterized by severe intracranial hypertension, profound lactic acidosis, hemodynamic instability, and MODS. It has been suggested that removal of the necrotic liver might improve the hemodynamic status of these patients and lower their ICP. In such extreme cases, a two-stage procedure has been performed: total hepatectomy with an end-to-side portacaval shunt, followed by liver transplantation when an allograft becomes available. In one large series,[46,47] 32 adult patients with toxic liver syndrome underwent total hepatectomy with a portacaval shunt. The patients were anhepatic for several hours (range, 6.5 to 41.4). Whereas 13 patients showed no signs of improvement after hepatectomy and soon died of MODS, 19 became more stable and underwent the full procedure. Only seven patients were alive at 46 months.

In the early 1990s, we used this approach to treat an 18-year-old female patient with uncontrollable cerebral edema secondary to FHF; she underwent total hepatectomy with a portacaval shunt, followed by orthotopic liver transplantation (OLT) 14 hours later.[48] During the anhepatic period, she was supported with the help of a bioartificial liver (BAL) [*see* Discussion, Bioartifical Liver Support System, *below*]. With artificial liver support, the severe neurologic dysfunction was reversed, ICP was normalized, and the serum ammonia level was reduced. The patient recovered completely, with no neurologic deficits. We subsequently used the same approach with another FHF patient in our unit, also successfully (unpublished data). It appears that for highly selected patients exhibiting severe toxic metabolic derangement and uncontrollable intracranial hypertension, total hepatectomy with a portacaval shunt—preferably accompanied by some form of artificial liver support—followed by OLT may be considered as a desperate salvage measure.

LIVER TRANSPLANTATION

With the introduction of OLT as a treatment modality for FHF patients, overall patient survival has improved from less than 20% to greater than 60%.[49,50] As more experience was gained with OLT, it became apparent that optimal patient selection is essential for successful outcome. FHF patients must be considered for OLT before irreversible brain injury, MODS, and sepsis develop. Patient selection should be based on a clear understanding of the natural history of the disease as well as of the underlying etiology and the likelihood of spontaneous recovery without transplantation. One of the most difficult aspects of the management of these patients is the lack of reliable prognostic indicators or criteria predicting outcome. In our experience, the King's College criteria are less sensitive and specific in determining prognosis for patients with acetaminophen-induced FHF than for patients with FHF from other causes (71% and 78% versus 96% and 100%).[51]

As a result of these imperfectly reliable criteria, a small number of patients who either might have recovered spontaneously or might have sustained irreversible brain damage undergo unnecessary or unwarranted liver transplantation. Given the severe shortage of organ donors as well as the cost and medical consequences of liver transplantation and a commitment to lifelong immunosuppression, this is a significant problem.

Chronic Liver Disease

Chronic liver disease usually develops as a result of long-standing, ongoing injury to one or more components of the liver, including the liver parenchyma, the biliary tree, and the hepatic and biliary blood vessels. 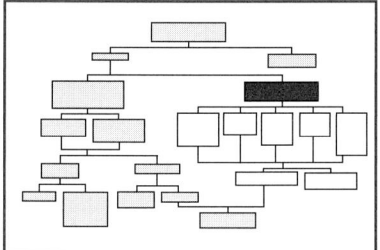 The repeated injury and the ensuing repair usually result in deposition of excessive amount of extracellular matrix (ECM), with or without accompanying inflammation. As the disease process progresses, excess ECM forms connective tissue bridges linking portal and central areas (so-called bridging fibrosis), which eventually lead to the formation of dense collagen bands enclosing nodules of hepatocytes—that is, to cirrhosis. Cirrhosis is an irreversible state that gives rise to significant physiologic impairment, including poor exchange of nutrients and metabolites between sinusoidal blood and hepatocytes. Eventually, the lobular architecture becomes distorted and blood flow altered, leading to portal hypertension and its numerous complications. In addition to portal hypertension, repeated parenchymal injury results in the loss of a large number of functioning hepatocytes and subsequently in hepatic failure.

ETIOLOGY

Like ALF, chronic liver disease is usually classified into various categories on the basis of the underlying causative process [*see* Table 4].

TREATMENT OF COMPLICATIONS

Chronic liver disease may be associated with a variety of complications, depending on the nature and extent of hepatocyte injury and regeneration. Most patients with chronic liver disease and possible cirrhosis are well compensated, maintain a relatively normal functional status, and remain essentially undiagnosed; however, a small percentage eventually become symptomatic. Hepatic failure secondary to cirrhosis is not an all-or-none phenomenon: patients may lose one or more specific liver functions while retaining the remainder. In addition to the hepatic effects, cirrhosis and hepatic failure can exert a wide range of extrahepatic effects that involve virtually every organ system, leading to MODS and death in most cases if appropriate therapy is not instituted promptly. Consequently, treatment of cirrhosis and chronic hepatic failure must focus on treating both the underlying primary disease and all of its extrahepatic manifestations and complications.

Table 4   Etiology of Chronic Liver Disease

Alcoholic liver disease (exclude acute alcoholic hepatitis)
Viral hepatitis
  Hepatitis B virus
  Hepatitis C virus
Biliary cirrhosis
  Primary biliary cirrhosis
  Primary sclerosing cholangitis
  Secondary sclerosing cholangitis
  Biliary atresia
Autoimmune hepatitis
Metabolic abnormalities
  Wilson disease
  α_1-Antitrypsin deficiency
  Hemochromatosis
  Inborn errors of metabolism
Cryptogenic cirrhosis
Miscellaneous
  Vascular anomalies (Budd-Chiari syndrome)
  Toxin- or drug-induced
  Inborn errors of metabolism
  Other

Portal Hypertension

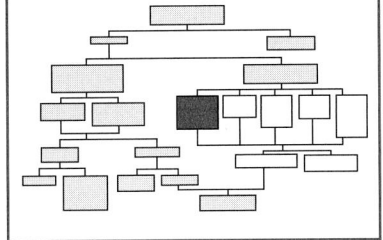

In the majority of patients with chronic liver disease and cirrhosis, portal hypertension (PHT) develops as a result of increased resistance to portal venous blood flow within the liver. PHT is defined as portal venous pressure higher than 12 mm Hg or a hepatic wedge venous pressure that exceeds the inferior vena cava pressure by more than 5 mm Hg. It is classified as prehepatic, hepatic, or posthepatic according to the anatomic site of increased portal venous resistance [*see Table 5*]. Hepatic PHT is further classified according to the functional relationship to the hepatic sinusoids. Sinusoidal obstruction is more frequently seen with postnecrotic cirrhosis (e.g., from HCV and HBV infection), whereas postsinusoidal obstruction is more common with alcoholic cirrhosis. Prehepatic and posthepatic causes of PHT are less often encountered in patients with cirrhosis; however, efforts should always be made to rule out such causes, because these conditions all require different therapeutic approaches.

PHT is associated with numerous complications, most of which are life-threatening if not diagnosed and treated promptly [*see Table 6*]. Generally, these complications result from adaptive physiologic responses to elevated portal venous pressure, which lead to the development of collateral vessels or shunts to decompress the portal venous system. The absence of valves within the portal venous system allows retrograde portal blood flow into the splenic and mesenteric circulation and rerouting of blood into the systemic circulation through newly formed collaterals. Several portosystemic venous collateral networks have been identified within the GI tract, the peritoneal cavity, the chest, the retroperitoneum, and subcutaneous tissue. Patients with cirrhosis frequently have one or more areas of collateral formation.

Variceal bleeding   The most dramatic and catastrophic complication of PHT is bleeding from esophageal and gastric varices.

Prompt diagnosis and management are vital. Since the early 1990s, management of variceal bleeding has evolved significantly, thanks to the advent of novel endoscopic therapies and nonoperative portosystemic shunt procedures.

Although the esophagus and the stomach are the most common sites of bleeding varices, other sites within the GI tract may be involved as well, including the duodenum, the jejunum, the rectum, and ileostomy and colostomy sites [*see Table 7*]. The diagnosis and management of gastrointestinal bleeding associated with varices are discussed in more detail elsewhere in this text [*see 3:6 Upper Gastrointestinal Bleeding*].

Ascites   Ascites—that is, leakage of lymph fluid into the peritoneal cavity—is one of the principal clinical manifestations of cirrhosis and PHT. Its appearance is indicative of advanced liver disease and is associated with a poor prognosis.[52] It is believed that increased hepatic sinusoidal pressure results in increased formation of lymph and causes hepatic lymph to weep from Glisson's capsule into the peritoneal cavity. As ascitic fluid accumulates, patients exhibit increasing abdominal distention, which causes abdominal pain, decreased appetite, dyspnea, and, occasionally, pleural effusion (so-called hepatic hydrothorax). Umbilical and inguinal hernias are common in patients with tense ascites.

Evaluation. Hepatic ascites should be distinguished from other types of ascites (e.g., chylous, malignant, or cardiac). All patients with ascites should undergo diagnostic paracentesis to characterize the fluid and rule out bacterial peritonitis (see below). In addition, therapeutic large-volume paracentesis (LVP) is indicated for patients who are symptomatic as a result of the large volume of ascitic fluid.

Ascitic fluid analysis should include a white blood cell count and a differential count, Gram stain and cultures, and measurement of total protein, albumin, glucose, lactic dehydrogenase (LDH), and

Table 5   Etiology of Portal Hypertension

Prehepatic obstruction
  Splenic vein thrombosis
  Portal vein thrombosis
  Partial nodular transformation
Hepatic obstruction
  Presinusoidal
    Idiopathic portal hypertension
    Schistosomiasis
    Congenital hepatic fibrosis
    Sarcoidosis
  Sinusoidal
    Nodular regenerative hyperplasia
    Most forms of cirrhosis
    Viral hepatitis
    Acute alcoholic hepatitis
  Postsinusoidal
    Alcoholic cirrhosis
    Veno-occlusive disease
Posthepatic obstruction
  Budd-Chiari syndrome
  IVC web
  Right-sided congestive heart failure/tricuspid valve insufficiency
  Constrictive pericarditis

IVC—inferior vena cava

Table 6 Complications of Portal Hypertension

Variceal bleeding
Portal hypertensive gastropathy
Ascites
    Spontaneous bacterial peritonitis
Spontaneous shunts
Encephalopathy
Hypersplenism

amylase concentrations. In addition, the serum albumin level should be measured at the same time so that the serum-ascites albumin gradient (SAAG) may be determined; this value has been shown to correlate directly with portal pressure.[53,54] Portal hypertensive ascitic fluid is characterized by a low albumin content, with a SAAG greater than 1.1 g/dl; non–portal hypertensive ascites fluid is characterized by a SAAG less than 1.1 g/dl.[55]

Spontaneous bacterial peritonitis. An elevated WBC count in the ascitic fluid provides immediate information about possible bacterial infection. Cell counts higher than 500/mm³ suggest bacterial peritonitis, especially when the absolute neutrophil count exceeds 250/mm³.[56] More than 20% of cirrhotic patients with ascites eventually manifest bacterial peritonitis—an occurrence known as spontaneous bacterial peritonitis (SBP). Patients with a low total protein level in their ascitic fluid (< 1.5 g/dl) appear to be at highest risk as a result of the reduced complement level and opsonic activity in the fluid. SBP should be considered in any cirrhotic patient with fever, abdominal pain, or worsening encephalopathy or renal function. Ascitic fluid analysis [see Table 8] allows SBP to be distinguished from secondary bacterial peritonitis, which develops as a consequence of an intra-abdominal abscess or a perforated viscus.

Once the diagnosis is made, empirical antibiotic therapy is employed until the final culture result becomes available. At present, cefotaxime (or a similar third-generation cephalosporin) is considered the treatment of choice. A dosage of 1 to 2 g I.V. every 6 to 8 hours (depending on renal function) is optimal. Therapy is continued for 14 days. The response to therapy should be monitored by repeating the paracentesis within 48 hours. Ciprofloxacin, either 200 mg I.V. every 12 hours for 7 days or 200 mg I.V. every 12 hours for 2 days followed by 500 mg orally every 12 hours for 5 days, has been shown to be effective as well.[57]

Currently, it is recommended that antibiotic prophylaxis for SBP (norfloxacin, 400 mg/day) be given only to patients with active GI bleeding and low protein levels in their ascitic fluid or to those who have had SBP before and are awaiting liver transplantation.[58] There is no good evidence to support antibiotic prophylaxis in patients whose ascitic fluid protein levels are low and who have never had SBP. Like ascites, SBP carries a grave prognosis: estimated 1-year survival is less than 50% without liver transplantation.[59,60]

Table 7 Ectopic Sites for Variceal Bleeding

Site	Frequency
Duodenum	17%
Jejunum and ileum	18%
Colon	15%
Rectum	9%
Ileostomy or colostomy	27%
Miscellaneous	14%

Medical management. Sodium retention is the pathophysiologic hallmark of ascites in cirrhotic patients, and the rate of fluid accumulation is directly related to the amount of sodium retained. Many patients excrete sodium at rates lower than 10 mmol/day, in which case even a modest sodium intake results in a positive sodium balance and continued accumulation of ascitic fluid. Therefore, to achieve effective control of ascites, dietary intake of sodium should be restricted to 1 to 2 g/day (43 to 87 mmol/day). With simple bed rest and salt restriction, ascites can be controlled in about 20% of patients.[61]

In addition to salt retention, patients with cirrhosis exhibit impaired free water excretion, which may cause hyponatremia. This state appears to be partially attributable to excessive secretion of antidiuretic hormone (ADH) caused by a reduced effective plasma volume. Water intake need not be restricted in all patients with ascites, because many will not become seriously hyponatremic. Water intake should be restricted (to 1.0 to 1.5 L/day) only in patients who become hyponatremic (serum sodium level < 130 mmol/L) and in those who continue to gain weight despite severe sodium restriction and diuretic therapy. Hyponatremia is associated with a variety of neurologic symptoms resembling those of hepatic encephalopathy. Severe hyponatremia (serum sodium < 120 mmol/L), on the other hand, is associated with seizure activity and should be corrected judiciously. Given the risk of the development of demyelinating lesions associated with rapid changes in the serum sodium concentration, it is recommended that correction of serum sodium—mainly by free water restriction to a serum sodium level between 120 and 130 mmol/L—be carried out gradually.

Diuretic therapy remains the cornerstone of management of cirrhotic ascites; however, it should be monitored carefully to ensure that intravascular volume depletion, development of prerenal azotemia, and electrolyte imbalances do not occur. The peritoneum can absorb no more than 700 to 900 ml of ascitic fluid a day; accordingly, vigorous diuresis in excess of this amount (in the absence of peripheral edema) results in intravascular volume depletion and renal failure.

The two groups of diuretic agents most commonly used to treat ascites are distal tubular–acting agents (e.g., spironolactone) and loop diuretics (e.g., furosemide). Spironolactone inhibits sodium reabsorption in the distal tubules by blocking the effect of serum aldosterone, which is usually elevated in patients with cirrhosis. A spironolactone dosage of 150 to 300 mg/day is sufficient for achieving effective natriuresis in many patients; however, larger dosages (up to 500 to 600 mg/day) may be preferable in certain patients with markedly elevated serum aldosterone concentrations. Adverse effects of spironolactone therapy include hyperkalemia and hyperchloremic acidosis. Tender gynecomastia is also an important side effect; if gynecomastia occurs, amiloride (20 to 40 mg/day) is a good alternative to spironolactone.

Furosemide therapy is usually started if the desired diuresis is not achieved with spironolactone or if the urinary sodium-potassium ratio is less than 1. A typical starting dosage is 40 to 80 mg/day, which is gradually increased until adequate diuresis is achieved. Because furosemide causes loss of urinary sodium and potassium, its use may lead to hypokalemia and metabolic alkalosis.

Surgical management. Despite large doses of diuretics, some patients become refractory to medical therapy and manifest tense ascites. Abdominal paracentesis is a safe and effective alternative to diuretic therapy and is currently used in patients with poor renal function who cannot tolerate aggressive diuresis and intravascular volume depletion. Most patients tolerate removal of large amounts of ascitic fluid (5 to 10 L) without significant adverse hemodynamic effects.[62] Albumin replacement (7 to 9 g/L) with LVP has been asso-

Table 8 Differentiation of Spontaneous Bacterial Peritonitis from Secondary Bacterial Peritonitis through Analysis of Ascitic Fluid

Fluid Assay	Spontaneous Bacterial Peritonitis	Secondary Bacterial Peritonitis
WBC (cells/mm³)	> 500	> 500
Total protein (g/dl)	< 1.0	> 1.0
Glucose (mg/dl)	> 50	< 50
Lactic dehydrogenase (U/L)	< 225	> 225
Gram stain	Monomicrobial	Polymicrobial

ciated with a significantly lower rate of complications (e.g., hyponatremia, encephalopathy, and renal insufficiency) and is recommended when repeated LVP is indicated.[63]

In performing paracentesis, one should avoid surgical scars and obvious large subcutaneous collaterals. In general, a point 1 to 2 cm below the umbilicus along the midline is an optimal site in patients with no previous surgical incisions. Ultrasonographic guidance is usually necessary for localization when the amount of fluid present is small and when the fluid is loculated because of earlier episodes of peritonitis or previous surgical procedures.

The most common complications of LVP are bleeding, peritonitis, perforated viscus, and intra-abdominal abscess. Other complications (e.g., renal failure and cardiovascular instability) are less common and can usually be prevented by means of albumin and colloid replacement and intravascular volume expansion.

A few patients with ascites either become refractory to medical therapy or have contraindications to diuretic therapy or LVP. The usual practice has been to treat these patients with a peritoneovenous shunt through which the ascitic fluid can be reinfused into the systemic circulation, so that effective plasma volume is not reduced. The early enthusiasm for these shunts and their potential advantages notwithstanding, it is clear that there are a number of major complications limiting their use—in particular, early shunt occlusion, disseminated intravascular coagulation (DIC), sepsis, and central venous thrombosis. These complications occur with widely varying degrees of frequency; overall, however, it is estimated that about half of all shunted patients die within 1 year of the operation.[64,65]

If ascites develops as a result of PHT, it is logical to assume that reduction of the portal pressure might relieve the stimulus for ascites and control its formation. Earlier experience with the side-to-side portacaval shunt showed that this approach effectively controlled ascites; however, about one third of the patients died of postoperative complications and liver failure.[66] More recently, the transjugular intrahepatic portosystemic shunt (TIPS) has proved effective in correcting portal hypertension and controlling acute variceal bleeding while carrying low morbidity and mortality.[67]

These results have led to increasing use of TIPS to manage refractory ascites. In most patients, ascites can be completely or partially controlled with TIPS.[68,69] Approximately two thirds of patients with refractory ascites exhibit significantly reduced fluid accumulation and improved renal function. There are, however, a number of complications. Some of these complications are technical (e.g., bleeding from the liver capsule caused by inadvertent puncture, hemobilia, contrast-induced renal failure, and stent malposition or migration). The most significant nontechnical complications associated with the use of TIPS are an increased incidence of encephalopathy

(seen in about 25% to 30% of patients),[70,71] hemolysis, and worsening jaundice.[72]

Stenosis or occlusion of the shunt that necessitates shunt revision is so frequent that it is considered the norm rather than a complication: in most series, 1-year patency rates range from 27% to 57%.[73] No long-term follow-up data are available; however, in one study, the overall survival rate was lower among patients who underwent TIPS placement than among those who received repeated LVP.[74] These data suggest that whereas TIPS is superior to LVP in controlling refractory ascites, it confers no survival advantage, and most patients will die of other complications of cirrhosis.

Hepatic Encephalopathy

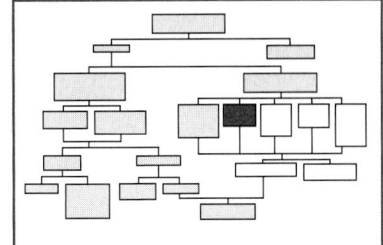

Hepatic encephalopathy is a complex neuropsychiatric syndrome that arises in patients with severe hepatic insufficiency and cirrhosis. It is characterized by progressive alteration of cognitive function and coordination and depression of consciousness, leading to deep coma. Hepatic encephalopathy takes two main forms: (1) acute encephalopathy associated with FHF and (2) portosystemic encephalopathy (PSE) associated with cirrhosis and portosystemic shunts. It is classified into four stages according to the severity and extent of CNS impairment [see Table 9].

For accurate diagnosis of hepatic encephalopathy, all other disorders that affect cerebral function—including fluid and electrolyte abnormalities, hypoglycemia, azotemia, metabolic acidosis or alkalosis, hypoxia, and plasma hyperosmolality—must be recognized and corrected. Sedatives and paralytic agents should be avoided during the initial assessment period if possible; if sedation or paralysis is required, the combination of poor hepatic function with the shunting of blood away from the liver may greatly lengthen drug elimination, thereby complicating patient assessment.

Management of PSE begins with treatment and reversal of all potential precipitating factors: sedatives and other drugs with CNS effects should be discontinued, fluid and electrolyte abnormalities should be corrected, GI bleeding should be controlled, and underlying infectious states (especially SBP) should be treated. Early elective tracheal intubation and airway protection may be necessary in patients with stage III or IV encephalopathy because of the high risk of aspiration and subsequent pneumonia.

The classic therapeutic objectives in the management of hepatic

Table 9 Grading of Hepatic Encephalopathy

Encephalopathy Stage	Neurologic Changes
Stage I	Mild confusion, euphoria or depression, decreased attention span, slowing of ability to perform mental tasks, irritability, disorder of sleep pattern
Stage II	Drowsiness, lethargy, gross deficit in ability to perform mental tasks, obvious personality changes, inappropriate behavior, intermittent and short-lived disorientation
Stage III	Somnolent but arousable, unable to perform mental tasks, disorientation with respect to time or place, marked confusion, amnesia, occasional fits of rage, speech present but incomprehensible
Stage IV	Coma

encephalopathy are (1) to minimize ammonia formation and (2) to augment ammonia elimination [*see* Discussion, Mechanism of Hepatic Encephalopathy, *below*]. Lactulose and certain antibiotics are commonly employed to achieve these ends. Lactulose is a synthetic disaccharide cathartic that can be delivered orally, through a nasogastric tube, or via a high enema and can be administered early in the course of the disease. The dosage should begin at 25 g/day and then be titrated to a level at which the patient can produce three or four loose bowel movements a day. Lactulose is neither absorbed nor metabolized in the upper GI tract. When it reaches the colon, the ensuing bacterial degradation acidifies the luminal contents and causes an intraluminal osmotic shift. The more acid environment that results inhibits coliform bacterial growth, thereby reducing ammonia production. Additionally, the low intraluminal gut pH causes ammonia to be converted to ammonium ions, which do not enter the bloodstream easily. Finally, the cathartic action of lactulose clears ammonium ions from the bowel. Aggressive lactulose therapy may induce volume depletion and electrolyte imbalances; metabolic acidosis is a rare occurrence.

Neomycin, an agent commonly used for bowel preparation, alters gut flora, especially *Escherichia coli* and other urease-producing organisms, and thereby causes production of ammonia to fall. Only about 1% of a neomycin dose is absorbed systemically; because of possible ototoxicity and nephrotoxicity, special care should be taken if it is administered on a continuous basis.[75] Other oral antibiotics used to treat hepatic encephalopathy are polymyxin B, metronidazole, and vancomycin; they affect gut flora in much the same fashion as neomycin.

Aromatic amino acids (AAAs) are known neurotransmitter precursors, and it has been suggested that their products interfere with the activity of true neurotransmitters. It has also been shown that the ratio of branched-chain amino acids (BCAAs) to AAAs in plasma decreases steeply with encephalopathy. Because AAAs and BCAAs compete for the same blood-brain barrier carrier transport sites, the relative paucity of BCAAs leads to increased cerebral uptake of AAAs, which in turn promotes synthesis of false neurotransmitters that then compete with the endogenous transmitters dopamine and norepinephrine.[76] Parenteral administration of BCAA-enriched formulas to patients with hepatic encephalopathy has been advocated, but it has not proved beneficial in comparison with administration of conventional parenteral amino acid solutions.[77]

Renal Failure

Liver disease and cirrhosis are commonly associated with functional renal failure—that is, impaired renal function in the absence of significant underlying renal pathology. The most common functional renal abnor- 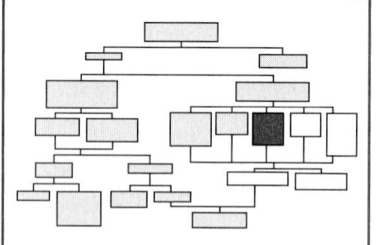 mality in cirrhotic patients is a condition known as hepatorenal syndrome (HRS). HRS is defined as a reversible state of renal failure characterized by azotemia, oliguria (< 500 ml/day), low urinary sodium excretion (< 10 mEq/L), and an increased urine-plasma osmolality ratio (U/P > 1.0) in the absence of urinary sedimentation. HRS occurs in 18% to 55% of cirrhotic patients with ascites and is characterized by intense renal vasoconstriction, a decreased glomerular filtration rate (GFR), preserved tubular function, and normal renal histology.[39,78] Although the exact etiology of HRS is not known, the evidence currently available suggests that it is multifactorial, involving systemic vasodilatation and reduced effective plasma volume along with increased activity of the renin-angiotensin-aldosterone system, which causes further reduction of the GFR. On clinical grounds,

Table 10 Differentiation of Hepatorenal Syndrome from Acute Tubular Necrosis

Criteria	Hepatorenal Syndrome	Acute Tubular Necrosis
Underlying liver disease	Advanced liver damage with jaundice and impaired synthetic function	Mild or severe liver disease
Precipitant	GI bleeding, diuretics, paracentesis, sepsis, or none	Shock, nephrotoxins, sepsis
Onset	Days to weeks	Hours to days
Urinalysis	Renal epithelial cells with or without pigmented granular cells	Pigmented granular casts with or without RBCs, WBCs
Urinary sodium concentration	< 10 mEq/L	> 10 mEq/L
Urinary osmolarity	> Serum osmolarity	Isotonic
Urinary volume	Oliguric	Variable
Course	Progressive, unremitting	Deterioration followed by improved renal function

HRS has been classified into two types: (1) type 1 HRS, in which renal failure is rapidly progressive, as defined by a doubling of the initial serum creatinine level to a value higher than 2.5 mg/dl or a 50% reduction in the initial creatinine clearance to a value lower than 20 ml/min in less than 2 weeks; and (2) type 2 HRS, in which renal failure takes a slower, more gradual course.

The prognosis for patients with HRS is poor: to date, all therapeutic approaches have proved unsuccessful. Pharmacologic therapy has consisted of correcting effective volume status and attempting to reverse renal vasoconstriction through I.V. administration of vasodilators (e.g., dopamine, misoprostol, and aminophylline) or drugs that inhibit the synthesis or the effects of endogenous vasoconstrictors (e.g., captopril and thromboxane inhibitors). These approaches have not yielded any effective and reproducible improvements in renal hemodynamics and renal function. Several investigators, however, have reported improved renal function after OLT.[79]

Subsequently, a newer approach to the management of HRS was introduced that aimed at correcting the primary underlying defect (i.e., systemic vasodilatation) instead of the secondary renal vasoconstriction. Two classes of drugs have been investigated, either individually or in various combinations: (1) agents that inhibit the effects of endogenous systemic vasodilators (e.g., prostacyclin, nitric oxide, and glucagon) and (2) agents that cause systemic vasoconstriction (e.g., ornipressin and terlipressin). In one small series of patients with type 1 HRS, a combination of an oral β-adrenergic drug with midodrine and octreotide led to improved renal function and better long-term outcome.[80]

Besides functional renal failure, various types of nonfunctional, or organic, renal failure (e.g., acute tubular necrosis [ATN], renal tubular acidosis [RTA], and drug-induced interstitial nephritis) may occur in patients with cirrhosis. ATN is especially common among patients with chronic liver disease or FHF and is usually seen in patients who are poorly resuscitated, have experienced prolonged hypotension, have undergone severe septic episodes, or have ingested hepatotoxins that are also nephrotoxic (e.g., acetaminophen). ATN is characterized by an abrupt rise in blood urea nitrogen (BUN) and serum creatinine levels accompanied by oliguria or anuria. Unlike HRS, ATN leads to impairment of the concentrating ability of the tubular system and to excessive urinary sodium excretion; accordingly, a urine sodium concentration higher than 10 mEq/L has been proposed as a diagnostic criterion for ATN in cirrhotic patients [see Table 10]. RTA is commonly seen in patients with primary biliary cirrhosis (PBC), autoimmune liver disease, and alcoholic cirrhosis. It is characterized by an inability of the renal tubules to acidify the urine in the presence of a normal GFR.

Management of renal failure is usually aimed at correcting the underlying precipitating causes. In patients with ascites, who experience ongoing loss of fluid and protein into the peritoneum, it is important to maintain an adequate intravascular volume. If intravascular volume is depleted, blood components, volume expanders, or both should be given. Given that the plasma albumin level is invariably low in these patients, salt-poor albumin solutions may be preferable to carbohydrate-based volume expanders. Albumin replacement has been effectively used for volume expansion after LVP.[63]

Because of the complex interaction between the liver and the kidneys, fluid and electrolyte management often proves exceptionally challenging. In particular, it is difficult to estimate the actual intravascular volume, which is depleted in most cirrhotic patients even though total body fluid volume is higher than normal. Sodium retention and free water retention are the two most common abnormalities of renal function that lead to ascites and dilutional hyponatremia. Typically, sodium retention is an early manifestation, whereas water retention and renal failure are late findings. Nephrotoxic drugs and I.V. contrast agents should be avoided, and dosages of antibiotics and other medications should be adjusted appropriately.

Hypernatremia and metabolic acidosis can develop secondary to excessive lactulose therapy and dehydration and cause renal function to deteriorate. Hypokalemia is also common; it develops secondary to increased serum aldosterone concentration, which leads to excessive excretion of potassium in exchange for sodium. Once renal failure develops, hyperkalemia, hypercalcemia, and hyperphosphatemia become significant problems, often necessitating dialysis.

Malnutrition

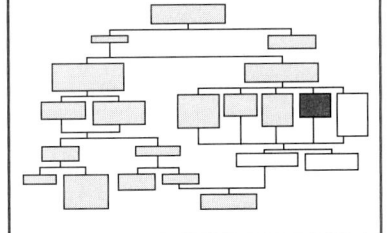

Most cirrhotic patients present with depleted glycogen stores, severe protein-calorie malnutrition, and wasting. Impaired hepatic synthetic activity, causing a deficiency of both visceral and structural proteins, is one of the hallmarks of advanced liver disease. In addition, poor appetite, tense ascites, abdominal pain, and excessive loss of protein through repeated LVP and overall increased energy expenditure tend to exacerbate malnutrition.

Excessive protein administration can induce hepatic encephalopathy; accordingly, protein intake should be limited to 1 to 1.2 g/kg/day. Glucose is the main energy source given to malnourished cirrhotic patients; however, its use is not without complications, in that these patients typically exhibit glucose intolerance. Lipid emulsion can be safely administered to most patients with liver failure and should be withheld only from patients with overt coma.[81] It is generally agreed that the ideal energy source should consist of a mixture of glucose and fat emulsion. Approximately 30% to 40% of all nonprotein calories can be provided in the form of fat. The total energy requirement should be in the range of 25 to 35 kcal/kg/day.

As noted [see Hepatic Encephalopathy, above], although AAAs have been implicated in the pathogenesis of hepatic encephalopathy,

administration of BCAA solutions has not proved helpful, and the evidence does not support their routine use.[77,82]

In general, the potential risks and complications associated with total parenteral nutrition (TPN) outweigh the benefits in patients with a functioning GI tract. When properly administered, enteral nutrition is safer, more physiologically correct, and significantly more cost-effective than TPN. It should therefore be considered the first choice for nutritional support in most patients with chronic liver disease unless a contraindication to enteral feeding is present.

Coagulopathy and Nonvariceal Bleeding

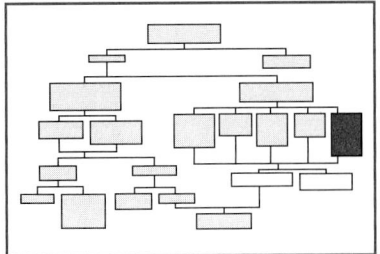

The spectrum of coagulation disorders in patients with liver disease varies from minor localized bleeding to massive life-threatening hemorrhage. Abnormal bleeding may be spontaneous in some patients, but it is more often the result of a hemostatic challenge (e.g., surgical wounds or procedures, gastritis, portal hypertensive gastropathy, gastric or duodenal ulcers, or ruptured varices). The underlying anatomic lesion is believed to be as responsible for bleeding as the hemostatic defect is; accordingly, therapy should be directed at correcting both.

Although most bleeding episodes are secondary to decreased synthesis of clotting factors, other causes of bleeding (e.g., defective or dysfunctional factor synthesis and increased consumption of clotting components) must always be ruled out [see 1:4 Bleeding and Transfusion]. In most patients, the decreased levels of clotting factors parallel the progressive loss of parenchymal cell function. Usually, the levels of the vitamin K–dependent factors (i.e., prothrombin, factor VII, factor IX, factor X, protein S, and protein C) fall first, followed by the levels of other factors as cirrhosis progresses. Factor V is synthesized independently of vitamin K availability, and its concentration is of special interest because the plasma factor V level seems to be a predictor of the extent of liver cell damage. Impaired synthesis of coagulation proteins also has an impact on antithrombin III (AT-III), protein C inhibitor, plasminogen, and α_2-antiplasmin as well as on several other inhibitors and activators of both the extrinsic coagulation pathway and the intrinsic pathway. The combination of decreased factor levels and impaired synthesis of coagulation proteins explains the prolongation of the PT, the activated partial thromboplastin time (aPTT), and the thrombin clotting time (TCT) in these patients.[83,84]

Given the complexity of hemostasis in cirrhotic patients, accurate diagnosis of a bleeding disorder is often hard to achieve. Several disorders and abnormalities may be present simultaneously, and one or more parameters of hemostasis and coagulation may be impaired. Therefore, any effective treatment approach should be broad-based and aimed at correcting several deficiencies or abnormalities at once. FFP contains all of the components of the clotting and fibrinolytic systems but lacks platelets. In most cases, transfusion of 6 to 8 units of FFP suffices to correct severe clotting factor defects; however, the excess volume may not be well tolerated. Cryoprecipitate, the precipitate formed when FFP is thawed at 4°C, is rich in factor VIII, von Willebrand factor, and fibrinogen but lacks the vitamin K–dependent factors. Therefore, it should be given only when the fibrinogen level is lower than 100 mg/dl. Prothrombin complex concentrates contain only the vitamin K–dependent factors and proteins, and their use can provoke serious thromboembolic complications, including disseminated intravascular coagulation (DIC). Therefore, their potential utility must be weighed carefully against the risk that thrombotic events may develop.[85]

Other major disorders of hemostasis in patients with chronic liver disease and cirrhosis involve platelets and are manifested as thrombocytopenia, abnormal platelet function (thrombocytopathy), or both. In most cases, thrombocytopenia is related to splenomegaly and hypersplenism (a common feature of PHT). Abnormal platelet function is attributed to many causes, including intrinsic platelet defects and abnormal interaction among platelets, endothelial surfaces, and clotting factors. It is manifested by a prolonged bleeding time, impaired platelet aggregation, and reduced adhesiveness. Some authorities attribute the inhibition of platelet aggregation to fibrin degradation products (FDPs); however, the FDP levels noted in the plasma of cirrhotic patients are not sufficient to impair platelet aggregation, nor do they correlate with the observed reductions in platelet aggregation.[86]

Platelets should be transfused whenever a patient with either a quantitative or a qualitative defect experiences active bleeding. A normal response is a rise of 10,000/mm³ with each unit transfused; however, in cases of hypersplenism and accelerated consumption, such a response is rare. Transfusion should be continued until all serious bleeding has ceased, with the therapeutic goal being the maintenance of a platelet count near 50,000/mm³. Platelet transfusion is also indicated before any surgical or invasive procedure (e.g., paracentesis or liver biopsy). Indications for prophylactic platelet transfusion are less clear, and any potential gains must be balanced against potential side effects and development of antibodies. Most patients with advanced cirrhosis and liver failure have platelet counts lower than 100,000/mm³; however, prophylactic platelet transfusion is usually not recommended until the count falls below 15,000 to 20,000/mm³, at which point the risk of spontaneous bleeding is considerably increased.

Another feature of severe liver disease is increased fibrinolytic activity, which may be either primary or secondary to DIC.[87] The exact causes of primary fibrinolysis and DIC remain unclear. Primary fibrinolysis appears to derive from increased activity of tissue plasminogen activator and decreased levels of α_2-antiplasmin.[88] DIC is believed to be triggered by the release of thromboplastic substances into the circulation as a consequence of liver cell damage or necrosis and by poor clearance of circulating activated tissue and clotting factors and FDPs by a defective reticuloendothelial system. Accelerated fibrinolysis is manifested by reductions in the whole blood clot lysis time and the euglobulin clot lysis time as well as by elevated levels of fibrinolysis products (e.g., FDPs and D-dimer). Although enhanced fibrinolysis is relatively common in patients with cirrhosis,

Table 11 Contraindications to Liver Transplantation

Absolute contraindications	Severe, irreversible brain damage
	HIV infection
	Extrahepatic malignancy
	Uncontrolled sepsis
	Severe pulmonary hypertension and advanced cardiopulmonary disease
	Active substance abuse or major psychosocial problems
	Extrahepatic portal vein thrombosis in patients with hepatocellular carcinoma
Relative contraindications	Elevated ICP or reduced CPP (in patients with FHF)
	Multiple organ dysfunction syndrome
	Hemodynamic instability
	Advanced age
	Portal vein thrombosis (except when secondary to hepatocellular carcinoma)

CPP—cerebral perfusion pressure   ICP—intracranial pressure

Table 12   Child-Turcotte-Pugh Scoring System

Points	1	2	3
Encephalopathy	None	Stage I or II	Stage III or IV
Ascites	Absent	Slight (or controlled by diuretics)	Moderate despite diuretic treatment
Bilirubin (mg/dl) Patients with PBC or PSC	< 2 < 4	2–3 4–6	> 3 > 6
Albumin (g/L)	> 3.5	2.8–3.5	< 2.8
PT (prolonged sec) INR	< 4 < 1.7	4–6 1.7–2.3	> 6 > 2.3

PBC—primary biliary cirrhosis   PSC—primary sclerosing cholangitis

most of the characteristic abnormalities can occur after many types of physiologic stress and are not necessarily accompanied by a bleeding tendency.

At present, no satisfactory method of managing DIC is available. An extensive workup must be completed to rule out underlying causes (e.g., sepsis, ARDS, and MODS). FFP, platelet concentrates, and, possibly, low-dose heparin (200 to 800 U/hr) may be given. AT-III concentrate has been used in an attempt to inhibit the action of thrombin, thereby decreasing procoagulant consumption, restoring normal levels of factors, and improving hemostasis. Clinical experience with AT-III therapy in this setting has been limited to a few case reports and a few small series; however, there is some evidence to suggest that AT-III may reduce the hemostatic abnormalities and help control bleeding.[89]

Antifibrinolytic agents (e.g., ε-aminocaproic acid and tranexamic acid) impede fibrinolysis and thus may be useful for treating bleeding in patients who have liver disease and show evidence of fibrinolysis.[90] In patients with DIC, however, administration of antifibrinolytic agents is contraindicated because of the potential for thrombotic complications. D-dimer levels should be determined to rule out DIC before use of these medications is considered. Because DIC is difficult to rule out in patients with liver disease, the use of antifibrinolytic agents in liver disease is limited.

LIVER TRANSPLANTATION

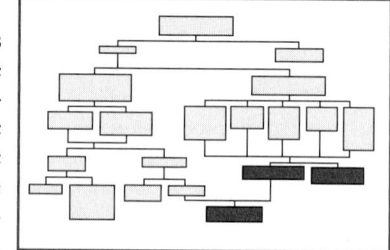

The standard indications for liver transplantation are well documented[91]: they include PHT, poor hepatic synthetic function, hepatic encephalopathy, progressive jaundice, severe malnutrition, and excessive fatigue. As noted [see Treatment of Complications, above], PHT is manifested by variceal bleeding, hypersplenism, thrombocytopenia, ascites, hepatic hydrothorax, and SBP. Poor synthetic function is usually manifested by a prolonged PT and low serum albumin and cholesterol levels. In general, any concurrent medical or psychosocial condition that prohibits a major surgical procedure or subsequent immunosuppression constitutes a contraindication to liver transplantation [see Table 11].

The United Network for Organ Sharing (UNOS) currently regulates organ allocation to transplant candidates. In January 1988, minimal listing criteria for liver transplantation were implemented.[92] These criteria are based on the Child-Turcotte-Pugh (CTP) scoring system [see Table 12], which includes five parameters: serum albumin and bilirubin levels, PT, ascites, and hepatic encephalopathy. To be listed for liver transplantation, a patient must have a CTP score of 7 or higher. In addition to the general listing criteria, various disease-specific criteria were developed for patients with alcoholic liver disease, patients with cholestatic liver disease (e.g., PBC or primary sclerosing cholangitis), and patients with hepatocellular carcinoma.

Discussion

Mechanisms of Hepatic Encephalopathy

The association between liver disease and altered mental status and consciousness has been recognized for centuries, but the exact underlying mechanisms remain unknown. It appears that this syndrome has a multifactorial etiology and is associated with a number of complex changes, which are manifested collectively as hepatic encephalopathy. It is generally believed that hepatocerebral dysfunction is caused by accumulation of cerebral toxins as a result of low hepatic clearance.[93]

Of all the physiologic factors thought to contribute to the development of encephalopathy, the best known is ammonia. Arterial ammonia levels are frequently elevated in persons with hepatic encephalopathy; however, the clinical severity of hepatic encephalopathy correlates poorly with the degree to which the ammonia level is elevated.[94] The precise contribution of ammonia to hepatic encephalopathy remains unclear; however, ammonia is known to inhibit the uptake of glutamate into the astrocytes, thereby causing a rise in the extracellular glutamate level that appears to downregulate the postsynaptic glutamate receptors, resulting in decreased neuronal excitation.[95]

Endogenous or exogenously ingested benzodiazepines may also play a role in the etiology of acute and chronic hepatic encephalopathy by interacting with the high-affinity γ-aminobutyric acid (GABA)–benzodiazepine receptor complexes. These substances are known to enhance inhibitory GABA-ergic tone. Animal studies suggest that the gut flora may contribute benzodiazepine ligand activity[96] as well as increased benzodiazepine receptor agonist activity.[97] Clinical studies of FHF patients show increased benzodiazepine receptor ligands with enhanced GABA-ergic tone in all stages of encephalopathy.[98] Ammonia-induced activation of peripheral-type benzodiazepine receptors on astrocytes may cause the release of neurosteroids that enhance GABA-ergic neurotransmission. Hence, neurosteroids may potentate the inhibitory actions of GABA at the receptor level as well as lengthen the period during which the GABA ligand remains in the synaptic cleft. Ammonia also acts directly to potentate GABA-ergic tone by enhancing the affinity of GABA for GABA-A receptors.[99]

Despite these seemingly compelling findings, there is no apparent correlation between benzodiazepine ligand activity and clinical stage of encephalopathy, nor is ligand elevation a consistent finding in all patients. Furthermore, clinical and animal studies in which a benzodiazepine receptor antagonist has been administered have not shown consistent effects. The anecdotal success of flumazenil, the principal benzodiazepine antagonist, has been ascribed to the antagonism of benzodiazepines ingested by patients. Support for the concept of so-called endogenous benzodiazepines arising from the intestine can be found in a number of sources, including studies of dogs with congenital portacaval shunts, which document ligand activity in stool samples.[100] Whether there is a causal relation to hepatic encephalopathy or whether this is merely a case of associated phenomena remains to be determined. Whatever the contribution of benzodiazepines to the pathophysiology of acute hepatic encephalopathy and cerebral edema, it appears likely that other mechanisms are involved.

Bioartificial Liver Support System

Despite the best management efforts, the morbidity and mortality associated with ALF remain exceptionally high. For most severe cases, liver transplantation is still the only effective therapeutic modality. Unfortunately, because of the severe organ donor shortage, the waiting period for transplantation is long, and patients consequently are at risk for the development of irreversible complications or contraindications to liver transplantation while awaiting a donor. In an effort to mitigate this problem, investigators have studied various artificial liver support systems designed to provide full metabolic, hemodynamic, and physiologic support until either the native liver regenerates or a liver becomes available for transplantation. From the 1970s to the 1990s, most therapeutic attempts focused primarily on detoxifying plasma. All such attempts either failed or had no significant impact on survival.[101]

The ongoing severe organ shortage has led several investigators to develop and test a number of xenogeneic-based liver support systems employing whole-organ perfusion or isolated hepatocytes. At our institution, we developed and tested a hybrid bioartificial liver (BAL) support system employing isolated porcine hepatocytes in an extracorporeal perfusion circuit. We subsequently initiated a clinical trial addressing the use of this system in patients with severe ALF as a bridge to either transplantation or spontaneous recovery.[102-104]

CLINICAL TRIAL

Study Design

Hepatocytes Methods of porcine hepatocyte isolation, purification, attachment to a collagen-coated matrix, cryopreservation,

Table 13 Neurologic Effects of BAL Treatment

Study Group	Results		
	Pre-BAL	Post-BAL	*P*
Group I			
ICP (mm Hg)	17.0 ± 1.5	10.9 ± 1.0	< 0.0002
CPP (mm Hg)	70 ± 2	75 ± 2	< 0.04
GCS	6.8 ± 0.4	7.4 ± 0.4	< 0.01
CLOCS	24.7 ± 1.2	32.0 ± 1.1	< 0.000001
Group II			
GCS	5.0 ± 1.1	7.0 ± 1.4	< 0.2
CLOCS	29.7 ± 7.4	31.7 ± 7.9	< 0.5
Group III			
ICP (mm Hg)	12.3 ± 0.9	14.0 ± 1.5	< 0.4
CPP (mm Hg)	85 ± 1	98 ± 8	< 0.3
GCS	8.2 ± 0.7	8.4 ± 0.7	< 0.4
CLOCS	29.7 ± 2.3	34.0 ± 1.7	< 0.001

BAL—bioartificial liver CLOCS—Comprehensive Level of Consciousness score
CPP—cerebral perfusion pressure GCS—Glasgow Coma Scale ICP—intracranial pressure

Table 14 Metabolic Effects of BAL Treatment

Study Group	Results		
	Pre-BAL	Post-BAL	*P*
Group I			
AST (U/L)	1,255 ± 261	879 ± 148	< 0.002
ALT (U/L)	1,075 ± 184	674 ± 120	< 0.000005
Total bilirubin (mg/dl)	17.9 ± 1.5	14.6 ± 1.2	< 0.000001
Glucose (mg/dl)	126 ± 5	175 ± 7	< 0.0000006
Ammonia (μmol/L)	160 ± 8	134 ± 6	< 0.0002
Lactate (mmol/L)	4.4 ± 0.7	4.2 ± 0.6	< 0.2
Albumin (g/dl)	3.12 ± 0.08	2.6 ± 0.1	< 0.0000006
Creatinine (mg/dl)	1.5 ± 0.2	1.1 ± 0.1	< 0.000001
Group II			
AST (U/L)	5,661 ± 2,613	2,821 ± 1,291	< 0.1
ALT (U/L)	2,139 ± 704	1,633 ± 544	< 0.05
Total bilirubin (mg/dl)	19.1 ± 2.2	14.7 ± 1.7	< 0.009
Glucose (mg/dl)	117 ± 26	144 ± 24	< 0.06
Ammonia (μmol/L)	81 ± 9	91 ± 13	< 0.03
Lactate (mmol/L)	13.1 ± 2.9	13.2 ± 2.2	< 0.9
Albumin (g/dl)	3.7 ± 0.3	2.7 ± 0.1	< 0.01
Creatinine (mg/dl)	1.6 ± 0.3	1.6 ± 0.3	< 1.0
Group III			
AST (U/L)	692 ± 374	723 ± 409	< 0.5
ALT (U/L)	349 ± 126	281 ± 114	< 0.06
Total bilirubin (mg/dl)	26.0 ± 2.7	21.6 ± 2.2	< 0.000003
Glucose (mg/dl)	141 ± 9	171 ± 11	< 0.001
Ammonia (μmol/L)	173 ± 31	131 ± 15	< 0.08
Lactate (mmol/L)	5.7 ± 1.1	5.6 ± 0.9	< 0.9
Albumin (g/dl)	3.0 ± 0.1	2.6 ± 0.1	< 0.00003
Creatinine (mg/dl)	2.8 ± 0.3	2.2 ± 0.2	< 0.00002

ALT—alanine aminotransferase   AST—aspartate aminotransferase   BAL—bioartificial liver

and storage were developed. Five to seven billion fresh or cryopreserved hepatocytes (70% to 90% viability) were used for each patient treatment.[103,104]

System characteristics The system was standardized and subsequently modified and is currently manufactured as the HepatAssist 2000 (Circe Biomedical, Inc., Lexington, Massachusetts). The main components are (1) a plasmapheresis unit, (2) an activated cellulose-coated charcoal column, (3) an oxygenator, (4) a blood warmer, and (5) a hollow-fiber module containing isolated microcarrier-attached porcine hepatocytes. The module consists of (a) an intracapillary chamber made of several porous, hollow 0.2 μm fibers through which plasma flows and (b) an extracapillary chamber surrounding the hollow fibers, where the microcarrier-attached hepatocytes are suspended. Plasma circulates through the fibers at a rate of 400 ml/min, with free exchange of macromolecules across the surface of the fibers driven by a transmembrane pressure gradient. When plasma and blood

cells return from the BAL, they are reconstituted and returned to the patient via the double-lumen venous dialysis catheter.

Patient population Three groups of patients were enrolled in the phase 1 trial. Group I patients (N = 24) had no previous history of liver disease, fulfilled all the diagnostic criteria of FHF, and were candidates for OLT at the time of admission. Group II patients (N = 3) had undergone OLT and exhibited primary nonfunction (PNF) of the transplanted liver in the immediate postoperative period with rapid deterioration. Group III patients (N = 10) presented with acute exacerbation of known underlying chronic liver disease and were not candidates for OLT at the time of study enrollment. Patients were enrolled in the study when stage III or IV encephalopathy developed in the course of optimal standard medical therapy.

Results

Of the 24 group I patients, 18 were candidates for OLT. Five additional patients with FHF secondary to acetaminophen toxicity who were treated with the BAL support system recovered fully without the need for liver transplantation. One patient with FHF secondary to heatstroke received BAL treatment while awaiting OLT; he died as a result of MODS after 21 days. All 18 OLT candidates in group I and all three patients in group II were successfully bridged to transplantation, experienced full neurologic and functional recovery, and were discharged from the hospital. Patients in group III experienced transient clinical improvement after BAL treatment. Two patients recovered enough native liver function to survive; they subsequently became candidates for OLT and underwent the procedure successfully. The remaining eight patients died 1 to 21 days (mean, 7.1 days) after their last BAL treatment as a result of variceal bleeding, sepsis, or MODS.

Treatment with the BAL support system gave rise to several neurologic and metabolic effects that were seen in all three groups of patients. Of these, the neurologic changes were the most dramatic. Patients with FHF (group I) exhibited remarkable neurologic improvement after BAL treatment, with the reversal of decerebrate posturing states, anisocoria, and sluggish pupillary reflexes. Both responsiveness to external stimuli and brain-stem function improved, as shown by a higher comprehensive level of consciousness score. There was a significant reduction in ICP with a concomitant increase in CPP; these changes were most dramatic in patients with ICP levels higher than 25 mm Hg [*see Table 13*]. In patients with PNF (group II), the impact of BAL treatment on neurologic status was difficult to assess because heavy sedation was used in the postanesthetic period; however, transient neurologic improvements were noted after BAL treatment, manifested primarily by increased responsiveness.

Additional metabolic effects of BAL treatment on liver function included improvements in renal function and hematologic and coagulation parameters [*see Table 14*]. There was a significant (*P* < 0.01) increase in the plasma BCAA-AAA ratio in plasma, which may be one of many possible reasons for the observed mitigation of encephalopathy. This increase was primarily due to a reduction in AAA levels.

References

1. Kotwal GJ, Baroudy BM, Kuramoto IK, et al: Detection of acute hepatitis C virus infection by ELISA using a synthetic peptide comprising a structural epitope. Proc Natl Acad Sci USA 89:4486, 1992

2. Polito AJ, DiNello RK, Quan S, et al: New generation RIBA hepatitis C strip immunoblot assays. Ann Biol Clin (Paris) 50:329, 1992

3. Bukh J, Purcell RH, Miller RH: Importance of primer selection for the detection of hepatitis C virus RNA with the polymerase chain reaction assay. Proc Natl Acad Sci USA 89:187, 1992

4. Trey C, Davidson CS: The management of fulminant hepatic failure. Prog Liver Dis 3:282, 1970

5. Bernuau J, Rueff B, Benhamou JP: Fulminant and

subfulminant liver failure: definitions and causes. Semin Liver Dis 6:97, 1986

6. Schiodt FV, Atillasoy E, Shakil AO, et al: Etiology and outcome for 295 patients with acute liver failure in the United States. Liver Transpl Surg 5:29, 1999

7. Ritt DJ, Whelan G, Werner DJ, et al: Acute hepatic

necrosis with stupor or coma: an analysis of thirty-one patients. Medicine (Baltimore) 48:151, 1969

8. Lettau LA, McCarthy JG, Smith MH, et al: Outbreak of severe hepatitis due to delta and hepatitis B viruses in parenteral drug abusers and their contacts. N Engl J Med 317:1256, 1987

9. Gimson AE, Tedder RS, White YS, et al: Serological markers in fulminant hepatitis B. Gut 24:615, 1983

10. Samuel D, Bismuth A, Mathieu D, et al: Passive immunoprophylaxis after liver transplantation in HBsAg-positive patients. Lancet 337:813, 1991

11. Govindarajan S, Chin KP, Redeker AG, et al: Fulminant B viral hepatitis: role of delta agent. Gastroenterology 86:1417, 1984

12. Smedile A, Farci P, Verme G, et al: Influence of delta infection on severity of hepatitis B. Lancet 2:945, 1982

13. Lichtenstein DR, Makadon HJ, Chopra S: Fulminant hepatitis B and delta virus coinfection in AIDS. Am J Gastroenterol 87:1643, 1992

14. Rakela J, Lange SM, Ludwig J, et al: Fulminant hepatitis: Mayo Clinic experience with 34 cases. Mayo Clin Proc 60:289, 1985

15. Castells A, Salmeron JM, Navasa M, et al: Liver transplantation for acute liver failure: analysis of applicability. Gastroenterology 105:532, 1993

16. Zimmerman HJ: Update of hepatotoxicity due to classes of drugs in common clinical use: non-steroidal drugs, anti-inflammatory drugs, antibiotics, antihypertensives, and cardiac and psychotropic agents. Semin Liver Dis 10:322, 1990

17. Carney FM, Van Dyke RA: Halothane hepatitis: a critical review. Anesth Analg 51:135, 1972

18. Floersheim GL: Treatment of human amatoxin mushroom poisoning. Myths and advances in therapy. Med Toxicol 2:1, 1987

19. Klein AS, Hart J, Brems JJ, et al: Amanita poisoning: treatment and the role of liver transplantation. Am J Med 86:187, 1989

20. Rector WG Jr, Uchida T, Kanel GC, et al: Fulminant hepatic and renal failure complicating Wilson's disease. Liver 4:341, 1984

21. McCullough AJ, Fleming CR, Thistle JL, et al: Diagnosis of Wilson's disease presenting as fulminant hepatic failure. Gastroenterology 84:161, 1983

22. Stremmel W, Meyerrose KW, Niederau C, et al: Wilson disease: clinical presentation, treatment, and survival. Ann Intern Med 115:720, 1991

23. Amon E, Allen SR, Petrie RH, et al: Acute fatty liver of pregnancy associated with preeclampsia: management of hepatic failure with postpartum liver transplantation. Am J Perinatol 8:278, 1991

24. O'Grady JG, Alexander GJ, Hayllar KM, et al: Early indicators of prognosis in fulminant hepatic failure. Gastroenterology 97:439, 1989

25. Bernuau J, Goudeau A, Poynard T, et al: Multivariate analysis of prognostic factors in fulminant hepatitis B. Hepatology 6:648, 1986

26. Saibara T, Onishi S, Sone J, et al: Arterial ketone body ratio as a possible indicator for liver transplantation in fulminant hepatic failure. Transplantation 51:782, 1991

27. Ranek L, Andreasen PB, Tygstrup N: Galactose elimination capacity as a prognostic index in patients with fulminant liver failure. Gut 17:959, 1976

28. Ware AJ, D'Agostino AN, Combes B: Cerebral edema: a major complication of massive hepatic necrosis. Gastroenterology 61:877, 1971

29. Silk DB, Trewby PN, Chase RA, et al: Treatment of fulminant hepatic failure by polyacrylonitrile-membrane haemodialysis. Lancet 2:1, 1977

30. Lidofsky SD: Fulminant hepatic failure. Crit Care Clin 11:415, 1995

31. Wijdicks EF, Plevak DJ, Rakela J, et al: Clinical and radiologic features of cerebral edema in fulminant hepatic failure. Mayo Clin Proc 70:119, 1995

32. Sidi A, Mahla ME: Noninvasive monitoring of cerebral perfusion by transcranial Doppler during fulminant hepatic failure and liver transplantation. Anesth Analg 80:194, 1995

33. Munoz SJ, Robinson M, Northrup B, et al: Elevated intracranial pressure and computed tomography of the brain in fulminant hepatocellular failure. Hepatology 13:209, 1991

34. Blei AT, Olafsson S, Webster S, et al: Complications of intracranial pressure monitoring in fulminant hepatic failure. Lancet 341:157, 1993

35. Aldersley MA, Juniper M, Richardson P, et al: Inability of intracranial pressure monitoring to select patients with acute liver failure for transplantation (abstract). Hepatology 22:208A, 1995

36. Davies MH, Mutimer D, Lowes J, et al: Recovery despite impaired cerebral perfusion in fulminant hepatic failure. Lancet 343:1329, 1994

37. Canalese J, Gimson AE, Davis C, et al: Controlled trial of dexamethasone and mannitol for the cerebral oedema of fulminant hepatic failure. Gut 23:625, 1982

38. Forbes A, Alexander GJ, O'Grady JG, et al: Thiopental infusion in the treatment of intracranial hypertension complicating fulminant hepatic failure. Hepatology 10:306, 1989

39. Ring-Larsen H, Palazzo U: Renal failure in fulminant hepatic failure and terminal cirrhosis: a comparison between incidence, types, and prognosis. Gut 22:585, 1981

40. Trewby PN, Warren R, Contini S, et al: Incidence and pathophysiology of pulmonary edema in fulminant hepatic failure. Gastroenterology 74(5 pt 1):859, 1978

41. Bailey RJ, Woolf IL, Cullens H, et al: Metabolic inhibition of polymorphonuclear leucocytes in fulminant hepatic failure. Lancet 1:1162, 1976

42. Imawari M, Hughes RD, Gove CD, et al: Fibronectin and Kupffer cell function in fulminant hepatic failure. Dig Dis Sci 30:1028, 1985

43. Rolando N, Harvey F, Brahm J, et al: Prospective study of bacterial infection in acute liver failure: an analysis of fifty patients. Hepatology 11:49, 1990

44. Rolando N, Harvey F, Brahm J, et al: Fungal infection: a common, unrecognised complication of acute liver failure. J Hepatol 12:1, 1991

45. O'Grady JG, Langley PG, Isola LM, et al: Coagulopathy of fulminant hepatic failure. Semin Liver Dis 6:159, 1986

46. Ringe B, Pichlmayr R, Lubbe N, et al: Total hepatectomy as temporary approach to acute hepatic or primary graft failure. Transplant Proc 20(1 suppl 1):552, 1988

47. Ringe B, Lubbe N, Kuse E, et al: Management of emergencies before and after liver transplantation by early total hepatectomy. Transplant Proc 25(1 pt 2):1090, 1993

48. Rozga J, Podesta L, LePage E, et al: Control of cerebral oedema by total hepatectomy and extracorporeal liver support in fulminant hepatic failure. Lancet 342:898, 1993

49. Ascher NL, Lake JR, Emond JC, et al: Liver transplantation for fulminant hepatic failure. Arch Surg 128:677, 1993

50. Emond JC, Aran PP, Whitington PF, et al: Liver transplantation in the management of fulminant hepatic failure. Gastroenterology 96:1583, 1989

51. Choi W-C, Arnaout WS, Villamil FG, et al: Comparison of the applicability of two prognostic indicator scores in patients with fulminant hepatic failure (abstract). Gastroenterology 118(suppl 2, pt 1):A896, 2000

52. Powell WJ, Jr., Klatskin G: Duration of survival in patients with Laennec's cirrhosis: influence of alcohol withdrawal, and possible effects of recent changes in general management of the disease. Am J Med 44:406, 1968

53. Pare P, Talbot J, Hoefs JC: Serum-ascites albumin concentration gradient: a physiologic approach to the differential diagnosis of ascites. Gastroenterology 85:240, 1983

54. Runyon BA: Paracentesis and ascitic fluid analysis. Textbook of Gastroenterology. Yamada T, Alpers D, Owyang C, et al, Eds. JB Lippincott Co, New York, 1991, p 2455

55. Runyon BA, Montano AA, Akriviadis EA, et al: The serum-ascites albumin gradient is superior to the exudate-transudate concept in the differential diagnosis of ascites. Ann Intern Med 117:215, 1992

56. Akriviadis EA, Runyon BA: Utility of an algorithm in differentiating spontaneous from secondary bacterial peritonitis. Gastroenterology 98:127, 1990

57. Terg R, Cobas S, Fassio E, et al: Oral ciprofloxacin after a short course of intravenous ciprofloxacin in the treatment of spontaneous bacterial peritonitis: results of a multicenter, randomized study. J Hepatol 33:504, 2000

58. Gines P, Rimola A, Planas R, et al: Norfloxacin prevents spontaneous bacterial peritonitis recurrence in cirrhosis: results of a double-blind, placebo-controlled trial. Hepatology 12(4 pt 1):716, 1990

59. Hoefs JC, Canawati HN, Sapico FL, et al: Spontaneous bacterial peritonitis. Hepatology 2:399, 1982

60. Mihas AA, Toussaint J, Hsu HS, et al: Spontaneous bacterial peritonitis in cirrhosis: clinical and laboratory features, survival and prognostic indicators. Hepatogastroenterology 39:520, 1992

61. Gregory PB, Broekelschen PH, Hill MD, et al: Complications of diuresis in the alcoholic patient with ascites: a controlled trial. Gastroenterology 73:534, 1977

62. Tito L, Gines P, Arroyo V, et al: Total paracentesis associated with intravenous albumin management of patients with cirrhosis and ascites. Gastroenterology 98:146, 1990

63. Gines P, Tito L, Arroyo V, et al: Randomized comparative study of therapeutic paracentesis with and without intravenous albumin in cirrhosis. Gastroenterology 94:1493, 1988

64. Bernhoft RA, Pellegrini CA, Way LW: Peritoneovenous shunt for refractory ascites: operative complications and long-term results. Arch Surg 117:631, 1982

65. Greig PD, Langer B, Blendis LM, et al: Complications after peritoneovenous shunting for ascites. Am J Surg 139:125, 1980

66. Welch HF: Prognosis after surgical treatment of ascites: results of side-to-side shunt in 40 patients. Surgery 56:75, 1964;

67. Burroughs AK, Patch D: Transjugular intrahepatic portosystemic shunt. Semin Liver Dis 19:457, 1999

68. Ochs A, Rossle M, Haag K, et al:. The transjugular intrahepatic portosystemic stent-shunt procedure for refractory ascites [published erratum appears in N Engl J Med 332:1587, 1995]. N Engl J Med 332: 1192, 1995

69. Trotter JF, Suhocki PV, Rockey DC: Transjugular intrahepatic portosystemic shunt (TIPS) in patients with refractory ascites: effect on body weight and Child-Pugh score. Am J Gastroenterol 93:1891, 1998

70. Rossle M: [Transjugular intrahepatic portasystemic shunt (TIPS)—indications and outcome]. Z Gastroenterol 35:505, 1997

71. Jalan R, Forrest EH, Stanley AJ, et al: A randomized trial comparing transjugular intrahepatic portosystemic stent-shunt with variceal band ligation in the prevention of rebleeding from esophageal varices. Hepatology 26:1115, 1997

72. Rouillard SS, Bass NM, Roberts JP, et al: Severe hyperbilirubinemia after creation of transjugular intrahepatic portosystemic shunts: natural history and predictors of outcome. Ann Intern Med 128:374, 1998

73. Sterling KM, Darcy MD: Stenosis of transjugular intrahepatic portosystemic shunts: presentation and management. AJR Am J Roentgenol 168:239, 1997

74. Lebrec D, Giuily N, Hadengue A, et al: Transjugular intrahepatic portosystemic shunts: comparison with paracentesis in patients with cirrhosis and refractory ascites: a randomized trial. French Group of Clinicians and a Group of Biologists. J Hepatol 25:135, 1996

75. Berk DP, Chalmers T: Deafness complicating antibiotic therapy of hepatic encephalopathy. Ann Intern Med 73:393, 1970

76. Soeters PB, Fischer JE: Insulin, glucagon, aminoacid imbalance, and hepatic encephalopathy. Lancet 2:880, 1976

77. DerSimonian R: Parenteral nutrition with branched-chain amino acids in hepatic encephalopathy: meta analysis. Hepatology 11:1083, 1990

78. Gines A, Escorsell A, Gines P, et al: Incidence, predictive factors, and prognosis of the hepatorenal syndrome in cirrhosis with ascites. Gastroenterology 105:229, 1993

79. Gonwa TA, Goldstein M, Holman M, et al: Orthotopic liver transplantation and renal function: outcome of hepatorenal syndrome and trial of verapamil for renal protection in nonhepatorenal syndrome. Transplant Proc 25:1891, 1993

80. Angeli P, Volpin R, Gerunda G, et al: Reversal of type 1 hepatorenal syndrome with the administration of midodrine and octreotide. Hepatology 29:1690, 1999

81. Nagayama M, Takai T, Okuno M, et al: Fat emulsion in surgical patients with liver disorders. J Surg Res 47:59, 1989

82. Gluud C: Branched-chain amino acids for hepatic encephalopathy? Hepatology 13:812, 1991

83. Mammen EF: Coagulopathies of liver disease. Clin Lab Med 14:769, 1994

84. Mammen EF: Coagulation defects in liver disease. Med Clin North Am 78:545, 1994

85. Mannucci PM, Franchi F, Dioguardi N: Correction of abnormal coagulation in chronic liver disease by combined use of fresh-frozen plasma and prothrombin complex concentrates. Lancet 2:542, 1976

86. Ballard HS, Marcus AJ: Platelet aggregation in portal cirrhosis. Arch Intern Med 136:316, 1976

87. Brophy MT, Fiore L, Deykin D: Hemostasis. Hepatology: A Textbook of Liver Disease. Zakim D, Boyer T, Eds. WB Saunders Co, Philadelphia, 1996, p 691

88. Hersch SL, Kunelis T, Francis RB Jr: The pathogenesis of accelerated fibrinolysis in liver cirrhosis: a critical role for tissue plasminogen activator inhibitor. Blood 69:1315, 1987

89. Riewald M, Riess H: Treatment options for clinically recognized disseminated intravascular coagulation. Semin Thromb Hemost 24:53, 1998

90. Bismuth H, Samuel D, Castaing D, et al: Liver transplantation in Europe for patients with acute liver failure. Semin Liver Dis 16:415, 1996

91. Rosen HR, Shackleton CR, Martin P: Indications for and timing of liver transplantation. Med Clin North Am 80:1069, 1996

92. Lucey MR, Brown KA, Everson GT, et al: Minimal criteria for placement of adults on the liver transplant waiting list: a report of a national conference organized by the American Society of Transplant Physicians and the American Association for the Study of Liver Diseases. Liver Transpl Surg 3:628, 1997

93. Butterworth RF: The neurobiology of hepatic encephalopathy. Semin Liver Dis 16:235, 1996

94. Ferenci P, Puspok A, Steindl P: Current concepts in the pathophysiology of hepatic encephalopathy. Eur J Clin Invest 22:573, 1992

95. Maddison JE, Watson WE, Dodd PR, et al: Alterations in cortical [3H]kainate and alpha-[3H]amino-3-hydroxy-5-methyl-4-isoxazolepropionic acid binding in a spontaneous canine model of chronic hepatic encephalopathy. J Neurochem 56:1881, 1991

96. Yurdaydin C, Walsh TJ, Engler HD, et al: Gut bacteria provide precursors of benzodiazepine receptor ligands in a rat model of hepatic encephalopathy. Brain Res 679:42, 1995

97. Jones EA, Basile AS, Skolnick P: Hepatic encephalopathy, GABA-ergic neurotransmission and benzodiazepine receptor ligands. Adv Exp Med Biol 272:121, 1990

98. Basile AS, Harrison PM, Hughes RD, et al: Relationship between plasma benzodiazepine receptor ligand concentrations and severity of hepatic encephalopathy. Hepatology 19:112, 1994

99. Takahashi K, Kameda H, Kataoka M, et al: Ammonia potentiates GABAA response in dissociated rat cortical neurons. Neurosci Lett 151:51, 1993

100. Aronson LR, Gacad RC, Kaminsky-Russ K, et al: Endogenous benzodiazepine activity in the peripheral and portal blood of dogs with congenital portosystemic shunts. Vet Surg 26:189, 1997

101. Demetriou AA, Watanabe F: Support of the Acutely Failing Liver, 2nd ed. RG Landes Co, Austin, Texas, 2000.

102. Rozga J, Holzman MD, Ro MS, et al: Development of a hybrid bioartificial liver. Ann Surg 217:502, 1993

103. Watanabe FD, Mullon CJ, Hewitt WR, et al: Clinical experience with a bioartificial liver in the treatment of severe liver failure: a phase I clinical trial. Ann Surg 225:484, 1997

104. Watanabe FD, Arnaout WS, Ting P, et al: Artificial liver. Transplant Proc 31:373, 1999

11 ENDOCRINE PROBLEMS

Robert H. Bartlett, M.D., F.A.C.S., and Preston B. Rich, M.D.

Patients scheduled for operation may be receiving treatment with insulin, oral hypoglycemics, corticosteroids, thyroid hormone, or estrogen. The presence of any state calling for such treatment must be taken into consideration in planning operative management and perioperative care. In addition, glucose intolerance may develop in otherwise normal patients after operation, and this possibility must be taken into account as well. In what follows, we describe an approach to preventing and managing common endocrine conditions that occur as complicating factors in the perioperative period. We do not, however, address perioperative problems related to operations for primary endocrine disease.

Diabetes Mellitus

Diabetics have a 50% chance of undergoing a surgical procedure during their lifetime.[1] In the past, operation in these patients was associated with a mortality of 4% to 13%,[2] usually attributed to cardiovascular complications—clearly a significant operative risk. Any subsequent improvement in diabetes-related operative mortality has probably been offset by the increasing age of patients with diabetes and the larger variety of procedures they undergo.

Perioperative management of diabetic patients [*see Figure 1*] is complicated both by the metabolic abnormalities of the disease and by the effects of any diabetic complications that may be present. There is also an increased risk of postoperative surgical site infection (SSI).

EVALUATION OF THE DIABETIC PATIENT

History and Physical Examination

In taking a preoperative history from a diabetic patient, attention should be directed to any recent fluctuation in blood glucose level as well as to the type of therapy used to control the condition. The timing and dosage of medication should be considered, especially if the patient is taking long-acting insulin or an oral hypoglycemic. The extent to which diabetes is controlled in the perioperative period, which has a significant impact on postoperative recovery, may be affected by certain medications (e.g., antihypertensive agents). The presence of diabetic complications (e.g., atherosclerotic disease, diabetic nephropathy, and autonomic neuropathy) should be documented because these conditions may have serious effects during and after operation.

Medications used to control diabetes include the various forms of insulin as well as oral hypoglycemic agents. The most commonly used oral hypoglycemics are sulfonylurea, which acts by stimulating insulin secretion, and metformin, which acts by decreasing intestinal absorption. Patients should stop taking oral hypoglycemics before major operations, and their blood glucose should be controlled with insulin if necessary. Because sudden discontinuance of sulfonylurea can lead to hypoglycemia, blood glucose levels should be carefully monitored in patients taking this medication who have experienced injury or undergone operation.

Laboratory Studies

The degree of control of diabetes can be assessed by recording blood glucose measurements at frequent intervals during fasting and at other times during the day and by determining what percentage of total hemoglobin is combined with carbohydrate (i.e., glycosylated). Normally, glycosylated hemoglobin (commonly called HbA_{1c}) accounts for 4% to 7% of total hemoglobin. HbA_{1c} levels increase when hyperglycemia occurs, and the increases are cumulative over time. The value of measuring HbA_{1c} in a preoperative patient known to be diabetic is that it gives the attending physicians some idea of how well hyperglycemic episodes are being controlled by insulin or oral hypoglycemics. Monthly measurements yield a good picture of the adequacy of glucose control over extended periods. HbA_{1c} percentages higher than 10% to 20% indicate that the hyperglycemic aspect of diabetes has been poorly controlled. Chronic diabetic complications are reduced when good control of blood glucose is maintained; diabetic patients are advised to measure their blood glucose levels frequently, which should result in normal HbA_{1c} levels. HbA_{1c} percentages higher than 15% suggest that the diabetes is quite brittle and that more frequent monitoring of blood glucose levels and closer control of insulin administration are indicated during and after operation. As long as the patient is carefully monitored, there is no evidence that high levels of HbA_{1c} are associated with any increased risk of impaired glucose control or complications after operation.

The other important laboratory study in diabetic patients is measurement of serum creatinine levels (or, perhaps, creatinine clearance) as an indicator of renal function. Renal insufficiency is a common complication of diabetes that may not be recognized during normal preoperative testing.

PREOPERATIVE MANAGEMENT

Metabolic Monitoring and Medications

All diabetic patients who are candidates for elective surgical procedures should undergo careful preoperative assessment, including metabolic monitoring. Ideally, glycemic control is achieved before a diabetic patient is admitted to the hospital. More realistically, however, admission may have to be scheduled for the day before the operation to allow time for optimizing metabolic control in all insulin-dependent patients as well as in non–insulin-dependent patients who have inadequate metabolic control. As a rule, target blood glucose levels before operation should be less than 125 mg/dl (6.9 mmol/L) during fasting and less than 180 mg/dl (10.0 mmol/L) postprandially. If emergency operation is required in patients with severe metabolic derangements (e.g., diabetic ketoacidosis or hyperosmolar nonketotic states), 6 to 8 hours of intensive treatment with insulin infusion

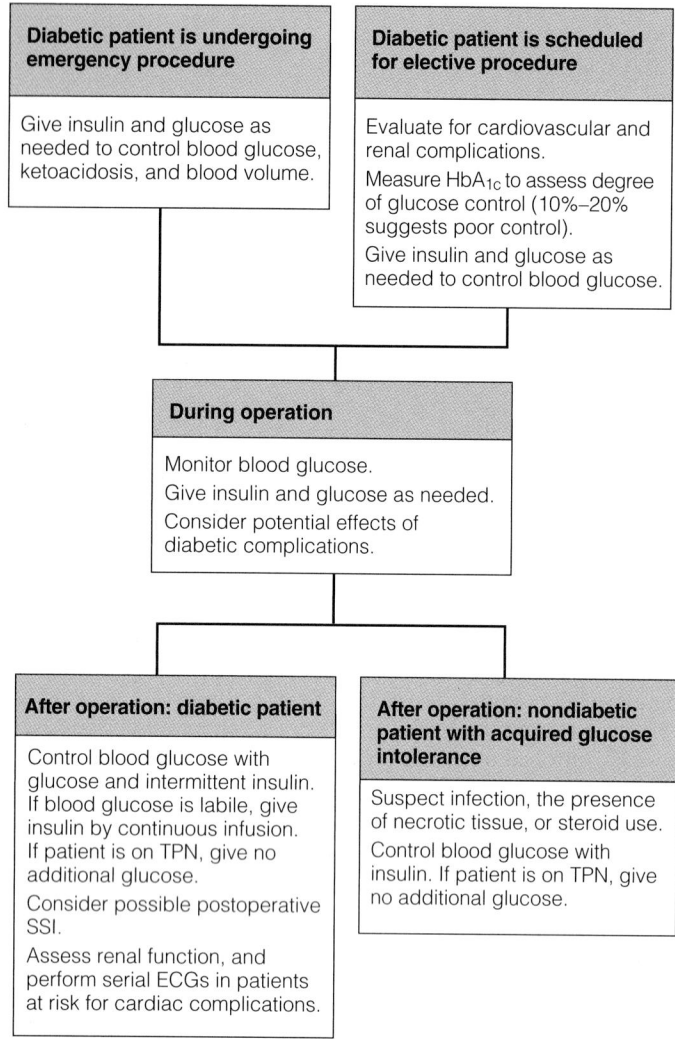

Diabetic patient is undergoing emergency procedure
Give insulin and glucose as needed to control blood glucose, ketoacidosis, and blood volume.

Diabetic patient is scheduled for elective procedure
Evaluate for cardiovascular and renal complications. Measure HbA$_{1c}$ to assess degree of glucose control (10%–20% suggests poor control). Give insulin and glucose as needed to control blood glucose.

During operation
Monitor blood glucose. Give insulin and glucose as needed. Consider potential effects of diabetic complications.

After operation: diabetic patient
Control blood glucose with glucose and intermittent insulin. If blood glucose is labile, give insulin by continuous infusion. If patient is on TPN, give no additional glucose. Consider possible postoperative SSI. Assess renal function, and perform serial ECGs in patients at risk for cardiac complications.

After operation: nondiabetic patient with acquired glucose intolerance
Suspect infection, the presence of necrotic tissue, or steroid use. Control blood glucose with insulin. If patient is on TPN, give no additional glucose.

Figure 1   **Shown is an algorithm outlining preoperative and postoperative management of the diabetic surgical patient.**

and volume restoration usually improves their general condition. This brief period permits clarification of the diagnosis in patients with acute abdominal pain, which may be the consequence of diabetic ketoacidosis rather than a so-called surgical abdomen.

In preparing diabetic patients for operation, all long-acting insulins (i.e., Ultralente preparations) should be replaced with intermediate-acting insulins (i.e., neutral protamine Hagedorn [NPH] or Lente preparations). If the patient has type 2 (non–insulin-dependent) diabetes mellitus, use of long-acting sulfonylureas (e.g., chlorpropamide and glyburide) should be stopped because of the risk of hypoglycemia; a short-acting preparation should be substituted. Use of metformin should be stopped because of the risk of lactic acidosis when renal function is impaired, as it may be during any procedure requiring anesthesia. Chronically hyperglycemic patients are frequently dehydrated, and this condition should be corrected before operation.

INTRAOPERATIVE MANAGEMENT

Metabolic Effects of Operation and Anesthesia

During anesthesia and operation, endogenous insulin secretion is suppressed, but the plasma levels of counterregulatory hormones (glucagon, epinephrine, cortisol, and growth hor-

mone) increase in nondiabetic as well as diabetic patients. Increased secretion of these hormones in the setting of low insulin levels stimulates hepatic production of glucose. In nondiabetic persons, major procedures are frequently associated with blood glucose levels of 150 to 200 mg/dl (8.3 to 11.1 mmol/L). In diabetic persons, the metabolic abnormality varies according to the extent and duration of the surgical procedure and the degree to which insulin secretion is impaired.

A study in patients with stable type 1 (insulin-dependent) diabetes mellitus showed that blood glucose levels rose from about 180 mg/dl (10.0 mmol/L) to about 270 mg/dl (15.0 mmol/L) postoperatively.[3] Ketone body levels increased by about 100%, as compared with levels in nondiabetic control subjects. Similar metabolic findings were reported even in patients with type 2 diabetes mellitus who underwent minor procedures that generated relatively little stress: blood glucose levels rose to 180 mg/dl (10.0 mmol/L), with higher than normal levels of ketone bodies and free fatty acids.[4]

Autonomic neuropathy can cause severe hypotension during induction of anesthesia. Diabetic nephropathy complicates fluid management and usually results in electrolyte abnormalities. All diabetic patients are at high risk for postoperative myocardial infarction, which is often asymptomatic. Poor nutrition and impaired phagocytosis make diabetic patients more susceptible to infection and slower to heal.

Insulin and Glucose Administration

Emergency procedures   Diabetic patients may be more likely than nondiabetic patients to undergo emergency operation, which can cause rapid metabolic decompensation with dehydration, hyperglycemia, and ketoacidosis. In addition, a surgical emergency can precipitate uncontrolled diabetes in patients with no history of diabetes. Appropriate management depends, to a large extent, on the patient's metabolic condition. When one is faced with a so-called surgical abdomen, it is crucial to determine whether there is a metabolic abnormality that may be causing the condition. Given this possibility, it is sensible to manage the patient conservatively at first, with an emphasis on metabolic correction. If the underlying problem is in fact metabolic, it should resolve or improve in 3 to 4 hours; if the problem is surgical, it should remain the same or worsen over this period.

Elective major procedures   In a patient undergoing general anesthesia, regardless of the duration of the operation, infusion of insulin and glucose is recommended if the patient is taking insulin for diabetes or is using drugs or diet therapy (or both) without achieving satisfactory control of type 2 diabetes mellitus.

Several methods of insulin administration may be used during the perioperative period. Most of the protocols include I.V. administration of short-acting insulin and 5% to 10% glucose. In some, glucose and insulin are administered together in a single infusion. The advantage of this approach is that if the glucose infusion is accidentally disconnected or obstructed, the insulin infusion is disconnected or obstructed as well, so that the risk of hypoglycemia is eliminated. The disadvantage of this method is that it is impossible to change the delivery rate of one agent without changing the delivery rate of the other. Administration of insulin and glucose in separate bags allows either infusion rate to be adjusted without the other being affected. The insulin infusion rate is progressively increased and the glucose infusion rate progressively decreased in accordance with the capillary blood glucose levels, measured hourly [*see Table 1*]. With this protocol,

Table 1 Representative Protocol for Insulin-Glucose Infusion during the Perioperative Period

1. Infuse 5% dextrose in water (D5W) I.V. via pump.

2. Make insulin solution with 0.5 U/ml of short-acting insulin (i.e., 250 U of regular insulin in 500 ml of normal saline). Administer in piggyback fashion via infusion pump into D5W infusion or through a separate I.V. site.

3. After initiating glucose-insulin infusion, stop all subcutaneous insulin therapy.

4. Measure capillary blood glucose levels every hour.

5. On the basis of hourly blood glucose levels, adjust each infusion according to the following schedule:

Blood Glucose (mg/dl)	Insulin Infusion		D5W Infusion (ml/hr)
	(ml/hr)	(U/hr)	
< 70*	1.0	0.5	150
71–100	2.0	1.0	125
101–150	3.0	1.5	100
151–200	4.0	2.0	100
201–250	6.0	3.0	100
251–300	8.0	4.0	75
> 300	12.0	6.0	50

*Give 10 ml D5W I.V. and repeat blood glucose measurement 15 min later.

a blood glucose level in the range of 125 to 200 mg/dl (6.9 to 11.1 mmol/L) can easily be maintained throughout the perioperative period. Close observation of blood glucose levels and prompt adjustment of insulin and glucose delivery are mandatory for achieving a stable blood glucose level. Electrolyte supplementation is administered via a separate infusion.

Minor procedures Diabetic patients who fast before minor operations (e.g., endoscopic procedures and operations performed with the patient under local anesthesia) should omit the morning dose of insulin or oral hypoglycemic agent, and their capillary blood glucose level should be measured every 2 to 4 hours. Supplemental subcutaneous short-acting insulin can be administered according to a variable insulin schedule, and the usual insulin or oral agent can be taken after the procedure [see Table 2]. This method of administration, which is associated with unpredictable absorption and variable plasma insulin levels, is restricted to surgical patients undergoing minor procedures and should not be used in those undergoing major operations.

POSTOPERATIVE MANAGEMENT

Insulin and Glucose Administration

After minor procedures, diabetic patients should receive I.V. glucose and insulin until their metabolic condition is stable and oral feeding can be tolerated. To prevent ketosis, the insulin and glucose infusions should be continued for at least 1 hour after the administration of subcutaneous short-acting insulin. After major procedures, patients should receive I.V. glucose and insulin until they are able to take solid food without difficulty. A regimen consisting of multiple subcutaneous injections of short-acting insulin before meals and intermediate-acting insulin twice

daily is recommended during the first 24 to 48 hours after cessation of the insulin and glucose infusions and before resumption of the patient's usual insulin regimen.

Total parenteral nutrition (TPN) [see 6:23 Nutritional Support], often required during the postoperative period, can cause serious metabolic derangements in diabetic patients. For a diabetic patient receiving TPN, a variable insulin infusion schedule [see Table 2] is recommended, with hourly determinations of blood glucose; however, additional glucose is not needed, because it is included in the TPN solution. Initially, the insulin should be given as a continuous infusion separate from the TPN solution. Once a stable dose of insulin is reached (usually within 24 to 48 hours), the total amount of insulin required over a 24-hour period can be added to the TPN bag. This amount may be high—often more than 100 units. At this point, capillary blood glucose levels can be measured every 2 to 4 hours.

Hypoglycemia can be difficult to detect in critically ill patients, in whom blood glucose levels are often elevated for any of a number of reasons. Accordingly, it has been common practice to accept blood glucose levels ranging from 150 to 200 mg/dl in these patients. This practice, however, was called into question by a 2001 randomized study of 1,548 ICU patients in which liberal glucose control (blood glucose level, 180 to 200 mg/dl) was compared with tight control (blood glucose level, 80 to 110 mg/dl).[5] ICU survival was significantly better in the tight control group (95.4%) than in the liberal control group (92%). In addition, the tight control group had a lower incidence of systemic infection, had less need of antibiotic therapy, required fewer transfusions, and were less subject to hypobilirubinemia. These findings support the view that tight regulation of glucose and insulin to maintain normal blood glucose levels is desirable in critically ill patients.

Cardiovascular and Renal Assessment

Serial postoperative electrocardiograms are recommended for older diabetic patients, those with long-standing type 1 diabetes mellitus, and those with known heart disease. Postoperative myocardial infarction, which may be silent, is associated with a high mortality. Careful monitoring of blood urea nitrogen and serum creatinine levels facilitates the detection of acute renal

Table 2 Management of Diabetes in Patients Undergoing Minor Surgical Procedures[30]

If patient fasted

1. Withhold morning dose of insulin or oral agent.

2. Measure capillary blood glucose level before procedure and every 2–4 hr thereafter.

3. Give short-acting insulin every 2–4 hr, as follows:

Blood Glucose (mg/dl)	Short-Acting Insulin (U)
< 150	0
151–200	2
201–250	3
251–300	5
> 300	6

4. After procedure, give usual dose of insulin or oral agent.

failure [*see 6.7 Renal Failure*]. If a contrast agent is used, the patient should be well hydrated before and after the procedure.

Infection

SSI is common in diabetic patients with poor metabolic control. Impaired granulocyte function resulting from hyperglycemia may predispose to bacterial infections. Autonomic neuropathy, if present, may lead to difficulty in postoperative voiding, which increases the risk of urinary tract infection. Poor circulation as a result of macroangiopathy or microangiopathy can also contribute to the likelihood of postoperative infection.

Tight metabolic control during the perioperative period can decrease the risk of postoperative infection. When SSIs do occur in the diabetic population, they are usually caused by mixed flora, including aerobic and anaerobic organisms such as *Escherichia coli*, Enterobacteriaceae, various streptococci, *Staphylococcus aureus*, and *Bacteroides fragilis*. Necrotizing infections (e.g., fasciitis, gangrene, and Fournier gangrene) are more common and spread more readily in diabetic patients.

Surgical debridement and drainage, if needed, should be performed early. Cultures should be obtained during drainage procedures. Ideally, antibiotic therapy awaits and is based on culture results; however, in practice, it is often preferable to initiate empirical therapy for the most likely organisms before the results are available. Swarming of *Proteus* organisms may obscure other pathogens on culture plates. Unless the patient is clearly manifesting a septic response, aminoglycosides should be avoided because of their nephrotoxicity and the likelihood that diabetic patients may have underlying renal disease. If severe infections do not respond to antibiotic therapy, the presence of *Candida* or other fungal species should be suspected.

Many factors play a role in the increased susceptibility of diabetics to infection, including macroangiopathy, microangiopathy, neuropathy, impaired neutrophil and lymphocyte function, increased capillary permeability, and impaired granulation and healing.[6] An obvious example of this interaction of multiple contributing factors is a chronically infected nonhealing ulcer on a neuropathic foot. A less obvious but more serious example is the failure of host defenses against peritonitis, soft tissue infection, and bacteremia that develops in diabetic patients. Chemotaxis, adherence, phagocytosis,[7] bacterial killing, and production of cytokines and complement are all impaired in patients with type 1 diabetes mellitus. The greater prominence of such abnormalities in patients with type 1 diabetes mellitus suggests that the most likely cause is related to chronic and irreversible glycosylation of many proteins, which limits the function of intracellular and intercellular messengers. The implication of this theory is that tight short- and long-term control of blood glucose should allow better control of infection.[5]

The impaired wound healing seen in diabetic patients clearly is related in part to increased susceptibility to infection; however, it is also observed with sterile wounds. Many animal studies have corroborated the clinical observation that skin, fascia, and bone all heal more slowly and with less strength in diabetic patients. Such studies have generally found that this impaired healing is partially mitigated by insulin control, which suggests that glycosylation of proteins is an important factor. A 1999 study indicated that the impaired healing is significantly mediated by endogenous corticosteroids.[8] Local application of inflammatory substances or growth factors (e.g., platelet-derived growth factor, tissue growth factor, bacterial by-products, growth hormone, and hyperosmotic sugar) has been shown to stimulate healing in diabetic animals.[6,9]

Adrenal Insufficiency

The anti-inflammatory properties of the glucocorticoid steroids [*see Table 3*] are commonly exploited to treat disease. Patients are often treated for long periods with large pharmacologic doses of steroids (commonly, prednisone by mouth) for inflammatory or autoimmune diseases such as arthritis, systemic lupus erythematosus, inflammatory bowel disease, and bronchial asthma. Primary failure of the hypothalamic-pituitary-adrenal (HPA) axis (as in Addison disease, Sheehan syndrome, and panhypopituitarism) is rare, but when it does occur, it must be treated with long-term administration of physiologic doses of corticosteroids. It is not uncommon for patients who are receiving such corticosteroid therapy to require operations, and this surgical population presents a unique perioperative management challenge [*see Figure 2*]. It is axiomatic that any patient treated with exogenous steroids may eventually manifest adrenal atrophy as a result of suppressed endogenous production of adrenocorticotropic hormone (ACTH). Actual or relative adrenal insufficiency may occur during or after a major operation, resulting in a syndrome whose manifestations can range from nausea, vomiting, fever, abdominal pain, and electrolyte abnormalities to complete circulatory collapse.

The adrenal cortex is central to the maintenance of homeostasis both at rest and during stress.[10] Cortisol, the predominant glucocorticoid hormone, is produced by the fascicular and reticular zones of the adrenal cortex. It is under the strict regulatory control of both the hypothalamus (via corticotropin-releasing hormone) and the anterior pituitary gland (via ACTH). Cortisol itself participates in its own regulation, imparting a potent negative feedback signal to both the hypothalamus and the ACTH-producing basophilic cells within the adenohypophysis of the pituitary. Together, these components, which constitute the HPA axis, form a finely regulated feedback loop for cortisol secretion.

Under unstressed physiologic conditions, the adrenal cortex constitutively produces approximately 20 to 25 mg of cortisol daily.[11] Cortisol secretion normally occurs in diurnal surges; consequently, simple measurements of serum cortisol levels in isolation generally do not suffice for accurate evaluation of the status of the HPA axis. Much of the daily variability in cortisol secretion can be tracked with 24-hour urinary measurements of the hydroxysteroid metabolites; however, there can be significant

Table 3 Selected Corticosteroid Preparations

Preparation	Equivalent Doses (mg)	Glucocorticoid Activity*	Mineralocorticoid Activity*
Short-acting (8–12 hr)			
Hydrocortisone	20	1	1
Cortisone	25	0.80	0.80
Intermediate-acting (12–36 hr)			
Prednisone	5	4	0.80
Prednisolone	5	4	0.80
Methylprednisolone	4	5	0
Triamcinolone	4	5	0
Long-acting (36–54 hr)			
Betamethasone	0.60	25	0
Dexamethasone	0.75	30	0
Mineralocorticoid			
Fludrocortisone	—	10	125

*Ranked on a scale rating hydrocortisone as 1.

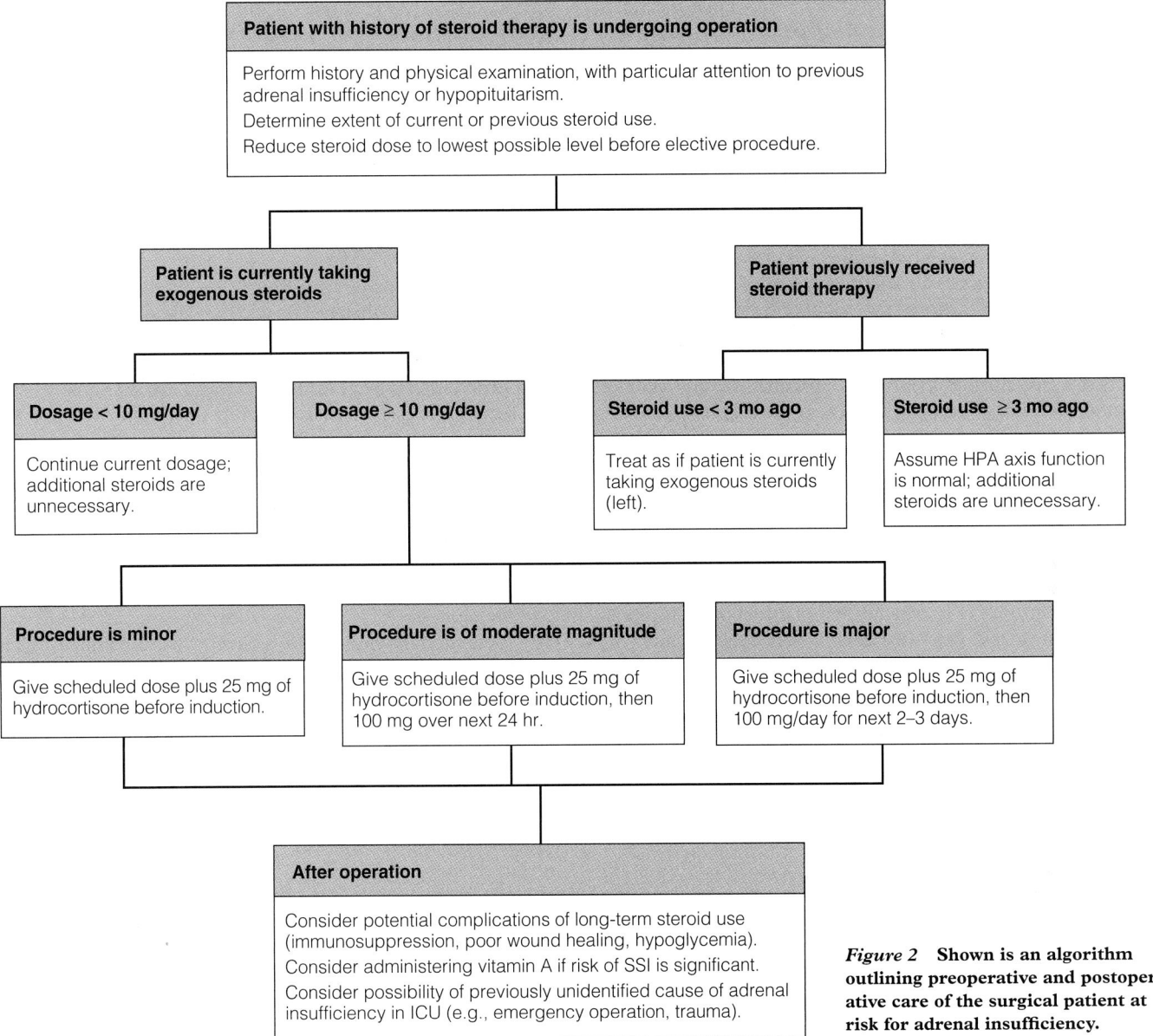

Patient with history of steroid therapy is undergoing operation

Perform history and physical examination, with particular attention to previous adrenal insufficiency or hypopituitarism.
Determine extent of current or previous steroid use.
Reduce steroid dose to lowest possible level before elective procedure.

Patient is currently taking exogenous steroids

Patient previously received steroid therapy

Dosage < 10 mg/day

Continue current dosage; additional steroids are unnecessary.

Dosage ≥ 10 mg/day

Steroid use < 3 mo ago

Treat as if patient is currently taking exogenous steroids (left).

Steroid use ≥ 3 mo ago

Assume HPA axis function is normal; additional steroids are unnecessary.

Procedure is minor

Give scheduled dose plus 25 mg of hydrocortisone before induction.

Procedure is of moderate magnitude

Give scheduled dose plus 25 mg of hydrocortisone before induction, then 100 mg over next 24 hr.

Procedure is major

Give scheduled dose plus 25 mg of hydrocortisone before induction, then 100 mg/day for next 2–3 days.

After operation

Consider potential complications of long-term steroid use (immunosuppression, poor wound healing, hypoglycemia).
Consider administering vitamin A if risk of SSI is significant.
Consider possibility of previously unidentified cause of adrenal insufficiency in ICU (e.g., emergency operation, trauma).

Figure 2 **Shown is an algorithm outlining preoperative and postoperative care of the surgical patient at risk for adrenal insufficiency.**

overlap between normal patients and those with clinical adrenal insufficiency.[12] Provocative testing of the HPA axis is based on the normal physiologic response of the adrenal gland to release cortisol in a receptor-mediated G-protein–coupled response to circulating ACTH.

Although there is some controversy regarding which laboratory evaluation is the best predictor of adequate adrenal response to a surgical stress, it is clear that ACTH stimulatory testing is more sensitive and specific than unprovoked steroid measurement alone. Hypoglycemia-induced release of ACTH in response to exogenous insulin infusion (the insulin tolerance test, or ITT) has long been considered the gold standard for determination of relative adrenal insufficiency, but various complications, including discomfort, seizures, and even death, limit its clinical usefulness as a routinely applied test.[13] In several studies, strong correlations have been observed between the ITT and adrenal stimulation with a synthetic corticotropin construct.[14,15] In this test, the plasma cortisol response is measured 0, 30, and 60 minutes after infusion of 250 μg of the ACTH analogue. Although there is no unanimously accepted cutoff value for stim-

ulated cortisol levels above which the HPA axis can be assumed to be intact, it has been suggested that a value higher than 600 mol/L at 30 minutes should be a sufficiently sensitive confirmation of an intact HPA axis.

Adrenal glucocorticoids are important modulators of the stress response: they play a complex role in the metabolic pathways for carbohydrates, fats, and proteins; modulate gluconeogenesis and lipolysis; mediate insulin resistance; and exert a host of well-documented effects on inflammation and wound healing. It is clear that physiologic stresses (e.g., burns, trauma, and iatrogenic tissue damage occurring during operations) result in an ACTH-induced surge in the adrenal steroid response.[16,17] Serum measurements reveal that this response can produce cortisol elevations several times greater than those produced under basal conditions. It is becoming apparent that although this exaggerated adrenal stress response may have conferred a certain evolutionary benefit, prolonged exposure to high doses of steroids may nonetheless have deleterious consequences. The potential complications of long-term or high-dose administration of glucocorticoids are well described: they include hypertension, cataracts, myopathy (especially when glucocorticoids are used in conjunction with nondepolarizing paralytic drugs), osteonecrosis (particularly on the femoral head), impaired wound healing, and immunosuppression.[18]

It was the observed (and presumably physiologic) magnitude of the cortisol response to stress that led to the long-held—albeit never corroborated—assumption that supraphysiologic levels of steroids were required to maintain homeostasis in the stressed environment. In the 1950s, two case reports were published that described perioperative deaths thought to result from untreated and unrecognized adrenal insufficiency.[19,20] Thereafter, it became common practice to supply supraphysiologic doses of exogenous steroids (i.e., doses two to three times that expected under basal conditions) to patients believed to be at risk for adrenal suppression and therefore unable to mount the expected cortisol surge during operation. Subsequently, this practice came under scrutiny. Primary studies suggested that although HPA suppression could occur as a result of long-term steroid use, normal physiologic replacement doses were sufficient to maintain perioperative homeostasis; supraphysiologic doses were unnecessary.[21] The concept that significantly lower doses of steroids are required to maintain homeostasis and normotension in the perioperative period than was once believed has been supported by prospective clinical studies in humans.[22]

It is clear that ACTH is not only stimulatory but also trophic for the adrenal cortex. There is evidence that if the adrenal cortex is not exposed to ACTH, it is subject to hyposecretion and anatomic atrophy. It was once thought that exposure to even low doses of steroids (< 10 mg of prednisone equivalent) was sufficient to suppress the endogenous release of ACTH and thus to result in a state of adrenal insufficiency. This belief led to the common practice of administering so-called stress-dose steroids to surgical patients who had received exogenous steroids even in small doses or as long ago as 1 year before operation. Provocative studies on patients previously exposed to steroids demonstrated that the HPA axis usually remains intact despite either ongoing exposure to small doses of exogenous steroids (< 10 mg of prednisone equivalent daily) or earlier steroid use (if the time since discontinuance was longer than 2 to 3 months).[23-26]

In summary, the glucocorticoids are essential components of human homeostasis both at rest and under stressful conditions such as occur during surgery. Complete or even relative adrenal insufficiency is preventable; when it does occur, it can have disastrous consequences if not recognized and appropriately treated. Exogenous administration of steroids in sufficient doses is generally adequate to prevent the syndrome of adrenal insufficiency. The decision to administer supplemental perioperative steroids should be based on the specific details of the history of steroid use as well as on the magnitude of the proposed operation.

Hormone Replacement

Many surgical patients are receiving thyroid or ovarian hormone replacement therapy. In addition, the use of growth hormone, growth hormone precursors, and anabolic steroids has become more common in general practice. The effects of these hormone medications must be taken into account in any patient undergoing an elective or emergency operation. Because all of these substances have long half-lives, replacement is not necessary for the first 2 weeks after operation; however, if the illness or the operation itself prevents oral intake for more than 2 weeks, the possibility of hypothyroidism or estrogen depletion should be considered. Postoperative weakness, lack of energy, depression, and sleeping disorders can all be caused by the lack of long-term hormone supplements.

Some patients exhibit decreased endogenous thyroid function after operation, either because their thyroid-stimulating hormone (TSH) levels are depressed as a consequence of long-term thyroid medication or because they experience complications and become critically ill. Critical illness typically leads to reduced blood levels of triiodothyronine (T_3) and thyroxine (T_4). In addition, glucocorticoids, radiopaque dyes, propranolol, and amiodarone all lower plasma T_4 levels,[27] and dopamine decreases TSH secretion directly.[28] Most critically ill patients, however, do not exhibit metabolic or hemodynamic changes indicative of hypothyroidism. Measurement of TSH is helpful for determining the significance of thyroid function in critically ill patients. If the serum TSH level is lower than 5 μU/ml and the patient is not on high-dose dopamine therapy, thyroid function is considered adequate regardless of other plasma markers. If the TSH level is higher than 20 μU/ml, replacement with thyroxine is indicated.[29]

References

1. Root HF: Preoperative medical care of the diabetic patient. Postgrad Med 40:439, 1966

2. Galloway JA, Shuman CR: Diabetes and surgery: a study of 667 cases. Am J Med 34:177, 1963

3. Walts LF, Miller J, Davidson MB, et al: Perioperative management of diabetes mellitus. Anesthesiology 55:104, 1981

4. Thompson J, Husband DJ, Thai AC, et al: Metabolic changes in the non-insulin-dependent diabetic undergoing minor surgery: effect of glucose-insulin-potassium infusion. Br J Surg 73:301, 1986

5. van den Berghe G, Wouters P, Weekers F, et al: Intensive insulin therapy in critically ill patients. N Engl J Med 345:1359, 2001

6. Kamal K, Powell RJ, Sumpio BE: The pathobiology of diabetes mellitus: implications for surgeons. J Am Coll Surg 183:271, 1996

7. Davidson NJ, Snowden JM, Fletcher J: Defective phagocytosis in insulin controlled diabetics: evidence for a reaction between glucose and opsonizing proteins. J Clin Pathol 37:783, 1984

8. Bitar MS, Farook T, Wahid S, et al: Glucocorticoid dependent impairment of wound healing in experimental diabetes: amelioration by adrenalectomy and RU486. J Surg Res 82:234, 1999

9. Qiu JG, Chang TH, Steinberg JJ, et al: Single local installation of Staphylococcus aureus peptidoglycan prevents diabetes impaired wound healing. Wound Repair Regen 6:449, 1998

10. Orth DN, Kovacs WJ: The adrenal cortex. Williams Textbook of Endocrinology, 9th ed. Wilson JD, Foster DW, Kronenberg HM, et al, Eds. WB Saunders Co, Philadelphia, 1998, p 517

11. White PC, Pescovitz OH, Cutler GB: Synthesis and metabolism of corticosteroids. Principles and Practice of Endocrinology and Metabolism, 2nd ed. Becker KL, Ed. JB Lippincott Co, Philadelphia, 1995, p 647

12. Moore A, Aitken R, Burke C, et al: Cortisol assays: guidelines for the provision of clinical biochemistry service. Ann Clin Biochem 22:435, 1985

13. Jacobs HS, Nabarro JDN: Tests of hypothalamic-pituitary-adrenal function in man. Q J Med 38:475, 1969

14. Kehlet H, Binder C: Value of an ACTH test in assessing hypothalamic-pituitary-adrenocortical function in glucocorticoid-treated patients. BMJ 2:147, 1973

15. Clayton RN: Short Synacthen test versus insulin stress test for assessment of the hypothalamo-pituitary-adrenal axis: controversy revisited. Clin Endocrinol 44:147, 1996

16. Chernow B, Alexander R, Smallridge RC, et al: Hormonal responses to graded surgical stress. Arch Intern Med 147:1273, 1987

17. Hume DM, Bell CC, Bartter F: Direct measurement of adrenal secretion during operative trauma and convalescence. Surgery 52:174, 1962

18. Dujovne CA, Azarnoff DL: Clinical complica-

tions of corticosteroid therapy: a selected review. Med Clin North Am 57:1331, 1973

19. Fraser CG, Preuss FS, Bigford WD: Adrenal atrophy and irreversible shock associated with cortisone therapy. JAMA 149:1542, 1952

20. Lewis L, Robinson RF, Yee J, et al: Fatal adrenal cortical insufficiency precipitated by surgery during prolonged continuous cortisone treatment. Ann Intern Med 39:116, 1953

21. Udelsman R, Ramp J, Gallucci WT, et al: Adaptation during surgical stress: a re-evaluation of the role of glucocorticoids. J Clin Invest 77:1377, 1986

22. Symreng T, Karlberg BE, Kagedal B, et al: Physiological cortisol substitution of long-term steroid-treated patients undergoing major surgery. Br J Anesth 53:949, 1981

23. Bromberg JS, Baliga P, Cofer JB, et al: Stress steroids are not required for patients receiving a renal allograft and undergoing operation. J Am Coll Surg 180:532, 1995

24. Bromberg JS, Alfrey EJ, Barker CF, et al: Adrenal suppression and steroid supplementation in renal transplant recipients. Transplantation 51:385, 1991

25. Livanou T, Ferriman D, James VHT: Recovery of hypothalamo-pituitary adrenal function after corticosteroid therapy. Lancet 2:856, 1967

26. LaRochelle G, LaRochelle AG, Ratner RE, et al: Recovery of the hypothalamic-pituitary-adrenal (HPA) axis in patients with rheumatic diseases receiving low-dose prednisone. Am J Med 95:258, 1993

27. Wartofsky L, Burman KD: Alterations in thyroid function in patients with systemic illness: "the euthyroid sick syndrome." Endocr Rev 3:164, 1982

28. Kaptein EM, Spencer CA, Kamiel MD, et al: Prolonged dopamine administration and thyroid hormone economy in normal and critically ill subjects. J Clin Endocrinol Metab 51:387, 1980

29. Burman KD: Thyroid hormones. Pharmacologic Approach to the Critically Ill Patient. Chernow B, Ed. Williams & Wilkins, Baltimore, 1983, chap 30

30. Surgery: practical guidelines for diabetes management. Clin Diabetes 5:49, 1987

12 COMA, SEIZURES, COGNITIVE IMPAIRMENT, AND BRAIN DEATH

Marike Zwienenberg-Lee, M.D., and J. Paul Muizelaar, M.D., Ph.D.

Management of the Patient with Altered Consciousness

Every clinician will at some point encounter a patient who is in an altered state of consciousness. Altered consciousness is not a disease per se but rather a symptom of some underlying process. It is variable in degree, ranging from mere confusion to deep coma.

Consciousness depends on both the reticular activating system (RAS), which is responsible for general alertness, and the cerebral cortex, which is responsible for the quality of behavior. The integrity of the cerebral hemispheres, the RAS, and the connections between them is essential for the maintenance of conscious behavior.

Coma is thought to result from a lesion to the hemispheres, the RAS, or both and may be caused by structural or toxic metabolic abnormalities. Specific causes of coma are numerous and include alcohol and drug intoxication, epilepsy, infection, uremia and other metabolic disorders, head injury, cerebral tumors, hypothermia, psychiatric disorders, and stroke and other vascular diseases. Accordingly, the management of coma is complex. In what follows, we discuss the various underlying causes of coma and provide general and specific guidelines.

Loss of consciousness associated with seizure activity is thought to result from a global disturbance of electrochemical activity that involves both hemispheres. Brain death represents the extreme end of the spectrum of altered consciousness and results when the loss of cerebral and brain-stem function is irreversible. Management of seizures and determination of brain death are discussed separately from management of coma.

Cognitive impairment is common in surgical patients, particularly in those who undergo major surgical procedures. The degree and nature of impairment are dependent on the underlying disease and the presence of precipitating factors, which may range from communication deficits, anxiety, and sleep deprivation to drug withdrawal, metabolic disturbances, and infection. Cornerstones of management include identification and alleviation of risk factors as well as recognition of frequent causes of cognitive impairment, such as delirium, depression, and dementia.

Often, little information is available about the circumstances leading to the disturbance in consciousness or about the patient's medical history. It is therefore essential that the surgeon follow a systematic management approach that quickly establishes the etiology and prevents unnecessary delay in initiating appropriate treatment.

Initial Management of the Comatose Patient

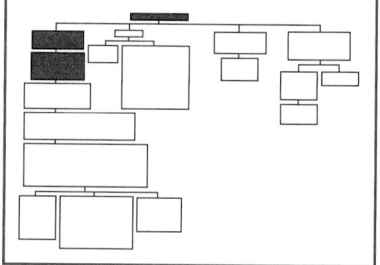

Initial management of the comatose patient is aimed at stabilization of the patient's condition and prevention of further central nervous system damage. The immediately occurring damage that is preventable results from cerebral hypoxia, ischemia, and low blood glucose levels. Therefore, initial evaluation and treatment of the comatose patient must be carried out simultaneously: the airway (A), breathing (B), and circulation (C) must be assessed and controlled, and hypoglycemia must be excluded or corrected. Attention should then be directed toward treatment of specific causes of coma, such as seizures, drug or alcohol overdose, head injury, or infection. Specific questions regarding medical history, recent changes in behavior, use of medications or drugs, recent trauma, and history of seizures must be asked so that the events leading to coma can be reconstructed. If the cause of coma remains elusive, the physical and neurologic examinations may yield clues that clarify the underlying etiology. In addition, laboratory tests and diagnostic imaging methods, such as computed tomography and magnetic resonance imaging, can provide important information for establishing a diagnosis and instituting proper treatment.

AIRWAY

To ensure adequate oxygenation and ventilation, the patient's airway must be cleared of all foreign material, the patency of the airway must be verified, and oxygen must be administered. The spontaneous rate and rhythm of respiration should be noted before they are obscured by therapeutic measures. The respiratory pattern is a good indicator of the depth of depression and the etiology of the coma [see Physical and Neurologic Examinations, below].

BREATHING

An oropharyngeal or nasopharyngeal airway may suffice in unresponsive patients who are breathing normally; however, endotracheal intubation is indicated in patients who are dyspneic, hypoventilating, or vomiting uncontrollably. Hyperventilation with a bag and mask and 100% oxygen should be performed before intubation to ensure adequate oxygenation during the procedure. If there is any possibility of a cervical spine injury, intubation should be delayed until fracture can be ruled out radiographically. If, however, the patient's condition is such that delay is inadvisable, intubation should be done without manipulation of the spine. In patients with head injury who are at risk for basilar skull fractures, the oropharyngeal route is preferred for intubation. In these patients, an aggressive approach to early intubation is usually indicated because hypoxia aggravates brain injury. In the Traumatic Coma Data Bank study, mortality was almost twice as high among hypoxic patients as among nonhypoxic patients (50% versus 27%).[1] It should be noted, however, that hypoxia alone adds little to mortality; it is the combination of ischemia and hypoxia that appears to be responsible for the increase in mortality.

CIRCULATION

Because substrate delivery to the brain is dependent on the cardiovascular system, circulation must be vigorously supported. A large-bore I.V. or central venous catheter is inserted, and blood volume is replenished with fluids or volume expanders. Solutions that contain free water (e.g., 5% dextrose in water) should be avoided, particularly in patients with head injury, because they may exacerbate brain edema. Vasoactive agents are infused if necessary. An electrocardiographic monitor is placed, and cardiac rate and rhythm are recorded. When vasopressor therapy is instituted, insertion of a pulmonary catheter is recommended in elderly patients or in patients with current or past cardiopulmonary disease. In patients suffering from head injury, hypotension and shock rarely result from a cerebral lesion; their presence should alert the physician to seek a source of extracorporeal or intracorporeal hemorrhage. However, when hypertension is present in these patients, it should be left untreated because it is likely to be an adaptive response (i.e., part of the Cushing response) of the brain to the increase in intracranial pressure (ICP) [see 5:2 Injuries to the Central Nervous System].

LABORATORY SCREENING

As soon as the venous line is in place, blood specimens are obtained for laboratory screening. The following tests and measurements should be performed:

1. Complete blood count.
2. Serum electrolyte (Na, K, Cl, CO_2, Ca, PO_4) levels.
3. Blood urea nitrogen level.
4. Creatinine level.
5. Glucose level.
6. Liver function tests.
7. Osmolarity.
8. Toxic screen (including drugs and alcohol).

GLUCOSE
ADMINISTRATION

Glucose is the basic substrate for cerebral metabolism. Even a transient decrease in oxidative metabolism of glucose may lead to an abrupt disruption of brain function. Blood glucose levels should be assessed by

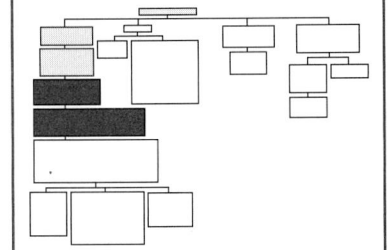

means of a rapid bedside technique and verified in the laboratory. If the bedside determination yields a low value (< 40 to 60 mg/dl) or cannot be done immediately, 50 mg of a 50% glucose solution is administered I.V., even if laboratory verification of the blood glucose

level is not yet available. The risk of hypoglycemic cerebral damage outweighs the risk of temporary worsening of the rare case of hyperosmolar coma. Many patients admitted to the emergency ward while in coma are chronic alcoholics or malnourished and thus are prone to Wernicke encephalopathy, which is caused by thiamine deficiency and can be precipitated by a large glucose load. To prevent acute symptomatic thiamine deficiency, 50 to 100 mg of thiamine should be given I.V. to all patients before glucose is administered. Afterward, 100 mg is given I.M. every day for 3 days.

Physical and Neurologic Examinations

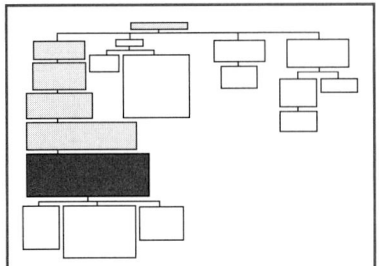

When the necessary resuscitative measures have been initiated, the next step is to perform basic physical and neurologic examinations. These examinations should be brief yet sufficiently thorough to yield the key information required for further evaluation and treatment. The physical examination should focus on signs of trauma, chronic disease (e.g., alcoholism or renal failure), infection, or self-administration of drugs. The neurologic examination should focus on diagnosing those conditions that call for rapid treatment, such as the following:

1. Lateralizing signs in trauma patients.
2. Signs of an increase in ICP.
3. Meningism.
4. Seizures.

LEVEL OF CONSCIOUSNESS

The patient's level of consciousness is assessed by means of the Glasgow Coma Scale (GCS), which is widely accepted as the standard method [see 5:2 Injuries to the Central Nervous System]. The GCS consists of three components: eye opening (E), motor function (M), and verbal response (V) [see Table 1]. The score on each component is assessed by recording the response of the patient to verbal or noxious stimuli, such as pressure on the supraorbital notch or compression of the distal interphalangeal joints; the total GCS score is the sum of the scores of these three components [see Table 1]. The maximum GCS score is 15, and the minimum score is 3. Coma is usually defined as a GCS score of 9 or less.

A persistent misconception about the GCS, which results from equating abnormal flexion with so-called decorticate rigidity and extensor response with so-called decerebrate rigidity, is that the type of motor response corresponds to the level of the lesion. In this view, decorticate rigidity would indicate a lesion affecting the hemispheres or the diencephalon, and decerebrate rigidity would suggest a lesion affecting the midbrain or the brain stem, as shown in the Sherrington preparations.[2,3] It is now clear, however, that in patients with head injury, decerebrate motor posturing and prolonged coma are not associated with brain-stem dysfunction but rather with dysfunction of the hemispheres.[4] Therefore, we prefer to use the terms abnormal flexion and extension or flexor and extensor posturing instead of the terms decorticate and decerebrate rigidity.

LOCALIZING OR LATERALIZING SIGNS

The presence of localizing or lateralizing signs suggests that the underlying abnormality of coma is structural (i.e., caused by a focal lesion) rather than metabolic. Rapid radiologic evaluation (CT scan) is essential in these cases, particularly in patients with head injuries who may harbor an expanding intracranial hematoma, for which

Patient is in state of altered consciousness

Patient is in coma

Coma is defined as a sleeplike state of continuous unarousable unresponsiveness in which there is no spontaneous activity.

Ensure adequate ventilation and circulatory support. Obtain specimens for laboratory screening:
- CBC
- Serum electrolytes
- BUN
- Creatinine
- Glucose
- Liver function tests
- Osmolarity
- Toxic screen

Administer glucose and thiamine

Assess glucose level by bedside technique. If level is low or not immediately obtainable, give 50 mg of 50% glucose solution I.V. immediately. Before glucose administration, give 50–100 mg of thiamine I.V., followed by 100 mg I.M. daily for 3 days.

Patient has seizure

Seizure is self-limited

Emergency treatment is not required.

Tonic-clonic seizure persists

Treat status epilepticus:
- Obtain quick history and perform physical examination while assistant draws blood and inserts venous line.
- Perform bedside blood glucose determination. If glucose < 60 mg/dl or not immediately available, infuse dextrose (50 ml of 50% solution for adults and 1–2 ml/kg of 25% solution for children).
- Give adult patients 100 mg thiamine I.V.
- Correct hyponatremia with 3% NaCl solution in slow I.V. infusion.
- Give calcium (1–2 ampules of calcium gluconate for 5–10 min) if necessary.

Administer anticonvulsants in the following sequence:
- Phenytoin
- Benzodiazepines
- Phenobarbital

Last resort: general anesthesia or pentobarbital-induced coma

Manage intoxication

Provide early intubation and respiratory support; maintain normal BP. Perform gastric lavage if
- Ingestion occurred within 4 hr (or within 10 hr for salicylates), or
- Patient has been in shock, or
- Time of ingestion is not known.

Excretion of toxins can be facilitated with catharsis, diuresis, dialysis, or charcoal hemoperfusion. Give antidotes (if known).

Perform basic physical and neurologic examinations

Physical: Search for signs of trauma, systemic illness, infection, or drug ingestion.
Neurologic: Ascertain cause of coma and site of impairment. Differentiate between anatomic and structural lesions:
- Presence of lateralizing signs suggests structural lesion.
- Presence of pupillary light response is an important feature of metabolic coma, except in cases of drug ingestion or prolonged anoxia.
- Absence of pulillary response to light suggests structural lesion.
- Decorticate posturing suggests structural lesion; decerebrate rigidity may be caused by structural or metabolic coma (posturing has little diagnostic value after the acute phase of the coma).
If structural coma is suspected, the clinical diagnosis may be confirmed by appropriate imaging studies (CT or MRI).

Metabolic coma

Restore acid-base balance.
Restore electrolyte balance.
Restore normal body temperature.

Treat underlying conditions:
- Hypoxia
- Hypoglycemia or hyperglycemia
- Infection
- Overdose
- Specific disease process

Structural coma

Treat structural lesions. Determine severity of symptoms and rapidity of their evolution as soon as possible.
If patient is stable, obtain CT scan or MRI urgently: perform contrast study (CT or MRI) if structural lesion is suspected on the basis of noncontrast studies. If patient is deeply comatose or symptoms are evolving rapidly, treat elevated ICP urgently:
- Hyperventilate patient to P_aco_2 of 25–30 mm Hg.
- Give osmotic diuretics (e.g., 0.25 –1.5 g/kg of 20% mannitol solution I.V.).
- If patient does not have severe intracranial hypertension, consider elevating head of bed 30°–50°.
- If patient does not respond to hyperventilation or mannitol, consider barbiturate administration or, if possible, ventriculostomy.

Other causes of coma and similar syndromes

Alternative causes of coma and coma-resembling states include hypothermia, psychiatric disorders, persistant vegetative states, and locked-in syndrome.
Treat causative conditions as appropriate.

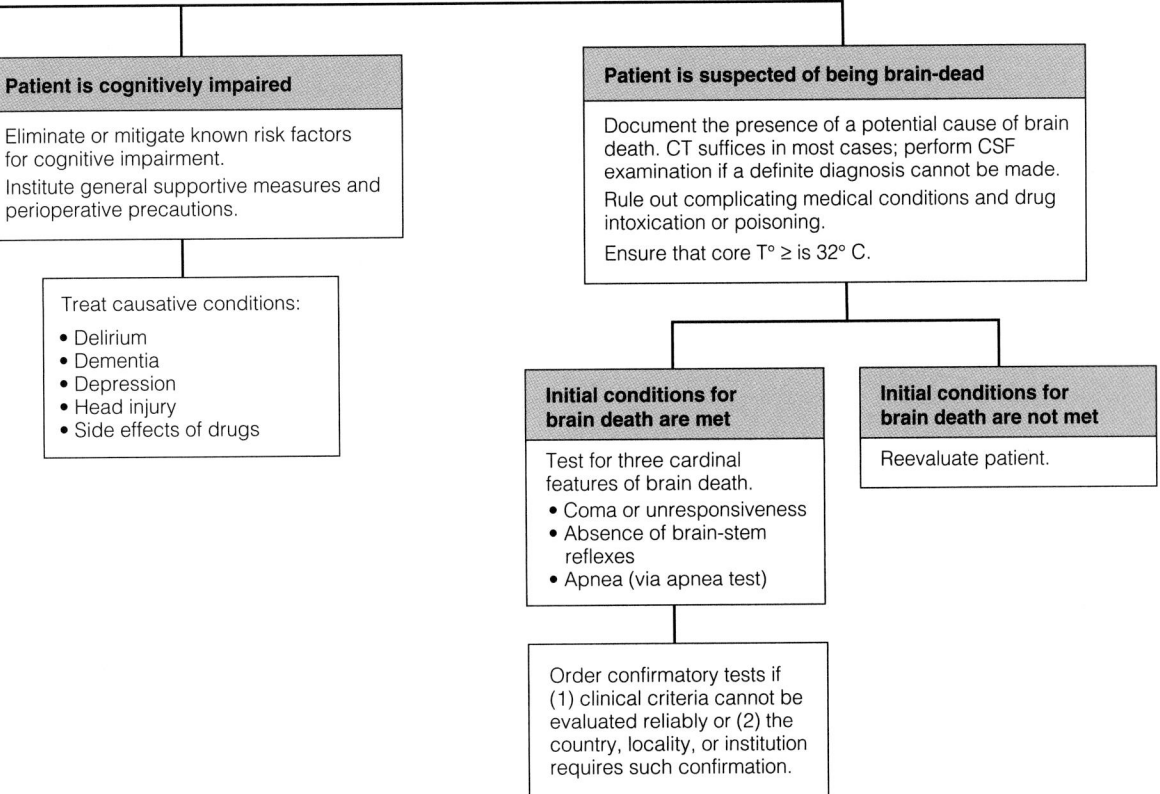

Patient is cognitively impaired

Eliminate or mitigate known risk factors for cognitive impairment.

Institute general supportive measures and perioperative precautions.

Treat causative conditions:
- Delirium
- Dementia
- Depression
- Head injury
- Side effects of drugs

Patient is suspected of being brain-dead

Document the presence of a potential cause of brain death. CT suffices in most cases; perform CSF examination if a definite diagnosis cannot be made.

Rule out complicating medical conditions and drug intoxication or poisoning.

Ensure that core T° ≥ is 32° C.

Initial conditions for brain death are met

Test for three cardinal features of brain death.
- Coma or unresponsiveness
- Absence of brain-stem reflexes
- Apnea (via apnea test)

Order confirmatory tests if (1) clinical criteria cannot be evaluated reliably or (2) the country, locality, or institution requires such confirmation.

Initial conditions for brain death are not met

Reevaluate patient.

Management of the Patient
with Altered Consciousness

Table 1 Glasgow Coma Scale[80]

Test	Response	Score
Eye opening (E)	Spontaneous	4
	To verbal command	3
	To pain	2
	None	1
Best motor response (arm) (M)	Obedience to verbal command	6
	Localization of painful stimulus	5
	Flexion withdrawal response to pain	4
	Abnormal flexion response to pain (decorticate rigidity)	3
	Extension response to pain (decerebrate rigidity)	2
	None	1
Best verbal response (V)	Oriented conversation	5
	Disoriented conversation	4
	Inappropriate words	3
	Incomprehensible sounds	2
	None	1
	Total (E + M + V)	3–15

rapid surgical intervention is indicated. Patients are observed for asymmetrical movements of the extremities, which may occur spontaneously or in response to noxious stimuli. They are also evaluated for asymmetry of tone and reflexes, with special attention paid to such signs as unilateral flaccidity, spasticity, clonus, or Babinski signs. Most comatose patients, however, will have bilateral Babinski signs regardless of the cause of their condition.

PUPILLARY SIZE AND RESPONSE

The pathways involved in the pupillary response to light are relatively resistant to most metabolic causes of coma; unless the patient is under the influence of certain drugs, this response is preserved until the near-terminal stages of metabolic coma. Consequently, the presence or absence of the pupillary light reflex is the most useful single sign for distinguishing metabolic causes of coma from structural causes. Both the size of the pupil and its direct and consensual response to light should be noted.

Bilateral reactive constricted pupils are most often seen in patients in metabolic coma. Pinpoint pupils are indicative of either a pontine lesion or an overdose of narcotics; the latter is more likely if the pupillary constriction is reversed when naloxone is administered. Fixed dilated pupils can be the result of an intrinsic midbrain lesion or, more commonly, damage to the parasympathetic fibers accompanying the third nerve in its intracranial course. Unilateral pupillary dilatation usually indicates an ipsilateral mass and is typically a sign of uncal herniation when associated with contralateral hemiplegia. Rarely, unilateral pupillary dilatation is associated with ipsilateral hemiplegia as a result of a mass that compresses the cerebral peduncle of the midbrain against the opposite tentorial margin (Kernohan's notch). Bilateral fixed dilated pupils indicate severe midbrain damage, usually from transtentorial herniation. Fixed midposition pupils are the result of injury at the midbrain level, which impairs both sympathetic (dilatation) and parasympathetic (constriction) outflow.

It has been suggested that a decrease in brain-stem blood flow, rather than direct mechanical compression of the third cranial nerve, may be a cause of mydriasis after severe head injury.[5] The investigators measured cerebral blood flow (CBF) in the brain stems of 162 patients with severe head injury and correlated these findings with pupillary response. Brain-stem blood flow was significantly lower in patients with bilateral nonreactive pupils than in patients with responsive pupils, indicating that decreased pupillary reactivity may be the result of brain-stem ischemia. This hypothesis is supported by a subsequent study documenting significantly decreased brain-stem CBF and absent pupillary response in the presence of transtentorial herniation, both of which findings were reversed after administration of hypertonic saline.[6]

EYE MOVEMENTS

Eye movements are of major importance in the physical diagnosis of coma because they involve pathways that stretch through a large part of the brain and the brain stem. In conscious patients, eye movements are either voluntary—that is, controlled by the hemispheres—or dictated by superimposed involuntary brain-stem reflexes (which in turn are influenced by afferent impulses from the labyrinth and the vestibular nuclei). In deeply comatose patients, spontaneous eye movements are usually absent; however, they may occur even in the absence of functioning frontal or occipital cortices, in which case they generally take the form of conjugate horizontal roving. This movement indicates that the midbrain and the pontine tegmentum are spared. Ocular bobbing, a brisk downward and slow upward conjugate motion of the globes, is an indication of bilateral pontine damage. Conjugate lateral deviation of the eyes suggests the presence of either an ipsilateral hemispheric lesion or a contralateral pontine lesion. Seizures may cause sustained eye deviation, in which the eyes look away from the seizure focus and exhibit rhythmic, jerky movements in the direction of the deviation.

In drowsy patients, divergence of eye positions in the horizontal plane is normal; it disappears when consciousness returns or the coma deepens. An adducted eye signals sixth-nerve palsy or pontine damage. Unilateral or bilateral sixth-nerve palsy may be associated with increased ICP. An abducted eye signals third-nerve palsy. Skew deviation, in which the eyes are not in the same horizontal plane, is usually the result of pontine or cerebellar damage.

BRAIN-STEM REFLEXES

If spontaneous eye movements are absent, the integrity of the brain stem can be assessed by means of the so-called doll's-eyes maneuver or the caloric test. These tests are based on the observation that brain-stem reflexes become hyperactive when they are released from hemispheric inhibitory influences, as in coma or sleep. The anatomic pathways involved in these brain-stem reflexes arise from the upper cervical spinal cord and the medulla (the sources of vestibular and proprioceptive input from head turning) and from the inner ear via the vestibular and sixth nerves. The fibers then pass through the contralateral medial longitudinal fasciculus to the level of the third nerve in the midbrain.

The doll's-eyes maneuver tests the oculocephalic reflex. When coma is caused by hemispheric disease and the brain stem is intact, the doll's-eyes maneuver yields horizontal conjugate deviation of the eye in the direction opposite the direction of rotation, flexion, or extension; thus, the gaze remains stationary as the head is turned. When the brain stem is dysfunctional, there is no such deviation of the eyes; thus, the gaze does not remain stationary but moves as the head is turned. The connection between the vestibular nuclei and the third, fourth, and sixth cranial nerves, which is termed the medial longitudinal fasciculus, is interrupted. As a result, the oculocephalic reflexes are impaired, so that patients with bilateral lesions are unable to maintain a stationary gaze as the head is turned and those with unilateral lesions are unable to turn their gaze toward the side on which the lesion is located.

The caloric test is used to evaluate the oculovestibular reflex. It yields much the same information as the doll's-eyes maneuver; however, it is a stronger stimulus to reflex eye movements and therefore should be performed only if the doll's-eyes maneuver yields negative results. The patient's head is elevated 30°, and the external auditory canal is irrigated with 20 to 50 ml of ice water. The ice-water injection generates convection currents in the endolymph of the labyrinth that inhibit the normal spontaneous firing of the vestibular nerve. If the coma is caused by hemispheric disease and the brain stem is intact, the normal response is sustained conjugate deviation of the eyes toward the side of the irrigated ear. Structural brain-stem lesions may abolish these responses, as may an overdose of a sedative, a hypnotic, or phenytoin. Disconjugate ocular deviation suggests the presence of either a unilateral brain-stem lesion or a metabolic depression of the brain-stem pathways. Failure of one or both eyes to adduct indicates that the lesion is located in the medial longitudinal fasciculus or the third cranial nerve. Failure to abduct signals a sixth-nerve lesion.

Other brain-stem reflexes are the corneal reflex and the gag reflex. The corneal reflex is mediated by the fifth and seventh cranial nerves and is elicited by briefly striking the corneal surface with a piece of cotton wool twisted to a point. Both eyes should blink quickly in response to this stimulus. Bilateral absence of the corneal reflex usually suggests a deep coma, and unilateral absence of the reflex indicates an ipsilateral lesion. The gag reflex is elicited by stimulating the back of the throat or by passing a suction tube down the endotracheal tube while the patient is intubated. In unconscious patients who are at risk for aspiration, this reflex should be elicited only when the airway is protected (i.e., when the endotracheal cuff is inflated). The sensory stimulus is relayed via the ninth cranial nerve, but the 10th cranial nerve mediates the resulting palatal movement. A depressed or absent gag reflex usually indicates significant brain-stem pathology.

RESPIRATION

Respiration is dependent on neural influences arising from nearly every level of the brain, from the forebrain to the upper cervical spinal cord. Oxygenation and acid-base balance are primarily regulated in the lower brain stem. If the function of the hemispheres or the thalamus is structurally or metabolically impaired, the respiratory response to carbon dioxide is reset, so that a higher level of carbon dioxide is required to trigger the respiratory drive. The resulting respiratory pattern, known as Cheyne-Stokes respiration, is characterized by periods of increasing hyperventilation alternating with apnea in a crescendo-decrescendo fashion. If more caudal regions at the level of the midbrain and the upper pons are injured, central neurogenic hyperventilation may result. This pattern of respiration, characterized by hyperventilation with forced and prolonged inspiration and expiration, is commonly seen in metabolic disorders such as hypoxia. In the lower brain stem, if the lower pons or the medulla is injured, any of several respiratory patterns may occur. Apneusis, a pattern in which long inspiration is followed by a pause lasting a few seconds and then by normal expiration, results from pontine lesions and occasionally from metabolic suppression. Cluster breathing, a pattern in which breaths are irregular and fall into groups, is associated with lower pontine lesions. Atactic breathing, characterized by irregular respiratory rate and amplitude, with gasps held in inspiration intermingling with periods of apnea, is associated with lower medullary lesions and may be indicative of a terminal respiratory pattern in severely brain-damaged patients.

Other patterns of respiration, such as slow and shallow but regular breathing, are suggestive of metabolic or drug-induced depression. Kussmaul respiration, a pattern of rapid, deep breathing that is also known as air hunger, occurs with metabolic acidosis.

ELEVATED INTRACRANIAL PRESSURE

An increase in ICP occurs when an increase in the volume of one of the three components of the intracranial cavity (i.e., blood, cerebrospinal fluid, and brain parenchyma) cannot be compensated for by a similar decrease in the volume of one of the other components.[7,8] Causes of increased intracranial volume include intracranial hematoma, hydrocephalus, tumor, vascular congestion, and cerebral edema. Cerebral edema is a nonspecific accompaniment of many disorders, such as head injury, tumor, stroke, and infection. Cerebral edema and increased ICP are particularly common after severe head injury and are important determinants of the prognosis of these patients[9-11] [see 5:2 Injuries to the Central Nervous System]. Signs and symptoms of rising ICP include increasing arterial blood pressure, slowing of the pulse rate, and slowing or periodic respiration. This so-called Cushing response has been related to brain-stem ischemia; however, brain-stem blood flow is not always decreased in the presence of a Cushing response.[12] Papilledema caused by raised ICP takes several weeks to develop and is usually not a presenting symptom in patients with rapidly rising ICP.

MENINGISM

Meningism, or neck stiffness, occurs when the meninges are irritated by inflammation (as in meningitis) or the presence of blood (as in subarachnoid hemorrhage). In addition to nuchal rigidity, signs of meningeal irritation include a positive Kernig sign (elicited by flexing the thigh to 90° with the knee bent and then straightening the knee; the sign is positive when this maneuver causes pain in the hamstrings) and a positive Brudzinski sign (elicited by flexing the neck in a supine patient, which results in involuntary flexion of the hip).

Differential Diagnosis of Coma: Metabolic, Structural, and Other Causes

The differential diagnosis of coma is complex. It is essential to differentiate coma of metabolic origin from coma caused by structural lesions. In addition, both of these varieties of coma must be distinguished from psychogenic and other causes of coma and similar states, such as a persistent vegetative state and locked-in syndrome. Each of these types of coma has a characteristic clinical presentation and evolution [see Table 2].

TOXIC METABOLIC COMA

General Considerations

Toxic metabolic coma results from derangement of metabolism, alteration in resting membrane potentials, or suppression of neurotransmission in the cerebral cortex or the brain stem. Both exogenous toxins, such as sedatives and alcohol, and endogenous toxins, such as those produced in the course of uremia and hepatic failure, may suppress metabolic and electrical processing in the brain. Hypoxia and hypoglycemia lead to acute deficiencies of metabolic substrates. Acid-base and electrolyte imbalance suppress neuronal excitability, as do osmolarity abnormalities. Metabolic causes of coma usually cannot be demonstrated by means of radiography; however, signs of cerebral edema or increased ICP may be apparent on CT scan.

The hallmark of metabolic coma is that it is difficult to attribute neurologic signs to a restricted region because not all levels of the CNS are depressed concurrently and equally; for example, pupillary responses may be normal, and consciousness and respiration may be suppressed. The preservation of the pupillary light reflex even in the presence of signs of lower brain injury is an important feature distinguishing metabolic from structural coma. This rule does not, however, hold true for patients who have ingested drugs or sustained anoxic damage. The ingestion of narcotics results in reactive pinpoint pupils; the ingestion of the anticholinergic agents atropine and scopolamine gives rise to fixed fully dilated pupils; and the ingestion of glutethimide yields moderately dilated pupils that are unequal in size and frequently fixed. Severe anoxia may lead to bilateral fixed dilated pupils. Profound barbiturate poisoning or hypothermia may cause pupils to be both fixed and dilated. Although asymmetry of motor function is rare in metabolic coma, it does occur, often fluctuating from side to side. Abnormal motor signs such as tremor, myoclonus, and asterixis are characteristic of a metabolic derangement.

Specific Causes

Hypoglycemic coma   Hypoglycemic coma is a serious complication of long-term insulin use, with a single episode occurring in at least one third of these patients at some point in their lives.[13] Tremor, tachycardia, sweating, blurring of vision, confusion, irritability, and abnormal behavior may precede the loss of consciousness, but in patients who are long-term insulin users, the premonitory symptoms may be absent and these patients may slip into a coma without any warning.

Diabetic ketoacidosis   Diabetic ketoacidosis is a metabolic acidosis that develops in diabetic patients as a result of raised levels of circulating ketone bodies.[13] It is a severe complication of uncontrolled diabetes that requires emergency treatment. Initially, these patients present with severe dehydration, compensatory hyperventilation (Kussmaul respiration), vomiting, depression of consciousness, and sometimes abdominal pain. Coma is not common.

Uncontrolled hyperglycemia   Nonketotic hyperosmolar coma results when uncontrolled hyperglycemia leads to dehydration and increased osmolality.[13] In this type of uncontrolled hyperglycemia, endogenous insulin secretion is still sufficient (and thus peripheral lipolysis and hepatic ketogenesis are inhibited), but hepatic glucose production, which is less sensitive to insulin control, is unrestrained. Patients with this disorder typically are in middle or later life and have been previously diagnosed with mild diabetes or have undiagnosed diabetes. Initial symptoms are profound dehydration and a decreased level of consciousness. The condition may be precipitated by an underlying infection or, in older patients, by vascular disease.

Hepatic and renal failure   Hepatic encephalopathy may occur in the setting of acute fulminant hepatitis, in which there is no history of liver disease, or after rapidly progressive chronic liver disease.[14] The exact cause of the encephalopathy is not known, but possible factors include the release of toxins from the damaged liver, failure to detoxify metabolic products, and alterations in cerebral neurotransmitters caused by amino acid imbalances. Initial symptoms include slowness of mentation and affect, fluctuant mild confusion, reversed sleep rhythm, slurred speech, alternating euphoria and depression, and untidiness. Additional clues to underlying liver disease include fetor hepaticus, flapping tremor (asterixis), and constructional apraxia. A progressive deterioration in mental status and behavior usually follows, leading eventually to coma. In the early stages of coma, patients hyperventilate and their pupils react sluggishly to light. There is a general muscle hypertonia, and a grasp reflex may be elicited. Deeper coma develops rapidly if no treatment is instituted, and extensor posturing, loss of oculovestibular reflexes, hypotension, cardiac arrhythmias, and respiratory arrest occur.

Untreated acute and chronic renal failure may lead to uremic encephalopathy, which is associated with a progressive decrease in the

Table 2   Etiology of Coma

Causes of structural coma	Tumor
	Vascular
	  Cerebrovascular accident
	  Subarachnoid hemorrhage
	  Arteriovenous malformation
	  Global ischemia (vasospasm)
	Trauma
	  Intracranial hematoma
	  Multiple contusions
	  Diffuse axonal injury
	Infection
	  Cerebral abscess
	  Meningoencephalitis

Causes of toxic metabolic coma	Hypoxia Hypercarbia Hypoglycemia Hepatic failure Renal failure Electrolyte disorders Endocrine abnormalities Poisons Drugs
Other causes of coma	Hypothermia Hypotension and shock Psychiatric disorders

level of consciousness, hyperventilation, asterixis, myoclonic jerking, tetany, and convulsions.[15] Higher mental functions are affected first, followed by motor symptoms. The onset of uremic encephalopathy depends on both the severity of the uremia and its rate of onset; rapid onset is associated with early CNS manifestations.

Electrolyte disturbances   Coma can result from disturbances in sodium, potassium, and magnesium homeostasis.[16] Hyponatremia (e.g., from renal or GI sodium loss) may cause coma when the plasma sodium concentration falls below 110 to 115 mmol/L, particularly when the fall is rapid. Hypernatremia occurs in a hyperosmolar nonketotic coma. The level of consciousness falls and convulsions develop when the plasma sodium concentration rises above 155 to 160 mmol/L. Hypokalemia usually does not produce a frank coma, but rather a decrease in the level of consciousness. Death in these patients is caused by ventricular tachycardia. Both hypomagnesemia (e.g., from severe vomiting and diarrhea) and hypermagnesemia (e.g., from renal failure) can produce coma. Increased irritability, hallucinations, convulsions, myoclonus, and chorea usually precede hypomagnesemia, whereas hypermagnesemia is preceded by increased lethargy and generalized weakness. Death in patients with hypermagnesemia results from respiratory paralysis.

STRUCTURAL COMA

General Considerations

Structural brain lesions produce coma either by destroying the brain parenchyma or by causing shifting or herniation of the brain within the rigid confines of the tentorium and skull [*see* Discussion, Pathophysiology of Coma, Herniation Syndromes, *below*]. Supratentorial lesions produce coma by causing a caudal shift of the cerebral contents beyond the confines of the tentorium, which results in compression of the brain stem and dysfunction of the ascending RAS. Infratentorial lesions produce coma by compressing the brain stem from either inside (i.e., intrinsic brain-stem lesions) or outside (i.e., cerebellar lesions).

As mentioned previously, the hallmark of a structural lesion underlying coma is the presence of localizing signs. In addition, unilateral pupillary abnormalities and unilaterally absent brain-stem reflexes are highly suggestive of an anatomic lesion. Some structural lesions (e.g., aneurysmal subarachnoid hemorrhage) often have a typical clinical presentation, and this may aid in the differential diagnosis. Specific structural causes of coma and their clinical presentation are discussed below.

Specific Causes

Cerebral tumor Coma is usually not the presenting symptom in patients with brain tumors. In most patients with cerebral tumors, a progressive neurologic deficit or focal seizure activity precedes the onset of coma, and their presence is an important clue in the differential diagnosis. Headache is also a common presenting symptom and is present in approximately 50% of patients with primary brain tumors or metastatic lesions. The classic headache associated with a brain tumor is described as being worse in the morning; exacerbated by coughing, straining, or bending forward; and accompanied by nausea and vomiting, which often afford relief for the patient. However, this classic pattern occurs only in a subset of patients. In a study of 111 patients with brain tumors, investigators showed that 77% of the patients had headaches that were similar to tension headaches, 9% had headaches that were migrainelike, and only 8% had the typical headache symptoms of a brain tumor.[17]

Signs and symptoms of supratentorial tumors include those caused by raised ICP (e.g., mass effect of the tumor or blockage of CSF drainage), focal deficits (e.g., destruction of the brain parenchyma; compression of the parenchyma by edema, mass, or hemorrhage; and compression of the cranial nerves), headache, seizures, mental status changes, transient ischemic attack symptoms (caused by vessel occlusion or hemorrhage into the tumor), and, in the case of pituitary tumors, endocrine symptoms and visual impairment. Patients with infratentorial tumors usually do not present with seizures, because such seizures are thought to arise from irritation of the cerebral cortex. Signs and symptoms of these lesions include headache, nausea, vomiting, papilledema, gait disturbances, vertigo, diplopia, and cranial nerve abnormalities and nystagmus when there is brain-stem involvement.

Stroke Stroke is categorized as cerebral infarction (thromboembolic or ischemic stroke), which signifies ischemic brain damage, or cerebral hemorrhage (hemorrhagic stroke), in which damage to the brain mainly consists of vascular rupture and extravasation of blood into the brain parenchyma. The hallmark of both types of stroke is the abrupt onset of a focal neurologic deficit. Whereas brain-stem infarcts can result in an immediate coma, ischemic stroke usually does not produce coma as a predominant symptom. In most cases, coma develops later, when edema develops in and around the infarct or when hemorrhagic conversion of the infarct results in the development of a massive hematoma that produces brain herniation.

In intracerebral hemorrhage (ICH), loss of consciousness is a prominent feature. The hallmarks of ICH are a rapidly developing neurologic deficit, vomiting, and a fluctuating level of consciousness. Coma usually indicates a large lobar or ganglionic hemorrhage (> 60 ml),[18] and coma is thought to result either from direct destruction or from herniation caused by the mass effect of the hemorrhage.

Both hemorrhagic and thromboembolic stroke predominantly affect the elderly. Diabetes, atherosclerosis, cardiac disease, hypertension, vasculitis, and hematologic disorders are important risk factors for ischemic stroke. The main causes of ICH include hyper-

tension, arteriovenous (AV) malformations, ruptured aneurysms, arteriopathies, tumors, coagulation or clotting disorders, venous or dural sinus thrombosis, abuse of drugs (e.g., cocaine or amphetamines), eclampsia, postsurgical complications (e.g., repair of congenital heart defects in children, hyperemia after carotid endarterectomy, or repair of AV malformation), and infection. Whether hypertension actually causes ICH is still subject to debate because 66% of patients older than 65 years are hypertensive, and the observed hypertension associated with ICH may in fact be part of the physiologic Cushing response and not a preexisting condition.[19]

Aneurysmal subarachnoid hemorrhage Subarachnoid hemorrhage (SAH) refers to bleeding within the subarachnoid space rather than the brain parenchyma and is the result of either a ruptured aneurysm (aneurysmal SAH) or a severe head injury (traumatic SAH). Aneurysmal SAH occurs most frequently in the fourth to sixth decades of life. The classic manifestations of aneurysmal SAH are headache of sudden onset (commonly described as the most severe headache ever experienced), a variable period of consciousness, meningism, photophobia, vomiting, and focal signs. The clinical severity of SAH is graded by using the Hunt and Hess Scale [*see Table 3*][20] or the World Federation of Neurological Surgeons Scale [*see Table 4*].[21]

Delayed cerebral ischemia or vasospasm is responsible for considerable morbidity and mortality and is an important cause of impaired consciousness and coma in patients with aneurysmal SAH. Vasospasm has a typical pattern of development. It generally occurs between day 5 and day 14 after aneurysmal SAH, with a peak incidence between day 7 and day 10. Clinical signs and symptoms include an insidious decrease in the level of consciousness and fluctuating neurologic signs. The diagnosis is confirmed by means of transcranial Doppler ultrasonography or cerebral angiography.

Table 3 Hunt and Hess Classification of Subarachnoid Hemorrhage[20]

Score*	Definition
0	Unruptured aneurysm
1	Asymptomatic; or mild headache and slight nuchal rigidity
1a	No acute meningeal/brain reaction, but with fixed neurologic deficit
2	Moderate to severe headache and nuchal rigidity; or CNS palsy (e.g., III, IV)
3	Lethargy or confusion; mild focal deficit
4	Stupor; moderate to severe hemiparesis
5	Deep coma, extensor posturing, moribund appearance

*Add one grade for serious systemic disease (e.g., hypertension, diabetes mellitus, severe atherosclerosis, chronic obstructive pulmonary disease) or severe vasospasm on arteriography.

Table 4 World Federation of Neurological Surgeons Committee on Universal Subarachnoid Hemorrhage Grading Scale[21]

Grade	GCS Score	Motor Deficit
I	15	Absent
II	13–14	Absent
III	13–14	Present
IV	7–12	Present or absent
V	3–6	Present or absent

GCS—Glasgow Coma Scale

Traumatic SAH is a common phenomenon in patients with severe head injuries. The diagnosis is made by means of CT. In a study from the National Institutes of Health Traumatic Coma Data Bank, traumatic SAH was identified in 39% of 753 patients with severe head injury.[22] Clinically, traumatic SAH is associated with signs and symptoms of vasospasm that are similar to those occurring with aneurysmal SAH. Vasospasm affects between 25% and 40% of patients with severe head injuries,[23] and the presence of traumatic SAH appears to be related to an unfavorable outcome.

Meningoencephalitis and cerebral abscess Bacteria, viruses, spirochetes, and fungi may infect the meninges and the subarachnoid space. In most cases, infection of the CNS results from an infection that originates somewhere else. For example, meningococcal meningitis is often a complication of meningococcal bacteremia; tuberculous meningitis is the result of breakdown of a tuberculous lesion or miliary tuberculosis; and herpes zoster, listeriosis, and cryptococcal meningitis are opportunistic CNS infections that typically occur with debilitating disease or altered immune status. After neurosurgery, gram-negative aerobic bacilli usually cause meningitis. Signs and symptoms of meningoencephalitis include fever, headache, raised ICP, meningism, photophobia, seizures, and focal signs. A depressed level of consciousness, sometimes progressing to a frank coma, is a relatively common clinical manifestation of CNS infection. About 50% of patients with acute meningitis have a depressed level of consciousness.[24] The exact mechanism behind depressed levels of consciousness in CNS infection is unknown. A direct effect of the organism or its toxins on the brain parenchyma has been suggested, but disturbance of the cerebral microcirculation and occlusion of the larger vessels through either vessel wall thickening or vasospasm have also been suggested.[25]

Cerebral abscesses commonly produce focal signs or seizures but may lead to brain herniation and coma when they expand. In the classic case, the presentation is acute, with fever followed by confusion and the development of focal signs over the course of days; however, a cerebral abscess may also develop gradually, without overt disease. Cerebral abscesses may be associated with sinusitis, otitis, cranial trauma, or disseminated infection.

Head injury Head injury is discussed in more detail elsewhere [see 5:2 Injuries to the Central Nervous System].

OTHER CAUSES OF COMA AND COMA-RESEMBLING SYNDROMES

Hypothermia

Hypothermia occurs when the body's core temperature is 35° C or lower. It can result from exposure (i.e., from cold stress exceeding the body's maximum heat production), exhaustion (i.e., from depletion of the body's available energy sources), or failure of central temperature regulation (mainly in elderly patients and newborns). Loss of consciousness by itself may result in hypothermia. Consciousness decreases when the core body temperature is at or below 32° C and progresses to coma with further temperature decline. Metabolic processes slow, and for each 1° C decrease in body temperature, CBF diminishes by about 6%. At 28° C, the metabolic rate is 50% of normal, and below 25° C, asystole and death occur. At this point, cerebral autoregulation fails, and CBF follows the systemic blood pressure in a pressure-passive manner.[26]

Psychiatric Disorders

Psychogenic coma is an uncommon cause of unresponsiveness. It may be observed in patients with psychiatric disorders such as conversion reactions, catatonic schizophrenia, severe psychotic depres-

sion, or frank malingering. In most cases, the physical examination reveals normal tone and reflexes, as well as normal oculocephalic and oculovestibular reflexes. Occasionally, EEG is necessary to demonstrate a normal waking pattern.

Persistent Vegetative State

A vegetative state is a syndrome of diffuse cortical damage in which brain-stem activity is preserved. Consequently, eye opening and muscle movements are observed, but there is no voluntary control of the movements. A vegetative state is usually a long-term and often a permanent state associated with injuries such as head trauma and global ischemia.

Locked-in Syndrome

The locked-in syndrome is a state in which quadriplegia and paralysis of the lower cranial nerves are present but the level of consciousness is normal. This syndrome is rare and usually results from thrombosis of the basilar artery, which is attributed to a variety of causes. Patients can communicate only by eye movements (e.g., blinking). Long-term survival is uncommon but has been reported.[27]

Radiologic Imaging

Radiologic imaging modalities depict the anatomic configuration of intracranial structures and play a crucial role in the evaluation of comatose patients, particularly when an adequate history cannot be obtained and the physical examination is inconclusive. They can be used to confirm or exclude the presence of clinically suspected abnormalities or, in some instances, to make a specific diagnosis, thereby greatly expediting treatment or intervention.

TYPES OF IMAGING MODALITIES

Plain Skull Radiography

Plain skull radiography is particularly useful in the evaluation of patients with head injuries. Bullets and bullet fragments can be easily detected, and the points of entry and exit can generally be determined with this method. In patients with closed head injuries, plain skull radiography is used to detect fractures of the cranial vault and base. It is important to obtain a skull radiograph in patients with head injuries because the presence of a fracture is related to intracranial hematoma and thus is an indication of the severity of head injury [see Table 5].

Computed Tomography and Magnetic Resonance Imaging

Both CT and MRI provide detailed information on brain anatomy, including the configuration and size of the ventricular chambers; the presence of midline displacements; the presence of subfalcial, transtentorial, or uncal herniations; and the position of vascular structures. CT is usually the first investigation performed in comatose patients. Compared with MRI, CT takes less time for a complete investigation, and the CT unit is much easier to access. These are significant advantages of CT in comatose patients, who are usually monitored with multiple electronic devices—a practice that, by itself, limits the use of MRI because of the effect of the magnetic field on these devices. In addition, CT is better at imaging bony structures than MRI is, it is an excellent method of demonstrating ICH, and it offers the best resolution for demonstrating SAH. MRI, however, offers the advantage of imaging in multiple planes, which allows accurate anatomic visualization of the lesion. Furthermore, it is more sensitive than CT in detecting intracranial abnormalities and thus is better able to find small lesions. In addition, the absence of bony artifacts makes MRI more useful for imaging lesions in the

Table 5 Relation between Presence of
Skull Fracture and Intracranial Hematoma in Patients
with Severe, Moderate, and Minor Head Injury[124]

Severity	Hematoma on CT	No Hematoma on CT	Total
Severe (GCS 8)			
Fracture	74 (44%)	94 (56%)	168
No fracture	43 (32%)*	91 (68%)	134
Moderate (GCS 9–12)			
Fracture	49 (29%)	118 (71%)	167
No fracture	25 (8%)†	299 (92%)	324
Minor (GCS 13–15)			
Fracture	42 (10%)	391 (90%)	433
No fracture	27 (1%)‡	2,549 (99%)	2,576
Total	260	3,542	3,802

*$P < 0.05$.   †$P < 0.001$.   ‡$P < 0.0001$.
GCS—Glasgow Coma Scale

posterior and temporal fossae. Overall, CT is preferred for initial evaluation of comatose patients. MRI should be reserved for patients who require less monitoring, who are able to remain still for prolonged examination, and in whom CT has not been beneficial or is inconclusive.

RADIOLOGIC DIAGNOSIS OF SPECIFIC CAUSES OF COMA

Cerebral Tumor

CT (with and without injection of contrast) is a useful and quick first investigation for detecting a tumor. It demonstrates mass effect, edema, calcifications, and accompanying disorders that may necessitate rapid intervention (e.g., hydrocephalus). Low-grade gliomas show a decreased density on CT scans that does not enhance with contrast. The surrounding edema is minimal. Calcifications may be present, particularly in certain subtypes (e.g., oligodendrogliomas). High-grade gliomas are usually large and enhance intensely after contrast administration [*see Figure 1*]. In most cases, the enhancement is irregular. A central area of low density may also be present, indicating necrosis. High-grade gliomas are usually surrounded by marked cerebral edema and compression of the ipsilateral ventricle by a hemispheric mass; alternatively, the surrounding edema may result in obstructive hydrocephalus with dilatation of the contralateral ventricle.

On MRI, low-grade gliomas may present as abnormal areas of decreased T_1 signal (spin-lattice or longitudinal relaxation time) and increased T_2 signal (spin-spin or transverse relaxation time), even in the absence of CT evidence of a tumor. High-grade gliomas characteristically have a low signal intensity on T_1-weighted images and a high signal on T_2-weighted images. Gadolinium enhancement is more likely to occur in high-grade gliomas. Metastatic lesions have a variable intensity on T_2-weighted images, and they commonly enhance with gadolinium. Meningiomas are hypointense to isointense on T_1 and hyperintense to isointense on T_2, and they enhance strongly with contrast. Nerve sheet tumors are isointense or hypointense on T_1 and hyperintense on T_2 and enhance intensely with contrast. Pituitary tumors are best visualized on T_1-weighted imaging. They are hypointense lesions within the intermediate intensity of the anterior lobe. Lymphomas are usually hypointense to isointense on T_1-weighted images and isointense to hyperintense on T_2-weighted images. These tumors enhance after I.V. injection of gadolinium.

Stroke

CT abnormalities can be detected a few hours after an ischemic stroke. In patients with a middle cerebral artery (MCA) stroke, CT findings include effacement of the sulci, loss of distinction of the caudate nucleus and lentiform nucleus, and loss of the insular ribbon. The hyperdense MCA sign, which is caused by the clot in the artery, is present in almost 50% of patients when a CT scan is performed within the first 2 hours.[28,29] The characteristic triangle-shaped hypodensity usually develops fully within 3 days, and the mass effect, caused by cerebral swelling as well as petechial hemorrhages and indicating hemorrhagic conversion, may be seen at this time. The likelihood of edema increases with the size of MCA infarcts; if the infarct size, as determined on CT scan within 5 hours after the insult, is larger than 50% of the MCA territory, significant edema develops in 85% of patients.[30]

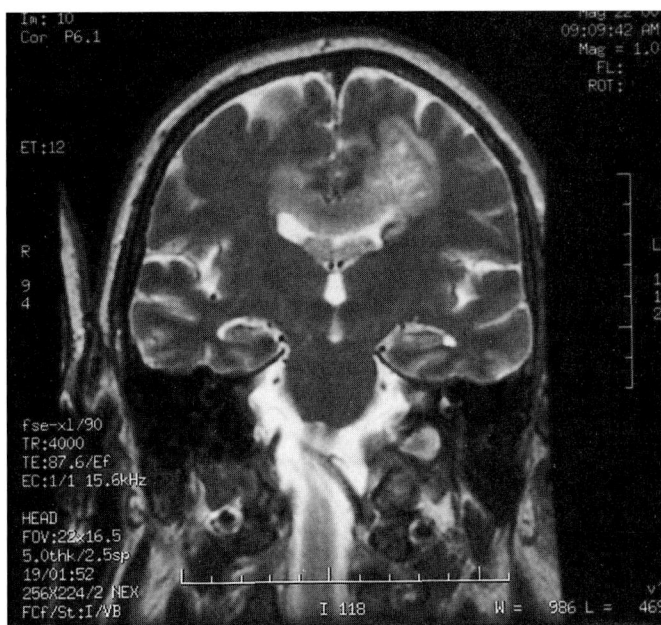

Figure 1 **Characteristic appearance of butterfly glioma is apparent on coronal T_1-weighted MRI. The tumor mass extends to the contralateral side across the corpus callosum.**

Table 6 Fisher CT Classification of Subarachnoid Hemorrhage[31]

| Grade | Amount of Blood on CT | No. of Patients | Angiographic Vasospasm | | DIND |
			Slight	Severe	
1	No SAH detected	11	2	2	0
2	Diffuse or vertical layers* < 1 mm	7	3	0	0
3	Localized clot and/or vertical layer > 1 mm	24	1	23	23
4	Intracerebral or intraventricular clot with diffuse or no SAH	5	2	0	0

*Vertical layers refer to blood within the vertical subarachnoid spaces, including the interhemispheric fissure, insular cistern, and ambient cistern.
DIND—delayed ischemic neurologic deficit   SAH—subarachnoid hemorrhage

Supratentorial, cerebellar, and brain-stem hemorrhages appear as hyperdense lesions on CT scan. Putaminal hemorrhages may extend into the thalamus and enter the ventricular system. Caudate hemorrhage may be difficult to detect because the ventricular extension may predominate. Lobar hematomas on CT scan may show compression of the sulci, midline shift, and compression of the lateral ventricle. MRI is a useful test for excluding metastasis, occult vascular malformations, previous hemorrhages associated with amyloid angiopathy, or cerebral venous thrombosis that is not detected with CT.

Cerebellar hematomas may cause significant compression and obliteration of the basal cisterns, resulting in CSF obstruction and hydrocephalus; these signs, together with the size of the hematoma,

are important determinants of further management. In patients with pontine hemorrhage, massive hemorrhages are most frequent, but small ones occur as well.

Subarachnoid Hemorrhage

Aneurysmal SAH is classified according to the Fisher CT classification, which relates severity of bleeding to prognosis [*see Table 6*].[31] The sensitivity of CT scanning for detecting SAH is very high, approximately 95%.[32,33] In many cases, there is a slight preponderance of blood deposited in the area of the ruptured aneurysm, which may aid in determining the location of the aneurysm or the location of multiple intracranial aneurysms. Cerebral angiography [*see Figure 2*] is the gold standard for evaluating the size and location of the aneurysm, though newer methods (e.g., MR angiography and CT angiography) are being used increasingly.[34-38]

Lumbar puncture is never the first choice of investigation for confirming a diagnosis of SAH. As noted, a mass lesion in the posterior fossa may closely mimic the signs and symptoms of SAH, and patients are at considerable risk for herniation if a lumbar puncture is performed. A CT scan usually yields the diagnosis, and a lumbar puncture is rarely necessary. If SAH is suspected and CT is not available, it is safer to transport the patient to a facility where CT scanning is available, particularly when the patient is rapidly deteriorating.[33] Lumbar puncture, however, must be used when the CT scan is negative and there is even a slight suspicion of aneurysmal SAH.

Meningoencephalitis and Cerebral Abscess

Other than diffuse basal dural enhancement on MRI, meningoencephalitis usually does not produce specific signs on CT or MRI. A CT scan is indicated in comatose patients, however, to rule out complications of meningitis such as hydrocephalus, subdural empyema, and abscess. On CT, a cerebral abscess appears as a smooth thin-walled lesion with a low-density center that enhances brightly after administration of contrast. In some cases, it is difficult to distinguish between a tumor and an abscess on CT, and stereotactic biopsy is essential to confirm the diagnosis [*see Figure 3*]. Diffusion-weighed MRI also may be useful in these cases.[39] MRI can show intracranial abscesses with a much greater resolution than CT scanning can, and it is excellent for detecting cerebritis and abscesses that are undetectable or uncertain on CT.[40]

Head Injury

Fractures of the cranial vault and base are sometimes difficult to detect, particularly by the inexperienced investigator. Depressed and linear fractures are the most common types [*see Figure 4*]. Types of ICH that are often seen after head injury and that can be detected with CT include contusions and epidural, subdural, subarachnoid, and intraparenchymal hemorrhages. An epidural hematoma

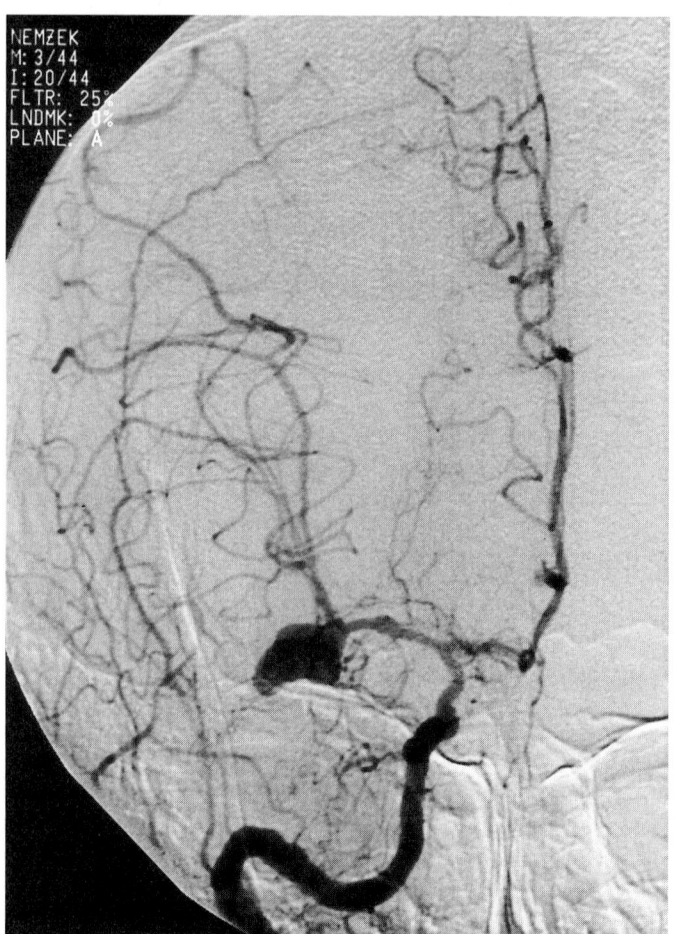

Figure 2 **Cerebral angiography shows a large right middle cerebral artery aneurysm.**

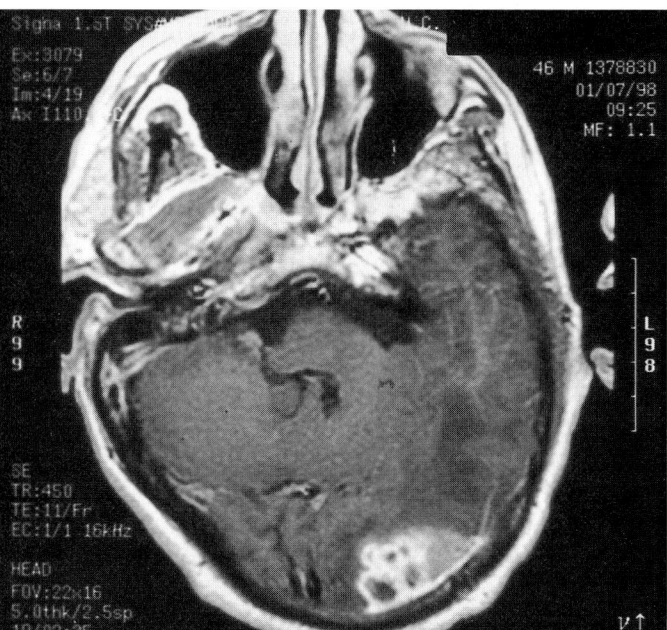

Figure 3 MRI reveals a cerebral abscess. Axial T_1-weighted image with gadolinium contrast medium shows multiloculated, brightly enhancing mass. Signal intensity is low at the abscess wall. There is significant surrounding edema and mass effect, which results in effacement of the ipsilateral occipital horn of the left lateral ventricle. Local involvement of the meninges is indicated by enhancement of the overlying meninges.

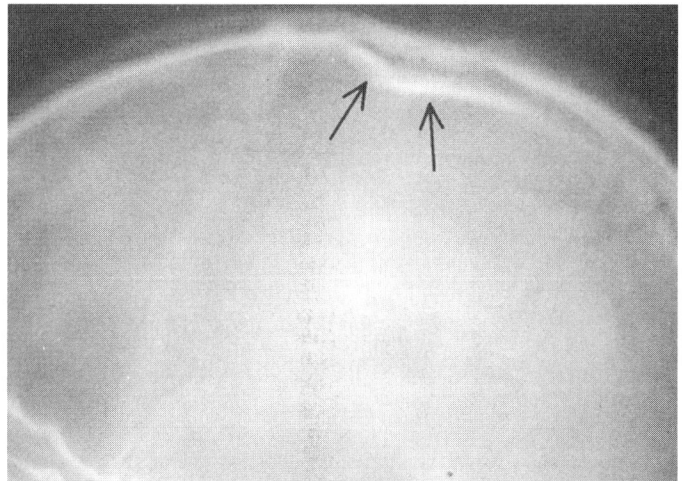

Figure 4 Conventional lateral radiograph shows a skull fracture.

characteristically appears as a biconvex hyperdense lesion [*see Figure 5*]. Epidural hematomas have been classified into three types on the basis of CT scan criteria.[41] Type I (acute) hematomas are characterized by a lucent swirl (unclotted blood) in a dense hematoma. Some investigators call these hematomas hyperacute extradural hematomas. Type II (subacute) hematomas appear as solid clots. Type III (chronic) hematomas appear as mixed-density or lucent hematomas with a contrast-enhanced membrane.

Subdural hematomas appear as convex-concave lesions on CT [*see Figure 6a, b*]. In many cases, subdural hemorrhage is accompanied by SAH, indicating severe injury.[42] The complex of subdural hematoma and adjacent contusion in the brain is sometimes referred to as a burst lobe. Acute subdural hematomas are hyperdense with

respect to the adjacent brain, subacute hematoma are hyperdense to isodense, and chronic hematomas [*see Figure 6c*] are hypodense.

Intraparenchymal lesions appear as an area of increased density on CT scans [*see Figure 7*]. The hematomas are usually associated with extensive lobar contusions, from which they are indistinguishable in many cases.[43,44] The amount of blood in a lesion determines whether the lesion is classified as a hematoma or a contusion. If blood accounts for at least two thirds of the lesion, the lesion is classified as an intracerebral hematoma. The remaining lesions are described as disrupted tissue with areas of microscopic hemorrhage.[45] A hemorrhagic mass should be considered an intracerebral hematoma when there is a homogeneous collection of blood with relatively well-defined margins. Multiple intracerebral hematomas are found in approximately 20% of cases.[46]

Contusions, appearing as small hyperdense lesions on CT, usually have a characteristic distribution, affecting the frontal poles, the orbital gyri, the cortex above and below the sylvian fissures, the temporal poles, and the lateral and inferior aspects of the temporal lobes. Over time, significant swelling may accompany these lesions, appearing as hypodense areas around the contusion.

Diffuse axonal injury is characterized by the presence of punctate hemorrhages or so-called Strich hemorrhages and indicates severe head injury.[47] Strich hemorrhages are most commonly found in the corpus callosum, the walls of the third ventricle (hypothalamus, columns of the fornix, and anterior commissure), the internal capsule, the basal ganglia, the dorsolateral brain stem, and the superior cerebellar peduncles.

Midline shift and compression of the subarachnoid space are parameters indicating the extent of mass expansion or cerebral swelling. The National Institutes of Health Traumatic Coma Data Bank introduced a classification of head injury based on initial CT findings [*see Table 7*].[48] This classification is commonly used in clinical trials investigating new treatments for severe head injury. Eisenberg and colleagues have shown a correlation between some of the CT scan characteristics after severe head injury (i.e., compression of the basal cisterns, the presence of SAH, and midline shift) and the frequency of raised ICP, mortality, and other outcomes.[22]

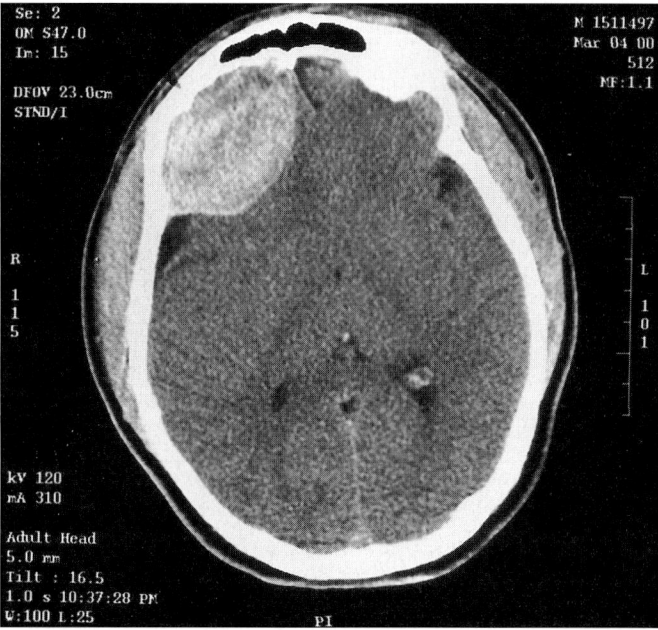

Figure 5 CT scan shows acute epidural hematoma. Note the characteristic biconvex hyperdense lesion.

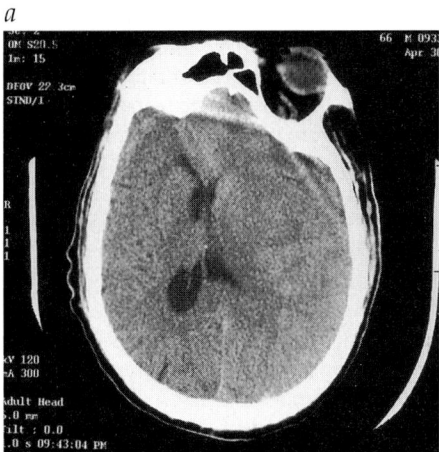
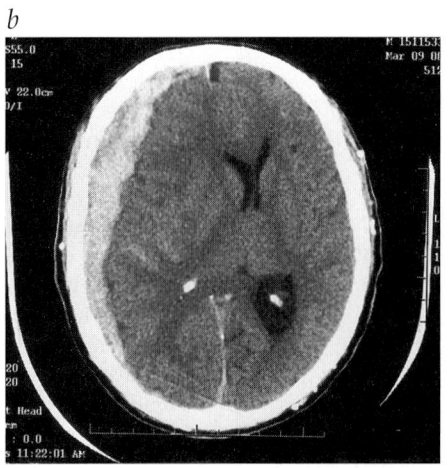
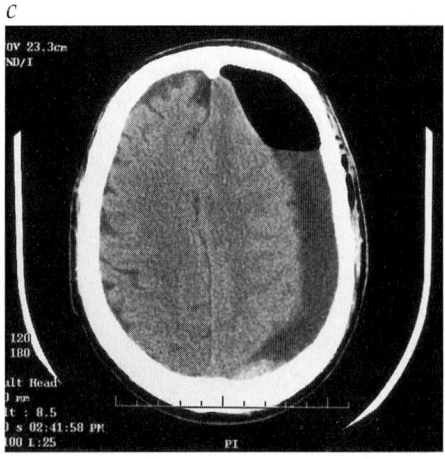

a   *b*   *c*

Figure 6   Shown are three examples of subdural hematoma: (*a*) hyperacute subdural hematoma (note that there is only a slight difference in density between the convex-concave hematoma and the brain parenchyma; the hematoma causes significant midline shift and ipsilateral brain compression), (*b*) acute subdural hematoma, and (*c*) chronic subdural hematoma after surgical evacuation.

Treatment of Coma

METABOLIC COMA

Management of Intoxication

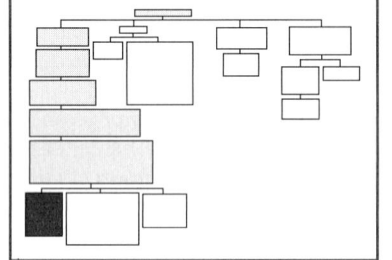

Many comatose patients who are seen in the emergency ward are suffering from an overdose of alcohol, narcotics, sedatives, or a combination thereof. Most of these drugs induce respiratory and cardiovascular depression, which is a major cause of mortality in comatose patients. Anticipation and early treatment of these complications may alleviate their effects.

Figure 7   CT scan shows intracerebral hematoma resulting from a cranial gunshot wound.

Early intubation, respiratory support, and maintenance of normal blood pressure are essential. Gastric lavage is effective when ingestion of a drug is discovered no more than 4 hours after the event, except in the case of salicylates, which may be removed in substantial amounts as long as 10 hours after ingestion. As a rule, little is gained by performing gastric lavage more than 4 hours after ingestion, unless the patient has been in shock and consequently manifests delayed gastric emptying and slowed absorption. In comatose or uncooperative patients, however, it is rarely possible to determine the exact time of ingestion; thus, gastric lavage is almost always indicated.

Patients are intubated with a cuffed endotracheal tube (to protect the airway from aspirated gastric contents) and then positioned on their left side (to allow pooling of the gastric contents) with the head down. Lavage is then performed with copious amounts of fluid until the return is clear. After evacuation, a slurry of 10 g of activated charcoal in 30 to 50 ml is instilled in the stomach via a nasogastric

Table 7   Classification of Head Injury Based on Initial CT Findings

Category	Definition
Diffuse injury I	No visible intracranial pathology on CT scan

Diffuse injury II	Cisterns present with midline shift of 0–5 mm and/or the following:
	    Lesion densities present
	    No high- or mixed-density lesion > 25 ml
	    May include bone fragments and foreign bodies

Diffuse injury III (swelling)	Cisterns compressed or absent, with midline shift of 0–5 mm; no high- or mixed-density lesion > 25 ml
Diffuse injury IV	Midline shift > 5 mm; no high- or mixed-density lesion > 25 ml
Evacuated mass lesion	Any lesion surgically evacuated
Nonevacuated mass lesion	High- or mixed-density lesion > 25 ml, not surgically evacuated

tube. After lavage, cathartic agents may be used to shorten the transit time through the GI tract and thus to decrease absorption of the ingested material. Diuresis (saline, ionized, or osmotic), dialysis, and charcoal hemoperfusion all facilitate the excretion of toxins. Specific antidotes exist for several common intoxicants; however, these antidotes are beyond the scope of the present discussion.

Hypoglycemic Coma

Initial treatment of hypoglycemic coma is discussed elsewhere [see Initial Management of the Comatose Patient, above]. In addition, treatment consists of prevention, in the form of education in the use of insulin and encouragement of patients to carry glucose tablets or sweets with them at all times. A supply of glucagon (1 g I.M.) that can be administered by relatives may also be stored at home.

Diabetic Ketotic Coma

Treatment must be initiated as soon as possible because these patients often present with profound dehydration. Key points in the management of diabetic ketoacidosis include the following:

1. Replace fluid losses (the average fluid loss is approximately 7 L).
2. Replace electrolytes and monitor potassium carefully.
3. Restore acid-base balance (with bicarbonate infusion only in severe cases).
4. Replace insulin deficiency (4 to 6 U/hr).
5. Replace energy losses (dextrose infusion with insulin cover until the patient can eat).
6. Look for an underlying cause (infection is common).

Hyperglycemic Hyperosmolar Nonketotic Coma

Management of hyperosmolar nonketotic coma does not differ from that of diabetic ketotic coma; however, meticulous rehydration should be performed, particularly because many patients with this condition are elderly.

STRUCTURAL COMA

Cerebral Tumor

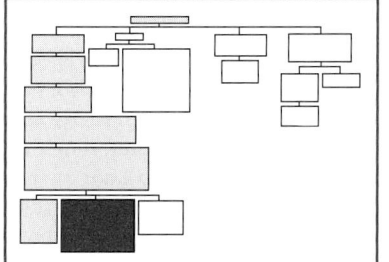

Management of brain tumors consists of surgery, radiotherapy, and other adjuvant treatments (e.g., chemotherapy). Ultimately, treatment of these lesions depends on both tumor characteristics (e.g., localization, malignancy, tumor spread, and associated edema) and patient characteristics (e.g., age, medical history, and personal beliefs). An in-depth discussion of the diverse treatment strategies, however, is beyond the scope of this chapter.

In the comatose patient, two interventions deserve particular consideration. First, to reduce cerebral edema, patients should be started on glucocorticosteroid therapy (e.g., dexamethasone), particularly when signs of elevated ICP are present. Second, coexisting hydrocephalus may be alleviated by the insertion of a ventricular catheter.

Stroke

In patients with thromboembolic stroke, coma is usually caused by brain swelling. Cerebral edema occurs in approximately 10% to 20% of patients with MCA stroke and in almost 100% of those with complete MCA occlusion.[49,50] It typically occurs after 2 to 7 days and is characterized by a gradual deterioration, though the level of consciousness may fluctuate in some patients. Measurement of ICP is indicated because it has been shown that ICP may predict the ultimate outcome of these patients[49] and thus can serve as a guide for patient management.[51] Administration of mannitol is initially selected to treat an increase in ICP. Acute episodes of impending herniation may be treated with hyperventilation if mannitol fails, and further clinical deterioration can be followed by decompressive surgery if the patient has no other significant disease and is relatively young. In addition, a ventriculostomy can be placed if significant contralateral hydrocephalus is present.

In patients with nondominant ischemic stroke, including comatose patients and patients with a fixed dilated pupil, decompressive surgery has been successful, though it has not been tested in a randomized clinical trial.[52-57] Moreover, it should be noted that although mortality may decrease substantially with decompressive surgery, it may not be desirable to salvage those patients who may end up with a severe disability or in a vegetative state. In a recent study of 32 surgically treated patients, mortality decreased by 35% in comparison with historic controls, but one in four patients experienced severe disability.[55]

Treatment of so-called supratentorial hypertensive intraparenchymal hemorrhage is still subject to considerable debate. No uniform treatment guidelines are available, and there is very little clinical evidence to support either a surgical or a conservative medical approach. In two randomized trials, no significant differences in outcome were found between surgical and medical management.[58,59] Stereotactic aspiration of the clot has achieved some degree of success, but to date, no comparative studies have been published.[60,61]

Subarachnoid Hemorrhage

Treatment of a ruptured aneurysm consists of either surgical clipping or endovascular treatment, depending on the location, size, and shape of the aneurysm and the age, clinical condition, and past medical history of the patient. Ideally, patients are treated within 48 hours of hemorrhage because the risk of rebleeding is highest early after the initial bleeding episode. The estimated frequency of repeat bleeding in untreated patients is 4% on day 1 and 1.5% from day 2 to day 14. Overall, 15% to 20% of patients experience repeat bleeding within 14 days, and 50% within 6 months; thereafter, the risk is 3% per year, with an annual mortality of 2%.[62,63] An advantage of clipping or coiling the aneurysm is that it allows the institution of so-called triple-H therapy (i.e., therapy for hypertension, hypervolemia, and hemodilution) and transluminal balloon angioplasty in the case of vasospasm. In a subset of patients (i.e., those with poor neurologic condition or those who present with symptomatic vasospasm), surgical treatment may be postponed, or the aneurysm may be treated by means of endovascular techniques.

Cerebral vasospasm is initially treated with ample fluid replacement and discontinuance of any antihypertensive or diuretic agents. When necessary, triple-H therapy and transluminal balloon angioplasty to dilate the vasospastic vessels are instituted.[64,65] Prevention of vasospasm by means of prophylactic transluminal balloon angioplasty is currently under investigation.[66]

Meningoencephalitis and Cerebral Abscess

If there is a strong suspicion of bacterial meningitis, I.V. antibiotics should be started immediately because this condition can be rapidly fatal. If there is a delay in obtaining the CSF, one should start treatment blind. Antibiotic selection depends on the initial expectation of the organism most likely to be involved, the results of Gram stain of the CSF, and the drug's ability to penetrate the CNS. Neurosurgical consultation is obtained in the case of a suspected cerebral abscess or hydrocephalus, both of which may require emergcncy drainage. Subdural empyema is a rare complication of meningitis that usually requires drainage. In the case of diffuse cerebral edema, management and monitoring of ICP are indicated.

Treatment of a cerebral abscess consists of identification of the bacterial organisms, institution of antibiotic therapy, and drainage or excision of the abscess through a craniotomy or bur hole.[67-70] Repeated aspiration of the abscess may be necessary. Surgical excision is considered if there is persistent reaccumulation of the abscess, if the abscess is in an accessible site or is located in the cerebellum, or if there is a well-formed fibrous capsule that fails to collapse despite repeated aspiration.

Head Injury

The main goal in the management of head injury is the prevention of secondary injury. Treatment of such injuries is addressed more fully elsewhere [see 5:2 Injuries to the Central Nervous System].

OTHER CAUSES OF COMA

Hypothermia

Early intubation and respiratory support facilitate oxygenation and rewarming. In the case of circulatory arrest, for every decrease of 1° C in body temperature, the time during which there is

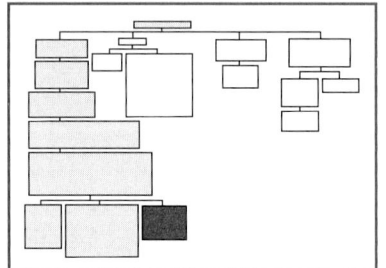

hope for recovery without cardiopulmonary resuscitation can be doubled (this applies only to patients with primary hypothermia, not to those who are hypothermic because of cardiac arrest). Hypothermia can cause considerable coagulation disturbances, which predispose the patient to bleeding. To detect these abnormalities, the physician should perform clotting tests at the patient's core body temperature rather than at 37° C.

External or surface rewarming by covering the patient, by conducting treatment in a warm room, and by giving warmed I.V. fluids and warmed humidified oxygen is indicated in patients with a core body temperature higher than 30° C. In patients with a core body temperature below 30° C, surface rewarming is contraindicated. In these patients, surface rewarming could cause shunting of the blood to the dilated skin vessels, thereby exacerbating hypotension and further decreasing the core temperature, both of which predispose these patients to ventricular fibrillation. Active core rewarming is therefore instituted in these patients, which consists of delivering warmed humidified gases and parenteral fluids, performing peritoneal dialysis (4 to 8 L/hr at a temperature of 37° to 42° C), circulating water at 42° C through a closed irrigation system inserted into the esophagus or stomach (3 L/hr), or performing hemodialysis with the blood flowing past a dialysis solution warmed to 40° C. Considerations in the management of hypothermia are discussed more fully elsewhere.[71-77]

Seizures

Seizures or epileptic attacks are episodes of transient disturbance of electrochemical activity within the brain, expressed as abnormal motor, sensory, or psychological behavior. Epilepsy is defined as a condition characterized by recurrent

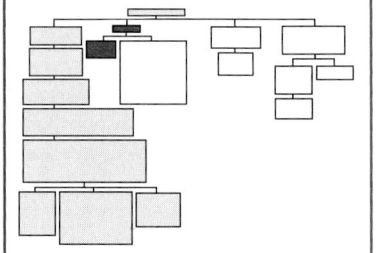

Table 8 Classification of Epilepsy

Generalized: bilaterally symmetrical; no local onset; loss of consciousness from onset
  Generalized tonic-clonic: idiopathic, no anatomic abnormality
  Absence (petit mal seizure): impaired consciousness with mild or no motor involvement
  Bilateral myoclonus: syndrome of three seizure types, including myoclonic jerks, generalized tonic-clonic seizures, and absence
  Infants and children: infantile spasms, atonic seizures, and tonic seizures

Partial: focal from onset
  Simple (usually no loss of consciousness)
  Complex (any alteration of consciousness, automatisms)
  Partial with secondary generalization

Unclassified epileptic seizures

unprovoked seizures. Traditionally, epileptic attacks are classified into three main groups [see Table 8]. Partial (focal) seizures are often associated with a structural abnormality, such as a scar, a tumor, or an AV malformation. Generalized seizures are a result of diffuse neuronal hyperactivity; there is usually no identifiable structural abnormality. Seizures that induce loss of consciousness may involve both cerebral hemispheres and may either be generalized from onset (primary generalized seizures) or begin focally and then spread to involve both hemispheres (secondary generalized seizures).

Several systemic and neurologic diseases can give rise to seizures. Head trauma, cerebrovascular disease, and CNS infections are common causes, as are metabolic imbalances such as hypoglycemia, hypoxia, hyponatremia, hypernatremia, hypocalcemia, and hypomagnesemia. In addition, hypothermia can induce seizures. Drugs and toxins, such as methylxanthines, tricyclic antidepressants, phenothiazine, cocaine, and local anesthetics (e.g., lidocaine), can lead to seizures. Withdrawal of a drug—particularly of a barbiturate, alcohol, or a hypnotic—can cause seizures if too abrupt.

Generalized tonic-clonic seizures are characterized by sudden loss of consciousness associated with tonic-clonic movements. There is no preceding aura, but occasionally, there may be preictal irritability or a rising epigastric sensation. During the seizure, the patient falls to the ground, sometimes with a cry; tongue biting and loss of sphincter control are often noted. After an initial period of tonic rigidity and short-lived apnea, clonic jerking of the neck, trunk, and extremities ensues. The clonic jerking gives way to flaccid relaxation accompanied by labored breathing, pallor, and hypersalivation. Consciousness, lost at the beginning of the seizure, is gradually regained, but postictal confusion and drowsiness may last for hours. Grand mal seizures may predispose the patient to serious bodily injuries, such as vertebral compression fractures, cerebral trauma, and drowning.

Status epilepticus occurs when the seizures follow one another without recovery of consciousness between episodes. Specifically, it is defined as more than 30 minutes of convulsive activity or repeated convulsions over the course of 30 minutes without return of consciousness in between. This arbitrary definition is related to the onset of cerebral metabolic and systemic consequences of prolonged seizure activity [see Discussion, Cellular, Metabolic, and Systemic Effects of Status Epilepticus, below]. Withdrawal of antiepileptic drugs is the most common cause of status epilepticus among patients with epilepsy. Status epilepticus can be classified into convulsive status epilepticus and nonconvulsive status epilepticus. Tonic-clonic status epilepticus is the most feared complication of epilepsy and is potentially lethal. The death rate approaches 60% in untreated patients; even with skilled management, the death rate is 10%.[78] In what follows, we focus on management of tonic-clonic status epilepticus.

MANAGEMENT OF STATUS EPILEPTICUS

General Management of Seizures

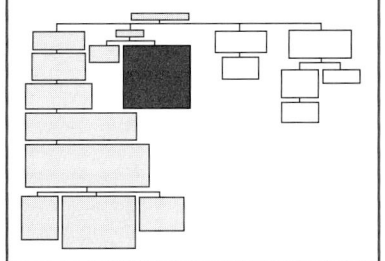

Most seizures are self-limited and therefore rarely require emergency treatment. When a seizure does not resolve quickly and spontaneously, treatment must be rapid and efficient. The primary goals of treatment are (1) to ensure adequate ventilation so as to prevent hypoxia and (2) to prevent complications such as aspiration and physical injuries. A quick history and physical examination are performed in an attempt to determine the underlying cause of the seizure, while an assistant begins drawing blood and inserting a venous line. Blood specimens are obtained for measurement of anticonvulsant drug levels, biochemical tests, a hemogram, and assessment of arterial blood gas pressures. Blood glucose level is determined by means of rapid bedside techniques; if it cannot be estimated immediately or is estimated to be lower than 60 mg/dl, dextrose is infused (50 ml of a 50% solution for adults and 1 to 2 ml/kg of a 25% solution for children). Adult patients are also given 100 mg of thiamine I.V. as a safeguard against an exacerbation of Wernicke encephalopathy, which is a relatively common disease among patients with status epilepticus. Thiamine is always given before dextrose is administered.

Patients with hyponatremia, whose condition may be associated with compulsive water drinking, fluid overload, or the syndrome of inappropriate antidiuretic hormone secretion, are given a hypertonic (3%) solution of sodium chloride by slow I.V. infusion. Half the calculated sodium deficit is administered, which is usually sufficient to stop seizures; the remaining deficit can be corrected by fluid restriction and diuresis. Excessively rapid correction of hyponatremia may result in cardiovascular overload or central pontine myelinosis. Patients with a recent history of thyroid or parathyroid surgery as well as a prolonged QT interval on the ECG should immediately be given I.V. calcium—1 to 2 ampules of calcium gluconate for 5 to 10 minutes—even if confirmatory laboratory results are not yet available. Because oxygenation, blood pressure, acid-base balance, and blood glucose may all be disturbed by prolonged convulsions, supportive medical care is just as important as anticonvulsant drug therapy.

Pharmacotherapy for Status Epilepticus

The three main drugs or drug classes used in the treatment of status epilepticus are the benzodiazepines, phenytoin, and the barbiturates. Usually a benzodiazepine is administered first, followed immediately by a loading dose of phenytoin. Benzodiazepines exert their effect by enhancing γ-aminobutyric acid (GABA) inhibition, whereas phenytoin interferes with sodium entry into the cell [see Discussion, below]. Among the benzodiazepines, lorazepam is the preferred drug. Because diazepam is redistributed rapidly in fatty tissue, seizures may recur within 10 to 20 minutes. Furthermore, diazepam appears to be less effective in aborting status epilepticus. A 1995 study showed that lorazepam aborted status epilepticus in 97% of cases and diazepam in only 68%.[79] A side effect of benzodiazepines is respiratory depression, which occurs in approximately 12% of patients. Lorazepam appears to cause less respiratory depression than diazepam. In adults, lorazepam is given I.V. in a dosage of 4 mg over 2 minutes; the dose may be repeated after 5 min-

utes. In pediatric patients, a dose of 0.1 mg/kg is used, up to a maximum of 5 to 6 mg.

In adult patients who are not already taking phenytoin, the loading dose is 20 mg/kg, infused at a maximum rate of 50 mg/min. In patients taking phenytoin, 0.74 mg/kg is given to raise the level by 1 μg/ml. If the phenytoin level is unknown, a loading dose of 500 mg is given. In pediatric patients, the loading dose is 20 mg/kg infused at a rate of 1 to 3 mg/kg/min.

If the seizures continue, the initial strategy is to give additional doses of phenytoin (5 mg/kg each, to a maximum of 30 mg/kg). Thereafter, phenobarbital is loaded (20 mg/kg in adults, to a maximum of 100 mg/minute; 5 to 10 mg/kg in pediatric patients every 20 to 30 minutes, to a maximum of 30 to 40 mg/kg), or diazepam is given (100 mg/500 ml drip at 40 ml/min). As a last resort, general anesthesia is instituted, usually with pentobarbital. EEG monitoring should be performed in these patients, and pentobarbital should be titrated until burst-suppression occurs. In addition, blood pressure should be monitored closely because hypotension may occur.

Cognitive Impairment

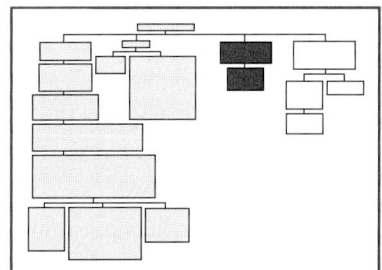

Cognitive functions include consciousness; attention; orientation to time, place, and person; immediate, recent, and remote memory; abstraction; language; praxis; and visuomotor ability. Cognitive impairment is a common consequence of coma, particularly in patients with structural lesions. It may also follow status epilepticus, though more likely as a result of underlying brain abnormalities than of status epilepticus itself.[80]

In surgical settings, however, cognitive impairment is most common in patients who undergo major operations. It is often the result of delirium but may also be associated with dementia, amnestic disorders, depression, and various other mental disorders. In addition, several drugs may cause cognitive impairment, especially when administered in combination. Early detection is important because patients with cognitive deficits have higher rates of perioperative morbidity and mortality, longer hospital stays, and higher rates of institutionalization than patients with normal cognitive function do.

PERIOPERATIVE CARE: RISK FACTORS AND PREVENTIVE MEASURES

Certain factors increase the risk that cognitive impairment will develop in a surgical patient [see Table 9].[81,82] It is important to iden-

---

Table 9   Risk Factors and Exacerbating Factors for Cognitive Impairment

Risk factors	Exacerbating factors
Age > 60 yr	Unfamiliar environment
Addiction to alcohol, narcotics, or both	Communication deficits
Cerebral damage or disease	Sensory deprivation or overload
Cardiac, renal, or hepatic disease	Sleep deprivation
Visual or auditory impairment	Immobilization
Preoperative depression	Anxiety
History of delirium or functional psychosis	Pain
Family history of psychosis	

Table 10 Precipitating Medical and Surgical Causes of Delirium

Drug intoxication
Alcohol, anesthesia, antianxiety agents, anticholinergics, anticonvulsants, antidepressants, antihistamines, antihypertensives, antiparkinsonian agents, cimetidine, clonidine, digitalis, insulin, lithium, neuroleptics, opiates, salicylates, sedative-hypnotics

Drug withdrawal
Alcohol, antianxiety agents, sedative-hypnotics

Metabolic disturbances
Electrolyte, fluid, or acid-base imbalance; endocrine disorders; hepatic or renal failure; hypoglycemia; hypothermia; hypoxia; paraneoplasm

Acute cerebral disorders
Edema, encephalitis, epilepsy, fat emboli, primary or metastatic neoplasm, stroke, transient ischemic attack, vasculitis

Infections
Bacterial endocarditis, meningitis, pneumonia, septicemia, urinary tract infection

Hemodynamic disturbances
Anemia, arrhythmia, congestive heart failure, hypertensive encephalopathy, hypotension, hypovolemia, myocardial infarction, orthostatic hypotension

Respiratory disorders
Pulmonary embolus

Nutritional and vitamin deficiency

Trauma
Burns, fractures, head injury

---

tify and, when possible, reduce these risk factors by adopting the following measures:

1. Simplify drug regimens.
2. Taper and discontinue unnecessary medications. Obtain psychiatric consultation for patients receiving monoamine oxidase (MAO) inhibitors to determine whether the drug can be discontinued 2 weeks before operation.
3. Ensure therapeutic blood levels of drugs such as digitalis, anticonvulsants, and lithium. Lithium should be discontinued 1 to 2 days before operation.
4. For patients dependent on alcohol, analgesics, or anxiolytic-sedatives, stabilize drug intake, make proper substitutions, or, if time permits, gradually withdraw the agent.
5. Ensure nutritional, thiamine, and multivitamin supplementation in alcoholic patients and in malnourished elderly patients.
6. Review the management of the patient's existing medical and psychiatric disorders and obtain early consultation to provide optimal preoperative management.
7. Correct visual and auditory deficits if possible.

In addition, general supportive measures should be instituted as early as possible, and factors that exacerbate cognitive impairment should be mitigated [*see Table 9*]. Patients with cognitive impairment should be further evaluated for suicidal intent and behavior. If the patient is at risk of suicide or exhibits dangerous behavior (e.g., wandering, falling, or acting aggressively), psychiatric consultation should be obtained immediately, the physical environment should be secured, and a sitter should be present when family and staff are absent. Pharmacologic management may be necessary and is usual-

ly preferable to physical restraints, which can increase agitation, decrease mobility, and damage soft tissue.

Meticulous intraoperative care can prevent or diminish postoperative delirium in high-risk and cognitively impaired patients. The following precautionary measures are recommended:

1. If the patient has received an MAO inhibitor within 2 weeks of operation, monitor blood pressure levels carefully. If hypotension develops, treat with a direct-acting sympathomimetic such as phenylephrine.[83]
2. Plan anesthesia and surgical interventions so as to minimize operative time, hypotension, tissue damage, and the use of psychoactive drugs.
3. Avoid premedication with highly anticholinergic drugs (e.g., scopolamine or atropine).
4. Schedule the operation to minimize waiting time, anxiety, and fasting.
5. Maintain normal body temperature, especially in an elderly patient.
6. Carefully monitor hemodynamic, cardiac, and metabolic functions.
7. Ensure that orienting procedures and the use of glasses and hearing aids are resumed in the recovery room.

In the postoperative period, measures to prevent medical and surgical causes of delirium include the following:

1. Administer essential medications, sufficient calories, and detoxification agents parenterally until oral intake can be resumed.
2. Avoid excessive analgesic administration or routine use of long-acting benzodiazepines (e.g., diazepam or flurazepam).
3. Initiate early and vigorous treatment of metabolic imbalances, infection, hemodynamic disturbances, respiratory failure, and trauma (e.g., from falls or bedsores).
4. Reduce factors that contribute to cognitive impairment by continuing the supportive measures that were initiated before the operation.
5. Preserve maximum possible visual input in eye-surgery patients; enhance tactile and auditory clues.
6. Encourage all patients to become mobile and to resume autonomous functioning as soon as physical and cognitive abilities permit.

DIAGNOSIS AND MANAGEMENT OF FREQUENT CAUSES OF COGNITIVE IMPAIRMENT

The Mini-Mental State Examination and the Confusion Assessment Method are useful, rapid tests for evaluating cognitive functions,[84-87] though their sensitivity largely depends on the experience and background of the investigator.[88] These tests should be repeated daily in patients with cognitive impairment and in high-risk patients. The most frequent causes of cognitive impairment are delirium, dementia, depression, head injury, and pharmacotherapy.

Delirium

An obvious deterioration in cognitive ability, behavior, or mood during the first week after operation is usually caused by delirium and signals the presence of potentially life-threatening disorders [*see Table 10*]. Delirium is a transient mental disorder characterized by acute onset of global impairment of cognitive functions and widespread disturbance of cerebral metabolism. Delirium may arise immediately after the operation but typically follows after an interval of several days. Early manifestations include restlessness, irritability, insomnia, lethargy, kinesthetic sensations, vivid and frightening dreams, illusions, difficulty in thinking, and thickening or slurring of speech. As

Table 11 DSM-IV Diagnostic Criteria for Delirium

Disturbance of consciousness (i.e., reduced clarity of awareness of environment) with reduced ability to focus or sustain or shift attention

Change in cognition (e.g., memory deficit, disorientation, language disturbance) or the development of a perceptual disturbance that is not better accounted for by a preexisting, established, or evolving dementia

Development of the disturbance over a short time (usually hours to days) and fluctuation during the course of the day

Evidence from the history, physical examination, or laboratory findings that the disturbance is caused by a general medical condition, substance intoxication, substance withdrawal, or more than one such cause

DSM-IV—Diagnostic and Statistical Manual of Mental Disorders, 4th edition.

Table 12 Laboratory Studies to Investigate Delirium

Routine procedures

Complete blood count

Blood chemistry tests for electrolytes; calcium, phosphate, and glucose; blood urea nitrogen; liver enzymes

Urinalysis

Erythrocyte sedimentation rate

Serologic test for syphilis

Chest x-ray

Electrocardiogram

Special procedures

Blood chemistry tests for creatinine, magnesium, vitamin B_{12}, folate, thyroxine, ammonia, serum proteins, osmolality, arterial blood gases, cortisol

Test for levels of medications in the blood

Blood and urine toxicology screens

Blood cultures

HIV antibody test

Lupus erythematosus preparation and antinuclear antibody test

Urine tests for osmolality, porphobilinogen, 5-hydroxyindoleacetic acid

CSF examination for cells, protein, glucose, culture, viral serology, pressure

Cranial CT scan or MRI

Electroencephalogram

the syndrome progresses, fluctuations in attention, perception, orientation, language, and intellectual functioning may become apparent. Sleep becomes fragmented, and day and night cycles may be reversed. Urinary incontinence, loss of motor coordination, focal neurologic signs, nystagmus, and various types of tremor may also be noted. Bilateral asterixis and multifocal myoclonus are highly suggestive of delirium. Current diagnostic criteria for delirium are given in the fourth edition of the *Diagnostic and Statistical Manual of Mental Disorders* (*DSM-IV*) [*see Table 11*].

When delirium is suspected on clinical grounds, appropriate laboratory studies should be performed to help identify precipitating organic causes [*see Table 12*]. Management of delirium includes treatment of precipitating factors [*see Table 9*], control of exacerbating factors [*see Table 9*], continuation of prophylactic measures, and management of agitation (see below).

Dementia

Dementia is a clinical syndrome that usually occurs in the elderly. Dementia has a protracted course that is characterized by loss of cognitive abilities, disorganization of personality, and decreased ability to perform activities of daily living. Consciousness is usually not disturbed, unless delirium is present. Dementia can be totally reversed in 10% to 15% of patients if detected early and treated appropriately, and it can be arrested or at least partially improved in 25% to 30%.[89,90] Of the many disorders that cause dementia [*see Table 13*], Alzheimer disease and vascular diseases (multi-infarct dementia) are most commonly implicated, accounting for, respectively, 40% to 60% and 10% to 25% of all cases.[89,90] The diagnosis of Alzheimer disease is based on the presence of a progressive dementia of insidious onset with prominent aphasia, apraxia, and cognitive impairment, but with relatively intact motor functions until the final stages of the disease.[91] A family history of the disease may be present. The diagnosis of vascular dementia is suggested by a sudden onset, a stepwise deteriorating course, focal neurologic signs and symptoms, and evidence of significant cerebrovascular disease from the history, clinical examination, or laboratory tests. Other causes of dementia are excluded by the history, clinical examination, and laboratory results.[90,92] *DSM-IV* also lists diagnostic criteria for dementia [*see Table 14*], and recommended investigations for suspected dementia are similar to those outlined previously [*see Table 12*]. In addition, psychological tests may be helpful in certain cases.[89,93,94]

Management of dementia includes treating underlying causes and superimposed delirium or coexisting depression, minimizing exacerbating factors for cognitive impairment [*see Table 9*], and alleviating common manifestations of dementia (e.g., intellectual impairment, depression, insomnia, wandering, agitation, immobility, motor instability, incontinence, iatrogenic conditions, and family

Table 13 Causes of Dementia

Degenerative

Senile dementia, Alzheimer disease, Pick disease, Huntington chorea, Parkinson disease, Creutzfeldt-Jakob disease, normal-pressure hydrocephalus, multiple sclerosis

Intracranial space-occupying lesions

Tumor, subdural hematoma

Trauma

Single severe head injury, repeated head injury (e.g., in boxers, football players)

Infections and related conditions

Encephalitis, neurosyphilis, cerebral sarcoidosis

Vascular

Multi-infarct dementia, occlusion of the carotid artery, cranial arteritis

Metabolic

Sustained uremia, liver failure, remote effects of carcinoma or lymphoma, renal dialysis

Toxic

Alcohol, poisoning with heavy metals (e.g., lead, arsenic, thallium)

Anoxia

Anemia, postanesthesia, carbon monoxide, cardiac arrest, chronic respiratory failure

Vitamin deficiency

Sustained lack of vitamin B_{12}, folic acid, thiamine

Table 14   DSM-IV Diagnostic Criteria for Dementia

Development of multiple cognitive deficits

Impaired memory (new and previously learned information)

One or more of the following: aphasia, apraxia, agnosia, and disturbed executive functioning (planning, organizing, sequencing, abstracting)

Each of the above cognitive deficits must cause significant social or occupational impairment and represent a significant decline from previous functioning

Deficits do not occur exclusively during the course of delirium

Additional criteria are required for diagnosis of one of the following dementia types

Dementia of Alzheimer type

Gradual onset and continuing cognitive decline; cognitive deficits resulting from other CNS conditions, systemic conditions, or substance-induced conditions not better accounted for by other axis I disorders

Vascular dementia

Focal signs and symptoms or laboratory evidence of cerebrovascular disases that are judged to be etiologically related

Dementia resulting from other general medical conditions

Evidence that the disturbance is a direct physiologic consequence of a general medical disorder (to be coded on axis III)

Substance-induced persistent dementia

Deficits present beyond the usual duration of substance intoxication or withdrawal. Evidence that deficits are etiologically related to the persisting effects of substance use.

Dementia resulting from multiple etiologies

Evidence that the disturbance has more than one cause

DSM-IV—Diagnostic and Statistical Manual of Mental Disorders, 4th edition.

---

burden). Specific patient management and pharmacologic interventions are discussed elsewhere.[95-102]

Depression

Features that suggest a depressive disorder underlying cognitive impairment include a history of affective disorder in the patient or the family, a clearly depressed mood, and an atypical recent history of cognitive deficit.[103-105] Depression may also be the result of a general medical condition or an underlying organic cause; in addition, medications, substance abuse, endocrinopathies, malignant disorders, head injury, infectious disorders, and metabolic disorders should always be considered. Furthermore, the depressive episode may continue even after the precipitating organic factor has been removed and may require the same treatment as a major depressive episode. *DSM-IV* outlines the criteria for a major depressive episode [*see Table 15*].

If the patient is currently depressed and is already receiving a maintenance regimen of antidepressants, the dose should be increased every 2 to 5 days until the maximum daily dose is reached, intolerable side effects occur, or a clinical response is achieved. If the patient is starting antidepressant therapy and there is no history of a good response to any particular drug in either the patient or the family, the treatment of choice should be a tricyclic antidepressant (TCA) with minimal anticholinergic properties (e.g., desipramine) or a selective serotonin reuptake inhibitor (SSRI) (e.g., fluoxetine or sertraline). In elderly patients, it is wise to initiate therapy with a low dose and to increase the dose gradually while watching for adverse effects, such as delirium or orthostatic hypotension with a TCA and nausea, anxiety, insomnia, or headache with an SSRI.[106-108]

A combined antidepressant-neuroleptic regimen or electroconvulsive therapy may be indicated in delusional patients. Electroconvulsive therapy is also indicated for severely depressed patients at risk of suicide or rapid physical decline. Depressed patients with a personal or family history of hypomania may need additional medication with lithium or anticonvulsant agents (i.e., carbamazepine or valproate). In these last three groups of patients, psychiatric consultation is advisable.

Head Injury

Cognitive impairment is common after severe head injury. The extent of cognitive impairment is not always clearly reflected in the Glasgow Outcome Scale (GOS) [*see Table 16*], however, which is one of the most popular scales used to assess outcome after head injury.[109,110] Many patients cannot function normally months or years after severe traumatic brain injury; common cognitive deficits include memory and behavior disturbances. In the group of patients with so-called GOS good recovery, a substantial number of patients undergo personality changes that interfere with their personal lives and careers.[111-113] In a study of 82 patients with severe head injury, the investigators monitored GOS scores and psychosocial reintegration (defined in terms of employment, interpersonal relationships, social contacts, and leisure interests) for 6 years after injury.[114] Of the 82 patients, 76% were classified as having poor or substantially limited reintegration; among the patients with favorable GOS scores (i.e., good recovery or moderate disability), only 50% were found to have good reintegration.

The severity of cognitive impairment is related to the severity of the initial injury (as reflected in the GCS), the time between injury and hospital admission, the type of brain lesion, the duration of coma, and the extent of posttraumatic amnesia.[115,116] In a study of 117 patients with severe head injuries, neuropsychological sequelae were ascertained from two examinations in 30 of the conscious survivors within the first year after injury and were related to CT examinations. CT findings included diffuse axonal injury, diffuse swelling,

---

Table 15   DSM-IV Diagnostic Criteria for Major Depressive Episodes

At least five of the following symptoms have been present during the same 2-week period and represent a change from previous functioning

and

either symptom 1 or 2 is present

and

symptoms are not caused by a general medical condition or by mood-incongruent delusions or hallucinations.

1. Depressed mood
2. Markedly diminished interest or pleasure
3. Significant gain or loss of weight or appetite
4. Insomnia or hypersomnia
5. Psychomotor agitation or retardation
6. Fatigue or loss of energy
7. Feelings of worthlessness or excessive or inappropriate guilt
8. Diminished ability to think, concentrate, or make decisions
9. Recurrent thoughts of death or suicide, suicide attempt, or suicide plan

Symptoms do not meet criteria for a mixed (with manic features) episode.

Symptoms cause clinically significant distress or impairment of functioning.

Symptoms do not result from a substance (e.g., drug or abuse of medication) or a general medical condition.

Symptoms are not explained by bereavement.

DSM-IV—Diagnostic and Statistical Manual of Mental Disorders, 4th edition.

Table 16 Glasgow Outcome Scale[110]

Description	Score
Good recovery	5
Moderate disability	4
Severe disability	3
Vegetative state	2
Death	1

and focal injuries. Neuropsychological outcome varied with the type of CT lesion and the function measured. Overall differences in memory and learning were found among the three categories of CT lesions, whereas differences in intelligence and visuomotor functions were not significant. Levels of memory, learning, and visuomotor speed were higher after diffuse swelling injuries, but less improvement was noted. Greater improvements in memory, learning, and visuomotor speed occurred after diffuse axonal injury. After focal injuries, visuomotor speed improved, but recall and learning did not improve.[117]

Cognitive Side Effects of Pharmacologic Therapy

Cognitive side effects may be produced by a variety of medications from multiple drug classes. As noted, multidrug pharmacotherapy is an important cause of cognitive impairment, and drug regimens should be carefully evaluated, particularly in elderly patients. Impaired renal and hepatic function and the use of medications that interfere with hepatic and renal drug excretion may predispose patients to untoward effects. Elderly patients are more susceptible to cognitive side effects than younger patients are because of age-related alterations in pharmacokinetics, increased use of medications, and an increased incidence of premorbid cognitive impairment. Cognitive impairment in demented patients may be exacerbated by medications, and dementia increases the risk of delirium by twofold to threefold.[118] A comprehensive review of the cognitive side effects of pharmacotherapy together with an excellent source of references is available elsewhere.[119]

MANAGEMENT OF AGITATION

Agitation is frequently seen in patients with cognitive impairment and may present as increased psychomotor activity, often accompanied by wandering, shouting, and verbal or physical aggression. Management includes treatment of underlying disorders and intervention to reduce symptoms. The first steps in management consist of removing any obvious causes of the behavior, orienting the patient, increasing levels of safe activity, and improving pain control, any or all of which may suffice. If these measures are inadequate or the situation becomes life-threatening, psychopharmacologic management is indicated.

In several delirium syndromes, an antipsychotic drug is not considered the treatment of choice. In anticholinergic delirium, anticholinergic drugs are discontinued and supportive care is provided. If the delirium is life-threatening (i.e., associated with coma, seizures, or cardiac arrhythmias), parenteral physostigmine may reverse the danger. Because of its side effects, however, this drug should be used with caution.[120] For hepatic encephalopathy, a short-acting benzodiazepine that requires little hepatic degradation is preferred (e.g., oral oxazepam 15 to 30 mg every 6 hours as required). For delirium caused by alcohol or benzodiazepine withdrawal, benzodiazepines are preferred to antipsychotics, which are epileptogenic and may cause akathisia (motor restlessness). For alcohol withdrawal, 50 to 100 mg of thiamine should also be admin-

istered.[121] In emergency situations, 50 mg of chlordiazepoxide, 10 mg of diazepam, or 2 mg of lorazepam may be given slowly by I.V. infusion every 1 or 2 hours until control is established. Alternatively, 4 mg of lorazepam may be given intramuscularly. In less urgent situations, 25 to 50 mg of chlordiazepoxide given I.M. or orally four times a day will suffice. As soon as the patient's condition is stable, the dosage can be tapered at a daily rate of about one tenth to one quarter of the initial dose.

Haloperidol is the drug of choice for most other causes of agitation, particularly if patients display psychosis, aggression, or both. Haloperidol is relatively free from anticholinergic, autonomic, and drug-interaction effects. Side effects of the drug include extrapyramidal syndromes (i.e., Parkinson-like symptoms, akathisia, dyskinesia, or dystonia) and neuroleptic malignant syndrome, which is a rare but life-threatening complication. Brief treatment, however, does not usually cause severe side effects.

Mild forms of agitation are managed with haloperidol dosages of 2 to 15 mg orally twice a day. In elderly patients, 0.5 to 3 mg/day is usually sufficient. In emergency situations, haloperidol should be administered I.V. in a dose of 1 to 5 mg, and the dose should be increased by 5 to 10 mg/hour until an effective dose is achieved. Use of single doses of 30 mg and maximum daily doses of 100 mg has been reported.[121] For refractory cases, 1 to 4 mg of I.V. lorazepam may be added. Once improvement occurs, the regimen may be continued via the I.M. or oral route. In less urgent situations, severely agitated patients will usually respond to haloperidol, 2 to 10 mg/hr I.M., up to a daily dose of 10 to 60 mg (one third of this dose in the elderly). Supplementary parenteral dosages of 2 to 10 mg/hr may be administered. When the patient's behavior is controlled, haloperidol should be continued orally; if no supplementary doses are necessary, the dosage should be decreased by one quarter each day until discontinuance.

For delirium, the total duration of treatment with haloperidol is usually 3 to 5 days. For agitation associated with psychoses, longer

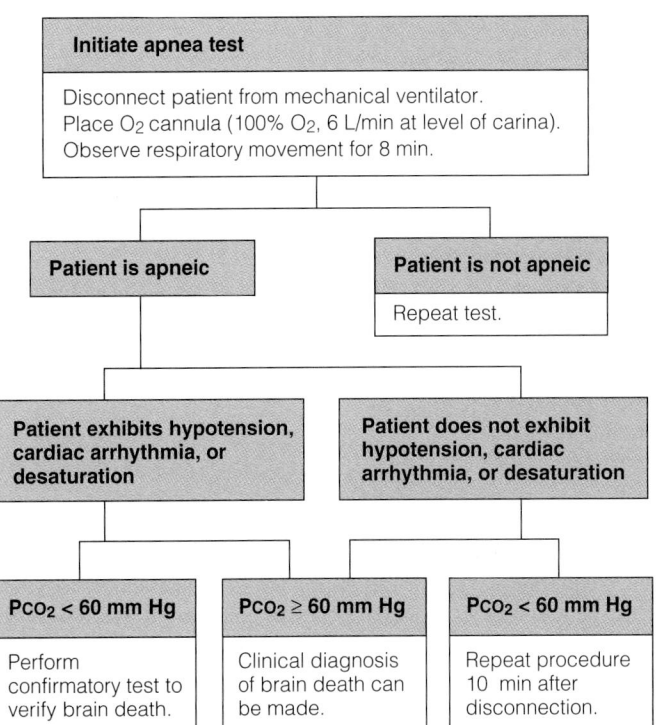

Figure 8 **Algorithm depicts the procedure for the apnea test in brain death.**[124]

treatment is usually required and psychiatric follow-up is advisable. Patients who cannot tolerate or fail to respond to haloperidol may respond to a phenothiazine antipsychotic such as chlorpromazine (25 to 50 mg I.M. every hour, followed by 25 to 100 mg orally every 4 to 6 hours). Side effects of chlorpromazine include hypotension, drowsiness, cardiac arrhythmias, seizures, respiratory depression, and coma.

Brain Death

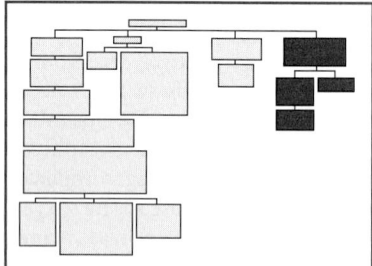

The term brain death implies irreversible cessation of activity in the cerebrum and brain stem. Brain death is frequently a consequence of severe head injury, (re)rupture of a cerebral aneurysm, or ICH[122,123]; less commonly, it is a consequence of fulminant encephalitis, bacterial meningitis, or anoxic-ischemic encephalopathy. A qualified physician should determine the occurrence of brain death, but legal requirements are different in various states and countries. Areas of concern include recognition of conditions that may mimic brain death, the procedure for the apnea test, indications for confirmatory tests, and management of physiologic changes associated with brain death. In addition, early identification of potential donor candidates is important, though selection of these candidates can proceed only after the clinical diagnosis of brain death has been established and family members have given their consent.

GUIDELINES FOR THE DETERMINATION OF BRAIN DEATH

The guidelines for determining brain death in adults and children have been published elsewhere[124]; accordingly, we provide here only a brief summary of the procedures involved. In most cases, the differences in the criteria for brain death from one state or country to another have to do with the type and number of confirmatory tests (see below) that are needed. The clinical diagnosis of brain death requires the following:

1. The presence of a cause that is compatible with brain death.
2. The absence of complicating medical conditions that may confound clinical assessment.
3. The absence of drug intoxication or poisoning.
4. A core temperature of at least 32° C.

In most patients, a CT scan will document an abnormality that is compatible with brain death. In patients with normal CT scans, the diagnosis should be reconsidered, unless there is a high certainty about the mechanism that has led to brain death (e.g., ischemic-anoxic brain death caused by cardiac arrest or asphyxia). CSF examination is indicated if a definite diagnosis cannot be made. Severe electrolyte, acid-base, and endocrine disturbances should be excluded, and a drug screen may be helpful to detect a specific drug or poison. In the presence of barbiturates, the diagnosis of brain death can likely be made when the levels are subtherapeutic; however, supportive data for this approach are available only for pediatric patients.[125] The core temperature should be at least 32° C because brain-stem reflexes are absent below 27° C.

If these conditions are met, clinical testing should follow. Three cardinal features of brain death are evaluated, as follows:

1. Coma or unresponsiveness.
2. Absence of brain-stem reflexes.
3. Apnea.

Coma or unresponsiveness is evaluated by assessing the motor response to painful stimuli, such as either supraorbital pressure or nail-bed pressure; this response should be absent. Pitfalls include the observation of spontaneous spinal motor responses (Lazarus sign), which may occur during pain stimuli, during the apnea test, and after recent administration of neuromuscular blocking agents. In the latter case, examination with a bedside nerve stimulator is required (so-called train-of-four monitoring). In a brain-dead patient, the pupils are typically in the middle position (4 to 6 mm) and fixed, although dilated pupils may be observed as well. Many drugs affect pupil size, but the light reflex usually remains intact. Topical ocular instillation of drugs, trauma to the cornea or the bulbus oculi, preexisting anatomic abnormalities, and previous surgical procedures should all be considered in the evaluation of the pupils and the pupillary response. The oculocephalic and caloric responses are then tested; these too should be absent. The caloric response can be diminished or abolished by a variety of drugs, including sedatives, TCAs, anticholinergics, antiepileptics, and chemotherapeutics. In addition, clotted blood or cerumen may occlude the external auditory canal, and fracture of the petrous bone may result in unilateral absence of a response. Finally, the corneal, pharyngeal, and tracheal reflexes are tested, all of which should be absent.

If all brain-stem reflexes are absent, the apnea test is performed [see Figure 8].[126] To minimize confounding factors, such as marked hypotension, severe cardiac dysrhythmias, and desaturations, the following precautions are taken[125]:

1. Core temperature must be 36° C or higher (rewarm the patient if temperature is lower).
2. Systolic BP must be 90 mm Hg or higher (use dopamine if BP is lower).
3. Fluid balance must be positive for 6 hours or longer (use vasopressin if this cannot be accomplished).
4. Arterial PCO_2 must be 40 mm Hg or higher (decrease minute ventilation if PCO_2 is lower).

Table 17   Guidelines for the Determination of Brain Death in Children

Historical criteria
 Determination of the proximate cause of coma
 Absence of remediable or reversible conditions such as toxins, drugs (sedatives, hypnotics, paralytics), metabolic disorders, surgically correctable conditions, hypotension, and hypothermia

Physical examination criteria
 Coexisting coma and apnea (standardized apnea test)
 Absence of brain-stem function
 Absence of hypothermia or hypotension
 Flaccid tone or absence of spontaneous or induced movements (except spinal cord events)
 Consistent examination findings throughout observation and testing periods

Observation periods and laboratory testing
 7 days to 2 months: two clinical examinations and apnea tests and two EEGs at least 48 hr apart
 2 to 12 months: two clinical examinations and apnea tests and two EEGs at least 24 hr apart*
 > 12 months: two clinical examinations and apnea tests at least 12 hr apart†

*Repeat examination and EEG are obviated by the absence of flow on cerebral angiogram.
†If hypoxic-ischemic encephalopathy is suspected, the observation period should be extended to 24 hr. Laboratory testing is not required if there is absence of a remediable or reversible condition.

5. Arterial PO_2 must be 200 mm Hg or higher (inspired oxygen fraction = 1.0 for 10 minutes).

CONFIRMATORY TESTS

Brain death is essentially a clinical diagnosis; it may be repeated after 6 hours to establish the final diagnosis. In most cases, this clinical diagnosis is sufficient; however, in cases in which the specific components of clinical testing cannot be evaluated reliably (e.g., as a result of drug intoxication, altered metabolic status, shock, or hypothermia), confirmatory tests may be indicated. Moreover, some countries require such confirmation by law, and many hospitals have their own policies for determining brain death. Generally accepted tests include EEG, cerebral angiography, single-photon emission CT, and, more recently, transcranial Doppler ultrasonography. In our experience, angiography not only is the most reliable and rapid way of establishing brain death but also occasionally shows that the cerebral circulation is normal and that further therapeutic efforts (such as hemicraniectomy) are justified. The tests are particularly important when organ and tissue donation are under consideration.

DETERMINATION OF BRAIN DEATH IN CHILDREN

Finally, a word is reserved for the determination of brain death in children. In children younger than 5 years, caution is indicated in applying the neurologic criteria for brain death. In comparison with adult brains, the brains of infants and young children have an increased resistance to cerebral damage that makes it easier for them to recover substantial functions, even after exhibiting unresponsiveness for longer than is possible in adults. Guidelines for the determination of brain death in children are available [see Table 17], but clear recommendations are lacking.[124,127,128]

Discussion

Pathophysiology of Coma

The pathophysiologic basis of coma is either a structural disruption of crucial areas in the cerebral hemispheres or brain stem (structural coma) or a diffuse depression of cerebral metabolism (metabolic coma). Cerebral metabolism is described in greater detail elsewhere [see 5:2 Injuries to the Central Nervous System]. Key variables for understanding the pathophysiology of coma include ICP, mean arterial pressure (MAP), cerebral perfusion pressure (CPP) (defined as MAP minus ICP), CBF (derived from CPP via the Poiseuille equation), the global arterial–jugular venous oxygen difference (A-VDO$_2$), and the cerebral metabolic rate of oxygen (CMRO$_2$) (derived via the Fick equation, CBF times A-VDO$_2$).

Because 95% of the energy in the normal brain is generated by oxidative metabolism, CMRO$_2$ is considered a sensitive measure of cerebral metabolism. Metabolic causes of coma predominantly interfere with CMRO$_2$, whereas structural causes of coma may interfere with both CMRO$_2$ and the supply of substrates. In patients with head injury, the observed depression in CMRO$_2$ has been related to impairment of mitochondrial function and consequently to depression of oxidative ATP generation.[129]

The resting CBF is approximately 55 ml/100 g/min, which is adequate for meeting normal metabolic demands and includes a modest safety margin to accommodate most physiologic changes. Between a CBF of 55 ml/100g/min and one of 25 ml/100 g/min, increased oxygen extraction compensates for the decrease in CBF, and CMRO$_2$ can be maintained. When the mean CBF drops below 25 ml/100 g/min, slowing of brain electrical activity is apparent on EEG, and a progressive depression of consciousness occurs clinically. This represents a stage of reversible brain dysfunction. Below a CBF of 18 ml/100 g/min, however, ATP generation is insufficient to support CMRO$_2$. Consequently, arrest of the sodium-potassium pump occurs, leading to membrane failure, cell swelling, and irreversible brain dysfunction. The resulting cell damage depends on both the duration and the amount of CBF depression.[130] In most circumstances, structural lesions affect CBF by their effect on the CPP.

Because CPP is defined as MAP minus ICP, it follows that CPP can be decreased by severe hypotension, which is a common complication in structural lesions such as head injuries, or by raised ICP, which may accompany any type of intracranial lesion.

As mentioned before, ICP is the product of a constantly changing interplay between CSF volume, brain tissue volume, and cerebral blood volume (CBV). These three compartments are enclosed within a rigid cranium, which implies that if ICP is to remain constant, any volume gained (e.g., from tumor, hematoma, or abscess) must be balanced by volume lost. In the presence of a cerebral mass, ICP can be maintained initially because CSF is displaced to the spinal compartment. At a certain volume, however, this compensatory mechanism is exhausted, and ICP rises rapidly [see Figure 9]. The resulting pressure-volume curve is exponential in shape; in other words, a relatively small increase in volume may cause only a small rise in ICP at the flat portion of the curve but a large increase in ICP at the steep portion. A small increase in volume (such as results from CO$_2$ retention [see below] or obstruction of venous outflow) can prove fatal to a patient with an elevated ICP.

Manipulation of CBV is an artificial method of compensating for raised ICP. CBV is determined by the total diameter of the vascular bed, and changes in diameter thus affect CBV. The cerebral vessels are sensitive to changes in the pH of the CSF and thus respond to changes in the partial pressure of CO$_2$ with caliber adjustments. CO$_2$ can be regulated by adjusting ventilatory settings, and hyperventilation (i.e., induction of hypocapnia) to induce vasoconstriction is a useful method to manage acute episodes of raised ICP. For longterm treatment of ICP, however, hyperventilation is not recommended [see 5:2 Injuries to the Central Nervous System].

Translocation of different parts of the brain produces specific herniation syndromes that have characteristic clinical presentations and temporal profiles. Brain herniation occurs in five major patterns.[1]

HERNIATION SYNDROMES

Subfalcial (Cingulate) Herniation

Mass lesions in the anterior or middle fossa may result in herniation of the cingulate gyrus under the free edge of the falx cerebri. Usually, patients with this condition are asymptomatic. If the herniation is severe, however, the pericallosal arteries may be compressed, resulting in unilateral or bilateral frontal infarcts in their region of distribution. Clinically, this may result in paresis of one or both legs.

Lateral (Uncal) Tentorial Herniation

Uncal herniation is caused by mass lesions in the lateral middle fossa or temporal lobe, which displace the medial edge of the uncus and hippocampal gyrus medially over the ipsilateral edge of the tentorium cerebelli. The uncus and the hippocampus thus herniate in the space between the midbrain and the tentorial edge, resulting in compression of the midbrain from side to side and elongation of its anteroposterior diameter. The ipsilateral cerebral peduncle and the

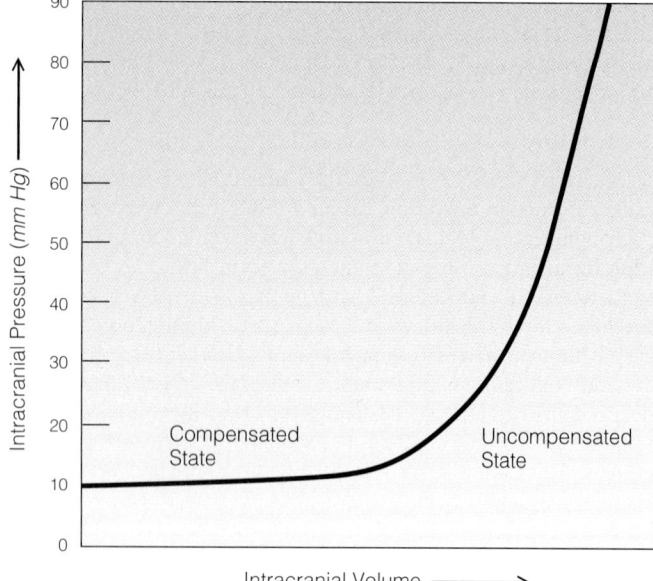

Figure 9 Depicted is the relation between ICP and intracranial volume.

oculomotor nerve are compressed, resulting in the classic syndrome of uncal herniation, which consists of contralateral hemiparesis, decreased consciousness (possibly caused by distortion or deafferentiation of the upper part of the RAS), and ipsilateral pupillary dilatation. In some cases, the herniation may cause compression of the contralateral cerebral peduncle against the tentorium, resulting in ipsilateral hemiparesis (Kernohan's notch). In these cases, the contralateral oculomotor nerve may also be stretched.

As uncal herniation progresses, it becomes clinically indistinguishable from central herniation. Early recognition of uncal herniation is important because deterioration may proceed rapidly once signs of herniation and brain-stem compression appear. In its initial stages, uncal herniation is fully reversible; however, as it evolves, neurologic recovery becomes progressively less likely.

Posterior (Tectal) Herniation

Posterior or tectal herniation may occur in patients who have purely frontal or occipital lesions or have bilateral lesions such as a bilateral chronic subdural hematoma. Under these circumstances, the medial temporal structures do not herniate between the tentorium and midbrain; instead, they herniate posteriorly or on both sides, thereby compressing the quadrigeminal plate at the level of the superior colliculi. Clinically, this results in findings resembling Parinaud syndrome. The patient has bilateral ptosis and an upward gaze paralysis in the presence of initially preserved pupillary response.

Central (Axial) Herniation

Central or axial herniation is defined as a downward shift of the entire brain stem toward the foramen magnum. Because of the downward herniation, the brain stem is elongated in its anteroposterior diameter, and stretching may occur in the central perforating branches of the basilar artery. This stretching is thought to produce ischemia and hemorrhage, although hemorrhage occasionally results from reversal of the displacement by operative decompression. Impaired consciousness has been related to this axial displacement. The Cushing response (arterial hypertension, bradycardia, and respiratory irregularity) has also been related to brain-stem ischemia.

Brain-stem blood flow is not always decreased in the presence of a Cushing response, however, and variant Cushing responses (e.g., hypotension) exist.[12,131]

The first clinical signs are reduced consciousness; symmetrical, small, reactive pupils; paresis of the upward gaze; signs of bilateral corticospinal tract dysfunction; and periodic breathing (Cheyne-Stokes respiration). As herniation progresses, flexor and eventually extensor posturing occurs, the pupils become fixed and dilated or remain in midposition, and hyperpnea results. At later stages, the lower pons and upper medulla are affected; this is characterized by fixed midposition pupils, limb flaccidity, bilateral Babinski responses, abolished oculovestibular reflexes, and shallow, regular breathing, often at an increased rate. Finally, medullary dysfunction occurs; patients display slow, irregular respiration interrupted by deep sighs and gasps. All reflexes disappear and the pupils become widely dilated.

Tonsillar Herniation

Prolapse of the cerebral tonsils through the foramen magnum can occur with either supratentorial or infratentorial masses or with a generalized increase in ICP. Tonsillar herniation causes obliteration of the cisterna magna and compression of the medulla oblongata, the latter resulting in apnea. The shape and size of the tentorial opening determine whether signs of tentorial or tonsillar herniation predominate with supratentorial mass lesions. When the opening is small, major symptoms are usually tentorial in nature; however, when the opening is large, tonsillar herniation may follow without any preceding signs of tentorial herniation.

Prognosis for the Comatose Patient

Even when optimal treatment is provided, the overall prognosis for the comatose patient is poor. Only about 40% of patients who are unconscious as a result of head trauma make a satisfactory recovery. In nontraumatic coma, the outcome is worse. In a study of 596 patients who were admitted for cardiac arrest (31%), cerebral infarction (36%), or ICH (36%), follow-up at 2 months showed that 69% had died, 20% survived with severe disability, 8% survived without severe disability, and 3% survived with unknown functional status.[132]

Outcome depends primarily on the etiology and the duration of coma, the initial clinical signs of neurologic damage, and the general medical condition and age of the patient. In patients with head injury, a motor score of 3 on admission, episodes of hypoxia ($PO_2 < 60$ mm Hg), hypotension (systolic blood pressure < 90 mm Hg), and raised ICP are important prognosticators of poor outcome.[133] Coma caused by depressant drug poisoning carries the most favorable prognosis if treated early: overall mortality is 1% to 5%.[134,135] Hypoxic-ischemic coma carries the worst prognosis: overall mortality is as high as 54%.[135,136] Most patients who recover from drug overdose suffer no residual brain damage, even after prolonged coma, whereas in one study, more than 50% of patients with hypoxic-ischemic coma who survived for at least 2 weeks remained comatose and suffered permanent brain damage.[135]

Cellular, Metabolic, and Systemic Effects of Status Epilepticus

The events that initiate status epilepticus are not known. The presence of an abnormally prolonged seizure has been attributed to excessive excitation, a failure of inhibition, or a combination of the two. However, relatively little is known about the cellular and molecular changes within a neuronal network that are responsible for persistent seizure activity. Excitation is a glutamate-dependent process and is initiated when the neurotransmitter glutamate binds to postsynaptic N-methyl-D-aspartate (NMDA) and non-NMDA glutamate receptors.[137] Initially, only non-NMDA channels are activated, resulting in the influx of sodium and depolarization. Ion flow through NMDA channels is blocked because of the presence of magnesium in the ion channel and because of GABA-mediated inhibitory mechanisms. In status epilepticus, however, GABA-mediated inhibition is suppressed, resulting in depolarization of the NMDA receptor, removal of magnesium from the ion channel, and influx of calcium, followed by further depolarization and intracellular calcium accumulation. Cell death after status epilepticus has been attributed to increased calcium accumulation, initiation of cell swelling, and calcium-mediated cell destruction.[138]

The effects of status epilepticus on cerebral metabolism and circulation can be divided into two phases, whereby the transition from phase 1 to phase 2 typically occurs at 30 to 60 minutes of continuous seizure activity.[138] In phase 1, an increase in CBF compensates for the increase in cerebral metabolic activity caused by the seizures, and the delivery of oxygen and glucose is maintained. In phase 2, the physiologic compensation mechanism (i.e., cerebral autoregulation) begins to fail because CBF is no longer sufficient to support the high metabolic demands of the epileptic tissue, and ischemia ensues.[139-141] Ischemia is further precipitated by systemic hypotension, which almost invariably occurs in phase 2 and which is in turn greatly exacerbated by I.V. antiepileptic drug therapy, particularly when these drugs are infused quickly. ICP can rise exponentially in late status epilepticus, and this rise, combined with hypotension, results in a decrease in CPP, which further compromises the cerebral circulation.

Other general metabolic and systemic effects of status epilepticus occurring in phase 1 include autonomic changes such as tachycardia, cardiac dysrhythmias, hypertension, apnea, pupillary enlargement, hypersecretion, sweating, incontinence, hyperglycemia, and lactic acidosis. In phase 2, changes include hypoglycemia, hyponatremia, hypokalemia or hyperkalemia, metabolic and respiratory acidosis, hepatic and renal dysfunction, diffuse intravascular coagulation, multiorgan failure, rhabdomyolysis, leukocytosis, hypoxia, hypotension, respiratory and cardiac impairment, and hyperpyrexia.[138]

Prognosis for the Patient in Status Epilepticus

Several factors determine the prognosis of status epilepticus. In tonic-clonic status epilepticus, the actual time that patients are seizing appears to be the most important determinant of outcome, followed by the nature of the underlying disease and the age of the patient. Furthermore, in adults it appears that intermittent status epilepticus has a better prognosis than continuous status epilepticus. The reported mortality from convulsive status epilepticus in several clinical series varied from 0% to 6% in children and from 0% to 10% in adults.[142] It should be noted that all of these cases were retrieved from hospital-based series and that these figures are estimates because it is sometimes difficult to establish whether death was caused by status epilepticus itself or by the underlying disease.

Status epilepticus in patients with head injury may represent a significant contribution to poor outcome, but sufficient clinical data are unavailable. Seizure prophylaxis is recommended in patients with head injuries, but no guidelines are currently available to indicate who should receive it (i.e., patients with severe head injuries only or those with moderate head injuries as well). In a recent study of 94 patients with moderate to severe head injuries who underwent continuous EEG monitoring, seizure activity was demonstrated in 22% of patients despite phenytoin prophylaxis. Six of them displayed status epilepticus, all of whom subsequently died; these results indicate that continuous evaluation for seizures or status epilepticus should be seriously considered in these patients, together with aggressive intervention.[143]

References

1. Miller J, Becker D: Pathophysiology of head injury. Neurological Surgery, 2nd ed. Youmans J, Ed. WB Saunders Co, Philadelphia, 1982, p 1896

2. Denny-Brown D: Selected Writings of Sir Charles Sherrington. Oxford University Press, Oxford, 1979

3. Eccles J, Gibson W: Sherrington, His Life and Thought. Springer International, Berlin, 1979

4. Greenberg RP, Stablein DM, Becker DP: Noninvasive localization of brain-stem lesions in the cat with multimodality evoked potentials: correlation with human head-injury data. J Neurosurg 54:740, 1981

5. Ritter AM, Muizelaar JP, Barnes T, et al: Brain stem blood flow, pupillary response, and outcome in patients with severe head injuries. Neurosurgery 44:941, 1999

6. Qureshi A, Wilson D, Traystman R: Treatment of elevated intracranial pressure in experimental intracerebral hemorrhage: comparison between mannitol and hypertonic saline. Neurosurgery 44:1055, 1999

7. Kellie G: On death from cold, and on congestions of the brain. An account of the appearances observed in the dissection of two of three individuals presumed to have perished in the storm of 3rd November 1821; with some reflections on the pathology of the brain. Trans Med Chir Soc Edinburgh 1:84, 1824

8. Monro A: Observations on the Structure and Function of the Nervous System. Creech and Johnson, Edinburgh, 1783

9. Chesnut RM, Marshall LF: Management of head injury. Treatment of abnormal intracranial pressure. Neurosurg Clin N Am 2:267, 1991

10. Eisenberg HM, Frankowski RF, Contant CF, et al: High-dose barbiturate control of elevated intracranial pressure in patients with severe head injury. J Neurosurg 69:15, 1988

11. Miller JD, Becker DP, Ward JD, et al: Significance of intracranial hypertension in severe head injury. J Neurosurg 47:503, 1977

12. Rowan JO, Teasdale G: Brain stem blood flow during raised intracranial pressure. Acta Neurol Scand Suppl 64:520, 1977

13. Souhami R, Moxham J: Textbook of Medicine. Churchill Livingstone, Edinburgh, 1990, p 747

14. Souhami R, Moxham J: Textbook of Medicine. Churchill Livingstone, Edinburgh, 1990, p 971

15. Souhami R, Moxham J: Textbook of Medicine. Churchill Livingstone, Edinburgh, 1990, p 806

16. Souhami R, Moxham J: Textbook of Medicine. Churchill Livingstone, Edinburgh, 1990, p 968

17. Forsyth PA, Posner JB: Headaches in patients with brain tumors: a study of 111 patients. Neurology 43:1678, 1993

18. Ropper A, Gress D: Computerized tomography and clinical features of large cerebral hemorrhages. Cerebrovasc Dis 1:38, 1991

19. Brott T, Thalinger K, Hertzberg V: Hypertension as a risk factor for spontaneous intracerebral hemorrhage. Stroke 17:1078, 1986

20. Hunt WE, Hess RM: Surgical risk as related to time of intervention in the repair of intracranial aneurysms. J Neurosurg 28:14, 1968

21. Drake C: Report of World Federation of Neurological Surgeons Committee on a universal subarachnoid hemorrhage grading scale. J Neurosurg 68:985, 1988

22. Eisenberg HM, Gary HE Jr, Aldrich EF, et al: Initial CT findings in 753 patients with severe head injury. A report from the NIH Traumatic Coma Data Bank. J Neurosurg 73:688, 1990

23. Martin NA, Doberstein C, Alexander M, et al: Post-traumatic cerebral arterial spasm. J Neurotrauma 12:897, 1995

24. Romer F: Difficulties in the diagnosis of acute bacterial meningitis: evaluation of antibiotic pretreatment and causes of admission to the hospital. Lancet 2:345, 1977

25. Bolton C: Infections of the central nervous system. Coma and Impaired Consciousness. Young G, Ropper A, Bolton C, Eds. McGraw-Hill Book Co, New York, 1998, p 228

26. Young G: Impaired consciousness and disorders of temperature. Coma and Impaired Consciousness. Young G, Ropper A, Bolton C, Eds. McGraw-Hill Book Co, New York, 1998, p 213

27. Katz RT, Haig AJ, Clark BB, et al: Long-term survival, prognosis, and life-care planning for 29 patients with chronic locked-in syndrome. Arch Phys Med Rehabil 73:403, 1992

28. Tomsick TA, Brott TG, Chambers AA, et al: Hyperdense middle cerebral artery sign on CT: efficacy in detecting middle cerebral artery thrombosis. AJNR Am J Neuroradiol 11:473, 1990

29. Tomsick T, Brott T, Barsan W, et al: Thrombus localization with emergency cerebral CT. AJNR Am J Neuroradiol 13:257, 1992

30. Wijdicks E: The Clinical Practice of Critical Care Neurology. Lippincott-Raven, Philadelphia, 1997, p 193

31. Fisher CM, Kistler JP, Davis JM: Relation of cerebral vasospasm to subarachnoid hemorrhage visualized by computerized tomographic scanning. Neurosurgery 6:1, 1980

32. Brouwers PJ, Wijdicks EF, Van Gijn J: Infarction after aneurysm rupture does not depend on distribution or clearance rate of blood. Stroke 23:374, 1992

33. Hillman J: Should computed tomography scanning replace lumbar puncture in the diagnostic process in suspected subarachnoid hemorrhage? Surg Neurol 26:547, 1986

34. Hashimoto H, Iida J, Hironaka Y, et al: Use of spiral computerized tomography angiography in patients with subarachnoid hemorrhage in whom subtraction angiography did not reveal cerebral aneurysms. J Neurosurg 92:278, 2000

35. Strayle-Batra M, Skalej M, Wakhloo AK, et al: Three-dimensional spiral CT angiography in the detection of cerebral aneurysm. Acta Radiol 39:233, 1998

36. Velthuis BK, Rinkel GJ, Ramos LM, et al: Subarachnoid hemorrhage: aneurysm detection and preoperative evaluation with CT angiography. Radiology 208:423, 1998

37. Harrison MJ, Johnson BA, Gardner GM, et al: Preliminary results on the management of unruptured intracranial aneurysms with magnetic resonance angiography and computed tomographic angiography. Neurosurgery 40:947, discussion 955, 1997

38. Wardlaw JM, White PM: The detection and management of unruptured intracranial aneurysms. Brain 123:205, 2000

39. Desprechins B, Stadnik T, Koerts G, et al: Use of diffusion-weighted MR imaging in differential diagnosis between intracerebral necrotic tumors and cerebral abscesses [see comments]. AJNR Am J Neuroradiol 20:1252, 1999

40. Miller ES, Dias PS, Uttley D: CT scanning in the management of intracranial abscess: a review of 100 cases. Br J Neurosurg 2:439, 1988

41. Zimmerman RA, Bilaniuk LT: Computed tomographic staging of traumatic epidural bleeding. Radiology 144:809, 1982

42. Gennarelli TA, Thibault LE: Biomechanics of acute subdural hematoma. J Trauma 22:680, 1982

43. Gudeman SK, Kishore PR, Miller JD, et al: The genesis and significance of delayed traumatic intracerebral hematoma. Neurosurgery 5:309, 1979

44. Ribas G, Jane J: Traumatic contusions and intracerebral hematomas. Central Nervous System Trauma Status Report 1991. J Neurotrauma 9[suppl 1]: S265, 1992

45. Becker D, Doberstein C, Hovda D: Craniocerebral Trauma: Mechanisms, Management, and the Cellular Response to Injury. Current Concepts. The Upjohn Co, Kalamazoo, Michigan, 1994

46. Chesnut R, Servadei F: Surgical treatment of post-traumatic mass lesions. Traumatic Brain Injury. Marion D, Ed. Thieme Medical Publishers, New York, 1999, p 81

47. Strich S: Shearing of nerve fibers as a cause of brain damage due to head injury: a pathological study of twenty cases. Lancet 2:443, 1961

48. Marshall LF, Marshall SB, Klauber MR, et al: The diagnosis of head injury requires a classification based on computed axial tomography. J Neurotrauma 9(suppl 1):S287, 1992

49. Ropper AH, Shafran B: Brain edema after stroke. Clinical syndrome and intracranial pressure. Arch Neurol 41:26, 1984

50. Shaw C, Alvord E, Berry R: Swelling of the brain following ischemic infarction with arterial occlusion. Arch Neurol 1:161, 1959

51. Schwab S, Aschoff A, Spranger M, et al: The value of intracranial pressure monitoring in acute hemispheric stroke. Neurology 47:393, 1996

52. Doerfler A, Forsting M, Reith W, et al: Decompressive craniectomy in a rat model of "malignant" cerebral hemispheric stroke: experimental support for an aggressive therapeutic approach. J Neurosurg 85:853, 1996

53. Forsting M, Reith W, Scheabitz WR, et al: Decompressive craniectomy for cerebral infarction: an experimental study in rats. Stroke 26:259, 1995

54. Rabb CH: Surgical treatment strategies in ischemic stroke. Neuroimaging Clin N Am 9:527, 1999

55. Rieke K, Schwab S, Krieger D, et al: Decompressive surgery in space-occupying hemispheric infarction: results of an open, prospective trial. Crit Care Med 23:1576, 1995

56. Sakai K, Iwahashi K, Terada K, et al: Outcome after external decompression for massive cerebral infarction. Neurol Med Chir (Tokyo) 38:131, 1998

57. Schwab S, Steiner T, Aschoff A, et al: Early hemicraniectomy in patients with complete middle cerebral artery infarction. Stroke 29:1888, 1998

58. McKissock W, Richardson A, Taylor J: Primary intracerebral hemorrhage: a controlled trial of surgical and conservative treatment in 180 unselected cases. Lancet 2:221, 1961

59. Juvela S, Heiskanen O, Poranen A, et al: The treatment of spontaneous intracerebral hemorrhage: a prospective randomized trial of surgical and conservative treatment. J Neurosurg 70:755, 1989

60. Kandel EI, Peresedov VV: Stereotaxic evacuation of spontaneous intracerebral hematomas. J Neurosurg 62:206, 1985

61. Kanno T, Nagata J, Nonomura K, et al: New approaches in the treatment of hypertensive intracerebral hemorrhage. Stroke 24(12 suppl):I96, 1993

62. Winn HR, Richardson AE, Jane JA: The long-term prognosis in untreated cerebral aneurysms: I. The incidence of late hemorrhage in cerebral aneurysm: a 10-year evaluation of 364 patients. Ann Neurol 1:358, 1977

63. Winn HR, Richardson AE, O'Brien W, et al: The long-term prognosis in untreated cerebral aneurysms: II. Late morbidity and mortality. Ann Neurol 4:418, 1978

64. Dorsch NW: Cerebral arterial spasm—a clinical review. Br J Neurosurg 9:403, 1995

65. Levy ML, Giannotta SL: Induced hypertension and hypervolemia for treatment of cerebral vasospasm. Neurosurg Clin North Am 1:357, 1990

66. Muizelaar JP, Zwienenberg M, Rudisill NA, et al: The prophylactic use of transluminal balloon angioplasty in patients with Fisher grade 3 subarachnoid hemorrhage: a pilot study. J Neurosurg 91:51, 1999

67. Dyste GN, Hitchon PW, Menezes AH, et al: Stereotaxic surgery in the treatment of multiple brain abscesses. J Neurosurg 69:188, 1988

68. Kala M: Aspiration or extirpation in cerebral abscess surgery? Neurosurg Rev 16:121, 1993

69. Mampalam TJ, Rosenblum ML: Trends in the management of bacterial brain abscesses: a review of 102 cases over 17 years. Neurosurgery 23:451, 1988

70. Tekkeok IH, Erbengi A: Management of brain abscess in children: review of 130 cases over a period of 21 years. Childs Nerv Syst 8:411, 1992

71. Ballester JM, Harchelroad FP: Hypothermia: an easy-to-miss, dangerous disorder in winter weather. Geriatrics 54:51, 1999

72. Gentilello LM: Advances in the management of hypothermia. Surg Clin N Am 75:243, 1995

73. Goodlock JL: Methods of rewarming the hypothermic patient in the accident and emergency department. Accid Emerg Nurs 3:114, 1995

74. Haskell RM, Boruta B, Rotondo MF, et al: Hypothermia. AACN Clinical Issues 8:368, 1997

75. Kofstad J: Blood gases and hypothermia: some theoretical and practical considerations. Scand J Clin Lab Invest Suppl 224:21, 1996

76. Lloyd EL: Accidental hypothermia. Resuscitation 32:111, 1996

77. McGowan J: Management of hypothermia in adults. Nursing Crit Care 4:59, 1999

78. Patten J: Attacks of Altered Consciousness, 2nd ed. Springer-Verlag, Berlin, 1996

79. Appleton R, Sweeney A, Choonara I, et al: Lorazepam versus diazepam in the acute treatment of epileptic seizures and status epilepticus. Dev Med Child Neurol 37:682, 1995

80. Dodrill CB, Wilensky AJ: Intellectual impairment as an outcome of status epilepticus. Neurology 40 (suppl 2):23, 1990

81. Lipowski Z: Delirium in surgery: historical introduction. Delirium: Acute Brain Failure in Man. Charles C Thomas, Springfield, Illinois, 1980, p 213

82. Fisher B, Gilchrist D: Postoperative delirium in the elderly. Ann R Coll Phys Surg Canada 26:358, 1993

83. El-Ganzouri A, Ivankovich A, Braverman B, et al: Monoamine oxidase inhibitors: should they be discontinued preoperatively? Anesth Analg 64:592, 1985

84. Grigoletto F, Zappalaa G, Anderson DW, et al: Norms for the Mini-Mental State Examination in a healthy population. Neurology 53:315, 1999

85. McDowell I, Kristjansson B, Hill GB, et al: Community screening for dementia: the Mini-Mental State Exam (MMSE) and Modified Mini-Mental State Exam (3MS) compared. J Clin Epidemiol 50:377, 1997

86. Rapp CG, Wakefield B, Kundrat M, et al: Acute confusion assessment instruments: clinical versus research usability. Appl Nurs Res 13:37, 2000

87. Wind AW, Schellevis FG, Van Staveren G, et al: Limitations of the Mini-Mental State Examination in diagnosing dementia in general practice. Int J Geriatr Psychiatry 12:101, 1997

88. Rolfson DB, McElhaney JE, Jhangri GS, et al: Validity of the confusion assessment method in detecting postoperative delirium in the elderly. Int Psychogeriatrics 11:431, 1999

89. Spar JE: Dementia in the aged. Psychiatr Clin N Am 5:67, 1982

90. Kaplan H, Sadock B, Grebb J: Dementia. Synopsis of Psychiatry. Williams & Wilkins, Baltimore, 1994, p 345

91. McKhann G, Drachman D, Folstein M, et al: Clinical diagnosis of Alzheimer's disease: report of the NINCDS-ADRDA Work Group under the auspices of Department of Health and Human Services Task Force on Alzheimer's Disease. Neurology 34:939, 1984

92. Cummings J: Neuropsychiatric aspects of Alzheimer's disease and other dementing illnesses. Textbook of Neuropsychiatry. Yudofsky S, Hales R, Eds. American Psychiatric Association, Washington, DC, 1992, p 605

93. McEvoy J: Organic brain syndromes. Ann Intern Med 95:212, 1981

94. Wells C: Organic syndromes: dementia. Comprehensive Textbook of Psychiatry. Kaplan H, Sadock B, Eds. William & Wilkins, Baltimore, 1985, p 851

95. Daly MP: Diagnosis and management of Alzheimer disease. J Am Board Fam Pract 12:375, 1999

96. Davis RE, Emmerling MR, Jaen JC, et al: Therapeutic intervention in dementia. Crit Rev Neurobiol 7:41, 1993

97. Diaz Brinton R, Yamazaki RS: Advances and challenges in the prevention and treatment of Alzheimer's disease. Pharm Res 15:386, 1998

98. Flint AJ, van Reekum R: The pharmacologic treatment of Alzheimer's disease: a guide for the general psychiatrist. Can J Psychiatry 43:689, 1998

99. Foy JM, Starr JM: Assessment and treatment of dementia in medical patients. Psychother Psychosom 69:59, 2000

100. Nyenhuis DL, Gorelick PB: Vascular dementia: a contemporary review of epidemiology, diagnosis, prevention, and treatment. J Am Geriatr Soc 46:1437, 1998

101. Rabins PV: Developing treatment guidelines for Alz-

heimer's disease and other dementias. J Clin Psychiatry 59(suppl 11):17, 1998

102. Scheltens P, van Gool WA: Emerging treatments in dementia. Eur Neurol 38:184, 1997

103. Sadavoy J: A review of pseudodementia. Mod Med Canada 39:319, 1984

104. Wells C: Pseudodementia. Am J Psychiatry 136:895, 1979

105. Yesavage J: Differential diagnosis between depression and dementia. Am J Med 94(suppl 5a):23s, 1993

106. Touringy-Rivard M: Treatment of depression in the elderly. Med North Am 1:56, 1986

107. Jenike M: Treatment of affective illness in the elderly with drugs and electroconvulsive therapy. Geriatr Psychiatry Neurol 22:77, 1989

108. Rosenberg D, Wright B, Gerson S: Depression in the elderly. Dementia 3:157, 1992

109. Jennett B, Snoek J, Bond MR, et al: Disability after severe head injury: observations on the use of the Glasgow Outcome Scale. J Neurol Neurosurg Psychiatry 44:285, 1981

110. Teasdale GM, Pettigrew LE, Wilson JT, et al: Analyzing outcome of treatment of severe head injury: a review and update on advancing the use of the Glasgow Outcome Scale. J Neurotrauma 15:587, 1998

111. Blyth B: The outcome of severe head injuries. N Z Med J 93:267, 1981

112. Gensemer IB, McMurry FG, Walker JC, et al: Behavioral consequences of trauma. J Trauma 28:44, 1988

113. Gensemer IB, Smith JL, Walker JC, et al: Psychological consequences of blunt head trauma and relation to other indices of severity of injury. Ann Emerg Med 18:9, 1989

114. Tate RL, Broe GA, Lulham JM: Impairment after severe blunt head injury: the results from a consecutive series of 100 patients. Acta Neurol Scand 79:97, 1989

115. Dikmen S, Temkin N, McLean A, et al: Memory and head injury severity. J Neurol Neurosurg Psychiatry 50:1613, 1987

116. Paniak CE, Shore DL, Rourke BP: Recovery of memory after severe closed head injury: dissociations in recovery of memory parameters and predictors of outcome. J Clin Exp Neuropsychol 11:631, 1989

117. Uzzell BP, Dolinskas CA, Wiser RF, et al: Influence of lesions detected by computed tomography on outcome and neuropsychological recovery after severe head injury. Neurosurgery 20:396, 1987

118. Francis J: Delirium in older patients. J Am Geriatr Soc 40:829, 1992

119. Meador KJ: Cognitive side effects of medications. Neurol Clin 16:141, 1998

120. Burns MJ, Linden CU, Grandins A, et al: A comparison of physostigmine and benzodiazepines for the treatment of anticholinergic poisoning. Ann Emerg Med 35:374, 2000

121. Tesar GE, Murray GB, Cassem NH: Use of high-dose intravenous haloperidol in the treatment of agitated cardiac patients. J Clin Psychopharmacol 5:344, 1985

122. Black PM: Brain death (pt 1). N Engl J Med 299:338, 1978

123. Black PM: Brain death (pt 2). N Engl J Med 299:393, 1978

124. Report of Special Task Force: Guidelines for the determination of brain death in children. Pediatrics 80:298, 1987

125. LaMancusa J, Cooper R, Vieth R, et al: The effects of the falling therapeutic and subtherapeutic barbiturate blood levels on electrocerebral silence in clinically brain-dead children. Clin Electroencephalogr 22:112, 1991

126. Wijdicks E: Precautions for the apnea test in brain death. Neurology of Critical Illness. FA Davis Co, Philadelphia, 1995, p 329

127. Lynch J, Eldadah MK: Brain-death criteria currently used by pediatric intensivists. Clin Pediatr 31:457, 1992

128. Mejia RE, Pollack MM: Variability in brain death determination practices in children [see comments]. JAMA 274:550, 1995

129. Verweij BH, Muizelaar JP, Vinas FC, et al: Mitochondrial dysfunction after experimental and human brain injury and its possible reversal with a selective N-type calcium channel antagonist (SNX-111). Neurol Res 19:334, 1997

130. Jones T: Thresholds of focal cerebral ischemia in awake monkeys. J Neurosurg 54:773, 1981

131. Marshiman L: Cushing's variant response (acute hypotension) after subarachnoid hemorrhage. Association with moderate intracranial hypertension and subacute cardiovascular collapse. Stroke 28:1445, 1997

132. Hamel MB, Goldman L, Teno J, et al: Identification of comatose patients at high risk for death or severe disability. SUPPORT Investigators. Understand Prognoses and Preferences for Outcomes and Risks of Treatments. JAMA 273:1842, 1995

133. Combes P, Fauvage B, Colonna M, et al: Severe head injuries: an outcome prediction and survival analysis. Intensive Care Med 22:1391, 1996

134. Ghodse A: Deliberate self-poisoning: a study in London casualty departments. Br Med J 1:805, 1977

135. Sacco RL, Van Gool R, Mohr JP, et al: Nontraumatic coma. Glasgow Coma Score and coma etiology as predictors of 2-week outcome. Arch Neurol 47:1181, 1990

136. Bertini G, Margheri M, Giglioli C, et al: Prognostic significance of early clinical manifestations in postanoxic coma: a retrospective study of 58 patients resuscitated after prehospital cardiac arrest. Crit Care Med 17:627, 1989

137. Fountain N, Bleck T: Mechanism of action of drugs for status epilepticus. Epilepsy Quarterly, winter 1996

138. Shorvon S: Status Epilepticus: Its Clinical Features and Treatment in Children and Adults. Cambridge University Press, Cambridge, 1994, p 54

139. Meldrum B: Metabolic factors during prolonged seizures and their relation to cell death. Status Epilepticus. Mechanisms of Brain Damage and Treatment, Vol 34. Delgado-Escueta A, Wasterlain C, Treiman D, et al, Eds. Raven Press, New York, 1986, p 261

140. Franck G, Sadzot B, Salmon F, et al: Regional cerebral blood flow and metabolic rates in human focal epilepsy and status epilepsy. Basic Mechanisms of the Epilepsies: Molecular and Cellular Approaches, Vol 44. Delgado-Escueta A Jr., Woodbury D, Porter R, Eds. Raven Press, New York, 1986, p 935

141. Siesjo B, Wieloch T: Epileptic brain damage: pathophysiology and neurochemical pathology. Basic Mechanisms of the Epilepsies: Molecular and Cellular Approaches, Vol 44. Delgado-Escueta A Jr., Woodbury D, Porter R, Eds. Raven Press, New York, 1986, p 813

142. Shorvon S: Status Epilepticus: Its Clinical Features and Treatment in Children and Adults. Cambridge University Press, Cambridge, 1994, p 296

143. Vespa P, Prins M, Ronne-Engstrom E, et al: Increase in extracellular glutamate caused by reduced cerebral perfusion pressure and seizures after human traumatic brain injury: a microdialysis study. J Neurosurg 89:971, 1998

Acknowledgments

Portions of this chapter are adapted from material contained in two chapters previously published in *Scientific American® Surgery:* "Coma, Seizures, and Brain Death," by Ehud Arbit, M.D., and George Krol, M.D., and "Cognitive and Sensory Deficits," by Richard Monks, M.D.

13 MULTIPLE ORGAN DYSFUNCTION SYNDROME

John C. Marshall M.D., F.A.C.S., F.R.C.S.(C)

Approach to Multiple Organ Dysfunction Syndrome

The multiple organ dysfunction syndrome (MODS)—also known as progressive systems failure,[1] multiple organ failure,[2] and multiple system organ failure[3]—is characterized by progressive but potentially reversible physiologic dysfunction of two or more organ systems that arises after resuscitation from an acute life-threatening event. The term MODS was introduced by a 1991 consensus conference of the American College of Chest Physicians (ACCP) and the Society of Critical Care Medicine (SCCM).[4] The designation of MODS as a syndrome emphasizes that dynamic alterations in physiologic function in critically ill patients may have common pathophysiologic underpinnings. However, MODS is as much a paradigm as a syndrome—that is, it represents an approach to the care of the critically ill patient that emphasizes intensive monitoring and support of organ system function over specific therapies for isolated disease processes and that focuses on preventing or minimizing iatrogenic injury resulting from ICU interventions.

MODS evolves in the wake of a profound disruption of systemic homeostasis.[5,6] It was originally described in patients with overwhelming infection, multiple injuries, or tissue ischemia; however, it has many overlapping risk factors [*see Table 1*]. Preexisting illness—in particular, chronic alcohol abuse[7]—predisposes to the development of organ dysfunction in patients exposed to these risk factors.

Clinical Definitions of Organ Dysfunction

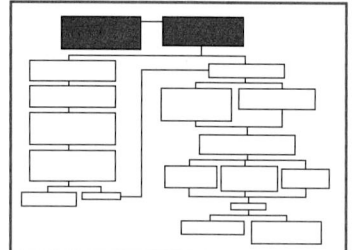

Although MODS is readily recognized by experienced clinicians, there is still no clear consensus on its description with respect to either the systems whose function is deranged, the descriptors that best measure that derangement, or the degree of derangement that constitutes organ dysfunction or failure.

A systematic review of 30 published clinical studies evaluated the organ systems and variables used to describe MODS.[8] Seven organ systems—the respiratory system (all 30 reports), the renal system (29 reports), the hepatic system (27 reports), the cardiovascular system (25 reports), the hematologic system (23 reports), the GI system (22 reports), and the CNS (18 reports)—were included in at least half of the studies. Scoring systems from both North America[9,10] and Europe[11,12] define MODS using six of these seven organ systems, eliminating the GI system because of the declining prevalence of stress-related upper GI bleeding and the lack of satisfactory measures of GI dysfunction. These scoring systems have many similarities [*see Table 2*].

In general terms, the dysfunction of a given organ system can be described in one of three ways:

1. As a physiologic derangement (e.g., an altered ratio of arterial oxygen tension [P_aO_2] to fractional inspiration of oxygen [F_IO_2] or an altered platelet count).
2. As the clinical intervention used to correct that derangement (e.g., mechanical ventilation or blood component replacement therapy).
3. As a discrete clinical syndrome incorporating several descriptive variables (e.g., acute respiratory distress syndrome [ARDS] or disseminated intravascular coagulation [DIC]).

Whichever of these three perspectives is adopted, common pathogenetic mechanisms underlie MODS, and common principles direct its prevention and management.

RESPIRATORY DYSFUNCTION

ARDS, initially described in the early 1960s,[13,14] is the prototypical expression of respiratory dysfunction in MODS.[15] In its

Table 1 Risk Factors for MODS

Infection	Peritonitis and intra-abdominal infections Pneumonia Necrotizing soft tissue infections
Inflammation	Pancreatitis
Injury	Multiple trauma Burn injury
Ischemia	Ruptured aneurysm Hypovolemic shock Mesenteric ischemia
Immune reactions	Autoimmune disease Transplant rejection Graft versus host disease
Iatrogenic factors	Delayed or missed injury Blood transfusion Injurious mechanical ventilation Total parenteral nutrition
Intoxication	Drug reactions Arsenic intoxication Drug overdose
Idiopathic factors	Thrombotic thrombocytopenic purpura Hypoadrenalism Pheochromocytoma

Table 2 Multiple Organ Dysfunction (MOD) Score[9]

Organ System	Indicator of Dysfunction	Degree of Dysfunction				
		None (0)	Minimal (1)	Mild (2)	Moderate (3)	Severe (4)
Respiratory	P_aO_2/F_IO_2 ratio	> 300	226–300	151–225	76–150	≤ 75
Renal	Serum creatinine level	≤ 100 µmol/L	101–200 µmol/L	201–350 µmol/L	351–500 µmol/L	> 500 µmol/L
Hepatic	Serum bilirubin level	≤ 20 µmol/L	21–60 µmol/L	61–120 µmol/L	121–240 µmol/L	> 240 µmol/L
Cardiovascular	Pressure-adjusted HR*	< 10.0	10.1–15.0	15.1–20.0	20.1–30.0	> 30.0
Hematologic	Platelet count	> 120,000/mm³	81,000–120,000/mm³	51,000–80,000/mm³	21,000–50,000/mm³	≤ 20,000/mm³
Neurologic	Glasgow Coma Scale score	15	13–14	10–12	7–9	≤ 6

*Calculated as the product of HR and central venous pressure (CVP), divided by mean arterial pressure (MAP): (HR · CVP)/MAP.

mildest form, respiratory dysfunction is characterized by tachypnea, hypocapnia, and hypoxemia. As lung injury evolves, a combination of worsening hypoxemia and increased work of breathing necessitates mechanical ventilatory support [see *6:6 Use of the Mechanical Ventilator*].

Increased capillary permeability and neutrophil influx are the earliest pathologic events in ARDS. As the acute inflammatory process resolves, further lung injury results both from the process of repair, which involves fibrosis and the deposition of hyaline material, and from further lung trauma, resulting from positive pressure mechanical ventilation.[16]

Lung involvement in ARDS is inhomogeneous, with areas of functional and aerated alveoli interspersed with areas of non-functional alveoli.[17] The distribution of injury reflects the sequelae of care in the intensive care unit: consolidation occurs in the posterior dependent regions of the lung, and cystic changes develop from overdistention by the ventilator in the antidependent regions.[18]

Impaired lung function is reflected in a reduced P_aO_2. To ensure adequate oxygen delivery to the tissues, mechanical ventilation must be instituted and F_IO_2 increased. The ratio of P_aO_2 to F_IO_2, therefore, provides a sensitive and objective measurement of the degree to which oxygenation is impaired and so is a reliable measure of physiologic respiratory dysfunction.[19] Mechanical ventilation reflects the clinical intervention triggered by impaired oxygenation, and the additional criteria for ARDS—bilateral lung infiltrates and a normal pulmonary capillary wedge pressure—serve to exclude such primary causes of acute hypoxemia as pulmonary embolism, atelectasis, and congestive heart failure. By consensus, ARDS is defined as a P_aO_2/F_IO_2 ratio lower than 200 mm Hg in association with bilateral fluffy pulmonary infiltrates and a pulmonary capillary wedge pressure lower than 18 mm Hg.[20]

ARDS is a robust model for the complex interactions that result in MODS. Lung injury in ARDS is the outcome of an interaction between an insult, a susceptible host, and the clinical therapeutic response, and its severity reflects not only the degree of the initial insult but also various poorly defined genetic influences in the host[21] and the inadvertent adverse consequences of the mode of respiratory support employed.[22]

RENAL DYSFUNCTION

Acute renal failure (ARF) [see *6:7 Renal Failure*] was first described as a significant clinical problem during World War II,[23]

but supportive care, in the form of dialysis, did not become available until the 1950s.

Clinical or subclinical renal dysfunction is common in MODS. Early-onset renal dysfunction typically results from hypotension and decreased renal blood flow. The etiology of late-onset renal failure is multifactorial and includes both prerenal factors (e.g., decreased cardiac output and hypovolemia) and the cumulative renal effects of nephrotoxic agents (e.g., medications and radiocontrast material).[24] Intrarenal vasoconstriction results in a reduction in the glomerular filtration rate, hypoxic or oxidative injury to tubular epithelial cells, and desquamation of injured cells into the tubules, causing leakage of filtrate back into the renal interstitium and evoking neutrophil-mediated inflammation that causes further local tissue injury.[25] Intrarenal shunting of blood flow, coupled with occlusion of the renal microvasculature by thrombi or aggregated blood cells, further contributes to ischemia and physiologic dysfunction. The situation may be further aggravated by renal circulatory changes resulting from vasoactive agents administered to treat shock and by increased intra-abdominal pressure consequent to massive fluid resuscitation. Histologic studies show acute tubular necrosis with disruption of the basement membrane, patchy necrosis of the renal tubules, interstitial edema, and tubular casts; these microscopic changes correlate poorly with functional impairment.[26] Activated neutrophils have also been implicated in the pathogenesis of ARF,[27,28] as has the induction of apoptosis in renal epithelial cells.[29]

Renal dysfunction in MODS is reflected physiologically in a decreased urine output, biochemically in a rising serum creatinine level, and therapeutically as the introduction of exogenous renal replacement therapy or dialysis.

HEPATIC DYSFUNCTION

Hepatic dysfunction after trauma, like ARF, was first described during World War II [see *6:10 Hepatic Failure*].[30] Two clinical syndromes have been described. The first, ischemic hepatitis, or shock liver, characteristically follows an episode of profound hypotension with splanchnic hypoperfusion. Early elevations of aminotransferase levels are striking and may be associated with an increased international normalized ratio and hypoglycemia; centrilobular necrosis is evident histologically. Successful resuscitation of the shock state results in rapid normalization of the biochemical abnormalities.[31] The second syndrome, ICU jaundice, is much more common than ischemic

Approach to Multiple Organ Dysfunction Syndrome

Recognize susceptible patient

Patients at high risk for multiple organ dysfunction syndrome (MODS) are those who have experienced a disruption of systemic homeostasis resulting from one or more of the following:

- Infection
- Inflammation
- Injury
- Ischemia
- Immune system activation
- Intoxication
- Iatrogenic factors

Minimal organ dysfunction

Prevent progression to MODS by optimizing support of hemodynamic, metabolic, and immunologic function, taking care to minimize iatrogenic injury during the provision of physiologic support.

Hemodynamic support

Maximize O_2 delivery to tissues by the following measures:

- Fluid replacement therapy
- Inotropic agents
- Vasoactive agents
- Mechanical ventilation

Metabolic support

Reverse catabolic state with definitive intervention, including the following:

- Debridement of devitalized tissue
- Burn wound excision and grafting
- Fixation of long bone fractures

Provide early nutritional support by the enteral route. If gut function is inadequate, parenteral nutrition should be employed.

Immunologic support

Prevent nosocomial infection, treat documented infection, and minimize the consequences of injurious host defense responses by such measures as the following:

- Timely and appropriate surgical intervention
- Limiting breaches of mucosal defenses
- Selective, targeted use of antibiotics

Organ function is preserved or restored

Patient survives. Discharge patient from ICU.

Organ function deteriorates

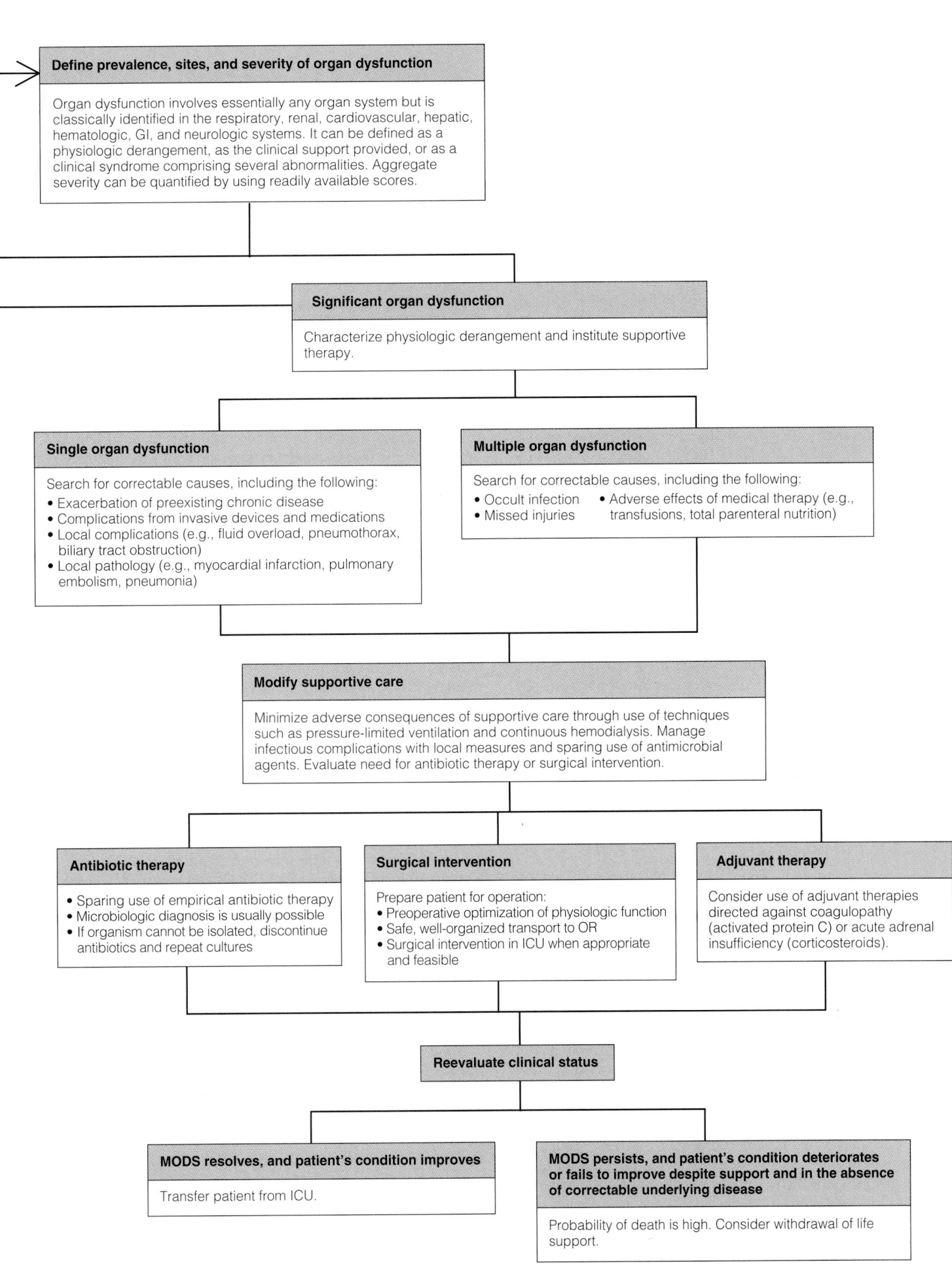

Define prevalence, sites, and severity of organ dysfunction

Organ dysfunction involves essentially any organ system but is classically identified in the respiratory, renal, cardiovascular, hepatic, hematologic, GI, and neurologic systems. It can be defined as a physiologic derangement, as the clinical support provided, or as a clinical syndrome comprising several abnormalities. Aggregate severity can be quantified by using readily available scores.

Significant organ dysfunction

Characterize physiologic derangement and institute supportive therapy.

Single organ dysfunction

Search for correctable causes, including the following:
• Exacerbation of preexisting chronic disease
• Complications from invasive devices and medications
• Local complications (e.g., fluid overload, pneumothorax, biliary tract obstruction)
• Local pathology (e.g., myocardial infarction, pulmonary embolism, pneumonia)

Multiple organ dysfunction

Search for correctable causes, including the following:
• Occult infection   • Adverse effects of medical therapy (e.g.,
• Missed injuries   transfusions, total parenteral nutrition)

Modify supportive care

Minimize adverse consequences of supportive care through use of techniques such as pressure-limited ventilation and continuous hemodialysis. Manage infectious complications with local measures and sparing use of antimicrobial agents. Evaluate need for antibiotic therapy or surgical intervention.

Antibiotic therapy

• Sparing use of empirical antibiotic therapy
• Microbiologic diagnosis is usually possible
• If organism cannot be isolated, discontinue antibiotics and repeat cultures

Surgical intervention

Prepare patient for operation:
• Preoperative optimization of physiologic function
• Safe, well-organized transport to OR
• Surgical intervention in ICU when appropriate and feasible

Adjuvant therapy

Consider use of adjuvant therapies directed against coagulopathy (activated protein C) or acute adrenal insufficiency (corticosteroids).

Reevaluate clinical status

MODS resolves, and patient's condition improves

Transfer patient from ICU.

MODS persists, and patient's condition deteriorates or fails to improve despite support and in the absence of correctable underlying disease

Probability of death is high. Consider withdrawal of life support.

1243

hepatitis and typically evolves many days after the inciting physiologic insult. Conjugated hyperbilirubinemia is a prominent feature, whereas elevation of aminotransferase levels and alterations of hepatic synthetic function are less pronounced.[32] Histologic features include intrahepatic cholestasis, steatosis, and Kupffer cell hyperplasia. The pathogenesis is multifactorial and includes ongoing hepatic ischemia, total parenteral nutrition (TPN)–induced cholestasis, and drug toxicity.

An increased serum bilirubin level is the most commonly recognized feature of the hepatic dysfunction of MODS. Although extracorporeal support devices have been used for patients with end-stage liver disease, the hepatic dysfunction of critical illness is not considered to be life-threatening in itself, and no specific supportive therapy is indicated.

CARDIOVASCULAR DYSFUNCTION

Both peripheral vascular and myocardial function are altered in MODS. Characteristic changes in the peripheral vasculature include a reduction in vascular resistance and an increase in microvascular permeability, resulting in a hyperdynamic circulatory profile and peripheral edema. Both alterations jeopardize tissue oxygenation—reduced vascular resistance by facilitating shunting in the microvasculature and edema by increasing the distance across which oxygen carried in the blood must diffuse to reach the cell. Shunting also occurs as a result of occlusion of the microvasculature by thrombi and aggregates of nondeformable red cells[33]; it is signaled by a reduction in arteriovenous oxygen extraction and an increase in mixed venous oxygen saturation ($S_{mv}O_2$). Biventricular dilatation with a reduction in the right and left ventricular ejection fractions has been described.[34] Right ventricular dysfunction is particularly prominent, perhaps as a consequence of increased pulmonary vascular resistance secondary to concomitant lung injury.[35] Finally, a loss of normal heart rate variability characterizes advanced cardiovascular dysfunction.[36]

The cardiovascular dysfunction of MODS is apparent clinically as increased peripheral edema with hypotension that is refractory to volume challenge and therapeutically in the use of vasoactive agents to support the circulation. Nitric oxide (NO) has been implicated in both the peripheral vasodilatation[37] and the myocardial depression[38] associated with critical illness.

NEUROLOGIC DYSFUNCTION

Abnormalities of both central and peripheral nervous system function are common in critical illness. CNS dysfunction occurs in as many as 70% of critically ill patients, typically presenting as a reduced level of consciousness without localizing signs. Its pathophysiology is incompletely understood. Postulated mechanisms include the direct effects of proinflammatory mediators on cerebral function, the development of vasogenic cerebral edema, areas of cerebral infarction related to hypotension, and alterations in the blood-brain barrier resulting in changes in the composition of the interstitial fluid.[39] Electroencephalography typically shows one of four patterns indicating increasingly abnormal activity: diffuse theta wave rhythms, intermittent rhythmic delta waves, triphasic delta waves, and suppression or burst-suppression patterns.[39] Peripheral nervous system dysfunction, also known as critical illness polyneuropathy, is also common in MODS, though its clinical presentation tends to be more subtle than that of CNS dysfunction.[40-42] Peripheral nervous system dysfunction may present as failure of weaning from mechanical ventilation[43] or as limb weakness with relative sparing of the cranial nerves. Endoneural edema and axonal hypoxia[44] contribute to its pathogenesis, as do the iatrogenic sequelae of neuromuscular blockade.[45]

HEMATOLOGIC DYSFUNCTION

The most common hematologic abnormality of critical illness is thrombocytopenia, which occurs in approximately 20% of all ICU admissions.[46,47] Causes include increased consumption, intravascular sequestration, and impaired thrombopoiesis secondary to suppression of bone marrow function. In addition, heparin-induced thrombocytopenia resulting from antibodies to complexes of heparin and platelet factor 4 develops in as many as 10% of patients receiving heparin.[48] The most fulminant expression of hematologic dysfunction in MODS is DIC, which is characterized by derangements in platelet numbers and clotting times and the presence of fibrin degradation products in plasma.[49] The coagulopathy of critical illness is complex, involving multiple alterations in the biochemical mediators of coagulation and resulting in a shift to a procoagulant state.[50]

Mild anemia is common in critical illness, though the nature of abnormalities in red cell production and removal are less well characterized in this setting.[51] Transient leukopenia may develop in response to an overwhelming inflammatory stimulus, but neutrophilia is much more commonly encountered; total lymphocyte counts are reduced. Abnormalities in white cell populations reflect, at least in part, altered expression of apoptosis, which is inhibited in the neutrophil[52] but accelerated in lymphoid cells.[53]

GASTROINTESTINAL DYSFUNCTION

Upper GI hemorrhage after burn injury was first described by Curling in 1842.[54] Stress bleeding was once a relatively common complication, but improved techniques of resuscitation and hemodynamic support, earlier diagnosis of infection, and the widespread use of stress ulcer prophylaxis have reduced the frequency of this event, to the point where it now is seen in fewer than 4% of ICU admissions.[55] Other manifestations of GI dysfunction in MODS include ileus and intolerance of enteral feeding,[56,57] pancreatitis,[58] and acalculous cholecystitis.[59]

OTHER ORGAN SYSTEM DYSFUNCTION

MODS is associated with functional abnormalities of virtually every organ system. Endocrine abnormalities include impaired glucose regulation with hyperglycemia and insulin resistance[60] and hypercortisolemia with impaired responsiveness to adrenocorticotropic hormone (ACTH) stimulation.[61,62] The sick euthyroid syndrome, characterized by reductions in serum T_3, with or without an increase in reverse T_3 levels and a normal T_4 level, is another manifestation of the endocrine dysfunction of MODS.[63]

Numerous derangements of immune function have been described in MODS patients. Cell-mediated immunity is impaired, as reflected by anergy to delayed hypersensitivity recall skin testing[64] and impaired in vitro lymphocyte proliferative responses.[65] The development of ICU-acquired infections caused by organisms of low intrinsic virulence can also be considered a manifestation of impaired immunity in MODS.[66]

Abnormal wound healing also occurs in MODS. Common manifestations of impaired wound healing are the failure of an open wound to develop satisfactory granulation tissue and the development of decubitus ulcers.[67]

Quantification of Organ Dysfunction

Physiologic instability is the major indication for ICU admission, and support of failing organ function is the ICU's raison d'être. The degree of physiologic derangement present at the time of ICU admission is a potent determinant of ICU survival,[68,69] and irreversible organ dysfunction is the preeminent

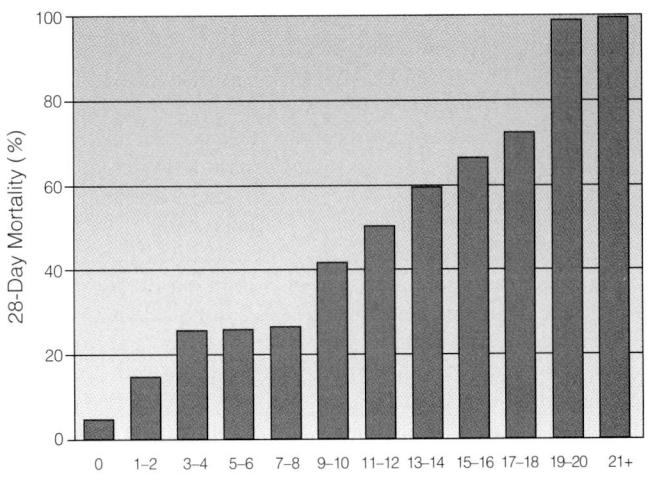

Figure 1 **Increasing severity of organ dysfunction is directly correlated with increasing ICU mortality.**

mode of ICU death.[6,70] Formal quantification of the severity of physiologic derangement or of the evolution of organ dysfunction over time is not generally incorporated into individual patient care in the ICU. However, validated scoring systems have proved invaluable in describing patient populations, stratifying patients for entry into clinical trials, and assessing ICU morbidity in patient groups.

There are a number of published systems for quantifying the severity of organ dysfunction in the critically ill.[9,10,12,66,71-74] These systems are all structurally similar, evaluating dysfunction in each of six or seven organ systems on a numerical scale in which more points are assigned for greater degrees of physiologic severity; they vary primarily with respect to the variables used to describe dysfunction. A representative example of such a scoring system is the Multiple Organ Dysfunction (MOD) score [*see Table 2*].[9]

The numerical scores can be obtained and applied in a variety of ways.[75] Scores can be calculated on the day of ICU admission or at the start of the institution of a novel therapy during the ICU stay; such scores provide a measure of baseline illness severity and correlate in a graded manner with the risk of ICU mortality [*see Figure 1*]. Scores can also be calculated daily, allowing the clinician to track net clinical improvement or deterioration over time[76] and to assess the progression or resolution of organ dysfunction (expressed as the area under the curve for the daily

scores).[77] Alternatively, the aggregate severity of organ dysfunction over time can be quantified by summing the worst values over time in each of the component systems. Such an approach permits quantitation of attributable ICU morbidity as the difference between the aggregate score and the score at baseline—thus identifying that component of ICU morbidity that can be prevented by an effective ICU intervention. Finally, morbidity and mortality can be combined into a single value by using a mortality-adjusted score that assigns a maximum number of points plus 1 to any patient who dies [*see Table 3*].

Prevention of Organ Dysfunction in Critically Ill Patients

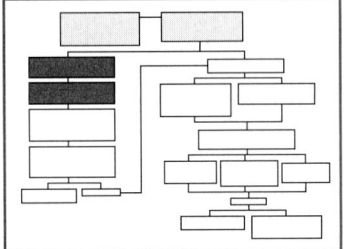

Acute organ dysfunction is the most common indication for admission to an ICU, and any patient with significant physiologic instability is at risk for MODS. A number of risk factors for the development of organ dysfunction have been identified [*see Table 1*]: these reflect a common pathogenesis for the syndrome through the activation of an innate immune response to tissue injury.

The first priority for optimal ICU care is to halt the progression of existing organ dysfunction while preventing the development of new organ dysfunction. Prevention of organ dysfunction is perhaps best approached from the perspective of optimization of hemodynamic, metabolic, and immune homeostasis. There are a number of interventions for which level 1 evidence of efficacy in reducing mortality or preventing organ dysfunction exists [*see Table 4*].

OPTIMIZING HEMODYNAMIC HOMEOSTASIS

The ability of the heart to pump blood is determined by (1) the preload delivered to the right atrium, (2) the intrinsic contractility of the myocardium, and (3) the afterload against which the heart must work—all of which may be deranged in critical illness. First, reduction of intravascular volume as a consequence of hemorrhage, third-space loss, and increased microvascular permeability reduces preload. Second, circulating mediators and NO depress myocardial contractility and thus impair the heart's intrinsic pumping ability. Third, reduced vascular tone, mediated by NO, reduces afterload. The first two abnormalities reduce cardiac output; the third increases it but may, by altering resistance gradients

Table 3 Approaches to Measuring Severity of MODS[75]

Objective	Approach	Uses
To quantify baseline severity of organ dysfunction	Calculate organ dysfunction score on day of admission (admission MODS)	To establish baseline severity (e.g., for entry criteria for a clinical trial) or to ensure comparability of study groups
To quantify severity of organ dysfunction at point in time	Calculate score on particular ICU day (daily MODS)	To determine intensity of resource utilization or evolution or resolution of organ dysfunction at discrete point in time
To measure aggregate severity of organ dysfunction over ICU stay	Sum individual worst scores for each organ system over defined time interval (aggregate MODS)	To determine severity of physiologic derangement over defined time interval (e.g., ICU stay)
To quantify new organ dysfunction arising after ICU admission	Calculate difference between aggregate and admission scores (delta MODS)	To measure organ dysfunction attributable to events occurring after ICU admission
To provide combined measure of morbidity and mortality	Adjust aggregate score so that all patients dying receive maximal number of points (mortality-adjusted MODS)	To create single measure that integrates impact of morbidity in survivors and mortality for nonsurvivors

Table 4 ICU Interventions That Reduce Mortality or Attenuate Organ Dysfunction

Objective	Intervention
Resuscitation	Early goal-directed resuscitation[243]
Prophylaxis	Selective digestive tract decontamination[90]
ICU support	Restrictive transfusion strategy[107] Low tidal volume ventilation[22] Daily wakening[144] Tight glucose control[60] Enteral feeding[86]
Mediator-targeted therapy	Activated protein C[146] Corticosteroids[148] Antibody to TNF[244]

in the microvasculature, alter nutrient flow to the tissues.

The first priority in supporting cardiovascular homeostasis, therefore, is to restore intravascular volume by administering fluids. There is no convincing evidence that any particular resuscitation fluid is superior in all patients, though crystalloid is associated with a lower mortality in trauma patients.[78] Either normal saline or lactated Ringer solution is an appropriate choice. The volume of fluid needed to restore optimal preload may be significant, reflecting not only acute losses but also the effective expansion of the vascular compartment because of vasodilatation and the loss of fluids into the extravascular compartment because of increased capillary permeability. Blood loss should be corrected by transfusing red cells, preferably in fresh, leukocyte-depleted blood. When hypotension is refractory to fluid administration, vasoactive agents, including vasopressors (e.g., dopamine and norepinephrine) and inotropes (e.g., dobutamine, epinephrine, and amrinone) may help increase blood flow to the tissues.[79]

Given that the goal of hemodynamic stabilization is to support organ function rather than to restore physiologic or biochemical normalcy, the best measures of the success of resuscitation are those that reflect either return of function (in particular, urine output) or adequate blood flow to the tissues (e.g., $S_{mv}O_2$ or lactate concentration). Each of these measures, however, has shortcomings of which the clinician must be aware. Urine output may be decreased because of intrinsic renal damage even in the face of adequate renal flow. $S_{mv}O_2$ may be artefactually high because of shunting and abnormalities of oxygen uptake in the microvasculature. Lactate concentration is relatively insensitive to mild degrees of inadequate oxygen delivery and may be elevated in patients with liver disease.

Gastric production of CO_2 as measured with a gastric tonometer has been proposed as a means of evaluating splanchnic blood flow, but the benefits of tonometry in improving outcome are unproven.[80] Microvascular flow can also be directly visualized in the tongue or another exposed mucosal surface by using orthogonal polarization spectral imaging.[81] Neither of these approaches has been widely used to guide resuscitation.

Blood pressure is widely used as an index of the initial adequacy of resuscitation, but pressure measurements may not reliably reflect flow in the microvasculature, particularly when systemic vascular resistance is low. Measurement of central venous or pulmonary capillary wedge pressures provides an estimate of the preload to the heart, though factors such as positive pressure ventilation, the extent of capillary leakage in the lungs, and

intrinsic myocardial dysfunction can all alter the pressure at which optimal preload is obtained.

In practice, resuscitation should be titrated to optimize the balance between several parameters rather than targeting any one parameter. It is sobering to recognize that current sophisticated approaches to resuscitation using the pulmonary arterial catheter have not been shown to yield net clinical benefit and may, in fact, cause harm [*see 6:4 Cardiopulmonary Monitoring*].[82]

Hemodynamic resuscitation is most effective when it is early and rapid. A randomized trial of goal-directed therapy for sepsis, using a protocol comprising fluid administration, transfusion, and vasoactive support titrated to $S_{mv}O_2$ as measured from the superior vena cava through a central venous catheter, found that mortality was reduced from 46.5% to 30.5% when patients were resuscitated according to protocol in the emergency department within hours of their initial presentation. On the other hand, studies of goal-directed therapy initiated in the ICU have generally failed to demonstrate any evidence of benefit.[83,84]

Optimization of oxygen delivery presupposes the ability to oxygenate blood adequately in the lungs. Increased pulmonary capillary permeability, atelectasis, altered consciousness, and intrinsic lung disease can all reduce oxygen uptake in acutely ill patients. Support can be provided through the administration of oxygen to the spontaneously breathing patient, through the use of positive pressure ventilation by mask, or through endotracheal intubation and mechanical ventilation. Positive pressure ventilation can cause further lung injury, however, particularly when the lung has been rendered vulnerable by early acute lung injury. Limiting tidal volume during mechanical ventilation to 6 ml/kg has been shown to improve survival in patients with early ARDS.[22]

OPTIMIZING METABOLIC HOMEOSTASIS

The acute response to stress and injury is a complex, coordinated process characterized by increases in levels of catecholamines, glucocorticoids, antidiuretic hormone, and hormones that regulate

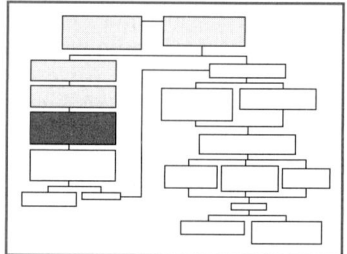

intermediary metabolism, including insulin, glucagon, and growth hormone [*see 6:22 Metabolic Response to Critical Illness*].[6] The activation of this response results in a predictable series of metabolic alterations, including retention of salt and water, increased production of glucose, enhanced lipolysis, increased protein catabolism, and an altered pattern of hepatic protein synthesis known as the acute-phase response, characterized by increased synthesis of C-reactive protein, alpha$_1$-anti-trypsin, and fibrinogen and reduced synthesis of albumin.

Metabolic prophylaxis of MODS is directed toward reversal of the stimuli responsible for the catabolic hormonal milieu and toward the provision of adequate biochemical substrate at a time of increased metabolic demand. Early definitive surgical therapy in the form of debridement of devitalized tissue, burn wound excision and grafting, and rigid fixation of long bone fractures can attenuate the postinjury hypermetabolic state and minimize the subsequent development of MODS, though the benefits of early definitive therapy must be weighed against the additional stress of blood loss and hemodynamic instability. In the face of overwhelming injury, a policy of damage control to permit stabilization of the patient in the ICU is associated with an improved clinical outcome.[85]

Nutritional support should be provided by the enteral route if possible [see 6:23 Nutritional Support]. Enteral nutrition is feasible in most patients, particularly if feedings are initiated early. The administration of even small quantities of enteral nutrition is considered advisable, even if it must be supplemented by some degree of parenteral nutrition. There is increasing evidence that immunologically enhanced enteral formulas can yield better clinical outcomes than standard enteral formulas.[86]

Close regulation of glucose levels in accordance with an intensive policy of monitoring and insulin administration has been shown to improve clinical outcome.[60] On the other hand, there is no evidence that administration of growth hormone offers any significant benefit.[87]

OPTIMIZING IMMUNOLOGIC HOMEOSTASIS

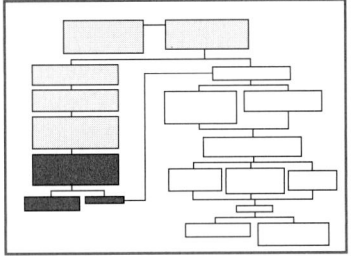

Infection is an important risk factor for MODS, but the converse is equally true: patients with MODS are at significantly increased risk for infection. This risk arises as a consequence both of impairment of normal host defense mechanisms and of colonization with potentially infectious nosocomial pathogens [see 6:17 Nosocomial Infection].

Of the numerous derangements of normal immune function with which critical illness is associated, impairment of mucosal defenses is probably the most important (and certainly the most preventable). Mucosal defenses are breached by surgical incisions and by invasive devices, including intravascular catheters, urinary catheters, and endotracheal and nasogastric tubes. Limiting the number of such devices in use and paying rigorous attention to their insertion and maintenance are important for minimizing nosocomial infection rates.[88] Gastric acid plays a primary role in maintaining the relative sterility of the stomach. Antacids ablate this defense and are a recognized risk factor for nosocomial pneumonia; they should not be used for stress ulcer prophylaxis. The declining incidence of clinically significant stress bleeding in the contemporary ICU suggests that prophylaxis should be limited to patients who are at increased risk for stress ulceration.[55] Cytoprotective agents (e.g., sucralfate) appear to have no significant advantages over H_2 receptor antagonists in reducing the risk of ventilator-associated pneumonia and are less efficacious in preventing bleeding[89]; accordingly, H_2 receptor antagonists appear to be the prophylactic agents of choice.

An alternative strategy for preventing pathologic gut colonization and nosocomial infection involves prophylactic administration of a combination of systemic antibiotics (e.g., cefotaxime) and topical nonabsorbed antibiotics (e.g., tobramycin, polymyxin, and amphotericin B). This approach, known as selective decontamination of the digestive tract (SDD), has proved effective in reducing nosocomial infection rates and even ICU mortality[90]; the effect is particularly evident in surgical patients who receive both systemic and topical therapy.[91]

Enteral feeding is beneficial in preventing nosocomial infection. Systemic antibiotics suppress the indigenous flora of mucosal surfaces, promoting pathologic colonization with resistant organisms.[92] Therefore, use of antimicrobial agents in critically ill patients must be selective and targeted, and the use of broad-spectrum empirical therapy should be minimized by regular reviews of culture and sensitivity results and restrictions on antibiotic prescription practices.

Although nosocomial infections in critically ill patients usually arise from endogenous reservoirs, pathogens may also spread from patient to patient and from environment to patient. Certain organisms—in particular, Acinetobacter, Xanthomonas, and Legionella—are transmitted through aqueous sources in the ICU, and the isolation of these organisms from a critically ill patient is evidence of a potential problem in environmental infection control. Hand washing is an important but underutilized mode of infection prevention in the ICU [see 1:2 Prevention of Postoperative Infection]. There is no clear evidence that protective isolation of critically ill patients warrants the increased costs and increased demands on nursing staff.

The role of immunomodulation in the prophylaxis of MODS remains undefined. At present, there is no defined role for chemoprophylaxis of MODS beyond the specific effects of drugs such as heparin (prevention of deep vein thrombosis [DVT]) and H_2 receptor antagonists (prevention of upper GI bleeding).

Evaluation of the Patient with Organ Dysfunction

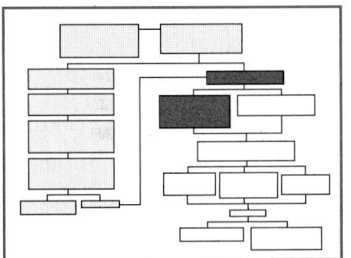

SINGLE ORGAN DYSFUNCTION

Single organ dysfunction suggests local disease and should trigger a search for potentially correctable causes in the organ system involved. Isolated organ dysfunction may reflect preexisting chronic disease or a local problem such as fluid overload, atelectasis, biliary tract obstruction, or elevated intracranial pressure. Complications related to invasive devices or the adverse effects of medications are common causes of single organ dysfunction; the diagnosis is often presumptive, established on the basis of clinical improvement after discontinuance of the agent or removal of the device. Finally, single organ dysfunction may indicate acute disease in the involved organ, such as myocardial infarction, pulmonary embolism, or bone marrow suppression.

Acute respiratory dysfunction, for example, may be caused by pneumonia, atelectasis, pleural effusion, pneumothorax, or pulmonary embolism. Central venous and pulmonary arterial catheters may induce tachyarrhythmias as a result of mechanical irritation of the conducting system. Isolated renal dysfunction may be a consequence of abdominal compartment syndrome or of the nephrotoxic effects of medications (e.g., acute tubular necrosis caused by aminoglycosides and interstitial nephritis caused by penicillins and cephalosporins). Occasionally, renal dysfunction arises from a postrenal cause, such as blockage of a Foley catheter.

Medications are important causes of liver dysfunction in the critically ill patient. Erythromycin, ketoconazole, and haloperidol, for example, can induce cholestatic liver injury. Thrombocytopenia is an important adverse effect of a number of medications, including heparin flushes to maintain the patency of arterial lines. A decreased level of consciousness is usually the result of the poorly characterized metabolic encephalopathy of critical illness; however, it is necessary to rule out local causes such as meningitis, encephalitis, brain abscess, and subdural hematoma. Excessive or prolonged use of narcotics or sedative-hypnotics may lead to sustained alterations in level of consciousness, particularly when hepatic or renal function is impaired. Nondepolarizing muscle relaxants (e.g., vecuronium) may cause prolonged neuromuscular blockade and peripheral neuropathy.[45]

MULTIPLE ORGAN DYSFUNCTION

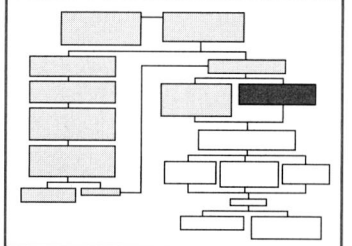

Although it has been suggested that there is a characteristic temporal sequence in the development of MODS [*see Table 5*],[3,9] the clinical course tends to be variable and depends in part on the criteria used to define organ system dysfunction (see above). The specific pattern of dysfunction is much less important than the course of the evolving syndrome. Resolution of dysfunction suggests an appropriate response to specific and supportive therapy. Worsening of dysfunction, on the other hand, should prompt a search for potentially correctable causes and a reevaluation of the methods of supportive care in use. Not infrequently, a treatable cause of evolving MODS is found; often, however, no cause is evident. When no specific cause of the deterioration can be identified, therapy should focus on optimizing supportive measures to limit iatrogenic injury either until the patient recovers or, alternatively, until a considered decision is made that continuing active care is futile.

Search for Correctable Causes

Occult infection Uncontrolled infection, particularly infection arising within the abdomen, is an important risk factor for MODS.[2,3,93] The development of otherwise unexplained organ dysfunction should trigger a careful radiologic search for an occult intra-abdominal focus.[94] However, MODS also develops in patients with pneumonia[58] and other life-threatening infections, and it sometimes evolves in patients in whom no infectious focus can be identified.[66,95]

When MODS develops in the postoperative period, a careful search for infection must be undertaken, concentrating in particular on the operative site and on any invasive devices used. With appropriate attention to the clinical possibilities, aided by ultrasonography and CT scanning, the presence or absence of significant intra-abdominal pathology can usually be established. Local wound exploration may suggest the possibility of occult intra-abdominal infection through the demonstration of impaired wound healing or fascial dehiscence or through the isolation of typical intestinal microflora from a wound infection. The diagnosis of pneumonia in intubated ICU patients is notoriously difficult; however, the use of quantitative techniques (e.g., protected specimen brush bronchoscopy

Table 5 Temporal Evolution of MODS[3,9]

System	Time from ICU Admission to Onset of Significant Dysfunction (days)
Respiratory	1–2
Hematologic	3
Central nervous	4
Cardiovascular	4
Hepatic	5–6
Renal	4–11
Gastrointestinal	10–14

and bronchoalveolar lavage) can aid in establishing or excluding the diagnosis.[96,97]

MODS is rarely caused by urinary tract infections or device-related bacteremias, though these conditions are common in patients with significant organ dysfunction. *Clostridium difficile* colitis or disseminated fungal infection may also present as deteriorating organ function in critically ill patients.[98]

Iatrogenic factors MODS can be considered the quintessential iatrogenic disorder, reflecting both the successes and the failures of contemporary ICU practice. On one hand, the syndrome arose only because the supportive care available today permits the prolonged survival of critically ill patients who, in an earlier era, would have died rapidly; on the other hand, potentially avoidable iatrogenic factors contribute prominently to the evolution of MODS.

Technical or judgmental errors often set the stage for MODS.[99-101] Whenever a patient manifests unexplained organ failure in the postoperative period, the surgeon must consider the possibility of an iatrogenic complication—for example, a missed intestinal perforation in a trauma victim, a leak from a tenuous anastomosis, or left colon ischemia after aneurysmectomy.

Many of the therapeutic interventions that are the mainstay of ICU care have the potential to cause local and remote organ injury. In the experimental setting, mechanical ventilation with high tidal volumes and low levels of positive end-expiratory pressure (PEEP) can induce both pulmonary injury and remote organ injury.[102,103] In a multicenter, randomized, controlled trial, it was confirmed that mechanical ventilation of patients with acute lung injury in accordance with a lung-protective strategy (i.e., a tidal volume of 6 ml/kg) significantly improves survival[22] and attenuates the local and systemic release of proinflammatory mediators [*see 6:6 Use of the Mechanical Ventilator*].[16] Oxygen in high concentrations can produce pulmonary damage, probably as a result of the generation of toxic oxygen intermediates.[104]

Blood transfusion has been implicated in the development of organ dysfunction, an effect that occurs independent of the effects of shock, blood loss, and fluid resuscitation.[105,106] A multicenter, randomized, controlled trial demonstrated a significant reduction in the severity of new organ dysfunction in a heterogeneous population of critically ill patients when transfusion was withheld unless the hemoglobin concentration was less than 70 g/L (7 g/dl).[107] The age of the blood administered may be an underappreciated factor in defining optimal transfusion strategies. The effects of blood transfusion on splanchnic blood flow as measured with a gastric tonometer are significantly dependent on the age of the transfused blood. Transfusion of blood that is more than 12 days old can have an adverse impact on oxygen delivery.[108]

TPN can also contribute to the de novo development of organ dysfunction. TPN-associated alterations in hepatic function with intrahepatic cholestasis and fatty infiltration are relatively common and are manifested by elevated aminotransferase and alkaline phosphatase levels.[109] TPN may also give rise to glucose intolerance and can aggravate ventilatory impairment through increased CO_2 production. In patients with borderline pulmonary function, this additional CO_2 production may prevent weaning from ventilatory support.[110] Parenteral nutrition is also associated with higher rates of postoperative and nosocomial infections after multiple trauma.[111]

Medications—in particular, analgesics, sedatives, and antibiotics—have also been associated with evolving organ dysfunction.

Support of Patients with Established Organ Dysfunction

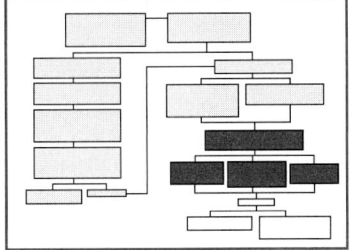

The fundamental challenge in providing intensive supportive care to patients with established organ dysfunction is how to support physiologic function while minimizing new iatrogenic organ dysfunction. As more is understood about the consequences of various treatment strategies, it is increasingly apparent that optimizing function is not synonymous with maximizing function and that the clinician must be acutely aware of the potential for causing more harm than good.

VENTILATORY SUPPORT

Although ventilatory support is generally provided by endotracheal intubation and mechanical ventilation, noninvasive positive pressure ventilation may be appropriate for patients with milder degrees of respiratory failure. A small randomized trial of patients with cardiogenic pulmonary edema found that when compared with conventional administration of oxygen by mask, noninvasive positive pressure ventilation shortened the time to resolution of respiratory failure and reduced the need for subsequent endotracheal intubation.[112] Whether this approach is useful in patients with early ARDS is less clear, however; it may be associated with a higher risk of complications.[113]

Endotracheal intubation and positive pressure ventilation constitute the mainstay of support for critically ill patients with respiratory failure. In unstable patients, it is best to use a controlled ventilatory mode (e.g., pressure control ventilation) rather than a spontaneous breathing mode (e.g., pressure support ventilation). Oxygenation can be optimized through the use of PEEP, a maneuver that may also decrease the accumulation of interstitial fluid and minimize ventilator-associated lung injury.[114] Ventilation with large tidal volumes and high peak inspiratory pressures contributes to lung injury, and it has been shown that the survival of ARDS patients can be improved by using low tidal volumes (~ 6 ml/kg).[22] Pressure-controlled ventilatory techniques limit peak airway pressures to a maximum predetermined level, optimizing gas exchange by inverting the inspiration-to-expiration ratio (I/E) from its normal value of 1:2 to 1:1 or higher and by changing the shape of the inspiratory flow curve (normally square) to one in which flow initially is rapid, then decelerates [*see 6:6 Use of the Mechanical Ventilator*].[115] Although oxygenation can be maintained with low tidal volumes, ventilation is jeopardized, with the result that CO_2 levels rise (so-called permissive hypercapnia).[116] Hypercapnia per se does not appear to be deleterious[117]; indeed, animal studies suggest that increased levels of CO_2 may be independently beneficial to critically ill patients.[118] For patients with refractory hypoxemia, high-frequency oscillation appears to be a promising ventilatory mode.[119,120]

Inhaled NO is selectively delivered to ventilated lung segments and may effect early improvement of oxygenation in ARDS patients[121]; whether this early physiologic effect translates into an improved clinical outcome is unknown. Extracorporeal lung support by means of extracorporeal membrane oxygenation or extracorporeal CO_2 removal can be lifesaving in patients with isolated severe respiratory failure that is refractory to other forms of respiratory support.[122,123] These techniques are resource intensive, however, and have not been convincingly shown to yield better outcomes than conventional mechanical ventilation.[124] If the patient remains hypoxemic despite optimization of ventilatory support, it may be necessary to accept an arterial oxygen saturation (S_aO_2) as low as 80%.

CARDIOVASCULAR SUPPORT

Tissue oxygen delivery ($\dot{D}O_2$) is a function of three variables—cardiac output, hemoglobin concentration, and S_aO_2 (oxygen dissolved in the plasma makes only a negligible contribution). Tissue oxygen consumption ($\dot{V}O_2$) is a function of cardiac output and oxygen extraction (defined as the difference between arterial and venous oxygen content). In practice, multiple factors can impair oxygen delivery and consumption, and it is important that the clinician recognize these.

Oxygen uptake in the tissues is an entirely passive process, resulting from the diffusion of oxygen toward the relatively hypoxic extravascular space along an oxygen saturation gradient that is highest in the microvasculature and lowest at the cell. This passive diffusion can be reduced if there is interstitial edema, which makes the concentration gradient less steep, or if blood flow through the microvasculature is rapid. Alternatively, a reduction in the resistance of small arterioles may impede the diversion of blood into the microvasculature. Moreover, nutrient vessels in the microcirculation may be occluded by aggregates of neutrophils, platelets, and aged (and thus less deformable) red blood cells. The net result of these abnormalities is the shunting of oxygenated blood from the arterial side of the circulation to the venous side. This phenomenon is readily detected through measurement of $S_{mv}O_2$, which is about 70% in normal persons but typically is much higher in patients with sepsis and organ dysfunction.

Paradoxically, each of the interventions commonly used to increase tissue oxygen delivery can also decrease it. Fluid resuscitation can increase cardiac output by increasing preload, but in patients with altered capillary permeability, it can create edema, thereby lengthening the distance across which oxygen must diffuse. Vasopressors can raise cardiac output by increasing peripheral vascular resistance, but at the cost of reducing flow through nutrient vessels in the microcirculation. Inotropes, on the other hand, directly increase cardiac output, albeit at the cost of increased myocardial oxygen consumption, but agents such as dobutamine may lead to further shunting by decreasing peripheral vascular resistance.

Currently, intensive invasive monitoring of critically ill patients with organ dysfunction is employed less frequently than it once was. The benefits of such monitoring remain somewhat uncertain. For example, a 1996 study suggested that the use of a pulmonary arterial catheter was associated with a 24% increase in mortality—not, presumably, because of complications of the catheter itself but rather because the decisions made on the basis of the data provided led to greater harm than benefit.[125] Although this estimate of harm may be exaggerated, there is little countervailing evidence of benefit to justify routine use of pulmonary arterial catheters. A 2003 study of 1,994 high-risk patients undergoing major elective surgery found that Swan-Ganz catheterization and preoperative optimization did not reduce mortality but was associated with a significant increase in the risk of pulmonary embolism.[84]

RENAL SUPPORT

Renal replacement therapy in critically ill patients with MODS serves three functions:

1. Regulation of fluid and electrolytes in patients in whom normal renal function is compromised and altered capillary permeability has led to total body fluid overload with edema.

2. Removal of products of metabolism, medications, and other toxins that the failing kidneys are unable to clear.
3. Removal of circulating mediators of inflammation.

The first two are classic indications for dialysis, though the therapeutic objectives may differ; the third lies more in the realm of promising experimental therapy.

Fluid overload is a common consequence of hemodynamic resuscitation during the early stages of acute illness. It results from increased capillary permeability, peripheral vasodilatation with expansion of the intravascular compartment, and impaired renal function. The use of continuous renal replacement therapies to titrate fluid balance and reduce uremia is conceptually appealing, but the benefits remain unproven. Both individual randomized trials[126,127] and a systematic review[128] failed to show that early and aggressive continuous renal replacement improved clinical outcome. On the other hand, a multicenter randomized trial of more than 400 ICU patients with ARF showed that high-flow ultrafiltration (at a rate of 35 ml/kg/hr or higher) increased survival,[129] and a prospective study demonstrated that daily (as opposed to alternate-day) intermittent hemodialysis improved survival and hastened the resolution of ARF.[130] Another systematic review suggested that imbalances between study groups might have masked a potential benefit of therapy associated with early continuous hemodialysis.[131]

Whether it significantly improves outcome or not, early continuous renal replacement therapy does facilitate early management of the patient with MODS by permitting the removal of fluid, and it is generally better tolerated by hemodynamically unstable patients than is intermittent hemodialysis. Evidence that dialytic therapy can accelerate the clearance of circulating mediators of sepsis is scant.[132]

SUPPORT OF OTHER ORGANS

Enteral nutritional support has been shown to reduce the rate of infectious complications in patients with multiple trauma[111,133] and in those with pancreatitis.[134] A systematic review of 15 randomized trials found that early enteral feeding reduced the infectious complication rate and shortened the ICU stay without affecting mortality.[135] The use of immunologically enhanced enteral formulas appears to be associated with a further reduction in infectious complications, ventilator days, and length of hospital stay.[136] Paralytic ileus makes the provision of enteral feeding more difficult. Erythromycin, which is a motilin secretagogue, can facilitate bedside placement of enteral feeding tubes[137] and accelerate gastric emptying.[138]

Techniques for extracorporeal support of the failing liver have been described, but their use is generally limited to a few centers with a particular interest in liver failure and organ transplantation.[139,140] Unlike primary liver failure, the hepatic dysfunction of MODS does not lead to life-threatening organ system insufficiency and rarely calls for specific support. Hypoalbuminemia is common in MODS, occurring as a consequence of increased vascular permeability, loss through the GI tract, and reduced hepatic synthesis from the activation of an acute-phase response. Although hypoalbuminemia is associated with increased ICU morbidity and mortality, there is no convincing evidence that albumin supplementation improves clinical outcome.[141]

A randomized trial of transfusion strategies in the ICU demonstrated that organ function was improved by a restrictive transfusion policy that withheld transfusion unless the hemoglobin level dropped below 70 g/L,[107] a conclusion supported by a large European multicenter observational study.[142] Benefit is also seen in patients with underlying cardiovascular disease.[143] Thrombocytopenia is corrected by transfusion of platelet concentrates, but this generally is done only if the platelet count drops below 20,000/mm^3. Coagulation factors can be replaced by giving fresh frozen plasma or cryoprecipitate.

Adequate analgesia and sedation are essential components of the care of MODS patients; however, the natural desire to alleviate pain and discomfort can lead to oversedation. A policy of daily awakening can reduce morbidity and shorten the ICU stay.[144]

PHARMACOLOGIC THERAPY TARGETING HOST RESPONSE

Experimental studies implicate an activated inflammatory response in the pathogenesis of MODS. Despite extensive evaluation of a variety of novel strategies to target the host response in sepsis, to date, only two approaches have demonstrated an ability to improve survival.

Activated protein C is an endogenous anticoagulant molecule that inhibits factors V and VIII; in addition to its anticoagulant activities, it exerts significant anti-inflammatory activity.[145] Activated protein C has been produced as a recombinant protein (drotrecogin alfa activated) and has been evaluated in a multicenter randomized trial involving 1,690 patients with severe sepsis. In this trial, treatment resulted in a 6.1% improvement in 28-day survival[146] and a more rapid resolution of cardiovascular, respiratory, and hematologic dysfunction.[147] The benefit appears to be greatest in patients who have more severe illness (reflected in an elevated APACHE II [Acute Physiology and Chronic Health Evaluation II] score or a greater number of dysfunctional organs), community-acquired infection, or coagulopathy.

Critical illness is associated with multiple abnormalities of endocrine function, including reduced responsiveness to endogenous glucocorticoids,[62] a state that predicts an increased risk of ICU mortality.[61] In a 2002 study, administration of pharmacologic doses of corticosteroids (50 mg of hydrocortisone every 6 hours and 50 μg of fludrocortisone) to patients with refractory septic shock and an impaired response to a short-course ACTH stimulation test reduced mortality by 10%.[148] In contrast, earlier studies of high-dose corticosteroids in more heterogeneous groups of patients with sepsis found no evidence of benefit.[149]

Systematic reviews have suggested that neutralization of tumor necrosis factor (TNF) or interleukin-1 (IL-1) can improve outcome in sepsis,[150] but neither of these approaches is clinically available at present. Other anticoagulant or anti-inflammatory strategies have been suggested but remain unproven.

MODS AND ICU-ACQUIRED INFECTION

Infection is a risk factor for organ dysfunction, but the converse is equally true: organ dysfunction is a risk factor for nosocomial infection, with the risk increasing as the severity of organ dysfunction increases.[66] The typical isolates are microbes of low intrinsic pathogenicity, including coagulase-negative *Staphylococcus*, *Enterococcus*, and *Candida* species and gram-negative organisms such as *Pseudomonas* and *Enterobacter*.[151] These organisms commonly colonize the upper GI tract of the critically ill patient,[152] they emerge under antibiotic pressures, and they form colonies on invasive devices—all of which may explain why they emerge as predominant infecting species in this setting. Studies of SDD have demonstrated that preventing such infections reduces ICU morbidity and mortality,[90,153] but there is scant evidence that aggressive antimicrobial therapy to treat suspected nosocomial infection improves outcome. In fact, two reports from 2000 suggested that a more restrictive approach to the prescription of antimicrobial agents reduced mortality and morbidity.[97,154] Worsening organ dysfunction should prompt a careful search for untreated foci of infection, but empirical therapy should be used cautiously; if such therapy is started, it should be discontinued promptly as culture data are obtained. Often, mere removal of a colonized device (e.g., a central line or a urinary catheter) amounts to definitive therapy for these infections.

The association of organ dysfunction with occult intra-abdominal infection[3,94] stimulated a period of enthusiasm for the practice of so-called blind laparotomy—that is, laparotomy undertaken to identify and treat an intra-abdominal infectious focus without radiographic evidence that infection is present.[155,156] The uniformly disappointing results of such intervention,[157] coupled with improvements in diagnostic imaging techniques, led to abandonment of this approach except in certain unusual circumstances (e.g., clinically compelling evidence of a surgically correctable problem, suspicion of visceral ischemia, or the absence of the appropriate imaging facilities). It goes without saying that the classic physical findings of peritonitis—particularly when no abdominal operation has been done—may be the sole indication for surgical exploration. Moreover, in a complicated postoperative patient transferred from another institution because of worsening organ dysfunction, repeat laparotomy may legitimately be considered a component of the admission physical examination.

Outcome

PROGNOSTIC INDICATORS

The prognosis of MODS is directly related to the severity of the underlying organ dysfunction, which can be expressed in terms of either the number of failing systems[3,73,158] [see Table 6] or the global severity of dysfunction as determined by an organ dysfunction score [see Figure 1]. It must be emphasized, however, that prognostic indicators reflect the expected outcome of a group of patients and are of limited use in making decisions about the care of an individual patient. Moreover, the prognostic weight of these scales reflects standards of care prevalent at a particular time and in a particular clinical setting. For example, at the time when Ranson's criteria were developed,[159] patients with pancreatitis and six or more

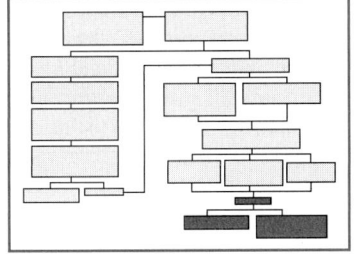

Table 6 Prognosis in MODS

Number of Failing Systems	Mortality (%)
0	3
1	15–30
2	50–60
3	60–100
4	70–100
5	100

positive indicators according to those criteria had a mortality of close to 100%; today, a majority of such patients survive.[93]

Organ dysfunction is potentially recoverable when the factors responsible for the persistence or progression of MODS can be reversed. Identifying these factors, treating them appropriately, and providing optimal physiologic support can prove a daunting challenge, and it is often advisable to consider seeking independent advice or transporting the patient to a center with the clinical expertise and facilities to manage the multidisciplinary problems faced by MODS patients. Given that MODS often evolves as a consequence of medical misadventure, early consultation or referral may be a sound approach from a medicolegal perspective as well. On the other hand, it is a common contemporary ICU scenario that MODS evolves and worsens despite optimal care, necessitating a decision whether to continue or discontinue active care.

WITHDRAWAL OF LIFE SUPPORT

The most common mode of death for a patient with advanced MODS is limitation or withdrawal of life support in the face of a persistent failure to respond to full, aggressive ICU care.[160] The decision to withdraw or withhold life support is a complex one, and there are considerable differences of professional opinion and practice regarding how best to make it.[161] Factors that must be taken into consideration include the nature of the underlying disease, the patient's premorbid health status, the wishes of the patient and the family regarding long-term ICU care, the patient's ultimate prospects for an independent existence, and the presence of active problems amenable to medical therapy. Although end-of-life deliberations may be difficult for medical staff and family alike, careful and realistic consideration of the expectations of all involved can facilitate a decision to discontinue active therapy in a manner that is dignified and humane rather than adversarial.

Discussion

MODS: Evolution of a Syndrome

The first ICU was established in Baltimore in the late 1950s.[162] Its development marked much more than a simple advance in medical technology. The improvements in fluid resuscitation achieved during World War II, followed by the development of techniques of positive pressure mechanical ventilation, hemodialysis, and central venous catheterization over the subsequent decade, had set the stage for an entirely new disease paradigm—that of a disease that arose only in patients who would have died in the absence of resuscitation and exogenous support. The need for that support to sustain life became the metaphor that described this new disorder, originally described as sequential systems failure[163] and now generally known as

MODS.[4] MODS is perhaps the classic instance of the new disease paradigm, in that it develops only in patients who would have died without medical intervention and evolves because of the inadvertent consequences of that intervention.

Earlier reports had described the physiologic failure of discrete organ systems after trauma or acute illness. Stress-related upper GI bleeding was described in 1842[54] and trauma-related renal[23] and hepatic[30] dysfunction during World War II. Description of respiratory failure awaited the widespread use of mechanical ventilators, but a process termed high-output respiratory failure was described in patients with peritonitis in 1963,[13] anticipating the classic description of ARDS 4 years later.[14] In each of these reports, however, the physiologic organ abnormality was viewed as an isolated problem of a single organ, albeit one that could have broader secondary consequences. The suggestion by Baue[1] in 1975 that each organ abnormality was simply the local manifestation of a systemic process set the stage for attempts to identify common systemic pathologic processes and hence to develop therapies that were not merely supportive but also targeted fundamental mechanisms in the pathogenesis of MODS. The search for such therapies is, admittedly, still in its infancy. Not only is the disease process complex, but our ability to describe and characterize it is limited as well.

MODS is invariably preceded by evidence of systemic activation of an adaptive host stress response to infection or tissue injury. This response, which includes changes in cardiorespiratory function, increased microvascular permeability, evidence of activation of innate immune mechanisms, and alterations in intermediary metabolism, is termed sepsis when caused by infection and the systemic inflammatory response syndrome (SIRS) when considered independent of cause.[4,164] SIRS is mediated through the release of a complicated network of host-derived mediator molecules (see below). The name notwithstanding, designation of SIRS as a syndrome may be somewhat presumptuous. There is no discrete or invariant pattern of clinical manifestations that identifies patients with activation of this complex response, nor is there convincing evidence that the response is common to all patients who meet the clinical criteria for SIRS.

It has been suggested that it is also possible to define a compensatory anti-inflammatory response syndrome (CARS) or a mixed acute response syndrome (MARS)[165]; however, these "syndromes" are more conceptual entities than they are diseases that can be diagnosed and treated.[166]

Theories of Pathogenesis

Organ dysfunction must ultimately be the consequence of the malfunctioning or death of cells in that organ. Although cellular derangements are readily documented under experimental conditions, it remains largely unknown how these derangements translate into the physiologic changes that define the clinical syndrome. Cellular dysfunction may reflect altered patterns of synthetic function, either because of activation of alternate patterns of gene expression or because of relative cellular oxygen deficiency from defective cellular respiration (so-called cytopathic hypoxia).[167] Mechanisms of fibrosis and repair may alter the normal cellular anatomic relationships and thereby impair function. Finally, cell death may result from mechanical or biochemical injury of sufficient severity to prevent oxidative metabolism and produce anatomic disruption of the cell or necrosis, but it may also occur through the activation of apoptosis (programmed cell death). Each of these abnormalities has been described in patients with sepsis, and each has multiple overlapping causes.

INFECTION AND HOST SEPTIC RESPONSE

The earliest descriptions of MODS emphasized its association with occult infection,[58,94] prompting the hypothesis that organ dysfunction arises through the direct effects of one or more microbial toxins. However, the observations that MODS could also develop in patients with no identifiable focus of infection[95] and that treatment of infection did not necessarily reverse the syndrome[168] suggested that infection may be a cause of organ dysfunction in critical illness but is not necessarily the fundamental mechanism.

Microbial products, independent of bacterial viability, can evoke the clinical features of sepsis. Injection of endotoxin, or lipopolysaccharide (LPS), derived from the cell wall of gram-negative bacteria reproduces the physiologic features of sepsis in human volunteers,[169] with larger doses producing life-threatening organ dysfunction.[170] Moreover, endotoxin can be detected in the circulation of patients at risk for MODS—not only patients with sepsis,[171,172] but also those who have experienced traumatic[173] or thermal injury[174] and those who are undergoing cardiopulmonary bypass or repair of an abdominal aortic aneurysm.[175]

Animal studies, however, have shown that the sequelae of endotoxemia are an indirect consequence of the activation of host innate immunity rather than a direct cytopathic effect of the endotoxin molecule. The C3h HeJ strain of mice arose through a spontaneous mutation of the parental C3h HeN strain, involving an alteration in a single gene product. This defect, later recognized as a point mutation in the gene encoding Toll-like receptor 4 (TLR4),[176] conferred complete resistance to endotoxin lethality in C3h HeJ mice. Studies involving bone marrow irradiation and crossover transplants of bone marrow cells between C3h HeN and C3h HeJ mice showed that endotoxin sensitivity was transferred with bone marrow cells[177] and confirmed that the sequelae of endotoxin challenge arose indirectly, through the activity of marrow-derived cells from the host. Microarray studies have demonstrated that literally hundreds of genes are expressed in macrophages, endothelial cells, and neutrophils after stimulation by LPS.[178,179] The importance of this enormously complex response is underlined by the observation that the lethality of murine endotoxemia can be prevented by neutralizing any one of several dozen of these gene expressions before endotoxin challenge.[145]

Endotoxin interacts with cells of the host innate immune system through TLR4. TLR4 is one of a family of 10 TLRs that have evolved to recognize danger signals in the extracellular environment and to activate cells to mount an appropriate response to a threat.[180] TLRs recognize not only microbial products (e.g., endotoxin) and components of the wall of gram-positive bacteria (e.g., lipoteichoic acid and peptidoglycan) (TLR2) but also bacterial DNA (TLR9) and even heat-shock proteins and structural components of damaged cells (TLR2) [see Table 7]. Thus, the response evoked appears not to be specific for the stimulus that elicited it, just as the clinical syndrome of systemic inflammation and organ dysfunction is not unique to patients with infection but can also be seen in association with other causes of tissue injury.[164,181]

The binding of endotoxin to TLR4 triggers a cascade of intracellular signaling pathways leading to the expression of hundreds of genes whose products mediate innate immunity [see Figure 2]. The resulting alterations in normal patterns of cellular protein synthesis are profound: not only does the initial stimulus trigger a complex response, but the newly synthesized protein products of this response also, in turn, are capable of acting on the cell to induce a further cascade of mediator molecules. Any attempt to classify the mediators involved is inevitably arbitrary and simplistic. It is useful, however, to consider the response as involving (1) early inflammatory mediators (e.g., TNF and IL-1), (2) late inflammatory mediators (e.g., macrophage inhibitory factor and high-mobility group box [HMGB]–1), (3) counterinflammatory and tissue repair mediators (e.g., IL-10 and transforming growth factor [TGF]–β), (4) enzymes involved in the regulation of nonprotein inflammatory mediators (e.g., inducible NO synthase, phospholipase A_2, and platelet-activating factor acetylhydrolase), (5) acute-phase reactants, and (6) cell surface adhesion or signaling molecules (e.g., intercellular adhesion molecule [ICAM]–1 and tissue factor).

Table 7 Toll-like Receptors and Their Ligands

Toll-like Receptor	Ligand(s)
TLR1	*Mycobacterium leprae* lipopeptide, *Borrelia* outer surface protein
TLR2	Peptidoglycan, lipoteichoic acid, bacterial lipoprotein, *Mycoplasma* lipopeptide, zymosan, CMV, *M. leprae* lipopeptide, lipoarabinomannans, injured cells
TLR3	Double-stranded RNA
TLR4	Endotoxin, HSP60, β-glucan, neutrophil elastase
TLR5	Flagellin
TLR6	*Mycoplasma* lipopeptide
TLR7	Imidazoquinolones, guanine ribonucleosides
TLR8	Unknown
TLR9	Bacterial CpG DNA
TLR10	Unknown

Blockade of any of these molecules prevents lethality in mice that are subsequently challenged with endotoxin. None of these mediators, however, is directly cytotoxic. This suggests that the role that these mediators play is to activate effector mechanisms of injury further downstream. The identity of those downstream mechanisms of cellular dysfunction or death is still a matter of speculation, though a number of attractive possibilities have been proposed.

GENETIC FACTORS IN HOST RESPONSE

A Scandinavian population-based study of causes of premature mortality in adoptees revealed that genetic factors play a significant role in the outcome of infection. When one of an adoptee's biologic parents died before the age of 50, the adoptee faced a six-fold increase in the risk of infectious mortality; this increased risk was substantially greater than that associated with premature death from cardiovascular disease or cancer.[182] It is now known that polymorphisms in genes for TLRs and cytokines are common in the general population[183] and are associated with both altered expression of the gene product and enhanced susceptibility to sepsis and organ dysfunction. A mutation in the gene for TLR4 has been associated with a significantly increased risk of gram-negative infection in ICU patients.[184,185] Polymorphisms in the genes for CD14,[186] TNF,[187,188] heat shock protein 70,[189] IL-10,[190] and IL-1 receptor antagonist[191] all have been associated with greater degrees of organ dysfunction and a worse clinical outcome in critical illness.

TISSUE INJURY MEDIATED BY PHAGOCYTIC CELLS OF INNATE IMMUNE SYSTEM

Polymorphonuclear neutrophils and monocytes form the first line of innate host defenses against invading microorganisms and injured tissue. Neutrophils are recruited to the site of tissue invasion or injury by locally released chemokines (e.g., IL-8). They adhere to the endothelium of the microvasculature through the interaction of the neutrophil adhesion molecule CD11b with ICAM-1 on the endothelial cell. Adherent neutrophils are then able to extravasate by degrading the tight junctions between endothelial cells, probably through the action of the neutrophil enzyme elastase; this process can cause injury to the cell as the neutrophil transits.[192] Once localized to the site of challenge, the neutrophil releases a variety of molecules (e.g., proteases and reactive oxygen intermediates) that directly injure microorganisms and host tissue alike. Opsonization of bacteria by immunoglobulin or complement enables the neutrophil to phagocytose and kill invading pathogens. Activated neutrophils have been implicated in the pathogenesis of pulmonary,[193,194] hepatic,[195] GI,[196] and renal[28] injury in experimental models of inflammation. Similarly, though ablation of fixed tissue macrophages increased the number of bacteria isolated from an animal model of peritonitis, it nonetheless reduced the severity of septic symptoms and improved survival.[197]

Other studies have implicated natural killer (NK) cells[198,199] and CD8-positive T cells[200] in the lethality of experimental sepsis, though it is unclear whether lethality is a consequence of direct cellular cytotoxicity or of the activation of other biologic processes by secreted products of these cells.[201]

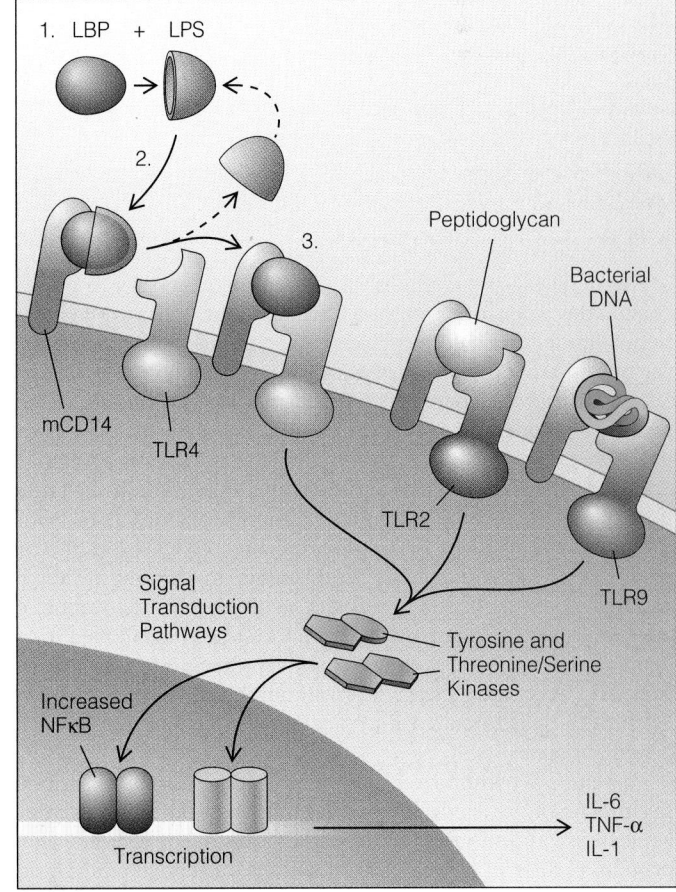

Figure 2 **During lipopolysaccharide (LPS) signaling, (1) LPS binds to LPS-binding protein (LPB). (2) This complex is delivered to membrane-bound CD14 (mCD14). (3) The CD14-LPS complex interacts with Toll-like receptor 4 (TLR4), which initiates the intracellular signal transduction pathway. The signal transduction pathway leads to NFκB translocation into the nucleus, with increased transcription of proinflammatory cytokines. TLR2 is known to signal membrane compounds of gram-positive bacteria such as peptidoglycan. TLR9 recognizes bacterial DNA. (IL—interleukin; NFκB—nuclear factor κB; TNF-α—tumor necrosis factor–α)**

ENDOTHELIAL INJURY

The network of endothelial cells lining the large and small vessels of the vascular tree is enormous, encompassing an area 600 times larger than that of the skin.[202] Far from being a passive conduit for blood cells and plasma, the endothelium contributes actively to the initiation, localization, and resolution of inflammation.[203] Circulating inflammatory mediators evoke an endothelial cell response characterized by upregulation of adhesion molecules such as ICAM-1 and vascular cell adhesion molecule (VCAM), expression of TLR2 and tissue factor, and shedding of endothelial cell thrombomodulin.[203,204] These changes result in neutrophil localization and local activation of coagulation with secondary tissue injury. In addition, healthy endothelial cells appear to play a role in limiting host injury during inflammation, as indicated by the observation that mice with a genetic deletion of syndecan-4 (a proteoglycan involved in endothelial cell adhesion and signaling) exhibit increased mortality and exaggerated release of IL-1 after endotoxin challenge.[205]

Postmortem studies of patients with ARDS show that ICAM-1 is upregulated throughout the lung, whereas VCAM is expressed in larger vessels,[206] and that circulating markers of endothelial activation are present in critically ill patients with organ failure.[207] Moreover, diffuse endothelial injury is suggested by the presence of circulating endothelial cells in the blood of patients in septic shock.[208] Therapeutic strategies that target the adhesive interactions of lymphocytes and endothelial cells have shown promise against inflammatory conditions such as psoriasis and Crohn disease; studies of agents targeting the interaction of neutrophils with endothelial cells have so far yielded disappointing results.[209]

INTRAVASCULAR COAGULATION

Although plasma contains all the factors necessary to induce coagulation and formation of a fibrin clot, intravascular coagulation is limited in healthy persons by the absence of a trigger and the presence of endogenous anticoagulant mechanisms. This balance is disrupted in persons experiencing systemic inflammation, resulting in microvascular coagulation and obstructing oxygen delivery to the cell. Injury and inflammation can upregulate endothelial cell tissue factor expression and activate the coagulation cascade by catalyzing the conversion of factor VII to factor VIIa. Sequential activation of circulating coagulation factors results in the conversion of prothrombin to thrombin and, in turn, the conversion of fibrinogen to fibrin. The activation of coagulation is inhibited by three important endogenous anticoagulant pathways: the protein C pathway, the antithrombin pathway, and the tissue factor pathway inhibitor (TFPI) pathway. Each of these is impaired in critical illness, leading to a net procoagulant state.

Protein C is synthesized in the liver and circulates as an inactive precursor. It is activated in the vascular tree through its interaction with thrombomodulin on the endothelial cell; activated protein C blocks thrombin generation through its inhibitory interactions with factors V and VIII.[210] Hepatic production of protein C is impaired in sepsis. Moreover, shedding of endothelial cell thrombomodulin results in a reduction in the activation of available protein C, whereas acute-phase reactants such as α_1-antitrypsin accelerate its degradation. The importance of this anticoagulant mechanism is underlined by a 2001 study of recombinant activated protein C in patients with severe sepsis, in which treated patients experienced a significant improvement in 28-day survival and those with the greatest degrees of organ dysfunction benefited most.[147]

Antithrombin is a serine protease inhibitor that binds to and inactivates thrombin and inhibits factors IXa, XIa, and XIIa. Levels of circulating antithrombin are reduced in sepsis. Administration of recombinant antithrombin failed to improve survival in a large multicenter study of patients with severe sepsis, though interaction with heparin may have masked a therapeutic effect.[211]

TFPI is synthesized by endothelial cells in response to cytokines and shear stress. It too is a serine protease inhibitor whose target is the complex of tissue factor, factor VIIa, and factor Xa that initiates the coagulation cascade. Recombinant TFPI has been evaluated as a therapy for sepsis; however, a large multicenter trial failed to show any survival benefit from such therapy.[212]

The interactions between coagulation and inflammation are complex. Protein C binds to a receptor expressed on endothelial cells and neutrophils, and prevention of this interaction results in a disseminated inflammatory process.[146] Binding of activated protein C to its receptor in brain endothelium inhibits endothelial cell apoptosis and is neuroprotective during cerebral ischemia.[213]

APOPTOSIS

Apoptosis, or programmed cell death, is a process through which cellular structural elements and DNA are degraded and residual cellular constituents are converted into membrane-bound vesicles (apoptotic bodies) that are cleared by macrophages. Phagocytosis of apoptotic bodies prevents the uncontrolled release of cellular constituents and so prevents an inflammatory response to the injured cell.[214] Apoptosis is also an intrinsically anti-inflammatory process, however, in that phagocytosis of an apoptotic cell by the macrophage evokes the expression of anti-inflammatory genes such as those for TGF-β and IL-10.[215,216] Apoptosis, like cell replication, is a physiologic process that is essential for normal growth and development; either excessive or inadequate apoptosis can produce disease.

Increased rates of apoptosis of colonic epithelial cells and splenic lymphocytes are seen in autopsy specimens from patients dying as a consequence of sepsis or multiple trauma.[217] Conversely, whereas circulating neutrophils survive less than a day in vivo in healthy persons, neutrophils isolated from the blood of patients with sepsis show both phenotypic features of activation and prolonged survival (a consequence of the inhibition of a constitutively expressed apoptotic program).[52] Animal studies have shown that inhibition of lymphoid cell apoptosis improves survival after septic challenge.[218] Conversely, induction of neutrophil apoptosis improved survival in a rodent model of intestinal ischemia-reperfusion injury.[219] The potential role of apoptosis in the pathogenesis of MODS is further suggested by animal studies of ventilator-induced lung injury, which demonstrated that injurious mechanical ventilation strategies can induce renal epithelial cell apoptosis and biochemical evidence of renal dysfunction.[220]

GASTROINTESTINAL DYSHOMEOSTASIS

Because MODS not infrequently evolves despite apparently adequate control of infection or other inciting triggers, it has been suggested that the GI tract may serve as the unseen motor of the pathologic state,[221-224] both as a reservoir of microorganisms and their products and as a mechanism for the evolution of inflammation.

The GI tract of a healthy human being harbors upward of 600 different microbial species, and bacteria outnumber human cells 10 to 1.[225] The composition of the GI flora is stable over a person's lifetime, but intercurrent disease can produce profound changes in bacterial numbers and patterns of colonization. In critically ill surgical patients, the normally sterile proximal GI tract becomes heavily colonized with the same organisms that predominate in nosocomial ICU-acquired infection—*Staphylococcus epidermidis*, *Pseudomonas*, *Candida*, and *Enterococcus*. Colonization is significantly associated with the development of nosocomial infection with the same organism.[152] Extensive studies in animal models have shown that acute insults (e.g., endotoxemia, peritonitis, pneumonia, trauma, burns, biliary tract obstruction, malnutrition, and lack of enteral feeding) can induce bacterial overgrowth in the gut and translocation of enteric bacteria to regional lymph nodes of the peritoneal cavity.[226] Similar stimuli result in translocation in humans,[227,228] and prevention of colonization with topical nonabsorbed antibiotics reduces the incidence of nosocomial infections, including bacteremias.[153] Detection of circulating endotoxin after burns[174] or major vascular surgery[175] suggests that endotoxin is also absorbed from the gut under conditions of altered gut barrier function.

The role of the gut in MODS is not limited to that of a microbial reservoir. The GI tract and adjacent structures constitute the largest aggregation of immune cells in the body. Normal interactions between the indigenous flora and the gut immune system serve to prevent the generation of immune responses to luminal antigens. Loss of these tonic inhibitory interactions may, in turn, contribute to a state of systemically activated inflammation. Accordingly, hemorrhagic shock results in significantly elevated levels of TNF and IL-6 in portal venous blood,[229] and portal endotoxemia replicates systemic features of MODS, such as hypermetabolism,[230] impairment of cell-mediated immunity,[231] and activation of coagulation.[232] Ablation of the hepatic Kupffer cell population has improved survival in animal models of peritonitis.[197] Mesenteric lymph has been shown to contain factors that can evoke inflammatory changes in organs remote from the gut.[233] Thus, dysfunction of normal microbiologic and immunologic homeostasis in the GI tract and the liver results in the gut serving as a secondary source of the stimuli that induce and perpetuate MODS.

A clinically relevant role for the gut in the pathogenesis of MODS is supported by the results of randomized trials of SDD.[153]

Table 8 Characteristics of Linear and Complex Systems[241]

Assumptions of Linear Systems	Assumptions of Complex Systems
Mediators have unique, consistent biologic effects	Mediators have redundant, variable, and context-dependent effects
Antagonism of effect is mediated by specific inhibitor	Antagonism of effect is not attributable to single mediator or process
Biologic processes occur sequentially	Biologic processes occur concurrently
Biologic response is reliably predicted by measurement of responsible mediator	Biologic response is not consistently predicted by measure of single mediator
Modulation of biologic process occurs in dose-dependent fashion; small intervention has small effect	Modulation of process is not predictably dose-dependent; small perturbation may have large effect
Normal behavior of system results in physiologic stability	Normal integrated behavior of system results in physiologic variability or oscillations over time

TWO-HIT HYPOTHESIS

A complementary hypothesis of MODS pathogenesis suggests that an acute insult, such as infection or trauma, primes the host so that a subsequent, relatively trivial, insult produces a markedly exaggerated host response.[234] Such a model would account for the severity of MODS developing late after multiple trauma[181] as well as the substantial morbidity associated with nosocomial infection in the ICU.[151] Studies in animal models have revealed that previous hemorrhagic shock leads to an exaggerated response to subsequent endotoxin challenge.[235]

MODS and Complexity Theory

None of the various theories of pathogenesis described so far is adequate to explain the evolution of the clinical syndrome of MODS. These models are not mutually exclusive; rather, they reflect differing perspectives on a profoundly deranged state of systemic homeostasis—one that has evolved only because the health care team has intervened to subvert an otherwise lethal process. The enormously complicated interactions among multiple predisposing patient factors, a series of physiologic insults, and an endogenous response effected via multiple cell types and many hundreds of biochemical mediators is best modeled by means of complexity theory.[236,237]

According to the precepts of complexity theory, a complex system cannot be understood through isolated analysis of its component parts: it can be understood only through an appreciation of the various interactions of those parts. The result of these multiple interactions is neither a state of anarchy nor a limitless series of unpredictable outcomes but, rather, a series of stable responses known as an emergent order. This stable order is dependent on the interactions of all its parts but is much more than their simple sum. It is characterized both by a resilience to potentially disruptive external influences and by a degree of intrinsic variability. Loss of intrinsic variability is a marker of a failing or diseased system. The healthy human heart exhibits normal variability in rate and rhythm, which is lost in patients with significant congestive heart failure.[238] Loss of intrinsic heart rate and blood pressure variability is also evident in patients with septic shock.[239,240]

The idea that concepts inherent in complex nonlinear systems can be applied to the understanding of MODS is compelling.[241] Clinicians are most familiar with linear models of disease, and the assumptions on which these models are based generally lead to effective clinical responses. For example, diabetes results from the deficiency of a single protein and is treated effectively by replacing that protein; cholangitis is the consequence of obstruction of the bile duct and is treated by relieving that obstruction. For linear diseases such as these, a single abnormality produces the clinical phenotype, and definitive therapy involves correcting that abnormality. Disorders of biologic pathways such as the coagulation cascade represent a somewhat more elaborate variation on the same theme. For example, pathologic coagulation resulting in DVT can be treated by means of a variety of different strategies aimed at disrupting the clotting cascade. Similarly, hypertension can be managed by means of various pharmacologic strategies that modify different aspects of the regulation of vasomotor tone.

Complex disorders such as MODS, however, are not so predictable, and the therapeutic modulation required is much more difficult [*see Table 8*]. The consequences of manipulating a particular mediator may be highly context dependent, varying with the nature of the insult, the predisposition of the host, and the timing of administration.[145] Moreover, intervention carries the potential cost of inadvertent iatrogenic harm. A sobering consequence of high-quality clinical trials performed in the ICU over the past decade has been the realization that making a normal or supranormal physiologic state the therapeutic target in a critically ill patient whose homeostasis is profoundly disrupted may, on occasion, be detrimental rather than beneficial.[22,107,242]

References

1. Baue AE: Multiple, progressive, or sequential systems failure: a syndrome of the 1970s. Arch Surg 110:779, 1975

2. Eiseman B, Beart R, Norton L: Multiple organ failure. Surg Gynecol Obstet 144:323, 1977

3. Fry DE, Pearlstein L, Fulton RL, et al: Multiple system organ failure: the role of uncontrolled infection. Arch Surg 115:136, 1980

4. Bone RC, Balk RA, Cerra FB, et al: ACCP/SCCM Consensus Conference. Definitions for sepsis and organ failure and guidelines for the use of innovative therapies in sepsis. Chest 101:1644, 1992

5. Deitch EA: Multiple organ failure: pathophysiology and potential future therapy. Ann Surg 216:117, 1992

6. Beal AL, Cerra FB: Multiple organ failure syndrome in the 1990's: systemic inflammatory response and organ dysfunction. JAMA 271:226, 1994

7. Moss M, Parsons PE, Steinberg KP, et al: Chronic alcohol abuse is associated with an increased incidence of acute respiratory distress syndrome and severity of multiple organ dysfunction in patients with septic shock. Crit Care Med 31:869, 2003

8. Marshall JC: Multiple organ dysfunction syndrome (MODS). Clinical Trials for the Treatment of Sepsis. Sibbald WJ, Vincent J-L, Eds. Springer-Verlag, Berlin, 1995, p 122

9. Marshall JC, Cook DJ, Christou NV, et al: Multiple organ dysfunction score: a reliable descriptor of a complex clinical outcome. Crit Care Med 23:1638, 1995

10. Bernard G: The Brussels score. Sepsis 1:43, 1997

11. Vincent JL: The sepsis-related organ failure assessment (SOFA) score. Intens Care Med 1996

12. Le Gall JR, Klar J, Lemeshow S, et al: The logistic organ dysfunction system—A new way to assess organ dysfunction in the intensive care unit. JAMA 276:802, 1996

13. Burke JF, Pontoppidan H, Welch CE: High output respiratory failure: an important cause of death ascribed to peritonitis or ileus. Ann Surg 158:581, 1963

14. Ashbaugh DG, Bigelow DB, Petty TL, et al: Acute respiratory distress in adults. Lancet 2:319, 1967

15. Kollef MH, Schuster DP: Medical progress: the acute respiratory distress syndrome. N Engl J Med 332:27, 1995

16. Ranieri VM, Suter PM, Tortorella C, et al: Effect of mechanical ventilation on inflammatory mediators in patients with acute respiratory distress syndrome: a randomized controlled trial. JAMA 282:54, 1999

17. Gattinoni L, Pesenti A, Bombino M: Relationships between lung computed tomographic density, gas exchange, and PEEP in acute respiratory failure. Anesthesiology 69:824, 1988

18. Pinhu L, Whitehead T, Evans T, et al: Ventilator-associated lung injury. Lancet 361:332, 2003

19. Murray JF, Matthay MA, Luce JM, et al: An expanded definition of the adult respiratory distress syndrome. Am Rev Respir Dis 138:720, 1988

20. Bernard GR, Artigas A, Brigham KL, et al: The American-European consensus conference on ARDS. Definitions, mechanisms, relevant outcomes, and clinical trial coordination. Am J Respir

Crit Care Med 149:818, 1994

21. Marshall RP, Webb S, Bellingan GJ, et al: Angiotensin converting enzyme insertion/deletion polymorphism is associated with susceptibility and outcome in acute respiratory distress syndrome. Am J Respir Crit Care Med 166:646, 2002

22. Brower RG, Matthay MA, Morris A, et al: Ventilation with lower tidal volumes as compared with traditional tidal volumes for acute lung injury and the acute respiratory distress syndrome. N Engl J Med 342:1301, 2000

23. Bywaters EGL, Beall O: Crush injuries with impairment of renal function. Br Med J 1:427, 1941

24. Morris JA Jr, Mucha P Jr, Ross SE, et al: Acute posttraumatic renal failure: a multicenter perspective. J Trauma 31:1584, 1991

25. Lameire N, Vanholder R: Pathophysiologic features and prevention of human and experimental acute tubular necrosis. J Am Soc Nephrol 12:S20, 2001

26. Tilney NL, Lazarus JM. Acute renal failure in surgical patients: causes, clinical patterns and care. Surg Clin North Am 63:357, 1983

27. Lauriat S, Linas SL: The role of neutrophils in acute renal failure. Semin Nephrol 18:498, 1998

28. Heinzelmann M, Mercer-Jones MA, Passmore JC: Neutrophils and renal failure. Am J Kidney Dis 34:384, 1999

29. Faraco PR, Ledgerwood EC, Smith KGC: Apoptosis and renal disease. Sepsis 2:31, 1998

30. Bywaters EGL: Anatomical changes in the liver after trauma. Clin Sci 6:19, 1946

31. Hawker F. Liver dysfunction in critical illness. Anaesth Intens Care 19:165, 1991

32. Schwartz DB, Bone RC, Balk RA, et al: Hepatic dysfunction in the adult respiratory distress syndrome. Chest 95:871, 1989

33. Langenfeld JE, Machiedo GW, Lyons M, et al: Correlation between red blood cell deformability and changes in hemodynamic function. Surgery 116:859, 1994

34. Parrillo JE, Parker MM, Natanson C, et al: Septic shock in humans. Advances in the understanding of pathogenesis, cardiovascular dysfunction, and therapy. Ann Intern Med 113:227, 1990

35. Vincent JL, Gris P, Coffernils M, et al: Myocardial depression characterizes the fatal course of septic shock. Surgery 111:660, 1992

36. Yien HW, Hseu SS, Lee LC, et al: Spectral analysis of systemic arterial pressure and heart rate signals as a prognostic tool for the prediction of patient outcome in the intensive care unit. Crit Care Med 25:258, 1997

37. Lorente JA, Landin L, Renes E, et al: Role of nitric oxide in the hemodynamic changes of sepsis. Crit Care Med 21:759, 1993

38. Finkel MS, Oddis CV, Jacob TD, et al: Negative inotropic effects of cytokines on the heart mediated by nitric oxide. Science 257:387, 1992

39. Bolton CF, Young GB, Zochodne DW: The neurological complications of sepsis. Ann Neurol 33:94, 1993

40. Bolton CF: Sepsis and the systemic inflammatory response syndrome: Neuromuscular manifesta-

tions. Crit Care Med 24:1408, 1996

41. Hund E: Neurological complications of sepsis: critical illness polyneuropathy and myopathy. J Neurol 248:929, 2001

42. de Letter MA, Schmitz PI, Viseer LH, et al: Risk factors for the development of polyneuropathy and myopathy in critically ill patients. Crit Care Med 29:2281, 2001

43. Coronel B, Mercatello A, Couturier JC, et al: Polyneuropathy: potential cause of difficult weaning. Crit Care Med 18:486, 1990

44. Bolton CF: Neuromuscular complications of sepsis. Intensive Care Med 19(suppl 2):S58, 1993

45. Segredo V, Caldwell JE, Matthay MA, et al: Persistent paralysis in critically ill patients after long-term administration of vecuronium. N Engl J Med 327:524, 1992

46. Baughmann RP, Lower EE, Flessa HC, et al: Thrombocytopenia in the intensive care unit. Chest 104:1243, 1993

47. Gando S, Nanzaki S, Kemmotsu O: Disseminated intravascular coagulation and sustained systemic inflammatory response syndrome predict organ dysfunctions after trauma: application of clinical decision analysis. Ann Surg 229:121, 1999

48. Aster RH: Heparin-induced thrombocytopenia and thrombosis. N Engl J Med 332:1374, 1995

49. van der Poll T, de Jonge E, Levi M, et al: Pathogenesis of DIC in sepsis. Sepsis 3:103, 1999

50. Marshall JC: Inflammation, coagulopathy, and the pathogenesis of the multiple organ dysfunction syndrome. Crit Care Med 29(suppl):S106, 2001

51. Todd JC III, Mollitt DL: Effect of sepsis on erythrocyte intracellular calcium homeostasis. Crit Care Med 23:459, 1995

52. Jimenez MF, Watson RWG, Parodo J, et al: Dysregulated expression of neutrophil apoptosis in the systemic inflammatory response syndrome (SIRS). Arch Surg 132:1263, 1997

53. Hotchkiss RS, Tinsley KW, Swanson PE, et al: Sepsis-induced apoptosis causes progressive profound depletion of B and CD4+ T lymphocytes in humans. J Immunol 166:6952, 2001

54. Curling TB: On acute ulceration of the duodenum in cases of burns. Med-Chir Tr London 25:260, 1842

55. Cook DJ, Fuller H, Guyatt GH, et al: Risk factors for gastrointestinal bleeding in critically ill patients. N Engl J Med 330:377, 1994

56. Chang RWS, Jacobs S, Lee B: Gastrointestinal dysfunction among intensive care unit patients. Crit Care Med 15:909, 1987

57. van der Spoel JI, Oudemans-van Straaten HM, Stoutenbeek CP, et al: Neostigmine resolves critical illness-related colonic ileus in intensive care patients with multiple organ failure—a prospective, double-blind, placebo-controlled trial. Intensive Care Med 27:822, 2001

58. Bell RC, Coalson JJ, Smith JD, et al: Multiple organ system failure and infection in adult respiratory distress syndrome. Ann Intern Med 99:293, 1983

59. Glenn F, Becker CG: Acute acalculous cholecystitis: an increasing entity. Ann Surg 195:131, 1982

60. Van den Berghe G, Wouters P, Weekers F, et al: Intensive insulin therapy in the surgical intensive

care unit. N Engl J Med 345:1359, 2001

61. Annane D, Sebille V, Troche G, et al: A 3-level prognostic classification in septic shock based on cortisol levels and cortisol response to corti-cotropin. JAMA 2834:1038, 2000

62. Cooper MS, Stewart PM: Corticosteroid insuffi-ciency in acutely ill patients. N Engl J Med 348:727, 2003

63. Vasa FR, Molitch ME: Endocrine problems in the chronically critically ill patient. Clin Chest Med 22:193, 2003

64. Christou NV, Meakins JL, Gordon J, et al: The delayed hypersensitivity response and host resis-tance in surgical patients—20 years later. Ann Surg 222:534, 1995

65. Grbic JT, Mannick JA, Gough DB, et al: The role of prostaglandin E_2 in immune suppression fol-lowing injury. Ann Surg 214:253, 1991

66. Marshall JC, Christou NV, Horn R, et al: The microbiology of multiple organ failure. The proxi-mal GI tract as an occult reservoir of pathogens. Arch Surg 123:309, 1988

67. Eachempati SR, Hydo LJ, Barie PS: Factors influ-encing the development of decubitus ulcers in critically ill surgical patients. Crit Care Med 29:1678, 2001

68. Knaus WA, Wagner DP, Lynn J: Short-term mor-tality predictions for critically ill hospitalized adults: science and ethics. Science 254:389, 1991

69. Lemeshow S, Le Gall JR: Modeling the severity of illness of ICU patients: a systems update. JAMA 272:1049, 1994

70. Vincent JL, De Mendonca A, Cantraine F, et al: Use of the SOFA score to assess the incidence of organ dysfunction/failure in intensive care units: results of a multicenter, prospective study. Crit Care Med 26:1793, 1998

71. Goris RJA, te Boekhorst TPA, Nuytinck JKS, et al: Multiple organ failure. Generalized autode-structive inflammation? Arch Surg 120:1109, 1985

72. Moore FA, Moore EE, Poggetti R, et al: Gut bac-terial translocation via the portal vein: a clinical perspective with major torso trauma. J Trauma 31:629, 1991

73. Hebert PC, Drummond AJ, Singer J, et al: A sim-ple multiple system organ failure scoring system predicts mortality of patients who have sepsis syn-drome. Chest 104:230, 1993

74. Vincent J-L, Moreno R, Takala J, et al: The SOFA (sepsis-related organ failure assessment) score to describe organ dysfunnction/failure. Intensive Care Med 22:707, 1996

75. Marshall JC: Charting the course of critical ill-ness: prognostication and outcome description in the intensive care unit. Crit Care Med 27:676, 1999

76. Cook RJ, Cook DJ, Tilley J, et al: Multiple organ dysfunction: baseline and serial component scores. Crit Care Med 29:2046, 2001

77. Ferreira FL, Bota DP, Bross A, et al: Serial evalu-ation of the SOFA score to predict outcome in critically ill patients. JAMA 286:1754, 2001

78. Choi PT, Yip G, Quinonez LG, et al: Crystalloids vs. colloids in fluid resuscitation: a systematic review. Crit Care Med 27:200, 1999

79. Dellinger EP: Cardiovascular management of sep-tic shock. Crit Care Med 31:946, 2003

80. Gomersall CD, Joynt GM, Freebairn RC, et al: Resuscitation of critically ill patients based on the results of gastric tonometry: a prospective, ran-domized, controlled trial. Crit Care Med 28:607, 2000

81. De Backer D, Creteur J, Preiser JC, et al: Microvascular blood flow is altered in patients with sepsis. Am J Respir Crit Care Med 166:98, 2002

82. Connors AF Jr, Speroff T, Dawson NV, et al: The

effectiveness of right heart catheterization in the initial care of critically ill patients. JAMA 276:889, 1996

83. Gattinoni L, Brazzi L, Pelosi P, et al: A trial of goal-oriented hemodynamic therapy in critically ill patients. N Engl J Med 333:1025, 1995

84. Sandham JD, Hull RD, Brant RF, et al: A ran-domized, controlled trial of the use of pulmonary-artery catheters in high-risk surgical patients. N Engl J Med 348:5, 2003

85. Pape HC, Giannoudis P, Krettek C: The timing of fracture treatment in polytrauma patients: rele-vance of damage control orthopedic surgery. Am J Surg 183:622, 2002

86. Heyland DK, Novak F, Drover JW, et al: Should immunonutrition become routine in critically ill patients? A systematic review of the evidence. JAMA 286:944, 2001

87. Takala J, Ruokonen E, Webster NR, et al: Increased mortality associated with growth hor-mone treatment in critically ill adults. N Engl J Med 341:785, 1999

88. Maki DG: Risk factors for nosocomial infection in intensive care: devices vs nature and goals for the next decade. Arch Intern Med 149:30, 1989

89. Cook DJ, Guyatt GH, Marshall JC, et al: A ran-domized trial of sucralfate versus ranitidine for stress ulcer prophylaxis in critically ill patients. N Engl J Med 338:791, 1998

90. D'Amico R, Pifferi S, Leonetti C, et al: Effec-tiveness of antibiotic prophylaxis in critically ill adult patients: systematic review of randomized controlled trials. Br Med J 316:1275, 1998

91. Nathens AB, Marshall JC: Selective decontamina-tion of the digestive tract in surgical patients. Arch Surg 134:170, 1999

92. Van Der Waaij D: The ecology of the human intes-tine and its consequences for overgrowth by pathogens such as Clostridium difficile. Annu Rev Microbiol 43:69, 1989

93. Le Mee J, Paye F, Sauvanet A, et al: Incidence and reversibility of organ failure in the course of ster-ile or infected necrotizing pancreatitis. Arch Surg 136:1386, 2001

94. Polk HC, Shields CL: Remote organ failure: a valid sign of occult intraabdominal infection. Sur-gery 81:310, 1977

95. Meakins JL, Wicklund B, Forse RA, et al: The sur-gical intensive care unit: current concepts in infec-tion. Surg Clin North Am 60:117, 1980

96. Heyland DK, Cook DJ, Marshall JC, et al: The clinical utility of invasive diagnostic techniques in the setting of ventilator-associated pneumonia. Chest 115:1076, 1999

97. Fagon J-Y, Chastre J, Wolff M, et al: Invasive and noninvasive strategies for management of suspect-ed ventilator-associated pneumonia: a randomized trial. Ann Intern Med 132:621, 2000

98. Nieto-Rodriguez JA, Kusne S, Mañez R, et al: Factors associated with the development of can-didemia and candidemia-related death among liver transplant recipients. Ann Surg 223:70, 1996

99. Henao FJ, Daes JE, Dennis RJ: Risk factors for multiorgan failure: a case control study. J Trauma 31:74, 1991

100. Muckart DJ, Thomson SR: Undetected injuries: a preventable cause of increased morbidity and mortality. Am J Surg 162:457, 1991

101. Davis JW, Hoyt DB, McArdle MS, et al: The sig-nificance of critical care errors in causing pre-ventable death in trauma patients in a trauma sys-tem. J Trauma 31:813, 1991

102. Muscedere JG, Mullen JBM, Gan K, et al: Tidal ventilation at low airway pressures can augment lung injury. Am J Respir Crit Care Med 149:1327, 1994

103. Slutsky AS, Tremblay LN: Multiple system organ failure. Is mechanical ventilation a contributing

factor? Am J Respir Crit Care Med 157(6 pt 1):1721, 1998

104. Deneke SM, Fanburg BL: Normobaric oxygen toxicity of the lung. N Engl J Med 303:76, 1980

105. Maetani S, Nishikawa T, Tobe T, et al: Role of blood transfusion in organ system failure follow-ing major abdominal surgery. Ann Surg 203:275, 1986

106. Sauaia A, Moore FA, Moore EE, et al: Early risk factors for postinjury multiple organ failure. World J Surg 20:392, 1996

107. Hebert PC, Wells G, Blajchman MA, et al: A mul-ticentre randomized controlled clinical trial of transfusion requirements in critical care. N Engl J Med 340:409, 1999

108. Marik PE, Sibbald WJ: Effect of stored blood transfusion on oxygen delivery in patients with sepsis. JAMA 269:3024, 1993

109. Grant JP, Cox CE, Kleinman LM, et al: Serum hepatic enzyme and bilirubin elevations during parenteral nutrition. Surg Gynecol Obstet 145:2398, 1977

110. Askanazi J, Rosenbaum SH, Hyman AI, et al: Respiratory changes induced by the large glucose loads of total parenteral nutrition. JAMA 243:1444, 1980

111. Moore FA, Feliciano DV, Andrassy RJ, et al: Early enteral feeding, compared with parenteral, reduces postoperative septic complications: the results of a meta-analysis. Ann Surg 216:172, 1992

112. Masip J, Betbese AJ, Paez J, et al: Non-invasive pressure support ventilation versus conventional oxygen therapy in acute cardiogenic pulmonary oedema: a randomised trial. Lancet 356:2126, 2000

113. Delclaux C, L'Her E, Alberti C, et al: Treatment of acute hypoxemic nonhypercapnic respiratory insufficiency with continuous positive airway pres-sure delivered by a face mask: a randomized con-trolled trial. JAMA 284:2352, 2000

114. Parker JC, Hernandez LA, Peevy KJ: Mechanisms of ventilator induced lung injury. Crit Care Med 21:131, 1993

115. Munoz J, Guerrero JE, Escalante JL, et al: Pressure-controlled ventilation versus controlled mechanical ventilation with decelerating inspira-tory flow. Crit Care Med 21:1143, 1993

116. Hickling KG, Henderson SJ, Jackson R: Low mortality associated with low volume pressure limited ventilation with permissive hypercapnia in severe adult respiratory distress syndrome. Intensive Care Med 16:372, 1990

117. Hickling KG, Walsh J, Henderson S, et al: Low mortality rate in adult respiratory distress syn-drome using low-volume, pressure-limited ventila-tion with permissive hypercapnia: a prospective study. Crit Care Med 22:1568, 1994

118. Laffey JG, Tanaka M, Engelberts D, et al: Therapeutic hypercapnia reduces pulmonary and systemic injury following in vivo lung reperfusion. Am J Respir Crit Care Med 162:2287, 2000

119. Derdak S, Mehta S, Stewart TE, et al: High-fre-quency oscillatory ventilation for acute respiratory distress syndrome in adults: a randomized, con-trolled trial. Am J Respir Crit Care Med 166:801, 2002

120. Ferguson ND, Stewart TE: The use of high-fre-quency oscillatory ventilation in adults with acute lung injury. Respir Care Clin North Am 7:647, 2001

121. Dellinger RP, Zimmerman JL, Taylor RW, et al: Effects of inhaled nitric oxide in patients with acute respiratory distress syndrome: results of a randomized phase II trial. Crit Care Med 26:15, 1998

122. Lewandowski K: Extracorporeal membrane oxy-genation for severe acute respiratory failure. Crit Care 4:156, 2000

123. Mols G, Loop T, Geiger K, et al: Extracorporeal membrane oxygenation: a ten-year experience. Am J Surg 180:144, 2000

124. Morris AH, Wallace CJ, Menlovet RL, et al: Randomized clinical trial of pressure-controlled inverse ratio ventilation and extracorporeal CO2 removal for adult respiratory distress syndrome. Am J Respir Crit Care Med 149:295, 1994

125. Connors AF Jr, Speroff T, Dawson NV, et al: The effectiveness of right heart catheterization in the initial care of critically ill patients. JAMA 276:889, 1996

126. Mehta RL, McDonald B, Gabbai FB, et al: A randomized clinical trial of continuous versus intermittent dialysis for acute renal failure. Kidney Int 60:1154, 2001

127. Bouman CS, Oudemans-van Straaten HM, Tijssen JG, et al: Effects of early high-volume continuous venovenous hemofiltration on survival and recovery of renal function in intensive care patients with acute renal failure: a prospective, randomized trial. Crit Care Med 30:2205, 2002

128. Tonelli M, Manns B, Feller-Kopman D: Acute renal failure in the intensive care unit: a systematic review of the impact of dialytic modality on mortality and renal recovery. Am J Kidney Dis 40:875, 2002

129. Ronco C, Bellomo R, Homel P, et al: Effects of different doses in continuous veno-venous haemofiltration on outcomes of acute renal failure: a prospective randomised trial. Lancet 356:26, 2000

130. Schiffl H, Lang SM, Fischer R: Daily hemodialysis and the outcome of acute renal failure. N Engl J Med 346:362, 2002

131. Kellum JA, Angus DC, Johnson JP, et al: Continuous versus intermittent renal replacement therapy: a meta-analysis. Intensive Care Med 28:29, 2002

132. Cole L, Bellomo R, Hart G, et al: A phase II randomized, controlled trial of continuous hemofiltration in sepsis. Crit Care Med 30:100, 2002

133. Kudsk KA, Croce MA, Fabian TC, et al: Enteral versus parenteral feeding: effects on septic morbidity after blunt and penetrating abdominal trauma. Ann Surg 215:503, 1992

134. McGregor CS, Marshall JC: Enteral feeding in acute pancreatitis: just do it. Curr Opin Crit Care 7:89, 2001

135. Marik PE, Zaloga GP: Early enteral nutrition in acutely ill patients: a systematic review. Crit Care Med 29:2264, 2003

136. Beale RJ, Bryg DJ, Bihari DJ: Immunonutrition in the critically ill: a systematic review of clinical outcome. Crit Care Med 27:2799, 1999

137. Griffith DP, McNally AT, Battey CH, et al: Intravenous erythromycin facilitates bedside placement of postpyloric feeding tubes in critically ill adults: a double-blind, randomized, placebo-controlled study. Crit Care Med 31:39, 2003

138. Berne JD, Norwood SH, McAuley CE, et al: Erythromycin reduces delayed gastric emptying in critically ill trauma patients: a randomized, controlled trial. J Trauma 53:422, 2002

139. Rozga J, Podesta L, LePage EA, et al: A bioartificial liver to treat severe acute liver failure. Ann Surg 219:538, 1994

140. Mitzner SR, Stange J, Klammt S, et al: Extracorporeal detoxification using the molecular adsorbent recirculating system for critically ill patients with liver failure. J Am Soc Nephrol 12(17 suppl):S75, 2001

141. Alderson P, Bunn F, Lefebvre C, et al: Human albumin solution for resuscitation and volume expansion in critically ill patients. Cochrane Database Syst Rev (1):CD001208, 2002

142. Vincent JL, Baron JF, Reinhart K, et al: Anemia and blood transfusion in critically ill patients. JAMA 288:1499, 2002

143. Hebert PC, Yetisir E, Martin C, et al: Is a low transfusion threshhold safe in patients with cardiovascular diseases? Crit Care Med 29:227, 2001

144. Kress JP, Pohlman AS, O'Connor MF, et al: Daily interruption of sedative infusions in critically ill patients undergoing mechanical ventilation. N Engl J Med 342:1471, 2000

145. Taylor FB Jr, Stearns-Kurosawa DJ, Kurosawa S, et al: The endothelial cell protein C receptor aids in host defense against Escherichia coli sepsis. Blood 95:1680, 2000

146. Bernard GR, Vincent J-L, Laterre PF, et al: Efficacy and safety of recombinant human activated protein C for severe sepsis. N Engl J Med 344:699, 2001

147. Vincent J-L, Angus DC, Artigas A, et al: Effects of drotrecogin alfa (activated) on organ dysfunction in the PROWESS trial. Crit Care Med 31:834, 2003

148. Annane D, Sebille V, Charpentier C, et al: Effect of treatment with low doses of hydrocortisone and fludrocortisone on mortality in patients with septic shock. JAMA 288:862, 2002

149. Cronin L, Cook DJ, Carlet J, et al: Corticosteroid treatment for sepsis: a critical appraisal and meta-analysis of the literature. Crit Care Med 23:1430, 1995

150. Marshall JC: Such stuff as dreams are made on: mediator-targeted therapy in sepsis. Nat Rev Drug Discov 2:391, 2003

151. Vincent JL, Bihari DJ, Suter PM, et al: The prevalence of nosocomial infection in intensive care units in Europe: results of the European Prevalence of Infection in Intensive Care (EPIC) Study. JAMA 274:639, 1995

152. Marshall JC, Christou NV, Meakins JL: The gastrointestinal tract: the "undrained abscess" of multiple organ failure. Ann Surg 218:111, 1993

153. Nathens AB, Marshall JC: Selective decontamination of the digestive tract (SDD) in surgical patients. Arch Surg 134:170, 1999

154. Singh N, Rogers P, Atwood CW, et al: Short-course empiric antibiotic therapy for patients with pulmonary infiltrates in the intensive care unit: a proposed solution for indiscriminate antibiotic prescription. Am J Respir Crit Care Med 162(2 pt 1):505, 2000

155. Ferraris VA: Exploratory laparotomy for potential abdominal sepsis in patients with multiple-organ failure. Arch Surg 118:1130, 1983

156. Hinsdale JG, Jaffe BM: Re-operation for intra-abdominal sepsis. Indications and results in modern critical care setting. Ann Surg 199:31, 1984

157. Bunt TJ: Non-directed relaparotomy for intraabdominal sepsis: a futile procedure. Am Surg 52:294, 1986

158. Knaus WA, Draper EA, Wagner DP, et al: Prognosis in acute organ system failure. Ann Surg 202:685, 1985

159. Ranson JHC, Rifkind KM, Turner JW: Prognostic signs and nonoperative peritoneal lavage in acute pancreatitis. Surg Gynecol Obstet 143:209, 1976

160. Prendergast TJ, Claessens MT, Luce JM: A national survey of end-of-life care for critically ill patients. Am J Respir Crit Care Med 158:1163, 1998

161. Cook DJ, Guyatt GH, Jaeschke R, et al: Determinants in Canadian health care workers of the decision to withdraw life support from the critically ill. JAMA 273:703, 1995

162. Safar P, DeKornfeld T, Pearson J, et al: Intensive care unit. Anesthesia 16:275, 1961

163. Tilney NL, Bailey GL, Morgan AP: Sequential system failure after rupture of abdominal aortic aneurysms: an unsolved problem in postoperative care. Ann Surg 178:117, 1973

164. Muckart DJJ, Bhagwanjee S: The ACCP/SCCM consensus conference definitions of the systemic inflammatory response syndrome (SIRS) and allied disorders in relation to critically injured patients. Crit Care Med 25:1789, 1997

165. Bone RC: Sir Isaac Newton, sepsis, SIRS, and CARS. Crit Care Med 24:1125, 1996

166. Marshall JC: Rethinking sepsis: from concepts to syndromes to diseases. Sepsis 3:5, 1999

167. Fink MP: Cytopathic hypoxia. Crit Care 6:491, 2002

168. Norton LW: Does drainage of intraabdominal pus reverse multiple organ failure? Am J Surg 149:347, 1985

169. Suffredini AF, Fromm RE, Parker MM, et al: The cardiovascular response of normal humans to the administration of endotoxin. N Engl J Med 321:280, 1989

170. Taveira Da Silva AM, Kaulach HC, Chuidian FS, et al: Brief report: shock and multiple organ dysfunction after self administration of salmonella endotoxin. N Engl J Med 328:1457, 1993

171. Danner RL, Elin RJ, Hosseini JM, et al: Endotoxemia in human septic shock. Chest 99:169, 1991

172. Bates DW, Parsonnet J, Ketchum PA, et al: Limulus amebocyte lysate assay for detection of endotoxin in patients with sepsis sydrome. Clin Infect Dis 27:582, 1998

173. Hoch RC, Rodriguez R, Manning T, et al: Effects of accidental trauma on cytokine and endotoxin production. Crit Care Med 21:839, 1993

174. Winchurch RA, Thupari JN, Munster AM: Endotoxemia in burn patients: Levels of circulating endotoxins are related to burn size. Surgery 102:808, 1987

175. Roumen RMH, Frieling JTM, van Tits HWHJ, et al: Endotoxemia after major vascular operations. J Vasc Surg 18:853, 1993

176. Poltorak A, He X, Smirnova I, et al: Defective LPS signaling in C3H/HeJ and C57BL/10ScCr mice: mutations in the Tlr4 gene. Science 282:2085, 1998

177. Michalek SM, Moore RN, McGhee JR, et al: The primary role of lymphoreticular cells in the mediation of host responses to bacterial endotoxin. J Infect Dis 141:55, 1980

178. Zhao B, Bowden RAS, Stavchansky SA, et al: Human endothelial cell response to gram-negative lipopolysaccharide assessed with cDNA microarrays. Am J Physiol Cell Physiol 281:C1587, 2001

179. Fessler MB, Malcolm KC, Duncan MW, et al: A genomic and proteomic analysis of activation of the human neutrophil by lipopolysaccharide and its mediation by p38 mitogen-activated protein kinase. J Biol Chem 277:31291, 2002

180. Aderem A, Ulevitch RJ: Toll-like receptors in the induction of the innate immune response. Nature 406:782, 2000

181. Faist E, Baue AE, Dittmer H, et al: Multiple organ failure in polytrauma patients. J Trauma 23:775, 1983

182. Sorenson TI, Nielsen GG, Andersen PK, et al: Genetic and environmental influences on premature death in adult adoptees. N Engl J Med 318:727, 1988

183. Lazarus R, Vercelli D, Palmer LJ, et al: Single nucleotide polymorphisms in innate immunity genes: abundant variation and potential role in complex human disease. Immunol Rev 190:9, 2002

184. Agnese DM, Calvano JE, Hahm SJ, et al: Human toll-like receptor 4 mutations but not CD14 polymorphisms are associated with an increased risk of gram-negative infections. J Infect Dis 186:1522, 2002

185. Lorenz E, Mira J-P, Frees KL, et al: Relevance of mutations in the TLR4 receptor in patients with

gram-negative septic shock. Arch Intern Med 162:1028, 2002

186. Gibot S, Cariou A, Drouet L, et al: Association between a genomic polymorphism within the CD14 locus and septic shock susceptibility and mortality rate. Crit Care Med 30:969, 2002

187. Mira J-P, Cariou A, Grall F, et al: Association of TNF2, a TNF-a promoter polymorphism, with septic shock susceptibility and mortality. JAMA 282:561, 1999

188. Appoloni O, Dupont E, Vandercruys M, et al: Association of tumor necrosis factor-2 allele with plasma tumor necrosis factor-α levels and mortality from septic shock. Am J Med 110:486, 2001

189. Schroder O, Schulte KM, Ostermann P, et al: Heat shock protein 70 genotypes HSPA1B and HSPA1L influence cytokine concentrations and interfere with outcome after major injury. Crit Care Med 31:73, 2003,

190. Reid CL, Perrey C, Pravica V, et al: Genetic variation in proinflammatory and anti-inflammatory cytokine production in multiple organ dysfunction syndrome. Crit Care Med 30:2216, 2003

191. Ma P, Chen D, Pan J, et al: Genomic polymorphism within interleukin-1 family cytokines influences the outcome of septic patients. Crit Care Med 30:1046, 2002

192. Ginzberg HH, Cherapanov V, Dong Q, et al: Neutrophil-mediated epithelial injury during transmigration: role of elastase. Am J Physiol Gastrointest Liver Physiol 281:G705, 2001

193. Yum HK, Arcaroli J, Kupfner J, et al: Involvement of phosphoinositide 3-kinases in neutrophil activation and the development of acute lung injury. J Immunol 167:6601, 2001

194. Lee WL, Downey GP: Leukocyte elastase. Physiological functions and role in acute lung injury. Am J Respir Crit Care Med 164:896, 2001

195. Jaeschke H, Smith CW. Mechanisms of neutrophil-induced parenchymal cell injury. J Leukoc Biol 61:647, 1997

196. Kubes P, Hunter J, Granger DN: Ischemia/reperfusion induced feline intestinal dysfunction: importance of granulocyte recruitment. Gastroenterology 103:807, 1992

197. Nieuwenhuijzen GAP, Haskel Y, Lu Q, et al: Macrophage elimination increases bacterial translocation and gut origin septicemia but attenuates symptoms and mortality rate in a model of systemic inflammation. Ann Surg 218:791, 1993

198. Carson WE, Yu H, Dierksheide J, et al: A fatal cytokine-induced systemic inflammatory response reveals a critical role for NK cells. J Immunol 162:4943, 1999

199. Badgwell B, Parihar R, Magro C, et al: Natural killer cells contribute to the lethality of a murine model of Escherichia coli infection. Surgery 132:205, 2002

200. Sherwood ER, Lin CY, Tao W, et al: b2 Microglobulin knockout mice are resistant to lethal intra-abdominal sepsis. Am J Respir Crit Care Med (in press)

201. Sempowski GD, Lee DM, Scearce RM, et al: Resistance of CD7-deficient mice to lipopolysaccharide-induced shock syndromes. J Exp Med 189:1011, 1999

202. Henneke P, Golenbock DT: Innate immune recognition of lipopolysaccharide by endothelial cells. Crit Care Med 30(5 suppl):S207, 2002

203. Aird WC: The role of the endothelium in severe sepsis and multiple organ dysfunction syndrome. Blood 101:3765, 2003

204. Faure E, Thomas L, Xu H, et al: Bacterial lipopolysaccharide and IFN-gamma induce Toll-like receptor 2 and Toll-like receptor 4 expression in human endothelial cells: role of NF-kappa B activation. J Immunol 166:2018, 2001

205. Ishiguro K, Kadomatsu K, Kojima TY, et al: Syndecan-4 deficiency leads to high mortality of lipopolysaccharide-injected mice. J Biol Chem 276:47483, 2001

206. Muller AM, Cronen C, Muller KM, et al: Heterogeneous expression of cell adhesion molecules by endothelial cells in ARDS. J Pathol 198:170, 2002

207. Ueno H, Hirasawa H, Oda S, et al: Coagulation/fibrinolysis abnormality and vascular endothelial damage in the pathogenesis of thrombocytopenic multiple organ failure. Crit Care Med 30:2242, 2002

208. Mutunga M, Fulton B, Bullock R, et al: Circulating endothelial cells in patients with septic shock. Am J Respir Crit Care Med 163:195, 2001

209. Harlan JM, Winn RK: Leukocyte-endothelial interactions: clinical trials of anti-adhesion therapy. Crit Care Med 30(suppl):S214, 2002

210. Esmon C: The protein C pathway. Crit Care Med 28(suppl):S44, 2000

211. Warren BL, Eid A, Singer P, et al: High-dose antithrombin III in severe sepsis: a randomized, controlled trial. JAMA 286:1869, 2001

212. Abraham E, Reinhart K, Opal S, et al: Efficacy and safety of tifacogin (recombinant tissue factor pathway inhibitor) in severe sepsis. JAMA 290:283, 2003

213. Cheng T, Liu D, Griffin JH, et al: Activated protein C blocks p53-mediated apoptosis in ischemic human brain endothelium and is neuroprotective. Nature Med 9:338, 2003

214. Thompson CB: Apoptosis in the pathogenesis and treatment of disease. Science 267:1456, 1995

215. Fadok VA, Bratton DL, Konowal A, et al: Macrophages that have ingested apoptotic cells in vitro inhibit proinflammatory cytokine production through autocrine/paracrine mechanisms involving TGFb, PGE2, and PAF. J Clin Invest 101:890, 1998

216. Byrne A, Reen DJ: Lipopolysaccharide induces rapid production of IL-10 by monocytes in the presence of apoptotic neutrophils. J Immunol 168:1968, 2002

217. Hotchkiss RS, Schmieg RE Jr, Swanson PE, et al: Rapid onset of intestinal epithelial and lymphocyte apoptotic cell death in patients with trauma and shock. Crit Care Med 28:3207, 2000

218. Hotchkiss RS, Tinsley KW, Swanson PE, et al: Prevention of lymphocyte cell death in sepsis improves survival in mice. Proc Natl Acad Sci USA 96:14541, 1999

219. Sookhai S, Wang JH, McCourt M, et al: A novel mechanism for attenuating neutrophil-mediated lung injury in vivo. Surg Forum 50:205, 1999

220. Imai Y, Parodo J, Kajikawa O, et al: Injurious mechanical ventilation and end-organ epithelial cell apoptosis and organ dysfunction in an experimental model of acute respiratory distress syndrome. JAMA 289:2104, 2003

221. Carrico CJ, Meakins JL, Marshall JC, et al: Multiple organ failure syndrome. The gastrointestinal tract: the 'motor' of MOF. Arch Surg 121:196, 1986

222. Marshall JC, Nathens AB: The gut in critical illness: evidence from human studies. Shock 6:S10, 1996

223. Deitch EA. The role of intestinal barrier failure and bacterial translocation in the development of systemic infection and multiple organ failure. Arch Surg 125:403, 1990

224. Fink MP: Gastrointestinal mucosal injury in experimental models of shock, trauma, and sepsis. Crit Care Med 19:627, 1991

225. Savage DC: Microbial ecology of the gastrointestinal tract. Annu Rev Med 31:107, 1977

226. Wells CL, Maddaus MA, Simmons RL: Proposed mechanisms for the translocation of intestinal bacteria. Rev Infect Dis 10:958, 1988

227. O'Boyle CJ, MacFie J, Mitchell CJ, et al: Microbiology of bacterial translocation in humans. Gut 42:29, 1998

228. MacFie J, O'Boyle C, Mitchell CJ, et al: Gut origin of sepsis: a prospective study investigating associations between bacterial translocation, gastric microflora, and septic morbidity. Gut 45:223, 1999

229. Deitch EA, Xu D, Franko L, et al: Evidence favoring the role of the gut as a cytokine generating organ in rats subjected to hemorrhagic shock. Shock 1:141, 1994

230. Arita H, Ogle CK, Alexander JW, et al: Induction of hypermetabolism in guinea pigs by endotoxin infused through the portal vein. Arch Surg 123:1420, 1988

231. Marshall JC, Ribeiro MB, Chu PTY, et al: Portal endotoxemia stimulates the release of an immunosuppressive factor from alveolar and splenic macrophages. J Surg Res 55:14, 1993

232. Sullivan BJ, Swallow CJ, Girotti MJ, et al: Bacterial translocation induces procoagulant activity in tissue macrophages: a potential mechanism for end-organ dysfunction. Arch Surg 126:586, 1991

233. Gonzalez RJ, Moore EE, Ciesla DJ, et al: Posthemorrhagic shock mesenteric lymph activates human pulmonary microvascular endothelium for in vitro neutrophil-mediated injury: the role of intercellular adhesion molecule-1. J Trauma 54:219, 2003

234. Moore FA, Moore EE: Evolving concepts in the pathogenesis of postinjury multiple organ failure. Surg Clin North Am 75:257, 1995

235. Fan J, Marshall JC, Jimenez M, et al: Hemorrhagic shock primes for increased expression of cytokine-induced neutrophil chemoattractant in the lung: role in pulmonary inflammation following lipopolysaccharide. J Immunol 161:440, 1998

236. Godin PJ, Buchman TG: Uncoupling of biological oscillators: a complementary hypothesis concerning the pathogenesis of multiple organ dysfunction syndrome. Crit Care Med 24:1107, 1996

237. Seely AJE, Christou NV: Multiple organ dysfunction syndrome: exploring the paradigm of complex non-linear systems. Crit Care Med 28:2193, 2000

238. Ivanov PC, Nunes Amaral LA, Goldberger AL, et al: Multifractality in human heartbeat dynamics. Nature 399:461, 1999

239. Korach M, Sharshar T, Jarrin I, et al: Cardiac variability in critically ill adults: influence of sepsis. Crit Care Med 29:1380, 2001

240. Annane D, Trabold F, Sharshar T, et al: Inappropriate sympathetic activation at onset of septic shock: a spectral analysis approach. Am J Respir Crit Care Med 160:458, 1999

241. Marshall JC: Complexity, chaos, and incomprehensibility: parsing the biology of critical illness. Crit Care Med 28:2646, 2000

242. Hayes MA, Timmins AC, Yau EHS, et al: Elevation of systemic oxygen delivery in the treatment of critically ill patients. N Engl J Med 330:1717, 1994

243. Rivers E, Nguyen B, Havstad S, et al: Early goal-directed therapy in the treatment of severe sepsis and septic shock. N Engl J Med 345:1368, 2001

244. Panacek EA, Marshall JC, Fischkoff S, et al: Neutralization of TNF by a monoclonal antibody improves survival and reduces organ dysfunction in human sepsis: results of the MONARCS trial. Chest 118:88S, 2000

14 CLINICAL AND LABORATORY DIAGNOSIS OF INFECTION

David C. Evans, M.D., F.A.C.S., and Jonathan L. Meakins, M.D., D.Sc., F.A.C.S.

Approach to Diagnosis of Surgical Infection

Surgical infection is a term that, though frequently used, is not clearly defined. In the strictest sense, it implies infection amenable to operative management through surgical source control, as in the case of complicated diverticulitis or necrotizing soft tissue infection. More generally, however, the term can refer to any infection commonly seen in surgical patients (e.g., central line infection or postoperative pneumonia). Both definitions are pertinent, in that the same diagnostic principles apply in each situation.

The presence of surgical infectious disease is usually determined clinically and confirmed microbiologically. Identification of an infection is rarely incidental: most often it is sought in response to a clinical signal. This signal is frequently fever but may be one or more of a number of other symptoms and signs.

Most surgical infections are outpatient conditions that are easily diagnosed and treated. Infections in hospitalized patients, whether related to the primary surgical disease or resulting from surgical therapy, are less easily managed. The greatest challenges in diagnosis and treatment of surgical infections arise in the perioperative and postoperative periods.

Terminology

Traditionally, the terms infection, sepsis, septicemia, bacteremia, endotoxemia, and septic shock have borne similar connotations; this imprecision of terminology has led to considerable confusion about the specific role of microbial infection as a cause of the common clinical presentation of fever, tachycardia, and occasional hypotension. The traditional tendency to conflate these distinct concepts in this simplistic and unrefined manner has had major implications for how antibiotics are used—or, more to the point, misused—in surgical patients.

The human body's physiologic response to systemic infection is well characterized and is often referred to as sepsis. However, infection and sepsis are distinct entities. The normal septic response to infection may, in fact, be completely absent in immunosuppressed patients. Most surgeons, for example, have encountered a patient receiving high doses of steroids who has a perforated intra-abdominal viscus and fecal peritonitis but whose leukocyte count, temperature, and blood pressure are all normal. Conversely, a systemic inflammatory response mimicking sepsis may be present in noninfected patients.[1,2] For example, patients with acute pancreatitis, tissue necrosis, or fractures may manifest physiologic and metabolic changes that are indistinguishable from those associated with bacteremia, even in the absence of infection. Animal studies have confirmed that a sepsislike syndrome can occur without microbial invasion of host tissues.[3]

Accordingly, several clinicians have used the term sepsis syndrome to refer to the group of signs, symptoms, and physiologic changes that result from a variety of sterile inflammatory processes as well as from systemic infection.[2,4] The problem with using the term in this way, however, is that it derives from a Greek word (*sepsis*, "decay") that implies infection with microorganisms. It is therefore not surprising that application of the term sepsis syndrome to noninfectious settings has led to some confusion.[5,6]

To clarify the relevant terminology and provide a common vernacular with which to discuss surgical infection, the American College of Chest Physicians and the Society of Critical Care Medicine held a joint consensus conference in 1991 that led to the publication in 1992 of the currently used terminology and definitions [*see Sidebar* Definitions of Key Concepts].[7] A key outcome was the definition of the nonspecific clinical picture of temperature, heart rate, respiratory rate, and white blood cell (WBC) count abnormalities as the systemic inflammatory response syndrome (SIRS). SIRS may or may not be due to infection; when it is, it is referred to as sepsis. When sepsis results in organ dysfunction, the ensuing state is referred to as severe sepsis; when it results in persistent cardiovascular decompensation, the ensuing state is referred to as septic shock.

Definitions of Key Concepts

- *Systemic inflammatory response syndrome (SIRS):* This response is manifested by the occurrence of two or more of the following conditions as a result of infection: (a) temperature higher than 38° C (100.4° F) or lower than 36° C (96.8° F), (b) heart rate greater than 90 beats/min, (c) respiratory rate greater than 20 breaths/min or arterial carbon dioxide tension less than 32 mm Hg, and (d) white blood cell count greater than 12,000/mm³ or less than 4,000/mm³, or immature (band) forms accounting for more than 10% of the neutrophils present.
- *Sepsis:* SIRS when specifically caused by infection.
- *Severe sepsis:* Sepsis associated with organ dysfunction, hypoperfusion, or hypotension. Hypoperfusion and perfusion abnormalities may include, but are not limited to, lactic acidosis, oliguria, or acute alteration of mental status.
- *Septic shock:* Sepsis with hypotension despite adequate fluid resuscitation, with persistent perfusion abnormalities that may include, but are not limited to, lactic acidosis, oliguria, or acute alteration of mental status. Patients receiving inotropes or vasopressors may not be hypotensive at the time perfusion abnormalities are measured.
- *Multiple organ dysfunction syndrome (MODS):* MODS is the presence of altered organ function in an acutely ill patient such that homeostasis cannot be maintained without intervention.

Approach to Diagnosis of Surgical Infection

Clinical signal of possible infection is noted

Assess patient characteristics and circumstances of presentation:
- Health of host
- Intensity of physiologic response
- Nature of pathogen

Host status is assessed: normal vs. compromised/complex

Response to infection in compromised or complex patients differs from that in normally responsive patients.

Patient is normally responsive

Cardinal signs of inflammation are
- Redness
- Heat
- Pain
- Swelling
- Loss of function

Other signals include
- New or persistent postoperative fever
- Tachypnea/tachycardia
- Confusion
- Ileus

Patient is compromised or complex

Risk factors include
- Advanced age
- Major trauma
- End-organ failure
- Thermal injury
- Chemotherapy
- ≥ 1 chronic disease

Cardinal signs may be present, but more often, infection is occult. Clinical manifestations may include
- Confusion
- Ileus
- Gastric bleeding
- Intermittent hypotension and septic shock
- Water retention
- Delayed wound healing

Laboratory signs of occult infection include
- Renal, hepatic, or respiratory failure
- Thrombocytosis or thrombocytopenia
- Hyperglycemia and insulin resistance
- Immune failure

Patient is evaluated for presence of infection

Begin with history and physical examination.

Perform laboratory assessment:
- Obtain Gram stain and cultures of wound tissue, sputum, urine, and drainage effluent
- Consider percutaneous aspiration and microbiologic examination of potentially infected fluid
- Obtain WBC and blood chemistry measurements
- Obtain chest x-ray; consider imaging of operative site

Therapy is initiated

Treatment is governed by health of host, nature of response to infection (local vs. SIRS; mild sepsis vs. septic shock/MODS), and nature of pathogen (suspected or proven).

Patient has SIRS or uncomplicated sepsis

Withhold antibiotics until definitive diagnosis is made, unless patient is compromised or situation is urgent.
Restore homeostasis (give fluids).
Identify and control source of infection.
Identify pathogen and give suitable antibiotics.

Patient has severe sepsis or is in septic shock

Simultaneously resuscitate, identify infectious focus, give empirical broad-spectrum antibiotics, and undertake source control if able.
Antibiotic choice should reflect (1) likely source of infection, (2) hospital- vs. community-acquired, (3) previous antibiotic therapy.

1261

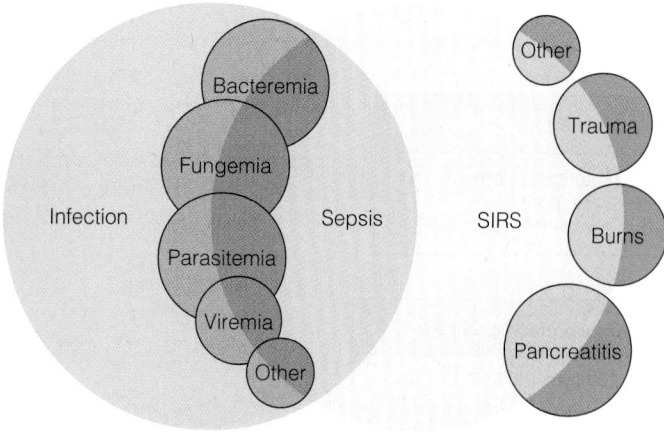

Figure 1 **Depicted are the interrelationships among infection, sepsis, and the systemic inflammatory response syndrome (SIRS).**

Clearly, SIRS includes all the signs, symptoms, and physiologic changes characteristic of the sepsis syndrome; however, use of the term SIRS avoids the idea that such manifestations are necessarily the product of infection. Sepsis may be thought of as a special case of SIRS—SIRS associated with infection [*see Figure 1*]. The term sepsis syndrome, although very useful in guiding clinical thinking, is insufficiently precise for our current needs and probably should no longer be used. The term septicemia should not be used either.

The crucial point is that infection and sepsis are conceptually distinct: infection is a process, and sepsis is the response to that process. The response provides the clinical signals that lead to diagnosis of the initiating process. As a rule, infection, once diagnosed, is easily treated with antibiotics and drainage. It is the management of sepsis that is difficult [*see 6:13 Multiple Organ Dysfunction Syndrome*].

General Approach to Diagnosis of Infection

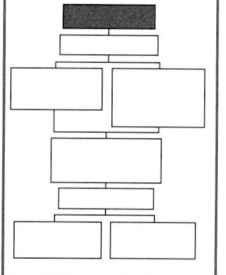

The search for an infection is prompted by a clinical signal indicating a problem in need of resolution [*see Table 1*]. The signal denotes the response of a patient to an infectious stimulus and is a function of the patient's physiologic ability to react to the endogenous and exogenous mediators liberated through the infectious process. A thorough history and physical examination are imperative and should be followed by selected laboratory tests. Normally responsive patients tend to show the classic signals, whereas compromised or complex patients often show more subtle signs that may only be noted as abnormalities on routine bloodwork.

The diagnostic approach to suspected infection must be modified according to patient characteristics and the circumstances of presentation; for example, the specific differential diagnosis for infection appearing on postoperative day 1 will clearly be different from that for infection appearing after 1 week in the ICU. There are three important elements at play when a surgical patient experiences an infection: (1) the health of the host, (2) the intensity of the physiologic response to infection, and (3) the nature of the pathogen. All three factors must be considered carefully in the diagnosis of surgical infection.

Host Status: Normally Responsive versus Compromised or Complex

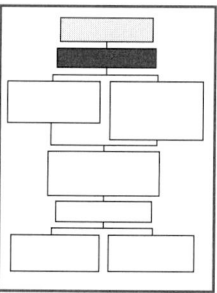

That signs and symptoms of infection in compromised or complex patients differ from those in normally responsive hosts has important diagnostic implications. Normally responsive patients, for whom the physician can obtain a history and perform a physical examination, respond to infection in the classic manner—typically, with fever, tachycardia, leukocytosis, malaise, and other appropriate symptoms. For many reasons—even simply if the infection is severe—normally responsive patients may become compromised. Compromised or complex patients are unable to meet inflammatory or infectious challenges in the normal manner. Hence, the clinical signals of infection in such patients differ from those in normally responsive patients, often being absent or developing at a later stage of infection. Indeed, a multitude of clinical conditions or physiologic states define compromised or complex patients. These include the extremes of age, immunosuppression as a result of either disease (e.g., HIV infection or lymphoma) or medication (e.g., chemotherapy), thermal injury, major trauma, acute end-organ failure in the ICU, and the presence of more than one chronic disease. The prevalence of such patients in modern hospital surgical practice is increasing steadily.

It must be kept in mind, however, that the normally responsive patient and the compromised or complex patient are merely extreme points on the clinical spectrum rather than categorically distinct populations.

Physiologic Response to Infection

NORMALLY RESPONSIVE PATIENTS

Cardinal Signs of Inflammation

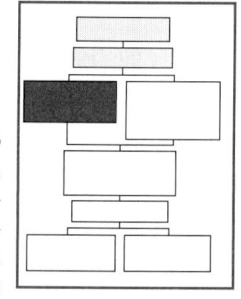

Rubor, calor, dolor, tumor, and functio laesa—that is, redness, heat, pain, swelling, and loss of function—have been considered the cardinal signs of localized inflammation since the times of Hippocrates and Galen. They remain the primary signals leading to medical consultation for outpatient surgical infections and for many of the infectious complications of operation. They are emblematic of the host's effort to contain infection locally, and they may signal the presence of infection even in cases where the primary site of infection is a deeply situated organ or tissue. Infections amenable to surgical intervention may present in this way; however, nosocomial infections complicating the course of surgical patients are generally signaled in more subtle ways.

Fever

Fever is perhaps the most common signal that an infectious process is present. Postoperative fever is a normal part of the recovery process; understanding the typical febrile course is important in differentiating normal from pathologic fever. It is unusual for a sudden, very high fever to be the first signal of an infection. Infection usually begins to manifest itself with a prodrome, recognition of which speeds diagnosis and therapy. Investigation should be started when the patient's temperature reaches 38° C (100.4° F) rather than 40° C (104° F). Although this point may seem obvious, many of the crisis intervention measures required

Table 1 Fundamental Approach to Diagnosis of Infection
Recognize clinical signal and observe its characteristics: 　Nature 　Intensity 　Rapidity of development Make best guess as to source and likely pathogen on the basis of 　History of surgical disease 　Physical examination 　Microbiologic examination of stained specimens 　Radiologic findings Confirm presence of infection by means of 　Laboratory results 　Observation of clinical course 　Invasive procedures (e.g., paracentesis, thoracentesis, 　　interventional radiology, operation)

in managing fevers could be avoided if the significance of more modest temperature elevations were recognized more often.

A fever that appears after the normal postoperative temperature elevation has resolved must not be ignored. To simply wait for such a fever to dissipate is to court disaster. In the absence of a clear diagnosis, a thorough physical examination of the patient, directed by laboratory tests and followed by reexamination as necessary, is required to identify occult infection.

Miscellaneous Signals

It is common wisdom that the signals communicating underlying infection in the compromised or complex host may be subtle. The astute clinician will be in tune with these and, with experience, will recognize when to undertake a diligent search for infection.

Altered heart rate　A heart rate that is either too high or too low may signal an infection. On rare occasions, a change in rhythm in the elderly (e.g., paroxysmal atrial tachycardia, flutter, or atrial fibrillation) indicates an infectious process. Gram-negative sepsis may produce a so-called relative bradycardia, meaning that the resulting tachycardia is not as pronounced as one might expect. An unexplained sustained increase in heart rate should not be ignored.

Tachypnea　Whereas tachypnea occurs commonly after operation in response to pain or poor pulmonary toilet, it may also signal either the prodrome of infection or the onset of SIRS. Because tachypnea may herald not only infection but also other important diagnoses (e.g., pulmonary embolism), it must be thoughtfully and methodically evaluated.

Pain　Pain that persists or is out of proportion to the expected response deserves attention. Whenever a surgical wound that was healing favorably for the first 5 to 7 days becomes more painful, a deep surgical site infection (SSI) must be suspected and ruled out, even if other signs are absent. Unexplained muscular pain is often the first harbinger of deadly necrotizing soft tissue infection caused by gram-positive bacteria (e.g., group A streptococci), the early recognition of which may be lifesaving and limb-preserving [*see 2:2 Soft Tissue Infection*]. Sometimes pain is referred, and the painful area appears normal on examination. Pneu-

monia that presents with abdominal findings is a classic example, as is the shoulder-tip pain with a normal range of motion seen in patients with a subphrenic abscess.

Confusion　Confusion is a common symptom of infection in the elderly; it is also an important signal in patients who had been well and fit. The physician's first response to confusion in an elderly patient in the postoperative period must be to seek a cause, not to order sedation.

Ileus　Ileus has many causes, some of which are not well understood. Prolonged ileus after abdominal operation—as well as almost any ileus after other operations—requires explanation. Infections at remote sites (e.g., SSI and pneumonia) can produce ileus, as if the bowel were a target organ such as the kidney, the liver, or the lung.

COMPROMISED OR COMPLEX PATIENTS

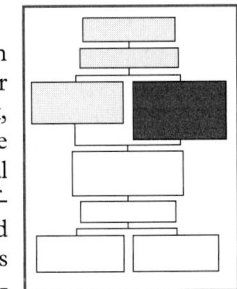

The presence of fever remains a common signal of infection in the compromised or complex patient; however, it may be absent, or the patient's temperature may already be elevated as a result of other causes. Cardinal signs of infection may be present. More often, however, the infection is occult, and classic signals are unrelated to the infectious focus. In some very ill immunocompromised patients, findings that usually signal an infection may already be present. Slight changes in clinical status (e.g., minor temperature elevations, increased fluid requirements, confusion, and ileus) or changes in laboratory findings (e.g., an elevated WBC count, glucosuria, and hyperglycemia) should trigger investigation.

Patients in whom the first signal of an infectious process is organ dysfunction or failure, rather than fever and tachycardia, are likely to be physiologically compromised and seriously ill; perhaps more important, however, is that they are a group whose diagnosis and management require expert clinical skills. Because the classic septic response may not be present, it is essential to be alert to the signs and symptoms of occult infection (see below). In these patients, the laboratory and the radiology suite become increasingly important in diagnosing and documenting the evolution of the infection.

Clinical Signs and Symptoms of Occult Infection

Subtle changes in temperature, mental status, pulse rate, or respiratory rate may signal occult infection, as may the development of pain or ileus.

Intermittent hypotension and septic shock　Septic shock, an important manifestation of an unrecognized focus of infection, is the original expression of multisystem failure. Fortunately, it rarely occurs without warning. The prodrome often includes fever and sometimes other signals. Recurring hypotension is the most characteristic signal; it usually is not catastrophic and responds quickly to fluid resuscitation. Oliguria may accompany the hypotension. If this clinical state is allowed to progress, the hypotension will lead to renal failure (see below), with substantial water retention. Septic shock will result if the infection is not identified and treated with appropriate antibiotics and source control as necessary.

Both clinical assessment and laboratory studies are necessary to confirm the presence of septic shock, although florid septic shock is easily recognized on clinical examination alone [*see 6:3*

Shock]. Any or all of the following findings may be present in varying degrees: tachycardia; tachypnea; hypotension; warm, dry extremities; generalized flushing; and other signs suggesting a hyperdynamic, hypermetabolic state. Swan-Ganz catheter measurements confirm high cardiac output and low peripheral vascular resistance.

Gastric hemorrhage   Gastric hemorrhage may be the presenting symptom of serious infection even if prophylactic measures against such hemorrhage have been taken. It is particularly suggestive of perigastric abscess resulting from anastomotic leakage after upper abdominal surgery. Gastric hyperacidity and bleeding generally respond to drainage of an abscess. Hemorrhagic gastritis must always be considered a signal of occult infection, which demands prompt diagnosis and treatment.

Delayed wound healing   The absence of wound healing can indicate the presence of a significant infection. Typically in such a case, wounds left for delayed primary closure or secondary closure do not exhibit the appropriate granulation tissue and appear pale, dry, and unhealthy. The development of good granulation tissue is a sign that infection is controlled.

Laboratory Signs of Occult Infection

Renal failure   Renal failure [*see 6:7 Renal Failure*] is identified by elevations in serum creatinine and blood urea nitrogen (BUN) levels, which can be highly sensitive signals of developing infection. A still more sensitive indicator is an alteration in creatinine clearance, a laboratory test underutilized in the ICU. Such alterations are generally evident before changes in serum levels. Creatinine clearance should be measured at an early stage in high-risk patients. In the presence of shock, renal failure can develop suddenly. Otherwise, loss of renal function is insidious, but it can usually be identified if sought before oliguria or anuria develops. Resolution of infection is associated with return of function.

Hepatic and respiratory failure   Hepatic failure [*see 6:10 Hepatic Failure*], primarily manifested as jaundice, and respiratory failure [*see 6:5 Pulmonary Insufficiency*], initially presenting as a falling arterial oxygen tension and subsequently marked by a need for mechanical ventilation [*see 6:6 Use of the Mechanical Ventilator*] or by a change in the fraction of inspired oxygen (F_IO_2) requirement, can behave in the same way as renal failure (i.e., with drainage and control of infection leading to restoration of function).

Abnormal platelet count   Thrombocytosis is often seen in association with infection, particularly with compromised hosts, in whom the infection may be occult. Thrombocytopenia may also indicate serious infection, though it is not a common signal. When this occurs in the context of sepsis, it is either because disseminated intravascular coagulation (DIC) has developed or because there is a diminution of all blood lines indicating marrow dysfunction. The cause of any abnormal platelet count should be identified promptly if possible.

Hyperglycemia and insulin resistance   Hyperglycemia and insulin resistance are often reliable signals of the presence of infection in diabetic patients as well as in nondiabetic patients. The degree of insulin resistance can reflect the severity of the infection as well as the effectiveness of infection control.

Immune failure   Severe infection is immunosuppressive.

The most clinically applicable measure of immune failure at present is probably delayed wound healing.

Evaluation for Presence of Infection

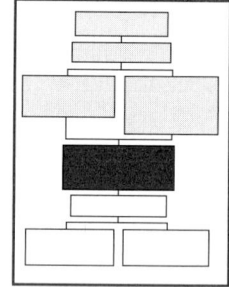

Once the surgeon has evaluated in which ways the patient may be compromised or susceptible to infection and to which degree the physiologic response is inappropriate or harmful (i.e., provokes multiple organ dysfunction or shock), then it is important to consider which microorganisms might be responsible for the presenting clinical picture. This obviously varies with the clinical situation and requires knowledge of specific condition-associated pathogens, as well as the prevalence of certain pathogens in a particular hospital or ICU.

The prevalence of resistant bacterial strains should be monitored in clinical settings in order to guide empirical therapy. Methicillin-resistant *Staphylococcus aureus* (MRSA), once an occasional finding, has become so common in some ICUs and chronic wards that surveillance and isolation programs are no longer employed. It is now the rule for extensive invasive monitoring and access devices to be used in the care of critically ill patients, who thereby become particularly predisposed to gram-positive infection; accordingly, it is important to appreciate the likelihood that MRSA will be encountered. The same is true of *Pseudomonas aeruginosa*, a ubiquitous commensal and a common gram-negative pathogen in hospitals. In compromised patients exposed to multiple antibiotics, *P. aeruginosa* readily acquires antibiotic resistance that usually necessitates the use of double-agent or broad-spectrum coverage for effective management.

Recognizing the virulence of certain pathogens is as important as appreciating their antibiotic susceptibilities. Enteroinvasive *Escherichia coli* 0157-H7, for example, may cause a rapidly progressive hemorrhagic enteritis and provoke a fatal septic syndrome marked by acute renal failure, bleeding, and coma. Necrotizing soft tissue infections, particularly when caused by gram-positive organisms, may be precipitously fatal. Early Gram stain microscopy to identify the specific pathogen is a critical step in the management of this condition.

Essentially the same clinical and laboratory assessments are used to evaluate normally responsive and compromised or complex patients for the presence of infection. There is, however, a significant difference in emphasis. In normally responsive patients, the diagnosis of infection is usually made on clinical grounds with laboratory support, whereas in compromised or complex patients, the diagnosis is usually made on the basis of laboratory findings with clinical support.

The ICU patient presents a particular conundrum. Nosocomial infection is identified in an estimated 20% of such patients.[8] Despite the frequency with which it is suspected and reported, it is difficult to prove unequivocally. The perceived prevalence of nosocomial infection has created a strong predisposition toward instituting empirical antibiotic therapy in ICU patients; however, the global value of this action in terms of both patient outcome and the impact on the ecology of the ICU is unconfirmed and requires validation. The enormous inconsistencies in how infections are diagnosed have a tremendous effect on our ability to assess the efficacy of therapy for infection. The current approach to diagnosing infection in surgical patients, particularly those who are critically ill or compromised, is still in great need of clarification and standardization.[9] Until these issues are resolved, the clinician must be familiar with the strengths and limitations of a variety of current diagnostic methodologies and then exercise thoughtfulness and disciplined diligence. The likelihood that a particular patient is infected (i.e., the pretest probability) is as important in the decision to treat as the fulfillment of any particular constellation of diagnostic criteria.

HISTORY AND PHYSICAL EXAMINATION

The history should include all comorbid conditions (e.g., diabetes, lung disease, cirrhosis, hepatitis, kidney disease necessitating dialysis, and previous important infections) as well as a hospitalization history that covers health status, surgical diagnosis and therapy, additional therapeutic interventions (including interventional radiology, monitoring devices, drains, and drugs), and other related variables.

In the early postoperative period (3 to 6 days after operation), the traditional causes of the signals of infection have their origin in the wound, intravascular lines, the urinary tract, and the lungs. Deep thrombophlebitis, with or without pulmonary embolism, may also initiate a systemic inflammatory response that mimics sepsis. The general physical examination is often unrewarding, but a number of specific examinations should be carefully performed, with emphasis given to (1) all wounds and surgical sites, (2) all invasive monitoring or therapeutic devices and surrounding areas (notably central and peripheral I.V. lines), (3) all drainage systems and surrounding tissue, with particular attention paid to the nature of the drainage and whether it has recently changed in character or volume (particularly if it has stopped), (4) the rectal examination (for pelvic or prostatic infection), (5) areas of potential decubitus ulcers, (6) the neck (for CNS infection), (7) intravascular lines, surrounding tissue, and proximal vessels, (8) the lungs, and (9) the legs. The physical examination is important as a guide for selecting specimens for microbiologic analysis, particularly when there have recently been significant changes in wounds or drainage. The decision to seek radiologic consultation may depend on the findings on physical examination.

DIAGNOSTIC TESTS

Hematologic and Biochemical Tests

After physical assessment, laboratory blood tests are routinely relied on to orient the surgeon toward or away from a clinical diagnosis of infection. Leukocytosis, particularly with an increase in band forms, is a usual but inconsistent marker for infection. The WBC count is widely used to follow the response of infection to therapy and thus has been adopted as a surrogate indicator of the success or failure of therapy. Surprisingly, however, the documentation supporting this ubiquitous practice is sparse.[10,11] Not only is the daily series of complete blood counts often ordered in conjunction with the initiation of antibiotic therapy wasteful and unpleasant for the patient, but it also typically tells the clinician little about the clinical course that cannot be gleaned at the bedside.

In more complex surgical patients, other biochemical cues are used to varying degrees as means of assessing the likelihood of infection. In addition to thrombocytosis, thrombocytopenia, hyperglycemia, and metabolic acidosis, which commonly reflect the stress of severe infection, changes in the erythrocyte sedimentation rate (ESR) and in blood levels of C-reactive protein (CRP), procalcitonin (PCT), interleukin-6 (IL-6), and tumor necrosis factor (TNF) have a significant association with the presence of clinical infection. Plasma CRP concentration, which has been extensively used in some

European countries to monitor the evolution of infection, has been found to be significantly elevated in patients with pulmonary aspiration that has induced bacterial infection, compared with patients with sterile pneumonitis.[12] Some investigators have suggested that because CRP concentration appears to be particularly responsive to bacterial infection, it may be useful as a monitor of the efficacy of antibiotic use, thereby guiding discontinuance of treatment.[13] A host of cytokines, cellular adhesion molecules, oxidants, and other biomolecules known to participate in systemic inflammation from numerous causes are being extensively investigated to establish both diagnostic and therapeutic functions. As yet, however, no single mediator of systemic inflammation has been validated as a reliable clinical tool for surveillance of the progression of infection or the response of infection to treatment.

Case Study: Clinical Picture of Sepsis without Infection

Infection is a process; sepsis is the response.

The difficulty of managing the patient who manifests the septic response in the absence of infection is illustrated by the following case.

A 55-year-old insulin-dependent man with peripheral vascular disease presented with evidence of infection in both feet. Hydration and antibiotic therapy did not prevent progression of the infection, and within 18 hours, it was apparent that amputation would be required for source control. In the course of the operation, gas gangrene, more extensive than had been clinically suspected, was discovered. The initial below-the-knee amputations were eventually followed by a hip disarticulation on one side and a high above-the-knee amputation on the other. Over the 36-hour period during which the infectious process was being controlled, classic septic shock, renal failure, coma, and respiratory failure developed. There was no change in the patient's hyperdynamic and hypermetabolic state after the amputations. During the next 3 weeks, he required ventilator support and daily hemodialysis or hemofiltration; became jaundiced and more deeply comatose; received fluids in amounts significantly in excess of output to maintain blood volume; was hyperglycemic despite receiving regular insulin in dosages of 3 to 5 U/hr; and remained in a hyperdynamic state. Shortly after the last operation, an ileus developed, accompanied by gross fluid retention, which further increased the patient's girth. This state of overt sepsis with hypermetabolism persisted while the wounds healed by primary closure, but no focus of infection could be found.

Antibiotic therapy was stopped for 10 days after operation; the patient's clinical status did not change. Frequent searches were made to ensure that no infection had been overlooked. Suggestions—seriously put forward—to explore the patient's abdomen because "there must be something there" were not heeded. At the end of the third week, for no obvious reason, the patient started to urinate, his ileus resolved, and he was gradually weaned from the ventilator. His level of consciousness improved, the massive edema cleared, and the high cardiac output and low peripheral resistance resolved over a period of 72 hours. He was discharged from the surgical ICU 1 day later and from the hospital in 3 weeks. Some noninfectious process that had maintained this patient's persistent septic response had disappeared or had been turned off, and the result was rapid resolution of the septic state and recovery of health.

As noted, initial control of infection, though difficult, was achieved relatively early. Subsequent therapeutic efforts involved providing hemodynamic, metabolic, and physiologic support of the patient's failing organs and organ systems while waiting for the septic response to resolve. The real problem in this case was not the infection but the patient's unremitting septic response, which was initiated by the infection but maintained in its absence.

Microbiologic Studies

As a rule, Gram stains and cultures of wound tissue, sputum, urine, and drainage effluent are useful studies. In some cases, a battery of cultures of potential sites of infection may be the only feasible approach. Culture techniques are discussed more thoroughly elsewhere [*see 6:15 Blood Cultures and Infection in the Patient with the Septic Response and 6:17 Nosocomial Infection*].

The use of polymerase chain reaction (PCR) technology to detect bacterial DNA is emerging as a useful alternative to microbiologic culture for determining the presence of infection. PCR identifies and amplifies a specific bacterial DNA sequence by means of a chemical proliferation process that may take no longer than a few hours. Unfortunately, the sensitivity and specificity of this powerful technique is highly variable. Although investigations have shown PCR to be a sensitive method of confirming the presence of bacteria in the blood of clinically septic ICU patients,[14] comparison of PCR results with blood culture results is problematic in that nonviable bacteria or bacterial debris are likely to create false positive results, leaving the clinician uncertain as to whether treatment is indicated. The accuracy of PCR thus remains to be established, but the rapidity with which it yields results makes it highly promising as a potential guide to therapeutic intervention.

Radiology

A chest x-ray is mandatory. Ultrasonographic examination of the operative site may be useful to evaluate the possibility of a deep abscess. Computed tomography of the operative site is often more useful than ultrasonography because the presence of wounds, dressings, and drainage tubes may obscure ultrasonographic findings. The possibility of acalculous cholecystitis must be kept in mind, though this is probably an overdiagnosed entity of unvalidated clinical significance [*see 6:18 Intra-abdominal Infection*]. In compromised or complex patients who have not recently undergone an operation, the medical and surgical history combined with the radiologic examination may be the only guide to the potential infectious focus (e.g., ulcer, diverticulitis, cholecystitis or cholangitis, or obstructed ureter). Percutaneous aspiration of potentially infected fluid should be considered, and this fluid should be microbiologically examined if possible.

Institution of Therapy

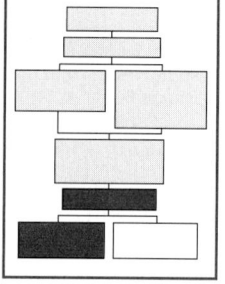

As noted, the response to infection occupies a continuum ranging from virtually no clinical expression in the immunosuppressed patient to full-blown septic shock. Sepsis, in its basic form, represents a mild to moderate response to infection that occurs in normally responsive patients as well as in many compromised or complex patients. On the basis of the results of clinical or laboratory tests, the clinician can evaluate the magnitude of the septic response and thus its clinical gravity.

It is therefore the magnitude of the host response, in combination with the health of the patient and the nature of the likely infecting organism, that directs the clinician's approach to therapy. The greater the degree of sepsis, the greater the clinical urgency of solving the two fundamental problems involved: resolution of the initiating process (i.e., treatment of the infection) and modulation of the response to that process (i.e., management of sepsis) [*see 6:13 Multiple Organ Dysfunction Syndrome*]. The therapeutic approach to a given patient is based on the need for speed.

As mentioned, SIRS was specifically defined in such a way as to emphasize that this common clinical syndrome frequently occurs without infection and does not routinely necessitate treatment, especially with empirical antibiotic therapy. As an illustration, simply climbing a set of stairs is often enough to enable a healthy individual to fulfill the diagnostic criteria for SIRS—albeit briefly.

The point that SIRS is not invariably associated with microbial invasion is especially relevant to critically ill and traumatized ICU patients, in whom it is not uncommon for clinical signs and symptoms indistinguishable from those of severe sepsis to arise or persist in the absence of any infection [*see Sidebar* Case Study: Clinical Picture of Sepsis without Infection]. Burn injury and pancreatitis are classic examples of conditions that can provoke such a response: both can give rise to a hyperdynamic, hypermetabolic clinical picture identical to that of sepsis or severe sepsis, even when no infection is present. Surgeons have learned not to give antibiotics unless there is evidence of infection. The instinctive reflex to do something must be held in check: "masterful inactivity" is the appropriate response until a specific source that can be controlled is identified.

UNCOMPLICATED SEPSIS

The approach to treatment of infection in both normally responsive and compromised patients with mild to moderate sepsis includes five steps: (1) resuscitation and reestablishment of homeostasis and organ function, if necessary; (2) identification of the focus of infection by clinical or radiologic examination; (3) source control, which implies removal, containment or control of the infectious focus (e.g., open drainage of an infected wound; resection of compromised bowel, as for appendicitis or advanced diverticulitis; or percutaneous drainage, as for pancreatic abscess); (4) microbiologic characterization of the offending pathogen by means of culture, Gram stain, or both; and (5) empirical or targeted treatment with antibiotics, depending on the clinical urgency.

In compromised patients, empirical antibiotic therapy is often started before diagnosis, and its efficacy gauged by the patient's subsequent clinical course [*see Discussion, below*]. In normal hosts with uncomplicated sepsis, many would consider it appropriate to withhold empirical therapy until source control has been effected and the pathogen or pathogens characterized. Adequate source control, when possible, is often all that is required for successful management of sepsis, particularly in healthy hosts. In such cases, antibiotic use for prophylaxis against complications such as SSIs is of proven benefit; however, there actually is little evidence to indicate that antibiotics are necessary to treat sepsis if mechanical source control has been definitively achieved.

Antibiotic Treatment

In the absence of convincing culture data, antibiotic treatment must be directed against a likely cause, as determined by recent history (particularly procedures), past history, and physical examination. Examples of likely causes are (1) urinary manipulation, which necessitates coverage against enterococci and gram-negative bacteria with ampicillin and an aminoglycoside; (2) colonic flora, which mandates wide coverage against anaerobes and aerobes; (3) infected vascular lines, which warrant coverage against gram-positive organisms; (4) cholangitis, which calls for coverage against aerobic gram-negative bacteria with ceftriaxone or an aminoglycoside; and (5) pneumonia, which necessitates coverage against gram-positive and gram-negative aerobes.

Drainage

The search for the focus of infection is important because drainage may resolve the entire problem. The clinical state can be changed dramatically by technical or mechanical management of pus behind an obstruction (e.g., in the biliary tree, the urinary tract, or the tracheobronchial tree) or pus under pressure (e.g., an abscess), by manipulation of a drain, or by removal of a foreign body (e.g., an intravascular line). Prompt elimination of all foci of infection that can be drained or are operable is critical. Needle aspiration of peritoneal or pleural fluid may be very helpful. Wounds must be reevaluated constantly and the presence of pressure sores ruled out. Drainage can often be performed either percutaneously (e.g., for pyelonephritis from ureteral obstruction or for subphrenic abscess) or endoscopically (e.g., for cholangitis). Antibiotics alone may suffice to treat small collections not accessible by means of percutaneous techniques.

SEVERE SEPSIS AND SEPTIC SHOCK

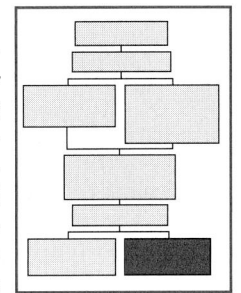

For assessment and management of severe sepsis and septic shock [*see Sidebar Definitions of Key Concepts*], the four steps in treatment—resuscitation, diagnosis of the infectious focus, antibiotic therapy, and drainage—must be performed concurrently. Specifically, I.V. administration of empirical antibiotics must be initiated promptly, before the diagnostic process is completed, and any potentially drainable focus must be identified via physical examination or radiologic imaging. The choice of antibiotic depends on (1) what the likely source of infection is (e.g., a lung, a perforated viscus, or the biliary tract), (2) whether the infection is hospital acquired (in which case antibiotic resistance must be considered), and (3) whether the patient has previously received antibiotic therapy.

Discussion

Approaches to Specific Infections in Complex Surgical Patients

The following infections may occur in all surgical patients. They are, however, much more difficult to identify in complex surgical patients, such as those admitted to the ICU. Because the signals of infection are less specific and extremely difficult to interpret after injury or operation, the approach to diagnosing and treating infection must be cautious and disciplined.

SURGICAL SITE INFECTION

SSIs include all infections occurring within the operative field, from the skin to the actual area of surgery [*see 1:2 Prevention of Postoperative Infection*].[15] The patient history should address previous diseases as well as issues concerning the operation itself, such as wound risk classification, duration, difficulty, urgency, use of drains, other details of the procedure, time elapsed since the operation, and whether the patient was immunosuppressed, experienced trauma, or received chemotherapy. Physical examination should focus on the cardinal signs of infection and the absence or presence of a healing ridge.

Deeper infections tend to become apparent later in the postoperative course, often after a period in which the patient appears to be recovering, and are associated with a variety of signals, some of which can appear suddenly. The physical examination is often useless or misleading because of discomfort associated with the operation. Surgical site pain that increases or fails to resolve in the 7 to 10 days following surgery is an important yet subtle marker for occult infection that calls for investigation. Rectal examination is important because it may detect abscess formation or bleeding. Return of ileus after an abdominal operation is a significant clue to the presence of abdominal infection.

Culture is essential because use of the correct antibiotics is particularly vital in treatment of compromised or complex patients. Knowledge of the organism and its sensitivities is the key to identifying epidemic or multiresistant strains.

URINARY TRACT INFECTION

Nearly all patients admitted to the ICU have a urinary catheter in place; of these, it is estimated that about 20% progress to urinary tract infection (UTI).[8] Bacteria adhere to urinary catheter surfaces, where they promote growth of a so-called biofilm composed of microorganisms, bacterial glycocalices, Tamm-Horsfall protein, and urinary salts. Eradication of this infectious nidus is essentially impossible without catheter removal.[16] The standard criterion for the diagnosis of UTI (10^5 bacteria/ml) is difficult to apply in catheterized patients because antibiotic therapy without removal of the catheter and the source of bacteriuria would be ineffective. Furthermore, it is well established that urine cultures demonstrating as few as 10^1 or 10^2 bacteria/ml increase 1,000-fold within 1 to 2 days[17]; effectively, therefore, any bacterial growth on a urine culture from a catheterized patient signals heavy colonization, if not infection.

More important than quantifying the degree of bacteriuria is determining whether there is any evidence of tissue invasion by urinary bacteria, which would present as pyelonephritis, cystitis, prostatitis, epididymitis, bacteremia, or sepsis. The patient history should determine whether a Foley catheter was used and for how long; how, when, and why it was inserted; instrumentation (e.g., a so-called in-and-out catheter, cystoscopy, or transurethral resection of the prostate); and whether the patient has had any previous UTIs. The physical examination should ascertain whether there is any costovertebral angle tenderness or evidence of prostatic or epididymal tenderness.

Laboratory tests should include gross and microscopic urinalysis, urine culture, and sensitivity tests. Blood culture is important because it may substantiate the diagnosis, identify the bacteria present, and determine the degree of invasiveness of the infectious process.

VASCULAR CATHETER INFECTION

The most frequent sites of infection postoperatively are I.V. catheters, particularly peripheral ones. Diagnosis of peripheral catheter infection is simple and is made on clinical grounds. Diagnosis of central venous catheter (CVC) infection is more difficult. Because hospitalized patients are increasingly being managed with monitoring or therapeutic modalities that depend on vascular access (e.g., total parenteral nutrition and dialysis), line infections have become more common, with an incidence ranging from two to 30 infections per 1,000 CVC days.[18] The combined pressures imposed by (1) the need to maintain vascular access in sicker and more complex patients and (2) the increasing predominance of gram-positive CVC infections observed since the late 1970s have led clinicians in many centers to administer empirical therapy without line removal to complex patients as a matter of course; some even advocate 10 to 21 days of vancomycin-based therapy. The problems associated with the latter approach—emerging vancomycin resistance, nephrotoxicity, and rash—are serious and relate specifically to the diagnostic strategy used to manage potential CVC infections. Distinguishing between contamination, colonization, and true infection is problematic; as a result, a number of diagnostic strategies have been advocated that are predicated more on practicality and cost-effectiveness than on microbiologic reality.

It is believed that CVC infection most commonly arises from invasion by skin microorganisms (*S. aureus* or *S. epidermidis* in about 80% of cases), which may manifest itself as exit-site purulence with or without local cellulitis, as a tunnel infection that may be clinically difficult to detect, or as catheter-related bloodstream infection (CR-BSI). Of these, CR-BSI, which complicates as many as 5% of line placements, is the most clinically important entity. It is strictly diagnosed by identification of the same microorganism (identical species and antibiogram) grown from both the catheter and a peripheral blood culture.

The catheter may be cultured in one of several ways, the most common of which is the roll-plate method [*see 6:17 Nosocomial Infection*]. Because it is theoretically possible that this technique may fail to detect bacteria harbored within the catheter lumen, some authorities advocate the more sensitive sonication method, in which the catheter segment is immersed and agitated in a medium to produce a broth that contains bacteria from both the internal and the external surfaces of the line. This technique is both more costly and more time consuming, in that it requires quantitative cultures that are deemed positive only when more than 10^3 colony-forming units are detected. More often, blood drawn through the CVC or cultured from an exit-site exudate is compared with peripheral cultures, and thus there is no need to remove the line. If quantitative cultures are done, a line blood culture showing five to 10 times more growth than the peripheral sample strongly suggests that the catheter is the source of the bacteremia. A less costly method that renders quantitative cultures unnecessary relies on the speed of bacterial growth: if growth in catheter-drawn blood is faster than that in peripherally drawn blood, a primary line infection is likely. On its own, a line blood culture is not sensitive or specific enough to be diagnostically useful.

PULMONARY INFECTION

Diagnosis and management of nosocomial pneumonia in surgical patients is addressed elsewhere [*see 6:17 Nosocomial Infection*]. The central issue is that there is no universal agreement as to how pneumonia—particularly ventilator-associated pneumonia—should be diagnosed. Of the innumerable diagnostic options, none can rely on demonstration of tissue invasion by microorganisms, as would be ideal: all are to some degree nonspecific, and any may be invoked to justify initiation of antibiotic therapy.[19] Randomized trials linking mode of diagnosis to therapeutic strategy and then to outcome are yet to resolve this issue.[20]

SINUSITIS

All patients undergoing prolonged nasogastric intubation are predisposed to sinus infection. Previous facial trauma and a history of sinusitis are potential contributing factors as well. (Otitis and pharyngitis, which are not often considered, occur in much the same group of patients.) Because maxillary or frontal area tenderness is nonspecific in very ill surgical patients, the diagnosis is usually based on CT demonstration of sinus opacification or air-fluid levels. As a first step, sinus drainage should be reestablished by removal of an unnecessary nasogastric tube. Some authorities advocate sinus aspiration for culture before empirical antibiotic therapy is begun in urgent cases.

PAROTITIS

Parotitis is an increasingly common clinical diagnosis in elderly patients. It is usually caused by *S. aureus* and diagnosed on the basis of the presence of the classic local signs of inflammation. Culture of Stensen's duct and blood culture are useful.

PROSTATITIS

Prostatitis (diagnosed by rectal examination) and epididymitis are clinical expressions of Foley catheter–related infection. The aid of prostatic massage is important in obtaining specimens for culture. It should be remembered that a blocked Foley catheter is the most common cause of hospital anuria. This obstruction can lead to devastating purulent cystitis and upper UTI.

PSEUDOMEMBRANOUS ENTEROCOLITIS

Antibiotic-associated pseudomembranous enterocolitis is diagnosed by obtaining specimens for serology and culture and performing proctosigmoidoscopy. *Clostridium difficile* is frequently identified as the causative pathogen. Although pseudomembranous colitis is rarely clinically impressive and is easy to overlook, it can be rapidly fatal. Initial appropriate antibiotic therapy is not always successful; therefore, reevaluation at the end of the treatment course is required.

Problems with Empirical Treatment of Infection

The frequent presence of SIRS in complex or critically ill surgical patients usually prompts a reflexive response to "pan-culture" the patient if no credible source of infection is apparent. When permissive or loose diagnostic criteria for infection are invoked, the inevitable result is the commencement of empirical antibiotic therapy for suspected infection, which is often, by default, continued for days, if not weeks, pending definitive culture results or clinical improvement. This strategy may seem reasonable and is understandably difficult to resist, but it is potentially deleterious in many ways, and there are many sound objections to its reflexive use.[21]

Empirical antibiotic therapy can obfuscate future cultures, predispose to the emergence of resistant organisms (which are associated with increased attributable mortality), promote derepression of homeostasis-maintaining endogenous flora, cause toxic reactions and secondary effects, alter the ecology of the unit in which it is used (as shown by the rising prevalence of MRSA and vancomycin-resistant enterococci in both European and North American centers), and raise the cost of patient care. This widely used strategy is largely unvalidated.[10,11] It must be emphasized that the paramount principle of therapy for infection is treatment focused on appropriate microbiologic cultures in the context of strict diagnostic criteria for infection.

Many authorities espouse streamlining of empirically begun broad-spectrum antibiotic therapy in response to microbiologic data once culture results are available; however, it is frequently difficult to discontinue antibiotics once they have been started. When strict diagnostic criteria for infection are not met or, more important, when antibiotic therapy based on nonmicrobiologic evidence of infection yields negligible results, strong consideration should be given to stopping the antibiotics, and an exhaustive effort should be made to identify and control any occult persistent cause of the inflammatory state. Of course, this is easier said than done. Moreover, positive cultures do not automatically confirm infection, and great discretion must be exercised in determining how the microbiologic information obtained should be used. For example, tracheal aspirates from intubated patients routinely reveal gram-negative flora, but this finding in no way confirms pneumonia. A single blood culture growing *S. epidermidis* is similarly difficult to interpret.

Despite ubiquitous use in surgical patients, there is not a great deal of evidence in the clinical literature to substantiate the effectiveness of either empirical or streamlined antibiotic therapy. Further efforts must be made to find such evidence because this practice could theoretically exact a substantial cost from both the patient and the environment in which the patient is cared for. In the meantime, clinicians must approach the development of SIRS or other nonspecific signs of infection in their patients by predicating antimicrobial use on carefully formulated diagnostic criteria for the presence of infection; CDC consensus definitions of infection are a good starting point.

Source Control for Management of SIRS

In the past, because the term sepsis was loosely used to describe any general systemic inflammatory state and because such states often arose as a result of infection, it was assumed that antimicrobial therapy was generally appropriate in the management of "septic" patients. Now that sepsis has been redefined exclusively as SIRS in a patient in whom a causative source of infection has been identified, it is clear that the use of antibiotics in "septic" (i.e., SIRS) patients should be more discriminating.

In the same vein, so-called source control was developed as a strategy for managing "septic" patients. Like the term sepsis, the term source control traditionally connotes management of infection rather than, more generally, management of a cause of inflammation. Classically, source control consists of a three-pronged approach employing measures to (1) eradicate a focus of infection, (2) eliminate ongoing microbial contamination, and (3) render the local environment inhospitable to microbial growth and tissue invasion. Diligent source control has long been considered pivotal to successful management of sepsis. Although this traditional approach addresses the infectious causes of local or systemic inflammation very well in a great variety of clinical situations, good judgment must not yield to dogmatism in deciding which processes are required to control infection and inflammation. Challenging convention, a surprising number of investigators have successfully managed many supposedly surgical conditions (e.g., appendicitis[22] and intra-abdominal abscess[23]) without intervention or by using only prolonged antibiotic therapy. Seasoned general surgeons are well aware that if acute cholecystitis is not operated on urgently, it may certainly harm the patient or cause recurring discomfort, but

it may also resolve completely on its own. What actually constitutes adequate source control and how this can be measured are critical questions and remain the subject of debate. These questions become particularly problematic with respect to ICU patients, in whom SIRS is highly nonspecific.

It would seem rational to take our current understanding of SIRS as encompassing both infectious and noninfectious pathology and extrapolate it to the concept of source control. Indeed, as regards more complex surgical patients, it may be appropriate to broaden the definition of source control to include control of all causes of SIRS, not merely infectious ones. For example, debriding devitalized injured tissue, removing a rejected allograft, and resolving postoperative atelectasis are all important for successfully abating a systemic inflammatory state that might easily be mistaken for a manifestation of infection. Deemphasizing infection as the predominant cause of SIRS and withholding antibiotic therapy until stricter, more focused diagnostic criteria for infection are met should make treatment paradigms for managing difficult surgical patients, if not altogether more effective, at least more evaluable.

If one assumes that source control is in fact a therapeutic response to the presence of SIRS, one may then think of it as being either assisted or unassisted. The therapeutic response is initiated by the host, with either complete or partial success. Only in the latter instance should one assist the host's efforts at source control by providing antibiotics or taking surgical measures. This is by no means to suggest that one should not search diligently for a correctable cause of infection or inflammation but rather to suggest that when such an effort yields negligible results, one should consider the possibility that SIRS may be not only appropriate but desirable and may represent the patient's own adequate management of the underlying physiologic insult. Thus, in certain situations, source control may be best regarded as an endogenous or unassisted event. For instance, when fever, tachycardia, and leukocytosis are observed in a surgical patient who is coping well, antibiotics should not necessarily be given automatically. Indeed, such "default therapy" should be actively discouraged. One should also keep in mind that some forms of injury or insult (e.g., some viral infections) not only are very well managed without intervention but may not even prompt clinically evident SIRS.

The notion that no intervention may be required is understandably difficult for many surgeons to embrace at the bedside. Nonetheless, extensive ongoing research elucidating the complex dynamic of circulating proinflammatory and counterinflammatory mediators (e.g., TNF, the interleukins, and a host of other cytokines) suggests that a poorly understood but highly sophisticated biologic apparatus exists for responding to injury and insult. Indeed, it is widely hypothesized (though yet unproved) that this systemic response can be manipulated to restore health in stressed or deteriorating surgical patients. The prospect of untangling the complex biology of systemic inflammation through advances in this field is truly engaging.

References

1. Marshall J, Sweeny D: Microbial infection and the septic response in critical surgical illness. Arch Surg 125:17, 1990

2. Meakins JL, Marshall JC: The gut as the motor of multiple system organ failure. Splanchnic Ischemia and Multiple Organ Failure. Marston A, Ed. Edward Arnold, London, 1989, p 339

3. Goris RJA, Boekhorst TAP, Nuytinck JKS, et al: Multiple organ failure: generalized autodestructive inflammation? Arch Surg 120:1109, 1985

4. Bone RC, Fisher CJ Jr, Clemmer TP, et al: Sepsis syndrome: a valid clinical entity. Crit Care Med 17: 389, 1989

5. Bone RC: Let's agree on terminology: definitions of sepsis. Crit Care Med 19:973, 1991

6. Sibbald WJ, Marshall J, Christou N, et al: "Sepsis"—clarity of existing terminology . . . or more confusion? Crit Care Med 19:996, 1991

7. American College of Chest Physicians/Society of Critical Care Medicine Consensus Conference: Definitions for sepsis and organ failure and guide-

lines for the use of innovative therapies in sepsis. Crit Care Med 20:864, 1992

8. Vincent J, Bihari DJ, Suter PM, et al: The prevalence of nosocomial infection in intensive care units in Europe: results of the European Prevalence of Infection in Intensive Care (EPIC) Study. JAMA 274:639, 1995

9. Casadevall A: Crisis in infectious diseases: time for a new paradigm? Clin Infect Dis 32:790, 1996

10. Lennard ES, Mineshew BH, Dellinger EP, et al: Leukocytosis at termination of antibiotherapy: its importance for intra-abdominal sepsis. Arch Surg 115:918, 1980

11. Stone HH, Bourneuf AA, Stinson LD: Reliability of criteria for predicting recurrent sepsis. Arch Surg 120:17, 1985

12. Adnet F, Borron SW, Vicault E, et al: Value of C-reactive protein in the detection of bacterial contamination at the time of presentation in drug-induced aspiration pneumonia. Chest 112:466, 1997

13. Young B, Gleeson M, Cripps AW: C-reactive protein: a critical review. Pathology 23:118, 1991

14. Cursons RTM, Jeyerajah E, Sleigh JW: The use of polymerase chain reaction to detect septicemia in critically ill patients. Crit Care Med 27:937, 1999

15. The Society for Hospital Epidemiology of America, the Association for Practitioners in Infection Control, the Centers for Disease Control, the Surgical Infection Society: Consensus paper on the surveillance of surgical wound infections. Infect Control Hosp Epidemiol 13:599, 1992

16. Stamm WE, Hooton TM: Management of urinary tract infection in adults. N Engl J Med 329:1328, 1993

17. Stark RP, Maki DG: Bacteriuria in the catheterized patient: what quantitative level of bacteriuria is relevant? N Engl J Med 311:560, 1984

18. Bullard KM, Dunn DL: Diagnosis and treatment of bacteremia and intravascular catheter infections. Am J Surg 172(suppl 6A):13S, 1996

19. American Thoracic Society: Hospital-acquired pneumonia in adults: diagnosis, assessment of severity, initial antimicrobial therapy, and preventive strategies: a consensus statement. Am J Respir Crit Care Med 153:1711, 1995

20. Sterling TR, Ho EJ, Brehm WT, et al: Diagnosis and treatment of ventilator-associated pneumonia-impact on survival. Chest 110:1025, 1996

21. Timsit M, Misset B, Renaud B, et al: Effect of previous antimicrobial therapy on the accuracy of the main procedures used to diagnose nosocomial pneumonia in patients who are using mechanical ventilation. Chest 108:1036, 1997

22. Eriksson S, Granstrom L: Randomized controlled trial of appendectomy versus antibiotic therapy for acute appendicitis. Br J Surg 82:166, 1995

23. Montgomery RS, Wilson SE: Intraabdominal abscess: image-guided diagnosis and therapy. Clin Infect Dis 23:28, 1996

15 BLOOD CULTURES AND INFECTION IN THE PATIENT WITH THE SEPTIC RESPONSE

Donald E. Fry, M.D., F.A.C.S.

Approach to Blood Cultures in Patients with the Septic Response

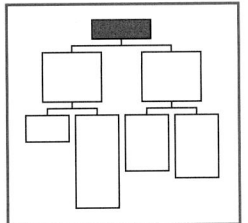

It has been well established that infection and sepsis are distinct events [*see 6:14 Clinical and Laboratory Diagnosis of Infection* and Discussion, *below*]. Infection is local activation of the human inflammatory response secondary to local proliferation and invasion of tissue by microorganisms. When infection reaches a critical threshold of severity, the inflammatory response may be activated at a systemic level. Systemic activation of inflammation is called the systemic inflammatory response syndrome (SIRS); when infection is the putative agent for SIRS, the resulting state is called sepsis.[1]

SIRS secondary to infection occurs when (1) whole microorganisms are disseminated from the primary site of infection, usually via the vascular or lymphatic system (e.g., bacteremia); (2) structural components of the cell wall (e.g., gram-negative endotoxin) or secreted exotoxins are systemically disseminated (as in toxic shock); or (3) normal autocrine and paracrine proinflammatory signals (e.g., tumor necrosis factor [TNF]) from a severe local inflammatory focus reach high systemic concentrations, activating SIRS by virtue of their exaggerated endocrine domain of action.

Although biologic factors other than infection may cause SIRS and provoke a syndrome that is virtually identical to that resulting from invasive infection, infection is the most common cause of SIRS in acutely ill surgical patients. Effective management of infection in these patients requires recognition of the primary site of infection, control of the source of microbial contamination and dissemination (i.e., source control); characterization of the causative microorganism or microorganisms); drainage and debridement of inflammatory exudates and necrotic tissue at the primary site; and antibiotic therapy specific for the pathogen.

Positive Blood Culture with Infection

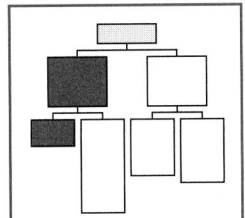

A positive blood culture in a patient with the septic response identifies the putative cause of the infection [*see Table 1*].[2] This identification not only permits institution of appropriate systemic antibiotic therapy [*see Figure 1*] but also facilitates assessment of potential primary sources of the infection because of the established associations between specific anatomic sites and specific microbial isolates. Although it is not always possible to identify

the microorganism or microorganisms responsible for the septic response, organization of the discussion according to the proven or suspected pathogen that may be recovered in a blood culture is a convenient way of addressing treatment options.

GRAM-POSITIVE COCCI

Staphylococci

The identification of gram-positive organisms from a blood culture immediately arouses suspicion that a *Staphylococcus* species is the likely pathogen. Because staphylococci ordinarily colonize the skin and integument, infection from those sources must be considered responsible for the bacteremia.

In surgical patients, a blood culture positive for staphylococci must be assumed to indicate infection arising from an intravascular device until proven otherwise [*see Table 2*].[3] Peripheral I.V. catheters, subclavian lines, Swan-Ganz catheters, systemic arterial lines, and even transvenous pacemaker wires are all documented sources of staphylococcal bacteremia [*see Table 3*]. All lines must be removed and their sites changed. The line and catheter tips should be cultured by semiquantitative methods[4] to document the role of the device in question [*see 6:19 Nosocomial Infection*]. Although this semiquantitative method uses a count of 15 colony-forming units as the threshold for a positive culture of the catheter, devices responsible for bacteremia will usually demonstrate a solid sheet of bacterial growth on the agar [*see Figure 2*].

Septic thrombophlebitis may occur at the site of a previously placed device even though the foreign body has been removed.[5,6] Pus within the vein becomes a source of persistent bacteremia

Table 1 Most Common Nosocomial Bacteremia Pathogens Isolated from All Sites in 12,243 Patients[2]

Pathogen	Prevalence (%)
Coagulase-negative staphylococci	31.9
Staphylococcus aureus	15.7
Enterococcus species	11.1
Candida species	7.6
Escherichia coli	5.7
Klebsiella species	5.4
Enterobacter species	4.5
Pseudomonas aeruginosa	4.4
Serratia species	1.4

Approach to Blood Cultures in Patients with the Septic Response

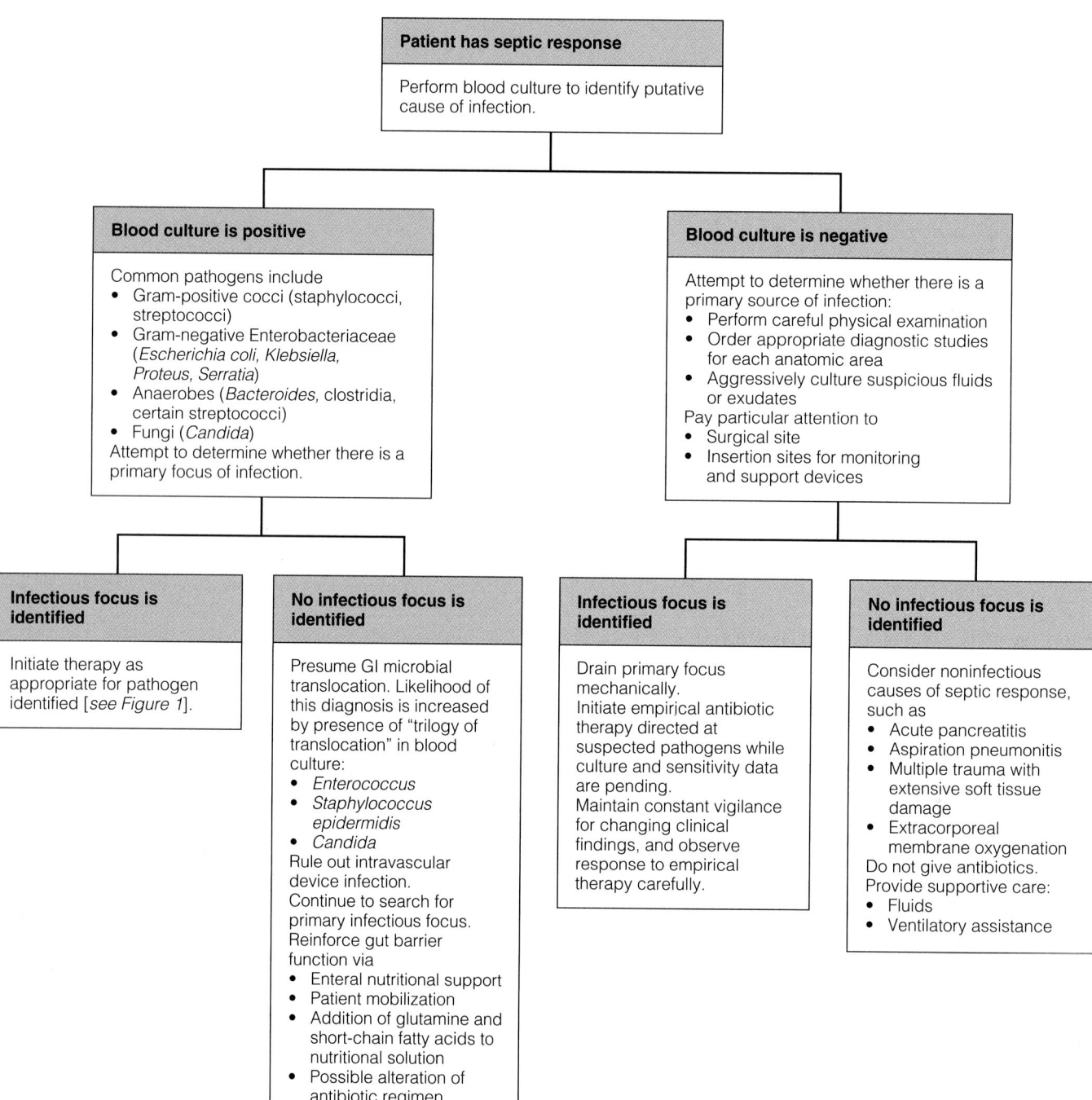

Patient has septic response

Perform blood culture to identify putative cause of infection.

Blood culture is positive

Common pathogens include
- Gram-positive cocci (staphylococci, streptococci)
- Gram-negative Enterobacteriaceae (*Escherichia coli, Klebsiella, Proteus, Serratia*)
- Anaerobes (*Bacteroides*, clostridia, certain streptococci)
- Fungi (*Candida*)

Attempt to determine whether there is a primary focus of infection.

Blood culture is negative

Attempt to determine whether there is a primary source of infection:
- Perform careful physical examination
- Order appropriate diagnostic studies for each anatomic area
- Aggressively culture suspicious fluids or exudates

Pay particular attention to
- Surgical site
- Insertion sites for monitoring and support devices

Infectious focus is identified

Initiate therapy as appropriate for pathogen identified [*see Figure 1*].

No infectious focus is identified

Presume GI microbial translocation. Likelihood of this diagnosis is increased by presence of "trilogy of translocation" in blood culture:
- *Enterococcus*
- *Staphylococcus epidermidis*
- *Candida*

Rule out intravascular device infection.

Continue to search for primary infectious focus.

Reinforce gut barrier function via
- Enteral nutritional support
- Patient mobilization
- Addition of glutamine and short-chain fatty acids to nutritional solution
- Possible alteration of antibiotic regimen

Infectious focus is identified

Drain primary focus mechanically.

Initiate empirical antibiotic therapy directed at suspected pathogens while culture and sensitivity data are pending.

Maintain constant vigilance for changing clinical findings, and observe response to empirical therapy carefully.

No infectious focus is identified

Consider noninfectious causes of septic response, such as
- Acute pancreatitis
- Aspiration pneumonitis
- Multiple trauma with extensive soft tissue damage
- Extracorporeal membrane oxygenation

Do not give antibiotics.

Provide supportive care:
- Fluids
- Ventilatory assistance

Positive blood culture identifies putative source of infection

Staphylococcus aureus

Causes soft tissue infection, commonly with a foreign body (e.g., intravascular device or prosthesis). Infected device will have to be removed; may have to excise infected vein.

Antibiotic selection:

If organism is methicillin sensitive, give either nafcillin, 1 g q. 4 hr; oxacillin, 1 g q. 4 hr; or cefazolin, 1–2 g q. 8 hr. If organism is methicillin resistant, give vancomycin, 0.5–1.0 g q. 6 hr.

Escherichia coli, Klebsiella species

Infection usually arises in peritoneal cavity, biliary tract, or urinary tract. Must ensure adequate drainage and debridement of primary focus of infection.

Antibiotic selection:

Choice of antibiotic is based on sensitivity data. Empirical therapy: gentamicin, 3–5 mg/kg (pharmacokinetically dosed), cefotaxime, 2 g q. 6–8 hr, or ceftizoxime, 2 g q. 8–12 hr.

Bacteroides species, clostridia, anaerobic streptococci

Intra-abdominal sepsis, polymicrobial soft tissue infection, or female genital tract infection is likely. Adequate drainage and debridement of primary site of infection is mandatory.

Antibiotic selection:

Give clindamycin, 900–1,200 mg q. 6–8 hr, or metronidazole, 500 mg q. 6 hr.

S. epidermidis

Infection of intravascular device is presumed until proved otherwise; remove infected foreign body. May need to excise infected vein.

Antibiotic selection:

S. epidermidis shows a high frequency of methicillin resistance; vancomycin, 0.5–1.0 g q. 6 hr, will likely be necessary.

Enterococcus

Infection of intravascular device (remove device), heart valve, or biliary tract is likely. May occur with *Candida* species as primary bacteremia without anatomic site of infection.

Antibiotic selection:

Give piperacillin, mezlocillin, or ticarcillin at 12–16 g/day; consider ampicillin-sulbactam.

Pseudomonas species, Serratia species

Pulmonary sepsis (usually with pulmonary failure), urinary tract sepsis, or infection of intravascular device is likely. Treatment requires aggressive pulmonary toilet, ensurance of unobstructed urinary tract, and removal of potentially infected devices.

Antibiotic selection:

Give gentamicin, 3–5 mg/kg/day, or amikacin, 15 mg/kg/day (depending on sensitivity; pharmacokinetically dosed). The addition of expanded-spectrum penicillin (ticarcillin, mezlocillin, or piperacillin, 12–16 g/day) may be desirable in severe infections.

Candida species

Primary source of infection is infected central catheters or gastrointestinal translocation. Remove catheters at risk.

Antifungal selection:

Give amphotericin B, 0.5 mg/kg/day (after test dose documents patient tolerance), or fluconazole, 200–800 mg/day.

Figure 1 **Identification of the putative cause of infection permits institution of appropriate antibiotic therapy.**

until appropriate therapy is employed. Persistent evidence of gram-positive bacteremia after removal of all intravascular lines gives rise to a high index of suspicion for suppurative thrombophlebitis. Previous I.V. sites must be examined for evidence of pus; suspicious sites may even have to be explored with the patient under local anesthesia. When identified, the entire length of septic vein must be surgically excised. Although many different species of bacteria may be responsible for suppurative thrombophlebitis, *S. aureus* is decidedly the most common.

The implantable synthetic prosthetic materials that are now such a major part of vascular, cardiac, and orthopedic surgery may become sources of bacteremia secondary to infections resulting from intraoperative contamination. When gram-positive organisms are identified in the blood of a patient at risk, the synthetic implant should be considered the source of blood-borne infection. As the use of synthetic devices has increased, the

delayed nature of some infections, particularly those involving *S. epidermidis*, has become more readily apparent. These indolent infections are consequences of intraoperative contamination but may not be clinically evident for months to years after implantation. Because selected species of *S. epidermidis* produce biofilm,[7] even culturing the microorganism from the infected prosthesis that has been removed can be very difficult, and recovery of the microorganism from a blood culture is quite uncommon in the period before the infection becomes clinically apparent.[8]

Diagnosis of arterial graft, heart valve, and total-joint arthroplasty infections can be very difficult. Once infection has been established, however, prompt removal of the prosthesis is mandatory. Removal of an actively infected prosthesis is invariably associated with major morbidity because the infection limits the reconstructive options available. Antibiotic therapy alone will not eradicate the infection, and it may lead to a delay in the decision to

Table 2 Pathogens in 159 Cases of Intravascular Device–Associated Bacteremia[3]

Organism	No. of Isolates
Staphylococcus aureus	78
S. epidermidis	33
Serratia marcescens	18
Klebsiella/Enterobacter species	16
Candida species	11
Enterococcus species	8
Proteus species	6
Others	6
Total	176*

*The total exceeds 159 because of polymicrobial isolates in several patients.

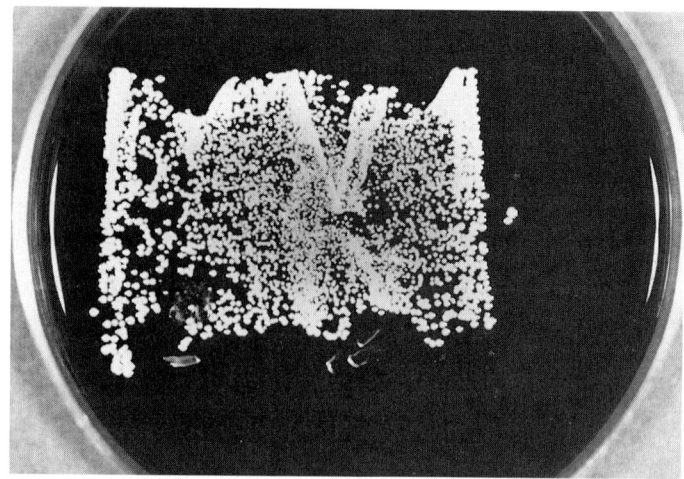

Figure 2 **Illustrated is a blood agar plate 24 hours after an infected catheter has been cultured by semiquantitative technique. Although colony counts higher than 15 are associated with a positive culture, the prolific growth shown here is commonly seen.**

remove the prosthesis; this can result in arterial graft failure (e.g., thrombosis or pseudoaneurysm), cardiac valvular insufficiency, or extensive arthroplasty infection (e.g., extrusion or osteomyelitis).

Because *S. epidermidis* normally colonizes skin, it is also a potential contaminant in the blood culture process. Accordingly, close attention to proper culturing technique is crucial for minimizing this potential diagnostic artifact. A frequent cause of false positive cultures of *S. epidermidis* is use of the arterial line or the central venous catheter for drawing blood samples instead of a separate and carefully prepared venopuncture site. When more than one culture shows *S. epidermidis* or when cultures taken at separate times show the same organism, however, the clinician must assume that the organism is participating in clinical infection.

Staphylococcal bacteremia is a preventable complication of indwelling devices and implants. Aseptic placement of intravascular devices cannot be compromised. Peripheral I.V. catheters should be changed routinely every 48 to 72 hours. Arterial lines that have been in place for more than 72 hours are at considerable risk for being foci for bacteremia. Catheters devoted to parenteral nutrition must receive ongoing care to prevent septic morbidity [*see 6:23 Nutritional Support*].

The primary therapy for device-related infection is removal of the infected device. Systemic antibiotics cannot overcome the adjuvant effects of the foreign body in supporting bacterial growth. Antimicrobial therapy thus becomes adjunctive to removal of the primary nidus of infection.

To prevent infection from prosthetic implants, efforts must be made to minimize development of a microenvironment in the wound that favors bacterial proliferation. Meticulous technique, appropriate hemostasis, conservative use of the electrocautery, judicious use of suture ligatures, and antibiotics given immediately before operation will reduce infectious morbidity. Cefazolin, 1 g preoperatively, administered either I.V. (by prefer-

Table 3 Sites of Intravascular Device–Associated Bacteremia in 159 Patients[3]

Site	No. of Patients
Peripheral I.V. catheter	72
Central venous catheter	49
Arterial line	18
Subclavian dialysis catheter	12
Swan-Ganz catheter	4
Broviac catheter	3
Transvenous pacemaker wire	1

ence) or intramuscularly, is the agent of choice [*see 1:2 Prevention of Postoperative Infection*]. With lengthy operations, repeat doses should be given at 4-hour intervals. Prolonged postoperative administration is of no value.

Methicillin-resistant staphylococci are becoming increasingly prevalent; in some series, they account for more than 50% of clinical isolates. Consequently, presumptive antimicrobial therapy for bacteremia arising from an intravascular or implantable device requires vancomycin, 1 g every 8 to 12 hours. If the patient is intolerant of or unresponsive to vancomycin, then either linezolid, 600 mg every 12 hours,[9] or quinupristin-dalfopristin, 7.5 mg/kg every 8 to 12 hours,[10] may be given instead. The antimicrobial choice may be modified when culture and sensitivity data subsequently become available. If methicillin-resistant species are not a concern, nafcillin, 1 g every 4 hours, is appropriate. Because of the risks of metastatic infectious complications from staphylococcal bacteremia, systemic antibiotics should be continued for a minimum of 7 days.

The toxic-shock syndrome, caused by *S. aureus*, gives the clinical impression of being a bacteremic illness.[11] However, positive blood cultures are uncommon with this syndrome because the SIRS is created by the exotoxin produced by the microorganism, not by bacteremia per se. Initially associated with vaginal tampons, the toxic-shock syndrome can be seen wherever body cavities or open wounds are filled with gauze or other packing. Diagnosis of this syndrome requires a high index of suspicion in the septic, hypotensive patient with body packing. Treatment requires removal of the packing, aggressive systemic supportive care of shock and associated organ failure, and systemic administration of suitable antibiotics.

Streptococci

Streptococcal bacteremia occurs less frequently than staphylococcal blood-borne infection, though some areas of the United States have experienced an apparent increase in these infections. Invasive group A streptococcal infections with bacteremia are seen in patients with necrotizing soft tissue infections, invasive pharyngeal infections, bone and joint infections, and severe and rapidly advancing pneumonia. About 20% of bacteremias with group A streptococci are without a primary source of infection[12] and probably arise from the oropharynx.

Necrotizing soft tissue infection is the most common setting for a positive blood culture with group A streptococci. These fulminant infections are seen after seemingly trivial cutaneous injuries but may also complicate chickenpox in children[13] and may even be seen as complications of elective surgical wounds. The necrotizing infection is characterized by pain, tenderness, and induration around a wound that is out of proportion to the size or mechanism of the injury. The infection dissects along the fascial plane and can evolve from injury to a fatal illness in 24 hours. The diagnosis requires a high index of suspicion in a toxic patient with rapidly advancing cellulitis. The induration of the advancing infection may be palpable in thin patients and serves to distinguish this condition from clostridial gas gangrene. Necrotizing soft tissue infections are associated with a toxic-shock–like syndrome, but unlike patients with true toxic shock, these patients usually have blood cultures that are positive for group A streptococci.[11] Unfortunately, the positive blood culture result is not available until the patient's fate has already been dictated by earlier clinical decisions.

Therapy requires aggressive local debridement of necrotic tissue, systemic antibiotic therapy, and systemic supportive therapy for the shock and organ failure characteristic of severe infections. The recommended antibiotic regimen includes both penicillin, 12 to 24 million U/day, and clindamycin, 900 to 1,200 mg every 6 hours in adult patients. The addition of clindamycin is believed to reduce toxin production by inhibiting protein synthesis in the rapidly multiplying bacteria. Another reason why clindamycin is useful is that large inocula of group A streptococci are believed not to express penicillin-binding proteins.[14]

α-Hemolytic streptococcal bacteremia is well known in patients with endocarditis and is generally associated with this condition when blood cultures are positive for these organisms. Echocardiographic confirmation of the diagnosis sets the stage for treatment with penicillin. Therapy is continued until there is conclusive evidence that the infection has been eradicated.

Other groups of streptococci may be noted in positive blood cultures, usually reflecting infections secondary to GI contamination. Group B streptococci, long identified as bacteremic pathogens in neonates, are now being seen with greater frequency in adults. In adult bacteremia, group D streptococci are identified in circumstances similar to those associated with group B pathogens. Gut-derived streptococcal pathogens are usually quite sensitive to penicillins.

Enterococci

Although there is disagreement regarding the true virulence and pathogenicity of *Enterococcus* when it is isolated as part of the polymicrobial microflora of a clinical exudate,[15,16] no one would deny the need for antimicrobial chemotherapy when it is isolated in blood cultures. Mortalities exceeding 40% clearly underscore the severity of enterococcal bacteremia, though it is likely that impaired host status contributes significantly to the poor outcome.

The primary foci of infection in enterococcal bacteremia include intravascular devices and the biliary and GI tracts. Enterococcal bacteremia ordinarily occurs in elderly or chronically ill patients receiving broad-spectrum antibiotics. Cephalosporins in particular have been implicated as favoring enterococcal overgrowth.[17] *Enterococcus* is usually associated with other bacterial species at the primary site of intra-abdominal or soft tissue infection, and a synergistic relation with other organisms may be part of its pathogenic expression.[18,19]

Therapy for enterococcal bacteremia requires definition of the primary infectious focus. When *Enterococcus* is a solitary isolate in

blood, I.V. devices should be changed and semiquantitatively cultured. Potential biliary sources must be evaluated, with all available clinical data, including those from ultrasound examination of the gallbladder [*see 6:18 Intra-abdominal Infection*], taken into account. Gangrenous acalculous cholecystitis must be kept in mind because of the type of patient likely to have enterococcal bacteremia.[20] Intra-abdominal abscesses and serious soft tissue infections are customarily associated with polymicrobial isolates, which may include *Enterococcus*. The urinary tract, however, appears to be an infrequent cause of enterococcal bacteremia in the absence of anatomic obstruction of urine flow.

Once the primary focus has been identified, removal of the foreign body, drainage and debridement of infected material, and specific antibiotic therapy are indicated. Piperacillin-tazobactam, 3.375 g every 6 hours, is recommended. Although ampicillin appears to have nearly uniform activity against *Enterococcus* in vitro, the production of β-lactamase by synergistic pathogens in the polymicrobial milieu raises serious questions about the effectiveness of this choice. Addition of sulbactam to ampicillin improves enterococcal coverage in mixed infections.

In about 40% of patients with blood cultures positive for *Enterococcus,* no primary site of infection can be identified.[21] This observation has led to considerable speculation as to whether this organism is a marker of microbial translocation from the gut [*see* Positive Blood Culture without Infection, *below*] or whether the infection derives from a clinically obscure primary focus (e.g., a catheter).

The emergence of vancomycin-resistant enterococci is a matter of great concern,[22] and considerable effort has been expended on finding newer agents that are effective against these organisms.[23] Both linezolid, 600 mg every 12 hours,[24] and quinupristin-dalfopristin, 7.5 mg/kg every 8 to 12 hours,[25] have been successfully used in small treatment groups. The addition of rifampin may enhance the therapeutic effect.[26] Vancomycin resistance is mediated by two separate genes, and there is substantial concern in the academic community regarding the possible transfer of these genes into staphylococci or other gram-positive organisms.

GRAM-NEGATIVE ENTEROBACTERIACEAE

The gram-negative Enterobacteriaceae represent a group of facultative bacteria that are associated with infections of the abdominal cavity, the biliary tract, and the genitourinary tract. Infections tend to be monomicrobial when the urinary and biliary tracts are involved[27,28] but are nearly always polymicrobial with peritonitis and intra-abdominal abscess.[29] The common gram-negative Enterobacteriaceae include *Escherichia coli*, *Klebsiella* species, *Enterobacter* species, and *Proteus* species. Because intra-abdominal infection is a polymicrobial process, bacteremia with one of these organisms in patients with such infection represents only the tip of the iceberg, with a polymicrobial flora presumed to be present at the focus [*see 6:18 Intra-abdominal Infection*].

In the surgical patient, eradication of gram-negative bacteremia requires identification of the primary focus. The intra-abdominal compartment must be the primary consideration. Ultrasound examination of the biliary tract may be useful. Abdominal computed tomography is approximately 90% accurate in defining abscess. Urinary cultures may be useful but must be cautiously interpreted because a well-drained urinary tract is an improbable focus for bacteremia. *P. vulgaris* is a urease-producing organism, and its presence in patients with ileal conduits or staghorn calculi strongly favors a urinary tract source. Gram-

Table 4 Expanded-Spectrum β-Lactam Antibiotics Effective against Enterobacteriaceae

Drug	Half-life (hr)	Dose Interval (hr)	Total 24-Hr Dose (g)
Cephalosporins			
Cefoxitin	0.7–1.0	4–6	12–18
Cefotetan	3.5	12	2–4
Cefotaxime	1.0	6	8–12
Ceftizoxime	1.5	8	6
Ceftazidime	2.0	8	6
Ceftriaxone	6.5–8.0	12–24	2–4
Penicillins			
Ampicillin-sulbactam	1.0	6	12
Ticarcillin-clavulanate	1.0	4	18.6
Piperacillin-tazobactam	1.0	6	13.5
Monobactams			
Aztreonam	2.0	8	6
Carbapenems			
Imipenem-cilastatin	1.0	6	2–4
Meropenem	1.0	6	2–4
Ertapenem	4.0	24	1

negative bacteremia from hospital-acquired pneumonitis is always a possibility but is less common with the Enterobacteriaceae than with *Pseudomonas* or *Serratia* species. In general, bacteremia from nosocomial pneumonia is relatively uncommon in surgical patients. *Klebsiella* and *Enterobacter* species are known pathogens for bacteremia from intravascular devices; appropriate cultures of the primary device are necessary to establish this potential source.

Mechanical treatment is necessary at the primary focus of infection.[30] Defects in the GI tract must be managed, pus drained, necrotic tissue debrided, urinary obstruction relieved, and infected catheters removed. Empirical exploration of the abdomen may be necessary in bacteremic patients with a high index of suspicion for an intra-abdominal source, though at present, it is infrequently required, thanks to ongoing improvements in the technology used to visualize the abdominal compartment (i.e., CT).

Considerable latitude surrounds appropriate antibiotic therapy for gram-negative bacteremia, particularly when the bacteremia is secondary to intra-abdominal infection. When the infectious process is community-acquired, an expanded-spectrum β-lactam antibiotic is appropriate [*see Table 4*]. Although anaerobic coverage is a necessary prerequisite in intra-abdominal infection, the expanded-spectrum β-lactam agents appear to yield results equivalent to those of drug combinations that might appear to have superior anaerobic activity. Furthermore, single-agent treatment with expanded-spectrum β-lactam antibiotics is less expensive than multiple-drug therapy and eliminates the toxicity and pharmacokinetic dosage complexities of the aminoglycoside alternatives.[31] Ertapenem, a newer carbapenem that can be given once daily, may become a desirable choice in the initial management of peritoneal infection.[32]

For patients with bacteremia from infections that are hospital-acquired or represent failures of previous antimicrobial therapy, specific treatment addressed to these more resistant isolates is required. Single antibiotics that may be chosen to cover hospital-acquired gram-negative bacteria include aminoglycosides, expanded-spectrum penicillins, ceftazidime, aztreonam, quinolones, and carbapenems. Even though the isolate may be sensitive

to lesser drugs, a combination of an expanded-spectrum penicillin with an aminoglycoside is commonly chosen [*see Table 5*] because of the synergism between these two types of agents. Culture and sensitivity data from the primary source of infection are particularly important for guiding modification of drug therapy. Because a complex patient in the surgical ICU typically has an expanded volume of distribution and an altered pattern of antibiotic excretion,[31] it is essential that aminoglycoside therapy be pharmacokinetically dosed. Considerable interest has been expressed regarding once-daily dosing of aminoglycosides for gram-negative hospital-acquired infections[33]; at present, however, there is only testimonial evidence to support this approach for intra-abdominal infection.

Nosocomial gram-negative bacteremia is a significant complication in surgical patients [*see 6:17 Nosocomial Infection*]. The principal sites are usually the respiratory and urinary tracts and intravascular devices; the surgical site is a common locus for nosocomial infection but is only infrequently responsible for the septic response or bacteremia.

ANAEROBES

The anaerobes of particular significance to surgeons as bacteremic pathogens are principally colonists of the human GI tract and the female genital tract. Oral and cutaneous anaerobes (e.g., diphtheroids) are rarely identified as bacteremic pathogens, though diphtheroids are common skin contaminants of the blood-culturing process. *Bacteroides* species, anaerobic streptococci, and *Clostridium* species are the anaerobic pathogens more commonly identified in blood.

Among all anaerobes, *Bacteroides* species, particularly *B. fragilis*, are the preeminent pathogens. They are customarily identified in infections involving distal ileal or colonic contamination. Intra-abdominal infection must be considered the primary focus of *B. fragilis* bacteremia.[34] Soft tissue infections may also be the source of *Bacteroides* bacteremia, particularly in the presence of a polymicrobial infection or necrotic tissue and especially in soft tissue infections of the perineum. In one series of patients with *B. fragilis* bacteremia, 80% required operative drainage and debridement as primary treatment.[34]

Selection of antimicrobial therapy for *B. fragilis* must be based on an understanding of the pathogenesis of anaerobic infections. Anaerobic infection in the abdomen and soft tissues is synergistic in that both anaerobic and aerobic organisms benefit from the polymicrobial environment. The aerobes reduce the oxidation-reduction potential of the environment, thereby optimizing condi-

Table 5 Expanded-Spectrum Penicillins and Aminoglycosides Used in Combination Regimens in Treatment of Nosocomial Gram-Negative Bacteremia

Drug		Half-life (hr)	Total 24-Hr Dose
Penicillins	Ticarcillin	1.0	16–18 g
	Mezlocillin	1.0	16–18 g
	Piperacillin	1.0	12–18 g
Aminoglycosides*	Gentamicin	2.0	3–5 mg/kg
	Tobramycin	2.0	3–5 mg/kg
	Amikacin	2.0	15–20 mg/kg

*Dosing interval and total dose per day are variable: pharmacokinetic dosing is required to prevent toxicity or underdosing.

tions for anaerobic proliferation. The anaerobes may then elaborate factors that accelerate the aerobes' growth cycle, or they may shed a portion of their capsular polysaccharide into the environment, thereby retarding phagocytosis of all components of the infection.[35] The complexity of this synergistic relation may be further compounded by interactions between *Enterococcus* and either the gram-negative rod[18] or the anaerobic organism.[19]

Antimicrobial therapy must address both halves of the synergistic pair, with coverage of the aerobic Enterobacteriaceae being a vitally important component of treatment for the anaerobe. The expanded-spectrum β-lactam antibiotics appear to provide adequate polymicrobial coverage. Clindamycin, 900 to 1,200 mg every 6 to 8 hours, or metronidazole, 500 mg every 6 hours, in combination with an aminoglycoside has been the traditional treatment but, as noted, poses special problems. *B. fragilis* bacteremia arising from unusual sites (e.g., endocarditis) or bacteremia in the face of β-lactam antibiotic therapy both call for specific clindamycin or metronidazole therapy. It is of the utmost importance that treatment of anaerobic bacteremia include complete drainage and debridement of the primary focus.

Peptostreptococci and, to a lesser degree, peptococci are anaerobic streptococcal species that may cause bacteremia from infection after GI contamination. More commonly, their presence should arouse suspicion that bacteremia may be arising from the female genital tract. Either of these anaerobes may participate in puerperal sepsis and pelvic inflammatory disease, with common gram-negative Enterobacteriaceae, enterococci, or both acting as synergistic partners in the infection. *Bacteroides* species may also participate in such infections.

Bacteremia with anaerobic streptococci secondary to infection in the female genital tract mandates a search for a drainable primary focus. For puerperal sepsis, dilatation and curettage may be required to eliminate retained products of conception. Pfannenstiel flaps may become sources of surgical site infection (SSI) that may cause bacteremia and thus must be drained and debrided. Pelvic inflammatory disease may be complicated by tubo-ovarian abscess or extrauterine abscess within the pelvis that will have to be drained.

Appropriate antibiotic therapy for anaerobic streptococcal bacteremia remains unclear. Most anaerobic species likely to cause infection in the female genital tract are sensitive to penicillin, with *Bacteroides* species being a notable exception. Therapy with an anaerobe-specific agent (e.g., clindamycin or metronidazole) in combination with an aminoglycoside, however, appears to offer better clinical results in puerperal infection. The role of the expanded-spectrum β-lactam agents remains poorly defined. Because *Enterococcus* is commonly identified in infections involving the female genital tract, ampicillin is frequently added to the antibiotic regimen, but this measure is of unproven value.

Clostridium species are gram-positive anaerobic rods that are relatively uncommon in blood cultures and are ordinarily associated with clostridial myonecrosis or cellulitis. Usually, the fulminant nature of the infection is readily identifiable at the primary soft tissue focus, and blood culture is of little assistance in diagnosis. Therapy consists of radical debridement of the primary site of infection and aggressive administration of penicillin [see *2:2 Soft Tissue Infection*].

Nonhistotoxic clostridial bacteremia has been identified with increased frequency. In a series of 47 patients with such bacteremia, only 25% had a focus of infection[36]; the remaining 75% had no clinically identifiable source. The patients in this latter group either were severely, chronically ill or were alcoholics; thus, the presence of a colonic anaerobe in blood may be evidence for primary bacteremia from the GI tract without a primary focus of infection, and nonhistotoxic clostridial bacteremia may be an expression of failed GI barrier function rather than infection in the classic sense.

FUNGI

Candida species are the most common fungal organisms cultured from the blood in surgical patients. Candidemia is typically seen in a severely ill patient who has had or continues to have bacterial infection and is being treated with a prolonged course (more than 7 days) of broad-spectrum antibiotics.[37,38] Parenteral nutrition and corticosteroid therapy are associated with candidemia. The bacterial microflora becomes suppressed, and colonization of the alimentary tract by *Candida* organisms becomes the reservoir for dissemination.

Candidemia appears to occur principally via two mechanisms. In the first, indwelling catheters (particularly central lines) become colonized. Catheter removal and appropriate culture will document the process and likewise be effective treatment. In the second, GI overgrowth with *Candida* leads to impairment of host barrier function and resultant fungemia.[38] Although peritonitis and intra-abdominal abscess with *Candida* organisms have been identified,[39] translocation of the organisms across the gut barrier is the probable source of contamination.

Prevention of candidemia requires aseptic care of catheters and prompt catheter removal when fungemia is suspected or documented. A reduction in the spectrum and duration of systemic antibiotic therapy is probably the most important method of reducing fungal overgrowth and subsequent risk of dissemination. Oral nystatin, ketoconazole, and fluconazole have been recommended for prophylaxis in patients at risk for candidemia but remain unproven.

Diagnosis and treatment of candidemia are discussed in detail elsewhere [see *6:19 Fungal Infection*].

Positive Blood Culture without Infection

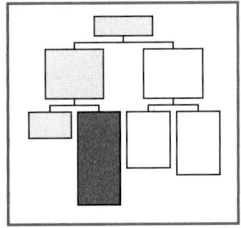

In the late 1950s, Jacob Fine proposed the theory that acute physiologic perturbations (e.g., hemorrhagic shock) could disrupt GI barrier function to the point where bacteria and their cellular products could escape from the gut reservoir[40-42] and contribute to clinical illness. In other words, the septic response could be triggered by bacteria or their products (e.g., endotoxin) in the absence of infection, as it is traditionally understood. Although this theory was discredited in the 1960s in germ-free rat experiments,[43,44] it enjoyed a considerable resurgence in the late 1980s, as both experimental[45-49] and clinical[50,51] studies demonstrated that GI microbial translocation appears to be a valid biologic event. Consequently, it has been proposed (although not universally accepted[52]) that some surgical patients may have the septic response secondary to microorganisms while lacking a primary infectious focus.

MECHANISMS OF GUT BARRIER FUNCTION

For microbial translocation to be clinically relevant, gut barrier function must be impaired. At its most distal site, the lumen of the human GI tract may contain as many as 10^{10} bacteria/g colon contents. The biologic partition that prevents microbes from escaping from this reservoir is complex and consists of anatomic, physiologic, and immunologic mechanisms.

The physical barrier of the gut consists of a contiguous layer of enterocytes and colonocytes. An intercellular matrix exists between the cells. Both types of cell appear to obtain a large part of the nutrients they need directly from the gut lumen. Enterocytes have a specific nutrient requirement for glutamine,[53] and colonocytes require short-chain fatty acids.[54] Deficiencies of these critical nutrients lead to atrophy of the gut lining, which results in a defective physical barrier.

The surface of the gut mucosal cells is covered with the glycoprotein mucin,[55] which is an important component of the gut barrier. The mucin layer has a nonspecific retarding effect on bacterial adherence to mucosal cells; in addition, it has a nonspecific inhibitory effect on bacterial proliferation at the mucosal cell surface, thereby helping prevent invasion by luminal bacteria.

Secretory IgA also prevents the binding of bacteria to mucosal cells.[56] Presumably produced as nonspecific antibody from submucosal gut lymphocytes, IgA does not fix complement and does not have cytotoxic effects on bacteria. Rather, it is thought to bind to bacteria and impede their binding to the mucosal cell lining. The IgA concentration is highest at the mucosal cell surface.

The normal microflora that colonizes the GI lumen appears to make a significant contribution to normal gut barrier function. Anaerobic bacteria play a positive role by virtue of their species-specific adherence to mucosal cell-binding sites and their ability to prevent more noxious aerobic species from adhering to mucosal cells via competitive inhibition.[57] This positive role creates a real dilemma for clinicians attempting to formulate antimicrobial regimens for critically ill patients.

Normal GI motility is perhaps the most important of the physiologic components of the gut barrier. Movement of luminal contents distally within the gut keeps intraluminal bacterial concentrations relatively low in the proximal gut and reduces the risk of adherence and translocation. There is, in fact, considerable evidence suggesting that ileus and intestinal obstruction may be important factors in the so-called gut origin septic response.[58]

FACTORS COMPROMISING BARRIER FUNCTION

In critically ill surgical patients, numerous associated clinical factors compromise the various components of barrier function. Critical illness and injury lead to disordered GI motility and ileus. Antibiotic therapy frequently covers the common aerobic and anaerobic members of the normal microflora, which results in overgrowth of the gut with resistant aerobic species. Parenteral nutrient solutions are characteristically deficient in glutamine and short-chain fatty acids, and sustained use of such solutions can cause atrophy of the mucosal barrier. IgA and mucin production may be compromised by the catabolism typical of severe illness. In essence, all of the components of the gut barrier are potentially vulnerable, and microbial translocation (and, subsequently, the systemic septic response) can result from impairment of any or all of them.

RECOGNITION AND MANAGEMENT OF MICROBIAL TRANSLOCATION

The clinical basis for the diagnosis of microbial translocation is imprecise: there is no distinctive clinical marker of this event. Essentially, the diagnosis is one of exclusion. When all conventional infectious sources for a septic response have been excluded by careful clinical evaluation, microbial translocation is considered to be the cause. This clinical diagnosis is a treacherous one and can only be made presumptively. Even when one is convinced that microbial translocation is operative, it is vital to

remain vigilant and continue to search for infectious foci that may be driving the septic response.

The presence of certain opportunistic microbes in blood cultures strongly implies that GI microbial translocation may have occurred. The organisms making up the so-called trilogy of translocation—namely, *Enterococcus, S. epidermidis,* and *Candida* species—are common overgrowth organisms after long-term broad-spectrum antibiotic therapy and are commonly identified together in blood cultures. Obviously, when blood cultures are positive for these organisms, any potential infectious source must be ruled out, particularly bacteremia from intravascular devices.

Fundamental to the prevention and treatment of microbial translocation is reinforcement of the gut barrier. Enteral rather than parenteral nutritional support is always recommended if the clinical circumstances permit [*see 6:23 Nutritional Support*].[59] Intraluminal nutrients are delivered directly to the mucosal cells and promote GI motility[60]; moreover, they foster proliferation of a more normal intestinal microflora. Mobilization of the patient from the recumbent position likewise promotes GI motility and is a critical feature of early fixation of long-bone fractures in multiple-trauma patients.[58,61] Immunonutritional regimens enhanced with glutamine, arginine, omega-3 fatty acids, and nucleotides have yielded encouraging results in prospective clinical trials.[62]

It is also important to reevaluate patterns of antibiotic use. Although anaerobes act synergistically with aerobes in intra-abdominal and soft tissue infections, the anaerobes in the GI tract are important components of the gut barrier.[63,64] Because anaerobes are seldom nosocomial pathogens, systemic antibiotics that act against anaerobes should not be used for ICU-acquired infections unless clearly necessary. Some clinicans advocate selective gut decontamination (SGD), in which intraluminal antibiotics are employed to reduce aerobic colonization of the gut while preserving the anaerobic species.[65,66] One meta-analysis found this technique to improve survival.[67] In the United States, however, concerns about potential resistance problems from using antibiotics in this way within the critical care environment has limited the use of SGD.

Negative Blood Culture with Infection

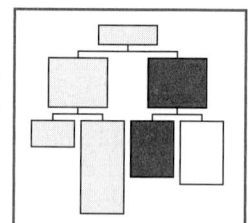

A positive blood culture is generally accepted as proof that microbial dissemination has occurred and that this process is the stimulus for the septic response (though, as noted [*see Positive Blood Culture without Infection, above*], such an assumption is not always warranted). However, most patients who manifest the septic response secondary to severe infection do not have positive blood cultures. In such cases, it is the septic response, rather than the blood culture itself, that is the most useful clinical indicator of a systemic reaction to infection.

REASONS FOR NEGATIVE CULTURE

Patients with the septic response secondary to infection may have negative blood cultures for any of several reasons. First, the septic response may have been activated by disseminated microorganisms that are sensitive to concurrently administered antibiotics. The patient may actually be bacteremic, but the presence of active antibiotic in the blood prevents bacterial growth in the culture. For certain antibiotics, there are laboratory methods for neutralizing the effects of their concurrent administration

Table 6 Common Bacteria Cultured from ICU Patients with Pneumonia: NNIS System Report, 1990–1999[70]

Organism	Type of ICU		
	Cardiothoracic (%)	General Surgery (%)	Trauma (%)
Pseudomonas aeruginosa	13.1	17.2	17.1
Enterobacter species	13.1	12.8	13.4
Staphylococcus aureus	11.3	17.0	18.1
Candida albicans	6.3	3.9	1.5
Klebsiella pneumoniae	5.9	7.2	7.0
Haemophilus influenzae	5.8	4.4	7.4
Escherichia coli	4.8	4.9	4.4
Enterococcus species	2.3	1.8	1.1
All others	37.4	30.9	29.9

(e.g., penicillinase), but for most, this is not the case. Second, it may have been dissemination of bacterial cellular products (most notably, endotoxin) rather than whole, viable microorganisms that activated the septic response. Third, the response may have been activated by systemic distribution of cytokine signals from an intense infectious focus (e.g., severe peritonitis), without dissemination of either bacteria or their products from the focus. Fourth, given that bacteremia is an episodic process and blood culture a random event, the culture sample may simply have been obtained at a time when the patient was temporarily nonbacteremic. The frequency of positive blood cultures in critically ill SICU patients is so low and the value of the occasional positive culture so minimal that several authors have recommended not even drawing blood samples for culture in this population.[68,69]

EVALUATION AND MANAGEMENT

Nonbacteremic patients who manifest the septic response must still be evaluated just as thoroughly as bacteremic patients would be, with the aim of ascertaining whether there is a primary source of infection. The lungs, the urinary tract, surgical or traumatic wounds, visceral compartments, and I.V. devices must all be sequentially evaluated. Careful physical examination, appropriate diagnostic studies for each anatomic area (e.g., CT scans for the abdomen), and aggressive culturing of suspicious fluids or exudates are indicat-

Table 7 Common Bacteria Cultured from ICU Patients with Urinary Tract Infections: NNIS System Report, 1990–1999[70]

Organism	Type of ICU		
	Cardiothoracic (%)	General Surgery (%)	Trauma (%)
Candida albicans	21.0	16.3	10.8
Pseudomonas aeruginosa	12.6	13.1	13.5
Escherichia coli	12.5	14.6	20.1
Enterococcus species	8.5	14.5	15.5
Klebsiella pneumoniae	6.1	6.1	4.5
Enterobacter species	5.9	6.2	6.5
Coagulase-negative staphylococci	1.6	1.9	3.5
Staphylococcus aureus	0.6	1.3	1.7
All others	31.2	26.0	23.9

ed. Special emphasis must be placed on the surgical site and on sites where invasive monitoring devices (e.g., a Foley catheter) or support instruments (e.g., an endotracheal tube) have been introduced into the patient. Nonbacteremic patients may indeed have the septic response without being infected [*see* Septic Response without Microorganisms, *below*], but this can only be determined after systematic evaluation for a primary infectious focus.

Once a presumptive source of infection has been identified, the primary focus should be drained mechanically, and empirical antimicrobial therapy directed toward the anticipated pathogens should be initiated while culture and sensitivity data are pending. For intra-abdominal infections, the antibiotic regimen must cover both enteric aerobes and anaerobes. For postoperative pulmonary infection, multiresistant gram-negative rods and *S. aureus* are the most common pathogens [*see Table 6*].[70] Postoperative urinary tract infections are usually caused by enteric aerobic gram-negative rods, but more and more often, they are being caused by *Candida* species [*see Table 7*]. Intelligent antibiotic selections for these infections requires a working knowledge of the antibiogram of the ICU.

Many critically ill patients who have undergone operation have already received antibiotic therapy at some point during management. Culture and sensitivity information must therefore be continuously obtained because the pathogens found in complex ICU patients with the septic response are often resistant to multiple conventional antibiotics.

Although in many cases the source of the infection and the attendant septic response is readily apparent, in many others the diagnosis can only be presumptive. Constant vigilance for changing clinical findings and careful observation of the response to empirical therapy are essential. For example, if a postoperative patient with the septic response has a urinary tract culture that is positive for *E. coli* at 10^5 colony-forming units/ml, it does not necessarily follow that the urinary tract is the source of the septic response. In my experience, a well-drained urinary tract is seldom the source of a postoperative septic response; other sources must be considered even when a positive urinary tract culture has been obtained.

In the absence of a diagnosis, it is generally difficult to handle either the infection or the septic response effectively; thus, continued intensive surveillance is essential. The objective of management is to control, by mechanical and pharmacologic means, the primary infectious source or sources of the disseminated whole microorganisms, microbial cellular products, or inflammatory cytokines that are responsible for the clinical septic response. Unfortunately, this objective is not equally appropriate for all nonbacteremic septic patients: as is now well established, the septic response can be activated by processes other than clinical infection.

Septic Response without Microorganisms

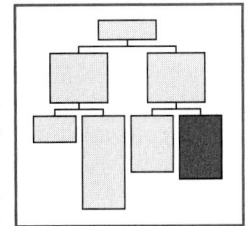

Traditional assumptions notwithstanding, there is no necessary association between the activation of the septic response and the presence of infection: any physiologic event that can trigger a severe local inflammatory response is potentially capable of activating the septic response.[71-73] Extreme local tissue inflammation without a microbial component can cause the release of inflammatory cytokines into the circulation in sufficient quantities to evoke the septic response. The clinical manifestations of the septic response are essentially the same whether it is caused by infection or not; thus, the diagnosis of the septic response secondary to sterile inflammation must be one of suspicion and exclusion.

Of the common clinical entities that can trigger the systemic septic response, perhaps the most notable is acute pancreatitis. The clinical course of severe acute pancreatitis managed with aggressive volume resuscitation includes loss of peripheral vascular resistance, elevated cardiac output, elevated white blood cell counts, and fever. Indeed, Ranson's criteria reflect characteristics of systemic inflammation, including end-organ damage to the lungs, the liver, and the kidneys.[74] Patients with severe acute pancreatitis often clearly illustrate the rapid physiologic progression from the septic response to the multiple organ dysfunction syndrome (MODS) [see 6:13 Multiple Organ Dysfunction Syndrome]. Other conditions that can activate the septic response are severe aspiration pneumonitis, which initially is a chemical event that evokes an intense inflammatory response, and multiple trauma with extensive soft tissue injury, necrosis at the injury site, and tissue hematoma. Even extracorporeal membrane oxygenation can be associated with acute activation of the complement cascade and a postoperative septic response leading to end-organ failure, without infection or bacteria being involved at all.

When the septic response occurs in one of these settings, the clinician often is anxious about the possibility of infection and is tempted to initiate antimicrobial therapy, at the very least. However, it is the response itself, rather than any infection, that is the fundamental problem to be dealt with in these patients. Obviously, then, antibiotic therapy will be ineffective in such cases, and specific treatment must be directed toward the septic response.

Effective supportive care is essential to the management of the septic response secondary to sterile inflammation. Volume support to maintain an adequate cardiac output and tissue perfusion is vital. The pulmonary microcirculation is the early target of the septic response; accordingly, support of systemic oxygenation with mechanical ventilation is often necessary.

A vexing problem associated with severe pancreatitis or aspiration pneumonia is that a number of separate stimuli capable of activating the septic response will present themselves during the course of protracted management. In a patient with severe pancreatitis, for example, the primary inflammatory focus gives rise to an initial septic response characterized by pulmonary failure. The patient is effectively resuscitated and appears clinically improved by the fourth or fifth day of hospitalization. By this point, however, an infectious focus, in the form of a pancreatic abscess, has often developed, and this infectious focus evokes a second septic response. Multiple operations and prolonged antibiotic therapy then set the stage for microbial translocation from the gut, which results in candidemia and a third septic response.

What is more, not only may a single pathologic condition give rise to various stimuli that can elicit the septic response, but severely ill surgical patients may also have additional separate inciting causes (which can occur either sequentially or simultaneously) during management, each of which may be associated with one or more septic stimuli. Indeed, a major challenge for the future—perhaps the major challenge—is the necessity of achieving better definition of clinical markers for specific stimuli of the septic response so that treatment can be better directed.

Discussion

Sepsis as Nonspecific Systemic Inflammatory Response

Infection has traditionally been viewed as a local inflammatory response within tissue that is initiated and perpetuated by microorganisms. It is generally agreed that the numerous elements of host defense are designed to both contain and eradicate the microbial provocateurs of this inflammatory process. It is also generally recognized that a threshold exists, the breaching of which results in the dissemination of the infectious process and the elicitation of a systemic inflammatory response. The precise point at which this threshold is passed has not been well defined clinically; however, the clinical expressions of this event are easily recognized [see 6:14 Clinical and Laboratory Diagnosis of Infection].

There is considerable evidence to support the theory that in the so-called septic patient, there occurs a generalized, systemic activation of the inflammatory cascade. The intricate inflammatory response to injury that is so salutary at the tissue level actually becomes a self-destructive process when activated at the systemic level.[75] Although these septic events have been associated most often with uncontrolled infection, it is now appreciated that the systemic inflammatory response is in fact a nonspecific host response in the same way that soft tissue inflammation is nonspecific.

We can now identify a changing perspective with respect to the stimuli of the septic response in the SICU. Current support technology permits sustained survival of critically ill and severely injured patients to a biologic point never before reached. As a result, the septic response may now be seen as a consequence of (1) microorganisms in the context of infection, (2) microorganisms in the absence of infection, and (3) inflammatory events not associated with either microorganisms or clinical infection.

Elements of the Septic Response

The septic response represents an evolution of multiple physiologic and metabolic changes. These changes do not constitute an either-or phenomenon but instead take place along an ever-changing continuum. Consequently, it is difficult to determine exactly when a patient ceases to manifest an appropriate stress response and begins to manifest a deleterious septic response. The key physiologic elements of the septic response are (1) reduced peripheral vascular resistance, (2) hyperdynamic cardiac performance, and (3) narrowing of the arteriovenous oxygen content difference. The metabolic features of the septic response are quite complex but can be simplified into five main elements: (1) hypermetabolism, (2) accelerated hepatic gluconeogenesis, (3) accelerated hepatic ureagenesis, (4) increased urinary nitrogen loss, and (5) insulin resistance. These metabolic changes are discussed in greater detail elsewhere [see 6:22 Metabolic Response to Critical Illness].

Reduced peripheral vascular resistance—contrasting dramatically with the increased resistance associated with hypovolemia and cardiac failure—is the sine qua non of the septic response.

Cardiac Output

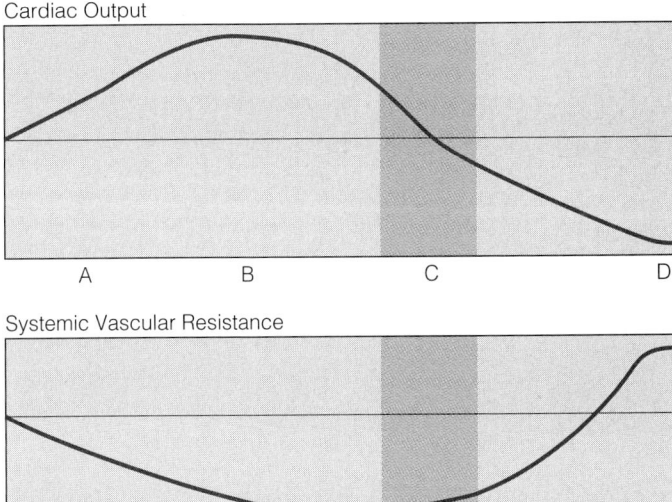

Systemic Vascular Resistance

Figure 3 **Illustrated is the relation of cardiac output to peripheral vascular resistance during the natural history of the septic response. The areas indicated by the light-red boxes are state C, reflecting the onset of clinical septic shock.**

(It must be emphasized that whereas resistance is reduced for the vascular system as a whole, this may not be the case for each individual tissue bed.) The loss of resistance is particularly interesting in light of the elevated catecholamine concentrations that are simultaneously identified in these patients. These elevations reflect the counterregulatory metabolic milieu of the septic response.[76,77] The alpha-adrenergic effects of the catecholamines are obviously overridden by other peripheral mechanisms.

The systemic vasodilatation appears to be caused primarily by nitric oxide from endothelial cells in the microcirculation.[78-81] Nitric oxide is a paracrine signal that mediates relaxation of vascular smooth muscle. Its synthesis and release are stimulated by several agonists, including endotoxin, bradykinin, and acetylcholine. Although prostacyclin and histamine are also potential mediators of vasodilatation, at present, nitric oxide appears to be the principal mechanism.

Hyperdynamic cardiac performance is the obligatory response of the left ventricle when peripheral vascular resistance declines. For cardiac output to increase, however, intravascular volume must be replenished, and the myocardium must possess sufficient physiologic reserve. Thus, elderly patients may not be able to meet the physiologic demands imposed by sepsis-induced afterload reduction, and such inability results in the hypodynamic septic shock state. Even in young, healthy patients, sustained hyperdynamism ultimately leads to ventricular failure and low cardiac output.

Narrowing of the arteriovenous oxygen content difference in the hyperdynamic patient is perhaps the most important of the critical mechanisms responsible for the septic response. Oxygen consumption is inadequate to meet the demands of hypermetabolism,[82,83] and lactate production is the result. When intravascular volume is fully expanded, further increases in cardiac output result in further narrowing of the arteriovenous oxygen content difference. Failure of peripheral oxygen utilization is fundamental to the septic process and underscores that this response is not characterized by inadequate myocardial performance until its very latest stages.

Natural History of the Septic Response

In the predominant view of the natural history of the septic response,[84] exaggeration of the fundamental stress response is the basis for deterioration of the patient from a compensated state (i.e., the stress response) to a decompensated state (i.e., the septic response). The key element in the natural history of the septic response is the relation between cardiac output and peripheral vascular resistance [*see Figure 3*].

State A represents the normal adaptive stress response, the first-order response to biologic insults. Cardiac output is modestly elevated, and peripheral vascular resistance is modestly reduced. Systemic oxygen consumption is increased, but lactate concentration is not. State A reflects the postresuscitative physiology of the injured or postoperative patient. The hemodynamic profile progressively returns to normal over several days, provided that there is no intercurrent insult (e.g., infection).

State B represents the exaggerated stress response and marks the transition to the beginning of biologic decompensation. Peripheral vascular resistance is profoundly reduced. A total peripheral vascular resistance lower than 800 dynes-sec/cm⁵ is the commonly recognized threshold for the septic response; resistance may decline to 400 dynes-sec/cm⁵ or even lower. The afterload reduction results in dramatic elevation of cardiac output. An acceptable arterial blood pressure can usually be sustained unless intrinsic myocardial disease or hypovolemia is present. The increased capacitance typical of state B necessitates considerable preload support, which often calls for aggressive fluid administration. Measurement of the pulmonary capillary wedge pressure is often necessary to facilitate the expansion of intravascular volume.

State B is also characterized by accumulation of lactate species in the blood before the evolution of frank clinical hypotension. Blood lactate concentrations reflect net lactate production in selected tissues minus lactate utilization in other tissues. Because not all tissues are necessarily affected equally by the septic response process, oxidation of lactate by selected well-perfused tissues may compensate for production of lactate by others. Lactic acidemia preceding lactic acidosis is usually seen in patients with sustained state B; compensatory mechanisms prevent acidosis until later in the process. These patients are actually in a state of shock, even though their arterial blood pressure is considered normal, because tissue oxygen utilization is clearly impaired.

State C heralds the beginning of septic shock as traditionally defined—that is, as hypotension in a nonhypovolemic patient that is secondary to severe infection. State C patients fulfill this definition: they have mild to severe hypotension, with systolic arterial blood pressure lower than 80 mm Hg. In this setting, however, septic shock is secondary to the severe and exaggerated loss of peripheral vascular resistance; although cardiac output may be normal or slightly increased (8 to 10 L/min), it is insufficient to compensate for this loss.

State C patients are in so-called hot shock. They are warm to the touch and usually show evidence of diaphoresis. Their cutaneous tissues appear well perfused, even though the arterial blood pressure is low. The loss of perfusion pressure acts synergistically with the peripheral defect in oxygen utilization to create a severe peripheral oxygen debt that is clearly reflected in the severe lactic acidosis seen in state C.

State D represents the final phase in the process, in which frank congestive heart failure emerges. Cardiac performance is considerably depressed. Autonomic mechanisms override the vasodilatory influences seen in state C, and peripheral vascular resistance is now increased. In state D, low cardiac output, peripheral vasoconstriction, and peripheral defects in oxygen utilization work simultaneously to produce profound tissue hypoxemia and lactic acidosis. In the absence of dramatic therapeutic and supportive measures, this is the preagonal period before death.

Pathophysiology of the Septic Response

Fundamental to our understanding of the septic response is the idea that its negative and destructive features are simply the systemic manifestations of what is otherwise a positive and beneficial local inflammatory response to tissue injury. This crucial point can be illustrated by considering the local events that attend soft tissue injury. These events, in essence, are the septic response in microcosm.

LOCAL EVENTS

Soft tissue injury triggers a local inflammatory response that includes disruption of blood vessels, exposure of the collagen matrix, extravasation of red blood cells and plasma proteins, activation of the coagulation cascade, aggregation of platelets, and activation of the complement cascade via the alternative pathway. It is likely that by-products of coagulation and complement activation, among other potential biochemical signals, stimulate mast cells to initiate the first phases of the inflammatory response; the specific cleavage products of complement proteins C3, C4, and C5 (the soluble anaphylatoxins C3a, C4a, and C5a) are known to be the most potent stimuli of mast cell degranulation.[85-87] The production of bradykinin from plasma protein precursors occurs via the stimulation of activated factor XII from the coagulation cascade. The activation of these five initiators of inflammation (coagulation cascade, platelets, complement proteins, mast cells, and bradykinin) have the specific effects of (1) local vasodilatation, which increases local flow but reduces flow velocity in the area of injury; (2) increased capillary permeability, which results in extravasation of protein-rich plasma into the injured area, thereby initiating edema formation; and (3) generation of numerous inflammatory enzyme and protein cleavage products, which act as chemoattractants.

Diffusion of the chemoattractant signals from the epicenter of injury begins the process of phagocytic infiltration of the injured area. Chemoattractants bind to specific receptor sites on vascular endothelial cells and initiate the interaction of the endothelial cell with the intravascular neutrophil. The gradient of chemoattractant signals from the epicenter of the injury then serves as a beacon to direct phagocytic diapedesis toward the site of injury and contamination. The severity of the injury, the extent of necrosis, and the degree of exogenous microbial contamination dictate the intensity of the summed chemoattractant signals that govern the rapidity and the quantity of neutrophil infiltration.

Approximately 24 hours after injury, macrophages infiltrate the area via the same mechanisms for margination and chemotaxis that mobilized the neutrophils. Macrophages orchestrate the severity of the inflammatory response. If necrotic tissue and foreign elements (e.g., bacteria) are minimally present in the area of injury, then the magnitude of the chemoattractant signal is small, macrophages are minimally activated, and the neutrophils proceed with phagocytosis in an orderly fashion. If, however, bacterial contamination is severe and there is considerable necrotic tissue, then the amplitude of chemoattractant effects will be great, which results in full activation of macrophages. Fully activated macrophages elaborate multiple proinflammatory signals that induce the neutrophils to enter a state of accelerated and enhanced phagocytic activity and elicit the extracellular release of

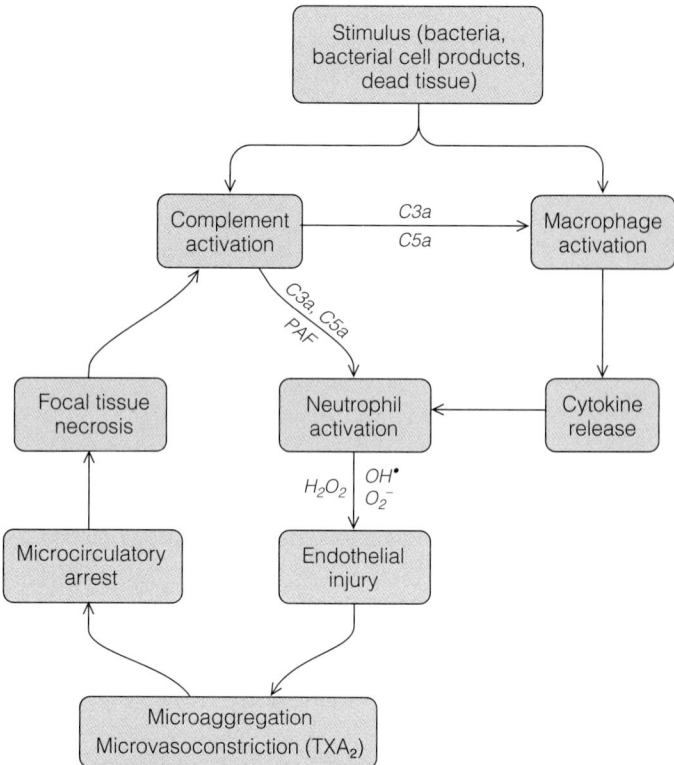

Figure 4   **Shown is the self-energized cycle of tissue-level injury that becomes the end-organ consequences of the septic response. Activation of the inflammatory cascade via several different stimuli results in neutrophil activation, which leads to autodestructive inflammation, tissue ischemia, tissue necrosis, and reactivation of the process.**

reactive oxygen intermediates and lysosomal enzymes. The accelerated phagocytic activity results in the death of the neutrophils and the formation of pus. Suppuration at the epicenter of the injury is further enhanced when the TNF signal diffuses into the adjacent microcirculation, where marginated neutrophils, recruited into the inflammatory focus, are fully activated, resulting in thrombosis of the adjacent microcirculation. This microcirculatory thrombosis is actually beneficial in that it prevents bacteria or their products from gaining systemic access. Indeed, the ultimate function of the inflammatory response is the containment and subsequent eradication of bacterial contaminants.

SYSTEMIC EVENTS

The systemic septic response comprises the same sequence of events just described, except that the activation of the inflammatory cascade is generalized and lacks the clear directional focus that characterizes the local response. In severe infection, dissemination of bacteria and endotoxins leads to systemic activation of the initiator pathways of inflammation. Systemic activation of coagulation, platelets, complement proteins, mast cells, and bradykinin results in generalized edema, systemic vasodilatation, and a generalized release of chemoattractant signals. Generalized neutrophil margination occurs. The upregulation of the generalized inflammatory response results in full activation of marginated neutrophils. From their intravascular and perivascular positions, the activated neutrophils subsequently release reactive oxygen intermediates and lysosomal enzymes. The resulting inflammatory injury to the microcirculation leads to aggregation of platelets, damage to the endothelial cells, and release of prostaglandin derivatives that promote vasoconstriction. The consequence of these events is a two-pronged injury comprising the biomechanical blockade caused by the inflammatory aggregate and the vasoconstriction caused by thromboxane A_2.

When an inflammatory focus is sufficiently severe (as, for example, in pancreatitis), it may release sufficient TNF to activate macrophages and neutrophils within the circulation. In these circumstances, in situ macrophage cells (e.g., alveolar macrophages and Kupffer's cells) can be activated, and a generalized inflammatory response is the result. The key point in this latter scenario is that this response does not depend on systemic dissemination of the pathogen or its cellular products but can be triggered simply by dissemination of the proinflammatory cytokine signal.

The microcirculatory arrest, in turn, leads to the formation of foci of necrotic tissue,[88] which evoke a local inflammatory response that eventually reactivates the septic response. A self-energized and futile cycle is created in which an initial injury elicits a local response, the local response expands into a systemic response, and the systemic response finally generates tissue-level injuries that start the whole process all over again [see Figure 4]. The progressive loss of microcirculatory units within the critical organ systems leads to MODS [see 6:13 Multiple Organ Dysfunction Syndrome] and ultimately to the death of the host.[89-91]

New Approaches to Management of the Septic Response

It is to be hoped that growing comprehension of the mechanisms involved in the evolution of the septic response and its end-organ effects will lead to new and better therapeutic regimens. Various treatments have already been examined in experimental studies, and a few of them have been used on an investigational basis in humans. These treatments have focused on the following seven basic approaches.

1. Neutralization of activation of inflammation. Efforts to neutralize or inhibit the provocative stimulation of SIRS have principally targeted bacterial endotoxin, a potent activator of the septic response. To this end, antiendotoxin antibody has been given to septic response patients in an attempt to neutralize the effects of endotoxin. Although some clinical studies found that certain patients benefited from administration of polyclonal sera[92-94] or the monoclonal antibody,[95,96] controversy continues to surround this proposed treatment. Initial favorable reports describing beneficial effects in specific subpopulations were not confirmed by later prospective studies specifically addressed to these same cohorts.[97,98] Because endotoxin is only one of numerous stimuli of the septic response, routine use of the very expensive monoclonal antiendotoxin antibody for all septic response patients would be difficult to justify. It appears unlikely that this treatment strategy will be generally deployed in clinical practice.
2. Inhibition of initiator signals. Numerous experimental investigations have explored inhibition of the initiators of inflammation: specifically, inhibition of coagulation,[99] coagulation and platelets,[100-102] bradykinin,[103] mast cell products,[104] and complement proteins.[105,106] Few of these approaches have been pursued in prospective clinical trials. A prospective,

multicenter trial of a promising bradykinin antagonist failed to demonstrate any clinical benefit.[107] However, a large prospective trial found that giving recombinant activated protein C (drotrecogin alpha) to septic response patients led to an absolute 6% increase in survival. This result raises hope that significant improvements can be achieved via modulation of the coagulation cascade.[108]
3. Inhibition of proinflammatory signals. A third major area of investigation has been the inhibition or alteration of effector mechanisms or consequences of activation of inflammation. Initially, specific neutralization of TNF[109,110] and receptor blockade of the effects of interleukin-1[111] were the most promising prospects; however, clinical trials of both failed to demonstrate any meaningful benefit.[112-116] Antibodies to prevent neutrophil-endothelial interaction have also been investigated,[117] as have platelet-activating factor antagonists.[118]
4. Neutralization of effector signals. The effector signals are the destructive consequences of the activation of inflammation. Antioxidant therapy aimed at neutralizing the effects of reactive oxygen intermediates has gone from laboratory experimentation to clinical application.[119] Experimentally, lazaroids[120] and nitrones[121] also appear to have promise as potential treatments.
5. Enhancement of the compensatory anti-inflammatory response syndrome (CARS). The exaggerated inflammatory response results in a counterinflammatory response (i.e., CARS) that modulates inflammatory effects.[122] Some would argue that SIRS may be understood as the consequence of inadequate CARS. Counterinflammatory signals produced by IL-4,[123] IL-10,[124] IL-13,[125] transforming growth factor-β,[126] and prostaglandin E[127] appear to offset or balance inflammation. Administration of these agents may play a role in future therapy for the septic response.
6. Management of immunosuppression. It has long been recognized that immunosuppression has long been recognized asis a consequence of severe injury and sepsis. Accordingly, enhancement of host responses has been explored as a potential therapy for the septic response. Interferon gamma,[128] levamisole,[129] muramyl dipeptide,[130] granulocyte colony-stimulating factor,[131] and granulocyte-monocyte colony-stimulating factor[132] have all been studied experimentally or clinically.
7. Gene therapy. Experimental studies have explored the use of viral vectors or liposomal delivery systems to enhance endogenous production of counterinflammatory signals,[133] antioxidants,[134] antiproteases,[135] and heat shock proteins.[136] Administration of antisense nucleotides to block excessive cellular production of proinflammatory signals has been examined as well.[137,138]

As the complexity of the host response comes to be better understood, the new knowledge gained generates an ever-increasing number of potential treatments. It is likely that multimodality therapy will receive increased attention in the treatment of sepsis, as such approaches have already done in the treatment of cancer. Balancing proinflammatory signals against counterinflammatory signals may well prove to be the key to modulating this complex human response.

References

1. Definitions for sepsis and organ failure and guidelines for the use of innovative therapies in sepsis. American College of Chest Physicians/Society of Critical Care Medicine Consensus Conference. Crit Care Med 20:864, 1992

2. Edmond MB, Wallace SE, McClish DK, et al: Nosocomial bloodstream infection in United States hospitals: a three-year analysis. Clin Infect Dis 29:234, 1999

3. Fry DE, Fry RV, Borzotta AP: Nosocomial blood-borne infection secondary to intravascular devices. Am J Surg 167:268, 1994

4. Maki DG, Weise CE, Sarafin HW: A semiquantitative culture method for identifying intravenous-catheter-related infection. N Engl J Med 296:1305, 1977

5. Stein JM, Pruitt BA Jr: Suppurative thrombophlebitis: a lethal iatrogenic disease. N Engl J Med 282:1452, 1970

6. Garrison RN, Richardson JD, Fry DE: Catheter-associated septic thrombophlebitis. South Med J 75:917, 1982

7. Gotz F: Staphylococcus and biofilms. Mol Microbiol 43:1367, 2002

8. Bandyk DF, Bergamini TM, Kinney EV, et al: In situ replacement of vascular prostheses infected by bacterial biofilm. J Vasc Surg 13:575, 1991

9. Zurenko GE, Gibson JK, Shinabarger DL, et al: Oxazolidinones: a new class of antibacterials. Curr Opin Pharmacol 1:470, 2001

10. Allington DR, Rivey MP: Quinupristin/dalfopristin: a therapeutic review. Clin Ther 23:24, 2001

11. Stevens DL: The toxic shock syndromes. Infect Dis Clin North Am 10:727, 1996

12. Davies HD, McGeer A, Schwartz B, et al: Invasive group A streptococcal infection in Ontario, Canada. Ontario Group A Streptococcal Study Group. N Engl J Med 335:547, 1996

13. Aebi C, Ahmed A, Ramilo O: Bacterial complications of primary varicella in children. Clin Infect Dis 23:698, 1996

14. Stevens DL, Gibbons AE, Bergstrom R, et al: The eagle effect revisited: efficacy of clindamycin, erythromycin, and penicillin in the treatment of streptococcal myositis. J Infect Dis 158:23, 1988

15. Barie PS, Christou NV, Dellinger EP, et al: Pathogenicity of the enterococcus in surgical infections. Ann Surg 212:155, 1990

16. Nichols RL, Muzik AC: Enterococcal infections in surgical patients: the mystery continues. Clin Infect Dis 15:72, 1992

17. Yu VL: Enterococcal superinfection and colonization after therapy with moxalactam, a new broad-spectrum antibiotic. Ann Intern Med 94:784, 1981

18. Fry DE, Berberich S, Garrison RN: Bacterial synergism between the enterococcus and Escherichia coli. J Surg Res 38:475, 1985

19. Onderdonk AB, Bartlett JG, Louie T, et al: Microbial synergy in experimental intra-abdominal abscess. Infect Immun 13:22, 1976

20. Fry DE, Cox RA, Harbrecht PJ: Gangrene of the gallbladder: a complication of acute cholecystitis. South Med J 74:666, 1981

21. Garrison RN, Fry DE, Berberich S, et al: Enterococcal bacteremia: clinical implications and determinants of death. Ann Surg 196:43, 1982

22. Eliopoulos GM: Vancomycin-resistant enterococci: mechanism and clinical relevance. Infect Dis Clin North Am 11:851, 1997

23. Linden PK: Treatment options for vancomycin-resistant enterococci infections. Drugs 62:425, 2002

24. Steinmetz MP, Vogelbaum MA, De Georgia MA, et al: Successful treatment of vancomycin-resistant enterococcus meningitis with linezolid: case report and review of the literature. Crit Care Med 29:2383, 2001

25. Moellering RC: Quinupristin/dalfopristin: therapeutic potential for vancomycin-resistant enterococcal infections. J Antimicrob Chemother 44(suppl A):25, 1999

26. Matsumura S, Simor AE: Treatment of endocarditis due to vancomycin-resistant Enterococcus faecium with quinupristin/dalfopristin, doxycycline, and rifampin: a synergistic drug combination. Clin Infect Dis 27:1554, 1998

27. Asher EF, Oliver BG, Fry DE: Urinary tract infections in the surgical patient. Am Surg 54:466, 1988

28. Fry DE, Cox RA, Harbrecht PJ: Empyema of the gallbladder: a complication in the natural history of acute cholecystitis. Am J Surg 141:366, 1981

29. Mosdell DM, Morris DM, Voltura A, et al: Antibiotic treatment for surgical peritonitis. Ann Surg 214:543, 1991

30. Bohnen JM, Marshall JC, Fry DE, et al: Clinical and scientific importance of source control in abdominal infections: summary of a symposium. Can J Surg 42:122, 1999

31. Niemiec PW Jr, Allo MD, Miller CF: Effect of altered volume of distribution on aminoglycoside levels in patients in surgical intensive care. Arch Surg 122:207, 1987

32. Solomkin JS, Choe KA, Christou NV, et al: A prospective, randomized, blinded study of ertapenem (ETP) vs. piperacillin/tazobactam (PTZ) for intraabdominal infection (IAI). Abstract 3. Presented at the 21st Annual Meeting of the Surgical Infection Society, May 3, 2001, Snowbird, Utah

33. Koo J, Tight R, Rajkumar V, et al: Comparison of once-daily versus pharmacokinetic dosing of aminoglycosides in elderly patients. Am J Med 101:177, 1996

34. Fry DE, Garrison RN, Polk HC Jr: Clinical implications in Bacteroides bacteremia. Surg Gynecol Obstet 149:189, 1979

35. Kasper DL, Hayes ME, Reinap BG, et al: Isolation and identification of encapsulated strains of Bacteroides fragilis. J Infect Dis 136:75, 1977

36. Fry DE, Klamer TW, Garrison RN, et al: Atypical clostridial bacteremia. Surg Gynecol Obstet 153:28, 1981

37. Dyess DL, Garrison RN, Fry DE: Candida sepsis: implications of polymicrobial blood-borne infection. Arch Surg 120:345, 1985

38. Stone HH, Kolb LD, Currie CA, et al: Candida sepsis: pathogenesis and principles of treatment. Ann Surg 179:697, 1974

39. Solomkin JS, Flohr AB, Quie PG, et al: The role of Candida in intraperitoneal infections. Surgery 88:524, 1980

40. Fine J, Frank ED, Ravin HA, et al: The bacterial factor in traumatic shock. N Engl J Med 260:214, 1959

41. Ravin HA, Fine J: Biological implications of intestinal endotoxins. Fed Proc 21:65, 1962

42. Schweinburg F, Fine J: Evidence for a lethal endotoxemia as the fundamental feature of irreversibility in three types or traumatic shock. J Exp Med 112:793, 1960

43. Zweifach BW: Hemorrhagic shock in germ free rats. Ann NY Acad Sci 78:315, 1959

44. Zweifach BW, Gordon HA, Wagner M, et al: Irreversible hemorrhagic shock in germfree rats. J Exp Med 107:437, 1958

45. Maejima K, Deitch EA, Berg RD: Bacterial translocation from the gastrointestinal tracts of rats receiving thermal injury. Infect Immun 43:6, 1984

46. Baker JW, Deitch EA, Li M, et al: Hemorrhagic shock induces bacterial translocation from the gut. J Trauma 28:896, 1988

47. Deitch EA, Winterton J, Li M, et al: The gut as portal of entry for bacteremia: role of protein malnutrition. Ann Surg 205:681, 1987

48. Deitch DE, Berg R, Specian R: Endotoxin promotes the translocation of bacteria from the gut. Arch Surg 122:185, 1987

49. Rush BF Jr, Sori AJ, Murphy TF, et al: Endotoxemia and bacteremia during hemorrhagic shock. Ann Surg 207:549, 1988

50. Deitch EA: Simple intestinal obstruction causes bacterial translocation in man. Arch Surg 124:699, 1989

51. Rush BF Jr, Redan JA, Flanagan JJ Jr, et al: Does bacteremia in hemorrhagic shock have clinical significance? A study in germ-free animals. Ann Surg 210:342, 1989

52. Lanser ME: An experimental phenomenon without clinical significance. Multiple System Organ Failure. Fry DE, Ed. Mosby-Year Book, Chicago, 1992, p 382

53. Wilmore DW, Smith RJ, O'Dwyer ST, et al: The gut: a central organ after surgical stress. Surgery 104:917, 1988

54. Roediger WE, Rae DA: Trophic effect of short chain fatty acids on mucosal handling of ions by the defunctional colon. Br J Surg 69:23, 1982

55. McNabb PC, Tomasi TB: Host defense mechanisms at mucosal surfaces. Annu Rev Microbiol 35:477, 1981

56. Tomasi TB Jr, Bienenstock J: Secretory immunoglobulins. Adv Immunol 9:1, 1968

57. Suegara N, Morotomi M, Watanabe T, et al: Behavior of the microflora in the rat stomach: adhesion of lactobacilli to the keratinized epithelial cells of the rat in vitro. Infect Immun 12:173, 1975

58. Border J, Hassett J, LaDuca J, et al: The gut origin septic states in blunt multiple trauma (ISS=40) in the ICU. Ann Surg 206:427, 1987

59. Moore FA, Moore EE, Jones TN, et al: TEN versus TPN following major abdominal trauma: reduced septic morbidity. J Trauma 29:916, 1989

60. Mochizuki H, Trocki O, Dominioni L, et al: Mechanism of prevention of postburn hypermetabolism and catabolism by early enteral feeding. Ann Surg 200:297, 1984

61. Seibel R, LaDuca J, Hassett JM, et al: Blunt multiple trauma (ISS 36), femur traction, and the pulmonary failure–septic state. Ann Surg 202:283, 1985

62. Kudsk KA, Minard G, Croce MA, et al: A randomized trial of isonitrogenous enteral diets following severe trauma: an immune-enhancing diet (IED) reduces septic complications. Ann Surg 224:531, 1996

63. Berg RD: Promotion of the translocation of enteric bacteria from the gastrointestinal tracts of mice by oral treatment with penicillin, clindamycin, or metronidazole. Infect Immun 33:854, 1981

64. Epstein MD, Tchervenkov JI, Alexander JW, et al: Effect of intraluminal antibiotics on the translocation of Candida albicans in burned guinea pigs. Burns 16:105, 1990

65. van der Waaij D: Colonization resistance of the digestive tract: clinical consequences and implications. J Antimicrob Chemother 10:263, 1982

66. Cerra FB, Maddaus MA, Dunn DI, et al: Selec-

tive gut decontamination reduces nosocomial infections and length of stay but not mortality or organ failure in surgical intensive care unit patients. Arch Surg 127:163, 1992

67. Nathens AB, Marshall JC: Selective decontamination of the digestive tract in surgical patients: a systematic review of the evidence. Arch Surg 134:170, 1999

68. Theuer CP, Bongard FS, Klein SR: Are blood cultures effective in the evaluation of fever in perioperative patients? Am J Surg 162:615, 1991

69. Henke PK, Polk HC Jr: Efficacy of blood cultures in the critically ill surgical patient. Surgery 120:752, 1996

70. Centers for Disease Control and Prevention: National Nosocomial Infections Surveillance (NNIS) system report: data summary from January 1990–May 1999. Issued June 1999. Am J Infect Control 27:520, 1999

71. Goris RJ, Boekholtz WK, van Bebber IP, et al: Multiple-organ failure and sepsis without bacteria: an experimental model. Arch Surg 121:897, 1986

72. Schirmer WJ, Schirmer JM, Naff GB, et al: Systemic complement activation produces hemodynamic changes characteristic of sepsis. Arch Surg 123:316, 1988

73. Schirmer WJ, Schirmer JM, Townsend MC, et al: Femur fracture with associated soft-tissue injury produces hepatic ischemia: possible cause of hepatic dysfunction. Arch Surg 123:412, 1988

74. Ranson JHC, Rifkind KM, Roses DF, et al: Prognostic signs and the role of operative management in acute pancreatitis. Surg Gynecol Obstet 139:69, 1974

75. Goris RJ, te Boekhorst TP, Nuytinck JK, et al: Multiple organ failure: generalized autodestructive inflammation? Arch Surg 120:1109, 1985

76. Bessey PQ, Watters JM, Aoki TT, et al: Combined hormonal infusion simulates the metabolic response to injury. Ann Surg 200:264, 1984

77. Watters JM, Bessey PQ, Dinarello CA, et al: Both inflammatory and endocrine mediators stimulate host responses to sepsis. Arch Surg 121:179, 1986

78. Moncada S, Palmer RMJ, Higgs EA: The discovery of nitric oxide as the endogenous nitrovasodilator. Hypertension 12:365, 1988

79. Ignarro LJ: Biological actions and properties of endothelium-derived nitric oxide formed and released from artery and vein. Circ Res 65:1, 1989

80. Ignarro LJ: Biosynthesis and metabolism of endothelium-derived nitric oxide. Annu Rev Pharmacol Toxicol 30:535, 1990

81. Vallance P, Collier J, Moncada S: Nitric oxide synthesized from L-arginine mediates endothelium dependent dilatation in human veins in vivo. Cardiovasc Res 23:1053, 1989

82. Siegel JH, Greenspan M, Del Guercio LRM: Abnormal vascular tone, defective oxygen transport and myocardial failure in human septic shock. Ann Surg 165:504, 1967

83. Siegel JH, Farrell EJ, Miller M, et al: Cardiorespiratory interactions as determinants of survival and the need for respiratory support in human shock states. J Trauma 13:602, 1973

84. Siegel JH, Cerra FB, Coleman B, et al: Physiological and metabolic correlations in human sepsis: invited commentary. Surgery 86:163, 1979

85. Gorski JP, Hugli TE, Muller-Eberhard HJ: Characterization of human C4a anaphylatoxin. J Biol Chem 256:2707, 1981

86. da Silva WD, Eisele JW, Lepow IH: Complement as a mediator of inflammation: III. Purification of the activity with anaphylatoxin properties generated by interaction of the first four components of complement and its identification as a cleavage product of C'3. J Exp Med 126:1027, 1967

87. Shin HS, Snyderman R, Friedman E, et al: Chemotactic and anaphylatoxic fragment cleaved from the fifth component of guinea pig complement. Science 162:361, 1968

88. Asher EF, Rowe RL, Garrison RN, et al: Experimental bacteremia and hepatic nutrient blood flow. Circ Shock 20:43, 1986

89. Townsend MC, Hapton WW, Haybron DM, et al: Effective organ blood flow and bioenergy status in murine peritonitis. Surgery 100:205, 1986

90. Schirmer WJ, Townsend MC, Schirmer JM, et al: Galactose elimination kinetics in sepsis: correlations of hepatic blood flow with function. Arch Surg 122:349, 1987

91. Haybron DM, Townsend MC, Hampton WW, et al: Alterations in renal perfusion and renal energy charge in murine peritonitis. Arch Surg 122:328, 1987

92. Lachman E, Pitsoe SB, Gaffin SL: Anti-lipopolysaccharide immunotherapy in management of septic shock of obstetric and gynaecological origin. Lancet 1:981, 1984

93. Baumgartner JD, Glauser MP, McCutchan JA, et al: Prevention of gram-negative shock and death in surgical patients by antibody to endotoxin core glycolipid. Lancet 2:59, 1985

94. Ziegler EJ, McCutchan JA, Fierer J, et al: Treatment of gram-negative bacteremia and shock with human antiserum to a mutant Escherichia coli. N Engl J Med 307:1225, 1982

95. Ziegler EJ, Fischer CJ, Sprung CL Jr, et al: Treatment of gram-negative bacteremia and septic shock with HA-1A human monoclonal antibody against endotoxin: a randomized, double-blind, placebo-controlled trial. N Engl J Med 324:429, 1991

96. Greenman RL, Schein RMH, Martin MA, et al: A controlled clinical trial of E5 murine monoclonal IgM antibody to endotoxin in the treatment of gram-negative sepsis. JAMA 266:1097, 1991

97. McCloskey RV, Straube RC, Sanders C, et al: Treatment of septic shock with human monoclonal antibody HA-1A: a randomized, double-blind, placebo-controlled trial. CHESS Trial Study Group. Ann Intern Med 121:1, 1994

98. Bone RC, Balk RA, Fein AM, et al: A second large controlled study of E5, a monoclonal antibody to endotoxin: results of a prospective, multicenter, randomized, controlled trial. The E5 Sepsis Study Group. Crit Care Med 23:994, 1995

99. Jansen PM, Pixley RA, Brouwer M, et al: Inhibition of factor XII in septic baboons attenuates the activation of complement and fibrinolytic system and reduces the release of interleukin-6 and neutrophil elastase. Blood 87:2337, 1996

100. Hau T, Simmons RL: Heparin in the treatment of experimental peritonitis. Ann Surg 187:294, 1978

101. O'Leary JP, Malik FS, Donahoe RP, et al: The effects of a minidose of heparin on peritonitis in rats. Surg Gynecol Obstet 148:571, 1979

102. Schirmer WJ, Schirmer JM, Naff GB, et al: Heparin's effect on the natural history of sepsis in the rat (abstr). Circ Shock 21:363, 1987

103. Ridings PC, Blocher CR, Fisher BJ, et al: Beneficial effects of a bradykinin antagonist in a model of gram negative sepsis. J Trauma 39:81, 1995

104. Leeper-Woodford SK, Carey D, Byrne K, et al: Histamine receptor antagonists, cyclooxygenase blockade, and tumor necrosis factor curing acute septic insult. Shock 9:89, 1998

105. Jansen PM, Eisele B, de Jong IW, et al: Effect of C1 inhibition on inflammatory and physiologic response patterns in primates suffering from lethal septic shock. J Immunol 160:475, 1998

106. Mohr M, Hopken U, Opperman M, et al: Effects of anti-C5a monoclonal antibodies on oxygen use in a porcine model of severe sepsis. Eur J Clin Invest 28:227, 1998

107. Fein AM, Bernard GR, Criner GJ, et al: Treatment of severe systemic inflammatory response syndromes and sepsis with a novel bradykinin antagonist, deltibant (CP-0127): results of a randomized, double-blind, placebo-controlled trial. CP-1027 SIRS and Sepsis Study Group. JAMA 277:482, 1997

108. Bernard GR, Vincent J-L, Laterre P-F, et al: Efficacy and safety of recombinant human activated protein C for severe sepsis. N Engl J Med 344:699, 2001

109. Beutler B, Milsark IW, Cerami AC: Passive immunization against cachectin/tumor necrosis factor protects mice from lethal effect of endotoxin. Science 229:869, 1985

110. Tracey KJ, Fong Y, Hesse DG, et al: Anti-cachectin/TNF monoclonal antibodies prevent septic shock during lethal bacteraemia. Nature 330:662, 1987

111. Wakabayashi G, Gelfand JA, Burke JF, et al: A specific receptor antagonist for interleukin 1 prevents Escherichia coli–induced shock in rabbits. FASEB J 5:338, 1991

112. Abraham E, Wunderink R, Silverman H, et al: Efficacy and safety of monoclonal antibody to human tumor necrosis factor alpha in patients with sepsis syndrome: a randomized, controlled, double-blind, multicenter clinical trial. JAMA 273:934, 1995

113. Cohen J, Carlet J: Intersept: an international, multicenter, placebo-controlled trial of monoclonal antibody to human tumor necrosis factor-alpha in patients with sepsis. International Sepsis Trial Study Group. Crit Care Med 24:1431, 1996

114. Reinhart K, Wiegard-Lohnert C, Grimminger F, et al: Assessment of the safety and efficacy of the monoclonal anti–tumor necrosis factor antibody-fragment, MAK 195F, in patients with sepsis and septic shock: a multicenter, randomized, placebo-controlled, dose-ranging study. Crit Care Med 24:733, 1996

115. Fisher CJ Jr, Dhainaut JF, Opal SM, et al: Recombinant human interleukin 1 receptor antagonist in the treatment of patients with sepsis syndrome: results from a randomized, double-blind, placebo-controlled trial. Phase III rhIL-1ra Sepsis Syndrome Study Group. JAMA 271:1836, 1994

116. Opal SM, Fisher CJ Jr, Dhainaut JF, et al: Confirming interleukin-1 receptor antagonist trial in severe sepsis: a phase III, randomized, double-blind, placebo-controlled, multicenter trial. The Interleukin-1 Receptor Antagonist Sepsis Investigation Group. Crit Care Med 25:1115, 1997

117. Walsh CJ, Carey D, Cook DJ, et al: Anti CD18 antibody attenuates neutropenia and alveolar capillary membrane injury during gram negative sepsis. Surgery 110:205, 1991

118. Fink MP: Therapeutic options directed against platelet activating factor, eicosanoids, and bradykinin in sepsis. J Antimicrob Chemother 41(suppl A):81, 1998

119. Nathens AB, Neff M, Jurkovich GJ, et al: Antioxidant supplementation in the critically ill surgical patient. Abstract 12. Presented at the 21st annual meeting of the Surgical Infection Society, May 3, 2001, Snowbird, Utah

120. Krysztopik RJ, Bentley FR, Spain DA, et al: Free radical scavenging by lazaroids improves renal blood flow during sepsis. Surgery 120:657, 1996

121. Pou S, Keaton L, Surichamorn W, et al: Can

nitric oxide be spin trapped by nitrone and nitroso compounds? Biochim Biophys Acta 1201:118, 1994

122. Bone RC, Grodzin CJ, Bulk RA: Sepsis: a new hypothesis for pathogenesis of the disease process. Chest 112:235, 1997

123. Maher DW, Davis I, Boyd AW, et al: Human interleukin-4: an immunomodulator with potential therapeutic application. Prog Growth Factor Res 3:43, 1991

124. De Waal Malefyt R, Abrams J, Bennet B, et al: Interleukin10 (IL-10) inhibits cytokine synthesis by human monocytes: an autoregulatory role of IL-10 production by monocytes. J Exp Med 174:1209, 1991

125. De Vries JE: Molecular and biological characteristics of interleukin-13. Chem Immunol 63:204, 1996

126. Wahl SM, McCartney-Francis N, Mergenhagen SE: Inflammatory and immunomodulatory roles of TGF-β. Immunol Today 10:258, 1989

127. Faist E, Schinkel C, Zimmer S: Update on the mechanisms of immune suppression of injury and immune modulation. World J Surg 20:454, 1996

128. Polk HC Jr, Cheadle WG, Livingston DH, et al: A randomized prospective clinical trial to determine the efficacy of interferon-gamma in severely injured patients. Am J Surg 163:191, 1992

129. Meakins JL, Christou NV, Shizgal HM, et al: Therapeutic approaches to anergy in surgical patients: surgery and levamisole. Ann Surg 190:286, 1979

130. Brown GL, Foshee H, Pietsch J, et al: Muramyl dipeptide enhances survival for experimental peritonitis. Arch Surg 121:47, 1986

131. O'Reilly M, Silver GM, Greenhalgh DG, et al: Treatment of intra-abdominal infection with granulocyte colony-stimulating factor. J Trauma 33:679, 1992

132. Stern AC, Jones TC: Role of human recombinant GM-CSF in the prevention and treatment of leukopenia with special reference to infectious disease. Diagn Microbiol Infect Dis 13:391, 1990

133. Xing Z, Ohkawara Y, Jordana M, et al: A transient transgenic model of IL-10 functional studies in vivo: adenoviral-mediated intramuscular IL-10 gene transfer inhibits cytokine responses in endotoxemia. Gene Therapy 4:140, 1997

134. Ezurum SC, Lemarchand P, Rosenfeld MA, et al: Protection of human endothelial cells from oxidant injury by adenovirus-mediated transfer of the human catalase cDNA. Nucleic Acids Research 21:1607, 1993

135. Canonico AE, Conary JT, Meyrick BO, et al: Aerosol and intravenous transfection of human alpha-1 antitrypsin gene to lungs of rabbits. Am J Respir Cell Mol Biol 10:24, 1994

136. De Maio A: The heat-shock response. New Horizons 3:198, 1995

137. Rojanasakul Y, Weissman DN, Shi X, et al: Antisense inhibition of silica-induced tumor necrosis factor in alveolar macrophages. J Biol Chem 272:3910, 1997

138. Maier JAM, Voulalas P, Roeder D, et al: Extension of the life-span of human endothelial cells by an interleukin-1 alpha antisense oligomer. Science 249:1570, 1990

16 ANTIBIOTICS

Nicolas V. Christou, M.D., F.A.C.S.

Antibiotic Therapy in Surgical Patients

Several important advances in antimicrobial therapy have been made since the early 1980s. Among these advances are (1) improved understanding of the microbiologic spectrum of so-called optimal therapy, (2) better application of pharmacokinetic principles to drug administration, (3) the development of several new classes of antibiotics, and (4) greater insight into the interplay among host resistance factors, microorganisms, and chemotherapy.

General Principles of Antimicrobial Therapy

EMPIRICAL THERAPY

Even with the most rapid bacteriologic tests currently available, it may not be possible to identify a pathogen in less than 24 hours, and antimicrobial sensitivities can rarely be obtained in less than 48 to 72 hours. In seriously ill patients, treatment cannot be delayed for 2 to 3 days until these data become available. If therapy is to be successful, it must be started as soon as a life-threatening infection is diagnosed or, in some patients, as soon as such an infection is suspected. Which antimicrobial agents are to be used depends on the suspected site of infection and on the organisms that are commonly pathogenic at this site. Therapy is initiated with an agent or combination of agents whose action is broad enough to cover all the suspected microbial pathogens. The application of such broad-spectrum antibiotic therapy in the absence of microbiologic confirmation is termed empirical therapy.

To make a rational decision regarding empirical therapy, the surgeon must be familiar with the organisms that are likely to be encountered when a particular infection (e.g., an intra-abdominal abscess) is suspected. Selection of the agent or agents is based on the history, the physical examination, where the infection was likely to have been acquired, the host defense status, the overall clinical severity of the infection, and the response of the host. Definitive therapy is initiated after the host response to the infection and to the empirical treatment has been monitored and the results from the microbiology laboratory—specifically, identification of the isolated organisms and the minimal inhibitory concentrations (MICs) of various antimicrobial agents—have been assessed.

LABORATORY TESTS

Many laboratory tests, if used in the proper context, can guide selection of optimal antimicrobial therapy.

In vitro susceptibility tests are indicated when the susceptibility of an organism is not completely predictable or when certain other specific problems arise, such as the necessity of determining whether resistance has developed during the course of therapy. An organism is generally considered susceptible if the concentration of antimicrobial agent necessary to inhibit its growth is lower than that usually attainable in body fluids, particularly blood, cerebrospinal fluid, or urine.

The disk diffusion method has been standardized by the National Committee for Clinical Laboratory Standards (NCCLS)[1] for in vitro susceptibility testing. Commercially available paper disks containing specific amounts of antimicrobial agents are placed on Mueller-Hinton agar plates that contain a standard bacterial inoculum. A zone of inhibition of bacterial growth develops around each active antibiotic after overnight incubation. The size of the zone determines the organism's susceptibility or resistance; prior studies have correlated zone sizes with MICs obtained through dilution tests. Arbitrary zone-size break points for susceptibility have been established by clinical and laboratory investigators on the basis of such additional factors as achievable serum levels, degree of protein binding, and toxicity.

The broth dilution method exposes an inoculum of bacteria to various concentrations of an antimicrobial agent during incubation. The MIC of an agent that inhibits growth can be determined, and this value can be correlated with blood, urine, or other body fluid levels of the antimicrobial agent. Moreover, those tubes that show inhibition of growth can be subcultured to an antimicrobial-free medium, and the minimal bactericidal concentration (MBC) can be determined. Unfortunately, this test is not well standardized at present, and its reproducibility is poor when it is subjected to intralaboratory and interlaboratory comparisons.[2]

The agar dilution method works in much the same way as the broth dilution method, except that the former employs agar plates that contain various dilutions of antimicrobial agents, and as many as 36 organisms can be efficiently inoculated on each plate by means of a replicator device. The MIC is determined by reading inhibition of colony growth on the agar surface. Agar dilution has the advantage of producing MIC data efficiently in a laboratory that performs large numbers of tests daily.

In the serum bactericidal test (SBT), samples of the serum of the treated patient are obtained and incubated with the infecting organism in doubling dilutions with broth to determine the highest dilution that is bactericidal. (Not all antimicrobial agents exhibit bactericidal activity; some exhibit only bacteriostatic activity [*see Table 1*].) The drawing of serum specimens can be timed to coincide with anticipated peak and trough antimicrobial levels. In effect, this test indirectly assesses both the susceptibility of the organism and the serum concentration of the antimicrobial agent, as well as the interactions between serum and organism and serum and drug. The NCCLS has developed proposed guidelines for the SBT.[3] A comprehensive review of the technical and clinical considerations associated with the SBT has been published.[4]

Factors Influencing Application of Antimicrobial Therapy

ROUTE OF ADMINISTRATION

Many antibiotics are absorbed sufficiently well via the oral route to provide effective blood levels in patients with normal GI function.[5] The enteral absorption of some antimicrobials is impeded by food and some medications (e.g., antacids). Many antibiotics cannot be given intramuscularly because of local pain or necrosis at the injection site. Intravenous administration must be used in the treatment of major and life-threatening infections such as suppurative diffuse peritonitis. In many cases, patients are clinically stable during intravenous treatment, and it is often possible to discharge them and to administer parenteral antibiotics on an outpatient basis. Supervision by special teams of physicians, nurses, and pharmacists is required[6]; antibiotics can be administered either in the hospital outpatient department or at home if competent family members are available. New antibiotics with long half-lives can be used with improved intravenous catheters and delivery devices in simplified regimens; this leads to substantial economic benefits, enhanced patient comfort, and good therapeutic results with few complications.[7]

HOST FACTORS

Hypersensitivity to Antibiotics

Because of widespread exposure to antimicrobial agents, many patients develop allergies to them.[8] A careful history of hypersensitivity should thus be obtained [*see Hypersensitivity Reactions, below*].

Concurrent Illnesses

Patients with immunosuppressive illnesses are vulnerable to opportunistic pathogens. These patients may require broader antimicrobial coverage as well as intense therapy for ordinary pathogens. The same is true to a lesser extent for patients with a chronic debilitating illness. Patients with renal insufficiency or liver disease may be unusually susceptible to direct drug toxicity.

Pregnancy

The administration of antimicrobial agents during pregnancy and in the postpartum period poses several problems. Foremost is the question of safety, both for the mother and the fetus or neonate. Although most antibiotics cross the placenta and enter maternal milk, the concentrations to which the fetus or neonate is exposed vary widely. Because the immature liver may lack the enzymes required to metabolize certain drugs, pharmacokinetics and toxicities in the fetus are often very different from those in older children and adults. Teratogenicity is a major concern when any drug is administered during pregnancy. Finally, it may be necessary to alter the dosage schedules of drugs that appear to be safe to use during pregnancy; increases in maternal blood volume, glomerular filtration rule (GFR), and hepatic metabolic activity often reduce the maternal serum levels of antimicrobials by 10% to 50%, especially late in pregnancy and in the early postpartum period. In some women, delayed gastric emptying may reduce the absorption of antibiotics that have been administered orally during pregnancy.

Even though 25% to 40% of women receive antibiotics during pregnancy, data regarding safety and efficacy in this setting are often scarce. Some general recommendations have been proposed, but they are intended only as a guide [*see Table 2*]; in all cases, therapy must be individualized, and both the indications for antibiotics and the possible risks to mother and fetus must be considered. Individual decisions are also required for lactating mothers; although most antimicrobials appear safe for breast-fed infants, chloramphenicol and the tetracyclines should be avoided.[9]

Advanced Age

Physiologic changes that occur with age can alter the pharmacokinetics of antimicrobial agents. For example, decreased gastric acidity and intestinal motility can impair drug absorption; increased body fat and decreased serum albumin levels can alter drug distribution; and decreased hepatic blood flow and enzymatic action can delay drug metabolism. Although these factors have not consistently affected antibiotic levels in the elderly, the decrease in GFR that occurs with age can lead to the accumulation of drugs excreted by the kidney. The high therapeutic index of the penicillins and cephalosporins obviates major changes in dosage schedules in elderly patients who have normal serum creatinine levels. However, in the case of aminoglycosides and vancomycin, decreased dosage schedules are often required; ideally, drug levels should be measured and renal function should be monitored when these agents are given. The dosage of amantadine and rimantadine should also be reduced in elderly patients.

Antibiotic Selection for Infections in Surgical Patients

The term surgical infection is difficult to define, but for the purposes of this chapter, it means infections that are related to surgical procedures or that require, in addition to antibiotic therapy, surgical debridement or control of the source of the infection. Such infections include infections of the soft tissues of the integument; muscles; bones; and body cavities (e.g., empyema, intra-abdominal infections, pyelonephritis, and infections of the retroperitoneum).

A framework for antibiotic selection for intra-abdominal infections is presented [*see Table 3*]; this framework can be modified for the selection of antibiotic for other types of surgical infection. A therapeutic regimen for the treatment of intra-abdominal infection should include agents that are active against *Staphylococcus aureus*, enteric gram-negative bacilli, and anaerobes, including *Bacteroides fragilis*. The regimen that has been regarded as the gold standard consists of an aminoglycoside, to cover the enteric gram-negative organisms, and clindamycin or metronidazole, to cover the anaerobes; other approaches, however, look promising.

A well-designed, controlled, prospective, randomized trial that compared imipenem therapy with acceptable aminoglycoside-based regimens supports the use of imipenem as monotherapy for intra-abdominal infections in which an enteric mixed flora is anticipated.[10] When the analysis was restricted to the residual effect of treatment assignment, a significant improvement in outcome was found in the patients receiving imipenem ($P = 0.043$).

Table 1 Bactericidal and Bacteriostatic Agents[155]

Bactericidal Agents	Bacteriostatic Agents
Aminoglycosides*	Chloramphenicol
Aztreonam	Clindamycin
Bacitracin	Erythromycin
Cephalosporins	Sulfonamides
Imipenem	Tetracyclines
Penicillins	Trimethoprim
Polymyxins†	
Quinolones‡	
Vancomycin	

*Including streptomycin, neomycin, kanamycin, gentamicin, tobramycin, amikacin, and netilmicin.
†Including polymyxin B and colistimethate.
‡Including norfloxacin and ciprofloxacin.

Table 2 Antibiotics in Pregnancy[155]

Drug	Major Toxic Potential		Pharmacology	
	Maternal	Fetal	Maternal Serum Levels	Excreted in Mother's Milk
Considered safe				
Cephalosporins	Allergies	None known	Decreased	Trace
Erythromycin base	Allergies, GI intolerance	None known	Decreased	Yes
Penicillins	Allergies	None known	Decreased	Trace
Spectinomycin	?	None known	?	?
Use with caution				
Aminoglycosides	Ototoxicity, nephrotoxicity	Ototoxicity	Decreased	Yes
Clindamycin	Allergies, colitis	None known	Unchanged	Trace
Ethambutol	Optic neuritis	Probably safe	?	?
Isoniazid	Allergies, hepatotoxicity	Neuropathy, seizures	Unchanged	Yes
Rifampin	Hypersensitivity, hepatotoxicity	Probably safe	Unchanged	Yes
Sulfonamides (contraindicated at term)	Allergies, crystalluria	Kernicterus (at term), hemolysis (G6PD deficiency)	Unchanged	Yes
Avoid if possible				
Metronidazole	Hypersensitivity, alcohol intolerance, neuropathy	None known (teratogenic in animals)	Probably unchanged	Yes
Contraindicated				
Chloramphenicol	Blood dyscrasias	Gray syndrome	Unchanged	Yes
Erythromycin estolate	Hepatotoxicity	None known	Decreased	Yes
Nalidixic acid	GI intolerance	Increased intracranial pressure	?	?
Nitrofurantoin	Allergies, neuropathy, GI intolerance	Hemolysis (G6PD deficiency)	Decreased	Trace
Norfloxacin, ciprofloxacin, ofloxacin, lomefloxacin	GI intolerance	Arthropathies in immature animals	?	?
Tetracyclines	Hepatotoxicity, renal failure	Tooth discoloration and dysplasia, impaired bone growth	Probably unchanged	Yes
Trimethoprim	Hypersensitivity	Teratogenicity	Unchanged	Yes

Meropenem was found to be as effective as imipenem for the treatment of moderately severe intra-abdominal infections.[11]

Ertapenem has a pharmacokinetic profile and an antimicrobial spectrum that support its use as a once-daily agent for the treatment of common mixed aerobic and anaerobic infections. A prospective, randomized, controlled, double-blind trial compared ertapenem with piperacillin-tazobactam as therapy following adequate surgical management of complicated intra-abdominal infections. The modified intent-to-treat population consisted of 633 patients, of whom 396 met all criteria for the evaluable population. Patients with a wide range of infections were enrolled. A prospective expert-panel review was conducted to assess the adequacy of surgical source control in patients in whom therapeutic failure was a component of evaluability. For the modified intent-to-treat groups, 245 of 311 patients treated with ertapenem (78.8%) were cured; 232 of 304 patients (76.3%) treated with piperacillin-tazobactam were cured. Of 203 microbiologically evaluable patients treated with ertapenem, 176 (86.7%) were cured; 157 of the 193 patients (81.3%) treated with piperacillin-tazobactam were cured. In this study, ertapenem, 1 g once a day, was equivalent to piperacillin-tazobactam, 3.375 g every 6 hours, in the treatment of a range of intra-abdominal infections. Ertapenem may be a useful option that could eliminate the need for combination therapy, multidose antibiotic regimens, or both for the empirical treatment of intra-abdominal infections.[12]

Appropriate surgical control of the source of the intra-abdominal infection is of utmost importance in determining outcome; antibiotics play a necessary but secondary role.[13,14] The controversies regarding the pathogenicity of enterococci have been addressed by guidelines published by members of the Surgical Infection Society.[15] The third-generation cephalosporins have been proposed as candidates for single-agent therapy for infection in the abdominal cavity because their spectra of activity encompass both the aerobic gram-negative bacilli and some of the anaerobic isolates that cause infection in this region. No cephalosporin, of any generation, has been shown to have a clear advantage over an aminoglycoside-clindamycin combination in the treatment of intra-abdominal infections.

Interpretation of overall results in intra-abdominal infections is difficult because of the numerous variables involved, including the diversity of the possible infectious processes, the variable quality of the surgical technique employed, the variety of the patient characteristics observed, the possibility of one or more underlying diseases, and the differing doses of antibiotics used in individual studies.[16] Most third-generation cephalosporins do not cover anaerobes well and should be used in conjunction with an antianaerobic agent, such as clindamycin or metronidazole, for empirical therapy for serious intra-abdominal infections. In a recent prospective, randomized, double-blind study, cefoxitin was found to be comparable to imipenem with regard to outcome (defined as survival); failure to cure infections was attributed to resistant organisms at the primary site in the cefoxitin arm of the trial.[17]

Adverse Reactions to Antimicrobial Agents

There are three general types of adverse reactions to antimicrobial agents: hypersensitivity reactions (which are not dose related), direct drug toxicity (which usually is dose related and

Table 3 Antibiotic Selection for Infections in Surgical Patients

Type of Infection	Expected Pathogen	First Choice I.V. Rx	Second Choice I.V. Rx	Switch to P.O. Choice
Brain infection (abscess, subdural empyema, intracranial suppurative thrombophlebitis)				
Traumatic brain injury	*Staphylococcus aureus,* Enterobacteriaceae, *Pseudomonas aeruginosa*	Cefepime, 2 g I.V. q. 8 hr	Meropenem, 1 g I.V. q. 8 hr	Not recommended
Postneurosurgical procedure	*S. aureus, S. epidermidis*	Nafcillin, 2 g I.V. q. 4 hr *or* Cefepime, 2 g I.V. q. 8 hr *or* If methicillin resistant: Linezolide, 600 mg I.V. q. 12 hr	Meropenem, 1 g I.V. q. 8 hr	Linezolid, 600 mg p.o., q. 12 hr
Vascular graft infection				
Arteriovenous graft/shunt	*S. aureus,* Enterobacteriaceae, enterococci	Vancomycin, 1 g I.V. *plus* Gentamicin, 240 mg I.V. and remove graft	Meropenem, 1 g I.V. q. 8 hr and remove graft	Moxifloxacin, 400 mg p.o. and remove graft
Aortic graft (treat with antibiotics until graft is replaced)	*S. aureus, S. epidermidis,* Enterobacteriaceae	Cefepime, 2 g I.V. q. 12 hr *or* Imipenem, 1 g I.V. q. 8 hr *or* Meropenem, 1 g I.V. q. 8 hr	Ceftizoxime, 2 g I.V. q. 8 hr *or* Cefotaxime, 2 g I.V. q. 6 hr	Levofloxacin, 500 mg p.o., q. 24 hr *or* Moxifloxacin, 400 mg p.o., q. 24 hr
Intra-abdominal infection (peritonitis, abscess)				
Gastric perforation (peptic ulcer disease)	*Candida,* oral anaerobes, *S. aureus*	Cefazolin, 1 g I.V. q. 8 hr	Ceftizoxime, 2 g I.V. q. 8 hr *or* Cefotaxime, 2 g I.V. q. 6 hr	Levofloxacin, 500 mg p.o., q. 24 hr *or* Moxifloxacin, 400 mg p.o., q. 24 hr
Gastric perforation (malignancy)	*S. aureus, S. epidermidis,* Enterobacteriaceae, *Candida*	Cefepime, 2 g I.V. q. 12 hr *or* Imipenem, 1 g I.V. q. 8 hr *or* Meropenem, 1 g I.V. q. 8 hr	Ceftizoxime, 2 g I.V. q. 8 hr *or* Cefotaxime, 2 g I.V. q. 6 hr	Levofloxacin, 500 mg p.o., q. 24 hr *or* Moxifloxacin, 400 mg p.o., q. 24 hr
Cholecystitis with gangrene/perforation	*Escherichia coli, Klebsiella,* enterococci	Piperacillin-tazobactam, 4.5 g I.V. q. 8 hr	Cefotaxime, 2 g I.V. q. 6 hr	Levofloxacin, 500 mg p.o., q. 24 hr *or* Moxifloxacin, 400 mg p.o., q. 24 hr
Emphysematous cholecystitis	*Clostridium perfringens*	Piperacillin-tazobactam, 4.5 g I.V. q. 8 hr	Ertapenem, 1 g I.V. q. 24 hr	Clindamycin, 300 mg p.o., q. 8 hr
Ascending cholangitis	*E. coli, Klebsiella,* enterococci	Imipenem, 1 g I.V. q. 8 hr *or* Meropenem, 1 g I.V. q. 8 hr	Cefoperazone, 2 g I.V. q. 12 hr	Levofloxacin, 500 mg p.o., q. 24 hr *or* Moxifloxacin, 400 mg p.o., q. 24 hr
Infected hemorrhagic/ necrotizing pancreatitis	Enterobacteriaceae, *Bacteroides fragilis*	Imipenem, 1 g I.V. q. 8 hr *or* Meropenem, 1 g I.V. q. 8 hr *or* Ertapenem, 1 g I.V. q. 24 hr	Piperacillin-tazobactam, 4.5 g I.V. q. 8 hr *or* Ampicillin-sulbactam, 3 g I.V. q. 6 hr	Clindamycin, 300 mg p.o., q. 8 hr *plus* Levofloxacin, 500 mg p.o., q. 24 hr *or* Moxifloxacin, 400 mg p.o., q. 24 hr
Liver abscess (bacterial)	Enterobacteriaceae, *B. fragilis*	Imipenem, 1 g I.V. q. 8 hr *or* Meropenem, 1 g I.V. q. 8 hr *or* Ertapenem, 1 g I.V. q. 24 hr	Metronidazole, 1 g I.V. q. 24 hr *plus* Levofloxacin, 500 mg I.V. q. 24 hr *or* Moxifloxacin, 400 mg I.V. q. 24 hr	Metronidazole, 500 mg p.o., q. 12 hr *plus* Levofloxacin, 500 mg p.o., q. 24 hr *or* Moxifloxacin, 400 mg p.o., q. 24 hr
Liver abscess (amebiasis)	*Entamoeba histolytica*	Metronidazole, 750 mg p.o., q. 8 hr	Tinidazole, 2 g/day p.o. in three divided doses	Not applicable

(continued)

Table 3 (continued)

Type of Infection	Expected Pathogen	First Choice I.V. Rx	Second Choice I.V. Rx	Switch to P.O. Choice
Intra-abdominal Infection (peritonitis, abscess) (continued)				
Distal small bowel, appendix, colon, rectum perforation in nonhospitalized patient (mild to moderate infection)	Enterobacteriaceae, enterococci, B. fragilis	Piperacillin-tazobactam, 4.5 g I.V. q. 8 hr *or* Ertapenem, 1 g I.V. q. 24 hr	Cefoxitin, 2 g I.V. q. 6 hr *or* Ampicillin-sulbactam, 3 g I.V. q. 6 hr	Ciprofloxacin, 250–750 mg p.o., q. 12 hr *plus* Metronidazole, 500 mg p.o., q. 12 hr
Distal small bowel, appendix, colon, rectum perforation in hospitalized patient (severe infection requiring ICU support)	Enterobacteriaceae, enterococci, B. fragilis, P. aeruginosa, Acinetobacter	Imipenem, 1 g I.V. q. 8 hr *or* Meropenem, 1 g I.V. q. 8 hr	Tobramycin, 5 mg/ kg loading dose, then 3 mg/kg I.V. q. 8 hr *plus* Clindamycin, 900 mg I.V. q. 8 hr	Moxifloxacin, 400 mg p.o., q. 24 hr
Spontaneous bacterial peritonitis	Enterobacteriaceae	Ciprofloxacin, 400 mg I.V. q. 12 hr	Cefepime, 2 g I.V. q. 12 hr	Ciprofloxacin, 250–750 mg p.o., q. 12 hr *plus* Metronidazole, 500 mg p.o., q. 12 hr
Pelvic inflammatory disease (tubo-ovarian abscess, salpingitis, endometritis, infected abortion)				
Mild to moderate infection (outpatients)	Enterobacteriaceae, B. fragilis, Neisseria gonorrhoeae, Chlamydia trachomatis	Moxifloxacin, 400 mg p.o., q. 24 hr	None	Ciprofloxacin, 250–750 mg p.o., q. 12 hr *plus* Doxycycline, 100 mg p.o., q. 12 hr
Severe infection (hospitalized patient)	Enterobacteriaceae, B. fragilis, N. gonorrhoeae, C. trachomatis	Doxycycline, 200 mg I.V. q. 12 hr *plus* Clindamycin, 600 mg I.V. q. 8 hr	Levofloxacin, 500 mg p.o., q. 24 hr *plus* Metronidazole, 1 g I.V. q. 24 hr	Moxifloxacin, 400 mg p.o., q. 24 hr

manifests in a single organ or, occasionally, in several organs), and microbial superinfection.

HYPERSENSITIVITY REACTIONS

A history of allergies should be taken before antimicrobial therapy is initiated in any patient. More information is available regarding allergies to the penicillins than allergies to other agents, but skin eruptions, drug fever, and even anaphylaxis may be produced by many antibiotics. Allergic reactions occur in 1% to 10% of patients who receive penicillin. Fatal anaphylactic reactions are much less frequent.

DIRECT DRUG TOXICITY

Although antimicrobials can produce damage to virtually all human organ systems, the potential for toxicity varies widely from drug to drug.[18] The principal antibiotics that are directly toxic to the kidney are aminoglycosides, polymyxins, and amphotericin B; azotemia and renal tubular damage may be caused by any of these drugs. Patients with preexisting renal insufficiency are at increased risk for toxic reactions to various antibiotics, including nephrotoxicity, coagulopathies and other hematologic toxicities, seizures, and ototoxicity and other neurotoxicities.

Penicillins, cephalosporins, tetracyclines, and rifampin can cause hemolytic anemia, thrombocytopenia, and leukopenia that involve an immune mechanism, but these reactions are uncommon. Macrolides and trimethoprim-sulfamethoxazole have been associated with agranulocytosis. Trimethoprim can produce anemia, leukopenia, and thrombocytopenia from folate deficiency; the effect is reversible with folinic acid. Amphotericin B commonly produces a reversible normocytic normochromic anemia,

probably secondary to injury to the red cell membrane. Flucytosine causes bone marrow suppression (leukopenia or pancytopenia) when its excretion is reduced by renal failure. Linezolid can also produce myelosuppression; although experience is limited, bone marrow function usually recovers when the drug is discontinued. Neutropenia can occur during therapy with penicillins, cephalosporins, or vancomycin. It may be severe, but it is self-limited; recovery occurs 1 to 7 days after the antibiotic is withdrawn. Penicillins inhibit platelet aggregation by adenosine diphosphate, which may account for the bleeding that occurs in some patients receiving these antibiotics in high doses. Various cephalosporins may produce coagulopathies by prolonging the prothrombin time; the methylthiotetrazole side chain present in cephalosporins such as cefotetan appears to be responsible.

Antibiotics may produce a wide range of toxic effects on the central and peripheral nervous systems. Ototoxicity, either vestibular or auditory, can be produced by any of the aminoglycosides; neuromuscular blockade is much less common. Minocycline has occasionally been reported to produce significant vestibular reactions. Vancomycin can cause auditory neurotoxicity. Intravenous administration of large doses of penicillin and other β-lactams may produce seizures, especially when administered in very high doses or when given to azotemic patients or to patients with underlying epilepsy.

Metronidazole can sometimes cause ataxia, encephalopathy, seizures, or peripheral neuropathies. Ofloxacin has been reported to cause seizures; mania has been attributed to clarithromycin. Optic neuritis, usually manifested by decreased visual acuity and decreased perception of the color green, may occur as a side effect of ethambutol.

Table 4 Antimicrobial Drugs of Choice for Various Infections in Adults[18]

	Causative Organism	Drug of Choice	Alternative Drugs
Gram-Positive Cocci	*Staphylococcus aureus* Methicillin-sensitive Methicillin-resistant[1]	Vancomycin,[2] with or without rifampin or gentamicin Penicillinase-resistant penicillin[5]	Linezolid; quinupristin-dalfopristin Trimethoprim-sulfamethoxazole (TMP-SMX),[2] with or without rifampin[2]; a fluoroquinolone[3]; a tetracycline[4] A cephalosporin,[6] clindamycin, vancomycin,[7] meropenem or imipenem,[8] ticarcillin–clavulanic acid, ampicillin-sulbactam, amoxicillin–clavulanic acid, piperacillin-tazobactam, a fluoroquinolone[3]
	Coagulase-negative staphylococci[9]	Vancomycin,[7] with or without rifampin[2] or gentamicin	Linezolid, quinupristin-dalfopristin, a cephalosporin, a penicillinase-resistant penicillin, meropenem or imipenem,[8] a fluoroquinolone[3]
	Anaerobic streptococcus (*Peptostreptococcus*)	Penicillin G[10]	Clindamycin, a cephalosporin,[6] vancomycin[7]
	Streptococcus bovis	Penicillin G[10,11]	A cephalosporin,[6] vancomycin[7]
	Groups A, G, and C streptococci	Penicillin G[10,12] or penicillin V	A cephalosporin,[6] vancomycin,[7] an erythromycin,[13] clindamycin, clarithromycin, azithromycin
	Group B streptococcus	Penicillin G[10,12] or ampicillin	A cephalosporin,[6] vancomycin,[7] an erythromycin
	S. pneumoniae (pneumococcus) Penicillin sensitive	Penicillin G[10,12] or penicillin V, amoxicillin	An erythromycin,[12,13] a cephalosporin,[6] meropenem or imipenem,[8] vancomycin,[7,12] azithromycin, clarithromycin, a fluoroquinolone; a tetracycline[4]
	Non–penicillin sensitive	Vancomycin; ceftriaxone or cefotaxime[6]; levofloxacin, moxifloxacin, or gatifloxacin[3]; linezolid; quinupristin-dalfopristin; imipenem or meropenem	—
	Viridans streptococcus	Penicillin G,[10,11] with or without gentamicin	A cephalosporin,[6] vancomycin[7]
	Enterococcus Endocarditis or other serious infection	Penicillin or ampicillin, plus gentamicin[14] or streptomycin	Vancomycin,[7] with gentamicin or streptomycin; linezolid; quinupristin-dalfopristin
	Uncomplicated urinary tract infection	Ampicillin or amoxicillin	A fluoroquinolone,[3] nitrofurantoin,[15] fosfomycin
Gram-Positive Bacilli	*Bacillus cereus, B. subtilis*	Vancomycin	Meropenem or imipenem,[8] clindamycin
	Bacillus anthracis	Penicillin G	Ciprofloxacin,[3] a tetracycline,[4] an erythromycin[2]
	Clostridium difficile	Metronidazole[16]	Vancomycin[16]
	C. perfringens	Penicillin G; clindamycin	Metronidazole, meropenem or imipenem,[8] chloramphenicol[7]
	C. tetani	Metronidazole	Penicillin G, a tetracycline[4]
	Corynebacterium diphtheriae	An erythromycin	Penicillin G
	Corynebacterium, JK group	Vancomycin	Penicillin G, with gentamicin; an erythromycin
	Listeria monocytogenes	Ampicillin, with or without gentamicin	TMP-SMX
	Propionibacterium	Penicillin G	Clindamycin, an erythromycin
Gram-Negative Cocci	*Moraxella* (formerly *Branhamella*) *catarrhalis*	Cefuroxime,[6] a fluoroquinolone[3]	TMP-SMX, amoxicillin–clavulanic acid, an erythromycin, a tetracycline, third-generation cephalosporins, clarithromycin, azithromycin
	Neisseria gonorrhoeae[17]	Ceftriaxone or cefixime,[6] ciprofloxacin, ofloxacin, or gatifloxacin[3]	Cefotaxime,[10] penicillin or ampicillin
	N. meningitidis Meningitis, bacteremia	Penicillin G	A third-generation cephalosporin,[6] TMP-SMX, a fluoroquinolone,[3] chloramphenicol[7]
	Carrier state	Rifampin	Minocycline, ciprofloxacin
Enteric Gram-Negative Bacilli	*Bacteroides* GI tract strains (*B. fragilis*)	Metronidazole or clindamycin	Cefoxitin, cefotetan, ceftizoxime, or cefmetazole; chloramphenicol[18]; imipenem or meropenem[8]; ticarcillin–clavulanic acid; ampicillin-sulbactam, piperacillin-tazobactam
	Respiratory tract strains	Penicillin G or clindamycin	Metronidazole, cefoxitin,[6] cefotetan, ceftizoxime, cefmetazole, chloramphenicol[7]
	Campylobacter fetus	Imipenem or meropenem[8]	Gentamicin
	C. jejuni	Azithromycin or an erythromycin	A fluoroquinolone,[3] a tetracycline,[4] gentamicin[7]
	Citrobacter	Imipenem or meropenem[8]	A fluoroquinolone,[3] amikacin; TMP-SMX; a tetracycline[4]; a third-generation cephalosporin[6]
	Enterobacter	Imipenem or meropenem[8]	A third-generation cephalosporin[6]; for serious infections, use with a fluoroquinolone[3] or gentamicin; gentamicin, tobramycin, amikacin, a fluoroquinolone,[3] a carboxypenicillin or acylaminopenicillin,[19] aztreonam[20]
	Escherichia coli	Ampicillin, a cephalosporin,[6] a fluoroquinolone,[3] TMP-SMX[22]	Gentamicin,[21] tobramycin, amikacin, imipenem or meropenem,[8] aztreonam[20]

Note: all superscript numbers refer to footnotes that follow table.

(continued)

Table 4 (*continued*)

	Causative Organism	Drug of Choice	Alternative Drugs
Enteric Gram-Negative Bacilli (continued)	*Helicobacter pylori*	Tetracycline with metronidazole and bismuth subsalicylate or omeprazole with amoxicillin and clarithromycin	Amoxicillin with metronidazole and bismuth subsalicylate; tetracycline with clarithromycin and bismuth subsalicylate; clarithromycin with omeprazole; amoxicillin with clarithromycin
	Klebsiella	A cephalosporin[6]	Imipenem or meropenem,[9] gentamicin,[23] tobramycin, amikacin, TMP-SMX,[21] a carboxypenicillin or acylaminopenicillin,[21] amoxicillin–clavulanic acid, ampicillin-sulbactam, ticarcillin–clavulanic acid, piperacillin-tazobactam, aztreonam,[20] a fluoroquinolone[3]
	Proteus mirabilis	Ampicillin	A cephalosporin, gentamicin or tobramycin, chloramphenicol,[7] a carboxypenicillin or acylaminopenicillin,[19] imipenem or meropenem,[8] TMP-SMX, aztreonam,[20] a fluoroquinolone[3]
	non-*mirabilis*, including *P. vulgaris*, *Morganella morganii*, and *Providencia rettgeri*	A third-generation cephalosporin[6]	Gentamicin, tobramycin, amikacin, a carboxypenicillin or acylaminopenicillin,[19] imipenem or meropenem,[8] aztreonam,[20] ampicillin-sulbactam, ticarcillin–clavulanic acid, piperacillin-tazobactam, amoxicillin–clavulanic acid, a fluoroquinolone[3]
	Providencia stuartii	A third-generation cephalosporin[6]	An aminoglycoside, TMP-SMX,[21] imipenem or meropenem,[8] aztreonam,[20] a carboxypenicillin or acylaminopenicillin,[19] a fluoroquinolone[3]
	Salmonella typhi	Ceftriaxone or a fluoroquinolone[3]	Chloramphenicol or ampicillin,[22] TMP-SMX
	Other *Salmonella* species	Ceftriaxone or cefotaxime or a fluoroquinolone[3]	Ampicillin or amoxicillin, TMP-SMX, chloramphenicol[7]
	Serratia	Imipenem or meropenem	A third-generation cephalosporin,[6] gentamicin or amikacin, a carboxypenicillin or acylaminopenicillin,[19] chloramphenicol,[7] aztreonam, a fluoroquinolone[3]
	Shigella	A fluoroquinolone[3]	TMP-SMX, ampicillin, ceftriaxone, azithromycin
Other Gram-Negative Bacilli	*Acinetobacter (Herellea)*	Imipenem or meropenem[8]	Tobramycin, gentamicin, amikacin, doxycycline, minocycline, a carboxypenicillin or acylaminopenicillin,[19] TMP-SMX, a fluoroquinolone,[3] ceftazidime
	Aeromonas hydrophilia	TMP-SMX[2]	A fluoroquinolone,[3] gentamicin, tobramycin, imipenem or meropenem[8]
	Bartonella henselae (cat-scratch disease)	Azithromycin	Ciprofloxacin,[3] TMP-SMX, gentamicin; rifampin, erythromycin
	Bartonella henselae (bacillary angiomatosis)	Erythromycin	Doxycycline, azithromycin
	Bordetella pertussis (whooping cough)	Erythromycin	TMP-SMX; azithromycin or clarithromycin
	Brucella	A tetracycline, with rifampin	A tetracycline with gentamicin or streptomycin; chloramphenicol,[7] with or without streptomycin; TMP-SMX[2] with or without gentamicin; ciprofloxacin[3] with rifampin
	Eikenella corrodens	Ampicillin	An erythromycin, a tetracycline,[4] amoxicillin–clavulanic acid, ampicillin-sulbactam, ceftriaxone
	Francisella tularensis (tularemia)	Streptomycin	Gentamicin, a tetracycline,[4] chloramphenicol,[7] ciprofloxacin[3]
	Fusobacterium	Penicillin	Clindamycin, metronidazole, chloramphenicol;[7] cefoxitin
	Gardnerella (formerly *Haemophilus*) *vaginalis*	Metronidazole[2] (oral)	Intravaginal metronidazole, intravaginal or oral clindamycin
	Haemophilus influenzae Bronchitis, otitis media	TMP-SMX	Ampicillin or amoxicillin; a tetracycline;[4] amoxicillin–clavulanic acid, cefuroxime axetil, ceftizoxime, clarithromycin, azithromycin, a fluoroquinolone[3]
	Meningitis, epiglottitis, life-threatening infections	Cefotaxime or ceftriaxone	Chloramphenicol,[24] meropenem[9]
	Legionella species	Azithromycin or a fluoroquinolone[3]	Erythromycin, rifampin,[25] TMP-SMX,[2] doxycycline[4]
	Pasteurella multocida	Penicillin G	A tetracycline,[4] a cephalosporin,[6] amoxicillin–clavulanic acid, ampicillin-sulbactam
	Calymmatobacterium granulomatis (granuloma inguinale)	TMP-SMX	A tetracycline;[4] ciprofloxacin with or without rifampin
	H. ducreyi (chancroid)	Ceftriaxone or azithromycin	A fluoroquinolone[3]
	Pseudomonas aeruginosa Urinary tract infections	Ciprofloxacin[3]	Levofloxacin; gentamicin or tobramycin; amikacin; ceftazidime,[6] with or without gentamicin or tobramycin; imipenem or meropenem;[8] aztreonam,[20] a carboxypenicillin or acylaminopenicillin[19]
	Other infections	Gentamicin or tobramycin, with or without a carboxypenicillin or acylaminopenicillin[19]; ceftazidime or cefipime; imipenem or meropenem;[8] aztreonam,[20] alone or with gentamicin or tobramycin	Amikacin, with or without a carboxypenicillin or acylaminopenicillin[19]; ciprofloxacin[7]
	P. cepacia	TMP-SMX	Chloramphenicol,[7] ceftazidime,[2] imipenem[2,8] or meropenem[8]
	Streptobacillus moniliformis (rat-bite fever)	Penicillin G	A tetracycline,[4] streptomycin

Note: all superscript numbers refer to footnotes that follow table.

(continued)

Table 4 (continued)

	Causative Organism	Drug of Choice	Alternative Drugs
Other Gram-Negative Bacilli (continued)	Vibrio cholerae	A tetracycline[4]	TMP-SMX, a fluoroquinolone[3]
	V. vulnificus	A tetracycline[4]	Cefotaxime
	Agents of Vincent stomatitis (trench mouth)	Penicillin G	A tetracycline,[4] an erythromycin
	Stenotrophomonas (formerly Xanthomonas) maltophilia	TMP-SMX	Minocycline, ceftazidime,[6] a fluoroquinolone[3]
	Yersinia enterocolitica	TMP-SMX[2]	A fluoroquinolone, gentamicin,[2] tobramycin,[2] amikacin, cefotaxime[2,6] or ceftizoxime[2,6]
	Y. pestis (plague)	Streptomycin with or without a tetracycline	A tetracycline,[4] chloramphenicol,[7] gentamicin,[2] TMP-SMX
Acid-Fast Bacilli	Mycobacterium avium complex	Clarithromycin or azithromycin plus one or more of the following: ethambutol, rifabutin, ciprofloxacin	Rifampin, amikacin
	M. fortuitum	Amikacin[2] with clarithromycin	Rifampin,[2] cefoxitin, a sulfonamide, doxycycline, ethambutol, linezolid
	M. kansasii	Isoniazid with rifampin, with or without ethambutol or streptomycin	Cycloserine, ethionamide, clarithromycin
	M. leprae	Dapsone[7] with rifampin, with or without clofazimine	Minocycline,[4] ofloxacin or sparfloxacin,[3] clarithromycin
	M. marinum (balnei)[26]	Minocycline	TMP-SMX, rifampin, clarithromycin, doxycycline
	M. tuberculosis[27]	Isoniazid with rifampin, and pyrazinamide with or without ethambutol or streptomycin	Ciprofloxacin or ofloxacin; third-line agent
Actinomycetes	Actinomyces israelii	Penicillin G	A tetracycline[4]; an erythromycin; clindamycin
	Nocardia	TMP-SMX	Minocycline, sulfisoxazole, imipenem or meropenem,[8] amikacin,[2] cycloserine, linezolid
Chlamydia	Chlamydia psittaci (psittacosis)	A tetracycline[4]	Chloramphenicol[7]
	C. trachomatis		
	Inclusion conjunctivitis	An erythromycin (oral or I.V.)	A sulfonamide (topical plus oral)
	Lymphogranuloma venereum	A tetracycline[4]	An erythromycin
	Pneumonia	An erythromycin	A sulfonamide
	Trachoma	Azithromycin	A tetracycline[4] (topical plus oral), a sulfonamide (topical plus oral)
	Urethritis or pelvic inflammatory disease	Doxycycline or azithromycin	Erythromycin, ofloxacin, amoxicillin
	C. pneumoniae	An erythromycin or clarithromycin or azithromycin; a fluoroquinolone	A tetracycline
Mycoplasma	Mycoplasma pneumoniae	An erythromycin, clarithromycin or azithromycin; a fluoroquinolone,[3] doxycycline[4]	—
	Ureaplasma urealyticum	An erythromycin	A tetracycline,[4] clarithromycin, or azithromycin; ofloxacin[3]
Rickettsia	Various rickettsial organisms Rocky Mountain spotted fever, epidemic and endemic (murine) typhus, rickettsial pox, Q fever, scrub typhus	Doxycycline[4]	Chloramphenicol,[7] a fluoroquinolone,[3] rifampin
Spirochetes	Borrelia burgdorferi (Lyme disease)	Doxycycline or amoxicillin or ceftriaxone	Penicillin, an erythromycin, clarithromycin, azithromycin, cefuroxime
	B. recurrentis (relapsing fever)	A tetracycline[4]	Penicillin G
	Leptospira	Penicillin G	A tetracycline,[4] an erythromycin
	Treponema pallidum	Penicillin G	A tetracycline,[4] an erythromycin, ceftriaxone

1. Some strains of S. aureus and most strains of coagulase-negative staphylococci are resistant to penicillinase-resistant penicillins; these strains are also resistant to cephalosporins.

2. Not approved for this indication by the FDA.

3. None of these drugs is recommended for children. In 1999, the FDA limited trovafloxacin to inpatient use for limb- or life-threatening infections.

4. Doxycycline is the safest tetracycline for treatment of extrarenal infections in renal insufficiency. Tetracyclines should be avoided in pregnant women and in children younger than 8 yr.

5. For severe infections, I.V. nafcillin or oxacillin should be used. For mild infections, oral cloxacillin, dicloxacillin, or oxacillin may be employed. Between 1% and 2% of S. aureus strains are resistant to penicillinase-resistant penicillins (and usually to cephalosporins) but are susceptible to vancomycin. High doses of penicillin G, ampicillin, amoxicillin, carbenicillin, or ticarcillin do not overcome the clinical resistance of penicillinase-producing staphylococci to these drugs.

6. Cephalosporins are sometimes used as alternatives to penicillin in patients with sus-

pected penicillin allergy but not in patients with serious hypersensitivity (especially immediate anaphylactic or accelerated urticarial reactions). Patients allergic to penicillin may be hypersensitive to cephalosporins. Only third-generation cephalosporins are effective in bacterial meningitis.

7. In view of the occurrence of adverse reactions, this drug should be used only for serious infections and when less toxic drugs are ineffective.

8. Imipenem and meropenem are β-lactam antibiotics that should be used with caution in patients who are allergic to penicillins and cephalosporins.

9. In vitro sensitivity testing with cephalosporins or penicillins may be misleading because of heteroresistance and because these antibiotics may be bacteriostatic only. For serious infections, vancomycin is preferred (see text).

10. Crystalline penicillin G is administered parenterally for serious infections. For less severe infections caused by pneumococci, group A streptococci, gonococci, or T. pallidum, procaine penicillin is administered I.M. once or twice daily. For mild infections caused by streptococci and pneumococci, oral penicillin V is preferable to oral penicillin G. Benzathine penicillin G is given I.M. (once monthly for the prophylaxis of rheumatic fever,

(continued)

Table 4   (continued)

a single injection for the treatment of group A streptococcal pharyngitis) when patients' compliance for oral medication is questionable and for treatment of syphilis, in one to three doses at weekly intervals, depending on the stage of the disease.

11. The combination of penicillin G with streptomycin for the first 2 wk of treatment of endocarditis caused by viridans streptococci is preferred by some.

12. In patients with major allergy to penicillin, erythromycin is the alternative for respiratory tract infections; chloramphenicol is the preferred alternative for meningitis. Occasional strains of pneumococci have high-level resistance to penicillin and to most other antibiotics except vancomycin.

13. Some strains of pneumococci and group A streptococci are erythromycin resistant.

14. Various aminoglycosides have been used in synergistic combination with penicillin or vancomycin. Because of the appearance of enterococcal strains resistant to the synergistic action with streptomycin (but not gentamicin), gentamicin is preferred for use in the combination.

15. Contraindicated in pregnancy or in the presence of renal insufficiency.

16. Antibiotics may be administered orally for antibiotic-associated pseudomembranous enterocolitis. Vancomycin and metronidazole are equally effective but metronidazole is much less expensive.

17. Large doses of penicillin G or ampicillin (or amoxicillin) may be required because some strains are resistant to these drugs. Penicillinase-producing gonococci, which are more resistant to penicillin, have appeared in the United States; spectinomycin is the treatment of choice for infections with such strains.

18. In CNS infection, metronidazole or chloramphenicol should be used.

19. The carboxypenicillins are carbenicillin and ticarcillin; the acylaminopenicillins are mezlocillin, azlocillin, and piperacillin. When one of these drugs is used for a severe infection, an aminoglycoside is often recommended as well.

20. Aztreonam is a β-lactam antibiotic; cross-sensitivity has not occurred, but use with caution in patients allergic to penicillins, cephalosporins, or imipenem.

21. Principally in treatment of uncomplicated urinary tract infections.

22. Ampicillin or amoxicillin may be effective in milder cases.

23. In severely ill patients, an aminoglycoside is combined with a cephalosporin.

24. Some encapsulated *H. influenzae* (type b) strains and some unencapsulated strains are resistant to ampicillin, and rare strains are resistant to chloramphenicol. Chloramphenicol plus ampicillin (or chloramphenicol alone) should be used for initial treatment of meningitis or epiglottitis in children until the organism is identified and its susceptibility is determined. For adults with meningitis of unknown etiology and an indeterminate Gram stain and in whom *H. influenzae* is suspected, chloramphenicol is added to ampicillin (or penicillin G) for the first 24 hr until the results of culture are available. Ampicillin is preferred when the infecting strain of *H. influenzae* is susceptible.

25. Not an FDA-approved use. Evidence for possible efficacy comes only from in vitro susceptibility testing and from treatment of infections in experimental animals. In both cases, *L. pneumophila* is highly susceptible to rifampin.

26. Most infections are self-limited without therapy.

27. Various combination treatments are available.

Trovafloxacin was restricted for use in seriously ill patients because of hepatotoxicity, but other fluoroquinolones have not been implicated. The tetracyclines can occasionally cause fatty liver; hepatotoxicity is most likely to occur in patients receiving 2 g or more daily by the intravenous route. Patients receiving high-dose β-lactam antibiotics may develop hepatitis or cholestasis, presumably as a result of hypersensitivity reactions. Nitrofurantoin may cause chronic active hepatitis in some patients. Erythromycins and sulfonamides have been associated with acute hepatitis, and a case of fatal hepatic necrosis has been attributed to fluconazole.

GI reactions to antibiotics result either from direct irritation by the drug, the occurrence of which is usually dose related, or from bacterial overgrowth.[19] Irritative GI side effects are usually produced when antibiotics are administered orally rather than parenterally. The predominant site of irritation varies from drug to drug; for example, erythromycin more commonly produces gastric irritation with epigastric distress and nausea, whereas tetracyclines may produce diarrhea as well as upper GI symptoms. Some qualitative and quantitative changes in the intestinal flora occur after antibiotic administration; they may contribute to flatulence and other lower GI symptoms, which are quite common when broad-spectrum antibiotics are administered orally. Selective overgrowth of *Clostridium difficile* can result in antibiotic-induced pseudomembranous enterocolitis.[20]

Antibiotics may cause various other toxicities. Erythromycin and other macrolides can cause prolongation of the QT interval and polymorphic ventricular tachycardia; in rare instances, this toxicity occurs in the absence of predisposing factors, but it is more likely to occur in patients with significant heart disease and in patients taking terfenadine, astemizole, or cisapride. Several fluoroquinolones, such as moxifloxacin, gatifloxacin, and sparfloxacin, can have similar effects on cardiac conduction.[21,22] All fluoroquinolones can cause tendinitis. Trimethoprim-sulfamethoxazole can cause hyperkalemia, particularly in azotemic patients. Sulfonamides, fluoroquinolones, and tetracyclines can produce photosensitivity.[23]

MICROBIAL SUPERINFECTION

Antimicrobial therapy reduces susceptible organisms from the normal flora of the skin, oral and genitourinary mucosae, and GI tract and exerts selective pressures that favor survival of drug-resistant organisms. Such resistant organisms can occasionally establish a superinfection, either at the site of the original infection or at remote sites.

Public Health Considerations

ANTIMICROBIAL RESISTANCE

The extensive use of antimicrobial agents, especially in ICUs[24] and other health care facilities, strongly favors the selection of resistant microbial species, particularly bacterial strains harboring plasmids that confer transmissible resistance.[25,26] Although antibiotics have played a major role in the treatment of such infections, the pathogens have responded to the antibiotic challenge, developing resistance to all available antimicrobial agents to a greater or lesser degree. Specific mechanisms of resistance are evident in the reduced permeability of cell wall membranes, changes in the target sites of antimicrobial agents, enzymatic inactivation of antibiotics, and the development of pathways bypassing antimicrobial targets.[27]

The widespread use of antibiotics for animals compounds the problem; about 50% of the 25,000 tons of antibiotics that are sold annually in the United States are used in agriculture and aquiculture.[28] Infections from highly resistant strains of *Enterococcus*, *Pneumococcus*, *Staphylococcus aureus*, *Gonococcus*, *Salmonella*, *Serratia*, *Klebsiella*, *Acinetobacter*, *Enterobacter*, and *Mycobacterium* have become important problems. Infections from resistant strains can spread rapidly, first within an institution, then throughout a community, and eventually even globally.[29] Although antibiotic resistance is a worldwide problem, control depends on local measures, beginning with the judicious prescription of antibiotics by individual practitioners[30] and with formulary restrictions that reinforce prudence.[31] Patients harboring resistant strains should be identified rapidly, treated appropriately, and isolated as needed to prevent the spread of infection.

The incidence of superinfection with cephalosporin therapy is actually quite low (< 5%); however, the organisms encountered are often more virulent and difficult to eradicate than the original infecting pathogen.[32] Commonly seen superinfecting pathogens include *Enterobacter* species, *Pseudomonas aeruginosa*, *S. aureus*, *Acinetobacter* species, enterococci, and *Candida* species. Because these organisms are generally multiresistant, therapy with antibiotic combinations, including aminoglycosides, is usually necessary. There appear to be no significant differences among the cephalosporins with respect to the incidence of superinfection or the types of superinfecting pathogens found.

The most worrisome resistance is that of vancomycin-resistant enterococci (VRE). Risk factors for bloodstream infection with VRE are an increasing APACHE II (Acute Physiology and

Table 5 Antimicrobial Drug Dosages for Treatment of Bacterial Infections in Adults with Normal Renal Function[155]

| Class of Agent | Specific Agent | Trade Names | Modest Infections* | | | |
| | | | Oral | | Intramuscular | |
			Daily Dose	Interval	Daily Dose	Interval
Penicillinase-susceptible penicillins	Penicillin G	Pentids, Crystifor, Pfizerpen, etc.	0.8–3.2 million units	6 hr	1.2 million units	8 hr
	Penicillin G benzathine	Bicillin	—	—	1.2–2.4 million units	See fn. 1
	Penicillin G procaine	Crysticillin, Duracillin, etc.	—	—	0.6–4.8 million units	6–24 hr
	Penicillin V	Pen-Vee K, V-Cillin K, etc.	0.8–3.2 million units (0.5–2.0 g)	6 hr	—	—
Penicillinase-susceptible penicillins with activity against gram-negative bacilli	Amoxicillin	Amoxil, Larotid, etc.	750–1,500 mg	8 hr	—	—
	Ampicillin	Omnipen, Polycillin, etc.	1–4 g	6 hr	1–2 g	6 hr
	Azlocillin	Azlin	—	—	—	—
	Carbenicillin indanyl sodium	Geocillin	—	—	—	—
	Mezlocillin	Mezlin	—	—	—	—
	Piperacillin	Pipracil	—	—	See fn. 3	See fn. 3
	Ticarcillin	Ticar	—	—	See fn. 4	See fn.4
Penicillinase-resistant penicillins	Cloxacillin	Tegopen	1–3 g	6 hr	—	—
	Dicloxacillin	Dynapen, Pathocil	1–2 g	6 hr	—	—
	Nafcillin	Nafcil, Unipen	2–4 g[5]	6 hr	2–3 g	4–6 hr
	Oxacillin	Bactocill, Prostaphlin	2–4 g	6 hr	1–2 g	6 hr
Penicillins with β-lactamase inhibitors	Amoxicillin-clavulanate	Augmentin	750 mg–1.5 g (amoxicillin)	8 hr	—	—
	Ampicillin-sulbactam	Unasyn	—	—	1 g (ampicillin)	6 hr
	Piperacillin-tazobactam	Zosyn	—	—	—	—
	Ticarcillin-clavulanate	Timentin	—	—	—	—
Cephalosporins	Cefaclor	Ceclor	750 mg–1.5 g	8 hr	—	—
	Cefadroxil	Duricef, Ultracef	500 mg–2g	12–24 hr	—	—
	Cefamandole	Mandol	—	—	2–4 g	6 hr
	Cefazolin	Ancef, Kefzol	—	—	750 mg–1.5 g	8 hr
	Cefdinir	Omnicef	600 mg	24 hr	—	—
	Cefditoren pivoxil	Spectracef	200–400 mg	12 hr	—	—
	Cefepime	Maxipime	—	—	—	—
	Cefixime	Suprax	400 mg	24 hr	—	—
	Cefmetazole	Zefazone	—	—	—	—
	Cefonicid	Monocid	—	—	See fn. 7,8	See fn. 7,8
	Cefoperazone	Cefobid	—	—	See fn. 7,8	See fn. 7,8
	Ceforanide	Precef	—	—	See fn. 7,8	See fn. 7,8
	Cefotaxime	Claforan	—	—	See fn. 7,8	See fn. 7,8
	Cefotetan	Cefotan	—	—	See fn. 7,8	See fn. 7,8
	Cefoxitin	Mefoxin	—	—	2–4 g	6 hr
	Cefpodoxime	Vantin	200–800 mg	12 hr	—	—
	Cefprozil	Cefzil	500 mg–1 g	12–24 hr	—	—
	Ceftazidime	Fortaz, Tazidime	—	—	See fn. 7,8	See fn. 7,8
	Ceftibutin	Cedax	400 mg	—	—	—
	Ceftizoxime	Cefizox	—	—	See fn. 7,8	See fn. 7,8
	Ceftriaxone	Rocephin	—	24 hr	See fn. 7,8	See fn. 7,8
	Cefuroxime	Zinacef, Ceftin (p.o.)	250–500 mg	12 hr	See fn. 7,8	See fn. 7,8
	Cephalexin	Keflex	1–4 g	6 hr	—	—
	Cephapirin	Cefadyl	—	—	2–3 g	6 hr
	Cephradine	Anspor, Velosef	1–4 g	6 hr	2 g	6 hr
	Loracarbef	Lorabid	400–800 mg	12 hr	—	—
Carbapenems	Imipenem-cilastatin	Primaxin	—	—	—	—
	Meropenem	Merrem	—	—	—	—
	Ertapenem	Ivanz	—	—	—	—

Note: all superscript numbers refer to footnotes following table.
*Infections of the upper respiratory tract, soft tissues, etc.

(continued)

Table 5 *(continued)*

Uncomplicated Urinary Tract Infections		Major and Systemic Infections†			
Oral		Intramuscular		Intravenous	
Daily Dose	Interval	Daily Dose	Interval	Daily Dose	Interval
—	—	—	—	4–24 million units	2–4 hr
—	—	—	—	—	—
—	—	—	—	—	—
—	—	—	—	—	—
750–1,500 mg	8 hr	—	—	—	—
2–4 g	6 hr	—	—	4-12 g	2–4 hr
—	—	—	—	12–18 g	4 hr
4–8 tablets²	6 hr	—	—	—	—
—	—	—	—	12–18 g	4 hr
—	—	See fn. 3	See fn. 3	12–18 g	4 hr
—	—	—	—	16–24 g	3–6 hr
—	—	—	—	—	—
—	—	—	—	—	—
—	—	—	—	4–12 g	4–6 hr
—	—	—	—	4–12 g	4–6 hr
750 mg (amoxicillin)	8 hr	—	—	—	—
—	—	1–2 g (ampicillin)	6 hr	1–2 g (ampicillin)	6 hr
—	—	—	—	12 g (piperacillin)	6 hr
—	—	—	—	12–18 g (ticarcillin)	4–6 hr
750 mg–1.5 g	8 hr	—	—	—	—
500 mg–2 g	12–24 hr	—	—	—	—
—	—	—	—	4–12 g	2–4 hr
See fn. 6	See fn. 6	2–3 g	6–8 hr	2–6 g	6–8 hr
—	—	—	—	—	—
400 mg	24 hr	—	—	2–6 g	8–12 hr
—	—	—	—	2–4 g	12 hr
—	—	—	—	4–8 g	6–12 hr
—	—	—	—	0.5–2.0 g	12–24 hr
—	—	—	—	2–12 g	6–8 hr
—	—	—	—	1–2 g	12 hr
—	—	—	—	2–12 g	4–6 hr
—	—	—	—	2–6 g	12 hr
—	—	—	—	4–12 g	4 hr
200 mg	12 hr	—	—	—	—
—	—	—	—	—	—
—	—	—	—	2–6 g	8–12 hr
400 mg	24 hr	—	—	—	—
—	—	—	—	2–6 g	8–12 hr
—	—	—	—	1–4 g	12–24 hr
—	—	—	—	3–6 g	6 hr
1–4 g	6 hr	—	—	—	—
—	—	—	—	4–12 g	2–4 hr
2 g	6 hr	—	—	3–8 g	4–6 hr
400 mg	12 hr	—	—	—	—
—	—	—	—	1–4 g	6–8 hr
—	—	—	—	3 g	8 hr
—	12 hr	—	—	1 g	24 hr

†Osteomyelitis, peritonitis, bacteremia, meningitis, endocarditis, etc.

(continued)

Table 5 (continued)

Class of Agent	Specific Agent	Trade Names	Modest Infections*			
			Oral		Intramuscular	
			Daily Dose	Interval	Daily Dose	Interval
Monobactams	Aztreonam	Azactam	—	—	1–2 g	8–12 hr
Aminoglycosides	Amikacin	Amikin	—	—	—	—
	Gentamicin	Garamycin	—	—	3–5 mg/kg[11]	8 hr
	Kanamycin	Kantrex	—	—	—	—
	Neomycin	—	See fn. 15	See fn. 15	—	—
	Netilmicin	Netromycin	—	—	4–6 mg/kg[11,12]	8 hr
	Streptomycin	—	—	—	1–2 g	12 hr
	Tobramycin	Nebcin	—	—	3–5 mg/kg[11]	8 hr
Tetracyclines	Demeclocycline	Declomycin	600 mg	6 hr	—	—
	Doxycycline	Vibramycin, etc.	100–200 mg[17]	12 hr	—	—
	Minocycline	Minocin	200 mg[19]	12 hr	—	—
	Oxytetracycline	Terramycin	1–2 g	6 hr	See fn. 21	See fn. 21
	Tetracycline	Achromycin, Panmycin, Sumycin, Tetracyn, etc.	1–2 g	6 hr	See fn. 21	See fn. 21
Macrolides	Azithromycin	Zithromax	500 mg day 1 250 mg days 2–5	24 hr	—	—
	Clarithromycin	Biaxin	500 mg–1 g	12 hr	—	—
	Dirithromycin	Dynabac	500 mg	24 hr		
	Erythromycin	E-Mycin, Erythrocin, Ilotycin	1–2 g	6 hr	See fn. 21	See fn. 21
	Erythromycin estolate[23]	Ilosone	1–2 g	6 hr	—	—
Sulfonamides	Sulfadiazine	—	2–4 g[24]	6 hr	—	—
	Sulfisoxazole	Gantrisin	2–6 g[24]	6 hr	—	—
	Trimethoprim-sulfamethoxazole	Bactrim, Septra	4 tablets[25]	12 hr	—	—
Miscellaneous antibacterial agents	Clindamycin	Cleocin	600 mg–1.8 g	6 hr	600 mg–1.2 g	6–8 hr
	Chloramphenicol	Chloromycetin	1.5–3.0 g	6 hr	See fn. 26	See fn. 26
	Metronidazole	Flagyl	250 mg	8 hr	—	—
	Spectinomycin	Trobicin	—	—	2 g[28]	Single injection
	Trimethoprim	Proloprim, Trimpex	200 mg	12 hr	—	—
	Vancomycin	Vancocin	2 g[29]	6 hr	—	—
Urinary tract disinfectants	Fosfomycin	Monurol	—	—	—	—
	Methenamine mandelate	Mandelamine	—	—	—	—
	Methenamine hippurate	Hiprex	—	—	—	—
	Nalidixic acid	NegGram	—	—	—	—
	Nitrofurantoin	Furadantin, Macrodantin	—	—	—	—
Antifungal drugs	Amphotericin B	Fungizone	—	—	—	—
	Fluconazole[31]	Diflucan	100–200 mg[32]	24 hr	—	—
	Flucytosine	Ancobon	50–150 mg/kg[33]	6 hr	—	—
	Itraconazole	Sporanox	100–400 mg	12 or 24 hr	—	—
	Ketoconazole	Nizorol	200 mg[33]	24 hr	—	—
	Miconazole	Monistat	—	—	—	—
	Nystatin	Mycostatin	1.5–3.0 million units[35]	8 hr	—	—
Fluoroquinolones[36]	Alatrofloxacin[36]	Trovan I.V.	—	—	—	—
	Ciprofloxacin	Cipro	500 mg	12 hr	—	—
	Levofloxacin	Levaquin	500 mg	24 hr	—	—
	Lomefloxacin	Maxaquin	400 mg	24 hr	—	—
	Norfloxacin	Noroxin	—	—	—	—
	Ofloxacin	Floxin	400–800 mg	12 hr	—	—
	Sparfloxacin	Zagam	400 mg first day, then 200 mg	24 hr	—	—
	Trovafloxacin[36]	Trovan	See fn. 36	See fn. 36	—	—
	Gatifloxacin	Tequin	400 mg	24 hr	—	—
	Moxifloxacin	Avelox	400 mg	—	—	—

(continued)

Table 5 (*continued*)

| Uncomplicated Urinary Tract Infections | | Major and Systemic Infections[†] | | | |
| Oral | | Intramuscular | | Intravenous | |
Daily Dose	Interval	Daily Dose	Interval	Daily Dose	Interval
—	—	—	—	3–8 g	6–8 hr
—	—	15 mg/kg[9]	8–12 hr	15 mg/kg[10]	8 hr
—	—	3–5 mg/kg	8 hr	3–5 mg/kg[12]	8 hr
—	—	15 mg/kg[13]	8–12 hr	15 mg/kg[14]	8 hr
—	—	—		—	
—	—	4–6 mg/kg	8 hr	4–6 mg/kg[16]	8 hr
—	—	1–2 g	12 hr	—	
—	—	3–5 mg/kg	8 hr	3–5 mg/kg[16]	8 hr
600 mg	6 hr	—	—	—	—
100–200 mg[17]	12 hr	—	—	100–200 mg[18]	12 hr
200 mg[19]	12 hr	—	—	200 mg[20]	12 hr
1–2 g	6 hr	—	—	—	—
1–2 g	6 hr	See fn. 21	See fn. 21	750 mg–1.0 g[22]	6–12 hr
—	—	—	—	—	—
—	—	—	—	—	—
—	—	—	—	—	—
—	—	See fn. 21	See fn. 21	2–4 g	6 hr
—	—	—	—	—	—
2–4 g[24]	6 hr	—	—	—	—
2–6 g[24]	6 hr	—	—	100 mg/kg[24]	4–6 hr
4 tablets[25]	12 hr	—	—	8–12 mg/kg[25] (trimethoprim)	6 hr[25]
—	—	1.2–2.4 g	6–8 hr	1.8–3.0 g	6–8 hr
1.5–2.0 g[27]	6 hr	See fn. 26	See fn. 26	2–4 g	6 hr
—	—	—	—	30 mg/kg	6 hr
—	—	—	—	—	—
200 mg	12 hr	—	—	—	—
—	—	—	—	1–2 g	6–12 hr
3 g	1 dose	—	—	—	—
4 g	6 hr	—	—	—	—
2 g	12 hr	—	—	—	—
2–4 g	6 hr	—	—	—	—
200–400 g	6 hr	—	—	Not recommended	—
—	—	—	—	0.25–1.0 mg/kg[30]	24 hr
—	—	—	—	200 mg[31]	24 hr
—	—	—	—	—	—
—	—	—	—	—	—
—	—	See fn. 32	See fn. 32	See fn. 32	See fn. 32
—	—	—	—	600 mg–3.6 g[34]	8 hr
—	—	—	—	—	—
—	—	—	—	200 mg	24 hr
200–500 mg	12 hr	—	—	400 mg	12 hr
500 mg	24hr	—	—	500 mg	24 hr
400 mg	24 hr	—	—	—	—
800 mg	12 hr	—	—	—	—
400 mg	12 hr	—	—	800 mg	12 hr
—	—	—	—	—	—
—	—	—	—	—	—
400 mg	24 hr	—	—	400 mg	24 hr
400 mg	24 hr	—	—	—	—

(*continued*)

Table 5 (continued)

| Class of Agent | Specific Agent | Trade Names | Modest Infections* | | | |
| | | | Oral | | Intramuscular | |
			Daily Dose	Interval	Daily Dose	Interval
Streptogramins	Quinupristin-dalfopristin	Synercid	—	—	—	—
Oxazolidinones	Linezolid	Zyvox	400 mg	12 hr	—	—

Note: all superscript numbers refer to footnotes following table.
*Infections of the upper respiratory tract, soft tissues, etc.
†Osteomyelitis, peritonitis, bacteremia, meningitis, endocarditis, etc.

1. Benzathine penicillin G is used primarily in three circumstances. (1) Treatment of streptococcal pharyngitis in cases in which patient compliance is questionable (a single dose of 1.2 million units I.M.). (2) Prophylaxis of rheumatic fever recurrences (1.2–2.4 million units I.M. once monthly). (3) Treatment of syphilis: for primary, secondary, or early (< 1 yr) latent syphilis, a single dose of 2.4 million units I.M.; for late syphilis (late latent, cardiovascular, neurosyphilis, etc.), 2.4 million units I.M. weekly for three doses has been recommended, but many authorities now treat neurosyphilis with high-dose I.V. penicillin.

2. Each tablet of carbenicillin indanyl sodium is equivalent to 382 mg of carbenicillin (usual dosage is one to two tablets p.o., q.i.d.).

3. Piperacillin is most often used in the treatment of serious infections caused by susceptible *Pseudomonas, Klebsiella, Enterobacter*, and non-*mirabilis Proteus* strains; the agent is given in maximal dosage (12–18 g I.V. daily). It is commonly used in synergistic combination with tobramycin or gentamicin for treatment of *Pseudomonas* infections. Occasionally, it is given in smaller dosages (1.0–1.5 g I.M. or I.V. q. 6 hr) to treat an uncomplicated urinary tract infection caused by the same organisms.

4. Ticarcillin, piperacillin, mezlocillin, and azlocillin are usually used in the treatment of serious infections caused by susceptible *Pseudomonas, Enterobacter*, and non-*mirabilis Proteus* strains and are given in maximal dosage (12–24 g I.V. daily). One of these agents is commonly used in synergistic combination with tobramycin or gentamicin for treatment of *Pseudomonas* infections. Occasionally, they are given in smaller dosages (1 g I.M. or I.V. q. 6 hr) to treat an uncomplicated urinary tract infection caused by the same organisms.

5. Nafcillin is not reliably absorbed by the oral route.

6. Cefazolin may be used in the treatment of acute uncomplicated urinary tract infections caused by susceptible gram-negative bacilli (*E. coli, P. mirabilis*, and *Klebsiella*). It is administered I.M. in a dosage of 2 g daily (given as aliquots q. 8 hr).

7. Although the second- and third-generation cephalosporins can be used for milder infections at the lower end of their recommended dosage range, these potent but expensive agents should generally be reserved for treatment of serious infections or for the treatment of resistant organisms when the alternative is a more toxic antimicrobial drug.

8. The I.M. route is acceptable for milder illnesses, but the I.V. route is recommended for serious infections, including bacteremias and meningitis. The range for the I.M. dosage is the same as that for the I.V. dosage.

9. Dosage must be reduced in the presence of renal insufficiency. The daily parenteral dose should not exceed 15 mg/kg, and the total daily amount administered should not exceed 1.5 g, regardless of the patient's weight.

10. The I.V. dose should be infused during a period of 30–60 min q. 8 hr.

11. For urinary tract infections caused by resistant organisms.

12. Dosage must be reduced in the presence of renal insufficiency. The I.V. dose should be administered for a period of 30–60 min q. 8 hr. In patients with meningitis caused by susceptible gram-negative bacilli, intrathecal gentamicin (5 mg for adults, 1–2 mg for infants) is often administered once daily along with parenteral gentamicin until CSF cultures are negative.

13. Dosage must be reduced in the presence of renal insufficiency. The daily parenteral dose should not exceed 15 mg/kg (daily dose should not exceed 1.5 g, regardless of the patient's weight); the total quantity administered in a therapeutic course should not exceed 15 g.

14. The I.V. route should be employed only when I.M. administration is not possible. The I.V. dose should be administered during a period of at least 60 min q. 8 hr.

15. There are no clinical indications for the parenteral administration of neomycin in view of its marked toxicity and the availability of safer alternative drugs. The drug is given p.o. or by nasogastric tube (4–6 g daily in 4 divided doses) to reduce the number of ammonia-forming bacteria in the intestine in the short-term treatment of acute hepatic coma. It is also given in a total daily dose of 2–3 g in long-term therapy for chronic hepatic encephalopathy or episodic hepatic coma. Nephrotoxicity and ototoxicity have followed prolonged high-dose therapy in hepatic coma, particularly in patients with some renal impairment. Neomycin is also used along with vigorous mechanical cleansing of the large bowel as preoperative prophylaxis for bowel surgery. In this situation, it is administered for 1–3 days preoperatively (40 mg/ kg p.o. daily in 6 divided doses).

16. Dosage must be reduced in the presence of renal insufficiency. The I.V. dose should be administered during a period of 30–60 min q. 8 hr.

17. Usually administered as 100 mg p.o. q. 12 hr on the first day of treatment, followed by 50 mg q. 12 hr. For more difficult infections, the dosage may be continued at 100 mg q. 12 hr.

18. Usually administered as 100 mg I.V. q. 12 hr on the first day of treatment. Thereafter, it may be given as 50–100 mg I.V. q. 12 hr. Each I.V. dose should be given during a period of 1–4 hr.

19. Usually administered initially as 200 mg p.o., followed by 100 mg q. 12 hr.

20. Usually given initially as 200 mg I.V., followed by 100 mg q. 12 hr. Maximum dose in any 24-hr period is 400 mg.

21. I.M. administration is generally unsatisfactory because of poor absorption and local irritation.

22. In special circumstances, it may be given in higher doses but not in excess of 500 mg q. 6 hr.

23. Cholestatic hepatitis may develop as a hypersensitivity response to erythromycin estolate but not to the other erythromycin preparations. For this reason, erythromycin base or erythromycin stearate is preferable.

24. A loading dose of one half the daily dose is given initially. In severe infections, the dosage of sulfonamide is adjusted to provide a blood level of 10–15 mg/dl. Sulfonamides must be used with caution in patients with renal insufficiency. Sulfisoxazole is the preferred sulfonamide.

25. Each tablet contains 80 mg trimethoprim and 400 mg sulfamethoxazole. Double-strength tablets are also available (usual dosage is 1 tablet q. 12 hr). Pediatric suspensions contain 40 mg trimethoprim and 200 mg sulfamethoxazole/5 ml. Trimethoprim-sulfamethoxazole has also been used in the treatment of typhoid fever in the same dosage as recommended for urinary tract infections. It has been used in a dosage of 4–8 standard tablets daily in the treatment of brucellosis. For pneumonia caused by *Pneumocystis carinii*, the oral dosage is 20 mg/kg trimethoprim and 100 mg/kg sulfamethoxazole/24 hr (equally divided doses q. 6 hr). The I.V. dosage of trimethoprim-sulfamethoxazole ranges from 8 mg/kg trimethoprim and 40 mg/kg sulfamethoxazole/24 hr to 20 mg/kg trimethoprim and 100 mg/kg sulfamethoxazole/24 hr. The lower dosage range is used in the treatment of urinary tract infections that require parenteral antimicrobial therapy and in the treatment of shigellosis; the larger dosage is employed in the treatment of *P. carinii* pneumonia.

26. Chloramphenicol sodium succinate, the parenteral preparation, should only be used I.V. It is ineffective when administered I.M.

27. Chloramphenicol should not be used in the treatment of a urinary tract infection that could

(continued)

Chronic Health Evaluation II) score, treatment with vancomycin, and a diagnosis of hematologic malignancy. Thus, severe illness, underlying disease, and the use of vancomycin are major risk factors for infection of the bloodstream with VRE.[33] Fueling the excessive use of broad-spectrum antimicrobial drugs is the lack of reliable tests that would permit physicians to discern when antimicrobial drugs are not needed. When antimicrobial therapy is needed, improved diagnostic tests would permit better targeting and thereby reduce the widespread administration of broad-spectrum drugs. Selective pressure exerted by widespread antimicrobial use is the driving force in the development of antibiotic resistance. The association between increased rates of antimicrobial use and resistance has been documented for nosocomial infections[34] and community-acquired infections in studies associating resistance patterns with rates of drug use on a regional or national basis.[35]

Resistance to antimicrobial drugs is a global problem. Multidrug-resistant pathogens travel not only locally but globally. Because of increased international travel and increased foreign trade in fresh-food products, the threat of global spread of antibiotic resistance is greater than ever. There is no national or global surveillance system for the monitoring of antibiotic resistance in animals or humans. New classes of antimicrobials are being developed to deal with drug resistance.

Table 5   (continued)

Uncomplicated Urinary Tract Infections		Major and Systemic Infections[†]			
Oral		Intramuscular		Intravenous	
Daily Dose	Interval	Daily Dose	Interval	Daily Dose	Interval
—	—	—	—	7.5 mg/kg	8 hr
—	—	—	—	600 mg (I.V. or p.o.)	12 hr

[†]Osteomyelitis, peritonitis, bacteremia, meningitis, endocarditis, etc.

be managed with another, safer, effective antimicrobial.

28. The only approved indication for the use of spectinomycin is in the treatment of anogenital and urethral gonorrhea in a penicillin-allergic patient or when the infecting organism is highly penicillin resistant. In geographic areas where antibiotic-resistant gonococci are prevalent, treatment with 4 g of spectinomycin (2 g in each gluteal region) may be indicated.

29. Vancomycin is not absorbed through the GI tract. Its use orally is for treatment of staphylococcal enterocolitis or antibiotic-associated enterocolitis.

30. The dry powder is reconstituted by addition of Sterile Water for Injection, USP, without a bacteriostatic agent. The solution is then added to a bottle of 5% Dextrose Injection, USP. The pH of the dextrose solution should first be checked to verify that it is above 4.2. If it is not, a buffer solution (as described in package insert) should be added. Amphotericin B solutions should be administered promptly after preparation and should be protected from light during administration. It is given once a day over 6 hr. (Later in the course of administration, double the daily dose is sometimes given on an alternate-day schedule.) Dosage is 1 mg on the first day and then increased in 5 mg increments each day until maintenance dosage is reached. The daily dose is determined by the susceptibility of the organism and the occurrence of toxic side effects. In some instances (e.g., cryptococcal meningitis), combination therapy with flucytosine p.o. may allow employment of smaller daily doses (0.3–0.4 mg/kg) of amphotericin B. In fungal meningitis, intrathecal administration may be necessary (0.1 mg initially, increased gradually to 0.5 mg q. 48–72 hr), depending on the evaluation of the patient's condition.

31. Fluconazole is very useful for the treatment of oropharyngeal, esophageal, and disseminated infections caused by Candida and for control of cryptococcus, especially chronic suppression of cryptococcal meningitis in patients with AIDS. To initiate therapy, a loading dose of twice the usual daily dose should be used. A daily dose of 400 mg can be used for cryptococcal meningitis, depending on the patient's response to therapy. The dose should be reduced in patients who have renal insufficiency.

32. Used in the treatment of urinary tract infections and visceral infections caused by Candida. Also used in cryptococcal infections in which amphotericin B is not tolerated. Resistance to flucytosine may develop during treatment of candidal and cryptococcal infections. Sometimes used in combination with amphotericin B to treat systemic fungal infections.

33. Ketoconazole is indicated in the treatment of patients with susceptible fungal infections that have failed to respond to amphotericin B or in the treatment of patients unable to tolerate the toxic effects of amphotericin B. In either role, it is generally preferred to therapy with miconazole when the patients can take oral medications. It is also the drug of choice in the long-term treatment of chronic mucocutaneous candidiasis. It has been useful in the treatment of histoplasmosis, coccidioidomycosis, chromomycosis, and paracoccidioidomycosis. In view of its poor penetration of the CSF, it should not be used in the treatment of coccidioidal or cryptococcal meningitis. Ketoconazole requires gastric acidity for dissolution and absorption. Antacids and cimetidine, if needed, should be given at least 2 hr after a dose of ketoconazole. The most frequent side effects have been nausea and vomiting. Several cases of liver injury of varying severity, possibly the result of idiosyncratic reactions, have occurred during ketoconazole therapy. Liver function tests, therefore, should be evaluated before and periodically during treatment, especially in patients who are on prolonged therapy or who have preexisting hepatic disease. Ketoconazole, in daily dosages of 200–1,800 mg p.o., is used in major and systemic fungal infections for which the mycotic agent is susceptible and amphotericin B cannot be employed.

34. Miconazole is available for parenteral therapy for systemic mycoses. Experience is relatively limited, and it should probably be reserved for patients who cannot tolerate or who do not respond to amphotericin B and flucytosine. Miconazole is metabolized by extrarenal mechanisms, and patients with fungal bladder infections require supplementary bladder irrigation with the drug. Side effects of miconazole include phlebitis, fever, rash, nausea and vomiting, anemia, thrombocytopenia, and transient hyperlipidemia caused by the diluent used.

35. Not absorbed from the GI tract. Use only in treatment of intestinal tract colonization by Candida species and not for any systemic mycotic infection. Nystatin suspension (400,000–600,000 units q.i.d.) is used as a mouthwash in treatment of oral thrush. The suspension can also be swallowed for use in the treatment of candidal esophagitis.

36. None of these drugs is recommended for children. In 1999, the FDA limited trovafloxacin to inpatient use for limb- or life-threatening infections.

Discussion

The antimicrobial agents of choice for various infections (e.g., community-acquired pneumonia[7-9]) in adults are well established [see Table 4], as are their dosages in patients with normal renal function [see Table 5]. Excellent reviews and practice guidelines have been published.[18,19]

Penicillins

Although the original penicillins are still useful against specific bacteria, there are some infections in which both they and the penicillinase-resistant semisynthetic penicillins are ineffective because of the emergence of penicillinase-producing staphylococci and methicillin-resistant staphylococci. The penicillins can be classified by structure, β-lactamase susceptibility, and spectrum of action [see Figure 1].

The action of the penicillins depends on the presence of a bacterial cell wall containing peptidoglycans that are accessible to the agent. In actively growing bacteria, interference with biosynthesis of the peptidoglycan structure—specifically, of the cross-linkages between the peptide chains—prevents the bacterium from developing its normal structural firmness, and this lack of firmness leads to lysis.

NATURAL PENICILLINS

Aqueous Crystalline Penicillin G

Aqueous crystalline penicillin G is used when a high serum concentration of the agent is required.[36] Its half-life is normally 30 minutes but may be as long as 10 hours in patients with anuria. Approximately 50% of penicillin G is bound to plasma proteins.

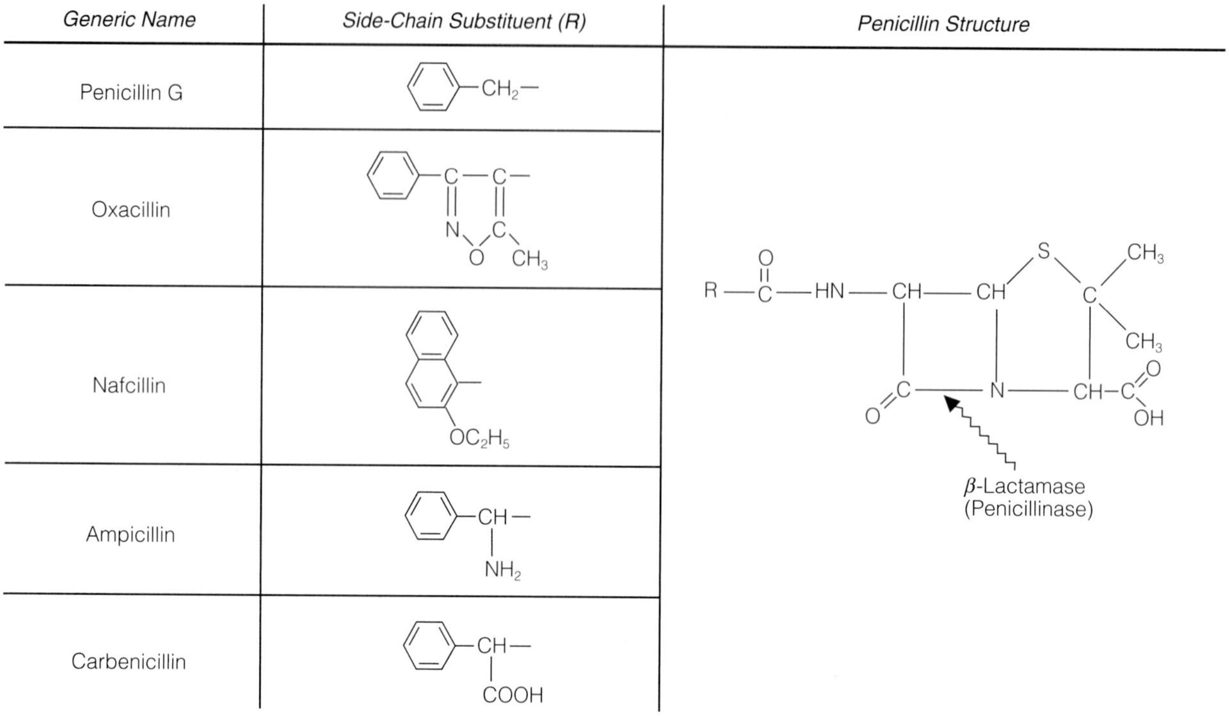

Generic Name	Side-Chain Substituent (R)	Penicillin Structure
Penicillin G	⟨phenyl⟩–CH₂–	
Oxacillin	⟨structure⟩	
Nafcillin	⟨structure⟩	
Ampicillin	⟨structure⟩	
Carbenicillin	⟨structure⟩	

β-Lactamase
(Penicillinase)

Figure 1 **Various semisynthetic penicillins have been produced by modifying the structure of the side chain (R) attached to the penicillin nucleus (right). In this way, penicillins have been developed that lack some of the drawbacks of penicillin G, such as poor gastrointestinal absorption, limited spectrum of antibacterial activity, and inactivation by penicillinase-producing microorganisms; for example, oxacillin and nafcillin are resistant to inactivation by penicillinase. This bacterial enzyme (also termed β-lactamase) cleaves the β-lactam ring of penicillin to form an inactive product; the site of action of penicillinase is shown at right.**

Penicillin G sodium contains approximately 2 mEq of sodium per one million units. Therefore, the potassium salt of penicillin G should be used except in patients with renal insufficiency, who may not be able to tolerate the 1.7 mEq of potassium contained in each one million units. This agent is destroyed by gastric acid when given orally.

Penicillin G Benzathine

Penicillin G benzathine, 1.2 to 2.4 million units I.M., is used in the definitive management of certain infections, such as streptococcal sore throat, and as prophylaxis for several conditions, such as rheumatic fever, in which reinfection by β-hemolytic streptococci is a constant threat.

Penicillin G Procaine

Penicillin G procaine is used intramuscularly when a long-acting preparation is preferred and high blood levels are not required. It is indicated for the treatment of pneumococcal pneumonia, uncomplicated cases of which are adequately treated by administration of one or two daily doses of 300,000 units, and for treatment of acute genitourinary gonorrhea, for which a dose of 4.8 million units is divided and injected at two sites and 1 g of probenecid is given orally before the injection.

Penicillin V

Phenoxymethyl penicillin, or penicillin V, is resistant to gastric acid and therefore reaches higher serum concentrations, when given orally, than penicillin G does at similar doses. Penicillin V should not be substituted for parenterally administered penicillin G when such therapy is needed, but it can be given orally to treat mild infections of the throat, the respiratory tract, or soft tissue in doses of 125 to 500 mg given four to six times daily.

PENICILLINASE-RESISTANT PENICILLINS

Methicillin

Methicillin is the least protein-bound of this group (39%); nafcillin (90%), oxacillin (94%), cloxacillin (95%), and dicloxacillin (98%) all have higher rates of protein binding. Methicillin was the first of the semisynthetic penicillinase-resistant penicillins.[37] It must be administered parenterally and is usually given every 4 to 6 hours in a total daily dose of 100 to 300 mg/kg body weight.

Oxacillin and Nafcillin

Oxacillin seems to be as effective as methicillin against staphylococcal infections, and it causes interstitial nephritis less often. For parenteral use, oxacillin or nafcillin can be given in dosages of 100 to 300 mg/kg/day for children and up to 4 to 12 g/day for adults.

Cloxacillin and Dicloxacillin

If penicillinase-producing organisms are identified or suspected and oral therapy is desired, cloxacillin or dicloxacillin, 1 to 2 g/day, can be given.

AMINOPENICILLINS

Ampicillin

Ampicillin is active against a variety of bacteria, including many strains of *Escherichia coli, Proteus mirabilis, Salmonella, Shigella,*

Listeria, and *Haemophilus influenzae.* Most strains of *Klebsiella* and all strains of *P. aeruginosa* are resistant.

Because it is stable in gastric juices, ampicillin is suitable for oral as well as parenteral use. When it is given orally, peak serum levels are reached in about 2 hours, but they seldom exceed 0.3 μg/ml. When it is given intramuscularly, peak serum levels are achieved in 1 hour, and they are both higher and more prolonged than the peak levels achieved after oral administration. About 10% of ampicillin is bound to plasma proteins. The recommended daily dose is 1 to 4 g; parenteral administration of up to 12 g/day is recommended for major systemic infections.

Amoxicillin

Amoxicillin is closely related to ampicillin, both in chemical structure and in spectrum of antibacterial activity.[38] Amoxicillin, however, is more completely absorbed than ampicillin: approximately 70% of a dose of amoxicillin is absorbed, compared with approximately 50% of a dose of ampicillin. Consequently, the blood levels attainable with a given dose of amoxicillin are usually about twice those attainable with a comparable dose of ampicillin. Amoxicillin is at least as effective as ampicillin in the treatment of respiratory disorders that are caused by susceptible bacteria, including otitis media, sinusitis, and bronchitis.

CARBOXYPENICILLINS

Carbenicillin

Carbenicillin has an antibacterial range similar to that of ampicillin, with the added benefit of activity against certain strains of *P. aeruginosa,*[39] indole-positive *Proteus* species, and *Enterobacter* species.[40] Because carbenicillin is inactivated by penicillinase, penicillinase-producing *S. aureus* is resistant to it. *Klebsiella* species are resistant to carbenicillin, as are many *Serratia* organisms. Carbenicillin is bactericidal and is recoverable from blood, urine, lymph, CSF, and most body tissues. About 50% of the drug is bound to serum proteins.[41]

Ticarcillin

The antibacterial spectrum of ticarcillin is similar to that of carbenicillin; however, it is two to four times more active against *P. aeruginosa.* It is frequently preferred to carbenicillin in the treatment of serious gram-negative infections because of its greater potency and the lower incidence of adverse effects.[42] The primary use of ticarcillin is in the treatment of proven or suspected *Pseudomonas* infections. The recommended dosage is 16 to 24 g/day.

UREIDOPENICILLINS

Mezlocillin, Azlocillin, and Piperacillin

Mezlocillin, azlocillin, and piperacillin are semisynthetic penicillins derived from the ampicillin molecule with side-chain adaptations. The ureidopenicillins are generally bactericidal and act primarily by inhibiting cell wall synthesis in dividing bacteria. In comparison with the carboxypenicillins carbenicillin and ticarcillin, the ureidopenicillins exhibit less pronounced plasma protein binding, a shorter serum half-life, and a greater volume of distribution.[43-45] They are minimally metabolized (10%) and are primarily excreted in an active form by glomerular filtration and tubular secretion. Unlike carbenicillin and ticarcillin, the ureidopenicillins achieve high concentrations in bile because of increased biliary excretion.

In vitro, the ureidopenicillins are active against streptococci, enterococci, most Enterobacteriaceae, *Pseudomonas,* β-lactamase–negative staphylococci, *Neisseria,* and *Haemophilus.*[46-48] β-Lactamase–producing staphylococci and *H. influenzae* are resistant. The major advantage the ureidopenicillins have over other penicillins in clinical use is their increased activity against *P. aeruginosa* and *Klebsiella.*

The recommended dosages of the ureidopenicillins are 6 to 16 g/day for mild to moderate infections and 18 to 24 g/day for severe to life-threatening infections. Small doses may be given intramuscularly, but large doses must be given intravenously. The dosing interval is usually 4 to 6 hours.

Cephalosporins

Cephalosporium acremonium was discovered in 1948. This fungus was found to produce cephalosporin C, from which cephalothin, the first cephalosporin to be introduced, was in turn derived. The basic cephalosporin structure consists of a dihydrothiazine ring fused to a β-lactam ring.

Substitutions at the acyl side chain have led to differences in antibacterial spectrum and β-lactamase stability. The side chains substituted at this position interfere with proper stereotactic binding of the molecule to the β-lactamase active site, thus preventing degradation of the cephalosporin. Some of the side effects involving platelet aggregation that have been observed with the use of moxalactam can be traced to substitutions at this position.

For convenience, cephalosporins are divided into four generations or groups according to the nature and extent of their antibacterial spectra. More specifically, the division into generations is based on the number of gram-negative bacterial species against which each cephalosporin demonstrates clinical activity. It must be remembered, however, that although the members of each generation are sufficiently similar to be grouped together, they also are different from one another in a number of ways [*see Table 6*].

FIRST-GENERATION CEPHALOSPORINS

First-generation cephalosporins have good activity against aerobic gram-positive cocci such as *S. aureus,* group B streptococci, and *Streptococcus pneumoniae.* In addition, they are effective against three aerobic gram-negative bacilli—*E. coli, K. pneumoniae,* and *P. mirabilis*—although even among these three, resistance is common, occurring in as many as 30% of cases. First-generation cephalosporins are also active against most anaerobic cocci and bacilli (other than *B. fragilis*). They have little or no activity against *Enterobacter, Serratia, Acinetobacter, Pseudomonas,* methicillin-resistant *S. aureus, S. epidermidis,* and enterococci. They are also inactive against *B. fragilis, Citrobacter, Listeria monocytogenes, Proteus* (except for *P. mirabilis*), and *Providencia.*

First-generation cephalosporins are used for infections caused by gram-positive cocci, such as skin infections and osteomyelitis, although penicillins are the agents of choice for all streptococcal infections and for infections proven by culture to be caused by susceptible staphylococci. The best use for first-generation cephalosporins is in surgical prophylaxis. For this application, cefazolin sodium is the preferred agent.

SECOND-GENERATION CEPHALOSPORINS

Second-generation cephalosporins possess the same spectrum of activity as the first-generation cephalosporins, with the addition of broader coverage of gram-negative organisms, including *H. influenzae, E. aerogenes,* and some *Neisseria* species. Fewer than

Table 6 Properties of Cephalosporins[155]

	Specific Agent	Trade Names	Comment*
First Generation	**Oral**		
	Cefadroxil	Duricef, Ultracef	Longer half-life
	Cephalexin	Keflex	Most experience with this agent
	Cephradine	Anspor, Velosef	Properties are similar to those of cephalexin
	Parenteral		
	Cefazolin	Ancef, Kefzol	Longer half-life; well tolerated when given I.M.
	Cephapirin	Cefadyl	Properties are similar to those of other first-generation cephalosporins
	Cephradine	Anspor, Velosef	Properties are similar to those of other first-generation cephalosporins
Second Generation	**Oral**		
	Cefaclor	Ceclor	Moderately active against *Haemophilus influenzae*
	Cefprozil	Cefzil	Active against *H. influenzae*
	Cefuroxime axetil	Ceftin	Active against *H. influenzae*
	Loracarbef	Lorabid	A carbacephem with properties and spectrum similar to those of cefuroxime
	Parenteral		
	Cefamandole	Mandol	Active against *H. influenzae*; may cause bleeding
	Cefmetazole	Zefazone	Spectrum and half-life similar to cefoxitin; may cause bleeding
	Cefonicid	Monocid	Spectrum similar to that of cefamandole
	Ceforanide	Precef	Spectrum similar to that of cefamandole
	Cefotetan	Cefotan	Spectrum similar to that of cefoxitin; longer half-life than cefoxitin; may cause bleeding
	Cefoxitin	Mefoxin	Active against *Bacteroides fragilis, Serratia, Neisseria gonorrhoeae*
	Cefuroxime	Zinacef, Kefurox	Active against *H. influenzae*; only second-generation drug approved for meningitis (selected pathogens)
Third Generation	**Oral**		
	Cefixime	Suprax	More active against gram-negative bacilli, gonococci, *Moraxella catarrhalis*, and *H. influenzae* than other oral cephalosporins but much less active against *Staphylococcus aureus*; not active against *Pseudomonas*
	Cefpodoxime	Vantin	Similar to cefixime but more active against *S. aureus*
	Ceftibuten	Cedax	Similar to cefixime but has poor activity against pneumococci and staphylococci
	Parenteral		
	Cefepime	Maxipime	Active against most gram-positive cocci (except enterococci and methicillin-resistant staphylococci), *Neisseria, Haemophilus*, enteric gram-negative bacilli, and *Pseudomonas*
	Cefoperazone	Cefobid	Increased activity against *Pseudomonas aeruginosa* but less against Enterobacteriaceae; may cause bleeding
	Cefotaxime	Claforan	More active against gram-positive cocci
	Ceftazidime	Fortaz, Tazidime, Tazicef	Most active against *Pseudomonas*
	Ceftizoxime	Cefizox	Properties are similar to those of cefotaxime
	Ceftriaxone	Rocephin	Longer half-life; less active against *Pseudomonas, B. fragilis*

Note: detailed information about the various cephalosporins is covered in the text.
*Agents are being compared with other members of the same generation of cephalosporins.

5% of *E. coli* and *Proteus* strains are resistant to second-generation cephalosporins. The activity of second-generation agents against *S. pyogenes* and *S. pneumoniae* is equal to that of the first-generation agents, but their activity against staphylococci is variable: the MIC ranges from 0.20 to 25 µg/ml. Of the second-generation agents, the most active against staphylococci is cefamandole, which has an MIC of 0.6 µg/ml for *S. aureus*. Cefotetan and cefoxitin have significant activity against *B. fragilis*. Cefoxitin is less active against *H. influenzae* and *E. aerogenes* than other second-generation cephalosporins, but it is more active against *Serratia* species. Cefoxitin by itself is effective in patients with community-acquired peritonitis who are unlikely to be infected with *Enterobacter* or *P. aeruginosa*.[49] Cefuroxime and cefamandole have been used with some success in empirical therapy for community-acquired pneumonia.[50] Cefotetan, a cephamycin introduced in 1986, has a spectrum of activity very similar to that of cefoxitin.[51] It is as active as cefoxitin against *B. fragilis* but is less active against other strains in the *B. fragilis* group. Unlike cefoxitin, cefotetan is active against *H. influenzae*. Cefotetan has proved effective and safe in a variety of clinical situations, including gynecologic infections and surgical prophylaxis.[52]

Cefprozil is an oral agent whose spectrum of activity includes gram-positive and gram-negative pathogens. It has achieved good results in patients with pharyngitis or tonsillitis.[53]

Loracarbef is an oral agent of the carbacephem class that is active in vitro against the common pathogens associated with skin infections, otitis media, sinusitis, bronchopulmonary infections, and urinary tract infections.[54]

THIRD-GENERATION CEPHALOSPORINS

In the third-generation cephalosporins, activity against gram-positive cocci is replaced by broader gram-negative coverage. This development is illustrated by susceptibility testing done on *S. aureus*: the MIC of first-generation cephalosporins is 1 µg/ml, that of second-generation cephalosporins is 2 µg/ml, and that of third-generation cephalosporins is 3 µg/ml. Third-generation cephalosporins are more active against the enteric gram-negative bacilli covered by first- and second-generation cephalosporins. Their spectrum of activity includes *Serratia* and *Citrobacter*. They are also highly active against *H. influenzae* and *N. gonorrhoeae* and moderately active against *P. aeruginosa* and some anaerobes. At first, the third-generation cephalosporins seemed capable of providing the same spectrum of activity as the aminoglycosides but without their inherent toxicity; however, they have failed to gain wide popularity in the treatment of high-risk patients or patients with extensive infections. The reasons for this failure include their incomplete spectra of activity against the range of organisms likely to be encountered in polymicrobial infections, their unexpected agent-specific toxicity, their suboptimal pharmacokinetic properties, and their high propensity for inducing resistance.

Cefixime, an orally absorbed iminomethoxyaminothiazolyl cephalosporin, inhibits 90% of *S. pneumoniae, H. influenzae,* and *H. parainfluenzae* strains, whether they produce β-lactamase or not, at concentrations of less than 0.25 mg/L. It inhibits 90% of *Moraxella catarrhalis* strains at concentrations of less than 1 mg/L.

Ceftibuten is an orally active third-generation cephalosporin that possesses increased potency against members of the Enterobacteriaceae.[55] Generally, it is about 16 times more active than cefuroxime, cefaclor, cephalexin, or amoxicillin-clavulanate; its activity is comparable to that of cefixime. Ceftibuten is ineffective against staphylococci and only partially effective against *S. pneumoniae. H. influenzae* and *Neisseria* species, however, are highly susceptible to this agent.

Pharmacokinetics

After I.V. administration, third-generation cephalosporins conform to an open, two-compartment model, characterized by an initial rapid distribution phase followed by a slower terminal elimination phase. The relatively long elimination half-lives of many of the newer β-lactam antibiotics make less frequent dosing possible. Most third-generation cephalosporins are primarily eliminated renally, with two exceptions: cefoperazone and ceftriaxone. Cefoperazone is primarily eliminated unchanged in the bile, and only about 25% of an administered dose is recovered in the urine after 24 hours.[56] Peak biliary concentrations of cefoperazone approach or exceed 2,000 μg/ml after a 2 g I.V. dose.[57] Fifty percent of an administered dose of ceftriaxone is eliminated in the bile; the rest is eliminated renally. Ceftriaxone elimination is decreased to a small extent in end-stage renal disease; however, because the drug is normally given every 12 to 24 hours, there is little accumulation and therefore no need to adjust the dose. In general, third-generation cephalosporins penetrate most tissue and fluid compartments in amounts that, though variable, usually exceed the MIC for most susceptible pathogens. Sputum concentrations in the range of 0.3 to 6.0 μg/ml are attained with all the agents, and higher concentrations are found in purulent sputum. Ascitic fluid concentrations ranging from 2.4 μg/ml with ceftizoxime to greater than 60 μg/ml with cefoperazone are seen in patients with peritonitis.[58]

Concentrations in excess of the MIC for susceptible aerobic and anaerobic organisms (except for *B. fragilis*) are achieved in female genital tissue with all these agents.[59] These compounds also appear to penetrate the prostate, the testes, the ureters, and renal tissue in significant amounts.[60]

With each of these agents, therapeutic concentrations can be obtained in the gallbladder wall; these concentrations may be as high as 60 μg/g with cefoperazone. Bone-penetration studies reveal penetration with each of these agents.[61]

Clinical Utility

Many studies have compared third-generation cephalosporins in an effort to establish a superior drug or drug combination for life-threatening infections; most have found no statistically significant differences. It is important to remember that even if there is a difference in efficacy between two or more antibiotics, that difference may not be apparent if the study group is not large enough. For example, if one agent fails in 10% of patients and another in only 5%, a study group of 250 to 500 patients would be required to show a statistical difference.[62,63] Most comparative antibiotic trials, however, have reported on fewer than 60 patients and thus have not been able to pinpoint small differences in effi-

cacy between antibiotics.[64] Many studies that find no difference between two regimens are in fact subject to this type of error.

Cefepime is an extended-spectrum parenteral cephalosporin that provides coverage against both gram-positive and gram-negative organisms, including *S. aureus* and *P. aeruginosa.* Cefepime, which is a zwitterion, has a net neutral charge that allows it to penetrate the outer membrane of gram-negative bacteria faster than third-generation cephalosporins. It is more stable against β-lactamases because of the lower affinity of the enzymes for cefepime when compared with third-generation cephalosporins. In comparison with third-generation cephalosporins, cefepime appears to be less likely to induce resistance, because of a lower rate of hydrolysis by β-lactamases, a low affinity for these enzymes, and more rapid permeation into the cell. It has been used to treat patients with pneumonia, with results comparable to those obtained with ceftazidime.[65] Because of its antibacterial coverage and proven tissue penetration in acute pancreatitis, cefepime should be studied in patients with severe acute pancreatitis.[66] However, it offers poor coverage against *Bacteroides* and must be combined with metronidazole or clindamycin. The combination of cefepime and metronidazole was found to be equivalent to imipenem in a prospective, randomized study of intra-abdominal infections.[67]

ADVERSE EFFECTS

Cephalosporins are associated with a number of adverse side effects. The adverse reactions associated with their use are similar to those associated with use of other β-lactam compounds, such as local pain and irritation, hypersensitivity reactions, positive Coombs reaction, leukopenia, thrombocytopenia, transient abnormalities in liver function enzyme levels, and GI disturbances.[68,69] These reactions are usually mild and reversible, except in those rare patients who manifest life-threatening hypersensitivity reactions. Cephalosporins may be administered to most patients who are allergic to penicillin, because only 5% to 15% of penicillin-allergic patients react adversely to cephalosporins.[70] An excellent review of cephalosporin allergy and its treatment has been published.[71]

Aminoglycosides

Aminoglycosides are composed of two or more amino sugars bound by glycosidic linkage to a central hexose (aminocyclitol) nucleus. Their highly polar, polycationic structure contributes to their poor GI absorption and their meager ability to penetrate the blood-brain barrier. They bind irreversibly to the 30S bacterial ribosome and interfere with protein synthesis. Aminoglycosides also disturb calcium homeostasis and induce cell death as a result of efflux of potassium, sodium, and other essential bacterial constituents. Unlike most other antimicrobial agents that inhibit protein synthesis, aminoglycosides are bactericidal.

All aminoglycosides share certain pharmacokinetic properties. Because they are poorly absorbed when given orally, adequate serum concentrations can be obtained only through parenteral administration. Protein binding is negligible,[72] and the volume of distribution approximates the volume of the extracellular space.[73] In adults with normal renal function, the aminoglycosides have a half-life of about 2 hours, but there is considerable variation between individual patients.[74] In patients with deteriorating renal function, the half-life of an aminoglycosides increases, often exceeding 24 hours in patients with end-stage renal disease.[75]

The prolonged half-lives of aminoglycosides are substantially shortened during hemodialysis[76]; these agents are much less efficiently removed by peritoneal dialysis.[77] The aminoglycosides do not penetrate the blood-brain barrier well, even in patients with meningeal inflammation.[78,79] Drug levels in pulmonary secretions are typically 20% to 40% of serum levels. Low concentrations of aminoglycosides in purulent fluids are probably related to local inactivation caused by DNA released from leukocytes[80] and by the low regional pH.

The aminoglycosides are rapidly excreted, primarily by glomerular filtration. Urine concentrations may be 100 times the serum level in patients with normal renal function. The aminoglycosides accumulate in the renal cortex; sensitive assay techniques can detect them in urine and serum for up to 10 days after cessation of therapy.

STREPTOMYCIN

Widespread resistance among Enterobacteriaceae has limited the usefulness of streptomycin. At present, streptomycin is almost always employed in combination with other antimicrobial agents. With penicillin or vancomycin, streptomycin is used to treat infective endocarditis caused by viridans streptococci or susceptible enterococcal streptococci. It may also be given in conjunction with other antituberculous drugs to treat mycobacterial diseases and in conjunction with tetracycline to treat brucellosis. Streptomycin is used alone in the treatment of tularemia and plague.

KANAMYCIN

Because of widespread resistance among Enterobacteriaceae and *P. aeruginosa*, kanamycin is rarely used today. It is occasionally used as a second-line agent in combination with other antibiotics in the treatment of tuberculosis.

GENTAMICIN

Gentamicin is used for serious hospital-acquired infections caused by Enterobacteriaceae and most strains of *P. aeruginosa* in institutions in which there is minimal background resistance to this agent (other *Pseudomonas* species are predictably resistant to aminoglycosides). Gentamicin is given with penicillin to treat enterococcal endocarditis and with vancomycin plus rifampin to treat prosthetic valve endocarditis caused by *S. epidermidis*.

TOBRAMYCIN

Tobramycin closely resembles gentamicin with respect to antimicrobial spectrum and pharmacokinetics. Tobramycin is more active against some strains of *A. calcoaceticus* but less active against *S. marcescens*. Although tobramycin has slightly greater intrinsic activity against *P. aeruginosa*, most gentamicin-resistant strains of this organism are also resistant to tobramycin. The difference in nephrotoxicity between gentamicin and tobramycin is clinically insignificant.[81-83]

AMIKACIN

Amikacin is a semisynthetic derivative of kanamycin. Its major advantage is its resistance to aminoglycoside-modifying enzymes, the production of which is the principal mechanism of bacterial resistance to aminoglycosides. Amikacin may therefore be used against gentamicin-resistant organisms, and it is clearly the aminoglycoside of choice where gentamicin resistance is prevalent. Fortunately, no substantial increase in amikacin resistance has been noted, even in medical centers where it has been used extensively.[84]

NETILMICIN AND SISOMICIN

Netilmicin, a semisynthetic derivative of sisomicin, is not metabolized by most of the aminoglycoside-modifying enzymes and therefore is active against some strains of Enterobacteriaceae that are resistant to gentamicin and tobramycin; however, it is less active against *P. aeruginosa*. Animal studies suggest that netilmicin may be less nephrotoxic than other aminoglycosides,[82,85] and human studies suggest that it is somewhat less likely to exert toxic effects on cranial nerve VIII.[82] Sisomicin is more active than gentamicin against Enterobacteriaceae and *P. aeruginosa*, but the nephrotoxicity it has exhibited in animal studies exceeds that of other aminoglycosides.[86]

ADVERSE EFFECTS

Unlike β-lactam antibiotics, aminoglycosides, have a narrow range between therapeutic and toxic levels and are thus more likely to cause side effects. Their ototoxicity is potentially more significant than their nephrotoxicity because it is often irreversible. Cochlear toxicity has been reported in 8% to 10% of patients and has been clinically evident in as many as 4% of patients treated with aminoglycosides for various infections.[87] Vestibular toxicity, as manifested by electronystagmographic changes, has been found in 5% to 10% of patients and has been clinically significant in 1% to 5%.[82] Vestibular toxicity is more frequently associated with streptomycin, gentamicin, and tobramycin, whereas auditory toxicity is more typical of kanamycin and amikacin. Ototoxicity and vestibular toxicity are difficult to monitor, particularly in hospitalized patients for whom formal audiometry and caloric testing may be cumbersome or uncomfortable. Because aminoglycoside-associated auditory toxicity generally affects the higher frequencies, early bedside detection is difficult. Toxic effects on cranial nerve VIII seem to be related to advanced age, previous aminoglycoside treatment, and excessive serum levels.

AMINOGLYCOSIDE PHARMACOKINETICS

Peak aminoglycoside concentrations higher than 5 μg/ml are associated with improved survival in patients with gram-negative infections.[88,89] With gram-negative pulmonary infections, peak concentrations of 8 to 10 μg/ml are necessary because of poor penetration of aminoglycosides into the lungs.[90,91] It has been shown that a loading dose of gentamicin or tobramycin of 2 mg/kg of lean body weight cannot guarantee adequate peak concentrations in acutely ill patients. The most likely explanation for the usually low peak serum concentrations of aminoglycosides in acutely ill patients is an expanded volume of distribution.[92-96] Dosage adjustments based on blood levels should be made as soon as possible after the beginning of therapy and after the steady state has been reached.

Once-Daily Dosing of Aminoglycosides

Efforts to improve the toxic-to-therapeutic ratio of aminoglycosides include once-daily dosing schedules and reevaluations of the recommended therapeutic ranges. In conventional administration of aminoglycosides to patients with normal renal function, divided doses are administered at 8- to 12-hour intervals. In an effort to improve efficacy and decrease toxicity and cost, once-daily regimens have been compared with conventional regimens. In most protocols, the total doses were equivalent in the single and divided-dose regimens. Two meta-analyses of such trials have concluded that once-daily dosing is as effective as divided dosing and has a lower risk of toxicity in patients with normal renal function.[97,98] Although most trials evaluated immunocompetent adults, similar trends were noted for children and for patients with febrile neutropenia. In elderly patients, however, the high peak serum concentrations that occur with once-daily dosing may increase the risk of nephrotoxicity,[99] probably because of diminished renal clearance. There are several excellent reviews of the subject in the literature.[100,101]

Tetracyclines

The tetracyclines act against microorganisms by inhibiting protein synthesis; their site of action is the bacterial ribosome. Resistance to the tetracyclines appears slowly and in a stepwise fashion and is mediated by plasmids. Plasmids impart resistance by coding for proteins that interfere with active transport of tetracycline through the cytoplasmic membrane. Microorganisms that acquire resistance to one tetracycline are usually resistant to the other tetracyclines as well.

At appropriate dosages, peak serum concentrations 1 hour after intravenous administration of tetracycline, doxycycline, or minocycline are typically 10 to 20 µg/ml. The newer semisynthetic tetracyclines—doxycycline, methacycline, and minocycline—have considerably longer serum half-lives than the older agents.

Tetracyclines are metabolized by the liver and concentrated in the bile. Biliary concentrations of these agents are, on average, five to 10 times higher than concurrent plasma concentrations. The tetracyclines penetrate body tissues well and are capable of entering the CSF even in the absence of inflammation of the meninges. They readily cross the placental barrier, and relatively high concentrations are found in human milk.

Tetracyclines are useful in the treatment of sexually transmitted diseases. Tetracyclines are also effective for the treatment of other chlamydial infections, such as lymphogranuloma venereum, psittacosis, inclusion conjunctivitis, and trachoma. A tetracycline may also be used in the treatment of gonococcal infections in patients who are unable to tolerate penicillin G. Other sexually transmitted diseases that may be treated with tetracyclines are chancroid and granuloma inguinale.

A tetracycline or erythromycin is the agent of choice for the treatment of *Mycoplasma pneumoniae* infection. Tetracyclines are also effective against rickettsial infections, tularemia, and cholera; in patients unable to tolerate penicillin, they may be used to treat actinomycosis. Doxycycline is useful as prophylaxis against traveler's diarrhea caused by toxicogenic strains of *E. coli*. Unfortunately, the widespread use of tetracyclines as additives to livestock feed has resulted in increasing bacterial resistance to these agents.

Macrolides

ERYTHROMYCIN

Erythromycin is a macrolide that contains a many-membered lactone ring to which one or more deoxy sugars are attached. Erythromycin and other macrolide antibiotics inhibit protein synthesis through reversible binding to the 50S ribosomal subunits of susceptible microorganisms.

Erythromycin is well absorbed from the GI tract. The presence of food in the stomach reduces absorption of the drug, except when it is in the estolate form.[102] Erythromycin is excreted primarily in the bile; only 2% to 5% of a given dose is excreted in the urine. Concentrations in the bile may be more than 10 times those in plasma. Erythromycin diffuses readily into most tissues, except for the brain and the CSF.

Erythromycin is the agent of choice for the treatment of *M. pneumoniae* and *Legionella* infections. It is also effective against infections caused by group A β-hemolytic streptococci or *S. pneumoniae*. Accordingly, it is the agent of choice for the treatment of community-acquired pneumonia in nonimmunosuppressed patients who do not require hospitalization and who are allergic to penicillin.[103] In addition, erythromycin may be used to treat gonorrhea and syphilis in patients who are unable to tolerate penicillin G or tetracycline. The incidence of serious erythromycin-related adverse effects is low.

CLARITHROMYCIN AND AZITHROMYCIN

Clarithromycin and azithromycin are new semisynthetic macrolides that are structurally related to erythromycin. They inhibit protein synthesis in susceptible organisms by binding to the 50S ribosomal subunit. Clarithromycin and azithromycin are well absorbed and widely distributed, with excellent cellular and tissue penetration. Both agents have a broader spectrum of activity than erythromycin does; in addition, they have fewer GI side effects (a major obstacle to compliance with erythromycin therapy).

Clarithromycin is several times more active against gram-positive organisms in vitro than erythromycin, whereas azithromycin is two to four times less potent than erythromycin. Azithromycin has excellent in vitro activity against *H. influenzae*; clarithromycin, although less active against *H. influenzae* according to standard in vitro testing, is metabolized into an active compound with twice the in vitro activity of the parent drug. Azithromycin and clarithromycin also are active against some unexpected pathogens (e.g., *Borrelia burgdorferi, Toxoplasma gondii, M. avium* complex, and *M. leprae*). At present, clarithromycin appears to be the more active of the two against atypical mycobacteria, giving new hope to surgeons faced with what has become a difficult group of infections to treat.

Superior pharmacodynamic properties distinguish these new macrolides from the prototypical macrolide, erythromycin. Azithromycin has a large volume of distribution, and although serum concentrations remain low, it concentrates readily within tissues, demonstrating a tissue half-life of approximately 3 days; a 5-day course of therapy will provide therapeutic tissue concentrations for at least 10 days. These properties allow novel dosing schemes. For instance, azithromycin can be given once daily for 5 days to treat respiratory tract and soft tissue infections, and administration of a single 1 g dose of azithromycin can effectively treat *Chlamydia trachomatis* genital infections; these more convenient dosing schedules improve patient compliance.

DIRITHROMYCIN

Dirithromycin is an oral macrolide antibiotic with an antibacterial spectrum similar to that of erythromycin; it can be administered once daily but has no other advantages over erythromycin. The drugs produce similar GI side effects, and dirithromycin is substantially more expensive.

Clindamycin

Clindamycin is a 7-deoxy-7-chloro derivative of lincomycin that consists of an amino acid attached to a sulfur-containing octose. Clindamycin binds exclusively to the 50S subunit of bacterial ribosomes and suppresses the synthesis of protein. Clindamycin, erythromycin, and chloramphenicol all act at the same site, and the binding of one of these antibiotics to the ribosome may inhibit the binding of the others. Plasmid-mediated resistance to clindamycin has been reported in *B. fragilis*; this may be caused by methylation of bacterial RNA found in the 50S ribosomal subunit.[104] Peak serum concentrations 1 hour after intravenous administration of a 600 mg dose are approximately 10 to 12 μg/ml. Clindamycin is metabolized by the liver and excreted in an inactive form in the urine. It readily penetrates most body tissues but not the CSF.[105]

Clindamycin is active against *B. fragilis* and other anaerobic microorganisms and is useful in the treatment of patients with intra-abdominal, pelvic, and pulmonary infections. It is associated with a modest number of adverse effects.

Chloramphenicol

Chloramphenicol is unique among antibiotics in that it contains a nitrobenzene moiety and is a derivative of dichloroacetic acid. Like clindamycin, it inhibits bacterial protein synthesis by binding reversibly to the 50S ribosomal subunit, thus keeping the amino acid–containing end of aminoacyl–transfer RNA (tRNA) from binding to the ribosome. Chloramphenicol is rapidly and completely absorbed from the GI tract, and absorption is not impaired by concomitant ingestion of food or administration of antacids. It is inactivated in the liver by glucuronyl transferase. Chloramphenicol and its metabolites are excreted rapidly in the urine. About 80% to 90% of a dose is excreted in this way, about 5% to 10% of which is in the biologically active form. The drug penetrates well into all tissues, including the brain; it also penetrates well into the CSF and the aqueous humor.

Because of the risk of serious or fatal bone marrow toxicity, chloramphenicol should be used only against those infections for which the benefits of its use outweigh the risks of its potential toxicity. It still plays a major role in the treatment of typhoid fever, although plasmid-mediated resistance of *S. typhi* to chloramphenicol has been reported. Chloramphenicol is effective therapy for bacterial meningitis and brain abscesses caused by susceptible microorganisms; in conjunction with penicillin, it is effective empirical therapy for brain abscesses.

Vancomycin

Vancomycin is a narrow-spectrum antibiotic derived from *Nocardia orientalis*. Vancomycin exerts its bactericidal effect by inhibiting the biosynthesis of the major structural cell wall polymer, peptidoglycan.[106] Vancomycin is about 55% protein bound. Its activity is not significantly affected by pH values between 6.5 and 8.0. It is poorly absorbed from the GI tract. Because patients invariably experience pain after intramuscular injections, parenteral administration is limited to the intravenous route. Vancomycin is primarily excreted by the kidneys; about 80% to 90% of the dose is eliminated in a 24-hour period. Its half-life is approximately 6 hours in patients with normal renal function. In anuric patients, the half-life may be prolonged to approximately 7 days.[107] Vancomycin is not removed by hemodialysis or peritoneal dialysis.

Vancomycin is mainly effective against gram-positive organisms. No cross-resistance has been demonstrated between vancomycin and other antibiotics, and resistance is uncommon. Vancomycin, given alone, is the agent of choice in the treatment of methicillin-resistant *S. aureus* infections.[108,109] Some strains of methicillin-resistant *S. aureus*, however, are resistant to vancomycin. If vancomycin therapy is ineffective against severe infections caused by such strains, the addition of either an aminoglycoside or rifampin, or both, should be considered. Several reports

have indicated that vancomycin is not bactericidal for enterococci.[110] Vancomycin is indicated for other serious infections caused by organisms with multiple antibiotic resistance, such as CSF shunt infections and prosthetic valve infection caused by *S. epidermidis* or *Corynebacterium diphtheriae*.[111] It is the agent of choice for infections caused by penicillin-resistant group JK corynebacteria[112] and is uniformly active against rare, multiply resistant strains of *S. pneumoniae*.[113] Given orally, vancomycin is also the agent of choice for *C. difficile*–associated enterocolitis,[114] although less expensive agents, such as bacitracin[115] and metronidazole,[116] may be as effective.

Anaphylactoid reactions to vancomycin have been reported since the earliest clinical trials. Such reactions can occur with the first dose; signs and symptoms range from mild pruritus to dramatic hypotension and cardiovascular arrest. The rapid intravenous infusion of vancomycin can cause a peculiar reaction consisting of pruritus; an erythematous or maculopapular rash involving the face, neck, and upper torso; and possible hypotension.

Metronidazole

Metronidazole acts by disrupting bacterial DNA and inhibiting nucleic acid synthesis[117]; it is bactericidal against almost all anaerobic gram-negative bacilli, including *B. fragilis*, and against most *Clostridium* species. Although true anaerobic streptococci are generally susceptible to it, microaerophilic streptococci as well as *Actinomyces* and *Propionibacterium* species are often resistant.

Metronidazole is excellent for anaerobic infections of the abdomen and pelvis. For serious anaerobic infections, the drug is administered intravenously; a loading dose of 15 mg/kg is given, followed by 7.5 mg/kg every 6 hours until the patient is well enough to take an oral dosage of 7.5 mg/kg every 6 hours. The dosage need not be reduced in azotemic patients, but it should be reduced in patients with hepatic insufficiency. Because of its bactericidal action and excellent tissue penetration, intravenous metronidazole may be the treatment of choice for *B. fragilis* endocarditis and central nervous system infections, both of which are uncommon. When metronidazole is administered orally, it is well absorbed and is widely distributed in body tissues, including those of the CNS.

Side effects of metronidazole include dry mouth (associated with a metallic taste) and nausea. Concurrent use of alcohol may cause a reaction similar to that produced when alcohol is ingested after taking disulfiram. Neurologic symptoms, including peripheral neuropathy and encephalopathic reactions, and neutropenia are uncommon. Pancreatitis has been reported,[118] but alternative drugs are available.

Carbapenems

Imipenem and meropenem were the first carbapenems available for clinical use in the United States; the third, ertapenem, was released in 2002. Like other β-lactam antibiotics, they are bactericidal and act by inhibiting bacterial cell wall synthesis.[119] Three properties account for the extraordinarily broad antibacterial spectrum of the carbapenems: there is no permeability barrier excluding the drugs from bacteria; they have high affinity for penicillin-binding protein 2, which is a crucial component of cell wall structure; and they are extremely resistant to hydrolysis by β-lactamases.

Carbapenems are extraordinarily active against gram-negative bacteria. Whereas imipenem tends to be more active against gram-positive cocci, meropenem appears to be more active against gram-negative bacilli. Virtually all Enterobacteriaceae are susceptible. *Haemophilus* and *Neisseria* species are also susceptible to carbapenems but at concentrations somewhat higher than those of third-generation cephalosporins. Acinetobacter, which is resistant to most other β-lactam antibiotics, is susceptible to imipenem and meropenem, as are *Serratia, Salmonella, Citrobacter, Yersinia,* and *Brucella* species. Gram-negative anaerobes, including *B. fragilis,* are susceptible. *P. aeruginosa* is also susceptible, but some resistant strains have emerged during therapy; as a result, imipenem or meropenem should probably be combined with a second antipseudomonal drug when they are used to treat serious pseudomonal infections. Certain nosocomial pathogens, such as *Stenotrophomonas maltophilia* and *P. cepacia,* are resistant, as are *Flavobacterium* species.

Imipenem is extensively degraded in the renal tubule, which results in low urinary levels of the drug. This drawback can be prevented by using cilastatin, an inhibitor of the brush-border enzyme dehydropeptidase-1. Cilastatin also appears to prevent the tubular damage that is occasionally observed in animals given imipenem alone in high doses. For clinical use, imipenem and cilastatin are administered simultaneously in equal doses.

Meropenem is pharmacologically similar to imipenem except that it is not susceptible to degradation by dehydropeptidase; as a result, it can be administered without cilastatin. About 70% of both meropenem and imipenem is excreted in the urine; the dosage should be reduced in azotemic patients. Like imipenem, meropenem is active against most clinically active gram-positive and gram-negative bacteria, including anaerobes; however, neither drug is active against methicillin-resistant staphylococci or *E. faecium.* Resistant strains of *P. aeruginosa* have emerged during therapy with each drug.

The clinical efficacy and toxicity of meropenem are similar to those of imipenem, except that meropenem appears more likely to be effective in meningitis and less likely to cause seizures.

Because the newest carbapenem, ertapenem, has a longer half-life than the other members of the group, it can be administered in a single daily intravenous dose.[120] Like the other carbapenems, ertapenem is excreted in the urine, and the dosage should be reduced in azotemic patients. The antibacterial spectrum of ertapenem is similar to that of meropenem, except that *Pseudomonas* and *Acinetobacter* strains are less susceptible, and *E. faecalis* is resistant.[121] Ertapenem appears effective against community-acquired pneumonias, intra-abdominal infections, complicated skin and soft tissue infections, and complicated urinary tract infections, but experience is limited.

The carbapenems have broader antibacterial spectrums than any other β-lactam antibiotics. They are active against most gram-positive bacteria—both aerobes and anaerobes. Exceptions include some enterococci; many *E. faecalis* strains are sensitive to imipenem and meropenem but not ertapenem, and most *E. faecium* strains are resistant to all three drugs. Some diphtheroids are resistant. Although most *S. aureus* strains are very sensitive, the susceptibility of methicillin-resistant *S. aureus* and coagulase-negative staphylococci is highly variable. Methicillin-resistant *S. aureus* and *Listeria* exhibit carbapenem tolerance. Finally, some strains of *C. difficile* are resistant.

Ertapenem has a spectrum of activity similar to that of meropenem, except that *Pseudomonas* and *Acinetobacter* strains are much less susceptible, and *E. faecalis* is resistant.

The safety of carbapenems seems comparable to that of other β-lactam antibiotics. Nausea and vomiting, local pain at injection sites, and hypersensitivity are the most common reactions. Seizures, although unusual, are a potential concern with imipen-

em; they have been observed in 0.9% of patients who have received the drug; risk factors for seizure include excessive dosages of the drugs, preexisting CNS lesions, epilepsy, and renal insufficiency. Meropenem is less likely to provoke seizures.[119] Transient elevations of liver enzymes and leukopenia can occur in patients who are given carbapenems. Antibiotic-associated pseudomembranous colitis has occurred.

Because the structure of the carbapenems resembles that of the penicillins and cephalosporins, there is potential for cross-reactivity in patients allergic to other β-lactam antibiotics. Clinical experience in this situation is limited, but it appears prudent to avoid carbapenems in patients with anaphylactic sensitivity to β-lactam drugs and to use them with caution in patients with milder allergies to penicillins or cephalosporins.[122]

Carbapenems have been used successfully in patients with pneumonia, intra-abdominal infections, urinary tract infections, endocarditis, bacteremia, osteomyelitis, cellulitis, and febrile neutropenia. The broad spectrum and apparent low toxicity of carbapenems is impressive, but they should be used selectively and with restraint.

Monobactams

The monobactams are monocyclic β-lactam antibiotics that lack the thiazolidine ring found in penicillins and the dihydrothiazine ring found in cephalosporins. Although there are several monobactams under investigation, only aztreonam has been approved for clinical use in the United States. It has been evaluated in open and comparative studies against a number of agents currently used to treat infections.[123,124] It inhibits only aerobic gram-negative species. It can be administered two or three times daily. It is a poor hapten and has been successfully administered to small numbers of patients with proven allergy to penicillins and cephalosporins.[125]

Aztreonam has been shown to be effective against bacteremia caused by *E. coli, K. pneumoniae, P. mirabilis, S. marcescens, P. aeruginosa, Enterobacter* species, *Proteus* species, and *Providencia* species.[126,127] It has also been used, alone or in combination with clindamycin, to treat gram-negative aspiration pneumonia, with results comparable or superior to those obtained with an aminoglycoside-clindamycin combination.[128,129]

Aztreonam has been advocated as directed therapy to obviate more toxic drugs. It seems possible that aztreonam could replace aminoglycosides in many situations in which they are combined with other agents.

β-Lactamase Inhibitors

A novel approach to antibacterial chemotherapy is the use of β-lactamase inhibitors with β-lactam agents. Clavulanate has been combined with both amoxicillin and ticarcillin. Because neither clavulanate nor sulbactam inhibits the β-lactamases that function primarily as cephalosporinases in *Enterobacter, Serratia,* and *P. aeruginosa* infections, the addition of clavulanate or sulbactam does not enhance ticarcillin's activity against *Pseudomonas.* The principal use of amoxicillin-clavulanate has been in the treatment of upper respiratory tract infections caused by β-lactamase–producing *H. influenzae* or *M. catarrhalis.* Ticarcillin-clavulanate has been used to treat pneumonia caused by *P. aeruginosa* and mixed β-lactamase–producing flora as well as intra-abdominal infections and gynecologic infections in which the infecting organisms often possess β-lactamases. In febrile neutropenic patients, its efficacy is comparable to that of other agents, but superinfections may be a problem.[130,131] Because some strains of *K. pneumoniae* are not adequately inhibited by ticarcillin-clavulanate, addition of an aminoglycoside would be appropriate in neutropenic patients. Sulbactam has also been combined with ampicillin.

Clavulanate, sulbactam, and tazobactam have all been combined with piperacillin in an attempt to enhance the agent's activity against β-lactamase–producing bacteria.[132,133] Tazobactam enhances the spectrum of action and potency of piperacillin to a greater extent than sulbactam does. Although piperacillin-clavulanate is more potent than piperacillin-tazobactam, the two combinations are effective against virtually the same spectrum of resistant β-lactamase–producing gram-negative organisms. Piperacillin-tazobactam is more potent than ticarcillin-clavulanate and is effective against a wider range of gram-negative enteric organisms. Combinations of piperacillin with tazobactam or clavulanate have a broader spectrum of activity than combinations of piperacillin with sulbactam against bacteria that produce characterized plasmid-mediated enzymes of clinical significance. In particular, piperacillin-tazobactam and piperacillin-clavulanate inhibit TEM-1, TEM-2, and SHV-1 β-lactamases, but piperacillin-sulbactam does not. In mice infected with β-lactamase–producing *E. coli*, *K. pneumoniae*, *P. mirabilis*, and *S. aureus*, both tazobactam and clavulanate have provided greater enhancement of the therapeutic efficacy of piperacillin than sulbactam has. Reviews of the TEM-type β-lactamases[134] and the piperacillin-tazobactam combinations[135] have been published.

Quinolones

The addition of a fluorine group and a piperazine substituent to the first quinolones has greatly improved the antibacterial spectrum of this class of drugs; the addition of a methyl group on the piperazine ring appears to further enhance the bioavailability of these compounds.

The fluoroquinolones are bactericidal compounds that act by inhibiting DNA gyrase, the bacterial enzyme responsible for maintaining the supertwisted helical structure of DNA; DNA topoisomerase IV is a secondary target.[136] The fluoroquinolones rapidly kill bacteria, probably by impairing DNA synthesis and possibly by mechanisms involving the cleaving of bacterial chromosomal DNA. Bacterial resistance to the fluoroquinolones depends on a change in their DNA gyrase. Bacterial strains that are resistant to one fluoroquinolone tend to be cross-resistant to related compounds; such resistance is usually mediated by chromosomes, but plasmid-mediated resistance raises the possibility of transferable resistance.

The fluoroquinolones are broad-spectrum antimicrobials. Most enteric gram-negative bacilli, including *E. coli*, *Proteus*, *Klebsiella*, and *Enterobacter*, are highly susceptible; common GI pathogens, such as *Salmonella*, *Shigella*, and *Campylobacter* species, are also very sensitive. Other gram-negative organisms that are killed by low concentrations of the fluoroquinolones are *N. gonorrhoeae* and *N. meningitidis*, *H. influenzae*, *P. multocida*, *M. catarrhalis*, and *Y. enterocolitica*. *Acinetobacter* and *Serratia* are somewhat less susceptible. *P. aeruginosa* is susceptible to ciprofloxacin and trovafloxacin; ofloxacin and levofloxacin are moderately active, but the other quinolones are not effective. *P. cepacia* and *S. maltophilia* are quinolone-resistant. Ciprofloxacin is the drug of choice for *Bacillus anthracis*; oflaxacin and levofloxacin are also active in vitro.[137] Among gram-positive cocci, methicillin-sensitive strains of *S. aureus* and coagulase-negative staphylococci are usually susceptible to quinolones, but methicillin-resistant *S. aureus* and enterococci are not. Lomefloxacin is not active against pneumococci and other streptococci; ciprofloxacin and ofloxacin are moderately active; and levofloxacin, sparfloxacin, gatifloxacin, moxifloxacin, and trovafloxacin are highly effective, even against non–penicillin-sensitive pneumococci. Even fastidious intracellular pathogens can be inhibited by the quinolones; *Chlamydia*, *Mycoplasma*, *Listeria*, *Legionella*, and *M. tuberculosis* are in this category. Only trovafloxacin is highly active against anaerobes. Levofloxacin, gatifloxacin, moxifloxacin, and sparfloxacin demonstrate some activity against anaerobes, but the other quinolones do not. *C. difficile* is resistant to quinolones.

The fluoroquinolones are rapidly absorbed from the GI tract. Penetration into body fluids and tissues is generally excellent; therapeutic concentrations are readily achieved in blister fluid, bile, urine, saliva and sputum, bone, and muscle. Excellent concentrations of these drugs are achieved in the prostate, and stool levels are extraordinarily high. The fluoroquinolones appear to penetrate the CSF in the presence of meningeal inflammation,[138] but experience in treating meningitis is scant.

Although serum protein binding is modest, the fluoroquinolones have long serum half-lives, which range from 3 to 4 hours for ciprofloxacin to 12 hours for moxifloxacin. Most fluoroquinolones are eliminated by glomerular filtration and tubular secretion, and their dosages should be reduced in the presence of moderately severe renal failure. Trovafloxacin and moxifloxacin, however, are excreted chiefly by the liver.

The fluoroquinolones appear to be very well tolerated, with mild GI side effects (nausea, vomiting, or anorexia), CNS side effects (light-headedness, dizziness, somnolence, or insomnia), or rash occurring in fewer than 10% of treated patients. Lomefloxacin and sparfloxacin can cause phototoxicity. Less common side effects include allergic intestinal nephritis, pseudomembranous colitis, and neutropenia. Sparfloxacin and moxifloxacin may cause QT interval prolongation and should not be used by patients who have conditions or are using drugs known to prolong the QT interval or predispose to arrhythmias.[139] Tendinitis has been reported; in severe cases, it has resulted in rupture of the tendons of the shoulder and hand and the Achilles tendon. Crystalluria has been reported after the use of very large doses. Because fluoroquinolones have caused arthropathy in young animals, these drugs should be avoided in children and in women who are pregnant or nursing. Ciprofloxacin is safe in long-term use; there is less long-term experience with the other fluoroquinolones.

The fluoroquinolones have been useful clinically in a variety of infections, including urinary tract, genital, prostatic, GI, respiratory tract, soft tissue, and bone infections. Because of its excellent activity against anaerobes, trovafloxacin was considered useful in intra-abdominal and pelvic infections, but concerns about serious hepatotoxicity have restricted its use to infections deemed life- or limb-threatening and for patients in whom the benefit of trovafloxacin outweighs its potential risks. If it must be used, liver function must be monitored carefully.

The fluoroquinolones, administered in various regimens ranging from a single dose to 5 days of therapy, are effective in preventing and treating traveler's diarrhea and shigellosis. They have been highly effective in the treatment of typhoid fever. However, prolongation of the carrier state limits their role in nontyphoidal *Salmonella* enteritis, and the development of resistance limits their role in *Campylobacter* enteritis. The fluoroquinolones may be useful in the empirical treatment of severe community-acquired gastroenteritis, particularly if treatment is started early.

Because of their extraordinarily broad antimicrobial activity, their favorable pharmacokinetics, and their low toxicity,[140] the fluoroquinolones are extremely valuable new drugs. Like all antimicrobials, however, fluoroquinolones should be used judiciously, especially in view of new concerns about resistance[141,142] and toxicity and practical considerations about expense.

ADVERSE EFFECTS

Adverse reactions to the quinolones are estimated to occur in 4% to 8% of cases.[143] Most such reactions are not severe: cessation of therapy has been necessary in only about 1% to 2% of patients, and in all cases, the reactions have been reversible. The most common adverse effects are gastrointestinal—namely, nausea, vomiting, and diarrhea. The next most common are CNS effects, which include dizziness, headache, insomnia, hallucinations, agitation, and seizures. (The last three have been attributed to coadministration of enoxacin and theophylline.) Other effects include skin rash, pruritus, photosensitivity (with ofloxacin and pefloxacin), and mild alterations in hematologic and biochemical laboratory values.

Streptogramins

Quinupristin and dalfopristin are two structurally distinct streptogramins that bind to separate sites on the bacterial 50S ribosomal subunit; they thus act synergistically to inhibit protein synthesis. The drugs are marketed together in a 30:70 ratio as Synercid.[144]

Although quinupristin-dalfopristin is active against a variety of bacteria, its major use is in the treatment of serious infections caused by vancomycin-resistant strains of *E. faecium*. The drugs may also be useful in occasional vancomycin-intolerant patients with severe infections caused by methicillin-resistant *S. aureus* or coagulase-negative staphylococci. Resistance to quinupristin-dalfopristin is emerging.[145]

Quinupristin-dalfopristin is administered intravenously; because of a high incidence of phlebitis, a central line should be used. Other adverse effects include arthralgias and myalgias, which may be severe, and elevated bilirubin levels. The antibiotic may elevate levels of drugs that are metabolized by the hepatic enzyme CYP3A4; nifedipine and cyclosporine are examples.

The usual dose of quinupristin-dalfopristin is 7.5 mg/kg given intravenously over 1 hour every 8 hours. The drug is metabolized by the liver, so no dose reduction is required in azotemic patients. Quinupristin-dalfopristin is extremely expensive.

Oxazolidinones

In 2000, linezolid became the first member of the oxazolidinone class to be approved for clinical use in the United States.[146] Linezolid is a synthetic antibiotic that inhibits protein synthesis by binding to a site on the bacterial 23S ribosomal RNA of the 50S subunit, thus preventing function of the initiation complex that is required for ribosomal function.[147] Because no other antibiotic acts in this way, bacteria that have developed resistance to other ribosomally active antimicrobials do not display cross-resistance to linezolid.

Linezolid is active against nearly all aerobic gram-positive cocci at concentrations of 4 mg/ml or less,[148] including penicillin-resistant pneumococci, methicillin-resistant staphylococci, and vancomycin-resistant enterococci; however, resistant strains have been isolated.[149] The drug is bacteriostatic against staphylococci and enterococci, but it is bactericidal against most streptococcal strains. Linezolid is also active against *L. monocytogenes*, *M. catarrhalis*, *H. influenzae*, *N. gonorrhoeae*, *Bordetella pertussis*, *Pasteurella*

multocida, and *Nocardia* species. *C. difficile*, *C. perfringens*, and *Bacteroides* species are susceptible, but enteric gram-negative bacilli and *Pseudomonas* species are not.[150]

Intravenous and oral preparations of linezolid are available; the oral form is absorbed rapidly and completely with 100% bioavailability that is not affected by meals. Linezolid is widely distributed in well-perfused tissues. Nonrenal mechanisms account for 65% of the drug's clearance. Patients with mild to moderate renal or hepatic insufficiency do not appear to require reduced doses; linezolid is removed by hemodialysis.

Linezolid is well tolerated. Adverse effects have been reported in about 2.8% of all patients[150]; nausea, vomiting, and headaches are the most common side effects, but reversible marrow suppression, including thrombocytopenia, leukopenia, and anemia, can also occur. Because linezolid is a reversible inhibitor of monoamine oxidase, patients taking linezolid may experience an exaggerated hypertensive response to sympathomimetic agents. In addition to avoiding decongestants, patients taking linezolid should avoid foods or beverages with a high tyramine content; aged cheeses, air-dried meats, tap beer, red wine, soy sauce, and sauerkraut are examples. Monoamine oxidase inhibitors and other antidepressants should not be administered during linezolid therapy.

Linezolid has been used successfully in the therapy of multidrug-resistant gram-positive bacterial infections.[146,147,151] The drug is approved for vancomycin-resistant enterococcal infections and for pneumonias and skin and soft tissue infections. The usual dosage is 600 mg every 12 hours (p.o. or I.V.); uncomplicated skin and soft tissue infections may be treated with 400 mg every 12 hours.

Linezolid is a very promising new antimicrobial agent, but clinical experience is still limited. Although resistance is uncommon, it can develop during therapy. As a result, it may be wise to reserve this unique antibiotic for serious infections in hospitalized patients; in particular, linezolid should be useful for infections caused by methicillin-resistant *S. aureus* or coagulase-negative staphylococci that do not respond to vancomycin, for penicillin-resistant pneumococcal infections that do not respond to other agents, and for vancomycin-resistant enterococcal infection. An excellent general review of the use of linezolid in serious gram-positive infections has been published.[152]

Fosfomycin

Fosfomycin is a broad-spectrum antibiotic that inhibits cell wall synthesis in infections caused by *E. coli*, *S. saprophyticus*, and many other common urinary tract pathogens.[153] Although it has been used parenterally in Europe for many years, the drug is approved in the United States only for the single-dose treatment of uncomplicated urinary tract infections in women. A 3 g dose is generally effective and well tolerated; diarrhea is the most common side effect. Because of its activity against vancomycin-resistant enterococci (VRE), fosfomycin may be a useful alternative to linezolid and quinupristin-dalfopristin in the treatment of VRE infections in certain clinical situations (e.g., uncomplicated urinary tract infections). In addition, the use of fosfomycin could limit the use of newer agents, thus reducing the chance of development of further resistance in the enterococci.[154]

Concerns for the Future

Despite a century of often-successful prevention and control efforts, infectious diseases remain an important global problem in public health, causing over 13 million deaths each year. Changes in society, technology, and the microorganisms themselves are contributing to the emergence of new diseases, the reemergence of diseases once controlled, and the development of antimicrobial resistance. Two areas of special concern in the 21st century are food-borne disease and antimicrobial resistance. The effective control of infectious diseases in the new millennium will require effective public health infrastructures that will rapidly recognize and respond to outbreaks and will prevent emerging problems.

Over the past 40 years, the search for new antibiotics has been largely restricted to well-known classes of compounds that are active against a standard set of drug targets. Although many effective compounds have been discovered, insufficient chemical variability has been generated to prevent a serious escalation in clinical resistance. Recent advances in genomics have provided an opportunity to expand the range of potential drug targets and have facilitated a fundamental shift from direct antimicrobial screening programs toward rational target-based strategies. The application of genome-based technologies such as expression profiling and proteomics will lead to further changes in the drug discovery paradigm by combining the strengths and advantages of both screening strategies in a single program.

References

1. Jones RN: NCCLS regulatory guidelines. Antimicrobic Newsletter 1:5, 1984

2. Murray PR, Jorgensen JH: Quantitative susceptibility test methods in major United States medical centers. Antimicrob Agents Chemother 20:66, 1981

3. Reller LB: The serum bactericidal test. Rev Infect Dis 8:803, 1986

4. Weinstein MP, Stratton CW, Ackley A, et al: Multicenter collaborative evaluation of a standardized serum bactericidal test as a prognostic indicator in infective endocarditis. Am J Med 78:262, 1985

5. Sensakovic JW, Smith LG: Oral antibiotic treatment of infectious diseases. Med Clin North Am 85:115, 2001

6. Hoffman-Terry ML, Fraimow HS, Fox TR, et al: Adverse effects of outpatient parenteral antibiotic therapy. Am J Med 106:44, 1999

7. Gilbert DN, Dworkin RJ, Raber SR, et al: Outpatient parenteral antimicrobial-drug therapy. N Engl J Med 337:829, 1997

8. Lee CE, Zembower TR, Fotis MA, et al: The incidence of antimicrobial allergies in hospitalized patients: implications regarding prescribing patterns and emerging bacterial resistance. Arch Intern Med 160:2819, 2000

9. Ito S: Drug therapy for breast-feeding women. N Engl J Med 343:118, 2000

10. Solomkin JS, Dellinger EP, Christou NV, et al: Results of a multicenter trial comparing imipenem/cilastatin to tobramycin/clindamycin for intra-abdominal infections. Ann Surg 212:581, 1990

11. Zanetti G, Harbarth JS, Trampuz A, et al: Meropenem (1.5 g/day) is as effective as imipenem/cilastatin (2 g/day) for the treatment of moderately severe intra-abdominal infections. Int J Antimicrob Agents 11:107, 1999

12. Solomkin JS, Yellin AE, Rotstein OD, et al: Ertapenem versus piperacillin/tazobactam in the treatment of complicated intraabdominal infections: results of a double-blind, randomized comparative phase III trial. Ann Surg 237:235, 2003

13. Nichols RL: Empiric antibiotic therapy for intraabdominal infections. Rev Infect Dis 5:S90, 1983

14. Lea AS, Feliciano DV, Gentry LO: Intra-abdominal infections: an update. J Antimicrob Chemother 9(suppl A):107, 1982

15. Barie PS, Christou NV, Dellinger EP, et al: Pathogenicity of the enterococcus in surgical infections. Ann Surg 212:155, 1990

16. Solomkin JS, Dellinger EP, Christou NV, et al: Design and conduct of antibiotic trials: a report of the Scientific Studies Committee of the Surgical Infection Society. Arch Surg 122:158, 1987

17. Christou NV, Turgeon P, Wassef R, et al: Management of intra-abdominal infections: the case for intra-operative cultures and comprehensive broad spectrum antibiotic coverage. Arch Surg 131:1193, 1996

18. Cunha BA: Antibiotic side effects. Med Clin North Am 85:149, 2001

19. Hogenauer C, Hammer HF, Krejs GJ, et al: Mechanisms and management of antibiotic-associated diarrhea. Clin Infect Dis 27:702, 1998

20. Barlett JG: Antibiotic-associated diarrhea. N Engl J Med 346:334, 2002

21. Gatifloxacin and moxifloxacin: two new fluoroquinolones. Med Lett Drugs Ther 42:1, 2000

22. Bertino JS Jr, Owens RC Jr, Carnes TD, et al: Gatifloxacin-associated corrected QT interval prolongation, torsades de pointes, and ventricular fibrillation in patients with known risk factors. Clin Infect Dis 34:861, 2002

23. Vassileva SG, Mateev G, Parish LC: Antimicrobial photosensitive reactions. Arch Intern Med 158:1993, 1998

24. Kollef MH, Fraser VJ: Antibiotic resistance in the intensive care unit. Ann Intern Med 134:298, 2001

25. Virk A, Steckelberg JM: Clinical aspects of antimicrobial resistance. Mayo Clin Proc 75:200, 2000

26. Moellering RC Jr: Antibiotic resistance: lessons for the future. Clin Infect Dis 27(suppl 1):S135, 1998

27. Jenkins SG: Mechanisms of bacterial antibiotic resistance. New Horizons 4:321, 1996

28. Tenover FC: Development and spread of bacterial resistance to antimicrobial agents: an overview. Clin Infect Dis 33(suppl 3):S108, 2001

29. Williams RJ: Globalization of antimicrobial resistance: epidemiological challenges. Clin Infect Dis 33(suppl 3):S116, 2001

30. de Man P, Verhoeven BAN, Verbrugh HA, et al: An antibiotic policy to prevent emergence of resistant bacilli. Lancet 355:973, 2000

31. Cunha BA: Effective antibiotic-resistance control strategies. Lancet 357:1307, 2001

32. Moellering RC Jr: Enterococcal infections in patients treated with moxalactam. Rev Infect Dis 4(suppl):S708, 1982

33. Shay DK, Maloney SA, Montecalvo M, et al: Epidemiology and mortality risk of vancomycin-resistant enterococcal bloodstream infections. J Infect Dis 172:993, 1995

34. McGowen JE: Antimicrobial resistance in hospital organisms and its relation to antibiotic use. Rev Infect Dis 5:1033, 1983

35. Baquero F, Martinez-Beltran J, Loza E: 1991: A review of antibiotic resistance patterns of *Streptococcus pneumoniae* in Europe. J Antimicrob Chemother 28(suppl C):31, 1991

36. Wormer DC, Martin WJ, Nichold DR, et al: Concentrations in serum of procaine and crystalline penicillin G administered orally or parenterally. Antibiotics in Medicine 1:589, 1955

37. Gilbert DN, Sanford JP: Methicillin: critical appraisal after a decade of experience. Med Clin North Am 54:1113, 1970

38. Amoxicillin. Med Lett Drugs Ther 16:49, 1974

39. Bodey GP, Whitecar JP Jr, Middleman E, et al: Carbenicillin therapy for *Pseudomonas* infections. JAMA 218:62, 1971

40. Hoffman TA, Bullock WE: Carbenicillin therapy of *Pseudomonas* and other gram-negative bacillary infections. Ann Intern Med 73:165, 1970

41. Butler K, English AR, Ray VA, et al: Carbenicillin: chemistry and mode of action. J Infect Dis 122(suppl):S1, 1970

42. Ticarcillin. Med Lett Drugs Ther 19:17, 1977

43. Tjandramaga TB, Mullie A, Verbesselt R, et al: Piperacillin: human pharmacokinetics after intravenous and intramuscular administration. Antimicrob Agents Chemother 14:829, 1978

44. Bergan T: Pharmacokinetics of mezlocillin in healthy volunteers. Antimicrob Agents Chemother 14:801, 1978

45. Bergan T, Brodwall EK, Wiik-Larsen E: Mezlocillin pharmacokinetics in patients with normal and impaired renal functions. Antimicrob Agents Chemother 16:651, 1979

46. Gentry LO, Jemsek JG, Natelson EA: Effects of sodium piperacillin on platelet function in normal volunteers. Antimicrob Agents Chemother 19:532, 1981

47. Fu KP, Neu HC: Azlocillin and mezlocillin: new ureido penicillins. Antimicrob Agents Chemother 13:930, 1978

48. Bodey GP, Le Blanc B: Piperacillin: in vitro evaluation. Antimicrob Agents Chemother 14:78, 1978

49. Tally FP, McGowan K, Kellum JM, et al: A randomized comparison of cefoxitin with or without amikacin and clindamycin plus amikacin in surgical sepsis. Ann Surg 193:318, 1981

50. Donowitz GR, Mandell GL: Empiric therapy for pneumonia. Rev Infect Dis 5(suppl):S40, 1983

51. Cefotetan disodium (Cefotan). Med Lett Drugs Ther 28:70, 1986

52. Orr JW Jr, Varner RE, Kilgore LC, et al: Cefotetan versus cefoxitin as prophylaxis in hysterectomy. Am J Obstet Gynecol 154:960, 1986

53. McCarty JM, Renteria A: Treatment of pharyngitis and tonsillitis with cefprozil: review of three multicenter trials. Clin Infect Dis 14(suppl 2):S224, 1992

54. Doern G: In vitro activity of loracarbef and effects of susceptibility test methods. Am J Med 92:7S, 1992

55. Wise R, Andrews JM, Ashby JP, et al: Ceftibuten: a new orally absorbed cephalosporin: in vitro activity against strains from the United Kingdom. Diagn Microbiol Infect Dis 14:45, 1991

56. Boscia JA, Korzeniowski OM, Snepar R, et al: Cefoperazone pharmacokinetics in normal subjects and patients with cirrhosis. Antimicrob Agents Chemother 23:385, 1983

57. Kemmerich B, Lode H, Borner K, et al: Biliary excretion and pharmacokinetics of cefoperazone in humans. J Antimicrob Chemother 12:27, 1983

58. Wittmann DH, Schassan HH: Distribution of moxalactam in serum, bone, tissue fluid, and peritoneal fluid. Rev Infect Dis 4(suppl):S610, 1982

59. Saito Y, Kushima T, Seimori T, et al: Absorption and excretion of cefotaxime and its levels in uterine arterial blood, female internal genital organ tissue and pelvic cavity fluid. Jpn J Antibiot 34:481, 1981

60. Grabe M, Andersson KE, Forsgren A, et al: Concentrations of cefotaxime in serum, urine, and tissues of urological patients. Infection 9:154, 1981

61. Kosmidis J, Stathakis C, Mantopoulos K, et al: Clinical pharmacology of cefotaxime including penetration into bile, sputum, bone and cerebrospinal fluid. J Antimicrob Chemother 6(suppl A):147, 1980

62. Watts JM, McDonald PJ, Woods PJ: Clinical trials of antimicrobials in surgery. World J Surg 6:321, 1982

63. Solomkin JS, Meakins JL Jr, Allo MD, et al: Antibiotic trials in intra-abdominal infections: a critical evaluation of study design and outcome reporting. Ann Surg 200:29, 1984

64. Feinstein AR: Clinical Biostatistics. CV Mosby Co, St Louis, 1977

65. Edelstein H, Chirurgi V, Oster S, et al: A randomized trial of cefepime (BMY-28142) and ceftazidime for the treatment of pneumonia. J Antimicrob Chemother 28:569, 1991

66. Gloor B, Worni M, Strobel O, et al: Cefepime tissue penetration in experimental acute pancreatitis. Pancreas 26:117, 2003

67. Barie PS, Vogel SB, Dellinger EP, et al: A randomized, double-blind clinical trial comparing cefepime plus metronidazole with imipenem-cilastatin in the treatment of complicated intra-abdominal infections. Cefepime Intra-abdominal Infection Study Group. Arch Surg 132:1294, 1997

68. Smith CR: Cefotaxime and cephalosporins: adverse reactions in perspective. Rev Infect Dis 4(suppl):S481, 1982

69. Parks D, Layne P, Uri J, et al: Ceftizoxime: clinical evaluation of efficacy and safety in the U.S.A. J Antimicrob Chemother 10(suppl C):327, 1982

70. Petz LD: Immunologic cross-reactivity between penicillins and cephalosporins: a review. J Infect Dis 137:S74, 1978

71. Kelkar PS, Li JT-C: Cephalosporin allergy. N Engl J Med 345:804, 2001

72. Gordon RC, Regamey C, Kirby WMM: Serum protein binding of the aminoglycoside antibiotics. Antimicrob Agents Chemother 2:214, 1972

73. Siber GR, Echeverria P, Smith AL, et al: Pharmacokinetics of gentamicin in children and adults. J Infect Dis 132:637, 1975

74. Walker JM, Wise R: The pharmacokinetics of amikacin and gentamicin in volunteers: a comparison of individual differences. J Antimicrob Chemother 5:95, 1979

75. Lockwood WR, Bower JD: Tobramycin and gentamicin concentrations in the serum of normal and anephric patients. Antimicrob Agents Chemother 3:125, 1973

76. McHenry MC, Wagner JG, Hall PM, et al: Pharmacokinetics of amikacin in patients with impaired renal function. J Infect Dis 134(suppl):S343, 1976

77. Regeur L, Colding H, Jensen H, et al: Pharmacokinetics of amikacin during hemodialysis and peritoneal dialysis. Antimicrob Agents Chemother 11:214, 1977

78. Goitein K, Michel J, Sacks T: Penetration of parenterally administered gentamicin into the cerebrospinal fluid in experimental meningitis. Chemotherapy 21:181, 1975

79. Briedis DJ, Robson HG: Cerebrospinal fluid penetration of amikacin. Antimicrob Agents Chemother 13:1042, 1978

80. Vaudaux P, Waldvogel FA: Gentamicin inactivation in purulent exudates: role of cell lysis. J Infect Dis 142:586, 1980

81. Smith CR, Lipsky JJ, Laskin OL, et al: Double-blind comparison of the nephrotoxicity and auditory toxicity of gentamicin and tobramycin. N Engl J Med 302:1106, 1980

82. Kahlmeter G, Dahlager JI: Aminoglycoside toxicity: a review of clinical studies published between 1975 and 1982. J Antimicrob Chemother 13(suppl A):9, 1984

83. Kumin GD: Clinical nephrotoxicity of tobramycin and gentamicin: a prospective study. JAMA 244:1808, 1980

84. Betts RF, Valenti WM, Chapman SW, et al: Five-year surveillance of aminoglycoside usage in a university hospital. Ann Intern Med 100:219, 1984

85. Luft FC, Yum MN, Kleit SA: Comparative nephrotoxicities of netilmicin and gentamicin in rats. Antimicrob Agents Chemother 10:845, 1976

86. Robbins G, Tettenborn D: Toxicity of sisomicin in animals. Infection 4(suppl 4):S349, 1976

87. Fee WE Jr: Gentamicin and tobramycin: comparison of ototoxicity. Rev Infect Dis 5(suppl 2):S304, 1983

88. Moore RD, Smith CR, Lietman PS: The association of aminoglycoside plasma levels with mortality in patients with gram-negative bacteremia. J Infect Dis 149:443, 1984

89. Noone P, Parsons TMC, Pattison JR, et al: Experience in monitoring gentamicin therapy during treatment of serious gram-negative sepsis. Br Med J 1:477, 1974

90. Alexander MR, Schoell J, Hicklin G, et al: Bronchial secretion concentrations of tobramycin. Am Rev Respir Dis 125:208, 1982

91. Moore RD, Smith CR, Lietman PS: Association of aminoglycoside plasma levels with therapeutic outcome in gram-negative pneumonia. Am J Med 77:657, 1984

92. Zaske DE, Cipolle RJ, Strate RJ: Gentamicin dosage requirements: wide interpatient variations in 242 surgery patients with normal renal function. Surgery 87:164, 1980

93. Kaye D, Levison ME, Labovitz ED: The unpredictability of serum concentrations of gentamicin: pharmacokinetics of gentamicin in patients with normal and abnormal renal function. J Infect Dis 130:150, 1974

94. Zaske DE, Cipolle RJ, Strate RG: Increased gentamicin dosage requirements: rapid elimination in 249 gynecology patients. Am J Obstet Gynecol 139:896, 1981

95. Dasta JF, Armstrong DK: Variability in aminoglycoside pharmacokinetics in critically ill surgical patients (abstr). Crit Care Med 14:393, 1986

96. Hassan E, Ober J: Predicted and measured aminoglycoside pharmacokinetic parameters in critically ill patients (abstr). Crit Care Med 14:394, 1986

97. Hatala R, Dinh T, Cook DJ: Once-daily aminoglycoside dosing in immunocompetent adults: a meta-analysis. Ann Intern Med 124:717, 1996

98. Barza M, Loannidis JPA, Cappelleri JC, et al: Single or multiple daily doses of aminoglycosides: a meta-analysis. BMJ 321:338, 1996

99. Koo J, Tight R, Rajkumar V, et al: Comparison of once-daily versus pharmacokinetic dosing of aminoglycosides in elderly patients. Am J Med 101:177, 1996

100. Schumock GT, Raber SR, Crawford SY, et al: National survey of once-daily dosing of aminoglycoside antibiotics. Pharmacotherapy 15:201, 1995

101. Preston SL, Briceland LL: Single daily dosing of aminoglycosides. Pharmacotherapy 15:297, 1995

102. Griffith RS, Black HR: Comparison of the blood levels obtained after single and multiple doses of erythromycin estolate and erythromycin stearate. Am J Med Sci 247:69, 1964

103. Washington JA II, Wilson WR: Erythromycin: a microbial and clinical perspective after 30 years of clinical use (pt 2). Mayo Clin Proc 60:271, 1985

104. Steigbigel NH: Erythromycin, lincomycin, and clindamycin. Principles and Practice of Infectious Diseases, 2nd ed. Mandell GL, Douglas RG Jr, Bennett JE, Eds. John Wiley & Sons, New York, 1985, p 224

105. Panzer JD, Brown DC, Epstein WL, et al: Clindamycin levels in various body tissues and fluids. J Clin Pharmacol 12:259, 1972

106. Sande MA, Mandell GL: Antimicrobial agents: tetracyclines, chloramphenicol, erythromycin, and miscellaneous antibacterial agents. Goodman and Gilman's The Pharmacological Basis of Therapeutics, 7th ed. Gilman AG, Goodman LS, Rall TW, et al, Eds. Macmillan Publishing Co, New York, 1985, p 1170

107. Moellering RC Jr: Pharmacokinetics of vancomycin. J Antimicrob Chemother 14(suppl D):43, 1984

108. Myers JP, Linnemann CC Jr: Bacteremia due to methicillin-resistant Staphylococcus aureus. J Infect Dis 145:532, 1982

109. Watanakunakorn C: Treatment of infections due to methicillin-resistant Staphylococcus aureus. Ann Intern Med 97:376, 1982

110. Harwick HJ, Kalmanson GM, Guze LB: In vitro activity of ampicillin or vancomycin combined with gentamicin or streptomycin against enterococci. Antimicrob Agents Chemother 4:383, 1973

111. Van Scoy RE, Cohen SN, Geraci JE, et al: Coryneform bacterial endocarditis: difficulties in diagnosis and treatment, presentation of three cases, and review of literature. Mayo Clin Proc 52:216, 1977

112. Riley PS, Hollis DG, Utter GB, et al: Characterization and identification of 95 diphtheroid (group JK) cultures isolated from clinical specimens. J Clin Microbiol 9:418, 1979

113. Liñares J, Perez JL, Garau J, et al: Comparative susceptibilities of penicillin-resistant pneumococci to co-trimoxazole, vancomycin, rifampicin and fourteen β-lactam antibiotics. J Antimicrob Chemother 13:353, 1984

114. Fekety R, Silva J, Armstrong J, et al: Treatment of antibiotic-associated enterocolitis with vancomycin. Rev Infect Dis 3(suppl):S237, 1981

115. Dudley MN, McLaughlin JC, Carrington G, et al: Oral bacitracin vs vancomycin therapy for Clostridium difficile–induced diarrhea: a randomized double-blind trial. Arch Intern Med 146:1101, 1986

116. Teasley DG, Gerding DN, Olson M, et al: Pro-

spective randomised trial of metronidazole versus vancomycin for *Clostridium difficile*–associated diarrhoea and colitis. Lancet 2:1043, 1983

117. Koch-Wesser J, Goldman P: Drug therapy: metronidazole. N Engl J Med 303:1212, 1980

118. Corey WA, Doebbeling BN, Dejong KJ, et al: Metronidazole-induced acute pancreatitis (note). Rev Infect Dis 13:1213, 1990

119. Hellinger WC, Brewer NS: Carbapenems and monobactams: imipenem, meropenem, and aztreonam. Mayo Clin Proc 74:420, 1999

120. Odenholt I: Ertapenem: a new carbapenem. Expert Opin Investig Drugs 10:1157, 2001

121. Livermore DM, Carter MW, Bagel S, et al: In vitro activities of ertapenem (MK-0826) against recent clinical bacteria collected in Europe and Australia. Antimicrob Agents Chemother 45:1860, 2001

122. McConnell SA, Penzak SR, Warmack TS, et al: Incidence of imipenem hypersensitivity reactions in febrile neutropenic bone marrow transplant patients with a history of penicillin allergy. Clin Infect Dis 31:1512, 2000

123. Barry AL, Thornsberry C, Jones RN, et al: Aztreonam: antibacterial activity, β-lactamase stability, and interpretive standards and quality control guidelines for disk-diffusion susceptibility tests. Rev Infect Dis 7(suppl 4):S594, 1985

124. Swabb EA: Clinical pharmacology of aztreonam in healthy recipients and patients: a review. Rev Infect Dis 7(suppl 4):S605, 1985

125. Adkinson NF Jr, Saxon A, Spence MR, et al: Cross-allergenicity and immunogenicity of aztreonam. Rev Infect Dis 7(suppl 4):S613, 1985

126. Scully BE, Henry SA: Clinical experience with aztreonam in the treatment of gram-negative bacteremia. Rev Infect Dis 7(suppl 4):S789, 1985

127. Pierard D, Boelaert J, Van Landuyt HW, et al: Aztreonam treatment of gram-negative septicemia. Antimicrob Agents Chemother 29:359, 1986

128. Rodriguez JR, Ramirez-Ronda CH, Nevárez M: Efficacy and safety of aztreonam-clindamycin versus tobramycin-clindamycin in the treatment of lower respiratory tract infections caused by aerobic gram-negative bacilli. Antimicrob Agents Chemother 27:246, 1985

129. Scully BE, Neu HC: Use of aztreonam in the treatment of serious infections due to multiresistant gram-negative organisms, including *Pseudomonas aeruginosa*. Am J Med 78:251, 1985

130. Meylan PR, Calandra T, Casey PA, et al: Clinical experience with Timentin in severe hospital infections. J Antimicrob Chemother 17(suppl C):127, 1986

131. Meunier F, Snoeck R, Lagast H, et al: Empirical antimicrobial therapy with Timentin plus amikacin in febrile granulocytopenic cancer patients. J Antimicrob Chemother 17(suppl C):195, 1986

132. Kuck NA, Jacobus NV, Petersen PJ, et al: Comparative in vitro and in vivo activities of piperacillin combined with the beta-lactamase inhibitors tazobactam, clavulanic acid, and sulbactam. Antimicrob Agents Chemother 33:1964, 1989

133. Fass RJ, Prior RB: Comparative in vitro activities of piperacillin-tazobactam and ticarcillin-clavulanate. Antimicrob Agents Chemother 33:1268, 1989

134. Knox J: Extended spectrum and inhibitor-resistant TEM-type β-lactamases: mutations, specificity, and three-dimensional structure. Antimicrob Agents Chemother 39:2593, 1995

135. Sanders E, Sanders C: Piperacillin/tazobactam: a critical review of the evolving clinical literature. Clin Infect Dis 22:107, 1996

136. Hooper DC: Mechanisms of action of antimicrobials: focus on fluoroquinolones. Clin Infect Dis 32(supp 1):S9, 2001

137. Swartz MN: Recognition and management of anthrax: an update. N Engl J Med 345:1621, 2001

138. Lipman J, Allworth A, Wallis SC: Cerebrospinal fluid penetration of high doses of intravenous ciprofloxacin in meningitis. Clin Infect Dis 31:1131, 2000

139. Gatifloxacin and moxifloxacin: two new fluoroquinolones. Med Lett Drugs Ther 42:15, 2000

140. Mandell LA, Ball P, Tillotson G: Antimicrobial safety and tolerability: differences and dilemmas. Clin Infect Dis 32(suppl 1):S72, 2001

141. Chen DK, McGeer A, de Azavedo JC, et al: Decreased susceptibility of *Streptococcus pneumoniae* to fluoroquinolones in Canada. N Engl J Med 341:233, 1999

142. Thomson CJ: The global epidemiology of resistance to ciprofloxacin and the changing nature of antibiotic resistance: a 10 year perspective. J Antimicrob Chemother 43:31, 1999

143. Halkin H: Adverse effects of the fluoroquinolones. Rev Infect Dis 10(suppl 1):S258, 1988

144. Quinupristin/dalfopristin. Med Lett Drugs Ther 41:109, 1999

145. Johnson AP, Livermore DM: Quinupristin/dalfopristin, a new addition to the antimicrobial arsenal. Lancet 354:2012, 1999

146. Linezolid (Zyvox). Med Lett Drugs Ther 42:1, 2000

147. Diekema DJ, Jones RN: Oxazolidinone antibiotics. Lancet 358:77, 2001

148. Cercenado E, García-Garrote F, Bouza E: In vitro activity of linezolid against multiply resistant gram-positive clinical isolates. J Antimicrob Chemother 47:77, 2001

149. Tsiodras S, Gold HS, Sakoulas G, et al: Linezolid resistance in a clinical isolate of *Staphylococcus aureus*. Lancet 358:207, 2001

150. Clemett D, Markham A: Linezolid. Drugs 59:815, 2000

151. Chien JW, Kucia ML, Salata RA: Use of linezolid, an oxazolidinone, in the treatment of multidrug-resistant gram-positive bacterial infections. Clin Infect Dis 30:146, 2000

152. Perry CD, Jarvis B. Linezolid: A review of its use in the management of serious gram-positive infections. Drugs 61:525, 2001

153. Fosfomycin for urinary tract infections. Med Lett Drugs Ther 39:66, 1997

154. Shrestha NK, Chua JD, Tuohy MH, et al: Antimicrobial susceptibility of vancomycin-resistant *Enterococcus faecium*: potential utility of fosfomycin. Scand J Infect Dis 35:12, 2003

155. Simon HB: XIV Antimicrobial chemotherapy. 7 Infectious Disease. WebMD Scientific American® Medicine. Dale DC, Federman DD, Eds. WebMD Inc. New York, 2003. http://www.samed.com. June 2003

17 NOSOCOMIAL INFECTION

E. Patchen Dellinger, M.D., F.A.C.S.

Approach to Postoperative Symptoms of Infection

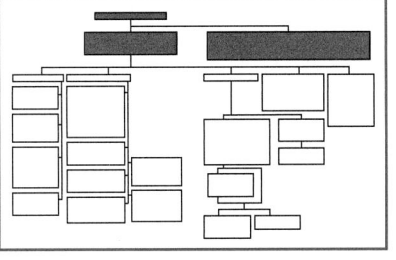

Nosocomial infections are a potential threat to all hospitalized patients. They increase morbidity and mortality, prolong hospital stay, increase patient care costs,[1-5] and occur in almost every body site.

At any time during hospitalization, but especially postoperatively, the onset of fever or an elevated white blood cell count may signal an infectious process. Fever that begins or persists after postoperative day 4 is more likely to represent true infection. Although an infection will not develop in many febrile postoperative patients [*see* Discussion, *below*], a careful, directed examination of the patient, guided by history and operative procedure, should be undertaken, including inspection of the ears and the pharynx. Laboratory tests and x-rays are complementary. The use of empirical antibiotics or the prolonged administration of perioperative prophylactic antibiotics in the absence of a specific diagnosis is rarely efficacious. In fact, either may confuse the clinical picture and may lead to separate toxic or allergic complications. Antibiotics alone rarely constitute an adequate response to infectious complications, especially in the early postoperative period.

Respiratory infections are the most common early infection, with most wound infections presenting between postoperative days 4 and 7 and urinary tract infections (UTIs) occurring throughout hospitalization. However, if a high fever (temperature > 38.9° C [102° F]) develops in a patient within 48 hours of an operation, three diagnoses are most likely: atelectasis [*see 6:5 Pulmonary Insufficiency*], peritonitis caused by a leaking viscus after intra-abdominal operation [*see 6:18 Intra-abdominal Infection*], and invasive wound infection. Of these, atelectasis is most often diagnosed. It is not serious if recognized and treated. Atelectasis can be diagnosed on the basis of decreased breath sounds, rales, or both on physical examination and on the basis of platelike densities or volume loss on chest x-ray. Atelectasis may be accompanied by hypoxemia and usually responds to standard physical measures. However, many patients with x-ray evidence of atelectasis are not febrile, and more than one third of patients with fever and no other apparent cause have no evidence of atelectasis.[6,7]

Clues to the diagnosis of peritonitis caused by a leaking viscus are knowledge of problems in the conduct of the operative procedure, evidence of the hemodynamic and fluid balance changes that usually accompany a leaking viscus, and suggestive findings on abdominal examination. Technical difficulties with anastomoses, excessive operative blood loss, and multiple bowel injuries can all increase the risk of leakage. Diffuse abdominal tenderness away from the incision, excessive fluid requirements in the early postoperative interval, and tachycardia all suggest iatrogenic peritonitis. Treatment always involves operative intervention and antibiotics. The least common cause of early high postoperative fever is an invasive wound infection, either with β-hemolytic streptococci or with clostridia. Diagnosis is made by local inspection of the wound and by a Gram stain of the wound's contents; treatment requires operative intervention in addition to antibiotics [*see* Infection Related to Operative Site or Injury, *below*].

Respiratory Infection

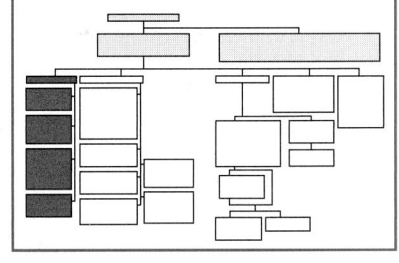

Pneumonia is the third most common nosocomial infection on surgical services and is the one most commonly associated with death.[8] Diagnosis is not usually difficult in a patient without respiratory failure who is breathing spontaneously. In a patient with acute respiratory distress syndrome (ARDS) who is intubated and being ventilated, however, the diagnosis may be extremely difficult.[9] This is because ARDS is associated with markedly abnormal chest x-ray findings and gas exchange abnormalities and may also include an elevated temperature without infection. A number of techniques for diagnosis, including bronchoalveolar lavage both with and without a bronchoscope and protected specimen brush cultures, have been reported to increase the sensitivity and specificity of diagnosis of pneumonia in this setting but have not been widely adopted.[10,11]

The prevention of pneumonia in ventilated patients would be the best alternative, but there is not widespread agreement about the best means of prevention. Recommendations include standard infection control measures, elevation of the head of the bed, and possibly the use of endotracheal tubes that permit the aspiration of subglottic secretions.[10,12-14]

The diagnosis of pneumonitis or atelectasis (see above) is frequently entertained during the workup of postoperative fever. It is important to remember that a common cause of basilar atelectasis and pleural effusion in the postlaparotomy patient is an inflammatory process below the diaphragm. Tracheitis or bronchitis, as indicated by purulent sputum in the absence of pul-

Approach to Postoperative Symptoms of Infection

Fever or an elevated WBC develops postoperatively

Fever begins or persists after 4th postoperative day

Identify source of infection:
- Perform physical examination guided by history and prior operations.
- Inspect all intravascular devices and urinary catheters.
- Order appropriate x-rays and laboratory tests.

Respiratory infection

Pneumonia, as suggested by ↑ WBC, ↑ temperature, purulent sputum, and lung infiltrate

Give appropriate antibiotics; provide supportive care.

Tracheitis or bronchitis, as suggested by purulent sputum, normal x-ray findings, and endotracheal or tracheostomy intubation

Give appropriate antibiotics if patient is febrile.

Paranasal sinusitis, as suggested by purulent nasal drainage, otitis media, and/or CT findings of fluid, air-fluid levels, and mucosal thickening

Identify pathogen via Gram stain and culture of sinus aspirate. Remove all nasal tubes; administer decongestants and appropriate antibiotics. Perform sinus irrigation or drainage for unresponsive cases.

Otitis media (associated with eustachian tube blockage from nasal tubes or inflammation)

Remove nasal tube, and give decongestants.

Infection related to operative site or injury

Wound infection (incisional SSI), as suggested by erythema, swelling, drainage, and increasing local pain and tenderness

Incise and drain. For minimal local soft tissue and systemic response, treat with dressing changes and no antibiotics. If antibiotics are required, give as follows. Clean wounds: Give cefazolin, 1 g I.V. q. 8 hr, or oxacillin, 1 g I.V. q. 6 hr. Other wounds: If infection is aggressive, give a third-generation cephalosporin or a quinolone plus clindamycin or metronidazole; or aztreonam plus clindamycin; or imipenem-cilastatin, meropenem, or piperacillin-tazobactam alone. If infection is less serious, give cefotetan, 1 g I.V. q. 12 hr, or cefoxitin, 1 g I.V. q. 6 hr. Invasive and necrotizing infection requires aggressive debridement. Stop antibiotics as soon as local inflammation and systemic signs of infection have resolved.

Intra-abdominal infection (organ/space SSI), as suggested by fever and abdominal tenderness

Confirm diagnosis by CT or ultrasonography. Perform appropriate operative or percutaneous procedure; give antibiotics.

Sternal and mediastinal infection, as suggested by sternal instability

Debride the sternum and affected mediastinal tissues. Consider transposition of viable soft tissue for wound closure.

Osteomyelitis (suggested by nonunion of a fracture, loosening of a prosthesis, or prolonged wound drainage)

Repeated operative debridement, prolonged use of antibiotics, and fracture stabilization may be required.

Empyema, as suggested by systemic signs and pleural effusion

Examine and culture pleural fluid. Drain pleural space. Give appropriate antibiotics. If empyema fails to resolve, consider thoracoscopy, thoracotomy, and decortication.

Posttraumatic meningitis (anticipate if there is a history of CSF rhinorrhea or otorrhea)

Perform lumbar puncture for examination and culture of CSF if unexplained fever, headache, spinal pain or stiffness, or changes in mental status develop. Give appropriate antibiotics.

High fever (> 38.9° C [102° F]) develops within 48 hr of operation

Consider:
- Atelectasis (suggested by decreased breath sounds or rales, or both, and by platelike densities or volume loss on x-ray): Manage via standard physical measures.
- Peritonitis from a leaking viscus (suggested by hemodynamic changes, diffuse abdominal tenderness, excessive early fluid requirements, and tachycardia): Treat with operative intervention and antibiotics.
- Invasive wound infection: Inspect wound and obtain Gram stain of wound contents; treat with operative intervention and antibiotics.

Infection related to intravascular devices

Catheter-associated urinary tract infection

Remove catheter as soon as possible.
Symptomatic bacteriuria:
Give appropriate antibiotics on the basis of culture and sensitivity results.
Asymptomatic bacteriuria: Treat with appropriate antibiotic for 1 day after catheter removal. Culture urine 1 wk later; if bacteriuria persists, give appropriate antibiotics for 7 to 10 days.

Enteric infection

Consider antibiotic-associated colitis in any patient with diarrhea.
Severe cases: Identify mucosal changes immediately via endoscopy.
All cases: Culture stool for *Clostridium difficile* and assay for *C. difficile* toxin.
Severe diarrhea with systemic manifestations: Discontinue antibiotics. Give metronidazole (500 mg p.o., t.i.d.); if unresponsive to metronidazole, give vancomycin (125 mg p.o., q.i.d.).
Mild cases: Discontinue antibiotics.

Systemic symptoms suggest catheter-related bacteremia

Peripheral catheters:
Remove and culture via semiquantitative technique.
Central venous catheters:
If local signs of infection are present, remove catheter and culture insertion site and catheter.
If local infection is not present:
- Consider placing a second catheter over a guide wire.
- Culture intracutaneous segment, or the intracutaneous segment and the distal tip, of first catheter semiquantitatively.

Infection is localized

Remove catheter promptly, and culture via semiquantitative technique. Place any new catheter in a different site.

Infection progresses to septic thrombophlebitis

Correct surgically.

Culture results are not available, or empirical treatment is required

Include antibiotic effective against methicillin-resistant *Staphylococcus aureus* (e.g., vancomycin) in therapy.

Culture results are positive

Give appropriate antibiotics. Remove any second catheter placed by guide wire; place any new catheter in a different site.

Culture results are negative

Second catheter may be left in place.

1317

monary infiltrate, is often seen in modern ICUs, most commonly in association with an endotracheal or tracheostomy tube. Pneumonia may or may not follow. There is often a febrile response, in which case antibiotics may be appropriate on the basis of culture and sensitivity information. Sorting out the cause of purulent secretions in intubated patients is not easy but is important. Other causes of fever should be sought and an overall judgment rendered regarding the probable cause. If tracheitis or bronchitis is suspected, it can be treated with a brief course of antibiotics. A 2000 report described empirical treatment of patients for suspected pneumonia, followed by reevaluation at 3 days.[15] By stopping antibiotic treatment at 3 days for patients without a confirmed diagnosis, the investigators were able to reduce antibiotic use threefold in that group, lower costs by more than half, and decrease the frequency with which resistant bacteria were isolated by more than half.

Paranasal sinusitis is a potentially lethal nosocomial infection, especially in ICU patients with nasogastric or nasotracheal tubes in place.[16-18] In one report, it accounted for 5% of all nosocomial infections.[16] The diagnosis of paranasal sinusitis should be considered in any febrile postoperative patient with nasal tubes or with facial fractures. Purulent nasal drainage is an important clue but may not be present. Plain films can be diagnostic but are often difficult to interpret in these patients because of superimposition of tubes, preexisting injuries, and suboptimal portable films. Fluid, air-fluid levels, and mucosal thickening are more easily detected by computed tomography. Diagnosis ultimately requires demonstration of white blood cells and bacteria on a Gram stain of sinus aspirate as well as culture for identification and sensitivity testing.

In one study of 67 patients with craniofacial injuries who underwent prospective otoscopy three times a week, 11 patients experienced either serous or purulent otitis media and were all found to have purulent paranasal sinusitis.[19] Eleven of 12 patients who were ultimately diagnosed as having purulent paranasal sinusitis had coexistent otitis media.

The spectrum of causative bacteria of paranasal sinusitis is similar to that of nosocomial pneumonia. Treatment includes removal of all nasal tubes and administration of decongestants and antibiotics. Occasionally, sinus irrigation, drainage, or both may be required. If empirical therapy must be initiated before specific culture results are known, the agents chosen should be effective against bacteria known to be present in sputum. The best method of prevention is to limit the number and the duration of use of nasal tubes.

Inflammation and infection of the nasopharyngeal mucosa can be significant in an ICU patient, though it is not often identified. Eustachian tube blockage, either from tubes or from inflammation, can be associated with either serous or infective otitis media. Prudent use of tubes is the most effective preventive measure. If clinical infection is recognized, tube removal and decongestants will usually provide adequate treatment.

Infection Related to Operative Site or Injury

SURGICAL SITE INFECTION

An infection of a surgical wound—that is, an incisional surgical site

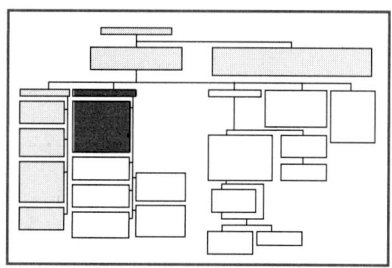

infection (SSI)—traditionally reflects on a surgeon's care and skill and is the classic surgical nosocomial infection [see 1:2 Prevention of Postoperative Infection] Such infections are diagnosed primarily on the basis of local findings. Erythema, swelling, and drainage, as well as increasing local pain and tenderness in a site at which pain should be decreasing, all suggest infection. Fever and an elevated white blood cell count may or may not be present. An incisional SSI develops most commonly in the subcutaneous layer, though animal studies fail to explain this observation.[20] In an obese patient, however, a thick, overlying layer of uninfected tissue may obscure evidence of infection and thus delay diagnosis. Presentation may also be delayed if the infection begins in anatomic layers below fascial and muscular barriers, as may be the case after a thoracotomy or an operation on the femur.

Whether an infection will occur in a wound is probably determined within the first few hours of wounding[21,22]; efforts to prevent wound infection are probably ineffective after this period.[23-27] The incidence of SSI is reduced with appropriate use of perioperative antibiotics.[28,29] However, there is no advantage to continuing prophylactic antibiotics beyond the perioperative period in response to fever or local wound erythema in the hope of preventing an overt SSI.[30-32]

The risk that an SSI will develop in an individual patient is best described by an index defined by the Centers for Disease Control and Prevention (CDC) in its National Nosocomial Infections Surveillance (NNIS) System. The index awards one point each for an American Society of Anesthesiologists (ASA) preoperative assessment score of III, IV, or V; an operation classified as either contaminated or dirty-infected; and an operation duration exceeding the 75th percentile for that procedure.[33,34] Examination of the NNIS data demonstrates that in patients undergoing procedures commonly performed laparoscopically, SSI rates are decreased to levels comparable to those reported in patients with a one point lower risk index who undergo equivalent open procedures.[35] The CDC definitions for SSI were agreed to by a consensus panel representing the CDC, the Society for Hospital Epidemiology of America, the Association for Practitioners in Infection Control, and the Surgical Infection Society.[34,36] In addition to appropriate use of prophylactic antibiotics, proper management of intraoperative temperature, oxygen concentrations, and blood glucose levels exerts a powerful influence on the risk of SSI and of other nosocomial infections.[37-41]

Primary treatment of an SSI consists of opening the wound. When an SSI is suspected, the patient should not be given antibiotics without the wound having been opened. In most cases, the infection is confined to the incision. If the infection is of a superficial wound and if no major systemic manifestations are present, antibiotic therapy is unnecessary. If the local reaction around an infected wound is severe or extensive, administration of antibiotics is advisable until the reaction subsides (which usually takes no more than 3 days). In clean wounds that are away from the perineum and that are not associated with an operation that entered the bowel, the likely pathogens are Staphylococcus aureus, streptococci, or both. In such cases, treatment with cefazolin, 1 g I.V. every 8 hours, or oxacillin, 1 g I.V. every 6 hours, is satisfactory. By contrast, SSIs in the perineum and those that occur after bowel operations often involve mixed aerobic and anaerobic bacterial flora. If the infection is not very serious, it can be treated with cefoxitin, 1 g I.V. every 6 hours, or with cefotetan, 1 g I.V. every 12 hours. For more aggressive infections accompanied by evidence of tissue invasion or necrosis beyond the immediate wound or by a severe systemic reaction, more comprehensive antibiotic treatment is indicated—that is, a third-generation cephalosporin or a quinolone combined with clindamycin or metronidazole; aztreonam combined with clindamycin; or imipenem-cilastatin, meropenem, or piperacillin-tazobactam alone. Infection of an abdominal incision may be a superficial manifestation of an underlying intra-abdominal abscess or of peritonitis.

Occasionally, infection is invasive and necrotizing. In surgical wounds, such an infection is most common after a GI procedure in which the wound was exposed to colonic microflora and in which wound closure was difficult. Necrotizing infection is also more likely in a patient who is seriously ill or who has evidence of multiple organ failure. Such infection should be suspected if there is undermining of the wound edges, extensive fascial necrosis, distant signs of infection, or a marked systemic response. It requires aggressive operative debridement and administration of antibiotics [see 2:2 Soft Tissue Infection].

Clostridium species, which can cause life-threatening postoperative necrotizing SSI, can also cause routine postoperative incisional infection limited to the wound and without myonecrosis.[42] Such infection is marked by the absence of the systemic symptoms associated with clostridial myonecrosis and by the presence of intact white blood cells on a Gram stain of the wound contents. (Clostridial myonecrosis, on the other hand, is characterized by a Gram stain that shows gram-positive rods but few or no white blood cells [see 2:2 Soft Tissue Infection].)

INTRA-ABDOMINAL INFECTION

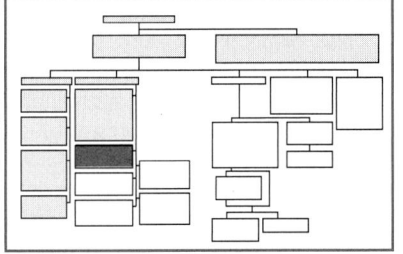

Intra-abdominal infections—that is, organ/space SSIs—are a major cause of postoperative morbidity and mortality, particularly when diagnosis is delayed.[43,44] Suspected intra-abdominal organ/space SSI in a patient with fever or abdominal tenderness, or both, after an abdominal procedure or injury should not be treated with antibiotics alone; after a specific diagnosis is made, the appropriate operative or percutaneous procedure must be performed [see 6:18 Intra-abdominal Infection].

EMPYEMA

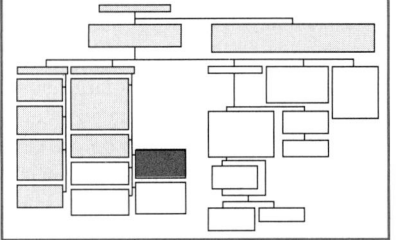

Empyema, which may follow thoracotomy or chest trauma necessitating tube thoracostomy, is a significant cause of posttraumatic infection.[45] Less commonly, empyema develops as a complication of pneumonia. Empyema should be suspected in any patient with systemic signs of infection, a pleural effusion, and no other obvious source of infection. Diagnosis requires thoracentesis of pleural fluid for a Gram stain and culture. The most common pathogen is *S. aureus,* though many other pathogens may be found as well. Initial treatment is by drainage with a chest tube and by administration of appropriate antibiotics based on the results of the Gram stain and culture. Because treatment is invasive, it should not be instituted until the diagnosis is confirmed.

Cases that do not resolve promptly and completely may ultimately require thoracoscopy or thoracotomy and decortication. Empyema after pulmonary resection or esophageal operation raises the possibility of a leaking bronchial closure or esophageal anastomosis. A leak is almost certain if an air-fluid level is present on chest x-ray. An esophageal leak is treated with repair or diversion.

STERNAL AND MEDIASTINAL INFECTION

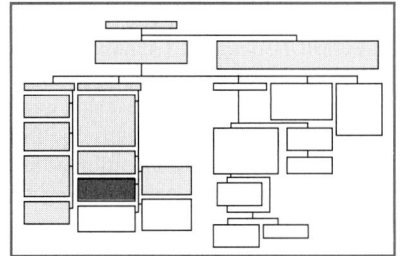

Sternal and mediastinal infections are the most serious infectious complications of operations that involve a median sternotomy.[46] The risk that a superficial infection will spread to involve the sternum and mediastinum is high because there is little soft tissue between the skin and the sternum. Infection may also start deep to the sternum without early superficial evidence. Sternal instability is an important indication of sternal infection. Computed tomography of the chest is sensitive and specific for the diagnosis of sternal osteomyelitis and mediastinitis.[47] All such infections require operative debridement of the sternum and of affected mediastinal tissues. Some wounds can then be closed. Many wounds require closure of the mediastinal space by transposition of viable soft tissue. Pectoralis or rectus muscle flaps, omental flaps, or both are commonly used.[48]

POSTTRAUMATIC MENINGITIS

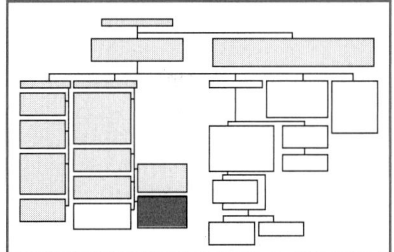

A basilar skull fracture with a cerebrospinal leak increases the risk of posttraumatic meningitis.[49] The most common pathogens are *Streptococcus pneumoniae, S. aureus,* other streptococcal species, and *Haemophilus influenzae,* but any oropharyngeal organism can be responsible.[50] Since the association between trauma and meningitis was first reported in 1970,[49] the appropriate use of antibiotics in these patients has been debated. Some researchers advocate prophylactic administration of antibiotics until any CSF leakage ceases,[51] whereas others advocate them for an arbitrary period after injury (usually 5 days); however, controlled studies have failed to support a specific protocol.[50] Furthermore, experience in other clinical settings suggests that prophylactic antibiotics would be as likely to promote the development of resistant oropharyngeal flora and subsequent meningitis as they are to prevent it.[52,53]

The ideal approach to patients with CSF rhinorrhea or otorrhea is to maintain a high index of suspicion for the development of meningitis. Fever not clearly attributable to another source or not immediately responsive to specific treatment for its presumed cause should prompt a lumbar puncture for examination and culture of spinal fluid. Lumbar puncture should also be performed to investigate headache, spinal pain or stiffness, or unexplained changes in mental status. Such an approach should result in a prompt diagnosis and permit early specific treatment of the responsible pathogen if meningitis is diagnosed.

OSTEOMYELITIS

Osteomyelitis is a relatively rare complication after elective orthopedic procedures. Its diagnosis and management are similar to those of infections involving other operative sites, but because the 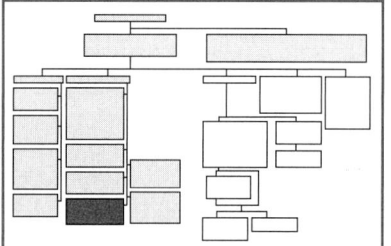 infection is deep and covered by muscular and fascial planes, diagnosis may be delayed. Nonunion of a fracture or loosening of a prosthesis may be the first sign of infection. Infection after open fractures is common; rates range from 5% to 50%.[54-56] The primary determinants of infection after open fracture are the degree of soft tissue damage surrounding the fracture and the surgeon's ability to stabilize the fracture fragments.[55] Other important factors include the patient's age and overall condition, the severity of other injuries, the interval between injury and definitive management, and the use of prophylactic antibiotics. A brief course of perioperative antibiotics may prevent subsequent infection as effectively as a more prolonged course.[30,57]

Treatment of osteomyelitis may require repeated operative debridement, prolonged use of specific antibiotics, and fracture stabilization. Pathogens include *S. aureus* for all grades of open fracture and, increasingly, gram-negative bacteria (e.g., *Pseudomonas aeruginosa* and *Klebsiella* and *Enterobacter* species) for grade III fractures.[57]

Infection Associated with Intravascular Devices

Every type and location of intravascular device has been associated with clinically significant nosocomial bloodstream infection. The inci- 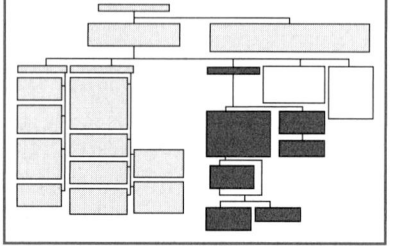 dence of infection is highest with central venous catheters used for monitoring purposes.[58,59]

It is important to specify the different definitions of catheter infection and catheter-related bloodstream infection (CRBSI). Infection at the catheter site is commonly defined as the presence of lymphangitis, purulence, or at least two of the following: erythema, tenderness, increased warmth, and a palpable thrombosed vein. However, many cases of phlebitis with no evidence of bacterial infection present with erythema and with tenderness, a palpable thrombosed vein, or both.[60] Few or no premonitory signs occur before phlebitis is obvious, and the first evidence of as many as 45% of phlebitis cases appears more than 24 hours after catheter removal. If a functional catheter remains in place for 12 hours after the onset of phlebitis symptoms, the duration and severity of symptoms increase markedly.[61]

CRBSI is characterized by (1) isolation of the same organism from the catheter and the blood, (2) clinical (or autopsy) and microbiologic data disclosing no other source of the bloodstream infection, and (3) clinical features of bloodstream infection (e.g., fever and leukocytosis).[62] For indwelling, long-term central venous catheters (e.g., Hickman, Broviac, and Groshong), infections have been classified as exit-site and tunnel infections. Infections at the exit site are defined as the presence of erythema, tenderness, induration, or purulence within 2 cm of the skin around the exit site. They are presumably confined to the portion of the catheter external to the subcutaneous Dacron cuff. Tunnel infections are defined as the presence of the same signs along the subcutaneous tract, at a distance more than 2 cm from the tract.[63,64] The importance of this distinction is that many infections at the exit site are successfully treated with antibiotic therapy and local wound care, whereas tunnel infections usually necessitate removal of the catheter.[63,64]

A semiquantitative technique for culturing intravascular catheters has been shown to distinguish between infection and contamination of the catheter and is more specific in the diagnosis of CRBSI than is broth culture of the catheter.[62] The catheter is removed from the patient after antiseptic cleansing of the insertion site to prevent contamination from surrounding skin. A 5 to 6 cm segment of the catheter is aseptically removed; transported to the laboratory in a dry, sterile tube; placed on the surface of an agar culture plate; and rolled at least four times across the surface of the plate [see Figure 1]. If the plate grows at least 15 colonies, the culture is positive. Most catheters associated with bloodstream infection actually grow more than 1,000 colonies [see Figure 1]. For peripheral catheters, the entire catheter is cultured. For central catheters that are longer than 6 cm, either the distal tip or both the intracutaneous segment and the distal tip should be cultured [see Figure 2].

The most common source of bacteria involved in catheter infection is the skin around the insertion site.[65,66] Patients who have a skin colonization at the insertion site of greater than 10^3 colony-forming units/25 cm^2 are 10 times more likely to have a catheter infection than those whose skin colonization is less. Of catheters that test positive with the semiquantitative culture technique, 16% to 44% appear to be primary sources of septicemia.[62,67-69]

The catheter hub and lumen are recognized as important routes of infection. Colonization at these sites is detected not by roll-plate cultures but by sonication culture of catheter segments or by simultaneous cultures of blood drawn through the suspect catheter and from a distant site. Either sonication cultures recovering more than 10^2 colonies or catheter cultures more than five times the number recovered from distant sites are sensitive and specific indicators of catheter infection.[70,71]

For catheters that are only locally infected and not responsible for CRBSI, removal is adequate treatment; the same is true for most catheters that cause bloodstream infection. If the patient's temperature and white blood cell (WBC) count return to normal within 24 hours after removal of the catheter and if local signs of inflammation at the catheter insertion site resolve within that period, antibiotics are not necessary. However, if the patient continues to show clinical signs of infection or has a documented bacteremia, a brief course of specific antibiotic therapy is indicated. Specific antibiotic therapy is also indicated if semiquantitative catheter culture reveals a large number of *S. aureus* organisms in conjunction with systemic signs of infection. If empirical therapy for CRBSI is undertaken before culture and sensitivity results are available, the antibiotic regimen should include vancomycin or another antibiotic known to be effective against methicillin-resistant *S. aureus* (MRSA): coagulase-negative staphylococci are the most commonly implicated pathogens,[58,70,72] and there is a high rate of methicillin resistance among these organisms. In candidemic patients with I.V. catheters in place, candidemia resolves an average of 3 days earlier if the catheters are removed at the time of diagnosis and initiation of antifungal therapy.[73]

For patients with documented catheter-associated bacteremia, treatment depends on the organism or organisms present. The available data on the necessary duration of treatment for coagulase-negative staphylococci are inconclusive. Often, good results

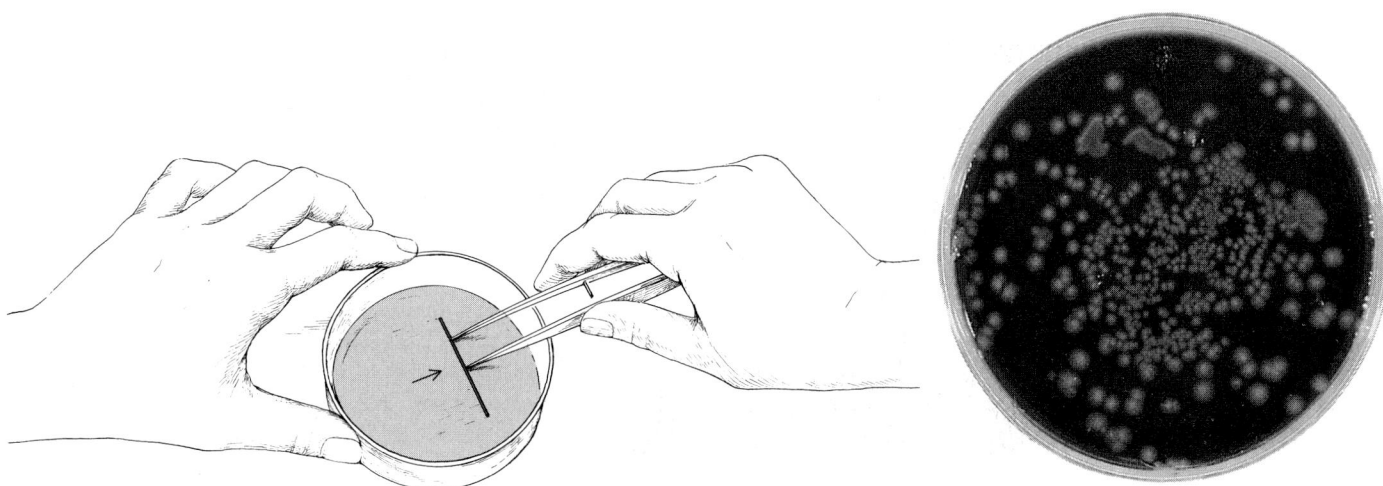

Figure 1 In a semiquantitative technique used to distinguish between infection and contamination of intravascular catheters, a 5 to 6 cm segment of the catheter is rolled at least four times across the surface of an agar culture plate (left). Typically, a positive culture grows far more than 15 colonies (right).

are achieved with catheter removal and either no antibiotics or a short course (1 to 3 days) of antibiotics; some experts recommend a 5- to 7-day course, but there is no compelling evidence that this is necessary. For *S. aureus* bacteremia, a 10- to 14-day antibiotic course is recommended if the infection is uncomplicated and a 4- to 6-week course if the infection is complicated. The relevant data on CRBSI caused by gram-negative bacilli or *Candida* are even sparser. Current recommendations call for antibiotic treatment lasting 10 to 14 days for gram-negative pathogens and 14 days or longer for *Candida*.[74]

In a small proportion of patients, local catheter-related infection may progress to a life-threatening condition characterized by the formation of microabscesses within the cannulated vein and by persistent bacteremia after catheter removal. Septic thrombophlebitis can occur in a broad range of hospitalized patients and should be suspected when clinical signs of systemic sepsis, local signs of inflammation, and positive blood cultures persist after removal of the catheter. A surgical approach to the affected vein is required. When possible, the vein should be excised over the affected area and the wound left open. The presence of gross pus within the vein wall is not necessary for the diagnosis. The wall of the affected vein may simply appear thickened, with inflammation surrounding it and an edematous, pale thrombus enclosed within it. Fungal peripheral thrombophlebitis may be especially difficult to diagnose because the local site often does not appear infected. In the presence of continued candidemia without an obvious source, any palpably thrombosed vein near a site of present or previous catheterization must be suspected. Gram staining and hematoxylin-eosin staining of the vein contents or the vein wall are significantly less sensitive than silver staining and culture.[59]

Even more rare is catheter-related septic central venous thrombosis. The diagnosis is made by the occurrence of (1)

thrombosis of the internal jugular, subclavian, or brachiocephalic vein proved by venography or duplex Doppler examination; (2) central venous catheter infection with positive catheter tip culture and positive peripheral blood cultures; and (3) persistent bacteremia or candidemia after catheter removal.[75,76] Initial therapy consists of catheter removal, systemic antibiotics based on sensitivity testing and administered in a quantity and duration appropriate to treatment of endocarditis, and systemic anticoagulation during the same period. Surgical excision or drainage is reserved for failure of nonoperative measures.

At one time, it was common practice for both central and peripheral venous catheters to be either completely changed or exchanged over a guide wire at fixed intervals to reduce the risk of infection. Data from randomized, controlled, prospective trials did not demonstrate any advantage to this policy.[60,70,77,78] These trials demonstrated that the risk of infection is linear, increasing with the duration of I.V. catheterization, whether one or multiple catheters are used.

Current practice is to change catheters when infection is suspected when the catheters are not working or not needed.[60,70,77,79,80] Clearly, any catheter that is a cause of bloodstream infection must be removed, as should infected catheters that may not yet have caused such infection. The practical problem is that not all infected catheters show external evidence of infection. In addition, catheter culture and the subsequent clinical course confirm infection in only a small proportion of patients with central venous catheters or pulmonary artery catheters in place who are suspected on clinical grounds of having CRBSI.[81] Changing central venous catheters over a guide wire circumvents most of the mechanical complications associated with central venous catheterization, saves time, and is more comfortable for the patient.[82] However, if a culture of the first catheter is positive, the second catheter should be removed immediately, and any new

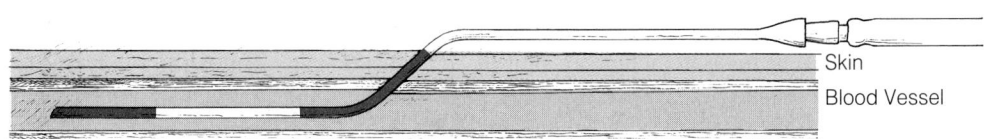

Skin
Blood Vessel

Figure 2 When a catheter is longer than 6 cm, either 5 to 6 cm of the catheter tip or both this segment and a 5 to 6 cm intracutaneous segment (red) can be cultured.

catheter should be placed in a different location.[60,70,77,79-81]

Recommendations for changing central venous and pulmonary artery catheters are as follows:

1. Signs of inflammation, skin irritation, or purulence at the insertion site should prompt immediate removal of the catheter. Any new catheter should be inserted in a different site. In a patient with systemic signs of infection (fever, leukocytosis, malaise), culture of the insertion site or of the catheter, or both, is indicated to identify potential pathogens and to direct therapy. In a patient without systemic signs of infection, culture is not necessary.

2. If a patient with a catheter experiences systemic signs and symptoms of infection without a readily apparent source, the catheter should be removed even in the absence of inflammation at the insertion site. In this setting, however, approximately 75% of catheters are not infected, and a new catheter can be inserted at the same site over a guide wire placed through the first catheter.[81,83-85] However, a catheter exchange places the new catheter in the old subcutaneous tunnel, which would be the most likely origin of catheter infection. The first catheter should be cultured semiquantitatively. If the culture is negative (i.e., < 15 colonies), the second catheter can be left in place. If the culture is positive (i.e., ≥ 15 colonies), the second catheter should be removed immediately, and any new catheter should be placed at a different site.

Sterile technique is always required for catheter insertion. However, most authorities advocate a surgical approach to preparation of the insertion site, with the operator wearing gown, gloves, mask, and hat for the procedure, if any of the following risk factors is present[70,86]: (1) the location is central, (2) catheterization will probably be long term, (3) the patient is seriously ill, or (4) parenteral nutrition is to be employed. Educational efforts to reinforce these guidelines in the hospital setting can reduce the incidence of catheter-related infections.[87]

Traditionally, central venous catheters have been inserted most commonly via either the subclavian or the internal jugular route. There is a well-demonstrated increase in infection risk when catheters are inserted by the jugular route instead of the subclavian.[69,80,88] The infection rate for the femoral route of insertion appears to be higher than that for the subclavian route and possibly higher than that for the internal jugular route[89]; however, it can be reduced by tunneling.[90] The femoral route can be used if other access routes are not available, but at the cost of a higher rate of thrombotic complications.[91]

A promising approach to prevention of catheter infection is antibiotic bonding of the entire catheter surface. Two trials reported fewer catheter and bloodstream infections in patients with antimicrobial-bonded catheters than in patients with unbonded catheters,[92,93] and one trial reported a lower infection rate with a catheter coated on both internal and external surfaces with minocycline and rifampin than with a catheter coated only on the external surface with chlorhexidine and silver sulfadiazine.[94]

The ideal method of caring for intravascular catheters after insertion is not firmly established. Sterile dressings of gauze and tape, as well as a variety of commercially available transparent dressings, have been advocated. The transparent dressings appear to save nursing time and permit the insertion site to be inspected without changing the dressing, but they promote bacterial growth on the underlying skin, as compared with gauze and tape dressings.[95] Transparent dressings have also been associated with an increased number of cases of catheter infection and CRBSI in

patients with central venous catheters.[96] Thus, use of transparent dressings is not recommended, at least for central lines.

In addition, there is no firm evidence that the use of polyantibiotic ointments or iodophor ointments at the insertion site prevents infection, though such ointments have not been associated with an increase in infections with resistant organisms. Catheter teams are recommended to care for vascular catheters. Regular inspection of insertion sites and adherence to a specific protocol for catheter care can result in acceptably low infection rates.[70]

Catheters with two or three internal lumina have become widely available and are often sold in kits that include equipment for guide-wire insertion. These catheters are more convenient when a patient requires multiple lines for monitoring and for delivery of intravenous medications and parenteral nutrition. However, these multiple-lumen lines may be associated with a higher incidence of catheter-associated bloodstream infection than are single-lumen catheters[97,98]; the data are inconclusive.[85,99] In one small study, the insertion of two single-lumen catheters did not result in a lower complication rate than the insertion of one double-lumen catheter.[100] A catheter with multiple infusion ports is likely to be manipulated more often than a single-lumen catheter, but it is unclear whether the extra manipulation results in a higher infection rate. In situations in which one lumen would suffice, the temptation to insert a multiple-lumen line in case additional lumina are needed later should be resisted. One study showed that 53% of all triple-lumen lines observed had only one lumen in use, indicating that multiple-lumen lines are often used unnecessarily.[97]

When long-term use of catheters is required, insertion of a Silastic catheter with a subcutaneous Dacron cuff (e.g., Broviac, Hickman, or Groshong) is associated with the lowest rate of catheter-associated infection and the longest useful catheter life.[63] In the largest reported study of these catheters, the incidence of infection was only 0.14 infection per 100 catheter-days (range, 0.0 to 0.8).[63] The study also showed that double-lumen catheters did not have a higher rate of infection than single-lumen catheters, but the rate of catheter infections was increased 10-fold in patients who had catheter-related thrombosis. The mean catheter life span in this report was greater than 120 days.

Very low infection rates and long catheter life are also reported with nontunneled Silastic catheters and with peripherally inserted central catheters (PICC).[70,101] The lowest infection rates are associated with totally implantable devices with subcutaneous reservoirs.[102]

Use of warfarin to prevent thrombosis may result in a reduced rate of catheter infection. A prospective trial found a clinically and statistically significant reduction in the incidence of catheter-associated thrombosis (from 38% to 10%) over 90 days with the administration of 1 mg of warfarin daily, beginning 3 days before catheter insertion.[103] Measured prothrombin times did not increase, and no bleeding complications occurred.

Urinary Tract Infection

The traditional definition of urinary tract infection in patients without urinary catheters specifies the presence of at least 10^5 organisms/ml, but this criterion is probably not appropriate for catheterized patients. Research has

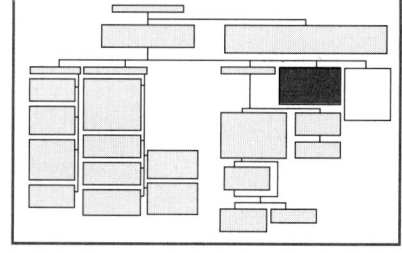

shown that of catheterized patients who have any detectable organisms in their urine (even < 10^2/ml), whose catheters remain in place, and who receive no specific antimicrobial therapy, 96% have organism counts higher than 10^5/ml within 3 days.[104] (By comparison, 27% of patients with sterile urine subsequently have colony counts higher than 10^5/ml before catheter removal.)

Although a catheter-associated UTI is a significant nosocomial infection with measurable morbidity and mortality [see Discussion, below], not all cases of bacteriuria should be treated with antibiotics. If a patient with bacteriuria is symptomatic, treatment should be initiated according to culture results and sensitivity testing. Although bacteriuria can sometimes be cleared without removal of the catheter, the risk of a new episode continues while the catheter is in place.[105] Ideally, the catheter should be removed as soon as possible. In one study, only 36% of untreated women with asymptomatic bacteriuria had sterile urine within 2 weeks after catheter removal, and 17% progressed to symptomatic bacteriuria; however, 81% of patients treated with a single dose of trimethoprim-sulfamethoxazole had sterile urine within 2 weeks after catheter removal.[106] Thus, it is prudent to obtain a culture at the time of catheter removal and to treat any bacteriuria detected.

A condom catheter is often used in male patients in place of a urethral catheter when neurologic injury or incontinence mandates long-term drainage. The available data are not sufficient to establish the ideal care of these devices and the true infection rate associated with their use. UTI rates as low as 0% in 79 patients managed with condom catheter drainage[107] and as high as 53%[105] to 63%[108] have been reported. Severe noninfectious local complications (e.g., ulceration and maceration of the penis) also can occur.[107,108]

Because indwelling urinary catheters are a major source of nosocomial infection, they should be employed only when necessary and removed as soon as practicable. The most effective method of reducing infections among patients with urinary catheters is to use completely closed urinary drainage systems and to limit breaks in the closed system.[109] The incidence of new infections doubles on any day in which a closed urinary drainage system is opened.[110] Urine samples for culture should be aspirated with a needle and syringe from the catheter lumen after antiseptic cleansing of the catheter sampling port. The catheter junction should not be disconnected to obtain a specimen. The use of a preconnected and sealed catheter and drainage bag system has been shown to result in a 2.7-fold reduction in the rate of catheter-associated UTIs and an adjusted risk ratio for death of 0.29.[111]

Antibiotic irrigation systems do not reduce infections, but they do increase the incidence of resistant organisms.[110] Systemic antibiotics reduce infections to a modest degree in the first 4 days of catheterization but at the expense of an increase in resistant organisms. The infection rate is higher in females than in males, in older patients than in younger ones, and in patients with critical illness than in those without critical illness.[109] Patients with nosocomial diarrhea and an indwelling bladder catheter have a ninefold higher risk of subsequent UTI than patients with an indwelling bladder catheter who do not have diarrhea.[112]

Although most UTIs acquired by hospitalized patients are assumed to be simple bladder infections, there is no strong correlation between location of infection and clinical symptoms.[113,114] Many patients with upper UTIs do not have flank pain, fever, or other signs of systemic infection, and patients with a bladder infection may not have dysuria or suprapubic tenderness. Many patients with upper UTIs are treated without the diagnosis ever being made. Systemic infection and associated bacteremia or complications such as intrarenal or perinephric abscesses occur more commonly in immunocompromised patients (e.g., those with urinary tract obstruction or diabetes).[115] In patients with a neurogenic bladder or indwelling bladder catheters, urinary sepsis may develop without symptoms referable to the urinary tract. However, symptoms of localized flank or low back pain, along with systemic signs, such as fever, rigors, sweats, and nausea, are relatively specific indicators of renal infection.[116]

If a patient has fever and bacteriuria during the postoperative period, the surgeon should perform a careful evaluation to determine whether he or she has pyelonephritis or a postoperative intra-abdominal infectious complication. Pyelonephritis can be treated solely with antimicrobial therapy in most cases, whereas all postoperative intra-abdominal infectious complications call for surgical intervention as well as antimicrobial therapy. No simple methods are available to distinguish between these diagnoses. The operating surgeon should carefully evaluate all of the patient's clinical signs and symptoms. A hospitalized patient with pyelonephritis should usually receive antimicrobial therapy for at least 14 days. An agent demonstrated to be effective against the causative organism by in vitro sensitivity testing should be used. In any patient who has severe signs of systemic infection or does not respond promptly to treatment, ultrasonography, renal scanning, or I.V. pyelography should be done to rule out obstruction. If obstruction is found, it must be corrected. If the patient has an indwelling bladder catheter, the catheter should be removed, appropriate therapy started, and a new, clean catheter inserted.[116]

Enteric Infection

Any organism that can cause food-borne enteric infection in the community can do so in the hospital,[117] but cultures for routine enteric pathogens are not useful for patients who have been hospitalized for more than 3 days.[118] The most important nosocomial enteric disease to confront most surgeons is antibiotic-associated diarrhea, which can range from trivial, self-limited episodes of diarrhea to fulminant disease with systemic signs of sepsis, collapse, and death.

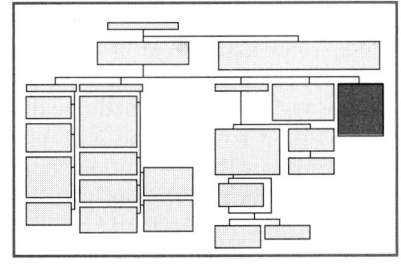

The first step in diagnosis is to consider antibiotic-associated colitis in any hospitalized patient with diarrhea. Mild cases may not be associated with any systemic signs or pathologic findings in the colon, and in the majority of mild episodes, there are no identifiable pathogens. More severe cases are marked by one or more of the following signs: nonspecific hyperemia, edema, granularity, or ulceration of colonic mucosa. The most severe cases are marked by pseudomembrane formation.

The single most efficient measure for detecting C. difficile–associated diarrhea is to send a stool sample for cytotoxin determination, a procedure that has a sensitivity of 70% to 100%. By sending a sample is sent for stool culture as well, one can increase sensitivity slightly (to 96%); however, if C. difficile is grown on the culture, the organism must still be tested for cytotoxin production, and this takes another day.[118,119] Rectal swab cultures transported in anaerobic containers are at least as sensitive as conventional stool cultures,[120] but they are not adequate for detection of cytotoxin.[119] Although it is possible that poly-

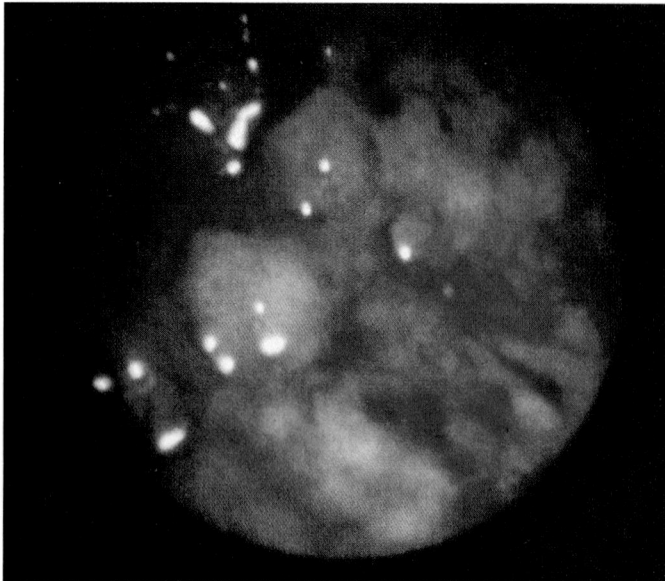

Figure 3   An endoscopic view of pseudomembrane formation is shown.

merase chain reaction assays for the cytotoxin gene in stool can eventually be developed, such assays are not available at present. Stool smears for detection of WBCs are not helpful.[118,119] Endoscopy to detect pseudomembranes is indicated if the patient is seriously ill and a prompt diagnosis and initiation of specific treatment are desired. Administration of empirical therapy until a specific pathogen is identified is appropriate in this circumstance.[119]

Severe and persistent cases of antibiotic-associated diarrhea are most commonly associated with the recovery of *C. difficile* by culture and of *C. difficile* toxin by tissue culture assay.[121] In more than 90% of patients who have pseudomembranous colitis, *C. difficile* toxin will be present on tissue culture assay. In antibiotic-associated diarrhea without pseudomembrane formation, positive toxin titers may be found in 70% of patients with signs of colitis and in 11% to 27% of patients without colitis.[122-124]

Pseudomembranes, present in about half of patients with *C. difficile*–associated diarrhea,[119] are elevated, whitish plaques that vary in size from a few millimeters to 1 to 2 cm and may coalesce and slough. Histologically, the plaques show epithelial debris, polymorphonuclear infiltrate, chronic inflammatory cells, and fibrin deposition.[121] The diagnosis of pseudomembrane formation is made by endoscopy [*see Figure 3*]. Most cases involve the rectum and the left colon, but as many as 25% may be missed by rigid sigmoidoscopy; by comparison, the false negative rate with flexible endoscopy is only 10%.[125] Although the great majority of cases involve only the colon, two fatal cases that primarily involved the ileum and the jejunum have been recorded.[126,127] The clinical picture of pseudomembranous colitis includes watery diarrhea in 90% to 95% of cases, with bloody diarrhea in the remaining cases. Abdominal cramps, leukocytosis, and elevated temperature are present in approximately 80% of cases.[121]

All commonly employed antibiotics have been implicated in cases of antibiotic-associated pseudomembranous colitis, including vancomycin[128-130] and antibiotics used for perioperative antibiotic prophylaxis, even in a single dose.[131] Treatment should include cessation of the offending antimicrobial agent, if possible. In mild cases, this step may be all that is necessary: in 23% of

such cases, resolution occurs within 2 to 3 days of discontinuance of antibiotic therapy.[119]

A patient with systemic symptoms should also receive one of the agents with proven efficacy against the disease. The agent with which there has been the most recorded experience is vancomycin, but it is more expensive than the alternatives. The usual dosage is 500 mg/day orally in four divided doses. Metronidazole, 500 mg three or four times daily for at least 10 days, is an effective alternative.[132] Bacitracin, 20,000 to 25,000 units four times daily, is also effective but should be considered the third choice.[119,132] The current recommendation is to begin therapy with metronidazole to reduce the risk of inducing vancomycin-resistant enterococci [*see* Pathogens, *below*].[119,133]

Relapses after treatment for *C. difficile* colitis are common, occurring in 5% to 30% of cases, perhaps because of persistence of the organism in spore form; 92% of these cases respond to a second course of treatment without relapse.[119,132] Cases that do recur involve both persistent infection and new reinfection.[132]

A profound ileus is sometimes associated with the severe form of the disease and may prevent the delivery of oral antibiotics to the site of infection. Limited experience suggests that parenteral metronidazole may be effective in these cases. However, there have been several cases of unsuccessful treatment of *C. difficile*–associated colitis with I.V. metronidazole and of the development of *C. difficile* colitis in patients receiving I.V. metronidazole alone or together with other antibiotics.[132,134] In the most severe cases, the clinical evolution resembles that of toxic colitis associated with inflammatory bowel disease, and the patient may require a colectomy if the disease is unresponsive to nonoperative management. If operative treatment proves necessary, subtotal colectomy is preferred to hemicolectomy.[132] In as many as 5% of cases, colitis may present as acute abdominal pain and tenderness and leukocytosis without diarrhea.[135,136] Any patient with acute abdominal symptoms who has received antibiotics within the past 2 months should be considered for the diagnosis of *C. difficile*–associated colitis.[132] If colitis is suspected because of previous antibiotic administration, sigmoidoscopy may facilitate the correct diagnosis and avert unnecessary abdominal exploration. CT may show thickening of the bowel wall, but operative exploration often does not yield significant findings.[136] Extraintestinal infections have also been reported.[137]

Transfusion-Associated Infection

The transfusion of blood would seem to be an excellent method for transmitting blood-borne diseases; however, transmission of disease by blood transfusion is rare.[138,139] Transfusion-associated malaria is occasionally reported in North America but occurs quite infrequently. The primary method for preventing malaria transmission is careful screening of donors by history. A handful of cases of babesiosis, Chagas disease, trypanosomiasis, toxoplasmosis, and infections with various herpesviruses, parvovirus, or West Nile virus have been reported over many years, but these are rare as well.[138-141]

In the early years of blood collection and transfusion, cases of syphilis related to blood transfusion were reported infrequently. The practice of refrigerating blood, which kills circulating spirochetes within 1 to 2 days, is probably responsible for the absence of transfusion-associated syphilis today. Unfortunately, refrigerating blood does not kill all potential pathogens. Bacterial pathogens that can survive blood storage and cause subsequent symptomatic infection include *Yersinia enterocolitica, Pseudomonas fluorescens, P. putida, Campylobacter jejuni, Escherichia coli, Serratia* species, *Salmonella* species, *Enterobacter* species, *Providencia* species, *S. aureus,* and streptococci. When transfusion-associated bacteremia or endotoxemia is suspected, the residual blood product in the bag should be examined by means of a hematologic stain, and the blood in the bag and samples of the recipient's blood should be cultured.

Bacterial contamination of transfused blood components accounted for 11% of all fatal transfusion reactions reported to the FDA between 1985 and 1999. In 2001, CDC investigators published a prospective survey of bacterial infections resulting from blood component transfusion in the United States between January 1998 and December 2000.[142] This survey covered approximately 60% to 70% of all transfusions recorded in the United States during that period. The investigators identified 34 confirmed cases of bacterial infection from transfused blood components, nine (27%) of which were responsible for deaths. The estimated rates of transfusion-transmitted bacteremia were one per 100,000 single or pooled units of platelets and one per 5 million units of red blood cells. The estimated fatality rates were one per 500,000 units of platelets and one per 8 million units of red blood cells.

Until recently, the most severe and most common disease transmitted by blood transfusion in North America was viral hepatitis [*see 6:20 Viral Infection*]. With the development of specific and sensitive tests for detecting hepatitis B surface antigen (HBsAg), the incidence of posttransfusion hepatitis B dropped from 25% to 30% of all cases of transfusion-associated hepatitis to 5% to 10%. However, the advent of serologic tests for hepatitis B did not result in an overall decrease in posttransfusion hepatitis (PTH), because 80% to 90% of cases of PTH were caused by hepatitis C virus (HCV). Since the development of sensitive antibody tests for HCV, the incidence of PTH has dropped dramatically, and since the introduction in 1999 of nucleic acid amplification technology (NAT) (e.g., PCR and transcription-mediated amplification), it has fallen even further, to the point where the current estimated risk is one per 1.9 million transfused units.[143]

The spread of AIDS [*see 6:21 Acquired Immunodeficiency Syndrome*] brought a new risk of transfusion-associated viral disease. The risk of acquiring transfusion-associated HIV infection is extremely low compared with posttransfusion hepatitis; transfusion-associated HIV infection is vastly less likely to occur and

has accounted for fewer deaths. Nevertheless, transfusion-associated AIDS is much more frightening to most patients and physicians than PTH because of its usually fatal prognosis. Prevention of HIV transmission during transfusion is accomplished by screening potential donors to eliminate those at high risk for infection and by testing all donated units for HIV with both antibody tests and NAT.[143-145] It has been estimated that predonation screening is 98% effective in eliminating donation of positive units and that postdonation antibody testing is more than 95% effective, for a combined effectiveness of approximately 99.9%.[144] Overall, posttransfusion HIV infections were reduced by 76% between 1985 and 1988, a time during which the overall prevalence of the condition was increasing.[144]

The continued concern about possible HIV transmission during transfusion arises from the so-called window of seronegativity between the time at which a potential donor becomes infected and the time at which the donor's antibody test becomes positive. A 1989 analysis of available data from most United States blood banks concluded that the risk of receiving a unit of blood that contained HIV but was negative for anti-HIV antibody in 1987 was approximately one per 153,000 transfusions on the basis of an average window period of 8 weeks.[144] A 2002 report, making use of data obtained since the introduction of NAT, established the current risk at one per 2.1 million transfusions.[143] In comparison, the risk of experiencing a fatal hemolytic transfusion reaction is one per 100,000 transfusions.[145] Thus, a transfusion recipient is much more likely to die of a hemolytic reaction than of infection.

Analysis of transfusion practices in the United States between 1982 and 1988 reveals a decrease in the number of blood, platelet, and plasma transfusions after 1986; before 1986, the number of these transfusions increased each year. In addition, between 1982 and 1987, the number of autologous units donated increased from 30,000 to 397,000 a year. In 1987, autologous units accounted for 3% of all blood transfused.[146] Since 1987, refinements of operative techniques have reduced the need for transfusion in many procedures, and research has demonstrated that in many cases, transfusion can safely be withheld until hemoglobin levels lower than 7 g/dl are reached [*see 1:4 Bleeding and Transfusion*].[147] In addition to the overall decline in transfusions since the late 1980s, the number of autologous units of blood transfused yearly has declined.[148]

Discussion

Postoperative Fever

Many patients experience fever in the postoperative period without infection. In a prospective study of 871 general surgery patients, 213 (24%) had a documented infection or an unexplained fever in the postoperative period.[149] The most common occurrence was unexplained fever in 81 cases (38%), followed by wound infection in 55 (26%), UTI in 44 (21%), respiratory tract infection in 27 (13%), and other infections in 6 (3%). Of all unexplained fevers, 72% occurred in the first 2 days, and of all occurrences in the first 3 days, 67 (71%) of 95 were unexplained, with only 18 (27%) representing true infection. In another study, 73 (45%) of 162 patients experienced unexplained fever after general surgical or orthopedic procedures; 25% of the unexplained fevers were at least 38.3° C (101° F).[150]

At Harborview Medical Center, 316 (98%) of 322 patients who underwent laparotomy for penetrating trauma had a temperature of at least 37.5° C (99.5° F) orally during the first 5 days after operation. Of these patients, however, only 67 (21%) actually acquired any infection during a 30-day follow-up. Even for the 80 patients whose temperatures were as high as 39° C (102.2° F) orally, only 48% actually acquired an infection before discharge. Fever that persisted or began after postoperative day 4 was more likely to represent true infection. Similarly, an elevated WBC count was nonspecific during the first 5 postoperative days: 89% of all patients had a WBC count greater than 10,000/mm³.[151,152] A high fever should prompt examination of the patient, but in the absence of systemic signs of sepsis, an extensive laboratory or radiologic workup during the first 4 to 5 days is usually unhelpful.[153]

Magnitude and Significance of Nosocomial Infection

An understanding of the prevalence of nosocomial infections and of the factors predisposing to their occurrence will help in prevention, diagnosis, and treatment. Since 1970, the NNIS system has collected and analyzed data on the frequency of nosocomial infections in a voluntary sample of hospitals (currently numbering 280) in the United States.[154] Although it has been suggested that the NNIS system underestimates the true incidence of nosocomial infections by 30% to 40%,[3,155,156] the large number of cases studied during consecutive years provides a useful description of the most frequently encountered infections, their relative incidences, and the responsible pathogens.

INCIDENCE

In the 1986 NNIS report, the overall incidence of nosocomial infection was 33.5 per 1,000 discharges; the range extended from 13.3 per 1,000 pediatric discharges to 46.7 per 1,000 surgical discharges. Generally, the rate of infection is highest in large teaching hospitals and lowest in nonteaching hospitals. The higher incidence of infection among surgical patients is largely attributable to SSI. SSIs are the most frequent adverse events reported for hospitalized surgical patients and account for 38% of all nosocomial infections in surgical patients.[157] Two thirds of SSIs are incisional infections, and one third are organ/space infections.[35,158] Some 38% of all SSIs result in readmission to the hospital.[35]

Across all services, UTIs are the most common infections, accounting for 38.5% of all nosocomial infections, followed by lower respiratory tract infections (17.8%), surgical wound infections (16.6%), primary bacteremias (7.5%), and cutaneous infections (5.8%). All other categories combined account for 13.8% of nosocomial infections. The total incidence of nosocomial infection from all sites on surgical services ranges from 30.8 to 59.3 per 1,000 discharges. The risk that a surgical patient will acquire any infection varies according to the type of procedure performed as well as to the patient's underlying risk.[159]

In the 1993 NNIS report, the most common nosocomial infections for surgical patients after an SSI were UTIs (27%), pneumonias (15%), primary bloodstream infections (7%), and all other sites combined (15%).[159] Of the infected surgical patients, 17% had more than one nosocomial infection, and 9% of surgical patients with nosocomial infections subsequently died; nosocomial infections were reported to have caused or contributed to 60% of the deaths. Of infections related to death, 38% were pneumonias, 21% occurred at the surgical site, and 20% were primary bloodstream infections. The likelihood that a specific infection will be related to death varies with the type of infection [see Table 1].

Urinary Tract Infection

With so many cases of bacteriuria occurring in catheterized patients, it would be easy to become complacent about the problem. Urinary tract catheterization is performed seven to eight million times a year in acute care hospitals in the United States.[160] Approximately 5% to 8% of catheterized, uninfected patients will acquire a urinary tract infection for each day of catheterization, leading to a cumulative infection rate of 40% to 50% after 10 days.[109] However, the great majority of catheterized patients with bacteriuria are asymptomatic.[109,161] It has been estimated that only 0.7% of catheterized patients will acquire a symptomatic infection and that 8% to 10% of patients will have bacteriuria after the catheter has been removed.[109]

In many of these patients, the bacteriuria resolves without specific therapy after the catheter has been removed. However, a

Table 1 Contribution of Nosocomial Infection to Death in Infected Surgical Patients Who Died[159]

Type of Nosocomial Infection	Probability That Infection Was Related to Death (%)
Organ/space surgical site infection	89
Primary bloodstream infection	79
Pneumonia	77
Other	48
Incisional surgical site infection	46
Urinary tract infection	22

careful study of more than 1,458 patients clearly demonstrated that mortality is higher in catheterized patients who acquire bacteriuria than in those who do not.[160] In this study, 9% of all catheterized patients acquired catheter-related UTIs; these infections were associated with a threefold increase in deaths occurring during hospitalization, even after correction for other factors (e.g., age, severity of illness, hospital service, duration of catheterization, and renal function). In surgical patients between 50 and 70 years of age with normal renal function and without a fatal underlying disease, a 3% increase in the death rate per patient per hospitalization was associated with the occurrence of a UTI. Of all deaths occurring in catheterized patients, 14% were associated with a UTI.[160] By extrapolation, this mortality suggests that as many as 56,000 deaths a year in the United States may be related to catheter-acquired UTI.

Although the risk of bacteremia is small for any individual patient with bacteriuria, the large number of hospitalized patients with bacteriuria means that many bacteremic episodes are seen in this population. UTI is the most commonly diagnosed source of gram-negative sepsis, and the rate of bacteremia secondary to urinary catheters is estimated to be between 0.7% and 2%.[109] In a case-matched study from 1978, a postoperative UTI was associated with a 2.4-day prolongation of hospital stay and an excess cost of more than $500.[162] A subsequent study revealed that 2.3% of postoperative patients with UTIs were subsequently diagnosed as having a wound infection caused by the same organism responsible for the UTI.[163] This finding accounted for 3.4% of the wound infections occurring during the study.

Infection Associated with Intravascular Devices

Nosocomial infection associated with intravascular devices, which are placed for either monitoring or therapeutic purposes, assumed increasing importance during the 1970s and 1980s. In the United States, central venous catheters are in place for approximately 15 million patient-catheter-days per year, resulting in approximately 250,000 catheter-associated bloodstream infections.[70] Of all cases of nosocomial bacteremia occurring in NNIS hospitals between September 1984 and July 1986, 82% were associated with intravascular devices[164]: 27% were associated with parenteral nutrition catheters and 55% with other vascular access devices. Reports from as early as 1963 called attention to the risk of serious systemic infections arising from peripheral I.V. catheters.[165] For ICU patients with bloodstream infections associated with central venous catheters, the attributable mortality is 25% to 35%, and the excess cost for survivors is $34,000 to $56,000 per patient, for a total annual cost of $296 million to $2.3 billion.[70]

In terms of infection risk, pulmonary arterial catheters are no different from central venous catheters, except for their potential to cause right-side heart lesions that could predispose to right-side endocarditis.[166] Pulmonary arterial catheters can be responsible for bloodstream infection, and they require as much attention during insertion and subsequent care as central venous catheters do.[68,167]

The arterial catheters used for monitoring purposes in the ICU have been thought to be less frequently associated with infection than central venous catheters are, but it is clear that life-threatening infections can originate with peripheral arterial lines.[168,169] In early studies of radial artery catheters in which nonquantitative culture techniques were employed, catheter contamination rates of 4% to 39% were recorded, but there were no cases of CRBSI or clinical infection in 605 catheterizations.[170] In these studies, the majority of catheters were removed from patients within 3 days.

Prospective studies of arterial catheters demonstrated that 18% to 35% of the lines were locally infected, as reflected in semiquantitative cultures of at least 15 colonies.[171] In one study, five cases of CRBSI occurred, representing an overall incidence of 4% and an incidence of 23% among locally infected catheters.[171] The incidence of CRBSI was increased in catheters that were inserted by cutdown rather than by percutaneous puncture and in catheters with signs of local inflammation. In another, the clinical features of bloodstream infection arising from an arterial catheter were indistinguishable from the clinical features of episodes arising from a central venous line, and 12%

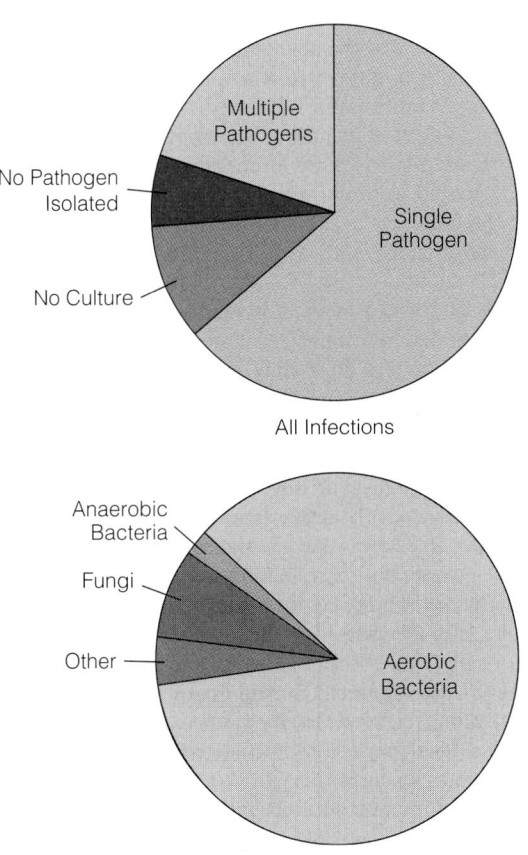

All Infections

Infections of Known Etiology

Figure 4 Illustrated is a breakdown of the etiology of 26,965 nosocomial infections from the National Nosocomial Infections Surveillance System.[173]

Table 2 Five Most Common Pathogens Isolated from Surgical Patients and Percentage of Total within Each Site[173]

Infection Site	Organism	Isolates at That Site (%)
Urinary tract infection	*Escherichia coli*	29
	Pseudomonas aeruginosa	16
	Enterococci	13
	Proteus species	7
	Klebsiella species	7
Surgical wound infection	*Staphylococcus aureus*	19
	Enterococci	12
	E. coli	12
	P. aeruginosa	10
	Coagulase-negative staphylococci	8
Lower respiratory infection	*P. aeruginosa*	17
	S. aureus	12
	Enterobacter species	11
	Klebsiella species	11
	Serratia species	7
Bacteremia	Coagulase-negative staphylococci	14
	S. aureus	10
	Enterobacter species	9
	Enterococci	9
	Klebsiella species	8
Cutaneous infections	*S. aureus*	19
	P. aeruginosa	13
	Enterococci	11
	Coagulase-negative staphylococci	10
	E. coli	8

of all nosocomial bacteremias in the ICU originated from an arterial catheter.[171] Clearly, arterial lines as well as venous lines must be considered in the examination of a patient for the source of fever or bloodstream infection in the ICU.[68,169,171,172] Twelve cases of radial artery rupture after arterial line infection have been reported. All but one were associated with *S. aureus* infection, and nearly all demonstrated systemic signs of infection for 2 days or longer after catheter removal.[169] Although there is no published experience with the use of guide wires to change and culture arterial lines in relation to possible catheter-related infection, the technique can be applied with the same rationale used for central venous catheters.

PATHOGENS

In 1984, the NNIS reported on 26,965 infections. Of these cases, 64% were caused by single pathogens, 20% were caused by multiple pathogens, 6% had no pathogen identified on culture, and 10% were not cultured [*see Figure 4*].[173] Of the 84% in which a pathogen was identified, 86% were caused by aerobic bacteria, 2% by anaerobes, and 8% by fungi [*see Figure 4 and Table 2*]. Overall on the surgical services, the most common pathogen isolated was *E. coli*, followed by *P. aeruginosa*, enterococci, *S. aureus*, *Enterobacter* species, *Klebsiella* species, coagulase-negative staphylococci, *Proteus* species, *Candida* species, and *Serratia* species. These 10 types of pathogens accounted for 84% of all isolates. Gram-negative rods were most common in UTIs and lower respiratory tract infections, though *S. aureus* was the second most common pathogen isolated in lower respiratory tract infections. *S. aureus* was the most common isolate from surgical wound infections, whereas coagulase-negative staphylococci, followed closely by *S. aureus,* were the pathogens most often responsible for primary bacteremias.

As a consequence of changing hospital practices, hospitalized patients today tend to be more severely ill than was once the case. Large amounts of antibiotics are being used in hospitals, and antibiotic-resistant pathogens have become increasingly problematic. Current NNIS data indicate that the frequency with which antibiotics are administered to hospitalized patients who are not in an ICU is approximately 468 defined daily doses (DDD) per 1,000 patient-days.[174] For hospitalized ICU patients, the frequency is between 800 and 1,031 DDD per 1,000 patient-days. MRSA accounts for 51% of total *S. aureus* isolates in ICU patients, 40% in non-ICU patients, and 24% in outpatients with nosocomial infections; the corresponding figures for quinolone-resistant *P. aeruginosa* in relation to total *P. aeruginosa* isolates are 37%, 27%, and 27%.[174] In 2002, the second clinical isolate of vancomycin-resistant *S. aureus* in the United States was reported.[175]

Nosocomial infections with resistant enterococci have become a serious problem. Enterococci were the third most common nosocomial bloodstream isolate reported by NNIS hospitals between 1990 and 1992.[176] The incidence of vancomycin-resistant enterococci (VRE) increased 26-fold between 1989 and 1993, from 0.3% to 7.9%, with a 34-fold rise in ICUs,[177] and the rate has continued to increase. The 2001 NNIS report stated that 13% of enterococci were resistant to vancomycin in ICU patients, 12% in non-ICU patients, and 5% in outpatients.[174] These strains arise from the patient's endogenous flora, but nosocomial spread within the hospital environment is also an important source.[177,178] The environment around infected patients is heavily contaminated with VRE, and gown and glove isolation techniques are required to stop transmission.[178] Strict application of hand hygiene is also important for reducing the spread of VRE and other nosocomial pathogens. According to the available data and current CDC recommendations, the use of alcohol-based hand-rub solutions is superior to washing with soap and water: it can be performed more rapidly and is less damaging to the skin.[179]

VRE are also highly resistant to other available antibiotics. Acquisition of VRE is significantly associated with prior hospitalization and with use of third-generation cephalosporins, vancomycin, or multiple antibiotics.[180,181] In one study, 16% of stool specimens submitted for testing for *C. difficile* toxin were colonized with VRE, and all surgical patients in that study had the same strain.[182]

High mortality can be associated with VRE infections. In a study comparing the outcome of patients having VRE bacteremia with the outcome of patients having bacteremia caused by vancomycin-sensitive enterococci (VSE), mortality was 2.3 times higher in those with VRE bacteremia, and 89% of patients with VRE bacteremia were colonized or infected with VRE at another site.[183] Prior treatment with third-generation cephalosporins is another risk factor for increased mortality.[176] Liver transplant patients with VRE bacteremia had a 92% higher mortality than comparable patients with VSE bacteremia, and those with VRE bacteremia also had a higher recurrence rate and greater need for invasive procedures.[184]

Current recommendations include decreased—and possibly restricted—use of vancomycin, as well as aggressive infection control measures whenever VRE are isolated in a hospitalized patient.[177] In particular, vancomycin should not be used as primary treatment for *C. difficile*–associated diarrhea and should be avoided for surgical prophylaxis unless the hospital has a specific problem with MRSA or the patient cannot receive other appropriate antibiotics.

ENTERIC INFECTION

C. difficile is often found in patients with severe antibiotic-associated enteric infections. In one report, 691 (2%) of 32,757 consecutive postoperative patients experienced watery diarrhea significant enough to stimulate a request for *C. difficile* toxin assay.[185] Of this number, 75 (11% of patients with diarrhea) had a positive toxin assay. All cases were associated with antibiotic administration. Approximately 94% of the patients had received a cephalosporin either alone or in combination with other antibiotics; 29% of these responded to cessation of antibiotics and supportive measures, and the remainder were treated with vancomycin, metronidazole, or bacitracin. Six (14%) of the patients who required specific therapy relapsed after initial response to treatment and were subsequently cured with one or more additional courses of treatment. Two patients died, and the overall hospital stay for the remaining patients was prolonged by an average of 50%.

Most patients with mild cases of antibiotic-associated diarrhea do not have either positive cultures for *C. difficile* or positive toxin assays, and the etiologic role of *C. difficile* is unclear. Many hospitalized patients without diarrhea also have *C. difficile* in the stool, with or without toxin production,[123,186] and the likelihood of isolating this pathogen increases with patients' increasing length of stay.[118] A nonpathogenic yeast, *Saccharomyces boulardii,* when administered by mouth to hospitalized patients receiving antibiotics, significantly reduced the occurrence of antibiotic-associated diarrhea without affecting the rate of acquisition of *C. difficile.*[123]

Some 3% of asymptomatic adults carry *C. difficile* in their stools, but 30% to 40% of healthy neonates may carry the organism. The rate of carriage declines after the age of 1 to 2 years. *C. difficile* can be spread in the hospital and has been isolated from 10% of inanimate objects in the environment of patients with *C. difficile* colonization, compared with 3% in hospital areas with no known cases.[187] In one report,[187] this organism was recovered from the hands of 13% of medical personnel working in a ward with affected patients; in another,[188] it was recovered from 60% of personnel immediately after they had cared for an affected patient. Soap-and-water washing was ineffective in preventing acquisition, but the combination of glove use and chlorhexidine washing was effective. In another medical center,[189] clusters of new nosocomial *C. difficile* diarrhea were prevented by screening all patients with diarrhea by active surveillance (using culture to identify *C. difficile* infection) and by instituting isolation precautions and daily disinfection of infected patients' rooms.

The prevalence of *C. difficile* in the environment is increased when a patient has diarrhea.[187,188] In one prospectively studied cohort, 21% of patients without *C. difficile* in their stools on admission acquired the organism during hospitalization, and 37% of these patients experienced diarrhea; no cases of colitis occurred.[187] Diarrhea was more common in patients who received antibiotics. The rate of acquisition of *C. difficile* was 73% higher if a patient had a roommate colonized with *C. difficile.*

COST

The cost of nosocomial infections, both in dollars and in morbidity, is high. According to one estimate, 8.7 million extra hospital days and $4.5 billion in hospital charges were attributable to nosocomial infections in United States hospitals in 1976.[190]

Estimates of the number of deaths caused by nosocomial infections run as high as 58,000 a year; 9,700 of these deaths and 36% of all costs attributed to nosocomial infections are due to wound infections.[190] The actual numbers may be even higher. Another study found that 63 of 200 consecutive patients dying in the hospital had nosocomial infections; 18 (29%) of the 63 were judged causal and 26 (41%) contributory.[8] Most of the causal and contributory infections were of the lower respiratory tract, and deaths were significantly associated with invasive devices (e.g., intra-arterial and central venous pressure monitoring devices and nasogastric tubes). Of the 57 deaths occurring on the surgical service, 27 (47%) were associated with nosocomial infections.

RISK

The risk of acquiring a nosocomial infection is clearly related to the reason for hospitalization as well as to the underlying disease.[8,191] Patients admitted to the hospital with a fatal underlying disease have a nosocomial infection rate of 24%, compared with 10% in patients with ultimately fatal disease and 2% in those with nonfatal disease. Among 100 consecutive trauma patients admitted to the ICU at Harborview Medical Center in 1986, 42 acquired 64 nosocomial infections, including 23 lower respiratory tract infections, 17 urinary tract infections, and 6 wound infections.[152] These 100 ICU admissions and 101 consecutive trauma admissions to the general ward were examined together. Of 153 patients admitted with injury severity scores of 25 or less, nosocomial infection occurred in 32 (21%). Of 48 patients with injury severity scores higher than 25, nosocomial infection occurred in 26 (54%).[152] A statewide survey of hospitals in Virginia from 1978 to 1982 found that infections in ICU patients accounted for 25% of all cases of nosocomial infections, although fewer than 10% of the beds were in ICUs.[192]

References

1. Haley RW, Schaberg DR, Crossley KB, et al: Extra charges and prolongation of stay attributable to nosocomial infections: a prospective interhospital comparison. Am J Med 70:51, 1981

2. Haley RW, Schaberg DR, Von Allmen SD, et al: Estimating the extra charges and prolongation of hospitalization due to nosocomial infections: a comparison of methods. J Infect Dis 141:248, 1980

3. Haley RW, Culver DH, White JW, et al: The nationwide nosocomial infection rate: a new need for vital statistics. Am J Epidemiol 121:159, 1985

4. Haley RW, White JW, Culver DH, et al: The financial incentive for hospitals to prevent nosocomial infections under the prospective payment system: an empirical determination from a nationally representative sample. JAMA 257:1611, 1987

5. Haley RW, Culver DH, Morgan WM, et al: Increased recognition of infectious diseases in US hospitals through increased use of diagnostic tests, 1970 to 197

6. Roberts J, Barnes W, Pennock M, et al: Diagnostic accuracy of fever as a measure of postoperative pulmonary complications. Heart Lung 17:166, 1988

7. Engoren M: Lack of association between atelectasis and fever. Chest 107:81, 1995

8. Gross PA, Neu HC, Aswapokee P, et al: Deaths from nosocomial infections: experience in a university hospital and a community hospital. Am J Med 68:219, 1980

9. Andrews CP, Coalson JJ, Smith JD, et al: Diagnosis of nosocomial bacterial pneumonia in acute, diffuse lung injury. Chest 80:254, 1981

10. Craven DE, Steger KA: Ventilator-associated bacterial pneumonia: challenges in diagnosis, treatment, and prevention. New Horizons 6:S30, 1998

11. Croce MA, Fabian TC, Schurr MJ, et al: Using bronchoalveolar lavage to distinguish nosocomial pneumonia from systemic inflammatory response syndrome: a prospective analysis. J Trauma 39:1134, 1995

12. Valles J, Artigas A, Rello J, et al: Continuous aspiration of subglottic secretions in preventing ventilator-associated pneumonia. Ann Intern Med 122:179, 1995

13. Fernandez-Crehuet R, Diaz-Molina C, de Irala J, et al: Nosocomial infection in an intensive-care unit: identification of risk factors. Infect Control Hosp Epidemiol 18:825, 1997

14. Guidelines for prevention of nosocomial pneumonia. Centers for Disease Control and Prevention. Respir Care 39:1191, 1994

15. Singh N, Rogers P, Atwood CW, et al: Short-course empiric antibiotic therapy for patients with pulmonary infiltrates in the intensive care unit: a proposed solution for indiscriminate antibiotic prescription. Am J Respir Crit Care Med 162:505, 2000

16. Caplan ES, Hoyt NJ: Nosocomial sinusitis. JAMA 247:639, 1982

17. Deutschman CS, Wilton P, Sinow J, et al: Paranasal sinusitis associated with nasotracheal intubation: a frequently unrecognized and treatable source of sepsis. Crit Care Med 14:111, 1986

18. Grindlinger GA, Niehoff J, Hughes SL, et al: Acute paranasal sinusitis related to nasotracheal intubation of head-injured patients. Crit Care Med 15:214, 1987

19. Christensen L, Schaffer S, Ross SE: Otitis media in adult trauma patients: incidence and clinical significance. J Trauma 31:1543, 1991

20. Roettinger W, Edgerton MT, Kurtz LD, et al: Role of inoculation site as a determinant of infections in soft tissue wounds. Am J Surg 126:354, 1973

21. Miles AA, Milles EM, Burke J: The value and duration of defence reactions of the skin to the primary lodgement of bacteria. Br J Exp Pathol 38:79, 1957

22. Burke JF, Miles AA: The sequence of vascular events in early infective inflammation. J Pathol Bacteriol 76:1, 1958

23. Burke JF: The effective period of preventive antibiotic action in experimental incisions and dermal lesions. Surgery 50:161, 1961

24. Alexander JW, Altemeier WA: Penicillin prophylaxis of experimental staphylococcal wound infections. Surg Gynecol Obstet 120:243, 1965

25. Edlich RF, Smith QT, Edgerton MT: Resistance of the surgical wound to antimicrobial prophylaxis and its mechanisms of development. Am J Surg 126:583, 1973

26. McKittrick LS, Wheelock FC: The routine use of antibiotics in elective abdominal surgery. Surg Gynecol Obstet 99:376, 1954

27. Barnes J, Pace WG, Trump DS, et al: Prophylactic postoperative antibiotics: a controlled study of 1007 cases. AMA Arch Surg 79:190, 1959

28. Dellinger EP, Gross PA, Barrett TL, et al: Quality standard for antimicrobial prophylaxis in surgical procedures. Clin Infect Dis 18:422, 1994

29. Page CP, Bohnen JMA, Fletcher JR, et al: Antimicrobial prophylaxis for surgical wounds: guidelines for clinical care. Arch Surg 128:79, 1993

30. Dellinger EP: Antibiotic prophylaxis in trauma: penetrating abdominal injuries and open fractures. Rev Infect Dis 13(suppl 10):S847, 1991

31. Fabian TC, Croce MA, Payne LW, et al: Duration of antibiotic therapy for penetrating abdominal trauma: a prospective trial. Surgery 112:788, 1992

32. McDonald M, Grabsch E, Marshall C, et al: Single- versus multiple-dose antimicrobial prophylaxis for major surgery: a systematic review. Aust N Z J Surg 68:388, 1988

33. Culver DH, Horan TC, Gaynes RP, et al: Surgical wound infection rates by wound class, operative procedure, and patient risk index: National Nosocomial Infections Surveillance System. Am J Med 91:152S, 1991

34. Consensus paper on the surveillance of surgical wound infections. The Society for Hospital Epidemiology of America, The Association for Practitioners in Infection Control, The Centers for Disease Control, The Surgical Infection Society. Infect Control Hosp Epidemiol 13:599, 1992

35. Gaynes RP, Culver DH, Horan TC, et al: Surgical site infection (SSI) rates in the United States, 1992-1998: the National Nosocomial Infections Surveillance System basic SSI risk index. Clin Infect Dis 33(suppl 2): S69, 2001

36. Horan TC, Gaynes RP, Martone WJ, et al: CDC definitions of nosocomial surgical site infections, 1992: a modification of CDC definitions of surgical wound infections. Am J Infect Control 20:271, 1992

37. Kurz A, Sessler DI, Lenhardt R: Perioperative normothermia to reduce the incidence of surgical-wound infection and shorten hospitalization. Study of Wound Infection and Temperature Group. N Engl J Med 334:1209, 1996

38. Greif R, Akca O, Horn EP, et al: Supplemental perioperative oxygen to reduce the incidence of surgical-wound infection. Outcomes Research Group. N Engl J Med 342:161, 2000

39. Furnary AP, Zerr KJ, Grunkemeier GL, et al: Continuous intravenous insulin infusion reduces the incidence of deep sternal wound infection in diabetic patients after cardiac surgical procedures. Ann Thorac Surg 67:352, 1999

40. Latham R, Lancaster AD, Covington JF, et al: The association of diabetes and glucose control with surgical-site infections among cardiothoracic surgery patients. Infect Control Hosp Epidemiol 22:607, 2001

41. van den Berghe G, Wouters P, Weekers F, et al:

Intensive insulin therapy in the surgical intensive care unit. N Engl J Med 345:1359, 2001

42. MacLennan JD: The histotoxic clostridial infections of man. Bacteriologic Reviews 26:177, 1962

43. Pitcher WD, Musher DM: Critical importance of early diagnosis and treatment of intra-abdominal infection. Arch Surg 117:328, 1982

44. Bohnen J, Boulanger M, Meakins JL, et al: Prognosis in generalized peritonitis: relation to cause and risk factors. Arch Surg 118:285, 1983

45. Caplan ES, Hoyt NJ, Rodriguez A, et al: Empyema occurring in the multiply traumatized patient. J Trauma 24:785, 1984

46. Milano CA, Kesler K, Archibald N, et al: Mediastinitis after coronary artery bypass graft surgery: risk factors and long-term survival. Circulation 92:2245, 1995

47. Gur E, Stern D, Weiss J, et al: Clinical-radiological evaluation of poststernotomy wound infection. Plast Reconstruct Surg 101:348, 1998

48. Pairolero PC, Arnold PG, Harris JB: Long-term results of pectoralis major muscle transposition for infected sternotomy wounds. Ann Surg 213:583, 1991

49. Hand WL, Sanford JP: Posttraumatic bacterial meningitis. Ann Intern Med 72:869, 1970

50. MacGee EE, Cauthen JC, Brackett CE: Meningitis following acute traumatic cerebrospinal fluid fistula. J Neurosurg 33:312, 1970

51. Leech PJ, Paterson A: Conservative and operative management for cerebrospinal-fluid leakage after closed head injury. Lancet 1:1013, 1973

52. Davis CH: Traumatic CSF fistula: investigation and treatment. Current Controversies in Neurosurgery. Morley TP, Ed. WB Saunders Co, Philadelphia, 1976, p 572

53. Petersdorf RG, Curtin JA, Hoeprich PD, et al: A study of antibiotic prophylaxis in unconscious patients. N Engl J Med 257:1001, 1957

54. Chapman MW, Mahoney M: The role of early internal fixation in the management of open fractures. Clin Orthop 138:120, 1979

55. Gustilo RB, Mendoza RM, Williams DN: Problems in the management of type III (severe) open fractures: a new classification of type III open fractures. J Trauma 24:742, 1984

56. Rittmann WW, Schibli M, Matter P, et al: Open fractures: long-term results in 200 consecutive cases. Clin Orthop 138:132, 1979

57. Dellinger EP, Miller SD, Wertz MJ, et al: Risk of infection after open fracture of the arm or leg. Arch Surg 123:1320, 1988

58. Sattler FR, Foderaro JB, Aber RC: Staphylococcus epidermidis bacteremia associated with vascular catheters: an important cause of febrile morbidity in hospitalized patients. Infect Control 5:279, 1984

59. Maki DG, Mermel LA: Infections due to infusion therapy. Hospital Infections, 4th ed. Bennett JV, Brachman PS, Eds. Lippincott-Raven Publishers, Philadelphia, 1998, p 689

60. Bregenzer T, Conen D, Sakmann P, et al: Is routine replacement of peripheral intravenous catheters necessary? Arch Intern Med 158:151, 1998

61. Hershey CO, Tomford JW, McLaren CE, et al: The natural history of intravenous catheter-associated phlebitis. Arch Intern Med 144:1373, 1984

62. Maki DG, Weise CE, Sarafin HW: A semiquantitative culture method for identifying intravenous-catheter-related infection. N Engl J Med 296:1305, 1977

63. Press OW, Ramsey PG, Larson EB, et al: Hickman catheter infections in patients with malignancies. Medicine (Baltimore) 63:189, 1984

64. Clarke DE, Raffin TA: Infectious complications of indwelling long-term central venous catheters. Chest 97:966, 1990

65. Maki DG, Cobb L, Garman JK, et al: An attachable silver-impregnated cuff for prevention of infection with central venous catheters: a prospective randomized multicenter trial. Am J Med 85:307, 1988

66. Conly JM, Grieves K, Peters B: A prospective, randomized study comparing transparent and dry gauze dressings for central venous catheters. J Infect Dis 159:310, 1989

67. Myers ML, Austin TW, Sibbald WJ: Pulmonary artery catheter infections: a prospective study. Ann Surg 201:237, 1985

68. Cooper GL, Hopkins CC: Rapid diagnosis of intravascular catheter-associated infection by direct Gram staining of catheter segments. N Engl J Med 312: 1142, 1985

69. Charalambos C, Swoboda SM, Dick J, et al: Risk factors and clinical impact of central line infections in the surgical intensive care unit. Arch Surg 133:1241, 1998

70. O'Grady NP, Alexander M, Dellinger EP, et al: Guidelines for the prevention of intravascular catheter-related infections. MMWR Recomm Rep 51:1, 2002

71. Sherertz RJ, Heard SO, Raad II: Diagnosis of triple-lumen catheter infection: comparison of roll plate, sonication, and flushing methodologies. J Clin Microbiol 35:641, 1997

72. Ponce de Leon S, Wenzel RP: Hospital-acquired bloodstream infections with Staphylococcus epidermidis. Am J Med 77:639, 1984

73. Rex JH, Bennett JE, Sugar AM, et al: Intravascular catheter exchange and duration of candidemia: NIAID Mycoses Study Group and the Candidemia Study Group. Clin Infect Dis 21:994, 1995

74. Mermel LA, Farr BM, Sherertz RJ, et al: Guidelines for the management of intravascular catheter-related infections. Clin Infect Dis 32:1249, 2001

75. Kaufman J, Demas C, Stark K, et al: Catheter-related septic central venous thrombosis: current therapeutic options. West J Med 145:200, 1986

76. Strinden WD, Helgerson RB, Maki DG: Candida septic thrombosis of the great central veins associated with central catheters: clinical features and management. Ann Surg 202:653, 1985

77. Cobb DK, High KP, Sawyer RG, et al: A controlled trial of scheduled replacement of central venous and pulmonary-artery catheters. N Engl J Med 327: 1062, 1992

78. Mermel LA: Prevention of intravascular catheter-related infections. Ann Intern Med 132:391, 2000

79. Cook D, Randolph A, Kernerman P, et al: Central venous catheter replacement strategies: a systematic review of the literature. Crit Care Med 25:1417, 1997

80. Reed CR, Sessler CN, Glauser FL, et al: Central venous catheter infections: concepts and controversies. Intens Care Med 21:177, 1995

81. Pettigrew RA, Lang SD, Haydock DA, et al: Catheter-related sepsis in patients on intravenous nutrition: a prospective study of quantitative catheter cultures and guidewire changes for suspected sepsis. Br J Surg 72:52, 1985

82. Newsome HH, Armstrong CW, Mayhall GC, et al: Mechanical complications from insertion of subclavian venous feeding catheters: comparison of de novo percutaneous venipuncture to change of catheter over guidewire. J Parenter Enteral Nutr 8:560, 1984

83. Sitzmann JV, Townsend TR, Siler MC, et al: Septic and technical complications of central venous catheterization: a prospective study of 200 consecutive patients. Ann Surg 202:766, 1985

84. Bozzetti F, Terno G, Bonfanti G, et al: Prevention and treatment of central venous catheter sepsis by exchange via a guidewire: a prospective controlled trial. Ann Surg 198:48, 1983

85. Norwood S, Ruby A, Civetta J, et al: Catheter-related infections and associated septicemia. Chest 99:968, 1991

86. Raad II, Hohn DC, Gilbreath BJ, et al: Prevention of central venous catheter-related infections by using maximal sterile barrier precautions during insertion. Infect Control Hosp Epidemiol 15:231, 1994

87. Sherertz RJ, Ely EW, Westbrook DM, et al: Education of physicians-in-training can decrease the risk for vascular catheter infection. Ann Intern Med 132:641, 2000

88. Richet H, Hubert B, Nitemberg G, et al: Prospective multicenter study of vascular-catheter-related complications and risk factors for positive central-catheter cultures in intensive care unit patients. J Clin Microbiol 28:2520, 1990

89. Goetz AM, Wagener MM, Miller JM, et al: Risk of infection due to central venous catheters: effect of site of placement and catheter type. Infect Control Hosp Epidemiol 19:842, 1998

90. Timsit JF, Bruneel F, Cheval C, et al: Use of tunneled femoral catheters to prevent catheter-related infection: a randomized, controlled trial. Ann Intern Med 130:729, 1999

91. Merrer J, De Jonghe B, Golliot F, et al: Complications of femoral and subclavian venous catheterization in critically ill patients: a randomized controlled trial. JAMA 286:700, 2001

92. Central venous catheters coated with minocycline and rifampin for the prevention of catheter-related colonization and bloodstream infections: a randomized, double-blind trial. The Texas Medical Center Catheter Study Group. Ann Intern Med 127:267, 1997

93. Maki DG, Stolz SM, Wheeler S, et al: Prevention of central venous catheter-related bloodstream infection by use of an antiseptic-impregnated catheter: a randomized, controlled trial. Ann Intern Med 127:257, 1997

94. Darouiche RO, Raad II, Heard SO, et al: A comparison of two antimicrobial-impregnated central venous catheters. N Engl J Med 340:1, 1999

95. Maki DG, Band JD: A comparative study of polyantibiotic and iodophor ointments in prevention of vascular catheter-related infection. Am J Med 70:739, 1981

96. Hoffman KK, Weber DJ, Samsa GP, et al: Transparent polyurethane film as an intravenous catheter dressing: a meta-analysis of the infection risks. JAMA 267:2072, 1992

97. Hilton E, Haslett TM, Borenstein MT, et al: Central catheter infections: single- versus triple-lumen catheters: influence of guidewires on infection rates when used for replacement of catheters. Am J Med 84:667, 1988

98. Pemberton LB, Lyman B, Lander V, et al: Sepsis from triple- vs single-lumen catheters during total parenteral nutrition in surgical or critically ill patients. Arch Surg 121:591, 1986

99. Miller JJ, Venus B, Mathru M: Comparison of the sterility of long-term central venous catheterization using single lumen, triple lumen, and pulmonary artery catheters. Crit Care Med 12:634, 1984

100. Powell C, Fabri PJ, Kudsk KA: Risk of infection accompanying the use of single-lumen vs. double-lumen subclavian catheters: a prospective randomized study. J Parenter Enteral Nutr 12:127, 1988

101. Raad I, Davis S, Becker M, et al: Low infection rate and long durability of nontunneled Silastic catheters: a safe and cost-effective alternative for long-term venous access. Arch Intern Med 153:1791, 1993

102. Groeger JS, Lucas AB, Thaler HT, et al: Infectious morbidity associated with long-term use of venous access devices in patients with cancer. Ann Intern Med 119:1168, 1993

103. Bern MM, Lokich JJ, Wallach SR, et al: Very low doses of warfarin can prevent thrombosis in central venous catheters: a prospective randomized trial. Ann Intern Med 112:423, 1990

104. Stark RP, Maki DG: Bacteriuria in the catheterized patient: what quantitative level of bacteriuria is relevant? N Engl J Med 311:560, 1984

105. Kunin CM: Genitourinary infections in the patient at risk: extrinsic risk factors. Am J Med 76:131, 1984

106. Harding GK, Nicolle LE, Ronald AR, et al: How long should catheter-acquired urinary tract infection in women be treated? A randomized controlled study. Ann Intern Med 114:713, 1991

107. Hirsh DD, Fainstein V, Musher DM: Do condom catheter collecting systems cause urinary tract infection? JAMA 242:340, 1979

108. Johnson ET: The condom catheter: urinary tract infection and other complications. South Med J 76: 579, 1983

109. Stamm WE: Urinary tract infections. Hospital Infections, 4th ed. Bennett JV, Brachman PS, Eds. Lippincott-Raven Publishers, Philadelphia, 1998, p 477

110. Warren JW, Platt R, Thomas RJ, et al: Antibiotic irrigation and catheter-associated urinary tract infections. N Engl J Med 299:570, 1978

111. Platt R, Polk BF, Murdock B, et al: Reduction of mortality associated with nosocomial urinary tract infection. Lancet 1:893, 1983

112. Lima NL, Guerrant RL, Kaiser DL, et al: A retrospective cohort study of nosocomial diarrhea as a risk factor for nosocomial infection. J Infect Dis 161:948, 1990

113. Jones SR, Smith JW, Sanford JP: Localization of urinary-tract infections by detection of antibody-coated bacteria in urine sediment. N Engl J Med 290:591, 1974

114. Latham RH, Stamm WE: Role of fimbriated Escherichia coli in urinary tract infections in adult women: correlation with localization studies. J Infect Dis 149:835, 1984

115. Anderson RU: Urinary tract infections in compromised hosts. Urol Clin North Am 13:727, 1986

116. Stamm WE, Stapleton AE: Approach to the patient with urinary tract infection. Infectious Disease, 2nd ed. Gorbach SL, Bartlett JG, Blacklow NR, Eds. WB Saunders Co, Philadelphia, 1998, p 943

117. DuPont HL, Ribner BS: Infectious gastroenteritis. Hospital Infections, 4th ed. Bennett JV, Brachman PS, Eds. Lippincott-Raven Publishers, Philadel-phia, 1998, p 537

118. Hines J, Nachamkin I: Effective use of the clinical microbiology laboratory for diagnosing diarrheal diseases. Clin Infect Dis 23:1292, 1996

119. Gerding DN, Johnson S, Peterson LR, et al: Clostridium difficile–associated diarrhea and colitis. Infect Control Hosp Epidemiol 16:459, 1995

120. McFarland LV, Coyle MB, Kremer WH, et al: Rectal swab cultures for Clostridium difficile surveillance studies. J Clin Microbiol 25:2241, 1987

121. George WL: Antimicrobial agent-associated colitis and diarrhea: historical background and clinical aspects. Rev Infect Dis 6:S208, 1984

122. Grube BJ, Heimbach DM, Marvin JA: Clostridium difficile diarrhea in critically ill burned patients. Arch Surg 122:655, 1987

123. Surawicz CM, Elmer GW, Speelman P, et al: Prevention of antibiotic-associated diarrhea by Saccha-romyces boulardii: a prospective study. Gastroente-rology 96:981, 1989

124. McFarland LV, Surawicz CM, Stamm WE: Risk factors for Clostridium difficile carriage and C. dif-ficile–associated diarrhea in a cohort of hospitalized patients. J Infect Dis 162:678, 1990

125. Tedesco FJ, Corless JK, Brownstein RE: Rectal

sparing in antibiotic-associated pseudomembranous colitis: a prospective study. Gastroenterology 83:1259, 1982

126. Dane TE, King EG: Fatal pseudomembranous enterocolitis following clindamycin therapy. Br J Surg 63:305, 1976

127. Cheung A, Tank RE, Dellinger EP: Antibiotic-associated enterocolitis involving the small bowel. Surgical Rounds 14:821,1991

128. Hecht JR, Olinger EJ: Clostridium difficile colitis secondary to intravenous vancomycin. Dig Dis Sci 34:148, 1989

129. Miller SN, Ringler RP: Vancomycin-induced pseudomembranous colitis (letter). J Clin Gastroenterol 9:114, 1987

130. Oliva SL, Guglielmo BJ, Jacobs R, et al: Failure of intravenous vancomycin and intravenous metronidazole to prevent or treat antibiotic-associated pseudomembranous colitis (letter). J Infect Dis 159:1154, 1989

131. Freiman JP, Graham DJ, Green L: Pseudomembranous colitis associated with single-dose cephalosporin prophylaxis (letter). JAMA 262:902, 1989

132. Gerding DN: Treatment of Clostridium difficile–associated diarrhea and colitis. Curr Top Microbiol Immunol 250:127, 2000

133. Recommendations for preventing the spread of vancomycin resistance. Hospital Infection Control Practices Advisory Committee. MMWR Morb Mortal Wkly Rep 44:1, 1995

134. Gerding DN, Olson MM, Johnson S, et al: Clostridium difficile diarrhea and colonization after treatment with abdominal infection regimens containing clindamycin or metronidazole. Am J Surg 159:212, 1990

135. Drapkin MS, Worthington MG, Chang TW, et al: Clostridium difficile colitis mimicking acute peritonitis. Arch Surg 120:1321, 1985

136. Chatila W, Manthous CA: Clostridium difficile causing sepsis and an acute abdomen in critically ill patients. Crit Care Med 23:1146, 1995

137. Byl B, Jacobs F, Struelens MJ, et al: Extraintestinal Clostridium difficile infections. Clin Infect Dis 22: 712, 1996

138. Infectious risks of blood transfusions. Transfusion Medicine Bulletin 4:1, 2001

139. Kahn RA, Barrios SDP: Diseases transmitted by blood transfusion. Transfusion Therapy: Principles and Procedures. Rutman RC, Miller WV, Eds. Aspen Publishers, Rockville, Maryland, 1985, p 311

140. Herwaldt BL, Kjemtrup AM, Conrad PA, et al: Transfusion-transmitted babesiosis in Washington State: first reported case caused by a WA1-type parasite. J Infect Dis 175:1259, 1997

141. Update: investigations of West Nile virus infections in recipients of organ transplantation and blood transfusion—Michigan, 2002. MMWR Morb Mortal Wkly Rep 51:879, 2002

142. Kuehnert MJ, Roth VR, Haley NR, et al: Transfusion-transmitted bacterial infection in the United States, 1998 through 2000. Transfusion 41:1493, 2001

143. Dodd RY, Notari EP, Stramer SL: Current prevalence and incidence of infectious disease markers and estimated window-period risk in the American Red Cross blood donor population. Transfusion 42:975, 2002

144. Cumming PD, Wallace EL, Schorr JB, et al: Exposure of patients to human immunodeficiency virus through the transfusion of blood components that test antibody-negative. N Engl J Med 321:941, 1989

145. Menitove JE: Current risk of transfusion-associated human immunodeficiency virus infection. Arch Pathol Lab Med 114:330, 1990

146. Surgenor DMacN, Wallace EL, Hao SH:

Collection and transfusion of blood in the United States, 1982– 1988. N Engl J Med 322:1646, 1990

147. Hebert PC, Wells G, Blajchman MA, et al: A multicenter, randomized, controlled clinical trial of transfusion requirements in critical care. Transfusion requirements in critical care investigators, Canadian Critical Care Trials Group. N Engl J Med 340:409, 1999

148. Goldman M, Savard R, Long A, et al: Declining value of preoperative autologous donation. Transfusion 42:819, 2002

149. Garibaldi RA, Brodine S, Matsumiya S, et al: Evidence for the non-infectious etiology of early postoperative fever. Infect Control 6:273, 1985

150. Dykes MH: Unexplained postoperative fever: its value as a sign of halothane sensitization. JAMA 216: 641, 1971

151. Dellinger EP, Wertz MJ, Oreskovich MR, et al: Specificity of fever and leukocytosis after laparotomy for penetrating abdominal trauma (abstr). J Trauma 23:633, 1983

152. Dellinger EP: Prevention and management of infections. Trauma, 2nd ed. Moore EE, Mattox KL, Feliciano DV, Eds. Appleton & Lange, Norwalk, 1988, p 231

153. Dellinger EP: Approach to the patient with postoperative fever. Infectious Diseases, 3rd ed. Gorbach S, Bartlett J, Blacklow N, Eds. WB Saunders Co, Philadelphia (in press)

154. Richards C, Emori TG, Edwards J, et al: Characteristics of hospitals and infection control professionals participating in the National Nosocomial Infections Surveillance System 1999. Am J Infect Control 29:400, 2001

155. Haley RW, Culver DH, White JW, et al: The efficacy of infection surveillance and control programs in preventing nosocomial infections in US hospitals. Am J Epidemiol 121:182, 1985

156. Haley RW, Hooton TM, Culver DH, et al: Nosocomial infections in US hospitals, 1975 to 1976: estimated frequency by selected characteristics of patients. Am J Med 70:947, 1981

157. Brennan TA, Leape LL, Laird NM, et al: Incidence of adverse events and negligence in hospitalized patients: results of the Harvard Medical Practice Study I. N Engl J Med 324:370, 1991

158. Mangram AJ, Horan TC, Pearson ML, et al: Guideline for prevention of surgical site infection, 1999. Hospital Infection Control Practices Advisory Committee. Infect Control Hosp Epidemiol 20:250, 1999

159. Horan TC, Culver DH, Gaynes RP, et al: Nosocomial infections in surgical patients in the United States, January 1986–June 1992: National Nosocomial Infections Surveillance (NNIS) System. Infect Control Hosp Epidemiol 14:73, 1993

160. Platt R, Polk BF, Murdock B, et al: Mortality associated with nosocomial urinary tract infection. N Engl J Med 307:637, 1982

161. Tambyah PA, Knasinski V, Maki DG: The direct costs of nosocomial catheter-associated urinary tract infection in the era of managed care. Infect Control Hosp Epidemiol 23:27, 2002

162. Givens CD, Wenzel RP: Catheter-associated urinary tract infections in surgical patients: a controlled study on the excess morbidity and costs. J Urol 124:646, 1980

163. Krieger JN, Kaiser DL, Wenzel RP: Nosocomial urinary tract infections cause wound infections postoperatively in surgical patients. Surg Gynecol Obstet 156:313, 1983

164. Dickinson GM, Bisno AL: Infections associated with indwelling devices: concepts of pathogenesis; infections associated with intravascular devices. Antimicrob Agents Chemother 33:597, 1989

165. Druskin MS, Siegel PD: Bacterial contamination of indwelling intravenous polyethylene catheters.

JAMA 185:966, 1963

166. Rowley KM, Clubb KS, Walker Smith GJ, et al: Right-sided infective endocarditis as a consequence of flow-directed pulmonary-artery catheterization: a clinicopathological study of 55 autopsied patients. N Engl J Med 311:1152, 1984

167. Hudson-Civetta JA, Civetta JM, Martinez OV, et al: Risk and detection of pulmonary artery catheter-related infection in septic surgical patients. Crit Care Med 15:29, 1987

168. Meakins JL: Infection associated with radial artery catheters (editorial). Can Med Assoc J 121:1564, 1979

169. Arnow PM, Costas CO: Delayed rupture of the radial artery caused by catheter-related sepsis. Rev Infect Dis 10:1035, 1988

170. Gardner RM, Schwartz R, Wong HC, et al: Percutaneous indwelling radial-artery catheters for monitoring cardiovascular function: prospective study of the risk of thrombosis and infection. N Engl J Med 290:1227, 1974

171. Band JD, Maki DG: Infections caused by arterial catheters used for hemodynamic monitoring. Am J Med 67:735, 1979

172. Kaye W, Wheaton M, Potter-Bynoe G: Radial and pulmonary artery catheter-related sepsis (abstr). Crit Care Med 11:249, 1983

173. Horan TC, White JW, Jarvis WR, et al: Nosocomial infection surveillance, 1984. CDC Surveillance Summaries. MMWR Morb Mortal Wkly Rep 35:17SS, 1986

174. National Nosocomial Infections Surveillance (NNIS) System Report, Data Summary from January 1992-June 2001, issued August 2001. Am J Infect Control 29:404, 2001

175. Vancomycin-resistant Staphylococcus aureus—Pennsylvania, 2002. MMWR Morb Mortal Wkly Rep 51:902, 2002

176. Stroud L, Edwards J, Danzing L, et al: Risk factors for mortality associated with enterococcal bloodstream infections. Infect Control Hosp Epidemiol 17:576, 1996

177. Recommendations for preventing the spread of vancomycin resistance: recommendations of the Hospital Infection Control Practices Advisory Committee (HICPAC). Centers for Disease Control and Prevention. MMWR Morb Mortal Wkly Rep 44(RR-12):1, 1995

178. Murray BE: What can we do about vancomycin-resistant enterococci? Clin Infect Dis 20:1134, 1995

179. Boyce JM, Pittet D: Guideline for hand hygiene in health-care settings. Recommendations of the Healthcare Infection Control Practices Advisory Committee and the HICPAC/SHEA/APIC/IDSA Hand Hygiene Task Force. Society for Healthcare Epidemiology of America/Association for Professionals in Infection Control/Infectious Diseases Society of America. MMWR Recomm Rep 51:1, 2002

180. Weinstein JW, Roe M, Towns M, et al: Resistant enterococci: a prospective study of prevalence, incidence, and factors associated with colonization in a university hospital. Infect Control Hosp Epidemiol 17:36, 1996

181. Tornieporth NG, Roberts RB, John J, et al: Risk factors associated with vancomycin-resistant Enterococcus faecium infection or colonization in 145 matched case patients and control patients. Clin Infect Dis 23:767, 1996

182. Rafferty ME, McCormick MI, Bopp LH, et al: Vancomycin-resistant enterococci in stool specimens submitted for Clostridium difficile cytotoxin assay. Infect Control Hosp Epidemiol 18:342, 1997

183. Edmond MB, Ober JF, Dawson JD, et al: Vancomycin-resistant enterococcal bacteremia: natural history and attributable mortality. Clin Infect Dis 23:1234, 1996

184. Linden PK, Pasculle AW, Manez R, et al: Differences in outcomes for patients with bacteremia due to vancomycin-resistant Enterococcus faecium or vancomycin-susceptible E. faecium. Clin Infect Dis 22:663, 1996

185. Rosenberg JM, Walker M, Welch JP, et al: Clostridium difficile colitis in surgical patients. Am J Surg 147:486, 1984

186. McFarland LV, Elmer GW, Stamm WE, et al: Correlation of immunoblot type, enterotoxin production, and cytotoxin production with clinical manifestations of Clostridium difficile infection in a cohort of hospitalized patients. Infect Immun 59:2456, 1991

187. Fekety R, Kim KH, Brown D, et al: Epidemiology of antibiotic-associated colitis: isolation of Clostridium difficile from the hospital environment. Am J Med 70: 906, 1981

188. McFarland LV, Mulligan ME, Kwok RY, et al: Nosocomial acquisition of Clostridium difficile infection. N Engl J Med 320:204, 1989

189. Struelens MJ, Maas A, Nonhoff C, et al: Control of nosocomial transmission of Clostridium difficile based on sporadic case surveillance. Am J Med 91(suppl 3B):138S, 1991

190. Martone WJ, Jarvis WR, Edwards JR, et al: Incidence and nature of endemic and epidemic nosocomial infections. Hospital Infections, 4th ed. Bennett JV, Brachman PS, Eds. Lippincott-Raven, Philadelphia, 1998, p 461

191. Britt MR, Schleupner CJ, Matsumiya S: Severity of underlying disease as a predictor of nosocomial infection: utility in the control of nosocomial infection. JAMA 239:1047, 1978

192. Wenzel RP, Thompson RL, Landry SM, et al: Hospital-acquired infections in intensive care unit patients: an overview with emphasis on epidemics. Infect Control 4:371, 1983

Acknowledgments

Figures 1 and 2   Carol Donner.
Figure 4   Albert Miller.

18 INTRA-ABDOMINAL INFECTION

Robert G. Sawyer, M.D., F.A.C.S., Jeffrey S. Barkun, M.D., F.A.C.S., Robert Smith, M.D., Tae Chong, M.D., and George Tzimas, M.D.

Recognition and Management of Intra-abdominal Infection

The basic principles of rapid diagnosis, timely physiologic support, and definitive intervention for intra-abdominal infections have remained unchanged over the past century. Specific management of these conditions, however, has been transformed of late as a result of numerous advances in technology. Improved radiologic and laboratory techniques have led to more precise preoperative diagnoses, and newer procedures have led to treatment algorithms that cause less morbidity and permit faster recovery. Whereas the pathophysiology of these infections remains largely unchanged, their management is now marked by an ever-growing complexity. It is no longer true that the diagnosis of intra-abdominal infection, even in association with a perforated viscus, necessitates urgent exploration, but it remains the case that decisions regarding the ultimate course of action for any individual patient are solely the responsibility of the surgeon.

Clinical Evaluation

HISTORY

The general approach to a patient suspected of having an intra-abdominal infection is much like that to a patient with any other acute surgical condition. Specific approaches to various intra-abdominal infections are addressed in more detail elsewhere [*see* Infections of the Upper Abdomen *and* Infections of the Lower Abdomen, *below*].

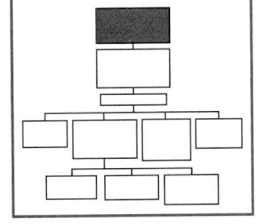

The first step is an accurate history. To begin with, cases of peritonitis are broadly classified as primary, secondary, or tertiary; this classification provides a useful framework for suggesting general approaches to treatment. Primary peritonitis arises spontaneously, without a demonstrable source of contamination, and is generally treated with antibiotics alone; an example is spontaneous bacterial peritonitis in the setting of ascites. Secondary peritonitis is caused by a breach in the GI tract that leads to contamination of a normally sterile space. Control of the source of infection via drainage, resection, diversion, or some combination thereof is imperative for optimizing outcome. Tertiary peritonitis is a poorly defined entity associated with recurrence of intra-abdominal infection after the treatment of secondary peritonitis. It frequently features a diffuse infection in a critically ill patient and may be caused by any of a long list of nosocomial pathogens (e.g., *Pseudomonas aeruginosa, Staphylococcus aureus,* and *Candida albicans*). Management of tertiary peritonitis is complex and must be individualized for each patient.

The acuteness and severity of the presenting symptoms may help localize the origin of the infection. More important, however, they allow appropriate triage of these patients, who are frequently seen in a crowded emergency department. For example, a patient with sudden onset of severe abdominal pain and physiologic derangement must take precedence over almost all other patients, whereas a stable patient presenting with a chronic complaint can be evaluated in a more deliberate fashion. The specifics of the presenting episode (e.g., the onset, location, and nature of the pain and any changes in bowel habits) are undeniably crucial, but the patient's medical and surgical histories, as well as any previous similar illnesses, are equally critical. Many medical problems and therapies are associated with abdominal pain or discomfort, and an accurate accounting of previous surgical manipulation of the abdomen is vital for refining the differential diagnosis, as well as for prioritizing further tests. The question of whether a patient has presented with similar symptoms before (particularly if those symptoms led to a diagnosis) may be important for determining the timing of any intervention, as well as for putting the current complaint in the context of an ongoing condition. In fact, many patients arrive for medical treatment with a strong (and frequently correct) concept of the nature of their disease.

PHYSICAL EXAMINATION

Once the history has been obtained, a thorough physical assessment is performed, with the emphasis on the abdomen, the pelvis (including the vagina), and the rectum. The usual sequence—inspection, auscultation, percussion, and palpation—should be followed as traditionally taught. This sequence need not be extensively reviewed here; however, certain points should be emphasized. With the advent of laparoscopy, inspection must include a careful search for scars indicating previous operations, given that any laparoscopic procedure can be undertaken by way of a variety of trocar sites. Auscultation, though occasionally helpful, is also probably the least specific form of examination. Percussion is valuable for assessing tenderness, as well as for differentiating abdominal distention caused by intraluminal gas or free air (signaled by tympany) from that caused by fluid in the peritoneum, such as ascitic fluid or blood (signaled by dullness).

Proper and humane assessment of the abdomen for tenderness via palpation can be learned only through extensive experience. Gaining the patient's trust is fundamental: an anxious or distressed examinee may respond in a hypersensitive manner, thereby hindering the acquisition of information. An individualized approach is essential as well. Palpation should not be performed in a uniform manner from patient to patient; rather, the amount of tenderness present ought to be judged by the degree of pressure or indentation required to cause a given patient significant discomfort. In the setting of severe abdominal pain, elicitation of rebound tenderness by means of deep palpation followed by rapid release of pressure usually does not improve diagnostic accuracy or alter subsequent evaluation and should therefore be discouraged. Finally, administration of small doses of narcotics to patients with abdominal pain is unlikely to alter an experienced examiner's diagnostic ability for the worse.

Occasionally, a young patient whose history and physical examination (including vital signs) fit the classic clinical picture of appendicitis may be taken to the OR without further assessment.

1333

Recognition and Management of Intra-abdominal Infection

Patient has suspected intra-abdominal infection

Obtain history, including previous surgical manipulation of abdomen.

Perform physical examination, focusing on abdomen, pelvis and vagina, and rectum (inspection, auscultation, percussion, palpation).

Order blood tests as appropriate.
- General tests of systemic response to infection
- Specific tests to localize source or focus of infection

On occasion, a young patient with classic presentation of appendicitis may be taken to OR without blood tests or imaging.

Order diagnostic imaging as appropriate.

Patient has "certain" appendicitis

Resuscitate, give antibiotics, and take to OR.

History and physical exam warrant exploration of abdomen for peritonitis, but confirmation (free air) is needed first; or index of suspicion for peritonitis is very low

Obtain plain abdominal films, including upright chest film.

Patient has upper abdominal pain, elevated bilirubin level or liver function test results, or history of biliary tract disease

Order upper abdominal US.
Treat specific infection as appropriate [see Figure 1].

All other patients

Order abdominal and pelvic CT scans.

Treat specific infection as appropriate [see Figure 9].

Free peritoneal air is present

Resuscitate, give antibiotics, and take to OR.

No free peritoneal air is present, and index of suspicion for peritonitis is low

Discharge from surgical care.

No free peritoneal air is present, but index of suspicion for peritonitis is high

Order abdominal and pelvic CT scans (see above, right).

Practically speaking, however, almost all patients with significant intra-abdominal infections undergo blood tests, and most also undergo some sort of radiologic evaluation.

Investigative Studies

LABORATORY TESTS

Blood work can be divided into two categories: (1) general tests designed to assess the systemic response to infection and (2) specific tests designed to localize the source or site of infection. The former 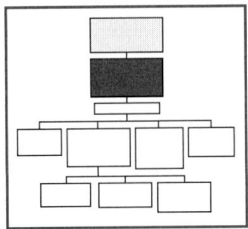 category includes serum chemistries and hematology studies. The latter category commonly includes amylase and lipase concentrations (in patients suspected of having pancreatitis), bilirubin levels and liver function tests (to evaluate hepatic or biliary tract disease), and lactate levels (when an ischemic bowel is suspected). These tests are discussed further elsewhere, in connection with specific infections (see below). Urinalysis, of course, is necessary whenever urinary tract infection or urolithiasis is a possibility.

DIAGNOSTIC IMAGING

The use of various radiologic studies in the diagnosis of intra-abdominal infection continues to evolve rapidly. Outside the setting of trauma, it is now very rare for patients to undergo operations or other major interventions without first undergoing imaging. At one time, plain films of the abdomen (including an 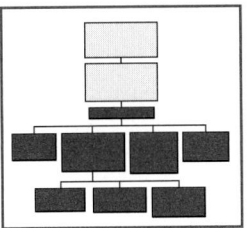 upright chest film) were routinely obtained whenever a significant intra-abdominal infection was suspected, principally to detect free peritoneal air, bowel obstruction, or fecaliths. Abdominal plain films proved to lack sensitivity, specificity, and anatomic definition in this setting and consequently have, in many cases, been supplanted by abdominal and pelvic computed tomographic scanning. There are, however, two circumstances in which plain films of the abdomen remain a reasonable first study for a patient with suspected peritonitis: (1) when the surgeon has almost decided, on the basis of the history and physical examination, to explore the patient yet needs confirming evidence of perforation (i.e., free air), and (2) when the index of suspicion for peritonitis is so low that the plain film studies are intended to rule out an unexpected positive finding and will not be followed by an abdominal CT scan if negative.

Ultrasonography for intra-abdominal infection is useful only for focused examination of specific organ systems; it is inferior to CT scanning for generalized surveillance of the abdomen because of the inability of sound waves to penetrate gas in the bowel. By far the best-delineated use of ultrasonography is in the diagnosis of liver and biliary tract disease, for which its ability to demonstrate cholelithiasis makes it superior to CT and for which it should almost always be the first radiologic test in the appropriate circumstances (e.g., a classic history of biliary colic or an elevated serum bilirubin level). Ultrasonography also visualizes the spleen, the kidneys, and the gynecologic pelvic organs well and has the additional benefit of using no ionizing radiation.

The abdominal and pelvic CT scan, appropriately, has become the key diagnostic test for evaluating patients with suspected peritonitis. This modality is widely available throughout much of the world, and newer scanners yield significantly higher resolution than older ones, with reduced scanning times and radiation exposure. CT is highly sensitive for free air, fluid collections, bowel wall abnormalities, and inflammatory changes. Now that significant intra-abdominal infections—perhaps even in the setting of a perforated viscus—are no longer automatically considered to mandate operative intervention, the ability of CT scanning to identify the source and assess the chronicity of an infection is critical to effective modern management. Multiple common conditions have now been defined for which an adequate CT scan allows nonoperative management either as definitive therapy (e.g., expectant treatment of a simple perforated duodenal ulcer) or as a means of temporizing (e.g., percutaneous drainage of a periappendiceal or peridiverticular abscess). In addition, in experienced hands, a negative CT scan of the abdomen and the pelvis virtually excludes any significant acute surgical illness.

It must be noted, however, that a CT scan is not necessary in all patients with abdominal pain, and the decision whether to obtain one should be made on the basis of predefined guidelines or with the input of a general surgeon. When the need for operative intervention has already been determined, as in a classic case of appendicitis, imaging is unnecessary. In addition, some patients with an intra-abdominal infection amenable to nonoperative management (e.g., simple, mild diverticular disease that can be treated with oral antibiotics on an outpatient basis) do not necessarily benefit from CT scanning.

In selected cases, other forms of imaging may be used. Magnetic resonance imaging, though usually more difficult to obtain in an emergency and logistically more complicated than CT scanning, yields excellent tomographic images and has the added benefit of imaging vascular structures and the pancreaticobiliary tree more precisely. Nonetheless, MRI has no significant role in the evaluation of acute peritonitis. Nuclear medicine scans and fluoroscopic studies, though occasionally useful adjuncts for evaluating biliary tract and upper GI disorders, also play no role in the assessment of acute peritonitis.

Options for Intervention

Once an intra-abdominal infection is diagnosed, there are multiple options for intervention. Not infrequently, an approach combining several modalities is warranted. Occasionally, administration of systemic antibiotics is all that is necessary (or practical), as in cases of spontaneous primary bacterial peritonitis or of multiple infected fluid collections that are small but too numerous to drain. Single abscesses, particularly those without thick or particulate contents, can be adequately treated with simple aspiration and a short course of antibiotics. For discrete infected fluid collections in almost any setting, placement of a percutaneous indwelling drain (most commonly under radiologic guidance) is currently the treatment of choice. Operative management, either open or laparoscopic, is employed for resection of damaged or inflamed and unsalvageable organs, diversion of enteric contents, or drainage of collections that are too thick or numerous for percutaneous drainage. Beyond these general guidelines, therapy for specific intra-abdominal infections must be individualized (see below).

Infections of the Upper Abdomen

Biliary tract and pancreatic infections present as a systemic septic response or as infections localized in the upper abdomen [see Figure 1]. Typical findings include abdominal pain, a tender upper abdominal mass, fever and leukocytosis, and jaundice. Various combinations of these symptoms may occur, but it is convenient to consider three common clinical presentations. In each of the presentations, one or two symptoms dominate: (1) upper abdom-

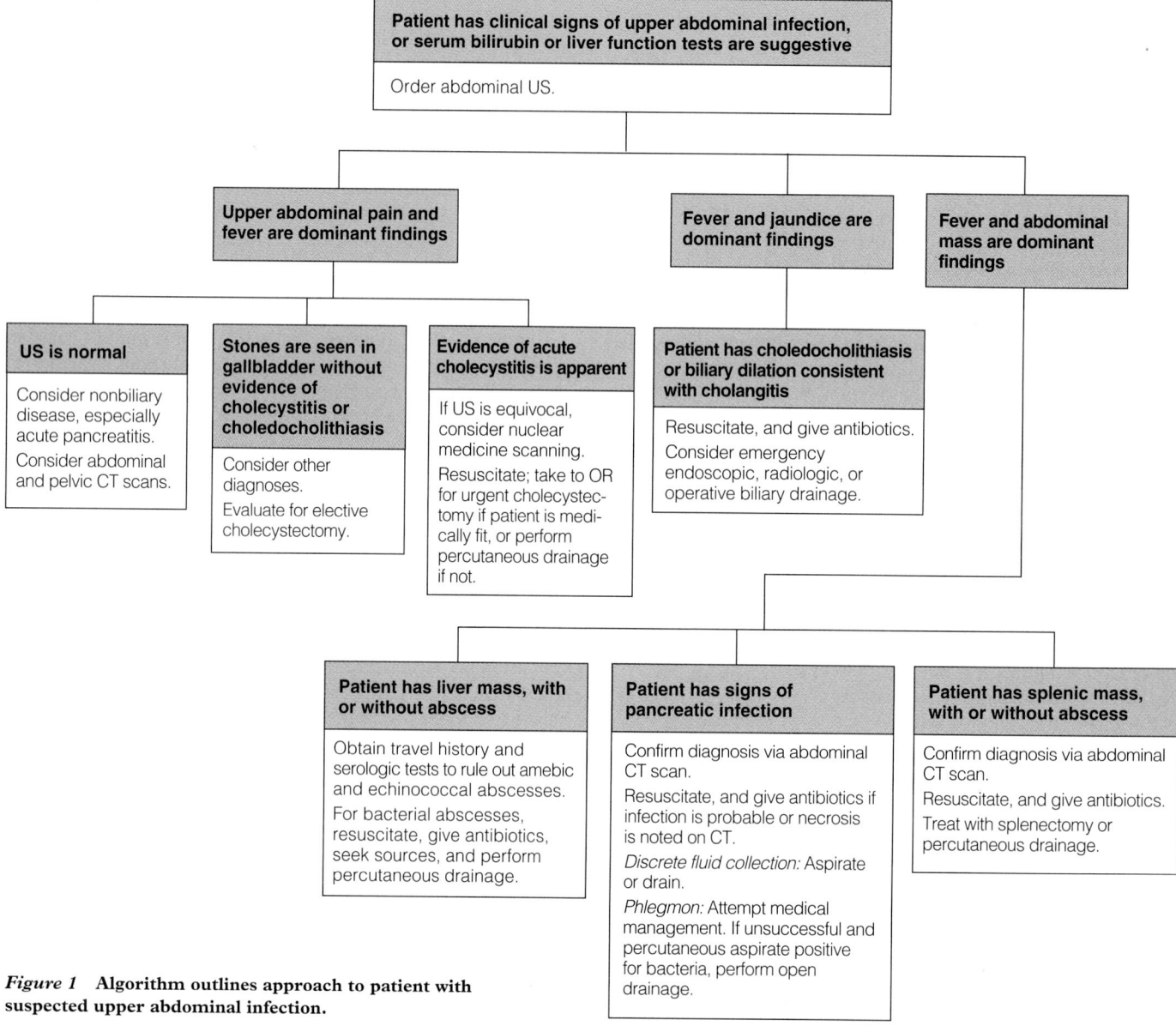

Figure 1 Algorithm outlines approach to patient with suspected upper abdominal infection.

inal pain and fever, (2) fever and jaundice, and (3) an upper abdominal mass and fever. These clinical findings signal the need for a battery of screening tests, including a complete blood count (CBC); routine blood tests of liver function; determination of serum amylase level, prothrombin time (PT), and partial thromboplastin time (PTT); blood culture; chest and abdominal x-rays; and abdominal ultrasonography. When considered together, the clinical findings and the test results allow early differentiation of the three most common disease entities: acute cholecystitis, acute cholangitis, and acute pancreatitis.

UPPER ABDOMINAL PAIN AND FEVER

Patients with upper abdominal sepsis may present with epigastric or right upper quadrant pain and fever. Only two thirds of these patients admitted with a working diagnosis of acute cholecystitis have acute biliary inflammation.[1] In some patients, nonsurgical conditions (e.g., pneumonia, acute hepatitis, familial Mediterranean fever, herpes zoster of the intercostal nerves, and gastroenteritis) can be distinguished clinically from biliary disease. The most important screening test for acute biliary infection is the abdominal ultrasound examination: an abnormal image of the gallbladder or bile ducts supports a biliary etiology [*see Figure 2*].

The differential diagnosis should include acute cholecystitis, biliary colic, acute pancreatitis, and acute cholangitis, each of which requires specific management [*see Table 1*]. For example, initial management of biliary colic and mild acute pancreatitis is usually nonoperative, whereas severe acute cholangitis and acute cholecystitis are treated by means of surgical, endoscopic, or radiologic intervention (see below). Clinical features and blood test results, though helpful, may be inconclusive. The abdominal ultrasonogram may provide specific clues. Stones appear in biliary colic [*see Figure 2*]; stones and thickening of the gallbladder wall, in acute cholecystitis; gallstones and dilatation of the common bile duct (CBD), in acute cholangitis; and pancreatic enlargement and sonolucency, in pancreatitis.

Pancreatitis

Diagnosis Differentiating acute pancreatitis from acute cholecystitis may be difficult. The serum amylase level lacks specificity, but if the clinical findings suggest acute pancreatitis, an ele-

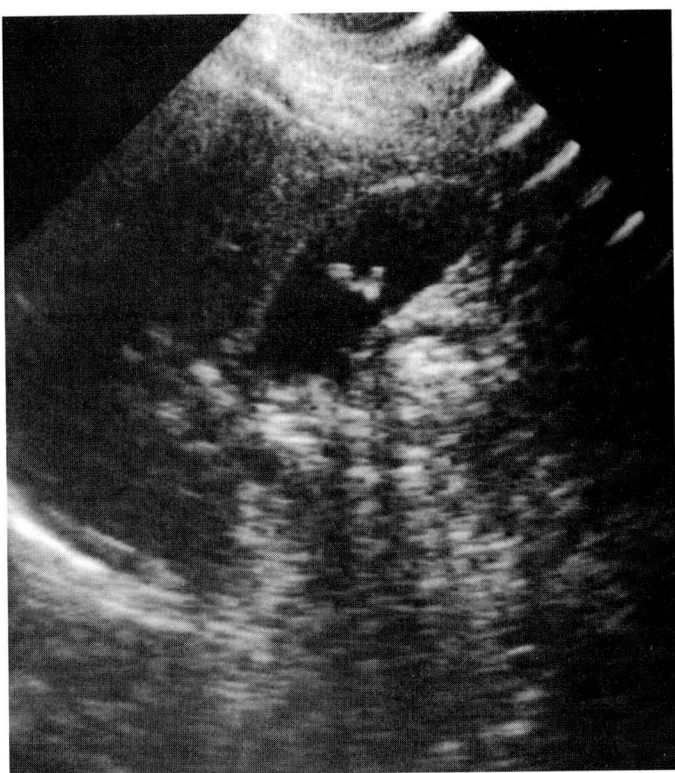

Figure 2 Abnormal abdominal ultrasound examination shows calculi in gallbladder casting shadows on underlying liver tissue.

vated level of serum amylase clinches the diagnosis. In one study, the initial laboratory results in 100 patients with acute pancreatitis were compared with those in 100 patients with acute abdominal pain caused by acute cholecystitis, perforated peptic ulcer, or acute appendicitis.[2] The serum amylase concentrations were elevated in 95% of patients with acute pancreatitis but were normal in 95% of patients with acute abdominal pain from other causes. These concentrations peak within the first 48 hours and are almost always elevated in biliary pancreatitis[3]; in fact, a serum amylase concentration above 1,000 U/L strongly suggests a biliary origin of the pancreatitis.[4] In addition, determination of serum lipase levels has been shown to be more specific than and at least as sensitive as determination of amylase levels for the detection of

Table 1 Diagnostic Indicators of Upper Abdominal Pain and Fever

	Biliary Colic	Acute Cholecystitis	Acute Pancreatitis
Duration	Short: 40% < 1 hr	Persistent	Persistent
Pathogenesis	Visceral	Somatic	Retroperitoneal
Signs	Tender	Guarding and spasm	Guarding and spasm
Laboratory tests Liver function tests	Occasionally abnormal	Abnormal	Abnormal
Serum amylase	Normal	Normal or slightly increased	Increased
Leukocyte counts	Often normal	Increased	Increased

Table 2 Ranson's Early Objective Signs of Severity of Acute Pancreatitis[2]

On Admission	After Initial 48 Hours
Age > 55 yr Glucose > 200 mg/dl WBC > 16,000/mm^3 LDH > 350 IU/L AST > 250 Sigma Frankel U/dl	Serum Ca^{2+} < 8 mg/dl Arterial PO_2 < 60 mm Hg Base deficit > 4 mEq/L BUN increase > 5 mg/dl Hematocrit fall > 10% Fluid sequestration > 6,000 ml

Note: < 3 signs = mild pancreatitis; ≥ 3 signs = severe pancreatitis.
AST—aspartate aminotransferase   BUN—blood urea nitrogen   PO_2—oxygen tension
WBC—white blood cell

acute pancreatitis.[5,6] Unless clinical findings and the results of biochemical tests and ultrasonography are unequivocal, a contrast-enhanced spiral abdominal CT scan is usually performed to establish the diagnosis and stage acute pancreatitis. It has been suggested, however, that CT scanning should be reserved for patients with clinically suspected severe acute gallstone pancreatitis, on the grounds that the results would not change the recommended course of action in other patients.[7] Occasionally, a very mild pancreatitis may give rise to no findings on a CT scan, and a normal technetium-99m (^{99m}Tc)–labeled HIDA (lidofenin) scan may help differentiate this condition from acute cholecystitis.

Treatment Given that pancreatitis encompasses a wide range of diseases with varying degrees of severity, treatment must be individualized for each patient. Possible therapeutic strategies range from outpatient management with temporary dietary modification (for very mild cases) to open debridement and complex intensive care (for severe cases). It is therefore useful to base possible treatment approaches in particular cases on the cause and severity of the pancreatitis.

Gallstone pancreatitis. Standard therapy for gallstone pancreatitis includes I.V. fluids and narcotic analgesics. Nasogastric suction is useful in patients with significant ileus but need not be used routinely.[8] The use of systemic antibiotics is controversial; they are of benefit in the 10% to 34% of patients who have concomitant cholangitis.[9] Other treatments suggested previously—including total parenteral nutrition (TPN) and various pharmacologic agents (e.g., cimetidine, somatostatin, glucagon, and insulin)—have not proved useful in all cases of gallstone pancreatitis.[10] Continuous intraduodenal infusion of an elemental diet has reduced exocrine pancreatic secretions in animal experiments.[11] Furthermore, enteral feeding has been shown to be beneficial and to decrease disease severity in patients with acute pancreatitis.[12-14]

In clinical practice, the need for further treatment depends on the severity of the acute pancreatitis. Severity determines both the risk of sepsis, which governs outcome, and the risk associated with early cholecystectomy [see 3:15 Laparoscopic Cholecystectomy]. The most commonly used clinical prognostic index in North America was developed by Ranson and reliably defines the severity of pancreatitis [see Table 2].[2] In mild pancreatitis, one or two Ranson signs are present; in more severe pancreatitis, three to five signs are present; and in very severe pancreatitis, more than five signs are present. This distinction serves to stratify further treatment. Other clinical prognostic scores, such as the APACHE-II (Acute Physiology and Chronic Health Evaluation II) and APACHE-III scores and the Balthazar score, have been shown to possess discriminatory value in identifying patients at high risk for complications.[15,16]

Mild pancreatitis usually subsides within 1 week of onset. Most surgeons defer cholecystectomy until then; urgent operation should be reserved for cases complicated by biliary sepsis, and it may reveal acute cholecystitis in as many as 31% of patients.[17]

An attack of acute gallstone pancreatitis is initiated by obstruction at the confluence of the lower end of the CBD and the pancreatic duct by a stone or by edema at the ampulla of Vater resulting from stone migration. These stones may be found and removed in 63% to 78% of patients who undergo operation within 72 hours of admission[17-19] [see 3:16 Biliary Tract Procedures]; by contrast, they are present in only 3% to 33% of patients explored after the first week.[18-22] A randomized trial exploring the optimal timing of surgery for gallstone pancreatitis showed that early surgery (within 48 hours after admission) was not associated with a significant increase in morbidity or mortality in patients with mild pancreatitis but did not change prognosis.[23]

Endoscopic retrograde cholangiopancreatography (ERCP). Early ERCP and sphincterotomy [see 3:8 Gastrointestinal Endoscopy] has been suggested as an alternative to surgery of the CBD in patients with mild pancreatitis. However, randomized trials comparing endoscopic treatment with conservative treatment within the first 72 hours in patients with mild pancreatitis did not find that urgent endoscopic sphincterotomy improved outcome in this group of patients.[24,25] Other studies showed that delaying surgery beyond 6 weeks may lead to a 32% to 57% risk of recurrent pancreatitis.[26,27] Therefore, cholecystectomy and cholangiography should be delayed only until just before patients are discharged from the hospital, 5 to 15 days after the onset of symptoms. Laparoscopic

cholecystectomy has facilitated this approach safely without prolonging hospital stay.

Severe pancreatitis. Patients with three or more Ranson signs are at particular risk for pancreatic sepsis.[28] Repeated clinical and radiologic evaluation is required in these patients to ensure early detection of complications, because the outcome of an episode of pancreatitis depends on whether sepsis supervenes. When infection occurs, operative debridement and drainage are required [see Fever and Abdominal Mass, below]. Some surgeons have attempted to alter the course of severe disease by early operation; however, urgent operation is associated with a high mortality in patients with more than three Ranson signs.[19,21,23,29] To avoid the mortality associated with early operative intervention, some clinicians advocate early diagnosis by ERCP [see Figure 3], followed by biliary decompression by means of endoscopic sphincterotomy and stone extraction. In a randomized trial comparing early ERCP and sphincterotomy with conservative therapy in patients with severe acute pancreatitis, ERCP and sphincterotomy decreased morbidity from 61% to 24% and lowered mortality from 18% to 4%.[24] The results of this trial, however, have been the subject of debate, and the success of this approach has been attributed by some authors to the treatment of a concomitant cholangitis rather than of the actual pancreatitis.[25] A well-conducted trial that excluded patients with concomitant cholangitis was published in 1997; unfortunately, this trial was unable to answer the question definitively, because too few patients with severe pancreatitis had been recruited.[30] It appears that ERCP is warranted mainly in cases of acute pancreatitis complicated by cholangitis and biliary sepsis.[31,32]

Use of peritoneal lavage in early severe pancreatitis was advocated in one study to decrease morbidity and mortality.[33] Use of standard lavage over a 2-day period did not improve patient outcome, but use of peritoneal lavage for 7 days (long peritoneal lavage) yielded some improvement in outcome.[34] Early use of antibiotics and selective decontamination have been proposed as a means of reducing septic complications, but neither has convincingly or reproducibly been shown to improve prognosis.[35,36] Although prophylactic antibiotics have been shown to decrease the rate of infectious complications in severe acute pancreatitis, they have not clearly been shown to reduce overall disease mortality.[35,37-40] Attempts have been made to modulate the initial systemic inflammatory response seen in early severe acute pancreatitis to reduce the risk of subsequent infection and improve overall prognosis; somatostatin has exhibited limited success in this regard.[41,42] Another drug in this category, the platelet-aggregating factor (PAF) inhibitor lexipafant, initially yielded promising results in animal models[43,44] and in phase II trials[45]; however, a 2001 trial using the same drug did not find it efficacious for treating severe acute pancreatitis.[46]

Acute Cholecystitis

Diagnosis Acute cholecystitis is the most common diagnosis in patients presenting with upper abdominal pain and fever and is characterized by the clinical finding of a midinspiratory arrest on palpation of the right upper quadrant (Murphy's sign). As noted (see above), with the widespread availability of ultrasonography, acute cholecystitis can usually be diagnosed rapidly on the basis of the findings of gallbladder wall thickening, pericholecystic fluid, and stones. Occasionally, more complex cases must be evaluated with nuclear medicine scanning to look for cystic duct obstruction. Concurrent acute obstructive cholangitis must also be considered in all patients with acute cholecystitis. Supportive laboratory data include a high serum bilirubin level and an increased

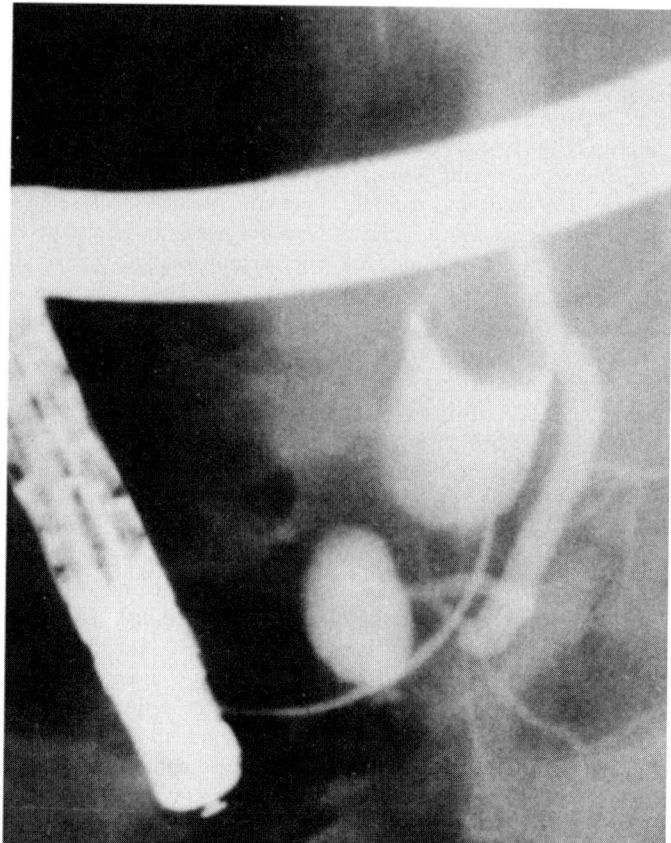

Figure 3 **Endoscopic retrograde cholangiopancreatography shows distal CBD stone in acute pancreatitis. Papillotome has been placed through sphincter of Oddi in preparation for endoscopic sphincterotomy.**

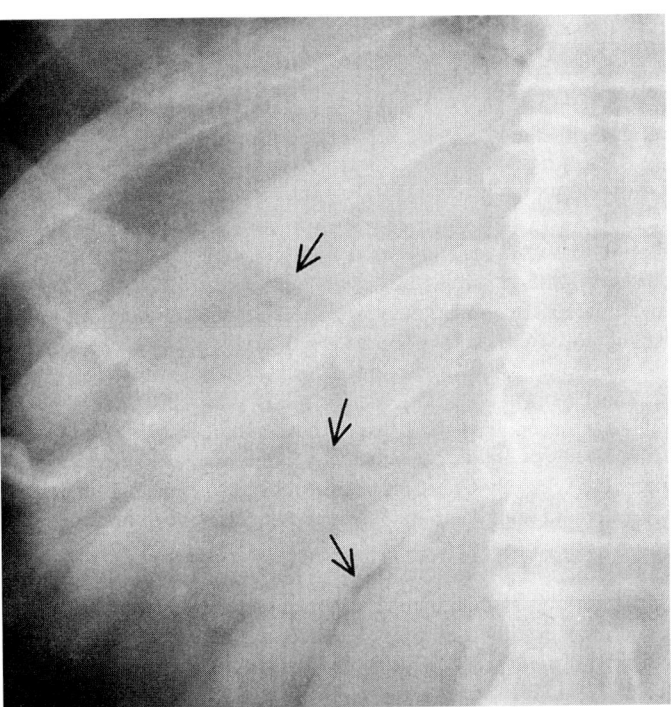

Figure 4 **Air outlines gallbladder and bile ducts in emphysematous cholecystitis.**

Table 3 Comparison of Acute Cholecystitis and Emphysematous Cholecystitis

	Emphysematous Cholecystitis	Acute Cholecystitis
Gender	70% male	70% female
Stones	70%	90%
Bile culture positive	95%	66%
Clostridia found	46%	1.2%
Gangrenous gallbladder	75%	2.5%
Perforation of gallbladder	20%	4%
Mortality at age < 60 yr	15%	1.5%
Pathogenesis	Ischemia, obstruction	Obstruction

alkaline phosphatase level. Positive blood cultures and dilated biliary ducts on abdominal ultrasonography usually confirm the diagnosis.

Emphysematous cholecystitis. An uncommon and insidious variant of acute cholecystitis, emphysematous cholecystitis is characterized by gas in the gallbladder lumen or wall or in the pericholecystic soft tissue and biliary ducts secondary to gas-forming bacteria. The key to the diagnosis is the presence of air on abdominal x-ray [*see Figure 4*] or ultrasound examination. Three stages of emphysematous cholecystitis have been defined: (1) gas is seen only in the lumen of the gallbladder, (2) a ring of gas is identified in the wall of the gallbladder, and (3) gas is seen in the tissues adjacent to the wall. Compared with ordinary acute cholecystitis, emphysematous cholecystitis is associated with a fivefold increase in the risk of gallbladder perforation, as well as a 10-fold increase in mortality in patients younger than 60 years [*see Table 3*].[47]

Studies from the 1960s noted an increased risk of gangrene and perforation of the acutely inflamed gallbladder in patients with diabetes mellitus.[48,49] The mortality for acute cholecystitis was also shown to be five to 10 times higher in patients with diabetes than in other patients. Later studies, however, did not show an increased mortality in patients with both diabetes and acute cholecystitis.[50,51] Nevertheless, one third of patients with emphysematous cholecystitis also have diabetes. This factor, coupled with the current tendency to perform cholecystectomy early in most patients with acute cholecystitis, may account for the disparity between previous studies and later reports.

Acute acalculous cholecystitis. Another variant of acute cholecystitis is acalculous cholecystitis; though still rare, it became more common from the 1950s through the 1990s. This disease was originally described as occurring after surgical treatment of unrelated disease but was subsequently identified in patients with multiple trauma, prolonged critical illness, and sepsis. Predisposing factors include gallbladder ischemia (in patients with shock or trauma) and biliary stasis (in prolonged fasting, hyperalimentation, and sustained narcotics therapy). In addition, focal inflammation may cause biliary colonization or may activate coagulation factor XII, thereby causing severe injury to the blood vessels in the gallbladder muscularis and serosa. A high index of suspicion is necessary. Acute acalculous cholecystitis should be considered in any postoperative or acutely ill patient with upper abdominal pain and fever or with unexplained fever and leukocytosis. It is particularly common 2 to 4 weeks after injury. The diagnosis is confirmed by findings on abdominal ultrasound examination [*see Figure 5*] and ^{99m}Tc-labeled HIDA scanning coupled with infusion of cholecystokinin and morphine.[52-54]

Treatment Standard treatment of acute cholecystitis consists of I.V. fluid administration, analgesics, and cholecystectomy. Although the timing of operation is somewhat controversial in ordinary acute cholecystitis, cholecystectomy should be performed at the earliest opportunity [*see 3:15 Laparoscopic Cholecystectomy*]. This approach has been confirmed by at least one randomized trial comparing early with late laparoscopic cholecystectomy.[55] The delayed-surgery group had a greater need for conversion to open cholecystectomy (23% versus 11%), as well as a longer

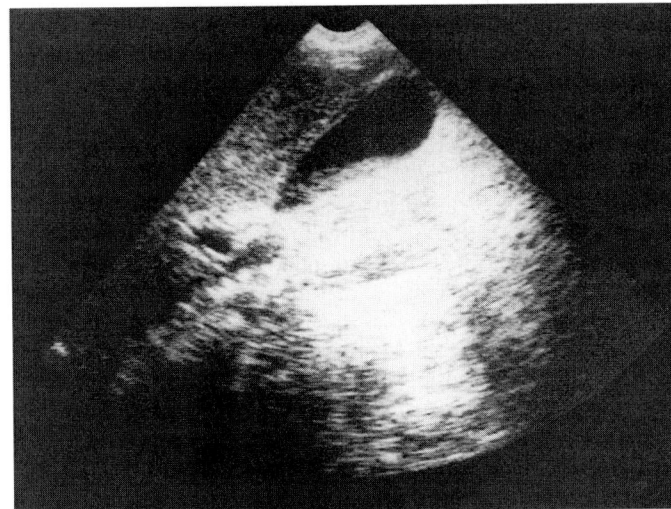

Figure 5 **Abnormal abdominal ultrasound examination confirms diagnosis of acute acalculous cholecystitis. When image is compared with that in Figure 2, thickening of gallbladder wall and intraluminal debris are obvious.**

average total hospital stay and convalescence. Administration of systemic antibiotics is not required; however, single-dose antibiotic prophylaxis (e.g., cefazolin, 2 g I.V.) can be given at the start of the operation [see 1:2 Prevention of Postoperative Infection].[56-58]

Some patients with acute cholecystitis are at high risk for gangrene and perforation of the gallbladder. It is crucial to identify these patients and perform cholecystectomy promptly because delay increases morbidity and mortality. Clinically, gangrene and perforation of the gallbladder in this high-risk population are suggested by marked systemic toxicity or by the radiologic demonstration of either emphysematous cholecystitis or acute acalculous cholecystitis.

With ordinary acute cholecystitis, body temperature is slightly increased in most patients—averaging 37.8° C (100.04° F)—but is normal in 20% of patients. By comparison, the risk of gangrene and perforation is reportedly higher in patients with marked systemic toxicity, manifested by a pulse rate greater than 120 beats/min, a body temperature higher than 39° C (102.2° F), and a left shift in the differential white blood cell count, showing more than 90% polymorphonuclear leukocytes. Unfortunately, findings of systemic toxicity are frequently absent in elderly patients.

Patients with acute cholecystitis who have signs of systemic toxicity, emphysematous cholecystitis, or acalculous cholecystitis are at high risk for gallbladder gangrene and perforation and therefore require prompt and aggressive treatment. I.V. antibiotic therapy with a single agent (e.g., ceftriaxone, piperacillin, or a quinolone such as ciprofloxacin or ofloxacin) can be given.[59,60] Early cholecystectomy is the treatment of choice. Unfortunately, mortality may be as high as 20% to 30% with the traditional surgical approach.[61] If perforation and gangrene are not suspected but medical illness poses a high risk of mortality from operation, nonoperative supportive therapy may suffice. If this fails, another treatment option is cholecystostomy.

Percutaneous transhepatic cholecystostomy has been recommended for these high-risk patients,[62] particularly where there is a low risk for perforation of the gallbladder.[63] To determine the risk of gallbladder perforation, a risk score can be assigned to each of seven findings that may be present on the preoperative abdominal ultrasound examination: pericholecystic fluid, 7 points; distention of the gallbladder, 4 points; intraluminal membrane, 4 points; intraluminal debris, 3 points; round gallbladder, 3 points; sonolucent zone in the gallbladder wall, 2 points; and a thick gallbladder wall (> 3.5 mm), 1 point.[63] A patient with a total risk score of 12 or more points requires urgent cholecystectomy; one with a lower score who does not respond to conservative treatment may be treated with percutaneous transhepatic cholecystostomy.

A 1997 review of 59 patients exhibiting the septic response who underwent successful percutaneous radiologic cholecystostomy defined predictors of a successful clinical outcome: localized right upper quadrant tenderness and gallstones, as well as gallstones and pericholecystic fluid on ultrasound examination.[64] Patients with more equivocal findings may derive greater benefit from more invasive techniques that can simultaneously be used for diagnostic purposes (e.g., laparoscopy, which can even be performed at the ICU bedside[65]).

A few patients with acute cholecystitis will have concurrent acute cholangitis. Cholecystostomy is contraindicated in these patients because of its high mortality; adequate drainage of the CBD is required in such cases [see Fever and Jaundice, below].

FEVER AND JAUNDICE

An alternative presentation of upper abdominal infection includes patients whose predominant symptoms are fever and jaundice, with pain a less marked component. Jaundice is almost always associated with obstruction of the biliary tree, either intrahepatic or extrahepatic. The combination of fever with jaundice always suggests acute cholangitis, a condition that can have a fulminant and fatal course if not treated promptly.

Acute Cholangitis

Diagnosis If a patient presents with a temperature higher than 38.5° C (101.3° F) in conjunction with jaundice [see 3:4 Jaundice], the possibility of acute cholangitis should always be investigated. If cholangitis is present, laboratory studies will reveal leukocytosis, and blood cultures will often be positive. A finding of gallstones and dilated biliary ducts on abdominal ultrasound examination supports the diagnosis. Reynolds' pentad is present in the full-blown syndrome.[66] This syndrome includes upper abdominal pain, fever and chills, jaundice, hypotension, and mental status changes. Acute cholangitis is usually related to choledocholithiasis, recent biliary manipulation, or biliary stenting performed for chronic obstruction.

Gallbladder infections. Gallbladder empyema can duplicate most of the findings associated with acute cholangitis. In this condition, acute cholecystitis is complicated by suppuration within the gallbladder, which then becomes the focus of generalized sepsis. The distended gallbladder may be palpable and tender. When jaundice is associated with empyema of the gallbladder, it is less likely to be obstructive than when it is associated with acute cholangitis. True empyema of the gallbladder is rare. Treatment includes administration of I.V. fluids, systemic antibiotic therapy, analgesics, and early cholecystectomy.

In some patients with jaundice and inflammation, a stone impacted in the cystic duct or in Hartmann's pouch may suggest choledocholithiasis, but preoperative diagnosis by ERCP shows an extrinsic compression of the duct known as Mirizzi syndrome. Two types of Mirizzi syndrome exist. In type I, a stone impacted in the cystic duct or Hartmann's pouch compresses the common hepatic duct and causes inflammation, thereby leading to jaundice. Treatment of this type consists of obliteration of the cystic duct and careful partial cholecystectomy, with the neck of the gallbladder left in place. In type II, protrusion of the stone into the hepatic duct erodes the septum between the cystic duct and the hepatic duct and causes a cholecystocholedochal fistula. Treatment of this type involves internal biliary drainage to the wall of the cholecystocholedochal defect, usually with a choledochojejunostomy [see 3:16 Biliary Tract Procedures], in addition to cholecystectomy.[67]

Primary sclerosing cholangitis. Patients with primary sclerosing cholangitis, especially those who have undergone internal or external biliary drainage, are at high risk for recurrent bouts of ascending cholangitis. Primary sclerosing cholangitis predominantly affects young males, particularly those with chronic ulcerative colitis. The diagnosis is suggested by the dominant cholestatic biochemical profile—that is, elevation of the serum bilirubin concentration, the serum alkaline phosphatase level, and aspartate aminotransferase activity. Because of the concomitant hepatic scarring, ultrasonography may not reveal the presence of dilated intrahepatic ducts. Definitive diagnosis requires visualization of the beaded appearance of the biliary tree by means of cholangiography. Cholangiocarcinoma and secondary sclerosing cholangitis in patients with Caroli disease or choledochal cysts may mimic these clinical, biochemical, and radiologic features, but this is an unusual occurrence and can be distinguished by careful follow-up of patients.

Currently, magnetic resonance cholangiopancreatography (MRCP) is the imaging modality of choice for elective management of patients with primary sclerosing cholangitis, in that it yields results comparable to those of ERCP without being invasive.[68-71]

Other causes of cholangitis. An uncommon cause of recurrent cholangitis in North America is Oriental cholangiohepatitis, which is characterized by intrahepatic duct scarring, biliary strictures, and hepatolithiasis, as demonstrated by cholangiography. Irreversible intrahepatic and extrahepatic liver damage may result because of the overwhelming propensity of these patients to form calcium bilirubinate stones.

A few patients with cholangiocarcinoma causing bile duct obstruction or liver metastases causing intrahepatic bile duct obstruction may also present with a clinical picture suggestive of cholangitis. CT followed by MRCP can delineate the diagnosis in most such cases. Treatment consists of I.V. antibiotics and biliary drainage by radiographic or surgical means.

Treatment Once acute cholangitis is diagnosed, resuscitation is started with I.V. fluids and antibiotics, such as fluoroquinolones, mezlocillin, cefoperazone, or piperacillin,[59,72-75] particularly in patients with marked hyperbilirubinemia, in whom treatment with aminoglycosides may contribute to renal toxicity in up to 33% of cases [see *6:7 Renal Failure*].[76] These antibiotics are required to deal with the various aerobic bacteria, of which *Escherichia coli*, *Klebsiella* species, and enterococci are the most frequently encountered in this setting. Anaerobes may be isolated in 15% to 30% of patients and are particularly likely to be present in diabetics, the elderly, and patients who have previously undergone biliary manipulation. In patients with indwelling catheters, *Enterobacter*, *Pseudomonas*, and *Candida* organisms are being isolated with increasing frequency. Indications of high risk include a serum bilirubin concentration higher than 3 mg/dl.

Approximately 75% of patients with acute cholangitis respond to conservative measures,[77] and supportive treatment is continued. Subsequent investigations usually include CT followed by MRCP.[78,79] Because of their invasive nature, ERCP and needle percutaneous transhepatic cholangiography (PTC) are reserved for cases in which a drainage procedure is anticipated or the information from the MRCP is deemed inadequate.

For the 25% of patients who do not respond to conservative treatment, early recognition may improve their prognosis. In one study, patients who did not respond immediately to antibiotics had a mortality of 62%, compared with a mortality of 1.5% in those who improved.[80] In another study, indicators of high risk were an arterial blood pH less than 7.4, a serum bilirubin concentration above 9 mmol/L, a blood platelet count below 150,000/mm³, and a serum albumin concentration lower than 3 g/dl.[102] These high-risk patients often have systemic hypotension, mental confusion, a temperature higher than 39° C (102.2° F), or hypothermia. Occasionally, acute cholangitis is complicated by disseminated intravascular coagulation (DIC), which manifests itself as a tendency to bruise and bleed or merely as prolongation of the PT and the PTT, together with a fall in the blood platelet count [see *1:4 Bleeding and Transfusion*]. If DIC is suspected, the diagnosis should be confirmed and treatment started before biliary decompression.

Patients with refractory cholangitis who do not improve within 24 hours require urgent biliary decompression. Urgent biliary decompression had traditionally been accomplished via surgical exploration of the CBD and T-tube drainage [see *3:16 Biliary Tract Procedures*]. Cholecystostomy is an inadequate and often fatal option in this context. Rarely, T-tube insertion alone may be life-saving in a desperately ill patient; generally, however, definitive internal decompression is preferable. Unfortunately, any surgical decompression in these critically ill patients can result in a mortality of 30% to 40%.[82-85] Furthermore, reoperation is required in one third of survivors because important diagnostic information is not available at the initial laparotomy. As a result, nonoperative methods of biliary decompression, including percutaneous transhepatic biliary drainage (PTBD) and endoscopic sphincterotomy at ERCP, have gained favor. PTBD was originally developed for preoperative management of biliary obstruction without cholangitis but has not been found to be beneficial in that setting. At present, it is mainly used for the management of proximal bile duct strictures or for the treatment of cases not amenable to ERCP; its complication rate is less than 10%.[86]

Although PTBD can reduce the mortality associated with initial biliary decompression, many patients still require a definitive operation. Consequently, endoscopic sphincterotomy [see *3:8 Gastrointestinal Endoscopy*] has been proposed for decompression of the biliary tree in patients with acute cholangitis from choledocholithiasis [see *Figure 6*]. In a study of 82 patients with acute cholangitis caused by CBD calculi, early operation was employed in 28 patients, endoscopic sphincterotomy in 43, and antibiotic therapy alone in 11.[87] Surgical mortality was 21% and morbidity 57%; by comparison, mortality for endoscopic sphincterotomy was 5% and morbidity 28%. Others confirmed these findings.[81] In patients whose gallbladder is still in place, endoscopic sphincterotomy alone, without cholecystectomy, may even be a reasonable long-term option. Of 23 patients whose gallbladders were left in situ,[87] only two required cholecystectomy in the 1- to 7-year follow-up period: one for empyema of the gallbladder and one for recurrent cholangitis.

An increasingly recognized cause of cholangitis is biliary sepsis after manipulation of the biliary tree with ERCP or PTBD. Treatment includes I.V. fluids and antibiotics. To prevent this complication, prophylactic antibiotics should be administered before every biliary manipulation.[88]

FEVER AND ABDOMINAL MASS

A third group of patients with upper abdominal infection present with fever and an upper abdominal mass identified either by clinical signs or through diagnostic imaging. Even if the mass is only vaguely palpable, the mass effect is demonstrable on ultrasound examination of the abdomen. If the abdominal ultrasound examination is technically unsatisfactory because of intestinal gas, contrast-enhanced CT of the abdomen will facilitate the diagnosis.

The differential diagnosis is aided by the location of the mass. A mass in the right upper quadrant usually indicates acute cholecystitis, though the possibility of a liver abscess must also be considered. A mass in the epigastrium or in the left upper quadrant usually signals a pancreatic infection; in rare instances, a solitary splenic abscess is found. Patients with an intra-abdominal abscess in the subphrenic space or an interloop abscess may also present in this manner.

Liver Abscess

Diagnosis In the setting of acute upper abdominal sepsis, a tender mass in the right upper quadrant is most likely an enlarged, inflamed gallbladder, possibly wrapped with omentum [see Upper Abdominal Pain and Fever, Acute Cholecystitis, *above*]. The next most common cause of fever and abdominal mass in the right upper quadrant, however, is liver abscess.

Pyogenic abscess. Today, pyogenic liver abscess is most commonly related to biliary tract obstruction from gallstones or malignant disorders (35% of cases), and the ultrasound examination may

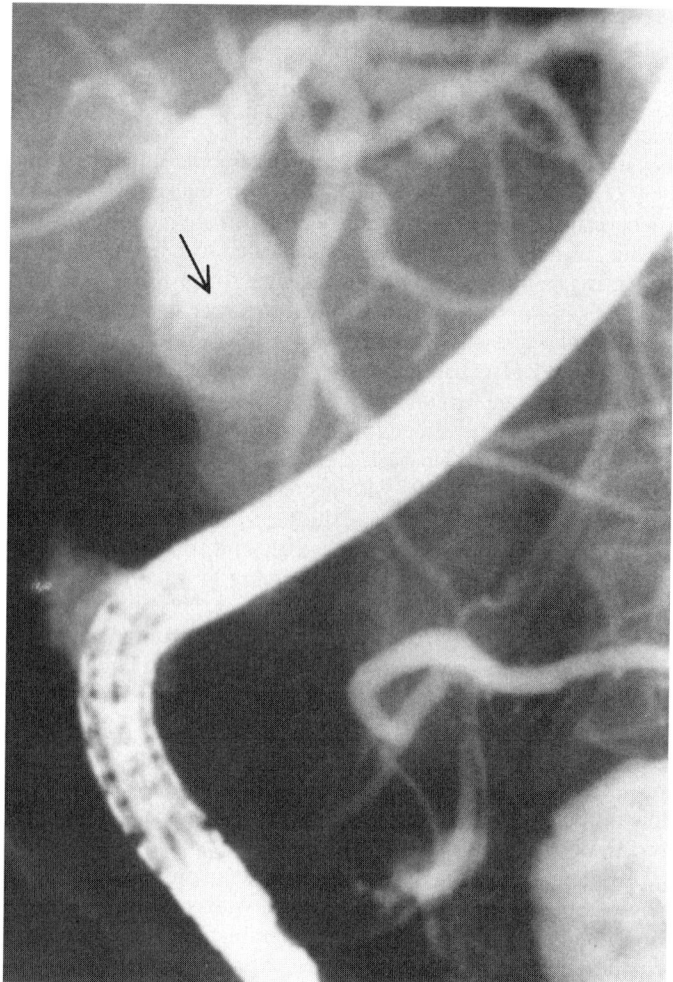 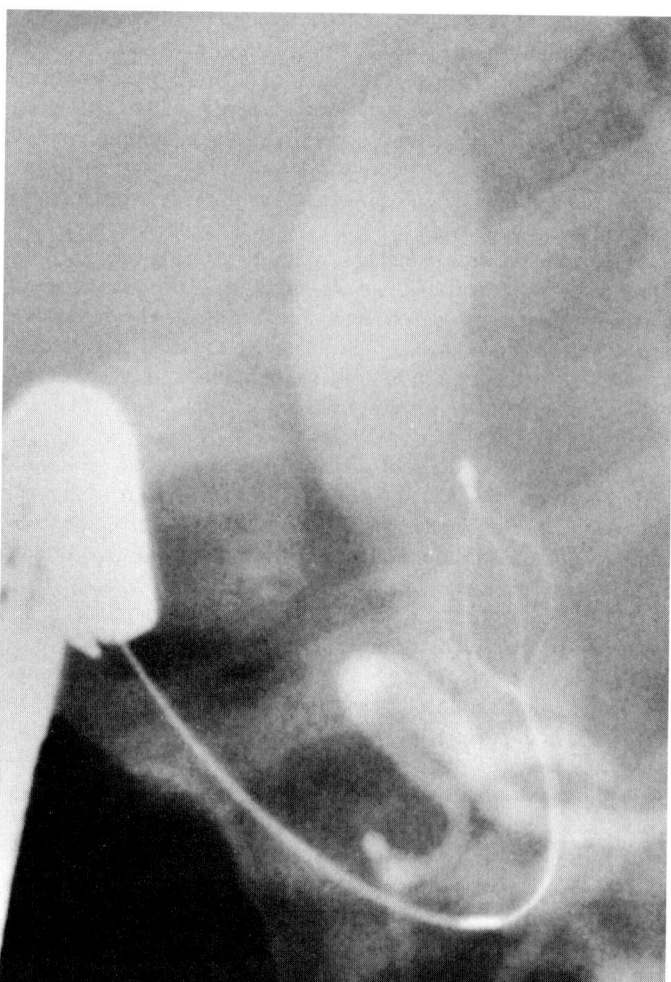

Figure 6 **Endoscopic sphincterotomy for acute biliary decompression in acute obstructive cholangitis is shown. At left, stone is visible in common hepatic duct, and papillotome has been passed through sphincter of Oddi. At right, stone is held within a Dormia basket before extraction.**

reveal both the abscess and the dilated biliary ducts. Previously, portal pyemia from diverticulitis, inflammatory bowel disease (IBD), or perforated appendicitis had been the most common cause; it now accounts for 20% of cases. Even less common is hematogenous spread via the hepatic artery. Approximately 20% of hepatic abscesses are cryptogenic. Ultrasonographic imaging of the liver may demonstrate lesions as small as 2 cm in the liver substance. CT scanning, however, is superior to ultrasonography for evaluating the presence of air and abscesses as small as 0.5 cm in diameter, especially near the hemidiaphragms.[89] Abdominal CT is also the diagnostic modality of choice in the postoperative patient.[90] ERCP and PTC are indicated only when gallstone disease or a biliary malignancy is the potential source of the abscess. Most liver abscesses occur in the right lobe: 40% are 1.5 to 5 cm in diameter, 40% are 5 to 8 cm in diameter, and 20% are greater than 8 cm in diameter.

Amebic abscess. Although pyogenic abscesses are commonly multiple, no imaging technique can reliably differentiate them from amebic abscesses. The best indication of a parasitic infection is a history of travel to an endemic area (e.g., Mexico, Central America, or Southeast Asia). However, when a hepatic abscess is detected by an imaging technique, serologic tests should be performed to rule out active amebiasis or echinococcal infection. Examination of stool for amebae is insensitive; consequently,

isoenzyme analysis, *Entamoeba histolytica*–specific antigen detection, or even polymerase chain reaction (PCR) is preferred to confirm the diagnosis of amebiasis.[91]

Echinococcal abscess. The diagnosis of echinococcal liver abscess can be confirmed by means of elevated indirect hemagglutination (IHA) titers (> 250). In the late 1980s, a combination of tests that included IHA for *Echinococcus granulosus* and enzyme-linked immunosorbent assay (ELISA) using *E. multilocularis* antigen yielded an 89% species-specific diagnosis of echinococcal disease.[92] Later work indicated that IgG ELISA and IHA were the best tests for follow-up after resection of the abscess. In patients with a favorable clinical outcome, the specific IgG level decreased toward the end of the first year, though in some cases, a positive serologic result persisted beyond 6 years.[93] Diagnostic aspiration is indicated when a diagnosis of pyogenic or amebic abscess is in doubt, but not in echinococcal disease. Aspiration may also be beneficial in patients with left-side abscesses and abscesses greater than 10 cm in diameter. The chest x-ray is abnormal in as many as 50% of cases of amebic abscess, and the plain abdominal x-ray may show calcification of an echinococcal cyst with secondary pyogenic infection.

It is essential to differentiate infected echinococcal cysts from pyogenic abscess: special precautions are required for drainage of echinococcal cysts because of the risk of spillage and anaphylaxis.

Blood cultures are positive in as many as 50% of patients with pyogenic abscess, particularly in those with multiple abscesses; in fact, the presence of *Streptococcus milleri* in the blood suggests a visceral abscess.

Treatment *Pyogenic abscess.* The preferred treatment of pyogenic abscess is closed continuous percutaneous drainage guided by CT or ultrasonography, provided that it is technically feasible and no other indication for laparotomy exists.[94] More than one catheter may be required for complete drainage. An alternative treatment is repeated percutaneous needle aspiration, the results of which are comparable to those of continuous drainage.[95] One advantage to repeated needle aspiration is the elimination of cumbersome, painful drainage tubes, which are prone to dislodgment. Although initial studies showed a good response rate with repeated needle aspiration,[96] the results were not duplicated in a subsequent randomized trial.[97]

The abscess cavity dimensions are followed by serial imaging until the cavity collapses, and the catheter can usually be removed 2 to 3 weeks later. Continuous percutaneous drainage has been associated with a complication rate of 4% and a failure rate of 15%.[98] However, operative drainage is the treatment of choice in patients with an identified intra-abdominal focus of infection and in patients in whom percutaneous drainage is not feasible or has failed.[99] Operative drainage, especially via a laparoscopic approach, is a highly effective treatment option that is associated with low mortality and morbidity.[100] In some patients, a limited hepatic resection [*see 3:17 Hepatic Resection*] may be required to eliminate multiple abscesses, particularly when an underlying intrahepatic stricture is the source.[101]

Treatment of pyogenic liver abscess should include systemic antibiotic therapy. Approximately 70% of pyogenic liver abscesses yield polymicrobial isolates,[102] and 25% to 45% of the organisms are anaerobic.[103] Multiple anaerobic isolates suggest the colon as a source, whereas a single isolate of *E. coli* suggests a nidus in the biliary tree. Antibiotic treatment should include initial coverage of both aerobes and anaerobes with either a single agent or multiple agents. The need to cover enterococci has been debated, but these organisms clearly are increasingly important nosocomial pathogens. An acceptable initial treatment regimen consists of a single broad-spectrum agent (e.g., ticarcillin-clavulanate or meropenem). It should be noted that significant changes have occurred in the etiology, bacteriology, and treatment of liver abscesses. There is a trend toward a higher incidence of pseudomonal and streptococcal infections, and the frequency of fungal infection is increasing as well.[104] The mortality from this disease remains high, and appropriate antibiotic coverage with drainage is of paramount importance.

The duration of antibiotic therapy is controversial[105]; according to one set of guidelines, antibiotics should be continued for 3 to 4 weeks when the abscess has been excised, 4 to 8 weeks when a solitary abscess has been drained, and 6 to 8 weeks when multiple macroscopic abscesses have been drained.[106] Multiple microscopic abscesses usually require that a biliary source also be treated.[85] The overall prognosis for multiple small hepatic abscesses is not as good as that for solitary abscesses, and the development of a pyogenic abscess in a patient with an underlying hepatobiliary or pancreatic malignancy has been identified as a preterminal event associated with a hospital mortality of 28% and survival of less than 6 months.[107]

Amebic abscess. Medical treatment is now the standard approach to management of amebic liver abscesses. Metronidazole, 750 mg orally three times a day for 10 days, is a highly effective regimen.[108] A favorable response to treatment occurs within 4 to 5 days, and a decrease in the size of the abscess is apparent within 1 week on ultrasonographic examination, though a small residual cavity may persist for as long as 2 years. If the patient's condition does not improve, needle aspiration and culture are indicated. Secondary infection is treated as a pyogenic abscess. Otherwise, oral emetine, 65 mg/day, is added for up to 10 days.

Echinococcal abscess. Symptomatic or secondarily infected echinococcal cysts are best treated by means of surgical excision or marsupialization. The use of oral anthelmintics (e.g., albendazole and mebendazole) has met with limited success. Nevertheless, preoperative treatment with albendazole or mebendazole for 1 month, combined with postoperative treatment, is indicated to reduce the risk of intraoperative seeding or postoperative recurrence.[109,110]

Pancreatic Infection

Diagnosis When the mass is located in the epigastrium or the left upper quadrant, a pancreatic source is most likely. Prompt and accurate diagnosis is crucial because severe pancreatic infection is fatal if left untreated. The key to successful treatment is early diagnosis of infected pancreatic necrosis, infected pseudocyst, and pancreatic abscess. A high index of suspicion is required to diagnose these three infectious processes and to differentiate them from a pancreatic inflammatory mass or phlegmon,[28] in which pancreatic edema and inflammation are present without necrosis or infection.

Correct diagnosis and treatment of infected pancreatic necrosis, infected pseudocyst, and pancreatic abscess require an understanding of their pathophysiology. It is generally assumed that infected pancreatic necrosis develops as a transmural, transductal, lymphatic, or hematogenous infection of a necrotic region of the pancreas. Infection develops in 40% of cases of pancreatic necrosis, usually in week 2 or 3 after development of the acute pancreatitis.[111] Surgical debridement is required in these cases to prevent death. Pancreatic abscesses form by liquefaction of infected necrosis. They usually occur after week 5 of pancreatitis, when the acute phase of the disease has subsided.[112] Pancreatic abscesses are associated with a lower mortality than infected pancreatic necrosis. Like pancreatic abscesses, infected pancreatic collections and pseudocysts present late in the course of pancreatitis. They are associated with a lower mortality than pancreatic abscesses. Caused by infection in 13% of localized collections resulting from ductal blowout, infected pancreatic collections and pseudocysts may occur in the pancreas itself, in contiguous peripancreatic tissue, or in remote (extrapancreatic) tissue.

Clinical evaluation alone is generally insufficient to diagnose pancreatic infection. A clearly defined upper abdominal mass is palpable in only 50% to 75% of cases.[28] In most patients, the screening battery of tests reveals leukocytosis with leukocyte counts greater than 15,000/mm^3. Blood cultures are positive in 50% of cases. CT-guided percutaneous aspiration with Gram stain and culture provides the best method of diagnosing pancreatic infection. In one study of 75 patients with clinical toxicity suggestive of pancreatic sepsis, infection was confirmed in only 40%.[113] In another study of 21 patients with pancreatic infection, only five had specific signs on abdominal CT scan.[114] CT-guided diagnostic needle aspiration leads to a correct diagnosis within 72 hours in two thirds of patients, and the mortality associated with operative intervention is 19%; however, CT-guided needle aspiration is beneficial only if pancreatic infection is suspected and if the technique is used early in the course of disease.

Several laboratory markers of pancreatic necrosis have been investigated, such as serum methemalbumin, serum ribonuclease, and C-reactive protein. Most of these markers are too insensitive for routine clinical practice. However, serum levels of C-reactive protein above 10 mg/dl have been reported to be 95% accurate in predicting necrosis.[115]

Currently, the best indicators of infected pancreatic necrosis or abscess are a combination of Ranson's objective prognostic signs [see Table 2] and dynamic abdominal CT scan findings. In Ranson's series, the pancreatic findings on CT were graded in five categories [see Figure 7][116]: (a) normal, (b) pancreatic enlargement alone, (c) inflammation of the pancreas and peripancreatic fat, (d) one peripancreatic fluid collection, and (e) two or more peripancreatic fluid collections. Only category e was associated with a high (61%) incidence of pancreatic abscess. The number of objective prognostic signs present also predicted the subsequent development of an abscess: fewer than three signs, 12.5%; three to five signs, 31.8%; and more than five signs, 80%. However, the value of this method was limited because only five of the 83 patients evaluated had more than five prognostic signs. By combining the objective prognostic signs with positive abdominal CT findings, the investigators identified 30 patients who had three or more objective signs and were graded as category c, d, or e on abdominal CT scan; in these patients, the incidence of pancreatic abscess was 56.7%. By contrast, no patient with fewer than three prognostic signs and graded as category a or b on abdominal CT scan had a pancreatic abscess.

Treatment Once pancreatic infection is diagnosed, supportive measures are initiated, including nasogastric suction, withholding of oral feedings, meticulous attention to respiratory care and fluid and electrolyte balance, systemic antibiotic therapy, and nutritional support. The key to successful treatment, however, is surgical, radiologic, or endoscopic drainage.

Pancreatic necrosis. Sterile pancreatic necrosis alone is not an indication for surgical debridement. In one prospective study, 11 patients with sterile pancreatic necrosis were all followed successfully with conservative treatment.[117] However, once infected pancreatic necrosis is confirmed by Gram stain or culture, surgical debridement is required to remove the characteristically thick necrotic material; radiologic or endoscopic methods alone are not as effective for this purpose.

The choice of drainage technique is nevertheless controversial. Many clinicians prefer operative debridement and sump drainage. The mortality associated with extensive operative debridement (so-called necrosectomy) and sump drainage may range from 30% to 40%,[118] and this technique may be associated with a 30% to 40% reoperation rate because of sepsis or GI complications.[28,119]

Open drainage. To reduce the frequency of reoperation and to lower mortality, some clinicians opt for open drainage or marsupialization of the infected pancreas. One modification involves the use of a prosthetic mesh and a zipper to facilitate reexploration in patients with severe intra-abdominal abscess.[120] A 1991 meta-analysis of published surgical studies on infected pancreatic necrosis found statistically better results with debridement and lavage or debridement and open packing than with extensive debridement and sump drainage.[121] However, surgical treatment should be customized for each patient. In one study, open packing was used for massive necrosis (more than 100 g removed by debridement at operation or CT evidence of at least 50% pancreatic necrosis) or for extrapancreatic necrosis, whereas conventional debridement and sump drainage were used in other cases; the overall mortality in this study was only 14%.[122]

Pancreatic abscess. Pancreatic abscess resulting from liquefaction of necrosis is also best treated by surgical drainage because residual necrosis may cause failure of treatment by percutaneous methods.[123] On the other hand, infected pancreatic fluid collections and pseudocysts can usually be treated nonoperatively. In one prospective study, percutaneous and surgical drainage were equally successful in treating infected pancreatic fluid collections and pseudocysts.[124] Clinical signs of progress rather than CT findings are the best indicators of the need for intervention, and nonoperative methods should be attempted before open surgery is planned.

Adjunctive procedures. In the past, debridement and sump drainage were accompanied by the so-called triple ostomy technique, which involved cholecystostomy, gastrostomy, and jejunostomy. The role of these ancillary procedures, however, is controversial at best, and currently, cholecystostomy is employed only if gallstones are detected.

Other operative procedures may be required to manage gastric or colonic complications. Gastric bleeding, gastric outlet obstruction, and gastric fistula necessitating reoperation are relatively infrequent in this setting. By contrast, colonic necrosis and fistula formation are relatively common and occur either spontaneously or as complications of treatment. The usual site of involvement is the splenic flexure or upper descending colon. Treatment consists of colonic resection or a diverting colostomy [see 3:27 Colorectal Procedures].

Antibiotic therapy. The role of systemic antibiotic therapy in the prophylaxis of pancreatic abscess is controversial. Experimental evidence suggests that antibiotics may sometimes decrease the severity of pancreatitis,[125] and endoscopic cannulation of the pancreatic duct has yielded bacteria in pancreatic secretions of patients with acute pancreatitis.[126] In patients with pancreatic abscess, bacteriologic cultures are usually polymicrobial, the most common organisms being *E. coli*, enterococci, *Klebsiella pneumoniae*, *P. aeruginosa*, *S. aureus*, *Bacteroides fragilis*, and *Clostridium perfringens*. There is a growing trend toward early use of prophylactic antibiotics in cases of pancreatic necrosis, even though there are no data that convincingly demonstrate a clinical benefit. This trend may be partly responsible for the increasing prevalence of *Candida* species in pancreatitis-related sepsis; a 1996 report stated that *Candida* infection was detected in 21% of patients.[127]

Nutrition. Nutritional support of patients with pancreatic abscesses usually consists of TPN, though small bowel feeding may be attempted occasionally. These patients have high metabolic demands and may experience glucose intolerance or hyperlipidemia. Nevertheless, they generally tolerate I.V. feeding well. A 10-fold increase in mortality (from 2.5% to 21%) was reported in patients in whom a positive nitrogen balance could not be achieved.[128]

Splenic Abscess

Diagnosis A splenic abscess should be considered in patients who present with fever and a left upper quadrant mass, though it remains a rare cause of these symptoms. Most splenic abscesses encountered in clinical practice are solitary; multiple abscesses are usually covert and are typically found at autopsy in patients with disseminated malignancy, collagen vascular disease, or chronic debility.

Because splenic abscess is rare, correct diagnosis requires a high index of suspicion. The main clue is the clinical setting: both bacteremia and local splenic disease are required to produce splenic abscess. In the preantibiotic period, this combination was seen most frequently in patients with bacterial endocarditis and typhoid. Even today, more than three quarters of splenic abscesses occur in patients who already have an infection elsewhere in the body; splenic abscesses can also occur in patients with splenic infarcts, splenic hematomas, or local splenic disease caused by hemoglobinopathies.

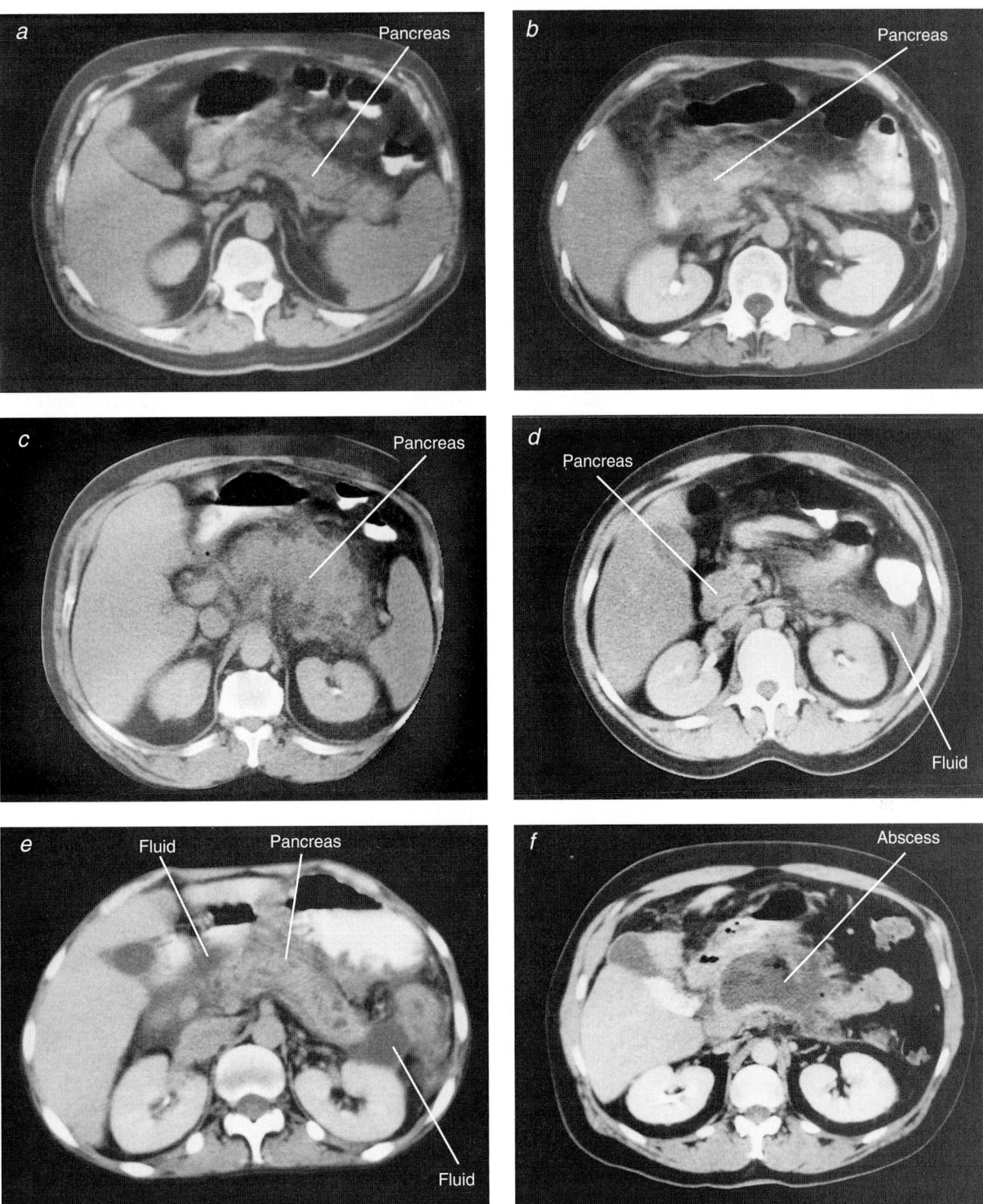

Figure 7 **Pancreatic findings on CT scan have been graded by Ranson into five categories: grade A—normal pancreas (*a*); grade B—diffuse enlargement of pancreas and nonhomogeneous density of gland (*b*); grade C—diffuse enlargement of pancreas associated with peripancreatic inflammation (*c*); grade D—high-density fluid collection in left anterior pararenal space (only head of pancreas is visualized at this level) (*d*); and grade E—diffuse enlargement of pancreas with several intrapancreatic small fluid collections and poorly defined fluid collections adjacent to tail and head of pancreas (*e*). In final CT scan (*f*), pancreatic abscess is demonstrated; partially encapsulated fluid collection containing bubbles of air represents large abscess.**

The diagnosis of splenic abscess may be supported by indirect radiologic signs, such as an elevated left hemidiaphragm or the finding of a left upper quadrant air-fluid level (mimicking the stomach). To clinch the diagnosis, an abdominal ultrasound examina-tion or abdominal CT scan is required. The abdominal CT scan, enhanced with I.V. or oral contrast material, is preferred [*see Figure 8*].[129] This technique provides a direct image of the spleen, on which abscesses appear as low-density areas that may contain gas.

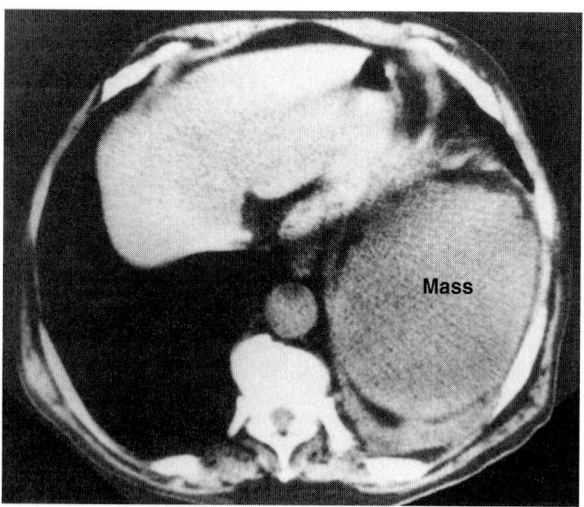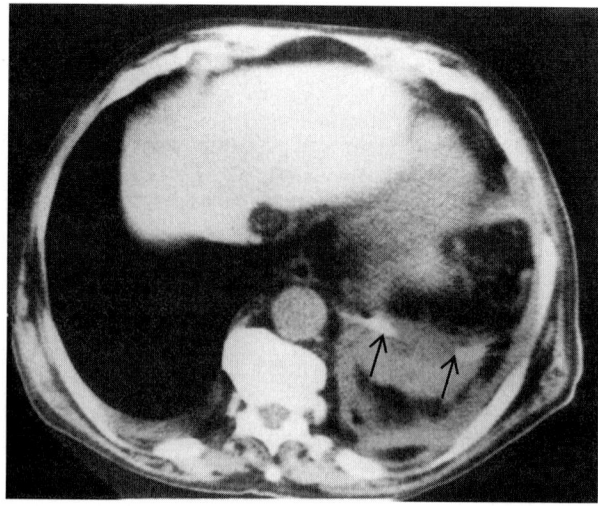

Figure 8   Abdominal CT scan, enhanced by contrast material, confirms diagnosis of splenic abscess.

Treatment   Treatment of splenic abscess includes I.V. administration of antibiotics and splenectomy [*see 3:19 Laparoscopic Splenectomy*]. The usual pathogenic organisms found are staphylococci and streptococci, though gram-negative bacilli and anaerobes may also be present. When splenic abscesses are not drained, mortality approaches 100%. At one time, splenotomy was the preferred operative treatment, but splenectomy is currently the preferred approach. Percutaneous catheter drainage is being performed with increasing frequency and appears to be as effective as operative drainage.[8,130,131]

Infections of the Lower Abdomen

Although enteric perforations, like pancreatitis and cholecystitis, present most commonly with pain and fever, their diagnosis differs from that of upper abdominal infections of the solid organs. The pain associated with enteric perforation frequently is not well localized; consequently, CT scanning is used more frequently than ultrasonography because it is superior for evaluating the entire abdomen [*see Figure 9*]. Moreover, a perforated viscus may present more acutely than other forms of infection do, and it is a common indication for emergency exploration. Thus, in the setting of a possible lower

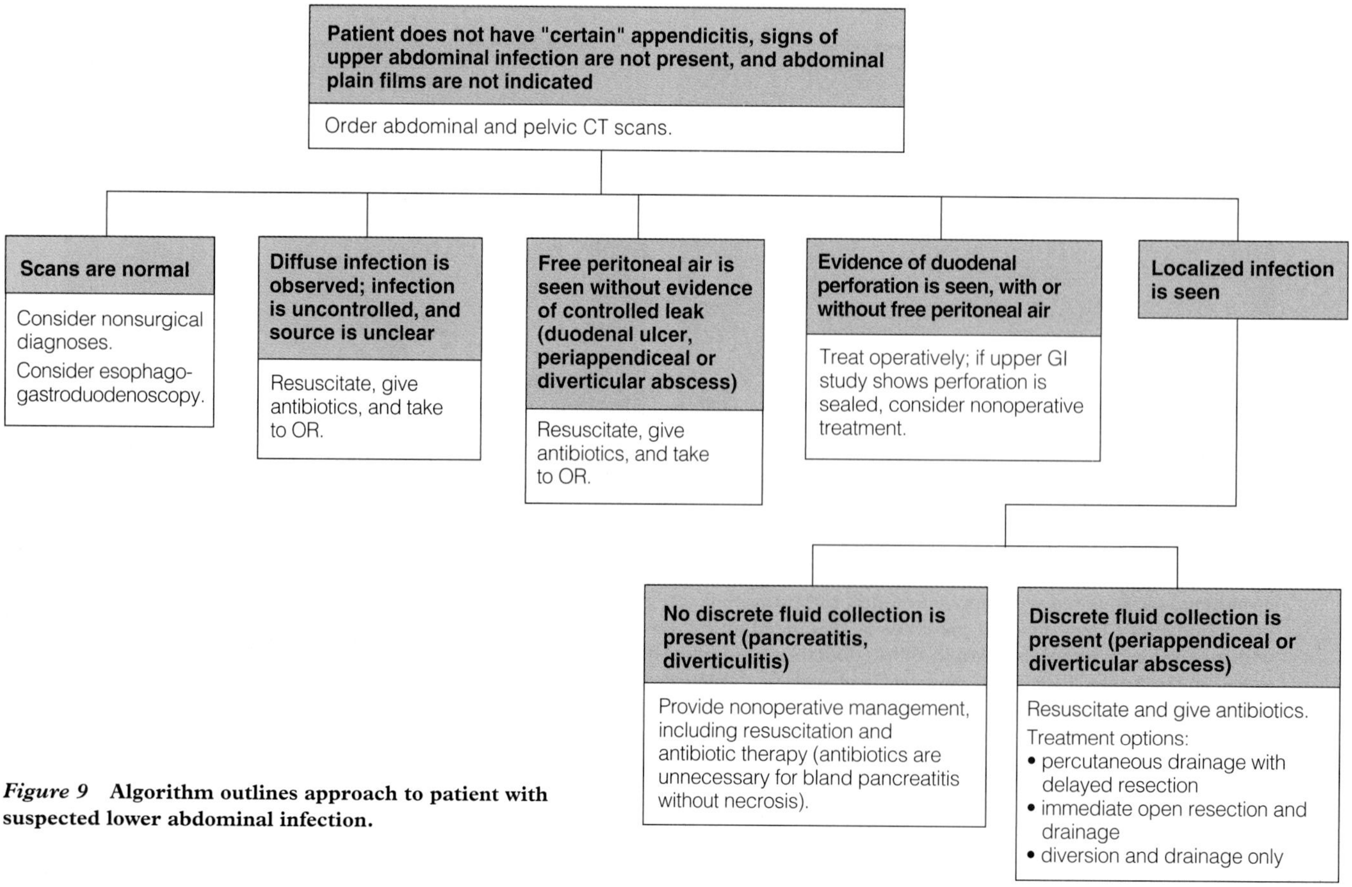

Patient does not have "certain" appendicitis, signs of upper abdominal infection are not present, and abdominal plain films are not indicated

Order abdominal and pelvic CT scans.

Scans are normal

Consider nonsurgical diagnoses.
Consider esophagogastroduodenoscopy.

Diffuse infection is observed; infection is uncontrolled, and source is unclear

Resuscitate, give antibiotics, and take to OR.

Free peritoneal air is seen without evidence of controlled leak (duodenal ulcer, periappendiceal or diverticular abscess)

Resuscitate, give antibiotics, and take to OR.

Evidence of duodenal perforation is seen, with or without free peritoneal air

Treat operatively; if upper GI study shows perforation is sealed, consider nonoperative treatment.

Localized infection is seen

No discrete fluid collection is present (pancreatitis, diverticulitis)

Provide nonoperative management, including resuscitation and antibiotic therapy (antibiotics are unnecessary for bland pancreatitis without necrosis).

Discrete fluid collection is present (periappendiceal or diverticular abscess)

Resuscitate and give antibiotics.
Treatment options:
• percutaneous drainage with delayed resection
• immediate open resection and drainage
• diversion and drainage only

Figure 9   Algorithm outlines approach to patient with suspected lower abdominal infection.

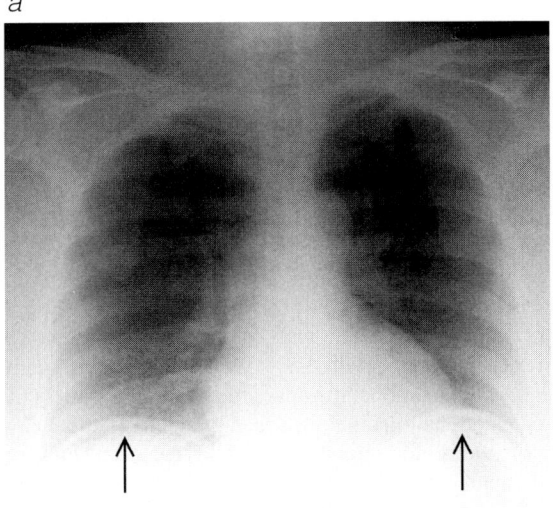

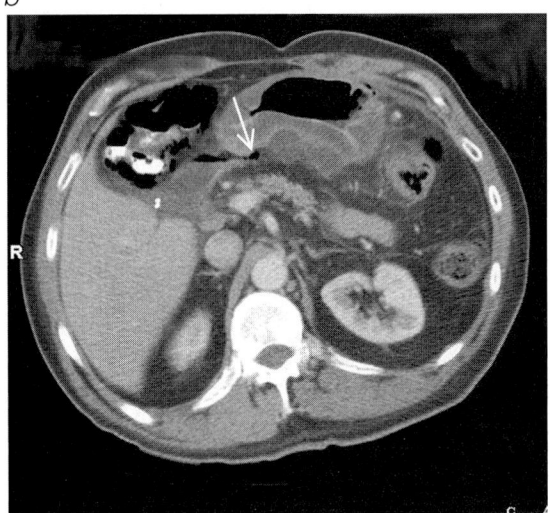

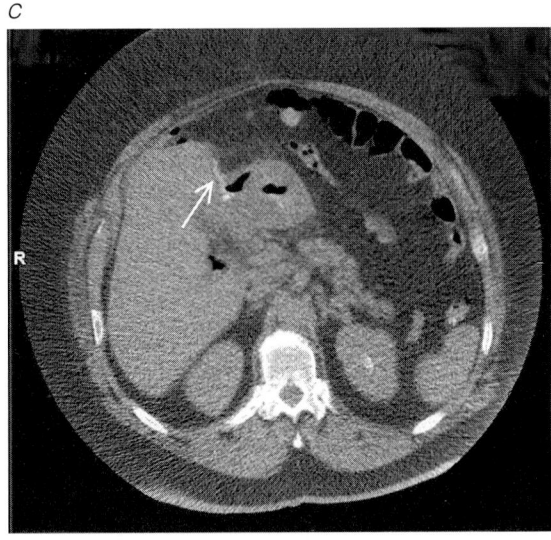

Figure 10 (*a*) Upright chest x-ray of patient with sudden onset of diffuse abdominal pain demonstrates free peritoneal air underneath both diaphragms (black arrows). Emergency exploration was carried out without further studies, and perforated gastric ulcer was excised. (*b*) Abdominal CT scan of patient with history of ulcer disease and 1-week history of increasing abdominal pain shows retrogastric fluid collection with air that appears to be in communication with duodenum (white arrow). Patient underwent laparotomy, and perforated duodenal ulcer was repaired. (*c*) Abdominal CT scan of patient with 2- to 3-day history of worsening abdominal pain demonstrates extravasation of oral contrast from anterolateral aspect of duodenum (white arrow). Patient underwent laparoscopic omental patch closure.

abdominal infection, the diagnostic emphasis is on confirming or ruling out the presence of an acute condition necessitating operation, rather than on fine localization of a more chronic illness.

PEPTIC ULCER PERFORATION

The incidence of peptic ulcer perforation has decreased significantly as a consequence of the changes in disease progression and incidence of intractable ulcers brought about by the advent of H_2 receptor antagonists and proton pump inhibitors (PPIs). Still, a significant percentage of all hospital admissions are secondary to perforated peptic ulcers, and the patient population is becoming older and more evenly balanced between men and women, presumably because of increased use of nonsteroidal anti-inflammatory drugs and cigarettes.[132]

Several studies found a high (80% to 92%) incidence of *Helicobacter pylori* infection in patients with perforated peptic ulcers.[133,134] Although the prevalence of *H. pylori* infection in this population is well established, the causal role that such infection plays in peptic ulcer perforations has been questioned.[135] In a 1999 study involving 50 patients with juxtapyloric perforations related to crack cocaine use who were successfully managed with simple omental patch closure, the investigators found that approximately 80% of the patients who underwent antral mucosal biopsy at the time of closure had a positive urease test, a finding that suggested

a role for *H. pylori* infection in the pathogenesis of these perforations as well.[136]

Diagnosis

A patient with a perforated peptic ulcer will complain of the sudden onset of intense abdominal pain and will often be able to pinpoint the exact time when the symptoms began. If the perforation has not spontaneously sealed or been managed with operative closure, the clinical picture can progress to florid sepsis and shock. Evidence of free air on plain upright and left lateral decubitus radiographs will be seen in as many as 70% of cases [*see Figure 10a*].[137] Endoscopy should be avoided in the evaluation of peptic ulcer perforation, but equivocal cases or spontaneously sealed perforations can be evaluated with water-soluble contrast studies. CT scanning can be used to localize an infection to the duodenum, particularly if communication of air or fluid with the duodenum is established [*see Figure 10b*] or if extravasation of contrast is seen [*see Figure 10c*].

Treatment

Surgical management centers on control of the site of perforation (via surgical closure or spontaneous sealing), with or without an acid-reducing procedure [*see 3:13 Gastroduodenal Procedures*]. Before this is done, I.V. fluids should be given, metabolic derangements corrected, appropriate antibiotics and an H_2 receptor blocker or PPI administered, and a nasogastric tube placed for decompression.

Operative versus conservative management Several studies have shown nonoperative management to be safe and effective for perforations that have sealed spontaneously. A 1989 study evaluated 35 patients with acute duodenal perforations—excluding those with a history of chronic ulcer disease who ultimately went on to primary repair and acid-reducing surgery—who were managed nonoperatively after evidence of a sealed perforation was noted on a water-soluble upper GI study. The investigators reported one death, in a patient with a history of metastatic breast cancer, and one intra-abdominal abscess.[138] In a 1989 prospective trial of 83 patients with perforated peptic ulcers randomly assigned to either conservative or operative management, the two groups experienced similar morbidity and mortality (~5%), and 73% of the patients in the conservatively managed group experienced full resolution of their symptoms.[139] The only significant difference between the groups was in the length of hospital stay. It has been suggested that patients with evidence of a sealed perforation confirmed by a Gastrografin upper GI study can be managed conservatively with a low incidence of reperforation and intra-abdominal abscess formation.[140] These patients must undergo repeated clinical examination and receive supportive therapy until clinical symptoms resolve.

Laparoscopic versus open repair A prospective, randomized trial of perforated peptic ulcers to either open or laparoscopic suture omental patch repair concluded that for perforations smaller than 10 mm, laparoscopic repair was associated with reduced operating times, less need for analgesics, fewer postoperative chest infections, earlier return to normal activities, and shorter hospitalizations.[141] An earlier study also demonstrated reduced analgesic times and earlier return to normal activities but reported longer operating times.[142] These studies confirm that small perforations can be adequately managed laparoscopically without exacerbation of bacterial sepsis. It must be emphasized, however, that biopsy of perforated gastric ulcers is critical for ruling out malignancies, and laparoscopic repair of the perforation may preclude biopsy.

Simple repair with medical management versus repair with acid-reducing procedure Definitive surgical management of ulcer disease during repair of a perforated peptic ulcer is contraindicated in patients who are hemodynamically unstable, have diffuse peritonitis, have an abscess, or have multiple underlying comorbid conditions.[143] The significant side effects associated with definitive surgery (dumping and diarrhea) and the success of medical management (PPIs, H_2 receptor blockers, and *H. pylori* eradication) have further contributed to the reduced popularity of proximal vagotomy at the time of repair. Now that fewer acid-reducing operations are being performed, there is some justifiable concern that younger surgeons will not be able to obtain the degree of training they would need to perform a definitive operation (highly selective vagotomy) in an urgent or emergency scenario.

A 1987 study found that simple closure with a Graham patch, without a concurrent operation to reduce ulcer recurrence, resulted in a higher recurrence rate than closure with proximal gastric vagotomy did (52% versus 16%; median follow-up, 54 months).[144] In a subsequent study of patients with acute perforations who were randomly assigned to undergo either simple closure or simple closure with proximal vagotomy, ulcer recurrence rates in the two groups after 2 years were 36.6% and 10.6%, respectively.[145]

Both of these studies, however, were performed before PPIs became routinely available.

Some 40% of patients with duodenal perforation treated with simple closure may experience recurrent duodenal ulcer. A 1995 series associated such recurrence with *H. pylori* infection.[146] To further study the role of *H. pylori* eradication in ulcer recurrence after peptic ulcer perforation, a randomized study was done in which patients with perforated duodenal ulcers and *H. pylori* infection after simple closure received either quadruple anti–*H. pylori* therapy (1 week of bismuth, tetracycline, and metronidazole with 4 weeks of omeprazole) or omeprazole alone.[133] After 1 year, 38.1% of patients managed with PPIs alone experienced ulcer recurrence, compared with 4.8% of patients managed with PPIs and *H. pylori* eradication. A similar study followed patients with perforated duodenal ulcers for up to 2 years after simple closure and randomization to either short-term H_2 receptor blockers or H_2 blockers with quadruple therapy; ongoing *H. pylori* infection correlated with recurrent ulcers for up to 2 years.[147]

On the basis of these findings, definitive acid-reducing procedures should be reserved for (1) patients in whom medical management of peptic ulcers and *H. pylori* fails, (2) patients whose ulcer symptoms have persisted for longer than 3 months, and (3) patients with otherwise complicated ulcers (e.g., lesions that are bleeding or causing obstruction).[148]

Antibiotic therapy In fasting persons, gastric juice contains as many as 10^3 organisms/ml. These organisms are typically facultative gram-positive salivary bacteria (e.g., lactobacilli and streptococci) and fungi (e.g., *Candida* species). In induced states of achlorhydria (e.g., from treatment with H_2 receptor blockers or PPIs), there is an increase in the total number of organisms, including enterococci and nitrate-reducing organisms. This phenomenon suggests a proliferation of salivary and enteric organisms, but its clinical relevance is unknown.[149]

Eradication of *H. pylori* in patients with uncomplicated ulcers and bleeding ulcers is now the standard of care.[150,151] Infection with this organism is associated with a 1% per year risk of peptic ulcer disease, a level of risk approximately 10 times that seen in uninfected patients. Eradication of *H. pylori* with medical management typically results in resolution of the ulcer, and recurrence is rare. Consequently, acid-reducing procedures are not often required.[152]

SMALL INTESTINAL PERFORATION

Diagnosis

Small intestinal perforation is a very difficult entity to diagnose, in large part because of its relative rarity. There are certain clinical scenarios (e.g., strangulated hernia and Crohn disease) in which the likelihood of this condition is heightened, but in the setting of blunt small intestinal injury, the low incidental occurrence of perforation (~1%[153]) and the complexity of the presentation frequently lead to a delay in diagnosis. Such delay is associated with increases in the morbidity and mortality directly attributable to the injury.[154] The radiographic modality most useful in diagnosis is CT scanning.[155]

Treatment

The basics of treatment are the same for small bowel perforation as for all perforations: isolation and control of the source of contamination. In the acute setting, this is accomplished through laparotomy and excision of the disease segment, whether the perforation is the result of ischemic necrosis, of blunt injury, or of IBD. Primary reanastomosis is generally accepted in these patients [*see 3:23 Intestinal Anastomosis*]. For patients with Crohn disease, perforation (usually presenting as a fistula) is a risk factor for postoperative disease recurrence[156]; accordingly, close postoperative follow-up is indicated.

There are two additional issues regarding small bowel perforations that warrant special mention. The first has to do with small bowel perforation secondary to obstruction. When this event occurs, it is important not only that the perforated segment be resected but also that the cause of obstruction be identified to prevent recurrence. The second issue has to do with anastomotic leakage. Not all leaks call for surgical intervention. If the leak is a late complication, it is likely to have walled itself off into an abscess, in which case CT-guided drainage of the abscess is the treatment of choice. Efforts at reducing the luminal transport are also made to improve healing.

Nutritional support plays a major supportive role in the treatment of patients with small bowel perforation. Many of these patients, either because of their underlying pathology (e.g., Crohn disease) or because of their hypermetabolic state (e.g., from trauma), lose some of their innate ability to heal and prevent anastomotic breakdown. The presence of a knowledgeable nutrition staff can dramatically enhance patient recovery in this setting.

Antibiotic therapy The small bowel flora is typically sparse (10^3 to 10^4/ml), with salivary organisms predominating. In conditions of stasis, obstruction, or impaired motility, however, colonic flora can proliferate, with *E. coli*, enterococci, and obligate anaerobes the dominant organisms. In the distal ileum, there are typically about 10^6 colony-forming units/ml, with an increasing proportion of enteric organisms and anaerobic bacteria, presumably as a result of backwash through the ileocecal valve.[157] Although there are generally far fewer bacteria in the small intestine than in the colon (which contains about 10^{12} organisms/ml), the standard antimicrobial therapy remains broad-spectrum coverage (e.g., fluoroquinolone plus an antianaerobic agent for 5 days).[158]

APPENDICITIS

Obstruction of the appendiceal lumen by a fecalith, a hyperplastic lymph node, or a foreign body is typically the inciting event in the pathogenesis of appendicitis. Luminal obstruction with continued secretion results in progressive distention, proliferation of luminal microorganisms, ischemia, gangrene, and subsequent perforation. The clinical history during this evolution is marked by diffuse epigastric pain with anorexia, nausea, and vomiting. The pain typically progresses first to the periumbilical region and then to the right lower quadrant (at McBurney's point). Patients have a low-grade fever and exhibit direct tenderness at McBurney's point but may also manifest rebound tenderness, guarding, rigidity, and marked temperature elevation if the appendix perforates and results in diffuse peritonitis. As the viscera and the omentum localize and sequester the perforation, the symptoms may subside to a degree, with localized pain and a palpable abdominal mass the primary manifestations remaining.

Diagnosis

Classically, the diagnosis of appendicitis has been made primarily through clinical examination, with laboratory tests consistent with inflammation (i.e., an elevated leukocyte count with a left shift and an elevated C-reactive protein level) serving as confirmation. In as many as 20% of patients with appendicitis, however, the incorrect diagnosis is made, and the incidence of removal of a normal appendix can approach 40%.[159-161] Early diagnosis of appendicitis can decrease the risk of postoperative complications

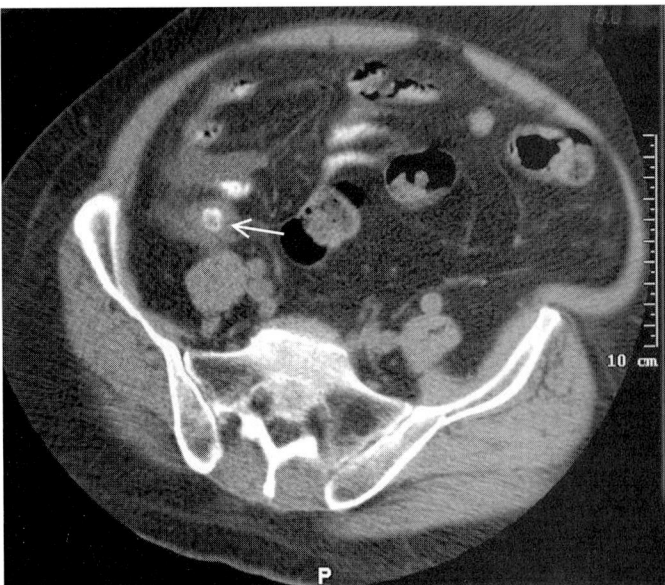

Figure 11 Pelvic CT scan of patient with distant history of right lower quadrant abdominal pain with recurrent acute attack demonstrates inflamed and thickened appendix with surrounding fat stranding (white arrow). Gangrenous appendix was removed laparoscopically.

from 39% to 8%, and one retrospective study found that the use of diagnostic CT lowered the rate of misdiagnosis to 7%.[162] CT scanning is reported to be 93% to 98% in diagnosing appendicitis, with significantly improved accuracy achieved by using an appendicitis protocol after retrograde water-soluble contrast administration.[163] CT findings suggestive of appendicitis [*see Figure 11*] include enlargement and dilation of the appendix (to > 6 mm), nonfilling of the appendix, and periappendiceal inflammation (fat stranding, abscess, phlegmon, and dependent fluid collections); these findings do not differ significantly between acute appendicitis and chronic, recurrent appendicitis.[164,165]

Current evidence supports the role of CT scanning in the diagnostic evaluation of patients with suspected appendicitis. Studies have demonstrated decreases both in the incidence of normal appendectomies and in the incidence of prolonged, unnecessary observations.[166,167] Furthermore, alterations in patient management attributable to diagnostic CT have been shown to decrease overall hospital and patient costs. Nevertheless, the utility of CT in young men whose history, physical examination, and laboratory test results fit the classic picture of appendicitis remains unproven; this subset of patients may be managed without confirmatory CT.[166] On the other hand, CT scanning appears to be quite useful for diagnosing appendicitis in women, in which setting it decreases the incidence of normal appendectomies and facilitates diagnosis of other causes of the symptoms.[168,169] Preoperative CT scanning assists in planning an operation, identifying a periappendiceal abscess that may delay immediate appendectomy, and recognizing other sources of intra-abdominal pathology.

Treatment

Initial management consists of fluid resuscitation, appropriate prophylactic antibiotics, and preparation for surgery. Currently, acute nonperforated appendicitis, gangrenous appendicitis, and perforated appendicitis without an associated abscess are managed with urgent appendectomy [*see 3:24 Appendectomy*]. The main dilemmas in management center on the appropriate use of laparoscopic appendectomy and the role of conservative management for periappendiceal masses with interval appendectomy.

Laparoscopic versus open appendectomy In several prospective, randomized clinical trials that compared laparoscopic with open appendectomy, the consensus was that the former was associated with a lower incidence of wound infection, decreased utilization of pain medication, earlier return to normal activities, and reduced cost of hospitalization (though the data were conflicting on this last point).[170-173] On the other hand, the trials found the laparoscopic approach to be associated with significantly longer operating time, equivalent duration of hospitalization, and a possible increased risk of abscess formation. A retrospective review published in 2000, however, found that when a dedicated laparoscopic service was established for patients with appendicitis, the rates of intra-abdominal abscess formation after laparoscopic appendectomy decreased to levels equivalent to those reported after open appendectomy.[174]

Although laparoscopic appendectomy is associated with a higher incidence of intra-abdominal abscess formation in the setting of perforated appendicitis, it is not associated with a higher incidence of wound infection or abscess in patients with gangrenous or nonperforated appendicitis.[175] Furthermore, a prospective, randomized trial found that laparoscopic appendectomy was associated with reduced overall cost of hospitalization, decreased use of pain medication, and earlier return to functional status in patients with uncomplicated appendicitis.[170]

Two groups of patients clearly benefit from laparoscopic appendectomy: women and obese patients. In women, laparoscopy aids in the diagnosis of other pelvic pathologic conditions and lowers the incidence of negative appendectomies; in obese patients, it results in less postoperative pain and a shorter recovery time, even though it does not significantly reduce the postoperative complication rate.[176,177] Patients who present with evidence of perforated or complicated appendicitis may be better managed with the traditional open approach to minimize the risk of postoperative abscess formation.[178] Improvements in laparoscopic techniques, however, may eventually reduce the incidence of this complication to a level comparable to that seen with open management.

Periappendiceal abscess and interval appendectomy The mainstays of conservative management have been parenteral antibiotics, supportive fluid resuscitation, and percutaneous drainage of radiographically amenable fluid collections. In a 2001 review of 155 patients with periappendiceal abscesses, the complication rate was 36% for patients managed with surgical incision and drainage and appendectomy, compared with 17% for patients managed nonoperatively.[179] The recurrence rate was 8% in the conservatively managed patients, and nonoperative management failed in five patients. Patients with perforated appendicitis and abscess or phlegmon diagnosed by CT scanning but without a palpable mass were safely managed with conservative therapy. In a 2002 study, immediate appendectomy was associated with a higher postoperative complication rate and an increased incidence of more extensive initial operations (e.g., ileocecal resection, right hemicolectomy, and temporary ileostomy).[180]

The recurrence rate after conservative management ranges from 10% to 20%. In one study of patients managed with interval appendectomy for periappendiceal mass, histologic evaluation revealed that a significant majority of samples had a patent appendiceal lumen and were at risk for recurrent appendicitis.[181] In a 2002 report, 45.8% of interval appendectomy pathologic samples showed evidence of chronic active inflammation.[182] The risk of re-

currence and progression to chronic appendicitis supports the use of interval appendectomy in young patients, but in adults, the decision algorithm must also consider the incidental diagnosis of tumor.

Interval appendectomy is typically performed between 6 weeks and 3 months after percutaneous intervention and clinical resolution [see Figure 12]. The risk of recurrence is greatest after the 6-month point in the clinical progression of acute appendicitis managed conservatively.[183] In several retrospective analyses, interval appendectomy proved to be a safe management plan, but to date, there have been no randomized, prospective trials evaluating its role in management.[184,185]

Antibiotic therapy The pathogenic organisms recovered in peritoneal cultures derive from the colon and consist of aerobic or facultative bacteria and anaerobes. The most frequently isolated organisms are *E. coli*, enterococci, viridans streptococci, *B. fragilis*, *Lactobacillus* species, *Prevotella melaninogenica*, and *Bilophila wadsworthia*.[186,187] It is noteworthy that the use of intraoperative peritoneal cultures has not been shown to affect the incidence of wound infection, abscess formation, or small bowel obstruction if patients are presumptively managed with antibiotics that cover gram-negative bacteria and enteric anaerobes.[188]

Appropriate coverage can be obtained with any of the following: ampicillin-sulbactam, piperacillin-tazobactam, ticarcillin-clavulanate, cefoxitin, cefotetan, and ciprofloxacin plus metronidazole.[189-192] In a trial involving children with perforated appendicitis, conversion to oral therapy after parenteral therapy was equivalent to parenteral therapy alone.[193] In a study of patients with acute nonperforated appendicitis, preoperative administration of cefoxitin was superior to placebo in reducing the incidence of wound infection.[190] In a study of children with acute nonperforated appendicitis, prolonged antibiotic administration (5 days) had no advantage over a single preoperative dose with respect to the incidence of wound infection or subsequent abscess formation.[194] The duration and timing of antibiotic administration in patients with nonperforated gangrenous appendicitis have not been shown to correlate with the wound infection rate.[195]

COLONIC PERFORATION

Diagnosis

Diagnostic strategies for identifying colon lesions associated with intra-abdominal infection follow the general approach outlined earlier [see Clinical Evaluation *and* Investigative Studies, *above*]. For unstable patients with generalized peritonitis, there is no need to delay operative intervention to wait for radiologic confirmation: the pathologic condition will be identified in the course of the operation. However, for patients who have localized peritonitis or those who are stable and whose physical examination is not conclusive for peritonitis, radiologic evaluation is pivotal in planning treatment.

Although plain films may reveal free air in the abdomen and prompt surgical intervention, CT scanning may be a more valuable first study because of its ability to delineate the bowel wall and surrounding soft tissues with remarkable accuracy. In a 2002 study comparing abdominal radiography with CT for the evaluation of acute nontraumatic abdominal pain in the ED, the former was not nearly as diagnostically sensitive as the latter (a nonspecific diagnosis in 68%, compared with a specific diagnosis in 80%).[196] The investigators concluded that CT was the initial radiographic modality of choice for patients with acute abdominal pain in the ED. Another study found that CT scans frequently changed physicians' initial diagnoses, increased diagnostic certain-

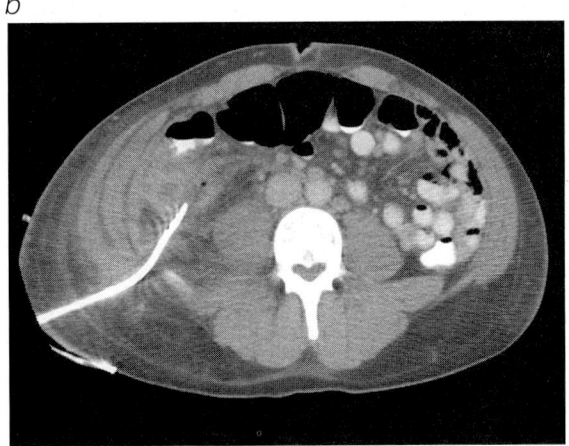

Figure 12 (*a*) **Pelvic CT scan of young patient with a 5-day history of right lower quadrant abdominal pain shows fluid collection containing air adjacent to appendix and consistent with appendiceal perforation and abscess formation (white arrow). (*b*) Pelvic CT scan of same patient after percutaneous ultrasound-guided placement of drainage catheter shows evacuation of air and much fluid. Patient underwent uneventful interval appendectomy 6 weeks later.**

ty, and led to more appropriate treatment in patients with acute abdominal pain in the ED.[197]

In view of the relatively high cost of CT scanning, the concomitant radiation exposure, and the use of I.V. contrast agents to enhance the scans, some have suggested using ultrasonography to make diagnoses. However, the well-documented dependency of this modality on the skill of the individual technician makes it less attractive to the broader health care community, where full-time sonographers are not always available. Finally, it should be noted that there is no role for MRI in the acute setting. Although it is both sensitive and specific, the logistic hindrances associated with its use greatly limit its applicability.

Treatment

Diverticulitis Diverticular disease ranges in severity from minor to serious. The focus of our discussion will be on management of complicated (perforated) diverticular disease, for which resection should be considered after only one attack.

In the past, treatment of perforated diverticular disease involved a multistage surgical approach whereby the patient underwent three separate procedures: one for fecal diversion and drainage of the infection, a second for resection of the diseased segment, and a third for closure of the colostomy. This three-stage approach proved to be associated with high morbidities, high cumulative mortalities, and prolonged hospitalizations.[198-200] Since then, CT-guided percutaneous drainage, primary resection of the diseased segment, and improved patient selection for resection and primary anastomosis have improved patient outcomes dramatically. Few adequately powered multicenter, prospective, randomized trials evaluating treatment of complicated diverticular disease have been done; accordingly, many of the current treatment standards have been derived by consensus on the basis of thorough review of the literature.

Therapy for perforated diverticular disease depends greatly on the patient's condition at the time of presentation and on the stage of the disease. The Hinchey staging system[201] [*see Table 4*] classifies perforated diverticular disease according to the associated inflammatory process and is used to guide and compare treatment options.[202-204]

In stage I disease, a small pericolic abscess [*see Figure 13a*] in a stable and otherwise healthy patient may resolve with conservative

management, including broad-spectrum antibiotics and bowel rest. The patient can be evaluated for definitive surgical treatment later, after the episode resolves and the patient is in better condition for surgery. For larger abscesses or stage II disease [*see Figure 13b*], the standard of care is CT-guided percutaneous abscess drainage, if feasible. After drainage, resuscitation, and bowel preparation, a one-stage colectomy can be done (resection of the diseased segment with primary anastomosis) so as to avoid the potential increased morbidity of a two-stage procedure.[205]

For patients who have abscesses that are inaccessible to percutaneous drainage or who experience persistent symptoms despite drainage, operative correction is required. If adequate bowel preparation can be carried out, primary anastomosis at the time of surgery should be considered. If adequate bowel preparation is not possible, a two-stage approach, including a Hartmann procedure and subsequent stoma reversal, should be considered. Alternatively, depending on the patient's condition, resection with primary anastomosis may be attempted. There is some evidence that employing intraoperative colonic lavage to reduce the fecal column and thus allow primary anastomosis may reduce morbidity, especially in patients with stage I or II disease.[206-208] However, the studies supporting this view are not conclusive enough for such a regimen to be considered standard; further investigation is warranted before it is generally accepted. Finally, whether to add a covering stoma to a primary anastomosis is a case-by-case decision that is usually guided by the presence of risk factors such as poor nutritional status, inadequate bowel preparation, blood loss, or intraoperative hypotension.[209]

Table 4 Hinchey System for Classification of Perforated Diverticulitis[201]

Stage	Description
Stage I	Pericolic or mesenteric abscess
Stage II	Pelvic or retroperitoneal abscess that is walled off
Stage III	Purulent peritonitis
Stage IV	Feculent peritonitis

a
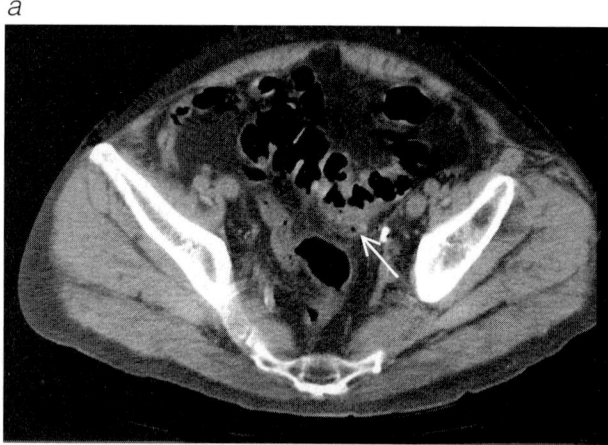

b
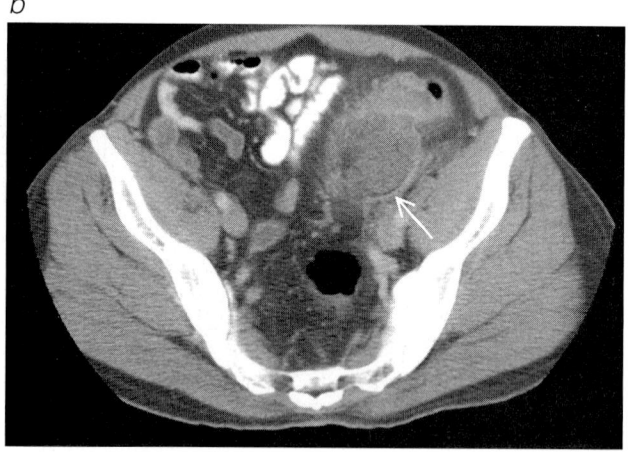

Figure 13 (*a*) Pelvic CT scan of elderly patient with left lower quadrant abdominal pain of 2 days' duration shows diverticulitis with small amount of extraluminal air (white arrow). Patient was treated acutely with resuscitation and antibiotics alone and was discharged home without complications. (*b*) Pelvic CT scan of middle-aged patient with 1-week history of constipation and moderate pelvic pain shows left lower quadrant fluid collection consistent with peridiverticular abscess (white arrow). Proximal bowel is seen anterior to abscess, distal bowel posterior. Percutaneous drain was placed, and elective colectomy with primary reanastomosis was performed 12 days later.

Stage III or IV diverticulitis is a surgical emergency that calls for prompt resuscitation and administration of broad-spectrum antibiotics, followed rapidly by surgical treatment. The Hartmann procedure is the most widely accepted operation for this presentation.[210-212] It is associated with a substantially lower mortality than drainage followed by colostomy as a separate, delayed procedure (12% versus 28%).[213] In certain circumstances, with appropriate patient selection and low feculent contamination, primary anastomosis, with or without a covering stoma, may be feasible.[214-216]

The goals of resection are to remove the focus of infection and to prevent recurrent attacks. Recurrent diverticulitis after resection is the result of incomplete removal of the diseased segment, especially at the rectosigmoid junction. Therefore, when the diseased segment is resected, the entire sigmoid must be removed, and the distal resection margin must extend below the confluence of the taeniae coli and onto pliable rectum.[217] Proximally, the colon is mobilized until a margin of uninflamed bowel is identified. It is not, however, necessary to remove the entire colon affected by diverticuli.

Laparoscopy. Laparoscopic treatment of diverticular disease is becoming more common but remains controversial. Many feel that there is no place for laparoscopic-assisted colectomy in the treatment of stage III or IV disease,[202] but there is growing acceptance of this approach in the treatment of stage I and II disease. A review of several small studies concluded that laparoscopic colectomy had a high potential for reducing hospitalization time and operative morbidity; however, the cost analysis data were conflicting, and some of the trials reported very high conversion rates.[218]

Right-side disease. Particular mention should be made of right-side diverticulitis. In the past, this condition was often misdiagnosed as appendicitis before exploration, but today, with the increased use of CT scanning, this error is less frequently made. Given that diagnosis is difficult and the disease is surgically curable, some authors suggest that it should be treated with aggressive resection, ranging from simple diverticulectomy to right hemicolectomy.[219,220] Others argue that the disease is relatively benign in the absence of perforation and suggest leaving the diseased bowel in situ, performing an incidental appendectomy, and then treating the patient conservatively.[221,222] There is no standard therapy for cecal diverticulitis, mainly because of the small number of patients

it affects annually, which translates into small series reported in the literature. In the course of follow-up, it is important that these patients undergo thorough evaluation for colon cancer.

Antibiotic therapy. Appropriate antibiotic administration is an integral part of standard therapy for diverticular disease and is started at diagnosis. The most frequently isolated organisms are anaerobes, including *Bacteroides, Peptostreptococcus, Clostridium,* and *Fusobacterium* species. Gram-negative aerobes (predominantly *E. coli*) and facultative gram-positive bacteria (predominantly streptococci) are also associated with these infections.[223] Parenterally administered broad-spectrum antibiotics are standard. A particularly common regimen is ciprofloxacin plus metronidazole, but there are other regimens that are equally efficacious for treatment. According to a 2002 report from the Surgical Infection Society, the duration of therapy for complicated intra-abdominal infections should be no longer than 5 to 7 days.[158] If ongoing infection is suspected at termination of treatment, investigation into a potential source of infection is warranted.

Other colon lesions associated with perforation and peritonitis A number of colonic conditions besides diverticular disease may be manifested by colonic perforation and secondary peritonitis. Whatever the specific cause, the general goals of therapy remain the same: (1) to identify and control the source of bacterial contamination, (2) to reduce the level of peritoneal contamination, and (3) to prevent recurrent infections.

Colon cancer. After diverticular disease, colon cancer is the next leading cause of colonic perforation in uninjured patients. In general, perforated colon cancer carries a high mortality,[224,225] and the operative technique of choice is controversial. Perforation typically occurs at the site of the lesion but can also occur proximally (e.g., at the cecum) as a result of luminal obstruction.

Generally, perforations at the site of cancer in the ascending and transverse colon are treated with primary resection and anastomosis, with or without a diverting stoma, regardless of whether localized or diffuse peritonitis is present. When perforations occur at the site of cancer in the descending and sigmoid colon, however, there is some debate over the appropriate surgical approach, with some advocating primary resection and others staged proce-

a

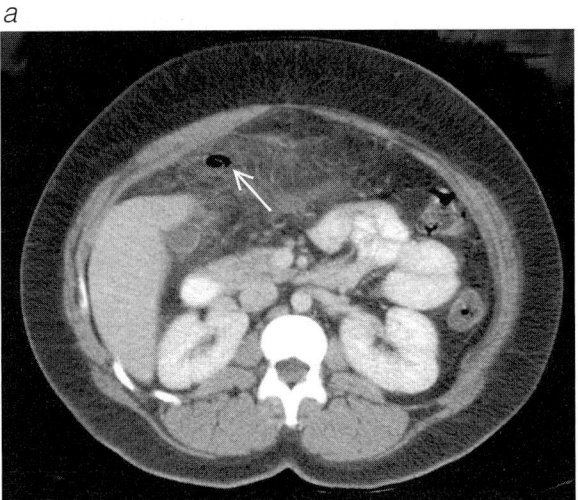

b

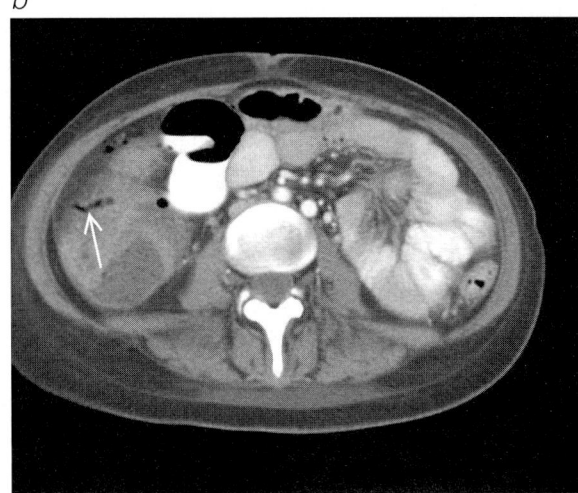

Figure 14 (*a*) Abdominal CT scan of elderly patient with history of vascular disease and worsening abdominal pain over a 3-day period shows diffuse inflammation and right upper quadrant extraluminal air (white arrow). Patient underwent emergency exploration, and ischemic perforation of cecum was found. Right hemicolectomy and temporary diverting ileostomy were performed. (*b*) Abdominal CT scan of patient with history of Crohn disease and worsening abdominal pain demonstrates thickening of colonic wall with both intramural and extramural air (white arrow). Patient was treated with emergency total abdominal colectomy for pancolitis with creation of temporary diverting ileostomy.

dures. Two studies from the early 1990s suggested improved long-term mortality after primary resection.[226,227] A subsequent study, however, suggested that the improved mortality associated with primary resection was secondary to preselection and therefore could not be considered conclusive proof of the superiority of this approach. The authors of this latter study concluded that primary resection was appropriate for a select patient population with minimal comorbidity and that staged resection was beneficial for patients with a high degree of acute illness and comorbidity (e.g., elderly patients).[228]

Less common causes of colonic perforation. Other diagnoses associated with colonic perforation and peritonitis (localized or diffuse) are ischemic necrosis as a result of vasculopathology [*see Figure 14a*] or volvulus, missed traumatic injury, and IBD [*see Figure 14b*]. Except for IBD, the standard therapy is excision of the affected segment and reanastomosis, with or without a covering stoma. For patients with numerous comorbidities, a high degree of feculent contamination, or very severe illness necessitating an extremely abbreviated operating time, a Hartmann procedure with a mucous fistula or an oversewn distal segment is the primary treatment. Because perforation associated with IBD is typically a self-limited disease, treatment is directed at the underlying pathophysiology and excision of the diseased segment is not always indicated.[229]

Other Abdominal Infections

PELVIC INFLAMMATORY DISEASE

Because of the diverse clinical presentations of pelvic inflammatory disease (PID) and the significant sequelae associated with delayed diagnosis, women with this condition can pose a major diagnostic dilemma in the ED. In 2002, the Centers for Disease Control and Prevention (CDC) updated their established diagnostic guidelines for initiating therapy in patients with suspected PID.[230] According to these guidelines, empirical treatment should be started if a young sexually active woman or any woman at risk for sexually transmitted diseases presents with minimal symptoms [*see Table 5*] that cannot be attributed to another cause. To reduce undue treatment-associated morbidity, additional criteria are supplied to aid in specifying precisely who should receive treatment.

Treatment of PID, according to the CDC, includes broad-spectrum antibiotics directed toward *Neisseria gonorrhoeae, Chlamydia trachomatis,* anaerobes, gram-negative facultative bacteria, and streptococci [*see Table 6*]. Hospitalization is suggested when surgical emergencies (e.g., appendicitis) cannot be excluded or when the patient is pregnant; does not respond clinically to oral antimicrobial therapy; cannot follow or tolerate an outpatient oral regimen; has severe illness, nausea and vomiting, or high fever; or has a tubo-ovarian abscess. Surgical intervention for PID is generally limited to patients with symptomatic pelvic masses, ruptured

---

Table 5 CDC Guidelines for Diagnosis of Pelvic Inflammatory Disease[230]

Minimal symptoms
Uterine/adnexal tenderness
Cervical motion tenderness

Additional supportive criteria (enhance specificity of minimal symptoms)
Oral temperature >101° F (> 38.3° C)
Abnormal cervical or vaginal mucopurulent discharge
Presence of white blood cells on saline microscopy of vaginal secretions
Elevated erythrocyte sedimentation rate
Elevated C-reactive protein
Laboratory documentation of cervical infection with *Neisseria gonorrhoeae* or *Chlamydia trachomatis*

Most specific criteria
Endometrial biopsy with histopathologic evidence of endometritis
Transvaginal sonography or magnetic resonance imaging techniques showing thickened, fluid-filled tubes with or without free pelvic fluid or tubo-ovarian complex
Laparoscopic abnormalities consistent with PID

Table 6 CDC Guidelines for Antibiotic Treatment of PID[230]

Parenteral Regimens

A	Cefotetan, 2 g I.V. q. 12 hr *or* Cefoxitin, 2 g I.V. q. 6 hr *plus* Doxycycline, 100 mg p.o. or I.V. q. 12 hr
B	Clindamycin, 900 mg I.V. q. 8 hr *plus* Gentamicin, loading dose I.V. or I.M. (2 mg/kg body weight) followed by maintenance dose (1.5 mg/kg) q. 8 hr; single daily dosing may be substituted
Alternative	Ofloxacin, 400 mg I.V. q. 12 hr *or* Levofloxacin, 500 mg I.V. s.i.d. *with or without* Metronidazole, 500 mg I.V. q. 8 hr *or* Ampicillin-sulbactam, 3 g I.V. q. 6 hr *plus* Doxycycline, 100 mg p.o. or I.V. q. 12 hr

Enteral Regimens

A	Ofloxacin, 400 mg p.o., b.i.d., for 14 days *or* Levofloxacin, 500 mg p.o., s.i.d., for 14 days *with or without* Metronidazole, 500 mg p.o., b.i.d., for 14 days
B	Ceftriaxone, 250 mg I.M. in single dose *or* Cefoxitin, 2 g I.M. in single dose, and probenecid, 1 g p.o. administered concurrently in a single dose *or* Other parenteral third-generation cephalosporin (e.g., ceftizoxime or cefotaxime) *plus* Doxycycline, 100 mg p.o., b.i.d., for 14 days *with or without* Metronidazole, 500 mg p.o., b.i.d., for 14 days

tubo-ovarian abscesses, or draining abscesses that do not respond to antibiotic therapy. Aspiration has also been considered as a treatment modality; it may limit morbidity and preserve fertility.[231]

PYELONEPHRITIS

Pyelonephritis is a complication of urinary tract infection; consequently, it affects women more often than men. The diagnosis is typically made on the basis of systemic symptoms in the setting of a known, bacteriologically confirmed urinary tract infection. Pyelonephritis may be classified as either complicated or uncomplicated, depending on patient factors (e.g., previous transplantation or an anatomic abnormality) and infectious characteristics (e.g., sepsis).

The typical pathogen in uncomplicated disease is *E. coli*, and outpatient treatment with trimethoprim-sulfamethoxazole or a fluoroquinolone usually suffices.[232] Complicated pyelonephritis, however, often is caused by microbes other than *E. coli*, including *Pseudomonas* species and enterococci. Hospitalization is required, and treatment usually involves parenteral administration of ceftriaxone and gentamicin[233] or piperacillin-tazobactam[234]; vancomycin is indicated if the patient is allergic to penicillin. More aggressive therapies, including percutaneous nephrostomy or abscess drainage, may be considered on a case-by-case basis.

SPONTANEOUS BACTERIAL PERITONITIS

In adult patients, primary peritonitis usually accompanies cirrhosis and ascites[235]; however, the presentation can be highly variable. To diagnose spontaneous bacterial peritonitis, paracentesis is performed and the fluid sent for Gram stain and culture; pH determination; measurement of glucose, protein, lactate, and lactic dehydrogenase levels; and a cell count with differential. According to a consensus statement from the International Ascites Club, diagnostic paracentesis is recommended for every cirrhotic patient with ascites upon admission to the hospital.[236] Empirical therapy is started if the neutrophil count is higher than 250/mm³, the pH is lower than 7.35, and the lactate concentration is greater than 32 ng/ml. If the results of other studies suggest peritonitis, radiographic evaluation is indicated to rule out potential causes of secondary peritonitis.

Treatment consists of cefotaxime at a minimum dosage of 2 g every 12 hours for 5 days, with follow-up paracentesis scheduled for 48 hours after the start of treatment.[237,238] If the neutrophil count does not decrease significantly (to < 25% of the pretreatment value), treatment may be assumed to have failed. Surgical intervention is undertaken if the patient is refractory to medical management, the ascitic fluid grows mixed aerobes and anaerobes, or radiographic studies suggest bowel perforation.

PERITONEAL DIALYSIS CATHETER–RELATED INFECTIONS

Peritonitis is a major cause of failure of peritoneal dialysis in long-term studies.[239] Peritonitis is especially difficult to diagnose in dialysis patients because the presentation is usually vague. Accordingly, it is critical to maintain a low threshold for testing. The definition of peritonitis in this population includes satisfaction of two of the following three criteria: (1) a Gram stain demonstrating microorganisms or a positive culture of the dialysis effluent, (2) a dialysate white blood cell count higher than 100/mm³, with at least 50% neutrophils, and (3) peritoneal signs or symptoms.[240] The microbes most commonly identified are *S. epidermidis* and *S. aureus* (~60% of isolates), followed by gram-negative bacteria (~30% of isolates); the remaining isolates are largely accounted for by fungi, anaerobes, and mycobacteria.

Treatment usually includes cefazolin and an aminoglycoside, with or without vancomycin (depending on local *S. aureus* resistance patterns). Antibiotics are administered via the catheter and allowed to dwell intraperitoneally. When treatment is complete, the antibiotic effluent is drained via the catheter. If infection continues despite antibiotic treatment, a recurrent infection with the same microbe is likely. If fecal contamination occurs, the catheter must be removed.

Discussion

Controversies and Special Cases

The controversies surrounding the management of intra-abdominal infections are numerous and ongoing, in large part because of the relative lack of well-organized, unbiased clinical evidence. There are several reasons for this information deficit.

First, although in the aggregate, peritonitis is a common problem seen by general surgeons, any given practitioner sees most of the life-threatening forms of the disease (e.g., free perforation from colon cancer) infrequently. Second, advances in nonsurgical medicine and technology (e.g., laparoscopy) have made new forms of treatment available and have improved outcomes from older techniques. As a result, conclusions drawn from older data may no longer be accurate. Third, many forms of intra-abdominal infection routinely present in such a complex and ill patient population (e.g., elderly patients with multiple comorbidities) that randomized studies with multiple exclusion criteria can rarely capture a high percentage of what is a highly heterogeneous group. Fourth, patients presenting with common causes of intra-abdominal infection that occur in relatively healthy and homogeneous populations (e.g., acute appendicitis and cholecystitis) tend to do well no matter what reasonable therapy is applied. Consequently, it is frequently difficult to detect any significant differences between therapeutic modalities. For example, despite multiple randomized trials, it is still unclear whether a laparoscopic approach has any long-term superiority over an open approach in patients with right lower quadrant pain and suspected appendicitis: outcomes are excellent with either method. Finally, for almost any given argument, sufficient supporting data, whether in the form of randomized trials or—equally valuable—of large observational studies performed with statistical rigor, simply do not exist at present. Even simple questions, such as the optimum duration of antibiotic treatment for a patient with a single well-drained liver abscess, lack good answers.

In the end, most controversies in this area are not so much a matter of precisely determining the right or the wrong intervention for a disease as they are a matter of making a judgment about which of many possible interventions is likely to result in the lowest morbidity and mortality. For example, the decision to perform a primary colon reanastomosis in a patient with a perforated colon cancer cannot be considered either universally correct or universally incorrect; rather, it is subject to the surgeon's opinion about the specific patient involved. In what follows, we focus on several controversial decision points and discuss important factors that ought to be considered in attempting to optimize patient care.

NEW CONCEPTS IN PATHOPHYSIOLOGY OF ACUTE BACTERIAL CHOLANGITIS

Longmire's widely accepted classification of acute bacterial cholangitis consists of five categories: acute nonobstructive, acute nonsuppurative, acute suppurative, acute obstructive suppurative, and acute suppurative with intrahepatic abscess. It implies that the severity of disease parallels the degree of obstruction of biliary ducts.[241] This suggestion is well founded. In acute nonobstructive cholangitis associated with acute cholecystitis, infection ascends along the intrahepatic and extrahepatic lymphatics. In obstructive cholangitis, the bile duct contains bacteria under pressure. When the pressure is at or above the normal secretion pressure (i.e., 200 mm Hg), bacteria pass into the lymphatic system. At a pressure greater than 250 mm Hg, bacteria may pass directly from the bile ductules through the spaces of Mall and Disse and into the hepatic sinusoids via cholangiovenous reflux.[242] One study confirmed the clinical significance of increasing ductal pressure by demonstrating a higher ductal pressure and a higher incidence of bacteremia in patients with proximal ductal obstruction, compared with those with distal malignant biliary obstruction.[243] However, no correlation exists between the degree of suppuration in the duct and the clinical or pathologic severity of obstructive cholangitis.[82] Therefore, the terms acute nonsuppurative cholangitis and acute suppurative cholangitis are purely descriptive and do not imply differing degrees of severity.

The source of bacteria in acute cholangitis is most often the duodenum. The ease with which organisms reflux from the duodenum depends on the degree of obstruction. Thus, in patients with malignant biliary obstruction, in whom obstruction is usually complete, bile culture is positive in only 10% to 15% of patients[244]; acute cholangitis is seldom spontaneous in this setting but often follows radiologic intervention.[245] By comparison, in patients with ductal stones or benign strictures, in whom biliary obstruction is often incomplete, bile cultures obtained on ERCP are positive in 64% to 87% of cases; in these patients, acute cholangitis occurs frequently, both spontaneously and after ductal manipulation.[246]

An alternative source of organisms in acute bacterial cholangitis is portal venous blood. In patients who have recurrent pyogenic cholangitis, which occurs frequently in the Far East, a 40% incidence of positive portal blood culture has been reported.[247] In studies of rats with ligated bile ducts, bacteria were shown to be effectively transmitted to the bile ducts and the liver through portal blood.[248] Finally, in nonobstructive cholangitis and acute cholecystitis, as well as in the early stages of obstructive cholangitis, infection ascends to the liver through the lymphatic system.

CHANGING BACTERIOLOGY OF ACUTE BILIARY INFECTION

Most biliary infections are polymicrobial. The organisms most frequently cultured are *E. coli*, *Klebsiella* species, *Enterobacter* species, and enterococci. Anaerobic bacteria are infrequently implicated in biliary infections. Peptostreptococci and clostridia are found occasionally; clostridia are especially common in patients with emphysematous cholecystitis.[47] Gram-negative anaerobic bacilli are rarely present in patients with biliary infection. In one study, only two of 28 patients with acute cholangitis had anaerobic bacteria in the bile; another investigator found anaerobic bacteria in 3% to 4% of cultures in similar patients.[83] However, a higher incidence of anaerobic bacteria has been reported in patients who have acute cholangitis and acute cholecystitis than in patients who have chronic cholecystitis and cholelithiasis.[249]

One investigator noted an increased incidence of anaerobic bacteria in biliary infection and suggested that *B. fragilis* may play a more important role in the polymicrobial flora of biliary tract infection than was previously appreciated.[250] These findings remain controversial. *Bacteroides* species are generally considered to be of limited importance in biliary tract infections, except in selected groups of patients. These groups include diabetics, the elderly,[251] and those with acute cholangitis who have previously undergone biliary operation[252,253]; in particular, malfunctioning biliary-intestinal anastomoses increase the risk of *Bacteroides* infection.[254]

NECESSITY OF DIVERSION AFTER EMERGENCY COLONIC PROCEDURES

The goal of safely repairing or resecting the colon in an emergency setting without leaving a patient with a temporary or permanent stoma for diversion has been pursued for decades. Through much of the 20th century, largely on the basis of wartime experience, diversion was routinely performed. Today, however, it is apparent that this approach is not always necessary either for trauma or for intrinsic colon disease. Thus, the question is no longer whether primary repair or reanastomosis can be achieved safely but, rather, in which individual patient a given treatment is prudent.

Traditionally, clinical studies have attempted to define patient characteristics associated with complications after attempted primary repair or reanastomosis. Not surprisingly, hypotension, blood loss, delay before treatment, and extensive contamination have all been associated with postoperative complications after primary repair; however, these risk factors are associated with complications after diversion as well. The nature of the colon injury is clearly an important consideration: multiple studies now support a one-step approach to traumatic colon injury in all except the most ill patients, but primary resection and reanastomosis for other causes of perforation (e.g., diverticulosis and cancer) remain controversial. Many nonrandomized studies have demonstrated that for nontraumatic causes of perforation, on-table lavage and primary resection yield outcomes equivalent to those of the Hartmann procedure, which suggests that both approaches are safe and that surgeons are capable of identifying the patients best suited to each one.

Perhaps more important than determining how likely a patient is to experience a complication after a given operation, however, is assessing how well the patient is likely to tolerate that complication in the early postoperative period. Thus, elderly patients with multiple comorbidities might be better off undergoing diversion and thus avoiding the potential significant physiologic stress posed by an anastomotic leak in the early postoperative period, even though they will face the additional risk associated with reoperation if they subsequently choose to have a stoma reversed.

ROLE OF LAPAROSCOPY IN MANAGEMENT OF PERITONITIS

Laparoscopy has altered the surgical landscape by offering a minimally invasive approach that reduces the morbidity associated with a large incision, generally decreasing convalescence time and hastening return to normal activity. Nonetheless, laparoscopic management of intra-abdominal infection is still hindered somewhat by the difficulty of inspecting the entire bowel, the decreased tactile sensation, and the significantly greater expertise required for laparoscopic resection and reanastomosis of the bowel. These obstacles notwithstanding, almost every intra-abdominal procedure used to treat infection has been performed laparoscopically with acceptable results.

The single most important factor in the decision whether to take a laparoscopic approach is the skill and experience of the surgeon. From a theoretical point of view, it is almost always possible to treat a patient with peritonitis laparoscopically; the real question is whether the attending surgeon can perform the procedure most safely and efficiently via an open or a minimally invasive approach. The answer to this question will rely to a large extent on preoperative imaging studies. In addition, even if the surgeon does not plan to complete the operation laparoscopically, initial placement of the scope may aid in planning the most appropriate open incision and procedure by localizing the lesion of interest.

MANAGEMENT OF ANASTOMOTIC LEAKS

Dehiscence of a gastrointestinal anastomosis is a common and too frequently fatal complication of modern GI surgery. Again, there is little debate regarding which therapeutic options are available to surgeons managing this problem. The options include the following: supporting the patient with medical care only, in the case of a tiny radiographically evident but clinically insignificant leak seen on fluoroscopic study; reoperating and performing primary repair and drainage, in the case of a small early leak from an enteroenterostomy with minimal soilage; performing percutaneous drainage, in the case of a moderately symptomatic leak presenting in a delayed manner with an abscess; and reexploring and performing a diverting procedure, in the case of complete disruption of an anastomosis with widespread fecal contamination. The only controversy has to do with which course (or combination of courses) to take in an individual patient.

Some general guidelines for the management of anastomotic dehiscence may be recommended, with the caveat that they have not yet been rigorously tested. Leaks diagnosed in the immediate postoperative period are easily approached because the relevant tissue planes have been dissected free. After 1 to 2 weeks, however, early adhesion formation makes reoperation more difficult, especially if the initial operation was for an infectious or inflammatory process, and increases the risk of complications, particularly inadvertent enterotomy and enterocutaneous fistula formation. Small, contained leaks, if accessible, frequently respond to percutaneous drainage and antibiotics alone, with the small fistula resolving spontaneously. Medical management in such cases generally includes TPN, though enteral nutrition is occasionally feasible if it is shown to have no effect on drain output. Larger leaks, on the other hand, are more likely to call for direct operative repair, resection and reanastomosis, or diversion. Once it is decided that surgical treatment is warranted and is not precluded by the state of the abdomen, definitive management should not be delayed. Exactly which operation is to be performed depends on the health of the bowel, the severity of abdominal contamination, and the level of overall physiologic dysfunction.

MANAGEMENT OF ENDOSCOPIC BOWEL PERFORATION

Large rents in a peritoneal portion of the bowel generally call for operative repair (most commonly to the colon), though it should be noted that simple repair or resection without diversion is almost always all that is required. Extraperitoneal or retroperitoneal perforations, however, can be managed nonoperatively with antibiotics and I.V. fluids if the patient is stable. This situation occurs most frequently after ERCP or with low rectal perforations. Typically, CT scanning demonstrates retroperitoneal air with minimal free peritoneal air. In these circumstances, patients can be safely observed as long as their condition does not deteriorate; oral intake can be restarted after 5 to 7 days. Endoscopic perforations of a normal distal esophagus can also be managed nonoperatively, though a perforation proximal to a tumor or stricture is unlikely to heal and almost always must be treated operatively.

NONOPERATIVE MANAGEMENT OF INFECTED FLUID COLLECTIONS

It is axiomatic that abscesses are best treated with drainage rather than with antibiotics, but there are certain circumstances in which drainage may not be possible. Pyogenic liver abscesses may not be amenable to either percutaneous or open drainage if they are multiple and involve both lobes. In such circumstances, aspiration or drainage of the largest abscess, followed by a long course of antibiotics, is generally successful. It has been argued that this approach works because of the liver's luxurious dual blood supply.

On the other hand, multiple peritoneal fluid collections (without a natural blood supply) are not infrequently seen even after successful management of diffuse or fecal peritonitis yet can occasionally be managed without drainage. Even if these collections are subsequently proved to be infected, they may be too numerous to approach percutaneously, and ongoing inflammation of the bowel may render an operative approach unsafe. Again, drainage of the largest accessible collection to establish a diagnosis and guide antibiotic management, followed by long-term antibiotic therapy, is the most feasible course. In this case, sampling is imperative because a hospital-acquired intra-abdominal infection is more likely to involve less common but more resistant pathogens, including fungi. Regardless of the situation, though, the optimal duration of antibiotic therapy for small undrained abscesses remains to be established.

ADJUNCTIVE MEDICAL THERAPIES

Until recently, it could be said that advances in surgical therapy for intra-abdominal infection were outpacing other aspects of patient management. Too often, operations were technically successful, yet patients died afterward as a result of their systemic response to the original insult. Such deaths are still attributed to overwhelming sepsis, to multiple organ dysfunction syndrome, or to any number of other terms used to describe an irreversible sequence of organ failure and death [see 6:13 Multiple Organ Dysfunction Syndrome].

Multiple attempts over the years to alter this downward trajectory by using novel therapies to target this generalized inflammatory response proved unsuccessful. In the past few years, however, both recombinant human activated protein C and corticosteroid replacement therapy (for those with sepsis-associated adrenal insufficiency) were shown to improve survival in randomized, placebo-controlled trials involving mixed populations of patients with sepsis. Although the number of patients with intra-abdominal infection was relatively small in each study, there was no indication that these agents would not be similarly effective in this specific subgroup. The overall benefit of each of these treatments appears to be small, but the results of these trials are highly encouraging in that they suggest that related agents might be able to achieve further decreases in mortality. These possibilities, combined with significant improvements in general critical care, portend a future in which significant reductions in mortality may be realized even in the most severely infected patients.

References

1. Schofield PF, Hulton NR, Baildam AD: Is it acute cholecystitis? Ann R Coll Surg Engl 68:14, 1986
2. Ranson JH: Acute pancreatitis. Curr Probl Surg 16:1, 1979
3. Winslet M, Hall C, London NJ, et al: Relation of diagnostic serum amylase levels to aetiology and severity of acute pancreatitis. Gut 33:982, 1992
4. Patti M, Pellegrini CA, Way LW: Serum amylase is useful in the differential diagnosis of acute abdominal pain. Gastroenterology 90:1580, 1986
5. Yadav D, Agarwal N, Pitchumoni CS: A critical evaluation of laboratory tests in acute pancreatitis. Am J Gastroenterol 97:1309, 2002
6. Smotkin J, Tenner S: Laboratory diagnostic tests in acute pancreatitis. J Clin Gastroenterol 34:459, 2002
7. Toosie K, Chang L, Renslo R, et al: Early computed tomography is rarely necessary in gallstone pancreatitis. Am Surg 63:904, 1997
8. Sarr MG, Sanfey H, Cameron JL: Prospective, randomized trial of nasogastric suction in patients with acute pancreatitis. Surgery 100:500, 1986
9. Bradley EL 3rd: Antibiotics in acute pancreatitis: current status and future directions. Am J Surg 158:472, 1989
10. Steinberg WM, Schlesselman SE: Treatment of acute pancreatitis: comparison of animal and human studies. Gastroenterology 93:1420, 1987
11. McArdle AH, Rosenberg M, Fried GM, et al: Pancreatic exocrine secretion in response to continuous and bolus feeding (abstract), 19th Annual Meeting, Association for Academic Surgery, Cincinnati, Ohio, 1985
12. Erstad BL: Enteral nutrition support in acute pancreatitis. Ann Pharmacother 34:514, 2000
13. Scolapio JS, Malhi-Chowla N, Ukleja A: Nutrition supplementation in patients with acute and chronic pancreatitis. Gastroenterol Clin North Am 28:695, 1999
14. Windsor AC, Kanwar S, Li AG, et al: Compared with parenteral nutrition, enteral feeding attenuates the acute phase response and improves disease severity in acute pancreatitis. Gut 42:431, 1998
15. Chatzicostas C, Roussomoustakaki M, Vardas E, et al: Balthazar computed tomography severity index is superior to Ranson criteria and APACHE II and III scoring systems in predicting acute pancreatitis outcome. J Clin Gastroenterol 36:253, 2003
16. Liu TH, Kwong KL, Tamm EP, et al: Acute pancreatitis in intensive care unit patients: value of clinical and radiologic prognosticators at predicting clinical course and outcome. Crit Care Med 31:1026, 2003
17. Stone HH, Fabian TC, Dunlop WE: Gallstone pancreatitis: biliary tract pathology in relation to time of operation. Ann Surg 194:305, 1981
18. Acosta JM, Rossi R, Galli OM, et al: Early surgery for acute gallstone pancreatitis: evaluation of a systematic approach. Surgery 83:367, 1978
19. Kelly TR: Gallstone pancreatitis: the timing of surgery. Surgery 88:345, 1980
20. Dixon JA, Hillam JD: Surgical treatment of biliary tract disease associated with acute pancreatitis. Am J Surg 120:371, 1970
21. Ranson JH: The timing of biliary surgery in acute pancreatitis. Ann Surg 189:654, 1979
22. Paloyan D, Simonowitz D, Skinner DB: The timing of biliary tract operations in patients with pancreatitis associated with gallstones. Surg Gynecol Obstet 141:737, 1975
23. Kelly TR, Wagner DS: Gallstone pancreatitis: a prospective randomized trial of the timing of surgery. Surgery 104:600, 1988
24. Neoptolemos JP, Carr-Locke DL, London NJ, et al: Controlled trial of urgent endoscopic retrograde cholangiopancreatography and endoscopic sphincterotomy versus conservative treatment for acute pancreatitis due to gallstones. Lancet 2:979, 1988
25. Fan ST, Lai EC, Mok FP, et al: Early treatment of acute biliary pancreatitis by endoscopic papillotomy. N Engl J Med 328:228, 1993
26. Williamson RC: Early assessment of severity in acute pancreatitis. Gut 25:1331, 1984
27. Srinathan SK, Barkun JS, Mehta SN, et al: The management of gallstone pancreatitis in the laparoscopic era. J Gastrointest Surg (in press)
28. Ranson JH, Spencer FC: Prevention, diagnosis, and treatment of pancreatic abscess. Surgery 82:99, 1977
29. Osborne DH, Imrie CW, Carter DC: Biliary surgery in the same admission for gallstone-associated acute pancreatitis. Br J Surg 68:758, 1981
30. Folsch UR, Nitsche R, Ludtke R, et al: Early ERCP and papillotomy compared with conservative treatment for acute biliary pancreatitis. The German Study Group on Acute Biliary Pancreatitis. N Engl J Med 336:237, 1997
31. Chang L, Lo S, Stabile BE, et al: Preoperative versus postoperative endoscopic retrograde cholangiopancreatography in mild to moderate gallstone pancreatitis: a prospective randomized trial. Ann Surg 231:82, 2000
32. Nitsche R, Folsch UR, Ludtke R, et al: Urgent ERCP in all cases of acute biliary pancreatitis? A prospective randomized multicenter study. Eur J Med Res 1:127, 1995
33. Kozarek RA, Patterson DJ, Ball TJ, et al: Endoscopic placement of pancreatic stents and drains in the management of pancreatitis. Ann Surg 209:261, 1989
34. Ranson JH, Berman RS: Long peritoneal lavage decreases pancreatic sepsis in acute pancreatitis. Ann Surg 211:708, 1990
35. Pederzoli P, Bassi C, Vesentini S, et al: A randomized multicenter clinical trial of antibiotic prophylaxis of septic complications in acute necrotizing pancreatitis with imipenem. Surg Gynecol Obstet 176:480, 1993
36. Luiten EJ, Hop WC, Lange JF, et al: Controlled clinical trial of selective decontamination for the

treatment of severe acute pancreatitis. Ann Surg 222:57, 1995

37. Sharma VK, Howden CW: Prophylactic antibiotic administration reduces sepsis and mortality in acute necrotizing pancreatitis: a meta-analysis. Pancreas 22:28, 2001

38. Golub R, Siddiqi F, Pohl D: Role of antibiotics in acute pancreatitis: a meta-analysis. J Gastrointest Surg 2:496, 1998

39. Uhl W, Warshaw A, Imrie C, et al: IAP Guidelines for the Surgical Management of Acute Pancreatitis. Pancreatology 2:565, 2002

40. Howard TJ, Temple MB: Prophylactic antibiotics alter the bacteriology of infected necrosis in severe acute pancreatitis. J Am Coll Surg 195:759, 2002

41. Fiedler F, Jauernig G, Keim V, et al: Octreotide treatment in patients with necrotizing pancreatitis and pulmonary failure. Intensive Care Med 22:909, 1996

42. Paran H, Neufeld D, Mayo A, et al: Preliminary report of a prospective randomized study of octreotide in the treatment of severe acute pancreatitis. J Am Coll Surg 181:121, 1995

43. de Souza LJ, Sampietre SN, Assis RS, et al: Effect of platelet-activating factor antagonists (BN-52021, WEB-2170, and BB-882) on bacterial translocation in acute pancreatitis. J Gastrointest Surg 5:364, 2001

44. Lane JS, Todd KE, Gloor B, et al: Platelet activating factor antagonism reduces the systemic inflammatory response in a murine model of acute pancreatitis. J Surg Res 99:365, 2001

45. Kingsnorth AN, Galloway SW, Formela LJ: Randomized, double-blind phase II trial of lexipafant, a platelet-activating factor antagonist, in human acute pancreatitis. Br J Surg 82:1414, 1995

46. Johnson CD, Kingsnorth AN, Imrie CW, et al: Double blind, randomised, placebo controlled study of a platelet activating factor antagonist, lexipafant, in the treatment and prevention of organ failure in predicted severe acute pancreatitis. Gut 48:62, 2001

47. Mentzer RM Jr, Golden GT, Chandler JG, et al: A comparative appraisal of emphysematous cholecystitis. Am J Surg 129:10, 1975

48. Turner RJ 3rd, Becker WF, Coleman WO, et al: Acute cholecystitis in the diabetic. South Med J 62:228, 1969

49. Turrill RL: Gallstones and diabetes: an ominous association. Am J Surg 102:184, 1961

50. Walsh DB, Eckhauser FE, Ramsburgh SR, et al: Risk associated with diabetes mellitus in patients undergoing gallbladder surgery. Surgery 91:254, 1982

51. Pickleman J: Controversies in biliary tract surgery. Can J Surg 29:429, 1986

52. Weissmann HS, Berkowitz D, Fox MS, et al: The role of technetium-99m iminodiacetic acid (IDA) cholescintigraphy in acute acalculous cholecystitis. Radiology 146:177, 1983

53. Chen CC, Holder LE, Maunoury C, et al: Morphine augmentation increases gallbladder visualization in patients pretreated with cholecystokinin. J Nucl Med 38:644, 1997

54. Cabana MD, Alavi A, Berlin JA, et al: Morphine-augmented hepatobiliary scintigraphy: a meta-analysis. Nucl Med Commun 16:1068, 1995

55. Lo CM, Liu CL, Fan ST, et al: Prospective randomized study of early versus delayed laparoscopic cholecystectomy for acute cholecystitis. Ann Surg 227:461, 1998

56. Koc M, Zulfikaroglu B, Kece C, et al: A prospective randomized study of prophylactic antibiotics in elective laparoscopic cholecystectomy. Surg Endosc, June 17, 2003, Epub

57. Higgins A, London J, Charland S, et al: Prophylactic antibiotics for elective laparoscopic cholecystectomy: are they necessary? Arch Surg 134:611, 1999

58. Illig KA, Schmidt E, Cavanaugh J, et al: Are prophylactic antibiotics required for elective laparoscopic cholecystectomy? J Am Coll Surg 184:353, 1997

59. Karachalios GN, Nasiopoulou DD, Bourlinou PK, et al: Treatment of acute biliary tract infections with ofloxacin: a randomized, controlled clinical trial. Int J Clin Pharmacol Ther 34:555, 1996

60. Krajden S, Yaman M, Fuksa M, et al: Piperacillin versus cefazolin given perioperatively to high-risk patients who undergo open cholecystectomy: a double-blind, randomized trial. Can J Surg 36:245, 1993

61. Skillings JC, Kumai C, Hinshaw JR: Cholecystostomy: a place in modern biliary surgery? Am J Surg 139:865, 1980

62. Klimberg S, Hawkins I, Vogel SB: Percutaneous cholecystostomy for acute cholecystitis in high-risk patients. Am J Surg 153:125, 1987

63. Miyazaki K, Uchiyama A, Nakayama F: New approach to the timing of operative intervention for acute cholecystitis: use of ultrasound risk score (abstr). 32nd World Conference of Surgery, Sydney, Australia, September 20–26, 1987

64. England RE, McDermott VG, Smith TP, et al: Percutaneous cholecystostomy: who responds? AJR Am J Roentgenol 168:1247, 1997

65. Orlando R 3rd, Crowell KL: Laparoscopy in the critically ill. Surg Endosc 11:1072, 1997

66. Reynolds BM, Dargan EL: Acute obstructive cholangitis: a distinct clinical syndrome. Ann Surg 150:299, 1959

67. Baer HU, Matthews JB, Schweizer WP, et al: Management of the Mirizzi syndrome and the surgical implications of cholecystcholedochal fistula. Br J Surg 77:743, 1990

68. Textor HJ, Flacke S, Pauleit D, et al: Three-dimensional magnetic resonance cholangiopancreatography with respiratory triggering in the diagnosis of primary sclerosing cholangitis: comparison with endoscopic retrograde cholangiography. Endoscopy 34:984, 2002

69. Ferrara C, Valeri G, Salvolini L, et al: Magnetic resonance cholangiopancreatography in primary sclerosing cholangitis in children. Pediatr Radiol 32:413, 2002

70. Chen JH, Chai JW, Chu WC, et al: Free breathing magnetic resonance cholangiopancreatography (MRCP) at end expiration: a new technique to expand clinical application. Hepatogastroenterology 49:593, 2002

71. Matos C, Nicaise N, Deviere J, et al: Choledochal cysts: comparison of findings at MR cholangiopancreatography and endoscopic retrograde cholangiopancreatography in eight patients. Radiology 209:443, 1998

72. Gerecht WB, Henry NK, Hoffman WW, et al: Prospective randomized comparison of mezlocillin therapy alone with combined ampicillin and gentamicin therapy for patients with cholangitis. Arch Intern Med 149:1279, 1989

73. Thompson JN, Edwards WH, Winearls CG, et al: Renal impairment following biliary tract surgery. Br J Surg 74:843, 1987

74. Thompson JE Jr, Pitt HA, Doty JE, et al: Broad spectrum penicillin as an adequate therapy for acute cholangitis. Surg Gynecol Obstet 171:275, 1990

75. Muller EL, Pitt HA, Thompson JE Jr, et al: Antibiotics in infections of the biliary tract. Surg Gynecol Obstet 165:285, 1987

76. Pitt HA, Postier RG, Cameron JL: Consequences of preoperative cholangitis and its treatment on the outcome of operation for choledocholithiasis. Surgery 94:447, 1983

77. Leung JW, Chung SC, Sung JJ, et al: Urgent endoscopic drainage for acute suppurative cholangitis. Lancet 1:1307, 1989

78. Lomanto D, Pavone P, Laghi A, et al: Magnetic resonance-cholangiopancreatography in the diagnosis of biliopancreatic diseases. Am J Surg 174:33, 1997

79. Becker CD, Grossholz M, Mentha G, et al: MR cholangiopancreatography: technique, potential indications, and diagnostic features of benign, postoperative, and malignant conditions. Eur Radiol 7:865, 1997

80. Gigot JF, Leese T, Dereme T, et al: Acute cholangitis: multivariate analysis of risk factors. Ann Surg 209:435, 1989

81. Lai EC, Tam PC, Paterson IA, et al: Emergency surgery for severe acute cholangitis: the high-risk patients. Ann Surg 211:55, 1990

82. O'Connor MJ, Schwartz ML, McQuarrie DG, et al: Acute bacterial cholangitis: an analysis of clinical manifestation. Arch Surg 117:437, 1982

83. Thompson JE Jr, Tompkins RK, Longmire WP Jr: Factors in management of acute cholangitis. Ann Surg 195:137, 1982

84. Bismuth H, Kuntziger H, Corlette MB: Cholangitis with acute renal failure: priorities in therapeutics. Ann Surg 181:881, 1975

85. Cho SR, Turner MA: Hepatic abscesses due to suppurative cholangitis. South Med J 75:488, 1982

86. Gould RJ, Vogelzang RL, Neiman HL, et al: Percutaneous biliary drainage as an initial therapy in sepsis of the biliary tract. Surg Gynecol Obstet 160:523, 1985

87. Leese T, Neoptolemos JP, Baker AR, et al: Management of acute cholangitis and the impact of endoscopic sphincterotomy. Br J Surg 73:988, 1986

88. Davis AJ, Kolios G, Alveyn CG, et al: Antibiotic prophylaxis for ERCP: a comparison of oral ciprofloxacin with intravenous cephazolin in the prophylaxis of high-risk patients. Aliment Pharmacol Ther 12:207, 1998

89. Saini S: Imaging of the hepatobiliary tract. N Engl J Med 336:1889, 1997

90. Bearcroft PW, Miles KA: Leucocyte scintigraphy or computed tomography for the febrile postoperative patient? Eur J Radiol 23:126, 1996

91. Haque R, Ali IK, Akther S, et al: Comparison of PCR, isoenzyme analysis, and antigen detection for diagnosis of Entamoeba histolytica infection. J Clin Microbiol 36:449, 1998

92. Auer H, Picher O, Aspock H: Combined application of enzyme-linked immunosorbent assay (ELISA) and indirect haemagglutination test (IHA) as a useful tool for the diagnosis and postoperative surveillance of human alveolar and cystic echinococcosis. Zentralbl Bakteriol Mikrobiol Hyg [A] 270:313, 1988

93. Force L, Torres JM, Carrillo A, et al: Evaluation of eight serological tests in the diagnosis of human echinococcosis and follow-up. Clin Infect Dis 15:473, 1992

94. Aeder MI, Wellman JL, Haaga JR, et al: Role of surgical and percutaneous drainage in the treatment of abdominal abscesses. Arch Surg 118:273, 1983

95. Ch Yu S, Hg Lo R, Kan PS, et al: Pyogenic liver abscess: treatment with needle aspiration. Clin Radiol 52:912, 1997

96. Giorgio A, Tarantino L, Mariniello N, et al: Pyogenic liver abscesses: 13 years of experience in percutaneous needle aspiration with US guidance. Radiology 195:122, 1995

97. Rajak CL, Gupta S, Jain S, et al: Percutaneous treatment of liver abscesses: needle aspiration versus catheter drainage. AJR Am J Roentgenol 170:1035, 1998

98. Gerzof SG, Johnson WC, Robbins AH, et al: Intrahepatic pyogenic abscesses: treatment by percutaneous drainage. Am J Surg 149:487, 1985

99. Seeto RK, Rockey DC: Pyogenic liver abscess: changes in etiology, management, and outcome. Medicine (Baltimore) 75:99, 1996

100. Herman P, Pugliese V, Montagnini AL, et al: Pyogenic liver abscess: the role of surgical treatment. Int Surg 82:98, 1997

101. Klatchko BA, Schwartz SI: Diagnostic and therapeutic approaches to pyogenic abscess of the liver. Surg Gynecol Obstet 168:332, 1989

102. Gyorffy EJ, Frey CF, Silva J Jr, et al: Pyogenic liver abscess: diagnostic and therapeutic strategies. Ann Surg 206:699, 1987

103. Sabbaj J, Sutter VL, Finegold SM: Anaerobic pyogenic liver abscess. Ann Intern Med 77:627, 1972

104. Huang CJ, Pitt HA, Lipsett PA, et al: Pyogenic hepatic abscess: changing trends over 42 years. Ann Surg 223:600, 1996

105. Schein M, Wittmann DH, Lorenz W: Duration of antibiotic treatment in surgical infections of the abdomen. Forum statement: a plea for selective and controlled postoperative antibiotic administration. Eur J Surg Suppl (576):66, 1996

106. Rubin RH, Swartz MN, Malt R: Hepatic abscess: changes in clinical, bacteriologic and therapeutic aspects. Am J Med 57:601, 1974

107. Yeh TS, Jan YY, Jeng LB, et al: Pyogenic liver abscesses in patients with malignant disease: a report of 52 cases treated at a single institution. Arch Surg 133:242, 1998

108. Cohen HG, Reynolds TB: Comparison of metronidazole and chloroquine for the treatment of amoebic liver abscess: a controlled trial. Gastroenterology 69:35, 1975

109. Turkcapar AG, Ersoz S, Gungor C, et al: Surgical treatment of hepatic hydatidosis combined with perioperative treatment with albendazole. Eur J Surg 163:923, 1997

110. Saimot AG: Medical treatment of liver hydatidosis. World J Surg 25:15, 2001

111. Stiles GM, Berne TV, Thommen VD, et al: Fine needle aspiration of pancreatic fluid collections. Am Surg 56:764, 1990

112. Bittner R, Block S, Buchler M, et al: Pancreatic abscess and infected pancreatic necrosis. Different local septic complications in acute pancreatitis. Dig Dis Sci 32:1082, 1987

113. Banks PA, Gerzof SG, Chong FK, et al: Bacteriologic status of necrotic tissue in necrotizing pancreatitis. Pancreas 5:330, 1990

114. Crass RA, Meyer AA, Jeffrey RB, et al: Pancreatic abscess: impact of computerized tomography on early diagnosis and surgery. Am J Surg 150:127, 1985

115. Buchler M, Malfertheiner P, Schoetensack C, et al: Sensitivity of antiproteases, complement factors and C-reactive protein in detecting pancreatic necrosis: results of a prospective clinical study. Int J Pancreatol 1:227, 1986

116. Ranson JH, Balthazar E, Caccavale R, et al: Computed tomography and the prediction of pancreatic abscess in acute pancreatitis. Ann Surg 201:656, 1985

117. Bradley EL 3rd, Allen K: A prospective longitudinal study of observation versus surgical intervention in the management of necrotizing pancreatitis. Am J Surg 161:19, 1991

118. Warshaw AL: Pancreatic abscesses. N Engl J Med 287:1234, 1972

119. Frey CF, Lindenauer SM, Miller TA: Pancreatic abscess. Surg Gynecol Obstet 149:722, 1979

120. Hedderich GS, Wexler MJ, McLean AP, et al: The septic abdomen: open management with Marlex mesh with a zipper. Surgery 99:399, 1986

121. D'Egidio A, Schein M: Surgical strategies in the treatment of pancreatic necrosis and infection. Br J Surg 78:133, 1991

122. Stanten R, Frey CF: Comprehensive management of acute necrotizing pancreatitis and pancreatic abscess. Arch Surg 125:1269, 1990

123. Rotman N, Mathieu D, Anglade MC, et al: Failure of percutaneous drainage of pancreatic abscesses complicating severe acute pancreatitis. Surg Gynecol Obstet 174:141, 1992

124. Lang EK, Paolini RM, Pottmeyer A: The efficacy of palliative and definitive percutaneous versus surgical drainage of pancreatic abscesses and pseudocysts: a prospective study of 85 patients. South Med J 84:55, 1991

125. Williams LF Jr, Byrne JJ: The role of bacteria in hemorrhagic pancreatitis. Surgery 64:967, 1968

126. Gregg JA: Detection of bacterial infection of the pancreatic ducts in patients with pancreatitis and pancreatic cancer during endoscopic cannulation of the pancreatic duct. Gastroenterology 73:1005, 1977

127. Farkas G, Marton J, Mandy Y, et al: Surgical strategy and management of infected pancreatic necrosis. Br J Surg 83:930, 1996

128. Grant JP, James S, Grabowski V, et al: Total parenteral nutrition in pancreatic disease. Ann Surg 200:627, 1984

129. Johnson JD, Raff MJ, Drasin GF, et al: Radiology in the diagnosis of splenic abscess. Rev Infect Dis 7:10, 1985

130. Sones PJ: Percutaneous drainage of abdominal abscesses. AJR Am J Roentgenol 142:35, 1984

131. Berkman WA, Harris SA Jr, Bernardino ME: Nonsurgical drainage of splenic abscess. AJR Am J Roentgenol 141:395, 1983

132. Espinoza R, Rodriguez A: Traumatic and nontraumatic perforation of hollow viscera. Surg Clin North Am 77:1291, 1997

133. Ng EK, Lam YH, Sung JJ, et al: Eradication of Helicobacter pylori prevents recurrence of ulcer after simple closure of duodenal ulcer perforation: randomized controlled trial. Ann Surg 231:153, 2000

134. Tokunaga Y, Hata K, Ryo J, et al: Density of Helicobacter pylori infection in patients with peptic ulcer perforation. J Am Coll Surg 186:659, 1998

135. Matsukura N, Onda M, Tokunaga A, et al: Role of Helicobacter pylori infection in perforation of peptic ulcer: an age- and gender-matched case-control study. J Clin Gastroenterol 25(suppl 1):S235, 1997

136. Feliciano DV, Ojukwu JC, Rozycki GS, et al: The epidemic of cocaine-related juxtapyloric perforations: with a comment on the importance of testing for Helicobacter pylori. Ann Surg 229:801, 1999

137. Cho KC, Baker SR: Extraluminal air: diagnosis and significance. Radiol Clin North Am 32:829, 1994

138. Berne TV, Donovan AJ: Nonoperative treatment of perforated duodenal ulcer. Arch Surg 124:830, 1989

139. Crofts TJ, Park KG, Steele RJ, et al: A randomized trial of nonoperative treatment for perforated peptic ulcer. N Engl J Med 320:970, 1989

140. Donovan AJ, Berne TV, Donovan JA: Perforated duodenal ulcer: an alternative therapeutic plan. Arch Surg 133:1166, 1998

141. Siu WT, Leong HT, Law BK, et al: Laparoscopic repair for perforated peptic ulcer: a randomized controlled trial. Ann Surg 235:313, 2002

142. Lau WY, Leung KL, Kwong KH, et al: A randomized study comparing laparoscopic versus open repair of perforated peptic ulcer using suture or sutureless technique. Ann Surg 224:131, 1996

143. Feliciano DV: Do perforated duodenal ulcers need an acid-decreasing surgical procedure now that omeprazole is available? Surg Clin North Am 72:369, 1992

144. Christiansen J, Andersen OB, Bonnesen T, et al: Perforated duodenal ulcer managed by simple closure versus closure and proximal gastric vagotomy. Br J Surg 74:286, 1987

145. Boey J, Branicki FJ, Alagaratnam TT, et al: Proximal gastric vagotomy: the preferred operation for perforations in acute duodenal ulcer. Ann Surg 208:169, 1988

146. Sebastian M, Chandran VP, Elashaal YI, et al: Helicobacter pylori infection in perforated peptic ulcer disease. Br J Surg 82:360, 1995

147. Kate V, Ananthakrishnan N, Badrinath S: Effect of Helicobacter pylori eradication on the ulcer recurrence rate after simple closure of perforated duodenal ulcer: retrospective and prospective randomized controlled studies. Br J Surg 88:1054, 2001

148. Kauffman GL Jr: Duodenal ulcer disease: treatment by surgery, antibiotics, or both. Adv Surg 34:121, 2000

149. Ruddell WS, Axon AT, Findlay JM, et al: Effect of cimetidine on the gastric bacterial flora. Lancet 1:672, 1980

150. Hosking SW, Ling TK, Chung SC, et al: Duodenal ulcer healing by eradication of Helicobacter pylori without anti-acid treatment: randomised controlled trial. Lancet 343:508, 1994

151. Sung JJ, Leung WK, Suen R, et al: One-week antibiotics versus maintenance acid suppression therapy for Helicobacter pylori–associated peptic ulcer bleeding. Dig Dis Sci 42:2524, 1997

152. Sung JJ, Chung SC, Ling TK, et al: Antibacterial treatment of gastric ulcers associated with Helicobacter pylori. N Engl J Med 332:139, 1995

153. Wisner DH, Chun Y, Blaisdell FW: Blunt intestinal injury: keys to diagnosis and management. Arch Surg 125:1319, 1990

154. Fakhry SM, Watts DD, Luchette FA: Current diagnostic approaches lack sensitivity in the diagnosis of perforated blunt small bowel injury: analysis from 275,557 trauma admissions from the EAST multi-institutional HVI trial. J Trauma 54:295, 2003

155. Malhotra AK, Fabian TC, Katsis SB, et al: Blunt bowel and mesenteric injuries: the role of screening computed tomography. J Trauma 48:991, 2000

156. Lautenbach E, Berlin JA, Lichtenstein GR: Risk factors for early postoperative recurrence of Crohn's disease. Gastroenterology 115:259, 1998

157. Walker AP, Krepel CJ, Gohr CM, et al: Microflora of abdominal sepsis by locus of infection. J Clin Microbiol 32:557, 1994

158. Mazuski JE, Sawyer RG, Nathens AB, et al: The Surgical Infection Society guidelines on antimicrobial therapy for intra-abdominal infections: an executive summary. Surg Infect (Larchmt) 3:161, 2002

159. Reynolds SL: Missed appendicitis in a pediatric emergency department. Pediatr Emerg Care 9:1, 1993

160. Rothrock SG, Green SM, Dobson M, et al: Misdiagnosis of appendicitis in nonpregnant women of childbearing age. J Emerg Med 13:1, 1995

161. Izbicki JR, Knoefel WT, Wilker DK, et al: Accurate diagnosis of acute appendicitis: a retrospective and prospective analysis of 686 patients. Eur J Surg 158:227, 1992

162. Rao PM, Rhea JT, Rattner DW, et al: Intro-

duction of appendiceal CT: impact on negative appendectomy and appendiceal perforation rates. Ann Surg 229:344, 1999

163. Rao PM, Boland GW: Imaging of acute right lower abdominal quadrant pain. Clin Radiol 53:639, 1998

164. Rao PM, Rhea JT, Novelline RA, et al: The computed tomography appearance of recurrent and chronic appendicitis. Am J Emerg Med 16:26, 1998

165. Rao PM, Rhea JT, Novelline RA: Sensitivity and specificity of the individual CT signs of appendicitis: experience with 200 helical appendiceal CT examinations. J Comput Assist Tomogr 21:686, 1997

166. Rao PM, Rhea JT, Novelline RA, et al: Effect of computed tomography of the appendix on treatment of patients and use of hospital resources. N Engl J Med 338:141, 1998

167. Walker S, Haun W, Clark J, et al: The value of limited computed tomography with rectal contrast in the diagnosis of acute appendicitis. Am J Surg 180:450, 2000

168. Rao PM, Feltmate CM, Rhea JT, et al: Helical computed tomography in differentiating appendicitis and acute gynecologic conditions. Obstet Gynecol 93:417, 1999

169. Wilson EB, Cole JC, Nipper ML, et al: Computed tomography and ultrasonography in the diagnosis of appendicitis: when are they indicated? Arch Surg 136:670, 2001

170. Long KH, Bannon MP, Zietlow SP, et al: A prospective randomized comparison of laparoscopic appendectomy with open appendectomy: clinical and economic analyses. Surgery 129:390, 2001

171. Pedersen AG, Petersen OB, Wara P, et al: Randomized clinical trial of laparoscopic versus open appendectomy. Br J Surg 88:200, 2001

172. Ortega AE, Hunter JG, Peters JH, et al: A prospective, randomized comparison of laparoscopic appendectomy with open appendectomy. Laparoscopic Appendectomy Study Group. Am J Surg 169:208, 1995

173. Frazee RC, Roberts JW, Symmonds RE, et al: A prospective randomized trial comparing open versus laparoscopic appendectomy. Ann Surg 219:725, 1994

174. Katkhouda N, Friedlander MH, Grant SW, et al: Intraabdominal abscess rate after laparoscopic appendectomy. Am J Surg 180:456, 2000

175. Krisher SL, Browne A, Dibbins A, et al: Intraabdominal abscess after laparoscopic appendectomy for perforated appendicitis. Arch Surg 136:438, 2001

176. Larsson PG, Henriksson G, Olsson M, et al: Laparoscopy reduces unnecessary appendicectomies and improves diagnosis in fertile women: a randomized study. Surg Endosc 15:200, 2001

177. Enochsson L, Hellberg A, Rudberg C, et al: Laparoscopic vs open appendectomy in overweight patients. Surg Endosc 15:387, 2001

178. Horwitz JR, Custer MD, May BH, et al: Should laparoscopic appendectomy be avoided for complicated appendicitis in children? J Pediatr Surg 32:1601, 1997

179. Oliak D, Yamini D, Udani VM, et al: Initial nonoperative management for periappendiceal abscess. Dis Colon Rectum 44:936, 2001

180. Tingstedt B, Bexe-Lindskog E, Ekelund M, et al: Management of appendiceal masses. Eur J Surg 168:579, 2002

181. Mazziotti MV, Marley EF, Winthrop AL, et al: Histopathologic analysis of interval appendectomy specimens: support for the role of interval appendectomy. J Pediatr Surg 32:806, 1997

182. Hoffmann J, Lindhard A, Jensen HE: Appendix mass: conservative management without interval appendectomy. Am J Surg 148:379, 1984

183. Samuel M, Hosie G, Holmes K: Prospective evaluation of nonsurgical versus surgical management of appendiceal mass. J Pediatr Surg 37:882, 2002

184. Lasson A, Lundagards J, Loren I, et al: Appendiceal abscesses: primary percutaneous drainage and selective interval appendicectomy. Eur J Surg 168:264, 2002

185. Lidar Z, Kuriansky J, Rosin D, et al: Laparoscopic interval appendectomy for periappendicular abscess. Surg Endosc 14:764, 2000

186. Bennion RS, Baron EJ, Thompson JE Jr, et al: The bacteriology of gangrenous and perforated appendicitis—revisited. Ann Surg 211:165, 1990

187. Bennion RS, Thompson JE, Baron EJ, et al: Gangrenous and perforated appendicitis with peritonitis: treatment and bacteriology. Clin Ther 12(suppl C):31, 1990

188. Bilik R, Burnweit C, Shandling B: Is abdominal cavity culture of any value in appendicitis? Am J Surg 175:267, 1998

189. Ferzoco LB, Raptopoulos V, Silen W: Acute diverticulitis. N Engl J Med 338:1521, 1998

190. Bauer T, Vennits B, Holm B, et al: Antibiotic prophylaxis in acute nonperforated appendicitis. The Danish Multicenter Study Group III. Ann Surg 209:307, 1989

191. Liberman MA, Greason KL, Frame S, et al: Single-dose cefotetan or cefoxitin versus multiple-dose cefoxitin as prophylaxis in patients undergoing appendectomy for acute nonperforated appendicitis. J Am Coll Surg 180:77, 1995

192. Salam IM, Abu Galala KH, el Ashaal YI, et al: A randomized prospective study of cefoxitin versus piperacillin in appendicectomy. J Hosp Infect 26:133, 1994

193. Rice HE, Brown RL, Gollin G, et al: Results of a pilot trial comparing prolonged intravenous antibiotics with sequential intravenous/oral antibiotics for children with perforated appendicitis. Arch Surg 136:1391, 2001

194. Gorecki WJ, Grochowski JA: Are antibiotics necessary in nonperforated appendicitis in children? A double blind randomized controlled trial. Med Sci Monit 7:289, 2001

195. Almqvist P, Leandoer L, Tornqvist A: Timing of antibiotic treatment in non-perforated gangrenous appendicitis. Eur J Surg 161:431, 1995

196. Ahn SH, Mayo-Smith WW, Murphy BL, et al: Acute nontraumatic abdominal pain in adult patients: abdominal radiography compared with CT evaluation. Radiology 225:159, 2002

197. Tsushima Y, Yamada S, Aoki J, et al: Effect of contrast-enhanced computed tomography on diagnosis and management of acute abdomen in adults. Clin Radiol 57:507, 2002

198. Rodkey GV, Welch CE: Surgical management of colonic diverticulitis with free perforation or abscess formation. Am J Surg 117:265, 1969

199. Byrne JJ, Garick EI: Surgical treatment of diverticulitis. Am J Surg 121:379, 1971

200. Graves HA Jr, Franklin RM, Robbins LB 2nd, et al: Surgical management of perforated diverticulitis of the colon. Am Surg 39:142, 1973

201. Hinchey EJ, Schaal PG, Richards GK: Treatment of perforated diverticular disease of the colon. Adv Surg 12:85, 1978

202. Kohler L, Sauerland S, Neugebauer E: Diagnosis and treatment of diverticular disease: results of a consensus development conference. The Scientific Committee of the European Association for Endoscopic Surgery. Surg Endosc 13:430, 1999

203. Farthmann EH, Ruckauer KD, Haring RU: Evidence-based surgery: diverticulitis—a surgical disease? Langenbecks Arch Surg 385:143, 2000

204. Wong WD, Wexner SD, Lowry A, et al: Practice parameters for the treatment of sigmoid diverticulitis—supporting documentation. The Standards Task Force. The American Society of Colon and Rectal Surgeons. Dis Colon Rectum 43:290, 2000

205. Ambrosetti P, Robert J, Witzig JA, et al: Incidence, outcome, and proposed management of isolated abscesses complicating acute left-sided colonic diverticulitis: a prospective study of 140 patients. Dis Colon Rectum 35:1072, 1992

206. Koruth NM, Krukowski ZH, Youngson GG, et al: Intra-operative colonic irrigation in the management of left-sided large bowel emergencies. Br J Surg 72:708, 1985

207. Lee EC, Murray JJ, Coller JA, et al: Intraoperative colonic lavage in nonelective surgery for diverticular disease. Dis Colon Rectum 40:669 1997

208. Murray JJ, Schoetz DJ Jr, Coller JA, et al: Intraoperative colonic lavage and primary anastomosis in nonelective colon resection. Dis Colon Rectum 34:527, 1991

209. Belmonte C, Klas JV, Perez JJ, et al: The Hartmann procedure: first choice or last resort in diverticular disease? Arch Surg 131:612, 1996

210. Nagorney DM, Adson MA, Pemberton JH: Sigmoid diverticulitis with perforation and generalized peritonitis. Dis Colon Rectum 28:71, 1985

211. Illert B, Engemann R, Thiede A: Success in treatment of complicated diverticular disease is stage related. Int J Colorectal Dis 16:276, 2001

212. Tucci G, Torquati A, Grande M, et al: Major acute inflammatory complications of diverticular disease of the colon: planning of surgical management. Hepatogastroenterology 43:839, 1996

213. Krukowski ZH, Matheson NA: Emergency surgery for diverticular disease complicated by generalized and faecal peritonitis: a review. Br J Surg 71:921, 1984

214. Gooszen AW, Gooszen HG, Veerman W, et al: Operative treatment of acute complications of diverticular disease: primary or secondary anastomosis after sigmoid resection. Eur J Surg 167:35, 2001

215. Maggard MA, Chandler CF, Schmit PJ, et al: Surgical diverticulitis: treatment options. Am Surg 67:1185, 2001

216. Wedell J, Banzhaf G, Chaoui R, et al: Surgical management of complicated colonic diverticulitis. Br J Surg 84:380, 1997

217. Benn PL, Wolff BG, Ilstrup DM: Level of anastomosis and recurrent colonic diverticulitis. Am J Surg 151:269, 1986

218. Wexner SD, Moscovitz ID: Laparoscopic colectomy in diverticular and Crohn's disease. Surg Clin North Am 80:1299, 2000

219. Fang JF, Chen RJ, Lin BC, et al: Aggressive resection is indicated for cecal diverticulitis. Am J Surg 185:135, 2003

220. Lane JS, Sarkar R, Schmit PJ, et al: Surgical approach to cecal diverticulitis. J Am Coll Surg 188:629, 1999

221. Oudenhoven LF, Koumans RK, Puylaert JB: Right colonic diverticulitis: US and CT findings—new insights about frequency and natural history. Radiology 208:611, 1998

222. Graham SM, Ballantyne GH: Cecal diverticulitis: a review of the American experience. Dis Colon Rectum 30:821, 1987

223. Brook I, Frazier EH: Aerobic and anaerobic microbiology in intra-abdominal infections associated with diverticulitis. J Med Microbiol 49:827, 2000

224. Runkel NS, Schlag P, Schwarz V, et al: Outcome after emergency surgery for cancer of the large intestine. Br J Surg 78:183, 1991

225. Welch JP, Donaldson GA: Perforative carcinoma of colon and rectum. Ann Surg 180:734, 1974

226. Nespoli A, Ravizzini C, Trivella M, et al: The choice of surgical procedure for peritonitis due to colonic perforation. Arch Surg 128:814, 1993

227. Anderson JH, Hole D, McArdle CS: Elective versus emergency surgery for patients with co-lorectal cancer. Br J Surg 79:706, 1992

228. Koperna T, Kisser M, Schulz F: Emergency surgery for colon cancer in the aged. Arch Surg 132:1032, 1997

229. Nathens AB, Rotstein OD: Therapeutic options in peritonitis. Surg Clin North Am 74:677, 1994

230. Sexually transmitted diseases treatment guidelines 2002. Centers for Disease Control and Prevention. MMWR Recomm Rep 51:1, 2002

231. Cohn DE, Rader JS: Gynecology. Surgery: Basic Science and Clinical Evidence. Surgery: Basic Science and Clinical Evidence. Norton JA, Bollinger RR, Chang AE, et al, Eds. Springer, New York, 2001, p 1923

232. Nickel JC: The management of acute pyelonephritis in adults. Can J Urol 8(suppl 1):29, 2001

233. Roberts JA: Management of pyelonephritis and upper urinary tract infections. Urol Clin North Am 26:753, 1999

234. Naber KG, Savov O, Salmen HC: Piperacillin 2 g/tazobactam 0.5 g is as effective as imipenem 0.5 g/cilastatin 0.5 g for the treatment of acute uncomplicated pyelonephritis and complicated urinary tract infections. Int J Antimicrob Agents 19:95, 2002

235. Conn HO: Spontaneous bacterial peritonitis: variant syndromes. South Med J 80:1343, 1987

236. Rimola A, Garcia-Tsao G, Navasa M, et al: Diagnosis, treatment and prophylaxis of spontaneous bacterial peritonitis: a consensus document. International Ascites Club. J Hepatol 32:142, 2000

237. Runyon BA, Antillon MR: Ascitic fluid pH and lactate: insensitive and nonspecific tests in detecting ascitic fluid infection. Hepatology 13:929, 1991

238. Felisart J, Rimola A, Arroyo V, et al: Cefotaxime is more effective than is ampicillin-tobramycin in cirrhotics with severe infections. Hepatology 5:457, 1985

239. Kawaguchi Y: Peritoneal dialysis as long-term treatment: comparison of technique survival between Asian and Western populations. Perit Dial Int 19(suppl 2):S327, 1999

240. Vas SI: Infections of continuous ambulatory peritoneal dialysis catheters. Infect Dis Clin North Am 3:301, 1989

241. Longmire WP: Suppurative cholangitis. Critical Surgical Illness. Hardy JD, Ed. WB Saunders Co, Philadelphia, 1971, p 400

242. Stewart L, Pellegrini CA, Way LW: Cholangio-venous reflux pathways as defined by corrosion casting and scanning electron microscopy. Am J Surg 155:23, 1988

243. Lygidakis NJ, Brummelkamp WH: Bacteremia in relation to intrabiliary pressure in proximal v. distal malignant biliary obstruction. Acta Chir Scand 152:305, 1986

244. Flemma RJ, Flint LM, Osterhout S, et al: Bacteriologic studies of biliary tract infection. Ann Surg 166:563, 1967

245. Weissglas IS, Brown RA: Acute suppurative cholangitis secondary to malignant obstruction. Can J Surg 24:468, 1981

246. Elson CO, Hattori K, Blackstone MO: Polymicrobial sepsis following endoscopic retrograde cholangiopancreatography. Gastroenterology 69:507, 1975

247. Ong GB: A study of recurrent pyogenic cholangitis. Arch Surg 84:199, 1962

248. Jackaman FR, Triggs CM, Thomas V, et al: Experimental bacterial infection of the biliary tract. Br J Exp Pathol 61:369, 1980

249. Lewis RT, Goodall RG, Marien B, et al: Biliary bacteria, antibiotic use, and wound infection in surgery of the gallbladder and common bile duct. Arch Surg 122:44, 1987

250. Finegold SM: Anaerobes in biliary tract infection. Arch Intern Med 139:1338, 1979

251. Shimada K, Inamatsu T, Yamashiro M: Anaerobic bacteria in biliary disease in elderly patients. J Infect Dis 135:850, 1977

252. Shimada K, Noro T, Inamatsu T, et al: Bacteriology of acute obstructive suppurative cholangitis of the aged. J Clin Microbiol 14:522, 1981

253. Lee WJ, Chang KJ, Lee CS, et al: Surgery in cholangitis: bacteriology and choice of antibiotic. Hepatogastroenterology 39:347, 1992

254. Bourgault AM, England DM, Rosenblatt JE, et al: Clinical characteristics of anaerobic bactibilia. Arch Intern Med 139:1346, 1979

Acknowledgments

Figures 2 through 5 Dr. L. Stein, Montreal, Quebec.

Figure 6 From "Computed Tomography and the Prediction of Pancreatic Abscess in Acute Pancreatitis," by J. H. C. Ranson, E. Balthazar, R. Caccavale, et al, in *Annals of Surgery* 201:656, 1985. Used by permission.

Figure 7 From "Nonsurgical Drainage of Splenic Abscess," by W. A. Berkman, S. A. Harris Jr., and M. E. Bernardino, in *American Journal of Roentgenology* 141:395, 1983. Used by permission.

19 FUNGAL INFECTION

Elias J. Anaissie, M.D., Albair B. Bishara, M.D., and Joseph S. Solomkin, M.D., F.A.C.S.

Approach to the Surgical Patient at Risk for Candidiasis

The infectious diseases that are most commonly encountered by surgeons are acute events in which fever, leukocytosis, and localized signs of inflammation develop in a reasonably healthy host. In this clinical situation, the presence of microorganisms in such normally sterile foci as blood and intra-abdominal sites indicates an infection and the need for antimicrobial chemotherapy.

The clinical setting in which *Candida* species are isolated from various body sites is generally much different. Patients harboring *Candida* infections frequently have had antecedent infections that were treated with antibacterial agents, have received therapy that suppressed their immunologic responses,[1] or have undergone extensive surgery or several operations, especially on the gastrointestinal tract. Such patients are generally long-term residents in acute care hospitals. Previous operative intervention may have left surgical wounds or drainage tracts. These circumstances favor colonization by various opportunistic pathogens, with the resultant risk of overgrowth or invasion by normal enteric microorganisms such as *Candida* species. In this setting, the elements that characterize most infectious processes (i.e., an acute change from wellness to illness and isolation of microorganisms from ordinarily sterile sites) no longer have great diagnostic value.

The problem of defining indications for administration of antifungal therapy in surgical patients is compounded by the limited data available, the difficulty of establishing a diagnosis, and the small number of effective antifungal agents. Although amphotericin B is currently the standard antifungal agent, fluconazole, a newer triazole antifungal that is generally well tolerated, appears to be effective in the treatment of serious *Candida* infections in surgical patients.

Noncandidal fungal infections, although still rare in surgical patients, may cause morbidity and mortality. Because infections such as aspergillosis and mucormycosis may be refractory to standard antifungal therapy, there is an urgent need to define the role of novel antifungal agents in surgical patients.

This chapter summarizes the current understanding of fungal infections, particularly candidiasis, in nonneutropenic surgical patients and provides recommendations for prophylaxis and therapy.

Magnitude of the Problem in the Surgical Patient

Whereas the high mortality associated with bacterial infections in surgical patients has been reduced by the early administration of antibacterial therapy, the incidence of fungal infections, particularly with *Candida* species, has dramatically increased.[2] In a 1984 nationwide survey of medical and surgical patients, *Candida* species were the eighth most common cause of nosocomial bloodstream infection.[3] In a similar survey conducted between October 1986 and December 1990, *Candida* species became the fourth

leading cause of nosocomial bloodstream infection, preceded only by coagulase-negative-staphylococci, *Staphylococcus aureus*, and enterococci.[3] According to the National Nosocomial Infections Surveillance (NNIS) system, the percentage of nosocomial infections caused by *C. albicans* increased from 2% in 1980 to an average of 5% over the 4-year period from 1986 through 1989.[4] Data from NNIS hospitals also show that between 1980 and 1989, the incidence of primary bloodstream infections attributable to *Candida* species increased by 487% in large teaching hospitals and by 219% in small (< 200 bed) hospitals.[5] In addition, the NNIS system reported that the rate of nosocomial fungal infection increased from 2.0 to 3.8 infections per 1,000 patients discharged between 1980 and 1990.[6] Current data from the SCOPE (Surveillance and Control of Pathogens of Epidemiologic Importance) system confirm that *Candida* species were the fourth leading cause of bloodstream infection.[7] These data are supported by the Surveillance Network–USA, which compiles information from more than 100 laboratories in the United States. Fungi including *Candida* species were isolated from 17% of 10,038 patients included in a European study of the prevalence of infection in patients in intensive care units.[8]

The most marked increase in candidiasis occurred in surgical patients, particularly in burn and trauma patients followed by cardiac surgery patients and general surgery patients. *Candida* species now account for 78% of all nosocomial fungal infections.[6]

Nosocomial bloodstream infections caused by *Candida* species are an independent predictor of risk of mortality (38% mortality directly attributable to candidiasis) and prolonged hospital stay (30 additional days in comparison with controls).[1] In a more recent prospective study, *Candida* species were the only microorganisms that independently influenced the outcome of nosocomial primary infections of the bloodstream (odds ratio for mortality, 1.84; 95% confidence interval [CI]) and were associated with the highest mortalities (35% at 28 days and 69% at discharge).[9] In properly conducted multivariate analyses, the most important prognostic factors in patients with hematogenous candidiasis include older age, poor performance status (on Acute Physiology and Chronic Health Evaluation [APACHE] or other measures), the presence and persistence of neutropenia, and dissemination of the infection to noncontiguous organs. Central venous catheter retention appears to play a minimal role.[8,10]

Definitions of Hematogenous *Candida* Infection Syndromes

In this chapter, the general term hematogenous candidiasis is used to identify all infections involving the bloodstream. Hence, hematogenous candidiasis refers to candidemia, disseminated candidiasis, or both.

CANDIDEMIA

Candidemia is defined as the isolation of any pathogenic species of *Candida* from at least one blood culture specimen. The recovery of *Candida* species from the bloodstream can be a significant observation in the absence of clinical signs and symptoms, especially if the patient is debilitated or uremic or is receiving adrenal corticosteroid therapy.

CATHETER-ASSOCIATED CANDIDEMIA

Catheter-associated candidemia is candidemia that occurs in a patient with an intravascular catheter and no other obvious origin of infection after careful clinical and laboratory evaluation. Several procedures have been developed to aid in the diagnosis of catheter-associated candidemia. If the catheter is removed, a quantitative culture of the tip should recover at least 15 colony-forming units (CFU) of the same *Candida* species as that found in blood culture by the roll-plate technique (or at least 100 CFU of the same *Candida* species as that found in blood culture by the sonication technique). If the catheter is not removed, a quantitative blood culture collected through a central catheter should contain at least a 10-fold greater concentration of *Candida* species than a simultaneously collected quantitative peripheral blood culture. Routine catheter tip cultures appear to be of no value.

ACUTE DISSEMINATED CANDIDIASIS

Patients who have several noncontiguous organs infected by *Candida* species have a disseminated infection acquired through hematogenous spread. For diagnosis, the organism must be identified by histologic analysis, culture of tissue samples obtained from at least one internal organ, or both; the patient should have radiographic, pathologic, or cultural evidence of infection in at least one other organ. Candidemia associated with *Candida* skin lesions or endophthalmitis consistent with a diagnosis of *Candida* infection also indicates a diagnosis of disseminated candidiasis.[11]

CHRONIC DISSEMINATED CANDIDIASIS

Chronic disseminated candidiasis, a chronic form of disseminated infection that is also known as hepatosplenic candidiasis, occurs in cancer patients who have been afflicted with protracted neutropenia.[12] This form of hematogenous candidiasis has not yet been described in the nonneutropenic surgical patient.

Characteristics of Surgical Patients at Risk for Candidiasis

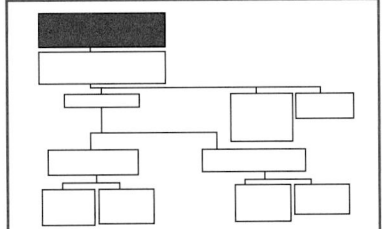

Fungal translocation that leads to hematogenous candidiasis is believed to be promoted by (1) colonization of the GI tract by *Candida* species, (2) physical disruption of the intestinal mucosal barrier, and (3) immunosuppression of the host leading to dissemination of the infection in the bloodstream and other organs [*see* Discussion, *below*].

Other important risk factors for hematogenous candidiasis include malignancies,[13] neutropenia and immunosuppressive therapy,[14] use of urinary catheters and diarrhea, prematurity,[15] heroin addiction,[16] abdominal surgery,[17] organ transplantation,[18] and extensive burns.[19]

The reported frequency of hematogenous candidiasis in burn patients ranges from 2% to 14%, depending on the reporting center and the study period.[19-21] Colonization by *Candida* species, hematogenous dissemination, and mortality caused by *Candida* infections have been found to correlate with the amount of body surface area burned and with the extent of full-thickness burn.

The pathogenesis, the incidence, and the microbial etiology of fungal infection vary in different groups of transplant recipients, depending on the organ transplanted, the donor source, the type of surgical procedure performed, and the recipient's age and general condition at the time of the procedure; other influential factors are the conditioning regimen, the type and duration of immunosuppressive therapy, and the presence or absence of organ rejection and graft versus host disease. In heart transplant recipients, for example, *Aspergillus* infection is a major problem, whereas in other organ transplant recipients, most fungal infections are attributable to *Candida*.[22] The infection is usually located at the site of the operation (e.g., an intra-abdominal abscess in liver[18] or pancreas[23] transplantation, the mediastinum or the lungs in heart[24] or heart-lung[25] transplantation, and the urinary tract in kidney[26] transplantation); however, dissemination from the primary site is common.

The central venous catheter has been reported as a risk factor in some studies but not in others,[10] particularly with *Candida parapsilosis*. This species, which may become part of the biofilm of intravascular catheters, may not respond to antifungal agents. Alternatively, *Candida* colonization of the catheter may result from gut-derived hematogenous seeding.[27,28]

Laboratory and Clinical Assessment of Candidiasis

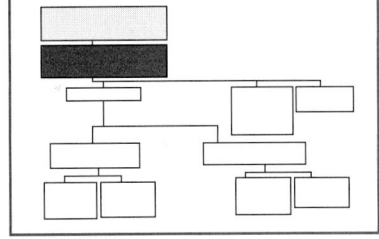

CULTURES

The workup of the surgical patient suspected of having hematogenous candidiasis begins with a complete set of cultures of sputum, oropharynx, stool, urine, all drain sites, and blood [*see Table 1*]. Candidiasis rarely develops in patients whose cultures show no evidence of *Candida* at some site. Obtaining more than six sets of blood cultures has little value, and there is no evidence to support arterial cultures.

The incidence of positive antemortem blood cultures in patients found to have candidiasis at autopsy is about 30% to 50%, possibly as a result of concomitant bacteremia, which may decrease the recovery of *Candida* species from the bloodstream. Because *Candida* species grow poorly under anaerobic conditions, venting the blood culture bottles is thought to improve the yield. The use of biphasic media also improves recovery of *Candida* species from the blood. Improved sensitivity and time to positivity of fungal blood cultures has been achieved with the development of new media, including biphasic media, automated radiometric and nonradiometric systems, and the lysis-centrifugation technique, a system that allows estimation of the number of *Candida* CFU/ml blood.[29] Commercial applications of these techniques include the BACTEC high-blood-volume fungal media system and the BacT/Alert system, both having comparable sensitivity to lysis-centrifugation. There is little evidence, however, that use of these newer methods provides a clinical advantage in the management of patients with hematogenous candidiasis. In a study by Berenguer and colleagues, the sensitivity of the lysis-centrifugation method increased with increasing numbers of involved organs but was still only 58% overall.[30]

Identify patient at risk for *Candida* infection

Major risk factors include
- Previous bacterial infection and therapy with multiple antibiotics.
- Isolation of *Candida* from ≥ 2 sites.
- Disruption of the intestinal mucosal barrier (total parenteral nutrition, severe diarrhea, colitis, major operation, trauma, or extensive burns).
- Immunosuppression (neutropenia, cancer, organ transplantation, hemodialysis, or extensive burns).

Other risk factors include
- Tunneled central venous catheters • Urinary catheters • Prematurity • Heroin addiction.

Initiate studies to diagnose candidiasis

Obtain cultures of sputum, oropharynx, stool, urine, drain sites, and blood.

Obtain 2 sets of blood cultures daily for 2 days (or longer if the patient remains febrile).

Consider serologic tests and histologic analyses (see text).

Look for findings that may signal hematogenous candidiasis:
- Endophthalmitis • Suppurative thrombophlebitis • High-grade candiduria without instrumentation of the bladder or the renal pelvis.

Exclude other possible causes of persistent fever.

Blood cultures are positive for *Candida*, or clinical or laboratory signal of potential hematogenous candidiasis is present

Patient is hemodynamically stable, does not have high-grade candidemia, and does not appear to have organ infection

Remove all venous catheters.

or

Leave venous catheter in place initially, and consider removal if clinical condition deteriorates or does not improve after 2 days of therapy.

Patient is infected or colonized by *C. albicans*, *C. tropicalis*, *C. parapsilosis*, or other germ tube–positive candidal organism

Give fluconazole, 600–800 mg/day I.V. for 2–3 days, then, if possible, lower dosage to 400 mg/day p.o.

Treat for 7–10 days (patient should be free of signs and symptoms of infection for 5 days before treatment is ended).

Patient is infected or colonized by *C. krusei*, *C. glabrata*, or *C. lusitaniae*

Give amphotericin B, 0.5–0.7mg/kg/day. (Consider adding flucytosine, 25 mg/kg/day p.o. in 2 divided doses, for *C. glabrata* and *C. lusitaniae*.)

Treat for 5–7 days (patient should be free of signs and symptoms of infection for 5 days before treatment is ended).

Approach to the Surgical Patient at Risk for Candidiasis

Blood cultures are negative for *Candida*, and no clinical or laboratory signal of potential hematogenous candidiasis is present, but *Candida* is isolated from ≥ 2 remote sites (≥ 1 site for *C. tropicalis*)

Give fluconazole, 400 mg/day I.V. for 2–3 days, then 400 mg/day p.o. If patient is colonized by *C. krusei*, *C. glabrata*, or *C. lusitaniae*, give amphotericin B, 0.5 mg/kg/day. (Consider adding flucytosine, 25 mg/kg/day p.o. in 2 divided doses, for *C. glabrata* and *C. lusitaniae*.)

Treat for 7–10 days (patient should be free of signs and symptoms of infection for 5 days before treatment is ended).

Blood cultures are negative for *Candida*, no clinical or laboratory signal of potential hematogenous candidiasis is found, and *Candida* is isolated from ≤ 1 remote site (0 sites for *C. tropicalis*)

Continue surveillance cultures weekly.

Patient is hemodynamically unstable, has high-grade candidemia, or shows evidence of organ infection

Remove all venous catheters.

Treat any associated syndromes of hematogenous candidiasis (e.g., endophthalmitis, pericarditis, suppurative thrombophlebitis, endocarditis).

Patient is infected or colonized by *C. albicans*, *C. tropicalis*, *C. parapsilosis*, or other germ tube–positive candidal organism

Give fluconazole, 800 mg/day I.V. (Consider adding flucytosine, 25 mg/kg/day p.o. in 2 divided doses. Also consider adding G-CSF, 300 µg/day.)

Treat for 10–14 days after disappearance of all signs and symptoms of infection.

Patient is infected or colonized by *C. krusei*, *C. glabrata*, or *C. lusitaniae*

Give amphotericin B, 0.7–1.0 mg/kg/day I.V. (Consider adding flucytosine, 25 mg/kg/day p.o. in 2 divided doses. Also consider adding G-CSF, 300 µg/day).

Treat for 10–14 days after disappearance of all signs and symptoms of infection.

Table 1 Clinical Presentation and Diagnostic Methods for Common Fungal Infections[139]

Host Fungus	Major Clinical Presentations	Diagnostic Methods
Normal host		
Aspergillus	Allergic bronchopulmonary	Serum IgE, precipitins
Blastomyces	Acute pneumonitis: chronic lung or skin	Culture, tissue
Candida	Vaginitis, thrush, candidemia, I.V. catheter	Culture/smear
Coccidioides	Acute pneumonitis, chronic cavitary, pulmonary nodule	Precipitins, complement fixation, culture
Cryptococcus	Pulmonary, meningitis	Culture, latex agglutination
Histoplasma	Acute pulmonary, progressive dissemination in infants and elderly, chronic cavitary in chronic airway obstruction	Culture, antigen detection
Compromised host		
Diabetes mellitus		
Candida	Disseminated, pyelonephritis, vaginitis	Culture/smear
Torulopsis	Pyelonephritis	Culture
Zygomycetes	Rhinocerebral, paranasal, pulmonary, gastrointestinal, cutaneous	Culture, tissue
Malignancy or corticosteroids		
Aspergillus	Invasive/lung, sinuses, disseminated	Culture, tissue
Candida	Fungemia, acute and chronic disseminated candidiasis	Culture, tissue
Coccidioides	Disseminated	Culture, precipitins, complement fixation
Cryptococcus	Pulmonary, meningeal, disseminated	Culture, latex agglutination, India ink preparation
Dematiaceous fungi	Lung, sinuses, brain, disseminated	Culture, tissue
Fusarium	Lung, sinuses, cellulitis at site of onychomycosis, disseminated	Culture, tissue
Histoplasma	Progressive disseminated	Culture, antigen detection
Torulopsis	Disseminated	Culture, tissue
Trichosporon	Disseminated	Culture, tissue
Zygomycetes	Rhinocerebral, paranasal, pulmonary, gastrointestinal, cutaneous, disseminated	Culture, tissue
Extensive surgery and previous antibiotic therapy		
Candida	Vaginitis, thrush, esophagitis, disseminated	Culture, tissue
Torulopsis	Disseminated	Culture

A rapid and inexpensive test is the germ tube test that can distinguish *C. albicans* (positive test) from other *Candida* species. More than 90% of *C. albicans* isolates produce germ tubes when incubated in serum for 2 to 3 hours at 37° C.

Several newer culture media allow the rapid identification of *C. albicans*. These include Albicans ID (bioMerieux, France), CandiSelect (Sanofi Diagnostics Pasteur, France), CHROMagar *Candida* (Becton Dickinson, USA), Fluoroplate *Candida* (Merck, Germany), Fongiscreen 4H (Sanofi Diagnostics Pasteur), and Murex *Candida albicans* (Murex Diagnostics, USA). CHROMagar and Fongiscreen 4H are also used for detection of other *Candida* species, including *C. glabrata*, *C. tropicalis*, and *C. krusei*. A recent study of 485 isolates (350 of *C. albicans* and 135 of other candidal species) evaluated the presumptive identification of *C. albicans* by comparing results of the germ-tube test to results of these six commercial tests. For *C. albicans*, the sensitivity and specificity of all six tests were greater than 97%. The sensitivity and specificity of the two tests that allow presumptive identification of other candidal species (CHROMagar *Candida* and Fongiscreen 4H) were lower, especially for *C. glabrata* and *C. tropicalis*.

Positive cultures from nonsterile sites (sputum, urine, and wound drainage) need to be interpreted with caution because of the frequent occurrence of *Candida* as a normal commensal of humans. Such cultures are useful mainly as an indication of colonization and, consequently, of the risk of infection in the appropriate setting.

ANTIBODY DETECTION

Previous studies have reported the use of incompletely characterized antigenic extracts of *C. albicans* to detect anticandidal antibodies in human sera. Difficulties with consistent production of uniform materials[31] have limited the usefulness of these tests. A variety of detection technologies (enzyme-linked immunosorbent assay [ELISA], immunodiffusion, and latex agglutination) have been used in attempts to detect antibodies directed toward defined purified antigen, but the sensitivity and specificity of these methods are low.[32] Methods using newly described antigens appear more promising.[33]

ANTIGEN DETECTION AND POLYMERASE CHAIN REACTION

Mannan, a polysaccharide component of the *Candida* cell wall, has the disadvantages of a short serum half-life and binding by antimannan antibody.[34] Although mannan can be detected by several methods,[35] complicated techniques are required to dissociate the mannan-antibody complex.[36] The sensitivity of mannan detection is approximately 70%.

A simple test available commercially (CAND-TEC *Candida* detection system, manufactured by Ramco Laboratories, USA) relies on the detection of a heat-labile antigen; however, its low sensitivity (as low as 19%) and specificity have limited its clinical use.[37] An antigen studied more recently is an immunodominant 48 kd cytoplasmic protein, *Candida* enolase. Because it is thought that cytoplasmic antigens are released during invasive infection, detection of this antigen may be able to distinguish between colonization and invasive infection.[33] A sensitivity of 54% was demonstrated in a study of 24 patients with invasive candidiasis,[38] but the sensitivity increases to 75% with the use of multiple samples. A sensitivity of 65% and a specificity of 97% were shown in a study assessing multiple samples.[39] Unfortunately, this test is not commercially available.

A commercial kit (Bichro-latex albicans) using monoclonal antibodies against cell wall extracts of *C. albicans* mannoprotein appears to have high sensitivity and specificity for *C. albicans*.[40]

Another antigen studied is (1-3)-β-D-glucan, an important cell wall constituent of fungi that is not shared with bacteria. Studies of this assay, which indicates the presence of fungi but does not identify the genus causing infection, have been promising in patients with fungal colonization. In these patients, its concentration remains lower than 20 pg/ml.

Amplification of the DNA of *Candida* species appears to be a quick and specific diagnostic tool. Although multiple approaches have been pursued,[41-43] several limitations need to be overcome before this method can be used routinely.[44]

METABOLITES

Systems based on the detection of D-arabinitol and mannose release by the fungus have been proposed,[45] but only those detecting D-arabinitol have been extensively developed. D-Arabinitol, a pentose produced by all of the major *Candida* species except *C. krusei* and *C. glabrata*, is excreted by the kidneys in the same rate as creatinine, and the ratio of D-arabinitol to creatinine must be used to interpret any observed concentration of D-arabinitol. Gas-liquid chromatographic as well as enzymatic methods are available for the detection of D-arabinitol, but gas-liquid chromatography is both technically demanding and expensive; it has been replaced by the recently developed enzymatic assay system. The sensitivity of the serum D-arabinitol–creatinine ratio for the diagnosis of invasive candidiasis, reported in the range of 40% to 83%, rises with repeated sampling.[46] Sensitivity is highest in patients with fungemia (74% to 83%) and lowest in patients with tissue-invasive *Candida* infections (40% to 44%). The magnitude of the D-arabinitol–creatinine ratio is strongly related to the degree of tissue invasion.[28,46] Although this assay may produce false positive results in some patients, it offers the promise of earlier detection of invasive candidiasis.[46]

Mannose, the other metabolite of *Candida* species that has been studied, can be detected only by a complicated gas-liquid chromatographic system. Initial estimates of its sensitivity (39%) have limited interest in this technique.[45]

HISTOLOGIC ANALYSES

Fungal smears are relatively insensitive methods of diagnosing candidiasis in otherwise sterile sites (e.g., joint fluid, peritoneal fluid, vitreous humor, or cerebrospinal fluid). Centrifugation of these fluids and examination of the sediment may improve the diagnostic yield. Conventional fungal stains, such as hematoxylin-eosin, periodic acid–Schiff (PAS), and Gomori methenamine-silver (GMS), are useful. The most sensitive stain is calcofluor white, but unfortunately, it requires fluorescent microscopy. Deep tissue biopsy provides a definitive diagnosis of candidiasis.

CLINICAL DIAGNOSIS

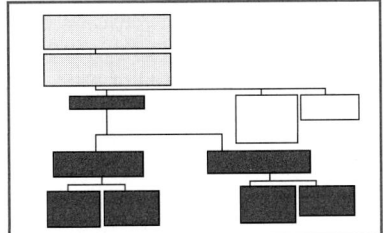

Hematogenous candidiasis has no characteristic clinical picture. Three clinical findings that may lead to an early diagnosis of hematogenous candidiasis in the surgical patient are candidal endophthalmitis, suppurative phlebitis, and candiduria in the absence of bladder instrumentation. A careful eye examination to identify the presence of candidal infection should be performed while the results of cultures of various sites are being awaited, and a repeat exam-

ination should be performed after therapy for proven candidemia. Candidal endophthalmitis may remain asymptomatic until late in the course of infection.

The presence of peripheral suppurative phlebitis that fails to yield bacteria or does not respond to antibacterial agents may be an early clue to the presence of hematogenous candidiasis. Gentle squeezing of the venous catheter exit site may express pus that yields *Candida* species on a smear or culture. Surgical excision of the infected vein usually reveals *Candida* infection in its lumen.

The presence of high-grade candiduria in surgical patients who have not had instrumentation of the renal pelvis or the bladder suggests hematogenous candidiasis and should prompt a workup for this infection. In this setting, candiduria may result from seeding of or filtering through the kidney.

Fever may be the only sign of infection but may be absent in patients who are receiving corticosteroids. Occasionally, a patient with hematogenous candidiasis presents with the systemic inflammatory response syndrome (SIRS) or septic shock. The diagnosis should be seriously considered in high-risk patients who are persistently febrile. Because of the high mortality associated with this infection, empirical antifungal therapy is recommended for early treatment of a clinical occult fungal infection or for the prevention of new fungal infections.

Management of Hematogenous Candidiasis

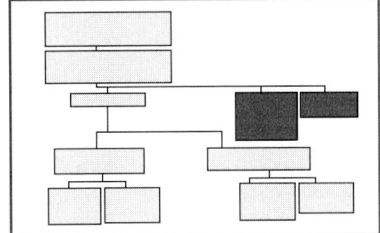

CANDIDEMIA AND ACUTE DISSEMINATED CANDIDIASIS

During the 1960s and the 1970s, the standard approach to managing candidemia was to classify patients according to degree of risk of disseminated candidiasis and to withhold antifungal treatment from those in whom dissemination appeared to be unlikely. This approach was based on unawareness of the magnitude of the problem in surgical patients and on acute awareness of the toxicities of amphotericin B, which was the only systemic antifungal agent available at the time; eventually, this type of management was found to be associated with a substantial mortality and a high incidence of long-term sequelae (e.g., deep-seated candidiasis presenting with endophthalmitis or other organ infection).[1] Consequently, it is now common practice to treat all candidemic patients except those who are afebrile, asymptomatic, or at low risk for disseminated candidiasis [*see Table 2*].

Candidates for empirical antifungal therapy are at high risk for candidiasis, colonized by *Candida* species (at one or more sites for *C. tropicalis* or at two or more for other candidal species), and unresponsive to broad-spectrum antibiotics in the absence of any other cause for their fever. Unresponsive patients may be characterized by rapid clinical deterioration, particularly if there is evidence of physical disruption of the intestinal mucosal barrier or immunosuppression.

The role of amphotericin B in the treatment of hematogenous candidiasis in surgical patients has been difficult to determine—first, because most of the studies that evaluated amphotericin B were retrospective trials with small sample sizes, and second, because few of the studies defined hematogenous candidiasis in the same way. In one study, treatment with amphotericin B had no effect on overall outcome in a mixed population of patients; however, the timing of therapy and the dose administered were not clearly stated.[47] In general, mortality was lower in patients who re-

Table 2 Antimicrobial Agents of Choice for Candidal Infections*

Infection	Agent of Choice	Alternative Agents	Comments
Hematogenous			
Candidemia and acute disseminated candidiasis	Fluconazole, or amphotericin B ± flucytosine	Lipid formulations of amphotericin B	Fluconazole should be given for *C. albicans*, amphotericin for all other *Candida* species; a 2-drug regimen should be given to hemodynamically unstable patients with persistent high-grade fungemia
Candida endophthalmitis	Fluconazole	Amphotericin B + flucytosine	Patients with vitral involvement require vitrectomy in addition to antifungal therapy
Suppurative phlebitis	Fluconazole + flucytosine	Amphotericin B + flucytosine	The central venous catheter should be removed and the infected vein excised
Endocarditis	Amphotericin B + flucytosine	—	Surgical replacement or repair of valves is essential to prevent death from embolization or cardiac failure; oral fluconazole should be given after successful completion of a prolonged course of amphotericin B therapy
Pericarditis	Amphotericin B	Fluconazole	
Prosthetic device–related infection	Fluconazole or amphotericin B	—	Removal of device is required for successful therapy
Arthritis	Fluconazole	—	—
Osteomyelitis	Amphotericin B	Fluconazole	Surgical drainage of pus is required
Meningitis	Amphotericin B + flucytosine	Fluconazole + flucytosine	—
Nonhematogenous			
Oropharyngeal			
Otherwise normal host	Nystatin	Ketoconazole, fluconazole, clotrimazole troches	—
Patients at risk for hematogenous infection (e.g., cancer patients, surgical patients)	Fluconazole	Ketoconazole	—
Deep candidiasis			
Esophagitis and GI candidiasis	Fluconazole	Amphotericin B	Amphotericin B should be reserved for cases of fluconazole failure without endoscopic evidence of other causes of disease
Peritonitis and intra-abdominal	Fluconazole	Amphotericin B	—
Wound	Fluconazole	Amphotericin B	Antifungal therapy should be given to patients who do not respond to antibacterial therapy
Urinary tract			
Cystitis	Fluconazole	Amphotericin B	Fluconazole is preferable because of its high drug concentration in urine and because it is better tolerated
Pyelitis			
Without papillitis	Fluconazole	—	—
With papillitis	Fluconazole + flucytosine	Amphotericin B	—
Pyelonephritis	Fluconazole + flucytosine	Amphotericin B	—

*Therapy is individualized on the basis of the patient's clinical condition and the infecting species.

ceived amphotericin B than in those who did not.[48] Significant amphotericin B–related nephrotoxicity may occur.

The discovery of the azole antifungal agents has changed the management of *Candida* infections. The first two azoles, clotrimazole and miconazole, were not, however, suitable for systemic use. As for ketoconazole, the lack of a parenteral formulation and the erratic bioavailability of the drug in patients receiving H$_2$ receptor blockers or antacids have limited its use in the treatment of hematogenous candidiasis in surgical patients.

Fluconazole is a well-tolerated triazole with good activity in hematogenous candidiasis. Data available from several clinical trials suggest that the drug is as effective as and better tolerated than amphotericin B. Overall, four comparative studies have been completed in various patient populations. Two were randomized,[49,50] one was prospective observational,[51] and one used matched cohorts.[50] Fluconazole dosages ranged from 200 to 800 mg/day, given orally or intravenously, while intravenous amphotericin B was given at doses of 0.3 to 1.2 mg/kg.

The first prospective, randomized study of fluconazole included 40 surgical patients with hematogenous candidiasis, of whom 20 received 300 mg/day of fluconazole and 20 received 0.5 mg/kg/day of amphotericin B plus flucytosine.[52] There were no significant differences in outcome between the two study groups.

A matched-pair study compared the outcomes of 45 candidemic cancer patients who were treated with fluconazole with the outcomes of 45 candidemic cancer patients who were treated with amphotericin B[53]; in several of the 90 patients, hematogenous candidiasis had developed after operation. This study demonstrated that fluconazole was as effective as and better tolerated than amphotericin B. In one prospective, randomized multicenter study, 164 patients with documented or presumed invasive candidiasis received either amphotericin B, 0.7 mg/kg/day, or fluconazole, 400 mg/day.[50] The response rate for fluconazole (62%) was virtually identical to that for amphotericin B (63%), and fluconazole was better tolerated. In another prospective, randomized multicenter study, 206 nonimmunocompromised candidemic patients received either amphotericin B or fluconazole.[49] Once again, the two drugs were comparable in their efficacy, and fluconazole had a better safety profile.

Newer therapeutic options have now become available with the advent of the lipid-associated formulations of amphotericin B, which are less nephrotoxic than the parent compound.[54] Thus far, three lipid products of amphotericin B have been marketed in Europe or the United States: Abelcet (amphotericin B lipid complex), Amphocil (amphotericin B colloidal dispersion), and AmBisome (liposomal amphotericin B). A prospective, randomized trial has shown that Abelcet is as efficacious as conventional amphotericin B in hematogenous candidiasis.[55]

All patients with candidemia should receive antifungal therapy. We recommend the administration of fluconazole, 600 to 800 mg/day I.V. for 3 days, particularly if the infecting organism is known to be or is likely to be *C. albicans*. If the patient responds rapidly to this regimen, the dosage may be decreased to 400 mg/day and administered orally. For patients with hematogenous candidiasis who are known to be colonized by *C. glabrata, C. krusei,* or *C. lusitaniae,* amphotericin B, 0.5 to 0.7 mg/kg/day, should remain the treatment of choice. For patients who are hemodynamically unstable and for those who have high-grade persistent fungemia, we recommend a two-drug antifungal regimen: the combination of fluconazole and flucytosine or the combination of amphotericin B and flucytosine, depending on the infecting strain.

Clinical data on the effect of itraconazole in hematogenous candidiasis are scant. Given that itraconazole has limited bioavailability in the presence of antacids and H_2 receptor blockers, it should not be used to treat hematogenous candidiasis in the critically ill. However, an I.V. formulation of itraconazole is now available, and it is possible that this formulation may prove effective in patients with hematogenous candidiasis.

Liposomal formulations of amphotericin B offer new therapeutic alternatives. Their substantial cost limits their routine use, but they are appropriate if the patient has renal failure and is infected with an azole-resistant strain. Of the three available formulations, AmBisome is the best tolerated and yields the highest blood levels of amphotericin B.

The duration of therapy depends on the extent and severity of the infection. Therapy can be limited to 7 to 10 days for patients with low-grade fungemia and no evidence of organ involvement or hemodynamic instability. Patients with high-grade fungemia and evidence of organ involvement or hemodynamic instability need to receive antifungal therapy for 10 to 14 days after resolution of all signs and symptoms of infection.

Catheter Management

Controversy remains concerning the role of central venous lines in patients' outcome in hematogenous candidiasis. According to Nguyen and colleagues,[51] patients with catheter-related candidemia had a more favorable prognosis than patients with candidemia from other sources, but the prognosis was worse in patients whose catheters were retained. In contrast, studies by Carroll and colleagues, Nucci and coworkers,[56] and Anaissie and associates[10] failed to show a major role for retention of central venous catheters in the outcome of hematogenous candidiasis. The study by Anaissie and associates[10] examined the impact of catheter management on outcome in 416 cancer patients with candidemia who had an indwelling catheter at the time of candidal infection. Catheter exchange within 0, 2, or 4 days of the first positive blood culture had no significant effect on outcome. A second analysis, performed in a subset of 363 patients who had a central venous catheter in place and received antifungal therapy, revealed that catheter exchange was associated with improved outcome (80% versus 54%; $P < 0.001$). However, the subset in which the catheter was not exchanged had higher APACHE III scores and were more likely to be neutropenic. By multivariate analysis, catheter retention was not found to significantly affect outcome.

In one study in noncancer patients, Rex and colleagues[57] showed that replacement of all vascular catheters shortened the duration of candidemia from 5.6 days to 2.6 days. This finding suggests that catheters may play a role in perpetuating infection in nonneutropenic patients. In neutropenic patients, however, the primary source of candidemia is usually the GI tract, not the intravenous catheter, and other factors (e.g., the severity of disease, visceral dissemination, and neutrophil recovery) appear to have more impact on the outcome of neutropenic patients with candidemia.

Given the available data, we recommend that physicians consider the removal of all intravascular catheters in inpatients who have candidemia with persistent fever, persistent or high-grade fungemia, or *C. parapsilosis* (which is more likely to be catheter related than infection with other *Candida* species).

Cytokine Therapy for Opportunistic Infections

Polymorphonuclear leukocytes and macrophages are the predominant host defense against candidal infections. Candidal antigens induce lymphocyte proliferation and cytokine synthesis (interferon gamma and tumor necrosis factor); tumor necrosis factor enhances the candidacidal activity of phagocytes,[58] probably through increased production of reactive oxygen radicals. Another mechanism by which interferon gamma may augment host defenses against candidal infections is modulation of endothelial cell phagocytosis of *C. albicans.*[59] Granulocyte colony-stimulating factor (G-CSF) and granulocyte-macrophage colony-stimulating factor (GM-CSF) activate phagocytic cells to restrict the growth of *C. albicans.*[60]

Recently, a multicenter, double-blind, randomized phase II trial examined the activity of G-CSF in combination with fluconazole for treatment of hematogenous candidiasis in nonneutropenic patients. Preliminary analysis (Kullberg BJ and associates, unpublished report, 2000) indicated that an increase in the number of circulating neutrophils strongly correlates with accelerated clearance of bloodstream infection and reduced mortality. Additional data are needed to confirm these findings.

Antifungal Prophylaxis

Prophylaxis may be considered in surgical patients at high risk for invasive candidiasis. To date, there have been few trials of antifungal prophylaxis, whether as part of selective bowel decontamination[61] or in the form of low-dose amphotericin B[62] or liposomal formulations of amphotericin B in surgical transplant recipients.[63]

Fluconazole prophylaxis has been shown to reduce the rate of superficial and systemic fungal infections in cancer patients undergoing chemotherapy (with or without bone marrow transplantation)[64,65] and oropharyngeal and esophageal candidiasis in patients infected with HIV.[66] A recent double-blind randomized trial showed that intravenous fluconazole prophylaxis was effective in preventing candidal colonization and invasive intra-abdominal candidal infections in high-risk surgical patients.[67]

A retrospective study in burn patients reported that topical nystatin in the wound dressing was associated with a significant decrease in yeast acquisitions in burn wounds and fungemia but with an increase in colonization and fungemia caused by nystatin-resistant, amphotericin B–susceptible *C. rugosa.*[68]

Invasive fungal infection is one of the most important causes of mortality in organ transplant recipients.[69] Antifungal prophylaxis has been recommended in organ transplant recipients undergoing immunosuppressive therapy, but there is controversy about which drug is most effective and least toxic. Some physicians use fluconazole prophylactically in organ transplant recipients, but others recommend itraconazole or liposomal amphotericin B.[1,70,71]

ORGAN INFECTIONS

Candida *Endophthalmitis*

The diagnosis of candidal endophthalmitis usually implies hematogenous spread to multiple organs and the need for systemic antifungal therapy. Patients with chorioretinitis alone respond better to drug therapy alone than do those with vitreal involvement. Because antifungal drugs do not penetrate the vitreous body as well as the other ocular compartments,[72] patients with vitreal involvement require early vitrectomy in addition to antifungal therapy. Fluconazole is currently the drug of choice because of its proven efficacy and its higher concentration (20% to 70% of the corresponding plasma level) in ocular tissue, including the vitreous body.[73] Thus, we recommend 800 mg/day of fluconazole until a major response is observed, at which time it may be possible to reduce the dose to 400 mg/day. Although endophthalmitis due to *C. albicans* is commonly seen, recent series have reported on the importance of endophthalmitis caused by other candidal species. If the infecting organism (especially *C. krusei*) is potentially resistant to fluconazole, the recommended therapy is amphotericin B, 0.7 to 1.0 mg/kg/day I.V., preferably in conjunction with flucytosine.[74] Intravitreal injection of amphotericin B is recommended for vitreal infections.

The optimal duration of therapy for endogenous endophthalmitis is unknown, but we recommend that treatment be continued for at least 10 to 14 days after complete resolution of all signs and symptoms of infection. Ophthalmologic consultation is critical in establishing the diagnosis, assessing the patient's response to therapy, detecting complications, and determining whether early vitrectomy is indicated to prevent loss of sight.[75]

Suppurative *Thrombophlebitis*

A rare but serious consequence of hematogenous candidemia is suppurative thrombophlebitis, which results from infection of a vessel traumatized by prolonged catheterization. Endothelial disruption exposes the basement membrane and leads to thrombus formation and propagation. Suppurative thrombophlebitis is particularly serious because intravascular infection results in a persistent high-density fungemia. Management of this disease consists of high-dose antifungal therapy, removal of the central venous catheter, and excision of the infected vein, when possible.[76] Typically, blood cultures remain positive for several days; sometimes, they remain positive for as long as 3 to 4 weeks despite appropriate antifungal therapy, if the infected vein is not excised.

Endocarditis

Hematogenous candidiasis may also lead to the establishment of endocarditis, particularly in patients with a prosthetic heart valve or with a previously damaged native valve. Intravenous drug abuse and central intravenous catheterization appear to be predisposing factors. Candidal endocarditis after permanent pacemaker implantation has also been reported. The clinical picture is similar in many respects to that of bacterial endocarditis, although embolic phenomena have been more commonly associated with fungal endocarditis. Transesophageal echocardiography is more sensitive than transthoracic echocardiography in detecting candidal vegetation. Mortality due to *Candida* prosthetic valve endocarditis (PVE) is high, especially when complicated by congestive heart failure and persistent fungemia. For uncomplicated PVE, the mortality for patients receiving antifungal therapy alone (40%) is no worse than that for patients receiving combined medical and surgical therapy (33%).

Candidal endocarditis is very difficult to treat. Surgical replacement or repair of valves is essential to prevent death from embolization or cardiac failure in patients with complicated PVE. Ampho-

tericin B, with or without flucytosine, has been the therapy of choice; however, neither the optimal dosage nor the optimal duration of therapy has been determined. There is anecdotal information on the successful use of fluconazole in this setting, primarily as long-term suppressive therapy after the initial administration of amphotericin B.[73,77] Because of the high risk of late relapse, long-term maintenance therapy with oral fluconazole should be begun after successful completion of a prolonged course of amphotericin B.

Pericarditis

Candidal pericarditis is a very rare complication of hematogenous candidiasis. The surgical patients at risk for purulent pericarditis caused by *Candida* species are those who have undergone a cardiac operation, those who have a malignancy and whose host defenses are impaired, and those who have a debilitating chronic disease.[78] High-dose amphotericin B therapy, with or without surgical drainage, is recommended in these cases.

Arthritis

Joint infections with *Candida* species have resulted from hematogenous spread from inadvertent direct inoculation during joint procedures or intra-articular injection of corticosteroids. These infections typically involve a single joint, most frequently the knee, and tend to occur in patients with rheumatoid arthritis or prosthetic joint devices.[79] Local symptoms of pain on weight bearing or on full extension may be present. Diagnosis is best achieved by visualizing or growing the organisms from the joint fluid. Early diagnosis and systemic antifungal therapy are important to prevent destruction of the cartilage or loosening of the prosthesis. Successful treatment with fluconazole has been reported in several patients with fungal arthritis.[80] We recommend a dose of 400 to 800 mg/day for 6 months. Fluconazole can be used in acute therapy, alone or in combination with surgery, as well as in long-term suppressive therapy in patients at risk for recurrence or those who cannot undergo surgical debridement.

Osteomyelitis

Except for sternal infections complicating median sternotomy, most cases of candidal osteomyelitis have followed hematogenous spread. Vertebral body involvement is common. Back pain and fever may be followed by radiculopathy. Surgical drainage of pus is essential for a good response; however, surgical debridement of bony lesions may not be needed. Although amphotericin B has been the standard drug of choice, fluconazole offers an alternative in the treatment of these cases.[81]

Meningitis

Candidal meningitis may follow hematogenous spread or be a complication of neurosurgery or the implantation of ventriculoperitoneal shunts.[82] The infection is insidious and may remain undiagnosed. Most patients have recently received antibacterial agents, and half have had antecedent bacterial meningitis. The overall mortality is around 10%. The standard therapy is amphotericin B with flucytosine. The combination of high-dose fluconazole (800 mg/day) and flucytosine (50 mg/kg/day) is a particularly attractive approach because of the high CSF concentrations achieved with both agents. Removal of the infected shunts is recommended when possible.[51,82] The duration of treatment should be based on clinical response and culture results.

Nonhematogenous Candidiasis

SUPERFICIAL INFECTION

Oral candidiasis (thrush) appears as a whitish, patchy pseudomembrane covering an inflamed oropharynx and commonly involves the tongue, the hard and soft palates, and the tonsillar pillars. Controlled trials have documented the efficacy of nystatin suspension, clotrimazole troches, oral ketoconazole, fluconazole, or itraconazole in eradicating the clinical symptoms of oral candidiasis.[83,84]

Nystatin should be given as a 10 to 30 ml suspension five times daily, and the patient should be instructed to swish it around the mouth before swallowing; alternatively, the patient may take one or two troches five times daily. Clotrimazole troches are given five times daily as a 10 mg troche that should be held in the mouth until dissolved. In surgical patients at risk for hematogenous infection, systemic therapy with ketoconazole (200 to 400 mg once daily), itraconazole (100 to 200 mg/day), or fluconazole (100 mg once daily) is preferred.[85] Antifungal therapy should be administered for 1 week, except for fluconazole therapy, which is likely to be effective when given for 2 or 3 days.

DEEP CANDIDIASIS

Esophagitis and Gastrointestinal Candidiasis

Superficial candidiasis involving only mucosal surfaces used to be a common finding at autopsy in surgical patients who had a protracted hospital stay characterized by recurrent sepsis. Such lesions may arise at any site in the GI tract but appear most commonly in the esophagus and the small bowel and may progress to hematogenous infection [see Figure 1].

In a minority of patients, the pathology of infection of the lower GI tract by *Candida* species may change from diarrhea without demonstrable tissue invasion to direct penetration into the submucosa, which eventually leads to pseudomembranous enterocolitis. Direct vascular invasion through the bowel wall has been reported only in patients receiving immunosuppressive chemotherapy.[86] These patients may have extensive involvement of the GI tract from mouth to anus. Nonneutropenic surgical patients exhibit more localized involvement.

The preferred therapy for esophageal candidiasis is fluconazole or itraconazole, 200 mg daily. In patients who remain symptomatic after 5 days of therapy, endoscopy is needed to rule out other causes of esophagitis. If endoscopy proves that esophagitis is caused by candidal infection, low-dose amphotericin B (0.4 mg/kg/day) should be administered. Therapy for esophageal candidiasis should be continued for at least 4 days after symptoms resolve; immunosuppressed patients generally require more extended therapy to prevent relapse.

Because stool cultures do not differentiate between colonization and infection, candidiasis in the lower gastrointestinal tract is usually a postmortem diagnosis; hence, there are no reliable criteria governing when and how to treat this condition. It has been reported, however, that patients who have diarrhea that can only be caused by heavy colonization with *Candida* species may respond dramatically to 2 to 4 days of nystatin therapy.[87]

Peritonitis and Intra-abdominal Abscess

Perhaps the most controversial aspect of *Candida* infectious syndromes in surgical patients is whether specific systemic therapy is required to eradicate the infection within intra-abdominal abscesses, peritoneal fluid, or fistula drainage. *Candida* is frequently cultured from intra-abdominal infectious foci but should be considered a serious threat only in high-risk patients. Four risk factors for intra-abdominal candidiasis are gastrointestinal perforations, anastomotic leakage, surgery for acute pancreatitis, and splenectomy.[88]

Patients with peritonitis and intra-abdominal abscesses should receive systemic antifungal therapy, usually in combination with antibacterial therapy, given that these infections are almost always polymicrobial in origin. The risk of dissemination is increased by

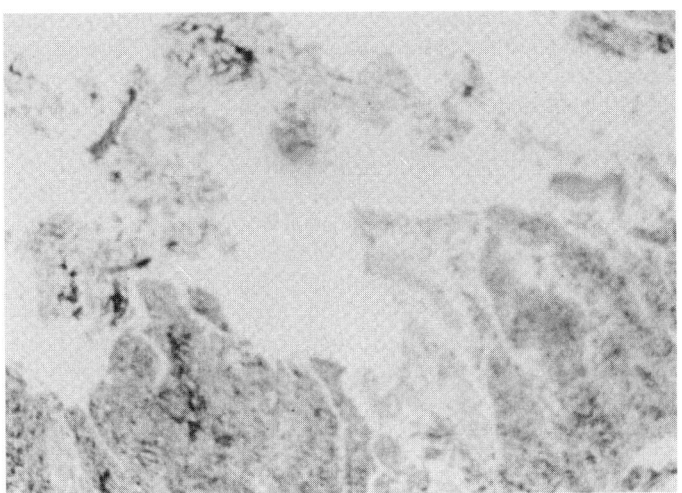

Figure 1 **Superficial candidiasis may be found at all levels of the GI tract. Here, the esophagus of a patient found at autopsy to have disseminated candidiasis shows disrupted epithelium, submucosal inflammation, and the presence of yeast in the submucosa.**

both the recurrence of intra-abdominal infections and the presence of extensive areas of communication between the abdominal cavity and the external environment via either fistulas or drain tracts.

On rare occasions, candidal peritonitis occurs after long-term ambulatory peritoneal dialysis. In such cases, the infection tends to remain localized and to manifest with low-grade fever and abdominal pain and tenderness. The peritoneal dialysate is usually cloudy and contains more than 100 neutrophils/mm³. Therapy consists of systemic antifungal therapy and removal of the peritoneal catheter. The abdominal pain caused by the addition of amphotericin B to the dialysate has raised concern that chemical peritonitis might give rise to adhesions and thus impair the efficacy of dialysis.

Because fluconazole is very safe and is capable of reaching high concentrations in peritoneal fluid, it is likely to be useful in the management of candidal peritonitis.[89] Fluconazole should be given at a dosage of 100 to 200 mg/day orally for 2 to 6 weeks. Immediate removal of the peritoneal catheter has been recommended. In one study, however, seven of nine patients treated with oral flucytosine responded to therapy without catheter removal.[90]

A prospective, randomized study in patients on continuous ambulatory dialysis found that successful prophylaxis for *Candida* peritonitis was achieved with oral nystatin (tablets containing 500,000 units given four times a day).[91]

Occasionally, *Candida* species may cause cholangitis, biliary tract disease, pancreatic abscess, or liver abscess. This problem is increasingly found in patients with percutaneously placed drainage catheters for malignancy. Such patients must be given systemic therapy for clinical evidence of infection, including candidemia, and the drainage catheter must be changed. Diverticulitis complicated by candidal pylephlebitis has also been reported.

Wound Infections

The diagnosis and treatment of candidal wound infections are problematic. Recovering *Candida* species from drains and wounds does not necessarily mean that this organism is causing tissue infection. Colonization of wounds by *Candida* species should not compel physicians to use systemic antifungal therapy. However, such therapy should be administered to those patients whose wound infections do not respond to appropriate antibacterial therapy, particularly if one *Candida* species is repeatedly isolated from the site and the patient is at high risk for hematogenous infection. Antifungal therapy should be administered to prevent the establishment of *Candida* osteomyelitis when sternal wound cultures obtained after coronary artery bypass surgery yield *Candida* species.

Urinary Tract and Genital Candidiasis

The recovery of *Candida* species from the urinary tract most commonly results from contamination from the perirectal or the genital area or from colonization of the bladder, which is usually seen in patients who have undergone prolonged catheterization or who have diabetes mellitus or another disease that leads to incomplete bladder emptying. In addition, *Candida* species usually colonize ileal conduits. Persistent candiduria in the surgical intensive care unit may, however, be an early marker of disseminated infection in critically ill high-risk patients.[92] In a study of 91 pediatric ICU patients who were clinically suspected of having disseminated candidiasis, the isolation of candidal species other than *C. albicans* from the urine was a better indicator of candidemia than was isolation of *C. albicans;* 60% of the patients whose urine contained candidal species other than *C. albicans* had candidemia, versus 33.3% of the patients whose urine contained *C. albicans*.[93]

Alkalization of the urine with oral potassium-sodium hydrogen citrate is a simple and effective method of treating candiduria in patients with an indwelling catheter.[94] Replacing or removing the bladder catheter is preferable. If *Candida* colonization persists, particularly if the patient has a risk factor for cystitis (e.g., diabetes mellitus or a disease that leads to incomplete bladder emptying) or for hematogenous dissemination (e.g., immunosuppression or manipulation of the genitourinary system), antifungal therapy should be considered. Amphotericin B bladder irrigation provides only temporary clearance of funguria, and systemic agents (a single I.V. dose of amphotericin B or a 5-day course of oral fluconazole) are usually needed.

The spectrum of urinary tract infection by *Candida* species includes cystitis, pyelitis (i.e., infection of the renal pelvis), fungus ball of the ureter, and renal abscesses. The diagnosis of cystitis is based on the presence of symptoms of cystitis, diffuse erythema or fungal plaques on cystoscopy, candiduria, and pyuria. *Candida* cystitis warrants therapy. If a triple-lumen catheter is in place, bladder irrigation with amphotericin B, 50 mg/L/day for 2 days, may be tried. Fluconazole, 200 mg once daily, is a more attractive approach because of the convenience, lower cost, and very high drug concentrations achieved in the urine.[95] Flucytosine is excreted in the urine in high concentrations and may be particularly useful against *C. glabrata* infection.

The management of pyelitis depends on whether the renal papillae are invaded or the ureter is obstructed with a fungus ball. Patients with no papillitis and an open ureter usually respond to irrigation with amphotericin B through a ureteral or percutaneous catheter. If papillitis is present, systemic antifungal therapy with fluconazole, 400 mg daily, is recommended. If fungus balls are present, surgical removal should be considered in addition to treatment with antifungal agents.

Hematogenous infections of the kidneys leading to multiple renal abscesses are treated as instances of hematogenous candidiasis. However, because both fluconazole and flucytosine are well tolerated, have good tissue diffusion, and are excreted in the urine in high concentrations, it is reasonable to assume that the combination of these two agents represents the therapy of choice for candidiasis that involves renal parenchyma.

Surgical patients are also at risk for vulvovaginal candidiasis. The diagnosis is based on the clinical findings and on the presence of pseudohyphae on a fungal smear. Various antifungal agents, including oral azoles and topical medications (suppositories, creams, and vaginal tablets) are effective in more than 80% of uncomplicated infections. Oral agents include fluconazole (150 mg in a single dose), ketoconazole (400 mg daily for 5 days), and itraconazole (200 mg in a single dose). However, women with four or more episodes of vulvovaginal candidiasis during a 12-month period and women with acute severe attacks of candidal vaginitis are less likely to respond to conventional therapy. Preventive measures include control of host factors such as diabetes mellitus, antifungal prophylaxis during the use of antibiotics and under other high-risk conditions, and the avoidance of systematic corticosteroids, oral contraceptives, and antibiotics if possible. Therapy with oral fluconazole, itraconazole, or ketoconazole is recommended for approximately 14 days to ensure clinical remission and negative fungal culture, followed by a maintenance regimen of fluconazole (150 mg once weekly for 6 months). Recurrence of vulvovaginal candidiasis is common, occurring in 30% to 40% of patients after cessation of the maintenance regime.[96]

Other Fungal Infections

ASPERGILLOSIS

Aspergillosis, a rare infection in the surgical patient, usually occurs in those who are markedly immunosuppressed after undergoing chemotherapy with cytotoxic agents or adrenal corticosteroids. Most cases of nosocomial aspergillosis are acquired via airborne transmission.[13,97] Colonization of the respiratory tract is followed by invasive disease if these predisposing factors are present. Sources of airborne fungi in microepidemics frequently are associated with construction within the hospital or at adjacent sites. Other modes of transmission of aspergillosis have been reported, including infections associated with foreign bodies, catheters, and bandages.

Acute invasive pulmonary aspergillosis is the most common form of *Aspergillus* infection in immunocompromised surgical patients. The organisms tend to invade blood vessels and cause thrombosis and infarction of the surrounding tissues. The infection may manifest itself in the form of acute vascular events such as pulmonary embolus or, more rarely, myocardial infarction, cerebral hemorrhage, or Budd-Chiari syndrome. Pulmonary *Aspergillus* infections include necrotizing bronchopneumonia and hemorrhagic pulmonary infarction, each accounting for about one third of these infections. Pulmonary aspergillosis may extend to contiguous organs or be disseminated. The rhinocerebral form of aspergillosis occurs less often than pulmonary infection. It originates in the sinuses and progresses through soft tissues, cartilage, and bone, causing lesions in the palate and the nose. Occasionally, the infection progresses through the base of the skull and involves the brain.

Diagnosis of *Aspergillus* infection is difficult and relies on identifying the organism in culture or histopathologic specimens.[13] The recovery of *Aspergillus* species from the respiratory tract culture of a surgical patient should be considered to represent contamination or colonization unless the patient is symptomatic and severely immunosuppressed. The standard therapy is high-dose amphotericin B (1 mg/kg/day) for a minimum of 2 g.[98] The addition of flucytosine may be useful. Liposomal formulations of amphotericin B and itraconazole offer additional treatment alternatives; at present, however, clinical experience with these new antifungal agents in patients with aspergillosis is limited.

ZYGOMYCOSIS (MUCORMYCOSIS)

Agents of zygomycosis have caused nosocomial infections in the surgical patient. The reservoir, the mode of transmission, the pathogenesis, and the clinical presentations are similar to those of *Aspergillus* species. In the surgical patient, the major risk factors include diabetic ketoacidosis, immunosuppression after cytotoxic chemotherapy, adrenocorticosteroid therapy, organ transplantation, skin damage (e.g., from adhesive tape, an arm board, or severe burns), and a prolonged postoperative stay.[99] Zygomycotic infections include rhinocerebral, paranasal, pulmonary, gastrointestinal, cutaneous, and, very rarely, disseminated disease.

Appropriate management of zygomycosis consists of extensive surgical debridement of infected areas, rapid correction of the underlying disease, and high-dose amphotericin B therapy up to a total dose of 2 to 3 g.

EMERGING PATHOGENS

Fungi such as *Fusarium* species, *Curvularia* species, *Alternaria* species, and *Trichosporon beigelii* were once thought to represent contamination or harmless colonization when isolated from tissue specimens. These and other newly recognized fungi have since been clearly shown to be potentially serious pathogens in immunosuppressed surgical patients.[100] In such patients, the recovery of any fungus from any site should prompt an evaluation by an infectious disease specialist to determine the clinical significance of the isolate.

Systemic Antifungal Agents

AMPHOTERICIN B

Amphotericin B is structurally similar to membrane sterols, and its major mechanism of action is believed to be through interaction with membrane sterols and creation of pores in the fungal outer membrane. The clinical usefulness of amphotericin B is believed to be attributable to the greater affinity of amphotericin B for ergosterol (found in fungal cell membranes) than for cholesterol (the principal sterol found in mammalian cell membranes). Oxidation-dependent amphotericin B-induced stimulation of macrophages is another proposed mechanism of action.[101] Most species of fungi that cause human infections are susceptible to amphotericin B.

Amphotericin B is supplied as a sterile lyophilized powder in vials containing 50 mg of amphotericin B, deoxycholate, and buffer. The contents are then diluted in 5% dextrose in water at a concentration of 10 mg/dl. Less precipitation occurs in saline solutions. The agent is stable at room temperature for 24 hours and is not sensitive to light. An acute infusion-related reaction, consisting of fever, hypotension, and tachycardia, occurs in about 20% of patients.[90] Premedication with acetaminophen may blunt this response. If this approach is unsuccessful, premedication with meperidine (25 to 50 mg I.V.) or hydrocortisone (25 to 50 mg I.V.) is recommended. Hypotension, hypertension, hypothermia, and bradycardia are other reported infusion-related toxic effects of amphotericin B deoxycholate. Ventricular arrhythmias have been associated with rapid infusion of amphotericin B deoxycholate and with administration of the agent to patients with severe hypokalemia or renal failure. Through inhibition of erythropoietic production secondary to nephrotoxicity, amphotericin B suppresses the production of red blood cells, causing a normocytic, normochromic anemia.

Common practice is to give a 1 mg test dose and observe the patient for 1 hour in the hope of identifying patients at risk for severe acute reactions. The full dose of the drug (0.6 to 1 mg/kg/day) is then infused over a period of 4 to 6 hours, although there is evidence to suggest that much shorter infusion times (e.g., 1 hour in patients with adequate cardiopulmonary and renal function) may be acceptable. The total dose depends on the extent of the infection and the patient's condition. Patients must be monitored carefully during the first day of therapy. The infusion should be discontinued if the patient becomes hemodynamically unstable.

If acute reactions limit the amount of drug that can be infused, patients are premedicated with hydrocortisone, 25 to 50 mg I.V., either alone or in combination with meperidine, 25 to 50 mg I.V., 30 minutes before amphotericin B infusion is begun.

The distribution of the drug after I.V. infusion does not directly correlate with the daily dose. This finding is consistent with the unusual pharmacokinetics of amphotericin B. The initial serum half-life of the drug is about 24 hours, and the terminal half-life is about 15 days.

Renal toxicity and hypokalemia are the primary toxicities of amphotericin B [see Table 3]. Amphotericin B-induced nephrotoxicity may be glomerular, characterized by a decrease in glomerular filtration rate and renal blood flow, or tubular, with urinary casts, hypokalemia, hypomagnesemia, renal tubular acidosis, and nephrocalcinosis.[102] All of these abnormalities occur to varying degrees in almost all patients receiving the drug. In most patients, renal dysfunction gradually resolves after discontinuance of therapy. Amphotericin B nephrotoxicity may be minimized by avoiding other agents with synergistic nephrotoxicity (e.g., aminoglycosides, vancomycin, cisplatin, and cyclosporine) and by the administration of sodium supplementation. The latter approach consists of I.V. infusion of 500 ml of 0.9% saline solution 30 minutes before the administration of amphotericin B and a second infusion of the same amount of saline after the amphotericin B infusion is completed.

If the serum creatinine level exceeds 3.5 mg/dl, amphotericin B should be discontinued and the serum creatinine level monitored twice weekly. Administration of amphotericin B may be resumed at 50% to 75% of the original dosage when the serum creatinine level falls below 3 mg/dl.

The combined use of amphotericin B deoxycholate and other nephrotoxic agents, such as cyclosporine, aminoglycosides, and foscarnet, may result in synergistic nephrotoxicity.[103] Less nephrotoxic lipid formulations of amphotericin B include amphotericin B lipid complex (Abelcet), amphotericin B colloidal dispersion (Amphotec), and liposomal amphotericin B (AmBisome). These preparations differ in the amount of amphotericin B and the type of lipid used as well as in the physical form, pharmacokinetics, and toxicities. Of the three formulations, AmBisome is the one that is best tolerated.

FLUCYTOSINE

Flucytosine can be useful for the treatment of hematogenous candidiasis; however, a high failure rate and secondary emergence of resistance have been reported when flucytosine was used alone, and serious concerns exist regarding its myelosuppressive potential. A review of the literature on the activity of flucytosine in acute disseminated candidiasis and candidemia indicates a good response rate.

The standard dosage for flucytosine is 37.5 mg/kg every 6 hours. On the basis of the pharmacokinetics of flucytosine and the in vitro susceptibility of *Candida* species to the drug, much lower dosages of flucytosine (e.g., 12.5 mg/kg every 12 hours) would probably maintain serum and tissue levels significantly above the minimal inhibitory concentration (MIC) needed for most susceptible strains throughout therapy. For example, giving 25 mg/kg/day at 12-hour intervals would result in peak and trough serum levels of about 25 and 5 µg/ml, respectively, given a steady state and normal kidney function in a 70 kg patient. Because the MIC of flucytosine for most susceptible *Candida* species is usually 1 µg/ml or less, such a dosage schedule will constitute

Table 3 Antifungal Chemotherapy[140]

Drug	Indications	Route of Administration	Major Side Effects
Amphotericin B	Hematogenous and deep-seated candidiasis; aspergillosis; blastomycosis; coccidioidomycosis; histoplasmosis; cryptococcosis	Intravenous, intrathecal	Anemia, headache, chills, fever, nausea, renal dysfunction, hypotension, tachypnea, hypokalemia, phlebitis
Clotrimazole	Oropharyngeal candidiasis	Oral	—
Flucytosine	Candidiasis (septicemia, endocarditis, and urinary tract infections); cryptococcosis	Oral	Leukopenia, thrombocytopenia, liver dysfunction, diarrhea
Fluconazole	Oropharyngeal and esophageal candidiasis; hematogenous candidal infection; other candidal infections (e.g., urinary tract infections, peritonitis); meningeal coccidioidomycosis; cryptococcosis	Oral, intravenous	Nausea and vomiting, skin rash, liver dysfunction
Itraconazole	Histoplasmosis; blastomycosis; aspergillosis	Oral	Nausea, vomiting, liver dysfunction
Ketoconazole	Candidiasis (chronic mucocutaneous candidiasis or oropharyngeal candidiasis); candiduria; blastomycosis; coccidioidomycosis; histoplasmosis; chromomycosis; paracoccidioidomycosis	Oral	Hepatotoxicity, nausea or vomiting, occasional suppression of adrenal function

appropriate therapy, given that the drug is used in combination with other antifungals. This approach may decrease the myelosuppressive potential that the drug usually exhibits at levels of 100 µg/ml, and it may lead to the drug's wider use.

Peak serum concentrations should be monitored and the dosage adjusted so as to maintain a peak level of about 25 µg/ml. Flucytosine is removed by hemodialysis and peritoneal dialysis. Patients undergoing hemodialysis should receive a 37.5 mg/kg dose of flucytosine after each dialysis session unless their initial peak serum concentration is higher than 25 µg/ml or their postdialysis concentration is higher than 10 µg/ml. Patients undergoing peritoneal dialysis should receive a single 37.5 mg/kg dose daily.

FLUCONAZOLE

The mechanism of action of fluconazole is preferential inhibition of cytochrome P-450 enzymes in fungal organisms. Fluconazole is active against several *Candida* species, including *C. tropicalis. C. krusei*, however, is highly resistant to this agent.[90] Fluconazole also does not appear to have good clinical activity against *Aspergillus* species. Fluconazole is available in either an oral form or an I.V. form, both of which are rapidly and almost completely absorbed from the GI tract. The serum concentrations after oral administration are almost identical to those achieved when the drug is administered intravenously. A major advantage of fluconazole over ketoconazole is its high degree of GI absorption, which is not affected by gastric acidity or the presence of food. Steady-state serum concentrations of fluconazole are obtained within 5 to 10 days. An initial loading dose that is twice the usual daily dose is recommended. Fluconazole is distributed evenly in body tissues, penetrates into the vitreous humor and the aqueous humor of the eye, and crosses the blood-brain barrier. The drug is excreted largely unchanged in the urine, with only minimal liver metabolism. Consequently, dosage schedules must be adjusted in patients with renal impairment. Hemodialysis significantly reduces the serum concentrations, and the drug appears also to be removed by peritoneal dialysis. A standard dose should be given after each course of dialysis.

The toxicities of fluconazole are similar to those of other azoles and include nausea and vomiting in about 2% of patients, as well as headache, fatigue, abdominal pain, and diarrhea[104]; exfoliative dermatitis also occurs, but very rarely. Transient abnormalities of liver function have been observed in 3% of patients receiving fluconazole. In addition, fatal hepatic necrosis developed in two patients who were receiving fluconazole, but it was unclear whether the agent played a causal role in this event. No significant hormonal abnormalities have been reported after administration of fluconazole.

Because fluconazole interacts with warfarin, phenytoin, and cyclosporine when given in a daily dose of 200 mg or more,[104] serum concentrations of these agents should be monitored.

ITRACONAZOLE

Itraconazole is the only available azole that has substantial activity against *Aspergillus* species. It exists in an oral capsule formulation, the bioavailability of which is approximately 55%. Absorption is enhanced by the presence of food in the stomach but is significantly reduced by the presence of antacids or H_2 receptor blockers. A new solution, which has significantly higher bioavailability, may not be well tolerated by patients. When erratic absorption is of concern, use of the I.V. formulation is recommended. The serum elimination half-life, 15 to 25 hours, increases to 34 to 42 hours after weeks of administration and with increasing itraconazole doses.

Metabolized by the liver, itraconazole is excreted as metabolites primarily in the feces (54%) and urine (35%). A hepatic metabolite, hydroxyitraconazole, has an antifungal spectrum similar to that of the parent compound. Because itraconazole is metabolized to a large degree in the liver, the dosage must be adjusted in patients with hepatic failure; however, its pharmacokinetics are not affected by renal impairment or hemodialysis. Serum concentrations of digoxin may increase when this agent is given with itraconazole,[105] and the metabolism of itraconazole may be accelerated when drugs that induce hepatic enzymes are given simultaneously.[106] Serum concentrations of itraconazole should therefore be measured in patients with invasive infections.

Itraconazole is generally well tolerated in dosages of up to 400 mg/day. The most common side effects are nausea, vomiting, diarrhea, and abdominal discomfort. Headaches, rash, pruritus, and dizziness occasionally occur. At higher doses, a mineralocorticoid excess syndrome (hypokalemia, hypertension, and edema) has been described, and hypokalemia develops in as many as 6% of patients who take 400 mg/day for several months.[107]

Itraconazole is available in 100 mg capsules and oral suspension (10 mg/ml). Because itraconazole may be teratogenic, it should be avoided in pregnant patients. A large number of drug interactions occur with itraconazole, many related to inhibition of the cytochrome P-450 enzyme system. Care should be taken in prescribing itraconazole with these agents. Itraconazole is currently approved for the treatment of blastomycosis, histoplasmosis, and aspergillosis but is also effective for the treatment of candidiasis and cryptococcosis.

KETOCONAZOLE

Ketoconazole is effective against yeast infections of the skin and the mucous membranes; however, it should not be used to treat hemato-

Table 4 Characteristics of Currently Available Azoles*[139]

	Ketoconazole	Fluconazole	Itraconazole
Spectrum	Narrow	Expanded	Expanded
Route(s) of administration	Oral	Oral, intravenous	Oral
Bioavailability	Erratic, requires gastric acidity	Excellent	Erratic, requires gastric acidity
Plasma half-life (hr)	6–9	30	20–40
Hepatotoxicity	Occasional	Occasional	Occasional
Gastrointestinal intolerance	Frequent	Occasional	Occasional
CSF penetration	No	Yes	No
Renal excretion	No	Yes	No
Interaction with other drugs	Frequent	Occasional	Frequent

*Intravenous miconazole is also available but offers no advantage over the currently available azoles.

genous candidiasis. Ketoconazole is not available in an intravenous form, and the serum levels it is capable of reaching depend largely on gastric acidity [*see Table 4*]. The same adverse events and drug-drug interactions observed with itraconazole occur with ketoconazole.

SPECIAL CONSIDERATIONS IN ORGAN TRANSPLANT RECIPIENTS

Intravenous amphotericin B (0.4 to 0.8 mg/kg/day) has been the mainstay of treatment in organ transplant recipients, but concerns have been expressed about increased nephrotoxicity, particularly in patients receiving cyclosporine or tacrolimus. The lipid formulations of amphotericin B (1 to 3 mg/kg/day) are less nephrotoxic, particularly liposomal amphotericin B (AmBisome). Fluconazole has a minimal effect on hepatic microsomal enzymes in comparison with ketoconazole and itraconazole and therefore is the drug of choice in organ transplant recipients who have candidiasis caused by fluconazole-susceptible strains.

Conclusion

Continued progress in supportive care, including the development of antibiotics with increasingly broad spectra of activity, has resulted in an increased incidence of fungal infections, particularly candidiasis. Because of the inadequacy of the available knowledge base, we do not fully understand the pathophysiology of these infections in surgical patients, nor can we be certain precisely when prophylaxis and therapy should be administered.

Despite these limitations, there is now sufficient information available to justify an aggressive therapeutic approach to suspected *Candida* infections. Now that less toxic agents are available (the newer triazoles, particularly fluconazole, and the lipid formulations of amphotericin B), the clinical approach to presumed fungal infections in surgical patients has been made far simpler.

Discussion

Microbiologic Characteristics of Pathogenic *Candida* Species

Candida species multiply by producing buds from ovoid yeast cells. They are differentiated from other yeasts (e.g., *Saccharomyces* species) by their ability to produce pseudohyphae on certain media and, in the case of *C. albicans*, true hyphae in serum [*see Figure 2*].

VIRULENCE FACTORS

Four virulence factors have been demonstrated for *Candida* species: adherence to mucosal epithelial cells; secretion of proteinases, which degrade connective tissue proteins, thereby allowing yeast to enter beyond connective tissue barriers; ambient pH[108]; and resistance to oxidative killing by neutrophils.

For *Candida* species to disseminate, the organisms must be able to adhere to the vascular system (i.e., endothelium, the basement membrane, or both), an ability that is probably receptor mediated.[109] In vitro, however, *Candida* adheres more avidly to the subendothelial extracellular matrix than to endothelial cells. This finding

may explain the increased risk of hematogenous candidiasis in patients receiving cytotoxic chemotherapy. Such therapy causes denudation of endothelium and consequent exposure of the basement membrane, to which *Candida* then readily adheres.

Genetic studies have evaluated the role of various virulence factors for *Candida* species, including ambient pH,[108] adherence mechanisms, and enzyme production. Mechanisms by which *Candida* species lose virulence include the following: gene dysregulation, stopping the switch from budding yeast to filamentous form; disruption of a gene that results in decreased hyphal growth, adherence, and virulence[110]; deficiency of *C. albicans* in mannosyl transferase, resulting in decreased adherence and virulence; and deletion of the gene that encodes the production of phospholipase leading to decreased cell wall penetration.

CHANGING MICROBIOLOGIC SPECTRUM OF *CANDIDA*

Although there are more than 100 described species of *Candida*, only four are commonly associated with infection: *C. albicans, C. tropi-*

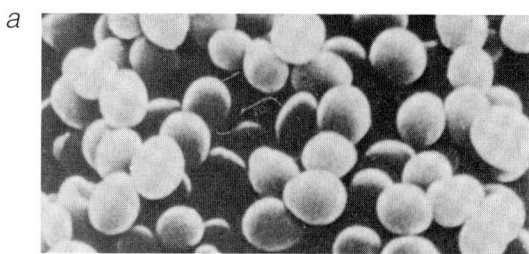

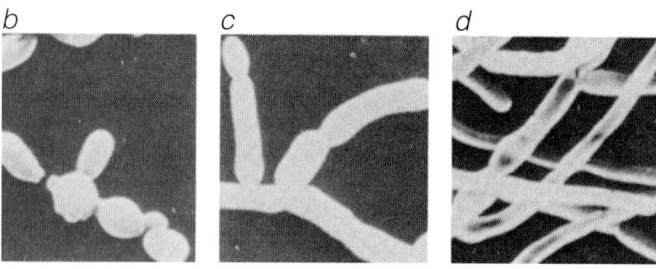

Figure 2   Candida **takes several forms as it grows. A blastospore is a unicellular form (*a*). Blastospores divide by budding, a process in which new cellular material grows from a site on the blastospore (*b*). Nuclear division then occurs, and a septum forms between the two new cells. A hypha is a long tube of several cells divided by septa (*c*). A mycelium is a cellular aggregate that includes a hypha and its branches (*d*). A pseudohypha differs from a true hypha in that it is composed of morphologically distinct, elongated blastospores.**

calis, C. parapsilosis, and *C. glabrata.*[10] Of these, *C. albicans* has been isolated from more than 60% of candidal infections; the other three major species are seen at rates varying from 5% to 20%. Mucosal colonization by *C. tropicalis,* a virulent organism, frequently leads to invasive infection. *C. glabrata* and *C. parapsilosis* appear to be relatively less virulent,[111] and the latter typically causes infection in association with prosthetic materials (e.g., catheters) or glucose-rich intravenous solutions.[10] Finally, *C. krusei* and *C. lusitaniae* rarely cause disease, being isolated from fewer than 1% of cultures.[10] The epidemiology of candidiasis has changed, with reduced rates of *C. albicans* in favor of other candidal species—in particular, *C. glabrata* and *C. krusei.*[112] This change is important because *C. krusei* and several strains of *C. glabrata* are highly resistant to the triazoles such as fluconazole and itraconazole.[10,112]

A study by the NNIS group evaluated 1,579 bloodstream isolates of *Candida* species obtained from more than 50 hospitals in the United States over a 7-year period (1992–1998) to detect trends in species distribution and susceptibility to fluconazole. *C. albicans* accounted for 52% of isolates, followed by *C. glabrata* (18%), *C. parapsilosis* (15%), *C. tropicalis* (11%), and *C. krusei* (2%). Since 1995, *C. glabrata* has been more prevalent than *C. parapsilosis.* The susceptibility of all *Candida* species to fluconazole has remained stable.[113]

Pathogenesis of Candidiasis in the Surgical Patient

COLONIZATION OF THE GUT BY *CANDIDA* SPECIES

That colonization is a necessary prelude to infection is supported by studies demonstrating (1) that 95% of neutropenic patients and 84% of nonneutropenic patients were infected with the same strains that had previously colonized them and (2) that infection was significantly less likely to develop in patients who were not colonized.[114,115] In a study investigating the sequence of colonization and candidemia in nonneutropenic patients, Voss and colleagues[114] found that the strains recovered from the initial colonized or infected site and from

the bloodstream were identical in patients with disseminated candidiasis; furthermore, nearly every patient was infected with a distinct or unique *Candida* strain. In another study, positive surveillance cultures were found to be highly predictive of systemic infection, whereas negative surveillance cultures correlated with a low risk of candidal dissemination.[116] Clinical studies of antifungal prophylaxis in neutropenic cancer patients have also suggested that antifungal regimens effectively prevent hematogenous infection when they can eliminate or reduce colonization by *Candida.*[117]

The density of colonization appears to be predictive of the risk of hematogenous candidiasis. In two large series of neutropenic cancer patients, hematogenous candidiasis almost never developed in noncolonized patients, compared with an infection rate of more than 30% in patients with multiple colonized sites.[115,118] In a study of patients with acute lymphocytic leukemia, a relatively high concentration of *Candida* organisms in the stools was found to be a significant risk factor for hematogenous candidiasis.[119] In 40 infants of very low birth weight, a value of 8×10^6 *Candida* CFU/g stool was established as a threshold, beyond which GI symptoms (attributed to *Candida*) developed in 50% of the infants and a systemic septic response in 28.5% during 1 to 3 weeks of heavy colonization.[120] In a prospective study of patients admitted to surgical and neonatal intensive care units, Pittet and coworkers demonstrated that the intensity of *Candida* colonization (as determined by a *Candida* colonization index) was significantly higher in patients who subsequently became infected than in those who did not.[121] Other case-control studies have demonstrated that colonization by *Candida* species at various body sites and exposure to several antibiotics were independent risk factors for candidemia.[122]

The normal endogenous intestinal flora inhibits GI colonization and overgrowth by potentially pathogenic bacteria and fungi by forming what may be thought of as living wallpaper in the large intestine. Suppression of endogenous microflora as a consequence of antimicrobial administration[123] may permit overgrowth of pathogenic strains in the GI tract and selection of resistant strains, which may result in enterocolitis, systemic infection, or the septic response.

PHYSICAL DISRUPTION OF THE INTESTINAL MUCOSAL BARRIER

In humans, as well as in animals, the GI tract is considered to be the most important portal of entry for microorganisms, including yeasts, into the bloodstream. The passage of endogenous fungi from the GI tract to extraintestinal sites can be referred to as fungal translocation (by analogy with bacterial translocation).

Although yeast cells have no intrinsic motility, they are able to translocate from the intestinal lumen within a few hours of ingestion. In a study conducted in the 1960s, two nonpathogenic yeasts were surgically instilled into the rat duodenum and were recovered from the cisterna chyli within 4 hours.[124] Even in the absence of disease, any marked increase in the intestinal population of *Candida* can lead to fungal translocation and subsequent hematogenous infection. That candidal species can translocate from the gut to the bloodstream was demonstrated in a study in which signs and symptoms of sepsis developed in a healthy volunteer 2 hours after ingestion of a suspension containing 10^{12} *C. albicans* organisms, and blood cultures taken 3 and 6 hours after ingestion were positive for *Candida.*[125] In addition, autopsy studies conducted in patients with hematogenous candidiasis found involvement of the GI tract and submucosal invasion in almost all patients.[86]

Microbial translocation has been demonstrated in several animal models and has been shown to be enhanced by several factors, including fasting, which induces complex changes in host defenses, and protein deficiency, which results in intestinal microbial overgrowth, increased intestinal absorption of intact proteins, and decreased intracellular killing of bacteria and fungi. In one study involving *C. albicans,* volatile fatty acids and secondary bile salts

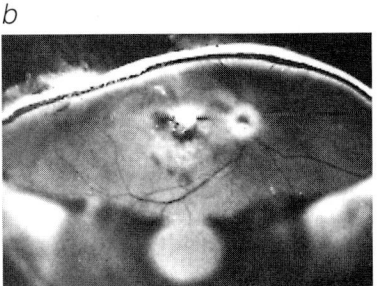
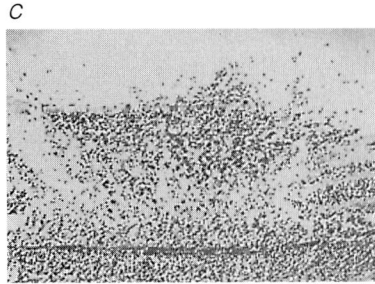

a *b* *c*

Figure 3 *Candida* endophthalmitis is common in patients with persistent fungemia. On funduscopy, a characteristic white, cotton-wool–like exudate can be seen (*a*). Cut section of an eye shows *Candida* retinitis (*b*). A microscopic view of *Candida* chorioretinitis is also provided (*c*).[138]

reduced fungal adhesion to the mucosa, colonization, and dissemination in mice by causing the formation of a dense layer of bacteria in the mucus gel; these bacteria successfully competed with the yeast cells for the same adhesion sites and produced various substances that inhibited fungal growth.[126] In another animal model, bile duct ligation resulted in bacterial translocation.[127] In yet another, splanchnic ischemia in guinea pigs increased fungal translocation.[128] Similar results were obtained in guinea pigs and rats that had burns covering 50% of their total body surface area. After the yeast cells penetrated the lamina propria, the cells were found either free in the lymphatic vessels and in the blood vessels or engulfed by macrophages.[129]

Microbial translocation has been shown to be clinically relevant in humans. Surveillance cultures from patients with leukemia have demonstrated an association between the bacterial biotype or serotype that was most prevalent in the patient's feces and the bacterial biotype or serotype that subsequently caused septicemia. Significant microbial translocation has been demonstrated in patients who underwent operation for colorectal carcinoma, intestinal obstruction, or Crohn disease. In addition, translocation is thought to occur as a result of flattening of the intestinal villi that results from the administration of total parenteral nutrition.[130]

Immunosuppression Leading to Dissemination of Candidiasis

Host defenses against *Candida* infections include T cell immunity, to prevent colonization and superficial invasion, and phagocytic immunity, to prevent deeper tissue invasion and hematogenous dissemination. Any condition that suppresses any of these arms of the immune system puts the patient at increased risk for candidiasis. Phagocytes ingest intestinal microbes. In a patient whose immune system has been compromised, these phagocytes transport microbes out of the intestine, fail to kill them, and finally liberate them in extraintestinal sites. Examples of immunosuppression include hematologic malignancy, bone marrow or organ transplantation, and immunosuppressive therapy such as cancer chemotherapy and corticosteroid therapy. Total parenteral nutrition (TPN) may result in immunosuppression. Transient hyperglycemia in patients receiving TPN causes an acceleration in the nonenzymatic glycosylation of immunoglobulin G, leading to its inactivation and impairment of complement fixation.[131] In a randomized, prospective study,[132] long-chain triglycerides in TPN significantly decreased the ratio of helper B cells to suppressor T cells. There is evidence that fat emulsions may impair polymorphonuclear and macrophage function.[133] In animal models, TPN induced macrophage suppression with decreased peritoneal macrophage superoxide production and *Candida* phagocytosis, associated with bacterial translocation to mesenteric lymph nodes.[134]

Pathology of *Candida* Colonization and Infectious Syndromes

The evolution of *Candida* microabscesses after hematogenous distribution has been studied in animal models. After intravenous infusion in nonneutropenic animals, the liver, the kidneys, the heart, the eyes, the brain, and the skin show a pattern of intracapillary fungi (yeasts and pseudohyphae) with an accumulation of neutrophils. In time, focal areas of necrosis occur, resulting in organ dysfunction that ultimately leads to death.

In nonneutropenic patients who are dying of candidiasis, a similar histologic picture and a similar pattern of organ involvement are seen. The organs most frequently involved are the brain, the heart, the kidneys, and the eyes. *Candida* produces microabscesses and, frequently, noncaseating granulomas. The histologic picture suggests that blood-borne fungi are lodged in the microvasculature, resulting in vasculitis. This multifocal microscopic disease explains the absence of localizing findings despite the progressive cerebral, renal, and cardiac dysfunction seen in infected persons.

The high incidence of cerebral involvement has been underscored by findings in an autopsy study of 41 nonneutropenic patients with tissue-verified deep candidiasis, of whom 26 (63%) had undergone major operations.[135] Nineteen (46%) were found to have cerebral candidal infections; all 19 individuals had antecedent proven or suspected gram-negative sepsis and had been treated with appropriate antibiotic therapy. In every patient studied, *Candida* organisms were identified at sites outside the brain, including the kidneys (90%) and the heart (80%). Candidiasis produced intracerebral microabscesses and noncaseating granulomas without diffuse leptomeningitis.

In a nearly identical autopsy series, 18 patients with disseminated candidiasis were found to have myocardial involvement.[136] This mycosis was characterized by myocardial microabscesses with yeasts and pseudohyphal elements. Noncaseating granulomas were seen in only one patient. Eight patients had recognized conduction disturbances, including alterations in both heart rate and heart rhythm.

As in the animal models, ocular involvement is a common finding in patients with disseminated candidiasis and by itself is an indication for systemic therapy. The eye pathology is a chorioretinitis with microabscess formation. Funduscopic examination, mandatory in patients suspected of having systemic *Candida* infection, reveals patchy, wool-like tufts [*see Figure 3*].

Despite the frequent finding of *Candida* in sputum cultures, primary *Candida* pneumonitis is extremely uncommon[137]; when it occurs, it usually follows aspiration of oropharyngeal contents. However, pulmonary involvement resulting from hematogenous seeding is common.

References

1. Wey SB, Mori M, Pfaller MA, et al: Hospital-acquired candidemia: the attributable mortality and excess length of stay. Arch Intern Med 148:2642, 1988

2. Pfaller M, Wenzel R: Impact of the changing epidemiology of fungal infections in the 1990s. Eur J Clin Microbiol Infect Dis 11:287, 1992

3. Jarvis WR, Martone WJ: Predominant pathogens in hospital infections. J Antimicrob Chemother 29:19, 1992

4. Schaberg DR, Culver DH, Gaynes RP: Major trends in the microbial etiology of nosocomial infection. Am J Med 91:72S, 1991

5. Banerjee SN, Emori TG, Culver DH, et al: Secular trends in nosocomial primary bloodstream infections in the United States, 1980-1989. National Nosocomial Infections Surveillance System. Am J Med 91(3B):86S, 1991

6. Beck-Sagué C, Jarvis WR: Secular trends in the epidemiology of nosocomial fungal infections in the United States, 1980-1990. National Nosocomial Infections Surveillance System. J Infect Dis 167:1247, 1993

7. Pfaller MA, Jones RN, Messer SA, et al: National surveillance of nosocomial blood stream infection due to Candida albicans: frequency of occurrence and antifungal susceptibility in the SCOPE Program. Diagn Microbiol Infect Dis 31:327, 1998

8. Vincent JL, Anaissie E, Bruining H, et al: Epidemiology, diagnosis and treatment of systemic Candida infection in surgical patients under intensive care. Intens Care Med 24:206, 1998

9. Pittet D, Li N, Woolson RF, et al: Microbiological factors influencing the outcome of nosocomial bloodstream infections: a 6-year validated, population-based model. Clin Infect Dis 24:1068, 1997

10. Anaissie EJ, Rex JH, Uzun O, et al: Predictors of adverse outcome in cancer patients with candidemia. Am J Med 104:238, 1998

11. Bodey GP, Luna M: Skin lesions associated with disseminated candidiasis. JAMA 229:1466, 1974

12. Anaissie E, Bodey GP, Kantarjian H, et al: Fluconazole therapy for chronic disseminated candidiasis in patients with leukemia and prior amphotericin B therapy. Am J Med 91:142, 1991

13. Anaissie E: Opportunistic mycoses in the immunocompromised host: experience at a cancer center and review. Clin Infect Dis 14:S43, 1992

14. Meunier F, Aoun M, Bitar N: Candidemia in immunocompromised patients. Clin Infect Dis 14:S120, 1992

15. Baley JE, Annable WL, Klegman RM: Candida endophthalmitis in the premature infant. J Pediatr 98:458, 1981

16. Dupont B, Drouhet E: Cutaneous, ocular, and osteoarticular candidiasis in heroin addicts: new clinical and therapeutic aspects in 38 patients. J Infect Dis 152:577, 1985

17. Eubanks PJ, de Virgilio C, Klein S, et al: Candida sepsis in surgical patients. Am J Surg 166:617, 1993

18. Castaldo P, Stratta RJ, Wood RP, et al: Clinical spectrum of fungal infections after orthotopic liver transplantation. Arch Surg 126:149, 1991

19. Prasad JK, Feller I, Thomson PD: A ten-year review of Candida sepsis and mortality in burn patients. Surgery 101:213, 1987

20. Desai MH, Rutan RL, Heggers JP, et al: Candida infection with and without nystatin prophylaxis: an 11-year experience with patients with burn injury. Arch Surg 127:159, 1992

21. Desai MH, Herndon DN: Eradication of Candida burn wound septicemia in massively burned patients. J Trauma 28:140, 1988

22. Paya CV: Fungal infections in solid-organ transplantation. Clin Infect Dis 16:677, 1993

23. Hesse UJ, Sutherland DE, Simmons RL, et al: Intra-abdominal infections in pancreas transplant recipients. Ann Surg 203:153, 1986

24. Hofflin JM, Potasman I, Baldwin JC, et al: Infectious complications in heart transplant recipients receiving cyclosporine and corticosteroids. Ann Intern Med 106:209, 1987

25. Brooks RG, Hofflin JM, Jamieson SW, et al: Infectious complications in heart-lung transplant recipients. Am J Med 79:412, 1985

26. Ramsey DE, Finch WT, Birtch AG: Urinary tract infections in kidney transplant recipients. Arch Surg 114:1022, 1979

27. Anaissie E, Samonis G, Kontoyiannis D, et al: Role of catheter colonization and infrequent hematogenous seeding in catheter-related infections. Eur J Clin Microbiol Infect Dis 14:134, 1995

28. Walsh TJ, Lee JW, Sien T, et al: Serum D-arabinitol measured by automated quantitative enzymatic assay for detection and therapeutic monitoring of experimental disseminated candidiasis: correlation with tissue concentrations of Candida albicans. J Med Vet Mycol 32:205, 1994

29. Brannon P, Kiehn TE: Large-scale clinical comparison of the lysis-centrifugation and radiometric systems for blood culture. J Clin Microbiol 22:951, 1985

30. Berenguer J, Buck M, Witebski F, et al: Lysis-centrifugation blood cultures in the detection of tissue-proven invasive candidiasis: disseminated versus single-organ infection. Diagn Microbiol Infect Dis 17:103, 1993

31. Ho YM, Ng MH, Teoh-Chan CH, et al: Indirect immunofluorescence assay for antibody to germ tube of Candida albicans—a new diagnostic test. J Clin Pathol 29:1007, 1976

32. Greenfield RA, Stephens JL, Bussey MJ, et al: Quantitation of antibody to Candida mannan by enzyme-linked immunosorbent assay. J Lab Clin Med 101:758, 1983

33. van Deventer AJM, van Vlient HJA, Hop WCJ, et al: Diagnostic value of anti-Candida enolase antibodies. J Clin Microbiol 32:17, 1994

34. Jones JM: Quantitation of antibody against cell wall mannan and a major cytoplasmic antigen of Candida in rabbits, mice, and humans. Infect Immun 30:78, 1980

35. Weiner MH, Coats-Stephen M: Immunodiagnosis of systemic candidiasis: mannan antigenemia detected by radioimmunoassay in experimental and human infections. J Infect Dis 140:989, 1979

36. Bailey JW, Sada E, Brass C, et al: Diagnosis of systemic candidiasis by latex agglutination for serum antigen. J Clin Microbiol 21:749, 1985

37. Fung JC, Donta ST, Tilton RC: Candida detection system (CAND-TEC) to differentiate between Candida albicans colonizations and disease. J Clin Microbiol 24:542, 1986

38. Walsh TJ, Hathorn JW, Sobel JD, et al: Detection of circulating Candida enolase by immunoassay in patients with cancer and invasive candidiasis. N Engl J Med 324:1026, 1991

39. Gutiérrez J, Maroto C, Piédrola G, et al: Circulating Candida antigens and antibodies: useful markers of candidemia. J Clin Microbiol 31:2550, 1993

40. Freydiere AM, Buchaille L, Guinet R, et al: Evaluation of latex reagents for rapid identification of Candida albicans and C. krusei colonies. J Clin Microbiol 35:877, 1997

41. Fujita S-I, Lasker BA, Lott TJ, et al: Microtitration plate enzyme immunoassay to detect PCR-amplified DNA from Candida species in blood. J Clin Microbiol 33:962, 1995

42. Sandhu GS, Kline BC, Stockman L, et al: Molecular probes for diagnosis of fungal infections. J Clin Microbiol 33:2913, 1995

43. Walsh TJ, Francesconi A, Kasai M, et al: PCR and single-strand conformational polymorphism for recognition of medically important opportunistic fungi. J Clin Microbiol 33:3216, 1995

44. Reiss E, Morrison CJ: Nonculture methods for diagnosis of disseminated candidiasis. Clin Microbiol Rev 6:311, 1993

45. de Repentigny L, Marr LD, Keller JW, et al: Comparison of enzyme immunoassay and gas-liquid chromatography for the rapid diagnosis of invasive candidiasis in cancer patients. J Clin Microbiol 21:972, 1985

46. Walsh TJ, Merz WG, Lee JW, et al: Diagnosis and therapeutic monitoring of invasive candidiasis by rapid enzymatic detection of serum D-arabinitol. Am J Med 99:164, 1995

47. Dyess DL, Garrison N, Fry DE: Candida sepsis: implications of polymicrobial blood-borne infection. Arch Surg 120:345, 1985

48. Rantala A, Niinikoski J, Lehtonen OP: Yeasts in blood cultures: impact of early therapy. Scand J Infect Dis 21:557, 1989

49. Rex JH, Bennett JE, Sugar AM, et al: A randomized trial comparing fluconazole with amphotericin B for the treatment of candidemia in patients without neutropenia. Candidemia Study Group and the National Institute. N Engl J Med 331:1325, 1994

50. Anaissie EJ, Vartivarian SE, Abi-Said D, et al: Fluconazole versus amphotericin B in the treatment of hematogenous candidiasis: a matched cohort study. Am J Med 101:170, 1996

51. Nguyen MH, Peacock JE Jr, Tanner DC, et al: Therapeutic approaches in patients with candidemia: evaluation in a multicenter, prospective, observational study. Arch Intern Med 155:2429, 1995

52. Kujath P, Lerch K, Kochendorfer P, et al: Comparative study of the efficacy of fluconazole versus amphotericin B/flucytosine in surgical patients with systemic mycoses. Infection 21:376, 1993

53. Van't Wout JW, Mattie H, van Furth R: A prospective study of the efficacy of fluconazole (UK-49,858) against deep-seated fungal infections. J Antimicrob Chemother 21:665, 1988

54. de Marie S, Janknegt R, Bakker-Woudenberg IA: Clinical use of liposomal and lipid-complexed amphotericin B. J Antimicrob Chemother 33:907, 1994

55. Walsh TJ, Hiemenz JW, Seibel NL, et al: Amphotericin B lipid complex for invasive fungal infections: analysis of safety and efficacy in 556 cases. Clin Infect Dis 26:1383, 1998

56. Nucci M, Colombo AL, Silveira F, et al: Risk factors for death in patients with candidemia. Infect Control Hosp Epidemiol 19:846, 1998

57. Rex JH, Bennett JE, Sugar AM, et al: Intravascular catheter exchange and duration of candidemia. NIAID Mycoses Study Group and the Candidemia Study Group. Clin Infect Dis 21:994, 1995

58. Stevenhagen A, van Furth R: Interferon-gamma activates the oxidative killing of Candida albicans by human granulocytes. Clin Exp Immunol 91:170, 1993

59. Fratti RA, Ghannoum MA, Edwards JE Jr, et al: Gamma interferon protects endothelial cells from damage by Candida albicans by inhibiting endothelial cell phagocytosis. Infect Immun 64:4714, 1996

60. Gaviria JM, van Burik JA, Dale DC, et al: Comparison of interferon-gamma, granulocyte colony-stimulating factor, and granulocyte-macrophage colony-stimulating factor for priming leukocyte-mediated hyphal damage of opportunistic fungal pathogens. J Infect Dis 179:1038, 1999

61. Gorensek MJ, Carey WD, Washington JA 2nd, et al: Selective bowel decontamination with quinolones and nystatin reduces gram-negative and fungal infections in orthotopic liver transplant recipients. Cleve Clin J Med 60:139, 1993

62. Mora NP, Cofer JB, Solomon H, et al: Analysis of severe infections (INF) after 180 consecutive liver transplants: the impact of amphotericin B prophylaxis for reducing the incidence and severity of fungal infections. Transplant Proc 23:1528, 1991

63. Tollemar J, Ringden O, Andersson S, et al: Randomized double-blind study of liposomal amphotericin B (AmBisome) prophylaxis of invasive fungal infections in bone marrow transplant recipients. Bone Marrow Transplant 12:577, 1993

64. Slavin MA, Osborne B, Adams R, et al: Efficacy and safety of fluconazole prophylaxis for fungal infections after bone marrow transplantation—a prospective, randomized, double-blind study. J Infect Dis 171:1545, 1995

65. Rotstein C, Bow EJ, Laverdiere M, et al: Randomized placebo-controlled trial of fluconazole prophylaxis for neutropenic cancer patients: benefit based on purpose and intensity of cytotoxic therapy. The Canadian Fluconazole Prophylaxis Study Group. Clin Infect Dis 28:331, 1999

66. Powderly WG, Finkelstein D, Feinberg J, et al: A randomized trial comparing fluconazole with clotrimazole troches for the prevention of fungal infections in patients with advanced human immunodeficiency virus infection. NIAID AIDS Clinical Trials Group. N Engl J Med 332:700, 1995

67. Eggimann P, Francioli P, Bille J, et al: Fluconazole prophylaxis prevents intra-abdominal candidiasis in high-risk surgical patients. Crit Care Med 27:1066, 1999

68. Dube MP, Heseltine PN, Rinaldi MG, et al: Fungemia and colonization with nystatin-resistant Candida rugosa in a burn unit. Clin Infect Dis 18:77, 1994

69. Torbenson M, Wang J, Nichols L, et al: Causes of death in autopsied liver transplantation patients. Mod Pathol 11:37, 1998

70. Lumbreras C, Cuervas-Mons V, Jara P, et al: Randomized trial of fluconazole versus nystatin for the prophylaxis of Candida infection following liver transplantation. J Infect Dis 174:583, 1996

71. Lorf T, Braun F, Ruchel R, et al: Systemic mycoses during prophylactical use of liposomal amphotericin B (AmBisome) after liver transplantation. Mycoses 42:47, 1999

72. Savani DV, Perfect JR, Cobo LM, et al: Penetration of new azole compounds into the eye and efficacy in experimental Candida endophthalmitis. Antimicrob Agents Chemother 31:6, 1987

73. Venditti M, De Bernardis F, Micozzi A, et al: Fluconazole treatment of catheter-related right-sided endocarditis caused by Candida albicans and associated with endophthalmitis and folliculitis. Clin Infect Dis 14:422, 1992

74. Moyer DV, Edwards JE Jr: Candida endophthalmitis and central nervous system infection. Candidiasis: Pathogenesis, Diagnosis, and Treatment. Bodey GP, Ed. Raven Press, New York, 1993, p 331

75. Martinez-Vazquez C, Fernandez-Ulloa J, Bordon J, et al: Candida albicans endophthalmitis in brown heroin addicts: response to early vitrectomy preceded and followed by antifungal therapy. Clin Infect Dis 27:1130, 1998

76. Yackee JM, Topiel MS, Simon GL: Septic phlebitis caused by Candida albicans and diagnosed by needle aspiration. South Med J 78:1262, 1985

77. Czwerwiec FS, Bilsker MS, Kamerman ML, et al: Long-term survival after fluconazole therapy of candidal prosthetic valve endocarditis. Am J Med 94:545, 1993

78. Kraus WE, Valenstein PN, Corey GR: Purulent pericarditis caused by Candida: report of three cases and identification of high-risk populations as an aid to early diagnosis. Rev Infect Dis 10:34, 1988

79. Cuende E, Barbadillo C, E-Mazzuchelli R, et al: Candida arthritis in adult patients who are not intravenous drug addicts: report of three cases and review of the literature. Semin Arthritis Rheum 22:224, 1993

80. Penk A, Pittrow L: [Status of fluconazole in the therapy of endogenous Candida endophthalmitis]. Mycoses 41(suppl 2):41, 1998

81. Tang C: Successful treatment of Candida albicans osteomyelitis with fluconazole. J Infect 26:89, 1993

82. Shapiro S, Javed T, Mealey J Jr: Candida albicans shunt infection. Pediatr Neurosci 15:125, 1989

83. Mascarenas CA, Hardin TC, Pennick GJ, et al: Treatment of thrush with itraconazole solution: evidence for topical effect. Clin Infect Dis 26:1242, 1998

84. Crutchfield CE 3rd, Lewis EJ: The successful treatment of oral candidiasis (thrush) in a pediatric patient using itraconazole (letter). Pediatr Dermatol 14:246, 1997

85. Tunkel AR, Thomas CY, Wispelwey B: Candida prosthetic arthritis: report of a case treated with fluconazole and review of the literature. Am J Med 94:100, 1993

86. Walsh TJ, Merz WG: Pathologic features in the human alimentary tract associated with invasiveness of Candida tropicalis. Am J Clin Pathol 85:498, 1986

87. Gupta TP, Ehrinpreis MN: Candida-associated diarrhea in hospitalized patients. Gastroenterology 98:780, 1990

88. Calandra T, Bille J, Schneider R, et al: Clinical significance of Candida isolated from peritoneum in surgical patients. Lancet 2:1437, 1989

89. Corbella X, Sirvent JM, Carratala J: Fluconazole treatment without catheter removal in Candida albicans peritonitis complicating peritoneal dialysis. Am J Med 90:277, 1991

90. Eisenberg ES, Leviton I, Soeiro R: Fungal peritonitis in patients receiving peritoneal dialysis: experience with 11 patients and review of the literature [published erratum appears in Rev Infect Dis 8:839, 1986]. Rev Infect Dis 8:309, 1986

91. Lo WK, Chan CY, Cheng SW, et al: A prospective randomized control study of oral nystatin prophylaxis for Candida peritonitis complicating continuous ambulatory peritoneal dialysis. Am J Kidney Dis 28:549, 1996

92. Huang CT, Leu HS: Candiduria as an early marker of disseminated infection in critically ill surgical patients (letter; comment). J Trauma 39:616, 1995

93. Chakrabarti A, Reddy TC, Singhi S: Does candiduria predict candidaemia? Ind J Med Res 106:513, 1997

94. Strassner C, Friesen A: [Therapy of candiduria by alkalinization of urine: oral treatment with potassium-sodium-hydrogen citrate]. Fortschr Med 113:359, 1995

95. Tacker JR: Successful use of fluconazole for treatment of urinary tract fungal infections. J Urol 148:1917, 1992

96. Sobel JD: Recurrent vulvovaginal candidiasis: a prospective study of the efficacy of maintenance ketoconazole therapy. N Engl J Med 315:1455, 1986

97. Walsh TJ, Dixon DM: Nosocomial aspergillosis, environmental microbiology, hospital epidemiology, diagnosis and treatment. Eur J Epidemiol 5:131, 1989

98. Denning DW, Stevens DA: Antifungal and surgical treatment of invasive aspergillosis: review of 2,121 published cases [published erratum appears in Rev Infect Dis 13:345, 1991]. Rev Infect Dis 12:1147, 1990

99. Anaissie E, Bodey GP: Nosocomial fungal infections: old problems and new challenges. Infect Dis Clin North Am 3:867, 1989

100. Anaissie E, Bodey GP, Kantarjian H, et al: New spectrum of fungal infections in patients with cancer. Rev Infect Dis 11:369, 1989

101. Sokol-Anderson ML, Brajtburg J, Medoff G: Amphotericin B-induced oxidative damage and killing of Candida albicans. J Infect Dis 154:76, 1986

102. Burgess JL, Birchall R: Nephrotoxicity of amphotericin B, with emphasis on changes in tubular function. Am J Med 53:77, 1972

103. Kennedy MS, Deeg HJ, Siegel M, et al: Acute renal toxicity with combined use of amphotericin B and cyclosporine after marrow transplantation. Transplantation 35:211, 1983

104. Zervos M, Meunier F: Fluconazole (Diflucan): a review. Int J Antimicrob Agents 3:147, 1993

105. McClean KL, Sheehan GJ: Interaction between itraconazole and digoxin (letter; comment). Clin Infect Dis 18:259, 1994

106. Drayton J, Dickinson G, Rinaldi MG: Coadministration of rifampin and itraconazole leads to undetectable levels of serum itraconazole (letter). Clin Infect Dis 18:266, 1994

107. Tucker RM, Haq Y, Denning DW, et al: Adverse events associated with itraconazole in 189 patients on chronic therapy. J Antimicrob Chemother 26:561, 1990

108. De Bernardis F, Muhlschlegel FA, Cassone A, et al: The pH of the host niche controls gene expression in and virulence of Candida albicans. Infect Immun 66:3317, 1998

109. Klotz SA: Fungal adherence to the vascular compartment: a critical step in the pathogenesis of disseminated candidiasis. Clin Infect Dis 14:340, 1992

110. Gale CA, Bendel CM, McClellan M, et al: Linkage of adhesion, filamentous growth, and virulence in Candida albicans to a single gene, INT1. Science 279:1355, 1998

111. Lecciones JA, Lee JW, Navarro EE, et al: Vascular catheter-associated fungemia in patients with cancer: analysis of 155 episodes. Clin Infect Dis 14:875, 1992

112. Abi-Said D, Anaissie E, Uzun O, et al: The epidemiology of hematogenous candidiasis caused by different Candida species [published erratum appears in Clin Infect Dis 25:352, 1997]. Clin Infect Dis 24:1122, 1997

113. Pfaller MA, Messer SA, Hollis RJ, et al: Trends in species distribution and susceptibility to fluconazole among blood stream isolates of Candida species in the United States. Diagn Microbiol Infect Dis 33:217, 1999

114. Voss A, Hollis RJ, Pfaller MA, et al: Investigation of the sequence of colonization and candidemia in nonneutropenic patients. J Clin Microbiol 32:975, 1994

115. Martino P, Girmenia C, Venditti M, et al: Candida colonization and systemic infection in neutropenic patients: a retrospective study. Cancer 64:2030, 1989

116. Pfaller M, Cabezudo I, Koontz F, et al: Predictive value of surveillance cultures for systemic infection due to Candida species. Eur J Clin Microbiol Infect Dis 6:628, 1987

117. Uzun O, Anaissie EJ: Antifungal prophylaxis in patients with hematologic malignancies: a reappraisal. Blood 86:2063, 1995

118. Martino P, Girmenia C, Micozzi A, et al: Fungemia in patients with leukemia. Am J Med Sci 306:225, 1993

119. Richet HM, Andremont A, Tancrede C, et al: Risk factors for candidemia in patients with acute lymphocytic leukemia. Rev Infect Dis 13:211, 1991

120. Pappu-Katikaneni LD, Rao KP, Banister E: Gastrointestinal colonization with yeast species and Candida septicemia in very low birth weight infants.

Mycoses 33:20, 1990

121. Pittet D, Monod M, Suter PM, et al: Candida colonization and subsequent infections in critically ill surgical patients. Ann Surg 220:751, 1994

122. Wey SB, Mori M, Pfaller MA, et al: Risk factors for hospital-acquired candidemia: a matched case-control study. Arch Intern Med 149:2349, 1989

123. Giuliano M, Barza M, Jacobus NV, et al: Effect of broad-spectrum parenteral antibiotics on composition of intestinal microflora of humans. Antimicrob Agents Chemother 31:202, 1987

124. Wolochow H, Hildebrand GJ, Lamanna C: Translocation of microorganisms across the intestinal wall of the rat: effect of microbial size and concentration. J Infect Dis 116:523, 1966

125. Krause W, Matheis H, Wulf K: Fungaemia and funguria after oral administration of Candida albicans. Lancet 1:598, 1969

126. Kennedy MJ, Volz PA: Ecology of Candida albicans gut colonization: inhibition of Candida adhesion, colonization, and dissemination from the gastrointestinal tract by bacterial antagonism. Infect Immun

49:654, 1985

127. Deitch EA, Sittig K, Li M, et al: Obstructive jaundice promotes bacterial translocation from the gut. Am J Surg 159:79, 1990

128. Gianotti L, Alexander JW, Fukushima R, et al: Translocation of *Candida albicans* is related to the blood flow of individual intestinal villi. Circ Shock 40:250, 1993

129. Alexander JW, Boyce ST, Babcock JF, et al: The process of microbial translocation. Ann Surg 212:496, 1990

130. Pappo I, Polacheck I, Zmora O, et al: Altered gut barrier function to Candida during parenteral nutrition. Nutrition 10:151, 1994

131. Hennessey PJ, Black CT, Andrassy RJ: Nonenzymatic glycosylation of immunoglobulin G impairs complement fixation. JPEN J Parenter Enteral Nutr 15:60, 1991

132. Gogos CA, Kalfarentzos FE, Zoumbos NC: Effect of different types of total parenteral nutrition on T-lymphocyte subpopulations and NK cells. Am J Clin Nutr 51:119, 1990

133. Gogos CA, Kalfarentzos F: Total parenteral nutrition and immune system activity: a review. Nutrition 11:339, 1995

134. Shou J, Lappin J, Minnard EA, et al: Total parenteral nutrition, bacterial translocation, and host immune function. Am J Surg 167:145, 1994

135. Parker JC Jr, McCloskey JJ, Lee RS: Human cerebral candidosis—a postmortem evaluation of 19 patients. Hum Pathol 12:23, 1981

136. Parker JC Jr: The potentially lethal problem of cardiac candidosis. Am J Clin Pathol 73:356, 1980

137. Haron E, Vartivarian S, Anaissie E, et al: Primary Candida pneumonia: experience at a large cancer center and review of the literature. Medicine (Baltimore) 72:137, 1993

138. Gaines JD, Remington JS: Disseminated candidiasis in the surgical patient. Surgery 72:730, 1972

139. Greenburg SB: Fungal and viral infections. Critical Care, 2nd ed. Civetta JM, Taylor RW, Kirby RR, Eds. JB Lippincott Co, Philadelphia, 1993, p 1055

140. Medoff G, Kobayashi GS: Systemic fungal infections: an overview. Hosp Pract 26(2):41, 1991

20 VIRAL INFECTION

Jennifer W. Janelle, M.D., and Richard J. Howard, M.D., Ph.D., F.A.C.S.

Approach to Viral Exposure

Compared with primary care physicians, such as internists, family physicians, and pediatricians, surgeons are seldom called on to treat viral infections. Viral infections nonetheless deserve the attention of surgeons because these infections can cause illness in patients after operation, albeit infrequently, and can spread to the hospital staff. Some viral infections (e.g., infections with the hepatitis viruses, HIV, and cytomegalovirus [CMV]) can result from administration of blood or blood products or can be transmitted to hospital personnel through needle-stick injury. Viral infections can also result from organ transplantation or trauma (e.g., rabies, which is transmitted by the bite of an infected animal). Some viruses, especially the herpesviruses, frequently infect immunosuppressed patients, in whom the viruses can cause severe illness and even death. In many surgical practices, there are increasing numbers of immunosuppressed patients, including organ transplant recipients; patients with cancer; patients receiving cancer chemotherapy, steroids, and other immunosuppressive drugs; the elderly; and the malnourished. Some viral infections can cause neoplastic disease for which operation may become necessary. Examples are hepatitis B virus (HBV) and hepatitis C virus (HCV), which are implicated in the etiology of hepatocellular carcinoma; Epstein-Barr virus (EBV), which can cause a lethal lymphoproliferative disorder in immunosuppressed patients; and human T cell lymphotropic virus type I (HTLV-I), which can induce a T cell leukemia. Viral infections very likely can cause other neoplasms as well.

Prevention of Transmission of HIV, Hepatitis B Virus, and Hepatitis C Virus

TRANSMISSION FROM PATIENTS TO HEALTH CARE WORKERS

The Centers for Disease Control and Prevention (CDC) has published extensive recommendations for preventing transmission of HIV, the etiologic agent of AIDS.[1-5] Applicable to clinical and laboratory staffs,[3,4] to workers in health care settings [see Table 1][1] and in other occupational settings,[1] and to health care workers performing invasive procedures,[1-5] these precautions are appropriate for preventing transmission not only of HIV but also of other blood-borne viruses, including HBV and HCV. The recommendations share the objective of minimizing exposure of personnel to blood and body secretions from infected patients, whether through needle-stick injury or through contamination of mucous membranes or open cuts.

Despite the apparently low risk of such exposure, the CDC recommends enforcement of these as well as other standard infection control precautions, regardless of whether health care workers or patients are known to be infected with HIV or HBV. The CDC has taken the position that blood and body fluid precautions should be used consistently for all patients because medical history and physical examination cannot reliably identify all patients infected with HIV or other blood-borne pathogens and because in emergencies there may be no time for serologic testing. If these universal precautions are implemented, as the CDC recommends,[1-5] no additional precautions should be necessary for patients known to be infected with HIV.

The CDC does not recommend routine HIV serologic testing for all patients.[1-5] HIV serologic testing of patients is recommended for management of health care workers who sustain parenteral or mucous membrane exposure to blood or other body fluids, for patient diagnosis and treatment, and for counseling associated with efforts to prevent and control HIV transmission in the community.[1-5]

Nevertheless, some hospitals and physicians are likely to perform serologic testing of patients if it is possible that health care workers will be exposed to the patients' blood or other body fluids, as would be the case with patients undergoing major operative procedures or receiving treatment in intensive care units. Those who favor routine preoperative testing of patients undergoing invasive procedures maintain that precautions are more likely to be followed and additional steps taken to lower the likelihood of virus transmission from patients to health care workers when it is known which patients are HIV positive.[6,7] If such policies are adopted, the CDC advocates certain principles: (1) obtain consent for testing, (2) inform patients of results and provide counseling to seropositive patients, (3) ensure confidentiality, (4) ensure that seropositive patients will not receive compromised care, and (5) prospectively evaluate the efficacy of the program in reducing the incidence of exposure of health care workers to blood or body fluids of patients who are infected with HIV.

Although possible acquisition of HIV infection is the major concern for any health care worker who is exposed to blood products in the workplace, acquisition of viral hepatitis is actually much more likely. From a single needle-stick exposure, the estimated average risk of HIV transmission is 0.3%, whereas that of HCV transmission ranges from 0% to 10%.[8] The risk that HBV will be transmitted from a single needle-stick exposure varies according to the hepatitis B e antigen (HBeAg) status of the source patient, ranging from 1% to 6% for HBeAg-negative patients to 22% to 40% for HBeAg-positive patients.[9-11] That health care workers are at increased risk for hepatitis B is indicated by the seroprevalence of HBV in this population, which is two to four times that in the general United States population (6% to 15% versus < 5%).[9,12] This seroprevalence is expected to decrease with the availability of the hepatitis B vaccine and the mandate from the Occupational Safety

Human immunodeficiency virus (HIV)

Health care worker is exposed to any patient's blood or body secretions by a needle stick or by a splash in the eye or mouth

The health care worker should be counseled about the risk of HIV infection and should follow U.S. Public Health Service recommendations for preventing HIV transmission.

Patient is judged on clinical and epidemiologic grounds to be a likely source of HIV infection

Ask the patient to consent to serologic testing for HIV.

Patient refuses to be tested

Follow state and local laws regarding testing for a nonconsenting patient's HIV source status.

Patient is seropositive

Evaluate the health care worker for clinical or serologic evidence of HIV infection as soon as possible after the exposure. Consider prophylaxis:
Low to moderate risk: AZT plus 3TC.
High risk: AZT plus 3TC plus indinavir.

Health care worker is seronegative

Repeat serologic testing 6 wk and 3, 6, 12 mo after exposure.

Patient is seronegative and has no other evidence of HIV infection

No further follow-up of the health care worker is necessary.

Patient is seronegative but has engaged in high-risk behavoirs

Perform baseline HIV testing of the health care worker. Repeat test 3 months and 6 months after exposure.

Rabies

All bites and wounds should be immediately and thoroughly cleansed with soap and water.

Bite of domestic animal (dog or cat)

Animal is healthy at time of attack

Observe the animal for 10 days. If the animal shows signs of rabies, proceed with treatment.

Animal shows signs of rabies

Animal escapes

Consult with public health officials to determine need for treatment.

Bite of wild animal (skunk, bat, fox, coyote, raccoon, bobcat, or other carnivore)

Regard as rabid unless proved negative by laboratory tests.

Bite of another animal (e.g., livestock)

Consult with public health officials to determine need for treatment.

Give the exposed person RIG (20 IU/kg). If anatomically feasible, infiltrate the full dose around the wounds. Infiltrate any remaining RIG I.M. at a site distant from that of vaccine administration. Also, administer 1.0 ml of HDCV into the deltoid muscle or, in children, the upper thigh on days 0, 3, 7, 14, and 28. If the animal is available, kill it and immediately examine its brain tissue for the presence of rabies by using fluorescent antibody tests. If the tests are negative, discontinue HDCV.

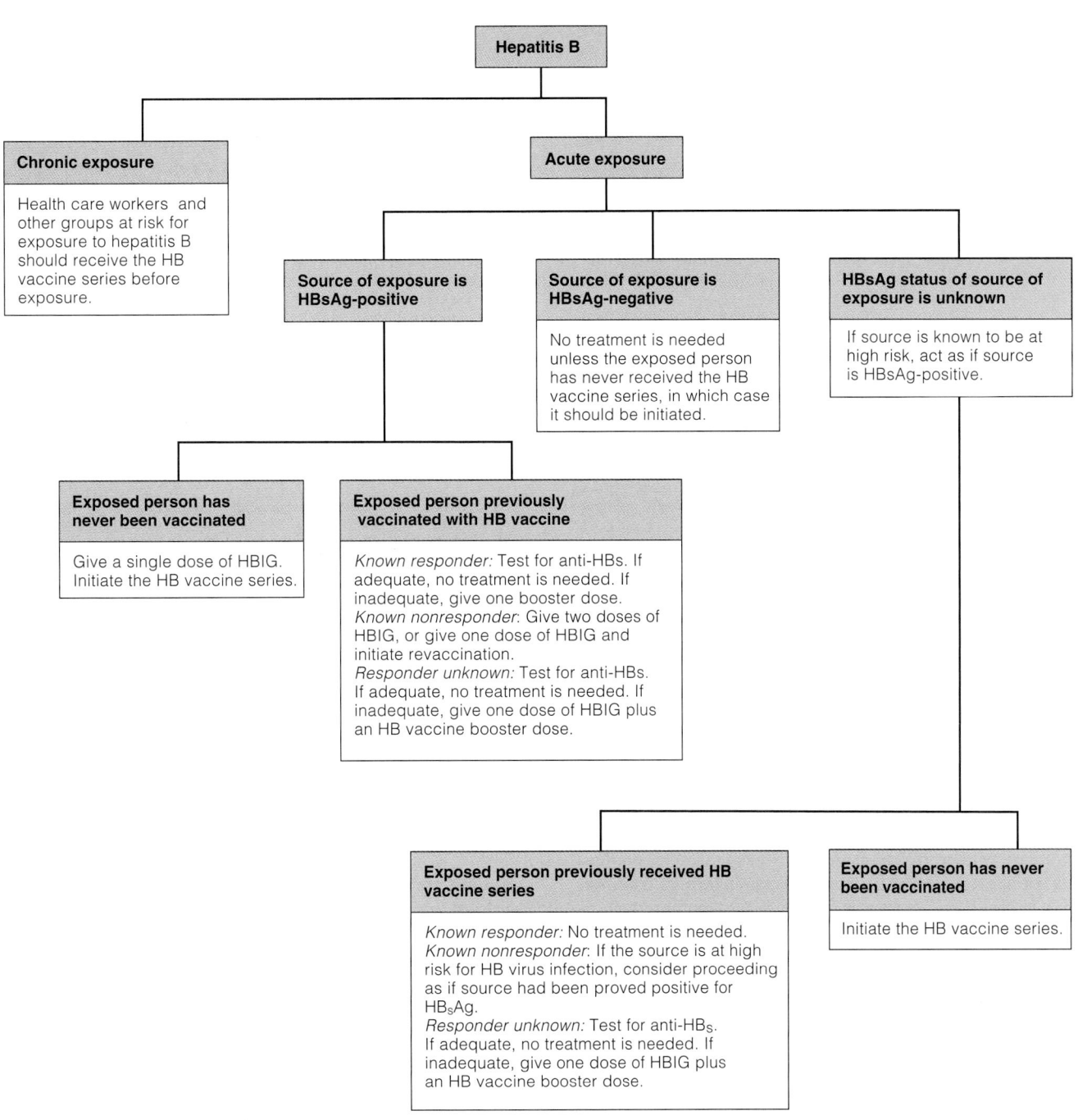

Hepatitis B

Chronic exposure

Health care workers and other groups at risk for exposure to hepatitis B should receive the HB vaccine series before exposure.

Acute exposure

Source of exposure is HBsAg-positive

Source of exposure is HBsAg-negative

No treatment is needed unless the exposed person has never received the HB vaccine series, in which case it should be initiated.

HBsAg status of source of exposure is unknown

If source is known to be at high risk, act as if source is HBsAg-positive.

Exposed person has never been vaccinated

Give a single dose of HBIG. Initiate the HB vaccine series.

Exposed person previously vaccinated with HB vaccine

Known responder: Test for anti-HBs. If adequate, no treatment is needed. If inadequate, give one booster dose.
Known nonresponder: Give two doses of HBIG, or give one dose of HBIG and initiate revaccination.
Responder unknown: Test for anti-HBs. If adequate, no treatment is needed. If inadequate, give one dose of HBIG plus an HB vaccine booster dose.

Exposed person previously received HB vaccine series

Known responder: No treatment is needed.
Known nonresponder: If the source is at high risk for HB virus infection, consider proceeding as if source had been proved positive for HB$_s$Ag.
Responder unknown: Test for anti-HB$_s$. If adequate, no treatment is needed. If inadequate, give one dose of HBIG plus an HB vaccine booster dose.

Exposed person has never been vaccinated

Initiate the HB vaccine series.

Approach to Viral Exposure

Hepatitis C

Perform serologic testing for ALT and HCV antibody at time of exposure and again at 6 months. If anti-HCV is detected, confirmatory testing with recombinant immunoblot is indicated. HCV immunoglobulin is no longer recommended.

Table 1 Precautions to Prevent Transmission of HIV[1]

Universal Precautions

1. All health care workers should use appropriate barrier precautions routinely to prevent skin and mucous membrane exposure when contact with blood or other body fluids of any patient is anticipated. Gloves should be worn for touching blood and body fluids, mucous membranes, or nonintact skin of all patients; for handling items or surfaces soiled with blood or body fluids; and for performing venipuncture and other vascular-access procedures. Gloves should be changed after contact with each patient. During procedures that are likely to generate aerosolized droplets of blood or other body fluids, masks and protective eyewear or face shields should be worn to prevent exposure of mucous membranes of the mouth, nose, and eyes. Gowns or aprons should be worn during procedures that are likely to generate splashes of blood or other body fluids.

2. Hands and other skin surfaces should be washed immediately and thoroughly if contaminated with blood or other body fluids. Hands should be washed immediately after gloves are removed.

3. All health care workers should take precautions to prevent injuries caused by needles, scalpels, and other sharp instruments or devices during procedures; when cleaning used instruments; during disposal of used needles; and when handling sharp instruments after procedures. To prevent needle-stick injuries, needles should not be recapped, purposely bent or broken by hand, removed from disposable syringes, or otherwise manipulated by hand. After they are used, disposable syringes and needles, scalpel blades, and other sharp items should be placed in puncture-resistant containers for disposal; the puncture-resistant containers should be located as close as practical to the area of use. Large-bore reusable needles should be placed in a puncture-resistant container for transport to the reprocessing area.

4. Although saliva has not been implicated in HIV transmission, to minimize the need for emergency mouth-to-mouth resuscitation, mouthpieces, resuscitation bags, or other ventilation devices should be available for use in areas in which the need for resuscitation is predictable.

5. Health care workers who have exudative lesions or weeping dermatitis should refrain from all direct patient care and from handling patient care equipment until the condition resolves.

6. Pregnant health care workers are not known to be at greater risk for contracting HIV infection than health care workers who are not pregnant; however, if a health care worker acquires HIV infection during pregnancy, the infant is at risk for infection resulting from perinatal transmission. Because of this risk, pregnant health care workers should be especially familiar with and strictly adhere to precautions to minimize the risk of HIV transmission.

Additional Precautions for Invasive Procedures

1. All health care workers who participate in invasive procedures must use appropriate barrier precautions routinely to prevent skin and mucous membrane contact with blood and other body fluids of all patients. Gloves and surgical masks must be worn for all invasive procedures. Protective eyewear or face shields should be worn for procedures that commonly result in the generation of aerosolized droplets, splashing of blood or other body fluids, or the generation of bone chips. Gowns or aprons made of materials that provide an effective barrier should be worn during invasive procedures that are likely to result in the splashing of blood or other body fluids. All health care workers who perform or assist in vaginal or cesarean deliveries should wear gloves and gowns when handling the placenta or the infant until blood and amniotic fluid have been removed from the infant's skin and should wear gloves during postdelivery care of the umbilical cord.

2. If a glove is torn or a needle-stick or other injury occurs, the glove should be removed and a new glove used as promptly as patient safety permits; the needle or instrument involved in the incident should also be removed from the sterile field. In the event of an injury, postexposure evaluation should be sought as soon as possible.

& Health Administration (OSHA) directing that all health care workers potentially exposed to blood or other potentially infectious material either be offered hepatitis B vaccine free of charge, demonstrate immunity to hepatitis B, or formally decline vaccination.[13] That vaccination has been effective in decreasing the incidence of hepatitis B in health care workers is shown by the decrease in infection rates from 174/100,000 in 1982 to 17/100,000 in 1995.[14] Most series have not found the seroprevalence of HCV to be higher in health care worker groups at risk than in the general population.[14] That hepatitis B and hepatitis C are much more common than HIV in health care workers is a strong argument for using universal precautions in all patients.

One reason why hepatitis B is so much more transmissible than HIV is the greater number of virus particles in the blood of hepatitis B carriers. These persons have blood concentrations of 10^8 to 10^9 virus particles/ml, compared with 10^2 to 10^4/ml for persons with HIV infection and 10^6/ml for persons with HCV infection.

The extensive guidelines that have been established by the CDC for the care of patients with HBV infection[4,15-17] also apply to patients with HIV infection. Patients known to have hepatitis B, hepatitis C, or AIDS need not be put in a private room unless they are fecally incontinent or are shedding virus in body fluids. Health care workers should wear gloves and gowns when they have contact with or may have contact with a patient's blood, feces, or other body fluids. Needles used for drawing blood should be disposed of with special care: they must not be reused, recapped, or removed from the syringe. Hands must be washed before and after direct contact with the patient or with items that have been in contact with the patient's blood, feces, or body fluids.

Published recommendations also provide guidelines for health care workers who are not directly involved in patient care (e.g., housekeeping personnel, kitchen staff, and laundry workers).[1-7]

No additional precautions are necessary for these individuals because their risk of acquiring HIV, HCV, or HBV is so low; in fact, transmission to them has not been documented. However, staff should be educated about appropriate procedures. Workers should wear gloves when handling blood and body fluids of all patients and should wear masks in areas where blood may spatter (e.g., the dialysis unit or the obstetrics unit).

TRANSMISSION FROM HEALTH CARE WORKERS TO PATIENTS

To date, there have been only two reports of HIV transmission from infected health care workers to patients. In one report, DNA sequence analysis linked a Florida dentist with AIDS to HIV infection in six of his patients.[18] In the other, an orthopedic surgeon in France may have transmitted HIV to one of his patients in the course of an operation.[19] Despite extensive investigation, no break in infection control precautions was documented in either case, nor was any clear-cut means of transmission identified.

HBV transmission from health care workers to patients is known to occur. Nineteen case reports have documented physician-to-patient transmission.[20-32] Eighteen of the 19 physicians were surgeons; seven of the surgeons were gynecologists, three were cardiac surgeons, and one was an orthopedic surgeon. All of the physicians were positive for HBeAg. Three of the gynecologists made a practice of handling needle tips. Of the 135 patients studied, 121 had clinical hepatitis B, and 14 had only serologic evidence of infection. Forty-one of the 135 patients were accounted for by the only nonsurgeon, a family practitioner from rural Switzerland. There are many additional cases of HBV having been transmitted by dentists and oral surgeons. In addition, three patients' relatives, two members of a surgeon's family, and one laboratory technician became infected.

In five studies, patients of 16 health care workers (including two surgeons) who were positive for hepatitis B surface antigen (HBsAg) were prospectively followed for evidence of hepatitis.[33-37] A total of 784 patients were followed and were compared with 656 patients cared for by health care workers who were HBsAg negative. None of the patients acquired overt hepatitis or became seropositive for HBsAg. Eight (1.02%) of the 784 patients cared for by HBsAg-positive health care workers developed antibody to HBsAg (anti-HBs), but so did six (0.91%) of the 656 patients cared for by health care workers who were negative for HBsAg. These reports suggest that the likelihood of infected surgeons' or other health care workers' transmitting HIV or HBV to their patients is extremely low. Chronic carriers of HBsAg who are seronegative for HBeAg are much less likely to transmit HBV than persons who are HBeAg positive.

Before the cases of transmission of HIV from the dentist to six of his patients were reported, the CDC had not taken a position on whether HBV- or HIV-infected surgeons should be allowed to continue practicing medicine. After these cases were reported, the CDC held meetings of health care professionals and other interested parties and published its recommendations on July 12, 1991.[38] These recommendations called for physicians not to perform "exposure-prone invasive procedures" unless they sought counsel from an expert review panel and were advised under what circumstances, if any, they might be allowed to continue to perform these procedures. Physicians would have to notify prospective patients of their seropositivity. These recommendations were strongly resisted by the medical community because at that time, only one health care worker, the dentist, had been implicated in transmitting HIV to his patients, no mechanism of transmission had been elucidated, no other patients had HIV transmitted by a health care worker, and invasive procedures that were "exposure prone" (exposing the patient to blood of the health care worker) were impossible to define. After subsequent meetings, the CDC abandoned its attempts to define exposure-prone procedures but did not alter its recommendations. Rather, it left it up to the states to define exposure-prone procedures. Subsequently, the President's Commission on AIDS recommended that HIV-infected health care workers should not have to curtail their practices or inform their patients of their infection.

Transmission of HCV from health care workers to patients has been reported. In one such case, a cardiac surgeon transmitted HCV to at least five patients during valve replacement surgery.[39] In another, an anesthesiologist in Spain may have infected more than 217 patients by first injecting himself with narcotics, then giving the remainder of the drugs to his patients.[40] At present, no recommendations exist for restricting the professional activities of health care workers with HCV infection.

Management of Viral Exposure

HIV

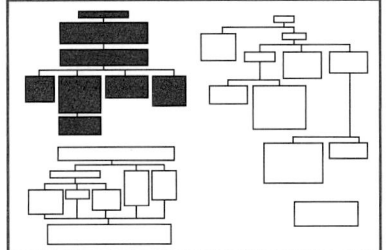

The CDC has issued recommendations for the management of potential exposure of health care workers to HIV.[1,4,41] If a health care worker is exposed by a needle stick or by a splash in the eye or mouth to any patient's blood or other body fluids, and the HIV serostatus of the patient is unknown, the patient should be informed of the incident and, if consent is obtained, tested for serologic evidence of HIV infection. If consent cannot be obtained, procedures for testing the patient should be followed in accordance with state and local laws. Testing of needles or other sharp instruments associated with exposure to HIV is not recommended, because it is unclear whether the test results would be reliable and how they should be interpreted.[41]

Health care workers exposed to HIV should be evaluated for susceptibility to blood-borne infection with baseline testing, including testing for HIV antibody. If the patient who is the source of exposure is seronegative and exhibits no clinical evidence of AIDS or symptoms of HIV infection, further follow-up of the health care worker is usually unnecessary.[41] If the source patient is seropositive or is seronegative but has engaged in high-risk behaviors, baseline and follow-up HIV-antibody testing of the health care worker at 6 weeks, 3 months, and 6 months after exposure should be considered.[41] Seroconversion usually occurs within 6 to 12 weeks of exposure; infrequently, it occurs considerably later. Three cases of delayed HIV seroconversion among health care workers have been reported.[42-44] In all three patients, an HIV antibody test yielded negative results at 6 months but positive results at some point during the following 1 to 7 months. In two cases, coinfection with HCV had occurred and took an unusually severe course. At present, it is unclear whether coinfection with these two viruses directly influences the timing or severity of either infection, but most experts recommend close monitoring for up to 1 year for health care workers exposed to both viruses in whom serologic evidence of HCV infection develops.

Treatment of the exposed health care worker should begin with careful washing of the exposure site with soap and water. Mucous membranes should be flushed with water. There is no evidence that either expressing fluid by squeezing the wound or applying antiseptics is beneficial, though antiseptics are not contraindicated. The use of caustic agents (e.g., bleach) is not recommended.

Any health care worker concerned about exposure to HIV should receive follow-up counseling regarding the risk of HIV transmission, postexposure testing, and medical evaluation, regardless of whether postexposure prophylaxis is given. HIV antibody testing should be performed at specified intervals for at least 6 months after the exposure (e.g., at 6 weeks, 3 months, and 6 months). The risk of HIV transmission is believed to depend on several factors: how much blood is involved in the exposure, whether the blood came from a source patient with terminal AIDS (thought to be attributable to the presence of large quantities of HIV), whether any host factors are present that might affect transmissibility (e.g., abnormal CD4 receptors for HIV), and whether the source patient carries any aggressive HIV viral mutants (e.g., syncytia-inducing strains). Factors indicating exposure to a large quantity of the source patient's blood (and thus a high risk of HIV transmission) include a device visibly contaminated with the patient's blood, a procedure that involved a needle placed directly in a vein or artery, and a deep injury.[45]

During the follow-up period, especially the first 6 to 12 weeks, exposed health care workers should follow the U.S. Public Health Service recommendations for preventing further transmission of HIV.[1-4] These recommendations include refraining from blood, semen, or organ donation and either abstaining from sexual intercourse or using measures to prevent HIV transmission during intercourse.[46]

The circumstances of the exposure should be recorded in the worker's confidential medical record and should include the following:

Table 2 Recommendations for Hepatitis B Prophylaxis after Percutaneous or Permucosal Exposure[15]

Hepatitis B Vaccination Status of Exposed Person	HBsAg Status of Source of Exposure		
	HBsAg-Positive	HBsAg-Negative	Untested or Unknown
Unvaccinated	Give single dose of HBIG Initiate HB vaccine series	Initiate HB vaccine series	Initiate HB vaccine series
Previously vaccinated Known responder	Test exposed person for anti-HBs If anti-HBs levels are adequate,* no treatment is needed; if they are inadequate, give an HB vaccine booster dose	No treatment is needed	No treatment is needed
Known nonresponder	*No response to three-dose vaccine series:* give two doses of HBIG or one dose of HBIG plus revaccination *No response to three-dose vaccine series plus revaccination:* give one dose of HBIG as soon as possible and a second dose 1 mo later	No treatment is needed	If source is at high risk for hepatitis B infection, consider proceeding as if source had been demonstrated to be HBsAg-positive
Response unknown	Test exposed person for anti-HBs If anti-HBs levels are adequate,* no treatment is needed; if they are inadequate, give one dose of HBIG plus an HB vaccine booster dose	No treatment is needed	Test exposed person for anti-HBs If anti-HBs levels are adequate,* no treatment is needed; if they are inadequate, initiate revaccination

*An adequate anti-HBs level is ≥ 10 mIU/ml, which is approximately equivalent to 10 sample ratio units (SRU) on radioimmunoassay or a positive result on enzyme immunoassay.

1. The date and time of the exposure.
2. Details of the exposure, including (a) where and how the exposure occurred, (b) the type and amount of fluid or other material involved, and (c) the severity of the exposure (for a percutaneous exposure, this would include the depth of injury and whether fluid was injected; for a skin or mucous membrane exposure, it would include the extent and duration of contact and the condition of the skin—chapped, abraded, or intact).
3. A description of the source of the exposure, including (if known) whether the source material contained HIV or other blood-borne pathogens, whether the source was HIV positive, the stages of any diseases present, whether the patient had previously received antiretroviral therapy, and the viral load.
4. Details about counseling, postexposure management, and follow-up.[41]

The data currently available on primary HIV infection indicate that systemic infection does not occur immediately. There may be a brief window of opportunity during which postexposure antiretroviral therapy may modify viral replication. Findings from animal and human studies provide indirect evidence of the efficacy of antiretroviral drugs in postexposure prophylaxis. The majority of these studies included zidovudine (AZT); consequently, all postexposure prophylaxis regimens now in use include AZT. Combination treatment regimens using nucleoside reverse transcriptase inhibitors and protease inhibitors have proved effective. Accordingly, most experts now recommend dual therapy with two nucleosides (zidovudine and lamivudine) for low- to moderate-risk exposures. For high-risk exposures, most experts would add a protease inhibitor (usually either indinavir or nelfinavir) to the two nucleoside reverse transcriptase inhibitors. These medications should be started as soon as possible after the exposure (within hours rather than days) and should be continued for 4 weeks.

An important component of postexposure care is encouraging and facilitating compliance with the lengthy course of medication. Therefore, careful consideration must be given to the toxicity profiles of the antiretroviral agents chosen. All of these agents have been associated with side effects, include GI (e.g., nausea or diarrhea), hematologic, endocrine (e.g., diabetes), and urologic effects (e.g., nephrolithiasis with indinavir). According to some early data, 50% to 90% of health care workers receiving combination regimens for postexposure prophylaxis (e.g., zidovudine plus 3TC, with or without a protease inhibitor) reported one or more subjective side effects that were substantial enough to cause 24% to 36% of the workers to discontinue postexposure prophylaxis.[47-49]

Whether antiretroviral agents should be chosen for postexposure prophylaxis on the basis of the resistance patterns of the source patient's HIV remains unclear. Transmission of resistant strains has been reported[50-52]; however, in the perinatal clinical trial that studied vertical transmission of HIV, zidovudine prevented perinatal transmission despite genotypic resistance of HIV to zidovudine in the mother.[53] Further study of the significance of genotypic resistance is necessary before definitive recommendations can be made.

HEPATITIS B

Both passive immunization with hepatitis B immune globulin (HBIG) and active immunization with hepatitis B vaccine (HB vaccine) are currently available for prophylaxis against hepatitis B [*see Table 2*].

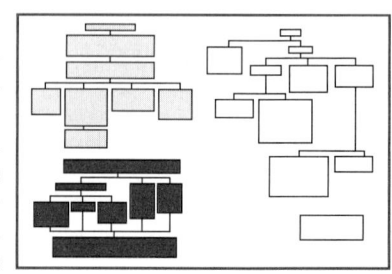

Passive Immunoprophylaxis

HBIG is prepared by Cohn ethanol fractionation from plasma selected to contain a high titer of anti-HBs; this process inactivates and eliminates HIV from the final product. In the United States, HBIG has an anti-HBs titer of at least 1:100,000 by radioimmunoassay.[54] HBIG provides temporary, passive protection. It is indicated after low-volume percutaneous or mucous membrane exposure to HBV; it is not effective for high-

Table 3 Candidates for Hepatitis B Vaccine[15]

Preexposure vaccination	Persons with occupational risk (e.g., health care workers, public safety workers)
	Clients and staffs of institutions for the developmentally disabled
	Hemodialysis patients
	Sexually active homosexual men
	Users of illicit injectable drugs
	Recipients of certain blood products (e.g., patients with clotting disorders who receive clotting factor concentrates)
	Household and sexual contacts of HBV carriers
	Adoptees from countries of high HBV endemicity
	Other contacts of HBV carriers (vaccination is usually not required unless there are special circumstances, such as biting or scratching, or medical conditions, such as severe skin disease, that facilitate transmission)
	Populations with high endemicity of HBV infection (e.g., Alaskan natives, Pacific islanders, and refugees from HBV-endemic areas)
	Inmates of long-term correctional facilities
	Sexually active heterosexual persons with multiple sexual partners
	International travelers who spend more than 6 mo in HBV-endemic areas and have close contact with the local population
	All infants born in the United States
	Adolescents 11 to 12 years old who have not previously been vaccinated
Postexposure vaccination	Perinatal exposure (infants born to HBsAg-positive mothers)
	Acute exposure to blood that contains (or might contain) HBsAg
	Sexual partners of persons with acute HBV infections
	Household contacts of persons with acute HBV infections (infants and older persons who have had identifiable blood exposure to the index patient)

volume exposure (e.g., blood transfusion). The recommended dose of HBIG for adults is 0.06 ml/kg I.M. Passive prophylaxis with HBIG should begin as soon as possible after exposure—ideally, within 24 hours.[54]

Active Immunoprophylaxis

Two types of HB vaccine are currently licensed in the United States, plasma-derived vaccine (Heptavax-B) and recombinant vaccine (Recombivax HB and Engerix-B). Heptavax-B contains alum-adsorbed 22 nm HBsAg particles purified from human plasma and processed to inactivate the infectivity of HBV and other viruses. Plasma-derived vaccine is no longer being produced in the United States, but similar vaccines are produced and used in China and other countries. In the United States, use of Heptavax-B is limited to persons allergic to yeast. Recombivax HB and Engerix-B are prepared by recombinant DNA technology in common baker's (or brewer's) yeast, *Saccharomyces cerevisiae*.

For primary vaccination, three I.M. injections (into the deltoid muscle in adults and children and into the anterolateral thigh muscle in infants and neonates) are given, with the second and third doses 1 and 6 months after the first dose.[54] The dose for Heptavax-B and Engerix-B is 20 µg (volume, 1.0 ml) for persons older than 11 years, and that for Recombivax HB is 10 µg (1.0 ml) for persons older than 19 years and 5 µg (0.5 ml) for persons 11 to 18 years of age. For immunologically impaired patients, including hemodialysis patients, the dose is 40 µg for all three vaccines. For postexposure prophylaxis with Engerix-B, a regimen of four doses given soon after exposure and 1, 2, and 12 months afterward has been approved.

HB vaccine is more than 90% effective at preventing infection or clinical hepatitis in susceptible persons. Protection is virtually complete in persons who develop adequate antibody. Routine testing for immunity after vaccination is not recommended, but testing should be considered for persons at occupational risk who require postexposure prophylaxis for needle-stick exposure.

Between 30% and 50% of persons who have been vaccinated will cease to have detectable antibody levels within 7 years, but protection against infection and clinical disease appears to persist.[54,55] The need for booster doses has not been established. Revaccination of individuals who do not respond to the primary series will produce adequate antibody in 15% to 25% of cases after one additional dose and in 30% to 50% after three additional doses.[56]

Although effective HB vaccines have been available since 1982, the incidence of hepatitis B in the United States continued to increase in the first decade of HB vaccine use. In 1991, the Advisory Committee for Immunization Practices (ACIP), citing the safety of the vaccine and the evidence of continuing spread of HBV, recommended universal vaccination of all infants born in the United States.[57]

Recommendations for Exposure to Blood That Contains (or May Contain) HBsAg

Acute exposure The U.S. Public Health Service has provided recommendations for hepatitis B prophylaxis after accidental percutaneous, mucous membrane, or ocular exposure to blood that contains (or may contain) HBsAg [see Table 2].[43] These recommendations are based on consideration of several factors: (1) whether the source of the blood is available, (2) the HBsAg status of the source, and (3) the hepatitis B vaccination and vaccination-response status of the exposed person. After exposure, a blood sample should be obtained from the person who was the source of the exposure and should be tested for HBsAg. The hepatitis B vaccination status and the anti-HBs response status (if known) of the exposed person should be reviewed. Because passive administration of antibody with HBIG does not inhibit the active antibody response to HB vaccine, the two can be given simultaneously.

Chronic exposure The U.S. Public Health Service recommends that persons who are at risk for exposure to HBV receive the HB vaccine series [see Table 3].[54] Health care workers who are at increased risk for acquiring hepatitis B include all physicians (especially surgeons), dentists, and laboratory and support personnel, such as nurses and technicians who work in the operating room or who have contact with infected patients, blood or blood products, or excreta. Because of their frequent exposure to blood and their high risk of hepatitis B, all surgeons should receive HB vaccine. As of 1994, however, only 50% of surgeons had been vaccinated, despite the proven efficacy and safety of the vaccine and surgeons' increased risk of exposure.[58] Hospital personnel who do not have frequent contact with blood or blood products (e.g., the janitorial, laundry, and kitchen staffs) need not be vaccinated.

Screening of personnel and patients for anti-HBs before vaccination is indicated only for individuals in high-risk groups; it has not been found to be cost-effective outside these groups.

HEPATITIS C

The only tests currently approved by the U.S. Food and Drug Administration for diagnosis of hepatitis C are those that measure antibody to HCV. These tests detect anti-HCV in at least 97% of infected patients, 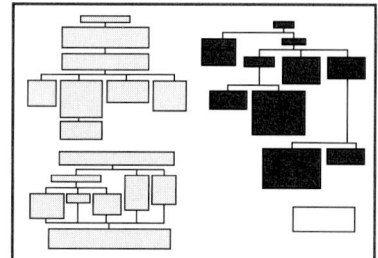 but they cannot distinguish between acute, chronic, and resolved infection.[59] The positive predictive value of enzyme immunoassay (EIA) for anti-HCV varies depending on the prevalence of the infection in the population. Therefore, supplemental testing of a specimen with a positive EIA result with a more specific assay (e.g., the recombinant immunoblot assay [RIBA]) may detect false positives, especially when asymptomatic persons are being tested. Qualitative polymerase chain reaction (PCR) testing for HCV RNA can also be used to identify HCV. This test can detect HCV at concentrations as low as 100 to 1,000 viral genome copies/ml, and it can detect HCV RNA in serum or plasma within 1 to 2 weeks after viral exposure and weeks before alanine aminotransferase (ALT) levels rise or anti-HCV appears.[59] Under optimal conditions, the reverse transcriptase PCR assay for HCV can identify 75% to 85% of persons who are anti-HCV–positive and more than 95% of persons with acute or chronic hepatitis C.[59] Quantitative assays for measuring HCV RNA are also available but are less sensitive and should not be used as primary tests for confirming or excluding the diagnosis of HCV infection or monitoring the end point of treatment.[59] The data currently available on prevention of HCV infection with immune globulin (IG) indicate that this approach is not effective as postexposure prophylaxis for HCV infection.[59] Interferon may have a role in the treatment of acute hepatitis C: several studies have shown that interferon may delay or prevent the onset of chronic hepatitis C in patients treated early in the course of acute HCV infection.[60-62]

RABIES

The CDC has made recommendations for the prevention of rabies in people bitten by animals [see Table 4].[63] Bite wounds should always be thoroughly scrubbed with soap and water. Postexposure anti- 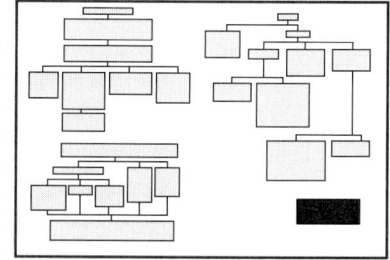 rabies treatment includes both rabies immune globulin (RIG) and human diploid cell (rabies) vaccine (HDCV). The decision to administer such treatment should be based on the following considerations.

Species and Availability of Biting Animal

In the United States, rabies is most commonly transmitted by skunks, raccoons, foxes, and bats. Livestock occasionally transmit the virus, but rodents and lagomorphs (i.e., rabbits and hares) are rarely infected.[64] In different parts of the country, different animals predominate in the transmission of the virus. The likelihood that domestic cats or dogs in the United States will be infected varies from region to region. The chances of rabies transmission by a domestic animal that has been properly immunized are minimal.

Whether an animal is available for observation after biting someone also influences the need for antirabies prophylaxis. In certain cases, an animal that bites a person must be killed and tissue from its brain checked for the presence of rabies by fluorescent antibody tests as soon as possible [see Table 4].

Type of Exposure

Infected animals transmit rabies primarily by biting, although licking may introduce the virus into open cuts in skin or mucous membranes. Transmission occasionally occurs as a result of aerosol exposure: the virus may be excreted in the urine and feces of infected bats, aerosolized during urination and defecation, and then inhaled, for example, by spelunkers exploring caves.

Table 4 Rabies Postexposure Prophylaxis[63]

	Animal Species	Condition of Animal at Time of Attack	Treatment of Exposed Person*
Domestic	Dog, cat	Healthy and available for 10 days of observation	None, unless animal develops rabies†
		Rabid or suspected rabid	RIG (20 IU/kg)‡ and HDCV§ (five 1.0 ml doses intramuscularly, on days 0, 3, 7, 14, and 28)
		Unknown (escaped)	Consult public health officials. If treatment is indicated, give RIG‡ and HDCV
Wild	Skunk, bat, fox, coyote, bobcat, raccoon, other carnivores	Regard as rabid unless proved negative by laboratory tests‖	RIG (20 IU/kg)‡ and HDCV (five 1.0 ml doses intramuscularly, on days 0, 3, 7, 14, and 28)
Other	Livestock, rodents, lagomorphs (rabbits and hares)	Consider individually. Local and state public health officials should be consulted on questions about the need for rabies prophylaxis. Bites of squirrels, hamsters, guinea pigs, chipmunks, gerbils, rats, mice, other rodents, and lagomorphs almost never call for antirabies prophylaxis.	

*All bites and wounds should immediately be thoroughly cleansed with soap and water. If antirabies treatment is indicated, both rabies immune globulin (RIG) and human diploid cell rabies vaccine (HDCV) should be given as soon as possible, regardless of the interval from exposure. (The administration of RIG is the more urgent procedure. If HDCV is not immediately available, start RIG and give HDCV as soon as it is obtained.) Local reactions to vaccines are common and do not contraindicate continuing treatment. Discontinue vaccine if fluorescent antibody tests of the animal are negative.

†During the usual holding period of 10 days, begin treatment with RIG and HDCV at first sign of rabies in a dog or cat that has bitten someone. The symptomatic animal should be killed immediately and tested.

‡The full dose should be infiltrated around the wounds; any remaining RIG should be given I.M. at a site distant from that of vaccine administration. If RIG is not available, use antirabies serum, equine (ARS). Do not use more than the recommended dosage of RIG or ARS.

§HDCV should be administered into the deltoid (not the gluteus) muscle in adults and adolescents. In children, it may be administered into the upper thigh.

‖The animal should be killed and tested as soon as possible. Holding for observation is not recommended.

Circumstances of the Bite

An unprovoked attack is more indicative of a rabid animal than is a provoked attack.

If the animal shows signs of rabies or the patient has been bitten by a wild animal that is not captured, the patient should be treated as soon as possible with both RIG and HDCV. The recommended dose of RIG for postexposure prophylaxis is 20 IU/kg.[63] If anatomically feasible, the entire dose of RIG should be infiltrated into the area around the wound.[65,66] Postexposure HDCV should be given I.M. in five 1.0 ml doses on days 0, 3, 7, 14, and 28.[63] Those with adequate preexposure immunization should receive two 1.0 ml doses of HDCV I.M. on days 0 and 3 but should receive no RIG. For adults, the vaccine should be administered in the deltoid area. For children, the anterolateral aspect of the thigh is also acceptable. The gluteal area should never be used for HDCV injections, because administration in this area results in lower neutralizing antibody titers.[63] HDCV must not be given in the same region as RIG.

The CDC recommends that preexposure immunization be considered for high-risk groups, such as animal handlers, certain laboratory workers and field personnel, and persons planning to stay for more than 1 month in areas where canine rabies is highly prevalent and access to appropriate medical care is limited. The recommended preexposure regimen is 0.1 ml of HDCV on days 0, 7, and 21 or 28.[67] Testing for adequate antibody response is not necessary for persons at low risk for exposure, but administration of booster doses every 2 to 3 years is recommended for those at high risk for exposure. Postexposure treatment for persons who have received preexposure immunization consists of 1 ml HDCV on days 0 and 3 only, without RIG.[68]

Although only a few cases of clinical rabies occur each year in the United States, approximately 30,000 persons a year are given postexposure prophylaxis. In 1992, 49 states, the District of Columbia, and Puerto Rico collectively reported 8,644 cases of animal rabies and one case of human rabies to the CDC.[69] The total expense associated with one rabid dog in California was $105,790, even though no human contracted rabies.[70] This amount represents the costs of human antirabies treatment, vaccination of other animals, and animal-containment programs.

Discussion

Size and Structure of Viruses

Viruses are among the smallest and simplest of microorganisms. Human viruses can be as small as 18 to 26 nm in diameter (parvoviruses) or as long as 300 nm (vaccinia virus), slightly longer than *Chlamydia* (a bacterium). Viruses do not have the complex enzyme systems required for synthesis of nucleic acid precursors, they lack ribosomes for protein synthesis, and they have no energy-generating mechanism. Consequently, they cannot replicate outside cells.

The core of a virus is made of either RNA or DNA, but never both. The nucleic acid can be either single stranded or double stranded. This nucleic acid core is surrounded by the capsid, which is a protein coat made up of capsomers, repetitive subunits consisting of one protein or at most a few. Because the viral nucleic acid must code for coat proteins, a limitation in the number of capsid proteins conserves viral nucleic acid. The capsid protects the nucleic acid from nucleases in the environment, serves as its vehicle of transmission from one host to another, and plays a role in the attachment of the virus to the receptor sites on susceptible cells. The complete nucleic acid–protein coat complex is termed the nucleocapsid. For many viruses, the nucleocapsid is the complete virus particle, the virion. Other viruses, such as herpesviruses, may acquire an envelope, an additional lipid-containing membrane coat around the nucleocapsid, by budding through a membrane of the host cell [*see Figure 1*]. Some viruses may also have an enzyme associated with their core that replicates the nucleic acid. Examples are the DNA polymerase of the HBV and the reverse transcriptase of retroviruses.

Classification of Viruses

Viruses, like other organisms, are classified into families, genera, and species, but most viral species do not have formal names and in practice are referred to by common names (e.g., cytomegalovirus, coxsackievirus, Norwalk virus, and varicella-zoster virus). Viruses can also be classified by chemical characteristics and by structural characteristics determined from electron microscopy (e.g., dimensions and site of assembly). Viruses are categorized into two broad groups depending on whether their nucleic acid is RNA or DNA. These two groups can be subdivided first according to whether the nucleic acid is single stranded or double stranded and then according to the presence or absence of an envelope. Single-stranded RNA viruses that replicate by means of a DNA step (i.e., retroviruses) are grouped separately from those that do not.

Identification of Viruses

Viruses can be identified by means of (1) serologic tests, (2) isolation of virus, (3) histologic examination, (4) detection of viral antigens, (5) detection of viral nucleic acid, and (6) electron microscopy. One or more of these techniques may be applicable to a given viral infection.

Specimens must be handled properly to maximize the likelihood of identifying the virus. If isolation of the virus is desired, blood and tissue samples should be taken promptly to the virology laboratory and inoculated onto the appropriate cell line. Samples obtained at night or on weekends can be placed in a balanced salt solution or tissue culture medium and kept in a refrigerator until taken to the laboratory. If microscopic identification of the virus is planned, specimens must be preserved appropriately. Routine preservation in formalin, for example, permits visualization of viral inclusions by routine staining and light microscopy. For identification of viral antigens by immunofluorescence techniques, the tissue specimen should be immediately frozen, preferably in liquid nitrogen. Specimens to be examined by electron microscopy must be placed in glutaraldehyde or another appropriate fixative.

SEROLOGIC TESTS

The antibody response to viral antigens can be detected in the serum of patients with viral infections. An IgM response usually indicates recent exposure to the virus, whereas the presence of IgG reflects past exposure.

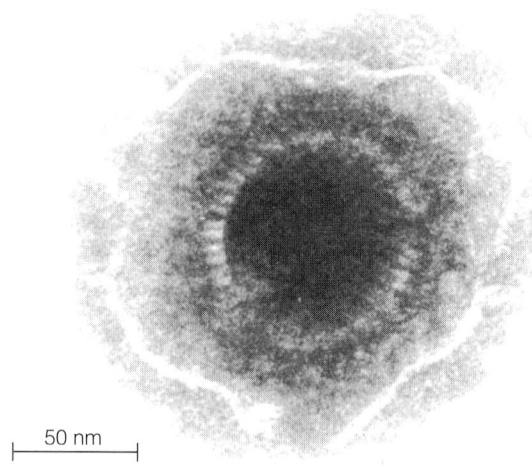

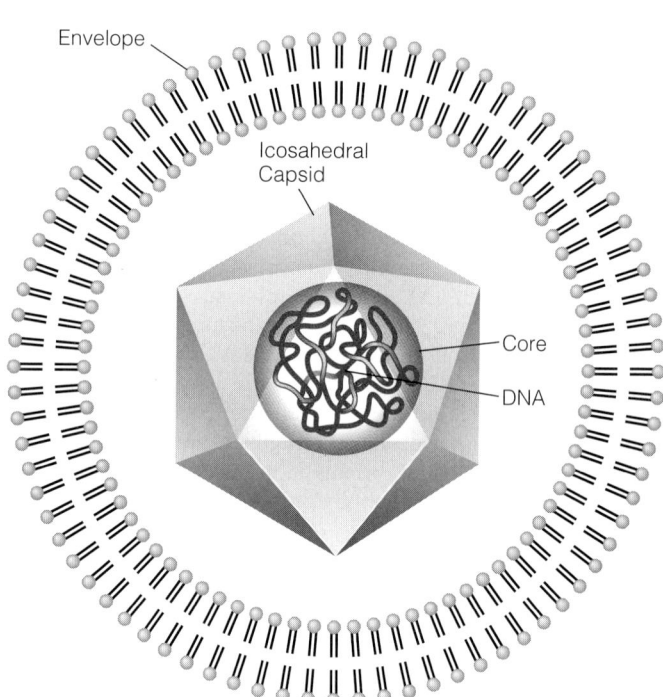

Figure 1 The capsomers and the irregularly shaped surrounding envelope of a cytomegalovirus are highlighted by negative staining with uranyl acetate (above). A typical herpesvirus (right) consists of a central core containing DNA; an icosahedral capsid, a surrounding layer of protein made up of 162 individual capsomers; and an envelope, a membrane coat acquired when the virus buds from the nuclear membrane of the host cell.

For most acute primary infections, serum obtained during late recovery or after recovery (convalescent serum) has an increased antibody titer, compared with serum obtained early in the course of the disease (acute serum). Most tests are performed on an initial serum dilution of 1:2 or 1:10 and on serial twofold dilutions thereafter. A fourfold increase in titer (indicated by reactivity of a two-tube dilution) usually represents a significant increase in antibody response and is considered to constitute seroconversion. An immunocompromised host may occasionally fail to mount an antibody response.

Some viruses are so common that patients may already have antibody titers when the disease is first suspected. Herpesviruses are ubiquitous and are present in many healthy people in latent form. At the onset of herpesvirus infections, patients may already have the corresponding antibody. Nevertheless, their antibody titer will almost always increase significantly after recovery.

A variety of serologic tests are available in the clinical laboratory: complement fixation, radioimmunoassay, enzyme-linked immunosorbent assay (ELISA), immunofluorescence, immune precipitation, immune blotting, latex agglutination, virus neutralization, indirect hemagglutination, immune adherence hemagglutination, and hemagglutination inhibition. None of these serologic tests is appropriate for identification of all viruses.

ISOLATION OF VIRUS

The isolation of virus requires appropriate specimen collection and inoculation into animals or onto appropriate cell lines. Blood sent for virus isolation should be unclotted because some viruses, such as herpesviruses, are found primarily in lymphocytes. If cell-associated viruses are suspected, lymphocytes should be inoculated directly onto target cells. Several types of cells are available for growing viruses, and no single cell line is appropriate for all of them. Therefore, it is helpful to the laboratory to know which virus the clinician suspects.

Viruses that grow in cell monolayers in tissue culture have cytopathic effects that can be recognized under the microscope (e.g., rounding, transformation, or death) [see Figure 2]. Some viruses, such as rubella, produce no direct cytopathic effects but can be

detected because they inhibit the cytopathic effects of a second test virus. This phenomenon is called viral interference. Other viruses (e.g., myxoviruses) cause changes in the cell membrane so that red blood cells adhere to the cell surface (hemadsorption). The identity of isolated viruses can be confirmed by use of specific antisera that are known to inhibit viral growth.

Tissue suspected of containing an encephalitis or other neurotropic virus can be minced and the extract injected intracerebrally into an infant mouse. If the mouse dies and bacteria cannot be cultured from the brain, the injected material presumably contained such a virus. If antiserum of known specificity neutralizes the virus, the specificity of the antiserum indicates the specific identity of the virus. The criterion for neutralization is that inoculation of neutralized virus will not kill the mouse.

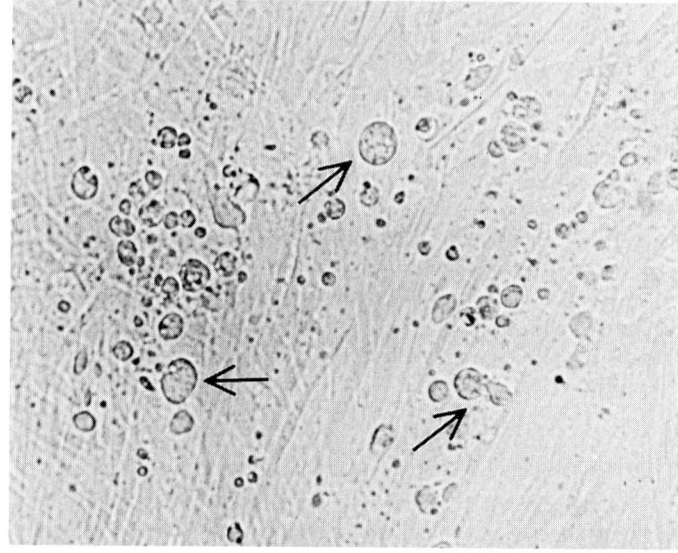

Figure 2 Cells infected with cytomegalovirus become large and round (arrows). Note the uniform appearance of adjacent uninfected cells.

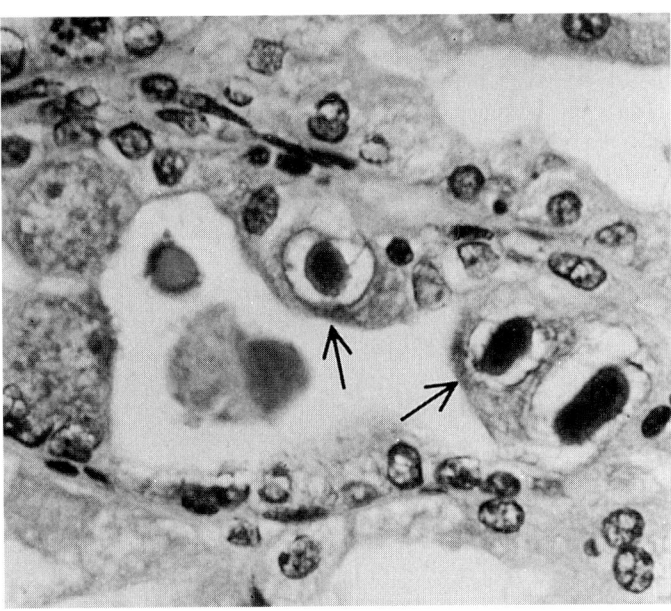

Figure 3 **Kidney biopsy shows cytomegalovirus-infected tubular epithelial cells (arrows). In such cells, a dark intranuclear inclusion is surrounded by a clear halo. Inclusions usually indicate sites of previous or current viral replication.**

HISTOLOGIC EXAMINATION

Histologic examination of biopsy and autopsy tissues may demonstrate changes that are typical of certain viruses. Members of the herpesvirus group can be characterized by intranuclear inclusions surrounded by a clear halo [*see Figure 3*]. RNA viruses usually produce inclusions in the cytoplasm; for instance, dark-staining intracytoplasmic inclusions in the brain tissue of animals or patients are diagnostic of rabies infection and are called Negri bodies. Inclusion bodies are either masses of closely packed virus particles or remnants of prior virus replication.

DETECTION OF VIRAL ANTIGENS

Viral antigens can be detected in tissues by techniques employing their corresponding antibodies. If virus is present, these antigens may be visible microscopically under ultraviolet light either by direct immunofluorescence (i.e., in tissue sections stained with fluorescein-labeled antiviral antibody) or by indirect immunofluorescence (i.e., in tissue sections exposed first to antiviral antibody and then to fluorescein-labeled anti–γ-globulin antibody). Fluorescence microscopy requires specimens that are fresh frozen (preferably in liquid nitrogen). Immunofluorescence staining of cells in tissue culture can detect viral antigens before cytopathic effects are evident. Viral antigens in formalin-fixed tissue can be identified by immunohistochemical microscopy (e.g., using peroxidase-labeled antibodies).

DETECTION OF VIRAL NUCLEIC ACID

Viral nucleic acids can be detected in body fluids and tissues at virus concentrations too low to be detected by other means. The PCR permits amplification of even a small number of copies of viral nucleic acid. In theory, even a single copy of a specific DNA can be detected by PCR. Before PCR is performed, DNA can be synthesized from viral RNA by means of reverse transcriptase. The PCR product can be detected by gel electrophoresis and compared with known viral DNA. This test is currently being used to diagnose CMV infection and is more sensitive than current serologic testing for HCV. Nucleic acid hybridization can detect viral nucleic acid in tissue specimens. Epstein-Barr virus genomes

can be detected in this way in EBV-related cancers and lymphoproliferative disorders.

ELECTRON MICROSCOPY

Although seldom used routinely, electron microscopy allows rapid identification (in a matter of hours) of viruses in body fluids, tissues, and tissue extracts. Identification of viruses in body fluids and tissue extracts by this method is easier if the samples are first concentrated by ultracentrifugation, evaporation, or ultrafiltration. HBV has been observed in specimens from hepatitis patients only after ultracentrifugation.

Epidemiology of Viral Infections of Interest to Surgeons

Viral infections are spread to humans via several patterns of transmission: (1) direct transmission from humans with symptomatic infection (e.g., HBV, HCV herpesviruses, and HIV), (2) transmission from asymptomatic human carriers (e.g., HBV, HCV, HIV, and varicella-zoster virus), (3) transmission from arthropods (e.g., encephalitis and dengue viruses), and (4) transmission from other animals (e.g., rabies virus).

Viral infections are common in immunosuppressed patients in general and especially in recipients of organ transplants, who must take immunosuppressive drugs to prevent rejection. The overwhelming majority of these infections are caused by members of the herpesvirus family (e.g., CMV, herpes simplex viruses, varicella-zoster virus, and EBV); infections with HBV and with papovaviruses (e.g., human papillomavirus, which causes warts, and BK virus) are also frequent.

Because surgical patients are frequently given transfusions of blood or blood products and because hospital staff often incur accidental needle-stick injury, viruses that can be transmitted by these routes are of prime interest to surgeons and their patients. Examples of such viruses are HBV, hepatitis D, HCV, HIV, HTLV-I, and the herpesviruses, including EBV and CMV. These viruses can also be transmitted by organ transplantation either from the cells of the organ itself (e.g., HBV in liver cells or CMV in kidney cells) or from blood that has not been completely removed from the organ. Changes in donor acceptance and screening policies over time have increased the safety of the blood supply and should continue to do so in the future [*see Table 5*].[71]

HIV

Two serotypes of HIV, HIV-1 and HIV-2, have been identified. Both can cause AIDS. HIV-1 accounts for virtually all cases of AIDS in the United States and equatorial Africa. HIV-2 is found almost exclusively in West Africa; only a few cases of HIV-2 infection have occurred in the United States.

Because AIDS patients are immunodepressed, they are susceptible to opportunistic infections and neoplasms, especially non-Hodgkin lymphoma, *Pneumocystis carinii* pneumonia, and Kaposi sarcoma. AIDS is most prevalent in the United States among male homosexuals, abusers of I.V. drugs, and hemophiliacs. Since the implementation of testing for blood-borne HIV and the near-elimination of HIV from blood products, the incidence of HIV infection in the hemophiliac population has diminished markedly; however, in recent years, the incidence in the heterosexual population has been increasing rapidly.

HIV can be transmitted by transfusion of whole blood, packed red cells, plasma, factor VIII concentrates, factor IX concentrates, and platelets. The likelihood that a person will become infected with HIV after receiving a single-donor blood product that tests

Table 5 Changes in Donor Acceptance and Screening Policies Instituted to Reduce the Risk of Transmitting Infectious Diseases[71]

Policy	Implementation Date
Screening for HBsAg	July 1972
Voluntary exclusion of persons at high risk for AIDS	March 1983
Redefinition of high-risk behavior to include men who have had sex with more than one man since 1979	December 1984
Testing for antibody to HIV-1	Spring 1985
Redefinition of high-risk behavior to include any man who has had sex with another man since 1977	September 1985
Implementation of a mechanism to allow donors to indicate confidentially that their donations should not be used for transfusion	October 1986
Testing for alanine aminotransferase (ALT, formerly SGPT)	Winter 1986–1987
Testing for anti-HBc	Spring 1987
Testing for antibody to HTLV-1	January 1990
Testing for antibody to HCV	May 1990
Testing for antibody to HIV-2	April 1992
Testing for HIV-1 antigen	March 1996

positive for HIV approaches 100%.[72-73] Before the advent of serologic testing for HIV in 1985, 0.04% of 1,200,000 blood donations in the United States were estimated to be HIV positive.[74] AIDS has developed in more than 8,500 recipients of blood transfusions, blood components, or transplanted organs or tissue.

Federal regulations now require that all prospective blood and plasma donors be screened for antibody to HIV by ELISA. Because this test yields a low rate of false positive results, assay by the more sensitive Western blot electrophoresis is always used to confirm positive ELISA results. Routine testing of blood donors has greatly reduced HIV transmission via blood transfusions, but infection can still occur if the donor has been infected with HIV but has not yet developed antibody.[75] The risk of HIV transmission via transfusion of screened blood that is negative for HIV is estimated to be one in 200,000 to one in 2,000,000 per unit transfused in the United States.[76] Antibody to HIV usually develops within 4 weeks to 6 months of HIV infection.[77] From the time of infection until the appearance of antibody, infected individuals will test negative by ELISA or Western blot, and their blood might still be used for transfusion.

HIV and AIDS can also be transmitted by organ transplantation.[78] So far, only a small number of patients have been found to be infected in this way, but more will undoubtedly be reported. These patients received transplants before HIV testing of potential donors became possible. All prospective organ and tissue donors now should be tested for HIV infection and other blood-borne viral infections.

HIV infection is also a potential problem in health care workers, who are exposed to a large and growing population of AIDS patients. In the United States, an estimated 1.0 to 1.5 million people are infected with HIV but as yet have no symptoms. HIV transmission from blood, tissue, or other body fluids can occur in the health care setting as a result of percutaneous injury (e.g., from needles or other sharp objects), contamination of mucous membranes or nonintact skin (e.g., skin that is chapped, abraded, or affected by dermatitis), prolonged contact with intact skin, or contamination involving an extensive area.[79] HIV infection may be contracted through a variety of sources including blood, semen, vaginal secretions, visibly bloody fluids, and a number of other fluids for which the precise risk of transmission is undetermined (e.g., cerebrospinal, synovial, pleural, peritoneal, pericardial, and amniotic fluid). Infection may also be contracted from concentrated HIV used in research settings.[79] The results of multiple prospective studies quantifying transmission risk associated with a discrete occupational HIV exposure indicate that the average risk of HIV transmission associated with needle punctures or similar percutaneous injuries is approximately 0.3%. The estimated risk of transmission from mucocutaneous exposure to HIV-contaminated material is 0.03%. As of December 1999, the CDC had received reports of 56 U.S. health care workers in whom documented HIV seroconversion was temporally related to occupational HIV exposure. Of these 56, 48 had percutaneous exposures, five mucocutaneous exposures, two both percutaneous and mucous membrane exposures, and one an unknown route of exposure.[80] Another 138 possible cases of occupational HIV transmission—six involving surgeons—have been reported in persons with no risk factors for HIV transmission other than workplace exposure; however, seroconversion after a specific exposure was not documented. There may be other health care workers who also have acquired HIV infection from needle-stick or mucous membrane exposure but have not been reported, either because they and their patients have not been tested or because they have other risk factors for HIV infection

The concentration of virus in the blood or serum of antigen-positive individuals is several orders of magnitude less for HIV than for HBV. The number of needle-stick exposures to HIV that have actually led to a positive test result for HIV has been extremely small, whereas hepatitis B occurs in as many as 40% of health care workers exposed to the virus by needle-stick injury. Despite this relatively low infectiousness, AIDS is much more feared than hepatitis B because AIDS is often fatal. Although hepatitis B is usually not fatal and is often of short duration, several health care workers die of hospital-acquired hepatitis B and hepatitis C each year.

Hepatitis

Several viruses can cause hepatitis. Hepatitis A virus (HAV) and HBV cause what were formerly known as infectious hepatitis and serum hepatitis, respectively. HCV is the major cause of parenterally transmitted non-A, non-B hepatitis. Hepatitis E virus is a common cause of epidemic non-A, non-B hepatitis, which is chiefly found in developing countries in Africa and Asia. Hepatitis D virus (HDV, formerly called the delta agent) is defective or incomplete and is pathogenic only in the presence of HBV. The hepatitis viruses are the most common infectious agents to which hospital personnel may be exposed. Herpesviruses can also cause serious and sometimes fatal hepatitis, especially in severely immunocompromised patients, such as recipients of organ or bone marrow transplants and patients receiving intensive chemotherapy for cancer.

HEPATITIS A

HAV is a small (27 nm), single-stranded RNA virus belonging to the enterovirus subgroup of picornaviruses. Its almost exclusive transmission by the fecal-oral route is enhanced by poor personal hygiene, poor sanitary conditions, and crowding. Transmission can be contained by careful hand washing and the isolation of excretions. Unlike other types of viral hepatitis, hepatitis A is rarely transmitted by blood, blood products, or needle sticks and is rarely transmitted among hemodialysis patients, health care workers, and I.V. drug abusers. The infrequent parenteral transmission of HAV is attributed in part to its lack of an asymptomatic carrier state. Hepatitis A can be transmitted percutaneously only during a brief period of viremia before the onset of symptoms and jaundice. The chance that an infected person will donate blood during this short period is small; also, patients are usually outside the hospital during this period.

HEPATITIS B

HBV is a member of the Hepadnaviridae family of DNA viruses. It is most prevalent in the Far East, the Middle East, Africa, and parts of South America, where as many as 15% of the general population are chronic carriers. Worldwide, the most common mode of transmission is from mother to child during the perinatal period. In the United States, however, sexual or parenteral transmission has been implicated in most infections. The high-risk groups for chronic HBV infection in the United States include I.V. drug users, men who have sex with men, other individuals with multiple sexual partners, household contacts and sexual partners of HBV carriers, health care workers, patients on long-term hemodialysis, and organ transplant recipients.[81]

Clinical Course

The clinical course of hepatitis B is extremely variable: infection ranges from the completely asymptomatic to the rapidly fatal. The incubation period averages 75 days but can last from 40 to 180 days. Exposure to HBV has five potential outcomes: (1) no infection occurs; (2) acute hepatitis develops, followed by clearance of infection; (3) acute fulminant infection develops, leading to hepatic necrosis and death; (4) acute hepatitis develops without clearance of infection, and a chronic carrier state ensues; and (5) no acute illness develops, but a chronic carrier state ensues.

Approximately 55% of adults infected with HBV have no symptoms despite serologic documentation of infection (see below), which explains why blood donors who seem to be in good health are capable of transmitting the virus. Other individuals infected with HBV may have such mild symptoms (e.g., slight malaise, fatigability, and loss of appetite) that they do not seek medical attention.

Approximately 45% of people infected with HBV experience typical acute, icteric hepatitis, which is characterized by fatigue, anorexia, nausea, vomiting, and hepatomegaly. In approximately 1% of adults infected with HBV, acute fulminant hepatitis develops. This condition is characterized by progressive hepatocellular destruction, encephalopathy, and deepening coma. Fulminant hepatitis causes death in approximately 80% of affected adults and 30% of affected children.

In approximately 5% to 10% of hepatitis B cases, the infection becomes chronic. Patients with chronic hepatitis may be asymptomatic or may have clinical and histologic evidence of the disease, as well as persistently elevated levels of serum aminotransferases [see Figure 4]. With time, many patients pass to an asymptomatic carrier state, and serum aminotransferase levels fall. The duration of the asymptomatic carrier state appears to be indefinite. Chronic HBV infection can result in hepatocellular carcinoma, which is especially common in China, Southeast Asia, and sub-Saharan Africa.

Because most patients remain asymptomatic until the development of end-stage liver disease, there are no specific clinical findings that are indicative of chronic HBV infection. There are, however, several clinical syndromes linked to HBV infection that may provide a clue to the presence of chronic HBV infection. These syndromes include polyarteritis nodosa, membranous or membranoproliferative glomerulonephritis, leukocytoclastic vasculitis, erythema nodosum, arthritis, and serum sickness.

Antigens

HBV has a diameter of 42 nm and contains circular, double-stranded DNA. The protein coat on its outer surface is termed hepatitis B surface antigen. HBsAg is made in quantities greatly exceeding the amount required to coat the nucleic acid. The excess surface antigen appears in the serum as spheres 22 nm in diameter or tubules of the same diameter and of varying length. These spheres and tubules contain no nucleic acid and hence are not infectious. They may persist in the serum for prolonged periods, even for life, and in great quantities, up to 10^{12} to 10^{14} surface antigen particles (500 μg protein) per milliliter.[82]

The hepatitis B virus also has a nucleocapsid core, the outside of which contains the hepatitis B core antigen (HBcAg). HBcAg is not detected in hepatitis B during acute infection, because its antigenic determinants are hidden by the outer surface antigen of the intact virion.

Inside the hepatitis B nucleocapsid is a DNA-dependent DNA polymerase and the hepatitis B e antigen, which is thought to be either an internal component or a degradation product of the core antigen. HBeAg is found only in the serum of individuals whose serum also contains HBsAg, and it appears in the serum of virtually all patients early in the course of HBV infection. The presence of HBeAg in serum is indicative of the presence of large numbers of circulating intact virions: serum containing HBeAg is estimated to be one million times more infectious than serum containing HBsAg but not HBeAg.

Serology

HBsAg can be detected in the serum within a few weeks of viral exposure [see Figure 5]. It usually persists throughout the symptomatic period and does not disappear until after recovery. Anti-HBs appears shortly after the disappearance of HBsAg [see Table 6]. During this window period, neither HBsAg nor anti-HBs is detectable [see Table 7]. Anti-HBs persists for years and is associated with immunity to reinfection. HBV can be differentiated into eight serotypes on the basis of determinants of the surface antigen.

Hepatitis B core antigen (HBcAg) is not found free in the serum, but antibody to HBcAg (anti-HBc) becomes detectable at an early stage in the course of acute infections, 1 to 2 weeks after the appearance of HBsAg. Titers of anti-HBc fall after the disappearance of HBsAg but persist for life. In patients with chronic hepatitis B, HBsAg remains detectable indefinitely, and titers of anti-HBc remain high. Years after infection, titers of anti-HBs may have fallen to undetectable levels, and anti-HBc may be the only marker of previous infection. HBeAg is detectable immediately after the appearance of HBsAg. Antibody to HBeAg (anti-HBe) appears just after HBeAg becomes undetectable (usually before the disappearance of HBsAg) and persists for 1 to 2 years [see Figure 5].

HEPATITIS D

HDV is a defective, 35 to 37 nm RNA virus that can infect only persons who are also infected with HBV, because it uses HBsAg for its structural protein shell. HDV is found worldwide and is especially prevalent in the Amazon basin, central Africa, southern Italy, and the Middle East.[83] HDV infection is less common in the United States and Western Europe, where it is generally associat-

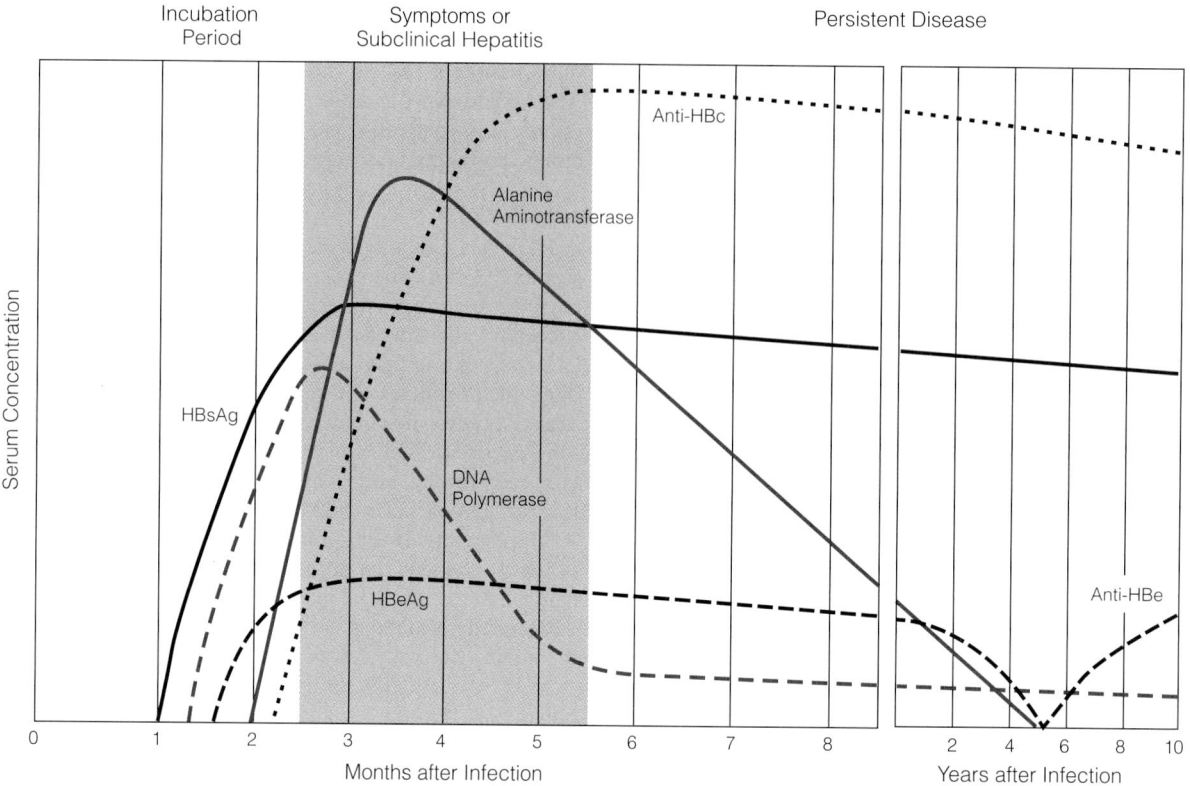

Figure 4 Schematic shows virologic, clinical, and serologic events of a hepatitis B infection that becomes persistent.

ed with parenteral blood exposure, typically in the setting of I.V. drug abuse or multiple transfusions.

Clinically, hepatitis D is found only in association with acute or chronic hepatitis B, and it cannot last longer than hepatitis B does. Depending on the state of the HBV infection, HDV infection appears either as a coinfection or a superinfection. Coinfection occurs when acute HDV infection and acute HBV infection are present simultaneously; superinfection occurs when acute HDV infection is superimposed on chronic HBV infection. Coinfection with HDV is associated with fulminant hepatitis and a mortality of 2% to 20%.[84] Fewer than 5% of cases of coinfection progress to chronic hepatitis D. In contrast, superinfection with HDV results in chronic HDV hepatitis, often with cirrhosis, in more than 70% of cases. The clinical and biochemical features of HDV infection resemble those of HBV infection alone. Chronic active hepatitis B progresses faster when hepatitis D is also present. Chronic HDV infection is more likely to result in severe morbidity and mortality than chronic HBV or HCV infection alone.

Diagnosis of acute HDV infection may be difficult: HDAg appears in the circulation only briefly and often goes undetected. Antibody to HDAg (anti-HD) of the IgM class subsequently appears in serum in low titers. Because no anti-HD IgG response occurs, no serologic marker of previous HDV infection may remain after recovery. Chronic HDV infection is easier to diagnose: high titers of anti-HD in the serum indicate ongoing HDV infection, and HDV antigen is detectable in the liver by means of immunohistochemical techniques. Moreover, IgM anti-HD remains detectable in serum.[83]

NON-A, NON-B HEPATITIS: HEPATITIS E AND HEPATITIS C

Non-A, non-B hepatitis is divided into two varieties, an epidemic form (hepatitis E) and a parenterally transmitted form (hepatitis C).[85] Hepatitis E is an acute, self-limited disease whose clinical features are similar to those of other types of hepatitis. Hepatitis E virus (HEV) is prevalent in the developing world, where it is spread by the fecal-oral route and has been associated with large outbreaks as well as sporadic cases. Outbreaks have been linked to contaminated water supplies. No cases of HEV infection acquired in the United States have been reported to date, but HEV acquisition has been reported in international travelers.

Hepatitis C is the most common cause of nonalcoholic liver disease in the United States. HCV is an RNA virus of the flavivirus family. It can be transmitted through parenteral exposure (usually in the setting of I.V. drug abuse), sexual contact, or the sharing of a household with an HCV-infected person; however, some persons with HCV infection have none of these risk factors, and there may be other means of transmission that have yet to be elucidated. Before the advent of antibody testing, HCV infection accounted for the majority (75% to 95%) of cases of posttransfusion hepatitis.[83] Since the spring of 1990, when a serologic test for HCV became available, all transfused blood has been screened for HCV, and the incidence of transfusion-associated hepatitis C has fallen precipitously. At present, however, I.V. drug use still accounts for a large proportion (60%) of HCV transmission in the United States.[59]

The presence of anti-HCV IgG appears not to be protective: blood donors with anti-HCV antibody can transmit hepatitis.[62] Surveys of HCV seropositivity indicate that 0.2% to 0.6% of volunteer blood donors carry anti-HCV IgG,[83] and the prevalence may be much higher among high-risk populations (e.g., residents of large inner-city communities). The prevalence of anti-HCV IgG is high among I.V. drug users, hemodialysis patients, and hemophiliacs.

Clinical Manifestations

The incubation period of hepatitis C averages 7 to 8 weeks in length but may be as short as 2 weeks or as long as 15. The clini-

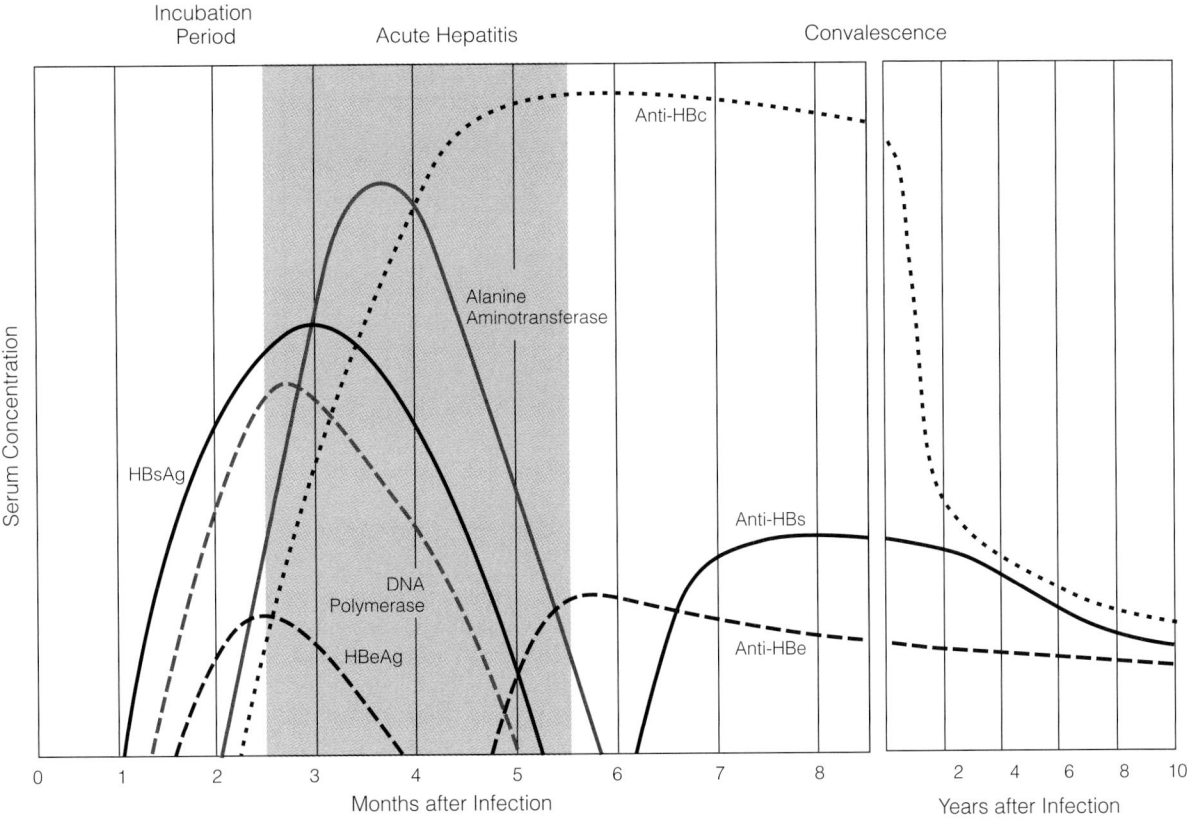

Figure 5 **Schematic shows virologic, clinical, and serologic events during acute hepatitis B infection.**

cal manifestations and biochemical alterations associated with acute hepatitis C are similar to but milder than those associated with hepatitis B. Serum aminotransferase levels can fluctuate widely; the peak levels are lower than those seen in hepatitis B (10 to 20 times normal as opposed to 20 to 50 times normal). Only about 25% of cases of acute HCV infection are icteric, and the mortality for acute infection is about 1%. Most patients have no acute illness suggestive of HCV infection. Antibody is not always present early in infection, and there are no clinically available assays for detecting IgM antibody to HCV. Thanks to improvements in the immunodetection of HCV, however, the interval before anti-HCV can be detected has decreased from the 6 to 12 months required with the first-generation tests to 8 to 12 weeks with the second-generation assays.[83]

The most striking feature of HCV infection is its tendency to become chronic in as many as 50% to 75% of cases. One study found that even among the 1% to 10% of individuals with HCV whose bloodstreams had been cleared of HCV according to RT-PCR assay, as many as 90% still had HCV in the liver.[86] It is estimated that in the United States, nearly four million people are seropositive for HCV, and more than 30% of liver transplantations are performed to treat end-stage liver disease related to chronic HCV infection. The presence of anti-HCV IgG does not distinguish acute from chronic hepatitis. Within 10 years, cirrhosis may develop in as many as 20% to 25% of patients with active hepatitis[87]; accordingly, these patients must be followed up carefully.

Chronic active hepatitis is characterized by elevated serum aminotransferase levels; however, other test results remain normal, and the patient is usually asymptomatic until end-stage liver disease develops. Liver biopsy shows inflammation around the portal triads. Recombinant interferons have been used to treat

chronic HCV infection, with mixed results: frequently, there is little response to treatment, or viremia returns after treatment. The combination of interferon with ribavirin has shown promise, however. Interferon treatment is generally reserved for patients who have chronic HCV infection and show evidence of active necroinflammatory liver disease with persistent ALT elevations.

HEPATITIS IN HOSPITAL PERSONNEL

Patients with hepatitis can infect hospital personnel with the

Table 6 Serologic Markers of Hepatitis B Infection

HBsAg	Present in acute and chronic infection Indicator that person is infectious
Anti-HBs	Appears 2 to 16 wk after HBsAg disappears from the serum Persists for years Confers immunity
HBcAg	Not present in the serum Found in the hepatocyte
Anti-HBc	Appears in serum with or shortly after HBsAg Persists for years May be only indicator of hepatitis B infection
HBeAg	Appears in the early acute phase Indicates serum is highly infectious Persistence beyond 10 wk suggests progression to chronic carrier state
Anti-HBe	Good prognosis for resolution of infection

virus via needle-stick injuries and other forms of accidental exposure. Conversely, physicians who are chronic carriers of HBV or HCV can infect their patients. According to a nationwide seroepidemiologic survey reported in 1978, approximately 19% of physicians have anti-HBs, compared with 3.5% of healthy volunteer blood donors [see Table 8].[88] Anti-HBs was found in 28% of surgeons, the highest prevalence in any medical specialty. For physicians, the likelihood of being positive for anti-HBs correlates with age and the number of years in practice. The risk of hepatitis is greatest among medical staff members in renal dialysis units, oncology units, and the clinical laboratory. Since 1978, when these data were reported, HBV vaccination has made it impossible to perform similar, more recent studies, because vaccination rather than previous infection would be responsible for the presence of antibodies.

Physicians and other staff members who care for hemodialysis patients with end-stage renal disease are at greater risk for acquiring HBV because of the high prevalence of hepatitis in such patients [see Table 9].[89,90] Transmission of HBV decreases in dialysis centers when close attention is paid to hygienic technique. Isolation of patients who are carriers of HBsAg also reduces the incidence of HBV in hemodialysis patients and staff.[91]

From 0.28% to 9.3% of health care workers have antibody to HCV.[92-94] In one study from Connecticut, five (12.5%) of 40 surgeons had antibody to HCV.[92] In another study, from New York City, eight (1.75%) of 456 dentists had anti-HCV antibody.[93] The highest prevalence among dentists was found to occur in oral surgeons (9.3%). As use of vaccines for HBV becomes more widespread [see Management of Viral Exposure, Hepatitis B, above], HCV may come to predominate over HBV as the cause of the rare cases of hepatitis transmitted from hospital personnel to patients.

EPIDEMIOLOGY OF POSTTRANSFUSION HEPATITIS

Both HBV and HCV can be transmitted by percutaneous and other routes.[89] Rare cases of hepatitis have been attributed to the infusion of immune globulin, although its preparation by ethanol fractionation normally destroys hepatitis virus (as well as HIV). Albumin is pasteurized by heating at 60° C for 10 hours, which destroys hepatitis virus.

Because of the current criteria for acceptable blood donors, elimination of payment for blood donation, and serologic testing for HBV and HCV, the risk of contracting hepatitis B from a blood transfusion is now much lower than it once was. In the United States, it is now rare for either HBV or HCV to be transmitted via blood transfusion. According to the latest estimates available, the risk of HCV transmission via this route is approximately 1/103,000 (95% CI, 28,000 to 288,000), and that of HBV transmission is 1/63,000 (95% CI, 31,000 to 147,000).[95]

HDV can also be passed by transfusion. In a study of 262 patients who had posttransfusion hepatitis and whose serum was positive for HBsAg, anti-HD was found in nine patients.[96] HDV can be detected in 24% of HBsAg-positive drug abusers and in approximately 50% of HBsAg-positive hemophiliacs.

LONG-TERM EFFECTS OF CHRONIC HEPATITIS

Chronic hepatitis can lead to problems requiring surgical intervention. It can cause cirrhosis, which in turn can cause portal hypertension and bleeding varices that necessitate portal systemic shunting. In addition, HBV and HCV predispose to hepatocellular carcinoma, the most prevalent visceral cancer in the world. The condition is especially prevalent in China, Southeast Asia, and sub-Saharan Africa. It is estimated that 25% of chronically infected persons die of cirrhosis or hepatocellular carcinoma.[97] HBV coinfec-

Table 7   Serologic Patterns of Hepatitis B Infection

HBsAg	Anti-HBs	Anti-HBe	Interpretation
+	−	−	Early acute hepatitis B
+	−	+	Late acute hepatitis B
−	−	+	Window period between disappearance of HBsAg and appearance of anti-HBs *or* Chronic carrier with low HBsAg level *or* Infection in the remote past
−	+	+	Past hepatitis B infection
−	+	−	Infection in the remote past *or* Immunization with hepatitis B vaccine *or* HBIG received within the past 1 to 2 mo

+ = detectable   − = not detectable

tion appears to increase the risk of hepatocellular carcinoma in HCV-infected persons. A widespread program of vaccination against HBV could greatly decrease the incidence of hepatocellular carcinoma. Epidemiology, molecular biology, and comparative pathology provide strong circumstantial evidence that hepatitis B is a significant factor in the etiology of hepatocellular carcinoma. The risk of primary hepatocellular carcinoma is more than 250 times greater in carriers of HBV than in noncarriers. HBV markers can be found in 80% to 90% of patients with hepatocellular carcinoma. Perhaps the best epidemiologic data indicating that hepatitis B precedes hepatocellular carcinoma were obtained in Taiwan from male civil servants between 40 and 60 years of age.[98] Approximately 3,500 HBsAg carriers were matched by age and place of birth (either mainland China or Taiwan) to 3,000 HBsAg-negative men, who served as control subjects. An additional group of 16,000 HBsAg-negative men between 40 and 60 years of age served as unmatched control subjects. After subjects were followed for 2 to 4 years, 50 cases of hepatocellular carcinoma were found, all but one of which occurred in chronic HBsAg carriers.

HCV is also associated with chronic infection in a high percentage (approximately 50%) of cases. In many countries, chronic HBV infection remains the leading factor in the development of hepatocellular carcinoma, whereas in Japan, Korea, and southern Europe, 50% to 75% of cases of hepatocellular carcinoma are

Table 8   Frequency of Antibody to Hepatitis B Surface Antigen (Anti-HBs) by Physician Specialty[88]

Specialty	Number of Patients Tested	Positive Results (%)
Surgery	176	50 (28)
Pathology	37	10 (27)
Pediatrics	63	13 (21)
Internal medicine	259	46 (18)
Anesthesiology	59	10 (17)
Obstetrics-gynecology	63	10 (16)
Family practice	341	54 (16)
Nonpatient care	25	1 (4)
All others combined	169	26 (15)
Total	1,192	220 (18.5)

Table 9   Prevalence of Hepatitis B Virus (HBV)
Serologic Markers in Various Populations[90]

Population		Prevalence of Serologic Markers of HBV Infection (%)	
		HBsAg	All Markers
High risk	Immigrants or refugees from areas where HBV is highly endemic	13	70–85
	Clients in institutions for the mentally retarded	10–20	35–80
	Users of illicit parenteral drugs	7	60–80
	Homosexually active men	6	35–80
	Household contacts of HBV carriers	3–6	30–60
	Hemodialysis patients	3–10	20–80
Intermediate risk	Health care workers with frequent blood contact	1–2	15–30
	Prisoners (male)	1–8	10–80
	Staffs of institutions for the mentally retarded	1	10–25
Low risk	Health care workers with no or infrequent blood contact	0.3	3–10
	Healthy adults (first-time volunteer blood donors)	0.3	3–5

associated with chronic HCV infection.[99] In Japan, mortality from hepatocellular carcinoma increased approximately twofold in the 1980s, a change that may be attributable to a higher incidence of HCV-associated liver cancer.[100]

Herpesviruses

CYTOMEGALOVIRUS

CMV is a member of the B herpesvirus family and is the largest virus known to infect humans. In some U.S. cities, the seroprevalence of CMV is 60% to 70%. Like other members of the herpesvirus family, CMV is capable of remaining within its host in a latent state, probably by down-regulating cell surface markers (e.g., HLA-1) and thus avoiding immune destruction. Latent CMV has been found in circulating mononuclear cells, polymorphonuclear cells, vascular endothelium, renal epithelial tissue, and pulmonary secretions. The virus may become reactivated in the setting of immunodeficiency, such as may arise with HIV infection, transplantation, or significant stress from operations or injuries. In non-immunocompromised patients, CMV typically causes a self-limited mononucleosis-like syndrome characterized by fever and mild hepatic transaminase abnormalities. In immunocompromised patients, however, CMV infection can be much more severe and even potentially life threatening, causing myelosuppression, pneumonitis, colitis, and retinopathy.

Posttransfusion Cytomegalovirus Infection (Posttransfusion or Postperfusion Syndrome)

The transmission of CMV by extracorporeal perfusion is responsible for the occasional development of a syndrome similar to mononucleosis in patients who have undergone open-heart operation. The syndrome characteristically appears 3 to 5 weeks after operation; its features are splenomegaly, fever, atypical lymphocytosis, and, occasionally, hepatomegaly, erythematous rash, and eosinophilia.[89] CMV can be isolated from the blood of virtually all patients with the typi-

cal posttransfusion syndrome and from the urine of half of these patients.[89] The condition is nonfatal and self-limited, but it may result in prolonged hospitalization and a long, expensive search for the source of fever. Although uncommon in adults 30 years of age and older, the syndrome can occur in as many as 10% of susceptible children and adults younger than 30 years.

This syndrome can also occur in patients who receive transfusions but who do not undergo open-heart operation. Occasional cases that develop postoperatively in patients who did not receive transfusions are thought to be the result of reactivation of latent infection. EBV can sometimes cause the syndrome.

The incidence of posttransfusion CMV infection is related to the kind of blood or blood product transfused. CMV is highly cell associated and is transmitted with leukocytes, which may be present in transfusions of packed red blood cells, platelets, or white blood cells; transmission from transfusion of fresh frozen plasma or cryoprecipitate has not been documented.[14] Therefore, efforts to decrease the number of white blood cells in the transfused blood would be expected to decrease the rate of transfusion-associated CMV infection. Approximately 50% of patients who receive whole blood seroconvert to CMV, whereas only 10% of those who receive washed packed red blood cells seroconvert. The risk of seroconversion to CMV is between 12% and 100% when whole blood, either fresh or stored, is transfused.[101] In one study, transfusion of frozen deglycerolized red blood cells resulted in seroconversion in only 3% of patients,[89] whereas in another, seroconversion occurred in 58% of 36 leukemic patients transfused with lymphocytes.[102]

The risk of posttransfusion CMV infection is also related to the volume of blood received. In one study, 7% of patients receiving a single unit of whole blood seroconverted, whereas anti-CMV antibody titers rose in 21% of patients receiving more than one unit.[103] The risk of infection per unit of blood transfused is estimated to range between 2.7% and 12%.[104]

Preexisting antibody to CMV does not protect transfusion recipients against reinfection. After transfusion of whole blood, titers of antibody to CMV will increase in 10% of recipients (an indication of reinfection) and in 19% of patients who did not have antibody to CMV before transfusion (an indication of infection). Whereas a seronegative recipient of CMV-positive blood has a 21% chance of seroconversion, the risk of seroconversion from the receipt of one unit of CMV-negative blood is only 2%.[89] However, the sensitivity of the serologic test for CMV is such that even when blood that tests seronegative is used, there is still a residual 0% to 6% risk of CMV transmission.[105]

Because so many patients receive blood transfusions during operation, it is understandable that evidence of posttransfusion CMV infection has been found in many patients postoperatively (e.g., after gynecologic surgery, cholecystectomy, appendectomy, lumbosacral fusion, splenectomy, and transplantation). It has also been found in surgical patients who are victims of trauma or burns.

However, it is surprising that infection with CMV, a ubiquitous virus, does not occur more frequently after transfusion. Between 30% and 54% of the adult population in the United States have antibody to CMV, an indication of previous infection.[89] Because infection with the virus is probably lifelong, a significant proportion of blood donors harbor the virus. The prevalence of antibody to CMV is 25% in units of blood from donors between 18 and 23 years of age and increases to 89% in blood from donors older than 60 years. The overall prevalence of seropositive blood donors is between 30% and 70%.

Cytomegalovirus in Transplant Recipients

CMV infection occurs not only in patients who have received blood transfusions but also in those who have suffered trauma, those receiving immunosuppressive therapy, and those with neoplastic disease. The groups at highest risk for CMV infection are probably recipients of organ transplants and of bone marrow transplants.[106-108] Numerous studies have documented the high incidence of CMV infection after organ transplantation: the rates range from 26% to 100%.[89,109,110] Primary CMV infection occurs in patients who do not have antibody to CMV before receiving transplants. Infections are considered to be reactivated if they occur in patients who did have antibody to CMV before receiving transplants. Rates of infection in patients receiving cardiac or bone marrow transplants are similar to those in patients receiving kidney transplants.

The high incidence of CMV infections after transplantation was recognized in the early days of such procedures. At autopsy of patients who died after renal transplantation, the intranuclear inclusions typical of CMV were found in tissue from the lungs, the parotid glands, the lymph nodes, the liver, the pancreas, the parathyroid, and the brain. CMV has been cultured repeatedly from the urine of transplant recipients, and the frequency of seroconversion among them has been high.

Likely sources of the virus are blood, because fresh blood can transmit CMV, and the organ transplant itself, because CMV can grow in renal tubular epithelial cells and can be transmitted as a latent virus. In several studies, recipients of kidney transplants had a much higher incidence of CMV infection when the donors had antibody to CMV than when the donors did not. In one study, 57% of recipients of kidneys from seropositive donors acquired CMV infection after transplantation, compared with 8% of recipients of kidneys from seronegative donors.[111] Even patients who have antibody to CMV can acquire new CMV infections as a result of transfusion or transplantation because there is more than one antigenic variety of the virus. Also, CMV that is latent in many patients who have antibody before transplantation may be reactivated after transplantation by host versus graft reactions, corticosteroids, or other immunosuppressive drugs. Hospital personnel, family members, and the environment play very small roles in transmission of CMV to transplant recipients.

Several systematic studies have demonstrated that CMV causes clinical illness in renal transplant recipients. In four studies, clinical illness developed in 83% of 76 patients with primary infection, compared with 44% of 268 patients with reactivation of a previous infection.[89,109,110]

Recipients of renal transplants in whom CMV causes clinical illness most commonly present with fever. Fever occurs in 95% of patients with CMV infection and may be prolonged. Patients with CMV infection also frequently present with anorexia, arthralgias, and leukopenia. Other clinical features of the disease are diffuse pulmonary infiltrates, pancreatitis, transplant malfunction, and systemic bacterial and fungal superinfections. Invasion of the GI tract by CMV may cause gastritis and ulcers in both the duodenum and the colon, which in turn may lead to hemorrhage and perforation. Biopsies demonstrate CMV inclusions at the base of the ulcers. The virus appears to invade the vascular endothelium, and bleeding is possibly a result of vascular occlusion and ischemic necrosis of the overlying tissue.

Lethal CMV disease is characterized by the presence of most of the features listed above. Liver dysfunction is found in 100% of patients with lethal disease but in only 50% to 75% of patients with mild or moderate infection, and CMV viremia occurs in 46% to 48% of patients with severe CMV infection but in only 26% to 28% of patients with mild to moderate infection. Leukopenia and the presence of atypical leukocytes also correlate with the severity of the disease. CMV infection after renal transplantation is also associated with pneumonia, hepatitis, encephalitis, and retinitis.

Whether or not CMV infection causes or leads to graft rejection is uncertain. Both the highest incidence of CMV infection (> 80%)[89,109,110] and the highest incidence of graft rejection occur within the first 3 months after transplantation. In several studies, young patients and recipients of second kidney transplants were at higher risk for graft loss if they had CMV than if they did not.[89,109,110] In most studies, however, it is extremely difficult to demonstrate a relation between CMV infection and graft rejection.

Of the multiple factors affecting the risk of CMV infection in transplant recipients, the most important are (1) the familial relation and HLA matching between the kidney donor and the recipient and (2) the CMV serology of both the donor and the recipient. The presence of antibody in transplant recipients before transplantation seems to offer a small amount of protection against fever caused by CMV but does not protect against more serious consequences of the infection, such as leukopenia, graft failure, and death.

CMV infection is also a major problem in liver, heart, and bone marrow transplant recipients.[106,108] In liver transplant recipients, CMV is a cause of hepatitis and liver dysfunction that can be confused with rejection or other causes of liver malfunction,[106] and it can lead to lethal infection. CMV pneumonitis in bone marrow transplant recipients is the most common life-threatening infectious complication after transplantation. The severity of infection in bone marrow transplant recipients may be attributable to the higher incidence of host versus graft disease in patients with CMV pneumonitis (82%) than in those without CMV pneumonitis (27%).[112]

Prevention and Treatment of Cytomegalovirus Infection

Several methods have been proposed to reduce the incidence of CMV infection after transfusion or transplantation. One method is to eliminate as many white blood cells as possible from transfused blood because CMV is almost certainly transmitted solely through these cells. From 90% to 100% of viable leukocytes in blood have been removed from frozen deglycerolized erythrocytes. In one study, transfusion of 24 hemodialyzed patients with leukocyte-free red blood cells from frozen deglycerolized blood prevented subsequent CMV infection.[104]

Another approach is to transfuse blood only from CMV-negative donors. Because the majority of posttransfusion CMV infections are asymptomatic, however, the increased cost of performing serologic tests on all donated units might be difficult to justify.

Storage of blood to reduce infectiousness of CMV is another approach, but storage from 48 to 72 hours does not significantly reduce transmission of CMV infection. Irradiating the blood to render the CMV noninfectious is unacceptable because it causes cell transformation in vitro. Furthermore, in one study, administration of leukocytes previously exposed to 1,500 cGy (1,500 rads) of gamma radiation resulted in an increased incidence of CMV infection among recipients of these cells.[102]

Because the incidence of CMV infection is higher in patients who receive kidney transplants from seropositive donors, some centers do not transplant kidneys from seropositive donors into seronegative recipients. However, no published reports indicate that this practice leads to a significant alteration in the outcome of renal transplantation with respect to graft rejection. Moreover, excluding kidneys from seropositive donors makes it more difficult to find kidneys for seronegative recipients.

Many attempts have been made to develop a CMV vaccine for administration before viral exposure by multiple passages of the virus in tissue culture. Two such vaccines have been used in clinical trials, one prepared from the AD169 strain and the other from the Towne 125 strain of the virus. Immunization with these vaccines can elicit both serum antibody and cell-mediated immunity. In one trial, the vaccine prepared from the Towne 125 strain lowered the incidence of clinical disease but not of infection, and the disease tended to be less severe in vaccinated patients than in control subjects who received placebo.[113]

Human IG has been administered after transfusion or transplantation in attempts to prevent associated CMV infection. In one study, it reduced life-threatening infection to a less severe form in most patients, but in other studies, not surprisingly, it provided no consistent benefit.[114-117] In patients who are already seropositive, the virus is latent inside their cells, where it is probably not accessible to serum antibody. Patients with primary infections may not benefit from antibody treatment, because herpesviruses seem to transfer from cell to cell without ever existing free in serum. Even CMV hyperimmune globulin has no clear benefit in patients with clinical CMV infection.[118] It may, however, help control severe infections, such as those seen in bone marrow transplant recipients.

Several antiviral agents have been used in attempts to reduce the incidence or lessen the effect of CMV infection. Among these agents are interferon, transfer factor, immune globulin, and nucleoside derivatives, such as cytarabine, vidarabine, and acyclovir (see below). Immune globulins, acyclovir, and ganciclovir are effective at preventing CMV infection in transplant recipients.[109,110,114,119,120] Ganciclovir and foscarnet are active against CMV in vitro. Ganciclovir is currently being used to treat CMV and is the most effective agent in organ transplant recipients (see below).[109,110,119-121]

EPSTEIN-BARR VIRUS

EBV is the herpesvirus responsible for infectious mononucleosis. It can be found in B cells in peripheral blood of infected patients and in tumor cells of patients with Burkitt lymphoma and nasopharyngeal carcinoma. It remains in a latent form in an infected host for years, probably for life. Most posttransfusion EBV infections are asymptomatic. Seroconversion to EBV will develop in approximately 8% of recipients transfused with between two and 14 units of blood. In as many as 5% of patients with preexisting antibody to EBV, significant elevations of antibody titers may develop, beginning

2 weeks after transfusion. These elevations indicate either reinfection or reactivation of a latent infection.[89] Because EBV is associated with cells and does not exist free in serum to any great extent, antibody to EBV in either donors or recipients is unlikely to provide substantial protection against infection resulting from blood transfusions or organ transplants. Among transfused patients who do not have preexisting antibody to EBV, the prevalence of EBV infection can reach 33% to 46%. In these patients, the absence of preexisting antibody presumably rules out reactivation of latent EBV infection as the source of infection.

EBV occurs worldwide. In the United States, nearly all adults and as many as 65% of persons of all ages have antibody to EBV. Infection is thought to occur in infancy, and as many as 17% of infants have antibody to EBV. By 5 years of age, 72% of children have antibody to EBV, and the prevalence in adults is similar.[122] Thus, the majority of blood donors in the United States have been previously infected with EBV and probably have latent virus in their leukocytes. Although it is clear that EBV can be transmitted by blood when the transfusion occurs within 3 days of donation, it is not known whether blood stored for longer periods can transmit the virus. Because EBV is predominantly intracellular, plasma and its derivatives do not transmit the virus.

The diagnosis of EBV infection is made serologically. Tests both for IgM antibody to capsid antigens and for IgG antibody to the early antigens of EBV or tests of serial samples for IgG antibody to capsid antigens must be used. The heterophil antibody test (the Paul-Bunnell test) and a rapid slide test that is equivalent (the monospot test) are also used in most clinical studies to screen for EBV infection before more specific diagnostic tests are performed.

In cases of posttransfusion infection, IgG antibody to EBV can be detected at least 10 days before the onset of symptoms, and EBV can be cultured from circulating lymphocytes 11 days before the onset of symptoms. In patients with acute infection, EBV is found in approximately three of every 10^4 peripheral blood lymphocytes.[123] In contrast, all recovered persons with antibodies to EBV are thought to have the virus in one of every 10^7 circulating lymphocytes.

EBV is strongly implicated in the etiology of a posttransplantation lymphoproliferative disorder (PTLD).[89,124,125] EBV has been isolated from the tissues of most cases of PTLD, but not all.[126,127] Non–EBV-related cases of PTLD typically occur later after transplantation, and their etiology has not been elucidated.

PTLD comprises three general clinical presentations: (1) a mononucleosis-like syndrome involving the tonsils and the peripheral lymph nodes, (2) a diffuse polymorphous B-cell infiltration in many visceral organs, and (3) localized extranodal tumors in the GI tract, the neck, the thorax, or other parts of the body. Patients whose disease is limited to a single organ or to lymph nodes often respond to a reduction in immunosuppression or antiviral therapy; however, once the infection becomes widespread, the disease progresses rapidly and is fatal in more than 75% of cases.[128] In solid organ transplant recipients, PTLD may be limited to the allograft. There is some evidence to suggest that PTLD may have organ-specific features that promote lymphoproliferation: allograft involvement has been reported in 17% of renal transplant recipients, 8.6% of liver transplant recipients, and as many as 60% to 80% of lung or intestinal transplant recipients.[128]

The persons at highest risk for PTLD are EBV-seronegative persons receiving EBV-positive organs or bone marrow. Most infections occur within the first 4 months after transplantation.[129] Several specific risk factors for the development of PTLD have been identified: a seropositive graft in a seronegative recipient, certain types of organ allografts (with intestinal transplants carrying the highest risk), any type of immunosuppression that blunts cellular immunity to EBV (with risk increasing as immunosuppression becomes more pronounced), and the presence of other infections (CMV in particular).

The optimal treatment of lymphoproliferative disorders remains unclear. Some early EBV-associated lymphoproliferative disorders in solid organ transplant recipients have regressed completely after reduction of immunosuppression.[130,131] Early PTLD may respond to antiviral therapy with acyclovir or ganciclovir, which may prevent infection of resting B cells, but such therapy is less likely to be effective in the face of high concentrations of latently infected circulating or tissue-invasive B cells. Some investigators also report resolution of PTLD after treatment with interferon alfa.[132,133]

Transmission of EBV can occur simultaneously with transmission of CMV or hepatitis virus. Although hepatitis accompanies EBV infections in sporadic cases, EBV alone has not been documented as a cause of posttransfusion hepatitis.

HERPES SIMPLEX VIRUS

Infection or reactivation of infection with herpes simplex virus type 1 (HSV-1) follows renal transplantation in 50% to 75% of patients, most often within 30 days after transplantation. Reactivation of infection is more common than primary infection: only 14% of patients who are seronegative before transplantation become infected, but infection is reactivated in 64% of patients who were already seropositive before transplantation.

Most cases of HSV-1 infection after transplantation are clinically inapparent and are indicated only by a significant rise in titer of antibody to the virus. The most prevalent clinical manifestation is herpes labialis, that is, fever blisters affecting not only the lips but also the mucous membranes of the oral cavity and the skin of the head and neck. Although these lesions are painful and may make eating, drinking, and taking oral medications difficult, they are usually self-limited and heal without treatment or reduction of immunosuppression. However, HSV-1 infection can take a much more malignant course, disseminating to cause pneumonitis, fulminant hepatitis, upper GI hemorrhage, encephalitis, aseptic meningitis, and death.

VARICELLA-ZOSTER VIRUS

Varicella-zoster virus (VZV), another herpesvirus, is the etiologic agent of herpes zoster and chicken pox. This virus resides in the dorsal root ganglia of adults who had primary varicella infection in childhood. Herpes zoster is more common in organ transplant recipients, in patients with cancer (especially those who have leukemia or lymphomas), in burn patients, and in patients receiving immunosuppressive drugs. Serologic evidence of VZV infection occurs in 8% to 16% of renal transplant recipients. The lesions of herpes zoster become evident 12 to 511 days after organ transplantation.

In children or adults who have not already had chicken pox and occasionally even in children who have, VZV can cause disseminated chicken pox in many organs, which may be fatal.

AGENTS EFFECTIVE AGAINST HERPESVIRUSES

Because the essential synthetic activities of viruses depend on the metabolic machinery of their host, it has been difficult to devise specific antiviral agents that interfere with viral replication but are not harmful to host cells.[134,135] Many antiviral agents are too toxic to be used clinically. In contrast, antibacterial agents that are both toxic to bacteria and safe for human cells are easier to design because the structure and metabolic machinery of bacteria are distinct from those of host cells.

Although intracellular processes unique to viral replication have

been identified and specifically targeted for chemotherapeutic attack, very few agents have been effective against human viruses. Among these is amantadine, which is used for both prophylaxis and treatment of influenza A. Agents that were found to be effective for prophylaxis against smallpox, such as methisazone, now have no use, because the disease has been eradicated.

There are few effective chemotherapeutic agents for hepatitis or most of the other major viral diseases that concern surgeons, but several agents have been used for the treatment of herpesvirus infections, especially in immunosuppressed patients [see Table 10]. These agents, derivatives of purines and pyrimidines, interfere with viral nucleic acid synthesis.

Acyclovir and Valacyclovir

Acyclovir (acycloguanosine) is a nucleoside derivative that is used to treat herpesvirus infections, especially herpes simplex and varicella-zoster infections in immunocompromised hosts. Valacyclovir is the L-valyl ester prodrug of acyclovir. In cases of mucocutaneous herpes simplex and herpes zoster, acyclovir can shorten the period of virus shedding, decrease pain, and promote more rapid scabbing and healing of lesions. Acyclovir is also the drug of choice for encephalitis caused by herpes simplex, but it is not effective in patients with established neurologic damage resulting from herpes simplex or varicella-zoster infections or in patients infected with CMV. Acyclovir inhibits the replication of EBV in actively replicating cells but does not affect latent or persistent infection.

The total daily dose of acyclovir is 10 to 25 mg/kg, given by I.V. infusion lasting 60 minutes. The recommended length of parenteral acyclovir therapy ranges from 5 to 10 days, depending on the indication. A major side effect of such therapy is phlebitis at the injection site; rash, leukopenia, and neurotoxicity may also occur. Acyclovir applied topically as a 5% ointment is effective in immunocompromised patients for the treatment of limited cutaneous herpes infections and in patients with normal immunity for the treatment of initial episodes (but not recurrent episodes) of genital herpes simplex infection. Oral acyclovir seems to be effective as prophylaxis against reactivated herpes simplex infection in recipients of bone marrow transplants and in patients immunosuppressed as a result of HIV infection.

Penciclovir and Famciclovir

Penciclovir is a nucleoside analogue that is similar to acyclovir with respect to spectrum of activity and potency against herpesviruses. Famciclovir is the diacetyl ester of penciclovir. Penciclovir requires thymidine kinase (TK) for phosphorylation and thus is inactive against thymidine kinase–deficient strains of HSV or VZV; however, it may be active against some TK-altered or polymerase mutants that are resistant to acyclovir as well as against some foscarnet-resistant HSV isolates. In experimental settings, topical, parenteral, and oral penciclovir and oral famciclovir have been effective against HSV infection.

Vidarabine

Vidarabine (ara-A) is effective against herpes simplex and varicella-zoster viruses as well as poxviruses, oncornaviruses, and rhabdoviruses. It is used mostly to combat herpesvirus infections in immunosuppressed patients. In these patients, vidarabine accelerates healing of cutaneous herpes zoster, decreases its rates of cutaneous dissemination and of visceral complications, and shortens the duration of postherpetic neuralgia. For systemic use, a daily dose of 10 to 15 mg/kg of vidarabine is administered I.V. over a period of 12 hours. The duration of therapy for herpes zoster is

Table 10   Antiviral Therapy of Clinical Benefit

Virus	Condition	Regimen
Herpes simplex virus	Keratitis	3% Acyclovir ointment *or* 1% Trifluridine solution *or* 3% Vidarabine ointment *or* 0.5% IDU ointment or 0.1% IDU drops
	Herpes labialis	Treatment usually not indicated; may use 1% penciclovir cream or topical acyclovir q. 2 hr while patient is awake for 4 days
	Genital herpes Primary	Acyclovir, 200 mg p.o. 5 times daily or 400 mg p.o., t.i.d., for 10 days, *or* Valacyclovir, 500 mg–1 g p.o., b.i.d., for 10–14 days, *or* Famciclovir, 250 mg p.o., t.i.d., for 10 days*
	Recurrent	Acyclovir, 200 mg p.o. 5 times daily or 400 mg p.o., t.i.d., for 5 days, *or* Valacyclovir, 500 mg p.o., b.i.d., for 5 days, *or* Famciclovir, 125 mg p.o., b.i.d., for 5 days
	Prophylaxis	Acyclovir, 400 mg p.o., b.i.d., *or* Valacyclovir, 500 mg–1 g p.o., q.d., *or* Famciclovir, 250 mg p.o., b.i.d.
	Encephalitis	Acyclovir, 10 mg/kg t.i.d. I.V. for 14–21 days
	Neonatal HSV	Acyclovir, 10 mg/kg I.V. q. 8 hr for 10–21 days (20 mg/kg I.V. q. 8 hr if neonate is premature)
	Immunocompromised host	Acyclovir, 5 mg/kg I.V. q. 8 hr for 7 days or 400 mg p.o. 5 times daily for 14–21 days, *or* Famciclovir, 500 mg p.o., b.i.d., for 7 days,* *or* Valacyclovir, 1 g p.o., t.i.d., for 7 days*
Varicella-zoster virus	Immunocompetent host Eye infections Shingles	3% Acyclovir ointment Acyclovir, 800 mg p.o. 5 times daily for 7–10 days, *or* Valacyclovir, 1 g p.o., t.i.d., for 7–10 days, *or* Famciclovir, 500 mg p.o., t.i.d., for 7–10 days
	Immunocompromised host	Acyclovir, 10–12 mg/kg I.V. q. 8 hr for 7 days (500 mg/m²)
Cytomegalovirus	Immunocompromised host Retinitis	Ganciclovir, 5 mg/kg I.V. q. 12 hr for 14–21 days,† *or* Foscarnet, 90 mg/kg (adjusted for renal function) I.V. q. 12 hr for 14–21 days, *or* Cidofovir, 5 mg/kg I.V. weekly for 2 weeks, then every other week
	CMV pneumonia	Ganciclovir, 2.5 mg/kg I.V. q.d. for 20 days

*Not approved by the FDA for this indication.
†An intraocular insert is also available.

5 days. Side effects include anorexia, weight loss, nausea, vomiting, weakness, anemia, leukopenia, thrombocytopenia, tremors, and thrombophlebitis at the site of administration.

Idoxuridine

Idoxuridine (5-iodo-2′-deoxyuridine) (IUdR, IDU) was the first clinically effective antiviral nucleoside. It is a halogenated pyrimidine that resembles thymidine in structure. Topical application of either a 0.1% solution or a 0.5% ointment of idoxuridine is effective treatment of herpes simplex keratitis but not of recurrent herpes labialis or localized zoster. In the United States, IDU is approved only for topical treatment of HSV keratitis. When combined with dimethyl sulfoxide (DMSO), IDU is active against herpes zoster and recurrent or primary genital HSV infection. In Europe, IDU is available in combination with DMSO for the treatment of herpes labialis, herpes genitalis, and herpes zoster.

Ganciclovir

Ganciclovir (DHPG, 2′-NDG, or BIOLF-62) is an acyclic nucleoside structurally related to acyclovir but with greater activity against CMV in vitro and in vivo. It is effective in treating CMV disease in transplant recipients and AIDS patients. The usual total daily dose of ganciclovir is 7.5 to 10 mg/kg, given in two or three divided doses. The dosage should be adjusted if the patient has decreased renal function. Myelosuppression is the principal dose-limiting toxic side effect.

Foscarnet

Foscarnet (trisodium phosphonoformate) is a pyrophosphate derivative that inhibits herpesvirus DNA polymerases and retroviral reverse transcriptases.[134-136] In the United States, it has been used for the prevention and treatment of CMV retinitis in patients with AIDS. For patients who have received renal or bone marrow transplants, foscarnet is given in a bolus injection of 9 mg/kg followed by infusion of 0.015 to 0.090 mg/kg/min I.V. for 7 days. Foscarnet is also used to treat acyclovir-resistant HSV infection. The major toxicity associated with foscarnet is nephrotoxicity; CNS side effects (e.g., headache, tremor, irritability, and seizures) can also occur.

Viral Infections from Animal and Human Bites

Surgeons are frequently called on to treat patients who have been bitten by either an animal or another person. Such bites can transmit several viruses and other infections. Certainly, rabies is the most feared viral infection transmitted in this way. Viruses that are found in saliva, such as HBV, herpesviruses, and possibly HIV, can be transmitted by a human bite, although such cases are most likely rare.

From zero to five cases of human rabies occur each year in the United States. Animal rabies is widespread and is found in every state except Hawaii. In 1992, more than 8,600 cases of animal rabies were reported to the CDC by 49 states, the District of Columbia, and Puerto Rico. The great majority of cases occur in wild animals.[69] Before 1950, more than 8,000 cases of rabies in dogs were reported each year in the United States; the number is now fewer than 150 a year.

Rabies proceeds from a prodrome of fever, malaise, and headache, to hyperactivity and diffuse cerebral dysfunction, and then to coma and death. From 5% to 20% of patients may also show progressive paralysis. Occasionally, there is no history of an animal bite. Diagnosis can be confirmed by culture of saliva, cerebrospinal fluid, or brain tissue; demonstration of rabies antigen in the cornea or skin; or measurement of serum antibody to rabies virus. At postmortem examination, typical intracytoplasmic inclusions (Negri bodies) can be seen in the brain cells.

Although the number of cases of human rabies is small, the disease is an important problem because of the large number of animal bites that occur each year. Surgeons may have to consider rabies prophylaxis in patients whom they treat for bite injuries [*see* Management of Viral Exposure, Rabies, *above, and 1:7 Acute Wound Care*]. Also, two fatal cases of rabies have occurred in recipients of corneal transplants from a patient whose cause of death was later found to be rabies.[137]

References

1. Recommendations for prevention of HIV transmission in health-care settings. MMWR Morb Mortal Wkly Rep 36(suppl 2):1S, 1987

2. Recommendations for preventing transmission of infection with human T-lymphocyte type III/lymphadenopathy-associated virus in the workplace. MMWR Morb Mortal Wkly Rep 34:681, 1985

3. Update: universal precautions for prevention of transmission of human immunodeficiency virus, hepatitis B virus, and other blood-borne pathogens in health-care settings. MMWR Morb Mortal Wkly Rep 37:377, 1988

4. Guidelines for prevention of transmission of human immunodeficiency virus and hepatitis B virus to health-care and public-safety workers. MMWR Morb Mortal Wkly Rep 38(suppl 6):1, 1989

5. Recommendations for HIV testing services for inpatients and outpatients in acute-care hospital settings and technical guidance on HIV counseling. MMWR Morb Mortal Wkly Rep 42(RR-2):1, 1993

6. Rhame F, Maki D: The case for wider use of testing for HIV infection. N Engl J Med 320:1248, 1989

7. Telford GL, Quebbeman EJ, Condon RE: A protocol to reduce risk of contracting AIDS and other blood-borne disease in the OR. Surg Rounds 10:30, 1987

8. Recommendations for follow up of health care workers after occupational exposure to hepatitis C. MMWR Morb Mortal Wkly Rep 46:603, 1997

9. Mast EE, Alter MJ: Prevention of hepatitis B virus infection among health-care workers. Hepatitis B Vaccines in Clinical Practice. Ellis RW, Ed. Marcel Dekker, New York, 1993, p 295

10. Werner BG, Grady GF: Accidental hepatitis B-surface-antigen-positive inoculations: use of e antigen to estimate infectivity. Ann Intern Med 97:367, 1982

11. Gerberding JL: Management of occupational exposures to blood-borne viruses. N Engl J Med 125:917, 1996

12. Sepkowitz KA: Occupationally acquired infections in health care workers (part II). Ann Intern Med 125:917, 1996

13. Department of Labor, OSHA: Occupational exposure to blood-borne pathogens. Final rule. Fed Regist 56:64175, 1991

14. Sepkowitz KA: Nosocomial hepatitis and other infections transmitted by blood and blood products. Principles and Practice of Infectious Disease, 5th ed. Mandell GL, Bennet JE, Dolin R, Eds. Churchill Livingstone, Philadelphia, 2000, p 3039

15. Protection against viral hepatitis: recommendations of the Immunization Practices Advisory Committee (ACIP). MMWR Morb Mortal Wkly Rep 39 (RR-2):1, 1990

16. Syndman DR, Bryan JA, Dixon RE: Prevention of nosocomial viral hepatitis, type B (hepatitis B). Ann Intern Med 83:838, 1975

17. Favero MS, Maynard JE, Leger RT, et al: Guidelines for the care of patients hospitalized with viral hepatitis. Ann Intern Med 91:872, 1979

18. Ciesielski C, Marianos D, Ou C-Y, et al: Transmission of human immunodeficiency virus in a dental practice. Ann Intern Med 116:798, 1992

19. Lot F, Seguier J, Fegeux S, et al: Probable transmission of HIV from an orthopedic surgeon to a patient in France. Ann Intern Med 130:1, 1999

20. Welch J, Webster M, Tilzey A, et al: Hepatitis B infections after gynecological surgery. Lancet 1:205, 1989

21. Lettau LA, Smith JD, Williams D, et al: Transmission of hepatitis B with resultant restriction of surgical practice. JAMA 255:934, 1986

22. Communicable Disease Surveillance Centre: Acute hepatitis B associated with gynaecological surgery. Lancet 1:1, 1980

23. Carl M, Frances DP, Blakey DL, et al: Interruption of hepatitis B transmission by modification of a gynaecologist's surgical technique. Lancet 1:731, 1982

24. Coutinho RA, Albrecht-van Lent P, Stoutjesdijk L, et al: Hepatitis B from doctors (letter). Lancet 1:345, 1982

25. Grob PJ, Bischof B, Naeff F: Cluster of hepatitis B transmitted by a physician. Lancet 2:1218, 1981

26. Meyers JD, Stamm WE, Kerr MM, et al: Lack of transmission of hepatitis B after surgical exposure. JAMA 240:1725, 1978

27. Haerem JW, Siebke JC, Ulstrup J, et al: HBsAg transmission from a cardiac surgeon incubating hepatitis B resulting in chronic antigenemia in four patients. Acta Med Scand 210:389, 1981

28. Acute hepatitis B following gynecological surgery. J Hosp Infect 9:34, 1987

29. Polakoff S: Acute hepatitis B in patients in Britain related to previous operations and dental treatment. Br J Med 293:33, 1986

30. Heptonstall J: Outbreaks of hepatitis B virus infection associated with infected surgical staff. Communicable Disease Report 1:R81, 1991

31. Surgeons who are hepatitis B carriers. BMJ 303:184, 1991

32. Jones D: Hepatitis leaves Halifax surgeon an operating room outcast. Can Med Assoc J 145:1345, 1991

33. Alter HJ, Chalmers TC, Freeman BM, et al: Health-care workers positive for hepatitis B surface antigen: are their contacts at risk? N Engl J Med 292:454, 1975

34. Williams SV, Pattison CP, Berquist KR: Dental infection with hepatitis B. JAMA 232:1231, 1975

35. Gerber MA, Lewin EB, Gerety RJ, et al: The lack of nurse-infant transmission of type B hepatitis in a special care nursery. J Pediatr 91:120, 1977

36. LaBrecque DR, Dhand AK: The risk of hepatitis B transmission from staff to patients in hemodialysis units—an overrated problem? Hepatology 1:398, 1981

37. LaBrecque DR, Muhs JM, Lutwick LI, et al: The risk of hepatitis B transmission from health care workers to patients in a hospital setting—a prospective study. Hepatology 6:205, 1986

38. Recommendations for preventing transmission of human immunodeficiency virus and hepatitis B virus to patients during exposure-prone invasive procedures. MMWR Morb Mortal Wkly Rep 40(RR-8), 1991

39. Esteban JI, Gomez J, Martell M, et al: Transmission of hepatitis C by a cardiac surgeon. N Engl J Med 334:555, 1996

40. Bosch H: Hepatitis C outbreak astounds Spain. Lancet 352:1415, 1998

41. Public Health Service guidelines for the management of health-care worker exposures to HIV and recommendations for post-exposure prophylaxis. MMWR Morb Mortal Wkly Rep 47:1, 1998

42. Chiarello LA, Gerberding JL: Human immunodeficiency virus in health care settings. Principles and Practice of Infectious Disease, 5th ed. Mandell GL, Bennett JE, Dolin R, Eds. Churchill Livingstone, Philadelphia, 2000, p 3052

43. Ciesielski CA, Metler RP: Duration of time between exposure and seroconversion in healthcare workers

with occupationally acquired infection with human immunodeficiency virus. Am J Med 102(suppl 5B): S115, 1997

44. Busch MP, Satten GA: Time course of viremia and antibody seroconversion following human immunodeficiency virus exposure. Am J Med 102(suppl 5B):S117, 1997

45. Cardo DM, Culver DH, Ciesielski CA, et al: A case-control study of HIV seroconversion in healthcare workers after percutaneous exposure. N Engl J Med 337:1485, 1997

46. Public Health Service Statement on management of occupational exposure to human immunodeficiency virus, including considerations regarding zidovudine postexposure use. MMWR Morb Mortal Wkly Rep 39 (RR-1):1, 1990

47. Wang SA, the HIV PEP Registry Group: Human immunodeficiency virus (HIV) postexposure prophylaxis (PEP) following occupational HIV exposure: findings from the HIV PEP Registry (abstract 482). Program and abstracts of the 35th Annual Meeting of the Infectious Diseases Society of America, Alexandria, Virginia, Sept 13–16, 1997, p 161

48. Steger KA, Swotinsky R, Snyder S, et al: Recent experience with post-exposure prophylaxis (PEP) with combination antiretrovirals for occupational exposure (OE) to HIV (abstract 480). Program and abstracts of the 35th Annual Meeting of the Infectious Diseases Society of America, Alexandria, Virginia, Sept 13–16, 1997, p 161

49. Beekmann R, Fahrner R, Nelson L, et al: Combination post-exposure prophylaxis (PEP): a prospective study of HIV-exposed health care workers (HCW) (abstract 481). Program and abstracts of the 35th Annual Meeting of the Infectious Diseases Society of America, Alexandria, Virginia, Sept 13–16, 1997, p 161

50. Imrie A, Beveridge A, Genn W, et al: Transmission of human immunodeficiency virus type 1 resistant to nevirapine and zidovudine. J Infect Dis 175:1502, 1997

51. Veenstra J, Schuurman R, Cornelissen M, et al: Transmission of zidovudine-resistant human immunodeficiency virus type 1 variants following deliberate injection of blood from a patient with AIDS: characteristics and natural history of the virus. Clin Infect Dis 21:556-60, 1995

52. Fitzgibbon JE, Gaur S, Frenkel LD, et al: Transmission from one child to another of human immunodeficiency virus type 1 with a zidovudine-resistance mutation. N Engl J Med 329:1835, 1993

53. Coombs RW, Shapiro DE, Eastman PS, et al: Maternal viral genotypic zidovudine (ZDV) resistance and infrequent failure of ZDV therapy to prevent perinatal transmission (abstract 17). Program and abstracts of the 35th Annual Meeting of the Infectious Diseases Society of America, Alexandria, Virginia, Sept 13–16, 1997, p 74

54. Protection against viral hepatitis. Recommendations of the Immunization Practices Advisory Committee (ACIP). MMWR Morb Mortal Wkly Rep 39(RR-2):1, 1990

55. Hadler SC: Are booster doses of hepatitis B vaccine necessary? Ann Intern Med 108:457, 1988

56. Hadler SC, Francis DP, Maynard JE, et al: Long-term immunogenicity and efficacy of hepatitis B vaccine in homosexual men. N Engl J Med 315:209, 1986

57. Hepatitis B virus: A comprehensive strategy for eliminating transmission in the United States through universal childhood vaccination. Advisory Committee for Immunization Practices. MMWR Morb Mortal Wkly Rep 40:PR-13, 1991

58. Barie PS, Dellinger EP, Dougherty SH, et al: Assessment of hepatitis B virus immunization status among North American surgeons. Arch Surg 129:27, 1994

59. Recommendations for prevention and control of hepatitis C virus (HCV) infection and HCV-related chronic disease. MMWR Morb Mortal Wkly Rep 47(RR-19):1, 1998

60. Noguchi S, Sata M, Suzuki H, et al: Early therapy with interferon for acute hepatitis C acquired through the needlestick. Clin Infect Dis 24:992, 1997

61. Vogen W, Graziadei I, Umlauft F, et al: High-dose interferon-α_{2b} treatment prevents chronicity in acute hepatitis C: a pilot study. Dig Dis Sci 41(suppl 12):81S, 1996

62. Ohnishi K, Nomura F, Nakano M: Interferon therapy for acute posttransfusion non-A, non-B hepatitis: response with respect to anti-hepatitis C virus antibody status. Am J Gastroenterol 86:1041, 1991

63. Rabies prevention—United States, 1991: recommendations of the Immunization Practices Advisory Committee (ACIP). MMWR Morb Mortal Wkly Rep 40:1, 1991

64. Fishbein DB, Robinson LE: Rabies. N Engl J Med 329:1632, 1993

65. Rabies prevention—United States, 1999: recommendations of the Immunization Practices Advisory Committee (ACIP). MMWR Morb Mortal Wkly Rep 48(RR-1):1, 1999

66. WHO Recommendations on Rabies Post-exposure Treatment and the Correct Technique of Intradermal Immunization against Rabies. World Health Organization, Geneva, 1997

67. Rabies prevention: supplementary statement on the preexposure use of human diploid cell rabies vaccine by the intradermal route. MMWR Morb Mortal Wkly Rep 35:767, 1986

68. Bleck TP, Rupprecht CE: Rabies virus. Principles and Practice of Infectious Disease, 5th ed. Mandell GL, Bennett JE, Dolin R, Eds. Churchill Livingstone, Philadelphia, 2000, p 1811

69. Krebs JW, Strine TW, Childs JF: Rabies surveillance in the United States during 1992. J Am Vet Med Assoc 203:1718, 1993

70. The cost of one rabid dog—California. MMWR Morb Mortal Wkly Rep 30:527, 1981

71. Bove JR: Transfusion-associated hepatitis and AIDS: what is the risk? N Engl J Med 317:242, 1987

72. Donegan E, Stuart M, Niland JC, et al: Infection with the human immunodeficiency virus type 1 (HIV1) among recipients of antibody-positive blood donations. Ann Intern Med 113:733, 1990

73. Ward JW, Deppe DA, Samson S, et al: Risk of human immunodeficiency virus infection from blood donors who later developed the acquired immunodeficiency syndrome. Ann Intern Med 106:61, 1987

74. Ward JW, Grindon AJ, Feorino PM, et al: Laboratory and epidemiologic evaluation of an enzyme immunoassay for antibodies to HTLV-III. JAMA 256:357, 1986

75. Ward JW, Holmberg AD, Allen JR, et al: Transmission of human immunodeficiency virus (HIV) by blood transfusions screened as negative for HIV antibody. N Engl J Med 318:473, 1988

76. Schreiber GB, Bush MP, Kleinman SH, et al: The risk of transfusion-transmitted viral infections: the retrovirus epidemiology donor study. N Engl J Med 334:1685, 1996

77. Horsburgh BR Jr, Ou C-Y, Jason J, et al: Duration of human immunodeficiency virus infection before detection of antibody. Lancet 2:637, 1991

78. Erice A, Rhame FS, Heussner RC, et al: Human immunodeficiency virus infection in patients with solid-organ transplants: report of five cases and review. Rev Infect Dis 13:537, 1991

79. Public Health Service guidelines for the management of health-care worker exposures to HIV and recommendations for post-exposure prophylaxis. MMWR Morb Mortal Wkly Rep 47:1, 1998

80. Guidelines for national human immunodeficiency virus case surveillance, including monitoring for human immunodeficiency virus infection and acquired immunodeficiency syndrome. MMWR Morb Mortal Wkly Rep 48(RR-13):1, 1999

81. Alter M, Mast E: The epidemiology of hepatitis in the United States. Gastroenterol Clin North Am 23:437, 1994

82. Kim CY, Tilles JG: Purification and biophysical characterization of the hepatitis B antigen. J Clin Invest 52:1176, 1973

83. Kawai H, Feinstone SM: Acute viral hepatitis. Principles and Practice of Infectious Diseases, 5th ed. Mandell GL, Bennett JE, Dolin R, Eds. Churchill Livingstone, Philadelphia, 2000, p 1279

84. Omata M: Treatment of chronic hepatitis B infection. N Engl J Med 339:114, 1998

85. Kuo G, Choo Q-L, Alter HJ, et al: An assay for circulating antibodies to a major etiologic virus of non-A, non-B hepatitis. Science 244:362, 1989

86. Hayden GH, Jarvis LM, Blair CS, et al: Clinical significance of intrahepatic hepatitis C virus levels in patients with chronic HCV infection. Gut 42:570, 1998

87. Koretz RL, Stone O, Gitnick GL: The long-term course of non-A, non-B post-transfusion hepatitis. Gastroenterology 79:893, 1980

88. Denes AE, Smith JL, Maynard JE, et al: Hepatitis B infections in physicians: results of a nationwide seroepidemiologic survey. JAMA 239:210, 1978

89. Howard RJ: Viral infections in surgery. Problems in General Surgery 1:522, 1984

90. Recommendations for protection against viral hepatitis. MMWR Morb Mortal Wkly Rep 34:313, 1985

91. Valent WM, Wehrle PP: Selected viruses of nosocomial importance. Hospital Infections, 2nd ed. Bennett JV, Brachman PS, Eds. Little, Brown & Company, Boston, 1986, p 531

92. Cooper BW, Krusell A, Tilton RC, et al: Seroprevalence of antibodies to hepatitis C virus in high-risk hospital personnel. Infect Control Hosp Epidemiol 13:82, 1992

93. Klein RS, Freeman K, Taylor PE, et al: Occupational risk for hepatitis C virus infection among New York City dentists. Lancet 338:1539, 1991

94. Zuckerman J, Clewley G, Griffiths P, et al: Prevalence of hepatitis C antibodies in clinical health-care workers. Lancet 343:1618, 1994

95. Schreiber GB, Busch MP, Kleinman SH, et al: The risk of transfusion-transmitted viral infections. N Engl J Med 334:1685, 1996

96. Rosina F, Saracco G, Rizzetto M: Risk of posttransfusion infection with hepatitis delta virus: a multicenter study. N Engl J Med 312:1488, 1985

97. Friedman LS, Dienstag JL: Recent developments in viral hepatitis. Dis Mon 32:320, 1986

98. Beasley PR, Lin CC: Hepatoma risk among HBsAg carriers. Am J Epidemiol 105:247, 1978

99. Edamoto Y, Tani M, Durata T, et al: Hepatitis C and B virus infections in hepatocellular carcinoma—analysis of direct detection of viral genome in paraffin embedded tissues. Cancer 77:1787, 1996

100. Kiyosawa K, Furuta S: Hepatitis C virus and hepatocellular carcinoma. Curr Stud Hematol Blood Transfus 61:98, 1994

101. Rook AH, Quinnan GV Jr: Cytomegalovirus infections following blood transfusions. Infectious Complications of Blood Transfusion. Tabor E, Ed. Academic Press, San Diego, 1982, p 45

102. Winston DJ, Ho WG, Howell CL, et al: Cytomegalovirus infections associated with leukocyte transfusions. Ann Intern Med 93:671, 1980

103. Prince AM, Szmuness W, Millins SJ, et al: A serological study of cytomegalovirus infections associated with blood transfusions. N Engl J Med 284:1125, 1971

104. Tolkoff-Rubin NE, Rubin RH, Keller EE, et al: Cytomegalovirus infection in dialysis patients and personnel. Ann Intern Med 89:625, 1978

105. Bowden RA: Transfusion-transmitted cytomegalovirus infection. Hematol Oncol Clin North Am 9:155, 1995

106. Paya CV, Hermans PE, Wiesner RH, et al: Cytomegalovirus hepatitis in liver transplantation: prospective analysis of 93 consecutive orthotopic liver transplantations. J Infect Dis 160:752, 1988

107. Barkholt LM, Ericzon BG, Ehrnst A, et al: Cytomegalovirus infections in liver transplant patients: incidence and outcome. Transplant Proc 22:235, 1990

108. Englehard D, Or R, Strauss N, et al: Cytomegalovirus infection and disease after T cell depleted allogeneic bone marrow transplantation for malignant hematologic disease. Transplant Proc 21:3101, 1989

109. Griffiths PD: Current management of cytomegalovirus disease. J Med Virol (suppl 1):106, 1993

110. Farrusia E, Schwab TR: Management and prevention of cytomegalovirus infection after renal transplantation. Mayo Clin Proc 67:879, 1992

111. Ho M, Suwansirikul S, Dowling JN, et al: The transplanted kidney as a source of cytomegalovirus infection. N Engl J Med 293:1109, 1975

112. Myers JD, Fluornoy N, Thomas ED: Risk factors for cytomegalovirus infection after human marrow transplantation. J Infect Dis 153:478, 1986

113. Balfour HH Jr, Sachs GW, Welo P, et al: Cytomegalovirus vaccine in renal transplant candidates: progress report of a randomized, placebo-controlled, double-blind trial. Birth Defects 20:289, 1984

114. Snydman DR, Werner BG, Heinze-Lacey B, et al: Use of cytomegalovirus immune globulin to prevent cytomegalovirus disease in renal-transplant recipients. N Engl J Med 317:1049, 1987

115. Martin M: Antiviral prophylaxis for CMV infection in liver transplantation. Transplant Proc 25(suppl 4):10, 1993

116. Steinmuller DR, Novick AC, Streem SB, et al: Intravenous immunoglobulin infusions for the prophylaxis of secondary cytomegalovirus infection. Transplant 49:68, 1990

117. Kasiske BL, Heim-Duthoy KL, Tortorice KL: Polyvalent immune globulin and cytomegalovirus infection after renal transplantation. Arch Intern Med 149:2733, 1989

118. Lautenschlager I, Ahonen J, Eklund B, et al: Hyperimmune globulin therapy of clinical cytomegalovirus infection in renal allograft recipients. Scand J Infect Dis 21:139, 1989

119. Balfour HH Jr: Prevention of cytomegalovirus disease in renal allograft recipients. Scand J Infect Dis Suppl 80:88, 1991

120. Snydman DR, Rubin RH, Werner BG: New developments in cytomegalovirus prevention and management. Am J Kidney Dis 21:217, 1993

121. Emanuel D: Treatment of cytomegalovirus disease. Semin Hematol 27(suppl 1):22, 1990

122. Tabor E: Epstein-Barr virus and blood transfusion. Infectious Complications of Blood Transfusion. Tabor E, Ed. Academic Press, San Diego, 1982, p 65

123. Rocchi G, de Felici A, Ragona G, et al: Quantitative evaluation of Epstein-Barr-virus-infected mononuclear peripheral blood leukocytes in infectious mononucleosis. N Engl J Med 296:132, 1977

124. Armitage JM, Kormos RL, Stuart RS, et al: Posttransplant lymphoproliferative disease in thoracic organ transplant patients: ten years of cyclosporine-based immunosuppression. J Heart Lung Transplant 10:877, 1991

125. Lager DJ, Burgart LJ, Slagel DD: Epstein-Barr virus detection in sequential biopsies from patients with a posttransplant lymphoproliferative disorder. Mod Pathol 6:42, 1993

126. Dotti G, Fiocchi R, Motta T, et al: Epstein-Barr virus-negative lymphoproliferative disorders in long-term survivors after heart, kidney, and liver transplant. Transplantation 69:827, 2000

127. Leblond V, Davi F, Charlotte F, et al: Posttransplant lymphoproliferative disorders not associated with Epstein-Barr virus: a distinct entity? J Clin Oncol 16:2052, 1998

128. Preiksaitis JK, Cockfield AM: Epstein-Barr virus and lymphoproliferative disorders after transplantation. Transplant Infections. Bowden RA, Ljungman P, Paya CV, Eds. Lippincott-Raven Publishers, Philadelphia, 1998, p 245

129. Breinig MK, Zitelli B, Ho M: Epstein-Barr virus, cytomegalovirus and other viral infections in children after liver transplantation. J Infect Dis 156:273, 1987

130. Starzl TE, Porter KA, Iwatsuki SK, et al: Reversibility of lymphomas and lymphoproliferative lesions developing under cyclosporine-steroid therapy. Lancet 1:583, 1984

131. Hanto DW, Frizzera G, Gajl-Peczalska KJ, et al: Epstein-Barr virus, immunodeficiency, and B cell lymphoproliferation. Transplantation 39:461, 1985

132. Shapiro RS, McClain K, Frizzera G, et al: Epstein-Barr virus associated B cell lymphoproliferative disorders following bone marrow transplantation. Blood 71:1234, 1988

133. Benkerru M, Durandy A, Fischer A: Therapy for transplant-related lymphoproliferative diseases. Hematol Oncol Clin North Am 7:467, 1993

134. Keating MR: Antiviral agents. Mayo Clin Proc 67:160, 1992

135. de Clercq E: Antivirals for the treatment of herpesvirus infections. J Antimicrob Chemother 32(suppl A):121, 1993

136. Oberg B: Antiviral effects of phosphonoformate (PFA, foscarnet sodium). Pharmacol Ther 40:213, 1989

137. Houff SA, Burton RC, Wilson RW, et al: Human-to-human transmission of rabies virus by corneal transplant. N Engl J Med 300:603, 1979

Acknowledgments

Figure 1 Micrograph courtesy of F. K. Lee, A. J. Nahmias, and S. Stagno, Emory University. Drawing by George V. Kelvin.

Figures 4 and 5 Albert Miller.

21 ACQUIRED IMMUNODEFICIENCY SYNDROME

Kathleen Casey, M.D., and John Mihran Davis, M.D., F.A.C.S.

Approach to Human Immunodeficiency Virus Infection

In June 1981, the Centers for Disease Control and Prevention (CDC) published a report of *Pneumocystis carinii* pneumonia (PCP) in five previously healthy homosexual men living in Los Angeles.[1] At that time, the CDC was the sole distributor of pentamidine, the only treatment for this rare pulmonary infection. This outbreak represented a unique cohort for PCP, which until then had been seen only in severely immunosuppressed patients who were receiving chemotherapy for disseminated cancer. Even in this select group, PCP was rare, and *P. carinii* was not considered pathogenic in otherwise healthy adults. The sudden increase in demand for pentamidine in one geographic area raised the prospect of a new disease process. In July 1981, the CDC reported a group of young homosexual men with Kaposi sarcoma.[2] Like PCP, Kaposi sarcoma was a rare lesion not commonly seen in young adults. Many of these Kaposi sarcoma patients also had severe infections caused by organisms associated with immunodeficiency, including PCP, toxoplasmosis, candidiasis, cryptococcosis, and cytomegalovirus (CMV) infections.

These two accounts represented the first recognition of AIDS. The cause of the severe immunodepression in these patients, who were not otherwise at risk for opportunistic infection, was controversial until late 1983 and early 1984, when the human immunodeficiency virus (HIV) was isolated in AIDS patients.[3] This retrovirus—formerly known as human T cell lymphotropic virus (HTLV) type III and lymphadenopathy-associated virus (LAV)—is now recognized as the agent that causes AIDS. Presumably, the patients in the 1981 reports had become infected with HIV at least 3 to 4 years earlier.

In September 1987, the definition of AIDS was expanded to include symptomatic HIV-infected patients suspected of having an opportunistic infection. This new definition precipitated a potentially misleading sudden increase in new cases.[4] Since 1986, the percentage of homosexual or bisexual AIDS patients has steadily declined, and the percentage of AIDS patients who are I.V. drug abusers or are heterosexual has increased.

June 1, 2001, marked the 20th anniversary of the AIDS epidemic. Over those 2 decades, more than 20 million people died of AIDS, leaving an estimated 36 million people infected.[5] No immediate end to the epidemic is in sight, but current therapies have significantly altered the course of the illness. Until the advent of highly active antiretroviral agents (HAART), it was believed that everyone with an opportunistic infection or tumor associated with AIDS (e.g., Kaposi sarcoma or non-Hodgkin lymphoma) would die as a direct result of severe immunosuppression; that is no longer the case.[6] HIV-infected persons are living longer, are less likely to die of opportunistic infections, and are more likely to present with relatively well-preserved immune function.[7] With this increase in the prevalence of HIV infection, it is all the more important that surgeons have a basic understanding of HIV disease and its treatment and be familiar with prophylaxis after occupational exposure.

Recognition of HIV Infection

PATHOGENESIS

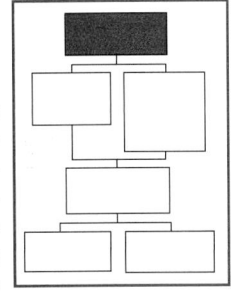

HIV is an oncovirus belonging to the retrovirus family. The potential of retroviruses to cause neoplasia was first recognized in 1911 by the American pathologist Rous, who associated them with certain malignant disorders in animals.[8] For example, HTLV-I, a retrovirus related to HIV, has been identified as a cause of leukemia in humans.[9]

One of the characteristic features of retroviruses is the presence of an enzyme called reverse transcriptase. This enzyme allows the virus to transcribe viral RNA to DNA. The virus can synthesize double-stranded DNA from single-stranded DNA that has been liberated from the RNA-DNA hybrid. This double-stranded DNA inserts itself into the nucleus of the host cell and serves as a template for viral replication. Thus, whenever the infected host cell divides, new HIV particles are also reproduced. HIV has been isolated in many cell types, but it is thought that helper T cells ($CD4^+$ cells) are most frequently infected. It is believed that when an HIV-infected $CD4^+$ cell is activated by a secondary infection, the virus is replicated, resulting in the dissemination of mature virions and the death of the cell.

The latency period between acquisition of HIV infection and onset of AIDS has been estimated to be about 5 years. This estimate is probably misleading because it is based on experience with patients in high-risk groups, who are frequently exposed to other infectious challenges. Exposure to these other pathogens activates the T cells that harbor HIV, which promotes dissemination of the virus throughout the host and significant impairment in cellular immunity. Because the incidence of concomitant infections is lower in the general population than in high-risk groups, the latency period of HIV infection is probably longer in the general population.

DIAGNOSTIC TESTS

The enzyme-linked immunosorbent assay (ELISA) and the Western blot assay are designed to detect the presence of HIV antibody in serum. ELISA is considered very sensitive (93% to 100%; i.e., its false negative rate is low). The specificity of a repeatedly reactive ELISA approaches 99%. The weakness of the ELISA is that some persons have antibodies that react with HIV antigens but are not specific for HIV.

The Western blot assay is more specific than ELISA but is cumbersome and less sensitive. It is therefore not a good screen-

Approach to Human Immunodeficiency Virus Infection

Potential HIV infection in surgical setting

Infection is diagnosed by ELISA or Western blot assay. SUDS ELISA results must be confirmed by Western blot.

Categorize patients according to CDC classification. Patients receiving HAART may not behave in accordance with CDC class.

Surgical issues in infected patients

General clinical problems:
- Immunosuppression   • Renal failure
- Cardiac dysfunction

Other problems include
- Splenomegaly or thrombocytopenia
- Central venous catheter infections
- GI disease   • Lymphadenopathy

Risk of HIV transmission to patient or medical personnel

Risk to patient comes from transfusion, transplantation, or, theoretically, transmission from surgical personnel (HBV transmission is a far more significant possibility).

Risk to health care workers (HCWs) comes from infected patients. All HCWs should take precautions to prevent HIV transmission with *all* patients, not only those with known or suspected HIV infection. Again, transmission of hepatitis is much more common.

Postexposure prophylaxis

Need for prophylaxis and choice of drugs are based on (1) risk assessment of exposure, (2) size of inoculum, (3) arterial vs. venous exposure, (4) intact or nonintact skin or mucous membrane exposure.

Consider possible HCV coinfection.

Source is HIV positive with low viral load; source is of unknown HIV status but high risk; or worker has minor skin or mucous membrane exposure

Initiate two-drug therapy (zidovudine and lamivudine) within 24 hr of exposure.

Source is HIV positive with high viral load, or worker has extensive skin or mucous membrane exposure

Initiate three-drug therapy (zidovudine, lamivudine, and indinavir or nelfinavir) within 24 hr of exposure.

ing test; it is used most effectively for confirming ELISA results. However, most blood banks will not use blood that has demonstrated a positive ELISA reaction, even if HIV antibody was not detected by Western blot testing.[10]

The Single-Use Diagnostic System (SUDS; Murex Diagnostics, Norcross, Georgia) provides a rapid ELISA technology that can yield a reliable result in 15 minutes. A positive SUDS result must still be confirmed by Western blot assay. SUDS is especially useful in occupational-injury investigation.

There is a window period of 25 days between infection with HIV and seroconversion detectable by ELISA. It has been estimated that since 1985, when all banked blood began to be tested for HIV, 35 persons in the United States have contracted HIV infection from transfusions containing blood collected from an HIV-infected individual during this window period.[11,12] For that reason, on August 8, 1995, the Food and Drug Administration recommended that all blood donated for transfusion be screened for the p24 antigen (the core structural protein of HIV).[13] Additional laboratory tests that may help in the diagnosis of patients believed to have HIV infection in whom HIV antibody screening yields negative results include DNA polymerase chain reaction (PCR), antigen testing after immune complex disruption, and RNA reverse transcriptase PCR.[14]

In February 2002, the FDA approved a nucleic acid test system that detects ribonucleic acid from HIV and hepatitis C virus (HCV) in whole blood and blood component donors, thus permitting earlier results than tests based on detection of antibodies or antigens (http://www.fda/gov/cber/approvltr/hivhcvgen022702L.htm). Like ELISA, the nucleic acid test has a window period during which the virus can be present but escape detection; however, this window period is substantially shorter than that associated with antibody-based tests (12 versus 22 days, on average, for HIV; 25 versus 82 days, on average, for HCV).

CDC Classification of HIV Infection

In 1993, the CDC revised the classification of the HIV-infected adult and adolescent [see Table 1]. In this classification, a CD4+ count below 200 cells/μl is considered an indicator of AIDS, regardless of the patient's symptoms. Once classified into a given group, a patient is not reclassified to a more favorable category, even if symptoms resolve or the CD4+ cell count rises. However, if the disease progresses or the CD4+ count falls, the patient is reclassified into the next less-favorable group. This system allows uniformity in patient classification for research trials and scientific communication and, of particular importance, facilitates formulation of health care policy and strategy.

Unfortunately, the system does not take into account the immune reconstitution that occurs with HAART. After successful treatment with HAART, patients originally classified as having AIDS (on the basis of their CD4+ count or level of immunocompromise) often will no longer have signs and symptoms in accordance with their original CDC classification. A number of studies have now shown that secondary prophylaxis for PCP, CMV retinitis, *Toxoplasma* encephalitis, and cryptococcal meningitis may be safely discontinued in patients whose CD4+ counts have risen and remained above 200 cells/μl because of HAART.[15] Similarly, recent studies of gynecologic procedures in HIV-infected patients have found that postoperative infection rates correlate only with the current CD4+ count. In these studies, a CD4+ level below 200 cells/μl at the time of the procedure was an independent risk factor for surgical complications, whereas the previous nadir had no influence on outcome.[14]

Surgical Issues

GENERAL

As a group, HIV-infected patients present the surgeon with three notable clinical problems: immunosuppression, renal failure, and cardiac dysfunction. Surgeons need to be aware of the immune status of their HIV-infected patients, because this has the greatest bearing on outcome. For example, in HIV-infected patients with 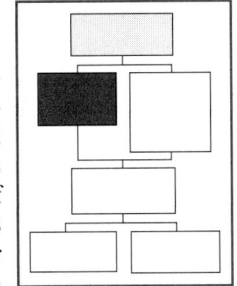 normal CD4+ counts, the risk of infectious complications after surgery for a perforated appendix is comparable to the risk in patients without HIV infection. In patients with AIDS (< 200 CD4+ cells/μl), the risk of infection is higher, though it is from opportunistic organisms associated with severe immunosuppression rather than common pathogens.[16-20]

Renal failure in HIV-infected patients can be the result of specific HIV-related nephropathy, which occurs in up to 10% of this population.[21] Another possible cause is drug toxicity from antiviral and antimicrobial medications: pentamidine, foscarnet, and aminoglycosides cause acute tubular necrosis; acyclovir, indinavir, and sulfadiazine cause intratubular obstruction.

Until recently, the risk of cardiac disease in HIV-infected patients had not been as well documented as that of renal failure. With HIV-infected patients living longer, the problems of acquired heart disease have been increasingly appreciated.[22-24]

In addition, malignancy has been increasingly recognized over the past 2 decades as a consequence of HIV infection. Initially, the occurrence of AIDS-defining tumors, such as B cell lym-

Table 1 1993 Revised Classification for HIV Infection and Expanded AIDS Surveillance Case Definition for Adolescents and Adults[81]

CD4+ T Cell Categories	Clinical Categories		
	A Asymptomatic, Acute (Primary) HIV, or PGL	B Symptomatic, Not A or C Conditions	C AIDS Indicator Conditions
≥ 500/μl	A1	B1	C1
200–499/μl	A2	B2	C2
< 200/μl AIDS-indicator T cell count	A3	B3	C3

PGL—persistent generalized lymphadenopathy

phoma and Kaposi sarcoma, was thought to relate to the immunosuppression of the host. Other tumors have now been associated with HIV infection, including squamous cell cancers of the cervix and anus and lung cancer. It is believed that at some point after infection with HIV, activation of oncogenes and loss of tumor suppressor genes give rise to microsatellite alterations. These are highly pleomorphic segments of DNA associated with the AIDS-defining malignancies.[25-27]

Treatment of patients with AIDS involves multimodal therapy and consultation with oncology and infectious disease specialists. It is beyond the scope of this discussion to describe the specific therapeutic approaches to the complications of HIV infections; however, three principal problems must be addressed. First, any opportunistic infection or secondary malignant disorder must be treated; second, the underlying immunodeficiency must be corrected; and finally, the cause—HIV infection—must be controlled. The role of the surgeon in the management of these chronically ill, and sometimes critically ill, patients includes performing diagnostic biopsies, giving supportive care, and managing complications of malignancy of infection.

SPLEEN

The role of splenectomy in patients with marked splenomegaly or with thrombocytopenia must be individualized. Some experts believe that coinfections such as HCV infection contribute to the development of HIV-related immune thrombocytopenic purpura (ITP). Thrombocytopenia occurs in AIDS patients as a result of the deposition of circulating immune complexes on platelets rather than as a result of a specific antiplatelet antibody.[28,29] Splenectomy has been extremely effective in the management of AIDS-related ITP, with a success rate of over 90%. Occasionally, patients who have debilitating fevers associated with significantly enlarged spleens experience dramatic palliation after splenectomy. Some data indicate that splenectomy favors a slower progression of HIV dissemination and progression to AIDS.[30,31] In patients with massive splenomegaly and fever, simple splenomegaly is sometimes difficult to distinguish from abscess or parenchymal necrosis, and splenectomy may be indicated to resolve the uncertainty. In addition, splenectomy may be indicated in instances in which there is merely a likelihood of injury and in those in which a large spleen compresses the stomach, thereby contributing to malnutrition.

IMPLANTABLE VENOUS ACCESS DEVICES

Placement of an indwelling central venous catheter is a request frequently directed to the general surgeon from the primary care physician, infectious disease consultant, or hematologist caring for an AIDS patient. Long-term venous access for treating fungal infections or, occasionally, for providing nutritional support in patients with debilitating diarrheal syndromes can enhance the care of these patients. However, lines are often placed when the patient is febrile, as a result of either the underlying infection or treatment with amphotericin B. Therefore, a close watch should be kept postoperatively to ensure that fevers are not related to a catheter infection. Although catheter-related infection develops in as many as 30% of AIDS patients with implanted lines, these infections do not increase mortality.[32] The high rate of infection relates in part to the high incidence of *Staphylococcus* colonization in these patients.

GASTROINTESTINAL DISEASES

Cryptosporidiosis and CMV infection of the biliary tree have been reported to cause both acute cholecystitis and acute cholan-

gitis, necessitating emergency surgical interventions.[12] Choledochoenteric bypass is thought to provide the best palliation in these patients. It is not known whether the biliary tree is ever cleared of the pathogens. *Candida* infection and Kaposi sarcoma have also caused cholangitis, necessitating bypass surgery.[17] The gallbladder is infected with unusual pathogens in over 50% of HIV-infected patients with cholangitis; therefore, the gallbladder wall should be sent for culture, and the pathologist should be alerted so that the tissue may be processed with special stains.[33-36]

Acute perforations of the GI tract from CMV infection, cryptosporidiosis, and candidiasis, as well as from necrotic lymphoma, have been reported in HIV-infected patients.[18,37,38] Obstruction of the GI tract by Kaposi sarcoma or lymphoma may also be an indication for resection, bypass, or colostomy. One study of AIDS patients requiring a laparotomy identified four distinct clinical syndromes that called for surgical intervention: (1) peritonitis secondary to CMV enterocolitis and perforation; (2) non-Hodgkin lymphoma of the GI tract (usually the terminal ileum), presenting as obstruction or bleeding; (3) Kaposi sarcoma of the GI tract; and (4) mycobacterial infection of the retroperitoneum or the spleen.[39]

Another GI lesion that has been increasingly associated with homosexual men who are infected with HIV is squamous cell carcinoma of the anus (SCCA). It is estimated that the risk of developing SCCA is nearly 25 times greater in HIV-infected homosexual men than in the general population. The underlying relationship is not well understood, because the development of SCCA is not related to the duration of the HIV infection. Some experts believe that human papillomavirus 16 (HPV-16) and HPV-18 are important cofactors in the evolution of SCCA.[40,41]

LYMPHADENOPATHY

Another group of HIV-infected patients defined by the CDC comprises those with persistent generalized lymphadenopathy—that is, palpable lymphadenopathy with nodes measuring greater than 1 cm in diameter in at least two extrainguinal sites and persisting for longer than 3 months. Before the introduction of HIV antibody testing, the relationship of such lymphadenopathy to systemic manifestations of immunosuppression (systemic symptoms, neurologic symptoms, secondary infections, or cancers) was not known. It is now clear that lymphadenopathy is part of the general clinical spectrum associated with HIV infection, and that opportunistic infection, Kaposi sarcoma, or large cell lymphoma will develop in some, if not all, patients with lymphadenopathy. The precise reason that lymphadenopathy occurs in some, but not all, patients with HIV infection is not known.

Lymph node biopsy in these patients is only of academic interest because of the development of serologic tests for HIV infection.[37] The histologic appearance of a clinically enlarged lymph node has prognostic value (see below); however, when the decision as to whether to perform a lymph node biopsy is being made, the value of the biopsy findings must be weighed against the value of the information that can be obtained by means of clinical staging with the ratio of helper T cells to suppressor T cells and the total lymphocyte count. The total number of helper T cells in the circulation has been correlated with the risk of AIDS in patients with generalized lymphadenopathy[20,42-44]; the Walter Reed classification provides the most detailed clinical staging system.[43,45] Should the clinical condition warrant, a lymph node biopsy may help in the diagnosis of an opportunistic infection. Performing a gallium scan to locate the most suspicious node can enhance the yield of the biopsy.

Four basic histologic patterns have been described in persistent generalized lymphadenopathy and have been correlated

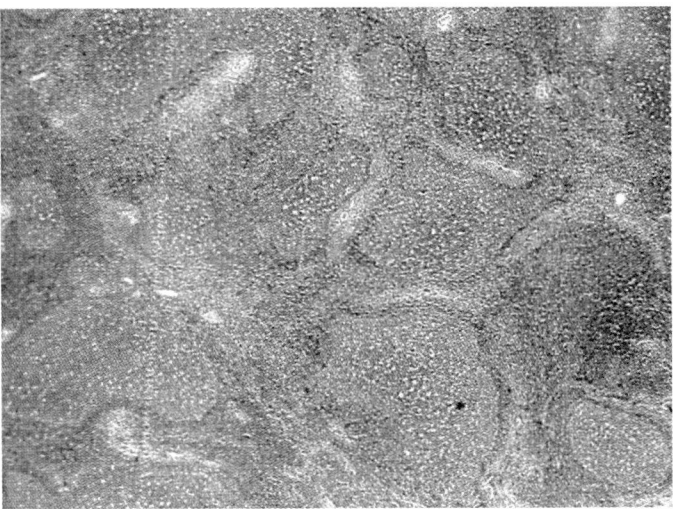

Figure 1 **Lymph node viewed under low power exhibits explosive follicular hyperplasia.**

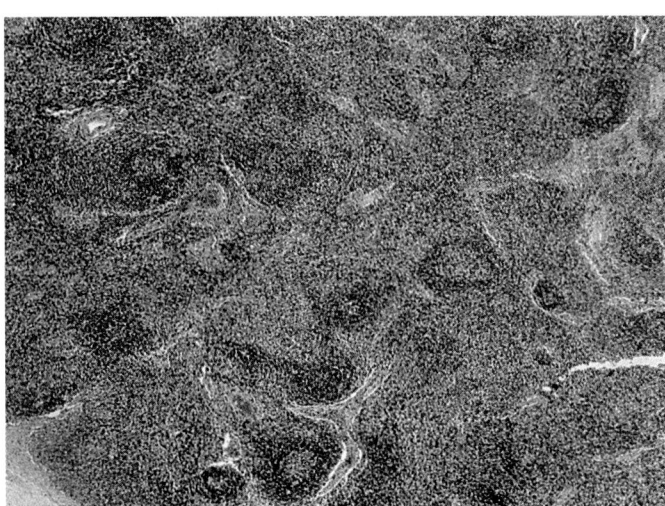

Figure 2 **Lymph node viewed under low power exhibits follicular involution.**

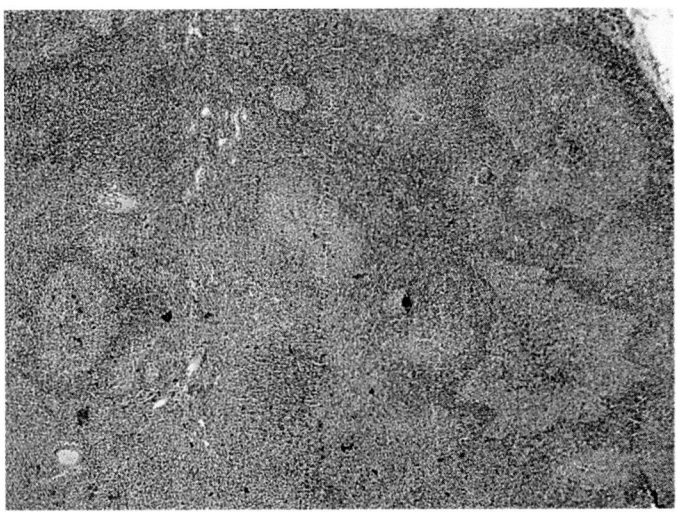

Figure 3 **Lymph node viewed under low power exhibits a mixed pattern of both explosive follicular hyperplasia and follicular involution.**

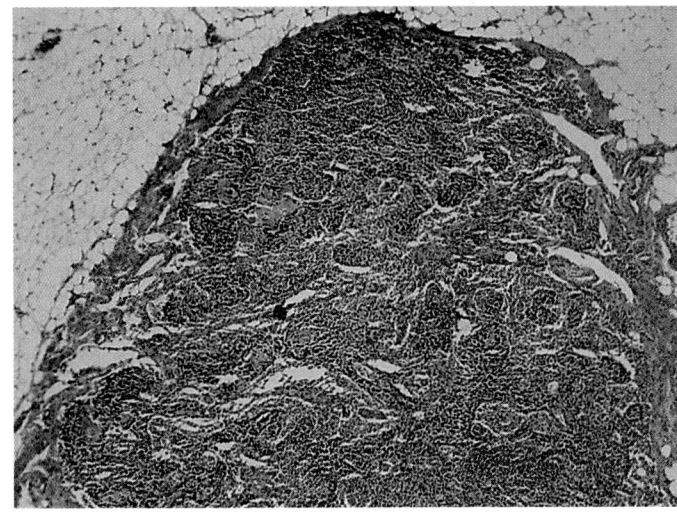

Figure 4 **Lymph node viewed under low power exhibits a pattern of lymphocyte depletion.**

with prognosis: explosive follicular hyperplasia, follicular involution, a mixed pattern, and a lymphocyte-depleted pattern. Explosive follicular hyperplasia describes a pattern of enlarged confluent follicles with disruption of the medullary zone of the lymph node [*see Figure 1*]. Follicular involution is associated with a hypocellular, frequently hyalinized follicle and with hyperplasia of the paracortical areas [*see Figure 2*]. The mixed pattern contains explosive follicular hyperplasia and follicular involution in the same lymph node [*see Figure 3*]. Finally, the lymphocyte-depleted pattern is characterized by the total absence of follicular and paracortical areas. The loss of lymphocytes in the lymph node is associated with the predominance of histiocytes and plasma cells [*see Figure 4*].

The presence of enlarged follicles is associated with a good immunologic response and slower progression of disease, whereas the presence of involuted, hyalinized follicles is more frequently associated with opportunistic infections, Kaposi sarcoma, and lymphoma. Evidence suggests that patients with either explosive follicular hyperplasia or the mixed pattern of explosive follicular hyperplasia and follicular involution have rather pro-

longed survival, even if they have Kaposi sarcoma. The presence of follicular involution in a lymph node is associated with a survival time of less than 1 year. Lymphocyte depletion was seen as a terminal finding in several autopsy cases, suggesting that the pattern represents the end stage of the hyperplastic process.[25] The pathologic findings reflect a progressive loss of the CD4[+]-bearing area of the lymph node.

After a lymph node is removed from an HIV-infected patient and before the tissue is removed from the operative field, representative specimens should be placed in sterile containers for routine bacterial culture, culture and smear for tuberculosis, fungal culture, and viral culture. Tissue from the same lymph node should then be delivered to the pathologist as quickly as possible. It is important that culture material from the same lymph node be examined microscopically, because granulomas or actual organisms may be detected before the culture results are available. Data from the pathologist may aid the microbiology laboratory staff in its handling of the cultures.

The pathologist needs to receive the fresh, gently handled specimen, in saline, as soon after the biopsy as possible, for two important reasons. First, because the tissue is not in formalin, it will rapidly autolyze if not processed immediately. Second, if the diagnosis is lymphoma, the pathologist must have the tissue when it is fresh to perform lymphocyte marker studies. Because different lymphomas respond to different chemotherapeutic regimens, the cell type of the lymphoma is critical. Most surgical pathology laboratories are equipped to perform membrane marker studies on lymph node tissue.

Prevention of Disease Transmission

GENERAL

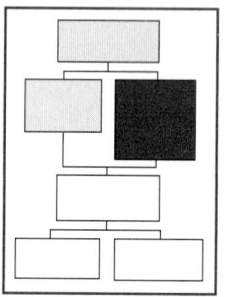

A key question for surgeons, operating room committees, infection control committees, and clinicians involved with endoscopy is how to effectively clean instruments, equipment, or other inanimate objects to be used with AIDS patients. Those agents that are effective against mycobacteria, the most resistant group of organisms encountered in this population, are also the agents considered most effective against other bacterial and viral pathogens.[46] A complete list of agents and their efficacies can be obtained from the Disinfectants Branch of the Office of Pesticides, United States Environmental Protection Agency, 401 M Street, S.W., Washington, DC 20460.

Agents are classified according to whether they are to be used for sterilization, disinfection, or antisepsis.[47] Agents that sterilize inanimate objects kill all microbial organisms as well as bacterial endospores. Disinfectants are not quite as effective, in that they are not capable of killing bacterial spores. In many cases, an agent may serve as a disinfectant when placed in contact for a short time with the object requiring cleansing and may be capable of sterilizing surgical instruments that are exposed to it for longer periods. Disinfectants are subclassified as having high-level, intermediate-level, or low-level germicidal activity. High-level agents are effective against bacterial spores. Intermediate-level disinfectants are less effective against spores but are mycobactericidal. Low-level disinfectants do not kill *Mycobacteria* and some fungi. Antiseptic agents are used on tissue and therefore must be less toxic than sterilants or disinfectants.

According to current CDC recommendations, agents classified by the United States Environmental Protection Agency as sterilants can be used for sterilization or high-level disinfection, depending on contact time. All instruments entering the bloodstream or other sterile tissues should be sterilized before use. Instruments that contact mucosal surfaces, such as endoscopes, should receive high-level disinfection, which can be achieved with solutions of glutaraldehyde (2%), hydrogen peroxide (3% to 6%), or formaldehyde (1% to 8%).

RISKS TO PATIENTS

Transfusions

Fresh whole blood, packed red blood cells, platelets, plasma, cryoprecipitate, and leukocytes can all carry HIV. In addition, clotting factor concentrates that are not generated by recombinant methods may also carry the virus. Some preparations of γ-globulin can temporarily cause a false positive ELISA result for HIV, but they do not contain the virus or transmit it to recipients. Albumin and plasma extracts (Plasmanate), although prepared from whole blood, do not carry HIV, hepatitis B virus (HBV), or

HCV, because the process by which they are purified inactivates the virus particles. Since adequate antibody testing became available in May 1985, the incidence of undetected HIV in transfused blood has been extremely low, and only anecdotal cases involving contaminated blood have been reported to the CDC. It is currently estimated that the risk of receiving a unit of blood that is contaminated with HIV is one in 150,000 (< 0.0007%).[48]

To minimize the risk of HIV being transmitted by transfusion, patients have increasingly requested the use of predeposited autologous blood donations (PAD) or blood donated by family members or friends (directed donations). This approach has been increasingly discouraged by blood bank and hospital administrators.[49] Both directed donations and PAD are very expensive methods of preserving homeostasis during surgery. Half of the PAD units of blood are discarded. In addition, the risk of an ABO mismatch error is as great as the risk of HIV transmission in standard bank blood. The use of intraoperative blood salvage and acute normovolemic hemodilution in combination with intravenous iron and erythropoietin provides a reasonable alternative to blood transfusion.[50]

Transplantation

Because it has been shown that HIV can be present in semen, blood, urine, tears, breast milk, cerebrospinal fluid, and saliva and because it is suspected that HIV can be present in all secretions and excretions, as well as all body tissues,[51] potential donors of tissue for transplantation must be tested for serum antibodies to HIV to prevent inadvertent transfer of the virus. Parenthetically, transmission of HIV by artificial insemination has also been documented, so this risk should be considered whenever artificial insemination is planned.[52]

Transmission from Surgical Personnel

An HIV-infected surgeon could theoretically transmit the virus to his or her patients. Although this concern has been well publicized,[53] there have been no documented reports of transmission from surgeon to patient. Furthermore, the CDC has not recommended restricting HIV-positive surgeons from operating.[54]

Unlike surgeon-to-patient transmission of HIV, HBV transmission from surgeon to patient is a significant concern. In a well-documented report involving a nonimmunized cardiac surgeon who acquired HBV infection in the workplace, transmission of the virus occurred in 19 of 122 patients (16%) on whom the surgeon operated over a 12-month period.[55] The surgeon's blood was positive for hepatitis B e antigen (HBeAg), and sweat from inside his glove was found to contain both HBV antigen and HBV DNA. No deficiencies were found in the surgeon's infection control practice by the CDC, which suggested that the virus might have spread through microperforations in his gloves. This case did not receive the same publicity that cases of HIV transmission have received in the lay press. However, its significance is clear: contact between health care workers who are HBV (HBeAg) positive and patients should be restricted.

RISKS TO HEALTH CARE WORKERS

The CDC now recommends that precautions to prevent HIV transmission be taken with all patients, not only those known to be infected with HIV or at high risk for such infection [*see 6:20 Viral Infection*].[18,20,38,39] It is important that any hospital personnel who come in contact with patients, their patients' tissues, or their blood, body fluids, or excreta know of the potential risk in

Table 2 Preventable Exposures to HIV among Health Care Workers*[49]

Circumstances of Preventable Exposure	Number of Health Care Workers (% of 938 Exposed Health Care Workers)
Recapping of needle	152 (16%)
Injury from improper disposal of needle or sharp object	119 (13%)
Contamination of open wound	93 (10%)
Use of needle-cutting device	9 (1%)
Total preventable exposures	373 (40%)

*The total sample under surveillance consisted of 938 health care workers exposed to blood or other body fluids of a patient with AIDS or an AIDS-related illness.

handling materials from these patients and take appropriate precautions. Patients in high-risk groups should be placed on enteric precautions to protect health care workers not only from HIV infection but also from HBV infection (up to 80% of such patients are HBV carriers). As part of any operative procedure on HIV-infected patients, all operating room, nursing, and anesthesia personnel, as well as employees of surgical pathology laboratories and any other laboratories, should employ universal precautions. Employees in ancillary areas, such as housekeeping and dietary services and the venipuncture team, need to be trained in the use of universal precautions.

Exposure to the virus in the workplace is considered to be preventable in many cases.[56] Most injuries result from carelessness in handling sharp objects, such as needles [see Table 2]. Self-inflicted puncture incurred in the course of recapping used needles is the most common cause of inadvertent exposure to HIV. Consequently, the most important rule to follow when handling used needles is to discard them uncapped in a container that is large enough to accommodate the attached syringe. Tissue specimens, wastes, soiled linen, blood samples, and sharp objects (e.g., surgical instruments, needles, and glassware) must be handled with extreme care. Dressings and other disposable materials should be discarded in specially marked containers and not with the regular hospital refuse.

The use of double gloves has been shown to minimize the possibility of contact with patient blood through small defects in the gloves, and it reduces the likelihood of blood contact with skin when a glove puncture occurs.[57,58] The following are additional precautions health care workers should take when handling any potentially infectious materials:

1. Wear gloves when handling body fluids.
2. Wear a gown to prevent contamination of clothing.
3. Wash hands after contact with body fluids.
4. Place fluid from a potentially contaminated host in two impervious containers.
5. Clean spills with either a 1:10 dilution of 5.25% sodium hypochlorite in water or with some other type of sterilant.
6. Wear masks and protective eyeglasses when there is a possibility of aerosolization of material.

Even health care workers who do not have exfoliative dermatitis or an open wound should wear gloves during patient care. Evidence suggests that the affinity of HIV for Langerhans cells may permit the virus to invade a host through intact skin or mucous membranes.[59]

RISKS TO SURGEONS

HIV Transmission

The risk that a surgeon will acquire an HIV infection while treating a patient who has undetected AIDS is quite low.[54,56] The CDC has prospectively evaluated nearly 1,500 health care workers who cared for AIDS patients. Serum samples were taken from these workers when they first began to work with AIDS patients and were stored in anticipation of a test for HIV. Of these workers, 666 were exposed to HIV through needlesticks or through cuts from sharp instruments. When tests were performed on these exposed individuals, none were found to have undergone seroconversion after their exposure to HIV. However, two health care workers for whom no baseline blood sample had been drawn did test positive for antibody to HIV after an injury. Because they did not belong to a known risk group for AIDS, they were believed to have generated antibody to HIV as a result of exposure in the workplace. On the basis of this study, the risk to a health care worker of acquiring HIV infection after an accidental needle-stick exposure was concluded to be 2 divided by 666, or 0.3%. A follow-up study found the rate of infection to be 0.5%.[60] Subsequent surveillance of health care workers identified 151 individuals who acquired HIV infection in the workplace [see Table 3]; 49 had proven seroconversion, and 102 were HIV positive but had no HIV-negative baseline serum sample.

The CDC conducted a serosurvey of 770 surgeons practicing in two inner-city areas where more than 3,000 cases of AIDS have been reported.[61] Accompanying the assay for HIV, HBV, and HCV was a questionnaire designed to elucidate the practice patterns of the surgeons tested. Of the 770 surgeons, 1 (0.13%) was HIV positive; he had practiced for more than 25 years and had performed more than 300 operations in the past year. The study did not specify how the surgeon acquired HIV, and it was noted that he did not participate in high-risk behavior. To date,

Table 3 Health Care Workers with Documented or Suspected HIV Infection[9]

Health Care Workers	No. of Workers	
	With Documented HIV (%)*	With Suspected HIV (%)†
Dental	0	7 (7%)
Mortician	0	3 (3%)
Emergency medical team/paramedic	0	9 (9%)
Health aide	1 (2%)	12 (12%)
Housekeeper	1 (2%)	7 (7%)
Laboratory technician	18 (37%)	15 (15%)
Nurse	19 (39%)	24 (24%)
Physician		
Surgeon	9	4 (4%)
Nonsurgeon	6 (12%)	10 (10%)
Respiratory therapist	1 (2%)	2 (2%)
Surgical technician	2 (4%)	1 (1%)
Other	1 (2%)	8 (8%)
Total	49	102

*Evidence of seroconversion after occupational exposure to HIV.
†HIV seropositivity in health care workers with occupational exposure to HIV who do not have behavioral or transfusion risks for HIV infection.

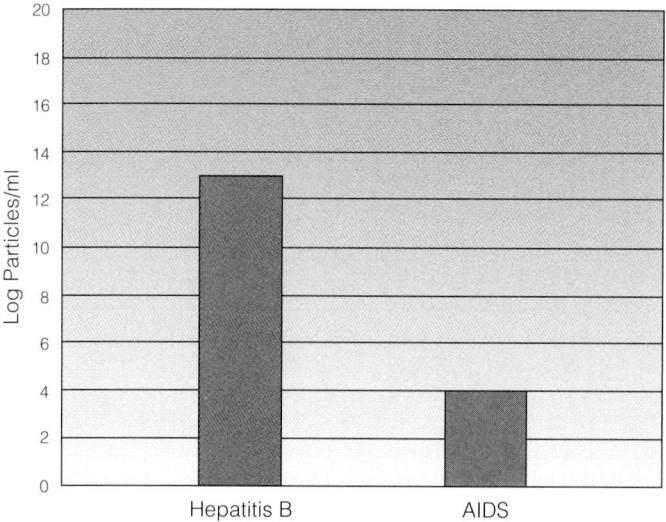

Figure 5 **The numbers of infectious viral particles per milliliter of blood in patients with active hepatitis B infections and in AIDS patients are compared.**[67]

there has been no documented seroconversion in operating room personnel after a solid-bore needle injury in the OR.

Transmission via skin contact with body fluids was documented in the case of a woman whose infant had received a transfusion from an HIV-infected donor at 3 months of age. The mother was closely involved in the baby's care and took no precautions against contact with the child's blood and body fluids. Seventeen months after the child received the contaminated blood, the mother tested positive on ELISA for HIV. No other risk factors accounted for the change in the mother's HIV antibody titer.[62]

Exposure to blood in the OR has been of great concern to all operating room personnel since the AIDS epidemic began. The average practicing surgeon has 30 parenteral exposures to blood a year.[63] The fact that hollow-bore needles carry more blood than solid-bore needles may be the reason that transmission in the operating room has not yet occurred. Four studies from the early 1990s established a blood-skin exposure rate of approximately 20% and a parenteral exposure rate of approximately 4% during surgical procedures.[46,64-66] Long operative procedures requiring transfusions are most likely to be associated with blood exposure. Types of procedures that pose a high risk of exposure to blood are cardiac surgery; obstetrics, especially cesarean sections; trauma surgery; and emergency surgery. Special care must be taken to minimize exposure in these procedures; eye protection and use of double gloves are barrier precaution measures that can reduce the likelihood of contact with the patient's blood.

Transmission of HIV to hospital workers is uncommon when compared with transmission of HBV because of the relatively low concentration of HIV in the blood of AIDS patients [*see Figure 5*]. The concentration of virus particles is estimated to be 10^4 particles/ml in an AIDS patient, whereas it is 10^{13} particles/ml in a patient who has an active HBV infection.[67]

Although HIV transmission is uncommon in the hospital environment, the risk to surgeons is very real. This is evidenced by the fact that even the lower reported rate of transmission by needle stick, 0.3%, is comparable to the 0.4% (1 in 250) rate of transmission by unprotected anal intercourse, which is considered high-risk behavior.[68,69] Three independent factors are important in determining a surgeon's risk of acquiring HIV infection: (1) the number of needle sticks or punctures contaminated with the patient's body fluids, (2) the percentage of HIV-infected patients in the surgeon's patient population, and (3) the number of years a surgeon is at risk for acquiring an HIV infection. If the risk of HIV transmission by a contaminated needle is 0.3% to 0.5%, if the HIV-infected population is 10%, if the number of needle sticks averages 30 a year, and if the surgeon has 40 years of exposure, then the lifetime risk of acquiring HIV infection can be as high as 60%.[70]

HEPATITIS TRANSMISSION

The primary health risk to surgeons caring for patients with HIV infection or AIDS is that of acquiring hepatitis B or hepatitis C. The hepatitis D virus (HDV) has been identified as posing an additional risk of death in patients with acute hepatitis; persons who are infected with both HBV and HDV have a higher mortality.[71]

The epidemiology of hepatitis B has been well studied because there are numerous antigen and antibody markers of the virus in the blood of chronic carriers. On the basis of data from assays of these markers, it is estimated that more than 200,000 persons in the United States acquire new HBV infections each year.[72] Of these 200,000, 25% will have symptoms of hepatitis, 5% will require hospitalization for their acute illness, and 1% to 2% of these hospitalized patients will develop fatal fulminant hepatitis [*see Figure 6*].

Between 5% and 10% of patients infected with HBV become chronic carriers—that is, they do not effectively clear the antigen from their systems, and they have a subclinical hepatic infection for prolonged periods. This group of patients is at risk for cirrhosis, with subsequent hepatic failure or hepatoma. Many chronic hepatitis carriers are unable to clear the infection because of immunosuppression as a result of another disease process, such as advanced HIV infection. AIDS patients are very likely to have had an HBV infection and to be chronic carriers. HIV-infected patients are also less likely to manifest an inflammatory response to hepatic infections. The CDC has estimated that as many as 80% of homosexual men, intravenous drug users, mentally retarded persons, and hemodialysis patients have serologic markers indicating a previous HBV infection.[73] Household contact or sexual relations with these high-risk individuals also involves a significant risk of acquiring HBV infection. It is estimated that up to 60% of such contacts have positive serology for HBV.

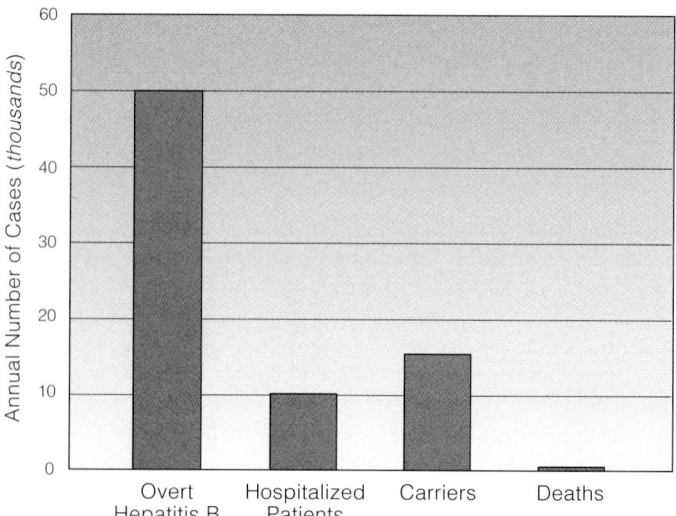

Figure 6 **The annual incidence of hepatitis B infection in the United States is 200,000 cases. Various subgroups of hepatitis B patients are shown.**[72]

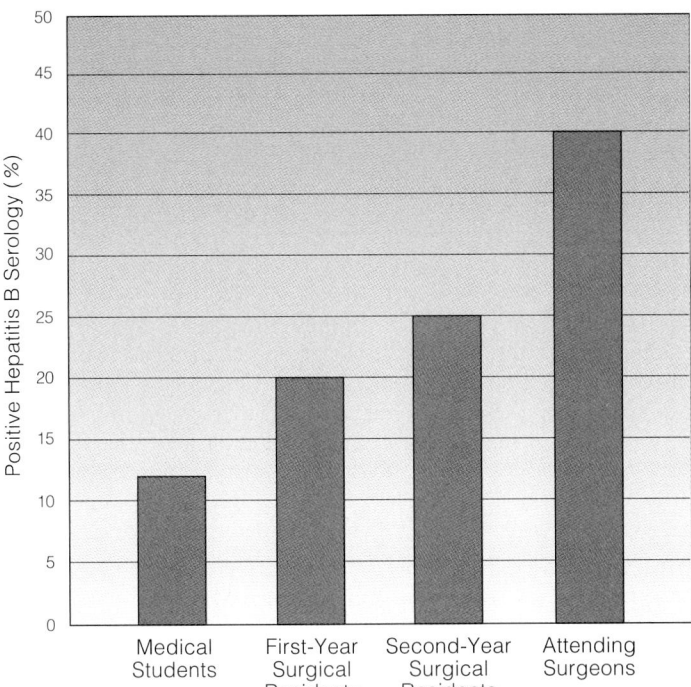

Figure 7 **The prevalence of positive serology for hepatitis B increases among individuals in successive stages of a surgical career.**[72]

Exposure to hepatitis carriers is a risk for health care workers, particularly for those who work with blood products [*see 6:20 Viral Infection*]. Physicians involved with direct patient care are at especially high risk.[74] Those in administrative situations who do not have clinical contact with patients have a relatively low risk of acquiring hepatitis, whereas surgeons, particularly cardiac surgeons and transplant surgeons, are at especially high risk. The risk of hepatitis infection also increases with age.[71,75] The incidence of positive hepatitis B serology is between 12% and 13% in students in their last year of medical school, nearly 20% in surgical residents at the end of their first year, and about 25% in surgical residents after the second year. During the course of an unimmunized senior surgeon's career, the risk of having hepatitis B approaches 50% [*see Figure 7*]. These risks are exceedingly high and emphasize the importance of widespread use of the hepatitis B vaccine [*see 6:20 Viral Infection*].

At least two studies have shown that there are numerous unimmunized practicing surgeons who finished medical school, training, or both before the hepatitis B vaccine first became available.[61,76] These surgeons are at substantial risk for HBV infection and consequently need to be immunized. Surgeons who were immunized 5 or more years ago should have their titers checked; if titers are low, a booster is advisable.

Postexposure Prophylaxis

MANAGEMENT AFTER EXPOSURE TO HIV

If a health care worker is injured by a sharp object that was contaminated by exposure to fluid or tissue from an HIV-positive patient, a series of blood samples should be drawn at the time of injury and again at 6 weeks and 3, 6, and 12 months after the injury to determine whether HIV

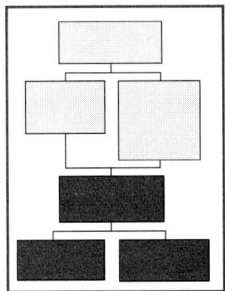

infection has occurred. Although administration of antiretroviral therapy is recommended,[77] to date, no prospective trials have been performed to confirm its effectiveness in humans. A retrospective case-control study published in 1996 supported the postexposure use of zidovudine.[78] The current recommendations for prophylaxis after a needle-stick injury are based on the likelihood of transmission from the incident.[79] In lower-risk situations, the risk of drug toxicity must be carefully weighed against the benefits of protection against HIV transmission.

The average risk of acquiring HIV after a percutaneous exposure is estimated to be 0.3%,[80] and the risk of acquiring HIV through mucocutaneous exposure approaches approximately 0.09%. It has been shown that the more blood transferred by a hollow-bore needle, the greater the likelihood of transmission. Clearly, patient factors such as viral burden and the presence of syncytia-inducing strains of virus will also influence the likelihood of seroconversion. Host factors such as cytotoxic T cell responses and perhaps T cell C3a/C5a receptors may also influence the outcome. With all this in mind, the CDC has formulated specific recommendations for postexposure prophylaxis (PEP).[81]

Because systemic infection after HIV exposure is thought not to occur immediately in primates, prompt initiation of antiretroviral therapy may sufficiently inhibit the initial replication to keep the inoculum of virus low and allow for effective immune clearance. Animal models are imperfect but have suggested that greatest efficacy of PEP was achieved when therapy was instituted within 24 hours of exposure. Overall efficacy of PEP is impossible to ascertain, because the incidence is fortunately low enough not to allow for a prospective study with sufficient statistical power to determine efficacy.

The current recommendations are based partly on the combination of simian studies, the experience with ziduvodine in a retrospective case-control study of health care workers, and collective experience with the prevention of vertical transmission through the use of antiviral prophylaxis. It is also recognized that as HIV-infected patients are increasingly likely to have been treated with a variety of retroviral agents, their likelihood of having multidrug-resistant strains of HIV increases correspondingly. Arbitrary selection of PEP agents may not be optimal; it is possible that knowledge of the patient's antiretroviral history and the results of genotypic antiretroviral resistance studies may need to be taken into account for optimal PEP selection. Whenever possible, physicians familiar with the source patient and local resistance patterns should be consulted on the choice of PEP regimens. However, institution of PEP should never be delayed for consultation, because the regimen can always be altered later if further information is obtained.

The choice of agents is largely empirical, but the need for PEP and the number of drugs to be used should be predicated on (1) the risk assessment of the injury, taking into account the source's HIV status (and, if the patient is HIV positive, the patient's clinical status and viral load); (2) solid-bore versus hollow-bore needle injury (large or small inoculum); (3) whether the source needle was used for arterial or venous puncture; and (4) whether the injury involved intact or nonintact skin or mucous membrane exposure.

A two-drug PEP regimen is probably adequate for situations in which the source is known to be HIV positive but thought to have a relatively low viral load, in which the source's HIV status is unknown but he or she is known to participate in high-risk activity, or in which the worker sustains either a minor percutaneous or mucous membrane exposure. A three-drug regimen would be advised with more severe percutaneous exposure, with

Table 4 Nucleoside Reverse Transcriptase Inhibitors

Agent	Toxicity
Zidovudine	Marrow suppression, myopathy, nausea
Stavudine	Peripheral neuropathy, pancreatitis, increased liver function tests
Lamivadine	Nausea, possible lipoatrophy, especially with concurrent stavudine
Didanosine	Pancreatitis, peripheral neuropathy, diarrhea
Abacavir	Life-threatening hypersensitivity reaction in approximately 5%

extensive exposure of intact skin or mucous membranes, or when the source is thought to have a high viral load. Because all the drugs used for PEP can have significant side effects, even in the short term, the potential risks of two-drug or three-drug therapy should be weighed against the likelihood of acquiring an HIV infection. With cases in which the source patient can be identified but the HIV status is unknown, a rapid HIV test such as the SUDS should be employed. If the results of such testing is negative, PEP should not be given. If rapid testing is not available, PEP can be offered until the source patient is proved to be HIV negative by conventional tests.

For the choice of agents, the 1998 CDC guidelines suggest zidovudine and lamivudine (3TC) for two-agent therapy, with the addition of indanivir or nelfinavir for three-drug therapy. Zidovudine and 3TC are now available in a combination pill that is taken twice a day, which makes it a more convenient alternative; however, the increasing prevalence of the 184 mutation that confers 3TC resistance makes this less likely to be effective in situations involving patients who have been treated with 3TC. Newer drugs such as efavirenz may offer more tolerable alternatives to adding a protease inhibitor, as was recommended in the past. The 2001 guidelines leave the choice more open to local expertise.

No discussion of occupational exposure is complete without mention of HCV coinfection. Approximately 40% of all HIV-infected patients are coinfected with HCV; in intravenous drug users, the incidence of HCV coinfection can be as high as 90%. Medical personnel exposed to HCV via occupational injury should undergo baseline testing for HCV antibodies and a baseline alanine transaminase (ALT) determination, with repeat testing in 4 to 6 months. There is no prophylactic regimen available, but some authorities recommend early intervention with HCV therapy (interferon alfa and ribavirin) if HCV remains detectable—a finding that would indicate persistence of infection.

TOXICITIES OF HIGHLY ACTIVE ANTIVIRAL THERAPY

Nucleoside Reverse Transcriptase Inhibitors

Long-term exposure to antiretroviral agents has not only improved survival but also introduced a variety of significant toxicities that physicians evaluating an HIV-infected patient must take into account. Nucleoside toxicities became apparent with the introduction of the first nucleoside reverse transcriptase inhibitor, zidovudine, 15 years ago, but a multitude of side effects are now known to be associated with all agents in this class. These agents appear to be toxic primarily through their ability to inhibit mitochondrial DNA synthesis. When critical levels of mitochondrial depletion are reached, the patient becomes symptomatic [*see Table 4*]. All the nucleoside transcriptase inhibitors have been associated with hepatotoxicity to some degree. All these agents may also cause increased levels of lactic acid, which may be asymptomatic or present as fulminant lactic acidosis and shock. Patients on combination therapy that includes both didanosine and stavudine seem to be at particular risk for severe lactic acidosis and hepatic steatosis. Patients may present with nausea, vomiting, abdominal pain, and diarrhea and become progressively more acidotic and hypotensive. Lactate levels in excess of 10 mmol/L are associated with multiorgan failure and a mortality of greater than 80%. Symptoms may develop gradually or suddenly and may occur from weeks to years after the start of antiretroviral therapy. Routine monitoring of lactic acid levels is of no benefit, because the results of such monitoring are not predictive of progression to symptomatic lactic acidemia. Once patients become asymptomatic, the keys to survival are early recognition, discontinuance of the offending drugs, and adequate oxygenation of tissues.

Nonnucleoside Reverse Transcriptase Inhibitors

The nonnucleoside reverse transcriptase inhibitors [*see Table 5*] are increasingly used in triple-drug regimens. They are known to cause rashes and have also been associated with hepatitis. Nevirapine has been implicated in fulminant hepatic failure in the setting of postexposure prophylaxis and in South African women. There is some concern that it may be more hepatotoxic in patients with hepatitis C infection.

Protease Inhibitors

The protease inhibitors [*see Table 6*] have been more frequently associated with metabolic syndromes involving alterations in fat metabolism, blood glucose, and lipids than with hepatitis or lactic acidemia. Hypercholesterolemia and hypertriglyceridemia have been associated with HAART, especially in regimens that include protease inhibitors. It is well recognized that there is a

Table 5 Nonnucleoside Reverse Transcriptase Inhibitors

Agent	Toxicity
Nevirapine	Rash, fever, hepatitis
Delavirdine	Rash, fever, hepatitis
Efavirenz	Rash, somnolence, insomnia, nightmares

Table 6 Protease Inhibitors

Agent	Toxicity
Indinavir	Nephrolithiasis, elevated bilirubin, fat redistribution, hyperglycemia, dry mouth
Nelfinavir	Diarrhea, abdominal pain
Ritonavir	Femoral numbness, diarrhea, hyperlipidemia
Saquinavir	Diarrhea, liver function abnormalities
Amprenavir	Diarrhea, nausea
Lopinavir/ritonavir	Diarrhea, hyperlipidemia

higher incidence of cardiac disease in HIV-infected patients receiving HAART than in age-matched control patients and that the presence of other traditional risk factors such as smoking and hypertension magnifies the risk. This has led most HIV practitioners to aggressively attempt to correct lipid abnormalities through the use of lipid-lowering agents. The increased risk of premature cardiac disease has also led physicians to consider

tests to attempt to identify occult coronary disease. Patients on protease inhibitors have been found to have insulin resistance even in the absence of overt diabetes, which also contributes to increased risk of coronary artery disease. For that reason, when HIV-infected patients with blood lipid abnormalities are being evaluated for elective surgical procedures, it is prudent to include a cardiac assessment.

References

1. Pneumocystis pneumonia—Los Angeles. MMWR Morb Mortal Wkly Rep 30:250, 1981

2. Kaposi's sarcoma and *Pneumocystis* pneumonia among homosexual men: New York City and California. MMWR Morb Mortal Wkly Rep 30:305, 1981

3. Barre-Sinoussi F, Chermann JC, Rey F, et al: Isolation of a T-lymphotropic retrovirus from a patient at risk for acquired immune deficiency syndrome (AIDS). Science 220:868, 1983

4. Current trends update: acquired immunodeficiency syndrome—United States, 1981–1988. MMWR Morb Mortal Wkly Rep 38:229, 1989

5. The global HIV and AIDS epidemic, 2001. MMWR Morb Mortal Wkly Rep 50:434, 2001

6. Institute of Medicine and the National Academy of Sciences: Mobilizing against AIDS: The Unfinished Story of a Virus. Harvard University Press, Cambridge, Massachusetts, 1986

7. Valdez H, Chowdhry TK, Asaad R, et al: Changing spectrum of mortality due to human immunodeficiency virus: analysis of 260 deaths during 1995–1999. Clin Infect Dis 32:1487, 2001

8. Rous T: Transmission of a malignant growth by means of a cell-free filtrate. JAMA 56:198, 1911

9. Robert-Guroff M, Nakao Y, Notake K, et al: Natural antibodies to human retrovirus HTLV in a cluster of Japanese patients with adult T-cell leukemia. Science 215:975, 1982

10. Barnes D: Keeping the AIDS virus out of blood supply. Science 233:514, 1986

11. U.S. Public Health Service guidelines for testing and counseling blood and plasma donors for human immunodeficiency virus type 1 antigen. MMWR Recomm Rep 45(RR-2):1, 1996

12. Persistent lack of detectable HIV-1 antibody in a person with HIV infections—Utah. MMWR Morb Mortal Wkly Rep 45:182, 1996

13. Recommendations for donor screening with a licensed test for HIV-1 antigen. US Department of Health and Human Services, Public Health Service, Food and Drug Administration, Center for Biologics Evaluation and Research, Rockville, Maryland, 1995

14. Grubert TA, Reindell D, Kastner R, et al: Rates of postoperative complications among human immunodeficiency virus–infected women who have undergone obstetric and gynecologic surgical procedures. Clin Infect Dis 34:822, 2002

15. Kirk O, Reiss P, Uberti-Foppa C, et al: Safe interruption of maintenance therapy against previous infection with four common HIV-associated opportunistic pathogens during potent antiretroviral therapy. Ann Intern Med 137:285, 2002

16. Margulis SJ, Honig CL, Soave R, et al: Biliary tract obstruction in the acquired immunodeficiency syndrome. Ann Intern Med 105:207, 1986

17. Robinson G, Wilson SE, Williams RA: Surgery in patients with acquired immunodeficiency syndrome. Arch Surg 122:170, 1987

18. Barone JE, Gingold BS, Arvanitis ML, et al: Abdominal pain in patients with acquired immunodeficiency syndrome. Ann Surg 204:619, 1986

19. Davis JM, Mouradian J, Fernandez RD, et al: Acquired immune deficiency syndrome: a surgical perspective. Arch Surg 119:90, 1984

20. Spach DH: HIV and AIDS. WebMD Scientific American Medicine, Section 7, Subsection XXIII. Dale DC, Federman DD, Eds. WebMD Inc, New York, 2001

21. Rao TK: Acute renal failure syndromes in human immunodeficiency virus infections. Semin Nephrology 18:370, 1998

22. Dube MP, Sprecher D, Henry WK, et al: Preliminary guidelines for the evaluation and management of dyslipidemia in adults infected with human immunodeficiency virus and receiving antiretroviral therapy: recommendations of the Adult AIDS Clinical Trial Group Cardiovascular Disease Focus Group. Clin Infect Dis 31:1216, 2000

23. Duong M, Cottin Y, Piroth L, et al: Exercise stress testing for detection of silent myocardial ischemia in human immunodeficiency virus–infected patients receiving antiretroviral therapy. Clin Infect Dis 34:523, 2002

24. Yunis NA, Stone VE: Cardiac manifestations of HIV/AIDS: a review of disease spectrum and clinical management. J Acquir Immune Defic Syndr Hum Retrovirol 18:145, 1998

25. Bedi GC, Westra WH, Farzadegan H, et al: Microsatellite instability in primary neoplasms from HIV + patients. Nat Med 1:65, 1995

26. Koblin BA, Hessol NA, Zauber AG, et al: Increased incidence of cancer among homosexual men, New York City and San Francisco, 1978–1990. Am J Epidemiol 144:916, 1996

27. Wistuba II, Behrens C, Milchgrub S, et al: Comparison of molecular changes in lung cancers in HIV-positive and HIV-indeterminate subjects. JAMA 279:1554, 1998

28. Morris L, Distenfeld A, Amorosi E, et al: Autoimmune thrombocytopenic purpura in homosexual men. Ann Intern Med 96:714, 1982

29. Walsh CM, Nardi MA, Karpatkin S: On the mechanism of thrombocytopenic purpura in sexually active homosexual men. N Engl J Med 311:635, 1984

30. Tsoukas CM, Bernard NF, Abrahamowicz M, et al: Effect of splenectomy on slowing human immunodeficiency virus disease progression. Arch Surg 133:25, 1998

31. Lord RV, Coleman MJ, Milliken ST: Splenectomy for HIV-related immune thrombocytopenia: comparison with results of splenectomy for non-HIV immune thrombocytopenic purpura. Arch Surg 133:205, 1998

32. Dega H, Eliaszewicz M, Gisselbrecht M, et al: Infections associated with totally implantable venous access devices (TIVAD) in human immunodeficiency virus–infected patients. J Acquir Immune Defic Syndr Hum Retrovirol 13:146, 1996

33. French AL, Beaudet LM, Benator DA, et al: Cholecystectomy in patients with AIDS: clinicopathological correlations in 107 cases. Clin Infect Dis 21:852, 1995

34. Kavin H, Jonas RB, Chowdhury L, et al: Acalculous cholecystitis and cytomegalovirus infection in the acquired immunodeficiency syndrome. Ann Intern Med 104:53, 1986

35. Benator DA, French AL, Beaudet LM, et al: *Isospora belli* infection associated with acalculous cholecystitis in a patient with AIDS. Ann Intern Med 121:663, 1994

36. Pol S, Romana CA, Richard S, et al: *Microsporidia* infection in patients with the human immunodeficiency virus and unexplained cholangitis. N Engl J Med 328:95, 1993

37. Nugent P, O'Connell TX: The surgeon's role in treating acquired immunodeficiency syndrome. Arch Surg 121:1117, 1986

38. Potter DA, Danforth DN Jr, Macher AM, et al: Evaluation of abdominal pain in the AIDS patient. Ann Surg 199:332, 1984

39. Wilson SE, Robinson G, Williams RA, et al: Acquired immune deficiency syndrome (AIDS): indications for abdominal surgery, pathology, and outcome. Ann Surg 210:428, 1989

40. Schecter WP: Human immunodeficiency virus and malignancy: thoughts on viral oncogenesis. Arch Surg 136:1419, 2001

41. Whiteford MH, Stevens KR Jr, Oh S, et al: The evolving treatment of anal cancer: how are we doing? Arch Surg 136:886, 2001

42. Fernandez R, Mouradian J, Metroka C, et al: The prognostic value of histopathology in persistent generalized lymphadenopathy in homosexual men. N Engl J Med 309:185, 1983

43. Redfield RR, Wright DC, Tramont EC: The Walter Reed staging classification for HTLV-III/LAV infection. N Engl J Med 314:131, 1986

44. Davis JM, Chadburn A, Mouradian JA: Lymph node biopsy in patients with human immunodeficiency virus infections. Arch Surg 123:1349, 1988

45. Redfield RR, Burke DS: HIV infection: the clinical picture. Sci Am 259:90, 1988

46. Farero MS: Disinfection, sterilization, and decontamination procedures. Occup Med 4(suppl):35, 1989

47. Jawetz E, Melnick JL, Adelberg EA: Antimicrobial chemotherapy. Review of Medical Microbiology, 15th ed. Adelberg EA, Melnick JL, Jawetz E, Eds. Lange Medical Publications, Los Altos, California, 1982, p 117

48. McCray E: Occupational risk of the acquired immunodeficiency syndrome among health care workers. N Engl J Med 314:1127, 1986

49. Gerberding JL, Littell C, Tarkington A, et al: Risk of exposure of surgical personnel to patients'

blood during surgery at San Francisco General Hospital. N Engl J Med 322:1788, 1990

50. Quebbeman EJ, Telford GL, Wadsworth K, et al: Double gloving: protecting surgeons from blood contamination in the operating room. Arch Surg 127:213, 1992

51. Braathen LR, Ramirez G, Kunze RO, et al: Langerhans cells as primary target cells for HIV infection (letter). Lancet 2:1094, 1987

52. Cumming PD, Wallace EL, Schorr JB, et al: Exposure of patients to human immunodeficiency virus through the transfusion of blood components that test antibody-negative. N Engl J Med 321:941, 1989

53. Moore SB: AIDS, blood transfusions, and directed donations. N Engl J Med 314:1454, 1986

54. Monk TG, Goodnough LT, Brecher ME, et al: A prospective randomized comparison of three blood conservation strategies for radical prostatectomy. Anesthesiology 91:24, 1999

55. Ho DD, Byington RE, Schooley RT, et al: Infrequency of isolation of HTLV-III virus from saliva in AIDS. N Engl J Med 313:1606, 1985

56. Morgan J, Nolan J: Risks of AIDS with artificial insemination. N Engl J Med 314:386, 1986

57. Gerbert B, Maguire BT, Hulley SB, et al: Physicians and acquired immunodeficiency syndrome: what patients think about human immunodeficiency virus in medical practice. JAMA 262:1969, 1989

58. Summary: recommendations for preventing transmission of infection with human T-lymphotropic virus type III/lymphadenopathy-associated virus in the workplace. MMRW Morb Mortal Wkly Rep 34:681, 1985

59. Harpaz R, Von Seidlein L, Averhoff FM, et al: Transmission of hepatitis B virus to multiple patients from a surgeon without evidence of inadequate infection control. N Engl J Med 334:549, 1996

60. Marcus R: Surveillance of health care workers exposed to blood from patients infected with the human immunodeficiency virus. N Engl J Med 319:1118, 1988

61. Serosurvey of human immunodeficiency virus, hepatitis B virus, and hepatitis C virus infection among hospital-based surgeons. Serosurvey Study Group. J Am Coll Surg 180:16, 1995

62. Apparent transmission of human T-lymphotropic virus type III/lymphadenopathy-associated virus from a child to a mother providing health care. MMWR Morb Mortal Wkly Rep 35:76, 1996

63. Howard RJ: Human immunodeficiency virus testing and the risk to the surgeon of acquiring HIV. Surg Gynecol Obstet 171:22, 1990

64. Popejoy SL, Fry DE: Blood contact and exposure in the operating room. Surg Gynecol Obstet 172:480, 1991

65. Panlilio AL, Foy DR, Edwards JR, et al: Blood contacts during surgical procedures. JAMA 265:1533, 1991

66. Tokars JI, Bell DM, Culver DH, et al: Percutaneous injuries during surgical procedures. JAMA 267:2899, 1992

67. Levy JA, Kaminsky LS, Morrow WJ, et al: Infection by the retrovirus associated with the acquired immunodeficiency syndrome: clinical, biological, and molecular features. Ann Intern Med 103:694, 1985

68. Lorian V: AIDS, anal sex, and heterosexuals. Lancet 1:1111, 1988

69. Update: acquired immunodeficiency syndrome and human immunodeficiency virus infection among health-care workers. MMWR Morb Mortal Wkly Rep 37:229, 1988

70. Hagen MD, Meyer KB, Kopelman RI, et al: Human immunodeficiency virus infection in health care workers: a method for estimating individual occupational risk. Arch Intern Med 149:1541, 1989

71. Parry MF, Brown AE, Dobbs LG, et al: The epidemiology of hepatitis B infection in housestaff. Infection 6:204, 1978

72. Alter HJ: The evolution, implications, and applications of the hepatitis B vaccine (editorial). JAMA 247:2272, 1982

73. Recommendation of the Immunization Practices Advisory Committee (ACIP). MMWR Morb Mortal Wkly Rep 34:313, 1985

74. Denes AE, Smith JL, Maynard JE, et al: Hepatitis B infection in physicians: results of a nationwide seroepidemiologic survey. JAMA 239:210, 1978

75. Lenimer JH: Hepatitis B as an occupational disease of surgeons. Surg Gynecol Obstet 159:91, 1984

76. Barie PS, Dellinger EP, Dougherty SH, et al: Assessment of HBV immunization status among North American surgeons. Arch Surg 129:27, 1994

77. Henderson DK, Gerberding JL: Prophylactic zidovudine after occupational exposure to the human immunodeficiency virus: an interim analysis. J Infect Dis 160:321, 1989

78. Case-control study of HIV seroconversion in healthcare workers after percutaneous exposure to HIV infected blood—France, United Kingdom and United States. MMWR Morb Mortal Wkly Rep 44:929, 1996

79. Update: provisional Public Health Service recommendations for chemoprophylaxis after occupational exposure to HIV. MMWR Morb Mortal Wkly Rep 45:468, 1996

80. 1993 Revised classification system for HIV infection and expanded surveillance case definition for AIDS among adolescents and adults. MMWR Morb Mortal Wkly Rep 41(RR-17):1, 1992

81. Updated U.S. Public Health Service guidelines for the management of occupational exposures to HBV, HCV, and HIV and recommendations for postexposure prophylaxis. MMWR Recomm Rep 50(RR-11):1, 2001

22 METABOLIC RESPONSE TO CRITICAL ILLNESS

Palmer Q. Bessey, M.D., F.A.C.S.

Metabolic Responses in Surgical Patients

Debility commonly accompanies surgical illness. It occurs in varying degrees after elective operations, major trauma, burns, infections, and other critical illnesses. Debility is caused by a variety of factors, including specific biochemical and physiologic alterations that usually occur in response to injury and disease, especially those that persist for a long time. Some aspects of surgical care that are common to almost all patients can also cause debility. This discussion will review these clinical factors and metabolic responses in critically ill surgical patients and will indicate how the clinician can manage them so as to minimize patient debility.

The metabolic responses to critical illness have been studied in a variety of critically ill patients, especially those with trauma, burns, or sepsis. The responses are often grouped into phases on the basis of their temporal relation to the injury or insult. The so-called ebb phase, which is the early phase of the injury response, is characterized by (1) an elevated blood glucose level, (2) normal glucose production, (3) elevated free fatty acid levels, (4) a low insulin concentration, (5) elevated levels of catecholamines and glucagon, (6) an elevated blood lactate level, (7) depressed oxygen consumption, (8) below-normal cardiac output, and (9) below-normal core temperature.[1] The subsequent phase, the so-called flow phase, is characterized by (1) a normal or slightly elevated blood glucose level, (2) increased glucose production, (3) normal or slightly elevated free fatty acid levels, with flux increased, (4) a normal or elevated insulin concentration, (5) high normal or elevated levels of catecholamine and an elevated glucagon level, (6) a normal blood lactate level, (7) elevated oxygen consumption, (8) increased cardiac output, and (9) elevated core temperature.[1]

The ebb phase is dominated by cardiovascular instability, alterations in circulating blood volume, impairment of oxygen transport, and heightened autonomic activity. Emergency support of cardiopulmonary performance is the paramount therapeutic concern. Shock [*see 6:3 Shock*] is the prototypical clinical manifestation of the ebb phase. After effective resuscitation has been accomplished and restoration of satisfactory oxygen transport has been achieved, the flow phase comes into play. These responses are marked by hyperdynamic circulatory changes, signs of inflammation, glucose intolerance, and muscle wasting. Surgical patients in the ICU usually exhibit these clinical features; these patients and the clinical challenge they pose are the focus of this chapter.

When wounds are closed and infection has resolved, repletion of lean tissue and fat stores and restoration of strength and stamina can begin. This final, anabolic phase often begins near the time of hospital discharge and may persist for months before the patient fully recovers.

Features of Critical Illness That Can Cause Debility

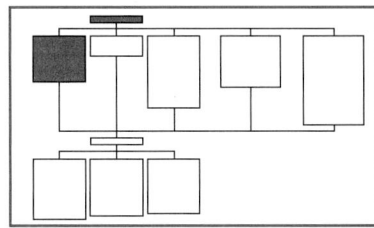

THE WOUND

The surgical wound is not only a site of tissue disruption but also a site of inflammation and repair [*see 1:7 Acute Wound Care*]. After resuscitation, the surgeon's principal task is to expedite and promote wound healing and restore tissue integrity. Because the wound is often the proximate cause of patient debility, providing optimal wound care amounts to providing the best patient care.

Wounds with necrotic or devitalized tissue (e.g., from ischemic necrosis, gangrene, or burns), foreign debris, or grossly contaminated material do not heal readily, if they heal at all. Necrotic tissue and eschar (slough) must be debrided, usually surgically, although application of enzymatic agents to wounds has also been effective in some cases. Foreign material must be removed by either hydrotherapy or debridement. Pus must be drained or removed by irrigation and dressing changes. Contaminated wounds are left open so that they can be repeatedly examined and further necrotic material can be removed. Open wounds should be covered with a dressing to prevent drying (i.e., tissue oxidation) and further tissue slough, to reduce bacterial contamination, and to prevent further mechanical injury. Unfortunately, none of the currently available dressing materials achieve all of these goals. Once it becomes apparent that the wound tissues are viable and uninfected, the wound should be closed primarily if possible or with a skin graft.

The cellular processes involved in wound healing are critically dependent on adequate perfusion and delivery of oxygen, glucose, and other essential nutrients. Inadequate perfusion may result in relative tissue ischemia and delay wound healing. A principal responsibility of the clinician is therefore to ensure adequate tissue perfusion during the entire period of wound healing. For instance, resuscitation from shock should be continued after blood pressure is stabilized and until there is clinical evidence of adequate flow—usually associated with warm extremities, pink nail beds, brisk capillary refilling, full peripheral pulses, urine output greater than 0.5 ml/kg/hr (50 to 70 ml/hr in adults), clear sensorium, and improving metabolic acidosis. Adequate oxygenation must also be ensured. Occasionally, invasive monitoring of cardiopulmonary performance [*see 6:4 Cardiopulmonary Monitoring*] and tissue oxygenation as well as pharmacologic support may be required to ensure adequate perfusion and oxygen delivery.

Patient problems that lead to debility

Wound

Debride necrotic tissue and foreign debris.
Drain pus.
Avoid drying of tissues.
Maintain satisfactory cardiopulmonary performance to optimize oxygen delivery.
Expedite wound closure.
For clean surgical wounds:
- Handle tissues gently.
- Use precise surgical technique and hemostasis.

Avoid contamination.
Use primary closure when possible.

Pain

Use systemic analgesics judiciously.
Consider patient-controlled analgesia.
Consider regional (epidural) anesthesia.

Inflammation

Fever
- If < 38.5° C (101.3° F), usually no treatment or evaluation is necessary.
- If ≥ 38.5° C (101.3° F), survey for source of infection; consider administering antipyretics.
- If > 41° C (105.8° F), increase antipyretics; consider use of cooling blankets, ice packs, etc.

Altered thermoregulation
- Maintain warm environment (26°–33° C [78.8°–91.4° F]) to achieve thermal comfort.

Anorexia
- Limit period of fasting to 3–4 days.

Immunosuppression
- Sterile technique for all procedures, including intravenous line manipulations, suctioning, etc.
- Universal precautions; change gloves, wash hands between patients.

Metabolic response to critical illness

Hyperdynamic or hypermetabolic state

Expect
- Tachycardia
- Widened pulse pressure
- Increased cardiac output
- Increased O_2 consumption
- Increased minute ventilation
- Increased energy expenditure
- Fever
- Sodium and water retention

Provide
- Volume and pharmacologic support of cardiovascular performance as appropriate
- Warm environment (26°–33° C)
- Increased water intake
- Increased caloric intake
- Judicious sedation and analgesia

Muscle wasting

Expect
- Rapid wasting of muscle and loss of strength and endurance
- Increased osmotic load filtered by kidney
- Increased formation and urinary loss of urea
- Increased urinary loss of potassium, phosphorus, and magnesium

Provide
- Increased protein or amino acid intake to 15%–20% of total energy
- Increased intake of potassium, phosphorus, and magnesium
- Massage, active and passive exercise, and early mobilization

Glucose intolerance

Expect
- Hyperglycemia that is aggravated by glucose intake, infection, and other stressors
- Relative insensitivity to insulin, which improves with recovery

Provide
- Glucose control
- Human insulin I.V. to maintain blood glucose in a target range of 110–160 mg/dl
- Maintenance nutritional support
- Glucose as 60%–75% of total energy (5–7 mg/kg/min or 7–10 g/kg/day)
- Lipid as 25%–40% of total energy

Infection	Hospital treatment
Initially diagnose by abrupt changes in fever, leukocytosis, hyperglycemia, pulmonary function, or pulse and blood pressure. Culture appropriately to establish micro-biologic diagnosis. Administer broad-spectrum antibiotics empirically to cover likely pathogens if signs of organ system dysfunction and of sepsis develop. Debride necrotic tissue. Establish drainage; remove catheters. Prevent contamination of different sites on same patient. Prevent cross-contamination between patients.	Bed rest: • Encourage frequent turning, coughing, and deep breathing. • Encourage active, assisted exercise in bed when feasible. • Move to chair as soon as possible. • Use incentive spirometer or similar device. • Practice good hygiene and skin care, and provide massage. Food deprivation: • Limit period of fasting to 3–4 days. • Begin nutritional support as soon as needed. • Provide enteral feeding when possible. Invasive devices: • Remove as soon as no longer required. • Remove I.V. lines placed under suboptimal conditions as soon as feasible. • Consider changing I.V. lines or rotating site every 2 or 4 days. • Change I.V. site if redness or inflammation develops. Sleep deprivation: • Reduce lighting and noise in ICU periodically, especially at night. • Orient patient frequently to time of day and situation. • Use sedation judiciously.

Metabolic Responses in Surgical Patients

Contused tissue, fractures, tissues surrounding an abscess or site of infection, inflammatory sites such as the pancreas in pancreatitis or the lung in acute respiratory distress syndrome (ARDS)—in fact, any mass of inflammatory tissue—can be considered to constitute the patient's wound because resolution of those focal sites of inflammation depends on the same basic cellular processes as does healing of an external wound.

Patients with a large total mass of inflammatory tissue—large wounds—usually are critically ill and clearly manifest most of the metabolic responses associated with critical illness [see Metabolic Responses That Can Cause Debility, below]. In contrast, patients with small wounds do not appear critically ill and are not significantly debilitated. Although elective operations result in wounds, the incisions are made under sterile, controlled conditions; there is minimal direct tissue injury, little contamination, no shock, and limited net loss of blood and fluid. The incisions are closed primarily and most often heal expeditiously. With the current proliferation of minimally invasive surgical techniques, operative incisions are now even more limited, patients recover more rapidly, and the resultant debility is minimal—often little more than a transient indisposition.

PAIN

Virtually all surgical patients experience some pain. Pain usually occurs in association with an incision or with a wound resulting from fracture, burn, contusion, or another type of injury. In ad-
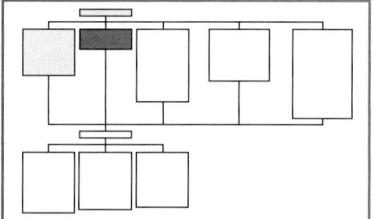
dition to creating an unpleasant subjective experience, pain often limits physical activities, such as turning in bed, deep breathing, coughing, and walking, and thereby directly interferes with recovery. A variety of techniques are available for pain management. However, each approach has side effects, the potential for abuse, or other features that limit its application.

Acute pain has traditionally been managed by intermittent parenteral administration of narcotic analgesics when requested by the patient or when the nurse perceives the patient to be in pain. The intravenous route is now preferred, because it does not require a painful injection and avoids potential uptake abnormalities. Intravenous analgesics have a short duration of action and must be given frequently to maintain good, sustained pain control; the dose also must be relatively small to minimize the side effects of sedation and impaired gastric motility. Thus, this approach to pain control is relatively labor intensive. Theoretically, this approach can prevent overuse of narcotics; in practice, it often results in inconsistent pain control and underdosing.

Continuous infusion of narcotic analgesics provides more consistent pain control and is common in the ICU. The dose should be adjusted upward before painful procedures but otherwise should be kept as low as possible to avoid ileus and prolonged sedation. Patient-controlled analgesia (PCA) is an extension of this approach. The patient controls a pump that administers a prescribed dose of the agent when activated; the clinician determines the amount of drug in each dose and the total dose permissible in a given period. This technique has been well accepted by patients who are awake and alert and are capable of controlling the system. One benefit is that the total amount of drug administered for pain relief is usually less than is given in a conventional as-needed dosing schedule.[2]

Administration of local anesthetics or narcotics into the epidural space may provide effective local pain relief without the sedating effects of parenteral narcotics. In addition, epidural anesthetics (but not opioids) reduce postoperative ileus.[3] Effective epidural analgesia can be maintained for several days and may have a beneficial effect

on pulmonary function in patients with rib fractures or truncal wounds.[4] This technique requires placement of a catheter in the epidural space.

Patients must be monitored closely, and the dosage schedule must be individualized. This technique is best suited to patients who will be relatively inactive for 24 to 36 hours postoperatively and who can be observed closely, such as patients in the ICU.

INFLAMMATION

Elevation of body temperature above normal, leukocytosis, and other signs of inflammation are common features of critical surgical illness and should be expected. The extent of temperature elevation is generally
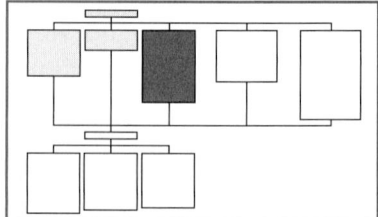
proportional to the severity of illness. In a patient with a major burn—an extreme example of critical surgical illness—body temperature may be as high as 39° C (102.2° F). The leukocyte count is also typically elevated and may be as high as 20,000 cells/ mm³ during satisfactory recovery. A normal or subnormal body temperature or white blood cell count is atypical and may indicate sepsis, drug-induced leukopenia, or limited physiologic reserve. For example, a critically ill elderly patient with a major injury or infection may be afebrile and have a white blood cell count in the normal range.

Fever, however, is also a cardinal sign of infection. It may be difficult to distinguish between a typical postoperative or posttraumatic fever and a fever caused by invasive infection. An acute elevation in rectal temperature of 1.0° to 1.5° C (1.8° to 2.7° F) that occurs within a short period or a rectal temperature higher than 38.5° C (101.3° F) should be considered indicative of infection and should be investigated thoroughly. Sputum, urine, and blood cultures should be obtained, and all wounds should be inspected carefully for signs of inflammation or infection. Devices commonly associated with nosocomial infection—intravenous cannulas, urinary catheters, and endotracheal tubes—should be removed as soon as feasible or else changed (see below).

Because inflammation is such a prominent feature of all critical illness, including that in patients with serious infectious complications of chronic diseases, several clinical syndromes have been defined in an effort to stratify patients according to the severity of their inflammatory responses [see Table 1].[5] These syndromes are associated with increased mortality, even in the absence of documented infection.[6] In the remainder of this chapter, I will refer repeatedly to the metabolic responses to critical illness; this term incorporates these inflammatory syndromes and more besides, and its use permits a more comprehensive discussion.

Mild elevation of body temperature is usually well tolerated and requires no specific treatment. However, a higher fever may impose significant stress on the patient, as indicated by pronounced tachycardia, tachypnea, malaise, and, occasionally, restlessness. Thus, a body temperature higher than 39° C (102.2° F) is usually treated with antipyretics (e.g., acetaminophen, aspirin, indomethacin, or ibuprofen).

The fever experienced by critically ill patients is an upward adjustment of the thermoregulatory center in the brain, the central thermostat. A consequence of this adjustment is that the patient usually prefers a warmer environmental temperature than do normal individuals. An ambient temperature in the hospital that is comfortable for the staff is often perceived as cool by the patient, who must generate extra heat to maintain the adjusted body temperature. Thus, patient areas of the hospital should be kept warm, usually in the range of 26° to 33° C (78.8° to 91.4° F). This temperature range will

Table 1 Components of Inflammatory Syndromes[5]

Systemic inflammatory response syndrome (SIRS)—two or more of the following are required:
Temperature > 38° C (100.4° F) or < 36° C (96.8° F)
Heart rate > 90 beats/min
Respirations > 20/min
WBC > 12,000/mm³, < 4,000 mm³, or > 10% bands

Sepsis
SIRS
Clinically likely source of infection (does not require bacteriologic confirmation)

Severe sepsis
Sepsis
Impaired cardiovascular performance necessitating fluid resuscitation

Septic shock
Severe sepsis
Impaired cardiovascular performance necessitating inotropic support

ment of oxygenation, and other signs associated with the septic response. The challenge for the clinician is to distinguish patients in whom this response is caused by established infection from those in whom it is not the result of an infectious focus. A temperature higher than 38.5° C (101.3° F) or an acute increase in temperature accompanied by an abrupt change in the white blood cell count should prompt investigation for a developing infection [see Figure 1], which would include appropriate cultures and other diagnostic studies. Other signs that suggest underlying infection include relative hypothermia, leukopenia, thrombocytopenia, abrupt elevation or depression of the blood glucose level, restlessness, lassitude, hyperpnea, and failure to progress as expected.

If the presence of infection is suggested by the clinical setting, the magnitude of fever, or any other systemic signs (such as renal or respiratory dysfunction, marked hyperglycemia or hypoglycemia, hypothermia, or hypotension), broad-spectrum antibiotic coverage should be instituted empirically before culture results are available [see 6:14 Clinical and Laboratory Diagnosis of Infection]. Specific antimicrobial therapy should be begun once the presence of infection has been confirmed and the microbiologic diagnosis has been established. Other therapeutic measures may also be necessary to treat the infection. Draining an abscess, debriding or excising necrotic tissue, removing indwelling catheters and placing new ones at other sites, performing therapeutic bronchoscopy to ensure drainage of major airways, or creating a tracheostomy in the patient who requires an airway for improved bedside pulmonary toilet may also be advisable.

Because all critically ill patients are at risk for infection, efforts directed at prevention are worthwhile. Medical and nursing personnel can prevent the transmission of organisms from one patient to another by effective hand washing between patient contacts. Gloves used by health care workers for their own protection whenever they have contact with patients must be changed between patients. Of course, sterile techniques should be used during invasive procedures.

promote patient comfort and reduce the physiologic demands of cold stress. When moved into the OR, radiology suite, or other typically cool environments, patients should be insulated, or the room should be warmed.

Attempts to treat a patient with fever by surface cooling (ice packs, alcohol rubs, cooling blankets) are not uncommon. Rather than addressing the altered physiology underlying the fever, however, surface cooling imposes a marked cold stress on an already critically ill and stressed patient. Except in the presence of hyperpyrexia (temperature ≥ 41° C [105.8° F]), surface cooling should be avoided; antipyretics should be administered first to reduce body temperature.

During acute surgical illness, patients typically have a poor appetite. Even when able to eat, they often do not consume sufficient nutrients even to approximate their needs. Accordingly, the clinician should initiate exogenous nutritional support early in the patient's course, especially if it is likely to be prolonged by the need for additional reparative procedures, such as fracture fixation or delayed wound closure.

Some degree of immunosuppression is also a common feature of inflammation. Thus, critically ill patients are more susceptible than normal to colonization and infection with a variety of microorganisms. Special attention to sterile technique during bedside procedures, the use of universal precautions, and hand washing after each patient encounter by all care providers should help reduce the risk of nosocomial infection.

INFECTION

Infections in hospitalized patients fall into two categories: they may be directly related to the patient's primary disease or injury (e.g., invasive burn wound sepsis, gangrene of an ischemic limb, or 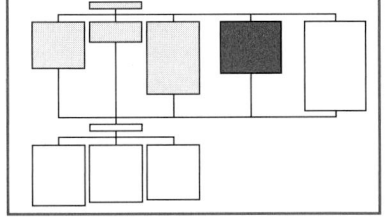 intra-abdominal abscess after perforated diverticulosis), or they may develop as a complication of physiologic support (e.g., pneumonia after prolonged mechanical ventilatory support).

Early diagnosis and treatment of infection in surgical patients can minimize debility. Most critically ill surgical patients experience fever, leukocytosis, tachycardia, widened pulse pressure (reduced vascular resistance), glucose intolerance, fluid retention, some impair-

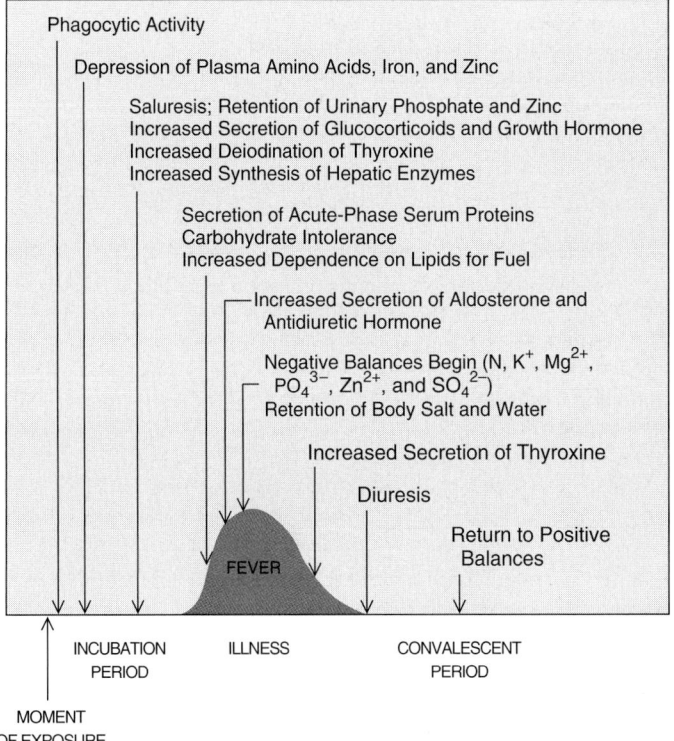

Figure 1 Illustrated is the time course of events that constitute the classic response to bacterial infection.[253]

Sites of insertion of intravascular cannulas should be inspected regularly, and the catheters should be moved to a new site if the skin becomes reddened or if pus is observed. Antibiotic-impregnated central venous catheters may reduce the incidence of catheter-related infection and thereby lower the frequency with which lines must be replaced.[7] The prophylactic use of antibiotics in the ICU is controversial[8-10] and cannot be encouraged at present.

IATROGENIC FACTORS

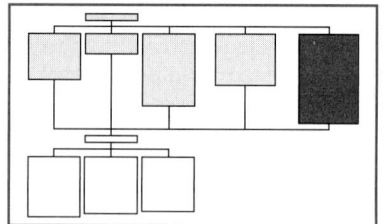

Bed Rest

Bed rest and inactivity both contribute to loss of muscle mass and strength. Immobility may result in progressive atelectasis, respiratory insufficiency, and pulmonary sepsis. If immobility is prolonged, open pressure sores may develop over bony prominences. Thus, patients should be turned frequently, and their position should be changed often. Patients who are able to participate actively in repositioning themselves should be encouraged to do so by helping to turn or lift themselves. They should be urged to take deep breaths and cough. An incentive spirometer is inexpensive and is often helpful in this regard. When patients are hemodynamically stable, they should be moved to a chair, provided that no musculoskeletal contraindications are present. This position improves ventilation and helps preserve postural reflexes. Patients should assist in sitting up as much as is feasible. Even simple actions such as standing in place or bearing weight during the transfer may be beneficial. Active and passive range-of-motion exercises can help maintain joint function. Proper positioning of the extremities may be necessary to prevent contractures and to preserve range of motion.

Skin integrity is preserved not only by frequent position changes but also by attention to hygiene. Patients should be bathed regularly, with special attention paid to intertriginous areas. Any soilage with blood, stool, urine, or other material should be removed and the skin thoroughly dried. Massage and application of moisturizing lotions are also helpful. The use of foam or air mattress pads that distribute body weight over a large area or low-air-loss beds may also benefit the patient confined to bed for a prolonged period. However, these devices are no substitute for good nursing care.

Food Deprivation

Food is commonly withheld from the patient before and during various diagnostic and therapeutic procedures as well as before operations or after injury. Starvation for several days appears to be well tolerated by patients who were relatively well nourished before their critical illness. However, if food deprivation is prolonged, the complications of starvation will compound the effects of critical surgical illness. Total starvation should usually be limited to a period no longer than 3 or 4 days. Nutritional support should be instituted via the most effective and safest route possible [see 6:23 Nutritional Support].

Invasive Devices

A variety of tubes, catheters, and drains are essential for the proper care and monitoring of critically ill patients. However, each of these devices transgresses a normal barrier to infection, and each is associated with infectious risks and other complications. An invasive device should be removed as soon as it is no longer required. Intravenous lines placed in the emergency room or under less than ideal conditions (e.g., at the scene of an accident or while the patient is en route to the hospital) should be removed as soon as possible and replaced, if necessary, with new devices by means of appropriate sterile

technique. Such lines should also be changed if the puncture site is red, inflamed, or purulent. With most of these devices, the risk of infectious complications increases after 3 or 4 days.[11] Regular replacement is commonly practiced, especially if the patient becomes febrile. Catheters impregnated with antibiotics appear not to require such frequent exchanges and may be safely used for longer periods.[7]

Sleep Deprivation

Normal sleep patterns are disturbed in ICU patients, in part because of the constant light and noise in the ICU and because of repetitive stimulation by the ICU staff. Such disturbances, in combination with other stresses associated with illness, often result in confusion, disorientation, anxiety, and, occasionally, frank psychosis. As many efforts as possible should be made to orient the patient, including the use of wall calendars, clocks, and other methods that serve as normal day-night indicators (e.g., turning the lights down at night). Even the personal activities of daily living, such as bathing and shaving, can serve as time cues. Patients should be reassured and reminded about the date, the time, their location, and the reason for their hospitalization. Sedatives and hypnotics may be useful in critically ill patients but occasionally have a paradoxically excitatory effect.

Metabolic Responses That Can Cause Debility

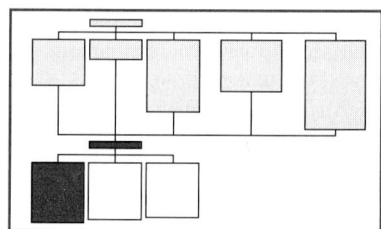

All of the clinical factors of surgical care contribute to or affect various physiologic and biochemical alterations that occur in response to critical illness; these physiologic and biochemical alterations collectively constitute the metabolic response to critical illness. The intensity and duration of this response determine debility. Current critical care management generally supports rather than modifies the response. Three major features of the metabolic response to critical illness affect clinical care: the hyperdynamic or hypermetabolic state, muscle wasting, and glucose intolerance.

HYPERDYNAMIC OR HYPERMETABOLIC STATE

In recovery from critical illness, several organ systems function at an accelerated pace. Principal among these is the cardiovascular system. Tachycardia and a widened pulse pressure are typically present and reflect cardiac output greater than that expected in a resting, healthy individual. The increased blood flow is distributed to most vascular beds, especially to inflammatory tissue or the wound, and supports increased cellular activity in the healing wound. In the kidneys, increased flow is associated with an elevated glomerular filtration rate. Thus, drug excretion may be accelerated, and increased dosages may be required to maintain therapeutic plasma concentrations.

Accompanying the increases in cardiac output and regional blood flow is an increase in oxygen delivery (transport) to the microcirculation. This increase in oxygen delivery supports the enhanced oxygen requirements of several organ systems. Total body oxygen consumption ($\dot{V}O_2$) is greater than normal because of the increased oxidation of body fuels—carbohydrates, fats, and amino acids—needed to provide the energy to drive the cellular machinery at this accelerated pace [see Figure 2]. These reactions produce heat. Heat production, also referred to as energy expenditure or metabolic rate, is increased in critically ill patients, who thus are said to be hypermetabolic.

The increase in $\dot{V}O_2$ is paralleled by increased carbon dioxide production ($\dot{V}CO_2$), which, under normal conditions, stimulates breathing and augments minute ventilation. For patients who require ventilatory assistance, the ventilator should be set to deliver a minute ventilation that is greater than normal.

As discussed earlier, critically ill patients typically have a fever and prefer warmer ambient temperatures than normal individuals. In these patients, metabolic rates increase in part to maintain a higher than normal core temperature. A warm environment may help blunt the patient's increased heat production and energy needs.

Associated with the hyperdynamic state of critical illness is expansion of the extracellular fluid (ECF) compartment. Total body water and total body sodium are increased. This expansion occurs perioperatively or with resuscitation after injury. Short-term changes in body weight reflect alterations in body water and in lean tissue mass. Slow, persistent expansion of the ECF may mask loss of tissue mass. Conversely, spontaneous diuresis of sodium and water during recovery may lead to pronounced weight loss in a patient who otherwise appears to be progressing well.

During critical illness, the daily loss of body water is increased in several ways. Fever accelerates insensible loss of body water, and renal loss may be greater than normal because of the increased osmotic load caused by the breakdown of lean tissue (see below). If there are open wounds, evaporative water loss is markedly increased, in proportion to the size of the open wound. Thus, maintenance water requirements may be greater than normal. It is often necessary to monitor both the intravascular fluid volume, using values for central venous or pulmonary arterial wedge pressures, and the ECF composition or tonicity, as indicated by changes in serum sodium concentrations.

The clinician should provide not only volume and possible pharmacologic support to maintain a hyperdynamic circulation but also an increased amount of calories to meet the patient's elevated energy needs. These needs can often be reliably estimated on the basis of the patient's age, sex, body size, and critical illness. Occasionally, it may be helpful to measure the patient's $\dot{V}O_2$ and $\dot{V}CO_2$ and to use these values to calculate daily caloric requirements.

In addition to providing cardiopulmonary and nutritional support to critically ill, hyperdynamic patients, the clinician should try to neutralize factors that may augment the hyperdynamic response to critical illness. Judicious analgesia and sedation provide metabolic benefits and relieve pain and anxiety. Providing a warm environment mitigates the hyperdynamic response by reducing cold stress. Antipyretics reduce the heart rate during periods of extreme fever.

MUSCLE WASTING

The distinguishing feature of the debility of critical illness is marked muscle wasting and weakness. Wasting is in part a consequence of accelerated muscle protein breakdown, which is gener-

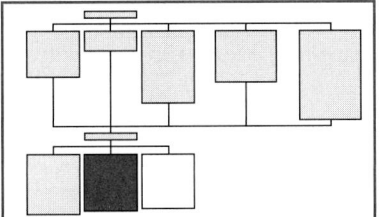

ally related to the severity of illness [see Figure 2]. The increased protein breakdown presumably serves to mobilize amino acids for synthesis of new protein in wounds; for proliferation of phagocytes, macrophages, and other cellular components involved in wound healing; and for synthesis of acute-phase proteins and glucose in the liver. The increased synthetic work and processing of amino acids in the liver result in increased production of urea, which is filtered and excreted by the kidneys. In the presence of renal dysfunction, blood urea nitrogen (BUN) may rise rapidly.

To reduce muscle wasting, additional exogenous protein or amino acids are provided through nutritional support. In general, protein needs increase in proportion to caloric requirements. However, for the critically ill surgical patient, it may be beneficial to provide at least

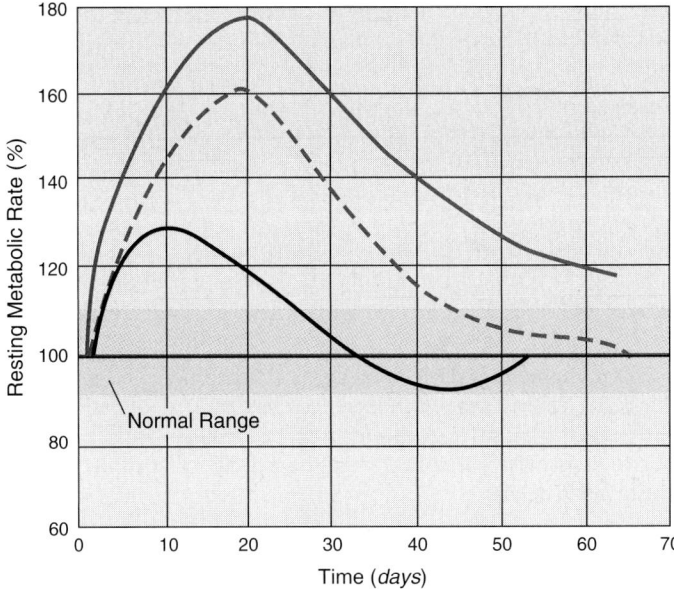

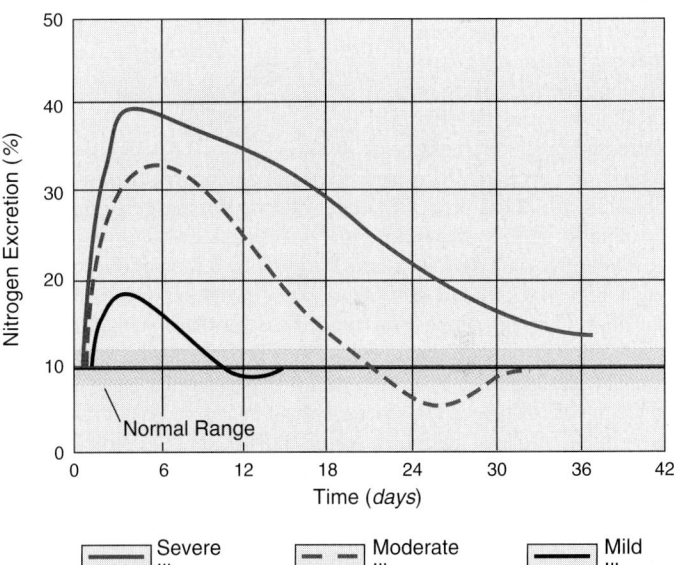

| | Severe Illness | | Moderate Illness | | Mild Illness |

Figure 2 Increased resting metabolic activity (hypermetabolism) and increased nitrogen loss are closely related during critical surgical illness. Both correlate with the severity of illness and return to normal as the patient recovers. Patients with severe illness are represented by the solid red line, those with moderate illness by the broken red line, and those with mild illness by the solid black line; the normal range is shown by the light-red bar.

20% to 25% of total calories as protein or amino acids. BUN may be higher than normal (at least 20 to 30 mg/dl) with this level of amino acid intake, even if renal function is normal.

In addition to amino acids, other intracellular constituents are released by these catabolic processes and subsequently excreted. Thus, metabolic alkalosis often develops, associated with mild hypochloremia and with reduction in total body potassium and magnesium. Repletion with potassium chloride and magnesium sulfate is usually effective. During nutritional support, generous amounts of potassium (≥ 100 mEq/day), magnesium (≥ 30 mEq/day), phosphate (20 to 30 mmol/day), and trace minerals should be provided to promote synthesis and restoration of intracellular proteins and other constituents.

Muscle mass is also lost as a result of disuse. The critically ill patient is usually confined to bed and may be further immobilized because of

Table 2 Blood Glucose and Insulin Concentrations in Burn Patients[1]

Group	N	Burn Size (% TBS)	Postburn Day Studied	Fasting Blood Glucose		Basal Insulin (µU/ml)
				(mmol/L)	(mg/dl)	
Control subjects	12	—	—	3.88 ± 0.11	69.8 ± 1.9	22 ± 3
Resuscitated burn patients	4	71	1	7.77 ± 0.61	139.9 ± 10.9	20 ± 6
Hypermetabolic burn patients	17	42	9	6.27 ± 0.28	112.9 ± 5.0	22 ± 2
Convalescing burn patients	5	56.5	69	4.05 ± 0.33	72.9 ± 5.9	14 ± 1
Septic burn patients	15	71	10	6.43 ± 0.55	115.8 ± 9.9	22 ± 4
Treated septic burn patients	4	72	11	6.11 ± 0.83	110.0 ± 15.9	12 ± 3

traction, monitoring devices, mechanical ventilation, and sedation. Massage, passive range-of-motion exercises, early mobilization, and limited bed exercises (e.g., moving from bed to chair, use of a trapeze bar to assist with positioning) may be helpful in reducing muscle wasting and debility.

GLUCOSE INTOLERANCE

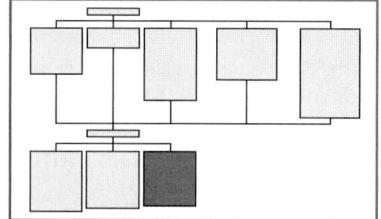

Critically ill patients usually exhibit glucose intolerance similar to that seen in diabetic patients [*see Table 2*]. Hyperglycemia during critical illness is a result of both increased production of glucose by the liver and decreased uptake of glucose by insulin-dependent tissues. These processes occur despite normal or exaggerated insulin responses to hyperglycemia.

Hyperglycemia may be marked, especially if the patient is receiving a large glucose load, such as might be provided with nutritional support. Hyperglycemia may exacerbate ventilatory insufficiency, contribute to hepatic dysfunction, and provoke osmotic diuresis, thereby leading to dehydration and a hyperosmolar state. Hyperglycemia has also been associated with an increased risk of postoperative infection, renal failure, increased transfusion requirements, and death in critically ill patients. Vigorous attempts to control the blood glucose concentration are therefore warranted.

The provision of safe amounts of glucose and the administration of exogenous recombinant human insulin are the mainstays of therapy for glucose control. Because insulin resistance is present in patients with critical illness, relatively large quantities of insulin may be required to control the blood glucose level. Intravenous administration of insulin provides rapid control and prevents unpredictable subcutaneous uptake caused by variations in blood flow. Because of its short half-life, intravenous insulin must be administered either in frequent intermittent doses or by continuous infusion. Both techniques can be used with a reasonable margin of safety. Blood glucose levels may be determined rapidly by using a portable glucose analyzer at the bedside on a small blood sample drawn every 1 or 2 hours. On the basis of the blood glucose value, a predetermined insulin dose may be administered (on a so-called sliding scale) or the infusion rate may be adjusted. Current data suggest that the optimal range for blood glucose values in critically ill surgical patients is 80 to 110 mg/dl (4.4 to 6.1 mmol/L).[12] One half to two thirds of the total insulin dose required to maintain blood glucose in this target range in a 24-hour period may be added to the intravenous feeding regimen on the next day. In this way, the blood glucose level is ultimately maintained in an acceptable range.

The degree of glucose intolerance will vary over the course of the critical illness. Therefore, regular monitoring of blood glucose concentrations is advisable, even after adequate control has been achieved. Further episodes of stress-inducing conditions, especially infection, may exacerbate glucose intolerance; an abrupt rise in blood glucose concentration may be the first indication of impending sepsis. As the patient recovers, glucose tolerance improves and the requirement for insulin decreases. When the patient is transferred from intravenous nutrition to enteral nutrition, insulin requirements often decrease despite similar nutrient intake.

Glucose remains an important fuel during critical illness, especially for healing wounds. However, the ability to utilize glucose effectively appears to be reduced. Most of the total energy administered in nutritional support should be provided by glucose (60% to 75% of total calories). The dose of glucose should, however, be limited if marked hyperglycemia cannot be readily controlled with insulin. The remaining calories can be provided by fat emulsion.

Discussion

The clinical features of all critical illnesses are similar, regardless of the type of insult sustained, be it injury, operation, or infection. Similar responses can be seen in a wide variety of animals that have been injured or challenged by invasive infection.[13,14] These responses to critical illness presumably evolved because they confer an advantage with respect to survival. In fact, it seems indisputable that when an individual organism acquires an enhanced ability to recover from an injury or infection, the species is thereby benefited. Accordingly, the metabolic responses to critical illness are often considered to be adaptive reactions that serve to promote recovery.

There is a cost for this benefit, however, and that is debility. In addition, the metabolic responses to critical illness can lead to organ system dysfunction. Critically ill patients also typically have immunologic abnormalities that may make them more susceptible to invasive infection by a variety of microorganisms, including those that are not usually pathogenic. The syndrome of multiorgan failure and sepsis that may develop in association with the metabolic responses to critical illness is often the final route to death [*see 6:13 Multiple Organ Dysfunction Syndrome*]. Thus, in some ways, certain metabolic responses seem maladaptive in that they retard recovery and lead to organ failure and death.

An improved understanding of the metabolic responses to critical illness may benefit patients in two ways. First, it may facilitate the development of improved supportive therapies. Much of current critical care practice is based on our understanding of these processes and has been designed to support them. Second, a better understanding of the mechanisms underlying the metabolic responses to critical illness may lead to strategies for altering the responses so as to stimulate those features that are beneficial and promote recovery and to suppress or limit those features that are debilitating or lead to organ system dysfunction.

Integrated Metabolic Response to Critical Illness

The metabolic responses to injury and critical illness occur simultaneously. They primarily involve the liver, skeletal muscle, the gut, the kidneys, and the wound or focus of inflammation [see Figure 3]. The heart also plays a major role by providing the motive force for the high rate of blood flow that is required to support increased exchange of nutrients and other substances between organs. The central and autonomic nervous systems and endocrine tissues are mainly involved in regulation of the responses.

The wound, which may include one or more foci of infection and other sites of inflammation in addition to external injuries, plays a principal role. It acts as a large arteriovenous shunt, robbing the host of blood supply and demanding increased cardiovascular work. The wound also induces and controls profound metabolic changes, which subside as the wound heals. Tissues are broken down, presumably to provide substrates for a variety of synthetic and energy-producing processes. The cost to the patient is increased metabolic work, elevated energy requirements, erosion of lean body tissue, and debility.

The healing wound is a site of intense metabolic activity. Dissolution and removal of necrotic tissue, containment and killing of bacteria, collagen synthesis and wound repair, cellular proliferation, and restoration of tissue integrity occur, often simultaneously. These processes require energy and a variety of substrates, particularly amino acids for protein synthesis. The microenvironment of a wound is often relatively hypoxic. However, inflammatory cells have a marked capacity for glycolytic metabolism,[15] in which adenosine triphosphate (ATP) can be generated without the consumption of oxygen. This capacity persists even when oxygen delivery is sufficient. Glucose is thus the principal fuel for the healing wound. It is metabolized to lactate, which is then released into the circulation for transport to the liver.

The liver produces the additional glucose that is required by the wound. It is capable of manufacturing glucose from lactate. In this manner, glucose is recycled between the liver and the wound, and there is no net gain or loss of carbon atoms. The liver also synthesizes glucose from amino acids, principally alanine, which comes from both skeletal muscle and the gut. This mechanism is termed gluconeogenesis. The nitrogen contained in the amino acids is converted to urea and excreted. The liver also synthesizes a variety of circulating proteins in response to inflammation and infection (so-called acute-phase proteins). All of these synthetic processes require energy, produced in part by fat oxidation, and therefore contribute to a general increase in energy utilization, heat production, and metabolic rate.

Skeletal muscle protein breaks down at an accelerated rate after injury and critical illness, releasing a variety of substances into the circulation, including creatine and creatinine, 3-methylhistidine, potassium, magnesium, and amino acids. The amino acids serve as precursors for protein synthesis in the wound and in the liver. The released amino acids do not reflect a simple dissolution of protein. Rather, alanine and glutamine are disproportionately released. Alanine can be readily converted to glucose in the liver. Glutamine serves both as a fuel—especially for the gut and for rapidly proliferating cells, including inflammatory cells and fibroblasts—and as a precursor for renal ammonia production, which is an important mechanism for neutralizing excreted acid loads.

Although muscle tissue in healthy persons is usually quite sensitive to insulin and commonly serves as a site of glucose storage, mus-

cle is resistant to insulin after injury or critical illness, and its capacity for glucose storage is reduced significantly. This response contributes to glucose intolerance and helps direct glucose to the healing wound.

The gut was long considered to be essentially inactive during convalescence, but it now appears to play a central role in the metabolic response to critical illness [see 6:23 Nutritional Support]. During critical illness, the gut utilizes glutamine as its principal fuel, converting glutamine to alanine, which is transported to the liver by the portal circulation. More important, perhaps, the gut can be a portal of entry for bacteria and bacterial toxins, which can worsen or perpetuate critical illness [6:13 Multiple Organ Dysfunction Syndrome].

The kidneys also contribute to the generalized increase in physiologic work and energy requirements that accompanies critical illness. The kidneys must excrete an increased solute load consisting of urea, potassium, magnesium, weak acids, and other intracellular constituents. In addition, many drugs and their metabolites depend on renal excretion. Production of ammonia from glutamine may be increased to neutralize acid loads. Many of these processes require energy.

All of these regional metabolic processes occur simultaneously. The net integrated metabolic response is evident clinically as increased energy expenditure and heat production, fever, accelerated nitrogen excretion and muscle wasting, and glucose intolerance. The wound appears to exert a controlling influence on the intensity and duration of the responses to critical illness or injury: the intensity is proportional to the size of the wound or the mass of inflammatory tissue. The larger the wound, the more intense the metabolic responses. As the wound heals and as inflammation subsides, the heightened metabolic demands abate. Expeditious wound closure and definitive treatment of infection are the most effective forms of anticatabolic therapy.

Hypermetabolism

Because humans maintain fairly constant body temperature, the heat generated by the body is equal to the heat lost in biochemical and physiologic processes and is an indicator of overall metabolic activity. This heat ultimately results from the oxidation of organic fuels. The rate of heat production, or metabolic rate (MR), is therefore related to $\dot{V}O_2$ and $\dot{V}CO_2$. It may be measured directly by means of direct calorimetry, or it may be calculated from measurements of $\dot{V}O_2$, $\dot{V}CO_2$, and body surface area (BSA) by means of indirect calorimetry:

$$\text{MR (kcal/m}^2\text{/hr)} = \frac{[(3.9 \times \dot{V}O_2 \text{ [L/min]}) + (1.1 \times \dot{V}CO_2 \text{ [L/min]})] \times 60 \text{ (min/hr)}}{\text{BSA (m}^2)}$$

A third term, $-3.3 \times$ urea nitrogen loss (g/time), is sometimes added to account for the heat produced by urea formation. However, it is usually a small factor, adjusting MR by only 2% to 3%.[16]

Values determined by direct and indirect calorimetry under steady-state conditions are comparable.[17] When metabolic rates of normal individuals are determined under controlled basal conditions, the values are reproducible and predictable ($\pm 12\%$) on the basis of age, sex, and body size.[18] When metabolic rates of critically ill patients with satisfactory hemodynamic function are determined under similar conditions, the rates are greater than predicted. Thus, patients are said to be hypermetabolic.

The degree of hypermetabolism is proportional to the severity of illness. This phenomenon was most dramatically demonstrated in careful studies of burn patients performed in the 1970s.[19] The increase in resting metabolic rate was proportional to the extent of tissue injury—that is, to the amount of the BSA that was burned. Hypermetabolism has also been demonstrated in a variety of other critically ill patients, but it has usually been less severe than that seen in patients with major burns.[20]

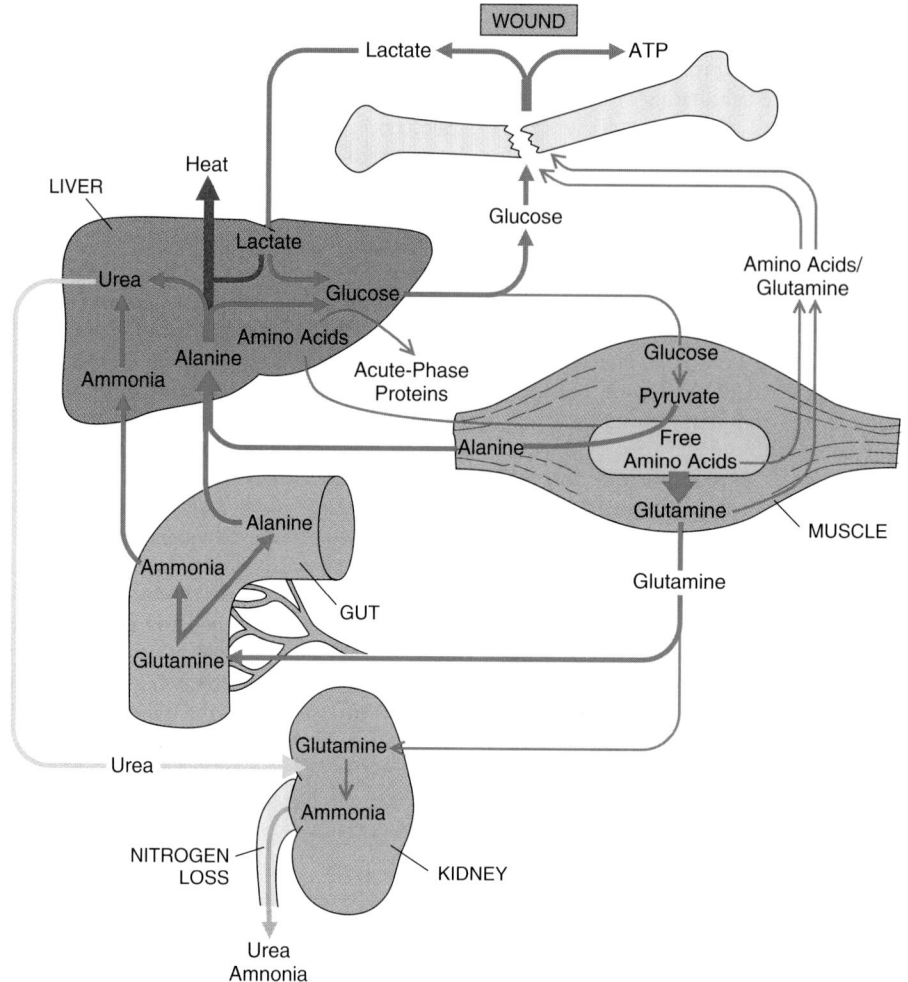

Figure 3 **The metabolic response to critical illness includes characteristic alterations in the exchange of substrates between organs. Presumably, these responses occur in support of the healing wound and are facilitated by a hyperdynamic circulation. The wound requires glucose (and probably glutamine) as a primary respiratory fuel. Glucose is converted to lactate; this conversion can occur in an aerobic environment. Lactate is transported to the liver for conversion back into glucose. The recycling of lactate to glucose is a major pathway that requires the input of energy and thereby contributes to increased energy utilization. Most of the glucose required for the healing wound (i.e., inflammatory tissue) is produced by the liver, not only from lactate but also from alanine and other glucogenic amino acids. These reactions require energy and also result in the formation of urea. Muscle is the major source of amino acids, which are used for protein synthesis both in the wound and in the liver. The most abundant amino acids released from muscle are alanine and glutamine. Glutamine serves as a primary fuel for the gut, producing ammonia and other products (e.g., alanine) that are processed by the liver. In addition, glutamine may help buffer filtered acid loads in the kidneys by the formation of ammonia. These metabolic processes contribute to the hypermetabolism, hyperdynamic circulation, increased nitrogen loss, and glucose intolerance that are clinically evident in critically ill patients.**

In the burn patients, moreover, there was a limit to the hypermetabolism: metabolic rates of patients with extensive burns were little different from those of patients with burns covering 50% to 60% of BSA.

These observations suggest that there is a limit to the metabolic activity that patients can support in response to critical illness. The difference between this limit and the magnitude of the patient's actual responses defines physiologic reserve [*see Figure 4*]. Physiologic reserve is presumably also affected by the patient's age and state of health before the critical illness. It reflects the patient's ability to meet additional complicating stresses, such as infection, volume loss, pain, anxiety, and cold ambient temperatures. For example, when patients are exposed to progressively colder ambient temperatures, the metabolic rate generally increases. However, when a group of patients

with very large burns were exposed to cold temperatures, their already high metabolic rates did not increase but actually fell.[19] None of these patients survived the injury, presumably because of inability to respond to new stresses. In another group of burn patients, the inability to increase metabolic rate to facilitate rewarming after skin grafting procedures also identified nonsurvivors.[21] When patients are cared for in a warm environment, hypermetabolism is reduced and physiologic reserve is increased.

Hypermetabolism refers to an increase in total body oxidative metabolism that is manifested by increases in total body $\dot{V}O_2$, cardiac output, and MR. Regional $\dot{V}O_2$ is generally increased throughout most tissue beds, but regional blood flow is not. The additional total body flow is directed largely to the wound or site of inflammation and to the splanchnic circulation, and it appears to supply the wound with increased amounts of glucose and other nutrients. In studies of patients who had sustained a large burn on one leg and no burn on the other, Wilmore and colleagues found that $\dot{V}o_2$ of both limbs was increased in proportion to the total BSA burned and represented a fairly constant 6% of total body $\dot{V}o_2$.[22] However, blood flow to the injured extremity was approximately twice that to the uninjured limb. Blood flow was proportional to the extent of the local injury and was directed to the surface wound.[23]

Oxygen consumption by the splanchnic and renal circulations also increases in proportion to total body $\dot{V}o_2$ and hence in proportion to total body injury.[24] Splanchnic flow increases in proportion to total body flow (cardiac output), and together with the blood flow to the wound, it accounts for a large part of the increase in cardiac output in critically ill patients.[25] The increase in renal blood flow correlates with solute load rather than with $\dot{V}o_2$. From these and other studies, it is possible to calculate how oxygen consumption and cardiac output are partitioned among different vascular beds.[26]

Altered Temperature Regulation

Body temperature is determined by the balance between heat production and heat loss. It is normally closely regulated and maintained within a narrow range. Critically ill patients typically have an elevated body temperature, even in the absence of clinical infection.[27] Heat production, as measured by metabolic rate, is increased in the critically ill patient. Heat loss may also be elevated in these patients.

It was once thought that increased evaporative heat loss was the driving force for hypermetabolism, at least in burn patients.[28,29] Barr and associates tested this assumption.[30] Although patients treated in warm, dry air showed substantially increased evaporation of water from the burn wound and more rapid drying of the wound surfaces than did patients exposed to normal ward conditions, they had reduced hypermetabolism and a smaller degree of weight loss.

Several other studies have examined the relation between thermoregulatory factors (evaporative heat loss and ambient temperature) and hypermetabolism. For example, the metabolic rates of burn patients were determined at several ambient temperatures, ranging from 19° to 33° C (66.2° to 91.4° F) [see Table 3].[31] Metabolic rate decreased as ambient temperature was increased, but core temperature remained elevated at all ambient temperatures, indicating that thermoregulation in these patients occurred in relation to an elevated central reference temperature. When febrile burn patients in another study were allowed to set the ambient temperature to achieve thermal comfort, they invariably preferred higher than normal temperatures, in the range of 30° to 33° C (86.0° to 91.4° F).[32] The patients' unburned skin remained relatively vasoconstricted at the higher temperatures as an additional way of maintaining the febrile state. However, even under these conditions of thermal comfort, the patients continued to maintain elevated metabolic rates. Thus, although thermoregulatory factors may influence hypermetabolism, the increased rate of heat production appears to be determined primarily by metabolic factors. Hypermetabolism is temperature sensitive but not temperature dependent.

Altered Protein Metabolism

MUSCLE WASTING, NITROGEN LOSS, AND ACCELERATED
PROTEIN BREAKDOWN

One of the most striking features of the metabolic response to critical illness is the marked degree of muscle wasting. This atrophy is associated with increased urinary excretion of nitrogen. Sir David Cuth-

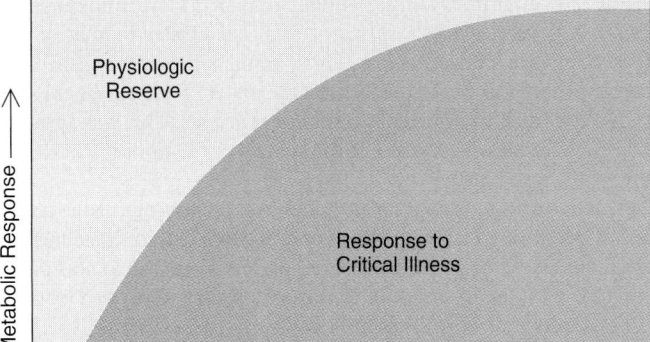

Figure 4 **The intensity of the metabolic response to critical surgical illness increases as a function of the severity of illness. In patients with extremely severe critical illness (e.g., patients with burns covering 60% of the body surface area), responses are near maximal, and physiologic reserves, with which patients respond to additional stressors (e.g., infection, hemorrhage, or cold exposure), are limited. Patients may also have limited physiologic reserves because of preexisting disease, starvation, or advanced age. Therapies that attenuate the stressors of critical surgical illness improve physiologic reserve.**

bertson first described this phenomenon in patients with long-bone fractures.[27] Similar observations were made by Howard and associates in the United States.[33] Cuthbertson concluded that injured and uninjured skeletal muscle was the source of the excreted nitrogen.[34,35] As skeletal muscle protein is degraded, a variety of markers are released into the circulation and then excreted by the kidneys. Increased excretion of several of these markers[36,37] has been observed in patients with trauma,[36,38] burns,[39] and infections.[40]

There are other sources of nitrogen loss in critically ill patients, including loss of tissue from slough or excision, loss of blood and exudate, and loss of mucosa from the GI tract. Cuthbertson estimated that in the first 10 days after a burn, the amounts of nitrogen lost as a result of direct tissue injury, wound exudation, generalized catabolism, and atrophy were roughly equivalent.[41] Moore and coworkers measured nitrogen loss in the wound exudate of burn patients. This wound loss accounted for as much as 20% to 30% of total nitrogen loss during the early postburn period.[42]

The time course of nitrogen excretion during critical illness is

Table 3 Effect of Ambient Temperature on Metabolic Rate and on Core and Skin Temperatures

Ambient Temperature (°C)	N	Core Temperature (°C)	Skin Temperature (°C)	Metabolic Rate (kcal/m²/hr)
Normal subjects				
21	3	36.7	30.0	41.2
25	4	36.8	31.4	35.6
33	4	36.8	34.2	36.3
Burn patients (45% TBS)				
21	9	38.1	32.1	83.7
25	20	38.5	33.1	63.5
33	20	38.0	36.2	62.0

distinctive. Cuthbertson observed that nitrogen excretion peaked several days after injury and gradually returned to normal during a period of several weeks.[34] The pattern was similar to that of increased oxygen consumption. Thus, both hypermetabolism and muscle proteolysis peak shortly after the onset of critical illness and gradually return to normal as recovery proceeds. This too appears to be a characteristic feature of the metabolic responses to critical illness [see Figure 2].[43-45]

Protein turnover is an indicator of overall protein metabolic activity. It is determined through use of tracers. Both extracellular and intracellular amino acids are considered part of a free amino acid pool. Nitrogen is added to this pool by nitrogen intake (diet) and by protein breakdown. Nitrogen is removed by protein synthesis and by conversion to urea. When a small quantity of a labeled amino acid is infused, the rate of appearance of nitrogen in the free amino acid pool can be determined. Under steady-state conditions, this appearance rate represents protein turnover and matches protein disappearance.[46] During critical illness, protein turnover is increased.[47] When nitrogen turnover data are combined with measurements of nitrogen intake and loss, rates of total body protein synthesis and catabolism can be estimated. These estimates indicate that protein catabolism is increased in critically ill patients.[48] Synthesis rates remain normal during fasting but increase to approach or match catabolic rates when feeding is adequate. Thus, the increase in net nitrogen loss during critical illness appears to result from an increase in protein breakdown. Decreased protein synthesis is less of a factor as long as nutritional intake is satisfactory [see Table 4].

ALTERED AMINO ACID METABOLISM

Protein synthesis and breakdown are processes that occur in cells and involve intracellular amino acids. It has been estimated that skeletal muscle contains as much as 80% of the free amino acid pool.[49] Intracellular concentrations of free amino acids in skeletal muscle are approximately 30 times greater than plasma concentrations of free amino acids.[50] Thus, the total muscle mass of a 70 kg man contains approximately 87 g of free amino acids in the intracellular water, whereas the extracellular pool contains only 1.2 g.

The relative amounts of individual free amino acids in cells differ from the proportions found in protein. Glutamine, a nonessential amino acid, accounts for only about 5% to 6% of protein, but it is the most abundant intracellular free amino acid, accounting for about 60% of the total intracellular free amino acid pool. In contrast, the eight essential amino acids together account for only 8.4% of the intracellular pool. The intracellular concentration of glutamine decreases under many catabolic conditions, including starvation, inactivity,[51] elective operation,[52] trauma,[53] and sepsis.[54] This decrease occurs early in the course of the acute illness, persists until late in convalescence, and appears to be related to the severity of illness.[55,56] The intracellular concentrations of phenylalanine, tyrosine, alanine, and the branched-chain amino acids (BCAAs)—leucine, isoleucine, and valine—typically increase after trauma and infection.[51,54] These levels return to normal during convalescence, usually before glutamine levels do.

Plasma concentrations of free amino acids generally decrease after operation, injury, or infection, largely because of a fall in the concentrations of the nonessential amino acids. Changes in extracellular concentrations of specific amino acids have been inconsistent between studies, presumably as a reflection of differences in patient selection, analytic methods, or treatment.[54]

The ECF compartment is important for amino acid transport between organs and between regions of the body. Aulick and Wilmore calculated amino acid release rates from peripheral tissues of burn patients on the basis of measurements of leg blood flow and of femoral arterial and venous plasma concentrations of 10 amino

Table 4 Alterations in Rates of Protein Synthesis and Catabolism That May Affect Hospitalized Patients

	Synthesis	Catabolism
Normal—starvation	↓	0
Normal—fed, bed rest	↓	0
Elective surgical procedure	↓	0
Injury/sepsis—I.V. dextrose	↑↑	↑↑↑
Injury/sepsis—fed	↑↑↑	↑↑↑

↓—decrease   ↑—increase   0—no change

acids.[57] The net release of amino acid nitrogen was five times greater in burn patients than in control subjects. Alanine was the only amino acid whose release rate was significantly elevated (glutamine concentration was not determined). Alanine release was related to total burn size (injury severity) and to total body $\dot{V}O_2$. In related studies, the accelerated peripheral amino acid release was matched by increased uptake across the splanchnic bed.[24] Alanine uptake was three to four times control values. This increased release of amino acids from the periphery and transport to splanchnic tissues appears to be another characteristic metabolic response to critical burn injury.

Garber and colleagues observed that glutamine and alanine together constituted as much as 70% of the amino acids released from skeletal muscle in vitro.[58] Furthermore, the release rates of alanine and glutamine reflected the net rates of formation from other amino acids.[59] Thus, during critical illness, skeletal muscle protein is broken down into amino acids that are largely converted to glutamine and alanine, which are then released into the ECF for transport. Although all amino acids are required for protein synthesis at remote locations, glutamine and alanine are the major nitrogen carriers from muscle. These two amino acids have other roles as well. Alanine is a precursor of glucose production in the liver. In that process, urea is also formed and subsequently excreted by the kidneys. Although there may be some minor recycling of urea nitrogen under certain conditions,[60] formation of urea is the final step in the loss of body protein, representing an irreversible loss of nitrogen.

Glutamine is a precursor for production of ammonia in the kidneys, an important buffering mechanism for excreted acid loads. Increased breakdown of intracellular constituents could result in such an acid load, and ammonia excretion is often increased after injury. Intracellular skeletal muscle glutamine may be an important determinant of net skeletal muscle protein breakdown.[61,62] After a standard operation in an animal model, net amino acid efflux from the hindquarter was increased as the glutamine concentration fell. However, if the intracellular glutamine concentration was maintained by the provision of exogenous glutamine, net efflux was reduced.

Glutamine also appears to be an important respiratory fuel for rapidly dividing cells. Glutamine can be converted to glutamate and then to α-ketoglutarate for participation in the citric acid cycle. The nitrogen of glutamine is used to form ammonia, alanine, and citrulline.[63] This process occurs in colonocytes, enterocytes, fibroblasts, and, possibly, inflammatory cells such as macrophages. Phagocytic cells are found in fixed locations in the GI tract, such as Peyer's patches and other regions containing Kupffer's cells, as well as in the wound, at other sites of inflammation, and in the bone marrow. Windmueller measured the nutrient requirements of the rat intestine using an isolated, perfused segment of small bowel.[63] The intestinal segment extracted large amounts of glutamine from the recirculated perfusate. Souba and Wilmore measured amino acid uptake by the gut in conscious animals and demonstrated that the consumption of glutamine by the gut was significantly increased after celiotomy, even though the circulating glutamine concentration was reduced (i.e., glutamine was actively taken up by the intestine).[64]

Dissolution of skeletal muscle protein during critical illness seems to serve many purposes. First, it provides amino acids to support protein synthesis at remote sites such as the wound, other inflammatory foci, and the liver. Proteolysis also provides amino acid precursors for glucose production by the liver and for production of ammonia in the kidneys. Finally, it provides glutamine, which appears to be a specific fuel for the gut and possibly for other tissues with rapid cell turnover, such as the wound, bone marrow, and fixed macrophages of the GI tract. This mobilization of amino acids from muscle protein, however, leads to an irretrievable loss of nitrogen in the form of urea, ammonia, creatinine, uric acid, and other compounds. The cost to the patient is rapid erosion of muscle mass and debility.

Altered Carbohydrate Metabolism

ACCELERATED ENDOGENOUS GLUCOSE PRODUCTION

The liver normally produces sufficient glucose to permit maintenance of the blood glucose concentration within narrow limits, even during periods of fasting. During critical illness, the rate of endogenous glucose production is increased.[24,65,66] Increased basal glucose production is matched by an increase in glucose uptake, so that glucose levels remain relatively stable. Thus, the mass flow, or turnover, of glucose is increased. In studies of patients with burns, glucose turnover was related to total body $\dot{V}o_2$ and thus to the size of the burn (i.e., to injury severity).[67] Regional uptake was closely related to regional blood flow and regional lactate release but not to regional $\dot{V}o_2$. Thus, glucose was directed by the circulation to the wound, where it was taken up and converted via glycolysis to lactate, even in the presence of adequate or increased oxygen delivery.

The liver produces glucose by a variety of mechanisms. Hydrolysis of hepatic glycogen mobilizes glucose rapidly to serve as an energy source in times of acute need. This mechanism is most important immediately after injury and during acute stress states, such as shock, fever, pain, and anxiety (ebb-phase responses). Glycogen reserves are limited, however, and glycogen is not the major source of hepatic glucose production during recovery from critical illness.

Glucose can also be formed from lactate and from alanine.[68] The conversion of lactate to glucose occurs via the Cori cycle in the liver. Lactate is formed from pyruvate, which is the end product of glycolysis. In critically ill patients with adequate oxygen delivery, the wound is a major source of lactate. Adenosine triphosphate (ATP) is formed during glycolysis and provides energy for the wound, but ATP is required to convert lactate back to glucose. The increased mass flow of glucose serves as a fuel for the healing wound. It may also reflect an inefficient biochemical cycle that requires energy but in which there is no net gain or loss of substrate. Accelerated glucose cycling has been documented both in burn patients and in blunt trauma patients.[69,70] The purpose of these so-called futile cycles is not clear. Because they result in the net generation of heat, they presumably contribute to hypermetabolism. That overall conversion requires net input of ATP and is thus another energy drain for the patient.

GLUCOSE INTOLERANCE AND INSULIN RESISTANCE

When glucose is administered to critically ill patients, hyperglycemia often results. Glucose tolerance tests typically yield abnormal results after injury.[71] During shock, immediately after injury or operation, and in the course of ebb-phase responses, the insulin response to hyperglycemia may be blunted. During the flow phase, however, after resuscitation and stabilization, the response to glucose is normal or even exaggerated.[72,73] Both glucose and insulin levels are higher in trauma patients than in control subjects [see Table 5], and the increase in insulin is proportionally greater than the rise in glucose.

Black and associates maintained a fixed level of hyperglycemia in patients recovering from trauma by adjusting a glucose infusion on the basis of bedside glucose readings and a negative-feedback algorithm.[74] Because the glucose concentration was at steady state, the glucose infusion rate reflected the rate of total body glucose uptake or disposal. Control subjects demonstrated continuously increasing glucose disposal over time; the glucose infusion rate was increased repeatedly to maintain fixed hyperglycemia. Glucose disposal was closely related to insulin concentration, which increased steadily during the 2-hour study. In contrast, glucose disposal in trauma patients was markedly lower than in control subjects, and it did not increase appreciably over time. The insulin concentrations did, however, increase throughout the study and were always greater than corresponding control values. The trauma patients were therefore less responsive (i.e., were resistant) to insulin.

These investigators also infused insulin into trauma patients and control subjects to maintain specific fixed levels of hyperinsulinemia. During these infusions, the glucose concentration was maintained at basal values (i.e., euglycemia). The glucose infusion rate again reflected total body glucose disposal, which was a function of tissue responsiveness to the insulin level. At all insulin levels, glucose disposal was lower in trauma patients than in control subjects. These studies quantitated posttraumatic insulin resistance and suggested that this response was caused by a postreceptor defect. In similar conditions, Brooks and associates demonstrated reduced forearm glucose uptake, indicating that peripheral tissue—principally skeletal muscle—was a major site of insulin resistance[75] [see Table 6].

ALTERED FUEL METABOLISM

The studies by Black and associates[74] demonstrated that in recovering trauma patients, there is an upper limit to glucose disposal of 5 to 6 mg/kg/min, despite hyperglycemia and hyperinsulinemia. Additional studies have confirmed that critically ill patients are limited in their ability to utilize glucose as a fuel. Long and coworkers studied the effect of increasing carbohydrate intake on net nitrogen loss in recovering burn patients.[76] They found that nitrogen loss was reduced as carbohydrate was increased to 60% to 70% of total caloric needs (also approximately 5 to 6 mg/kg/min). Very little additional reduction in nitrogen loss was observed with higher carbohydrate levels. Wolfe and associates used isotope-labeled glucose to measure glucose oxidation in postoperative[77] and burn patients[66,78] and found that both groups exhibited an upper limit of glucose oxidation. These studies also suggested that maximum glucose oxidation is inversely related to injury severity.

Lipid metabolism is also affected by critical illness. In an elegant series of kinetic studies performed in blunt trauma patients, Shaw and Wolfe[70] documented a greater than twofold increase in glycerol turnover, reflecting an accelerated rate of triglyceride hydrolysis to form free fatty acid (FFA) and glycerol. They also demonstrated a doubling of FFA oxidation rate; however, the measured turnover of FFA was only 30% greater than the control value, which suggested that some of the FFA released from triglyceride was oxidized in the

Table 5   Basal Glucose and Insulin Concentrations*

	N	Plasma Glucose (mg/dl)	Serum Insulin (μU/ml)
Normal subjects	49	98 ± 1	12 ± 1
Trauma patients	19	104 ± 2	17 ± 2
P		< 0.02	< 0.01

*Mean ± SEM.

cell and did not enter the circulating pool. These studies further demonstrated a high rate of FFA recycling, a phenomenon also described in burn patients.[69]

Askanazi and associates studied the metabolic effects of hypercaloric, glucose-based total parenteral nutrition (TPN) on starved patients.[79] Patients who were nutritionally depleted but were not critically ill showed an increase in $\dot{V}_{CO_2}$ and an increase in the respiratory quotient (RQ, the ratio of $\dot{V}_{CO_2}$ to $\dot{V}_{O_2}$) to 1.0 or greater. These findings indicated that these patients were able to meet all of their energy needs with glucose and that fat oxidation was suppressed. Patients who were depleted and also manifested hypermetabolic responses showed an increase not only in $\dot{V}_{CO_2}$ but also in $\dot{V}_{O_2}$, and the RQ remained below 1.0; therefore, these critically ill patients could not meet all of their energy needs by oxidation of glucose. Not only was there a limit to the ability of these critically ill patients to use glucose as a metabolic fuel, but the high glucose load intensified hypermetabolism as well. Thus, overfeeding with glucose can aggravate critical illness. The mechanisms of this phenomenon are not clear, but they may involve the futile cycling of glucose via fructose 1,6-diphosphate and its associated heat generation.[69]

In addition to protein, nutritional support of critically ill patients often consists of a mixture of carbohydrate and fat to meet energy requirements. In such a system, exogenous carbohydrate is oxidized directly, but exogenous lipid is added to body fat stores.[80] Lipid is mobilized from these endogenous stores for oxidation. Such a mixed-fuel preparation should provide sufficient glucose for those tissues that require it (i.e., central nervous system, renal medulla, hematopoietic cells, and inflammatory cells), prevent excessive hyperglycemia, stimulate insulin elaboration, and approach nitrogen equilibrium.

Systemic Mediators

It was once generally thought that the metabolic alterations associated with injury and critical illness were derived from some harmful substance (e.g., a toxin) or dysfunctional process (e.g., a deranged endocrine mechanism). We now appreciate that the regulatory mechanisms affecting these processes are intricate and highly complex and depend on the actions of a myriad of mediators that influence the proliferation, development, and behavior of cells. It is hard to judge which, if any, of these mediators is maladaptive or harmful: those that seem to have harmful effects that exacerbate debility and organ dysfunction in some settings often promote healing and recovery in others.

These mediators may be synthesized by one or many cell types. Some mediators may affect the cell that made them, thus exerting an autocrine effect. Others may affect cells in close proximity, thus exerting a paracrine effect. If they gain access to the ECF, they can be transported via the circulation and affect cells far removed from their site of origin, thus exerting an endocrine effect. Most interact with a specific receptor, usually on the surface of the target cell. This molecular interaction can influence the cell's biology in a number of ways.

First, it may alter the cell membrane, affecting its permeability to certain substances or changing the availability or affinity of other receptors for interaction with their specific mediators. Second, it may alter the structural organization of the cell, making certain intracellular constituents more or less available to exert their effects on cell behavior. Finally, it may initiate one of several intracellular molecular mechanisms that ultimately affect the nucleus, thereby altering gene expression for protein synthesis or DNA replication and cell proliferation.

These mediators have been categorized as endocrine hormones, inflammatory mediators, and growth factors. But as our knowledge about them has grown, it has become apparent that the distinctions are not always clear-cut, and some mediators can fit in more than one category. For example, the hormone insulin exerts definite endocrine metabolic effects that are well known, but it is also an important growth factor. Insulin receptors have been identified in embryos and in plants, and insulin is an important constituent of many cell culture media.[81] Insulin may also affect certain inflammatory responses. In a 2002 study, otherwise normal subjects manifested enhanced and prolonged hemodynamic and cytokine responses to endotoxin under conditions of hyperinsulinemia and euglycemia.[82]

The metabolic response to critical illness is a clinical phenomenon that dominates the clinical presentation and course of critically ill patients. It involves alterations that affect either the whole body or specific organ systems. In what follows, I discuss several ways in which these clinical events may be regulated.

HORMONES

During critical illness, the concentrations of several hormones are altered. The levels of the counterregulatory or so-called stress hormones—cortisol, glucagon, and the catecholamines epinephrine and norepinephrine—are typically increased. These hormones have several direct and indirect effects and appear to function as important regulating signals in the response to critical illness.

The sympathetic-adrenal axis is one of the major systems by which the body initiates responses to critical illness. It also modifies the elaboration and effects of other hormones and thus serves as a link between the central nervous system and the endocrinologic organs. Many of the changes in vital signs observed during critical illness, such as tachycardia, tachypnea, and widened pulse pressure, are ascribed to adrenergic and catecholamine effects; in addition, many of the signs of shock indicate autonomic overactivity. The catecholamine levels are increased in proportion to the severity of injury.[83] During the flow phase of critical illness, concentrations of the catecholamines may be persistently elevated; catecholamine turnover after burn injury is markedly increased.[44,84] $\dot{V}_{O_2}$ and metabolic rate have been directly related to the excretion of catecholamines. In one study, alpha- and beta-adrenergic blockade significantly reduced the metabolic rate in burn patients, although the rate did not return to control levels.[19] This effect was not produced by alpha-adrenergic blockade alone, which indicates that beta-adrenergic stimulation

Table 6 Glucose Disposal and Forearm Glucose Uptake during Hyperinsulinemia and Euglycemia

Target Dose	N	Plasma Glucose Concentration (mg/dl)	Serum Insulin Concentration (μU/ml)	Glucose Disposal Rate (mg/kg/min)	Arterial–Deep Venous Glucose Difference (mg/dl)	Forearm Glucose Uptake (mg/dl/min)
Normal subjects						
100 μU/ml	7	92 ± 2	106 ± 6	9.32 ± 1.04	21 ± 3	0.76 ± 0.12
200 μU/ml	6	92 ± 2	183 ± 19	8.91 ± 0.78	26 ± 4	1.10 ± 0.11
Injured patients						
200 μU/ml	4	97 ± 1	145 ± 11	5.29 ± 0.80	8 ± 4	0.36 ± 18
500 μU/ml	1	117	506	5.79	2	0.20

predominates in the flow phase of the response to critical illness.

The sympathetic-adrenal axis also affects the endocrine pancreas. Porte and Robertson determined that the insulin response to glucose in normal individuals was reduced substantially with alpha-adrenergic stimulation but was enhanced with beta-adrenergic stimulation.[85] Catecholamines may also modulate the peripheral action of insulin. When epinephrine was infused into normal individuals at doses low enough to allow beta-adrenergic effects to predominate, insulin resistance was observed in uninjured forearm tissue.[86] Despite its apparent catabolic effects on metabolic rate and insulin resistance, epinephrine alone reduces the release of amino acid from skeletal muscle in vitro.[87]

Cortisol[88] and glucagon[89] levels are elevated after major injury and during critical illness. The degree of elevation appears to be related to the extent or severity of the injury. An increased cortisol level is associated with glucose intolerance.[90] Patients with Cushing's syndrome manifest reduced muscle mass and loss of protein from the skin. Owen and Cahill administered hydrocortisone to starved obese patients.[91] Although they observed an increase in ammonia excretion and a decrease in urea excretion, there was no net change in total nitrogen loss. Glucagon promotes gluconeogenesis.[92] This effect may be overcome by increased concentrations of insulin.[93] Wolfe and colleagues administered glucagon to fasting normal individuals and observed a slight increase in nitrogen excretion, primarily as urea.[94] However, net nitrogen loss from peripheral tissues did not increase.

Although injury and critical illness clearly affect hormone levels, it has not been possible to ascribe all of the physiologic responses observed in patients to the known actions of individual hormones. A number of studies, however, have identified interacting effects by altering more than one hormone level simultaneously. For example, when Shamoon and coworkers infused a combination of hydrocortisone, glucagon, and epinephrine, they observed a synergistic effect on glucose production.[95]

Bessey and associates extended these observations.[96] In an attempt to simulate the endocrine environment of injured patients, they infused the same combination of hormones for 3 days in normal individuals. The infusion maintained elevated catabolic hormone levels, similar to those observed in patients with mild to moderate injury. The investigators monitored a variety of metabolic parameters and compared these results with measurements obtained in a control study of the same individuals, in which the patients received an infusion of saline. The alteration in the hormonal environment increased the resting heart and respiratory rates, widened the pulse pressure, and slightly elevated the rectal temperature. In addition, hypermetabolism, a negative potassium balance, increased endogenous glucose production, insulin resistance, sodium retention, and leukocytosis were observed [see Table 7]. During the control study, the individuals maintained nitrogen equilibrium, but during the triple-hormone infusion, they were in persistently negative nitrogen balance, even though nutritional intake was identical in the two studies. Whole body protein turnover, as measured by ^{15}N kinetics, was increased in the subjects who received the hormone infusion because of an increase in protein catabolism. These changes, which are typically seen in critically ill patients, occurred in the absence of a wound or inflammatory focus.

The negative nitrogen balance and increased turnover of whole body protein observed during the triple-hormone infusion were also associated with a significant decrease in total intracellular amino acid nitrogen in skeletal muscle.[97] This decrease was caused primarily by a fall in the intracellular glutamine level. Although these changes suggest that the posttraumatic hormonal environment plays a causative role in increasing net muscle proteolysis, the triple-hormone infusion did not appreciably alter either whole blood amino acid concentra-

tions or amino acid efflux from the forearm. A potential explanation for these findings is that the triple-hormone infusion, particularly the glucagon component, may have affected processing of amino acid by the liver, thereby reducing the net retention of dietary amino acids.[98]

The endocrine environment in critically ill patients, however, is not static. Although catabolic hormone levels may be persistently elevated, insulin is often suppressed during the early phases of critical illness but elevated later, during the flow phase. Bessey and Lowe attempted to simulate this changing hormonal environment in normal subjects by administering a somatostatin analogue during the first 24 hours of a 3-day infusion of catabolic hormones so as to inhibit the elaboration of insulin in response to hyperglycemia.[99] They compared the findings to those obtained from studies of the same individuals during triple-hormone infusion, when insulin levels were allowed to rise unchecked. Early whole body nitrogen loss was increased in the studies with the somatostatin analogue, but there was no difference in forearm nitrogen release at 24 hours; however, 2 days later, when glucose and insulin concentrations were similar in the two studies, total body nitrogen loss was equivalent, but forearm nitrogen release was increased in the patients receiving the somatostatin analogue. Coadministration of exogenous insulin with somatostatin prevented this acceleration of net muscle protein breakdown (P. Q. Bessey, K. A. Lowe, D. C. Blake; unpublished data). Thus, the interacting effects of multiple hormones and the changing relationships among them over time appear to be capable of inducing, at least qualitatively, most of the metabolic responses to critical illness.

Several investigators have attempted to modulate the catabolic responses of critical illness by altering the endocrine environment. For example, Hulton and colleagues monitored hind-leg amino acid efflux after abdominal operation in an animal model.[100] The accelerated efflux of skeletal muscle amino acids observed postoperatively was attenuated by complete alpha- and beta-adrenergic blockade or by thoracic epidural anesthesia. Both pharmacologic techniques are known to attenuate the hormonal response to operative stress. Brandt and coworkers measured hormonal and protein catabolic responses after abdominal hysterectomy.[101] In the patients who underwent epidural anesthesia, concentrations of cortisol and catecholamines were lower and nitrogen loss was less than in patients who received general anesthesia alone. Tsuji and associates reported similar findings.[102] Subsequent studies have shown that perioperative management of patients with high thoracic epidural analgesia and intravenous somatostatin and etomidate to inhibit elaboration of glucagon and cortisol prevents the typical postoperative increases in amino acid clearance and urea synthesis.[103]

In summary, the altered endocrine environment characteristically

Table 7 Effect of Infusion of Cortisol, Glucagon, and Epinephrine on Metabolism

	Saline	Hormones*
Metabolic rate (kcal/m²/hr)	32.24 ± 1.05	38.42 ± 1.31
Nitrogen balance (g/day)	−0.2 ± 0.4	−3.2 ± 0.4
Protein catabolic rate (g nitrogen/day)	38.4 ± 1.9	46.5 ± 2.5
Plasma glucose (mg/dl)	94 ± 2	133 ± 4
Serum insulin (μU/ml)	8 ± 1	22 ± 3
Glucose production rate (mg/kg/min)	2.08 ± 0.06	2.55 ± 0.06
Insulin-mediated glucose disposal (mg/kg/min)	8.62 ± 0.51	3.22 ± 0.51
Insulin-mediated forearm glucose uptake (mg/dl/min)	1.03 ± 0.09	0.48 ± 0.12

*All significantly different from control values.

associated with critical illness and the influence of the sympathoadrenal axis appear to play a major role in mediating the metabolic responses observed in critically ill surgical patients. Simple alteration of the stress hormonal environment in healthy individuals is capable of inducing many of these metabolic changes; however, the magnitude of these changes is generally less than that observed in critically ill patients. Blunting of the stress hormonal changes after operation or injury can modulate acute catabolic responses.

Although changes in stress hormones seem to dominate the clinical picture, characteristic alterations of other endocrine hormones also occur. Levels of thyroxine (T_4) and triiodothyronine (T_3) are typically reduced after critical illness, and levels of an inactive form of T_3, reverse T_3 (rT_3), are elevated; however, administration of thyroxine to critically ill patients seems to have little clinical effect.[104] Hormones of the gonadal axis are typically suppressed during critical illness. Levels of testosterone are decreased in men, as are levels of luteinizing hormone, follicle-stimulating hormone, and estradiol in women, apparently in proportion to injury severity.[105-107] These changes interrupt the menstrual cycle and decrease libido. Although growth hormone (GH) levels are increased after injury, patients demonstrate muscle wasting and weight loss.[108] The anabolic effects of GH depend on the synthesis and elaboration of insulinlike growth factor–1 (IGF-1), whose activity is affected also by the presence of various IGF-binding proteins (IGFBPs).[109] Despite elevation of circulating GH levels, IGF-1 concentrations are reduced, as are IGFBP-3 levels.

Taken together, all of these endocrine changes (1) mobilize amino acids and fuel substrates to support wound healing, resolution of inflammation, and tissue repair and (2) turn down anabolism and growth in the rest of the body. This response to acute illness would seem to be an adaptive one: wounds heal and patients recover, despite a transient loss of lean tissue. However, patients with protracted critical illnesses, who have been maintained for weeks or months in the ICU, may present a different clinical picture. Despite closure of the wound, drainage of pus, provision of nutrients, and treatment of infection, they remain catabolic and are extremely slow or unable to recover. Current evidence suggests that this syndrome may reflect a different endocrine pattern. Many of the anterior pituitary hormones (e.g., adrenocorticotropic hormone, thyroid-stimulating hormone, and GH) are present in reduced concentrations, or the pattern of their secretion is altered.[110] These alterations may reflect a change in hypothalamic function; infusion of various releasing factors can restore normal hormone responsiveness in the thyrotropic, somatotropic, and gonadotropic axes.[111]

CYTOKINES

A number of cell types appear in a healing wound soon after injury.[112] These cells are actively involved in angiogenesis, production and remodeling of collagen, scavenging of necrotic debris, and engulfment and killing of bacteria. Many of them release substances that influence cellular proliferation, development, and function and so regulate local inflammation and wound healing. These substances, collectively known as cytokines, can be produced by and interact with a wide variety of cells in addition to inflammatory cells and appear to be major mediators of multiple cellular responses to injury and infection.

Some cytokines primarily stimulate inflammatory responses and thus are known as proinflammatory cytokines, whereas others retard these responses and thus are known as anti-inflammatory cytokines. In addition, specific receptor antagonists have been identified that interfere with the interaction between a cytokine and its cellular receptor. Finally, there are specific soluble receptors, unassociated with a cell, that can effectively neutralize the cytokine before it interacts with

a target cell. Both proinflammatory and anti-inflammatory mechanisms may be stimulated together in acute illness.[113] The balance and interactions between them determine the course of the inflammatory process.

The major proinflammatory cytokines, tumor necrosis factor (TNF), interleukin-1 (IL-1), and IL-6, are closely related in that they are elaborated in a characteristic pattern (or cascade) in response to an inflammatory stimulus, such as trauma[114] or endotoxin.[115] TNF appears first, followed by IL-1 and then IL-6. The elaboration of TNF and IL-1 is relatively brief, but IL-6 persists longer.

Cytokines appear to regulate cell recruitment, proliferation, development, and other cellular events that occur in the wound, but how and to what extent they exert systemic effects and modulate the metabolic responses to critical illness is less clear. One conceptual model proposes that when local cytokine production is particularly abundant, owing to extensive wounds or uncontrolled infection, certain cytokines spill over into the circulation and then affect tissues at distant sites [see Figure 5]. Although elevated circulating cytokine levels have been detected in critically ill patients, only IL-6 has been consistently associated with severe illness and outcome.[116,117]

TNF can initiate the cytokine cascade, ultimately producing fever, leukocytosis, and other signs and symptoms of critical illness.[118] To characterize the role of TNF in proteolysis associated with endotoxin or sepsis, Michie and coworkers analyzed the responses of both animals and humans during prolonged infusions of TNF.[119] Negative nitrogen balance was related to the onset of anorexia and reduced food intake and not to the development of hypermetabolism. Mealy and associates performed adrenalectomies and abrogated the increase in nitrogen loss associated with TNF infusion.[120] Hall-Angeras and colleagues found that a steroid antagonist prevented the increase in myofibrillar protein breakdown usually seen in an animal model of intra-abdominal sepsis.[121] These observations suggest that even though TNF may be a major initiating signal for a variety of cellular events in critical illness, other mediators are required for the full development of the metabolic responses to injury and infection.

IL-1 was one of the first fever-producing cytokines, or pyrogens, to be identified.[122,123] Early in vitro studies appeared to present conflicting findings,[124-126] but the preponderance of the data currently available indicate that IL-1 can increase proteolysis, especially in intact animals. For example, Zamir and colleagues measured increased muscle protein breakdown in vitro after administration of IL-1 to intact animals.[127] In another study, they were able to reduce but not prevent the increased proteolysis that followed endotoxin administration by pretreating animals with IL-1 receptor antagonist (IL-1ra).[128]

To characterize the metabolic effects of IL-1 in vivo, Watters and associates gave daily intramuscular injections of etiocholanolone to normal individuals.[129] (This steroid stimulates the development of an inflammatory focus and the production of IL-1.) The subjects manifested an acute-phase response: fever, leukocytosis, increased concentrations of acute-phase proteins, and hypoferremia. They were not hypermetabolic, however, and they remained in nitrogen equilibrium when fed a standard diet. The concentrations of catabolic hormones were not affected by this treatment. When hydrocortisone, glucagon, and epinephrine were administered in conjunction with etiocholanolone, however, both inflammatory and metabolic responses were observed.[130] These healthy subjects exhibited the same clinical features as did patients with infection. These findings suggested that both endocrine and cytokine mechanisms influence the responses to critical illness.

IL-6 can induce many of the components of the acute-phase response[131] and may be measured in the blood of patients experiencing trauma,[132] sepsis,[133] pancreatitis,[134] or other critical illnesses (e.g., myocardial infarction).[135] Mateo and associates identified IL-6 in wound fluid from both animals and humans, and they found that the capacity of wound macrophages to produce IL-6 increased with time.[136] Thus, IL-6 might be one mechanism by which the wound influences critical illness. Persistent measurable levels of IL-6 have been related to mortality in both trauma[116] and burn[117] patients.

Stouthard and associates infused recombinant IL-6 (rIL-6) into uninjured cancer patients for 4 hours, then measured glucose and lipid kinetics, metabolic rate, and hormonal profiles during the infusion and during a saline control infusion.[137] IL-6–induced hypermetabolism and energy expenditure increased by 25%. Glucose production, lipolysis, and fatty acid oxidation also increased. Glucose clearance was also increased; serum glucose concentrations were not significantly affected by IL-6 infusion. Tsigos and colleagues administered increasing doses of IL-6 subcutaneously to healthy subjects and demonstrated a dose-response relationship between IL-6 dose and circulating level and glucose concentration.[138] In both of these studies, IL-6 also induced elevations in circulating stress hormone levels.

IL-6 also affects protein metabolism. Transgenic mice that overexpress IL-6 exhibit retarded growth and muscle atrophy. These observations have been correlated with reduced circulating concentrations of insulinlike growth factor–1 (IGF-1).[139] In another report, a specific IL-6 receptor antibody administered to the young IL-6 transgenic mice restored muscle growth to normal.[140] The muscle atrophy in these studies was associated with an increase in the synthesis and activity of several enzymes that catalyze muscle protein breakdown, and these changes too were blocked by IL-6 receptor antibody. The effects of IL-6 on long-term protein accretion in humans have not yet been elucidated, but severely burned children who survive after a long period of critical illness often experience growth retardation.[141]

Both endocrine and inflammatory mediators affect metabolic responses in critically ill patients. In fact, the two systems are closely linked—perhaps inseparably—and probably influence each other.[130] For example, Bornstein and colleagues identified IL-6 messenger RNA (mRNA) expression in the steroid-producing cells of the adrenal gland, which were located not only in the cortex but also in the medulla, adjacent to catecholamine-producing cells.[142] In a subsequent study, they detected IL-6 and IL-6 receptor expression in adrenal cell cultures, both with macrophages present and with macrophages absent.[143] They also found that IL-6 stimulated release of steroid hormones, aldosterone, cortisol, and androgens in vitro in a dose-dependent manner; however, these effects developed over a period of 24 hours. These findings indicate not only that IL-6 exerts autocrine and paracrine effects on adrenal cellular synthetic function but also that it is probably involved in the long-term regulation of adrenal steroidogenesis rather than being responsible for acute changes in adrenal function.

On the other hand, glucocorticoids have long been known to exert anti-inflammatory effects. They interfere with the proliferation and function of leukocytes and other immune cells, and they inhibit the synthesis and cellular action of cytokines and other molecules important for cellular responses.[144] In a clinical study, Barber and colleagues demonstrated that glucocorticoid administration led to a dose- and time-dependent reduction in TNF production and symptoms in response to endotoxin.[145]

Cytokines and hormones may also affect metabolic responses at the end-organ level via different mechanisms. For example, skeletal muscle protein breakdown can occur via any of at least four intracellular proteolytic systems.[146] One of the major pathways affecting myofibrillar proteins is energy dependent (i.e., ATP-dependent) and involves the cytosolic peptide cofactor ubiquitin. In animals, glucocorticoids stimulate an ATP-dependent proteolytic system and increase the expression of ubiquitin.[147] Zamir and colleagues administered a gluco-

corticoid antagonist to rats with intraperitoneal sepsis and demonstrated that it reduced but did not eliminate the increased muscle proteolysis.[127] In a subsequent study, they induced accelerated skeletal muscle proteolysis by injecting IL-1 intraperitoneally.[128] Previous adrenalectomy, which eliminated glucocorticoid elaboration, had little effect on the proteolysis observed.[148] These observations suggest

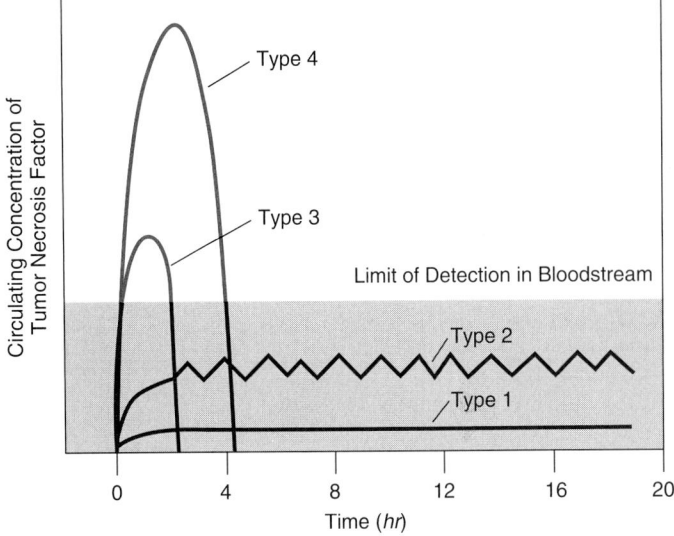

Figure 5 **Different infectious states are likely to be associated with different patterns of cytokine release into the circulation.[254] Type 1 in this figure could be considered to represent localized cellulitis, such as might be present at an infected intravenous catheter infusion site. Generation of tumor necrosis factor (TNF) and other cytokines occurs locally to produce local responses that aid host defense and tissue repair. Overspill into the circulation is minimal.**

The second type might represent the responses ensuing from appendiceal abscess. There is local generation of cytokines, and as bacteria or their endotoxins leak into the circulation, circulating mononuclear cells also elaborate cytokines and give rise to moderate systemic responses. The low level of persistent endotoxemia is reflected in the cytokine response. Because only a small number of cytokine-producing cells are stimulated at any one time, the responses of these cells, although of long duration, are not strong enough to be detectable in the bloodstream. However, this signal is sufficient to generate systemic manifestations of the localized infection.

A third type of infection might be one that follows manipulation of a catheter in the biliary tree or urinary bladder to resolve an obstruction. A few cytokine-producing cells simultaneously elaborate TNF to produce a high-amplitude signal. Because the endotoxemia is transient, both the signal and the host responses are short-lived. Clinical features include a brief episode of hyperpyrexia with rigors and severe symptoms, but the cytokine response is too short and of insufficient amplitude to give rise to life-threatening, irreversible host alterations.

A fourth type of infection might be precipitated by sudden dehiscence of a colonic anastomosis or by meningococcal septicemia. An acute, massive entry of endotoxins into the circulation stimulates virtually every cytokine-producing cell in the body. A very high amplitude signal occurs, but its duration is short, despite the host's continuing exposure to endotoxin. The short duration of the strong signal is caused by the quick disappearance of cytokines from the circulation; their half-life is short, and the cytokine-producing cells become refractory after their simultaneous explosive response to the initial, lethal signal. This high-amplitude signal is misinterpreted by the host, causing the entire body to behave as if it were a massive wound. The entire vascular tree shows increased permeability and vasodilatation, resulting in the clinical state of irreversible shock. These situations have been reversed or prevented by the use of TNF antibodies in animals and occasionally by the use of plasmapheresis in humans.

that both glucocorticoid-dependent and glucocorticoid-independent proteolytic mechanisms can be activated during critical illness.

Role of the Central Nervous System

The CNS plays a major role in the regulation of the metabolic response to critical illness. Hume and Egdahl were among the first to demonstrate its role in mediating early responses to injury.[149] They measured the rise in 17-hydroxycorticosteroids in adrenal venous blood in response to a burn to the lower limb of an animal under anesthesia. The limb was almost completely separated from the body, so that the only connections between the limb and the rest of the animal were the femoral vessels and the sciatic nerve. The prompt rise in the venous adrenocorticoid concentration after the burn could be prevented by sectioning of the sciatic nerve or of any portion of the CNS up to the level of the midbrain.

To characterize the role of the CNS in the regulation of later hypermetabolic flow-phase responses, Wilmore and associates administered inert gas anesthesia to hypermetabolic burn patients and demonstrated reduced core temperature and metabolic rates.[150] Fried and coworkers studied patients with head injuries during barbiturate coma.[151,152] Metabolic rate and nitrogen excretion were reduced to basal values during barbiturate administration. Given that its global suppression reduces the intensity of hypermetabolic responses, the CNS appears to be necessary for the full expression of both the ebb phase and the flow phase of the metabolic response to critical illness.

The CNS has long been considered part of a neuroendocrine reflex arc,[153] a view that has proved useful for explicating underlying regulatory mechanisms. According to this concept, there must be afferent input whereby (1) the body is alerted to an injury or any other threat to its integrity and (2) the wound or inflammatory focus signals its presence, its extent, and its resolution or closure. After reception and interpretation of this input, the CNS generates efferent signals that regulate the regional and systemic metabolic alterations observed clinically. This model is most obviously relevant to the early phase of the response to critical illness (the ebb phase). The hypothalamus, the peripheral and spinal neural pathways, and the adrenals all participate in the classic fright-fight-flight syndrome. Pain, hypovolemia, acidosis, and hypoxia stimulate neural afferent signals to the CNS. The importance of these neural pathways in transmitting afferent signals to the CNS during hypermetabolism is less clear. For example, when lidocaine was applied to burn wounds to anesthetize them, no decrease in hypermetabolism was observed.[154]

The CNS may play a role in a variety of immunologic and inflammatory responses.[155] Early studies demonstrated that a small amount of IL-1 injected intrathecally elicited the same increase in body temperature as a much larger dose administered intravenously. This suggested that IL-1 could act centrally and that it might function as an afferent signal from the wound to the CNS.[156] Demonstration of IL-1 immunoreactivity in the hypothalamus of humans lent weight to this suggestion.[157] Later studies, however, showed that astrocytes and microglia could express cytokines and cytokine receptors themselves.[158,159] In addition, these cells increased expression of IL-1 and IL-6 in vitro in response to hypoxia or endotoxin in vitro,[160,161] and systemic administration of endotoxin to intact animals increased cytokine expression in the CNS.[162,163]

Hill and colleagues used an animal model to assess the metabolic effects of IL-1 continuously infused either subcutaneously or into the lateral ventricle for 6 days.[164] Subcutaneous IL-1 was given in different doses, which induced fever, anorexia, increased protein catabolism, and weight loss in a dose-dependent manner. Intracerebroventricular (ICV) IL-1 evoked qualitatively similar responses.

Subcutaneous IL-1, however, resulted in a greater leukocytosis and a more pronounced acute-phase response than did ICV IL-1, even though the other systemic alterations were quantitatively similar. Thus, IL-1 produced in the CNS may not have the same physiologic consequences as IL-1 produced in other anatomic sites.

In another study, Hill and colleagues pair-fed control animals with animals receiving ICV IL-1.[165] They observed that the pair-fed animals also lost weight, but the weight loss was significantly less severe than in the animals receiving ICV IL-1. Long-term ICV IL-1 infusion also caused increased adrenal gland weight and corticosteroid levels in comparison with values in both pair-fed and chow-fed controls. The ICV IL-1–induced catabolic changes were not, however, attenuated by previous adrenalectomy. This finding indicates that the protein-catabolic effects induced by ICV IL-1 may involve not only glucocorticoid-dependent ATP-ubiquitin proteolysis but also systems that are independent of glucocorticoids. Such a conclusion is consistent with the finding by Zamir and associates that intraperitoneal IL-1 increased total and myofibrillar proteolysis in both adrenalectomized animals and sham controls.[148] Thus, the CNS may be able to influence metabolic responses via both endocrine pathways and other mechanisms that do not involve endocrine activation.

Elaboration of IL-6 typically follows elaboration of IL-1, and IL-6 is a potent activator of corticosteroid synthesis and release.[115,166] Long-term IL-1 infusion leads to increased muscle protein breakdown and nitrogen loss over and above what is attributable to reduced food intake, and it results in elevated circulating levels of IL-6.[167] When Hill and associates infused IL-6 into the CSF of rats, it had no effect, unlike ICV IL-1.[165] Reyes and Coe followed the appearance of IL-6 in CSF in primates after intravenous injection of IL-1α, IL-1β, and IL-6.[168] All three cytokines raised the circulating levels of IL-6, IL-1ra, and cortisol, but only IL-1β raised the CSF level of IL-6. Furthermore, IL-6 appeared in CSF from the lumbar region 2 hours after it peaked in CSF from the cervical region. These data suggest that the IL-6 in the CSF after the appearance of IL-1 in the periphery is elaborated by the brain.

Romero and colleagues gave an ICV injection of IL-1β to rats and measured IL-6 concentrations in CSF and in blood from the superior sagittal sinus and the aorta.[169] IL-6 was elevated in all three compartments, and the concentration gradient between the sagittal sinus and the aorta was widened in comparison with the control value. Both adrenergic pathways and adrenal activation are known to be stimulated by IL-1 administration, but the changes observed in this study were not affected by sympathetic blockade. In addition, ICV corticotropin-releasing hormone did not result in alterations in IL-6 levels in CSF or in blood. The investigators concluded that the IL-6 that appeared in both the CSF and the blood was derived from the brain.

Injury and inflammation also appear to affect nerve function. Compounds elaborated by platelets, neutrophils, and other inflammatory cells can alter the phenotype of neurons, affecting their growth, function, and electrical properties.[170] The complex of IL-6 and its receptor can activate specific neuronal signal transduction systems on sensory neurons and so affect gene expression and protein synthesis.[171] Sensory nerve injury induces the expression of IL-6 and IL-6 receptor in more central neurons, and this may influence nerve repair.[172] Current studies further suggest that IL-1, IL-6, and other proinflammatory cytokines may play a key role in generating pain syndromes associated with inflammation.[173] Inflammatory activation of sensory neurons, as opposed to strictly neural mechanisms of activation, also requires the participation of spinal cord astrocytes and microglia. Persistent inflammation, rather than altered neural properties, thus may be the major mechanism responsible for complex regional pain syndromes (e.g., reflex sympathetic dystrophy and causalgia) after injury.[174]

Thus, pain, acidosis, hypoxia, and hypovolemia, as well as cytokines and other substances produced by inflammatory cells, generate afferent signals to the CNS through a variety of mechanisms. Some signals may elicit a rapid effector response, whereas others appear to induce mechanisms that result in delayed and more prolonged end-organ functional alterations. The CNS affects both metabolic and inflammatory processes, and it may do so in multiple complementary but largely independent ways. Activation of the hypothalamic-pituitary-adrenal axis is one of these mechanisms, but the CNS also appears to be able to induce catabolic responses without this intervention. The CNS may also be a source of mediators that are released into the circulation for systemic distribution, thus acting as an endocrine organ.

Role of the Gut

Although the idea that endotoxin absorbed from the gut lumen during shock states might result in irreversible critical illness was first proposed more than 40 years ago,[175,176] most clinicians thought that the gut was inert after operation and injury until recently. It is now generally recognized that the gut plays an important role in augmenting or perpetuating the response to critical illness.[177]

Gram-negative pathogens are the predominant infectious organisms in the ICU, and the gut appears to be a major source of contamination. The gut lumen forms a large reservoir for gram-negative enteric bacteria, but the normal GI mucosa protects the host from intraluminal bacteria and their toxins. The maintenance of tight intracellular junctions between epithelial cells prevents the transepithelial migration of bacteria.[178] The GI tract is also richly supplied with macrophages and fixed immune cells. The elaboration of surface immunoglobulins (e.g., IgA) aids in the recognition of foreign antigens.[179] Finally, the liver and the spleen serve as backup systems for trapping bacteria and neutralizing absorbed toxins. The combination of an intact gut mucosa and a normally functioning immune system provides maximal barrier function. Even in immunosuppressed states, the mucosa can still maintain an effective barrier to infection. This suggests that cell-mediated immunity is secondary in importance to an intact intestinal epithelial lining.

When the barrier function of the GI epithelium is impaired, intraluminal bacteria and toxins can invade the host. In one set of experiments in rabbits, fatal endotoxic shock was observed after temporary occlusion of the superior mesenteric artery or a 30% scald burn[180]; however, if the enteric flora was reduced, the animals did not die. Endotoxemia has been observed in patients with a variety of critical illnesses.[176] Wellmann and associates reported that whole gut lavage with saline reduced the concentration of circulating endotoxin and improved the clinical outcome in a large group of patients with inflammatory bowel disease that was unresponsive to medical therapy.[181] Moreover, bacteremia in portal blood has been observed at the time of operation in as many as 30% of patients with noninflammatory bowel disease.[182] Ambrose and associates cultured both intestinal serosa and mesenteric lymph nodes during abdominal operation.[183] In patients without inflammatory bowel disease, the incidence of positive cultures was low, but in patients with Crohn disease, the incidence increased markedly, to approximately 30%.

Bacterial translocation is the migration of bacteria across the bowel wall to invade the host. In a review of the available animal and human data on this process, Berg identified three conditions that appear to promote translocation: altered permeability of the intestinal mucosa, decreased host defenses, and an increased number of bacteria within the intestinal lumen.[184] Deitch and colleagues observed this phenomenon in animals after a variety of insults, including burns,[185] hemorrhagic shock,[186] and endotoxin administration.[180] Malnutrition alone did not lead to translocation, but it made the gut barrier more susceptible to endotoxin.[187]

The extent of bacterial translocation in critically ill patients is not well defined. Moore and colleagues obtained both portal venous and systemic venous blood cultures in patients at risk for multiorgan failure after laparotomy for severe trauma.[188] Only 2% of cultures were positive in the first 5 days, which suggests that translocation of bacteria in sufficient quantities to cause portal vein bacteremia is not a major determinant of organ failure soon after injury.

Subsequent studies focused on the gut as a source of cytokines. Even the normal gut contains a large number of intestinal lymphocytes that elaborate proinflammatory cytokines, and these are counteracted by expression of anti-inflammatory cytokines in a state of so-called controlled inflammation.[189] Guy-Grand and colleagues detected measurable levels of TNF, IL-6, and interferon gamma in proximal small bowel secretions in humans.[190] The presence of bacterial overgrowth, especially colonic-type bacteria, however, was associated with increased IL-6 concentrations. Wyble and associates investigated the cytokine response to intestinal ischemia-reperfusion in ex vivo perfused segments of human intestine.[191] Concentrations of TNF and IL-1 increased in the venous effluent after reperfusion. The investigators subsequently exposed cultured human endothelial cells to physiologic concentrations of TNF and IL-1 that were lower than those observed after ischemia-reperfusion. The cytokines upregulated expression of E-selectin and intercellular adhesion molecule–1 (ICAM-1), which are thought to mediate the adhesion of neutrophils in the microcirculation and their transmigration across the capillary membrane into tissue, thus initiating tissue inflammation.

Mainous and colleagues produced sterile peritonitis with both a nonlethal and a median lethal dose (LD_{50}) of zymosan.[192] They detected increased IL-6 and TNF in both blood and lymph, but these changes did not correlate with zymosan dose or with bacterial translocation. Thus, the gut appears capable of producing cytokines in response to an inflammatory insult, and this may occur even in the absence of bacterial translocation.

Mochizuki and associates were among the first to demonstrate the importance of enteral feedings in maintaining gut mucosal integrity and modulating catabolic responses in critical illness.[193] They measured intestinal mucosal weight and several metabolic parameters in experimental animals after a standard burn injury. In one group of animals, feedings were delivered through a gastrostomy tube and were begun soon after the burn injury, whereas in a second group, feedings were oral and were begun after a 72-hour fast. Mucosal weight was preserved in the first group but reduced in the second group. In the animals that fasted, postburn hypermetabolism developed, but this response was attenuated in the ones that received early enteral feedings. Intravenous feeding did not preserve mucosal mass or modify postburn metabolic responses.[194] In an early clinical study, Alexander and colleagues documented improved survival in children with burns who were nourished enterally.[195] Furthermore, Border and associates found that the provision of enteral protein was one of only two factors statistically associated with improved survival in a large group of severely injured patients.[196]

Ogle and colleagues extended these observations by comparing intestinal and splenic cytokine expression in animals nourished by parenteral nutrition but allowed no oral intake with cytokine expression in control animals allowed food ad libitum.[197] After 7 days of infusion, mRNA expression for IL-1, IL-6, and TNF was increased in the intestine and decreased in the spleen. Lyoumi and associates also reported that protein malnutrition alone enhances intestinal IL-6 expression and acute-phase responses.[198] These findings suggest that augmented intestinal cytokine production is responsible, in part, for the earlier clinical observations that bowel rest or inadequate enteral protein amplifies the responses to critical illness and may adversely affect outcome.

The presence of food in the gut lumen is known to be a major stimulus for mucosal cell growth. Mucosal atrophy is observed in the absence of enteral nutrition (as occurs during starvation[199] or periods of parenteral nutrition[200]) and in defunctionalized intestinal segments.[201] Enteral feeding not only provides nutrients but also stimulates the elaboration of trophic hormones for the intestinal mucosa.[202,203] In addition to luminal bulk, specific nutrients (e.g., glutamine and butyrate) are important for the growth of gut mucosa. Glutamine is a major respiratory fuel for the gut, especially during critical illness (see above). Colonocytes also utilize butyrate, a short-chain fatty acid that is produced by bacterial fermentation of polysaccharides in the colonic lumen. In solution, glutamine decomposes into toxic substances; it is therefore not included in any commercially available parenteral amino acid solutions or in most enteral nutrition products. When glutamine was added to parenteral nutrition in place of other nonessential amino acids, however, increased mucosal cellularity was observed in the jejunum, ileum, and colon in an animal model.[204,205] In other studies, the toxic effects of methotrexate were alleviated and mucosal cellularity and nitrogen balance improved when parenteral solutions containing glutamine were used.[206]

Endotoxin, Bacteria, Inflammation, and Organ Failure

Endotoxin is a lipopolysaccharide component of bacterial cell walls that can reproduce the syndrome of sepsis and shock when given to animals or humans.[207] The presence of endotoxin is considered a major determinant of the clinical sequelae of bacterial infection. A low continuous dose of endotoxin in animals produces a hypermetabolic state that exhibits all of the features of the response to critical illness.[208]

Revhaug and associates administered *Escherichia coli* endotoxin to normal individuals under controlled conditions of activity and diet and compared the metabolic responses with those of subjects given only saline.[209] About 2 to 4 hours after administration of endotoxin, the subjects experienced headache, chills, malaise, nausea, fever, tachycardia, and an increased respiratory rate. In these and subsequent studies, endotoxin injection was also associated with leukocytosis, mild glucose intolerance, an increased metabolic rate, and elevated concentrations of adrenocorticotropic hormone, cortisol, catecholamines, and growth hormone.

Michie and colleagues found that the symptoms that followed a single dose of endotoxin in normal subjects were preceded by an abrupt and transient rise in circulating TNF concentration.[210] The symptoms developing after endotoxin injection were similar to those developing during TNF infusion, but they appeared 60 to 90 minutes after injection, in contrast with the appearance of symptoms 30 minutes after the start of TNF infusion.[118] In these studies, IL-1 was not detected, but Fong and associates detected both a peak rise in TNF and a later peak of IL-1 after administration of a lethal dose of bacteria in primates.[211] In those studies, death was prevented by an anti-TNF antibody. Thus, TNF is the first in a characteristic cascade of cytokines that mediate the physiologic responses to endotoxin.

Circulating endotoxin can be detected in patients who have experienced trauma[116] or burns[117] and even in those who have undergone cardiopulmonary bypass.[212] In healthy persons, repeated doses of endotoxin result in tolerance. In injured or critically ill patients, however, the responses to sustained or repeated doses of endotoxin have not been well characterized.

O'Dwyer and associates measured intestinal permeability in healthy human volunteers after a single dose of *E. coli* endotoxin or saline.[213]

Lactulose and mannitol were administered orally as markers of intestinal permeability. (Lactulose is not absorbed to any significant extent under normal conditions.) After endotoxin administration, the urinary excretion of lactulose was increased almost twofold, which indicated that intestinal permeability was markedly altered. This change was closely associated with increases in norepinephrine and cortisol levels, which suggested that these hormonal changes or other systemic responses induced by endotoxin were responsible for the change in permeability. If alteration of the gut barrier led to increased absorption of endotoxin, that could be another mechanism by which the systemic responses to critical illness were amplified and perpetuated.

Patients with infectious disease (e.g., typhoid fever or malaria)[214,215] manifest many of the clinical features observed in critically ill surgical patients; however, these phenomena are less intense in patients with infectious disease. Surgical patients with uninfected wounds also usually manifest relatively mild responses to injury; those with infected wounds exhibit the most intense metabolic alterations. The infection may be associated with the wound (e.g., surgical site infection, mature abscess, or ARDS and pulmonary sepsis), or it may be remote (e.g., pneumonia in a patient with multiple fractures). Peak catabolic responses in surgical patients often occur several days after operation or injury. This period corresponds to the development of the cellular phase of wound healing[112] and to colonization of the wound or another site.

Aulick and colleagues examined the possible contribution of bacteria or bacterial products to the metabolic response to injury in animals.[216] They measured $\dot{V}O_2$ and core temperature in animals for up to 3 weeks after a standard scald burn. Some of the wounds were seeded with bacteria (virulent and nonvirulent *Pseudomonas aeruginosa* and *Staphylococcus epidermidis*), and some of the infected wounds were treated with topical antibacterial agents. The use of topical antibiotics was associated with a reduction in hypermetabolism. In addition, in animals that became bacteremic, the degree of hypermetabolism was at least twice that in nonbacteremic animals. The metabolic effects of infection thus appear to be proportional to the severity and invasiveness of the infection. In analogous studies, Wilmore and associates examined burn patients with and without bacteremia.[24] Although total body $\dot{V}O_2$ and cardiac index were already elevated, the onset of bacteremia resulted in further increases in these parameters. In addition, hepatic glucose production and splanchnic uptake of lactate and alanine were significantly increased in patients with systemic infection. Hypermetabolism decreased, however, once organ failure occurred.

Bacteria are ubiquitous in both health and critical illness. The mechanisms by which bacteria become infective and invade host tissues and produce physiologic responses have yet to be fully elucidated. In part, these involve intracellular regulatory systems that respond to complex reciprocal interactions with the host and that can modify bacterial virulence. Guo and associates investigated the dual peptide system PhoP-PhoQ in *Salmonella*.[217] PhoP-PhoQ regulates genes required for the synthesis of lipid A, the active component of endotoxin. It is capable of modifying the structure of lipid A, and this structurally modified lipid A can affect the expression both of adhesion molecules by host endothelial cells and of TNF by neighboring monocytes. This capability may be a mechanism by which bacteria can not only increase their chances of survival in host tissues but also affect the character or intensity of host inflammatory responses to the infection. PhoP-PhoQ and other intracellular systems respond to characteristics of the host environment, such as pH, PO_2, and ionic composition.[218] Thus, the condition of the patient may influence the virulence characteristics of resident bacteria, and these characteristics, in turn, may modulate the patient's responses to critical illness.

The cellular response to localized injury or other inflammatory stimuli initially consists of the recruitment and proliferation of neutrophils. This process appears to be mediated in part by the expression of adhesion molecules by endothelial cells. These molecules capture passing circulating neutrophils and facilitate their passage through the capillary wall.[219] Neutrophils, macrophages, and other inflammatory cells have the capacity to engulf and dispose of necrotic debris and to kill bacteria. These same properties also make them potentially toxic to normal cells. Neutrophil infiltration of specific organs, such as the lung, appears to be a first step in the development of organ failure after shock, endotoxin, and other insults.[220] This finding suggests that neutrophils activated by potent inflammatory stimuli can invade unaffected tissues and so contribute to organ dysfunction in critically ill patients.

Not surprisingly, anti-inflammatory mechanisms exist to limit the intensity and toxicity of inflammatory processes. One such mechanism is apoptosis, or programmed cell death, which is thought to participate in the clearing of inflammatory cells as the wound heals and the inflammatory process subsides. Biffl and colleagues demonstrated that IL-6 inhibited apoptosis in human neutrophils in vitro.[221] They proposed that circulating IL-6 in critically ill patients retarded neutrophil apoptosis and thus enhanced and prolonged the toxic effects of the neutrophils. This could be another mechanism by which the responses to critical illness could be prolonged and lead to worsening organ failure and death.

Several investigators have sought to understand how neural mechanisms might also influence physiologic responses to infection and inflammation. The vagus nerve has been of particular interest because its fibers are widely distributed, especially in organs that contain large amounts of inflammatory cells (e.g., the liver, the spleen, the lungs, the thymus, the GI tract, and the lymph nodes). Niijima gave varying doses of IL-1β to rats by portal vein injection.[222] He observed a dose-dependent increase in the afferent activity of the hepatic branch of the vagus nerve. He also detected efferent signals in autonomic nerves to the spleen and the thymus after intraportal administration of IL-1. Because these signals were eliminated by vagotomy, they appeared to be the result of reflex activation. These findings suggested that there may be sensors in the hepatoportal system of vagal origin that can detect IL-1 and other inflammatory mediators and generate neural afferent activity, stimulating the brain to generate signals that affect host defense and other responses.

Maier and colleagues sought also to understand how the vagus nerve might influence the neural and behavioral changes associated with sickness.[223] Subdiaphragmatic vagotomy blocked or ameliorated many of the responses to intraperitoneal endotoxin or IL-1β that could be detected physiologically and behaviorally, as well as certain biochemical changes within the brain. Hansen studied the pyrogenic effects of different doses of intraperitoneal IL-1β.[224] Vagotomy abolished the fever after a low dose, reduced it after a medium dose, and had no effect after a high dose. Circulating IL-1β levels were increased only after the medium and high doses. Romanovsky also found the vagus nerve to be sensitive to low doses of IL-1β and suggested that prostaglandins mediated the communication in the periphery.[225] These data support the concept that peripherally elaborated cytokines may signal the brain either via the bloodstream or via the nervous system.

Goehler and associates used a labeled form of IL-1ra to try to identify IL-1 receptors associated with the vagus.[226] There was no specific binding to neural tissue, but there was intense binding to tissues closely surrounding the vagal fibers. These tissues consist primarily of chromaffin tissue and were formerly thought to serve primarily as chemosensors for oxygen and carbon dioxide tension in both the abdomen and the lung. These investigators further demonstrated that endotoxin administration induced IL-1β expression in dendritic cells and macrophages within the connective tissues associated with the abdominal vagus nerve, which suggested that these cells

were the source of proinflammatory cytokines that could initiate afferent signals to the brain via the vagus.[227]

The vagus nerve also contains efferent fibers that are widely distributed. Tracey and colleagues performed bilateral cervical vagotomies in rats and stimulated the distal nerves electrically before and after administering a lethal dose of endotoxin.[228] Stimulation of the distal vagus attenuated endotoxic shock and blunted the rise in circulating TNF. Electrical stimulation also resulted in decreased TNF in homogenates of liver, which suggested that vagal efferent activity diminished hepatic TNF elaboration in response to endotoxin.

These investigators also established primary cultures of human macrophages. These cells, in response to lipopolysaccharide, elaborated IL-1, TNF, and other proinflammatory cytokines, as well as the anti-inflammatory cytokine IL-10. Incubation with the parasympathetic neurotransmitter acetylcholine substantially reduced the endotoxin-stimulated synthesis of the proinflammatory cytokines but not that of IL-10. This group subsequently identified an acetylcholine receptor on human macrophages.[229] Thus, efferent parasympathetic vagal activity appears to dampen inflammation by suppressing elaboration of proinflammatory cytokines by tissue macrophages.

Thus, there is an emerging appreciation of a role for the parasympathetic arm of the autonomic nervous system, especially the vagus. Proinflammatory cytokines produced at the site of the inflammatory process may induce afferent neural activity that directly signals the brain, independent of any change in circulating cytokine levels. If the localized inflammatory response is intense or extensive enough, however, perhaps as a result of invasive infection or systemic bacteremia, locally produced cytokines may spill over into the circulation and also reach the brain via the bloodstream. The afferent branches of the vagus terminate in the nucleus tractus solitarius in the medulla. From there, neural fibers traverse the brain stem, terminating on specific cells in the hypothalamus. Thus, parasympathetic nerves may provide neural circuitry by which a focus of inflammation can signal the brain and activates the hypothalamic-pituitary-adrenal (HPA) axis.

Activation of the HPA axis, whether by neural signaling or by elevation of circulating cytokine levels, may result in sympathetic efferent activity, the characteristic elaboration of classic stress hormones, and alteration of the thyrotropic, somatotropic, and gonadotropic endocrine axes. These neuroendocrine responses induce systemic and metabolic alterations that serve to promote wound healing, such as increased blood flow, mobilization of amino acids from muscle, glucose intolerance, and insulin resistance. In addition, efferent parasympathetic activity may modulate the intensity of the inflammatory processes at specific sites of inflammation. Thus, neural mechanisms enable the CNS and the brain to direct and regulate the physiologic responses to injury, infection, inflammation, and critical illness.

Manipulating the Response to Critical Illness

The metabolic response to critical illness has survival value. Young patients are able to mount more intense hypermetabolic responses than elderly persons and in general have higher survival rates. However, these responses are debilitating in all patients and may be associated with organ failure and death. Many have sought to develop therapeutic strategies that would reduce the debilitating aspects of these responses, accelerate recovery, or both.

The endocrine response to injury or operation has been attenuated by adrenergic blockade or regional anesthesia (see above). These maneuvers are associated with an improved postoperative nitrogen balance[101,102] and decreased muscle protein breakdown.[100] Herndon and colleagues reported that continuous administration of propranolol to children with burns reduced cardiac work without adversely affecting mortality, postburn course, or wound healing.[230] This technique may benefit elderly, critically ill patients with limited cardiovascular reserve.

Several studies have evaluated the effectiveness of combined neural and humoral blockade in inhibiting the metabolic responses to operative injury. Schulze and associates compared the responses of patients receiving morphine and acetaminophen for pain control after colonic surgery with those of patients managed with methylprednisolone pretreatment, thoracic epidural analgesia, intrathecal anesthesia, and intravenous indomethacin.[231] In the patients receiving combined therapy, postoperative pain and fever were prevented, pulmonary function was improved, and fatigue was reduced. Synthesis of acute-phase proteins and IL-6 was reduced. Similarly, Heindorff and coworkers prevented the typical increases in amino acid clearance and urea synthesis with a combination of intravenous somatostatin and etomidate (to inhibit the elevation of glucagon and cortisol levels) and high thoracic epidural analgesia (to provide neural blockade).[103]

Advances in cell and molecular biology have led to an extraordinary expansion of knowledge about the mechanisms involved in the many local and systemic responses to injury, sepsis, and other critical illness. Developments in technology have also led to the formulation of novel strategies for inhibiting various components of these responses that were thought to be particularly deleterious. Thus, antibodies to endotoxin, IL-1, and TNF were developed and studied in clinical trials, along with receptor antagonists and other compounds designed to interfere with systemic inflammatory responses. None of these demonstrated clinical benefit in controlled trials.[232] Given that the regulatory mechanisms are highly complex and that the same ones that may be harmful in some cases promote recovery in others, it is not surprising that blockade of one component of the response might offer no net benefit.

An alternative strategic approach is to enhance or accelerate those components of the response to critical illness that seem to be primarily restorative and lead to wound healing and recovery.

Nutritional support of critically ill patients is important both for promoting protein synthesis and other anabolic processes essential to recovery and for reducing the net drain on the patient's fuel and protein stores. Enteral nutrition is preferred, but the availability of effective intravenous techniques allows the clinician to provide appropriate nutrition to virtually all patients. Exercise and mobility have clear anticatabolic effects and should be initiated as early as is practicable.

Previously, provision of glutamine to critically ill patients had not been possible; glutamine had not been included in most commercial nutrient preparations because of its instability in aqueous solutions. When added to standard TPN, however, glutamine can promote nitrogen retention in postoperative patients.[233] Ziegler and associates demonstrated that glutamine-supplemented TPN improved nitrogen balance, diminished clinical infection, and shortened hospital stay in a group of critically ill patients recovering from bone marrow transplantation.[234] Enteral preparations enriched with glutamine are now commercially available.

Kudsk and associates randomly selected patients with moderately severe injuries to receive either an enteral formulation enriched with glutamine, arginine, omega-3 fatty acids, and nucleotides or a standard formula that provided an isonitrogenous, isocaloric diet.[235] In both cases, protein content was moderately high (2 g/kg/day). Infectious complications in patients surviving to recovery were less frequent in those receiving the enhanced formula than in those receiving the standard diet.

Growth hormone, when administered to normal subjects, improves nitrogen balance, even if caloric intake is less than energy expenditure.[236] Jiang and associates administered growth hormone and hypocaloric parenteral nutrition perioperatively to patients undergoing elective abdominal operations.[237] They monitored a variety of metabolic parameters and compared the results with those from a

Table 8   Factors Affecting Metabolic Response to Critical Illness and Patient Outcome

Factors that *cannot* be directly controlled or influenced at present
  Patient's genetic makeup and premorbid state of health
  Gene transcription and translation
  Expression of hormones, cytokines, and growth factors
  Expression of hormone, cytokine, growth factor, and other specific cell receptors
  Expression of secondary messengers
  Generation of nitric oxide and other reactive oxygen intermediates
  Signal transduction mechanisms
  Intracellular transporters and other regulatory peptides and organelles
  CNS neural pathway traffic and cytokine expression
  Futile cycles
  Enzymes controlling protein synthesis and breakdown
  Bacterial virulence factors
  Expression of adhesion molecules
  Inflammatory and noninflammatory cell proliferation
  Apoptosis
  Wound-healing biology

Factors that *can* be directly controlled or influenced at present
  Whole-body oxygenation
  Whole-body perfusion
  Pain, anxiety
  Body temperature
  Acid-base balance
  ECF electrolyte composition and balance
  Nutrient supply
  Glucose concentration
  Anabolic factors
  Gut mucosal integrity
  Focal infection and bacteremia
  Wound repair and closure

control group of patients receiving parenteral nutrition alone. Growth hormone markedly reduced cumulative nitrogen loss. Although both groups of patients lost weight, those receiving growth hormone lost less. Bioelectric impedance data indicated that most of the weight lost by patients receiving growth hormone came from fat mass and not from the muscle compartment. Growth hormone also preserved muscle strength.

Herndon and colleagues administered growth hormone to severely burned children in a randomized trial.[238] Growth hormone accelerated donor site healing, allowing earlier reharvesting of skin. As a result, the time between skin graft procedures and the total length of time required for the children's recovery were both reduced. Knox and associates gave growth hormone to a group of severely burned adults and compared their outcome with that of a similar group of patients cared for without growth hormone in the immediately preceding years[239]; mortality was lower in the growth hormone group.

The favorable results reported in burn patients and patients who have undergone elective abdominal operations have not been duplicated in more diverse groups of surgical patients.

Two large multi-institutional randomized trials were conducted in Europe. They included trauma patients, patients who had undergone cardiac procedures, and patients with other acute surgical illnesses. The combined mortality of the patients receiving growth hormone was 42%, more than twice the 18% mortality in the control subjects. Although the reasons for this adverse outcome have not yet been fully elucidated, the manufacturer of the recombinant product issued a safety statement recommending that recombinant growth hormone not be used in catabolic patients.[240]

An anabolic steroid, oxandrolone, was introduced over 50 years ago as an adjunct to restoring weight loss. It has a good margin of safety and may play a beneficial role in critical illness by promoting nitrogen retention and accelerating recovery. Combined with a high-protein diet (2 mg/kg/day), oxandrolone promoted weight gain and functional improvement in a randomized study of burn patients who had recovered sufficiently to enter a rehabilitation program.[241] Hart and associates demonstrated improved efficiency of protein synthesis in nutritionally depleted burned children who received oxandrolone.[242] They observed the same benefit in patients who had received appropriate nutritional support from the time of injury.[243] In this group, oxandrolone was also associated with an improvement in lean body mass and increased expression of genes for several functional muscle proteins.

Insulin attenuates cortisol-induced breakdown of skeletal muscle protein in vitro.[244] Inculet and associates demonstrated improved nitrogen utilization in patients receiving TPN and insulin after operation.[245] The apparent mild beneficial effects of TPN enriched with branched-chain amino acids may be caused by increased insulin elaboration.[246] Bessey and Lowe induced accelerated skeletal muscle protein catabolism in normal subjects by blocking insulin elaboration during the first day of a 3-day infusion of stress hormones,[99] thereby simulating the typical hormonal profiles of injured patients. When insulin elaboration was allowed to rise unchecked or when exogenous insulin was administered to limit the rise of blood glucose, net muscle protein breakdown did not increase.

Although some degree of hyperglycemia may facilitate glucose uptake by the inflammatory cells in the wound, excessive elevations—in excess of 10 mmol/L (180 mg/dl)—have been associated with a variety of adverse effects, including impaired phagocytosis and immune function, increased CO_2 production and ventilatory requirements, increased vascular tone and reduction of regional blood flow, and altered collagen formation. Gore and associates demonstrated an association between hyperglycemia and increased net breakdown of muscle.[247] Thus, close control of blood glucose concentration with insulin therapy may not only prevent these effects but also exert a beneficial effect on net protein loss. The insulin resistance in critically ill patients blunts the hypoglycemic effects of insulin, so that it may be administered continuously and regulated safely at the bedside by means of a standardized algorithm (sliding scale).[248] Using two such algorithms, van den Berghe and colleagues administered insulin to a large group of critically ill patients (N = 1,548) to maintain blood glucose either in a normal range (80 to 110 mg/dl) or in a moderately hyperglycemic range (180 to 200 mg/dl).[12] Maintenance of normoglycemia was associated with a reduction in mortality from 8.0% to 4.6%. In a subsequent analysis, the investigators further showed that the benefit was related to the glucose concentration, not to the insulin dose.[249] Patients with mild hyperglycemia (110 to 150 mg/dl) had worse outcomes than those maintained in the normal range.

One of the most effective means of manipulating the metabolic response to critical surgical illness, however, remains excellent surgical care. Such care is directed toward reducing, limiting, preventing, or neutralizing the signals that initiate these debilitating responses. Aggressive and prompt resuscitation, restoration of tissue oxygenation, debridement of necrotic tissue, drainage of pus, and wound repair all should have a high priority in the early management of a critically ill patient. Maintenance of effective cardiopulmonary function and tissue oxygenation, provision of a warm environment, preservation of GI tract integrity, and control of infection are clinical objectives of later management.

Over the course of the past few decades, close attention to these details has resulted in improved outcome for critically ill patients. For example, Pruitt and Mason analyzed a population of over 8,000 burn patients treated at the US Army Burn Unit from 1950 through 1991.[250] Since the mid-1970s, the burn size associated with a 50% mortality steadily rose from 57% of BSA to 77%. Similarly, Milberg and colleagues demonstrated a reduction in ARDS-related mortality from nearly 70% to 30% between 1983 and 1993.[251]

In a 1995 study, Kelleman and colleagues determined the effect of burn size on resting energy expenditure.[252] This study reproduced that of Wilmore done at the same institution almost 20 years before. In the earlier study, the resting metabolic rate increased steadily with burn size and plateaued at about twice the basal level with burns larger than 50% of BSA. Kelleman found that energy expenditure plateaued at only 1.5 times the basal level with burns of about 25% of BSA or more. This dramatic change in the relationship between burn size (injury severity) and metabolic activity (hypermetabolism) probably reflects the combined effects of improvements in all aspects of burn care, including resuscitation, cardiopulmonary and metabolic support, wound care, nursing practice, occupational and physical therapy, and reduced time to excision and grafting and wound closure. Improvements in care have thus reduced the metabolic cost of critical surgical illness.

Conclusion

The physiologic impact of major trauma, burns, intra-abdominal catastrophe, sepsis, or other critical illness reverberates throughout the body and affects all organ systems. Knowledge about the mechanisms that regulate this comprehensive and commanding response is growing at an exponential rate. These mechanisms are intricate, interrelated, and redundant. Where we once looked for a simple, direct answer, we now see dizzying complexity. The critically ill patient is a true example of controlled inflammation, suspended between anabolic and catabolic forces and between inflammatory and anti-inflammatory forces.

Unfortunately, our ability to apply our improved understanding to the care of critically ill patients still lags far behind. When the patient is not progressing well, we lack the ability to make a specific bedside diagnosis that will pinpoint the part of the system that is out of balance. Even if we could make such a diagnosis, however, we still lack the accurately targeted therapies that would allow us to intervene precisely.

Thus, a wide variety of factors and processes, with both beneficial and adverse effects, appear to be involved in the metabolic response to critical illness, but we are unable to affect many of them directly with the means currently available [see Table 8]. We can remove necrotic tissue, repair wounds, and drain pus. We can also usually ensure excellent cardiovascular performance and maintain extracellular electrolyte and nutrient composition and acid-base balance. We can often suppress bacteremia and can treat some infections effectively with antibiotics. We can prevent many additional insults to and stresses on our patients. These measures may seem unsophisticated and clumsy in the light of our contemporary understanding of the biology of convalescence, but they clearly are capable of nudging the metabolic response to critical illness toward a successful outcome. At present, such measures constitute the essentials of excellent comprehensive care of critically ill patients, and they give these patients their best hope for recovery.

References

1. Wilmore DW: Metabolic Management of the Critically Ill. Plenum Press, New York, 1980

2. Patient-controlled analgesia (editorial). Lancet 1:289, 1980

3. Kehlet H: Multimodal approach to control postoperative pathophysiology and rehabilitation. Br J Anaesth 78:606, 1997

4. MacKersie RC, Shackford SR, Hoyt DB, et al: Continuous epidural fentanyl analgesia: ventilatory function improvement with routine use in treatment of blunt chest injury. J Trauma 27:1207, 1987

5. Bone RC, Balk RA, Cerra FB, et al: Definitions for sepsis and organ failure and guidelines for the use of innovative therapies in sepsis. Chest 101:1644, 1992

6. Rangel-Frausto MS, Pittet D, Costigan M, et al: The natural history of the systemic inflammatory response syndrome (SIRS): a prospective study. JAMA 273:117, 1995

7. Civetta JM, Hudson-Civetta J, Bell S: Decreasing catheter-related infection and hospital costs by continuous quality improvement. Crit Care Med 24:1660, 1996

8. Mandal AK, Monturo J, Thadepelli H: Prophylactic antibiotics and no antibiotics compared in penetrating chest trauma. J Trauma 25:639, 1985

9. Stoutenbeek CP, van Saene HKF, Miranda DR, et al: The effect of oropharyngeal decontamination using topical nonabsorbable antibiotics on the incidence of nosocomial respiratory tract infections in multiple trauma patients. J Trauma 27:357, 1987

10. Goldman DA, Weinstein RA, Wenzel RP, et al: Strategies to prevent and control the emergence and spread of antimicrobial-resistant microorganisms in hospitals: a challenge to hospital leadership. JAMA 275:234, 1996

11. Sise MJ, Hollingsworth P, Brimm JC, et al: Complications of the flow-directed pulmonary artery catheter. Crit Care Med 8:272, 1980

12. van den Berghe G, Wouters P, Weekers F, et al: Intensive insulin therapy in critically ill patients. N Engl J Med 345:1359, 2001

13. Cuthbertson DP: Surgical metabolism: historical and evolutionary aspects. Metabolism and the Response to Injury. Wilkinson AW, Cuthbertson DP, Eds. Year Book Medical Publishers, Chicago, 1977, p 1

14. Thomas L: The Lives of a Cell. Viking Press, New York, 1974, p 75

15. Im MJC, Hoopes JE: Energy metabolism in healing skin wounds. J Surg Res 10:459, 1970

16. Ben-Porat M, Sideman S, Bursztein S: Energy metabolism rate equation for fasting and postabsorptive subjects. Am J Physiol 244:R764, 1983

17. Atwater WO, Benedict FG: Experiments on the metabolism of matter and energy in the human body. US Department of Agriculture Office of Experimental Stations Bulletin, publication No. 136, 1903

18. Dubois EF: Basal Metabolism in Health and Disease. Lea & Febiger, Philadelphia, 1936, p 163

19. Wilmore DW, Long JM, Mason AD Jr, et al: Catecholamines: mediator of the hypermetabolic response to thermal injury. Ann Surg 180:653, 1974

20. Wilmore DW: Metabolic Management of the Critically Ill. Plenum Medical, New York, 1977, p 33

21. Shiozaki T, Kishikawa M, Hiraide A, et al: Recovery from postoperative hypothermia predicts survival in extensively burned patients. Am J Surg 165:326, 1993

22. Wilmore DW, Aulick LH, Mason AD, et al: Influence of the burn wound on local and systemic responses to injury. Ann Surg 186:444, 1977

23. Aulick LH, Wilmore DW, Mason AD Jr, et al: Muscle blood flow following thermal injury. Ann Surg 188:778, 1978

24. Wilmore DW, Goodwin CW, Aulick LH, et al: Effect of injury and infection on visceral metabolism and circulation. Ann Surg 192:491, 1980

25. Aulick LH, Goodwin CW Jr, Becker RA, et al: Visceral blood flow following thermal injury. Ann Surg 193:112, 1981

26. Wilmore DW, Aulick LH: Metabolic changes in burned patients. Surg Clin North Am 58:1173, 1978

27. Cuthbertson DP: The disturbance of metabolism produced by bony and non-bony injury, with notes on certain abnormal conditions of bone. Biochem J 24:1244, 1930

28. Monafo WW: Wound care: physiologic concepts. Treatment of Burns: Principles and Practice. Monafo WW, Pappalardo C, Eds. Warren H Green, Inc, St Louis, 1971, p 111

29. Caldwell FT Jr, Osterholm JL, Sower ND, et al: Metabolic response to thermal trauma of normal and thyroprivic rats at three environmental temperatures. Ann Surg 150:976, 1959

30. Barr PO, Birke G, Liljedahl SO, et al: Oxygen consumption and water loss during treatment of burns with warm dry air. Lancet 1:164, 1968

31. Wilmore DW, Mason AD Jr, Johnson DW, et al: Effect of ambient temperature on heat production and heat loss in burn patients. J Appl Physiol 38:593, 1975

32. Wilmore DW, Orcutt TW, Mason AD Jr, et al: Alterations in hypothalamic function following thermal injury. J Trauma 15:697, 1975

33. Howard JE, Parson W, Stein KE, et al: Studies on fracture convalescence: I. Nitrogen metabolism after fracture and skeletal operations in healthy males. Johns Hopkins Hospital Bulletin 75:156, 1944

34. Cuthbertson DP: Observations on disturbance of metabolism produced by injury to the limbs. Q J Med 25:233, 1932

35. Cuthbertson DP, McGirr JL, Robertson JSM: The effect of fracture of bone on the metabolism of the rat. Quarterly Journal of Experimental Physiology 29:13, 1939

36. Threlfall CJ, Stoner HB, Galasko CSB: Patterns in the excretion of muscle markers after trauma and orthopedic surgery. J Trauma 21:140, 1981

37. Young VR, Munro HN: N^γ-methylhistidine (3-methylhistidine) and muscle protein turnover: an overview. Federal Proceedings 37:2291, 1978

38. Williamson DH, Farrell R, Kerr A, et al: Muscle protein catabolism after injury in man as measured by urinary excretion of 3-methylhistidine. Clin Sci Molec Med 52:527, 1977

39. Bilmazes C, Kien CL, Rohrbaugh DK, et al: Quantitative contribution by skeletal muscle to elevated rates of whole-body protein breakdown in burned children as measured by N^γ-methylhistidine output. Metabolism 27:671, 1978

40. Long CL, Schiller WR, Blakemore WS, et al: Muscle protein catabolism in the septic patient as measured by 3-methylhistidine excretion. Am J Clin Nutr 30:1349, 1977

41. Cuthbertson DP: The physiology of convalescence after injury. Br Med Bull 3:96, 1945

42. Moore FD, Langohr JL, Ingebretsen M, et al: The role of exudate losses in the protein and electrolyte imbalance of burned patients. Ann Surg 132:1, 1950

43. Soroff HS, Pearson E, Artz CP: An estimation of the nitrogen requirements for equilibrium in burned patients. Surg Gynecol Obstet 112:150, 1961

44. Wilmore DW: Nutrition and metabolism following thermal injury. Clin Plast Surg 1:603, 1974

45. Kinney JM: Energy deficits in acute illness and injury. Proceedings of a Conference on Energy Metabolism and Body Fuel Utilization. Morgan AP, Ed. Harvard University Press, Cambridge, Massachusetts, 1966, p 174

46. Picou D, Taylor-Roberts T: The measurement of total protein synthesis and catabolism and nitrogen turnover in infants on different amounts of dietary protein. Clin Sci 36:283, 1969

47. Birkhahn RH, Long CL, Fitkin D, et al: Effects of major skeletal trauma on whole body protein turnover in man measured by L-[1,^{14}C]-leucine. Surgery 88:294, 1980

48. Kien CL, Young VR, Rohrbaugh DK, et al: Increased rates of whole body protein synthesis and breakdown in children recovering from burns. Ann Surg 187:383, 1978

49. Munro HN: Free amino acid pools and their role in regulation. Mammalian Protein Metabolism, Vol 4. Munro HN, Ed. Academic Press, New York, 1970, p 299

50. Bergström J, Fürst P, Noree L-O, et al: Intracellular free amino acid concentration in human muscle tissue. J Appl Physiol 36:693, 1974

51. Askanazi J, Elwyn DH, Kinney JM, et al: Muscle and plasma amino acids after injury: the role of inactivity. Ann Surg 188:797, 1978

52. Vinnars E, Bergström J, Fürst P: Influence of the postoperative state on the intracellular free amino acids in human muscle tissue. Ann Surg 182:665, 1975

53. Fürst P, Bergström J, Chao L, et al: Influence of amino acid supply on nitrogen and amino acid metabolism in severe trauma. Acta Chir Scand 494(suppl): 136, 1979

54. Askanazi J, Carpentier YA, Michelson CB, et al: Muscle and plasma amino acids following injury: influence of intercurrent infection. Ann Surg 192:78, 1980

55. Askanazi J, Fürst P, Michelsen CB, et al: Muscle and plasma amino acids after injury: hypocaloric glucose vs. amino acid infusion. Ann Surg 191:465, 1980

56. Wilmore DW, Black PR, Muhlbacher F: Injured man: trauma and sepsis. Nutritional Support of the Seriously Ill Patient. Winters RW, Greene HL, Eds. Academic Press, New York, 1983, p 33

57. Aulick LH, Wilmore DW: Increased peripheral amino acid release following burn injury. Surgery 85:560, 1979

58. Garber AJ, Karl IE, Kipnis DM: Alanine and glutamine synthesis and release from skeletal muscle: I. Glycolysis and amino acid release. J Biol Chem 251:826, 1976

59. Garber AJ, Karl IE, Kipnis DM: Alanine and glutamine synthesis and release from skeletal muscle: II. The precursor role of amino acids in alanine and glutamine synthesis. J Biol Chem 251:836, 1976

60. Close JH: The use of amino acid precursors in nitrogen-accumulation diseases. N Engl J Med 290:663, 1974

61. Johnson DJ, Jiang ZM, Colpoys M, et al: Branched chain amino acid uptake and muscle free amino acid concentrations predict postoperative muscle nitrogen balance. Ann Surg 204:513, 1986

62. Rennie MJ, Hundal HS, Babij P, et al: Characteristics of a glutamine carrier in skeletal muscle have important consequences for nitrogen loss in injury, infection, and chronic disease. Lancet 2:1008, 1986

63. Windmueller HG: Glutamine utilization by the small intestine. Adv Enzymol 53:201, 1982

64. Souba WW, Wilmore DW: Postoperative alteration of arteriovenous exchange of amino acids across the gastrointestinal tract. Surgery 94:342, 1983

65. Long CL, Spencer JL, Kinney JM, et al: Carbohydrate metabolism in man: effect of elective operations and major injury. J Appl Physiol 31:110, 1971

66. Wolfe RR, Durkot MJ, Allsop JR, et al: Glucose metabolism in severely burned patients. Metabolism 28:1031, 1979

67. Wilmore DW, Mason AD, Pruitt BA Jr: Alterations in glucose kinetics following thermal injury. Forum on Fundamental Surgical Problems 26:81, 1975

68. Ruderman MB: Muscle amino acid metabolism and gluconeogenesis. Annu Rev Med 26:245, 1975

69. Wolfe RR, Herndon DN, Jahoor F, et al: Effect of severe burn injury on substrate cycling by glucose and fatty acids. N Engl J Med 317:403, 1987

70. Shaw JHF, Wolfe RR: An integrated analysis of glucose, fat, and protein metabolism in severely traumatized patients: studies in the basal state and the response to total parenteral nutrition. Ann Surg 209:63, 1989

71. Howard JM: Studies of the absorption and metabolism of glucose following injury: the systemic response to injury. Ann Surg 141:311, 1955

72. Allison SP, Hinton P, Chamberlain MJ: Intravenous glucose-tolerance, insulin, and free–fatty-acid levels in burned patients. Lancet 2:1113, 1968

73. Wilmore DW, Mason AD Jr, Pruitt BA Jr: Insulin response to glucose in hypermetabolic burn patients. Ann Surg 183:314, 1978

74. Black PR, Brooks DC, Bessey PQ, et al: Mechanisms of insulin resistance following injury. Ann Surg 196:420, 1982

75. Brooks DC, Bessey PQ, Black PR, et al: Post-traumatic insulin resistance in uninjured forearm tissue. J Surg Res 37:100, 1984

76. Long JM III, Wilmore DW, Mason AD Jr, et al: Effect of carbohydrate and fat intake on nitrogen excretion during total intravenous feeding. Ann Surg 185:417, 1977

77. Wolfe RR, O'Donnell TF Jr, Stone MD, et al: Investigation of factors determining optimal glucose infusion rate in total parenteral nutrition. Metabolism 29:892, 1980

78. Burke JF, Wolfe RR, Mullany CJ, et al: Glucose requirements following burn injury: parameters of optimal glucose infusion and possible hepatic and respiratory abnormalities following excessive glucose intake. Ann Surg 190:274, 1979

79. Askanazi J, Carpentier YA, Elwyn DH, et al: Influence of total parenteral nutrition on fuel utilization in injury and sepsis. Ann Surg 191:40, 1980

80. Goodenough RD, Wolfe RR: Effect of total parenteral nutrition on free fatty acid metabolism in burned patients. JPEN J Parenter Enteral Nutr 8:357, 1984

81. Roth J, LeRoith D, Lesniak MA, et al: Molecules of intercellular communication in vertebrates, invertebrates, and microbes: do they share common origins? Prog Brain Res 68:71, 1986

82. Soop M, Duxbury H, Agwunobi AO, et al: Euglycemic hyperinsulinemia augments the cytokine and endocrine responses to endotoxin in humans. Am J Physiol Endocrinol Metab 282:E1276, 2002

83. Davies CL, Newman RJ, Molyneux SG, et al: The relationship between plasma catecholamines and severity of injury in man. J Trauma 24:99, 1984

84. Harrison TS, Seaton JF, Feller I: Relationship of increased oxygen consumption to catecholamine excretion in thermal burns. Ann Surg 165:169, 1967

85. Porte D Jr, Robertson RP: Control of insulin secretion by catecholamines, stress, and the sympathetic nervous system. Fed Proc 32:1792, 1973

86. Bessey PQ, Brooks DC, Black PR, et al: Epinephrine acutely mediates skeletal muscle insulin resistance. Surgery 94:172, 1983

87. Garber AJ, Karl JE, Kipnis DM: Alanine and glutamine synthesis and release from skeletal muscle: IV. β-Adrenergic inhibition of amino acid release. J Biol Chem 251:851, 1976

88. Vaughan GM, Becker RA, Allan JP, et al: Cortisol and corticotrophin in burned patients. J Trauma 22:263, 1982

89. Wilmore DW, Lindsey CA, Moylan JA, et al: Hyperglucagonaemia after burns. Lancet 1:73, 1974

90. Baxter JD, Forsham PH: Tissue effects of glucocorticoids. Am J Med 53:573, 1972

91. Owen OE, Cahill GF Jr: Metabolic effects of exogenous glucocorticoids in fasted man. J Clin Invest 52:2596, 1973

92. Felig P, Wahren J, Hendler R: Influence of physiologic hyperglucagonemia on basal and insulin-inhibited splanchnic glucose output in normal man. J Clin Invest 58:761, 1976

93. Ferrannini E, DeFronze RA, Sherwin RS: Transient hepatic response to glucagon in man: role of insulin and hyperglycemia. Am J Physiol 242:E73, 1982

94. Wolfe BM, Culebras JM, Aoki TT, et al: The effects of glucagon on protein metabolism in normal man. Surgery 86:248, 1979

95. Shamoon HM, Hendler R, Sherwin RS: Synergistic interactions among anti-insulin hormones in the pathogenesis of stress hypoglycemia in humans. J Clin Endocrinol Metab 52:1235, 1981

96. Bessey PQ, Watters JM, Aoki TT, et al: Combined hormonal infusion simulates the metabolic response to injury. Ann Surg 200:264, 1984

97. Bessey PQ, Jiang Z-M, Johnson DJ, et al: Post-traumatic skeletal muscle proteolysis: the role of the hormonal environment. World J Surg 13:465, 1989

98. Vilstrup H, Hansen BA, Aldal T: Glucagon enhances hepatic efficacy for urea production. Clinical Nutrition 7(suppl):35, 1988

99. Bessey PQ, Lowe KA: Early hormonal changes affect the catabolic response to trauma. Ann Surg 218:476, 1993

100. Hulton N, Johnson DJ, Smith RJ, et al: Hormonal blockade modifies post-traumatic protein catabolism. J Surg Res 39:310, 1985

101. Brandt MR, Fernandes A, Mordhorst R, et al: Epidural analgesia improves postoperative nitrogen balance. Br Med J 1:1106, 1978

102. Tsuji H, Shirasaka C, Asoh T, et al: Effects of epidural administration of local anaesthetics or morphine on postoperative nitrogen loss and catabolic hormones. Br J Surg 74:421, 1987

103. Heindorff H, Schulze S, Morgensen T, et al: Hormonal and neural blockade prevents the postoperative increase in amino acid clearance and urea synthesis. Surgery 111:543, 1992

104. Vaughan GM, Pruitt BA: Thyroid function in critical illness and burn injury. Semin Nephrol 13:359, 1993

105. Lephart ED, Baxter CR, Parker CR: Effect of burn trauma on adrenal and testicular steroid hormone production. J Clin Endocrinol Metab 64:842, 1987

106. Spratt DI, Cox P, Orav J, et al: Reproductive axis suppression in acute illness is related to disease severity. J Clin Endocrinol Metab 76:1548, 1993

107. Noel GI, Suh JK, Stone SJG, et al: Human prolactin and growth hormone release during surgery and other condtions of stress. J Clin Endocrinol Metab 35:840, 1972

108. Saito H: Anabolic agents in trauma and sepsis: repleting body mass and function. Nutrition 14:554, 1998

109. Baxter RC: Insulin-like growth factor (IGF)-binding proteins: interactions with IGF's and intrinsic bioactivities. Am J Physiol Endocrinol Metab 278:E967, 2000

110. van den Berghe G, de Zegher F, Bouillon R: Acute and prolonged critical illness as different neuroendocrine paradigms. J Clin Endocrinol Metab 83:1827, 1998

111. van den Berghe G, Baxter RC, Weekers F, et al: The combined administration of GH-releasing peptide-2 (GHRP-2), TRH, and GnRH to men with prolonged critical illness evokes superior endocrine and metabolic effects compared to treatment with GHRP-2 alone. Clin Endocrinol 56:655, 2002

112. Hunt TK: Physiology of wound healing. Trauma, Sepsis, and Shock: The Physiological Basis of Therapy. Clowes GHA Jr, Ed. Marcel Dekker, New York, 1988, p 443

113. Dinarello CA: Proinflammatory and anti-inflammatory cytokines as mediators in the pathogenesis of septic shock. Chest 112:321S, 1997

114. Cinat M, Waxman K, Vaziri ND, et al: Soluble cytokine receptors and receptor antagonists are sequentially released after trauma. J Trauma 39:112, 1995

115. Akira S, Hirano T, Taga T, et al: Biology of multifunctional cytokines: IL-6 and related molecules (IL-1 and TNF). FASEB J 4:2860, 1990

116. Jiang JX, Tian KL, Chen HS, et al: Plasma cytokines and endotoxin levels in patients with severe injury and their relationship with organ damage. Injury 28:509, 1997

117. Drosst AC, Burleson DG, Cioffi WG Jr, et al: Plasma cytokines following thermal injury and their relationship with patient mortality, burn size, and time postburn. J Trauma 35:335, 1993

118. Michie HR, Spriggs DR, Manogue KR, et al: Tumor necrosis factor and endotoxin induce similar metabolic responses in human beings. Surgery 104:280, 1988

119. Michie HR, Sherman ML, Spriggs DR, et al: Chronic TNF infusion causes anorexia but not accelerated nitrogen loss. Ann Surg 209:19, 1989

120. Mealy K, van Lanschot JJB, Robinson BG, et al: Are the catabolic effects of tumor necrosis factor mediated by glucocorticoids? Arch Surg 125:42, 1990

121. Hall-Angeras M, Angeras U, Zamir O, et al: Effect of the glucocorticoid receptor antagonist RU 38486 on muscle protein breakdown in sepsis. Surgery 109:468, 1991

122. Dinarello CA: Interleukin-1. Rev Infect Dis 6:51, 1984

123. Dinarello CA: An update on human interleukin-1: from molecular biology to clinical relevance. J Clin Immunol 5:287, 1985

124. Baracos V, Rodemann HP, Dinarello CA, et al: Stimulation of muscle protein degradation and prostaglandin E_2 release by leukocytic pyrogen (interleukin-1): a mechanism for the increased degradation of muscle proteins during fever. N Engl J Med 308:553, 1983

125. Sobrado JL, Moldawer LL, Dinarello CA, et al: Effect of ibuprofen on fever and metabolic changes induced by leukocytic pyrogen (interleukin-1) and endotoxin. Infect Immun 42:997, 1983

126. Moldawer LL, Svaninger G, Gelin J, et al: Interleukin-1 and tumor necrosis factor do not regulate protein balance in skeletal muscle. Am J Physiol 253:C766, 1987

127. Zamir O, Hasselgren P-O, von Allmen D, et al: The effect of interleukin-1 alpha and the glucocorticoid receptor blocker RU 38486 on total and myofibrillar protein breakdown in skeletal muscle. J Surg Res 50:579, 1991

128. Zamir O, Hasselgren P-O, O'Brien WO, et al: Muscle protein breakdown during endotoxemia in rats and after treatment with interleukin-1 receptor antagonist (IL-1ra). Ann Surg 216:381, 1992

129. Watters JM, Bessey PQ, Dinarello CA, et al: The induction of interleukin-1 in humans and its metabolic effects. Surgery 98:298, 1985

130. Watters JM, Bessey PQ, Dinarello CA, et al: Both inflammatory and endocrine mediators stimulate host responses to sepsis. Arch Surg 121:179, 1986

131. Koj A: The role of interleukin-6 as the hepatic stimulating factor in the network of inflammatory cytokines. Ann NY Acad Sci 557:1, 1989

132. Biffl WL, Moore EE, Moore FA, et al: Interleukin-6 in the injured patient: marker of injury or mediator of inflammation? Ann Surg 224:647, 1996

133. Casey LC, Balk RA, Bone RC: Plasma cytokines and endotoxin levels correlate with survival in patients with the sepsis syndrome. Ann Intern Med 119:771, 1993

134. de Beaux AC, Ross JA, Maingay JP, et al: Proinflammatory cytokine release by peripheral blood mononuclear cells from patients with acute pancreatitis. Br J Surg 83:1071, 1996

135. Guillen I, Blaines M, Gomez-Lechon MJ, et al: Cytokine signaling during myocardial infarction: sequential appearance of IL-1β and IL-6. Am J Physiol 269:R229, 1995

136. Mateo RB, Reichner JS, Albina JE: Interleukin-6 activity in wounds. Am J Physiol 266:R1840, 1994

137. Stouthard JM, Romijn JA, van der Poll T, et al: Endocrinologic and metabolic effects of interleukin-6 in humans. Am J Physiol 268:E813, 1995

138. Tsigos C, Papanicolaou DA, Kyrou I, et al: Dose-dependent effects of recombinant human interleukin-6 on glucose regulation. J Clin Endocrinol Metab 82:4167, 1997

139. De Benedetti F, Alonzi T, Moretta A, et al: Interleukin-6 causes growth impairment in transgenic mice through a decrease in insulin-like growth factor–1. J Clin Invest 99:643, 1997

140. Tsujinaka T, Fujita J, Ebisui C, et al: Interleukin-6 receptor antibody inhibits muscle atrophy and modulates proteolytic systems in interleukin-6 transgenic mice. J Clin Invest 97:244, 1996

141. Rutan RL, Herndon DN: Growth delay in postburn pediatric patients. Arch Surg 125:392, 1990

142. Gonzalez-Hernandez JA, Bornstein SR, Ehrhart-Bornstein M, et al: Interleukin-6 messenger ribonucleic acid expression in human adrenal gland in vivo: new clue to a paracrine or autocrine regulation of adrenal function. J Clin Endocrinol Metab 79:1492, 1994

143. Path G, Bornstein SR, Ehrhart-Bornstein M, et al: Interleukin-6 and the interleukin-6 receptor in the human adrenal gland: expression and effects on steroidogenesis. J Clin Endocrinol Metab 82:2343, 1997

144. Bone RC, Fisher CJ, Clemmer TP, et al: A controlled clinical trial of high-dose methylprednisolone in the treatment of severe sepsis and septic shock. N Engl J Med 317:653, 1987

145. Barber AE, Coyle SM, Maranao MA, et al: Glucocorticoid therapy alters hormonal and cytokine responses to endotoxin in man. J Immunol 150:1999, 1993

146. Hasselgren P-O: Protein Metabolism in Sepsis. RG Landes Co, Austin, Texas, 1993, p 82

147. Wing SS, Goldberg AL: Glucocorticoids activate the ATP-ubiquitin–dependent proteolytic system in skeletal muscle during fasting. Am J Physiol 264:E668, 1993

148. Zamir O, Hasselgren P-O, von Allmen D, et al: In vivo administration of interleukin-1α induces muscle proteolysis in normal and adrenalectomized rats. Metabolism 42:204, 1993

149. Hume DM, Egdahl RH: The importance of the brain in the endocrine response to injury. Ann Surg 150:697, 1959

150. Taylor JW, Hander EW, Skreen R, et al: The effect of central nervous system narcosis on the sympathetic response to stress. J Surg Res 20:313, 1976

151. Dempsey DT, Guenter P, Crosby LO, et al: Barbiturate therapy and energy expenditure in head trauma. Presented at the 42nd Annual Meeting of the American Association for the Surgery of Trauma, Colorado Springs, 1982

152. Fried R, Dempsey D, Guenter P: Barbiturates improve nitrogen balance in patients with severe head trauma (abstr). JPEN J Parenter Enteral Nutr 4:86, 1984

153. Wilmore DW, Long JM, Mason AD, et al: Stress in surgical patients as a neurophysiologic reflex response. Surg Gynecol Obstet 142:257, 1976

154. Wilmore DW, Taylor JW, Handler EW, et al: Central nervous system function following thermal injury. Metabolism and the Response to Injury. Wilkinson AW, Cuthbertson DP, Eds. Year Book Medical Publishers, Chicago, 1977, p 274

155. Chrousos GP: The hypothalamic-pituitary-adrenal axis and immune-mediated inflammation. N Engl J Med 332:1351, 1995

156. Turchik JB, Bornstein DL: Role of the central nervous system in acute-phase responses to leukocyte pyrogen. Infect Immun 30:439, 1980

157. Breder CD, Dinarello CA, Saper CB: Interleukin-1 immunoreactive innervation of the human hypothalamus. Science 240:321, 1988

158. Cunningham ET, Wada E, Carter DB, et al: In situ localization of type I interleukin-1 receptor messenger RNA in the central nervous system, pituitary, and adrenal gland of the mouse. J Neurosci 12:1101, 1991

159. Schöbitz R, DeKloet ER, Sutanto W, et al: Cellular localization of interleukin-6 mRNA and interleukin-6 receptor RNA in rat brain. Eur J Neurosci 5:1426, 1993

160. Lieberman AP, Pitha PM, Shin HS, et al: Production of tumor necrosis factor and other cytokines by astrocytes stimulated with lipopolysaccharide or a neurotrophic virus. Proc Natl Acad Sci USA 86:6348, 1989

161. Maeda Y, Matsumoto M, Hori O, et al: Hypoxia/ reoxygenation-mediated induction of astrocyte interleukin-6: a paracrine mechanism potentially enhancing neuron survival. J Exp Med 180:2297, 1994

162. Klir JJ, McClellan JL, Kluger MJ: Interleukin-1β causes the increase in anterior hypothalamic interleukin-6 during LPS-induced fever in rats. Am J Physiol 266:R1845, 1994

163. Nakamori T, Morimoto A, Yamaguchi K, et al: Interleukin-1β production in the rabbit brain during endotoxin-induced fever. J Physiol Lond 476:177, 1994

164. Hill AG, Hiegel J, Rounds J, et al: Metabolic responses to interleukin-1: centrally and peripherally mediated. Ann Surg 225:246, 1997

165. Hill AG, Jacobson L, Gonzalez J, et al: Chronic central nervous system exposure to interleukin-1β causes catabolism in the rat. Am J Physiol 271:R1142, 1996

166. Mastorakos G, Chrousos GP, Weber JS: Recombinant interleukin-6 activates the hypothalamic-pituitary-adrenal axis in humans. J Clin Endocrinol Metab 77:1690, 1993

167. Ling PR, Schwartz JH, Jeevanandam M, et al: Metabolic changes in rats during a continuous infusion of recombinant interleukin-1. Am J Physiol 270:E305, 1996

168. Reyes TM, Coe CL: The proinflammatory cytokine network: interactions in the CNS and blood of rhesus monkeys. Am J Physiol 274:R139, 1998

169. Romero LI, Kakucska I, Lechan RM, et al: Interleukin-6 (IL-6) is secreted from the brain after intercerebroventricular injection of IL-1β in rats. Am J Physiol 270:R518, 1996

170. Senba E, Kashiba K: Sensory afferent processing in multi-responsive DRG neurons. Prog Brain Res 113:387, 1996

171. Thompson SW, Priestley JV, Southall A: gp130 cytokines, leukemia inhibitory factor, and interleukin-6 induce neuropeptide expression in intact adult rat sensory neurons in vivo: time-course, specificity, and comparison with sciatic nerve axotomy. Neuroscience 84:1247, 1998

172. Hirota H, Kiyama H, Kishimoto T, et al: Accelerated nerve regeneration in mice by upregulated expression of interleukin (IL) 6 and IL-6 receptor after trauma. J Exp Med 183:2627, 1996

173. Watkins LR, Maier SF: Implications of immune-to-brain communication for sickness and pain. Proc Natl Acad Sci USA 96:771, 1999

174. Watkins LR, Maier SF: Beyond neurons: evidence that immune and glial cells contribute to pathological pain states. Physiol Rev 82:981, 2002

175. Ravin HA, Rowley D, Jenkins C, et al: On the absorption of bacterial endotoxin from the gastro-intestinal tract of the normal and shocked animal. J Exp Med 112:783, 1960

176. Caridis DT, Reinhold RB, Woodruff PW, et al: Endotoxaemia in man. Lancet 1:1381, 1972

177. Wilmore DW, Smith RJ, O'Dwyer ST, et al: The gut: a central organ after surgical stress. Surgery 104:917, 1988

178. Marin ML, Greenstein AJ, Geller SA, et al: A freeze fracture study of Crohn's disease of the terminal ileum: changes in epithelial tight junction organization. Am J Gastroenterol 78:537, 1983

179. Dobbins WO III: Gut immunophysiology: a gastroenterologist's view with emphasis on pathophysiology. Am J Physiol 242:G1, 1982

180. Deitch EA, Berg R, Specian R: Endotoxin promotes the translocation of bacteria from the gut. Arch Surg 122:185, 1987

181. Wellmann W, Fink PC, Schmidt FW: Whole-gut irrigation as antiendotoxinaemic therapy in inflammatory bowel disease. Hepatogastroenterology 31:91, 1984

182. Schatten WE, Desprez JD, Holden WD: A bacteriologic study of portal-vein blood in man. Arch Surg 71:404, 1955

183. Ambrose NS, Johnson M, Burdon DW, et al: Incidence of pathogenic bacteria from mesenteric lymph nodes and ileal serosa during Crohn's disease surgery. Br J Surg 71:623, 1984

184. Berg RD: Translocation of indigenous bacteria from the intestinal tract. Human Intestinal Microflora in Health and Disease. Hentges DJ, Ed. Academic Press, New York, 1983

185. Deitch EA, Winterton J, Berg R: Thermal injury promotes bacterial translocation from the gastrointestinal tract in mice with impaired T-cell–mediated immunity. Arch Surg 121:97, 1986

186. Baker JW, Deitch EA, Li M, et al: Hemorrhagic shock induces bacterial translocation from the gut. J Trauma 28:896, 1988

187. Deitch EA, Winterton J, Li M, et al: The gut as a portal of entry for bacteremia: role of protein malnutrition. Ann Surg 205:681, 1987

188. Moore FA, Moore EE, Poggetti R, et al: Gut bacterial translocation via the portal vein: a clinical perspective with major torso trauma. J Trauma 31:629, 1991

189. O'Farrely C: Just how inflamed is the normal gut? Gut 42:603, 1998

190. Guy-Grand E, DiSanto JP, Henchoz P, et al: Small bowel enteropathy: role of intraepithelial lymphocytes and of cytokines (IL-12, IFN-γ, TNF) in the induction of epithelial cell death and renewal. Eur J Immunol 28:730, 1998

191. Wyble CW, Desai TR, Clark ET, et al: Physiologic concentrations of TNFα and IL-1β released from reperfused human intestine upregulate E-selectin and ICAM-1. J Surg Res 63:333, 1996

192. Mainous MR, Ertel W, Chaudry IH, et al: The gut: a cytokine-generating organ in systemic inflammation? Shock 4:193, 1995

193. Mochizuki H, Trocki O, Dominioni L: Mechanism of prevention of postburn hypermetabolism and catabolism by early enteral feeding. Ann Surg 200:297, 1984

194. Saito H, Trocki O, Alexander JW: The effect of route of nutrient administration on the nutritional state, catabolic hormone secretion, and gut mucosal integrity after burn injury. JPEN J Parenter Enteral Nutr 11:1, 1987

195. Alexander JW, MacMillan BG, Stinnett JD: Beneficial effects of aggressive protein feeding in severely burned children. Ann Surg 192:505, 1980

196. Border JR, Hassett J, La Duca J: The gut origin septic states in blunt multiple trauma (ISS = 40) in the ICU. Ann Surg 206:427, 1987

197. Ogle CK, Zuo L, Mao JX, et al: Differential expression of intestinal and splenic cytokines after parenteral nutrition. Arch Surg 130:1301, 1995

198. Lyoumi S, Tamion F, Petit J, et al: Induction and modulation of acute-phase response by protein malnutrition in rats: comparative effect of systemic and localized inflammation on interleukin-6 and acute-phase protein synthesis. J Nutr 128:166, 1998

199. Steiner M, Bourges HR, Freedman LS, et al: Effect of starvation on the tissue composition of the small intestine in the rat. Am J Physiol 215:75, 1968

200. Clarke RM: Evidence for both luminal and systemic factors in the control of rat intestinal epithelial replacement. Clin Sci Mol Med 50:139, 1976

201. Gleeson MH, Dowling RH, Peters TJ: Biochemical changes in intestinal mucosa after experimental small bowel by-pass in the rat. Clin Sci 43:743, 1972

202. Johnson LR, Lichtenberger LM, Copeland EM, et al: Action of gastrin on gastrointestinal structure and function. Gastroenterology 68:1184, 1975

203. Sagor GR, Ghatei MA, Al-Mukhtar MYT, et al: Evidence for a humoral mechanism after small intestinal resection: exclusion of gastrin but not enteroglucagon. Gastroenterology 84:902, 1983

204. Hwang TL, O'Dwyer ST, Smith RJ, et al: Preservation of small bowel mucosa using glutamine-enriched parenteral nutrition. Forum on Fundamental Surgical Problems 37:56, 1986

205. Jacobs DO, Evans DA, O'Dwyer ST, et al: Trophic effects of glutamine-enriched parenteral nutrition on colonic mucosa. JPEN J Parenter Enteral Nutr 12 (suppl):6S, 1988

206. O'Dwyer ST, Smith RJ, Scott T: Glutamine enriched nutrition decreases intestinal injury and increases nitrogen retention. Br J Surg 74:1162, 1987

207. Young LS, Stevens P, Kaijser B: Gram-negative pathogens in septicaemic infections. Scand J Infect Dis 31(suppl):78, 1982

208. Fish RE, Spitzer JA: Continuous infusion of endotoxin from an osmotic pump in the conscious, unrestrained rat: a unique model of chronic endotoxemia. Circ Shock 12:135, 1984

209. Revhaug A, Michie HR, Manson JM, et al: Inhibition of cyclooxygenase attenuates the metabolic response to endotoxin in humans. Arch Surg 123:162, 1988

210. Michie HR, Manogue KR, Spriggs DR, et al: Detection of circulating tumor necrosis factor after endotoxin administration. N Engl J Med 318:1481, 1988

211. Fong Y, Tracey KJ, Moldawer LL, et al: Antibodies to cachectin/tumor necrosis factor reduce interleukin 1β and interleukin 6 appearance during lethal bacteremia. J Exp Med 170:1627, 1989

212. Riddington DW, Venkatesh B, Boivin CM, et al: Intestinal permeability, gastric intramucosal pH, and systemic endotoxemia in patients undergoing cardiopulmonary bypass. JAMA 275:1007, 1996

213. O'Dwyer ST, Michie HR, Ziegler TR, et al: A single dose of endotoxin increases intestinal permeability in healthy humans. Arch Surg 123:1459, 1988

214. Coleman W, DuBois EF: Calorimetric observations on the metabolism of typhoid patients with and without food. Arch Intern Med 15:887, 1915

215. Beisel WR, Sawyer WD, Ryll ED, et al: Metabolic effects of intracellular infections in man. Ann Intern Med 67:744, 1967

216. Aulick LH, McManus AT, Mason AD Jr, et al: Effects of infection on oxygen consumption and core temperature in experimental thermal injury. Ann Surg 204:48, 1986

217. Guo L, Lim KB, Gunn JS, et al: Regulation of lipid A modifications by Salmonella typhimurium virulence genes phoP-phoQ. Science 276:250, 1997

218. Mekalanos JJ: Environmental signals controlling expression of virulence determinants in bacteria. J Bacteriol 174:1, 1992

219. Springer TA: Traffic signals for lymphocyte recirculation and leukocyte emigration: the multistep paradigm. Cell 76:301, 1994

220. Demling RH: Adult respiratory distress syndrome: current concepts. New Horizons 1:388, 1993

221. Biffl WL, Moore EE, Moore FA, et al: Interleukin-6 delays neutrophil apoptosis via a mechanism involving platelet-activating factor. J Trauma 40:575, 1996

222. Niijima A: The afferent discharges from sensors for interleukin-1β in the hepatoportal system in the anesthetized rat. J Autonom Nerv Sys 61:287, 1996

223. Maier SF, Goehler LE, Fleshner M, et al: The role of the vagus nerve in cytokine-to-brain communication. Ann NY Acad Sci 840:289, 1998

224. Hansen MK, O'Connor KA, Goehler LE, et al: The contribution of the vagus nerve in interleukin-1b induced fever is dependent on dose. Am J Physiol Reg Interg Comp Physiol 280:R929, 2001

225. Romanovsky AA, Ivanov AI, Szekely M: Neural route of pyrogen signaling to the brain. Clin Infect Dis 31(suppl 5):S162, 2000

226. Goehler LE, Gaykema PA, Nguyen KT, et al. Interleukin-1b in immune cells of the abdominal vagus nerve: a link between the immune and nervous systems? J Neurosci 19:2799, 1999

227. Goehler LD, Gaykema RP, Hansen MK, et al: Vagal immune-to-brain communication: a visceral chemosensory pathway. Auton Neurosci 85:49, 2000

228. Borovikova LV, Ivanova S, Zhang, M, et al: Vagus nerve stimulation attenuates the systemic inflammatory response to endotoxin. Nature 405:458, 2000

229. Wang H, Yu M, Ochani M, et al: Nicotinic acetylcholine receptor α7 subunit is an essential regulator of inflammation. Nature 421:384, 2003

230. Herndon DN, Barrow RE, Rutan TC, et al: Effect of propranolol administration on hemodynamic and metabolic responses of burned pediatric patients. Ann Surg 208:484, 1988

231. Schulze A, Sommer P, Bigler D, et al: Effect of combined prednisolone, epidural analgesia, and indomethacin on the systemic response after colonic surgery. Arch Surg 127:325, 1992

232. Vincent J-L: New therapies in sepsis. Chest 112:330S, 1997

233. Hammarqvist F, Wernerman J, Ali R, et al: Addition of glutamine to total parenteral nutrition after elective abdominal surgery spares free glutamine in muscle, counteracts the fall in muscle protein synthesis, and improves nitrogen balance. Ann Surg 209:455, 1989

234. Ziegler TR, Young LS, Benfell K, et al: Clinical and metabolic efficacy of glutamine-supplemented parenteral nutrition after bone marrow transplantation: a randomized, double blind, controlled study. Ann Intern Med 116: 821, 1992

235. Kudsk KA, Minard G, Croce MA, et al: A randomized trial of isonitrogenous enteral diets after severe trauma: an immune-enhancing diet reduces septic complications. Ann Surg 224:531, 1996

236. Manson JM, Wilmore DW: Positive nitrogen balance with human growth hormone and hypocaloric intravenous feeding. Surgery 100:188, 1986

237. Jiang Z-M, He G-Z, Zhang S-Y, et al: Low dose growth hormone and hypocaloric nutrition attenuate the protein-catabolic response following major operation. Ann Surg 210:513, 1989

238. Herndon DN, Barrow RE, Kunkel KR, et al: Effects of recombinant human growth hormone on donor-site healing in severely burned children. Ann Surg 212:424, 1990

239. Knox J, Demling R, Wilmore D, et al: Increased survival after major thermal injury: the effect of growth hormone therapy in adults. J Trauma 39:526, 1995

240. Pharmacia & Upjohn: Safety statement from Pharmacia & Upjohn regarding the use of recombinant somatropin (Genotropin/Genotonorm) for treatment of acute catabolism in critically ill patients. Kalamazoo, Michigan, 1997

241. Demling RH, DeSanti L: Oxandrolone, an anabolic steroid, significantly increases the rate of weight gain in the recovery phase after major burns. J Trauma 43:47, 1997

242. Hart DW, Wolf SE, Ramzy PI, et al: Anabolic effects of oxandrolone after severe burn. Ann Surg 233:556, 2001

243. Wolf SE, Thomas SJ, Dasu MR, et al: Improved net protein balance, lean mass, and gene expression changes with oxandrolone treatment in the severely burned. Ann Surg 237:801, 2003

244. Tishler ME, Leng E, Al-Kanhal M, et al: Metabolic response of muscle to trauma: altered control of protein turnover. Clinical Nutrition and Metabolic Research: Proceedings of the 7th Congress of ESPEN, Munich 1985. Dietze D, Grünert A, Kleinberger G, et al, Eds. S Karger, Basel, 1986, p 40

245. Inculet RI, Finley RI, Duff JH, et al: Insulin decreases muscle protein loss after operative trauma in man. Surgery 99:752, 1986

246. Bower RH, Muggia-Sullam M, Vallgren S, et al: Branched chain amino acid–enriched solutions in the septic patient: a randomized prospective trial. Ann Surg 203:13, 1986

247. Gore DC, Chinkes DL, Hart DW, et al: Hyperglycemia exacerbates muscle protein in catabolism in burn-injured patients. Crit Care Med 30:2438, 2002

248. Cole M, Lipp J, Bessey PQ: Effective glucose control in the critically ill using a bedside, algorithm controlled insulin infusion (in preparation).

249. Van den Berghe G, Wouters PJ, Bouillon R, et al: Outcome benefit of intensive insulin therapy in the critically ill: insulin dose versus glycemic control. Crit Care Med 31:359, 2003

250. Pruitt BA Jr, Mason AD Jr: Epidemiological, demographic and outcome characteristics of burn injury. Total Burn Care. Herndon DN, Ed. WB Saunders Co, London, 1996, p 5

251. Milberg JA, Davis DR, Steinberg KP, et al: Improved survival of patients with acute respiratory distress syndrome (ARDS) 1983–1993. JAMA 273:306, 1995

252. Kelleman JJ 3rd, Cioffi WG Jr, Mason AD Jr, et al: Effect of ambient temperature on metabolic rate after thermal injury. Ann Surg 223:406, 1996

253. Beisel WR: Magnitude of host nutritional responses to infection. Am J Clin Nutr 30:1237, 1977

254. Michie HR, Wilmore DW: Sepsis, signals, and surgical sequelae. Arch Surg 125:531, 1990

Acknowledgments

Figures 1 and 5   Al Miller.

Figure 3   Nancy Lou Makris.

23 NUTRITIONAL SUPPORT

Rolando H. Rolandelli, M.D., F.A.C.S., Dipin Gupta, M.D., and Douglas W. Wilmore, M.D., F.A.C.S.

Nutritional Management of Hospitalized Patients

Evaluation of the Need for Nutritional Support

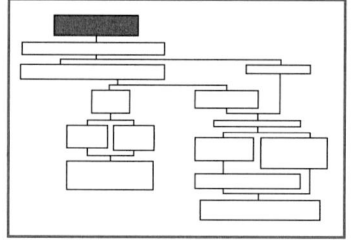

INDICATIONS FOR NUTRITIONAL INTERVENTION

Nutritional support is required in patients who fall into one of the following general categories:

1. The patient has been without nutrition for 10 days. In a well-nourished individual, body stores are generally adequate to provide nutrients during shorter periods of stress without compromising physiologic functions, altering resistance to infection, or impairing wound healing. Provision of nutrients becomes more important as body stores become eroded because of inadequate food intake and accelerated catabolism. In general, deficits occur in surgical patients after 7 to 10 days of partial starvation; nutritional intervention should be initiated before this time.
2. The duration of illness is anticipated to be longer than 10 days. In this context, nutritional support should be considered essential care. Thus, individuals with severe peritonitis or pancreatitis, major injury (injury severity score > 15), or extensive burns (> 20% total body surface area) are candidates for nutritional support because of the known duration of their ill-

ness. (The duration of illness in chronically malnourished patients also would be expected to exceed 10 days.)

3. The patient is malnourished (loss of > 10% of usual body weight over 3 months). In general, weight loss can be used as an index of nutritional deficiency, and recovery may be compromised in patients who lack adequate body nutrient stores because of an existing nutritional deficit [*see Figure 1*]. The patient should receive nutritional support when weight loss approaches or exceeds 15% of usual body weight:

$$\% \text{ Weight loss} = \frac{\text{Usual weight} - \text{present weight}}{\text{Usual weight}} \times 100$$

Patients who do not meet one of these three general indications should be reassessed after 7 days to identify individuals in whom complications develop after hospital admission and who require nutritional support. Serum proteins with a short half-life, such as prealbumin, transferrin, or retinol-binding protein, are useful markers for assessing response to therapy.

PRIORITY OF CARDIOPULMONARY FUNCTION

Intensive care unit patients are frequently candidates for nutritional support but often have complex medical and surgical problems that may take precedence. In decreasing order of importance, the priori-

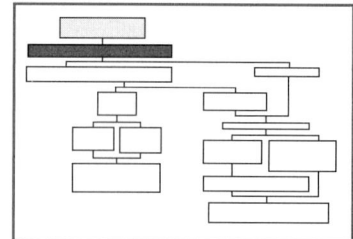

ties are to maintain airway patency, breathing, circulation, tissue oxygenation, acid-base neutrality, normal electrolyte concentrations, and adequate nutrition. The six functions that take priority over nutrition are usually impaired by acute and potentially life-threatening disorders that are often correctable over the short term. To optimize nutrient metabolism, circulation and tissue oxygenation must be adequate. In addition, hydrogen ion and electrolyte concentrations should be near normal in the extracellular fluid compartment, as reflected by blood or serum measurements.

If cardiopulmonary function is abnormal, nutrient administration may create additional problems. For example, in a patient with respiratory insufficiency, infusion of moderate quantities of carbohydrate could increase carbon dioxide tension (P_{CO_2}) and lower serum potassium concentration, thereby potentially initiating a life-threatening cardiac arrhythmia. The need for nutritional support in the ICU patient should always be evaluated with respect to other care problems; acute disorders of cardiorespiratory function, disturbed acid-base status, and altered electrolyte

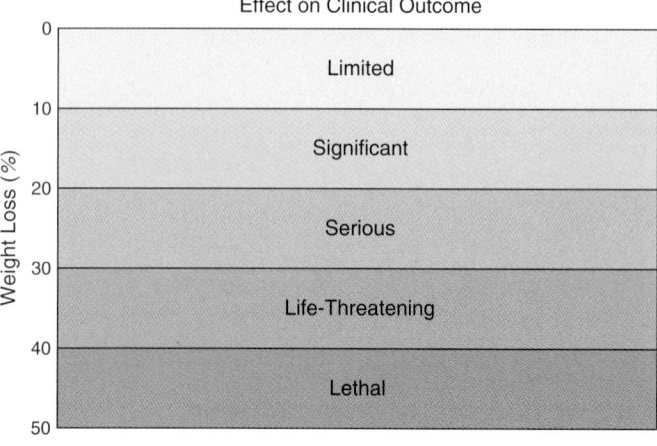

Figure 1 **The magnitude of weight loss is a rough predictor of its effect on clinical outcome.**

Table 1 Alterations in Metabolic Rate

Patient Condition	Basal Metabolic Rate
No postoperative complications Fistula without infection	Normal
Mild peritonitis Long-bone fracture or mild to moderate injury	25% above normal
Severe injury or infection in ICU patient Multiorgan failure	50% above normal
Burn of 40%–100% of TBS	100% above normal

concentrations should generally be corrected before nutritional support is initiated.

NUTRIENT REQUIREMENTS

Individual energy requirements are primarily related to body size, age, sex, and energy expenditure of activity (muscular work). In hospitalized patients who are generally inactive, the basal metabolic rate (BMR) accounts for the greatest amount of energy expenditure. The BMR in normal individuals is about 25 kcal/kg/day but can be calculated more precisely according to the Harris-Benedict formulas:

$$\text{Males: BMR (kcal/day)} = 66 + (13.7 \times \text{weight [kg]}) + (5 \times \text{height [cm]}) - (6.8 \times \text{age [yr]})$$

$$\text{Females: BMR (kcal/day)} = 665 + (9.6 \times \text{weight [kg]}) + (1.7 \times \text{height [cm]}) - (4.7 \times \text{age [yr]})$$

The BMR is influenced by the disease process. Hypermetabolism occurs in surgical patients with moderate to severe infection or injury, and the magnitude of the increase in the BMR depends on the extent of injury or infection. Patients generally fall into one of four categories according to their metabolic requirements [see Table 1].

Estimates that are based on normal basal metabolic requirements and adjusted only for disease state reflect the energy needs of patients requiring mechanical ventilation or those at bed rest. Further adjustments, however, are necessary for individuals who are out of bed and physically active. To meet the energy needs of such patients, who are in a nonbasal state, calculated requirements should be increased by an additional 15% to 20%. The metabolic response to stress and critical illness is complex and is mediated by interactions between the neuroendocrine system and circulating cytokines. This interaction produces a metabolic milieu in which the body cannot utilize supranormal amounts of nutritional substrates (i.e., hyperalimentation). In fact, administering excessive nutrients in an attempt at acute correction of nutrient deficits is often harmful, leading to an abnormal accumulation of hepatic glycogen, enhancing total energy expenditure, and causing increased urea production and elevation of the blood urea nitrogen (BUN).

Weight gain usually should not be a priority for ICU patients. Complications of nutrient delivery are minimized and nutrient metabolism generally optimized if only the energy necessary for weight maintenance is given. For most general surgical patients admitted to the ICU for non–trauma-related care, this amount is typically no more than 35 kcal/kg body weight/day. With resolution of the disease process, the hormonal environment is altered to favor anabolism. In addition, increases in spontaneous activity and in planned exercise stimulate rebuilding of lean body mass.

Protein

After energy requirements are determined, protein needs are calculated. For most patients, the protein requirement is 0.8 g/kg body weight/day (about 60 to 70 g/day). Critically ill patients, however, may need 1.5 to 2.0 g/kg/day (about 100 to 150 g/day). Most standard enteral and parenteral feeding mixtures provide this increased quantity of protein if enough formula is delivered to meet patients'

Table 2 Vitamin Requirements

Vitamin	Units	Recommended Dietary Allowance (RDA) for Daily Oral Intake	Daily Requirement of the Moderately Injured	Daily Requirement of the Severely Injured	Amount Provided by One Vitamin Pill	Daily Amount Provided by Standard Intravenous Preparations
Vitamin A (retinol)	IU	1,760 (females)–3,300 (males)	5,000	5,000	10,000	3,300 (retinal)
Vitamin D (ergocalciferol)	IU	200	400	400	400	200
Vitamin E (tocopherol)	mg TE	8–10	unknown	unknown	15	10 IU*
Vitamin K (phylloquinone)	μg	20–40†	20	20	0	0‡
Vitamin C (ascorbic acid)	mg	60	75	300	100	100
Thiamine (vitamin B₁)	mg	1.0–1.5	2	10	10	3.0
Riboflavin (vitamin B₂)	mg	1.2–1.7	2	10	10	3.6
Niacin	mg	13–19	20	100	100	40
Pyridoxine (vitamin B₆)	mg	2.0–2.2	2	40	5	4.0
Pantothenic acid	mg	4–7 (adults)†	18	40	20	15
Folic acid	mg	0.4	1.5	2.5	0	0.4
Vitamin B₁₂	μg	3.0	2	4	5	5
Biotin	μg	100–200†	unknown	unknown	0	60

*Equivalent to RDA. †Estimated to be safe and adequate dietary intakes. ‡Must be supplemented in peripheral venous solutions.

Give nutritional support if any of the following conditions is present:
- Patient has been without nutrition for 7–10 days
- Expected duration of illness > 10 days
- Patient is malnourished (weight loss > 15% of usual weight)

If nutritional intervention is not indicated initially, reassess patient after 5 days.

Initiate nutritional support only if tissue perfusion is adequate and PO_2, PCO_2, electrolyte concentrations, and acid-base balance are near normal

Estimate requirements for fluid, calories, protein, minerals, trace elements, and vitamins according to BMR, disease state, and activity level.

Abdominal distention, diarrhea, massive GI hemorrhage, obstruction, and hemodynamic instability are absent

Use existing nasogastric tube for enteral nutrition. Verify location of NG tube by aspiration of GI contents or by x-ray. Select balanced or disease-specific diet; deliver 30 ml/hr continuously at isotonicity for 24 hr. Elevate head during and after feeding to prevent regurgitation. Assess feeding tolerance.

Enteral feeding is tolerated

Assess risk for aspiration. Risk factors include depressed sensorium, gastroesophageal reflux, and history of aspiration or regurgitation.

Risk for aspiration is low

Give continuous gastric feedings of an isotonic formula at 30 ml/hr. Increase rate daily by 30 ml/hr. Increase tonicity after increasing volume.

Risk for aspiration is high

Pass feeding tube into jejunum; verify tube location by x-ray. Give formulas of 300 mOsm/kg at an initial rate of 30 ml/hr. Increase rate daily by 30 ml/hr. Increase tonicity after volume is fully increased.

Monitor patient; prevent and treat complications as necessary

Irrigate tube routinely with 20–25 ml normal saline or water.
If tube is blocked, clear by injection of a small volume of carbonated beverage.
For persistent diarrhea, give kaolin-pectin, 30 ml q. 3 hr.
To prevent peptic ulcers and bleeding, titrate gastric pH to 4.5–6.5 with antacids if necessary.
If nasoenteric tube dislodgment is recurrent, consider tube enterostomy.
If enterostomy tube leaks persistently, replace with tube of larger diameter.

Nutritional Management of Hospitalized Patients

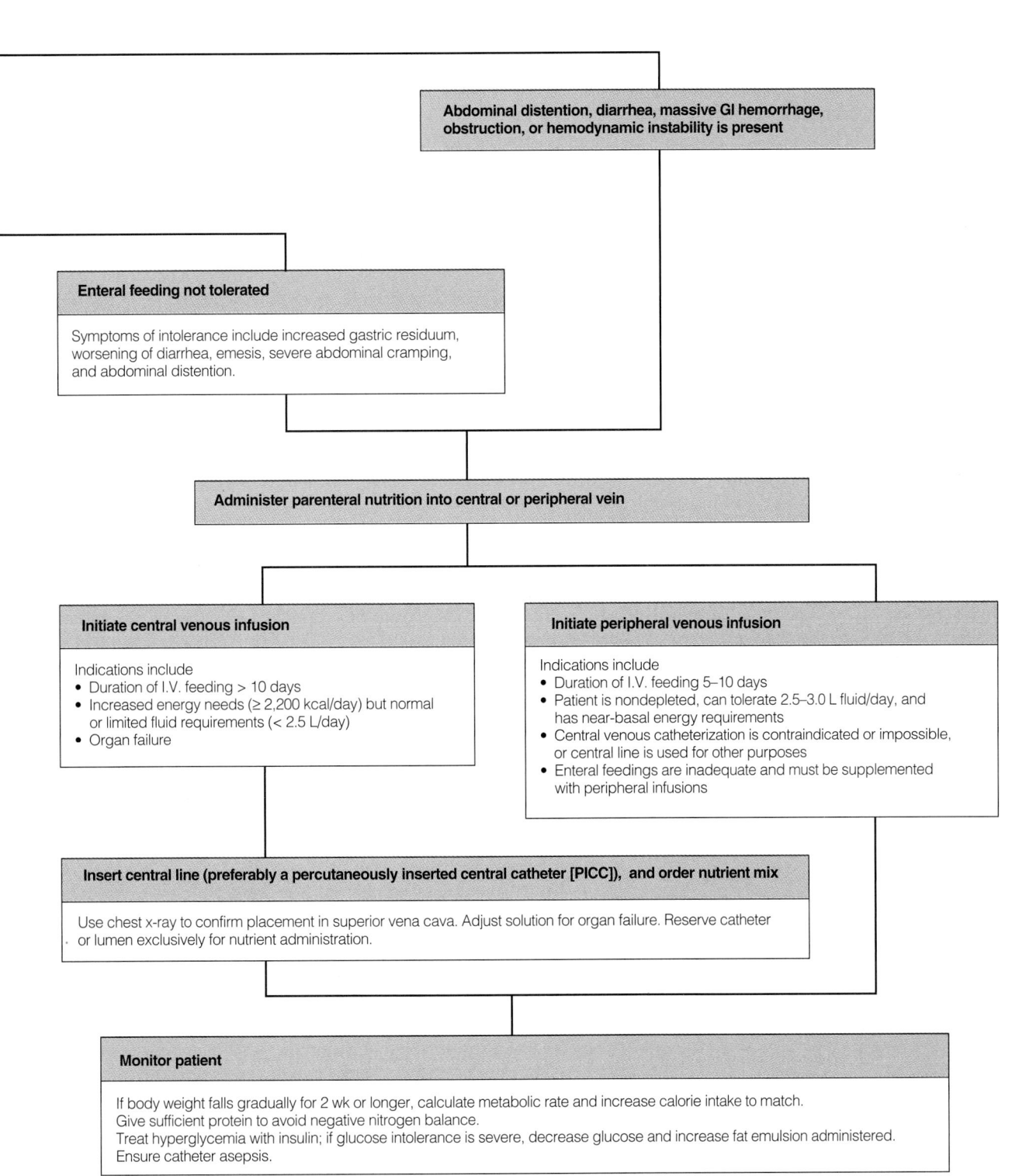

Abdominal distention, diarrhea, massive GI hemorrhage, obstruction, or hemodynamic instability is present

Enteral feeding not tolerated

Symptoms of intolerance include increased gastric residuum, worsening of diarrhea, emesis, severe abdominal cramping, and abdominal distention.

Administer parenteral nutrition into central or peripheral vein

Initiate central venous infusion

Indications include
- Duration of I.V. feeding > 10 days
- Increased energy needs (≥ 2,200 kcal/day) but normal or limited fluid requirements (< 2.5 L/day)
- Organ failure

Initiate peripheral venous infusion

Indications include
- Duration of I.V. feeding 5–10 days
- Patient is nondepleted, can tolerate 2.5–3.0 L fluid/day, and has near-basal energy requirements
- Central venous catheterization is contraindicated or impossible, or central line is used for other purposes
- Enteral feedings are inadequate and must be supplemented with peripheral infusions

Insert central line (preferably a percutaneously inserted central catheter [PICC]), and order nutrient mix

Use chest x-ray to confirm placement in superior vena cava. Adjust solution for organ failure. Reserve catheter or lumen exclusively for nutrient administration.

Monitor patient

If body weight falls gradually for 2 wk or longer, calculate metabolic rate and increase calorie intake to match.
Give sufficient protein to avoid negative nitrogen balance.
Treat hyperglycemia with insulin; if glucose intolerance is severe, decrease glucose and increase fat emulsion administered.
Ensure catheter asepsis.

Table 3 Trace Mineral Requirements

Mineral	Recommended Dietary Allowance (RDA) for Daily Oral Intake (mg)	Suggested Daily Intravenous Intake (mg)	Daily Amount Provided by a Commercially Available Mixture (mg)
Zinc	15	2.5–5.0*	5.0
Copper	2–3†	0.5–1.5	1.0
Manganese	2.5–5.0†	0.15–0.8	0.5
Chromium	0.05–0.2†	0.01–0.015	0.1
Iron	10 (males)–18 (females)	3	—

*Burn patients require an additional 2 mg. †Estimated to be safe and adequate dietary intakes.

increased caloric requirements. The nitrogen-to-calorie ratio for most feeding formulas prepared for surgical patients is 1:150 (i.e., 1 g of nitrogen for every 150 kcal).

The contraindications to this increased quantity of protein are renal failure before dialysis (BUN > 40 mg/dl) and hepatic encephalopathy. Patients with systemic inflammatory response syndrome (SIRS) often require increased quantities of dietary protein [*see 6:13 Multiple Organ Dysfunction Syndrome*]. Nutritional support reduces net nitrogen losses in such patients, but positive or even neutral nitrogen balance is generally not achieved because of the disturbance in metabolism and reduced intake of dietary protein.

Vitamins and Minerals

The requirements for vitamins, minerals, and trace elements are usually met when adequate volumes of balanced nutrient formulas are provided [*see Tables 2 and 3*]. The requirements for most of the major minerals (sodium, potassium, chloride, phosphorus, magnesium, and zinc) are satisfied by monitoring serum concentrations of these elements and adjusting intake to maintain levels within the normal range. Some minerals and electrolytes are restricted in patients with renal failure. Although serum concentrations may not directly reflect total body deficits, sufficient quantities of these nutrients are available to support normal cellular functions if adequate blood concentrations are maintained. Most premixed enteral formulas provide adequate quantities of these substances if caloric needs are met. Vitamins and trace elements must be added to parenteral solutions.

Pharmacologic recommendations for stress in surgical patients The doses of vitamins given are often not the recommended dietary allowance (RDA) but rather some multiple thereof;

Table 4 Safety Levels of Vitamins[2]

Safety Level	Vitamin
At least 50 to 100 times RDA	Vitamin B₁ Vitamin B₂ Niacin Vitamin C Vitamin E Biotin Folic acid Pantothenic acid
10 times RDA	Vitamin A Vitamin B₆ Vitamin D Vitamin K

for example, stressed patients usually receive three to 10 times the normal RDA.

The prescription of vitamins and minerals for therapeutic use should be based on the patient's nutritional history as well as on estimated requirements for the current disease state. These considerations are particularly important for fat-soluble vitamins, which are stored in body fat and thus may become toxic at high levels. Current recommendations stipulate that therapeutic dosages of vitamins should not exceed 10 times the RDA[1]; however, it has been suggested that some vitamins may be safe if given at dosages 50 to 100 times the RDA [*see Table 4*].[2] Vitamins and minerals are sometimes given in large dosages to exert antioxidant effects. Vitamins A, C, and E and the minerals zinc and selenium can attenuate the tissue-damaging effects of free radicals. One randomized, prospective trial, primarily involving trauma patients, demonstrated a significant reduction in organ failure with the administration of vitamins C (1,000 mg) and E (1,000 IU).[3] Many physicians are giving these vitamins and minerals as supplements to injured and infected patients[4]; supplementation with glutamine should also be considered [*see* Discussion, *below*].

Electronic Ordering to Optimize Nutritional Support

In hospital settings, nutritional care is often standardized to optimize formula composition and delivery. A useful electronic approach to nutritional prescription is available on the Internet (http://epen.kumc.edu).

Enteral Nutrition

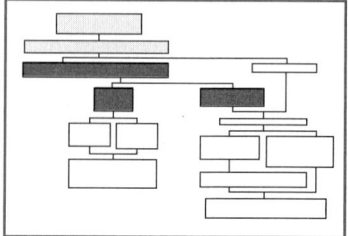

Enteral nutrition is the provision of liquid-formula diets by mouth or tube into the GI tract. It is the preferred method of feeding critically ill patients; however, it cannot be used safely in patients who are hemodynamically unstable or who have abdominal distention, intestinal obstruction, or massive GI bleeding [*see Table 5*]. For those who are able to receive enteral nutrition, either a balanced or a modified diet is selected on the basis of diagnosis and nutritional requirements. An isotonic (approximately 300 mOsm/kg) diet is given continuously for a trial period of 24 hours. If the patient tolerates this regimen but is at increased risk for aspiration, feeding is delivered into the jejunum rather than into the stomach. A standard protocol is helpful in reducing complications.

SAFE USE OF THE GI TRACT FOR FEEDING

Enteral nutrition should be prescribed only if safety and a low complication rate can be ensured. To determine whether enteral

Table 5 Indications for Enteral Nutrition (Partial Listing)

Considered Routine Care in the Following:

Protein-calorie malnutrition with inadequate oral intake of nutrients for the previous 5–7 days

Normal nutritional status but < 50% of required oral intake of nutrients for the previous 7–10 days

Severe dysphagia

Major full-thickness burns

Low-output enterocutaneous fistulas

Major trauma

Usually Helpful in the Following:

Radiation therapy

Mild chemotherapy

Liver failure and severe renal dysfunction

Massive small bowel resection (> 50%) in combination with administration of total parenteral nutrition

Of Limited or Undetermined Value in the Following:

Intensive chemotherapy

Immediate postoperative period or poststress period

Acute enteritis

> 90% resection of small bowel

Contraindicated in the Following:

Complete mechanical intestinal obstruction

Abdominal distention

Ileus or intestinal hypomotility

Severe diarrhea

Severe GI bleeding

High-output external fistulas

Severe, acute pancreatitis

Shock

Case of aggressive nutritional support not desired by the patient or legal guardian and respect of such wish being in accordance with hospital policy and existing law

Prognosis not warranting aggressive nutritional support

---

nutrition is feasible, a clinical assessment of intestinal function is performed. If GI output—defined as the volume of effluent from a nasogastric tube, an ostomy, or a rectal tube—is less than 600 ml/24 hr, enteral nutrition is likely to be well tolerated. Examples of conditions in critically ill patients that produce excessively high (> 600 ml/24 hr) GI outputs and therefore preclude the use of enteral nutrition are gastroparesis, intestinal obstruction, paralytic ileus, high-output enteric fistulas, antibiotic-induced colitis, severe idiopathic diarrhea, and the initial phase of short bowel syndrome. Selected patients with enteric losses exceeding 600 ml/24 hr may receive enteral nutrition, however, if carefully monitored by an experienced team.

Massive GI bleeding may also cause increased GI output. Conditions that produce bleeding of this magnitude include peptic ulcer disease, esophageal varices, diverticulosis, and angiodysplasia of the colon. Mild bleeding (e.g., that produced by stress gastritis) may actually resolve with the delivery of enteral nutrition into the stomach because the liquid diet buffers gastric acid.[5] Enteral nutrition does not exacerbate mild lower intestinal bleeding.

Although commonly used at the bedside as indicators of intestinal function, bowel sounds and passage of flatus are nonspecific and are unrelated to the eventual tolerance of enteral nutrition.

In the absence of excessively high GI output, abdominal distention, and massive GI bleeding, a trial of enteral nutrition is warranted to determine if the GI tract can be used safely for feeding.

SELECTION OF DIET

Before delivery of enteral nutrition, the appropriate diet must be selected on the basis of the patient's nutrient requirements [see Indications for Nutritional Intervention, above]. Most liquid-formula diets consist of either a balanced or a modified formula.

Balanced diets contain carbohydrates, proteins, and fats in complex (polymeric) forms in proportions similar to those of a regular Western diet. Frequently, however, the fat content is reduced to 10% to 15% of total calories, and the carbohydrate content is increased. Carbohydrates are present as oligosaccharides, polysaccharides, or maltodextrins; fats consist of medium-chain triglycerides (MCTs) or long-chain triglycerides (LCTs). The nitrogen source is a natural protein, which may be either intact or partially hydrolyzed. In general, balanced diets are isotonic, lactose free, and available in ready-to-use, liquid form. Flavored balanced diets can be used for oral supplementation as well as for enteral tube feeding.

Selection of a balanced diet is based on nutrient and fluid requirements. The caloric density of balanced diets can be 1.0, 1.5, or 2.0 kcal/ml; the largest number of commercially available diets provide 1.0 kcal/ml. Nonprotein caloric content is derived from either carbohydrates or lipids. Balanced diets formulated with carbohydrates as the main caloric source have higher osmolarity than isocaloric diets containing lipids. These carbohydrate-based diets are well tolerated when administered directly into the stomach and may be helpful for patients with steatorrhea. Fat-based balanced diets may be more appropriate for patients with diarrhea caused by diet hyperosmolarity, especially when feedings are infused directly into the small intestine. However, fat malabsorption is common in critically ill patients when the fat content of the diet exceeds 30% of total calories.

In modified formulas (also known as elemental or chemically defined diets), the proportions and types of nutrients differ from those of a regular Western diet. Such diets may be characterized according to the conditions for which they are formulated: stress, immunomodulation, and hepatic, renal, respiratory, or GI dysfunction [see Table 6]. Modified diets contain crystalline amino acids or short peptides in compositions that differ from the reference composition of proteins of high biologic value (e.g., egg albumin). The fat-to-carbohydrate ratio of modified diets varies depending on the purpose of the modification. The source of carbohydrate is either dextrose or oligosaccharides; fats are usually in the form of MCTs, essential fatty acids, or both. Because they are not palatable, modified diets are rarely used as oral supplements.

Diets for patients with GI dysfunction have modified nitrogen and fat composition. Transport of dietary nitrogen across the intestinal mucosa is enhanced when nitrogen is provided in the form of short peptides rather than free amino acids. It is also well documented that small bowel mucosa utilizes glutamine as the preferred fuel [see Discussion, below]. Consequently, some modified diets contain nitrogen in the form of short peptides, whereas others contain extra glutamine. MCTs are more easily absorbed and metabolized than LCTs are; accordingly, diets modified for improved absorption contain a higher proportion of MCT oil. These diets may be efficacious when used during the transition phase after a period of prolonged bowel rest or when the intestine is inflamed. Controlled trials are necessary to verify their clinical efficacy. Stress formulas are indicated for hypercatabolic patients whose nitrogen balance continues to be negative despite increased intake of a balanced diet; these diets usually contain more nitrogen and frequently have an altered amino acid composition. Little evidence supports the use of diets that provide branched-chain amino acids (BCAAs) in concentrations higher than 20% to 25% of total amino acid content for stressed patients.

The fat sources used for enteral diets are primarily omega-6 fatty acids. Supplementation with omega-3 fatty acids results in the synthesis of eicosanoids that enhance the immune response. Enteral diets may also include other substances believed to have immunomodulatory effects [see Discussion, below].

ASSESSMENT OF FEEDING TOLERANCE

The selected formula is started at isotonicity and delivered continuously at 30 ml/hr for 24 hours. During this initial trial, the formula is delivered via a previously inserted Salem sump or rubber nasogastric (Levin) tube. If a nasogastric tube is not already in place, a soft tube made of either silicone rubber or polyurethane is inserted (see below).

Feeding tolerance is assessed for the first 24 hours. Poor tolerance is indicated by vomiting and severe abdominal cramps, a gastric residuum greater than 50% of the volume administered during the previous 4-hour feeding period, increased abdominal distention (particularly in patients who are comatose or undergoing mechanical ventilation), and worsening diarrhea. If any of these conditions is present, parenteral nutrition is recommended. If there is no evidence of feeding intolerance, the patient is assessed for the aspiration risk.

ASSESSMENT OF RISK OF ASPIRATION

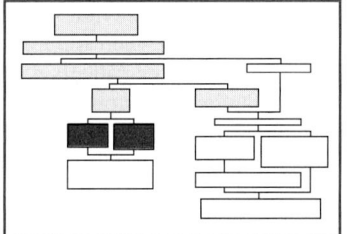

Aspiration is a major complication in patients receiving enteral nutrition. The propensity to aspirate enteral feedings is often related to the patient's primary disease and neurologic status as well as to the site of GI access and the method of delivery.

Important factors in assessing risk of aspiration include depressed sensorium, increased gastroesophageal reflux, and history of previously documented episodes of aspiration. Depressed sensorium in the critical care setting is secondary to organic lesions of the central nervous system, metabolic encephalopathies, or medications. Head trauma, hypoxemia, hepatic and septic encephalopathies, and the use of H_2 receptor blockers are common causes of depressed sensorium in critically ill patients. Increased gastroesophageal reflux may be present in individuals with reduced lower esophageal sphincter (LES) pressure and increased intragastric pressure. Many medications used in the ICU, such as theophylline, anticholinergics, calcium channel blocking agents, beta-adrenergic agonists, and alpha-adrenergic antagonists, cause a reduction in LES pressure. Finally, a history of aspiration places the patient at increased risk for recurrent episodes.

For most enterally fed patients, safety demands that the head be elevated at feeding time and for some period thereafter to prevent regurgitation. If this is not possible, an alternative nutrient delivery site should be considered. Nasogastric intubation, in particular, requires elevation of the head because the tube may render the upper and lower esophageal sphincters incompetent and liable to reflux. Even the presence of a tracheostomy or endotracheal tube does not ensure that regurgitated gastric contents will not be aspirated. Aspiration of liquid formulas can be verified if a bit of food coloring or methylene blue is included in the feeding mixture and subsequently detected in pharyngeal and tracheal secretions.[6]

ACCESS FOR FEEDING

In most general and thoracic surgical patients, access for feeding is most commonly obtained via the stomach or the jejunum. Methods of access for intragastric feedings include nasogastric tubes and feeding gastrostomies placed through a laparotomy or percutaneously with the aid of endoscopy, fluoroscopy, or laparoscopy.

Nasogastric tubes are the most commonly used access method for gastric feeding. Polyurethane or silicone rubber tubes are preferred because they are soft, nonreactive, and generally well tolerated; they are also less corrosive to the nasopharynx than rubber or polyvinyl chloride tubes. This very softness, however, often makes them hard to insert into critically ill patients and precludes checking of gastric residuum. Difficulties of tube passage into the stomach are increased when thin, floppy tubes are inserted into obtunded patients. Useful aids include stylets, judicious use of gravity and positioning, and designation of especially experienced and certified nursing personnel to assist in this task [see Table 7].

Passage of a tube through the pylorus into the jejunum may be necessary if the patient is at increased risk for aspiration (see above). Our practice is to place the tube into the stomach, to position the patient on the right side for several hours once or twice in the next 24 hours, and then to obtain an abdominal roentgenogram. If the tube has not passed, metoclopramide, 10 mg I.V., is given while the patient is still in the radiology department, and the roentgenogram is repeated. If the location of the feeding tube is not evident, a small amount of contrast material can be administered through the tube to verify its position. If the tube still has not passed through the pylorus, the aid of the fluoroscopist is enlisted. Finally, if all else has failed and no alternative route is appropriate, the endoscopist can capture the

Table 6 Composition of Modified Diets

Formula	Protein (g/L)	Carbohydrate (g/L)	Fat (g/L)	Ratio of Nitrogen (g) to Nonprotein Calories (kcal)	Caloric Density (kcal/ml)	Product* (Manufacturer)
Elemental	50	127	34	1:100	1.0	Subdue (Mead Johnson Nutritionals)
	40	127	39	1:131	1.0	Peptamen (Nestlé Clinical Nutrition)
Stress	56	130	28	1:71	1.0	Impact (Novartis)
	66	177	37	1:97	1.3	Perative (Ross Laboratories)
Hepatic	44	168	36	1:148	1.2	Hepatic Aid II (B. Braun Medical Inc.)
Renal	19	365	46	1:800	2.0	Amin-Aid (R&D Laboratories)

*Partial listing.

Table 7 Procedure for Inserting Nasoenteric Tubes

Provide privacy.

Explain procedure and its purpose.

Place patient in sitting position with neck flexed slightly and head of bed elevated to 45°.

Lubricate stylet and insert into feeding tube.

Inspect nares and determine optimal patency by having the patient breathe through one nostril while the other is temporarily occluded.

Estimate the length of tubing required to reach into the stomach by measuring the distance from the tip of the nose to the earlobe and then from the earlobe to the xiphoid process. Add 25 cm to this length for nasoduodenal intubation.

If the patient seems uncooperative, instill generous amounts of lidocaine jelly into the nares and nasopharynx before tube insertion. Lubricate the end of the tube and pass it posteriorly. Ask a cooperative patient to swallow water to facilitate passage of the tube.

Once the tube is beyond the nasopharynx, allow the patient to rest.

Have the patient continue neck flexion and swallowing while the tube is advanced.

If the patient begins to cough, withdraw the tube into the nasopharynx and then reattempt passage.

Confirm passage into the stomach by obtaining an abdominal x-ray.

Remove stylet.

Secure tube to bridge of nose or upper lip with nonallergenic tape and prevent undue pressure on external nares.

tube tip in the stomach with the biopsy forceps of the flexible endoscope (aided by a suture through the tube end) and guide the tube through the pylorus.

When any type of nasoenteric tube is placed for enteral nutrition, its location must be confirmed before feedings are started. The simplest means of accomplishing this is to aspirate gastric contents, the source of which can be determined by measuring the pH of the aspirate. Because small-bore, soft tubes tend to collapse under high negative pressure, a small syringe should be used to aspirate gastric contents. If gastric contents cannot be aspirated, radiographic confirmation of tube location is mandatory. Because feeding tubes are often radiopaque, a simple plain film of the abdomen may be adequate. If the exact location of the tube is still in doubt, a small amount of contrast material can be injected through the tube. Placement of the distal tip of the tube in the duodenum is usually confirmed by abdominal roentgenogram before transpyloric feedings are started. The tube should be inserted to a length sufficient to permit migration into the proximal jejunum.

Simple insufflation of air into the tube is not sufficient to verify its position. Auscultation over the stomach can detect sound transmitted through a tube that has been inadvertently passed into the bronchial tree. Many of these tubes are small enough to pass through the glottis and the trachea without markedly interfering with phonation or respiration. Enteral formulas delivered into the bronchial tree through a misplaced tube can cause severe pneumonitis and death.

The development of percutaneous techniques for the placement of gastrostomies has been a major contribution to enteral nutrition. Percutaneous endoscopic gastrostomy (PEG) [see 3:8 Gastrointestinal Endoscopy] and Witzel techniques for these procedures are well documented.

Concurrent decompression of the stomach and feeding into the small intestine have been used to reduce the risk of aspiration in critically ill patients. This combination of procedures requires either insertion of a multilumen nasojejunal tube, surgical placement of combined gastrojejunal tubes, modification of PEG, or insertion of a nasogastric tube in conjunction with a surgical jejunostomy. Such access to the GI tract also provides a route for the delivery of crushed medications and the option to provide cyclic nocturnal enteral nutrition with gastric decompression (i.e., the patient receives nutrients by mouth during the day).

FEEDING REGIMENS

If the patient tolerates the initial trial of enteral nutrition, then the delivery site for future feeding is chosen according to the risk of aspiration, and the feeding regimen is gradually intensified. If the risk of aspiration is minimal, intragastric feedings are preferred: they are better tolerated physiologically, easier to administer, and less restrictive for the patient than continuous feeding into the small intestine. Patients fed into the stomach receive an isotonic formula delivered continuously at a rate of 30 ml/hr; the delivery rate is increased daily by 30 ml/hr [see Table 8]. If the risk of aspiration is increased, feedings are delivered via nasoduodenal or nasojejunal tubes. Patients fed into either the duodenum or the jejunum receive formulas of 300 mOsm/kg delivered at an initial rate of 30 ml/hr with the aid of a peristaltic pump; the rate is increased daily by 30 ml/hr [see Table 8]. Only isotonic feedings should be administered into the small bowel: hypertonic formulations have been associated with small bowel injury and necrosis.

MONITORING AND PREVENTION OF COMPLICATIONS

Patients receiving enteral nutrition require careful monitoring similar to that required by patients receiving parenteral nutrition. Particular attention is directed to metabolic 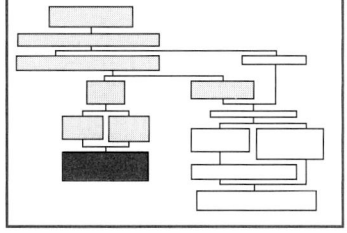 status and fluid and electrolyte balance. A protocol should be established and followed to ensure that nutritional goals are met and complications minimized. A standard checklist is helpful and prevents omission of important details [see Table 9].

Four types of complications are related to enteral nutrition: GI, mechanical, metabolic, and infectious. The first two are the most common.

The most frequent GI complication is diarrhea, which may occur in as many as 75% of critically ill patients receiving enteral nutrition. Diarrhea is best defined as stool weight greater than 300 g/24 hr or volume greater than 300 ml/24 hr. Given that such measurements are impractical and difficult to obtain, a more practical definition is more than three loose bowel movements during a 24-hour period. There are many causes of diarrhea in critically ill patients receiving enteral nutrition; the most frequent association is with antibiotic therapy [see Figure 2]. The desired therapeutic approach is to adjust the enteral nutrition regimen as necessary

Table 8 Suggested Starter and Advancement Regimens for Intragastric and Intrajejunal Feeding

Feeding Regimen	Days			
	1	2	3	4
Intragastric				
mOsm/kg	300	300	300	480
ml/hr	30	60	90	90
Intrajejunal				
mOsm/kg	300	300	300	300
ml/hr	30	60	90	90

Table 9 Standard Orders for Enteral Nutrition

Obtain abdominal x-ray to confirm tube location before feeding.

Elevate head of bed 45° when feeding into the stomach.

Record type and strength of diet and rate of infusion.

Check gastric residuum every 4 hr in patients receiving gastric feedings. Withhold feedings for 4 hr if residuum is 50% greater than ordered volume. Notify physician if two consecutive measurements detect excessive residuum.

Check for abdominal distention. Check frequency, consistency, and volume of stool output.

Weigh patient on Monday, Wednesday, and Friday. Record weight on graph.

Record intake and output daily. For every shift, chart volume of formula administered separately from water or other oral intake.

Change administration tubing and cleanse feeding bag daily.

Irrigate feeding tube with 20 ml of water at the completion of each intermittent feeding, when tube is disconnected, after the delivery of crushed medications, of if feeding is stopped for any reason.

When patient is ingesting oral nutrients, ask the dietitian to provide calorie counts daily for 5 days, then weekly thereafter.

On a weekly basis, obtain complete blood count with red blood cell indices, SMA-12, serum iron, and serum magnesium.

Obtain SMA-6 every Monday and Thursday.

Once a week, collect urine for 24 hours, starting at 8:00 A.M., and analyze for urea nitrogen.

rather than to discontinue it completely. Only one variable of the feeding regimen (i.e., osmolality, volume, rate, or type of diet) should be altered at a time. In our experience, critically ill patients tolerate continuous feeding better than intermittent feeding. If the patient still has diarrhea when receiving 150 to 300 mOsm/kg at 30 ml/hr, antidiarrheal treatment is indicated.

In many instances, antidiarrheal medication is given without a definite diagnosis; therefore, it is essential to select medications with both a wide therapeutic range and a low incidence of side effects. For these reasons, we prefer kaolin-pectin over opiates such as paregoric. Every 3 hours, 30 ml of kaolin-pectin solution is given through the feeding tube, followed by 25 ml of normal saline for irrigation. If this regimen is unsuccessful after 48 hours and opiates are not contraindicated, paregoric is added at a dose of 1 ml/100 ml formula [*see Figure 2*]. Opiates act by slowing intestinal motility. Because the normal motility pattern is a defense against bacterial growth in the small bowel, administering opiates to patients with a contaminated small bowel can lead to bacterial overgrowth and worsen diarrhea. In addition, opiates are respiratory depressants and are contraindicated in patients with infectious diarrhea.

Several diagnostic methods may help identify the cause of diarrhea associated with enteral nutrition, including the assaying of stool for *Clostridium difficile* enterotoxin, analysis of stool for fat malabsorption, the D-xylose test for carbohydrate malabsorption, and breath H_2 analysis for bacterial overgrowth. The D-xylose test and breath H_2 analysis are more commonly used in non–critically ill patients.

To prevent peptic ulcers and bleeding, gastric acidity is controlled with H_2 receptor blockers in critically ill patients. Although these drugs help control hyperacidity, which is a cause of diarrhea, they also lead to bacterial overgrowth in the intestine.[7] Therefore, they should not be used in patients who receive intragastric feedings, because the liquid formula in the stomach already provides a physiologic means of buffering acid. If necessary, antacids rather than H_2 receptor blockers should be used to titrate gastric pH to 4.5 to 6.5. Glutamine is also used to prevent or treat ulceration of the upper GI tract.

The most common mechanical complications related to enteral nutrition are tube dislodgment, clogging of the tube, and leakage of enteric contents around the tube's exit site. Tube dislodgment occurs more frequently in agitated patients and hypoxic patients. Inadvertent tube removal can usually be prevented by adequate taping or, in agitated patients, by suturing the tube or using a Velcro abdominal wall binder.

Clogging or plugging of the tube often results from failure to use saline irrigation after intermittent feedings or inadvertent delivery of crushed medications through a small-bore tube. The incidence of this complication is reduced by routine irrigations of 20 to 25 ml of normal saline or water after each intermittent feeding. Liquid medications may also help prevent this complication, though such medications are frequently hyperosmolar and may produce discomfort

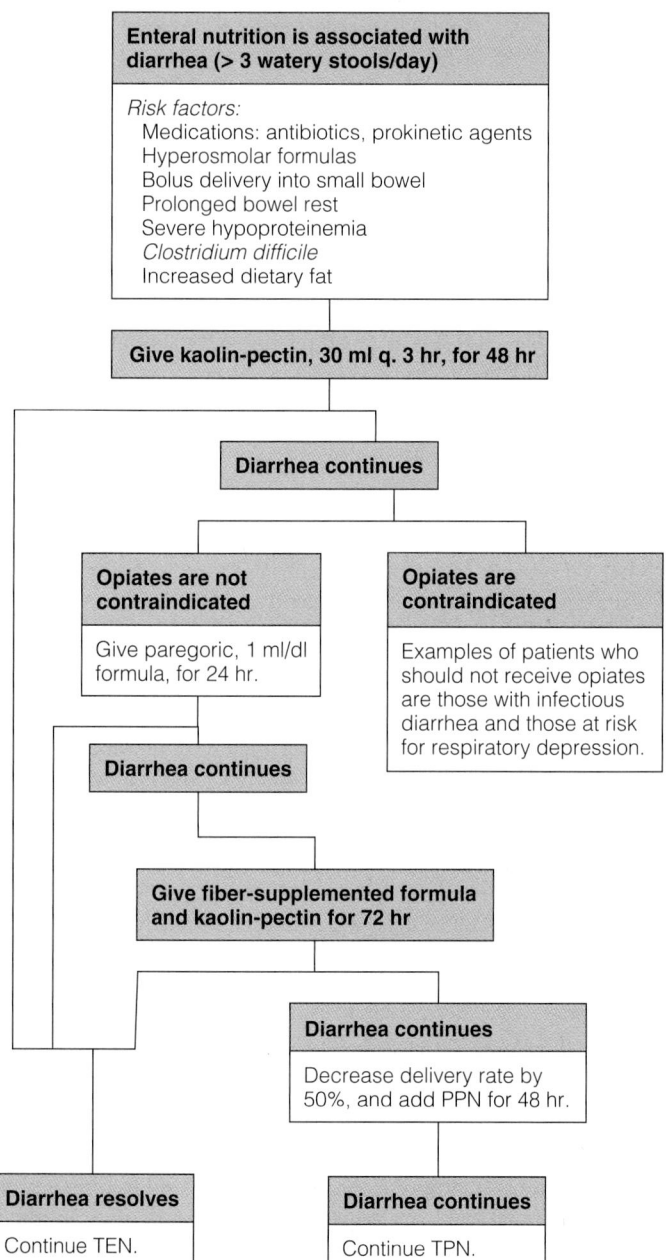

Figure 2 Shown is the decision-making approach for pharmacologic and dietary treatment of diarrhea associated with enteral nutrition.

and diarrhea when delivered rapidly into the jejunum. The injection of a small volume of a carbonated beverage into a plugged tube often clears the blockage. Occasionally, a guide wire and the help of the interventional radiologist will be needed.

Leakage of enteric contents onto the skin around the exit site is often uncomfortable for the patient and may produce a moderate amount of skin irritation. One cause of such leakage is inadequate approximation of the end of the tube to the gastric wall. Leakage around a tube is prevented by proper fixation of the end of the tube with a retention disk or bumper at the skin level. The aid of an enterostomal therapist is often useful, as are products such as karaya gum, zinc oxide, Stomahesive, and locally applied antacid. Also problematic is the inappropriate use of urinary catheters for enteral access; these devices were not designed to function as gastrostomy or enterostomy tubes.

Parenteral Nutrition

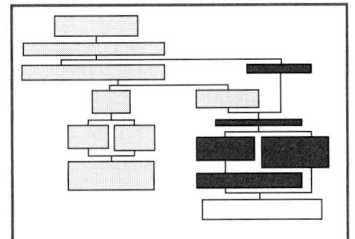

CENTRAL VENOUS VERSUS PERIPHERAL VENOUS INFUSIONS

Central venous infusions [see 4:15 Vascular and Peritoneal Access] are indicated in most critically ill patients who receive parenteral nutrition, because (1) patients in the ICU often require increased quantities of energy and cannot tolerate large fluid volumes and (2) solutions of much greater caloric density and tonicity can be infused into central veins than into peripheral veins. Nonetheless, peripheral venous infusions [see Peripheral Venous Nutrient Infusion, below] may be indicated in certain situations [see Table 10].

CENTRAL VENOUS NUTRIENT INFUSION

Hypertonic nutrient solutions are infused into the superior vena cava, where they are rapidly diluted. Usually, such solutions contain hypertonic glucose (25%), amino acids (5%), and other essential nutrients. Their tonicity (> 1,900 mOsm/kg) is so great that administration into peripheral veins would cause severe thrombophlebitis and venous sclerosis. These solutions contain at least 1 kcal/ml, and thus, infusion of 2.0 to 2.5 L/day provides 2,000 to 2,500 kcal and all essential nutrients. This calorie load is sufficient to meet energy requirements in more than 90% of surgical patients.

Once positioned, the catheter is used exclusively for administering the hypertonic nutrient solution: drawing blood, monitoring central venous pressure, and administering medication through this dedicated lumen are to be avoided. If a multiple-lumen central venous catheter is used, as is the case in most patients today, at least one port should be devoted solely to the infusion of hypertonic nutrient solutions. Some reports have suggested that the incidence of catheter-related infection is higher with multiple-lumen than with single-lumen feeding catheters[8,9]; others have not found such differences.[10] It appears that multiple-lumen catheters can be used in the ICU for central venous nutrient infusions if strict protocols are maintained to ensure that one lumen is dedicated to nutrient infusion, that other lumens are handled safely, and that catheters are removed when no longer required.

Occasionally, infusion of a hypertonic nutrient solution may be required in a situation where percutaneous puncture of central veins is impossible or contraindicated. In such cases, catheterization of an antecubital vein and insertion of a peripherally inserted central catheter (PICC) with the tip positioned in the superior vena cava should be considered. These catheters are readily insert-

ed by the interventional radiologist, and they eliminate the complications associated with subclavian and internal jugular vein insertions. The PICC line has become the primary route of central venous access in many institutions.

Silastic catheters have been safely kept in place for extended periods and provide an additional option for central venous access. Catheterization of the femoral vein may provide a route for central venous access in some situations. Because of the high density of skin pathogens in the groin area, these catheters should be replaced every 2 to 3 days. If the catheter tip is positioned in the iliac vein or the inferior vena cava, the concentration of solution infused through the catheter should not exceed 15%. Strict care of the entrance site should be maintained because of the high complication rate associated with lines placed in the groin.

Central Venous Solutions

Central venous solutions are formulated in the hospital pharmacy. They are commonly combinations of 500 ml of 50% dextrose and 500 ml of a 10% amino acid mixture [see Table 11] to which electrolytes, vitamins, and trace elements are added (see below). Each day, 2 L of the solution can be infused. Administration of fat emulsion (500 ml, 20%) 1 day each week meets essential fatty acid requirements. Alternatively, the three major nutrients may be mixed together in a 3 L bag (triple mix or three-in-one) and the entire contents of the single bag infused over the 24-hour period [see Table 11]. In addition, an automated mixing device may be used to compound various proportions of 70% glucose, 10% amino acids, and 20% fat emulsions into 3 L bags. Such devices allow the hospital pharmacy to manufacture a variety of nutrient combinations with minimal effort. More concentrated solutions can be made, and the computer will generate a label for the bag that allows nurses to verify the order.

Electrolytes and minerals are added to the base formula as required [see Table 12]. Sodium and potassium salts are added as chloride or acetate, depending on the acid-base status of the patient. The solution should usually consist of approximately equal quantities of chloride and acetate; if chloride losses from the body are increased, as in a patient requiring nasogastric decompression, the solution should contain proportionately more chloride. Sodium bicarbonate is incompatible with the nutrient solutions; if additional base is re-

---

Table 10 Indications for Central Venous or Peripheral Venous Infusions

Central Venous Infusions

To provide adequate intravenous nutritional support for 10 days or more

To satisfy nutrient requirements in patients with increased energy needs and normal or decreased fluid requirements

To support the patient with single- or multiple-organ failure by infusing modified nutrient solutions in a limited fluid volume

Peripheral Venous Infusions

To provide initial feeding (< 5 days) before catheter insertion in a patient who will require central venous feedings

To infuse less concentrated solutions via a multiuse central catheter (i.e., a line for blood drawing, medication, and nutrients) into an individual in whom other venous access cannot be easily or safely obtained

To supplement enteral feedings that are inadequate because of gastrointestinal dysfunction

To satisfy energy requirements that are near basal (1,500–1,800 kcal/day) in a nondepleted patient who can tolerate 2.5–3.0 L I.V. solution each day

Table 11 Composition of Central Venous Solutions

	Standard Solution	Triple-Mix Solution
Volume		
Amino acids 10% (ml)	500	1,000
Dextrose 50% (ml)	500	1,000
Fat emulsion 20% (ml)	—	250
Total (ml)	1,000	2,250
Contents		
Amino acids (g)	50	100
Dextrose (g)	250 (25%)	500
Total nitrogen (g)	8.4	16.8
Total calories (kcal)	1,050	2,600
Ratio of nitrogen to calories	1:125	1:154
Caloric density (kcal/ml)	1.0	1.15
Osmolarity (mOsm/kg)	≈1,970	≈1,900

quired, acetate, which generates bicarbonate when metabolized, is given. Phosphate is usually given as the potassium salt; if potassium phosphate is contraindicated, sodium phosphate is given. Phosphate is also present in fat emulsions.

Commercially available preparations of vitamins, minerals, and trace elements are also added to the nutrient mix for daily administration unless they are contraindicated. A solution containing both fat- and water-soluble vitamins should be added. Vitamin K_1 (phytonadione), 10 mg, is given once a week but is contraindicated in patients receiving warfarin.

Trace elements are given daily. Usual requirements are satisfied by adding commercially available mixtures either to 1 L of standard solution or to the triple-mix bag each day. Trace elements are indicated for all patients receiving central venous nutrient solutions, except those with chronic renal failure or severe liver disease. At especially high risk for zinc deficiency are alcoholics and patients with pancreatic insufficiency with malabsorption, massive small bowel resection, renal failure with dialysis, or nephrotic syn-

Table 12 Electrolytes Added
to Central Venous Solutions

	Usual Electrolyte Concentration	Usual Range of Electrolyte Concentration
Sodium (mEq/L)	30	0–150
Potassium (mEq/L)	30	0–80
Phosphate (mmol/L)	15	0–20
Magnesium (mEq/L)	5	0–15
Calcium* (mEq/L)	4.7	0–10
Chloride (mEq/L)	50	0–150
Acetate (mEq/L)	70	70–220

*As gluconate.

drome; at high risk for copper deficiency are patients with short-bowel syndrome, jejunoileal bypass, malabsorptive conditions with severe diarrhea, or nephrotic syndrome. Copper and manganese are excreted primarily via the biliary tract. Therefore, in patients with biliary tract obstruction, excess retention of these elements should be prevented by decreasing intake of these ions, monitoring blood levels, or both. Although the main excretory route for zinc and chromium is via the feces, renal excretion minimizes dangers from modest excesses of these elements. In patients with renal insufficiency, however, daily zinc and chromium administration may be contraindicated. ICU patients usually do not require iron. Iron supports bacterial growth and thus is contraindicated in patients with systemic infection. It may be required to treat iron deficiency anemia, particularly during convalescence from this condition, but rarely does the anemia associated with chronic disease and inflammation respond to iron therapy during its active stages.

Like other invasive therapies, total parenteral nutrition (TPN) is associated with potential complications deriving from either central venous access or the composition of the formula. Most such complications are preventable with appropriate attention to detail [*see Table 13*].

PERIPHERAL VENOUS NUTRIENT INFUSION

Slightly hypertonic nutrient solutions (approximately 600 to 900 mOsm/kg) can be prepared for peripheral venous infusion from commercially available amino acid mixtures (5%), dextrose solutions (10%), and fat emulsions (20%). These nutrient mixtures have a low caloric density (approximately 0.3 to 0.6 kcal/ml) and thus provide only 1,200 to 2,300 kcal in 2,000 to 3,500 ml of solution. Such solutions are particularly useful in patients whose tube feedings are insufficient and who need additional nutrients.

These dilute nutrient mixtures can be infused through plastic cannulas placed in large-bore peripheral veins. The catheter insertion site and the surrounding tissue should be inspected periodically for signs of phlebitis or infiltration, and the infusion site should be rotated every 48 to 72 hours to prevent thrombophlebitis. Only fat emulsion can be administered simultaneously through the same I.V. site as a peripheral venous solution. The nutrient solution should be temporarily stopped if the catheter is used for administration of antibiotics, chemotherapeutic agents, blood, or blood products. The infusion line should then be flushed with saline and nutrient infusion resumed.

If the fat emulsion is infused in a piggyback manner, administration should take place over a period of 8 to 12 hours and be concluded in the early morning hours (e.g., 3:00 A.M.) to allow clearance of the emulsion from the bloodstream. Blood sampling should be avoided during short-term fat infusion because the associated hypertriglyceridemia will interfere with many of the serum measurements. In patients who are receiving peripheral venous solutions by triple mix, hypertriglyceridemia is rare because the rate of infusion is reduced and infusion extended over a 24-hour period.

Patients receiving peripheral venous feedings should be monitored in much the same fashion as those receiving central venous feedings (see below). Mechanical and infectious complications are uncommon. Fluid imbalances and alterations in serum electrolyte concentrations are similar to those seen with standard I.V. support, and corrections are made by altering the volume of the infusion or adding or omitting electrolytes. Hyperglycemia and glycosuria are rarely observed unless the patient is diabetic.

Table 13 Diagnosis, Treatment, and Prevention of Potential Mechanical
and Metabolic Complications Associated with Total Parenteral Nutrition

	Complications	Diagnosis	Treatment	Prevention
Mechanical	Pneumothorax	Dyspnea, chest x-ray	Tube thoracostomy Observation	Avoid emergency procedures Trendelenburg's position
	Hemothorax	Dyspnea, chest x-ray	Remove catheter Observation	Insert catheter using appropriate technique
	Venous thrombosis	Inability to cannulate	Remove catheter Heparin therapy	Use silicone catheters Add heparin to solution
	Air embolism	Dyspnea, cyanosis, hypotension, tachycardia, precordial murmur	Trendelenburg's position Left lateral decubitus position	Trendelenburg's position Valsalva maneuver Tape intravenous connections
	Catheter embolism	Sheared catheter	Fluoroscopic retrieval	Never withdraw catheter through needle
	Arrhythmias	Catheter tip in right atrium	Withdraw catheter to superior vena cava	Estimate distance to SVC before insertion; confirm position with x-ray
	Subclavian artery injury	Pulsatile red blood	Remove needle Apply pressure Chest x-ray	Review anatomy
	Catheter tip misplacement	Chest x-ray	Redirect with a guide wire	Direct bevel of needle caudally
Metabolic	Hyperglycemic, hyperosmolar, nonketotic coma	Dehydration with osmotic diuresis, disorientation, lethargy, stupor, convulsions, coma, glucose 1,000 mg/dl, osmolarity 350 mOsm/kg	Discontinue TPN; infuse D5 in 0.45% S at 250 ml/hr Insulin 10–20 U/hr Bicarbonate Monitor glucose, potassium, pH	Monitor glucose
	Hypoglycemia	Headache, sweating, thirst, convulsions, disorientation, paresthesias	D50W I.V.	Taper TPN by 1/2 for 12 hr; then 12 hr of D5W at 100 ml/hr
	CO_2 retention	Ventilator dependence, high respiratory quotient	Taper glucose	Provide 30%–40% of calories with fat
	Azotemia	Dehydration, elevated BUN	Increase nonprotein calories	Monitor fluid balance
	Hyperammonemia	Lethargy, malaise, coma, seizures	Discontinue amino acid infusions Infuse arginine	Avoid casein or fibrin hydrolysate
	Essential fatty acid deficiency	Xerosis, hepatomegaly, impaired healing, bone changes	Fat administration	Provide 25–200 mg/kg/day of essential fatty acids
	Hypophosphatemia	Lethargy, anorexia, weakness	Supplemental phosphate	Treat causative factors: alkalosis, gram-negative sepsis, vomiting, malabsorption Provide 20 mEq/kcal
	Abnormal liver enzymes	Fatty infiltrate in liver	Evaluate for other causes	Provide balanced TPN solution
	Hypomagnesemia	Weakness, nausea, vomiting, tremors, depression, hyporeflexia	Infuse 10% $MgSO_4$	Supply 0.35–0.45 mEq/kg/day
	Hypermagnesemia	Drowsiness, nausea, vomiting, coma, arrhythmia	Dialysis Infuse calcium gluconate	Monitor serum levels

PATIENT MONITORING:
OPTIMIZING NUTRITIONAL
SUPPORT, PREVENTING
COMPLICATIONS, AND
RESOLVING COMMON
PROBLEMS

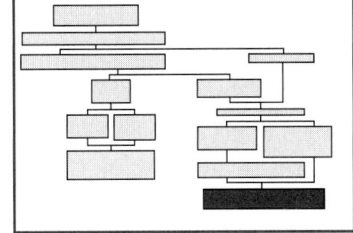

General Measures

Patients receiving central venous feedings should be weighed daily, and accurate intake and output records should be maintained. Blood glucose should be monitored daily. If levels are persistently elevated, a more stringent schedule of monitoring blood glucose should be instituted and specific therapy initiated.

The quantity of energy administered to most ICU patients should minimize the loss of lean body mass and adipose tissues. Thus, variations in body weight usually reflect alterations in fluid balance. If sustained weight loss occurs (as characterized by a gradual fall in body weight over a period of 2 weeks or more), caloric intake may be inadequate. Additional calories (500 to 1,000 kcal/day) should be administered to maintain weight. Alternatively, the metabolic rate can be calculated from oxygen consumption ($\dot{V}O_2$) and calorie intake, then matched to equal energy expenditure:

$$\text{Metabolic rate (kcal/hr)} = \dot{V}O_2 \text{ (ml/min)} \times 60 \text{ min/hr} \times 1 \text{ L}/1{,}000 \text{ ml} \times 4.83 \text{ kcal/L}$$

This calculation is required in only 5% of our patients.

Sample Calculation of Nitrogen Balance

A 65-year-old man with an infected aortic graft and ileus is receiving 2.2 L triple-mix solution containing 16.8 g nitrogen each day. His UUN is 500 mg/dl, and his urine output is 2,000 ml/day. Is he receiving adequate nitrogen?

24-hour UUN = 500 mg/dl × 2,000 ml/day × 1 g/1,000 mg
              × 1 dl/100 ml
            = 10 g/day

Nitrogen output
            = 24-hr UUN + (0.20 × 24-hr UUN) + 2 g/day
            = 10 g/day + (0.20 × 10 g/day) + 2 g/day
            = 14 g/day

Nitrogen balance
            = 16.8 g/day (N intake) − 14 g/day (N output)
            = 2.8 g/day

The patient is in positive nitrogen balance, retaining approximately 2 to 3 g nitrogen/day. If positive nitrogen balance had not been achieved, his protein and caloric intake would have had to be increased and the nitrogen balance recalculated.

In non–ventilator-dependent patients, oxygen consumption and, in turn, the metabolic rate can be derived from measurements of respiratory gas exchange. In patients with a Swan-Ganz catheter in place, oxygen consumption can be calculated from cardiac output, mixed venous oxygen content ($C_{mv}O_2$), and arterial oxygen content (C_aO_2):

$$\dot{V}O_2 \text{ (ml/min)} = \text{cardiac output (L/min)} \times (C_aO_2 \text{ [ml/dl]} - C_{mv}O_2 \text{ [ml/dl]}) \times 1 \text{ L/10 dl}$$

Another objective of nutritional support in the ICU patient is the maintenance of lean body mass, reflected by nitrogen balance equilibration or positive nitrogen balance. Although complete nitrogen balance determination is a complex and sophisticated study, nitrogen equilibration can be estimated by simply subtracting total nitrogen loss (or output) from total nitrogen intake [*see Sidebar* Sample Calculation of Nitrogen Balance]. Calculation of total nitrogen loss requires several steps. The urine urea nitrogen (UUN) concentration is multiplied by the total urine output during a given day to yield the 24-hour UUN (i.e., the total amount of urea excreted during that period). Because urea accounts for only approximately 80% of the nitrogen excreted in the urine, the value for the 24-hour UUN is then increased by an additional 20%. This quantity and an additional 2 g/day are added to the value for the 24-hour UUN to account for nonurea nitrogen, stool, and integumentary losses:

$$\text{24-hour UUN (g/day)} = \text{UUN (mg/dl)} \times \text{urine output (ml/day)} \times 1 \text{ g/1,000 mg} \times 1 \text{ dl/100 ml}$$

$$\text{Total nitrogen loss (g/day)} = \text{24-hour UUN (g/day)} + (0.20 \times \text{24-hour UUN [g/day]}) + 2 \text{ g/day}$$

Metabolic Monitoring

A wide variety of metabolic complications may occur during parenteral feeding [*see Table 14*]. They are minimized by frequent monitoring [*see Table 15*] and appropriate adjustment of nutrients in the infusion.

The most common metabolic problems in ICU patients are hyperglycemia and glucosuria. The combination of excessive counterregulatory hormone release and overproduction of tumor necrosis factor (TNF)–α, interleukin (IL)-1, and IL-6 character-istic of critical illness is a major cause of stress-induced hyperglycemia in nondiabetic hosts.[11] Hypergylcemia has been associated with infectious complications,[12,13] worsened outcome after head injury and stroke,[14] and increased proteolysis.[15] Moreover, prevention of hyperglycemia by means of aggressive insulin treatment has been associated with reduced mortality in ICU patients.[16] Initially, elevated blood glucose levels should be treated by administering insulin (5.0 U s.c. every 4 to 6 hours for glucose 200 to 250 mg/dl; 7.5 U for 250 to 300 mg/dl; 10.0 U for 300 to 350 mg/dl). When the nutritional solution is ordered for the next 24-hour period, half of the quantity of insulin administered subcutaneously is added to the mixture. The initial insulin dose should be least 10 U of regular insulin/L of solution, and in some cases, as much as 40 U/L may be required. If larger doses of insulin are needed (> 100 U/day), a separate insulin infusion or drip should be employed.

In most patients with severe glucose intolerance, the rate of glucose administration should not exceed 5 mg/kg/min (~ 500 g/day). Additional calories should be administered as fat emulsion. The commercially available fat emulsions are all generally well tolerated by critically ill patients. Triglyceride levels should be monitored, and the emulsion should be administered at a reduced rate or temporarily discontinued if levels exceed 500 mg/dl. Fat emulsion should be used with caution in patients with known hypertriglyceridemia or in those with gram-negative bloodstream infection that is associated with hyperlipidemia.

Infusion of excess glucose or lipid may alter pulmonary function and in some patients prevent weaning from a mechanical ventilator. Excessive carbohydrate loads (usually > 500 g/day) increase CO_2 production. If more CO_2 is produced than the lungs can excrete, hypercapnia results. Fat emulsion may also interfere with diffusion of gas across the alveolar membranes. This interference is generally related to the concentration of the emulsion in the bloodstream; hence, it can be minimized by monitoring triglyceride levels and preventing hypertriglyceridemia.

Catheter Care and Catheter Infection

The most serious problem associated with central venous feedings is catheter infection [*see 6:17 Nosocomial Infection*]. Primary catheter infection is defined as the signs and symptoms of infection (usually a febrile episode), with the indwelling catheter being the only anatomic infectious focus; after removal of the catheter, the symptoms usually attenuate. Cultures of the catheter tip with semiquantitative techniques yield at least 10^3 organisms,[17] and the organisms are the same as those recovered in blood drawn from a peripheral vein during initial evaluation of the infection. Secondary catheter infection is associated with a primary infectious focus that causes bacteremia and thus seeds or contaminates the catheter; the infection clears after specific treatment of the primary infection. The microorganisms cultured from the catheter tip are similar to those cultured from the primary source.

Primary catheter infection is prevented or at least greatly reduced by following strict protocols governing use and manipulation of the central venous feeding catheter and by employing a systematic method of care and surveillance of the catheter entrance site. Usually, catheter care and its supervision and certification are performed by a nurse with expertise in maintenance of long-term I.V. access. Every 48 to 72 hours, the dressing covering the entrance site of the catheter is removed, the site inspected, the area around the entrance site cleaned, a topical antibiotic or antiseptic ointment applied, and the site redressed with a new sterile dressing. This procedure is documented in the clinical

Table 14 Metabolic Complications of Total Parenteral Nutrition

Problems	Possible Causes	Solutions
Glucose		
Hyperglycemia, glycosuria, osmotic diuresis, hyperosmolar nonketotic dehydration and coma	Excessive total dose or rate of infusion of glucose; inadequate endogenous insulin; increased glucocorticoids; sepsis	Reduce amount of glucose infused; increase insulin; administer a portion of calories as fat emulsion
Ketoacidosis in diabetes mellitus	Inadequate endogenous insulin response; inadequate exogenous insulin therapy	Give insulin; reduce glucose input
Postinfusion (rebound) hypoglycemia	Persistence of endogenous insulin production secondary to prolonged stimulation of islet cells by high-carbohydrate infusion	Administer 5%–10% glucose before infusate is discontinued
Fat		
Pyrogenic reaction	Fat emulsion, other solutions	Exclude other causes of fever
Altered coagulation	Hyperlipidemia	Restudy after fat has cleared bloodstream
Hypertriglyceridemia	Rapid infusion, decreased clearance	Decrease rate of infusion; allow clearance before blood tests
Impaired liver function	May be caused by fat emulsion or by an underlying disease process	Exclude other causes of hepatic dysfunction
Cyanosis	Altered pulmonary diffusion capacity	Discontinue fat infusion
Essential fatty acid deficiency	Inadequate essential fatty acid administration	Administer essential fatty acids in the form of one 500 ml bottle of fat emulsion every 2–3 days
Amino Acids		
Hyperchloremic metabolic acidosis	Excessive chloride and monohydrochloride content of crystalline amino acid solutions	Administer Na^+ and K^+ as acetate salts
Serum amino acid imbalance	Unphysiologic amino acid profile of the nutrient solution; differential amino acid utilization with various disorders	Use experimental solutions if indicated
Hyperammonemia	Excessive ammonia in protein hydrolysate solutions; deficiency of arginine, ornithine, aspartic acid, or glutamic acid, or a combination of these deficiencies in amino acid solutions; primary hepatic disorder	Reduce amino acid intake
Prerenal azotemia	Excessive amino acid infusion with inadequate calorie administration; inadequate free water intake, dehydration	Reduce amino acid intake; increase glucose calories; increase intake of free water
Calcium and Phosphorus		
Hypophosphatemia	Inadequate phosphorus administration; redistribution of serum phosphorus into cells or bones, or both	Administer phosphorous ($\geq$ 20 mEq potassium dihydrogen phosphate/1,000 I.V. calories); evaluate antacid or calcium administration, or both
Hypocalcemia	Inadequate calcium administration; reciprocal response to phosphorus repletion without simultaneous calcium infusion; hypoalbuminemia	Administer calcium
Hypercalcemia	Excessive calcium administration with or without high doses of albumin; excessive vitamin D administration	Decrease calcium or vitamin D
Vitamin D deficiency; hypervitaminosis D	Inadequate or excessive vitamin D	Alter vitamin D administration
Miscellaneous		
Hypokalemia	Potassium intake inadequate relative to increased requirements for protein anabolism; diuresis	Alter nutrient administration
Hyperkalemia	Excessive potassium administration, especially in metabolic acidosis; renal failure	Alter nutrient administration
Hypomagnesemia	Inadequate magnesium administration relative to increased requirements for protein anabolism and glucose metabolism; diuresis; cisplatin administration	Alter nutrient administration
Hypermagnesemia	Excessive magnesium administration; renal failure	Alter nutrient administration
Anemia	Iron deficiency; folic acid deficiency; vitamin B_{12} deficiency; copper deficiency; other deficiencies	Alter nutrient administration
Bleeding	Vitamin K deficiency	Alter nutrient administration
Hypervitaminosis A	Excessive vitamin A administration	Alter nutrient administration
Elevations in AST (formerly SGOT), ALT (formerly SGPT), and serum alkaline phosphatase	Enzyme induction secondary to amino acid imbalance or to excessive deposition of glycogen or fat, or both, in the liver	Reevaluate status of patient

record; if drainage or crusting appears at the entrance site, appropriate cultures are taken. In addition, the dressing is changed if it becomes wet or soiled or no longer remains intact. In patients who have either draining wounds in close proximity to the catheter entrance site or tracheostomies, the entire dressing may be covered with a transparent barrier drape to minimize contamination.

If signs and symptoms of infection develop in a recipient of central venous parenteral nutrition, a history should be taken and a physical examination performed [*see Figure 3*]. Appropriate tests (e.g., complete blood count and urinalysis) and diagnostic studies (including roentgenogram) should also be performed. If blood cultures are needed, samples should be drawn from a peripheral vein. If trained nurses have maintained the catheter and there is no evidence of infection at the exit site, the dressing should not be removed, and the catheter should not be manipulated. Blood cultures should never be taken through the catheter—except, possibly, when the initial presentation of infection is characterized by marked hyperpyrexia or hypotension, in which case, contamination of the catheter is immaterial because the catheter will be removed. If no other infectious focus is identified, the physician may elect to remove all indwelling lines, including the feeding catheter. In addition, either drainage around the catheter or a previous positive culture from the catheter exit site may

Table 15 Variables to Be Monitored during Intravenous Alimentation and Suggested Frequency of Monitoring

Variables	Suggested Monitoring Frequency	
	First Week	Later
Energy Balance		
Weight	Daily	Daily
Metabolic Variables		
Blood measurements		
Plasma electrolytes (Na⁺, K⁺, Cl⁻)	Daily	3 × weekly
Blood urea nitrogen	3 × weekly	2 × weekly
Plasma osmolarity*	Daily	3 × weekly
Plasma total calcium and inorganic phosphorus	3 × weekly	2 × weekly
Blood glucose	Daily	3 × weekly
Plasma transaminases	3 × weekly	2 × weekly
Plasma total protein and fractions	2 × weekly	Weekly
Blood acid-base status	As indicated	As indicated
Hemoglobin	Weekly	Weekly
Ammonia	As indicated	As indicated
Magnesium	2 × weekly	Weekly
Triglycerides	Weekly	Weekly
Urine measurements		
Glucose	Daily	Daily
Specific gravity or osmolarity	Daily	Daily
General measurements		
Volume of infusate	Daily	Daily
Oral intake (if any)	Daily	Daily
Urinary output	Daily	Daily
Prevention and Detection of Infection		
Clinical observations (activity, temperature, symptoms)	Daily	Daily
WBC and differential counts	As indicated	As indicated
Cultures	As indicated	As indicated

*May be predicted from 2 × Na concentration (mEq/L) + (blood glucose [mg/dl] ÷ 1).

also indicate immediate removal. If another primary source of infection is diagnosed, specific therapy should be instituted and parenteral nutrition continued. If no source of infection is identified, the catheter should be removed and the catheter tip cultured [see 6:17 Nosocomial Infection].

A dilemma arises if another source of infection is identified and if signs and symptoms of infection persist despite what appears to be appropriate therapy. If blood cultures are positive, we favor removal of the catheter to avoid the complications associated with a contaminated indwelling catheter. If, however, peripheral blood cultures are negative, the catheter can be changed over a guide wire and the catheter tip cultured; central venous feeding can be continued during this interval. If the cultured catheter tip is positive (≥ 10⁵ organisms), the catheter should be removed.

Changing the central venous catheter over a guide wire can aid in the diagnosis of primary catheter infection.[18] Because most ICU patients have multiple potential sources for infection, this technique allows culture of the catheter tip but minimizes the risks associated with reinsertion of a new central catheter. With strict care of catheters, the incidence of catheter infection should be less than 6%.[19] Catheter-related bloodstream infection (CRBSI) is most commonly caused by growth and invasion of organisms along the catheter tract. Occasionally, bacteria are infused through the catheter because of a breach in sterility during care of the infusion apparatus. The most common bacterial organisms causing catheter sepsis are *Staphylococcus epidermidis*, *S. aureus*, *Klebsiella pneumoniae*, and *Candida albicans*. In some rare cases, the I.V. solutions may be contaminated. Moreover, most patients requiring central venous alimentation are immunocompromised hosts; their resistance is lowered further by disease, severe malnutrition, or treatment or by some combination of these factors. Coexisting conditions such as urinary tract infection, abscess, pneumonia, or mucositis secondary to chemotherapy predispose to bacteremia, which may contaminate the central venous catheter.

Immunosuppressed critically ill patients receiving multiple broad-spectrum antibiotics are also at risk for *Candida* CRBSI. Blood cultures positive for *C. albicans* in an ICU patient are an indication for catheter removal and treatment with fluconazole. An ophthalmologist should examine the eyegrounds of patients with proven candidemia to exclude the possibility of metastatic *Candida* ophthalmitis [see 6:19 Fungal Infection].

Home Nutritional Support

HOME PARENTERAL NUTRITION

Home parenteral nutrition is indicated for patients who are unable to eat and absorb enough nutrients for maintenance. Most of the adult surgical patients who require home parenteral nutrition suffer from short-bowel syndrome caused by (1) extensive Crohn disease, (2) mesenteric infarction, or (3) severe abdominal trauma. Pseudo-obstruction, radiation enteritis, carcinomatosis, necrotizing enterocolitis, and intestinal fistulas are other indications for home parenteral nutrition. Patients with these conditions cannot receive adequate nutrition enterally, though sometimes compensatory mucosal growth occurs that may reduce or eventually eliminate the need for continued home parenteral nutrition.

Patients must receive extensive evaluation, teaching, and training during hospitalization if home parenteral nutrition is to prove successful. These services should be provided by a team consisting of a physician, a nurse, a dietitian, a pharmacist, and a social worker. The team's instructions should cover the basic principles of parenteral nutrition as well as provide mechanical guidelines for catheter care, asepsis, and use of infusion pumps. Patients should be objectively evaluated before discharge to ensure that they adequately understand the principles of I.V. nutrition and can carry out home parenteral nutrition properly.

Once a patient is judged to be a suitable candidate for home TPN, a Silastic catheter is placed that is designed for more permanent use than the central venous catheter employed during hospitalization. Typically, the catheter is 90 cm long, with a thin 55 cm intravascular segment that is inserted either by venous cutdown into the internal or external jugular vein or the cephalic vein or by venipuncture directly into the subclavian vein. Its intravascular portion is cut so that the tip will lie at the junction of the superior vena cava and the right atrium.

Catheter placement is done in the OR with the patient under local anesthesia (1% lidocaine) and adequate sedation. The catheter is tunneled subcutaneously from a small incision lateral to the sternum to the site of venous insertion. The exit site is chosen on the basis of the patient's sex, physique, and hand dominance. In women, lower paraxiphoid or upper abdominal exit sites permit a more natural appearance. If coagulation status is abnormal, the cephalic vein is isolated in the deltapectoral groove and tied distally, and the catheter is inserted proximally by means of venotomy; otherwise, it is inserted into the subclavian vein percutaneously. Proper position-

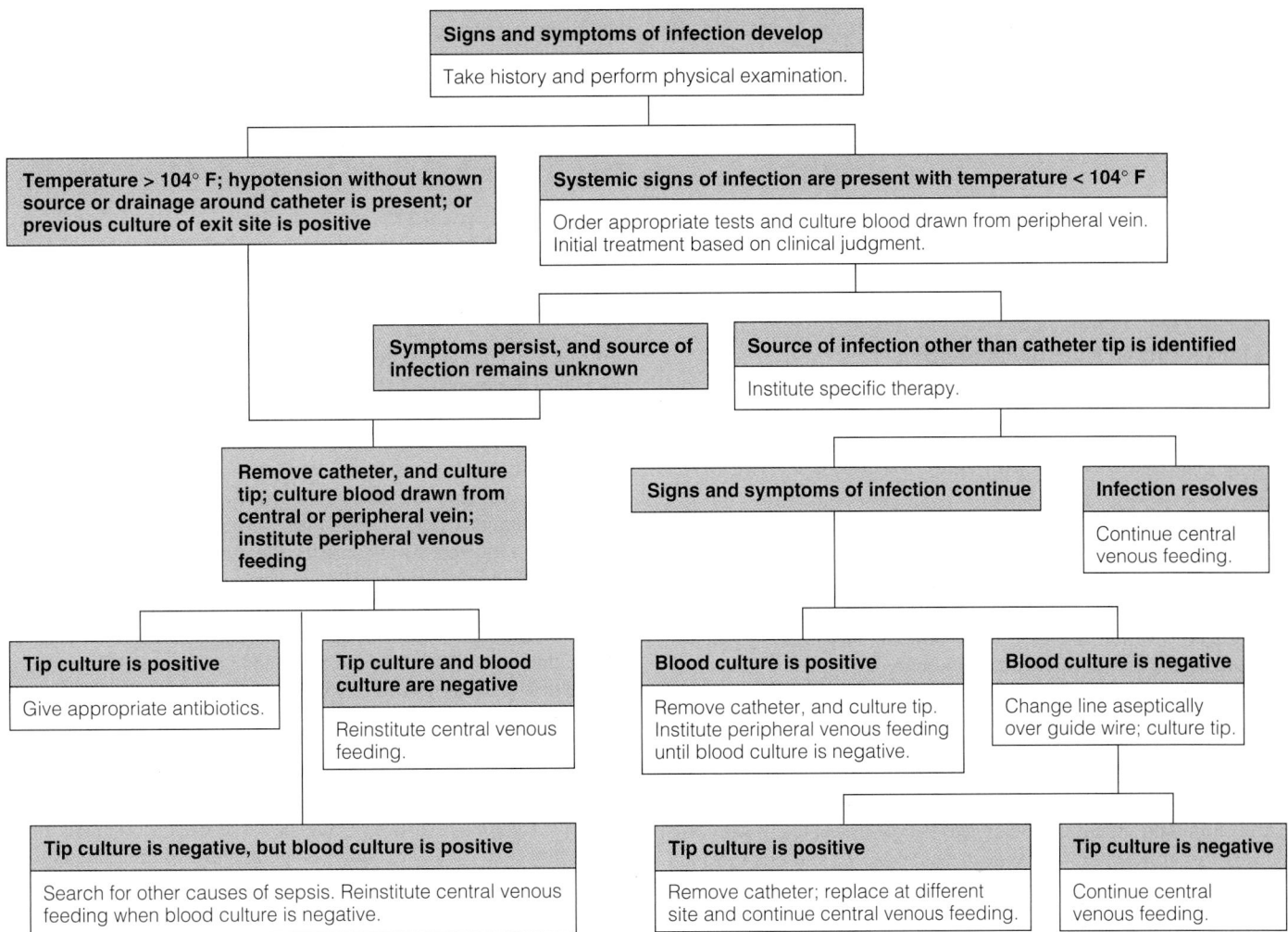

Figure 3 **Shown is an algorithm for evaluating a febrile patient receiving central venous parenteral nutrition.**

ing of the catheter is confirmed by fluoroscopy, and the incisions are closed with absorbable sutures. The catheter is sutured to the exit site, and the sutures are left attached for at least 2 weeks while tissue ingrowth into the cuff takes place. After the sutures are placed, sterile dressings are applied.

Calorie, protein, and fluid needs are carefully estimated for each patient, and the administration schedule is arranged so that the total volume may be infused nocturnally over 10 to 12 hours. Electrolytes, micronutrients, and trace minerals are added as indicated. Fat emulsions may be given either separately or admixed with glucose and protein and are used to reduce the requirement for dextrose calories and to prevent essential fatty acid deficiency.

The complications of home TPN are much the same as those of in-hospital TPN and may be divided into four categories: mechanical, infectious, metabolic, and psychosocial. Mechanical complications, which are generally easy to remedy, include catheter occlusion and dislodgment and damage to the external portion of the catheter. Infectious complications superficial to the cuff usually respond well to antibiotics. Catheter infections may necessitate removal of the device after the diagnosis is confirmed by blood cultures, but the usual therapeutic approach is to initiate a trial of parenteral antibiotics. Metabolic complications related to individual nutrient deficiencies may be corrected by adding the appropriate substance to the solution. The role of serum levels of trace minerals

and micronutrients in delineating nutrient deficiency states is unclear. In patients receiving insulin, hyperinsulinemia after infusion may be prevented by reducing the rate of administration gradually over the last hour of infusion. Psychosocial complications may vary from slight depression to suicidal tendencies, which must be treated with appropriate counseling.

The costs of a home TPN program may also be divided into four categories: patient training, equipment, supplies, and follow-up. It has been estimated that the average annual cost of home TPN is 70% less than that of in-hospital TPN. The growth of private companies that deliver equipment and supplies to the home, maintain inventory, bill patients, and help with health insurance reimbursement has considerably facilitated home care.

HOME ENTERAL NUTRITION

Home enteral nutrition is frequently used as either the sole source or a partial source of nutritional support. It is the preferred method when GI tract function is adequate. In patients undergoing surgery of the aerodigestive tract for cancer, jejunostomy feedings can supplement oral feedings, especially during adjuvant chemotherapy and radiation treatment. Patients are taught to cycle feedings over 12-hour periods, using an enteral pump system to provide 20 to 30 kcal/kg/day. Use of an appropriate feeding tube and immediate flushing of the tube after use reduce the incidence of clogging at home. If blockage occurs, proteases or carbonated beverages can be introduced into the tube in an attempt to open it. Jejunostomy feedings reduce the risk of aspiration and help maintain nutritional status during periods of inadequate oral intake. Use of inexpensive nutritionally complete commercial formulas is encouraged. For patients with more permanent disabilities that prevent adequate oral intake, a gastrostomy (or PEG [see 3:8 Gastrointestinal Endoscopy]) may be preferable; this reduces the GI complications of feeding by making use of the reservoir and admixing functions of the stomach.

Discussion

Evidence-Based Nutritional Support

EARLY ORAL FEEDINGS AFTER ELECTIVE OPERATIONS

Anesthetics, prolonged bed rest, and fluid shifts make the intestine susceptible to ileus after most operations, particularly abdominal ones. In the past, patients commonly underwent gastric decompression with a nasogastric tube until they showed obvious signs of bowel function. Over the past 10 years, however, several authors have questioned the necessity of postoperative nasogastric decompression.[20,21] Others have suggested not only that nasogastric decompression is unnecessary but also that perhaps patients should be fed earlier than is usually done.[22-24]

The traditional approach to postoperative feeding has been to start with a clear liquid or full liquid diet, continue this until the appearance of consistent flatus or bowel movements, and then switch to a regular diet. There is, however, no evidence that such a stepwise progression is necessary or leads to better outcomes. In fact, a 2002 study found no significant differences in time to diet tolerance, complications, or hospital stay between this approach and one in which postoperative feeding started with a regular diet.[25]

Use of opioids can have significant deleterious effects on nutrition. Opioid-induced constipation can lead to lower abdominal discomfort, fecal impaction, diarrhea, nausea, and inadequate absorption of oral drugs. The ensuing bowel dysfunction is a consequence both of CNS-mediated alteration of autonomic flow to the gut[26] and of a direct local opioid effect on the bowel.[27] Opioid receptor antagonists (e.g., naloxone and naltrexone) can reverse these changes, but at the cost of some reduction in analgesia. Newer agents (e.g., methylnaltrexone) are poorly lipid soluble and unable to penetrate the CNS and thus do not antagonize the central effects of opioids.[28] A 1996 study suggested, however, that I.V. methylnaltrexone could prevent opioid-induced delay in bowel motility without affecting analgesia.[29] Such drugs may be particularly useful as adjuncts, minimizing the side effects of opioids when these agents must be given.

Finally, early feeding has been combined with other therapies to enhance recovery. Patients who undergo epidural anesthesia, receive early oral feedings, and take part in an active exercise program experience much shorter convalescent recovery periods and require less hospitalization.[30]

DATA ON NUTRITIONAL SUPPORT IN SPECIFIC SETTINGS

Preoperative TPN

A number of studies have been conducted to evaluate the effect of preoperative TPN; most have involved patients with GI cancer who were considered at least moderately malnourished. A pooled analysis of the data showed that in patients who received preoperative TPN, the complication rate dropped from approximately 40% to 30%; in five studies, the differences reached statistical significance.[31] The pooled analysis found no significant difference in mortality between the TPN groups and the control groups.

Intraoperative TPN

Although not yet tested in clinical trials, intraoperative TPN should be avoided. The stress associated with surgery and anesthesia results in hyperglycemia even without the infusion of dextrose. When infused during surgery the dextrose in the TPN solution can increase blood glucose levels severalfold, and these extreme increases have been associated with impaired immune function. Furthermore, it appears that hypotension or cardiac arrest during concentrated dextrose infusion can result in more irreversible damage to the CNS.

Postoperative TPN

TPN in the immediate postoperative period without preoperative TPN has been evaluated in multiple trials—again, mostly involving GI cancer patients who were considered at least moderately malnourished.[31] In contrast to the pooled analysis of the preoperative data, a pooled analysis of the postoperative data showed that in patients who received TPN after operation, the complication rate rose from approximately 30% to 40%.

Perioperative Enteral Nutrition

Two studies compared preoperative enteral nutrition with an ad libitum oral diet,[32,33] and in one,[32] postoperative complications were significantly lower in patients who received enteral tube feeding. Other studies compared early postoperative jejunal tube feeding with a standard oral diet that was advanced as tolerated and found no consistent differences in postoperative morbidity or mortality.[34-37] Yet another evaluated the use of postoperative jejunostomy tube feeding with a special formula enriched with arginine, ribonucleic acids, and omega-3 fatty acids after operation for upper GI tract cancer.[38] When only successfully fed patients were evaluated, those who received the enriched formula had fewer complications and a shorter hospital stay than those who received the standard formula.

Nutrition in Cancer Patients

Trials addressing perioperative nutritional support have been conducted in patients undergoing surgery for pancreatic, hepatocellular, and upper GI malignancies. In one, patients undergoing major pancreatic resection were randomly assigned either to a group that received TPN on postoperative day 1 or to a non-TPN group.[39] Patients in the TPN group derived no demonstrable benefit and experienced more complications (primarily infectious). It was concluded that routine postoperative TPN could not be recommended for patients undergoing major pancreatic resection for malignancy.

Another trial examined the effects of cyclic versus continuous enteral nutrition on postoperative gastric function after pylorus-preserving pancreaticoduodenectomy.[40] Patients were evaluated with respect to gastric emptying, resumption of normal diet, and length of hospital stay. Cyclic nutrition was associated with shorter periods of nasogastric intubation, earlier resumption of normal diet, and reduced hospital stay. It was concluded that cyclic enteral nutrition was clinically efficacious in this selected group of patients.

Nutritional support has been shown to reduce the catabolic response, improve protein synthesis, and enhance liver regeneration. In a 1994 study, 124 patients undergoing hepatectomy for hepatocellular carcinoma were randomly assigned either to a control group or to a group receiving perioperative I.V. nutritional support in addition to their oral diet.[41] The overall postoperative morbidity rate was reduced in the perioperative nutrition group (34% versus 55%), mainly because the rate of infection-related complications was lower (17% versus 37%). These benefits were mainly seen in patients with underlying cirrhosis who underwent major hepatectomy. It was concluded that perioperative nutritional support can reduce complications after major hepatectomy in such patients.

Early Postoperative Enteral Nutrition

In a nonrandomized, uncontrolled study of 38 patients who underwent colorectal surgery over a 3-month period,[42] the 31 patients who were able to tolerate an early feeding regimen had shorter postoperative stays (5.7 versus 10.6 days); the seven who were not had longer operative procedures and lost more blood intraoperatively (possibly as a result of a more difficult operation, which itself might lead to prolonged recovery and decreased tolerance of early enteral feeding). The investigators concluded (1) that early postoperative feeding is safe and is tolerated by the majority of patients and (2) that if early feeding is tolerated, it shortens hospital stay and may decrease health care costs.

In another study, 28 patients undergoing esophagectomy or pancreaticoduodenectomy received either immediate postoperative enteral feeding via jejunostomy or no feedings during the first 6 days after operation.[43] Postoperative vital capacity and forced expiratory volume in 1 second (FEV_1) were consistently lower in the fed group than in the unfed group, but there were no significant differences in grip strength and maximal inspiratory pressure between the two groups. Patients in the fed group were less mobile after operation and tended to recover less rapidly; however, there were no significant differences in fatigue or vigor between the two groups. The investigators concluded that immediate postoperative jejunal feeding is associated with impaired respiratory mechanics and postoperative mobility and does not influence the loss of muscle strength or the increase in fatigue occurring after major surgery; they further concluded that immediate postoperative enteral feeding should not be routine in well-nourished patients who are at low risk for nutrition-related complications.

Another trial evaluated early enteral feeding after resection of upper GI malignancies with the aim of determining whether early postoperative enteral feeding with an immune-enhancing formula supplemented with arginine, RNA, and omega-3 fatty acids could decrease morbidity, mortality, and length of hospital stay.[44] A total of 195 patients with upper GI cancer were randomly selected to receive either the immune-enhancing formula via jejunostomy or standard I.V. crystalloid solutions. There were no significant differences between the two groups with respect to number of minor, major, or infectious wound complications; length of hospital stay; or mortality.

In yet another trial, 43 patients with nontraumatic intestinal perforation and peritonitis were randomly assigned after laparotomy either to a control group or to a study group that received a feeding jejunostomy, with enteral feeding started 12 hours after operation.[45] Mortality was high in both the control group and the study group

(18% versus 19%).[45] The control group had more infectious complications (22 versus 8).

Nutrition in ICU Patients

A meta-analysis of 26 relevant randomized clinical trials involving 2,211 patients cared for in ICUs demonstrated that parenteral nutrition did not reduce morbidity or mortality, though the data did suggest that the most malnourished groups of patients might derive some benefit.[46] Therefore, use of this expensive therapy in the ICU should be carefully limited to patients who have specific nutritional needs and cannot accept enteral feedings.

Conclusions

Parenteral and enteral nutritional support is a valuable adjunctive—and sometimes lifesaving—therapy in selected surgical patients. It is generally agreed that patients who cannot ingest adequate nutrients for a prolonged period require nutritional therapy. It is not entirely clear, however, precisely how "adequate" and "prolonged" should be defined. In practice, definitions are likely to vary from patient to patient, depending on the amount of body energy stores and lean body mass, the presence or absence of preexisting medical illnesses, the number and severity of postoperative complications, and the nature of the surgical procedure.

Summation of data from numerous trials suggests that giving nutritional support for 7 days before operation decreases postoperative complications. Severely malnourished patients (defined on the basis of percentage of body weight lost or nutritional risk index score) may derive greater clinical benefit from preoperative nutritional support, but support for this view comes largely from retrospective analysis of prospective data. In addition, certain subsets of patients may derive particular benefit from nutritional support (e.g., patients undergoing hepatic resection for hepatocellular carcinoma and elderly patients with hip fractures). The increased complication rates in patients receiving postoperative TPN and the case reports of small bowel necrosis in patients receiving early postoperative enteral nutrition are evidence that nutritional support has risks and should not be given indiscriminately.

Nutritional Pharmacology and Immunonutrition

The role of nutrient administration to surgical patients has evolved from maintenance of a positive energy and nitrogen balance to modulation of tissue metabolism and organ system function. This new role is referred to as nutrition pharmacotherapy. Like other forms of adjuvant therapy, nutrition pharmacotherapy is usually a multitargeted therapeutic modality. For instance, one form of nutrition pharmacotherapy, immunonutrition, makes use of combinations of specific amino acids, fatty acids, and, in some enteral formulas, nucleotides. Another form, so-called bowel rehabilitation, uses an amino acid (glutamine) in combination with growth hormone and a modified diet. Inclusion of a specific nutrient as part of a plan of nutrition pharmacotherapy is based either on clinical studies or, more often, on extrapolations from experimental observations. In what follows, we discuss each of the nutrients used, or proposed for use, in nutrition pharmacotherapy, with emphasis on chemical characteristics, physiologic effects, available forms for exogenous administration, and, if available, clinical data supporting its use for this purpose.

GLUTAMINE

Glutamine is the most abundant amino acid in the body and appears to be the most versatile. Most free glutamine is synthesized and stored in skeletal muscle.[47] Skeletal muscle releases net glutamine for transport to the gut, immune cells, and the kidneys. The cells of the gut and the immune system proliferate rapidly, and glutamine acts as their main fuel source and as a biosynthetic precursor. One of the compounds derived from glutamine is glutathione, a tripeptide with potent antioxidant effects. Finally, glutamine participates in acid-base regulation via release of ammonia, which combines with H^+ to form NH_4^+ and is lost in urine.

Catabolism induced by major injury, surgery, sepsis, or burns results in increased release of glutamine from skeletal muscle.[48] This output of glutamine into the circulation is associated with increased uptake and consumption by the gut, the immune system, the liver, and the kidneys. The net effect is a profound fall in intracellular muscle stores of glutamine. This deficit exceeds all other amino acid deficits and persists even when stores of all other amino acids have already been replenished.[49]

Standard amino acid formulations have always included all of the essential amino acids and most of the nonessential ones. For a long time, glutamine was excluded from parenteral formulations because of its instability in aqueous solutions. However, the pharmaceutical industry has now begun to develop ways of keeping glutamine stable in an aqueous solution. For instance, Glamin (Pharmacia & Upjohn, Sweden), an amino acid formulation that is commercially available in Europe, includes the dipeptide glycyl-L-glutamine, which is readily hydrolyzed to free glutamine in plasma and tissues. These dipeptide formulations are not yet approved for use in the United States.

Several clinical studies of supplementation of parenteral formulas with glutamine have been published. Striking results have been reported in patients undergoing bone marrow transplantation. A randomized, double-blind, controlled study from 1992 investigated the effects of glutamine on metabolic parameters and clinical outcome in 45 adult patients undergoing bone marrow transplantation for hematologic malignancies.[50] Patients were randomly selected to receive either a formula supplemented with L-glutamine or a standard glutamine-free isonitrogenous formula for an average of 4 weeks after operation. The patients who received the glutamine-supplemented formula had a better nitrogen balance than the control group; more important, they also had a lower incidence of microbial colonization and clinical infection and a shorter hospital stay. These findings were subsequently confirmed by a study performed by a different group of investigators.[51]

Equally striking results have been reported in patients with the short-bowel syndrome that develops after massive small bowel resection. Although the advent of parenteral nutrition has improved survival for many patients with this syndrome, it has also created a dependency on such therapy, which in the long term can have life-threatening complications. For this reason, many surgical scientists have searched for ways of augmenting these patients' intestinal absorption capacity so as to reduce or eliminate the need for parenteral nutrition. A growing understanding of the roles of glutamine, dietary fiber, short-chain fatty acids, and growth factors in the process of intestinal adaptation led to clinical trials aimed at evaluating the effects of supplementation of these substances on patients with this syndrome.

In a randomized, double-blind, prospective multicenter trial, 41 patients with short-bowel syndrome were given an optimal diet and then randomly selected to receive oral glutamine, 30 g/day, plus placebo growth hormone; placebo glutamine plus growth hormone (GH), 0.1 mg/kg/day; or the two active agents together.[52] Patients were weaned from TPN according to standard criteria. At the end of 4 weeks, all subjects had decreased I.V. nutrient requirements, with the glutamine-GH group showing a greater reduction than the GH group, which in turn showed a greater reduction than the glutamine-placebo group.

The studies just cited were all conducted according to research protocols that used L-glutamine, which is not practical for I.V. administration, rather than the dipeptide form now commercially available (in Europe), which is stable in an aqueous solution. A meta-analysis of all the appropriate studies involving I.V. glutamine showed a significant reduction in postoperative infection associated with a decreased length of stay.[53] Reduced long-term (6 month) mortality was noted in critically ill patients—a finding that has not been recently associated with the administration of other specific nutrients.

ARGININE

Arginine is a nitrogen-dense amino acid that is considered semiessential because it is required for growth.[54] Its effect on growth seems to be mediated by its role in polyamine and nucleic acid synthesis. In addition, it is a potent secretagogue of growth hormone, insulin, glucagon, prolactin, and somatostatin[55-57]; when this effect is abolished by hypophysectomy, the stimulatory effect on wound healing is lost.[58] Supplemental dietary arginine has thymotrophic effects and enhances the responsiveness of thymic lymphocytes to mitogens in rats.[59] A similar response occurs in peripheral blood mononuclear cells of healthy human volunteers[60] and postoperative patients,[61] as evidenced by an enhanced response to concanavalin A and phytohemagglutinin.

Arginine enhances cellular immunity, as demonstrated by an increased delayed hypersensitivity response in animals with burns.[62] Dietary supplementation with arginine improves the response to dinitrofluorobenzene (DNFB) and enhances the survival of guinea pigs with 30% body surface burns. However, in a model of acute peritonitis in guinea pigs, supplemental arginine did not improve DNFB response or survival.[63]

Studies of arginine in humans have not been conclusive, because this substance is often administered with other active substances (e.g., RNA and omega-3 fatty acids). However, oral arginine supplementation has enhanced markers of wound healing in human volunteers,[64] and both enteral and parenteral arginine administration have improved immunologic measures.[65] Although arginine has antitumor properties in animals, the only relevant study done to date in humans found that arginine supplementation stimulated growth of breast cancer.[66] Because there is now controversy over increased mortality in critically ill patients receiving arginine [see Enteral Formulations to Counteract Immunosuppression, below], careful patient selection and full informed consent are necessary with this agent.

NUCLEOTIDES

Purines and pyrimidines are precursors of DNA and RNA, which are essential for cell proliferation. Purines and pyrimidines are synthesized by the liver de novo from amino acids and reutilized by salvage pathways. Reduction of dietary nucleotides results in suppression of cellular immune responses and prolongation of allograft survival.[67] The mechanism of this immunosuppression seems to be an inability of T cells to undergo blastogenesis. Dietary supplements containing RNA or uracil (but not adenine) maintain resistance to infection by C. albicans or S. aureus in rodents.[68,69] However, they do not enhance the immune response in comparison with a standard control diet.

On the basis of the immunosuppressive effect of dietary nucleotide restriction, it has been postulated that nucleotide supplementation could provide an immunostimulant effect. This postulate has been tested in studies of the RNA–fish oil–arginine formula now available [see Enteral Formulations to Counteract Immunosuppression, below].

FATTY ACIDS

Fatty acids in the systemic circulation can be used in two forms: as fuels to be stored and oxidized as needed by the organism and as precursors for other essential compounds, such as eicosanoids (prostaglandins, leukotrienes, and thromboxanes). Fatty acids may be classified in several different ways. One classification is based on chain length: short (two to five carbons), medium (six to 11 carbons), and long (12 to 26 carbons). Another classification is based on the presence of double bonds in the carbon chain: those with double bonds are called unsaturated and are further subclassified as either monounsaturated fatty acids or polyunsaturated fatty acids (PUFAs), depending on the number of double bonds. Another classification is the omega classification, which indicates where the first double bond is located when carbons are counted from the noncarboxyl end of the chain (e.g., omega-3, omega-6).

Humans can synthesize only fatty acids with double bonds at position 7 (counting from the noncarboxyl end toward the carboxyl end). Therefore, omega-6 or omega-3 fatty acids must be supplied exogenously. Because linoleic acid and α-linolenic acid can be elongated and desaturated to produce the remaining omega-6 and omega-3 PUFAs, these are considered the essential fatty acids. Requirements for omega-6 PUFAs exceed those for omega-3 PUFAs by a ratio of approximately 5:1. Omega-6 PUFAs are abundant in vegetable oils, whereas omega-3 PUFAs are abundant in fish oils and seed oils.

The availability of 20-carbon PUFAs—arachidonic acid in the omega-6 series and eicosapentaenoic acid in the omega-3 series—is the determining factor for the synthesis of eicosanoids. Cells obtain arachidonic acid and eicosapentaenoic acid from degradation of phospholipids by phospholipase A_2 and phospholipase C or by elongation and desaturation of linoleic acid and α-linolenic acid. Because mature immune cells (e.g., monocytes, macrophages, lymphocytes, and polymorphonuclear cells) lack an enzyme needed for transformation of 18-carbon PUFAs into 20-carbon PUFAs,[70] availability of precursors for eicosanoid synthesis in such cells is largely dependent on their lipid composition. The lipid composition of immune cells, in turn, is influenced by lipid intake, and thus, the type of PUFAs ingested can affect the immune response.[71,72]

Eicosanoids, especially prostaglandin E_2 (PGE_2), leukotriene B_4 (LTB_4), 5-hydroxyeicosatetraenoic acid (5-HETE), and 15-hydroxyeicosatetraenoic acid (15-HETE), are immunomodulatory; when produced in excess (as in posttraumatic states), they are generally immunosuppressive.[73] Dietary supplementation with omega-3 PUFAs has improved survival of endotoxic shock in guinea pigs.[74] Reduced intake of omega-6 PUFAs seems to be as important as increased intake of omega-3 PUFAs. When animals are made deficient in linoleic acid, mortality after endotoxin challenge is only 24%; however, when arachidonic acid is given 2 days before endotoxin challenge, mortality reaches 100%.[75] Similar results were reported in guinea pigs recovering from flame burns covering 30% of body surface area.[76] Compared with animals fed dietary safflower oil (74% linoleic acid) or linoleic acid alone, animals fed fish oil had less weight loss, better skeletal muscle mass, lower resting metabolic expenditure, better cell-mediated immune responses, better opsonic indices, higher splenic weight, lower adrenal weight, higher serum transferrin levels, and lower serum C3 levels.

The fat emulsions currently available for I.V. use in the United States are made with LCTs derived either from soybean oil alone or from soybean oil and safflower oil. All of the fatty acids in LCTs are in the form of PUFAs. Intravenously administered LCT emulsions are cleared in part through the reticuloendothelial system (RES).[77] When such emulsions are used as a calorie source, they may impair the ability of the RES to clear bacteria if given too rapidly or in excessively large amounts. Moreover, the PUFAs in LCT emulsions require carnitine-mediated transport to cross the mitochondrial membrane for oxidation. During sepsis, urinary excretion of free carnitine rises significantly, and the plasma acylcarnitine level falls.[78] One way of circumventing these problems is to use emulsions that contain MCTs.

MCT-containing emulsions possess an absorptive advantage over LCT-containing emulsions: whereas LCTs are absorbed via lacteals and the lymphatic system, MCTs are absorbed via the portal system. MCTs are obtained from coconut oil and contain saturated fatty acids (with octanoic acids predominating). Because MCTs are smaller than LCTs, they are more water soluble; they are also poorly bound to albumin and diffuse more easily across body compartments. Several reports on the use of I.V. administered MCT fat emulsions have been published. One study evaluated the effect of a 75% MCT/25% LCT emulsion on RES function as demonstrated by ^{99m}Tc-sulfur colloid (Tc-SC) clearance. Tc-SC clearance was significantly higher after 3 days of MCT/LCT administration than after 3 days of LCT administration.[79] Another study investigated the metabolic effects of MCT-containing emulsions on surgical patients.[80] Its main finding was the appearance of β-hydroxybutyrate in association with MCT infusion, which was indicative of a ketogenic effect. A tendency toward improved nitrogen balance was also observed but was not statistically significant.

In summary, specific fatty acids have significant potential for use in nutrition pharmacotherapy. Omega-6 fatty acids are potential immunosuppressants, whereas omega-3 fatty acids are potential immunostimulants. A reduction in the intake of omega-6 PUFAs appears prudent in patients who are immunocompromised or in posttraumatic states. Formulas for nutritional support should include omega-3 PUFAs, though the exact amount of omega-3 PUFAs and the precise ratio of omega-6 to omega-3 remain to be determined.

In the United States, the only emulsions commercially available for I.V. use at present are made of LCTs containing omega-6 PUFAs. MCTs offer some metabolic advantages over LCTs and obviate the side effects resulting from an excess of omega-6 PUFAs. Enteral diets containing omega-3 PUFAs appear to benefit stressed surgical patients, particularly those who are immunosuppressed as a result of therapy for cancer.

ENTERAL FORMULATIONS TO COUNTERACT IMMUNOSUPPRESSION

Impact (Sandoz Nutrition, Minneapolis, MN), a commercially available enteral formula enriched with omega-3 PUFAs, arginine, and RNA, was shown to reduce infectious complications in postoperative patients[81,82] and in some critically ill patients.[83] It was also shown to reduce hospital stay in selected patient groups.[84] However, concern was raised by the publication of data from a large meta-analysis of studies using this formula, which suggested that its use led to increased mortality.[85] The investigators suggested that the immunomodulation associated with this diet might be beneficial in some patients (generally the less seriously ill) but harmful in others (generally the more critically ill patients who require nutritional support).[86] Until this issue is resolved, patient selection is extremely important if this diet is to be administered to surgical patients.

Nutritional Support Guidelines

In 2002, the American Society for Parenteral and Enteral Nutrition (ASPEN) published an updated version of guidelines for use of nutritional support.[87] These guidelines are also available on the Internet (http://www.nutritioncare.org/publications/2002guidelines.pdf).

References

1. Vitamin preparations as dietary supplements and as therapeutic agents. Council on Scientific Affairs. JAMA 257:1929, 1987
2. Marks J: The safety of vitamins: an overview. Int J Vitam Nutr Res 30(suppl):12, 1989
3. Nathens AB, Neff MJ, Jurkovich GJ, et al: Randomized, prospective trial of antioxidant supplementation in critically ill surgical patients. Ann Surg 236:814, 2002
4. Demling R, LaLonde C, Saldinger P, et al: Multiple-organ dysfunction in the surgical patient: pathophysiology, prevention, and treatment. Curr Probl Surg 30:345, 1993
5. Pingleton SK, Hadzima SK: Enteral alimentation and gastrointestinal bleeding in mechanically ventilated patients. Crit Care Med 11:13, 1983
6. Treolar DM, Stechmiller J: Pulmonary aspiration in tube-fed patients with artificial airways. Heart Lung 13:667, 1984
7. Du Moulin GC, Paterson DJ, Hedley-White J, et al: Aspiration of gastric bacteria in antacid-treated patients: a frequent cause of postoperative colonization of the airway. Lancet 1:242, 1982
8. Pemberton LB, Lyman B, Lander V, et al: Sepsis from triple- vs single-lumen catheters during total parenteral nutrition in surgical or critically ill patients. Arch Surg 121:591, 1986
9. Miller JJ, Venus B, Mathru M: Comparison of the sterility of long-term central venous catheterization using single lumen, triple lumen, and pulmonary artery catheters. Crit Care Med 12:634, 1984.
10. Belliveau K: Catheter infection rate using multiple lumen catheters. Read before the National Intravenous Therapy Association, New Orleans, April 1986
11. McCowen KC, Malhotra A, Bistrian BR, et al: Endocrine and metabolic dysfunction syndromes in the critically ill—stress-induced hyperglycemia. Crit Care Clin 17:107, 2001
12. Fietsam R Jr, Bassett J, Glover JL: Complications of coronary artery surgery in diabetic patients. Am Surg 57:551, 1991
13. Schloerb PR: TPN or intravenous food poisoning? Nutrition 17:680, 2001
14. O'Neill PA, Davies I, Fullerton KJ, et al: Stress hormone and blood glucose response following acute stroke in the elderly. Stroke 22:842, 1991
15. Flakoll PJ, Hill JO, Abumrad NN: Acute hyperglycemia enhances proteolysis in normal man. Am J Physiol 265:E715, 1993
16. Van der Berghe G, Wouters P, Weekers F, et al: Intensive insulin therapy in critically ill patients. N Engl J Med 345:1359, 2001
17. Maki DG, Weise CE, Sarafin HW: A semiquantitative culture method for identifying intravenous-catheter-related infection. N Engl J Med 296:1305, 1977
18. Pettigrew RA, Lang SDR, Haydock DA, et al: Catheter-related sepsis in patients on intravenous nutrition: a prospective study of quantitative catheter cultures and guidewire changes for suspected sepsis. Br J Surg 72:52, 1985
19. Williams WW: Infection control during parenteral nutrition therapy. JPEN J Parenter Enteral Nutr 9:735, 1985
20. Pearl ML: A randomized controlled trial of postoperative nasogastric tube decompression in gynecologic oncology patients undergoing intraabdominal surgery. Obst Gynecol 88:399, 1996
21. Friedman SG: A prospective randomized study of abdominal aortic surgery without post-operative nasogastric decompression. Cardiovasc Surg 4:492, 1996
22. Reissman PR, Teoh TA, Cohen SM, et al: Is early oral feeding safe after elective colorectal surgery? A prospective randomized trial. Ann Surg 222:73, 1995
23. Behrns KE, Kircher AP, Galanko JA, et al: Prospective randomized trial of early initiation and hospital discharge on a liquid diet following elective intestinal surgery. J Gastrointest Surg 4:217, 2001
24. Pearl ML, Valea FA, Fischer M, et al: A randomized controlled trial of early post-operative feedings in gynecologic oncology patients undergoing intra-abdominal surgery. Obstet Gynecol 92:94, 1998
25. Pearl ML: A randomized controlled trial of a regular diet as the first meal in gynecologic oncology patients undergoing intraabdominal surgery. Obstet Gynecol 100:230, 2002
26. Shook JE, Pelton JT, Hruby VJ, et al: Peptide opioid antagonist separates peripheral and central opioid anti-transit effects. J Pharm Exp Ther 243:492, 1987
27. Manara L, Bianchi G, Ferretti P, et al: Inhibition of gastrointestinal transit by morphine in rats results primarily from direct action on gut opioid sites. J Pharm Exp Ther 237:945, 1986
28. Foss JF: A review of the potential role of methylnaltrexone in opioid bowel dysfunction. Am J Surg 182(5A suppl):19S, 2001
29. Yuan FS, Foss JF, O'Connor M, et al: Methylnaltrexone prevents morphine-induced delay in oral-cecal transit time without affecting analgesia: a double-blind randomized placebo-controlled trial. Clin Pharm Ther 59:469, 1996
30. Kehlet H, Wilmore DW: Multimodal strategies to improve surgical outcome. Am J Surg 183:630, 2002
31. Klein S, Kinney J, Jeejeebhoy K, et al: Nutrition support in clinical practice: review of published data and recommendations for further research directions. JPEN J Parenter Enteral Nutr 21:133, 1997
32. von Meyenfeldt MF, Meijrink WJHJ, Rouflart MMJ, et al: Perioperative nutritional support: a randomized clinical trial. Clin Nutr 11:180, 1992
33. Shukla HS, Rao RR, Banu N, et al: Enteral hyperalimentation in malnourished surgical patients. Ind J Med Res 80:339, 1984
34. Sagar S, Harland P, Shields R: Early postoperative feeding with elemental diet. Br Med J 1:293, 1979
35. Ryan JA, Page CP, Babcock L: Early postoperative jejunal feeding of elemental diet in gastrointestinal surgery. Am Surg 47:393, 1981
36. Smith RC, Hartemink RJ, Holinshead JW, et al: Fine bore jejunostomy feeding following major abdominal trauma: a controlled randomized clinical trial. Br J Surg 72:458, 1985
37. Tovinelli G, Marsili I, Varrassi G: Nutrition support after total laryngectomy. JPEN J Parenter Enteral Nutr 17:445, 1993
38. Daly JM, Lieberman MD, Goldfine J, et al: Enteral nutrition with supplemental arginine, RNA and omega-3 fatty acids in patients after operation: immunologic, metabolic and clinical outcome. Surgery 112:56, 1992
39. Brennan MF, Pisters PW, Posner M, et al: A prospective randomized trial of total parenteral nutrition after major pancreatic resection for malignancy. Am Surg 220:436, 1994
40. Van Berge Henegowen M, Akkermans L, van Gulik T, et al: Prospective, randomized trial on the effect of cyclic versus continuous enteral nutrition on postoperative gastric function after pylorus-preserving pancreatoduodenectomy. Ann Surg 226:677, 1997
41. Fan ST, Lo CM, Lai E, et al: Perioperative nutritional support in patients undergoing hepatectomy for hepatocellular carcinoma. N Engl J Med 331:1547, 1994
42. Bufo A, Feldman S, Daniels G, et al: Early postoperative feeding. Dis Colon Rectum 37:1260, 1994
43. Watters JM, Kirkpatrick SM, Norris SB, et al: Immediate postoperative enteral feeding results in impaired respiratory mechanics and decreased mobility. Ann Surg 226:369, 1997
44. Heslin MJ, Latkany L, Leung D, et al: A prospective, randomized trial of early enteral feeding after resection of upper gastrointestinal malignancy. Ann Surg 226:567, 1997
45. Singh G, Ram RP, Khanna SK: Early postoperative enteral feeding in patients with non-traumatic intestinal perforation and peritonitis. J Am Coll Surg 187:142, 1998
46. Heyland DK, MacDonald S, Keefe L, et al: Total parenteral nutrition in the critically ill patient: a meta-analysis. JAMA 280:2013, 1998
47. Souba WW, Herskowitz K, Augstgen TR, et al: Glutamine nutrition: theoretical considerations and therapeutic impact. JPEN J Parenter Enteral Nutr 14:237S, 1990
48. Furst P, Albers S, Stehle P: Stress-induced intracellular glutamine depletion. Contr Infusion Ther Clin Nutr 17:117, 1987
49. Lacey JM, Wilmore DW: Is glutamine a conditionally essential amino acid? Nutr Rev 48:297, 1990
50. Ziegler TR, Young LS, Benfell K, et al: Clinical and metabolic efficacy of glutamine-supplemented parenteral nutrition after bone marrow transplantation. Ann Intern Med 116:821, 1992
51. Schloerb PR, Amare M: Total parenteral nutrition with glutamine in bone marrow transplantation and other clinical applications. JPEN J Parenter Enteral Nutr 17:407, 1993
52. Byrne TA, Morrissey T, Naltakom T, et al: Growth hormone, glutamine and a modified diet enhance nutrient absorption in patients with severe short bowel syndrome. JPEN J Parenter Enteral Nutr 19:296, 1995
53. Novak F, Heyland DK, Avenell A, et al: Glutamine supplementation in serious illness: a systematic review of the evidence. Crit Care Med 30:2022, 2002
54. Barbul A: Arginine and immune function. Nutrition 6:53, 1990
55. Rakoff JS, Siler TM, Sinha YN, et al: Prolactin and growth hormone release in response to sequential stimulation by arginine and synthetic TRF. J Clin Endocrinol Metab 37:641, 1973
56. Palmer JP, Walter RM, Ensinck JW: Arginine-stimulated acute phase of insulin and glucagon secretion: I. In normal man. Diabetes 24:735, 1975
57. Utsumi M, Makimura H, Ishihara K, et al: Determination of immunoreactive somatostatin in rat plasma and responses to arginine, glucose and glucagon infusion. Diabetologia 17:319, 1979
58. Barbul A, Rettura G, Levenson SM, et al: Wound healing and thymotropic effects of arginine: a pituitary mechanism of action. Am J Clin Nutr 37:786, 1983
59. Barbul A, Wasserkrug HL, Seifter E, et al: Immunostimulatory effects of arginine in normal and injured rats. J Surg Res 29:228, 1980
60. Barbul A, Sisto DA, Wasserkrug HL, et al: Arginine stimulates lymphocyte immune res-

ponse in healthy human beings. Surgery 90:244, 1981

61. Daly JM, Reynolds J, Thom A, et al: Immune and metabolic effects of arginine in the surgical patient. Ann Surg 208:512, 1988

62. Saito H, Trocki O, Alexander JW, et al: The effect of route of nutrient administration on the nutritional state, catabolic hormone secretion, and gut mucosal integrity after burn injury. JPEN J Parenter Enteral Nutr 11:1, 1987

63. Gonce SJ, Peck MD, Alexander JW, et al: Arginine supplementation and its effect on established peritonitis in guinea pigs. JPEN J Parenter Enteral Nutr 14:237, 1990

64. Kirk SJ, Hurson M, Regan MC, et al: Arginine stimulates wound healing and immune function in elderly human beings. Surgery 114:155, 1993

65. Daly JM, Reynolds J, Sigal RK, et al: Effect of dietary protein and amino acids on immune function. Crit Care Med 18:S86, 1990

66. Park KGM, Heys SD, Blessing K, et al: Stimulation of human breast cancers by dietary L-arginine. Clin Sci 82:413, 1992

67. Van Buren CT, Kim E, Kulkarni AD, et al: Nucleotide-free diet and suppression of immune response. Transplant Proc 19:57, 1987

68. Fanslow WC, Kulkarni AD, Van Buren CT, et al: Effect of nucleotide restriction and supplementation on resistance to experimental murine candidiasis. JPEN J Parenter Enteral Nutr 12:49, 1988

69. Kulkarni AD, Fanslow WC, Drath DB, et al: Influence of dietary nucleotide restriction on bacterial sepsis and phagocytic cell function in mice. Arch Surg 121:169, 1986

70. Chapkin RS, Somers SD, Erickson KL: Inability of murine peritoneal macrophages to convert linoleic acid into arachidonic acid. J Immunol 140:2350, 1988

71. Johnston DV, Marshall LA: Dietary fat, prostaglandins and the immune response. Prog Food Nutr Sci 8:3, 1984

72. Meade CJ, Mertin J: Fatty acids and immunity. Adv Lip Res 16:127, 1978

73. Kinsella JE, Lokesh B: Dietary lipids, eicosanoids, and the immune system. Crit Care Med 18(suppl):S94, 1990

74. Mascioli E, Leader L, Flores E, et al: Enhanced survival to endotoxin in guinea pigs fed IV fish oil emulsions. Lipids 23:623, 1988

75. Cook JA, Wise WC, Knapp DR, et al: Essential fatty acid deficient rats: a new model for evaluating arachidonate metabolism in shock. Adv Shock Res 6:93, 1981

76. Alexander JW, Saito H, Trocki O, et al: The importance of lipid type in the diet after burn injury. Ann Surg 204:1, 1986

77. Seidner DL, Mascioli EA, Istfan NW, et al: Effects of long-chain triglyceride emulsions on reticuloendothelial system function in humans. JPEN J Parenter Enteral Nutr 13:614, 1989

78. Nanni C, Pittiruti M, Giovannini I, et al: Plasma carnitine levels and urinary carnitine excretion during sepsis. JPEN J Parenter Enteral Nutr 9:483, 1985

79. Jonsen GL, Mascioli EA, Seidner DL, et al: Parenteral infusion of long- and medium-chain triglycerides and reticuloendothelial system function in man. JPEN J Parenter Enteral Nutr 14:467, 1990

80. Jiang Z, Zhang S, Wang X, et al: A comparison of medium-chain and long-chain triglycerides in surgical patients. Ann Surg 217:175, 1993

81. Daly J, Weintraub F, Shou J, et al: Enteral nutrition during multimodality therapy in upper gastrointestinal cancer patients. Ann Surg 221:127, 1995

82. Daly J, Lieberman M, Goldfine J, et al: Enteral nutrition with supplemental arginine, RNA, and omega-3 fatty acids in patients after operation: immunologic, metabolic, and clinical outcome. Surgery 112:56, 1992

83. Bower R, Lavin P, LiCari J, et al: A modified enteral formula reduces hospital length of stay (LOS) in patients in intensive care units (ICU). Crit Care Med 21(supp 4):S275, 1993

84. Galban C, Montejo JC, Mesejo A: An immune-enhancing enteral diet reduces mortality rate and episodes of bacteremia in septic intensive care unit patients. Crit Care Med 28:643, 2000

85. Heyland DK, Novak F, Drover JW, et al: Should immunonutrition become routine in critically ill patients? A systematic review of the evidence. JAMA 286:944, 2001

86. Suchner U, Heyland DK, Peter K: Immune-modulatory actions of arginine in the critically ill. Br J Nutr 87:S121, 2002

87. ASPEN Board of Directors and the Clinical Guidelines Task Force: Guidelines for the use of parenteral and enteral nutrition in adult and pediatric patients. JPEN J Parenter Enteral Nutr 26:62SA, 2002

Acknowledgments

Figure 2   Talar Agasyan.
Figure 4   Carol Donner.

INDEX

A

Aaron sign, 264t
Abciximab, preoperative
    discontinuance of, 37t
Abdomen
    fluid collections in, nonoperative
        management of, 1356-1357
    great vessels of, traumatic injury
        to, 947-957
        AAST injury scale for, 947, 948t
        aortic compression device for,
            949, 949f
        celiac axis in, 950
        complications of, 957
        damage-control laparotomy in,
            957
        iliac artery in, 955-956, 950t,
            955f
        iliac vein in, 956, 952t
        inferior vena cava in, 951-953,
            952t, 953f
        inframesocolic, 951-953
        infrarenal aorta in, 951, 953f,
            950t
        intra-abdominal hematoma in,
            947, 947f-948f
        left medial visceral rotation
            for, 947-948, 949f
        perirenal hematoma in, 953-954,
            953f-954f
        porta hepatis in, 956, 956f
        proximal renal artery in, 950-
            951, 950t
        PTFE prosthetic graft for, 949-
            950, 950f
        renal artery in, 953-955, 954f,
            950t
        renal vein in, 953-955, 952t
        retrohepatic area in, 956-957
        superior mesenteric artery in,
            950, 951f-952f, 950t
        superior mesenteric vein in,
            951, 952t
        supramesocolic, 947-951
        survival rate after, 950, 950t
        zone 1, 947-953

zone 2, 953-955
zone 3, 955-956
reconstructive flaps for, 168t,
    170
Abdominal compartment syndrome, in
    acute renal failure, 1139
Abdominal injury, 939-946
    blunt, nonoperative management of,
        924-925
    bowel in, damaged or devitalized,
        943-944
    closure in, 945-946
        general technique for, 945-946
        open fascial closure in, 945,
            944f
        "quick outs" and damage control
            in, 945-946, 945f
        skin closure in, 945
    contamination in, control of, 942
    hemorrhage control in, 942, 943f
    incision in, 939
    initial exploration in, 939-940
    management of, priorities in, 942-
        945
    operative exposure in, 940-942
        for aorta, 940, 941f
        for biliary tract, 942
        for duodenum, 942
        for pancreas, 942
        for vena cava, 940-942, 941f,
            943f
    patient preparation in, 939
    retroperitoneal hematoma in, 940,
        940f
    retroperitoneal injury repair in,
        944-945
    vascular repair in, 942-943
Abdominal mass, 269-279
    angiography in, 274
    barium studies, 274
    biopsy in, 275-278
        endoscopic ultrasound-guided,
            277-278
        image-guided percutaneous, 275-
            277, 276f
        laparoscopic, 278
    clinical history in, 269
    computed tomography in, 275, 275f
    differential diagnosis in, 272

evaluation of, *Algorithm,* 270-271
excretory urography in, 274
exploratory laparotomy in, 278
investigative studies in, 273-278
laboratory studies in, 273
magnetic resonance imaging in, 274
physical examination in, 272-273
plain abdominal radiography in,
    274
pulsatile, 680-695. *See also*
    Aortic aneurysm, abdominal
    clinical evaluation of, 680-684
    history in, 680-681, 681t, 681f
    physical examination in, 681-
        684, 684f
    preoperative evaluation for
        nonemergency patients, 688-
        692
    presentation in, 680
    rare causes of, 693, 692f
    stable patient and, 684-688
        aneurysm is absent, 685
        aneurysm is present, 685-688
    ultrasonography for, 684-685,
        685f, 686t
    unstable patient and, 684
radiographic studies in, 273-
    275, 274f-275f
radionucleotide scan in, 274
ultrasonography in, 274-275
working diagnosis in, 273
Abdominal procedures, antibiotic
    prophylaxis for, 22, 23
Abdominal radiography
    in abdominal mass, 274
    in intestinal obstruction, 306-
        307, 307f-310f
Abdominal wall, anatomy of, 546-
    548, 547f-548f
    blood supply, 547-548
    fascia, 549
    innervation, 547, 548f
    musculature, 546-547, 547f
Abdominal wall hernia
    classification of, 545-546, 546t-
        547t
    prevalence of, 545, 545f
Abdominoperineal resection, 646-648
    complications of, 647-648

operative planning in, 646
operative technique in, 646-647,
    647f
outcome in, 648
Abortion, infected, antibiotic
    selection in, 1291t
Abrasion, in extremity trauma, 987
Abscess
    breast, 132
    cerebral, coma in, 1222
        treatment of, 1227-1228
    cutaneous
        confined, 142
        pathogens in, 153
    hepatic, 1341-1343
    renal, candidal, 1372
    splenic, 1344-1346, 1346f
    tubo-ovarian, antibiotic selection
        in, 1291t
Accident(s), motorcycle, acute wound
    management after, 104
Acetabular fracture, 981-982
Acetaminophen
    suggested dosing for, 82t
    toxicity, in acute hepatic
        failure, 1192
Acetaminophen with codeine,
    suggested dosing for, 81t
Acetic acid, contraindicated in
    acute wound care, 107
Achalasia, esophageal, reoperation
    for, 388-389
Acid(s)
    causing chemical burns, 992t, 1030
    renal excretion of, 1170, 1171f-
        1173f
Acid-base disorder(s), 1170-1180
    in cardiac arrest, 1046t
    postoperative, 86-87
    in trauma patient, sodium
        bicarbonate and, 863
Acid-base physiology, normal,
    1170, 1170f-1173f
Acinetobacter infection,
    antimicrobial agents for, 1293t
Acquired immunodeficiency syndrome
    (AIDS), 1405-1416
    central venous catheterization in,
        1408

I

R